AMERICAN JOURNAL OF
DISEASES OF CHILDREN

AJDC

Index to

Volume 145

January through December 1991

SUBSCRIPTION RATES—The subscription rates for the American Journal of Diseases of Children are as follows:$58 for one year, $101 for two years in the United States and US Possessions; all other countries, one year, $73; two years, $131 for surface delivery. For expedited air delivery to most countries, add $15 surcharge for one year subscription, $30 for two years. (Rates for subscriptions for delivery to Japan or South Korea are available through exclusive agents–contact the publisher.) ***Special rates for residents and medical students in the United States and US Possesions are available.*** Address inquiries to the American Medical Association, Circulation and Fulfillment Division, 515 N State St, Chicago, Il 60610. Phone: (312) 464-0183.

AJDC, American Journal of Diseases of Children (ISSN 0002-922X) is published monthly by the American Medical Association, 515 N State St, Chicago, IL 60610, and is an official publication of the Association. Second-class postage paid at Chicago and at additional mailing office.

CHANGE OF ADDRESS—POSTMASTER, send all address changes to AMERICAN JOURNAL OF DISEASES OF CHILDREN, Attention: Subscription Department, 515 N State St, Chicago, IL 60610. Notification of address change must be made at least six weeks in advance. Include both old and new addresses, a recent mailing label, and your new zip code.

Please address communications concerning accepted or published communications to AMA Specialty Journals, 515 N State St, Chicago, Il 60610.

AMERICAN JOURNAL OF DISEASES OF CHILDREN

AJDC

Vol 145 **No. 1** **JANUARY 1991**

EDITORIAL

AJDC Is 80 Years Old: From Pedology to Pediatrics 11
Vincent A. Fulginiti, MD, New Orleans, La

THE PEDIATRIC FORUM

1991 Annual Meeting 26

Characteristics of Perinatal Cocaine-Exposed Infants With Necrotizing Enterocolitis 26
Gregory J. Downing, DO; Stanley R. Horner, DO; Howard W. Kilbride, MD, Kansas City, Mo

Current Social Practices Leading to Water Intoxication in Infants 27
Annabelle Schaeffer, MD, Stuart Ditchek, MD, Brooklyn, NY

Alkaline Urine Is Associated With Eating Disorders 28
Martha R. Arden, MD; Lauren Budow, MD; Douglas W. Bunnell, PhD; Michael P. Nussbaum, MD; I. Ronald Shenker, MD; Marc S. Jacobson, MD, New Hyde Park, NY

Major Congenital Neurologic Malformations 30
CPT Brian D. Ryals, MC, USA, Thomas E. Wiswell, MD, Washington, DC

EDITORIALS

Status Report on Phenylketonuria Treatment: 1990 33
C. Charlton Mabry, MD, Lexington, Ky

Development, Growth, and Cardiac Surgery 33
John E. Mayer, Jr, MD, Boston, Mass

Continued on page 5.

AMERICAN JOURNAL OF DISEASES OF CHILDREN

ARTICLES

Intellectual Development in 12-Year-Old Children Treated for Phenylketonuria 35
Colleen G. Azen, MS; Richard Koch, MD; Eva Gross Friedman, Los Angeles, Calif; Stanley Berlow, MD, Madison, Wis; James Coldwell, MD, Tulsa, Okla; Wilma Krause, MD, Iowa City, Iowa; Reuben Matalon, MD, PhD, Chicago, Ill; Edward McCabe, MD, PhD, Denver, Colo; Margaret O'Flynn, MD, Los Angeles, Calif; Raymond Peterson, MD, San Diego, Calif; Bobbye Rouse, MD, Galveston, Tex; C. Ronald Scott, MD, Seattle, Wash; Bernice Sigman, MD, David Valle, MD, Baltimore, Md; Robert Warner, MD, Buffalo, NY

Follow-up of Patients Who Underwent Arterial Switch Repair for Transposition of the Great Arteries 40
Julita C. Mendoza, MD; Shirley A. Wilkerson, MD, PhD; Anabel H. Reese, MEd, Louisville, Ky

Elevated Plasma Norepinephrine Levels in Infants of Substance-Abusing Mothers 44
Sally L. Davidson Ward, MD; Sally Schuetz, RN, CPNP; Laura Wachsman, MD; Xylena D. Bean, MD; Daisy Bautista; Sue Buckley; Sabitha Sehgal, MD; David Warburton, MB, MRCP, Los Angeles, Calif

SPECIAL CONTRIBUTION

Women in Medicine: Fantasies, Dreams, Myths, and Realities 49
Catherine DeAngelis, MD, Baltimore, Md

ARTICLES

Lumbar Puncture Frequency and Cerebrospinal Fluid Analysis in the Neonate 54
Jeffrey Schwersenski, MD; Lester McIntyre, MD; Charles R. Bauer, MD, Miami, Fla

Family History Fails to Identify Many Children With Severe Hypercholesterolemia 61
Thomas J. Starc, MD; Peter F. Belamarich, MD; Steven Shea, MD; Beth E. Dobrin-Seckler, RD; Ralph B. Dell, MD; Welton M. Gersony, MD; Richard J. Deckelbaum, MD, New York, NY

Acute Osteomyelitis in Children: Reassessment of Etiologic Agents and Their Clinical Characteristics 65
Howard Faden, MD, Mauro Grossi, MD, Buffalo, NY

Pneumococcal Osteomyelitis and Arthritis in Children: A Hospital Series and Literature Review 70
Norman M. Jacobs, MD, Chicago, Ill

Influence of Otitis Media on the Correlation Between Rectal and Auditory Canal Temperatures 75
Thomas E. Terndrup, MD, Agnes Wong, MD, Syracuse, NY

EDUCATIONAL INTERVENTIONS

School Health Training During Pediatric Residency 79
Virginia N. Niebuhr, PhD; David P. McCormick, MD; Stephen E. Barnett, MD, Galveston, Tex

Continued on page 6.

AMERICAN JOURNAL OF DISEASES OF CHILDREN

ARTICLES

Nevus Flammeus: Discordance in Monozygotic Twins 85
Raanan Shamir, MD; Gertrude Kohn, MD;
Aryeh Metzker, MD, Tel Aviv, Israel

Neural Arch Stenosis and Spinal Cord Injury in Thanatophoric Dysplasia 87
Ona Marie Faye-Petersen, MD, A. S. Knisely, MD, Salt Lake City, Utah

Marfanoid Children: Etiologic Heterogeneity and Cardiac Findings 90
Shawky Tayel, MD; Thaddeus W. Kurczynski, MD, PhD;
Marc Levine, MD; Ernest Brookfield, MD; Robert Ehrlich, MD;
James R. Hennessy, MD; Martin M. DeBeukelaer, MD, Toledo, Ohio

Differences in Expression of Cystic Fibrosis in Blacks and Whites 94
Susanna A. McColley, MD; Beryl J. Rosenstein, MD;
Garry R. Cutting, MD, Baltimore, Md

Cat-Scratch Disease: Acute Encephalopathy and Other Neurologic Manifestations 98
Hugh A. Carithers, MD, Jacksonville, Fla;
A. M. Margileth, MD, Bethesda, Md

Surfactant Replacement Therapy in Respiratory Distress Syndrome: Meta-analysis of Clinical Trials of Single-Dose Surfactant Extracts 102
Halim M. Hennes, MD; Martha B. Lee, PhD;
Alfred A. Rimm, PhD, Milwaukee, Wis;
Donald L. Shapiro, MD, Rochester, NY

Gallstones in Children: Characterization by Age, Etiology, and Outcome 105
Shimon Reif, MD, Buffalo, NY; Daniel G. Sloven, MD, St Louis, Mo;
Emanuel Lebenthal, MD, Philadelphia, Pa

SPECIAL FEATURES

Radiological Case of the Month 111
CPT Michael E. Ruff, MC, USA;
MAJ W. Michael Southgate, MC, USA, Hawaii;
Beverly P. Wood, MD, Los Angeles, Calif

Picture of the Month 113
Jeffrey L. Loughead, MD; Francis Mimouni, MD;
Sue Schilling, RN, Cincinnati, Ohio;
Murray Feingold, MD, Brighton, Mass

1990 Reviewers for AJDC 115

REGULAR DEPARTMENTS

Index to Advertisers 4

Information for Authors 110

Classified Advertising 122

EDITORIAL POLICY

The JOURNAL is meant to provide physicians in all specialties who practice pediatric medicine a complete and accurate synthesis of all current research developments and clinical topics pertinent to their practice, as well as an open forum for dialogue on scientific, educational, ethical, and humanistic issues of concern to any intellec-tual committed to the practice of pediatrics.

All articles published, including editorials, letters, and book reviews, represent the opinions of the authors and do not reflect the official policy of the American Medical Association, the Editorial Board, or the institution with which the author is affiliated, unless this is cleary specified.

SUBSCRIPTION RATES—The subscription rates for the AMERICAN JOURNAL OF DISEASES OF CHILDREN are as follows:$58 for one year, $101 for two years in the United States and US Possessions; all other countries, one year, $73; two years, $131 for surface delivery. For expedited air delivery to most countries, add $15 surcharge for one year subscription, $30 for two years. (Rates for subscriptions for delivery to Japan or South Korea are available through exclusive agents–contact the publisher.) ***Special rates for residents and medical students in the United States and US possesions are available.*** Address inquiries to the American Medical Association, Circulation and Fulfillment Division, 515 N State St, Chicago, IL 60610. Phone: (312) 464-0183.

The AMERICAN JOURNAL OF DISEASES OF CHILDREN (ISSN 0002-922X) is published monthly by the American Medical Association, 515 N State St, Chicago, IL 60610, and is an official publication of the Association. Second-class postage paid at Chicago and at additional mailing office.

CHANGE OF ADDRESS—POSTMASTER, send all address changes to AMERICAN JOURNAL OF DISEASES OF CHILDREN, Attention: Subscription Department, 515 N State St, Chicago, IL 60610. Notification of address change must be made at least six weeks in advance. Include both old and new addresses, a recent mailing label, and your new ZIP code.

Please address communications concerning accepted or published communications to AMA Specialty Journals, 515 N State St, Chicago, IL 60610.

AMERICAN JOURNAL OF DISEASES OF CHILDREN

AJDC

Vol 145 No. 2 FEBRUARY 1991

THE PEDIATRIC FORUM

1991 Annual Meeting 125

Impetigo 125
Nancy B. Esterly, MD; David B. Nelson, MD;
W. Michael Dunne, Jr, PhD, Milwaukee, Wis

Diagnosis of Child Sexual Abuse in Children With Genital Warts 126
Laura T. Gutman, MD; Marcia Herman-Giddens, PA, MPH;
Neil S. Prose, MD, Durham, NC; Alan S. Boyd, MD, Lubbock, Tex

Rickets Caused by Vitamin D Deficiency in Breast-fed Infants in the Southern United States 127
Samar K. Bhowmick, MD; Kevin R. Johnson, MD, Keesler, Miss;
Kenneth R. Rettig, MD, Mobile, Ala

THE EDITORIAL BOARD SPEAKS

Tell the Whole Story 135
John D. Johnson, MD, Albuquerque, NM

ARTICLES

Human Immunodeficiency Virus Transmission by Child Sexual Abuse 137
Laura T. Gutman, MD; Karen K. St Claire, MD; Chris Weedy, MSW;
Marcia E. Herman-Giddens, PA, MPH; Barbara A. Lane, MSN;
Jeanne G. Niemeyer, MSW; Ross E. McKinney, Jr, MD, Durham, NC

Sexual Maturation and Blood Pressure Levels of a Biracial Sample of Girls 142
Claudia A. Kozinetz, PhD, MPH, Houston, Tex

Lipoprotein Profiles in Hypercholesterolemic Children 147
Richard E. Garcia, MD, Douglas S. Moodie, MD, Cleveland, Ohio

Outpatient Assessment of Infants With Bronchiolitis 151
Kathy N. Shaw, MD, MS; Louis M. Bell, MD;
Nancy H. Sherman, MD, Philadelphia, Pa

Increased Transient Tachypnea of the Newborn in Infants of Asthmatic Mothers 156
Michael Schatz, MD; Robert S. Zeiger, MD, PhD; Clement P. Hoffman, MD;
Brian S. Saunders, MD; Kathleen M. Harden, RN, San Diego, Calif;
Alan B. Forsythe, PhD, Costa Mesa, Calif

Continued on page 123.

Landmark study concludes: Enuretic children may lack diurnal rhythm of ADH common in non-enuretic children[1]

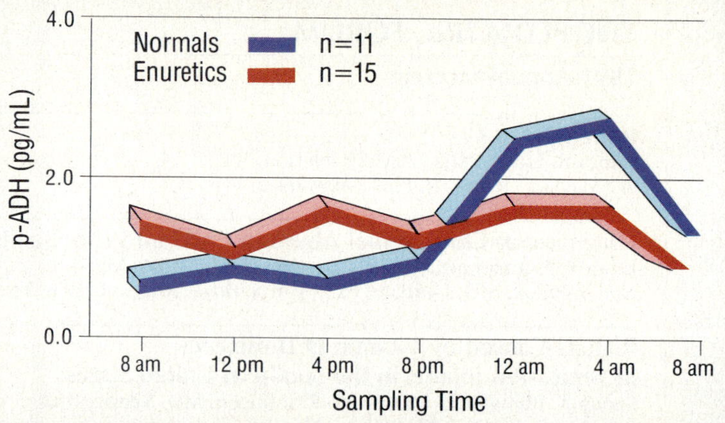

Mean diurnal variation in plasma antidiuretic hormone (p-ADH) between normal and enuretic children[1]

The ADH Deficit

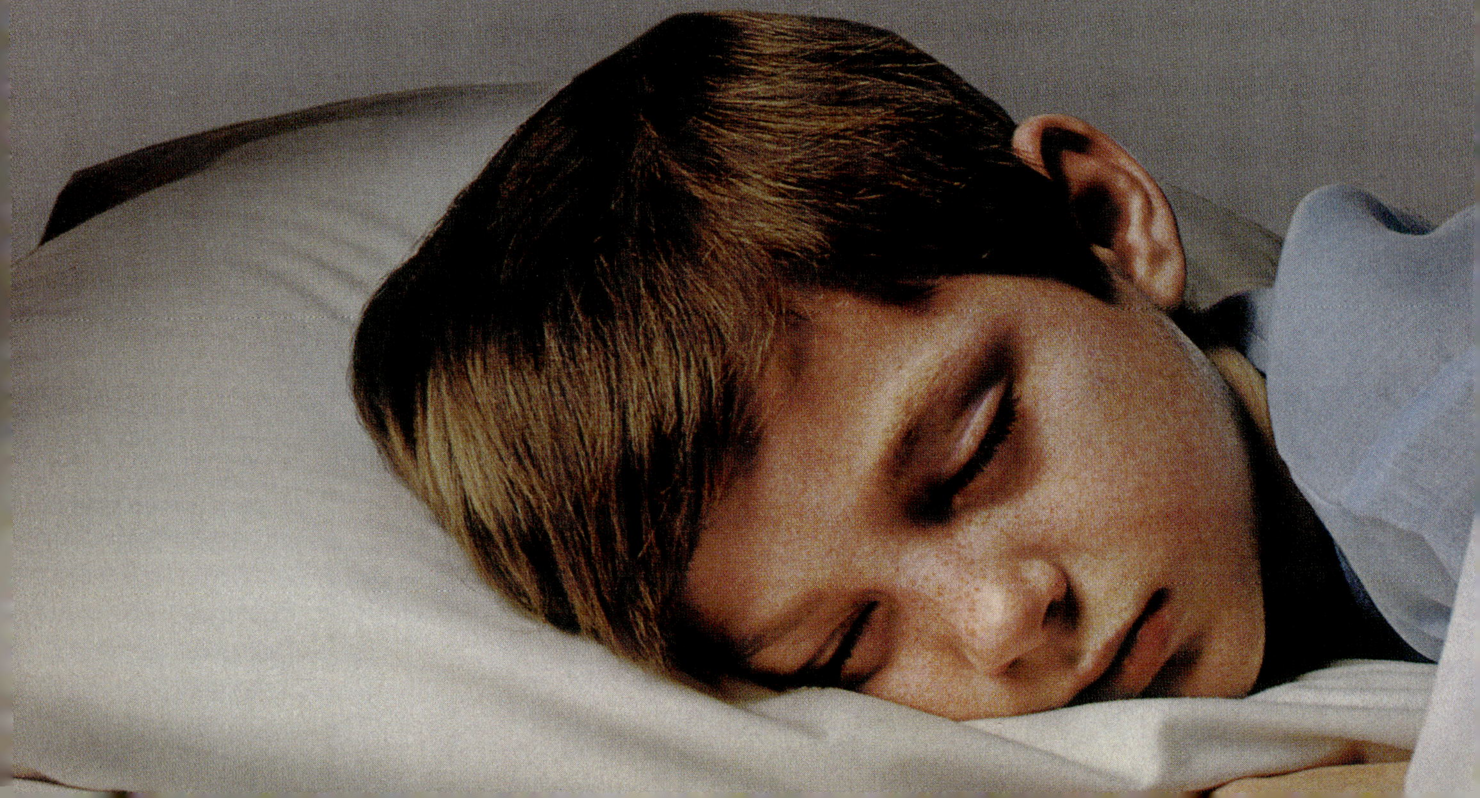

AMERICAN JOURNAL OF DISEASES OF CHILDREN

EDUCATIONAL INTERVENTION

A Medical Ethics Issues Survey of Residents in Five Pediatric Training Programs 161
Bruce David White, DO, JD; Gerald B. Hickson, MD; Rosemary Theriot, EdD; Richard M. Zaner, PhD, Nashville, Tenn

ARTICLES

Intraosseous Infusion of Dobutamine and Isoproterenol 165
John F. Bilello, MD, Kevin C. O'Hair, DVM, El Paso, Tex; William C. Kirby, MD; LTC John W. Moore, MC, USA, Washington, DC

Effectiveness of Growth-Promoting Therapies: Comparison Among Growth Hormone, Clonidine, and Levodopa 168
Cecilia Volta, MD; Lucia Ghizzoni, MD; Gaetano Muto, MD; Raffaella Spaggiari, MD; Raffaele Virdis, MD; Sergio Bernasconi, MD, Parma, Italy

Age-Related Patterns of Thyroid-Stimulating Hormone Response to Thyrotropin-Releasing Hormone Stimulation in Down Syndrome 172
Teresa Sharav, MBBS, MPH, Heddy Landau, MD, Jerusalem, Israel; Zvi Zadik, MD, Rehovot, Israel; Thomas R. Einarson, PhD, Toronto, Ontario

SPORTS MEDICINE

Sudden Cardiac Death in Young Athletes: A Review 177
Francis M. McCaffrey, MD, Augusta, Ga; LCDR David S. Braden, MC, USNR, Portsmouth, Va; William B. Strong, MD, Augusta, Ga

ARTICLES

Tattooing Behavior in Adolescence: A Comparison Study 184
James A. Farrow, MD, Seattle, Wash; Richard H. Schwartz, MD, Falls Church, Va; Joop Vanderleeuw, MD, Seattle, Wash

Skateboarding Injuries in Children: A Second Wave 188
Joel Retsky, MD; David Jaffe, MD; Katherine Christoffel, MD, MPH, Chicago, Ill

Differences in Infant Mortality by Race, Nativity Status, and Other Maternal Characteristics 194
Joel C. Kleinman, PhD; Lois A. Fingerhut, MA; Kate Prager, ScD, Hyattsville, Md

Retinopathy of Prematurity in Infants With Cyanotic Congenital Heart Disease 200
Karla J. Johns, MD; James A. Johns, MD; Stephen S. Feman, MD; Debra A. Dodd, MD, Nashville, Tenn

Unsuspected Cocaine Exposure in Young Children 204
Sigmund J. Kharasch, MD; Deborah Glotzer, MD; Robert Vinci, MD; Michael Weitzman, MD; James Sargent, MD, Boston, Mass

Continued on page 124.

AMERICAN JOURNAL OF DISEASES OF CHILDREN

SPECIAL FEATURES

Radiological Case of the Month 209
Kathlene S. Waller, MD, Jennifer Johnson, MD, Oklahoma City, Okla; Beverly P. Wood, MD, Los Angeles, Calif

Picture of the Month 211
Jeffrey R. Schneider, MD, Howard Fischer, MD, Detroit, Mich; Murray Feingold, MD, Brighton, Mass

ARTICLES

Late Cholangitis After Successful Surgical Repair of Biliary Atresia 213
Frederic Gottrand, MD; Olivier Bernard, MD; Michelle Hadchouel, MD; Daniele Pariente, MD; Frederic Gauthier, MD; Daniel Alagille, MD, Le Kremlin-Bicêtre, France

Factors Affecting Outcome in Meningococcal Infections 218
Louis J. Tesoro, MD, Steven M. Selbst, MD, Philadelphia, Pa

Antibody Responses to Four *Haemophilus influenzae* Type b Conjugate Vaccines 223
H. Kayhty, PhD; J. Eskola, MD; H. Peltola, MD; P-R. Ronnberg, RN; E. Kela, RN; V. Karanko, RN; L. Saarinen, MSc, Helsinki, Finland

Focal Scleroderma and Severe Cardiomyopathy: Patient Report and Brief Review 229
Ellen C. Moore, MD; Flossie Cohen, MD; Zia Farooki, MD; Chung-Ho Chang, MD, Detroit, Mich

Chronic Neutropenia During Childhood: A 13-Year Experience in a Single Institution 232
Olafur G. Jonsson, MD, George R. Buchanan, MD, Dallas, Tex

CORRECTION

Acquired Methemoglobinemia: The Relationship of Cause to Course of Illness 158
Jeffrey R. Avner, MD; Fred M. Henretig, MD; Constance M. McAneney, MD, Philadelphia, Pa

BOOK REVIEWS

Fasting Girls: History of Anorexia Nervosa 146
George D. Comerci, MD, Tucson, Ariz

Pediatric Intensive Care 175
J. Michael Dean, MD, Salt Lake City, Utah

REGULAR DEPARTMENTS

Index to Advertisers 118

Information to Authors 236

Classified Advertising 237

PUBLICATION STAFF

EDITORIAL POLICY

The Journal is meant to provide physicians in all specialties who practice pediatric medicine a complete and accurate synthesis of all current research developments and clinical topics pertinent to their practice, as well as an open forum for dialogue on scientific, educational, ethical, and humanistic issues of concern to any intellectual committed to the practice of pediatrics.

All articles published, including editorials, letters, and book reviews, represent the opinions of the authors and do not reflect the official policy of the American Medical Association, the Editorial Board, or the institution with which the author is affiliated, unless this is clearly specified.

SUBSCRIPTION RATES—The subscription rates for the AMERICAN JOURNAL OF DISEASES OF CHILDREN are as follows: $58 for 1 year, $101 for 2 years in the United States and US possessions; all other countries, 1 year, $73; 2 years, $131 for surface delivery. For expedited air delivery to most countries, add $15 surcharge for 1-year subscription, $30 for 2 years. (Rates for subscriptions for delivery to Japan or South Korea are available through exclusive agents—contact the publisher.) ***Special rates for residents and medical students in the United States and US possesions are available.*** Address inquiries to the American Medical Association, Circulation and Fulfillment Division, 515 N State St, Chicago, IL 60610. Phone: (312) 464-0183.

The AMERICAN JOURNAL OF DISEASES OF CHILDREN (ISSN 0002-922X) is published monthly by the American Medical Association, 515 N State St, Chicago, IL 60610, and is an official publication of the Association. Second-class postage paid at Chicago and at additional mailing office.

CHANGE OF ADDRESS—POSTMASTER, send all address changes to AMERICAN JOURNAL OF DISEASES OF CHILDREN, Attention: Subscription Department, 515 N State St, Chicago, IL 60610. Notification of address change must be made at least 6 weeks in advance. Include both old and new addresses, a recent mailing label, and your new ZIP code.

Please address communications concerning accepted or published communications to AMA Specialty Journals, 515 N State St, Chicago, IL 60610.

AMERICAN JOURNAL OF DISEASES OF CHILDREN

AJDC

Vol 145 No. 3 MARCH 1991

THE PEDIATRIC FORUM

1991 Annual Meeting 249

More on the *P* Value 249
David M. Coulter, MD, Salt Lake City, Utah

In Reply 249
George W. Brown, MD, Los Lunas, NM

Multiple Comparisons and *P* Values 250
Thomas B. Newman, MD, MPH;
Warren S. Browner, MD, MPH, San Francisco, Calif

***P* Values** 250
Ted Byrt, Parkville, Australia

Clavicular Fractures in Neonates: Frequency vs Significance 251
Michael J. O'Halloran, Eau Claire, Wis

In Reply 251
Paul R. Joseph, MD, Mineola, NY

Clavicular Fractures in Neonates 251
Gloria Carter, RN, PNP; J. W. Park, MD, Odessa, Tex

In Reply 252
Paul R. Joseph, MD; Warren Rosenfeld, MD, Mineola, NY

What About Gay Teenagers? 252
Charles R. Fikar, MD; Mary Koslap-Petraco, BSN, RN, Deer Park, NY

EDITORIALS

Pediatric Legal Medicine: A New Venture 255
Peggy C. Ferry, MD, Tucson, Ariz

Pediatric Perspectives: Vistas and Vantage Points 256
Alan D. Bedrick, MD, Tucson, Ariz

THE EDITORIAL BOARD SPEAKS

Your Child's Best Friend: TV or Not TV 257
E. Richard Stiehm, MD, Philadelphia, Pa

Continued on page 245.

AMERICAN JOURNAL OF DISEASES OF CHILDREN

ARTICLES

Standardized Percentile Curves of Body-Mass Index for Children and Adolescents 259
Lawrence D. Hammer, MD; Helena C. Kraemer, PhD; Darrell M. Wilson, MD; Philip L. Ritter, PhD; Sanford M. Dornbusch, PhD, Palo Alto, Calif

Improved Speed and Accuracy of Calculations With a Programmable Calculator in Pediatric Emergency Scenarios 264
Marlene Melzer-Lange, MD; David Wyatt, MD; Christine Walsh-Kelly, MD; Douglas Smith, MD; Mary A. Hegenbarth, MD; Carl S. L. Eisenberg, MD, Milwaukee, Wis

Psychosocial Predictors of Maternal and Infant Health Among Adolescent Mothers 267
W. Thomas Boyce, MD; Elizabeth A. Chesterman; Marilyn A. Winkleby, PhD, San Francisco, Calif

Physicians, Formula Companies, and Advertising: A Historical Perspective 282
Frank R. Greer, MD, Rima D. Apple, PhD, Madison, Wis

Ventriculitis in Newborns With Myelomeningocele 287
Edward B. Charney, MD; Jeanne B. Melchionni, RN; Donna L. Antonucci, MD, Philadelphia, Pa

Stimulant Medication and Attention Deficit Disorder: The Child's Perspective 291
Jennifer Bowen, MBBS; Terence Fenton, PhD; Leonard Rappaport, MD, Boston, Mass

Capillary Refilling (Skin Turgor) in the Assessment of Dehydration 296
Jose M. Saavedra, MD; Glenn D. Harris, MD; Song Li, MD; Laurence Finberg, MD, Brooklyn, NY

Neonatal Hepatitis and Extrahepatic Biliary Atresia Associated With Cytomegalovirus Infection in Twins 302
Michael H. Hart, MD; Stuart S. Kaufman, MD; Jon A. Vanderhoof, MD; Rodney S. Markin, MD; Robert Kruger, MD; Dean L. Antonson, MD, Omaha, Neb

Breast-feeding Initiation in a Triethnic Population 306
David E. Bee, PhD; Tom Baranowski, PhD; David K. Rassin, PhD; C. Joan Richardson, MD, Augusta, Ga; William Mikrut, MS, Galveston, Tex

Esophageal Motility in Children With Hirschsprung's Disease 310
Annamaria Staiano, MD, Naples, Italy; Enrico Corazziari, MD, Rome, Italy; Maria Rosaria Andreotti, MD, Naples, Italy; Ray E. Clouse, MD, St Louis, Mo

Adipsic Hypernatremia in Two Sisters 321
Giorgio Radetti, MD; Francesco Rizza, MD; Giuseppe Mengarda, MD; Klaus Pittschieler, MD, Bolzano, Italy

Continued on page 247.

EDITORIAL POLICY

The Journal is meant to provide physicians in all specialties who practice pediatric medicine a complete and accurate synthesis of all current research developments and clinical topics pertinent to their practice, as well as an open forum for dialogue on scientific, educational, ethical, and humanistic issues of concern to any intellectual committed to the practice of pediatrics.

All articles published, including editorials, letters, and book reviews, represent the opinions of the authors and do not reflect the official policy of the American Medical Association, the Editorial Board, or the institution with which the author is affiliated, unless this is clearly specified.

AMERICAN JOURNAL OF DISEASES OF CHILDREN

Anergy in Pediatric Head Trauma Patients 326
Nevin W. Wilson, MD, La Jolla, Calif; Ann Gooding, MD; Bradley Peterson, MD; John F. Bastian, MD, San Diego, Calif

Endocrine Function in Children With Human Immunodeficiency Virus Infection 330
Lisa J. Schwartz, DO, Bronx, NY; Yolaine St Louis, MD, Brooklyn, NY; Richard Wu, MD; Andrew Wiznia, MD; Arye Rubinstein, MD; Paul Saenger, MD, Bronx, NY

LEGAL MEDICINE

Photographing the Physically Abused Child: Principles and Practice 275
Lawrence R. Ricci, MD, Waterville, Me

EDUCATIONAL INTERVENTION

Practice Management Training for Pediatric Residents 299
Janice P. Piatt, MD; Douglas L. Bartley, MD; Albert D. Jacobson, MD; Mary E. Rimsza, MD, Phoenix, Ariz

PERSPECTIVES

Cortical Resection for Children With Epilepsy: Perspectives in Pediatrics 314
Elaine Wyllie, MD, Cleveland, Ohio

SPECIAL FEATURES

Radiological Case of the Month 339
Michele K. Holloway, MD; Suman Wason, MD, MBA; J. Paul Willging, MD; Charles M. Myer III, MD, Cincinnati, Ohio; Beverly P. Wood, MD, Los Angeles, Calif

Picture of the Month 341
Diane E. Friedman, MEd; Richard J. Pines, DO; Matthew Shelley, MD; Pamela Fisher, MD; G. Michael Silberbach, MD, Portland, Ore; Murray Feingold, MD, Brighton, Mass

REGULAR DEPARTMENTS

Index to Advertisers 244

Instructions for Authors 248

Classified Advertising 345

Instructions for Authors

New Manuscript Procedure

On January 1, 1988, *AJDC* initiated a new procedure. Manuscripts submitted to *AJDC* will NO LONGER BE RETURNED, except in the case of accepted manuscripts or those undergoing author revision. Original artwork and photographs will be returned.

General Information.—Please send manuscripts and correspondence by first-class mail *(do not use registered, certified, or express mail)* to the Editor, Vincent A. Fulginiti, MD, *AJDC*, Dean's Office, Room 1529, Tulane University, School of Medicine, 1430 Tulane Avenue, New Orleans, LA 70112. All accepted manuscripts are subject to copy editing. The corresponding author will receive an edited typescript and layout for approval. Forms for ordering reprints are included with the edited typescript. Reprints are shipped six to eight weeks after publication. Proofs will be sent for approval *if requested* by the author and if printing deadlines permit. The author is responsible for all statements in his/her work, including changes made by the copy editor.

Conforming with all of the steps listed below will facilitate the editorial processing of your manuscript.

Step 1.—*Cover Letter.*—All manuscripts must be accompanied on submission by a cover letter giving the name, address, affiliation, and telephone number of the corresponding author. The letter must include ALL of the following statements SIGNED BY ALL AUTHORS (ORIGINAL SIGNATURES):

1. *Copyright Release.*— "In consideration of the American Medical Association's taking action in reviewing and editing this submission, the author(s) undersigned hereby transfer(s), assign(s), or otherwise convey(s) all copyright ownership to the AMA in the event that this work is published by the AMA."

2. *Statement of Affirmation.*—"This manuscript has not been published anywhere in any language and is not under simultaneous consideration by another publication. This manuscript is original and ALL authors have seen and approve of its contents."

3. *Financial Disclosure.*—List all affiliations with or financial involvement in organizations or entities with a direct financial interest in the subject matter or material of the research discussed in the manuscript (eg, employment consultancies, stock ownership) OR include a statement disclaiming any such involvement. All such information will be held in confidence during the review process. Should the manuscript be accepted, the Editor will discuss with the author the extent of disclosures appropriate for publication. All accepted manuscripts become the permanent property of the publisher (AMA) and may not be published elsewhere without written permission from the AMA. After publication certain articles may appear in translation in the foreign-language edition(s) of *AJDC*.

Step 2.—*Manuscript Format.*—All articles submitted should have the following features:

1. Four copies of the manuscript should be submitted; three are for transmission to referees and one is to be retained in the editorial office. We prefer an original and three copies.

2. Manuscripts should be typed in triple-spaced format on heavy-duty white bond paper, 21.6×27.9 cm (8 ½×11 in) with 2.5-cm (1-in) margins. *Do not use justified right margins.*

3. Title should be no more than 75 characters.

4. Authors should be limited to six, all of whom have contributed to the study and manuscript preparation, are familiar with its substance, and are able to defend its conclusions.

5. The title page should give full names, degrees, and academic affiliations of all authors, address for request of reprints, and, if the manuscript was presented at a meeting, the organization, place, and exact date on which it was read.

6. Writing style should conform to proper English usage and syntax; consult the *American Medical Association Manual of Style*, available from Williams & Wilkins, 428 E Preston St, Baltimore, MD 21202.

7. Abstract should be limited to 135 words or less.

8. Each table should be typed, with a title, on a separate sheet of paper, with each line, including headings, *double-spaced*. Continuations should be on a second sheet with all headings repeated.

9. Use Système International (SI) measurements throughout the manuscript.

10. Illustrations should be high-contrast, glossy prints, in quadruplicate, unmounted and untrimmed; lettering should be legible after reduction to column size. Figure number, name of first author, and arrow indicating "top" should be typed on a gummed *label* and affixed on the back of each illustration. *Do not write directly on the print.*

Magnification and stain should be provided for histologic sections. Full-color illustrations should be submitted as 35-mm, positive color transparencies, mounted in cardboard and carefully packaged. Do not submit glass-mounted transparencies or color prints. Fee is $400 for up to six square-finished color illustrations that fit on one page. A letter of intent to pay the fee must accompany submission.

All photographs in which there is a possibility of patient identification should be accompanied by a signed statement of consent from both parents (or guardians). Covering eyes to mask identity is not sufficient.

11. References should be listed in order of their appearance in the text, type double-spaced, and in AMA format. Please follow the exact order of information and punctuation in the examples below. Note: List all authors and/or editors up to six; if more than six, list the first three and "et al."

Journal articles: Scott GB, Buck BE, Leterman JG, Bloom FL, Parks WP. Acquired immunodeficiency syndrome in infants. N Engl J Med. 1984;310:76-81.

Books: Naeye RL. How and when does antenatal hypoxia damage fetal brains? In: Kubli F, Patel N, Schmidt W, Linderkamp O, eds. *Perinatal Events and Brain Damage in Surviving Children.* New York, NY: Springer Verlag NY Inc; 1988:83-91.

Unpublished data, personal communications, or manuscripts "in preparation" or "submitted" should not be included in the list of references. Such material, if essential, may be incorporated in the body of the article.

Authors are responsible for the accuracy of the references.

12. Investigations involving human subjects require a specific statement in the "Methods" section that an appropriate institutional review board approved the project and/or that informed consent was obtained from both legal guardians and/or child, if appropriate.

13. Illustrations and tables from other publications should be suitably acknowledged, with written permission from *publisher* and *author.* Brief acknowledgements to specific contributors directly involved in the content of the manuscript may be placed at the end of the text, before the references. General acknowledgements will be deleted.

Step 3.—*Special Departments.*—Criteria for several special departments are given below.

1. *The Pediatric Forum.*— This is the place for comment, criticism, observations, and discussion of "issues of current concern and importance for children's health," in addition to letters that comment on articles in previous issues of *AJDC*. The Editor reserves the right to conduct review of and to edit all submissions. THE READER SHOULD SUBMIT TRIPLE-SPACED COPY CLEARLY MARKED 'FOR PUBLICATION' AND SIGNED BY ALL AUTHORS. REFERENCES, IF INCLUDED, SHOULD CONFORM TO THE USUAL AMA FORMAT. Copyright assignment, signed by all authors, must accompany the original submission.

2. *From Reseach to Relevance.*—PURPOSE: To focus on significant research that has a high probability of being translated into clinical usefulness.

3. *Educational Interventions.*—PURPOSE: To share information concerning any educational efforts in the broad field of pediatrics.

4. *Sports Medicine.*—PURPOSE: To provide current information related to the medical needs of young athletes, as pertinent to counseling young athletes and their parents regarding sports participation and practices contributing to the health maintenance of the athlete, as well as current concepts in the prevention, diagnosis, and treatment of sports-related illnesses and injuries.

5. *Picture of the Month.*—Submissions should be sent directly to Murray Feingold, MD, National Birth Defects Center, Kennedy Memorial Hospital, 30 Warren St, Brighton, MA 02135, and should conform to the format for original articles in terms of the text, references and illustrations.

6. *Radiological Case of the Month.*—Submissions should be sent directly to Beverly P. Wood, MD, University of Rochester Medical Center, 601 Elmwood Ave, PO Box 648, Rochester, NY 14642. Submissions should conform to the format for original articles in terms of the text, references, and illustrations.

Author's Checklist

___ 1. Cover letter with name, address, and telephone number of corresponding author.
___ 2. Copyright transmittal, affirmation, and financial statements signed by ALL authors.
___ 3. Original typed manuscript plus three copies.
___ 4. Triple-spacing; double-spacing for tables and legends.
___ 5. Right margins UNJUSTIFIED.
___ 6. Title 75 characters or less.
___ 7. Abstract included.
___ 8. References in proper format, cited in numerical order.
___ 9. Four sets of illustrations.
___ 10. Four sets of legends for illustrations.
___ 11. Proper consent forms for patient photographs.
___ 12. Permission forms for illustrations previously published elsewhere.

SUBSCRIPTION RATES—The subscription rates for the AMERICAN JOURNAL OF DISEASES OF CHILDREN are as follows: $58 for 1 year, $101 for 2 years in the United States and US possessions; all other countries, 1 year, $73; 2 years, $131 for surface delivery. For expedited air delivery to most countries, add $15 surcharge for 1-year subscription, $30 for 2 years. (Rates for subscriptions for delivery to Japan or South Korea are available through exclusive agents--contact the publisher.) ***Special rates for residents and medical students in the United States and US possessions are available.*** Address inquiries to the American Medical Association, Circulation and Fulfillment Division, 515 N State St, Chicago, IL 60610. Phone: (312) 670-SUBS.

The AMERICAN JOURNAL OF DISEASES OF CHILDREN (ISSN 0002-922X) is published monthly by the American Medical Association, 515 N State St, Chicago, IL 60610, and is an official publication of the Association. Second-class postage paid at Chicago and at additional mailing office.

CHANGE OF ADDRESS—POSTMASTER, send all address changes to AMERICAN JOURNAL OF DISEASES OF CHILDREN, Attention: Subscription Department, 515 N State St, Chicago, IL 60610. Notification of address change must be made at least 6 weeks in advance. Include both old and new addresses, a recent mailing label, and your new ZIP code.

Please address communications concerning accepted or published communications to AMA Specialty Journals, 515 N State St, Chicago, IL 60610.

GST tax number: R 126 225 556

AMERICAN JOURNAL OF DISEASES OF CHILDREN

AJDC

Vol 145 **No. 4** **APRIL 1991**

AMBULATORY PEDIATRIC ASSOCIATION:

PROGRAM AND ABSTRACTS 365

Annual Meeting of the Ambulatory Pediatric Association 383

THE PEDIATRIC FORUM

1991 Annual Meeting 425

Diphtheria and Tetanus Toxoids and Pertussis Vaccine Litigation 425
Howard Lokietz, MD, Arcadia, Calif

In Reply 425
Vincent A. Fulginiti, MD, New Orleans, La

Antibody Response to MMR Vaccination in Children Who Received IVIG as Neonates 425
Jeanne W. Ruderman, MD, Los Angeles, Calif;
Noori Barka, PhD,
James B. Peter, MD, PhD, Santa Monica, Calif;
E. Richard Stiehm, MD, Los Angeles, Calif

Vaccine Myth and Physician Handouts 426
Thomas P. Lynch, MD, Darien, Ill

In Reply 426
James D. Cherry, MD, Los Angeles, Calif

In Reply 427
Vincent A. Fulginiti, MD, New Orleans, La

Continued on page 355.

American Medical Association
Physicians dedicated to the health of America

The AMERICAN JOURNAL OF DISEASES OF CHILDREN is a member of the consortium of AMA journals listed below. The Archives reaches more than 40030 readers in 85 countries each month. The complete text of all AMA journals is available on the MEDIS database from Mead Data Central, Dayton, Ohio.

JAMA The Journal of the American Medical Association
AJDC American Journal of Diseases of Children
archives of Dermatology
archives of General Psychiatry
archives of Internal Medicine
archives of Neurology
archives of Ophthalmology
archives of Otolaryngology–Head & Neck Surgery
archives of Pathology & Laboratory Medicine
archives of Surgery

AMERICAN JOURNAL OF DISEASES OF CHILDREN

Exhibitor 'Giveaways': A Curmudgeon's View 427
Lawrence R. Berger, MD, MPH, Albuquerque, NM

New York State Health Code 405 Update 428
Gerald E. Daigler, MD; Robert C. Welliver, MD; F. Bruder Stapleton, MD, Buffalo, NY

THE EDITORIAL BOARD SPEAKS

Complex Problem: Complex Solutions 429
Elizabeth McAnarney, MD, Rochester, NY

ARTICLES

Acquired Immunodeficiency Syndrome and Adolescents: Knowledge, Attitudes, and Behaviors of Runaway and Homeless Youths 431
Susan Tucker Sugerman, MD, MPH; Albert C. Hergenroeder, MD; Mariam R. Chacko, MD; Guy S. Parcel, PhD, Houston, Tex

The Total Iron-Binding Capacity in Iron Poisoning: Is It Useful? 437
Milton Tenenbein, MD, FRCPC, FAAP, Randall W. Yatscoff, PhD, FCACB, Winnipeg, Manitoba

Improving the Use of Early Follow-up Care After Emergency Department Visits: A Randomized Trial 440
Eliot W. Nelson, MD; Susan Van Cleve, RN, MSN, PNP; Martha K. Swartz, RN, MSN, PNP; William Kessen, PhD; Paul L. McCarthy, MD, New Haven, Conn

Influenza Vaccination in the Prevention of Acute Otitis Media in Children 445
Terho Heikkinen, MD; Olli Ruuskanen, MD; Matti Waris, MSc; Thedi Ziegler, PhD; Mikko Arola, MD; Pekka Halonen, MD, Turku, Finland

Mineral Metabolism and Calcitriol Therapy in Idiopathic Juvenile Osteoporosis 457
Giuseppe Saggese, MD; Silvano Bertelloni, MD; Giampiero I. Baroncelli, MD; Giuseppe Perri, MD; Andrea Calderazzi, MD, Pisa, Italy

Continued on page 358.

AMERICAN JOURNAL OF DISEASES OF CHILDREN

Evaluation of Bayesian Forecasting for Individualized Gentamicin Dosage in Infants Weighing 1000 g or Less 463
Kei Lui, MBBS, FRACP;
Scott M. Bryson, MScPharm;
Danica B. Irwin, BScPharm;
Simon Costello, MBBS, FRACP, Toronto, Ontario

EDUCATIONAL INTERVENTION

The Pediatric Program Director: An Analysis of the Role and Its Problems 449
Jeffrey C. Weiss, MD, Philadelphia, Pa;
Robert A. Doughty MD, Wilmington, Del;
Richard Lampe, MD, Washington, DC

SPECIAL FEATURES

Radiological Case of the Month 471
Janice W. Allison, MD;
Carol A. Stephenson, MD;
Teresita L. Angtuaco, MD;
Charles M. Glasier, MD, Little Rock, Ark;
Beverly P. Wood, MD, Los Angeles, Calif

Picture of the Month 473
Zvi Laron, MD;
Beatrice Klinger, MD;
Michael Grunebaum, MD, Tel Aviv, Israel;
Murray Feingold, MD;
Walter P. Tunnessen, MD, Brighton, Mass

BOOK REVIEW

Current Concepts in Childhood Spinal Muscular Atrophy 462
Peggy C. Ferry, MD, Tucson, Ariz

REGULAR DEPARTMENTS

Index to Advertisers 354

Instructions for Authors 424

Classified Advertising 477

Please address communications concerning accepted or published communications to AMA Specialty Journals, 515 N State St, Chicago, IL 60610.

References: 1. Chandra RK, Singh G, Shridhara B: *Ann Allergy* 63:102–106, 1989.† 2. Vandenplas Y, Malfroot A, Dab I: *Immunology & Allergy Practice* XI:17–24, 1989.† 3. Lönnerdal B, Forsum E: *Am J Clin Nutr* 41:113–120, 1985. 4. Billeaud C, Guillet J, Sandler B: *European Journal of Clinical Nutrition* 44:577–583, 1990.

†Carnation GOOD START has been shown to be better tolerated than standard cow's-milk formula when fed exclusively from birth to infants with a positive family history of allergy.

*GOOD START Infant Formula should not be confused with highly-processed casein-based hydrolysate formulas advertised for the treatment of cow's-milk allergy. In cases of suspected milk allergy, all infant formulas should be used only under the supervision of a physician.

AMERICAN JOURNAL OF DISEASES OF CHILDREN

AJDC

Vol 145 **No. 5** **MAY 1991**

EDITORIALS

Far From the Ideal: The Plight of Poor Children in the United States — 489
Vincent A. Fulginiti, MD, New Orleans, La

Youth Alienation as an Emerging Pediatric Health Care Issue — 491
James A. Farrow, MD, Seattle, Wash

THE PEDIATRIC FORUM

New Initiatives in Adolescent Health Promotion — 495
Arthur B. Elster, MD, Chicago, Ill

ARTICLES

Redoing the Health Care Quilt: Patches or Whole Cloth? — 499
William W. Cleveland, MD, Miami, Fla

A Regional Pediatric Approach to the Epidemic of Social Ills Within Our Cities — 505
Waldo E. Nelson, MD, Philadelphia, Pa

Poverty and the Health of American Children: Implications for Academic Pediatrics — 507
Richard B. Johnston, Jr, MD, Philadelphia, Pa

Improving Health Care Provision to Neonates in the United States — 510
Mildred T. Stahlman, MD, Nashville, Tenn

Child Abuse and Neglect: Critical First Steps in Response to a National Emergency: The Report of the US Advisory Board on Child Abuse and Neglect — 513
Richard D. Krugman, MD, Denver, Colo

Continued on page 483.

SUBSCRIPTION RATES—The subscription rates for the AMERICAN JOURNAL OF DISEASES OF CHILDREN are as follows: $58 for 1 year, $101 for 2 years in the United States and US possessions; all other countries, 1 year, $73; 2 years, $131 for surface delivery. For expedited air delivery to most countries, add $15 surcharge for 1-year subscription, $30 for 2 years. (Rates for subscriptions for delivery to Japan or South Korea are available through exclusive agents–contact the publisher.) ***Special rates for residents and medical students in the United States and US possessions are available.*** Address inquiries to the American Medical Association, Circulation and Fulfillment Division, 515 N State St, Chicago, IL 60610. Phone: (312) 670-SUBS.

The AMERICAN JOURNAL OF DISEASES OF CHILDREN (ISSN 0002-922X) is published monthly by the American Medical Association, 515 N State St, Chicago, IL 60610, and is an official publication of the Association. Second-class postage paid at Chicago and at additional mailing office.

CHANGE OF ADDRESS—POSTMASTER, send all address changes to AMERICAN JOURNAL OF DISEASES OF CHILDREN, Attention: Subscription Department, 515 N State St, Chicago, IL 60610. Notification of address change must be made at least 6 weeks in advance. Include both old and new addresses, a recent mailing label, and your new ZIP code.

Please address communications concerning accepted or published communications to AMA Specialty Journals, 515 N State St, Chicago, IL 60610.

GST registration number: R 126 225 556

American Medical Association

Physicians dedicated to the health of America

The AMERICAN JOURNAL OF DISEASES OF CHILDREN is a member of the consortium of AMA journals listed below. The Archives reaches more than 40030 readers in 85 countries each month. The complete text of all AMA journals is available on the MEDIS database from Mead Data Central, Dayton, Ohio.

JAMA The Journal of the American Medical Association

AJDC American Journal of Diseases of Children

archives of Dermatology

archives of General Psychiatry

archives of Internal Medicine

archives of Neurology

archives of Ophthalmology

archives of Otolaryngology–Head & Neck Surgery

archives of Pathology & Laboratory Medicine

archives of Surgery

AMERICAN JOURNAL OF DISEASES OF CHILDREN

Children in and of the Streets: Health, Social Policy, and the Homeless Young 516
James D. Wright, PhD, New Orleans, La

A Survey of the Health of Homeless Children in Philadelphia Shelters 520
Ruth M. Parker, MD, Atlanta, Ga; Leslie A. Rescorla, PhD, Bryn Mawr, Pa; Jonathan A. Finkelstein, MD, Boston, Mass; Nathaniel Barnes, MD, Durham, NC; John H. Holmes, MS, Paul D. Stolley, MD, MPH, Philadelphia, Pa

Pediatric Acquired Immunodeficiency Syndrome, Poverty, and National Priorities 527
Margaret C. Heagarty, MD, New York, NY

Pediatric Human Immunodeficiency Virus Infection and the Acquired Immunodeficiency Syndrome: A Health Care Crisis of Children and Families 529
Russell B. Van Dyke, MD, New Orleans, La

The American Academy of Pediatrics Response to the Growing Health Needs of Children 536
James E. Strain, MD, Elk Grove Village, Ill

The Growing Neglect of American Children 540
Harold M. Maurer, MD, Salt Lake City, Utah

The Challenge of Care for the Poor Child: The Research Agenda 542
Steve Kohl, MD, San Francisco, Calif

Serving the Underserved: Impact on Resident Education 544
Carol D. Berkowitz, MD, McLean, Va

The Challenge of Care for the Poor and Underserved in the United States: An American College of Obstetricians and Gynecologists Perspective on Access to Care for Underserved Women 546
Ezra C. Davidson, Jr, MD; Charles E. Gibbs, MD; Janet Chapin, MPH, Washington, DC

Poverty and Cardiac Disease in Children 550
Hugh D. Allen, MD; Kathryn A. Taubert, PhD; Richard J. Deckelbaum, MD; David Driscoll, MD; Ann Dunnigan, MD; Samuel S. Gidding, MD; Paul Herndon, MD; Rae-Ellen W. Kavey, MD; Charles Mullins, MD; A. Rebecca Snider, MD; William B. Strong, MD; Reginald Washington, MD, Dallas, Tex

Continued on page 487.

Please address communications concerning accepted or published communications to AMA Specialty Journals, 515 N State St, Chicago, IL 60610.

All articles published, including editorials, letters, and book reviews, represent the opinions of the authors and do not reflect the official policy of the American Medical Association, the Editorial Board, or the institution with which the author is affiliated, unless this is clearly specified.

AMERICAN JOURNAL OF DISEASES OF CHILDREN

The Challenge of Caring for Indigent Children With Rheumatologic Diseases 554
Michael L. Miller, MD, San Antonio, Tex; Patience H. White, MD, Washington, DC

What Will It Take to Fully Protect All American Children With Vaccines? 559
Alan R. Hinman, MD, MPH, Atlanta, Ga

Improving Health Care for Underserved Infants, Children, and Adolescents: The Robert Wood Johnson Foundation's Experience 565
Michael P. Beachler, Princeton, NJ

Care of the Poor and Underserved in America: Older Adolescents: A Group at Special Risk 569
Robert J. Haggerty, MD, New York, NY

Health Care for Pregnant Women and Young Children 572
Richard E. Behrman, MD, Carol S. Larson, JD, Los Altos, Calif

Children's Services in an Era of Budget Deficits 575
Barbara B. Blum, Susan Blank, New York, NY

The Caring Program for Children: The Michigan Experience 579
Marianne Udow, MHSA; Vernon K. Smith, PhD; Margaret H. Mason, MHSA, Detroit, Mich

CORRECTION

Lipoprotein Profiles in Hypercholesterolemic Children 515
Richard E. Garcia, MD, Douglas S. Moodie, MD, Cleveland, Ohio

BOOK REVIEWS

Seizures and Epilepsy in Childhood: A Guide for Parents 539
Peggy C. Ferry, MD, Tucson, Ariz

Difficult Diagnosis in Pediatrics 541
Robert Kamei, MD, San Francisco, Calif

REGULAR DEPARTMENTS

Instructions for Authors 488

Classified Advertising 583

Index to Advertisers 588

INSTRUCTIONS FOR AUTHORS

General Information.—Please send manuscripts and correspondence to the Editor, Vincent A. Fulginiti, MD, *AJDC*, Dean's Office, Tulane University School of Medicine, 1430 Tulane Ave, New Orleans, LA 70112. *AJDC no longer returns nonaccepted manuscripts. Original artwork and photographs will be returned.* Manuscripts are considered with the understanding that they have not been published previously and are not under consideration by another publication.

Type of Manuscripts Suitable for Submission

Original Articles.—New observations that have not been submitted or published elsewhere.

Pediatric Forum.—A mixture of brief, peer-reviewed observations or investigations *and* letters to the editor and other short commentaries.

From Research to Relevance.—Significant research that has a high probability of being translated into clinical usefulness.

Educational Intervention.—Information concerning any educational efforts in the broad field of pediatrics.

Pediatric Legal Medicine.—A forum for discussion of broad issues relating to children and the law in today's environment.

Pediatric Perspectives.—Current information on clinical and scientific pediatric medical advances and analyses of current controversies in pediatrics.

Sports Medicine.—Current information relating to the medical needs of young athletes, as well as current concepts in the prevention, diagnosis, and treatment of sports-related illnesses and injuries.

Picture of the Month.—Submissions should be sent directly to Walter W. Tunnessen, Jr, MD, Children's Hospital of Philadelphia, Room 2143, 34th and Civic Center Blvd, Philadelphia, PA 19104.

Radiological Case of the Month.—Submissions should be sent directly to Beverly P. Wood, MD, Childrens Hospital of Los Angeles, Department of Radiology, 4650 Sunset Blvd, Los Angeles, CA 90054-0700.

AJDC Archives.—Occasional revivals of classic *AJDC* articles with contemporary commentary.

Pediatric Reviews.—Timely, comprehensive, well-referenced topics.

Conforming with all of the steps listed below will facilitate the editorial processing of your manuscript.

Step 1.—*Cover Letter.*—All manuscripts must be accompanied on submission by a cover letter giving the name, address, affiliation, and telephone and fax number of the corresponding author. The letter must include ALL of the following statements SIGNED BY ALL AUTHORS (ORIGINAL SIGNATURES):

1. Authorship Responsibility.—"I certify that I have participated sufficiently in the conception and design of this work and the analysis of the data (when applicable), as well as the writing of the manuscript, to take public responsibility for it. I believe the manuscript represents valid work. I have reviewed the final version of the manuscript and approve it for publication. Neither this manuscript nor one with substantially similar content under my authorship has been published or is being considered for publication elsewhere, except as described in an attachment. Furthermore, I attest that I shall produce the data upon which the manuscript is based for examination by the editors or their assignees if requested."

2. Financial Disclosure.—"I certify that affiliations (if any) with or involvement in any organization or entity with a direct financial interest in the subject matter or materials discussed in the manuscript (eg, employment, consultancies, stock ownership, honoraria, expert testimony) are disclosed below."

Research or project support should be listed in an acknowledgment.

3a. Copyright Transfer.—"In consideration of the action of the American Medical Association (AMA) in reviewing and editing this submission, the author(s) undersigned hereby transfer(s), assign(s), or otherwise convey(s) all copyright ownership to the AMA in the event that such work is published by the AMA."

3b. Federal Employment.—"I was an employee of the US federal government when this work was investigated and prepared for publication; therefore, it is not protected by the Copyright Act and there is no copyright of which the ownership can be transferred."

Editing.—Accepted manuscripts are copy edited according to AMA style and returned to the author for approval. Authors are responsible for all statements made in their work, including changes made by the copy editor and authorized by the corresponding author.

All accepted manuscripts become the permanent property of the AMA and may not be published elsewhere without written permission from both the author(s) and the AMA. After publication, certain articles may appear in translation in the foreign-language editions of *AJDC*. The corresponding author will receive typeset pages for approval. Forms for ordering reprints are included with the typeset pages. Reprints are shipped 6 to 8 weeks after publication.

Step 2.—*Manuscript Format.*—All articles submitted should have the following features:

1. Four copies of the manuscript should be submitted; three are for transmission to referees and one is retained in the editorial office. We prefer an original and three copies.
2. Manuscripts should be typed in double-spaced format throughout, including title page, abstracts, text, acknowledgments, references, legends for illustrations, and tables. Please number pages. *Do not use justified right margins.*
3. Title should be no more than 75 characters.
4. Authors should be limited to six, all of whom have contributed to the study and manuscript preparation, are familiar with its substance, and are able to defend its conclusions.
5. The title page should give full names, degrees, and academic affiliations of all authors, address for requests of reprints, and, if the manuscript was presented at a meeting, the organization, place, and exact date on which it was read.
6. Writing style should conform to proper English usage and syntax; consult the *American Medical Association Manual of Style*, available from Williams & Wilkins, 428 E Preston St, Baltimore, MD 21202.
7. Abstract should be limited to 135 words or less.
8. Each table should be typed, with a title, on a separate sheet of paper, with each line, including headings, *double-spaced*. Continuations should be on a second sheet with all headings repeated.
9. Use Système International (SI) measurements throughout the manuscript.
10. Illustrations should be high-contrast, glossy prints, in quadruplicate, in a proportion of 5x7 in. Figure number, name of first author, and arrow indicating "top" should be typed on a gummed *label* and affixed on the back of each illustration. *Do not write directly on the print.*

Full-color illustrations should be submitted as 35-mm, positive color transparencies, mounted in cardboard, and carefully packaged. Fee is $400 for up to six square-finished color illustrations that fit on one page. A letter of intent to pay the fee must accompany submission.

All photographs in which there is a possibility of patient identification should be accompanied by a signed statement of consent from both parents (or guardians). Covering eyes to mask identity is not sufficient.

11. References should be listed in order of their appearance in the text, typed double-spaced, and in AMA format. Please follow the exact order of information and punctuation in the examples below. Note: List all authors and/or editors up to six; if more than six, list the first three and "et al."

Journal articles: Bier DM, Fulginiti VA, Garfunkel JM, et al. Duplicate publication and related problems. *AJDC*. 1990;144:1293-1294.

Books: Naeye RL. How and when does antenatal hypoxia damage fetal brains? In: Kubli F, Patel N, Schmidt W, Linderkamp O, eds. *Perinatal Events and Brain Damage in Surviving Children.* New York, NY: Springer Verlag NY Inc; 1988:83-91.

Unpublished data, personal communications, or manuscripts "in preparation" or "submitted" should not be included in the list of references. Such material, if essential, may be incorporated in the body of the article.

Authors are responsible for the accuracy of the references.

12. Investigations involving human subjects require a specific statement in the "Methods" section that an appropriate institutional review board approved the project and/or that informed consent was obtained from both legal guardians and/or child, if appropriate.
13. Illustrations and tables from other publications should be suitably acknowledged, with written permission from *publisher* and *author.* Brief acknowledgments to specific contributors directly involved in the content of the manuscript may be placed at the end of the text, before the references.

Patient Reports: Reports of patient descriptions that do not contain sufficient new information are discouraged; normally, these will be returned without review. If new information is provided, such manuscripts will be submitted for critical review and may be published as a full original article or as a brief report in the Pediatric Forum.

SUBSCRIPTION RATES—The subscription rates for the AMERICAN JOURNAL OF DISEASES OF CHILDREN are as follows: $58 for 1 year, $101 for 2 years in the United States and US possessions; all other countries, 1 year, $73; 2 years, $131 for surface delivery. For expedited air delivery to most countries, add $15 surcharge for 1-year subscription, $30 for 2 years. (Rates for subscriptions for delivery to Japan or South Korea are available through exclusive agents—contact the publisher.) ***Special rates for residents and medical students in the United States and US possessions are available.*** Address inquiries to the American Medical Association, Circulation and Fulfillment Division, 515 N State St, Chicago, IL 60610. Phone: (312) 670-SUBS.

The AMERICAN JOURNAL OF DISEASES OF CHILDREN (ISSN 0002-922X) is published monthly by the American Medical Association, 515 N State St, Chicago, IL 60610, and is an official publication of the Association. Second-class postage paid at Chicago and at additional mailing office.

CHANGE OF ADDRESS—POSTMASTER, send all address changes to AMERICAN JOURNAL OF DISEASES OF CHILDREN, Attention: Subscription Department, 515 N State St, Chicago, IL 60610. Notification of address change must be made at least 6 weeks in advance. Include both old and new addresses, a recent mailing label, and your new ZIP code.

Please address communications concerning accepted or published communications to AMA Specialty Journals, 515 N State St, Chicago, IL 60610.

GST registration number: R 126 225 556

AMERICAN JOURNAL OF DISEASES OF CHILDREN

AJDC

Vol 145 No. 6 JUNE 1991

THE PEDIATRIC FORUM

Comments on Life After Residency 597
Robert L. Brent, MD, PhD, Philadelphia, Pa

How Much Iron Is Enough? 598
William B. Rogers, MD, Cuyahoga Falls, Ohio

In Reply 598
Laurence Finberg, MD, Brooklyn, NY

Acute Glossitis and Bacteremia Caused by *Streptococcus pneumoniae*: Case Report and Review 598
Jeffrey J. Stoddard, MD, Jayant K. Deshpande, MD, Baltimore, Md

Puncture Wound — Induced *Achromobacter xylosoxidans* Osteomyelitis of the Foot 599
David M. Hoddy, MD, St Louis, Mo, Leslie L. Barton, MD, Tucson, Ariz

Condylomata Acuminata: Still Usually a Sexually Transmitted Disease in Children 600
John M. Goldenring, MD, MPH, Redlands, Calif

In Reply 601
Alan S. Boyd, MD, Lubbock, Tex

Lead Poisoning in Children With Developmental Disabilities 602
Stephen B. Sulkes, MD, Rochester, NY,
Dennis W. O'Connor, MD, Bath, NY

Neurodevelopmental Outcome of Offspring of the Diabetic Mother: Need for Further Research 602
Esther Goldstein, PhD; Basil Porter, MBBCh;
Aharon Galil, MD, Beer Sheva, Israel

Albuterol Inhalations in Acute Chest Syndrome 603
Edward Handelsman, MD, New Hyde Park, NY,
Debra Voulalas, MD, Philadelphia, Pa

Penile Vasculitis With Impending Necrosis Treated With Prostaglandin E_1 Infusion 604
Anthony A. Horner, MD; Karen Dunn, MD;
E. Richard Stiehm, MD, Los Angeles, Calif

THE EDITORIAL BOARD SPEAKS

Losing Time 607
Albert W. Pruitt, MD, Augusta, Ga

Continued on page 595.

AMERICAN JOURNAL OF DISEASES OF CHILDREN

EDITORIAL

Parental Alcoholism: A Neglected Pediatric Responsibility 609
Donald Ian Macdonald, MD, Bethesda, Md

ARTICLES

Detection of Alcoholism in Hospitalized Children and Their Families 613
Anne K. Duggan, ScD; Hoover Adger, Jr, MD, MPH; Eileen M. McDonald; Emma J. Stokes, PhD; Richard Moore, MD, MHS, Baltimore, Md

The Causes of Hospital-Treated Acute Lower Respiratory Tract Infection in Children 618
Hanna Nohynek, MD; Juhani Eskola, MD; Eija Laine, MD, Helsinki, Finland; Pekka Halonen, MD, Turku, Finland; Petri Ruutu, MD; Pekka Saikku, MD; Marjaana Kleemola, MD; Maija Leinonen, PhD, Helsinki, Finland

Influenza Type A and B Infections in Hospitalized Pediatric Patients: Who Should Be Immunized? 623
Janet R. Serwint, MD; Ross M. Miller, MD; Barbara M. Korsch, MD, Los Angeles, Calif

Pediatric Cardiac Rehabilitation 627
Ian C. Balfour, MBBS; Ami M. Drimmer, PhD; Soraya Nouri, MBBS; D. Glenn Pennington, MD; Carol L. Hemkens, RN; Linda L. Harvey, RN, St Louis, Mo

Dietary Calcium and Bone Mineral Status of Children and Adolescents 631
Gary M. Chan, MD, Salt Lake City, Utah

Percentile Curves for Various Hematologic Measurements at Birth in Arab Preterm Babies of Different Gestational Ages 645
Khalid N. Haque, FRCP, DCH, Hassan M. Bahakim, MD, Riyadh, Saudi Arabia

Meconium for Drug Testing 650
Edward C. Maynard, MD, Worcester, Mass; Louis P. Amoruso, PhD, Mansfield, Mass; William Oh, MD, Providence, RI

Guidelines for Safe Transportation of Children in Wheelchairs 653
Kathleen M. DiGaudio, RN, MSN, PNP, Michael E. Msall, MD, Buffalo, NY

Osteochondrodysplasia in Fryns Syndrome 656
Matthew M. Kershisnik, MD; Catherine M. Craven, MD; A. L. Jung, MD; John C. Carey, MD; A. S. Knisely, MD, Salt Lake City, Utah

Autosomal Recessive Lethal Infantile Cytochrome C Oxidase Deficiency 661
Gideon Eshel, MD; Eliezer Lahat, MD; Kalman Fried, MD, PhD; Josef Barr, MD, Tel Aviv, Israel; Varda Barash, MD; Alisa Gutman, MD, Jerusalem, Israel; Salvatore DiMauro, MD, New York, NY; Mordechei Aladjem, MD, Tel Aviv, Israel

***Escherichia coli* Bacteremia in Children: A Review of 91 Cases in 10 Years** 671
William A. Bonadio, MD; Douglas S. Smith, MD; Elisabeth Madagame, MD; Jane Machi, MD; Narendra Kini, MD, Milwaukee, Wis

Continued on page 596.

AMERICAN JOURNAL OF DISEASES OF CHILDREN

Factors Associated With Umbilical Catheter-Related Sepsis in Neonates 675
Susan Landers, MD; Alicia A. Moise, MD; J. Kennard Fraley, MPH; E. O'Brian Smith, PhD; Carol J. Baker, MD, Houston, Tex

A 50-Year Follow-up of Childhood Plumbism: Hypertension, Renal Function, and Hemoglobin Levels Among Survivors 681
Howard Hu, MD, MPH, ScD, Boston, Mass

Brain and Ocular Abnormalities in Infants With In Utero Exposure to Cocaine and Other Street Drugs 688
Rodrigo Dominguez, MD; Antonio Aguirre Vila-Coro, MD; John M. Slopis, MD; Timothy Bohan, MD, PhD, Houston, Tex

A Preliminary Report of Prenatal Cocaine Exposure and Respiratory Distress Syndrome in Premature Infants 696
Barry Zuckerman, MD; Edward C. Maynard, MD; Howard Cabral, MPH, Boston, Mass

EDUCATIONAL INTERVENTION

Chief Resident Training: Developing Leadership Skills for Future Medical Leaders 639
Robert A. Doughty, MD, PhD; Patricia D. Williams, MD; Charles N. Seashore, PhD, Wilmington, Del

SPORTS MEDICINE

Tracking of Elevated Blood Pressure Values in Adolescent Athletes at 1-Year Follow-up 665
Jeffrey L. Tanji, MD, Sacramento, Calif

SPECIAL FEATURES

Radiological Case of the Month 699
David Ponder, MD; Gary S. Marshall, MD; Gerard P. Rabalais, MD, Louisville, Ky; Beverly P. Wood, MD, Los Angeles, Calif

Picture of the Month 701
Merlin G. Butler, MD, PhD, Sarah Hassell, MD, Nashville, Tenn; Murray Feingold, MD, Walter W. Tunnessen, Jr, MD, Brighton, Mass

REGULAR DEPARTMENTS

Index to Advertisers 594

Classified Advertising 706

Instructions for Authors (See May 1991 issue, p 488.)

COVER CREDIT

Last month's cover art, "Baby in Red Chair," artist unknown, was courtesy of the Abby Aldrich Rockefeller Folk Art Center, Williamsburg, Va.

Please address communications concerning accepted or published communications to AMA Specialty Journals, 515 N State St, Chicago, IL 60610.

SUBSCRIPTION RATES—The subscription rates for the AMERICAN JOURNAL OF DISEASES OF CHILDREN are as follows: $58 for 1 year, $101 for 2 years in the United States and US possessions; all other countries, 1 year, $73; 2 years, $131 for surface delivery. For expedited air delivery to most countries, add $15 surcharge for 1-year subscription, $30 for 2 years. (Rates for subscriptions for delivery to Japan or South Korea are available through exclusive agents—contact the publisher.) ***Special rates for residents and medical students in the United States and US possessions are available.*** Address inquiries to the American Medical Association, Circulation and Fulfillment Division, 515 N State St, Chicago, IL 60610. Phone: (312) 670-SUBS.

The AMERICAN JOURNAL OF DISEASES OF CHILDREN (ISSN 0002-922X) is published monthly by the American Medical Association, 515 N State St, Chicago, IL 60610, and is an official publication of the Association. Second-class postage paid at Chicago and at additional mailing office.

CHANGE OF ADDRESS—POSTMASTER, send all address changes to AMERICAN JOURNAL OF DISEASES OF CHILDREN, Attention: Subscription Department, 515 N State St, Chicago, IL 60610. Notification of address change must be made at least 6 weeks in advance. Include both old and new addresses, a recent mailing label, and your new ZIP code.

Please address communications concerning accepted or published communications to AMA Specialty Journals, 515 N State St, Chicago, IL 60610.

GST registration number: R 126 225 556

AMERICAN JOURNAL OF DISEASES OF CHILDREN

AJDC

Vol 145 **No. 7** **JULY 1991**

THE PEDIATRIC FORUM

More on a Myth
Jose Roman, Jr, MD, El Paso, Tex — 717
In Reply
Vincent A. Fulginiti, MD, New Orleans, La — 717

The Fallacy of the Hemorrhagic Shock and Encephalopathy Syndrome — 718
Millard Bass, DO, MPH, ScD, New York, NY

Hyperpyrexia, Hemorrhagic Shock and Encephalopathy, and Creatinine Phosphokinase — 719
C. Randall Dupee, MD, Los Angeles, Calif

Hemorrhagic Shock and Encephalopathy: An Entity Similar to Heatstroke — 720
Edward E. Conway, Jr, MD, Lewis P. Singer, MD, Bronx, NY

The 'H' in Hemorrhagic Shock and Encephalopathy Syndrome — 720
COL John D. Roscelli, MC, Tripler AMC, Hawaii

Fetal Alcohol Syndrome: Misplaced Emphasis
Karl W. Hess, MD, FAAP, Cleveland, Ohio — 721
In Reply
Bert Little, PhD; Larry C. Gilstrap III, MD; Laura M. Snell, MPH; Charles R. Rosenfeld, MD, Dallas, Tex — 721

Herpes Zoster Oticus
Mobeen H. Rathore, MD; Allan D. Friedman, MD, MHP, St Louis, Mo; Leslie L. Barton, MD, Tucson, Ariz; Lisa M. Dunkle, MD, Wallingford, Conn — 722

Laparoscopic Cholecystectomy Under Continuous Epidural Anesthesia in Patients With Cystic Fibrosis — 723
David S. Edelman, MD, Miami, Fla

War Souvenir Poisoning
Elizabeth Secord, MD; Shari Claude, MD; Charles Newton, MD, Brooklyn, NY — 724

Word Choice
Gary M. Gorlick, MD, MPH, Los Angeles, Calif — 724
In Reply
Richard Hong, MD, Madison, Wis — 724

EDITORIAL

Saving Money With Home Care
Robert A. Schoumacher, MD, Birmingham, Ala — 725

Continued on page 711.

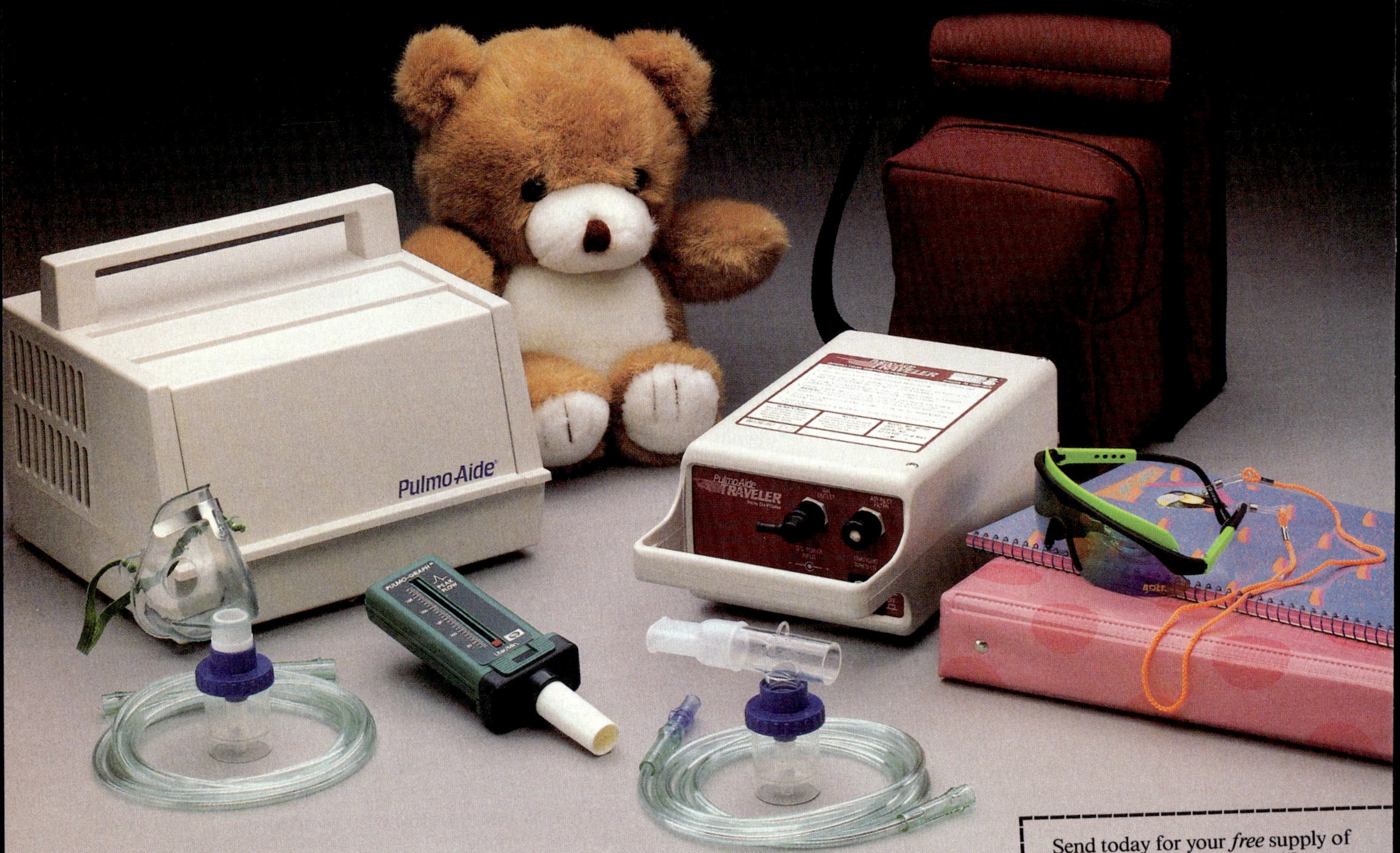

Pulmo-Aide
TRAVELER

AMERICAN JOURNAL OF DISEASES OF CHILDREN

THE EDITORIAL BOARD SPEAKS

Buddy, Can You Paradigm? 727
George W. Brown, MD, Los Lunas, NM

ARTICLES

Home Care Cost-effectiveness for Respiratory Technology—Dependent Children 729
Alan I. Fields, MD; Alan Rosenblatt, MBA, Millersville, Md; Murray M. Pollack, MD, Washington, DC; Joanne Kaufman, RN, MS, Millersville, Md

A Comparative Trial of the Reactogenicity and Immunogenicity of Takeda Acellular Pertussis Vaccine Combined With Tetanus and Diphtheria Toxoids: Outcome in 3- to 8-Month-Old Infants, 9- to 23-Month-Old Infants and Children, and 24- to 30-Month-Old Children 734
Mikio Kimura, MD; Harumi Kuno-Sakai, MD, Isehara, Japan; Yuji Sato, PhD, Tokyo, Japan; Hitoshi Kamiya, MD, Ritsue Nii, MD, Tsu, Japan; Shin Isomura, MD, Nagoya, Japan; Kiyoshi Horiuchi, MD, Utsunomiya, Japan; Tatsuo Kato, MD; Masanori Deguchi, MD, Omura, Japan; Hiroaki Saikusa, MD, Sasebo, Japan; Edward A. Mortimer, Jr, MD, Cleveland, Ohio; James D. Cherry, MD, Los Angeles, Calif

Dose-Related Immunogenicity of *Haemophilus influenzae* Type b Capsular Polysaccharide—*Neisseria meningitidis* Outer Membrane Protein Conjugate Vaccine 742
Victor K. Wong, MD; Rory Quagliata, MPH, RN; Robert Adler, MD; Kwang Sik Kim, MD, Los Angeles, Calif

Apparent Decreased Risk of Invasive Bacterial Disease After Heterologous Childhood Immunization 746
Steven B. Black, MD, Oakland, Calif; James D. Cherry, MD, Los Angeles, Calif; Henry R. Shinefield, MD; Bruce Fireman, MS, Oakland, Calif; Peter Christenson, PhD, Los Angeles, Calif; Dominique Lampert, MS, Oakland, Calif

DTP Immunization and Susceptibility to Infectious Diseases: Is There a Relationship? 750
Michael Davidson, MD, MPH; G. William Letson, MD, Anchorage, Alaska; Joel I. Ward, MD, Torrance, Calif; Angela Ball, MD; Lisa Bulkow, MS, Anchorage, Alaska; Peter Christenson, PhD; James D. Cherry, MD, MSc, Los Angeles, Calif

Seasonal Variation in Growth During Growth Hormone Therapy 769
Mary C. J. Rudolf, MD, Haifa, Israel; Zvi Zadik, MD, Rehovot, Israel; Shai Linn, MD, PhD; Zeev Hochberg, MD, DSc, Haifa, Israel

A Survey of Antiemetic Use in Children With Cancer 773
Jack van Hoff, MD, New Haven, Conn; Marilyn J. Hockenberry-Eaton, MSN, PNP, Atlanta, Ga; Katherine Patterson, MN, Kansas City, Kan; John J. Hutter, MD, Tucson, Ariz

Injuries and Poisonings in Out-of-Home Child Care and Home Care 779
Walter J. Gunn, PhD; Paul F. Pinsky, MPH; Jeffrey J. Sacks, MD, MPH; Lawrence B. Schonberger, MD, MPH, Atlanta, Ga

A Longitudinal Study of Birth Weight and Being Overweight in Late Adolescence 782
Daniel S. Seidman, MD; Arie Laor, MD, Hashomer, Israel; Rena Gale, MD, Jerusalem, Israel; David K. Stevenson, MD, Stanford, Calif; Yehuda L. Danon, MD, Tel-Aviv, Israel

Continued on page 713.

Please address communications concerning accepted or published communications to AMA Specialty Journals, 515 N State St, Chicago, IL 60610.

AMERICAN JOURNAL OF DISEASES OF CHILDREN

The Effect of Low-Dose Dopamine Infusion on Cardiopulmonary and Renal Status in Premature Newborns With Respiratory Distress Syndrome 799
Lily Cuevas, MD; Tsu F. Yeh, MD; Eunice G. John, MD; Danilo Cuevas, MD; Rosita S. Plides, MD, Chicago, Ill

Effect of Necrotizing Enterocolitis on Urinary Epidermal Growth Factor Levels 804
Susan M. Scott, MD; Cathy Rogers; Pam Angelus, RN; Conra Backstrom, RN, Albuquerque, NM

Neutropenia in an Extremely Premature Infant Treated With Recombinant Human Granulocyte Colony-Stimulating Factor 808
Robert L. Roberts, MD, PhD; Cynthia M. Szelc, MD; Steven M. Scates, MD; Maria T. Boyd, RN, MN, Los Angeles, Calif; Ken M. Soderstrom; Mark W. Davis, MS; John. A. Glaspy, MD, Los Angeles, Calif

Predictors of Neurodevelopmental Outcome Following Bronchopulmonary Dysplasia 813
Jean M. Luchi, MD; Forrest C. Bennett, MD; J. Craig Jackson, MD, Seattle, Wash

EDUCATIONAL INTERVENTION

Objective Structured Clinical Examination in a Pediatric Residency Program 757
Bahman Joorabchi, MD, MEd, Pontiac, Mich

SPORTS MEDICINE

Effects of Obesity on Aerobic Fitness in Adolescent Females 764
Thomas W. Rowland, MD, Springfield, Mass

REVIEW

Guidelines for Auditing Pediatric Blood Transfusion Practices 787
Victor S. Blanchette, FRCP(UK), FRCP(C), Toronto, Ontario; Heather A. Hume, FRCPC, Montreal, Quebec; Gary J. Levy, MD, Shreveport, La; Naomi L. C. Luban, MD, Washington, DC; Ronald G. Strauss, MD, Iowa City, Iowa

SPECIAL FEATURES

Radiological Case of the Month 821
Ahmed H. Al-Salem, FRCSI, FICS, Chris Grant, FRCS, Al-Khobar, Saudi Arabia; Beverly P. Wood, MD, Los Angeles, Calif

Picture of the Month 823
Walter W. Tunnessenn, Jr, MD, Philadelphia, Pa

BOOK REVIEW

The H. L. Mencken Baby Book 817
Peggy C. Ferry, MD, Tucson, Ariz

REGULAR DEPARTMENTS

Instructions for Authors 714

Classified Advertising 826

Index to Advertisers 820

INSTRUCTIONS FOR AUTHORS

General Information.—Please send manuscripts and correspondence to the Editor, Vincent A. Fulginiti, MD, *AJDC*, Dean's Office, Tulane University School of Medicine, 1430 Tulane Ave, New Orleans, LA 70112. *AJDC no longer returns nonaccepted manuscripts. Original artwork and photographs will be returned.* Manuscripts are considered with the understanding that they have not been published previously and are not under consideration by another publication.

Type of Manuscripts Suitable for Submission

Original Articles.—New observations that have not been submitted or published elsewhere.

Pediatric Forum.—A mixture of brief, peer-reviewed observations or investigations *and* letters to the editor and other short commentaries.

From Research to Relevance.—Significant research that has a high probability of being translated into clinical usefulness.

Educational Intervention.—Information concerning any educational efforts in the broad field of pediatrics.

Pediatric Legal Medicine.—A forum for discussion of broad issues relating to children and the law in today's environment.

Pediatric Perspectives.—Current information on clinical and scientific pediatric medical advances and analyses of current controversies in pediatrics.

Sports Medicine.—Current information relating to the medical needs of young athletes, as well as current concepts in the prevention, diagnosis, and treatment of sports-related illnesses and injuries.

Picture of the Month.—Submissions should be sent directly to Walter W. Tunnessen, Jr, MD, Children's Hospital of Philadelphia, Room 2143, 34th and Civic Center Blvd, Philadelphia, PA 19104.

Radiological Case of the Month.—Submissions should be sent directly to Beverly P. Wood, MD, Childrens Hospital of Los Angeles, Department of Radiology, 4650 Sunset Blvd, Los Angeles, CA 90054-0700.

AJDC Archives.—Occasional revivals of classic *AJDC* articles with contemporary commentary.

Pediatric Reviews.—Timely, comprehensive, well-referenced topics.

Conforming with all of the steps listed below will facilitate the editorial processing of your manuscript.

Step 1.—*Cover Letter.*—All manuscripts must be accompanied on submission by a cover letter giving the name, address, affiliation, and telephone and fax number of the corresponding author. The letter must include ALL of the following statements SIGNED BY ALL AUTHORS (ORIGINAL SIGNATURES):

1. Authorship Responsibility.—"I certify that I have participated sufficiently in the conception and design of this work and the analysis of the data (when applicable), as well as the writing of the manuscript, to take public responsibility for it. I believe the manuscript represents valid work. I have reviewed the final version of the manuscript and approve it for publication. Neither this manuscript nor one with substantially similar content under my authorship has been published or is being considered for publication elsewhere, except as described in an attachment. Furthermore, I attest that I shall produce the data upon which the manuscript is based for examination by the editors or their assignees if requested."

2. Financial Disclosure.—"I certify that affiliations (if any) with or involvement in any organization or entity with a direct financial interest in the subject matter or materials discussed in the manuscript (eg, employment, consultancies, stock ownership, honoraria, expert testimony) are disclosed below."

Research or project support should be listed in an acknowledgment.

3a. Copyright Transfer.—"In consideration of the action of the American Medical Association (AMA) in reviewing and editing this submission, the author(s) undersigned hereby transfer(s), assign(s), or otherwise convey(s) all copyright ownership to the AMA in the event that such work is published by the AMA."

3b. Federal Employment.—"I was an employee of the US federal government when this work was investigated and prepared for publication; therefore, it is not protected by the Copyright Act and there is no copyright of which the ownership can be transferred."

Editing.—Accepted manuscripts are copy edited according to AMA style and returned to the author for approval. Authors are responsible for all statements made in their work, including changes made by the copy editor and authorized by the corresponding author.

All accepted manuscripts become the permanent property of the AMA and may not be published elsewhere without written permission from both the author(s) and the AMA. After publication, certain articles may appear in translation in the foreign-language editions of *AJDC*. The corresponding author will receive typeset pages for approval. Forms for ordering reprints are included with the typeset pages. Reprints are shipped 6 to 8 weeks after publication.

Step 2.—*Manuscript Format.*—All articles submitted should have the following features:

1. Four copies of the manuscript should be submitted; three are for transmission to referees and one is retained in the editorial office. We prefer an original and three copies.

2. Manuscripts should be typed in double-spaced format throughout, including title page, abstracts, text, acknowledgments, references, legends for illustrations, and tables. Please number pages. *Do not use justified right margins.*

3. Title should be no more than 75 characters.

4. Authors should be limited to six, all of whom have contributed to the study and manuscript preparation, are familiar with its substance, and are able to defend its conclusions.

5. The title page should give full names, degrees, and academic affiliations of all authors, address for requests of reprints, and, if the manuscript was presented at a meeting, the organization, place, and exact date on which it was read.

6. Writing style should conform to proper English usage and syntax; consult the *American Medical Association Manual of Style*, available from Williams & Wilkins, 428 E Preston St, Baltimore, MD 21202.

7. Abstract should be limited to 135 words or less.

8. Each table should be typed, with a title, on a separate sheet of paper, with each line, including headings, *double-spaced.* Continuations should be on a second sheet with all headings repeated.

9. Use Système International (SI) measurements throughout the manuscript.

10. Illustrations should be high-contrast, glossy prints, in quadruplicate, in a proportion of 5x7 in. Figure number, name of first author, and arrow indicating "top" should be typed on a gummed *label* and affixed on the back of each illustration. *Do not write directly on the print.*

Full-color illustrations should be submitted as 35-mm, positive color transparencies, mounted in cardboard, and carefully packaged. Fee is $400 for up to six square-finished color illustrations that fit on one page. A letter of intent to pay the fee must accompany submission.

All photographs in which there is a possibility of patient identification should be accompanied by a signed statement of consent from both parents (or guardians). Covering eyes to mask identity is not sufficient.

11. References should be listed in order of their appearance in the text, typed double-spaced, and in AMA format. Please follow the exact order of information and punctuation in the examples below. Note: List all authors and/or editors up to six; if more than six, list the first three and "et al."

Journal articles: Bier DM, Fulginiti VA, Garfunkel JM, et al. Duplicate publication and related problems. *AJDC.* 1990;144:1293-1294.

Books: Naeye RL. How and when does antenatal hypoxia damage fetal brains? In: Kubli F, Patel N, Schmidt W, Linderkamp O, eds. *Perinatal Events and Brain Damage in Surviving Children.* New York, NY: Springer Verlag NY Inc; 1988:83-91.

Unpublished data, personal communications, or manuscripts "in preparation" or "submitted" should not be included in the list of references. Such material, if essential, may be incorporated in the body of the article.

Authors are responsible for the accuracy of the references.

12. Investigations involving human subjects require a specific statement in the "Methods" section that an appropriate institutional review board approved the project and/or that informed consent was obtained from both legal guardians and/or child, if appropriate.

13. Illustrations and tables from other publications should be suitably acknowledged, with written permission from *publisher* and *author.* Brief acknowledgments to specific contributors directly involved in the content of the manuscript may be placed at the end of the text, before the references.

Patient Reports: Reports of patient descriptions that do not contain sufficient new information are discouraged; normally, these will be returned without review. If new information is provided, such manuscripts will be submitted for critical review and may be published as a full original article or as a brief report in the Pediatric Forum.

SUBSCRIPTION RATES—The subscription rates for the AMERICAN JOURNAL OF DISEASES OF CHILDREN are as follows: $58 for 1 year, $101 for 2 years in the United States and US possessions; all other countries, 1 year, $73; 2 years, $131 for surface delivery. For expedited air delivery to most countries, add $15 surcharge for 1-year subscription, $30 for 2 years. (Rates for subscriptions for delivery to Japan or South Korea are available through exclusive agents—contact the publisher.) ***Special rates for residents and medical students in the United States and US possessions are available.*** Address inquiries to the American Medical Association, Circulation and Fulfillment Division, 515 N State St, Chicago, IL 60610. Phone: (312) 670-SUBS.

The AMERICAN JOURNAL OF DISEASES OF CHILDREN (ISSN 0002-922X) is published monthly by the American Medical Association, 515 N State St, Chicago, IL 60610, and is an official publication of the Association. Second-class postage paid at Chicago and at additional mailing office.

CHANGE OF ADDRESS—POSTMASTER, send all address changes to AMERICAN JOURNAL OF DISEASES OF CHILDREN, Attention: Subscription Department, 515 N State St, Chicago, IL 60610. Notification of address change must be made at least 6 weeks in advance. Include both old and new addresses, a recent mailing label, and your new ZIP code.

Please address communications concerning accepted or published communications to AMA Specialty Journals, 515 N State St, Chicago, IL 60610.

GST registration number: R 126 225 556

AMERICAN JOURNAL OF DISEASES OF CHILDREN

AJDC

Vol 145 No. 8 AUGUST 1991

THE PEDIATRIC FORUM

Child Welfare: The Phantom of the Health Care System 843
Frank S. Pidcock, MD, Philadelphia, Pa

Resident and Nurse Practitioners: Responding to Education and Patient Care Needs 843
Angelo Giardino, MD, MSEd, Eileen Giardino, PhD, RN, Philadelphia, Pa

Priorities in Academic Pediatrics 845
Stephen E. Jacobs, MD, Modesto, Calif

In Reply 845
Boyd W. Goetzman, MD, PhD, Davis, Calif

Thumb-Sucking 845
John P. Lubicky, MD, Chicago, Ill

In Reply 846
Patrick C. Friman, PhD, Philadelphia, Pa

The 80-Hour Workweek and Residency Programs: Closing Arguments 846
Alan D. Bedrick, MD, Tucson, Ariz

Child Sexual Abuse and Human Immunodeficiency Virus Transmission 847
James A. Monteleone, MD, St Louis, Mo

In Reply 847
Laura T. Gutman, MD; Karen St Claire, MD; Marcia Herman-Giddens, MPH; Ross E. McKinney, Jr, MD, Durham, NC

Anal Fissure Produced by Examination for Sexual Abuse 848
Robert B. Baker, MD, Bonita, Calif

In Reply 849
Jan Bays, MD, Portland, Ore; Carole Jenny, MD, Denver, Colo

Gilding the Lily 849
Harris C. Faigel, MD, Waltham, Mass

In Reply 849
Charles M. Myer III, MD, John Grosso, MD, Cincinnati, Ohio

Continued on page 835.

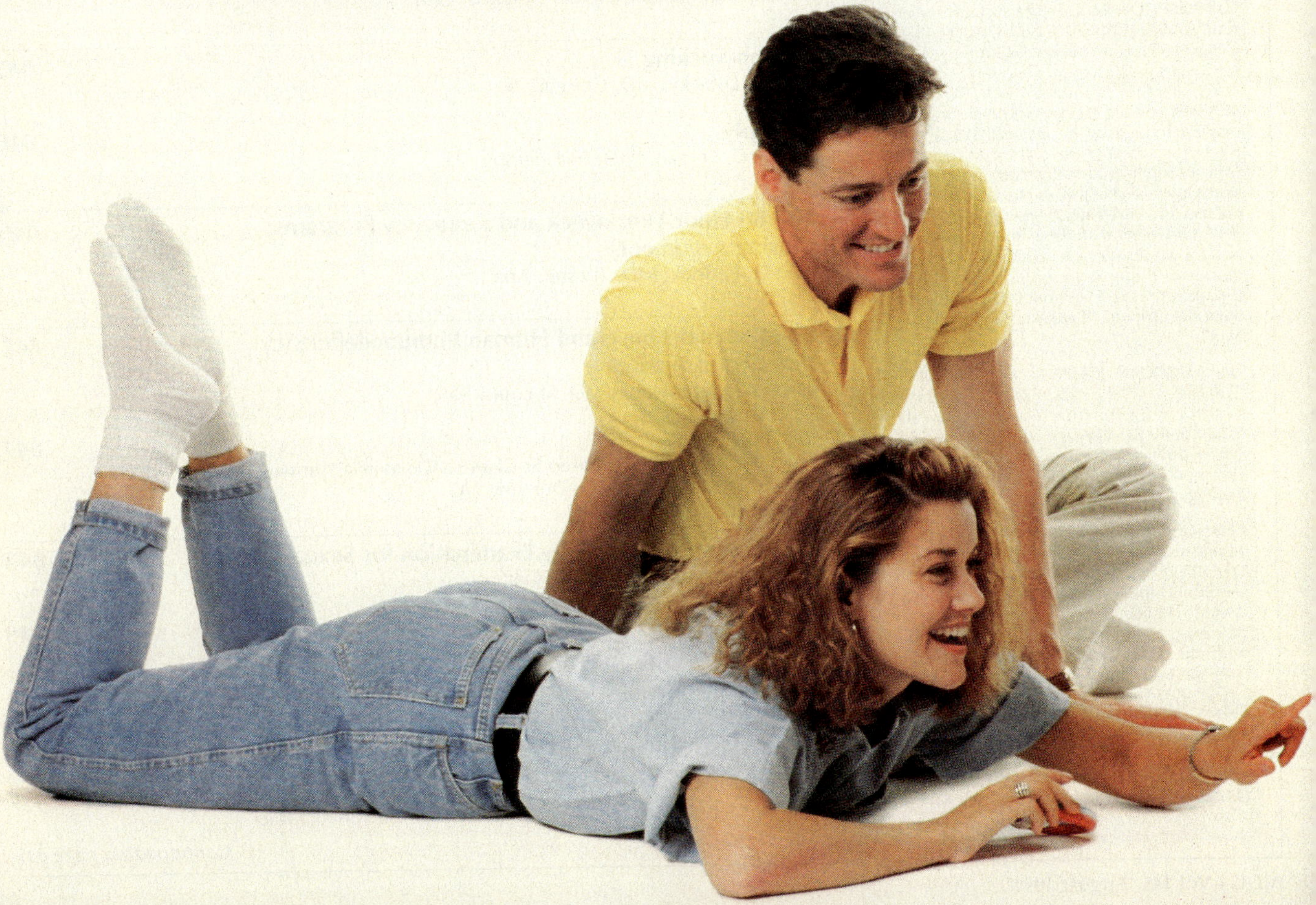

AMERICAN JOURNAL OF DISEASES OF CHILDREN

EDITORIAL

Jack Metcoff Festschrift 851
John E. Lewy, MD, New Orleans, La

THE EDITORIAL BOARD SPEAKS . . .

Part-time Peg: Who, Me? 852
Peggy C. Ferry, MD, Tucson, Ariz

ARTICLES

Zinc Deficiency: A Public Health Problem? 853
Harold H. Sandstead, MD, Galveston, Tex

Paleonephrology and Reflux Nephropathy: From the 'Big Bang' to End-Stage Renal Disease 860
Ronald J. Kallen, MD, Park Ridge, Ill

X-linked Hypophosphatemia: Genetic and Clinical Correlates 865
James D. Hanna, MD; Kazuhiko Niimi, MD; James C. M. Chan, MD, Richmond, Va

Studies in Fetal Malnutrition 871
Warren M. Crosby, MD, Oklahoma City, Okla

Partial Hypoparathyroidism: A Variant of Transient Congenital Hypoparathyroidism 877
Sang Whay Kooh, MD, FRCPC, Ann Binet, BScN, RN, Toronto, Ontario

Immunization Response Varies With Intensity of Acute Lymphoblastic Leukemia Therapy 887
Derry Ridgway, MD; Lawrence J. Wolff, MD, Portland, Ore; Adamadia Deforest, PhD, Philadelphia, Pa

Immunogenicity of Tetravalent Rhesus Rotavirus Vaccine Administered With Buffer and Oral Polio Vaccine 892
Donna J. Ing, MPH; Roger I. Glass, MD; Patricia A. Woods; Murri Simonetti; Mark A. Pallansch, PhD; Wallace D. Wilcox, MD, Atlanta, Ga; Bruce L. Davidson, MD, Philadelphia, Pa; Alan J. Sievert, MD, Decatur, Ga

Response of 7- to 15-Month-Old Infants to Sequential Immunization With *Haemophilus influenzae* Type b-CRM_{197} Conjugate and Polysaccharide Vaccines 898
Edward P. Rothstein, MD; Ruth P. Schiller, MD; Joseph A. C. Girone, MD; Thomas J. Hipp, MD; Ronald L. Souder, MD; Henry H. Bernstein, DO, Sellersville, Pa; Dace V. Madore, PhD; Cynthia L. Johnson; David H. Smith, MD, Rochester, NY

Testing the Psychogenic Vomiting Diagnosis: Four Pediatric Patients 913
Joseph Gonzalez-Heydrich, MD; John Alan Kerner, Jr, MD; Hans Steiner, MD, Stanford, Calif

A Practical Guide to Successful Breast-feeding Management 917
Gary L. Freed, MD; Susan Landers, MD; Richard J. Schanler, MD, Houston, Tex

Continued on page 839.

AMERICAN JOURNAL OF DISEASES OF CHILDREN

Predicting Risk of *Pneumocystis carinii* Pneumonia in Human Immunodeficiency Virus–Infected Children 922
Richard M. Rutstein, MD, Philadelphia, Pa

Measurement of Serum Granulocyte Colony-Stimulating Factor in a Patient With Congenital Agranulocytosis (Kostmann's Syndrome) 925
Lewis Glasser, MD; Burris R. Duncan, MD; James J. Corrigan, Jr, MD, Tucson, Ariz

Rice Solution and World Health Organization Solution by Gastric Infusion for High Stool Output Diarrhea 937
Felipe Mota-Hernández, MD, PhD; Daniel Bross-Soriano, MD; Maria L. Pérez-Ricardez, MD, PhD; Luis Velásquez-Jones, MD, PhD, Mexico City, México

Serum Calcium and High Parathyroid Hormone Levels in Neonates Fed 'Humanized' Cow's Milk–Based Formula 941
Bonny L. Specker, PhD; Reginald C. Tsang, MBBS; Mona L. Ho, MS; Theresa M. Landi, MSN; Teresa L. Gratton, MS, Cincinnati, Ohio

Evaluation of Intraosseous vs Intravenous Antibiotic Levels in a Porcine Model 946
David G. Jaimovich, MD, Chicago, Ill; Ashir Kumar, MD, PhD, Lansing, Mich; Steve Francom, Kalamazoo, Mich

EDUCATIONAL INTERVENTION

Clinic-Based Intervention to Promote Literacy: A Pilot Study 881
Robert Needlman, MD; Lise E. Fried, MSPH; Debra S. Morley, MA; Sunday Taylor; Barry Zuckerman, MD, Boston, Mass

REVIEW

Transfusion Therapy in Neonates 904
Ronald G. Strauss, MD, Iowa City, Iowa

SPECIAL CONTRIBUTION

Use of Infant Walkers 933
Board of Trustees, Chicago, Ill

BOOK REVIEW

An Introduction to Clinical Research 945
Jessie R. Groothuis, MD, Denver, Colo

REGULAR DEPARTMENTS

Index to Advertisers 932

Classified Advertising 950

Instructions for Authors — See July 1991 issue, p 714.

SUBSCRIPTION RATES—The subscription rates for the AMERICAN JOURNAL OF DISEASES OF CHILDREN are as follows: $58 for 1 year, $101 for 2 years in the United States and US possessions; all other countries, 1 year, $73; 2 years, $131 for surface delivery. For expedited air delivery to most countries, add $15 surcharge for 1-year subscription, $30 for 2 years. (Rates for subscriptions for delivery to Japan or South Korea are available through exclusive agents—contact the publisher.) ***Special rates for residents and medical students in the United States and US possessions are available.*** Address inquiries to the American Medical Association, Publishing Operations Division, 515 N State St, Chicago, IL 60610. Phone: **(312) 670-SUBS** (670-7827).

The AMERICAN JOURNAL OF DISEASES OF CHILDREN (ISSN 0002-922X) is published monthly by the American Medical Association, 515 N State St, Chicago, IL 60610, and is an official publication of the Association. Second-class postage paid at Chicago and at additional mailing office.

CHANGE OF ADDRESS—POSTMASTER, send all address changes to AMERICAN JOURNAL OF DISEASES OF CHILDREN, Attention: Subscription Department, 515 N State St, Chicago, IL 60610. Notification of address change must be made at least 6 weeks in advance. Include both old and new addresses, a recent mailing label, and your new ZIP code.

Please address communications concerning accepted or published communications to AMA Specialty Journals, 515 N State St, Chicago, IL 60610.

GST registration number: R 126 225 556

AMERICAN JOURNAL OF DISEASES OF CHILDREN

AJDC

Vol 145 No. 9 SEPTEMBER 1991

THE PEDIATRIC FORUM

Family Physicians and Neonatology 963
Floyd L. McIntyre, MD, South Dennis, Mass
In Reply 963
John DiTraglia, MD, Portsmouth, Ohio

Your Child's Best Friend: TV or Not TV? 963
Max Bader, MD, Lake Oswego, Ore
In Reply 963
E. Richard Stiehm, MD, Los Angeles, Calif

Misdiagnosis of Reye's-like Illness 964
Brian W. Forsyth, MB, ChB; Eugene D. Shapiro, MD; Ralph I. Horwitz, MD; Catherine M. Viscoli, PhD; Denise Acampora, MPH, New Haven, Conn

Syringomas in Down Syndrome 966
Murray Feingold, MD, Boston, Mass

Congenital Syphilis Associated With Negative Results of Maternal Serologic Tests at Delivery 967
Pablo J. Sanchez, MD; George D. Wendel, MD; Michael V. Norgard, PhD, Dallas, Tex

Response of Seronegative Adults to Measles Immunization 969
Herbert Braunstein, MD; Susan Thomas MT(ASCP); Ray Ito, MT(ASCP); Carole Jarman, MA, RN, San Bernardino, Calif

Improvement of Leukemic Hyperleukocytosis With Only Fluid and Allopurinol Therapy 969
André D. Lascari, MD, Albany, NY

Myopathy Associated With Ketoconazole Treatment 970
Ben-Zion Garty, MD; Rivka Kauli, MD; Ella Livni, MD; Zvi Laron, MD; Menachem Nitzan, MD, Petah Tiqva, Israel

Gallstones in Children 971
David J. Todd, MRCP(UK), Belfast, Northern Ireland

Obesity and Body-Mass Index 972
Albert C. Hergenroeder, MD, Houston, Tex
In Reply 972
Lawrence D. Hammer, MD; Darrell M. Wilson, MD; Helena C. Kraemer, PhD; Philip L. Ritter, PhD; Sanford M. Dornbusch, PhD, Palo Alto, Calif

Continued on page 957.

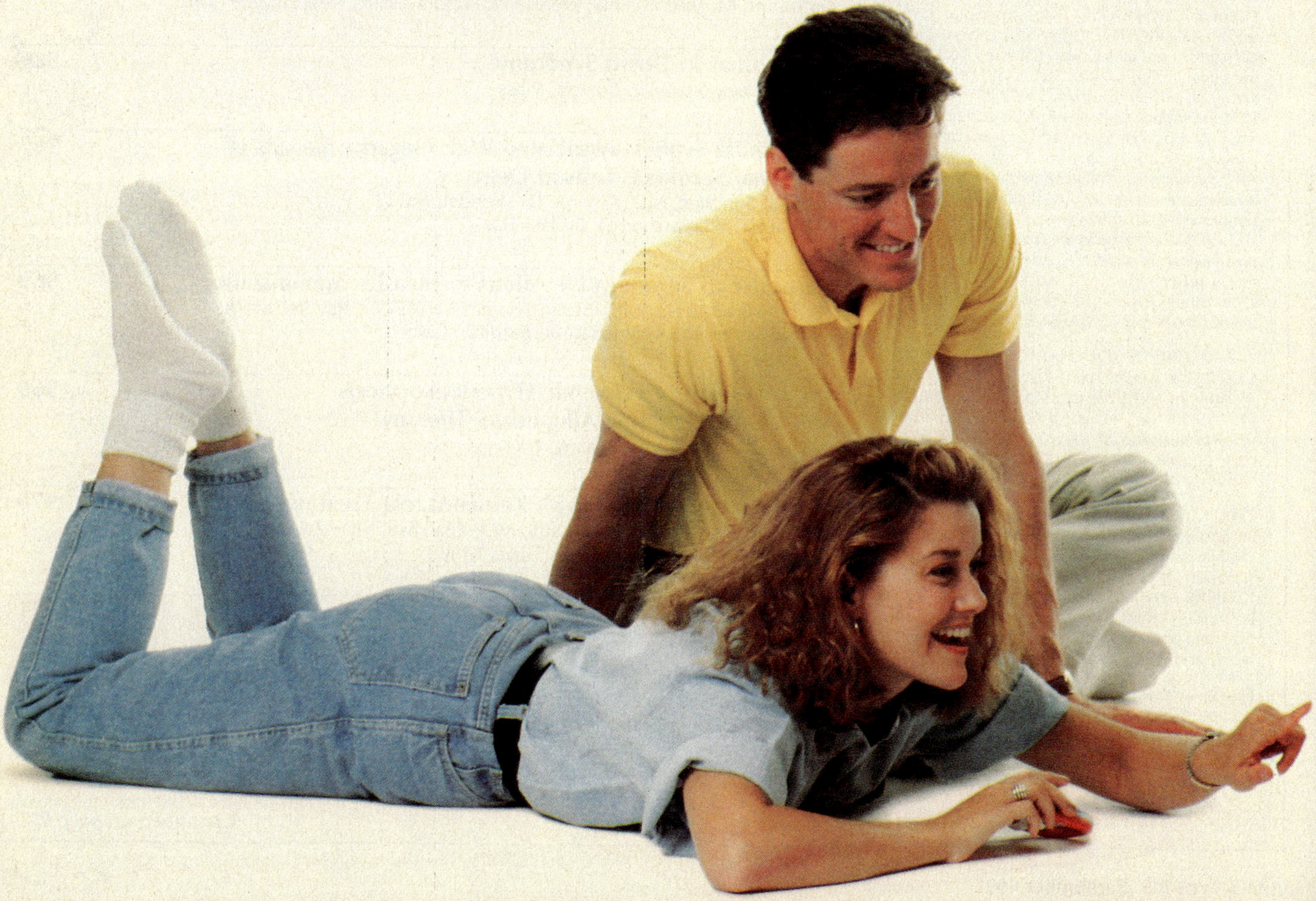

American Medical Association
Physicians Dedicated to the health of America

The AMERICAN JOURNAL OF DISEASES OF CHILDREN is a member of the consortium of AMA journals listed below. The Archives reaches more than 36 000 readers in 85 countries each month. The complete text of all AMA journals is available on the MEDIS database from Mead Data Central, Dayton, Ohio.

The Journal of the American Medical Association (JAMA)

American Journal of Diseases of Children (AJDC)

Archives of Dermatology

Archives of General Psychiatry

Archives of Internal Medicine

Archives of Neurology

Archives of Ophthalmology

Archives of Otolaryngology—Head & Neck Surgery

Archives of Pathology & Laboratory Medicine

Archives of Surgery

AMERICAN JOURNAL OF DISEASES OF CHILDREN

THE EDITORIAL BOARD SPEAKS

The Clinic Attending: Teaching Strategies for Patient Encounters 977
Barton Schmitt, MD, Denver, Colo

EDITORIAL

Water Intoxication: A Prevalent Problem in the Inner City 981
Laurence Finberg, MD, Brooklyn, NY

ARTICLES

Oral Water Intoxication in Infants: An American Epidemic 985
James P. Keating, MD, MSci(Epidem); Gregory J. Schears, MD; Philip R. Dodge, MD, St Louis, Mo

Vasopressin Levels in Infants During the Course of Aseptic and Bacterial Meningitis 991
Guadalupe Padilla, MD; M. Gore Ervin, PhD; Michael G. Ross, MD; Rosemary D. Leake, MD, Torrance, Calif

Demographic and Risk Factors Associated With Chronic Dieting in Adolescents 994
Mary Story, PhD; Kim Rosenwinkel, MPH; John H. Himes, PhD; Michael Resnick, PhD; Linda J. Harris; Robert Wm. Blum, MD, PhD, Minneapolis, Minn

The Effect of Valproic Acid on Plasma Carnitine Levels 999
Grzegorz Opala, MD, PhD; Susan Winter, MD; Carol Vance, MD; Hugh Vance, PhD; H. Terry Hutchison, MD, PhD; Lawrence S. Linn, Fresno, Calif

Optimal Positioning of Endotracheal Tubes for Ventilation of Preterm Infants 1007
Avi Rotschild, MD; David Chitayat, MD; Martin L. Puterman, PhD; Min S. Phang, MB; Emily Ling, MB, BS; Virginia Baldwin, MD, Vancouver, British Columbia

Evaluation of Auditory Brain-stem Response in Full-term Infants of Cocaine-Abusing Mothers 1013
Ronald P. Carzoli, MD; Suzanne P. Murphy, PhD; Judy Hammer-Knisely, MA, CCC-A; Jean Houy, ARNP, Jacksonville, Fla

Ductal Patency in Neonates With Respiratory Distress Syndrome: A Randomized Surfactant Trial 1017
Mark D. Reller, MD; Donald C. Buffkin, MD; Michael A. Colasurdo, MD; Mary J. Rice, MD; Robert W. McDonald, RCPT, RDMS, Portland, Ore

Decreasing Severity of Chronic Uveitis in Children With Pauciarticular Arthritis 1026
David D. Sherry, MD; Elizabeth D. Mellins, MD; Ralph J. Wedgwood, MD, Seattle, Wash

Family History of Myocardial Infarction and Hemodynamic Responses to Exercise in Young Black Boys 1029
Frank A. Treiber, PhD; William B. Strong, MD, Augusta, Ga; Frederick W. Arensman, MD, Louisville, Ky; Thomas Forrest, MD; Harry Davis, MS, Augusta, Ga; Linda Musante, PhD, Tampa, Fla

Continued on page 959.

AMERICAN JOURNAL OF DISEASES OF CHILDREN

Physiologic Responses to Playing a Video Game 1034
Karen R. Segal, EdD, William H. Dietz, MD, PhD, New York, NY

Arterial Catheter–Related Infections in Children: A 1-Year Cohort Analysis 1037
Susanna Furfaro, MD; Marie Gauthier, MD; Jacques Lacroix, MD; Daniel Nadeau, MD; Lucette Lafleur, MD; Sylvain Mathews, MD, Montreal, Quebec

A Variant Form of Thrombasthenia 1053
Michael D. Tarantino, MD; James J. Corrigan, Jr, MD; Lewis Glasser, MD; Claire M. Payne, PhD; Monette A. Jeter, PhD, Tucson, Ariz

Lichen Sclerosus et Atrophicus in Children 1058
Vera Loening-Baucke, MD, Iowa City, Iowa

Treatment of Ulcerated Hemangiomas With the Pulsed Tunable Dye Laser 1062
Joseph G. Morelli, MD, Denver, Colo; O. T. Tan, MD, Boston, Mass; William L. Weston, MD, Denver, Colo

EDUCATIONAL INTERVENTION

Support Services for Pediatric Trainees: A Survey of Training Program Directors 1002
Anne Sturmthal Bergman, LCSW, DrPH, Robert Adler, MD, MSEd, Los Angeles, Calif

SPORTS MEDICINE

Safety of a Preadolescent Basketball Program 1023
Margaret E. Gutgesell, MD, MPH, Charlottesville, Va

SPECIAL FEATURES

Radiological Case of the Month 1045
George P. Giacola, MD, Tulsa, Okla; Beverly P. Wood, MD, Los Angeles, Calif

Picture of the Month 1047
Luis A. Vera, MD; Nayere Zaeri, MD; Hallam Hurt, MD, Philadelphia, Pa; Murray Feingold, MD, Brighton, Mass; Walter W. Tunnessen, Jr, MD, Philadelphia, Pa

BOOK REVIEW

Parenteral Nutrition in Infants and Children: Basic Principles and Practical Guidelines 1025
Carol J. Rollins, MS, RD, PharmD, Tucson, Ariz

CORRECTION

Effect of Necrotizing Enterocolitis on Urinary Epidermal Growth Factor Levels 982
Susan M. Scott, MD; Cathy Rogers; Pam Angelus, RN; Conra Backstrom, RN, Albuquerque, NM

REGULAR DEPARTMENTS

Instructions for Authors—See July 1991 issue, p 714.

Classified Advertising 1069

Index to Advertisers 975

SUBSCRIPTION RATES—The subscription rates for the AMERICAN JOURNAL OF DISEASES OF CHILDREN are as follows: $58 for 1 year, $101 for 2 years in the United States and US possessions; all other countries, 1 year, $73; 2 years, $131 for surface delivery. For expedited air delivery to most countries, add $15 surcharge for 1-year subscription, $30 for 2 years. (Rates for subscriptions for delivery to Japan or South Korea are available through exclusive agents—contact the publisher.) ***Special rates for residents and medical students in the United States and US possessions are available.*** Address inquiries to the American Medical Association, Publishing Operations Division, 515 N State St, Chicago, IL 60610. Phone: **(312) 670-SUBS** (670-7827).

The AMERICAN JOURNAL OF DISEASES OF CHILDREN (ISSN 0002-922X) is published monthly by the American Medical Association, 515 N State St, Chicago, IL 60610, and is an official publication of the Association. Second-class postage paid at Chicago and at additional mailing office.

CHANGE OF ADDRESS—POSTMASTER, send all address changes to AMERICAN JOURNAL OF DISEASES OF CHILDREN, Attention: Subscription Department, 515 N State St, Chicago, IL 60610. Notification of address change must be made at least 6 weeks in advance. Include both old and new addresses, a recent mailing label, and your new ZIP code.

Please address communications concerning accepted or published communications to AMA Specialty Journals, 515 N State St, Chicago, IL 60610.

GST registration number: R 126 225 556

AMERICAN JOURNAL OF DISEASES OF CHILDREN

AJDC

Vol 145 **No. 10** **OCTOBER 1991**

THE PEDIATRIC FORUM

Call for Abstracts 1085

Health Care for Uninsured and Underinsured Children 1085
Joseph H. Davis, MD, Menlo Park, Calif; Barbara S. Kirschner, MD, Chicago, Ill; Stephen James Pearson, MD, Toppenish, Wash; James A. Hecker, MD, Cheyenne, Wyo; Lewis A. Barness, MD, Madison, Wis

Parental Drinking Habits 1087
Joseph J. Wells, MD, Phoenix, Ariz; Michael A. Villani, MD, Philadelphia, Pa

Cholesterol Testing in the Physician's Office: Accuracy Assessment 1087
Nader Rifai, PhD; Mariet Iosefsohn, MS; Jocelyn M. Hicks, PhD, Washington, DC

Formula Companies and the Medical Profession 1088
H. William Fink, MD, Norfolk, Va; Jack Newman, MD, FRCPC, Toronto, Ontario

In Reply 1090
Frank R. Greer, MD, Rima D. Apple, PhD, Madison, Wis

Scoring Systems for Accurate Prognosis of Patients With Meningococcal Infections 1090
Francis Leclerc, MD; Valérie Hue, MD; Alain Martinot, MD; Florence Delepoulle, MD, Lille, France

Association of Alkaline Urine With Eating Disorders 1091
William Lane M. Robson, MD, FRCPC, Alexander K. C. Leung, MBBS, FRCPC, FRCP(Edin), Calgary, Alberta

In Reply 1091
Martha R. Arden, MD; Michael P. Nussbaum, MD; Marc S. Jacobson, MD, New Hyde Park, NY

Reexpansion Pulmonary Edema 1092
David S. Jardine, MD, Seattle, Wash

Nintendo Enuresis 1092
Julian C. Schink, MD, Chicago, Ill

THE EDITORIAL BOARD SPEAKS . . .

Mitral Valve Prolapse: Back to the Basics 1095
Hugh D. Allen, MD, Columbus, Ohio

Continued on page 1079.

American Medical Association
Physicians dedicated to the health of America

The AMERICAN JOURNAL OF DISEASES OF CHILDREN is a member of the consortium of AMA journals listed below. The Journal reaches more than 36 000 readers in 85 countries each month. The complete text of all AMA journals is available on the MEDIS database from Mead Data Central, Dayton, Ohio.

The Journal of the American Medical Association (JAMA)

American Journal of Diseases of Children (AJDC)

Archives of Dermatology

Archives of General Psychiatry

Archives of Internal Medicine

Archives of Neurology

Archives of Ophthalmology

Archives of Otolaryngology—Head & Neck Surgery

Archives of Pathology & Laboratory Medicine

Archives of Surgery

AMERICAN JOURNAL OF DISEASES OF CHILDREN

ARTICLES

Endotoxin Concentrations in Cerebrospinal Fluid Correlate With Clinical Severity and Neurologic Outcome of *Haemophilus influenzae* Type B Meningitis 1099
Jussi Mertsola; William A. Kennedy; David Waagner; Xavier Sáez-Llorens; Kurt Olsen; Eric J. Hansen; George H. McCracken, Jr, Dallas, Tex

House Staff Work Hours and Moonlighting: What Do Residents Want?: A Survey of Pediatric Residents in California 1104
Tina L. Cheng, MD, MPH, San Francisco, Calif

Barriers to Medical Care for Homeless Families Compared With Housed Poor Families 1109
David Wood, MD, MPH; R. Burciaga Valdez, PhD, MHSA, Los Angeles, Calif

Gastroesophageal Reflux and Apnea in Prematurely Born Infants During Wakefulness and Sleep 1132
Mikel de Ajuriaguerra, MD; Marie-France Radvanyi-Bouvet, MD; Catherine Huon, MD; Guy Moriette, MD, Paris, France

Oxygen Saturation by Pulse Oximetry in Healthy Infants at an Altitude of 1610 m (5280 ft): What Is Normal? 1137
Elizabeth H. Thilo, MD; Beverly Park-Moore, CRTT; Edward R. Berman, MD; Bonita S. Carson, MD, Denver, Colo

Posthemorrhagic Hydrocephalus: Use of an Intravenous-Type Catheter for Cerebrospinal Fluid Drainage 1141
Peter J. Marro, MD; Douglas A. Dransfield, MD; Stephen H. Mott, MD; Walter C. Allan, MD, Portland, Me

How Much Vitamin D for Neonates? 1147
William B. Pittard III, MD; Kitty M. Geddes, RN, BSN; Thomas C. Hulsey, MSPH, ScD; Bruce W. Hollis, PhD, Charleston, SC

Growth Hormone Therapy in Hypophosphatemic Rickets 1165
Darrell M. Wilson, MD, Stanford, Calif; Phillip D. K. Lee, MD, Denver, Colo; Alan H. Morris, MD, Duarte, Calif; Edward O. Reiter, MD, Springfield, Mass; Joseph M. Gertner, MB, MRCP, New York, NY; Robert Marcus, MD, Stanford, Calif; Valerie E. Quarmby, PhD, Calabasas Hills, Calif; Ron G. Rosenfeld, MD, Stanford, Calif

Multilevel Model to Assess Appropriateness of Pediatric Serum Drug Concentrations 1171
Donna M. Kraus, PharmD, Chicago, Ill; Ina Lee Stile Calligaro, PharmD, Philadelphia, Pa; Hind T. Hatoum, PhD, Chicago, Ill

The Association of Pauciarticular Juvenile Arthritis and Myasthenia Gravis 1176
John B. Glass, MD; Phyllis K. Sher, MD, Minneapolis, Minn; Vanda A. Lennon, MD, PhD, Rochester, Minn; Warren E. Regelmann, MD, Minneapolis, Minn

Epidemic Nephropathy in Children 1181
Pentti Lautala, MD, Matti Uhari, MD, Oulu, Finland

Continued on page 1080.

AMERICAN JOURNAL OF DISEASES OF CHILDREN

Minor Malformations, Hyperactivity, and Learning Disabilities 1184
Pasquale J. Accardo, MD; Terry Tomazic, PhD; Jill Morrow, MD; Carol Haake, MS; Barbara Y. Whitman, PhD, St Louis, Mo

Hand Washing in Pediatric Ambulatory Settings: An Inconsistent Practice 1198
Jacob A. Lohr, MD, Charlottesville, Va; David L. Ingram, MD, Chapel Hill, NC; Sharon M. Dudley, MT; Elizabeth L. Lawton, RN, PNP; Leigh G. Donowitz, MD, Charlottesville, NC

Immersion Events in Residential Swimming Pools: Evidence for an Experience Effect 1200
Garen J. Wintemute, MD, MPH; Christiana Drake, PhD; Mona Wright, Sacramento, Calif

Natural History of Hematuria Associated With Hypercalciuria in Children 1204
Clotilde D. Garcia, MD, Buffalo, NY; Leslie A. Miller, MLT; F. Bruder Stapleton, MD, Memphis, Tenn

SPORTS MEDICINE

Adolescents' Attrition From School-Sponsored Sports 1119
Robert H. DuRant, PhD; Robert A. Pendergrast, MD, MPH; Josh Donner, MD, MPH; Carolyn Seymore, MD; Gregory Gaillard, Augusta, Ga

EDUCATIONAL INTERVENTIONS

Sun Protection in Newborns: A Comparison of Educational Methods 1125
Jean L. Bolognia, MD; Marianne Berwick, PhD; Judith A. Fine; Pamela Simpson, MPH; Marjorie Jasmin, RN, New Haven, Conn

Resident, Faculty, and Residency Program Development: An Integrated Approach Through Annual Retreats 1191
Robert J. Winter, MD; Sharon M. Unti, MD; Jeffrey S. Rubenstein, MD, Chicago, Ill; Fredric D. Burg, MD, Philadelphia, Pa; James A. Stockman III, MD, Chicago, Ill

PEDIATRIC LEGAL MEDICINE

Legalization of Drugs of Abuse and the Pediatrician 1153
Richard H. Schwartz, MD, Falls Church, Va

SPECIAL FEATURES

Radiological Case of the Month 1159
K. Kozlowski, MD, M. Glasson, MD, New South Wales, Australia; Beverly P. Wood, MD, Los Angeles, Calif

Picture of the Month 1161
Walter W. Tunnessen, Jr, MD, Philadelphia, Pa

REGULAR DEPARTMENTS

Index to Advertisers 1078

Instructions for Authors 1081

Classified Advertising 1208

SUBSCRIPTION RATES—The subscription rates for the AMERICAN JOURNAL OF DISEASES OF CHILDREN are as follows: $58 for 1 year, $101 for 2 years in the United States and US possessions; all other countries, 1 year, $73; 2 years, $131 for surface delivery. For expedited air delivery to most countries, add $15 surcharge for 1-year subscription, $30 for 2 years. (Rates for subscriptions for delivery to Japan or South Korea are available through exclusive agents—contact the publisher.) ***Special rates for residents and medical students in the United States and US possessions are available.*** Address inquiries to the American Medical Association, Publishing Operations Division, 515 N State St, Chicago, IL 60610. Phone: **(312) 670-SUBS** (670-7827).

The AMERICAN JOURNAL OF DISEASES OF CHILDREN (ISSN 0002-922X) is published monthly by the American Medical Association, 515 N State St, Chicago, IL 60610, and is an official publication of the Association. Second-class postage paid at Chicago and at additional mailing office.

CHANGE OF ADDRESS—POSTMASTER, send all address changes to AMERICAN JOURNAL OF DISEASES OF CHILDREN, Attention: Subscription Department, 515 N State St, Chicago, IL 60610. Notification of address change must be made at least 6 weeks in advance. Include both old and new addresses, a recent mailing label, and your new ZIP code.

Please address communications concerning accepted or published communications to AMA Specialty Journals, 515 N State St, Chicago, IL 60610.

GST registration number: R 126 225 556

AMERICAN JOURNAL OF DISEASES OF CHILDREN

AJDC

Vol 145 No. 11 NOVEMBER 1991

THE PEDIATRIC FORUM

Call for Abstracts 1223

Sudden Cardiac Death 1223
William Pearl, MD, El Paso, Tex

***Staphylococcus aureus* in Impetigo** 1223
Ron Dagan, MD, Beer-Sheva, Israel
In Reply 1223
James W. Bass, MD, Honolulu, Hawaii

Treatment Withdrawal in Neonates 1223
Paul Byrne, MB, CHB, FRCPC,
R. Welch, MB, CHB, MRCP, Edmonton, Canada

Exacerbation of Tinea Corporis During Treatment With 1% Clotrimazole/0.05% Betamethasone Diproprionate (Lotrisone) 1224
Ronald D. Reynolds, MD, New Richmond, Ohio;
Susan Boiko, MD, Anne W. Lucky, MD, Cincinnati, Ohio

Mediterranean Visceral Leishmaniasis: A Frequently Unrecognized Imported Disease 1225
Ludo M. Mahieu, MD, Karel J. Van Acker, MD, PhD, Antwerpen, Belgium

Send Linus to Me 1227
Harriet Szonyi, Toronto, Ontario
In Reply 1227
Patrick C. Friman, PhD, Philadelphia, Pa

A Markedly Immature Lecithin-Sphingomyelin Ratio at Term and Congenital Hypothyroidism 1227
Gary R. Cohen, MD; James Thorp, MD; John D. Yeast, MD;
Bruce A. Meyer, MD; Richard O'Kell, MD;
Candace Macy, Kansas City, Mo

EDITORIAL

Is Prophylaxis of Neonates With Intravenous Immunoglobulin Beneficial? 1229
Harvy R. Hill, MD, Salt Lake City, Utah

ARTICLES

Efficacy and Pharmacokinetics of Intravenous Immune Globulin Administration to High-Risk Neonates 1233
Janet Kinney, MD; Lucinda Mundorf, RN; Christine Gleason, MD;
Carlton Lee, PharmD; Timothy Townsend, MD; Roshelle Thibault, RPh;
Anna Nussbaum, MD; Helen Abby, PhD; Robert Yolken, MD, Baltimore, Md

Continued on page 1217.

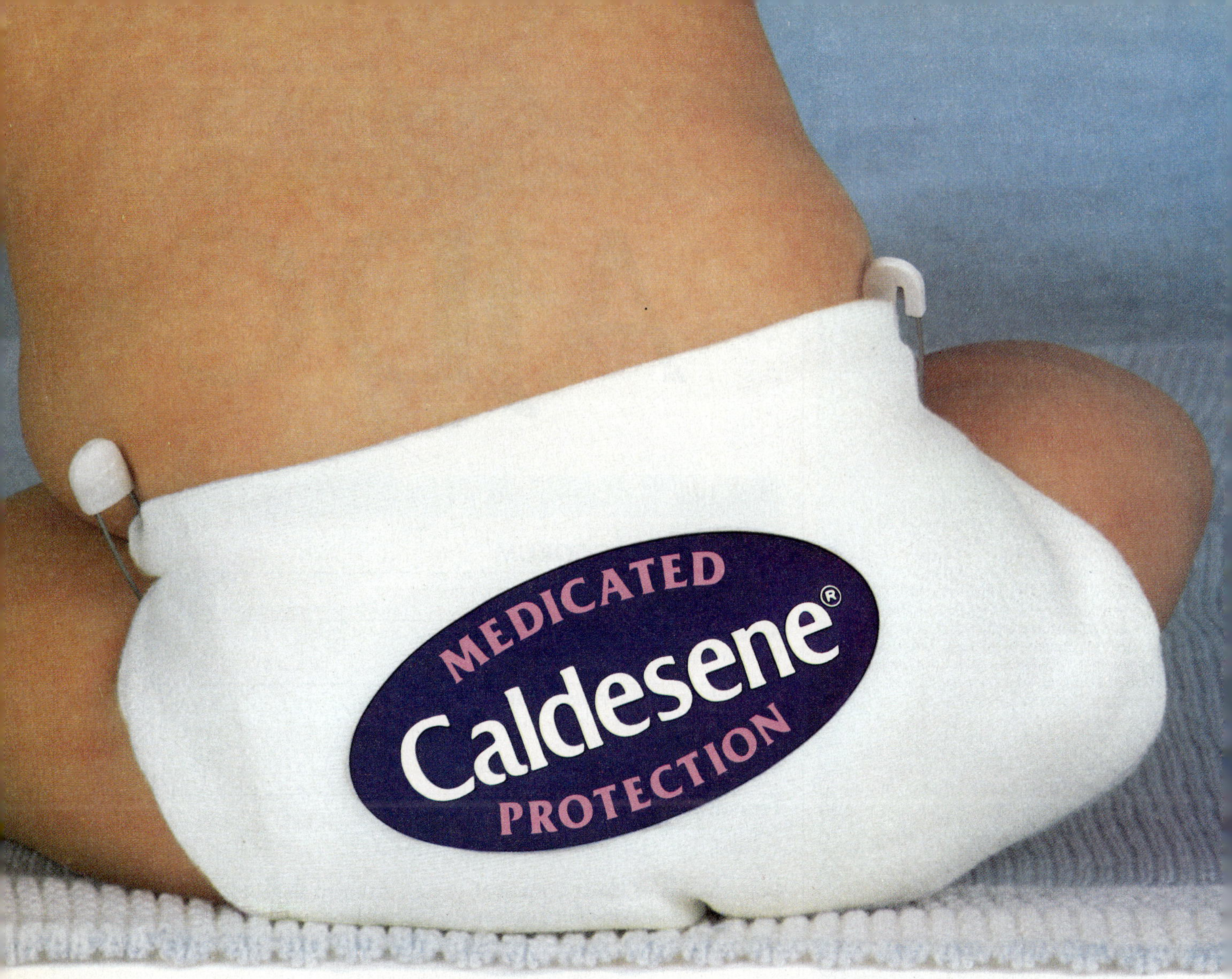
MEDICATED
Caldesene®
PROTECTION

American Medical Association
Physicians dedicated to the health of America

The AMERICAN JOURNAL OF DISEASES OF CHILDREN is a member of the consortium of AMA journals listed below. The Journal reaches more than 38 600 readers in 85 countries each month. The complete text of all AMA journals is available on the MEDIS database from Mead Data Central, Dayton, Ohio.

The Journal of the American Medical Association (JAMA)

American Journal of Diseases of Children (AJDC)

Archives of Dermatology

Archives of General Psychiatry

Archives of Internal Medicine

Archives of Neurology

Archives of Ophthalmology

Archives of Otolaryngology—Head & Neck Surgery

Archives of Pathology & Laboratory Medicine

Archives of Surgery

James S. Todd, MD, Executive Vice President
Kenneth E. Monroe, Deputy Executive Vice President
Larry E. Joyce, Senior Vice President
George D. Lundberg, MD, Editor-in-Chief, Scientific Publications
Robert L. Kennett, Vice President, Publishing
John P. Cahill, Advertising Sales Manager
Nawin Gupta, PhD, Director, Publishing Operations Division
Michael D. Springer, Associate Publisher

Please address communications concerning accepted or published communications to AMA Specialty Journals, 515 N State St, Chicago, IL 60610.

AMERICAN JOURNAL OF DISEASES OF CHILDREN

Vertical Transmission of Human Immunodeficiency Virus From Seronegative or Indeterminate Mothers 1239
John P. Johnson, MD; Peter E. Vink, MD; Susan E. Hines, MS, C PNP; Barbara Robinson, RNC; John C. Davis, Jr, MD; Prasanna Nair, MD, Baltimore, Md

Child Survival and Perinatal Infections With Human Immunodeficiency Virus 1242
John V. Bennett, MD, Martha F. Rogers, MD, Atlanta, Ga

Clinical and Endocrinologic Manifestations in Perinatally Human Immunodeficiency Virus Type 1–Infected Children Aged 5 Years or Older 1248
Philippe Lepage, MD; Philippe Van de Perre, MD; Guy Van Vliet, MD, PhD; François Nsengumuremyi, MD; Christiaan Van Goethem, MD; Philippe Kestelyn, MD, Brussels, Belgium; Philippe Msellati, MD, Bordeaux, France; Deo-Gratias Hitimana, MD, Brussels, Belgium

Obesity Among Mescalero Preschool Children: Association With Maternal Obesity and Birth Weight 1262
Margaret M. Gallaher, MD, Fern R. Hauck, MD, MS, Atlanta, Ga; Miranda Yang-Oshida, RD, MPH, Mescalero, NM; Mary K. Serdula, MD, MPH, Atlanta, Ga

Serum Lipid Concentrations in Subjects With Phenylketonuria and Their Families 1266
Terry J. DeClue, MD; Jim Davis, MD; Dawn M. Schocken, MPH; Ruth Kangas, RD; Steve A. Benford, Tampa, Fla

Adolescent Pelvic Examination: An Effective Practical Approach 1269
Hyman C. Tolmas, MD, New Orleans, La

Acellular Pertussis Vaccines: Efficacy and Evaluation of Clinical Case Definitions 1285
William C. Blackwelder, PhD, Bethesda, Md; Jann Storsaeter, MD; Patrick Olin, MD, PhD; Hans O. Hallander, MD, PhD, Stockholm, Sweden

Cardiopulmonary Exercise Testing in Children Following Surgery for Tetralogy of Fallot 1290
Teresa L. Tomassoni, PhD; Frank M. Galioto, Jr, MD, Washington, DC; Paul Vaccaro, EdD, College Park, Md

Pediatric Germ Cell and Human Chorionic Gonadotropin–Producing Tumors: Clinical and Laboratory Features 1294
Anna T. Englund, MD; Mitchell E. Geffner, MD; Ronald A. Nagel, MD; Barbara M. Lippe, MD; Glenn D. Braunstein, MD, Los Angeles, Calif

Direct Bilirubin Measurements in Jaundiced Term Newborns: A Reevaluation 1305
Thomas B. Newman MD, MPH, Sylvia Hope, PhD, San Francisco, Calif; David K. Stevenson MD, Stanford, Calif

Continued on page 1219.

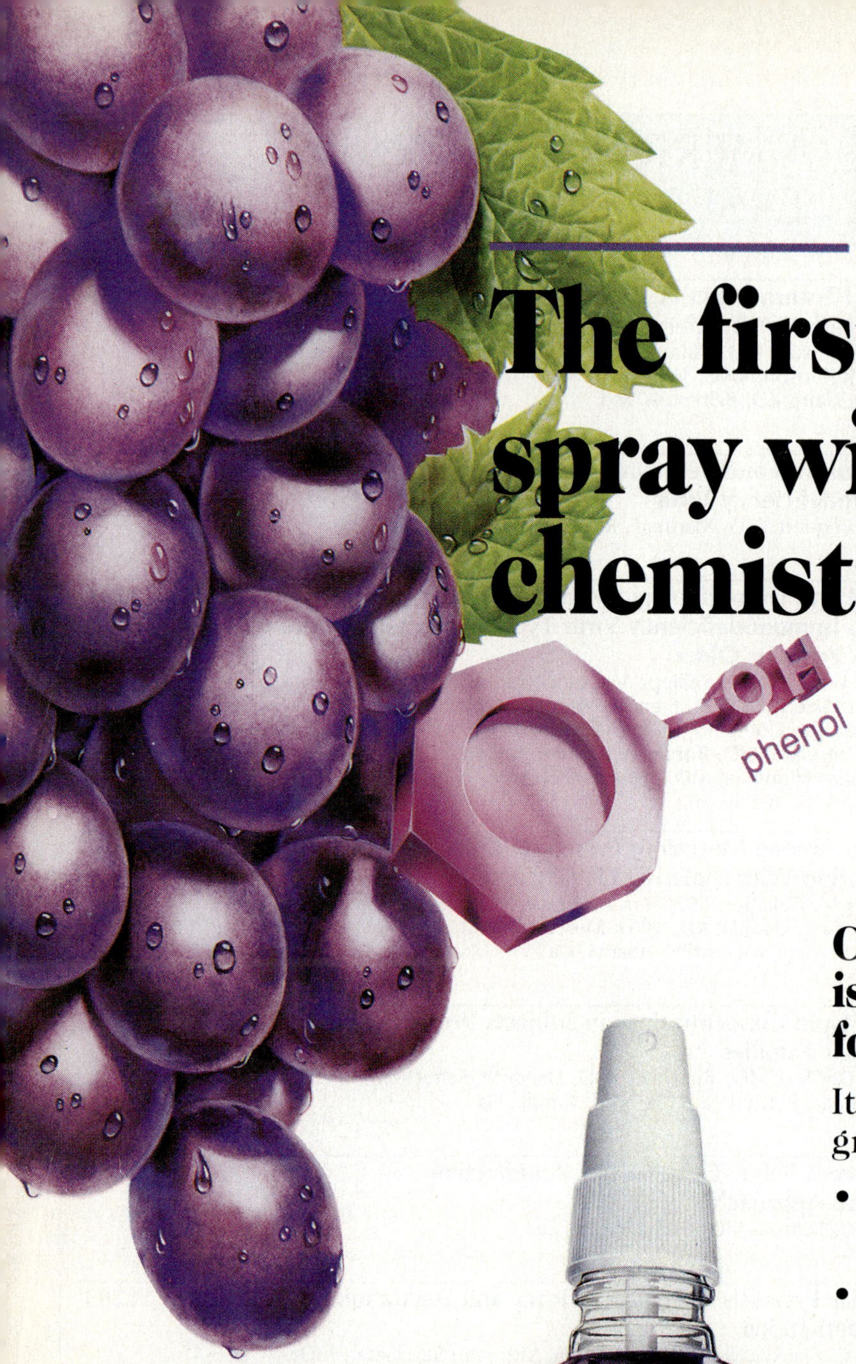

NEW!

The first sore throat spray with the right chemistry for kids.

Children's Chloraseptic® Spray is fast, effective, and especially for kids.

It tastes grape! But don't let that great taste fool you...

- 0.5% Phenol – a unique "child-strength" formula
- Rapidly penetrates irritated nerve endings – for fast relief
- Safe and effective for ages 2 and up
- Alcohol-free/sugar-free

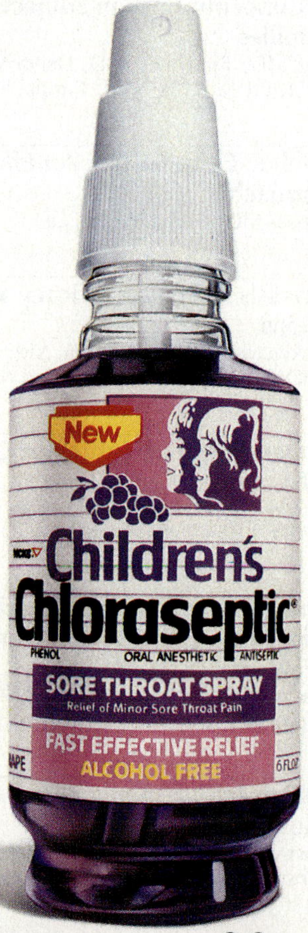

NEW Children's Chloraseptic®

SPRAY

Alcohol-free/Sugar-free

VICKS
RICHARDSON-VICKS INC.
A PROCTER & GAMBLE COMPANY

Fast, effective, great-tasting

AMERICAN JOURNAL OF DISEASES OF CHILDREN

Bone Mineral Content of Healthy, Full-term Neonates: Effect of Race, Gender, and Maternal Cigarette Smoking 1310
Pankaja S. Venkataraman, MBBS;
James C. Duke, PhD, Oklahoma City, Okla

Prevalence of Birth Defects Among Low-Birth-Weight Infants: A Population Study 1313
Fatima Mili, MD, MPH; Larry D. Edmonds, MSPH;
Muin J. Khoury, MD, PhD; Anne B. McClearn, Atlanta, Ga

Sudden Deaths and Apparent Life-Threatening Events in Hospitalized Neonates Presumed to Be Healthy 1319
David J. Burchfield, MD, Gainesville, Fla;
D. Jim Rawlings, MD, Jacksonville, Fla

EDUCATIONAL INTERVENTIONS

Comparison of a Computer Tutorial With Other Methods for Teaching Well-Newborn Care 1255
Larry W. Desch, MD; Maria T. Esquivel, MD;
Sharon K. Anderson, MA, Columbia, Mo

Current Trends in Pediatric Residency Training 1272
Carol Carraccio, MD, Alice Ackerman, MD, Baltimore, Md

SPORTS MEDICINE

Commotio Cordis: The Single, Most Common Cause of Traumatic Death in Youth Baseball 1279
Thomas J. Abrunzo, MD, Tampa, Fla

REVIEW

How Much of Neonatal Encephalopathy Is due to Birth Asphyxia? 1325
Karin B. Nelson, MD, Bethesda, Md; Alan Leviton, Boston, Mass

SPECIAL FEATURES

Radiological Case of the Month 1299
William G. Bennett, MD, Little Rock, Ark;
Beverly P. Wood, MD, Los Angeles, Calif

Picture of the Month 1301
Philip R. Cohen, MD, Adelaide A. Hebert, MD, Houston, Tex;
Murray Feingold, MD, Brighton, Mass;
Walter W. Tunnessen, Jr, MD, Philadelphia, Pa

CORRECTION

Intraosseous Infusion of Dobutamine and Isoproterenol 1312
John F. Bilello, MD, Washington, DC;
Kevin C. O'Hair, DVM, El Paso, Tex;
William C. Kirby, MD; John W. Moore, MD, Washington, DC

Evaluation of Intraosseous vs Intravenous Antibiotic Levels in a Porcine Model 1241
David G. Jaimovich, MD, Chicago, Ill; Ashir Kumar, MD, Lansing, Mich;
Steve Francom, PhD, Kalamazoo, Mich

REGULAR DEPARTMENTS

Instructions for Authors 1220

Classified Advertising 1334

Index to Advertisers 1214

INSTRUCTIONS FOR AUTHORS

General Information.—Please send manuscripts and correspondence to the Editor, Vincent A. Fulginiti, MD, *AJDC*, Dean's Office, Tulane University School of Medicine, 1430 Tulane Ave, New Orleans, LA 70112. *AJDC no longer returns nonaccepted manuscripts. Original artwork and photographs will be returned.* Manuscripts are considered with the understanding that they have not been published previously and are not under consideration by another publication.

Type of Manuscripts Suitable for Submission

Original Articles.—New observations that have not been submitted or published elsewhere.

Pediatric Forum.—A mixture of brief, peer-reviewed observations or investigations *and* letters to the editor and other short commentaries.

From Research to Relevance.—Significant research that has a high probability of being translated into clinical usefulness.

Educational Intervention.—Information concerning any educational efforts in the broad field of pediatrics.

Pediatric Legal Medicine.—A forum for discussion of broad issues relating to children and the law in today's environment.

Pediatric Perspectives.—Current information on clinical and scientific pediatric medical advances and analyses of current controversies in pediatrics.

Sports Medicine.—Current information relating to the medical needs of young athletes, as well as current concepts in the prevention, diagnosis, and treatment of sports-related illnesses and injuries.

Picture of the Month.—Submissions should be sent directly to Walter W. Tunnessen, Jr, MD, Children's Hospital of Philadelphia, Room 2143, 34th and Civic Center Blvd, Philadelphia, PA 19104.

Radiological Case of the Month.—Submissions should be sent directly to Beverly P. Wood, MD, Childrens Hospital of Los Angeles, Department of Radiology, 4650 Sunset Blvd, Los Angeles, CA 90054-0700.

AJDC Archives.—Occasional revivals of classic *AJDC* articles with contemporary commentary.

Pediatric Reviews.—Timely, comprehensive, well-referenced topics.

Conforming with all of the steps listed below will facilitate the editorial processing of your manuscript.

Step 1.—*Cover Letter.*—All manuscripts must be accompanied on submission by a cover letter giving the name, address, affiliation, and telephone and fax number of the corresponding author. The letter must include ALL of the following statements SIGNED BY ALL AUTHORS (ORIGINAL SIGNATURES):

1. Authorship Responsibility.—"I certify that I have participated sufficiently in the conception and design of this work and the analysis of the data (when applicable), as well as the writing of the manuscript, to take public responsibility for it. I believe the manuscript represents valid work. I have reviewed the final version of the manuscript and approve it for publication. Neither this manuscript nor one with substantially similar content under my authorship has been published or is being considered for publication elsewhere, except as described in an attachment. Furthermore, I attest that I shall produce the data upon which the manuscript is based for examination by the editors or their assignees if requested."

2. Financial Disclosure.—"I certify that affiliations (if any) with or involvement in any organization or entity with a direct financial interest in the subject matter or materials discussed in the manuscript (eg, employment, consultancies, stock ownership, honoraria, expert testimony) are disclosed below."

Research or project support should be listed in an acknowledgment.

3a. Copyright Transfer.—"In consideration of the action of the American Medical Association (AMA) in reviewing and editing this submission, the author(s) undersigned hereby transfer(s), assign(s), or otherwise convey(s) all copyright ownership to the AMA in the event that such work is published by the AMA."

3b. Federal Employment.—"I was an employee of the US federal government when this work was investigated and prepared for publication; therefore, it is not protected by the Copyright Act and there is no copyright of which the ownership can be transferred."

Editing.—Accepted manuscripts are copy edited according to AMA style and returned to the author for approval. Authors are responsible for all statements made in their work, including changes made by the copy editor and authorized by the corresponding author.

All accepted manuscripts become the permanent property of the AMA and may not be published elsewhere without written permission from both the author(s) and the AMA. After publication, certain articles may appear in translation in the foreign-language editions of *AJDC*. The corresponding author will receive typeset pages for approval. Forms for ordering reprints are included with the typeset pages. Reprints are shipped 6 to 8 weeks after publication.

Step 2.—*Manuscript Format.*—All articles submitted should have the following features:

1. Four copies of the manuscript should be submitted; three are for transmission to referees and one is retained in the editorial office. We prefer an original and three copies.
2. Manuscripts should be typed in double-spaced format throughout, including title page, abstracts, text, acknowledgments, references, legends for illustrations, and tables. Please number pages. *Do not use justified right margins.*
3. Title should be no more than 75 characters.
4. Authors should be limited to six, all of whom have contributed to the study and manuscript preparation, are familiar with its substance, and are able to defend its conclusions.
5. The title page should give full names, degrees, and academic affiliations of all authors, address for requests of reprints, and, if the manuscript was presented at a meeting, the organization, place, and exact date on which it was read.
6. Writing style should conform to proper English usage and syntax; consult the *American Medical Association Manual of Style,* available from Williams & Wilkins, 428 E Preston St, Baltimore, MD 21202.
7. Abstract should be limited to 135 words or less.
8. Each table should be typed, with a title, on a separate sheet of paper, with each line, including headings, *double-spaced.* Continuations should be on a second sheet with all headings repeated.
9. Use Système International (SI) measurements throughout the manuscript.
10. Illustrations should be high-contrast, glossy prints, in quadruplicate, in a proportion of 5x7 in. Figure number, name of first author, and arrow indicating "top" should be typed on a gummed *label* and affixed on the back of each illustration. *Do not write directly on the print.*

Full-color illustrations should be submitted as 35-mm, positive color transparencies, mounted in cardboard, and carefully packaged. Fee is $400 for up to six square-finished color illustrations that fit on one page. A letter of intent to pay the fee must accompany submission.

All photographs in which there is a possibility of patient identification should be accompanied by a signed statement of consent from both parents (or guardians). Covering eyes to mask identity is not sufficient.

11. References should be listed in order of their appearance in the text, typed double-spaced, and in AMA format. Please follow the exact order of information and punctuation in the examples below. Note: List all authors and/or editors up to six; if more than six, list the first three and "et al."

Journal articles: Bier DM, Fulginiti VA, Garfunkel JM, et al. Duplicate publication and related problems. *AJDC.* 1990;144:1293-1294.

Books: Naeye RL. How and when does antenatal hypoxia damage fetal brains? In: Kubli F, Patel N, Schmidt W, Linderkamp O, eds. *Perinatal Events and Brain Damage in Surviving Children.* New York, NY: Springer Verlag NY Inc; 1988:83-91.

Unpublished data, personal communications, or manuscripts "in preparation" or "submitted" should not be included in the list of references. Such material, if essential, may be incorporated in the body of the article.

Authors are responsible for the accuracy of the references.

12. Investigations involving human subjects require a specific statement in the "Methods" section that an appropriate institutional review board approved the project and/or that informed consent was obtained from both legal guardians and/or child, if appropriate.
13. Illustrations and tables from other publications should be suitably acknowledged, with written permission from *publisher* and *author.* Brief acknowledgments to specific contributors directly involved in the content of the manuscript may be placed at the end of the text, before the references.

Patient Reports: Reports of patient descriptions that do not contain sufficient new information are discouraged; normally, these will be returned without review. If new information is provided, such manuscripts will be submitted for critical review and may be published as a full original article or as a brief report in the Pediatric Forum.

SUBSCRIPTION RATES—The subscription rates for the AMERICAN JOURNAL OF DISEASES OF CHILDREN are as follows: $80 for 1 year, $145 for 2 years in the United States and US possessions; all other countries, 1 year, $95; 2 years, $175 for surface delivery. For expedited air delivery to most countries, add $20 surcharge for 1-year subscription, $40 for 2 years. (Rates for subscriptions for delivery to Japan or South Korea are available through exclusive agents—contact the publisher.) ***Special rates for residents and medical students in the United States and US possessions are available.*** Address inquiries to the American Medical Association, Publishing Operations Division, 515 N State St, Chicago, IL 60610. Phone: **(312) 670-SUBS** (670-7827).

The AMERICAN JOURNAL OF DISEASES OF CHILDREN (ISSN 0002-922X) is published monthly by the American Medical Association, 515 N State St, Chicago, IL 60610, and is an official publication of the Association. Second-class postage paid at Chicago and at additional mailing office.

CHANGE OF ADDRESS—POSTMASTER, send all address changes to AMERICAN JOURNAL OF DISEASES OF CHILDREN, Attention: Subscription Department, 515 N State St, Chicago, IL 60610. Notification of address change must be made at least 6 weeks in advance. Include both old and new addresses, a recent mailing label, and your new ZIP code.

Please address communications concerning accepted or published communications to AMA Specialty Journals, 515 N State St, Chicago, IL 60610.

GST registration number: R 126 225 556

AMERICAN JOURNAL OF DISEASES OF CHILDREN

AJDC

Vol 145 No. 12 DECEMBER 1991

PEDIATRIC FORUM

Call for Abstracts 1345

1992 Pediatric Cardiology Examination 1345

1992 Pediatric Hematology-Oncology Examination 1345

The 1992 General Pediatrics Certifying Examination of the American Board of Pediatrics 1345

Medical Management of Postobstructive Polyuria 1345
William E. Smoyer, MD, Philadelphia, Pa

A Third Pattern of Disease Progression in Children Infected With Human Immunodefiency Virus 1348
Ben Z. Katz, MD, James G. McNamara, MD, New Haven, Conn

In Reply 1349
Stephane Blanche, MD; Anne-Marie Duliege, MD; Christine Rouzioux, MD; Françoise Le Deist, MD; Ken Fukunaga, MD; Maurizio Caniglia, MD; Christine Jacomet, MD; Claude Griscelli, MD; Marc Tardieu, MD, Paris, France

Hydrocele in Kawasaki Disease: Importance in Early Recognition of Atypical Disease 1349
Amin Kabani, MD, FRCPC; Ari Joffe, MD; Taj Jadavji, MD, FRCPC, FAAP, Calgary, Alberta

Tiny Tim Remembered 1355
MAJ Charles W. Callahan, Jr, DO, MC, USAR, Philadelphia, Pa

THE EDITORIAL BOARD SPEAKS. . . .

"Grampa, Can I Get Something That I'd Like?" 1355
William B. Strong, MD, Augusta, Ga

EDITORIALS

Cautionary Note on the Use of Empiric Ceftriaxone for Suspected Bacteremia 1359
Ellen R. Wald, MD, Barry Dashefsky, MD, Pittsburgh, Pa

Continued on page 1341.

American Medical Association
Physicians dedicated to the health of America

The AMERICAN JOURNAL OF DISEASES OF CHILDREN is a member of the consortium of AMA journals listed below. The Journal reaches more than 38 600 readers in 85 countries each month. The complete text of all AMA journals is available on the MEDIS database from Mead Data Central, Dayton, Ohio.

The Journal of the American Medical Association (JAMA)
American Journal of Diseases of Children (AJDC)
Archives of Dermatology
Archives of General Psychiatry
Archives of Internal Medicine
Archives of Neurology
Archives of Ophthalmology
Archives of Otolaryngology—Head & Neck Surgery
Archives of Pathology & Laboratory Medicine
Archives of Surgery

Please address communications concerning accepted or published communications to AMA Specialty Journals, 515 N State St, Chicago, IL 60610.

AMERICAN JOURNAL OF DISEASES OF CHILDREN

Adolescents With Chronic Illness — 1361
James M. Perrin, MD, Boston, Mass

The Evolution of Surgical Treatment for Congenital Cardiac Disease — 1362
John D. Pigott, MD, New Orleans, La

ARTICLES

Prevalence and Impact of Chronic Illness Among Adolescents — 1367
Paul W. Newacheck, DrPH, San Francisco, Calif;
Margaret A. McManus, MHS, Hariette B. Fox, MSS, Washington, DC

The Role of Corticosteroid Therapy in Children With Pneumococcal Meningitis — 1374
William A. Kennedy, MD; Martha Jean Hoyt, RN;
George H. McCracken, Jr, MD, Dallas, Tex

***Haemophilus* b Disease After Vaccination With *Haemophilus* b Polysaccharide or Conjugate Vaccine** — 1379
Carl E. Frasch, PhD; Elizabeth E. Hiner, RPh;
Thomas P. Gross, MD, MPh, Bethesda, Md

Comparison of Maternal and Infant Serologic Tests for Syphilis — 1383
Sarah A. Rawstron, MB, BS, Kenneth Bromberg, MD, Brooklyn, NY

Breathing Patterns and Heart Rates at Ages 6 Weeks and 2 Years — 1393
Christian F. Poets, MD; Valerie A. Stebbens;
John R. Alexander, MSc, FSS MIS;
David P. Southall, MD, FRCP, London, England

Cardiac Care for Infants: Determinants of Hospital Charges for Acute Care — 1397
Gail D. Pearson, MD, ScD; Langford Kidd, MD, FRCP; Timothy M. Beittel;
Catherine A. Neill, MD, FRCP, Baltimore, Md

Taurine Decreases Fecal Fatty Acid and Sterol Excretion in Cystic Fibrosis: A Randomized Double-blind Trial — 1401
Lesley J. Smith, MD; Florence Lacaille, MD; Guy Lepage, MSc;
Nancy Ronco, RT; André Lamarre, MD;
Claude C. Roy, MD, Montréal, Québec

Respirosonography in Infants With Acute Bronchiolitis — 1405
Asher Tal, MD, Beersheba, Israel; Ignacio Sanchez, MD,
Hans Pasterkamp, MD, Winnipeg, Manitoba

Value of Subject Height in Predicting Lower Esophageal Sphincter Location — 1423
Annamaria Staiano, MD, Ray E. Clouse, MD, St Louis, Mo

Continued on page 1343.

AMERICAN JOURNAL OF DISEASES OF CHILDREN

Trimethoprim-Sulfamethoxazole Oral Desensitization in Hemophiliacs Infected With Human Immunodeficiency Virus With a History of Hypersensitivity Reactions **1428**
Morris Kletzel, MD; Suzanne Beck, MD; Joe Elser, MD; Nikki Shock, MSS; Wesley Burks, MD, Little Rock, Ark

Occult Cocaine Exposure in Children **1430**
Norman M. Rosenberg, DO; Kathleen L. Meert, MD; Stephen R. Knazik, DO; Hugh Yee, PhD; Ralph E. Kauffman, MD, Detroit, Mich

Frequency of Infections Associated With Implanted Systems vs Cuffed, Tunneled Silastic Venous Catheters in Patients With Acute Leukemia **1433**
Carlos Severien, MD, John D. Nelson, MD, Dallas, Tex

EDUCATIONAL INTERVENTIONS

How Are Pediatric Training Programs Preparing Residents for Practice? **1389**
Larrie W. Greenberg, MD; Pamela Getson, PhD; Cynthia Brasseux; Evan G. Pattishall III, MD; Sudesh Kataria, MD; Glen S. Bartlett, MD, PhD; Susan B. Tully, MD; Daniel Shea, MD, Washington, DC

REVIEW

Neuroblastoma Screening Data: An Epidemiologic Analysis **1415**
Steven N. Goodman, MD, MHS, PhD, Baltimore, Md

SPECIAL FEATURES

Radiological Case of the Month **1439**
Michael P. Mah, MD; Jonathan S. Fain, MD; Sue L. Hall, MD; Beverly P. Wood, MD, Los Angeles, Calif

Picture of the Month **1441**
Walter W. Tunnessen, Jr, MD, Philadelphia, Pa

REGULAR DEPARTMENTS

Instructions for Authors **1344**

Index to Advertisers **1358**

Index to Volume 145 **1443**

Classified Advertising **1470**

INSTRUCTIONS FOR AUTHORS

General Information.—Please send manuscripts and correspondence to the Editor, Vincent A. Fulginiti, MD, *AJDC*, Dean's Office, Tulane University School of Medicine, 1430 Tulane Ave, New Orleans, LA 70112. *AJDC no longer returns nonaccepted manuscripts. Original artwork and photographs will be returned.* Manuscripts are considered with the understanding that they have not been published previously and are not under consideration by another publication.

Type of Manuscripts Suitable for Submission

Original Articles.—New observations that have not been submitted or published elsewhere.

Pediatric Forum.—A mixture of brief, peer-reviewed observations or investigations *and* letters to the editor and other short commentaries.

From Research to Relevance.—Significant research that has a high probability of being translated into clinical usefulness.

Educational Intervention.—Information concerning any educational efforts in the broad field of pediatrics.

Pediatric Legal Medicine.—A forum for discussion of broad issues relating to children and the law in today's environment.

Pediatric Perspectives.—Current information on clinical and scientific pediatric medical advances and analyses of current controversies in pediatrics.

Sports Medicine.—Current information relating to the medical needs of young athletes, as well as current concepts in the prevention, diagnosis, and treatment of sports-related illnesses and injuries.

Picture of the Month.—Submissions should be sent directly to Walter W. Tunnessen, Jr, MD, Children's Hospital of Philadelphia, Room 2143, 34th and Civic Center Blvd, Philadelphia, PA 19104.

Radiological Case of the Month.—Submissions should be sent directly to Beverly P. Wood, MD, Childrens Hospital of Los Angeles, Department of Radiology, 4650 Sunset Blvd, Los Angeles, CA 90054-0700.

AJDC Archives.—Occasional revivals of classic *AJDC* articles with contemporary commentary.

Pediatric Reviews.—Timely, comprehensive, well-referenced topics.

Conforming with all of the steps listed below will facilitate the editorial processing of your manuscript.

Step 1.—*Cover Letter.*—All manuscripts must be accompanied on submission by a cover letter giving the name, address, affiliation, and telephone and fax number of the corresponding author. The letter must include ALL of the following statements SIGNED BY ALL AUTHORS (ORIGINAL SIGNATURES):

1. Authorship Responsibility.—"I certify that I have participated sufficiently in the conception and design of this work and the analysis of the data (when applicable), as well as the writing of the manuscript, to take public responsibility for it. I believe the manuscript represents valid work. I have reviewed the final version of the manuscript and approve it for publication. Neither this manuscript nor one with substantially similar content under my authorship has been published or is being considered for publication elsewhere, except as described in an attachment. Furthermore, I attest that I shall produce the data upon which the manuscript is based for examination by the editors or their assignees if requested."

2. Financial Disclosure.—"I certify that affiliations (if any) with or involvement in any organization or entity with a direct financial interest in the subject matter or materials discussed in the manuscript (eg, employment, consultancies, stock ownership, honoraria, expert testimony) are disclosed below."

Research or project support should be listed in an acknowledgment.

3a. Copyright Transfer.—"In consideration of the action of the American Medical Association (AMA) in reviewing and editing this submission, the author(s) undersigned hereby transfer(s), assign(s), or otherwise convey(s) all copyright ownership to the AMA in the event that such work is published by the AMA."

3b. Federal Employment.—"I was an employee of the US federal government when this work was investigated and prepared for publication; therefore, it is not protected by the Copyright Act and there is no copyright of which the ownership can be transferred."

Editing.—Accepted manuscripts are copy edited according to AMA style and returned to the author for approval. Authors are responsible for all statements made in their work, including changes made by the copy editor and authorized by the corresponding author.

All accepted manuscripts become the permanent property of the AMA and may not be published elsewhere without written permission from both the author(s) and the AMA. After publication, certain articles may appear in translation in the foreign-language editions of *AJDC*. The corresponding author will receive typeset pages for approval. Forms for ordering reprints are included with the typeset pages. Reprints are shipped 6 to 8 weeks after publication.

Step 2.—*Manuscript Format.*—All articles submitted should have the following features:

1. Four copies of the manuscript should be submitted; three are for transmission to referees and one is retained in the editorial office. We prefer an original and three copies.
2. Manuscripts should be typed in double-spaced format throughout, including title page, abstracts, text, acknowledgments, references, legends for illustrations, and tables. Please number pages. *Do not use justified right margins.*
3. Title should be no more than 75 characters.
4. Authors should be limited to six, all of whom have contributed to the study and manuscript preparation, are familiar with its substance, and are able to defend its conclusions.
5. The title page should give full names, degrees, and academic affiliations of all authors, address for requests of reprints, and, if the manuscript was presented at a meeting, the organization, place, and exact date on which it was read.
6. Writing style should conform to proper English usage and syntax; consult the *American Medical Association Manual of Style,* available from Williams & Wilkins, 428 E Preston St, Baltimore, MD 21202.
7. Abstract should be limited to 135 words or less.
8. Each table should be typed, with a title, on a separate sheet of paper, with each line, including headings, *double-spaced.* Continuations should be on a second sheet with all headings repeated.
9. Use Système International (SI) measurements throughout the manuscript.
10. Illustrations should be high-contrast, glossy prints, in quadruplicate, in a proportion of 5x7 in. Figure number, name of first author, and arrow indicating "top" should be typed on a gummed *label* and affixed on the back of each illustration. *Do not write directly on the print.*

Full-color illustrations should be submitted as 35-mm, positive color transparencies, mounted in cardboard, and carefully packaged. Fee is $400 for up to six square-finished color illustrations that fit on one page. A letter of intent to pay the fee must accompany submission.

All photographs in which there is a possibility of patient identification should be accompanied by a signed statement of consent from both parents (or guardians). Covering eyes to mask identity is not sufficient.

11. References should be listed in order of their appearance in the text, typed double-spaced, and in AMA format. Please follow the exact order of information and punctuation in the examples below. Note: List all authors and/or editors up to six; if more than six, list the first three and "et al."

Journal articles: Bier DM, Fulginiti VA, Garfunkel JM, et al. Duplicate publication and related problems. *AJDC.* 1990;144:1293-1294.

Books: Naeye RL. How and when does antenatal hypoxia damage fetal brains? In: Kubli F, Patel N, Schmidt W, Linderkamp O, eds. *Perinatal Events and Brain Damage in Surviving Children.* New York, NY: Springer Verlag NY Inc; 1988:83-91.

Unpublished data, personal communications, or manuscripts "in preparation" or "submitted" should not be included in the list of references. Such material, if essential, may be incorporated in the body of the article.

Authors are responsible for the accuracy of the references.

12. Investigations involving human subjects require a specific statement in the "Methods" section that an appropriate institutional review board approved the project and/or that informed consent was obtained from both legal guardians and/or child, if appropriate.
13. Illustrations and tables from other publications should be suitably acknowledged, with written permission from *publisher* and *author.* Brief acknowledgments to specific contributors directly involved in the content of the manuscript may be placed at the end of the text, before the references.

Patient Reports: Reports of patient descriptions that do not contain sufficient new information are discouraged; normally, these will be returned without review. If new information is provided, such manuscripts will be submitted for critical review and may be published as a full original article or as a brief report in the Pediatric Forum.

Editorial

AJDC Is 80 Years Old

From Pedology to Pediatrics

In 1911, the *American Journal of Diseases of Children* was initiated. The editorial board consisted of Abraham Jacobi (often referred to as the Father of Pediatrics), Frank Spooner Churchill, John Lovett Morse, William Fitch Cheney, Edwin E. Graham, and John Howland. If one looks at the first year of operation of the journal, one is struck with the similarity between the issues with which the pediatricians of that day were concerned and those that we deal with today. For example, in those first issues, meningitis, streptococcal infections, genetic disorders, nutritional topics, developmental research, hypertension, hemorrhagic diseases, and "modern" instrumentation for diagnosis and treatment were all present.

The biologic knowledge base was imperfect, and scant by our standards, but the questions asked were strikingly similar. What pathophysiologic processes underlie disease states? What is the best way to make a diagnosis? What is the best management for a given disorder? What is the best way to feed infants to ensure proper nutrition? What causes these odd disorders that develop in infants and children? What is the course of bone development? Each of these questions is at the base of the articles that appeared 80 years ago; they are still the basis of articles 80 years later, in this issue and in the remaining issues of this year. We continue the quest for new information, and *AJDC* continues in its perceived mission to disseminate answers to these pertinent questions to the best of our authors' knowledge.

In his introduction to the first issue in 1911, Dr Jacobi wrote, "Our present copious pediatric literature dates from about the middle of the last century. Extracts, reviews, and original contributions became plentiful; our weeklies, monthlies and quarterlies contained much that was and much that still is of value." I could have written those words today with a slight change in time frame! Dr Jacobi also lauded the development of a new discipline, pedology, which he defined as ". . . the science of the child age. . . . " He further directed readers to ". . . look on pediatrics not as a specialty, . . . but as that part of internal medicine and surgery which cannot be measured by the knowledge derived from and applied to the adult. . . ." Pediatrics has succeeded in that separation in the 80 years since Jacobi wrote that passage, and we have learned repeatedly that principles of biology and medicine are unique to the developing child and cannot be extrapolated from experience with adults. Dr Jacobi emphasized growth and development as singular characteristics that the budding specialty was to focus on and that the journal would give visibility to—he was again correct and prophetic. This fact seems second nature to us now, but in his day it was considered heretical by some.

AJDC played a role in that evolution by stressing observations and investigations that focused on the unique characteristics of childhood. For example, in the first issue, Fetterolf and Gittings of Philadelphia, Pa, focused on those thoracic anatomic features that conditioned the physical examination of a child in contrast to an adult. They outlined the enormous size of the thymus, the thinness of the chest wall, the relatively enlarged heart in the child's thorax than in the adult, and so on. Martha Wollstein of New York, NY, attempted to cultivate "influenza bacilli" from the cerebrospinal fluid of children with meningitis and inoculate mice, guinea pigs, rabbits, and monkeys. She produced meningitis in the simian model and detailed the factors that led to virulence, immune response, and disease production. Issac Abt described a child with "amaurotic family idiocy," complete with autopsy findings, which helped to define what we now know as Tay-Sachs disease. These all are examples of what Dr Jacobi was referring to when he defined pedology.

History is important to all of us; we ignore it at our peril. We need to know where we have been to know where we want to go. All of us connected with *AJDC* are proud that we are part of a historical thread that stretches back these 80 years, and that our journal has played its role in the development of "pedology" into the science and art of pediatrics. So we say "happy birthday to *AJDC*" and as temporary custodians of this important part of our discipline, we will strive to continue the tradition that Dr Jacobi and others inaugurated in January 1911. In celebration of that birthday and to remind us of our origins, we are reprinting Dr Jacobi's "Introduction" and the "Table of Contents" of the 1911 issues of *AJDC*.

Vincent A. Fulginiti, MD
Editor, *AJDC*
Dean's Office
Tulane University
School of Medicine
1430 Tulane Ave
New Orleans, LA 70112

American Journal of Diseases of Children

Vol. 1 JANUARY, 1911 No. 1

INTRODUCTION

The literature connected with pedology—the science of the child age —has undergone vast changes since Thomas Thacher's "A Brief Rule to Guide the Common People of New England How to Order Themselves and Theirs in the Small Pocks or Measles" (Jan. 21, 1677-78). This "Broadside," twelve inches by seventeen in size, has been followed by many more broadsides; indeed by roars of broadsides. "The History of American Pediatrics Before 1800," it is true, fills only twenty-five pages of *"Janus,* 1902." It contains, however, mention of the previous and classical treatise of Samuel Bard, "An Enquiry into the Nature, Cause, and Cure of the Angina Suffocativa, or Throat Distemper, as it is commonly called by the Inhabitants of this City and Colony. New York, 1771."

The Nineteenth Century yields a long series of magazine articles and text-books. Dewees, Stewart, Eberle, Condie, Charles D. and Fordyce Meigs were physicians of fame, and their manuals were highly appreciated. Toward the end of the century (1889) W. V. Keating began his five volumes of a "Cyclopedia of the Diseases of Children," which has exerted a great influence in enhancing the taste for the study of healthy and diseased child-life, similar to what C. Gerhardt's epoch-making "Handbuch"—a modest title for a vast achievement—accomplished for Germany since 1877, and Grancher and Comby's "Maladies des Enfants" for France since 1898.

The first systematic instruction in pedology was furnished by the small New York Medical College in East Thirteenth street. In its reorganization of 1860, a full professorship was established. It carried the title of "Infant Pathology and Therapeutics." Subsequent imitations in later times and in other schools of medicine contented themselves with "Pediatrics," the *treating* of children, or the "Diseases of Children," only. The college closed its doors in 1864, during the blights of the Civil War. Meanwhile, the newly founded Bellevue Hospital Medical College organized in 1861 a "Clinical Professorship" for the diseases of children. In that chair Dr. J. Lewis Smith displayed great industry and enthusiasm, and did much to enlighten the profession in regard to both the difficulties and the importance of the comparatively new doctrine. Another clinical professorship of the same nature was established in 1865 by the University Medical College, and in 1870 by the College of Physicians and Surgeons.

Since that time, the example given by New York has been followed by a large number of the medical schools in the country. Very few of them founded full professorships endowed with the full rights and duties awarded to the rest of the teachers who connected themselves with a medical school or the medical faculty of a university. Harvard was the first to see the light. Though the recognition came late and is far from being universal, we are still ahead of the present status of pedology in the curricula of most European medical schools. Germany, to this day, has few full professorships for instruction in the diseases of children. Indeed, its great teacher and classical writer, Eduard Henoch (1881) closed in 1893 his academic career with the title of a mere "Extraordinary Professor." When, a few weeks ago, however, he was taken away, 90 years old, he had the satisfaction of knowing that there was at last a breach in the short-sighted conservatism of German universities, and that at last a few full chairs of pedology had been established.

Great men like him are scarce in any part of medicine. To excel in close observation, logical reasoning, and elegant and precise diction, together with the faculty of teaching, is given to few men. Charles West in England (1848), Rilliet and Barthez in Switzerland and France (1843), belong to that class and deserve with Henoch the name of classical authors and instructors. They have passed away, but they have been followed by successors, few, it is true, of equal rank, but very numerous and many of them meritorious writers. If but few approach them, the multitude of those who have something to say—and the much greater multitude who say it anyhow—have made the study of the child and its diseases popular and interesting. If it so happens that too much is published, that is only a repetition of the experience of other doctrines in our science and art. Guttenberg's art could not have been discovered by everybody who is satisfied with utilizing or abusing it.

Our present copious pediatric literature dates from about the middle of the last century. Extracts, reviews, and original contributions became plentiful; our weeklies, monthlies, and quarterlies contained much that was and much that still is of value. The first extensive American papers on diphtheria (1860) and acute rheumatism (1875) were published in magazines. The first volumes of the *American Journal of Obstetrics and the Diseases of Women and Children* (founded in 1869) were almost entirely filled with subjects connected with the anatomy, physiology, and therapeutics of the young. But though the Germans had a special journal since 1843, the first American journal, the *Archives of Pediatrics,* was published by the enthusiastic Watson in 1884 and *Pediatrics* by Dillon Brown in 1896. My readers know that both have rendered good service, both by disseminating knowledge and rousing interest and enthusiasm. At the same time our weeklies have vied with them in supplying the practitioners of the country with information of increasing value.

What all of us have learned is to look on pediatrics not as a specialty, such as ophthalmology or otology, which concern single organs, but as that part of internal medicine and surgery which cannot be measured by the knowledge derived from and applied to the adult; it requires special study and research in order to become both scientific and practical. We learned that there is no uniformity of structure and function in the human organism between conception and death; that childhood must be studied, not from the point of view of reproduction only, but of reproduction *and growth;* that pediatrics does not deal with miniature men and women, with reduced doses and the same class of diseases in smaller bodies, but has its own independent range and horizon, and gives as much to general medicine as it has received from it; that there are anomalies and diseases which are encountered in the infant and child only. On the other hand, there are those which are *mostly* found in children, or with a symptomatology and course peculiar to them; and those, finally, which affect both the young and the old, with such varieties, however, in both symptoms and course, as depend on the size or anatomic structure of the afflicted organ or organism, or the difference in the degree of irritability.[1]

To learn and to teach all that—and many more things—the cooperation of many interests was required. The general practitioner—the majority of whose patients are young—since the belief ceased to be prevalent that the diseases of the small child are "small things," wanted more opportunities to learn than those which his college schooling had pro-

1. Arch. Pediat., November, 1889.

vided for him. The colleges themselves have not been slow in recognizing the advanced condition of pediatrics and the necessities of the physicians of the country.

The increased number of medical magazines—suggested by medical men and published by business men eager to profit by subscriptions and by ethical and unethical advertisements—and text-books—a few excellent, some good, many more, however, mere compilations, most of them with ample sales—have disseminated knowledge which without them would not have been accessible. Even inferior books will convey it and render their owners amenable to the consciousness of their defects and the longing for something more that is not only new but better. For, indeed, the latest is not necessarily the best.

The number of special journals dedicated to pedology or to pediatrics has become quite large. Germany began its oldest and most exclusive *"Journal für Kinderkrankheiten,"* in 1843; it has six or seven such magazines at present; another one appeared lately on account of the large amount of material offered, swamping those in existence. France, England, Spain, Italy, Turkey, and America, all have their special journals. Meanwhile the large weeklies and monthlies have continued to contribute information to those who are interested in pediatrics. In Germany, however, where special pediatric magazines are most numerous and widely appreciated, the pediatric contributions to general journals are becoming less predominant.

The same process of spontaneous exclusiveness will keep on when pediatric journals are published in sufficient numbers and of such a character as to justify and tempt authors to select them for their contributions. But journals are not all of the same standard. Mere compilations will find many grateful readers; a single interesting case accompanied by intelligent culling will prove as acceptable to many a subscriber as it is pleasing to the eye of the writer; discussions in medical societies will frequently add more to the knowledge of a given subject than a labored article on a topic studied up for the instruction, at least, of the author; extracts from the current literature of all nations, particularly when full and systematized, are eagerly sought for and enjoyed.

This new journal of ours, the American Journal of Diseases of Children, however, the first number of which we herewith offer to the profession, is not published to compete with those already in existence.

For some time it has been noted, however, that the pediatric material offered to *The Journal of the American Medical Association* is rapidly increasing in quantity, and also in the size of the articles. Writers were often annoyed by the delay encountered in the publication of their essays; it has even happened that after a delay of many months, authors of the very highest standing were requested to shorten their articles—in many instances an impossible task. Such occurrences suggested the publication of a new special organ. Even those who insisted on the right of the practitioners of the country—members of the Association—to be amply supplied with pediatric teaching by their own journal, receded from the stand taken by them when convinced by the fact that a new journal would not curtail the printing of pediatric contributions in *The Journal of the American Medical Association* and many others of high standing. On the contrary, with the increasing number of physicians interested and working in the field of pedology, there will be more than merely a vast number of papers; there will be more profundity and research. These our new journal is to gather in, and it is to be the companion and ally of the *Archives of Internal Medicine.* It may rarely give a mere case, still more rarely a prescription; it is to be a receptacle, however, of the very latest in the very best of American and European literatures. But extracts will be few in proportion. Reviews, carefully prepared by competent critics, will be offered from time to time. The bulk of the contents, however, will be original; anatomy—both embryonal and postnatal—physiology, biochemistry, nosology, and therapeutics will come to their own, and will be welcomed as our sources of actual progress. Thus, THE AMERICAN JOURNAL OF DISEASES OF CHILDREN is expected to be one of the number of strictly scientific magazines which, since the first appearance of the *Journal of Experimental Medicine* and its followers, have given American medical journalism its standing as an equal coworker in the modern world of Medicine. *Quod felix faustumque sit.*

A. JACOBI.

CONTENTS OF VOLUME I

JANUARY, 1911. NUMBER 1

PAGE

Introduction. A. Jacobi, M.D., New York 1

Some Anatomic Features of the Child's Thorax and Their Practical Application in Physical Diagnosis. George Fetterolf, M.D., and J. Claxton Gittings, M.D., Philadelphia 6

Observations on Three Hundred Cases of Acute Meningitis in Infants and Young Children. L. Emmett Holt, M.D., New York 26

The Constant Presence of Tubercle Bacilli in the Cerebrospinal Fluid of Tuberculous Meningitis. Josephine Hemenway, M.D., New York. 37

Influenzal Meningitis and its Experimental Production. Martha Wollstein, M.D., New York 42

Amaurotic Family Idiocy. Isaac A. Abt, M.D., Chicago 59

Atypical Scarlet Fever. C. Gilmore Kerley, M.D., New York 70

Progress in Pediatrics 73

FEBRUARY, 1911. NUMBER 2

Congenital Pyloric Stenosis. A. D. Bevan, M.D., Chicago 85

Cerebrospinal Meningitis, its Etiology, Diagnosis, Prognosis and Treatment. Charles Hunter Dunn, M.D., Boston 95

Some Investigations Concerning the Relation Between Carpal Ossification and Physical and Mental Development. Eli Long, M.D., and E. W. Caldwell, M.D., New York 113

Frequency and Significance of Albumin in the Urines of Normal Children. Samuel McClintock Hamill, M.D., Philadelphia, and Kenneth D. Blackfan, M.D., Cambridge, N. Y. 139

Progress in Pediatrics 164

MARCH, 1911. NUMBER 3

Physiology and Pathology of the Digestion of Fat in Infancy. Fritz B. Talbot, M.D., Boston 173

The Bacteriology of the Blood in Early Life. Frank Spooner Churchill, M.D., and Charles P. Clark, M.D., Chicago 193

The Metabolism of Nitrogen, Phosphorus and the Purin Substances in the New-Born; with Special Reference to the Causation of the Uric Acid Infarcts of the Kidney. Oscar M. Schloss, M.D., New York, and James L. Crawford, M.D., Troy, Texas 203

CONTENTS OF VOLUME I

PAGE

THE NON-SPECIFICITY OF THE CYTO-FINDINGS IN THE SPINAL FLUID IN VARIOUS MENINGEAL CONDITIONS, ESPECIALLY IN CHILDREN, FROM AN EXAMINATION OF OVER FIVE HUNDRED SPECIMENS. WILLIAM PALMER LUCAS, M.D., BOSTON 230

PROGRESS IN PEDIATRICS 238

APRIL, 1911. NUMBER 4

INFLUENZAL MENINGITIS, WITH ESPECIAL REFERENCE TO ITS PATHOLOGY AND BACTERIOLOGY. DAVID JOHN DAVIS, M.D., CHICAGO 249

THE TREATMENT OF CHRONIC INFANTILE PARALYSIS. MAX STRUNSKY, M.D., NEW YORK 266

A STUDY OF BLOOD-PRESSURE IN NORMAL CHILDREN. MAY MICHAEL, M.D., CHICAGO 272

SPONTANEOUS HEMORRHAGE IN THE NEW-BORN. OSCAR M. SCHLOSS, M.D., NEW YORK, AND LEO J. J. COMMISKEY, M.D., BROOKLYN 276

INFLAMMATORY CHANGES IN THE APPENDIX DURING EARLY INFANCY. GEORGE M. SMITH, M.D., ST. LOUIS 299

PROGRESS IN PEDIATRICS 310

MAY, 1911. NUMBER 5

STUDIES ON INFANT NUTRITION: I. METABOLISM IN CHRONIC MALNUTRITION. ANGELIA M. COURTNEY, NEW YORK 321

THE ETIOLOGY AND NATURE OF HARD CURDS IN INFANTS' STOOLS. JOS. BRENNEMANN, M.D., CHICAGO 341

A DUODENAL TUBE FOR INFANTS. ALFRED F. HESS, M.D., NEW YORK 360

SPASM OF THE PYLORUS IN INFANCY. J. L. MORSE, A.M., M.D., BOSTON 366

BLOOD TRANSFUSION IN INFANTS BY MEANS OF GLASS TUBES. BETH VINCENT, M.D., BOSTON 376

PROGRESS IN PEDIATRICS 382

JUNE, 1911. NUMBER 6

THE DIAGNOSIS OF INFANTILE TETANY, WITH A REPORT OF EXPERIMENTAL TETANY IN DOGS. HERBERT B. WILCOX, M.D., NEW YORK 398

TWO CASES OF INFLUENZAL MENINGITIS. PATIENTS TREATED WITH HEXAMETHYLENAMIN. WALTER V. BREM, M.D., AND A. H. ZEILER, M.D., CRISTOBAL, CANAL ZONE 416

THE DIAGNOSTIC VALUE OF A BLOOD-EXAMINATION IN PERTUSSIS. JOHN ALBERT KOLMER, M.D., PHILADELPHIA 431

PROGRESS IN PEDIATRICS 440

CONTENTS OF VOLUME II

JULY, 1911. NUMBER 1 — PAGE

The Treatment of Sepsis in Scarlatina with Antistreptococcus Serum. Matthias Nicoll, M.D., New York 1

Accessory Sinus Suppuration in Scarlatina. Thomas Hubbard, M.D., Toledo, O. 11

Studies in the Metabolism of Atrophic Infants. Charles A. Fife, M.D., and Borden S. Veeder, M.D., Philadelphia 19

A Preparatory Study of the Bacillus Acidophilus in Regard to Its Possible Therapeutic Use. Thomas Morgan Rotch, M.D., and Arthur I. Kendall, Ph.D., Boston 30

Anaphylaxis in Its Relation to Pediatrics. Godfrey R. Pisek, M.D., and Marshall C. Pease, M.D., New York 39

The Fundamental Requirements of an Infant's Nutrition. John Howland, M.D., St. Louis 49

Progress in Pediatrics 55

AUGUST, 1911. NUMBER 2

The Occurrence of Infantile Paralysis in the United States and Canada in 1910. Robert W. Lovett, M.D., Boston 65

The Cerebral Forms of Poliomyelitis. Henry Koplik, M.D., New York .. 75

Infantile Paralysis: Spinal Form. John Lovett Morse, A.M., M.D., Boston 92

The Control of Epidemic Poliomyelitis. Simon Flexner, M.D., New York 96

Infantile Paralysis. The Most Promising Outlook for Improvement in Treatment from the Standpoint of the Pediatrician. J. H. M. Knox, Jr., M.D., Baltimore 102

The Rôle of Mineral Salts in the Metabolism of Infants. B. Raymond Hoobler, M.D., New York 107

Progress in Pediatrics 141

SEPTEMBER, 1911. NUMBER 3

A Case of Scaphocephalus with Retinal Changes. Arthur Willard Fairbanks, M.D., Boston 149

Muscular Hypertrophy of the Pylorus in Infancy. Henry Larned Keith Shaw, M.D., and Thomas Ordway, M.D., Albany, N. Y. 159

Albumin-Milk in Infant Feeding. Clifford G. Grulee, M.D., Chicago .. 180

Protein Metabolism in Infants and Children. Herman Schwarz, M.D., New York 189

A Case of Infection of the New-Born. Louise Tayler-Jones, M.D., Washington, D. C. 210

Progress in Pediatrics 212

CONTENTS OF VOLUME II

OCTOBER, 1911. NUMBER 4

PAGE

Epidemiologic and Etiologic Studies of Acute Poliomyelitis in Pennsylvania. Samuel G. Dixon, M.D., Harrisburg 221

Relationship of Gastric to Pancreatic Fat Digestion in Infants. J. P. Sedgwick, M.D., and F. W. Schlutz, M.D., Minneapolis 243

Hippuric Acid in the Urine of Normal Breast-Fed Infants. Samuel Amberg, M.D., and J. H. Mason Knox, Jr., Baltimore 248

Further Observations on the Acid Control of the Pylorus in Infants. David Murray Cowie, M.D., and William Lyon, M.D., Ann Arbor ... 252

The Relation of Meat Ingestion to Indicanuria in Children. E. Charles Fleischner, M.D., San Francisco 262

The Treatment of Chronic Nephritis in Children by the Edebohls Operation. Henry Koplik, M.D., New York 267

Progress in Pediatrics 281

NOVEMBER, 1911. NUMBER 5

A Discussion of Mikulicz' Disease with Report of a Case of Lymphatic Leukemia in a Child with Marked Enlargement of the Salivary Glands. Wilder Tileston, M.D., New Haven, Conn. 293

A Study of the Caloric Needs of Premature Infants. Julius H. Hess, M.D., Chicago 302

The Use of Malt Sugar and High Percentages of Casein in Infant Feeding. John Lovett Morse, M.D., Boston 315

A Note on the Bacteriologic Examination of Lymphatic Glands in Scarlet Fever. John Albert Kolmer, M.D., Philadelphia 329

The Intestinal Infantilism of Herter. R. G. Freeman, M.D., New York. 332

Myatonia Congenita: A Report of a Case with Autopsy. W. T. Councilman, M.D., and Charles Hunter Dunn, M.D., Boston 340

Progress in Pediatrics 356

DECEMBER, 1911. NUMBER 6

Infantile Paralysis with Especial Reference to Its Occurrence in Massachusetts, 1907-1910. Robert W. Lovett, M.D., and Mark W. Richardson, M.D., Boston 369

Pyloric Stenosis in Older Children, with Report of a Case of Pyloric Spasm Ending Fatally. Edwin E. Graham, A.B., M.D., Philadelphia 407

An Apparatus for the Collection of the Excreta of Infants. Eugene F. DuBois, M.D., New York 415

A Metabolism Bed for Infants. John Howland, M.D., St. Louis, and Robert A. Cooke, M.D., New York 419

Progress in Pediatrics 422

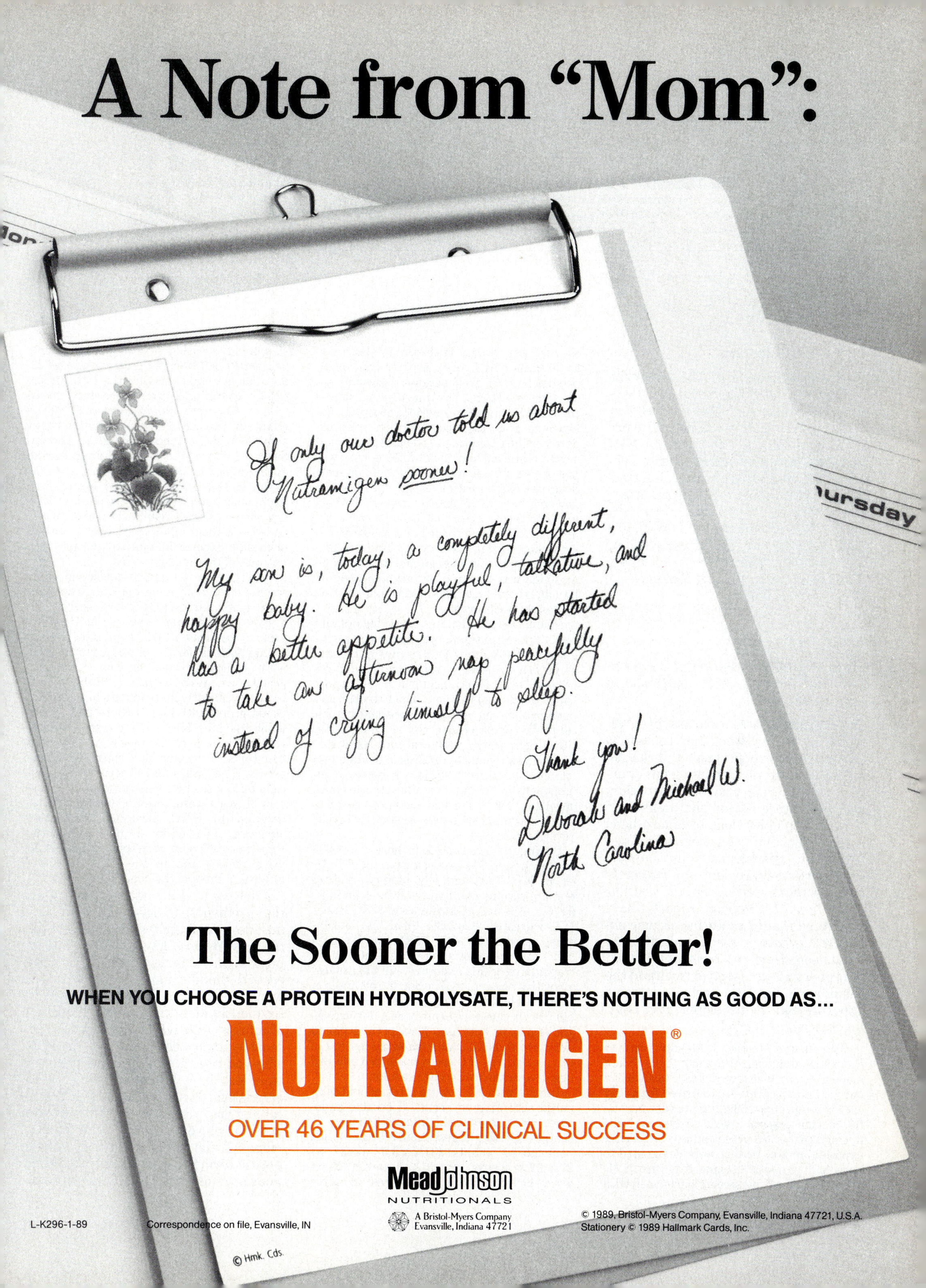
A Note from "Mom":
ursday
If only our doctor told us about
Nutramigen sooner!
My son is, today, a completely different,
happy baby. He is playful, talkative, and
has a better appetite. He has started
to take an afternoon nap peacefully
instead of crying himself to sleep.
Thank you!
Deborah and Michael W.
North Carolina
The Sooner the Better!
WHEN YOU CHOOSE A PROTEIN HYDROLYSATE, THERE'S NOTHING AS GOOD AS...
NUTRAMIGEN®
OVER 46 YEARS OF CLINICAL SUCCESS
Mead Johnson
NUTRITIONALS
A Bristol-Myers Company
Evansville, Indiana 47721
L-K296-1-89
Correspondence on file, Evansville, IN
© 1989, Bristol-Myers Company, Evansville, Indiana 47721, U.S.A.
Stationery © 1989 Hallmark Cards, Inc.
© Hmk. Cds.

The Pediatric Forum

This department of AJDC *is reserved for comment, criticism, observation, and discussion of "issues of current concern and importance for children's health." The Editor encourages our readers to express themselves on a variety of topics and issues. Further, we encourage the submission of unique and brief clinical and scientific observations that do not fulfill the criteria for original articles.*

1991 Annual Meeting

The annual meeting of The American Pediatric Society, The Society for Pediatric Research, and The Ambulatory Pediatric Association will be held April 29 through May 2, 1991, at the New Orleans (La) Hilton and Rivergate Convention Center. For further information, contact the APS/SPR Association Headquarters, 2650 Yale Blvd SE, Suite 104, Albuquerque, NM 87106; (505) 764-9099; FAX (505) 842-8227; or the Ambulatory Pediatric Association, 6728 Old McLean Village, McLean, VA 22101; (703) 556-9222.

Characteristics of Perinatal Cocaine-Exposed Infants With Necrotizing Enterocolitis

Sir.—Recently, attention has been directed at the complications related to cocaine use during pregnancy, including placental abruption, spontaneous abortion, intrauterine growth retardation, and premature labor and delivery.[1,2] Neonatal complications have also been noted, including neurobehavioral disturbances, microcephaly, intrauterine cerebrovascular accidents, and possibly malformations secondary to vascular disruptions.[3-5] Previous reports have suggested that intrauterine cocaine exposure may also be associated with neonatal necrotizing enterocolitis (NEC).[6,7] We report a retrospective review of the relationship between perinatal cocaine exposure and the development of NEC in the newborn period.

Patients and Methods.—All admissions to the neonatal intensive care unit (NICU) at a medical center that provides care to an urban indigent population were reviewed from July 1987 through June 1989. Infants with perinatal cocaine exposure who developed NEC during this period were compared with nonexposed infants. Infants were designated to have had perinatal cocaine exposure if (1) maternal urine drug screens performed with the mother's consent in the prenatal clinic or at the time of delivery were positive, or (2) newborn urine drug screens indicated cocaine metabolites at the time of admission to the NICU. During this period, maternal and newborn urine toxicologic studies were ordered at the discretion of the attending physician. Maternal and newborn screening was performed if there was a history of maternal drug use or compatible life-style, or if the newborn had unexplained neurologic (lethargy, jitteriness, agitation, or hypertonicity) or respiratory (tachypnea or nasal stuffiness) symptoms within the first 48 hours of life. Urinary excretion of ecgonine and benzoylecgonine was detected by enzyme modified immunoassay technique with confirmation by gas chromatography.

Infants were designated as having definite NEC if they had signs, symptoms, and roentgenographic findings consistent with those of stage IIA or greater of the modified Bell's criteria.[8] All infants included in this report had abdominal distention, bloody stools, and pneumatosis intestinalis roentgenographically. We compared descriptive characteristics (Apgar scores, umbilical cord blood gases, and gestational age), clinical course, and intrauterine growth variables between infants with and without cocaine exposure who developed NEC. We also compared risk factors and complications associated with NEC between groups.

During the 2-year period, there were 5937 live births and 794 admissions to the NICU. Of the NICU patients who underwent drug testing, cocaine metabolites were seen in 69 (8.7%). The overall incidence of NEC (stage IIA or greater) was 3.3% (26 of 794). Thirty-eight percent (10 of 26) of the infants with NEC had documentation of antenatal or intrapartum cocaine exposure. All infants had a positive screen result prior to the onset of NEC. Other drugs identified included cannabinoids (in one case) and opiate derivatives and alcohol (in one case). None of the other 16 infants with NEC had a maternal history of drug use; three of these were tested and had negative urine drug screen results.

Infants with NEC were grouped and compared according to perinatal cocaine exposure. Cocaine-exposed infants had significantly greater gestational age than nonexposed infants (31.2 ± 3.5 weeks vs 27.3 ± 2.4 weeks; $P<.01$); however, there were no significant differences in birth weight (1490 ± 646 g vs 1098 ± 817 g). Thirty percent (3 of 10) of the cocaine-exposed infants had a weight less than the 10th percentile for gestational age. There were no extremely-low-birth-weight (less than 800 g) infants in the cocaine-exposed group, while 44% (7/16) of the nonexposed group had low birth weights ($P=.03$). No differences existed in gender or route of delivery. Two patients in the cocaine-exposed group were term infants admitted to the well-baby nursery with no known risk factors for NEC. In addition to those infants with NEC, two other cocaine-exposed infants had multiple atretic areas of the small intestine.

Cocaine-exposed infants developed symptoms of NEC at a younger postnatal age than the nonexposed group (Figure). Three of the cocaine-exposed infants had not had feedings prior to the onset of NEC symptoms. Selected risk factors[8] for the development of NEC were compared between the cocaine-exposed and nonexposed groups (Table). There were significantly more infants in the nonexposed group with one or more risk factors associated with NEC. There were no significant differences in the incidence of positive blood or cerebrospinal fluid cultures between groups. The cases of NEC occurred sporadically during the period reviewed and no clusters of cases were noted. Complications attributed to NEC including perforation, stricture, and need for surgical intervention were not different between groups. There were two deaths in the cocaine-exposed group and three in the nonexposed group.

Comment.—Perinatal complications that predispose to development of NEC include prematurity, respiratory distress syndrome, low birth weight, asphyxia, and arterial occlusion associated with umbilical artery catheters.[8] As would be expected, these factors were frequently identified among the group of infants with NEC who did not have cocaine exposure. Infants with NEC who had intrauterine cocaine exposure were less likely to have known antecedent risk factors. Two infants in the cocaine group were low-risk infants born at term, who did not have prior feeding. None of the cocaine-exposed infants born at term had colonization with infectious organisms that might have predis-

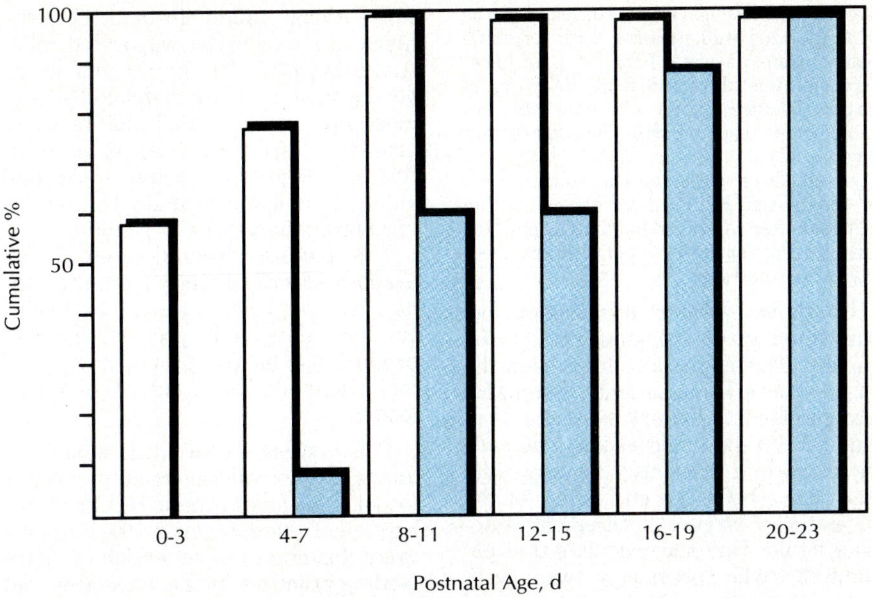

Cumulative percentage of infants developing NEC during first 23 days of life grouped according to cocaine exposure. Mean age at onset of NEC symptoms was significantly younger for the cocaine-exposed group ($P<.001$). Open bars represent the cocaine-exposed group (mean age, 4.5 ± 2.9 days), and tinted bars, the nonexposed group (mean age, 13.8 ± 6.8 days).

Selected Risk Factors for Necrotizing Enterocolitis	Cocaine-Exposed (n=10)	Non-exposed (n=16)
Respiratory distress syndrome	4	8
5-minute Apgar <8	2	8*
Cord pH <7.20	2	7
Preterm (<37 wk)	7	15
Umbilical vessel catheters	3	10
Polycythemia (hematocrit ≥0.65)	1	2
≥1 risk factor	3	13*

*$P<.01$.

posed to development of NEC.

Previous reports have indicated that perinatal cocaine use may cause ischemic injuries of the fetus and newborn—particularly cerebrovascular accidents and cerebral leukomalacia.[9,10] Necrotizing enterocolitis in cocaine-exposed infants who otherwise have no known risk factors suggests that fetal cocaine exposure may cause gastrointestinal ischemic injury. Early onset of NEC symptoms in the cocaine-exposed infants provides additional evidence that the injury was the result of an antenatal event. Intestinal atresia, which may also be the result of vascular insufficiency, was diagnosed in two additional cocaine-exposed infants, further documenting this reported association.[5,7]

There are several possible mechanisms for cocaine-induced gastrointestinal ischemia. Maternal hemodynamic responses include reduced uterine blood flow via vasoconstriction resulting in fetal hypoxemia, tachycardia, and hypertension.[11-13] Chronic placental insufficiency may result in intrauterine fetal growth retardation and/or altered circulation to nonvital organs, including the gastrointestinal tract. Diminished splanchnic circulation may also occur as a consequence of decreased cardiac output in the newborn, recently associated with perinatal cocaine use.[14] In addition, after maternal administration, cocaine may cross the placenta[11] and directly lead to fetal vasoconstriction possibly by a calcium-regulated mechanism.[15]

Our study is limited in interpretation because we only performed urine testing in mothers or infants based on history or clinical suspicion. We identified apparently low-risk infants who developed NEC following perinatal cocaine exposure; however, because we did not test universally, we may have misclassified some of the "nonexposed" infants. Additionally, multiple drug use is common and unrecognized agents may have been responsible for or had additive effects in predisposing to NEC in these infants. However, only two infants with NEC were identified who had excretion of drugs or metabolites other than cocaine.

We suggest that perinatal cocaine exposure be considered a risk factor for the development of NEC in infants. Accordingly, awareness of this association may lead to altered interpretation of feeding difficulties and related symptoms in cocaine-exposed newborns.

GREGORY J. DOWNING, DO
STANLEY R. HORNER, DO
HOWARD W. KILBRIDE, MD
Children's Mercy Hospital
University of Missouri–Kansas City School of Medicine
2401 Gillham Rd
Kansas City, MO 64108-9898

1. Chasnoff IJ, Burns WJ, Schnoll SH, Burns KA. Cocaine use in pregnancy. *N Engl J Med.* 1985;313:666-669.
2. MacGregor SN, Keith LG, Chasnoff IJ, et al. Cocaine use during pregnancy: adverse perinatal outcome. *Am J Obstet Gynecol.* 1987;157:686-690.
3. Oro A, Dixon S. Perinatal cocaine and methamphetamine exposure: maternal and neonatal correlates. *J Pediatr.* 1987;111:571-578.
4. Madden JD, Payne TF, Miller S. Maternal cocaine abuse and effect on the newborn. *Pediatrics.* 1986;77:209-211.
5. Hoyme HE, Jones KL, Dixon SD, et al. Prenatal cocaine exposure and fetal vascular disruption. *Pediatrics.* 1990;85:743-747.
6. Telsey AM, Merritt TA, Dixon SD. Cocaine exposure in a term neonate: necrotizing enterocolitis as a complication. *Clin Pediatr.* 1988;27:547-550.
7. Zauk A, Rosen TS. Consequences of in utero exposure to 'crack' in the premature infant. *Pediatr Res.* 1989;27:237. Abstract.
8. Walsh ME, Kliegman RM. Necrotizing enterocolitis: treatment based on staging criteria. *North Am Clin Pediatr.* 1986;33:179-202.
9. Chasnoff IJ, Bussey ME, Savich R, Stack CM. Perinatal cerebral infarction and maternal cocaine use. *J Pediatr.* 1986;108:456-459.
10. Dixon SD, Bejar R. Echoencephalographic findings in neonates associated with maternal cocaine and methamphetamine use: incidence and clinical correlates. *J Pediatr.* 1989;115:770-778.
11. Woods JR, Plessinger MA, Scott K, Miller RK. Prenatal cocaine exposure to the fetus: a sheep model for cardiovascular evaluation. *Ann N Y Acad Sci.* 1989;562:267-279.
12. Woods JR, Plessinger MA, Clark KE. Effect of cocaine on uterine blood flow and fetal oxygenation. *JAMA.* 1987;257:957-961.
13. Moore TR, Sorg J, Miller L, Key TC, Resnik R. Hemodynamic effects of intravenous cocaine on the pregnant ewe and fetus. *Am J Obstet Gynecol.* 1986;155:883-888.
14. Van derBor M, Walther FJ, Ebrahimi M. Decreased cardiac output in infants of mothers who abused cocaine. *Pediatrics.* 1990;85:30-32.
15. Chokski SK, Isner JM. Cocaine and vasospasm. *N Engl J Med.* 1989;321:1604-1606.

Current Social Practices Leading to Water Intoxication in Infants

Sir.—We recently treated three children with water intoxication who were receiving evaporated milk formula. During that same period (1985 to 1989), there were 14 instances of admissions to our institution for water intoxication, which we have already noted as having become more frequent than in the recent past.[1] Ordinarily, one would expect infants receiving evaporated milk formulas to be vulnerable to hypernatremia.[2] We tried to find a reason for this unexpected outcome.

In each instance, the problem was related to improper feeding practices. The mothers, all of whom were participants in the Women, Infants, Children (WIC) program at our institution, were either excessively diluting the milk or using small amounts of properly reconstituted evaporated milk to supplement larger quantities of relatively electrolyte-free fluids such as diluted fruit juices or water.

The parents of the infants enrolled in the WIC program are carefully instructed in the proper use of the conventional infant formulas for which they are issued redemption coupons. They receive four coupons weekly each month on which the name of a commonly used commercial infant formula is clearly written.

We investigated the circumstances of intoxication, since the frequency of water intoxication exceeded our prior experience and, given the usual feeding practices in the community, should not have occurred.

Subjects and Methods.—In the winter of 1988/1989, three patients receiving evaporated milk were admitted to the hospital with convulsions. Each had histories of feeding that revealed excessive water intake.

Patient 1 was age 4 months and had been admitted for seizures and diarrhea. Chemical analyses of serum revealed the following values: sodium, 128 mmol/L; potassium, 5 mmol/L; chloride, 105 mmol/L; bicarbonate, 9 mmol/L; glucose, 8.2 mmol/L; and urea nitrogen, 1.4 mmol/L. His recent daily food intake consisted of 7 oz of evaporated milk (two parts water and one part evaporated milk) every 3 to 4 hours, 16 oz of juice, and 8 oz of water.

Patient 2 was age 10 months and had been admitted for seizures. Chemical analyses of serum revealed the following values: sodium, 115 mmol/L; potassium, 4.1 mmol/L; chloride, 90 mmol/L; bicarbonate, 10 mmol/L; glucose, 7.2 mmol/L; and urea nitrogen, 3.9 mmol/L. His food intake consisted of more than 20 oz of evaporated milk (diluted with an equal part of water) 16 oz of water, 8 oz of grape juice diluted with water, and table food.

Patient 3 was age 6 months and had been admitted for seizures. Chemical analyses of serum revealed the following values: sodium, 113 mmol/L; potassium, 5.0 mmol/L; chloride, 86 mmol/L; bicarbonate, 13 mmol/L; glucose, 8.2 mmol/L; and urea nitrogen, 3.2 mmol/L. His food intake consisted of 6 oz of evaporated milk (diluted with an equal part of water) every 4 hours, 4 oz of juice, strained vegetables and fruit, and 6 oz of water. (Dietary history was unreliable because there were multiple caretakers that day.)

In all three patients, the sodium level in the serum returned to normal within 36 hours after restricted fluid intake and was sustained at that level when ordinary feedings were reinstated.

Comment.—Water intoxication occurs when water without solute is given rapidly. This appears to have been the case for these three patients. Even with a vague feeding history, one must conclude that a sodium level of 113 mmol/L in serum in a previously healthy child must have been the end result of the ingestion of large quantities of solute-poor liquid. One may calculate that patient 3, who previously was well, weighed 5.91 kg, and had a sodium level of 113 mmol/L and convulsions must have ingested 700 to1000 mL of water in a brief period of time to have brought the sodium level down to that level.

As early as 1923, investigators have referred to the complex of neurologic symptoms and signs resulting from the rapid decrease in the osmolality of extracellular fluid as water intoxication.[3]

The convulsions in water intoxicated infants are a manifestation of a rapid drop in extracellular solute concentration causing osmolal equilibration with the central nervous system to be achieved by movement of water from plasma to cerebrospinal fluid and neurons. The dominant solute of extracellular fluid, sodium and chloride ions, crosses the brain capillaries more slowly than water molecules because the endothelial cells of these capillaries (unlike most others) form a barrier layer from the tight junctions between adjacent cells.[4] The diffusion of water along an osmolal gradient causes brain swelling, which produces water intoxication and its symptoms.

We tried to find the causes of water intoxication in our patients. The nutrition educators of the WIC program at our hospital provided the appropriate information and described correct infant feedings. There appear to be several concomitant factors that set the stage for improper feeding. Many of our patients' families have emigrated from Caribbean countries where evaporated milk is commonly used in the kitchen, such as in coffee and cooking. It became apparent that a number of food store operators within the community are exchanging WIC coupons designated for conventional infant formula for the much less expensive evaporated milk. As an incentive for the consumer, the vendor includes more merchandise (eg, more cans of evaporated milk or extra groceries). In our experience, however, this exchange is not equal to the real value of the infant formula, thus creating a profit margin for the vendor.

The patient, having received the evaporated milk directly from the vendor, has not been educated by health care providers on the proper use of this product nor on the proper balance of milk, nonmilk fluids, and other infant foods.

Conclusions.—Clinicians should be aware that convulsions related to water intoxication may be direct results of corruption of the WIC infant feeding program, leading to a perversion of infant feeding practices by inexperienced and unsophisticated care givers, themselves meaning well.

Annabelle V. Schaeffer, MD
Stuart Ditchek, MD
Children's Medical Center of Brooklyn
Health Science Center
450 Clarkson Ave, Box 49
Brooklyn, NY 11203-2098

1. Finberg L. Too little water has become too much. *AJDC*. 1986;140:524.
2. Finberg L, Kravath RE, Fleischman AR. *Water and Electrolytes in Pediatrics*. Philadelphia, Pa: WB Saunders Co; 1982:190.
3. Rountree LG. Water intoxication. *Arch Intern Med*. 1923;32:157.
4. Goldstein GW. Pathogenesis of brain edema and hemorrhage. *Pediatrics*. 1979;64:357-360.

Alkaline Urine Is Associated With Eating Disorders

Sir.—Alkaline urine has traditionally been associated with *Proteus* urinary tract infections.[1] In the absence of an infection, clinical findings might suggest other diagnoses, but these are rare in adolescents. The following are some of the traditional causes of alkaline urine[2]: (1) urinary tract infection (*Proteus* and others); (2) metabolic alkalosis (pyloric stenosis and others); (3) failure of acidification (renal tubular acidosis, chronic renal failure, or aldosterone abnormalities); (4) ingestion (salicylate, sodium bicarbonate, acetazolamide, etc); and (5) respiratory alkalosis (hyperventilation).

After noticing alkaline urine in a number of otherwise healthy patients with eating disorders, we prospectively examined urine pH in a hospital-based adolescent medicine practice to determine

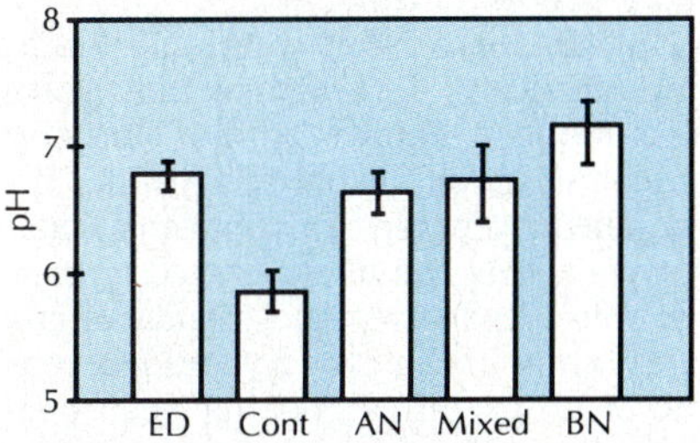

Urine pH (mean ± SE) in outpatients presenting to the adolescent medicine division. The difference between control subjects and patients with eating disorders was highly significant, at $P<.001$. ED indicates patients with eating disorders (n = 46); Cont, control subjects (n = 28); AN, patients with anorexia nervosa (n = 28); Mixed, mixed patients with (nonspecific) eating disorders (n = 9); and BN, patients with bulimia nervosa (n = 9).

if elevated urine pH is associated with eating disorders.

Patients and Methods.—All female patients presenting to a suburban New York adolescent medicine outpatient division during a 5-week period were asked to participate in this study of urine pH. Informed consent was obtained, and subjects were classified as patients with eating disorders (n = 46) or control subjects (n = 28) by their physicians according to the criteria given by the *Diagnostic and Statistical Manual of Mental Disorders–Revised Third Edition* for the diagnoses of anorexia nervosa (without self-induced vomiting), bulimia nervosa, and nonspecific (mixed) eating disorders.[3] Patients recovering from eating disorders were included, even if they no longer met the strict criteria (ie, percentage of weight lost or frequency of vomiting) for their diagnosis at the time of the study.

The control subjects presented for a variety of reasons, including general and gynecologic health maintenance, acute illness (such as viral syndrome), and emergency room or inpatient follow-up. Patients with urinary tract infections or renal disease were excluded (n = 2). None of the patients in either group had any of the known causes of alkaline urine listed above, and none was hypertensive or showed signs of adrenal dysfunction.

Patients with eating disorders completed a questionnaire about the frequency and duration of eating and purging behaviors before examination. Although they were told that this information would be used only for the study and would not affect their treatment, it is possible that the responses of some patients were not accurate. Physicians recorded clinical data at the time of the visit. Urinalysis was performed by a physician or nurse on freshly voided specimens, using the multitest reagent strips for urinalysis (Ames Labstix dipstick). These individuals were not blinded, but in all cases the result of the dipstick test was easily determined, so bias was not likely to have occurred. All samples were obtained on weekday afternoons during the summer of 1988.

Distribution of Alkaline Urine by Diagnosis*

	Urine pH Value, No.	
	≤7	>7
Patients with eating disorders	29	17
Control subjects	27	1

*$P = .001$ by χ^2 analysis. Specificity was 96%; sensitivity, 37%; and positive predictive value, 94%.

Statistical analysis was performed using the Mann-Whitney rank sum test, χ^2 analysis, or Spearman's correlation method, as appropriate. Bonferroni's adjustment was used to correct for multiple comparisons.

Results.—The urine pH of patients with eating disorders (mean ± SD, 6.8 ± 0.8) was significantly higher than that of control patients (5.9 ± 0.8; $P<.001$). This difference remained when patients were classified by specific diagnosis (Figure), but there were no significant differences among the diagnostic groups.

Alkaline urine, defined as urine with a pH value over 7, was found significantly more often in patients with eating disorders ($P = .001$) (Table). Seventeen of 46 patients with eating disorders had alkaline urine, while only one of 28 controls did. The specificity of alkaline urine for eating disorders was 96%, but sensitivity was only 37%. In our population, with a large number of patients with eating disorders (58% of female patient visits), the positive predictive value of alkaline urine for eating disorders was 94%.

Using χ^2 analysis, a number of clinical variables were examined for association with alkaline urine. Patients who weighed less than 85% of ideal body weight were significantly more likely to have alkaline urine ($P<.05$). Patients who reported vomiting within the previous month were also more likely to have alkaline urine ($P<.05$), but there was no association with reports of vomiting in the preceding week or distant past.

There was no association between the presence of alkaline urine and a number of other clinical variables, including change in weight during the previous week or month; urine ketones, protein, or specific gravity; duration of disease or amenorrhea; or self-report of the use of diuretics, laxatives, or salt. The patient's perception of the success of treatment was not associated with high urine pH, and there was also no association between urine pH and blood pressure.

In longitudinal examination of three patients individually, no correlation was found between weight and urine pH in a series of 10 to 30 weekly visits.

Comment.—Eating disorders are not traditionally included in the differential diagnosis of alkaline urine. This study demonstrates that alkaline urine is found in a substantial number of adolescents with eating disorders, while it is almost never found in those with other diagnoses. In our suburban adolescent patient population, in whom eating disorders are much more common than *Proteus* urinary tract infections, renal or adrenal diseases, or acute ingestions, the most likely diagnosis in a patient with alkaline urine is an eating disorder. Using the simple dipstick method, no special laboratory equipment was required to detect alkaline urine in our patients.

The presence of alkaline urine is not used in our adolescent medicine practice to make the diagnosis of an eating disorder; we rely on our experience with these conditions and consultation with psychologists, social workers, and nutritionists. However, the general pediatrician who rarely sees patients with eating disorders may use alkaline urine as a "flag" to signify the possibility of an eating disorder or to supplement clinical impressions. While the low sensitivity of the urine dipstick pH test for eating disorders precludes its use in ruling out the diagnosis, it may prove useful as a quick and inexpensive marker for the presence of these disorders in the clinician's office.

Elevation of urine pH was seen in all types of eating disorders, but was most common in two groups: the self-described vomiters and the most malnourished patients. Self-induced vomiting has been associated with alkaline urine in previous reports[4] due primarily to loss of acid in the vomitus. It is possible that elevated urine pH levels may be a marker for surreptitious vomiting, but other abnormalities in patients with eating disorders, listed below, may also cause alterations of net acid balance that increase urine pH levels: (1) self-induced vomiting (gastrointestinal acid loss)[4]; (2) "alkaline tide" (caused by release of bicarbonate into the gastric venous drainage after large meals are eaten in anticipation of weigh-in)[5]; (3) diet low in meat, high in vegetables, citrus fruits, and dairy products (decreased acid metabolites from meat[6] with increased organic acids and calcium salts[7] lead to abnormal net alkali balance); (4) osteoporosis (release of hydroxyapatite, a basic compound, during demineralization[8] from estrogen deficiency); and (5) hypochloremic alkalosis (from hyperaldosteronism or contraction alkalosis,[9] due to diuretic or laxative abuse).

Most likely, several of these mechanisms occur in patients with eating disorders, and because more than one mechanism may be present in a single patient, it is difficult to assess an individual's progress using urine alkalinity as a marker. Further study of patients with eating disorders under more controlled inpatient settings, in which the numerous variables that may contribute to the formation of alkaline urine can be monitored, is necessary to determine which factors are most important. Nonetheless, the finding of alkaline urine in an adolescent is significant and should always be investigated.

MARTHA R. ARDEN, MD
LAUREN BUDOW, MD
DOUGLAS W. BUNNELL, PHD
MICHAEL P. NUSSBAUM, MD
I. RONALD SHENKER, MD
MARC S. JACOBSON, MD
Division of Adolescent Medicine
Schneider Children's Hospital
Long Island Jewish Medical Center
Albert Einstein College of Medicine
New Hyde Park, NY 11042

1. Epstein M, Oster JR. Acid-base disturbances: the role of the kidney. In: Halsted JA, Halsted CH, eds. *The Laboratory in Clinical Medicine: Interpretation and Application.* 2nd ed. Philadelphia, Pa: WB Saunders Co; 1981:304-312.

2. Fischbach F. *A Manual of Laboratory Diagnostic Tests.* 3rd ed. Philadelphia, Pa: JB Lippincott; 1988:133-135.

3. American Psychiatric Association, Committee on Nomenclature and Statistics. *Diagnostic and Statistical Manual of Mental Disorders–Revised Third Edition.* Washington, DC: American Psychiatric Association; 1987:65-71.

4. Mars DR, Anderson NH, Reggall FC. Anorexia nervosa: a disorder with severe acid-base derangements. *South Med J.* 1982;75:1038-1042.

5. Narins RG, Jones ER, Townsend R, Gookin DA, Shay RJ. Metabolic acid-base disorders: pathophysiology, classification and treatment. In: Arieff AI, DeFronzo RA, eds. *Fluid, Electrolyte, and Acid-Base Disorders.* New York, NY: Churchill Livingstone Inc; 1985:335-384.

6. Lemann J Jr, Relman AS. The relation of sulfur metabolism to acid-base balance and electrolyte excretion: the effects of DL-methionine in normal man. *J Clin Invest.* 1959;38:2215-2223.

7. Lennon EJ, Lemann J Jr, Litzow JR. The effects of diet and stool composition on the net external acid balance of normal subjects. *J Clin Invest.* 1966;45:1601-1607.

8. Relman AS, Lennon EJ, Lemann J Jr. Endogenous production of fixed acid and the measurement of the net balance of acid in normal subjects. *J Clin Invest.* 1961;40:1621-1630.

9. Seldin DW, Rector FC Jr. The generation and maintenance of metabolic alkalosis. *Kidney Int.* 1972;1:306-321.

Major Congenital Neurologic Malformations

Sir.—I applaud the attempt by Wiswell et al[1] to estimate the current incidence of major congenital neurologic malformations. One factor may have caused an underestimate of the reported incidence. Many military posts are located in remote locations. When these malformations are discovered in utero, the mother is usually given the option of delivering in the nearest civilian institution with appropriate treatment capabilities or traveling a long distance to a major military medical center. Often, travel to the military facility is very inconvenient and requires a separation of the family. Many mothers elect to deliver in a civilian hospital. These patients are apparently not accounted for in the study, since it only contains infants born in US Army hospitals. The true current incidence of these malformations is probably higher then estimated in the study.

CPT BRIAN D. RYALS, MC, USA
Department of Child Neurology
Walter Reed Army Medical Center
Washington, DC 20307

1. Wiswell TE, Tuttle DJ, Northam RS, Simonds GR. Major congenital neurologic malformations: a 17-year study. *AJDC.* 1990;144:61-72.

In Reply.—I appreciate Dr Ryals' comments regarding the incidence of major congenital neurologic malformations that we recently reported.

Having spent many years as a military physician, I recognize that pregnant women known to be carrying fetuses with malformations are not infrequently referred to civilian hospitals. However, this has likely played a minimal role in affecting the results of our study. Only in the past 2 years has routine α-fetoprotein screening been performed on all pregnant woman in the major army medical centers, a period subsequent to the dates of the study. In addition, most of the smaller military hospitals do not have this capability. Furthermore, ultrasound study is not routinely performed on pregnant women. Although they have been commonly performed since the mid-1980s, the minority of women undergo ultrasound studies.

α-Fetoprotein levels in amniotic fluid have been evaluated since the mid-1970s. However, these evaluations were performed only in women with prior histories of having a child with a neural tube defect. Fewer than 5% of all infants with neural tube defects have siblings with the same defect. Thus, during the period of the study, the vast majority of women who delivered babies with such defects were unlikely to have undergone such screening.

We suspect that the incidence of neural tube defects from 1971 to 1987 was minimally affected by prenatal diagnosis and referral to civilian hospitals for either abortion or delivery. It is noteworthy that many investigators in Great Britain have found the enormous decline in the occurrence of these malformations during the past two decades more likely to have been influenced by unknown factors than by prenatal screening.

THOMAS E. WISWELL, MD
Neonatology Service
Department of Pediatrics
Walter Reed Army Medical Center
Washington, DC 20307-5001

Status Report on Phenylketonuria Treatment: 1990

In this issue of *AJDC*, the Writing Committee of the Collaborative Study of Children Treated for Phenylketonuria reports the status of 95 of these children who have reached age 12 years, a milepost age in the study.[1] At this point in the study, there were no surprises. However, the study has documented even more conclusively that (1) the sooner the low phenylalanine diet is begun, the better the outcome; (2) the longer a normal blood phenylalanine level is maintained, the better the outcome; and (3) termination of the diet has a deleterious effect. Because this collaborative study appears to be ending, I fear that it will be terminated prematurely.

See also p 35.

This carefully designed study was straightforward in concept and adequate for the knowledge and psychologic testing instruments of 1967. The planners underestimated the difficulty of maintaining near-normal blood phenylalanine levels in the 200 or more affected patients. This led to fewer patients in the continuously controlled group.

The current basic biochemical research and new understanding of the biochemical defects of phenylketonuria could not have been fully anticipated in 1967. We now know that the apoenzyme (phenylalanine hydroxylase) and generation of the cofactor (tetrahydrobiopterin) had several defects, most causing different clinical expressions. Most expressions of these defects would have allowed children with different molecular defects to be included in the study. Thus, it has been a study of several hyperphenylalanemias and not of a single disorder.

Use of a low-phenylalanine diet is still the only practical, available mode of treatment, and the experiences of most clinics today are similar to those documented in this study. However, the study in its original design does not address the late findings that are surfacing in the phenylketonuric patients. The fact is that these patients usually are not truly normal. This is hinted at in the committee's report that the children show deficiencies in mathematic performance. Others have revealed that older, well-treated patients have performance deficits in conceptual, visuospatial, and language skills. In light of these findings, the study now could be redesigned to include the newer and more revealing neuropsychologic testing instruments as well as the traditional instruments employed in the study. This is an important cohort of patients that should be followed up for at least another decade.

C. Charlton Mabry, MD
University of Kentucky
Department of Pediatrics
Endocrinology & Metabolism
800 Rose St
Lexington, KY 40536-0084

Reference

1. Azen CG, Koch R, Gross Friedman E, et al. Intellectual development in 12-year-old children treated for phenylketonuria. *AJDC*. 1991;145:35-39.

Development, Growth, and Cardiac Surgery

In this issue of *AJDC*, Mendoza and coworkers report the results of neurodevelopmental testing and somatic growth in 24 of 27 late survivors of arterial switch operations for transposition of the great arteries performed at Korsair Children's Hospital, Louisville, Ky. Six early deaths (18.2%) occurred among the 33 patients who underwent arterial switch operations, and three patients did not undergo follow-up testing. The data show that 18 (75%) had normal growth, while six had small head circumference. Developmental scores were within one SD of normal for 18 patients. Of the remaining six, three had scores between one and two SDs below normal, and three had scores that were greater than two SDs below normal. Previous reports[1,2] provide some information about developmental outcomes of patients who underwent cardiac repairs in infancy, but very little information about patients who underwent neonatal repair. In the report by Mendoza et al, all but three of the patients for whom follow-up data were available were neonates.

See also p 40.

The factors affecting neurodevelopment (and perhaps, indirectly, body size and head circumference) after neonatal cardiac surgery are undoubtedly complex, but likely involve the interactions of preoperative, intraoperative, and postoperative factors. There is no reason to believe that in utero neurologic development is impaired in patients with transposed great arteries, and one study[1] suggests that most patients undergoing early atrial level repair have normal results of neurologic development tests. I believe the authors are correct to point out the importance of preoperative events in determining neurologic outcome. Review of their data shows that four of the six patients with less favorable outcomes had either preoperative seizures (two patients) or sufficiently severe acidosis and/or hypoxia to require an emergency balloon atrial septostomy (one patient) or an emergency arterial switch operation (one patient).

Intraoperative events related to cardiopulmonary bypass, such as air or particulate embolism, time of circulatory arrest, and use of hypothermia alone, have been thought to affect postoperative outcome.[3] Unfortunately, the report by Mendoza et al contains only data on the depth of hypothermia (16°C to 18°C) and the average time of cardiopulmonary bypass. Neither were related to outcome in this study. Many surgical groups, including our own, use deep hypothermia with periods of circulatory arrest of up to 60 minutes for neonatal repairs of various defects.[3-6] However, hypothermia alone was initially thought to have a markedly adverse impact on neurologic outcome in reports by Bjork and Hultquist[7] and Egerton et al.[8] Other theoretically important factors during bypass may include acid-base (carbon dioxide) management during hypothermia,[9-11] perfusion pressure (particularly after a period of ischemia),[12,13] and pharmacologic interventions such as α-adrenergic blockade,[14] pretreatment with corticosteroids,[15] and use of mannitol (as a free radical scavenger).[16] All three of these pharmacologic interventions as well as the "alpha-stat" strategy of pH and P_{CO_2} management during hypothermia are used in our institution, although clear-cut data supporting their use is lacking. Undoubtedly, many other intraoperative variables may effect outcome, either alone or in combination.

Finally, the effect of postoperative events on outcome is demonstrated in patient 8 in the report by Mendoza et al. It is equally noteworthy, however, that seizures alone did not predict outcome. Only one of the three patients in this study who had postoperative seizures showed a subsequent developmental abnormality. This experience is similar to that generally quoted in current texts.[3]

These comments are offered primarily to emphasize that multiple preoperative, intraoperative, and postoperative variables may influence neurologic outcome in a complex manner. Multivariate analyses should generally be employed to assess the impact of any single variable or combination of variables. The report by Mendoza et al contains neither sufficient numbers of patients nor sufficient data on potentially important variables such as those outlined above to conduct a multivariate analysis. Therefore, the effect of any of the variables described in this report on the ultimate neurologic outcome cannot be assessed with certainty. It is to be emphasized that as many details as possible concerning the management of bypass and circulatory arrest, including both physical and pharmacologic interventions, should be included in reports such as these. The early poor experience with deep hypothermia[7,8] was probably due, in retrospect, to the failure to employ as simple a measure as hemodilution during hypothermic perfusion. Because our understanding of the complex events occurring during cardiopulmonary bypass and deep hypothermia (with or without circulatory arrest) is incomplete, reporting the details of perfusion management may allow both insights into pathophysiologic mechanisms and meaningful comparisons of the experiences at different centers. Despite many such details being excluded from this report, the descriptive data on outcome will be a useful basis for comparison in subsequent studies. Much more extensive data on neurologic outcome after neonatal cardiac surgery is necessary before any firm conclusion as to its safety can be reached, but these follow-up data are encouraging and confirm my own clinical impression that neonatal cardiac operations using cardiopulmonary bypass and deep hypothermia are associated with good neurologic outcome in most instances. As the potential benefits of early primary correction of congenital heart defects are now becoming clearer,[4] better understanding of the techniques of hypothermic cardiopulmonary bypass and circulatory arrest that are necessary to effect such repairs in neonates now assume even greater importance. More reports, such as that by Mendoza et al, will (I hope) further our knowledge in this important area.

John E. Mayer, Jr, MD
The Children's Hospital
Department of Cardiovascular Surgery
300 Longwood Ave
Boston, MA 02115

References

1. Newburger JW, Silbert AR, Buckley LP, Fyler DC. Cognitive function and age at repair of transposition of the great arteries in children. *N Engl J Med.* 1984:310:1495-1499.

2. Clarkson PM, MacArthur BA, Barratt-Boyes BG, Whitlock RM, Neutze JM. Developmental progress after cardiac surgery in infancy using hypothermia and circulatory arrest. *Circulation.* 1980;62:855-861.

3. Kirklin JW, Barratt-Boyes B. Hypothermia, circulatory arrest, and cardiopulmonary bypass. In: Kirklin JW, Barratt-Boyes B, eds. *Cardiac Surgery.* New York, NY: John Wiley & Sons Inc; 1986:29-82.

4. Castaneda AR, Mayer JE, Jonas RA, Lock JE, Wessel DL, Hickey PR. The neonate with critical congenital heart disease: repair, a surgical challenge. *J Thorac Cardiovasc Surg.* 1989;98:869-875.

5. Tharion J, Johnson DC, Celermajer JM, Hawker RM, Cartmill TB, Overton JH. Profound hypothermia with circulatory arrest. *J Thorac Cardiovasc Surg.* 1982;94:66-72.

6. Blackwood MJA, Haka-Ikse K, Steward DJ. Developmental outcome in children undergoing surgery with profound hypothermia. *Anesthesiology.* 1986;65:437-440.

7. Bjork VO, Hultquist G. Contraindications to profound hypothermia in open heart surgery. *J Thorac Cardiovasc Surg.* 1962;44:1-13.

8. Egerton N, Egerton WS, Kay JH. Neurologic changes following profound hypothermia. *Ann Surg.* 1963;157:366-382.

9. Becker Heinz MD, Vinten-Johansen J, Buckbery GD, et al. Myocardial damage caused by keeping pH 7.40 during systemic deep hypothermia. *J Thorac Cardiovasc Surg.* 1981;82:810-820.

10. Siemkowicz I, Gjedde A. Postischemic coma in rat: effect of different perischemia blood glucose levels on cerebral metabolic recovery after ischemia. *Acta Physiol Scand.* 1980;110:225-232.

11. White FN. A comparative physiological approach to hypothermia. *J Thorac Cardiovasc Surg.* 1981;82:821-831.

12. Fujiwara T, Kurtts T, Silvera M, Mayer JE. Physical and pharmacological manipulation of reperfusion conditions in neonatal myocardial preservation. *Circulation.* 1988;78(suppl II):I-444.

13. Sawatari K, Kadoba K, Bergner KA, Daitch JA, Mayer JE. Effect of reperfusion pressure after hypothermic cardioplegia on endothelial modulation of coronary tone in neonatal lambs: impaired coronary vasodilator response to acetylcholine. *J Thorac Cardiovasc Surg.* In press.

14. Nayler WG, Gordon M, Stephens DJ, Sturrock WJ. The protective effect of prazosin on the ischemic and reperfused myocardium. *J Mol Cell Cardiol.* 1985;17:685-699.

15. Cavarocchi NC, Pluth JR, Schaff HV, et al. Complement activation during cardiopulmonary bypass. *J Thorac Cardiovasc Surg.* 1986;91:252-258.

16. Gardner TJ, Stewart JR, Casale AS, Downey JM, Chambers DE. Reduction of myocardial ischemic injury with oxygen-derived free radical scavengers. *Surgery.* 1983;94:423-427.

Articles

Intellectual Development in 12-Year-Old Children Treated for Phenylketonuria

Colleen G. Azen, MS; Richard Koch, MD; Eva Gross Friedman; Stanley Berlow, MD; James Coldwell, MD; Wilma Krause, MD; Reuben Matalon, MD, PhD; Edward McCabe, MD, PhD; Margaret O'Flynn, MD; Raymond Peterson, MD; Bobbye Rouse, MD; C. Ronald Scott, MD; Bernice Sigman, MD; David Valle, MD; Robert Warner, MD

• Intelligence and achievement test scores were evaluated for 95 12-year-old children with phenylketonuria who had begun dietary therapy during the neonatal period. Dietary control of blood phenylalanine below 900 μmol/L was maintained beyond age 10 years in 23 children; 72 others had blood phenylalanine persistently above that level at ages ranging from 18 months to 10 years. Test scores at age 12 years were negatively correlated with the age at initiation of diet and with blood phenylalanine levels from ages 4 to 10 years, and positively correlated with parent IQ scores and the age at loss of dietary control. Children who maintained phenylalanine levels below 900 μmol/L beyond age 10 years showed no deficits in test scores, except for arithmetic, the scores of which declined between ages 6 and 12 years in 90% of the children in this study. These data strongly support a recommendation that dietary restriction of phenylalanine should be maintained through adolescence.

(*AJDC*. 1991;145:35-39)

Early diagnosis and treatment of children with phenylketonuria (PKU) has been regarded as a model of successful intervention in the prevention of mental retardation. Treatment consists of initiating a restricted phenylalanine (PHE) diet as early as possible after birth and maintaining blood PHE levels between 120 and 600 μmol/L. Discontinuation or relaxation of the PHE-restricted diet at ages varying from 4 to 10 years had been common practice in the United States for many years. However, a change in this approach has been occurring since 1977/1978, when Cabalska et al[1] and Smith et al[2] reported deteriorating IQ scores in children with PKU after diet termination. In 1980, Waisbren et al[3] reviewed 19 published studies of diet discontinuation, nine of which reported significant declines in intelligence test scores of children with PKU when diet therapy was discontinued.

A report from the Collaborative Study of Children Treated for Phenylketonuria (PKUCS) by Holtzman et al[4] in 1986 showed strong correlations between the age at loss of dietary control and cognitive test scores at ages 8 and 10 years. Fishler et al[5] found that, in this same group of children with PKU, those who stayed on diet had higher reading and spelling scores at age 10 years in comparison with diet discontinuers, but that arithmetic, language, and perceptual test scores declined uniformly for both groups from ages 6 to 10 years. Subsequent data from Germany,[6] Ireland,[7] and the United States[8] support the efficacy of maintaining dietary restriction of PHE throughout childhood and adolescence. However, in France, where diet discontinuation remains common, a recent study[9] found no evidence of deteriorating IQ when therapy was discontinued at 5 to 8 years, although perceptual motor dysfunction and learning disabilities were noted. Koch et al[10] reported higher scores on most intelligence and academic achievement tests in 12-year-old PKUCS patients who maintained dietary restriction of PHE through age 8, in contrast to those who had lost dietary control at earlier ages. In this report, we further investigate the relationship between test scores in 12-year-old PKUCS children and a number of other factors describing the diagnosis and treatment history of children with PKU, as well as their social and intellectual environment.

PATIENTS AND METHODS

Study Design and Patients

The Collaborative Study of Children Treated for PKU was initiated in 1967 at 16 treatment centers throughout the United States to investigate prospectively the effects of dietary restriction of PHE on the growth and development of children with PKU. Details of the study design and results have been published.[4,5,11-14] All patients were identified by newborn screening and began dietary therapy before age 120 days. Sample acquisition was completed in 1972 with the enrollment of 167 children with classic PKU. Ninety-five PKUCS patients whose psychologic test scores were available at age 12 years were evaluated for this report.

The study was conducted in two phases. During phase A, each child was randomly assigned to maintain average blood PHE levels either between 60 and 332 μmol/L or between 330 and 599 μmol/L until age 6 years. In phase B, children were randomly assigned at age 6 years either to continue the diet therapy to maintain blood PHE levels ideally below 720 μmol/L, or to discontinue diet therapy, with annual follow-up evaluations. Due to parental consent requirements, this randomization was disrupted by some parents choosing to either continue or discontinue diet therapy regardless of assignment. However, no child was dropped from the study because of failure to comply with randomization.

Throughout phases A and B, dietary compliance was assessed by monitoring blood PHE levels as follows: weekly during the first year of life and monthly thereafter, with quarterly assessments obtained after diet termination. For each child, the median PHE

Accepted for publication November 6, 1989.

From the Division of Medical Genetics, Children's Hospital of Los Angeles, Calif (Mss Azen and Friedman and Dr Koch); the universities of Wisconsin, Madison, (Dr Berlow), Colorado, Denver (Dr McCabe), Texas, Galveston (Dr Rouse), Iowa, Iowa City (Dr Krause), Washington, Seattle (Dr Scott), Maryland, Baltimore (Dr Sigman), and Illinois, Chicago (Dr Matalon); Children's Medical Center, Tulsa, Okla (Dr Coldwell); Children's Hospital, Los Angeles (Dr O'Flynn); Children's Hospital Health Center, San Diego, Calif (Dr Peterson); the Johns Hopkins Hospital, Baltimore, Md (Dr Valle); and Children's Hospital, Buffalo, NY (Dr Warner).

A complete list of institutions participating in this research study appears on page 39.

Reprint requests to Maternal PKU Collaborative Study, Division of Medical Genetics, Children's Hospital of Los Angeles, 4650 Sunset Blvd, Los Angeles, CA 90027 (Ms Azen).

level during each 6-month period constituted an index of dietary control (IDC) for that period.

Variables Used in Analyses

Outcome variables selected for evaluation in this report were Wechsler Intelligence Scale for Children–Revised (WISC-R)[15] IQ scores and Wide Range Achievement Test (WRAT)[16] standard scores at age 12 years. We also evaluated the change in test scores between ages 6 and 12 years, and the difference between the 12-year IQ scores of children with PKU and those of their parents. Scores for children with PKU at 6 years were measured by the 1972 norms of the Stanford-Binet Intelligence Scale,[17] and parental IQ was assessed with the Wechsler Adult Intelligence Scale (WAIS).[18] When IQ scores were available for both parents, their average scores were used as parent IQ; otherwise, the single available parent's scores were used.

Independent variables describing the diagnosis and treatment of the child with PKU included maximum diagnostic PHE level; maximum and 48-hour blood PHE levels during PHE challenges at ages 3 months and 1 year; age at initiation of diet; IDCs for 6-month periods ending at ages 2, 4, 6, 8, and 10 years; average IDC before age 4 years; average IDC between ages 4 and 6 years; average IDC between ages 6 and 10 years; and the age at which dietary control was lost. Loss of dietary control was defined in an earlier PKUCS report[4] as the age at the beginning of the first of three consecutive 6-month periods during which the IDC exceeded 900 µmol/L, regardless of whether the child was still receiving a PHE-restricted diet. Blood PHE levels after age 10 years were unavailable for one third of the sample, and were excluded from those multivariate analyses requiring complete data for all cases, to maintain maximum sample sizes. Most children with no reported PHE levels after age 10 years had discontinued treatment before that age. Levels after 10 years were comparable with 10-year levels in those for whom these data were available. Variables describing the environment of the child with PKU were parents' WAIS IQ scores, Hollingshead two-factor index of socioeconomic status (Hollingshead AB, unpublished data, 1957), and the family coping pattern, which was assessed by consensus of the clinic team on a four-point scale from adequate to dysfunctional.

Although the study was designed as a randomized trial, considerable deviation from dietary group assignments occurred toward the end of phase A and throughout phase B. Those who maintained their random assignment (65%) were comparable with those who declined or switched groups (35%) on the basis of sex, birth order, parental age, and IQ. There was a tendency for families who did not accept randomization to have higher socioeconomic status and better family coping pattern scores.

Table 1.—Multiple Regression Analyses for Cognitive and Achievement Test Scores in Children With Phenylketonuria*

	WISC-R IQ Scores (n=91)			WRAT Standard Scores (n=84)		
	Verbal	Performance	Full Scale	Reading	Spelling	Arithmetic
Partial correlation coefficient for:						
Parent IQ	0.36 (<.01)	0.47 (<.01)	0.47 (<.01)	0.39 (<.01)	0.33 (<.01)	0.33 (<.01)
Age when first treated	−0.17 (.04)	−0.23 (.01)	−0.22 (.01)	−0.17 (.07)	−0.28 (<.01)	−0.18 (.08)
Age at loss of dietary control	0.18 (.14)	0.22 (.01)	0.31 (<.01)	0.38 (<.01)	0.26 (.01)	0.10 (.36)
IDC between 4 and 6 y	−0.27 (.03)	...	...	...	...	...
R^2	.43	.38	.45	.36	.29	.17

*Numbers in parentheses are *P* values. WISC-R indicates Weschler Intelligence Scale for Children–Revised; WRAT, Wide Range Achievement Test; and IDC, index of dietary control.

Statistical Analysis

Test scores at age 12 years were evaluated as data from an observational study, ie, one group of children with PKU with varying degrees of dietary control throughout childhood along with other factors that may affect cognitive development. Probability values reported for statistical tests should be interpreted accordingly. Results were considered statistically significant at $P<.05$. While it is recognized that performing many statistical tests increases the risk of erroneously detecting significant results, the majority of significant results in this report had probability values too small to be explained by this factor alone.

For each outcome variable, stepwise regression was used to identify a subset of diagnostic, treatment, and social factors that contributed significantly to 12-year test scores. Multiple regression was then employed to evaluate the relative importance of each significant predictor variable to each of the outcome variables. A logarithmic transformation was applied to the age at initiation of treatment since the transformed data better fit a normal distribution.

Comparisons among three subgroups, defined on the basis of age at loss of dietary control, were made by one-way analysis of variance, with Bonferroni adjustment of probability values for pairwise group comparisons. Within each group, paired *t* tests were used to compare test scores at ages 6 and 12 years, and to compare the IQ scores of the child with PKU with those of his or her parents. Nonparametric tests were also employed where appropriate. Statistical analyses were performed using the Statistical Analysis System (SAS Institute, Cary, NC)[19] and BMDP computer programs (BMDP Statistical Software, Los Angeles, Calif).[20]

RESULTS

Families of children who participated in this study were primarily middle-class, with a shift toward the lower end of the Hollingshead Scale (62% fell in the two lowest categories; 14% in the two upper categories). Parents' WAIS IQ scores were above average (mean ± SD, 108 ± 11). The majority (56%) of these families were judged to have adequate coping skills by their respective clinic teams, 28% were considered to have minor coping problems, 14% had major problems in fulfilling marital or parental roles, and one family was judged dysfunctional.

All patients who remained active in the study through age 12 years had started receiving therapy prior to age 65 days (median, 17 days; range, 3 to 64 days). Maximum diagnostic PHE levels ranged from 1380 to 5340 µmol/L (mean ± SD, 2760 ± 720 µmol/L). Mean IDC values for the group rose from 402 ± 174 µmol/L at age 1 year to 714 ± 270 µmol/L at age 6 years. During phase B, the average IDC for children continuing therapy was 750 ± 318 µmol/L. Children who discontinued therapy exhibited a sharp rise in PHE, to a mean IDC level of 1584 ± 354 µmol/L.

Stepwise regression for each outcome variable showed that parent IQ was the strongest predictor of test scores at age 12 years. After entering parent IQ into

Table 2.—Treatment History of 12-Year-Old Children With Phenylketonuria Grouped by Age at Loss of Dietary Control*

	Group 1 (n=23)	Group 2 (n=47)	Group 3 (n=25)
Age first treated, d			
Median	23	17	14
Range	3-55	5-64	4-54
Maximum diagnostic phenylalanine levels, μmol/L			
Mean	2820	2820	2520
SD	780	720	660
Average blood phenylalanine levels between specified ages, μmol/L			
Diagnosis to 4 y			
Mean	576	462	354
SD	150	90	108
4 to 6 y			
Mean	912	564	462
SD	192	120	150
6 to 10 y			
Mean	1554	1326	600
SD	282	324	144
After 10 y	n=8	n=32	n=20
Mean	1554	1368	750
SD	372	342	270

*Group 1 includes patients who lost dietary control prior to age 6 years; group 2, between ages 6 and 10 years; and group 3, after age 10 years.

Table 3.—Mean 12-Year WISC-R, WRAT, and Parent WAIS IQ Scores for PKUCS Children Grouped by Age at Loss of Dietary Control*

	Group 1	Group 2	Group 3	ANOVA P
WISC-R IQ Scores	n=23	n=47	n=25	...
Verbal	85±15	95±14	101±11	.0004
Performance	92±15	95±14	101±11	.0499
Full scale	87±14	96±14	101±11	.0028
WRAT standard scores	n=22	n=46	n=20	...
Reading	92±13	97±11	105±12	.0029
Spelling	87±17	92±13	98±17	.0452
Arithmetic	80±11	82±11	84±10	.6033
Parent WAIS IQ scores	n=23	n=43	n=25	...
Full scale	104±10	109±9	108±14	.1905

*Group 1 includes patients who lost dietary control prior to age 6 years; group 2, between ages 6 and 10 years; and group 3, after age 10 years. WISC-R indicates Weschler Intelligence Scale for Children–Revised; WRAT, Wide Range Achievement Test; and WAIS, Weschler Adult Intelligence Scale; and PKUCS, Collaborative Study of Children Treated for Phenylketonuria. Values are means±SDs.

the regression equation, age at initiation of treatment was the next most significant predictor of dependent variables—spelling, arithmetic, and performance IQ scores—followed by age at loss of dietary control. When the dependent variable was reading, verbal IQ, or full scale IQ score, the order of entry into the regression equation was as follows: parent IQ, age at loss of dietary control, and age at initiation of treatment. Average IDC between 4 and 6 years had additional predictive power for verbal IQ. No other variables significantly improved any of the regression equations.

Table 1 summarizes multiple regression analyses for each outcome variable regressed on parent IQ and other variables identified by the stepwise procedure as contributing significantly to outcome. The partial correlation coefficients indicate the strength of the relationship between outcome and each independent variable after the remaining independent variables have been entered into the regression equation. For example, the correlation between age when first treated and full scale IQ after controlling for parent IQ and age at loss of dietary control was −.22 (P=.01). Among this set of variables, parent IQ had the highest partial correlation with each of the outcome variables, although age at loss of dietary control was nearly as highly correlated with reading. The percent of total variation in the outcome variables explained by the predictor variables (R^2) ranged from 17% for arithmetic to 45% for WISC-R full-scale IQ.

Further analyses were performed for the following three groups of PKUCS children: those who lost dietary control prior to age 6 years (group 1), between ages 6 and 10 years (group 2), and after age 10 years or not at all (group 3). The groups did not differ in age first treated or maximum diagnostic PHE (Table 2), but IDCs were consistently higher in group 1 than in groups 2 and 3 before age 4 years, between ages 4 and 6 years, and after age 6 years. Group 2 IDCs were also higher than those in group 3 at all ages.

Twelve-year WISC-R and WRAT mean test scores for groups 1, 2, and 3 are shown in Table 3. In all cases, group 1 had the lowest mean scores; group 3, which maintained dietary control at least through age 10 years, had the highest scores; and group 2 had mean scores falling between those of groups 1 and 2. Statistically significant differences by one-way analysis of variance were noted across groups for all of the 12-year test scores with the exception of arithmetic. The differences were primarily between groups 1 and 3, with significant differences also noted between groups 1 and 2 on WISC-R verbal and full-scale IQ scores, and between groups 2 and 3 on reading. Groups 2 and 3 did not differ significantly on any of the other 12-year test scores.

Scores on the WISC-R for children with PKU at age 12 years were compared with WAIS scores of their parents as an indication of the cognitive development of the child with PKU relative to other family members. Statistically significant deficits were observed on all three scales for all of the groups. The greatest differences were for group 1, followed by groups 2 and 3 (Table 4). Some of the apparent discrepancy may be attributed to the use at age 12 years of the revised WISC, which, on average, has been shown to produce scores approximately eight points lower than those attained by the same children on the unrevised WISC.[21]

Table 4.—Differences Between WISC-R Scores in 12-Year-Old Children With PKU and Their Parents on Comparable WAIS IQ Scales*

IQ Scale	Group 1 (n=23)	Group 2 (n=43)	Group 3 (n=25)
Verbal	−19±14 (.0001)	−13±12 (.0001)	−7±15 (.0191)
Performance	−12±16 (.0014)	−11±12 (.0001)	−7±11 (.0047)
Full	−17±14 (.0001)	−13±11 (.0001)	−8±12 (.0027)

*Group 1 includes patients who lost dietary control prior to age 6 years; group 2, between ages 6 and 10 years; and group 3, after 10 years. WISC-R indicates Weschler Intelligence Scale for Children–Revised; PKU, phenylketonuria; and WAIS, Weschler Adult Intelligence Scale. Values are mean (±SD) child minus parent differences. Numbers in parentheses are *P* values.

Table 5.—Changes in Test Scores Between Ages 6 and 12 Years for PKUCS Children Grouped by Age at Loss of Dietary Control*

IQ Test	Group 1	Group 2	Group 3
WISC-R vs Stanford-Binet	n=22 −4±6 (.0187)	n=47 −4±11 (.0085)	n=25 −1±10 (.6653)
WRAT	n=22	n=46	n=19
Reading	−6±14 (.0446)	−10±13 (.0001)	0±14 (.9501)
Spelling	−5±21 (.3136)	−8±14 (.0006)	1±16 (.7262)
Arithmetic	−11±15 (.0023)	−18±11 (.0001)	−16±12 (.0001)

*Group 1 includes patients who lost dietary control prior to age 6 years; group 2, between ages 6 and 10 years; and group 3, after age 10 years. PKUCS indicates collaborative study of Children Treated for Phenylketonuria; WISC-R, Weschler Intelligence Scale for Children–Revised; and WRAT, Wide Range Achievement Test. Values are mean (±SD) 12-years minus 6-years differences. Numbers in parentheses are *P* values.

At age 6 years, groups 2 and 3 had comparable mean scores on all tests (IQ, 100±14 vs 101±14; reading, 106±17 vs 105±13; spelling, 100±15 vs 99±13; and arithmetic, 100±13 vs 100±9), but mean scores for group 1, which had already lost dietary control, were six to 10 points lower (IQ, 91±15; reading, 99±20; spelling, 91±23; and arithmetic, 92±17). The differences in mean 6-year scores between group 1 and groups 2 and 3 combined were statistically significant for IQ ($P=.01$), spelling ($P=.01$), and arithmetic ($P=.03$), and approached significance for reading ($P=.05$).

Between ages 6 and 12 years, both groups of children who had lost dietary control had statistically significant drops in all areas, with the exception of spelling for group 1 (Table 5). The greatest overall declines were seen in group 2, the patients who lost control between ages 6 and 10 years. All groups showed significant declines in arithmetic scores.

COMMENT

For children with PKU, these data clearly show an association between exposure to high PHE levels prior to age 12 years and loss of cognitive and academic performance as measured by the WISC-R and WRAT tests. In this group of children, test scores at 12 years of age were negatively correlated with the age at which PHE restriction was begun. After treatment was begun, longer exposure to levels above 900 μmol/L was also associated with lower test scores at age 12 years.

It should be noted that the selection of PHE levels consistently above 900 μmol/L as an operational definition of loss of dietary control does not imply that any level up to that cutoff is safe, particularly at earlier ages. Indeed, Holtzman et al,[4] in their study of PKUCS children at ages 8 and 10 years, found similar results using 780 μmol/L as a cutoff for dietary control. They further pointed out that the small number of PKUCS children whose PHE levels exceeded 600 μmol/L after initiation of diet in the first years of life made it difficult to adequately assess lower thresholds at early ages. A similar problem was encountered in the present analyses in attempting to distinguish between 8 and 10 years as a critical age for maintaining dietary control. Only five children were in good control at age 8 years, but not at age 10 years—too few to form a separate group for analysis. Their pattern of test scores was similar to that of children who lost dietary control between ages 6 and 8 years and, hence, they were included with that group.

The greatest deficits at age 12 years were seen in those children whose levels exceeded 900 μmol/L before age 6 years. Test scores of these children were reduced at age 6 years and continued to decline until age 12 years. Children who maintained dietary control until age 6 years, but lost dietary control between ages 6 and 10 years, showed no differences in 6-year test scores compared with those who never lost dietary control. However, at age 12 years, they had significantly lower test scores and greater deviations from parent IQ. The greatest decreases in test scores between ages 6 and 12 years were seen in this group of children.

Some of the difference between IQ scores at ages 6 and 12 years may reflect different test content between the Stanford-Binet and the WISC-R, as well as a real decline in general cognitive ability. Nevertheless, children who maintained PHE levels below 900 μmol/L at least through age 10 years had the highest scores at age 12 years, showed little or no change in test scores between ages 6 and 12 years (except for arithmetic), and had 12-year mean IQ scores nearly comparable with those of their parents. In fact, an upward adjustment of WISC-R scores by the six-point difference reported between WISC-R and WAIS scores in nonretarded individuals[21] would have eliminated most of the child-parent IQ deficit in this group of children, but not in the other two groups.

Arithmetic was the only area of cognitive functioning evaluated at age 12 years for which maintaining dietary control of PHE below 900 μmol/L had no apparent beneficial effect. Mean scores declined significantly in all groups. In fact, all but eight of these children had lower arithmetic scores at age 12 years than at age 6 years. More than two thirds experienced a drop in arithmetic scores of 10 or more points. This finding is consistent with an earlier report of scores on arithmetic, perception, and linguistic tests declining between ages 6 and 10 years at similar rates for PKUCS children on and off diets.[5] The decline in arithmetic scores may be due to some aspect of test content at age 12 years that is particularly sensitive to even moderate elevations in PHE levels. A pilot study by Pennington et al[22] found children with PKU treated early to be deficient in certain cognitive and visuospatial skills that would be included in achievement tests at age 12 years but not at age 6 years.

The pattern of cognitive test scores observed in PKUCS children at age 12 years indicates that optimal intellectual and academic achievement are obtained by the earliest possible initiation of treatment and strict control of blood PHE levels throughout childhood. This conclusion is supported by the recent studies by Krause and coworkers[23] and Lou et al.[24] They independently demonstrated significant psychoneurologic changes associated with elevated blood levels of PHE. Another reason for continuation or resumption of dietary therapy, based on clinical experience with older off-diet individuals with PKU, is the devastating effects on offspring of untreated pregnant women with PKU.[25]

It is estimated that some 2700 women with PKU will be of childbearing age in the next two decades. In fact, Kirkman[26] has projected that unless a therapeutic remedy is developed soon, the beneficial results of the newborn screening programs for PKU will be neutralized by the birth of mentally retarded children to women with PKU. The problem of maternal PKU is now the subject of a national study sponsored by the National Institute of Child Health and Human Development.[27] The project encompasses all US states and Canadian provinces, and will ascertain whether therapy with the PHE-restricted diet protects fetal development and improves outcome so that physicians can properly advise the women with PKU approaching reproductive age.

The clinician now has data to recommend continuation of a diet restricted in PHE through age 12 years. While extended therapy is exceedingly important, particularly for women during their reproductive years, it certainly is not easily accomplished. In fact, many teenagers with PKU literally remove themselves from dietary therapy despite medical advice to the contrary. Attempts to reinstitute the PHE-restricted diet for prolonged periods have met with limited success.[28] Individuals with PKU, as well as their families, should receive counseling and support from the clinic team to facilitate the maintenance of extended therapy.

This study was funded in part by grant 4-RO1-HD-09543 and contract NO1-HD-4-3807 from the National Institute of Child Health and Human Development, Department of Health and Human Services, Bethesda, Md.

Gratitude is expressed and acknowledgement given to the many people who made important contributions to the Collaborative Study of Children Treated for Phenylketonuria, including project staff, laboratory directors, clinic directors, and consultants. We also thank Rita Kelly for her assistance in the preparation of this article.

Participating Centers

Project Staff.—Richard Koch, MD, Medical Director; Malcolm Williamson, PhD, Codirector; Eva Gross Friedman, Associate Director; Colleen Azen, MS, Coordinator, biostatistics.

Laboratory Directors.—Samuel Bessman, MD, Director, Serum/Blood Reference Laboratory, University of Southern California, Los Angeles; Kenneth Shaw, PhD, Director, Urine Chromatography Reference Laboratory, Childrens Hospital of Los Angeles.

Consultants.—*Nutrition:* Phyllis Acosta, DrPH, Florida State University, Tallahassee; *Education:* Robert Henderson, EdD, University of Illinois, Champaign; *Genetics:* Neil A. Holtzman, MD, MPH, Johns Hopkins University School of Medicine, Baltimore, Md; *Biostatistics:* Richard Kronmal, PhD, University of Washington, Seattle; *Psychology:* William van Doorninck, PhD, University of Colorado, Denver.

Clinic Directors.—Stanley Berlow, MD, University of Wisconsin, Madison; James Coldwell, MD, Childrens Medical Center, Tulsa, Oklahoma; Edward McCabe, MD, PhD, University of Colorado, Denver; Bobbye Rouse, MD, University of Texas, Galveston; Wilma Krause, MD, University of Iowa, Iowa City; Carol Shear, MD, University of Miami (Fla); C. Ronald Scott, MD, University of Washington, Seattle; Richard Koch, MD, Childrens Hospital, Los Angeles; Margaret O'Flynn, MD, Childrens Memorial Hospital, Chicago, Ill; Raymond Peterson, MD, Childrens Hospital Health Center, San Diego, Calif; Bernice Sigman, MD, University of Maryland School of Medicine, Baltimore; David Valle, MD, The Johns Hopkins Hospital, Baltimore; Robert Warner, MD, Childrens Hospital, Buffalo, NY; Reuben Matalon, MD, PhD, University of Illinois Hospital, Chicago.

References

1. Cabalska B, Duczynska N, Borzymowska J, Zorska, K, Koslacz-Folga A, Bozkowa K. Termination of dietary treatment in phenylketonuria. *Eur J Pediatr.* 1977;126:253-262.
2. Smith I, Lobascher ME, Stevenson JE, et al. Effect of stopping low-phenylalanine diet on intellectual progress of children with phenylketonuria. *BMJ.* 1978;2:723-726.
3. Waisbren SE, Schnell RR, Levy HL. Diet termination in children with phenylketonuria: a review of psychological assessments used to determine outcome. *J Inherited Metab Dis.* 1980;3:149-153.
4. Holtzman NA, Kronmal RA, van Doorninck W, Azen C, Koch R. Effect of age at loss of dietary control on intellectual performance and behavior of children with phenylketonuria. *N Engl J Med.* 1986;314:593-598.
5. Fishler K, Azen C, Henderson R, Friedman EG, Koch R. Psychoeducational findings among children treated for phenylketonuria. *Am J Ment Defic.* 1987;92:65-73.
6. Schmidt H, Mahle M, Michel U, et al. Continuation vs discontinuation of low-phenylalanine diet in PKU adolescents. *Eur J Pediatr.* 1987;146 (suppl):17-19.
7. Naughten ER, Kiely B, Saul I, Murphy D. Phenylketonuria: outcome and problems in a "diet-for-life" clinic. *Eur J Pediatr.* 1987;146(suppl):23-24.
8. Waisbren SE, Mahon BE, Schnell RR, Levy HL. Predictors of intelligence quotient and intelligence quotient change in persons treated for phenylketonuria early in life. *Pediatrics.* 1987;79:351-355.
9. Saudubray JM, Rey F, Ogier H, et al. Intellectual and school performance in early-treated classical PKU patients: the French collaborative study. *Eur J Pediatr.* 1987;146(suppl):20-22.
10. Koch R, Azen C, Hurst N, Friedman EG, Fishler K. The effects of diet discontinuation in children with phenylketonuria. *Eur J Pediatr.* 1987;146(suppl):12-16.
11. Williamson ML, Dobson JC, Koch R. Collaborative study of children treated for phenylketonuria: study design. *Pediatrics.* 1977;60:815-821.
12. Williamson ML, Koch R, Azen C, Chang C. Correlates of intelligence test results in treated phenylketonuric children. *Pediatrics.* 1981;68:161-167.
13. Koch R, Azen CG, Friedman EG, Williamson ML. Preliminary report on the effects of diet discontinuation in PKU. *J Pediatr.* 1982;100:870-875.
14. Koch R, Azen C, Friedman EG, Williamson ML. Paired comparisons between early treated PKU children and their matched sibling controls on intelligence and school achievement test results at eight years of age. *J Inherited Metab Dis.* 1984;7:86-90.
15. Wechsler D. *Wechsler Intelligence Scale for Children–Revised.* New York, NY: Psychological Corp; 1974.
16. Jastak J. *Wide Range Achievement Test.* Wilmington, Del: Story Press; 1946.
17. Thorndike RL. *Stanford-Binet Intelligence Scale 1972 Norms, Tables, Form LM.* Boston, Mass: Houghton Mifflin Co; 1972.
18. Wechsler D. *Wechsler Adult Intelligence Scale.* New York, NY: Psychological Corp; 1955.
19. SAS Institute Inc. *SAS User's Guide: Statistics.* Version 5 ed. Cary, NC: SAS Institute Inc; 1985.
20. Dixon WJ, Brown MB, Engelman L, Jennrich RI, eds. *BMDP Statistical Software 1985 Printing.* Berkeley, Calif: University of California Press; 1985.
21. Flynn JR. Wechsler intelligence tests: do we really have a criterion for mental retardation? *Am J Ment Defic.* 1985;90:236-244.
22. Pennington BF, van Doorninck WJ, McCabe LL, McCabe ERB. Neuropsychologic deficits in early treated phenylketonuric children. *Am J Ment Defic.* 1985;89:467-474.
23. Krause W, Halminski M, McDonald L, et al. Biochemical and neuropsychological effects of elevated plasma phenylalanine in patients with treated phenylketonuria. *J Clin Invest.* 1985;75:40-48.
24. Lou HC, Güttler F, Lykkelund C, Bruhn P, Niederwieser A. Decreased vigilance and neurotransmitter synthesis after discontinuation of dietary treatment for phenylketonuria in adolescents. *Eur J Pediatr.* 1985; 144:17-20.
25. Lenke RR, Levy HL. Maternal phenylketonuria and hyperphenylalaninemia: an international survey of the outcome of untreated and treated pregnancies. *N Engl J Med.* 1980;303:1202-1208.
26. Kirkman NH. Projections of a rebound in frequency of mental retardation from phenylketonuria. *Appl Res Ment Retard.* 1982;3:319-328.
27. Koch R, Friedman EG, Wenz E, Jew K, Crowley C, Donnell GN. Maternal phenylketonuria. *J Inherited Metab Dis.* 1986;9(suppl):159-168.
28. Michals K, Dominik M, Schuett V, Brown E, Matalon R. Return to diet therapy in patients with phenylketonuria. *J Pediatr.* 1985;106:933-936.

Follow-up of Patients Who Underwent Arterial Switch Repair for Transposition of the Great Arteries

Julita C. Mendoza, MD; Shirley A. Wilkerson, MD, PhD; Anabel H. Reese, MEd

• Thirty infants underwent arterial switch for transposition of the great arteries within the first week of life (mean age, 2.8 days). An additional three patients underwent repair at 5½, 8, and 9½ months of age. Six (18.2%) of 33 patients died. All the survivors were not receiving cardiac medications or diuretics at the time of the last follow-up visit. Examination of 24 of 27 survivors at 1 to 5 years of age revealed normal growth in 75% of the patients. Two patients had height, weight, and head circumference below the fifth percentile for age. Four patients had height and weight appropriate for age but head circumference below the fifth percentile. Neurodevelopmental testing yielded normal findings in 18 patients. Three patients were considered suspect and an additional three were abnormal neurodevelopmentally. Head circumference less than the fifth percentile, abnormalities on computed tomographic scans of the brain, and emergency balloon atrial septostomy or emergency switch operation were more likely to occur in patients who had low neurodevelopmental scores. We conclude that the majority of patients who undergo arterial switch repair demonstrate normal growth and development and no impairment of cardiovascular function. However, significant morbidity in the form of neurodevelopmental problems may occur.

(*AJDC.* 1991;145:40-43)

Transposition of the great arteries (TGA) is one of the most common cyanotic congenital heart defects, occurring in 1 in 2300 to 1 in 5000 live births.[1] Without intervention, the mortality rate is 90% before 6 months of age.[2,3] The use of prostaglandin E_1 to maintain patency of the ductus[4-6] and the performance of balloon atrial septostomy (BAS)[7] at the time of cardiac catheterization permit mixing of the pulmonary and systemic circulations, resulting in increased arterial oxygen saturation, thereby improving the general status and increasing the chances of survival before corrective surgery in these critically sick neonates.

Infants with TGA usually present shortly after birth with cyanosis and respiratory distress. A number of them have severe hypoxia and metabolic acidosis and will die unless their arterial oxygen saturation is improved. In our institution, infants undergo an arterial switch operation for simple TGA. We performed this study to determine the outcome in the first 33 infants who underwent this corrective procedure and to describe its effects on the growth and neurodevelopment of the survivors.

Accepted for publication March 5, 1990.

From the Division of Neonatology, Department of Pediatrics, University of Louisville (Ky).

Read before the annual meeting of the Southern Society for Pediatric Research, New Orleans, La, February 2, 1989.

Reprint requests to the Department of Pediatrics, School of Medicine, University of Louisville, Louisville, KY 40292 (Dr Wilkerson).

PATIENTS AND METHODS

Patients

Thirty-three patients with TGA underwent an arterial switch operation between November 1983 and October 1988 (Table 1). The gestational ages of the infants ranged from 36 to 41 weeks (mean, 39.8 weeks) and the birth weight ranged from 2.3 to 4.2 kg (mean, 3.48 kg). All the infants had weight, length, and head circumference within or above the normal range for gestational age at birth. Twenty-seven patients had simple TGA (with an intact ventricular septum) and six had TGA associated with a ventricular septal defect.

Preoperative Evaluation and Management

All patients underwent echocardiography on admission to the intensive care nursery, and all underwent cardiac catheterization before operation. Balloon atrial septostomy was performed in 24 patients (72.7%) at the time of catheterization, five of which were performed emergently due to severe hypoxia and metabolic acidosis. Prostaglandin E_1 was administered preoperatively in 30 patients.

The patients with simple TGA underwent repair within the first week of life, at a mean age of 2.8 days. Among the six patients with TGA and a ventricular septal defect, three had a moderate to large septal defect and were operated on at 5½, 8, and 9½ months of age. Five patients underwent emergency arterial switch operation due to severe hypoxia and acidosis despite prostaglandin E_1 infusion and BAS.

The operation was performed with the use of cardiopulmonary bypass and deep systemic hypothermia with core cooling to 16°C to 18°C. Duration of bypass surgery ranged from 50 minutes to 6 hours (mean, 2.4 hours). Aortic cross-clamp time was generally less than 60 minutes. The procedure consisted of the arterial switch repair introduced by Jatene et al[8] in 1975 and modified by Castaneda et al[9] and Mavroudis,[10] with excision of the two coronary arteries from the aorta and their implantation to the pulmonary artery, transection of the aorta and the pulmonary artery, and, finally, anastomoses between the pulmonary artery stump and the distal aorta and between the stump of the aorta and the distal end of the pulmonary artery. The Lecompte maneuver[11] was also employed, passing the ascending aorta posterior to the pulmonary artery birfurcation. Pericardial tissue was used as necessary in the arterial reconstruction.

All patients underwent ventilation for 2 to 27 days (mean, 7.4 days) after the operation and all required inotropic support. Nine patients were treated with digoxin and/or a diuretic agent until 4 to 18 months of age.

Follow-up

In addition to their cardiology follow-up, the survivors were seen in our neonatal follow-up clinic. Growth variables (weight, height, and head circumference) were plotted. Physical and neurologic examinations were performed by a neonatologist or neonatal fellow. Neurodevelopmental progress was evaluated by an experienced developmental psychologist with use of the Bayley Scales of Infant Development[12] for patients up to 2 years of age and the Stanford-Binet Intelligence Scale[13] and Denver Developmental Screening Test[14] for those older than 2 years. Functional cardiac status was also determined from cardiology records.

RESULTS

Mortality

Six (18.2%) of the 33 patients died (Table 2). Two deaths occurred among the first 15 patients who underwent the arterial switch procedure; the other

Table 1.—Characteristics of Infants Who Underwent Arterial Switch Repair for Transposition of the Great Arteries (TGA)*

Variable	Value
Total No. of patients	33
Birth weight, g	3476.0±512
Gestational age, wk	39.8±0.9
Sex	
M	24 (72.7)
F	9 (27.3)
Preoperative evaluation	
Echocardiography	33 (100)
Cardiac catheterization	33 (100)
With BAS	24 (72.7)
Without BAS	9 (27.3)
PGE_1 infusion	30 (90.9)
Diagnosis	
TGA with IVS	27
TGA with VSD	6
Age at surgery, d	
TGA with IVS or small VSD	2.8±1.7
TGA with moderate/large VSD	230.6±61.1

*Values represent number (percent) or mean±SD. BAS indicates balloon atrial septostomy; PGE_1, prostaglandin E_1; IVS, intact ventricular septum; and VSD, ventricular septal defect.

Table 2.—Details of Six Deaths After Arterial Switch Repair*

Patient	Timing of Death	Age at Death, d	Cause of Death
1	Early postoperative period	4	Pulmonary hypertension
2	Intraoperatively	6	MI, kinked coronary artery
3	Intraoperatively	2	Prolonged CPB; abnormal orientation of PA cusps
4	Late postoperative period	51	MI, obstruction of transposed left coronary artery
5	Intraoperatively	2	MI, abnormal coronary artery
6	Early postoperative period	3	Arrhythmia

*MI indicates myocardial infarction; CPB, cardiopulmonary bypass; and PA, pulmonary artery.

four occurred in the last 18 patients included in this report. There were three intraoperative deaths: two from myocardial infarction related to unusual coronary artery anatomy and the other after prolonged cardiopulmonary bypass (>6 hours) and technical difficulty due to abnormal orientation of the pulmonary artery cusps. Two patients died during the early postoperative period due to pulmonary hypertension and intractable arrhythmia. There was one late death at 51 days after repair secondary to myocardial infarction from occlusion of the transposed left coronary artery. Three of the nonsurvivors underwent an emergency switch operation due to persistent hypoxia and acidosis despite BAS and prostaglandin E_1 infusion.

Functional Status

No survivor was receiving cardiac medications or diuretics at the time of the last follow-up visit (Table 3). Detailed studies consisting of echocardiography, cardiac catheterization, and 24-hour electrocardiography showed a very low incidence of postoperative sequelae, such as supravalvular pulmonary stenosis, valvular insufficiency, and symptomatic arrhythmias.

Growth and Development

Among the 27 survivors, growth and developmental follow-up was performed in 24 between 1 and 5 years of age (mean, 2.1 years). Normal growth was seen in 18 (75%) of the patients. Two patients showed poor growth with all measurements below the fifth percentile for age. One of these two patients had a diagnosis that included a ventricular septal defect and aortic coarctation in addition to the TGA that had been repaired at 8 months of age. The other growth-retarded patient had a left-sided cerebral infarct and severe neurodevelopmental delay. Six patients had head circumference below the fifth percentile, two of whom also had weight and height that were below the fifth percentile, as described above. The other four patients had weight and height appropriate for age.

Neurodevelopmental Follow-up

Results of the neurodevelopmental testing showed normal scores (≥84 or <1 SD below the mean) in 18 (75%) of the patients. Three patients were considered suspect, with scores ranging from 68 to 83 (between 1 and 2 SDs below the mean). Three had scores below 68 (>2 SDs below the mean) and were considered to be abnormal neurodevelopmentally. In two of the latter three patients, central nervous system damage was noted on head computed tomographic scans, as were persistent severe mental and psychomotor delay; one had hypotonia at the 1-year follow-up visit but had grossly normal growth and development by parental report, except for some articulation problems at 3 years of age.

Among the six patients who had head circumference below the fifth percentile, four had neurodevelopmental scores suspicious for or indicative of abnormal neurodevelopment (Table 4). Four patients had major abnormalities seen on computed tomographic scans of the head. One patient had a left-sided posterior parietal hemorrhage that was noted on follow-up computed tomography to be resolved and had normal scores on neurodevelopmental testing. Two patients had a left-sided cerebral infarct with right-sided hemiparesis and language delay on follow-up. The fourth patient had a right-sided posterior parietal hemorrhage, mental retardation, and cortical blindness. Perioperative seizures were observed in 22% of the patients identified as having normal scores on neurodevelopmental testing compared with half of those with low scores. Head circumference below the fifth percentile, abnormalities noted on head computed tomographic scans, and emergency BAS or surgery for severe hypoxia and/or metabolic acidosis were more likely to occur in patients who had low scores on neurodevelopmental testing. Table 5 lists the details of the growth and neurodevelopmental outcome of the 24 survivors of arterial switch surgery.

COMMENT

The natural history of TGA is dismal, with only 10% of affected infants surviving the first year of life.[2] Measures that improve intracardiac mixing by means of BAS, introduced by Rashkind and Miller[7] in 1966, and the use of prostaglandin E_1 infusion[4-6] have substantially increased short-term survival but do not allow long-term survival.

Two types of repair are advocated in the surgical management of TGA. Physiologic repair by intra-atrial rerouting of venous return was first introduced by

Senning[15] in 1959, followed later by another procedure described by Mustard[16] in 1964. Both atrial switch procedures have low operative mortality,[17-19] but the occurrence of right ventricular dysfunction, tricuspid insufficiency, venous inflow obstructions, and symptomatic arrythmias[20-21] associated with these operations complicate their long-term results and limit their acceptability. These complications could be obviated by performance of anatomic or arterial switch repair, the first successful report of which was described by Jatene et al[8] in 1975 and which since then has been used with various modifications and improving survival rate.[22-24]

Evaluation of the two management strategies for TGA should not only focus on the surgical outcome and hemodynamic results of each procedure but also consider the quality of growth and development of the survivors. Only a few of the literature reports include the growth and neurologic outcome of TGA survivors. To our knowledge, this is the first report of detailed growth and neurodevelopmental follow-up in patients who have undergone the arterial switch procedure.

Our data indicate that the majority of

Table 3.—Outcome of Arterial Switch Repair Survivors (n=24)*

Variable	No. (%)
Functional status: no cardiac medicines or diuretics	24 (100)
Growth	
Normal weight, height, HC for age	18 (75.0)
Weight, height, HC <5th percentile	2 (8.3)
Weight <5th percentile	2 (8.3)
Height <5th percentile	2 (8.3)
HC <5th percentile	6 (25.0)
Neurodevelopmental follow-up (score)	
Normal (>84)	18 (75.0)
Suspect (68-83)	3 (12.5)
Abnormal (<68)	3 (12.5)

*HC indicates head circumference.

Table 4.—Factors Associated With Low Neurodevelopmental Scores*

Factor	No. (%) Normal (n=18)	No. (%) Suspect/Abnormal (n=6)
HC <5th percentile†	2 (11.1)	4 (66.7)
Abnormal head CT scan†	1 (5.6)	3 (50.0)
Emergency catheterization/repair‡	2 (11.1)	3 (50.0)
Seizures	4 (22.2)	3 (50.0)

*HC indicates head circumference; CT, computed tomographic.
†*P*<.04.
‡*P*<.08.

Table 5.—Growth and Neurodevelopmental Outcome of Arterial Switch Repair Survivors*

Patient	Follow-up Percentiles: Weight	Follow-up Percentiles: Height	Follow-up Percentiles: HC	Bayley: MDI	Bayley: PDI	S-B	Comment
1	45	20	**<5**	...	...	**81**	Seizures preoperatively, L hemispheric infarct, R hemiparesis, language delay
2	60	50	50	...	...	97	...
3	18	23	**<5**	...	...	**83**	Emergency catheterization
4	40	25	48	...	...	113	...
5	20	25	**<5**	125	96	...	Bradycardia, hypotension, CPR postoperatively
6	65	30	25	...	...	110	...
7	**<5**	**<5**	**<5**	**52**	**29**	...	Emergency catheterization, seizures preoperatively, L cerebral infarct, R hemiparesis, language delay
8	25	15	**<5**	**29**	**58**	...	Seizures postoperatively, R posterior parietal bleed, MR, cortical blindness
9	40	25	25	...	...	110	Seizures postoperatively, normal CT scan
10	70	78	98	130	87	...	L posterior parietal bleed, resolved
11	15	24	35	101	104	...	...
12	30	45	35	112	110	...	Seizures postoperatively, small IVH
13	58	75	50	112	111	...	...
14	8	50	20	**67**	**75**	...	Emergency repair, hypotonia
15	17	7	7	117	98	...	Emergency repair
16	95	77	20	131	111	...	...
17	**<5**	**<5**	**<5**	117	89	...	...
18	55	50	45	...	...	120	...
19	58	55	40	123	105	...	Emergency catheterization, seizures postoperatively
20	25	23	8	106	99	...	...
21	7	25	15	98	**81**	...	Increased tone in lower extremities
22	95	77	10	96	98	...	...
23	30	30	55	112	110	...	...
24	75	40	45	103	111	...	CPR×20 s in OR, seizures postoperatively

*HC indicates head circumference; MDI, Mental Developmental Index; PDI, Psychomotor Developmental Index; S-B, Stanford-Binet test; CPR, cardiopulmonary resuscitation; MR, mental retardation; CT, computed tomographic; IVH, intraventricular hemorrhage; and OR, operating room. Values in bold type are considered abnormal.

patients demonstrate normal growth and development and no impairment of cardiovascular function for up to 5 years following arterial switch repair. At least 90% of the patients were growing normally with respect to weight and height at the time of follow-up. This figure compares favorably with the 79% reported to have normal weight following the arterial switch operation (Quaegebeur et al[24]). Of concern, however, is the lack of head growth in a few of the survivors, 67% of whom have suspicious or abnormal neurodevelopmental outcome. Other factors associated with low neurodevelopmental scores include abnormal head computed tomographic scans and emergency BAS or repair. These risk factors are presumably related to the severe hypoxia and acidosis that characterize the clinical presentation of some of the patients.

At least one fourth of the survivors of arterial switch surgery demonstrate some abnormality on neurologic or developmental evaluation, although only three patients had major neurologic sequelae (hemiparesis, cortical blindness, and mental retardation). Rubay et al[25] described five of 100 patients with TGA who sustained neurologic damage, three of whom were diagnosed before the Senning operation and one of whom was diagnosed after surgery. Williams et al[26] described 10 of 115 patients with TGA who had significant neurologic damage; in five the damage was evident before the Mustard operation and in the remaining five the damage was noted immediately after repair. The inability of BAS to reliably prevent death before repair is well documented.[1,25,27] Ten to fifteen percent of patients who underwent BAS died or had a cerebrovascular accident while waiting for baffle repair.[1] The occurrence of prolonged or severe hypoxia and acidosis in patients with TGA certainly places them at increased risk for neurodevelopmental sequelae. Intraoperative factors, such as cardiopulmonary bypass, circulatory arrest, and hypothermia, may also contribute to neurologic morbidity[28-30]; however, there was no significant difference in the duration of bypass and degree of hypothermia between our patients who had normal outcome and those who had adverse outcome. Whether the type of surgical intervention itself increases the risk is unclear. There is evidence that chronic hypoxemia due to older age at the time of corrective repair of TGA by the Mustard operation may be associated with greater impairment of cognitive function.[31] Five of our patients required emergency switch operation due to progressive hypoxia and acidosis despite prostaglandin E_1 infusion and BAS. Because of the risk of major neurologic complications, early recognition, diagnosis, and intervention are mandatory. Detailed growth and neurodevelopmental follow-up, in addition to cardiac function determination, are important in the evaluation of any major cardiac surgery and should be particularly included in clinical trials that involve new procedures or techniques. It is imperative that follow-up assessment through early school age be performed in the evaluation of these procedures.

Our Neonatal Follow-up Program is partially funded by the Division of Maternal and Child Health, Kentucky Department of Health and Human Resources.

We thank our cardiologists, Francisco Elbl, MD, Robert Solinger, MD, Allan Rees, MD, and Juan Villafane, MD, and our cardiovascular surgeon, Constantine Mavroudis, MD. We also thank Judy Kantlehner for her help in gathering the data.

References

1. Gutgesell HP, Garson A, McNamara DG. Prognosis for the newborn with transposition of the great arteries. *Am J Cardiol*. 1979;44:96-100.

2. Liebman J, Cullum L, Belloc N. Natural history of transposition of the great arteries: anatomy and birth and death characteristics. *Circulation*. 1969;40;237-262.

3. Campbell M. Incidence of cardiac malformations at birth and later, and neonatal mortality. *Br Heart J*. 1973;35:189-200.

4. Hallidie-Smith KA. Prostaglandin E_1 in suspected ductus dependent cardiac malformation. *Arch Dis Child*. 1984;59:1020-1026.

5. Freed MD, Heymann MA, Lewis AB, Roehl SL, Kensey RC. Prostaglandin E_1 in infants with ductus arteriosus–dependent congenital heart disease. *Circulation*. 1981;64:899-905.

6. Lang PL, Freed MD, Bierman FZ, Norwood WI, Nadas AS. Use of prostaglandin E_1 in infants with *d*-transposition of great arteries and an intact ventricular septum. *Am J Cardiol*. 1979;44:76-81.

7. Rashkind WJ, Miller WW. Creation of an atrial septal defect without thoracotomy: a palliative approach to complete transposition of the great arteries. *JAMA*. 1966;196:991-992.

8. Jatene AD, Fontes VF, Paulista PP, et al. Successful anatomic correction of transposition of the great vessels: a preliminary report. *Arg Bras Cardiol*. 1975;28:461-464.

9. Castaneda AR, Norwood WI, Jonas RA, Colon SD, Sanders SP, Lang P. Transposition of the great arteries and intact ventricular septum: anatomical repair in the neonate. *Ann Thorac Surg*. 1984;38:438-443.

10. Mavroudis C. Anatomical repair of transposition of the great arteries with intact ventricular septum in the neonate: guidelines to avoid complications. *Ann Thorac Surg*. 1987;43:495-501.

11. Lecompte Y, Zannini L, Hazan E, et al. Anatomic correction of transposition of the great arteries—new technique without the use of a prosthetic conduit. *J Thorac Cardiovasc Surg*. 1981;82:629-631.

12. Bayley N. *Bayley Scales of Infant Development*. New York, NY: The Psychological Corp; 1969.

13. Terman LM, Merrill MA. *Stanford-Binet Intelligence Scale*. Chicago, Ill: Riverside Publishing Company; 1973.

14. Frankenburg WK, Dodds JB. The Denver Developmental Screening Test. *J Pediatr*. 1967; 71:181-191.

15. Senning A. Surgical correction of transposition of the great vessels. *Surgery*. 1959;45:966-980.

16. Mustard WT. Successful two-stage correction of transposition of the great arteries. *Surgery*. 1964;55:469-472.

17. Bender HW Jr, Graham TP, Boucek RJ, Walker WE, Boerth RG. Comparative operative results of the Senning and Mustard procedures for transposition of the great arteries. *Circulation*. 1980;62(2 pt 2):I197-I203.

18. Trusler GA, Williams WG, Duncan KF. Results of the Mustard operation in simple transposition of the great arteries 1963-1985. *Ann Surg*. 1987;206:251-260.

19. George BL, Laks H, Klitzner TS, Friedman WF, Williams RG. Results of the Senning procedure with simple and complex transposition of the great arteries. *Am J Cardiol*. 1987;59:426-430.

20. Trusler GA, Williams WG, Duncan KF, et al. Results with the Mustard operation in simple transposition of the great arteries. *Ann Surg*. 1987;206:251-260.

21. Warnes CA, Somerville J. Transposition of the great arteries: late results in adolescents and adults after the Mustard procedure. *Br Heart J*. 1987;58:148-155.

22. Norwood WI, Dobell AR, Freed MD, Kirklin JW, Blackstone EH, Congenital Heart Surgeons Society. Intermediate results of the arterial switch repair: a 20-institution study. *J Thorac Cardiovasc Surg*. 1988;96:854-863.

23. Idriss FS, Ilbawi MN, DeLeon SY, et al. Arterial switch in simple and complex transposition of the great arteries. *J Thorac Cardiovasc Surg*. 1988;95:29-36.

24. Quaegebeur JM, Rohmer J, Ottenkamp J, Buis T, Kirklin JW, Blackstone EH. The arterial switch operation: an eight-year experience. *J Throac Cardiovasc Surg*. 1986;92:361-384.

25. Rubay J, de Leval M, Bull C. To switch or not to switch? the Senning alternative. *Circulation*. 1988;78(5 pt 5):III1-III4.

26. Williams WG, Trusler GA, Kirklin JW, et al. Early and late results of a protocol for simple transposition leading to an atrial (Mustard) repair. *J Thorac Cardiovasc Surg*. 1988;95:717-726.

27. Castaneda AR, Trusler GA, Paul MH, Blackstone EH, Kirklin JW, Congenital Heart Surgeons Society. The early results of treatment of simple transposition in the current era. *J Thorac Cardiovasc Surg*. 1988;95:14-28.

28. Ferry PC. Neurologic sequelae of cardiac surgery in children. *AJDC*. 1987;141:309-312.

29. Ehyai A, Fenichel GM, Bender HW Jr. Incidence and prognosis of seizures in infants after cardiac surgery with profound hypothermia and circulatory arrest. *JAMA*. 1984;252:3165-3167.

30. Wells FC, Coghill S, Caplan HL, Lincoln C, Kirklin JW. Duration of circulatory arrest does influence the psychological development of children after cardiac operation in early life. *J Thorac Cardiovasc Surg*. 1983;86:823-831.

31. Newburger JW, Silbert AR, Buckley LP, Fyler DC. Cognitive function and age at repair of transposition of the great arteries in children. *N Engl J Med*. 1984;310:1495-1499.

Elevated Plasma Norepinephrine Levels in Infants of Substance-Abusing Mothers

Sally L. Davidson Ward, MD; Sally Schuetz, RN, CPNP; Laura Wachsman, MD; Xylena D. Bean, MD; Daisy Bautista; Sue Buckley; Sabitha Sehgal, MD; David Warburton, MB, MRCP

•Infants of substance-abusing mothers (ISAM) have significant growth and neurodevelopmental abnormalities. The origin of these abnormalities is unknown. We postulated that ISAM have increased sympathetic nervous system tone and altered catecholamine levels. Therefore, we measured plasma norepinephrine, epinephrine, and dopamine levels and the number and receptor affinity of β-adrenoreceptor binding sites on lymphocytes and α-adrenoreceptor binding sites on thrombocytes in 22 otherwise healthy ISAM (age, 2.1 ± 0.5 months; mean ± SD) and 15 healthy controls (age, 2.5 ± 0.8 months). Norepinephrine levels in venous blood were 1.8-fold higher in ISAM than in control infants (6.30 ± 3.85 nmol/L vs 3.55 ± 2.45 nmol/L). There were no differences in plasma epinephrine or dopamine levels. There were no differences in the number of binding sites or receptor affinity for β- and α-adrenoreceptors. We conclude that ISAM have elevated circulating norepinephrine levels compared with controls. We speculate that this is associated with increased sympathetic nervous system tone in ISAM and that the absence of adrenoreceptor down-regulation may create catecholamine suprasensitivity.

(*AJDC.* 1991;145:44-48)

Perinatal substance abuse among women of childbearing age has become a serious health problem in the United States. A recent survey of American households by the National Institute on Drug Abuse estimated that of 56 million women of childbearing age, 8 million, or 15%, are current abusers of illicit drugs. The same survey estimated that there are 750 000 cocaine-abusing women with children in this country.[1]

Infants of substance-abusing mothers (ISAM) have been reported to have a number of significant health problems. Infants exposed to either opiates or cocaine in utero have been reported to have lower birth weights, signs of neonatal abstinence syndrome, and abnormal scores on the Brazelton Neonatal Behavioral Assessment Scale.[2-8] In addition to growth and neurodevelopmental abnormalities, ISAM also have an increased risk for sudden infant death syndrome (SIDS)[9-13] and for having abnormalities of the ventilatory pattern during sleep recorded by pneumogram technique (overnight recordings of heart rate and ventilatory pattern).[13-16]

The mechanism by which cocaine and/or opiate exposure acts during fetal development to create abnormalities in infants is unknown. The pharmacologic action of cocaine is to block the reuptake of released monoamines (dopamine, serotonin, and norepinephrine) at the synaptic junction.[17,18] This leads to depletion of these neurotransmitters and their precursors and to catecholamine receptor suprasensitivity.[17] Animal studies of opiate exposure in utero revealed alterations in the neurochemical development of catecholaminergic systems in both central and peripheral nervous tissues of neonatal rats.[19] Opiate addiction and withdrawal alter brain catecholamine neurotransmitter and receptor function.[20,21]

Alterations in central and sympathetic nervous system neurotransmitters and receptors induced by intrauterine drug exposure could be associated with the neurodevelopmental and ventilatory pattern abnormalities in ISAM. Although direct measurements of central nervous system neurotransmitter systems cannot be made in infants, sympathetic nervous system activity can be inferred from measurements of plasma catecholamine levels.[22,23] In addition, changes in adrenoreceptor binding on circulating lymphocytes and platelets have been postulated to reflect changes in adrenoreceptors in other tissues.[24] We hypothesized that ISAM have elevated sympathetic nervous system tone, which would be reflected by alterations in circulating catecholaminergic neurotransmitters and receptors. Therefore, we measured plasma epinephrine, dopamine, and norepinephrine, α- and β-receptor binding sites, and receptor affinities on platelets and lymphocytes, respectively, in 22 ISAM and 15 healthy control infants for comparison.

PATIENTS AND METHODS

Infants of substance-abusing mothers were referred from either the state-funded clinic caring for infants born to substance-abusing mothers at Los Angeles County–University of Southern California Medical Center or from the Perinatal Substance Abuse Project at Martin Luther King, Jr, General Hospital, Los Angeles, Calif. They were identified by a positive maternal drug abuse history and/or positive urine toxicologic test at birth. Infants of substance-abusing mothers were excluded from study if they had a history of premature birth (gestation < 37 weeks based on physical assessment by Dubowitz examination[25]), required neonatal intensive care, or were requiring any medications. Assessment of gestational age was performed by two investigators (Drs Bean and Sehgal) for eight infants and was obtained by review of neonatal records for the remaining infants. They were required to be free from cardiac, pulmonary, or neurologic complications other than neonatal abstinence syndrome and to be growing appropriately. Infants who were born at term but were

Accepted for publication April 9, 1990.

From the Division of Neonatology and Pediatric Pulmonology, Childrens Hospital of Los Angeles (Drs Ward and Warburton and Mss Bautista and Buckley); Los Angeles County–University of Southern California Medical Center (Drs Ward, Wachsman, and Warburton, and Ms Schuetz), Department of Pediatrics, University of Southern California School of Medicine (Mss Bautista and Buckley); and Martin Luther King, Jr, General Hospital, Charles R. Drew Postgraduate Medical School (Drs Bean and Sehgal), Los Angeles, Calif.

Read before the New York Academy of Sciences Conference on Prenatal Abuse of Licit and Illicit Drugs, Bethesda, Md, September 9, 1988.

Reprint requests to Division of Neonatology and Pediatric Pulmonology, Childrens Hospital of Los Angeles, 4650 Sunset Blvd, Bin 83, Los Angeles, CA 90027 (Dr Ward).

small for gestational age were not excluded. Records were reviewed for signs of neonatal abstinence syndrome and were scored using a system proposed by Finnegan.[26] Control infants were recruited from well-baby clinics and the general population. Control infants were required to have been full term (≥ 37 weeks by maternal history and/or Dubowitz examination[25]), healthy and growing, without a personal or family history of apnea or a family history of SIDS, and requiring no medication. Control infants were not exposed to illicit drugs, tobacco, or excessive alcohol intake based on the history obtained from parents and/or the referring provider.

All infants were studied between 1.0 and 4.0 months of age. This age was chosen to coincide with the peak age for SIDS deaths.[27,28] Infants of substance-abusing mothers have been shown to have an increased risk for SIDS with a mean age at time of SIDS death of about 3 months.[28]

Informed consent was obtained from the caretaker of each infant studied. The study was approved by the Committee on Clinical Investigations (Institutional Review Board) at Childrens Hospital of Los Angeles.

Each infant underwent phlebotomy for 5 mL of blood from an antecubital vein as rapidly and atraumatically as possible with the infant supine. All samples were obtained between 8 and 9 AM. Four milliters of blood was placed in a tube containing ethylene glycol-bis (beta-aminoethyl ether) *N*, *N*'-tetraacetic acid (EGTA) as an anticoagulant for immediate lymphocyte and thrombocyte separation and adrenergic receptor analysis. The remaining milliliters of blood were placed on ice in a tube containing EGTA as an anticoagulant and glutathione as an antioxidant for catecholamine analysis.

PREPARATION AND β-RECEPTOR BINDING ASSAY OF LYMPHOCYTES

Lymphocytes were immediately isolated from the blood using a modification of the method described by Boyum.[29] The blood was diluted with an equal volume of phosphate-buffered saline at a pH of 7.4. The mixture was layered on 3 mL of lymphocyte separation medium (Boehringer, Mannheim, West Germany). Tubes were centrifuged at 400*g* at 20°C for 40 minutes. After removal of the thrombocyte-rich plasma, the lymphocyte band was washed twice with an equal volume of phosphate-buffered saline and recentrifuged at 100*g* at 20°C for 10 minutes. The resulting pellet was resuspended in 3 mL of buffer A containing 12 mmol/L of TRIS hydrochloride, 154 mmol/L of sodium chloride , 30 mmol/L of phentolamine hydrochloride, and 0.55 mmol/L of ascorbic acid at a pH of 7.4. Phentolamine was added to inhibit α-receptor binding and ascorbic acid was added to prevent oxidation. The cells were counted and checked for viability by trypan blue staining.

β-Receptors were assayed on intact lymphocytes using a modification of the method described by Brodde et al.[30] One hundred microliters of the lymphocyte suspension (5×10^5 cells) was incubated with 50 μL of buffer A and six different concentrations of cyanopindolol labeled with iodine I 125 (^{125}I)(8140×10^{10} Bq·mmol, 5 to 200 pmol/L, New England Nuclear, Boston, Mass) for 60 minutes at 37°C. The reaction was stopped by adding 10 mL of buffer B containing 12 mmol/L of TRIS and 157 mmol/L of sodium chloride, at a pH of 7.4, at 37°C to the incubation mixture. The mixture was filtered over 25-mm glass fiber filters (Whatman GF/C, Whatman International, Maidstone, England). Each filter was rapidly washed with an additional 10 mL of buffer B. The radioactivity of the dry filters was determined using a gamma counter (Berthold LP 2101) at an efficiency of 84%.

PREPARATION AND α-RECEPTOR BINDING ASSAY OF THROMBOCYTES

The thrombocyte-rich plasma, which was obtained after removal of the lymphocyte band, was centrifuged at 1800*g* at 20°C for 10 minutes. The sedimented thrombocytes were washed three times with buffer C containing 50 mmol/L of TRIS, 100 mmol/L of sodium chloride, 0.5 mmol/L of edetic acid, and 0.8 mmol/L of ascorbic acid, at a pH of 7.5.

α-Receptors were assayed on intact thrombocytes using a modification of the method described by Motulsky et al.[31] Approximately 2×10^7 thrombocytes in 50 μL of buffer C were incubated with 100 μL of six different concentrations of tritiated yohimbine (333×10^{10} Bq·mmol, 0.5 to 25 nmol/L; New England Nuclear, Boston, Mass) for 30 minutes at 25°C. At the end of the incubation, 10 mL of buffer D containing 50 mmol/L of TRIS, 100 mmol/L of sodium chloride, and 5 mmol/L of edetic acid was added. The mixture was rapidly filtered through glass filters (Whatman GF/C 25 mm). Each filter was rapidly washed with an additional 10 mL of buffer D. The dry filters were transferred to vials containing scintillation fluid (Research Product International, 3a70), and the radioactivity was measured in a scintillation counter (Beckman LS 3H01, Irvine, Calif).

EVALUATION OF SPECIFIC BINDING

Nonspecific binding of ^{125}I-cyanopindolol and yohimbine was defined as the amount of radioactivity bound to membranes that was not displaced by high concentrations of propranolol and phentolamine, respectively. Specific binding of ^{125}I-cyanopindolol and yohimbine was defined as the total radioactivity minus nonspecific binding and amounted to 70% for ^{125}I-cyanopindolol and 65% for yohimbine. For calculation of the receptor affinity and the binding sites, the Scatchard[32] plot was used.

A linear slope ($r = .9$) was obtained in each assay, indicating one class of binding sites. The binding sites per lymphocyte or the binding sites per thrombocyte were determined by dividing the total number of receptors by the number of the appropriate cells.

CATECHOLAMINE ASSAY

One milliter of blood from the 5 mL taken for the receptor assays was drawn into specimen tubes (Vacutainer) containing EGTA as an anticoagulant and glutathione as an antioxidant (Upjohn Diagnostic, Kalamazoo, Mich). The tubes were placed on ice and were centrifuged shortly afterward. The plasma was then rapidly frozen and stored at −70°C for future analysis. Plasma dopamine, epinephrine, and norepinephrine levels were measured by radioenzymatic assay using a modification of the method described by Passon and Peuler[33] with the CAT-A-KIT (catecholamine tritiated radioenzymatic) Assay Kit (Amersham Corp, Arlington Heights, Ill).

DATA ANALYSIS

The investigator who performed all the biochemical analyses was unaware of the subject's diagnosis. All assays were performed in duplicate with an agreement within 3% for acceptability. Results are expressed as mean ± SD. The Behrens Fisher independent *t* test was used to allow for variance heteroge-

Table 1.—Comparison of Plasma Catecholamine Levels in Infants of Substance-Abusing Mothers (ISAM) and Control Infants

	ISAM	Control Infants
Norepinephrine, nmol/L (pg/mL)		
n	22	15
Mean ± SD	6.30 ± 3.85 (1065 ± 651)*	3.55 ± 2.45 (600 ± 414)
Range	1.75-16.08 (296-2721)	0.28-9.30 (48-1574)
Epinephrine, pmol/L (pg/mL)		
n	22	13
Mean ± SD	911 ± 704 (167 ± 129)	846 ± 835 (155 ± 153)
Range	213-3264 (39-598)	109-3215 (20-589)
Dopamine, pg/mL		
n	22	11
Mean ± SD	122 ± 175	88 ± 73
Range	5-833	24-251

*$P<.025$.

Table 2.—Comparison of the Number (B_{max}) of β-Receptor Binding Sites on Lymphocytes (BS/L) and α-Receptor Binding Sites on Thrombocytes (BS/T) With Respective Receptor Affinities (K_d) Between Infants of Substance-Abusing Mothers (ISAM) and Control Infants*

	ISAM	Control Infants
β-Receptors		
n	18	11
B_{max} (BS/L)	854 ± 222	846 ± 315
Range	501-1179	375-1359
K_d (pmol/L)	35 ± 14	44 ± 28
α-Receptors		
n	14	7
B_{max} (BS/T)	238 ± 34	234 ± 58
Range	172-293	159-318
K_d (pmol/L)	2.9 ± 0.9	2.3 ± 1.3
Range	1.5-4.0	1.3-4.1

*Data are expressed as number of subjects (N), mean ± SD, and range.

neity in the comparisons of age, birth weight, catecholamine levels, adrenoreceptor binding sites, and affinity constants. A χ^2 analysis was used to compare sex, socioeconomic, and racial differences between groups. Two-way analysis of variance was used to assess the impact of significant confounding variables.[34]

RESULTS

The mean (± SD) age of the control infants at the time of study was 2.5 ± 0.8 months, with a range of 1.0 to 4.0 months; seven (46%) of 15 were female. The mean age of the ISAM was 2.1 ± 0.5 months, with a range of 1.3 to 3.0 months; nine (41%) of 22 were female. The mean ages and sex distributions of the control and ISAM groups were not significantly different. Eight control infants were Hispanic, five were non-Hispanic white, one was black, and one was Asian. Seven ISAM were Hispanic, three were non-Hispanic white, and 12 were black. There was a higher proportion of black infants in the ISAM group ($P<.02$). Six control families were receiving public assistance, whereas all but one ISAM family was receiving public assistance ($P<.01$).

All infants were born at term as defined in the "Patients and Methods" section. The mean birth weight for the controls was 3297 ± 570 g, compared with 2703 ± 410 g for the ISAM group ($P<.01$). Six (27%) of the ISAM weighed between 2100 and 2500 g; one control infant weighed less than 2500 g. All infants in both groups were thriving at the time of study, with no difference in the rate of growth between the two groups; all were free of intercurrent illnesses and required no medications.

All ISAM were exposed to cocaine for either all or part of gestation (range, 3 to 9 months). Five ISAM were also exposed to opiates, two were exposed to phencyclidine, four were exposed to alcohol, and eight were exposed to tobacco. Nine ISAM had a history of positive urine toxicologic tests for cocaine at the time of birth in mother and/or baby. One ISAM had a positive methadone toxicologic test. Ten ISAM were judged to have signs of neonatal abstinence syndrome using a scoring system proposed by Finnegan.[6,26] One ISAM required chlorpromazine for symptoms of neonatal abstinence for the first 48 hours of life.

Samples for dopamine, epinephrine, and norepinephrine analyses were successfully obtained and analyzed from all 22 ISAM. Analysis was performed for β-adrenergic receptors on 18 ISAM and for α-adrenergic receptors on 14 ISAM. Samples for norepinephrine were obtained and analyzed from 15 control infants, for epinephrine from 13 infants, for dopamine from 11 infants, for β-receptors from 11 infants, and for α-receptors from seven infants.

The mean plasma norepinephrine level was 1.8-fold higher in the ISAM than in control infants ($P<.025$). There were no significant differences in the mean plasma dopamine or epinephrine levels (Table 1). There were no significant differences in the number of binding sites or receptor affinity for either β- or α-adrenergic receptors (Table 2).

The range of postnatal ages was somewhat greater for control infants than for ISAM. However, there was no significant difference in the norepinephrine levels between the 21 infants 2 months or younger (ISAM plus controls) vs the 16 infants 2 months or older (4.97 ± 2.78 nmol/L vs 5.47 ± 4.66 nmol/L, respectively). There were more black infants and infants with a birth weight of less than 2500 g in the ISAM group. However, no significant differences were revealed by comparing results between the 13 total blacks and the 24 total nonblacks (6.32 ± 3.61 nmol/L vs 4.57 ± 3.61 nmol/L) or by comparing the seven total low-birth-weight infants with the 30 higher-birth-weight infants (7.78 ± 4.74 nmol/L vs 4.58 ± 3.14 nmol/L).

Almost all ISAM (21 of 22) were receiving public assistance as compared with six of 15 controls. There were significant independent effects of both a history of maternal substance abuse ($P<.025$) and socioeconomic status ($P<.01$) on mean plasma norepinephrine levels demonstrated by two-way analysis of variance. The mean plasma norepinephrine level was 6.12 ± 3.61 nmol/L for all 27 infants requiring public assistance (ISAM plus controls) vs 2.65 ± 2.51 nmol/L for the 10 infants who did not require public assistance.

There were no differences between

ISAM who had positive vs negative urine toxicologic tests (6.53±4.24 nmol/L vs 6.10±3.47 nmol/L) or between those who experienced neonatal abstinence syndrome vs those who did not (6.53±4.31 nmol/L vs 6.93±2.83 nmol/L).

COMMENT

Perinatal substance abuse results in a number of significant consequences for the newborn, including an increased likelihood of premature birth, growth retardation, abnormalities of sleep-related respiratory control, increased incidence of SIDS, and neurodevelopmental abnormalities.[2-16,28] We have shown that ISAM between 1 and 3 months of age have an elevated mean plasma norepinephrine level. This finding is suggestive of increased sympathetic nervous system tone. This is consistent with clinical descriptions by Dixon[6] of a prolonged withdrawal syndrome in cocaine-exposed infants witnessed between 2 and 8 weeks of age.

The development of catecholaminergic neurons in the human fetus occurs between the seventh and 17th weeks of gestation.[35] This is an early-appearing system that has been hypothesized to play a role in the regulation of neural cell proliferation and differentiation and in the organization of specific neural circuitry.[36] Kellogg and Guillet[37] have hypothesized that interference with specific neurotransmitter function during fetal development could have profound consequences on subsequent brain function, although they state that precisely how a drug will influence developing neurons is difficult to predict.

The mechanism of action of cocaine is to increase neurotransmitter concentrations at the noradrenergic, serotonergic, and dopaminergic synapses by blocking reuptake. This leads to depletion of these neurotransmitters and their precursors.[17,18] With long-term cocaine exposure and neurotransmitter depletion, postsynaptic suprasensitivity develops.[17] Studies of animals following cocaine withdrawal reveal increases in brain α- and β-adrenergic and dopaminergic receptor sensitivity.[17] Opiate addiction results in an increase in the number of brain α_2- and β-adrenergic receptors.[21] Although we could not measure brain adrenergic receptor function in ISAM, changes in adrenoreceptor binding on circulating lymphocytes and platelets have been postulated to reflect changes in adrenoreceptors in other tissues.[24] Several studies have demonstrated decreases or down-regulation in lymphocyte β-adrenoreceptor binding in response to β-agonists or increased endogenous catecholamines.[38-40] We found no difference in adrenergic receptor density or affinity in ISAM despite elevated levels of circulating norepinephrine. It is possible that a lack of receptor down-regulation may enhance adrenergic activity in ISAM.

Infants from families with a lower socioeconomic status, as indicated by a requirement for public assistance, had a higher mean plasma norepinephrine level than infants with a higher socioeconomic status, independent of maternal substance abuse history. Therefore, environmental factors may be associated with alterations in sympathetic nervous system function. However, nurturing ISAM in a quiet, calm environment is the first line of treatment for neonatal abstinence syndrome.[6-8] All of the caretakers of the ISAM in this study received careful education by the hospital discharge unit and follow-up clinic in limiting environmental stimuli. Therefore, it is unlikely that the independent effect of maternal substance abuse on plasma norepinephrine levels can be explained by environmental factors. The impact of socioeconomic status and environment on sympathetic nervous system function in infants requires further study, as do the physiologic responses of ISAM to stressful environments.

Although the ISAM were thriving at the time of study, they were smaller at birth than control infants, despite being similar in estimated gestational age. We did not find a difference in catecholamine levels in the ISAM with a birth weight less than 2500 g vs ISAM with higher birth weights. However, newborn infants who are small for gestational age have been described as having a number of physiologic differences in metabolism and endocrine functions.[41] Another possible alteration in the fetal environment induced by cocaine exposure in particular is chronic hypoxia. Studies of cocaine exposure in pregnant ewes demonstrate contraction of uterine blood vessels, suggesting exposure to chronic hypoxia is present in cocaine-exposed infants.[42] Chronic hypoxia during fetal development may have contributed to our findings, as all of the ISAM in this study were exposed to cocaine. Shaul and coworkers[43] have demonstrated impaired release of catecholamines in an animal model of intrauterine growth retardation induced by fetal hypoxia. They did not, however, find a difference in baseline plasma norepinephrine levels.[43] Whether the differences in circulating norepinephrine that we have shown are a direct effect of maternal substance abuse or are secondary to an indirect effect, such as growth retardation or hypoxia, is not clear.

Infants of substance-abusing mothers are at an increased risk of dying of SIDS and have been reported to have abnormalities of their ventilatory patterns during sleep.[9-16,28] All ISAM and control infants included in this study were between 1 and 4 months of age, which coincides with the age of peak risk for SIDS.[27,28] Infants with unexplained apnea (apnea of infancy), another group of infants at increased risk for SIDS, have also been shown to have elevated levels of circulating catecholamines.[44,45] Studies of infants who have died of SIDS have shown increased concentrations of dopamine and norepinephrine in their carotid bodies at postmortem examination.[46] Both norepinephrine and dopamine have been postulated to be central respiratory inhibitors.[47-49] Norepinephrine and dopamine do not cross the blood-brain barrier, and, therefore, our findings in ISAM and the studies of infants with apnea of infancy are only relevant to the function of the sympathetic nervous system. However, the relationship between the abnormalities of sleep-related respiratory control, increased risk for SIDS, and central catecholamine neurotransmitter systems in ISAM and infants with apnea of infancy may be an important avenue for future research.

In summary, we have demonstrated a higher mean plasma norepinephrine level in a group of infants exposed to substances of abuse during fetal development. This finding is consistent with increased sympathetic nervous system tone and may be associated with the neurodevelopmental abnormalities seen in ISAM. Whether this is a direct consequence of drug exposure or is mediated via a secondary effect such as growth retardation or chronic hypoxia is not known.

This research was supported, in part, by grants from American Lung Association of Los Angeles County; National Institutes of Health Biomedical Research Support grant 2 SO7 RRO5469-27 (Childrens Hospital of Los Angeles); the Greater Los Angeles and Washington State Chapters of the National Sudden Infant Death Foundation; the Los Angeles County, Orange County, and Inland Empire Chapters of the Guild for Infant Survival; Junior Women's Club of Orange; and the Ruth and Vernon Taylor Foundation.

Thomas G. Keens, MD, gave thoughtful comments, and Gary Williams assisted in preparation of the manuscript.

References

1. *National Household Survey on Drug Abuse: Population Estimates, 1985.* Rockville, Md: Department of Health and Human Services; 1987. US Dept of Health and Human Services publication 871539.

2. Zuckerman B, Frank DA, Hingson E, et al. Effects of maternal marijuana and cocaine use on fetal growth. *N Engl J Med.* 1989;320:762-768.

3. Chasnoff IJ, Burns WJ, Schnoll SH, Burns KA. Cocaine use in pregnancy. *N Engl J Med.* 1985;313:666-669.

4. Doberczak TM, Shanzer S, Senie RT, Kandall SR. Neonatal, neurologic and encephalographic effects of intrauterine cocaine exposure. *J Pediatr.* 1985;113:354-358.

5. Oro AS, Dixon SD. Perinatal cocaine and methamphetamine exposure: maternal and neonatal correlates. *J Pediatr.* 1987;111:571-578.

6. Dixon SD. Effects of transplacental exposure to cocaine and methamphetamine on the neonate. *West J Med.* 1989;150:436-442.

7. Deren S. Children of substance abusers: a review of the literature. *J Subst Abuse Treat.* 1986;3:77-94.

8. Rosen TS, Johnson HL. Children of methadone-maintained mothers: follow-up to 18 months of age. *J Pediatr.* 1982;101:192-196.

9. Chavez CJ, Ostrea EM, Styker JC, Smialek Z. Sudden infant death syndrome among infants of drug-dependent mothers. *J Pediatr.* 1979;95:407-409.

10. Pierson PS, Howard P, Kleber HD. Sudden death in infants born to methadone-maintained addicts. *JAMA.* 1972;220:1733-1734.

11. Rajegowda BK, Kandall SR, Falciglia H. Sudden infant death (SIDS) in infants of narcotic-addicted mothers. *Pediatr Res.* 1976;10:334. Abstract.

12. Finnegan LP, Reeser DS. The incidence of sudden death in infants born to women maintained on methadone. *Pediatr Res.* 1978;12:405. Abstract.

13. Chasnoff I, Hunt C, Kletter R, Kaplan D. Prenatal cocaine exposure is associated with respiratory abnormalities. *AJDC.* 1989;143:582-587.

14. Ward SLD, Schuetz S, Krishna V, et al. Abnormal sleeping ventilatory pattern in infants of substance abuse mothers. *AJDC.* 1986;140:1015-1020.

15. Braniff K, Sotomayor JL. Pneumograms in infants of cocaine abusing mothers: asymptomatic vs ALTE. *Pediatr Pulmonol.* 1989;5:260. Abstract.

16. Riley JG, Porat R. Abnormal pneumograms (PNG) in infants with in utero cocaine exposure. *Pediatr Res.* 1987;21:262A. Abstract.

17. Dackis CA, Gold MS. New concepts in cocaine addiction: the dopamine depletion hypothesis. *Neurosci Biobehav Rev.* 1985;9:469-477.

18. Wise RA. Neural mechanisms of the reinforcing action of cocaine. In: Grabowski J, ed. *Cocaine: Pharmacology, Effects and Treatment of Abuse.* Rockville, Md: National Institute on Drug Abuse; 1984;50:15-33. NIDA Research Monograph.

19. Lau C, Bartolme M, Slotkin TA. Development of central and peripheral catecholaminergic systems in rats addicted perinatally to methadone. *Neuropharmacology.* 1977;16:473-478.

20. Mulder AH, Schoffelmeer ANM. Catecholamine and opiate receptors, presynaptic inhibition of CNS neurotransmitter release and adenylate cyclase. *Advances in Cyclic Nucleotide and Protein Phosphorylation Research.* 1985;19:273-285.

21. Hamburg M, Tallman JF. Chronic morphine administration increases the apparent number of $\alpha_2$adrenergic receptors in rat brain. *Nature (London).* 1981;291:493-495.

22. Linsell CR, Lightman SL, Mullen PE, Brown MJ, Causon RC. Circadian rhythms of epinephrine and norepinephrine in man. *J Clin Endocrinol Metab.* 1985;60:1210-1215.

23. Cryer PE. Physiology and pathophysiology of the human sympathoadrenal neuroendocrine system. *N Engl J Med.* 1980;303:436-444.

24. Motulsky HJ, Insel PA. Adrenoreceptors in man. *N Engl J Med.* 1982;307:18-29.

25. Lubchenco LO, Koops BL. Assessment of weight and gestational age. In: Avery GB, ed. *Neonatology, Pathophysiology and Management of the Newborn.* Philadelphia, Pa: JB Lippincott Co; 1987:235-257.

26. Finnegan LP. Neonatal abstinence. In: Nelson M, ed. *Current Therapy in Neonatal-Perinatal Medicine 1985-86.* Burlington, Ontario: BC Decker; 1986:262-270.

27. Shannon DC, Kelly DH. SIDS and near SIDS. *N Engl J Med.* 1982;306:1022-1028.

28. Ward SLD, Bautista DB, Derry MK, et al. Incidence of SIDS in infants of substance abuse mothers. *Pediatr Res.* 1989;24:106A. Abstract.

29. Boyum A. A one-stage procedure for isolation of granulocytes and lymphocytes from human blood. *Scand J Clin Lab Invest.* 1986;97(suppl):51-89.

30. Brodde OE, Engel G, Hoyer D, Boch KO, Weber F. The beta-adrenergic receptor in human lymphocytes: subclassification by the use of new radioligand (^{125}I)-cyanopindolol. *Life Sci.* 1981;29:2189-2198.

31. Motulsky HJ, Shattil SJ, Insel PA. Characterization of alpha-adrenergic receptors on human platelets using (^{3}H) yohimbine. *Biochem Biophys Res Commun.* 1980;97:1562-1570.

32. Scatchard G. The attractions of proteins for small molecules and ions. *Ann N Y Acad Sci.* 1949;51:660-672.

33. Passon PG, Peuler JD. A simplified radiometric assay for plasma norepinephrine and epinephrine. *Anal Biochem.* 1973;51:618-631.

34. Snedecor DW, Cochran WG. *Statistical Methods.* 6th ed. Ames, Iowa: Iowa State University Press; 1967.

35. Miller RK, Kellogg CK, Saltzman RA. Reproductive and perinatal toxicology. In: Berndt WO, Haley W, eds. *Fundamentals of Toxicology.* Washington, DC: Hemisphere Publishing Corp; 1987:159-309.

36. Coyle JT, Henry D. Catecholamines in fetal and newborn rat brain. *J Neurochem.* 1973;18: 2061-2075.

37. Kellogg CK, Guillet R. Developmental effects of neuroactive drugs. In: Scarpelli DG, Migaki G, eds. *Transplacental Effects on Fetal Health.* New York, NY: Alan R Liss Inc; 1988:265-277.

38. Brodde OE, Brinkmann M, Schmeuth R, O'Hara W, Daul A. Terbutaline-induced desensitization of human lymphocyte beta$_2$ adrenoreceptor responses: accelerated restoration of beta adrenoreceptor responsiveness by prednisone and ketotifen. *J Clin Invest.* 1985;76:1096-1110.

39. Fraser J, Nadeau J, Robertson D, Wood AJJ. Regulation of human leukocyte beta receptors by endogenous catecholamines: relationship of leukocyte beta receptor density to the cardiac sensitivity to isoproterenol. *J Clin Invest.* 1981;67:1777-1784.

40. Reinhardt D, Becker B, Nagel-Hienke M, et al. Influence of beta receptor-agonist and glucocorticoids on alpha and beta adrenoreceptors of isolated blood cells from asthmatic children. *Pediatr Pharmacol.* 1983;3:293-302.

41. Cassady G, Strange M. The small for gestational age (SGA) infant. In: Avery GB, ed. *Neonatology: Pathophysiology and Management of the Newborn.* Philadelphia, Pa: JB Lippincott Co; 1987:299-331.

42. Woods JR, Plessinger MA, Clark KE. Effects of cocaine on uterine blood flow and fetal oxygenation. *JAMA.* 1987;257:957-961.

43. Shaul PW, Cha CM, Oh W. Neonatal sympathoadrenal response to acute hypoxia: impairment after experimental intrauterine growth retardation. *Pediatr Res.* 1989;25:466-472.

44. Rodriguez T, Warburton D, Keens T. Elevated catecholamines and absent hypoxic arousal responses in apnea of infancy. *Pediatrics.* 1987; 79:269-274.

45. Bader D, Keens TG, Buckley S, Warburton D. Decreased lymphocyte beta-adrenergic receptor binding and increased serum norepinephrine in persistent apnea of infancy. *Pediatr Res.* 1987; 21:209A. Abstract.

46. Perrin DG, Becker LE, Madapallimatum A. Sudden infant death syndrome: increased carotid-body dopamine and noradrenaline content. *Lancet.* 1984;2:535-537.

47. Welsh MJ, Heistad DD, Abboud FM. Depression of ventilation by dopamine in man: evidence for an effect on the chemoreceptor reflex. *J Clin Invest.* 1978;61:708-713.

48. Feinsilver SH, Barrows AA, Mair RG, McEntee WJ. Increased CO_2 responses in Korsakoff's syndrome: evidence for the role of the noradrenergic system in respiratory controls in humans. *Am Rev Respir Dis.* 1985;131:A298. Abstract.

49. Rosen JM, Feinsilver SH, Friedman JH. Increased CO_2 responsiveness in Parkinson's disease: evidence for a role of CNS dopamine in ventilatory control. *Am Rev Respir Dis.* 1985;131:A297. Abstract.

Special Contribution

Women in Medicine

Fantasies, Dreams, Myths, and Realities

Catherine DeAngelis, MD

When little girls and young women discuss their thoughts about medical careers, listeners often consider the thoughts to be fantasies. The same thoughts of little boys and young men are considered to be dreams. The difference in reactions to illusions or capricious images (fantasies) vs conceived possibilities or probabilities (dreams) has stymied the budding careers of many women. These reactions, added to the myths regarding women and men, threaten the future of the medical profession in the United States. I hope to convince you of this by reviewing the current status of women in medicine and proposing alternatives to alleviate the problem.

The gender gap in pay and occupations has narrowed during three periods of American history: the industrial revolution (1820 to 1850), the period from 1900 to 1930 in which there was a dramatic increase in white collar jobs, and now.[1] The current trend involves women entering higher-paying jobs and professions, such as business—which is the first choice of women and men—law, and medicine.

There are many indications that this trend will continue. According to the US Bureau of Labor Statistics, women have been earning more bachelor degrees than men since the mid-1980s. The current ratio is 1.1:1.0. Further, women now earn one third of all professional degrees, compared with fewer than 5% in 1960. Thirty percent of working women are professionals or managers, which is the same proportion as men. Women represent 30% of all physicians, a marked increase from the 5% between 1900 and 1960. There is every indication that this rise will continue. According to Bickel,[2] the number of women entering medical schools peaked at 12 476 in 1984 and has slightly declined since then to a level of 10 411 in 1987. On the other hand, the number of male applicants peaked in 1974 at 33 912 and has been declining dramatically since then, with 17 712 applying in 1987.

At least three major reasons account for the drastic rise of women in the general work force. First, there are more jobs available than capable men to fill them. This has been true in all fields, including science and the military. Second, the expectations of women and, to some degree, men have been elevated with advanced education and experience. Third, discrimination is decreasing, although it is still prevalent. Currently, blatant discrimination is not well tolerated in many areas, but it has been replaced by innuendo.

One example of how discrimination still exists in medicine is that while 37% of new entrants to medical schools in 1987 were women, the range was from 11% to 60%. The proportion of women in southern and north central medical schools has been consistently lower than in other schools.[3] However, the responsibility for the difference has not been determined. Is this difference a reflection of regional differences in women's attitudes regarding medicine as a career and/or the beliefs of the admissions committees?

The drastic influx of women into the medical profession has caused some anxiety and a great deal of discussion at many levels. Some of the anxiety is based on long-held myths and some on long-standing social mores. It is worthwhile to explore some of those that have had a great impact on medicine.

SCHOLARSHIP

One common myth, ie, something existing only in the imagination, is that thinking and reasoning are gender specific. Some persons act as if they actually believe in distinct testicular thoughts and ovarian ideas. Further, men generally are seen as assertive, dominant, worldly, tough, and nonemotional, while women are generally perceived as servile, gullible, weak, and emotionally labile.[4] In fact, thinking and reasoning is at most gender *related*, not gender *specific*. Crossovers are possible and desirable.

There has always been little difference between men and women in academic performance in medical school,[5] and the rate of attrition never has been significantly different.[6] While women's performances are slightly lower on standardized tests in the first 2 years of medical school, there is no significant difference in the last 2 years or during residency. Women are just as likely as men to be selected to honor societies.

Norcini et al[7] reported that women specializing in internal medicine were less likely to pass the certifying examinations, but this difference narrowed markedly to a level of 80% for women and 86% for men in 1986, the last year

Accepted for publication July 11, 1990.
From the Department of Pediatrics, The Johns Hopkins University, Baltimore, Md.
Presented as the Armstrong Award Address, Ambulatory Pediatrics Association, Anaheim, Calif, May 10, 1990.
Reprint requests to The Johns Hopkins School of Medicine, Administration 106, 720 Rutland Ave, Baltimore, MD 21205 (Dr DeAngelis).

data were examined. Further, this variance has been shown to be related to age and the quality of the medical school, and proportionally there are more female than male graduates of foreign medical schools in the United States. Certifying examination data from other specialties, including pediatrics and family medicine, show little or no differences between women and men.[8,9]

Interestingly, in one study, the best predictors of men's clerkship grades were their cognitive characteristics, but noncognitive characteristics contributed more to predicting women's subsequent performance.[10] One can only conjecture about differences in the evaluators' expectations of the students.

SPECIALTY CHOICES

Women generally choose different specialties than men, with the primary care specialties predominating. For instance, 65% of pediatric residents are women and comparable figures for other specialties are 46% in obstetrics-gynecology and 41% in psychiatry. On the other hand, only 4% of surgical residents are women.[11,12] Is this a reflection of believed capabilities and/or of acceptance in these specialties?

FINANCIAL ISSUES

Generally, women graduate from medical school in more debt than men. The difference in 1987 was $3000. Further, women make less money than men in comparable positions.[13] In 1986, the median female physician's earnings were $73 100 vs $118 000 for men. However, this does represent an improvement from 1983, when the comparable figures were $57 000 and $110 000, respectively. This phenomenon is probably related to specialty choices, total number of hours worked, number of patients seen, and relative nonassertiveness in negotiating salaries.

Female physicians are less likely to be self-employed (52% vs 77%). They also see fewer patients per week (12 vs 99), but care for more new patients and spend more time with all patients. Women work fewer hours per week on average than men (52.5 vs 58.2), but recent trends show a convergence with men.[14] Also, there is less difference in hours worked with advancing age, and this difference will dissipate as the proportion of older female physicians increases.[15] Finally, physicians on average live longer than other Americans, and female physicians live 4 to 5 years longer than male physicians. It is sad that we waste so much of the extra years waiting in line to enter women's restrooms.

CHILDBEARING AND CARING

Another common myth is that making a baby is "man's work," while bearing and caring for the child is "woman's work." This particular myth is responsible, at least in part, for some interesting behaviors among male and female physicians. Approximately two thirds of female physicians are married, compared with 90% of all women and 90% of male physicians. The divorce rate is approximately 10% for female physicians, which is far lower than the national average, but double that of male physicians. Only about two thirds of married female physicians have children, compared with 90% of male physicians.[16] Further, they have fewer children and are older when they have them.[16,17] This is especially interesting because in a study conducted at the end of medical school, 85% to 90% of men and women said they wanted to have children.[18] Consider what a terrible waste of human genetic potential this represents.

Many studies and commentaries in the literature deal with maternity leave. Most have found that female physicians are at increased risk of adverse pregnancy outcome.[19-22] This increased risk probably reflects, at least in part, the long working hours and psychological stress endured by pregnant physicians.

In a study by Levinson et al,[23] the median amount of time off for pregnancy was 6 weeks post partum, with 72% of women taking no time off before delivery and 83% returning to work within 12 weeks. Interestingly, I could find nothing in the literature about the amount of time missed by male physicians because of cardiovascular or other common male health issues. We apparently react more rationally and compassionately to issues related to male biology.

Men and women have different roles in household and child caring responsibilities. For example, in a study of family practitioners, 95% to 99% of husbands of physicians worked outside the home, regardless of whether the couple had children, compared with 70% of the wives of physicians with no children and 25% of those with children.[24]

Female physicians must rely on full-time household help, day care, and relatives to provide child care.[25] Fewer than 5% of husbands of physicians take major responsibilities, compared with 50% of wives of physicians taking full responsibilities and an additional 33% making a major contribution to child care.[17,24] There are some indications that this is changing, but it is happening slowly and there is still a great deal of feeling about the subject. For example, a recent study showed that 30% of physicians felt "a significant risk to the optimal functioning of a department that hired a female of childbearing age."[26]

There can be no doubt that child care has had a profound effect on female physicians. Although pregnancies during residencies are common and usually planned, most institutions are unprepared for them.[27] Many programs have no specific maternity leave policies and I could find none with a specific plan for covering the work load of women on leave. In one recent study, no men but 44% of female physicians said they had changed career plans because of family responsibilities.[17] In another study, women said they specifically sought shorter, regular working hours because of family responsibilities.[28] While it is absolutely true that children need mothers, it is not true that the nurturing role must be totally assumed by women.

ACADEMIC PRODUCTIVITY

For the past 30 years, women have been more likely than men to enter academic medicine. However, they have not achieved the same success as men. In the only published national study that I could find, female faculty members in internal medicine were less involved in research than were men except at the professorial level. Zuckerman[29] reported that male residents publish about twice as many articles as their female counterparts. In another study, women in internal medicine had less research funding from the National Institutes of Health despite the same proportion of time reportedly devoted to research.[30] Based on my experience, I wonder if the devoted research time was eroded equally among men and women by administrative and service demands.

Also, there is evidence that education and support are different for women and that gender biases remain. For example, Beaty et al[31] found that 16% of men but 29% of women faculty members had no research training. Requests for support to attend professional development conferences were granted more often to men despite identical justification and credentials.[32] Women in internal medicine are less likely to have assigned research space.[30] Finally, when college students were asked to review articles that were identical except for the fictitious names of the authors, those with male authors were consistently rated more positively.[33] These college students might well reflect tomorrow's leaders in medicine.

ACADEMIC SUCCESS

All phases of medical practice are highly dependent on medical school, residency, and fellowship education and training. Therefore, emphasis must be placed on the academic centers, and much work is needed. While the absolute numbers and proportions of female faculty members have increased dramatically during the past two decades, there is still great discrepancy in ranks. The problem of nonpromotion appears to lie primarily at the level of the chairman rather than with the promotion committees. Interestingly, there is no association between family size and academic rank.[34]

ADMINISTRATIVE LEADERSHIP

A profound lack of female physicians in academic leadership positions exists. In 1988, two (1.6%) of 127 deans, 11% of associate deans, 22% of assistant deans, and 3% of chairpersons were women. Nine (13%) of these chairs were in pediatrics. This is a self-perpetuating problem since people are generally more comfortable in situations in which there are more than a few of a similar kind or type.[35] Also, academic leaders make the rules, and the rules must be changed.

MOLDERS, MODELS, AND MENTORS

The roles of molders, models, and mentors cannot be overemphasized. A *molder* is one who shapes. This shaping begins at birth and is greatly influenced by parents and others with whom the child has consistent contact. General social molding of a child depends a great deal on gender stereotypes. While the pace for change is increasing, a great deal of gender stereotyping exists. Gender stereotypes are still widespread and deeply ingrained in society, such as in children's books,[36] commercials,[37,38] and comic strips.[39] This is unfortunate since such stereotyping is a vehicle for discrimination against women and restricts personal fulfillment for both men and women.[40]

Models are generally persons who have skills or traits that are lacking in others and from whom one can learn by observation and comparison.[41] It is vital for female physicians to have female role models who lead successful professional and personal lives.

Mentors are generally older, more experienced professionals who sponsor, encourage, and support younger members and their career advancement.[42] It is necessary for female physicians to have female mentors. In one study, female physicians with lower-ranking female mentors received more advice and had fewer problems retaining their autonomy. However, the mentors' academic or administrative rank was the chief determinant of sponsoring effectiveness. Success was unrelated to gender.[43] This is encouraging data owing to the relative paucity of female mentors. However, data emphasize the importance of male academic leaders assuming the responsibility for being mentors (not tormentors) of promising young female physicians. This must occur at least until a "critical mass" of female mentors is available who will, it is hoped, serve long afterwards as mentors for young men as well as women.

The thought of a woman becoming a successful physician changes from a fantasy to a dream when gender stereotyping disappears. I am convinced that the most effective method of altering the gender stereotyping of a male physician is for him to have a talented daughter who wants to enter the medical profession. This whole issue would be moot within one generation if all male physicians had no sons and at least one daughter interested in medicine. Of course, this is ludicrous, and other, more rational strategies exist. I propose the following six steps:

1. For the long term, we must begin with our own children, grandchildren, and patients to engender the similarities in intellect, creativity, and general abilities in men and women. Medicine needs the talents of both.
2. For the short term, those in higher ranks (mostly men) need to be mentors for deserving women as well as men.
3. It is vitally important to have a critical mass of female leaders. To achieve this end, women must receive equal promotions, salaries, scientific training, and research space as comparable men. This requires a specific plan or program in every medical school.
4. The clock for academic training and promotions must be altered to meet the biologic needs of the human race. Childbearing is *not* a "woman's problem." It is an issue for everyone.
5. Insurance to hire people to fill in for those on maternity or illness leave must be built into every program.
6. Appropriate child-care facilities must be made available to all physicians. Again, this is *not* a woman's issue. More male physicians are becoming involved in the care of their children, and whether or not they are, the care of children affects all of us.

Most importantly, the special biologic needs of women must not be seen as *women's* issues but rather as basic human qualities of importance to both men and women. Only when highly talented women, unencumbered by unnecessary social constraints, can join the ranks of highly talented men can the success of the medical profession be ensured. Otherwise, a dwindling proportion of only half the human potential will be available to medicine.

References

1. Goldin C. *Understanding the Gender Gap: An Economic History of American Women.* New York, NY: Oxford University Press Inc; 1990.
2. Bickel J. Women in medical education. *N Engl J Med.* 1988;319:1579-1584.
3. Jacobson SJ, Rimm AA. Regional differences in the proportion of women among first year medical students in the United States. *J Med Educ.* 1986;61:911-913.
4. Spence JT, Helmreich RL, Holahan CK. Neg-

ative and positive components of psychological masculinity and femininity and their relationship to self reports of neurotic and acting out behaviors. *J Pers Soc Psychol.* 1979;37:1973-1982.

5. Harward DH, Lyons CM, Porter CQ, Hunter RS. A comparison of the performance of male and female medical students and residents. *J Med Educ.* 1981;56:853-855.

6. Barondess JA. Are women different? Some trends in the assimilation of women in medicine. *J Am Med Wom Assoc.* 1981;36:95-104.

7. Day SC, Norcini JJ, Shea JA, Benson JA Jr. Gender differences in the clinical competence of residents in internal medicine. *J Gen Intern Med.* 1989;4:309-312.

8. Brownlee RC, Butzin DW. Are women that different? *J Am Med Wom Assoc.* 1981;36:378.

9. Ellsbury KR, Schneeweiss DE, Montano KC, Gordon KC, Kuykendall D. Gender differences and practice characteristics of graduates of family medicine residency. *J Med Educ.* 1987;162:895-903.

10. Calkins EV, Arnold LM, Willoughby TL. Gender differences in predictors of performance in medical training. *J Med Educ.* 1987;62:682-685.

11. Crowley AE, Etzel SI. Graduate medical education in the United States. *JAMA.* 1988; 260:1093-1101.

12. Roback G. Randolph L, Seidman B, Mead D. *Physician Characteristics and Distribution in the US, 1986.* Chicago, Ill: American Medical Association; 1987.

13. Brown S. Why the gender gap in earnings remains huge. *Med Econ.* 1985;62:173-186.

14. American Medical Association Center for Health Policy Research. *Socioeconomic Monitoring System Report.* Chicago, Ill: American Medical Association; 1987.

15. Kletke PR, Marder WD, Silberger AB. The growing proportion of female physicians: implications for US physician supply. *Am J Public Health.* 1990;80:300-304.

16. Schermerhorn GR, Colliver JA, Verhulst ST, Schmidt EL. Factors that influence career patterns of women physicians. *J Am Med Wom Assoc.* 1986;41:74-78.

17. Nadelson LL, Notman MT, Lowenstein P. The practice patterns, life styles and stresses of women and men entering medicine: a follow-up study of Harvard Medical School graduates from 1967-1977. *J Am Med Wom Assoc.* 1979;34:400-406.

18. Heins M. Women in medicine: two points of view, II: medicine and motherhood. *JAMA.* 1983; 249:209-210.

19. Gregant MA, Fletcher SW. Housestaff pregnancy in internal medicine residencies. *Ann Intern Med.* 1985;102:123-125.

20. Grunebaum A, Minkoff H, Blake D. Pregnancies among obstetricians: a comparison of births before, during and after residency. *Am J Obstet Gynecol.* 1987;157:79-83.

21. Miller NH, Katz VL, Cefalo RC. Pregnancies among physicians. *J Reprod Med.* 1989;34: 790-796.

22. Phelan ST. Pregnancy during residency: the decision 'to be or not to be.' *Obstet Gynecol.* 1988;72:425-436.

23. Levinson W, Tolle S, Lewis C. Women in academic medicine. *N Engl J Med.* 1989;321:1511-1517.

24. Ogle KS, Henry RC, Durda K, Zivick JD. Gender specific differences in family practice graduates. *J Fam Pract.* 1986;23:357-360.

25. Sinal S, Weavil P, Camp MG. Child care choices of women physicians. *JAMA.* 1989;44:183-184.

26. Franco K, Evans CL, Best AP, Zrull JP, Pizza GA. Conflicts associated with physicians' pregnancies. *Am J Psychiatry.* 1983;140:902-904.

27. Sayres M, Wyshak G, Denterlein G, Apfel R, Shore E, Federman D. Pregnancy during residency. *N Engl J Med.* 1986;314:418-423.

28. Ferrier BM, Woodward CA. Career choices, work patterns, and preceptors of undergraduate education of McMaster medical graduates: comparison between men and women. *Can Med Assoc J.* 1982;126:1411-1414.

29. Zuckerman H. Persistence and change in the careers of men and women scientists and engineers: a review of current research. In: Dix LS, ed. *Women: Their Underrepresentation and Career Differentials in Science and Engineering: Proceedings of a Conference.* Washington, DC: National Academy of Sciences; 1987:127-157.

30. Levey BA, Gentile NO, Jolly HP, Beaty HN, Levey GS. Comparing research activities of women and men faculty in departments of internal medicine. *Acad Med.* 1990;65:102-106.

31. Beaty HN, Babbott D, Higgins EJ, Jolly D, Levey GS. Research activities of faculty in academic departments of medicine. *Ann Intern Med.* 1986;104:90-97.

32. Rosen B, Jerdee THE. The influence of sex role stereotypes on evaluations of male and female supervisory behavior. *J Appl Psychol.* 1973;57:44-48.

33. Paludi MA, Strayer LA. What's in an author's name? Differential evaluations of performance as a function of author's name. *Sex Roles.* 1985;12:353-361.

34. Graves PL, Thomas CB. Correlates of midlife career achievement among women physicians. *JAMA.* 1985;254:781-787.

35. Ivey ES. Recruiting more women into science and engineering. *Issues Sci Technol.* 1987;4;83-87.

36. Weitzman LJ. Sex role socialization in picture books for preschool children. *Am J Social.* 1972;77:1125-1150.

37. Geis FL, Brown V, Jennings J, Walstedt JJ, Porter N. TV commercials as achievement scripts for women. *Sex Roles.* 1984;10:513-525.

38. Schwartz LA, Markham WT. Sex stereotypes in children's toy advertisements. *Sex Roles.* 1985;12:157-170.

39. Chavez D. Perpetuation of gender inequality: a content analysis of comic strips. *Sex Roles.* 1985;13:93-103.

40. Huston AC. Sex typing. In: Mussen PH, ed. *Handbook of Child Psychology.* 4th ed. New York, NY: John Wiley & Sons Inc; 1983.

41. Kemper T. Reference groups, socialization and achievement. *Am Soc Rev.* 1968;33:31-45.

42. Speizer JJ. Role models, mentors and sponsors: the elusive concepts. *Signs.* 1981;6:692-712.

43. Ochberg RL, Barton GM, West AN. Women physicians and their mentors. *J Am Med Wom Assoc.* 1989;44:123-126.

In Other AMA Journals

ARCHIVES OF INTERNAL MEDICINE

Testing for Uncommon Conditions: The Heroic Search for Positive Test Results

Steven Woolf, MD, MPH, Douglas B. Kamerow, MD, MPH (*Arch Intern Med.* 1990;150:2451-2458)

ARCHIVES OF OTOLARYNGOLOGY—HEAD & NECK SURGERY

Why Pediatric Otolaryngology?

Steven D. Handler, MD (*Arch Otolaryngol Head Neck Surg.* 1990;116:1377)

The Efficacy of Oral Steroids in the Treatment of Persistent Otitis Media With Effusion

Ludwig Podoshin, MD; Milo Fradis, MD; Yacov Ben-David, MD; David Faraggi, PhD (*Arch Otolaryngol Head Neck Surg.* 1990;116:1404-1406)

Lumbar Puncture Frequency and Cerebrospinal Fluid Analysis in the Neonate

Jeffrey Schwersenski, MD; Lester McIntyre, MD; Charles R. Bauer, MD

• A prospective study was performed to assess the frequency and diagnostic utility of lumbar punctures in neonates both during their first week of life and thereafter. During the two 6-month periods from January 1, 1985 to June 30, 1985, and February 1, 1986 to July 31, 1986, 712 neonates underwent 728 lumbar punctures during their first week of life primarily as part of the evaluation for suspected infection, either congenital or postnatal. There were eight patients with positive spinal fluid cultures in the first week of life, but only one patient simultaneously had a positive blood culture and a clinical course consistent with meningitis. In contrast, a considerably higher yield, approximating five times that of the first week of life, was obtained in patients undergoing a lumbar puncture after the first week of life.

(*AJDC.* 1991;145:54-58)

Lumbar punctures are considered a routine part of the evaluation of neonates who are thought to exhibit signs of generalized infection. The signs of sepsis, particularly in the preterm neonate, are vague and less specific than in the term neonate or older patient. The preterm neonate is thus more likely to have a course of antibiotic treatment instituted because of clinical signs of sepsis or because of the presence of risk factors that are known to be associated with an increased incidence of sepsis. In many such cases, the lumbar puncture is often delayed because of the neonate's "unstable" condition, and antibiotic administration is begun empirically, or else the procedure is performed with the attendant risks involved. Complications of the procedure that have been described include trauma, introduction of infection, spinal epidermoid tumors, brain-stem herniation in older children, and contamination of cerebrospinal fluid (CSF) with bone marrow cells.[1-7] The use of techniques for the continuous, noninvasive monitoring of measures such as Po_2 and Pco_2 and oxygen saturation has demonstrated that significant hypoxemia occurs during handling for routine procedures, especially in sick, preterm neonates. The manipulation and positioning required for lumbar punctures have been associated with rapid clinical deterioration in neonates.[8-10]

Sepsis, with or without meningitis, is one of the more commonly encountered problems in the newborn. The incidence of systemic bacterial infection is reported to vary between one and eight per 1000 live births.[11,12] Meningitis can coexist in up to one third of neonates with sepsis. During the first month of life, the mortality for sepsis is reported to be between 10% and 30% but exceeds 30% when meningitis is superimposed. Statistically, however, the highest risk of death occurs during the first week of life, when mortality associated with infection may approach 50%.[11,12]

To evaluate the frequency and diagnostic utility of lumbar puncture and CSF analysis in the newborn, this prospective study was undertaken. The study was approved by the Subcommittee for the Protection of Human Subjects in Research at the University of Miami (Fla)/Jackson Memorial Medical Center.

PATIENTS AND METHODS

All neonates born at or transferred to the University of Miami/Jackson Memorial Medical Center who, during the two 6-month periods from January 1, 1985 to June 30, 1985, and February 1, 1986 to July 31, 1986, underwent a lumbar puncture were identified and enrolled in the study. Ventricular and shunt taps were excluded. The clinical course and treatment of the neonates were prospectively followed up. Daily records were kept of diagnoses and the results of hematologic, bacteriologic, and other significant laboratory data. Total cell counts were performed on a hemocytometer on unspun, unstained CSF specimens. Differential cell counts were performed on spun specimens, and the sediment was stained with gentian violet. The cerebrospinal fluid protein level was determined by the trichloroacetic acid method (Dupont ACA Instrument, Dupont Co, Wilmington, Del). The glucose level was measured using a glucose oxidase method (Beckman Astra Instrument, Beckman Instruments, Inc, Brea, Calif). Cerebrospinal fluid was inoculated onto thioglycolate broth, chocolate agar, 5% sheep blood agar, and an enriched 5% sheep blood agar plate. The chocolate agar plates were incubated in 4% carbon dioxide, blood agar plates were incubated aerobically, and the enriched blood agar plates were incubated anaerobically. All cultures were incubated for 72 hours before a final negative report was generated.

The neonates who underwent lumbar punctures were subclassified into two groups determined by their age at the time of the procedure: within the first week of life and thereafter.

RESULTS

During these two 6-month periods, there were a total of 11 035 admissions to the newborn services at the University of Miami/Jackson Memorial Medical Center. Of these, 826 neonates, or 7.5% of all neonatal admissions, underwent 1104 lumbar punctures. Eighty-six percent of these neonates received their lumbar punctures during the first week of life. The remaining 14%, who had their first lumbar puncture after 7 days of age, averaged slightly more than

Accepted for publication June 4, 1990.

From the Division of Neonatology, Department of Pediatrics, University of Miami, Fla.

Read in part before the Southern Society for Pediatric Research, New Orleans, La, February 7,1986.

Reprint requests to Department of Pediatrics (R-131), University of Miami, PO Box 016960, Miami, FL 33101 (Dr Bauer).

three lumbar punctures per patient (Table 1). Forty-three percent of the neonates studied during the first week were of low birth weight (≤2500 g), with 17.6% being of very low birth weight (≤1500 g) (Table 2). These low-birth-weight neonates not only represent those at greatest risk for sepsis but are also those in whom the chances of adverse effects due to the procedure are most likely.

Of the lumbar punctures performed during the first week of life, approximately 63% were done on the first day, with the percentage increasing to 91% within the first 72 hours (Table 2). Irrespective of age, suspected infection was the overwhelming indication for performing a lumbar puncture, accounting for 90% of the procedures in the first week of life and for 93% in those patients older than 1 week. In the group less than 1 week of age, the remaining lumbar punctures were performed predominantly because of a positive serologic test for syphilis. In those older than 1 week, posthemorrhagic hydrocephalus with raised intracranial pressure was the indication in the remaining cases (Table 3).

In the first week of life, it should be noted that an amount of CSF adequate for culture only was obtained in 103 patients, who were 14.5% of the total number of neonates studied. This was usually because of technical difficulties, which occurred most often (51.5%) in neonates of low birth weight. An additional 98 patients (13.8%) had a "bloody" CSF sample, which was defined using the criteria of Visser and Hall,[13] that is, having a red blood cell count higher than 10×10^9/L. This finding was again more frequent in the low-birth-weight neonates, accounting for 63.1% of the total cases (Table 4).

Of the total of 712 patients having a lumbar puncture performed during the first week of life, only nine CSF cultures were positive. This represents a yield (by patients) of 1.3% (Table 5). Of these nine positive cultures, six yielded *Staphylococcus epidermidis*. In all of them, this was believed to be a contaminant, as the neonates had neither cytologic results consistent with infected CSF nor a clinical course consistent with meningitis. Four of the neonates whose cultures yielded *S epidermidis* were treated with intravenous antibiotics for 3 days; the other two neonates were treated for 7 and 10 days, respectively. None of the six neonates had a simultaneously positive blood culture.

The remaining three cultures yielded *Streptococcus viridans* in one case, group B *Streptococcus* in another, and a *Bacillus* species in one of the neonates whose culture yielded *S epidermidis* 24 hours later on a repeated CSF culture. Cytologic results in two of these neonates were not consistent with an infected CSF, and simultaneous blood cul-

Table 1.—Patients Undergoing Lumbar Puncture and Age at Initial Lumbar Puncture

	Study Period 1, Jan 1 to Jun 30, 1985	Study Period 2, Feb 1 to Jul 31, 1986	Total
Total No. of admissions	5423	5612	**11 035**
No. (%) of patients undergoing lumbar puncture	355 (6.5)	471 (8.4)	**826** (7.5)
No. of lumbar punctures performed	484	620	**1104**
Age, d			
≤7			
Patients, No. (%)	298 (84)	414 (88)	**712** (86)
Lumbar punctures, No.	304	424	**728**
>7			
Patients, No. (%)	57 (16)	57 (12)	**114** (14)
Lumbar punctures, No.	180	196	**376**

Table 2.—Patients in First Week of Life by Birth Weight and by Age at Initial Lumbar Puncture*

	Study Period 1 (n=298)	Study Period 2 (n=414)	Total (n=712)
Birth weight, g			
>2500	156 (52.3)	248 (59.9)	**404** (56.7)
≤2500	142 (47.7)	166 (40.1)	**308** (43.3)
1501-2500	80 (26.8)	103 (24.9)	**183** (25.7)
≤1500	62 (20.8)	63 (15.2)	**125** (17.6)
Age, h			
0-24	175 (58.7)	273 (65.9)	**448** (62.9)
25-72	94 (31.5)	106 (25.6)	**200** (28.1)
>72	29 (9.7)	35 (8.5)	**64** (9.0)

*Values are number (percent).

Table 3.—Indications for Lumbar Puncture

		Age, d				
		≤7				>7
Indication	Study	0-24 h	25-72 h	>72 h	Total	
Suspected infection	1	170	59	23	**252**	51
	2	269	85	32	**386**	55
	Total	**439**	**144**	**55**	**638** (90%)	**106** (93%)
Positive serologic study	1	1	29	4	34	0
	2	3	18	2	23	0
	Total	**4**	**47**	**6**	**57** (8%)	**0**
Both	1	4	6	2	12	0
	2	1	3	1	5	0
	Total	**5**	**9**	**3**	**17** (2%)	**0**
Raised intracranial pressure	1	0	0	0	0	6
	2	0	0	0	0	2
	Total	**0**	**0**	**0**	**0**	**8** (7%)

Table 4.—Inadequate Specimens in First Week of Life by Birth Weight Groupings

Birth Weight Group, g	Study 1 (n=298)	Study 2 (n=414)	Total (n=712)
Culture Only			
Total in group	**43** (14.4)	**60** (14.5)	**103** (14.5)
>2500	15 (34.9)	35 (58.3)	**50** (48.5)
≤2500	28 (65.1)	25 (41.7)	**53** (51.5)
1501-2500	11 (25.6)	15 (25)	**26** (25.2)
≤1500	17 (39.5)	10 (16.7)	**27** (26.2)
Bloody Specimen			
Total in group	**39** (13.1)	**59** (14.3)	**98** (13.8)
>2500	13 (33.3)	33 (55.9)	**46** (46.9)
≤2500	26 (66.7)	26 (44.1)	**52** (53.1)
1501-2500	17 (43.6)	16 (27.1)	**33** (33.7)
≤1500	9 (23.1)	10 (17.0)	**19** (19.4)

Table 5.—Lumbar Puncture Yields

	Age, d					
	≤7			>7		
	Study 1	Study 2	Total	Study 1	Study 2	Total
No. of patients	248	414	**712**	57	57	**114**
No. of lumbar punctures	304	424	**728**	180	196	**376**
No. of positive cultures	3	6	**9**	4	4	**8**
% yield by patient	1.2	1.4	1.3	7.0	7.0	7.0
% yield by procedure	1.0	1.4	1.2	2.2	2.0	2.1
Organisms	1 group B *Streptococcus*,*, 6 *Staphylococcus epidermidis*, 1 *Streptococcus viridans*, 1 *Bacillus* species			2 *S epidermidis* (1*), 1 group B *Streptococcus*,*, 1 *Serratia marcescens*,*, 1 *Corynebacterium* species, 1 *Acinetobacter*, 1 *Pseudomonas aeruginosa*, 1 combined *S epidermidis* and *Corynebacterium* species		

*Infants in whom both cerebrospinal fluid and blood cultures were simultaneously positive.

tures were negative. These two neonates were treated with antibiotics for 5 and 3 days, respectively. In the third neonate, group B *Streptococcus* grew in cultures from both the blood and the CSF; this patient had an increased CSF white blood cell count, a positive urine Wellcogen (latex particle agglutination for B-hemolytic *Streptococcus*), and clinical signs consistent with a central nervous system infection (Table 6).

Of the 712 neonates who underwent lumbar punctures in the first week of life, 63 (8.8%) had mothers who had been treated with antibiotics immediately preceding delivery. One of these neonates had a culture positive for *S epidermidis*, but this was thought to be a contaminant, as the cytologic study results and clinical status of the neonate were benign. All of these neonates were treated for 7 to 18 days with broad-spectum antibiotics because of the maternal indication, as well as the lack of culture reliability due to circulating maternal antibiotics.

In contrast, after the first week of life, 376 lumbar punctures were performed in 114 patients. There were eight positive CSF cultures in this group, giving a yield of 7.0%, more than five times that observed during the first week of life (Table 5). Three of these eight cultures had simultaneously positive blood cultures (group B *Streptococcus*, *Serratia marcescens*, and *S epidermidis*).

The one patient with group B streptococcal meningitis had three documented episodes of sepsis with this organism. The meningitis was associated with the second episode. The neonate with *S epidermidis* infection had a clinical and hematologic course consistent with sepsis and received a 21-day course of antibiotic therapy. The patient with *Serratia* infection died within 24 hours of the diagnosis and shortly after the initiation of treatment. Of the remaining five patients with negative blood cultures, four were considered to have contaminated specimens. The fifth patient was clinically symptomatic at the time of the positive culture and received antibiotic therapy. Symptoms and signs in this patient included seizures, apnea, and increases in both CSF white blood cell count and CSF protein level (Table 6).

COMMENT

A number of lumbar punctures are performed in most neonatal special care centers for indications such as suspected sepsis, positive serologic results, and relief of increased intracranial pressure in neonates with posthemorrhagic hydrocephalus. Often the procedure is performed by transient or junior nursery staff who may not yet fully appreciate the risks involved in performing the procedure. In addition, the procedure often provides fluid sufficient for culture only, or a blood-contaminated specimen. These problems have been reported in some series to account for up to 50% of specimens, thereby potentially reducing the amount of information that may help in reaching diagnostic and therapeutic conclusions.[13] In this study, approximately 28% of the samples obtained within the first week of life were limited by either the amount of fluid obtained or blood contamination.

We did not design the study to evaluate the risk-benefit ratio of this procedure. We did not specifically monitor neonates clinically or electronically during or after the procedure to determine their tolerance. Hence, we cannot comment on the incidence of complications in this population as compared with previously reported occurrences.

If, indeed, the co-occurrence of meningitis and sepsis in the neonate approaches 30%, the performance of a lumbar puncture as part of the complete evaluation for infection can be readily justified. In this series, however, the incidence of meningitis associated with sepsis, particularly in the first week of life, was extremely low. Even in the nine instances where positive spinal fluid cultures had been obtained in neonates who were in their first week of

Table 6.—Positive CSF Cultures*

Patient No./Gestational Age, wk/Birth Weight, g	Indication for Workup	Laboratory Results	Outcome
		Patients ≤7 d Old	
1/40/3360	Maternal temperature 39°C, 1 dose ampicillin before delivery; C section for fetal distress	CSF (culture only): *Staphylococcus epidermidis;* gastric aspirate: group B *Streptococcus;* urine Wellcogen: positive; blood culture: negative	Ampicillin sodium and gentamicin sulfate for 7 d
2/38/3170	2 cyanotic episodes after birth with opisthotonus; R/O seizures	CSF: *Bacillus* species, WBCs 3×10^6/L (100% monocytes), glucose 2.2 mmol/L, protein 0.92 g/L; CBC count: normal; urine Wellcogen: negative; blood culture: negative	Ampicillin and gentamicin for 3 d
	Repeated workup 24 h after stopping antibiotic administration	CSF: *S epidermidis,* WBCs 3×10^6/L (100% monocytes), protein 0.24 g/L, glucose QNS	Vancomycin hydrochloride for 3 d; repeated LP: WBCs 6×10^6/L, culture negative
3/43/4045	Prolonged ruptured membranes 45 h 30 min	CSF: *S epidermidis,* WBC 11×10^6/L (100% monocytes), glucose 2.5 mmol/L, protein 0.47 g/L	Ampicillin and gentamicin for 3 d
4/38/3435	Tachypnea, lethargy, opisthotonus at 24 h, R/O seizures	CSF: group B streptococcus, WBCs 689×10^6/L (27% PMNs), glucose 0.0 mmol/L, protein 2.56 g/L; urine Wellcogen: positive; blood culture: group B *Streptococcus*	Penicillin sodium for 14 d
5/40/2750	Maternal temperature 32.3°C before delivery	CSF: *S epidermidis* (broth only), RBCs $81\,000 \times 10^6$/L, WBCs 68×10^6/L	Ampicillin and gentamicin for 3 d
6/40/3760	Tachypnea, hypoxemia, acidosis at 24 h	CSF: *S epidermidis,* bloody tap; CBC count: left shift; blood culture: negative	Ampicillin and gentamicin for 10 d
7/40/3840	Maternal temperature 38.9°C before delivery	CSF: *Streptococcus viridans* (broth only), bloody tap; blood culture: negative	Ampicillin and gentamicin for 5 d; repeated CSF: WBCs 0×10^6/L, culture negative
8/40/3360	Marked tachypnea after birth, R/O pneumonia	CSF: *S epidermidis* (broth only); WBCs 1×10^6/L (100% monocytes), glucose 2.0 mmol/L, protein 0.93 g/L; urine Wellcogen: negative; blood culture: negative	Ampicillin and gentamicin for 3 d
		Patients >7 d Old	
1/31/950	1 mo old: apnea and bradycardia, abdominal distention, hypoactive; required intubation	CSF: *Serratia;* gram-negative rods; blood culture: *Serratia*	Seizures: died within 24 h; treated with oxacillin sodium, amikacin sulfate, and cefotaxime sodium
2/28/830	6 w old: apnea, pallor, bulging fontanelle; required intubation; group B *Streptococcus* sepsis at birth	CSF: group B *Streptococcus,* WBCs 349×10^6/L (14% PMNs); blood culture: group B *Streptococcus;* CBC count: neutropenia	Penicillin for 21 d
3/26/930	5 mo old; chronic lung disease, grade 4 IVH on daily LPs, increasing apnea, left shift on CBC count	CSF: *Corynebacterium* (broth only), WBCs 5×10^6/L (100% monocytes), glucose 3.4 mmol/L, protein 1.24 g/L (*Pseudomonas* grew from ET tube culture)	Oxacillin and tobramycin sulfate for 7 d; repeated CSF: culture negative
	6 mo old: asymptomatic on daily LPs	CSF: *Acinetobacter,* RBCs 162×10^6/L, WBCs 1×10^6/L (100% monocytes), glucose 4.2 mmol/L, protein 1.20 g/L	Cefotaxime sodium for 3 d; repeated CSF: culture negative
4/32/1500	2½ wk old: apnea and bradycardia, seizures; required intubation	CSF: *Pseudomonas,* WBCs 4500×10^6/L (78% monocytes), glucose 0.2 mmol/L, protein 5.41 g/L	Tobramycin for 21 d; CSF after 48 h: negative
5/27/840	28 d old: apnea and bradycardia, abdominal distention, pneumatosis of intestine	CSF: *S epidermidis* (broth only), WBCs 5×10^6/L (100% monocytes), glucose 12.0 mmol/L, protein 1.96 g/L	Ampicillin, gentamicin, and oral kanamycin sulfate for 9 d; perforated NEC; died
6/28/900	2 mo old: abdominal distention, necrotizing enterocolitis	CSF: *S epidermidis* and *Corynebacterium* (late growth), WBCs 13×10^6/L (100% monocytes), glucose 1.3 mmol/L, protein 0.26 g/L	Ampicillin, gentamicin, and oral kanamycin for 14 d
7/26/800	8 d old: lethargy, acidosis, carbon dioxide retention	CSF: *S epidermidis,* WBCs 4×10^6/L (98% monocytes), glucose 6.8 mmol/L, protein 2.31 g/L; CBC count: left shift; blood culture: *S epidermidis* and *Enterobacter*	Vancomycin hydrochloride for 21 d

*CSF indicates cerebrospinal fluid; C section, cesarean section; R/O, rule out; WBCs, white blood cells; CBC, complete blood cell; QNS, quantity not sufficient; LP, lumbar puncture; PMNs, polymorphonuclear leukocytes; RBCs, red blood cells; IVH, intraventricular hemorrhage; ET, endotracheal; and NEC, necrotizing enterocolitis.

life, eight were considered to be contaminated. None of these eight patients had simultaneously positive blood cultures, nor were they treated specifically for meningitis. After the first week of life, three neonates had simultaneously positive blood and spinal fluid cultures, accounting for a 2.5% incidence of coexisting sepsis and meningitis in this study.

Group B streptococcal sepsis is a frequently reported cause of very early neonatal sepsis that often results in significant morbidity and mortality.[14] Early-onset disease occurs in one to four per 1000 live births, the incidence and mortality being higher in smaller, premature neonates. It also has a reportedly high incidence of coexistent meningitis. In this study, only one of the lumbar punctures done in the first week of life yielded a group B *Streptococcus*, although there were 27 cases of blood culture–proved group B streptococcal sepsis in the first week, accounting for 24.3% of all positive blood cultures. In only one neonate with a positive blood culture performed after the first week of life did the culture yield group B *Streptococcus*, and this patient also had coexisting meningitis.

In summary, during two separate 6-month periods, nine of 712 patients undergoing lumbar puncture during the first week of life had positive cultures. On the other hand, eight of 114 patients undergoing lumbar puncture after the first week of life had positive cultures, most of which were clinically significant, although only three were accompanied by simultaneously positive blood cultures. This fivefold difference in incidence might be explained by the neonatal vs the maternal indication for the sepsis evaluation. The percentage of neonatal infections masked by maternal antibiotic treatment could not be determined and may have an impact on the interpretation of these data.

The results of this study suggest that the routine inclusion of lumbar puncture, performed in the first week of life as part of the workup for suspected infection in the asymptomatic but at-risk neonate, may not be indicated or justified. In contrast, when a lumbar puncture is performed for specific clinical indications in the older neonate to rule out an acquired infection, the yield is significant. The problems of blood contamination, inadequate amounts of fluid, and administration of antibiotics to the mother limit the interpretation of the results. The routine use of lumbar puncture as a part of the workup for infection during the first week of life in an asymptomatic neonate should be reassessed.

This project was supported in part by a grant from the Division of Children's Medical Services, State of Florida Department of Health and Rehabilitative Services.

We are grateful to Eduardo Bancalari, MD, and Gwendolyn Scott, MD, for their review and suggestions, and to Rose Wesley for preparation of the manuscript.

References

1. Hildebrand WL, Stevens DC, Gosling CG, Sternecker CL, Schreiner RL. Lumbar puncture in infants. *Am Fam Physician.* 1983;27:157-159.

2. Choremis C, Economos D, Papadatos C, Gargoulas A. Intraspinal epidermoid tumours (cholesteatomas) in patients treated for tuberculous meningitis. *Lancet.* 1956;2:437-439.

3. Shaywitz BA. Epidermoid spinal cord tumors and previous lumbar punctures. *J Pediatr.* 1972;80:638-640.

4. Batnitzky S, Keucher TR, Mealey J Jr, Campbell RL. Iatrogenic intraspinal epidermoid tumors. *JAMA.* 1977;237:148-150.

5. Teele DW, Dashefsky B, Rakusan T, Klein JO. Meningitis after lumbar puncture in children with bacteremia. *N Engl J Med.* 1981;305:1079-1081.

6. Kruskall MS, Carter SR, Ritz LP. Contamination of cerebrospinal fluid by vertebral bone-marrow cells during lumbar puncture. *N Engl J Med.* 1983;308:697-700.

7. Lane PA, Githens JH. Contamination of cerebrospinal fluid with bone marrow cells during lumbar puncture. *N Engl J Med.* 1983;309:434-435.

8. Long JG, Philip AGS, Lucey JF. Excessive handling as a cause of hypoxemia. *Pediatrics.* 1980;65:203-207.

9. Speidel BD. Adverse effects of routine procedures on preterm infants. *Lancet.* 1978;1:864-865.

10. Weisman LE, Merenstein GB, Steenbarger JR. The effect of lumbar puncture position in sick neonates. *AJDC.* 1983;137:1077-1079.

11. Remington JS, Klein JO. *Infectious Diseases of the Fetus and Newborn Infant.* Philadelphia, Pa: WB Saunders Co; 1983:680-687.

12. Gnehm H, Klein JO. Management of neonatal sepsis and meningitis. *Pediatr Ann.* 1983;12:195-204.

13. Visser VE, Hall RT. Lumbar puncture in the evaluation of suspected neonatal sepsis. *Pediatrics.* 1980;96:1063-1067.

14. Pyati SP, Pildes RS, Jacobs NM, et al. Penicillin in infants weighing two kilograms or less with early-onset group B streptococcal disease. *N Engl J Med.* 1983;308:1383-1389.

In Other AMA Journals

JAMA

The Efficacy of Preemployment Drug Screening for Marijuana and Cocaine in Predicting Employment Outcome
C. Zwerling; J. Ryan; E. J. Orav (*JAMA.* 1990;264:2644)

Legal Interventions During Pregnancy
AMA Board of Trustees Report (*JAMA.* 1990;264:2663)

Another Side Effect of NSAIDs
G. R. Gay (*JAMA.* 1990;264:2677)

Family History Fails to Identify Many Children With Severe Hypercholesterolemia

Thomas J. Starc, MD; Peter F. Belamarich, MD; Steven Shea, MD; Beth E. Dobrin-Seckler, RD; Ralph B. Dell, MD; Welton M. Gersony, MD; Richard J. Deckelbaum, MD

• Optimal strategies for identifying children with hypercholesterolemia have not been established. Several groups have advocated that testing of serum cholesterol levels be limited to those children who have family histories of hyperlipidemia or premature coronary heart disease. We studied the ability of comprehensive family histories to identify children with hyperlipidemia in a group of 114 children (mean age, 8 ± 4 years) who were referred for treatment of hypercholesterolemia. A positive family history was defined according to guidelines of the American Academy of Pediatrics. The mean fasting total cholesterol in the children was 5.74 ± 1.42 mmol/L (222 mg/dL). Family history was negative for hypercholesterolemia or premature coronary heart disease in 22 (22%) of 100 children with total cholesterol levels greater than the 75th percentile for their ages, in 13 (18.3%) of 71 children with total cholesterol levels greater than the 95th percentile for their ages, and in four (11.8%) of 34 children with presumed heterozygous familial hypercholesterolemia. Of the 78 children who had both hypercholesterolemia and positive family histories, hyperlipidemia was reported in 72 families, whereas premature heart disease was reported in only 27. We conclude that in a population of children referred because of known hypercholesterolemia, a detailed family history not only fails to identify many children with mild hypercholesterolemia, but also fails to identify a significant proportion of children with markedly elevated cholesterol levels. Additionally, in families of children with hypercholesterolemia, a history of hyperlipidemia is more common than a history of premature heart disease.

(*AJDC.* 1991;145:61-64)

Optimal strategies for cholesterol screening in children have not been established. Currently, both the American Academy of Pediatrics[1] and the American Heart Association[2] advocate that testing of serum cholesterol levels be limited to those children with family histories of either hyperlipidemia or premature coronary heart disease. Recently, several authors[3-7] have suggested that such limited testing may fail to identify a substantial number of children with hypercholesterolemia. There are limited data to determine if screening by family history will miss just children with mildly elevated cholesterol levels, or if it will also miss children with severe hypercholesterolemia or heterozygous familial hypercholesterolemia. Furthermore, in previous studies, family histories were usually obtained from written questionnaires completed by family members or from telephone interviews.[3-7] We do not know if a comprehensive family history, using both a questionnaire and a detailed personal interview, would identify more children with hypercholesterolemia.

Our purpose was to determine if screening recommendations based on detailed family histories would have identified children with elevated plasma cholesterol levels in a population of children referred to us with moderate to severe hypercholesterolemia. Using a selected population of children with severe hypercholesterolemia, we tested the hypothesis that currently recommended screening strategies would detect children with hypercholesterolemia.

Accepted for publication March 5, 1990.

From the Divisions of Pediatric Cardiology (Drs Starc and Gersony) and Gastroenterology and Nutrition (Drs Belamarich, Deckelbaum, and Dell and Ms Dobrin-Seckler) of the Department of Pediatrics and the Department of Medicine and School of Public Health (Dr Shea), Children's Cardiovascular Health Center, Columbia University, College of Physicians and Surgeons, New York, NY.

Presented in part at the annual meeting of the American Heart Association, New Orleans, La, November 12, 1989.

Reprint requests to Columbia Presbyterian Medical Center, Babies Hospital, Room 102A, 630 W 168th St, New York, NY 10032 (Dr Starc).

PATIENTS AND METHODS

Setting and Subjects

The study population comprised 114 children who were referred for evaluation of hypercholesterolemia to the Children's Cardiovascular Health Center at the Columbia Presbyterian Medical Center, New York, NY, between October 1987 and March 1989. The subjects were selected from a group of 151 children referred to the center for evaluation of risk factors for atherosclerotic heart disease. Children found to have hypercholesterolemia associated with other conditions (eg, renal disease and hypothyroidism) or who were referred for other causes (eg, obesity, hypertension, and hypertriglyceridemia) were excluded from this analysis.

All children were identified by their referring physicians as having elevated plasma cholesterol levels before enrollment in our center. The original cholesterol tests were performed by the referring physicians for a variety of reasons, including family history of hyperlipidemia or early heart disease, routine cholesterol screening on all children in that pediatrician's practice, parental concern about cardiovascular disease, recommendation of the parent's physician that the child be tested, or diagnostic evaluation for some other condition.

The mean age of the children in the study was 8.4 ± 3.7 years (range, 2 to 18 years). Seventy-three percent of the children were white, 15% were Hispanic, 7% were black, and 5% were Asian. Most children were from middle- and upper-middle–class families and were referred by private pediatricians.

The mean total cholesterol of the study group prior to referral to our center was 6.74 ± 1.64 mmol/L (range, 4.53 to 12.93 mmol/L). Methods varied for obtaining the cholesterol values prior to referral to our center and included fasting, nonfasting, finger-stick, and venous blood samples.

Table 1.—Fasting Lipid Values*

	All Children (n=114)	Positive History (n=86)	Negative History (n=28)
Lipid level, mmol/L (mean ± SD)			
Total cholesterol	5.74±1.44	5.94±1.53	5.11±0.80†
LDL-cholesterol	4.03±1.46	4.23±1.57	3.43±0.82†
HDL-cholesterol	1.21±0.32‡	1.21±0.33§	1.18±0.29
Triglycerides	1.17±0.64‡	1.17±0.63§	1.14±0.64

*LDL indicates low-density lipoprotein; and, HDL, high-density lipoprotein.
†$P<.02$, positive vs negative history.
‡n=113.
§n=85.

Measures

Family History.—Prior to their first visits to the center, parents were asked to answer comprehensive family history questionnaires. During the first visit, the family history was reviewed in detail with the physician and, if necessary, was completed at that time. A bilingual (Spanish-English) physician was present to assist in completion of the questionnaire when necessary. History and age of onset of myocardial infarction, coronary artery surgery, or sudden cardiac death and history of hypercholesterolemia or hypertriglyceridemia were obtained regarding each child's parents, grandparents, aunts, and uncles.

Following the recommendations of the American Academy of Pediatrics, the history of coronary heart disease was recorded as positive if a child's parent stated that a family member had a myocardial infarction, heart attack, coronary bypass surgery, or sudden cardiac death before age 50 years in men and before age 60 years in women. History of hyperlipidemia was considered positive if a parent stated that a family member had hyperlipidemia. If the family member's total cholesterol level was known and reported by the parent to be greater than 6.21 mmol/L (240 mg/dL), that family member was classified as having hypercholesterolemia regardless of whether the parent stated that the family member had hyperlipidemia.

Blood Lipids.—A fasting venous blood sample was obtained on the morning of each child's first visit to the center. Levels of plasma total cholesterol, high-density lipoprotein cholesterol (HDL-cholesterol), and triglycerides were determined using standard Lipid Research Clinics methodology[8] calibrated to Centers for Disease Control standards. Low-density lipoprotein cholesterol (LDL-cholesterol) was calculated using the following equation in which LDL-Cholesterol = [Total Cholesterol − HDL-Cholesterol − (Triglycerides/5)].[9] None of the children in the study had a triglyceride level greater than 4.52 mmol/L (400 mg/dL). One child did not undergo HDL-cholesterol testing owing to a laboratory error. Therefore, 113 HDL-cholesterol and LDL-cholesterol values were available for this analysis.

Children were classified as having hypercholesterolemia if their total cholesterol levels were greater than the 75th or the 95th percentile for their age and sex based on the "Visit 2, Random Sample" from *The Lipid Research Clinics Population Studies Data Book*.[10] We applied values from white males and females to all children because values were not published in "Visit 2, Random Sample" for blacks, Asians, or Hispanics. Because values for cholesterol distributions for 2- and 3-year-old children were also missing from the study data, we applied values for 4- to 9-year-old children to this age group. We also analyzed the data using three suggested fixed cutoff points for total cholesterol levels in children: 4.40 mmol/L (170 mg/dL),[11] 4.53 mmol/L (175 mg/dL, the approximate 75th percentile for 2- to 18-year-old children), and 5.17 mmol/L (200 mg/dL, the approximate 95th percentile for 2- to 18-year-old children).[10]

Some children have elevated total cholesterol levels because of high HDL-cholesterol levels and would be incorrectly identified as being at risk for early heart disease.[12] Therefore, we also analyzed the data using the age- and sex-specific values for LDL-cholesterol for the 75th and 95th percentiles. A subset of children was identified as having probable heterozygous familial hypercholesterolemia based on LDL-cholesterol levels of greater than 4.24 mmol/L (164 mg/dL).[13]

The HDL-cholesterol level was classified as low if it was less than or equal to the 10th percentile for age and sex based on distributions in the Lipid Research Centers' prevalence study.[10] Because values of HDL-cholesterol distributions for 2- and 3-year-old children were not among the study data, we applied values for 4- to 9-year-old children to this age group.

Statistical Analysis

Data are reported as the mean (±SD). Comparisons of lipoprotein values between those children with positive family histories and those with negative family histories were performed using Student's t test. We calculated the proportions of children with elevated cholesterol levels who had either positive or negative family histories. Differences in proportions were compared with the χ^2 test. Confidence intervals (CIs) for single proportions were calculated according to the method of Fleiss.[14]

RESULTS

The mean fasting total cholesterol level using Lipid Research Clinics methods in the 114 children was 5.74±1.44 mmol/L (222±56 mg/dL, range, 3.28 to 10.32 mmol/L)(Table 1). The mean LDL-cholesterol was 4.03±1.46 mmol/L (156±57 mg/dL). Both total cholesterol and LDL-cholesterol levels were higher in children with positive family histories for either premature heart disease or hyperlipidemia than in children with negative family histories for these conditions ($P<.02$) (Table 1). The HDL-cholesterol and triglyceride levels were similar in children with or without family histories of premature heart disease or hypercholesterolemia. Lipid values in children with family histories of premature ischemic heart disease were not statistically different from lipid values in children without family histories of ischemic heart disease.

Family history was negative for either hyperlipidemia or premature coronary heart disease in 22 (22%) of 100 (95% confidence interval, 14% to 30%) children with total cholesterol levels greater than the 75th percentile for their ages (Table 2). Among those children with total cholesterol levels greater than the 95th percentile for their ages, family history was negative in 13 (18.3%) of 71 (95% confidence interval, 9% to 27%) children. Similarly, family history was negative in 22 (22.9%) of 96 children with LDL-cholesterol levels greater than the 75th percentile for their ages and in 13 (20.3%) of 64 children with LDL-cholesterol levels greater than 95th percentile for their ages (Table 2).

Thirty-four children were presumed to have familial heterozygous hypercholesterolemia (LDL-cholesterol>4.24

Table 2.—Percent of Children With Negative Family Histories of Hyperlipidemia or Premature Atherosclerotic Heart Disease*

Cholesterol Levels	Total No. of Children	No. (%) With Negative History
TC ≥75th percentile	100	22 (22.0)
TC ≥95th percentile	71	13 (18.3)
TC ≥4.40 mmol/L	98	22 (22.4)
TC ≥4.53 mmol/L	95	20 (21.1)
TC ≥5.17 mmol/L	68	14 (20.6)
LDL-C ≥75th percentile	96	22 (22.9)
LDL-C ≥95th percentile	64	13 (20.3)
LDL-C ≥4.24 mmol/L	34	4 (11.8)
HDL-C ≤10th percentile	38	12 (31.6)

*TC indicates total cholesterol; LDL-C, low-density lipoprotein cholesterol; and, HDL-C, high-density lipoprotein cholesterol.

Table 3.—Family Histories in Children With Positive Family Histories and Total Cholesterol ≥75th Percentile for Age

Condition	No. (%) of Children (n=78)
Premature myocardial event	
Parent	13 (16.7)
Grandparent	16 (20.5)
Parent or grandparent	27 (34.6)
Hyperlipidemia	
Parent	51 (65.4)
Grandparent	53 (67.9)
Parent or grandparent	72 (92.3)

mmol/L or 164 mg/dL).[13] The mean total cholesterol level in this group was 7.50±1.29 mmol/L (290±50 mg/dL). Family history was negative in four (11.8%) of 34 children with presumed familial hypercholesterolemia, compared with 18 (27.2%) of 66 children with other causes of hypercholesterolemia ($P>.05$).

Some families had more than one hypercholesterolemic child in the study. Consequently, we also analyzed the data allowing only one child per family history. Family history was negative in 21 (23.9%) of 88 families that had at least one child with a total cholesterol level greater than the 75th percentile for the child's age.

Thirty-eight (33.6%) of the 113 children tested had HDL-cholesterol levels less than or equal to the 10th percentile for their ages. Family history was negative in 12 (31.6%) of these children. Only one child with a total cholesterol level above the 75th percentile and a negative family history had a high HDL-cholesterol level and an LDL-cholesterol level that was below the 75th percentile.

There were 78 children with positive family histories and total cholesterol levels greater than the 75th percentile. Hyperlipidemia was reported in the families of 72 of these children (Table 3), while premature heart disease was reported in the families of only 27 of these children.

COMMENT

Our study differs from others[4-7] in that it examined children referred to a cardiovascular health program who had been diagnosed with moderate to severe hypercholesterolemia. Our study did not screen a normal pediatric population. Rather than developing predictive values for current cholesterol screening recommendations in the general population, our study serves as a test of the effectiveness of current cholesterol screening guidelines in a group of high-risk children.

Family history is often used as a predictor of coronary heart disease, in part because of familial aggregation of several risk factors, including hyperlipidemia, hypertension, and diabetes mellitus.[15-16] We found that current cholesterol testing recommendations based on family histories of early heart disease or hyperlipidemia would have failed to identify approximately 20% of children with moderate or severe hypercholesterolemia, 12% of children with presumed heterozygous familial hypercholesterolemia, and 31% of children with HDL-cholesterol levels less than the 10th percentile for their ages.

Despite a well-defined relationship between a family history of early heart disease and childhood hypercholesterolemia,[17-19] our data and those of others,[3-17,20,21] indicate that a family history of early heart disease or hyperlipidemia is not as accurate a predictor of hyperlipidemia in children as might be expected. In the Bogalusa Heart Study,[20] a history of paternal or maternal heart disease was not a useful marker of elevated total cholesterol levels or LDL-cholesterol levels in children. By using a positive parental history of heart disease as a marker, approximately 60% of white children and 80% of black children with elevated LDL-cholesterol levels would not have been identified.[3,20] Other studies also suggest that if a family history of heart disease or hyperlipidemia were used as a marker, 20% to 60% of hypercholesterolemic children would not be detected.[4-7,21]

Differences in methods for obtaining family histories may explain the wide discrepancy in the effectiveness of family history–based cholesterol screening that is seen between various studies.[4-5] We used both questionnaires and personal interviews by physicians to obtain our detailed family histories. Others have used written questionnaires[3-7] or a combination of written questionnaires and telephone interviews[3,7] to obtain family histories. It is likely that a more extensive family history may have contributed to a somewhat higher proportion of hypercholesterolemic children being identified in this study. Furthermore, our data indicate that a family history of hyperlipidemia more accurately predicts the presence of hypercholesterolemia in children than does a family history of premature heart disease. This may, in part, explain why studies that used a family history of heart disease as the only screening measure[3,20] identified a smaller proportion of hyperlipidemic children than studies that also used a family history of hyperlipidemia as a screening measure. However, because we studied a select group of children who had already been identified as having hypercholesterolemia, our results should not be strictly compared with findings based on studies using nonselect populations. Current guidelines[1,2] for using family histories would have failed to identify 22 hypercholesterolemic children in our study. In four of these children, the family histories of one or both parents were not known in detail. For seven of the 22 children, atherosclerotic heart disease occurred in a family member, but did not fit the standard definition of "premature." In the remaining 11 children, no particular predisposing factor could be identified.

When initially studied at our center, 14 of the 114 children who had been previously diagnosed by their pediatricians as having hypercholesterolemia had fasting total cholesterol values below the 75th percentile for their ages. Many explanations for lower total cholesterol values at the time of referral can be offered: (1) the majority of children had modified their diets prior to their first visits to our center. (2) The Lipid Research Center techniques used in our laboratory to measure blood cholesterol levels have been demonstrated to produce consistently lower cholesterol values compared with two commonly used clinical laboratory instruments, the Technicon SMAC (Technicon Instruments Corp, Tarrytown, NY) and the Du Pont Automatic Clinical Analyzer (Du Pont Co, Wilmington, Del).[22] (3) We used fasting venous blood samples in contrast to nonfasting or fingerstick samples used by some of the referring physicians. These findings emphasize the importance of using standard techniques and obtaining several cholesterol determinations prior to identifying a child as having hypercholesterolemia.

Testing strategies for detecting hypercholesterolemia in children continue to be based on consensus and expert recommendations. It was not our purpose to address the broad issues of cost effectiveness of cholesterol screening and treatment in children. However, our work, together with studies based on less strictly selected populations,[3-7] raises questions about the effectiveness of current screening policies. If it is considered beneficial to identify every child with even mild hypercholesterolemia, testing for all children should be required, and recommendations for cholesterol testing should reflect this goal. On the other hand, if screening programs should focus on identifying only high-risk individuals, more reliable screening methods will be required.

This study was supported in part by grants from the William H. Donner Foundation, New York, NY, and Wyeth Laboratories Healthy Heart Program, Philadelphia, Pa.

The authors would like to thank Pauline Fusco for her secretarial assistance and Minnie Myers, Jim Lopez, and Henry Ginsberg, MD, for performing the blood lipid determinations.

References

1. American Academy of Pediatrics Committee on Nutrition. Indications for cholesterol testing in children. *Pediatrics.* 1989;83:141-142.

2. Position statement of American Heart Association: diagnosis and treatment of primary hyperlipidemia in childhood. *Circulation.* 1986;74:1181A-1188A.

3. Dennison BA, Kikuchi DA, Srinivasan SR, Webber LS, Berenson GS. Parental history of cardiovascular disease as an indication for screening for lipoprotein abnormalities in children. *J Pediatr.* 1989;115:186-194.

4. Meyerson DA, Santanello NC. Family oriented cardiovascular risk screening and intervention. *Maryland Med J.* 1988;37:395-398.

5. Davidson DM, Bradley BJ, Landry SM, Iftner CA, Bramblett SN. School based cholesterol screening. *J Pediatr Health Care.* 1989;3:3-8.

6. Griffin TC, Christoffel KK, Binns HJ, McGuire PA, and the Pediatric Practice Research Group. Family history evaluation as a predictive screen for childhood hypercholesterolemia. *Pediatrics.* 1989;84:365-373.

7. Garcia RE, Moodie DS. Routine cholesterol surveillance in childhood. *Pediatrics.* 1989;84:751-755.

8. Lipid Research Clinics Program. *Manual of Laboratory Operations, I: Lipid and Lipoprotein Analysis.* Washington, DC: National Institutes of Health; 1974. US Dept of Health, Education, and Welfare publication NIH 75-628.

9. The Expert Panel. Report of the National Cholesterol Education Program Expert Panel on detection, evaluation and treatment of high blood cholesterol in adults. *Arch Int Med.* 1988;148:36-69.

10. *The Lipid Research Clinics Population Studies Data Book, I: The Prevalance Study.* Washington, DC: US Government Printing Office; July 1980. US Dept of Health and Human Services publication NIH 80-1527.

11. NIH Consensus Development Conference statement: lowering blood cholesterol to prevent heart disease. *JAMA.* 1985;253:2080-2086.

12. Kwiterovich PO Jr, Heiss G, Johnson N, Chase GA, Tamir I, Rifkind B. Assessment of plasma total cholesterol as a test to detect elevated low density (beta) lipoprotein cholesterol levels (type IIa hyperlipoproteinemia) in young subjects from a population-based sample. *Am J Epidemiol.* 1982; 115:192-204.

13. Kwiterovich PO Jr. Pediatric implications of heterozygous familial hypercholesterolemia: screening and dietary treatment. *Arteriosclerosis.* 1989;9(suppl 1):I-111-I-120.

14. Fleiss JL. *Statistical Methods for Rates and Proportions.* 2nd ed. New York, NY: John Wiley & Sons Inc; 1981:13-15.

15. Shea S, Ottman R, Gabrieli C, Stein Z, Nichols A. Family history as an independent risk factor for coronary artery disease. *J Am Coll Cardiol.* 1984;4:793-801.

16. ten Kate LP, Boman H, Daiger SP, Motulsky AG. Familial aggregation of coronary heart disease and its relation to known genetic risk factors. *Am J Cardiol.* 1982;50:945-953.

17. Moll PP, Sing CF, Weidman WH, et al. Total cholesterol and lipoproteins in school children: prediction of coronary heart disease in adult relatives. *Circulation.* 1983;67:127-134.

18. Lee J, Lauer RM, Clarke WR. Lipoproteins in the progeny of young men with coronary artery disease: children with increased risk. *Pediatrics.* 1986;78:330-337.

19. Glueck CJ, Fallat RW, Tsang R, Buncher CR. Hyperlipidemia in progeny of parents with myocardial infarction before age 50. *AJDC.* 1974;127:70-75.

20. Shear CL, Webber LS, Freedman DS, Srinivasan SR, Berenson GS. The relationship between parental history of vascular disease and cardiovascular disease risk factors in children: the Bogalusa Heart Study. *Am J Epidemiol.* 1985;122:762-771.

21. Shea S, Basch CE, Irigoyen M, et al. Failure of family history to predict high blood cholesterol in Hispanic preschool children. *Prev Med.* 1990;19:443-455.

22. Blank DW, Hoeg JM, Kroll MH, Ruddel ME. The method of determination must be considered in interpreting blood cholesterol levels. *JAMA.* 1986;256:2767-2770.

Acute Osteomyelitis in Children

Reassessment of Etiologic Agents and Their Clinical Characteristics

Howard Faden, MD, Mauro Grossi, MD

• One hundred thirty-five children with acute osteomyelitis were identified by chart review during a 7-year period, January 1, 1980, through December 31, 1986. Bacteriologic causes were detected in 75 (55%) of the patients. *Staphylococcus aureus, Haemophilus influenzae* type b, and *Pseudomonos aeruginosa* were identified in 34 (25%), 16 (12%), and eight (6%) children, respectively. *Staphylococcus aureus* occurred in all age groups, *H influenzae* type b occurred only in children younger than 3 years and was the number one cause of disease in this group. *Pseudomonas aeruginosa* occurred exclusively in children older than 9 years. Children with *H influenzae* type b had clinical and laboratory findings that were almost indistinguishable from a matched group of children with osteomyelitis due to other known bacteria, although children with *H influenzae* type b tended to have more joint effusions (63% vs 27%), less lower extremity disease (22% vs 70%), and fewer positive cultures from bone or joint aspirates (41% vs 89%). Unlike most pediatric cases of osteomyelitis, the ones due to *P aeruginosa* did not represent the hematogenous route of infection; penetrating injury to the foot was present in every case. Children with *P aeruginosa* infections were older than 9 years (100%), predominantly male (88%), often afebrile (83%), and never bacteremic. These data provide guidelines for the initial work-up and management of osteomyelitis in children.

(*AJDC.* 1991;145:65-69)

Accepted for publication June 4, 1990.

From the Divisions of Infectious Diseases and Hematology/Oncology, Department of Pediatrics, State University of New York, School of Medicine at Buffalo, and Children's Hospital of Buffalo (NY).

Reprint requests to Division of Infectious Diseases, Children's Hospital of Buffalo, 219 Bryant St, Buffalo, NY 14222 (Dr Faden).

Osteomyelitis continues to be a common problem in children. Although various bacteria have been identified as causal agents in osteomyelitis, *Staphylococcus aureus* has been the single most frequent identifiable cause for more than 50 years.[1-10] Scattered reports over the past 10 to 20 years have identified *Haemophilus influenzae* type b as a potential pathogen in bone infections of young children.[11-14] However, evidence for a major role of *H influenzae* type b in osteomyelitis has been lacking.[9,10]

We reviewed a 7-year experience of 135 children with acute osteomyelitis in which specific bacterial agents were identified in 75 children. *Haemophilus influenzae* type b was the cause in 16 patients and was the number one cause of disease in children younger than 3 years.

PATIENTS, MATERIALS, AND METHODS

Population

The records of all patients discharged from a children's hospital with the diagnosis of acute osteomyelitis between January 1, 1980, and December 31, 1986, were reviewed. The diagnosis of osteomyelitis must have included clear evidence of bone involvement, ie, bone lesion on plain roentgenogram or an abnormal isotopic scan, as well as evidence of infection, ie, fever, local signs, including erythema or warmth, and an elevated erythrocyte sedimentation rate (ESR). One hundred thirty-five cases were selected after exclusion of patients with previous surgical orthopedic procedures, chronic osteomyelitis, or insufficient evidence to confirm the diagnosis of acute osteomyelitis.

Data Collected

Epidemiologic and clinical data were recorded. Laboratory data included white blood cell (WBC) count; ESR; cultures of blood, bone, joint, and soft tissue; bacterial antigen (*H influenzae* type b and *Streptococcus pneumoniae*) detection; plain roentgenogram; and bone scan with technetium Tc99m pyrophosphate or gallium Ga 67.

Statistics

Student's unpaired t test, χ^2, and Fisher's Exact Test were used to analyze the data.

RESULTS

Population

One hundred thirty-five cases were evaluated. Eighty-one patients were male and 54 were female (male-female ratio = 1.5:1). Subjects ranged in age from 1 day to 22 years (mean[± SD], 5.9 ± 5.1 years). Half of the subjects were younger than 5 years. The highest occurrence rate was in the first year of life (Fig 1). One hundred six children (79%) were white, 23 (17%) were black, and six (4%) were of other races. This proportion approximately represented the racial distribution of the population in the County of Erie, New York (white, 84%; black, 13%; and other races, 3%) ($P>.05$).

Clinical Characteristics

Pain, the most common presenting complaint in 127 (94%) of the subjects, was manifested differently according to age and site of involvement (Table 1). Pain was verbalized in 88 subjects (65%), manifested by decreased range of motion in 70 subjects (52%), by limping in 47 subjects (35%), and by refusal to bear weight in 47 subjects (35%) or walk in 24 subjects (18%). One hundred fifteen children (85%) were febrile. The temperature at the time of hospital admission ranged from 36°C to 41°C (mean[± SD], 38.6°C ± 1.1°C). Local

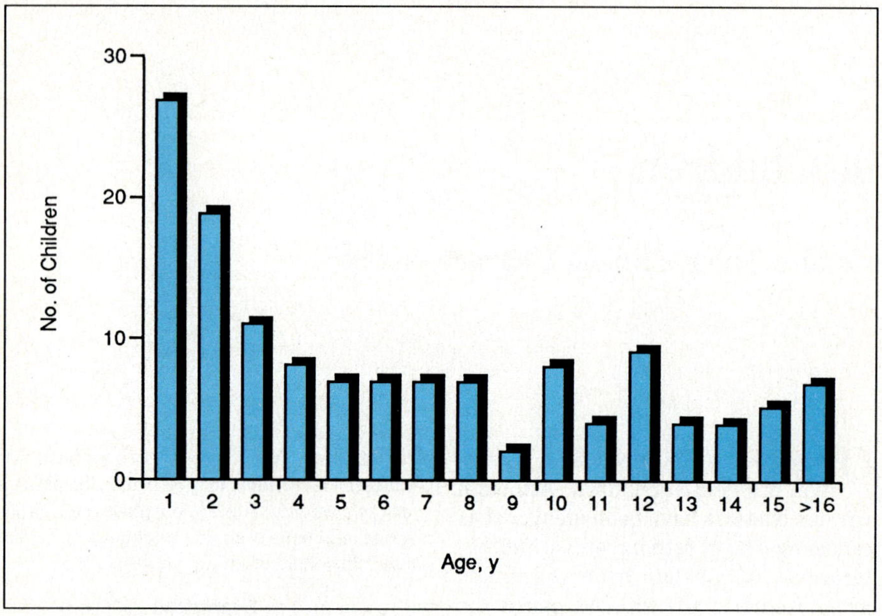

Fig 1.—Age distribution of 135 children with acute osteomyelitis.

Table 1.—Clinical Characteristics of Children With Acute Osteomyelitis

Signs and Symptoms	No. (%)
Pain	127 (94)
Fever	115 (85)
Local changes	93 (69)
Irritability	16 (12)
Anorexia	13 (10)
Lethargy	5 (4)
Vomiting	4 (3)

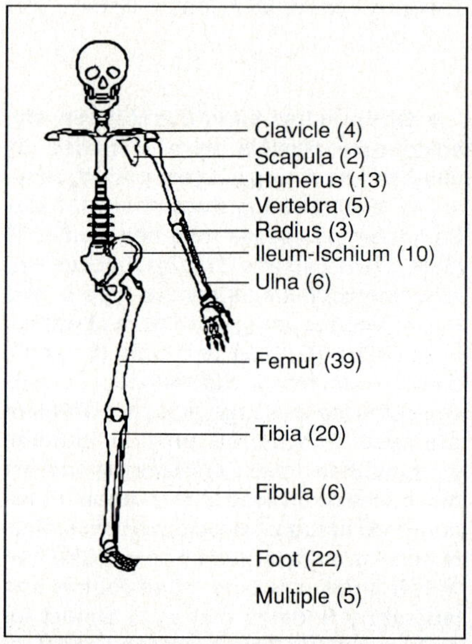

Fig 2.—Bone involvement in acute osteomyelitis.

signs and symptoms were evident in 93 children (69%).

These changes included swelling in 73 patients (54%), tenderness in 47 patients (35%), warmth in 37 patients (27%), and erythema in 35 patients (25%). Anorexia, lethargy, and vomiting were less common complaints.

The sites of infection are depicted in Fig 2. The femur was the most commonly involved bone, occurring in 39 patients, followed by the tibia in 20 patients, humerus in 13 patients, and pelvis in 10 patients. Bones of the foot were involved on 22 occasions; eight of these occurred in the calcaneous. Thus, infections of the lower extremity occurred in half of the subjects, while infections of the upper extremity occurred in less than one fifth of the subjects.

Five (3.7%) of the 135 children had infections in more than one bone. The multiple infections consisted of femur and foot in two children, humerus and clavicle, humerus and femur, and tibia and femur in one child each.

Laboratory Data

At the time of hospital admission, the WBC count was elevated in 42 patients (31%). The WBC count ranged from 2.4 to 45.5×10^9/L (mean[±SD], $13.1 \pm 6.4 \times 10^9$/L). The ESR was increased in 120 patients (89%). The ESR ranged from 4 to 132 mm/h (mean [±SD], 61±30 mm/h). Four children had both a normal WBC count and ESR at the time of hospital admission.

A causal diagnosis was sought by cultures of blood (129 patients), bone (43 patients), joint (41 patients), and soft tissue (six patients), and by determination of bacterial antigen in the urine or joint fluid (44 patients) (Table 2). Thirty-nine blood cultures (30%) were positive. Aspirates of bone, joint, and soft tissue yielded bacteria in 22 (51%), 15 (37%), and four cultures (67%), respectively. Antigen detection was positive in six samples(14%); however, the six positive results occurred in children younger than 24 months for a positive rate of 23% in infants. Overall, a bacteriologic diagnosis was confirmed in 75 (55%) of the cases.

Ten different genera of bacteria were identified as causal agents. *Staphylococcus aureus* was identified in 34 cases (25%), *H influenzae* type b was identified in 16 patients (12%), *Pseudomonas aeruginosa* was identified in eight patients (6%), group A *Streptococcus* was identified in five patients (4%), coagulase-negative *Staphylococcus* was identified in five patients (4%), and *Streptococcus pneumoniae* was identified in three patients (2%). *Escherichia coli*, *Kingella kingae*, *Neisseria meningitidis*, and group B *Streptococcus* were each isolated once. No causal agent could be identified in 60 (45%) of the subjects.

Table 2.—Results of Bacterial Culture and Antigen Detection Assay

Test	No. Tested	No. Positive (%)
Culture		
Blood	129	39 (30)
Bone	43	22 (51)
Joint fluid	41	15 (37)
Soft tissue	6	4 (67)
Antigen detection*	44	6 (14)

*Six of 25 children younger than 24 months had positive assays.

The causal agents exhibited an age-related distribution (Fig 3). Four infants younger than 30 days were infected with either *E coli*, group B *Streptococcus*, or *S aureus* (two cases). As seen in Fig 3, *S aureus* was distribut-

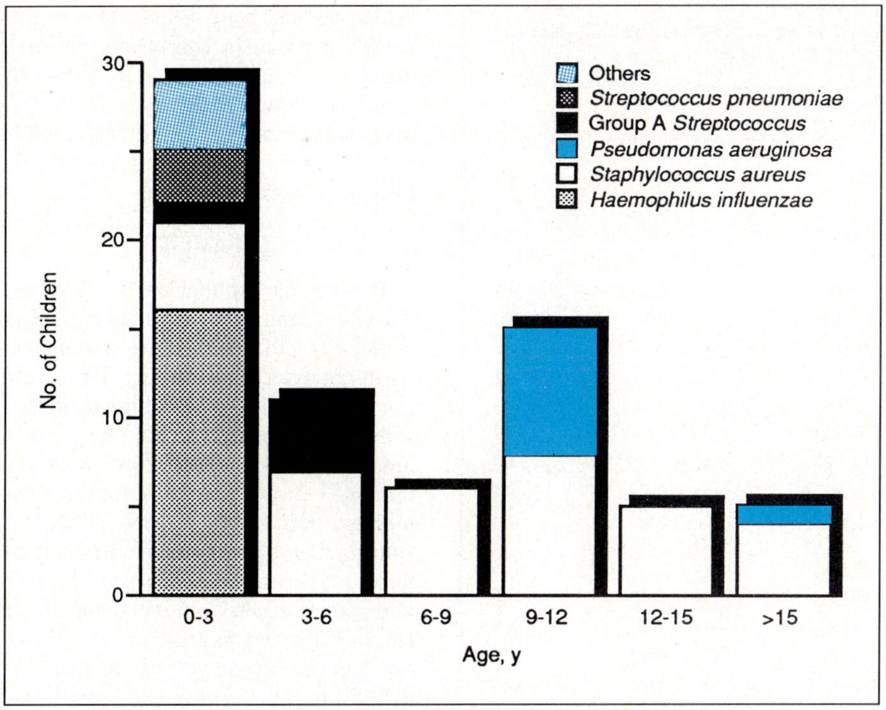

Fig 3.—Bacterial causes of acute osteomyelitis distributed by age of subject.

ed throughout the various age groups; however, *H influenzae* type b and *P aeruginosa* had rather distinctive age predilections. *Haemophilus influenzae* type b occurred only in children younger than 3 years; actually, all but one of the 16 children were younger than 2 years. However, *P aeruginosa* occurred only in children older than 9 years.

The causal agents also seemed to infect specific bony sites. For example, upper extremity osteomyelitis occurred in only 10% of the patients due to *S aureus*. In contrast, 38% the of children infected with *H influenzae* type b had upper extremity disease. In addition, *H influenzae* type b infection resulted in multiple bone involvement in three children; only five children in the entire group had multiple bone disease.

Ten children presented with osteomyelitis and obvious evidence of septic arthritis; another 36 had osteomyelitis with minimal but sufficient changes in their joints to warrant aspiration of the joint space. Joint fluids were examined in 43 of these 46 individuals and 15 (35%) proved to be infected. While 10 (29%) of 34 children with *S aureus* osteomyelitis had development of joint effusions, 10 (63%) of 16 children with *H influenzae* type b had development of joint effusions. In contrast, 60% of the staphylococcal effusions and 30% of the *Haemophilus* effusions were culture positive. Thus, 18% of children in either group had infected joints.

Roentgenographic studies were obtained on every patient. One hundred thirty-two subjects initially had plain roentgenograms. Abnormal findings were evident in 76 subjects (58%). These findings included soft-tissue swelling in 58 subjects (44%) and periosteal reaction, bony erosion, or lytic lesion in 35 subjects. Thus, 26% of the children had a bony lesion evident on presentation to the hospital. Isotopic bone scans were also performed. Of 126 technetium Tc99m pyrophosphate bone scans, 125 (99%) were abnormal. The bone scan detected osteomyelitis in 15 (94%) of 16 patients in whom the plain roentgenogram demonstrated only soft-tissue swelling. Gallium scans were also performed in 16 patient; 15 (94%) were abnormal. Every subject had at least one roentgenographic study that was consistent with osteomyelitis.

Characteristics of *H influenzae* Type b Osteomyelitis

Haemophilus influenzae type b was the second most frequent identifiable cause of osteomyelitis, comprising 21% of the identifiable organisms. All of the children were younger than 3 years (range, 5 months to 31 months; mean ± SD, 14.3 ± 7.5 months). Nine of the children with *H influenzae* type b were female and seven were male. Twelve of them were white, three were black, and one was an American Indian. All of the children were febrile at the time of hospital admission with temperatures ranging between 38.0°C and 39.9°C (mean, 38.9 ± 0.6°C). Fourteen children (89%) exhibited signs of pain. Local changes included swelling in 14 children (89%), erythema in nine children (56%), and warmth in six children (38%). One child each was irritable and lethargic. Other sites of infection were evident among 11 subjects: six had upper respiratory tract infections; two had meningitis; and three had otitis media. Of the 13 children with single bone infections due to *H influenzae* type b, six occurred in the upper extremity, three occurred in the lower extremity, and four occurred in the calcaneous. The three other children had multiple bone involvement (femur and metatarsal in two children, and femur and humerus in one child).

The WBC count was elevated in 15 (94%) of 16 children and ranged between 10 and 25.3×10^9/L (mean[± SD], $19.3 \pm 5.0 \times 10^9$/L). The ESR was abnormal in all patients. It ranged between 46 and 131 mm/h (mean[± SD], 77 ± 25 mm/h). Plain roentgenograms were abnormal in 14 (100%) of 14 children. Distinct bony lesions were seen in two (14%) of 14 children. Bone scans were abnormal in the other subjects. Blood cultures were positive in seven subjects, aspirates of bone, joint, or soft tissue were positive in five subjects, and antigen was detected in six subjects. The six positive antigen assays were the only positive tests in those six children to establish the diagnosis of *H influenzae* type b disease.

To describe the differences that might exist between *H influenzae* type b osteomyelitis and disease due to other organisms, epidemiologic, clinical, laboratory, and roentgenographic factors were compared in Table 3. A comparative group consisted of 11 children in the study who were in the same age group as those with *H influenzae* type b and

Table 3.—Characteristics of *Haemophilus influenzae* Type b Osteomyelitis Compared with Control

Characteristics*	*H influenzae* Type b (n=16)	Control (n=11)	*P*
Epidemiologic			
Age, mo	14.25±7.5	10.6±7.0	.22
Sex, M:F	7:9	6:7	.50
Race, W:B:C	12:3:1	9:2:0	.53
Clinical			
Pain	14/16	10/11	.64
Fever	16/16	10/11	.40
Local changes	15/16	7/11	.07
Joint effusion	10/16	3/11	.18
Laboratory tests			
WBC, $\times 10^9$/L	19.3±5.0	19.6±10.7	.90
ESR, mm/h	77±25	81±22	.57
Blood culture	7/16	6/11	.44
Aspirates (bone, joint, soft tissue)	5/12	8/9	.06
Bone involvement			
Extremity			
Upper	6/13	2/10	.20
Lower	3/13	7/10	.06
Foot	4/13	0/10	.08
Multiple	3/13	1/10	.40
Roentgenogram with bony lesion	2/16	4/11	.64

*W indicates white; B, black; O, other race; WBC, white blood cell count; and ESR, erythrocyte sedimentation rate.

for whom there was a definitive bacteriologic cause for the bone disease (*S aureus* in three children, *S pneumoniae* in three children, coagulase-negative staphylococci in two children, *K kingae* in one child, and *N meningitidis* in one child). As can be seen, the two groups were similar in most respects with several exceptions: joint effusions (63% vs 27%, *P*=.18) and local signs (94% vs 64%, *P*=.07) tended to occur more frequently in those with *H influenzae* type b. Cultures of aspirates from bone, joint, or soft tissue tended to be positive less often (43% vs 89%, *P*=.06) and involvement of the lower extremity occurred less often (23% vs 70%, *P*=.06) in the *H influenzae* type b group. Thus, when matched with an appropriate control group, *H influenzae* type b osteomyelitis was not unusually distinctive in most respects.

Characteristics of *P aeruginosa* Osteomyelitis

Pseudomonas aeruginosa was the third most common cause of osteomyelitis, comprising 11% of the identifiable organisms. All of the cases occurred in children older than 9 years (range, 9.2 to 17 years; mean±SD, 10.8±2.5 years) and seven of the eight children were between 9.2 and 11 years. This age group differed markedly from that seen with *H influenzae* type b and *S aureus* that occurred in children younger than 3 years and throughout all age groups, respectively. Seven of the children with *P aeruginosa* were male and one was female. Six of the children were white and two were black. All of the children had experienced penetrating injuries to the foot. Only one of the children was febrile. All of the children complained of pain. Local swelling was also evident in every subject. Local signs of erythema and warmth were present in five children (62%) and three children (37%), respectively. Seven of eight infections occurred in the foot (toe, three; calcaneous, two; and metatarsal, two).

The WBC count was rarely elevated. It ranged between 5.1 and 16.2 $\times 10^9$/(mean, $10.3\pm3.4\times10^9$/L). The ESR was elevated in each case and ranged between 18 and 103 mm/h (mean[±SD], 56±25 mm/h). Six (75%) of eight plain roentgenograms were abnormal at the time of hospital admission. Five of the roentgenograms revealed distinct bony lesions. Bone scans were abnormal in the other two children. The diagnosis was established by direct aspiration of the bone in six children, soft tissue in one child, and joint in one child. Six blood cultures were obtained; all were negative.

COMMENT

This report summarizes a 7-year experience, January 1, 1980, through December 31, 1986, with acute osteomyelitis in children. The current data, as in the past, demonstrated a high incidence of osteomyelitis in the first few years of life. Bacteriologic diagnoses were established in 55% of the children. The highest identification rate, 75%, resulted when blood culture and bone aspiration were used concurrently. Antigen detection was uniquely beneficial in establishing the diagnosis of *H influenzae* type b osteomyelitis. In fact, six (37.5%) of the 16 cases were confirmed by antigen detection alone. The latex agglutination test for detection of the capsular polysaccharide of *H influenzae* type b has been shown to be sensitive and when performed properly has few, if any, false-positive reactions.[15] A single report has suggested that antigen excretion in the urine may be detected by a more sensitive technique, such as enzyme-linked immunoabsorbent assay, in carriers of *H influenzae* type b.[16]

Staphylococcus aureus continued to be the major cause of osteomyelitis. It was recovered from 25% of the individuals, represented 47% of the identifiable causes of disease, and distributed throughout all age groups. Most surprising was the frequent recovery of *H influenzae* type b from the children. It was found only among children younger than 3 years and was the number one causal agent in this age group. Several studies demonstrated that *H influenzae* type b was an uncommon isolate in osteomyelitis prior to 1960.[1-6] During the subsequent 30 years, several reports identified *H influenzae* type b as a cause of osteomyelitis in children.[11-14] However, the importance of *H influenzae* type b as a major cause of osteomyelitis had not been substantiated previously.[6-8,10] Lebel and Nelson[10] reviewed a 28-year experience, 1958 through 1986, of 365 children with osteomyelitis and concluded that *H influenzae* type b caused less than 5% of all cases and 13% of the cases in children 1 to 24 months of age. In contrast, in our review of 135 cases during 7 years, 1980 through 1986, *H influenzae* type b caused 12% of all cases and 33% of the cases in children 1 to 24 months of age. The differences in the two studies cannot be readily explained except that antigen detection by latex agglutination permitted diagnosis in six (37.4%) of 16 of our patients while antigen detection by countercurrent immunoelectrophoresis, a less sensitive technique, contributed to the diagnosis in one (6.3%) of 16 patients in the Dallas study[10] ($\chi^2=2.06$, Fisher's Exact Test, $P=.15$).

In addition to the age restriction of *H influenzae* type b disease, several clinical characteristics of children with *H influenzae* type b osteomyelitis deserve mention. Earlier studies had noted a predisposition for upper extremity involvement[13,14] and a high incidence of concurrent joint disease.[9,10,13,14] Multiple bone involvement had also been observed previously.[10] Our study similarly noted a trend toward more joint effusions and upper extremity disease as well as multiple bone involvement; however, when the *H influenzae* type b group was compared with a group of children in the same age category with different bacterial causes, no statistical differences were observed.

Pseudomonas aeruginosa was the third most common etiologic agent in our series. It was isolated exclusively from children older than 9 years all of whom suffered penetrating injuries. This feature alone distinguishes *P aeruginosa* osteomyelitis from other types that predominantly represent hematogenous forms of osteomyelitis. A total of 22 cases of osteomyelitis of the foot were identified and only eight proved to be due to *P aeruginosa* (these eight were the only ones secondary to penetrating injuries of the foot). Earlier studies had documented the important role of injury as an antecedent event in *Pseudomonas* osteomyelitis.[17-20] The organism apparently resides within the sole of sneakers.[21] As observed previously, children with *P aeruginosa* osteomyelitis were likely to be male, and they were rarely febrile or bacteremic.[18]

The information generated from this study may provide guidelines to the approach and treatment of children with acute osteomyelitis. The data suggest that *S aureus* remains the most important causal agent in osteomyelitis. However, in children younger than 3 years, *H influenzae* type b is the number one concern. All cases of osteomyelitis of the foot following penetrating injuries through sneakers must be considered due to *P aeruginosa*; however, the presence of fever should cause one to think of other agents as well. The basic work-up of a child with a clinical picture of osteomyelitis should include a complete blood cell count with differential cell count, an ESR, and a blood culture. Joint fluid should be aspirated and cultured whenever available. In children younger than 3 years, urine should be checked for *H influenzae* type b capsular antigen. If these initial studies fail to yield the cause of the infection, a bone aspirate should be obtained.

References

1. Self EB. Acute hematogenous osteomyelitis. *Pediatrics.* 1948;1:617-626.
2. Blanche DW. Osteomyelitis in infants. *J Bone Joint Surg Am.* 1952;34:71-85.
3. Green M, Nyhan WL Jr, Fousek MD. Acute hematogenous osteomyelitis. *Pediatrics.* 1956; 17:368-381.
4. Waldvogel FA, Medoff G, Swartz MN. Osteomyelitis: a review of clinical features, therapeutic considerations and unusual aspects (first of three parts). *N Engl J Med.* 1970;282:198-206.
5. Blockley NJ, Watson JT. Acute osteomyelitis in children. *J Bone Joint Surg Br.* 1970;52:77-87.
6. Mollan RAB, Piggot J. Acute osteomyelitis in children. *J Bone Joint Surg Br.* 1977;59:2-7.
7. Anderson JR, Scobie WG, Watt B. The treatment of acute osteomyelitis in children: a 10-year experience. *J Antimicrob Chemother.* 1981;7:43-50.
8. Cole WG, Dalziel RE, Leitl S. Treatment of acute osteomyelitis in childhood. *J Bone Joint Surg Br.* 1982;64:218-223.
9. LaMont RL, Anderson PA, Dajani AS, Thirumoorthi MC. Acute hematogenous osteomyelitis in children. *J Pediatr Orthop.* 1987;7:579-583.
10. Lebel MH, Nelson JD. *Haemophilus influenzae* type b osteomyelitis in infants and children. *Pediatr Infect Dis.* 1988;7:250-254.
11. Ravn H. Acute haematogenous osteomyelitis due to type-b *Haemophilus influenzae. Lancet.* 1966;1:517-518.
12. Granoff DM, Sargent E, Jolivette D. *Haemophilus influenzae* type b osteomyelitis. *AJDC.* 1978;132:488-490.
13. Schwartz RH, Reing CM. Acute hematogenous osteomyelitis secondary to *Hemophilus influenzae. J Pediatr Orthop.* 1982;1:385-389.
14. Rotbart HA, Glode MP. *Haemophilus influenzae* type b septic arthritis in children: report of 23 cases. *Pediatrics.* 1985;75:254-259.
15. Ward JI, Siber GR, Scheifele DW, Smith DH. Rapid diagnosis of *Hemophilus influenzae* type b infections by latex particle agglutination and counterimmunoelectrophoresis. *J Pediatr.* 1978; 93:37-42.
16. Murphy TV, Clements JF, Granoff DM. Concentrations of *H influenzae* type b (HIB) polysaccharide (PRP) in urine of healthy HIB carriers and patients with disease as measured by ELISA. *Pediatr Res.* 1989;25:185A. Abstract.
17. Green NE, Bruno J III. *Pseudomonas* infections of the foot after puncture wounds. *South Med J.* 1980;73:146-149.
18. Elliott SJ, Aronoff SC. Clinical presentation and management of *Pseudomonas* osteomyelitis. *Clin Pediatr.* 1985;24:566-570.
19. Minnefor AB, Olson MI, Carver DH. *Pseudomonas* osteomyelitis following puncture wounds of the foot. *Pediatrics.* 1971;47:598-601.
20. Jacobs RF, McCarthy RE, Elser JM. *Pseudomonas* osteochondritis: complicating puncture wounds of the foot in children: a 10 year evaluation. *J Infect Dis.* 1989;160:657-661.
21. Fisher MC, Goldsmith JF, Gilligan PH. Sneakers as a source of *Pseudomonas aeruginosa* in children with osteomyelitis following puncture wounds. *J Pediatr.* 1985;106:607-609.

Pneumococcal Osteomyelitis and Arthritis in Children

A Hospital Series and Literature Review

Norman M. Jacobs, MD

• Twenty-nine children with pneumococcal osteomyelitis and/or arthritis, 11 of whom had osteomyelitis, were treated at Cook County Hospital, Chicago, Ill, in the past 20 years. They were mostly normal children with a single focus of infection. They represented more than 5% of the hospitalized children with a systemic pneumococcal infection. Most of the pneumococcal isolates were serotyped; serotype 19, in particular, seemed to be unusually common in these children. Twenty-three of the 29 children with pneumococcal osteomyelitis and/or arthritis had been hospitalized in the past 15 years. These 23 children were compared with 161 hospitalized children who had bone and joint infections with other isolated bacteria. The children with pneumococcal osteomyelitis and/or arthritis were indistinguishable from most of the other children, except by age. All but three of the children with pneumococcal osteomyelitis and/or arthritis were between the ages of 3 and 24 months. In this age group, *Pneumococcus* was the common isolate from children with osteomyelitis, and second only to *Haemophilus influenzae* from children with bacterial arthritis. Pneumococcal osteomyelitis and/or arthritis has never been rare; the medical literature describes at least 245 other children, most of whom were younger than 2 years.

(*AJDC.* 1991;145:70-74)

According to Bulkley,[1] the first patient with pneumococcal arthritis was identified in 1888, and by 1914 Bulkley could review 173 reported cases. Of these, more than one-third were children. Subsequent literature reviews of pneumococcal arthritis in 1964[2] and 1973[3] included few additional children, which suggested that pneumococcal arthritis in children had become less common. Likewise, other than the 1926 monograph on osteomyelitis by Lawford[4] and a few recent case reports,[5-7] little attention has been given to pneumococcal osteomyelitis. Thus, not surprisingly, most current pediatric textbooks say little about pneumococcal osteomyelitis and arthritis.

This article gives observations on 29 children with pneumococcal osteomyelitis and/or arthritis (PnOA), including how these children presented, how they differed from other children with bone and joint infections, and the relative prevalence of these pneumococcal infections. An attempt was made to document and review all previous reports of children with PnOA to establish the consistency of these observations.

PATIENTS AND METHODS

Patients

The children included in this article were hospitalized at Cook County Children's Hospital, Chicago, Ill, from 1967 to 1987. From 1974, the children with possible bacterial bone-joint infections and the children with other systemic bacterial infections were identified during their stay in the hospital by a member of the Pediatric Infectology Service. Before 1974, such children were identified from the records of the hospital's Microbiology Laboratory (1967 to 1974) and/or the hospital's Medical Records Department (1972 to 1974).

Comparisons

To show the relative prevalence of PnOA in the hospitalized children, these infected children were compared with two different groups of children: all other children hospitalized with a systemic pneumococcal infection (1967 to 1986) and all other children hospitalized with bacterial osteomyelitis and/or arthritis (1972 to 1987). Ages were compared using medians and semi-interquartile ranges. Medians were used because the age distributions were asymmetric, and the semi-interquartile range was used because it is a meaningful measure of variability about the median. The semi-interquartile range is equal to half of the interval from the first quartile to the third quartile of a distribution.[8]

Definitions

The children identified as having a *systemic bacterial infection* were those who had a recognized bacterial pathogen isolated from blood, bone, joint, or other normally sterile body fluid. The children identified as having *osteomyelitis* were so diagnosed by a radiologist from the roentgenograms or nuclear bone scans, or by an orthopedic surgeon after direct visualization of bone. The children identified as having *arthritis* were those who had pus drained from a joint, or those who had a systemic bacterial infection with swelling about a major joint in the absence of osteomyelitis. Children who had osteomyelitis with sterile joint effusions, obtained before antimicrobial therapy, were *not* considered to have arthritis. Excluded were children whose infections occurred in the proximity of, and following, an open wound. Thus, these children had *hematogenous* osteomyelitis and/or arthritis.

Table 1.—Children With Pneumococcal Osteomyelitis Recognized at Cook County Hospital, Chicago, Ill, 1967 to 1987

Patient/ Age/Sex	Local Disease Presentation	Culture*		Serotype	Roentgenographic Bone Site (Time, d†)
		Blood	Site		
1/7 wk/M	Elbow swelling	−	+	3	Humoral periosteum (20)
2/4 mo/F	Elbow arthritis	+	+	23	Humoral periosteum (14)
3/4 mo/F	Elbow arthritis	+	+	9	Humoral periosteum (14)
4/3 mo/M	Knee swelling	−	+	19	Tibial metaphysis (13)
5/4 mo/F	Hip arthritis	−	+	19	Femoral metaphysis (6)
6/10 mo/M	Hip arthritis	−	+	14	Femoral metaphysis (15)
7/14 y/F	Shin pain	−	+	31	Tibial metaphysis (24)
8/13 mo/F	Forearm swelling	+	ND	14	Radial diaphysis (21)
9/3 mo/M	Chest abscess	+	+	19	Sternal diaphysis (32)
10/5 mo/M	Chest abscess	ND	+	19	Costal diaphysis (6)
11/12 mo/M	Chest abscess	−	+	14	Costal diaphysis (6)

*ND indicates not done.
†Time from onset of disease until recognized bone changes.

Accepted for publication June 5, 1990.
From the Departments of Pediatrics, Cook County Hospital and University of Illinois School of Medicine, Chicago.
Reprint requests to Department Pediatrics, Cook County Hospital, 700 S Wood St, Chicago, IL 60612 (Dr Jacobs).

The bacteria isolated were identified by the hospital laboratory by using the standard microbiologic methods in practice at the time of isolation; these methods changed over the course of the reported period. Most of the pneumococci isolated were serotyped by the quellung reaction with antiserum samples from the Statens Seruminstut, Copenhagen, Denmark.[9] Recently isolated streptococci were serogrouped with commercial latex agglutination kits; older isolates were identified presumptively by the methods recommended at that time. All *Haemophilus influenzae* isolated after 1974 were serotyped with commercial antiserum samples by slide agglutination.

Literature Review

The medical literature was reviewed by searching for all reports in English from 1915 to 1987 that identified children with PnOA; one German article[10] was also included. An attempt was made to exclude reports that duplicated the same children.

RESULTS

In the 20-year period from 1967 through 1987, twenty-nine children with PnOA were identified among children admitted to Cook County Hospital. Their ages ranged from 44 days to 14 years; 16 were male.

Pneumococcal Arthritis

Twenty-two of the children had purulent arthritis. The oldest child was aged 23 months. Nineteen of the children were apparently normal, two had histories consistent with an immunodeficiency disease (recurrent bacterial infections), and one had spherocytosis. All the children presented with fever (temperature, >38.5°C) and signs of an acutely inflamed joint. All had involvement of only a single joint: the hip (10 children), knee (five), shoulder (three), elbow (two), or ankle (two). Pus was recovered from all joints, and pneumococci were isolated from all but one joint, that of a child who had received penicillin before the joint was aspirated. He and six other children in this series had pneumococcal bacteremia; one other child had *Staphylococcus aureus* isolated from a blood culture. Two children had other sites of infection: one had meningitis and the other had pneumonia.

Pneumococcal Osteomyelitis

Eleven children, four with purulent arthritis and seven others, had roentgenographic osteomyelitis (Table 1). Eight of the 11 children were apparently normal. The other three had cyanotic congenital heart disease, systemic lupus erythematosus, or sickle-cell disease (patients 6 through 8, respectively, in Table 1). All 11 children also presented with fever and inflammatory signs overlying the involved bone. Three children presented with chest-wall abscesses overlying their costal or sternal osteomyelitis. Five others had destructive long-bone lesions, including a Brodie abscess in the girl with systemic lupus erythematosus. The remaining three children had only small localized periosteal reactions. The bone lesions were detected roentgenographically from 6 to 32 days after the onset of clinical signs; only four children had these changes when admitted to the hospital. Only the child with sickle-cell disease had a second site of infection; he also had pneumonia.

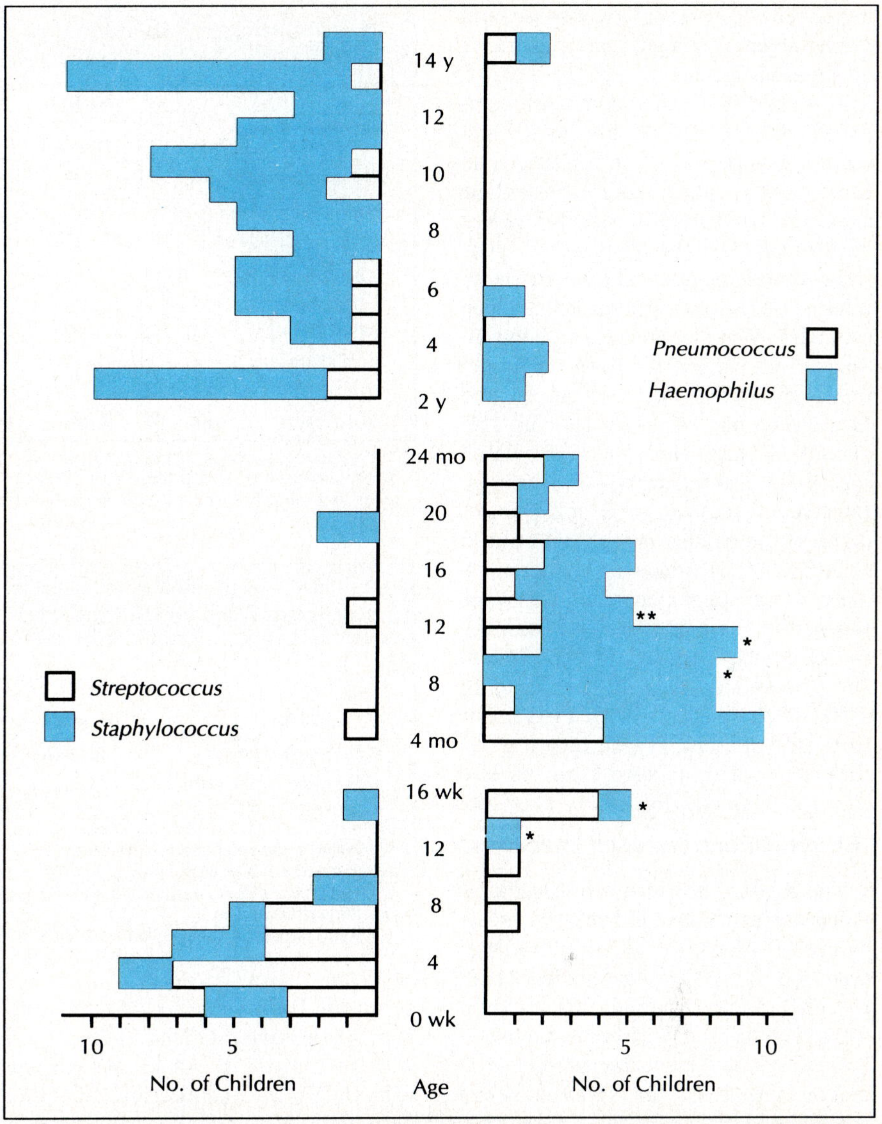

Age distribution of children with bacterial osteomyelitis and/or arthritis at Cook County Hospital, 1972 to 1987. Data for children with *Pneumococcus* and *Haemophilus* infections are on the right, and for those with *Streptococcus* and *Staphylococcus* infections, on the left. Asterisks indicate data for the six other children with pneumococcal osteomyelitis and/or arthritis, 1967 to 1972.

Systemic Pneumococcal Infections

In this 20-year period, 532 children were hospitalized with a systemic pneumococcal infection. The 29 children with PnOA accounted for more than 5% of these children. Of the remaining children, 166 had pneumonia, 137 had meningitis, 25 had another focal disease, and 175 had bacteremia with otitis media or no apparent focus.

The children with PnOA were compared with the other children with systemic pneumococcal infections, and three comparisons are of interest: their ages, the frequency they had detected bacteremia, and the serotypes of their isolated pneumococci. The age distributions of these two groups of children coincided. The median ages (±semi-interquartile ranges) of those with and those without PnOA were 11±6 and 11±8 months, respectively. The frequency of bacteremia and the isolated serotypes differed in the two groups. Bacteremia was detected in only nine (31%) of the children with PnOA but in 454 (90%) of the remaining children. Finally, two pneumococcal serotypes were more commonly isolated from the children with PnOA. Serotypes 14 and 19 were isolated from 10 (34%) and 10 (34%) of the children with PnOA, but from only 21% and 11% of the other 489 children with a serotyped isolate ($\chi^2=19.77$, $df=2$, $P<.001$).

Bacterial Bone and Joint Infections

The relative prevalence of the *Pneumococcus* as a cause of bacterial osteomyelitis and/or arthritis in children was assessed for a 15-year period (1972 to 1987). In that period, 184 children were hospitalized with an established (hematogenous) bacterial osteomyelitis and/or arthritis. The *Pneumococcus* was isolated from 23 (13%) of these children. The other commonly isolated bacteria were *S aureus*, *H influenzae* type b, and *Streptococcus* groups A through C (Table 2).

Table 2.—Numbers of Children With Bacterial Osteomyelitis (OS) and/or Arthritis (AR) at Cook County Hospital, Chicago, Ill, 1972 to 1987

Bacterial Isolates	Total	All Ages OS	All Ages OS+AR	All Ages AR	Aged 3-24 mo OS	Aged 3-24 mo OS+AR	Aged 3-24 mo AR	Blood Culture, No. Positive/No. Obtained
Pneumococcus	23	5	4	14	3	4	13	6/20
Staphylococcus aureus	71	48	12	11	3	0	0	39/56
Haemophilus influenzae type b	46	3	2	41	3	2	35	36/43
*Streptotoccus**	29	9	6	14	0	0	2	9/21
Meningococcus	5	0	0	5	0	0	3	4/5
Other†	10	10	0	0	2‡	0	0	5/10
All isolates	184	75	24	85	11	6	53	99/155

**Streptococcus* groups A (11), B (17), and C (one).
†*Salmonella* (six), *Serratia* (three), and *Brucella* (one).
‡Children with sickle-cell and chronic granulomatous diseases.

Table 3.—Ages of Children With Osteomyelitis and/or Arthritis vs Ages of Their Cohorts With Other Systemic Infections at Cook County Hospital, Chicago, Ill

Infection Sites	Median Age±SIQR* (No. of Children): *Pneumococcus*†	*Haemophilus*‡	Group B *Streptococcus*§
Osteomyelitis/arthritis	11±6 mo (29)	9±5 mo (46)	25±17 d (17)
Other systemic infections	11±8 mo (503)	10±7 mo (391)	21±16 d (164)
Total	... (532)	... (437)	... (181)

*SIQR indicates semi-interquartile range.
†Pneumococcal infections (1967 to 1987).
‡*Haemophilus influenzae* infections (1972 to 1987, excluding 20 children with epiglottitis and infants under the age of 3 days).
§Group B streptococcal infections (1972 to 1987, excluding infants under the age of 3 days).

Among the several population characteristics examined, age was the most useful predictor of the bacterial cause in these infected children. The children with pneumococcal and *Haemophilus* infections had a unimodal age distribution, with most (87%) occurring between the ages of 3 and 24 months, whereas the children with staphylococcal and streptococcal infections had a bimodal age distribution, with most (95%) occurring outside this age range (Figure). The *Pneumococcus* was isolated from 20 of the 70 children aged 3 to 24 months. In this age group, only *Haemophilus* was isolated more commonly (Table 2). However, the *Pneumococcus* was the common isolate (seven of 17 [41%]) from those with osteomyelitis. As in the children with PnOA, the age distribution of children with *Haemophilus* and group B streptococcal bone and joint infections coincided with the age distribution of their respective cohorts who had other systemic infections (Table 3).

Observations, other than age, were less useful predictors of the bacterial cause. The children's sex, clinical presentation, and peripheral blood counts were not useful. The blood culture, however, usually proved to be diagnostic. Among those children for whom a blood culture was obtained, however, only a minority of those with pneumococcal infections had detectable bacteremia. Conversely, most of the children with staphylococcal, *Haemophilus*, and meningococcal infections had detectable bacteremia (Table 2). Finally, the anatomic site of infection generally was not predictive of the bacterial cause of these infections. One exception, relative to the pneumococcal infections, was chest-wall osteomyelitis. Besides the three children with pneumococcal costal/sternal osteomyelitis noted above (Table 1), similar nonpneumococcal infections were observed in only two other children, both of whom had sickle-cell disease.

COMMENT

Since Bulkley's 1914 literature review,[1] which included 66 children under the age of 16 years, reports have noted 179 additional children with PnOA. Table 4 summarizes 16 reports[10-25] in which more than half of these children were described. Children with PnOA have been identified worldwide and in all decades since Bulkley's review. In 33 additional reports, the remaining 40 children with pneumococcal arthritis[7,26-42] and 35 with osteomyelitis[4-7,42-54] are described.

In the children in this study, pneumo-

Table 4.—Summary of 16 Hospital Reports of Osteomyelitis (OS) and/or Arthritis (AR), Including 37 Children With Pneumococcal Osteomyelitis and 67 With Pneumococcal Arthritis

				Isolate, No. of Children		
Source, y	Location	Age, y	Disease	*Staphylococcus* and/or *Streptococcus*	*Haemophilus*	*Pneumococcus*
Johnson,[11] 1921	New York, NY	<3	AR	21	3	14
Paschlau,[10] 1933	Berlin, Germany	<3	OS	41	0	9
Inge and Leibolt,[12] 1935	New York	<3	AR	9	0	2
		≥3	AR	19	0	1
Green and Shannon,[13] 1936	Boston, Mass	<2	OS	70	0	3
Self,[14] 1948	New York	All	OS	109	0	3
White and Dennison,[15] 1952	Glasgow, Scotland	All	OS	209	0	3
Samilson et al,[16] 1958	New York	<2	AR	14	2	4
		≥2	AR	12	1	1
Borella et al,[17] 1963	Memphis, Tenn	All	AR	25	6	3
Gillespie,[18] 1973	Toronto, Ontario	<3	AR	12	2	3
		≥3	AR	48	0	0
Nade,[19] 1977	Sydney, Australia	All	OS	78	3	5
		All	AR	40	14	0
Griffin and Green,[20] 1978	Boston	All	AR	38	4	9
Anderson et al,[21] 1980	Edinburgh, Scotland	All	OS	101	1	3
Fink and Nelson,[22] 1986	Dallas, Tex	<2	AR	38	133	14
		≥2	AR	112	16	3
		<2	OS	46	12	6
		≥2	OS	174	2	0
Welkon et al,[23] 1986	Philadelphia, Pa	<2	AR	9	24	8
		≥2	AR	11	4	0
Barton et al,[24] 1987	St Louis, Mo	<2	AR	14	14	3
		≥2	AR	34	6	2
LaMont et al,[25] 1987	Detroit, Mich	<2	OS	18	7	5
		≥2	OS	59	0	0

coccal bone and joint infections were found predominantly among those aged 3 to 24 months. This age group is not identifiable in most reports. Table 4 is arranged to show that most of the described children with PnOA were under the age of 2 to 3 years, and in these young children the *Pneumococcus* was a relatively common isolate. Where the age could be determined in Bulkley's review[1] and in the other reports describing children with pneumococcal arthritis[7,26-37] and pneumococcal osteomyelitis,[4-7,43-50] about two thirds of the children also were under the age of 24 months. Presumably this age association is related to the age when pneumococcal bacteremia is most common in children (Table 3).

More than 5% of the hospitalized children with systemic pneumococcal infections in this series had osteomyelitis and/or arthritis, and only two serotypes (14 and 19) accounted for 20 of these 29 infections. It is difficult to confirm either of these observations. Most reviews of serious pneumococcal infections in children are confined to those with bacteremia, and detectable bacteremia was uncommon in the untreated children with PnOA in this study. There are two reports[41,42] of children with systemic pneumococcal infections, one in 1933 and one in 1979, in which 10 (3%) and three (2%) of the children, respectively, had arthritis or osteomyelitis. Likewise, only three other described children with PnOA had their pneumococcal isolates serotyped[28,43]; none was serotype 14 or 19. However, in adults with pneumococcal arthritis,[33,55] four of 19 serotyped isolates were serotype 19. Serotype 19 also is the common isolate from children with otitis media,[56-58] an infection of a bone-lined, bone-filled cavity. Therefore, it may be that serotype 19, at least, is attracted to paraosteal tissues.

Most of the children with PnOA in this study had only a single site of infection, and most were otherwise normal children. Only three of the children had a second site of infection (pneumonia or meningitis), whereas in the preantimicrobial era, multiple infection sites were common.[1,4,11,26] However, recent cases of PnOA have been described in children compromised by malnutrition,[7] hemophilia,[35,37] immunodeficiency states,[33,49] and sickle-cell disease.[6,45,48,59] Again, only four of the children with PnOA in this study had similar problems. Sickle-cell disease, in particular, did not seem to predispose these children to PnOA. In the 20 years of the study, only one such infection was found among 40 childhood episodes of pneumococcal bacteremia occurring in 37 children with sickle-cell disease.

Differentiating the children with pneumococcal bone, joint, and deep subcutaneous infections proved to be difficult. Altering the definitions used in this report would have increased or decreased the numbers. The children presenting with pneumococcal chest-wall abscesses who proved to have costal-sternal osteomyelitis are a good example of this. This may be important because the literature review revealed that the *Pneumococcus* was the common isolate from children with costal osteomyelitis, with six other children described.[4,6,43,60,61]

CONCLUSION

The *Pneumococcus* is, and appears always to have been, a relatively common cause of bacterial osteomyelitis and/or arthritis in normal young children. The age of these children coincides with that age when pneumococcal bacteremia is most frequent. These children with PnOA may not be identified because most of them are not bacteremic when they are seen, and because many receive effective antibacterial therapy before the site of infection is cultured. Unfortunately, they are clinically indistinguishable from the children with type b *Haemophilus* arthritis, which is more common in children of the same age. As *Haemophilus* infections become less frequent because of effective vaccination, PnOA will probably become more apparent, if not more frequent.

I thank the many pediatric and orthopedic residents whose dedication and thoroughness made this study possible.

References

1. Bulkley K. Pneumococcic arthritis. *Ann Surg.* 1914;59:71-100.

2. Argen RJ. Suppurative pneumococcic arthritis. *N Y State J Med.* 1964;64:2573-2579.

3. Torres J, Rathbun HK, Greenough WB III. Pneumococcal arthritis: report of a case and review of the literature. *Johns Hopkins Med J.* 1973;132:234-241.

4. Lawford KR. *Inflammatory and Toxic Diseases of Bone.* New York, NY: William Wood and Co; 1926:39-41.

5. Lakhani U. Pneumococcal osteomyelitis and arthritis in an infant: report of a case and a brief review of the literature. *Conn Med.* 1977;41:479-483.

6. Chusid MJ, Sty JR. Pneumococcal arthritis and osteomyelitis in children. *Clin Pediatr.* 1981;20:105-107.

7. Hadari I, Dagan R, Gedalia A, Jeanine N, Moses S. Pneumococcal osteomyelitis, an unusual cluster of cases. *Clin Pediatr.* 1985;24:143-145.

8. Phillips JL Jr. *Statistical Thinking: A Structural Approach.* 2nd ed. New York, NY: WH Freeman & Co; 1982:29-30.

9. Jacobs NM, Lerdkachornsuk S, Metzger WI. Pneumococcal bacteremia in infants and children: a ten-year experience at the Cook County Hospital with special reference to the pneumococcal serotypes isolated. *Pediatrics.* 1979;64:296-300.

10. Paschlau G. Die Besonderheiten der Osteomyelitis im fruehen Kindesalter. *Monatschr Kinderheilkd.* 1933;55:280-306.

11. Johnson FE. A study of seventy-three cases of acute arthritis in infants. *AJDC.* 1921;21:170-175.

12. Inge GAL, Leibolt FL. The treatment of acute suppurative arthritis: report of thirty-six cases treated by operation. *Surg Gynecol Obstet.* 1935;60:86-101.

13. Green WT, Shannon JG. Osteomyelitis of infants: a disease different from osteomyelitis of older children. *Arch Surg.* 1936;32:462-493.

14. Self EB. Acute hematogenous osteomyelitis. *Pediatrics.* 1948;1:617-626.

15. White M, Dennison WM. Acute haematogenous osteitis in childhood: a review of 212 cases. *J Bone Joint Surg Br.* 1952;34:608-623.

16. Samilson RL, Bersani FA, Watkins MB. Acute suppurative arthritis in infants and children: the importance of early diagnosis and surgical drainage. *Pediatrics.* 1958;21:798-803.

17. Borella L, Goobar JE, Summitt RL, Clark GM. Septic arthritis in childhood. *J Pediatr.* 1963;62:742-747.

18. Gillespie R. Septic arthritis of childhood. *Clin Orthop.* 1973;96:152-159.

19. Nade S. Choice of antibiotics in management of acute osteomyelitis and acute septic arthritis in children. *Arch Dis Child.* 1977;52:679-682.

20. Griffin PP, Green WT Sr. Hip joint infections in infants and children. *Orthop Clin North Am.* 1978;9:123-134.

21. Anderson JR, Orr JD, Maclean DA, Scobie WG. Acute haematogenous osteitis. *Arch Dis Child.* 1980;55:953-957.

22. Fink CJ, Nelson JD. Septic arthritis and osteomyelitis in children. *Clin Rheum Dis.* 1986;12:423-435.

23. Welkon CJ, Long SS, Fisher MC, Alburger PD. Pyogenic arthritis in infants and children: a review of 95 cases. *Pediatr Infect Dis.* 1986;5:669-676.

24. Barton LL, Dunkle LM, Habib FH. Septic arthritis in childhood: a 13-year review. *AJDC.* 1987;141:898-900.

25. LaMont RL, Anderson PA, Dajani AS, Thirumoorthi MC. Acute hematogenous osteomyelitis in children. *J Pediatr Orthop.* 1987;7:579-583.

26. Sever JW. Pneumococcic arthritis, with report of six cases. *Bost Med Surg J.* 1915;173:387-391.

27. Eggers GWN. Suppurative arthritis of the knee joint. *Tex State J Med.* 1936;31:623-626.

28. Tucker JL, Tepper WR. Intra-articular penicillin treatment of suppurative arthritis in infants and children. *J Pediatr.* 1946;29:711-720.

29. Nicholson JT. Pyogenic arthritis with pathologic dislocation of the hip in infants. *JAMA.* 1949;141:826-830.

30. Baitch A. Recent observations of acute suppurative arthritis. *Clin Orthop.* 1962;22:157-165.

31. Stetson JW, DePonte RJ, Southwick WO. Acute septic arthritis of the hip in children. *Clin Orthop.* 1968;56:105-116.

32. Almquist EE. The changing epidemiology of septic arthritis in children. *Clin Orthop.* 1970;68:96-99.

33. Kauffman CA, Watanakunakorn C, Phair JP. Pneumococcal arthritis. *J Rheumatol.* 1976;3:409-419.

34. Wiley JJ, Fraser GA. Septic arthritis in childhood. *Can J Surg.* 1979;22:326-330.

35. Hoffman A, Wyatt R, Bybee B. Septic arthritis of the knee in a 12 year-old hemophiliac. *J Pediatr Orthop.* 1984;4:498-499.

36. Peltola H, Vahvanen V. A comparative study of osteomyelitis and purulent arthritis with special reference to aetiology and recovery. *Infection.* 1984;12:75-79.

37. Fajardo JE, Mickunas VH, deTriquet JM. Suppurative arthritis and hemophilia. *Pediatr Infect Dis.* 1986;5:593-594.

38. Harris RI. Acute suppurative arthritis in children. *J Bone Joint Surg.* 1925;23:849-872.

39. Aitken J, Laird AP. Pyogenic arthritis of the hip in childhood. *Z Kinderchir.* 1970;8:143-154.

40. Goldenberg DL, Cohen AS. Acute infectious arthritis: a review of patients with nongonococcal joint infections (with emphasis on therapy and prognosis). *Am J Med.* 1976;60:369-377.

41. Gray BM, Converse GM III, Dillon HC Jr. Serotypes of *Streptococcus pneumoniae* causing disease. *J Infect Dis.* 1979;140:979-983.

42. Blacklock JWS, Guthrie KJ. Pneumococcal infections in infancy and childhood. *J Pathol Bacteriol.* 1933;36:349-368.

43. Green M, Nyhan WL Jr, Fousek MD. Acute hematogenous osteomyelitis. *Pediatrics.* 1956;17:368-381.

44. Boyes J, Bremner AE, Neligan GA. Haematogenous osteitis in the newborn. *Lancet.* 1957;1:544-548.

45. Barrett-Connor E. Bacterial infection and sickle cell anemia: an analysis of 250 infections in 166 patients and a review of the literature. *Medicine.* 1971;50:97-112.

46. Edwards MS, Baker CJ, Wagner ML, Taber LH, Barrett FF. An etiologic shift of infantile osteomyelitis: the emergence of group B *Streptococcus. J Pediatr.* 1978;93:578-583.

47. Dan M. Septic arthritis in young infants: clinical and microbiologic correlations and therapeutic implications. *Rev Infect Dis.* 1984;6:147-155.

48. Rao SP, Miller S, Solomon N. Acute bone and joint manifestations of sickle cell disease in children. *N Y State J Med.* 1986;86:254-260.

49. Gottsegen DN. Pneumococcal osteomyelitis associated with IgG2 subclass deficiency. *Pediatr Infect Dis J.* 1987;6:281-284.

50. Hellerstein A, Wiedermann BL. Pneumococcal sacroiliitis in an infant. *Pediatr Infect Dis J.* 1987;6:759-761.

51. Blanche DW. Osteomyelitis in infants. *J Bone Joint Surg Am.* 1952;34:71-84.

52. Gilmore WN. Acute haematogenous osteomyelitis. *J Bone Joint Surg Br.* 1962;44:841-853.

53. Jacobs JC. Acute osteomyelitis: medical management in children. *N Y State J Med.* 1978;78:910-912.

54. Gillespie WJ, Mayo KM. The management of acute haematogenous osteomyelitis in the antibiotic era: a study of the outcome. *J Bone Joint Surg Br.* 1981;63:126-131.

55. Finland M, Barnes MW. Changes in occurrence of capsular serotypes of *Streptococcus pneumoniae* at Boston City Hospital during selected years between 1935 and 1974. *J Clin Microbiol.* 1977;5:154-166.

56. Kamme C, Ageberg M, Lundgren K. Distribution of *Diplococcus pneumoniae* types in acute otitis media in children and influence of the types on the clinical course in penicillin V therapy. *Scand J Infect Dis.* 1970;2:183-190.

57. Austrian R, Howie VM, Ploussard JH. The bacteriology of pneumococcal otitis media. *Johns Hopkins Med J.* 1977;141:104-111.

58. Gray BM, Dillon HC Jr. Clinical and epidemiologic studies of pneumococcal infection in children. *Pediatr Infect Dis.* 1986;5:201-207.

59. Syrogiannopoulos GA, McCracken GH Jr, Nelson JD. Osteoarticular infections in children with sickle cell disease. *Pediatrics.* 1986;78:1090-1096.

60. Voelcker AF, Handley WS. A case of multiple pneumococcal epiphysitis; recovery. *Lancet.* 1906;2:1436.

61. Coutts JA. A case of general pneumococcal infection, with acute necrosis of bone. *Lancet.* 1907;1:1648-1649.

Influence of Otitis Media on the Correlation Between Rectal and Auditory Canal Temperatures

Thomas E. Terndrup, MD, Agnes Wong, MD

• In a noninterventional, controlled, single-blinded trial, 251 children were examined in a university hospital emergency department setting to study the influence of acute otitis media on the relationship between rectal and auditory canal temperatures. Bilateral auditory canal temperatures were measured using an infrared detection probe and microprocessor by nursing staff blinded to the presence of acute otitis media. Correlation between rectal and auditory canal temperatures in children with (r=.81) and without (r=.75) acute otitis media were not significantly different. There was no significant difference between infected (38.1°C ± 1.0°C) and uninfected ears (38.0°C ± 1.0°C) with unilateral otitis (n=75). Although significantly higher than in uninfected children, auditory canal temperatures of children with acute otitis media reflected elevated rectal temperatures and not differences in auditory canal temperatures between ears.

(*AJDC.* 1991;145:75-78)

Childhood febrile illnesses account for a majority of telephone calls, unscheduled office visits, and trips to the emergency department (ED).[1,2] Fever may be the only objective indication of serious infection such as meningitis or bacteremia, particularly in infants.[3,4] Accurate determination of body temperature is essential for the differential diagnosis of acute illness. The accepted method for accurate determination of body temperature in nonneonatal ambulatory children is by inserting a thermometer into the rectum to obtain a rectal temperature (RT).[5] However, RT measurement is inconvenient, invasive, time consuming, and potentially painful; exposes personnel to contagious disease; and may lead to uncooperative behavior in some children.[6] Recent advances in thermometry technology allow body temperature to be measured as a function of infrared emissions.[7,8] Auditory canal temperature (ACT) measurement, obtained as a function of these emissions, appears to be accurate in adults and possibly in children when compared with RT obtained with standard digital electronic thermometers.[6,9-13] The use of ACT measurements would provide a noninvasive, rapid, and safe method of measuring body temperature.

Since acute otitis media (AOM) results in hyperemia, infrared emissions are increased and may influence the accuracy of ACT readings during AOM.[11] One author[14] stated that "[the ACT] . . . reading is invalidated by acute otitis media" and " . . . bilateral acute otitis media prohibits use of this method." Further, some authors have found that ACT measurements may be inaccurate in children.[10,13]

We examined the relationship between RT and bilateral ACT in children presenting for medical care in the ED. By controlling for the presence of AOM, the influence of AOM on this relationship was examined. We also sought to determine the influence of age on the accuracy of ACT measurements and the value of ACT measurements as a screening test for fever.

SUBJECTS AND METHODS

Children less than 16 years of age, who underwent either routine or physician-requested RT measurement while in the ED, were eligible for the study. Subjects were recruited by the triage or pediatric ED nurse following informed consent. The study was approved by the State University of New York Institutional Review Board for the Protection of Human Subjects. This study was carried out from November 16 through December 3, 1989.

Subjects underwent RT measurement with a calibrated digital electronic thermometer (Diatek, San Diego, Calif) and bilateral ACT measurement using an infrared emission detection probe and microprocessor (First Temp, Intelligent Medical Systems, Carlsbad, Calif). Rectal temperatures were obtained in the monitor mode, allowing at least 3 minutes for equilibration. Participating pediatric ED nurses were given a brief inservice on the use of the probe and microprocessor. They were instructed to retract the external ear posteriorly and place the probe snugly into the ostia of each auditory canal. Digital readings were obtained after approximately 2 seconds. Physicians, pediatric residents, or pediatric ED attending physicians then evaluated and treated each patient in the standard fashion, "blinded" to ACT measurements.

Following patient discharge, the physician recorded the presence or absence of AOM based on the presence of three or more of the following criteria: (1) rapid onset of fever and/or ear pain and/or irritability, (2) bulging or full tympanic membrane, (3) opaque or erythematous tympanic membrane, (4) limited or no mobility of tympanic membrane.[15] Auditory canal temperature readings of patients who could not be adequately evaluated were eliminated from analysis.

Temperature calibrations of the digital electronic thermometer, performed against a water bath, were found to be accurate within ±0.1°C (SD) at the beginning and end of the experimental period. The probe and microprocessor have an internal, self-adjusting calibration system and were operated in the rectal mode.

The relationship between RT and ACT for all patients was described using linear regression. The difference between RT and

Accepted for publication May 13, 1990.

From the Departments of Pediatrics (Drs Terndrup and Wong) and Critical Care and Emergency Medicine (Dr Terndrup), State University of New York Health Science Center at Syracuse.

Read before the Section III Ambulatory Pediatric Association Meeting of the American Pediatric Association, March 9, 1990, Rochester, NY.

Reprint requests to Critical Care and Emergency Medicine, SUNY Health Science Center, 750 E Adams St, Syracuse, NY 13210 (Dr Terndrup).

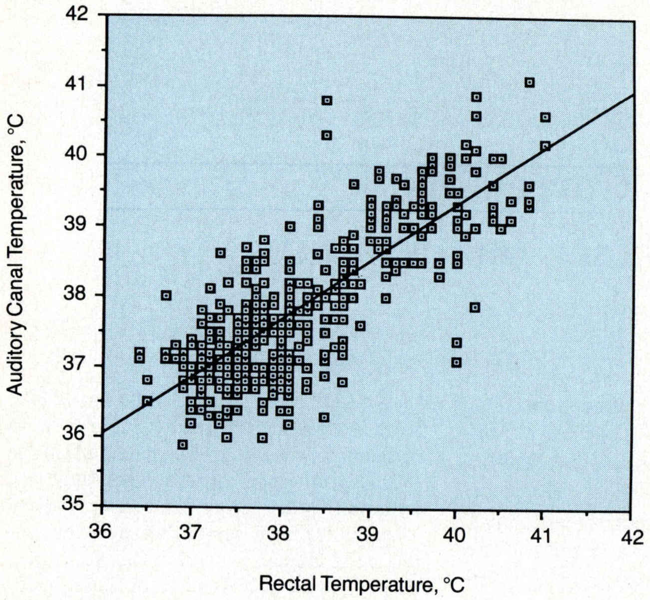

Fig 1.—Scattergram of 496 pairs of rectal and auditory canal temperatures.

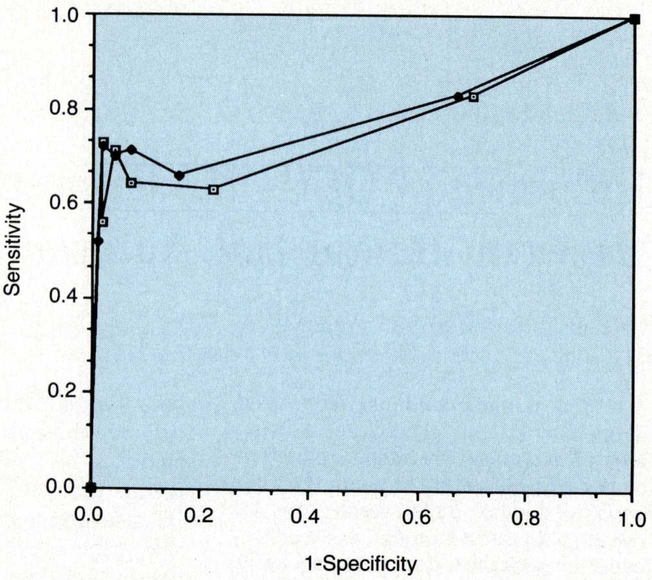

Fig 2.—Receiver operating characteristic curves for right (squares) and left (diamonds) auditory canal temperatures compared with rectal temperatures using five cutoffs for fever.

ACT was assessed using the two-tailed Student t test for all subjects, subjects with or without AOM, and for patients with unilateral AOM. Significant differences in the correlation between RT and ACT for ears with and without AOM were examined by calculating a Z value for homogeneity of the Pearson correlation coefficient. Significance was considered to be achieved at $P<.05$.

RESULTS

During the 2-week study period, 251 subjects were evaluated. Six patients whose ACTs could not be fully evaluated for the criteria of AOM were eliminated. Patients were young (mean age ±SD, 21.4±22 months), with 53% being male. Rectal temperature (mean±SD, 38.2°C±0.9°C; range, 36.4°C to 41°C) was significantly higher than ACT (37.8°C±1.0°C; range, 35.9°C to 41°C) for all subjects. Acute otitis media was seen in 35.5% (176/496) of ears. Using linear regression, the relationship between RT and ACT is described as follows: ACT=0.811(RT)+6.836 (Fig 1).

Rectal temperature was significantly greater than ACT in patients with and without AOM (Table 1). The correlation between RT and ACT was not significantly different for patients with (r=.81) and without (r=.75) AOM. Both the mean ACTs and RTs were greater in patients with AOM than in those without AOM. Patients with unilateral AOM (n=75) had no significant difference in the ACT of infected ears (38.1°C±1.0°C) vs uninfected ears (38.0°C±1.0°C), reflecting elevated body temperature and no unilateral ACT elevation in patients with AOM.

Table 1.—Influence of Otitis Media on Rectal and Auditory Canal Temperatures*

	Otitis Media	No Otitis Media	P
No. of ears	176	320	. . .
Age, mo	18.5±14.1	23.1±25.0	<.05
Temperature,°C			
Rectal	38.5±1.0	38.0±0.9	<.05
Tympanic	38.2±1.1	37.6±0.9	<.05
Rectal minus tympanic	0.3±0.6	0.4±0.6	NS
γ	.81	.75	NS†

*Data are means±SDs and Pearson correlation coefficient. NS indicates not significant.
†z test for homogeneity of correlation coefficient.

To examine the effectiveness of the device in fever screening, sensitivity, specificity, positive predictive values, and negative predictive values were calculated at four different RT readings (Table 2). By plotting sensitivity vs 1-specificity, a receiver operating characteristic curve is constructed (Fig 2). The receiver operating characteristic curve shows the relationship of sensitivity and specificity for a given ACT as a predictor of RT, using various cutoff points for fever. By choosing the point on the receiver operating characteristic curve that is farthest from the line of equivalence between X and Y values (ie, 39.0°C), the greatest value of the ACT test for fever screening information is obtained. Using an ACT of greater than or equal to 39.0°C to define fever, the sensitivity is found to be 73%, and the specificity is 98% (Table 2). Using an ACT of greater than or equal to 38.0°C to define fever, the sensitivity is found to be 68% and specificity is 93%.

Age less than 29 months had little influence on the relationship between ACT and RT(Table 3). The correlation between ACT and RT is not significantly different for age groups below 29 months. There is a significant reduction in the correlation coefficient for subjects older than 29 months compared with the group younger than 29 months ($P<.05$; Z test for homogeneity of the Pearson correlation coefficient).

COMMENT

The results of this study suggest that AOM does not significantly alter the relationship between RT and ACT in ambulatory children. Although children with infected ears had significantly higher temperatures than children with uninfected ears, this reflected elevated body temperature and not differences in ACTs between ears. In patients with unilateral AOM, there was no significant difference between the ACT of the infected vs the uninfected ear. The elevation of ACT during AOM was due to increased body temperature and not due to the effects of local inflammation. Using ACT measurements for fever screening is specific but not sensitive enough to allow for reliable screening. The accuracy of ACT readings was significantly poorer for active toddlers compared with younger ED patients.

Other investigators have performed limited comparisons between RT and ACT measurement during AOM in children. Lobbes,[16] in an unblinded trial, studied 30 children with unilateral AOM and 30 uninfected control subjects. She found that an ear with AOM was significantly warmer than the contralateral healthy ear, with a mean difference of 0.1°C (0.26°F). No significant differences between ears were seen in controls. She concluded that the increased ACT measurement reflected the effects of the local inflammation and might serve as a predictor of AOM. Weir and Weir[11] found in an unblinded, uncontrolled study of 62 children with unilateral AOM that infected ears were an average of 0.09°C±0.4°C warmer than uninfected ears. The results of this study support the conclusion that the differences between the ACTs of infected and uninfected ears is not large enough to interfere with the accuracy of the probe and microprocessor used to estimate body temperature in patients with AOM.

Other authors have examined the relationship between RT and ACT measurements with the use of the probe and microprocessor in children. Treloar and Muma[10] compared the relationship between axillary temperature, ACT, and RT in 224 children younger than 3 years of age in the ED. They found that AOM did not significantly change the relationship between the ACT and RT. The correlation between the RT and ACT was high overall ($r=.81$) but was lower for temperatures less than 38.0°C ($r=.12$) and greater than 39.5°C ($r=.24$). The overall specificity was 100%, but the sensitivity was only 54%. Ros[13] studied the correlation between temperatures measured with glass mercury thermometers and ACTs in 102 ambulatory children. He found that the mean (±SD) difference between the two methods was 0.3°C±0.7°C, which is nearly identical to our study. However, both oral temperatures and RTs were compared with ACT readings (no calibration of thermometers is mentioned) and inadequate equilibration times were used with the mercury thermometers for oral temperature measurement, making his results difficult to interpret.

Our study found that the age of the patients influenced the correlation between the RT and the ACT. For patients younger than 29 months of age, there was no difference in the correlation coefficients. However, there was a significant reduction in the correlation coefficient for patients older than 29 months of age. This difference may reflect the difficulty in positioning the auditory canal probe in active, less compliant toddlers. One group showed that there was a poor correlation in young patients less than 2 months of age.[10] They attributed this to the smaller size of the external auditory canal relative to the size of the temperature probe. By

Table 2.—Fever Screening Using Different Rectal Temperature Cutoffs*

Rectal temperature cutoff, °C	≥37.5	≥38.0	≥38.5	≥39.0	≥39.5
Sensitivity, %	65	68	71	73	54
Specificity, %	81	93	96	98	99
Positive predictive value, %	93	89	84	91	84
Negative predictive value, %	37	78	88	94	94
Prevalence, %	81	48	31	20	13

*Sensitivity=true positive/(true positive + false negative); specificity=true negative/(true negative + false positive); positive predictive value=true positive/(true positive + false positive); and negative predictive value=true negative/(true negative + false negative).

Table 3.—Influence of Age on the Relationship Between Rectal and Auditory Canal Temperatures*

Age range, mo	0-3	4-6	7-12	13-18	19-28	29-42	43-180
No. of Patients, %	26	34	47	36	42	38	28
Otitis media, %	15	40	51	36	35	38	24
Male, %	46	62	47	44	57	58	54
Temperature, °C							
Rectal	38.1±.6	38.5±1.2	38.2±.9	38.4±1	38.2±.9	38.0±.9	38.0±.7
Tympanic	37.4±.7	38.1±1.1	37.8±1	38.0±1	38.0±.9	37.6±.8	37.5±.8
Rectal minus tympanic	0.4±.4	0.4±.6	0.4±.6	0.4±.6	0.3±.5	0.3±.8	0.4±.7
γ	.81	.86	.83	.82	.84	.59	.57

*Data are the percent of patients in each age group with acute otitis media, means±SDs, and Pearson correlation coefficient.

slightly retracting the external ear and orienting the probe anteriorly, the impact of smaller size may have been overcome in this study.

The infrared tympanic thermometer has also been studied in various clinical situations in adults. Shinozaki et al[9] performed 260 comparisons of ACTs with RTs and pulmonary artery vascular temperature in adult patients who underwent postoperative coronary artery bypass surgery. Over a broad temperature range (34°C to 39.5°C), the correlation between the ACTs and the pulmonary artery temperatures was excellent ($r=.98$). Terndrup et al[6] found an excellent correlation between 107 pairs of RTs and ACTs ($r=.90$) in hospitalized adults. In 22 volunteers, ingestion of hot or cold liquids produced significant changes in oral temperature, but there was no significant change in ACTs. Green et al[12] found an excellent correlation between RTs and ACTs ($r=.90$) in 411 ambulatory adults. There was no significant difference between RTs and ACTs in their study.

Experimental work that supports using the tympanic membrane for temperature measurement comes from several sources. Using a thermistor placed in the esophagus and against the tympanic membrane, Wilson et al[7] found the latter to be equally sensitive during thermogenic stress in 44 burned children. Others have reported that tympanic thermistor measurement of body temperature was equally or more reliable during temperature changes in surgical patients than rectal or esophageal measures.[17,18] Infected tympanic membrane temperatures were not significantly different from uninfected contralateral ears in an experimental model of AOM in chinchillas.[12]

Using rectal temperature as the "gold standard" to assess ACTs for accuracy may have created falsely low sensitivity and specificity values for actual core body temperature. Rectal temperature has been shown to change slowly during rapid temperature changes, possibly due to vascular insulation from relatively poor blood flow to the normal rectum.[20] However, the rectum is the preferred measurement site in ambulatory children since it is unaffected by factors known to spuriously affect oral temperature, such as hyperventilation and recent ingestion of hot or cold liquids.[6] Axillary temperature measurement and liquid crystal forehead strips have been shown to be unreliable estimates of body temperature.[21-23] Esophageal and vascular thermistors are too invasive for routine temperature measurement in ambulatory patients.

This study has several limitations. Since nursing personnel were not blinded to ACT measurements, the potential for nursing bias was introduced. The standardized criteria for AOM may have been unreliable but are used by most pediatricians in evaluating children with AOM. This study did not seek to measure whether children older than 29 months of age were less cooperative. Other factors such as thermometer probe orientation or canal size may have accounted for the lesser accuracy in this age group.

In clinical practice, we find that ACT measurements are usually reliable. They are well accepted by children, parents, and nursing staff.[24] The probe and microprocessor has been shown to be easy to use, has excellent reproducibility, good acceptance by children and parents, is unaffected by factors influencing oral temperatures, and is a better indicator of RT than oral thermometers in adults.[6,12] Measurement of ACT appears to be a more appropriate temperature screening device than oral, axillary, or liquid crystal display thermometers. Occasionally there are patients who appear to have a 2°C- to 2.5°C-difference between RT and ACT measurements. Although some of these appear to be due to a low ambient temperature without adequate time for equilibration with a warmer environment, others are unexplained. We recommend further study in children before ACT systems replace RT systems when body temperature measurement is crucial.

We express our grateful appreciation to all the nurses, house staff, and faculty who participated in data collection and to Anne Milewski, RN, for staff orientation.

References

1. Long SS. Approach to the febrile patient with no obvious focus of infection. *Pediatr Rev.* 1984; 5:305-315.

2. Henretig FM. Fever. In: Fleisher GR, Ludwig S, eds. *Textbook of Pediatric Emergency Medicine.* Baltimore, Md: Williams & Wilkins; 1988:163-170.

3. Pantell RH, Naber M, Lamar R, Dias JK. Fever in the first six months of life: risks of underlying serious infection. *Clin Pediatr.* 1980;19:77-82.

4. Waskerwitz S, Berkelhamer JE. Outpatient bacteremia: clinical findings in children under two years with initial temperatures of 39.5° or higher. *J Pediatr.* 1981;99:231-233.

5. Tandberg D, Sklar D. Effect of tachypnea on the estimation of body temperature by an oral thermometer. *New Engl J Med.* 1983;308:945-946.

6. Terndrup TE, Allegra JR, Kealy JA. A comparison of oral, rectal, and tympanic membrane-derived temperature changes after ingestion of liquids and smoking. *Am J Emerg Med.* 1989;7:150-154.

7. Wilson RD, Knapp C, Traber DL, Priano LL. Tympanic thermography: a clinical and research evaluation of a new technic. *South Med J.* 1971; 64:1452-1455.

8. Hughes WT, Patterson GG, Thornton D, Williams BJ, Lott L, Dodge R. Detection of fever with infrared thermometry: a feasibility study. *J Infect Dis.* 1985;152:301-306.

9. Shinozaki T, Deane R, Perkins FM. Infrared tympanic thermometer: evaluation of a new clinical thermometer. *Crit Care Med.* 1988;16:148-150.

10. Treloar D, Muma B. Comparison of axillary, tympanic membrane, and rectal temperatures in young children. *Ann Emerg Med.* 1988;17:435. Abstract.

11. Weir MR, Weir TE. Are 'hot' ears really hot? *AJDC.* 1989;143:763-764.

12. Green MM, Danzl DF, Praszkier H. Infrared tympanic thermography in the emergency department. *J Emerg Med.* 1989;7:437-440.

13. Ros SP. Evaluation of a tympanic membrane thermometer in an outpatient clinical setting. *Ann Emerg Med.* 1989;18:1004-1006.

14. Hancock LA. First temp. *J Pediatr Health Care.* 1987;1:163-164.

15. Bluestone CD. State of the art: definitions and classifications. In: Lim DJ, Bluestone CD, Klein JO, Nelson JD, eds. *Recent Advances in Otitis Media With Effusion.* Philadelphia, Pa: BC Decker Inc; 1984:1-4.

16. Lobbes JM. *External Auditory Canal Temperatures as a Predictor of Acute Otitis Media.* Orlando, Fla: University of Florida/Humana-Lucerne Hospital; 1989. Thesis.

17. Benzinger M. Tympanic thermometry in surgery and anesthesia. *JAMA.* 1969;209:1207-1211.

18. Webb GE. Comparison of esophageal and tympanic temperature during cardiopulmonary bypass. *Anesth Analg.* 1973;52:729-733.

19. Fisch RO, Eaton BG, Giebink GS. Tympanic membrane temperature during experimental otitis media due to *Streptococcus pneumoniae* in chinchillas. *Lab Anim Sci.* 1982;32:278-279.

20. Molnar GW, Read RC. Studies during open-heart surgery on the special characteristics of rectal temperature. *J Appl Physiol.* 1974;36:333-336.

21. Kresch MJ. Axillary temperature as a screening test for fever in children. *J Pediatr.* 1984;104:596-599.

22. Reisinger KS, Kao J, Grant DM. Inaccuracy of the Clinitemp skin thermometer. *Pediatrics.* 1979;64:4-6.

23. Lewit EM, Marshall CL, Salzer JE. An evaluation of a plastic strip thermometer. *JAMA.* 1982;247:321-325.

24. Barber N, Kilmon CA. Reactions to tympanic temperature measurement in an ambulatory setting. *Pediatr Nurs.* 1989;15:477-481.

Hugh D. Allen, MD, Columbus, Ohio
Fredric Burg, MD, Philadelphia, Pa
Harold Levine, MPA, Galveston, Tex
Barbara Starfield, MD, Baltimore, Md
Larrie W. Greenberg, MD, Washington, DC

Purpose.—This department is intended to share information concerning educational efforts in the broad field of pediatrics. We welcome studies on the following topics: undergraduate and graduate education in medicine and allied health occupations; continuing education of health professionals; education of patients and families; and health education for the general public, the community, and organizations that contribute to the promotion and improvement of the health of children.

Editorial Comment.—*All year long, pediatricians are inundated with school health questions and problems. These present a unique focus of attention, yet few of us were trained in school health issues. The authors of this report discuss such an aspect of their training program and its success.*—H.D.A.

School Health Training During Pediatric Residency

Virginia N. Niebuhr, PhD; David P. McCormick, MD; Stephen E. Barnett, MD

• Pediatricians are becoming increasingly concerned about reaching beyond the office or clinic to help solve problems of child and family health. The physician's ability to interact with school personnel and communities is one important approach to this outreach effort. School health training has been a required 6-month component of the pediatric residency curriculum at the University of Texas Medical Branch, Galveston, since 1979, with second-year residents providing weekly on-site consultations to public school districts and participating in a weekly school health seminar series. In this study, graduates from this program were surveyed to determine their evaluations of the training and extent of current school involvement and to use their evaluations for curriculum evaluation. Residents who participated in the school consultation from 1979 through 1988 were surveyed. Seventy-eight pediatricians responded, a 79% return rate. Ratings by the graduates reveal that both pediatric generalists and subspecialists highly value their training experiences. Ratings were not related to the specific site to which the resident consultant had been assigned. Of these pediatricians, 41% are currently consulting with school personnel. These findings are discussed as they relate to other reports of physician involvement in schools and provide clues to curriculum design for school health training in pediatric residency.

(*AJDC.* 1991;145:79-84)

Just as physicians in the 1800s and early 1900s went into schools to stem infectious epidemics,[1] pediatricians of today need to return to the school setting to address the "new morbidities" of children and adolescents.[2-4] Traditional office management of the child and family has had little impact on the present-day problems of drug use, adolescent pregnancy and sexually transmitted disease, poor nutrition and lack of exercise, serious behavioral and emotional disorders, and learning disabilities and attentional disorders. If change is to be effected, it is imperative that health care professionals address these problems through interaction with school personnel and community systems.

More than 10 years ago, in a monograph entitled "The Future of Pediatric Education,"[5] it was predicted that *all* pediatricians would soon be expected to manage child health in the context of the community. If pediatricians are to function effectively in schools and communities, they must be trained to do so. Pediatricians need to learn the structure of school systems, effective communication with schools, and consultative techniques. To this day, however, much of pediatric training continues to focus on hospital care, and to a lesser degree on outpatient clinical practice—all primarily within the context of the patient, and sometimes the family, rather than the school or community.

Prior to the mid-1970s there were no training programs or curricula to prepare pediatricians for potential new roles in school settings. In response to this void, several school health training programs were initiated during the 1970s,[6-10] including one at the University of Texas Medical Branch (UTMB) in Galveston. We describe herein the current design of this program and report on a follow-up of graduates who trained in this program during the past 10 years.

BACKGROUND AND PROGRAM DESCRIPTION

Since the mid 1970s, the UTMB school health training program has evolved from an elective for physicians,

Accepted for publication June 15, 1990.
From the Department of Pediatrics, the University of Texas Medical Branch, Galveston.
Presented in part before the annual meeting of the American School Health Association, Chicago, Ill, October 20, 1989.
Reprints not available.

fellows, and residents[11-13] to a 6-month ambulatory core requirement for all second-year pediatric residents.[14,15] The major components of the program include weekly public school consultations, weekly school health/community pediatrics seminars, and clinical assessment and management of school-related problems in specialty teaching clinics.

Five Galveston County school districts currently contract with UTMB-Pediatrics for consultative services. Each second-year resident is assigned to spend one half day per week with a school district for 4 to 5 months in either a fall/winter or winter/spring rotation. School Health faculty provide back-up and act as mentors.

A major goal of the physician consultant program is for pediatricians in training to learn something of the environment in which their patients spend much of their time. Many pediatric residents do not have school-aged children and, indeed, have not been in a school since their own schooldays, yet the patient care they deliver often results from school referral, requires school involvement (eg, medication at school), or affects school performance (eg, behavioral effects of medical intervention and absence rates due to illness). Resident consultants are encouraged to visit a variety of regular and special education classes, to observe the most handicapped students served by the district, to teach a health-related topic to a class, and to interact with school nurses, administrators, and teachers.

A second major goal of the physician consultant program is for residents to learn about consultative processes. Residents are encouraged to consult rather than to provide direct patient care. Table 1 includes a list of potential activities of the consultants.

Resident consultants and their mentors meet to share consultative experiences and plan consultative activities. A weekly seminar series is designed to present a variety of school health and community pediatrics issues, using presenters from the UTMB faculty and staff and from the community. A sampling of topics that have been presented is included in Table 2.

Each resident is required to make a presentation during the rotation on a topic related to school health, a specific project developed through the consultation experience, or an individual case. In recent years, these presentations have included topics such as drugs, violence, pregnancy, discipline, and the impact of chronic handicaps, abuse, and prematurity.

School-related problems presented in general and specialty clinics at our health center are often complex and can easily overwhelm a resident during a busy day. Our child development clinic, behavioral pediatrics clinic, and chronic care clinic are specifically designed to handle complex school-related problems in a teaching climate (ie, opportunity to observe faculty, opportunity to be observed, and at least hour-long appointments). In these clinics, the residents judge what services they can provide vs when to refer, how to build and use referral networks, and how to include school personnel to facilitate assessment and management.

The purposes of the current project were to assess how valuable our school health training program has been to graduates, to document their current school-related activities, and to use their input for curriculum evaluation. Resident graduates were requested to rate the overall value of their consultation training experiences and the importance of specific curriculum components. They were also asked about their current school involvement.

A major question was whether there were discernible relationships between value ratings for school health training and subsequent school-related activity. We predicted that those who highly valued the training would be more likely to be currently involved in school consultation. In addition, comparisons were made between pediatric generalists and subspecialists to determine differences in their value ratings or in their current school-related practices.

Table 1.—Possible Contributions of the Resident Consultant in the Schools

Individual case consultation
Consultation regarding students with special needs
Explaining medical conditions
Instructing teachers and staff about special equipment or procedures
Assisting teachers in explaining conditions to other students
Facilitation of referrals
Interpretation of medical records
Liaison between school personnel and other physicians
Assistance in determination of eligibility for special education services
Participation in planning conferences to develop strategies for students with special needs
Program consultation
Provision of updated medical information to school nurses
Help with health screenings: planning, implementing, or evaluating
Involvement in health curriculum planning and implementation
In-service education of faculty and staff

Table 2.—Selected Topics Included in the School Health Seminar Series

Anatomy and physiology of schools
Consultation models and potential roles of a school health consultant
Special education laws and services
Attention-deficit–hyperactivity disorder
Intellectual and educational assessment
School health screening
The school consultants role concerning chronic illness
Community-oriented primary care: a model for needs assessment and program planning
Health promotion/health education

METHODS

Between 1979, when the School Health Training Program became a required component of UTMB residency, and 1988, 100 residents participated in the program. Questionnaires were sent to 99 of these graduates (one is deceased), and a second mailing went to nonrespondents 5 months later.

On a five-point Likert scale with anchor phases, respondents indicated the overall value of their school consultation experiences. On a set of four-point Likert scales, respondents rated the importance of various curriculum components: school visits, consultation training, interaction with school nurses, and evaluation of school problems. On another set of four-point Likert scales, respondents indicated how well prepared they felt for interacting with school personnel, understanding the structure of schools, understanding the role of school nurses, being able to contribute to health education in schools, and assessing normal development.

Respondents indicated whether they were currently consulting with schools, either informally or through formal contract. Finally,

Table 3.—Frequencies of High and Low Value Ratings for Overall Experience and Curriculum Components*

	Value of Overall Training (n=73)		Making School Visits (n=76)		Learning to Evaluate School Problems (n=76)		Consultation Training (n=76)		Opportunities to Interact With School Staff (n=76)	
	High	Moderate	High	Low	High	Low	High	Low	High	Low
No. of respondents										
Generalists	37	18	49	6	53	2	46	9	35	20
Specialists	8	10	12	9	17	4	16	5	15	6
Test for comparison	$P=.084$		$P=.0003$		$P=.004$		$P=.45$		$P=.52$	

*Some of the 78 respondents did not answer all questions.

they identified which of the following activities were part of their current professional work: interaction with school administrators, interaction with school nurses, assessment of normal development, and involvement in health education.

Data were analyzed using statistical software (SAS, SAS Institute, Inc, Cary, NC). For nominal data, χ^2 analyses were used when expected counts were greater than five, and Fisher's exact tests (two-tailed) were used when expected counts were less than five. Analyses of variances were made for comparisons of interval data.

RESULTS

After both mailings, 78 questionnaires were returned, a return rate of 79%. The mean (±SD) number of years out of residency was 4.6±2.8 (range, 1 to 9 years) and nearly equal numbers of women (n=40, 51.3%) and men (n=38, 48.7%) responded. Pediatric generalists constituted 73% of the respondents (n=57), and 27% were pediatric subspecialists (n=21). Of the three pediatricians in public health, two identified themselves as generalists and one as a specialist in behavioral/developmental pediatrics.

The mean overall value rating was 1.55±0.82, where one means very valuable ("I am glad I had the experience") and two means only moderately valuable ("It was okay, but I also could have done without it"). One respondent indicated no strong opinion, three indicated it was not very valuable, and one indicated it was definitely not valuable. Since the frequencies for the "no opinion" and low ratings were so small, only the high and moderate ratings were used in subsequent analyses. Frequencies of high and moderate overall ratings are presented in the first column of Table 3. For their overall experiences, generalists gave more high-value than moderate-value ratings, and specialists gave more moderate-value than high-value ratings, although these differences are not statistically significant ($\chi^2=2.99$, $P=.084$).

Agencies with which these respondents had consulted during their residencies included seven independent school districts, one state school for handicapped students, and two community agencies (Head Start and Children's Protective Services). Most residents (n=54, 69%) had consulted at one of four school districts or Children's Protective Services. Analysis of variance reveals no significant differences in overall value ratings among these sites ($F=.46$, $df=4$, $P=.76$).

For analyses of the value ratings of the four curriculum components, the four-point Likert scales were collapsed into two categories: "high" (important) and "low" (unimportant). Frequencies of high and low ratings for generalists and specialists are presented in Table 3. High value ratings were given more often than low value ratings for all four curriculum components. Some differences emerged between ratings from generalists and specialists: generalists were more likely than specialists to highly value "making school visits" (Fisher's exact test, two-tailed, $P=.0003$) and "learning to evaluate school problems" (Fisher's exact test, two-tailed, $P=.004$). There were no differences between generalists' and specialists' value ratings of "consultation training during residency" ($\chi^2=.56$, $P=.45$) or "interactions with school nurses during residency" ($\chi^2=.41$, $P=.52$).

Preparedness ratings were collapsed into two categories (one and two indicated low preparedness, and three and four indicated high preparedness). Frequencies of high and low preparedness ratings for generalists and specialists are presented in Table 4. Comparison of preparedness ratings between generalists and specialists yielded significant differences only in the category of "able to contribute to health education." Generalists were more likely than specialists to believe themselves highly prepared (Fisher's exact test, two-tailed, $P=.007$). Ratings did not differ between groups for preparedness to interact with school personnel, understanding of the structure of schools, understanding of the role of the school nurse, or ability to assess normal development.

Table 5 shows the numbers of generalists and specialists who are currently consulting with schools, with and without formal contracts. School or community consultation is provided by 41% of the total sample (n=32), 47% of the generalists (n=27), and 24% of the specialists (n=5). The five specialists who consult represent the following areas: allergy (one), adolescent medicine (one), behavioral/developmental pediatrics (two), and neonatology (one), who indicated her consultation was in her role as a parent, not through her role as a neonatologist).

The likelihood of current consultation is not related to a high vs moderate value rating for the training experience ($\chi^2=1.50$, $P=.22$). That is, those pediatricians currently consulting were no more likely to have rated their experiences as highly valuable than moderately valuable.

Comparison of generalists and specialists on likelihood of current consultation yields no statistically significant difference ($\chi^2=3.52$, $P=.06$). Comparison of generalists and specialists on other specific school-related activities is

Table 4.—Frequencies of High and Low Preparedness Ratings (n=70)*

	Contribution to Health Education		Interaction With School Personnel		Understanding of School Structure		Understanding Role of School Nurse		Assessment of Normal Development	
	High	Low	High	Low	High	Low	High	Low	High	Low
No. of respondents										
Generalists	46	8	46	8	43	11	50	4	51	3
Specialists	10	6	11	5	10	6	14	2	13	3
Test for comparison	$P=.007$		$P=.96$		$P=.95$		$P=.87$		$P=.98$	

*Some of the 78 respondents did not answer all questions.

Table 5.—Graduates Currently Involved in School Consultation

	Formal Consultation, With a Contract	Informal Consultation, Without Contract	Total No. Consulting
No. of respondents			
Generalists (n=57)	14	18	27*
Specialists (n=21)	0	5	5
Total (N=78)	**14**	**23**	**32**

*Five generalists are simultaneously involved in formal and informal consultations with two or more agencies; therefore, this total is not a sum.

Table 6.—Comparisons of Generalists and Specialists on Current School-Related Activities

	Generalists, No. (%) (n=55)*	Specialists, No. (%) (n=21)	χ^2	P
Interaction with school administrators	24 (43.6)	4 (19.1)	3.95	.047
Interaction with school nurses	45 (81.8)	5 (23.8)	22.72	.0001
Assessment of development	51 (92.7)	12 (57.1)	13.57	.00007
Involvement in health education	26 (47.3)	6 (28.6)	2.18	Not significant

*Data incomplete.

summarized in Table 6. Neither group is very likely to interact with school administrators, although generalists are more likely to do so than specialists ($\chi^2=3.95$ $df=1$, $P=.047$). Generalists are more likely than specialists to interact with school nurses, and more than 80% of the generalists do so ($\chi^2=22.72$, $df=1$, $P<.0001$). Generalists are very likely to be involved in the assessment of development (93%), and they are more likely to do so than are specialists ($\chi^2=13.57$, $P<.0001$). Fewer than half of the physicians in both groups are involved in health education at more than the individual patient level, and generalists and specialists do not differ in the likelihood of this activity ($\chi^2=2.18$, $df=1$, $P=.14$).

Twenty-five percent (n=14) of the generalists consult by contract, and none of the specialists do. Thirty-two percent (n=18) of the generalists and 24% (n=5) of the specialists consult without contract. Physicians with school-aged children are more likely to consult than those without school-aged children ($\chi^2=6.48$, $df=1$, $P=.011$).

COMMENT

One major purpose of this study was to retrospectively evaluate school health training based on the perceptions of graduated residents. Overall, our graduates highly valued their school health training experience; very few perceived the experience as not valuable. Specifically, the graduates have indicated that they valued the opportunities to visit schools, to interact with school nurses, and to receive consultation training. On an open-ended optional question asking for comments about the school health training program, 69% (n=54) of the respondents answered, and the comments were generally positive or constructive. Several respondents encouraged continuation of the program. Many acknowledged the importance of learning to deal with the school-related issues of their patients and reported frustration at not having learned even more.

The 79% return rate is high, but there remains the question of how nonrespondents might have evaluated the training experience. Perhaps those who valued the experience the least were also the least likely to respond to a survey, thus skewing the results in a more positive direction. Ratings could also be positively skewed by factors such as wording of the Likert scale anchors or respondents' eagerness to look good or reluctance to be critical.

The program faculty expected variations in ratings between different consultation sites. However, value ratings did not differ between sites, indicating that the training experience can be valuable despite individual site differences. In the open-ended questions, respondents shared some of the frustrations of their school health training experiences, yet highly valued those experiences overall. We contend that even frustrating experiences can be valuable for learning about the consultative process.

A second major purpose of our survey was to determine the respondents' current school involvement. In our sample, 41% indicated that they currently consult with school personnel. In Chilton's[16] sample of pediatricians in the Southwest 10 years ago, 65.6% provided some school health services. Ten years later, in reports based on a national sample of pediatricians, Nader[17] and Black et al[18] noted that 77% are involved in school-related activities.

The apparently higher rates of school involvement in Chilton's and Nader's samples compared to ours may reflect these investigators' broader definitions of school health involvement. We queried specifically for consultation activities. The differences in rates may also reflect regional differences in school health activities. Finally, the highest involvement rate, reported by Nader and Black et al, may be inflated by a lower return rate (46%). Respondents may have been more likely than nonrespondents to be involved in schools.

One of our initial questions was whether there is a relationship between perceived value of training and subsequent school involvement. Nearly all of the respondents, either currently consulting or not, gave high or moderately high ratings for the training. Those currently consulting gave ratings that showed no statistical differences between the high and moderately high categories. In addition, although nearly all the graduates valued the training, not all are currently involved with schools. That is, valuing the training does not necessarily result in current involvement. This suggests that the relationship between perceived value of training and subsequent school involvement is not direct.

Chilton discusses the relationship between presence or absence of school health training and subsequent school involvement. He suggests that training in school health arouses a pediatrician's interest in interacting with school personnel. Of his sample, 22% had received school health training, but 65.5% were involved in schools. In the studies by Black et al and Nader, 18% of the physicians had received school health training, but 77% were involved in schools. Although all of our subjects had received school health training, only 41% reported current involvement. Taken together, these three sets of data suggest little direct relationship between presence or absence of school health training and current school involvement. We conclude that neither the perceived value of the training nor school health training per se results in pediatricians interacting with school personnel. The findings of Chilton and Black et al indicate that many pediatricians will become involved with schools even without specific training in school health. Perhaps this is because of increasing community needs or demands for pediatricians' involvement to help solve the complex problems of children and adolescents.

We also conclude that the important question is not whether school health training creates school health involvement, but how we can best prepare pediatricians for this involvement. This question leads directly to examination of our school health curriculum. We have identified three elements of our curriculum that need further attention: training in administrative issues, health education in schools, and school health as it relates to both general and subspecialty pediatric practices.

The few formal contracts obtained by our repondents (25% of generalists and no specialists) and the infrequency of their current interaction with school administrators (43.6% of generalists and 19.1% of specialists) could reflect lack of skill or confidence in contract negotiation and dealing with school administrators. These findings suggest that increasing the emphasis on these aspects of school consultation in our curriculum would be beneficial.

Disappointingly few physicians in our sample indicated involvement in health education beyond the individual patient level, despite their perception that they were well prepared for such involvement. Generalists believed themselves better prepared than specialists, but were no more likely than specialists to be involved in this activity. We must examine how effectively we teach residents about their potential role in school and community health education, raise the valence for pediatricians' involvement in health promotion, and cultivate a realization that schools can be ideal environments for promoting healthy habits and life-styles for children.

Nearly one fourth of the specialists and nearly half of the generalists are currently consulting with school personnel, although generalists and specialists did not differ in their overall value ratings of school health and consultation training. These findings emphasize our need to integrate school health issues into both primary care and subspecialty care and to continue to provide school health training for all pediatric residents, even those heading for subspecialties.

One difference that did emerge between generalists and subspecialists was that subspecialists were much less likely than generalists to interact with school nurses in their current work. The infrequency of specialists' current contact with school nurses is disappointing, since presumably many specialists could use the school nurse to help implement complex treatment plans, communicate with families, and monitor patients' daily functioning. We conclude that a stronger emphasis is needed on the potential interactions of pediatric subspecialists school staffs for the care of students with special health problems. This might be accomplished through greater involvement in the school health training program by the subspecialty faculty.

To provide more effective training in school health, we need to identify factors that promote or inhibit pediatricians' participation in school health. It was not surprising that among our respondents the likelihood of school involvement increased if the pediatrician had children in school. Unfortunately, we did not obtain data on when in their pediatric careers our graduates began consulting with schools. This leaves unanswered the question of whether pediatricians use school interactions as practice-builders or branch into school consultation after their practices are well established and they are searching for diversity.

Investigations of incentives, reinforcements, and remunerations for physician involvement with schools might help reveal how pediatricians can become more involved with schools. Investigations of how physician involvement in schools is affected by attitudes of school health personnel toward physician interaction may also be useful, as might investigations of whether requests for medical consultation are related to the absence or presence of school nurses and health educators in school systems.

For continued improvement of school health training for physicians, other questions need investigation. What do practicing pediatricians identify as important knowledge and skills for effective work with schools? How can continuing medical education at the postresidency level be used to provide training in school consultation? We intend to use our graduates' evaluations to further develop and refine our training program in hopes that we can better prepare pediatricians to meet the challenges of pediatrics through interactions with school personnel.

The authors wish to acknowledge the major contributions of Phil Nader, MD, Guy Parcel, PhD, Nathalie Vanderpool, MA, and Gregg Wright, MD, to the development of the UTMB School Health Program, and to Patricia Beach, MD, Mary Owen, MD, and Alma Golden, MD, for their involvement in the current implementation of the program. We also wish to express our gratitude to Charles Daeschner, Jr, MD, for his unwavering support of this program from its beginnings.

References

1. Kort M. The delivery of primary health care in American public schools: 1890-1980. *J Sch Health.* 1984;54:453-457.
2. Haggerty RJ, Roghmann KJ, Pless IB, eds. *Child Health and the Community*. New York, NY: John Wiley & Sons Inc; 1975:94-116.
3. Nader PR, Ray L, Brink SG. The new morbidity: use of school and community health care resources for behavioral, educational, and social-family problems. *Pediatrics.* 1981;67:53-60.
4. Porter PJ. School health is a place, not a discipline. *Pulse Am Sch Health Assoc.* Spring 1988:23-25.
5. Kempe CH, ed. *The Future of Pediatric Education.* Elk Grove, Ill: American Academy of Pediatrics; 1978:23.
6. Nader PR, ed. *Options for School Health.* Germantown, Md: Aspen Systems Corp; 1978:44-54.
7. McAnarney E. The pediatrician in an innovative public school health program. *Clin Pediatr.* 1971;10:86-89.
8. Nader PR. Community schools and pediatrics. *Clin Pediatr.* 1971;10:90-95.
9. Novak SF, Rockowitz RJ, Zastowny T, Stebbins WC, Burns C. In-school resident training for management of school problems. *N Y State J Med.* 1978: 1109-1112.
10. Vanderpool NA, Wright GF, Gilman SB. *Curriculum Guide for School Health and Community Pediatrics.* Galveston, Tex: University of Texas Medical Branch; 1980.
11. Vanderpool NA, Wright GF. Guidelines in Community Training for Pediatric Residents. Presented at the Annual Meeting of the Ambulatory Pediatrics Association; April 1978; New York, NY. Abstract.
12. Vanderpool NA, Wright GF. Evaluation of Resident Training in School and Community Pediatrics. Presented at the Annual Meeting of the Ambulatory Pediatrics Association; April 1979; Atlanta, Ga. Abstract.
13. Vanderpool NA, Wright GF, Nader PR. The pediatrician and the schools. *Pediatrics.* 1979; 63:681.
14. Vanderpool NA, Wright GF, Parcel GS. Residency Training in School Consultation. Presented at the Annual Meeting of the Ambulatory Pediatrics Association; April 1980; San Antonio, Tex. Abstract.
15. Vanderpool NA, Wright GF, Brink SG. Training Pediatricians to Serve as Consultants to Community Organizations. Presented at the Annual Meeting of the Ambulatory Pediatrics Association; April 1980; San Antonio, Tex. Abstract.
16. Chilton LA. School health experience before and after completion of pediatric training. *Pediatrics.* 1979;63:565-568.
17. Nader PR. School Health: 2000: First Annual Lectureship in School Health. Presented to the American Academy of Pediatrics; October 1989; Chicago, Ill.
18. Black JL, Nader PR, Broyles S, Nelson J. Pediatric training and activities in school health. In: *Ambulatory Pediatrics Association Abstracts.* McLean, Va: Ambulatory Pediatrics Association; 1990. Abstract 26.

In Other AMA Journals

JAMA

HIV Infection, Pregnant Women, and Newborns
Working Group on HIV Testing of Pregnant Women and Newborns (*JAMA.* 1990;264:2416)

A Formal Audit of Continuing Medical Education Activity for License Renewal
J. K. Stross; T. J. DeKornfeld (*JAMA.* 1990;264:2421)

Continuing Medical Education at a Crossroads
Dennis K. Wentz (*JAMA.* 1990;264:2425)

The Federal Regulation of Prescription Drug Advertising and Promotion
D. A. Kessler, W. L. Pines (*JAMA.* 1990;264:2409)

Nevus Flammeus

Discordance in Monozygotic Twins

Raanan Shamir, MD; Gertrude Kohn, MD; Aryeh Metzker, MD

• Nevus flammeus has been described as an inherited vascular anomaly. We report two cases of nevus flammeus, each appearing in one of two monozygotic twins. This finding supports the idea that nevus flammeus results from embryologic mishap rather than genetic transmission.
(*AJDC.* 1991;145:85-86)

Nevus flammeus (NF), or port-wine stain, is a pink to purple vascular nevus, located anywhere on the skin, but occurring most often on the face. It persists throughout life and has an incidence of 0.5%.[1] The psychological burden to a child with such a blemish is obvious. Apprehensive parents of a child with NF often voice their reluctance to have more children because of the fear that NF, as an inheritable phenomenon, might recur. Publications that describe familial NF and suggest an autosomal dominant inheritance with irregular penetrance give credence to this fear.[2-5]

Our study of two pairs of monozygotic twins provides evidence that NF is not transmitted genetically.

PATIENT REPORTS

PATIENT 1.—A 3-year-old girl, an identical twin, was seen in the Pediatric Dermatology Clinic of Beilinson Medical Center, Petah Tiqva, Israel, for a light purple discoloration on her left cheek. This patch appeared as a typical NF and had not changed since birth, except that it became slightly more pronounced in color. The girl was otherwise well, and results of her physical examination were normal.

Her twin sister had no such discoloration and was well in every respect. The two girls resembled each other remarkably (Fig 1). Their dermatoglyphic patterns were almost identical. Their HLA alleles (A2, B38, B39, B42, and W7, with identical response to 120 antisera) and blood groups and subgroups (0+, E+, C+, M+, and N−) were identical.

PATIENT 2.—A 13-year-old boy, an identical twin, was seen in Beilinson Medical Center's Pediatric Dermatology Clinic for a large NF covering half of the nape (Fig 2). Results of his physical examination were normal. His twin brother did not have an NF, but the two brothers otherwise resembled each other remarkably (Fig 3). The two brothers were monochorionic and monoamniotic, and had identical blood groups and subgroups (AB+, C+, M+, and N+) and identical HLA alleles (A1, A24, B57, B35, W4, DR5, DR6, DQw1, DQw3, and DRw52). Their parents' HLA alleles were not identical.

COMMENT

To the best of our knowledge, these cases are the first reported occurrences of NF appearing in only one of two identical twins.

The occurrence of an NF in only one of two monozygotic twins indicates that such a nevus is not part of the genetic code. All twins in our report strikingly resembled their twins and had the same HLA alleles and blood groups as their twins. All these factors render remote the possibility of their not being monozygotic sets of twins.

Nevus flammeus is a localized ectasia of capillaries in the upper dermis caused

Fig 1.—Identical twin sisters (case 1). One has a nevus flammeus on her left cheek.

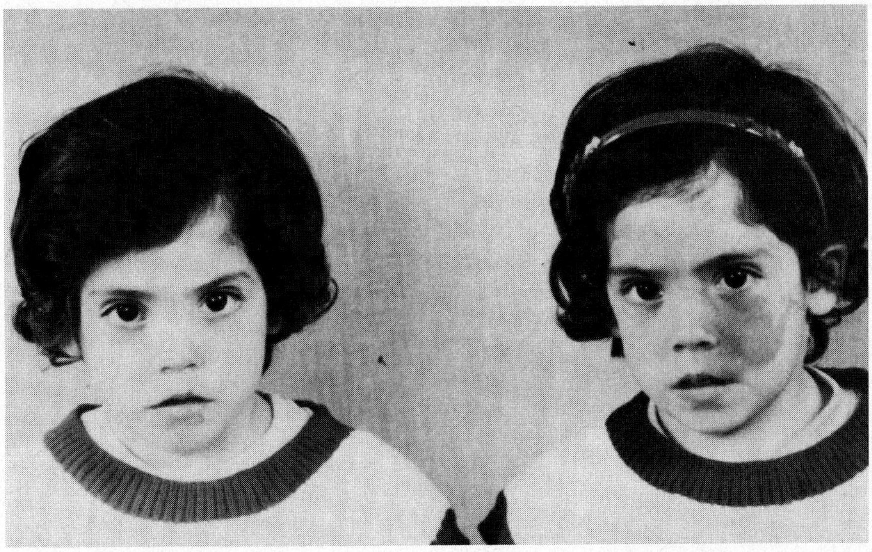

Accepted for publication June 27, 1990.
From the Units of Pediatric Dermatology (Drs Shamir and Metzker) and Medical Genetics (Dr Kohn), Beilinson Medical Center, Petah Tiqva, Israel, and Sackler School of Medicine, Tel Aviv (Israel) University.
Reprint requests to Pediatric Dermatology Unit, Beilinson Medical Center, Petah Tiqva 49 100, Israel (Dr Metzker).

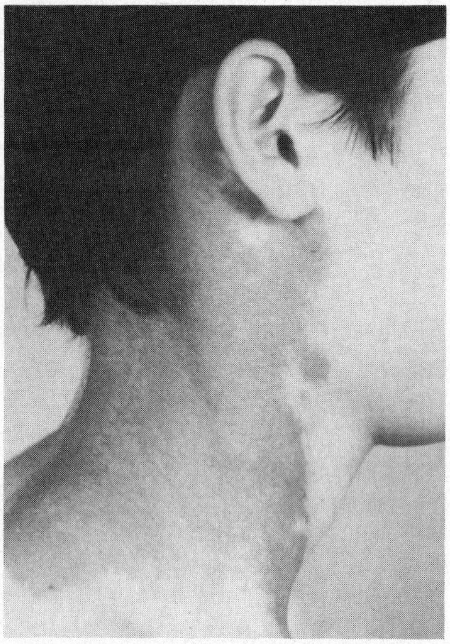

Fig 2.—Nevus flammeus on the neck and nape (case 2).

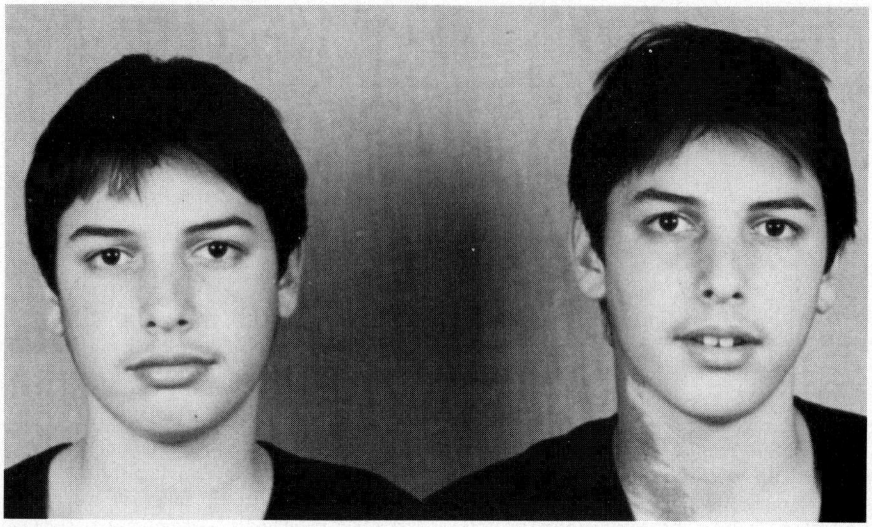

Fig 3.—Identical twin brothers (case 2). One has a nevus flammeus on his nape.

by a circumscribed nervous dysfunction of the vascular plexus or loss of sympathetic neurons.[6] The relatively high incidence of NF makes reappearance of NF likely in the same family. Curiously enough, two reports[2,4] refer to multiple NFs, which are uncommon. Nevertheless, the appearance of such a nevus in siblings and their parents is not sufficient to suggest a dominant inheritance, as claimed in those two reports.

Two other authors[3,5] describe familial NF of the forehead. A clear distinction between true NF, which persists throughout life, and NF simplex, which is mostly transient, is called for. Nevus flammeus simplex combines erythema nuchae, alias "stork bite," and the salmon patch of face, alias "angel kiss." Nearly 50% of newborns have NF simplex. The salmon patch clears, in most cases, during the first year, but shades of it might persist into adulthood. The stork bite is slower in disappearing. It seems likely that Selmanowitz[3] and Merlob and Reisner[5] were describing cases of persistent salmon patch.

It might be possible that monozygotic twins, discordant for a cryptogenic trait, have a genetic cause for their disorder; this could be explained by heterogenic monozygocity.[7] For all practical purposes, the occurrence of NF in only one of two identical twins attests either to absence of a genetic factor in this disorder or to a new mutation not present in the parental DNA. Both suggest embryologic mishap as a cause of NF. Further, despite extensive literature on Sturge-Weber syndrome, which also involves NF, no evidence for genetic tendency can be found.

Today, the psychological distress caused by NF can sometimes be alleviated by lightening the stain with tunable pulsed-dye laser therapy.[8] Nevertheless, anxious parents with NF or parents of children with NF may be reassured that another case of NF is probably no more likely to occur in their families than in the general population. If inherited at all, NF may be a rare phenomenon based on multifactorial inheritance.

References

1. Metzker A. Congenital vascular lesions. *Semin Dermatol.* 1988;7:9-16.
2. Shelley WB, Livinghood CS. Familial multiple nevi flammei. *Arch Dermatol Syphilol.* 1949;59:343-345.
3. Selmanowitz VJ. Nevus flammeus of the forehead. *J Pediatr.* 1968;73:755-757.
4. Shuper A, Merlob P, Garty BA, Varsano I. Familial multiple nevi flammei. *J Med Genet.* 1984;21:112-113.
5. Merlob P, Reisner SH. Familial nevus flammeus of the forehead and Unna's nevus. *Clin Genet.* 1985;27:165-166.
6. Rosen S, Smoller BR. Port-wine stains: a new hypothesis. *J Am Acad Dermatol.* 1987;17:164-166.
7. Cantu J. Heterogenic monozygocity: evidence for the transmission of half chromatid mutations in humans? *Am J Hum Genet.* 1976;28:190-191.
8. Tan OT, Sherwood K, Gilchrest BA. Treatment of children with port wine stain using the flash-lamp–pulsed tunable dye laser. *N Engl J Med.* 1989;320:416-421.

Neural Arch Stenosis and Spinal Cord Injury in Thanatophoric Dysplasia

Ona Marie Faye-Petersen, MD, A. S. Knisely, MD

• Bony abnormalities caused by thanatophoric dysplasia affect the base of the skull and the vertebrae as well as the ribs and appendicular long bones. We present our findings in a full-term infant with thanatophoric dysplasia in whom the posterior fossa, the rostral vertebral column, and the neuraxis at and adjoining the craniovertebral junction were studied by dissection, roentgenography, and histologic examination. In this infant, malformations of the vertebral laminae, most prominent in the basiocciput and atlas vertebra, led to compression of the rostral cervical spinal cord, causing gliosis and focal necrosis. Stenosis of the foramen magnum and spinal canal may contribute to the ventilatory insufficiency that often causes death in patients with thanatophoric dysplasia. We suggest that the causes of death in patients with thanatophoric dysplasia and other severe forms of osteochondrodysplasia should be sought in neuraxial injury rather than attributed solely to pulmonary hypoplasia.

(*AJDC.* 1991;145:87-89)

In thanatophoric dysplasia (TD), the limbs are short, the thorax is small, and the clivus and posterior fossa are hypoplastic.[1-3] These deformities result from disordered endochondral ossification.[4] Reduced thoracic dimensions in TD are frequently associated with moderate pulmonary hypoplasia,[5] to which, at least in part, death is generally ascribed.[1] The vertebral laminae, components of the neural arch, are endochondrally formed, and stenosis of the foramen magnum has long been recognized in TD.[2,3] We examined the basiocciput, vertebrae, and spinal cord of a full-term infant with TD. We found malformations, deformation, and potentially significant neuraxial injury, principally at the level of the atlas vertebra, that may have contributed to ventilatory failure.

Accepted for publication June 18, 1990.

From the Department of Pathology, Primary Children's Medical Center (Dr Faye-Petersen) and the Departments of Hematology and Pathology, University of Utah Medical Center (Dr Knisely), Salt Lake City.

Reprint requests to Department of Pathology, Children's Hospital of Pittsburgh, One Children's Pl, Pittsburgh, PA 15213-3417 (Dr Knisely).

PATIENT REPORT

Clinical History

A 19-year-old woman presented for initial evaluation in the 42nd week of gestation by dates. She described the pregnancy, her fourth, as uncomplicated. The family history was unremarkable. Sonography identified short-limbed osteochondrodysplasia and breech presentation. After a short period of spontaneous labor, a male infant was born by cesarean section. Thick meconium was in the amniotic fluid. Craniomegaly, short limbs, and poor ventilatory effort were noted at birth. Endotracheal intubation was performed for pulmonary toilet; ventilatory support was continued pending evaluation. Skeletal roentgenograms showed short, curved femora, squared iliac bones, platyspondylisis, and subperiosteal juxtaphyseal spurring. These findings were consistent with TD. After consultations with the parents, ventilatory support was discontinued on the third postnatal day, and the infant died within 5 minutes. Skin fibroblasts from the infant were cultured and banked (National Institute of General Medical Sciences Human Genetic Mutant Cell Repository GM10749, Coriell Institute for Medical Research, Camden, NJ).

Necropsy Techniques

After standard necropsy evisceration, the posterior fossa and rostral spinal column were excised en bloc, including the in situ neuraxis distal to the obex.[6] The posterior fossa and vertebrae C-1 through T-1, with the encased length of spinal cord in situ, were fixed in 10% phosphate-buffered formaldehyde solution. Individual vertebrae were separated at the levels of the intervertebral disks using sharp dissection. Roentgenograms of the posterior fossa with basiocciput and of vertebrae C-1 through T-1 were exposed with the specimens in contact with the cassette to avoid magnification. The vertebrae and fossa were decalcified in 8% sulfosalicylic acid, hemisected transversely, and embedded in paraffin. Whole-mount sections were stained with hematoxylin-eosin, Masson's trichrome, periodic acid–Schiff, Luxol fast blue–cresyl violet, Bodian, and immunoperoxidase. A portion of the spinal cord at the level of the atlas vertebra was postfixed and routinely processed for transmission electron microscopy.

Necropsy Results

Findings included megalencephaly (brain weight, 577 g; normal, 7362 ± 55 g) with temporal-lobe gyral abnormalities characteristic of TD,[5] posterior-fossa hypoplasia, and rostral herniation of the cerebellum through the tentorial leaflets. The lungs were hypoplastic on gross examination and weighed 29 g together (normal lung weight,[7] 56 ± 15 g). Aspirated meconium without pneumonitis was seen on microscopic examination. The cartilaginous framework of the larynx, trachea, and bronchi was unremarkable grossly; on microscopic examination, however, architectural immaturity and chondrocyte disarray were apparent. Sections of iliac crest and costal physes showed the effects of TD.[4] Stenosis of the midportion of the ductus arteriosus, without typical postnatal proliferative changes, and right ventricular hypertrophy also were noted.

Contact roentgenograms and tissue sections showed malformations of the vertebral laminae, which were shortened and bowed ventrally and medially, with periosteal bony spurring and disordered ossification at the physes. Malformation was most pronounced in the basiocciput, which showed stenosis and ventral displacement of the foramen magnum (Fig 1), and in the C-1 vertebra. The

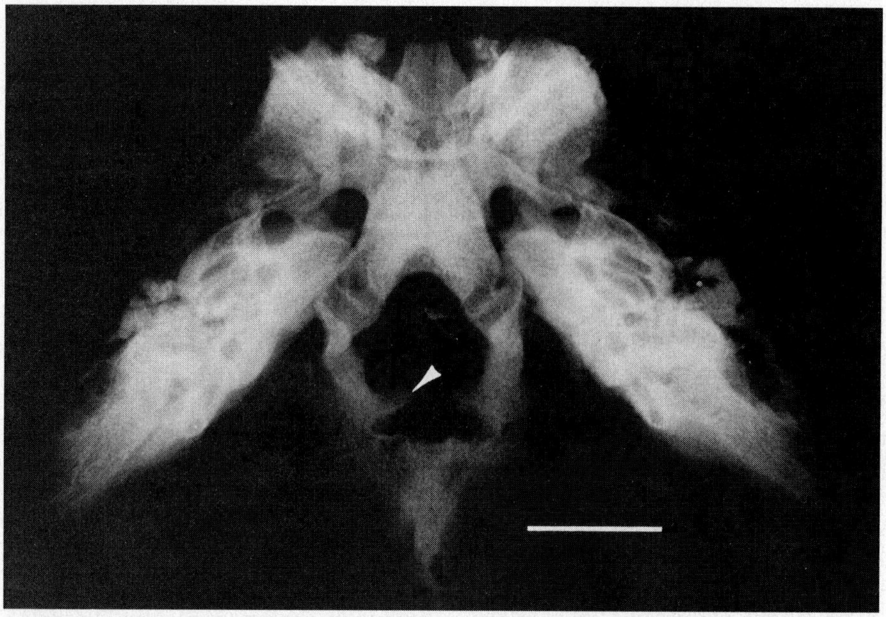

Fig 1.—Contact roentgenogram of the posterior fossa of the patient. The contours of the foramen magnum of an infant without osteochondrodysplasia are smooth[12]; here, the occipital laminae are shortened and incurved, and the lumen of the foramen magnum is irregularly narrowed by bony protuberances that represent the physes of the occipital laminae.[2,3] Note the juxtaphyseal bone spurs, one of which is indicated by an arrowhead, in the occipital laminae and body. Similar spurring is well recognized at proximal femoral physes in thanatophoric dysplasia (original magnification ×2; bar equals 1 cm).[4]

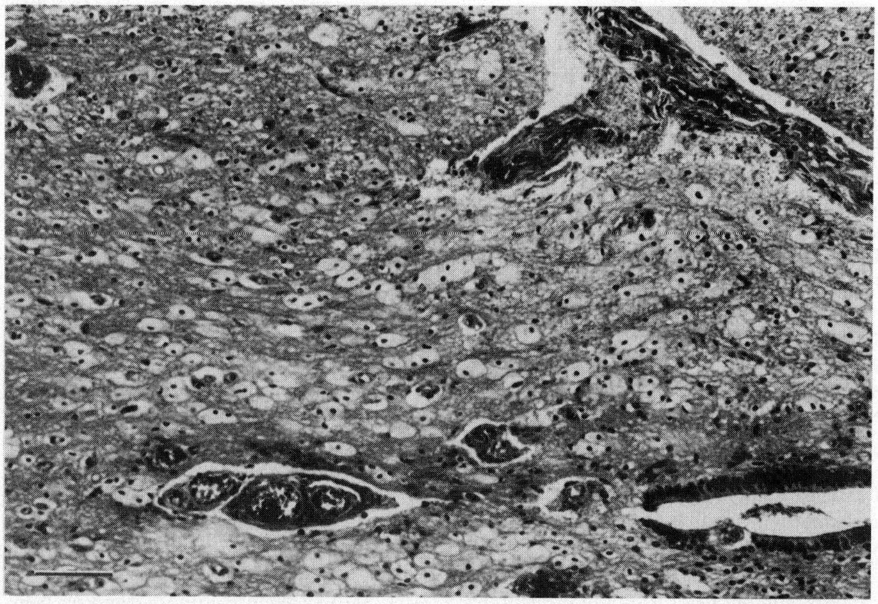

Fig 2.—Swollen immature astroglial cells in the central gray matter of the spinal cord at the C-1 level. The central canal, which is flattened anteroposteriorly, is at the lower right, and the tortuous anterior spinal vessels are at the upper right (Luxol fast blue-cresyl violet, original magnification ×180; bar equals 80 μm).

spinal cord was deformed at all levels, fitting snugly within the triangular lumen of the spinal canal, and was rotated 45° to the right at the L-1 level.

Injury, as opposed to deformation, of the spinal cord was present from the foramen magnum through the C-3 level. It was most conspicuous at the C-1 level, where swollen immature astroglial cells[8] (Fig 2) were identified ventral to the central canal and in the uncrossed corticospinal tracts. Vascular congestion with endothelial reactive changes was marked. Axonal swellings and gliosis with mature reactive astrocytes also were present (Fig 3), but were more numerous at the C-2 and C-3 levels. Gliosis with reactive astrocytes and small clusters of lipid-laden macrophages (gitter cells) were seen at the level of the foramen magnum. Gliosis was not observed caudal to the C-4 level or in the medulla immediately above the level of the foramen magnum. Reactive astrocytes stained well for glial fibrillary acid protein, while the cytoplasm of enlarged immature astroglial cells stained only faintly. Neuronal loss, degenerative changes, and pyknosis were not apparent. Transmission electron micrographs showed only advanced autolytic change that precluded meaningful ultrastructural analysis.

COMMENT

This infant with TD had abnormally short and incurved vertebral and modified vertebral (basioccipital) laminae, with consequent stenosis of the spinal canal and foramen magnum. The entire spinal canal was stenotic, but was relatively less narrowed caudally to C-1. Our dissection did not identify a cause for rotation of the lumbar spinal cord within the spinal canal.

The neural arch fit closely around the distal medulla and the rostral cervical spinal cord, which showed marked compressive deformity and injury manifested as necrosis, gliosis, and unusual cytoplasmic changes in immature astroglial cells. The lesions affected predominantly the ventral cord and were essentially limited to the region immediately caudal to the craniovertebral junction; we propose that this suggests compression of the cord against the dens of the axis vertebra (body of the atlas vertebra) during flexion of the head and neck. The injury seen could have led to impaired diaphragmatic function and, hence, to impaired ventilation. Gliosis, vacuolation, and macrophages in the cervical spinal cord, as documented here, have been observed in at least one other newborn with TD,[5] and are consistent with antenatal onset of injury. These findings may be correlated not only with ventilatory failure but also with polyhydramnios[9] (possibly due to impaired swallowing) and decreased fetal motion,[10] which are both commonly

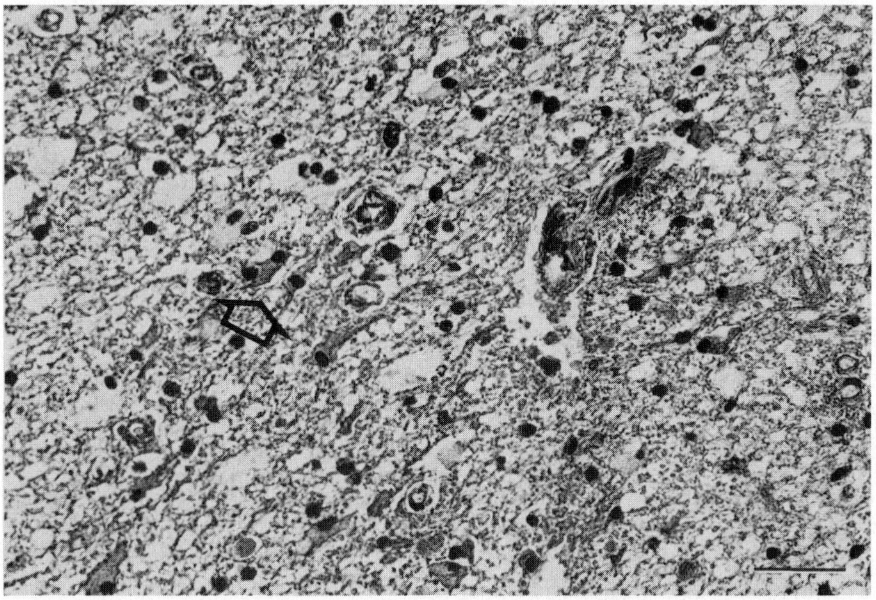

Fig 3.—Mature reactive astrocytes (arrow) and rare swollen immature astroglial cells in uncrossed corticospinal tract at the C-2 level (hematoxylin-eosin, original magnification × 575; bar equals 30 μm).

associated with TD.

Neural arch malformation with neuraxial deformation is recognized in other forms of osteochondrodysplasia,[11-14] in which it is associated with ventilatory dysfunction that can be surgically relieved.[14] Release of the neuraxis by suboccipital craniectomy has allowed two individuals with TD and ventilatory dysfunction to survive for several years; one of them had evidence of brainstem compression on measurement of auditory evoked potentials. These children remained ventilator dependent.[15] Our findings indicate that compressive deformity at C-1 and foramen magnum levels may be a significant complication of TD. If potentially lifesparing surgery is performed to combat the effects of TD, it may be necessary to unroof the neuraxis in the rostral spinal canal as well as at the craniovertebral junction. Evaluations of thoracic wall mechanics, pulmonary function, and brain-stem and phrenic evoked potentials (to assess the extent to which abnormalities in thoracic and diaphragmatic conformation, anatomy of the cartilaginous airways, and neuraxial injury may contribute to ventilatory insufficiency) should perhaps precede such procedures. To our knowledge, these studies have yet to be performed in individuals with TD.

Thoracic malformations, abnormalities in lung mesenchyme, and neuraxial injury all may be present in osteochondrodysplasia. These lesions may produce both pulmonary hypoplasia and ventilatory insufficiency of multifactorial cause.[16-18] Assessment of skeletal and neuraxial abnormalities at the craniovertebral junction and in the rostral cervical spine and spinal cord, as performed in this patient, facilitates study of the contributions of thoracic, pulmonary, and neural-arch malformations to the ventilatory insufficiency seen in many forms of osteochondrodysplasia.

This study was supported in part by grant 5T32 DK07115 from the National Institutes of Health.

We thank Mary W. Ambler, MD, Margaret G. Norman, MD, and Bernd W. Scheithauer, MD, for assistance in interpreting neuropathologic findings. Kelly C. Bowles, HT(ASCP), Maurine A. Peterson, HT(ASCP), and Susan L. Wall, HT(ASCP), performed outstanding histotechnical work. Don Morse helped greatly with photography.

References

1. Jones KL. *Smith's Recognizable Patterns of Human Malformation.* 4th ed. Philadelphia, Pa: WB Saunders Co; 1988:290-291.

2. Potter EL, Craig JM. *Pathology of the Fetus and the Infant.* 3rd ed. Chicago, Ill: Year Book Medical Publishers Inc; 1975:552-554.

3. Marin-Padilla M, Marin-Padilla TM. Developmental abnormalities of the occipital bone in human chondrodystrophies (achondroplasia and thanatophoric dwarfism). In: Bergsma D, Lowry RB, Gorlin RJ, Doran TA, Paul NW, eds. *Embryology and Pathogenesis and Prenatal Diagnosis: Part D of Annual Review of Birth Defects, 1976.* New York, NY: Alan R Liss Inc; 1977;13:7-23.

4. Horton WA, Hood OJ, Machado MA, Ahmed S, Griffey ES. Abnormal ossification in thanatophoric dysplasia. *Bone.* 1988;9:53-61.

5. Knisely AS, Ambler MW. Temporal-lobe abnormalities in thanatophoric dysplasia. *Pediatr Neurosci.* 1988;14:169-177.

6. Knisely AS, Singer DB. A technique for necropsy evaluation of stenosis of the foramen magnum and rostral spinal canal in osteochondrodysplasia. *Hum Pathol.* 1988;19:1372-1375.

7. Gruenwald P, Minh HN. Evaluation of body and organ weights in perinatal pathology, I: normal standards derived from autopsies. *Am J Clin Pathol.* 1960;34:247-253.

8. Privat A. Postnatal gliogenesis in the mammalian brain. *Int Rev Cytol.* 1975;40:281-323.

9. Thompson BH, Parmley TH. Obstetric features of thanatophoric dwarfism. *Am J Obstet Gynecol.* 1971;109:396-401.

10. Tóth Z, Vachter J, Szeifert G, et al. Antenatally diagnosed thanatophoric dysplasia. *Acta Paediatr Hung.* 1982;23:423-430.

11. Pauli RM, Scott CI, Wassman ER Jr, et al. Apnea and sudden unexpected death in infants with achondroplasia. *J Pediatr.* 1984;104:342-348.

12. Knisely AS, Steigman CK. Stenosis of the foramen magnum and rostral spinal canal, with spinal cord deformity, in Jeune's asphyxiating thoracic dystrophy. *Pediatr Pathol.* 1989;9:299-305.

13. Pauli RM, Gilbert EF. Upper cervical cord compression as cause of death in osteogenesis imperfecta type II. *J Pediatr.* 1986;108:579-581.

14. Reid CS, Pyeritz RE, Kopits SE, et al. Cervicomedullary compression in young patients with achondroplasia: value of comprehensive neurologic and respiratory evaluation. *J Pediatr.* 1987; 110:522-530.

15. MacDonald IM, Hunter AGW, MacLeod PM, MacMurray SB. Growth and development in thanatophoric dysplasia. *Am J Med Genet.* 1989;33:508-512.

16. Cunningham M, Stocks J. Werdnig-Hoffmann disease: the effects of intrauterine onset on lung growth. *Arch Dis Child.* 1978;53:921-925.

17. Wigglesworth JS, Desai R. Effects on lung growth of cervical cord section in the rabbit fetus. *Early Hum Dev.* 1979;3:51-65.

18. Shapiro JR, Burn VE, Chipman SD, et al. Case report: pulmonary hypoplasia and osteogenesis imperfecta type II with defective synthesis of alpha I(1) procollagen. *Bone.* 1989;10:165-171.

Marfanoid Children

Etiologic Heterogeneity and Cardiac Findings

Shawky Tayel, MD; Thaddeus W. Kurczynski, MD, PhD; Marc Levine, MD; Ernest Brookfield, MD; Robert Ehrlich, MD; James R. Hennessy, MD; Martin M. DeBeukelaer, MD

• The clinical, cardiac, and echocardiographic test results of 20 children with marfanoid features are reviewed. Fifteen were diagnosed as having Marfan syndrome, two had "possible" Marfan syndrome, and three had other diagnoses. On first evaluation, eight patients with Marfan syndrome (53%) had mitral regurgitation and none had aortic regurgitation. Echocardiography showed aortic root enlargement in 12 (80%) of 15 patients and mitral valve prolapse in 12 (80%) of 15. None had a normal echocardiogram. At follow-up examination, one patient had developed aortic root enlargement, and one patient, mitral valve prolapse. Thus, although aortic root enlargement is usually present in early childhood in patients with Marfan syndrome, it is not considered specific because in this study it also occurred in one child with Alport's syndrome and in one with marfanoid features. Four patients with aortic root enlargement were treated with propranolol and their echocardiograms showed no further increase in the aortic root diameter for several years. We recommend echocardiography in the diagnosis and routine management of children in whom Marfan syndrome is suspected.

(*AJDC.* 1991;145:90-93)

A marfanoid appearance consisting of a variable combination of a tall slender body build, long extremities and digits, pectus deformity, scoliosis, and myopia is relatively common. When such children seek medical attention, the question of Marfan syndrome is often raised. This specific autosomal-dominantly inherited disorder of connective tissue has important cardiovascular manifestations but is only one of the causes of a marfanoid appearance.[1-4] No specific diagnostic test is yet available, and since various marfanoid features are age dependent, the diagnosis of Marfan syndrome may be more difficult in young children. Clinical criteria, however, have been established.[2] In this study, we present a retrospective analysis of the clinical and echocardiographic findings of 20 marfanoid children, 15 of whom met the criteria for the diagnosis of Marfan syndrome and were followed up for at least 6 months.

PATIENTS AND METHODS

We reviewed the medical records of all children under 17 years of age evaluated between 1980 and 1987 at the Medical College of Ohio Hospitals, Toledo, with a suspected diagnosis of Marfan syndrome. The diagnosis of Marfan syndrome was based on the presence of abnormalities in three or more of the following four categories: skeletal, ocular, cardiovascular, and family history.[2]

Skeletal and Connective Tissue
- Tall stature
- Dolichostenomelia
- Arachnodactyly
- High arched palate
- Joint laxity
- Anterior chest deformity (pectus excavatum or carinatum or a combination)
- Scoliosis
- Pes planus
- Inguinal hernia

Ocular
- Myopia
- Lens subluxation (ectopia lentis)
- Flat cornea (less than 42 by keratometer)
- Retinal detachment

Cardiovascular
- Aortic root dilatation
- Mitral valve prolapse
- Mitral regurgitation
- Aortic regurgitation
- Aortic dissection

Positive Family History

Children with skeletal findings and abnormalities in fewer than three categories were considered marfanoid. All subjects underwent complete clinical examination and detailed M-mode and two-dimensional echocardiographic studies. Aortic regurgitation (AR) and mitral regurgitation (MR) were detected clinically, since complete Doppler evaluation was not available for many of the patients. Nine patients were followed up for an average of 34 months (range, 6 to 60 months). Four patients were treated with propranolol to prevent aortic root enlargement (ARE) and dissection.[4,5]

Echocardiography was performed using standard techniques.[6] Left ventricular diastolic dimension, aortic root dimension, and left atrial dimension were measured as described by Sahn et al.[6] Mitral valve prolapse (MVP) was defined as deflection of a mitral leaflet posterior to the "C" point by at least 2 mm throughout systole or beginning of diastole. Each measurement was plotted as a linear function of body surface area, with normal values defined as those falling within 95% of predicted values for normal children as described by Henry et al.[7]

RESULTS

The clinical features of the 20 patients are summarized in the Table. The most frequent skeletal abnormality was a pectus deformity in 16 patients (80%).

Accepted for publication June 27, 1990.

From the Department of Pediatrics, Medical College of Ohio, Toledo.

Presented at the First International Symposium on the Marfan Syndrome, Baltimore, Md, July 9, 1988.

Reprint requests to Department of Pediatrics, Medical College of Ohio, CS 10008, Toledo, OH 43699 (Dr Kurczynski).

Clinical Findings of 20 Marfanoid Children*

Patient No./Sex	Age at Last Evaluation, y	Age at Diagnosis, y	Skeletal Features: Ara	Dol	Sco	PD	PP	JL	HAP	IH	Ocular Features: EL	Myo	Cardiac Features: MR	MVP	AR	ARE	LVE	LAE	Family History	Diagnosis
1/M	15	6	+	+	+	−	−	−	+	−	+	+	+	+	−	+	−	−	−	MS
2/M	10	7	+	+	+	+	−	−	+	−	+	+	+	+	−	+	−	−	Mo	MS
3/F	15	8	−	+	+	+	−	+	+	−	−	−	−	−	−	+	−	−	Fa	MS
4/F	13	7	+	−	−	+	−	−	+	+	+	+	+	+	−	+	+	−	−	MS
5/F	11	7	−	−	−	+	−	−	−	−	−	+	−	+	−	−	−	−	Fa	MS
6/F	15	13	−	+	−	−	−	−	+	−	−	+	+	−	−	−	+	−	−	MS
7/M	9	2	−	+	+	+	−	−	+	+	−	+	+	+	−	+	+	+	Fa	MS
8/M	9	4	−	−	−	+	+	+	−	−	−	+	+	+	−	+	−	−	Mo	MS
9/F	17	12	+	−	+	+	−	−	+	−	−	+	−	+	−	+	−	−	Mo	MS
10/M	14	10	+	−	+	+	−	+	−	−	+	+	+	+	−	+	−	+	Mo	MS
11/M	10	8	+	−	−	+	−	−	−	−	+	+	+	+	−	+	+	+	−	MS
12/M	16	15	+	−	−	−	+	−	−	−	−	+	−	+	+	+	+	+	−	MS
13/F†	15	14	−	+	+	+	+	+	−	−	−	−	−	+	−	+	−	−	Fa	MS
14/F†	9	9	−	+	+	+	+	+	−	−	−	−	−	+	−	+	−	−	Fa	MS
15/M†	12	12	−	+	+	+	+	+	−	−	−	−	−	+	−	+	+	−	Fa	MS
16/F	14	7	+	−	+	+	−	+	+	−	−	−	+	+	+	+	−	−	−	MA
17/M	14	11	−	−	+	−	−	−	+	−	−	−	+	+	−	+	+	+	NA	MA
18/F	12	11	−	+	+	+	−	−	−	−	−	+	−	+	−	−	−	−	−	MA with neurofibromatosis
19/M	15	10	−	+	+	+	−	−	−	−	−	−	−	−	+	+	+	−	−	MA with Alport's syndrome
20/M‡	17	13	−	+	+	+	+	+	+	+	−	+	+	+	−	+	+	−	−	Marfanoid syndrome with craniosynostosis[10]

*Ara indicates arachnodactyly; Dol, dolichostenomelia; Sco, scoliosis; PD, pectus deformity; PP, pes planus; JL, joint laxity; HAP, high arched palate; IH, inguinal hernia; EL, ectopic lentis; Myo, myopia; MR, mitral regurgitation; MVP, mitral valve prolapse; AR, aortic regurgitation; ARE, aortic root enlarged; LVE, left ventricle enlarged; LAE, left atrium enlarged; Mo, mother; Fa, father; MS, Marfan syndrome; MA, marfanoid appearance; NA, not available; plus signs, presence of listed features; and minus signs, absence of listed features.

†These patients are siblings.

‡Patient died suddenly of aortic dissection.

The least frequent findings were inguinal hernia and pes planus, present in three patients (15%). Myopia was seen in 13 patients (65%) while only five patients (25%) had ectopia lentis. Ten patients had a parent with Marfan syndrome, in nine patients the disease was sporadic, and one patient was adopted, with unknown family history.

Fifteen of the children were diagnosed as having Marfan syndrome. Two children, patients 9 and 17, were considered possible patients with Marfan syndrome because they met two of the four criteria, including the presence of ARE and MVP.

Patients 18, 19, and 20 were marfanoid with other diagnoses. Patient 18 was a black girl who was referred for genetic evaluation at age 12 years because of multiple cafe au lait spots and marfanoid features. There was also a history of learning disability. Her examination showed significant findings: a slender appearance, dolichostenomelia, myopia, an alternating exotropia, multiple cafe au lait spots, axillary freckling, a probable neurofibroma of the left heel, pectus excavatum, scoliosis, a systolic click, an enlarged thyroid, and mild incoordination. Echocardiography showed MVP but no ARE. She was diagnosed as having hyperthyroidism and treated with propylthiouracil. The family history was negative for cafe au lait spots, neurofibromatosis, or marfanoid features.

Patient 19 was a boy with Alport's syndrome. He had progressive renal insufficiency and sensory neural hearing loss. At age 15 years, he was 187 cm tall and weighed 67.3 kg. Skeletal abnormalities included a tall, slender appearance, dolichostenomelia, maxillary hypoplasia, a prominent mandible, pectus carinatum, and scoliosis. There was no arachnodactyly or ectopia lentis. Echocardiography and cardiac catheterization performed to rule out a possible aortic root dissection demonstrated ARE (aortic root diameter, 4.4 cm; normal, 2.1 to 2.8 cm), and he was treated with propranolol. He received a renal transplant at 16 years of age. At this writing, he was 18 years old, was mildly hypertensive, and had a well-functioning kidney graft. There has been no further ARE. The family history was significant in that his mother and three brothers also had Alport's syndrome. His two other brothers required kidney transplants at ages 13 and 15 years, respectively. One of his brothers had been receiving long-term hemodialysis when he died at age 13 years of a dissecting aortic aneurysm. Although this patient never had an echocardiogram done, his autopsy revealed a normal aortic root diameter. One brother was nearsighted and had mild pectus excavatum, and the other had scoliosis and mild pectus excavatum. None of the family members had a marfanoid appearance, and their echocardiographic studies showed no cardiac abnormalities.

Patient 20 was a boy who died at 17 years of age of a dissecting aortic aneurysm. He had features typical of Marfan syndrome, such as dolichostenomelia, scoliosis, pectus carinatum, myopia, and recurrent inguinal hernia. There were, however, atypical anomalies such as craniosynostosis, ptosis of the eyelids, hypospadias, and spondylolisthesis. Ectopia lentis was absent. He was the only one in the family affected and had four normal siblings. He was previously described as a patient with a new marfanoid syndrome.[8]

The cardiovascular features of the 20 patients are summarized in the Table. On initial examination, five patients had a midsystolic click, 11 had a pansystolic apical murmur of MR, and one had a murmur of AR. The most frequent abnormalities at the initial echocardiographic examination were ARE, present in 15 patients (75%), and MVP, present in 16 patients (80%). Increased left ventricular diastolic dimension was detected initially in nine patients (45%); six of these patients had MR, one had AR, and two had neither MR nor AR.

During the period of the study, four additional patients developed a systolic click and two developed combined MR and AR. Eight patients had progression of mitral valve dysfunction defined by the appearance of a new systolic click, an increase in the murmur of MR by at least two grades, the appearance of left ventricular enlargement in the absence of AR.

Repeated echocardiograms were available for nine patients who were followed up for an average of 34 months (range, 6 to 60 months). Seven of these patients were initially found to have ARE at a mean age of 11.8 years (range, 4 to 15 years), and the other two developed it during the period of study (at 8 and 13 years of age). No patient developed ARE greater than 4.6 cm over the period of the study. Six of the nine patients had MVP initially at a mean age of 8.5 years (range, 4 to 14 years), two more patients developed it during the study period (at 17 and 16 years of age), and one patient did not develop it.

In one third (5 of 15) of the children diagnosed with Marfan syndrome, the disease was sporadic. When first examined, four (80%) of the five sporadic patients with cases had MR compared with three (30%) of of the 10 patients with familial cases. On echocardiographic examination, ARE and MVP were found to be similar in both groups. The mean paternal age for sporadic cases was 34.4 years (range, 29 to 38 years), whereas the mean paternal age at the time of birth of familial cases was 26.3 years (range, 19 to 33 years).

Four patients with ARE (patients 8, 9, 10, and 19) were treated with propranolol for an average of 4.2 years. One patient (patient 8) showed no further increase in the aortic root diameter for 1 year, another patient (patient 9) showed no increase for 5 years, and a third patient (patient 10) showed no increase for 3 years. None of these three patients experienced left ventricular enlargement. The fourth patient (patient 19) showed left ventricular enlargement because of preexisting mild hypertension due to renal failure, but his aortic root diameter did not increase during a 2.5-year follow-up.

COMMENT

Marfan syndrome is usually suspected when children with a marfanoid appearance are referred for medical evaluation. The presence of associated cardiac abnormalities such as mitral valve regurgitation and ARE may raise a strong suspicion of Marfan syndrome. These cardiac features, however, are not specific or certain evidence of the diagnosis in the absence of a positive family history or other system involvement. Three of our patients were found to have other diagnoses in spite of a marfanoid appearance and characteristic cardiac findings. Patient 17, with neurofibromatosis, in fact had MVP and myopia and, therefore, based on meeting three of four positive criteria, was diagnosed as having Marfan syndrome. Myopia and MVP, however, although common in Marfan syndrome, are relatively weak diagnostic features because of their high frequency in the general population. Therefore, the ultimate classification of marfanoid children and a definitive diagnosis of Marfan syndrome will likely await the discovery of the primary genetic defect or associated molecular markers. In the meantime, detailed clinical assessments must serve to distinguish other disorders with concomitant marfanoid features.

The cardiovascular system was involved in all 20 children with marfanoid features, of whom 15 (75%) were thought to have Marfan syndrome. Whether this high association of cardiac findings and marfanoid appearance is due to a selected sample will require prospective or population-based studies to evaluate. In any case, marfanoid children may have potentially serious cardiac findings and will require the same careful follow-up as those diagnosed with Marfan syndrome.

In the subset of the 15 children with diagnosed Marfan syndrome, pectus deformity and myopia were common findings. Similar observations were made by Geva et al.[9] In contrast, however, ectopia lentis was present in only 30% of our children, compared with 60% of those studied by Geva et al.[9] The absence of ectopia lentis, therefore, does not exclude the diagnosis. It is of interest, however, that we did not find ectopia lentis in any marfanoid child who was not thought to have Marfan syndrome.

In one third of our children diagnosed with Marfan syndrome, the disease was sporadic and had a greater frequency of MR than in the familial cases. The sporadic patients also had older fathers. These findings are consistent with previous reports[1,2] showing that in one third of patients with Marfan syndrome, the disease is sporadic and that sporadic cases tend to be more severely affected.[1] It has also been previously reported that there is a higher frequency of MR in sporadic cases than in familial ones (75% vs 29.4%).[9] The advanced paternal age of sporadic cases is related to the increased chance of new mutations.[10]

There are few reports of the cardiac manifestations of Marfan syndrome in young children that include echocardiography.[9,11-13]

These studies and our data indicate that aortic dilatation may appear early in life, precede the appearance of AR probably in all cases, and not be detectable by clinical examination or chest roentgenography. Aortic root enlargement was found in 12 (80%) of our 15 patients with Marfan syndrome. Only three patients had AR detected by auscultation. Moreover, the aortic root progressively enlarges throughout childhood, a process that, when accelerated, may lead to AR before adolescence. Involvement of the mitral value is almost as common as ARE in Marfan syndrome and may be severe in children.[14-20] In a longitudinal review of 120 patients younger than 22 years, mitral valve dysfunction in Marfan syndrome presented as MVP and, as opposed to idiopathic MVP, progressed clinically in about half.[21]

Therefore, periodic clinical and echocardiographic evaluation of children with Marfan syndrome is mandatory to establish the optimal time for surgical intervention. Gott et al[22] suggest elective aortic graft surgery when the aortic root diameter reaches 6 cm. Aortic root enlargement is progressive and most likely due to the strain of ventricular ejection; thus, chronic reduction in inotropy might retard the rate of ARE and prevent or delay complications.[23] In our study, none of the four patients treated with propranolol showed an increase in the aortic root diameter or experienced left ventricular enlargement. This finding is consistent with those of Pyeritz,[24] who suggested that long-term propranolol treatment reduces the rate of ARE and the development of severe complications in Marfan syndrome. Long-term, prospective, and controlled studies, however, are necessary to evaluate the effectiveness of this treatment in children.

References

1. McKusick VA. *Heritable disorders of connective tissue.* St Louis, Mo: CV Mosby Co; 1972: 61-223.
2. Pyeritz RE, McKusick VA. The Marfan syndrome: diagnosis and management. *N Engl J Med.* 1979;300:772-777.
3. Murdoch JL, Walker BA, Halpern BL, Kuzma JW, McKusick VA. Life expectancy and causes of death in the Marfan syndrome. *N Engl J Med.* 1972;286:804-808.
4. Pyeritz RE. Diagnosis and management of cardiovascular disorders in the Marfan syndrome. *J Cardiovasc Med.* 1980;5:759-769.
5. Halpern BL, Char F, Murdoc TL, Horton WB, McKusick VA. A prospectus on the prevention of aortic rupture in the Marfan syndrome with data on survivorship without treatment. *Johns Hopkins Med J.* 1971;129:123-129.
6. Sahn DT, DeMaria A, Kisslo T, Weyman A. Recommendations regarding quantitation in M-mode echocardiography: results of a survey of echocardiographic measurements. *Circulation.* 1978; 58:1072-1083.
7. Henry WL, Ware T, Gardin JM, Hepner SI, McKay J, Weiner M. Echocardiographic measurements in normal subjects. *Circulation.* 1979; 57:278-285.
8. Furlong J, Kurczynski TW, Kennessy RJ. New marfanoid syndrome with craniosynostosis. *Am J Med Genet.* 1987;26:599-604.
9. Geva T, Hegesh J, Frand M. The clinical course and echocardiographic features of Marfan's syndrome in childhood. *AJDC.* 1987;141:1179-1182.
10. Pyertiz RE. The Marfan syndrome. *Am Fam Physician.* 1986;34:83-94.
11. Sisk HE, Zahka KG, Pyeritz RE. The Marfan syndrome in early childhood: analysis of 15 patients diagnosed at less than 4 years of age. *Am J Cardiol.* 1983;52:352-358.
12. Brown OR, DeMots H, Kloster FE, Roberts A, Menashe VJ, Beals RK. Aortic root dilatation and mitral valve prolapse in Marfan's syndrome. *Circulation.* 1975;52:651-657.
13. Spangler RD, Nora TT, Lortscher RH, Wolfe RR, Orkin JT. Echocardiography in Marfan's syndrome. *Chest.* 1976;69:72-78.
14. Salle V. Über einen Fall von angeborener abnormalen Grösse der Extremitäten mit einem an Akromegalie erinnernden Symptomen Komplex. *Jahrb Kinderheilk.* 1912;75:540-548.
15. Tung HL, Liebow AA. Marfan's syndrome. *Lab Invest.* 1952;1:382-406.
16. Papaionnou AC, Agustsson MH, Gasul BM. Early manifestations of the cardiovascular disorders in Marfan's syndrome. *Pediatrics.* 1961; 27:255-268.
17. Bowden H, Favara BE, Donahoe TL. Marfan's syndrome. *Am Heart J.* 1965;69:96-99.
18. Phornphutkul C, Rosenthal A, Nadas AS. Cardiac manifestations of Marfan syndrome in infancy and childhood. *Circulation.* 1973;47:587-596.
19. Simpson TW, Nora TT, McNamara DG. Marfan syndrome and mitral valve disease: acute surgical emergencies. *Am Heart J.* 1969;77:96-99.
20. Caves PK, Panech M. Replacement of the mitral valve, aortic valve, and ascending aorta with coronary transplantation in a child with the Marfan syndrome. *Thorax.* 1972;27:58-65.
21. Pyeritz RE, Wappel MA. Mitral valve dysfunction in the Marfan syndrome: a clinical and echocardiographic study of prevalence and natural history. *Am J Med.* 1983;74:797-807.
22. Gott VL, Peperitz RE, Magovern GJ, et al. Surgical treatment of aneurysms of the ascending aorta in the Marfan syndrome. *N Engl J Med.* 1986;314:1070-1074.
23. Koenigsberg M, Factor S, Cho S, Herskowitz A, Nitowsky H, Morecki R. Fetal Marfan syndrome: prenatal ultrasound diagnosis with pathologic confirmation of skeletal and aortic lesions. *Prenat Diagn.* 1981;1:241-247.
24. Pyeritz RE. Propranolol retards aortic root dilatation in the Marfan syndrome. *Circulation.* 1983;68(suppl):III-365.

Differences in Expression of Cystic Fibrosis in Blacks and Whites

Susanna A. McColley, MD; Beryl J. Rosenstein, MD; Garry R. Cutting, MD

• The recent identification of the cystic fibrosis (CF) gene confirms that genetic heterogeneity occurs in CF. A three-base-pair deletion in exon 10 resulting in a loss of the phenylalanine residue at amino acid position 508 of the gene product, termed the *CF conductance regulator protein*, accounts for 70% of cases of CF in white subjects. However, this gene defect occurs in only 37% of affected blacks. Analysis of CF genes from American blacks has revealed a number of mutations, most of which are unique to that population. We therefore searched for potential differences in expression of CF between 24 black and 48 white patients with CF matched for birth date and gender. Black patients more frequently presented with only respiratory symptoms (38% vs 10%). Black patients had fewer hospitalizations for pulmonary exacerbations (2 vs 6.9), a better mean forced vital capacity (77% vs 62% of predicted), and higher chest roentgenogram scores (18.2 vs 14.4) than white patients. Complication rates were similar except for a higher incidence of hyponatremic dehydration (21% vs 2%) and peptic ulcer disease (13% vs 0%) in blacks. Survival time appeared to be longer in blacks, but the difference was not statistically significant. We conclude that phenotypic differences exist between black and white patients with CF, which may be due to the genetic heterogeneity between these two populations.

(*AJDC*. 1991;145:94-97)

Accepted for publication June 27, 1990.

From the Eudowood Division of Pediatric Respiratory Sciences (Drs McColley and Rosenstein) and the Division of Pediatric Genetics (Dr Cutting), Department of Pediatrics, The Johns Hopkins University School of Medicine, Baltimore, Md. Dr McColley is a fellow of the American Lung Association of Maryland, Inc.

Read before the Society for Pediatric Research Annual Meeting, Washington, DC, May 3, 1989.

Reprint requests to Department of Pediatrics, The Johns Hopkins Hospital, CMSC 1-141, 600 N Wolfe St, Baltimore, MD 21205 (Dr McColley).

Localization of the gene for cystic fibrosis (CF) to chromosome 7 was reported in 1985.[1-3] Before the discovery of the gene, several DNA markers were linked to the CF gene. Patterns of these markers, called haplotypes, were identified. It was discovered that the haplotype most highly associated with CF in white subjects was only weakly associated with CF in blacks, suggesting genetic heterogeneity between these populations.[4,5] The gene responsible for CF was recently identified and is predicted to encode a 1480-amino acid protein termed the *CF conductance regulator protein*.[6-8] One common mutation, resulting in a loss of the phenylalanine residue at amino acid position 508 of the CF conductance regulator protein (delta F508), accounts for 70% of CF gene mutations in whites but for only 37% of CF gene mutations in American blacks.[8-10] This confirms that the incidence of CF in American blacks is not due to genetic admixture alone. Analysis of CF genes from American blacks has revealed a number of mutations, most of which appear to be unique to that population.[10]

Cases of CF have been reported in blacks since 1954.[11] Early reports suggested that the prognosis for blacks was poor, with all patients dying by the age of 6 months in one retrospective study,[12] and 75% dying before the age of 5 years in another.[13] A subsequent study found that black patients experienced more severe gastrointestinal manifestations but less severe respiratory disease than white patients and had a longer survival.[14] Others have not observed differences in the clinical course.[15,16]

Since the genotypes of most American black and white patients differ, we compared the clinical course of patients from these two groups to detect any differences in phenotype. We reviewed the presenting features, clinical course, and survival of patients with CF followed up at The Johns Hopkins Hospital (JHH), Baltimore, Md.

PATIENTS AND METHODS

The charts of all 24 black patients with CF seen at JHH from 1971 to 1986 and 48 matched white patients were reviewed. The diagnosis of CF was based on characteristic clinical features and two positive pilocarpine iontophoresis sweat tests. Fourteen of the black patients were subjects of haplotype and subsequent gene analysis, reported previously.[5,10]

Two white patients with CF were selected for each black patient. Matching was by birth date and, when possible, by gender. Birth dates of the white patients were within 10 months of those of the black patients. In four cases, there were no white patients of the same gender born within 10 months, or charts could not be located. For these cases, opposite-sex patients matched for birth date were selected.

Patients were seen in the JHH CF clinic at 3-month intervals. One physician (B.J.R.) the CF center director, coordinated care for all subjects and was chiefly responsible for patient treatment decisions. Respiratory tract cultures and measurements of height and weight were obtained at each visit. Chest roentgenograms were obtained at least yearly, and more frequently if clinically indicated. Spirometry was done at each visit on patients who could perform forced expiratory maneuvers. Results were compared with predicted values calculated according to height, gender, and race.[17,18] Routine management included chest physiotherapy and aggressive nutritional support. Use of pancreatic enzymes, antibiotics, and bronchodilators was individualized according to the results of clinical, roentgenographic, and laboratory findings.

Outpatient and inpatient medical records were reviewed for clinical data, including sweat chloride concentrations, presenting features, diagnostic delay, colonization with *Pseudomonas aeruginosa*, use of pancreatic enzymes and bronchodilators, complications, hospitalizations, and growth measures. Diagnostic delay was defined as the interval between the onset of symptoms suggestive of CF and the first positive sweat test. The patients' most recent chest roentgenograms were reviewed by one of us (B.J.R.), who was unaware of the patient's identity at the time of the review. Roentgenograms were scored by the method of Brasfield et al[19]; 25 represents a maximum score, with points subtracted for air trapping, linear markings, nodular-cystic lesions, large lesions, and general severity. Roentgenograms were available for 23 of 24 black patients and 42 of 48 white patients. Data on survival and withdrawal from the clinic were compiled, and life-table analyses and survival curves were generated using standard techniques.[20]

To determine whether the matched white patients were representative of our entire white population with CF, we abstracted data on presenting features for the 206 white patients with CF followed up at JHH between 1971 and 1986 who were not included in the study population.

Statistical analysis was performed using Mann-Whitney *U* tests for data that were not normally distributed and Fisher's Exact Test for comparing clinical data. Survival curves were compared using the log likelihood test. A *P* value of .05 was considered significant.

RESULTS

The presenting features of the 24 black and 48 matched white patients are given in Table 1. Black patients were diagnosed later and had a longer diagnostic delay, but the differences were not significant. Black patients were more likely to present with only respiratory symptoms.

Data related to the clinical course of the black and matched white patients are given in Table 1. Mean follow-up was 8.0 years for black patients and 10.9 years for white patients, with a total follow-up of 192 and 501 patient-years, respectively. Mean age at last follow-up was 12.5 years for black patients and 13.3 years for white patients. Three white and four black patients were unavailable for follow-up at a mean age of 11.7 and 8.4 years, respectively. Black patients had fewer total hospitalizations, but there was no difference in the number of hospital days per year of follow-up. This discrepancy was due to two black patients who had prolonged hospitalizations for respiratory symptoms early in life and who died at ages 3 years 11 months and 5 years, respectively. Age at first colonization with *P aeruginosa*, as well as colonization rates, were similar for both groups. Pulmonary function testing showed no difference in forced expiratory volume in 1 second, but a higher mean forced vital capacity in blacks. Significantly more white patients received bronchodilator therapy because of symptoms and clinical findings consistent with reactive airways disease. Chest roentgenogram scores were significantly higher in blacks, indicating less severe roentgenographic changes. Age at most recent chest roentgenogram and pulmonary function testing was similar for both groups. The percentage of subjects who took pancreatic enzyme supplements was the same for both groups. There was no difference in the incidence of growth failure, defined as height or weight less than the fifth percentile for age.

The incidence of nasal polyps, hemoptysis, rectal prolapse, diabetes mellitus, pneumothorax, cirrhosis, and distal intestinal obstruction syndrome (meconium ileus equivalent) was similar in both groups. Blacks had a significantly higher incidence of hyponatremic dehydration and of peptic ulcer disease (Table 1).

Characteristics at presentation of the 206 white patients not included in the study were similar to those of the 48 white patients selected for study, except that more of the nonstudy patients had presenting features other than meconium abnormalities or gastrointestinal and respiratory symptoms (Table 2). Most of these patients were asymptomatic siblings of patients with CF; others had a variety of manifestations, including anemia and edema, fat-soluble vitamin deficiencies, liver disease, or salty taste.

Survival curves of the black and white study patients are shown in the Figure. The configuration is similar to the curves of Stern et al.[14] Although black survival appears to be longer, there were few deaths and a relatively large number of patients unavailable for follow-up, and the difference was not statistically significant.

Table 1.—Characteristics, Clinical Course, and Complications in 24 Black and 48 White Patients with CF*

	Black	White
Characteristics		
Sex		
M	12 (50)	28 (58)
F	12 (50)	20 (42)
Family history	2 (8)	14 (29)†
Sweat chloride, mmol/L	108 (27)	100 (32)
Mean (SD) age at diagnosis, mo	58 (80)	24 (42)
Diagnostic delay, mo [mean (SD)]	34 (40)	16 (31)
Features at presentation		
Meconium abnormality‡	6 (25)	10 (21)
GI symptoms	3 (13)	7 (15)
Respiratory symptoms	9 (38)	5 (10)§
Both GI and respiratory symptoms	5 (21)	21 (44)
Other	1 (4)	5 (10)
Clinical course		
Mean (SD) hospitalizations	2.0 (3.5)	6.9 (12.6)†
Hospital d/y [mean (SD)]	6.1 (10.6)	6.6 (10.8)
Bronchodilator use	5 (21)	42 (88)†
Pancreatic enzyme use	21 (88)	42 (88)
Colonization with *Pseudomonas aeruginosa*		
Cumulative	15 (63)	36 (75)
Mean (SD) age colonized, y	5.8 (5.6)	5.7 (5.9)
FEV_1, % predicted [mean (SD)]	64 (27)	52 (32)
FVC, % predicted [mean (SD)]	77 (18)	62 (29)†
FEV_1:FVC [mean (SD)]	0.72 (0.19)	0.62 (0.16)
Mean (SD) age at last PFT, y	16.2 (5.2)	16.6 (6.1)
Mean (SD) chest roentgenogram score	18.2 (3.2)	14.4 (5.6)§
Mean (SD) age at last chest roentgenogram, y	15.7 (5.6)	12.5 (8.1)
Height <5th percentile	8 (33)	12 (25)
Weight <5th percentile	9 (38)	20 (42)
Complications		
Nasal polyps	4 (17)	5 (10)
Hemoptysis	3 (13)	6 (13)
Pneumothorax	1 (4)	4 (8)
DIOS	3 (13)	7 (15)
Diabetes mellitus	1 (4)	3 (6)
Cirrhosis	0 (0)	2 (4)
Peptic ulcer	3 (13)	0 (0)†
Hyponatremic dehydration	5 (21)	1 (2)‡

*CF indicates cystic fibrosis; GI, gastrointestinal; FEV_1, forced expiratory volume in 1 second; FVC, forced vital capacity; PFT, pulmonary function testing; and DIOS, distal intestinal obstruction syndrome. Values are number (percent) or mean (SD).

†$P<.05$.

‡Meconium abnormality includes meconium ileus or meconium plug syndrome.

§$P<.01$.

Table 2.—Characteristics of 206 White Patients with CF Not Studied*

	Value
Characteristics	
Age at diagnosis, mo	31±60
Diagnostic delay, mo	25±55
Features at presentation	
Meconium abnormality†	28 (14)
GI symptoms only	20 (10)
Respiratory symptoms only	27 (13)
Both GI and respiratory symptoms	77 (37)
Other	54 (26)‡

*CF indicates cystic fibrosis; GI, gastrointestinal. Values are mean±SD or number (percent).
†Meconium abnormality includes meconium ileus or meconium plug syndrome.
‡$P<.05$ compared with white patients studied.

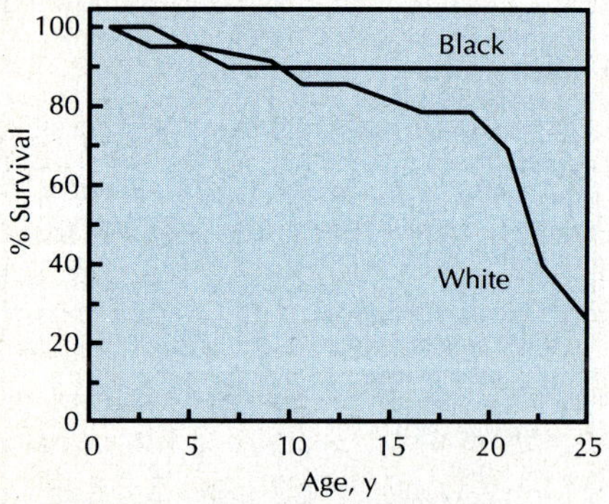

Survival of 24 black and 48 white patients with cystic fibrosis. The difference in survival is not statistically significant.

COMMENT

Cystic fibrosis is the most common lethal genetic disease in the white population, with an incidence of approximately 1:2200.[21-24] The incidence is lower in blacks, estimated at 1:17 000.[12] In 1987, among 14 026 patients reported to the Cystic Fibrosis Foundation registry, 2.9% were black.[25] At the JHH CF center, 8% of patients are black, possibly reflecting the racial composition of our referral area. This has allowed us the opportunity to study a larger group of black patients with CF than has been previously reported. We chose to compare their clinical course with that of white patients matched for birth date to eliminate confounding factors related to changing standards of care over time.

Significantly more black than white patients had only respiratory symptoms at diagnosis. This differs from the findings of Kulczycki et al[13] who found both respiratory and gastrointestinal symptoms at diagnosis in most blacks and from those of Stern el al[14] who found a preponderance of gastrointestinal symptoms at diagnosis in blacks. Our findings are similar to those of Prapphal et al[26] who found only respiratory symptoms at diagnosis in 40% of black patients with CF. The finding that fewer black patients had gastrointestinal manifestations at diagnosis, but that an equal percentage required pancreatic enzyme supplements, suggests that the onset of pancreatic insufficiency may be delayed in this population.

Complications were similar in our black and white patients except for the higher incidence of hyponatremic dehydration and peptic ulcer disease in blacks. Hyponatremic dehydration occurs in CF secondary to excessive losses of sodium and chloride in the sweat. The higher frequency of dehydration in black patients cannot be explained by a difference in sweat electrolyte concentrations, which were similar in both groups. We are not aware of data regarding comparative sweating rates in blacks and whites. It is possible that the higher incidence of hyponatremic dehydration in blacks was secondary to socioeconomic factors such as less use of air conditioners. Peptic ulcer disease has been previously reported as a complication in adolescent blacks with CF.[27] The 13% incidence is much higher than expected for the general pediatric and young adult population.[28-30] Unlike Stern et al,[14] we did not observe a higher incidence of distal intestinal obstruction syndrome in our black patients.

Our results suggest that respiratory disease is milder in black patients with CF. Although *P aeruginosa* colonization rates were similar between black and white patients, blacks had higher forced vital capacities, better chest roentgenogram scores, less bronchodilator use, and fewer hospitalizations for pulmonary exacerbations. Chest roentgenogram scores have been shown to correlate with clinical scores, pulmonary function, and morbidity.[19] Airway hyperreactivity has been shown to correlate with more rapid respiratory deterioration.[31] Although the retrospective nature of our study did not allow for formal testing of airway reactivity, it is likely that those patients who took bronchodilators had some component of reversible airways obstruction.

Our data suggest that survival may be better in blacks; this has been suggested by Stern et al[14] and by data from the Cystic Fibrosis Foundation.[32] However, a larger series with longer follow-up will be necessary to analyze this trend further.

Prognostic indicators have been previously reported in patients with CF.[33-38] Early *Pseudomonas* colonization, female gender, pancreatic insufficiency, and presentation with pulmonary manifestations suggest a worse prognosis, while diagnosis at an early age has been associated with less rapid progression of pulmonary disease.[39] These factors do not account for the milder pulmonary course in our black patients. Black patients were older at diagnosis, more frequently presented with pulmonary manifestations, and had a sex ratio, incidence of pancreatic insufficiency, and mean age at first *Pseudomonas* colonization similar to those of our white patients.

Cystic fibrosis is a disease with marked phenotypic heterogeneity.[40] Genetic heterogeneity between black and white patients with CF may account for the observed differences in the clinical course. Analysis of genes from a number of black patients, including 14 who were a part of this study, showed a high frequency of non–delta F508 mutations.[10] Genotypic variation may produce a different, perhaps milder, phenotype in some black patients than that commonly observed in the white population. Because a number of mutations were found and only a relatively small number of subjects had gene analysis, we were unable to correlate specific gene mutations with disease severity. Previous reports have suggested that different haplotypes may be associated with milder disease in other populations with CF[41,42] and that pancreatic sufficiency in white patients with CF may be the result of multiple different mutations of the CF gene.[8,43] The success in identifying the most common gene mutation resulting in CF should allow investigators to continue defining other gene mutations, further delineating genetic differences between populations. Larger, multicenter studies of black patients with CF may then be useful for further characterizing differences in clinical course and survival.

We express our appreciation to Alan Gittlesohn, PhD, and David Mellits, ScD, for assisting with life-table and statistical analysis, and to Leon Gordis, MD, Frank Oski, MD, Haig Kazazian, Jr, MD, and Gerald Loughlin, MD, for their review of the manuscript.

References

1. Knowlton RG, Cohen-Haguenauer O, Van Cong N, et al. A polymorphic DNA marker linked to cystic fibrosis located on chromosome 7. *Nature.* 1985;318:380-382.
2. Wainwright BJ, Scambler PJ, Schmidtke J, et al. Localization of cystic fibrosis locus to human chromosome 7cen-q22. *Nature.* 1985;318:384-385.
3. White R, Woodward S, Leppert M, et al. A closely linked genetic marker for cystic fibrosis. *Nature.* 1985;318:382-384.
4. Estivill X, Scambler PJ, Wainwright BJ, et al. Patterns of polymorphism and linkage disequilibrium for cystic fibrosis. *Genomics.* 1987;1:254-263.
5. Cutting GR, Antonarakis SE, Buetow KH, Kasch LM, Rosenstein BJ, Kazazian HH. Analysis of DNA polymorphism haplotypes linked to the cystic fibrosis locus in North American black and caucasian families support the existence of multiple mutations of the cystic fibrosis gene. *Am J Hum Genet.* 1989;44:307-318.
6. Rommens JM, Ianuzzi MC, Kerem B, et al. Identification of the cystic fibrosis gene: chromosome walking and jumping. *Science.* 1989;245:1059-1065.
7. Riordan JR, Rommens JM, Kerem B, et al. Identification of the cystic fibrosis gene: cloning and characterization of complementary DNA. *Science.* 1989;245:1066-1073.
8. Kerem B, Rommens JM, Buchanan JA, et al. Identification of the cystic fibrosis gene: genetic analysis. *Science.* 1989;245:1073-1080.
9. Lemna WK, Feldman GL, Kerem B, et al. Mutation analysis for heterozygote detection and the prenatal diagnosis of cystic fibrosis. *N Engl J Med.* 1990;322:291-296.
10. Cutting GR, Kasch LM, Rosenstein BJ, et al. A cluster of cystic fibrosis mutations in the first nucleotide binding domain of the cystic fibrosis conductance regulator protein. *Nature.* 1990;346:366-369.
11. Senecal JJ, Toury M, Camain R. Deux cas de fibrose cystique du pancreas chez l'enfant Africain realisant le syndrome de kwashiorkor. *Bull Med Afr Occidentale Fr.* 1954;11:95-99.
12. Kulczycki LL, Schauf V. Cystic fibrosis in blacks in Washington, D.C. *AJDC.* 1974;127:64-67.
13. Kulczycki LL, Guin GH, Mann N. Cystic fibrosis in negro children: results of a search. *Clin Pediatr.* 1964;3:692-705.
14. Stern RC, Doershuk CF, Boat TF, Tucker AS, Primiano FP, Matthews LW. Course of cystic fibrosis in black patients. *J Pediatr.* 1976;89:412-417.
15. Heffer ET. Cystic fibrosis in black children. *J Pediatr.* 1977;90:324-325.
16. Kulczycki LL. Cystic fibrosis in black children revisited. *J Pediatr.* 1978;92:855.
17. Polgar G, Promadhat V. *Pulmonary Function Testing in Children: Techniques and Standards.* Philadelphia, Pa: WB Saunders Co; 1971.
18. Hsu KHK, Jenkins DE, Hsi BP, et al. Ventilatory functions of normal children and young adults: Mexican-American, white, and black, I: spirometry. *J Pediatr.* 1979;95:14-23.
19. Brasfield D, Hicks G, Soong S, Tiller R. The chest roentgenogram in cystic fibrosis: a new scoring system. *Pediatrics.* 1979;63:24-29.
20. Cox RR, Oakes D. *Analysis of Survival Data.* London, England: Chapman & Hall; 1984.
21. Nadler HL, Ben-Yoseph Y. Genetics. In: Taussig LM, ed. *Cystic Fibrosis.* New York, NY: Thieme-Stratton Inc; 1984:10-11.
22. Hammond KB, Reardon MC, Accurso FJ, et al. Early detection and follow-up of cystic fibrosis in newborns: the Colorado experience. In: Carter T, Willy AM, eds. *Genetic Disease: Screening and Management.* New York, NY: Alan R Liss Inc; 1986:81-101.
23. Wilcken B, Brown ARD, Urwin R, Brown DA. Cystic fibrosis screening by dried blood spot trypsin assay: results in 75,000 newborn infants. *J Pediatr.* 1983;102:383-387.
24. Allan JL, Robbie M, Phelan PD, Danks DM. The incidence and presentation of cystic fibrosis in Victoria 1955-1978. *Aust Paediatr J.* 1980;16:270-273.
25. *Patient Registry.* Rockville, Md: Cystic Fibrosis Foundation; 1987.
26. Prapphal N, Fitzpatrick SB, Getson P, Fink R, O'Donnell R, Chaney M. Cystic fibrosis in blacks in Washington, D.C.: fifteen years experience. *J Natl Med Assoc.* 1989;81:263-267.
27. Rosenstein BJ, Perman JA, Kramer SS. Peptic ulcer disease in cystic fibrosis: an unusual occurrence in black adolescents. *AJDC.* 1986;140:966-969.
28. Sutz SA, Schlesinger ER, Feldman JG, et al. The epidemiology of peptic ulcer in childhood. *Am J Public Health.* 1970;60:492-498.
29. Miranti JP. A review of experience with peptic ulcer in adolescents and young adults in a university health service. *J Am Coll Health.* 1970;18:381.
30. Robb JDA, Thomas PS, Orszulok J, Odling-Smee GW. Duodenal ulcer in children. *Arch Dis Child.* 1972;47:688-696.
31. Eggleston PA, Rosenstein BJ, Stackhouse CM, Alexander MF. Airway hyperreactivity in cystic fibrosis. *Chest.* 1988;94:360-365.
32. Wood RE. Prognosis. In: Taussig LM, ed. *Cystic Fibrosis.* New York, NY: Thieme-Stratton Inc; 1984:434-460.
33. Kulczycki LL, Murphy TM, Bellanti JA. Pseudomonas colonization in cystic fibrosis. *JAMA.* 1978;240:30-34.
34. Wilmott RW, Tyson SL, Matthew DJ. Cystic fibrosis survival rates. *AJDC.* 1985;139:669-671.
35. Katz JN, Horowitz RI, Dolan TF, Shapiro ED. Clinical features as predictors of functional status in children with cystic fibrosis. *J Pediatr.* 1986;108:352-358.
36. Gaskin K, Gurwitz D, Durie P, Levison H, Forstner G. Improved respiratory prognosis in patients with cystic fibrosis with normal fat absorption. *J Pediatr.* 1982;100:857-862.
37. Kraemer R, Hadorn B, Ross E. Classification at time of diagnosis and subsequent survival in patients with cystic fibrosis. *Helv Paediatr Acta.* 1977;32:107-114.
38. Hudson I, Phelan PD. Are sex, age at diagnosis, or mode of presentation prognostic predictors for cystic fibrosis? *Pediatr Pulmonol.* 1987;3:288-297.
39. Orenstein DM, Boat TF, Stern RC, et al. The effect of early diagnosis and treatment in cystic fibrosis. *AJDC.* 1977;131:973-975.
40. Gurwitz D, Corey M, Francis PW, Crozier D, Levison H. Perspectives in cystic fibrosis. *Pediatr Clin North Am.* 1979;26:603-615.
41. Estivill X, del Rio E, Casals T, Volpini V, Bazet M. Linkage disequilibrium for cystic fibrosis in Spanish families. *Pediatr Pulmonol.* 1988;S.2:96. Abstract.
42. Witt M, Erickson RP, Sing CF, Howatt WF, Farquhar S. The relationship of XV2c, KM19 and J3.11 haplotypes to clinical heterogeneity of cystic fibrosis. *Pediatr Pulmonol.* 1988;S.2:98. Abstract.
43. Kerem B, Buchanan JA, Durie P, et al. DNA marker haplotype association with pancreatic sufficiency in cystic fibrosis. *Am J Hum Genet.* 1989;44:827-834.

Cat-Scratch Disease

Acute Encephalopathy and Other Neurologic Manifestations

Hugh A. Carithers, MD, A. M. Margileth, MD

• Seventy-six patients with neurologic complications of cat-scratch disease are discussed. Encephalopathy occurred in 61, while 15 had either cranial or peripheral nerve involvement. The average age of the patients with encephalopathy was 10.6 years (range, 1 to 66 years), and almost twice as many males as females were affected in contrast to patients with uncomplicated cat-scratch disease, in which the ratio was almost equal. Fever was not documented in 50% of patients with encephalopathy and only 26% had temperatures higher than 39°C. Convulsions occurred in 46% and combative behavior in 40%. Lethargy with or without coma was accompanied by variable neurologic signs. Results of laboratory studies, including imaging of the central nervous system, were inconsistent and nondiagnostic. Biopsy tissue from 14 patients showed histopathologic findings compatible with cat-scratch disease. The "English-Wear bacillus" was demonstrated by the Warthin-Starry stain in 10 of 14 skin or lymph node specimens. Of the 15 patients without encephalopathy, two children with facial nerve paresis displayed cranial nerve symptoms and/or signs, 10 patients had cat-scratch disease neuroretinitis, and three women had peripheral neuritis. All 76 patients recovered within 12 months; 78% recovered within 1 to 12 weeks. There were no neurologic sequelae. Treatment consisted of control of convulsions and supportive measures. Commonly used antibiotics administered to more than half of the patients were apparently ineffective.

(*AJDC.* 1991;145:98-101)

Accepted for publication June 27, 1990.

From the Jacksonville Health Education Program, University of Florida (Dr Carithers), and Department of Pediatrics, Uniformed Services University of the Health Sciences, Bethesda, Md (Dr Margileth).

Reprint requests to 2121 Park St, Jacksonville, FL 32204 (Dr Carithers).

Cat-scratch disease (CSD) is a universally encountered infection caused by a pleomorphic gram-negative bacillus.[1] Its most serious clinical feature is an encephalopathy that was first described by Stevens[2] 2 years after the first description of CSD by Debre et al.[3] A review of the world literature in 1967 revealed 20 patients with diverse central nervous system manifestations.[4] Lyon[5] collected 18 patients from the English literature in 1974 and added a case of his own. In 1986, Lewis and Tucker[6] described 38 cases with diverse neurologic manifestations, including those previously mentioned, and added two new patients with encephalopathy; four of these patients had predominantly myelopathic involvement without encephalopathy.

Cat-scratch disease encephalopathy (CSDE) ranks with chicken pox, herpes simplex, Lyme disease, Rocky Mountain spotted fever, and Kawasaki disease in frequency of neurologic complications. This coincides with a recent reduction in the number of patients with measles and mumps encephalitis due to vaccination, and with the increasing rarity of insect-borne encephalitis.[7] It is not known whether the CSDE is due to direct invasion of the brain by the bacillus or some other mechanism such as cerebral vasculitis.[8] We describe herein the course, unique clinical features, and outcomes of CSDE in 61 patients, and describe the cranial and peripheral nerve involvement in an additional 15 patients.

PATIENTS AND METHODS

All patients presented or were reported to us between 1959 and 1987, a period in which we observed approximately 3000 patients with CSD.[9,10] We observed 25 of the 76 patients in this report; the remaining 41 with encephalopathy were reported to us by their physicians, who supplied details of the clinical course, laboratory findings, and follow-up. We provided antigen for skin testing to confirm the diagnosis.

The diagnosis was confirmed in all 76 patients when three of the following four criteria were met: (1) single or regional lymphadenopathy without obvious signs of cutaneous or throat infection; (2) contact with a cat, usually an immature one; (3) detection of an inoculation site; and (4) a positive skin test result for CSD. The finding of the bacteria causing CSD might be considered a single valid criterion; however, this mode of diagnosis is almost never necessary, is unreliable except in experienced hands, and requires general anesthesia for most patients. We, therefore, do not include it as a criterion. One of us (A.M.M.) usually includes the elimination of other causes of lymphadenopathy as a criterion for diagnosis, but routine laboratory work is inconsistent and most cases can be readily diagnosed without it.

The age range of the 61 patients with CSDE was 1 to 66 years (mean, 10.6 years). In a previous report of 34 patients with CSDE, the range was 3 to 48 years (mean, 13 years).[6] The Table compares the ages of these two combined groups (95 patients) with those of 1200 patients with CSD described by Carithers.[9] Of the 95 patients with CSDE, 37% were female and 63% male. In two studies of uncomplicated CSD, the male-female ratio showed only a slight increase in males (54% and 56%).[9,10] The patients with CSDE resided in 15 states representing all geographic areas delineated for reporting purposes by the United States Public Health Service. Of the 15 patients without encephalopathy seen between 1972 and 1987, five were males and 10 females, and the age range was 1.5 to 54 years (mean, 21 years).

RESULTS

Clinical Data

The manner in which our data were collected does not provide an accurate

Age Distribution of Patients With Cat-Scratch Disease (CSD)[9] and CSD Encephalopathy (CSDE)*

Age, y	Patients With CSD, % (n=1200)	Patients With CSDE, % (n=95)
1 to 6	41.0	20.0
7 to 12	42.0	48.0
13 to 18	7.3	17.0
≥18	9.7	15.0

*Patients with CSDE included 61 patients from current study and 34 from the study by Lewis and Tucker.[6]

estimate of the incidence of encephalopathy in patients with CSD. However, it is a rare complication. One of us examined over 1800 patients and diagnosed only three with CSDE, for an incidence of 0.17%, while the other author (A.M.M.) included patients seen directly or by consultation and diagnosed CSDE in 31 of 1500 patients, for an incidence of 2%. On a percentage basis, encephalopathy occurs more commonly among adolescents and adults.

The interval between onset of CSD and the first sign of central nervous system involvement is impossible to determine accurately from the data in the present study. Since CSD is characteristically benign, often undiagnosed, it makes the determination of its onset questionable. The histories of these patients allowed us to conclude that encephalopathic complications may occur from a few days to as long as 2 months after detection of illness, usually in the form of a mildly tender lymphadenopathy. It cannot be assumed that patients who present with convulsions are at the onset of CSD. All three patients in this study who presented in this manner had been infected for more than a week.

All patients had a history of cat contact, usually with an immature cat. All but one patient had a positive cat-scratch skin test result and most had a negative tuberculin skin test result.

Fever was not a characteristic feature; 30 (50%) had no recognized fever with temperatures less than 38.3°C, 14 (23%) had fever not exceeding 39°C, and 16 (26%) had fever between 39°C and 40°C. These closely approximate the percentages seen in a previous study of 1200 patients with CSD.[9]

The lymph nodes involved in the 61 patients were detected in approximately the same locations as in patients with typical CSD.[9,10] There were no indications suggesting that affected lymph nodes around the head and neck predisposed to central nervous system involvement.

Convulsions in 28 (46%) of 61 patients varied from mild twitching of extremities to status epilepticus of 3 to 4 hours' duration. One infant had generalized tonic-clonic seizures, each lasting 1 minute and occurring one to 21 times daily for 6 weeks. She was comatose for 7 weeks. Developmental delay and deafness both resolved after 8 months. No patient had absence seizures. Patients without convulsions may have depression of the central nervous system varying from lethargy to coma.

Transient combative behavior occurred in 24 (39%) of 61 patients who were comatose or semiconscious during the "recovery" phase of a convulsive episode, occasionally during the twitching phase and rarely in a quiet postictal state. The patients acted out by hitting, pushing away, and vocally protesting. This was typically provoked by parents as well as medical staff on touching the patient, especially around the head and neck. To our knowledge, this behavior with this frequency is undocumented in any other type of encephalopathy.

Of other signs and symptoms, headache, usually generalized and persistent, was the most common. Lethargy and malaise lasting 1 to many weeks were common, as is the case in uncomplicated CSD. Persistent ataxia lasting 1 to 8 weeks following the acute phase of encephalopathy was noted in four patients. Less common findings (occurring in only one patient each) were bilateral sixth nerve palsy, aphasia lasting several days, transient hemiplegia, and profound hearing loss lasting 8 months. We do not believe that the severity of CSD is related to development of encephalopathy. Confirming this impression, the presence and degree of elevation of fever are approximately the same in patients with uncomplicated CSD and in those with encephalopathic complications.

Laboratory and Other Studies

The cerebrospinal fluid findings in 51 patients were neither consistent nor characteristic. Sixteen (31%) patients had white blood cell counts of more than 5×10^6/L; the range was 5 to 33×10^6 and 70% to 100% were lymphocytes. Protein concentration was normal in 33 patients (65%) and ranged between 0.41 and 0.93 g/L in 18 (35%). Cerebrospinal fluid glucose was abnormally low in one patient. Routine cultures of cerebrospinal fluid were negative for aerobic, anaerobic, fungal and mycobacterial organisms. Peripheral blood counts in 60 patients were not helpful in diagnosis or prognosis. In 15 patients, the white blood cell count was more than 12×10^9/L, ranging from 12.2 to 37×10^9/L. Two patients had counts below 6×10^9/L. Elevated sedimentation rates occurred in 21 (46%) of 46 patients tested.

Computed tomographic scans performed on 33 patients were not diagnostic and were usually normal or revealed transient abnormalities. Electroencephalography performed during the acute phase of the disease showed background slowing consistent with encephalopathy in 36 (80%) of 46 patients. Follow-up electroencephalograms after 3 to 18 months were normal in all patients.

Cranial magnetic resonance imaging was performed on six patients, five of whom showed normal findings, but one patient had focal changes in the occipital area, also noted on the computed tomographic scan. Carotid arteriography performed on two patients showed normal results.

Fifty-nine of 60 skin tests with cat-scratch antigen had positive results.[11] One patient who was tested elsewhere had a questionable reaction. Another patient who did not undergo a skin test showed a positive reaction to Warthin-Starry stain on lymph node biopsy. Serologic tests for cytomegalovirus, Epstein-Barr virus, toxoplasmosis, and fungi; blood chemistries; cultures of blood or cerebrospinal fluid; tests for mononucleosis; toxic screens; tuberculin tests; and skull films showed normal findings.

Pathologic Findings

Histopathologic study was performed on tissue from 14 patients by Wear et al,[1] who discovered the cat-scratch bacillus in 1983. Biopsies of 13 lymph nodes, two primary skin inoculation lesions, and one conjunctival granuloma were performed. Stellate or inflammatory granulomas were detected in six lymph nodes, and focal or multiple areas of necrosis with vasculitis were found in seven patients' nodes or skin. The cat-scratch bacillus was detected by the Warthin-Starry silver stain in 10 of the 14 patients. Only three specimens were unfixed and fresh enough for culture studies, and all results were negative.

Pathologic sections of nodes removed from patients with CSD may show abscesses and/or granulomas. These changes can occur in other diseases and are not diagnostic of CSD, but when both abscesses and granulomas are observed in the same specimen, the findings are consistent with CSD.

COMMENT

Diagnosis

Cat-scratch disease encephalopathy is readily diagnosed when signs and symptoms of central nervous system dysfunction develop during the course of CSD. In patients not identified as having CSD, a convulsion is usually the first symptom of CSDE.[9,11] Typical of this group was a 9-year-old boy who was brought to the emergency room with generalized convulsions and a temperature of 38°C. He was admitted to the intensive care unit and the convulsions were controlled after 30 minutes with diazepam. A spinal tap showed no abnormalities; a complete blood cell count showed a white blood cell count of 16×10^9/L, 72% of which were polymorphonuclear. Drug screening showed normal findings, as did biochemical studies, skull and chest roentgenograms, computed tomographic scan of the brain, and ultrasound study of the abdomen. The patient was initially examined by an emergency room physician, a pediatric resident, and two intensive care attending physicians. An electroencephalogram was normal. The patient was combative and unconscious throughout the next 12 hours, becoming more responsive but remaining querulous for 2 days. Twelve hours after admission, another resident found a large inguinal lymph node measuring 2×3 cm. A red papule, more firm than a mosquito bite, was found on the ankle on the same side as the lymphadenopathy. The presence of a 4-month-old kitten in the patient's home was established. The cat-scratch skin test showed positive results in 48 hours and the boy was discharged on the fifth hospital day, having entirely recovered. Follow-up for several months showed no residual effects of the illness.

Cat-scratch disease encephalopathy should be considered when a young patient presents with a sudden onset of coma and/or convulsions. One should probe for a history of cat exposure even though the parents and child deny such contact. Children may express denial due to feared parental disapproval or through forgetfulness. A thorough search should be made for lymphadenopathy and presence of a regional inoculation papule or conjunctival granuloma. An almost certain diagnosis of CSD can be made if these signs are found. The diagnosis of CSD can be confirmed if a cat-scratch skin test shows positive results at 48 to 72 hours.[11] Removal of the lymph node involved is rarely necessary.[12] The processing of biopsied tissue requires several or more days, compared with cat-scratch skin testing, which is more diagnostic.[8,9,11] Granulomatous or necrotic changes found in lymph nodes due to CSD are nonspecific.[1] Unless the organism causing CSD is found in the biopsy tissue, the study will not be conclusive. Special stains such as the Warthin-Starry stain are not available in most clinical laboratories and, at times, are difficult to interpret.[13]

Differential considerations include viral or Lyme encephalitis, drug intoxication, poisonings, bacterial infections such as meningitis, Rocky Mountain spotted fever, Kawasaki disease, and Reye's syndrome. The viral encephalitides seen in this country include those associated with common contagious diseases that are disappearing, except for varicella, herpes, arboviruses, and enteroviruses. Central nervous system involvement may rarely be encountered with acute disseminated encephalomyelitis, acute hemorrhagic leukoencephalopathy, granulomatous arteritis, and the so-called slow viruses—conventional and unconventional.[7]

Treatment

It is believed that antibiotics do not modify the course of CSD. This opinion was based on the observation that the lymph nodes involved often continue to enlarge or progress to suppuration despite the oral or intravenous administration of several commonly used antibiotics. Not included in this group of drugs are gentamicin sulfate and third generation cephalosporins.[13] Recently, Bogue and associates[14] reported that signs and symptoms of systemic CSD promptly disappeared in three acutely ill patients after intravenous treatment with gentamicin sulfate. We are not aware of any patient with CSDE being treated with intravenous gentamicin sulfate. However, in the severely ill patient, we recommend the intravenous administration of 5 to 7 mg/kg per day of gentamicin sulfate at 8-hour intervals.[14] Duration of treatment would be based on response and the knowledge that recovery from CSDE is usually prompt (4 to 14 days) in the natural course of the disease. Recently, Collipp[15] reported excellent response to trimethoprim-sulfamethoxazole in 11 patients with CSD.

In addition to the control of convulsions and respiratory support, the most important aspect in the treatment of patients with encephalopathy is to establish the diagnosis as quickly as possible. This might avoid extensive and unrewarding studies that will disturb the patient. During coma, we recommend supportive measures with appropriate nursing care and close observation of the patient.

Prognosis

There were no deaths in this series. Reports of seven deaths due to CSDE[4] did not meet our diagnostic criteria for the disease. Although it is often difficult to determine the exact duration of illness in childhood, we believe the acute phase of encephalopathy associated with CSD is usually short. Approximately two thirds of the patients recovered fully in 4 weeks and none showed evidence of encephalopathy after 1 year. Patients of all ages may complain of lethargy, headache, fatigue or weakness, and anorexia for several weeks or months. These symptoms also appear in uncomplicated CSD.[8,9,11]

Follow-up data ranging from 3 months to 22 years were available in all 61 patients in this series. Over 50% of patients were followed up for more than 2 years. To date, no lasting neurologic impairment due to CSDE developed in these 61 patients. This form of encephalopathy is probably the least hazardous of any caused by direct central nervous system infection or serious response of the central nervous system to infection or toxins.

Neurologic Symptoms and Signs in Patients With CSD Without Encephalopathy

Transient dysfunction of cranial and/or peripheral nerves occurred in 15 of 1471 patients with CSD observed by one of us (A.M.M.) during the last 15 years. Two children aged 18 months and 8 years had temporary facial nerve paresis (Bell's palsy) associated with CSD oculoglandular syndrome lasting 4 to 5 weeks. These patients have not been studied as exhaustively as have the patients with CSDE and some are still under observation. We are including them in this presentation to alert physicians to the recent recognition of peripheral nerve disease associated with CSD.

Three women aged 26, 27, and 54 years had peripheral neuritis lasting 1 to 4 months. The 26-year-old had unilateral paresthesia with a transient Babinski sign and leg edema associated with inguinal lymphadenitis lasting 4 weeks. The 27-year-old patient developed severe neuralgia and myalgia of the left shoulder shortly after the onset of lymphadenitis of the left anterior and posterior cervical chains. The paresthesia, myalgia, and adenopathy slowly resolved over 4 to 5 months. The 54-year-old woman was hospitalized for 2 months with severe headaches; facial, eye, parietal, and temporomandibular painful swelling; and multiple cat scratches with bilateral cervical lymphadenitis.[16] The neuralgia and cephalgia persisted for 6 weeks, during which results of multiple diagnostic studies were normal or nondiagnostic. Treatment with several antibiotics and prednisone was ineffective. A diagnosis of oculoglandular syndrome of Parinaud due to CSD was confirmed, and all symptoms and signs abated after 3 months.

Ten patients (seven adults, one adolescent, and two children) with neuroretinitis and CSD were observed during the past 3 years.[17] Each patient presented with a sudden onset of blindness in one eye associated with regional lymphadenitis and cat scratches. All 10 recovered slowly during 4 to 12 months with subsequent visual acuity of 20/20 to 20/50 in the affected eye. Therapy with several antibiotics and/or prednisone was apparently ineffective.

Since preparation of this article, we have been consulted concerning an additional 14 patients with probable CSDE. Although follow-up has been brief, their clinical courses were similar to those of the 61 patients described. Presentation of an exhibit by R. Sawyer, MD; J. Teahan, MD; and A. M. Margileth, MD, on CSD neuroretinitis at the annual meeting of the American Academy of Ophthalmology has led to an increasing number of diagnoses of this condition in widespread areas of this country.

We are grateful to Douglas J. Wear, MD, for performing pathologic studies in 14 patients; Harold Stevens, MD, and Gerald M. Fenichel, MD, for their critical review of the article; and to the following physicians who referred patients and supplied follow-up studies: W. Bernstein, MD; S. Birnbaum, MD; John B. Black, MD; Dean A. Blumberg, MD; Bartley Cilento, MD; Richard Cohen, MD; Thomas Curtin, MD; D. D. Demicco, MD; Depue H. Duffey, MD; Joel B. Edman, MD; Gerald Fenichel, MD; Albert Fink, MD; Margaret C. Fisher, MD; C. Fowler, MD; Sandy Glikin, MD; W. F. J. Gordon, MD; Andrea Gravatt, MD; Stephen A. Green, MD; Melvin Greer, MD; Art Guarinello, MD; Michael Gurney, MD; Caroline B. Hall, MD; Harvey J. Hamrick, MD; Mark Helfaer, MD; W. M. Hufstetter, MD; Richard Kalm, MD; Margaret Keller, MD; Anthony P. Lamantia, MD; Myron Levin, MD; Jack Lynch, MD; J. Marcidas, MD; James McDowall, MD; Tracy Middlebrooks, MD; Richard Moriarty, MD; Larry Nester, MD; L. D. Penny Jr, MD; R. H. Pollen, MD; Robert Prouty, MD; John Ritrosky, MD; William A. Rodriguez, MD; Lorry Rubin, MD; Ralph Sawyer, MD; George Schwartz, MD; D. M. Tardiff, MD; C. H. Wharten, MD; Paul Wherle, MD; Marvin Weil, MD; Elliot Wilner, MD; and Celeste Woodward, MD.

References

1. Wear DJ, Margileth AM, Hadfield TL, Fischer G, Schagel C, King F. Cat-scratch disease: a bacterial infection. *Science.* 1983;221:1403-1405.

2. Stevens H. Cat-scratch fever encephalitis. *AJDC.* 1952;84:218-222.

3. Debre R, Lamy M, Jamment ML, et al. La maladie des griffes de chat. *Sem Hop Paris.* 1950;26:1895-1904.

4. Warwick WJ. The cat scratch syndrome: many diseases or one disease? *Prog Med Virol.* 1967;9:256-301.

5. Lyon LW. Neurologic manifestations of cat scratch disease. *Arch Neurol.* 1971;25:23-27.

6. Lewis DW, Tucker SH. Central nervous involvement in cat-scratch disease. *Pediatrics.* 1986;77:714-721.

7. Booss J, Esiri M. *Viral Encephalitis: Pathology, Diagnosis and Management.* Boston, Mass: Blackwell Scientific Publications Inc; 1986:32-69.

8. Selby G, Walker GL. Cerebral arteritis in cat scratch disease. *Neurology.* 1979;29:1413-1418.

9. Carithers HA. Cat-scratch disease: an overview based on a study of 1200 patients. *AJDC.* 1985;139:1124-1133.

10. Margileth AM. Dermatologic manifestations and update of cat-scratch disease. *Pediatric Dermatol.* 1988;5:1-9.

11. Moriarty RA, Margileth AM. Cat-scratch disease. *Infect Dis Clin North Am.* 1987;1:575-590.

12. Knight PJ, Muline AF, Vassy LE. When is lymph node biopsy indicated in children with enlarged peripheral nodes? *Pediatrics.* 1982;69:391.

13. English CK, Wear DJ, Margileth AM, et al. Cat-scratch disease: isolation and culture of the bacterial agent. *JAMA.* 1988;259:1347-1352.

14. Bogue CW, Wise JD, Gray GF, Edwards KM. Antibiotic therapy for cat-scratch disease? *JAMA.* 1989;262:813-816.

15. Collipp PJ. Cat-scratch disease therapy. *AJDC.* 1989;143:1261.

16. Flessner MF. A tough diagnosis in a neutropenic patient: it's cat-scratch disease. *JAMA.* 1989;261:991.

17. Schlossberg D, Morad Y, Krouse TB, et al. Culture-proved disseminated cat-scratch disease in acquired immunodeficiency syndrome. *Arch Intern Med.* 1989;149:1437-1439.

Surfactant Replacement Therapy in Respiratory Distress Syndrome

Meta-analysis of Clinical Trials of Single-Dose Surfactant Extracts

Halim M. Hennes, MD; Martha B. Lee, PhD; Alfred A. Rimm, PhD; Donald L. Shapiro, MD†

• Replacement therapy with surfactant extracts in premature infants with respiratory distress syndrome has been evaluated in several clinical trials. The results of individual trials do not provide conclusive evidence that administration of a single dose of surfactant improves morbidity or mortality. Meta-analysis is a statistical method to combine the results of such clinical trials, and combined analysis provides a means to overcome the problem of not being able to detect significant small differences in individual trials due to these small sample sizes. Seven clinical trials (277 patients treated with nonhuman surfactant extract and 263 controls) met the criteria for analysis; five outcome measurements (mortality, patent ductus arteriosus, pneumothorax, intraventricular hemorrhage, and bronchopulmonary dysplasia) were selected to estimate the treatment effect. The meta-analysis showed that a single dose of surfactant administered before the first breath or within 15 hours of birth significantly decreased the mortality rate (95% confidence interval = −0.19 to −0.03) and the risk of developing pneumothorax (95% confidence interval = −0.28 to −0.14) in infants with respiratory distress syndrome. Further clinical trials are needed to evaluate other aspects of surfactant replacement therapy in premature infants because inconsistent results were observed among the seven analyzed studies.

(*AJDC.* 1991;145:102-104)

Neonatal respiratory distress syndrome (RDS) is a major cause of morbidity and mortality in premature infants.[1] Continuing advances in the respiratory care of infants and animal studies provide evidence that deficiency of lung surfactant is the primary underlying cause of RDS.[1,2] In 1978, Adams et al[2] showed that surfactant replacement in premature lambs resulted in improved aeration and prevented atelectasis. In 1980, Fujiwara et al[3] reported that treatment with exogenous surfactant (an extract of bovine lung) improved oxygenation and reduced the need for ventilatory support in premature infants with severe RDS. Since then, several clinical trials have been undertaken to evaluate the efficacy of surfactant replacement therapy using various surfactant preparations in the treatment or prevention of RDS.[4-18] The individual results of this group of trials have not provided conclusive evidence that surfactant replacement significantly improves morbidity or mortality of premature infants. Differences in study design, type of surfactant and dose used, and delivery technique may explain the variability in the reported results.

Meta-analysis is a statistical method designed to analyze and combine results from different clinical trials.[19-21] The objective of such analysis is to obtain a stable estimate of treatment effect, examine variability between trials, and resolve the uncertainty of conflicting results.[20] Selected trials should be of like design, have a similar study population, use the same or similar therapy, and measure the same outcome variables. To evaluate the treatment effect of surfactant replacement therapy on morbidity and mortality of premature infants with RDS, we performed a meta-analysis of seven published randomized clinical trials that used a single dose of nonhuman surfactant extract.

Accepted for publication April 19, 1990.

From the Departments of Pediatrics (Dr Hennes) and Biostatistics and Clinical Epidemiology (Drs Lee and Rimm), Medical College of Wisconsin and Children's Hospital of Wisconsin, Milwaukee, and the Department of Pediatrics (Neonatology) and Specialized Care Center of Research for Respiratory Distress in Neonates, University of Rochester (NY) Medical Center (Dr Shapiro).

†Dr Shapiro died October 15, 1989.

Reprint requests to Department of Pediatrics, Children's Hospital of Wisconsin, PO Box 1997, MS 756, Milwaukee, WI 53201 (Dr Hennes).

MATERIALS AND METHODS

Selection of Trials

A computer search of the English language literature was performed on surfactant replacement therapy used between January 1975 and May 1989 in premature infants with RDS. The bibliographies of the articles obtained by computer search were also reviewed. All studies were reviewed by all investigators and only randomized, controlled trials that used a single dose of nonhuman surfactant extract administered within the first 24 hours after birth were selected for meta-analysis. Inclusion criteria included (1) randomized controlled trials; (2) single dose nonhuman surfactant extract administered either at birth or within the first 24 hours; and (3) documentation of outcome which included survival, development of patent ductus arteriosus, pneumothorax, intraventricular hemorrhage, and bronchopulmonary dysplasia.

Statistical Analysis

Data were abstracted from the selected trials by one investigator (H.M.H.) and reviewed by two additional investigators (M.B.L. and D.L.S.) in a blinded fashion. Disagreements were resolved by group consensus. To evaluate the constancy of treatment effect across studies, a test of homogeneity[22] (the Cochran's Q) was used. The rate difference (rate in the treatment group minus rate in control group) was calculated for each of the five selected outcomes in each study. Results of all trials were then combined using the method described by DerSimonian and Laird[19] that allows each study to have its own treatment effect and incorporate any among-study differences that may cause variability in treatment effect. The mean effect of treatment (combined rate differences) can be estimated by a weighted average of rate differences. A negative value of this estimate would indicate a benefit from treatment. The 95% confidence interval (CI) was calculated for the combined rate difference. When the 95% CI includes zero, it suggests that there is no statistically significant difference between treatment and control groups.

RESULTS

Sixteen clinical trials were located: two nonrandomized trials[3,4] were excluded, as were trials using synthetic surfactant[6,14] or human surfactant.[5,7,11] One duplicate report[9] and one trial[18] that included patients from a pilot study were excluded from the analysis. Seven randomized clinical trials[8,10,12,13,15-17] re-

Table 1.—General Characteristics of Selected Trials

Source, y	No. of Patients: Treatment	No. of Patients: Control	Average Gestational Age, wk: Treatment	Average Gestational Age, wk: Control	Average Birth Weight, kg: Treatment	Average Birth Weight, kg: Control	Blinded	Placebo	Total Dose, mg	Time of Administration, h
Enhorning et al,[8] 1985	39	33	27.4	27.2	976	974	Yes	Air	75-100	0*
Kwong et al,[10] 1985	14	13	26.7	26.2	971	892	Yes	Saline	90	0*
Gitlin et al,[12] 1987	18	23	29	29	1214	1214	No	Saline	100†	<8
Raju et al,[13] 1987	17	13	28.4	27.6	1119	1096	Yes	Saline	100†	<6
Kendig et al,[15] 1988	34	31	28.8	28.4	1057	996	Yes	Saline	90	0*
European,[16] 1988	77	69	28.8	28.4	1246	1182	No	No	200†	2-15
Horbar et al,[17] 1989	78	81	28.5	28.2	1119	1160	Yes	Air	100†	<8

*Zero hour indicates at birth.
†Dose in milligrams per kilogram.

Table 2.—Effect of Surfactant Replacement on the Outcome in the Selected Trials*

Study	Mortality, %: S	Mortality, %: C	RD, %	PDA, %: S	PDA, %: C	RD, %	Pneumothorax, %: S	Pneumothorax, %: C	RD, %	IVH, %: S	IVH, %: C	RD, %	BPD, %: S	BPD, %: C	RD, %
Enhorning et al[8]	3	18	−15†	46	58	−12	15	33	−18	28	61	−33†	56	67	−11
Kwong et al[10]	7	14	−7	50	29	21	43	50	−7	36	28	8	43	64	−21
Gitlin et al[12]	17	26	−9	78	65	13	17	57	−40†	89	74	15	22	30	−8
Raju et al[13]	18	47	−29	71	23	48†	12	47	−35†	47	62	−15	24	92	−68†
Kendig et al[15]	29	29	0	27	16	11	9	23	−14	24	16	8	35	36	−1
European[16]	31	51	−20†	60	46	14	18	35	−17†	47	55	−8	16	26	−10
Horbar et al[17]	17	17	0	1	48	−7	10	30	−20†	24	25	−1	45	44	1

*RD indicates rate difference; PDA, patent ductus arteriosus; IVH, intraventricular hemorrhage; S, surfactant group; C, controls; and BPD, bronchopulmonary dysplasia.
†Indicates that the results were statistically significant ($P<.05$).

mained for the meta-analysis that included 277 infants treated with surfactant and 263 controls. The general characteristics of these trials are summarized in Table 1. There were no significant differences in gestational age or birth weights among those in the selected trials. All studies were randomized; five were blinded and six were placebo controlled. Surfactants were various bovine surfactant extracts in six studies and porcine in one[16] instilled into the lungs as a single dose. The lowest total dose used was 75 mg/kg[8] and the highest dose was 200 mg/kg.[16] Surfactant was administered before the first breath in three trials[8,10,15] and within 15 hours of birth in four trials.[12,13,16,17]

Table 2 summarizes the occurrence rates and risk differences for each outcome during the neonatal period in these trials. Although the rate difference for mortality ranged from 0% to −29%, only two studies[8,16] reported a significant decrease in mortality rate among the treatment group. For patent ductus arteriosus, the risk difference was −12% to 48%. Raju et al[13] found significantly fewer cases of patent ductus arteriosus in the surfactant group. Four trials[12,13,16,17] indicated that pneumothorax was observed less frequently in treated infants (rate difference, −7% to −40%). Surfactant treatment was also associated with statistically significant decreases in the occurrence rate of intraventricular hemorrhage in one trial[8] and the development of bronchopulmonary dysplasia in another.[13] The test of homogeneity (Cochran's Q) for treatment effect indicated lack of homogeneity across the studies for patent ductus arteriosus and bronchopulmonary dysplasia; hence, we used the method described by DerSimonian and Laird[19] that estimates the magnitude of heterogeneity and assigns a greater variability to the estimate of overall treatment effect to account for such heterogeneity (Table 3). Results of the combined analysis are summarized in Table 4. The combined rate differences for four of the five outcomes (mortality, pneumothorax, intraventricular hemorrhage, and bronchopulmonary dysplasia) were

Table 3.—Results of Cochran's Q Test of Homogeneity

Outcome*	Q	P Value
Death	6.57	.36
PDA	13.58	.03
Pneumothorax	3.86	.69
IVH	11.55	.07
BPD	24.29	.001

*PDA indicates patent ductus arteriosus; IVH, intraventricular hemorrhage; and BPD, bronchopulmonary dysplasia.

Table 4.—The Combined Analysis of Treatment Effect for All Selected Trials*

Diagnosis	No. of Events/No. of Patients (%) Treatment	Control	Treatment Effect	95% CI	*P* Value
Death	55/277 (20)	78/263 (30)	−0.105	−0.19/−0.03	.01
PDA	135/277 (49)	117/263 (44)	0.073	−0.06/0.2	.26
Pneumothorax	43/277 (16)	98/263 (37)	−0.214	−0.28/−0.14	.0001
IVH	103/277 (37)	112/263 (43)	−0.051	−0.16/0.06	.35
BPD	95/277 (34)	115/263 (44)	−0.062	−0.14/0.03	.11

*PDA indicates patent ductus arteriosus; IVH, intraventricular hemorrhage; BPD, bronchopulmonary dysplasia; and CI, confidence interval.

negative in the direction of a treatment benefit. Only two of those differences, however, were statistically significant. For mortality, the combined rate difference was −0.105 and the corresponding 95% CI was −0.19 to −0.03 (*P*=.01). For pneumothorax, the combined rate difference was −0.214 and the corresponding 95% CI was −0.28 to −0.14 (*P*=.0001).

COMMENT

When performing meta-analysis, the selected trials should be randomized, placebo controlled, double blind, evaluate the same therapy in a comparable group of patients, and evaluate the same outcome variables. Of the seven selected clinical trials, two were not blinded[11,15] and one used no placebo.[15] However, all trials used objective outcome measurements (arterial blood gas values, ventilator requirements, etc) to determine treatment benefit. Accordingly, it is unlikely that the results were subject to observer bias. While no placebo was used in the collaborative European study, both treatment and control groups were subjected to the same protocol. To avoid the variability in reporting the results of pulmonary functions among these trials, we selected five binary outcomes to measure the treatment effect.

We were unable to determine from the available data if a specific surfactant dose or the time of administration significantly affected the observed results. Currently, the dose is based on the available theoretical data that 100 mg/kg will cover the entire lung surface, and we have no knowledge regarding the number of doses that should be given to maintain a stable physiological surfactant level. Shapiro et al[9] demonstrated that using multiple doses of surfactant significantly improved the survival rate among a high-risk group of infants. The timing of surfactant administration does not appear to be crucial since we observed no consistent difference between the trials that administered surfactant before the first breath and those that delayed administration for several hours. One disadvantage in administering surfactant prior to the first breath is the possibility of giving it to infants who do not need it, which may bias the observed results.

The detection of a statistically significant decrease in mortality rate and pneumothorax suggests that a single dose of nonhuman surfactant extract administered before the first breath or within 15 hours of birth to premature infants with RDS is beneficial. Leviton et al,[23] in a recent review, examined the association between RDS and the development of intraventricular hemorrhage using the results of the surfactant replacement trials. They concluded that these trials provided no evidence that surfactant replacement lowered the incidence of intraventricular hemorrhage. Therefore, further clinical trials are needed to evaluate specific aspects of surfactant replacement therapy such as repeated dosing, time of administration, potency and safety of various surfactants, and differences in response to surfactant by different patients.

Frances Sommer provided assistance in the preparation of the manuscript.

This article is dedicated to the memory of Donald L. Shapiro, MD.

References

1. Stahlman MT. Acute respiratory disorders in the newborn. In: Avery GB, ed. *Neonatology Pathophysiology and Management of the Newborn.* 3rd ed. Philadelphia, Pa: JB Lippincott; 1987:418-445.

2. Adams FH, Towers B, Osher AB. Effect of tracheal instillation of natural surfactant in premature lambs: clinical and autopsy findings. *Pediatr Res.* 1978;12:841-848.

3. Fujiwara T, Chida S, Watabe Y, Maeta H, Morita T, Abe T. Artificial surfactant therapy in hyaline membrane disease. *Lancet.* 1980;1:55-59.

4. Morley CJ, Miller N, Bangham AD, Davis JA. Dry artificial surfactant and its effect on very premature babies. *Lancet.* 1981;1:64-68.

5. Hallman M, Merritt A, Schneider H, et al. Isolation of human surfactant from amniotic fluid and a pilot study of its efficacy in respiratory distress syndrome. *Pediatrics.* 1983;71:473-481.

6. Halliday H, Reid M, Meban C, et al. Controlled trial of artificial surfactant to prevent respiratory distress syndrome. Lancet. 1984;1:476-478.

7. Hallman M, Merritt A, Jarvenpaa AL, et al. Exogenous human surfactant for treatment of severe respiratory distress syndrome: a randomized prospective clinical trial. *J Pediatr.* 1985;106: 963-969.

8. Enhorning G, Shennon A, Possmayer F, Dunn M, Chen C, Milligan J. Prevention of neonatal respiratory distress syndrome by tracheal instillation of surfactant: a randomized clinical trial. *Pediatrics.* 1985;76:145-153.

9. Shapiro D, Notter R, Morin III FC, et al. Double-blind randomized trial of a calf lung surfactant extract administered at birth to very premature infants for prevention of respiratory distress syndrome. *Pediatrics.* 1985;76:593-599.

10. Kwong M, Egan E, Notter RH, Shapiro DL. Double-blind clinical trial of calf lung surfactant extract for the prevention of hyaline membrane disease in extremely premature infants. *Pediatrics.* 1985;76:585-592.

11. Merritt T, Hallman M, Bloom BT, et al. Prophylactic treatment of very premature infants with human surfactant. *N Engl J Med.* 1986;315: 785-790.

12. Gitlin JD, Soll RF, Parad RB, et al. Randomized controlled trial of exogenous surfactant for the treatment of hyaline membrane disease. *Pediatrics.* 1987;79:31-37.

13. Raju TNK, Bhat R, McCulloch KM, et al. Double-blind controlled trial of single-dose treatment of bovine surfactant in severe hyaline membrane disease. *Lancet.* 1987;1:651-656.

14. Ten Center Study Group. Ten center trial of artificial surfactant in very premature babies. *BMJ.* 1987;294:991-996.

15. Kendig JW, Notter RH, Cox C, et al. Surfactant replacement therapy at birth: final analysis of a clinical trial and comparisons with similar trials. *Pediatrics.* 1988;82:756-762.

16. Collaborative European Group. Surfactant replacement therapy for severe neonatal respiratory distress syndrome: an international randomized clinical trial. *Pediatrics.* 1988;82:683-691.

17. Horbar J, Soll R, Sutherland JM, et al. A multicenter randomized placebo-controlled trial of surfactant therapy for respiratory distress syndrome. *N Engl J Med.* 1989;320:959-965.

18. Charon A, Taeusch W, Fitzgibbon C, Smith G, Treves T, Phelps D. Factors associated with surfactant treatment response in infants with severe respiratory distress syndrome. *Pediatrics.* 1989;83:348-354.

19. DerSimonian R, Laird N. Meta analysis in clinical trials. *Controlled Clin Trials.* 1986;7:177-188.

20. Jenicek M. Meta analysis in medicine. *J Clin Epidemiol.* 1989;42:35-44.

21. Sacks H, Berrier J, Reitman D, Ancona-Berk V, Chalmers T. Meta analysis of randomized controlled trials. *N Engl J Med.* 1987;316:450-455.

22. Cochran WG. The combination of estimates from different experiments. *Biometrics.* 1954;10: 101-129.

23. Leviton A, VanMarter L, Kuban KCK. Respiratory distress syndrome and intracranial hemorrhage: cause or association ? inference from surfactant clinical trials. *Pediatrics.* 1989;84:915-922.

Gallstones in Children

Characterization by Age, Etiology, and Outcome

Shimon Reif, MD; Daniel G. Sloven, MD; Emanuel Lebenthal, MD

• Fifty children and adolescents were found to have gallstones at Children's Hospital of Buffalo (NY) during a period of 10 years. The mean (±SD) age was 12.2±6.2 years, with 21 boys and 29 girls. The majority of patients could be categorized into four groups: hemolytic disease (18 patients), parenteral nutrition (eight patients), adolescent pregnancy (seven patients), and idiopathic (10 patients), while seven patients had a variety of other etiologies. Right upper quadrant pain was the most common symptom (32 patients), followed by jaundice (15 patients), vomiting (13 patients), and nonspecific abdominal complaints (13 patients). Ten patients presented with jaundice and underlying hemolytic disease; seven patients were asymptomatic. Clinical presentation was found to vary with age and factors associated with the development of gallstones. Ultrasonography was the mode of diagnosis in 48 patients. Cholecystectomy was performed in 36 patients. In contrast to gallstones in adults, after exclusion of the patients with adolescent pregnancy, there was no female predominance. Pancreatitis was the most common complication, occurring in 8% of the patients; cholecystitis and cholangitis were absent.

(*AJDC.* 1991;145:105-108)

Gallstones have been regarded as an uncommon problem in children.[1-5] Reports since the advent of ultrasonography have identified groups of children not previously known to be at risk for gallbladder disease, such as patients with spinal injury and spinal surgery,[6,7] immunodeficiency,[8] and parenteral nutrition.[9] In this study, we discuss all patients having gallstones diagnosed at Children's Hospital of Buffalo (NY) from 1979 to 1989 to determine the clinical presentation, method of diagnosis, and modality of treatment in regard to the different age groups and factors associated with the development of gallstones.

Accepted for publication June 4, 1990.

From the Division of Gastroenterology and Nutrition and Colucci Memorial Liver Research Center, Children's Hospital of Buffalo (NY) (Dr Reif); the Department of Pediatrics, St John's Mercy Medical Center, St Louis, Mo (Dr Sloven); and the Department of Pediatrics, Hahnemann School of Medicine, Philadelphia, Pa (Dr Lebenthal).

Reprint requests to Department of Pediatrics (402), Hahnemann University School of Medicine, Broad and Vine Streets, Philadelphia, PA 19102-1192 (Dr Lebenthal).

PATIENTS AND METHODS

All charts of inpatients and outpatients with gallstones diagnosed radiographically or surgically at Children's Hospital of Buffalo from 1979 to 1989 were reviewed. Sonographic diagnosis of gallstones was based on the presence of mobile echogenic foci in the gallbladder lumen or in the region of the gallbladder fossa. Acoustic shadowing was not required for sonographic diagnosis because it is not always present when the foci are small.[10] Roentgenographic diagnosis of gallstones required calcifications in the right upper quadrant to be present in more than one view. Patients with previous biliary tract surgery, acalculus cholecystitis, and biliary tract disease without proven gallstones were excluded from our study.

Fifty patients met the criteria of the study. Patients were characterized by age, associated conditions, clinical presentation, laboratory studies, method of diagnosis, therapy, and outcome. A univariate analysis was conducted looking for a correlation between age, race, sex, clinical presentation, laboratory studies, therapy, and factors associated with gallstones by χ^2 analysis.

RESULTS

Fifty children with gallstones were identified at Children's Hospital of Buffalo from 1979 to 1989 with ages ranging from prenatal to 20 years. The mean (±SD) age at presentation was 12.2±6.2 years, with 21 boys and 29 girls. There were 29 whites, 17 blacks, and four Hispanics.

The age distribution is presented in the Figure. The tendency toward female predominance was noted only after 15 years of age. Diagnosis was most frequent after age 15 years; however, 8 patients were 5 years old or less. Conditions associated with the development of gallstones are shown in Table 1. Several of our patients had more than one associated factor. The majority of the patients could be categorized in one of four main groups: hemolytic disease (18 patients), parenteral nutrition (eight patients), adolescent pregnancy (seven patients), and idiopathic (10 patients). Seven patients who were not included in the four main groups had a variety of other etiologies.

Clinical presentations and the relationship between age and clinical presentation are shown in Table 2. While right upper quadrant pain was the most common symptom in 32 patients, 13 patients had nonspecific abdominal symptoms, including poorly localized abdominal pain, nausea, and chest pain; only one patient had fever. Seven patients were asymptomatic, including one patient diagnosed in utero by a routine maternal ultrasound study. The majority of patients had more than one symptom.

Right upper quadrant pain predominated in patients ages 6 years and older. No patients less than 6 years old presented with jaundice. Fatty food intolerance was observed only in patients older than 6 years old, and asymptomatic presentations predominated in younger patients. Nonspecific abdominal pain and vomiting showed no specific age distribution.

Ultrasonography was used to diagnose 48 patients. Other diagnostic methods included plain films (for four patients), abdominal computed tomography (for three patients), and oral cho-

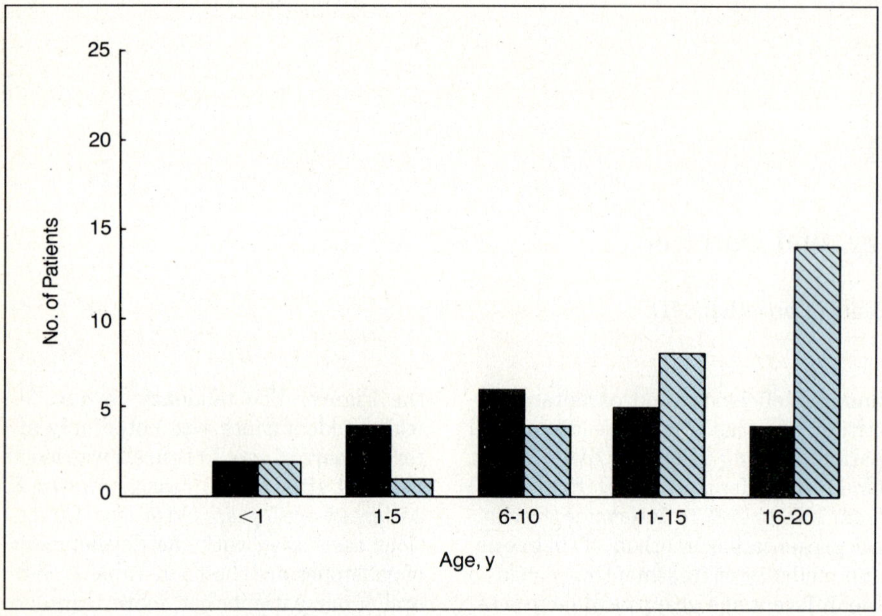

Age and sex distribution of children with gallstones. The highest incidence is noted between 16 and 20 years of age. The female predominance was noted only in the second decade. Solid bar indicates males (n=21); and hatched bar, females (n=29).

Table 1.—Conditions Associated With Gallstones in 50 Children*

Associated Conditions	No. of Patients
Hemolysis	18
Sickle cell anemia	11
Spherocytosis	3
Autoimmune	2
Thalassemia major	1
Pyruvate kinase deficiency	1
Parenteral nutrition	8
Adolescent pregnancy	7
Ileal resection	4
Obesity†	3
Sepsis	3
Nectrotizing enterocolitis	2
Spinal cord disease	2
Transverse myelitis	1
Spina bifida	1
Other	
Hemobilia	1
Chronic intestinal pseudo-obstruction	1
Chylous ascites	1
Muscular dystrophy	1
Sarcoidosis	1
Systemic lupus erythematosus	1
Hyperlipidemia	1
Cystic fibrosis	1
Hepatitis type B	1
Dysgammaglobulinemia	1
Prolonged ceftriaxone therapy	1
Idiopathic	10

*Children with gallstones could be categorized into four main groups: patients with hemolysis (18), patients with parenteral nutrition (8), adolescent pregnancy (7), and patients with other predisposing factors (7). More than one predisposing factor was present in some patients.

†Obesity is defined as weight divided by height, 95th percentile.

langiogram (for two patients). One patient was diagnosed at laparotomy for a small-bowel obstruction; some patients had more than one diagnostic study.

The relationship between associated factors and age, sex, racial distribution, symptoms, laboratory studies, and therapy is shown in Table 3. The patients with parenteral nutrition were significantly younger than the average age at presentation ($P<.05$), and the pregnant adolescent patients were significantly older ($P<.01$). After exclusion of the adolescent pregnancy group, female predominance was observed only in the miscellaneous group, while the hemolytic, parenteral nutrition, and idiopathic groups had nearly equal sex distributions. Right upper quadrant pain was the chief presenting symptom in all groups except the patients with parenteral nutrition. Jaundice was seen mainly in the hemolytic group. No hemolytic or pregnant adolescent patients were asymptomatic. Leukocytosis was not present in the parenteral nutrition group and was present most commonly in the adolescent pregnancy and hemolytic groups. Elevated serum transaminase levels were seen in all the pregnant patients and half of the hemolytic patients. Cholecystectomy was performed in 36 patients and was the main therapy in all groups except the patients with parenteral nutrition, for whom conservative treatment was preferred.

Complications of gallstones occurred in six patients,including pancreatitis (4 patients), retained duct stone (one patient), and recurrence (one patient). No patient with pancreatitis was found to have a stricture of the Vater's ampulla or other obstruction of the pancreatic duct. The only death occurred in a patient with sickle cell anemia presenting with repeated episodes of biliary colic. The patient's parents refused preoperative transfusions due to religious beliefs.

COMMENT

According to the experience at Children's Hospital of Buffalo and other institutions,[1,5,11] gallstones are currently being diagnosed more frequently in children. This apparent increase in incidence may be attributed to improved diagnostic modalities with their extensive use in abdominal illness, prematurity, and adolescent pregnancy. Alternatively, a true increase in gallstones, which could be confirmed only by a general population–based survey, may be occurring. As more cases of gallstones in children are recognized, there is evidence of associations and clinical manifestations distinct from those cases found in adults.

The female predilection for gallstones in adults was present in our study; however, when the adolescent pregnant patients were excluded, the sexual distribution was equal: 22 females and 21 males. This concurs with other studies.[11-13] The emergence of female predominance starting from puberty supports the hypothesis of a hormonal influence rather than genetic predisposition in the female preponderance seen in adult gallstones.[14]

The mean age of our patients was 12.2 years, which is in accordance with the reports by others[12,13] of a peak incidence between ages 10 and 15 years. Because Children's Hospital of Buffalo is a tertiary neonatal center, our study may include larger numbers of complicated neonates than expected. Eight percent of our cases occurred in patients less than 1 year old, including one case diagnosed in utero by maternal ultrasound

Table 2.—Clinical Presentation in Relation to Age in 50 Children With Gallstones

Symptom	Age, y: 1	1-5	6-10	11-15	16-20	Total
Right upper quadrant pain	1	0	9	7	15	**32**
Jaundice	0	0	6	6	3	**15**
Vomiting	0	2	2	2	7	**13**
Nonspecific (abdominal pain, nausea, chest pain)	0	3	1	3	6	**13**
Fatty food intolerance	0	0	3	2	1	**6**
Fever	0	0	0	1	0	**1**
Asymptomatic	3	2	0	0	1	**6**

Table 3.—The Relationship Between Predisposing Factors and Age, Race, Sex, Clinical Presentation, Laboratory Studies, and Therapy in 50 Children With Gallstones

	All Patients	Hemolytic	Parenteral Nutrition	Adolescent Pregnancy	Idiopathic	Other
No. of patients	50	18	8	7	10	7
Age, y (mean ± SD)	12.2 ± 6.2	12.6 ± 4.1	6.3 ± 6.9*	18.1 ± 1.6*	10.6 ± 6.7	17.1 ± 2.0
Race						
White	29	7	6	2	9	5
Black	17	11	2	2	1	1
Hispanic	4	0	0	3	0	1
Sex, No. M/F†	21/29	9/9	5/3	0/7	5/5	2/5
Clinical presentation‡						
Right upper quadrant pain	32	11	3	6	7	5
Jaundice	15	12	0	1	1	1
Vomiting	13	0	3	6	1	3
Nonspecific	13	5	2	2	2	2
Fatty food intolerance	6	1	0	1	2	2
Fever	1	1	0	0	0	0
Asymptomatic	6	0	3	0	2	1
Laboratory studies§						
Leukocytosis	16	7	0	4	2	2
Elevated transaminases	22	9	2	7	2	2
Elevated amylase	8	2	0	3	1	2
Therapy						
Conservative	15	3	5	4	3	0
Cholecystectomy	35	15	3	3	7	7

*The patients with parenteral nutrition were significantly younger than the group taken as a whole ($P<.05$), while the adolescent pregnancy patients were significantly older than the group as a whole ($P<.01$).

†After exclusion of the adolescent pregnancy group, the sex distribution was equal in the patients as a whole.

‡Jaundice was largely confined to the patients with hemolytic disease. Nonspecific abdominal complaints included poorly localized pain, nausea, and chest pain.

§Leukocytosis was defined as white blood cell count $>14 \times 10^9$; elevated transaminase levels defined as alanine aminotransferase >20 U/L, or aspartate aminotransferase >20 U/L; elevated amylase levels defined as >125 U/L.

study. We found that the mean age of the hemolytic patients was 12.6 years, which is compatible with the other reports of congenital hemolytic disease occurring with gallstones in late childhood,[12,13] although the mean age in our study was slightly older. The mean age of the patients with parenteral nutrition was significantly younger than the average age of presentation for all patients in our study ($P<.05$). The idiopathic patients were also younger than the group taken as a whole, but the differences were not statistically significant.

Like other studies,[13] the most common predisposing factor was hemolytic disease, including two patients with autoimmune hemolysis and one patient with pyruvate kinase deficiency. Because adolescent pregnancy is increasing dramatically in the United States,[15] and because pregnant or postpartum teenagers accounted for 14% of the patients in our study, this group merits more consideration from pediatricians. Patients receiving parenteral nutrition are at risk of developing gallstones due to bile stasis,[16] especially those patients not receiving oral supplementation.[17] In addition, patients receiving parenteral nutrition may be further predisposed toward biliary disease by their underlying disease state, such as necrotizing enterocolitis,[18] ileal resection, and ileal disease.[19,20] Determination of the relative importance of each associated factor in these patients is beyond the scope of our study.

Only one patient had cystic fibrosis. This scarcity can be explained by early diagnosis and prompt pancreatic supplementation.[14] Spinal surgery and spinal cord injury have been associated with gallstones in adults[6] and children[7]; our series included one patient with transverse myelitis and one patient with spina bifida. Hemobilia is a rare cause of gallstones in adults[21]; in our series, one patient presented with gallstones 1 year after posttraumatic liver laceration. Finally, only 20% of our patients had no conditions associated with gallstones, which is less than in early reports by Harned and Babbitt[22] and Spahr.[23]

The classic adult presentation of gallstones as biliary colic applies best to children over 15 years of age. The younger patients, especially the patients less than 5 years of age, tended to present with nonspecific symptoms. The ability to localize pain to the right upper quadrant or to relate symptoms to fatty foods depended on the patient's age. Irritability, particularly when occurring after feedings, should suggest the possibility of gallstones, especially in premature infants or infants with a history of parenteral nutrition or necrotizing enterocolitis.

Nearly half of the preschool children were asymptomatic. Diagnosis of gallstones in the asymptomatic young child was often incidental, eg, by ultrasound study performed for recurrent urinary tract infections. The finding of a fever in only one patient underscores the rarity of cholecystitis and cholangitis in children with gallstones.[11]

Jaundice can be related either to common bile duct obstruction or to inflammation in the presence of gallstones confined to the gallbladder. Like other series,[11,24] choledocholithiasis in children was found to be rare, without a single case among our 50 patients. Twelve patients with jaundice had underlying hemolytic disease, and only three patients with jaundice did not have underlying hemolysis, suggesting that biliary obstruction was not the mechanism for the jaundice.

Ultrasonography proved to be a noninvasive, accurate method of diagnosis with no false-positive results in our study. Other methods of diagnosis should be employed when the ultrasonographic findings are not conclusive or when biliary tract anomalies or complications are suspected.

In contrast to adults, in whom cholecystitis, choledocholithiasis, cholangitis, and perforation are the most common complications of gallstones, such complications are rare in children.[11] Pancreatitis was found to be the most common complication, occurring in 8% of the patients, and no patient was documented to have a stricture of the ampulla of vater. One patient with sickle cell anemia died postoperatively. Mortality was attributed to the postoperative complications of the hemolytic disease rather than complications of the gallstones. As in other studies[25] when preoperative transfusions were performed, mortality from cholecystectomy in patients with sickle cell anemia was low. Current medical ethics would favor preoperative transfusion despite parental objection in a patient with sickle cell disease.

The decision between cholecystectomy and conservative management depended on patient age and severity of symptoms; the cause did not have a major impact on the method of treatment. In general, infants and patients with parenteral nutrition were managed more conservatively, and all were managed without specific medical or surgical therapy directed to the stones. Management of asymptomatic gallstones in children is controversial and beyond the scope of our study.

Our results indicate that gallstones in children have a variety of associated factors and presentations. The classic clinical picture, as well as the laboratory confirmation in adults, does not apply to children. Therefore, more attention must be paid to the possibility of gallstones in the evaluation of children with nonspecific abdominal symptoms, especially in children with associated conditions.

References

1. Sorge DV. Cholecystitis and cholelithiasis in children. *Pediatrics.* 1962;29:46-51.
2. Walker CHM. Aetiology of cholelithiasis in childhood. *Arch Dis Child.* 1955;32:293-297.
3. Seiler I. Gallbladder disease in children. *AJDC.* 1960;99:662-666.
4. Graivier L, Dorman GW, Votteler TP. Gallbladder disease in infants and children. *Surgery.* 1968;68:690-696.
5. Goodman DB. Cholelithiasis in persons under 25 years old. *JAMA.* 1976;236:1731-1732.
6. Apstein MD, Chipperfield KD. Spinal cord injury is a risk factor for gallstone disease. *Gastroenterology.* 1987;92:966-968.
7. Teele RT, Nussbaum AR, Wyly JB, Allred EN, Emans J. Cholelithiasis after spinal fusion for scoliosis in children. *J Pediatr.* 1987;111:851-860.
8. Danon Y, Dinari G, Garty BZ, Horodniceanu C, Nitzan M, Grunebaum M. Cholelithiasis in children with immunoglobulin A deficiency: a new gastroenterologic syndrome. *J Pediatr Gastroenterol Nutr.* 1983;2:663-666.
9. Roslyn JJ, Berquist WE, Pitt HA, et al. Increased risk of gallstone in children receiving total parenteral nutrition. *Pediatrics.* 1983;71:784-789.
10. Greenberg M, Kangarloo H, Cochran ST, Sample WE. The transographic diagnosis of cholecystitis and choledocholithiasis in children. *Radiology.* 1980;137:745-749.
11. MacMillan RW, Schullinger JN, Santuli TV. Cholelithiasis in childhood. *Am J Surg.* 1974;127:689-692.
12. Heschke CI, Teele RL. Cholelithiasis in children: recent observation. *Ultrasound Med Biol.* 1983;2:481-484.
13. Pokorny WJ, Saleem M, Ogrorman R, McGill C, Harberg FJ. Cholelithiasis and cholecystitis in childhood. *Am J Surg.* 1984;148:742-744.
14. Scott M, Kalser S. Highlights of the meeting on prevention of gallstones. *Hepatology.* 1987;7:946-951.
15. McAnarney ER, Hendee WR. Adolescent pregnancy and its consequences. *JAMA.* 1989;262:74-77.
16. Roslyn JJ, Pitts HA, Mann LL, Ament ME, DenBelsten L. Long-term parenteral nutrition induces gallbladder disease. *Gastroenterology.* 1981;80:1264.
17. Pitt HA, King W, Mann LL. Increased risk of cholelithiasis with prolonged parenteral nutrition. *Am J Surg.* 1983;145:106-112.
18. Whittington, PF, Black DD. Cholelithiasis in premature infants treated with parenteral nutrition and furosemide. *J Pediatr.* 1980;97:647-649.
19. Pellerin D, Bertin P, Nihoul-Fecetec C, Ricout CI. Cholelithiasis and ileal pathology in childhood. *J Pediatr Surg.* 1975;10:35-41.
20. Hill GL, Mair WS, Goligher JC. Gallstones after ileostomy and ileal resection. *Gut.* 1975;16:932-936.
21. Luzuy F, Reinberg O, Kauszlaric D, et al. Biliary calculi caused by hemobilia. *Surgery.* 1987;102:886-889.
22. Harned RK, Babbitt DP. Cholelithiasis in children. *Radiology.* 1975;117:391-393.
23. Spahr RC. Calculous cholecystitis without underlying disease in adolescents. *Clin Pediatr Phila.* 1978;17:908-909.
24. Ulin AW, Nosal JL, Martin WL. Cholecystitis in childhood: associated obstructive jaundice. *Surgery.* 1952;31:312-326.
25. Rutledge R, Croom RD, Davis JW, Berkowitz LR, Orringer EP. Cholelithiasis in sickle cell anemia: surgical considerations. *South Med J.* 1986;79:28-30.

Radiological Case of the Month

CPT Michael E. Ruff, MC, USA; MAJ W. Michael Southgate, MC, USA *(Contributors)*;
Beverly P. Wood, MD *(Section Editor)*

A term, 3740-g newborn was admitted for suspected sepsis. Rupture of the membranes had occurred 18 hours prior to delivery and was associated with a maternal temperature of 38.1°C. Apgar scores were eight and nine at 1 and 5 minutes, respectively. A white blood cell count was 14.7×10^9/L, with the following differential cell count: polymorphonuclear cells, 0.16; band cells, 0.31; lymphocytes, 0.21; monocytes, 0.25; and eosinophils, 0.02. An admission blood culture was positive for group B *Streptococcus*. The infant received intravenous ampicillin and gentamicin.

The patient did well until the fourth day after birth when he developed bile-stained emesis. His temperature was 36.8°C. The heart rate was 131 beats per minute. Respirations were 52 per minute. The blood pressure was 77/61 mm Hg. The physical examination revealed a distended abdomen that was tender to palpation and moderately tense. Bowel sounds were hypoactive. The hematocrit was 0.40; the platelet count was 3.78×10^{11}/L. The white blood cell count was 5.6×10^9/L and the differential cell count was as follows: polymorphonuclear cells, 0.23; band cells, 0.17; lymphocytes, 0.41; monocytes 0.08; and atypical cells, 0.10. An abdominal roentgenogram was obtained (Fig 1). A nasogastric tube was placed and a large amount of bilious fluid was drained from the stomach. An upper gastrointestinal tract series with normal results was followed by barium enema examination (Fig 2). The infant was then taken to surgery for an exploratory laparotomy.

Accepted for publication January 22, 1990.
Contributed from the Department of Pediatrics, Tripler Army Medical Center, Hawaii.
Reprint requests to the Department of Radiology, Childrens Hospital of Los Angeles, 4650 Sunset Blvd, Los Angeles, CA 90027 (Dr Wood).

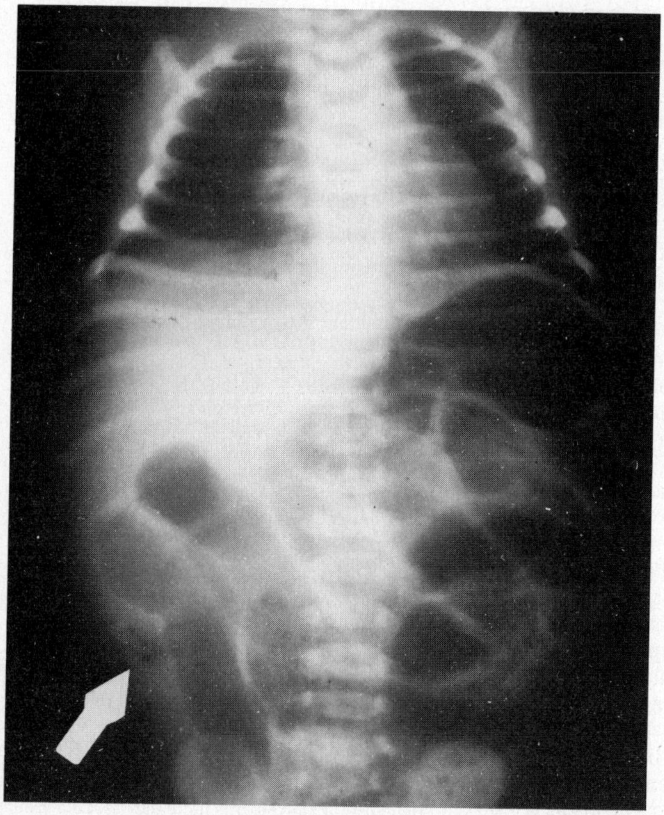

Figure 1.

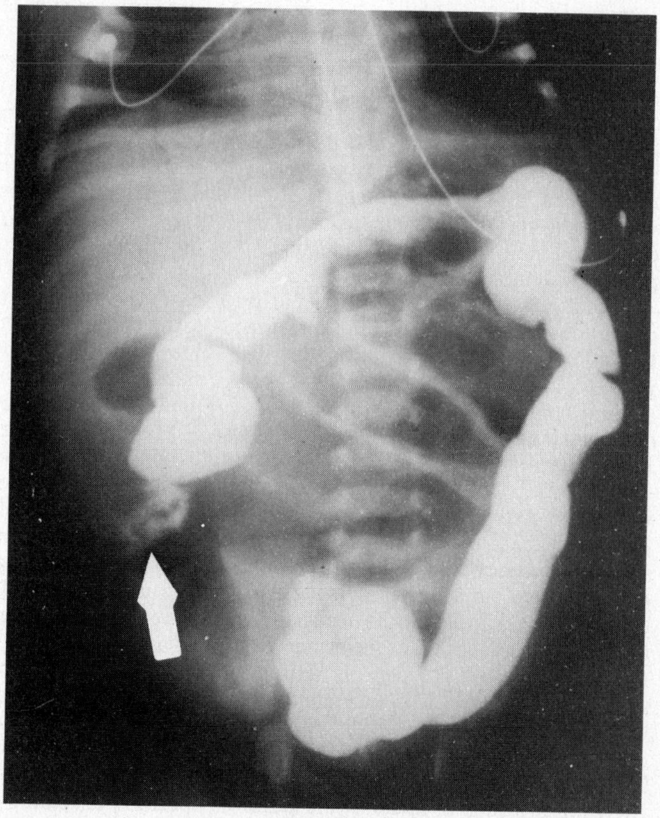

Figure 2.

Denouement and Discussion

Neonatal Appendicitis With Perforation

Fig 1.—Supine roentgenogram of the abdomen demonstrates multiple long dilated loops of bowel with a fixed collection of apparently extraluminal gas in the right lower quadrant of the abdomen. (arrow).

Fig 2.—Contrast enema demonstrates a colon of normal appearance and caliber distal to the ascending colon. Extravasated barium is present at the cecum (arrow).

Fig 3.—Surgical specimen shows acute suppurative appendicitis with perforation (arrow).

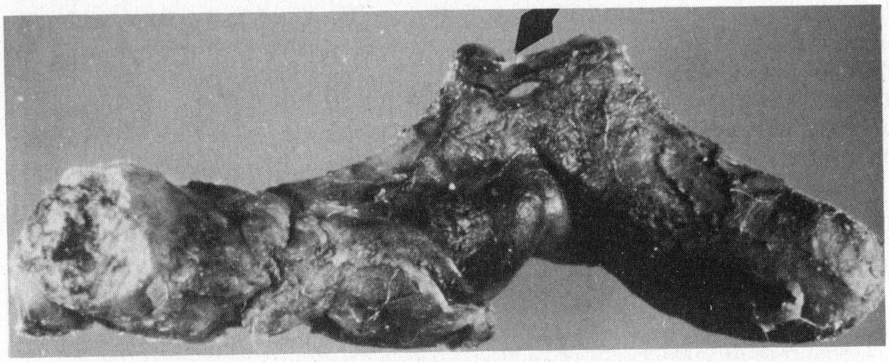

Figure 3.

At laparotomy, there was a large amount of seropurulent fluid in the abdomen. The cecum was indurated and an acutely inflamed appendix, with perforation at its midportion, was present. A culture of the peritoneal fluid was positive for *Klebsiella pneumoniae*. After surgery, the patient received intravenous antibiotics for 7 days. The patient was discharged home on the 18th postoperative day.

Less than 2% of all children treated for appendicitis are younger than 2 years of age.[1,2] Neonatal appendicitis is extremely rare.[3] Diess, as cited by Hemalatha and Spitz,[4] described the first case in 1903. Subsequently, there have been 120 cases reported in the English literature.[5]

The rarity of appendicitis in infancy is primarily ascribed to the conical shape of the infantile appendix, decreasing the likelihood of its obstruction. The appendix assumes its adult vermiform configuration between 1 and 2 years of age.[1] Other factors cited include the soft diet of neonates and the decreased incidence of viral-induced appendiceal lymphoid hyperplasia.[6]

Although earlier diagnosis of the acute abdomen in neonates and improved postoperative care have contributed to increased survival, there are several reasons why neonatal appendicitis continues to have a high mortality.[3] First, there is a high incidence of perforation. This is attributed to the thin wall of the neonatal appendix as well as the fact that the cecum does not distend easily in infancy and therefore cannot help decompress the appendix.[5] Perforated neonatal appendicitis occurs with increased incidence in association with obstructive lesions, such as Hirschsprung's disease.[7,8] The second factor that contributes to the high mortality of patients with this disease is the very limited ability of the neonate to combat the complications of appendiceal perforation. This is due to an immature immune system and an underdeveloped omentum, which is short and thin and has little capacity to wall off infection.[9]

The clinical presentations of neonatal appendicitis are abdominal distention (80%) and vomiting (60%).[3] Other less consistent findings are irritability, anorexia, fever, cellulitis, abdominal tenderness, hypoperistalsis, and leukocytosis.[3] In addition, 27 (29%) of the 94 patients described by Srouji and Buck[10] presented with a hernial mass. This manifestation of the disease process leads to earlier recognition and surgical intervention. Isolation of the inflammatory process within the hernial sac contributes to decreased mortality.[10]

Unique to this case is the history of group B streptococcal sepsis. The possibility of an antecedent bacteremia as a pathologic agent in neonatal appendicitis has not been previously reported to our knowledge, and we postulate that it was coincidental in this case.

In the roentgenographic evaluation of a neonate with suspected appendicitis, an acute abdominal series is useful in establishing the diagnosis but is not specific.[11] A contrast enema examination may be of value by demonstrating nonfilling of the appendix or, as in our patient, revealing extravasation of contrast near the cecum.[3]

The differential diagnosis of neonatal appendicitis includes sepsis, necrotizing enterocolitis, pancreatitis, intestinal atresia, meconium ileus, and Hirschsprung's disease.

References

1. Snyder WH Jr, Chaffin L. Appendicitis during first two years of life. *Arch Surg.* 1952; 64:549-560.
2. Grosfeld JL, Weinberger M, Clatworthy HW Jr. Acute appendicitis in the first two years of life. *J Pediatr Surg.* 1973;8:285-293.
3. Buntain WL, Krempe RE, Kraft JW. Neonatal appendicitis. *Ala J Med Sci.* 1984;21:295-299.
4. Hemalatha V, Spitz L. Neonatal appendicitis. *Clin Pediatr.* 1979;18:621-622.
5. Massad M, Srouji M, Awdeh A, Slim M, Tamer M, Tabbara M. Neonatal appendicitis. *Z Kinderchir.* 1986;41:241-243.
6. Walker RH. Appendicitis in the newborn infant. *J Pediatr.* 1957;51:429-434.
7. Martin LW, Perrin EV. Neonatal perforation of the appendix in association with Hirschsprung's disease. *Ann Surg.* 1967;166:799-802.
8. Newman B, Nussbaum A, Kirkpatrick JA Jr, Colodny A. Appendiceal perforation, pneumoperitoneum, and Hirschsprung's disease. *J Pediatr Surg.* 1988;23:854-856.
9. Firor HV, Myers HA. Perforating appendicitis in premature infants. *Surgery.* 1964;56:581-583.
10. Srouji MN, Buck BE. Neonatal appendicitis. *J Pediatr Surg.* 1978;13:177-179.
11. Wilkinson RH, Bartlett RH, Eraklis AJ. Diagnosis of appendicitis in infancy. *AJDC.* 1969; 118:687-690.

Picture of the Month

Jeffrey L. Loughead, MD; Francis Mimouni, MD; Sue Schilling, RN (*Contributors*);
Murray Feingold, MD (*Section Editor*)

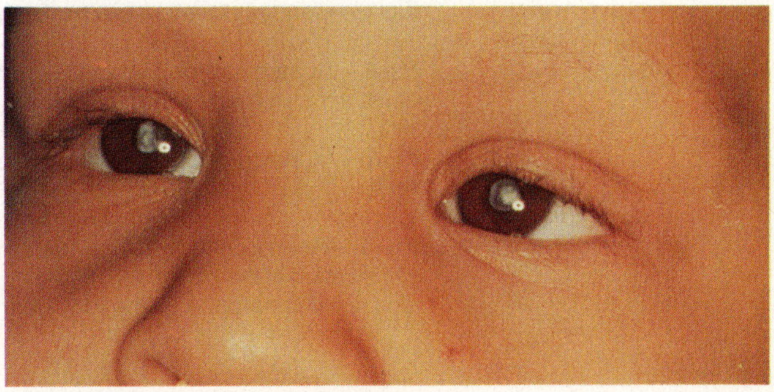

Figure 1.

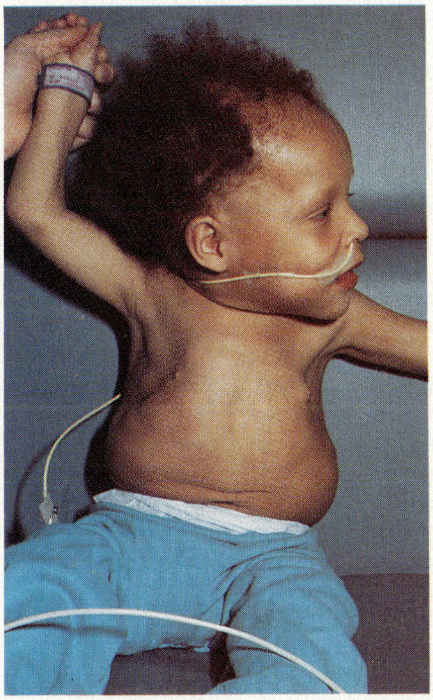

Figure 2.

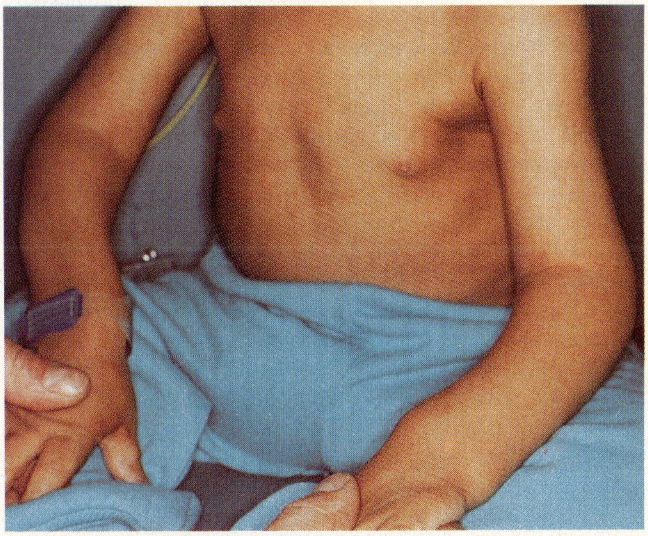

Figure 3.

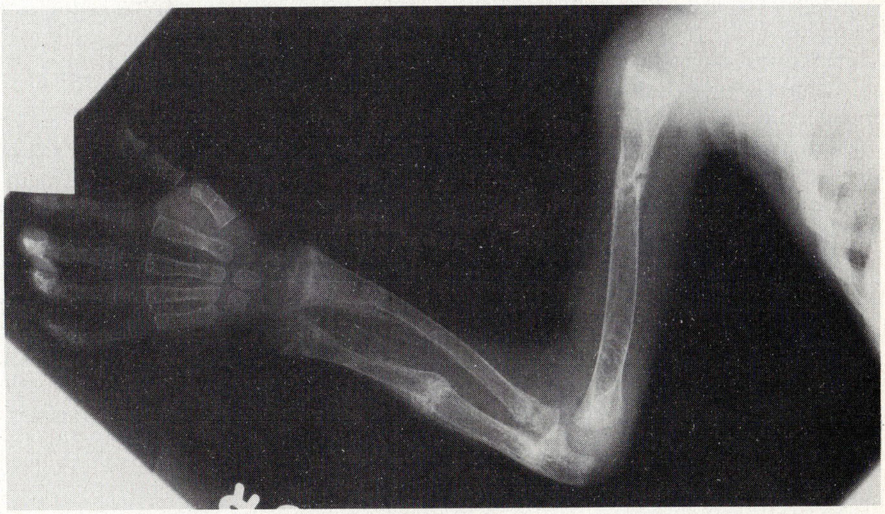

Figure 4.

Accepted for publication April 12, 1990.
From the Division of Neonatology, Department of Pediatrics, University of Cincinnati, Ohio.
Reprint requests to National Birth Defects Center, Franciscan Children's Hospital, 30 Warren St, Brighton, MA 02135 (Dr Feingold).

Denouement and Discussion

Lowe's Syndrome

Fig 1.—Centrally located, bilateral cataracts.

Fig 2.—Sparse hair, bell-shaped chest with rachitic rosary, thin limbs with decreased muscle mass, and signs of hypotonia.

Fig 3.—Marked bowing of forearms and prominent metaphyseal enlargement of left wrist.

Fig 4.—Roentgenographic examination of the right arm showing markedly poor calcification of the bones with splaying and cupping of the metaphyses of the radius, ulna, and humerus. Also present are multiple fractures in various stages of healing.

Lowe's syndrome, or oculocerebrorenal syndrome, is an X-linked hereditary disease characterized by congenital ocular disease, renal tubular dysfunction, hypotonia, moderate to severe bone disease, and mental retardation. It is present in all races, with a predominance in those with Caucasian and Asian ancestries.

The disease has three identifiable stages. The first, during the newborn period, is characterized by ocular pathologic features. Nearly all affected individuals have congenital, centrally located cataracts that are frequently associated with glaucoma and a miotic pupil. Asymptomatic aminoaciduria is usually found during this stage and a generalized aminoaciduria develops by age 1 year. This is often accompanied by varying degrees of proteinuria.

The second stage occurs during early childhood and is dominated by metabolic acidosis. The underlying basis for the disturbances is not known, but central to many of the symptoms appears to be a renal tubular dysfunction that results in urinary loss of bicarbonate, glucose, calcium, phosphorus, and protein. As a result of this serum metabolic acidosis and losses of calcium and phosphorus, secondary hyperparathyroidism occurs. Severe rickets and demineralization may develop leading to frequent fractures, pain, and delay or loss of normal motor physical development. The severe hypophosphatemia may lead to weakness and lethargy.

In the third stage, the metabolic disturbances of early childhood may continue or become progressively less severe, and have even been reported to resolve entirely. The prominent manifestations of this period are largely related to the sequelae of the previous two stages. This includes blindness from a combination of glaucoma and cataracts and orthopedic disabilities associated with the severe bone disease. Mental retardation has been described as moderate to severe and is of unknown origins. Computed tomography shows confluent irregular lucencies in the cerebral white matter, especially in the periventricular areas, and magnetic resonance imaging reveals patchy areas of white-matter demyelination. Electroencephalograms often demonstrate nonspecific abnormalities; however, some may show overt seizure activity. Auditory acuity is generally normal.

Genetics

The etiologic and biochemical basis of this syndrome is yet unknown. The inheritance pattern appears to be X-linked recessive and recent gene mapping, using tightly linked flanking markers, has placed the probable gene site at Xq24-26. The carrier state is identifiable through family history, ophthalmic examination, and genetic mapping. Slit-lamp examination of carriers has revealed increased numbers of punctate lenticular opacifications as early as the second decade of life. These lenticular opacifications appear to be the only clinical manifestation in the carrier. Prenatal diagnosis using flanking gene markers is now theoretically possible with a high degree of accuracy.

Treatment

Therapy consists mainly of supportive care. The renal tubular acidosis and rickets respond well to a combination of sodium-potassium citrate and phosphorus replacement. Vitamin D supplement therapy may be of benefit. Close attention to general nutrition and ophthalmic disease are important to enhance development. Despite treatment, the prognosis for mental development is guarded and death often occurs in the second decade of life. Genetic counseling should be provided.

References

1. Abbassi V, Lowe CU, Calcagno PL. Oculo-cerebro-renal syndrome: a review. *AJDC*. 1986; 15:145-168.

2. Cibis GW, Waeltermann JM, Whitcraft CT, Tripathi RC, Harris DJ. Lenticular opacities in carriers of Lowe's syndrome. *Ophthalmology*. 1986;93:1041-1045.

3. Wadelius C, Fagerholm P, Petterson U, Anneren G. Lowe oculocerebrorenal syndrome: DNA-based linkage of the gene to Xq24-q26, using tightly linked flanking markers and a correlation to lens examination and carrier diagnosis. *Am J Hum Genet*. 1989;44:241-247.

1990 Reviewers for *AJDC*

Few of our readers and authors recognize the enormous contributions that reviewers make to the process of publishing articles in AJDC. These women and men give unselfishly, and without compensation, of their time, effort, and consideration to the analysis, judgment, and evaluation of the multitude of manuscripts that are submitted to us each year. This is the only public opportunity that we have to commend and thank them. Listed below are those reviewers active from November 1989 through October 1990.

Our special appreciation is extended to each person on this list for his or her efforts on behalf of our readers, authors, and editorial staff.

—ED.

John Aase
Charles Abildgaard
Frank Accurso
Phyllis Agran
Charles Ahlfors
Kirk Aleck
E. Russell Alexander
Hugh D. Allen
Bruce Alpert
Arthur Ammann
James Arens
Adriano Arguedas
Milton Arnold
Antonio Arrieta
Mary Ellen Avery
Ellis Avner

Robert Baehner
Michael Bailie
Thomas Balkany
William Banner
Oped Bar-Or
Thomas Baranowski
Lewis Barness
James Bass
Frederick Battaglia
Robert Beckerman
J. Bruce Beckwith
Alan Bedrick
Stephen Beitler
David Bell
James Bennett
Charles Berde
Walter Berdon
Gerald Berenson
Lawrence Berger
Melvin Berger
Roger Bernier
Larry Beutler
Charles Bluestone
Richard Blumberg
Thomas Boat
William Bonadio
aurence Boxer
V. Thomas Boyce
Anne Manon Brenner
imothy Bricker
Ielen Britton
en Brouhard
urnell Brown
eorge W. Brown
hillip Brunnel
obert Brunner
ebecca Buckley
redric Burg
ergio Bustamante

Bonnie Camp
Robert Cannon
Daniel Caplan
Susanne Cassidy
Evan Charney
Robert Chen
James Cherry
Russell Chesney
Katherine Christoffel
David Clark
Stephen Cochi
Michael Cohen
George Comerci
Louis Cooper
Marvin Cornblath
James J. Corrigan
Peter Crowe
Nancy Cummings
Kirk Cureton

Beverly Dahms
Alan Daneman
Robert Daum
Ronald David
Patricia Davis
Scott Davis
Catherine De Angelis
Michael Dean
Susan Denson
Michael DeVoe
Hugh C. Dillon
N. Daisy Dodd
Phillip Dodge
Wendy Dorchester
Amanda M. Dove
Stewart Duban
Hosea Ducote III
Anne Marie Duncan
Burris Duncan
Clare Dykewicz
Paul Dyment

Allan Eisenbaum
M. Jocelyn Elders
Elliot Ellis
George Ellis, Jr
Victor Elsberry
E. Jean Emans
Blackwell Evans
John Ey

Debra Fanurik
Michael Farrell
Rosanne Farris
Ralph Feigin
Murray Feingold
Gerald Fenichel
Patricia Ferrieri
Peggy C. Ferry
Laurence Finberg
Jan Goddard Finegold
Loretta Finnegan
Howard Fishbein
David Fixler
Alan Fleischman
Samuel Fomon
Marc Forman
Lawrence Fox
Douglas Frasier
Patty Freedson
Johnette Frentz
Gilbert Friday
Allan Friedman
John Fulginiti

Robert Garner
Michael Gerber
Anne Gershon
Ira Gessner
Joan Gibson
Louis Gibson
Samuel Gidding
Scott Giebink
Enid Gilbert-Barness
William Gill
Charles Ginsberg
Paul Glezen
Mary Glode
Boyd W. Goetzman
Michael Gold
Stanley Goldberg
Gerald Golden
Jay Goldsmith
Edward Goldson
W. Manford Gooch
Morris Green
Larrie Greenberg
Robert Greenberg
Harry Greene
Alan Grogono
Jay Grosfeld
Lindsey Grossman
Melvin Grumbach
Michael Grunstein
Joyce Gryboski
Yezid Gutierrez

Carmen Hadley
Robert Haggerty
Barrett Haik
Caroline Hall
Michael Hambidge
Sherril Hammar
Margaret Hammerschlag
Ronald Hansen
Thomas Hansen
William Hardin
Rita Harper
Gail Harrison
William Hathaway
William Hay
Thomas Hazinski
Margaret Heagarty
Frederick Hecht
Karen Hein
Marilyn Heins
Ray Helfer
Bettina Hilman
Alan Hinman
Paul Hletko
Joan Hodgman
J. Roger Hollister
Richard Hong
Robert Hopkins
Margaret Hostetter
H. Eugene Hoyme
Walter Hughes
James Humbert
Carl Hunt
John Hutter

Charles Irwin
Kenneth Iserson

Hillel Janai
Jerri Jenista
John Johnson
James Jones
Nancy R. Joye

Bryna Kane
William Kanto
Selma Kaplan
Michael Kappy
Karol Katenbach
John Kattwinkel
Michael Katz
James Keating
H. William Kelly
Michael Kiernan
Dahlia Kirkpatrick
John Kirkpatrick
C. Thomas Kisker
Marshall Klaus
Jerome Klein
Katherine Knight
Otakar Koldovsky
Charles Koopmann
Arthur Kopelman
Rowena Korobkin
Richard Kreipe
Richard Krugman
Saul Krugman

Geoffrey Kurland

Maurice Landers
Benjamin Landing
Gary Larsen
William Lavia
Ruth Lawrence
Peter Lee
Richard Levenson
Harold Levine
Melvin Levine
John Lewy
Elmer Lightner
Barbara Lippe
Iris Litt
Katherine Lobach
Jennifer Loggie
Sarah Long
Bo Lönnerdal
Gerald Loughlin
Frederick Lovejoy
Stephen Ludwig

C. Charlton Mabry
Ian Macdonald
Cecile Many
Edgar Marcuse
Melvin Marks
Gary Marshall
Gerald Marx
Francis Mather
Alvin Mauer
Robert Mauro
Elizabeth McAnarney
Edward McCabe
Paul McCarthy
Richard McClead
Kenneth McConnochie
George McCracken
Dan McNamara
Marian Melish
Walter Meyer
Lyle Micheli
Claude Migeon
Susan Millard
Bruce Miller
Dennis Miller
Randy Miller
Robert Miller
Jere Mitchell
James Moller
Michael Moran
Beverly Morgan
Wayne Morgan
Richard Moriarty
Ted Mortimer

Etsuro Motoyama
David Mrazek

Joseph Nadell
Henry Nadler
Richard Naeye
S. H. Naqvi
Marianne Neifert
John Nelson
Karin Nelson
Phillip Nieburg
Allen Niems
Jackie Noonan

April O'Quinn
William Oh
Walter Orenstein
James Orlowski
Frank Oski
George Owen

Lu Ann Papile
Jack Paradise
Robert A. Parker
John Parks
J. C. Partin
Russell Pate
Patti Patterson
David Pearlman
Robert Penny
James Perry
Roderic Phibbs
Anthony Philipps
Alistair Phillip
William Pierson
Philip Pizzo
Leslie Platnick
Stanley Plotkin
Stephen Polmar
Bernard Portnoy
Albert Pruitt

George Rab
Ronald Rabinowitz
Gary Rachelefsky
A. H. Ragab
Richard Rapkin
Albert Rauber
C. George Ray
David Rice
Thomas Riemenschneider
Mary Ellen Rimsza
Kenneth Roberts
William Robertson
Arvin Robinson
Uros Roessmann
Allen Root

Patricia Rosen
Arlan Rosenbloom
Walter Rosenfeld
Robert Rosenfield
Mitch Ross
Alan Roth
Leslie Rothenberg
Marc Rowe
Claude Roy
Robert Ruben
Arye Rubenstein
Barry Rumack

David Sahn
Robert Sargent
James Sayre
Emilie Scarpelli
Julius Schachter
Richard Schieken
Barton Schmitt
Kenneth Schonberg
Michael Schumacher
Richard Schwartz
James Schwarz
William Scott
Steven Selbst
Elsa Sell
John Sever
Penelope Shackelford
Daniel Shannon
Michael Shannon
Emmanuel Shapira
Gail Shapiro
Ziad Shehab
Stephen Shelov
Jack Shonkoff
Stanford Shulman
Stanley Shulman
Gary Smith
Hilary Smith
Margaret Smith
Thomas F. Smith
Charles Spencer
Adrain Spitzer
Alan Spitzer
E. T. Sproles
S. R. Srinivasan
Sergio Stagno
Mildred Stahlman
Thomas Stanisic
Carl Stanitski
Barbara Starfield
Mark Steele
Janet Stewart
E. Richard Stiehm

James Stockman
Sylvan Stool
James Storer
Daniel Stowens
Victor Strasburger
John Straus
William Strong
Harris R. Stutman
John Stutman
Siva Subramanian
Philip Sunshine
Robert Suskind
Stanley Szefler

Larry Taber
Lynn Taussig
David Teele
Anthony Temple
Douglas Teske
Samuel Tilden
James Todd
Edward Tronick
William Truog

John Udall

Russell Van Dyke
Robert Vannucci
Yvonne Vaucher
Victor Vaughn
Donald Vernon
Joseph Volpe

Ellen Wald
Philip Walson
Nell Pape Waring
Reginald Washington
John Watkins
William Weil
Barry Weiss
William Weston III
William L. Weston
Susanne White
Rick Williams
Jack Wilmore
Mark Windome
Don Witzke
Beverly Wood
James Wright
Peter Wright

Alayne Yates

Lonnie Zeltzer
Paul Zeltzer
Barry Zuckerman

1991 Annual Meeting

The annual meeting of The American Pediatric Society, The Society for Pediatric Research, and The Ambulatory Pediatric Association will be held April 29 through May 2, 1991, at the New Orleans (La) Hilton and Rivergate Convention Center. For further information, contact the APS/SPR Association Headquarters, 2650 Yale Blvd SE, Suite 104, Albuquerque, NM 87106; (505) 764-9099; FAX (505) 842-8227; or the Ambulatory Pediatric Association, 6728 Old McLean Village, McLean, VA 22101; (703) 556-9222.

Impetigo

Sir.—Issues relating to the management of impetigo, a common pediatric problem, continue to be discussed in these pages.[1,2] Although orally administered antibiotics have been considered optimal therapy for many years, the advent of a novel topical antibiotic, mupirocin, has prompted several clinical trials comparing the efficacy, compliance, cost, and safety of these two treatment modalities. In many of these trials, erythromycin has been used as the prototypic oral agent.[3-6]

We recently completed a study of 48 patients with impetigo randomized to receive mupirocin or erythromycin therapy. Twenty-five children received mupirocin and 23, erythromycin. We were interested not only in the comparative efficacy of these drugs, but also in the microbiologic data and antibiotic sensitivities of the bacteria cultured, as recent studies have suggested that *Staphylococcus aureus* is now the most common cause of impetigo and that a large number of these strains may be resistant to erythromycin.

Patients and Methods.—Both groups in our study comprised mainly urban black children (64% of the mupirocin group and 74% of the erythromycin group). Mean ages were 3.7 years in the mupirocin group (range, 3 months to 10 years) and 4.9 years in the erythromycin group; (range, 5 months to 14 years). Lesions ranged in number from one to 20 (the mupirocin group) and one to 15 (the erythromycin group) per child and were vesicobullous in 32% and 48% of patients in the mupirocin and erythromycin groups, respectively. The mean duration of infection prior to enrollment was 8.5 days in the mupirocin group and 11.6 days in the erythromycin group. The range for both groups was 1 to 30 days. Initial cultures yielded *S aureus* in only 33% of patients, *S aureus* and group A β-hemolytic *Streptococcus* in 41%, group A *Streptococcus* in 12%, and group B *Streptococcus* plus *S aureus* in 4%. In vitro resistance to erythromycin was noted in 10.5% of *S aureus* isolates (five patients). Of these five patients with erythromycin-resistant strains, cultures from four yielded both group A *Streptococcus* and *S aureus*. Three were randomized to the mupirocin group, and a fourth in the erythromycin group who was not followed up could not be evaluated. The fifth patient, with *S aureus* only on culture, was initially in the erythromycin group but was switched to the mupirocin group because of noncompliance in taking oral medication.

Three patients in each of our study groups failed to return for follow-up and therefore could not be evaluated. Of those who were evaluated, 21 (95%) in the mupirocin group and 18 (90%) in the erythromycin group were clinically cured or improved on follow-up. The one patient in the mupirocin group who did not improve had continued spread of lesions and was switched to erythromycin because his culture yielded erythromycin-sensitive *S aureus*. No side effects of medication were encountered in the mupirocin group. Two patients in the erythromycin group were switched to mupirocin, one because of noncompliance and the other because of reported "hysterical attacks" after ingestion of the drug. Two others completed their courses of oral antibiotics, but one complained of stomach pain and nausea and the other, vomiting and irritability. Thus, the incidence of side effects was none in the mupirocin group and 14% (three of 21) in the erythromycin group. Rice et al[6] also documented a higher incidence of side effects with erythromycin, but, unlike our study, found that noncompliance was greater in the mupirocin group.

Nine patients had draining lesions that were recultured at the first follow-up visit; of those nine cultures, two were positive for the same organisms as in the initial cultures. A second culture of another patient was positive for *S aureus* with a different antibiogram.

Comment.—Of particular interest is evidence of group A streptococcal cause in more than half of our cases (53%). Until the early 1980s, impetigo was considered primarily a streptococcal infection; however, during the past decade, several studies have documented a shift to a predominantly staphylococcal cause. In a study of 243 children from Sydney, Australia, with impetigo, Rogers et al[7] cultured *S aureus* from 86% of cases (69.6% of cultures yielded *Staphylococcus* only; 15.2% yielded *S aureus* and β-hemolytic streptococci). Less than 50% of these strains were sensitive to erythromycin. Barton and Friedman[2] identified *S aureus* in cultures from 75% of cases in three consecutive studies of a total of 268 patients, but erythromycin resistance was detected in only 14% of strains. In Barton and Friedman's three series, *S aureus* only was grown from 62%, 46%, and 51% of patients, whereas mixed organisms were grown from 30%, 25%, and 29% of patients. Goldfarb et al[4] found *S aureus* in 59 (95%) of 62 patients with impetigo. Cultures from nine (14.5%) of these patients yielded mixed organisms. Of the 59 original isolates, 58 (98%) were erythromycin-sensitive in vitro. Eells et al[8] cultured *S aureus* from 94% of cases in a study reported in 1986.

It is noteworthy that this latter group of investigators identified group A β-hemolytic streptococci (45% in combination with *S aureus*) from cultures of 71% of patients with impetigo in a study 3 years later.[5] Although 50% of the *S aureus* isolates were erythromycin-resistant, these

This department of *AJDC* is reserved for comment, criticism, observation, and discussion of "issues of current concern and importance for children's health." The Editor encourages our readers to express themselves on a variety of topics and issues. Further, we encourage the submission of unique and brief clinical and scientific observations that do not fulfill the criteria for original articles.

patients responded well when given erythromycin. This indicates that when cultures yielded both organisms, the *Streptococcus* was the likely causative agent. In view of the resurgence of other streptococcal diseases during the past few years, one might speculate that recent impetigo studies documenting a high percentage of group A streptococci on culture may indicate a reversal in the trend of increasing numbers of cutaneous infections caused by *S aureus*.

As in other studies, we found these drugs to be equally efficacious. However, the issue of drug resistance must be considered when selecting an antibiotic. Fortunately, mupirocin resistance appears to be uncommon.[9]

Nancy B. Esterly, MD
Departments of Pediatrics and Dermatology
David B. Nelson, MD
Department of Pediatrics
W. Michael Dunne, Jr, PhD
Departments of Pediatrics and Pathology
Medical College of Wisconsin
Milwaukee, WI 53226

1. Bronfin DR. Increasing the antibiotic spectrum in the treatment of impetigo. *AJDC.* 1990;144:274.
2. Barton LL, Friedman AD. Etiology and therapy of impetigo: reconsidered. *AJDC.* 1990;144:274.
3. Barton LL, Friedman AD, Sharkey A, Schneller DJ, Swierkosz EM. Impetigo contagiosa, III: comparative efficacy of oral erythromycin and topical mupirocin. *Pediatr Dermatol.* 1989;6:134-138.
4. Goldfarb J, Crenshaw D, O'Horo J, Lemon E, Blumer JL. Randomized clinical trial of topical mupirocin versus oral erythromycin for impetigo. *Antimicrob Agents Chemother.* 1988;32:1780-1783.
5. Mertz PM, Marshall DA, Eaglstein WH, Piovanetti Y, Montalvo J. Topical mupirocin treatment of impetigo is equal to oral erythromycin therapy. *Arch Dermatol.* 1989;125:1069-1073.
6. Rice TD, Duggan AK, DeAngelis C. Cost effectiveness of erythromycin versus mupirocin. *AJDC.* 1990;144:443-444. Abstract.
7. Rogers M, Dorman DC, Gapes M, Ly J. A three-year study of impetigo in Sydney. *Med J Aust.* 1987;147:63-65.
8. Eells LD, Mertz PM, Piovanetti Y, Pekoe GM, Eaglstein WH. Topical antibiotic treatment of impetigo with mupirocin. *Arch Dermatol.* 1986;122:1273-1276.
9. Cookson BD. Mupirocin resistance in staphylococci. *J Antimicrob Chemother.* 1990;25:497-503.

Diagnosis of Child Sexual Abuse in Children With Genital Warts

Sir.—We appreciate the review by Boyd[1] on condylomata acuminata in children in the July issue of *AJDC*. This review of the results of the various forms of therapy of genital warts in children was helpful in emphasizing the need for more data regarding the immediate and late results of therapy.

We are writing, in part, to comment on the data regarding the prevalence of sexual abuse in children who develop genital warts. While presenting a case report of any medical condition, the justification for the diagnosis and any critical negative results should be given in sufficient detail to allow the reader to appreciate the basis of the diagnosis. The medical diagnosis of child sexual abuse has been the subject of very active research during the past decade, and the methods for adequate assessment of sexual abuse in a child now include each of the following areas: (1) assessments of medical and behavioral indicators of abuse; (2) a medical examination to identify physical indications of abuse; (3) a microbiologic assessment of other sexually transmittable diseases; and (4) age-appropriate interviews of the child and caretakers by skilled personnel. Some reviews and descriptions of these techniques are given in references 2 through 5.[2-5]

Children with genital warts have only infrequently received an assessment employing these techniques, and the methods used in the assessments of children with genital warts have not been described in most previously published reports. The reason for the scarcity of data regarding abuse is that many reports were published prior to the development of adequate diagnostic methods. In one study in which adequate methods were used, 10 (91%) of 11 children with genital warts who presented after the first year of life were proved to have been sexually abused.[6] The data included proof of abuse in three of the four children who were younger than 3 years at presentation.

We recommend that reports and reviews of children with genital warts that attempt to identify the status of the child regarding abuse should include only those cases in which the assessment methods which were used are described in detail and which meet current diagnostic standards. Other cases are truly "unknown" and should not appear in the denominator. On this basis, Boyd's conclusion that only 27% of the children had been abused is probably inaccurate. Most of the cases cited were not presented in sufficient detail to allow the reader to determine the adequacy of the evaluation.

The diagnosis and management of child sexual abuse is a rapidly evolving pediatric discipline. Physicians who care for children should be encouraged to establish a relationship with their colleagues in this area so that their patients with genital warts may have the services of a skilled child protection team. Certainly all children with genital warts should be carefully evaluated for sexual abuse.

Laura T. Gutman, MD
Marcia Herman-Giddens, PA, MPH
Neil S. Prose, MD
Duke University Medical Center
Box 3971
Durham, NC 27710

1. Boyd AS. Condylomata acuminata in the pediatric population. *AJDC.* 1990;144:817-823.
2. Herbert CP. Expert medical assessment in determining probability of alleged child sexual abuse. *Child Abuse Negl.* 1987;11:213-221.
3. Goff CW, Burke KR, Rickenbach KC, Buebendorf DP. Vaginal opening reassessment in prepubertal girls. *AJDC.* 1989;143:1366-1368.
4. Herman-Giddens ME, Frothingham TE. Prepubertal female genitalia: examination for evidence of sexual abuse. *Pediatrics.* 1987;80:203-208.
5. Tipton AC. Child sexual abuse: physical examination techniques and interpretation of findings. *Adolesc Pediatr Gynecol.* 1989;2:10-25.
6. Herman-Giddens ME, Gutman LT, Berson NL, Duke Child Protection Team. Association of coexisting sexually transmitted diseases and multiple abusers in female children with genital warts. *Sex Transm Dis.* 1988;15:63-67.

In Reply.—I am indebted to Gutman et al for their careful and critical analysis of this work.[1] They may or may not be correct when they propose that the 27% incidence rate of sexual abuse found in this review was too low. As stated in the article, many authors believe that the presence of condylomata acuminata in children is all but pathognomonic of sexual assault.[2-4] Conflicting evidence has also recently been presented.[5,6] It should be noted that, while admirable, it was not the point of my article to apply the criteria for child abuse discussed in it to the cases currently in the literature.

The consideration of sexual contact should be entertained when any child presents with venereal warts. As Herman-Giddens[2] has previously noted, those physicians who deal with pediatric venereal warts are hampered by the fact that methods for ascertaining the means of their acquisition are not foolproof. In fact, one of the references[7] cited by Gutman et al noted that in almost 21% of their pediatric patients suspected of having been sexually abused, no definite determination could be made, and in an additional 57% it was only "probable." Conversely, the incidence of "benign" venereal wart transmission is also unknown. The pleas of Gutman et al for complete assessment of children with condylomata acuminata and the observation that their presence may portend the existence of other sexually transmitted diseases should be self-evident.

Alan S. Boyd, MD
Department of Dermatology
Texas Tech University
Health Sciences Center
Lubbock, TX 79430

1. Boyd AS. Condylomata acuminata in the pediatric population. *AJDC.* 1990;144:817-823.

2. Herman-Giddens M. Condylomata acuminata in children and sexual abuse. *Genitourin Med.* 1985;61:68.

3. Schachner L, Hankin DE. Assessing child abuse in childhood condyloma acuminatum. *J Am Acad Dermatol.* 1985;12:157-160.

4. Goldenring JM. Condylomata acuminata in the evaluation of child sexual abuse. *Arch Dermatol.* 1987;123:1265-1266.

5. Obalek S, Jablonska S, Favre M, Walczak L, Orth G. Condolymata acuminata in children: frequent association with human papillomavirus responsible for cutaneous warts. *J Am Acad Dermatol.* 1990;23:205-213.

6. Cohen BA, Honig P, Androphy E. Anogenital warts in children. *Arch Dermatol.* 1990;126:1575-1580.

7. Herbert CP. Expert medical assessment in determining probability of alleged child sexual abuse. *Child Abuse Negl.* 1987;11:213-221.

Rickets Caused by Vitamin D Deficiency in Breast-fed Infants in the Southern United States

Sir.—Rickets caused by vitamin D deficiency in breast-fed infants is rarely reported in patients from the southern part of the United States. Milder winters, a perennially sunny climate, and liberal vitamin D supplementation are the most likely reasons for this low incidence. We report four cases of rickets in breast-fed black infants who received no vitamin D supplementation. Except for one patient, there was no history of patients being overdressed or deprived of sunlight exposure. Lack of familiarity with the disease, stemming from the rarity of its occurrence in warm climates,

Fig 1.—*Growth chart of patient 1 before and after vitamin D therapy.*

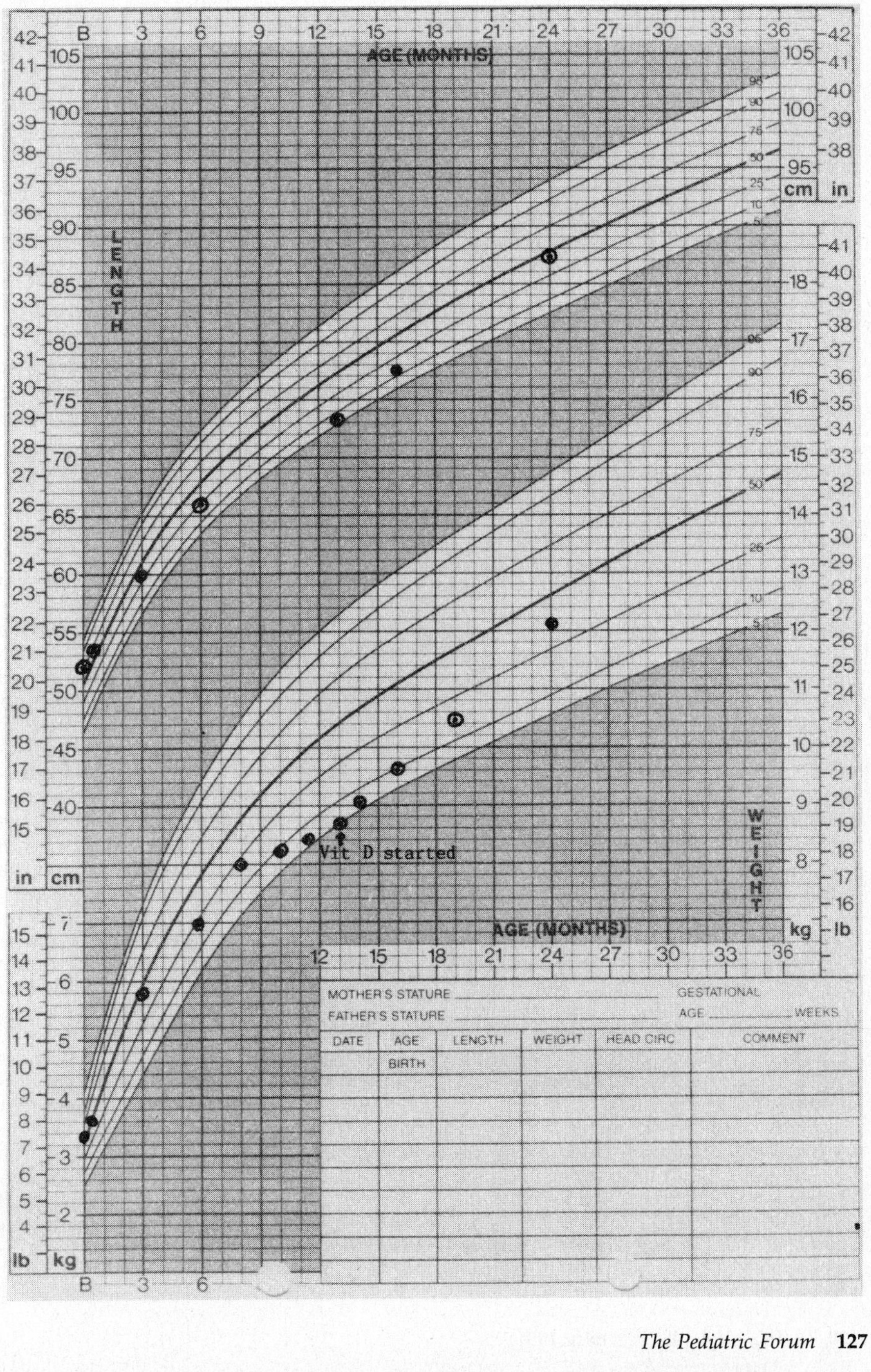

Pertinent Clinical and Biochemical Data*

Case No.	Age at Diagnosis, mo	Duration of Breast-Feeding, mo	Ca, mmol/L (2.25-2.7)	P, mmol/L (1.45-2.1)	ALP (<300 IU/L)	25OHD, nmol/L (37-137)	PTH, C-Terminal (<340 ng/L)	Clinical/Radiologic Findings
1	13	12	2.25	1.1	1868	12	456	FTT at 9 months; inability to walk, muscle weakness at 12 months; rickets diagnosed at 13 months; roentgenogram consistent with rickets
2	16	13	2.27	1.0	952	10	434	Diagnosed with motor neuron disease at 13 months; walked at 14 months; significant bowing of leg, enlargement of knee and wrist at diagnosis of rickets, 16 mo; roentgenogram consistent with rickets
3	8	6	2.50	1.5	2797	NA	450	FTT at 8 months; roentgenogram consistent with rickets
4	12	8	2.50	1.4	392	22	NA	FTT, bowing of leg at 1-y physical examination; walked at 10 months; roentgenogram consistent with healing rickets

*No vitamin D supplements were taken by the patients. Normal ranges and values are shown in parentheses. Ca indicates calcium; P, phosphate; ALP, alkaline phosphatase; 25OHD, 25-hydroxycholecalciferol; PTH, parathormone; FTT, failure to thrive; and NA, not available.

probably delayed the diagnosis in two cases.

Patient Reports.—PATIENT 1.—A 13-month-old black boy presented to the Pediatric Clinic of the United States Air Force (USAF) Medical Center, Keesler Air Force Base, Miss, with failure to thrive, inability to walk, and muscle weakness. He had been delivered after a full-term pregnancy. He had visited the clinic many times for the treatment of upper respiratory and ear infections. At 9 months, he fell from the growth chart for both height and weight and continued to fall from the weight curve at a subsequent visit (Fig 1). At age 13 months, parental concern was heightened by the patient's failure to thrive and inability to walk.

The infant was breast-fed for 1 year, and his diet was intermittently supplemented with formula. No vitamin supplement was prescribed; solid food was introduced at age 6 months, but the infant was described as a "very picky eater." There was no history of undue restriction from sunlight. Pertinent physical findings included hypotonia, proximal muscular weakness, minimal bowing of the legs, an open anterior fontanelle, and rachitic rosary. He was at the 5th percentile for his age for height and weight. Roentgenographic examination of the leg and wrist revealed classic rachitic changes; biochemical data are provided in the Table. Vitamin D, administered in a dosage of 4000 IU/d, was prescribed initially and gradually reduced to a maintenance dosage of 400 IU/d after 3 months. Alkaline phosphatase (ALP) returned to normal levels within 3 months, and significant healing of the rickets (as demonstrated on roentgenography) and satisfactory weight gain were noted after 1 month of therapy (Fig 1).

PATIENT 2.—A 16-month-old black girl was referred to the Pediatric Endocrine Clinic of the USAF Medical Center because of significant bowing of the legs, weakness, "funny gait," enlargement of the wrists and knees, and poor weight gain.

The child had been delivered after a full-term pregnancy and was breast-fed for 13 months; solid food was introduced at age 6 months. Because of hypotonia and inability to walk at age 13 months, she was taken to a neurologist, who considered the diagnosis of muscle disease/motor neuron disease. However, the patient started walking at age 14 months. At age 16 months, the parents noted significant bowing of the legs, which prompted the visit.

Results of a physical examination revealed a child at the 5th percentile for her age for both weight and height. Pertinent positive findings were significant bowing of the legs, enlargement of both the wrists and knees, rachitic rosary, waddling gait, and low muscle mass with mild weakness and hypotonia. Biochemical and roentgenographic findings were consistent with rickets caused by vitamin D deficiency (Fig 2 and Table). The child was administered 4000 U of vitamin D daily. Levels of ALP returned to normal by 8 weeks after initiation of therapy with satisfactory healing of the bone (as demonstrated on roentgenography) by that time. Increases in height and weight were noted in follow-up visits. Vitamin D intake was gradually reduced to 400 IU/d by 10 weeks after initiation of therapy.

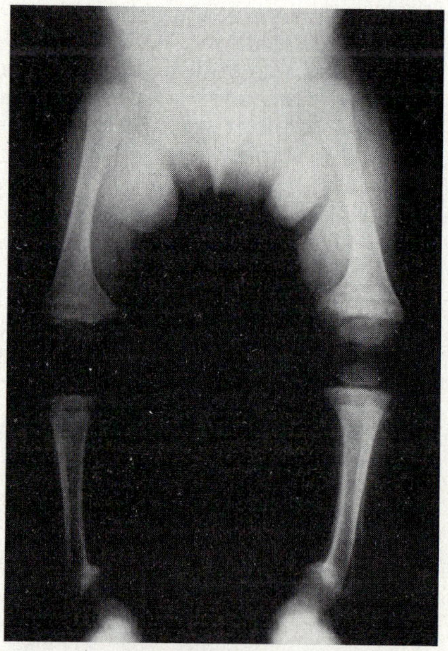

Fig 2.—*A roentgenogram of patient 2 shows symmetrical marked metaphyseal flaring and irregularities involving both lower extremities in association with a metaphyseal band of lucency. There is also significant deformity of the lower tibia.*

PATIENT 3.—An 8-month-old black girl was brought to her pediatrician because of poor weight gain (her height and weight were below the 5th percentile for her age). She had been delivered after an uncomplicated 37-week gestation and was breast-fed until age 6 months without vitamin D supplementation; solid food was introduced at 5 months, but her intake was poor. Results of physical examination were unremarkable. Laboratory and roentgenographic findings were consistent with rickets. The patient was administered a multivitamin drop (400 U of vitamin D) with iron daily. At age 10½ months, the infant returned to the clinic. Weight gain was not satisfactory and her ALP level remained elevated (1339 IU/L). The vitamin D dosage was increased to 1000 U/d. On a follow-up visit at age 12 months, a 1.5-kg weight gain and a significant increase in height were noted. Her ALP level had fallen to 486 IU/L and there was near complete healing of the rickets (as demonstrated on roentgenography).

PATIENT 4.—A 12-month-old black boy was taken to the Pediatric Clinic of the USAF Medical Center for a routine physical examination. He was a twin delivered after 38 weeks' gestation. His dietary history was remarkable for breast-feeding through the first 8 months of life without vitamin D supplementation. Solid foods were introduced at age 4 months. His mother reported restricted sun exposure during his first 8 months of life; the patient walked at age 10 months.

Results of physical examination were remarkable for bilateral bowing of the legs; height and weight were at the 5th percentile for the patient's age. Results of the remainder of the examination were within normal limits. Roentgenographic and biochemical findings were consistent with resolving rickets.

The child was administered 400 IU of vitamin D per day. At follow-up 3 weeks later, a 0.9-kg weight gain was noted and his ALP level had fallen from 392 to 251 IU/L.

Comment.—Breast-feeding has increased during the past decade in the United States.[1] Nevertheless, controversy exists concerning the development of rickets in the breast-fed infant. There are articles recommending[2,3] and disputing[4,5] routine vitamin D supplementation in the breast-fed infant. Human milk contains adequate quantities of calcium and phosphorous for bone mineralization and skeletal growth of full-term infants.[2] However, the vitamin D content of breast milk is generally low.[2,5] Despite this, breast-fed infants usually do not develop nutrition-related rickets. The American Academy of Pediatrics[6] recommends that breast-fed infants receive vitamin D supplements if they do not receive adequate sunlight exposure or if the maternal diet is low in vitamin D. However, sporadic cases of nutrition-related rickets continue to appear in the American literature. Most of the reports are from the North and Northeast, and the majority of the patients are black.[7] There are only rare reports of rickets in the South.

Several studies[8,9] have emphasized the importance of environmental and other risk factors in the development of nutrition-related rickets. These include darkly pigmented skin, dwelling in the inner city, excessive clothing, restricted sunlight exposure, and maternal vegetarian or other unusual diet. Identifiable risk factors for all of our patients included dark skin, prolonged breast-feeding without vitamin D supplementation, and poor intake of solid foods.

Three of our patients had adequate sunlight exposure, but each still developed rickets. This emphasizes the fact that breast-fed black infants without vitamin D supplementation require much more exposure to sunlight to prevent rickets than originally estimated by Specker et al.[10] They estimated that an infant wearing a diaper needs only 30 minutes of sunshine per week to maintain normal levels of 25-hydroxycholecalciferol, while a fully clothed infant without a hat needs 2 hours of sunlight exposure per week. However, black infants in their study had significantly lower serum 25-hydroxycholecalciferol levels than their white counterparts. This finding may be explained by high melanin concentrations in dark-skinned people.[11] High melanin concentrations may limit vitamin D synthesis by competing with 7-dehydrocholesterol for UV photons.[11,12] Clemens et al[12] have demonstrated that blacks may need six times more exposure to UV light than whites to maintain similar levels of vitamin D.

Adequate vitamin D in the diet and/or vitamin D supplementation to the lactating mother are also important factors in the prevention of rickets in the breast-fed infant.[11] The vitamin D levels of the mothers of our patients were not known, although two gave histories of taking multivitamins during breast-feeding. The amount of vitamin D necessary for a lactating mother to prevent rickets in her breast-fed infant may vary with different geographic locations.[13] However, the Food and Nutrition Board of the National Academy of Science recommends 600 IU of vitamin D daily in an adolescent who is pregnant or lactating.[14]

Another effective strategy in the prevention of nutrition-related rickets is direct supplementation of the infant's diet. Reasons for not providing supplementary vitamin D were not clear in two of our patients. In the other patients, however, pediatricians did not believe vitamin D supplementation necessary because the patients lived in warm climates. This trend is not uncommon among young physicians. In one survey taken in San Diego, Calif, 29% of pediatricians did not routinely prescribe vitamin D supplements to breast-fed infants, and those in practice for fewer than 10 years were even less likely to do so.[9] The fact that diagnosis was delayed in two of these infants even though they were receiving regular pediatric supervision illustrates the lack of awareness in the medical profession about this condition. Two of these described infants presented with classic features of rickets (ie, growth failure, hypotonia, muscle weakness, and delayed motor development[15]), yet this diagnosis was not considered until the skeletal manifestations of rickets were evident. In the third patient, rickets was correctly diagnosed, but treatment was inadequate. The fourth patient was diagnosed to have rickets, but only after healing had already begun. Rickets is a systemic disease[16]; the standard pediatric textbooks, however, emphasize mainly the skeletal manifestations of rickets. Many times, however, skeletal manifestations lag behind other signs. Failure to recognize these signs will lead to misdiagnosis and late diagnosis of rickets, as these patient reports illustrate.

Although rickets caused by vitamin D deficiency is rare, it still exists, and subclinical rickets may be more frequent than is generally recognized. Patients may not present with the classic signs and symptoms of rickets; therefore, physicians caring for infants and children must be familiar with the early manifestations of rickets to provide an early diagnosis of the condition. Because the disease is preventable, prevention should be the goal. Although it may be true that some breast-fed infants do not routinely need vitamin D supplements, we do recommend 400 IU of supplementary vitamin D per day in all breast-fed black infants regardless of geographic location. This dose of vitamin D is safe,[7,17] cost-effective,[7] and proven adequate to prevent rickets caused by vitamin D deficiency in breast-fed infants.

Samark K. Bhowmick, MD
Kevin R. Johnson, MD
Pediatric Endocrinology
and Metabolism
USAF Medical Center
Keesler, MS 39534-5300

Kenneth R. Rettig, MD
Pediatric Endocrinology
University of South Alabama
1005 Medical Science Bldg
Mobile, AL 36688

Reprint requests to USAF Medical Center, Pediatric Department, Keesler AFB, MS 39534-5300 (Dr Bhowmick).

We wish to thank Sandra Amidon for her typing expertise, which made the manuscript possible.

The views expressed in this article are those of the authors and do not reflect the official policy or position of the Air Force, the Department of Defense, or the US government.

1. Lawrence RA. Practices and attitudes toward breast feeding among medical professionals. *Pediatrics.* 1982; 70:912-920.

2. Howard RB, Winter HS. *Nutrition and Feeding of the Infant and Toddler.* Boston, Mass; Little Brown & Co Inc; 1984:89.

3. Finberg L. Human milk feeding and vitamin D supplement. *J Pediatr.* 1981;99:228-229.

4. Birkbeck JA, Scott HF. 25 Hydroxycholecalciferol serum levels in breast fed infants. *Arch Dis Child.* 1980;55:691-695.

5. Greer FR, Marshall S. Bone mineral content, serum vitamin D metabolite concentration and ultraviolet B light exposure in infants fed human milk with and without Vitamin D_2 supplements. *J Pediatr.* 1989;114:204-212.

6. American Academy of Pediatrics Committee on Nutrition. Nutrition and lactation. *Pediatrics.* 1981;68:435-443.

7. Cosgrove L, Dietrich A. Nutritional rickets in breast fed infants. *J Fam Pract.* 1985;21:205-209.

8. Bachrach S, Fisher J, Parks JS. An outbreak of vitamin D deficiency rickets in a susceptible population. *Pediatrics.* 1977;64:871-877.

9. Hayward I, Stein MT, Gibson MI. Nutritional rickets in San Diego. *AJDC.* 1987;141:1060-1062.

10. Specker BL, Valaris B, Hertzberg V. Sunshine exposure and serum 25-hydroxy vitamin D concentration in exclusively breast fed infants. *J Pediatr.* 1985;107:372-376.

11. Belton NR. Rickets—not only the 'English disease.' *Acta Paediatr Scand Suppl.* 1986;323:68-75.

12. Clemens TL, Adams JS, Henderson SL, Holick MF. Increased skin pigmentation reduces the capacity of skin to synthesize vitamin D_3. *Lancet.* 1982;1:74-76.

13. Ala-Houhala M, Koskinen T, Terho A, Koivula T, Visakorpi J. Maternal compared with infant vitamin D supplementation. *Arch Dis Child.* 1986;61:1159-1163.

14. Forbes GB, Woodruff CW, eds. *Pediatric Nutrition Handbook.* Elk Grove, Ill: Committee on Nutrition, American Academy of Pediatrics; 1985:350-356.

15. Torres CF, Forbes GB, Decancq GH. Muscle weakness in infants with rickets: distribution, course and recovery. *Pediatr Neurol.* 1986;2:95-98.

16. Rudolf M, Arulanantham K, Greenstein RM. Unsuspected nutritional rickets. *Pediatrics.* 1980;66:72-76.

17. Chesney RW. Requirements and upper limits of vitamin D intake in the term neonate, infant and older child. *J Pediatr.* 1990;116:159-166.

THE EDITORIAL BOARD SPEAKS...

Tell the Whole Story

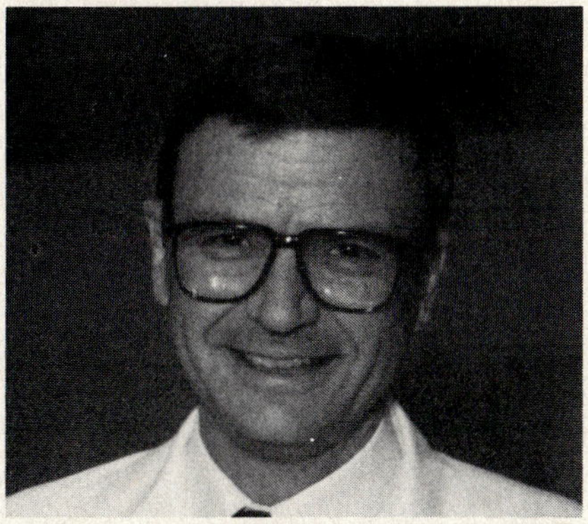

John D. Johnson

John Johnson has been a faithful member of our editorial board for 6 years. He has been a stalwart in refereeing manuscripts in neonatology, an area in which we receive more articles than any other. In every instance, his opinion has been insightful, appropriately critical, and often of great help to authors. It is fitting that his essay in this issue deals with observations that he has made in this process.

John is currently professor and chairperson of the Department of Pediatrics at the University of New Mexico in Albuquerque, and pediatrician-in-chief at Children's Hospital of New Mexico. He has received many teaching, clinical, and research awards. He has also been active in regional, national, and international organizations. Most recently, he was elected chief of staff at the University of New Mexico Medical Center (1989-1991), and was named an ex-officio member of the Board of Trustees of the University of New Mexico Hospital (1989-1990). He is a current recipient of a research grant from the National Institutes of Health, Bethesda, Md, to the Rocky Mountain Center for the Biology of Development (1990-1995). He recently reported on fetal hyperinsulinemia and protein turnover in a rat model and on increasing breast milk for premature infants using a unique relaxation imagery audio tape.

As my term on the editorial board of *AJDC* draws to a close, a series of observations and experiences prompts me to make some recommendations to authors and to university administrators, tenure and promotions committees, department chairpersons, and National Institutes of Health (NIH) administrators. During the past several years, I have served on promotions committees and as a department chairperson, and have reviewed numerous manuscripts submitted to *AJDC* as a member of the editorial board. This combination of experiences has convinced me that changes are needed in the academic milieu that would benefit faculty members aspiring to promotions and tenure, and provide promotions committees and deans with more objective and valid indexes when considering the research productivity of faculty members as one of the three legs of our academic tripartite stool. My observations are as follows:

1. Authors often present an *incomplete* "story" when submitting manuscripts. Results of a single study are "presented" to the medical literature as a series of related overlapping studies. A single piece of research is broken down into a series of reports, each of which, to quote Broad,[1] is the "least publishable unit." The coherent whole is frequently missed unless readers are diligent in tracking the authors' publications. This fragmentation of information detracts from the overall message the authors have to provide, and has significant economic implications for publishers, libraries, and indexes.

2. Such fragmentation is, in fact, *encouraged* by the "weight" that tenure and promotions committees give to the quantity rather than the quality of publications. With some exceptions, it is easier for these committees to weigh or count the number of publications than to critically *identify* and *assess the importance* of the candidates' best research efforts. The same is true for study sections of the NIH and other granting agencies.

3. Deans and department chairpersons have not, for the most part, insisted on change in this archaic system. Their passive acceptance of this process only accentuates the anxieties of faculty aspiring to promotions and tenure and, in turn, promotes the fragmentation existing within the biomedical literature that I deplore.

My recommendations follow logically:

1. Authors should be encouraged to "tell the whole story" in each of their publications. The critical readers will appreciate and acknowledge the wisdom of this approach.

2. Promotions and tenure committees should set very specific criteria for evaluation of research productivity, eg, considering *only* those three to five publications that the nominee and his or her chairperson consider most significant. Weight and quantity should be disregarded. Thereby, members of these committees could concentrate their own efforts on a critical evaluation of this small number of publications. This same recommendation extends to study sections of the NIH, National Science Foundation, and other agencies.

3. Chairpersons and deans must buy into this process and agree to *instruct* the promotions and tenure committees that *more* is not necessarily better. Instructions to the committees and to chairpersons by deans must stress *quality* rather than *quantity*.

These suggestions are not novel. Some, but very few, academic institutions have already adopted such policies. Angell[2] has made similar suggestions in the internal medicine literature. I only wish to make a similar plea to academic pediatrics—authors should be allowed and encouraged to tell the whole story and the policies of universities and granting agencies should, in fact, *require* them to do so.

References

1. Broad WJ. The publishing game: getting more for less. *Science.* 1981;211:1137-1139.
2. Angell M. Publish or perish: a proposal. *Ann Intern Med.* 1986;104:261-262.

We're introducing a change... without changing a thing about our formulas

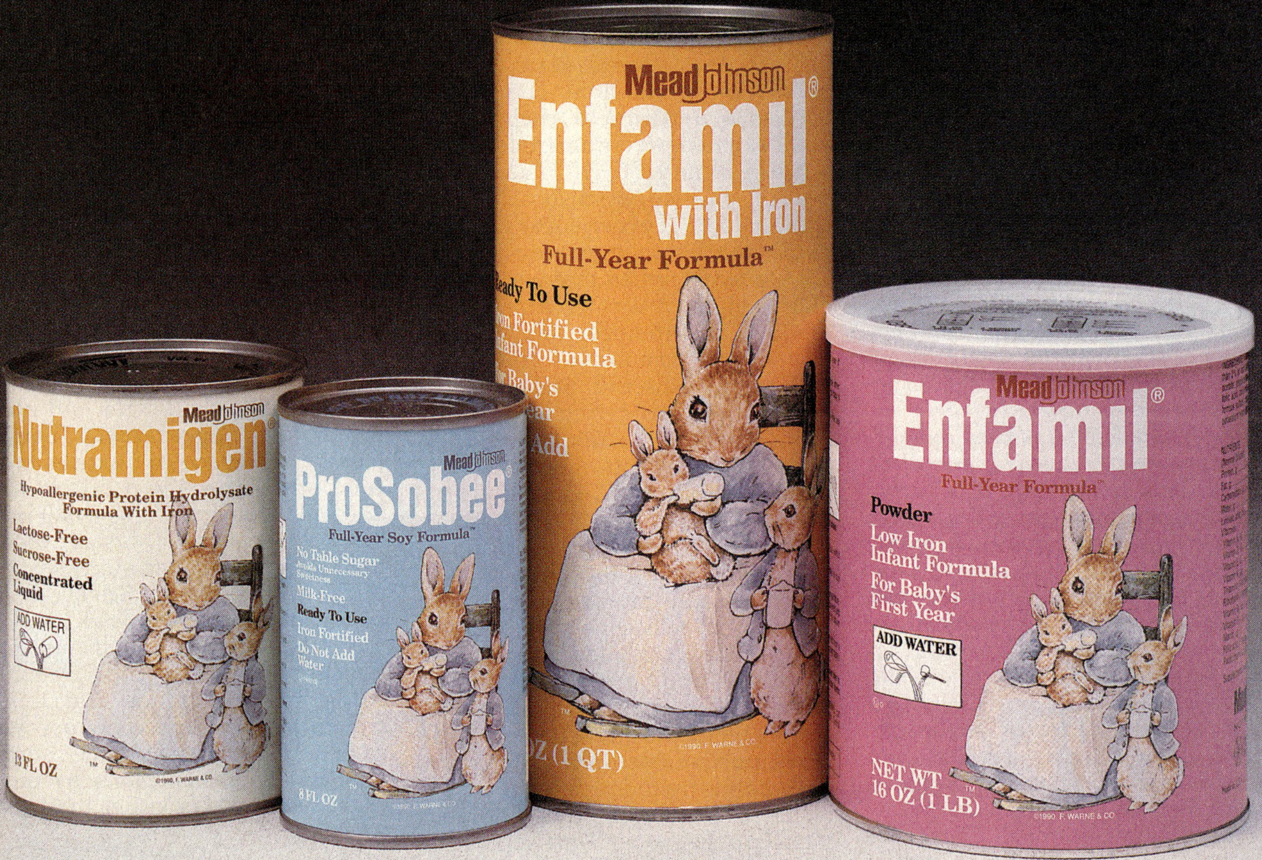

Our new labels convey warmth and tradition in an updated way. And they're appropriate for all ethnic backgrounds. The formulas inside, though, haven't changed at all. They still offer the same good nutrition for babies that physicians have trusted over the years.

At Mead Johnson Nutritionals, our look is new, but our commitment to helping you provide excellent infant nutrition continues.

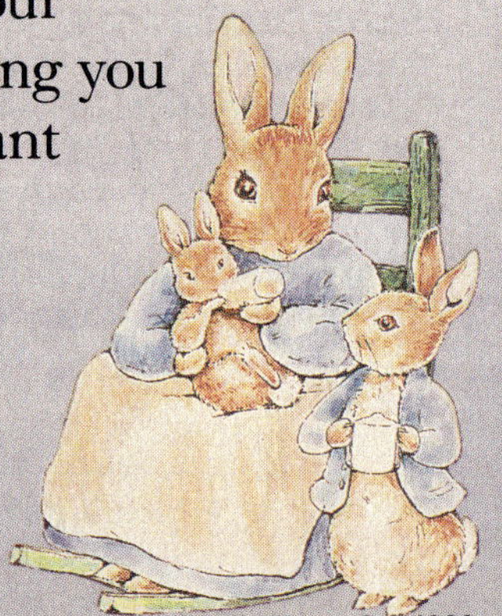

Mead Johnson
NUTRITIONALS

L-K332

Human Immunodeficiency Virus Transmission by Child Sexual Abuse

Laura T. Gutman, MD; Karen K. St Claire, MD; Chris Weedy, MSW; Marcia E. Herman-Giddens, PA, MPH; Barbara A. Lane, MSN; Jeanne G. Niemeyer, MSW; Ross E. McKinney, Jr, MD

• During 1987-1989, 14 (14.6%) of the 96 children who tested positive for the human immunodeficiency virus (HIV) and were followed up by the Duke University (Durham, NC) pediatric acquired immunodeficiency syndrome team were confirmed to have been sexually abused. Every sexually abused child was evaluated for each of five modes of HIV transmission, and in nine children the pathway was identified. Four of the study children acquired HIV from child sexual abuse and in six, abuse was a possible source. Transmission by child sexual abuse was the most frequent of the proven modes of acquisition of HIV in this population. The other proven modes of acquisition were vertical transmission (n=3) and HIV–contaminated blood transfusion (n=2). Twelve males were identified (n=8) or suspected (n=4) of being perpetrators. Three knew themselves to have HIV at the time of an assault and eight were aware that the child had HIV at the time of an assault. There was no indication from any child that "safe sex" precautions had been observed. Children with HIV infection had multiple risk factors for abuse or neglect. The sociological descriptors of the lives of the 14 abused children showed multiple known risk factors for sexual abuse that also overlapped with known risk factors for or sequelae of the acquisition of HIV infection. These included drug abuse and alcoholism in the home, prostitution of a parent, lack of parenting, poverty, and chronic illness of the child. Prevention efforts should recognize that children as well as adults are at risk for sexually transmitted HIV infection.

***(AJDC.* 1991;145:137–141)**

The Duke University (Durham, NC) pediatric acquired immunodeficiency sydrome (AIDS) team began accepting pediatric patients in 1987 and by December 1989 had a census of 96 patients who showed positive results to the human immunodeficiency virus (HIV) antibody test and were known to the AIDS team social worker. These children were at all stages of HIV-related illness and ranged in age from newborn to 17 years. All children received integrated multidisciplinary services that delivered optimal therapy and treatment of the complex problems that characterize children with AIDS.

During this period, 14 children from the AIDS population were confirmed to have been sexually abused. The medical and social conditions of the lives of the abused children were reviewed for known risk factors for the acquisition of HIV and for child sexual abuse (CSA). This study describes the results of the evaluation of the sexually abused children, the circumstances surrounding the abusive experiences, the perpetrators, and the data regarding the means by which the children had acquired HIV.

PATIENTS AND METHODS

Evaluation Process

All children seen by the AIDS team who presented with or developed indications of possible abuse or neglect were referred to the child protection team for evaluation. Data for this study were collected at the time of the assessment of each child and represent cumulative information regarding the child's environment from the family, child, child protection team, AIDS team, social service agencies, schools, and, often, charitable agencies. Child sexual abuse was defined in 1977 as the involvement of dependent developmentally immature children and adolescents in sexual activities that they do not fully comprehend, to which they are unable to give informed consent, or that violate the social taboos of family roles.[1] Child sexual abuse includes rape, pedophilia, child prostitution, child pornography, child sex rings, and incest.

Multiple issues often led to referral to the child protection team. The instigating events included (1) the suspicion of or disclosure of CSA volunteered by the child or a caretaker (n=2); (2) abnormal genital findings revealed by routine medical examination (n=5); (3) suspected physical abuse or neglect, or a chaotic family environment (n=3); (4) medical or behavioral histories indicative of CSA (n=5); (5) children older than 6 years at onset of HIV disease, or with no known risk factor for HIV (n=3); and (6) the child was an HIV-positive sibling of a sexually abused child (n=1). All of the children were known to be infected with HIV prior to the diagnosis of CSA.

Evaluation for CSA

The evaluation of a child for CSA began with a family interview regarding the family constellation, patterns of care for the child, interactions of family members, behavioral characteristics of the child, and concerns or knowledge that the caretaker may have had regarding possibly abusive events. The following five groups of data needed for adequate evaluation of possible CSA were then obtained: (1) a review of the behavioral history of the child; (2) a review of the medical history of the child; (3) diagnostic interview(s) with the child; (4) results of physical examination; and (5) assessment for other sexually transmitted diseases.[2-4]

The diagnostic interviews followed a standard format. Draw-

Accepted for publication November 6, 1990.

From the Department of Pediatrics, Duke University Medical Center, Durham, NC.

Presented in part at the annual meeting of the Society for Pediatric Research, Anaheim, Calif, May 11, 1990.

Reprint requests to Box 3971, Duke University Medical Center, Durham, NC 27710 (Dr Gutman).

ings and anatomically correct dolls were available for use when appropriate.[5] In the present study, "disclosure" refers to the disclosure by the child or witness of a specific sexually abusive act. Perpetrators were "identified" if the child or a caretaker had specifically identified the person as an assailant. Perpetrators were considered "suspected" if the interview or historical information indicated sexually inappropriate interactions with the study child or another child and unsupervised access to the study child.

Each child received a complete physical examination and external genital examination using standard techniques.[6,7] For the girls, genital examinations included identification of hymenal type and contour, measurement of the horizontal diameter of the hymenal opening, and anal examination.[8,9] Samples of vaginal secretions were examined for indicators of bacterial vaginosis and *Trichomonas.* Cultures of the introitus or vaginal canal of girls and of the anus of boys for *Neisseria gonorrheae* and *Chlamydia trachomatis* were taken unless the child was receiving antimicrobial therapy. Cultures of other sites and assessments for other infectious diseases were made when indicated.

Sexual abuse was confirmed if there was a detailed account from the child or a witness, a sexually transmitted disease in addition to HIV was found, the genital examination showed abnormal findings clearly indicative of abuse as defined at the 1985 National Child Sexual Abuse Summit meeting[10] and subsequently updated,[2,11,12] serial genital examinations showed significant changes, or the abuse was acknowledged by the perpetrator.

Mode of Acquisition of HIV by Study Children

The five possible routes of transmission of HIV that were separately assessed for each child were vertical transmission, transfusion, clotting factor concentrates, intravenous drugs, and sexual abuse (including child prostitution).

Data regarding vertical transmission included date(s) and result(s) of maternal HIV serologic tests relative to the birth of the child or HIV-related illness of the child. Data regarding transfusion-transmitted HIV included dates of transfusion to the child and the results of retrospective blood-bank HIV surveillance. None of the children in the study had received clotting factor concentrate therapy or had engaged in intravenous drug abuse. Data regarding transmission by sexual abuse included available information on the HIV status of the perpetrator(s) and the type of abuse.

Since many of the abused children had multiple possible modes of acquisition of HIV, the influence of each on the transmission of the HIV infection was stratified into categories of "proven," "possible," "disproven," and "unknown."

The following criteria were used to define the categories for vertical transmission: proven, the mother was HIV positive prior to or within 6 months of giving birth, or was first shown to be HIV positive 6 or more months after delivery and the child had an opportunistic infection or lymphocytic interstitial pneumonia by the age of 2 years; possible, the mother was first known to be HIV positive 6 or more months after delivery; disproven, the mother was HIV negative 6 or more months after delivery; and unknown, the mother's HIV seroactivity was unknown.

Criteria to define the categories for transmission by transfusion were as follows: proven, the mother was HIV negative at or after delivery and the child was known to have received an HIV-contaminated transfusion; possible, the mother was first known to be HIV positive 6 or more months after delivery and the child received an HIV positive transfusion; disproven, the child either received no transfusion, or it was HIV negative; and unknown, the child received a transfusion and retrospective surveillance was not able to trace the unit.

The criteria to define the categories for transmission of HIV through CSA were as follows: proven, either all other risk factors were disproven or the child was older than 12 years when HIV was first diagnosed, sexual contact had involved high risk for HIV, and no other factor had been proven; possible, the perpetrator was either HIV positive or unknown, and no other risk factor was proven; disproven, identified perpetrator was HIV negative; and unknown: an additional risk factor was proven. Inclusion in this report required that sexual abuse of the child had been confirmed. A conservative definition of proven transmission of HIV by CSA gave priority to other known modes of transmission.

Table 1.—Forms of Child Sexual Abuse

	Female Children (n = 11)	Male Children (n = 3)
Genital-vaginal	7	Not applicable
Digital-vaginal	2	Not applicable
Genital-rectal	4	1
Genital-oral	3	0
Unknown	4	2

Sociological Setting

The social settings of the subjects were evaluated for five sociological risk factors for CSA identified from the 1987 National Survey of Children.[13] In that study, a significantly greater incidence of CSA was experienced by girls who had lived apart from their biological parents before age 16 years; had been raised in poverty; had an emotional, physical, or mental handicap; and had family members who were alcoholic or drug abusers.

Other aspects of the social setting that were recorded in the present study included prostitution by adults in the home; the presence of multiple, unrelated, and frequently changing live-in visitors to the household; significant personality disorder of a caretaker; and AIDS encephalopathy or other AIDS-related disability of a caretaker.

RESULTS

Fourteen HIV-positive children were confirmed to have been sexually abused. The children included three boys and 11 girls (79% female) whose ages at the time of the diagnosis of CSA ranged from 3.5 to 13 years and whose mean age was 6.2 years. Thirteen of the 14 children were classified as P-2 based on Centers for Disease Control (CDC) criteria at the time they were diagnosed to be HIV positive. Eleven children were black, two were white, and one was Native American.

Diagnosis of CSA

Each of the 14 children with confirmed CSA either had disclosed sexual abuse, had genital or anal findings strongly indicative of CSA, or both. All of the 11 girls had abnormal examinations of the introital area and/or hymen. Two of the three boys had abnormal anal examination results. The genital findings indicative of abuse were scars or healed lesions of the posterior fourchette, (n = 4); scars, tears, notches, or significant distortions of the hymen (n = 5); recurrent or persistent vaginal discharge and odor or vaginal bleeding (n = 6); hymenal opening size greater than or equal to 8 mm in a prepubertal child or a significant change in the genital examination results on serial evaluations (n = 8); -perianal scars (n = 2); significant and rapid anal dilation (n = 4); and perianal lesions (n = 1). Neither *N gonorrheae* nor *C trachomatis* was isolated from the vagina, throat, or rectum of any study child. Three children had a sexually associated disease other than HIV; two had bacterial vaginosis[14]; and one had condylomata acuminatum.[15]

Eight children were able to disclose their abuse. Two made partial disclosure and four were unable to disclose. The forms of sexual abuse described by the eight children who were able to disclose are listed in Table 1.

All identified or suspected perpetrators were male. The number of known or suspected assailants and their relationship to the child when information was available are

Table 2.—Relation of Identified and Suspected Perpetrator(s) to an Assaulted Child

Relation	No. Identified	No. Suspected
Brother	1*	...
Father	1	3
Uncle	2	1*
Grandfather	2*	...
Foster father	1*	...
Foster brother	1*	...
Nonrelated assailant of child prostitute	7*	...

*One of multiple identified or suspected assailants of a single child.

Table 3.—Assessed Mode of Acquisition of Human Immunodeficiency Virus in Sexually Abused Children (n = 14)*

Mode of Acquisition	Proven	Possible	Disproven	Unknown
Child sexual abuse	4	6	...	4
Vertical transmission	3	5	5	1
Transfusion	2	...	12	...

*Acquisition of human immunodeficiency virus by clotting factor concentrate and by intravenous drug use was disproven in all cases.

shown in Table 2. For four children, the number and identity of perpetrator(s) was unknown. A single perpetrator was identified for three children, and for three children multiple perpetrators were identified. For two children a single perpetrator was suspected. For one child, one perpetrator was identified and additional perpetrators were also suspected. For another child, one perpetrator was suspected while the multiple perpetrators known to have abused the child were unidentified.

Acquisition of HIV

Using the criteria stated in the "Patients and Methods" section, an assessment was made of the mode of transmission of HIV when all data were considered. The results are shown in Table 3. For four (29%) of the 14 children, CSA was the only means of transmission of HIV to the child. A brief synopsis of the histories of these children follows. To protect the identities of the children, gender identification is not provided.

CASE 1.—The child was an emotionally abused, physically healthy child who lived in fear of the stepfather. At age 13 years, the child ran away from home and lived as a child prostitute for 3 months, during which time sexual practices included unprotected anal-receptive intercourse with multiple high-risk adults. Intravenous drugs were never used. The child had never had a transfusion and was not hemophilic. The mother was not tested but had no risk factors for HIV. At age 15 years, the child requested an HIV assay because of the high-risk history. Results of enzyme-linked immunosorbent assay (ELISA) and Western blot were positive, and the disease was CDC class P-1, subclass B. It was concluded that the child had acquired HIV as a child prostitute.

CASE 2.—At age 3 years 9 months, this child was HIV positive based on ELISA and Western blot test results; the disease was CDC class P-2, subclass A. The child's mother was HIV negative. The child had not received a transfusion or blood products and was not hemophilic. Genital examination results were abnormal and included condyloma acuminatum, which had first been noted at age 3 years and 3 months. After partial disclosure it was concluded that the abuse had occurred during a chaotic family episode when numerous caretakers had had access to the child, and that the child had acquired HIV during the abuse.

CASE 3.—This child was aged 2 years 2 months when diagnosed to be HIV positive by ELISA and confirmed by Western blot; the disease was CDC class P-2, subclass F. The mother was HIV negative by ELISA, Western blot, and HIV culture. Although the child had received a transfusion, the donor was HIV negative. The child was not hemophilic. Genital examination was positive for traumatic abuse. Although verbal disclosure was obtained, identification of the assailant was not made, and a suspected assailant refused HIV testing. Because of the disclosure and the fact that another child had been sexually abused in the same home, the child was removed from the household and restricted from contact with the suspected perpetrator. Further abuse was subsequently documented by the development of new physical signs and symptoms, but specific identification of the perpetrator again could not be made. It was concluded that the child had acquired HIV during abuse by multiple perpetrators.

CASE 4.—This child was diagnosed at age 6 years and 2 months to be HIV positive by ELISA and Western blot, and classified as CDC P-2 subclass C. At the time of the diagnosis, the mother was HIV-negative, the child had never had a transfusion, and the child was not hemophilic. The genital examination revealed definitive evidence of traumatic abuse, as did the medical history. Two assailants were identified, one of whom was known to be HIV positive. It was concluded that the child had acquired HIV infection during child sexual abuse by an HIV-positive assailant.

Knowledge by the Assailant of the Possibility of HIV Transmission to or From the Child

Three of the assailants who were identified or suspected were HIV positive and knew of their HIV status at the time they assaulted the child. There was no indication from the children that "safe sex" precautions had been taken.

Eight identified or suspected assailants were aware that the child was HIV positive at the time of the assault. Five of these eight were themselves either HIV negative or their status was unknown when the child was assaulted. Again, there was no indication from the children that "safe sex" precautions had been taken.

COMMENT

In a recent review of the data from the 1987 National Survey of Children, social settings were identified that increased the risk of CSA.[13] All but one child in the present study had two or more of these risk factors, and the proportion of children who had a given risk factor ranged from 43% to 71%, as shown below.

Social Conditions	No. (%) of Children
Lived apart from both biological parents	6 (43)
Raised in poverty*	10 (71)
Child was handicapped†	9 (64)
Alcoholic family member*	7 (50)
Drug abusing family member*	10 (71)
Prostitution at home	4 (29)
Transient adults living at home	8 (57)
Mentally ill caretaker	5 (36)
AIDS-related disability of caretaker	2 (14)

*Risk factors for CSA identified by National Survey of Children.[13]
†Handicap was probably apparent before onset of CSA.

In the National Survey of Children, 6% of girls with no risk factor, 9% of girls with one risk factor, 26% of girls with two risk factors, and 68% of girls with three or more risk factors had been sexually abused as children. In the present study, five of these identified factors were assessed, and 11 (78%) of 14 children had three or more of these risk factors each, demonstrating that the living circumstances of the abused children in the present study included previously described indicators for increased risk of sexual abuse.

Many of the circumstances surrounding the sexual abuse of these children are also previously identified risk factors for adult HIV transmission. First, promiscuous sexual activity with multiple partners is a well-defined risk factor for adult HIV infection.[16] In the present series, seven (50%) of 14 children were known or suspected to have been assaulted by multiple perpetrators, eight children (57%) lived in homes in which casual adult acquaintances frequently slept in the home, thereby creating opportunities to abuse a vulnerable child, and four of these eight homes were also the sites for prostitution by adult caretakers. One of the children in the study had turned to child prostitution, itself a form of CSA.[17] A second risk factor for adult HIV infection is sexual contact that is physically traumatic or involves impaired mucosal barriers. Both anal-receptive and oral-receptive sex have been associated with increased rates of transmission of HIV in adults, and were acts that these children described.[18-20] Furthermore, the children in the study had an unusually high incidence of physical signs of genital injury compared with usual groups of sexually abused children. A third risk factor for adult HIV infection is sexual intercourse without barrier protection. Assailants of children in this study practiced high-risk and unprotected sex even when the assailant knew himself to be HIV infected or when he knew the child to be HIV infected. A fourth risk factor for adult HIV infection, which was also found in most children in the study, is genital mucosal lesions as evidenced by vaginal bleeding, discharge, infections, and scars, perianal infections, lesions, and scars, and other sexually transmitted diseases.[21] Finally, the adult population with whom many children lived were at increased risk of HIV from the use of illicit drugs. Use of drugs and alcohol by caretakers may also have diminished their ability to protect the child and lowered their threshold for sexual aggression.[22,23] Consequently, these children were subjected to forms of sexual intercourse that were known from adult studies to be especially hazardous regarding transmission of HIV, and the children lived in family and social settings in which many adults who were their caretakers were at increased risk of being HIV infected.

In spite of the multiple risk factors for CSA that characterize the lives of many children with HIV, acquisition of HIV by children through abusive sexual assault has been infrequently considered or reported in the medical literature. Although individual case reports have provided evidence that this route of transmission should be examined for children with HIV,[24,25] few medical reviews of the routes of transmission of HIV or of unsolved epidemiologic problems with HIV allude to transmission through CSA.[2,26-29] For example, the exposure categories for reporting cases of childhood HIV infection by the Centers for Disease Control do not include the category of exposure through sexual contact. The lack of data and the need for policies on the testing of abused children for HIV has been the subject of a recent review.[30] The present study indicates that at least four (4.2%) of 96 children with HIV and four (29%) of 14 sexually abused children with HIV acquired the infection through CSA. These represent the minimal percentages of pediatric HIV disease that can be attributed to CSA, since the abused children were identified during standard, nondirected pediatric interactions rather than by specific screening for abuse. In addition, children who also had other "possible" modes of transmission, such as maternal HIV, could not be proven to have acquired their disease through CSA. It was notable that four of the five children for whom vertical transmission of HIV was assessed to have been "possible" because the mother was HIV positive were older than 3 years when AIDS-like illness first began. This would be a long incubation period for perinatally transmitted HIV,[31] and some of these children may instead have acquired their disease through CSA. This situation is exemplified by one of the study cases, in which the HIV-positive man who was identified as the perpetrator of a child's abuse was also the source of the mother's HIV infection.

The diagnosis of CSA in children who have AIDS or who are in a high-risk environment is of particular importance because some immediate and delayed behavioral sequelae of CSA may put the adolescent and adult survivor at increased risk of exposure to HIV or transmission of HIV to others if they are infected. First, high-risk sexual behaviors that may characterize female survivors of CSA include early entry into sexual activities, sexual promiscuity, and a particular vulnerability to further abuse and sexual exploitation, including prostitution and unintended pregnancy at an early age.[32-40] Male victims of CSA may develop a cycle of sexual behavior in which the child victim becomes a sexual aggressor of other children, either immediately or in adulthood.[41] Multiple victims may be involved.[42] The consequences of the intersection of child sexual abuse with immediate and delayed risk factors for acquisition of HIV are dramatically highlighted in the "street" children of New York, NY.[43] Many of these children were sexually abused in earlier childhood, presumably providing their motivation for leaving their homes at a highly vulnerable, adolescent age.

In conclusion, this study has demonstrated that child sexual abuse was the proven mode of transmission in at least 4% of all study children with HIV followed up by the pediatric AIDS team, and may have been the mode of transmission for a considerably larger proportion of cases. The abused children lived in circumstances that put them at high risk for both CSA and HIV infection, and these risk factors often overlapped. Assailants were known to have abused children in spite of knowing themselves or the child to be HIV positive. Prevention of HIV transmission in populations of children and adolescents cannot be successful without the development of policies and resources to identify and eliminate the underlying sexual abuse to which these children are exposed. Sexual abuse and its consequences provide a major mechanism for the introduction of HIV to children and adolescents.

We are grateful for funding from the National Institutes of Allergy and Infectious Disease for the Duke University Pediatric AIDS Treatment and Evaluation Unit, Durham, NC.

References

1. Kempe HC. Sexual abuse, another hidden pediatric problem: the 1977 C. Anderson Aldrich Lecture. *Pediatrics.* 1978;62:382-389.

2. Herbert CP. Expert medical assessment in determining probability of alleged child sexual abuse. *Child Abuse Negl.* 1987;11:213-221.

3. Sargent DA, Blumberg M, Broughton D, et al. AMA diagnostic and treatment guidelines concerning child abuse and neglect. *JAMA.* 1985;254:796-800.

4. Berson N, Herman-Giddens M, eds. *Duke University Medical Center Child Protection Team Manual 1990*. Durham, NC: Duke University Medical Center Child Protection Team; 1986.
5. Berkowitz CD. Sexual abuse of children and adolescents. *Adv Pediatr.* 1987;34:275-312.
6. Finkel MA. The medical evaluation of child sexual abuse. In: Schetky D, Green A, eds. *Child Sexual Abuse*. New York, NY: Brunner-Mazel Inc; 1988:82-103.
7. McCann J, Voris J, Simon M, Wells R. Comparison of genital examination techniques in prepubertal girls. *Pediatrics.* 1990;85:182-187.
8. Goff CW, Burke KR, Rickenback C, Buebendorf DP. Vaginal opening measurement in prepubertal girls. *AJDC.* 1989;143:1366-1368.
9. Herman-Giddens ME, Frothingham TE. Prepubertal female genitalia: examination for evidence of sexual abuse. *Pediatrics.* 1987;80:203-208.
10. Tipton AC. Child sexual abuse: physical examination techniques and interpretation of findings. *Adolesc Pediatr Gynecol.* 1989;2:10-25.
11. Emans SJ, Woods E, Flagg M, Freeman A. Genital findings in sexually abused symptomatic and asymptomatic girls. *Pediatrics.* 1987;79:778-785.
12. White ST, Ingram DL, Lyner PR. Vaginal introital diameter in the evaluation of sexual abuse. *Child Abuse Negl.* 1989;13:217-224.
13. Moore KA, Nord CW, Peterson JL. Nonvoluntary sexual activity among adolescents. *Fam Plann Perspect.* 1989;21:110-114.
14. Hammerschlag MR, Cummings M, Doraiswamy B, Cox P, McCormack WM. Nonspecific vaginitis following sexual abuse in children. *Pediatrics.* 1985;75:1028-1031.
15. Herman-Giddens ME, Gutman LT, Berson NL, Duke Child Protection Team. Association of coexisting sexually transmitted disease and multiple abusers in female children with genital warts. *Sex Transm Dis.* 1988;15:63-67.
16. Pape JW, Liautaud B, Thomas F, et al. The acquired immunodeficiency syndrome in Haiti. *Ann Intern Med.* 1985;103:674-678.
17. Cohen MI. Effective low enforcement strategies for handling juvenile prostitution. *Nat Sheriff.* 1988;40:49-52.
18. Fischl MA, Dickinson GM, Scott GB, Klimas N, Fletcher MA, Parks W. Evaluation of heterosexual partners, children, and household contacts of adults with AIDS. *JAMA.* 1987;257:640-644.
19. Padian N, Marquis L, Francis DP, et al. Male-to-female transmission of human immunodeficiency virus. *JAMA.* 1987;258:788-790.
20. Frederick W, Olopoenia L, Delapenha R, Barnes S, Saxinger C, Greaves W. Sexual practices associated with HIV transmission among female sexual partners of HIV seropositive men. Presented at the 29th International Conference on Antimicrobial Agents and Chemotherapy; September 18, 1989; Houston, Tex.
21. Greenblatt RM, Lukehart SA, Plummer FA, et al. Genital ulceration as a risk factor for human immunodeficiency virus infection. *AIDS.* 1988;2:47-50.
22. Browning DH, Boatman B. Incest: children at risk. *Am J Psychiatry.* 1977;134:69-72.
23. Famularo R, Stone K, Barnum R, Wharton R. Alcoholism and severe child mistreatment. *Am J Orthopsychiatry.* 1986;56:481-485.
24. Leiderman IZ, Grimm KT. A child with HIV infection. *JAMA.* 1986;256:3094.
25. Gellert GA, Durfee MJ. HIV infection and child abuse. *N Engl J Med.* 1989;321:685.
26. Gellert GA, Mascola L. Rape and AIDS. *Pediatrics.* 1989;83(suppl):644-645.
27. Fuller AK, Bartucci RJ. HIV transmission and childhood sexual abuse. *JAMA.* 1988;259:2235-2236.
28. Osterholm MT, MacDonald KL. Facing the complex issues of pediatric AIDS: a public health perspective. *JAMA.* 1987;258:2736-2737.
29. Novick BE, Rubinstein A. AIDS: the pediatric perspective. *AIDS.* 1987;1:3-7.
30. Gellert GA, Durfee MJ, Berkowitz CD. Developing guidelines for HIV antibody testing among victims of pediatric sexual abuse. *Child Abuse Negl.* 1990;14:9-17.
31. Johnson JP, Nair P, Hines SE, et al. Natural history and serologic diagnosis of infants born to human immunodeficiency virus–infected women. *AJDC.* 1989;143:1147-1153.
32. Browne A, Finkelhor D. Impact of child sexual abuse: a review of the research. *Psychol Bull.* 1986;99:66-77.
33. Briere J, Runtz M. Post sexual abuse trauma: data and implications for clinical practice. *J Interpers Violence.* 1987;2:367-379.
34. Miller J, Moeller D, Kaufman A, Divasto P, Pathak D, Christy J. Recidivism among sexual assault victims. *Am J Psychiatry.* 1978;135:1103-1104.
35. Sedney MA, Brooks B. Factors associated with a history of childhood sexual experience in a nonclinical female population. *J Am Acad Child Psychiatry.* 1984;23:215-218.
36. Finkelhor D, Browne A. The traumatic impact of child sexual abuse: a conceptualization. *Am J Orthopsychiatry.* 1985;55:530-541.
37. Bagley C, McDonald M. Adult mental health sequels of child sexual abuse, physical abuse and neglect in maternally separated children. *Can J Commun Ment Health.* 1984;3:15-26.
38. Silbert MH, Pines AM. Sexual child abuse as an antecedent to prostitution. *Child Abuse Negl.* 1981;5:407-411.
39. James J, Meyerding J. Early sexual experience and prostitution. *Am J Psychiatry.* 1977;134:1381-1385.
40. Gershenson HP, Musick JS, Ruch-Ross HS, Magee V, Rubino KK, Rosenberg D. The prevalence of coercive sexual experience among teenage mothers. *J Interpers Violence.* 1989;4:204-219.
41. Longo R. Sexual learning and experience among adolescent sexual offenders. *Int J Offender Ther Comp Crimonol.* 1982;26:235-241.
42. Abel GG, Becker JV, Mittelman M, Cunningham-Rathner J, Rouleau JL, Murphy WD. Self-reported sex crimes of nonincarcerated paraphiliacs. *J Interpers Violence.* 1987;2:3-25.
43. Stricof R, Novick LF, Kennedy J, Weisfuse I. HIV seroprevalence of adolescents at Convenant House/under 21, New York City. Presented at the American Public Health Association Conference; November 1988; Boston, Mass.

Sexual Maturation and Blood Pressure Levels of a Biracial Sample of Girls

Claudia A. Kozinetz, PhD, MPH

• A cross-sectional survey of 142 black and 361 white girls was performed to investigate whether differences in the timing of maturation account for blood pressure differences between same-aged subjects. Data were collected on blood pressure, anthropometric parameters, socioeconomic status, and secondary sex characteristics. Analysis of covariance was used to determine whether blood pressure for black and white girls differed significantly after adjusting for the confounding effects of different body size and sexual maturation distributions of the two groups. Advanced sexual maturation of the black girls contributed as much as the larger body sizes of the black girls to the blood pressure differences found between the black and white girls. Assessment of an individual's stage of sexual maturation at blood pressure measurement should be considered as important as the measurement of height and weight.

(*AJDC.* 1991;145:142–147)

The underlying mechanism of the development of blood pressure level during childhood and adolescence is unknown. This is due, in part, to the many physical, physiological, and hormonal changes; the variability between and within individuals and populations of the onset and rate of sexual maturation; and the rate of growth that occurs during childhood and adolescence.

The association of height and weight with blood pressure during childhood has been well documented.[1,2] As a result of those findings, the Second Task Force on Blood Pressure Control in Children[3] revised its recommendations from its first report[4] to include consideration of the child's height and weight at the measurement of blood pressure. However, an important variable not considered or evaluated for those blood pressure standards was sexual maturation. Many of the data sets used for the task force report did not have data available on sexual maturation, preventing its inclusion in the analyses. The current second task force age- and sex-specific blood pressure standards, however, include adolescents in various stages of sexual maturation. This variability in maturation possibly obscures the isolated effect of puberty on blood pressure level.

A number of studies on blood pressure and sexual maturation have produced conflicting results.[5,6] Londe et al[6] concluded from their study of 189 measurements among girls 10 to 14 years of age that there is no relationship between blood pressure level and sexual maturation. The authors based their findings, however, on single determinations of the cyclic luteinizing and follicle-stimulating hormones. The daily intraindividual variation of these hormones precludes their use as cross-sectional, single-determination, independent variables. The authors did not control for possible confounding effects or covariance. They also seemed to misunderstand the strength of longitudinal studies for the investigation of development, as evidenced by their statement, "since blood pressure increases with age, longitudinal studies are unsatisfactory, because rise in pressure may be due to age rather than sexual maturation."

It is not known whether sexual maturation contributes to blood pressure during childhood and adolescence independently of chronological age or body size. Thus, it is logical to compare blood pressure levels of two groups that have different ages of onset of and, possibly, different rates of sexual maturation. A more sexually mature population would be expected to have a higher mean blood pressure than a comparison population of the same chronological age but sexually less mature. Black youths are known to enter into puberty at a younger chronological age than white youths.[7]

The objective of this study was to investigate whether differences in the timing of maturation account for blood pressure differences between same-aged black and white girls. Specifically, this study analyzed the data to answer the following questions: (1) Are there differences in systolic and diastolic blood pressure between black and white girls? (2) Are there differences in height, weight, body-mass index, socioeconomic status, and timing of sexual maturation between black and white girls? (3) Are observed patterns of differences in blood pressure associated with differences in height, weight, body-mass index, socioeconomic status, and timing of sexual maturation?

SUBJECTS AND METHODS

Participants were recruited from female students enrolled in a public school district in central Texas for a cross-sectional study of blood pressure and maturation. The school district was large, so schools were selected using a multistage sampling method with initial stratification of schools according to the enrolled students' socioeconomic status. A census tract for each eligible student was determined using the student's address. The median income levels associated with eligible students' census tracts, as

Accepted for publication October 26, 1990.

From the Department of Pediatrics, Baylor College of Medicine, Houston, Tex.

Reprint requests to Baylor College of Medicine, 6560 Fannin, Suite 920, Houston, TX 77030 (Dr Kozinetz).

Table 1.—Sociodemographic Characteristics of the Study Population

	Race, No. (%)	
	Black	White
Age category, y*		
7-9	59 (41.5)	123 (34.1)
10-12	47 (33.1)	160 (44.3)
13-15	27 (19.0)	67 (18.6)
16-18	9 (6.3)	11 (3.0)
Median income index†		
1	6 (4.4)	58 (16.3)
2	62 (45.9)	192 (54.1)
3	29 (21.5)	46 (13.0)
4	18 (13.3)	34 (9.6)
5	20 (14.8)	25 (7.0)

*The age distribution did not differ significantly between the races.
†The median income index, derived from the US Census, was missing for seven black and six white girls. $\chi^2=22.40$, $df=4$, $P=.0001$.

published by the US Census Bureau, were combined and averaged to determine a representative median income level for each school.

The schools were categorized into four income level groups, from low to high. Four elementary schools (grades 2 through 5), two middle schools (grades 6 through 8), and the health classes from two high schools (grades 9 through 12) were randomly selected. Students from these selected schools volunteered for participation in this study.

Informed consent and assent were obtained from the parent or guardian and student, respectively. This project was approved by the institutional review board of the University of Texas Health Science Center, Houston.

Sample size calculations were done to determine the number of black and white girls necessary to detect a minimum difference in mean blood pressure levels of 4 mm Hg. With an α level of .05 and 90% power, a minimum of 118 girls in each racial group was required.

The highest participation rate occurred in the elementary schools (63%) and the lowest rate occurred in the high schools (16%). Hence, this was largely a study of the younger age groups. To examine possible nonresponse bias, addresses of the nonresponders were abstracted from official school records. The addresses were categorized by census tract and rank-ordered by the socioeconomic level of the census tract. The socioeconomic status distribution did not differ between responders and nonresponders. In addition, the ethnic group distribution of the responders was similar to that of the nonresponders. There appeared to be no biases that would cause serious concerns when studying the relationship of blood pressure and the characteristics of the study population.

The subject's upper-arm circumference was measured with a steel tape to select a cuff of appropriate bladder width, ie, a cuff with a bladder that could completely encircle the circumference of the arm. The same trained and certified observer performed blood pressure measurements on the right arm of all subjects after they had been seated for approximately 5 minutes. A standard desktop mercury sphygmomanometer (Baumanometer, W. A. Baum Co Inc, Copiague, NY) was used to measure the systolic and fourth- and fifth-phase diastolic blood pressures. Three measurements were performed; the last two were averaged and used in the analyses.

Trained observers followed standard methods for the anthropometric measurements.[8] Height was measured with the subject wearing no shoes, standing with arms at sides, legs straight, feet together (toes and heels), knees together, eyes looking straight ahead, and shoulders, buttocks, and heels against a steel tape firmly attached to a wall. The zero mark of the tape was placed at foot level.

Table 2.—Distribution of Secondary Sex Characteristics by Race

	Secondary Sex Characteristics, %			
	Breast*		Pubic Hair†	
Stage	Black	White	Black	White
1	22	22	21	34
2	16	26	15	19
3	23	24	15	16
4	25	22	37	22
5	14	6	12	9

*$\chi^2=14.97$, $df=4$, $P=.005$.
†$\chi^2=15.63$, $df=4$, $P=.004$.

The edge of a plastic right angle was placed on the top of a subject's head to form a 90° angle with the wall. The measurement was read to the nearest millimeter. Weight was measured on a beam balance scale. Without shoes and in light clothing, the subject stood still in the middle of the platform. The observer first moved the biggest balance weight, then the smaller upper balance, until the indicator on the balance stabilized at zero. The measurement was read to the nearest 0.1 kg. The scale was calibrated each day with dead weights matching the expected weights of the participants. The body-mass index (kg/m^2) was calculated on the basis of the height and weight measurements. The ratio of weight to the square of height was used to estimate total body fat.[9]

To determine the stage of sexual development as described by Tanner,[10] each subject self-assessed her secondary sex characteristics according to drawings of the breast and pubic hair maturation stages.[11] Pearson correlation coefficients of 0.63 and 0.81 for breast and pubic hair stages, respectively, were reported by Morris and Udry[11] from a validity study of the self-assessment method. Their study population consisted of 12- to 16-year-olds. Frankowski et al[12] investigated the ability of children aged 7 through 12 years to perform self-assessment from drawings of the maturation stages. There was a strong correlation with physician ratings for breast stage ($r=.75$) and pubic hair stage ($r=.88$). Because of the success of the self-assessment method in these studies, it was used in the current study.

Smoking history, menstrual history, and oral contraceptive use were obtained from each participant during a standard interview with a research assistant. All items were close-ended.

Subject and parental health histories, subject medication use, and parental education and occupation were collected by means of a questionnaire that was mailed, with instructions for completion, to the parents of each subject. All questions were close-ended. Whether the mother, father, or both parents completed the interview was not determined.

Comparisons of blood pressure, height, weight, and body-mass index between the black and white girls were based on two-tailed t tests. The χ^2 test was used to compare the distributions of socioeconomic status and sexual maturation between the two race groups. Analysis of covariance was used to compare the mean blood pressure levels of the black and white girls, adjusting for possible confounding effects due to differing independent variable distributions in the two groups. Because misleading results can be obtained if inappropriate variables are used to adjust blood pressure differences between groups, only variables that were significantly associated with the dependent variable, systolic or diastolic blood pressure, were included as covariates in the analysis.

RESULTS

Race Differences in Socioeconomic Status, Anthropometric Parameters, and Sexual Maturation

The study population comprised 142 black girls and 361 white girls (Table 1). The mean age of the black girls (10.6±2.7 years) did not differ from that of the white girls

Table 3.—Median Ages at Entry to Sexual Maturation Stages

	Median Age by Race, y	
	Black	White
Breast stage		
2	8.47	9.28
3	9.65	11.00
4	11.85	12.91
Pubic hair stage		
2	8.36	9.69
3	9.51	11.25
4	10.71	12.61

Table 4.—Mean Blood Pressure by Race and Age

Age Category, y	Blood Pressure, mm Hg: Race, White	Black	Difference Between Means (95% Confidence Interval)
Systolic			
7-9	100.3 (7.86)	98.1 (8.87)	2.2 (−0.52 to 4.92)
10-12	108.1 (11.21)	102.7 (9.86)	5.4 (2.01 to 8.78)
13-15	113.3 (9.64)	109.4 (9.67)	3.9 (−0.50 to 8.30)
16-18	113.4 (9.54)	111.6 (10.59)	1.8 (−7.33 to 10.93)
Fourth-Phase Diastolic			
7-9	66.0 (6.66)	64.1 (6.89)	1.9 (−0.26 to 4.06)
10-12	71.9 (6.93)	68.1 (6.16)	3.8 (1.69 to 5.91)
Fifth-Phase Diastolic			
13-15	69.9 (6.92)	67.2 (7.02)	2.7 (−0.49 to 5.89)
16-18	74.2 (7.81)	69.8 (5.90)	4.4 (−1.74 to 10.54)

*Values are mean (SD).

(10.7±2.3 years). There was, however, a significant difference in the socioeconomic status distributions. The majority of the white girls were in the top two socioeconomic status categories, whereas the majority of the black girls were in the second and third socioeconomic status categories. However, in a univariate regression analysis of socioeconomic status and blood pressure, socioeconomic status was not significantly associated with systolic or diastolic blood pressure.

The black girls were significantly taller (by an average of 6 cm) and heavier (by an average of 6 kg) than the white girls at ages 7, 9, and 12 years and significantly taller (but not heavier) at ages 10 and 14 years. The body-mass index was used as an indicator of body fat. Body mass did not differ between the black and white girls at any age.

A significantly larger percentage of the black girls were at the more advanced stages (Tanner stages 4 and 5) of sexual maturation than the white girls (Table 2). For breast stage, 39% of the black girls were at either stage 4 or 5 compared with 28% of the white girls. For pubic hair stage, 49% of the black girls were at either stage 4 or 5 compared with 31% of the white girls.

The Spearman-Karber procedure was used in a manner similar to that of Villarreal et al[13] to estimate the median age at entry into the breast and pubic hair stages. This procedure allows the use of cross-sectional data. Black girls had younger median ages of entry into all stages compared with white girls (Table 3).

All girls were questioned about their menstrual status. A larger percentage of the black girls (36%) had reached menarche than the white girls (24%, $P<.01$), even though the age distributions and mean ages were the same.

Race Differences in Blood Pressure

Table 4 presents the mean (SD) systolic and diastolic blood pressures for participants classified by racial group and age. Black girls had higher mean systolic and diastolic blood pressures than white girls in every age category. These differences were statistically significant only in the 10- to 12-year-old age category. However, the 95% confidence intervals around the differences in mean blood pressure between the black and white girls for the age categories of 7 through 9 and 13 through 15 years were close to not including the null value.

The unadjusted means for systolic and fourth- and fifth-phase diastolic blood pressure differed significantly between the black and white girls (Table 5). Fourth-phase diastolic blood pressures were compared for the girls less than 13 years of age in accordance with the recommendations of the Second Task Force on Blood Pressure Control in Children.[3] As indicated by the 95% confidence intervals, the mean blood pressure differences ranged between 1.4 and 5.6 mm Hg. The mean levels of the black girls were significantly higher than the mean levels of the white girls.

Race Differences in Adjusted Blood Pressure

Height, weight, and maturation stage were included in analysis of covariance models to test the differences in blood pressure between the black and white girls. The mean systolic and diastolic blood pressures for each ethnic group, unadjusted and adjusted for each covariate, are shown in Table 6. Correcting for the covariates of height, weight, or pubic hair stage did not change the pattern of differences in blood pressure between the black and white groups. The mean blood pressure remained higher for the black girls than the white girls, but the differences were no longer significant. Adjusting for sexual maturation (pubic hair or breast stage) produced results similar to those after adjusting for body size (height or weight).

COMMENT

This study examined blood pressure levels and the timing of sexual maturation among young black and white female participants in a cross-sectional survey. At the time of the survey, same-aged black girls were more sexually mature than white girls. The black girls also had entered each stage of breast development and pubic hair growth at a younger median age. Black participants had higher mean systolic and diastolic blood pressure levels in all age categories and as a group. Adjustment for body size, represented by height or weight, and adjustment for sexual maturation, represented by secondary sex characteristics, equally reduced the blood pressure differences. Thus, the stage of sexual maturation may play a significant role in the assessment of blood pressure level during adolescence. Recording the stage of sexual maturation of a subject at blood pressure measurement may be as important as recording height and weight.

Sexual maturation is a complex process represented by many physical, physiologic, and hormonal changes, some of which could be related to blood pressure patterns. Because body size, represented by height and/or weight, is highly correlated with the stage of maturation, it is difficult

Table 5.—Differences in Unadjusted Mean Blood Pressure Between Black and White Girls

	Blood Pressure, mm Hg		
	Race*		Difference Between Means
	Black	White	(95% Confidence Interval)
Systolic	106.2	102.7	3.5 (1.4 to 5.6)
Fourth-phase diastolic	70.4	67.5	2.9 (1.5 to 4.4)
Fifth-phase diastolic	66.0	63.1	2.9 (1.4 to 4.6)

*Values are means.

Table 6.—Mean Blood Pressure Adjusted by Covariates

	Blood Pressure by Race, mm Hg*	
	Black	White
	Systolic	
Unadjusted	106.18	102.67
Adjusted by		
Weight	105.12±0.71	103.09±0.44
Height	105.08±0.75	103.10±0.47
Pubic hair†	105.00±0.81	103.14±0.50
	Fourth-Phase Diastolic	
Unadjusted	70.41	67.50
Adjusted by		
Weight	69.79±0.53	67.75±0.33
Height	69.71±0.53	67.78±0.33
Pubic hair†	69.61±0.56	67.81±0.35
	Fifth-Phase Diastolic	
Unadjusted	66.04	63.15
Adjusted by		
Weight	65.44±0.57	63.38±0.36
Height	65.34±0.56	63.42±0.36
Pubic hair†	65.25±0.59	63.46±0.37

*Values are mean±SD.
†Similar results were generated when breast stage was entered into the model.

to separate these two effects on blood pressure.[14] However, analysis of covariance suggested that their individual effects on blood pressure were similar.

This study was large enough to guard against chance alone being responsible for the differences in mean blood pressure level between the black and white girls. However, the girls in this study may not be representative of a same-aged sample of girls from the US population; thus, the results may not be generalizable to the US population.

The use of the self-assessment method for estimating sexual maturation may be questioned by some. However, several studies have demonstrated that this is a valid method for the assessment of sexual maturation.[11,12] Also, it does not seem reasonable that the black girls would systematically report a higher stage of sexual maturation than the white girls. The median age of entry to each stage linearly increased with chronological age for both the black and white girls; this supports the biologic plausibility of the method.

Additional potential confounding variables not considered in this study were nutritional status and physical activity and fitness of the girls. A confounding variable is a factor associated with both the dependent and independent variables under study. Undernutrition has been reported to be associated with the rate of maturation; however, its association with blood pressure level is unknown. There are data regarding diet composition and blood pressure level; however, the relationship of diet with sexual maturation is unknown. Reliable methods of recording diets during childhood and adolescence are still being developed, so data are difficult to collect. Accurate methods of recording physical activity and fitness during childhood and adolescence are also still being developed. Perhaps the results of and methods developed for the Childhood and Adolescence Trial of Cardiovascular Health, funded by the National Heart, Lung, and Blood Institute at four US field centers, will provide us with reliable and valid methods for assessing cardiovascular risk factors during childhood and adolescence.

Because of the cross-sectional design of this study, it could not be determined whether a difference in the rate of puberty of the black girls compared with the white girls had an influence on the blood pressure level. A longitudinal design would be necessary to observe the rate of maturation. There are, however, no current longitudinal studies that observe rates of sexual maturation by race.

Inherent metabolic differences in maturation between ethnic groups may account for the differences in mean blood pressure level. Perhaps the onset of sexual maturation at an earlier age in black girls produces a more striking blood pressure response than the onset of sexual maturation at a later age in white girls. However, remarkably little is known about the anthropometric and physiologic correlates of sex hormones and the possible effects of increased hormone production during adolescence on blood pressure for either black or white girls. In the United States, the prevalence of essential hypertension in adults is considerably higher among blacks than whites.[15]

Investigating the blood pressure levels of two groups of girls with a different distribution of sexual maturation stages led to the conclusion that the stage of sexual maturation should be taken into consideration at routine blood pressure measurements. Early maturers could be at a higher risk of hypertension as adults.

References

1. Voors AW, Webber LS, Berenson GS. Time course studies of blood pressure in children: the Bogalusa Heart Study. *Am J Epidemiol.* 1979;109:320-334.
2. Gillum RF, Prineas RJ, Horibe H. Maturation vs age: assessing blood pressure by height. *J Natl Med Assoc.* 1982;74:43-46.
3. National Heart, Lung, and Blood Institute's Task Force on Blood Pressure Control in Children. Report of the Second Task Force on Blood Pressure Control in Children. *Pediatrics.* 1987;79:1-25.
4. National Heart, Lung, and Blood Institute's Task Force on Blood Pressure Control in Children. Report of the Task Force on Blood Pressure Control in Children. *Pediatrics.* 1977;59:797-820.
5. Weir MR, Stafford EM, Gregory D, Lawson MA, Pearl W. The relationship between sexual maturity rating, age and increased blood pressure in adolescents. *J Adolesc Health Care.* 1988;9:465-469.
6. Londe S, Johanson A, Kronemer NS, Goldring D. Blood pressure and puberty. *J Pediatr.* 1975;87:896-900.
7. Marshall WA, Tanner JM. Puberty. In: Falkner F, Tanner JM, eds. *Human Growth: A Comprehensive Treatise.* New York, NY: Plenum Press; 1986;2(*Postnatal Growth Neurobiology*):171-209.
8. *A Guide to Pediatric Weighing and Measuring.* Atlanta, Ga: Centers for Disease Control; 1981. US Dept of Health and Human Services.
9. Cronk CE, Roche AF. Race and sex specific reference data for triceps and subscapular skinfolds and weight/stature. *Am*

J Clin Nutr. 1982;35:347-354.
10. Tanner JM. *Growth at Adolescence.* 2nd ed. Boston, Mass: Blackwell Scientific Publications Inc; 1986.
11. Morris WM, Udry JR. Validation of a self-administered instrument to assess stage of adolescent development. *J Youth Adolesc.* 1980;9:271-279.
12. Frankowski B, Duke-Duncan P, Guillot A, McDougal D, Wasserman R, Young P. Young adolescents' self-assessment of sexual maturation. *AJDC.* 1987;141:385-386. Abstract.
13. Villarreal, SF, Martorell R, Mendoza F. Sexual maturation of Mexican-American adolescents. *Am J Hum Biol.* 1989;1:87-95.
14. Frischancho AR, Housh CH. The relationship of maturity rate to body size and body proportions in children and adults. *Human Biol.* 1988;60:759-770.
15. Joint National Committee. The 1988 report of the Joint National Committee on detection, evaluation, and treatment of high blood pressure. *Arch Intern Med.* 1988;148:1023-1038.

BOOK REVIEW

Fasting Girls: The History of Anorexia Nervosa

By Joan Jacobs Brumberg, 370 pp, with illus, $9.95, New York, NY, A Plume Book, New American Library, Division of Penguin Books USA, 1989.

Students of anorexia nervosa and those responsible for treating patients with eating disorders continue to struggle with the question of the cause of this biopsychosocial condition. Perhaps out of frustration and the inherent management difficulties many physicians are quick to embrace the concept of a biologic vulnerability as the organic cause of the disorder. While not dismissing the importance of biologic determinants and the possibility that anorexia nervosa may be a manifestation of an underlying hypothalamic defect, Brumberg builds a convincing case against this simplistic biomedical model. As physicians, we would very much welcome a breakthrough proving that the unusual eating behaviors of patients with eating disorders are somehow the result of an imbalance, deviance, or abnormality of biological processes. If such were the case, it might be prevented by a vaccine for those with a strong family history of eating disorders or treated with a specific hormone or chemical that quickly would alleviate the problem, much like that used for schizophrenia and bipolar and depressive disorders. Stressing the sociocultural influences on the development of anorexia nervosa, the author argues for a multifactorial and asks why, if the cause is primarily organic, there is a predominance of the condition in middle and upper social class women, and why recently there has been an increase in the incidence of this and other eating disorders. Brumberg forced me to reconsider my bias toward accepting the easy answer of biologic predisposition or vulnerability.

In Western society, fasting and purging have been an important part of Judeo-Christian religious practices. In *Fasting Girls* the author traces the history of food refusal from the medieval period, when between 1200 and 1500 the practice was considered to be a characteristic of medieval spirituality. A discussion of female saints, for whom fasting was basic to the model of female holiness, is presented in an early chapter. The emphasis, however, is on the "fasting girls" of the 19th and 20th centuries and the heated debate between physicians on the one side and religious leaders and spiritualists on the other. Increasingly, scientifically minded physicians objected to the idea of a miraculously inspired loss of appetite (anorexia mirabilis). According to Brumberg, "Among certain segments of the Victorian religious community, fasting girls and the fiction of total food abstinence became a way of sustaining belief itself." The 19th-century Victorian family, with its rigidity and possessiveness and its use of food as a reward and punishment, is identified as a major determinant of modern-day anorexia nervosa. In the case of anorexia mirabilis ("holy anorexia"), the quest for purity through self-sacrifice and the belief that there are other forms of sustenance, such as prayer and the Christian Eucharist, provided the driving force for fasting. In making a case that the self-imposed starvation of the saints and of 19th- and 20th-century adolescent women took place under different conditions, the author underscores her belief that to a great extent cultural factors determine the manifestations of this illness.

A fascinating chapter deals with the history of anorexia nervosa and its early introduction into the medical literature. In 1694 Richard Morton, in *Phthisologia; or, a Treatise on Consumptions,* described two cases of "nervous consumption" considered by many to be the first reported cases of anorexia nervosa. Brumberg challenged that assumption and introduced William Stout Chipley (1810 to 1880), who published in the *American Journal of Insanity* the first American description of sitomania, a "phase of insanity" characterized by an "intense dread of food." A discussion of institutionalized patients who rejected food is interesting, but most delightful is the close look at Sir William Withey Gull (1816-1890) who, in 1868 at the annual meeting of the British Medical Association, first made reference to the condition. A most prestigious consultant and physician to Queen Victoria and her family, he was held in high esteem. Nevertheless, it was a Paris neurologist, Charles Lasegue (1816-1883), who preempted Gull's use of the term *anorexia* rather than *apepsia* (indigestion) and emphasized the importance of psychological and family factors, whereas Gull's approach was much more simplistic. The detailed description of the cases of Sarah Jacob, the "Welsh Fasting Girl," and Mollie Fancher, known as the "Brooklyn Enigma," and the raging controversy involving the "feisty" leading neurologists of the day, including William Hammond and George Beard, and eccentric believers (such as spiritualists), pious clergy, and physicians of "secondary status" are most informative and very fascinating.

Brumberg has a nice writing style, which makes it difficult to put the book down. She has made an important contribution to the history of medicine and psychology. It should be required reading for serious students of eating disorders and all those who are actively involved in their diagnosis and treatment.

George D. Comerci, MD
Section of Adolescent/
Young Adult Medicine
Department of Pediatrics
University of Arizona
College of Medicine
Tucson, AZ 85724

Lipoprotein Profiles in Hypercholesterolemic Children

Richard E. Garcia, MD, Douglas S. Moodie, MD

• Atherosclerosis is a process that begins in early life. Coronary heart disease is the result of complex interactions among a variety of risk factors of which hypercholesterolemia is but one. During routine screening, 500 children were identified with total cholesterol levels above the 95th percentile of 5.2 mmol/L (200 mg/dL). Lipoprotein profiles were then performed to confirm and delineate their lipid abnormalities. A definable lipid disorder was present in 85% of such children. Abnormal lipoprotein patterns included 292 children with type IIa, 99 with type IIb, and 25 with type IV phenotypes. An abnormally low high-density lipoprotein cholesterol level of less than 0.9 mmol/L (35 mg/dL) was observed in 20 children. Only 5% of patients were identified as being hypercholesterolemic because they had high-density lipoprotein cholesterol levels above the 95th percentile of 1.8 mmol/L (70 mg/dL). Thirty-two percent of children with total cholesterol levels above 5.2 mmol/L had a family member (sibling, parent, uncle, aunt, or grandparent) with a myocardial infarction prior to 55 years of age. Data from this study support universal cholesterol testing after 3 years of age and lipoprotein profiles for those with levels above 5.2 mmol/L.

(*AJDC.* 1991;145:147–150)

There is increasing evidence that routine cholesterol testing of children after 2 to 3 years of age is both appropriate and productive.[1-3] When a child is identified as having hypercholesterolemia, it is not uncommon to discover a lipid disorder in other family members. Increasing numbers of pediatricians are performing cholesterol screening at early ages,[4] and they are more consistently advising patients and their families to avoid high-risk coronary life-style behaviors such as dietary excess, physical inactivity, and smoking.

A recent cholesterol surveillance study[5] of 6500 children found nearly twice the expected number to have cholesterol levels above the Lipid Research Clinics' 90th percentile of 4.8 mmol/L (185 mg/dL).[6] The present report concerns 500 children from the same study who had lipoprotein profiles performed because they had cholesterol levels above 5.2 mmol/L (200 mg/dL) detected by an earlier screening test. Recognizable types of lipoprotein abnormalities in this population of children and their lipoprotein profile data are presented.

Accepted for publication October 1, 1990.

From the Department of Pediatrics, Cleveland (Ohio) Clinic Foundation.

Reprint requests to Cleveland Clinic Foundation, One Clinic Center, 9500 Euclid Ave, Cleveland, OH 44195-5223 (Dr Garcia).

PATIENTS AND METHODS

The private pediatric practice in which this study was carried out consists of six pediatricians and a pediatric nurse practitioner and is located in Parma Heights, Ohio. The children studied were at least 3 years old, white, and residents of southwest Cleveland suburbs. During routine health care visits, nonfasting total cholesterol levels were observed to be above 5.2 mmol/L (200 mg/dL). The original cholesterol screening was carried out on a fingerstick blood specimen using a reflectance photometer (Reflotron, Boehringer Mannheim Diagnostics, Indianapolis, Ind). An arbitrary decision was made, for purposes of this report, to study prospectively 500 consecutive children on whom lipoprotein profiles were then performed. Ninety percent of the studied population had lipoprotein profiles performed within 1 month of the original cholesterol screening test.

Lipoprotein samples were collected by venipuncture and analyzed with a Dupont Analyst instrument (Dupont Co, Wilmington, Del). Patients were scheduled for the procedure during early morning office hours after an overnight 12-hour fast. The instrument was calibrated daily according to manufacturer's recommendations and control serum samples were used regularly to check for precision and accuracy. Twice weekly, two trained office nurses performed the venipunctures and ran the lipoprotein profiles. The laboratory instrument is an automated microprocessor that photometrically measures the results of enzymatic cleavage of cholesterol ester and hydrolysis of triglycerides. Low-density lipoprotein (LDL) cholesterol was calculated using the standard formula[7]: LDL Cholesterol = Total Cholesterol − High-Density Lipoprotein Cholesterol (HDL) − Triglycerides/5.

The normal distribution of plasma lipid levels in children 3 to 19 years of age is shown in Table 1. The data are derived from the Lipid Research Clinics[8] and the Bogalusa Heart Study.[9] For purposes of this report, lipid levels above the 95th percentile and/or below the 5th percentile are defined as *abnormal.*

RESULTS

Five hundred children had lipoprotein profiles performed in the described pediatric office setting between August 1, 1986, and July 1, 1988. The mean age of the studied population was 8.1 years (range, 3 to 21 years), and the male-female ratio was 1:1 (251:249). Table 2 contains the descriptive statistics for the entire group of patients.

Figure 1 depicts the distribution of the 500 children according to important LDL cholesterol cutoff points as defined by the National Cholesterol Education Program for adults.[10] Similar LDL cholesterol reference data and treatment recommendations for children are currently being considered by a panel of experts at the National Heart, Lung, and Blood Institute. Figures 2 through 5 are histograms showing the frequency distribution of LDL cholesterol, HDL cholesterol, and triglyceride levels for the 500 children who had lipoprotein analyses. The mean LDL-HDL ratio for the group was 2.9 (range, 0.9 to 9.5) compared with a normal value of 1.6 in a population of

Table 1.—Expected Distribution of Serum Lipid Levels for Children 3 to 19 Years of Age*			
Serum Lipid Levels	Distribution: 5th Percentile	95th Percentile	Mean
TC	3.1	5.2	4.1
LDL-C	1.7	3.4	2.6
HDL-C	0.9	1.8	1.4
TG	0.4	1.3	0.9

*All values are in millimoles per liter. TC indicates total cholesterol; LDL-C, low-density lipoprotein cholesterol; HDL-C, high-density lipoprotein cholesterol; and TG, triglycerides.

Table 2.—Descriptive Statistics of 500 Hypercholesterolemic Children Whose Lipoprotein Profiles Were Tested*

Variable	Minimum	Maximum	Mean ± SD
Age, y	3	21	8.1 ± 4
TC	3.7	9.6	5.7 (220.9) ± 0.8 (29.9)
HDL	0.7	2.7	1.4 (54.4) ± 0.3 (12.7)
LDL	2.1	8.1	3.9 (149.4) ± 0.8 (30.3)
TG	0.3	5.6	1.1 (94.4) ± 0.6 (50.1)
LDL-HDL ratio	0.9	9.5	2.9 ± 1

*All lipid levels are in millimoles per liter. TC indicates total cholesterol; HDL, high-density lipoprotein; LDL, low-density lipoprotein; and TG, triglycerides.

8000 school-age children in Bogalusa, La.[11]

The frequency of recognizable abnormal lipoprotein patterns in these 500 patients based on the classification of hyperlipoproteinemia types described by Fredrickson et al[12] was as follows. There were 292 patients (58%) classified as type IIa with LDL levels higher than 3.4 mmol/L (130 mg/dL) and triglyceride levels higher than 1.3 mmol/L (110 mg/dL); 99 patients (20%) as type IIb with LDL levels higher than 3.4 mmol/L and triglyceride levels lower than 1.3 mmol/L; 25 patients (5%) as type IV with LDL levels lower than 3.4 mmol/L and triglyceride levels higher than 1.3 mmol/L; 20 (4%) as "low HDL" with HDL levels lower than 0.90 mmol/L (35 mg/dL), who were further divided into two groups of those with LDL levels higher than 3.4 mmol/L (n = 13) and those with levels lower than 3.4 mmol/L (n = 7). More information regarding lipid disorders in family members is required to make specific genotypic diagnoses. Familial hyperlipidemias may become evident as careful pedigrees are constructed for these children.

Twenty-three percent (n = 116) of the children who originally had total cholesterol levels above the 95th percentile of 5.2 mmol/L (200 mg/dL) had LDL cholesterol levels lower than the 95th percentile of 3.4 mmol/L (130 mg/dL) when they had lipoprotein profiles performed. Fifty-six of the children whose total cholesterol levels were greater than 5.2 mmol/L had LDL cholesterol levels below the 95th percentile because they had high HDL cholesterol and/or triglyceride levels. Similarly, 60 children had LDL cholesterol levels below the 95th percentile because their total cholesterol levels had fallen below 5.2 mmol/L (Fig 6). Only 15 patients (3%) who had lipoprotein profiles performed were found to have total cholesterol levels lower than the 75th percentile of 4.4 mmol/L (170 mg/dL).

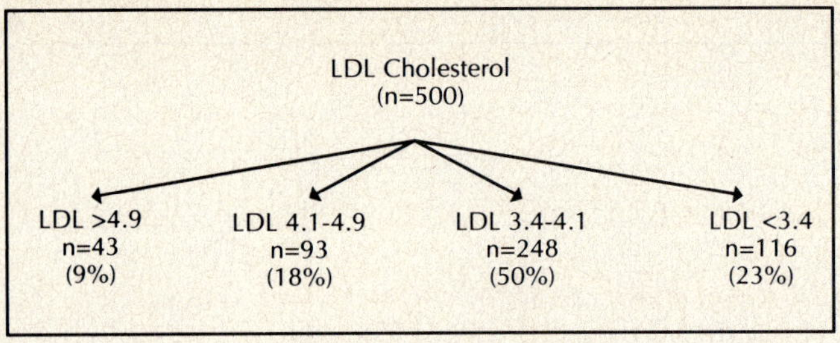

Fig 1.—*Distribution of 500 hypercholesterolemic children who underwent a lipid profile test, according to low-density lipoprotein (LDL) cholesterol levels. All values are in micromoles per liter.*

COMMENT

Evidence is overwhelming that atherosclerosis begins early in life.[13-15] Coronary artery disease results from complex interactions among various well-recognized risk factors, of which hypercholesterolemia is but one.[16] Heredity (genetic disorders of lipoprotein metabolism) as well as environment (poor nutritional behaviors, sedentary lifestyle, and smoking) play important roles in the evolution of the disease process. Cholesterol surveillance in childhood allows the pediatrician to identify some, but not all, genetic disorders of lipid metabolism in early life. Not uncommonly, an identified hypercholesterolemic child serves as the index case to uncover a familial lipid disorder. For purposes of this report, the term *family member* includes siblings, parents, grandparents, aunts, and uncles.

Excessive dietary saturated fat and cholesterol, familial hypercholesterolemia, familial combined hyperlipidemia, and polygenic hypercholesterolemia can all be responsible for the isolated high levels of LDL cholesterol characteristic of type IIa hyperlipidemia. Type IIb hyperlipidemia is present when both LDL cholesterol and triglyceride levels are elevated and familial combined hyperlipidemia is the usual cause. Elevation of the triglyceride level alone characterizes the type IV phenotype that can be caused by familial hypertriglyceridemia, familial combined hyperlipidemia, or the nonfasting state. More complete family history and lipoprotein profile data are gradually being gathered from family members of these hypercholesterolemic children, and will enable genotypic classification, genetic counseling, and more specific treatment.

Accuracy and consistency of blood lipid measurements in the office setting have been issues of concern.[17] There was remarkable agreement between cholesterol levels from one period to another in this group of patients despite using two different instruments to perform the test. Only 3% (n = 15) of the population identified by routine screening had a normal cholesterol level (<75th percentile) at the time of subsequent lipoprotein analysis, and 93% had levels above the 90th percentile of 4.8 mmol/L (185 mg/dL). Similarly, 77% of children who were determined to be hypercholesterolemic by routine screening had LDL cholesterol levels above the 95th percentile, and only 2.5% had levels below the mean of 2.6 mmol/L (100 mg/dL). With careful attention to quality control, the instruments used for office lipid measurements have been shown to be 97% accurate.[18] On the basis of office lipoprotein analyses alone, it is important to note that no treatment was provided for these children other than advice regarding diet and risk factor avoidance. Patients with more severe or complex hyperlipidemia and those for whom drug therapy became a consideration were candidates for referral to pediatric lipid clinics for evaluation and treatment. Children with LDL cholesterol levels above 4.1 mmol/L (160

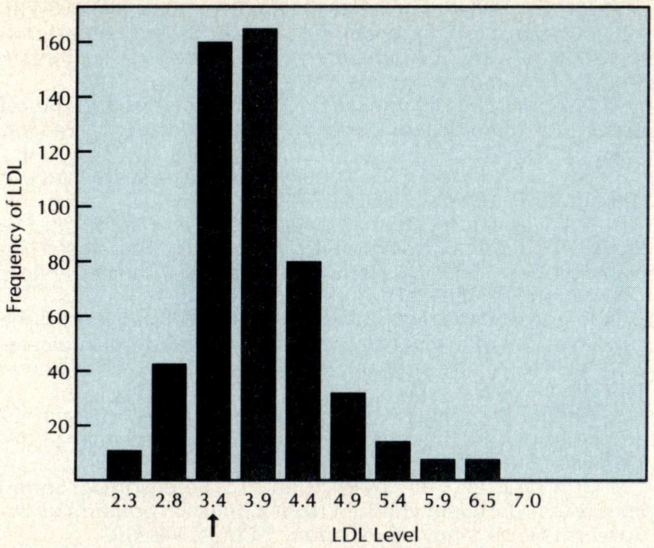

Fig 2.—*Distribution of 500 patients according to low-density lipoprotein (LDL) cholesterol levels. Arrow indicates 95th percentile for age. All values are in micromoles per liter.*

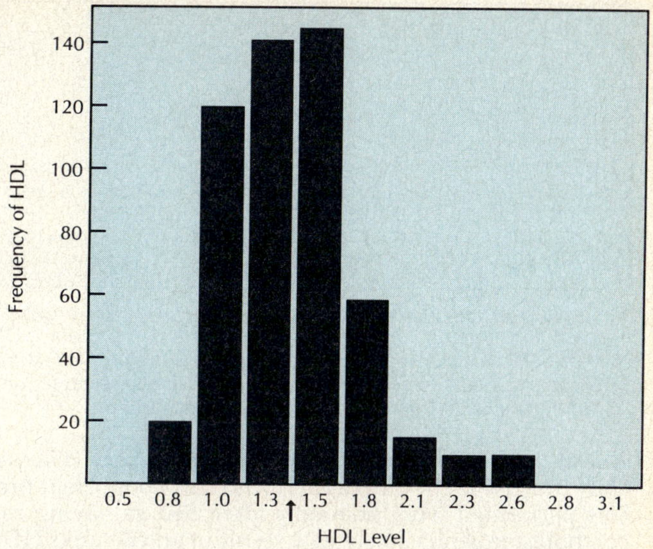

Fig 4.—*Distribution of 500 patients according to high-density lipoprotein (HDL) cholesterol levels. Arrow indicates mean HDL cholesterol level. All values are in micromoles per liter.*

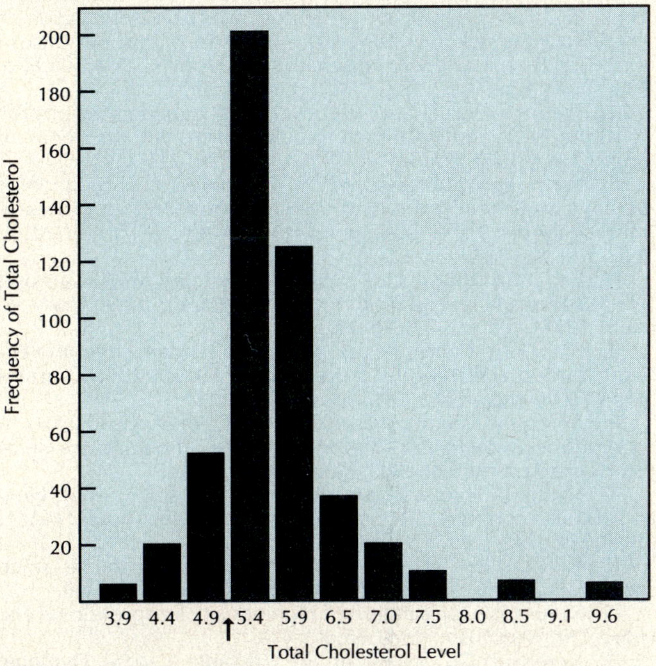

Fig 3.—*Distribution of 500 patients according to total cholesterol levels. Arrow indicates 95th percentile for age. All values are in micromoles per liter.*

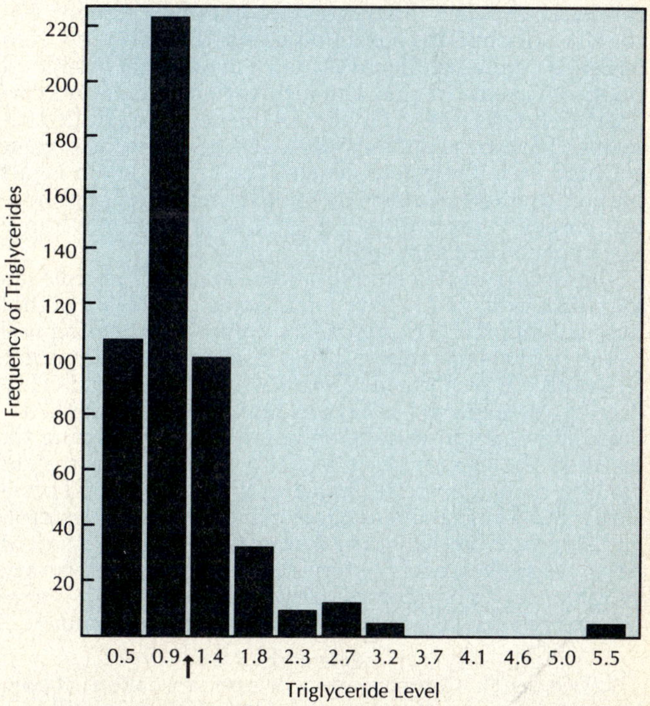

Fig 5.—*Distribution of 500 patients according to triglyceride levels. Arrow indicates 95th percentile for age. All values are in micromoles per liter.*

mg/dL) despite appropriate dietary changes, especially with a family history of premature coronary heart disease, were considered for referral.

An elevated HDL cholesterol level is antiatherogenic, and a low level is an independent risk factor for coronary artery disease.[19] High-density lipoprotein cholesterol levels are not predictive of adult levels, however, until puberty, according to the Bogalusa Heart Study.[20] Fifty-three (10.6%) of the 500 patients studied were found to have HDL cholesterol levels above the 95th percentile of 1.8 mmol/L (70 mg/dL). Thirty-seven families could be contacted for questioning, and 11 (30%) reported a family member who had a myocardial infarction prior to 55 years of age. An abnormally low HDL cholesterol level of less than 0.9 mmol/L (35 mg/dL) was observed in 20 children (4%), and seven of the 15 families contacted similarly reported a family member with premature myocardial infarction. The mean LDL cholesterol levels in these two groups of patients were 3.4 mmol/L (132 mg/dL) and 4.0 mmol/L (153 mg/dL), respectively, both well above the 95th percentile. High-density lipoprotein cholesterol levels in the studied population do not appear to be as important a predictor of coronary artery disease in their families as do LDL cholesterol levels. Children can have total cholesterol levels above the 95th percentile because their HDL cholesterol levels are very high. They are protected

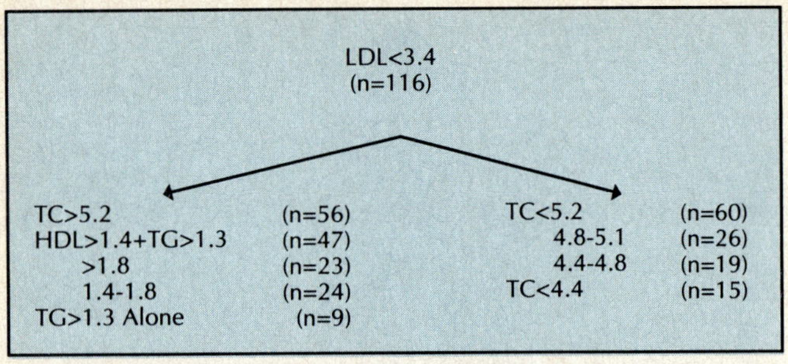

Fig 6.—*Distribution of causative factors to explain why 116 originally hypercholesterolemic children had low-density lipoprotein (LDL) cholesterol levels below the 95th percentile on lipid profile testing. TC indicates total cholesterol; HDL, high-density lipoprotein; and TG, triglycerides. All values are in micromoles per liter.*

and at reduced risk for future coronary artery disease. Only 5% (n = 23) of the children who had lipoprotein profiles performed were originally identified as having hypercholesterolemia solely as a result of an elevated HDL cholesterol level.

Fifty percent of children found to have LDL cholesterol levels above the 95th percentile of 3.4 mmol/L (130 mg/dL) had no known family history of premature coronary heart disease or hypercholesterolemia. Of the 500 families of the children who had lipoprotein profiles performed, 374 could be reached for questioning and 123 (32%) reported having a family member who had a myocardial infarction prior to 55 years of age. The incidence of premature coronary heart disease in families of the children studied remained fairly constant regardless of the magnitude of their elevated LDL cholesterol levels. The Framingham Heart Study[21] predicts an approximate 15% incidence of premature coronary heart disease in families of children who are not hypercholesterolemic.

The results of this study indicate that 85% of children identified with nonfasting total cholesterol levels higher than 5.2 mmol/L (200 mg/dL) by universal screening will have a definable phenotypic lipid disorder when a lipoprotein profile is performed. Thirty-two percent of such children can be expected to have a family member with a myocardial infarction prior to 55 years of age. Screening for elevated cholesterol levels leads to discussion of weight control, regular exercise, smoking avoidance, blood pressure monitoring, and reduction of dietary salt, cholesterol, and saturated fat. Advice and example regarding prudent life-style choices, early dietary intervention, and, in an appropriate few, pharmacotherapy surely will reduce the incidence of coronary heart disease in years to come.

References

1. Wynder EL. Coronary artery disease prevention: cholesterol, a pediatric perspective. *Prev Med.* 1989;18:323-409.
2. Wappner RS, Brandt IK. Inborn errors of metabolism, disorders of lipoproteins. In: Oski FA, ed. *Principles and Practice of Pediatrics.* Philadelphia, Pa: JB Lippincott Co; 1990:108-110.
3. Kwiterovich P, Berenson GS. Pediatrics and cholesterol-related issues. In: *A Lipid Letter.* New York, NY: Healthmark Medical Education Programs; 1989;6.
4. Jacobson NS, Lillienfeld DE. Current literature and clinical issues: the pediatrician's role in atherosclerosis. *J Pediatr.* 1988;112:836-841.
5. Garcia RE, Moodie DS. Routine cholesterol surveillance in childhood. *Pediatrics.* 1989;84:751-755.
6. Lipid Research Clinics. *Population Studies Data Book: The Prevalence Study.* Washington, DC: US Dept of Health and Human Services; 1980. US Dept of Health and Human Services publication NIH 80-1527.
7. Friedewald WT, Levy RI, Fredrickson DS. Estimation of the concentration of low density lipoprotein cholesterol in plasma without use of the preparative ultracentrifuge. *Clin Chem.* 1972;18:499-502.
8. Rifkind BM, Segal P. Lipid Research Clinics Program reference values for hyperlipidemia and hypolipidemia. *JAMA.* 1983;250:1869-1872.
9. Srinivasan SR, Frerichs RR, Weber LS, Berenson GS. Serum lipoprotein profile in children from a biracial community: the Bogalusa Heart Study. *Circulation.* 1976;54:309-318.
10. The Expert Panel. Report of the National Cholesterol Education Program Expert Panel on detection, evaluation, and treatment of high blood cholesterol in adults. *Arch Intern Med.* 1988;148:36-61.
11. Berenson GS, Webber LS, Srinivasan SR, Cresanta JL, Frank GC, Farris RD. Black-white contrasts as determinants of cardiovascular risk in childhood: precursors of coronary artery and primary hypertensive diseases. *Am Heart J.* 1984;108:672-683.
12. Fredrickson DS, Levy RI, Lees RS. Fat transport in lipoproteins: an integrated approach to mechanisms and disorders. *N Engl J Med.* 1967;276:34-44, 94-103, 148-156, 215-225.
13. Newman WP, Freedman DS, Voors AW, et al. Relation of serum lipoprotein levels and systolic blood pressure to early atherosclerosis: the Bogalusa Heart Study. *N Engl J Med.* 1986;314:138-144.
14. Enos WF, Holmes RH, Boyer J. Coronary disease among United States soldiers killed in action in Korea: preliminary report. *JAMA.* 1953;152:1090-1093.
15. Stary HC. Macrophages, macrophage foam cells, and eccentric internal thickening in the coronary arteries of young children. *Atherosclerosis.* 1987;64:91-108.
16. Berenson GS, Srinivasan SR, Mac D, et al. Risk factors in early life as predictors of adult heart disease: the Bogalusa Heart Study. *Am J Med Sci.* 1989;298:141-151.
17. Kaufman HW, McNamara JR, Anderson KA, et al. How reliably can compact chemistry analyzers measure lipids? *JAMA.* 1990;263:1245-1249.
18. Burke JJ II, Fischer PM. A clinician's guide to the office measurement of cholesterol. *JAMA.* 1988;259:3444-3448.
19. Krauss RM. Regulation of high density lipoprotein levels. *Med Clin North Am.* 1982;66:403-418.
20. Berenson GS, Srinivasan SR, Cresanta JL, et al. Dynamic changes of serum lipoproteins in children during adolescence and sexual maturation. *Am J Epidemiol.* 1981;113:157-170.
21. Castelli WP. Cholesterol and lipids in the risk of coronary artery disease: the Framingham Heart Study. *Can J Cardiol.* 1988;4;(supplA):5-10.

Outpatient Assessment of Infants With Bronchiolitis

Kathy N. Shaw, MD, MS; Louis M. Bell, MD; Nancy H. Sherman, MD

• Two hundred thirteen infants younger than 13 months with bronchiolitis were prospectively followed up to identify the historical, physical, and laboratory clues at initial emergency department evaluation that would help to predict disease severity. Based on their total course of illness, the patients were classified as having mild (139 patients) or severe (74 patients) disease, and the initial emergency department evaluation findings of these two groups were compared. Six independent clinical and laboratory findings were identified that were strongly associated with more severe illness: (1) "ill" or "toxic" general appearance; (2) oxygen saturation less than 95%, as determined by pulse oximetry; (3) gestational age, younger than 34 weeks; (4) respiratory rate, 70/min or greater; (5) atelectasis on a chest roentgenogram; and (6) age, younger than 3 months. The infant's oxygen saturation as determined by pulse oximetry was the single best objective predictor of more severe disease.

(*AJDC.* 1991;145:151–155)

Physicians are often faced with evaluating infants with bronchiolitis and deciding which infants have more severe disease that may require hospitalization. Respiratory syncytial virus (RSV) is probably the most important respiratory pathogen among young children and may cause serious morbidity and mortality.[1-6] Approximately 50% of infants will acquire RSV infection during the first epidemic that they experience, and approximately 13 infants per 1000 require hospitalization in lower income populations.[6-9] Of particular concern is that hypoxemia is often present and may not correlate with the clinical impression of the severity of the disease.[10] In addition, the risk factors for morbidity have been identified only among infants who have been already hospitalized and who represent the "tip of the iceberg" of this disease.[7,10-21] The purpose of our study was to identify at the *initial* outpatient evaluation those historical, physical, and laboratory clues that may predict more severe disease.

Accepted for publication August 17, 1990.

From the Section of Emergency Medicine, Divisions of General Pediatrics (Drs Shaw and Bell) and Infectious Diseases (Dr Bell), Department of Pediatrics, and the Department of Radiology (Dr Sherman), The Children's Hospital of Philadelphia (Pa). Dr Sherman is now with the Department of Medical Imaging, Alfred I. DuPont Institute, Wilmington, Del.

Presented in part at the Annual Meeting of the Ambulatory Pediatric Association, Washington, DC, May 3, 1988.

Reprint requests to Department of Emergency Medicine, The Children's Hospital of Philadelphia, 34th Street and Civic Center Boulevard, Philadelphia, PA 19104 (Dr Shaw).

PATIENTS AND METHODS

All children who presented to The Children's Hospital of Philadelphia (Pa) Emergency Department during the 1987 epidemic season for RSV bronchiolitis (January through April) and who were (1) younger than 13 months, (2) had signs of lower airway disease such as tachypnea, rales, or wheezing, and (3) had a history of a preceding upper respiratory tract infection were eligible for the study. Following routine emergency department evaluation and treatment by the resident physician and senior-level supervising physician, a disposition was made.

At this point, the infant's condition was reassessed by the emergency department attending staff who were present 24 hours per day, and study data were obtained. The severity of respiratory distress was assessed by using the Clinical Asthma score.[22] General appearance was judged as "well appearing," "ill—not toxic," or "toxic" and also was quantified by using the Yale Observation Scale (YOS).[23] The infant's oxygen saturation in room air, both while the infant was quiet and while he or she was sucking on a bottle, was determined by using pulse oximetry. The oxygen saturation was read when the pulse oximeter (Nellcor Inc, Hayward, Calif) correctly reflected the infant's heart rate. Measurement of oxygen saturation was not part of the infant's routine evaluation.

Laboratory evaluation included anteroposterior and lateral chest roentgenograms that were subsequently read by a staff radiologist (N.H.S.) who was blinded to the clinical presentation of the patient. Nasopharyngeal aspirates were sent to the laboratory for viral isolation in tissue culture and for testing with a rapid immunoassay, RSV enzyme-linked immunosorbent assay[24,25] (Abbott Laboratories, North Chicago, Ill), that detects the presence of RSV in respiratory secretions.

Infants enrolled in the study were scheduled for reevaluation by the primary investigators (K.N.S. and L.M.B.) 24 to 72 hours after the emergency department visit, and additional follow-up visits or telephone calls were made until the patient was judged to be clinically "well." After resolution of the symptoms, the enrolled infants were divided into "mild disease" or "severe disease" groups. Infants were judged to have had mild disease if they remained alert and active and were well hydrated while they were taking fluids orally throughout their illness. The *initial* emergency department evaluation findings of these two groups of infants were compared to establish which historical, physical examination, and laboratory clues were associated with severity of disease.

Only study information with an 80% or greater response or completion rate was included in the data analysis. The χ^2, Mann-Whitney *U*, or *t* test was used to determine which individual components of the initial emergency department evaluation were associated with severity of disease, and the relative risk (RR) of having severe disease was calculated for each of these findings. Discriminant analysis was then used to determine a model of clinical and laboratory findings that would best predict illness severity. An a priori level of statistical significance was chosen at .05. The study protocol was approved by the hospital's Human Subjects Committee.

Table 1.—Historical Information Associated With Severity of Disease*

	%				
	Total (N=213)	Severe Disease (n=74)	Mild Disease (n=139)	RR	95% Confidence Intervals
History of cyanosis or apnea	5	12	1†	2.76	2.02-3.77
Gestational age, wk					
<34	5	27	13†	2.55	1.86-3.50
<37	25	43	15†	2.31	1.63-3.27
Age, <3 mo	24	38	16†	1.93	1.36-2.74
Decreased PO intake	65	77	58‡	1.82	1.15-2.90
Perinatal complications	41	54	34‡	1.70	1.18-2.46
URI symptoms, ≤3 d	48	58	43§	1.48	1.02-2.16

*RR indicates relative risk; PO, oral (by mouth); and URI, upper respiratory tract infection.
†$P<.001$.
‡$P<.01$.
§$P<.05$.

Table 2.—Physical Examination: Findings and Observations Associated With Severity of Disease*

	%				
	Total (N=213)	Severe Disease (n=74)	Mild Disease (n=139)	RR	95% Confidence Intervals
General appearance—"ill" or "toxic"	41	76	24†	4.56	2.71-7.69
Yale Observation Scale score, ≥10	24	52	12†	3.30	2.24-4.85
Accessory muscle use	46	72	33†	3.01	1.94-4.66
Clinical Asthma Score, ≥2	50	73	38†	2.68	1.71-4.21
Respiratory rate, per minute					
≥70	14	29	5†	2.60	1.90-3.57
≥60	37	54	28†	2.01	1.39-2.90
Rales	24	40	16†	2.09	1.44-3.02

*RR indicates relative risk.
†$P<.001$.

RESULTS

Study Population and Outcome

Of the 228 study infants with bronchiolitis who were evaluated in our emergency department, 213 had adequate follow-up to judge eventual outcome and severity of illness. Of the 148 patients (65%) who were initially discharged from the emergency department, 89 returned for follow-up appointments. The parents of an additional 44 patients were reached by telephone and were not requested to return because they reported improvement with normal oral feeding and activity. Ninety patients were admitted at some point during their illness (80 directly and 10 at follow-up visits).

Based on their total course of illness, the patients were classified into two groups: (1) 139 patients with mild disease (16 who were judged to be hospitalized inappropriately based on results of follow-up evaluations, and 123 who were discharged from the emergency department with resolution of their illness), and (2) 74 patients with more severe disease (64 who were hospitalized initially and 10 who were hospitalized at follow-up). Of these 74 patients with more severe disease, 59 (80%) received oxygen therapy, 13 (18%) were admitted to the intensive care unit, and eight (11%) underwent mechanical ventilation.

Historical Information

The average±SD age of the babies in the study was 5.6±3.1 months. Most of the patients were black (86%) and male (62%). This was a largely lower socioeconomic group, with 79% either having no medical insurance or receiving medical assistance.

Historical factors associated with more severe disease and their RRs are presented in Table 1. The sex of the infant, a history of exposure to a smoker in the family (66%), whether the baby had been breast-fed (14%), a history (37%) or family history (71%) of wheezing, and the parental report of the duration of wheezing (median, 4 days) were not associated with disease severity.

Physical Examination Findings

Most infants were described as "well appearing" on physical examination and were afebrile (68%, <38.3°C). Eighty-six percent had a YOS score less than 10 (scale, 6 through 30), and 50% scored less than 2 on the Clinical Asthma Score (scale, 0 through 10).

Physical examination findings associated with disease severity and their RRs are given in Table 2. The presence (86%) or degree of wheezing on auscultation, the infant's temperature, the presence of a cough (91%) or nasal discharges (82%), and subjective response to epinephrine hydrochloride.

Laboratory Evaluation

The RSV enzyme-linked immunosorbent assay test and viral-culturing techniques were able to identify a viral pathogen or chlamydia in approximately half of patients (48%). Respiratory syncytial virus constituted 42%, and parainfluenza (type III), enterovirus, and chlamydia constituted 2% each.

Infants with more severe disease had lower oxygen saturations as determined by pulse oximetry. Clinical judgment of a baby's color, which is used in the YOS, correlated with oxygen saturations below 95% in only 45% of the cases. Chest roentgenograms of the babies with more severe illness were more likely to show atelectasis and hyperaeration, but not peribronchial thickening. Respiratory syncytial virus was also subsequently identified more often in patients with more severe disease (Table 3).

Multiple-Factor Analysis

Discriminant analysis identified six clinical and laboratory findings that were independently and strongly associated with more severe disease: (1) general appearance of the infant, (2) oxygen saturation as determined by pulse oximetry, (3) gestational age, (4) respiratory rate, (5) presence of atelectasis on a chest roentgenogram, and (6) current age ($r=.67$, $R^2=.45$, F=21.5 [6, 158]). The combination of these six variables maintained good specificity

Table 3.—Laboratory Findings Associated With Severity of Illness*

		%			
	Total (N=213)	Severe Disease (n=74)	Mild Disease (n=139)	RR	95% Confidence Intervals
Pulse oximetry—while quiet					
Oxygen saturation, <97%	25	54	11†	3.44	2.38-4.98
Oxygen saturation, <95%	12	32	2†	3.28	2.42-4.43
Pulse oximetry—while sucking					
Oxygen saturation, <97%	32	71	14†	5.19	2.71-9.97
Oxygen saturation, <95%	18	58	0†	6.31‡	3.83-10.39‡
Chest roentgenograms					
Atelectasis	9	21	2†	2.70	1.97-3.70
Hyperaeration	58	69	52§	1.58	1.03-2.42
Viral isolation					
RSV	42	52	35§	1.53	1.06-2.20

*RR indicates relative risk; RSV, respiratory syncytial virus.
†$P<.001$.
‡Estimated.
§$P<.05$.

Table 4.—Model of Six Independent Factors Associated With Severity of Illness: Sensitivity, Specificity, and Predictive Value

	%			
			Predictive Value	
	Sensitivity	Specificity	Positive	Negative
General appearance "ill" or "toxic"	76	76	60	87
Pulse oximetry—while quiet				
<97%	54	89	72	79
<95%	32	98	87	73
Gestational age, <34 wk	27	95	74	71
Respiratory rate, ≥70/min	29	95	75	71
Chest roentgenogram with/without atelectasis	21	98	82	70
Age, <3 mo	38	83	55	72
Six-variable model	76	91	81	88

(91%) with higher sensitivity (76%) when compared with any individual factor (Table 4). The predictive values, positive and negative, were 81% and 88%, respectively. When only those infants with documented RSV infection were included, this group of findings was still good ($r=.68$, $R^2=.46$, $F=8.43$ [6, 59]) with a sensitivity and specificity of 86% and 91%, respectively, and predictive values (positive and negative, respectively) of 86% and 91%.

In an attempt to utilize only clinical observations during outpatient evaluation, as would occur in office practice, pulse oximetry and roentgenograms were removed from the regression equation and replaced with the "color" observation item on the YOS, which was strongly correlated ($r=.66$) with pulse oximetry results, but not as sensitive in discriminating low oxygen saturations. No individual clinical finding correlated well with atelectasis on a chest roentgenogram. This model ($r=.64$, $R^2=.41$, $F=23.7$ [5, 172]) was less sensitive in discerning severity of illness (65%), but maintained specificity (90%). Predictive values, positive and negative, were 74% and 85%, respectively.

Clinical Judgment at Initial Evaluation

Overall, clinical judgment, as reflected by the decision to admit babies to the hospital, was good in our emergency department, which has attending physician supervision at all times. However, too much importance may have been attributed to a history of prematurity in the presence of a benign evaluation, as the 16 infants who were hospitalized but had mild disease were more likely to have had a history of prematurity (42% vs 17%; $P<.04$). Otherwise, the initial outpatient assessment of this group was indistinguishable from those infants with mild disease who were never hospitalized. A review of their hospital course found that none of these infants received oxygen, had apnea or bradycardia, or were observed for more than 48 hours.

The 10 babies who were initially thought to have mild disease at their initial emergency department assessment, but subsequently experienced more severe disease, were early in their course of illness as determined by the duration of their upper respiratory tract infection symptoms (3.8 vs 6.3 days; $P<.04$). They were also subsequently found to have RSV bronchiolitis as determined by enzyme-linked immuosorbent assay or culture (70% vs 34%; $P<.04$) compared with other infants who had mild illness and never required hospitalization.

COMMENT

This prospective study identifies several important components of the initial outpatient evaluation that can be used to assess severity of disease in babies with bronchiolitis. These results are contrary to findings of the retrospective study by McMillan et al,[17] which stated that clinical parameters are ineffective in establishing the severity of disease in infants with bronchiolitis.

Our investigation suggests that the infant's gestational age at birth, more than the chronologic age, is the historical factor most strongly associated with illness severity. Although infants born prematurely may have a higher incidence of perinatal complications such as bronchopulmonary dysplasia and congenital lung or cardiac abnormalities, and, therefore, more severe bronchiolitis,[7,16,17,20] gestational age at birth overshadowed the parental history of perinatal complications in predicting disease severity at initial outpatient assessment. Young postnatal age, although less important, also increased the infant's RR of having more severe bronchiolitis in our study and has been associated with increased risk of apnea,[11-13] hypoxemia,[10] and respiratory failure[14,17] among infants hospitalized for RSV. Other historical and demographic factors that have been reported to increase the infant's likelihood of acquiring RSV or parainfluenza bronchiolitis, such as crowding or presence of older siblings,[15] cigarette smoking in the household,[7,15] a family history of allergies or asthma,[7,15,18] a medical history of wheezing,[18] male sex of the child,[5,6] and lack of breast-feeding,[18,21] were not associated with disease severity in our study.

On physical examination, the simple clinical description of the infant's general appearance ("well appearing," "ill— not toxic," or "toxic") by an attending physician was better at predicting illness severity in this group of patients than the Clinical Asthma Score,[22] which was designed to evaluate persons with asthma, or the YOS,[23] which was initially designed to assess serious illness in febrile babies. Tachypnea, but not the presence or degree of wheezing, was also found to be a helpful measure in assessing the degree of illness. Although McMillan et al[17] did not find that the degree of tachypnea at the time of hospital admission was associated with a prolonged hospital stay, the study was retrospective and included patients who had endotracheal tubes at the time of evaluation.

Lobar or streaky atelectasis on a chest roentgenogram was highly associated with more severe disease. Wildin et al[26] noted a significant correlation between lobar atelectasis and severity of illness in children hospitalized with RSV, parainfluenza, influenza, and adenovirus infections. In addition, Outwater and Crone[14] noted that atelectasis or pneumonia was present on chest roentgenograms in all 15 of their study infants who had respiratory failure that required intubation. Although a chest roentgenogram may not be necessary in all outpatients with bronchiolitis, roentgenographic information can be a useful adjunct to clinical decision making and diagnosis.

We found the infant's oxygen saturation, as determined by pulse oximetry, to be the single best predictor of illness severity. Low oxygen saturation is often not clinically apparent. In one study, pulse oximetry that was done shortly after admission to the hospital on babies with RSV bronchiolitis found a mean oxygen saturation of 87%, with little correlation between clinical assessments of degree of hypoxia.[10] Pulse oximeters give rapid, continuous, noninvasive, and valid measurements of oxygen saturation.[27-30] Their rapid response time was able to detect changes in saturation that occurred when the infant was feeding.

A broad definition of mild and severe disease was used in classifying severity of illness in our study. Strict objective criteria (such as respiratory rate or pulse oximetry results) were not chosen to avoid preselecting for the parameters that we wished to evaluate at initial outpatient assessment. Without strict criteria, children with more moderate disease may have been included into either category. However, these infants would tend to bias the findings by making it more difficult (not less difficult) to distinguish differences between the two groups. Additionally, since severity of illness was based on eventual outcome during the course of illness, rather than a hospital admission decision, no infant who was initially discharged and experienced more severe disease was missed, and those infants with very mild disease who were admitted were identified.

We studied all infants with bronchiolitis and not just those with proved RSV infections, because at first evaluation, the viral cause is not often known. For this reason, and because no patients who bypassed the emergency department and were directly admitted were included, the severity of illness may have been lower than in other studies that have reported higher incidences of apnea[11-13] and longer lengths of hospitalization.[10,16,17] However, the percentage of our hospitalized patients who required intensive care and mechanical ventilation was similar to that reported by other studies.[7,10,16]

In summary, we were able to identify a group of six clinical and laboratory findings at initial outpatient evaluation that may aid in identifying infants with bronchiolitis who are at risk for having or experiencing more severe disease: (1) "ill or toxic" general appearance; (2) oxygen saturation less than 95% by pulse oximetry; (3) gestational age, younger than 34 weeks; (4) respiratory rate, 70/min or greater; (5) atelectasis on chest roentgenograms, and (6) postnatal age, younger than 3 months. We would highly recommend that emergency department evaluation of infants with bronchiolitis include pulse oximetry, as this simple and noninvasive test is the single best predictor of illness severity.

References

1. Hall CB. When to suspect respiratory syncytial virus. *J Respir Dis.* 1980;1:18-22.
2. Medical Research Council Subcommittee on Respiratory Syncytial Virus Vaccines. Respiratory syncytial virus infection: admissions to hospital in industrial, urban, and rural areas. *BMJ.* 1978;2:796-798.
3. Paisley JW, Lauer BA, McIntosh K, Glode MP, Schachter J, Rumack C. Pathogens associated with acute lower respiratory tract infection in young children. *Pediatr Infect Dis.* 1984;3:14-19.
4. Chanock RM, Parrott RH. Acute respiratory disease in infancy and childhood: present understanding and prospects for prevention. *Pediatrics.* 1965;36:21-39.
5. Henderson FW, Clyde WA, Collier AM, et al. The etiologic and epidemiologic spectrum of bronchiolitis in pediatric practice. *J Pediatr.* 1979;95:183-190.
6. Glezen WP, Denny FW. Epidemiology of acute lower respiratory disease in children. *N Engl J Med.* 1973;288:498-505.
7. Eriksson M, Forsgren M, Sjoberg S, von Sydow M, Wolontis S. Respiratory syncytial virus infection in young hospitalized children: identification of risk patients and prevention of nosocomial spread by rapid diagnosis. *Acta Paediatr Scand.* 1983;72:47-51.
8. Parrott RH, Kim HW, Brandt CD, Chanock RM. Respiratory syncytial virus in infants and children. *Prev Med.* 1974;3:473-480.
9. Glezen WP, Paredes A, Allison JE, Taber LH, Frank AL. Risk of RSV infection for infants from low-income families in relationship to age, sex, ethnic group and maternal antibody level. *J Pediatr.* 1981;98:708-715.
10. Hall CB, Hall WJ, Speers DM. Clinical and physiological manifestations of bronchiolitis and pneumonia. *AJDC.* 1979;133:798-802.
11. Anas N, Boettrich C, Hall CB, Brooks JG. The association of apnea and respiratory syncytial virus infection in infants. *J Pediatr.* 1982;101:65-68.
12. Church NR, Anas NG, Hall CB, Brooks JG. Respiratory syncytial virus—related apnea in infants. *AJDC.* 1984;138:247-250.
13. Bruhn FW, Mokrohisky ST, McIntosh K. Apnea associated with respiratory syncytial virus infection in young children. *J Pediatr.* 1977;90:382-386.
14. Outwater KM, Crone RK. Management of respiratory failure in infants with acute viral bronchiolitis. *AJDC.* 1984;138:1071-1075.
15. McConnochie KM, Roghmann KJ. Parental smoking, presence of older siblings, and family history of asthma increase risk of bronchiolitis. *AJDC.* 1986;140:806-812.
16. MacDonald NE, Hall CB, Suffin SC, Alexson C, Harris PJ, Manning JA. RSV infection in infants with congenital heart disease. *N Engl J Med.* 1982;307:397-400.
17. McMillan JA, Tristram DA, Weiner LB, Higgins AP, Sandstorm C, Brandon R. Prediction of the duration of hospitalization in patients with RSV infection: use of clinical parameters. *Pediatrics.* 1988;81:22-26.

18. Welliver RC, Wong DT, Sun M, McCarthy N. Parainfluenza virus bronchiolitis. *AJDC.* 1986;140:34-40.
19. Hall CB, Kopelman AE, Douglas RG, Geiman JM, Meagher MP. Neonatal RSV infection. *N Engl J Med.* 1979;300:393-396.
20. Hall CB, Powell KR, MacDonald WE, et al. RSV infection in children with compromised immune function. *N Engl J Med.* 1986;315:77-81.
21. Pullan CR, Toms GL, Martin AJ, Gardner PS, Webb JKG, Appleton DR. Breast-feeding and respiratory syncytial virus infection. *BMJ.* 1980;281:1034-1036.
22. Wood DW, Downes JJ, Lecks HI. A clinical scoring system for the diagnosis of respiratory failure. *AJDC.* 1972;123:227-228.
23. McCarthy PL, Sharpe MR, Spiegel SZ, et al. Observation scales to identify serious illness in febrile children. *Pediatrics.* 1982;70:802-809.
24. McIntosh K, Hendry RM, Fahnestock ML, Pierik L. Enzyme-linked-immunoabsorbent assay for detection of RSV infection: application to clinical samples. *J Clin Microbiol.* 1982;16:329-333.
25. Braffman M, Bacheson M, Forrer C, Friedman H. Superiority of ELISA for rapid diagnosis of respiratory syncytial virus. In: Program and abstracts of the 26th Interscience Conference on Antimicrobial Agents and Chemotherapy; September 28-October 1, 1986; New Orleans, La. Abstract 1986.
26. Wildin SR, Chonmaitree T, Swischuck LE. Roentgenographic features of common pediatric viral respiratory tract infections. *AJDC.* 1988;142:43-46.
27. Fanconi S, Doherty P, Edmonds JF, Barker GA, Bohn DJ. Pulse oximetry in pediatric intensive care: comparison with measured saturations and transcutaneous oxygen tension. *J Pediatr.* 1985;107:362-366.
28. Southall DP, Bignall S, Stebbens VA, Alexander JR, Rivers RPA, Lissauer T.Pulse oximeter and transcutaneous arterial oxygen measurements in neonatal and paediatric intensive care. *Arch Dis Child.* 1987;62:882-888.
29. Kulick RM. Pulse oximetry. *Pediatr Emerg Care.* 1987;3:127-130.
30. Swedlow DB, Stern S. Continuous non-invasive oxygen saturation monitoring in children with a new pulse oximeter. *Crit Care Med.* 1983;11:228. Abstract.

Increased Transient Tachypnea of the Newborn in Infants of Asthmatic Mothers

Michael Schatz, MD; Robert S. Zeiger, MD, PhD; Clement P. Hoffman, MD; Brian S. Saunders, MD; Kathleen M. Harden, RN; Alan B. Forsythe, PhD

• ***Objective:*** **To compare the incidence of transient tachypnea of the newborn (TTN) in infants of asthmatic vs nonasthmatic mothers.**
Research Design: **Case-control analysis.**
Setting: **Group model health maintenance organization.**
Patients: **A volunteer sample of 294 pregnant asthmatic women and 294 pregnant nonasthmatic women with normal pulmonary function test results, matched on the basis of age and smoking status. All subjects entered the study before their third trimester of pregnancy. Subjects with multiple gestations and abortions (<20 weeks' gestation) were excluded.**
Intervention: **Asthma was treated in the allergy department. Routine obstetric, neonatal, and pediatric care was provided to all patients by staff physicians.**
Measurements/Results: **Transient tachypnea occurred in 11 infants (3.7%) of asthmatic women and in one control infant (0.3%). There were no significant differences between asthmatic and matched control subjects in previously defined TTN risk factors, such as the occurrence of longer labors, failure to progress, cesarean sections, premature births, male sex, Apgar scores of less than 7 at 1 minute, or birth weight greater than 4 kg. Although infants of asthmatic mothers were more likely to exhibit wheezing by age 15 months compared with control infants (12.0% vs 3.2%), none of the infants with TTN manifested wheezing by age 15 months. No relationships could be identified in the asthmatic cohort between the occurrence of TTN and asthma severity or medication use (during the pregnancy in general or during labor and delivery in particular).**
Conclusion: **Although the mechanism is uncertain, maternal asthma appears to increase the risk of infant TTN.**
(*AJDC.* 1991;145:156–158)

Transient tachypnea of the newborn (TTN) was first described in 1966[1] and is a common cause of respiratory distress in the newborn.[2] It is typically associated with radiologic characteristics of so-called wet lung disease,[3] but its exact etiology and pathogenesis remain obscure. Although TTN is usually benign and self-limited,[1] recent reports emphasize that affected infants may experience substantial morbidity,[4-7] including profound hypoxemia, and may need mechanical ventilation. In an attempt to further understand this condition, recent studies have attempted to identify maternal, obstetric, and neonatal characteristics associated with TTN.[7,8] We suggest that maternal asthma should be added to the list of conditions that increase the risk of TTN.

Accepted for publication September 4, 1990.

From the Departments of Allergy (Drs Schatz and Zeiger and Ms Harden), Obstetrics/Gynecology (Dr Hoffman), and Pediatrics (Dr Saunders), Kaiser-Permanente Medical Center, San Diego, Calif, and the Department of Biostatistics, Viratek Inc, Costa Mesa, Calif (Dr Forsythe).

Reprint requests to the Department of Allergy, Kaiser-Permanente Medical Center, 7060 Clairemont Mesa Blvd, San Diego, CA 92111 (Dr Schatz).

SUBJECTS AND METHODS

Subjects

Subjects for this study were participants in the Kaiser-Permanente Prospective Study of Asthma During Pregnancy, conducted at Kaiser-Permanente Medical Center, San Diego, Calif, the design of which has been previously described.[9,10] Briefly, all asthmatic patients registering for prenatal care before their third trimester were recruited and matched with nonasthmatic (control) subjects according to age and smoking status. Asthma was defined as a history of chest wheezing, chest tightness, or chest cough that could be precipitated by infection, exercise, and/or allergens and could be relieved either spontaneously or by bronchodilator medication. The medical history was substantiated by demonstration of reversible airway obstruction (as previously defined[10]) on pulmonary function tests or by documentation of auscultatory wheezing during tidal breathing. All subjects completed pulmonary function tests at 7 months' gestation and/or after birth. Control subjects with abnormal pulmonary function test results were excluded from the study. The study was approved by the Kaiser-Permanente Institutional Review Board, and informed consent was obtained from all subjects.

Asthma was treated by an allergist (M.S.) who attempted to prevent acute asthmatic episodes and asthma symptoms that interfered with sleep or normal activity. Data were evaluated from singleton pregnancies ending in birth between June 1978 and December 1984. Subjects undergoing abortions (<20 weeks' gestation) were excluded. Asthmatic patients (n = 66) for whom suitable controls were not available were not included in the analysis. The final cohort included 294 asthmatic subjects and 294 matched controls. Fifteen-month follow-up data were available for 217 infants of asthmatic mothers and for 218 control infants.

Measurement of Variables

Perinatal outcome data were extracted from the standard obstetric and nursery medical records and 15-month infant data were taken from the pediatric medical records by a research nurse (K.M.H.) who did not know at the time of data collection to which group (asthma vs control) the subject belonged. The diagnosis of TTN was made by the attending neonatologist based on the

A Comparison of the Prevalences of Transient Tachypnea of the Newborn (TTN) and Other Relevant Perinatal Variables in the Pregnancies/Infants of Asthmatic Patients vs Matched Control Subjects

	Incidence, %	
Parameter	Asthmatic Group (N=294)	Control Group (N=294)
TTN	3.7	0.3
Maternal age >35 y	2.0	2.0
Maternal smoking	5.4	5.4
Multiparas	58.5†	34.4
Longer labor	50.9	49.1
Failure to progress	1.4	2.0
Cesarean section	20.1	19.0
Premature birth (<37 weeks' gestation)	5.8	3.4
Male sex	50.7	54.1
Apgar score <7 at 1 min	9.4	8.7
Birth weight >4 kg	8.5	12.9
Infant respiratory distress syndrome	1.0	0.7

*P=.003. Remains significant at the 5% level when the type 1 error is adjusted for multiple comparisons using Bonferroni's significance level.

†P<.001. Remains significant at the 5% level when the type 1 error is adjusted for multiple comparisons using Bonferroni's significance level.

following criteria: (1) onset of tachypnea (respiratory rate >60 breaths per minute) within 6 hours after birth; (2) persistence of tachypnea for at least 12 hours; (3) chest roentgenographic abnormalities consistent with TTN (ie, mild cardiomegaly, increased perihilar markings, perivascular cuffing, fluid in the lung fissures, and hyperinflation); and (4) exclusion of infant respiratory distress syndrome, meconium aspiration, air leak, congenital pulmonary abnormalities, and significant congenital heart disease. A wheezing episode in the first 15 months of life was defined as wheezing on chest auscultation documented in the pediatric records on at least one occasion.

The following perinatal variables were also evaluated: maternal age greater than 35 years (at entry to study), maternal smoking (>10 cigarettes per day for at least 1 month of pregnancy), parity (primipara vs multipara), labor longer than the median from this series (excluding births by cesarean section, with the median for primiparas and multiparas calculated separately), failure to progress, cesarean section, premature birth (<37 weeks' gestation), male sex, Apgar score of less than 7 at 1 minute, birth weight greater than 4 kg, and infant respiratory distress syndrome. In addition, the following asthma severity and gestational medication variables were assessed: overall severity (medication requirements), emergency treatment requirements, mean gestational forced expiratory volume in 1 second, and medication use any time during the pregnancy or specifically during labor and delivery (eg, inhaled bronchodilators, theophylline, or corticosteroids).

Statistical Methods

For all analyses, two-tailed statistical significance was set at the 5% level. In the case-control analyses, the prevalences of the perinatal variables were compared between asthmatic patients and matched controls by χ^2 analysis when the minimum expected value was greater than or equal to 5 and by Fisher's Exact Test otherwise.

In the asthmatic cohort, the relationship of the occurrence of TTN to the maternal asthma severity and medication variables described above were evaluated by χ^2 analysis for linear trend.[11] This type of analysis identifies linear relationships between an increasing prevalence of TTN and an increasing intensity of the asthma severity and medication variables. The relationship of the occurrence of TTN to maternal asthma medication use during labor and delivery was evaluated in the asthmatic cohort by Fisher's Exact Test.

RESULTS

The prevalences of TTN and other potentially relevant perinatal variables in asthmatic vs matched control subjects are shown in the Table 1. Transient tachypnea of the newborn occurred in 11 (3.7%) of 217 asthmatic subjects, but in only one (0.3%) of 294 control infants (P=.003). Multiparity was also significantly more common in asthmatic vs control subjects. However, when primiparas and multiparas were considered separately, the prevalence of TTN in the infants of asthmatic primiparas (5.0%) was significantly greater (P=.003) than the prevalence in control primiparas (no instances of TTN), and the prevalence in asthmatic multiparas (2.9%) was higher than that in control multiparas (1.0%), although this difference did not reach statistical significance.

Two of the infants with TTN were premature. However, the lung profile of one of them (lecithin-sphingomyelin ratio >5, phosphatidylglycerol present) was not consistent with surfactant deficient respiratory distress syndrome. Although a lung profile of the second infant was not available, the clinical course and oxygen requirements were consistent with TTN rather than infant respiratory distress syndrome.

Infants of asthmatic mothers were much more likely to experience a wheezing episode by age 15 months (12.0%) than were infants of control mothers (3.2%) (P<.001). However, none of the infants with TTN manifested wheezing by age 15 months. There were no significant relationships between any of the asthma severity or medication variables and the occurrence of TTN in asthmatic mothers (data not shown).

COMMENT

The Kaiser-Permanente Prospective Study of Asthma During Pregnancy was designed to evaluate obstetric and infant outcomes in prospectively treated asthmatic subjects compared with matched, simultaneously followed nonasthmatic controls. Although there was no significant increase in the occurrence of respiratory distress syndrome in the infants of asthmatic vs control subjects, a significant increase in the incidence of TTN was observed in infants of asthmatic mothers (Table). Although four prior studies have compared outcomes in the infants of asthmatic vs control mothers,[12-15] none of these reports mentioned TTN.

Since the exact etiology of TTN is unclear and because TTN can be a cause of substantial neonatal morbidity,[4-7] recent studies have attempted to identify maternal, obstetric, and neonatal characteristics that may be associated with TTN. Gross et al[7] compared 55 pregnancies in which the neonate developed TTN with 355 pregnancies in which infant respiratory distress did not occur. Of 14 parameters evaluated, negative amniotic fluid phosphatidylglycerol levels, premature delivery, and an Apgar score of less than 7 at 1 minute each made an independent contribution to the overall characterization of infants at risk for TTN. Rawlings and Smith[8] compared clinical data from 100 neonates with TTN with data from 100 healthy neonates. The prevalence of male sex and macrosomia were significantly higher in the infants with TTN, and the obstetric histories of mothers of infants with TTN were characterized by longer labor, a higher prevalence of failure to progress in labor, and a higher proportion of cesarean sections.

The increased occurrence of TTN in infants of asthmatic mothers that was observed in this study could not be explained by differences in the occurrence of previously defined risk factors between the asthmatic and control groups (Table). Although the asthmatic and control groups were not well matched for parity, parity has not been previously defined as a risk factor for TTN, and the incidence of TTN remained higher in infants of asthmatic vs control subjects when primiparas and multiparas were evaluated separately.

The occurrence of TTN in infants of asthmatic mothers was not related to maternal asthma severity, degree of control (ie, occurrence of acute episodes and gestational pulmonary function), or medication use (during the pregnancy in general or during labor and delivery in particular). However, the relatively small number of infants manifesting TTN makes the power of this analysis small.

Although infants of asthmatic mothers were significantly more likely to wheeze during the first 15 months of life than were infants of nonasthmatic mothers, the occurrence of TTN in infants of asthmatic mothers was not associated with subsequent wheezing within this period. This, of course, does not preclude an increased risk of asthma developing later in infants with TTN. Indeed, a recent study of 58 children evaluated at ages 4 to 5 years who demonstrated TTN at birth revealed significantly more clinical findings consistent with asthma than in 58 controls who did not demonstrate TTN at birth.[16]

One potential mechanism for both increased instances of TTN and subsequent asthma in infants of asthmatic mothers would be a genetic predisposition to β-adrenergic hyporesponsiveness, since animal studies suggest that the β-adrenergic system is important in the increased pulmonary fluid absorption and decreased production that normally occurs after birth,[17] and β-adrenergic hyporesponsiveness[18] associated with a reduction in the number of β-adrenergic receptors[19] may be important in the pathogenesis of asthma. Further studies are necessary to establish the mechanisms of the relationships between maternal asthma, infant TTN, and childhood asthma. However, our current results suggest that maternal asthma is an independent risk factor for the development of infant TTN.

This is the fourth report from the Kaiser-Permanente Prospective Study of Asthma During Pregnancy. The study was supported in part by grant AI 20426 from the Allergy and Asthma Branch of the National Institute of Allergy and Infectious Diseases, Bethesda, Md, and by grants from William H. Rorer—Dooner Laboratories, Ft Washington, Pa, and Kaiser Foundation Hospitals, San Diego, Calif.

We thank Linda M. Chilingar for performing the statistical analysis, and Richard P. Porreco, MD, and Abram S. Benenson, MD, for reviewing the manuscript. We also thank Tamara Haydon and Patricia Stanwood for typing the manuscript and the staff from the Kaiser Foundation Hospital Medical Library for their assistance with the references.

References

1. Avery ME, Gatewood OB, Brumley G. Transient tachypnea of the newborn. *AJDC.* 1966;111:380-385.

2. Miller LK, Calenoff L, Boehm JJ, Riedy MJ. Respiratory distress in the newborn. *JAMA.* 1980;243:1176-1179.

3. Wesenberg RL, Graven SN, McCabe EB. Radiologic findings in wet lung disease. *Radiology.* 1971;98:69-74.

4. Buccirelli RL, Egan EA, Gessner IH, Eitzman DV. Persistent fetal circulation: one manifestation of transient tachypnea of the neonate. *Pediatrics.* 1976;58:192-197.

5. Tudehope DI, Smyth MH. Is 'transient tachypnea of the newborn' always a benign disease? Report of 6 babies requiring mechanical ventilation. *Aust Paediatr J.* 1979;15:160-165.

6. Halliday HL, McClure G, McCreid M. Transient tachypnea of the newborn: two distinct clinical entities? *Arch Dis Child.* 1981;56:322-325.

7. Gross TL, Sokol RJ, Kwong MS, Wilson M, Kuhnert DM. Transient tachypnea of the newborn: the relationship to preterm delivery and significant neonatal morbidity. *Am J Obstet Gynecol.* 1983;146:236-241.

8. Rawlings JS, Smith FR. Transient tachypnea of the newborn: an analysis of neonatal and obstetric risk factors. *AJDC.* 1984;138:869-873.

9. Schatz M, Harden K, Forsythe A, et al. The course of asthma during pregnancy, postpartum and with successive pregnancies: a prospective analysis. *J Allergy Clin Immunol.* 1988;81:509-517.

10. Schatz M, Zieger RS, Harden KM, et al. The safety of inhaled beta agonist bronchodilators during pregnancy. *J Allergy Clin Immunol.* 1988;62:686-695.

11. Cochran WG. Some methods for strengthening the common chi square test. *Biometrics.* 1954;10:417-441.

12. Schaefer G, Silverman F. Pregnancy complicated by asthma. *Am J Obstet Gynecol.* 1961;82:182-191.

13. Gordon M, Niswander KR, Berendes H, Kantor AG. Fetal morbidity following potentially anoxigenic obstetric conditions, VII: bronchial asthma. *Am J Obstet Gynecol.* 1970;106:421-429.

14. Bahna SL, Bjerkedal T. The course and outcome of pregnancy in women with bronchial asthma. *Acta Allergol.* 1972;27:397-406.

15. Stenius-Aarniala B, Piirila P, Teramo K. Asthma and pregnancy: a prospective study of 198 pregnancies. *Thorax.* 1988;43:12-18.

16. Shohat M, Levy G, Levy I, Schonfeld T, Merlob P. Transient tachypnea of the newborn and asthma. *Arch Dis Child.* 1989;64:277-279.

17. Wyszogrodski I, Taeusch HW Jr, Avery ME. Isoxuprine-induced alterations of pulmonary pressure-volume relationships in premature rabbits. *Am J Obstet Gynecol.* 1974;119:1107-1111.

18. Larsson K. Studies of sympatho-adrenal reactivity and adrenoceptor function in bronchial asthma. *Eur J Respir Dis.* 1985;66(suppl):1-52.

19. Barnes PJ. Endogenous catecholemines and asthma. *J Allergy Clin Immunol.* 1986;77:791-795.

Correction

Errors in Table

In the article by Avner et al entitled "Acquired Methemoglobinemia," published in the November 1990 issue of *AJDC* (1990;144:1229-1230), there were errors in the Table. On page 1230 in the Table, in the entries under the column headed "**Methemoglobin** ," no decimal points should appear.

A Medical Ethics Issues Survey of Residents in Five Pediatric Training Programs

Bruce David White, DO, JD; Gerald B. Hickson, MD; Rosemary Theriot, EdD; Richard M. Zaner, PhD

• Few pediatric training programs offer formal instruction or have ethics consultants to assist residents with ethical dilemmas. Moreover, even if such assistance were available, it is not clear that educators have an adequate understanding of (1) the range and frequency of possible ethical dilemmas residents may encounter, (2) residents' most troublesome concerns, (3) their use of resources to resolve issues, and (4) their own ethics belief systems. A sample of convenience (51 residents) at five midsouth residency programs was queried during 25-minute open-ended interviews to answer ethical questions; there were no refusals to participate. The "most troublesome" cases cited by the residents were related to life-and-death issues (withholding and withdrawing life support), child abuse and neglect cases, and disputes regarding patient care that arise between services. Two thirds of those surveyed indicated that they are still somewhat troubled by these difficult ethical problems. Surprisingly, residents stated that they relied on their peers more often than their attending physicians for effective assistance in resolving their most troublesome dilemmas. We support continuing education and research efforts to help residents and educators feel "more comfortable" in resolving ethical dilemmas.

(*AJDC.* 1991;145:161–164)

Residents and residency educators should seek to identify and evaluate the moral problems and ethical dilemmas that they expect to encounter in the practice of medicine for two practical reasons. First, residency training represents a highly stressful time for young physicians.[1,2] A principal stressor is the recognition that one becomes personally responsible for the care and well-being of patients. Many believe that "caring for patients" means more than attending to a patient's immediate physical needs. Anxieties may arise within any physician confronted by the moral problems with which patients may present. Simultaneous attempts to treat physical maladies and resolve ethical dilemmas can prove to be especially overwhelming to those with little training in clinical medicine or ethics.[3] Second, the increase in medical litigation may be due to physicians' failure to communicate thoroughly and adequately with their patients.[4] This communication problem is particularly troublesome, perhaps approaching one of avoidance, when physicians are uncomfortable in dealing with the ethical dilemmas that arise during the course of patient care.[5]

Residency program directors attempt to prepare physicians-in-training for the medical problems that they may encounter in practice, yet few programs incorporate patterned instruction for the resolution of ethical dilemmas (C. Strong, J. E. Connelly, unpublished data, 1989). There may be several reasons for this posture. Some attending physicians believe that they lack the necessary training to adequately discuss ethical issues, maintain that certain ethical problems cannot be solved or that methods of resolution cannot be instilled, or sense that it takes too long (on rounds or in a busy clinic) to properly address such issues. Some attending physicians believe that "ethics cannot be taught" in the limited time available for residency education.[6] Whatever the reasons, residents often complete their training without satisfactory medical ethics instruction during the course of their graduate medical education.

This may be changing. Several medical ethicists have suggested a range of topics and goals for undergraduate medical ethics education, including "the ability to identify the moral aspects of medical practice," "the ability to obtain a valid consent or a valid refusal of treatment," "the ability to decide when it is morally justified to withhold

Accepted for publication May 1, 1990.

From The Center for Clinical and Research Ethics, Vanderbilt University Medical Center (Drs White, Hickson, and Zaner), and The Clinical Research Center, Meharry Medical College (Dr White and Ms Theriot), Nashville, Tenn.

Read before the annual meeting of the Residency Interest Group of the Society for Health and Human Values, Washington, DC, October 27, 1989.

Reprint requests to The Center for Clinical and Research Ethics, Vanderbilt University Medical Center, Nashville, TN 37232 (Dr White).

Purpose.—*This department is intended to share information concerning educational efforts in the broad field of pediatrics. We welcome studies on the following topics: undergraduate and graduate education in medicine and allied health occupations; continuing education of health professionals; education of patients and families; and health education for the general public, the community, and organizations that contribute to the promotion and improvement of the health of children.*

Editorial Comment.—*How do we train our residents in issues dealing with ethical decisions? Whom do they rely on for advice? White et al offer some interesting insights into these issues and offer suggestions for our training programs. Maybe ethics can be taught.*—H.D.A.

information frompatients," and "a knowledge of the moral aspects of the care of patients with a poor prognosis [including patients who are terminally ill]."[7] Others have proposed remedies that involve the introduction of ethics training through lectures, discussions, conferences, and courses[8] in pediatrics,[9] neonatology,[10] perinatology,[11] and obstetrics.[12] Recently, some medical centers have established medical ethics consult services to provide ethics instruction on a case-by-case basis within the acknowledged context of direct consultative patient care.[13]

In light of previous deficiencies and an increasing interest in medical ethics education, it was believed that a descriptive study should precede any curricula recommendations for our own institutions. We therefore conducted a survey to identify (1) the moral problems or ethical dilemmas that pediatric residents had confronted in their episodic training experiences, (2) each resident's single most troublesome ethical challenge, (3) the resources they had used to assist them in coping with these dilemmas, and (4) whether these issues were resolved. Perhaps a medical ethics instruction program focused on residents' experiences and needs will be better accepted by pediatric educators and physicians-in-training.[15]

MATERIALS AND METHODS

An open-ended questionnaire was developed specifically to gather the information described above and included questions to ascertain residents' sociodemographic characteristics. The instrument was reviewed by philosophers and pediatric educators and was compared with similar survey questionnaires.[15]

Continuity-care clinic directors and chief residents at five midsouth pediatric training sites were contacted about the possibility of administering the survey at their institutions. All five of the following centers agreed to participate: Hubbard Hospital of Meharry Medical College, Nashville, Tenn; Kosair Children's Hospital (a teaching hospital of the University of Louisville [Ky]); LeBonheur Children's Medical Center (a teaching hospital of the University of Tennessee [Memphis]); Metropolitan Nashville General Hospital; and Vanderbilt Children's Hospital, Nashville. One of us (B.D.W.) visited the five sites and administered the questionnaires to all participants. The sample of convenience included pediatric and combined medicine-pediatric program residents who held their continuity-care clinics on either Wednesdays or Thursdays at the various sites. Each resident was informed about the purpose of the study, was asked to participate, and gave oral consent. Fifty-two residents agreed to participate; none refused. One resident was called away before the interview was completed.

Resident responses were recorded by the interviewer and were repeated to each resident to ensure recording accuracy. Interviews averaged 25 minutes each. We categorized the responses to the open-ended questions to aid in conceptualization and data analysis. Consistency in categorization was verified by two consultants (a philosopher and a nurse clinician).

RESULTS

To identify the single greatest moral and ethical dilemma that each resident had faced and to document the wide range of moral and ethical problems that they might encounter in the future, a series of questions were posed. In answer to the question "What ethical dilemmas have *you* confronted in practice?" the 51 residents offered 109 total responses, or 2.14 responses each. The majority involved the life-and-death issues of withdrawing care (57%) or withholding life support (9%). Other responses included dealing with teenage pregnancies, birth control, and abortions (16%); facing the economic, legal, and social conflicts that arise in medical practice (9%); genetic counseling (4%); managing personal and societal uncertainties when reporting abuse and neglect (4%); and balancing professional responsibilities with family life (1%).

Table 1.—Respondents' Most Frequently Cited Troublesome Cases*

Category 1: Life and Death Issues (88%)
"Terminating care" or electing to discontinue "extraordinary care" in severely ill patients with an expected poor prognosis (24/47 [47%])
Withdrawing support from a patient in the neonatal intensive care unit (10/47 [20%])
Withholding life support in the extremely premature neonate (gestational age, ≤26 weeks) (often with or expected intracranial hemorrhage) in the delivery room (7/47 [21%])
Category 2: Abuse Cases (8%)
Reporting a physical or sexual abuse case encountered in the outpatient clinic or emergency department (4/47 [8%])
Category 3: Service Conflicts Cases (4%)
"Mediating between various services" with different opinions regarding treatment (2/47 [4%])

*Forty-seven (92%) of 51 residents responded.

Respondents were asked to review their lists and to identify the one case that had presented their single "most troublesome" ethical dilemma; 47 residents (92%) complied. In Table 1, the residents' most troublesome cases are divided into three categories. The vast majority of these cases (88%) involved life-and-death issues. There were, however, three subgroups with clearly distinguishing features. The two largest of these (67%) involved residents' concerns about withdrawing care (most often related to the process of actually removing life support, meaning extubation of a terminally ill patient with imminent cessation of all bodily functions) in either a neonate or an older child. The other subgroup (21%) included cases in which the resident had to decide, often within the confines of a delivery room, whether an extremely premature infant was actually viable and if, in retrospect, he or she had made the "right" decision. This subgroup also included the decisions that had to be made when faced with the birth of a seriously handicapped newborn, such as a child with trisomy 13 or 18. The second category (8%) involved questionable physical and sexual abuse cases, with residents asking how certain anyone could be that documented injuries actually occurred as a result of abuse. The remaining cases (4%) concerned professional conflicts that occurred when two services disagreed in their concurrent care for a terminally ill child.

Residents were then asked the following question: "Why do these issues become moral problems or ethical dilemmas?" The responses (110 total responses, or 2.16 per resident) included the following: these issues deal with the essence of medical practice in the physical care for the ill and show that decision making in treating patients cannot be separated from resolving ethical dilemmas (28%); these issues mark the tolerance one must accept with the uncertainties inherent in medical practice (18%); these issues prove the necessity to balance patient and societal as well as personal interests in medical practice that may conflict (17%); these issues illustrate the application of fundamental ethical principles, such as honesty, goodness, and justice (16%); these issues document that a number of external factors beyond the physician's control influence medical practice considerations (12%); these issues show that personal and staff conflicts may arise in medical practice (6%); and these issues demonstrate a lack of training in dealing with moral problems or ethical dilemmas (3%).

Respondents were also asked whether the most troublesome case identified was now "completely settled" in their own minds or if there were aspects of the case that were still of occasional concern. Thirty-six residents (71%)

Table 2.—Reasons 36 Respondents Gave as to Why Their Most Important Ethical Dilemma Was Not Resolved
Physician-Oriented
The dilemma recurs; it is a widely prevalent problem; each case must be individualized.
"I wonder if what we did was appropriate; was right."
"I have trouble talking to parents in these cases."
"The physician is helpless to effect any change."
It is painful for caregivers to see the consequences of treatment.
There are legal consequences to what we did.
Patient and Family-Oriented
"We caused pain and discomfort" and did not appear to affect the ultimate outcome.
"What quality of life have we obtained; did we do any good?"
"We created false hopes."
"Parents did not take an active role [in decision making]."
"The mother and siblings are innocent victims [now too]."
"I feel sorry for the parents and family who live with the consequences."
The decisions are made in an emotional, stressful climate.
Disease-Oriented
"The prognosis was hopeless."
"The prognosis is still uncertain in these cases."

indicated that their most troublesome case was not resolved for the reasons given in Table 2. Nine (18%) indicated that their most troublesome case was now resolved. Examples of their reasons included the following: "we did all that could be done"; "we did the right thing"; "I've accepted the consequences"; and "the child survived." Six respondents (12%) did not answer this question.

In an attempt to assess how residents strive to deal with these issues, each respondent was asked if assistance had been sought from other individuals or services to resolve this most troublesome case. If assistance was requested, the residents were asked to list the relationship of the individual or the service to the case and then to rate the overall perceived effectiveness of that assistance on a five-point Likert scale (with 1 indicating "detrimental," 5 indicating "beneficial," and 3 being "neutral"). Forty-one residents (79%) indicated that they sought assistance from 106 sources (2.6 sources per resident). Some of the more frequently cited individuals and services are shown in Table 3, with the total number of times assistance was sought along with mean ratings. Attending physicians participated in 83% of these cases with a mean rating of 3.74, and peers participated in 51% of the cases with a mean rating of 4.14.

RESPONDENTS' CHARACTERISTICS

The 51 responding residents represented 29% of the total house staff serving in the participating residency programs. Most (n=41) had graduated from medical school after 1985. They were almost equally divided among first-year (n=17), second-year (n=12), and third-year (n=20) residents. One was a fourth-year medicine-pediatrics resident, and one respondent did not indicate level of training. About half were male (n=26), and most were white (n=37), married (n=29), and without children (n=38). Sixty-one percent (n=30) were Protestant, 14% (n=7) were Catholic, 12% (n=6) were Jewish, and 14% (n=7) indicated another or no religious preference. Eighty-two percent indicated that religion was either "important" or "very important" in their lives. Sixty-seven percent (n=34) indicated that they had previously taken a course in "medical ethics." Thirty-seven percent (n=19) said that

Table 3.—Effectiveness of Those Whom 41 Respondents Asked for Assistance*

	No. of Times Listed	No. Listed as "Beneficial" (Rating >3)	Mean Rating
Physicians			
Attending physician	34	24	3.74
Supervising resident and peers†	21	18	4.14
Supporting staff			
Nursing staff and social services staff†	12	9	4.16
Patient and family			
Patient and patient's parents and family†	4	4	4.75
Others			
Resident's spouse/ significant other†	12	10	4.08

*Responses were rated on a scale of 1 (detrimental) to 5 (beneficial).
†Combined categories.

Table 4.—Sources of Respondents' Ethics Belief System*

Source	Rating
Family	4.55
Personal study and reflection	4.52
Religious teachings	4.20
Clinical experience	3.82
Some decisive personal experiences	3.82
Teachers	3.80
Personal understanding of societal needs	3.63
Peers	3.40
Societal contacts	3.10

*Responses were rated on a scale of 1 (added nothing) to 5 (added greatly).

they had been on at least one service team that had requested a "medical ethics consult" concerning one of their assigned patients.

Participants were asked to rate the degree to which a number of identified sources (for example, "family," "teachers," or "religious teachings") had contributed to their individual belief systems. The mean ratings are shown in Table 4.

COMMENT

Patterned educational efforts in medical ethics instruction might be better received if proportionately channeled into already identified problematic areas. An obvious purpose of our study is to illustrate the importance that residents attach to these issues (as shown by the insightfulness of their responses) and to serve as a marker for topic and resource allocation. For example, discussions of the withdrawal of life support (mentioned as a possible dilemma by more than half of the respondents) would appear to be a principal focus for life-and-death discussions. Ethics topics, however, like other points in most medical subject areas, should be selected for other reasons as well. Instructors would be ill-advised to teach and discuss *only* the problems that residents identified from their still rather limited practice perspective to the exclusion of other issues that are widely recognized because of history, principle, and anticipated future effect.

Residents stated that they turned to attending physicians for assistance and support in resolving the ethical dilemmas presented by their most troublesome cases (83% [34/41]). They also sought assistance from supervising residents (17% [7/41]), peers (34% [14/41]), and fellows (5% [2/41]), but to a lesser degree than attending physicians. It seems curious then that the rating for attending physicians (3.74) was low compared with that for supervising residents (4.14), peers (4.14), and fellows (4.00); in fact, some might have expected the reverse given the fact that residents stated that teachers contributed to their belief systems to a higher degree (3.80) than did peers (3.40). Some might wonder whether this is so because the attending physician is a little more "distant" from the patient's bedside than are the residents. (This may be supported by the fact that the residents rated patients [4.50 mean rating from two responses] and families [5.00 mean rating from two responses] higher than any other source in assisting in the resolution of those most troublesome cases. Residents' spouses, however, scored higher than attending physicians as well [4.09 mean rating from 12 responses]. Perhaps the important factor here is whether the attending physician is "distant" from the residents' perception or discussion of the case.) In the defense of the attending physician, one should recall that ultimate legal (and moral) responsibility of patient care does not lie with the residents. Residents may often lack the "big picture" of overall patient care because of their limited hospital involvement and have varied expectations of their attending physicians' abilities and responsibilities. Efforts directed to increase attending physician "effectiveness"—or better yet to eliminate their "detrimental assistance"—and to increase peer involvement might enhance the resolution of moral problems in practice (or at least the residents' understanding of resolution).

Residents indicated that "clinical experience" (rated 3.82), "decisive personal experiences" (rated 3.82), and "teachers" (rated 3.30) contribute to their ethics systems. These answers show that residents' systems can at least be influenced in these areas by theoretical and practical education.

Our survey was somewhat limited for the purposes expressed herein. As with almost any survey, one may question the motives and appropriateness of the respondents' answers and the editorial control exercised by the authors in the formulation of outlines and answer categorizations. The size of the sample population is relatively small (approximately 180 total residents in the programs selected), about one third of whom were interviewed. Even with the open-ended questions, there may be a failure to reflect the "real world" of medicine in the instrument—accentuating the economic, legal, and social aspects of health care—in any ethical decision-making discussions. This may suggest that the survey should be administered in other areas of the country and among different specialty groups.[16]

A CLOSING SUGGESTION

Our results document the unique perspective of a representative sample of pediatric residents to a number of propounded open-ended questions about ethics issues. Some may feel that those results raise more questions than they actually answer. Our study definitely identifies the need for further investigation in this area. However, this inquiry demonstrates that perhaps "ethics can be taught" or at least influenced. Residents indicated that teachers contribute greatly to their ethics belief systems and residents also evidenced their willingness to turn to attending physicians and peers in search of "solutions" to moral problems in medicine. With greater educational efforts and attempts on the part of staff, physicians-in-training would perhaps learn to feel "more comfortable" and more at ease in resolving ethical dilemmas as they do "more routine" medical practice concerns.

This work was supported in part by grant RR08198 from the GCRC and MBRS Branches of the Division of Research Resources, National Institutes of Health, Bethesda, Md.

The encouragement of Mary Ann South, MD, Director of the Clinical Research Center at Meharry Medical College, and the assistance of the continuity care clinic directors and the chief residents of the participating training programs are gratefully acknowledged. The editorial assistance of Martin E. Hamner, PhD, is deeply appreciated.

References

1. Colford JM, McPhee SJ. The ravelled sleeve of care: managing the stresses of residency training. *JAMA.* 1989;261:889-893. Special Communication.
2. Hoekelman RA. Stress experienced during pediatric residency. *AJDC.* 1989;143:177-189.
3. Pellegrino ED. Clinical ethics: biomedical ethics at the bedside. *JAMA.* 1988;260:837-838. Editorial.
4. Danzon P. The frequency and severity of malpractice claims: new evidence. *Law and Contemporary Problems.* 1986;49:57-72.
5. Graber GC, Beasley AD, Eaddy JA. *Ethical Analysis of Clinical Medicine.* Baltimore, Md: Urban & Schwarzenberg; 1985:113-117.
6. Zaner RM. 'Capstone' conference workshops: a reflection on the state of the art. In: Pellegrino ED, McElhinney TK, eds. *Teaching Ethics, the Humanities, and Human Values in Medical Schools: A Ten-Year Overview.* Washington, DC: Institute on Human Values in Medicine and the Society for Health and Human Values; 1981:58-65.
7. Culver CM, Clouser KD, Gert B, et al. Basic curricular goals in medical ethics. *N Engl J Med.* 1985;312:253-256. Special Report.
8. Veatch RM, Sollitto S. Medical ethics teaching: report of a national medical school survey. *JAMA.* 1976;235:1030-1033.
9. Fleischman A. Teaching medical ethics in a pediatric training program. *Pediatr Ann.* 1981;10:411-413.
10. Subramanian KNS, McCullough LB. A common framework for perinatal and neonatal medical ethics. *Semin Perinatol.* 1987;11:288-290.
11. Fleischman AR, Arras J. Teaching medical ethics in perinatology. *Clin Perinatol.* 1987;14:395-402.
12. Elkins TE, Strong C, Dilts PV Jr. Teaching bioethics within a residency program in obstetrics and gynecology. *Obstet Gynecol.* 1986;67:339-403.
13. LaPuma J, Stocking C, Silverstein MD, DiMartini A, Siegler M. An ethics consultation service in a teaching hospital: utilization and evaluation. *JAMA.* 1988;260:808-811.
14. McElhinney TK, ed. *Human Values Teaching Programs for Health Professionals.* Ardmore, Pa: Whitmore Publishing Company; 1981.
15. Tiberius RG, Cleave-Hogg D. Changes in undergraduate attitudes toward medical ethics. *Can Med Assoc J.* 1984;130:724-729.
16. Jacobson JJ, Tolle SW, Stocking S, Siegler M. Internal medicine residents' preferences regarding medical ethics education. *Acad Med.* 1989;64:760-764.

Intraosseous Infusion of Dobutamine and Isoproterenol

John F. Bilello, MD; Kevin C. O'Hair, DVM; William C. Kirby, MD; John W. Moore, MD

• Intraosseous infusion has been advocated as an emergency route in sick infants and children when intravenous access is not readily obtainable. Dobutamine hydrochloride and isoproterenol hydrochloride are useful emergency drugs that have not been studied when administered into the bone marrow. In a swine model, we compared the physiologic responses (heart rate, arterial pressure, and cardiac output) of dobutamine and isoproterenol infusions delivered intravenously and intraosseously during 20-minute intervals. We observed statistically significant effects of both dobutamine and isoproterenol delivered by the intraosseous route. In addition, the effects resulting from intraosseous infusion were statistically similar to those resulting from intravenous administration of these drugs. We conclude that the intraosseous infusion of dobutamine and isoproterenol is an effective and useful method for emergency administration of these medications.

(*AJDC*. 1991;145:165–167)

Delayed intravascular access has been recognized as a substantial obstacle to the successful resuscitation of pediatric patients in impending or frank cardiopulmonary arrest or shock. A recent study from a pediatric emergency department showed that it took more than 10 minutes to obtain venous access in 24% of cases of cardiac arrest. Intravenous access was never achieved in 6% of cases.[1]

Therapeutic intraosseous infusion was described in 1934 for injection of a liver preparation in the treatment of pernicious anemia.[2] Tocantins et al[3,4] described rapid absorption of various substances into the systemic circulation via the bone marrow. Several authors subsequently published reports of successful intraosseous infusions with few complications.[5-12] In 1977, Valdes[13] published his personal experience with emergency fluid administration via the bone marrow. Intraosseous infusion has continually been supported as an appropriate means of intravascular access in emergency situations.[14-16] Berg[17] published a case report of continuous infusion of dopamine and dobutamine in a pediatric patient, and Hodge[18] reviewed the methods and complications of pediatric intraosseous infusions.

Controlled studies of intraosseous infusions in animal models have supported the efficacy and potential benefit of emergency medications infused through the bone marrow when intravenous access is not available.[19-22] To our knowledge, no controlled study of the intraosseous infusion of either dobutamine or isoproterenol has been reported. The purpose of this study was to determine whether the intraosseous delivery of these drugs is as effective as the intravenous administration.

Accepted for publication July 2, 1990.

From the Department of Pediatrics (Dr Bilello) and the Section of Pediatric Cardiology (Drs Kirby and Moore), Walter Reed Army Medical Center, Washington DC, and the Departments of Pediatrics (Dr Bilello) and Clinical Investigation (Dr O'Hair), William Beaumont Army Medical Center, El Paso, Tex.

The opinions expressed are those of the authors and are not to be construed as official or as reflecting the views of the Department of the Army or the Department of Defense.

Reprint requests to Chief, Section of Pediatric Cardiology, Walter Reed Army Medical Center, Washington, DC 20307-5001 (Dr Moore).

MATERIALS AND METHODS

The experimental protocol was reviewed and approved by the Department of Clinical Investigation review board at the William Beaumont Army Medical Center, El Paso, Tex. Domestic swine weighing 10 to 20 kg were initially sedated with an intramuscular injection of ketamine hydrochloride before induction with intramuscular fentanyl citrate and droperidol. After an aural intravenous line was started, the animals were given intravenous pentathol sodium. General anesthesia was maintained with 1% to 3% halothane (2-bromo-2-chloro-1,1,1-trifluoroethane) to effect, 55% to 60% nitrous oxide, and 40% to 45% oxygen.

The animals were divided into two groups: intravenous and intraosseous. There were six runs per group, for a total of 12 runs. Two of the animals were used in both the intravenous and intraosseous trials at two separate times, for a total of 10 animals. All animals were treated in a humane fashion and recovered with adequate pain control after the procedure.

After intubation, all animals were continuously monitored with electrocardiography. All animals underwent a surgical procedure for placement of both a femoral artery catheter and a 7F Swan-Ganz catheter into the femoral vein. The venous catheter tip was advanced with continuous pressure monitoring through the heart to the pulmonary artery, where wedge pressures were identified. The intravenous group had a long intravenous catheter placed into the right femoral vein next to the Swan-Ganz catheter for delivery of dobutamine hydrochloride and isoproterenol hydrochloride. Both catheters were secured at their entry site with nylon suture. The intraosseous group had a bone marrow biopsy needle placed into the left tibial bone marrow space at the upper medial aspect of the tibia just below the tubercle. Placement into the bone marrow space was confirmed by both aspiration of bone marrow and demonstration of visible bone spicules. A pressure transducer was attached to the femoral arterial catheter to measure diastolic, systolic, and mean arterial pressures. Cardiac outputs were measured by the thermal dilution technique (American Edwards Laboratory Cardiac Output Computer, American Edwards Laboratory, Santa Ana, Calif). Intravenous and intraosseous infusions were delivered with Harvard infusion pumps.

Both dobutamine and isoproterenol were delivered at rates of 20 μg/kg per minute intraosseously or intravenously. Heart rate, mean

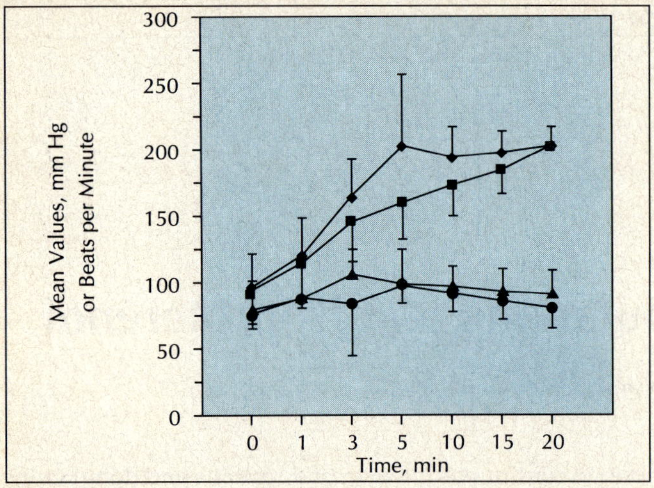

Fig 1.—*Effect of dobutamine hydrochloride on heart rate (in beats per minute) and arterial pressure (in millimeters of mercury). Mean values with 1 SD are given for both variables. Circles indicate arterial pressure with intravenous infusion; triangles, arterial pressure with intraosseous infusion; squares, heart rate with intravenous infusion; and diamonds, heart rate with intraosseous infusion.*

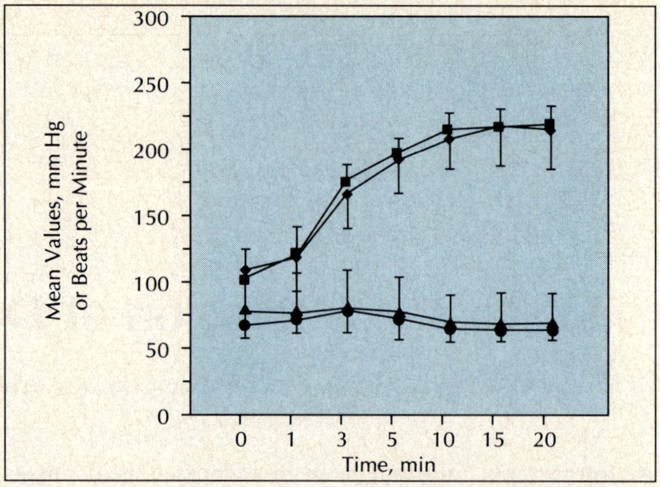

Fig 3.—*Effect of isoproterenol hydrochloride on heart rate (beats per minute) and arterial pressure (in millimeters of mercury). Mean values with 1 SD are given for both variables. See Fig 1 for explanation of symbols.*

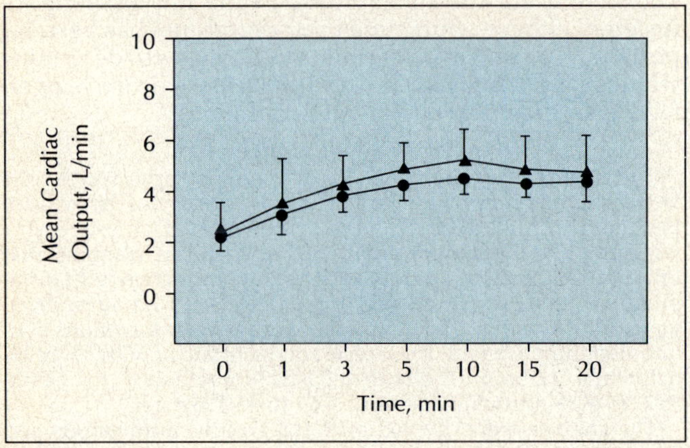

Fig 2.—*Effect of dobutamine hydrochloride on cardiac output. Values are means with 1 SD. Circles indicate intravenous infusion; triangles, intraosseous infusion.*

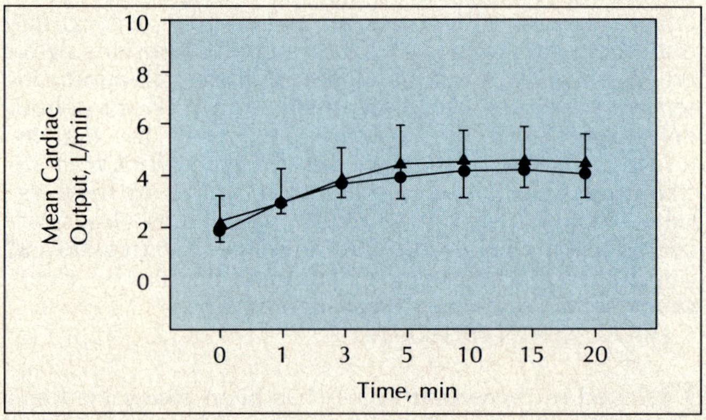

Fig 4.—*Effect of isoproterenol hydrochloride on cardiac output. Values are means with 1 SD. Circles indicate intravenous infusion; triangles, intraosseous infusion.*

arterial pressure, and cardiac output (average of three trials) were measured at 0, 1, 3, 5, 10, 15, and 20 minutes. Zero time data were recorded immediately before the onset of infusion. During all trials, the drug infusions were flushed to the ends of the tubing (to the hub of the bone biopsy needles or intravenous catheters).

For each animal, dobutamine was delivered first. The isoproterenol infusion trials were performed when both heart rate and blood pressure returned to within 5% of their original baseline values or after 30 minutes, whichever occurred first.

RESULTS

In the dobutamine studies, baseline values (mean±1 SD) of heart rate (intraosseous group vs intravenous group, 91±24 vs 95±24 beats per minute), arterial pressure (intraosseous group vs intravenous group, 75±8 vs 78±20 mm Hg), and cardiac output (intraosseous group vs intravenous group, 2.2±0.5 vs 2.4±1.0 L/min) were statistically similar ($P>.10$). The results of the heart rate, arterial pressure, and cardiac output determinations at each time interval are illustrated in Figs 1 and 2. The values for each variable at each time point were compared with use of a paired *t* test. All results were similar between the intraosseous and intravenous groups, with the exception of heart rate at 5 minutes. Heart rate for the intraosseus group at 5 minutes was greater than that for the intravenous group without apparent explanation. Moreover, statistically significant ($P<.05$) increases were noted in heart rates and cardiac outputs as a result of dobutamine infusions. Both heart rate and cardiac output essentially doubled by 20 minutes whether dobutamine was infused via a vein or into the bone marrow. Arterial pressure did not demonstrate a significant difference from its baseline in either group, regardless of the route of administration.

In the isoproterenol studies, baseline values of heart rate (intravenous group vs intraosseous group, 101±20 vs 107±22 beats per minute), arterial pressure (intravenous group vs intraosseous group, 65±8 vs 77±23 mm Hg), and cardiac output (intravenous group vs intraosseous group, 1.7±0.4 vs 2.1±0.9 L/min) were statistically similar ($P>.10$). The results of the heart rate, arterial pressure, and cardiac output determinations at each time interval are illustrated in Figs 3 and 4. The values for each variable at each time point were compared with use of a paired *t* test. All results were similar between the intraosseous and intravenous groups. In addition, statistically significant ($P<.05$) increases were noted in heart rates and cardiac outputs as a result of isoproterenol infusions. Both heart rate and cardiac output approximately doubled by 20 minutes whether isoproterenol was infused by the intravenous or the intraosseous route. Arterial pressure, on the other hand, showed no clear trend in either group.

COMMENT

In this study, the infusions of dobutamine and isoproterenol through the bone marrow were as effective as intravenous infusions of these drugs. Our data suggest that the emergency intraosseous infusion of dobutamine and isoproterenol may be successfully employed should achievement of intravenous access be delayed.

With our present data, the list of drugs for the treatment of cardiac arrest that have been studied with the use of intraosseous infusion continues to expand and now includes epinephrine, sodium bicarbonate, hypertonic glucose, dopamine, dobutamine, and isoproterenol. With the exception of sodium bicarbonate,[21] studies have involved observations made in animals under normal hemodynamic conditions. Although sodium bicarbonate was effectively administered by bone marrow infusion during circulatory collapse and cardiopulmonary resuscitation, the available animal data do not guarantee that the other drugs will be effective under such dire circumstances.

In addition, clinicians who employ intraosseous infusions must keep in mind that this method is simply a temporary measure until reliable and adequate intravenous infusion routes are established. Intraosseous infusion should be discontinued at the first available opportunity. Osteomyelitis has been cited as a serious complication of intraosseous infusion. In his study of almost 1000 intraosseous infusions, Heinild et al[11] documented osteomyelitis in 10% of hypertonic glucose infusions. Osteomyelitis is primarily associated with prolonged continuous infusion, especially longer than 24 hours.[10,11,18] A review by Rossetti et al[23] revealed that among 4270 cases of intraosseous infusions in humans, only 27 cases (0.6%) of osteomyelitis were reported. Osteomyelitis usually occurred with prolonged intraosseous infusion at a single site and in the bacteremic patient. The risk of osteomyelitis from an intraosseous line, therefore, should be weighed against the risks of impending or untreated cardiovascular collapse if immediate intravascular access is not obtained. Although the possibility of fat embolism has also been considered, it has not been reported to result from tibial infusions in humans, probably due to the relative lack of fat in the bone marrow of children.[24]

Our data provide further substantiation that intraosseous infusion should be regarded as an effective emergency technique for the administration of emergency drugs and fluids, especially dobutamine and isoproterenol.

References

1. Rossetti V, Thompson EM, Aprahamian C, Darin JC, Mateer JR. Difficulty and delay in intravascular access in pediatric arrests. *Ann Emerg Med.* 1984;13:406. Abstract.
2. Josefson A. A new method of treatment: introssal injections. *Acta Med Scand.* 1934;81:550-564.
3. Tocantins LM. Rapid absorption of substances injected into bone marrow. *Proc Soc Exp Biol Med.* 1940;45:292-296.
4. Tocantins LM, O'Neill JF, Jones HW. Infusions of blood and other fluids via the bone marrow. *JAMA.* 1941;117:1229-1234.
5. Papper EM. The bone marrow route for injecting fluids and drugs into the general circulation. *Anesthesiology.* 1942:3:307-317.
6. Macht DI. Studies on intraosseous injection of epinephrine. *Am J Physiol.* 1943;138:269-272.
7. Turkel H, Bethell FH. A new and simple instrument for administration of fluids through the bone marrow. *War Med.* 1944;5:222-225.
8. Arbeiter HI, Greengard J. Tibial bone marrow infusions in infancy. *J Pediatr.* 1944;25:1-12.
9. Meola F. Bone marrow infusions as a routine procedure in children. *J Pediatr.* 1944;25:13-16.
10. Quilligan JJ, Turkel H. Bone marrow infusion and its complications. *AJDC.* 1946;71:457-465.
11. Heinild S, Sondergaard J, Tuvdad F. Bone marrow infusions in childhood: experiences from a thousand infusions. *J Pediatr.* 1947;30:400-411.
12. Tarrow AB, Turkel H, Thompson CS. Infusions via the bone marrow and biopsy of the bone and bone marrow. *Anesthesiology.* 1952;13:501-509.
13. Valdes MM. Intraosseous fluid administration in emergencies. *Lancet.* 1977;1:1235-1236.
14. Intraosseous infusion. *JAMA.* 1953;151:1108. Editorial.
15. Turkel H. Intraosseous infusion. *AJDC.* 1983;137:706.
16. Orlowski JP. My kingdom for an intravenous line. *AJDC.* 1984;138:803.
17. Berg RA. Emergency infusion of catecholamines into bone marrow. *AJDC.* 1984;138:810-811.
18. Hodge D. Intraosseous infusions: a review. *Pediatr Emerg Care.* 1985;1:214-218.
19. Shoor PM, Berryhill RE, Benumof JL. Intraosseous infusion: pressure flow relationship and pharmacokinetics. *J Trauma.* 1979;19:772-774.
20. Thompson BM, Rossetti V, Miller J, Mateer JR, Aprahamian C, Darin JC. Intraosseous administration of sodium bicarbonate: an effective means of pH normalization in the canine model. *Ann Emerg Med.* 1984;13:405-409.
21. Spivey WH, Lathers CM, Malone DR, et al. Comparison of intravenous, central, and peripheral routes of sodium bicarbonate administration during CPR in pigs. *Ann Emerg Med.* 1985;14:1135-1140.
22. Neish SR, Macon MG, Moore JW, Graeber GM. Intraosseous infusion of hypertonic glucose and dopamine. *AJDC.* 1988;142:878-880.
23. Rossetti VA, Thompson BM, Miller J, Mateer JR, Aprahamian C. Intraosseous infusion: an alternative route of pediatric intravascular access. *Ann Emerg Med.* 1985;14:885-888.
24. Fiser DH. Intraosseous infusion. *N Engl J Med.* 1990;322:1579-1581.

Effectiveness of Growth-Promoting Therapies

Comparison Among Growth Hormone, Clonidine, and Levodopa

Cecilia Volta, MD; Lucia Ghizzoni, MD; Gaetano Muto, MD; Raffaella Spaggiari, MD; Raffaele Virdis, MD; Sergio Bernasconi, MD

• The ability of growth hormone, clonidine, and levodopa to stimulate growth was compared in short and slowly growing children randomly assigned to different treatment regimens for 6 months. There were 10 children in each group, and 10 additional subjects served as controls. Growth hormone improved mean height velocity, height velocity SD score, and height SD score. The mean height velocity and height velocity SD score were significantly increased by clonidine, while levodopa only enhanced the mean height velocity SD score of the treated children. Moreover, in nine patients (90%) receiving growth hormone, two (20%) receiving clonidine, and one (10%) receiving levodopa, the height velocity was raised by more than 2 cm/y. The increments in height velocity and height SD score were greatest in the growth hormone group. Clonidine induced an increase in height velocity significantly different from that in control children only. In the control group, there was a significant reduction of height SD score with time.

***(AJDC.* 1991;145:168–171)**

In 1981, Rudman et al[1] showed that short-term growth hormone (GH) treatment was effective in improving height velocity (HV) in a group of short and slowly growing children with normal pituitary function. Since then several other studies[2-7] have demonstrated that a high percentage of short normal children show a sustained clinical benefit from GH therapy. However, the important factors in predicting the response to treatment have not yet been clearly defined.[8]

Increasing knowledge of the neuroendocrine mechanisms regulating GH secretion has led to the use of substances known to acutely stimulate GH release from the pituitary, such as clonidine[9-11] and levodopa,[12,13] for the treatment of short stature. The results of these studies are extremely discordant, probably due to the heterogeneity of clinical features and the small number of subjects studied.

To evaluate and compare the growth-promoting effects of GH, clonidine, and levodopa, we analyzed the growth response to long-term administration of these agents in a group of short children with the same auxological features. The results obtained were compared with those in a group of subjects receiving no medication.

MATERIALS AND METHODS

Forty children (eight girls and 32 boys) with short stature were evaluated at the Growth Clinic of the Department of Pediatrics of the University of Parma, Italy. Inclusion criteria for entry in the study are reported in Table 1. The value of −0.8 for HV SD score (HVSDS) was chosen because it is the lowest value at which prepubertal children can grow at the third percentile.[14]

Patients were randomly assigned to the following groups: group 1 (n = 10), no medication; group 2 (n = 10), levodopa (Larodopa, LaRoche Inc, Basel, Switzerland), 60 mg/kg per day by mouth three times per day up to 25 kg, with a constant dosage of 1500 mg/d thereafter, for 6 months; group 3 (n = 10), clonidine (Catapresan, Boehringer, Mannheim, Germany), 75 $\mu g/m^2$ by mouth twice per day, one third in the morning and two thirds in the evening, for 6 months; and group 4 (n = 10), GH (Somatomorm, KabiVitrium Inc, Stockholm, Sweden), 13 IU/m^2 per week, subdivided in six subcutaneous daily injections, for 6 months.

Informed consent was obtained from parents, and the study was approved by the ethical committee of the Department of Pediatrics of the University of Parma. Standard auxological assessment (height, weight, height velocity, and pubertal staging) was performed at 3-month intervals for 6 months. Kidney, liver, and thyroid function was checked in all children at baseline, and, in the groups under treatment, after 3 and 6 months; in addition, an oral glucose tolerance test and glycosylated hemoglobin evaluation were performed before and after treatment in group 4 only. A roentgenogram of the left hand for bone age evaluation was performed at baseline and at the end of the study period.

Height was measured with a wall-mounted Harpender stadiometer; bone age was determined by an experienced examiner using the standards of Greulich and Pyle.[15] The HV before the study was calculated based on measurements taken in the preceding year and expressed as the HVSDS corrected for bone age. An increase in HV greater than 2 cm/y was considered significant, because this approximates 2 SDs of the variation that occurs in whole-year HVs in normal prepubertal children.[16] Serum GH, levothyroxine, triiodothyronine, thyroid-stimulating hormone, free thyroxine, and free triiodothyronine levels were measured as previously described.[13,17]

All results are expressed at mean±SD. For statistical analysis, we used the paired *t* test for comparisons within groups and the Newman-Keuls test for multiple comparisons among independent groups of data; correlations were evaluated by linear regression analysis.

Accepted for publication August 6, 1990.

From the Department of Pediatrics, University of Parma, Italy.

Presented in part at the Third Joint Meeting of the European Society for Pediatric Endocrinology and the Lawson Wilkins Pediatric Endocrinology Society, Jerusalem, Israel, October 31, 1989.

Reprint requests to Clinica Pediatrica, Università degli Studi di Parma, Via Gramsci 14, 43100 Parma, Italy (Dr Bernasconi).

Table 1.—Inclusion Criteria for Entry in the Study

Birth weight appropriate for gestational age
No evidence of systemic diseases, malnutrition, dysmorphic syndromes, or psychosocial disturbances
Tanner stage 1 of pubertal development
Height SD score < −2
Whole-year height velocity SD < −0.8
Growth hormone response to pharmacological stimuli >10 μg/L (insulin hypoglycemia, 0.1 U/kg intravenously, or clonidine, 100 μg/m² by mouth)
Normal thyroid function

RESULTS

At inclusion, mean chronological age, bone age, HV, height SD score (HSDS), and HVSDS corrected for bone age were similar in all groups (Table 2). There were also no differences in mean midparental height (group 1, 160.4.±4 cm; group 2, 157.5±4 cm; group 3, 157.3±6 cm; and group 4, 157.9±6 cm).

Results at the end of the study period are shown in Table 2 and Fig 1 and can be summarized as follows:

Group 1.—The HV and HVSDS did not significantly change in the 6-month follow-up. However, there was a significant decrease in the HSDS (−2.3±0.4 vs −2.4±0.4, $P<.05$).

Group 2.—Levodopa administration significantly improved the mean HVSDS only (−0.9±1.1 vs −2±0.8, $P<.05$); the mean HV and HSDS were similar to the baseline values. Only one patient had an increase in HV greater than 2 cm/y (from 3.6 to 7 cm/y).

Group 3.—The mean HV and HVSDS were significantly increased by clonidine therapy (5±1 vs 3.8±1 cm/y, $P<.005$; and −1.1±0.9 vs −2.4±1, $P<.005$, respectively). However, only two patients had an improvement in HV (from 4.6 to 6.8 cm/y and from 3 to 5.8 cm/y).

Group 4.—Administration of GH significantly improved HV (6.8±1 vs 3.9±0.6 cm/y, $P<.001$) and HVSDS (1.9±1.3 vs −1.9±0.8, $P<.001$) as well as HSDS (−2.8±0.5 vs −3.1±0.6, $P<.01$). Nine patients (90%) had an increase in HV greater than 2 cm/y.

The bone age/chronological age ratio did not change in any group, and all the children remained prepubertal throughout the study. When the baseline individual HV, HVSDS, and HSDS values of all subjects were plotted with respect to the corresponding values after therapy, no correlation was found.

Comparisons among independent groups after 6 months of either therapy or clinical follow-up showed that the mean posttreatment HV was significantly higher ($P<.05$) in group 4 than in all other groups (6.8±1 [group 4] vs 3.5±0.6 [group 1], 4.5±1.3 [group 2], and 5.1±1.1 [group 3] cm/y), and the value in group 3 was significantly higher ($P<.05$) than in group 1. Figure 2 shows the increment in HV. Growth hormone therapy resulted in an improvement in HV greater than that in all other groups (2.9±0.9 [group 4] vs −0.16±0.9 [group 1], 0.6±1.6 [group 2], and 1.2±0.8 [group 3] cm/y), while clonidine induced an increase in HV significantly greater than that in control children only. Levodopa seems not to be able to induce remarkable improvements in HV.

The changes in HVSDS and HSDS are also shown in Fig 2. The change in HVSDS was significantly greater ($P<.05$) in group 4 (3.9±1.4) than in all other groups (−0.13±1 [group 1], 0.88±1 [group 2], and 1.25±0.7 [group 3]), and the changes in HVSDS were significantly greater in groups 2 and 3 than in group 1. The change in HSDS was significantly greater in group 1 (−0.09±0.05) than in all other groups (0.001±0.1 [group 2], 0.08±0.1 [group 3], and 0.23±0.1 [group 4]), confirming that the HSDS worsened in the untreated children, and the change in HSDS was significantly greater in group 4 than in groups 2 and 3.

Table 2.—Auxological Data Before and After the Study Period

	Group			
	Control	Levodopa	Clonidine	Growth Hormone
No. of subjects	10	10	10	10
Chronological age, y				
Before study period	9.4±2.1	9.7±1.8	8.9±2.1	10.9±1.7
After study period	9.9±2.1	10.2±1.8	9.4±2.1	11.4±1.7
Bone age, y				
Before study period	6.89±2.1	7.70±2.2	6.51±2.1	8.75±1.9
After study period	7.88±1.8	8.21±2.4	7.12±1.9	9.57±1.9
Height velocity, cm/y				
Before study period	3.7±1.2	3.9±0.6	3.8±1.0*	3.9±0.6*
After study period	3.5±0.6	4.5±1.3	5.0±1.1*	6.8±1.0*
Height SD Score				
Before study period	−2.3±0.4*	−2.5±0.4	−2.6±0.6	−3.1±0.6*
After study period	−2.4±0.4*	−2.5±0.4	−2.5±0.7	−2.8±0.5*
Height velocity SD score corrected for bone age				
Before study period	−2.4±1.4	−2±0.8*	−2.4±1.0*	−1.9±0.8*
After study period	−2.5±0.9	−0.9±1.1*	−1.1±0.9*	1.9±1.3*

*$P<.05$ for before vs after the study period.

Thyroid, kidney, and liver function and oral glucose tolerance test results were normal in all subjects. The only side effects reported were slight transitory sleepiness in four children receiving clonidine and occasional nausea and vomiting in six patients receiving levodopa.

COMMENT

In recent years, the virtually unlimited supply of recombinant GH has led to renewed interest in treating short children who do not fulfill the classic criteria of GH deficiency. Even if the results of many studies seem encouraging, the long-term safety and efficacy of GH treatment are still unknown. Moreover, the ethics of treating disease-free children are still under debate, and the high cost of the drug places a heavy economic burden on the family and/or society.[18,19]

These problems together with expanded knowledge of the neuroregulatory mechanisms of GH secretion have led to the use of alternative agents, such as clonidine and

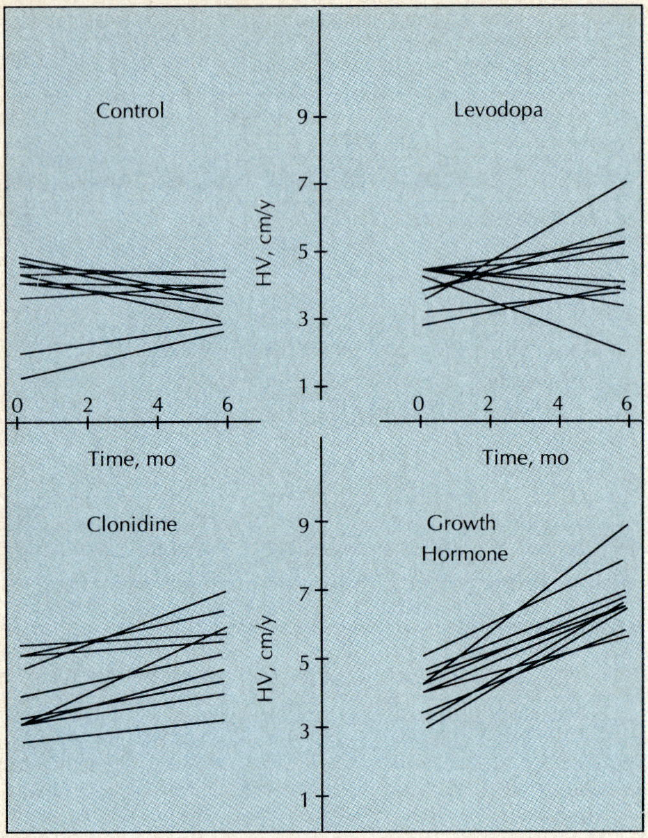

Fig 1.—*Individual height velocities (HVs) of children in groups 1 (no medication), 2 (levodopa), 3 (clonidine), and 4 (growth hormone).*

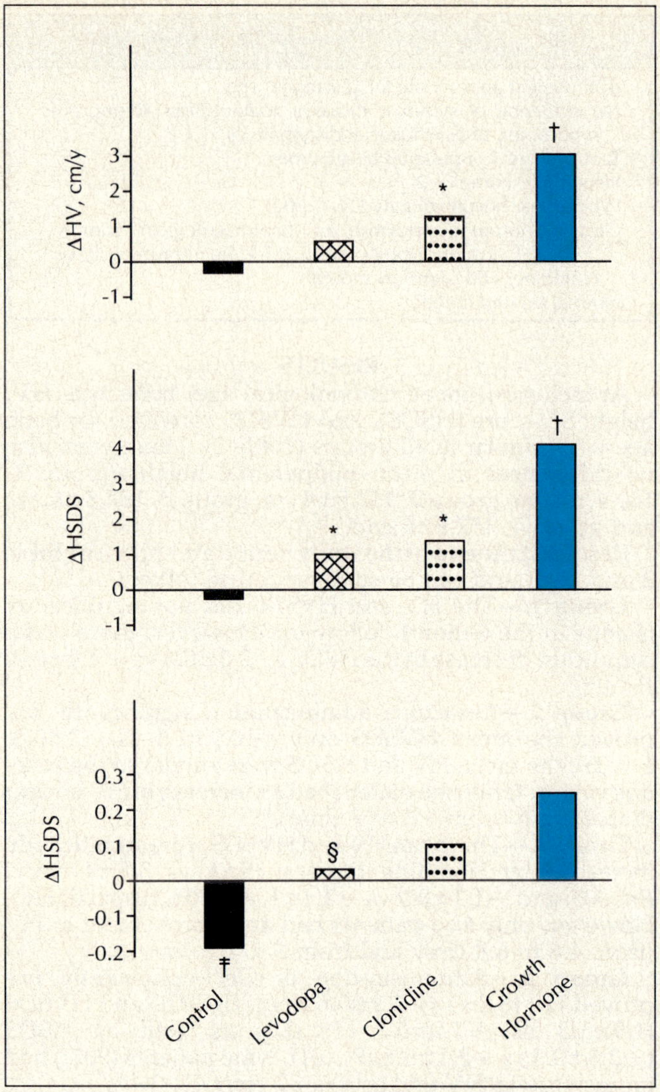

Fig 2.—*Changes in height velocity (ΔHV), HV SD score (ΔHVSDS), and height SD score (ΔHSDS). Asterisk indicates* $P<.05$ *compared with the control group; dagger,* $P<.05$ *compared with the control, levodopa, and clonidine groups; double dagger,* $P<.05$ *compared with the levodopa, clonidine, and growth hormone groups; and section mark,* $P<.05$ *compared with the growth hormone group.*

levodopa, that are able to stimulate GH production from the pituitary. The mechanism of action of these drugs is not yet completely clear. There is indirect evidence that the GH secretion induced by levodopa is due to the release of GH releasing hormone, while clonidine seems to predominantly act through inhibition of the somato-statinergic tone.[20]

Several trials with these agents have been conducted in different subpopulations of short normal children. However, to our knowledge, no studies have examined the different growth-stimulating efficacy of these drugs in children with similar clinical and auxological features. For this reason we compared the ability of GH, clonidine, and levodopa to enhance growth in a homogeneous group of short and slowly growing children.

The findings of the present study indicate that GH is effective in improving the growth of short normal children. The administration of levodopa for 6 months did not induce positive changes in the auxologic parameters analyzed, while the results obtained with clonidine were intermediate between those with GH and levodopa. However, despite the absence of remarkable improvements, both clonidine and levodopa were able to prevent the reduction of HSDS that occurred in the control group.

The results summarized above demonstrate that GH was the most effective growth-promoting agent we used. This observation is in agreement with studies in which a high percentage of short children receiving short-term GH therapy had an improvement in both HV and HSDS.[1-7] The lack of correlation between pretreatment and posttreatment values of all the auxologic parameters analyzed indicates that these factors were not important in predicting response to treatment. Therefore, a short-term therapeutic trial with GH seems to be the only way to identify the children who might benefit from this therapy.[21,22]

Huseman[12] reported evidence for dopaminergic stimulation of growth in GH-deficient subjects and in children with intrauterine growth retardation, microcephaly, and psychomotor delay. In addition, it has been shown that levodopa potentiates the effects of GH treatment in some children with growth hormone deficiency.[23] The results we obtained treating short normal children with levodopa are not as encouraging as those mentioned above. Only one child, in fact, had an improvement in HV greater than 2 cm/y. It should be pointed out, however, that the heterogeneity of clinical characteristics of the patients examined in the different studies makes comparisons unsuitable.

The potential usefulness of clonidine as a growth-promoting agent in the treatment of non–GH-deficient short stature has been shown in three studies. The most encouraging study reported on 16 prepubertal children from San Salvador, El Salvador, who were treated with a single nightly dose of clonidine, 0.15 mg/m^2, for 1 year.[10] All 16 children had a rise in HV during treatment. The other two reports were by Pintor et al,[9,24] who treated 34 short normal children with clonidine, 0.1 mg/m^2 daily in two doses. The majority of children responded to the treatment regimen, although HV increased by more than 2 cm/y in only 21 subjects. In contrast to these studies, Pescovitz and Tan[11] found no sustained increases in GH production or improvements in HV in a placebo-controlled trial with administration of a single daily dose of clonidine, 0.1 mg/m^2.

In the present investigation, despite the improvement in mean HV and HVSDS, clonidine raised HV by more than 2 cm/y in only two children, results that approximate those of Pescovitz and Tan.

The most significant differences among these studies are those in patient selection and clonidine dosing. This is why it was important to test the efficacy of these drugs in subjects with similar clinical characteristics randomly assigned to different treatment regimens.

The absence or inadequacy of controls is a major limit of many reports, particularly when the purpose of the study is the evaluation of drug efficacy. In our study the follow-up of the control children showed a significant reduction in HSDS with time, probably related to the persistence of low HV throughout. This finding is partially at variance with the results of Pescovitz and Tan[11] in children treated with placebo. However, the baseline HV in this group of children treated with placebo was higher than in our patients, which might explain the divergent growth patterns of the two groups. The fact that HSDS was not reduced in the children treated with levodopa and clonidine indicates that these drugs did positively affect growth; at least growth did not deteriorate in these subjects, as it did in untreated subjects.

In conclusion, GH appears to be the most effective drug tested in this study in promoting growth in short normal children with the above-mentioned auxological features. However the effect on growth showed by clonidine and, to a lesser degree, by levodopa, although not sufficient to counsel treatment with these drugs, could lead to new ways of treatment, such as with newer GH-stimulating substances.

References

1. Rudman D, Kutner MH, Blackston RD, Cushman RA, Bain RP, Patterson JH. Children with normal-variant short stature: treatment with human growth hormone for 6 months. *N Engl J Med.* 1981;305:123-131

2. Frazer T, Gavin JR, Daughaday WH, Hillman RE, Weldon VV. Growth hormone–dependent growth failure. *J Pediatr.* 1982;101:12-15.

3. Plotnick LP, Van Meter QL, Kowarski AA. Human growth hormone treatment of children with growth failure and normal growth hormone levels by immunoassay: lack of correlation with somatomedin generation. *Pediatrics.* 1983;71:324-327.

4. Van Vliet G, Styne DM, Kaplan SL, Grumbach MM. Growth hormone treatment for short stature. *N Engl J Med.* 1983;104:12-15.

5. Gertner JM, Genel M, Gianfredi SP, et al. Prospective clinical trial of human growth hormone in short children without growth hormone deficiency. *J Pediatr.* 1984;104:172-176.

6. Hindmarsh PC, Brook CDG. Effect of growth hormone on short normal children. *BMJ.* 1987;295:573-577.

7. Raiti S, Kaplan SL, Van Vliet G, Moore WV. Short-term treatment of short stature and subnormal growth rate with human growth hormone. *J Pediatr.* 1987;110:357-361.

8. Penny R. Growth retardation: impaired height velocity. *AJDC.* 1989;143:1269-1270.

9. Pintor C, Cella SG, Corda R, et al. Clonidine accelerates growth in children with impaired growth hormone secretion. *Lancet.* 1985;1:1482-1485.

10. Castro-Magana M, Angulo M, Fuentes B, Castelar ME, Canas A, Espinoza B. Effect of prolonged clonidine administration on growth hormone concentrations and rate of linear growth in children with constitutional growth delay. *J Pediatr.* 1986;109:784-787.

11. Pescovitz OH, Tan E. Lack of benefit of clonidine treatment for short stature in a double-blind placebo-controlled trial. *Lancet.* 1988;2:874-877.

12. Huseman CA. Growth enhancement by dopaminergic therapy in children with intrauterine growth retardation. *J Clin Endocrinol Metab.* 1985;61:514-518.

13. Ghizzoni L, Volta C, Buono T, et al. L-DOPA treatment of children with short stature: preliminary results. In: Bierich JR, Cacciari E, Raiti S, eds. *Growth Abnormalities: Serono Symposia.* New York, NY: Raven Press; 1989:321-325.

14. Hindmarsh PC, Matthews DR, Brook CGD. Growth hormone secretion in children determined by time series analysis. *Clin Endocrinol.* 1988;29:35-44.

15. Greulich WW, Pyle SJ. *Radiographic Atlas of Skeletal Development of the Hand and Wrist.* 2nd ed. Stanford, Calif: Stanford University Press; 1959.

16. Tanner JM, Whitehouse RH, Hughes PCR, Vince FP. Effect of human growth hormone treatment for 1 to 7 years on growth of 100 children, with growth hormone deficiency, low birthweight, inherited smallness, Turner's syndrome, and other complaints. *Arch Dis Child.* 1971;46:745-782.

17. Bernasconi S, Vanelli M, Nori G, et al. Serum TSH, T_4, T_3, FT_4, FT_3, rT_3 and TBG in youngsters with non ketotic insulin dependent diabetes mellitus. *Horm Res.* 1984;20:213-217.

18. Lantos J, Siegler M, Cuttler L. Ethical issues in growth hormone therapy. *JAMA.* 1989;261;1020-1024.

19. Alternatives to growth hormone. *Lancet.* 1989;1:820-822.

20. Tapanainen P, Knip M, Lautala P, et al. Variable plasma growth hormone (GH)–releasing hormone and GH responses to clonidine, L-dopa and insulin in normal men. *J Clin Endocrinol Metab.* 1988;67:845-849.

21. Milner RDG. Which children should have growth hormone therapy? *Lancet.* 1986;1:483-485.

22. Bercu BB. Growth hormone treatment and the short child: to treat or not to treat? *J Pediatr.* 1987;110:991-995.

23. Huseman CA, Hassing JM, Sibilia MG. Endogenous dopaminergic dysfunction: a novel form of human growth hormone deficiency and short stature. *J Clin Endocrinol Metab.* 1986;62:484-490.

24. Pintor C, Cella SG, Loche S, et al. Clonidine treatment for short stature. *Lancet.* 1987;1:1226-1230.

Age-Related Patterns of Thyroid-Stimulating Hormone Response to Thyrotropin-Releasing Hormone Stimulation in Down Syndrome

Teresa Sharav, MBBS, MPH; Heddy Landau, MD; Zvi Zadik, MD; Thomas R. Einarson, PhD

• Thyroid function in subjects with Down syndrome was studied using the thyrotropin-releasing hormone test. Forty-seven infants and children with Down syndrome were investigated. Ages ranged from 1 month to 7 years; there were 26 boys and 21 girls. Fourteen of the subjects with Down syndrome who had an exaggerated thyroid-stimulating hormone response to thyrotropin-releasing hormone stimulation had two or more annual follow-up tests. The remaining 33 subjects who only underwent one thyrotropin-releasing hormone test were compared with 22 age-matched controls (11 boys and 11 girls). Mean basal thyroxine 4 and triiodothyronine 3 values were in the normal ranges. All thyroid antibody titers were negative. Mean basal thyroid-stimulating hormone levels of subjects with Down syndrome were significantly higher than those of controls for all ages, even though there was a decline in thyroid-stimulating hormone levels in both groups. Peak thyroid-stimulating hormone response levels were significantly greater in the subjects with Down syndrome than in the controls. Longitudinal study of the 14 children with Down syndrome with an exaggerated thyroid-stimulating hormone response showed that the response remained exaggerated until the third year of life, when it declined to normal levels. Thyroid dysfunction during the growth spurt of infancy or delayed maturation of the hypothalamic pituitary thyroid axis are proposed mechanisms.

***(AJDC.* 1991;145:172–175)**

An increased prevalence of disorders of the hypothalamic pituitary thyroid axis in children with Down syndrome has been described. Autoimmune thyroiditis in cases of pubescent and postpubescent Down syndrome is well known.[1-4] The prevalence of congenital hypothyroidism in neonates with Down syndrome has been reported to be 28 times greater than that in normal neonates.[5] Higher mean basal thyroid-stimulating hormone (TSH) levels in patients with Down syndrome compared with controls has been shown to occur throughout the age spectrum, including infancy. This phenomenon has been termed *thyroid dysfunction*.[6,7] However, these high mean basal TSH levels are accompanied by normal mean thyroxine (T_4) and triiodothyronine (T_3) levels. The meaning of the high basal TSH levels in association with normal T_4 and T_3 levels in patients with Down syndrome has yet to be explained.

Infants with Down syndrome with high TSH levels have been shown to be smaller than those with lower TSH levels.[8] This observation has been noted in infancy, mainly before age 4 years. Some children with hypothalamic pituitary disorders have high basal TSH levels and an exaggerated TSH response to the administration of exogenous thyrotropin-releasing hormone (TRH) in the presence of normal T_3 and T_4 levels.[9,10] The present study, using the TRH stimulating test, was undertaken to further elucidate thyroid dysfunction in infants and children with Down syndrome.

Accepted for publication May 18, 1990.

From the Jerusalem (Israel) Child Development Center (Dr Sharav); the Department of Pediatrics and Clinical Endocrinology, Hadassah University Hospital, Jerusalem (Dr Landau); the Department of Pediatric Endocrinology, Kaplan Hospital, Rehovot, Israel (Dr Zadik); and the Faculty of Pharmacy and Department of Health Administration, Faculty of Medicine, University of Toronto, Ontario (Dr Einarson).

Reprint requests to the Jerusalem Child Development Center, 24 Strauss St, Jerusalem, Israel 95142 (Dr Sharav).

PATIENTS AND METHODS

Forty-seven infants and children with Down syndrome were included in the study. Chromosomal analysis showed that a trisomy 21 was present in 45 children; one other case was a translocation and another was a mosaic. Ages ranged from 1 month to 7 years; there were 26 girls and 21 boys. Thirty-seven of the patients were from the Jerusalem (Israel) Child Development Center to which all infants with Down syndrome born in Jerusalem are referred. Ten patients were from the Rehovot area of Israel. Initially, the patients were included as they came for routine follow-up; they ranged in age from 1 month to 7 years. However, as new infants were born they were studied within 3 months of birth; consequently, there were more infants in the youngest age category. All the infants included in the study were born within 3 weeks of term, all were in good health, and none had clinical goiter.

Patients were examined after an overnight fast or, in infants, 4 hours after their early morning feeding. The TRH stimulation test was performed by injecting an intravenous 4-μg/kg bolus of synthetic TRH (Roche, F. Hoffman La Roche Ltd, Basle, Switzerland); serum TSH levels were determined before injection and 15, 30, and 60 minutes after injection. The higher of the 15 and 30 minute values was designated as the peak value. Total T_4 and T_3 levels were measured in unextracted serum by radioimmunoassay (Seralute Ames Co, Elkhart, Ind; T3 RIA Kit, Amersham, Arlington Heights, Ill). Serum TSH levels were measured by radioimmunoassay[11] with a sensitivity of 0.5 to 1.0 mU/L.

Antibody titers to thyroglobulin and thyroidal microsomal antibodies were measured by immunofluorescence. The Jerusalem

Table 1.—Thyroxine (T_4) Values and Levels of TSH Response to TRH Injection in Patients With Down Syndrome and Controls by Age Groups*

Group	No.	T_4, nmol/L	Basal TSH, mU/L†	Peak TSH, mU/L (15 or 30 min)‡	TSH, mU/L (60 min)§
Overall					
Down syndrome	3	126±35	7.3±6.9	25.8±11.4	18.2±11.4
Control	22	142±19	2.5±1.8	14.7±5.7	10.8±5.4
<1 y					
Down syndrome	19	126±42	10.2±7.7	30.5±11.3	23.2±13.5
Control	7	138±19	4.0±2.3	18.0±4.2	15.5±5.3
1 to 3 y					
Down syndrome	7	127±23	4.2±3.9	23.9±8.1	15.3±4.4
Control	6	133±19	2.3±1.1	17.5±5.4	10.9±3.9
3 to 7 y					
Down syndrome	7	116±22	2.7±0.6	14.9±4.8	9.6±3.6
Control	9	153±21	1.3±0.8	9.0±2.4	5.9±1.7

*Numbers are means±SDs. TSH indicates thyroid-stimulating hormone; and TRH, thyrotropin-releasing hormone.
†Using analysis of variance (ANOVA), $f=4.1$; $P<.05$.
‡Using ANOVA, $f=11.9$; $P<.001$.
§Using ANOVA, $f=4.0$; $P<.05$.

and Rehovot laboratories used the same kits and standard measurements. The normal adult ranges for the laboratory values are as follows: T_4, 59 to 154 nmol/L; T_3, 1.23 to 3.1 nmol/L; and TSH, 0.5 to 6 mU/L. A peak TSH response of above 20 mU/L is classified as exaggerated. Fisher's criteria[12] were used to diagnose hypothyroidism as a function of age. The values were as follows: from 1 to 12 months, T_4, 80 to 198 nmol/L; T_3, 1.6 to 3.4 nmol/L; and TSH, 0.5 to 6.5 mU/L; from 1 to 6 years, T_4, 68 to 171 nmol/L; T_3, 1.5 to 3.4 nmol/L; and TSH, 0.6 to 6.3 mU/L; and from 7 to 12 years, T_4, 62 to 160 nmol/L; T_3, 1.3 to 3.2 nmol/L; and TSH, 0.6 to 6.3 mU/L. The TSH responses to TRH stimulation in the infants with Down syndrome were compared with those of the controls.

An age-matched control group of 22 infants and children (11 boys and 11 girls) was obtained from the Pediatric Endocrinology Departments of the Jerusalem and Rehovot Hospitals. These were children who, during the period of the study, underwent the TRH test for various clinical reasons and in whom no subsequent biologic or endocrine abnormality was found. Thirty-three of the children with Down syndrome who underwent only one TRH test were compared with the controls. The children with Down syndrome and the controls were grouped according to age.

There were insufficient numbers of subjects tested to group by year, so the grouping was as follows: younger than 1 year; 1 to 3 years of age; and older than age 3 years. The remaining subgroup of 14 children with Down syndrome who had an initial exaggerated response to TRH stimulation was analyzed separately. All 14 patients had a TRH test performed again after approximately 1 year, and six patients had three annual TRH tests performed. Eighteen of the tests were performed on children younger than 1 year, 11 on children between ages 1 and 3 years, and five on children older than 3 years.

For statistical analysis, a repeated-measures analysis of variance (ANOVA) was performed to examine differences between children with Down syndrome and controls at varying age groups.[13,14] For the group of 14 children with Down syndrome who had follow-up repeated TRH tests performed, Duncan's Multiple Range Test was used. This was used to partition the effects of age within subject variation and across subject variation in TSH.

RESULTS

Mean T_4 and T_3 values were within the normal range in both the Down syndrome and control groups. All thyroid antibody study results were negative. Using Fisher's criteria,[12] none of the infants with Down syndrome had T_4 levels sufficiently low to be designated clearly as hypothyroid. Table 1 shows T_4 values in relation to basal, peak, and 1-hour TSH levels in subjects with Down syndrome and controls. Repeated-measures ANOVA showed that mean basal TSH levels of subjects with Down syndrome were significantly higher than those of age-matched controls ($f=4.1$; $P<.05$). The peak TSH response was significantly higher in the Down syndrome population than in the control group ($f=11.9$; $P<.001$). The mean 1-hour TSH level was also significantly higher in the subjects with Down syndrome than in the controls ($f=4.0$; $P<.05$). This difference between patients with Down syndrome and controls held true for all age categories, even though the basal and peak TSH levels of the children with Down syndrome declined to levels that would be considered normal for age. The subgroup of 14 subjects with Down syndrome who had an initial exaggerated TSH response to TRH stimulation was studied longitudinally.

Table 2.—Basal and Peak TSH Levels in a Group of 14 Patients With Down Syndrome Studied Longitudinally*

	Age, y		
	<1†	1-3†	3-7
No. of tests	11	18	5
Basal TSH level, mU/L‡	8.1±4.9	6.8±3.9	2.1±1.0
Peak TSH level, mU/L§	35.9±7.1	36.4±10.1	24.3±13.6

*Unless otherwise indicated, numbers are means±SDs. TSH indicates thyroid-stimulating hormone.
†Values for patients younger than 1 year and between 1 and 3 years are not statistically different.
‡Using Duncan's Multiple Range Test, $f=3.45$ and $P<.05$.
§Using Duncan's Multiple Range Test, $f=3.96$ and $P<.05$.

Duncan's Multiple Range Test (Table 2) showed a significant difference of basal TSH and peak TSH levels between the two younger age groups compared with the oldest age category ($P<.05$). The mean peak TSH response remained at a level of 36.4 mU/L until the third year, after which it declined to approximately normal levels.

COMMENT

The concentrations of serum thyroid hormones vary with age, and norms as a function of age have been derived.[12] Our baseline results were compared with these norms as well as with levels in the controls used in the study. Although the number of controls in the present study was small because the TRH test is not a routine procedure, when control group peak TSH values were compared with those of a larger study, the values were compatible.[15] For children younger than 1 year, our control group peak TSH level was 18 mU/L compared with 17 mU/L for a larger study group; between 1 and 3 years, 17.5 mU/L compared with 14.1 mU/L; and between 3 and 6 years, 9.0 mU/L compared with 9.7 mU/L.

Using Fisher's criteria,[12] none of our patients with Down syndrome showed clear-cut hypothyroidism, but they had persistently higher basal TSH levels than did normal controls, which were associated with T_4 and T_3 levels appropriate for age. This higher basal TSH level was accompanied by a significantly greater TSH response than in the controls. With increasing age, there was a decline in both basal TSH and peak TSH responses to what could be considered normal levels, although they continued to be higher than those of the controls ($P<.001$). The subgroup of 14 patients with Down syndrome who, on initial testing, had an exaggerated TSH response maintained the exaggerated peak TSH response until the third year of life.

Transiently elevated TSH levels have been observed in premature infants, and are associated with jaundice and respiratory and fetal distress.[16,17] The cause of the thyroid insufficiency remains unknown. The suggested hypothesis is that it is due to low thyroidal content of iodine in newborn infants and delayed maturation of enzymatic mechanisms of intrathyroidal hormonogenesis. Although none of the infants or children with Down syndrome studied were premature or ill, the above hypothesis could be considered in the etiology. Thyrotropin levels are physiologically high in newborns. Levels decline to normal by age 4 days and even transiently high TSH levels return to normal by age 2 months.[17] In the infant with Down syndrome, prolongation of this physiologically high TSH could be an expression of immaturity of the hypothalamic pituitary axis. This could result in the secretion of a thyrotropin of low biologic activity, which, in turn, may be an expression of a TRH deficiency.[18,19] Other hypothalamic factors involved in TSH regulation, such as dopamine or somatostatin levels, may be involved.

Delayed maturation of the hormone somatomedin has been shown to occur in children with Down syndrome,[20] with incomplete switching from the fetal form of somatomedin to the growth hormone–related insulin growth factor. With increasing age, the basal TSH and peak TSH responses declined to normal levels. As metabolic needs decline with age, so the biochemical expression of thyroid dysfunction as expressed by TSH measurements improves. Other compensatory mechanisms may come into play, such as the reduction in the pituitary threshold for the feedback of TSH.[21,22] However, both the basal and peak TSH levels in patients with Down syndrome are consistently higher than those in the controls, which may suggest a different mechanism. The relatively high TSH levels were associated with normal T_4 and T_3 values. Paradoxically high TSH levels in the presence of normal T_4 and T_3 values have been described in a small number of heterogeneous thyroid disorders and have been termed *inappropriate secretion of TSH*.[23] Proposed mechanisms are of peripheral resistance to thyroid hormones or central disorders of TSH secretion. Down syndrome cell membranes are known to have abnormal biochemical, physiologic, and receptor functions.[24,25] These altered cell membrane properties could possibly have some effect on thyroid hormone receptor functions.

Since the biochemical findings are not of clear-cut hypothyroidism and only of dysfunction that appears to improve with age, one is prompted to ask if there are any clinical implications. Until now, empirical thyroid treatment without clinical or biochemical evidence of hypothyroidism has not proved to be of much value[26] and has only created false hopes in the parents of these children. However, it has been shown that children with Down syndrome who are younger than 4 years and who have elevated TSH levels showed growth retardation compared with children with lower TSH levels.[8]

Furthermore, thyroid supplement treatment of a number of infants with hypopituitarism who had normal T_4 values associated with high basal TSH levels and an exaggerated response to TRH led to an increased growth rate during the period of treatment.[9] Hence, these findings may warrant a trial of thyroid supplementation in those infants with Down syndrome who have high TSH secretion. Ideally, this should be done under double-blind conditions and the follow-up continued until adulthood. The key question remains that even if there is increased short-term growth velocity, is there significant long-term growth improvement? Criteria for improvement in growth and other areas of development will need to be established.

We express our appreciation to the Balint Foundation, London, England, for its financial support.

We also thank J. Gross, MD, and A. Russel, MD, for their advice and encouragement and Shoshana Shanan for her untiring help in doing the testing.

References

1. Murdoch JC, Ratcliffe WA, McLarty DG, Rodger JC, Ratcliffe JG. Thyroid function in adults with Down's syndrome. *Biol Psychiatry*. 1979;14:463-471.
2. Baxter RG, Larkins RG, Martin FIR. Down's syndrome and thyroid function in adults. *Lancet*. 1975;2:794-796.
3. Sare Z, Ruvalcaba RH, Kelly VC. Prevalence of thyroid disorders in Down's syndrome. *Clin Genet*. 1978;14:154-158.
4. Loudon MM, Day RE, Duke EMC. Thyroid dysfunction in Down's syndrome. *AJDC*. 1985;60:1149-1151.
5. Fort P, Lifshitz R, Bellisario R, et al. Abnormalities of thyroid function in infants with Down syndrome. *J Pediatr*. 1984;104:545-549.
6. Pueschel SM, Pezzulo JC. Thyroid dysfunction in Down syndrome. *AJDC*. 1985;139:636-638.
7. Cutler T, Benezra-Obeiter R, Brink SJ. Thyroid function in young children with Down syndrome. *AJDC*. 1986;140:479-483.
8. Sharav T, Collins RM, Baab PJ. Growth studies in infants and children with Down's syndrome and elevated levels of thyrotropin. *AJDC*. 1988;142:1302-1306.
9. Grunesco de Papendieck L, Iorcansky S, Rivarols MA, Heinrich JJ, Bergada C. Patterns of TSH response to TRH in children with hypopituitarism. *J Pediatr*. 1982;100:387-392.
10. Illig R, Krawczynska H, Torresani T, Prader A. Elevated plasma TSH and hypothyroidism in children with hypothalamic hypopituitarism. *J Clin Endocrinol Metab*. 1977;44:453-458.
11. Patel YC, Burger HG, Hudson B. Radioimmunoassay of serum thyrotropin: sensitivity and specificity. *J Clin Endocrinol Metab*. 1971;31:768-773.
12. Fisher AD. Thyroid physiology and function tests in infancy and childhood. In: Wermer SC, Ingabar SH, eds. *The Thyroid: A Fundamental and Clinical Text*. New York, NY: Harper & Row Publishers Inc; 1978:375-383.
13. *SAS/STAT Guide for Personal Computers, Version 6*. Cary, NC: SAS Institute Inc; 1985:56-82.
14. Cole JWL, Grizzle JE. Application of multivariate analysis of variance of repeated measurements. *Biometrics*. 1966;122:810-828.
15. Wolter R, Bourdoux R, Ermans AM. TSH response to TRH according to age. *Pediatr Res*. 1982;16:896.
16. Delange F, Dodion J, Walter R, et al. Transient hypothyroidism in the newborn infant. *J Pediatr*. 1978;92:974-976.
17. Barmasch M, Kuschiner A, Fontana O, Starface R, Velasquez B, Degrossi OJ. Elevated neonatal thyrotropin (TSH)

values in non-hypothyroid newborns: differentiation with congenital hypothyroidism: iodine deficiency disorders and congenital hypothyroidism. In: Proceedings of the Satellite meeting 9th International Thyroid Congress. Sao Paulo, Brazil; May 1985;276-283.
18. Faglia G, Bitensky L, Pinchera A, et al. Thyrotropin secretion in patients with central hypothyroidism: evidence for reduced activity in immunoreactive thyrotropin. *J Clin Endocrinol Metab.* 1979;48:989-996.
19. Beck-Peccoz P, Amr S, Menezes-Ferreira M, Faglia G, Weintraub BD. Decreased receptor binding of biologically inactive thyrotropin in central hypothyroidism. *N Engl J Med.* 1985;312:1085-1090.
20. Sara V, Gustavson KH, Anneren G, Hall K, Wetterberg L. Somatomedins in Down's syndrome. *Biol Psychiatry.* 1983;18:803-811.
21. Sato T, Sluzuki J, Takentani T, Ishiguro K, Nakajima H. Age-related change in pituitary threshold for TSH release during thyroxine replacement therapy for cretinism. *J Clin Endocrinol Metab.* 1977;44:553-559.
22. Schultz RM, Glassman MS, MacGillivary MH. Elevated threshold for thyrotropin suppression in congenital hypothyroidism. *AJDC.* 1980;134:19-20.
23. Weintraub BD, Gershengorn MD, Ione A, Kourides IA, Fein H. Inappropriate secretion of thyroid-stimulating hormone. *Ann Intern Med.* 1981;95:339-351.
24. Scott BS, Petit TL, Becker LE, Edwards BAV. Abnormal electric membrane properties of Down's syndrome DRG neurones in cell culture. *Dev Brain Res.* 1982;2:257-270.
25. McSwiggan JD, Hanson DR, Lubiniecki A, Heston LL, Sheppard JR. Down syndrome fibroblasts are sensitive to beta-adrenergic stimulation. *Proc Natl Acad Sci U S A.* 1981;78:7670-7673.
26. Koch R, Share J, Graliker B. The effects of Cytomel on young children with Down syndrome (mongolism): a double blind longitudinal study. *J Pediatr.* 1965;66:776-778.

BOOK REVIEW

Pediatric Intensive Care

2nd ed, edited by Eliezer Nussbaum, 964 pp, $155, Mount Kisco, NY, Futura Publishing Co, 1989.

This second edition is another entry in the burgeoning area of textbooks addressing topics of the intensive care unit. It bears little similarity to the first edition, being markedly better (and larger) in all respects.

The text is generally well written and covers most subjects in adequate detail for pediatric house officers and practitioners. Its 50 chapters have many excellent features. Most of the pulmonary section is superb. Roentgenographic evaluation of respiratory problems is dealt with nicely in numerous chapters. Several short chapters detail specific entities such as pneumothorax and pleural effusion. These are useful and well-written chapters that provide much valuable information to the bedside clinician. However, some areas are covered only superficially. The chapter on Reye's syndrome is six pages long; it has numerous typographical errors and covers the topic inadequately. Poisoning and drug ingestion also are covered weakly—tricyclic antidepressants and aspirin intoxication are not mentioned, for instance. Details concerning the implementation of technologies such as pulmonary artery catheters, intracranial pressure monitoring, and mechanical ventilation are scarce. Mechanical ventilators are discussed in 5½ pages. Most of the subjects in the section on neurointensive care are described briefly. Finally, issues concerning nursing receive only token attention.

Certain sections of this textbook are excellent. Michael Radetsky has written a beautiful presentation of medical ethics in the pediatric intensive care unit. The entire section is written eloquently; is readable for physicians, nurses, and students; and encapsulates subjects that are often inadequately covered in textbooks of pediatrics or critical care. The chapter by Drs Royall and Levin on adult respiratory distress syndrome is very good, presenting the perfect level of detail.

How does this book fit into our libraries? Dr Nussbaum has assembled a group of respected authors, and this single-volume text seems a compromise between bedside handbooks and two-volume tomes on the subject. This is not an encyclopedic work and it would be inadequate preparation for subspecialty examinations of critical care. It exceeds the limits of bedside handbooks, and it can be read in several weeks. In short, the textbook succeeds admirably in its purpose, bridging the gap between these two extremes. It should find a welcome spot in many personal libraries.

J. Michael Dean, MD
Division of Critical Care
Department of Pediatrics
University of Utah
Medical Center
100 N Medical Dr
Salt Lake City, UT 84113

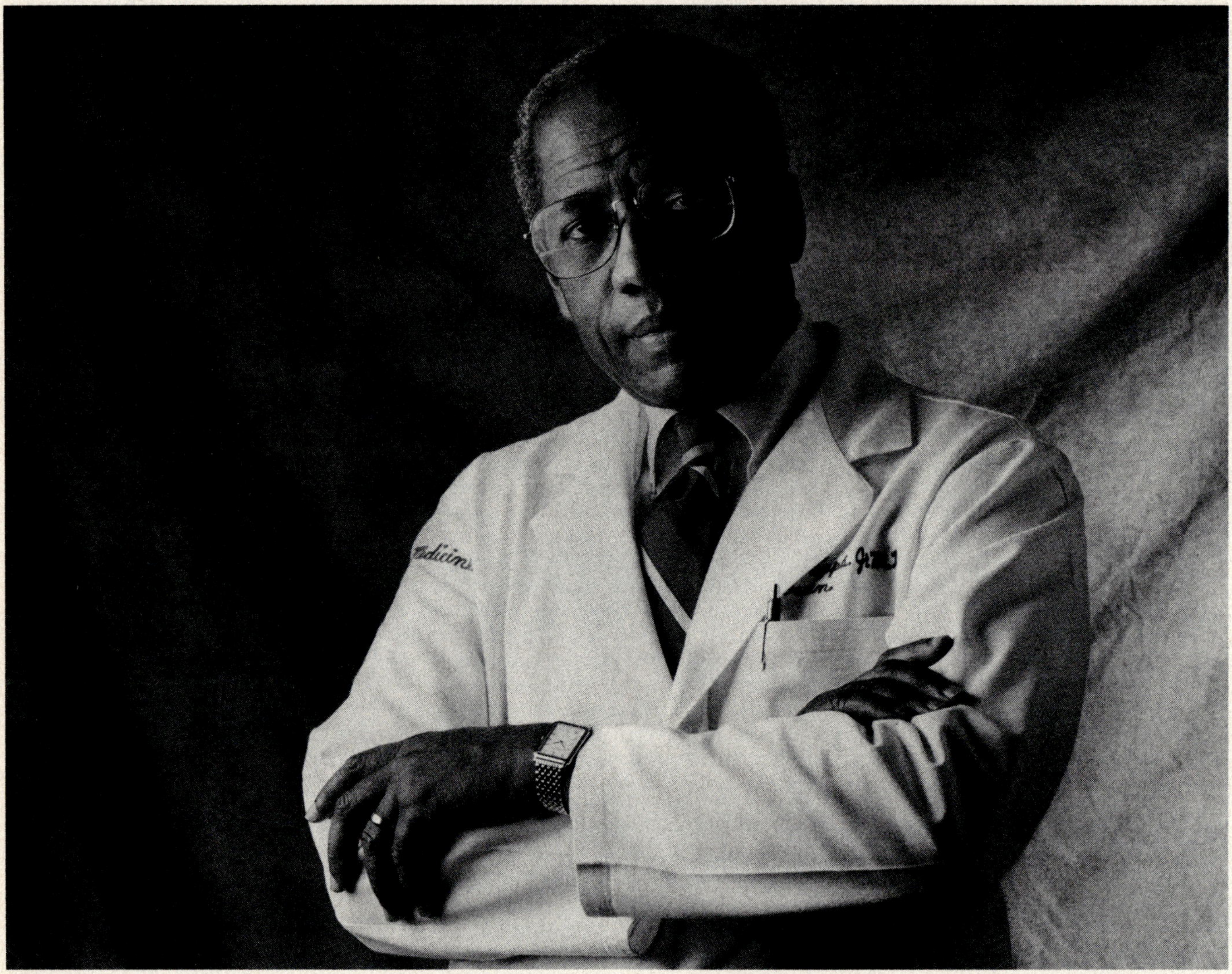

Sudden Cardiac Death in Young Athletes

A Review

Francis M. McCaffrey, MD; LCDR David S. Braden, MC, USNR; William B. Strong, MD

Death on the court: Loyola Marymount's Hank Gathers was at the top one minute, the next, he collapsed and lay dying as his mother stood mournfully by him." This was the lead story in the March 12, 1990, issue of *Sports Illustrated* (pp 14-17). *USA Today* (March 6, 1990:1A) carried the story of Hank Gathers' death for 4 days, including the front-page headline, "Athletes at risk: many put health, even life on the line to play." The tragic death of a national sports celebrity gaining front-page coverage is not unusual. Such events hold a morbid fascination and create undue fear among parents, coaches, community leaders, and physicians involved in the care of young athletes. This review will attempt to place sudden cardiac death in a previously asymptomatic young athlete in perspective while providing recommendations for identifying the athlete who may be at risk.

Sudden *unexpected* death (SUD) has been defined as death caused by cardiac arrest up to 6 hours after the initial onset of symptoms or collapse in individuals who have not been previously recognized to have cardiovascular disease.[1] In the following discussion, individuals with known, predisposing cardiac lesions will not be discussed.[2-4] Concern for SUD in athletes is out of proportion to the actual incidence (*Augusta Chronicle*. September 12, 1988:1B), which is estimated to be one to two cases per 200 000 athletes per year.[5,6] Epstein and Maron[5] have estimated that five in 100 000 young athletes may have a condition that makes them vulnerable to sudden death, and of those at risk, 10%, or one in 200 000 athletes, will die suddenly and unexpectedly. Between 1983 and 1988, there were less than 60 reported cases of sudden cardiac death among high school athletes, approximately 12 per year in the United States. The incidence of SUD in grade school athletes is less. After excluding trauma, cardiac death is the most frequent cause of sports-related death in young athletes.[1] Few studies are limited to SUD in young athletes.[1,7-9] However, if one reviews these studies and those involving youth, activity, and SUD, a fairly reproducible group of conditions are reported (Table 1).

Accepted for publication October 18, 1990.

From the Section of Pediatric Cardiology, Department of Pediatrics, The Medical College of Georgia, Augusta (Drs McCaffrey and Strong), and the Division of Pediatric Cardiology, Naval Hospital Portsmouth (Va) (Dr Braden).

Reprint requests to Section of Pediatric Cardiology, Department of Pediatrics, The Medical College of Georgia, 1120 15th St, Augusta, GA 30912 (Dr McCaffrey).

HYPERTROPHIC CARDIOMYOPATHY

Whether known as hypertrophic cardiomyopathy (HCM), or by almost 80 other names,[10] including idiopathic hypertrophic subaortic stenosis or hypertrophic obstructive cardiomyopathy, this disease process is the leading cause of SUD among young athletes.[2,11,12] Hypertrophic cardiomyopathy is characterized by a hypertrophied but nondilated left ventricle in the absence of systemic disease or left-sided obstruction capable of producing left ventricular hypertrophy (Table 2).[10,13] Muscular hypertrophy reduces left ventricular chamber size and volume and impairs diastolic filling.[14,15] Obstruction to left ventricular outflow may occur secondary to the hypertrophy of the subaortic septum[16,17] and to systolic anterior motion of the mitral valve.[18] In addition to inflow restriction and outflow obstruction, areas of localized hypertrophy other than the septum serve as potential arrhythmogenic foci. Most often, ventricular tachycardia leading to fibrillation is cited as the cause of death,[19,20] although supraventricular arrhythmias leading to secondary ventricular fibrillation may also occur.[20]

Prognostic factors for sudden death suggested in patients with HCM are a family history of sudden death,[21] ventricular tachycardia,[22] and a young age at onset of symptoms.[21,23] For patients known to have HCM, the annual mortality rate ranges from 2% to 3%. However, the annual mortality rate increases to 8% in those patients with a documented episode of ventricular tachycardia.[22]

The inheritance of HCM is autosomal dominant with a high degree of penetrance found on echocardiographic examination.[17,18,24] Therefore, if HCM is confirmed, all first-degree relatives should be examined echocardiographically.

Commonly, there are no symptoms, or the initial symptom is sudden death (Table 2).[22] Except for syncope and severe dyspnea,[25] symptoms are not predictive of SUD.[10,13,17,20]

The classic physical examination (Table 2) in patients with HCM includes an increased left ventricular impulse that may

Table 1.—Athletes Aged 30 Years or Younger With Sudden Unexpected Cardiac Death*

Disease	Total No. (%)	With Exercise	Nonexercise	Exercise Unknown
Hypertrophic cardiomyopathy	**20** (24)	5	1	14†
Coronary artery abnormalities	**15** (18)	12	0	3
Coronary artery disease	**12** (14)	9	0	3
Myocarditis	**10** (12)	9	1	0
Marfan's syndrome	**3** (4)	3	0	0
Dysrhythmias	**2** (2)	2	0	0
Mitral valve prolapse	**3** (4)	3	0	0
Other	**9** (11)	4	0	5
No cause identified	**10** (12)	6	3	1

*Studies reviewed for this table involved reports of athletes only (Tsung et al,[7] Thomas and Cantwell,[8] Maron et al,[11] Cantwell,[50] and James et al[76]) or of athletic endeavors (Topaz and Edwards,[9] and Lynch[37]). "Other" category primarily included idiopathic concentric cardiac hypertrophy or acute rheumatic heart disease.

†Most of the subjects were actively exercising.

Table 2.—Signs and Symptoms Associated With Hypertrophic Cardiomyopathy

Signs and Symptoms
Symptoms
Sudden death
Dyspnea
Fatigue
Syncope
Angina
Seizures
Physical examination
Palpation
4th heart sound
Brisk carotid upstroke
Pulsus bifieriens
Double apical impulse
Auscultation
Harsh left precordial ejection murmur
Murmur diminishes with squatting
Murmur increases with standing
Laboratory examination
Echocardiographic changes
Asymmetric septal hypertrophy with septal–free wall ratio >1.3
Diminished left ventricular cavity
Systolic anterior motion of the anterior leaflet of the mitral valve
Discrete (nonseptal) areas of hypertrophy
Diastolic dysfunction (impaired filling)
Cardiomegaly on chest roentgenogram
Electrocardiographic changes
Left ventricular hypertrophy
Repolarization abnormalities
Dysrhythmias

be double, a palpable fourth heart sound, pulsus bifieriens,[18] and a systolic murmur at the lower left sternal border to apex that diminishes on squatting and increases in intensity on assuming a standing position.[26] Occasionally, the highly conditioned athlete may have some findings that mimic HCM. The differentiation of this "athlete's heart" (Table 3) from HCM should be made by a cardiologist.

When the findings from a family history or physical examination are suggestive of HCM, the diagnosis is confirmed by two-dimensional and M-mode echocardiographic examination (Table 2).[13] The electrocardiogram is not diagnostic but is usually abnormal,[13,18,27,28] and cardiomegaly is often found on a chest roentgenogram.[19] Twenty-four– and 48-hour ambulatory monitoring is abnormal in a very high percentage of patients[29] and has potential prognostic significance.[22]

The athlete with HCM should be restricted from strenuous sports, dynamic or static, but may be permitted a light-exercise regimen.

CORONARY ARTERY ABNORMALITIES

Aberrant Coronary Arteries

Normal coronary artery anatomy is demonstrated in Fig 1 (top). Aberrant origin of the left coronary artery from the right sinus or the right coronary artery from the left sinus coursing between the aorta and the right ventricular outflow tract have been associated with SUD (Fig 1, center and bottom).[4,30] Other coronary anomalies have more rarely been associated with SUD.[30-37] The most frequent cause of SUD resulting from aberrant coronary origin is the left coronary artery originating at an acute angle from the right sinus of Valsalva or from the right coronary artery (Fig 1, center).[30] In the necropsy study by Cheitlin and colleagues,[30] 97% of subjects with an SUD attributed to left coronary artery aberrancy were younger than 22 years, and 78% of them died during exercise or immediately thereafter. Other authors have also found an association with an aberrant right coronary artery, exercise, and sudden death.[36] A tragic outcome may also result when the myocardium is supplied by a single coronary artery.[32]

Symptoms of aberrant coronary arteries include those symptoms associated with myocardial ischemia, ie, anginal chest pain and especially syncope with exertion.[6] However, as with HCM, sudden death may be, and often is, the presenting symptom, and the results of physical examination are usually entirely normal.

Any patient with syncope *during exercise* should have a cardiology consultation, and the cardiologist is obligated to address the possibility of coronary aberrancy. An aberrant left coronary artery coursing between the aorta and right ventricular outflow tract should be corrected. It is our experience that, once corrected, it may be possible to return to full athletic activity under medical supervision.

Kawasaki Disease

The authors are unaware of SUD in an athlete secondary to Kawasaki disease. However, a medical student at our institution did require coronary artery bypass surgery in adolescence as a result of Kawasaki disease as a child. Myocardial infarction and sudden death are well-recognized complications of Kawasaki disease.[38-40] Coronary stenosis

Table 3.—Hypertrophic Cardiomyopathy vs 'Athlete's Heart'*		
Echocardiographic Findings	**Hypertrophic Cardiomyopathy**	**Athlete's Heart**
Left ventricular cavity size	Diminished	Normal or increased
Septal–posterior wall thickness ratio	>1.3	<1.3
Diastolic function	Diminished left ventricular compliance and diastolic filling	Normal left ventricular compliance and filling
Evidence of inheritance (via echocardiogram)	Yes	No

*Echocardiographic signposts are listed that distinguish hypertrophic cardiomyopathy from athlete's heart, which results from intensive athletic training (see text).

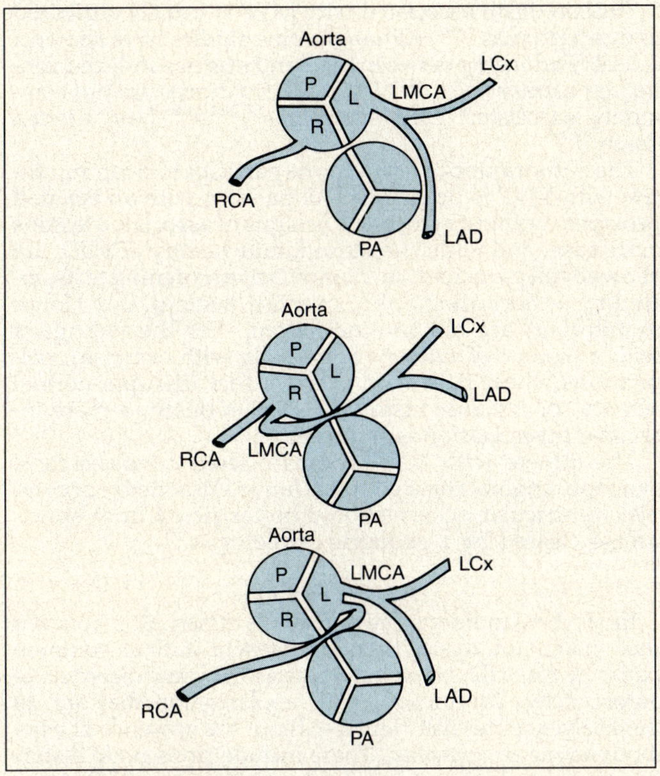

Fig 1.—*Normal and aberrant coronary anatomy. Top, Normal origin and course of the coronary arteries. Center and bottom, Two most common congenital coronary artery aberrations associated with sudden unexpected cardiac death. PA indicates pulmonary artery; RCA, right coronary artery; LMCA, left main coronary artery; LAD, left anterior descending coronary artery; LCx, left circumflex coronary artery; and P, R, and L, posterior, right, and left aortic cusps, respectively.*

may be severe and asymptomatic.[40] Approximately 25% of all myocardial infarctions in a nationwide study in Japan occurred several years after the initial disease. Although the majority of children in whom coronary artery stenosis will develop have coronary abnormalities by echocardiographic examination at the time of the initial disease, a small percentage may have a normal echocardiogram, and later, coronary artery stenosis will develop.[40]

The authors would recommend that any child with a history of Kawasaki disease, who at the time of initial disease had echocardiographically documented coronary changes, prolonged fever, or congestive heart failure without subsequent documentation of normal coronary arteries, should be seen by a cardiologist before athletic participation.

ATHEROSCLEROTIC CORONARY ARTERY DISEASE

While sudden cardiac death in adults older than 35 years is almost exclusively secondary to atherosclerotic coronary artery disease, children and young adults rarely die of coronary artery disease (Table 1).

Premature atherosclerotic coronary artery disease, resulting in a myocardial infarction or symptoms of ischemia in the second or early third decade of life, is usually the result of a severe familial dyslipidemia, most commonly severe heterozygous type II[41] or homozygous type II hypercholesterolemia. The gene for this is present in one of every 500 people.[41] Therefore, the statistical likelihood of the homozygous state occurring is only one per million. Nevertheless, a component of the preparticipation assessment should include a family history of premature cardiovascular death or hypercholesterolemia. A fasting lipoprotein profile should be measured on all individuals with a positive family history.

MYOCARDITIS

Active, acute myocarditis is an inflammation of the myocardium that is demonstrated on a biopsy specimen by lymphocytic infiltration of the myocardium associated with focal necrosis. Sudden cardiac death has been reported at rest and during exercise with both acute and chronic myocarditis.[12,37,42,44,45] Noren et al observed histologic evidence of myocarditis in 17% of SUDs in children younger than 16 years, while in a similar cohort of traumatic deaths, only 2% were observed to have myocarditis.[42] The proportion of sudden cardiac death ascribed to myocarditis has been reported to range from 18% to 29%.[2,12,43]

Myocarditis, sudden death, and exercise, are probably secondary to conduction system inflammation.[44,45]

Signs of myocarditis may range from only a mild but persistently elevated heart rate to ectopy, cardiomegaly, and signs of congestive heart failure. The electrocardiogram may show diffusely low voltages, ST-segment abnormalities, ventricular ectopy, fixed coupling, and/or heart block.[43,46,47]

Without symptoms or signs suggestive of myocardial involvement, the diagnosis of myocarditis is exceedingly difficult, if not impossible, to make. To restrict participation on the basis of a low-grade fever, or to recommend evaluation of such noncardiac symptoms by a cardiologist, is both impractical and unrealistic. Many athletes "play through" a cold or mild febrile illness, especially if they are highly competitive. For the athlete who does not feel well because of a febrile illness, participation should be restricted. For the athlete who has signs or symptoms suggestive of myocardial involvement (as listed above), restriction in athletic participation and a cardiovascular evaluation are recommended.

MARFAN SYNDROME

Marfan syndrome is a constellation of physical signs that primarily involve the musculoskeletal, ocular, and cardiovascular systems as a result of connective tissue derangement. The overall incidence of Marfan syndrome in its

Table 4.—Signs and Symptoms of Marfan's Syndrome*

Signs and Symptoms
Musculoskeletal
Arachnodactyly
Pectus deformity
High narrow palate
Height >95th percentile
Hyperextensible joints
Vertebral column deformities
Pes planus
Striae distensae
Inguinal hernia
Cardiovascular
Mitral valve prolapse
Aortic root dilation
Mitral regurgitation
Aortic regurgitation
Congestive heart failure
Infective endocarditis
Aortic dissection
Ocular
Upward ectopia lentis
Myopia
Iridodonesis
Glaucoma
Retinal detachment

*Findings are listed from most common to least common from top to bottom for each section (adapted from Missri and Swett[49]).

clinically diagnosable form is five to eight persons per 100 000.[48] It is inherited as an autosomal dominant with variable expression. It may occur sporadically in approximately 15% of cases.[49]

There have been recent and well-publicized reports of athletes[50] dying suddenly of complications of this syndrome, and most necropsy reviews of sudden cardiac death in young athletes have included cases of Marfan syndrome (Table 1).[1,2,12]

One or more musculoskeletal findings are seen in all patients (Table 4) although no one particular finding is found in all patients.[49] Other signs of musculoskeletal involvement, not listed in Table 4, include protrusion of the thumb across the palm when the thumb is enclosed in a fist and the overlap of the tip of the thumb and proximal interphalangeal joint of the third finger when the thumb and third finger are wrapped around the opposite wrist.

Cardiovascular findings include signs associated with mitral valve prolapse (MVP) and, less frequently, aortic insufficiency. Echocardiographic findings include up to a 100% incidence of MVP.[50,51] There is also a high percentage of aortic root dilation[51] early in the clinical course. Other echocardiographic findings are noted in Table 4.

Ocular abnormalities are found in 70% of patients,[49] with the most common finding being ectopia lentis, whereas myopia, iridonenesis, and secondary glaucoma are less common (Table 4).

As a syndrome, diagnosis is based on physical findings with supportive laboratory evidence. According to Pyeritz and McKusick,[52] two of four major findings are necessary for diagnosis. These include: (1) a positive family history, (2) ectopia lentis, (3) aortic root dilation, and (4) either severe kyphoscoliosis or anterior thorax deformities.

If the diagnosis is suspected, a cardiologist should be consulted. We reexamine our patients every 6 to 12 months, depending on the severity and stability of the cardiac findings. If the aortic root measurements are normal, strenuous, and dynamic, but not static or isometric, sports may be performed. Other family members should be examined, and genetic counseling is mandatory.

MVP

Isolated MVP may occur with or without mitral insufficiency. It has been reported to occur in less than 1% of males and 6% of females.[53]

Although some authors believe MVP is never associated with SUD in children,[54-56] there are at least six reported cases that list MVP as the cause of death in children.[7,57,58] In two of the six cases cited,[9,57] there was a strong family history of sudden cardiac death at a young age with an autosomal dominant–type inheritance. Autopsies on these family members who died suddenly did not reveal MVP in the majority of cases, leading one to suspect that while a genetic predisposition to sudden death existed, it was unrelated to MVP.

Sudden death associated with MVP is usually attributed to dysrhythmias.[59-61] Although some studies have shown a causal relationship between MVP and exercise-induced ventricular extrasystoles,[54,62,63] the dysrhythmias are not commonly associated with symptoms[57,59,62,64-69] or sudden death.[53,61]

The authors' approach to sports participation for the athlete with MVP is pragmatic. All patients with an isolated prolapse, without symptoms or signs of associated lesions or disease, and with a negative family history of SUD, are allowed full participation. Noninvasive screening tests, including echocardiography, exercise testing, and Holter monitoring, are not routinely done. For the youngster with a history of syncope (especially with exercise), palpitations, chest pain with exercise that disrupts normal activity, or a family history of sudden death, a more intensive investigation is indicated.

The athlete with MVP and associated *exercise-induced* syncope, anginal chest pain that limits full activity, or complex ventricular ectopy should be restricted from sports unless cleared by a pediatric cardiologist.[53]

DYSRHYTHMIAS

In all the conditions previously discussed, it is believed that malignant dysrhythmias represent a final common pathway for SUD. However, there are primary disorders of automaticity, conduction, and repolarization that are, of themselves, potentially lethal without the presence of a hemodynamic abnormality. These include sinus node disturbances,[70,71] exercise-induced ventricular ectopy,[72-74] disorders of conduction[75-77] such as in the Wolff-Parkinson-White syndrome, and repolarization abnormalities such as the the long QT syndrome[78] that occurs in an autosomal dominant form, the Jervell and Lange-Nielsen syndrome, and an autosomal recessive form, the Romano-Ward syndrome.

Syncope is the most common symptom of serious rhythm disturbances,[78] and exercise may increase the likelihood of both syncope[79] and sudden death.[60]

The American College of Cardiology guidelines for athletic participation[79] recommend restrictions of athletes with syncope, presyncope, or worsening arrhythmia. Patients with structural heart disease in association with sinus node dysfunction, junctional escape rhythm associated with syncope or exercise intolerance, and poorly regulated supraventricular tachycardia should also be restricted. Patients with Wolff-Parkinson-White syndrome with a family history of sudden death, documented episodes of supraventricular tachycardia, or premature ventricular complexes exacerbated by exercise are also discouraged from strenuous sports particpation, especially if they are not controlled medically. Conversely, without syncope, structural heart disease, or exercise exacerbation of dysrhythmias, these rhythm disturbances do not preclude full activity. In fact, endurance athletes often demonstrate "benign" dysrhythmias, such as marked sinus

PREPARTICIPATION HEALTH EXAMINATION RECORD

(1-4) ☐☐☐☐ (Office use only)

School ______________ ☐☐ (5-6)

Grade ______ ☐☐ (7-8)

Last Name   First Name   Middle Initial

(9-10) Age ☐☐ ______ (11) Race: ☐ Black ☐ White ☐ Other (1, 2, 3) (12) Sex: Male ☐ 1 Female ☐ 2

This application to compete in interscholastic athletics is entirely voluntary on my part and is made with the understanding that I have not violated any of the eligibility rules and regulations of the State Association.

Date ______________ Signature of Student ______________

Parent's or Guardian's Permission & Release

"I hereby give my consent for the above named student to represent his or her school in the athletic activities except those indicated on this form by the examining physician provided that such athletic activities are approved by the State Association. I also give my consent for the student to accompany the school team on any of its local or out-of-town trips."

The Richmond County Board of Education has no responsibility to provide first aid at any of the games and the parents understand that the risk of injury is assumed by the student and parents when they are executing this form. However, in the event physicians, physical therapists, physician's assistants, nurses or other persons trained in the rendering of first aid are available, as volunteers or otherwise, and render aid to any student injured during the course of any such activities or travel, then the parents do hereby release and forever discharge such persons and the Richmond County Board of Education from any liability arising out of any first aid or immediate treatment of injuries.

Typed or Printed Name of Parent or Guardian ______________ Signature of Parent or Guardian ______________

Address ______________ Phone ______________ Date ______________

HEALTH HISTORY

(To be completed by Student and Parents **prior to examination**)

(13-24)	1 Yes	2 No	**Has this student had any:**	(25-36)	1 Yes	2 No	**Does this student:**
1.	☐	☐	Chronic or recurrent illness?	13.	☐	☐	Wear eyeglasses or contact lens?
2.	☐	☐	Illness lasting over one week?	14.	☐	☐	Wear dental bridges, braces, plates?
3.	☐	☐	Hospitalizations?	15.	☐	☐	Take any medication?
4.	☐	☐	Surgery other than tonsillectomy?				**Is there any history of:**
5.	☐	☐	Missing organs (eye, kidney, testicle)?	16.	☐	☐	Injuries requiring MD treatment?
6.	☐	☐	Allergy to any medication?	17.	☐	☐	Neck injury?
7.	☐	☐	Problems with heart or blood pressure?	18.	☐	☐	Knee injury?
8.	☐	☐	Chest pain with exercise?	19.	☐	☐	Knee surgery?
9.	☐	☐	Dizziness or fainting with exercise?	20.	☐	☐	Ankle injury?
10.	☐	☐	Dizziness, fainting, frequent headaches, or convulsions?	21.	☐	☐	Other serious joint injury?
				22.	☐	☐	Broken bones (fractures)?
11.	☐	☐	Concussion or unconsciousness?	23.	☐	☐	Is there any reason why this student should not participate in sports?
12.	☐	☐	Heat exhaustion, heat stroke, or other problems with heat?	24.	☐	☐	Has any family member died suddenly at less than 40 years of age of causes other than an accident?

Date of last known Tetanus (lock jaw) shot: ______________

Use this space to **explain** any of the **above numbered YES answers** or to provide any additional information:

PHYSICAL EXAMINATION

Card two (1-4) ☐☐☐☐ (Office use only)

Date ______________

Height ☐☐ (37-38)

Weight ☐☐☐ (39-41)

Pulse rate ☐☐☐ (42-44)

Blood pressure ☐☐☐/☐☐☐ (45-47) (48-50)

Vision: Right ☐☐☐/☐☐☐ (5-7) (8-10)

Left ☐☐☐/☐☐☐ (11-13) (14-16)

(17) (CHECK ONE) Normal 1 ☐ without glasses; 2 ☐ with glasses; Abnormal 3 ☐ without glasses; 4 ☐ with glasses

(51-70)	1 Normal	2 Abnormal	3 Not Examined	Comments	Examiner	Problem Code (18-57)
1. Eyes						
2. Ears, Nose, Throat						
3. Mouth and Teeth						
4. Neck (soft tissue)						
5. Cardiovascular						
6. Chest and Lungs						
7. Abdomen						
8. Genitalia-Hernia						
9. Sexual Maturity						
10. Skin and Lymphatics						
11. Neck						
12. Spine						
13. Shoulders						
14. Arms and Hands						
15. Hips						
16. Thighs						
17. Knees						
18. Ankles						
19. Feet						
20. Neurological						

Based on this history and physical exam, the following abnormalities were found and may need treatment:

1. ______________
2. ______________
3. ______________

(71) **PARTICIPATION RECOMMENDATIONS**

1. ☐ There were no history or physical findings on this exam which would prohibit this student from participating in competeitive athletics.
2. ☐ This student should have the following health problems evaluated or treated prior to participating in competitive athletics: ______________
3. ☐ This student has health problems which would **prohibit** him or her from participating in competitive athletics.

______________ PHYSICIAN

Fig 2.—*Left and right, Preparticipation screening forms. These forms (devised by the Richmond County, Georgia, Medical Society and adopted by the American Academy of Pediatrics, Elk Grove Village, Ill) are recommended for pre–sports participation screening of young athletes (used with permission of the American Academy of Pediatrics[86]).*

bradycardia and type I second-degree atrioventricular block as a result of conditioning.[63] In general, supraventricular and ventricular premature beats are not worrisome if they are unifocal and if they abolish or diminish with exercise. Even ventricular couplets appear to be benign in the context of an otherwise normal heart.[80] First-degree and second-degree Mobitz type 1 heart blocks without syncope, structural heart disease, or exacerbation with exercise need no restriction. Because there is variability in approach to these rhythm disturbances, a cardiologist familiar with children and sports should be consulted before such a youngster is allowed to participate.

ADDITIONAL ISSUES

Almost all children who die suddenly with aortic stenosis have severe disease.[2,81-83] The probability of a child with severe aortic stenosis slipping through a well-conducted sports physical examination undetected is highly unlikely. In a series that reported sudden death, virtually all patients were symptomatic before their final episode.[81-83] However, as the severity of the aortic stenosis can sometimes not be accurately gauged by noninvasive testing, youngsters with aortic stenosis should be examined by their pediatric cardiologist.[84] Those children with severe or symptomatic aortic stenosis should never participate in sports unless their obstruction is relieved.

Hank Gathers' death has raised the issue of having a courtside defibrillator for those athletes at risk for ventricular fibrillation. While not unheard of, to have a defibrillator and personnel trained in its use present at all games and practices cannot be routinely justified except under extraordinary and clearly understood conditions. All parties must be aware that the athlete has a potentially lethal condition. The legal and financial implications and responsibilities must be developed on a case-by-case basis.

PREVENTION

In the Epstein and colleagues[5] report of sudden cardiac death in young, highly competitive athletes, only 25% had signs and symptoms suggestive of a cardiac abnormality, and of those with such signs and symptoms, most of the athletes were misdiagnosed. Other authors suggest that for the more common lesions already discussed, the potential of diagnosing these patients' conditions by history and physical examination alone ranges from 0% to 25%. The authors of this review do not accept this pessimistic outlook. They believe that with a competent screening history and physical examination, as recommended by the American Academy of Pediatrics (Fig 2), most patients with a significant cardiac lesion can and should be identified and referred for accurate diagnosis and management.

Unfortunately, this screening process has not been uniformly adopted, and many states do not require more than a physician's signature on a preparticipation form.[85]

SCREENING

An ideal screening evaluation should be based solely on history and physical examination results. It should require a modest amount of equipment and time. It should only be performed in a reasonably quiet environment and never in the locker-room atmosphere. Locker-room evaluations are perfunctory and potentially dangerous because they may provide a false sense of security.

The history can most efficiently be taken via a preparticipation questionnaire, such as the one used in the Richmond County, Georgia, school system[86] and recommended by the American Academy of Pediatrics Committee on Practice (Fig 2). Syncope (question 9) is often the most common symptom before death[87] and should prompt referral to a cardiologist for a thorough evaluation. A positive family history of sudden unsuspected cardiac death is also important (question 24). It is well known that seizures may be the initial and only manifestation of the prolonged QT syndrome,[88] and prolongation of the corrected QT interval should be looked for in any child with a history of seizures. The physical examination, like the history, should be complete but need not be extensive. The examination is based on the traditional methods of inspection, palpation, and auscultation[6] and, of course, should always include carefully measured vital signs. The authors have previously discussed the absolute impracticality of the echocardiogram as a screening method for SUD.[6] The electrocardiogram costs much less as a screening tool but, in the authors' opinion, is equally impractical, insensitive, and even less specific.

THE YOUNG ATHLETE AT KNOWN INCREASED RISK

What are the responsibilities toward the young athlete (and his or her family) who is identified as having a potentially lethal defect? Whose responsibility is it to provide emergency treatment if the athlete is allowed continued participation?

The authors believe it is the primary responsibility of the athlete and his or her parents to comprehend the cardiac lesion involved and the limitations required. Obviously, the consulting cardiologist and referring physician must work closely with the family and team and league officials to ensure that all vital information is accurately and clearly communicated. It seems reasonable to the authors to recommend that all coaches be trained in basic cardiopulmonary resuscitation and first aid.

CONCLUSIONS

Sudden unexpected death in otherwise healthy children and adolescent athletes is a source of concern and anxiety for physicians, parents, and coaches. However, the concern is out of proportion to the scope of the problem. The cardiac lesions that may result in sudden cardiac death include hypertrophic cardiomyopathy, coronary artery anomalies, Marfan syndrome, and primary arrhythmias. A concise, directed screening history and physical examination should identify the majority of the athletes with these lesions.

References

1. Maron BJ, Epstein SE, Roberts WC. Causes of sudden death in competitive athletes. *J Am Coll Cardiol.* 1986;7:204-214.
2. Lambert EC, Vijayan AM, Wagner HR, Vlad P. Sudden unexpected death from cardiovascular disease in children, a cooperative international study. *Am J Cardiol.* 1974;34:89-96.
3. Mitchell JH, Maron BJ, Epstein SE. 16th Bethesda Conference: cardiovascular abnormalities in the athlete: recommendations regarding eligibility for competition. *J Am Coll Cardiol.* 1984;6:1186-1224.
4. Strong WB, Alpert BS. The child with heart disease: play, recreation, and sports. *Curr Probl Cardiol.* 1981;6:1-37.
5. Epstein SE, Maron BJ. Sudden death and the competitive athlete: perspectives on preparticipation screening studies. *J Am Coll Cardiol.* 1986;7:220-230.
6. Braden DS, Strong WB. Preparticipation screening for sudden cardiac death in high school and college athletes. *Phys Sports Med.* 1988;16:128-140.
7. Tsung SH, Haung TY, Chang HH. Sudden death in young athletes. *Arch Pathol Lab Med.* 1982;106:168-170.
8. Thomas RJ, Cantwell JD. Sudden death during basketball games. *Phys Sports Med.* 1990;18:75-78.
9. Topaz O, Edwards JE. Pathologic features of sudden death in children, adolescents and young adults. *Chest.* 1985;87:476-482.
10. Maron BJ, Bonow RO, Cannon RO, Leon MB, Epstein SE. Hypertrophic cardiomyopathy: interrelations of clinical manifestations, pathophysiology, and therapy, I. *N Engl J Med.* 1987;316:780-789.
11. Maron BJ, Roberts WC, McAllister HA, Rosing DR, Epstein SE. Sudden death in young athletes. *Circulation.* 1980;62:218-229.
12. Kramer MR, Drori Y, Lev B. Sudden death in young soldiers, high incidence of syncope prior to death. *Chest.* 1988;93:345-347.
13. St John Sutton MG, Lie JT, Tajik AJ, Giuliani ER, Danielson GK, Frye RL. Hypertrophic obstructive cardiomyopathy. *Heart Failure.* July/August 1985:152-178.
14. Sanderson JE, Gibson DG, Brown DJ, Goodwin JF. Left ventricular filling in hypertrophic cardiomyopathy: an angiographic study. *Br Heart J.* 1977;39:661-670.
15. Spirito P, Maron BJ. Relation between extent of left ventricular hypertrophy and diastolic filling abnormalities in hypertrophic cardiomyopathy. *J Am Coll Cardiol.* 1990;15:808-813.
16. Kishel JC, Virmaru R. Pathologic features of sudden cardiac death: an overview. *South Med J.* 1987;80:487-493.
17. Maron B. Hypertrophic cardiomyopathy: the leading edge. *Cardiology.* 1988;2:1-12.
18. Malone R, Covitz W, Lovett EJ. Hypertrophic cardiomyopathy in childhood, II. *J Med Assoc Ga.* 1985;74:172-175.
19. Nicod P, Poliker R, Peterson KL. Hypertrophic cardiomyopathy and sudden death. *N Engl J Med.* 1988;318:1255-1256.
20. McKenna WJ, England D, Doi YL, Deanfield JE, Oakley C, Goodwin JF . Arrhythmia in hypertrophic cardiomyopathy: influence on prognosis. *Br Heart J.* 1981;46:168-172.
21. Maron BJ, Lipson LC, Roberts WC, Savage DD, Epstein SE. 'Malignant' hypertrophic cardiomyopathy: identification of families with unusually frequent premature death. *Am J Cardiol.* 1978;41:1133-1140.
22. Maron BJ, Savage DD, Wolfson JK, Epstein SE. Prognostic significance of 24 hour ambulatory electrocardiographic monitoring in patients with hypertrophic cardiomyopathy: a prospective study. *Am J Cardiol.* 1981;48:252-257.
23. Maron BJ, Roberts WC, Epstein SE. Sudden death in hypertrophic cardiomyopathy: a profile of 78 patients. *Circulation.* 1982;65:1388-1394.
24. Clark CE, Henry WL, Epstein SE. Familial prevalence and genetic transmission of idiopathic hypertrophic subaortic stenosis. *N Engl J Med.* 1973;289:709-714.
25. Romeo F, Cianfrocca C, Pelliccia F, Colloriai V, Cristofani R, Reale A . Long term prognosis in children with hypertrophic cardiomyopathy: an analysis of 37 patients aged ≤ 14 years at diagnosis. *Clin Cardiol.* 1990;13:101-107.
26. Strong WB. The young athlete with a heart murmur. In: Smith MJ, ed. *Common Problems in Pediatric Sports Medicine.* Chicago, Ill: Year Book Medical Publishers Inc; 1989:96-104.
27. Iida K, Sugishita Y, Yukisada K, Ito I. Diurnal change of giant negative T wave in patients with hypertrophic cardiomyopathy. *Clin Cardiol.* 1990;13:272-278.
28. Alfonso F, Nihoyannopoulos P, Stewart J, Dickie S, Lemery R, McKenna WJ . Clinical significance of giant negative T waves in hypertrophic cardiomyopathy. *J Am Coll Cardiol.* 1990;15:965-971.
29. Canedo MI, Frank MJ, Abdulla AM. Rhythm disturbances in hypertrophic cardiomyopathy: prevalence, relation to symptoms, and management. *Am J Cardiol.* 1980;45:848-855.
30. Cheitlin MD, DeCastro CM, McAllister HA. Sudden death as a complication of anomalous left coronary origin from the anterior sinus of Valsalva. *Circulation.* 1974;50:780-787.
31. Cohle SD, Graham MA, Pounder DJ. Nonatherosclerotic sudden coronary death. *Pathol Annu.* 1986;21(pt 2):217-249.
32. VanCamp SP, Choi JH. Exercise and sudden death. *Phys Sports Med.* 1988;16:49-52.
33. Morales AR, Romanelli R, Boucek RJ. The mural left anterior descending coronary artery, strenuous exercise and sudden death. *Circulation.* 1980;62:230-237.
34. Cheitlin MD. The intramural coronary artery: another cause of sudden death with exercise? *Circulation.* 1980;62:238-239.

35. Engle HJ, Torres C, Page HL Jr. Major variations in anatomical origin of the coronary arteries: angiographic observations in 4,250 patients without associated congenital heart disease. *Cathet Cardiovasc Diagn.* 1975;1:157-169.
36. Roberts WC, Siegel RJ, Zipes DP. Origin of the right coronary artery from the left sinus of Valsalva and its functional consequences: analysis of 10 necropsy patients. *Am J Cardiol.* 1982;49:863-868.
37. Lynch P. Soldiers, sport and sudden death. *Lancet.* 1980;1:1235-1237.
38. Kato H, Ichinose E, Kawasaki T. Myocardial infarction in Kawasaki disease: clinical analyses in 195 cases. *J Pediatr.* 1986;108:923-927.
39. Turner-Gomes S, Rose V, Brezina A, Smallhorn J, Rowe RD. High persistence rate of established coronary artery lesions secondary to Kawasaki disease among panethnic Canadian population. *J Pediatr.* 1986;108:928-932.
40. Pahl E, Ettedgui J, Neches WH, Park SC.The value of angiography in the follow-up of coronary involvement in mucocutaneous lymph node syndrome (Kawasaki disease). *J Am Coll Cardiol.* 1989;14:1318-1325.
41. Goldstein JL, Brown MS. Low density lipoproteins and atherosclerosis. *Cardiovasc Rev Rep.* 1982;3:1041-1049.
42. Noren GR, Staley NA, Kaplan EL. Non-rheumatic inflammatory disease. In: Adams FH, Emmanouillides GC, Riemenschneider TA, eds. *Moss' Heart Disease in Infants, Children, and Adolescents.* 4th ed. Baltimore, Md: Williams & Wilkins; 1989:730-746.
43. Koskenvuo K. Sudden death among Finnish conscripts. *BMJ.* 1976;2:1413-1415.
44. Burch GE, Sun SC, Chu KC, Sohal RS, Colcolough HL. Interstitial coxsackie virus B myocarditis in infants and children. *JAMA.* 1968;203:55-62.
45. Noren GR, Staley NA, Brandt CM, Kaplan EL. Occurrence of myocarditis in sudden death in children. *J Forensic Sci.* 1977;22:188-196.
46. Rose KD. Which cardiovascular 'problems' should disqualify athletes? *Phys Sports Med.* 1975;3:62-68.
47. Grody KL, Costanzo-Nordin MR. Myocarditis: review of a clinical enigma. *Heart Lung.* 1989;18:347-353.
48. Pierpont MEM, Moller JH. Cardiac manifestations of systemic disease. In: Adams FH, Emmanouillides GC, Fiemenschneider TA, eds. *Moss' Heart Disease in Infants, Children, and Adolescents.* 4th ed. Baltimore, Md: Williams & Wilkins; 1989:792-796.
49. Missri JC, Swett DD. Marfan syndrome: a review. *Cardiovasc Rev Rep.* 1982;3:1648-1653.
50. Cantwell JD. Marfan's syndrome: detection and management. *Phys Sports Med.* 1986;14:51-55.
51. Geva T, Hegesh J, Frand M. The clinical course and echocardiographic features of Marfan's syndrome in childhood. *AJDC.* 1987;141:1179-1182.
52. Pyeritz RE, McKusick VA. The Marfan syndrome: diagnosis and management. *N Engl J Med.* 1979;300:772-777.
53. Jeresaty RM. Mitral valve prolapse: definition and implications in athletes. *J Am Coll Cardiol.* 1986;7:231-236.
54. Bisset GS, Schwartz DC, Meyer RA, James PW, Kaplan S. Clinical spectrum and long-term follow-up of isolated mitral valve prolapse in 119 children. *Circulation.* 1980;62:423-429.
55. Leatham AL, Wallace B. Mild mitral regurgitation and the mitral prolapse fiasco. *Am Heart J.* 1980;99:659-664.
56. Garson A, McNamara DG. Sudden death in a pediatric cardiology population, 1958 to 1983: relation to prior arrhythmias. *J Am Coll Cardiol.* 1985;5:134B-137B.
57. Pocock WA, Bosman CK, Chesler E, Barlow JB, Edwards JE. Sudden death in primary mitral valve prolapse. *Am Heart J.* 1984;107:378-382.
58. Gingell RL, Vlad P. Mitral valve prolapses. In: Keith J, Rowe R, Vlad P, eds. *Heart Disease in Infancy and Childhood.* New York, NY: Macmillan Publishing Co Inc; 1978:810-827.
59. Chesler E, King RA, Edwards JE. The myxomatous mitral valve and sudden death. *Circulation.* 1983;67:632-638.
60. Anderson RC. Idiopathic mitral valve prolapse and sudden death. *Am Heart J.* 1980;100:941-942.
61. McNamara D. Idiopathic benign mitral leaflet prolapse. *AJDC.* 1982;136:152-156.
62. Kavey RW, Sondheimer HM, Balckman MS. Detection of dysrhythmia in pediatric patients with mitral valve prolapse. *Circulation.* 1980;3:582-587.
63. Coelho A, Palileo E, Ashley W, et al. Tachyarrhythmias in young athletes. *J Am Coll Cardiol.* 1986;7:237-243.
64. Campbell RWF, Godman MG, Fiddler GI, Marquis RM, Julian DG. Ventricular arrhythmias in syndrome of balloon deformity of mitral valve: definition of possible high risk group. *Br Heart J.* 1976;38:1053-1057.
65. Kavey RW. Mitral valve prolapse: not always benign. *Contemp Pediatr.* 1986;3:58-70.
66. Pocock WA, Barlow JB. Post exercise arrhythmias in the billowing posterior mitral leaflet syndrome. *Am Heart J.* 1970;9:740-745.
67. Stasberg B, Caspi A, Jusmiec J, Lewin RF, Sclarovsky S, Agmon J. Ventricular fibrillation in a patient with 'silent' mitral valve prolapse. *Cardiology.* 1988;75:149-153.
68. Koch FH, Hancock FW. Ten year follow-up of forty patients with the mid-systolic click/late systolic murmur syndrome. *Am Heart J.* 1976;37:149. Abstract.
69. Winkle RA, Lopes MG, Fitzgerald JW, Goodman DJ, Schroeder JS, Harrison DC. Arrhythmias in patients with mitral valve prolapse. *Circulation.* 1975;52:73-81.
70. Bharati S, Bauernfiend R, Miller LB, Stasberg B, Lev M. Sudden death in three teenagers: conduction system studies. *J Am Coll Cardiol.* 1983;1:879-885.
71. James TN, Froggatt P, Marshall TK. Sudden death in young athletes. *Ann Intern Med.* 1967;67:1013-1021.
72. Benson DW, Benditt DG, Anderson RW, et al. Cardiac arrest in young, ostensibly healthy patients: clinical, hemodynamic, and electrophysiologic findings. *Am J Cardiol.* 1983;52:65-69.
73. Palileo EV, Ashley WW, Swiryn S, et al. Exercise provacable right ventricular outflow tract tachycardia. *Am Heart J.* 1982;104:185-193.
74. Rocchini AP, Chun PO, Dick M. Ventricular tachycardia in children. *Am J Cardiol.* 1981;47:1091-1097.
75. Coslo FG, Benson DW Jr, Anderson RW, et al. Onset of atrial fibrillation during antidromic tachycardia: association with sudden cardiac arrest and ventricular fibrillation in a patient with Wolff-Parkinson-White syndrome. *Am J Cardiol.* 1982;50:353-359.
76. James TN, Jordan JD, Riddick L, Bargeron LM. Subaortic stenosis and sudden death. *J Thorac Cardiovasc Surg.* 1988;95:247-254.
77. Thiene G, Pennelli N, Ross L. Cardiac conduction system abnormalities as a possible cause of sudden death in young athletes. *Hum Pathol.* 1983;14:704-709.
78. Suryard RD, Wengor N. Long QT syndrome. *Prim Cardiol.* 1989;15:13-16.
79. Zipes DP, Cobb LA, Garson A Jr, et al. Task Force VI: arrhythmias. *J Am Coll Cardiol.* 1985;6:1225-1232.
80. Paul T, Marchal C, Garson A. Ventricular couplets in the young: prognosis related to underlying substrate. *Am Heart J.* 1990;119:577-581.
81. Braverman JB, Gibson S. The outlook for children with congenital aortic stenosis. *Am Heart J.* 1957;53:487-493.
82. Peckman GB, Keith JD, Evan JR. Congenital aortic stenosis: some observations on the natural history and clinical assessment. *Can Med Assoc J.* 1964;91:639-643.
83. Glew RH, Varghese PJ, Krovete LJ, Dorst JP, Rowe RD. Sudden death in congenital aortic stenosis: a review of eight cases with an evaluation of premonitory clinical features. *Am Heart J.* 1969;78:615-625.
84. James FW, Schwartz DC, Kaplan S, Spilkin SP. Exercise electrocardiogram, blood pressure, and work capacity in young patients with valvular or discrete subaortic stenosis. *Am J Cardiol.* 1982;50:769-775.
85. Feinstein RD, Soileau EJ, Daniel WA. A national survey of preparticipation physical examination requirements. *Phys Sports Med.* 1988;16:57-59.
86. Hulse E, Strong WB. Preparticipation evaluation for athletics. *Pediatr Rev.* 1987;9:1-10.
87. Kulangara RJ, Strong WB, Miller MD. Differential diagnosis of heart murmurs in children. *Postgrad Med.* 1982;72:219-228.
88. Garson A Jr. Medicolegal problems in the management of cardiac arrhythmias in children. *Pediatrics.* 1987;79:84-88.

Tattooing Behavior in Adolescence

A Comparison Study

James A. Farrow, MD; Richard H. Schwartz, MD; Joop Vanderleeuw, MD

• We characterize associations with and motivations for tattooing in adolescents through data from a controlled, three-group comparison of adolescents from a substance abuse treatment program, detention center, and private pediatric practice. We surveyed 474 adolescents (12 to 18 years old) with tattoos (12%) and without tattoos (88%). The private pediatric practice was the control site. A 34-item questionnaire was used to profile the three groups and their primary associations with tattooing with respect to race, drug use, school attendance, school grades, parental marital status, family income, tattooing by family members, criminal activity, and involvement with satanic rituals. Tattooing was significantly (*P*<.005) associated with all of these variables in the ways described, as was knowledge of its association with human immunodeficiency virus infection. No interventions were made. Tattooing is common in adolescents and is associated with low self-esteem, delinquency, drug abuse, family and peer modeling, and participation in satanic rituals. Addressing the behavior as a health problem is discussed.

(*AJDC*. 1991;145:184–187)

Tattooing is common among some adolescents. Whether the tattooing is of the more common, amateur variety, or scribed by a professional tattoo artist, the motivations for such behavior and its health implications for adolescents have not been clearly delineated. Tattooing has many potential medical complications.[1] Tattooing is practiced by adolescents in solitude, among peers, and, occasionally, as part of rituals.[2-4] In some instances, tattooing is deliberate self-harm akin to the "carving" behaviors seen in suicidal and depressed adolescents.[5,6] Most tattooing during adolescence is not, however, indicative of psychosis or self-destructive tendencies.[7] As with carving, adolescents may use tattooing as a way of displaying affection for a boyfriend, girlfriend, or popular rock music group.[5] The purpose of this three-group comparison study was to better characterize and delineate the motivation for tattooing among adolescents, a subject that is often misunderstood or misinterpreted by pediatricians.

Accepted for publication September 4, 1990.

From the Division of Adolescent Medicine and Department of Pediatrics, University of Washington, Seattle (Drs Farrow and Vanderleeuw), and the Department of Pediatrics, Fairfax Hospital, Falls Church, Va (Dr Schwartz).

Reprint requests to Division of Adolescent Medicine, Department of Pediatrics, CDMRC WJ-10, University of Washington, Seattle, WA 98195 (Dr Farrow).

SUBJECTS AND METHODS

A convenience sample of 474 adolescents with a mean age of 15.9 years (range, 14.9 to 17.1 years) responded to a 34-item questionnaire. Respondents included 160 adolescents (71% male) in a residential drug and alcohol treatment program in suburban Washington, DC, 102 juvenile detainees (80% male) in the King County (Washington) Juvenile Detention Center in Seattle, and 212 control subjects (43% male) from a private pediatric practice in a middle-class community in suburban Virginia. Questionnaires were administered to the cohort undergoing treatment for chemical dependency and the control subjects with explicit parental consent, and to the population of detainees with a letter of explanation to the child's parent or guardian. The questionnaire was pilot-tested for understandability and readability. Areas covered by the survey included sex, race, parents' marital status, family education and income, highest school year completed, grade point average (GPA), school attendance/dropout status, criminal behavior, drug use, participation in satanic rituals, and tattooing behavior by family, friends, and boyfriends or girlfriends. Tattooing-behavior questions included age at first tattoo, use of a professional tattoo artist, mental state during tattooing, identification of tattoos with satanic symbolism (Fig 1), and knowledge of the relationship between acquired immunodeficiency syndrome and needle use.

Characteristics of the subject populations were analyzed using standard statistical methods. Statistical methods employed in the data analysis consisted of analyses of variance for the continuous measures and χ^2 analyses for the evaluation of differences of frequencies between groups. Means were derived using Student's *t* test.

RESULTS

Table 1 profiles subjects by study groups and summarizes subject profiles with respect to race, parental marital status and education, subject's GPA, drug use, involvement in satanic rituals, and tattooing. Among all respondents, the parents of 172 (36%) were divorced or separated, with detainees having the highest incidence of this (64 subjects, 63% of all juvenile detainees). Ninety-six subjects (60%) from the drug abuse treatment program and 100 detainees (98% of all detainees) had been arrested. Drug use was highest overall among subjects in the drug treatment program.

Of all respondents, 54 (11.4%) had some experience with satanic rituals. Adolescents from the drug treatment program were more involved in this activity than adolescents from the other two groups. Fifty-eight (12.2% of all subjects) had tattoos or had engaged in tattooing behaviors. These behaviors consisted of intentional inscription of letters or symbols with and without indelible substances. Data describing tattooing among peers and family members are presented in Table 1.

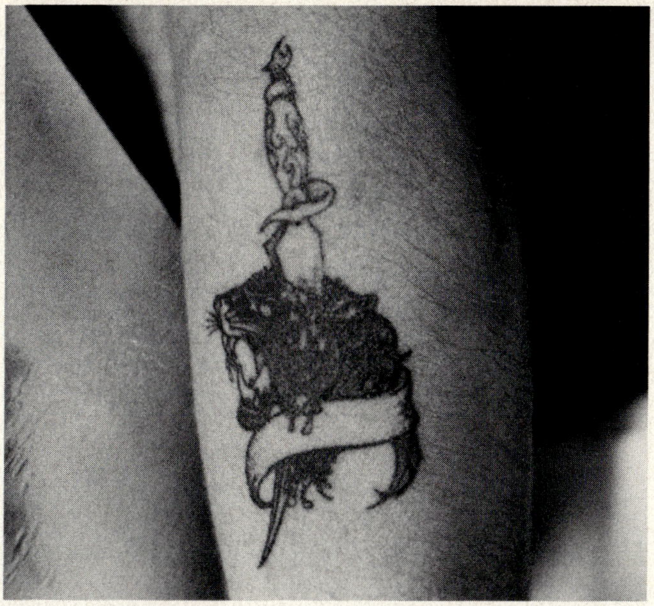

Fig 1.—*A symbol inscribed by a professional.*

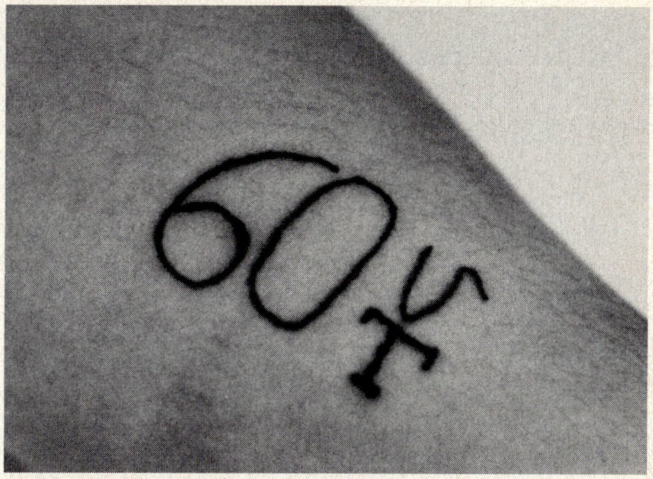

Fig 2.—*A self- or peer-inscribed tattoo.*

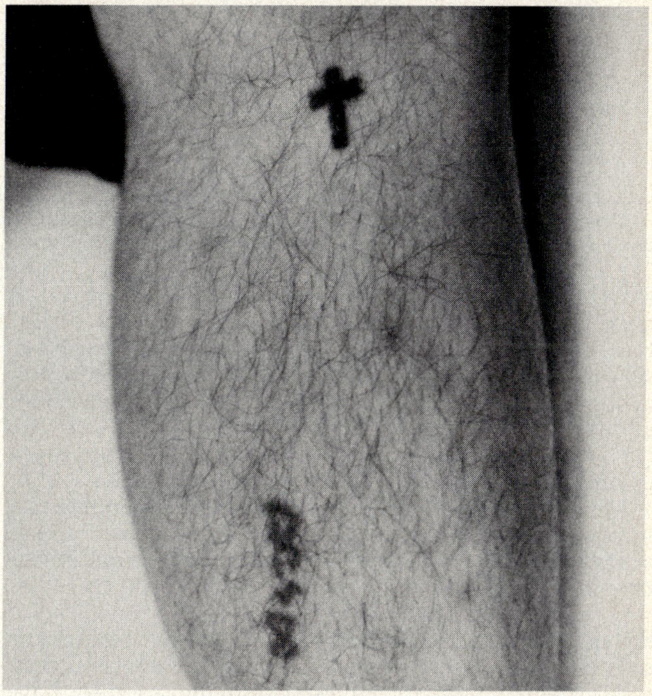

Fig 3.—*A self- or peer-inscribed tattoo.*

Table 1.—Subject Profiles by Study Group (N = 474)*

	Drug Abuse Group (n = 160)	Juvenile Detention Group (n = 102)	Control Group (n = 212)
Race, No. (%)			
White	143 (89)	38 (37)	198 (93)
Black	16 (10)	42 (41)	8 (4)
Hispanic	0	4 (4)	3 (1)
Asian	0	1 (1)	2 (0.9)
Other	1 (.6)	17 (17)	1 (.5)
Family history, No. (%)			
Parents divorced or separated	65 (41)	64 (63)	43 (20)
Father a college graduate	57 (36)	13 (13)	68 (32)
Family income more than $40 000 per year	9 (6)	32 (31)	84 (40)
Family member has a tattoo	26 (16)	30 (29)	13 (6)
Mean grade point average	2.5/4.0	2.0/4.0	3.0/4.0
Subject history, No. (%)			
Arrested	96 (60)	100 (98)	7 (3)
Participated in satanic rituals	41 (26)	12 (12)	1 (0.5)
Used marijuana weekly	135 (84)	56 (55)	11 (5)
Ever used phencyclidine	84 (53)	1 (1)	7 (3)
Drunk more than 10 times	DNA	10 (10)	10 (5)
Best friend has a tattoo	36 (23)	54 (53)	4 (2)
Girlfriend or boyfriend has a tattoo	29 (18)	22 (22)	5 (2)
Subject has a tattoo	21 (13)	34 (33)	3 (1)

*In descriptions of race, percentages may not total 100 because of rounding. DNA indicates data not available.

Eight (14%) of the 58 subjects with tattoos had more than one tattoo. The ages at which their first tattoos were engraved were fairly evenly distributed through age groups. Only 10 (17%) of the 58 had had the tattoos applied by a professional (Fig 1); the remainder were self- or peer-inscribed (Figs 2 and 3). Most tattoos were on the arms (42); other locations of tattoos included the face (two), hands (13), legs (three), chest (five), and back (one). A satanic symbol was identified on one subject (not shown). Eleven subjects (19%) were intoxicated when their tattoos were applied. Only six (10%) wanted the tattoo removed when surveyed. Seven (12%) of the tattooed adolescents had shared needles when the tattoo was created.

Table 2 profiles subjects with tattoos and notes differences between them and subjects without tattoos. Differences with respect to race, parental marital status, GPA, school attendance, arrest history, drug use, and tattooing by peers and family members were significant. Tattooing behavior was greater in children of fathers who had not graduated from college.

Most tattooed adolescents (50 subjects, 86%) came from middle-income families. Academic achievement was lower in the group with tattoos (mean GPA, 2.2 on a 4.0

Table 2.—Summary of Significant Associations With Tattooing in Adolescents*

	Group With Tattoos, No. (%) (n=58)	Group Without Tattoos, No. (%) (n=416)	χ^2	*df*
Male/female	46 (79)/12 (21)	237 (57)/179 (43)	9.3	1
Race	...	...	17.5	5
White	38 (66)	338 (81)	...	...
Black	10 (17)	54 (13)	...	...
Family history				
Parents divorced or separated	32 (55)	139 (33)	18.4	4
Father a college graduate	10 (17)	128 (31)	19.5	5
Family member has a tattoo	25 (43)	85 (20)	60.5	15
Subject history				
School dropout	25 (43)	72 (17)	19.7	1
Arrested	41 (71)	85 (20)	21.8	1
Used marijuana weekly	37 (64)	163 (39)	120.6	2
Ever used phencyclidine	12 (21)	49 (12)	8.5	1
Ever used lysergic acid diethylamide	33 (57)	136 (33)	19.5	4
Drunk more than 10 times	25 (43)	63 (15)	108.5	4
Received treatment for drug use	33 (57)	141 (34)	9.7	1
Participated in satanic rituals	15 (26)	38 (9)	14.2	1
Best friend has a tattoo	41 (71)	52 (13)	102.5	1
Girlfriend or boyfriend has a tattoo	23 (40)	32 (8)	48.4	1

*P values were significant ($P<.005$) for all associations. The group with tattoos had a mean grade point average of 2.2 on a 4.0 scale, and the group without tattoos had a mean grade point average of 3.0 on the same scale.

scale) than in the group without tattoos (mean GPA, 3.0 on a 4.0 scale, $P=.002$). Twenty-five (43%) of the 58 tattooed subjects had dropped out of school. With respect to school attendance, only one of the control subjects had dropped out of school, while 48 (47%) of the juvenile detainees had quit school. Of the 58 subjects with tattoos, 41 (71%) had arrest records. The relationship between types of offense and having a tattoo was nonsignificant.

Most drug and alcohol use was significantly related to having a tattoo, although a selection bias is inherent in the study population for adolescents who abuse drugs. A history of having received treatment for drug use was likewise associated with tattooing ($P=.002$). Fifteen (26%) of the tattooed adolescents had been involved in satanic rituals. Tattooing behavior was significantly associated with a best friend, girlfriend, boyfriend, or family member having a tattoo ($P<.001$).

No significant differences were evident between the responses of males and females with tattoos, although the male-female ratio was greater in the group with tattoos than in the group without tattoos. No significant difference existed among comparison groups with respect to knowing the relationship between human immunodeficiency virus (HIV) infection and tattooing. The correct relationship was acknowledged most often by the group of detainees (136 subjects, 85%). Of all subjects, 300 (63%) indicated that they knew HIV infection was related to tattooing. Eight tattooed subjects (14%) were unaware of the association. No significant difference was shown between groups with tattoos and groups without tattoos with respect to knowledge about the relationship between tattoos, needles, and acquired immunodeficiency syndrome.

COMMENT

This study reaffirms reports that tattooing is a common practice among adolescents[5,8-10] and attempts to characterize which adolescents are most likely to engage in this behavior. It does not define psychopathology in the study population. While many adolescents who engage in self-destructive behavior such as carving or tattooing suffer from significant psychiatric dysfunction, many also engage in the behavior because of low self-esteem or peer and family modeling and as an immediate reaction to drug and alcohol disinhibition.[3,5-7,11,12] Further, adolescents with tattoos appear to have also experienced family dysfunction, poor academic performance, poor school attendance, delinquent or gang-related behavior, heavier drug and alcohol use, and sometimes drug dealing.

Some of these associations have been noted previously.[6,7,12-14] To some extent, these youth are more alienated from family, school, and social institutions than their peers without tattoos. They are significantly more likely to be involved in satanic rituals. To what degree participation in satanic rituals promoted tattooing is unknown, and this study does not answer that question. Among our study population, tattooing appears to occur more from impulse than as part of any ritualistic activity.

Black adolescents were slightly more likely to have a tattoo than the general study population, with the highest proportion of black subjects coming from the detention population (42 subjects, 41%; Table 1).

All three groups appeared to be knowledgeable about the association between HIV infection and the use of needles for tattooing.[15] However, a large minority (175 subjects, 37%) of the total population was not aware of the potential for transmitting HIV infection through contaminated tattooing apparatus.[16] Adolescents with tattoos were not significantly less knowledgeable about this risk than those without tattoos. In general, our results indicate the need for more education of all adolescents about the relationship between HIV infection and tattooing.

Our findings have implications for how tattooing of adolescents is viewed in the clinical setting. Clinicians with tattooed adolescent patients should use these findings as a stimulus for discussions about self-care and disease prevention. Although tattooing is most often associated with underlying family modeling, low self-esteem, an impulsive personality style, and deviant behaviors, it should be addressed outright as a health issue. Physicians should also recognize that some tattoos symbolize involvement in satanic activities or indicate a state of depression and self-destructive tendencies. They should follow up on the behavior by investigating these possibilities. This study also confirms an association between tattooing and drug abuse. Tattooing, therefore, can be seen as another indicator of the deleterious nature of chemical dependency in this age group. All clinicians should be aware of the potential significance and underlying motivations of tattooing in adolescence and discuss the behavior while providing guidance to young patients.

References

1. Goldstein N. Complications from tattoos. *J Dermatol Drug Oncol.* 1979;5:869-877.
2. Roenigk HH. Tattooing: history, techniques, complications, removal. *Cleve Clin Q.* 1971;38:179-186.
3. Buhich N, Morris G. Significance of tattoos in male psychiatric patients. *Aust N Z J Psychiatry.* 1982;16:185-189.
4. Bennahum DA. Tattoos of heroin addicts in New Mexico. *Rocky Mt Med J.* 1971;68:63-66.
5. Schwartz RH, Cohen P, Hoffman NG, Meeks JB. Self-harm behaviors (carving) in female adolescent drug abusers. *Clin Pediatr (Phila).* 1989;28:340-346.
6. Fried RI. The psychodynamics of tattooing: a review. *Pediatr Rounds.* 1983;50:289-242.
7. Girumet GW. Psychodynamic implications of tattoos. *Am J Orthopsychiatry.* 1983;53:482-492.
8. Verberne TJP. The personality traits of tattooed adolescent offenders. *Br J Criminol.* 1969;9:172-175.
9. Burma JA. Self-tattooing among delinquents: a research note. *Sociol Soc Res.* 1959;43:341-345.
10. Harry B. Tattoos, body experience, and body image boundary among violent male offenders. *Bull Am Acad Psychiatry Law.* 1987;15:171-178.
11. Thomson W, McDonald JCH. Disfigurement by design. *Nurs Mirror.* 1984;158:40-41.
12. Newman G. The implications of tattooing in prisoners. *J Clin Psychiatry.* 1982;43:231-234.
13. Thomson W, McDonald JCH. Self-tattooing by school children. *Lancet.* 1983;2:1243-1244.
14. Buhrich N. Significance of tattoos in narcotic abusers. *Drug Alcohol Depend.* 1983;11:389-394.
15. Doll DC. Tattooing in prison and HIV infection. *Lancet.* 1988;1:66-67.
16. Phoon W, Fong N, Lee J. History of blood transfusion, tattooing, acupuncture and risk of hepatitis B among Chinese men in Singapore. *Am J Public Health.*1988;78:938-940.

Skateboarding Injuries in Children

A Second Wave

Joel Retsky, MD; David Jaffe, MD; Katherine Christoffel, MD, MPH

• **Motivated by a number of skateboard-related injuries seen in an emergency department, we undertook an investigation of skateboarding injuries in the mid-1980s. We studied US Consumer Product Safety Commission injury frequency estimates, which indicated a resurgence of these injuries: 19 182 in 1984 and 37 180 in 1985. Children 10 to 14 years old were injured with greatest frequency. Nontrivial injuries were more common among children younger than 5 years old, reflecting a larger proportion of head and neck injuries. Boys sustained more frequent and more severe skateboard-related injuries. Observed injury patterns (head and neck injuries in younger children, extremity injuries in older children, and more severe head and neck injuries in older children) probably reflect the role of psychomotor development on both risk exposure and biomechanics. Likely prevention strategies include warnings against skateboard use by children younger than 5 years, prohibition of skateboards on streets and highways, and the promotion of use of helmets and other protective gear.**

(*AJDC*. 1991;145:188–193)

Skateboarding is a visible activity of modern childhood whose popularity has waxed and waned since skateboards were first marketed in the 1960s. It provides pleasure and entertainment, yet also is a source of injury. The number of injuries related to skateboards peaked in 1977 and then declined through the early 1980s. During the several subsequent years, we noticed a rising number of skateboard injuries in the Children's Memorial Hospital emergency department, Chicago, Ill. Review of the US Consumer Product Safety Commission (CPSC) data indicated that such injuries were again rising in incidence nationally. We undertook an investigation of skateboard injuries in the 1980s with the following objectives: (1) to characterize the 1980s outbreak, (2) to compare certain aspects of this outbreak with that which occurred in the 1970s, and (3) to identify preventable causes of contemporary skateboarding injuries.

Accepted for publication August 6, 1990.

From the Department of Pediatrics, Children's Memorial Hospital and Northwestern University Medical School, Chicago, Ill. Dr Jaffe is now with The Hospital for Sick Children, Toronto, Ontario.

Read before the Annual Meeting of the Midwest Society for Pediatric Research, Chicago, Ill, November 11, 1987, and the National Meeting of the American Public Health Association, Boston, Mass, November 14, 1988.

Reprint requests to Department of Emergency Pediatrics, The Hospital for Sick Children, 555 University Ave, Toronto, Ontario M5G 1X8 (Dr Jaffe).

MATERIALS AND METHODS

Data were obtained from the CPSC Injury Information Clearinghouse in Washington, DC, concerning injuries associated with skateboard use (CPSC code 1333) during 1976 and 1977 (the peak years of the last outbreak) and 1984 and 1985 (the two most recent years about which complete data were available at the time of data collection). The data reviewed included the following:

(1) Age and sex-specific *injury frequency estimates* were obtained from the National Electronic Injury Surveillance System (NEISS) database. The NEISS estimates are derived from surveillance of statistically representative emergency departments in the United States (119 in 1976 and 1977; 73 in 1984; and 64 in 1985). These data consist of age- and sex-specific injury information, including body part injured, disposition, location, and severity. The CPSC severity coding scheme was developed by a panel of authorities (epidemiologists and other physicians) during the 1970s. Injuries were assigned severity ratings based on subjective opinions of the panel of authorities (Bart McDonald, CPSC spokesman, oral communication, 1989). The frequency estimate data reviewed included a brief description of each skateboard injury reported during the period studied. Injury frequency estimates are derived from NEISS reports using weightings for each recorded visit, based on the representativeness of the emergency department in which it originated. (2) *Summaries of cases* were reported to the CPSC by news clippings, consumers' complaints, the medical examiners' and coroners' alert program, government agency referral, and other sources during the years studied. (3) Brief reports of *in-depth investigations* were gathered by the CPSC staff of selected injury cases from 1977 through 1979 and 1983 through 1985. (4) *Information on deaths* from 1984 through 1987 was compiled by the CPSC from state health department death certificates. (5) Finally, CPSC *product summary reports* (on hundreds of products) were collected for 1976 through 1986.

Until 1979, 119 hospitals gathered NEISS data. In 1980, 11 large hospitals were added but, owing to financial constraints, the total number of reporting hospitals was reduced later that same year to 74 (nine of the 11 large hospitals remained). The estimated sampling error increased only slightly over what it was in the 1970s, ie, prior to the addition of the large hospitals. A further reduction in the number of reporting hospitals occurred in 1984 (reducing the total to 65); again the sampling error was estimated to have increased only slightly because the reductions affected mainly smaller hospitals (which were effectively substituted for by larger hospitals) (Bart McDonald, CPSC spokesman, oral communication, 1989).

To permit calculations of age-specific injury incidence rate estimates, data were obtained on age-specific population counts from the 1980 US census and on population projections for 1976, 1977, 1984, and 1985.[1] Information about skateboard manufacturing regulations, industry safety standards, and protective gear was obtained by personal communication with the CPSC, skate-

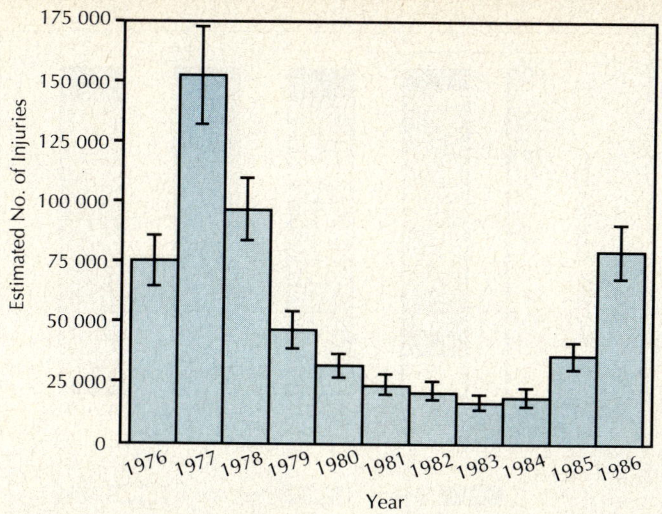

Fig 1.—*The number of injuries.*

board manufacturers, manufacturers of protective gear for skateboarding, and skateboard competition promotional organizations (oral communication with spokespersons from the Powell Corp, Santa Barbara, Calif, and the Pro Tech Corp, Belleview, Wash, which are manufacturers of skateboard equipment, and from the National Skateboard Association, San Bernardino, Calif, 1988).

Data were analyzed on a computer (IBM System 38). The strength of bivariate relationships between categorical variables was evaluated using the χ^2 statistic, with the level of significance set at P being less than .01.

RESULTS

The Current Outbreak

Number of Injuries.—More than 150 000 skateboard-related injuries occurred in the peak year of 1977, after which the incidence declined through 1983 (16 836). It then began to rise again (Fig 1): 19 182 injuries were reported in 1984 and 37 180 injuries were reported in 1985. Data concerning 1986, released after the data reported herein had been analyzed, showed an incidence of 81 000—a 120% increase from the year before.

Demographic Analysis. — Of all skateboard related injuries in the 1980s, 88% occurred to persons younger than 20 years, and 83% occurred among boys (range, 65% in boys 5 years old to 100% in boys younger than 1 year). For most analyses, we grouped data according to standard age groupings and labeled these groups as follows: 0 to 4 year olds, infants and toddlers; 5 to 9 year olds, young children; 10 to 14 year olds, young adolescents; and 15 to 19 year olds, older adolescents. Table 1 compares the estimated number of injuries by age group in the 1970s and the 1980s. A greater proportion of children 9 years old or younger were injured in the 1980s ($P<.001$). The largest number of injuries occurred among young adolescents. This age group, which represents 24% of the pediatric population and 6.5% of the total population, accounted for 45% of all injuries in the 1980s. The standard groupings obscure the fact that the incidence of injury and sex distribution for 15-year-old children seem to follow patterns for 10 to 14 year olds more closely than for 16 to 19 year olds, as seen in Fig 2, which displays incidence by year of age.

Body Part Injured.—Reported injuries were grouped into three anatomic regions: head and neck, extremities, and trunk. Almost 75% of all injuries involved the extremities. Greater than 90% of all injuries involved either the extremities or the head and neck.

There was a strong interaction between age and injured body part (Fig 3). With each increasing age group, the proportion of head injuries decreased while the proportion of extremity injuries increased ($P<.001$).

Table 1.—Injury Frequency by Age Grouping, 1970s and 1980s, Estimated Number of Injuries

Age, y	1976-1977, No. (%)	1984-1985, No. (%)
0-4	3272 (1.5)	2384 (4.2)
5-9	33 654 (14.9)	10 386 (18.4)
10-14	120 054 (53.3)	25 402 (45.1)
15-19	40 739 (18.1)	11 582 (20.5)
>20	27 679 (12.3)	6608 (11.7)

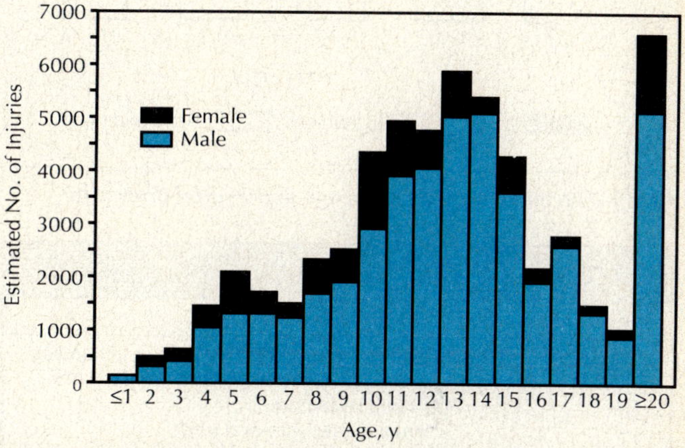

Fig 2.—*The incidence of injury and sex distribution.*

Severity of Injury.—Six levels of severity (1 = low to 6 = high) were coded by the CPSC (Table 2). We collapsed these to create three categories of severity: mild (1 to 2), moderate (3 to 4), and severe (5 to 6). Moderate injuries were the most frequent in every age group younger than 20 years, and most head injuries in all age groups were classified as moderate. No extremity injuries were scored as severe.

Severity and Age.—Overall, the proportion of mild injuries increased with increasing age (Fig 4). However, the proportion of mild head and neck injuries decreased with increasing age group (Fig 5) ($P<.001$), with the proportion of head injuries that were severe being largest (almost 23%) among young adolescents. The distribution of mild and moderate extremity injuries was nearly constant across age groups.

Location of Injury.—We collapsed the nine different injury occurrence location codes used by NEISS to form three groupings: home (home, apartment, condominium, farm), streets and highways (streets and highways), and other public places (school, industrial, and sports or recreational places). Almost 80% of all injuries occurred either at or near the home (49%) or on streets and highways (30%).

Location and Age.—Among infants and toddlers, 15% were injured on streets and highways compared with 23% for young children and more than 30% for adolescents ($P<.001$).

Injury Circumstances. — In-depth investigation of 218 skateboard injuries revealed information about injury circumstances. Although a large proportion of these investigations reported a nonspecific cause of injury (such as "fell from skateboard" or "lost control"), several recurrent scenarios were found in the 102 cases (47%) with more information. The most common specific circumstance was

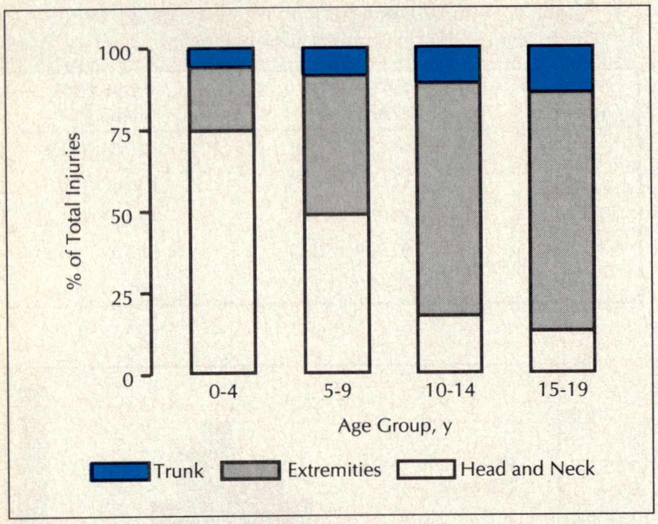

Fig 3.—*The interaction between age and injured body part.*

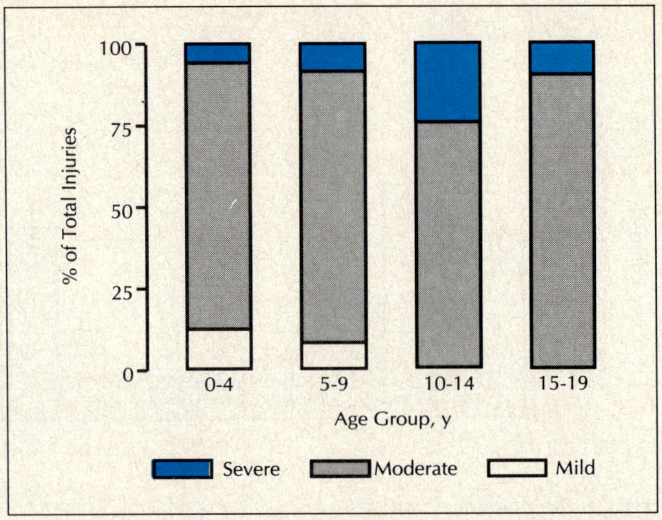

Fig 5.—*The proportion of mild head and neck injuries decreased with increasing age.*

Table 2.—Gradation of Severity

Severity	Examples
1	Sprained foot (mild injuries to small areas)
2	Contusion to lower trunk; dislocated arm, hand; puncture
3	Arm fracture; sprained neck
4	Finger crushing; head laceration; punctured eye
5	Concussion; fractured neck
6	Amputation; anoxia; arm crushing

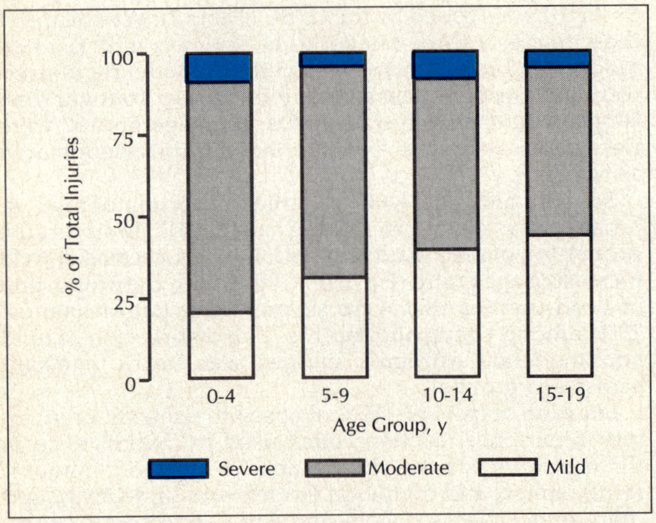

Fig 4.—*The proportion of mild injuries increased with increasing age.*

reported in 37 cases (17%): a moving skateboard hit an obstacle that caused a sudden cessation of the skateboard's forward motion, resulting in the rider's falling forward and off the skateboard. The obstacles encountered included sticks, stones, cracks, and bumps on the riding surface. Motor vehicles were involved in six injuries (3%) and bicycles were involved in another five injuries (2%). Nine injuries (4%) were attributed to skateboard failure.

Case reports concerning infants in the 0- to 2-year-old age range revealed additional circumstances of injury, including tripping over a stationary skateboard at home and being pushed off a skateboard by an older sibling (sometimes after having been placed on the board by the sibling). Most reports for children 3 to 4 years old indicated circumstances similar to those for school-age children (eg, skateboard wheel hits a small object). An additional factor in this age group may be poorer balance, as suggested by case reports of falling backwards off the board for no apparent reason.

Deaths.—According to the Reported Incident File of the CPSC, there were 36 deaths associated with skateboard use from June 1984 through August 1987. Of these, 21 (58%) involved motor vehicles. Severe head injury was the cause of death for all patients whose cause of death was reported, but the cause of death was reported in only 20% of the cases. Data from 1976 through 1979 indicate that of the 29 skateboard-related deaths reported, 90% were associated with severe head injury.

Age and Deaths.—Of the 36 deaths reported that were studied, 16 (44%) occurred in younger adolescents and 15 (42%) occurred in older adolescents. In addition, the deaths included one toddler, one young child, and three persons 20 years or older.

Changes From Past Outbreak.—Most of the patterns of injury found in the 1980s were similar to those in the 1970s. There were, however, some notable changes (Table 3). The proportion of boys among all injured children was higher. Younger children experienced a greater proportion of skateboard injuries. Hospitalization rates diminished. Finally, fewer injuries occurred at home in the 1980s, and more injuries occurred in the streets and on the highways.

Skateboard Safety Practices

The following information about skateboard safety was obtained in 1988 through oral communication with spokespersons from the Powell Corp, the Pro Tech Corp, and the National Skateboard Association. There are no skateboard manufacturing regulations, but US manufacturers report that they have set self-imposed industry standards to guard the market against lower-quality imported products. Many manufacturers produce or distribute protective gear, such as helmets, clothing, and pads, specifically designed for skateboarding. The proportion of skateboarders using protective equipment depends on the type of skateboarding practiced. Those engaged in vertical skating, such as skating on steep ramps, reportedly use protective gear most often. Vertical skating competition

Table 3.—Changes From Past Outbreak*

	1970s, No. (%)	1980s, No. (%)
Male subjects	159 378 (71)	46 160 (83)
Children younger than 10 y	36 926 (16)	12 689 (23)
Hospitalization rate	9155 (4)	1416 (2.5)
Injuries in streets and highways	15 243 (13)	15 357 (30)
Injuries occurring at home	86 878 (72)	24 162 (48)

*All $P<.001$ by χ^2.

events reportedly require skaters to wear helmets and knee and elbow pads. Freestyle skaters wear protective gear 50% to 70% of the time, depending on the spokesperson questioned. Street skaters, who are the most numerous, wear protective gear least often.

COMMENT

In the mid-1980s, skateboards were once again associated with a large number of injuries, some fatal. The available information, based on NEISS data, indicates that of the tens of thousands of children injured annually, most were preadolescent boys.

Because the number of hospitals surveyed by NEISS decreased during the years studied, confidence in the representativeness of the demographic composition of the sample from the 1980s may be decreased as compared with that of the 1970s. However, injury patterns in NEISS data from each period are still known to be valid for other types of injuries (eg, all terrain vehicles, L. Robertson, oral communication, 1988). As the best information available, the NEISS data remain instructive regarding the relationships between maturational levels and patterns of injury. However accurate they may be as estimates of emergency department visits, the NEISS estimates are underestimates of total injury frequency, because not all injured children are brought to emergency departments. In light of this, the estimated number of injuries is all the more striking.

Injury and Development

Age and injury were related in a discernible pattern. Younger children tended to sustain more severe injuries and more head injuries. In fact, these two observations are related because the CPSC tended to rank head injuries as more severe than extremity injuries. Overall, injuries to adolescents were milder, and they included more extremity injuries and fewer head injuries than those to younger children. However, when adolescents did sustain head injuries, they tended to be more severe. Finally, adolescents were more commonly injured on streets and highways than were younger children.

Several behavioral and developmental hypotheses concerning the mechanisms of skateboard injuries emerge from the data (Table 4). Because of immature motor coordination, young children may be unable to break falls with their arms. Their disproportionately large heads (as compared with adolescents) makes their heads the leading body part in falls from skateboards. These factors combine to cause young children to have more head injuries as compared with older children. However, because most injuries in young children probably occur at low speeds while using skateboards at home, the head injuries sustained are generally not severe. As children grow older, they develop increasing motor coordination and become better able to break falls with outstretched arms, thereby preferentially injuring extremities. However, older children also tend to

Table 4.—Psychomotor Development and Injury Characteristics

Age, y	Developmental Characteristics	Exposure	Injuries
0-4	High center of gravity; poor motor coordination; light weight; inexperienced riders	Low speed; home	Head > extremities Head: mild-moderate
5-9	Lower center of gravity; fair motor coordination; heavier weight; some risk taking	Higher speed; streets	Extremities = head Head: moderate
10-19	Lowest center of gravity; good motor coordination; heaviest weight; much risk taking; experienced riders	Highest speed; streets and highways	Extremities > head Head: moderate-severe

engage in increasingly risky behavior, often away from home. Consequently, they sustain more injuries on streets and highways where high-speed injuries are more prevalent. When head injuries occur under these circumstances, they are apt to be more severe.

Product Factors

Several product factors contribute to the danger associated with skateboarding today. Skateboards have small wheels as compared with bicycles, tricycles, and other children's vehicles. These small wheels are easily affected by small interruptions in the riding surface, such as sticks, stones, and cracks. The fact that these commonly cause skateboard mishaps has previously been recognized.[2-4] In addition, current construction uses urethane wheels and low rotational friction of the axles, enabling skateboards to achieve speeds of greater than 64 to 80 km/h (40 to 50 mph).[5-7] Skateboards are designed for high maneuverability at the expense of balance and control. Slight shifts in the rider's center of gravity cause great directional changes in the skateboard's motion, necessitating considerable skill for successful operators. This, coupled with the high speed of travel and the sensitivity of the wheels to irregularities in the riding surface, contributes to skateboard hazard.

Injury Prevention

The findings reported concerning age-related skateboard injury patterns suggest several strategies for injury prevention. Children younger than 5 years lack the motor coordination and judgment to operate skateboards safely. Use by children in this age group results in severe injury and, therefore, should be vigorously discouraged.

The most serious injuries, including deaths, involve severe head injury. Therefore, protective headgear should be used at all times, as recommended by various investigators.[2,4,7-11] Most injuries occurring to older children involve the extremities. Appropriately designed padding should prevent at least some soft-tissue injuries. The portions of the body that can be expected to sustain most of these injuries, such as knees, elbows, and palms, could be protected with elbow pads, knee pads, and gloves. Some studies have questioned the effectiveness of such protective gear[3,12] because the force of impact may be transmitted through protective clothing to cause fractures, whereas unprotected soft tissue may absorb the brunt of the injury. Appropriately designed gear should reduce this risk. Perhaps a more likely danger is that protective gear may give skateboarders a false sense of security, fostering more dangerous "tricks."

Because the worst injuries affected older children, who tended to ride in streets and highways, skateboard use in these areas should be prohibited, preferably by state or federal statute. Use of skateboards in the streets and highways poses a high risk of serious injury for at least three reasons. First, and most important, is the proximity to high-speed motor vehicles. That contact with these is likely to result in injuries of high severity is demonstrated by the fact that at least 58% of the CPSC-recorded skateboard-related deaths involved motor vehicles. Second, when skateboarders are in the roadway, traffic speeds are likely to encourage high-speed skating, which increases the chance of serious injury in the case of a tumble or collision. Third, roadways commonly have surface irregularities that readily affect the travel of small skateboard wheels, increasing the likelihood of falls and consequent injury (with or without motor vehicle contact).

Implications

Emergency department physicians need to be aware of the current pattern of skateboard use in the community and of the associated injuries. Continuing expansion of this outbreak would suggest a need for public awareness and perhaps local regulation.

While skateboarding is not a leading cause of death or disability, its prevalence—with a low but real risk of serious injury—merits preventive attention. Recognizing the age-related patterns reported in this study, pediatricians can help prevent serious injury by (1) promoting use of protective gear, (2) discussing skateboard safety with parents and children, (3) discouraging the use of skateboards by infants and toddlers, and (4) lobbying for CPSC and local government regulations, including age-related use guidelines and prohibitions on the use of skateboards on streets and highways.

Data from this study were shared with legislators and concerned citizens during a series of meetings to decide on the content of skateboarding regulations in the home town of one of the authors (K.C.). Several issues arose that are likely to come up in other settings as well, and so they bear mention herein.

A number of people were uncomfortable applying national data to our particular locale. Even more were dismayed that local data are not readily available: about either the prevalence of skateboarding or the prevalence of skateboard-related injuries. The basis of these concerns was that while it is important to prevent serious injuries, enforcement of an elaborate effort to prevent extremely uncommon injuries could not be justified in terms of the costs involved (mainly police effort and skateboarders' perceptions of harassment). Some tried to use bicycling data to argue for skateboarding in the streets (like bikes). It was helpful to point out (1) that policy must be based on the best available data, even when those data are imperfect, (2) that the injury scenarios that emerged from the national data match ones reported by local skateboarders (eg, a concussion from toppling in traffic after a wheel hit a pebble in the street), and (3) that the causal sequences are different for injuries from (large, flexible-wheeled) bikes and (small, hard-wheeled) skateboards.

Other issues related to the nature of skateboarders, most of whom are predriving adolescents. Parents and legislators identified the need for a variety of organized recreational opportunities for early teens, perhaps including a skateboard park. However, it is fairly expensive to construct an up-to-date facility that would be usable by skaters at a variety of skill levels, which was particularly relevant as it was not clear how many people would use such a facility. Liability issues were also a concern. A number of youngsters reported that they use their skateboards for transportation (eg, from school to work), and argued that avoiding street skating would interfere with this type of use (because local sidewalks are often cracked). Both the adults and teens agreed that any requirements that are both likely to be violated and difficult to enforce uniformly (eg, helmet wearing) are likely to be ineffective; they also could antagonize skaters if the rules are unevenly or punitively enforced. All agreed that the goal must be to set safe skateboarding guidelines that teens can follow and to avoid "criminalizing" any aspect of this basically wholesome pastime.

A final area of concern was the effect of skateboarding on pedestrians, which would be maximized by banning skateboarding in the streets. (It was an interaction with pedestrians that led to the arrest of some skateboarders under an ordinance passed during the skateboard injury outbreak of the 1970s, that generated the legislative activity in 1989.)

The outcome of these discussions was revision of the relevant local ordinance to regulate skateboard and rollerskate use in three ways. (1) Such activities cannot collect a crowd. (2) Skaters cannot enter the streets except to cross them (at which time they are considered pedestrians). (3) Sidewalk skating is limited to residential (ie, not business or commercial) areas. No mention is made of helmets. No action has yet been taken on the idea of a skateboard park.

Leon Robertson, PhD, provided helpful comments; Robert Tanz, MD, reviewed the manuscript; and Wanda Harold, Zsazanna Taborn, and Laura R. Gannott gave secretarial support.

References

1. US Bureau of the Census. *Current Population Reports, United States Population Estimates, by Age, Sex and Race: 1980 to 1987.* Series P-25, No. 1022. Washington, DC: US Bureau of the Census; 1988.
2. Hawkins RW, Lyne ED. Skateboard fractures. *Am J Sports Med.* 1981;9:99-102.
3. Illingworth CM, Jay A, Noble D, Collick M. Two hundred twenty-five skateboard injuries in children. *Clin Pediatr.* 1978;17:781-789.
4. Allum RL. Skateboard injuries: a new epidemic. *Injury.* 1978;10:152-153.
5. Jacobs RA, Keller EL. Skateboard accidents. *Pediatrics.* 1977;59:939-942.
6. Maddox D. Skateboards zip- and zap-riders once again. *Physician Sports Med.* 1976;4:24-25.
7. Kemm I. Skateboard injuries. *BMJ.* 1978;1:894.
8. Hawkins RW, Lyne ED. Skeletal trauma in skateboard injuries. *AJDC.* 1978;132:751-752.
9. Maddox D. Skateboarding: the spill-and-skill sport. *Physician Sports Med.* 1978;6:108-114.
10. Cook S, O'Hare P. Skateboard injuries. *Med J Aust.* 1976;2:733-734.
11. Fyfe IS, Guion AJ. Skateboard injuries. *Injury.* 1978;10:149-151.
12. Morgan WJ, Galloway DJ, Patel AR. Prevention of skateboard injuries. *Scott Med J.* 1980;25:39-40.

Differences in Infant Mortality by Race, Nativity Status, and Other Maternal Characteristics

Joel C. Kleinman, PhD; Lois A. Fingerhut, MA; Kate Prager, ScD

• The objective of this study was to examine the effects of nativity status (native vs foreign born) and other maternal characteristics (age, parity, education, and marital status) on infant, neonatal, and postneonatal mortality among white and black mothers. The design of this nonrandomized cohort study was based on birth and death certificates. The setting involved live births among US residents (excluding California, Texas, and Washington) in 1983 and 1984. The participants included white mothers with 4.4 million births and black mothers with 926 000 births in single deliveries. There were no interventions. With regard to measurements (the main results), after adjusting for other risk factors, neonatal mortality risk was 22% lower among the black foreign-born mothers than among the black native-born mothers, while among white infants, there was no risk difference by nativity. Relative risks were more similar for postneonatal mortality, ie, 24% lower among black foreign-born mothers and 20% lower among white foreign-born mothers. Combining the several categories of risk factors into three broad maternal risk groups, there was a near-doubling of black and near-tripling of white infant mortality rates between the low and high levels of maternal risk. We concluded that if the infant mortality rate in the low-risk groups could be achieved by the moderate- and high-risk groups, there would be a 30% reduction in infant deaths within each race. Since the black infant mortality rate is twice the white infant mortality rate and black foreign-born mothers have much lower rates than black native-born mothers, it is likely that further improvement is possible among black infants.
(*AJDC.* 1991;145:194–199)

Racial differences in infant mortality and in low birth weight have been the focus of many epidemiologic analyses. Maternal risk factors responsible for differences in low birth weight among white and black infants were examined in a recent study with the use of 1983 national data.[1] The analysis showed large racial differences even among mothers at low risk of poor pregnancy outcome. Furthermore, the effects of each of several maternal risk factors were found to be stronger among whites than among blacks. With the recent availability of national files of linked births and infant deaths, we are able in this article to extend the previous analysis to infant mortality. In addition, we focus on another maternal characteristic that has not received much attention—nativity status—that is, whether the mother was foreign born or native born.

Previous reports of pregnancy outcome among foreign-born mothers have been limited to relatively select population subgroups.[2-6] The 1971 through 1973 New York City, NY, data reported by Valanis and Rush[2,3] showed that black foreign-born women had a lower proportion of low-birth-weight infants than black native-born women. The study by Kessner[4] used New York City data for 1968 to show significantly higher mean birth weights and lower infant mortality rates among black foreign-born women than black native-born women. In a recent analysis of black foreign- and native-born women in Boston, Mass,[5] it was observed that the infants of foreign-born mothers experienced greater intrauterine growth than those of native-born mothers. In a 1979 analysis of data from Sweden, Smedby and Ericson[6] found that the perinatal mortality rate among children born to immigrant mothers was lower than the rate among children born to Swedish mothers. In this study, we used national linked birth and infant death files for 1983 and 1984 to examine racial differences in the effects of maternal sociodemographic risk factors, including nativity status, on infant, neonatal, and postneonatal mortality.

MATERIALS AND METHODS

We combined the 1983 and 1984 national files of linked birth and infant death certificates to investigate the relationships between maternal risk factors and infant mortality. The data were classified by maternal race and place of birth into four categories—black foreign- and native-born mothers and white foreign- and native-born mothers. Mothers who were born outside the 50 United States or the District of Columbia were classified as foreign born. All others (including the 0.2% with an unknown place of birth) were coded as native born. Births in California, Texas, and Washington where education is not on the birth certificate were omitted from the analysis. By excluding these births, 21% of the births to white native-born mothers, 16% of those to black native-born mothers, 49% of the births to white foreign-born mothers, and 12% of the births to black foreign-born mothers were omitted from the analysis. Most of the omitted white foreign-born mothers were of Mexican descent. Despite the large proportion of births excluded, the infant mortality rates based on all births were very similar to those based on births to mothers with known education. For example, the infant mortality rate among white

Accepted for publication August 17, 1990.

From the Division of Analysis (Dr Kleinman and Ms Fingerhut) and Mortality Statistics Branch, Division of Vital Statistics (Dr Prager), National Center for Health Statistics, Centers for Disease Control, Hyattsville, Md.

Reprint requests to Division of Analysis, National Center for Health Statistics, 6525 Belcrest Rd, Room 1080, Hyattsville, MD 20782 (Dr Kleinman).

foreign-born mothers was 7.9 per 1000 live births overall compared with 8.1 for those mothers with known education.

In 1983 and 1984, black foreign-born women who resided in large metropolitan counties (population, ≥250 000) accounted for 93% of the births to black foreign-born mothers. This compares with 63% of the births to black native-born mothers, 78% to white foreign-born mothers, and 43% to white native-born mothers. To ensure that residence was not a confounding factor, this variable (large metropolitan areas vs all other counties) was included as a covariate in the regression analysis. Furthermore, the analysis was repeated for the large metropolitan areas only. Since the results for the restricted analysis were nearly the same as the results for the entire United States, only the latter results are presented.

Only live births in single deliveries (98% of all births) and of known birth order (99.5% of all births) were included in the analysis. The low- and very-low-birth-weight rates were based on births with known birth weights (99.9% of all births).

Multiple logistic regression was used to estimate the effects of each of the maternal characteristics after controlling for the others. Separate analyses were carried out by using five different dependent variables: infant, neonatal, and postneonatal mortality; very low birth weight (<1500 g); and low birth weight (<2500 g). However, because the birth weight results are very similar to those presented earlier,[1] only the detailed results for the three mortality rates are presented in this article. Detailed birth weight results are available on request to the authors. The BMDP logistic regression programs were used.[7] For comparison with previous results on birth weight,[1] the results of the logistic regressions with mortality as the dependent variable are summarized by presenting directly standardized rates that were determined with the use of the fitted rates from the models and the combined distribution of all births as the standard population. These standardized rates provided an average risk of neonatal, postneonatal, or infant mortality for each maternal characteristic after adjustment for all the other characteristics in the model.

To maintain comparability with previous work,[1] other variables included in this analysis are as follows: maternal education (<12, 12, 13 through 15, and 16 or more years); marital status (married or not married); age (<18, 18 and 19, 20 through 29, and 30 years or older); and parity (primiparas or multiparas). High parity was defined as third- or higher-order births to women younger than 25 years and fourth- or higher-order births to women aged 25 years or older. All other multiparous births were considered to be of low parity.

The following three categories of maternal risk summarize these variables: (1) *Low-risk* mothers consisted of married mothers with at least 13 years of education who were either primiparas aged 20 through 29 years or low-parity multiparas aged 20 years or older. (2) *High-risk* mothers included unmarried mothers with less than 12 years of education who were either teenagers, primiparas aged 30 years or older, or high-parity multiparas. (3) The *moderate-risk* group of mothers included all other combinations of maternal characteristics.

RESULTS

Maternal Risk and Nativity

In 1983 and 1984, 7% of both white and black births were to foreign-born mothers. The distribution of births by maternal risk shows that, overall, 11% of black and 28% of white births were at low risk, while 22% of black and 4% of white births were at high risk of poor pregnancy outcome (Table 1). However, the black foreign-born mothers were more likely than the black native-born mothers to be at low risk, ie, 18% compared with 10%, and were much less likely to be at high risk, ie, 10% vs 23%. Among white births, the differences by nativity status were smaller and in the opposite direction. Twenty-nine percent of the births to white native-born mothers vs 23% of the births to white foreign-born mothers were at low risk, and only 4% of the births to white native-born mothers and 7% of the births to white foreign-born mothers were at high risk. Detailed distributions of births by the variables that were included in the risk categories are given in Table 2.

Table 1.—Distribution of Live Births by Maternal Race, Risk, and Nativity Status: United States, 1983 and 1984 Birth Cohorts*

Maternal Risk	All Mothers (%)	Foreign-born Mothers (%)	Native-born Mothers (%)
Black			
Low	10.6	17.6	10.1
Moderate	67.1	72.3	66.8
High	22.2	10.1	23.1
Total	**100.0**	**100.0**	**100.0**
White			
Low	28.3	22.6	28.7
Moderate	67.3	70.7	67.1
High	4.4	6.7	4.2
Total	**100.0**	**100.0**	**100.0**

*The number of black mothers was as follows: all, 926 118; foreign born, 61 900; and native born, 864 218. The number of white mothers was as follows: all, 4 401 338; foreign born, 286 229; and native born, 115 109.

Black foreign-born women had a 36% lower incidence of low-birth-weight infants and a 32% lower incidence of very-low-birth-weight infants than black native-born women (Table 3). Among white women, the differences in the incidence of low-birth-weight infants by nativity status were smaller and in the opposite direction. The incidence of very-low-birth-weight infants was 11% higher among the foreign- than the native-born women (Table 3).

Black foreign-born mothers also had 28% lower infant mortality rates than the black native-born mothers; 12.4 vs 17.3 deaths per 1000 live births (Table 4). The nativity difference was larger for postneonatal than for neonatal mortality, ie, 37% vs 23%. Among white mothers, however, there was virtually no difference in infant mortality by nativity status, ie, 8.1 vs 8.2 deaths per 1000 live births for foreign- and native-born mothers, respectively—the net result of 6% higher neonatal mortality and 10% lower postneonatal mortality among white foreign- than native-born mothers.

Differences in infant mortality rates by maternal risk categories were larger than differences by nativity status. Among blacks, the infant mortality rate for high-risk mothers was 84% higher than the rate for low-risk mothers, ie, 21.4 vs 11.6 per 1000 live births (Table 4). Among whites, the differences were even larger; the rate for high-risk mothers was 2.7 times the rate for low-risk mothers, ie, 15.4 vs 5.7 per 1000 live births. As a result, the black-white ratio decreased from 2.0 among low-risk mothers to 1.4 among high-risk mothers. For both black and white infants, differences between the low- and high-risk categories were much larger for postneonatal than for neonatal mortality. The postneonatal mortality rates for high-risk mothers, both black and white, were more than three times the rates for low-risk mothers (9.7 vs 3.1 for blacks and 6.5 vs 1.8 for whites). Although the black-white ratio in neonatal mortality was greater among low-risk (2.2) than high-risk (1.3) mothers, for postneonatal mortality, there was only a small difference in the ratios: 1.7 for low-risk vs 1.5 for high-risk mothers (Table 4).

Infant mortality rates for the variables that were included in the risk categorization are shown in Table 5.

Table 2.—Distribution of Live Births by Selected Maternal Characteristics According to Race and Nativity Status of Mother: United States, 1983 and 1984 Birth Cohorts

	Black		White	
	Foreign Born	Native Born	Foreign Born	Native Born
Total No. (%)	61 900 (100.0)	864 218 (100.0)	286 229 (100.0)	115 109 (100.0)
Age and parity				
Primaparas, y				
<18	2.1	9.4	2.1	3.2
18-19	3.6	7.8	3.9	5.2
20-29	21.1	14.0	21.7	23.5
≥30	5.1	1.4	5.2	4.2
Multiparas, y				
<18	0.4	2.6	0.6	0.5
18-19	2.0	6.5	2.2	2.4
20-29	39.1	44.2	39.0	41.3
≥30	26.8	14.0	25.4	19.6
Parity				
Primaparity	31.7	32.6	32.9	36.1
Low multiparity	40.9	36.6	43.5	45.0
High multiparity	27.3	30.7	23.6	18.8
Marital status				
Married	60.0	37.6	82.4	88.1
Not married	40.0	62.4	17.6	11.9
Educational attainment, y				
<12	30.9	34.2	32.9	17.5
12	37.1	42.9	35.3	43.9
13-15	19.0	16.5	16.6	20.6
≥16	13.1	6.3	15.2	18.1
Metropolitan residence status				
Metropolitan counties (250 000+ population)	93.0	62.5	78.1	42.9
All other counties	7.0	37.5	21.9	57.1
Mothers aged 20 y or older				
Total No. (%)	56 936 (100.0)	637 602 (100.0)	261 283 (100.0)	3 647 029 (100.0)
Educational attainment, y				
<12	28.7	23.3	29.4	12.0
12	37.0	47.0	36.1	44.9
13-15	20.0	21.2	17.8	22.8
≥16	14.2	8.6	16.6	20.4

Regression Analysis

Multiple logistic regression analysis was used to examine the effects of individual risk factors after adjusting for all the others. Previous regression results with the use of birth weight as the dependent variable (which did not include nativity status) showed that the effects of individual risk factors—education, marital status, age and parity—were generally stronger among whites than among blacks.[1] The results of multiple logistic regression on birth weight, which included residence and nativity status, were similar (detail not included here). Nativity status was the only factor that had stronger effects among blacks. Black foreign-born women were 36% less likely than black native-born women to have a low-birth-weight baby, whereas the risk of a white foreign-born woman having a low-birth-weight infant was only 10% less than for a white native-born woman (Table 6). Among black mothers, the risk of having a very-low-birth-weight baby was 31% lower for the foreign-born mothers than for the native-born mothers, while among white mothers, there was no difference by nativity status in the risk of having a very-low-birth-weight infant (Table 6).

Similarly, the effects of nativity status on infant mortality were considerably larger for blacks than for whites. The risk of an infant death was 23% lower among the black foreign-born mothers and 8% lower among the white foreign-born mothers as among the native-born mothers. Black foreign-born mothers had 22% lower neonatal and 24% lower postneonatal mortality than their native-born counterparts. Among white mothers, the likelihood of a neonatal death was equal among the foreign- and native-born women, while the risk of a postneonatal death was 20% lower among the foreign-born women (Table 6).

The effects of the other maternal risk factors—education, age, parity, and marital status—on neonatal and postneonatal mortality, unlike those found in the previous

Table 3.—Low- and Very-Low-Birth-Weight Rates by Race and Nativity Status of Mother: United States, 1983 and 1984 Birth Cohorts

	Rate/1000 Live Births*			
	Black		White	
	Foreign Born	Native Born	Foreign Born	Native Born
Low birth weight	75.4	117.4	49.5	47.8
Very low birth weight	15.4	22.6	8.3	7.5

*With known birth weight.

Table 4.—Infant Mortality Rates by Maternal Nativity Status and by Maternal Risk According to Race and Age at Death: United States, 1983 and 1984 Birth Cohorts

	Rate/100 Live Births					
	Black			White		
	Infant	Neonatal	Postneonatal	Infant	Neonatal	Postneonatal
All infants	17.0	10.6	6.3	8.2	5.2	3.0
Maternal nativity status						
Foreign born	12.4	8.3	4.1	8.1	5.5	2.7
Native born	17.3	10.8	6.5	8.2	5.2	3.0
Maternal risk						
Low	11.6	8.4	3.1	5.7	3.9	1.8
Moderate	16.3	10.6	5.7	8.8	5.5	3.3
High	21.4	11.7	9.7	15.4	8.9	6.5

birth weight analysis,[1] were not consistently greater among whites than blacks (Table 7). In particular, controlling for all other factors, the effects of education on postneonatal mortality were similar for whites and blacks: mothers with less than 12 years of education were twice as likely as those with 16 or more years to have a postneonatal death. The neonatal mortality risk ratios between the lowest and highest educational levels were smaller: 1.4 for whites vs 1.1 for blacks.

Age and parity effects on neonatal and postneonatal mortality were not consistent among whites and blacks. Standardized neonatal mortality rates were high among white and black multiparous teenagers younger than 18 years and primiparas aged 30 years or older. White primiparas younger than 18 years and multiparas aged 18 and 19 years also had high rates. Excess risks among teenagers (relative to 20- to 29-year-old multiparas) were greater among whites than blacks. On the other hand, excess risk was greater for black than white primiparas aged 30 years or older.

Standardized postneonatal mortality rates were highest for multiparous teenagers in both race groups, with excess risk greater for whites than blacks. Furthermore, in contrast to neonatal mortality, both white and black primiparous mothers aged 30 years or older had among the lowest standardized postneonatal mortality rates. It is of interest to note that primiparous teenagers aged 18 and 19 years had the lowest standardized neonatal and postneonatal rates among blacks.

High parity generally showed similar effects on neonatal and postneonatal mortality for whites and blacks (relative risk [RR] range, 1.3 to 1.4). The effects of marital status on neonatal and postneonatal mortality were slightly larger

Table 5.—Infant Mortality Rates by Race and Other Maternal Factors: United States, 1983 and 1984 Birth Cohorts

	Rate/1000 Live Births					
	Black			White		
	Infant	Neonatal	Postneonatal	Infant	Neonatal	Postneonatal
Total	17.0	10.6	6.3	8.2	5.2	3.0
Age and parity						
Primaparas, y						
<18	17.7	10.7	7.0	14.0	8.6	5.4
18-19	13.9	9.1	4.9	10.3	6.4	3.9
20-29	14.1	9.9	4.1	6.6	4.5	2.1
≥30	19.0	15.7	3.3	7.2	5.4	1.8
Multiparas, y						
<18	29.1	15.9	13.1	20.5	11.0	9.5
18-19	22.9	12.1	10.7	15.4	7.8	7.6
20-29	17.1	10.2	6.9	9.0	5.5	3.6
≥30	15.9	11.3	4.6	7.2	5.0	2.2
Parity						
Primiparity	15.3	10.2	5.0	7.9	5.2	2.6
Low multiparity	15.7	9.8	5.9	7.4	4.7	2.8
High multiparity	20.3	12.1	8.2	10.7	6.5	4.2
Marital status						
Married	14.0	9.4	4.6	7.5	4.9	2.7
Not married	18.9	11.4	7.4	13.0	7.8	5.2
Educational attainment, y						
<12	20.2	11.2	9.0	12.6	7.0	5.6
12	16.2	10.6	5.6	8.1	5.3	2.8
13-15	14.3	10.2	4.1	6.7	4.5	2.2
≥16	12.1	9.2	2.9	5.7	4.0	1.7
Metropolitan residence status						
Metropolitan counties (250 000+ population)	17.0	10.7	6.2	7.9	5.2	2.8
All other counties	16.9	10.4	6.5	8.4	5.3	3.2
Mothers aged 20 y or older						
Total	16.3	10.5	5.8	7.6	4.9	2.7
Educational attainment, y						
<12	20.1	10.9	9.1	11.6	6.4	5.2
12	16.1	10.7	5.4	7.8	5.1	2.6
13-15	14.2	10.1	4.1	6.7	4.5	2.2
≥16	12.1	9.2	2.9	5.7	4.0	1.7

Table 6.—Adjusted Odds Ratios Among Foreign-born Mothers for Birth Weight and Infant Mortality: United States, 1983 and 1984 Birth Cohorts*

	Black			White		
		95% CI			95% CI	
	Odds Ratio†	Lower	Upper	Odds Ratio†	Lower	Upper
Low birth weight	0.64	0.62	0.66	0.90	0.89	0.92
Very low birth weight	0.69	0.65	0.74	0.99	0.95	1.03
Infant mortality	0.77	0.72	0.83	0.92	0.88	0.96
Neonatal mortality	0.78	0.71	0.86	0.99	0.94	1.05
Postneonatal mortality	0.76	0.67	0.86	0.80	0.74	0.86

*CI indicates confidence interval.

†Odds ratios are for foreign-born mothers; reference group is native-born mothers. Variables included in the adjustment are age, parity, education, marital status, and metropolitan status.

for white than for black mothers (RR range, 1.4 vs 1.2 to 1.3). There were no differences by metropolitan residence in the risk of neonatal death. However, whites outside the large metropolitan areas had a somewhat greater risk of a postneonatal death (RR, 1.1).

COMMENT

In this analysis, the 1983 and 1984 national linked files of births and infant deaths were used to examine the differentials in infant mortality by race, nativity status, and other maternal characteristics. Black foreign-born mothers had 23% lower neonatal and 37% lower postneonatal mortality rates than their native-born counterparts. After adjustment for age, parity, education, marital status, and residence, the differential remained about the same for neonatal mortality but was reduced to 24% for postneonatal mortality. Among white women, the foreign-born mothers had 6% higher neonatal mortality and 10% lower postneonatal mortality rates. After adjustment for other risk factors, white foreign-born women had a 20% lower risk for postneonatal mortality, but similar risks for neonatal mortality compared with that for white native-born women.

The low risk of postneonatal death for both white and black foreign-born women raises the possibility of underreporting. It is possible, for example, that foreign-born mothers with sick infants return to their countries of origin before the infant's death. It is difficult to investigate this possibility, but it does not seem entirely plausible. Although access to preventive care may be problematic, treatment of life-threatening illness is probably as readily available in the United States as in most countries from which the foreign-born mothers have migrated.

Data from the 1983 Current Population Survey show that the black foreign-born population was of a higher socioeconomic status than the black native-born population, but that the reverse was true for the white population.[8] Median annual earnings were 22% higher for the black foreign-born mothers than for the black native-born mothers; family incomes of more than $35 000 were reported more by black foreign-born mothers than by black native-born mothers (30% vs 17%) Consistent with what the birth certificate data showed, there were proportionately more foreign-born mothers than native-born mothers who attained the higher levels of education. Among the white population, the differences were somewhat smaller and were in the opposite direction.

Table 7.—Standardized Infant Mortality Rates by Race and Other Maternal Factors: United States, 1983 and 1984 Birth Cohorts*

	Rate/1000 Live Births					
	Black			White		
	Infant	Neonatal	Postneonatal	Infant	Neonatal	Postneonatal
Nativity status						
Foreign born	12.7	8.6	4.1	7.7	5.1	2.6
Native born	16.4	11.0	5.4	8.4	5.1	3.3
Age and parity						
Primaparas, y						
<18	15.9	11.1	4.8	10.4	6.8	3.6
18-19	13.6	9.4	4.2	9.3	5.7	3.6
20-29	15.6	11.1	4.6	7.5	4.8	2.7
≥30	23.4	19.1	4.3	9.0	6.3	2.7
Multiparas, y						
<18	24.6	16.0	8.7	15.1	8.7	6.4
18-19	19.5	11.8	7.7	12.2	6.5	5.8
20-29	15.9	10.2	5.7	8.2	4.8	3.5
≥30	16.1	11.8	4.3	7.7	5.0	2.7
Parity						
Low	15.2	10.3	4.9	7.8	4.8	3.0
High	19.6	12.9	6.7	10.5	6.4	4.1
Marital status						
Married	15.2	10.3	4.9	7.8	4.8	3.0
Not married	19.1	12.5	6.5	10.8	6.6	4.2
Educational attainment, y						
<12	17.4	9.9	7.5	10.9	6.0	4.9
12	15.6	10.3	5.3	8.6	5.5	3.0
13-15	14.4	10.1	4.3	7.5	4.9	2.6
≥16	12.9	9.3	3.7	6.6	4.3	2.2
Metropolitan residence status						
Metropolitan counties (250 000+ population)	16.1	11.0	5.1	8.3	5.1	3.1
All other counties	15.9	10.7	5.2	8.5	5.2	3.3

*Rates are directly standardized by using the distribution of all live births and the fitted values from multiple logistic regression analyses of neonatal and postneonatal mortality.

Behavioral, cultural, and nutritional factors that might account for the lower infant mortality among the black foreign-born mothers are difficult to ascertain. One study of women receiving prenatal care in Boston (Mass) City Hospital[5] showed that the black foreign-born women were less likely than the black native-born women to smoke cigarettes or to abuse drugs. Unfortunately, there are no national data available to determine whether smoking prevalence differs by nativity and race. It is known, however, that smoking rates in the Caribbean countries (where most black foreign-born women are from) are relatively low compared with that in the United States.[9] Assuming that this positive health practice continues after the women migrate to the United States, reduced smoking could explain some portion of the differences by nativity in infant mortality and low birth weight.

The study of migrant populations is difficult because their health status could introduce opposing types of bias. First, the fact that they left their country of origin suggests that migrants may be healthier (both physically and mentally) than those remaining in their country or even their counterparts in the country to which they migrate. On the other hand, the stresses of migration itself are not inconsequential and may adversely affect the migrant population's health.[10] In any case, it is of interest to note that black foreign-born women in this country are not generally recent immigrants. Based on our analysis of 1980 census data, about 60% of the black foreign-born women aged 15 to 24 years and 70% of those aged 25 to 34 years lived in the United States for more than 5 years.[11] Further study of the black foreign-born population could yield valuable clues for prevention strategies.

With respect to the other risk factors examined, there are several points that are worth noting. In particular, black primiparas aged 18 and 19 years had the lowest infant mortality rates of all the age-parity groups for black mothers. Even black primiparas younger than 18 years did not have unusually high rates. It is the multiparous teenagers, both black and white, who have the highest rates, but they account for only a small proportion (9% of black and 3% of white) of births. Thus, although teenage childbearing represents a serious social problem, it does not account for the twofold black-white differential in infant mortality. If all teenage births are excluded, the black infant mortality rate would decline by 4%, while the white infant mortality rate would decline by 7%, thereby slightly increasing the black-white ratio.

Combining the several categories of risk factors into three broad maternal risk groups, there was a near-doubling of black and near-tripling of white infant mortality rates between the low and high levels of maternal risk. If the infant mortality rate in the low-risk groups could be achieved by the moderate- and high-risk groups, there would be a 30% reduction in infant deaths within each race. Since the black infant mortality rate is twice the white rate and foreign-born black mothers have much lower rates than native-born black mothers, it is likely that further improvement is possible among blacks.

One of the important differences among these maternal risk groups is their access to preventive health care during the prenatal and infant period. Data from birth certificates show that 91% of the low-risk white women and 82% of the low-risk black women began prenatal care in the first trimester compared with 47% and 44% among the high-risk white and black women, respectively. Data on health care utilization during infancy also show large differentials by mother's education.[12] Interventions to reduce the disparities in infant mortality need to include improving access to care during these critical periods. Yet, the large social class differentials in infant mortality, even in countries with universal access to health care,[13-15] suggest that having access to services is not sufficient. Aggressive outreach and educational efforts are also needed to prevent infant deaths in disadvantaged groups.

References

1. Kleinman JC, Kessel SS. Racial differences in low birth weight. *N Engl J Med.* 1987;317:749-753.
2. Valanis BM, Rush D. A partial explanation of superior birth weights among foreign-born women. *Soc Biol.* 1979;26:198-210.
3. Valanis BM. Relative contributions of maternal social and biological characteristics to birth weight and gestation among mothers of different childhood socioeconomic status. *Soc Biol.* 1979;26:211-225.
4. Kessner DM. *Infant Deaths: An Analysis by Maternal Risk and Health Care.* Washington, DC: National Academy of Sciences; 1973.
5. Cabral H, Fried LE, Levenson S, Amaro H, Zuckerman B. Foreign-born and US-born black women: differences in health behaviors and birth outcomes. *Am J Public Health.* 1990;80:70-72.
6. Smedby B, Ericson A. Perinatal mortality among children of immigrant mothers in Sweden. *Acta Paediatr Scand Suppl.* 1979;275:41-46.
7. Dixon WJ, Brown MB, Engelman L, Hill MA, Jennrich RI. *BMDP Statistical Software.* Los Angeles, Calif: University of California Press; 1988:2.
8. Sehgal E. Foreign born in the U.S. labor market: the results of a special survey. *Mon Labor Rev.* July 1985;108:18-24.
9. Masironi R, Rothwell K. Tendances et effets du tabagisme dans le monde. *World Health Stat Q.* 1988;41:228-241.
10. MacMahon B, Pugh TF. *Epidemiology Principles and Methods.* Boston, Mass: Little Brown & Co Inc; 1970.
11. US Bureau of the Census. *Census of Population and Housing, 1980: Public-Use Microdata Sample (A Sample),* machine-readable data file, prepared by the Bureau of the Census. Washington, DC: US Government Printing Office; 1983.
12. Kessel SS. Postneonatal mortality: a performance indicator of the child health care system. *Pediatrics.* In press.
13. Rodrigues L, Botting B. Recent trends in postneonatal mortality in England. *OPSC (Office of Population, Censuses and Survey).* 1989;55:7-15.
14. Knudsen L, Kamper-Joegensen F. Influence of social factors on pregnancy outcome in Denmark. Presented at the annual meeting of the American Public Health Association; October 25, 1989; Chicago, Ill.
15. Bakketig L, Arntzen A, Magnus P. Socioeconomic differentials and perinatal and infant survival in Norway. Presented at the annual meeting of the American Public Health Association; October 25, 1989, Chicago, Ill.

Retinopathy of Prematurity in Infants With Cyanotic Congenital Heart Disease

Karla J. Johns, MD; James A. Johns, MD; Stephen S. Feman, MD; Debra A. Dodd, MD

• We undertook a study of premature infants with cyanotic congenital heart disease to determine whether these infants develop retinopathy of prematurity despite a persistent hypoxemic state. Using the computerized registry of the neonatal intensive care unit of Vanderbilt University Medical Center, Nashville, Tenn, we identified six premature infants (<37 weeks' gestational age, with birth weights of 1100 to 2050 g) with cyanotic congenital heart disease who survived the neonatal period and underwent ophthalmologic evaluation. Review of their charts revealed that three of six infants developed retinopathy of prematurity (two had grade 1 and one had grade 3 disease), but none required treatment. Our data support the findings of other investigators that elevated arterial oxygen tension is not the sole factor leading to the development of retinopathy of prematurity. Premature infants with cyanotic congenital heart disease can develop retinopathy of prematurity despite persistent hypoxemia. Cyanotic premature infants should be screened for retinopathy of prematurity with the same thoroughness as other premature infants.

(*AJDC.* 1991;145:200–203)

Retinopathy of prematurity (ROP) remains a common cause of blindness and serious visual impairment in premature infants.[1] The etiology of ROP appears to be multifactorial, and investigators have identified such diverse risk factors as sepsis, gestational age, apnea, ambient light levels, reduced vitamin E levels, and xanthine administration.[2-8] The role of oxygen in the etiology of this disease remains controversial. Since the 1942-1954 epidemic of ROP, a relationship has been assumed between arterial oxygen tension and this disorder, but the nature of this relationship has been difficult to confirm in prospective clinical studies. Premature infants with cyanotic congenital heart disease (CCHD) are unable to develop elevated arterial oxygen tensions despite supplemental oxygen. For this reason, the risk of ROP in premature infants with CCHD has been thought to be very low, and only two isolated cases have been reported.[9,10]

The combination of CCHD and prematurity is uncommon, and the number of patients available for study is further reduced by the fact that many premature infants with CCHD do not survive. The objective of this study was to identify premature infants with CCHD who have been cared for in the neonatal intensive care unit of Vanderbilt University Medical Center, Nashville, Tenn, and to determine the incidence of ROP in these patients.

PATIENTS AND METHODS

The computerized registry of the neonatal intensive care unit at Vanderbilt University Medical Center was used to identify premature infants under 37 weeks' gestational age.[11] A total of 6401 premature infants were admitted to the neonatal intensive care unit over a 15-year period from January 1, 1974, through December 31, 1988. Of this population, 86 infants were identified as having congenital heart defects (other than patent ductus arteriosus). Of the 86 premature infants identified with congenital heart disease, 64 were acyanotic and 22 were cyanotic. Five of these cyanotic infants died in the early postnatal period. Seventeen infants survived the early neonatal period, and, of these, 11 had such a high birth weight (>2000 g) that ophthalmologic consultation was not requested. In one case, ophthalmologic consultation was requested in a patient with a birth weight of 2050 g. Although 2050 g is greater than the usual birth-weight criterion at our institution (2000 g), the neonatologist thought ophthalmologic evaluation was indicated because of the large amount of supplemental oxygen this infant required.

Six infants underwent complete ophthalmologic evaluation between the sixth and ninth weeks of life by a retinal specialist (S.S.F.) trained in the recognition of ROP. In patients found to have any features consistent with ROP or incomplete retinal vascular development, serial examinations were performed every 2 to 3 weeks. Because many of these infants were critically ill and required cardiac surgery, the exact timing of the examination was dependent on the cardiovascular stability of the infants. The medical records of these six patients were reviewed.

RESULTS

The clinical findings are summarized in the Table. The birth weights in our study group ranged from 1100 to 2050 g, with a mean of 1500 g. The gestational ages of the infants ranged from 26 to 34 weeks, with a mean of 30 weeks. There were four male and two female infants. Each of the infants had a cyanotic congenital heart lesion, resulting in a mean arterial oxygen tension lower than 55 mm Hg despite the administration of supplemental oxygen. All the infants required intubation and mechanical ventilation. All six infants underwent a palliative procedure,

Accepted for publication October 2, 1990.

From the Department of Ophthalmology (Drs K. J. Johns and Feman) and the Division of Pediatric Cardiology (Drs J. A. Johns and Dodd), Vanderbilt University Medical Center, Nashville, Tenn.

Presented in part at the Annual Meeting of the Association for Research in Vision and Ophthalmology, Sarasota, Florida, May 3, 1989, and at the Third World Congress of Pediatric Cardiology, Bangkok, Thailand, November 30, 1989.

Reprint requests to D-5217 Vanderbilt Medical Center North, Nashville, TN 37232-2540 (Dr K. J. Johns).

Clinical Findings in Infants With Cyanotic Congenital Heart Disease With and Without ROP*

Patient No./Sex	Birth Weight, g	Gestational Age, wk	Cardiac Diagnosis	Cardiac Procedure	Duration of Oxygen Supplementation, d	Fraction of Inspired Oxygen, %	Po_2, mm Hg†	Pco_2, mm Hg†	pH†	No. of Blood Gas Determinations	Ophthalmologic Findings
1/M	1400	29	Transposition of the great arteries, ventricular septal defect	Ballon atrial septostomy at age 1 d	33	30 to 100	46±12	37±10	7.41±0.08	57	No ROP; examinations at 8 and 11 wk
2/M	1100	26	Transposition of the great arteries	Atrial septectomy at age 3 wk	42	24 to 100	45±14	39±10	7.39±0.08	164	No ROP; examinations at 8 and 12 wk
3/F	1400	34	Tricuspid atresia, ventricular septal defect	Aorta to pulmonary artery shunt at age 2 wk	35	30 to 100	38±12	37±10	7.41±0.09	59	No ROP; examinations at 6 and 12 wk
4/M	1400	30	Transposition of the great arteries, ventricular septal defect	Ballon atrial septostomy at age 8 wk	40	30 to 100	38±12	44±22	7.38±0.13	172	Stage 1 ROP at 7 wk, resolved at 9 wk
5/M	2050	33	Tricuspid atresia, ventricular septal defect	Aorta to pulmonary artery shunt at age 1 mo	31	30 to 100	49±12	44±9	7.35±0.08	42	Stage 1 ROP at 6 wk, resolved at 8 wk
6/F	1650	28	Transposition of the great arteries, coarctation of the aorta	Repair of coarctation of the aorta and placement of pulmonary artery band at age 1 wk	42	25 to 100	55±29	44±10	7.36±0.06	109	Stage 3 ROP at 8 wk, patient died before another examination could be performed

*ROP indicates retinopathy of prematurity.
†Values are mean ± SD.

either surgical or with interventional catheterization, intended to improve oxygenation and/or congestive heart failure. Following these palliative procedures, arteriovenous mixing persisted and the infants remained hypoxemic. None of the infants had sustained hyperoxia, which we defined as arterial oxygen tension greater than 100 mm Hg.

Of the six patients in the study group, four had transposition of the great arteries with or without ventricular septal defects and two had tricuspid atresia.

Three patients developed ROP and three did not. In each group there were two infants with transposition and one with tricuspid atresia, and in each group there were two male and one female infants. Birth weights of the patients who developed ROP were 1400, 1650, and 2050 g; birth weights of the patients who did not develop ROP were 1100, 1400, and 1400 g.

During the initial evaluation of the three patients who did not develop ROP, incomplete retinal vascular development was found, and the patients were examined serially until each reached vascular maturity. Three patients did develop ROP. Patient 4 was noted, 7 weeks after birth, to have arteriovenous anastamoses posterior to the ora serrata and a demarcation line in both eyes, placing the retinopathy at stage 1 by the international classification of ROP.[12] When the patient was reexamined at age 9 weeks, the ROP had resolved and the retinal vasculature had reached maturity. Patient 5 was found to have a demarcation line in zone 3 of each eye at age 6 weeks, consistent with stage 1 disease. When the patient was reexamined at 8 weeks, the demarcation line had resolved and the retinal vasculature had completed its development. Patient 6 was first examined at 8 weeks of age. She was found to have peripheral arteriovenous anastamoses in the right eye. In the left eye there were arteriovenous anastamoses and neovascular tufts in the superotemporal retina, classifying this as stage 3 retinopathy. The patient died before another examination could be performed. The eyes were not available for postmortem examination.

The mean arterial oxygen tension of the study patients ranged from 38 to 54 mm Hg (Figure). The infants who developed ROP had mean arterial oxygen tensions similar to those of infants who did not develop ROP (47.2 vs 43.1 mm Hg). The duration of supplemental oxygen administration varied from 30 to 50 days, with the fraction of inspired oxygen ranging from 100% oxygen to room air in all patients. The mean duration of oxygen administration was 38±6 days in infants who developed ROP and 37±5 days in infants who did not develop ROP. The mean arterial P_{CO_2} of the study patients ranged from 36 to 44 mm Hg. The mean arterial carbon dioxide levels of the infants who developed ROP and those who did not were similar (43.2±2.3 vs 37.7±1.4 mm Hg). Mean pH values of these patients ranged from 7.35 to 7.41. The mean pH values were similar for infants who did and did not develop ROP (7.36±0.02 vs 7.40±0.02).

All patients received supplemental vitamin E therapy. All patients underwent transfusions as needed to maintain a hematocrit of at least 0.40 to maximize oxygen delivery.

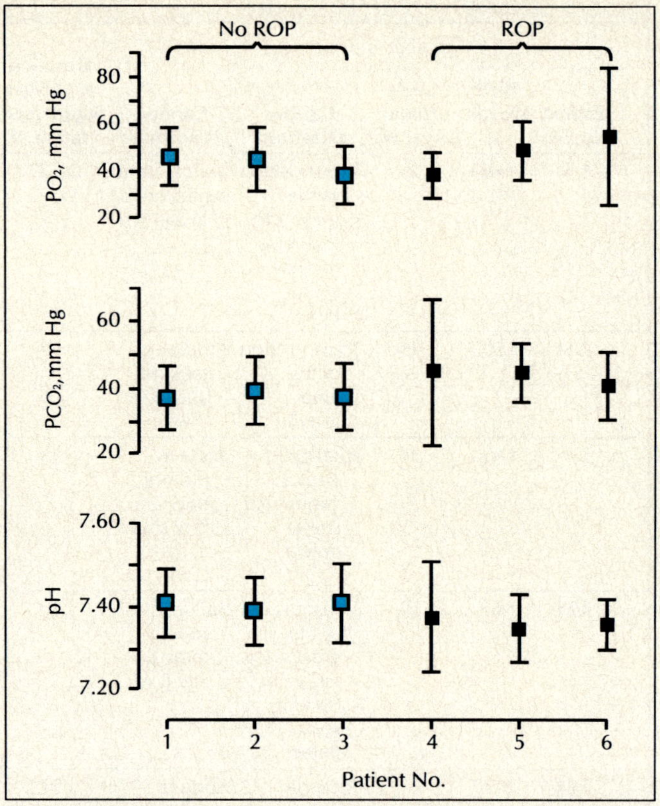

Mean arterial oxygen and carbon dioxide tensions and pH of six premature infants with cyanotic congenital heart disease with (patients 1 through 3) or without (patients 4 through 6) retinopathy of prematurity (ROP).

COMMENT

Since Terry[13] initially described the cicatricial stages of ROP (formerly known as retrolental fibroplasia) in 1942, there have been extensive efforts to identify the agent or agents responsible for this blinding process. Since the middle 1950s, the administration of oxygen has been implicated as one potential causative factor in the development of ROP.[2,14,15] The incidence of ROP has been found to correlate more closely with the duration of oxygen administration than with the concentration of inspired oxygen.[16]

In the Cooperative Study of Retrolental Fibroplasia and the Use of Oxygen, Kinsey and coworkers[16,17] found that the incidence of ROP increased with duration of exposure to oxygen. In that prospective multicenter clinical trial, premature infants with birth weights under 1500 g were assigned to receive either "routine oxygen" therapy, 28 days of supplemental oxygen with fractions of inspired oxygen exceeding 50%, or "curtailed oxygen" therapy, supplemental oxygen with fractions of inspired oxygen below 50%, administered only as needed to relieve anoxia. The incidence of ROP was significantly greater in the routine oxygen group. Although arterial oxygen tension measurement techniques were not in use at the time the study was conducted, it is reasonable to assume that the infants in the routine oxygen group had elevated arterial oxygen tensions. Thus, a relationship has been presumed between elevated arterial oxygen and the incidence of ROP.

Since the advent of routine clinical arterial oxygen tension measurement, there have been attempts to correlate arterial oxygen levels and the development of ROP, but the results have been contradictory. In a case-control study of 14 very-low-birth-weight infants (<1500 g), Yu and coworkers[18] found that the development of ROP was not related to arterial oxygen tension by intermittent sampling. In contrast, Shahinian and Malachowski[19] reported a correlation between the severity of ROP and duration of elevated capillary oxygen tension after the first week of life. In a prospective study, Prendiville and Schulenburg[20] noted that episodes of hyperoxia were significantly associated with the development of ROP.

The role of oxygen in the development of ROP has also been studied in animal models. Patz et al and[21] Ashton et al[22,23] have characterized the response of the retinal blood vessels of the immature retina in a kitten model of ROP. In a hyperoxic environment, the immature retinal blood vessels of the kitten undergo profound constriction and vaso-obliteration. When the experimental animal is then returned to room air, a secondary response of vasoproliferation and neovascularization occurs. This process has been considered analagous to the early stages of ROP. However, the cicatricial, advanced stages of ROP are not seen in this experimental model. Gole et al[24] and other investigators have noted important differences between the kitten model of oxygen-induced retinopathy and human ROP. Flower,[25] studying a beagle puppy model of ROP, produced cicatricial ROP when the animals were pretreated with a prostaglandin-synthetase inhibitor, which blocked the constriction of blood vessels caused by hyperoxia.

Oxygen exposure and hyperoxia have been considered important antecedents to the development of ROP. The occasional reports of this disease in premature and full-term infants who have not received supplemental oxygen[26-28] and in infants with CCHD[9,10] have been difficult to reconcile with these concepts.

The fetus with a cyanotic congenital heart lesion has a normal arterial oxygen level because the placenta, rather than the lungs, supplies oxygenated blood. Shortly after birth, however, the nascent functioning of the lungs combined with the closure of the ductus arteriosis and the foramen ovale completes the transformation to the postnatal circulation. At this time the infant with a cyanotic congenital heart lesion develops cyanosis.

In infants with CCHD, the blood flowing out through the aorta to the body is a mixture of deoxygenated blood from the systemic venous return and oxygenated blood from the pulmonary venous return. When these infants are given supplemental oxygen, the oxygen tension in the blood returning from the lungs may be increased, but, because of the mixing with desaturated blood, the aortic oxygen tension rises only slightly. For the arterial Po_2 to rise above 100 mm Hg, the hemoglobin must be more than 96% saturated with oxygen. Admixture with even a small amont of desaturated blood precludes arterial oxygen tensions over 100 mm Hg. Thus, in infants with CCHD, despite oxygen supplementation, the arterial oxygen tension remains lower than normal. In contrast, in infants with normal hearts, the systemic blood flow consists solely of blood returning from the lungs, and supplemental oxygen can raise the arterial oxygen concentrations well above normal.

There is some evidence that episodes of hypoxemia may be a risk factor for the development of ROP. Katzman and colleagues[29] compared a group of patients who had severe ROP with a group of patients who had less severe ROP and found that the patients with the more severe disease had a significantly higher number of hours with a Po_2 below 50 mm Hg. Flynn and coworkers[28] reported that retinal arteriolar constriction was more commonly found in hypoxic premature infants than in hyperoxic infants. Shohat and coworkers,[3] in a retrospective multivariant analysis, identified an association between the number of episodes of hypoxemia and the development of ROP in infants weighing less than 1250 g.[3] However, an association between hypoxia and ROP has not been demonstrated in all clinical studies.

Episodes of both hypercarbia and hypocarbia were found by Shohat and coworkers[3] to be associated with the development of ROP. Hypercarbia was also noted to be a risk factor for the development of ROP in a retrospective multivariate analysis by Bauer and Widmayer.[30] However, in a subsequent study, Brown and coworkers[31] found that Pco_2 was not a risk factor. Acidosis was also identified as a risk factor by Prendiville and Schulenburg.[20]

Premature infants with CCHD present a unique opportunity to study the possibility that hyperoxia is only one of a complex array of factors that lead to the development of ROP. The anatomic cardiac abnormalities in these infants preclude prolonged episodes of hyperoxia, despite supplemental oxygen administration and mechanical ventilation. The infants in our study population were persistently hypoxemic, but in general they had normal arterial carbon dioxide levels and pH values. Despite prolonged hypoxemia, three of six infants developed ROP. We speculate that hypoxemia alone, identified as a risk factor for the development of ROP by Katzman et al[29] and Shohat et al,[3] may have contributed to the development of ROP in these cyanotic infants.

The persistent hypoxemia of CCHD does not appear to protect an infant from the development of ROP. Premature infants with CCHD should be monitored for the development of ROP just as are premature infants with normal hearts. Our data support the finding of other investigators that arterial oxygen tension is not the sole factor leading to the development of ROP.

This study was supported in part by an unrestricted grant from Research to Prevent Blindness Inc, New York, NY.

We thank Robert Cotton, MD, and Susan Bigham for their assistance.

References

1. Phelps DL. Vision loss due to retinopathy of prematurity. *Lancet.* 1981;1:606.
2. Ben-Sira I, Nissenkorn I, Kremer I. Retinopathy of prematurity. *Surv Ophthalmol.* 1988;33:1-16.
3. Shohat M, Reisner SH, Krikler R, Nissenkorn I, Yassyur Y, Ben-Sira I. Retinopathy of prematurity: incidence and risk factors. *Pediatrics.* 1983;72:159-163.
4. Gunn TR, Easdown J, Outerbridge EW, Aranda JV. Risk factors in retrolental fibroplasia. *Pediatrics.* 1980;65:1096-1100.
5. Purohit DM, Ellison C, Zierler S, Miettinen OS, Nadas AS. Risk factors for retrolental fibroplasia: experience with 3025 premature infants. *Pediatrics.* 1985;76:339-344.
6. Hammer ME, Mullen PW, Ferguson JG, Pai S, Cosby C, Jackson KL. Logistic analysis of risk factors in acute retinopathy of prematurity. *Am J Ophthalmol.* 1986;102:1-6.
7. Lucey JF, Dangman B. A reexamination of the role of oxygen in retrolental fibroplasia. *Pediatrics.* 1984;73:82-96.
8. Biglan AW, Cheng KP, Brown DR. Update on retinopathy of prematurity. *Int Ophthalmol Clin.* 1989;29:2-9.
9. Naiman J, Green WR, Patz R. Retrolental fibroplasia in hypoxic newborn. *Am J Ophthalmol.* 1979;88:55-58.
10. Kalina RE, Hodson A, Morgan BC. Retrolental fibroplasia in a cyanotic infant. *Pediatrics.* 1972;50:765-768.
11. Lindstrom D, Cotton R. Use of computers in the newborn intensive care unit. *Clin Perinatol.* 1983;10:195-203.
12. Committee for the Classification of Retinopathy of Prematurity. An international classification of retinopathy of prematurity. *Arch Ophthalmol.* 1984;102:1130-1134.
13. Terry TL. Extreme prematurity and fibroblastic overgrowth of persistent vascular sheath behind each crystalline lens. *Am J Ophthalmol.* 1942;25:203-204.
14. Lanman JT, Guy LP, Dancis J. Retrolental fibroplasia and oxygen therapy. *JAMA.* 1954;155:223-225.
15. Patz A, Hoeck LE, DeLaCruz E. Studies on the effect of high oxygen administration in retrolental fibroplasia, I: nursery observations. *Am J Ophthalmol.* 1952;35:1248-1252.
16. Kinsey VE, Arnold HJ, Kalina RE, et al. PaO_2 levels and retrolental fibroplasia: a report of the cooperative study. *Pediatrics.* 1977;60:655-668.
17. Kinsey VE. Retrolental fibroplasia. *Arch Ophthalmol.* 1956;56:481-529.
18. Yu VYH, Hookham DM, Nave JRM. Retrolental fibroplasia-controlled study of 4 years' experience in a neonatal intensive care unit. *Arch Dis Child.* 1982;57:247-252.
19. Shahinian L, Malachowski N. Retrolental fibroplasia. *Arch Ophthalmol.* 1978;96:70-74.
20. Prendiville A, Schulenburg WE. Clinical factors associated with retinopathy of prematurity. *Arch Dis Child.* 1988;63:522-527.
21. Patz A, Eastham A, Higgenbottom DH, Kleh T. Oxygen studies in retrolental fibroplasia in experimental animals. *Am J Ophthalmol.* 1953;36:1511-1522.
22. Ashton N, Ward B, Serpell G. Role of oxygen in the genesis of retrolental fibroplasia: a preliminary report. *Am J Ophthalmol.* 1953;37:513-520.
23. Ashton N, Cook C. Direct observation of the effect of oxygen on developing vessels: preliminary report. *Am J Ophthalmol.* 1954;38:433-440.
24. Gole GA, Gannon BJ, Goodyer AM. Oxygen induced retinopathy: the kitten model reexamined. *Aust J Ophthalmol.* 1982;10:223-232.
25. Flower RW. Physiology of the developing ocular vasculature. *Birth Defects.* 1988;24:129-146.
26. Schulman J, Jampol LM, Schwartz H. Peripheral proliferative retinopathy without oxygen therapy in a full-term infant. *Am J Ophthalmol* 1980;90:509-514.
27. Harper RG, Sia CG. Retrolental fibroplasia in a full-term infant. *Am J Ophthalmol.* 1975;80:106-108.
28. Flynn JT, Cassady J, Essner D, et al. Fluorescein angiography in retrolental fibroplasia: experience from 1969-1977. *Trans Am J Ophthalmol Otolaryngol.* 1979;86:1700-1723.
29. Katzman G, Satish M, Krishnan V, Marcus D, Bovino J. Comparative analysis of lower and higher stage retrolental fibroplasia (RLF). *Pediatr Res.* 1982;16(suppl 2):294A.
30. Bauer CR, Widmayer SM. A relationship between $PaCO_2$ and retrolental fibroplasia (RLF). *Pediatr Res.* 1981;15:649.
31. Brown DR, Milley JR, Ripepi UJ, Biglan AW. Retinopathy of prematurity. Risk factors in a 5-year cohort of critically ill premature neonates. *AJDC.* 1987;141:154-160.

Unsuspected Cocaine Exposure in Young Children

Sigmund J. Kharasch, MD; Deborah Glotzer, MD; Robert Vinci, MD; Michael Weitzman, MD; James Sargent, MD

• ***Objective:*** **To determine the prevalence of cocaine exposure among preschool children with clinically unsuspected signs and/or symptoms.**
Design: **Prevalence study.**
Setting: **Pediatric emergency department in an inner-city hospital.**
Participants: **250 children aged 2 weeks to 5 years who underwent urine assays for cocaine prior to discharge from the emergency department.**
Interventions: **None.**
Measurements/Main Results: **Six (2.4%) of the 250 urine assays (95% confidence interval, 0.5% to 4.3%) were positive for benzoylecgonine, the major urinary cocaine metabolite. Four of the positive urine assays were from children younger than 1 year and all children with positive urine assays were younger than 24 months. None of these children presented with a complaint or was identified as having clinical problems currently associated with childhood exposure to cocaine. Possible exposure routes include breast-feeding, intentional administration, accidental ingestion of cocaine or cocaine-contaminated household dust via normal hand-to-mouth activity, and passive inhalation of "crack" vapors.**
Conclusion: **Among the inner-city children served by this hospital, significant numbers of infants and young children are being exposed to cocaine, and this exposure occurs in a clinically unsuspected population.**
(*AJDC.* 1991;145:204–206)

Cocaine use has increased dramatically during the past decade. While the medical complications of cocaine use have been frequently reported in the adult population, problems arising from cocaine exposure in young children have only recently been recognized. While many reports have focused on complications of prenatal exposure,[1-6] several recent reports have identified complications of exposure, including seizures,[7] arrhythmias,[8] and hypertension,[9] in infants and young children.

Data on the prevalence of cocaine exposure in the pediatric population are only now appearing. The National High School Senior Survey[10] in 1987 revealed a prevalence of cocaine use of 15% to 20%. In a recent retrospective review of clinically indicated serum and urine toxicologic screens of 1120 patients at a children's hospital, 52 patients (4.6%) had specimens that contained cocaine and/or cocaine metabolite.[11] Intrauterine exposure to cocaine is occurring with especially high frequency. Seventeen percent of pregnant women enrolled in prenatal care at Boston (Mass) City Hospital were found to have used cocaine at least once during pregnancy.[12]

In reports that describe clinical problems associated with cocaine exposure among young children, the routes of exposure include breast-feeding,[9] accidental ingestion,[8,13] and intentional administration.[7] Passive inhalation of crack vapors in children who are in close proximity to aerosolized cocaine has also been implicated as a possible exposure route.[14] While clinical cocaine toxicity may occur from environmental exposure, cases of asymptomatic children with positive cocaine screens have also been reported by the above routes.[11,15]

To our knowledge, no studies have systematically evaluated the prevalence of cocaine exposure in young children beyond the perinatal period. Given the high prevalence of cocaine use in adults at our hospital, we hypothesized that cocaine exposure may occur in significant numbers of young children and may occur in patients with clinically unsuspected signs and/or symptoms.

Accepted for publication September 4, 1990.

From the Department of Pediatrics, Boston (Mass) City Hospital, and Boston University School of Medicine.

Presented in part at the 30th Annual Meeting of the Ambulatory Pediatric Association, Anaheim, Calif, May 10, 1990.

Reprint requests to the Department of Pediatrics, Talbot 106, Boston City Hospital, 818 Harrison Ave, Boston, MA 02118 (Dr Kharasch).

PATIENTS AND METHODS

This study was conducted in the pediatric emergency department at Boston City Hospital during a 6-week period. Boston City Hospital is a 434-bed acute-care teaching hospital. There are approximately 24 000 annual visits to the pediatric emergency department, which provides service to patients aged 17 years or younger.

Parents and their children aged 2 weeks to 5 years who presented to the pediatric emergency department for care were eligible for this study. Children were excluded if they presented with any of the following: (1) acute life-threatening emergencies; (2) any history suggestive of cocaine exposure, ie, seizures, chest pain, or cocaine use by a caretaker; or (3) severe diaper rash precluding use of a urine bag. All eligible patients had the following data abstracted from their medical records: age, race, vital signs, insurer status, chief complaint, history of breast-feeding, and final diagnosis.

Parents were requested to participate in a study of children's exposure to environmental toxins, and anonymity was assured. If parents asked what environmental toxins were being investigated, they were informed that we were studying children's exposure to cocaine and antibiotics (antibiotics were being investigated as part of a concurrent emergency department study). Anonymity was ensured by a preassigned study number. Verbal consent was obtained for all children entered into the study. It was not possible to identify any child after the urine was assayed.

Characteristics of Patients With Positive Cocaine Screens					
		Vital Signs			
Patient No./Age, mo	Complaint	Temperature,°C	Pulse, Beats/Min	Respiratory Rate, Breaths/Min	Diagnosis
1/1	Cough	36.7	120	40	Pneumonia
2/4	Wheezing	37.9	120	32	Reactive airway disease
3/5	Social evaluation*	37.7	132	32	Otitis media
4/9	Fever	39.8	168	52	Bronchiolitis
5/22	Fever	39.3	160	36	Acute febrile illness
6/19	Trauma	37.6	140	36	Laceration

*Physical examination for placement by the Department of Social Services.

The study was approved by the Human Studies Committee of Boston City Hospital.

The urine samples were refrigerated overnight and transported to a commercial laboratory for analysis. All urine samples were screened within 24 hours by the enzyme-multiplied immunoassay technique for benzoylecgonine, the major metabolite of cocaine, in accordance with the quality assurance guidelines of the American College of Pathology.[16] All positive urine sample findings were confirmed by gas chromatography/mass spectrometry, thin-layer chromatography, or repeated enzyme-multipled immunoassay technique, depending on the quantity of urine obtained. The threshold for detection of benzoylecgonine in urine is 300 ng/mL.

We performed χ^2 analysis and Fisher's Exact Test to test the statistical significance of differences in response rates and rates of cocaine positivity by characteristics of the children.

RESULTS

Four hundred ninety-four patients were eligible for the study. The parents of 18 of these children refused participation. Of the 476 who agreed to participate, urine was obtained from 250 children (53%) prior to discharge from the emergency department. There were no significant differences between those children whose parents refused to participate and those who participated or between children who voided and those who did not with regard to race, gender, breast-feeding history, insurer status, or diagnosis (respiratory vs nonrespiratory illness). The mean age of the children from whom urine was obtained was 23 months (age range, 2 weeks to 5 years; 40% were younger than 1 year); 59% were male and 53% were black. Six (2.4%) of the 250 urine samples (95% confidence interval [CI], 0.5% to 4.3%) tested positive for benzoylecgonine (one result was reconfirmed by gas chromatography/mass spectrometry, one by thin-layer chromatography, and four by repeated enzyme-multiplied immunoassay technique). The characteristics of the patients with positive urine sample findings are shown in the Table. The cocaine-positive and cocaine-negative groups did not differ with regard to race, gender, breast-feeding history, insurer status, or diagnosis. Although rates of cocaine positivity did not differ significantly by age, the trend was for younger children to have higher rates of exposure (3.8% of children aged 2 weeks to 1 year; 4.4% of children aged 1 to 2 years; and no children aged 2 to 5 years). Of the children with positive urine assays, only one child, a 1-month-old boy, was currently being breast-fed.

COMMENT

In this study, 2.4% of infants and young children presenting to the pediatric emergency department of an urban, public hospital had laboratory evidence of cocaine exposure at the time of the visit. The observed rate of cocaine exposure in these young children was likely due, in large part, to the prevalence of cocaine use among their caretakers. A recent study documented that as many as one in five inner-city women seeking prenatal care at the same institution used cocaine during pregnancy.[12]

Although rates of cocaine positivity did not vary significantly by age, four of six children in this study with positive urine assays for cocaine were younger than 1 year and all were younger than 24 months. The lack of a significant association between cocaine positivity and children's age may well reflect sample size constraints. Younger children, being less mobile, may be at increased risk for exposure to parents smoking crack nearby or may be at increased risk for accidently ingesting cocaine or cocaine-contaminated household dust by virtue of normal hand-to-mouth activities of children of this age. It is also possible that cocaine was intentionally administered to some or all of these children. While these children did not have symptoms, younger children have less plasma cholinesterase to metabolize cocaine and are also at greater risk for cocaine toxicity at a given exposure level.[17] Passive inhalation has been suggested as the route of exposure in recent anecdotal reports,[14,15] and the aerosolized route of exposure is known to occur with other drugs, including marijuana and nicotine.[18-20]

Children with a history or clinical presentation suggestive of cocaine exposure were excluded from participation in this study so that the findings were limited to unsuspected exposures. None of the participants presented with currently recognized signs of cocaine exposure in children. It is possible, however, that infants and young children exposed to cocaine may suffer from subtle, less noticeable, or unrecognized problems, such as undetected cardiac dysrhythmias, altered gastrointestinal functioning, or neurobehavioral changes. In addition, these findings raise many critical unanswered questions regarding the possible long-term effects of repeated cocaine exposure on the physical, cognitive, and behavioral development of preschool children. Until the consequences of acute and chronic cocaine exposure are more completely understood, it is difficult to determine the implications for clinical practice and social policy of the unexpectedly high rates of exposure to cocaine found in this study.

Public debate, based at least in part on further research, must be directed toward explicating the social service implications of identifying an asymptomatic child with laboratory evidence of cocaine exposure. In Massachusetts, there are no uniform guidelines or practices for health and social service professionals to follow when confronted with documented cocaine exposure in an asymptomatic child. Further study on the physiologic and socioenvironmental effects of cocaine exposure in preschool children is needed to help direct rational and sound policy decisions on this issue.

Our findings suggest that significant numbers of infants and young children are being exposed to cocaine, and this exposure can occur in the absence of overt clinical signs. The clinical and public health implications of these findings, which are unknown at this time, are pressing topics in need of elucidation by subsequent surveillance and study.

This research was supported in part by Trustees of Health and Hospitals of the City of Boston Inc, BRSG 9057-09-00.

We thank the nursing staff of the Boston (Mass) City Hospital pediatric emergency department for their help in collecting urine samples and their continued efforts in our research projects. We also thank Howard Bauchner, MD, Marca Wilk, and Mary Grassley for their editorial assistance.

References

1. MacGregor SN, Keith LQ, Chasnoff IJ, et al. Cocaine use during pregnancy: adverse perinatal outcome. *Am J Obstet Gynecol.* 1987;157:686-690.

2. Zuckerman B, Frank DA, Hingson R, et al. Effects of maternal marijuana and cocaine use on fetal growth. *N Engl J Med.* 1989;320:762-768.

3. Chasnoff IJ, Burns WJ, Schnoll SH, Burns KA. Cocaine use in pregnancy. *N Engl J Med.* 1985;313:666-669.

4. Chasnoff IJ, Bussey ME, Savich R, Stack CM. Perinatal cerebral infarction and maternal cocaine use. *J Pediatr.* 1986;108:456-459.

5. Telsey AM, Merrit TA, Dixon SD. Cocaine exposure in a term neonate: necrotizing enterocolitis as a complication. *Clin Pediatr.* 1988;27:547-550.

6. Acker D, Sachs BJ, Tracey KJ, Wise WE. Abruptio placentae associated with cocaine use. *Am J Obstet Gynecol.* 1983;146:220-221.

7. Ernst AA, Sanders WM. Unexpected cocaine intoxication presenting as seizures in children. *Ann Emerg Med.* 1989;18:774-777.

8. Garland JS, Smith DS, Thomas B, Siker D. Accidental cocaine intoxication in a nine month old infant: presentation and treatment. *Pediatr Emerg Care.* 1989;5:245-247.

9. Chasnoff IJ, Lewis DE, Squires L. Cocaine intoxication in a breast fed infant. *Pediatrics.* 1987;80:836-838.

10. Johnston LD, O'Malley PM, Bachman JG. Illicit drug use, smoking, and drinking by America's high school students. *NIDA Res Monogr.* 1987;87:1535.

11. Shannon M, Lacouture PG, Roa J, Woolf A. Cocaine exposure among children seen at a pediatric hospital. *Pediatrics.* 1989;83:337-342.

12. Frank DA, Zuckerman BS, Amaro H, et al. Cocaine use during pregnancy: prevalence and correlates. *Pediatrics.* 1988;82:888-895.

13. Rivkin M, Gilmore H. Generalized seizures in an infant due to environmentally acquired cocaine. *Pediatrics.* 1989;84:1100-1102.

14. Bateman DA, Heagarty MC. Passive freebase cocaine ('crack') inhalation by infants and toddlers. *AJDC.* 1989;143:25-27.

15. Heideman SM, Goetting MG. Passive inhalation of cocaine by infants. *Pediatr Emerg Care.* 1989;5:283.

16. American Medical Association, Council on Scientific Affairs. Scientific issues in drug testing. *JAMA.* 1987;257:3110-3114.

17. Stewart OJ, Inaba T, Lucassen M. Cocaine metabolism: cocaine and norcocaine hydrolysis by liver and serum esterases. *Clin Pharmacol Ther.* 1979;25:464-468.

18. Morland J, Bugge A, Skuterud B, Steen A. Cannabinoids in blood and urine after passive inhalation of cannabis smoke. *J Forensic Sci.* 1985;30:997-1002.

19. Cone EJ, Johnson RE. Contact highs and urinary cannabinoid excretion after passive exposure to marijuana smoke. *Clin Pharmacol Ther.* 1986;40:247-256.

20. Greenberg RA, Bauman KE, Glover LH. Ecology of passive smoking by young infants. *J Pediatr.* 1989;114:774-780.

Radiological Case of the Month

Kathlene S. Waller, MD, Jennifer Johnson, MD (Contributors); *Beverly P. Wood, MD* (Section Editor)

A previously healthy 15-year-old white boy presented with a 4-week history of cough and fever. At admission, he had a productive cough with thick, yellow sputum; intermittent daily temperatures of 38.5°C; night sweats; malaise; anorexia; and weight loss of approximately 4.5 kg. At the onset of illness, three siblings had had sore throats, but he had no history of a sore throat, recent travel, or exposure to animals. He had been smoking one pack of cigarettes per day for 2 years. Three months before admission, he was diagnosed as having mild asthma, and intermittently used inhaled epinephrine. He reported exposure to a friend who was diagnosed with tuberculosis the previous year and was receiving antituberculosis medications.

Vital signs on admission to the hospital were as follows: temperature, 39.4°C; heart rate, 120 beats per minute; respiratory rate, 32/min; and blood pressure, 110/60 mm Hg. Physical examination revealed a pale, thin, ill-appearing male in moderate respiratory distress with anterior and posterior cervical adenopathy, but no other enlarged lymph nodes. Breath sounds were decreased and egophony was noted in the right upper and middle lobes. Expiratory wheezes were present bilaterally. There was no cyanosis or clubbing of the digits.

Chest roentgenograms were obtained (Figs 1 and 2). Initial laboratory results showed a white blood cell count of 25.9×10^9/L, with 0.73 segmented neutrophils, 0.08 band cells, 0.09 lymphocytes, 0.09 reactive lymphocytes, and 0.01 eosinophils. An arterial blood gas determination while the patient was breathing room air showed a pH of 7.49, Pco_2 of 34 mm Hg, and Po_2 of 52 mm Hg. A Gram's stain of sputum showed white blood cells; gram-positive cocci in pairs, chains, and clusters; and rare gram-negative bacilli. The original sputum culture yielded normal flora and moderate growth of β-hemolytic group C *Streptococcus*. No acid-fast bacilli were found. A purified protein derivative skin test using five tuberculin units was placed and was nonreactive in 48 hours. The mumps virus and *Candida* antigen were placed as controls and were also nonreactive. Antibiotic therapy was begun, but because the patient did not improve, he underwent bronchoscopy during his fourth day in the hospital. Much purulent material was recovered from the anterior, apical, and posterior segments of the right upper lobe. There was no obstructive lesion or inflammation in any other part of the bronchial tree.

Accepted for publication January 22, 1990.

Contributed from the Department of Pediatrics, Children's Hospital of Oklahoma, Oklahoma City.

Reprint requests to the Department of Radiology, Childrens Hospital of Los Angeles, 4650 Sunset Blvd, Los Angeles, CA 90027 (Dr Wood).

Figure 1.

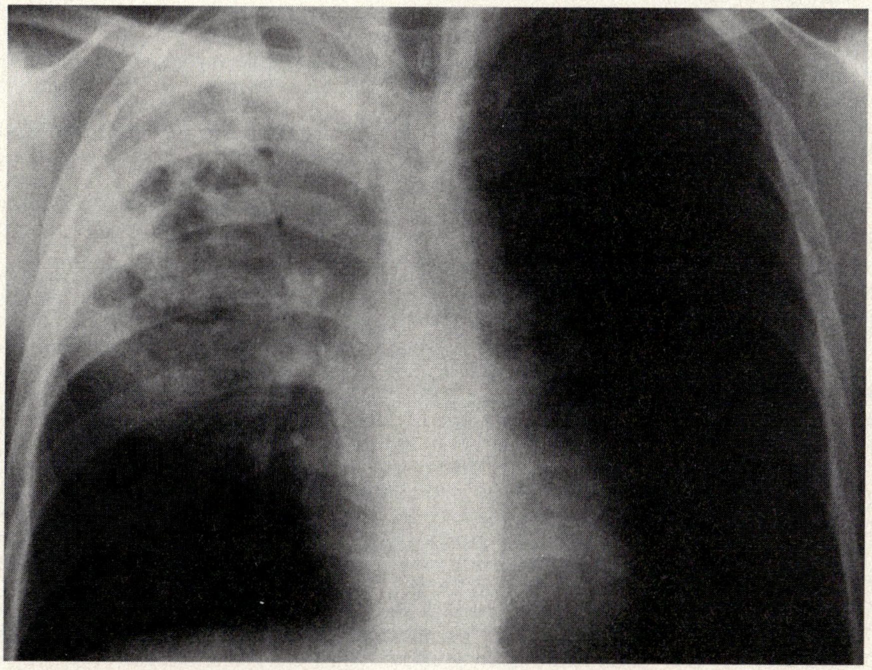

Figure 2.

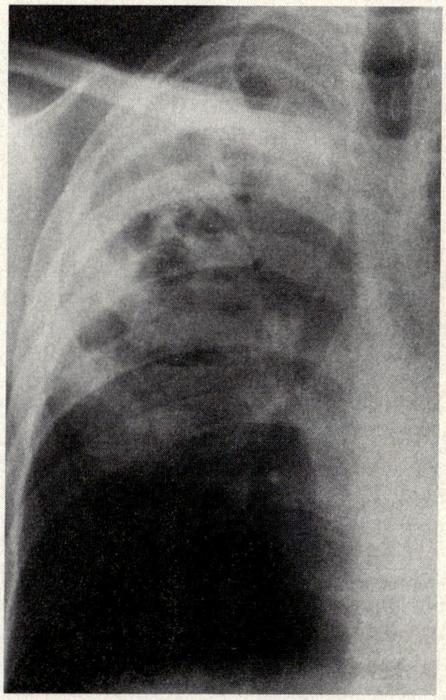

Denouement and Discussion

Cavitary Pneumonia due to *Arcanobacterium hemolyticum*

Fig 1.—*Posteroanterior chest roentgenogram shows consolidation of the right upper lobe and upper portions of the right middle and lower lobes.*

Fig 2.—*Coned view shows multiple cavitary areas with air-fluid levels and an air bronchogram in the consolidated lobes. Mediastinal adenopathy is present.*

The chest roentgenogram taken on admission showed pulmonary consolidation and cavities with air-fluid levels, suggesting parenchymal abscesses or necrosis. Initial antibiotic therapy included treatment for gram-positive species, such as *Staphylococcus* species, and gram-negative species. The patient's history and roentgenogram were suggestive of tuberculosis, although a stain of the sputum showed no acid-fast bacilli, and the patient was anergic. Because the patient did not show clinical improvement, antituberculosis therapy was begun 6 days after admission to the hospital. Later that day, a rapidly growing organism, which had previously been reported as group C *Streptococcus*, was correctly identified as *Arcanobacterium hemolyticum*. The therapeutic regimen was changed to penicillin G and antituberculosis medications only. The boy showed marked improvement within 48 hours, with resolution of fever, decreased white blood cell count, and improved pulmonary aeration, as determined roentgenographically. Antituberculosis therapy was discontinued 10 days after admission to the hospital, and the patient was intravenously administered penicillin G for 4 weeks.

Cavitary pneumonia is an uncommon manifestation of pulmonary infection in children and young adults, but is associated with debilitating illness. Organisms causing lung abscesses include *Staphylococcus aureus*, *Streptococcus pyogenes*, *Klebsiella*, *Bacteroides*, *Mycobacterium tuberculosis*, and *Fusobacterium*.[1] This report illustrates the need also to consider *Arcanobacterium hemolyticum* as a pathogen in cavitary pneumonia.

Corynebacterium hemolyticum was recognized as a human pathogen in 1946, when it was isolated from infections of the nasopharynx and skin of American soldiers and natives of southwest Pacific islands.[2] This organism was considered a mutant of *Corynebacterium pyogenes*,[3,4] and believed to be a purely human pathogen until it was isolated from a pneumonic sheep.[5] This gram-positive, facultatively anaerobic organism appears initially as a slender, irregular bacillus, but with growth changes morphologically and appears as a small, irregular coccus. In 1982, the organism was removed from the *Corynebacterium* genus and reclassified under a new genus named *Arcanobacterium*.[6]

Arcanobacterium hemolyticum causes pharyngitis in young, healthy adults.[7-11] A scarlatiniform skin rash frequently accompanies the pharyngitis, which usually resolves in a few days, regardless of antibiotic therapy. Localized skin lesions, another common manifestation of *A hemolyticum* infection, are frequently ulcerative.[2,8,9]

The organism also causes opportunistic infections in immunosuppressed patients. *Arcanobacterium hemolyticum* has caused vertebral osteomyelitis in a diabetic patient,[12] septicemia in an adolescent girl with infectious mononucleosis,[13] and empyema in a woman with breast cancer.[14]

Serious infections in previously healthy hosts include peritonsillar abscess,[15,16] endocarditis,[17] septicemia,[18] brain abscess,[19] and bacteremia,[20] but this is the first reported case of cavitary pneumonia. Because of the rarity of serious infection in immunologically normal hosts, this patient was evaluated for immunodeficiency. Results of all tests were normal, except B-cell subsets had decreased slightly both 10 days and 1 month after admission to the hospital.

References

1. Bartlett JG. Lung abscess. In: Wyngaarden JB, Smith LH Jr, eds. *Cecil Textbook of Medicine*. Philadelphia, Pa: WB Saunders Co; 1988:435-438.
2. MacLean PD, Liebow AA, Rosenberg AA. Hemolytic *Corynebacterium* resembling *Corynebacterium ovis* and *Corynebacterium pyogenes* in man. *J Infect Dis.* 1946;49:69-90.
3. Barksdale WL, Li K, Cummins CS, Harris H. The mutation of *Corynebacterium pyogenes* to *Corynebacterium haemolyticum*. *J Gen Microbiol.* 1957;16:749-758.
4. Patocka F, Mara M, Soucek A, Souckova A. Observations on the biological properties of atypical haemolytic Corynebacteria isolated from man as compared with *Cor haemolyticum*, *Cor pyogenes bovis* and *Cor ovis*, I: in vivo investigations. *J Hyg Epidemiol Microbiol Immunol.* 1962;6:1-12
5. Roberts RJ. Isolation of *Corynebacterium haemolyticum* from a case of ovine pneumonia. *Vet Rec.* 1969;84:490.
6. Collins MD, Jones D, Schofield GM. Reclassification of '*Corynebacterium haemolyticum*' (MacLean, Liebow & Rosenberg) in the genus *Arcanobacterium* gen nov as *Arcanobacterium haemolyticum* nom rev, comb nov. *J Gen Microbiol.* 1982;128:1279-1281.
7. Ryan WJ. Throat infection and rash associated with an unusual *Corynebacterium*. *Lancet.* 1972;2:1345-1347.
8. Fell HWK, Nagington J, Naylor GRE, Olds RJ. *Corynebacterium haemolyticum* infections in Cambridgeshire. *J Hyg.* 1977;79:269-274.
9. Wickremesinghe RSB. *Corynebacterium haemolyticum* infections in Sri Lanka. *J Hyg.* 1981;87:271-276.
10. Miller RA, Brancato F, Holmes KK. *Corynebacterium hemolyticum* as a cause of pharyngitis and scarlatiniform rash in young adults. *Ann Intern Med.* 1986;105:867-872.
11. Banck G, Nynam M. Tonsillitis and rash associated with *Corynebacterium haemolyticum*. *J Infect Dis.* 1986;154:1037-1040.
12. Ceilley RI. Foot ulceration and vertebral osteomyelitis with *Corynebacterium haemolyticum*. *Arch Dermatol.* 1977;113:646-647.
13. Goudswaard J, van de Merwe DW, van der Sluys P, Doorn H. *Corynebacterium haemolyticum* septicemia in a girl with mononucleosis infectiosa. *Scand J Infect Dis.* 1988;20:339-340.
14. Chlosta EM, Richards GK, Wagner E, Holland JF. An opportunistic infection with *Corynebacterium pyogenes* producing empyema. *Am J Clin Pathol.* 1970;53:167-170.
15. Miller RA, Brancato F. Peritonsillar abscess associated with *Corynebacterium hemolyticum*. *West J Med.* 1984;140:449-451.
16. Kovatch AL, Schuit KE, Michaels RH. *Corynebacterium hemolyticum* peritonsillar abscess mimicking diphtheria. *JAMA.* 1983;249:1757-1758.
17. Worthington MG, Daly BDT, Smith FE. *Corynebacterium hemolyticum* endocarditis on a native valve. *South Med J.* 1985;78:1261-1262.
18. Jobanputra RS, Swain CP. Septicaemia due to *Corynebacterium haemolyticum*. *J Clin Pathol.* 1975;28:798-800.
19. Washington JA, Martin WJ, Spiekerman RE. Brain abscess with *Corynebacterium hemolyticum*: report of a case. *Am J Clin Pathol.* 1971;56:212-215.
20. Chandrasekar PH, Molinari JA. *Corynebacterium hemolyticum* bacteremia with fatal neurologic complication in an intravenous drug addict. *Am J Med.* 1987;82:638-640.

SPECIAL FEATURE

Picture of the Month

Jeffrey R. Schneider, MD, Howard Fischer, MD (Contributors); *Murray Feingold, MD* (Section Editor)

Figure 1.

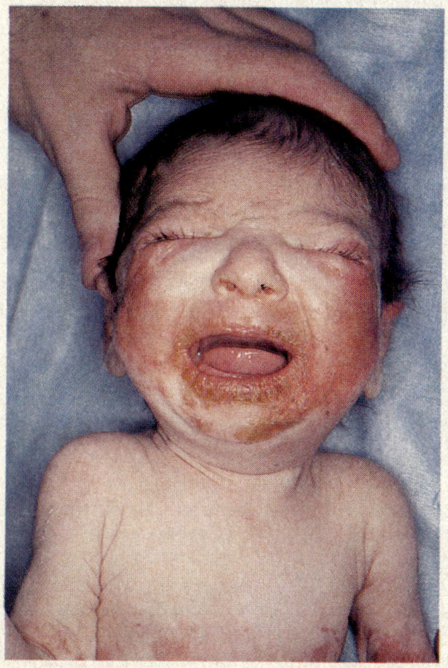

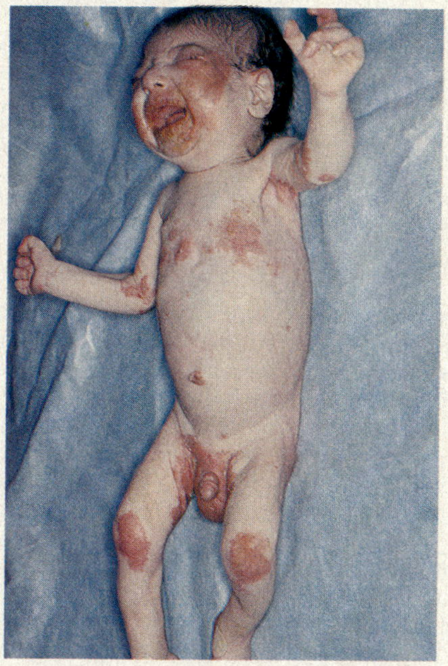

Figure 2.

Figure 3.

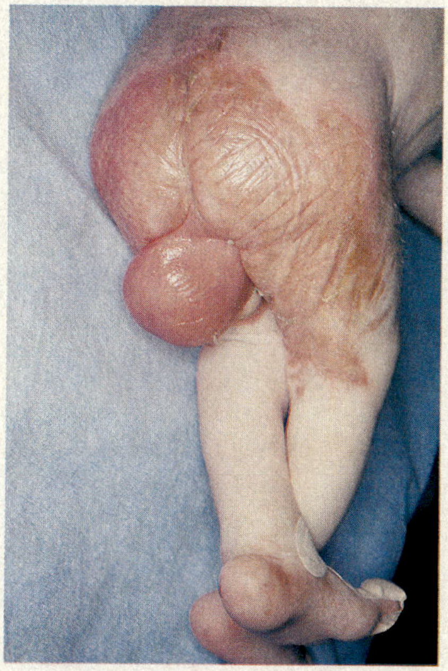

Accepted for publication August 15, 1990.

Contributed from the Department of Pediatrics, Children's Hospital of Michigan, and the School of Medicine, Wayne State University, Detroit, Mich.

Reprint requests to National Birth Defects Center, Franciscan Children's Hospital, 30 Warren St, Brighton, MA 02135 (Dr Feingold).

Denouement and Discussion

Acrodermatitis Enteropathica

Fig 1.—*Erosive lesions around eyes and mouth.*

Figs 2 and 3.—*Emaciated infant with rash surrounding body orifices and a symmetric distribution of lesions on the extremities.*

Manifestations

Acrodermatitis enteropathica is a rare hereditary disorder affecting zinc metabolism that is characterized by dermatitis, alopecia, gastrointestinal disturbances, eye infections, and growth failure. Poor wound healing and impaired cellular immunity have also been described as manifestations of this disorder. Acrodermatitis enteropathica was so named because of the acral distribution of skin lesions and the severe gastrointestinal disturbances it causes.

The classic triad of dermatitis, diarrhea, and alopecia is often seen in newborns and in early infancy. Symptoms may appear within 2 weeks of weaning from breast milk to cow's milk. Infants with acrodermatitis enteropathica typically are listless and anorexic and many have a wasted appearance with little subcutaneous fat. Skin manifestations begin with small, moist, erythematous lesions localized around body orifices (mouth, nose, ears, eyes, and perineum) and progress to a vesicobullous eruption with erosions. Symmetrically distributed lesions occur on the buttocks, the extensor surfaces of major joints, and the fingers and toes.

Later, the vesicobullous eruptions become dry, hyperkeratotic, and psoriasisform in appearance. Diarrhea in this disorder is severe, with steatorrhea, lactose intolerance, and progressive malabsorption. Eye manifestations include blepharitis, conjunctivitis, photophobia, and corneal opacities. Secondary monilial or bacterial skin infections occur frequently. The infections and severe malnutrition may lead to marasmus and death within 1 to 3 years in the untreated patient.

The diagnosis is established by the clinical findings and laboratory evidence of zinc deficiency. Plasma zinc levels are often below 7.7 μmol/L (normal levels are 10.7 to 16.8 μmol/L). Other useful laboratory findings include deficiency of certain zinc-dependent enzymes, such as alkaline phosphatase, and marked alterations of the fatty acid profile of plasma lipids. Skin biopsy is not diagnostic of this disorder.

Genetics

The mode of inheritance is considered to be autosomal recessive. The basic defect is presumed to be related to gastrointestinal malabsorption of zinc, but the exact mechanism is not yet understood.

Treatment

The treatment of choice is oral administration of zinc, usually in the sulfate or gluconate form. It is usually well tolerated, safe, inexpensive, effective, and expedient in rapidly reversing the manifestations of the disease. For many years, acrodermatitis enteropathica was treated empirically with iodoquinol and breast milk, a now outdated treatment.

References

1. Packman S. Zinc metabolism. In: Rudolph AM, Hoffman JIE, eds. *Pediatrics.* 18th ed. East Norwolk, Conn: Appleton & Lange; 1987:326-327.

2. Esterly NB. Vesicobullous disorders. In: Behrman RE, Vaughn VC, Nelson WE, eds. *Nelson Textbook of Pediatrics.* 13th ed. Philadelphia, Pa: WB Saunders Co; 1987:1399-1404.

3. Hurwitz S. *Clinical Pediatric Dermatology.* Philadelphia, Pa: WB Saunders Co; 1981:31-33.

4. Nelder KH, Hambidge KM, Walravens PA. Acrodermatitis enteropathica. *Int J Dermatol.* 1978;17:380-387.

Late Cholangitis After Successful Surgical Repair of Biliary Atresia

Frederic Gottrand, MD; Olivier Bernard, MD; Michelle Hadchouel, MD; Danièle Pariente, MD; Frederic Gauthier, MD; Daniel Alagille, MD

• Bacterial cholangitis is a frequent complication of successful surgical repair of biliary atresia, occurring in 93% of patients before the age of 1 year, but thought to be rare after 2 years of age. Among 76 children free of jaundice more than 5 years after operation, four presented with late cholangitis (7 to 13.5 years old), consisting of fever, jaundice, and abdominal pain with biochemical features of an inflammatory process and cholestasis. Liver biopsy specimens consistently demonstrated histological features of cholangitis, growth of microorganisms, or both. Cholangitis subsided spontaneously in one patient or in response to intravenous administration of antibiotics. Cholangiography consistently demonstrated biliary abnormalities but no definite obstruction to the bilioenteric anastomosis. All the children had good hepatic function 3 weeks to 4 years after the episode of cholangitis. These results suggest that cholangitis may occur several years after surgery but does not seem to alter prognosis.

(*AJDC*. 1991;145:213–215)

Bacterial cholangitis is a frequent complication of surgery for biliary atresia, occurring in about 30% of patients.[1] This frequency increases after successful hepatoportoenterostomy to above 50%.[1-3] It occurs most often within the first months after surgery, 93% of patients being observed before the age of 1 year.[1] Early cholangitis may worsen the prognosis, with increase in mortality, secondary failure of restoration of bile flow, and possible exacerbation of portal hypertension.[1,3-8] However, the frequency of cholangitis decreases with age and is considered rare after 2 years.[1] Indeed, only a few reports briefly note the possibility of late occurrence of cholangitis.[3,7,9-14]

We report the clinicopathological histories of four children operated on successfully for biliary atresia who presented with acute cholangitis at the ages of 7 to 13 years.

Accepted for publication September 5, 1990.

From the Units of Hepatology (Drs Gottrand, Bernard, and Alagille), Institut National de la Santé et de Recherche Médicale U56 (Dr Hadchouel), Radiology (Dr Pariente), and Surgery (Dr Gauthier), Department of Pediatrics, Bicêtre Hospital, Le Kremlin-Bicêtre, France.

Presented as a brief oral communication before the French Society of Gastroenterology and Paediatric Nutrition, Grenoble, France, April 29, 1988.

Reprint requests to Department of Pediatrics, Claude Huriez Hospital, University Hospital of Lille, 59037 Lille Cédex, France (Dr Gottrand).

PATIENT REPORTS

Between 1970 and 1982, 207 children who were operated on for biliary atresia were followed up at Bicêtre Hospital, Le Kremlin-Bicêtre, France. Seventy-six patients became free of jaundice. Among these, four children presented with late cholangitis, defined as follows: occurrence more than 2 years after surgery; exclusion of extrahepatic causes for fever; and a liver biopsy specimen either demonstrating histopathological signs of cholangitis or yielding several organisms on bacterial culture. Their histories follow.

PATIENT 1.—This girl was operated on at the age of 41 days for biliary atresia of the hepatic ducts. A hepatic portocholecystostomy was placed initially because of a patent gallbladder and choledochus. Postoperative choleperitonitis made it necessary to perform a hepatic portoenterostomy with external jejunostomy at the age of 67 days. Bile excretion was observed on the 11th postoperative day, and she became free of jaundice. Acute bacterial cholangitis developed 2 months after the last operation, which subsided in response to intravenous antibiotics. One year later, ultrasonography showed a cystic cavity 2 cm in diameter in the left lobe of the liver. Percutaneous transhepatic cholangiography was performed at the age of 2 years and showed the cystic cavity communicating with a patent portoenterostomy. The intrahepatic bile ducts were irregular. The external jejunostomy was closed at the age of 2.5 years. She remained free of jaundice for several years, with normal liver function test results. The liver was enlarged and firm and displayed histological features of micronodular cirrhosis. Ultrasonography and fibroscopy showed no portal hypertension. Repeated ultrasonography at the age of 8 years did not show any cyst or bile duct dilatation.

At the age of 8.5 years, fever, jaundice with clay-colored stools, abdominal pain, and vomiting developed, with abnormal laboratory findings (Table). Liver histological study (needle biopsy specimen) showed cholangitis with a polymorphonuclear cell infiltration around and inside the bile ducts. Liver and blood cultures remained negative. Intravenous cefotaxime sodium and amikacin sulfate were given for 3 weeks. Fever disappeared within 2 days, and jaundice disappeared gradually. Three months later, liver function test results were normal (Table).

PATIENT 2.—This boy was operated on at the age of 56 days for biliary atresia. A biliary cystic cavity at the porta hepatis was communicating with the intrahepatic bile ducts. A Roux-en-Y jejunal anastomosis to the cyst was performed. Normal-colored stools were seen 10 days later, and the boy became free of jaundice. Acute bacterial cholangitis developed 7 months later and was successfully treated by intravenous administration of antibiotics. He remained free of jaundice for several years, with normal laboratory liver function test results. The liver was not enlarged but showed histological features of moderate portal

Clinical and Laboratory Features in Four Cases of Late Cholangitis*

Signs	On Admission	On Follow-up: 1-4 wk Later	On Follow-up: 4 mo to 4 y Later
Clinical features			
Fever	4/4	0/4	0/4
Jaundice	4/4	0/4	0/4
Abdominal pain	4/4	0/4	0/4
Abnormal laboratory features			
WBC count	1/4	0/4	0/4
ESR	3/4	0/3	0/3
CRP	2/2	0/2	0/2
Bilirubin	4/4	0/4	0/4
γ-Glutamyltransferase	4/4	4/4	1/4†
Alkaline phosphatase	3/4	3/4	1/4†
ALT	4/4	4/4	1/4†

*WBC indicates white blood cell; ESR, erythrocyte sedimentation rate; CRP, C-reactive protein; and ALT, alanine aminotransferase.
†Patient 3.

fibrosis (needle biopsy specimen). There was no ultrasonographic or endoscopic evidence of portal hypertension. Ultrasonography did not show any cavity or dilatation of the bile ducts.

At the age of 8.5 years, fever, jaundice, and abdominal pain developed, all suggestive of cholangitis, but liver histological study and cultures were negative. Percutaneous transhepatic cholangiography showed abnormal intrahepatic bile ducts with stenosis and dilatations but an early opacification of the gut. Antibiotics were administered and fever and jaundice cleared.

At the age of 13.5 years, he again presented with fever, jaundice, and abdominal pain, with abnormal laboratory findings (Table). Liver histological study showed cholangitis with a polymorphonuclear cell infiltrate around and inside the bile ducts (Fig 1). Liver and blood cultures were negative. Symptoms resolved spontaneously within a few days. Repeated percutaneous transhepatic cholangiography demonstrated the same abnormalities of the intrahepatic bile ducts with rapid opacification of the gut (Fig 2).

At the age of 15.5 years, he again presented with the same symptoms. Liver histological study and culture were negative. Antibiotics were given for three weeks, and clinical and biological features resolved. He is 17 years old and has normal growth, no jaundice, no liver or spleen enlargement, normal liver function test results, and no signs of portal hypertension.

PATIENT 3.—This girl was operated on at the age of 112 days for biliary atresia, and a hepatic portoenterostomy with external jejunostomy was performed. She had normal-colored stools 1 month later, and her bilirubin level was normal 2 months later. The external jejunostomy was closed at the age of 2 years.

She remained free of jaundice for several years but with persisting biochemical signs of cholestasis (total bilirubin, 16 μmol/L; alkaline phosphatase, 490 U/L; γ-glutamyltransferase, 155 U/L). The liver was enlarged and firm with moderate splenomegaly, and a liver needle biopsy specimen showed histological features of micronodular cirrhosis. There were no endoscopic or ultrasonographic signs of portal hypertension. Ultrasonography did not show any intrahepatic bile duct abnormalities.

At the age of 7 years, she had fever, jaundice, and abdominal pain with abnormal laboratory findings (Table). *Escherichia coli* and *Enterococcus* species were isolated by cultures of the liver obtained by needle biopsy. The liver had moderate polymorphonuclear cell infiltrate around the bile ducts but none within the ducts themselves. Intravenous trimethoprim-sulfamethoxazole and netilmicin sulfate were given for 3 weeks, and clinical and biological features resolved (Table). An attempt at percutaneous transhepatic cholangiography failed. She is 9.5 years old and has normal growth, no jaundice, but persistently increased γ-glutamyltransferase and alkaline phosphatase levels. There were no esophageal varices, but at ultrasonography the lesser omentum was enlarged.

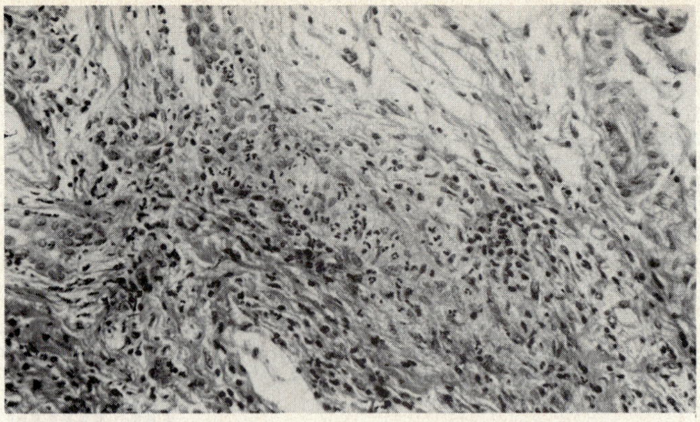

Fig 1.—*Detail of a fibrous portal area showing polymorphonuclear leukocytes inside and around a bile duct (hematein-eosin, ×170).*

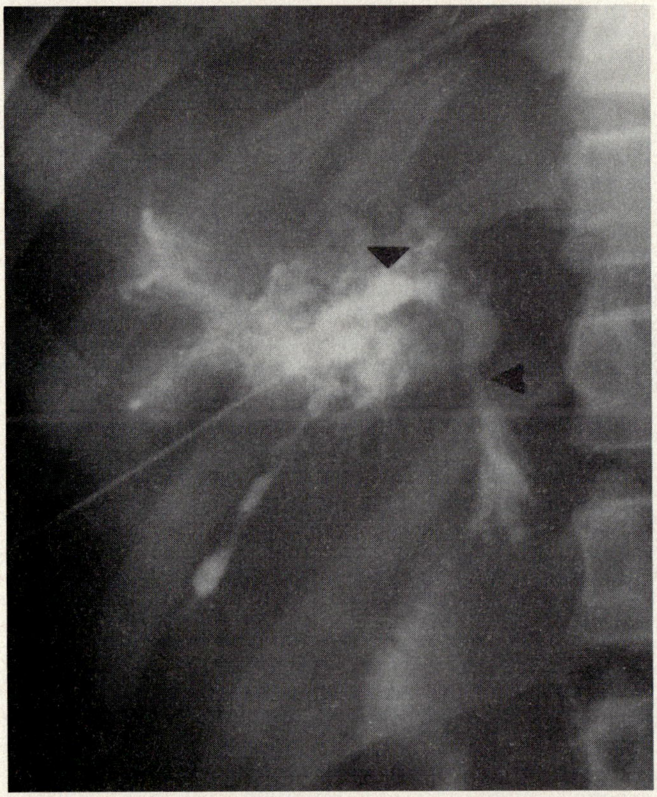

Fig 2.—*Percutaneous transhepatic cholangiography (patient 2) showing irregularly dilated intrahepatic ducts (higher arrow) and a patent anastomosis (lower arrow).*

PATIENT 4.—This boy was operated on for biliary atresia at the age of 57 days, and a hepatic portoenterostomy with external jejunostomy was performed. He had normal-colored stools in a few days and normal bilirubin values 2 months later.

Two episodes of acute cholangitis occurred 2.5 and 4.5 months after surgery. He then remained free of jaundice. Percutaneous transhepatic cholangiography performed at 1 year of age demonstrated narrowed and irregular intrahepatic bile ducts with rapid opacification of the gut. The external jejunostomy was closed at the age of 2 years. He was healthy, with normal laboratory liver function test results. The liver and spleen were not enlarged, but liver histological study (needle biopsy specimen) showed portal fibrosis. There was no sign of portal hypertension. At the age of 7 years he had fever, jaundice, and abdominal pain with abnormal laboratory findings (Table). Liver histological study showed cholangitis with a polymorphonuclear cell infiltrate around and inside the bile ducts. Cultures of blood and a liver biopsy specimen were negative. Ultrasonography showed no cavity or bile duct dilatation. Intravenous trimethoprim-sulfamethoxazole and amikacin were given for 3 weeks. Fever disappeared in 3 days, and he was anicteric on discharge from the hospital (Table). Four months later, he was healthy, with no jaundice or signs of portal hypertension, and had normal growth.

COMMENT

Late cholangitis is a rare complication of surgery for biliary atresia not mentioned in several large series with more than 5 years of follow-up.[4,7,8,15] Lilly and Hitch[12] report five cases of cholangitis occurring 1 to 2 years after operation. Nevertheless, we were only able to find five patients with cholangitis presenting after 2 years.[9-11,14,16] Three of them occurred after hepatoportoenterostomy,[9,14,16] one after choledochoduodenostomy,[11] and one after hepaticoduodenostomy.[10] Late cholangitis occurred at the age of 2.5 to 16 years. Clinical features, when described, consisted of fever, jaundice, and abdominal pain, as in the patients described here. Early cholangitis was absent in two children,[10,11] as in our patient 3. When there was obstruction of the bilioenteric conduit[10,12] or severe intestinal obstruction,[14,16] cholangitis was refractory to treatment or relapsed. However, no definite mechanical obstruction to the bilioenteric system was found in the report of Werlin et al,[9] as well as in our four patients. However, when cholangiograms were performed, abnormalities of intrahepatic bile ducts, ie, narrow or dilated ducts, draining and nondraining cysts, were always seen,[9,11,14] as in our report.

From our patient reports, the main characteristics of late cholangitis after successful surgery for biliary atresia may be summarized as follows: (1) Late cholangitis may occur several years after operation, even if there was no previous episode of early cholangitis. (2) It occurs in children with a healthy appearance; normal liver function test results (three cases) despite liver fibrosis (two) or cirrhosis (two); no or mild portal hypertension (one). (3) Late cholangitis was only seen in children with good bile flow, supporting the concept of a direct ascending cholangitis from intestinal bacteria. Biliary stasis secondary to narrow intrahepatic bile ducts and tiny bilioenteric anastomoses may contribute to cholangitis. Nevertheless, there was no definite mechanical obstruction to the bilioenteric system. The partial obstruction of intrahepatic bile ducts may resolve spontaneously. (4) Features of cholangitis resolve rapidly with use of intravenous antibiotics or spontaneously, as in one of these cases. Late cholangitis does not seem to alter the evolution of the liver condition but may relapse.[14,17] However, Kasai et al[14,16] describe a patient operated on successfully for biliary atresia who died at the age of 29 years after several episodes of late cholangitis. In a few patients, late cholangitis refractory to antibiotic therapy may require liver transplantation.

From the data reported herein, we suggest that children with features of late cholangitis after successful surgery for biliary atresia first have blood cultures taken and be observed for 3 to 4 days, clinical condition permitting. If fever continues and blood cultures are negative, liver needle biopsy should be performed and a 3-week regimen of intravenous antibiotics started. If fever subsides spontaneously, careful follow-up is necessary until all biochemical abnormalities of the liver function tests and inflammatory signs return completely to normal. This approach should prevent unnecessary treatment of a cholangitic episode that can resolve spontaneously; however, antibiotic treatment and follow-up could prevent an ongoing inflammatory process of the intrahepatic bile ducts, with the subsequent risk of complete obstruction, cyst formation, or refractory cholangitis. Should cholangitis recur, a percutaneous cholangiography should be performed in search of obstruction of the bilioenteric anastomosis.[9,18]

References

1. Ecoffey C, Rothman E, Bernard O, Hadchouel M, Valayer J, Alagille D. Bacterial cholangitis following surgery for biliary atresia. *J Pediatr.* 1987;111:824-829.
2. Akiyama H, Saeki M, Ogata T, Takamatsu H, Noguchi H, Tahara H. Ascending cholangitis after hepatic portoenterostomy (original Roux-en-Y) for biliary atresia. In: Ohi R, ed. *Proceedings of the 4th International Symposium on Biliary Atresia.* Tokyo, Japan: Professional Postgraduate Service; 1986:156-160.
3. Kobayashi A, Itabashi F, Ohbe Y. Long-term prognosis in biliary atresia after hepatic portoenterostomy: analysis of 35 patients who survived beyond 5 years of age. *J Pediatr.* 1984;195:243-246.
4. Psacharopoulos HT, Howard ER, Portmann B, Mowat AP. Extrahepatic biliary atresia: preoperative assessment and surgical results in 47 consecutive cases. *Arch Dis Child.* 1980;55:851-856.
5. Millar AJ, Davies MR, Rode H, Brown RA, Cywes S. Biliary atresia: surgical management: a 10 years review. *S Afr Med J.* 1986;69:288-293.
6. Ohi R, Mochizuki I, Komatsu K, Kasai M. Portal hypertension after successful hepatic portoenterostomy in biliary atresia. *J Pediatr Surg.* 1986;21:271.
7. Kasai M, Ohi R. Long-term follow-up results of patients with biliary atresia. *Indian J Pediatr.* 1983;50:209-217.
8. Chen WJ. Recent results of surgical treatment for biliary atresia. In: Ohi R, ed. *Proceedings of the 4th International Symposium on Biliary Atresia.* Tokyo, Japan: Professional Postgraduate Service; 1986:145-148.
9. Werlin SL, Sty JR, Starshak RJ, Glicklich M, Nathan R. Intrahepatic biliary tract abnormalities in children with corrected extrahepatic biliary atresia. *J Pediatr Gastroenterol Nutr.* 1985;4:537-541.
10. Caccia G, Dessanti A, Alberti D. Clinical results in 90 patients with biliary atresia: 2-10 years. In: Ohi R, ed. *Proceedings of the 4th International Symposium on Biliary Atresia.* Tokyo, Japan: Professional Postgraduate Service;1986:281-286.
11. Kimura S, Togon H, Sakai H. Histological studies of the liver in long-term survivors. In: Ohi R, ed. *Proceedings of the 4th International Symposium on Biliary Atresia.* Tokyo, Japan: Professional Postgraduate Service; 1986:299-303.
12. Lilly JR, Hitch DC. Postoperative ascending cholangitis following portoenterostomy for biliary atresia: measures for control. *World J Surg.* 1978;2:581-587.
13. Kuhls T, Jackson MA. Diagnosis and treatment of the febrile child following hepatic portoenterostomy. *Pediatr Infect Dis.* 1985;4:487-490.
14. Kasai M, Ohi R, Chiba T, Hayashi Y. A patient with biliary atresia who died 28 years after hepatic portojejunostomy. *J Pediatr Surg.* 1988;23:430-431.
15. Saeki M, Ogata T, Nakano M. Problems in long-term survivors of biliary atresia. In: Ohi R, ed. *Proceedings of the 4th International Symposium on Biliary Atresia.* Tokyo, Japan: Professional Postgraduate Service; 1986:287-293.
16. Kasai M, Ohi R, Chiba T. Long term survivors after surgery for biliary atresia. In: Ohi R, ed. *Proceedings of the 4th International Symposium on Biliary Atresia.* Tokyo, Japan: Professional Postgraduate Service; 1986:277-280.
17. Akiyama H, Sawaguchi S, Nakajo T. Late complication after surgery for biliary atresia. In: *Cholestasis in Infancy.* Tokyo, Japan: Japan Medical Research Foundation; 1980:413-423.
18. Kimura K, Hashimoto S, Nishijima E, Muraji T, Tsugawa C, Matsutmo Y. Percutaneous transhepatic cholangiodrainage after hepatic portoenterostomy for biliary atresia. *J Pediatr Surg.* 1980;15:811-816.

For most infants,

Predictable

PedvaxHIB®

(Haemophilus b Conjugate Vaccine [Meningococcal Protein Conjugate] | MSD)

INDICATIONS AND USAGE: PedvaxHIB is indicated for routine immunization against invasive disease caused by *Haemophilus influenzae* type b in infants and children 2 to 71 months of age.

PedvaxHIB will not protect against disease caused by *Haemophilus influenzae* other than type b or against other microorganisms that cause invasive disease, such as meningitis or sepsis.

Revaccination: Infants completing the primary two-dose regimen before 12 months of age should receive a booster dose (see DOSAGE AND ADMINISTRATION).

Use with Other Vaccines: Studies have been conducted in which PedvaxHIB has been administered concomitantly with the primary vaccination series of DTP and OPV, or concomitantly with M-M-R® II (Measles, Mumps, and Rubella Virus Vaccine Live, MSD) (using separate sites and syringes), or with a booster dose of OPV plus DTP (using separate sites and syringes for PedvaxHIB and DTP). No impairment of immune response to individual tested vaccine antigens was demonstrated. The type, frequency, and severity of adverse experiences observed in these studies with PedvaxHIB were similar to those seen when the other vaccines were given alone.

PedvaxHIB IS NOT RECOMMENDED FOR USE IN INFANTS YOUNGER THAN 2 MONTHS OF AGE.

CONTRAINDICATIONS: Hypersensitivity to any component of the vaccine or the diluent.

WARNINGS: USE ONLY THE ALUMINUM HYDROXIDE DILUENT SUPPLIED. If PedvaxHIB is used in persons with malignancies or in those who are receiving immunosuppressive therapy or who are otherwise immunocompromised, the expected immune response may not be obtained.

PRECAUTIONS: ***General:*** As for any vaccine, adequate treatment provisions, including epinephrine, should be available for immediate use should an anaphylactoid reaction occur. As with other vaccines, PedvaxHIB may not induce protective antibody levels immediately following vaccination. As with any vaccine, vaccination with PedvaxHIB may not result in a protective antibody response in all individuals given the vaccine. As reported with Haemophilus b polysaccharide vaccine and another Haemophilus b conjugate vaccine, cases of Haemophilus b disease may occur in the week after vaccination, prior to the onset of the protective effects of the vaccines. There is insufficient evidence that PedvaxHIB given immediately after exposure to natural *Haemophilus influenzae* type b will prevent illness. Any acute infection or febrile illness is reason for delaying use of PedvaxHIB except when, in the opinion of the physician, withholding the vaccine entails a greater risk.

Laboratory Test Interactions: Sensitive tests (e.g., Latex Agglutination Kits) may detect PRP derived from the vaccine in urine of some vaccinees for up to seven days following vaccination with PedvaxHIB; in clinical studies with PedvaxHIB, such children demonstrated normal immune response to the vaccine.

Carcinogenesis, Mutagenesis, and Impairment of Fertility: PedvaxHIB has not been evaluated for its carcinogenic or mutagenic potential or for its potential to impair fertility.

Pregnancy: *Pregnancy Category C:* Animal reproduction studies have not been conducted with PedvaxHIB. It is also not known whether PedvaxHIB can cause fetal harm when administered to a pregnant woman or can affect reproduction capacity. PedvaxHIB is not recommended for use in pregnant women.

ADVERSE REACTIONS: In early clinical studies involving the administration of 8,086 doses of PedvaxHIB alone to 5,027 healthy infants and children 2 months to 71 months of age, PedvaxHIB was generally well tolerated. No serious adverse reactions were reported. During a two-day period following vaccination with PedvaxHIB in a subset of these infants and children, the most frequently reported adverse reactions, excluding those shown in the first table, in decreasing order of frequency, included: irritability, sleepiness, respiratory infection/symptoms, and ear infection/otitis media. Urticaria was reported in two children. Thrombocytopenia was seen in one child. A cause-and-effect relationship between these side effects and the vaccination has not been established.

Selected objective observations reported by parents over a 48-hour period in infants and children 2 to 71 months of age following primary vaccination with PedvaxHIB alone are summarized in the first table.

In The Protective Efficacy Study, 4,459 healthy Navajo infants 6 to 12 weeks of age received PedvaxHIB or placebo. Most of these infants received DTP/OPV concomitantly. No differences were seen in the type and frequency of serious health problems expected in this Navajo population or in serious adverse experiences reported among those who received PedvaxHIB and those who received placebo, and none was reported to be related to PedvaxHIB. Only one serious reaction (tracheitis) was reported as possibly related to PedvaxHIB and only one (diarrhea) as possibly related to placebo. Seizures occurred infrequently in both groups (9 occurred in vaccine recipients, 8 of whom also received DTP; 8 occurred in placebo recipients, 7 of whom also received DTP) and were not reported to be related to PedvaxHIB. The frequencies of fever and local reactions occurring in a subset of these infants during a 48-hour period following each dose were similar to those seen in early clinical studies (see first table).

As with any vaccine, there is the possibility that broad use of PedvaxHIB could reveal adverse reactions not observed in clinical trials.

Potential Adverse Reactions: The use of Haemophilus b polysaccharide vaccines and another Haemophilus b conjugate vaccine has been associated with the following additional adverse effects: early onset of Haemophilus b disease and Guillain-Barré syndrome. A cause-and-effect relationship between these side effects and the vaccination was not established.

Fever or Local Reactions in Subjects 2 to 71 Months of Age Vaccinated with PedvaxHIB Alone: Other Clinical Studies

		Dose 1				Dose 2			
Age (Months)	Reaction	Number of Subjects Evaluated	6 hr.	24	48	Number of Subjects Evaluated	6 hr.	24	48
2-14*	Fever >38.3°C (101°F) Rectal	532	2.4%	3.8%	1.9%	329	3.0%	4.3%	3.6%
	Erythema >2.5 cm diameter	1,026	0.2%	1.0%	0.4%	585	0.9%	1.2%	0.7%
	Swelling/ Induration >2.5 cm diameter	1,026	0.6%	1.5%	1.6%	585	0.9%	2.8%	3.7%
15-71**	Fever >38.3°C (101°F) Rectal	149	4.0%	4.0%	6.7%				
	Erythema >2.5 cm diameter	572	0.0%	0.3%	0.2%				
	Swelling/ Induration >2.5 cm diameter	572	0.9%	2.1%	1.4%				

*Additional complaints reported following vaccination with the first and second dose of PedvaxHIB, respectively, in the indicated number of subjects were: nausea, vomiting, and/or diarrhea (101, 41), crying for more than one-half hour (43, 15), rash (16, 17), and unusual high-pitched crying (4, 4).

**Additional complaints reported following vaccination with one dose of PedvaxHIB in the indicated number of subjects were: nausea, vomiting, and/or diarrhea (44), crying for more than one-half hour (19), rash (12), and unusual high-pitched crying (0).

DOSAGE AND ADMINISTRATION:

FOR INTRAMUSCULAR ADMINISTRATION. DO NOT INJECT INTRAVENOUSLY.

2 to 14 Months of Age: Infants 2 to 14 months of age should receive a 0.5-mL dose of vaccine ideally beginning at 2 months of age followed by a 0.5-mL dose 2 months later (or as soon as possible thereafter). When the primary two-dose regimen is completed before 12 months of age, a booster dose is required (see text and second table).

15 Months of Age and Older: Children 15 months of age and older previously unvaccinated against Haemophilus b disease should receive a single 0.5-mL dose of vaccine.

Booster Dose: In infants completing the primary two-dose regimen before 12 months of age, a booster dose (0.5 mL) should be administered at 12 months of age but not earlier than 2 months after the second dose.

DATA ARE NOT AVAILABLE REGARDING THE INTERCHANGEABILITY OF OTHER HAEMOPHILUS b CONJUGATE VACCINES AND PedvaxHIB® (Haemophilus b Conjugate Vaccine [Meningococcal Protein Conjugate], MSD).

Vaccination Regimens by Age Group
(see text for details)

Age (Months) at First Dose	Primary	Age (Months) at Booster Dose
2-10	2 doses, 2 months apart	12
11-14	2 doses, 2 months apart	—
15-71	1 dose	—

TO RECONSTITUTE, USE ONLY THE ALUMINUM HYDROXIDE DILUENT SUPPLIED.

First, agitate the diluent vial; then, using sterile technique, withdraw the entire volume of aluminum hydroxide diluent into the syringe to be used for reconstitution. Inject all the aluminum hydroxide diluent in the syringe into the vial of lyophilized vaccine, and agitate to mix thoroughly.

Withdraw the entire contents into the syringe and inject the total volume of reconstituted vaccine (0.5 mL) intramuscularly, preferably into the anterolateral thigh or the outer aspect of the upper arm.

It is recommended that the vaccine be used as soon as possible after reconstitution. Store reconstituted vaccine in the vaccine vial at 2° to 8°C (36° to 46°F) and discard if not used within 24 hours. Agitate prior to injection.

Parenteral drug products should be inspected visually for extraneous particulate matter and discoloration prior to administration whenever solution and container permit. Aluminum hydroxide diluent and PedvaxHIB when reconstituted are slightly opaque white suspensions.

Special care should be taken to ensure that the injection does not enter a blood vessel.

It is important to use a separate sterile syringe and needle for each patient to prevent transmission of hepatitis B or other infectious agents from one person to another.

HOW SUPPLIED: No. 4792—PedvaxHIB is supplied as a single-dose vial of lyophilized vaccine, NDC 0006-4792-00, and a vial of aluminum hydroxide diluent.

No. 4797—PedvaxHIB is supplied as follows: a box of 5 single-dose vials of lyophilized vaccine, NDC 0006-4797-00, and 5 vials of aluminum hydroxide diluent.

Storage: Before reconstitution, store PedvaxHIB at 2° to 8°C (36° to 46°F). Store reconstituted vaccine in the vaccine vial at 2° to 8°C (36° to 46°F) and discard if not used within 24 hours.

DO NOT FREEZE the aluminum hydroxide diluent or the reconstituted vaccine.

For more detailed information, consult your MSD Representative or see Prescribing Information.

Merck Sharp & Dohme, Division of Merck & Co., INC., West Point, PA 19486.

MSD MERCK SHARP & DOHME

MAKING VACCINES THAT MAKE HISTORY

JOVA08(802)

Factors Affecting Outcome in Meningococcal Infections

Louis J. Tesoro, MD, Steven M. Selbst, MD

• A prognostic score for evaluating meningococcal infections in patients consists of the following five features that indicate a poor prognosis: onset of petechiae within 12 hours of presentation; shock; normal or low peripheral leukocyte count; normal or low erythrocyte sedimentation rate; and absence of meningitis. Based on our experience and some published data, we suspected that the score may no longer be reliable. We reviewed the charts of 73 children with meningococcal infection from December 19, 1979 to December 19, 1987 and applied the prognostic score mentioned previously. Our findings indicate that although a low score is generally associated with a good outcome, a higher score is less predictive of poor outcome than previously suggested. A rash with petechiae or purpura, the presence of shock, and a normal or low peripheral leukocyte count continue to be predictors of poor outcome. Erythrocyte sedimentation rate was not evaluated owing to a limited amount of data. The absence of meningitis did not correlate with a worse outcome in our patients. Most patients who died had evidence of meningeal involvement at the time of presentation. Instead, altered mental status at presentation, particularly obtundation or coma, was an ominous sign. We conclude that absence of meningitis is not a good predictor of outcome, as was previously thought. Altered mental status at the time of presentation may prove to be a stronger indicator of poor outcome.

***(AJDC.* 1991;145:218–220)**

A review of 63 cases of meningococcal disease in 1966 by Stiehm and Damrosch[1] identified five factors that were highly correlated with bad outcome. They were onset of petechiae within 12 hours prior to hospital admission, shock, normal or low leukocyte (WBC) count, normal or low erythrocyte sedimentation rate, and absence of meningitis. The presence of three or more of these features indicated a poor prognosis. Niklasson et al[2] found similar results in Sweden during the 1960s. We reviewed 73 cases of meningococcal infection in patients seen from December 1979 to December 1987 to reexamine the prognostic factors noted by Stiehm and Damrosch and others.

PATIENTS, MATERIALS, AND METHODS

Patients were identified for the study in two ways. Microbiology laboratory records were reviewed from December 19, 1979, to December 19, 1987, and all patients with cultures of cerebrospinal fluid (CSF), blood, or joint fluid positive for meningococcal infections were included. Also, medical record hospital discharge code books from the same period were reviewed, and all patient charts with hospital discharge codes indicating meningococcal disease were examined. Seventy-three patients were included in the study. Of those, 68 had positive CSF or blood cultures for meningococcus, two had positive CSF latex agglutination and a typical course of meningococcal disease, two had a typical course of meningococcal disease with gram-negative diplococci in the CSF, and one had a typical course of meningococcal disease plus a positive joint culture. One patient with a positive blood culture was excluded because he was transferred to another hospital and was unavailable for follow-up. Multiple factors were analyzed to see if they were associated with mortality.

Data were analyzed using the Statistical Package for the Social Sciences. Unless otherwise indicated, $P<.05$ is considered significant.

Accepted for publication July 8, 1990.

From the Division of General Pediatrics, The Children's Hospital of Philadelphia, University of Pennsylvania School of Medicine, Philadelphia. Dr Tesoro is now in private practice in Princeton, NJ.

Reprint requests to the Emergency Department, Children's Hospital of Philadelphia, Philadelphia, PA 19104 (Dr Selbst).

RESULTS

Seven deaths occurred among 73 patients for a fatality rate of 10%. This is not significantly different from the 19% fatality rate in the Stiehm-Damrosch[1] study. Although 42 (57%) of the cases occurred between December and April, there was no month or year with a higher mortality rate. The patients were usually male (79%) and white 46 (63%); fatality was not related to gender or race. The ages of patients ranged from 1 month to 15 years. Two (5%) of 40 who were younger than 2 years died, whereas five (15%) of 33 patients between the ages of 2 and 15 years died. The difference does not vary significantly from the expected outcome. These results are similar to those reported by other authors.[2-5]

The relationship between the five significant Stiehm-Damrosch[1] variables and fatality was examined for our 73 patients. First we compared the absence of meningitis with fatality (Table 1). We used the definition established by Stiehm and Damrosch for meningococcal meningitis ($>20\times10^6$/L WBCs in CSF with positive CSF culture or with negative culture if pretreated with antibiotics) and meningococcemia (positive blood culture or petechiael rash with negative blood culture if pretreated). Our table excludes five patients who did not have a lumbar puncture performed or five patients who did not fit the Stiehm-Damrosch definitions. Fatality was not significantly related to the presence or absence of meningitis. One (4%) of 26 patients with meningitis only died compared with one (5%) of 20 with both meningitis and meningococcemia and two (12%) of 17 with meningococcemia only.

However, this definition of meningitis excluded some patients with positive CSF cultures just because they had less than 20×10^6/L WBCs, as well as those with significant pleocytosis greater than 20×10^6/L WBCs in CSF, with pos-

Table 1.—Relationship of Death From Meningococcemia With the Presence of Meningitis (as Defined by Stiehm and Damrosch[1])

Illness Present	n	Died	%	P
Meningitis only (positive CSF culture, negative blood culture, CSF pleocytosis)	26	1	4	>.05
Meningitis and meningococcemia (positive CSF culture, positive blood culture, CSF pleocytosis)	20	1	5	>.05
Meningococcemia only (negative CSF culture, positive blood culture, no CSF pleocytosis)	17*	2	12	>.05

*Includes eight patients with positive cerebrospinal fluid (CSF) cultures but less than 20×10^6/L leukocytes (WBCs) in the CSF; and one patient with negative CSF cultures but more than 20×10^6/L WBCs. These patients did not have meningitis by the Stiehm-Damrosch strict criteria.

Table 2.—Relationship of Death From Meningococcemia and Presence of Cerebrospinal Fluid (CSF) Pleocytosis (>20×10^6/L White Blood Cells)*

	Pleocytosis	
	Present	Absent
n	48	18
Died	4	2
%	8	11
P	. . .	>.05

*Excluded are five patients who did not have lumbar puncture and two patients with unknown CSF cell counts.

Table 3.—Relationship of Death From Meningococcemia With Any Meningeal Involvement*

	Meningeal Involvement	
	Present	Absent
n	60	8
Died	7	0
%	12	0
P	<.05	. . .

*Positive cerebrospinal fluid (CSF) culture or Gram stain, positive CSF latex agglutination, or CSF pleocytosis.

Table 4.—Relationship of Death From Meningococcemia and the Presence of Petechiae/Purpura

	Petechiae/Purpura	No Rash
n	37	36
Died	7	0
%	19	0
P	. . .	<.01

Table 5.—Relationship of Death From Meningococcemia and Peripheral Leukocytes (WBCs)

WBC, $\times 10^9$/L	n	Died	%	P
≤5	12	5	42	<.01
5-10	16	0	0	. . .
10-15	17	0	0	. . .
>15	27	2	7	. . .

itive blood culture and negative CSF culture. No significant difference in fatality rate (Table 2) was noted when those with pleocytosis greater than 20×10^6/L WBCs were compared with those without pleocytosis. Next, we looked at meningeal involvement, including the presence of a positive CSF culture, a positive CSF Gram stain, a positive CSF latex agglutination, or CSF pleocytosis. Patients with these findings were evaluated for fatality (Table 3). Of the seven patients who died, all had evidence of meningeal involvement. Eight patients with normal CSF survived. Five additional patients (not listed) who did not require lumbar punctures as part of their evaluation also survived. Thus, our results do not support the notion that absence of meningitis results in increased mortality.

Next, we evaluated the relationship between death and the presence of a petechiael or purpuric rash within 12 hours prior to presentation. Unlike Stiehm and Damrosch,[1] we did not find a relationship between time of onset of the rash and death, probably because so few presented with such a rash after 12 hours. No patients (none of eight patients) with petechiae/purpura noted more than 12 hours into the illness died, but seven of 36 with early onset of this rash (<12 hours) died. This was not significantly different. However, the *presence* of this nonblanching rash on initial physical examination was important. Seven (19%) of 37 with petechiae, purpura, or purpura fulminans died, whereas none of 36 died if they had no petechiae or purpura ($P<.01$) (Table 4).

Next, we compared the relationship between death and the initial peripheral WBC count (Table 5). There is a high mortality rate associated with a WBC count less than 5×10^9/L, but no deaths are associated with a WBC count between 5.1 and 15×10^9/L. Only nine erythrocyte sedimentation rates were recorded; these were not analyzed.

Shock was present in 19 patients at time of presentation, and six (32%) of these patients died (Table 6). Only one (2%) of 53 patients who did not present with shock died ($P<.01$). This death was related to rapidly progressive cerebral edema. In 12 patients, shock persisted despite aggressive fluid resuscitation and pressor therapy was started. Six (50%) of 12 patients who received pressors died, compared with only one (2%) of 61 patients who did not require pressors.

We compared several clinical factors and laboratory values with outcome. Several factors are not related to death from meningococcemia, including the following: history of previous severe infection; duration of illness prior to presentation; duration of rash prior to presentation; history of fever; presence of bulging fontanelle; joint involvement; serum sodium concentration; hemoglobin value; differential cell count (peripheral blood); CSF WBC count, differential cell count, red blood cell count, protein concentration, glucose concentration, or Gram's stain (initial); blood culture results; absence of meningitis; and choice of antibiotic. Several factors that are related to death from meningococcemia ($P<.01$) are as follows: presentation to another hospital prior to transfer; change in mental status; coma; shock; nonblanching rash; purpura fulminans; peripheral WBC count; elevated serum creatinine value; prolonged prothrombin time or partial thromboplastin time; severe dissemintated intravascular coagulation; need for intubation; and need for pressors. Presenting to another hospital prior to transfer to our hospital was one factor associated with higher mortality. Those who required transfer to our center may have been more ill to begin with

Table 6.—Relationship of Death From Meningococcemia to Presence of Shock

	Shock	
	Absent	Present
n	53	19
Died	1	6
%	2	32
P	...	<.01

Table 7.—Relationship of Death From Meningococcemia to Mental Status

	Mental Status	
	Normal, Irritable, or Lethargic	Obtunded, Coma
n	56	17
Died	0	7
%	0	41
P	...	<.01

or may have had a delay in definitive treatment. Of those factors studied, however, we found that a change in mental status is most closely associated with mortality in meningococcal infection. None of 56 patients who had normal mental status or only irritability or lethargy died, whereas seven (41%) of 17 of the patients who were obtunded or comatose at the time of presentation died (*P*<.01) (Table 7). Five (83%) of six patients who presented in coma died.

We applied the Stiehm-Damrosch[1] factors associated with poor outcome (excluding erythrocyte sedimentation rate) to our patients (Table 8). Only one (2%) of 50 patients with a score of 1 or 0 died, whereas six (26%) of 23 with scores greater than 1 died. Five (55%) of nine patients with the highest scores survived.

Table 8.—Stiehm-Damrosch[1] Prognostic Score Applied to Our Patients*

Prognostic Score	n	Died	%
0	24	0	0
1	26	1	4
2	14	2	14
3	7	4	57
4	2	0	0

*One point each for normal or low peripheral leukocyte count, shock, onset of petechiae within 12 hours of presentation, and absence of meningitis. Erythrocyte sedimentation rate was not evaluated.

COMMENT

We examined each of the Stiehm-Damrosch[1] factors associated with poor prognosis in meningococcal infections (except erythrocyte sedimentation rates). We found that the absence of meningitis, as defined by Stiehm and Damrosch or defined by the absence of CSF pleocytosis, or the absence of meningeal involvement of any kind, are unimportant predictors of mortality. The reason for the discrepancy between the findings of Stiehm and Damrosch and ours regarding this issue is unclear.

Although peripheral WBC count continues to be associated with poor outcome, we discovered that a suppressed WBC count rather than a normal WBC count in the face of meningococcal infection is significant. Shock remains a significant marker for mortality. Furthermore, we found that the *presence* of nonblanching rash is a sensitive indicator of fatality. We could not determine if the early onset of this rash is important.

Despite some shortcomings, the Stiehm-Damrosch[1] score still identifies patients with a good outcome. It is less reliable for poor outcome. This could be due to the fact that in the last three decades, we have become better able to treat the severely ill child with meningococcal infection. Five (55%) of nine critically ill patients, those with the highest Stiehm-Damrosch scores, survived. All of these were treated aggressively with intensive care, intubation, pressors, and steroids. We suggest that this treatment altered the outcome of these patients and may have rendered the Stiehm-Damrosch score less useful in predicting poor outcome than when it was developed 30 years ago.

Inspired by these results, yet challenged by the fact that we could not demonstrate a reduced mortality rate overall, we looked for other factors that predict poor outcome. Of those we examined, we discovered that altered mental status at the time of presentation, particularly coma, was associated with a grave prognosis. We suggest that the presence of altered mental status, like the presence of shock, low peripheral WBC count, and nonblanching rash, become a "red flag" to the practitioner of the likelihood of poor prognosis. Table 9 compares the Stiehm-Damrosch[1] criteria with the proposed criteria found useful herein. Of course, these factors should be tested prospectively on other patients to see if they reliably predict fatality.

Table 9.—Comparison of Stiehm-Damrosch[1] Criteria to New Factors Associated With Poor Outcome

Stiehm-Damrosch	Proposed New Factors
Shock	Shock
Normal or low WBC*	Low WBC*
Rash within 12 h	Rash
Absent meningitis	Altered mental status
Low erythrocyte sedimentation rate	

*WBC indicates white blood cell count.

CONCLUSION

Presumably because of our improved ability to treat patients with meningococcal infection, prognostic factors developed 30 years ago may no longer be as helpful in predicting outcome. The absence of meningitis does not correlate with a poor outcome. Different criteria, including changes in mental status, shock, presence of nonblanching rash, and low peripheral WBC count may be better predictors of those patients at greatest risk for death from meningococcemia.

Pat Parkinson provided assistance with preparation of the manuscript.

References

1. Stiehm ER, Damrosch DS. Factors in the prognosis of meningococcal infection. *J Pediatr.* 1966;68:457-467.
2. Niklasson P, Lundbergh P, Strandell T. Prognostic factors in meningococcal disease. *Scand J Infect Dis.* 1971;3:17-25.
3. Edwards S, Baker CJ. Complications and sequelae of meningococcal infections in children. *J Pediatr.* 1981;99:540-545.
4. Floyd FW. Meningoccoccemia and meningoccoccal infections: review of 45 cases. *Clin Proc Child Hosp.* 1963;19:119-127.
5. Griffin JW, Daeschner CW. Meningococcal infections: with particular reference to fulminating meningococcemia (Waterhouse-Friderichsen syndrome) treated with cortisone and norepinephrine. *J Pediatr.* 1954;45:264-272.

Antibody Responses to Four *Haemophilus influenzae* Type b Conjugate Vaccines

H. Käyhty, PhD; J. Eskola, MD; H. Peltola, MD; P-R. Rönnberg, RN; E. Kela, RN; V. Karanko, RN; L. Saarinen, MSc

• **Serum antibody responses to four *Haemophilus influenzae* type b capsular polysaccharide-protein conjugate vaccines (PRP-D, HbOC, C7p, and PRP-T) were studied and compared in 175 infants, 85 adults, and 140 2-year-old children. Antibodies to the H influenzae type b polysaccharide vaccines were determined with a Farr-type radioimmunoassay. The infants received two doses of vaccine at the ages of 4 and 6 months. After the first dose of vaccine, the geometric mean antibody concentration measured at the age of 6 months was 0.09 to 0.10 mg/L, only marginally higher than that measured before immunization in all infants who had received PRP-D, HbOC, or C7p but increased to 0.82 mg/L in those who had received PRP-T. One month after the second dose, the geometric mean antibody concentration was increased in all vaccine groups. No significant differences were noted between recipients of HbOC, C7p, or PRP-T (geometric mean antibody concentrations, 4.32, 3.10, and 6.10 mg/L, respectively), whereas the PRP-D recipients had a significantly lower geometric mean antibody concentration (0.63 mg/L). In contrast, PRP-D, HbOC, C7p, and PRP-T were all highly immunogenic in adults, with no differences noted among them. The 2-year-old children also responded to one dose of these vaccines with a high antibody concentration.**

(*AJDC*. 1991;145:223–227)

Haemophilus influenzae type b (Hib) is the most common cause of bacteremic infections in infants and young children.[1,2] Although mortality due to these diseases has decreased to less than 5% as a result of efficient treatment, the occurrence of severe sequelae in survivors remains high.[3-5] A vaccine that could prevent this morbidity would therefore be welcome.

Early in this century, covalent coupling of the capsular polysaccharide (PS) of *Pneumococcus* to a protein carrier was described.[6,7] Many variations of such conjugate vaccines are possible depending on the protein carrier, the length of the PS chain, the linker, and the coupling procedure. Several groups and manufacturers have produced vaccines against Hib that incorporate some of these variations. Thus, PRP-D is composed of PS coupled to diphtheria toxoid via an adipic acid linker, as described originally by Schneerson et al[8] and Gordon.[9] A related preparation (PRP-T) that employs tetanus toxoid instead of diphtheria toxoid was originally described by Chu et al.[10] HbOC contains oligosaccharides (OSs) directly coupled by reductive amination to a nontoxic variant diphtheria toxin, CRM197; the OSs are activated biterminally so that they can bind to the protein at both ends.[11] Porter Anderson (University of Rochester [NY]) has prepared a series of vaccines, eg, C7p, in which uniterminally activated OSs are coupled to the protein (either diphtheria toxoid or CRM197) at one end.[12] In PRP-OMP, PS is coupled by a bigeneric linker to an outer membrane protein -complex isolated from *Neisseria meningitidis* group B, type 2a.[13]

All of these vaccines have been shown to be immunogenic in human infants.[11,14-18] A comparison of the vaccines is difficult based on the published data, as there are no standardized assays for anti-Hib PS and results from different laboratories may not be directly comparable.[19-21] Separate studies, however, suggest differences in immunogenicity. Furthermore, the extent to which the immunogenicity of the vaccines in adults or older children would predict immunogenicity in infants is unclear.

To consolidate the data base, we have compared, under similar conditions, the immunogenicity and reactogenicity of four Hib conjugate vaccines in infants immunized at 4 and 6 months of age, adults, and 2-year-old children; some of the data have been previously published,[22,23] but they are presented herein together with the new data to facilitate comparison.

PATIENTS AND METHODS

Vaccines, Vaccinees, and the Vaccination Schedules

The Hib vaccines used are listed in Table 1. The vaccination protocol was approved by the Ethical Committee of the National Public Health Institute, Helsinki, Finland. Informed consent was obtained from the adult vaccinees or from the parents of children and infants.

Healthy infants were recruited at the age of 3 months from the child health centers of two towns: Joensuu and Kerava. Seventy-two infants received PRP-D, 46 received HbOC, 32 received C7p, and 25 received PRP-T at the ages of 4 and 6 months. At the age of 4 months, they also received their second dose of diphtheria-pertussis-tetanus vaccine (National Public Health Institute); at the age of 6 months, they received their first dose of poliomyelitis vaccine (inactivated poliovirus vaccine; RIVM, Bilthoven, the Netherlands). The Hib vaccines were given intramuscularly into the right buttock, and the diphtheria-pertussis-tetanus and inactivated poliovirus vaccines were administered intramuscularly into the left buttock.

Healthy, mostly female young adults received intramuscular injections into the left arm of PRP-D (n = 27), HbOC (n = 19), C7p

Accepted for publication May 30, 1990.
From the Department of Bacteriology, National Public Health Institute, Helsinki, Finland.
Reprint requests to National Public Health Institute, Mannerheimintie 166, 00300 Helsinki, Finland (Dr Eskola).

Table 1.—*Haemophilus influenzae* Type (Hib) Vaccines Used in a Comparative Immunogenicity Trial Among Infants, Children, and Adults.

Vaccine	Lot No.	Manufacturer	Type of Saccharide	Spacer	Amount of Hib Polysaccharide per Dose, μg	Protein-to-Polysaccharide Ratio
PRP-D	5L294 4102, 4163*	Connaught Laboratories Inc, Swiftwater, Pa	Sized polysaccharide†	6 carbon	20	1.25
HbOC	BrH-5-12, 6174‡	Praxis Biologics Inc, Rochester, NY	20-unit oligosaccharide	None	10	2.5
C7p	1 lot	Porter Anderson, Rochester, NY	7-unit oligosaccharide	None	5	5.0
PRP-T	S-1890	Institute Merieux, Lyons, France	Native polysaccharide	6 carbon	10	1.88

*Lot 4163 was used in infants and lots 5L294 and 4102 were used in adults and children.
†The molecular weight of the polysaccharide is heat sized to 200 to 2000 kd.
‡Lot 6174 was used in infants and lots BrH-5-12 and 6174 were used in adults and children.

(n=18), or PRP-T (n=21). No other vaccinations were given at the same time. Children were immunized intramuscularly into the right buttock at 23 to 25 months of age with PRP-D (n=54), HbOC (n=56), or C7p (n=30). The children in the PRP-D group also received bivalent (groups A and C) meningococcal vaccine (Connaught Laboratories Inc, Swiftwater, Pa) and/or 23-valent pneumococcal vaccine (Pneumovax, Merck Sharp & Dohme, West Point, Pa); these vaccines have been shown to have no effect on the response to a Hib conjugate vaccine or to Hib CPS vaccine.[22,24]

Serum Samples

Blood samples were obtained from infants before the first and second doses and 1 month after the second dose, ie, at 4, 6, and 7 months of age. Blood samples were obtained from children and adults before and 1 month after vaccination. The samples were preserved at −20°C until testing.

Follow-up of Adverse Reactions

The vaccinees were observed for at least 15 minutes after each vaccination. The vaccinees or their parents were given a special form to be completed 6, 12, 24, and 48 hours after vaccination. The rectal temperature, any systemic reaction, and description of local reactions at the injection site were recorded on this form.

Serologic Methods

Antibodies to the Hib PS were measured by a Farr-type radioimmunoassay[25] with the use of a tyramine derivative of Hib PS prepared by Rachel Schneerson (National Institutes of Health, Bethesda, Md) for iodination. The reference serum was also received from Rachel Schneerson.

Statistical Analysis

The geometric mean antibody concentrations (GMCs) were calculated with 0.06 mg/L as the lower and 320 mg/L as the higher limit of detection. Analysis of variance, Duncan's test at $P=.05$ (both tests need log-transformed data), and χ^2 test were used for differences in the anti–Hib PS antibody concentrations at each sampling point.

RESULTS

Reactogenicity of the Hib Vaccines

Irritability was the most common adverse effect among infants, reported in 41% to 60% of the vaccinees after the first dose and in 16% to 32% after the second dose. Fever was uncommon, detected in 2% to 5% of infants, regardless of age at the time of vaccination. Local soreness was also uncommon. No significant differences were noted between the vaccine groups regarding the frequency of reactions.

None of the adults or 2-year-old children had a fever after any of the vaccines. Local redness was reported in three children, and local soreness was reported in 14 children, all of whom had received the PRP-D vaccine together with meningococcal vaccine and most of whom (n=11) had also received the Pneumovax vaccine. These reactions were probably due to the latter vaccine.[22]

Immunogenicity in Infants

Infants were immunized at 4 and 6 months of age. The preimmunization anti–Hib PS concentrations were similar (0.07 to 0.09 mg/L) in each group (Fig 1); few children actually had measurable antibody levels (Fig 2).

Two months after the first dose, at the age of 6 months, the anti–Hib PS concentrations differed significantly in the four vaccine groups ($P<.001$). The GMCs were only marginally higher than those measured before vaccination in the groups that had received either PRP-D, HbOC, or C7p vaccines (0.10, 0.09, and 0.10 mg/L, respectively). However, those who had received PRP-T showed an increase in anti–Hib PS concentration up to a GMC of 0.82 mg/L (Fig 1). At this time, only a few infants in the PRP-D, HbOC, and C7p vaccine groups but half of those in the PRP-T vaccine group had serum anti–Hib PS concentrations above 1 mg/L, and almost one fifth of the infants in the PRP-T group had concentrations higher than 4 mg/L (Fig 2).

At 7 months of age, 1 month after the second dose, the anti–Hib PS concentrations in the four groups differed significantly ($P<.001$). The GMCs in the HbOC, C7p, and PRP-T groups were similar (4.32, 3.10, and 6.10 mg/L, respectively), whereas the children who had received the PRP-D vaccine had a significantly lower GMC (0.63 mg/L; Fig 1). Most infants in the HbOC, C7p, and PRP-T groups had anti–Hib PS concentrations greater than 1 mg/L, and more than half of the infants had concentrations greater than 4 mg/L (Fig 2).

Immunogenicity in Adults and 2-Year-Old Children

All four vaccines listed in Table 2 elicited equally high anti–Hib PS antibody responses in adults. Among children immunized at 23 to 25 months of age, the postimmunization GMC was significantly higher after HbOC vaccine ($P<.01$) than after the other two vaccines. The recipients of the HbOC vaccine also had a significantly ($P<.05$) increased incidence of high antibody concentrations, exceeding 4.0 mg/L.

COMMENT

Significant differences were found between different Hib PS-protein conjugate vaccines given during infancy. Thus, the anti-Hib PS response was lower after two doses

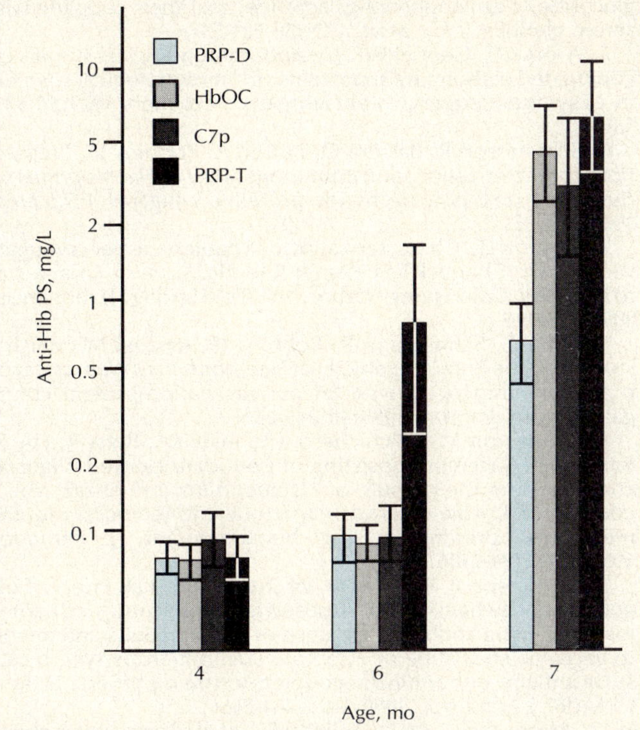

Fig 1.—*Geometric mean antibody concentrations and their 95% confidence intervals (vertical lines) of serum anti–*Haemophilus influenzae *type b capsular polysaccharide (anti-Hib PS) in infants before (at age 4 months) and after (at ages 6 and 7 months) the first and second doses of one of the four conjugate vaccines against* H influenzae *type b (PRP-D, HbOC, C7p, or PRP-T). The vaccines were administered at 4 and 6 months of age.*

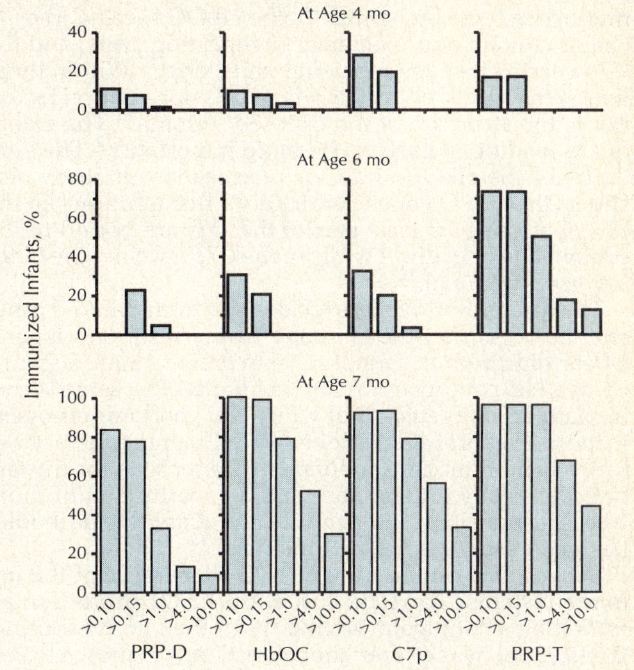

Fig 2.—*Percentages of infants with anti–*Haemophilus influenzae *type b antibody concentrations above a set of indicated limits before and after the first and second doses of one of the four* H influenzae *type b conjugate vaccines (PRP-D, HbOC, C7p, or PRP-T). The samples and vaccinations are as shown in Fig 1.*

of PRP-D than after two doses of the three other vaccines. Only the PRP-T vaccine gave rise to a significant antibody increase after the first dose given at age 4 months. In this respect, PRP-T may behave like PRP-OMP, which has also been reported to induce a response after one dose given at 2 to 6 months of age.[18]

The properties of a conjugate vaccine that determine its immunogenicity are unknown. The PRP-D and PRP-T vaccines proved to differ in immunogenicity despite the similarity of the PS and the coupling to protein; the protein partner was either diphtheria or tetanus toxoid.[9,10] In the PRP-D vaccine, the protein was modified by incorporation of the adipic dihydrazide linker before the addition of the PS,[9] whereas the linker in the PRP-T vaccine was first conjugated to the PS, which was then allowed to react with the protein.[10] The increased immunogenicity of the PRP-T vaccine may thus be related to a more native protein structure; however, in both cases the protein was detoxified by formaldehyde before coupling. The quality of the protein carrier in the Hib PS- or OS-conjugate vaccine may also be important—in human infants, a conjugate prepared with CRM197 proved to be superior to one prepared with diphtheria toxoid,[26] and in infant rhesus monkeys conjugates with cholera toxoid were superior to those with tetanus toxoid or horseshoe crab hemocyanin.[27] Furthermore, the ratio of protein to PS in a PS-protein conjugate can influence its immunogenicity[28]; the higher the ratio, the better the response, provided sufficient PS is present in one dose of vaccine. In our study, little difference was noted in the

Table 2.—Geometric Mean Anti–*Haemophilus influenzae* Type b Polysaccharide (Anti-Hib PS) Antibody Concentrations Before and After Immunization of Adults and 2-Year-Old Children With *H influenzae* Type b Conjugate Vaccines*

	Anti-Hib PS, mg/L					
	Adults			Children		
Vaccine	No.	Before	After	No.	Before	After
PRP-D	27	1.53 (0.97-2.42)	72.0 (45.3-114)	54	0.15 (0.11-0.20)	9.72 (6.72-14.1)
HbOC	19	2.58 (1.35-4.80)	85.5 (44.8-163)	56	0.19 (0.14-0.26)	30.6 (20.7-45.3)
C7p	18	1.90 (0.97-3.73)	63.3 (38.8-103)	30	0.14 (0.09-0.21)	11.2 (5.85-21.5)
PRP-T	21	0.86 (0.48-1.56)	29.8 (19.0-46.8)	...	...	...

*Values in parentheses indicate 95% confidence intervals.

ratio of protein to PS between the PRP-D and PRP-T vaccines (Table 1).

The HbOC and C7p vaccines both contain OS derived from Hib PS. Animal studies suggest that OS conjugates are more potent immunogens than PS conjugates.[29] These and several other studies on human infants[11,15,16,26] have shown that the Hib OS conjugate vaccines are good immunogens, even in infants. In the HbOC vaccine, the OS chains contain approximately 20 repeating units, and the C7p vaccine is seven repeating units long.[12] Within these limits, the length of the OS probably is not a critical factor, nor is the structure of the exposed termini.[12] The extent of OS loading is likely to be more important.[12] The similarity of the HbOC and C7p vaccines in our study also shows that the OS does not require a free terminus; in the HbOC vaccine, at least part of the OSs are bound to the protein biterminally,[11] while in the C7p vaccine, the binding is uniterminal.[12]

The disappointing message derived from this and other studies[11,12] is that the antibody responses in adults and 2-year-old children cannot reliably predict immunogenicity of a Hib conjugate vaccine in infants. The same is true of plain PS antigens, all of which are good immunogens in those 2 years of age or older, but only conjugate vaccines serve as immunogens in infants. The reasons for this are not completely understood, but late maturation of those B cells responsible for the production of anti-PS antibodies has been suggested to be important.[30]

It is also far from clear which characteristics of the immune response correlate best with clinical protection afforded by a conjugate vaccine. With the Hib PS vaccine, the situation was clearer: the protection was shown to correlate with the concentration of specific serum antibodies, and a concentration greater than 1 mg/L of anti–Hib PS was calculated to predict long-lasting protection after vaccination.[31,32] In contrast, the PRP-D vaccine has been shown to be highly protective among Finnish infants,[33,34] despite the relatively low antibody concentrations detected. In the field trial that showed protection in infants, the anti–Hib PS GMC at 7 months, after the course of three doses of PRP-D vaccine, was below 0.42 mg/L.[33] The best correlate of protection in that study was a measurable response of any magnitude (at least 0.1 mg/L of anti–Hib PS) obtained after the primary series of vaccinations in the infants. By this criterion, the PRP-D vaccine would be expected to be 80% to 90% protective vs 90% to 100% protection for the other vaccines (Fig 2) with the dosage and schedule used in our study.

This study was supported by Connaught Laboratories Inc, Swiftwater, Pa, Praxis Biologics Inc, Rochester, NY, and Institut Merieux, Lyons, France.

We thank the personnel in the Child Health Centers of Joensuu and Kerava for their valuable cooperation and the vaccinees and their parents for taking part in our study. We also thank P. Helena Mäkelä, MD, and Simon Kroll, MD, for fruitful discussions and their critical reading of the manuscript. The skillful assistance of Hannele Lehtonen and Sirkka-Liisa Wahlman and the help of Mari-Anna Berg, MSc, and Panu Rekola, MSc, in the handling of the data is gratefully acknowledged.

References

1. Dajani AS, Asmar BI, Thirumoorthi MC. Systemic *Haemophilus influenzae* disease: an overview. *J Pediatr.* 1979;94:355-364.
2. World Health Organization. Bacterial meningitis: United Kingdom. *Weekly Epid Rec.* 1985;60:146-147.
3. Lindberg J, Rosenthal U, Nylen O, Ringer A. Long-term outcome of *Haemophilus influenzae* meningitis related to antibiotic treatment. *Pediatrics.* 1977;60:1-6.
4. Sell SHW, Merrel RE, Pate JE, Doyne EO. Psychological sequelae to bacterial meningitis: two controlled studies. *Pediatrics.* 1972;49:212-217.
5. Sproles ET, Azerrad J, Williamson C, Merril RE. Meningitis due to *Haemophilus influenzae*: long-term sequelae. *J Pediatr.* 1969;75:782-788.
6. Goebel WF, Avery OT. Chemo-immunological on conjugated carbohydrate-proteins. I: the synthesis of *p*-aminophenol-glucoside, *p*-aminophenol-galactoside, and their coupling with serum globulin. *J Exp Med.* 1929;50:521-531.
7. Avery OT, Goebel WF. Chemo-immunological studies on conjugated carbohydrate-proteins. II: immunological specificity of synthetic sugar-protein antigens. *J Exp Med.* 1929;50:533-550.
8. Schneerson R, Barrera O, Sutton A, Robbins JB. Preparation, characterization, and immunogenicity of *Haemophilus influenzae* type b polysaccharide-protein conjugates. *J Exp Med.* 1980;152:361-376.
9. Gordon LK. Characterization of a hapten-carrier conjugate vaccine. In: Chanock RM, Lerner RA, eds. *Modern Approaches to Vaccines.* Cold Spring Harbor, NY: Cold Spring Harbor Press; 1984:393-396.
10. Chu C, Schneerson R, Robbins JB, Rastogi SC. Further studies on the immunogenicity of *Haemophilus influenzae* type b and pneumococcal type 6A polysaccharide-protein conjugates. *Infect Immun.* 1983;40:245-256.
11. Anderson PW, Pichichero ME, Insel RA, Betts R, Eby R, Smith DH. Vaccines consisting of periodate-cleaved oligosaccharides from the capsule of *Haemophilus influenzae* type b coupled to a protein carrier: structural and temporal requirements for priming in the human infant. *J Immunol.* 1986;137:1181-1186.
12. Anderson P, Pichichero ME, Stein EC, et al. Effect of oligosaccharide chain length, exposed terminal group, and hapten loading on the antibody response of human adults and infants to vaccines consisting of *Haemophilus influenzae* type b capsular antigen uniterminally coupled to the diphtheria protein CRM197. *J Immunol.* 1989;142:2464-2468.
13. Marburg S, Jorn D, Tolman RL, et al. Bimolecular chemistry of macromolecules: synthesis of bacterial polysaccharide conjugates with *Neisseria meningitidis* membrane protein. *J Am Chem Soc.* 1986;108:5282-5287.
14. Eskola J, Käyhty H, Peltola H, et al. Antibody levels achieved in infants by course *Haemophilus influenzae* type b polysaccharide/diphtheria toxoid conjugate vaccine. *Lancet.* 1985;1:1184-1186.
15. Anderson P, Pichichero M, Edwards K, Porch CR, Insel R. Priming and induction of *Haemophilus influenzae* type b capsular antibodies in each infancy by Dpo20, an oligosaccharide-protein conjugate vaccine. *J Pediatr.* 1987;111:644-650.
16. Anderson P, Pichichero ME, Insel RA. Immunization of 2-month-old infants with protein-coupled oligosaccharides derived from the capsule of *Haemophilus influenzae* type b. *J Pediatr.* 1985;107:346-351.
17. Reinert P, Olivier C, Palestro B, et al. Immune response to *H. influenzae* type b (Hib) capsular polysaccharide (PRP)–tetanus antigen conjugate vaccine (PRP-T) in 3-month-old infants. In: Program and abstracts of the 28th Interscience Conference on Antimicrobial Agents and Chemotherapy; October 23-26, 1988; Los Angeles, Calif. Abstract 1030.
18. Lenoir AA, Granoff PH, Granoff DM. Immunogenicity of *Haemophilus influenzae* type b polysaccharide: *Neisseria meningitidis* outer-membrane protein conjugate vaccine in 2- to 6-month-old infants. *Pediatrics.* 1987;80:283-287.
19. Ward JI, Greenberg DP, Anderson PW, et al. Variable quantitation of *H. Influenzae* type b anticapsular antibody by radioantigen binding assay. *J Clin Microbiol.* 1988;26:72-78.
20. Anderson P, Insel RA, Porcelli S, Ward JI. Immunochemical variables affecting radioantigen-binding assays of antibody to *Haemophilus influenzae* type b capsular polysaccharide in childrens' sera. *J Infect Dis.* 1987;156:582-590.
21. Edwards KM, Decker MD, Palmer P, et al. Lack of comparability between commonly used serological assays of immune response to *Haemophilus influenzae* vaccine. *J Infect Dis.* 1987;155:283-291.
22. Eskola J, Käyhty H, Takala AK, Rönnberg PR, Kela E, Peltola H. Reactogenicity and immunogenicity of combined vaccines for bacteremic diseases caused by *Haemophilus influenzae* type b, meningococci and pneumococci in 24-month-old children. *Vaccine.* 1990;8:107-110.
23. Käyhty H, Peltola H, Eskola J, Mäkelä PH. Immunogenicity

of *Haemophilus influenzae* oligosaccharide-protein (HbOC) and polysaccharide-protein (PRP-D) conjugate vaccines at 4, 6 and 14 months of age. *Pediatrics.* 1989;84:995-999.
24. Ambrosino DM, Siber GR. Simultaneous administration of vaccines for *Haemophilus influenzae* type b, pneumococci and meningococci. *J Infect Dis.* 1986;154:893-896.
25. Mäkelä PH, Peltola H, Käyhty H, et al. Polysaccharide vaccines of group A *Neisseria meningitidis* and *Haemophilus influenzae* type b: a field trial in Finland. *J Infect Dis.* 1977;136:S43-S50.
26. Anderson P, Pichichero ME, Insel RA. Immunogens consisting of oligosaccharides from the capsule of *Haemophilus influenzae* type b coupled to diphtheria toxoid or the toxin protein CRM197. *J Clin Invest.* 1985;76:52-59.
27. Schneerson R, Robbins JB, Chu C, et al. Serum antibody responses of juvenile and infant rhesus monkeys injected with *Haemophilus influenzae* type b and pneumococcus type 6A capsular polysaccharide-protein conjugates. *Infect Immun.* 1984;45:582-591.
28. Lepow ML, Barkin RM, Berkowitz CD, et al. Safety and immunogenicity of *Haemophilus influenzae* type b polysaccharide–diphtheria toxoid conjugate vaccine (PRP-D) in infants. *J Infect Dis.* 1987;156:591-596.
29. Mäkelä O, Peterfy F, Outschoorn IG, Richter AW, Seppälä J. Immunogenic properties of α-(1-6)-dextran, its protein conjugates and conjugates of its breakdown products in mice. *Scand J Immunol.* 1984;19:541-550.
30. Paul WE, Kung J, Ahmed A, et al. B lymphocyte subpopulations and responses to polysaccharide antigens. In: Sell SH, Wright PF, eds. Haemophilus influenzae: *Epidemiology, Immunology and Prevention of Disease.* New York, NY: Elsevier Science Publishing Co Inc; 1982:121-128.
31. Käyhty H, Peltola H, Karanko V, Mäkelä PH. The protective level of serum antibodies to the capsular polysaccharide of *Haemophilus influenzae* type b. *J Infect Dis.* 1983;147:1100.
32. Anderson P. The protective level of serum antibodiesto the capsular polysaccharide of *Haemophilus influenzae* type b. *J Infect Dis.* 1984;149:1034.
33. Eskola J, Peltola H, Takala AK, et al. Efficacy of *Haemophilus influenzae* type b polysaccharide–diphtheria toxoid conjugate vaccine in infancy. *N Engl J Med.* 1987;317:717-722.
34. Eskola J, Kayntz H, Takala TK, et al. A randomized, prospective field trial of a conjugate vaccine in the protection of infants and young children against invasive *Haemophilus influenzae* type b disease. *N Engl J Med.* 1990;323:1381-1387.

In Other AMA Journals

ARCHIVES OF GENERAL PSYCHIATRY

Heterogeneity in the Inheritance of Alcoholism: A Study of Male and Female Twins

Roy W. Pickens, PhD; Dace S. Svikis, PhD; Matt McGue, PhD; David T. Lykken, PhD; Leonard L. Heston, MD; Paula J. Clayton, MD
(*Arch Gen Psychiatry.* 1991;48:19-28)

Hyperactive Boys Almost Grown Up, V: Replication of Psychiatric Status

Salvatore Mannuzza, PhD; Rachel G. Klein, PhD; Norreen Bonagura, MSW; Patricia Malloy; Tina L. Giampino; Kathy A. Addalli
(*Arch Gen Psychiatry.* 1991;48:77-83)

Focal Scleroderma and Severe Cardiomyopathy

Patient Report and Brief Review

Ellen C. Moore, MD; Flossie Cohen, MD; Zia Farooki, MD; Chung-Ho Chang, MD

• A 21-month-old infant presented with simultaneous localized scleroderma and severe cardiomyopathy with heart failure. Cardiac abnormalities and serological changes (positive rheumatoid factor assay, elevated IgM and IgG levels, and elevated erythrocyte sedimentation rate) reverted to normal with prednisone therapy, and there was substantial, though incomplete, resolution of her skin changes during the same period. To our knowledge, this is the first patient with definite, clinically significant cardiac involvement associated with focal scleroderma. The possibility of internal organ involvement, including cardiac involvement, must be considered with focal scleroderma as well as with progressive systemic sclerosis.

(*AJDC.* 1991;145:229–231)

Focal scleroderma is a rare disorder, more commonly encountered in children than in adults.[1] It is usually benign, without apparent systemic involvement, but does form a continuum with generalized scleroderma (progressive systemic sclerosis [PSS]), where involvement of organs other than skin is common. Involvement of brain,[2] gastrointestinal tract[2] (especially the esophagus[3,4]), lung,[3,4] muscle,[4,5] and kidney[4] has been reported rarely in focal scleroderma. Serological abnormalities[6-11] also suggest this disorder is not limited to skin and underlying tissues.

In PSS, involvement of the heart may occur in up to 81% of the cases,[12] although it is clinically apparent only in about 15% and may be more common in children than in adults.[13] Two of three patients with morphea studied by echocardiography[14] also showed cardiac abnormalities, and sclerodermatous myocardial involvement on autopsy was found in an elderly patient with morphea described by Rodnan and Fennel[3] (case 4), though it is unclear whether her cardiac symptoms were due to the scleroderma per se, as she also had had multiple myocardial infarctions. To our knowledge, the infant described herein is the first patient with definite, clinically significant cardiac involvement associated with focal scleroderma.

Accepted for publication July 16, 1990.

From the Divisions of Clinical Immunology and Rheumatology (Drs Moore and Cohen), Pediatric Cardiology (Dr Farooki), and Surgical Pathology (Dr Chang), Children's Hospital of Michigan, and the Departments of Pediatrics (Drs Moore, Cohen and Farooki) and Pathology (Dr Chang), Wayne State University School of Medicine, Detroit.

Reprint requests to Division of Clinical Immunology and Rheumatology, Children's Hospital of Michigan, 3901 Beaubien Blvd, Detroit, MI 48201 (Dr Moore).

PATIENT REPORT

In a previously well Mexican-American girl, at 19 months of age, white blotches developed over her axillae, legs, and buttocks, and she gradually became unable to extend her legs fully. Her weight decreased from 14.0 to 11.7 kg. At 21 months, when she came for medical attention, she had white, hard, plaquelike skin in both axillae and similar, more confluent lesions on her legs and ankles (Fig 1). This skin was tense and adherent to the underlying structures, with loss of subcutaneous tissue and muscle atrophy. The remainder of her skin was normal. Marked flexion contractures were noted bilaterally on her knees and hips. Her right foot was fixed in equinus position with a limited range of motion. The left foot was somewhat more mobile than the right foot, but also had an equinus deformity, with a high arch because of the tight, adherent skin.

She was mildly febrile (temperature, 37.8°C), tachycardic (heart rate, 160 beats per minute), and tachypneic (respirations, 28 to 35 per minute). No significant murmur was heard, but a soft S_3 gallop was present. Her liver was palpable 3 cm below the costal margin, and pedal edema was present. Her hemoglobin level was 102 g/L. White blood count cell was 14.0×10^9/L, with granulocytes, 0.33; lymphocytes, 0.60; eosinophils, 0.04; and basophils, 0.03. Erythrocyte sedimentation rate (ESR) (Wintrobe) was elevated, IgG and IgM levels high, and rheumatoid factor assay (Organon) positive (Table). Antinuclear antibody assay was negative on peripheral blood and HEp-2 cells.

Chest roentgenography showed a generally enlarged heart (cardiothoracic ratio, 0.6) with vascular congestion. Echocardiographic examination revealed a moderately enlarged and nonhypertrophied left ventricle with depressed contractility (Table). Her left atrium was also enlarged. No pericardial effusion was noted. The electrocardiogram showed slightly decreased voltages, nonspecific T-wave changes, and sinus tachycardia. Anti–streptolysin O titer, anti-DNase, and antibodies to Epstein-Barr virus, toxoplasma, and varicella zoster were not detected. Only low titers of antibody were found to rubella, adenovirus, and cytomegalovirus. Acute and convalescent titers to coxsackievirus B1 through 6 showed no significant interval change.

Biopsy of the affected area of her legs (Fig 2) showed varying degrees of perivascular lymphocytic infiltration around the dermal capillaries and interstitial fibrosis. Increased cellularity was also noted around dermal appendages. The fascia and subcutaneous fat were severely inflamed, with some inflammation of the muscle itself, and diffuse interstitial fibrosis accompanied by hypertrophy of muscular arteries in the fibrofatty tissue around the muscle. Several small vessels in the perimysium showed mild perivascular lymphocytic infiltration. Immunofluorescent staining for immunoglobulin deposition and C3 was negative, and electron microscopy showed no immune complexes or viruslike structures.

During the next month, with 2 mg/kg per day of prednisone

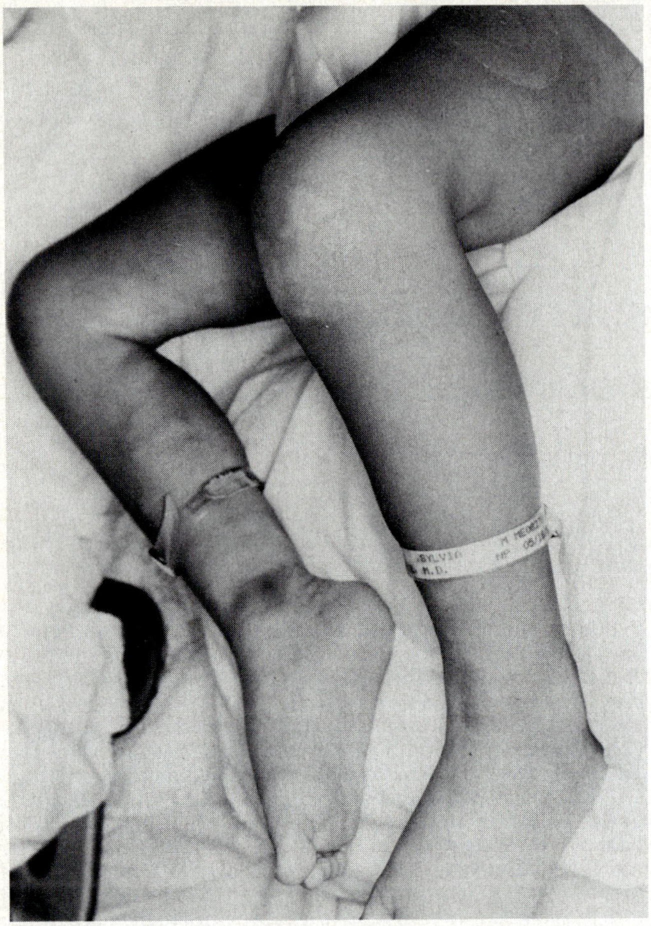

Fig 1.—*The patient at 21 months. The involved areas are hypopigmented and indurated. Contractures are present in knees, hips, and ankles.*

given as 9 mg orally three times daily, digoxin (Lanoxin), and physical therapy to her legs, the patient became less irritable and had some increase in range of motion. Her cardiac gallop disappeared, and her left atrium and ventricle decreased in size, though severely depressed left ventricular function remained. A right-sided Horner's syndrome developed. The initially positive rheumatoid factor assay became negative, and the ESR became normal during the first month.

After 6 weeks, the dose of prednisone was slowly tapered. The IgM level, which initially increased to 7.70 g/L after 6 weeks of therapy, decreased over several months. The elevated IgG level became normal after about 2.5 months. The ESR rose again in the third month, when the mother inadvertently and abruptly decreased the steroid dose. The ESR promptly returned to normal as prednisone therapy was resumed. By 4 months after the initiation of treatment, the child had a completely normal heart by clinical examination, chest roentgenography, and echocardiogram (Table) and had regained sufficient mobility of her legs to resume walking.

The digoxin therapy was discontinued at 15 months and the prednisone therapy at 16 months. The abnormal skin in the axillary areas became normal to the touch and hyperpigmented rather than white.

Although the skin on her legs remained tight, it became less hard and hyperpigmented rather than white (Fig 3). Her right ankle remained essentially fused in equinus and required later surgical release to improve her gait. The Horner's syndrome became inapparent, though the mother has reported occasional drooping of the child's eyelid. Seven years after presentation, the child has had no further internal organ involvement, and her skin disease has shown no further progression.

Cardiac and Laboratory Findings Initially and After 4 mo of Therapy

	Initial Findings	At 4 mo
L ventricular end-diastolic volume index, mL/m²	162	75
shortening fraction	0.17	0.36
ejection fraction	0.35	0.67
Aortic preejection time/ejection time	0.56	0.32
Cardiothoracic ratio	0.6	0.51
Erythrocyte sedimentation rate (Wintrobe)	44	8
IgG, g/L	31.00	8.60
IgM, g/L	4.26	2.80 (at 7 mo)
Rheumatoid factor	1:80	Negative
Antinuclear antibody	Negative	Negative

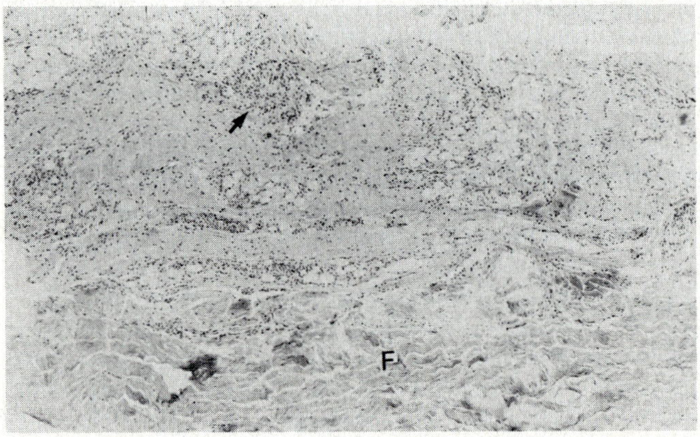

Fig 2.—*Microphotograph of perifascial tissue. Note the diffuse fibrosis of perifascial subcutaneous tissue with chronic inflammatory infiltrates (arrow; F indicates fascia; hematoxylin-eosin, × 40).*

COMMENT

A coincidental viral myocarditis in this patient cannot be totally excluded; also, that a viral agent may have initiated both processes must be considered, though we did not succeed in identifying a candidate virus for this role. However, the reports of echocardiographic changes with focal scleroderma,[14] the sclerodermatous changes in the heart in the patient of Rodnan and Fennel,[3] and the rarity of both cardiomyopathy and focal scleroderma suggest that the association of the two in our patient may be more than coincidental.

It may be debated that internal organ involvement together with any type of skin finding of scleroderma should be considered PSS, but the morphea plaques in the axillae and the involvement of the skin, subcutaneous tissue, and muscle of the legs and feet in our patient were characteristic of linear scleroderma[5,15] and unlike the skin changes in PSS. Also, there has been no subsequent involvement of internal organs in 7 years of observation, and her skin involvement has not progressed further.

Focal scleroderma, if sufficiently localized, often requires no specific treatment and may undergo spontaneous remission or arrest, with approximately 80% of patients no longer having persistent or recurrent activity after the first 2 years.[1] Children with limb contractures

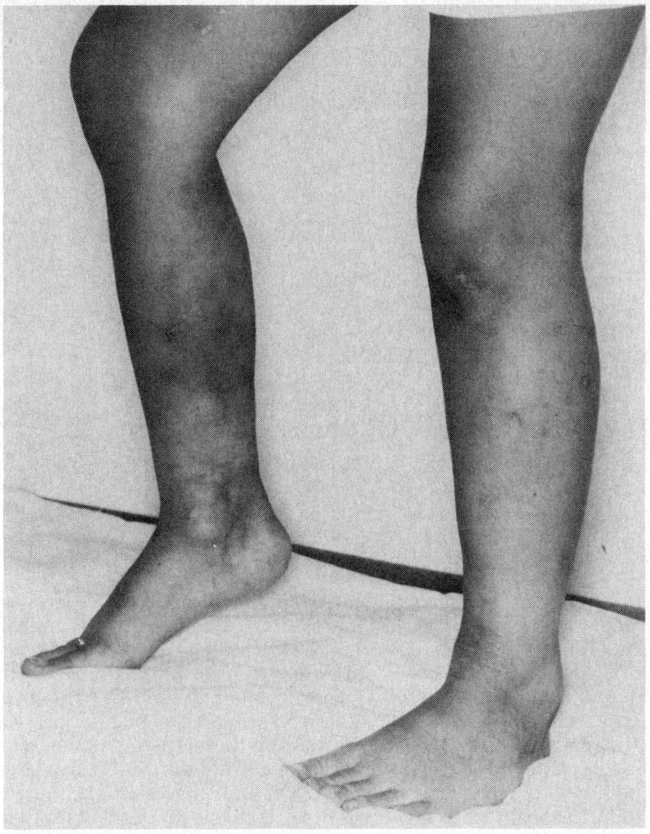

Fig 3.—*At 36 months, the skin had become hyperpigmented rather than white. Contractures are limited to the ankles. There has been further loss of subcutaneous tissue, particularly on the right lower leg and the medial side of the left foot.*

may benefit from an intensive physical therapy program to decrease residual deformity, and some patients later require surgery to improve function.

In some instances, where the disease is progressive and appears likely to be cosmetically or functionally disastrous, or both, or is associated with some form of systemic involvement, definitive treatment would be desirable. As in PSS, no really definitive treatment is known.

Corticosteroids are generally found ineffective, though in some cases[2,15-19] improvement is reported. Improvement is thought more likely where inflammation (rather than fibrosis) is more pronounced and more acute.[16] This child had a short history and had laboratory evidence of inflammation. Though it cannot be proved that the prednisone was responsible for her improvement, her prompt response in the face of severe illness makes it likely. The brief flare-up in her ESR in the third month when her mother inadvertently and markedly decreased the dose also suggests the effect of prednisone. Although it cannot yet be predicted which patients with focal scleroderma might respond, a trial of steroids may be warranted in the more severely afflicted patients, especially when the disease appears to be acute and inflammatory.

Other agents that have been proposed for the treatment of focal scleroderma include sulfasalazine,[20] etretinate,[21] and penicillamine.[22] The last drug, which appears the most promising, has received several recent favorable reports regarding its use in PSS.[1] It interferes with the intramolecular cross-linking of collagen and is also immunosuppressive. It may be worth trying when progressive fibrosis is likely to cause severe morbidity. This drug has multiple potential side effects, however, and must be carefully monitored.

In summary, we report the case of an infant with focal scleroderma and cardiomyopathy. The possibility of internal organ involvement, including cardiac involvement, must be considered with focal scleroderma as well as with PSS.

References

1. Medsger T. Systemic sclerosis (scleroderma), localized scleroderma, eosinophilic fascitis, and calcinosis. In: McCarty DJ, ed. *Arthritis and Allied Conditions.* 11th ed. Philadelphia, Pa: Lea & Febiger; 1989.
2. Leinwand J, Duryee AW, Richter MN. Scleroderma (based on a study of over 150 cases). *Ann Intern Med.* 1954;41:1003-1041.
3. Rodnan GP, Fennel RH. Progressive systemic sclerosis in scleroderma. *JAMA.* 1962;180:665-670.
4. Bourgeois-Droin C, Fouroine R. Sclerodermie en plaques. Perturbation immunologiques et viscerales. *Ann Med Interne.* 1978;129:107-112.
5. Stern LZ, Payne CM, Alvarez JT, Hannapel LK. Myopathy associated with linear scleroderma: a histochemical and electron microscopic study. *Neurology.* 1975;25:114-119.
6. Hanson V, Kornreich H, Drexler E. Some immunological consideration in focal scleroderma and progressive systemic sclerosis in children. *Pediatr Res.* 1974;8:806-809.
7. Warin AP. Acute scleroderma (morphea) with myositis. *Proc R Soc Med.* 1973;66:621-623.
8. Hanson V, Drexler E, Kornreich H. Rheumatoid factor (antigamma-globulins) in children with focal scleroderma. *Pediatrics.* 1974;53:945-947.
9. Stogmann W, Sandhofer M, Fritz J. Immunological studies in childhood scleroderma. *Eur J Pediatr.* 1977;124:223-230.
10. Sainan EM, Peachey RDG. Vitiligo and morphea. *Clin Exp Dermatol.* 1979;4:103-106.
11. Scarole JA, Shulman LE. Serologic abnormalities and their significance in localized scleroderma. *Arthritis Rheum.* 1975;18:526.
12. D'Angelo WA, Fries JF, Masi AT, Shulman LE. Pathologic observation in systemic sclerosis (scleroderma): a study of 58 autopsy cases and 58 matched controls. *Am J Med.* 1969;46:428-440.
13. Suarez-Almazor ME, Catoggio LJ, Maldonado-Cocco JA, Cuttica R, Garcia-Marteo D. Juvenile progressive systemic sclerosis: clinical and serological findings. *Arthritis Rheum.* 1985;28:699-702.
14. Gottdiener JS, Moutsopoulos CM, Decker JL. Echocardiographic identification of cardiac abnormality in scleroderma and related disorders. *Am J Med.* 1979;66:391-398.
15. Jablonska S. *Scleroderma and Pseudoscleroderma.* 2nd ed. Warsaw, Poland: Polish Medical Publishers; 1975.
16. Person JR, Daniel WP. Subcutaneous morphea: a clinical study of sixteen cases. *Br J Dermatol.* 1979;100:371-380.
17. Hazen PG, Walker AE, Carney JF, Stewart JJ. Cutaneous calcinosis of scleroderma: successful treatment with intralesional adrenal steroids. *Arch Dermatol.* 1982;118:366-367.
18. Rowell NR. Lupus erythematosus, scleroderma and dermatomyositis: the 'collagen' or 'connective-tissue' diseases. In: Rook A, Wilkinson DA, Ebling FJG, eds. *Textbook of Dermatology.* 3rd ed. Boston, Mass: Blackwell Scientific Publications Inc; 1979;2:1205.
19. Oka M, Ruotski A. Positive immuno-reactions in a case of unilateral scleroderma or progressive hemiatrophy. *Acta Rheum Scand.* 1969;15:29-34.
20. Czarbecki DP, Toft EH. Generalized morphea successfully treated with salazopyrine. *Acta Derm Venereol.* 1982;62:81-82.
21. Neuhofer J, Fritsch P. Treatment of localized scleroderma and lichen sclerosis with etretinate. *Acta Derm Venereol.* 1984;64:171-174.
22. Moynahan EJ. Morphea (localized cutaneous scleroderma) treated with low-dosage penicillamine (4 cases, including coup de sabre). *Proc R Soc Med.* 1973;66:1083-1085.

Chronic Neutropenia During Childhood

A 13-Year Experience in a Single Institution

Olafur G. Jonsson, MD, George R. Buchanan, MD

• To evaluate the clinical course and characteristics of children with chronic neutropenia, we reviewed the charts of all such patients seen at our center during a 13-year period. A total of 50 patients with chronic neutropenia were identified. Three patients had documented congenital neutropenia, and two siblings had cyclic neutropenia. The remaining 45 children had chronic neutropenia of unknown origin. All children except two had a remarkably benign course despite markedly reduced granulocyte counts. Of six girls in this group who had abscess or cellulitis of the labia majora, it was a presenting manifestation in three. Resolution of neutropenia was documented in 23 (62%) of 37 patients for whom follow-up information was available, with a median duration of neutropenia of 19 months. No differences were evident between patients with positive antineutrophil antibody test results and those in whom the test yielded negative results or was not performed. Chronic neutropenia in childhood is a relatively uncommon entity, characterized by a benign course and eventual resolution in the majority of patients.

(*AJDC*. 1991;145:232–235)

The chronic neutropenias of childhood are a group of disorders with a variable clinical course, ranging from death in early infancy to a benign condition often discovered incidentally.[1-3] The etiology, pathogenesis, natural history, and relative incidence of childhood neutropenia have been unclear, as reflected by confusing nomenclature[4,5] and a lack of general reviews of chronic neutropenia describing overall experiences at a single institution. We have noted that some children initially diagnosed as having congenital neutropenia subsequently had spontaneous and permanent remissions, seemingly inconsistent with the diagnosis.[6] In an attempt to clarify some of these uncertainties regarding chronic neutropenia and to identify common features among these patients, we reviewed the charts of patients with neutropenia seen at our center during a 13-year period. We found that most children with chronic idiopathic neutropenia had a relatively benign course that was indistinguishable from that described previously for patients with autoimmune neutropenia.

Accepted for publication March 19, 1990.

From the Department of Pediatrics, University of Texas Southwestern Medical Center, and the Children's Medical Center, Dallas.

Reprint requests to the Department of Pediatrics, 5323 Harry Hines Blvd, Dallas, TX 75235-9063 (Dr Buchanan).

PATIENTS AND METHODS

All patients referred for consultation to the Division of Hematology-Oncology at the Children's Medical Center of Dallas, Tex, from January 1, 1977, to December 31, 1989, with the primary diagnosis of neutropenia were identified from departmental files. Patients with other primary diagnoses known to cause neutropenia (eg, leukemia, preleukemic states, aplastic anemia, collagen-vascular disease, and hypersplenism) were not included in this listing even though neutropenia might have been noted at some time during their illnesses. Inpatient and outpatient charts on all patients were reviewed, with particular attention directed to the duration and severity of neutropenia, possible underlying diseases, frequency and severity of infection, and exposure to drugs. Physical findings were recorded, as were results of serial complete blood cell counts, serum immunoglobulin measurements, and antineutrophil antibody tests. Results of bone marrow examinations were obtained from pathology reports. Serum antineutrophil antibody levels were measured at the University of Michigan, Ann Arbor, using an indirect immunofluorescence assay.[7] Every effort was made to obtain follow-up information on patients by contacting their primary physicians.

Neutropenia was defined as an absolute neutrophil count (absolute neutrophil count equals the percent of neutrophils and band cells times the total white blood cell count divided by 100) of less than 1.5×10^9/L.[8] Chronic neutropenia was defined as neutropenia lasting more than 8 weeks. Patients were classified as having congenital neutropenia only when a complete blood cell count documenting neutropenia was available before age 3 months and the neutropenia persisted.

RESULTS

During this 13-year period, 101 patients were listed as having a primary diagnosis of neutropenia, as shown in Table 1. Fifty of these patients had chronic neutropenia and 51 had transient neutropenia. We will not discuss the patients with transient neutropenia.

Two siblings had cyclic neutropenia. One of them died at age 5 years of *Staphylococcus aureus* septicemia; the other was alive at age 6 years with relatively few infectious complications. Only several familial cases of cyclic neutropenia have been described previously.[9,10]

Three patients had congenital neutropenia. One of them had *S aureus* septicemia as an infant but has done well except for frequent episodes of otitis media, skin infections, and gingivitis. He remained profoundly neutropenic at age 16 years, but recently was treated with recombinant granulocyte colony-stimulating factor, with normalization of his neutrophil count.[11] The other two patients with congenital neutropenia are identical twins who were both noted to be neutropenic at birth. They were

Table 1.—All Patients With a Primary Diagnosis of Neutropenia Seen at Children's Medical Center of Dallas, 1977 Through 1989	
Type of Neutropenia	**No. of Patients**
Chronic	
Congenital	3
Cyclic	2
Severe	2
Other (benign)	43
Total	**50**
Transient	
Viral infection	16
Drugs	12
Underlying disease	8
Neonatal	7
Other	8
Total	**51**

aged 9 years at the time of this report and remained neutropenic (absolute neutrophil count, approximately 0.5×10^9/L) but have had few infectious complications.

Clinical Features

The remaining 45 patients are the main subjects of this report. They were generally healthy infants who came to medical attention because of fever and recurrent minor infections and were then found to be neutropenic. Only two patients had severe and recurrent infectious complications; both had measurable antineutrophil antibodies in their serum. One patient was a 6-year-old white girl with massive lymphadenopathy and hepatosplenomegaly and recurrent mouth ulcers; her bone marrow aspirate showed maturation arrest at the promyelocyte stage. She continued to be severely neutropenic despite various therapeutic interventions, including corticosteroids, intravenous immunoglobulin, and granulocyte-macrophage colony-stimulating factor, but at age 9 years the neutropenia had resolved concomitantly with cyclosporin A treatment. The other severely affected patient was an 8-year-old boy with profound neutropenia whose bone marrow aspirate showed granulocyte aplasia[12] but otherwise normal elements. He responded temporarily to prednisone therapy but remained markedly neutropenic and died of pneumonia and sepsis 6 weeks after the administration of antithymocyte globulin at another institution.

The median age of these 45 patients at the onset of neutropenia was 12 months (range, 3 to 144 months). Thirty-six (80%) of the 45 patients were younger than age 24 months when neutropenia was diagnosed. The male-female ratio was 1:1. Infections were frequent in this group of patients but they were generally mild (eg, upper respiratory infections, otitis media, and skin infections). One patient had periorbital cellulitis and another had one episode of pneumonia.

As listed in Table 2, six of the 23 girls in this patient population had an abscess or cellulitis involving the labia majora at some time during the duration of neutropenia. This infection was a presenting manifestation in three of these patients. *Pseudomonas aeruginosa* was cultured from three of these children. One patient had recurrent *Pseudomonas* labial infections. Invasive bacterial infections other than those mentioned above were not observed.

The physical examination was unremarkable in most patients with chronic neutropenia, with the exception of mild splenomegaly in six patients. One of the two severely affected patients had massive hepatosplenomegaly, and

Table 2.—Cellulitis or Abscess Involving the Labia Majora in Girls With Chronic Idiopathic Neutropenia

Patient	Age, mo*	Duration of Neutropenia*	Organism	Antineutrophil Antibody Test Results
1	15	At onset	Unknown	Negative
2	66	12 mo	*Pseudomonas aeruginosa* (with positive blood culture)	Positive
3	11	3 mo	Unknown	Not performed
4	9	At onset	*P aeruginosa*	Not performed
5	6	At onset	*P aeruginosa* (three episodes)	Positive
6	7	2 mo	Unknown	Positive

*When labial lesion occurred.

prominent lymphadenopathy was noted in four children. Recurrent gingivitis or mouth ulcers were a significant complaint in only three patients.

Laboratory Studies

Neutrophil counts were extremely low in all patients. The lowest recorded absolute neutrophil count was unmeasurable in nine patients; less than 0.2×10^9/L in 34 (76%) of 45 children; and less than 0.5×10^9/L in all but two patients. The median lowest value for the group was 0.1×10^9/L. Very low absolute neutrophil counts persisted in most patients, with temporary fluctuations into the normal range observed only occasionally.

An increased percentage of circulating blood monocytes was noted intermittently, but the number of monocytes did not clearly correlate with the degree of neutropenia or the presence of infection.

The median hemoglobin level at presentation was 118 g/L (range, 90 to 138 g/L). The hemoglobin concentration was more than 100 g/L in all but four patients, one of whom had β-thalassemia trait and two of whom had documented iron deficiency. Platelet counts were normal or mildly elevated in all patients.

Quantitative serum immunoglobulin levels were measured in 23 of the 45 patients and were within normal limits in 12 patients and only slightly elevated in another nine patients. One of the severely affected patients had a low IgA level and a high IgM level, and another patient had low IgG levels.

Serum antineutrophil antibody measurements, performed in 28 of the 45 patients, were positive in 13 patients and negative in 15 patients. There was no relationship between the severity of symptoms of neutropenia and the presence or absence of antineutrophil antibodies. As indicated in Table 3, no other differences could be detected between groups when patients were classified according to the antineutrophil antibody test result.

Bone marrow aspiration was carried out in 31 patients. In 28 of these patients the bone marrow was entirely normal or had only decreased numbers of neutrophils. Both of the severely affected patients described above had maturation arrest at an early stage in granulocyte development. Only one mildly affected patient had an early granulocyte maturation arrest.

Characteristic	All Patients (N=45)	Antineutrophil Antibody Results: Positive (n=13)	Negative (n=15)	Not Performed (n=17)
Male-female ratio	22:23	5:8	9:6	8:9
Mean age (range) at diagnosis of neutropenia, mo	12 (3-144)	10 (3-92)	16 (6-144)	12 (6-132)
Mean age (range) at resolution, mo	38 (10-114)	38 (10-114)	38 (21-86)	34 (15-72)
Mean duration (range) of neutropenia, mo	19 (6-64)	19 (7-45)	27 (11-61)	14 (6-64)
Mean (range) lowest recorded absolute neutrophil count, $\times 10^9$/L	0.1 (0-0.52)	0.1 (0-0.27)	0.1 (0-0.34)	0.12 (0-0.52)
No. of patients with splenomegaly	7	2	2	3
No. of patients with normal or near normal* bone marrow	28	8	11	9
No. of patients for whom resolution of neutropenia was documented	23	9	6	8
No. of patients in whom neutropenia did not resolve	13	0	7	6

Table 3.—Characteristics of Patients With Chronic Idiopathic Neutropenia

*Reduced number of neutrophils the only abnormality.

Treatment and Outcome

All of these children were treated with supportive measures and antibiotics (usually oral) for febrile illnesses. Only two patients received prophylactic antibiotic treatment at the decision of the referring physician. It is noteworthy that bacterial pneumonia was diagnosed in just one of 43 patients; the two severely affected patients had several episodes of lower respiratory tract infections. The only other cases of invasive bacterial infections included one episode of periorbital cellulitis and infections of the labia majora in six girls. The frequency of minor infections lessened with age in almost all patients.

Excluding the two severely affected patients, only 12 of the 43 children with chronic neutropenia were hospitalized, for a total of 18 admissions. Eleven of these hospitalizations were for initial diagnostic evaluation.

Four patients were treated with corticosteroids. The two severely affected patients described above responded poorly. One of the two other patients did not respond, but the other had partial resolution of neutropenia and healing of mouth ulcers, which recurred when prednisone therapy was discontinued. Intravenous immunoglobulin preparations were given to the two severely affected patients without response.

Follow-up information was available on 37 children, as outlined in Table 3. In 23 (62%) of these children, resolution of the neutropenia was documented, with a median duration of neutropenia of 19 months. The median age at resolution was 38 months. Thirteen children were still neutropenic at last contact, with a median period from diagnosis to last available blood cell count of 18 months. Three of these 13 patients had normal blood cell counts documented before the onset of neutropenia. One patient died, and follow-up information was not available on the eight remaining patients. Excluding the two severely affected patients, the remaining 35 children on whom follow-up information was available were in good health.

COMMENT

Although neutropenia during childhood has many definable causes, there exists a large group of patients in whom no clear cause can be identified. It has been recognized that many of these patients with chronic idiopathic neutropenia have a benign clinical course, and only a minority of patients have severe recurrent infections.[4,13-16] Bacterial infections, although increased in frequency, are generally mild and usually respond well to antibiotic treatment; mortality is low or absent.[4,13-16] Such a benign course was evident in most of our patients with chronic neutropenia.

Autoimmune neutropenia has been recognized increasingly during the past several years.[16] An ill-defined entity called "chronic benign neutropenia" is very similar in presentation and clinical course to autoimmune neutropenia.[15,16] It has been suggested that most of these cases are actually autoimmune in origin and pathogenesis even though antineutrophil antibodies may not always be demonstrated.[15] Technical difficulties in performing antineutrophil antibody tests are well recognized, and the sensitivity and specificity of these assays have not been well defined.[7] No apparent difference existed in this study between patients with chronic neutropenia who did and did not have antineutrophil antibodies detectable in their serum. Thus, it seems possible that most children with chronic neutropenia of unclear origin have a disorder caused by immune mechanisms despite negative antineutrophil test results.

To our knowledge, cellulitis involving the perirectal area, groin, or face caused by *Pseudomonas* has been reported just once in association with chronic neutropenia.[6] Two additional reports mentioned an infection of the vulva or Bartholin's gland, but the offending organism was not stated.[2,15] It is noteworthy that six (26%) of the 23 girls in our series had abscess or cellulitis involving the labia majora at one time or another during the course of their disease. In three patients, *P aeruginosa* was documented as the offending organism. This is a very unusual infection in healthy girls and clearly should lead to the suspicion of neutropenia when encountered clinically.

Maturation arrest at an early stage of granulopoiesis has been described in the bone marrow of some patients with chronic neutropenia.[7,12] Bone marrow examination in our patients usually showed normal myeloid maturation except for decreased numbers of segmented neutrophils, a feature previously noted to be associated with autoimmune neutropenias.[4,15,16] Our data suggest that infants with the typical features of chronic idiopathic (presumably autoimmune) neutropenia may not require a routine bone marrow aspiration for purposes of diagnosis and treatment. However, the presence of any other abnormalities on the complete blood cell count should definitely prompt a bone marrow examination to exclude acute leukemia, aplastic anemia, or a myelodysplastic state.

All of our patients responded well to standard supportive measures. Intravenous γ-globulin and corticosteroids have been reported to induce temporary remissions in some children with autoimmune neutropenia,[16,17] but treatment with these agents should probably be reserved for those rare patients who manifest severe or especially frequent infectious complications. Recombinant hematopoietic growth factors, such as granulocyte-macrophage colony-stimulating factor or granulocyte colony-stimulating factor, may, in the near future, play an important role in the treatment of severely affected patients with congenital and other forms of neutropenia,[11] but will not be required for most children with chronic neutropenia.

This review does not allow an accurate estimate of the incidence of chronic neutropenia in childhood, but it does suggest that it is a relatively uncommon condition, since only 45 patients were diagnosed during a 13-year period in the only pediatric hematology referral center serving a population of 3.5 million people. Congenital neutropenia is an uncommon entity and may be overdiagnosed. Young children incidentally found to be neutropenic are more likely to have an autoimmune disorder than a congenital neutropenic state. Only one of our patients with congenital neutropenia had features consistent with Kostmann's syndrome or infantile genetic agranulocytosis.[3]

Most children with chronic neutropenia, irrespective of antineutrophil antibody test results, have a remarkably benign disorder that often eventually resolves. We propose that most such patients have an autoimmune disorder rather than a congenital neutropenic state.

This work was supported in part by the Children's Cancer Fund of Dallas, Tex.

We thank Dawn Miller and Patricia Ellisor for their expert secretarial assistance, and physicians in North Texas for referring their patients and providing follow-up information.

References

1. Stahlie TD. Chronic benign neutropenia in infancy and early childhood. *J Pediatr.* 1956;48:710-721.
2. Zuelzer WW, Bajoghli M. Chronic granulocytopenia in childhood. *Blood.* 1964;23:359-374.
3. Kostmann R. Infantile genetic agranulocytosis: a review with presentation of ten new cases. *Acta Pediatr Scand.* 1975;64:362-368.
4. Dale DC, DuPont G IV, Wewerka JR, Bull JM, Chusid MJ. Chronic neutropenia. *Medicine.* 1979;58:128-143.
5. Pincus SH, Boxer LA, Stossel TP. Chronic neutropenia in childhood: analysis of 16 cases and a review of the literature. *Am J Med.* 1976;61:849-860.
6. Parmley RT, Crist WM, Ragab AH, et al. Congenital dysgranulopoietic neutropenia: clinical, serologic, ultrastructural, and in vitro proliferative characteristics. *Blood.* 1980;56:465-475.
7. Madyastha PR, Fudenberg HH, Glassman AB, Madyastha KR, Smith CL. Autoimmune neutropenia in early infancy: a review. *Ann Clin Lab Sci.* 1982;12:356-367.
8. Curnutte JT, Boxer LA. Disorders of granulopoiesis and granulocyte function. In: Nathan DG, Oski FA, eds. *Hematology of Infancy and Childhood.* Philadelphia, Pa: WB Saunders Co; 1987:797-847.
9. Morley AA, Carew JP, Baikie AG. Familial cyclic neutropenia. *Br J Haematol.* 1967;13:719-739.
10. Wright DG, Dale DC, Fauci AS, Wolff SM. Human cyclic neutropenia: clinical review and long-term follow-up of patients. *Medicine.* 1981;60:1-12.
11. Bonilla MA, Gillio AP, Ruggeiro M, et al. Effects of recombinant human granulocyte colony-stimulating factor on neutropenia in patients with congenital agranulocytosis. *N Engl J Med.* 1989;320:1574-1580.
12. Levitt LJ, Ries CA, Greenberg PL. Pure white-cell aplasia: antibody-mediated autoimmune inhibition of granulopoiesis. *N Engl J Med.* 1983;308:1141-1146.
13. Greenberg PL, Mara B, Steed S, Boxer LA. The chronic idiopathic neutropenia syndrome: correlation of clinical features with in vitro parameters of granulopoiesis. *Blood.* 1980;55:915-920.
14. Ducos R, Madyastha PR, Warrier RP, Glassman AB, Shirley LR. Neutrophil agglutinins in idiopathic chronic neutropenia of early childhood. *AJDC.* 1986;140:65-68.
15. Conway LT, Clay ME, Kline WE, Ramsay NKC, Krivit W, McCullough J. Natural history of primary autoimmune neutropenia in infancy. *Pediatrics.* 1987;79:728-733.
16. Lalezari P, Khorshidi M, Petrosova M. Autoimmune neutropenia of infancy. *J Pediatr.* 1986;109:764-769.
17. Bussel J, Lalezari P, Hilgartner M, et al. Reversal of neutropenia with intravenous gammaglobulin in autoimmune neutropenia of infancy. *Blood.* 1983;62:398-400.

Instructions for Authors

New Manuscript Procedure

On January 1, 1988, *AJDC* initiated a new procedure. Manuscripts submitted to *AJDC* will NO LONGER BE RETURNED, except in the case of accepted manuscripts or those undergoing author revision. Original artwork and photographs will be returned.

General Information.—Please send manuscripts and correspondence by first-class mail *(do not use registered, certified, or express mail)* to the Editor, Vincent A. Fulginiti, MD, *AJDC*, Dean's Office, Room 1529, Tulane University, School of Medicine, 1430 Tulane Avenue, New Orleans, LA 70112. All accepted manuscripts are subject to copy editing. The corresponding author will receive an edited typescript and layout for approval. Forms for ordering reprints are included with the edited typescript. Reprints are shipped six to eight weeks after publication. Proofs will be sent for approval *if requested* by the author and if printing deadlines permit. The author is responsible for all statements in his/her work, including changes made by the copy editor.

Conforming with all of the steps listed below will facilitate the editorial processing of your manuscript.

Step 1.—*Cover Letter.*—All manuscripts must be accompanied on submission by a cover letter giving the name, address, affiliation, and telephone number of the corresponding author. The letter must include ALL of the following statements SIGNED BY ALL AUTHORS (ORIGINAL SIGNATURES):

1. *Copyright Release.*— "In consideration of the American Medical Association's taking action in reviewing and editing this submission, the author(s) undersigned hereby transfer(s), assign(s), or otherwise convey(s) all copyright ownership to the AMA in the event that this work is published by the AMA."

2. *Statement of Affirmation.*—"This manuscript has not been published anywhere in any language and is not under simultaneous consideration by another publication. This manuscript is original and ALL authors have seen and approve of its contents."

3. *Financial Disclosure.*—List all affiliations with or financial involvement in organizations or entities with a direct financial interest in the subject matter or material of the research discussed in the manuscript (eg, employment consultancies, stock ownership) OR include a statement disclaiming any such involvement. All such information will be held in confidence during the review process. Should the manuscript be accepted, the Editor will discuss with the author the extent of disclosures appropriate for publication. All accepted manuscripts become the permanent property of the publisher (AMA) and may not be published elsewhere without written permission from the AMA. After publication certain articles may appear in translation in the foreign-language edition(s) of *AJDC*.

Step 2.—*Manuscript Format.*—All articles submitted should have the following features:

1. Four copies of the manuscript should be submitted; three are for transmission to referees and one is to be retained in the editorial office. We prefer an original and three copies.

2. Manuscripts should be typed in triple-spaced format on heavy-duty white bond paper, 21.6×27.9 cm (8 ½×11 in) with 2.5-cm (1-in) margins. *Do not use justified right margins.*

3. Title should be no more than 75 characters.

4. Authors should be limited to six, all of whom have contributed to the study and manuscript preparation, are familiar with its substance, and are able to defend its conclusions.

5. The title page should give full names, degrees, and academic affiliations of all authors, address for request of reprints, and, if the manuscript was presented at a meeting, the organization, place, and exact date on which it was read.

6. Writing style should conform to proper English usage and syntax; consult the *American Medical Association Manual of Style*, available from Williams & Wilkins, 428 E Preston St, Baltimore, MD 21202.

7. Abstract should be limited to 135 words or less.

8. Each table should be typed, with a title, on a separate sheet of paper, with each line, including headings, *double-spaced*. Continuations should be on a second sheet with all headings repeated.

9. Use Système International (SI) measurements throughout the manuscript.

10. Illustrations should be high-contrast, glossy prints, in quadruplicate, unmounted and untrimmed; lettering should be legible after reduction to column size. Figure number, name of first author, and arrow indicating "top" should be typed on a gummed *label* and affixed on the back of each illustration. *Do not write directly on the print.*

Magnification and stain should be provided for histologic sections. Full-color illustrations should be submitted as 35-mm, positive color transparencies, mounted in cardboard and carefully packaged. Do not submit glass-mounted transparencies or color prints. Fee is $400 for up to six square-finished color illustrations that fit on one page. A letter of intent to pay the fee must accompany submission.

All photographs in which there is a possibility of patient identification should be accompanied by a signed statement of consent from both parents (or guardians). Covering eyes to mask identity is not sufficient.

11. References should be listed in order of their appearance in the text, type double-spaced, and in AMA format. Please follow the exact order of information and punctuation in the examples below. Note: List all authors and/or editors up to six; if more than six, list the first three and "et al."

Journal articles: Scott GB, Buck BE, Leterman JG, Bloom FL, Parks WP. Acquired immunodeficiency syndrome in infants. N Engl J Med. 1984;310:76-81.

Books: Naeye RL. How and when does antenatal hypoxia damage fetal brains? In: Kubli F, Patel N, Schmidt W, Linderkamp O, eds. *Perinatal Events and Brain Damage in Surviving Children.* New York, NY: Springer Verlag NY Inc; 1988:83-91.

Unpublished data, personal communications, or manuscripts "in preparation" or "submitted" should not be included in the list of references. Such material, if essential, may be incorporated in the body of the article.

Authors are responsible for the accuracy of the references.

12. Investigations involving human subjects require a specific statement in the "Methods" section that an appropriate institutional review board approved the project and/or that informed consent was obtained from both legal guardians and/or child, if appropriate.

13. Illustrations and tables from other publications should be suitably acknowledged, with written permission from *publisher* and *author*. Brief acknowledgements to specific contributors directly involved in the content of the manuscript may be placed at the end of the text, before the references. General acknowledgements will be deleted.

Step 3.—*Special Departments.*—Criteria for several special departments are given below.

1. *The Pediatric Forum.*— This is the place for comment, criticism, observations, and discussion of "issues of current concern and importance for children's health," in addition to letters that comment on articles in previous issues of *AJDC*. The Editor reserves the right to conduct review of and to edit all submissions. THE READER SHOULD SUBMIT TRIPLE-SPACED COPY CLEARLY MARKED 'FOR PUBLICATION' AND SIGNED BY ALL AUTHORS. REFERENCES, IF INCLUDED, SHOULD CONFORM TO THE USUAL AMA FORMAT. Copyright assignment, signed by all authors, must accompany the original submission.

2. *From Reseach to Relevance.*—PURPOSE: To focus on significant research that has a high probability of being translated into clinical usefulness.

3. *Educational Interventions.*—PURPOSE: To share information concerning any educational efforts in the broad field of pediatrics.

4. *Sports Medicine.*—PURPOSE: To provide current information related to the medical needs of young athletes, as pertinent to counseling young athletes and their parents regarding sports participation and practices contributing to the health maintenance of the athlete, as well as current concepts in the prevention, diagnosis, and treatment of sports-related illnesses and injuries.

5. *Picture of the Month.*—Submissions should be sent directly to Murray Feingold, MD, National Birth Defects Center, Kennedy Memorial Hospital, 30 Warren St, Brighton, MA 02135, and should conform to the format for original articles in terms of the text, references and illustrations.

6. *Radiological Case of the Month.*—Submissions should be sent directly to Beverly P. Wood, MD, University of Rochester Medical Center, 601 Elmwood Ave, PO Box 648, Rochester, NY 14642. Submissions should conform to the format for original articles in terms of the text, references, and illustrations.

Author's Checklist

___ 1. Cover letter with name, address, and telephone number of corresponding author.
___ 2. Copyright transmittal, affirmation, and financial statements signed by ALL authors.
___ 3. Original typed manuscript plus three copies.
___ 4. Triple-spacing; double-spacing for tables and legends.
___ 5. Right margins UNJUSTIFIED.
___ 6. Title 75 characters or less.
___ 7. Abstract included.
___ 8. References in proper format, cited in numerical order.
___ 9. Four sets of illustrations.
___ 10. Four sets of legends for illustrations.
___ 11. Proper consent forms for patient photographs.
___ 12. Permission forms for illustrations previously published elsewhere.

1991 Annual Meeting

The annual meeting of The American Pediatric Society, The Society for Pediatric Research, and The Ambulatory Pediatric Association will be held April 29 through May 2, 1991, at the New Orleans (La) Hilton and Rivergate Convention Center. For further information, contact the APS/SPR Association Headquarters, 2650 Yale Blvd SE, Suite 104, Albuquerque, NM 87106; (505) 764-9099; FAX (505) 842-8227; or the Ambulatory Pediatric Association, 6728 Old McLean Village, McLean, VA 22101; (703) 556-9222.

More on the *P* Value

Sir.—Brown's discussion[1] on the *P* value continues his elegant series of lucid dissertations on medical statistics. A brief clarification is needed, however, concerning the issue of multiple statistical tests and the risk of type I error. Such corrections to compensate for multiple tests on the same data set are important during "data dredging" expeditions, explorations of a data set in search of statistical differences that were not anticipated by the original study design or hypothesis. As Brown points out, there is one chance in 20 that any such comparison will be significant at the $P = .05$ level. The corrected *P* values also protect against the type I error, which can occur when "in examining the treatment means we notice a combination that we did not intend to test but which seems unexpectedly large."[2]

In contrast to the data dredger is the investigator who designs a prospective study to test specific hypotheses that involve comparisons of several end points. As long as the comparisons made were planned in advance and address variables that might reasonably be expected to change with the intervention under study, it is probably inappropriate to employ corrections of *P* values. For example, a study of the effects of a pressor drug would test the hypothesis that treatment would improve systemic blood pressure, cardiac output, and left ventricular contractility. It would be appropriate to define the significance of these changes as $P = .05$. Applying the Bonferroni correction to each would needlessly increase the possibility of missing real differences. However, if this investigator later decides to review the data to compare the incidence of acne, borborygmi, and divorce in the treated and control groups, outcomes not anticipated in the study design and unsupported by a specific hypothesis prior to examining the data, correction of these *P* values *would* be appropriate.

Although it is difficult to make hard and fast rules that apply in all situations, Armitage's conclusions[3] seem reasonable. Multiple comparison methods "are appropriate only when means are being compared in an exploratory way to see what might 'turn up.' When comparisons are made which flow naturally from the plan of the experiment or survey, the usual *t* test is appropriate."

The carefully crafted prospective study is a refined instrument to test hypotheses. Arbitrary application of statistical correction needlessly blunts this instrument. Data dredging is a clumsy but effective way to generate hypotheses. Conclusions derived from these fishing trips deserve correction and appropriate skepticism.

DAVID M. COULTER, MD
The University of Utah
Department of Pediatrics
Eighth Avenue and C Street
Salt Lake City, UT 84143

1. Brown GW. *P* values. *AJDC.* 1990;144:493-495.
2. Snedecor GW, Cochran WG. *Statistical Methods.* 7th ed. Ames, Iowa: Iowa State University Press; 1980:232.
3. Armitage P. *Statistical Methods in Medical Research.* Boston, Mass: Blackwell Scientific Publications Inc; 1971:207.

In Reply.—The essay on *P* values was meant to alert readers to possible adverse *numeric* consequences of repeated, mindless, automatic grinding out of statistical tests. (This kind of unplanned data dredging might employ an automaton named Robostat.) I also wanted to point out the usefulness of the binomial expansion $[(p+q)^n = 1.0]$ in some ordinary biomedical situations.

Dr Coulter raises an interesting technical issue in *hypothesis testing.* Hypothesis formation and testing are somewhat different, and much more complex, subjects than those addressed in the essay on *P* values. Research hypotheses involve elements that are much more "scientific" than mere probability phenomena. Researchers incorporate many elements into their hypotheses, elements such as prior experience, extrinsic knowledge, biologic plausibility, subjective judgments, and so on.

For example, the essay on *P* values omitted discussion of one-tailed vs two-tailed statistical tests. The decision whether to use a one-tailed or a two-tailed test depends on the judgment of the researcher; the algebra is incidental.

The letter mentions comparisons "planned in advance" that address variables that ". . . might *reasonably* be expected to change . . ." (emphasis added). Reasonableness is a function of hypothesis formation, not of algebra; the numbers are neutral.

It is not universally agreed among biostatistical authorities that no adjustment of separate *P* values is needed if the hypotheses are stated in advance of evaluating the observations. For example, Fleiss[1] discusses

This department of *AJDC* is reserved for comment, criticism, observation, and discussion of "issues of current concern and importance for children's health." The Editor encourages our readers to express themselves on a variety of topics and issues. Further, we encourage the submission of unique and brief clinical and scientific observations that do not fulfill the criteria for original articles.

the Bonferroni adjustment in comparisons ". . . specified before the data are examined. . . ."

There is general agreement that statistical tests are more credible when used to evaluate hypotheses stated prior to examing the data. A pioneer in pediatric research, William Silverman, MD, tells of the rifleman who displays his bullet lodged in the center of a bull's eye drawn on the side of a barn. Was the target there before the shot was fired, or was the shot fired, and then the target drawn around the bullet?

George W. Brown, MD
PO Box 1269
Los Lunas, NM 87031

1. Fleiss JL. *The Design and Analysis of Clinical Experiments*. New York, NY: John Wiley & Sons Inc; 1986:104.

Multiple Comparisons and *P* Values

Sir.—We would like to comment on the multiple-comparisons problem posed by Brown[1] in his recent contribution about *P* values. The problem is: why should an investigator who wishes to compare treatments A and B be required to demonstrate a greater level of statistical significance if he or she studies treatment C at the same time? On the one hand, there is an apparent need to protect against the increased risk of a type I error associated with making multiple comparisons. On the other hand, it is counterintuitive that the conclusion for the comparison between A and B differs depending on whether the investigator had the resources to study treatment C at the same time.

Brown suggested leaving this enigma to experts in probability. While we do not claim such expertise, we have offered an explanation of this apparent contradiction that some of our colleagues have found helpful.[2] The multiple-comparisons problem in statistics has a ready analogy in clinical medicine: the problem of interpreting a serum chemistry panel. It is true that a chemistry panel with 20 independent tests has a probability of about 64% of including at least one value outside of the "normal" (95%) range in a normal person. What a clinician usually needs to know, however, is not the probability of finding an abnormality in a normal person, but the probability that a person is abnormal, given an abnormal test result. That probability does not depend on how many other tests were done at the same time, but on the other characteristics of the patient, which determine his or her "prior probability" of having a particular disease.

In a patient with oliguria, for example, an elevated serum creatinine level is just as likely to indicate renal disease if it was ordered as part of a 20-test panel, as if it was ordered as a single test. The reason that so many laboratory abnormalities that turn up on chemistry panels do not represent real disease is that few of the tests were ordered because of a clinical suspicion of abnormality. In general, when we order a panel of 20 tests, we may be fishing for abnormalities we have no reason to suspect, whereas when we perform just one test on a patient, it is because we are suspicious that results from that particular test will be abnormal.

The same general principle holds for multiple statistical comparisons: often, the more comparisons investigators make, the less they know about what they are looking for.[3] The problem is not with the multiple comparisons themselves, but with the hypotheses being tested, which start out less likely to be true (low prior probability). Even with a statistically significant result, the evidence often remains unconvincing. Thus, when interpreting *P* values, as when evaluating patients, any "significant" results must be interpreted in the context of other evidence.

Thomas B. Newman, MD, MPH
Division of General Pediatrics
Department of Pediatrics
School of Medicine
University of California
74 New Montgomery St,
Suite 600
San Francisco, CA 94105

Warren S. Browner, MD, MPH
Division of General
Internal Medicine
Department of Medicine
School of Medicine
University of California
74 New Montgomery St,
Suite 600
San Francisco, CA 94105

1. Brown GW. *P* values. *AJDC*. 1990;144:493-495.
2. Browner WS, Newman TB. Are all significant *P* values created equal?: the analogy between diagnostic tests and clinical research. *JAMA*. 1987;257:2459-2463.
3. Rothman KJ. No adjustments are needed for multiple comparisons. *Epidemiology*. 1990;1:43-46.

P Values

Sir.—In his article on *P* values[1] published in the April 1990 issue of *AJDC*, Brown has made some very helpful comments on the meaning of *P* values and has drawn attention to the difficulties associated with performing repeated statistical comparisons on the same set of subjects. However, twice in his article he does not pay sufficient heed to his own advice.

First, he correctly points out that when a *t* test is used to compare the birth weights of two groups of infants and the significant *P* value is set at .05, the random variation in birth weights among the infants would suggest, wrongly, in about one comparison of 20, that an important difference between the two groups in average weight was present. He goes on to consider what happens when a second test, eg, on head circumference, is performed on the same group, and says "The chance of 'significant' [it should read, "nonsignificant"] on the first test is .95. The chance on both the first and second is $.95 \times .95$. The chance of 'significant' on either the first or second or both is $1 - .95^2 = .0975$."

However, the probability on both the first and second is $.95 \times .95$ if the two tests are independent, which is most unlikely in the example given. Actually, the chance on both the first and second could have any value between .05 and .10 depending on the extent of dependence between the two events. Herein is a difficulty Brown has not mentioned: we do not know the effective change in *P* value when we perform a second test on the same group of individuals, because we do not know the extent of dependence between the two tests. It is because of this uncertainty that biostatisticians prefer a simultaneous evaluation that involves a *P* value that is known.

The purpose of these comments is not the trivial one of pointing out that there is a small statistical error in Brown's calculations, but the vital one of emphasizing his message even more strongly—that researchers must be wary of performing repeated tests on the same data. If they select a significance level of .05, the first test they perform *will* be at the .05 level,

The Pediatric Forum

but subsequent tests *will not* be at that level, and decisions based on them are likely to be erroneous.

Second, Brown refers to a conundrum by O'Brien: "Suppose a clinical investigator at MegaClinic conducts a clinical trial on treatments A, B, and C in three groups of patients. At the conclusion of the trial, the data analyst might perform *three* comparisons: A vs B, A vs C, and B vs C. The well-trained analyst would see that the *P* value for each comparison should be adjusted downward from the overall $P \leq .05$. That is, he/she would penalize himself/herself for doing three statistical tests."

The point is that when the analyst, X, performs the first comparison (A vs B), there is no difficulty. When the second comparison, A vs C, is made, X is using the same group A as in the first comparison, and it is likely that the two comparisons are mutually dependent. The extent of dependence is unknown, and the *P* value effectively decreases by an unknown amount. When X performs the third comparison, B vs C, X is performing a test that is likely to have dependence with the first test, which used group B, and with the second test, which used group C. Hence, the *P* value should be adjusted, to an unknown extent, downward from the overall $P \leq .05$. The analyst *should* penalize himself/herself for doing three statistical tests.

On the other hand, "suppose that out in Podunk a study was conducted of just A vs B. Another investigator in Boondock studied A vs C. A third researcher in Foozball studied B vs C. They each used, quite appropriately, $P \leq .05$ for evaluating their two sample results. . . . Why should the investigator who has the most comprehensive overview of treatments A, B, and C be punished with an adjustment to the *P* value that is not imposed on the separate studies done in three less elaborate trials?" The answer is that, in the three separate studies, there is presumably no dependence between the tests performed and in the single study, there is likely to be unknown dependence.

If each group referred to in the "conundrum" consisted of 100 patients, altogether, 300 patients are in the first study. In the separate studies, each of the three comparisons involves 200 patients (ie, 600 patients altogether). As fewer patients are involved, we would expect the first investigation to be disadvantaged in some way compared with the second.

Analysts should heed Brown's warning that repeated statistical tests on the same elements or subjects introduce an increase in the risk of a type I error. In the same vein, Dr David Kleinbaum commented during a course on epidemiology held last year in Sydney, Australia, that "if you torture data sufficiently, they will eventually confess to something."

Ted Byrt, MEd
Clinical Epidemiology
and Biostatistics Unit
Royal Children's Hospital
Flemington Rd
Parkville, Victoria 3052,
Australia

1. Brown GW. *P* values. *AJDC*. 1990; 144:493-495.

Clavicular Fractures in Neonates: Frequency vs Significance

Sir.—I wish to thank Drs Joseph and Rosenfeld[1] for their evaluation of the frequency and presentation of clavicular fractures in newborns. This is useful information for "frontline" pediatricians like myself, but I would like to make the following comments.

The fact that the occurrence of newborn clavicular fractures has remained stable in the Western world during the past 85 years suggests to me that the New York State Health Department may be on the wrong track if it thinks that this is "an indicator of the quality of care."

Also, it seems that clavicular fractures are benign occurrences that virtually always heal well without intervention. The only reason then to diagnose clavicular fracture would be to explain irritability with motion or asymmetric Moro's reflexes. That suggests to me that, in children without these symptoms, there may be no reason to make a significant effort to make this diagnosis.

Michael J. O'Halloran, MD
Midelfort Clinic Ltd
733 W Clairemont Ave
Eau Claire, WI 54702-1510

1. Joseph PR, Rosenfeld W. Clavicular fractures in neonates. *AJDC*. 1990; 144:165-167.

In Reply.—Dr O'Halloran points out that the New York State Health Department may be on the wrong track in using frequency of newborn clavicle fracture as a guideline for quality of care. By and large, we think he may be correct. In addition, the requirement for reporting newborn clavicle fractures in New York State may lead to unnecessary documentation and costs without any effect on the quality of care.

Dr O'Halloran also points out that the only reason to diagnose newborn clavicle fractures would be to explain symptoms, such as unexplained irritability. Another reason to diagnose newborn clavicle fractures is to prevent embarrassment at the first office visit when a large callus is felt covering the healthy broken clavicle. Additionally, we would prefer to make the diagnosis rather than to have the parent bring the callus to our attention on or before the first visit.

Paul R. Joseph, MD
Warren Rosenfeld, MD
Department of Pediatrics
Winthrop-University Hospital
259 First St
Mineola, NY 11501

Clavicular Fractures in Neonates

Sir.—We read with interest the article by Joseph and Rosenfeld[1] in the February 1990 issue of *AJDC*. We have noticed an increased occurrence of clavicular fractures in our institution during the last 6 months (12 [1.48%] of 812 newborns). We looked at different variables, including maternal age, parity, infant's weight, maternal diabetes, length of labor, oxytocin (Pitocin) induction, delivery methods, local anesthesia, episiotomy, delivery time, and delivering physician (house staff or attending staff) to find the common factor(s) in these infants.

The only common factor for seven of the affected infants was a shorter second stage of labor (mean, 11.4 minutes). In contrast to the authors' observation that only one of the 18 infants showed "classic" physical findings, we diagnosed fractures in 11 of 12 infants by the palpation of instability or crepitation over the fracture site. Roentgenography was used to confirm our clinical diagnosis. In one case, two of us (G.C. and J.P.) and an orthopedist felt a subtle crepitation at the distal end of one clavicle; however, roentgenography failed to reveal a clear fracture.

We noticed that a small number of

our patients (3 of 12) required two examinations (the second examination on the second day of life) to make a diagnosis, whereas most of Joseph and Rosenfeld's patients were diagnosed on the second day. The exact frequency of clavicular fracture in the neonatal period is not known, but the rates reported by Farkas and Levine[2] (1.7%) and Enzler[3] (2.6%) seem to be reasonable estimations.

We would like to remind readers that clavicular fractures are not limited to large infants, who may require a prolonged second stage of labor. On the contrary, more than half of the affected infants in our institution were born after a rather precipitous labor. We believe a daily, thorough physical examination in the nursery, instead of a superficial examination in a hasty fashion, would enable us to detect almost all of the clavicular fractures while the infant is still in the nursery.

Gloria Carter, RN, PNP
Jay W. Park, MD
Department of Pediatrics
Charles Tarvin, MD
Department of Obstetrics/Gynecology
Texas Tech University Health Sciences Center
Regional Academic Health Center at Odessa
Odessa, TX 79763

1. Joseph PR, Rosenfeld W. Clavicular fractures in neonates. *AJDC*. 1990;144:165-167.
2. Farkas R, Levine S. X-ray incidence of fractured clavicle in vertex presentation. *Am J Obstet Gynecol*. 1950;59:204-206.
3. Enzler A. Die Claviculafraktur als Geburtsverletzung des Neugeborenen. *Schweiz Med Worchenschr*. 1950;80:1280-1283.

In Reply.—Carter et al make several excellent points. The most interesting is the observation that the second stage of labor was short for seven of the 12 newborns with clavicle fractures. It would be interesting to know the length of the second stage of labor for the other 800 infants without clavicle fractures. Unfortunately, we did not analyze our data with regard to the length of second stage of labor.

We also found it interesting that at one institution, Carter et al clinically found a high incidence (12 [1.5%] of 812 newborns) of newborn clavicle fractures. It would be interesting to know whether the 800 infants without clavicle fractures had been examined for evidence of clavicle callus at approximately 2 to 4 weeks of age.

Paul R. Joseph, MD
Warren Rosenfeld, MD
Department of Pediatrics
Winthrop-University Hospital
259 First St
Mineola, NY 11501

What About Gay Teenagers?

Sir.—We read with great interest and careful attention the two articles[1,2] that appeared in the June issue of *AJDC* highlighting preventive aspects of pediatric injury, including suicide. Both of these well-written and researched reports placed great emphasis on the preventability of injury, as well as intervention strategies and suggestions for further research. Indeed, such emphasis is a most significant aspect of pediatric and adolescent medical practice, and much of our office time is devoted to the education of children, teenagers, and their parents.

During our study of these articles, we found the omission of a most important topic, one that brings into focus the existence of the gay (homosexual) teenager. Although adolescent suicide, including the causes and suggestions for prevention, is discussed, the gay adolescent was not mentioned.

Gay teenagers most certainly exist. At least 10% of our country's population is gay, and there are approximately 2.9 million gay adolescents in the United States.[3] Not only do gay youth exist, but they are made quite vulnerable by prevailing societal attitudes toward gays. Some feel so badly about their sexuality and about themselves that suicide can become a possible solution to perceived problems.[4,5] According to the US Public Health Service,[6] gay youths are estimated to be two to three times more likely to attempt suicide as their heterosexual peers, and it is believed that as many as 30% of suicides annually are those of gay teenagers. This is obviously a most significant problem.

As health care providers, we need to be concerned about these teenagers. If health professionals can prevent just one adolescent suicide or help just one gay teenager feel good about himself or herself, then they will be doing well. Therefore, we wish to include the topic of the gay adolescent for serious consideration in intervention and research on the problem of adolescent suicide. This should include methods of helping health professionals recognize the existence and legitimacy of gay youth and to behave in ways that demonstrate to gay teenagers that they are valid and wholesome human beings.

We strongly believe that professionals in the field of pediatric and adolescent medicine should attempt to communicate to all their patients a humanistic acceptance of and respect for alternate life-styles and to treat gay teenagers with the dignity and respect they so justly deserve. We all need to convey the message that it is perfectly acceptable to be gay.

A network of community resources needs to be identified, including organizations and educational materials whose aim is to communicate to our youth that they are not alone, and that the very special feelings that our gay youth need to confront are valid and quite wholesome and good.

We hope that more research will be done and more articles written about ways to decrease pediatric and adolescent morbidity and mortality. We also hope that these reports will discuss and describe ways for health professionals to reduce the grave injury being done to 10% of our youth, much of which is fostered by societal silence and neglect.

Charles R. Fikar, MD
Mary Koslap-Petraco, BSN, RN
PO Box 306
Deer Park, NY 11729

1. Division of Injury Control, Center for Environmental Health and Injury Control, Centers for Disease Control. Childhood injuries in the United States. *AJDC*. 1990;144:627-646.
2. Holinger PC. The causes, impact, and preventability of childhood injuries in the United States: childhood suicide in the United States. *AJDC*. 1990;144:670-676.
3. Sladkin KR, Krajeski J, Owen WF. The gay adolescent. *Audio-Digest Pediatrics*. 1984;30:1-4.
4. Remafedi G. Adolescent homosexuality: psychosocial and medical implications. *Pediatrics*. 1987;79:331-337.
5. Kourany RFC. Suicide among homosexual adolescents. *J Homosex*. 1987;13:111-116.
6. Gibson P. Gay male and lesbian youth suicide. In: *Report of the Secretary's Task Force on Youth Suicide*. Washington, DC: US Public Health Service; 1989:3-110–3-142.

EDITORIAL

Pediatric Legal Medicine

A New Venture

Medicine can no longer insist on dealing only with issues that relate to health and disease. Our educational, practice, and research efforts take place in a societal milieu that both reflects what we do and comments on it. Ethical, economic, social, and legal issues abound in society and affect us directly or indirectly. AJDC *has attempted to reflect these societal trends and influences by accepting or soliciting articles, editorials, letters, and commentaries on such topics. As Dr Ferry indicates in the following editorial,* AJDC *now is prepared to formalize one of these sets of issues, the legal environment in which we exist. As she states, this new department will be broad-based, not narrowly focused on any single issue. Articles will highlight some of the major legal issues in our communities. We look forward both to the inclusion of such information in the pages of our journal and to your responses as involved readers.*—V.A.F.

With this issue, *AJDC* inaugurates a new column, "Pediatric Legal Medicine." The stimulus for this column was a lunch in Bethesda, Md, in the fall of 1989, when my respected colleague Karin Nelson, MD, suggested, "Isn't it time a leading pediatric journal had a specific column on legal issues affecting children and pediatricians?" Both of us agreed that, over the years, legal considerations have had a serious impact on the practice of pediatrics.

As noted in a recent textbook, *Legal Aspects of Medicine*, "There is hardly a physician who has not been deeply troubled by legal problems professionally, economically, and, most important of all, psychologically."[1]

The concept was presented to the *AJDC* Editorial Board at its Spring 1989 meeting in Chicago, Ill, and enthusiastically endorsed. Strong caveats were issued, however, that the new forum should not just be a "malpractice column" but should reflect broader issues relating to children and the law in today's society.

See also p 275.

To assist in the development of this new enterprise, I have asked a small sub-board of knowledgeable individuals to assist me. These include Eileen Ouellette, MD, a pediatric neurologist at Massachusetts General Hospital, Boston, who recently completed her law degree and will specialize in medicolegal issues affecting children; Lynn D. Fleisher, PhD, JD, a Chicago attorney/geneticist who has written previously in *AJDC* on wrongful births and liability for prenatal injury[2]; and Robert L. Brent, MD, from the Department of Pediatrics, Jefferson Medical College, Philadelphia, Pa, who has written and spoken out forcefully on a number of medicolegal issues, particularly the inappropriate expert witness.[3] In addition, I have asked William O. Robertson, MD, from the Department of Pediatrics, University of Washington Medical School, Seattle, to serve as liaison between the new column and the Medical-Legal Section of the American Academy of Pediatrics, Elk Grove Village, Ill.

Topics for further discussion in the new forum include the rights of children and whether they are being met, emerging trends in the legal aspects of child abuse, management of children in persistent vegetative states, current aspects of "baby Doe" legislation, handgun legislation, child care legislation, problems of drug abuse (rights of children vs mothers), and discussion of pediatric malpractice cases (review of expert witness testimony, psychological aspects of the pediatrician being sued, etc).

In addition, we will offer periodic book reviews, editorial commentaries, and other relevant material as deemed appropriate. We welcome readers' suggestions, comments, and ideas. The main purpose of the new forum is to provide education and improve knowledge and communication about this important area of the practice of pediatrics and the care of children and families.

Peggy C. Ferry, MD
Department of Pediatrics
University of Arizona
Health Science Center
1501 N Campbell
Tucson, AZ 85724

References

1. Vevaina JR. Preface. In: Vevaina JR, Bone RC, Kassoff E, eds. *Legal Aspects of Medicine: Including Cardiology, Pulmonary Medicine, and Critical Care Medicine.* New York, NY: Springer-Verlag NY Inc; 1989:vii.
2. Fleisher LD. Wrongful births: when is there liability for prenatal injury? *AJDC.* 1987;141:1260-1265.
3. Brent RL. The irresponsible expert witness: a failure of biomedical graduate education and professional accountability. *Pediatrics.* 1982;70:754-762.

EDITORIAL

Pediatric Perspectives

Vistas and Vantage Points

According to *Webster's*, a perspective affords one the opportunity to make an accurate evaluation by observing things in their true relationships. Perhaps this includes a new view, a vista, from which the observer can stand back, observe, and get unique, refreshing new insights into common (and not so common) occurrences.

Pediatric Perspectives is a relatively new addition to *AJDC*'s special departments, which include Research to Relevance, Educational Interventions, Sports Medicine, and others. In this department, we hope to provide our readers with new insights into, and innovative ways of viewing, pediatric medical topics while providing learned treatises on current forces and issues that affect the everyday practice of pediatrics by all physicians, from the general practitioner to the teacher/clinician to the research scientist. For example, in this issue of *AJDC*, Elaine Wyllie, MD, discusses advances in diagnosis of and therapies for seizure disorders as they relate to central nervous system surgery.

per·spec·tive (per-spek´ tiv), adj. [ME. <LL. *perspectivus* <L. *perspicere*, to look through <*per*, through + *specere*, to look.] **1.** the art of picturing objects or a scene in such a way, eg, by converging lines as to show them as they appear to relative distance or depth **2.** the appearance of objects or scenes as determined by their relative distance and positions **3.** the relationship or proportion of the parts of a whole, regarded from a particular standpoint or point in time **4.** a specific point of view in understanding or judging things or events, esp. one that shows them in their true relation to one another b) the ability to see things in a true relationship[1]

See also p 314.

Pediatrics in the 1990s faces many issues that require immediate attention. For example, the exponential increase in knowledge of biochemical genetics has allowed prenatal detection of a number of inherited metabolic diseases, such as Tay-Sachs disease. Perhaps soon, medical practices will incorporate new therapies, such as genetically engineered prenatal treatment (eg, insertion of particular genes into a developing embryo's existing genetic material).

As neonatal intensive care becomes increasingly refined and complex, we may see the end of classic respiratory distress syndrome as a pathophysiologic entity because of the use of exogenous surfactant, but has this medical advance allowed the smallest, most fragile infants to survive who otherwise might have died? Are increasing numbers of infants living, but with long-term, chronic disabilities, such as retinopathy of prematurity or neurologic impairment?

Issues such as these are representative topics that can be addressed in Pediatric Perspectives. We invite pertinent "state-of-the-art" reviews. We also invite scholarly opinion pieces—those that provide unique approaches to difficult or common issues. Pediatric Perspectives is a medium for bringing readers up to date on new advances and for providing refreshing observations from new vantage points.

Alan D. Bedrick, MD
Department Editor,
Pediatric Perspectives *AJDC*

Reference

1. Guralnik D, ed. *Webster's New World Dictionary*. 2nd ed. New York, NY: Simon and Schuster Inc Publishers; 1982:1062.

Your Child's Best Friend: TV or Not TV

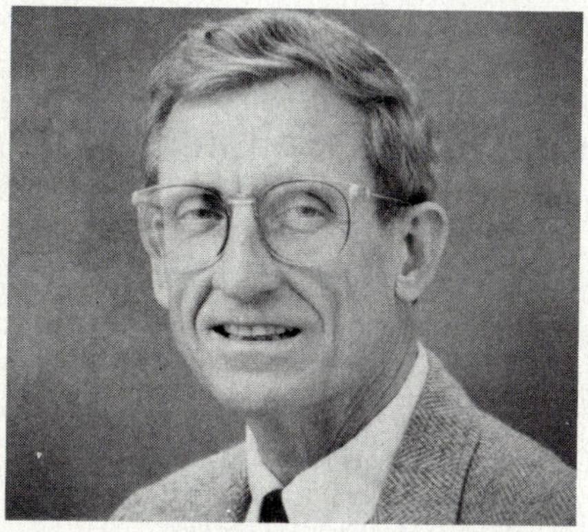

E. Richard Stiehm, MD

"Dick" Stiehm and I have been colleagues and friends for a long time, dating back to the golden days at Philadelphia (Pa) General Hospital, when we were both interns. We have authored a text together and dealt with similar issues in our research careers. Dick has been a valuable contributor to AJDC, *offering his insightful critiques on articles, suggesting ways that the journal could be improved, soliciting state-of-the-art articles for us, and offering nonmedical observations that stimulate our readers to respond. His contribution at right continues this last-named tradition.*

Dick is one of the most respected pediatric immunologists in the world. He is regarded as an expert in many areas, and his work has influenced the use of immunoglobulin therapy, particularly the newer intravenous preparations. He has contributed to our understanding of congenital and acquired immunodeficiencies, to our knowledge and use of vaccines, and to the unraveling of basic immunologic mechanisms. He is a prolific contributor to medical literature, both in scientific publications and in educational materials, such as the third edition of the textbook **Immunologic Disorders in Infants and Children** *(Philadelphia, Pa: WB Saunders Co; 1989). This is the definitive text in this area and Dick's skillful editing and writing have made it the most up-to-date, authoritative source for basic immunologic understanding and clinical applications.*

Would you like your children's best friend to monopolize 3 to 4 hours of their time every single day, discourage their participation in sports, prevent them from playing the piano or learning anything about classical music, interfere with their homework, and steal every book that they might want to read?

Well, I did not like my three daughters' best friend at all. Moreover, I had grave doubts about their friend's attitudes on sex, drugs, violence, and materialism. So I got rid of it. I banished TV!

All surviving parents have a list of things they believe they did right with their children, and a larger list, often repressed, of minor "boo-boos" and major catastrophes. The latter are too painful for me to resurrect. But three things I (we) did right were (1) to insist on music lessons; (2) to use a "magic apple" to cure all nightmares and bedtime insomnia (an apple slice anointed with the magic properties of "putting you to sleep within 10 minutes"); and (3) to abolish all TV privileges. My only concession was 1 hour on Friday and Saturday nights, and the nightly network news (which they did not watch).

I did it, in part, for selfish reasons. I wanted to listen to my music at night. But more importantly, I had the feeling that my first two daughters were shortchanging their schoolwork, their reading, and their music for their allotted nightly half-hour, "PTA-approved" TV program. And I was endlessly monitoring their viewing: "No, it's not my half hour, it's Carrie's!" "Why are these people killing each other?" "Jamie won't let me watch my program." "Why can't we have a Mercedes and a swimming pool?" About the time my two oldest girls were 12 and 10 years of age, I said, "Enough! No more TV!"

I was immediately branded the "meanest and strictest father in Santa Monica." Some wise pediatrician once told me that if your children do not think you are the strictest parent in the neighborhood, you are not strict enough. I reminded my girls that their piano teacher and her husband, who had three children too, did not even *have* a TV.

After a month or so, my girls realized I was not giving in, so they stopped sulking and started to do other things, like their schoolwork, playing the piano, reading, banging tennis balls against the garage door, and—would you believe it—listening to Brahms and liking it!

Our Saturdays did not start with 2 hours of cartoons. After their assigned chores, they were out all day playing tennis or soccer or spending time with real live friends (possibly at their house watching TV!). At any rate I did not have to put up with the banality of those awful, often violent, cartoons.

Our third and youngest daughter, who grew up with a "no TV" policy, never had TV withdrawal. She thought TV broadcasting stopped at 7:30 PM after the Evening News With Dan Rather and did not resume until Friday night.

There are a few disadvantages to a "no TV" policy. For one thing, you (the parents) cannot watch; for another, your children will be unable to answer the questions in the entertainment category of Trivial Pursuit (but they will be better at every other category); third, you will have to endure their stories about how excluded they felt from their friends' conversation at school about the previous night's programs; finally, *you* will have to pay more attention to your children because their best friend is not monopolizing all their time. But these are minor disadvantages compared with the multiple advantages.

My grown daughters, now in their 20s, today acknowledge that they got along "OK" without their best friend and do not want that friend for their own children.

Standardized Percentile Curves of Body-Mass Index for Children and Adolescents

Lawrence D. Hammer, MD; Helena C. Kraemer, PhD; Darrell M. Wilson, MD; Philip L. Ritter, PhD; Sanford M. Dornbusch, PhD

• **Weight-for-height indexes are often used in the clinical assessment of obesity in children and adolescents. The direct measurement of adiposity, using hydrostatic weighing and other techniques, is not feasible in studies involving young children or with large numbers of older subjects. Ratios of weight relative to height, such as the body-mass index (weight/height²), may be used as indirect measures of obesity and correlate with more direct measures of adiposity. Using data from the First National Health and Nutrition Examination Study, 1971 to 1974, standardized percentile curves of body-mass index for white children and adolescents were developed. These curves may be used to monitor the body-mass index of white children and adolescents longitudinally and for comparing an individual with others of the same sex and age.**

(*AJDC.* 1991;145:259-263)

Obesity is a significant health problem, with medical and psychological consequences for children and adolescents.[1-3] Obesity is best defined as a condition of excessive adiposity. Several methods are available for estimating adiposity, including measurement of body density using underwater weighing, estimation of lean body mass using deuterium distribution, and estimation of lean body mass by measurement of potassium 40 levels. Although these methods are considered to be "gold standards," they are based on assumptions regarding body density and lean body mass inferred from studies largely involving adults. Limitations in the validity of these methods are reviewed by Lohman.[4] Furthermore, these techniques are technically difficult to apply to children and are impractical in most clinical settings. Therefore, "indirect" measures of adiposity, such as skinfold thickness and weight-for-height indexes, are often used as proxy measures of adiposity or as criteria for defining obesity.[5]

Inconvenience and inaccuracy in the measurement of skinfold thickness and variability in the distribution of subcutaneous fat limit the use of this measure in many clinical settings.[6,7] The body-mass index (BMI), known also as the Quetelet Index,[8] is often used as an index of overweight in children[9,10] and is more easily obtained than measurement of skinfold thickness. For any index of overweight to be meaningful in the pediatric age group, there must be standards defined by age, sex, and race, since adiposity is known to vary with these factors.[11] We therefore developed percentile curves of BMI for white males and females, aged 1 to 19 years, using data from a national sample, representative of the noninstitutionalized population of the continental United States.

Accepted for publication October 29, 1990.

From Stanford University School of Medicine, Palo Alto, Calif.
Reprint requests to Children's Hospital at Stanford, 520 Sand Hill Rd, Palo Alto, CA 94304 (Dr Hammer).

SUBJECTS AND METHODS

The First National Health and Nutrition Examination Survey, 1971 to 1974 (NHANES I), was conducted for the purpose of gathering data regarding the nutritional and health status of the American population.[12] NHANES I includes data from a stratified probability sample, representative of the noninstitutionalized civilian population of the continental United States. These data were made available on computer tape from the National Center for Health Statistics, through the Interuniversity Consortium for Political and Social Research. Included in NHANES I are data from 5679 white individuals, aged 1 to 19 years. Only whites were included in the following analyses, since the distribution of BMI varies by race,[13] and the data set does not include a sufficient number of nonwhite children aged 1 through 19 years to allow development of age- and gender-specific standardized percentile curves.

Each subject in NHANES I underwent a complete physical examination, a detailed medical and nutritional history, and a variety of laboratory tests. Included in the physical examination were measurements of height and weight. The methods for obtaining these measurements are described in detail elsewhere.[12,13]

Each subject was assigned a Poverty Index score, based on the family's income and size[12]; we used this score as an index of social class. The effect of social class on BMI was examined and the correlation between social class and BMI was found to be nonsignificant in each age group and for the overall sample. For this reason, the group percentiles within each social class were not calculated and BMI distributions were not adjusted for social class.

Smoothed percentile curves of BMI by age were developed using raw data from the NHANES I (Figs 1 and 2). These curves were drawn by fitting unique quadratic models for the lower (males aged 1 to 11 years, females aged 1 to 13 years) and upper (males aged 8 to 19 years, females aged 6 to 19 years) portions of each curve. These quadratic models were then spliced and smoothed separately for males and females (males spliced at age 10 years, females at age 7 years). All procedures were done using the SAS.[14]

RESULTS

The Table contains the smoothed percentile values of BMI for white males and females, for ages 1 to 19 years, based on data from the NHANES I survey. Smoothed percentile curves of these data are presented in Figs 1 and 2.

Percentile Values of Body-Mass Index, NHANES I*

Age, y	Percentile 5	10	25	50	75	90	95
Males							
1	14.6	15.4	16.1	17.2	18.5	19.4	19.9
2	14.4	15.0	15.7	16.5	17.6	18.4	19.0
3	14.0	14.6	15.3	16.0	17.0	17.8	18.4
4	13.8	14.4	15.0	15.8	16.6	17.5	18.1
5	13.7	14.2	14.9	15.5	16.3	17.3	18.0
6	13.6	14.0	14.7	15.4	16.3	17.4	18.1
7	13.6	14.0	14.7	15.5	16.5	17.7	18.9
8	13.7	14.1	14.9	15.7	17.0	18.4	19.7
9	14.0	14.3	15.1	16.0	17.6	19.3	20.9
10	14.2	14.6	15.5	16.6	18.4	20.3	22.2
11	14.6	15.0	16.0	17.2	19.2	21.3	23.5
12	15.1	15.5	16.5	17.8	20.0	22.3	24.8
13	15.6	16.0	17.1	18.4	20.8	23.3	25.8
14	16.1	16.6	17.7	19.1	21.5	24.4	26.8
15	16.6	17.1	18.4	19.7	22.2	25.4	27.7
16	17.2	17.8	19.1	20.5	22.9	26.1	28.4
17	17.7	18.4	19.7	21.2	23.4	27.0	29.0
18	18.3	19.1	20.3	21.9	24.0	27.7	29.7
19	19.0	19.7	21.1	22.5	24.4	28.3	30.1
Females							
1	14.7	15.0	15.8	16.6	17.6	18.6	19.3
2	14.3	14.7	15.3	16.0	17.1	18.0	18.7
3	13.9	14.4	14.9	15.6	16.7	17.6	18.3
4	13.6	14.1	14.7	15.4	16.5	17.5	18.2
5	13.5	14.0	14.6	15.3	16.3	17.5	18.3
6	13.3	13.9	14.6	15.3	16.4	17.7	18.8
7	13.4	14.0	14.7	15.5	16.7	18.5	19.7
8	13.6	14.2	15.0	16.0	17.2	19.4	21.0
9	14.0	14.5	15.5	16.6	18.0	20.8	22.7
10	14.3	15.0	15.9	17.1	19.0	21.8	24.2
11	14.6	15.3	16.2	17.8	19.8	23.0	25.7
12	15.0	15.6	16.7	18.3	20.4	23.7	26.8
13	15.4	16.0	17.1	18.9	21.2	24.7	27.9
14	15.7	16.4	17.5	19.4	21.8	25.3	28.6
15	16.1	16.8	18.0	19.9	22.4	26.0	29.4
16	16.4	17.1	18.4	20.2	22.8	26.5	30.0
17	16.9	17.6	18.9	20.7	23.3	27.1	30.5
18	17.2	18.0	19.4	21.1	23.7	27.4	31.0
19	17.5	18.4	19.8	21.4	24.0	27.7	31.3

*NHANES I indicates National Health and Nutrition Examination Survey, 1971 to 1974.

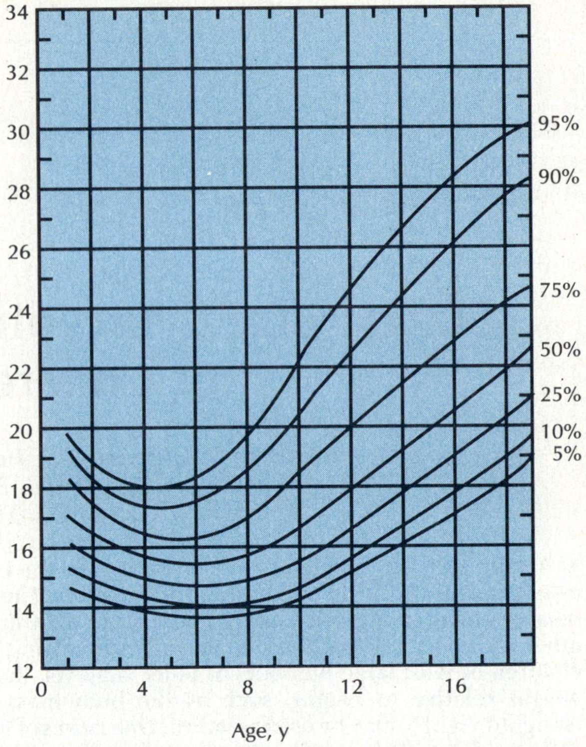

Fig 1.—*Body-mass index for white males aged 1 to 19 years. Percentiles were computed using data from the First National Health and Nutrition Examination Survey, 1971 to 1974.*

Fig 2.—*Body-mass index for white females aged 1 to 19 years. Percentiles were computed using data from the First National Health and Nutrition Examination Survey, 1971 to 1974.*

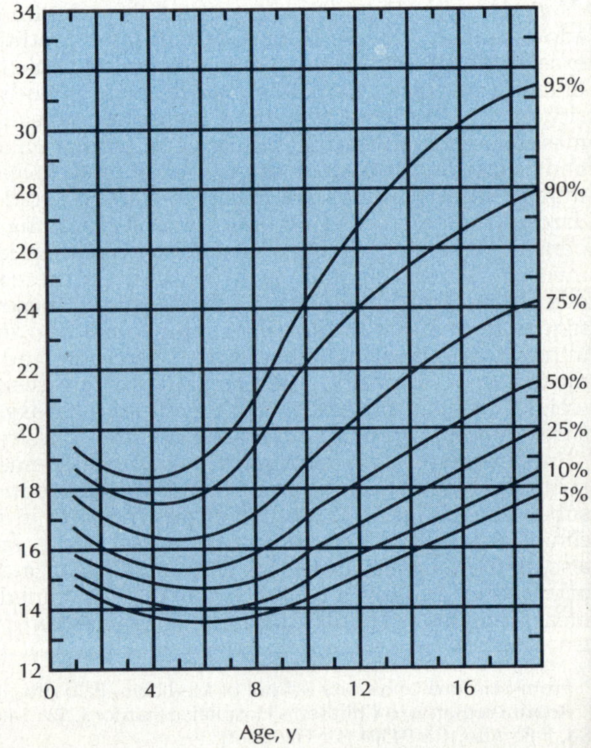

As previously reported, changes in BMI in early childhood are similar for males and females.[8,13] The BMI decreases from the age of 1 year until 4 to 6 years, when a trough occurs, after which BMI increases again.

Although the shapes of the curves for males and females are similar, the percentile values for BMI differ considerably in males and females at some ages. For the fifth to 75th percentiles, BMI values for males and females differ by less than 0.5 kg/m^2 between the ages of 1 and 14 years. After age 14 years, the fifth to 75th percentile values of BMI for males exceed those for females by as much as 1.5 kg/m^2.

The upper percentiles (90th to 95th) at the age of 1 year are higher for males than for females. From the age of 2 through 5 years, male-female differences in BMI are again less than 0.5 kg/m^2 at these upper percentiles. From age 6 years to 14 years, values of BMI for females exceed those for males, at these upper percentiles, by more than 0.5 kg/m^2. This trend continues in the 15- to 19-year age group, at the 95th percentile, with females having greater values of BMI than males.

COMMENT

Indicators of overweight are useful in the diagnosis and management of obesity in childhood and adolescence. An index of overweight that can be employed across all age groups would be ideal. Direct measures of adiposity, such as hydrostatic weighing, total body potassium determination, and deuterium distribution, are of only limited usefulness, owing to their cost, risk, inconvenience, and questionable validity, especially when applied to children and adolescents. On the other hand, BMI has been shown to have utility as an index of obesity during childhood[9] and adult life[13] and to be predictive, in childhood, of later obesity.[15] In a two-decade follow-up study, Rolland-Cachera et al[16] found that correlations between measures of BMI performed annually from 1 through 16 years of age and BMI at follow-up (18 to 25 years of age) exceeded the correlations between measures of skinfold thickness at four sites (individually or combined) taken annually during childhood and at follow-up, both for males and for females.

Skinfold thickness has often been used as a measure of adiposity in children and adolescents. Some investigators have used skinfold thickness as a gold standard against which other measures of obesity have been judged[17]; however, there are problems with skinfold thickness as a measure of either adiposity or obesity. Skinfold thickness is usually measured at only a limited number of sites and only reflects site-specific subcutaneous fat deposition[18]; moreover, the distribution of subcutaneous fat varies widely by age, sex, race, and body habitus.[19,20] Reference standards for skinfold thickness are available for only a limited number of sites. Furthermore, measurement of skinfold thickness in children, even when performed by trained personnel, may be unreliable, owing to interobserver error[21] and technical difficulty, especially in young children.[13] Measurements made using different types of calipers may also differ significantly.[22,23] The validity of skinfold measures as measures of adiposity or obesity may be even lower in obese subjects, in whom accuracy of measurement has not been adequately studied.[21] Finally, variation in subcutaneous fat distribution limits skinfold thickness as a predictor of risk secondary to obesity.[24]

Height and weight measurements are routinely performed in the clinical care of children and are monitored throughout childhood and adolescence as indicators of health and disease.[25] Accurate measurements of height and weight can be obtained using readily available instrumentation such as the stadiometer or, for children less than 3 years of age,[25] a supine measuring table for length and an appropriately calibrated scale for weight.[26] Furthermore, the impact of error in height measurement is minimized in the calculation by using height expressed in meters, since any error is placed in the second decimal column.

Although BMI ratios using various values of the exponent P in the ratio weight/height^P have been studied, where P may vary with gender, race, or other characteristics, noninteger values of P are clumsy to use in calculating weight/height^P in the clinical setting and offer little advantage over the ratio weight/height^2.[26] The BMI calculated as weight/height^2 is highly correlated with skinfold thickness in adult men and women[27] and in children and adolescents 4 through 17 years of age.[28] Despite the limitations of BMI as a measure of adiposity,[29] BMI remains a clinically useful index of weight relative to stature.[23] That BMI may reflect increased lean body mass as well as body fat[29] is appropriate, given that individuals who are fatter are likely to have more lean body mass and to be taller than individuals who are thinner, a pattern often observed during childhood and adolescence.[30]

The BMI is an easily calculated index. However, a nomogram for determining BMI has been previously published,[31] and tables for determining BMI (as kilograms per square meter) from measures of height and weight in inches and pounds are also available.[24]

The standardized curves of BMI offer an opportunity to monitor an individual's degree of obesity from childhood through adolescence. The Table contains the smoothed values of BMI used in plotting Figs 1 and 2. These values are similar to those published previously for males and females over the age of 6 years[13] and include newly smoothed values for children under 6 years of age. Although based on cross-sectional data, these curves follow the developmental pattern observed in longitudinal studies of BMI.[9,15] These curves may be used clinically as a means of monitoring relative change in BMI over time, as is routinely done in clinical practice for weight, height, and head circumference.[32] Use of a single computed measure simplifies the process of monitoring change in weight relative to change in height. Limitations in the use of cross-sectionally derived weight and height curves would also apply to these BMI curves.

The pattern of BMI over time has clinical significance. Longitudinal studies in childhood have demonstrated a developmental pattern of BMI. The age at which the trough in BMI occurs (4 to 8 years) is a potent predictor of later obesity, with children having an increased risk of later obesity if their BMI trough ends and the adiposity rebound begins before 5.5 years.[15] Though these BMI curves have been derived from cross-sectional data, the trough in the upper percentiles occurs earlier than the trough in the lower percentiles. This would suggest that children whose BMI falls in the upper percentiles may be more likely to have their adiposity rebound occur early. Furthermore, BMI has predictive value in adults with respect to morbidity and mortality.[24]

It is known that with the onset of adolescence and puberty, the adiposity of males and females increases, with females becoming increasingly fat compared with males. The use of skinfold thickness as a measure of body fatness may exaggerate the difference in adiposity between males and females,[33] since that difference can be partly explained by differences in fat distribution (including internal-external fat ratio) and gender-specific essential fat.[21]

The absence of large differences in BMI for males and females at each age may be due to the higher correlation of BMI with total body fat than with percentage of body fat[31]; total body fat is known to increase in both males and females through adolescence.[34,35] Higher values of BMI for males than females older than 14 years of age in the fifth through 75th percentiles may also be explained by the greater increase in lean body mass seen in males in this age group.

Percentile values for precisely defining obesity based on BMI or other measures remain to be determined. These cutoff points should be based on levels of BMI above which the morbidity related to obesity is known to occur. Though any degree of overweight may carry risk,[24] a definition of obesity based on BMI would be most useful if levels of BMI (by age and sex) that carry increased risk can be specified. For example, it has been suggested that adult men with BMI greater than 27.2 and adult women with BMI greater than 26.9 are at increased risk for morbidity and mortality.[24] These curves of BMI provide a clinical tool for monitoring BMI as children approach adult life. Further research is needed to provide a clearer picture of the relative risks associated with increased BMI at each age level for boys and girls. An additional use of the BMI as an index of obesity would arise from longitudinal research demonstrating the relative risk of long-term obesity associated with increased levels of BMI at particular ages in childhood.

The NIH Consensus Development Conference on Obesity has recommended use of the 85th percentile (weight for height) as a cutoff point for obesity in adults. For clinical purposes, we have found the 95th percentile BMI to be a conservative cutoff point for defining obesity in childhood. Following the BMI pattern provides more useful clinical information, however, than any single measurement of BMI. Further studies are needed to define useful criteria for defining obesity using BMI in childhood and adolescence. These studies should consider the morbidity associated with increasing percentile levels of BMI, including increased risk for long-term obesity.

A potential criticism of this study is that it relies on data from a national survey that oversampled from among lower socioeconomic groups in the United States. The effect of social class on BMI in this sample was examined and found to be nonsignificant within each age group and for the overall sample. For this reason, the group percentiles within each social class were not recalculated, nor were the distributions of BMI adjusted for social class.

CONCLUSION

Standardized curves of BMI were developed for white males and females by smoothing data from a large, stratified sample of 1- through 19-year-olds in the United States. These curves may be used to monitor the development of obesity as well as changes in BMI associated with treatment of obesity in childhood and adolescence. Since the pattern of BMI has been shown to be a predictor of long-term obesity in childhood, and to predict morbidity and mortality in adulthood, it is recommended that clinicians routinely measure height and weight and monitor BMI in caring for children and adolescents. Using appropriate data sets, such curves should also be developed for other racial groups. Further studies are needed to define appropriate cutoff points of BMI for more precisely defining obesity in childhood and adolescence.

Support for this work was provided by the Stanford Center for the Study of Families, Children, and Youth, Palo Alto, Calif.

We wish to acknowledge Leonard Epstein, PhD, for his review of the manuscript, and Pam Juanes for her assistance and tireless effort in its completion.

References

1. Brownell KD. Obesity: understanding and treating a serious, prevalent, and refractory disorder. *J Consult Clin Psychol.* 1982;50:820-840.

2. Lauer RM, Clarke WR, Beaglehole R. Level, trend, and variability of blood pressure during childhood: the Muscatine Study. *Circulation.* 1984;69:242-249.

3. Drash A. Relationship between diabetes mellitus and obesity in the child. *Metabolism.* 1973;22:337-344.

4. Lohman TG. Research progress in validation of laboratory methods of assessing body composition. *Med Sci Sports Exerc.* 1984;16:596-603.

5. Seltzer CC, Mayer J. A simple criterion of obesity. *Postgrad Med.* 1965;38:A101-A107.

6. Wormersley J, Durnin JVGA. An experimental study on variability of measurements of skinfold thickness on young adults. *Hum Biol.* 1973;45:281-292.

7. Brook CGD. Determination of body composition of children from skinfold measurements. *Arch Dis Child.* 1971;46:182-184.

8. Billewicz WZ, Kemsley FF, Thomson AM. Indices of adiposity. *Br J Prev Soc Med.* 1962;16:183-188.

9. Rolland-Cachera MF, Sempe M, Guilloud-Bataille M, Patois E, Pequignot-Guggenbuhl F, Fautrad V. Adiposity indices in children. *Am J Clin Nutr.* 1982;36:178-184.

10. Fomon SJ, Rogers RR, Ziegler EE, Nelson SE, Thomas LN. Indices of fatness and serum cholesterol at age eight years in relation to feeding and growth during early infancy. *Pediatr Res.* 1982;18:1233-1238.

11. Garn SM, Clark DC. Nutrition, growth, development, and maturation: findings from the 10-state nutrition survey of 1968-1970. *Pediatrics.* 1975;56:306-319.

12. National Center for Health Statistics. Plan and operation of the Health and Nutrition Examination Survey, United States, 1971-73. *Vital Health Stat 1.* 1973;No. 10a and 10b.

13. Cronk CE, Roche AF. Race- and sex-specific reference data for triceps and subscapular skinfolds and weight/stature^2. *Am J Clin Nutr.* 1982;35:347-354.

14. SAS Institute. *SAS User's Guide: Statistics.* 2nd ed. Cary, NC: SAS Institute Inc; 1982.

15. Rolland-Cachera MF, Deheeger M, Bellisle F, Sempe M, Guilloud-Bataille M, Patois E. Adiposity rebound in children: a simple indicator for predicting obesity. *Am J Clin Nutr.* 1984;39:129-135.

16. Rolland-Cachera MF, Bellisle F, Sempe M. The prediction in boys and girls of the weight/height^2 index and various skinfold measurements in adults: a two-decade followup study. *Int J Obes.* 1989;13:305-311.

17. Michielutte R, Diseker R, Corbett WT, Schey HM, Ureda JR. The relationship between weight-height indices and the triceps skinfold thickness measure among children age 5 to 12. *Am J Public Health.* 1984;74:604-606.

18. McClaren DS, Ajans ZA, Awdeh Z. Composition of human adipose tissue, with special reference to site and age differences. *Am J Clin Nutr.* 1965;17:171-176.

19. Edwards DAW. Differences in the distribution of subcutaneous fat with sex and maturity. *Clin Sci.* 1951;10:305-315.

20. Garn SM. Relative fat patterning: an individual characteristic. *Hum Biol.* 1955;27:75-98.

21. Pollack ML, Jackson AS. Research progress in validation of clinical methods of assessing body composition. *Med Sci Sports Exerc.* 1984;16:606-613.

22. Lohman TG, Pollack ML, Slaughter MH, Brandon LJ, Bolieau RA. Methodological factors and the prediction of body fat in female athletes. *Med Sci Sports Exerc.* 1984;16:92-96.

23. Jung E, Kaufman JJM, Narins DC, Kaufman GE. Skinfold measurements in children. *Clin Pediatr.* 1984;23:25-28.

24. Burton BT, Foster WR, Hirsch J, Van Italie TB. Health implications of obesity: an NIH consensus development conference. *Int J Obes.* 1985;9:155-169.

25. Forbes GB, Woodruff CW, eds. *Pediatric Nutrition Handbook.* Elk Grove Village, Ill:American Academy of Pediatrics,

Committee on Nutrition; 1985:190-191.
26. Cameron N. The methods of auxological anthropometry. In: Falkner F, Tanner JM, eds. *Human Growth 2.* New York, NY: Plenum Press; 1978:35-90.
27. Micozzi MS, Albanes D, Jones DY, Chumlea WC. Correlations of body mass indices with weight, stature, and body composition in men and women in NHANES I and II. *Am J Clin Nutr.* 1986;44:725-731.
28. Spyckerelle Y, Gueguen R, Guillemot M, Tosi E, Deschamps JP. Adiposity indices and clinical opinion. *Ann Hum Biol.* 1988;15:45-54.
29. Garn SM, Leonard WR, Hawthorne VM. Three limitations of the body mass index. *Am J Clin Nutr.* 1986;44:996-997.
30. Micozzi MS, Albanes D. Three limitations of the body mass index. *Am J Clin Nutr.* 1987;46:376-377.
31. Roche AF, Siervogel RM, Chumlea WC, Webb P. Grading body fatness from limited anthropometric data. *Am J Clin Nutr.* 1981;34:2831-2838.
32. Hamill PVV, Drizd TA, Johnson CL, Reed RB, Roche AF, Moore WM. Physical growth: National Center for Health Statistics percentiles. *Am J Clin Nutr.* 1979;32:607-629.
33. Cronk CE, Mukherjee D, Roche AF. Changes in triceps and subscapular skinfold thickness during adolescence. *Hum Biol.* 1983;55:707-721.
34. Rauh JL, Schumsky DA. Lean and nonlean body mass estimates in urban school children. In: Cheek DB, ed. *Human Growth*. Philadelphia, Pa: Lea & Febiger; 1968:242-252.
35. Haschke F. Body composition of adolescent males, II: body composition of male reference adolescent. *Acta Paediatr Scand Suppl.* 1983;307:13-23.

In Other AMA Journals

ARCHIVES OF DERMATOLOGY

Capillary Hemangiomas and Treatment With the Flash Lamp–Pumped Pulsed Dye Laser

Robin Ashinoff, MD, Roy G. Geronemus, MD (*Arch Dermatol.* 1991;127:202-205)

Acne Vulgaris in Early Adolescent Boys: Correlations With Pubertal Maturation and Age

Anne W. Lucky, MD; Frank M. Biro, MD; Gertrude A. Huster, MS; John A. Morrison, PhD; Nancy Elder, RN (*Arch Dermatol.* 1991;127:210-216)

Intralesional Bleomycin Sulfate Therapy for Warts: A Novel Bifurcated Needle Puncture Technique

Walter B. Shelley, MD, PhD, E. Dorinda Shelley, MD (*Arch Dermatol.* 1991;127:234-236)

A Plea for a Biologic Approach to Hemangiomas of Infancy

John B. Mulliken, MD (*Arch Dermatol.* 1991; 127:243-244)

Improved Speed and Accuracy of Calculations With a Programmable Calculator in Pediatric Emergency Scenarios

Marlene Melzer-Lange, MD; David Wyatt, MD; Christine Walsh-Kelly, MD; Douglas Smith, MD; Mary A. Hegenbarth, MD; Carl S. L. Eisenberg, MD

• Both mathematical and selection errors may occur when ordering drug or fluid therapy in a busy emergency department. In an attempt to improve the speed and accuracy of such calculations, we programmed a hand-held calculator to assist in drug and intravenous fluid therapy dosages and rates for three emergency situations: diabetic ketoacidosis, asthma, and asystole. Performance by 58 subjects at various levels of training was compared when using either the programmable calculator or standard materials and methods. When standard methods were used, an average of 30.6 minutes was needed to complete the three scenarios, with an accuracy of 73%; by contrast, use of programmable calculator resulted in a significant decline in time needed to calculate doses (an average of only 8.5 minutes), with an improved accuracy of 98%. The use of a programmable calculator can result in a significant improvement in both speed and accuracy of drug and fluid selection and dosage and rate calculations, regardless of the level of the subject's medical training.

***(AJDC.* 1991;145:264-266)**

Pediatric emergencies present special challenges to the physician. Children vary widely in weight, age, and biological maturity. These variables influence the selection of drug and fluid therapy. Initial selection and subsequent rate and dose calculations for therapy of the critically ill child can be especially difficult under the pressure of an emergent situation. Through experience, the pediatric emergency specialist may develop the facility to effectively handle the great majority of such emergencies; for other physicians or residents caring for children in a general emergency department, these calculations may be more difficult due to unfamiliarity.

Several authors have presented guidelines to simplify this situation. *The Harriet Lane Handbook*[1] is a traditional pediatric reference that has long given standards for fluid and drug therapies for children. Losek and Garland[2] published *The First Five Minutes,* which lists precalculated doses of drugs used to resuscitate critically ill children based on patients' body weights. Computerization of such guidelines has also been developed. Kelly et al[3] described the use of a programmable calculator for calculation of pediatric vasopressor drugs. Yamamoto and Wiebe[4] devised a computer program (for an IBM-PC compatible computer) that gives guidelines and calculates weight-appropriate doses for adult and pediatric patients.

We compared the use of a programmable calculator with more traditional methods for calculating weight and age doses of specific fluids and medications used in three common pediatric emergencies. The intention of this study is to examine whether a programmable calculator aids physicians in their capacity to rapidly and accurately calculate fluid and drug doses for common pediatric emergencies.

METHODS

Fifty-eight physicians and medical students took two sequential written tests. Each test consisted of a set of three common pediatric emergency scenarios: asystole, acute asthma, and diabetic ketoacidosis. Each scenario consisted of a brief case history and used a fill-in-the-blank or short answer format. The scenarios in each test set were of comparable difficulty, varying only in details such as patient's age and weight. The asystole scenario required calculation of resuscitation and maintenance fluids; endotracheal tube size; a single dose of epinephrine hydrochloride, atropine sulfate, and sodium bicarbonate; and instructions for preparation of a dopamine hydrochloride infusion. The asthma scenario required calculation of maintenance fluids, an intravenous aminophylline bolus based on the patient's weight and serum aminophylline level, a maintenance aminophylline infusion based on the patient's age, a methylprednisolone bolus infusion, and mixing instructions and flow rate for an isoproterenol hydrochloride infusion. The diabetic ketoacidosis scenario required calculation of the initial 2 hours of replacement fluid (amount and type), insulin infusion (amount and type), and serum osmolalities.

Each subject took one test set using the programmable calculator and one test set using a pocket calculator, a *Harriet Lane Handbook,*[1] and the Children's Hospital of Wisconsin guidelines routinely available to all physicians who have rotations in the emergency department. Ranges of correct answers to all questions were based on these standard therapeutic guidelines. To negate any potential bias due to learning effects, subjects were randomly assigned to first use either the programmable calculator or the standard materials. Randomization was performed by sequential assignment to a list of computer-generated random numbers. The tests were administered without interruption to single subjects under supervision either in a room with tape-recorded emergency department background noise or in the emergency department itself. Times required for each test set were recorded.

The programmable calculator (model 42S, Hewlett-Packard Company, Corvallis, Ore) (Figure) is a small 140-g hand-held, battery-operated model with 7 kilobytes of memory and more

Accepted for publication August 17, 1990.

From the Medical College of Wisconsin, Children's Hospital of Wisconsin, Milwaukee.

Reprint requests to Department of Pediatrics, 9000 W Wisconsin Ave, MS 756, Milwaukee, WI 53226 (Dr Melzer-Lange).

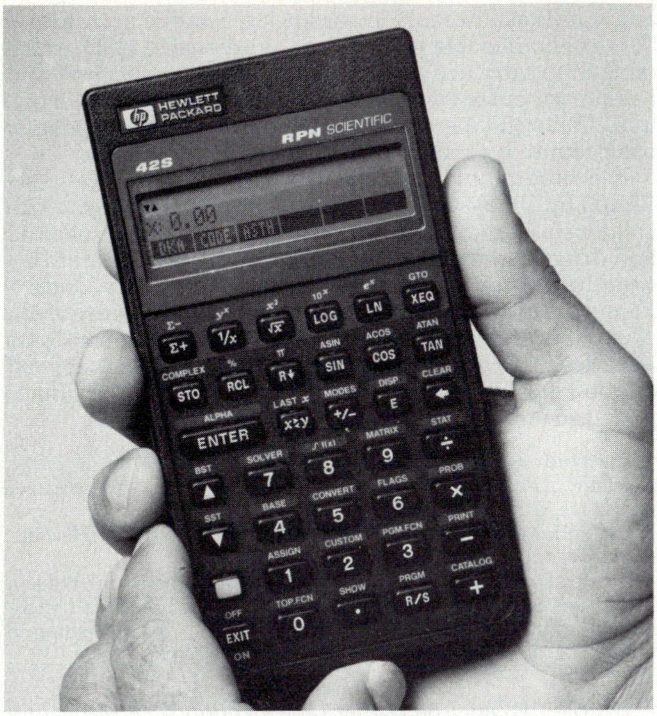

Programmable calculator with menu display.

than 350 internal functions. It has an automatic four-level memory stack, can store both α-strings and numeric variables, is capable of program branching, and can accept and test user input from the keyboard. The two-line liquid crystal display is 22 characters wide, can display both uppercase and lowercase letters with punctuation, and can show a customized menu. This allows effective prompting of the user, and the calculator program can lead the subject through the questions in each of the scenarios. The subject chooses the scenario from a menu and provides input as requested in the display. The program pauses after each calculation is displayed and is restarted by the user after the answer has been noted. Subjects quickly learn to use the calculator after a standard 2-minute demonstration.

For statistical comparison, subjects were divided into seven groups based on the degree and type of training: private practice pediatricians, first-year (PL-1) and third-year (PL-3) pediatric residents completing their respective year of training, emergency medicine residents at all levels of training, second-year family practice residents, third-year medical students on their first pediatric rotations, and fourth-year medical students on elective pediatric rotations.

Numerical answers were considered correct if they were within 10% of the expected value. Failure to indicate a fluid or insulin type, incorrect fluid type, or no answer given were considered incorrect answers. There were 27 questions in each test set. Scores were calculated as the percentage of correct answers.

Analysis of variance techniques were used to evaluate differences in mean times between the seven subject groups for each method. Statistical analysis was also performed for the difference in total time required between the two methods for each individual physician. Two-sided paired t tests were used to test the significance of this difference within each physician group. Analysis of variance was performed to assess overall significant difference between physician groups with Tukey-Sidak's tests employed for pairwise comparisons between these groups. We used χ^2 tests to evaluate differences in accuracy between the methods.

RESULTS

The PL-3 group had the shortest time required to complete the test set using standard methods. One subject in the PL-1 group was excluded from the study; the prolonged time (103.9 minutes) required to complete the calculations using the standard method was 6 SDs beyond the mean. There was an overall significant difference for time among the subject groups using the standard method ($P=.0427$), with a significant difference between the PL-1 and PL-3 groups (Table 1). There were no significant differences for time among the subject groups using the programmable calculator. In addition, there was an overall significant difference between the time required to complete the scenarios with the programmable calculator vs the standard method ($P=.0067$), as well as a significant difference between the PL-3 group and both the PL-1 group and attending physicians. This means that the improved time in both the PL-1 and attending physician groups was significantly greater than in the PL-3 group. There was no significant difference in mean times based on method first employed. Failure to show significance could be due to small sample sizes. Each subject group showed significant speed improvements with the programmable calculator. Accuracy was also significantly improved using the calculator (Table 2). Ninety-eight percent of the answers were correct with the programmable calculator vs 73% of the responses using standard methods ($P<.0001$).

Table 1.—Time (Minutes) Needed to Complete Calculations*

Group†	No. of Subjects	Standard Method	Calculator	Difference
MS-3	10	35.1±9.9	9.89±2.6	25.3±9.4
MS-4	10	31.9±9.4	9.0±4.1	22.9±9.4
FP-2	9	30.0±10.1	8.5±1.9	21.6±10.3
PL-1	6	27.9±12.5	8.4±2.7	19.4±10.2
PL-3	9	16.6±7.1	6.9±1.1	9.7±6.6
EMR	7	27.9±8.9	7.7±1.4	20.2±7.9
PRV	6	36.9±11.8	8.2±1.2	28.7±10.6
All subjects	**57**	29.4±11.2	8.4±2.5	21.0±10.4

*All calculator times are significantly less than standard method times at $P<.0067$; paired t tests. Values are mean±SD.

†MS-3 indicates third-year medical student on first pediatric rotation; MS-4, fourth-year medical student on elective pediatric rotation; FP-2, second-year family practice resident; PL-1, first-year pediatric resident; PL-3, third-year pediatric resident; EMR, emergency medicine resident; and PRV, private practice pediatrician.

Table 2.—Accuracy Scores (% Correct, Range) by Method of Calculation*

Group†	No. of Subjects	Standard Method, %	Programmable Calculator, %
MS-3	10	72 (59-81)	98 (96-100)
MS-4	10	74 (56-89)	98 (96-100)
FP-2	9	80 (56-93)	99 (96-100)
PL-1	6	69 (59-81)	99 (96-100)
PL-3	9	77 (59-93)	96 (85-100)
EMR	7	71 (33-93)	97 (92-100)
PRV	6	65 (44-92)	99 (96-100)
All subjects	**57**	73 (33-93)	98 (85-100)

*All calculator scores show significantly more accuracy than standard method scores ($P<.0001$).

†MS-3 indicates third-year medical student on first pediatric rotation; MS-4, fourth-year medical student on elective pediatric rotation; FP-2, second-year family practice resident; PL-1, first-year pediatric resident; PL-3, third-year pediatric resident; EMR, emergency medicine resident; and PRV, private practice pediatrician.

Errors using traditional methods included mathematical errors, decimal point errors, erroneous fluid types, failure to designate fluid types, erroneous endotracheal tube size, erroneous pressor mixtures and infusion rates, and omitted answers. Many participants did not complete the problems for vasopressor mixtures and rates in the standard methods test. All of these errors would have been considered clinically significant. The only errors seen with the programmable calculator involved not designating fluid or insulin type in the diabetic ketoacidosis scenario and a single incorrect dopamine rate in the asystole scenario. These errors occurred because the subject incorrectly or incompletely transcribed the information supplied by the programmable calculator. No errors using the programmable calculator involved entering incorrect numbers.

COMMENT

This study highlights the difficulty that medical students, house staff, and attending physicians may have with drug and fluid management in pediatric emergencies. Even with the "open book" approach used for the standard method scenarios, erroneous calculations were frequent, and calculations took significantly longer compared with those made using the programmable calculator. These problems occurred in a simulated setting, without the pressures and distractions of procedures and medication administration that accompany a true emergency.

The significantly decreased time and improvement in accuracy of calculations seen with the use of the programmable calculator should be helpful in caring for ill children. This program not only calculates drug doses but also offers guidelines for the type of fluids, drugs, and endotracheal tube sizes for various pediatric problems. The rare error made using the programmable calculator could have been avoided with the use of a printer or by improving the graphic display in our program. Students and physicians at all levels of training were able to use the calculator readily after a brief instruction period. Although few subjects had extensive computer expertise, most were enthusiastic about using the programmable calculator in their medical practices.

From a medical education standpoint, the study produced several interesting observations during the testing period. When approached about volunteering as a subject for our study, many subjects were somewhat wary and reluctant. Although our testing was done anonymously and with reference materials, our subjects verbalized concern that they would be unable to do an adequate job. In the group of subjects who used the programmable calculator for the first half of testing, many verbalized frustration with the manual calculations required with the second set of scenarios; although not statistically significant, this group tended toward slightly longer times for the standard calculations than those who had used the standard method first. Many of the test subjects wanted to review the calculations after testing was completed and to check their manual calculations with the programmable calculator. The study prompted many questions from subjects on all levels regarding drug dose calculations specifically and patient care in general. The fact that students, residents, and staff using the programmable calculator could produce quick, accurate orders without a statistical difference regardless of training level is definitely an asset.

Others have also noted the usefulness of computers in medical education[5,6] and in emergency medicine.[4,7-9] Programmable calculators have been used by others for drug pharmacokinetics,[10-12] in calculating hyperalimentation and nutritional needs,[13] in anesthesia,[14] and in pediatrics.[15] This programmable calculator is inexpensive ($85), small enough to carry in a pocket or to attach to a clipboard, and has printer output available with a cordless infrared signal to a small roll-tape printer ($100). It offers an inexpensive compromise compared with a large microcomputer.

The programmable calculator was enthusiastically accepted by almost every subject. Routine use of such a calculator should result in more error-free, standardized fluid and drug therapy. Such a goal is especially difficult to accomplish when physicians staffing emergency departments differ greatly in their training and experience level. The ability of this program not only to calculate drug doses but also to provide types of drugs, intravenous fluids, and endotracheal tube sizes offers many applications to clinical pediatric and emergency medicine practices.

This study was supported in part by a grant from the American Academy of Pediatrics Memorial and Endowment Fund for Children, Elk Grove Village, Ill.

The authors do not have a financial or other interest in Hewlett-Packard Company.

Frances Sommer assisted with manuscript preparation, William Bonadio assisted with manuscript review, and the house staff, medical students, and attending physicians assisted by participating in the testing procedure.

References

1. Cole CH, ed. *The Harriet Lane Handbook: A Manual for Pediatric House Officers.* 11th ed. Chicago, Ill: Year Book Medical Publishers Inc; 1987.
2. Losek J, Garland J. *The First Five Minutes.* 6th ed. Milwaukee, Wis: Maxishare; 1989.
3. Kelly KJ, Neu J, Rice TB, Crim W, Eisenberg CS. Efficacy of a programmed calculator for constant-infusion medication calculations. *Pediatrics.* 1984;73:68-70.
4. Yamamoto LG, Wiebe RA. Pediatric and adult emergency management assistance using computerized guidelines. *Am J Emerg Med.* 1989;7:791-796.
5. Diserens D, Schwartz MW, Guenin M, Taylor LA. Measuring the problem-solving ability of students and residents by microcomputer. *J Med Educ.* 1986;61:461-466.
6. McDonald CJ. Protocol-based computer reminders, the quality of care and the non-perfectibility of man. *N Engl J Med.* 1976;295:1351-1355.
7. Edwards FH, Davis RS. The hand-held computer in critical care medicine. *Am Surg.* 1986;52:452-455.
8. Johnson S, Cramer R. Individualized microcomputer-generated emergency pediatric dosing guidelines. *Am J Hosp Pharm.* 1986;43:1507-1508.
9. Enderlin GM, Summerfield MR, Burney MT. Use of a microcomputer in a pediatric hospital. *Am J Hosp Pharm.* 1987;44:565-568.
10. Hochstrasser DF, Fleck RJ, Hull JH, Sarubbi FA. A pocket calculator program for pharmacokinetic dosing of drugs exhibiting single compartment first-order elimination and zero-order or first-order absorption. *Comput Biomed Res.* 1984;17:27-37.
11. Mitsuoka JC, Fleck RJ. Individualized estimation of clearance following a loading dose and continuous intravenous infusion using a programmable calculator. *Comput Methods Programs Biomed.* 1983;16:21-26.
12. Mitsuoka JC, Fleck RJ. A system for individualized dosing of intravenous aminophylline using a programmable calculator. *Pediatrics.* 1984;73:64-67.
13. Neu J, Crim W, Kien CL, Kelly K. Calculator assisted monitoring of nutrition, fluids and electrolytes. *Crit Care Med.* 1982;10:461-462.
14. Haddad M, Reiss R, Lilos P, Fuchs C. TI-59 programmable calculator program for calculating predicted operative mortality in general surgery. *Comput Biol Med.* 1986;16:445-452.
15. Milazzo CF. A pocket computer program for common calculation in clinical pediatrics. *Comput Biomed Res.* 1985;15:41-55.

Psychosocial Predictors of Maternal and Infant Health Among Adolescent Mothers

W. Thomas Boyce, MD; Elizabeth A. Chesterman; Marilyn A. Winkleby, PhD

• **Past work suggests that stressful life events and social support are significantly associated with a broad range of child health outcomes. Such associations have remained, however, generally modest in magnitude, suggesting that stress and support may be only proxy measures for a deeper, more central aspect of childhood psychosocial experience. One aspect of young people's lives that could plausibly mediate the effects of stress and social support on health is the sense of stability and "permanence" in ongoing life experience. We developed a standardized psychometric instrument for measuring a "sense of permanence" and employed the measure in a prospective 1-year study of health outcomes among 89 adolescent mothers and their infants. Psychosocial and demographic factors were significantly predictive of maternal, but not infant, health outcomes, and the sense of permanence appeared to operate as a "final common pathway" in the influence of psychosocial variables on health and illness end points. Results of the study underscore the importance of continuity and stability in childhood and suggest that changes in an individual's sense of permanence may underlie the previously documented health effects of stressful life events and social support.**

(*AJDC.* 1991;145:267-273)

Over the past two decades, a substantial body of work has evolved examining the association between psychosocial stressors and child health. Studies of acute and chronic stressors in the lives of children have demonstrated significant, but modest, associations between environmental stressors and childhood illness.[1,2] The generally low magnitude of such associations has been attributed, in part, to the countervailing effects of supportive and protective aspects of social experience that have often gone unmeasured in studies of stress and disease. When measured, positive features of the social environment, such as social support, have been shown to have significant beneficial effects on illness end points in diverse populations of children.[3-5]

The underlying biological mechanisms that may explain a relationship between psychosocial factors and health have been elucidated by new knowledge regarding the physiologic correlates of emotion and social experience. Data from a variety of animal and human studies suggest that both positive and negative aspects of psychosocial experience can affect physiologic response.[6-10] Stressors in laboratory and natural settings have been shown to influence hormone secretion,[8,10,11] cardiovascular measures such as blood pressure and heart rate,[12-15] and immunocompetence.[16-19] In addition, there is evidence that the salutary effects of social support may arise from an activation of central nervous system centers controlling affective and emotional experience.[20] Taken together, these and other studies suggest credible physiologic mechanisms that may underlie the epidemiologic observations of a connection between psychosocial processes and disease.

Despite the accumulation of significant findings, current work on psychosocial factors in child health has been impeded by the following two related problems: (1) the consistently low magnitude of reported associations, and (2) the lack of a coherent, unifying theory that could account for the diverse, and sometimes opposing, effects of psychosocial variables. One explanation for the failure of social factors to account for a greater share of the variance in childhood illness outcomes is the possibility that measures of stress and social support are only markers for a deeper, more central aspect of a child's psychosocial experience. We have proposed in past reports[21,22] that the effects of both stressful and protective social factors might be usefully viewed as acting on child health through their capacity to undermine or sustain a child's sense of permanence and continuity in ongoing life experience. We defined "a sense of permanence" as the belief or perception that certain central, valued elements of life experience are stable and enduring, and we developed a reliable and valid psychometric instrument to measure this construct using a self-report questionnaire.[21] Our previous work provided preliminary cross-sectional evidence that the sense of permanence was significantly related to neonatal complications and maternal affect in a population of unmarried, adolescent mothers.

Antonovsky[23,24] and Syme[25] have similarly proposed that stress and social support (as well as other social factors) exert their effects through underlying influences on an individual's sense of coherence or control. However, missing to date from such unifying theories is a *prospective* test of the hypothesized relationships. In this article, we report the results of a longitudinal prospective study of adolescent mothers and their infants during the year following delivery. The study examined the specific hypoth-

Accepted for publication November 8, 1990.

From the Division of Behavioral and Developmental Pediatrics, University of California, San Francisco.

Reprint requests to Division of Behavioral and Developmental Pediatrics, University of California, A203, 400 Parnassus Ave, San Francisco, CA 94143 (Dr Boyce).

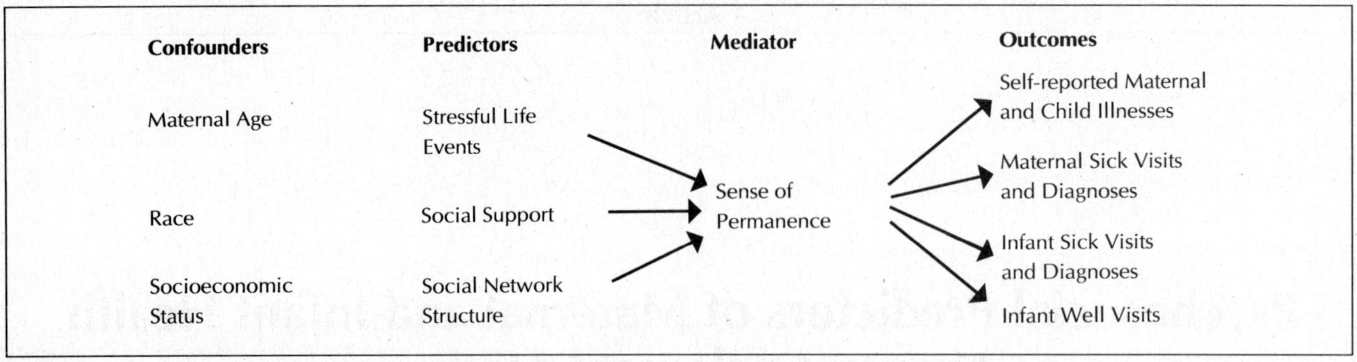

Fig 1.—*Theoretical model of effects on maternal and child health outcomes.*

esis that the effects of stressful and supportive experience on maternal and child health outcomes would be mediated, or accounted for, by underlying effects on the mother's sense of permanence.

SUBJECTS AND METHODS

A sample of convenience comprising 89 unmarried pregnant adolescents was recruited in Pima County, Arizona, from a variety of settings including schools, teenage-parent programs, clinics, and hospitals. All subjects were younger than 19 years, spoke English, and planned to retain primary responsibility for their babies' care following delivery. Subjects were offered free pediatric care for themselves and their infants during the 1-year study period as an incentive to enrollment. All subjects were recruited in their third trimester of pregnancy, and none who were approached regarding enrollment in the study refused to participate.

Figure 1 displays the independent and outcome variables assessed, the timing of variable measurements, and the theoretical ordering of their hypothesized relationships. Age, race, and socioeconomic status (SES) were viewed as potential confounders and are listed in the first tier of variables as factors to be controlled for in testing the principal study hypotheses. Stressful life events, social support, and social network structure were viewed as predictor variables and are shown in the second tier of the causal chain. All six of the variables in the first two tiers were assessed as baseline measures in the perinatal period, within 2 weeks before or after delivery. Sense of permanence was regarded as a more distal mediator variable and was measured in the fourth postpartum month. The outcome variables—self-reported maternal and infant illnesses, maternal/infant "sick visits" and diagnoses, and infant "well visits"—were assessed prospectively from the fifth through the 12th postpartum months using biweekly completion of home health diaries and medical record reviews. It is important to note that one of the study's methodologic strengths was the prospective, sequential measurement of variables, which replicated the theoretical ordering of the hypothesized causal relationships. Age, race, SES, stressful life events, social support, and social network structure were thus viewed as causally antecedent to a sense of permanence and were measured prior to the assessment of sense of permanence. Sense of permanence, in turn, was regarded as antecedent to the health outcomes and was measured in the month prior to the prospective collection of outcome data.

Based on subject response, race was coded as black, white, Hispanic, or Native American. Socioeconomic status was scored using a modification of Green's index[26] of social position, which was based on the income of the household in which the subject lived and the occupation of the main wage earner.

Stressful life events were assessed for the 4-month period preceding delivery using a set of 50 life event items compiled from the studies by Coddington,[27] Holmes and Rahe,[28] and Monaghan et al.[29] Previous work with life event instruments[30,31] has confirmed strong reliability and validity characteristics and has suggested that consensus weightings of events account for little, if any, additional variance in health outcomes. Because of this, scores in this study were calculated as the simple, unweighted frequency of reported life events.

Social network structure and social support were measured using an instrument drawn from the work of Berkman and Syme[32] and others.[33-35] Consistent with current work distinguishing structural and functional aspects of social affiliation,[36] two measures were employed: one describing and counting existing social ties and the other ascertaining the degree to which members of the social network served particular supportive functions. Social network was operationally defined as those relatives and friends with whom subjects made planned contacts at a frequency of once or more per month. The measure of social network structure was scored as a sum based on the following: (1) marital status (0, unmarried; 1, married to person other than infant's father; 2, married to infant's father), (2) the number of network members (0 to 2, lowest three deciles on social network size; 3, all others), and (3) the subject's relationship to the person(s) with whom she was living (0, alone or with other adults; 1, subject's parents or infant's father). Social support was defined as benefits derived from interactions with network members and was scored based on functional questions regarding the provision of favors and assistance by individuals (equally weighted subscores for "special favors," "gone out of the way to help," "discussed personal problem," and "really count on").

Sense of permanence was assessed using a previously reported 40-item scale.[21] Items were generated to reflect perceptions and experiences theoretically consistent with a sense of permanence. These included (1) an awareness of *self* as reliable and consistent, (2) the perception of stability in important interpersonal *relationships*, (3) the identification of certain *places* as special points of reference, (4) the awareness of behavioral patterns and *routines* in day-to-day activities, and (5) a consciousness of religious or *spiritual principles* that suggest a universal order. Five of the original 40 items had insufficient variation in responses and were excluded. Factor analysis was applied to the remaining 35 items, and the 19 items that loaded together in the first factor were used as the final measure of sense of permanence (Table 1). Assessment of the measure's reliability demonstrated high internal consistency with Cronbach $\alpha = .81$. (In the only previous use of the instrument measuring sense of permanence, 277 randomly selected men and women ranging in age from 15 to 92 years were administered the questionnaire in two family medicine clinics. There were no significant age or sex differences in scores, and the internal consistency of the scale [Cronbach $\alpha = .84$] was as high as that found in our study.)

As noted above, self-reported maternal and infant illnesses were measured using a home health diary that was completed every 2 weeks from the fifth through the 12th postpartum month. Diaries included reports on symptoms of illness for both mother and infant, number of sick days in the 2-week period, and general well-being on a 10-point Likert scale. Maternal and infant sick visits, maternal and infant diagnoses, and infant well visits were compiled from medical record reviews. Since free medical care was provided to the mothers and their infants, a large majority of the care was given at a single site, the Pediatric Clinic at the University of Arizona Health Sciences Center, Tucson. Emergency department and weekend care was occasionally sought at other sites. In every known case, however, visits outside the university clinic were reported to study personnel by the subject,

Table 1.—Sense of Permanence Scale*

Score	Statements Describing People's Feelings About Themselves, the World, and People Closest to Them
+1	I feel sure of my family's love for me
+2	I have friends I can really count on
+3	Despite all the problems in the world, I feel pretty hopeful about life
+4	I am a fairly stable person
−5	My family is sometimes inconsistent in the way they respond to the things I do
−6	My relationship to my family feels pretty uncertain some of the time
−7	It does not take much to upset me
−8	Nothing is very permanent
−9	My friendships tend to come and go
+10	I have great faith in the person who is closest to me
−11	Sometimes I really think the world is falling apart
−12	I am not always sure where I stand in my closest relationship
+13	I feel pretty settled in my home right now
−14	I do not feel very connected to any special place right now
−15	Even the person you are closest to cannot always be counted on
−16	Sometimes it seems like everything is changing too fast around here
−17	My reactions to new situations are fairly unpredictable
−18	I am never really sure how some of my friends feel about me
−19	Something always interrupts the routines I try to follow

*To compute sense of permanence score, a score of 1 is assigned to each positive item circled and 1 to each negative item *not* circled. A score of 0 is assigned to the remaining items. Then the sum of item scores is added for the total score. Pluses and minuses were not included in subject's version.

Table 2.—Frequency Distributions for Independent and Outcome Variables

Variable	Mean ± SD	Range
Maternal age, y	16.5 ± 1.2	14-18
Maternal race*	. . .	. . .
Socioeconomic status	101.7 ± 17.0	58-141
Stressful life events	17.6 ± 6.3	7-33
Social support	29.2 ± 14.5	5-77
Social network structure	3.0 ± 1.1	0-4
Sense of permanence	11.6 ± 4.2	3-19
Maternal days sick†	10.6 ± 8.1	0-45
Infant days sick†	18.2 ± 8.3	1-37
Maternal symptoms†	42.1 ± 20.5	10-122
Infant symptoms†	67.9 ± 20.4	20-120
General well-being†	100.5 ± 22.5	34-143
Maternal sick visits†	1.2 ± 2.2	0-12
Maternal diagnoses†	1.5 ± 2.1	0-12
Infant sick visits†	3.8 ± 3.9	0-17
Infant diagnoses†	4.5 ± 3.8	0-17
Infant well visits†	2.4 ± 1.1	0-5

*Forty-three percent were white, 37% Hispanic, 18% black, and 2% Native American.

†Principal-components analysis of these 10 variables identified four factors that served as the outcome variables for the subsequent test of study hypotheses. For each factor, scores on component variables were standardized and summed to derive the outcome variable score. The four outcomes were designated self-reported maternal and infant illnesses; maternal sick visits and diagnoses; infant sick visits and diagnoses; and infant well visits.

thereby allowing review of all medical records and a comprehensive summary of medical care utilization. All outcome data were gathered by study personnel who had no knowledge of subjects' prior responses on measures of independent variables.

Statistical analyses first examined frequency distributions for independent and outcome measures and Pearson correlation coefficients for the bivariate relationships among pairs of variables. The hypothesized relationships depicted in Fig 1 were tested with path analysis using a series of standard multiple regression equations.[37] In this path analytic approach, each variable in the second through the fourth tiers in the causal model was regressed on all antecedent variables. Stressful life events were therefore regressed on maternal age, race, and SES; sense of permanence was regressed on all six of the variables in the first and second tiers, and so on. The resultant path model provided a summary estimate of the degree to which data conformed to Fig 1, the hypothesized set of causal associations.

RESULTS

Table 2 presents the frequency distributions for all independent and outcome variables. The mean age of study subjects was 16.5 years, with a range of 14 to 18 years. The distribution of the study population by race was 18% black, 43% white, 37% Hispanic, and 2% Native American. These distributions were comparable with those of the Pima County population of adolescent mothers from which the sample was drawn, except that mothers younger than 15 years were slightly overrepresented (7% vs 3%) and Native American mothers were underrepresented (2% vs 17%).[21] Socioeconomic status had a broad and representative range.

The average number of life events reported in the perinatal period was 18, reflecting the tumult and change that often accompany a teenage pregnancy and birth. Among the events most frequently reported were "change to a different school," "change in the way friends treat me," "not making it into an extracurricular activity I wanted to be involved in (ie, athletic team, band, etc)," "change in my financial situation," and "move to a new house or apartment." The measures of functional and structural social support, as well as the sense of permanence score, showed extensive variability around generally normal distributions.

Table 2 also displays the frequency distributions for component variables within the four outcome measures. Over the 8-month follow-up period between the infant's fifth and 12th month of life, mothers reported an average of 11 sick days for themselves and 18 sick days for their infants. These periods of illness resulted in a mean of 1.2 physician visits for mothers and 3.8 visits for infants, indicating as expected that an infant illness was more likely to result in a medical visit than a maternal illness. The number of well child visits over the first year of life—an index of maternal use of preventive pediatric care—averaged only 2.4, a number substantially below the five or six well child visits generally recommended.

Not shown in Table 2 is the finding that correlations between serial measures of the sense of permanence over approximately 4-month intervals averaged about 0.70. It is consistent with our theoretical view of this construct that the correlations demonstrate a reasonably high level of temporal stability, but a significant influence of changing life circumstances as well.

Initial analysis of bivariate relationships among pairs of independent variables (ie, confounders, predictors, and mediator) and outcome variables revealed several significant findings. The tabulation below displays correlation

Table 3.—Bivariate Relationships Among Psychosocial Variables and Maternal and Infant Health Outcomes (Pearson Correlation Coefficients)

Psychosocial Variables	Self-reported Maternal and Infant Illnesses	Maternal Sick Visits and Diagnoses	Infant Sick Visits and Diagnoses	Infant Well Visits
Stressful life events	.39*	.27*	.06	−.01
Social support	−.14	−.04	−.09	.10
Social network structure	−.21†	−.09	−.02	.09
Sense of permanence	−.44*	−.24†	.01	.14

*$P<.01$.
†$P<.05$.

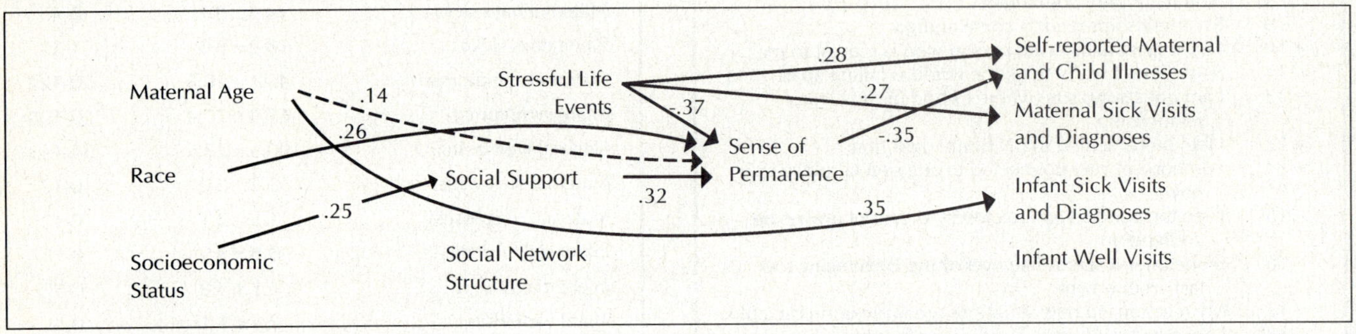

Fig 2.—*Path model of effects on maternal and child health outcomes.* P≤*.01 for all solid paths;* P<*.10 for broken path. Numbers represent standardized regression coefficients.*

coefficients for the associations found between predictor variables and the score of sense of permanence.

Predictor Variables	**Sense of Permanence Score, Pearson *r* (*P*)**
Stressful life events	.31 (<.01)
Social support	.29 (<.01)
Social network structure	.23 (<.05)

As predicted by our theoretical model, higher sense of permanence was significantly related to fewer stressful life events, higher perceived social support, and a larger social network structure.

Table 3 shows bivariate associations among predictor, mediator, and outcome variables. Stressful life events were significantly related to self-reported maternal and infant illnesses and to maternal sick visits and diagnoses, with higher numbers of events associated with higher levels of each of these illness outcomes. Perceived social support was unrelated to any outcome, and network structure was associated only with self-reported illnesses. Sense of permanence, on the other hand, was significantly related both to self-reported illnesses and to maternal sick visits and diagnoses. The strongest of all examined bivariate relationships was the inverse association between sense of permanence and self-reported maternal and infant illnesses, indicating that subjects with a high sense of permanence reported fewer illnesses for both themselves and their infants ($r=-.44$, $P<.01$).

It is important to note that the only significant bivariate associations with psychosocial variables were those found for outcomes based on *maternal* rather than infant data. Five of eight correlations with maternal outcomes were significant, whereas none of eight with infant outcomes reached significance. Stressful life events and sense of permanence were significantly related only to self-reported illnesses (a variable based on the mother's perceptions) and maternal sick visits and diagnoses (a variable based on the mother's clinical illness experience). Examination of bivariate associations thus offered preliminary support for the proposed theoretical model (Fig 1), but only for end points derived from *maternal* perceptions and experiences.

Multivariate analyses were required to test hypotheses regarding causal ordering and to assess the independent effects of predictor and mediator variables while controlling for the potential confounding effects of maternal age, race, and SES. Figure 2 displays path analysis data derived from the three sequential multiple regression procedures corresponding to the variables in the second, third, and fourth tiers of the theoretical model. Only significant or borderline significant paths identified by the regression models are displayed. Maternal age, race, and SES were significantly related to various predictor, mediator, and outcome variables. Maternal age, for example, was strongly associated with infant sick visits and diagnoses such that older maternal age was predictive of more infant sick visits and diagnoses. Stressful life events were related to sense of permanence and two of the outcome variables, self-reported illnesses and maternal sick visits and diagnoses.

Sense of permanence appeared to operate as the final common pathway for a number of antecedent confounder and predictor variables, including maternal age, race, stressful life events, and perceived support. Each of these variables was predictive of self-reported maternal and infant illnesses, but *through* their influence on the mother's sense of permanence. Sense of permanence scores remained strongly and inversely associated with self-reported illnesses, even after adjustment for the effects of demographic and other psychosocial measures. It is again important to note that, although the sense of permanence and other psychosocial variables were strongly related to health outcomes, the significant relationships found in this regression model were almost exclusively those with end points derived from maternal, rather than infant, experience.

COMMENT

This study confirmed, in part, the hypothesized relationships of psychosocial factors to health outcomes over the first year following an adolescent pregnancy. The data presented provide evidence that (1) an adolescent mother's stressful and supportive social experience is a significant prospective predictor of maternal health outcomes during the first year of her infant's life; (2) a young mother's sense of permanence, defined as her perception of stable continuous aspects of ongoing life experience, is significantly determined by demographic factors, such as her age and race, and by psychosocial factors, such as stressful events and social support; and (3) psychosocial factors have both direct and indirect effects on maternal health outcomes, with indirect effects operating *through* the young woman's sense of permanence.

While not all aspects of our theoretical model were confirmed by these data, several important elements of the model were strongly supported. Results of the path analysis indicate, for example, that virtually all demographic and psychosocial variables affected the young mother's sense of permanence, and the influence of these variables on health outcomes operated almost entirely through intervening effects on the sense of permanence. Furthermore, the strongest association found in the study was the inverse relationship between scores of sense of permanence and self-reported illnesses, so that subjects with a weaker sense of permanence recorded significantly higher rates of illness for both themselves and their babies. Note that it is impossible, using these data, to disentangle actual maternal and infant illness experience from the mother's *perception* of illness events. Nonetheless, the findings support the general conclusion that a young mother's sense of permanence and stability exert significant influences on her illness experience, her subjective appraisal of illness symptoms, or both.

Several aspects of the proposed theoretical model were *not* confirmed, however, by data derived from the study. In particular, predicted relationships were not found between the sense of permanence and the more objective, medically based measures of sick visits and diagnoses. The bivariate association, for example, between scores of sense of permanence and maternal sick visits and diagnoses did not reach significance after adjustment for the effects of confounder and predictor variables. Further, no significant associations were found between psychosocial variables and infant, as opposed to maternal, health outcomes. The only significant relationship with infant outcomes was that noted between maternal age and infant sick visits and diagnoses. Taken together, these findings indicate that, in the setting of adolescent pregnancy and parenthood, the sense of permanence and other psychosocial factors may have stronger effects on maternal than on infant outcomes and be more highly correlated with self-reported appraisals of health status.

Several shortcomings in the design of the study and in the character of the data should be taken into account in evaluating the reported findings. First, the study sample is relatively small and was not chosen at random from a larger population of adolescent mothers. Inspection of the sample's demographic characteristics nevertheless indicates moderate comparability with the population of teenage mothers in Pima County, where subjects were recruited. Second, three of the psychosocial variables employed in the study—social support, social network structure, and sense of permanence—were assessed using instruments designed for this study, on which only limited psychometric information is currently available. The reliability of the measure of sense of permanence is supported by the findings of strong internal homogeneity and high stability over time. Construct validity of the measure is undergirded by the significant associations found, in the expected direction, between sense of permanence and both stressful life events and social support. Finally, the finding that sense of permanence was related only to *self-reported* health status and not to more objective measures of medically generated diagnoses raises the issue of a "response-set," which could create spurious associations among subjective, self-report measures. There is thus the possibility that some characterologic feature of certain subjects could create a tendency to underestimate experiences of stability and continuity and to overestimate experiences of illness. Such a process occurring in a subset of subjects could potentially result in a biased association between the sense of permanence and self-appraised health status.

On the other hand, past independent observations and research findings similarly suggest the importance of a child's experiences of continuity and stability. Developmental theory, for example, has emphasized the significance of object relations in early childhood and the child's "search for constancy" in the establishing of social bonds. Bank and Kahn[38] wrote that "A young child needs a stable, reliable environment or 'object constancy' . . . the child who can fuse or merge with another person will feel more whole, more integrated, and less vulnerable to the vagaries of an uncertain world."

Similarly, Erikson[39] suggested that the development of "basic trust" in the first year of life depends, in part, on "an outer predictability (the mother) becoming an inner certainty," the process by which the infant maps parental dependability onto the larger arena of ongoing life experience. Others[40,41] have noted children's use of treasured transitional objects from infancy to adolescence as another source of familiarity and a symbol of constancy during moments of fear, discomfort, or difficult change.

Even in adult life, the stable presence of other persons can be a meaningful source of comfort and solace during times of stress. Kennell et al,[42] for example, found that for pregnant women the presence of a supportive companion during labor resulted in a significant decrease in the need for medical interventions such as cesarean or forceps deliveries or epidural anesthesia. Medical and biological effects of a supportive social environment have become increasingly well known,[36] but what is remarkable about the study by Kennell et al is that much of the protective effect persisted when the labor companion *only observed* without interacting with the mother. This finding suggests that simply the stability and continuity inherent in having another person in the room throughout labor was itself a protective social factor.

In work suggesting the relevance of an even more mundane aspect of social experience, Boyce and colleagues[43,44] have demonstrated that family rituals and routines can provide children with a stable point of reference during times of unsettling change in the life of the family. In one study, respiratory illnesses among preschool children were more prolonged and more severe in children whose families had fewer and less predictable routines. The notion that ritual behavior may have important influences on health has been further advanced by the work of Ehlers et al,[45] indicating that disruption of social rhythms may result in unstable biological rhythms and trigger the onset of major depressive episodes in adult subjects. It is important to note in these studies that the presence of rituals and routines is one component of the sense of permanence construct.

Related to the experience of routines, predictability appears to be a salient central dimension of social experience during times of major stress. The animal study by Weiss[46] demonstrated that unpredictable shock was many times more pathogenic than predictable shock of equal intensity in producing gastrointestinal lesions in laboratory animals. Similarly, Seligman[47] has shown that inescapable, uncontrollable shock results in a state of helplessness and slow learning that mimics clinical depression. In their work with chronically ill children, Jessop and Stein[48] have pointed out the importance of uncertainty and unpredictability in patients' experiences of illness. Further, Mechanic's[49] study of illness behavior in adolescence indicates that discontinuities in family life and social experience tend to exacerbate the perception of bodily symptoms, while stability and predictability tend to protect against preoccupation with self-perceived symptoms.

Finally, paralleling our proposal here, a number of other investigators have proposed that a central, underlying construct might account for the health effects of diverse psychosocial factors such as life events, social support, or styles of coping. Our theoretical frame of reference and research findings are highly convergent, for example, with the work of Antonovsky[23,24] on the "sense of coherence." Citing a variety of evidence, he proposes that underlying an individual's capacity to resist disease is a "way of seeing the world," a perception of life experiences as predictable, understandable, and ordered. Rodin,[50] in addition, sees the individual's "sense of control" as the central psychological attribute determining health and resilience, and Syme[25] has proposed that one's "control of destiny" is perhaps the most salient aspect of health-altering psychosocial experience.

In conclusion, we have offered a perspective in which the various effects of psychosocial factors in *childhood* are seen as operating through the child's evolving belief in the stability and continuity of life experience. For a contemporary child, the already tumultuous changes inherent in growth and maturation are magnified by a set of powerful societal forces that include divorce, poverty, residential mobility, family isolation, violence, and a host of others. It is our hope, in presenting the data reviewed above, to underscore for those who care for the health of children the critical importance of permanence and stability in the lives of the patients they treat.

This work was supported by a research grant from the WT Grant Foundation of New York and a Biomedical Research Support Grant from the University of Arizona.

We are grateful to Professor S. Leonard Syme, PhD, who played a critical, encouraging role in the development of the ideas on which the article is based. We also appreciate the helpful comments and suggestions of our colleagues, John Jemerin, MD, and Lane Tanner, MD, regarding earlier drafts of the manuscript.

References

1. Haggerty RJ. Life stress, illness and social supports. *Dev Med Child Neurol.* 1980;22:391-400.
2. Boyce WT. Stress and child health: an overview. *Pediatr Ann.* 1985;14:539-542.
3. Boyce WT, Chesterman E. Life events, social support, and cardiovascular reactivity in adolescence. *J Dev Behav Pediatr.* 1990;11:105-111.
4. Pascoe JM, Earp JA. The effect of mothers' social support and life changes on the stimulation of their children in the home. *Am J Public Health.* 1984;74:358-360.
5. Shonkoff JP. Social support and the development of vulnerable children. *Am J Public Health.* 1984;74:310-312.
6. Boyce WT, Jemerin JJ. Psychobiological differences in children stress response, I: patterns of illness and susceptibility. *J Dev Behav Pediatr.* 1990;11:86-94.
7. Gunnar MR. Psychobiological studies of stress and coping: an introduction. *Child Dev.* 1987;58:1403-1407.
8. Axelrod J, Reisine T. Stress hormones: their interaction and regulation. *Science.* 1984;224:452-459.
9. Hofer MA. Early social relationships: a psychobiologist's view. *Child Dev.* 1987;58:633-647.
10. Rose RM. Endocrine responses to stressful psychological events. *Psychiatr Clin North Am.* 1980;3:251-276.
11. Asterita MF. *The Physiology of Stress.* New York, NY: Human Sciences Press; 1985.
12. Matthews KA, Woodall KL. Childhood origins of overt type A behaviors and cardiovascular reactivity to behavioral stressors. *Ann Behav Med.* 1988;10:71-77.
13. Murphy JK, Alpert BS, Willey ES, Somes GW. Cardiovascular reactivity to psychological stress in healthy children. *Psychophysiology.* 1988;25:144-152.
14. Krantz DS, Manuck SB. Acute psychophysiological reactivity and risk of cardiovascular disease: a review and methodologic critique. *Psychol Bull.* 1984;96:435-464.
15. Jemerin JJ, Boyce WT. Psychobiological differences in childhood stress response, II: Cardiovascular markers of vulnerability. *J Dev Behav Pediatr.* 1990;11:140-150.
16. Ader R. *Psychoneuroimmunology.* Orlando, Fla: Academic Press Inc; 1981.
17. Jemmott JB, Locke SE. Psychosocial factors, immunologic mediation, and human susceptibility to infectious diseases: how much do we know? *Psychol Bull.* 1984;78:78-108.
18. Kiecolt-Glaser JK, Glaser R. Psychosocial moderators of immune function. *Ann Behav Med.* 1987;9:16-20.
19. Palmblad JEW. Stress and human immunologic competence. In: Guillemin R, ed. *Neural Modulation of Immunity.* New York, NY: Raven Press; 1985.
20. Bovard EW. Brain mechanisms in effects of social support on viability. *Perspect Behav Med.* 1985;2:103-129.
21. Boyce WT, Schaefer C, Uitti C. Permanence and change: psychosocial factors in the outcomes of adolescent pregnancy. *Soc Sci Med.* 1985;21:1279-1287.
22. Chesterman E, Boyce WT, Winkleby MA. Psychosocial predictors of maternal and infant health: a 'sense of permanence' as a mediating variable. Presented at the Society of Behavioral Medicine Annual Meeting. April 1, 1989; San Francisco, Calif. Abstract.
23. Antonovsky A. The sense of coherence as a determinant of health. In: Matarazzo J, ed. *Behavioral Health: A Handbook of Health Enhancement and Disease Prevention.* New York, NY: John Wiley & Sons Inc; 1984:114-129.
24. Antonovsky A. *Unraveling the Mystery of Health: How People Manage Stress and Stay Well.* San Francisco, Calif: Jossey-Bass; 1987.
25. Syme SL. Control and health: an epidemiologic perspective. In: Schaie KW, Rodin J, Schroeder C, eds. *Control and Health: An Epidemiologic Perspective.* Hillsdale, NJ: Erlbaum; 1990:213-229.
26. Green LW. Manual for scoring socioeconomic status for research on health behavior. *Public Health Rep.* 1970;85:815.
27. Coddington RD. Life events associated with adolescent pregnancies. *J Clin Psychiatry.* 1979;40:180-185.
28. Holmes TH, Rahe RH. The social readjustment rating scale. *J Psychosom Res.* 1967;11:213.
29. Monaghan JH, Robinson JO, Dodge JA. The children's life events inventory. *J Psychosom Res.* 1979;23:63-68.
30. Rabkin JG, Struening EL. Life events, stress and illness. *Science.* 1976;194:1013-1020.
31. Dohrenwend BS, Dohrenwend BP. *Stressful Life Events and Their Contexts.* New Brunswick, NJ: Rutgers University Press; 1981.
32. Berkman LF, Syme SL. Social networks, host resistance, and mortality: a nine-year follow-up study of Alameda County residents. *Am J Epidemiol.* 1979;109:186.
33. Jones LM, Fisher CS. *Studying Egocentric Networks by Mass Survey.* Berkeley, Calif: University of California Press;

1978: working paper No. 284.
34. Salloway JC, Dillon PB. A comparison of family network and friend networks in health care utilization. *J Comp Fam Studies.* 1973;4:131.
35. Pilisuk M, Frolund C. Kinship, social networks, social support and health. *Soc Sci Med.* 1978;12:273.
36. Cohen S, Syme SL. *Social Support and Health.* Orlando, Fla: Academic Press Inc; 1985.
37. Pedhazur EJ. *Multiple Regression in Behavior Research: Explanation and Prediction.* New York, NY: Holt Rinehart & Winston; 1982.
38. Bank SP, Kahn MD. *The Sibling Bond.* New York, NY: Basic Books; 1982.
39. Erikson EH. *Childhood and Society.* New York, NY: Norton; 1963.
40. Sherman M, Hertzig M, Austrian R, Shapiro T. Treasured objects in school-aged children. *Pediatrics.* 1981;68:379-386.
41. Shafii T. The prevalence and use of transitional objects: a study of 230 adolescents. *J Am Acad Child Psychiatry.* 1986;25:805-808.
42. Kennell J, Klaus M, McGrath S, Robertson S, Hinkley C. Medical intervention: the effect of social support during labor. *Pediatr Res.* 1988;23:211. Abstract.
43. Boyce WT. Interaction between social variables in stress research. *J Health Soc Behav.* 1981;22:194-195.
44. Boyce WT, Jensen EW, Cassel JC, Collier AM, Smith AH, Ramey CT. Influence of life events and family routines on childhood respiratory tract illness. *Pediatrics.* 1977;60:609-615.
45. Ehlers CL, Frank E, Kupfer DJ. Social zeitgebers and biological rhythms. *Arch Gen Psychiatry.* 1988;45:948-952.
46. Weiss JM. Somatic effects of predictable and unpredictable shock. *Psychosom Med.* 1968;32:397-408.
47. Seligman MEP. Anxiety and unpredictability. In: Seligman MEP, ed. *Helplessness: On Depression, Development, and Death.* San Francisco, Calif: WH Freeman; 1975:107-159.
48. Jessop DJ, Stein REK. Uncertainty and its relation to the psychological and social correlates of chronic illness in children. *Soc Sci Med.* 1985;20:993-999.
49. Mechanic D. Adolescent health and illness behavior: review of the literature and a new hypothesis for the study of stress. *J Hum Stress.* 1983;9:4-13.
50. Rodin J. Aging and health: effects of the sense of control. *Science.* 1986;233:1271-1276.

ONLY NIX.™ ONLY ONCE.

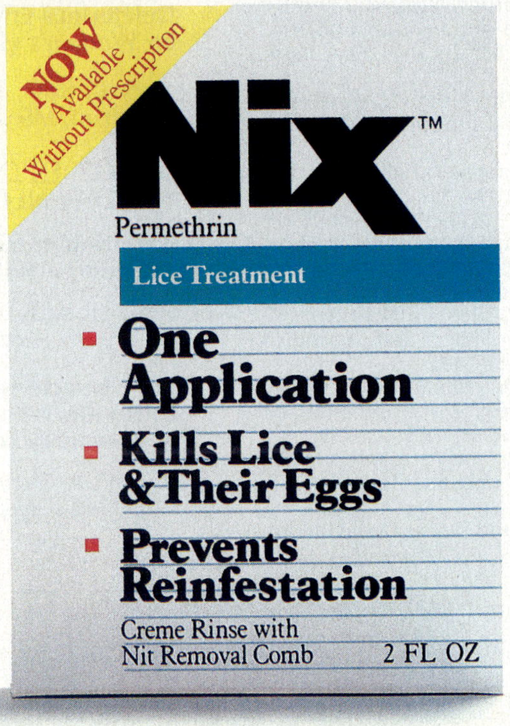

Only Nix™ Creme Rinse has been proved up to 99% effective with a single 10-minute application.[1]

Only Nix protects against reinfestation for up to two weeks.

And the active ingredient in Nix has been tested for safety in children as young as two months.[2]

Until now, only products with pyrethrins were available OTC.

Now Nix, with the unique ingredient permethrin, is available without a prescription.

Put anxious parents at ease. Recommend Nix. It's the best way–Rx or OTC–to kill lice and nits.

1. Brandenburg K, Deinard AS, DiNapoli J, Englender SJ, Orthoefer J, Wagner D. 1% permethrin cream rinse vs 1% lindane shampoo in treating pediculosis capitis. *Am J Dis Child.* 1986;140:894-896. 2. Data on file, Burroughs Wellcome Co., 1990.

Nix™
CREME RINSE

The best way to kill lice and nits.

Call 1-800-FOR-LICE to report outbreaks in your community.

Photographing the Physically Abused Child

Principles and Practice

Lawrence R. Ricci, MD

• Photographic documentation of significant findings is an important part of any child abuse evaluation. High-quality photographs of significant physical findings may be important in helping courts to adjudicate whether child abuse has taken place. The physician evaluating abused children should ensure adequate photographic documentation of visible lesions. Physicians who care for abused children should be familiar with the basic principles and techniques of clinical photography. These include good equipment, adequate lighting, and planned composition. Equally important is a working knowledge of camera equipment, film procedure, and medicolegal implications. This review outlines for the practicing physician the basic concepts and techniques of photographing abused children.

***(AJDC.* 1991;145:275-281)**

Photographic documentation of significant findings is an important part of any child abuse evaluation.[1-6] The American Medical Association's diagnostic and treatment guidelines for the abused child recommend that all visible lesions be photographed.[2] High-quality photographs of significant physical findings may be important in helping courts to adjudicate whether child abuse has taken place.[7]

See also pp 255 and 256.

This review outlines for the practicing physician the basic concepts and techniques of photographing abused children. The focus of the review will be on the physically abused child; however, the principles apply equally to the sexually abused child. A detailed review of photographing sexually abused children is presented elsewhere.[5] Although some institutions have access to professional photographic staff either inside the institution via a media department or outside via law enforcement, many do not.[1] It is incumbent on physicians evaluating abused children to ensure adequate photographic documentation of visible lesions either by taking the photographs themselves or by guaranteeing that they are taken by someone else. Indeed, many states require that reasonable efforts be made by the reporting hospital staff member to take or cause to be taken color photographs of any areas of visible trauma on the child.[1] Every physician who cares for abused children should be familiar with the basic principles and techniques of clinical photography.

These principles include good equipment, adequate lighting, and planned composition. The key equipment concerns are camera, lens, lighting, and film. A high-quality lens, adequate flash, and proper technique are of far greater importance than the brand or features of a camera.[8] No particular system is best. Decisions should be based on the needs of the photographer and the cost of the system.

CAMERAS

Camera systems recommended for photographing the abused victim range from expensive and sophisticated 35-mm close-up systems[5,6,9-11] to less expensive and simpler instant or self-developing camera systems.[3] Although new technologies, including videotape and computer-based digital image manipulation, are emerging, 35-mm slide and print photography remains the standard for patient documentation.[12]

Specific camera types available include instant-processing cameras, fixed-focus lens "point and shoot" 35-mm cameras, traditional 35-mm single lens reflex (SLR) cameras, and "bridge" cameras, a new generation of 35-mm cameras offering the simplicity of a fixed-focus lens camera and the versatility of a 35-mm SLR camera.

Instant-processing cameras have the advantage of simple operation and low initial cost. Their disadvantages include poor resolution and poor color rendition compared with 35-mm cameras and film.[1] This is particularly a problem when photographing subtle or faded bruises. Instant-processing cameras also have minimal close-up capability and require expensive film that is difficult to reproduce and store. The best argument for using an instant-processing camera is that the print develops just after the photograph is taken, guaranteeing at least some form of documentation. One compromise, particularly when there is a need for immediate documentation, is to take both instant and 35-mm photographs.

Fixed-focus lens "point and shoot" 35-mm cameras are inexpensive and easy to use, yet, much like instant-processing cameras, in the past they have offered limited close-up capability and expandability. Newer "point and shoot" cameras, however, have a variable focal length and often a modicum of macro capability (see below, the section on "bridge" cameras).

Accepted for publication September 6, 1990.

From the Diagnostic Program for Child Abuse, Mid-Maine Medical Center, Waterville.

Reprint requests to the Diagnostic Program for Child Abuse, Mid-Maine Medical Center, Waterville, ME 04901 (Dr Ricci).

Edited by Peggy C. Ferry, MD

Serious medical photography requires a camera that offers control over aperture, focusing, and shutter speed. The camera should also be able to accept a variety of lenses and other attachments. The 35-mm format offers an unrivaled choice of cameras, lenses, and accessories and, hence, excellent close-up capability and resolution. The most widely used 35-mm camera is the 35-mm SLR camera. A reflex camera is one whose viewing system employs a mirror to reflect the image onto the viewing screen. The mirror swings out of the way to expose the film when the shutter is released. A 35-mm SLR camera uses 35-mm film and a single lens for both viewing and recording the image. The photographer sees the same image as the lens and the film; this is important when using close-up or zoom lenses.

The most versatile system for the relatively skilled photographer utilizes a 35-mm SLR camera body with a series of lenses (eg, 50-mm, 105-mm, 35- to 105-mm zoom, and macro lenses) and both hotshoe and ring flashes.[5] The accessories may be used in various combinations depending on the clinical circumstances. Combining a 35- to 105-mm zoom lens with a 105-mm macro lens offers the most versatility. Attached to a 35-mm camera, a macro lens or a standard lens with close-up adapters allows photographs of fine anatomic detail otherwise not easily documented.[5] A colposcope mount may be useful for magnifications greater than life size, particularly of the genitalia.[6] Although adaptable to most clinical photographic situations, a traditional 35-mm SLR camera may be expensive and technically demanding.

The simplest system for a multiuser environment or for those unable to master a 35-mm SLR camera is a so-called "bridge" camera. These cameras combine the simplicity and ease of use of (bridge the gap between) a point and shoot camera with the versatility, expandability, and close-up capability of a 35-mm SLR camera.

LENSES

Lens quality, more than anything else, determines picture quality. Lenses come in three basic types: normal focal length, wide angle, and long or telephoto. The description of a particular focal length is dictated by the format (negative or transparency image size) of the camera. A normal lens is one in which the focal length approximately equals the diagonal measurement of the camera film format. For a 35-mm camera, a normal focal length would be 50 to 55 mm. A wide-angle lens would be 28 to 35 mm, while a long lens would be 80 mm or greater. Thirty-five–millimeter film is supplied in sprocketed rolls of variable length depending on the number of photographs on the roll. In all cases the width of the film on the roll is 35 mm. The image on the film, however, is 24×36 mm. The diagonal of the image size determines the lens classification.

The ideal lens for medical photography should have good optics, medium telephoto focal length (85 to 105 mm) to minimize distortion, and macro or close-up capability up to ×1 (the image on the negative or transparency is magnified to life size).

Magnification is the ratio of image size on the negative or transparency to actual object size (m = image size/object size). It can be expressed as a ratio (1:2), a fraction (1/2), a decimal (×0.5), or a percentage (50%). Close-up magnification is ×0.1 to ×0.5, extreme close-up magnification is ×0.5 to ×1, and true macro magnification is ×1 to ×35. For example, photographing an 8-year-old child using a 35-mm format would produce the following views on the print or slide at different magnifications: ×0.05, full body; ×0.1, half body; ×0.2, face or hand; ×0.5, ear, lips, and eye; and ×1, fingernail or hymen.

The maximum magnification of a lens can be checked by focusing the camera on a metric ruler at the closest focusing distance of the lens. With a 35-mm SLR camera, the viewfinder screen and film are both 36 mm wide. Thus, if the screen or the film "sees" a 36-mm segment of ruler horizontally (at the closest working distance of the lens), the magnification is ×1. If the screen sees 72 mm, the magnification is ×0.5 (m = 36 mm/No. of millimeters "seen" horizontally on the viewfinder screen).

The lens focal length dictates lens-to-subject distance, which in turn determines image distortion. A 90- to 110-mm lens is recommended for close-up work, particularly facial work, when using a 35-mm camera.[13] Long lenses compress or flatten perspective. This flattening is advantageous in face shots, because features such as the nose are less distorted. For torso or full-length photography, a 50- or 55-mm lens is adequate.[12] In general, a medium telephoto lens, such as a 105-mm lens, is best for everything from ×0.2 to ×1 (from the head and neck down to the fingernails), while a wider (55-mm) lens should be used for full- and half-body length photographs only (×0.05 to ×0.1).[1,14]

An additional advantage of a longer focal length is greater working distance. A typical 50-mm lens at a magnification of ×0.1 has a close working distance of 25 cm. A 100-mm lens doubles this working distance. Children may be less fearful if the camera is further away, ie, if the subject-to-lens distance is increased. In addition, flash illumination is more uniform as the distance increases.[11]

For very close work, magnifications greater than ×0.5, a macro lens provides the best solution. A macro lens is one capable of providing a magnification of ×1 or greater, although the term *macro* is often used to describe any close-focusing lens. Lenses sold as "zoom with macro focusing" are not true macro lenses and often magnify only up to ×0.25. True macro lenses have their barrels embossed with magnifications, especially from ×0.5 to ×1.[15]

A relatively inexpensive alternative to a macro lens for close-up work is a set of close-up or supplementary lenses. These are lens attachments placed over the normal lens to magnify the image. These auxiliary lenses provide magnification up to ×0.5. However, using close-up lens attachments to achieve magnifications greater than ×0.5 significantly reduces image quality. Beyond ×0.5, a macro lens offers the best option. Bellows and extension tubes, although cumbersome and difficult to use, are another option. Colposcopic camera attachments use the extension-tube principle to achieve magnifications of ×1 or greater.

Zoom lenses offer variable focal length. This allows one lens to be used for both close-up and distant work. By changing the focal length, zoom lenses allow the photographer to remain stationary while changing the magnification. Some zoom lenses provide macro capability up to ×0.25.

A particular problem in close-up work is narrow depth of field. Depth of field is the zone of acceptable sharpness extending in front of and behind the center of focus. It is determined by aperture, lens focal length, and subject-to-lens distance. The aperture or opening within the lens that limits the amount of light reaching the film can be varied by means of a diaphragm. The opening is measured by an f-number. The larger the aperture (ie, the smaller the f-number), the narrower the depth of field. In the close-up range, depth of field can be quite narrow (a typical 105-mm macro lens focusing at ×1 magnification at f-22 has a maximum depth of field of 4 to 6 mm). This can particularly be a problem with deep cavities, such as the rectum, where the pathology may have a greater depth than the depth of field of the camera. This problem may necessitate a series of photographs, each focused at different points near and far, none of which captures the entire area. When depth of field is a problem it is important not only to focus carefully but also to try to position the subject and/or the camera so that all of the important parts to be photographed fall in a plane parallel to the film. A powerful flash can improve depth of field by allowing a smaller aperture.

LIGHTING

Lighting is the single aspect that most directly affects the quality and usefulness of a medicolegal photograph. Proper lighting can show texture, color, depth, and contours. Improper lighting can hide details in shadow, wash out bruises, and even misrepresent evidence.[1,14,15]

Short of three-source studio lighting, electronic flash offers the best light for indoor color medical photography.[12,15] There are two basic types of electronic flash units, a traditional point-source flash mounted to one side or on top of the camera and a ring flash that encircles the camera lens.

A ring flash provides the best overall lighting in the form of shadowless, uniform illumination. This is particularly useful when photographing cavities and recesses, such as the mouth, vagina, and rectum. Shadowing for detail, important in black-and-white photography, is less important when using color film, which utilizes varying colors and hues to separate detail.

With modern through-the-lens (TTL) metering systems, flash use has become quite simple. The flash may be connected to the shutter for synchronization either through a coaxial cable or directly through a shoe fitting on the camera (hotshoe). Many electronic flash guns have automatic exposure control. Light from the flash is reflected from the subject back to a sensing cell. When sufficient light has been reflected, the cell cuts off the current and the light is switched off. The light-producing power of a flash is measured by its guide number (for a given film speed the guide number equals the f-number chosen multiplied by the lens-to-subject distance). A higher guide number represents a more powerful flash. A more powerful flash allows a smaller aperture and, hence, a greater depth of field.

Limitations of electronic flash include reflections, particularly from mucous membranes; loss of three-dimensional quality of textured areas, such as abrasions; washout of subtle colors by overexposure; and inadequate lighting, especially if the flash is blocked by the lens.[1,14] When using an electronic flash, it is important to remove or neutralize other light sources, such as shadow-producing operative lights or sunlight, which may only illuminate a portion of the subject and create exposure imbalance.

Flash recycle time, the time it takes the flash capacitor to recharge and be ready to fire again, is especially important when photographing children. The difference between 3 to 5 seconds and 20 to 30 seconds may be the difference between a good photograph and none at all with a child who is unwilling to sit still for the several seconds it takes a slow flash to recycle. As batteries discharge, recycle time lengthens; thus, fresh batteries should always be used.

FILM

Thirty-five–millimeter color slide film, sometimes called color transparency or color reversal film, remains the standard for medical use.[12,15] Color film offers a distinct advantage over black-and-white film, in that color film uses the various hues of the subject to separate details much more effectively than shades of grey.[1] Color slides are relatively inexpensive, quickly developed, and easy to file and can be converted into satisfactory color prints if necessary.[12,15] Although color negative or print film offers greater exposure and contrast latitude and, hence, is more forgiving of exposure mistakes, color slide film offers a distinct advantage by providing a first-generation image that can be projected. Because color negative film necessitates a second-generation conversion into a print, the color balance may be distorted. Conversion of color negatives to slides also usually results in loss of sharpness and color balance.

Table 1.—Photography Shooting Tips

Take a photograph with landmarks and one close-up of the lesion alone
Magnify in the original, not in a blowup
Arrange the subject so the surface of interest is parallel to film
Take several shots from different angles and distances
Compose the picture the way you normally look at the area
Keep the photographer and subject at the same level
Bracket shots if the correct exposure is uncertain
Shoot more slides rather than planning to duplicate
Shoot a face to identify the patient
Take a photograph of the patient's name
Use an uncluttered, neutral-colored background
Shoot only one patient per roll

Duplicating slides or prints may significantly alter color and resolution and should be avoided if at all possible.[1] Rather, two or three sets of slides should be shot initially, ie, each view should be photographed twice. One set can be used in court, while the others are retained with the child's record. Also, magnification should be accomplished in the original photograph by varying camera distance and/or focal length, not in the print- or slide-making process. As a rule, only one patient should be photographed on each roll of film. Even if a roll has only a few exposures, it should be developed rather than kept in the camera, where a mistake might either expose the film or lead to a mix-up of subjects.

Film speed is the sensitivity of the film emulsion to light, as measured by the International Standards Organization (ISO) rating. A film rated at 400 ISO is twice as light-sensitive or "fast" as one rated at 200 ISO. Slower film (with a lower ISO rating) offers a finer grain, which means greater sharpness and definition. However, slower film requires more light, a larger aperture, and, hence, narrower depth of field. Film should be fast enough to provide an aperture of f-11 or f-16. Medium-speed (100 ISO) daylight film allows a smaller aperture for greater depth of field yet minimum grain.[15] This is particularly true if a powerful flash is used.

A flash should always be used when shooting indoors with daylight film. Daylight film is color film balanced to give accurate color rendition in average daylight. The color temperature of daylight is 5000°K. Normal indoor lighting has a color temperature of 3000°K and will create significant color distortion if daylight film is used without a flash. Electronic flash is standardized to the same color temperature as average daylight.[16] A standardized color bar, although awkward, may be placed in the photographic plane for comparison with the subject color. However, if color is a significant concern, as when trying to age a bruise, it is far more useful to carefully document the coloring in writing than to rely on the photograph.

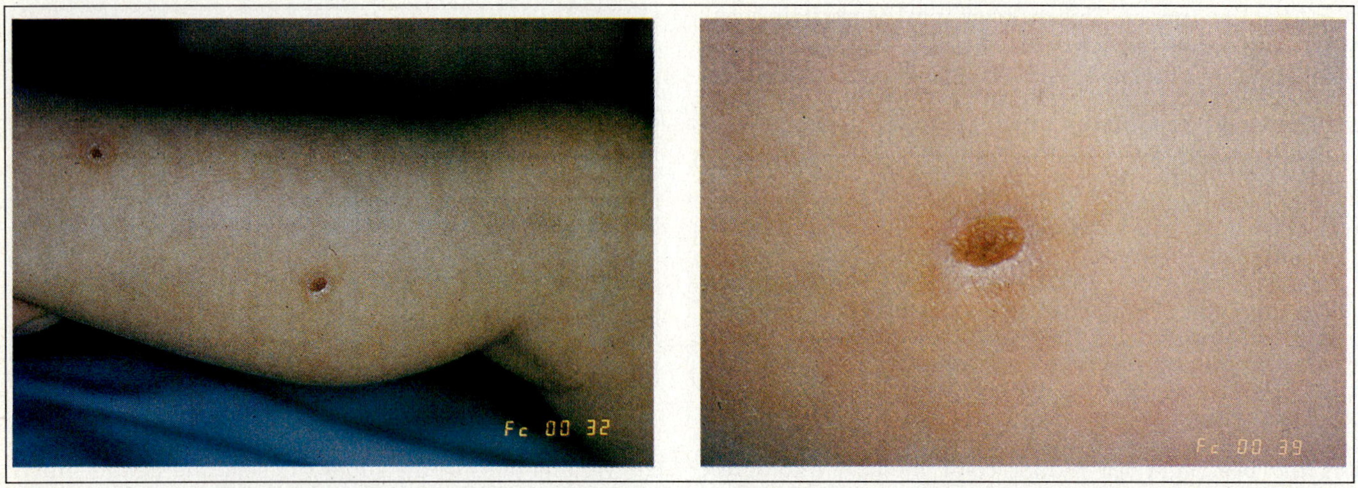

Fig 1.—*Six-week-old male infant with 10-day-old lesions on the outer aspect of the left lower leg, thought to be due to nonaccidental cigarette burns. A 35-mm single lens reflex camera with a 105-mm macro lens and a ring flash was used. Left, The lesions in relation to each other and neighboring anatomy at ×0.2 magnification. Right, The more proximal lesion at ×1 magnification, demonstrating the deeply punched out oval eschar. The eschar has a diameter of 4 mm, while the ill-defined halo of surrounding redness extends the diameter to 8 mm, the size of a cigarette. Note the databack identification code in the lower right corner.*

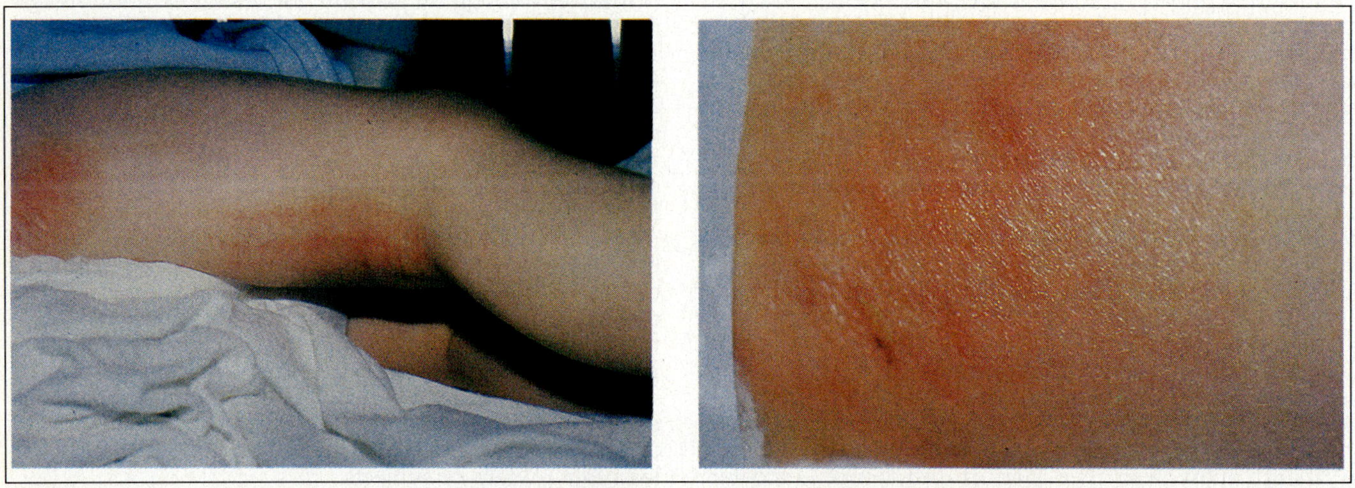

Fig 2.—*Two-year, 6-month-old male infant reported by his mother to have fallen down a set of stairs. The camera used was an auto-focus 35-mm camera with a built-in 35- to 80-mm zoom lens, macro capability up to ×0.25, and built-in flash. Left, Two abraded areas on the right posterior thigh at ×0.1 magnification. The neighboring anatomy is clearly identified, although the viewpoint is not quite parallel and the foreground is cluttered. Right, The more proximal abrasion at ×0.25 magnification, demonstrating obliquely directed linear streaking. The directional orientation of this abrasion is different from that of the distal abrasion, which appears to be oriented either horizontally or vertically. The child's mother subsequently admitted hitting the child with a rolled scatter rug.*

Some centers refrigerate or freeze film to prolong its effective shelf life. Film that is refrigerated requires 3 hours at room temperature to reach a usable temperature. If film is frozen it must be left at room temperature for 24 hours before use.[16]

Differences may be noted between film laboratories and even at the same laboratory with successive roles of film if quality control of the development process is not maintained.[15] The use of a standard commercial processing laboratory for color film is an assurance of quality control and standardization.[17]

After the film is developed, each image should be reviewed both for technique and content. No photographs, even poor ones, should be discarded. This could be misconstrued as destruction of evidence.[12,18]

A storage/filing system should be established in a cool, dry location with low light. Each slide should be stored in a clear plastic sheet to minimize handling and to allow viewing and easy storage. Kodak (Rochester, NY) slides last many years with proper use, care, and storage.[16] However, a slide used for lectures or left out in the light will fade (a washout of 1 f-stop) after only a few years.[19]

PHOTOGRAPHIC COMPOSITION

Composition is the proper arrangement of the elements in a photograph. The compositional goal of medical photography is to accurately document the patient's condition. Artistic composition is less important than consistency of technique and reproducibility of results. A technically excellent photograph or series of photographs may not be admissible as evidence if they do not establish both the scale and the anatomic location of the trauma.[1] Perspective (viewpoint), scale, and background all must be carefully considered.

Table 2.—Sample Checklist for Camera Operation
Secure lens to camera body
Remove lens cap
Secure flash to camera hotshoe
Load film
Set film speed on camera and flash
Set lens aperture (usually to automatic)
Check flash setting and turn on flash
Focus and compose the picture
Shoot
Check to be sure flash has fired
Advance film
Check to be sure film is advancing
Rewind film when done shooting
Only then open back to remove film

Medical photography must show injuries as realistically as possible and should not be used to enhance or exaggerate trauma. It is useful to photograph burns, dirty abrasions, or even unkempt children both before and after cleaning. As they change over time, lesions should be rephotographed.[1] Just as varying perspective can add a three-dimensional quality to photographic representation, so photographs of the same child over time can add a fourth dimension.

Perspective or viewpoint refers to the depiction of the relationships between objects at different distances from the camera as well as the angle from which the objects are viewed. Proper perspective as viewed in a print is very important in accurately depicting a scene. Perspective can be altered by subject-to-lens distance, lens focal length, magnification, point of view, size of the final photograph, and even the distance from which the photograph is viewed.[18] The following compositional principles should be kept in mind when photographing abused children (Table 1).

1. At least one if not several pictures should contain an anatomic landmark (Figures 1 and 2). The inclusion of an elbow or knee allows the viewer to identify the anatomic location of a wound. Anatomic or background material unnecessary to the photograph, however, should be left out. If the photographer follows this principle, the main subject will occupy a larger portion of the picture and will be easier to study. In addition, unneeded and possibly confusing visual information will be omitted.[8,15,20]

2. At least two photographs should be taken of each finding, one including identifying landmarks and one close-up with the lesion filling the frame. Magnification should be obtained in the original, not from a blowup (Figures 1 and 2).

3. The subject should be arranged in a manner that allows the surface of interest to be parallel to the film. This is done by making sure the back of the camera, the film plane, is parallel to the pathology. Likewise, the photographer and the subject should be at the same level.[8,15,20]

4. Varying perspective, taking a number of shots from different angles and distances, is quite useful, particularly since electronic flash may produce unpredictable reflections.[15,17] Additionally, since the skin is a curved surface, some lesions may require several photographs to fully reveal the pathology.

5. The picture should be composed the way an examiner would normally look at that anatomic area. The horizontal format should be primarily used. However, when necessary, such as for full-body shots, the vertical format may be used.

6. The size of lesions should, if possible, be documented on the photograph by using some measuring device, such as a metric ruler.[1,18] Photographs are no substitute, however, for clearly written and detailed descriptions of the dimension, shape, color, size, and location of lesions. Color along with size may be distorted in the photograph.

7. It is desirable but not always possible to have a standard set of views for each area of the body photographed.[14] The four cardinal anatomic positions, anteroposterior, posteroanterior, right lateral, and left lateral, should be kept in mind when photographing children. However, young children may not cooperate with such positioning plans, reinforcing the usefulness of multiple views from varying perspective.

8. Forensic bite mark photography is a specialized branch of medical photography and is best left to a forensic dentist or pathologist. The basic objective of photographing bites is the accurate recording of all aspects of the mark. Size, shape, color, depth of indentations, and three-dimensional contours must be preserved. No one medium is suitable for all these functions. Photographs, both black-and-white and color, can record the first three, whereas dental impressions show the last two. Ultimately, the photographs may be enlarged to life size and compared with representations of the suspect's teeth.[17]

9. Recording photographic data (date, time, location, case number, camera, lens, aperture, film, light source, and subject distance) helps reconstruct cases, particularly for courtroom verification, aids learning and teaching, and encourages consistent technique if more photographs are required later.

10. Background is important.[12,14,20] The background wall should be nonreflective, ideally a neutral gray, green, or blue in a matte finish. Glossy background surfaces can produce a glare. A cluttered room makes a poor background for medical photographs. Materials unnecessary for the photograph should be removed. A backdrop may be useful.

11. Before photographing children in clinical settings it is important to establish both a protocol and a checklist for operation (Table 2). Clearly identify who will take the photographs and how the film will be handled after picture taking. Always shoot a test roll first when using a new camera setup.

COMMON PHOTOGRAPHIC ERRORS

Despite the advent of simple and sophisticated electronic cameras, a number of traditional camera operation errors continue to occur.

1. The subject is blurred. This is usually caused by improper focusing, often because the photographer attempted to get closer than the minimum focusing distance of the lens to magnify the image. Sometimes, movement of the subject or camera, particularly with shutter speeds slower than 1/90 second, will also cause this, although with high-speed electronic flash this is usually not a problem.

2. The negative is clear or the transparency is black. Most likely the film was never exposed, because it did not advance in the camera. The most common cause of this is failure to properly load the film. It is important to load film correctly and ensure that the film is being transported through the camera by checking that the rewind knob turns as the film is advanced. Because of this problem, some centers recommend shooting a backup set of prints using an instant-picture Polaroid (Clifton, NJ) camera.[12]

3. The film is overexposed or underexposed. Incorrect exposure continues to be a common problem in photography despite advances in automatic exposure control. Exposure is dependent on the brightness of the image, the

camera aperture, the time the photographic material is exposed, and film speed. The usual cause of incorrect exposure is incorrect setting of the aperture, film speed, shutter speed, or flash. Camera and flash settings should be carefully checked. An exposure technique some professionals use to avoid overexposure or underexposure is bracketing. If the final combination of film and flash indicates an aperture of f-16, three frames are exposed, one at a setting of f-16, the second overexposed at f-11, and the third underexposed at f-22. One of the three will be perfectly exposed.[15,17]

4. The print or slide has distorted color, often yellow or green. This most commonly occurs because color daylight film is used indoors without a flash. Always use a flash indoors, even if the room is very bright.

PHOTOGRAPHING CHILDREN

When photographing children it is important to explain to the child what is going to happen in language the child will understand.[21] Allowing children to try out the camera and flash often aids in gaining their trust.[14] Children should be allowed to assume a position of comfort. It is far better to have a cooperative child somewhat out of optimal photographic position yet still rather than an uncooperative, moving child.

Correct anatomic relationships are not always possible with children. It is thus helpful to take many pictures in different poses. If the child will not move, the photographer should. Besides affording greater opportunity for a satisfactory photograph, multiple views add a three-dimensional quality to a two-dimensional medium.

It is often useful to involve a trusted support person in the photographic session. Apart from being a comfort to the child in unfamiliar surroundings, such a person provides an extra pair of hands.[21]

Film-advancing motor drives are extremely useful when photographing children, as are a fast-recycling flash with fresh batteries and a single zoom-macro lens.

Most critically, the photographer must remain cognizant of the potential traumatic effect of photographs on the abused child, both with regard to the photographic process itself and with regard to the use of these photographs in court.

LEGAL ISSUES

In child abuse litigation, photographs of the injured child may play an important role in helping prove nonaccidental injury. For photographs to be used as court evidence they must be properly verified and relevant.[22]

Verification requires that the photographer or physician testify that the pictures accurately portray the findings.[1] From a medicolegal perspective, photographs of abused children should convey a fair and accurate representation of the scene. The photographer should also be able to state how the photograph was taken. Pictures that are inadmissible because of technical error (out of focus, distorted, unidentifiable, too dark, etc) must be avoided.[23]

To help verify that the photographs are actually of a particular child, one picture can be taken of the child's name and one of the child's face. An identifying sign may be placed in front of the patient for each picture. The inclusion in the photograph of such signs or labels with the patient's name and date, however, is time-consuming and distracting.[8] An alternative for identification of the film is the use of a camera databack. Many 35-mm cameras have available databack attachments that imprint the time, date, and an identifying code on each frame. Another advantage of a databack is that, since the imprint is always located in the bottom right of the transparency or negative, right-left and top-bottom orientation are made simpler (Fig 1).

Once processed, the slides or prints should be labeled. Each print or slide should contain the name of the child, age, date of birth, date and time of photograph, hospital number, name of photographer, and name of physician. If confidentiality is a concern, each print or slide should, at a minimum, be labeled with a medical record number and the date the photographs were taken.[5]

Relevance is a judicial decision.[24] Photographs may have evidentiary value yet be deemed prejudicial to the defendant. Whether the probative value outweighs the prejudicial danger is a decision each trial judge must make with each case. Photographs are generally considered admissible, however, if they shed light on the issue, enable a witness to better describe the objects portrayed, permit the jury to better understand the testimony, or corroborate testimony. Courts generally permit physicians to explain and illustrate their testimony with a photograph.

The laws of a number of states refer to taking photographs in cases of suspected abuse.[1] Indeed, many states require that reasonable efforts be made by the reporting hospital staff member to take or cause to be taken color photographs of any areas of visible trauma on the child. Many states provide for immunity from civil or criminal prosecution for the reporting institution and for the person arranging for or taking photographs if done in good faith. However, a survey of professional medical photographers suggested a lack of awareness of the statutes that require photographs and provide immunity.[1]

Each institution should have a policy for both the handling and release of photographs.[1] Although an unbroken chain of evidence may be important in a criminal proceeding, in a civil case, where the photographer's testimony can verify that the photographs are representative of a particular subject, such a chain of evidence may be less critical. For an unbroken chain of evidence, film should change hands as infrequently as possible. With each transfer, the signature of an authorized recipient should be affixed to a list of the materials received, along with the date, time, and place. Outside laboratory processing may be acceptable even if the laboratory does not sign for the film, if sending film out is the normal business procedure for the institution.[18] Courts usually accept film sent to a standard commercial processing laboratory via first-class mail as an unbroken chain of custody.[25] These laboratories will, on request, enclose an affidavit ensuring the receipt, correct processing, and return of the film. The use of a standard commercial processing laboratory for color film assures quality control, standardization, and legal acceptability.

SUMMARY

The principles of medical photography are good equipment, adequate lighting, and planned composition. Equally important is a working knowledge of camera equipment, film procedure, and medicolegal implications.

Since photographs offer the only certain method of preserving often perishable findings, they may serve several useful purposes. Photographs can be reviewed after the examination to double-check findings or perhaps even to discover previously unnoticed findings. If the magnification is precisely known, measurements can be obtained directly from the photograph. Photographic findings can be discussed among colleagues and consultants. Photographs taken during an initial examination can provide a standard for subsequent comparison. Should a second opinion be required, photographs may save the child from the trauma of a repeated examination. In court, photographs can provide a powerful and convincing statement where a simple verbal description might fail. Even when not directly used in court, photographs may serve to enhance testimony by jogging the examiner's memory of specific findings.[5]

Whether child abuse has occurred and who is responsible is a legal issue for the courts to decide.[10] Corroborative physical evidence photographically documented can, however, be an important adjunct to the legal process. Physicians who perform medicolegal examinations of abused children must have access to adequate photographic equipment and a working knowledge of photographic techniques.

The author wishes to thank Martin Finkl, DO, and Robert Reece, MD, for manuscript review.

References

1. Ford RJ, Smistek, BS. Photography of the maltreated child. In: Ellerstein NS, ed. *Child Abuse and Neglect: A Medical Reference.* New York, NY: John Wiley & Sons Inc; 1981:315-325.

2. Council on Scientific Affairs. AMA diagnostic and treatment guidelines concerning child abuse and neglect. *JAMA.* 1985;254:796-800.

3. Baum E, Grodin MA, Alpert JJ, Glantz L. Child sexual abuse, criminal justice, and the pediatrician. *Pediatrics.* 1987;79:437-439.

4. Ford RJ, Smistek, BS, Glass JT. Photography of suspected child abuse and maltreatment. *Biomed Commun.* July 1975;3:12-17.

5. Ricci LR. Medical forensic photography of the sexually abused child. *Child Abuse Negl.* 1988;12:305-310.

6. Woodling BA, Heger A. The use of the colposcope in the diagnosis of sexual abuse in the pediatric age group. *Child Abuse Negl.* 1986;10:111-114.

7. Ladson S, Johnson CF, Doyt RE. Do physicians recognize sexual abuse? *AJDC.* 1987;141:411-415.

8. Sebben JE. Office photography from the surgical viewpoint. *J Dermatol Surg Oncol.* 1983;9:763-768.

9. Teixeira WRG. Hymenal colposcopic examination in sexual offenses. *Am J Forensic Med Pathol.* 1981;2:209-215.

10. Woodling B, Kossoris P. Sexual misuse: rape, molestation and incest. *Pediatr Clin North Am.* 1981;28:481-499.

11. Cordell W, Zollman W, Karlson H. A photographic system for the emergency department. *Ann Emerg Med.* 1980;9:210-214.

12. Gilmore J, Miller W. Clinical photography utilizing office staff: methods to achieve consistency and reproducibility. *J Dermatol Surg Oncol.* 1988;14:281-286.

13. Morello D, Converse J, Allen D. Making uniform photographic records in plastic surgery. *Plast Reconstr Surg.* 1977;59:366-372.

14. Williams AR. Positioning and lighting for patient photography. *J Biol Photogr.* 1985;53:131-143.

15. Weiss CH. Dermatologic photography of nail pathologies. *Dermatol Clin.* 1985;3:543-556.

16. Freehe CL. Photography in dentistry: equipment and technique. *Dent Clin North Am.* 1983;27:3-73.

17. Bernstein ML. The application of photography in forensic dentistry. *Dent Clin North Am.* 1983;27:151-170.

18. Spring GE. Evidence photography: an overview. *J Biol Photogr.* 1987;55:129-132.

19. Eaton GT. Proper storage of photographic images. *J Audiov Media Med.* 1985;8:94-98.

20. Whitesell J. The basics of medical photography in plastic surgery. *J Plast Reconstr Surg Nursing.* 1981;1:89-92.

21. Reeves C. Pediatric photography. *J Audiov Media Med.* 1986;9:131-134.

22. Flower MS. Photographs in the courtroom: getting it straight between you and your professional photographer. *N Kent State Law Forum.* 1974;2:184-211.

23. Scott CC. *Photographic Evidence.* 2nd ed. St Paul, Minn: West Publishing Co; 1969.

24. Myers JEB, Carter LE. Proof of physical child abuse. *Missouri Law Rev.* 1988;53:189-224.

25. Luntz LL, Luntz P. *Handbook for Dental Identification: Techniques in Forensic Dentistry.* Philadelphia, Pa: JB Lippincott Co; 1973.

Physicians, Formula Companies, and Advertising

A Historical Perspective

Frank R. Greer, MD, Rima D. Apple, PhD

• The recent advent of new advertising campaigns for infant formulas aimed at the general public via television commercials, newspapers, free formula coupons, and lay periodicals has disrupted a comfortable symbiotic relationship between infant food manufacturers and the medical profession that has endured for more than 50 years. In the late 19th century, physicians were concerned about the advertising claims of these products and generally felt that indications and directions for their use should be the province of the physician. Between 1929 and 1932, the American Medical Association, through its Committee on Foods and "Seal of Acceptance," essentially required the entire formula industry to advertise only to the medical profession. Since 1932, the US formula industry has developed into a $1.6 billion market. In 1988, Nestlé (absent from the US infant formula industry since the 1940s) acquired the Carnation Company and launched an advertising campaign to the general public for its formula products. Bristol Myers/Mead Johnson, in cooperation with Gerber Products Company, quickly followed suit. These actions threaten to once again remove the realm of infant feeding from the exclusive supervision of the medical profession. The new multimedia public advertising campaigns may increase the cost of infant formula to the general public and have a negative impact on the incidence of breast-feeding. In addition, formula advertising campaigns will likely increase the danger of advertising hyperbole and affect the level of financial support by formula companies for scientific meetings, medical research, education, and social events at medical meetings.

***(AJDC.* 1991;145:282-286)**

In October 1989, millions of television viewers throughout the United States saw 30-second advertising spots extolling the advantages of Gerber Baby Formula. Earlier that year, Nestlé-Carnation launched a similar television advertising campaign to promote its formula product, Good Nature (the name was recently changed to Follow-up Formula). These commercial presentations conflicted directly with the medical profession's longstanding and effective opposition to the advertising of infant formula to the general public, and disrupted a comfortable symbiotic relationship between infant food manufacturers and the profession that had lasted for more than 50 years.

Since the early decades of this century, the formula companies have advertised to the medical profession by promoting their products extensively in professional journals and displaying them at state and national medical meetings, which they also financially supported. After 1960, they also supplied free formula to physician-dominated hospitals, including starter packs for new mothers to bring home. Additionally, during this period, infant formula manufacturers funded medical research in pediatric nutrition, particularly when the studies were related to product development.

The medical profession's negative response to the new advertising campaigns was swift. The American Academy of Pediatrics (AAP) announced a new policy refusing contributions from formula companies who marketed their products directly to the public rather than exclusively to health care providers, and the Executive Board of the AAP subsequently rejected $760 000 in pledged contributions from Mead Johnson Nutritionals and Gerber Products Company (written communication from Donald W. Schiff, MD, AAP president, to membership, September 27, 1989).[1] There were also scattered reports that Mead Johnson formula products had been stricken from hospital formularies. What were the events that led to the 50-year advertising understanding between formula companies and physicians? What factors precipitated its demise?

In the 1870s, the vast majority of American babies were fed human milk. Mothers were expected to breast-feed and the few available alternatives were considered poor and risky substitutes. During the next 75 years, however, the US infant food and formula industry developed rapidly, accompanying a dramatic shift from breast-feeding to artificial or bottle feeding. Developments in technology, science, and medicine, along with social and economic changes, fueled the transformation in infant feeding practices and established the infant formula industry. In the 1940s and 1950s, this now safe and alternative method to breast-feeding rapidly gained popularity among physicians and consumers.[2] Indeed, by 1958, 63% of all newborns were fed formula exclusively before being discharged from the hospital.[3]

Many proprietary infant foods appeared in the United States in the last decades of the 19th century. Early manufacturers usually produced a variant of the formula developed by Justus von Liebig in Germany in the 1860s.[4] In Switzerland, Henri Nestlé created his variant of Liebig's

Accepted for publication October 25, 1990.

From the Departments of Pediatrics (Dr Greer) and History of Medicine (Dr Apple), University of Wisconsin, Madison.

Reprint requests to the Wisconsin Perinatal Center, 202 S Park St, Madison, WI 53715 (Dr Greer).

formula combining condensed milk, sugar, and wheat flour. The first Nestlé's Milk Food plant opened in 1868, and by 1873 the formula was sold in the United States and 16 other countries.[5] Companies also formed on this side of the Atlantic. James Horlick, a pharmacist, formulated another Liebig-type formula, Horlick's Malted Milk, in Racine, Wis, in 1882.[6] During the early years of the industry, manufacturers solicited the broadest audience possible, advertising both to the general public and to physicians. As is still the practice today, the inclusion of medical testimonials by the profession in the advertising copy added a veneer of "scientific" and medical respectability. In addition, the companies distributed brochures and free samples at medical conventions and advertised in medical journals.[2] During this early period, promotions in nonmedical journals advised mothers to write in for free samples and brochures.

From the beginning of the infant food industry, physicians expressed concern about direct advertising to the public. Dr Thomas Morgan Rotch, on the staff of Harvard Medical School, believed that infant foods produced and advertised by "commercial men" rather than the medical profession contributed to the high infant mortality rate.[7] Dr Rotch demanded that pediatrics "rescue" infant feeding from "the pretensions of proprietary foods."[7] Thus, despite the 19th-century manufacturers' attention to physicians, the medical profession resisted and debated the use of infant formula products and opposed their direct advertisement to laypersons. Undoubtedly, these physicians believed that the indications and guidelines for the use of these products were the province of the medical profession.

An 1888 American Medical Association (AMA) Subcommittee on Infant Feeding clearly documented a lack of uniformity among physicians regarding infant feeding,[8] but most physicians unquestionably preferred breast-feeding, with bottle feeding being strongly associated with the high infant mortality rates. In fact, the ward for artificially fed infants of the New York (NY) Foundling Asylum was known as the "ward of the dying babies."[4] During this period, a growing proportion of general medical practice concerned the safe feeding of infants and the specialty of pediatrics emerged as a group of physicians particularly interested in promoting good infant nutrition and hygiene.

Between 1890 and 1910, these early pediatric researchers advocated the cleanup of infant milk supplies, including improving the quality and care of dairy herds, the establishment of infant milk depots and clinics for the distribution of "clean milk" to the public, and the founding of milk laboratories.[2] The latter change was a direct result of the dominant theory of infant feeding of the period, Rotch's percentage method.[9] He insisted that infants were to be fed a certain percentage of each known food element (ie, fat, protein, and carbohydrate) in proportions dictated by the individual's needs. Rotch believed that minute variations (as little as 0.1%) in the composition of the food could make a difference in its digestibility and healthfulness. As many as 19 formulations were recommended for healthy infants during the first year of life. Minute changes were made on weekly and even daily bases and elaborate tables and mathematical formulas were published to optimize Rotch's principles. Therefore, the need for laboratories to compound the required formulations developed. By 1910, growing numbers of studies in infant nutrition demonstrated the inadequacy of the percentage method. The most important data of this research supported the caloric method of infant feeding, the method that persists to this day.[10]

Despite continued medical criticism of commercial foods, a significant and increasing number of physicians did advise their patients to use these products. Physicians, rather than ignoring all commercial foods, became mediators between manufacturers and consumers. Henry Tuley, MD, writing in *JAMA* in 1899, concluded, "The method of artificial feeding which will prove most popular with the laity must embody two requisites: cheapness and ease of preparation. On the physician devolves the great burden of educating people beyond the indiscriminate use of proprietary foods, and the importance of accuracy in the preparation of the food prescribed."[11] Thus, given the complexities inherent in these early infant "percentage" formulas, both for the physician to calculate and for the mother to prepare, it was easier for busy practitioners to give up the whole program in despair and "resort to the use of the patent baby foods as the easiest way out of the difficulty," opined Eugene Darling, MD, in 1911.[12] Unfortunately, once this occurred, the mother could follow the printed instructions on the product and did not need to return to the physician for further supervision. Such a situation could be physically unhealthy for the infant and potentially economically harmful to the physician.

In 1910, J. S. Leopold, MD, returning to New York City from Germany, reported that the German use of dextrin and maltose in infant formulas resulted in improved tolerance and digestibility. Unable to find a source of this sugar in the United States, he convinced the Mead Johnson Company to manufacture and distribute Dextri-Maltose.[13] Dextri-Maltose was evaluated at the Babies Ward of New York (NY) Postgraduate Hospital, and was the first example of an infant food product developed through the cooperation of an investigative pediatric researcher and a private company. With its initial promotional efforts, Mead Johnson began a trend in the industry by deciding that gaining the respect and goodwill of the medical community could be potentially more profitable than marketing the product directly to the public.

Accordingly, the company unveiled Dextri-Maltose at the 1912 AMA convention and promoted this milk modifier, as well as its later infant feeding products, exclusively to the medical profession. No directions appeared on the package. Wheel "feeding calculators" and formula prescription blanks imprinted with the physician's name and address were supplied to physicians. Such prescriptions told the mother how to mix the formula and feed it to her child, and reminded her to bring the baby back to the physician for a checkup and new formula on a specified date. Mead Johnson announced its policy in many of its advertisements and brochures for physicians, frequently stressing that "when Dextri-Maltose is used as the added carbohydrate of the baby's food, the physician himself controls the feeding problems."[14]

Following Mead Johnson's success, other companies emulated the company's so-called "ethical" policy of infant food advertising. In 1915, H. J. Gerstenberger, MD, of Western Reserve University, Cleveland, Ohio, formulated an infant milk food that was closer to human milk than any other popular artificial feeding product of its day. In this product, human milk fat was approximated for the first time by a blend of homogenized vegetable and animal fats. Gerstenberger presented this infant food at the 1915 meeting of the American Pediatric Society after testing it at the Babies Dispensary and Hospital in Cleveland.[15] The Laboratory Products Company (eventually bought by

Wyeth Laboratories) subsequently produced and distributed Gerstenberger's formulas under the name S.M.A. (Synthetic Milk Adapted) and directed its advertising campaign primarily toward physicians. Although a few advertisements did appear in the early years in lay journals such as *Hygeia*, actually published by the AMA, the advertising copy typically stated that S.M.A. was "to be used only under the direction of the physician."

The commercial success of Dextri-Maltose and S.M.A., both produced by companies new to the infant feeding industry, demonstrated to other companies that such advertising policies could result in a satisfactory compromise between the needs of the manufacturers to sell their products and the desires of physicians to control the distribution and use of infant foods. Although the Nestlé Company, unlike Mead Johnson and Laboratory Products, continued to advertise its milk food in lay journals and to offer mothers free samples and booklets, the company announced a new product, Lactogen, in 1924 "sold only on the prescription or recommendation of a physician. No feeding instructions appear on the trade package." At about the same time, the Horlick Company developed its Horlick's Milk Modifier, which was "offered for sale on physician prescription only."[2]

Another aspect of the infant food industry, the manufacture and promotion of evaporated milk formulas, showed a similar pattern. In 1929, W. M. Marriott, MD, of Washington University, St Louis, Mo, published a controlled study comparing evaporated milk formula, human milk, and bottled cow's milk formula.[16] The infants fed evaporated cow's milk formula showed better weight gain during the first week of life than the other infants; moreover, over the long term, those infants fed evaporated cow's milk formula grew as well as those fed human milk or bottled cow's milk formula. The evaporated milk industry quickly cited Marriott's studies in advertising and informational brochures for physicians. The Pet Milk Company even hired Marriott as a consultant to show the company's sales personnel the right and wrong ways to contact physicians.[17] By 1935, evaporated milk formulas dominated infant feeding and as late as 1956, 80% of all formulas used in hospital nurseries in the United States were some dilution of evaporated milk.[18]

Clearly, the apparent success of companies such as Mead Johnson and Laboratory Products resulted in the willingness of the infant food manufacturers to forego public advertising and to direct their attention to the medical profession. Additionally, direct pressures from the medical profession spurred the demise of promotions to the laity. In 1923, the Philadelphia Pediatric Society urged the AMA to halt infant food advertising in its lay journal *Hygeia*. Such advertising, the society contended, implied recommendations by the members of the American Medical Association "[which] will tend to undo all the work which thousands of members of the medical profession have been trying to accomplish in the education of the public to the fact that infants cannot be fed in this indiscriminate manner."[19]

Although advertisements continued to appear, in 1924 the Section on Diseases of Children of the AMA established a committee "to investigate the general question of advertising of proprietary foods in medical journals and to the laity."[20] In its 1925 report, the committee acknowledged the significance of infant food products in medical practice and concluded that "it is impractical at the present time to dispense entirely with all proprietary foods." While stressing the nutritional importance of breast-feeding and "the dangers of artificial feeding of infants, particularly when carried out without supervision of medical men," it found heartening the "disposition on the part of many manufacturers of proprietary foods to cooperate with the medical profession and its medical journals."[21]

Four years later, the AMA established its Committee on Foods, within the Council on Pharmacy and Chemistry, to approve the composition and advertising claims of food products in general. Infant food companies, including evaporated milk producers, quickly presented their products for AMA approval and its "Seal of Acceptance." In 1932, the committee published specific advertising guidelines for infant foods. These insisted that "every infant, breast-fed, and doubly so, the artificially fed should be under the supervision of the physician who is experienced and skilled in the care and feeding of infants."[22] The new rules sought to restrain manufacturers from distributing directions for formulas to nonmedical personnel, reasoning that "The feeding of an infant by routine feeding formulas and instructions distributed by food manufacturers, or according to directions, printed material, or advice of any person other than the attending physician who can personally observe the condition of the baby, may seriously endanger the health of the infant. The promulgation of feeding formulas in advertising to the laity is considered to be in conflict with the best experience, authoritative judgment, and basic principles in infant feeding, and is not permissible."[22]

Nestlé did not have to change its Lactogen promotions, but the company did stop advertising Nestlé's Milk Food to the general public and limited distribution of feeding directions to physicians only.[2] Most, but not all, other companies and evaporated milk producers followed suit. The labels and advertising for Horlick's Malted Milk continued to "present explicit infant feedings formulas for infants age one week to 12 months." Despite the committee's recommendation that the company alter its advertising copy, Horlick's refused. The committee stated, "The manufacturer when informed of these opinions expressed himself unwilling to remove the feeding formulas from advertising addressed to the public for merchandising reasons. The acceptance of Horlick's Malted Milk is being withdrawn for the preceding reasons; the product will therefore no longer be listed among the committee's accepted foods."[23]

The withdrawal of the AMA's previous acceptance of Horlick's Malted Milk meant that the company could no longer advertise in AMA publications or participate in AMA meetings. Furthermore, many medical journals, such as the *New England Journal of Medicine*, received advertising contracts through AMA's Cooperative Medical Advertising Bureau.[24] This group would approve copy only for "drugs, therapeutic agents and food which are acceptable to the respective approving committees of the American Medical Association." As a result, withdrawal of the Committee on Foods' acceptance further limited Horlick's promotional activities by preventing the company from advertising in other major medical journals.

The subsequent demise of Horlick's in the United States is more complex than this analysis suggests, but it is true that the action of the committee significantly lessened the use of Horlick's products in infant feeding. Companies that allowed the AMA committee to approve their promotional material fared much better. As Mead Johnson cogently explained, "When mothers in America feed their babies by lay advice, the control of your pediatric cases passes out of your hands, doctor. Our interest in this important phase of medical economics springs, not from any motive of altruism, philanthropy or paternalism, but rather from a spirit of enlightened self-interest and cooperation because [our] infant diet materials are advertised only to you, never to the public."[25]

By the 1930s, simplified, standardized, and inexpensive artificial infant food products were widely available in this country. They contained appropriate amounts of nutrients, were free of pathogenic bacteria, and were generally accepted by the medical profession as a safe alternative to breast-feeding. Also, by this time, physicians and infant food companies had established a beneficial, reciprocal relationship.[26] In 1933, a Pennsylvania practitioner counted no fewer than 17 advertisements for infant foods in a single issue of *JAMA*.[27] Elaborate presentations by infant food manufacturers appeared at medical conventions. Ties between the formula companies and academic medicine were also well established through the funding of scientific meetings and the open support of published infant nutritional research. What happened to change this advantageous 50-year association between physicians and the formula companies?

In the late 1960s and 1970s, world attention was focused on the declining incidence of breast-feeding and the associated increasing infant mortality in some third world countries. This decline was in part attributed by physicians and laypersons to the marketing and advertising of infant formulas by international companies to the mothers in these countries. Families were often unable to maintain adequate supplies of formula without making severe economic sacrifices and lacked the necessary sanitary facilities for formula preparation and storage. Furthermore, many mothers were unable to read and/or follow the directions for safe formula preparation. In truth, no scientific data were ever presented that could separate the effects of marketing infant formulas from other causes for the decline in breast-feeding in these countries. These factors included the negative overall influence of western culture with its acceptance of formula feeding, the increasing urbanization of the population, the economic necessity for mothers to work outside the home in urban areas, and the negative effects of government health services in those countries distributing free milk powder and Western ways of infant medical care in general.[28]

Ultimately, Nestlé was singled out and an international boycott of its products was organized by INFACT (Infant Formula Action Coalition), a group that drew on existing organizations committed to curbing infant formula promotions in third world countries.[29] The controversy led to US Senate hearings in 1978, chaired by Sen Edward Kennedy (D, Mass), on the subject.[29] The World Health Organization became involved and adopted its *International Code of Marketing of Breast-Milk Substitutes* in 1981.[30] Article 5.1 of the code stated that "There should be no advertising or other form of promotion to the general public of products within the scope of this Code." Subsequently, the formula companies largely complied with these guidelines for marketing their products in third world countries. Ironically, all countries endorsed this code except the United States, citing concerns about possible restraint of trade infringements and violations of the US Constitution.

Closer to home, by the 1970s and 1980s, notwithstanding the nationwide surge in the incidence of breast-feeding, the vast majority of infants aged 3 months and older were receiving commercial formula preparations as the US infant formula industry evolved into a $1.6 billion market. In 1988, Abbott Laboratories (parent company of Ross Laboratories) and Bristol Myers (parent company of Mead Johnson Nutritionals) had a virtual lock on this lucrative market. Nestlé, absent from the United States since the 1940s, was poised to reestablish its presence. As a first step, the company acquired the Carnation Company and its image of the "Carnation baby," familiar to millions of Americans who had been fed Carnation evaporated milk formula in the 1940s and 1950s (*Wall Street Journal*. February 16, 1989:A-1).

In June 1988, Nestlé-Carnation introduced two infant formulas to the United States market. The first, Good Start H.A., was a "hypoallergenic" product for the sensitive, colicky newborn. Its advertising, which the company called an "informational campaign," was directed to the general public and made no specific mention of the formula, yet its scientific benefits were pushed vigorously to the medical profession. The second formula, Good Nature (now Follow-up Formula), was designed for older infants weaned from the breast and would, in theory, not discourage breast-feeding. It became the first infant formula marketed directly to the public on US television. Additionally, for the first time in half of a century, an infant formula, Good Nature (Follow-up Formula), was widely advertised in lay journals and newspapers. Within a short time, Nestlé-Carnation captured between 2% and 4% of the US formula market, although its proportion has since fallen somewhat (*Wall Street Journal*. June 15, 1989:B-3).[1]

Subsequently, Good Start H.A. has fallen on hard times. Public advertising has been discontinued since the product was found to be not so "hypoallergenic," and reports of severe allergic reactions to the formula appeared in the press. However, although the company has discontinued television advertising and despite extensive pressure from the medical profession and most prominently the AAP, Follow-up Formula continues to be advertised in lay journals.

With the sudden success of Nestlé-Carnation in the United States, Bristol Myers entered into an agreement with Gerber Food Company to produce Gerber Baby Formula and to market it directly to the public (*Wall Street Journal*. June 15, 1989:B-3). Not only was the product promoted on US television, but free formula coupons and free formula samples were mailed to 1.6 million new mothers throughout the United States.[31] The company argued that this was no different from supplying mothers with take-home samples of their competitors' products at the time of discharge from the hospital. Interestingly, the Gerber Baby Formula is a former Mead Johnson product that was discontinued in the early 1980s in favor of a new "superior" and heavily advertised product.

This new marketing strategy has resulted in strong reactions from the American medical community. Although the AMA has a smaller role in setting infant nutrition policies than it did 50 years ago, it recently confirmed its opposition to the direct advertising of infant formula in the United States.[32] An official statement was made by the AAP before the US Senate Judiciary Subcommittee on Antitrust, Monopolies and Business Rights at its May 29, 1990, hearing on "Advertising of Infant Formula." In this statement, the academy officially opposed any form of direct advertising to the public for the following reasons: (1) negative effect on breast-feeding; (2) interference with the patient-physician relationship regarding nutritional advice; (3) advertising hyperbole leading to consumer confusion; and (4) the impact of large-scale public advertising on the cost of infant formula.[33] The AAP did not comment, however, on the negative impact that large-scale advertising might have on the financial support that the formula industry has made available to physicians for scientific meetings, medical research, education, and social events.

It does not take a crystal ball to predict that if Gerber, Bristol Myers, and Nestlé-Carnation are successful with their new marketing strategies, then other infant formula manufacturers may follow with direct public advertising. This will once again remove the realm of infant feeding from the supervision of the physician and will likely have a negative impact on the incidence and duration of breast-feeding. Of importance economically is the potential effect of new multimedia, public advertising campaigns on the cost of infant formula. Although the new marketing strategy will not have the economic impact on medical practice it would have had 50 or more years ago, it will permanently alter the mutually beneficial relationship between the medical profession and the infant formula industry.

References

1. Oski FA. Heating up the bottle battle. *The Nation.* 1989;249:665, 683-684.
2. Apple RA. 'To be used only under the direction of a physician': commercial infant feeding and medical practice, 1870-1940. *Bull Hist Med.* 1980;54:402-417.
3. Meyer HF. Infant feeding practices in hospital maternity nurseries. *Pediatrics.* 1958;21:288-296.
4. Cone TE Jr. *History of American Pediatrics.* Boston, Mass: Little Brown & Co Inc; 1979:131-148.
5. Heer J. *World Events, 1866-1966: The First Hundred Years of Nestlé.* Lausanne, Switzerland: Nestl´e; 1966:29-35, 39-43, 58-64, 78-79.
6. Campbell P. Typescript history of Horlick's Corp. Available in: Horlick's Corp papers, 1873-1974, State Historical Society of Wisconsin, Division of Archives and Manuscripts, Madison.
7. Rotch TM. The general principles underlying all good methods of infant feeding. *Boston Med Surg J.* 1893;129:505-506.
8. Report of subcommittee on infant feeding (1888 AMA meeting). *Boston Med Surg J.* 1888;118:504-505.
9. Rotch TM. *Pediatrics: The Hygienic and Medical Treatment of Children.* 3rd ed. Philadelphia, Pa: JB Lippincott Co; 1901:276-281.
10. Lackner E. Huebner's system of infant feeding based on calories. *Arch Pediatr.* 1907;24:549-553.
11. Tuley HE. Progress in pediatrics. *JAMA.* 1899;33:997-1001.
12. Darling EA. The use of whole milk and fat diminished milk in infant feeding. *Boston Med Surg J.* 1911;165:747-754.
13. A glimpse of Mead Johnson. 1971:8-9. Available in: Mead Johnson Company Business Records (1895-1971), Indiana State University, Evansville, Special Collection.
14. Ashley HF. *History of Mead Johnson and Company* [slide presentation]. Evansville, Ind: Mead Johnson & Co; 1968.
15. Gerstenberger HJ. Studies in the adaptation of an artificial food to human milk. *AJDC.* 1915;10:249-265.
16. Marriott WM, Schoenthal L. An experimental study of the use of unsweetened evaporated milk for the preparation of infant feeding. *Arch Pediatr.* 1929;46:135-148.
17. Bell ML. *A Portrait of Progress: A Business History of Pet Milk Company From 1885 to 1960.* St Louis, Mo: Pet Milk Co; 1962:101-102.
18. Meyer HF. *Infant Foods and Feeding Practice.* Springfield, Ill: Charles C Thomas Publisher; 1960:95.
19. Communication from Philadelphia Pediatric Society on advertising of infant foods. *JAMA.* 1923;81:36.
20. Minutes of Section on Diseases of Children. *JAMA.* 1924;82:2042.
21. Resolutions from Section on Diseases of Children. *JAMA.* 1925;84:1743-1744.
22. Committee on foods. *JAMA.* 1932;99:391.
23. Committee on foods. *JAMA.* 1933;100:1175.
24. Advertisement. *N Engl J Med.* 1938;218:940-941. Editorial.
25. Mead Johnson advertisement. *JAMA.* 1930;95:22.
26. Apple RA. *Mothers and Medicine: A Social History of Infant Feeding, 1890-1950.* Madison, Wis: University of Wisconsin Press; 1987.
27. Crawford WH. Infant feeding and summer care. *Arch Pediatr.* 1933;50:642-645.
28. Jelliffe D, Jelliffe EFP. *Human Milk in the Modern World. Psychosocial, Nutritional and Economic Significance.* New York, NY: Oxford University Press Inc; 1978:211-240.
29. McClomas M, Fookes G, Taucher G. *The Dilemma of Third World Nutrition: Nestlé and the Role of Infant Formula.* Nestlé SA; 1985:3-20.
30. *International Code of Marketing of Breast-Milk Substitutes.* Geneva, Switzerland: World Health Organization; 1981.
31. Fleischman D. AAP raps Gerber for delivering formula samples. *AAP News.* 1990;6:1.
32. *American Medical Association Proceedings of the House of Delegates.* Report of Council on Scientific Affairs. 138th annual meeting; June 1989. Resolution 9:343.
33. *Statement Submitted to United States Senate Committee on the Judiciary Subcommittee on Antitrust, Monopolies and Business Rights on Advertising of Infant Formula.* May 29, 1990. American Academy of Pediatrics, Dept of Government Liaison, Washington, DC.

Ventriculitis in Newborns With Myelomeningocele

Edward B. Charney, MD; Jeanne B. Melchionni, RN; Donna L. Antonucci, MD

• It has frequently been cited that a delay in back closure of beyond age 48 hours in newborns with myelomeningocele is associated with an increased risk of ventriculitis. It has been suggested that antibiotic therapy prior to surgery might minimize this risk. We reviewed our experience with ventriculitis in newborns with myelomeningocele and its relationship to antibiotic usage and time of back closure. Of 186 newborns, ventriculitis developed in 13 (7%), and there was no observed difference by time of back closure, clinical severity of infant at birth, status of myelomeningocele sac at birth, or type of delivery. There was a significant association between antibiotic usage and ventriculitis among the infants with delayed surgery, of which only one (1%) of 73 receiving broad-spectrum antibiotic prophylactic therapy developed ventriculitis compared with five (19%) of the 27 who did not receive antibiotics. Our data support the suggestion that antibiotic treatment is effective in minimizing the risk of ventriculitis among infants with myelomeningocele undergoing surgery after 48 hours of age.

(*AJDC.* 1991;145:287-290)

It is often stated that surgical closure of the back lesion in a newborn with myelomeningocele is an emergency, and a delay of more than 48 hours is associated with significant increase in mortality and morbidity.[1-5] An often-cited risk of delayed surgery has been the increase in ventriculitis, with reports of an 8% incidence of central nervous system infection with immediate surgery compared with a 25% to 40% incidence among infants with surgery delayed for more than 48 hours.[6] In a previous study,[7] we concluded that surgical intervention for newborns with myelomeningocele was not an emergency because, irrespective of whether surgery was done on day 1 or day 7 of life, there was no difference in mortality or morbidity. Our data suggested that the use of prophylactic antibiotics might be effective in minimizing the previously reported increased risk of central nervous system infection or ventriculitis during that period. We wanted to assess further what factors might influence the development of neonatal ventriculitis among infants with myelomeningocele receiving surgical intervention, and whether antibiotic use prior to surgical closure of the back lesion is protective.

Accepted for publication September 19, 1990.

From the Department of Pediatrics, University of Pennsylvania School of Medicine, Philadelphia, and the Division of Child Development and Rehabilitation, Children's Seashore House at the Children's Hospital of Philadelphia.

Reprint requests to the Children's Hospital of Philadelphia, 34th St and Civic Center Blvd, Philadelphia, PA 19104 (Dr Charney).

PATIENTS AND METHODS

We reviewed the hospital records of 186 consecutive newborns with myelomeningocele surgically treated at the Children's Hospital of Philadelphia (Pa) between 1978 and 1987. Data collected included the following: level of motor paralysis; type of delivery (vaginal or cesarean section); associated adverse criteria[8] (gross paralysis of the legs with, at most, active hip flexors; clinically evident kyphosis or scoliosis; congenital hydrocephalus with head circumference greater than the 95% percentile; birth injury; or other severe birth defects) to reflect clinical severity at birth; status of sac (leaking or intact) overlying the neural tube defect; time of back closure ("early" defined as within 48 hours, "delayed" defined as between 3 and 7 days, and "late" defined as after 1 week); time of ventricular shunt procedure; use of broad-spectrum antibiotics prior to back closure (type or combination and duration of treatment); and the occurrence of ventriculitis as defined by culture-positive ventricular fluid within the first month of life. The data were analyzed by χ^2 two-way contingency tables with Yates' correction for continuity, with statistical significance being defined as $P<.05$.

RESULTS

Patient Population

All infants were transferred to the Children's Hospital of Philadelphia for their initial treatment within the first 24 hours of life with local back care consisting of sterile saline–soaked gauze applications. Of the 186 infants with myelomeningocele receiving neurosurgical intervention, 74 (40%) had high lumbar or thoracic paralysis, 47 (25%) had midlumbar paralysis, and 65 (35%) had low lumbar or sacral paralysis. Sixty-seven (36%) were delivered by cesarean section, and 119 (64%) were vaginal deliveries. One hundred twelve (60%) had no adverse criteria at birth, whereas 51 (27%) had one, and 23 (12%) had two or more. The sac was intact in 82 (44%) and leaking in 104 (56%). No sac that was initially intact leaked prior to surgical closure. One hundred sixty-two (87%) received ventricular shunts for hydrocephalus within the first 8 weeks of life.

Of the 186 infants, 86 (46%) had early surgical closure of the back lesion, 78 (42%) had delayed closure, and 22 (12%) had late closure, based on time of parental consent for surgical management. Of the 82 infants with intact sacs, 41% had early, 48% had delayed, and 11% had late surgery compared with the 104 infants with leaking sacs, of whom 50% had early, 38% had delayed, and 12% had late surgery. Of the 119 infants delivered vaginally, 50% had early, 42% had delayed, and 8% had late surgery compared with the 67 infants delivered by cesarean section, of whom 39% had early, 43% had delayed, and 18% had late surgery. These differences were not significant. There was, however, a significant difference ($P<.05$) between those infants with no adverse criteria and those with one or more with regard to time of surgery. Of the 112 infants

Infants With Ventriculitis*

Infant No.	Type of Delivery	No. of Adverse Criteria	Status of Sac	Time of Back Closure, d	Time of Ventricular Shunt, d	Age at Positive CSF Culture, d	Antibiotics (Duration in Days)	Organism
1	Vaginal	2	Intact	4	6,14	17	Ampicillin sodium, gentamicin sulfate (7)	*Escherichia coli*
2	C-Section	0	Intact	2	42	9	Ampicillin sodium, gentamicin sulfate (4)	*E coli*
3	Vaginal	1	Intact	2	2	2	Oxacillin sodium, gentamicin sulfate (4)	*E coli*
4	C-Section	0	Leaking	1	4	16	Ampicillin sodium, gentamicin sulfate (6)	enterococcus
5	Vaginal	0	Intact	1	14	28	Ampicillin sodium, gentamicin sulfate (3)	*Staphylococcus aureus*
6	C-Section	0	Leaking	1	3	8	Ampicillin sodium, gentamicin sulfate oxacillin sodium (5)	*Staphylococcus epidermidis*
7	Vaginal	0	Leaking	4	8	13	. . .	*E Coli*
8	Vaginal	0	Intact	3	. . .	4	. . .	*E Coli*
9	Vaginal	0	Intact	2	24	11	. . .	*E Coli*
10	Vaginal	0	Intact	2	29	6	. . .	*E Coli*
11	C-Section	3	Leaking	19	14	25	. . .	Group B *Streptococcus*
12	Vaginal	0	Intact	19	14	25	. . .	Group B *Streptococcus*
13	C-Section	0	Intact	4	18	24	. . .	*Klebsiella pneumoniae*

*CSF indicates cerebrospinal fluid, and C-Section, cesarean section.

with no adverse criteria, 61 (54%) had early surgery compared with 24 (32%) of the 74 infants with one or more adverse criteria.

Antibiotic Use

A total of 131 newborns (70%) received antibiotic prophylaxis within the first 24 hours of life and prior to surgical closure of their back lesion, at the discretion of the neurosurgeon, without apparent influence of type of delivery, status of sac, or clinical severity of the condition. Antibiotics were received by 79 (66%) of 119 infants delivered vaginally and 52 (78%) of 67 infants delivered by cesarean section; by 55 (67%) of 82 infants with intact sacs and 76 (73%) of 109 infants with leaking sacs; and by 77 (69%) of 112 infants with no adverse clinical criteria and 54 (73%) of 74 infants with one or more adverse criteria at birth.

Fifty-nine (69%) of the early surgery group, 61 (78%) of the delayed group, and 11 (50%) of the late surgical group received therapy. Mean durations of therapy for the early, delayed, and late groups were 4.6 days (range, 1 to 14 days), 6.1 days (range, 1 to 14 days), and 8.5 days (range, 1 to 18 days), respectively. These differences were not significant. Antibiotic usage included a combination of ampicillin sodium (100 mg/kg per 24 hours in two divided doses) and gentamicin sulfate (5 mg/kg per 24 hours in two divided doses) in 92 infants (70%); oxacillin sodium (100 mg/kg per 24 hours in two divided doses) and gentamicin sulfate in 21 infants (16%); and vancomycin hydrochloride (20 mg/kg per 24 hours in two divided doses) and gentamicin in six infants (5%). Other antibiotic regimens included use of nafcillin sodium, kanamycin sulfate, tobramycin hydrochloride (20 mg/kg per 24 hours in two divided doses) and gentamicin in six infants (5%). Other antibiotic regimens included use of nafcillin, kanamycin, and tobramycin sulfate.

Ventriculitis

Thirteen (7%) of 186 infants developed ventriculitis within the first month of life (Table). All but one (infant 3) underwent a clinical deterioration (eg, lethargy and fever) that necessitated cerebrospinal fluid culture for diagnostic evaluation. The age at which culture-positive ventricular fluid was obtained varied from 2 to 28 days, with a mean of 14 days. Isolated organisms among the 13 infants included: *Escherichia coli* in seven, group B *Streptococcus* in two, *Staphylococcus epidermidis* in one, *Staphylococcus aureus* in one, *Klebsiella pneumoniae* in one, and enterococcus in one. In vitro resistance to ampicillin sodium was noted in three of the seven *E coli* isolates and to gentamicin sulfate in the *S epidermidis* isolate. Positive ventricular fluid cultures were obtained prior to the insertion of a ventricular shunt in six infants, whereas seven had organisms isolated within 4 to 14 days after a ventricular shunting procedure. Of these seven, all but one (infant 6) had organisms that were typical for sac colonization rather than for acquisition during a shunting procedure. Positive cultures were obtained between 3 and 10 days after antibiotics were discontinued in infants 1 (10 days), 2 (5 days), 4 (10 days), and 6 (3 days). Infant 3 had a positive cerebrospinal fluid culture on 2 of the 4 days of antibioti coverage, whereas infant 5 had a positive culture 25 days after a 3-day course of antibiotics was discontinued.

As shown in the tabulation below, there was no observed significant difference in the occurrence of ventriculitis by type of delivery, clinical severity of infant (associated adverse criteria), status of myelomeningocele sac at birth, or time of back closure.

Variables (No.)	No. (%) of Infants With Ventriculitis
Type of Delivery	
Cesarean section (67)	5 (7)
Vaginal (119)	8 (7)
Adverse Criteria	
None (112)	9 (8)
One (51)	2 (4)
More than two (23)	2 (9)
Status of sac	
Intact	9 (11)
Leaking (104)	4 (4)
Time of back closure	
Early (86)	7 (8)
Delayed (78)	5 (6)
Late (22)	1 (15)
Antibiotic prophylaxis	
Early surgery	
Yes (59)	5 (8)
No (27)	2 (7)
Delayed or late surgery ($P = .005$)	
Yes (73)	1 (1)
No (27)	5 (19)

Antibiotic use did not significantly affect the development of ventriculitis among the infants with early surgery; however, of the 100 infants with delayed or late surgery, only one (1%) of 73 receiving broad-spectrum antibiotic prophylactic therapy developed ventriculitis compared with five (19%) of the 27 who did not receive such therapy. This difference is highly significant at $P = .005$ by χ^2 testing with Yates' correction for continuity. Of the five infants with early surgery and ventriculitis, mean duration of therapy was 4.4 days compared with a mean of 4.6 days among the 54 infants with early surgery and no ventriculitis. Infant 11, with delayed surgery and ventriculitis, initially received antibiotics for 7 days, compared with a mean of 6.1 days for the 60 infants with delayed surgery and no ventriculitis.

COMMENT

Central nervous system infection in any neonate is associated with high morbidity and mortality, even in those infants receiving early and appropriate treatment at the time of diagnosis. Most of the investigative work in evaluating various strategies to prevent this condition has focused on early-onset group B streptococcal disease with trials of chemoprophylaxis in selected mothers and/or infants.[9,10] All infants with myelomeningocele are at an increased risk of central nervous system infection, as the abnormally covered neural elements of their backs are exposed to the normal intrapartum bacteria and postpartum nosocomial skin colonization. The factors that influence the conversion from bacterial colonization to disease in the normal newborn are not well understood, and little investigation has been done in evaluating strategies for preventing infection in the myelomeningocele newborn population.

The development of ventriculitis in our population of newborns with myelomeningocele was found not to be associated with the timing of surgical intervention for the back lesion, status of the back lesion, clinical severity of the condition, or the type of delivery. There were, however, data to support our earlier suggestion[7] that broad-spectrum antibiotic prophylaxis is effective in minimizing the risk of ventriculitis among infants receiving surgical intervention after 48 hours of age. This observation is contrary to the often-cited argument advocating a need for early surgery to avoid ventriculitis. Since there was no apparent influence of type of delivery, status of sac, or clinical severity of the condition on whether antibiotic prophylaxis was received, it appears that clinical bias for antibiotic usage, which might have influenced our final results, did not exist.

The development of ventriculitis in the six infants with chemoprophylaxis requires further comment and speculation. Infants 2 and 5 had bacterial organisms (*E coli* and *S aureus*, respectively) that were resistant to ampicillin sodium but sensitive to gentamicin sulfate, which has relatively poor cerebrospinal fluid penetration.[11] Infant 6 had *S epidermidis*, which was resistant to all three antibiotics used for chemoprophylaxis. Infant 3 had an *E coli* organism sensitive to both ampicillin sodium and gentamicin sulfate isolated at 2 days of age, and may have had in utero-acquired disease rather than postpartum colonization-conversion to disease.

On the basis of our data, we conclude and recommend that chemoprophylaxis should be used routinely in newborns with myelomeningocele, especially in those for whom there may be a delay in surgical management. This is particularly relevant for hospital delivery settings in which the newborn may require transport to a hospital with a multidisciplinary team specialized in the care of children with myelomeningocele and their families. In our review of the factors that might have influenced the timing of surgical intervention, we observed that a delay in surgery was more common among infants with one or more adverse criteria. Since the time of surgery was based on time of parental consent, we may assume that for many of the parents with more severely involved infants, additional time was necessary to make a decision regarding surgical management. It is for these families that a "decision making process is best handled in an atmosphere wherein feelings of emergency or urgency are minimized and time for parental discussion is maximized."[7]

The finding that some infants developed ventriculitis in spite of chemoprophylaxis allows us to suggest some modification in therapeutic strategy. First, trials of a more effective chemoprophylactic regimen may be indicated, since three of our six "failures" had organisms that were not effectively treated by the ampicillin sodium and gentamicin sulfate regimen. The use of a third-generation cephalosporin, such as cefotaxime sodium, with its broad spectrum of activity against both gram-positive and gram-negative organisms, high-level resistance to hydrolysis by β-lactamase, enhanced blood-brain barrier penetration, and cerebrospinal fluid bactericidal activity,[12] in combination with vancomycin hydrochloride for *S epidermidis* coverage may provide more effective chemoprophylaxis. In addition to use during the first week of life, similar chemoprophylaxis might be reinstituted just before and several days after any neurosurgical procedure during the first month. The aforementioned interventions are speculative and require additional investigative work before specific guidelines may be established. We hope that implementation of such guidelines might further minimize the risk for ventriculitis in all newborns with myelomeningocele.

References

1. Sharrard WJW, Zachary RB, Lorber J, Bruce AM. A controlled trial of immediate and delayed closure of spina bifida cystica. *Arch Dis Child.* 1963;38:18-22.
2. Brocklehurst G, Gleave JRW, Lewin WS. Early closure of myelomeningocele with special reference to leg movement. *Dev Med Child Neurol.* 1967;13(suppl):51-56.
3. Sharrard WJW, Zachary RB, Lorber J. Survival and paralysis in open myelomeningocele with special reference to the time of repair of the spinal lesion. *Dev Med Child Neurol.* 1967;13(suppl):35-50.
4. Foltz EL, Kromal R, Shurtleff DB. To treat or not to treat: a neurosurgeon's perspective of myelomeningocele. In: Wilkins RH, ed. *Clinical Neurosurgery.* Baltimore, Md: Williams & Wilkins; 1973:147-163.
5. McClone DG. Technique or closure of myelomeningocele. *Child's Brain.* 1980;6:65-75.
6. Fernandez-Serrats AA, Guthkelch AN, Parker SA. The prognosis of open myelocele with a note on a trial of Laurence's operation. *Dev Med Child Neurol.* 1967;13(suppl):65-74.
7. Charney EB, Weller S, Sutton LN, Bruce DA, Schut L. Myelomeningocele newborn management: time for a decision making process. *Pediatrics.* 1985;75:58-64.
8. Lorber J. Spina bifida cystica: results of treatment of 270 consecutive cases with criteria for selection for the future. *Arch Dis Child.* 1972;47:854-873.
9. Boyer KM, Gadzala CA, Kelly PD, Gotoff SP. Selective intrapartum chemoprophylaxis of neonatal group B streptococcal early onset disease, III: interruption of mother to infant transmission. *J Infect Dis.* 1983;148:810-816.
10. Gotoff SP. Chemoprophylaxis of early onset group B streptococcal disease. *Pediatr Infect Dis.* 1984;3:401-403.
11. Stutman HR. Therapy for bacterial meningitis: which drugs, and for how long? *J Pediatr.* 1987;110:812-814.
12. Mullaney DT, John JF. Cefotaxime therapy: evaluation of its effect of bacterial meningitis, CSF drug levels and bactericidal activity. *Arch Intern Med.* 1983;143:1705-1708.

In Other AMA Journals

ARCHIVES OF PATHOLOGY & LABORATORY MEDICINE

Cancer Patient Staging: A Perspective

Donald Earl Henson, MD (*Arch Pathol Lab Med.* 1991;115:120-121)

Steroid Cell Tumor of the Ovary in a Child

Alan C. Harris, MD; Paul E. Wakely, Jr, MD; Paul B. Kaplowitz, MD; Robert D. Lovinger, MD (*Arch Pathol Lab Med.* 1991;115:150-154)

The Anatomy of a Gene: C-*myc*

Dennis W. Ross, MD, PhD (*Arch Pathol Lab Med.* 1991;115:193-194)

ARCHIVES OF NEUROLOGY

Results of Surgery for Extratemporal Partial Epilepsy That Began in Childhood

John Adler, MD; Giuseppe Erba, MD; Ken R. Winston, MD; Keasley Welch, MD; Cesare T. Lombroso, MD, PhD (*Arch Neurol.* 1991;48:133-140)

Stimulant Medication and Attention Deficit–Hyperactivity Disorder

The Child's Perspective

Jennifer Bowen, MBBS; Terence Fenton, PhD; Leonard Rappaport, MD

• Fifty-eight children receiving stimulant medication for attention deficit–hyperactivity disorder at referral clinics for learning disabilities at two teaching hospitals in Massachusetts were invited to participate in a study of their knowledge and attitudes. The 45 respondents and parents completed separate questionnaires concerning how they felt about receiving stimulant medication. Eighty-nine percent of the children felt that the medication was helpful and 78% liked or were indifferent to it despite a high rate (85%) of reported side effects. The five children (11%) who responded that they would stop taking stimulant medication if they could were more likely to perceive the medication as unhelpful and were receiving standard methylphenidate hydrochloride rather than a long-acting preparation. We conclude that children's perspectives on medication should be elicited directly and sustained-release medication may be more acceptable to children with attention deficit–hyperactivity disorder.

(*AJDC.* 1991;145:291-295)

Stimulant medication has been used in the treatment of children with attention deficit–hyperactivity disorder (ADHD) for over 50 years,[1] yet its use still causes intermittent controversy and adverse publicity in the media.[2] There is, however, a general consensus among physicians that stimulant medication is useful in the treatment of ADHD,[3] particularly as part of a multimodal approach to treatment.[4,5]

Ideally, children who are treated with stimulant medication are allowed to be active participants in their own treatment, yet response to treatment is usually determined by asking parents and teachers about changes in the child's behavior. To our knowledge, only a few studies[6-9] have assessed children's perceptions of the effects of stimulant medication and how children feel about receiving such treatment. These studies have shown that children are generally knowledgeable about the purpose of their medication, but have mixed feelings about taking it. Many children have been found to dislike taking stimulant medication even if they feel that it is helping them. Few studies, however, have examined in detail the differences between children who dislike medication and those who like, or are indifferent to, taking medication.

Recent studies[10-12] have shown that compliance in the use of stimulant medication is poor, and it has been suggested that this may be a factor in the relatively poor long-term outcomes in some studies of children treated with stimulant medication. Because a child's dissatisfaction with stimulant medication may have significant implications for compliance, it seems important to increase our knowledge of factors associated with children's attitudes toward stimulant medication. The purposes of the current study were to: (1) assess the general feelings, knowledge, and attitudes of children with ADHD who are being treated with stimulant medication as part of a multimodal approach to treatment; (2) assess the impact of recent adverse media publicity on these children; (3) compare the children's perceptions concerning the effects of the medication with those of their parents; and (4) examine factors that may distinguish children who generally dislike taking stimulant medication from other children.

PATIENTS AND METHODS

Questionnaires were sent by mail to 58 children with ADHD and their parents. The children were all between ages 8 and 18 years, were receiving stimulant medication, and had been doing so for at least 6 months. The children were all patients in programs for children with problems at school at Children's Hospital, Boston, Mass, or the Franciscan Children's Hospital, Boston. The children had been diagnosed as having ADHD by a multidisciplinary team consisting of a pediatrician, a psychoeducational specialist, and a child psychologist or psychiatrist. Diagnoses were made on the basis of parent interview, parent and teacher ANSER questionnaires, and neurodevelopmental, psychoeducational, psychological, and medical assessments. This protocol was approved by the committee on human investigation.

All children in the study met with the *Diagnostic and Statistical Manual of Mental Disorders, Revised Third Edition*[13] criteria for moderate or severe ADHD. All were in at least the average range of intelligence and none had gross neurologic damage or psychosis. As reported by parents and teachers, all the children had shown a positive response to stimulant medication (methylphenidate hydrochloride or dextroamphetamine sulfate). In addition to the stimulant medication, children were receiving a variety of other services as part of a multimodal approach to treatment based on findings at the time of the initial assessment. Children were reviewed every 3 to 6 months by their physician and other members of the assessment team.

The children's questionnaires were designed to assess their

Accepted for publication August 28, 1990.

From the Division of Ambulatory Pediatrics, Children's Hospital, Boston, Mass.

Reprint requests to Children's Hospital, Fegan 6, 300 Longwood Ave, Boston, MA 02115 (Dr Rappaport).

Table 1.—Comparison of Children who Returned Questionnaires With Those Who Did Not

Characteristics	Respondents (n=45)	Nonrespondents (n=13)	P
1. Age, y (mean ± SD)	11.9 ± 2.4	12.5 ± 2.7	.82*
2. Duration of medication, y	3.3 ± 2.0	3.7 ± 1.5	.47*
3. Males	41 (91.1%)	12 (93.3%)	.89†
4. Sustained-release medication‡	28 (62.3%)	8 (61.5%)	.92†

**t* test for differences between independent variables.
†χ^2 statistic for differences between expected frequencies.
‡Sustained-release methylphenidate or dextroamphetamine.

Table 2.—General Feelings of Children Regarding Stimulant Medication

Child's Feelings	No. (%)
Helpfulness of medication	
Very helpful	22 (48.9)
A little helpful	18 (40.0)
Not helpful	5 (11.1)
Child's feelings about medication	
Liked taking medication	15 (33.3)
Neither liked nor disliked medication	20 (44.4)
Disliked medication	10 (22.2)
Would child keep taking medication?	
Every day	21 (46.7)
Some of the time	19 (42.2)
Stop taking medication	5 (11.1)

understanding of why they were receiving the stimulant medication; their attribution of the cause of their problems; the benefits and side effects that they perceived as being due to the stimulant medication; other medication-related complaints or worries; general feelings about its helpfulness; whether they liked, were indifferent to, or disliked taking the stimulant medication; and whether they would continue taking the medication if it was entirely up to them. Children were also asked about their responses to recent media publicity concerning the use of stimulant medication.

Questions were developed through a survey of currently available rating scales for children with ADHD, and the format was based on the ANSER System Self-Administered Student Profile.[14,15] Each child's questionnaire used the name of the child's own medication (methylphenidate hydrochloride [Ritalin] or dextroamphetamine sulfate [Dexedrine])as listed below.

Sample Items From the Children's Questionnaire

1. Before starting Ritalin, I had trouble sitting still in the classroom (circle one):
   a. very true for me
   b. a little true for me
   c. not true for me
2. Now that I am taking Ritalin, I find getting to sleep at night is (circle one):
   a. easier
   b. no different
   c. harder
3. What would you do if you were told that it was entirely up to you whether you took your Ritalin (circle one):
   a. I would keep taking Ritalin every day
   b. I would take it sometimes but not all the time
   c. I would stop taking Ritalin

In addition, the children were asked to complete the Perceived Competence Scale for Children,[16] a self-report questionnaire that measures a child's perception of cognitive, social, and physical competence, as well as general sense of self-worth. Children were asked to complete all questionnaires as independently of parent involvement as possible.

The parents' questionnaire included questions about their children identical to those in the children's questionnaire. In addition, the parents were asked to provide demographic data, stimulant dosage, and medical and developmental histories, including provision of academic and nonacademic support services. Current behavior was described using the Conners' Abbreviated Parent Rating Scale.[17,18]

RESULTS

Demographics

Of the 58 children recruited for the study, both parent and child questionnaires were completed by 45 (77.5%). Table 1 shows that the children who completed the questionnaires did not differ significantly from the children who failed to do so with respect to their age, sex, length of time receiving stimulant medication, or type of medication.

Of those who completed the questionnaires, 36% were receiving standard methylphenidate (mean dose, 16.4 mg/d; range, 5 to 27.5 mg/d; mean dose by weight per day, 0.33 mg/kg per day), 26% were receiving slow-release methylphenidate (mean dose, 23.3 mg/d; range, 20 to 60 mg/d; mean dose by weight per day, 0.53 mg/kg per day), and 38% were receiving dextroamphetamine (mean dose, 12.9 mg/d; range, 10 to 30 mg/d; mean dose by weight per day, 0.28 mg/kg per day); 93% were of middle or upper-middle class socioeconomic background (by Hollingshead's classification[19]); 84% were receiving academic support services at school, 80% were receiving individual or family counseling or psychotherapy, and 38% were involved in a behavior treatment program either at home or at school.

Children's Perceptions

General Feelings.—The majority of children (88.9%) felt that the stimulant medication was helpful to them and most (77.7%) reported that they liked or felt indifferent to taking stimulant medication (Table 2). The vast majority of children (88.9%) also reported that they would keep taking the medication some or all of the time if it were completely up to them.

Attributions.—In general, children had a good understanding of why they were receiving stimulant medication, with a majority of them reporting poor concentration (81.8%) and trouble sitting still in the classroom (71.1%) as reasons for starting the treatment. A significant number of children (31.8%), however, also reported that they did not know why they were receiving stimulant medication in spite of the fact that all had listed at least two specific reasons (Table 3). Most children (72.7%) attributed their ADHD to physiologic causes ("just something I was born with"), although many children also reported that external factors (schoolwork, teachers, or other students) played a role; a smaller number felt that they were partly to blame for their difficulties ("my fault because I'm lazy") (Table 4).

Medication Effects (Table 5).—The most frequently reported benefits were improved concentration (80%) and improved ability to sit still in the classroom (73.3%). Overall, 97.8% of children reported at least one positive benefit. Many children also reported side effects or other complaints or worries related to the medication. In total, 82.2%

Table 3.—Reasons Given by Parents and Children for Commencing Stimulant Medication

Reasons	Children (n=45), %*	Parents (n=45), %*	% of Agreement†
Poor concentration	81.8	97.7	79.5
Difficulty sitting still	71.1	86.7	66.7
School work too hard	71.1	84.4	82.2
Trouble getting along at home	71.1	80.0	82.2
Poor control of temper	51.1	42.2	73.3
Trouble with friends	48.9	77.8	57.8
Always in trouble at school	43.2	47.7	77.3
Do not know why	31.8	2.3	69.7

*Percentage of children and parents responding "very true" or "a little true" for each reason given. More than one reason could be given for each subject; therefore, percentages do not add up to 100%.

†Percent of agreement between children's and parents' perceptions.

Table 4.—Attributions of Cause of Attention-Deficit Disorder

Cause Attributions	Children (n=45), %*	Parents (n=45), %*	% of Agreement†
Physiologic factors			
"Something I was born with"	72.7	91.3	70.7
"Injury or illness as child"	9.5	16.8	85.4
External factors			
"School work was too hard"	40.9	22.5	68.2
"Other kids caused trouble"	27.3	18.3	75.0
"The teacher didn't like me"	24.4	14.2	82.2
Personal factors			
"My fault because I'm lazy"	22.8	12.2	77.3

*Percentage of children and parents responding "very true" or "a little true" for each attribution. More than one attribution could be given by each subject; therefore, percentages do not add up to 100%.

†Percent of agreement between children's and parents' perceptions.

of children reported at least one negative aspect of receiving medication. The most commonly reported side effects were difficulty getting to sleep and decreased appetite.

Adverse Media Reports.—Only 13 children (28.9%) were aware of adverse media reports about stimulant medication. Of these, only three reported that the media reports had made them feel worse about receiving stimulant medication and 10 children stated that the reports had made no difference to the way they felt.

Agreement Between Children's and Parents' Perceptions

Parents and children tended to agree in identifying the children who disliked receiving stimulant medication (86.7% agreement, Phi coefficient, 0.79) and those who would stop taking medication if it were up to them (88.6% agreement, $\varphi = .80$).

Although the majority of children and parents gave poor concentration and trouble sitting still as reasons for commencing stimulant medication, children's and parents' responses differed somewhat (Table 3). Children were less likely than their parents to report poor concentration, trouble sitting still in the classroom, and trouble getting along with friends as reasons for commencing stimulant medication and were more likely to report that they did not know why they were receiving medication. While the majority of children and parents attributed the child's ADHD to physiologic factors (Table 4), a greater number of children than parents attributed their problems to external causes. Although there was reasonable agreement between parents and children regarding the major benefits (improved concentration) and specific side effects (sleep, appetite, etc; Table 5), there was less agreement about more abstract effects such as ability to get along at home or with peers, and feeling "different" or "not in control" while receiving the medication.

Table 5.—Perceived Effects of Medication Noted by Children and Parents

Effects of Medication	Children (n=45), %*	Parents (n=45), %*	% of Agreement†
Benefits of medication			
Improved concentration	80.0	97.8	82.2
Better able to sit still	73.3	86.7	73.3
School work easier	58.1	69.8	69.8
Less time in trouble	51.1	51.1	64.4
Better control of temper	44.4	46.7	75.5
Get along better with friends	29.5	47.7	59.1
Get along better at home	37.2	39.5	55.8
Side effects of medication			
Harder getting to sleep	31.0	28.6	71.1
Decreased appetite	31.0	28.6	78.6
Less energy	17.8	13.3	86.7
Sad more often	11.6	14.0	83.7
Increased nervousness	11.6	11.6	90.9
New onset of tics/twitches	4.6	2.3	97.6
Other complaints or worries			
Child feels "different"	48.9	62.2	51.1
Feels "something must be wrong with me"	44.4	60.0	57.8
Worried about long-term effect	35.6	13.3	68.9
Feels "not in control"	26.7	22.2	64.4
Embarrassed about medication	26.7	40.0	64.4
Kids tease about medication	11.1	11.1	91.1

*Percentage of children and parents who noted each effect. More than one effect could be noted for each subject; therefore, percentages do not add up to 100%.

†Percent of agreement between children's and parents' perceptions.

Factors Related to Children's Attitudes Regarding Stimulant Medication

Comparisons between children who disliked receiving stimulant medication and those who were not averse to the treatment showed no significant differences in respect to (1) the age of the child, (2) the duration of medication, (3) the presence of other support services, (4) parental occupation or education, (5) the child's awareness of recent adverse newspaper reports regarding stimulant medication, or (6) the child's self-esteem as measured on the Perceived Competence Scale for Children.

A number of factors were found to be related to whether a child would continue taking the stimulant medication if given a choice (Table 6). The five children who said they would stop taking the medication disliked taking it, were more likely to find it unhelpful, were taking standard

Table 6.—Factors Related to Children Who Would Stop Taking Stimulant Medication

Factors	Would Continue Medication	Would Cease Medication	P
Attitude to medication (No. [%])			
Like/indifferent to medication	35 (87.5)	0	<.001*
Dislike receiving medication	5 (12.5)	5 (100)	<.001
Perceived helpfulness of medication (No. [%])			
Helpful	38 (95)	2 (40)	. . .
Unhelpful	2 (5)	3 (60)	<.001*
Type of medication (No. [%])			
Standard methylphenidate†	12 (30)	5 (100)	. . .
Sustained-release medication	28 (70)	0	.002*
Medication dose, mg/kg per day (mean ± SD)			
Standard methylphenidate	0.33 ± 0.16	0.28 ± 0.11	NS
Slow-release methylphenidate	0.52 ± 0.18	. . .	. . .
Slow-release dextroamphetamine	0.32 ± 0.11	. . .	. . .
Conners' Abbreviated			
Parent Rating Scale Score (mean ± SD)	19.8 ± 5.8	28.4 ± 4.2	.003‡

*χ^2 statistic.
†Sustained-release methylphenidate or dextroamphetamine.
‡Two-tailed *t* test.

methylphenidate, and were more likely to receive a score on the Conners Abbreviated Parent Rating Scale indicating activity and attentional problems while receiving medication. There was no significant difference in the dose per kilogram of methylphenidate prescribed to children who would stop taking stimulant medication compared with those who would continue taking stimulant medication, although the dose per kilogram of standard methylphenidate was relatively low for both these groups of children.

To examine the factors that influence a child's attitude toward receiving medication, we used a logistic regression model in which liking vs disliking medication was predicted by its perceived positive and negative effects on the children. These analyses employed a backward stepwise procedure in which all variables measuring the perceived effects of the medication were entered into the model on an initial step; those failing to contribute significantly to the accuracy of prediction were removed on subsequent steps. Preliminary analyses were performed separately on variables measuring children's and parents' perceptions. In each case, the analyses revealed two variables exhibiting unique and significant relationships with feelings toward receiving stimulant medication. The significant children's variables were a perception that the medication makes them feel as if something is wrong with them ($P = .038$) and feelings of embarrassment about receiving the medication ($P = .029$). The significant parent variables also included a perception that the children who disliked medication were embarrassed about taking it ($P = .042$) and that these children also had more difficulty getting to sleep at night ($P = .015$).

On a subsequent analysis, these four variables, as well as a number of covariates including age, type of medication, and the Abbreviated Conners' scores, were entered into a similar logistic model. Here, only the two parent variables (embarrassment and sleep difficulties) remained statistically significant. However, the type of medication being taken by the child was also marginally significant, with children who disliked taking medication more often taking standard methylphenidate than long-acting stimulant medication ($P = .060$). A model that includes these three variables (embarrassment, sleep difficulties, and type of medication) was able to predict whether a child liked or disliked taking medication, with an overall accuracy of 88.9%, a sensitivity of 97.1%, and a specificity of 60%.

COMMENT

These results show that the majority of children with ADHD who received stimulant medication for more than 6 months as part of a multimodal approach to therapy found the stimulant medication helpful. In contrast to previous studies,[2,3] we found that the majority of children (77.8%) reported that they liked or were indifferent to receiving the medication.

The high rate of acceptance of stimulant medication by children in this study may have been due to a number of factors, including the multimodal approach to the treatment of these children in which education of the child regarding his or her problems is stressed; flexibility of medical treatment regimens so that the type of medication could be more closely tailored to the child's needs; a higher percentage of children receiving long-acting stimulant medication than in previous studies; and the fact that all children in this study were receiving stimulant medication and had been for at least 6 months. Other factors that may have influenced the level of reported acceptance include: (1) possible sampling bias in the group of children who completed the questionnaire compared with those who did not (although the high rate of returned questionnaires and demographic similarities between the two groups makes this less likely); (2) association of the study team with the clinic team; and (3) the forced choice format of the questionnaire.

Although children and parents generally agreed in identifying children who disliked receiving stimulant medication, there was somewhat less agreement in identifying the specific reasons for commencing the medication and in assessing its benefits and adverse effects. Many of these children have been receiving stimulant medication for a number of years, and it is likely that they do not have a clear recollection of why they started receiving it. In addition, problems for which such medication is often prescribed involved concepts such as concentration, attention, and relationships with others, which are relatively abstract and may be difficult for many of the children to fully grasp. Agreement concerning positive and negative effects was greatest over major benefits (improved concentration) and concrete side effects that were evident at home as well as at school. There was less agreement over more subjective or abstract concepts, such as ability to get on with others and feeling "different" or "not in control" while receiving the stimulant medication. These findings are consistent with those of previous studies[20] concerning the correlation between parent and child reports. Differing perceptions may be due to lack of knowledge by the parents about how the child is performing at school, a true difference of opinions between parents and children, or the child's cognitive limitations in handling more abstract questions.

These differences between parents' and children's perspectives illustrate the importance of asking children about their perceptions. The child may express concerns or worries about which the parent is unaware, and which may be important in providing a successful treatment regimen.

Our findings suggest that children's negative attitudes toward stimulant medication are often due to a perception of adverse effects or lack of effectiveness. Although all of these children had been reported by their parents and teachers to be responsive to stimulant medication, they were all receiving a relatively low total daily dose of methylphenidate (mean, 0.28 mg/kg per day). It is possible that this may account for the persistent symptomatic behavior among the children and may explain their perceptions that the medication was not helpful.[21,22] This suggests that children's reports may provide information useful in evaluating the potential benefits of changing either the dosage or type of medication.

The fact that all of the children who would have stopped taking stimulant medication if they could were taking standard methylphenidate rather than a sustained-release preparation suggests that the need to take stimulant medication while at school may be an important factor in the child's attitude or that sustained-release medication may be more effective than standard methylphenidate.[23] Previous studies[24] have shown that compliance for prescribed therapies can be improved by decreasing the complexity or inconvenience of the therapy regimen. The need to take stimulant medication at school not only adds to the complexity of the drug regimen, but also increases the likelihood of embarrassment on the part of the child. Taken together, these factors may contribute to the child's dislike of the medication and decreased compliance.

The findings of this study emphasize the importance of asking children how they feel about receiving stimulant medication and of employing a flexible approach that matches medication regimens to the needs of the children.

This research was supported in part by a grant from the Dyson Foundation, New York, NY.

We thank William Kent, MD, and the Franciscan Children's Hospital, Boston, for their collaboration on the project, and Judith Palfrey, MD, Alan Woolf, MD, MPH, and Marie McCormick, MD, ScD, for their thoughtful review of the article.

References

1. Bradley C. The behavior of children receiving benzedrine. *Am J Psychiatry.* 1937;94:577-585.
2. Cowart VS. The Ritalin controversy: what's made this drug's opponents hyperactive? *JAMA.* 1988;259:2521-2523.
3. American Academy of Pediatrics Council on Child Health. Medication for children with an attention deficit disorder. *Pediatrics.* 1987;80:758-760.
4. Hansen CR, Cohen DJ. Multimodality approaches in the treatment of attention deficit disorders. *Pediatr Clin North Am.* 1984;31:499-513.
5. Satterfield JH, Satterfield MS, Cantwell DP. Three year multimodality treatment study of 100 hyperactive boys. *J Pediatr.* 1981;98:650-655.
6. Baxley GB, Turner PF, Greenwold WE. Hyperactive children's knowledge and attitudes concerning drug treatment. *J Pediatr Psychol.* 1978;8:172-176.
7. Henker B, Whalen CK. The many messages of medication: hyperactive children's perceptions and attributions. In: Salzinger S, ed. *The Ecosystem of the 'Sick Child': Implications for Classification and Intervention for Disturbed and Mentally Retarded Children.* Orlando, Fla: Academic Press Inc; 1980:141-165.
8. Cohen NJ, Thompson L. Perceptions and attitudes of hyperactive children and their mothers regarding treatment with methylphenidate. *Can J Psychiatry.* 1982;27:40-42.
9. Sleator EK, Ullmann RK, Von Neumann A. How do hyperactive children feel about taking stimulants and will they tell the doctor? *Clin Pediatr.* 1982;21:474-479.
10. Firestone P. Factors associated with children's adherence to stimulant medication. *Am J Orthopsychiatry.* 1982;52:447-457.
11. Brown RT, Borden KA, Clingerman MS. Adherence to methylphenidate therapy in a pediatric population: a preliminary investigation. *Psychopharmacol Bull.* 1985;21:28-36.
12. Brown RT, Borden KA, Wynne ME, Spunt AL, Clingerman SR. Compliance with pharmacological and cognitive treatments for attention deficit disorder. *J Am Acad Child Adolesc Psychiatry.* 1987;26:521-526.
13. American Psychiatric Association, Committee on Nomenclature and Statistics. *Diagnostic and Statistical Manual of Mental Disorders–Revised Third Edition.* Washington, DC: American Psychiatric Association; 1987:50-53.
14. Levine MD. *The ANSER System: Interpreters Guide.* Cambridge, Mass: Educators Publishing Service; 1980:33-38.
15. Rappaport L, Levine MD, Aufseeser MS, Incerto RA. Children's descriptions of their developmental dysfunctions. *AJDC.* 1983;137:369-374.
16. Harter S. The perceived competence scale for children. *Child Dev.* 1982;53:87-97.
17. Conners CK. A teacher rating scale for use in drug studies with children. *Am J Psychiatry.* 1969;126:884-888.
18. Conners CK, Barkley RA. Rating scales and checklists for child psychopharmacology. *Psychopharmacol Bull.* 1985;21:809-843.
19. Hollingshead AB, Redlich FC. *Social Class and Mental Illness: A Community Study.* New York, NY: John Wiley & Sons Inc; 1958: 390-396.
20. Pantell RH, Lewis CC. Measuring the impact of medical care on children. *J Chronic Dis.* 1987;40(suppl):995-1085.
21. Sprague RL, Sleater EK. Methylphenidate in hyperkinetic children: differences in dose effects on learning and social behavior. *Science.* 1977;198:1274-1276.
22. Sebrechts MM, Shaywitz SE, Shaywitz BA, Jatlow P, Anderson GM, Cohen DJ. Components of attention, methylphenidate dosage and blood levels of children with attention deficit disorder. *Pediatrics.* 1986;77:222-228.
23. Pelham WE Jr, Greenslade KE, Vodde-Hamilton M, et al. Relative efficacy of long-acting stimulants on children with attention deficit-hyperactivity disorder: a comparison of standard methylphenidate, sustained-release methylphenidate, sustained-release dextroamphetamine, and pemoline. *Pediatrics.* 1990;86:226-237.
24. Becker MH. Patient adherence to prescribed therapies. *Med Care.* 1985;23:539-555.

Capillary Refilling (Skin Turgor) in the Assessment of Dehydration

Jose M. Saavedra, MD; Glenn D. Harris, MD; Song Li, MD; Laurence Finberg, MD

• This study was undertaken to evaluate the usefulness of skin turgor or capillary refilling in estimating the degree of dehydration in infants with diarrhea. After initial standardization of the technique, capillary filling time was found to be more reproducible when measured in the fingernail bed after applying just the amount of pressure necessary to blanch the nail bed. Capillary refilling time in 30 normal infants 2 to 24 months of age was 0.81±0.31 seconds. Capillary filling time was then measured in 32 infants with diarrhea admitted to the hospital and correlated to the degree of dehydration as estimated from the difference in weight from the time of hospital admission to the weight after rehydration. A turgor time of 1.5 seconds or less was found to be indicative of a less than 50-mL/kg deficit or of a normal infant; 1.5 to 3.0 seconds suggests a deficit between 50 and 100 mL/kg, and more than 3 seconds suggests a deficit of more than 100 mL/kg.

(*AJDC.* 1991;145:296-298)

The decrease of skin *elasticity* (the delayed return of skin to its original state after it is pinched into folds) and the loss of skin *turgor* or increased capillary refilling time (the slow return of color to the skin after pressure has been applied) are signs commonly used by pediatricians in the evaluation of dehydration, particularly in infants younger than 2 years.[1,2] For many years, one of us (L.F.) has used turgor times learned during his residency; however, to our knowledge, no studies have standardized the technique of timing skin turgor or evaluating its accuracy as a predictor of the degree of dehydration in infants. Accordingly, we set out to obtain data correlating the state of hydration in infants by timing capillary refilling.

MATERIALS AND METHODS

Study 1

Study 1 was performed to standardize the technique of measurement of capillary refilling (turgor time). Three different observers used a stopwatch to time the capillary refilling in three normal infants 6, 9, and 14 months of age, at two different sites (nail bed and heel), on three separate occasions, a total of six times per patient per observer per site.

To measure capillary refilling time in each instance, the observer applied pressure with his right thumb at the site chosen: nail bed of the right thumb or the right heel. Also, in each instance the measurement was made with two "degrees" of pressure applied: one degree of pressure was enough only to blanch the site ("light") and the other was "moderate" pressure. The pressure was maintained for 1 to 2 seconds and the capillary refilling was timed with a stopwatch from the moment of release to total recovery of color of the blanched area. Occasionally, a second person was necessary to gently immobilize the child's limb.

The types of measurements performed included nail bed with light pressure applied, nail bed with moderate pressure applied, heel with light pressure applied, and heel with moderate pressure applied. The times thus obtained were compared among observers, subjects, degrees of pressure applied, and sites.

Additionally, one of the investigators measured the nail bed refilling time applying light pressure in 30 apparently healthy infants seen in an outpatient clinic for a routine "well child" visit and immunization. The only criterion for selection was that they had had no apparent illness for the last 2 weeks prior to the visit.

Study 2

Study 2 was performed to evaluate capillary refilling (turgor time) as an estimate of the degree of dehydration. Any patient admitted to the infant ward at Kings County Hospital, Brooklyn, NY, with a history of diarrhea, with or without clinical evidence of dehydration, was enrolled in the study.

On admission to the ward and at regular intervals (usually after 4, 12, and 24 hours, and twice daily thereafter), the patients' conditions were reassessed for their hydration status. Weight and capillary refilling time were determined simultaneously at the time of admission to the ward. Particular attention was given to weighing the patients accurately. Infants were weighed on a digital scale, without clothes or diapers, and possible sources of error were accounted for (eg, intravenous equipment, armboards, etc).

Given the results in study 1, detailed below, capillary refill times were measured in the nail bed with light pressure applied. The times measured in the heel were not considered. The degree of dehydration of the patients (in milliliters per kilogram of body weight) was determined by the difference in weight from the time of hospital admission to "stable weight" once the infant had no clinical signs of dehydration. Stable weight was defined as the mean of two consecutive daily weights with a difference no greater than 2% of the highest of these two weights. The extent of dehydration thus calculated was correlated with the capillary refilling time at the time of hospital admission.

RESULTS

Study 1

Figure 1 shows the capillary refilling times found in three healthy, well-hydrated infants by three different observers. There were six observations per patient per observer for a total of 54 measurements per site per degree of pressure applied (nail bed with light pressure, nail bed with moderate pressure, heel with light pressure, and heel

Accepted for publication June 4, 1990.

From the Department of Pediatrics, SUNY Health Science Center at Brooklyn (NY).

Reprint requests to Box 49, 450 Clarkson Ave, Brooklyn, NY 11203 (Dr Finberg).

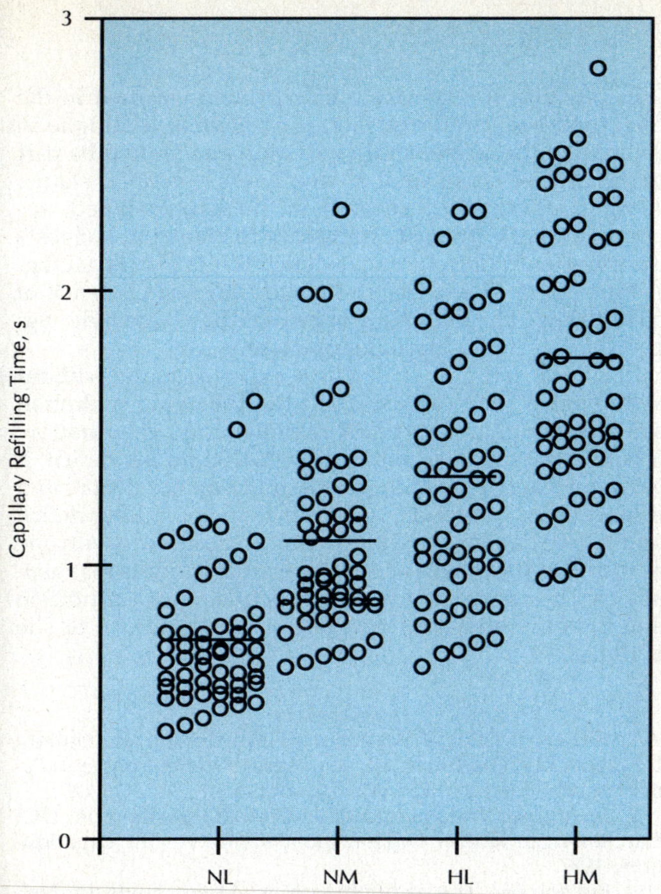

	NL	NM	HL	HM
Mean	0.73	1.09	1.32	1.76
±SD	±0.25	±0.37	±0.45	±0.49

Fig 1.—*Scattergram of 54 measurements of capillary refilling time (turgor time) in three normal infants in two sites and applying two degrees of pressure: "light," just enough to produce blanching and "moderate" pressure. NL indicates fingernail bed with light pressure applied; NM, fingernail bed with moderate pressue applied; HL, heel with light pressure applied; and HM, heel with moderate pressure applied. Measurement of capillary filling in the nail bed using light pressure was the most reproducible.*

with moderate pressure). The means and SDs for turgor time in each site with different pressure applied are shown. The shortest times were obtained in the nail bed of the hand; the longest times were obtained in the heel. In both sites, an increase in the amount of pressure applied, moderate vs light, prolonged turgor time. The least scatter with the smallest SD was also smaller in the nail bed as compared with the heel. For this reason, refilling time measured in the nail bed applying light pressure was the technique used in study 2. For the three observers who participated in the study, the interobserver coefficients of variation for 54 measurements done on three separate occasions were 28%, 36%, and 25%, and the intraobserver coefficients of variation in the same opportunities were 25%, 35%, and 32%.

Using the same technique, 30 healthy infants had their conditions evaluated. Their median age was 6 months, with a range of 2 to 24 months. Fifteen were male and 15 were female. Refilling time in this group was 0.81±0.31 seconds.

Study 2

A total of 32 patients (16 male and 16 female infants) were studied. Median age was 6 months, with a range from 1 week to 26 months.

Figure 2 shows the correlation of the refilling times at hospital admission with degree of dehydration. Of the 24 patients with a deficit greater than 50 mL/kg, only one

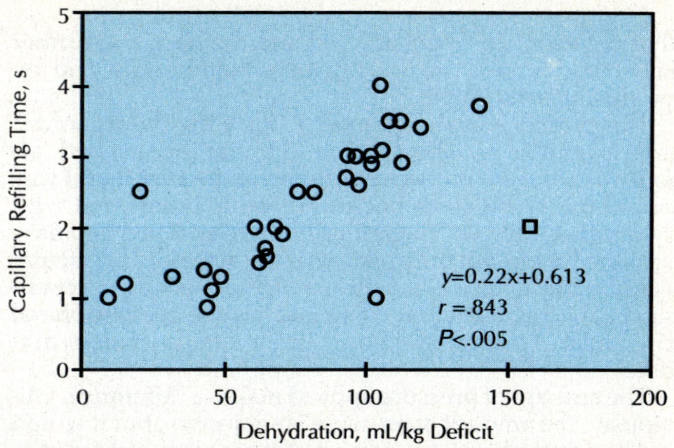

Fig 2.—*Correlation of capillary refilling time and degree of dehydration at the time of admission to the hospital. A square was not used in the regression analysis.*

(4.2%) had a refilling time of less than 1.5 seconds. Only one (11.1%) of nine patients with a refilling time of less than 1.5 seconds had a deficit greater than 50 mL/kg. Thirteen (76.5%) of 17 patients with a refilling time between 1.5 and 3 seconds had deficits between 50 and 100 mL/kg. Of the 11 patients with more than 100 mL/kg of deficit, 10 (90.9%) had refilling times greater than 1.5 seconds and seven (63.6%) had refilling times greater than 3.0 seconds. The correlation coefficient of .843 was significant ($P<.005$).

COMMENT

Skin turgor (capillary refilling) and skin elasticity are useful clinical signs in the assessment of dehydration.[1] Unfortunately, the terms have been used interchangeably in the literature leading to considerable confusion.

Elasticity is the physical property a body has to return to an original shape after it has been compressed, bent, or otherwise distorted. Thus, skin elasticity is the characteristic of the skin to spring back to its original shape after a fold of skin has been pinched up.[3-7] The loss of elasticity is also referred to as "tenting." The term *turgor*, on the other hand, refers to the fullness or resiliency of living animal or plant cells, and *turgor vitalis* refers to the normal fullness of the blood vessels or capillaries. It is preferable, then, to reserve the use of the term *skin turgor* to allude to the filling of the vascular bed of the skin. Turgor time is commonly referred to as *capillary refilling time*, the term we have chosen to use herein to avoid confusion.

Many sources use the terms *turgor* and *elasticity* interchangeably,[8,9] and others advocate the use of only skin elasticity in the clinical assessment of dehydration.[10,11] Laron and Crawford[12] showed a significant correlation between dehydration and skin elasticity (which they called turgor) as measured by timing the return of a pinched skin fold to its original contour. A time of 0.5 seconds was found with a weight loss of 2.5% to 5% and a time of 1 to 2.5 seconds was found with a weight loss of 5% to 8% in infants with diarrhea. Skin elasticity, while altered in dehydrated patients, can be affected significantly in the presence of malnutrition, obesity, or edema.

The presence of skin turgor is a sign of circulatory adequacy, since the speed of refilling of the capillary bed is responsible for the rapid return of color of the skin after the area has been blanched by pressure. The time for this refilling can be influenced by a number of factors, including the site, presence of edema, characteristics of the skin, temperature, and cardiovascular status. The nail bed, the thenar surface, and the heel are the usual preferred sites, particularly in dark-skinned infants. Our results suggest that between the fingernail bed and the heel, the former is better, because the color is more readily seen and reproducibility is better.

The presence of the glomus body, a highly organized arteriovenular anastomosis found under the nail bed, offers a practically direct visualization of the peripheral vascular bed. The glomus bodies are richly innervated with sympathetic fibers. Theoretically then, nail bed capillary refilling time is not only related to the actual intravascular volume but is also a sensitive reflection of the compensatory mechanisms that come into play in the peripheral circulation (vasoconstriction) during states of dehydration.

The amount of pressure applied makes a difference. Obviously, the amount of pressure is subjective, but it would not be practical to standardize it using mechanical devices. From our findings it appears that applying the minimal pressure necessary to produce blanching will yield more reproducible measurements. We did not assess the effect of maintaining the pressure for different periods before releasing, although probably the shorter time in which this is done, the less variability will be introduced. Timing can be done with a simple and usually inexpensive stopwatch, but with practice these times can be reasonably estimated without the need of a watch.

The average refilling time obtained in the nail bed in the normal infants studied was 0.81 ± 0.31 seconds. This would imply that refilling time in normal children can be expected to be as high as 1.43 seconds (mean+2 SDs) or 1.5 seconds for practical purposes. This is in agreement with the fact that in study 2 refilling time was 1.3 ± 0.5 seconds in the children with diarrhea but with a deficit of less than 50 mL/kg. The values for normal infants are also close to those of Schriger and Baraff[13] who reported an average capillary refilling time of 0.9 ± 0.5 seconds using the pulp of the distal phalanx in children 1 month to 12 years old. In adults, the average increased to 1.3 ± 0.7 seconds. From our measurements also, refilling time in the heel could be as high as 2.7 seconds in normal infants without any fluid deficit.

Capillary refill time correlated well with the degree of dehydration of the patients admitted to the hospital for diarrhea. It is apparent that a refilling time of 1.5 seconds or less is indicative of a less than 50-mL/kg deficit or of a normal infant; a refilling time of 1.5 to 3.0 seconds suggests a deficit between 50 and 100 mL/kg, and a refilling time greater than 3 seconds suggests a deficit of more than 100 mL/kg.

Certain clinical situations not evaluated in this study could alter capillary filling time. Hypothermia, hyponatremia, and cardiac failure may prolong it. Fever may have the opposite effect, and hypernatremic states clearly do so. Similarly, hypernatremia appears to preserve skin elasticity to a certain degree in the presence of dehydration.[14] The clinician must bear both of these complications in mind when making a quantitative judgment. The influence of nutritional status on capillary refilling time was not assessed in this study. In our experience, a marasmic state would not affect the results unless complicated by cardiac malfunction. In the presence of edema (kwashiorkor), capillary filling times might be less reliable.

In conclusion, capillary refilling time measured in the fingernail bed (preferred site) is a valuable technique in estimating the degree of dehydration and should be part of the clinical assessment of an infant's hydration status. A value less than 1.5 seconds in the fingernail bed, applying only the pressure necessary to blanch it, suggests a normal hydration status or a deficit of less than 50 mL/kg. A time of 1.5 to less than 3 seconds suggests a deficit of 50 to 100 mL/kg, and a time of greater than 3 seconds suggests a deficit of 100 mL/kg or more.

In clinical settings, with a little experience and without a stopwatch, one can ascertain the following hydration status: if less than 2 seconds, minimal or no dehydration; if between 2 and 3 seconds, a 50- to 100-mL/kg deficit; if between 3 and 4 seconds, a 100- to 120-mL/kg deficit; and if more than 4 seconds, a greater than 150-mL/kg deficit and urgent danger. As with all clinical signs, even with one as useful as this, there will be occasional variants that usually can be anticipated by the patient's overall condition and the environmental circumstance in which he or she is found.

References

1. Finberg L. Clinical evaluation of dehydration. In: Finberg L, Kravath RE, Fleischman AR, eds. *Water and Electrolytes in Pediatrics.* Philadelphia, Pa: WB Saunders Co; 1982:115-120.
2. Manual de Tratamiento de la Diarrea. Washington, DC: Pan American Health Organization, World Health Organization; 1987.
3. Robson AM. The pathophysiology of body fluids. In: Nelson WE, Behrman RE, Vaughan VC, eds. *Nelson Textbook of Pediatrics.* 12th ed. Philadelphia, Pa: WB Saunders Co; 1983:233-236.
4. Kokko JP, Tannen RL. Fluids and Electrolytes. Philadelphia, Pa: WB Saunders Co; 1986:83-86.
5. Olson R, Riddle I. Fluid balance in infants and children. In: Metheny NM, ed. *Fluid and Electrolyte Balance, Nursing Considerations.* Philadelphia, Pa: JB Lippincott; 1987:333-335.
6. Engquist A. Fluids, Electrolytes, Nutrition. Copenhagen, Denmark: Munksgaard International Publishers Ltd; 1985:30-31.
7. Groër ME. *Physiology and Pathophysiology of the Body Fluids.* St Louis, Mo: CV Mosby Co; 1981:132-146.
8. Shoemaker WC, Walker WF. *Fluid-Electrolyte Therapy in Acute Illness.* Chicago, Ill: Year Book Medical Publishers Inc; 1970:92,189.
9. Goldberger E. *A Primer of Water, Electrolyte and Acid-Base Syndromes.* Philadelphia, Pa: Lea & Febiger; 1986:31-35,76-78.
10. Siegel NJ, Lattanzi WE. Fluid and electrolyte therapy in children. In: Arieff AI, DeFronzo RA, eds. *Fluid, Electrolyte and Acid-Base Disorders.* New York, NY: Churchill Livingstone Inc; 1985:1211-1217.
11. Treatment and Prevention of Dehydration in Diarrhoel Diseases: A Guide for Use at the Primary Level. Geneva, Switzerland: World Health Organization; 1976.
12. Laron Z, Crawford JD. Skin turgor as a quantitative index of dehydration in children. *Pediatrics.* 1957;19:810-815.
13. Schriger DL, Baraff LJ. Determination and comparison of normal capillary refill between healthy children and adults. *Pediatr Res.* 1988;23:236. Abstract.
14. Laron Z. Skin turgor as a quantitative index of dehydration in rats. *Pediatrics.* 1957;19:810-815.

Practice Management Training for Pediatric Residents

Janice P. Piatt, MD; Douglas L. Bartley, MD; Albert D. Jacobson, MD; Mary E. Rimsza, MD

• In 1986, a practice management training program was developed for pediatric house staff. In conjunction with this program, pediatric residents for the following 2 years completed questionnaires regarding their career goals, interests, and perceived competence in practice management. Postgraduate level–3 residents who completed the program felt more competent than postgraduate level–1 residents in all areas of practice management and were more likely to take an active role in managing their practice. There was a significant difference between postgraduate level–1 and level–3 residents who completed the program in several areas: feelings of overall competence in office management, choosing a practice location, office staff, appointment system, billing system, office computer, fee schedules, telephone management, and setting up an office laboratory. Exposure to a practice management program during residency training may better prepare future pediatricians for a successful practice.

(*AJDC.* 1991;145:299-301)

The clinical practice of medicine continues to become more complex with expanding technology and increasing specialization. The business aspects of practice are also becoming more demanding, with tighter regulations, third-party restrictions, and increasing litigation.

Although most pediatric residents will ultimately work in a private practice after completion of their training, they are rarely exposed to the issues that are important in managing a practice. To meet these needs, an educational program was designed to provide residents with training in practice management.

In April 1986, one of us (A.D.J.) attended a meeting sponsored by the American Academy of Pediatrics (AAP) on practice management training for residents. Following this meeting, a faculty curriculum committee was established and the practice management program was initiated in October 1986. The goals of the program were as follows: (1) to familiarize pediatric residents with different types of office settings, including small and large group private practices, closed-panel health maintenance organizations (HMOs), and private pediatric subspecialty practices; (2) to increase residents' knowledge and thus feelings of competence in managing a practice; (3) to increase residents' knowledge and thus competence in establishing their own practices; and (4) to provide residents with practical information on private practice experiences that can aid them in establishing their own career goals.

Our program relied heavily on the guidelines set forth by the Committee on Practice and Ambulatory Medicine of the AAP. This committee produced a manual on practice management and developed a sample course outline using both didactic lectures and office preceptorships. The committee believed that the major objectives of a practice management program should be to familiarize pediatric trainees with the major issues in practice management, to provide an opportunity for the trainee to observe the mechanics of practice management in an office setting, and "to observe the unique relationship between practitioner and patient in the private office setting and discover how this relationship influences the context of practice."[1]

At the beginning of the program, the residents were asked to complete a questionnaire regarding their career goals, interest in practice management, and perceived competence in various aspects of practice management. The questionnaire was repeated at the completion of each academic year for the next 2 years. The purpose of the questionnaire was to try to evaluate how career goals and attitudes about practice management change from postgraduate level (PL)–1 to PL-3. We also were interested in evaluating whether PL-3 residents who had participated in the practice management program felt more competent in establishing and managing a practice than the PL-1 residents. This report discusses the practice management

Accepted for publication August 20, 1990.

From the Departments of Pediatrics, Maricopa Medical Center, Phoenix, Ariz (Drs Bartley and Rimsza), and Phoenix Children's Hospital (Dr Piatt). Dr Jacobson is in private practice in Phoenix.

Presented at the Region IX Annual Meeting of the Ambulatory Pediatric Association, Carmel, Calif, February 6, 1989.

Reprint requests to Department of Pediatrics, Maricopa Medical Center, PO Box 5099, Phoenix, AZ 85010 (Dr Rimsza).

Editorial Comment.—*During their training, we spend several months teaching our residents how to adjust ventilators in the neonatal intensive care unit, a technique they are then permitted to watch after residency as practitioners at the same hospital. At the same time, do we teach them how to run their practice, a real and necessary skill? This article describes a successful practice management training program that may have importance for your training programs.*—H.D.A.

program used in our residency program and the results of the practice management questionnaire that was completed by the house staff.

DESCRIPTION OF PROGRAM

The practice management program was developed by a private practitioner (A.D.J.) and full-time faculty member (M.E.R.) based on the recommendations of the AAP Committee on Practice Management and Ambulatory Care. The program consisted of didactic lectures and office preceptorships. Six didactic lectures on practice management topics were added to the core curriculum lecture series for residents. Topics for these lectures included "Insurance," "Selecting Accountants/Attorneys," "Practice Location," "Types of Practice (HMO or Small Group)," and "Personnel Management." Additionally, arrangements were made for outside experts on practice management to provide two half-day seminars for our house staff biannually.

The most important part of the program was the office preceptorship. Five pediatric offices that represented different types of practice experiences as listed below were asked to participate. An outline of areas to be covered during each session was given to the participating private pediatrician.

- Small group practice 1
  - Introduction to small group practice
  - Marketing and satellite office
  - Printed materials
  - Current procedural terminology codes, medical records
  - Telephone management
- Small group practice 2
  - Laboratory
  - Fees and compensation
  - Financial planning
  - Professional courtesy
- Large primary-care group
  - Introduction to large group practice
  - Office personnel
  - Accounting, legal, and management services
  - Time conservation and peer and community relations
- HMO
  - Introduction to HMOs
  - Office equipment
  - Computers in practice
  - Appointment system
- Subspecialty practice
  - Introduction to subspecialty practice
  - Fees and compensation
  - Risk management
  - Business office and payment systems

Each resident was assigned to spend one half-day per week in each practice management office preceptorship during five 1-month elective rotations. This program was offered to second- and third-year pediatric residents. Four PL-3 chief residents each year did not participate. Since our PL-2 and PL-3 residents normally have three elective experiences per year, they completed the entire practice management program by the completion of their third year of residency. Most preceptors had residents assigned to them for 30 half-day sessions per year. The residents' reading assignments for the course included the AAP's *Management of Pediatric Practice*[1] and other materials provided by the participating private practitioners and lecturers. Each office designed its own program using specific guidelines. The sessions usually began with an office tour and discussion about the assigned topics prior to regular office hours. Most offices involved their business managers and office staff in the teaching program as well. The residency program was unable to directly reimburse the participating pediatricians for their teaching efforts, but did make arrangements for these physicians to attend our hospital-sponsored continuing medical education programs without charge.

METHODS

At the start of the program, and for the next 2 years, incoming PL-1 residents completed a questionnaire regarding their career goals, interests, perceived competence, and knowledge of various aspects of practice management. This questionnaire was also administered to third year (PL-3) residents who had participated in the practice management curricula at the end of their PL-3 year in 1987 and 1988.

Comparison of Responses to Questions of Perceived Competence by PL-1 Residents vs PL-3 Residents*

Perceived Competence in:	PL-1	PL-3	P<
Office management	2.45	4.80	.0001
Selecting a practice location	2.97	6.00	.0001
Designing an office	2.98	4.53	.006
Choosing office staff	3.15	5.13	.001
Choosing appointment system	1.96	4.80	.0001
Choosing billing system	1.66	4.46	.0001
Selecting a computer system	1.72	3.93	.0001
Telephone management	2.42	5.46	.0001
Setting up fees	2.30	4.93	.0001
Setting up laboratory	2.27	4.93	.0001

*Residents were asked to rate their feelings of competence on a scale of 1 (no competence) to 9 (very competent). Values are means. PL indicates postgraduate level.

RESULTS

Thirty-four (85%) of 40 PL-1 residents and 15 (83%) of 18 eligible PL-3 residents completed the questionnaire. Most PL-1 residents (56%) expected to enter a subspecialty area of pediatrics. However, 86% of the PL-3 residents planned to enter general pediatrics and only 7% chose a subspecialty. (The percentages do not add up to 100 because some residents did not complete the question or did not know their preference.)

Residents were asked to indicate what type of practice they preferred (private, academic, HMO, hospital-based, or unknown). The majority (85%) of the PL-3 residents preferred to work in a private practice setting, usually in a small group. Thirty percent of the PL-1 residents also chose private practice, but 35% did not know what type of practice they preferred. Residents were asked the following question:

I prefer to have the business aspects of my practice handled by

(a) a partner;
(b) a business manager;
(c) me;
(d) an institution that employs me.

The majority of the PL-1 and PL-3 residents preferred to use the services of a business manager. No resident wanted his or her partner to run the office and only one resident chose an institution. Only 15% of the PL-1 residents wanted to manage the office themselves, while 33% of the PL-3 residents wanted to manage their own offices or use their own skills in addition to a manager.

The questionnaire also asked residents to select the type of practice they thought would provide the easiest call schedule. Sixty-five percent of the PL-1 house staff thought the call schedule would be easiest for them in an HMO. Twenty-one percent chose a hospital-based practice and 12% chose private practice. However, 44% of the PL-3 residents believed that their call would be easiest in a private group practice and 38% felt it would be easiest in an HMO.

The residents were also asked to rate the importance of call schedule, patient population, and problems managing the business aspects of practice in their decisions about choice of practice. Seventy-six percent of the PL-1 residents and 80% of the PL-3 residents rated the type of patient they would see as important in their decision. Forty-seven percent of the PL-1 residents and 33% of the PL-3 residents thought the call schedule was important. Forty-one percent of the PL-1 residents believed that their choice of practice would be based on their *dislike* for handling the business aspects, and only 6% believed that their choice would be based on the fact that they *enjoyed* managing the business aspects of practice. In contrast, only three PL-3 residents (20%) believed that their choice of type of practice would be based on their *dislike* for handling the business aspects of practice and 20% felt that their choice would be based on their enjoyment of handling the business aspects of practice. (These numbers are greater than the number of respondents, since residents were asked to circle all answers that applied.)

Residents were asked to rate their feelings of competence in practice management issues in a series of questions using a scale of 1 to 9, with 1 representing a low competence and 9 a high competence. The results were analyzed statistically using Student's *t* test on a computerized software program (Table). There was a statistically significant difference between PL-1 and PL-3 residents who had completed the practice management course in the following areas: perceived competence in office management, choosing a practice location, office design, choosing office staff, appointment systems, billing systems, computer systems, and deciding fee schedules. There was also a statistically significant difference between PL-1 and PL-3 residents' confidence in telephone management and setting up an office laboratory. There was no significant difference between PL-1 and PL-3 residents' level of interest in practice management issues, perceived relevance of a practice management course, or desire to learn more about practice management (average scores, 6.5 to 8.0).

The PL-3 residents were also asked to evaluate the program. Comments were generally quite favorable. Residents found the sessions with office managers and the discussions with private practitioners to be especially useful. The only complaint about the program was that the practice management sessions were taken out of elective time. Most residents would have preferred to have the practice management experience as part of other rotations. The practice management experience has now been moved to a third-year clinic rotation. Residents may also elect to spend time in practice management during ambulatory electives as well. The office preceptors in general enjoyed working with our house staff.

COMMENT

The PL-3 residents who participated in our practice management program felt more competent in all areas of practice management than the PL-1 residents. Perhaps because of this greater sense of competence, 33% of the PL-3 residents were planning to take an active role in managing the business aspects of their practice.

Despite a large number of PL-1 residents (56%) who expected to practice a subspecialty, most of our PL-3 residents had opted for general pediatrics by the completion of their third year of residency. During the past 13 years, approximately 26% (similar to the national average)[2] of our residents have continued their training in either a pediatric subspecialty or other residency after their PL-3 year. Thus, the number of residents (86%) entering general pediatric practice immediately after the PL-3 year during the study period was slightly high for our program.

It is possible that the practice management experience influenced our pediatric residents to choose a career in general pediatrics over a subspecialty, but without the benefit of a "control" group of PL-3 residents who had not participated in practice management and completed their residencies during the same academic year, this question could not be answered. Perhaps some residents enter fellowship training because they are fearful of starting a practice and thus wish to defer assuming this responsibility until a later date by working in a hospital or university setting.

We suspect that the change in our resident's perception of call schedule differences was directly related to their practice management experience. Again, however, this change, may be unique to our community and may relate to the call schedules of the private practitioners who participated in our practice management program. None of the reference materials we provided, including the AAP guidebook *Management of Pediatric Practice*,[1] discussed the types of practice that had the easiest call schedules.

A practice management program can easily be incorporated into pediatric residency training with the help of community pediatricians. Previous authors have shown that office pediatric rotations are helpful in reducing misconceptions about private practice and can be beneficial to both the resident and the practitioner.[3-5] Residents are very interested in learning more about practice management and developing skills that will be essential to their success in the private community. In addition, knowledge about practice management issues "can lower the business stresses a physician faces, permitting them to devote more energy to the practice of medicine."[3] Therefore, pediatric training programs should consider adding practice management lectures and experiences to residency training.

We would like to thank the following physicians and their office staff for their help in making the practice management program possible: Richard S. Reznick, MD, and associates; Mary McGee, MD, and associates; Howard S. Kandell, MD, and associates; Robert Hellmers, MD, and associates; and Jesse Cohen, MD, and associates.

References

1. Saltzman EJ, Shea DW, eds. *Management of Pediatric Practice*. Elk Grove Village, Ill: American Academy of Pediatrics; 1986.
2. Sehring DA. *1988 US and Canadian PL-3 Pediatric Resident Survey*. Columbus, Ohio: Ross Laboratories; 1988.
3. Altemeier WA, St Petery L, Schiebler GL. The demonstration of private practice to pediatric residents through office rotations. *J Med Educ*. 1976;51:138-140.
4. Greenberg LW. Teaching primary care pediatrics to pediatric residents through an office rotation. *J Med Educ*. 1979;54:340-347.
5. McCue JD. Training internists: insights from private practice. *Am J Med*. 1981;71:475-479.

Neonatal Hepatitis and Extrahepatic Biliary Atresia Associated With Cytomegalovirus Infection in Twins

Michael H. Hart, MD; Stuart S. Kaufman, MD; Jon A. Vanderhoof, MD; Steven Erdman, MD; James Linder, MD; Rodney S. Markin, MD; Robert Kruger, MD; Dean L. Antonson, MD

• **Prenatally acquired cytomegalovirus infection in twins was temporally associated with a discordant development of neonatal hepatitis and extrahepatic biliary atresia. This case presents evidence suggesting an association between perinatal cytomegalovirus infection and selected extrahepatic biliary atresia and neonatal hepatitis. Congenital cytomegalovirus infections and cytomegalovirus hepatitis are also discussed.**

(*AJDC.* 1991;145:302-305)

Extrahepatic biliary atresia (EHBA) occurs in approximately one of 10 000 live births. It is a disease of unknown origin that has been variably attributed to genetic,[1-4] toxic,[5] or infectious[6-8] causes. Concordance[9] and discordance[5,10-12] of biliary atresia have been described in newborn twins. The variable expression of biliary atresia in these infants supports a multifactorial cause of the pathogenesis of EHBA and Landing's[6] hypothesis that neonatal hepatitis and EHBA are a continuum of the same disease.

Cytomegalovirus (CMV) infection occurs in approximately 1% to 2% of newborns,[13-15] with greater than 90% of infected newborns being asymptomatic.[16] Although CMV infection can cause neonatal hepatitis and has been associated with EHBA,[17-19] a causal relationship with the latter has never been documented. We describe a set of twins with prenatal CMV infection and discordant development of neonatal hepatitis and EHBA. Albeit circumstantial, the data from our report support the concept of neonatal hepatitis and EHBA as different expressions of a similar disease process. This case also supports a possible causal association between CMV infection and the pathogenesis of selected cases of EHBA.

PATIENT REPORTS

Twin A.—Twin A was born after 35 weeks' gestation and weighed 2100 g. He was not identical to his twin, as determined by human leukocyte antigen typing, and had an Apgar score of 6/9 at 1 and 5 minutes. Both twins had normal karyotypes (46,XY).

Accepted for publication November 8, 1990.

From the Departments of Pediatrics (Drs Hart, Kaufman, Vanderhoof, Erdman, and Antonson) and Pathology (Drs Linder, Markin, and Kruger), Creighton University School of Medicine, University of Nebraska Medical Center, Omaha.

Reprint requests to the Division of Pediatric Gastroenterology and Nutrition, Creighton University School of Medicine, 601 N 30th St, Omaha, NE 68131 (Dr Hart).

Maternal history included a culture-negative pharyngitis with adenopathy and malaise 4 weeks before delivery. Hyperbilirubinemia was noted in the infant on day 2, when total bilirubin measured 242 μmol/L, and direct bilirubin, 94 μmol/L. A urine culture on day 2 was positive for CMV. γ-Glutamyl transpeptidase measured 748 U/L on day 6 and 596 U/L on day 10. The serum α_1-antitrypsin level was normal, measuring 1.07 g/L. Results of tests for possible infectious and metabolic causes of hepatitis with conjugated hyperbilirubinemia were negative. Abdominal ultrasonography revealed an enlarged liver with a normal-appearing spleen. The gallbladder wall was slightly thickened, and no gallstones were found. The common bile duct appeared normal. Levels of bilirubin (total and direct), aspartate aminotransferase, alanine aminotransferase, and γ-glutamyl transpeptidase were elevated (Table). A urine culture again yielded CMV. A hepatobiliary scan using diisopropylimido acetic acid showed good dye uptake by the liver, with delayed excretion into the gallbladder and bowel. A biopsy of a liver specimen was positive for CMV by viral culturing and immunoperoxidase staining. Microscopic examination of a liver specimen showed expanded portal areas with dense, mixed cellular, inflammatory infiltrate. Some neutrophils had infiltrated ductal epithelium. Bile ducts were present in most portal areas, and only occasional proliferative-appearing ductules were found. The lobule was moderately disorganized, with prominent multinucleated hepatocytes and giant-cell transformation. Trichrome staining showed mild portal fibrosis with portal bridging and fine bands of fibrosis tissue extending into hepatic parenchyma. No regenerative nodules were identified. The patient has done well since, and has had normal, age-appropriate weight gain. At age 1 year, his hepatosplenomegaly had resolved and serum and urine values had normalized (Table).

Twin B.—Twin B, a male, weighed 1890 g and had an Apgar score of 3/6 at 1 and 5 minutes. On day 1, the patient was identified with hemodynamically significant coarctation of the aorta and a tracheoesophageal fistula with esophageal atresia (Gross type C). The coarctation was repaired on day 1 with concomitant placement of a gastrostomy tube. Definitive surgical correction of the tracheoesophageal fistula/esophageal atresia was performed on day 4. On day 2, the infant had hyperbilirubinemia, with a total bilirubin level of of 208 μmol/L and a direct bilirubin level of 64 μmol/L. A culture of urine collected on day 2 yielded CMV. Results of a VDRL test were negative, as were results of titers for herpes, toxoplasmosis, and rubella, and serologic tests for hepatitis A and B. Levels of γ-glutamyl transpeptidase on day 6 were elevated to 396 U/L. Levels of serum α_1-antitrypsin were normal (1.37 g/L) (Table). Abdominal ultrasonography revealed a persistent ductus venosus and nonvisualization of the gallbladder. Liver and spleen were otherwise unremarkable. On day 13, the patient underwent a duodenal duodenostomy secondary to an obstructive annular pancreas. At surgery, a normal-appearing, bile-filled gallbladder was identified, as was a normal-appearing extrahepatic biliary system. Biopsy of a liver specimen revealed several large portal areas showing bile ducts, blood vessels, and

Enzyme Levels in Twins With Extrahepatic Biliary Atresia

Substance	Twin	Day 2	Day 6	Day 10	Day 25	Day 56	Day 73	Day 83	Day 90	Day 150
Aspartate aminotransferase, U/L	A	...	...	204	...	...	...	...	158	129
	B	...	...	256	...	...	...	...	253	192
Alanine aminotransferase, U/L	A	...	...	145	...	...	...	...	176	151
	B	...	...	176	...	...	...	...	135	156
Total bilirubin/direct bilirubin, μmol/L	A	242/94	208/54	174/82	...	...	...	...	50/38	8/2
	B	208/64	266/126	166/104	84/70	132/98	140/98	116/86	166/152	128/94
γ-Glutamyl Transpeptidase, U/L	A	...	748	596	...	...	...	...	761	460
	B	...	396	...	378	828	1140	1056	1302	1051

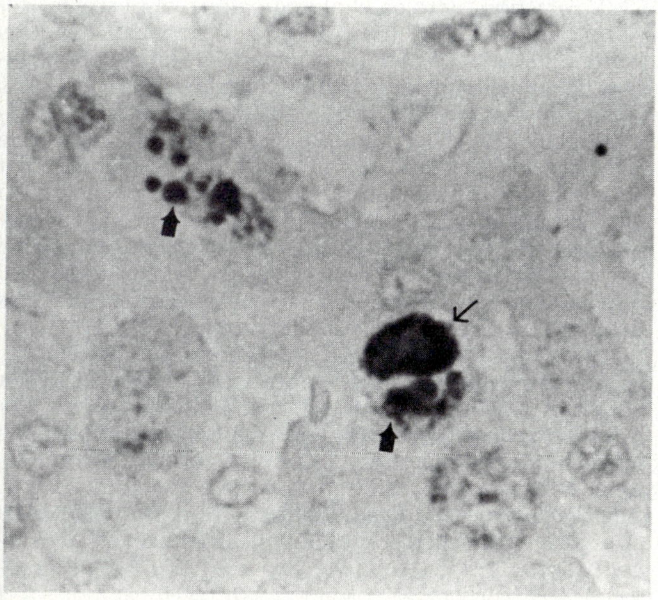

Fig 1.—*Complementary DNA probe of a liver biopsy in twin B shows intranuclear (thin arrow) and intracytoplasmic (wide arrows) staining (original magnification ×400).*

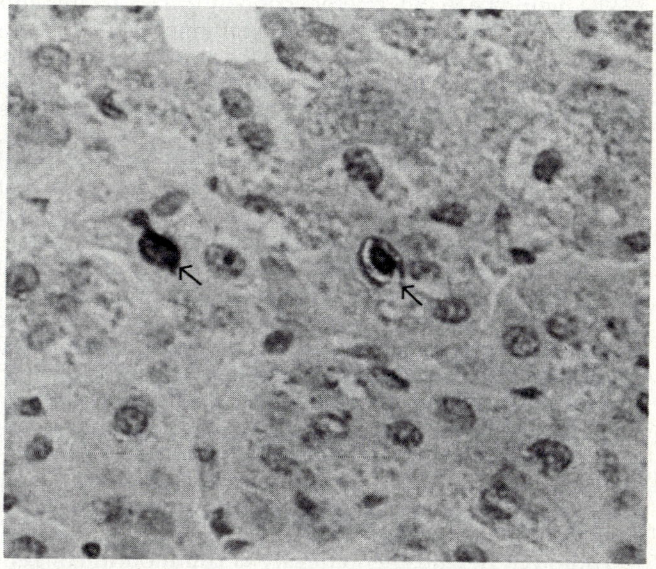

Fig 2.—*Immunoperoxidase stain for cytomegalovirus (arrows) in a liver biopsy specimen of twin B (original magnification ×400).*

focally prominent inflammatory infiltrates of histiocytes and scattered neutrophils. The hepatic parenchyma was moderately disorganized. Hepatocyte cytoplasm showed granular and vacuolar degeneration associated with abundant intracytoplasmic and intracanalicular bile pigment. Gomori's stains showed significant fibrosis extending from portal areas. No cholangiolar proliferation was noted. Bile ducts were adequate, ruling out syndromic paucity of biliary ducts. A complementary-DNA probe for CMV[20] and viral cultures were negative. A hepatobiliary scan using diisopropylimido acetic acid on day 27 showed good dye uptake and no biliary excretion for up to 24 hours. A second liver biopsy was performed on day 29, revealing histologic changes similar to those of the biopsy on day 13. A complementary DNA probe for CMV was positive (Fig 1), as was a CMV-specific immunoperoxidase stain[21] (Fig 2). Exploratory laparotomy was performed on day 42. During surgery, obliteration of a previously normal extrahepatic biliary system was noted, and a fibrous atretic cord was identified in lieu of a common hepatic duct. An operative cholangiogram showed no hepatic radicles. While no dye was initially excreted, follow-up films suggested that dye had passed into the duodenum. A Kasai procedure and liver biopsy were performed. This biopsy showed prominent cholestasis, which was primarily centrolobular and focally panlobular. Hepatocytes, ductules, and Kupffer's cells contained bile. Binucleated hepatocytes were seen occasionally, although giant-cell transformation was not present. Focal collections of neutrophils were present in the lobule without associated necrosis. In contrast to results of a previous biopsy, portal tracts showed variable ductular proliferation, and a trichrome stain indicated periportal fibrosis. Three cystic duct sections showed patent ducts surrounded by smaller ductular structures and mononuclear cells. Bile was not seen in the lumen. The fourth duct showed a smaller, stenosed lumen with epithelial sloughing. Each section taken from the porta hepatis exhibited a compressed cut with considerable sloughing of biliary epithelium. Deeper sections showed multiple smaller branches replacing the larger duct. These structures were surrounded by fibrous tissue and mononuclear cells. The gallbladder lumen did not contain bile. The lining of the epithelium was tall and columnar with some cytoplasmic vacuolization and intracellular bile staining. A complementary DNA probe, an immunoperoxidase stain, and a viral culture were all negative for CMV. Postoperatively, the patient did not have significant bile flow. Bilirubin values at age 2 months remained elevated (Table). At age 4 months, the patient experienced apnea and cyanosis associated with a viral pneumonitis. Cytomegalovirus was cultured from bronchial washings, and intracytoplasmic inclusions were noted in bronchial epithelium cells. Treatment with dihydroxypropylmethyl guanine was initiated. The patient responded to treatment and was in good condition at discharge from the hospital. Because of progressive end-stage liver disease, orthotopic liver transplantation was performed at age 2 years. Pathologic evaluation of the intact liver confirmed previous histologic findings of extrahepatic biliary atresia. Viral cultures, a complementary DNA probe, and an immunoperoxidase stain were negative for CMV at transplantation. At age 7 weeks, both twins tested positive for IgG to CMV (≥1:640; maximal dilution) and negative for IgM to CMV (<1:10). Maternal titers of antibodies to CMV were 1:16 for IgG and nondetectable for IgM.

COMMENT

Before 1974, neonatal hepatitis and EHBA were generally considered separate entities. In 1974, Landing[6] proposed that neonatal hepatitis, EHBA, and choledochal cysts were different expressions of a continuum of "infantile obstructive cholangiopathy." The discordant expression of EHBA and neonatal hepatitis in twins associated in part with CMV infection, as described herein, supports the concept of EHBA and neonatal hepatitis as a continuum of expression of infantile obstructive cholangiopathy.

Cytomegalovirus infection is the most common congenital viral infection. Prevalence rates for congenital CMV infection vary from 0.5% to 2.4% of live births.[13-16] Fewer than 10% of infected infants are symptomatic.[16] Frequent abnormalities associated with symptomatic congenital CMV infection are petechiae (79%), hepatosplenomegaly (74%), jaundice (63%), microencephaly (50%), height and weight below normal for gestational age (41%), prematurity (34%), inguinal hernia (26%), and chorioretinitis (12%).[22] Results of laboratory tests of infected newborns include increased cord IgM (84%), atypical lymphocytosis (80%), elevated aspartate aminotransferase level (79%), thrombocytopenia (61%), and increased cerebrospinal fluid protein (47%).[22] Our patients did have evidence of hepatosplenomegaly and jaundice, although they did not exhibit microencephaly, chorioretinitis, thrombocytopenia, petechiae, or intracranial calcifications. These infants apparently were infected prenatally, most probably 1 month before delivery, when maternal symptoms were noted. In this instance, the classic findings of congenital CMV infection would not necessarily be present. Twin B did have other congenital anomalies that were not attributed to CMV infection. In all likelihood, the other congenital anomalies were merely coincidental, although their presence and the clinical course that ensued may have modified the host response of the infant to the CMV infection.

Although hepatosplenomegaly is common in congenitally CMV-infected infants, chronic hepatitis and its resultant sequelae are rare.[15,23-25] Typically, the biochemical and histologic evidence of CMV-associated hepatic injury resolves within a couple of months. One child had residual mild hepatic fibrosis on biopsy of a liver specimen at age 4 years.[26] A recent article described a symptomatic, congenitally infected infant who died at age 3 months of end-stage liver disease secondary to diffuse hepatic fibrosis.[27] In this case, the biliary epithelium was not affected by the infection.

Although relatively rare, severe liver disease has been reported following CMV infection. Oppenheimer and Esterly[18] described an infant with cystic fibrosis and congenital CMV infection who also had cholestasis and paucity of bile ducts. Hepatic lesions in CMV-infected infants include hepatic fibrosis, hepatic necrosis, giant-cell transformation, cholestasis, extrahepatic hematopoiesis, and large intranuclear inclusions.[17,27] Previous reports have documented concomitant CMV infection and biliary atresia,[17-19] but a convincing cause-effect relationship has yet to be documented. Finegold and Carpenter[28] described a fetus at 24 weeks' gestation with obliterative intrahepatic cholangitis associated with CMV infection, and proposed that similar in utero CMV infection might play a role in the development of some cases of EHBA. Undoubtedly, host factors affect the expression of CMV infection in the developing fetus and newborn infant. This could certainly account for the discordant presence of liver disease in the infants in our study, despite similar exposure to CMV.

Compared with CMV infection in adults, congenital infection results in more variable findings. Typically, it causes more extensive hepatocellular injury. Widespread multinucleated giant cells with or without bile duct proliferation, areas of fatty metamorphosis, cholangitis, interstitial fibrosis, and periportal fibrosis are frequently seen.[17,25,29] Intranuclear and cytoplasmic inclusions are often seen in the hepatocytes, with endothelial cells, and in bile duct epithelium. Functional obstruction of bile ducts is not uncommon, and is presumably mediated by mechanical obstruction of the canalicular lumen by edematous CMV-infected cells.[30-33] Using electron microscopy of tissues from a congenitally infected infant, Balazs[34] found viral particles or inclusions in bile duct cells (both at nuclear and cytoplasmic locations) and intraluminally in the bile duct and the duodenum.

Our infants exhibited evidence of prenatally acquired CMV infection, with an evolving pattern of postnatal development of EHBA (twin B) and of neonatal hepatitis (twin A). The postnatal development of signs of progressive hepatocellular injury with cholestasis in twin B was temporally associated with CMV infection, as documented by a positive immunoperoxidase stain, a positive cDNA probe, and a viral culture of liver specimens that yielded CMV. Subsequent cultures of liver specimens on day 35 did not yield CMV. The occurrence of EHBA coincident with primary CMV infection suggests a causative role of CMV in the evolution of hepatocellular injury and the development of EHBA. It should be clarified that this does not confirm the role of CMV in EHBA.

Although CMV infection is a quite common congenitally acquired infection, the development of CMV and EHBA is rare in newborns. Although prenatally acquired CMV infection is associated with EHBA and neonatal hepatitis in the infants in our study, most cases of EHBA and neonatal hepatitis occur without associated viral infections. The discordance in disease expression is probably most accurately attributed to unknown differences in host responses.

References

1. Shim WKT, Kasai M, Spence MA. Racial influence on the incidence of biliary atresia. *Prog Pediatr Surg.* 1974;6:53-62.

2. Thaler MM, Gellis SS. Studies in neonatal hepatitis and biliary atresia, III: progression and regression of cirrhosis in biliary atresia. *AJDC.* 1968;116:271-284.

3. Nevin NC, Bell M, Frazer MJL, Froggatt P. Congenital extrahepatic biliary atresia in two brothers. *J Med Genet.* 1969;6:379-381.

4. Danks DM, Bodian M. A genetic study of neonatal obstructive jaundice. *Arch Dis Child.* 1963;38:378-390.

5. Strickland AD, Shannon K. Studies in the etiology of extrahepatic biliary atresia: time-space clustering. *J Pediatr.* 1982;100:749-753.

6. Landing BH. Considerations of the pathogenesis of neonatal hepatitis, biliary atresia and choledochal cyst: the concept of infantile obstructive cholangiopathy. *Prog Pediatr Surg.* 1974;6:113-138.

7. Danks DM, Campbell PE, Jack I, Rogers J, Smith AL. Studies of the aetiology of neonatal hepatitis and biliary atresia. *Arch Dis Child.* 1977;52:360-367.

8. Morecki R, Glaser GH, Cho S, Balisteri WF, Horwitz MS. Biliary atresia and reovirus type 3 infection. *N Engl J Med.* 1982;307:481-484.

9. Strickland AD, Shannon K, Coln CD. Biliary atresia in two sets of twins. *J Pediatr.* 1985;107:418-420.

10. Hyams JS, Glaser JH, Leichtner AM, Morecki R. Discordance for biliary atresia in two sets of monozygotic twins. *J Pediatr.* 1985;107:420-422.

11. Werlin SL. Extrahepatic biliary atresia in one of twins. *Acta Paediatr Scand.* 1981;70:943-944.

12. Morris BD, Nuss D, Winship WS. Biliary atresia in a twin. *S Afr Med J.* 1977;51:469-470.

13. Stagno S, Pass FR, Alford CA. Perinatal infections and maldevelopment. *Birth Defects.* 1981;17:31-50.

14. Hanshaw JB. Congenital cytomegalovirus infection: a 15-year perspective. *J Infect Dis.* 1971;123:555-561.
15. Panjvani ZFK, Hanshaw JB. Cytomegalovirus in the perinatal period. *AJDC.* 1981;135:56-60.
16. Stagno S, Pass RF, Cloud GF, et al. Primary cytomegalovirus infection in pregnancy: incidence, transmission to fetus, and clinical outcome. *JAMA.* 1986;256:1904-1908.
17. Lang DJ, Marshall WC, Pincott JR, Stern H. Cytomegalovirus: an association with neonatal hepatitis and biliary atresia. In: Javitt NB, ed. *Neonatal Hepatitis and Biliary Atresia.* Bethesda, Md: US Dept of Health, Education, and Welfare; 1977:33-41.
18. Oppenheimer EH, Esterly JR. Cytomegalovirus infection: a possible cause of biliary atresia. *Lancet.* 1973;2:1031-1032.
19. Stern H, Tucker SM. Cytomegalovirus infection in the newborn and in early childhood: three atypical cases. *Lancet.* 1965;2:1268-1271.
20. Masih AS, Linder J, Shaw BH, et al. Rapid indentification of cytomegalovirus in liver allograft biopsies by *in situ* hybridization. *Am J Surg Pathol.* 1988;12:362-367.
21. Przepiorda D, Myerson D. A single step silver enhancement method permitting rapid diagnosis of cytomegalovirus infection in formalin-fixed, paraffin-embedded tissue sections by *in situ* hybridization and immunoperoxidase detection. *J Histochem Cytochem.* 1986;34:1731-1734.
22. Pass RF, Stagno S, Myers GJ, Alford CA. Outcome of symptomatic congenital cytomegalovirus infection: results of long-term longitudinal follow-up. *Pediatrics.* 1980;66:758-762.
23. Berenberg W, Nankervis G. Long-term follow-up of cytomegalic inclusion disease of infancy. *Pediatrics.* 1970;46:403-410.
24. Henson DE, Grimley PM, Strano AJ. Postnatal cytomegalovirus hepatitis. *Hum Pathol.* 1974;5:93-96.
25. Toghill PJ, Williams R, Stern H. Cytomegalovirus infection in chronic liver disease. *Gastroenterology.* 1969;56:936-937.
26. McCracken GH, Shonefield HR, Cobb R. Congenital cytomegalic inclusion disease: a longitudinal study of 20 patients. *AJDC.* 1969;117:522-539.
27. Zuppen CW, Bai HD, Grill BG. Diffuse hepatic fibrosis in congenital cytomegalovirus infection. *J Pediatr Gastroenterol Nutr.* 1986;5:489-491.
28. Finegold MJ, Carpenter RJ. Obliterative cholangitis due to cytomegalovirus: a possible precursor of paucity of extrahepatic bile ducts. *Hum Pathol.* 1982;13:662-666.
29. Lurie M, Elmalach I, Schuger L, Weintraub Z. Liver findings in infantile cytomegalovirus infection: similarity to extrahepatic biliary obstruction. *Histopathology.* 1987;11:1171-1180.
30. Khige RC, Widesman RS, Weller TH. Cytomegalic inclusion disease of the newborn: report of a case with persistent viruria. *Pediatrics.* 1960;25:35-39.
31. Odierre M. Cholostase intra-hepatique par obstruction des voies biliaires interlobulaires au cours d'une maladie generalisée des inclusions cytomegaliques chez une nouveau-né. *Arch Fr Pediatr.* 1970;27:211-214.
32. Weller TH, Hanshaw JB. Virological and clinical observations on cytomegalic inclusion disease. *N Engl J Med.* 1962;266:1233-1244.
33. Medearis DN. Observations concerning human cytomegalovirus infection and disease. *Bull Johns Hopkins Hosp.* 1964;114:181-211.
34. Balazs M. Electron microscopic examination of congenital cytomegalovirus hepatitis. *Virchows Arch (A).* 1984;405:119-129.

Breast-feeding Initiation in a Triethnic Population

David E. Bee, PhD†; Tom Baranowski, PhD; David K. Rassin, PhD; C. Joan Richardson, MD; William Mikrut, MS

• The influence of sociodemographic factors on the initiation of breast-feeding was evaluated in a triethnic population from Galveston, Tex. Breast-feeding rates were 44.3% among Anglo-Americans, 13.5% among blacks, and 26.6% among Mexican-Americans. Mexican ethnicity, education levels among Anglo-Americans, and marital status were associated with the initiation of breast-feeding. Odds ratios for breast-feeding were 1.94 (95% confidence interval, 1.10 to 3.43) times higher in Mexican-American compared with black women, and 1.94 (95% confidence interval, 1.34 to 2.83) times higher in married than unmarried women. Anglo-American ethnicity and education, as main effects, were not significantly associated with breast-feeding, but their interaction was. Among Anglo-American women (in comparison with black women), the odds ratios of breast-feeding increased with education level, ranging from 1.84 for those with less than an eighth grade education to 7.46 for those with some college. In contrast to recent findings suggesting that education was more important than ethnicity in predicting breast-feeding, the odds of breast-feeding among Anglo-American compared with black women depended on the level of maternal education, but the odds of breast-feeding for Mexican-American vs black women did not depend on education.

(*AJDC.* 1991;145:306-309)

The prevalence of breast-feeding at the time of discharge from the hospital in the United States has declined over the last few years to about 55% in 1988 after reaching a high of about 62% in 1984[1-3] (Gilbert A. Martinez, MBA, Ross Labs, Columbus, Ohio, unpublished report, November 23, 1988). This recent decline represents a reversal of the trend to increased breast-feeding incidence that started in the early 1970s, when only about 25% of babies were breast-fed on discharge from the hospital. The recent decline in breast-feeding incidence has taken place despite efforts by professional groups[4,5] and the Surgeon General of the United States[6] to encourage a greater incidence of breast-feeding. Better understanding of the factors that influence breast-feeding should serve to promote this important health behavior.

A number of demographic factors, such as education, income, age, parity, working status, and ethnicity,[1-3,7,8] have been bivariately associated with breast-feeding. Ethnicity has been consistently highly associated with breast-feeding.[3,7,9,10] For example, in 1985, 64% of white, 51% of Hispanic, and 29% of black mothers in the United States were breast-feeding their infants at discharge from the hospital.[3] These ethnic group differences were magnified within the southern and central regions of the United States.[3] Kurinij and colleagues,[11] however, reported that when using more sophisticated statistical techniques, ie, logistic regression, differences in education were more important than differences in ethnicity as a predictor of breast-feeding. Ethnic group differences suggest that cultural differences across the ethnic groups, eg, in expectancies[12,13] or social support,[14] affect the decision to breast-feed. The fact that education was an important predictor suggests that some aspect of social class characteristics affects the initiation of breast-feeding. As a result, whichever factor is more important will affect the kind of program designed to promote breast-feeding. Since little is known about demographic predictors of breast-feeding using multivariate data analysis techniques, the relative influence of ethnicity and education was reexamined in a large triethnic data set using log-linear and logistic regression techniques.

SUBJECTS AND METHODS

Demographic and initial infant-feeding characteristics of participants from two previous studies (August 1981, August 1983, and January 1984)[9,13] were combined to permit a sufficiently large sample to address the research questions. Both studies were reviewed and approved by the University of Texas Medical Branch (Galveston) Institutional Review Board. Data on maternal ethnicity, age, education, employment status, marital status, income, and gravidity were obtained from 881 completed questionnaires. These questions were worded using a standard format[15] adapted to local use. Breast-feeding initiation as a variable was defined to include breast-feeding in the hospital at the time of the survey. Breast-feeding status was both self-reported and verified with the nursery nurse. In all cases, there was perfect agreement between mother and nurse. Fifty subjects were deleted from the analysis, leaving 831 with complete information for the demographic variables of interest. Twenty-seven of the 50 deleted subjects were classified in another ethnicity group and 23 had at least one missing observation for the variables of interest.

Data analyses were conducted in two stages. First, a log-linear analysis[16] was conducted to determine the nature of potential relationships (ie, potential interactions) among the categorical demographic variables and breast-feeding initiation. The classic χ^2 analysis for a two-dimensional contingency table can be thought of as a test for a two-factor interaction between the rows and columns of the table. That is, a significant observed χ^2 value implies that the pattern of cell frequencies across columns (rows)

Accepted for publication May 13, 1990.

From the Department of Pediatrics, Georgia Prevention Institute, Medical College of Georgia, Augusta (Dr Baranowski); and the Division of Perinatal Pediatrics (Drs Rassin and Richardson) and the Office of Academic Computing and Biostatistics (Mr Mikrut and Dr Bee), The University of Texas Medical Branch, Galveston.

†Deceased.

Reprint requests to Medical College of Georgia, Georgia Prevention Institute, Augusta, GA 30912-3710 (Dr Baranowski).

Table 1.—Frequency Distributions by Demographic Characteristics of All Mothers and Mothers Breast-feeding*

Variables	No. (%) in Study Group	No. (%) Breast-feeding	χ^2 *(df), P*
Maternal ethnicity			
Anglo-American	402 (46.3)	178 (44.3)	
Black	266 (30.7)	36 (13.5)	73.5 (3), <.001
Mexican-American	173 (19.9)	46 (26.6)	
Other	27 (3.1)	11 (40.7)	
Age (y)			
Adolescent (13-17)	135 (15.6)	33 (24.4)	
Young (18-21)	293 (34.0)	87 (29.7)	8.7 (3), .033
Adult (22-25)	243 (28.2)	75 (30.9)	
Older (26-43)	192 (22.3)	75 (39.1)	
Marital status			
Married	558 (64.2)	215 (38.5)	
Single	222 (25.6)	38 (17.1)	39.5 (2), <.001
Other	89 (10.2)	18 (20.2)	
Employment status			
Unemployed	495 (56.9)	149 (30.1)	0.7 (1), .395
Employed	375 (43.1)	123 (32.8)	
Education			
Grade 8 or less	123 (14.2)	35 (28.5)	
Some high school	298 (34.3)	76 (25.5)	
Graduate of high school and/or technical school	281 (32.3)	80 (28.5)	29.2 (3), <.001
Some college	167 (19.2)	81 (48.5)	
Annual income, $†			
<5000	165 (36.3)	48 (29.1)	
5000 to 15 000	203 (44.6)	77 (37.9)	12.5 (2), .002
>15 000	87 (19.1)	45 (51.7)	
Gravidity			
First	291 (33.6)	101 (34.7)	
Second	245 (28.3)	74 (30.2)	2.5 (2), .293
Third or more	330 (38.1)	96 (39.1)	

*Statistical tests are for equality of breast-feeding proportions.
†Data were not reported for 426 mothers.

is not the same for all rows (columns). The log-linear analysis (while not using the χ^2 test for two categories) extends the notion of testing for interaction to tables of higher dimensions with potentially higher-order interactions. For example, a four-dimensional contingency table (subjects classified by four criteria) could exhibit a statistically significant four-factor interaction, as well as significant three- and two-factor interactions. Higher-order interactions can be difficult to interpret. Different combinations of possible effects are combined into models and tested for goodness of fit. The G^2 statistic provides the goodness of fit of a log-linear model. The G^2 statistic should be nonsignificant for the fit of a model to be considered good. The log-linear analysis permits the estimation of cell effects, which aids in the interpretation of significant higher-order interactions. Interactions are described by *u* terms, which reflect the relative strength of relationships among variables.

For this analysis, education level, defined by years of schooling completed, was dichotomized into low and high groups. Mothers in the high category had at least a high school diploma or equivalent. Age was partitioned into four categories, representing adolescent (13 to 17 years), postadolescent (18 to 21 years), young adult (22 to 25 years), and older (26 to 43 years) mothers. A base

Table 2.—Estimated Interaction *u* Terms Corresponding to Estimated Expected Values From Log-Linear Analysis of Breast-feeding, Ethnicity, and Education

		Breast-feeding	
Ethnicity	Education Level	No	Yes
Anglo-American	Low	0.162	−0.162
	High	−0.162	0.162
Black	Low	−0.084	0.084
	High	0.084	−0.084
Mexican-American	Low	0.078	−0.078
	High	−0.078	0.078

model strategy was employed using the CATMOD procedure of SAS[17] to obtain G^2 goodness-of-fit statistics and model parameter estimates. The G^2 statistic has an approximate χ^2 distribution and is equal to 0 if estimated cell frequencies are exactly equal to observed cell frequencies (a perfect fit of the model). The base model consisted of ethnicity, marital status, categorized age, categorized education, and all possible interactions among these four main effects.

The second stage used linear logistic regression to predict initiation of breast-feeding (no, yes). The logistic model included the main effects (specific demographic variables) and interactions suggested by the log-linear analysis. Age was considered at this second stage as a continuous variable, while education was coded as a four-category ordinal response, where 1 is grade 8 or less, 2 is some high school, 3 is graduate of high school and/or technical school, and 4 is at least some college. The base model strategy was also used in the logistic analysis.[18,19] For example, if an interaction term between two explanatory variables had a statistically significant coefficient ($P \leq .05$ as a stepwise entrance criterion), then both explanatory variables were included in the model regardless of their level of significance. Adjusted odds ratios and corresponding confidence limits are based on the estimated parameters of the linear logistic regression model.[18]

RESULTS

Pairwise Associations

Frequency distributions of demographic characteristics and their pairwise relationships with breast-feeding status are given in Table 1. Differences in sample size across characteristics are due to missing information. Statistical significance of the pairwise associations (as assessed by χ^2 analysis) indicates that the initiation of breast-feeding was not independent of maternal ethnicity, marital status, education, or income. The association between age and breast-feeding initiation ($P = .033$), however, is weak and would not be considered statistically significant if an experimentwise error rate of $\alpha = .05$ is to be achieved. That is, with seven tests, each individual inference should be made with an error rate set at $.05/7 = .0071$. The combined data set revealed the same pattern of breast-feeding responses as observed in the two previous studies.[9,13]

Relative to ethnicity, the highest proportion of women breast-feeding was observed for the Anglo-American group (44.3%) compared with a low of 13.5% for blacks. Older women (26 to 43 years) exhibited the highest incidence of breast-feeding (39.1%) among the four age categories, and married women and women with a higher education showed the highest proportion of breast-feeding in their respective categories (38.5% and 48.5%).

Log-Linear Analysis

The initial log-linear analysis revealed that categorized age in the presence of marital status, ethnicity, and education was not significantly related to breast-feeding initiation. Thus, age was dropped from the base model and

Table 3.—Adjusted Odds Ratios for Breast-feeding Initiation (n = 831)

Terms in Logistic Regression Model	Odds Ratio	95% Confidence Limits
Anglo-American vs black for		
Grade 8 or less	1.84	0.82, 4.11
Some high school	2.93	1.73, 4.98
Graduate of high school and/or technical school	4.68	3.05, 7.19
Some college	7.46	4.11, 13.57
Mexican-American vs black	1.94	1.10, 3.43
Marital status	1.94	1.34, 2.83

a new analysis was initiated. This search resulted in a model with excellent fit ($G^2 = 2.04$, $df = 5$, $P = .8430$) that contained a significantly nonzero three-factor interaction ($P = .0183$) for breast-feeding, ethnicity, and education. In keeping with the base model approach, each of the three variables and all two-factor interactions among these three variables were also included in the model. Of these, all were significantly nonzero ($P < .0001$), with the exceptions of education ($P = .8004$) and the interaction of breast-feeding and education ($P = .1106$). A two-factor interaction between breast-feeding and marital status was also significantly nonzero ($P = .0003$). The three-factor interaction component is displayed in Table 2. The magnitude and direction of the *u* terms revealed that Anglo-American women who had not graduated from high school were less likely to initiate breast-feeding than their more highly educated Anglo-American counterparts. Mexican-American women followed the same pattern as the Anglo-Americans, but the strength of the association was only about half as great. Black women, however, exhibited an opposite pattern, with higher-educated women less likely to initiate breast-feeding.

Linear Logistic Regression Analysis

Blacks were used as a reference category for coding purposes to estimate odds ratios for ethnicity. Anglo-Americans and Mexican-Americans, marital status, education (coded as a four-level ordinal variable), and two two-factor interactions identified by the log-linear analysis (ethnicity by education, ethnicity by marital status) were analyzed as potential explanatory variables for breast-feeding. Age, as a continuous variable, was incorporated in the logistic model as a main effect as well as in two-factor interaction terms with all other variables. This was done to verify that the categorization of age in the log-linear analysis had not disguised a potential age effect. As in the log-linear analysis, age in the presence of the other main effects showed no ability to predict breast-feeding initiation either as a main effect or in any two-factor interaction with other main effects. Thus, age was deleted from the base model. From a stepwise search procedure, the final model consisted of main effects (Anglo-American, Mexican-American, education, marital status) and one two-factor interaction (Anglo-American by education). The model χ^2 value was 117.7 ($df = 5$, $P < .0001$). Sensitivity and specificity of the model were 42.4% and 87.5%, respectively. The total correct classification rate for the complete original sample was 73.5%. The interaction in the model (Table 3) revealed that the odds ratio for Anglo-American women vs black women was an increasing function of the level of education, while the same was not true for Mexican-Americans. That is, as education increased, the disparity in breast-feeding proportions between Anglo-American and black mothers increased, but the odds of Mexican-American women vs black women initiating breast-feeding did not depend on education.

COMMENT

Rassin et al[9] reported that ethnicity was the variable most closely associated with breast-feeding initiation, with the implication that something about cultural practices or relationships was strongly affecting this important infant feeding practice. Kurinij et al[11] reported that education was more closely associated with breast-feeding initiation than was ethnicity, implying that social class was the primary determining factor. The current reanalysis of combined earlier data sets[9,12] using more sophisticated statistical procedures revealed an interaction between education and ethnicity: education is an important factor, but only among Anglo-American in comparison with black mothers. As education increased, Anglo-American mothers were more likely to breast-feed in comparison with black mothers. Education was independent of breast-feeding initiation for Mexican-American mothers, with Mexican-American mothers being 1.94 times as likely to initiate breast-feeding as black mothers, regardless of education level.

Several reasons could explain the differences between the results of Kurinij et al and the current findings, including regional differences, characteristics of the samples, and methods of analysis. Martinez and Krieger[3] reported regional differences in breast-feeding prevalence. Regional differences in associations among variables are equally comprehensible, if difficult to interpret. What it is about the regions that might induce different associations requires further thought and research.

Sociodemographic characteristics of the current sample indicate a young triethnic group with a low to moderate level of education and high unemployment. Of incomes reported (455 of 881 subjects), only 19.1% were above $15 000 per year. The educational attainment in the current black and Anglo-American samples was equivalent, in contrast to the lower educational attainment of the black population reported on by Kurinij et al.[11] The Mexican-American group generally had a lower education level than the other two groups. Breast-feeding rates, regardless of ethnicity, were lower in the current sample than those reported by Kurinij et al[11] or Martinez and Krieger.[3] Perhaps the predominantly lower social class composition of the present sample accounted for these differences.

Another important difference between the present study and that of Kurinij and coworkers was in the analysis procedure itself. Their technique for determining odds ratios did not include potential interaction terms among the demographic variables. If interactions involving specified risk factors are significant, the adjusted odds ratios must be modified accordingly.

The Anglo-American–by-education interaction revealed that as the education level of mothers increased, the proportion of Anglo-American mothers who breast-fed increased relative to the proportion of black mothers. Since education level is most clearly interpreted as a proxy variable for social class, it is apparent that the norm for breast-feeding significantly differs between the middle class of the two groups. Perhaps middle-class blacks have a greater pressure to return to work (which has been shown to affect breast-feeding patterns[8]), or perhaps the message about the extensive benefits of breast-feeding has not permeated the black middle class. Why Mexican-American mothers were more likely than black mothers to breast-feed is unclear but may be related to acculturation processes.[20] These issues require further, more intensive analysis in future studies.

Specificity for the predictive model was relatively strong (87.5%), while sensitivity was relatively weak (42.4%). Thus, the ability to predict mothers who did not initiate breast-feeding was reasonably good, but the ability to predict mothers who did breast-feed was poor. This indicates that demographic characteristics provide an important first approximation to understanding breast-feeding initiation, but these variables must be supplemented with other, more closely related variables. For example, Baranowski et al[13] have shown that attitudes toward infant-feeding vary by ethnicity, and Baranowski et al[14] have shown that sources of social support vary by ethnicity, both of which may account for some of these ethnic group differences.

A limitation of the current study is that it deals exclusively with the initiation of breast-feeding. Many mothers stop breast-feeding soon after they leave the hospital, which is not taken into account in these analyses. However, if mothers do not initiate breast-feeding, they cannot maintain it, and the factors maintaining breast-feeding may differ from those leading to its initiation.[21] Another limitation is that this study includes a sample of generally lower-income mothers from one Southwestern city. The results may not be generalizable to other samples. Finally, some statisticians prefer that a model developed on one sample be shown to have predictive value in a second independent sample before concluding that an interaction term is significant. Further research must be conducted to validate the current interaction terms.

All prospective mothers should receive messages encouraging breast-feeding to promote the health and well-being of their infants. If the findings of the current study are verified at other sites, a stronger message must be addressed to black mothers in general, and middle-class black mothers in particular. The content of this message, or other approaches to intervention, should emerge as further research delineates the roles of cultural factors in these ethnic groups.

References

1. Martinez GA, Nalezienski JP. 1980 update: the recent trend in breastfeeding. *Pediatrics.* 1981;67:260-263.

2. Martinez GA, Dodd DA, Samatgedes JA. Milk feeding patterns in the United States during the first 12 months of life. *Pediatrics.* 1981;68:863-868.

3. Martinez GA, Krieger FW. 1984 milk-feeding patterns in the United States. *Pediatrics.* 1985;76:1004-1008.

4. Nutrition Committee of the Canadian Pediatric Society and the Committee on Nutrition of the American Academy of Pediatrics. Breast-feeding: a commentary in celebration of the International Year of the Child, 1979. *Pediatrics.* 1978;62:591-601.

5. European Society for Pediatric Gastroenterology and Nutrition Committee on Nutrition. Guidelines on infant nutrition, I: recommendations for the composition of an adopted formula. *Acta Paediatr Scand Suppl.* 1977;262:3-20.

6. *Report of the Surgeon General's Workshop on Breastfeeding and Human Lactation.* Washington, DC: Public Health Service; 1984. US Dept of Health and Human Services.

7. Hendershot GE. Trends in breast-feeding. *Pediatrics.* 1984;74(suppl):591-602.

8. Simopoulos AP, Grave GD. Factors associated with the choice and duration of infant-feeding practice. *Pediatrics.* 1984;74(suppl):603-614.

9. Rassin DK, Richardson J, Baranowski T, et al. Incidence of breastfeeding in a low sociodemographic group of mothers in the United States: ethnic patterns. *Pediatrics.* 1984;73:132-137.

10. Farris RP, Frank GC, Webber LS, Srinivasan SR, Berenson GS. Influence of milk source on serum lipids and lipoproteins during the first year of life: Bogalusa heart study. *Am J Clin Nutr.* 1982;35:42-49.

11. Kurinij N, Shiono PH, Rhoads GC. Breastfeeding incidence and duration in black and white women. *Pediatrics.* 1988;81:365-371.

12. Baranowski T, Rassin DK, Richardson CJ, Brown JP, Bee DE. Attitudes toward breastfeeding. *J Dev Behav Pediatr.* 1986;7:367-372.

13. Baranowski T, Rassin DK, Bee DE, et al. Expectancies of infant-feeding methods among mothers in three ethnic groups. *Psychol Health.* 1990;5:59-75.

14. Baranowski T, Bee DE, Rassin DK, et al. Social support, social influence, ethnicity, and the breastfeeding decision. *Soc Sci Med.* 1983;17:1599-1611.

15. Sudman S, Bradburn NM. *Asking Questions, A Practical Guide to Questionnaire Design.* San Francisco, Calif: Jossey-Bass Inc Publishers; 1982.

16. Feinberg SE. *The Analysis of Cross-Classified Categorical Data.* Cambridge, Mass: MIT Press; 1977.

17. *SAS User's Guide: Statistics.* Version 5. Cary, NC: SAS Institute Inc; 1985:171-253.

18. Hosmer DW Jr, Lemeshaw S. *Applied Logistic Regression.* New York, NY: John Wiley & Sons Inc; 1989.

19. *SAS User's Group International (SUGI).* Version 5. Cary, NC: SAS Institute Inc; 1986:269-293.

20. Rassin DK, Markides K, Baranowski T, et al. Acculturation and breastfeeding on the United States–Mexico border. *Pediatr Res.* 1990;27:97A. Abstract.

21. Brodwick M, Baranowski T, Rassin D. Infant feeding patterns in three ethnic groups. *J Am Diet Assoc.* 1989;89:1129-1132.

Esophageal Motility in Children With Hirschsprung's Disease

Annamaria Staiano, MD; Enrico Corazziari, MD; Maria Rosaria Andreotti, MD; Ray E. Clouse, MD

• Esophageal motility was studied in 12 children with Hirschsprung's disease to see if extracolonic motor dysfunction was present in this disorder. Manometric tracings were compared with those from eight children with idiopathic megacolon and from 10 children without esophageal disease or constipation. Amplitude of esophageal contraction waves was significantly higher in children with Hirschsprung's disease than in the other two groups. Swallows that were followed by simultaneous contractions or double-peaked waves were also more common in the group with Hirschsprung's disease (subjects with Hirschsprung's disease, subjects with megacolon, and controls: 57%, 10%, and 8%, respectively). Lower esophageal sphincter characteristics did not differ among the three groups. The increase in simultaneous contractions and double-peaked waves persisted in those children who were reexamined following surgery for Hirschsprung's disease, whereas wave amplitudes fell to a level similar to that observed in the other groups. These data suggest that gastrointestinal motor dysfunction in persons with Hirschsprung's disease is not restricted to the colon, and that some of the observed abnormalities in esophageal motility do not reflect nonspecific responses to megacolon or colonic obstruction.

***(AJDC.* 1991;145:310-313)**

It is well recognized that Hirschsprung's disease may directly or indirectly affect neuromuscular function throughout the colon, but little attention has been given to gastrointestinal motility proximal to this organ.[1] Although any observed abnormalities in extracolonic motor dysfunction could be secondary to megacolon or colonic obstruction, it is clinically recognized that children with this disease often have more severe gastrointestinal distress (including anorexia and failure to thrive) than other children with megacolon and constipation.[1,2] The aim of our investigation was to study esophageal motility in children with Hirschsprung's disease in the preoperative and postoperative setting and compare the findings with those of studies from subject groups with idiopathic megacolon or with no esophageal or colonic complaints.

Accepted for publication August 13, 1990.

From the Department of Pediatrics, II School of Medicine, University of Naples (Italy) (Drs Staiano and Andreotti), the Division of Gastroenterology I, Second Medical Clinic, La Sapienza University, Rome, Italy (Dr Corazziari), and the Division of Gastroenterology, Washington University School of Medicine, St Louis, Mo (Dr Clouse).

Presented at the 21st Annual Meeting of the European Society for Paediatric Gastroenterology and Nutrition, Budapest, Hungary, June 1, 1989.

Reprint requests to Dipartimento di Pediatria, II Facolta' di Medicina e Chirurgia, Via S Pansini, 5, 800131 Naples, Italy (Dr Staiano).

SUBJECTS AND METHODS

The study population consisted of 12 children with Hirschsprung's disease (11 boys; mean±SEM age, 2.4±0.5 years [age range, 0.5 to 5 years]) and two control groups, ie, eight children with idiopathic megacolon (seven boys; mean±SEM age, 7.4±1.6 years [age range, 3 to 13 years]) and 10 children without esophageal or bowel complaints matched for age to the children with Hirschsprung's disease (six boys; mean±SEM age, 2.0±0.5 years [age range, 0.5 to 5 years]). All subjects were recruited from Naples, Italy. Further clinical characterization of the two subject groups with colonic disease is described in Table 1.

Hirschsprung's disease and idiopathic megacolon were diagnosed by findings from a barium enema, anorectal manometry, and suction biopsy (Noblett capsule), or deep rectal biopsy. In eight of 12 children with Hirschsprung's disease, a barium enema revealed a narrowed segment that was limited to the rectum and rectosigmoid. In one other subject, this segment extended to the transverse colon, and in the remaining three subjects, colonic dilatation extended to the anus without an apparent narrowed segment. In each subject with Hirschsprung's disease, the rectal inhibitory reflex was absent by anorectal manometry, and ganglion cells were not found on rectal biopsy specimens. All children with Hirschsprung's disease underwent surgery, and six were available for repeated manometric examination 3 months after the operation when symptoms had disappeared or had significantly improved.

Children with idiopathic megacolon had abnormal stool frequency (<4/wk) for more than 1 year in all cases. In three of eight children, the onset of constipation occurred in the first year of life; in the remaining five subjects, the onset of symptoms was between 2 and 4 years of age. Dilatation of the rectum and sigmoid was present on barium enema examination in all eight children. A normal rectoanal response (consisting of three successive pressure falls immediately following rectal distention and a transient pressure fall during prolonged rectal distention), as well as normal ganglion cells on superficial rectal biopsy specimens, were required for this diagnosis.

Ten additional control subjects were children who were being investigated for symptoms that originally suggested gastroesophageal reflux. None of these subjects were ultimately found to have any esophageal (including esophagitis) or colonic disorders. Final diagnoses in this group were as follows: overfeeding vomiting (two children), upper respiratory tract infection (four children), and urinary tract infection (four children).

Esophageal Manometry

Manometry was performed in fasting children without sedation according to a previously described method.[3] In brief, sub-

Table 1.—Clinical Features in Children With Hirschsprung's Disease and With Idiopathic Megacolon

	No. (%) of Children	
Sign or Symptom*	Hirschsprung's Disease (n=12)	Idiopathic Megacolon (n=8)
Constipation	12 (100)	8 (100)
Delayed passage of meconium	3 (25)	0 (0)
Recurrent fecal impaction	12 (100)	3 (38)
Vomiting	6 (50)	1 (12)
Failure to thrive	5 (42)	1 (12)
Abdominal distention	12 (100)	4 (50)
Palpable stool in rectal ampulla	3 (25)	8 (100)

*As defined according to Tunnessen.[19]

Table 2.—Manometric Features of the LES in the Three Subject Groups*

	Mean±SEM	
Subject Group	Basal LES Pressure, mm Hg	LES Relaxation, % of Basal LES Pressure
Hirschsprung's disease (unoperated)	24.1±1.5	99±1
Idiopathic megacolon	23.2±1.9	98±1
Control children	24.4±2.1	99±1

*LES indicates lower esophageal sphincter.

jects in a supine position were studied with the use of a triple-lumen polyvinyl catheter (outside diameter, 2.4 mm) with radially oriented side openings that were spaced at 2.5 cm. The lumina were perfused with a low-compliance pneumohydraulic system at a rate of 0.5 mL/min. The recording probe was initially placed so that all side openings were in the stomach, and then, it was withdrawn at 0.5-cm intervals through the esophagus. Lower esophageal sphincter (LES) pressure was measured as the maximal midrespiratory pressure by using mean intragastric pressure as the zero reference (slow pull-through technique). The mean of the three luminal determinations was reported. Manometry of the esophageal body was performed with the distal side hole placed immediately above the LES. To assess peristaltic activity, only waves that were induced by wet swallows (1 to 2 mL of 5% dextrose), preceded by 30 seconds or more of absent motor activity, were used. Contraction wave parameters (amplitude and duration) were only measured from the distal esophagus. All constipated children underwent esophageal manometry during continuous treatment with daily enemas to avoid fecal impaction. Medications were withheld for at least 24 hours before manometry in all subjects.

Tracings were coded and analyzed in our conventional way[3] by one of the authors (M.R.A.) who was unaware of the clinical status of the child. The following esophageal motility parameters were recorded: basal LES pressure, LES relaxation with swallowing (as a percentage), distal contraction wave amplitude, distal contraction wave duration, and number of abnormal motor responses (as a percentage of assessable swallows). Abnormal motor responses consisted of simultaneous contraction sequences (velocity, >6.25 cm/s) and double-peaked waves.[4] Manometric measurements were taken from 10 wet swallows in each subject. In all cases, informed written consent for participation in this study was obtained from the parents, and this investigation was approved by the Ethical Board of the University of Naples (Italy).

Statistical Methods

Data are reported as mean±SEM throughout. Mean values across patient groups were compared by using a one-way analysis of variance. If the one-way analysis of variance revealed significant differences, an unpaired, two-tailed Student's *t* test was applied for individual comparisons. In all cases, a *P* value of less than .05 was required for statistical significance. A paired *t* test was used for presurgery and postsurgery data comparisons.

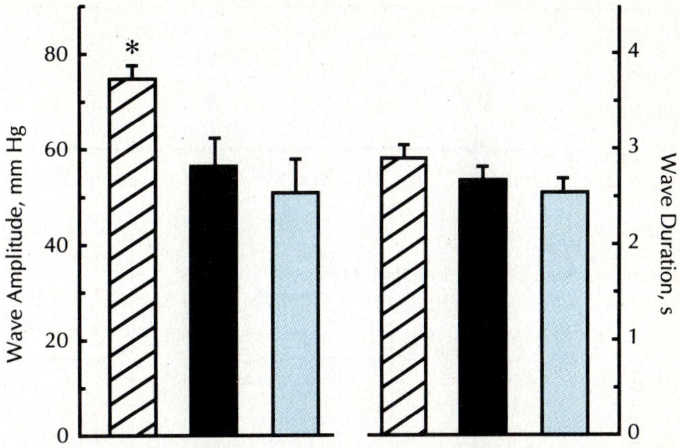

Fig 1.—*Contraction wave amplitudes and durations in the three subject groups. A significant elevation in wave amplitude was noted for children with Hirschsprung's disease prior to operation (hatched bars) when compared with the other two subject groups. (One-way analysis of variance for all groups: wave amplitude, P<.01; wave duration, P=.03.) Asterisk indicates P<.05 compared with each of the other two groups; solid bars, subjects with idiopathic megacolon; and open bars, control children.*

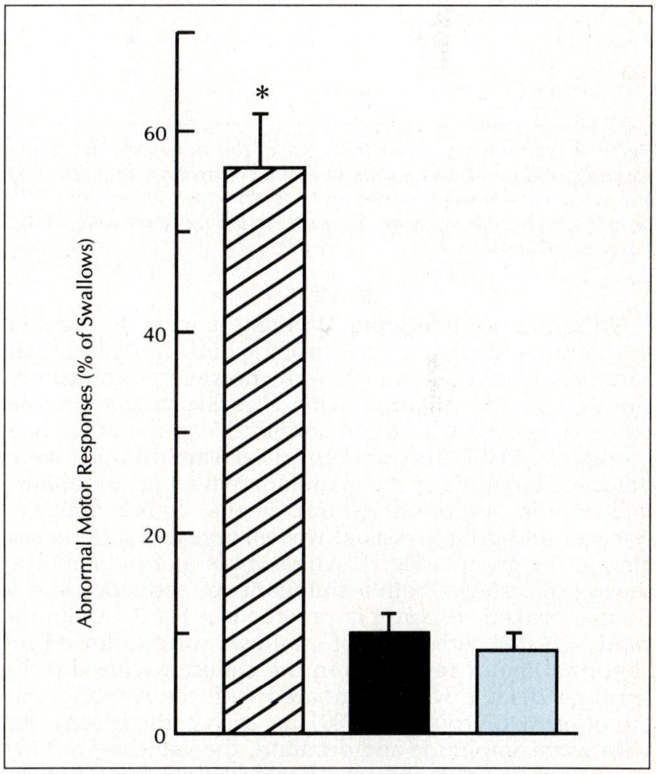

Fig 2.—*Frequency of abnormal motor responses (simultaneous sequences and double-peaked contraction waves) following swallows for each subject group. Abnormal motor responses were more commonly seen in children with Hirschsprung's disease prior to operation (hatched bar) than in each of the other two subject groups. (One-way analysis of variance for all groups P<.001.) Asterisk indicates P<.001 when compared with each of the other two groups; solid bar, subjects with idiopathic megacolon; and open bar, control children.*

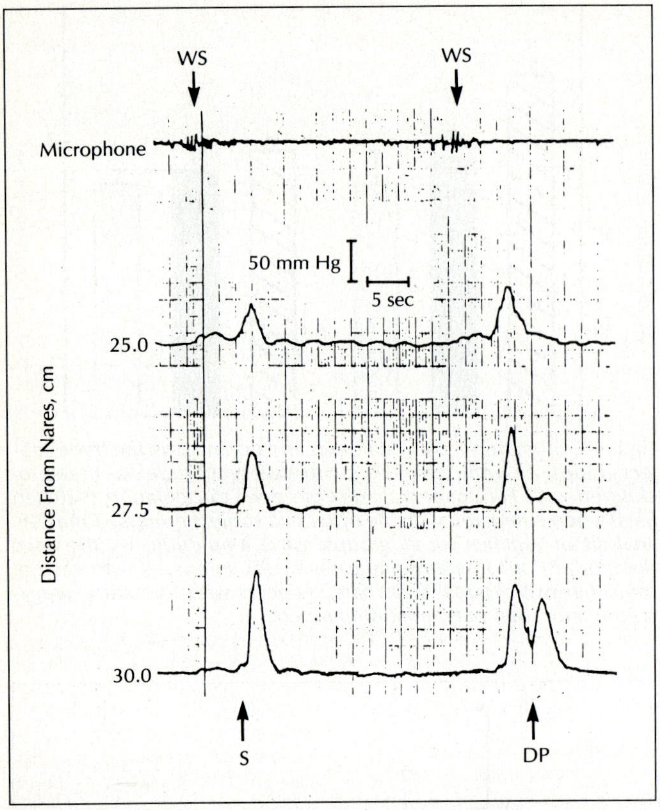

Fig 3.—*A manometric tracing from one of the subjects with Hirschsprung's disease shows a simultaneous contraction sequence (S) following one wet swallow (WS) and a double-peaked response (DP) on the subsequent swallow. All three recording ports were in the distal esophagus.*

RESULTS

No significant intergroup differences were detected in the manometric characteristics of the LES (Table 2). Distal contraction wave amplitudes were, however, significantly elevated in the children with Hirschsprung's disease when compared with those amplitudes in the other two groups (Fig 1). No differences in distal wave duration were detected. Analysis of the manometric tracings for abnormal motor responses (simultaneous contraction sequences and double-peaked waves) revealed differences among the groups (Fig 2). An example of a manometric tracing that shows both a simultaneous sequence and a double-peaked response is provided in Fig 3. A significantly greater percentage of swallows were followed by abnormal motor responses in the children with Hirschsprung's disease when compared with the responses in the other two groups ($P<.001$ for each comparison). As with wave amplitude and duration, the subjects with idiopathic megacolon did not differ from the control group.

Manometric results before and after operative treatment of Hirschsprung's disease are shown for six subjects in Fig 4. The Soave procedure was performed in three children, the Duhamel procedure was performed in two, and anorectal myectomy was performed in one. Findings in the control children are included in Fig 4 for comparison. Contraction wave amplitude significantly decreased in the postoperative period ($P<.05$), such that differences between subjects with Hirschsprung's disease and the control children were no longer evident (Fig 4). However, the increased frequency of abnormal motor responses was not influenced by operative correction of Hirschsprung's disease (Fig 4, bottom).

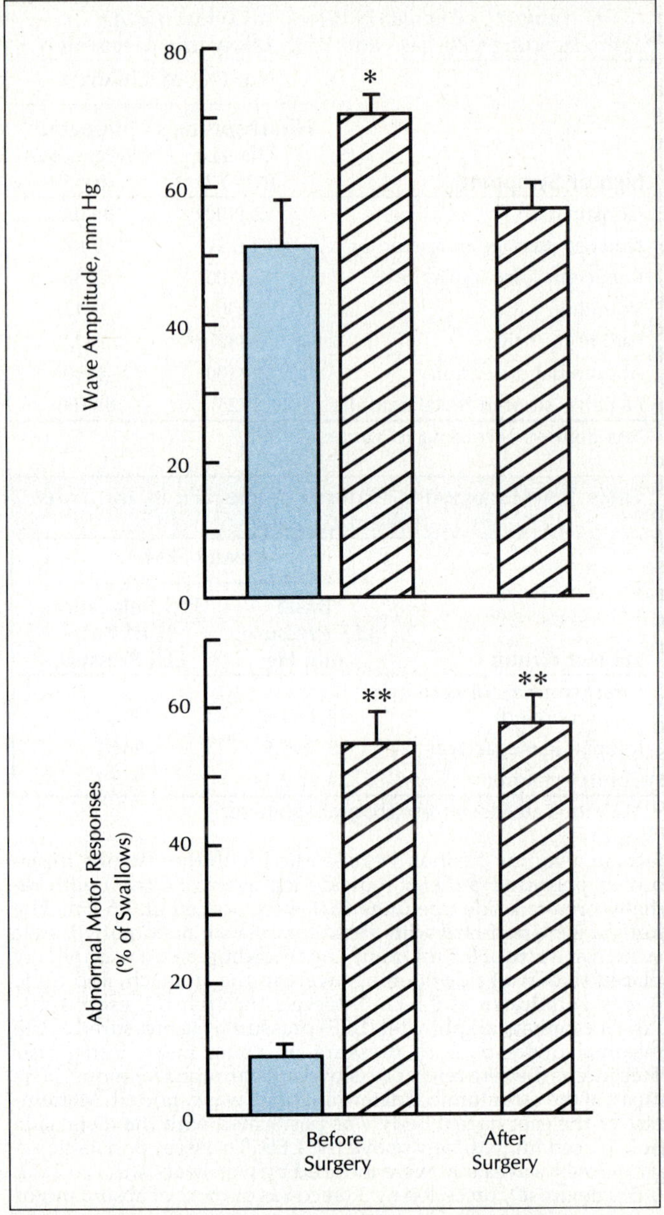

Fig 4.—*Manometric findings in six children before and 3 months after operative treatment of Hirschsprung's disease (hatched bars). Findings in the control children (open bars) are included on the figure for comparison. One asterisk indicates* $P<.05$*; double asterisks,* $P<.001$ *when compared with control children.*

COMMENT

These data demonstrate that motor abnormalities are detected in the esophagi of children with Hirschsprung's disease who have not yet undergone operations; some of these abnormalities do not resolve with surgical treatment of the colonic disorder. Previous reports of this disease have focused only on neuromuscular dysfunction of the colon. However, it would appear that more diffuse gastrointestinal motor dysfunction may be subclinically present. Esophageal motor abnormalities were not related to the extent of colonic aganglionosis in our subjects, and previous studies have suggested an inconsistent correlation between the degree of colonic involvement and the clinical course.[5,6]

The high prevalence of abnormal motor responses to swallows, findings that may relate to esophageal neural dysfunction,[7] were not nonspecific findings related to colonic disease or to an obstructed state. These abnormalities were not found in the children with idiopathic megacolon and persisted following surgical correction of Hirschsprung's disease. In contrast, the wave amplitudes normalized following surgical correction, making the finding of elevated amplitudes in untreated children of lesser significance. A neuropathologic explanation for these findings is not apparent. To our knowledge, esophageal neural abnormalities have not been described in subjects with Hirschsprung's disease, and results of detailed microscopic examination of the esophagus have not been included in reports of this disease. Contiguous involvement to the stomach has been found in a case of total intestinal aganglionosis,[8] but extreme cases of aganglionosis differ from cases of typical Hirschsprung's disease. At present, Hirschsprung's disease is considered a neurogenic developmental disorder with a heterogeneous origin and some heterogeneity in neuropathologic characteristics.[9,10] Chromosomal and genic defects (as well as other undefined factors) are invoked in producing aganglionosis and subsequent functional errors in excitatory and inhibitory neural transmission.[9,11] Whether these basic defects also produce less severe abnormalities in extracolonic myenteric nervous function remains unknown.

We could not show that esophageal motility in children with idiopathic megacolon differed from findings in children without esophageal or colonic disease. Previous studies in some adult subjects with severe idiopathic constipation with and without megacolon have demonstrated diffuse gastrointestinal motor dysfunction with esophageal involvement in many cases.[12-14] An identifiable pathologic condition in extracolonic bowel segments has been found in the neuromuscular apparatus of some of these adult subjects.[14] Although motor dysfunction has been well demonstrated in the distal colon of some children with idiopathic forms of constipation,[15,16] extracolonic motor abnormalities have not been reported and were not found in the present study. The adult and childhood varieties of severe idiopathic constipation differ also in other regards: in the former, symptom onset is rarely in the first decade of life, females predominate, and the conditions of many adults improve only after colectomy.[13] In the latter, onset is in early childhood, males predominate, and surgery is rarely needed.[17]

Distinct esophageal complaints are not recognized as a component of Hirschsprung's disease.[18] However, it is clinically acknowledged that children with this disorder frequently have more gastrointestinal complaints (including anorexia and failure to thrive) than other subjects with megacolon.[1,2] The present data suggest that neuromuscular dysfunction in this disease may be more diffuse within the gastrointestinal tract than previously had been appreciated, and further systematic studies of extracolonic motility appear to be merited. Besides potential clinical importance, this concept is relevant when considering the pathogenesis of Hirschsprung's disease.

Preliminary data from this work were published in abstract form in *Pediatric Research* (1989;26:269).

References

1. Perman JA. The gastrointestinal tract: clinical presentation. In: Rudolph AM, ed. *Pediatrics*. East Norwalk, Conn: Appleton & Lange; 1987:900-901.
2. Behrman RE, Vanghan VC. *Nelson Textbook of Pediatrics*. Philadelphia, Pa: WB Saunders Co; 1987:783-785.
3. Cucchiara S, Staiano A, Di Lorenzo C, et al. Esophageal motor abnormalities in children with gastroesophageal reflux and peptic esophagitis. *J Pediatr*. 1986;108:907-910.
4. Clouse RE, Staiano A. Contraction abnormalities of the esophageal body in patients referred for manometry: a new approach to manometric classification. *Dig Dis Sci*. 1983;28:784-791.
5. Arhan P, Devroede G, Davis K, et al. Viscoelastic properties of the rectal wall in Hirschsprung's disease. *J Clin Invest*. 1978;62:82-86.
6. Stone WD, Hendrix TR, Schuster MM. Aganglionosis of the entire colon in an adolescent. *Gastroenterology*. 1965;48:636-641.
7. Diamant NE. Physiology of the esophagus. In: Sleisenger MH, Fordtran JS, eds. *Gastrointestinal Disease: Pathophysiology, Diagnosis, and Management*. 4th ed. Philadelphia, Pa: WB Saunders Co; 1989:548-557.
8. Senyuz OF, Danismend N, Erdogan E, Ozbay G, Buyukunal C. Total intestinal aganglionosis with involvement of the stomach. *Pediatr Surg Int*. 1988;3:74-75.
9. Passarge E. The genetics of Hirschsprung's disease: evidence for heterogeneous etiology and a study of sixty-three families. *N Engl J Med*. 1967;276:138-143.
10. Christensen J. Motility of the colon. In: Johnson LR, Christensen J, eds. *Physiology of the Gastrointestinal Tract*. New York, NY: Raven Press; 1987:685-686.
11. Kubota M, Ito Y, Ikeda K. Membrane properties and innervation of smooth muscle cells in Hirschsprung's disease. *Am J Physiol*. 1983;244:G406-G415.
12. Reynolds JC, Ouyang A, Lee CA, Baker L, Sunshine AG, Cohen S. Chronic severe constipation: prospective motility studies in 25 consecutive patients. *Gastroenterology*. 1987;92:414-420.
13. Leon SH, Krishnamurthy S, Schuffler MD. Subtotal colectomy for severe idiopathic constipation: a follow-up study of 13 patients. *Dig Dis Sci*. 1987;32:1249-1254.
14. Krishnamurthy S, Schuffler MD, Rohmann CA, Pope CE. Severe idiopathic constipation is associated with a distinctive abnormality of the colonic myenteric plexus. *Gastroenterology*. 1985;8:26-34.
15. Meunier P, Louis D, DeBeaujeu MJ. Physiologic investigation of primary chronic constipation in children: comparision with the barium enema study. *Gastroenterology*. 1984;87:1351-1357.
16. Loening-Beucke V. Abnormal rectoanal function in children recovered from chronic constipation and encopresis. *Gastroenterology*. 1986;87:1233-1241.
17. Abrahamian PP, Lloyd Still JD. Chronic constipation in childhood: a longitudinal study of 186 patients. *J Pediatr Gastroenterol Nutr*. 1984;3:460-467.
18. Swenson O. Sherman JO, Fisher JH. Diagnosis of congenital megacolon: an analysis of 501 patients. *J Pediatr Surg*. 1973;8:587-591.
19. Tunnessen WW. *Signs and Symptoms in Pediatrics*. 2nd ed. Philadelphia, Pa: JB Lippincott; 1988.

Cortical Resection for Children With Epilepsy

Perspectives in Pediatrics

Elaine Wyllie, MD

The potential of cortical resection for epilepsy was first demonstrated by Penfield and Jasper[1] at the Montreal Neurologic Institute (Montreal, Quebec) in the 1940s and 1950s. The application of this technique in children was emphasized in the 1960s and 1970s[2-8]; since then, it has become apparent that early surgery in selected cases may enable children to become seizure free for a normal transition into adulthood. This may prevent some of the difficult psychosocial problems that occur in adults with long-standing epilepsy, including dependency, poor self-esteem, and long-term vocational disability.[9] In addition, if epilepsy surgery enables a child to discontinue antiepileptic medication, years of exposure to these drugs can

For editorial comment see p 256.

be avoided. As pediatricians become better acquainted with surgical options, patients are benefiting from earlier referral for surgery. The purpose of this review is to inform children's physicians about the indications for referral and new approaches to surgical management of pediatric epilepsy.

TEMPORAL LOBECTOMY

Selection of Candidates

Clinical Features.—Temporal lobectomy can successfully control seizures in children and adults with temporal lobe epilepsy. Patients typically have complex partial seizures,[10] with or without secondarily generalized tonoclonic convulsions, and the electroencephalogram (EEG) shows focal epileptiform discharges from the temporal lobe (Fig 1).

The seizures of temporal lobe epilepsy typically begin in middle childhood or adolescence but may occur earlier. Epilepsy surgery series note onset of seizures in children as young as 2 or 3 years old; in one study of pediatric patients with temporal lobe epilepsy, 16% had onset of seizures before age 2 years.[11] However, the duration from onset of seizures until epilepsy surgery is often many years. In one series, the average delay until operation was 13.6 years from onset of seizures and 11.3 years from onset of medical intractability.[12] This delay is often due to delayed referral to special centers.

Complex partial seizures in children older than 6 or 7 years often involve clinical features similar to those seen in adulthood. They may begin with an unusual sensation (aura) preceding loss of consciousness or may proceed directly to alteration of awareness, unresponsiveness, and repetitive semipurposeful automatic movements.[13-16] The automatisms may be oral, gestural, or ambulatory and are often stereotyped for individual patients from one seizure to another. Seizures may also involve emotional expressions, such as anger, laughing, or fear; afterward, the child may seem agitated and upset due to postictal confusion. Patients have at least partial amnesia for ictal events. Some have secondarily generalized tonic-clonic convulsions, but others with temporal lobe epilepsy have only complex partial seizures for many years.

In infants and young children, the clinical manifestations of complex partial seizures may be subtle, making the diagnosis more difficult.[11,13,14] If an aura occurs, it may not be appreciable in the nonverbal child unless he or she is able to run to the parents for help at the onset of an attack. Staring, altered awareness, and oral automatisms may be difficult to distinguish from background behavior, especially in infants; the more complex gestural and ambulatory automatisms that are prominent in adulthood are typically absent in younger patients.[17,18] Few studies have addressed the clinical symptoms of complex partial seizures in infants based on video-EEG recording,[17,18] and further research in this area will be important.

Noninvasive EEG Findings.—The EEG hallmark of temporal lobe epilepsy is epileptiform discharges from the temporal lobe (Figs 1 and 2). However, this finding may be less common in young children than in adults, and routine EEGs may be normal.[15,18,19] Definitive diagnosis may require intensive video-EEG monitoring during an attack. An EEG seizure pattern arising from the temporal lobe during a complex partial seizure can confirm the diagnosis (Fig 3).

Origin.—Temporal lobe epilepsy may be due to a slow-growing neoplasm, vascular malformation,trauma, infarction, or previous infection. The epilepsy may also be caused by developmental disturbances, such as cortical dysplasia, with abnormal migration and maturation of neurons during early brain development or by mesial-temporal sclerosis with damage to hippocampal neurons, sometimes secondary to an early hypoxic or ischemic insult. Because of the high incidence of structural lesions, especially in children,[11,20] neuroimaging is important. Magnetic resonance imaging is the test of choice because

Accepted for publication August 8, 1990.

From the Pediatric Epilepsy Program, The Cleveland (Ohio) Clinic Foundation.

Reprint requests to the Pediatric Epilepsy Program, The Cleveland Clinic Foundation, One Clinic Center, 9500 Euclid Ave, Cleveland, OH 44195-5221 (Dr Wyllie).

Department Editor.—*Alan D. Bedrick, MD, Tucson, Ariz*

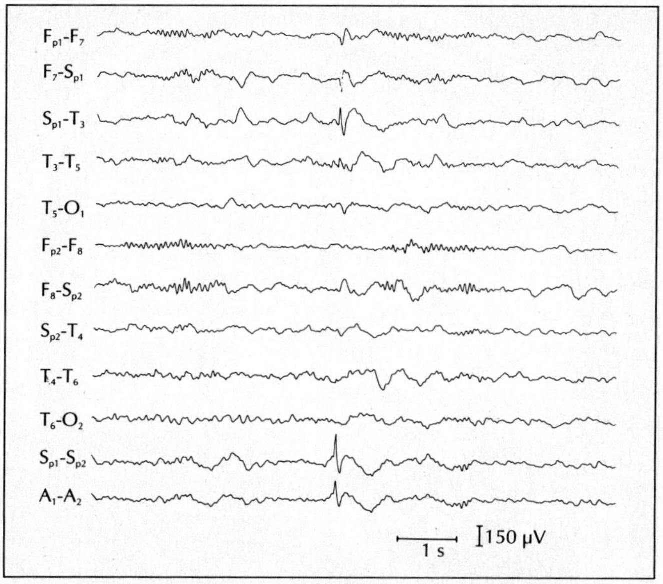

Fig 1.—*Electroencephalogram with an interictal sharp wave in the center of the tracing. The discharge was from the left anterior temporal region, maximal at the sphenoidal (S_{p1}) electrode. This 13-year-old boy had complex partial seizures arising from that area since the age of 7 years and a large low-grade astrocytoma in the same region.*

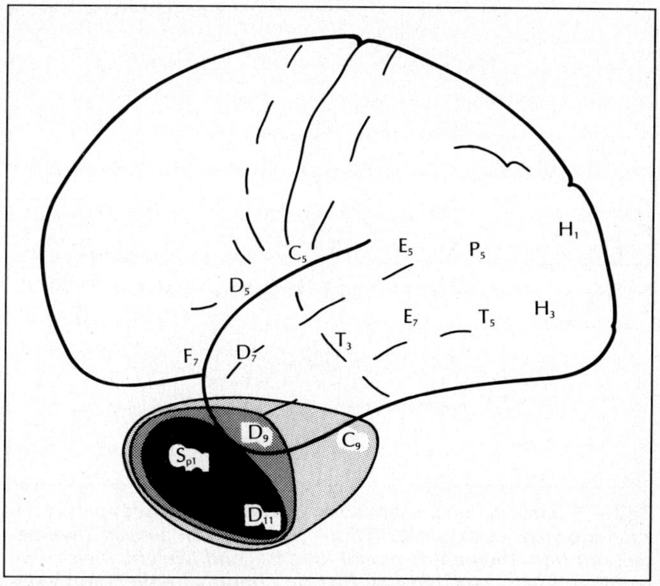

Fig 2.—*Distribution of the electrical field of the epileptiform discharges shown in Fig 1, mapped with the use of special closely spaced surface electrodes. The isoelectric lines indicate the relative voltage of the discharge at each of the electrodes. The amplitude was highest at S_{p1}, 80% as high at D_{11}, 70% as high at D_9, and 60% as high at C_9.*

of its increased sensitivity compared with computed tomography. The presence of a structural lesion on a preoperative magnetic resonance imaging scan may help to direct treatment plans for epilepsy surgery, if the location is concordant with findings seen on the EEG. Additional localizing information may sometimes be gained from positron emission tomography.[21] In cases in which neuroimaging findings are not concordant with EEG localization, the decision to operate is difficult and should be handled on a case-by-case basis.

Intractability, Disability, and Duration.—Issues in the selection of children for epilepsy surgery include medical intractability, degree of disability due to seizures, and lack of realistic hopes for spontaneous remission.

Confirmation of medical intractability requires thorough trials of all major antiepileptic medications, first singly and then in two-drug combinations, to the point of clinical toxicity. The medications most likely to be effective for complex partial seizures include carbamazepine, phenytoin sodium, primidone or phenobarbital, and valproic acid or diralproex sodium. Systematic exploration of these drug regimens is important to rule out the possibility that surgery may not be necessary. The observation time necessary to demonstrate intractability may vary among patients, depending on the baseline seizure frequency. However, most investigators believe that each drug should be used at maximum tolerated dosages for at least 1 month without success, preferably longer, before it is abandoned. Therefore, it usually takes several months to demonstrate medical intractability before epilepsy surgery.

If seizures persist despite maximum tolerated doses of the major medications, further consideration for epilepsy surgery should include careful assessment of the degree of disability caused by the seizures. This may not be solely dependent on absolute seizure frequency or on the presence or absence of secondarily generalized tonic-clonic convulsions. For example, a 6-year-old child with one complex partial seizure a month may be able to have a relatively normal life-style despite the attacks, but the same problem in an older child or adolescent may be severely disabling because of complications for peer relations, driving, dating, sports, employment, and college. On the other hand, one complex partial seizure per week might not add significantly to the disability of a mentally retarded adolescent if seizures do not interfere with lifestyle and employment in a sheltered setting, whereas the same patient's quality of life might be adversely affected by the same frequency of secondarily generalized tonic-clonic convulsions.

The decision whether to proceed to surgery, therefore, must be weighed in the context of the degree of disability due to seizures for each child. However, it should be recognized that for all children, recurrent, unpredictable attacks of altered consciousness may have damaging effects on self-esteem, confidence, and independence. Persistent psychosocial problems are not uncommon in children with uncontrolled complex partial seizures, complicated by parental overprotection and decreased expectations of teachers.[9] These problems may be alleviated by good seizure control after surgery.

Another serious consideration is the chance for spontaneous remission of seizures in children with temporal lobe epilepsy. Adults may present with an intractable seizure disorder that has not changed clinically in 10 or 15 years, and in this setting the likelihood of spontaneous remission is remote. With children, the period of observation is typically shorter, and population data about natural history are more sparse. Previous studies have suggested that childhood-onset epilepsy is more likely than adult-onset epilepsy to remit.[14,22-29] However, these series often did not rigorously exclude patients with benign partial epilepsy of childhood, generalized absence epilepsy, or psychogenic seizures. Only recently have data been collected specifically about children with EEG-documented temporal lobe epilepsy; in these series, the rate of spontaneous remission was low, in the range of 10% to 18%.[11,30]

For selected patients with temporal lobe epilepsy, surgery should be considered before late adolescence.[14,31] If

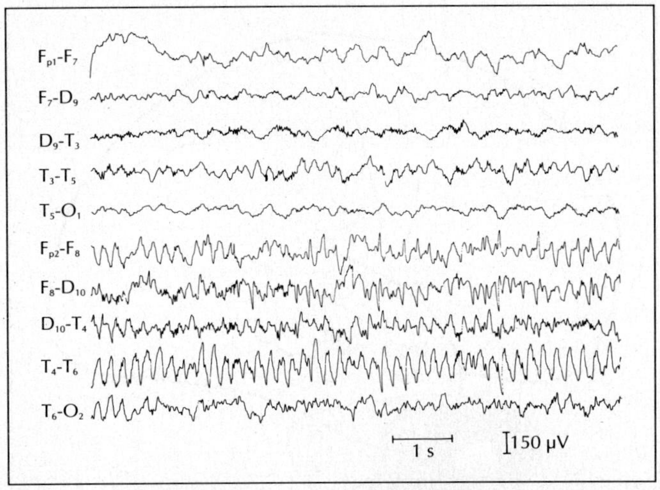

Fig 3.—*Electroencephalogram obtained during a complex partial seizure showing paroxysmal rhythmic epileptiform activity (five per second) from the right temporal lobe (second five channels of recording). This 2-year-old boy had no abnormal epileptiform discharges between seizures, so this recorded seizure pattern was the first electrographic evidence of his epilepsy.*

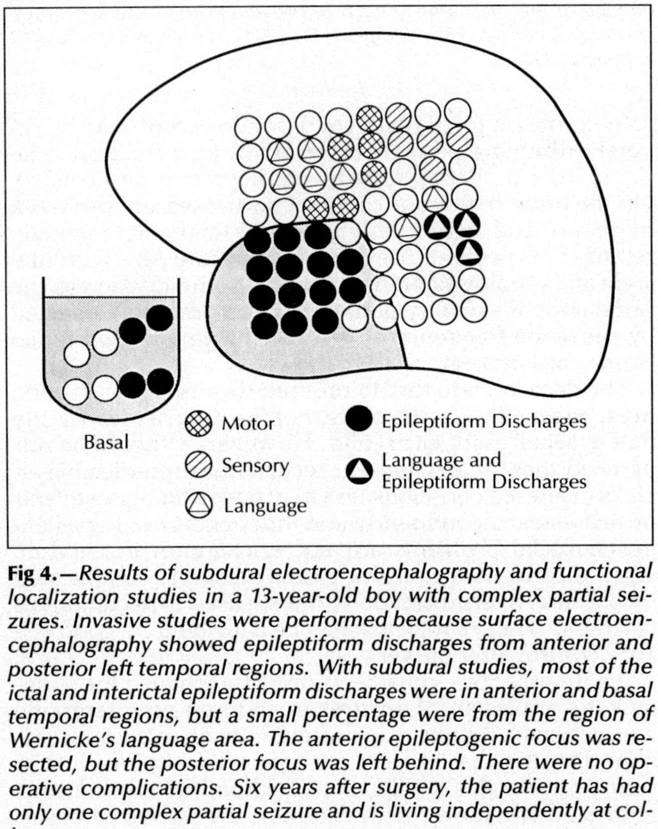

Fig 4.—*Results of subdural electroencephalography and functional localization studies in a 13-year-old boy with complex partial seizures. Invasive studies were performed because surface electroencephalography showed epileptiform discharges from anterior and posterior left temporal regions. With subdural studies, most of the ictal and interictal epileptiform discharges were in anterior and basal temporal regions, but a small percentage were from the region of Wernicke's language area. The anterior epileptogenic focus was resected, but the posterior focus was left behind. There were no operative complications. Six years after surgery, the patient has had only one complex partial seizure and is living independently at college.*

other selection criteria are satisfied, then earlier surgery may be appropriate. Because temporal lobe epilepsy tends not to manifest as an intractable, disabling problem until at least age 7 or 8 years, it is uncommon for children to present for consideration of epilepsy surgery before that age. This is in contrast to extratemporal epilepsy, which may present as a devastating problem as early as infancy because of many seizures every day.[32]

When referring a child for possible epilepsy surgery, it is important to select an institution with experience in this specialized field. Epilepsy surgery in children requires a team of pediatric neurologists, neuropsychologists, electroencephalographers, and neurosurgeons, as well as a large number of support and technical personnel. These resources are usually centralized at specialized medical centers.

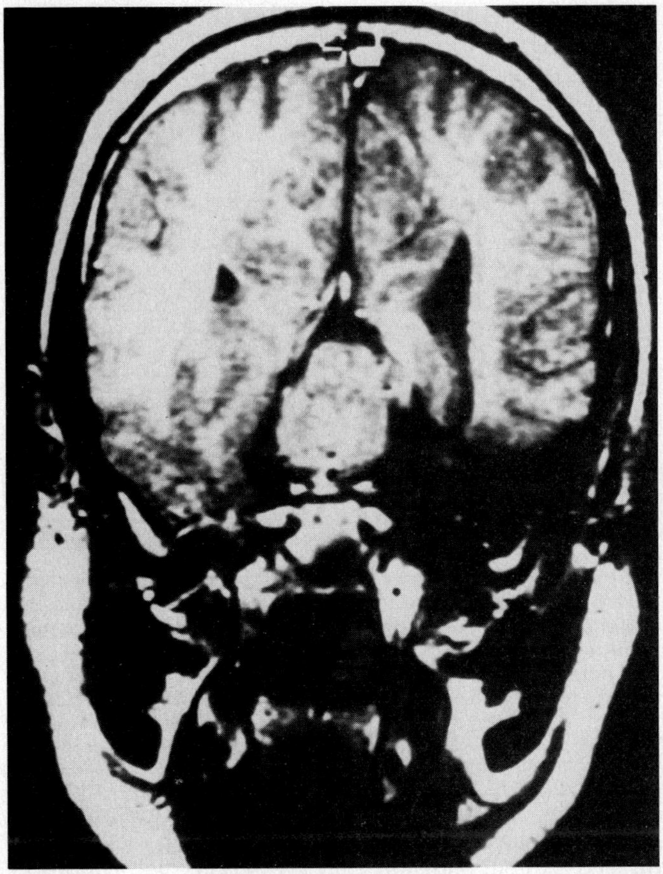

Fig 5.—*T_1-weighted magnetic resonance image after right temporal lobectomy, including resection of the amygdala and hippocampus. This 18-year-old male adolescent had intractable daily complex partial seizures starting in infancy. Since surgery, he has been seizure free for 2 years.*

Presurgical Neurophysiologic Evaluation

Careful video-EEG evaluation with scalp electrodes is the cornerstone of planning for epilepsy surgery; special additional scalp electrodes may be added over the area of interest. For patients with possible temporal lobe epilepsy, sphenoidal electrodes may also be helpful (Figs 1 and 2).[33] Sphenoidal electrodes are thin wires that are inserted inside a lumbar puncture needle into the muscles of the face, between the zygomatic process and the angle of the mandible. The lumbar puncture needle is withdrawn, and the electrode wires may remain in place near the region of the foramen ovale, recording epileptiform discharges from the basal temporal region. The sphenoidal electrodes may remain in place for several days or weeks, with minimal discomfort or risk. Placement of sphenoidal electrodes is painful, so sedation in children may be helpful during the procedure.[34]

Video EEG recording of clinical seizures is a critical part of the presurgical evaluation. One technique involves a split video screen displaying the real-time EEG along with the clinical seizure, and another technique involves display of a computer-generated time code on the video screen and the EEG paper printout. Both of these techniques permit precise correlation of ictal clinical and EEG events to enable better understanding of the location of seizure onset. Results are correlated with findings from neuropsychological testing, MRI, and PET to give a complete picture of the epileptogenic tone.

When surface and sphenoidal EEG clearly indicates onset of seizures from the anterior mesial or basal region of one temporal lobe, it may be appropriate to proceed to surgery without invasive study.[12,35] However, if findings are more complex, then further investigation may be necessary.

One such situation is the identification of the origin of seizure onset in the middle or posterior portion of the temporal lobe in the language-dominant hemisphere. The side that is dominant for language and memory function can be determined by the intracarotid amobarbital procedure, in which each cerebral hemisphere is separately anesthetized while the functioning hemisphere is tested for language and memory function. When seizures begin in the middle or posterior portion of the temporal lobe on the dominant side, invasive EEG and electrical stimulation studies may be helpful to map Wernicke's language area in relation to the epileptogenic zone, so that language function can be protected during resection (Fig 4). Cortical stimulation studies can be performed in the operating room after craniotomy with the patient under local anesthesia, but this may be arduous for younger patients.[36,37] Cortical EEG and functional localization studies can be performed outside the operating room, with implanted epidural[38] or subdural[20,39] electrodes. With this technique, arrays of electrodes embedded in sheets of Silastic are placed directly over the dura mater or surface of the brain. Language, motor, and sensory regions can be mapped by passing a small electric current into single subdural or epidural electrodes, with careful observation for signs and symptoms, such as transient interference with language function or tingling or involuntary movement of a part of the body.

Possible complications of subdural electrodes include wound infection or increased intracranial pressure. Wound infection is especially troublesome, with symptoms ranging from transient incision drainage to osteomyelitis. For this reason, subdural electrode grids are only used when detailed neurophysiologic information is necessary for a safe and effective resection. Smaller subdural electrode strips, inserted through burr holes, may have a lower incidence of infection than larger grids placed after craniotomy.

Cortical mapping techniques may be highly successful in older children, adolescents, and adults. However, these techniques may be difficult in young children with limited language abilities and attention span. Under age 5 or 6 years, it may be difficult to map language or sensory regions; rolandic motor regions can still be localized by cortical stimulation or evoked potential responses to median or posterior tibial nerve stimulation.[32] In addition, children under age 2 or 3 years may not show motor responses with the cortical stimulation techniques used in adults for reasons that are unclear.[32,38] Therefore, with current techniques, cortical localization findings in infants may be limited to results of evoked potential studies.[32] New stimulation techniques are needed to achieve better localization of functional areas in the youngest patients.

Other techniques available to selected epilepsy surgery candidates include flexible epidural peg electrodes,[40] foramen ovale electrodes,[41,42] and depth electrodes.[43-45] Each may be helpful in certain circumstances when the area for resection is unclear. Depth electrodes are the most commonly used of these invasive techniques.

Depth electrodes are especially useful when the question is which temporal lobe to resect or whether to resect the frontal or temporal lobe on one side, in the setting of epileptiform discharges from both areas. These needle electrodes are placed stereotactically, with the patient under general anesthesia, through small burr holes. The electrode contacts are implanted directly into the brain and may help to determine which area is generating the majority of seizures. Infrequent complications of depth electrodes include intracerebral hematoma or infection.

Operation

The plan for temporal lobectomy is determined individually for each patient based on EEG and neuroimaging results. When EEG suggests that seizures arise from the mesial-basal temporal lobe, this area is targeted for resection (Fig 5). This can be accomplished in several ways: (1) selective amygdalohippocampectomy with use of microsurgical techniques as developed by Wieser and Yasargil[46]; (2) a "keyhole" resection of the amygdala and hippocampus under direct vision after resection of the anterior temporal tip; or (3) a larger "standard" temporal resection of the amygdala and hippocampus plus several centimeters of lateral temporal cortex, more on the side that is nondominant for language. Controlled, prospective series are needed to evaluate the comparative efficacy and adverse effects of these three surgical approaches.

Complications

The most frequent complication of temporal lobectomy is homonymous superior quadrantanopia due to resection of visual fibers in Meyer's loop in the anterior temporal lobe. This complication most commonly occurs when the resection is extensive. In one series, it occurred in 60% of cases overall.[47] However, in the vast majority of cases, the visual field defect is asymptomatic and discovered only with perimetric testing.[47]

Mild dysphasia may occur after left-sided temporal lobectomy, even with resection only of anterior regions of the temporal lobe. In one adult series, mild dysphasia occurred in 17% of patients who underwent left temporal lobectomy.[47] Memory dysfunction may also occur, especially after left-sided temporal lobectomy in adults with high preoperative memory function.[48-50] The exact incidence of postoperative dysphasia and memory dysfunction in children is unknown, but it has been noted that children and adolescents who become seizure free after temporal lobectomy typically experience improved rather than decreased school performance due to dysphasia or memory dysfunction.

Other rare, persistent adverse effects of temporal lobectomy include hemiparesis or other focal neurologic deficits due to infection, infarction, or bleeding.

Outcome

The overall percentage of children and adolescents with excellent outcome after temporal lobectomy, with either no seizures, rare seizures, or auras only, has ranged from 57% to 100%.[6-8,20,36,38,51-54] Among the subgroup in which EEG and neuroimaging had been performed and in which clinical evidence of epileptogenicity was noted only in the anterior portion of one temporal lobe, the frequency of good outcome has reportedly been as high as 91%.[55] The results generally appear to be at least as good in children and adolescents as in adults.[20]

Many patients who undergo temporal lobectomy are eventually able to discontinue medications. It is possible for some patients to achieve a totally normal life-style after surgery. When this major change occurs early in life, before the development of chronic disability, the chances for normal psychosocial maturation are maximized. The ultimate definition of good outcome includes not only seizure control but also normal integration into the social and vocational fabric of society. It appears that for selected patients, the benefits of temporal lobectomy far outweigh the risks.

EXTRATEMPORAL RESECTION

Selection of Candidates

Temporal lobectomy is overall the most common epilepsy surgery procedure. However, among the small subgroup of infants and very young children who undergo epilepsy surgery, extratemporal resections are more common, especially frontal lobectomy.[32] Factors resulting in earlier surgery for infants and children with frontal, parietal, or occipital lobe epilepsy include earlier onset and a higher frequency of daily seizures.[32]

The seizures of extratemporal epilepsy are characterized by various signs and symptoms depending on which cortical regions are affected.[13] They may appear similar to the complex partial seizures of temporal lobe epilepsy or there may be additional signs or symptoms suggesting an extratemporal onset, such as a visual or somatosensory aura or early, prominent focal motor phenomena. Noninvasive EEG may show focal spikes or sharp waves from the affected area or the epileptogenic zone may be identified with MRI or PET. Causative findings may be similar to those in temporal lobe epilepsy. Cortical dysplasia is a common pathologic finding in pediatric patients.[32]

Presurgical Neurophysiologic Evaluation

The techniques of intensive noninvasive and invasive EEG evaluation are similar to those used in the evaluation of temporal lobe epilepsy. Functional localization studies may be important if epileptogenic regions are closely related to functional areas.

Operation

A variety of operations can be performed, including frontal or occipital lobectomy or parietal topectomy.[13] Complications may include focal neurologic deficit due to infection, infarction, bleeding, or resection of functional areas within the epileptogenic zone.

Outcome

Few series are available for analysis, but it appears that the likelihood of becoming totally seizure free after extratemporal resection is lower than that after temporal resection.[56,57] In one series of children and adults, only 17% were seizure free after extratemporal resection, while approximately 70% had a significant reduction in seizure frequency.[57] Therefore, extratemporal resection was more often "palliative" than "curative." However, in the setting of many seizures every day, chronic drug toxicity, and a resultant plateau in neurologic development, it may be appropriate to recommend extratemporal resection with the hope of a major reduction in seizure frequency. Occasional persistent seizures after surgery may not be considered a good outcome for patients with temporal lobe epilepsy and preoperative seizure frequencies of one or two per week, but it may be an extremely gratifying outcome for an infant with extratemporal epilepsy and many seizures every day.[32]

HEMISPHERECTOMY

Selection of Candidates

Since the 1950s, hemispherectomy has been performed for patients with infantile hemiplegia and frequent, debilitating, intractable focal-onset seizures arising from multiple areas within one hemisphere.[58-64] These patients have epileptogenic areas that are too many and too extensive for focal excision of a single lobe. In patients with seizures arising from a severely damaged or malformed hemisphere, hemispherectomy may yield complete seizure control with no new neurologic deficits in addition to preexisting hemiplegia, homonymous hemianopia, and mental retardation. More recently, hemispherectomy has also been successfully performed in children with Rasmussen's focal chronic encephalitis who have progressive hemiparesis, hemispheric atrophy, and focal-onset seizures[65] and in small numbers of infants with infantile spasms and focal abnormalities seen on positron emission tomographic scans.[66]

Presurgical EEG Evaluation

Once it is clear that seizures arise from within the damaged hemisphere and that the epileptogenic zone is too extensive for a more limited cortical resection, further intensive neurophysiologic studies may not be necessary. Most patients proceed to surgery based primarily on results of scalp EEG, neuroimaging, and clinical assessment.

Operation

Early operations included en bloc removal of the entire hemisphere down to the basal ganglia.[59,61] However, in the 1970s it became clear that some patients had serious late-onset complications after hemispherectomy, with progressive neurologic deterioration and often death.[58,64] The incidence of these late complications 1 to 20 years after operation ranged from 17% to 35%, with 44% mortality.[58] The mechanism for these late complications is unclear but may be related to alteration of cerebrospinal fluid dynamics between the ventricular system and the large subdural cavity. These problems led to the development of new operative approaches,[59] including the following: (1) complete hemispherectomy with suturing of the dura mater to reduce the size of the subdural cavity[63]; (2) subtotal hemispherectomy with one or more transected cortical areas left in place as a mechanical buffer[58]; (3) hemicorticectomy, with sparing of white matter around the ventricles; and (4) complete hemispherectomy with placement of shunt tubing from the subdural cavity into the intraperitoneal space. Long-term follow-up data are so far limited to the subtotal hemispherectomies reported by Rasmussen,[58] but at least with this modification it appears that late complications are decreased with no loss of efficacy.

Outcome

Complete or near-complete seizure control after hemispherectomy is in the range of 85%.[58] This operation is therefore one of the most effective, albeit radical, forms of epilepsy surgery with regard to seizure control.

FUTURE DIRECTIONS

With the growing experience with epilepsy surgery in children, it appears that patients should be referred for consideration for possible cortical resection at specialized centers when there are intractable, disabling partial or secondary generalized seizures and focal spikes or sharp waves on EEG, with or without focal abnormalities on neuroimaging studies or neurologic examination. For selected children, a greatly improved life-style with a low risk for serious adverse effects is possible.

Many questions remain. Areas for continued research include the following: (1) better definition of the natural history of focal-onset epilepsy in infants and young children, with more longitudinal prospective follow-up studies of well-documented cases into adolescence and adulthood; (2) better understanding of the clinical and EEG findings in infants with focal-onset seizures, based on results of careful video-EEG evaluation and positron emission tomography; (3) new neuropsychologic testing methods for infants and young children to better quantify the psychosocial impact of epilepsy and epilepsy surgery; and (4) basic science investigations into the pathophysiologic mechanisms of epilepsy beginning early in life. Continued exploration in these areas will expand our understanding of optimal selection criteria and timing for epilepsy surgery in children. I thank my colleagues in the Section of Epilepsy and Clinical Neurophysiology, the Section of Pediatric Neurology, and the Department of Neurosurgery at The Cleveland (Ohio) Clinic Foundation, who have collaborated extensively in the development of the concepts behind our pediatric epilepsy surgery program.

References

1. Penfield W, Jasper H. Surgical therapy. In: *Epilepsy and the Functional Anatomy of the Human Brain.* Boston, Mass: Little Brown & Co Inc; 1954:739-817.
2. Falconer MA, Hill D, Meyer A, Mitchell W. Treatment of temporal-lobe epilepsy by temporal lobectomy: a survey of findings and results. *Lancet.* 1955;2:827-835.
3. Falconer MA, Serafetinides EA. A follow-up study of surgery in temporal lobe epilepsy. *J Neurol Neurosurg Psychiatry.* 1963;26:154-165.
4. Falconer M. Significance of surgery for temporal lobe epilepsy in childhood and adolescence. *J Neurosurg.* 1970;33:233-252.
5. Falconer M. Temporal lobe epilepsy in children and its surgical treatment. *Med J Aust.* 1972;1:1117-1121.
6. Davidson S, Falconer M. Outcome of surgery in 40 children with temporal-lobe epilepsy. *Lancet.* 1975;2:1260-1263.
7. Polkey CE. Selection of patients with intractable epilepsy for resective surgery. *Arch Dis Child.* 1980;55:841-844.
8. Lindsay J, Ounsted C, Richards P. Long-term outcome in children with temporal lobe seizures, V: indications and contraindications for neurosurgery. *Dev Med Child Neurol.* 1984;26:25-32.
9. Holmes GL. Psychosocial factors in childhood epilepsy. In: *Diagnosis and Management of Seizures in Children: Major Problems in Clinical Pediatrics.* Philadelphia, Pa: WB Saunders Co; 1987:30, 112-124.
10. Commission on Classification and Terminology of the International League Against Epilepsy. Proposal for revised clinical and electroencephalographic classification of epileptic seizures. *Epilepsia.* 1981;22:489-501.
11. Harbord MG, Manson JI. Temporal lobe epilepsy in childhood: reappraisal of etiology and outcome. *Pediatr Neurol.* 1987;3:263-268.
12. Lüders H, Dinner DS, Morris HH, Wyllie E, Godoy J. EEG evaluation for epilepsy surgery in children. *Cleve Clin J Med.* 1989;56(suppl):S53-S61.
13. Wyllie E, Lüders H, Rothner D. Partial seizures in children: clinical features, medical treatment, and surgical considerations. *Pediatr Clin North Am.* 1989;36:343-364.
14. Wyllie E, Lüders H. Complex partial seizures in children: clinical manifestations, and identification of surgical candidates. *Cleve Clin J Med.* 1989;56(suppl):S43-S52.
15. Holmes GL. Partial complex seizures in children: an analysis of 69 seizures in 24 patients using EEG FM radiotelemetry and videotape recording. *Electroencephalogr Clin Neurophysiol.* 1984;57:13-20.
16. Holmes GL. Partial seizures in children. *Pediatrics.* 1986;77:725-731.
17. Duchowny MS. Complex partial seizures of infancy. *Arch Neurol.* 1987;44:911-914.
18. Yamamoto N, Watanabe K, Negoro T, et al. Complex partial seizures in children: ictal manifestations and their relation to clinical course. *Neurology.* 1987;37:1979-1982.
19. Dinner DS, Lüders H, Rothner AD, Erenberg G. Complex partial seizures of childhood onset: a clinical and encephalographic study. *Cleve Clin Q.* 1984;51:287-291.
20. Wyllie E, Lüders H, Morris HH, et al. Subdural electrodes in the evaluation for epilepsy surgery in children and adults. *Neuropediatrics.* 1988;19:80-86.
21. Engel J, Kuhl DE, Phelps ME, Crandall PH. Comparative localization of epileptic foci in partial epilepsy by PCT and EEG. *Ann Neurol.* 1982;12:529-537.
22. Glaser GH. Limbic epilepsy in childhood. *J Nerv Ment Dis.* 1967;114:391-397.
23. Currie S, Heathfield KWG, Henson RA, et al. Clinical course and prognosis of temporal lobe epilepsy: a survey of 666 patients. *Brain.* 1971;94:173-190.
24. Lindsay J, Ounsted C, Richards P. Longterm outcome in children with temporal lobe seizures, I: social outcome and childhood factors. *Dev Med Child Neurol.* 1979;21:285-298.
25. Sofijanov NG. Clinical evolution and prognosis of childhood epilepsies. *Epilepsia.* 1982;23:61-69.
26. Loiseau P, Dartigues JF, Pestre M. Prognosis of partial epileptic seizures in the adolescent. *Epilepsia.* 1983;24:472-481.
27. Sillanpää M. Social functioning and seizure status of young adults with onset of epilepsy in childhood: an epidemiological 10-year follow-up study. *Acta Neurol Scand.* 1983;68:8-77.
28. Schmidt D, Tsai JJ, Janz D. Generalized tonic-clonic seizures in patients with complex partial seizures: natural history and prognostic relevance. *Epilepsia.* 1983;24:43-48.
29. Deonna T, Ziegler AL, Despland PA, et al. Partial epilepsy in neurologically normal children: clinical syndromes and prognosis. *Epilepsia.* 1986;27:241-247.
30. Kotagal P, Rothner AD, Erenberg G, Cruse R, Wyllie E. Complex partial seizures of childhood onset: a five-year follow-up study. *Arch Neurol.* 1987;44:1177-1180.
31. Rasmussen T. Cortical resection in children with focal epilepsy. In: Parsonage M, et al, eds. *Advances in Epileptology: XIVth Epilepsy International Symposium.* New York, NY: Raven Press; 1983:249-254.
32. Nespeca M, Wyllie E, Lüders H, et al. Subdural electrodes in infants and young children. *J Epilepsy.* In press.
33. Lesser RP, Dinner DS, Lüders H, Morris HH. Differential diagnosis and treatment of intractable seizures. *Cleve Clin Q.* 1984;51:227-240.
34. Wyllie E, Wyllie R, Kotagal P, Lüders H, Kanner A. Sphenoidal electrodes in children and adolescents. *Epilepsia.* 1990;31:521-523.
35. Morris HH, Kanner A, Lüders H, et al. Can sharp waves localized at the sphenoidal electrode accurately identify a mesial temporal epileptogenic focus? *Epilepsia.* 1989;30:532-539.
36. Rasmussen TB. Surgical aspects. In: Wise G, ed. *Topics in Child Neurology.* Englewood Cliffs, NJ: Spectrum Publishers; 1977:143-153.
37. Rapport RL, Ojemann GA, Wyler AR, Ward AA. Surgical management of epilepsy. *West J Med.* 1977;127:185-189.
38. Goldring S, Gregorie EM. Surgical management using epidural recordings to localize the seizure focus: review of 100 cases. *J Neurosurg.* 1984;60:457-466.
39. Lüders H, Lesser RP, Dinner DS, et al. Chronic intracranial recording and stimulation with subdural electrodes. In: Engel J Jr, ed. *Surgical Treatment of the Epilepsies.* New York, NY: Raven Press; 1987:297-321.
40. Wyllie E, Burgess R, Awad I, Barnett G, Lüders H. Flexible epidural peg electrodes for chronic EEG recording. *Ann Neurol.* 1989;26:424.
41. Wieser HG, Elger CE, Stodieck SRG. The 'foramen ovale electrode': a new recording method of the preoperative evaluation of patients suffering from mesio-basal temporal lobe epilepsy. *Electroencephalogr Clin Neurophysiol.* 1985;61:314-322.

42. Meglio M, Cioni B, Cruccu G, Inghilleri M. The 'foramen ovale electrode': a safe tool to study temporal lobe epilepsy. *Electroencephalogr Clin Neurophysiol.* 1987;66:327-330.
43. Bancaud J. Surgery of epilepsy based on stereotactic investigations: the plan of SEEG investigations. *Acta Neurochir (Wien).* 1980;30(suppl):25-34.
44. Lieb JP, Engel J, Gevins A, Crandall P. Surface and deep EEG correlates of surgical outcome in temporal lobe epilepsy. *Epilepsia.* 1981;22:515-538.
45. Spencer SS. Depth electroencephalography in selection of refractory epilepsy for surgery. *Ann Neurol.* 1981;9:207-214.
46. Wieser HG, Yasargil MG. Selective amygdalohippocampectomy as a surgical treatment of mesiobasal limbic epilepsy. *Surg Neurol.* 1981;17:445-457.
47. Katz A, Awad IA, Kong AK, et al. Extent of resection in temporal lobectomy for epilepsy, II: memory changes and neurologic complications. *Epilepsia.* 1989;30:763-771.
48. Wyllie E, Naugle R, Awad I, et al. The intracarotid amobarbital procedure (Wada test), I: prediction of modality-specific memory decline after temporal lobectomy. *Epilepsia.* In press.
49. Milner B. Disorders of learning and memory after temporal lobe lesions in man. *Clin Neurosurg.* 1972;19:421-446.
50. Rausch R, Babb T, Brown JW. A case of amnesic syndrome following selective amygdalohippocampectomy. *J Clin Exp Neuropsychol.* 1985;7:643.
51. Jensen I, Vaernet K. Temporal lobe epilepsy: follow-up investigation of 74 temporal lobe resected patients. *Acta Neurochir (Wien).* 1977;37:173-200.
52. Green JR. Surgical treatment of epilepsy during childhood and adolescence. *Surg Neurol.* 1977;8:71-80.
53. Whittle IR, Ellis HJ, Simpson DA. The surgical treatment of intractable childhood and adolescent epilepsy. *Aust N Z J Surg.* 1981;51:190-196.
54. Meyer FB, Marsh WR, Laws ER, Sharbrough FW. Temporal lobectomy in children with epilepsy. *J Neurosurg.* 1986;64:371-376.
55. Wyllie E, Lüders H, Morris HH, et al. Clinical outcome after complete or partial cortical resection for intractable epilepsy. *Neurology.* 1987;37:1634-1641.
56. Ludwig BI, Ajmone Marsan C, Van Buren J. Depth and direct cortical recording in seizure disorders of extratemporal origin. *Neurology.* 1976;26:1085-1099.
57. Van Ness PC, Estes ML, Salanova V, Morris HH, Lüders HO. Seizure reduction and pathologic findings in 37 operated patients with suspected neocortical epilepsy. *Epilepsia.* 1989;30:728.
58. Rasmussen T. Hemispherectomy for seizures revisited. *Can J Neurol Sci.* 1983;10:71-78.
59. Goodman R. Hemispherectomy and its alternatives in the treatment of intractable epilepsy in patients with infantile hemiplegia. *Dev Med Child Neurol.* 1986;28:251-258.
60. Rasmussen T, Villemure JG. Cerebral hemispherectomy for seizures with hemiplegia. *Cleve Clin J Med.* 1989;56 (suppl): S62-S68.
61. Krynauw R. Infantile hemiplegia treated by removing one cerebral hemisphere. *J Neurol Neurosurg Psychiatry.* 1950;13:243-267.
62. Wilson PJE. Cerebral hemispherectomy for infantile hemiplegia. *Brain.* 1970;93:147-180.
63. Adams CBT. Hemispherectomy: a modification. *J Neurol Neurosurg Psychiatry.* 1983;46:617-619.
64. Oppenheimer DR, Griffith HB. Persistent intracranial bleeding as a complication of hemispherectomy. *J Neurol Neurosurg Psychiatry.* 1966;29:229-240.
65. Dalos N, Vining EPG, Carson B, Freeman JM. Rasmussen's encephalitis: clinical recognition and surgical management. *Ann Neurol.* 1986;20:434.
66. Chugani HT, Shields WD, Shewmon DA, Olson DM, Phelps ME, Peacock WJ. Infantile spasms, I: PET identifies focal cortical dysplasia in cryptogenic cases for surgical treatment. *Ann Neurol.* 1990;27:406-413.

In Other AMA Journals

ARCHIVES OF DERMATOLOGY

Intercellular IgA Dermatosis of Childhood: Selective Deposition of Monomer IgA1 in the Intercellular Space of the Epidermis

Yuichi Teraki, MD; Naoko Amagai, MD; Takashi Hashimoto, MD; Toshio Kusunoki, MD; Takeji Nishikawa, MD (*Arch Dermatol.* 1991;127:221-224)

The Challenge of Limiting the Spread of Human Immunodeficiency Virus by Controlling Other Sexually Transmitted Diseases

Philip K. Kirby, MD; Titus Munyao, MD, ChB; Joan Kreiss, MD, MSPH; King K. Holmes, MD, PhD (*Arch Dermatol.* 1991;127:237-242)

Adipsic Hypernatremia in Two Sisters

Giorgio Radetti, MD; Francesco Rizza, MD; Giuseppe Mengarda, MD; Klaus Pittschieler, MD

• We describe two sisters with chronic hypernatremia, lack of thirst, and inappropriate osmoregulated vasopressin secretion. Only one sister, who presented with microcephaly and developmental delay, showed signs of dysplasia of the midline structures (ie, septum pellucidum and corpus callosum) and a large intracranial cyst. Neither sister showed any signs of thirst, even when osmolality exceeded 337 mmol/kg. In both patients, the vasopressin secretion did not respond to either osmotic or nonosmotic stimuli or was suppressed by a water load. Plasma osmolality values returned to normal after treatment with forced hydration and a vasopressin analogue, desamino-D-arginine vasopressin. These findings indicate a severe defect in the hypothalamic osmoreceptors that control thirst and vasopressin secretion. To our knowledge, this is the first report of such a disorder in two sisters.

(*AJDC.* 1991;145:321-325)

Adipsic hypernatremia is an uncommon disorder caused by a defect in the osmoregulation of thirst, leading to chronic hyperosmolality of body fluids.[1] In affected patients, adipsia is often associated with an abnormality in osmoregulated vasopressin secretion.[2] Different types of intracranial lesions are usually present and are thought to have damaged the hypothalamic osmoreceptors for thirst and vasopressin secretion. We describe two sisters with inappropriate lack of thirst and vasopressin secretion in the presence of chronic plasma hyperosmolality. Only one sister had a well-defined pathologic hypothalamic lesion.

PATIENT REPORTS

Patient 1.—Patient 1 was born after a 36-week uncomplicated pregnancy and normal delivery. Birth weight was 2.530 kg (50th percentile), length was 47 cm (50th percentile), and head circumference was 31 cm (50th percentile). The parents were nonconsanguineous. A maternal aunt had died at the age of 3 months of an undiagnosed illness; she was microcephalic and had a cleft lip and palate. The patient was first admitted to our hospital at the age of 3 months with meningococcal meningitis. She responded well to antibiotic therapy and was discharged after 15 days. On admission, laboratory values were as follows: plasma sodium, 144 mmol/L; potassium, 4.7 mmol/L; urea nitrogen, 4.8 mmol/L; creatinine, 70 μmol/L; glucose, 4.7 mmol/L; and plasma osmolality, 277 mmol/kg. During hospitalization, electrolyte levels were always within the normal range. The patient was then readmitted at the age of 10 months because of failure to thrive. On admission, the mother indicated that since the age of 5 months her daughter had been drinking very little. Laboratory values were as follows: plasma sodium, 173 mmol/L; potassium, 5.4 mmol/L; chloride, 125 mmol/L; calcium, 2.45 mmol/L; urea nitrogen, 9.6 mmol/L; creatinine, 79 μmol/L; glucose, 4.7 mmol/L; and plasma osmolality, 334 mmol/kg (normal range, 280 to 295 mmol/kg). Urinalysis showed an osmolality of 290 mmol/kg, a specific gravity of 1008, and a pH of 5. Neither proteinuria nor glycosuria was noted. Intravenous fluid therapy for 36 hours resulted in a gradual decrease in the serum concentration of sodium (to 143 mmol/L) and plasma osmolality (to 292 mmol/kg), with no convulsions and optimal weight gain. Two days after the intravenous fluid administration was stopped, the plasma sodium and osmolality values increased to 169 mmol/L and 322 mmol/kg, respectively. Plasma renin activity was 52.65 $ng \cdot L^{-1} \cdot s^{-1}$ (normal range, 0.27 to 1.08 $ng \cdot L^{-1} \cdot s^{-1}$ μg/L per hour) and the plasma aldosterone concentration was 1900 pmol/L (normal range, 20 to 440 pmol/L). The patient never showed any sign of thirst, even when the plasma osmolality was 334 mmol/kg.

Adipsic hypernatremia was suspected, and the patient underwent an extensive evaluation of the anterior and posterior portions of the hypophysis, with special interest in vasopressin secretion.

Apart from vasopressin investigation, all endocrinologic investigations were performed when the patient had good metabolic control (see "Materials and Methods" section).

Levels of serum prolactin and thyroid hormones and the thyrotropin response to thyrotropin releasing hormone were all within the normal range, as were growth hormone, cortisol, and corticotropin responses to insulin-induced hypoglycemia. Gonadotropin response to gonadotropin-releasing hormone was not tested because of the patient's young age.

Computed tomography of the skull and magnetic resonance imaging showed no parenchymal abnormalities. After water metabolism investigations were completed, the patient was discharged while receiving intranasal desamino-D-arginine vasopressin (DDAVP) (0.05 mL twice daily) and forced hydration. Although this allowed the child to grow and gain weight, every minor illness was accompanied by a recurrence of hypertonic dehydration and the need for hospitalization. The child is now 3 years old and is mentally normal.

Patient 2.—Patient 2, the sister of patient 1, was the product of an uncomplicated full-term pregnancy. Birth weight was 3.350 kg (50th percentile), length was 50 cm (50th percentile), and head circumference was 32 cm (10th percentile); in addition to microcephaly, a cleft lip and palate were evident.

The patient was admitted to our hospital at the age of 4 months because of seizures. Head circumference at that time was below the third percentile (37.5 cm), while the length and weight were still at the 50th percentile. The serum biochemical profile was as follows: sodium, 159 mmol/L; potassium, 4.9 mmol/L; chloride, 119 mmol/L; creatinine, 44 μmol/L; glucose, 4.7 mmol/L; calcium, 2.52 mmol/L; urea nitrogen, 8.9 mmol/L; bicarbonate, 17 mmol/L; and plasma osmolality, 309 mmol/kg. The urine specific gravity was 1005, osmolality was 120 mmol/kg, pH was 5, and no proteinuria or glycosuria was detected. Like her sister, she showed no sign of thirst.

Accepted for publication July 8, 1990.

From the Department of Pediatrics (Drs Radetti, Mengarda, and Pittschieler) and the Laboratory Unit (Dr Rizza), Regional Hospital of Bolzano (Italy).

Reprint requests to the Department of Pediatrics, Regional Hospital, via Lorenz Boehler 5, 39100 Bolzano, Italy (Dr Radetti).

Laboratorty Values at Varying States of Hydration*

State of Hydration	Plasma Sodium, mmol/L	Plasma Urea Nitrogen, mmol/L	Plasma Osmolality, mmol/kg	Urine Osmolality, mmol/kg	Plasma Vasopressin ng/L	PRA, $ng \cdot L^{-1} \cdot s^{-1}$	Aldosterone, pmol/L	Specific Gravity
Ad libitum A	155	5.7	298	110	3.5	8.1	600	1005
Water loading	149	7.1	299	123	2.50	8.37	800	1006
Ad libitum B	167	11	335	186	1.50	20.79	1200	1010
Normal Range	135-143	1.8-7.1	280-295	See text	See text	0.27-1.08	20-440	1002-1030

PRA indicates plasma renin activity; ad libitum A, ad libitum fluid intake on admission; and ad libitum B, fluid intake after a water load and discontinuation of hydration, when body weight decreased by more than 5%.

Antibodies against rubella, herpesvirus, *Toxoplasma*, *Treponema pallidum*, or cytomegalovirus were not detected. Karyotype was 46,XX. The electroencephalogram showed a hypsarrhythmic pattern. Computed tomography of the brain revealed dysplasia of the septum pellucidum and corpus callosum and a large cyst occupying the third and lateral ventricles. Magnetic resonance imaging confirmed these findings.

Adipsic hypernatremia was suspected, and a full endocrinologic evaluation of the anterior and posterior portions of the hypophysis was performed.

The total serum thyroxine concentration was 120 nmol/L (normal range, 56 to 154 nmol/L), free thyroxine concentration was 12 pmol/L (normal range, 9.2 to 28.3 pmol/L), triiodothyronine concentration was 1.7 nmol/L (normal range, 0.8 to 2.7 nmol/L), free triiodothyronine concentration was 4.5 pmol/L (normal range, 3.8 to 9.2 pmol/L), and reverse triiodothyronine concentration was 0.54 nmol/L (normal range, 0.14 to 0.54 nmol/L). The thyrotropin responses to an injection of 100 μg of thyrotropin releasing hormone were 1.6, 23.3, 24.7, and 25.8 mU/L at 0, 20, 40, and 60 minutes, respectively. The thyrotropin value did not return to baseline, which was interpreted as a sign of hypothalamic dysfunction. The serum prolactin level was normal, as were the responses of growth hormone, cortisol, and corticotropin to insulin-induced hypoglycemia. After water metabolism studies were completed, the patient was discharged while receiving intranasal DDAVP (0.05 mL twice daily) and forced hydration. With this regimen, satisfactory growth and weight gain were achieved, but every minor illness led to dehydration and the need for hospitalization.

At the age of 12 months, a diagnosis of West syndrome was made; at 2 years of age, the patient is severely mentally retarded.

MATERIALS AND METHODS

Informed parental consent was obtained for all the investigations performed. The patients were on an unrestricted diet and were taking no medications. For vasopressin determination, blood was collected from the antecubital vein into a chilled tube containing edetic acid, and 500 kallikrein inactivating units of aprotinin (Trasylol) was added per milliliter of blood; the blood was centrifuged at 4°C and stored at −20°C. The assay was performed within 2 months by radioimmunoassay with a commercial kit (Clonesystem, Euro Diagnostic, Apeldoorn, Holland). The assay is calibrated against the first World Health Organization Standard, 77/501: 410 IU/mg (1 ng of antidiuretic hormone per liter is equal to 0.41 μIU/mL). In a group of control patients, vasopressin values of up to 8 ng/L were found. The sensitivity of the assay is 0.8 ng/L. The plasma and urine osmolalities were calculated from the following formula: osmolality = 1.86 × (sodium + potassium) + (glucose/18) + (urea nitrogen/2.8). Blood samples for the determination of plasma renin activity and aldosterone concentration were added to edetic acid, placed on ice, centrifuged, and stored at −20°C until assay. The Diagnostic Products Corp (Los Angeles, Calif) and the SORIN (SORIN Biomedica, Saluggia, Italy) commercial kits were used for the determination of aldosterone values and renin activity, respectively. Growth hormone, cortisol, thyrotropin, prolactin, corticotropin, triiodothyronine, thyroxine, free triiodothyronine, free thyroxine, and reverse triiodothyronine levels were determined by standard radioimmunoassays.

Patient 1.—To test osmoreceptor function, during the first 2 hours, 20 mL/kg of a 5% dextrose solution was administered intravenously, followed by an additional 16 mL/kg in the third hour. During the test, 100 mL of water was administered orally to sustain diuresis. On a separate day, 0.85 mol/L of saline solution was infused at a rate of 0.05 mL/kg per minute for 3 hours.

During both tests, blood was taken from the opposite arm at 30-minute intervals for determination of plasma renin activity, plasma aldosterone concentration, vasopressin secretion, plasma osmolality, and sodium concentration. Urine specimens were also collected at the same time, via a catheter, for determination of osmolality, sodium level, and potassium level.

To test baroreceptor function, on a separate day, the effect of orthostasis on vasopressin secretion was studied while the patient was receiving 5% dextrose solution (150 mL/kg per day) intravenously for the previous 24 hours to achieve adequate hydration. At 9 AM, after basal samples of blood and urine were obtained while the patient was in the recumbent position, the patient was allowed to stand and walk, and samples of blood were taken hourly for determination of vasopressin secretion, plasma renin activity, plasma aldosterone level, sodium level, potassium level, and plasma osmolality. At the same time, urine specimens were collected for determination of osmolality and sodium and potassium concentrations. To maintain adequate diuresis, 20 mL/kg per hour of water was administered orally. Blood pressure was monitored at 30-minute intervals.

Other endocrine investigations were performed when the child was in a stable condition. We determined the response of vasopressin to other nonosmotic stimuli, such as insulin-induced hypoglycemia (during the insulin tolerance test) and emesis (15 mL of ipecac syrup given orally and blood samples taken every 10 minutes for 40 minutes).

Patient 2.—Due to the younger age of this patient, it was impossible to perform the same investigations as were performed in patient 1. Values of serum electrolytes, urea nitrogen, plasma and urine osmolality, plasma renin activity, plasma aldosterone, vasopressin, and urine specific gravity were measured during different states of hydration (Table): first on admission, when the patient was receiving fluids ad libitum, and then after a water load (intravenous infusion for 2 days with 100 mL/kg of 5% dextrose with 0.25% saline solution and forced oral hydration), and also after hydration was discontinued and body weight decreased by more than 5%.

RESULTS

Patient 1.—During the water load (Fig 1), plasma renin activity decreased from 58.32 to 27 $ng \cdot L^{-1} \cdot s^{-1}$, plasma aldosterone level decreased from 2000 to 500 pmol/L, sodium level decreased from 180 to 159 mmol/L, and osmolality decreased from 350 to 337 mmol/kg, while vasopressin secretion did not change (3.6 ng/L before water loading and 3 ng/L after water loading). Plasma vasopressin concentrations in relation to plasma osmolality were greatly reduced compared with normal values.[1] Urine osmolality at the beginning of the test was 387 mmol/kg, and specific gravity was 1017. Excretion of water load was delayed 180 minutes, at which time urine osmolality was 200 mmol/kg and specific gravity was 1009.

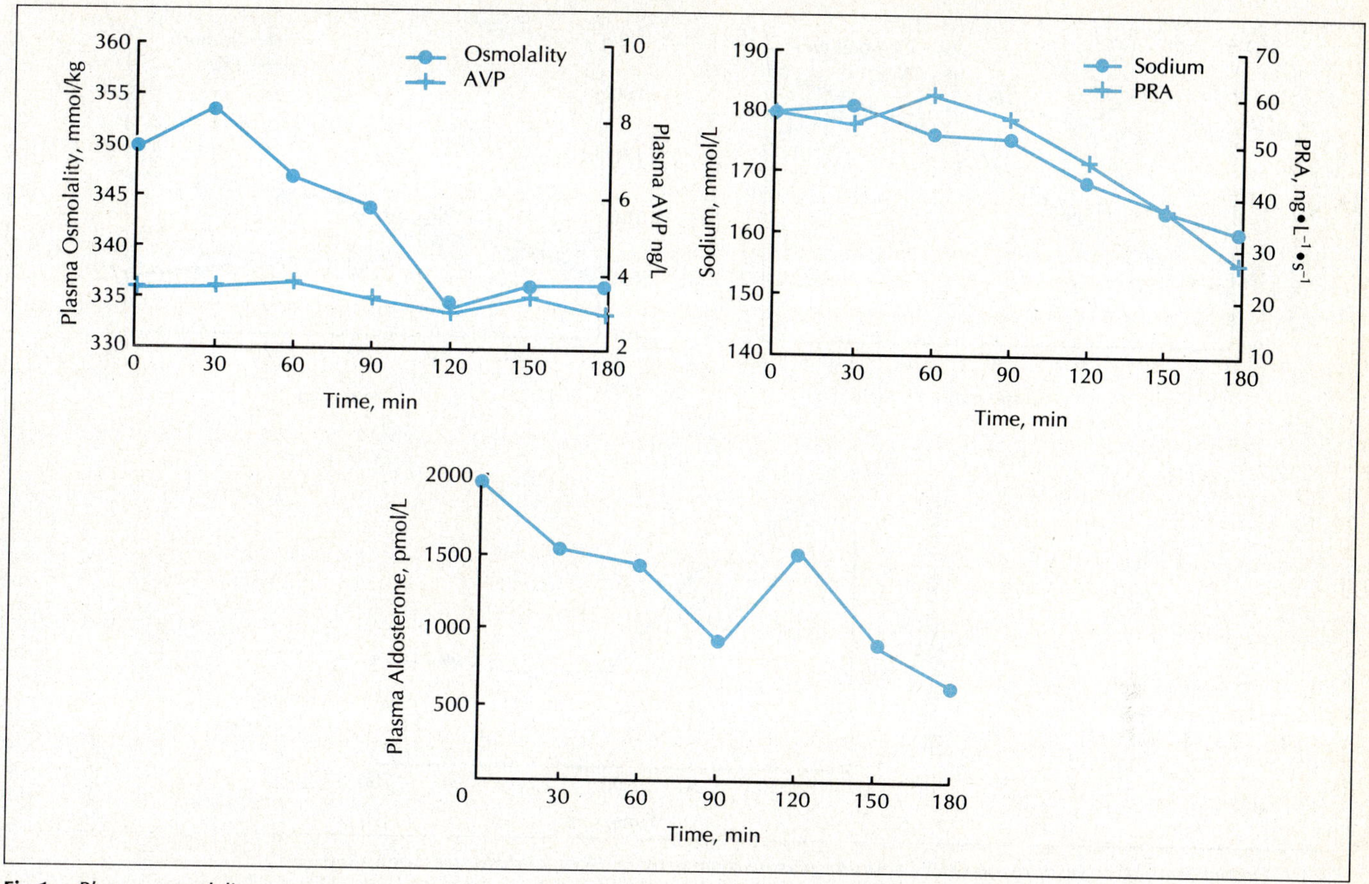

Fig 1.—*Plasma osmolality, vasopressin (AVP), sodium, plasma renin activity (PRA), and aldosterone values during water loading.*

During saline infusion (Fig 2), plasma renin activity and plasma aldosterone level decreased from 12.15 to 8.77 $ng \cdot L^{-1} \cdot s^{-1}$ and from 500 to 200 pmol/L, respectively, in response to volume expansion, while sodium level and plasma osmolality increased from 153 to 165 mmol/L and from 302 to 326 mmol/kg, respectively. Vasopressin excretion decreased from 5.2 to 3.9 ng/L. Urinary excretion of sodium began at 180 minutes. Urine specific gravity and osmolality were 1002 and 224 mmol/kg, respectively, at the beginning of the test and 1002 and 248 mmol/kg, respectively, at the end of the study.

During orthostasis (Fig 3), plasma renin activity and plasma aldosterone level increased from 15.66 to 22.95 $ng \cdot L^{-1} \cdot s^{-1}$ from 400 to 600 pmol/L, respectively; sodium level and plasma osmolality remained unchanged, as did vasopressin secretion, which was 5 ng/L at the beginning of the test and 4.2 ng/L at the end. Urinary osmolality ranged between 72 and 56 mmol/kg.

Other endocrine investigations were also performed. During the insulin-induced hypoglycemia, the vasopressin concentration increased from 3.9 to 5.2 ng/L, which is negligible after the administration of ipecac syrup, however, this value remained unchanged (from 2 to 2.8 ng/L).

Patient 2.—When patient 2 (Table) was receiving ad libitum fluid intake, the plasma sodium level ranged from 155 to 167 mmol/L; osmolality, from 298 to 335 mmol/kg; urea nitrogen level, from 5.7 to 11 mmol/L; plasma renin activity, from 8.1 to 20.79 $ng \cdot L^{-1} \cdot s^{-1}$; and plasma aldosterone, from 600 to 1200 pmol/L. Plasma vasopressin concentration was 3.5 and 1.5 ng/L, a very low value for the corresponding osmolality.[1] Concurrent urine specific gravity and osmolality were always very low compared with plasma osmolality, ranging from 1005 to 1010 and from 110 to 186 mmol/kg, respectively. The more normal biochemical measurements observed while the patient was receiving fluids ad libitum were obtained on the first day of admission, making it possible that the parents forced the child to drink at home due to fear of dehydration. We believe that the state during which fluid intake was ad libitum after a water load and discontinued hydration, as described above, reflects a more accurate basal state, as it occurred during hospitalization.

After a water load, the plasma sodium level was 149 mmol/L, osmolality was 229 mmol/kg, plasma renin activity was 8.37 $ng \cdot L^{-1} \cdot s^{-1}$, plasma aldosterone level was 800 pmol/L, urea nitrogen level was 7.1 mmol/L, and vasopressin concentration was 2.5 ng/L. Concurrent urine specific gravity was 1006 and urine osmolality 123 mmol/kg.

Investigations were also performed in the parents. Serum electrolyte levels, plasma renin activity, plasma aldosterone level, plasma osmolality, urine osmolality, and specific gravity measured in the basal state were normal. A computed tomographic scan of the skull was also normal in both parents.

COMMENT

Adipsic hypernatremia is an uncommon disease associated with a lack of thirst and often with an abnormal secretion of vasopressin. The disease includes four degrees of severity, as reviewed recently by Baylis and Thompson,[3] that are based on the thirst patterns and vasopressin secretion following an infusion of hypertonic saline solution.

In the most severe form, which is probably due to the complete destruction of hypothalamic osmoreceptors,

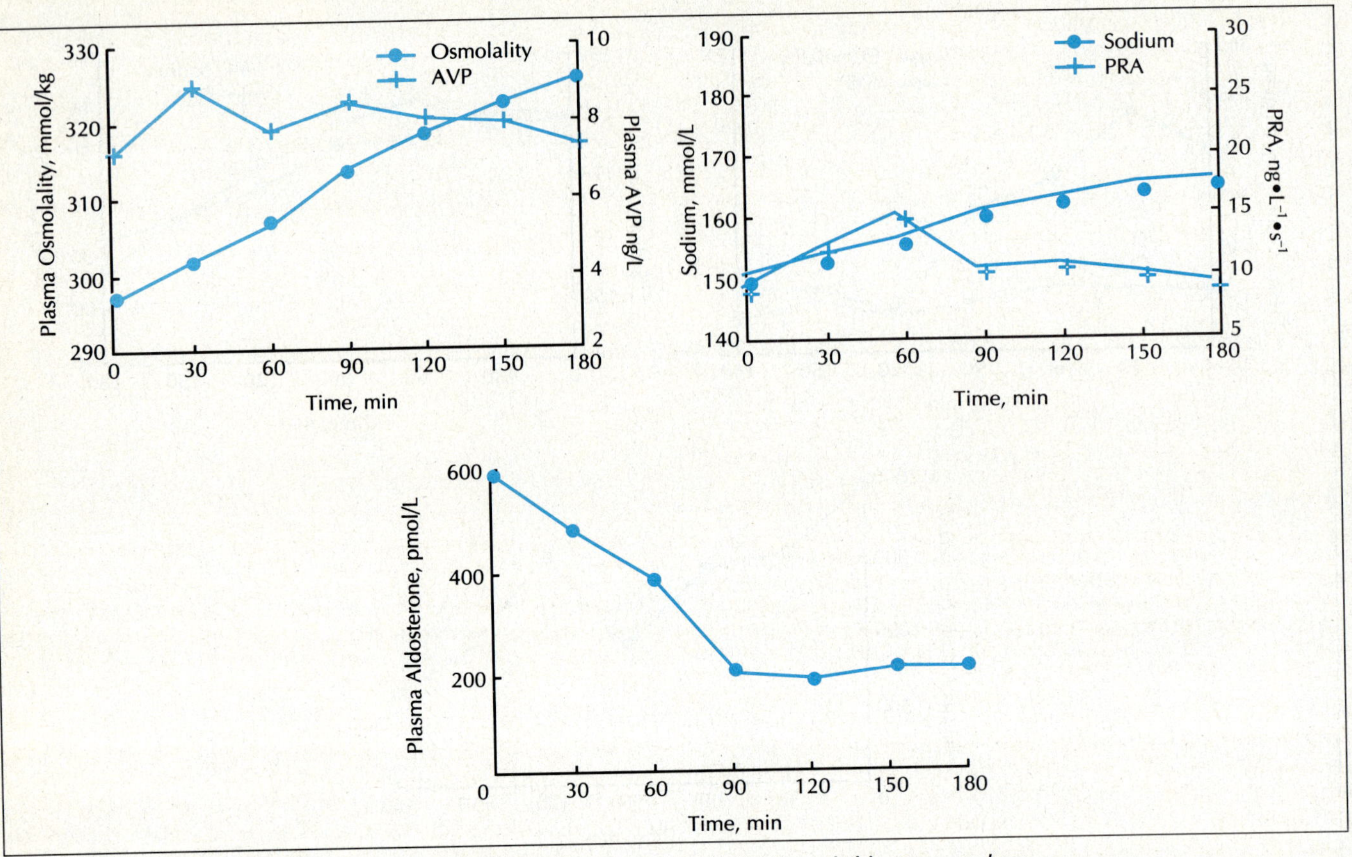

Fig 2.—*Plasma osmolality, vasopressin (AVP), sodium, plasma renin activity (PRA), and aldosterone values during hypertonic saline solution infusion.*

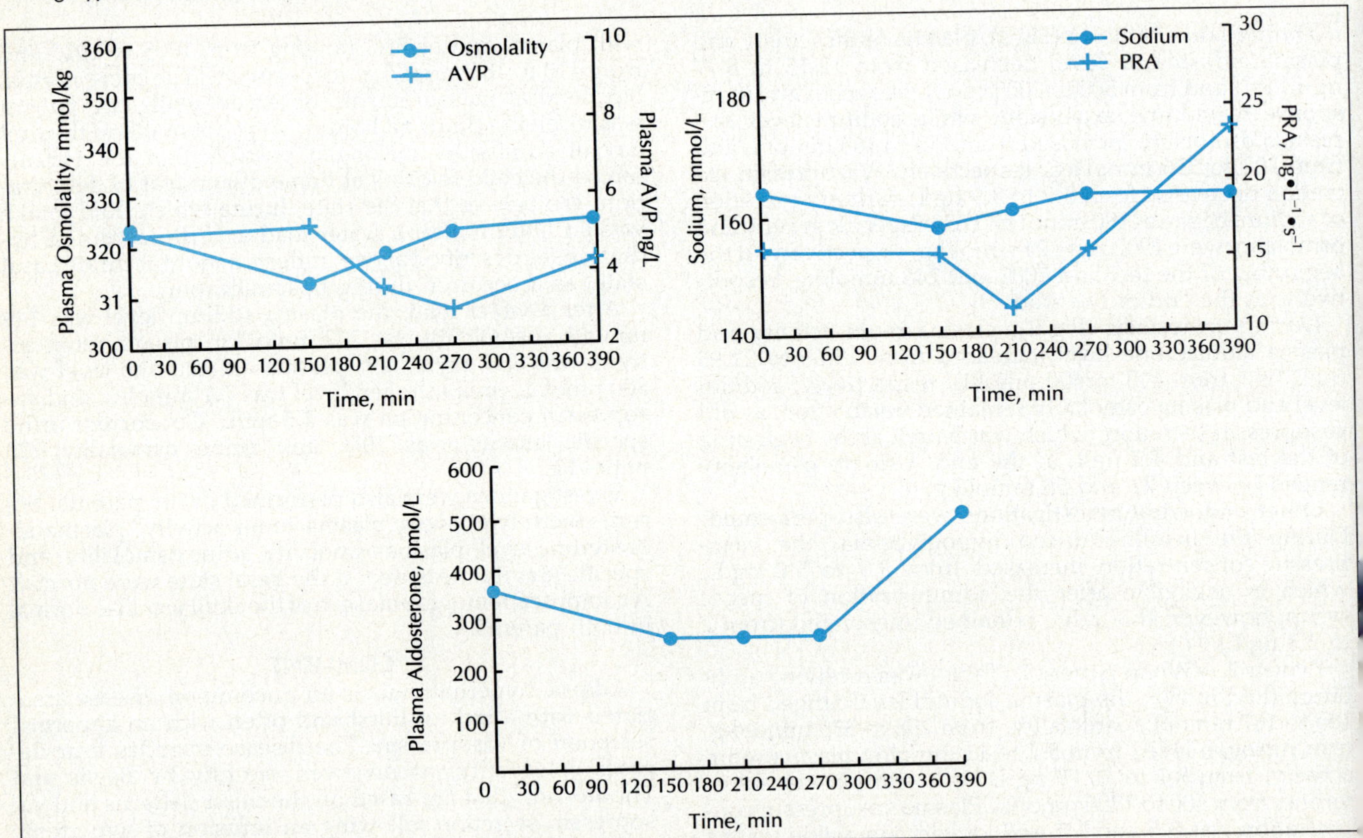

Fig 3.—*Plasma osmolality, vasopressin (AVP), sodium, plasma renin activity (PRA), and aldosterone during baroreceptor stimulation.*

neither thirst nor vasopressin response occurs irrespective of plasma osmolality; vasopressin is secreted continuously, albeit in small quantities. Herein, we describe two sisters with adipsic hypernatremia. In only one of these sisters could a diffuse alteration of the brain structure be found.

In these two patients, the lack of thirst was evident both in basal conditions and in response to osmotic stimuli, irrespective of plasma osmolality. It is well known that an increase in plasma osmolality to greater than 300 mmol/kg leads to severe thirst[4]; however, this never occurred in our patients.

Basal vasopressin secretion was evaluated in both patients and was always inappropriately low for the corresponding level of plasma osmolality.[1] A water load failed in both patients to further suppress the vasopressin secretion, and osmotic stimuli had no effect on vasopressin secretion. Moreover, following hemodynamic stimuli during orthostasis in patient 1, no response of plasma vasopressin was shown, even if the test was appropriate in light of the increase in plasma renin activity and aldosterone level. The response of vasopressin to nonosmotic stimuli such as hypoglycemia[5] (in both patients) and emesis[6] (only in the older sister) was then investigated with a negligible response. We conclude that, in our patients, vasopressin is continuously secreted and that it is neither stimulated by osmotic and nonosmotic stimuli nor suppressed by a water load. We therefore believe that both sisters suffer from the most severe form of adipsic hypernatremia; in our patients, nonosmotic stimuli had no effect on vasopressin secretion, contrary to previously reported cases.[7]

Urine osmolality was always very low in both patients when compared with plasma osmolality and especially the plasma vasopressin level.[1] In patient 1, urine osmolality never rose above 312 mmol/kg, although the vasopressin value was as high as 5.2 ng/L, which would normally cause maximal antidiuresis.[1] In patient 2, when the plasma vasopressin concentration was 3.5 ng/L, we found a corresponding urinary osmolality of only 110 mmol/kg.

We could speculate that some kind of peripheral resistance to endogenous vasopressin was present, which is supported by the normal urinary osmolality values found in both sisters (610 mmol/kg in patient 1 and 362 mmol/kg in patient 2) after the initiation of therapy with the synthetic analogue DDAVP, together with a normal plasma osmolality.

There are two possible explanations for this: either the vasopressin assay was not sufficiently sensitive or the patients' vasopressin was radioimmunologically but not biologically active, probably due to an abnormal molecule. It is also possible that antibodies to vasopressin were present, which could interfere with the radioimmunologic assay.

Adipsic hypernatremia is a rare disorder that is due to a defect in the hypothalamic osmoreceptors for thirst and vasopressin, which, to our knowledge, has not previously been reported within the same family. The sisters were affected by the same disease, although apparently caused in different ways: in the first patient, the symptoms appeared abruptly 2 months after the onset of meningitis, while in the second patient the disease was apparently due to diffuse brain abnormalities. The family history was remarkable for a maternal aunt who died at 2 months of age of an unknown disease and who had a cleft lip and palate and microcephaly, making her case very similar to that of patient 2.

References

1. Robertson GL, Aycinena P, Zerbe RL. Neurogenic disorders of osmoregulation. *Am J Med.* 1982;72:339-353.
2. Robertson GL. Abnormalities of thirst regulation. *Kidney Int.* 1984;25:460-469.
3. Baylis PH, Thompson CJ. Osmoregulation of vasopressin secretion and thirst in health and disease. *Clin Endocrinol.* 1988;29:549-576.
4. Thompson CJ, Bland J, Burd J, Baylis PH. The osmotic thresholds for thirst and vasopressin release are similar in healthy man. *Clin Sci.* 1986;71:651-656.
5. Baylis PH, Zerbe RL, Robertson GL. Arginine vasopressin response to insulin-induced hypoglycemia in man. *J Clin Endocrinol Metab.* 1981;53:935-940.
6. Rowe JW, Shelton RL, Helderman JH, Vestal RE, Robertson GL. Influence of the emetic reflex on vasopressin release in man. *Kidney Int.* 1979;16:729-735.
7. De Robertis FR, Michelis MF, Beck N, Field JB, Beck BB. Essential hypernatremia due to ineffective osmotic and intact volume regulation of vasopressin secretion. *J Clin Invest.* 1971;50:97-111.

Anergy in Pediatric Head Trauma Patients

Nevin W. Wilson, MD; Ann Gooding, MD; Bradley Peterson, MD; John F. Bastian, MD

• To assess cellular immune function in children following severe blunt trauma, 25 children (mean: age, 7.1 years; Injury Severity Score, 34.9; and Glascow Coma Score, 5.6) admitted with severe trauma were examined with the use of the CMI Multitest system (Merieux Institute, Miami, Fla) to test delayed-type hypersensitivity. Patients were monitored for evidence of infection for the next 3 weeks. Ten children (mean: age, 6.2 years; Injury Severity Score, 31.2; and Glascow Coma Score, 5.4) admitted with severe trauma had the percentage of circulating lymphocyte subpopulations (pan–T cell marker T101, CD4, CD8, and B cells) measured on day 1 and then weekly for 3 weeks. Fourteen (56%) of the 25 children had no reaction to any of the skin tests (anergic). Eleven (79%) of 14 anergic patients became infected, while three (27%) of 11 of the nonanergic children became infected. There were no significant changes in pan–T cell marker T101, CD4, or CD8 lymphocyte populations in the 3 weeks following injury; however, absolute numbers of circulating B cells dropped significantly by day 7. These data indicate that children with severe trauma who are anergic are significantly more susceptible to infection. Unlike the results reported previously in adult trauma patients, these children had no significant fluctuations in T-cell populations; however, there was a significant decrease in circulating B cells in the first week. The use of the delayed-type hypersensitivity skin test can aid in identifying which patients are at an increased risk for nosocomial infection.

***(AJDC.* 1991;145:326-329)**

Infection is one of the major complications of severe trauma and is a primary cause of prolonged hospitalizations and death among these patients.[1] Suppression of the immune system after major blunt trauma has been implicated in adults as a cause of increased secondary infection.[2] In children, blunt trauma is responsible for more than 80% of the serious injuries,[3] with head injuries occurring more often in children than adults.[4] Additionally, there are notable differences in the immune function of young children when compared with adults. While there has been extensive research concerning the response of the immune system after severe thermal and nonthermal trauma in adults, very little information is available on severely injured children.

Accepted for publication November 5, 1990.

From the Division of Pediatric Immunology and Allergy, Department of Pediatrics, University of California–San Diego, La Jolla (Dr Wilson), and the Divisions of Critical Care (Drs Gooding and Peterson) and Allergy and Immunology (Dr Bastian), The Children's Hospital and Health Center, San Diego, Calif.

Reprint requests to Division of Pediatric Immunology and Allergy, Department of Pediatrics/0609D, University of California–San Diego, La Jolla, CA 92093 (Dr Wilson).

Measurement of delayed-type hypersensitivity (DTH) to commonly encountered antigens is a well-accepted method of assessing cell-mediated immunity.[5,6] Evaluation of DTH has been used to predict immunologic failure in adult trauma patients.[7] In this study, we describe the effect of severe head injury on circulating T cells, B cells, and T-cell subsets, as well as the use of the DTH skin test, to predict the risk of infection in critically injured children.

PATIENTS

All children in these studies were kept paralyzed with nondepolarizing muscle relaxants and sedated with fentanyl citrate while they were intubated. All children had central venous catheters, arterial catheters, and intracranial pressure monitors placed. Techniques used for the management of increased intracranial pressure included hyperventilation, mannitol treatment, and, for some patients, thiopental sodium (Pentothal). None of the children received steroids.

The protocol for this study was approved by the Children's Hospital–San Diego (La Jolla, Calif) Institutional Review Board, and written informed consent was obtained from each family.

DTH Skin Tests

Delayed-type hypersensitivity skin tests were placed on 25 children between the ages of 2 and 14 years (mean age, 7.1 years) who were admitted to the intensive care unit (ICU) at Children's Hospital–San Diego with a diagnosis of major trauma. Criteria for admission to the study included a Trauma Score less than 15 and Injury Severity Score (ISS)[8] greater than 15. The mean ISS for these patients was 34.9 (range, 17 to 50); the mean Glascow Coma Score was 5.6 (range, 3 to 11). An ISS score of 30 has a predicted mortality of 20%. Severe head injuries were the primary trauma in all 25 children. All children had immunization histories that were up to date for age. Controls consisted of 10 children (mean age, 5.5 years) who were seen in the clinic for an allergic or upper respiratory tract disorder.

T- and B-Cell Enumeration

T- and B-cell numbers were obtained on 10 children between the ages of 2 months and 14 years (mean age, 6.2 years) who were admitted with a diagnosis of major trauma. They were enrolled into the study within 36 hours of admission to the ICU (day 1). The mean ISS for these patients was 31.2 (range, 17 to 48), and the mean Glascow Coma Score was 5.4 (range, 3 to 9). Severe head injuries constituted the primary trauma in all 10 of these children.

METHODS

DTH Skin Tests

Delayed-type hypersensitivity skin reactions were measured with the use of the CMI Multitest (Merieux Institute, Miami, Fla). This is a plastic disposable puncture device that simultaneously applies seven antigens and a negative glycerin-saline control. The seven antigens were tetanus, diphtheria, *Streptococcus*, tuberculin, *Candida*, *Trichophyton*, and *Proteus*. This device has been

Table 1.—Types of Infections

Infection	No.
Anergic patients	11
Sepsis	
Pseudomonas	1
Staphylococcus aureus	1
Candida albicans	1
Pneumonia–tracheal aspirate	
Staphylococcus epidermidis	5
Haemophilus influenzae	4
Candida species	3
S aureus	3
Pseudomonas species	2
Pneumococcus	1
Sinusitis	3
Stomatitis	
Herpes simplex virus	1
Nonanergic patients	3
Brain abscess	
Enterococcus	1
Meningitis	
Streptococcus viridans	1
Cellulitis	1
Pneumonia–tracheal aspirate	
Klebsiella	1
No organism	1

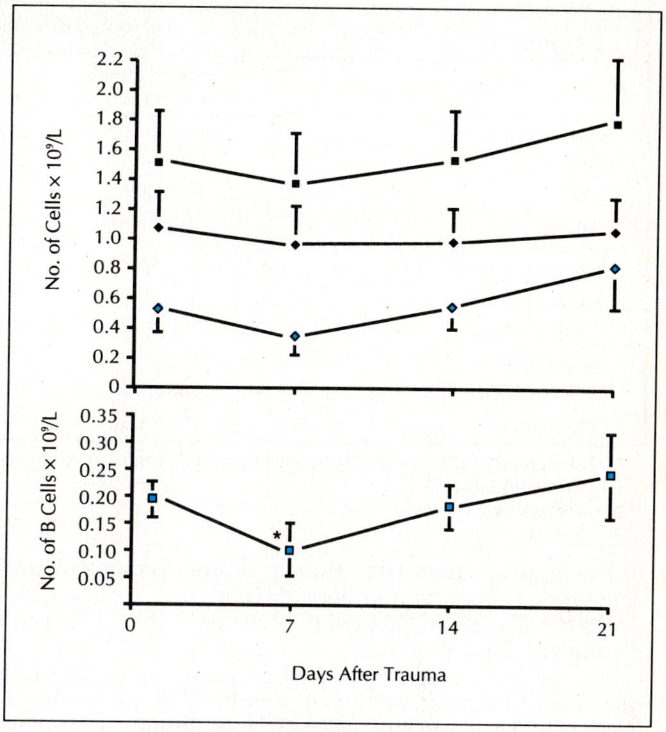

Changes in numbers of circulating T cells (closed squares), CD4+ cells (closed diamonds), CD8+ cells (open diamonds), and B cells (open squares) following trauma. Error bars signify 1 SEM; asterisk, $P = .05$ compared with that on day 1.

shown to assess DTH accurately in normal infants and preschool-age children.[9] This device was placed on the volar surface of one forearm within 24 hours of admission to the ICU. Skin induration was measured in two perpendicular dimensions with the use of calipers at 24 and 48 hours. All measurements were made by one observer (N.W.W.). Only reactions that were 2 mm or larger were considered to be positive. Anergy was defined as an absence of expression of DTH skin test reactivity to any of the antigens tested.[5]

Criteria for infection were defined as follows: (1) pneumonia—new or changing infiltrates on a chest roentgenogram with evidence of a systemic inflammatory response (temperature, >39°C; and leukocytosis); and (2) sepsis—positive blood culture for a commonly accepted pathogen with clinical evidence of sepsis, ie, as temperature greater than 39°C, hypotension, cardiovascular instability, elevated white blood cell count with increased neutrophils, or disseminated intravascular coagulation. Other infections were defined with use of criteria from the Centers for Disease Control, Atlanta, Ga.[10]

T- and B-Lymphocyte Enumeration, T-Cell Subsets, and Absolute Monocyte and Granulocyte Counts

Peripheral blood, collected at 1, 7, 14, and 21 days after the injury, was diluted 1:2 in phosphate-buffered saline solution and then placed over equal amounts of Ficoll-Hypaque (Pharmacia Laboratories, Piscataway, NJ). This was centrifuged for 15 minutes at 400*g*. The peripheral blood mononuclear cells were collected at the interface and then washed with RPMI 1640 with glutamine medium (Cell Culture Facility, University of California–San Diego) two times.

T-cell subsets were analyzed with standard methods,[11] by using monoclonal antibodies to pan-T cell marker T101 (Hybritech Inc, San Diego, Calif) and CD4 and CD8 that were obtained from a manufacturer (Becton Dickinson & Co, Mountain View, Calif). B lymphocytes were identified with the use of polyclonal goat $F(ab')_2$ anti–human immunoglobulins antibody (Tago, Burlingame, Calif). The peripheral blood mononuclear cells were counted on a flow cytometer (Ortho Immunology Systems, Westwood, Mass).

Absolute numbers of monocytes and granulocytes were monitored at 1, 7, 14, and 21 days after the injury.

RESULTS

Fourteen (56%) of the 25 children met criteria for at least one infection. Three patients died: two of complications of pneumonia and one of increased intracranial pressure. There were 13 patients with pneumonia, three patients with documented sepsis, three patients with sinusitis, one patient with meningitis, one patient with a brain abscess, one patient with cellulitis, and one patient with herpes simplex stomatitis. Infections commonly occurred 5 to 10 days after admission. Table 1 lists the types of infections that were seen in the anergic and nonanergic patients.

DTH Skin Tests

Results of DTH skin tests are shown in Table 2. There were no significant differences in age, ISS, or Glascow Coma Score between the anergic and nonanergic patients. There was no difference between our controls and published values for the CMI Multitest in children.[9]

Fourteen (56%) of the 25 children were anergic with no reactions at either 24 or 48 hours. Eleven (79%) of 14 anergic patients became infected, while three (27%) of 11 nonanergic children became infected ($P = .013$ by Fisher's Exact Test). Anergic children averaged 17 days longer in the ICU and 31 days longer in the hospital than nonanergic children. All 11 nonanergic children reacted to tetanus toxoid. Diphtheria toxoid was the second most common positive reaction, with six of 11 children reacting.

There was a significant difference in the number of skin tests that were positive ($P = .02$ by unpaired *t* test) between the nonanergic trauma patients and controls. This suggested that all of the trauma patients had some degree of anergy.

T- and B-Lymphocyte Enumeration, T-Cell Subsets, and Absolute Monocyte and Granulocyte Counts

Changes in the absolute number of T cells, T-cell subsets, and B cells for the 10 children after trauma are shown

Table 2.—Results of DTH Skin Tests*

	Anergic Patients (n=14)	Nonanergic Patients (n=11)	Controls (n=10)	P†
Mean ± SD				
Age, y	6.5±3.5	7.8±3.2	5.5±5.5	.34
ISS	35.14±9.6	34.6±12.4	...	.9
GCS	4.86±2.9	6.55±2.7	...	.15
No. of positive skin tests	0	1.73±0.8	2.6±0.8	.02
Sum of induration, mm	0	5.55±2.77	8.6±3.7	.03
No. infected	11	3	...	.01‡
Mean ± SD				
Hospital days	66.6±52	35.4±28	...	.09
ICU days	30.6±30	13.8±14	...	.1

*DTH indicates delayed-type hypersensitivity; ISS, Injury Severity Score; GCS, Glascow Coma Score; and ICU, intensive care unit.
†By unpaired *t* test.
‡By Fisher's Exact Test.

in the Figure. There were no significant changes in percentages or absolute numbers of circulating T cells, CD4-positive cells, and CD8-positive cells or in the T4-T8 ratio during the 3-week period.

Nine of the 10 patients showed decreases in the absolute number and the percentage of peripheral blood mononuclear cells that were surface immunoglobulin positive between days 1 and 7 ($P=.05$ by paired t test). The number of B cells then increased at 14 and 21 days to levels similar to that of day 1.

There were no significant changes noted in the absolute monocyte count or absolute granulocyte count during the 3-week period.

COMMENT

Nosocomial infections remain a major cause of increased morbidity and mortality in the severely injured patient. Sepsis accounts for 78% of all nonneurologic deaths following nonthermal trauma in adults.[1] In one study, 42% of adults admitted to an ICU with multiple trauma experienced a secondary infection.[12] This was significantly higher than for other diagnostic categories. Breaux et al[13] reported that 12% of all pediatric patients admitted for trauma experienced infectious complications.

This high nosocomial infection rate has been attributed to suppression of the immune system following severe injury.[2] Abnormalities in cellular immune function after severe nonthermal trauma in adults include depressed DTH skin tests,[7] decreased response of lymphocytes to mitogens,[14] decreases in number of T cells and helper T cells,[15] and decreased production of interleukin 2.[16] Much less is known about the effects of severe blunt trauma on the immune system of infants and children. We have recently reported that pediatric trauma patients make an abnormally low primary antibody response to a T cell–dependent neoantigen but are able to respond with normal antibody production to recall antigens, such as tetanus and diphtheria.[17]

A DTH skin reaction is a complex series of events and requires a previously sensitized subject. It requires processing of the antigen by antigen-processing cells, such as macrophages or Langerhans cells, and then presentation of this antigen to previously sensitized T cells. Production of lymphokines by these T cells induces migration of granulocytes and mononuclear cells to the site of inflammation. These cells and various soluble factors produce the vasculitis and edema that are visible in 1 to 2 days. A defect in any of these events would produce anergy.

While anergy is a marker for increased susceptibility to infection in these patients, the relationship of anergy to susceptibility remains unknown. There may exist a causal relationship, ie, trauma causes immune deficiency, which results in an increased infection rate. There may also be a noncausal relationship. Some unknown covariate(s) may cause anergy but cause increased susceptibility by a mechanism independent of anergy. Further studies are needed to elucidate the mechanism of anergy in these patients. If a causal relationship to susceptibility is present, then correction of the defect may decrease the risk of infection.

Many adults do not respond to DTH skin tests during the posttrauma period. Meakins et al[7] studied 53 adults with blunt trauma for responses to five recall antigens at admission. Twenty-two of the 53 patients were completely anergic, with 13 of 22 patients becoming septic and three deaths. Twenty-six patients had normal responses, of whom four became septic and none died. They found that the incidence of anergy depended on age and the extent of trauma. Hoyt et al[18] placed CMI Multitests on 30 adults with blunt trauma and found all 30 to be anergic. Our results are different probably because of the much shorter time period between the last immunization and testing. In our study, tetanus and diphtheria antigens were, by far, the most common positive tests in both the patients and controls.

Unlike the results that we have reported in traumatized children, adults have been shown to have decreases in the numbers of circulating T cells, as well as shifts in the T4-T8 ratio.[18] O'Mahony et al[14] studied 31 adults (mean: age, 31 years; ISS, 22) with multiple trauma and found significant decreases in circulating CD3-positive cells, as well as increases in CD8-positive cells, in the first 2 weeks after trauma.

Until recently, it has been generally thought that the effects of severe blunt trauma on intrinsic B-cell function were minor when compared with the effect on T cells.[2] Few studies have examined changes in circulating B-lymphocyte populations. Hoyt et al[18] reported no significant changes in the lymphocyte surface marker B1 in 30 adults following blunt trauma. Faist et al[19] also showed no decrease in the number of circulating B cells, but did demonstrate a decrease in the number of B cells that bore cytoplasmic immunoglobulin following injury. This suggested that impaired terminal B-cell maturation into plasma cells occurs after severe trauma in adults.

Various strategies have been proposed to help reduce the nosocomial infection rate in the severely ill, mechanically ventilated patient, such as the pediatric head trauma patient. These include the prophylactic use of intravenous immunoglobulin[20] and protective isolation.[21] Since it would be less feasible to institute these measures in all such patients, the ability to predict which patients are at a higher risk for infection would be valuable. The CMI Multitest may be useful for this purpose since it is easy to use, provides reproducible results, is relatively inexpensive, and provides a battery of seven antigens and a negative control.

We conclude that there is a significant depression of DTH reactions after severe trauma in infants and children. Furthermore, this depression correlates with the subsequent development of secondary infection. Unlike the results reported previously in adult blunt trauma patients, these children had no significant fluctuation in T-cell populations; however, there was a significant decrease in circulating B cells in the first week. The use of the DTH skin test may aid in predicting which patients are at increased risk for nosocomial infection.

This study was supported by a grant from Sandoz Pharmaceuticals, East Hanover, NJ.

References

1. Baker CC, Oppenheimer L, Stephens B, Lewis FR, Trunkey DD. Epidemiology of trauma deaths. *Am J Surg.* 1980;140:144-148.

2. Munster AM. Immunologic response of trauma and burns. *Am J Med.* 1984;76:142-145.

3. Haller JA. An overview of pediatric trauma. In: Touloulian RJ, ed. *Pediatric Trauma.* New York, NY: John Wiley & Sons Inc; 1978:3-19.

4. Haller JA. Problems in children's trauma. *J Trauma.* 1970;10:269-271.

5. Palmer DL, Reed WP. Delayed hypersensitivity skin testing, II: clinical correlates and anergy. *J Infect Dis.* 1974;130:138-143.

6. Turk JL. *Delayed Hypersensitivity.* 3rd ed. New York, NY: Elsevier Science Publishing Co Inc; 1980:111-145.

7. Meakins JI, McLean APH, Kelly R, Buenik O, Pietsch JB, Maclean LD. Delayed hypersensitivity and neutrophil chemotaxis: effect of trauma. *J Trauma.* 1978;18:240-246.

8. Baker SP, O'Neill B, Haddon W, Long WB. The Injury Severity Score: a method for describing patients with multiple injuries and evaluating emergency care. *J Trauma.* 1974;14:187-196.

9. Kniker WT, Lesourd BM, McBryde JL, Corriel RN. Cell-mediated immunity assessed by Multitest CMI skin testing in infants and preschool children. *AJDC.* 1985;139:840-845.

10. Centers for Disease Control. *Outline for Surveillance and Control of Nosocomial Infections.* Atlanta, Ga: Centers for Disease Control; 1972.

11. Reinherz EZ, King PC, Goldstein G, Schlossman SF. Separation of functional subsets of human T cells by monoclonal antibody. *Proc Natl Acad Sci U S A.* 1979;76:4061-4065.

12. Potgieter P, Linton D, Oliver S, Forder A. Nosocomial infections in a respiratory intensive care unit. *Crit Care Med.* 1987;15:495-498.

13. Breaux CW, Smith G, Georgeson KE. The first two years; experience with major trauma at a pediatric trauma center. *J Trauma.* 1990;30:37-43.

14. O'Mahony JB, Palder SB, Wood JJ, et al. Depression of cellular immunity after multiple trauma in the absence of sepsis. *J Trauma.* 1984;24:869-875.

15. Faist E, Kupper TS, Baker CC, Chandry IH, Dwyer J, Baue AE. Depression of cellular immunity after major injury. *Arch Surg.* 1986;121:1000-1005.

16. Roderick ML, Wood JJ, O'Mahony JB, et al. Mechanisms of immunosuppression associated with severe nonthermal traumatic injuries in man: production of IL-2. *J Clin Immunol.* 1986;6:310-318.

17. Wilson NW, Ochs HD, Peterson B, Hamburger RN, Bastian JF. Abnormal primary antibody response in pediatric trauma patients. *J Pediatr.* 1989;115:424-427.

18. Hoyt DB, Ozkan AN, Ninnemann JL. Immunological monitoring of infection risk in trauma patients: research questions and an approach to the problem. *J Burn Care Rehabil.* 1987;8:549-553.

19. Faist E, Ertel W, Baker CC, Heberer G. Terminal B-cell maturation and immunoglobulin synthesis in vitro in patients with major injury. *J Trauma.* 1989;29:1-9.

20. Glinz W, Grob PH, Nydegger UE, et al. Polyvalent immunoglobulins for prophylaxis of bacterial infections in patients following multiple trauma. *Intensive Care Med.* 1985;11:288-294.

21. Klein BS, Perloff WH, Maki DG. Reduction of nosocomial infection during intensive care by protective isolation. *N Engl J Med.* 1989;320:714-721.

Endocrine Function in Children With Human Immunodeficiency Virus Infection

Lisa J. Schwartz, DO; Yolaine St Louis, MD; Richard Wu, MD; Andrew Wiznia, MD; Arye Rubinstein, MD; Paul Saenger, MD

• **We sought to determine if failure to thrive in pediatric patients with the human immunodeficiency virus could be explained based on endocrine dysfunction. Fourteen human immunodeficiency virus–infected pediatric patients, all of whom had adequate nutritional status, underwent endocrine evaluation. Growth hormone and cortisol responses to glucagon stimulation were adequate. Despite this, eight of the 12 subjects had low somatomedin C levels. Although all patients were clinically and biochemically euthyroid, 36% (5/14) demonstrated elevated baseline and peak thyrotropin levels in response to thyroid releasing hormone, suggesting a state of compensated hypothyroidism. Although the importance of these findings is unclear, it is possible that subtle alterations of thyroid regulation may contribute to failure to thrive in some pediatric patients infected with human immunodeficiency virus and may represent a potentially correctable defect.**

***(AJDC.* 1991;145:330-333)**

The effects of the human immunodeficiency virus (HIV) are widespread and generally the result of either opportunistic infections or neoplastic processes. Endocrine involvement, though previously described, has received less attention than many other organ systems, probably because of its often subtle manifestations. In addition, most of the information available on endocrine function in HIV infection is based on either pathologic findings at autopsy[1-4] or tests of endocrine function in adult populations.[5-8] Little attention with regard to hormonal regulation has been directed toward the pediatric population infected with HIV. However, these children are often small for gestational age at birth and continue to exhibit poor weight gain and growth through infancy and childhood.[9] By assessing the hypothalamic-pituitary axis and adrenal and thyroid function, we sought to determine if hormonal deficiencies are responsible for the failure to thrive syndrome often seen in pediatric patients known to be infected with HIV.

Accepted for publication July 26, 1990.

From the Division of Pediatric Endocrinology, Department of Pediatrics (Drs Schwartz, Wu, and Saenger), and the Division of Allergy and Immunology (Drs Wiznia and Rubinstein), Albert Einstein College of Medicine, Bronx, NY; and the Department of Pediatrics (Dr St Louis), Interfaith Medical Center, Brooklyn, NY.

Reprint requests to Division of Pediatric Endocrinology, Department of Pediatrics, Montefiore Medical Center of the Albert Einstein College of Medicine, 111 E 210th St, Bronx, NY 10467 (Dr Saenger).

PATIENTS AND METHODS

Subjects were selected from the group of patients followed up at the Albert Einstein College of Medicine–affiliated hospitals, Bronx, NY (n = 12), and the Interfaith Hospital, Brooklyn, NY (n = 2), who met the following criteria: (1) HIV seropositivity determined by enzyme-linked immunosorbent assay and Western blot analysis; (2) prepubertal status; (3) no active opportunistic infections or neoplastic processes when tested; (4) no known past or present endocrinopathy; and (5) no systemic therapy with glucocorticoids within 6 months of participation. All patients were classified by the Centers for Disease Control criteria for HIV infection in children.[10]

Patient characteristics are given in Table 1. Fourteen subjects (eight females and six males) were enrolled between November 1987 and August 1988. There were eight female and six male patients. Ages ranged from 6 months to 10.5 years, with a mean (±SD) of 4.8±2.8 years. The mean height was 2.23±1.2 SDs below the norm; mean weight was 1.12±1.26 SDs below the norm; and mean growth velocity was 1.84±2.34 SDs below the norm. All patients, though free of active infection when tested, were classified as P2, ie, symptomatic infection had been noted previously. Subclassifications of P2 disease states according to the Centers for Disease Control Criteria[10] are given in Table 1. Six patients were receiving intravenous gamma globulin (300 mg/kg; Cutter Immune Globulin, Cutter Biologicals, Division of Miles, Westhaven, Conn, or Sandoglobulin, Sandoz Pharmaceuticals, East Hanover, NJ) biweekly, and these subjects were tested at least 1 week after infusion.

Endocrine Assessment

All subjects underwent the protirelin stimulation test to evaluate the hypothalamic-pituitary-thyroid axis. Protirelin was administered intravenously at a dose of 7 μg/kg. Thyrotropin response was measured by radioimmunoassay (RIA) at 0, 30, 60, 90, and 120 minutes. Baseline samples were also obtained for antithyroglobulin and antimicrosomal antibodies. Thyroxine (T_4) and triiodothyronine (T_3) levels were measured by RIA.

Glucagon (0.1 mg/kg) was administered intramuscularly. Cortisol (fluorescent polarization immunoassay) and growth hormone (RIA double-antibody technique, Cambridge Medical Diagnostics, Billerica, Mass) responses were measured at 0, 60, 90, 150, and 180 minutes. Baseline somatomedin C values (Smith Kline Bioscience Laboratories, Van Nuys, Calif, and Roche Biomedical, Raritan, NJ) were obtained as well.

All subjects were assessed at baseline and at 6 months with measurement of standing height (centimeters, Harpenden Stadiometer, Seritex, Carlstadt, NJ) and weight (kilograms). Nutritional assessment included measurement of serum transferrin (RIA, Nichols Institute, San Juan Capistrano, Calif) and serum albumin levels.

Statistical analysis was performed by a two-tailed Student *t* test. Informed consent was obtained from parents or guardians

Table 1.—Patient Characteristics*

Patient No./Age, y/mo/Sex	Height	Weight	Growth Velocity	Disease Stage	Albumin, g/L	Transferrin, g/L	CD4 Count	Gamma Globulin Therapy	Somatomedin C, ng/mL
1/6/9/F	−2.5	−1.3	−4.74	P2D1	40	2.60	35	No	...
2/5/8/F	−3.0	−1.78	−0.70	P2B	32	2.00	112	Yes	13 (L)
3/5/10/F	−3.0	−1.23	0	P2D	35	2.65	897	Yes	13 (L)
4/5/5/F	0	0	−3.50	P2A	42	3.48	712	No	60 (N)
5/3/7/M	−1.0	+0.34	+1.30	P2D1	41	3.60	1108	Yes	19 (N)
6/2/10/F	−2.0	−1.4	−1.85	P2D1	30	...	774	No	0.25 U/mL (N)
7/1/10/M	−4.0	+3.3	−3.16	P2D1	35	...	143	No	0.52 U/mL (N)
8/6/1/F	−1.5	+1.29	−3.08	P2D1	35	3.36	10	Yes	13 (L)
9/10/4/F	−3.5	−0.9	+0.22	P2D1	30	2.43	104	Yes	22 (L)
10/4/2/F	−1.0	+.036	−2.60	P2D2	45	3.16	512	No	<5 (L)
11/3/0/M	−1.8	−1.67	+1.16	P2F	29	3.32	79	Yes	7 (L)
12/0/5/M	−3.4	−2.78	−5.80	P2A	37	2.86	212	No	7 (L)
13/10/6/M	−1.0	−1.0	−1.50	P2D2	41	3.66	280	No	95 (L)
14/1/5/M	−3.6	−2.35	−4.00	P2D1	29	...	479	No	...

*Height, weight, and growth velocity are given in SDs from the norm. For explanation of disease stages, see Centers for Disease Control.[10] Normal range for albumin is 35 to 50 g/L. Normal range for transferrin is 2.04 to 2.60 g/L. CD4 count is absolute number of T-helper lymphocytes per minute. Except for patients 6 and 7, somatomedin C values are in nanograms per milliliter. Patients 6 and 7 had values measured in a different laboratory, where they are given in units per milliliter. As normal range for somatomedin C levels are age and sex specific, each value in the table is accompanied by N (normal) or L (low).

Table 2.—Thyrotropin Response to Protirelin Stimulation Test*

Patient No.	Thyrotropin, mU/L Baseline (0 min)	Peak (30 min)	Final (120 min)
1	3.5	26.0	13.0
2	9.6	>60.0	20.1
3	2.0	17.7	3.5
4	2.2	21.2	5.4
5	3.4	25.1	4.6
6	2.0	21.2	4.8
7	36.3	>45.0	>45.0
8	<1.0	22.9	9.5
9	2.8	15.5	8.0
10	5.8	17.9	12.6
11	2.7	11.5	2.0
12	12.9	56.0	34.4
13	12.2	60.2	33.6
14	11.7	55.7	20.0

*For details of protirelin administration, see text.

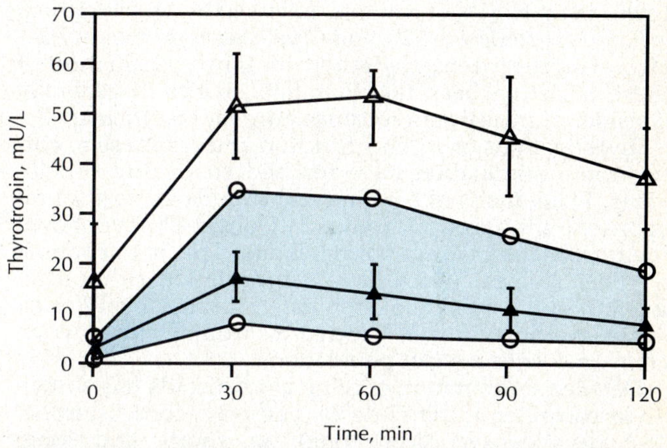

Thyrotropin response to protirelin stimulation. Shaded area between circles represents range of normal values obtained in a control population. Closed triangles indicate study subjects (n=9) with a normal protirelin response (mean±SD); open triangles, subjects (n=5) with abnormal protirelin responses (mean±SD). See text for details.

for all subjects participating in the study. This study was approved by the institutional review board.

RESULTS

All subjects were clinically euthyroid, with normal T_3 and T_4 levels; no antimicrosomal or antithyroglobulin antibodies were detected. However, five (36%) of 14 subjects had abnormal thyrotropin responses to protirelin stimulation as defined by initial thyrotropin values greater than 5 mU/L and peak values greater than 35 mU/L.[11] These responses failed to decline to normal levels by 120 minutes after stimulation (Table 2 and Figure). When this group was analyzed separately, they were shorter (2.99±1.17 vs 1.8±1.08 cm below the norm) and had slower growth velocities (3.03±1.81 SDs vs 1.45±2.07 SDs below the norm), although the differences were not statistically significant when compared with subjects with normal thyrotropin responses.

Twelve of 14 subjects had glucagon stimulation tests. All subjects tested had adequate growth hormone responses (>10 μg/L), with a mean peak of 24.2±12.1 μg/L. In contrast, somatomedin C levels were low in eight (67%) of 12 subjects when compared with age-appropriate standards. The pituitary-adrenal axis as assessed by cortisol response to glucagon was intact in all 12, with a mean response of 830±320 nmol/L.

All subjects who had serum transferrin levels measured

(n = 12) had normal values, and most had albumin levels that were normal or slightly below normal. Gamma globulin therapy did not alter hormonal responses, as those subjects receiving gamma globulin, when analyzed separately, did not demonstrate any differences.

COMMENT

Failure to thrive is a common finding in the pediatric acquired immunodeficiency syndrome. These patients are often small for gestational age and have persistent growth failure throughout infancy and childhood.[9] The general clinical status, including the persistence and severity of infection, does not consistently have a good correlation with the patient's growth.[9] Therefore, we sought to determine if the growth disturbance in pediatric patients infected with HIV could be related to hormonal dysfunction.

Endocrine complications of the acquired immunodeficiency syndrome, although not prominent features of the disease, are being increasingly recognized in adults with HIV infection. Initial attention was directed toward autopsy studies, which have demonstrated opportunistic infections and the presence of Kaposi's sarcoma in the adrenal, pituitary, and thyroid glands.[3,4,12-15]

Prompted by reports of hyponatremia, hyperkalemia, and hypotension, adrenal involvement has received the most attention to date.[16-18] Invasion by opportunistic infection, when specifically searched for, has been reported in the adrenal in up to 81% of patients examined.[3] Cytomegalovirus is the most commonly noted pathogen, found in up to 51% of patients, followed by *Mycobacterium avium-intracellulare* in 12% and *Cryptococcus* species in 7%.[3] However, the extent of adrenocortical necrosis in most of these cases has been less than 50%, which is generally considered insufficient to cause adrenal insufficiency.[3]

Investigations of adrenal function and response to corticotropin stimulation have reached conflicting conclusions. Evaluations of baseline and stimulated cortisol responses by our group as well as by Dobs et al[6] have shown them to be well within normal limits. This is in contrast to other studies, which have demonstrated either a reduction in the maximum stimulated cortisol level[19] or elevated baseline cortisol[5,20] and corticotropin[20] values when compared with control populations.

Detailed examination of mineralocorticoids has shown an impairment of the 17-deoxy pathway (corticosterone, 18-hydroxydeoxycorticosterone) on short- and long-term corticotropin stimulation, with no alteration in the end products of the pathway (aldosterone, 18-hydroxycorticosterone).

Although histopathologic abnormalities of the pituitary have been reported to be unusual,[21] involvement has been demonstrated in up to 23% of patients with HIV.[13] Again, most of these lesions are infectious in origin, although vascular anomalies, including ischemic necrosis and microthrombosis of the neurohypophyseal vessels, were seen as well.

Given these lesions of the pituitary, it is appealing to attempt to correlate the growth abnormalities in HIV-infected patients with pituitary dysfunction. An isolated case of growth hormone deficiency was reported in a 6-year, 10-month-old girl who was HIV positive and had a 2-year history of growth failure.[22] However, our data, and those of Rappaport et al,[23] could find no correlation between growth or growth velocity and hormonal measures, such as growth hormone and/or somatomedin C level.

In this study, we examined an unselected population of HIV-positive pediatric patients who had no known active opportunistic infection but demonstrated as a group short stature and abnormally low growth velocities. When we specifically examined pituitary and adrenal unresponsiveness to glucagon stimulation, we were unable to demonstrate any abnormality in growth hormone or cortisol secretion. However, despite normal growth hormone and normal visceral protein synthetic capabilities, as measured by transferrin level,[24] most of these patients had depressed somatomedin C levels. Low somatomedin C level has also been observed in patients with hemophilia and HIV infection.[25]

The thyroid gland has also been demonstrated to be involved with opportunistic infectious processes. Again, cytomegalovirus appears frequently in studies of pathologic specimens, but Kaposi's sarcoma, *Pneumocystis carinii*, and *Cryptococcus* species have also been reported.[26]

To date, evaluation of thyroid function has yielded conflicting results. Initial studies reported normal measures of thyroid function, including normal thyrotropin responses to protirelin stimulation.[6] Others, however, found changes in thyroid function commonly associated with nonthyroidal illness, ie, the sick euthyroid syndrome.[7] LoPresti et al[8] reported unique alterations in thyroid function in patients with acquired immunodeficiency syndrome: a progressive decline in reverse T_3 value and elevation in T_4-binding globulin level that accompanied advancing HIV infection. They postulated that perhaps the persistence of a normal T_3 value in the setting of a severe systemic illness may play a role in facilitating the weight loss and wasting syndrome often seen in HIV-positive patients even in the absence of an active infectious or neoplastic process.

We have found that all subjects examined in this study had normal T_3 and T_4 levels. However, we identified a subset of individuals in whom not only growth measures were abnormal, but who also manifested an abnormal thyrotropin response to protirelin stimulation. These subjects had elevated baseline thyrotropin levels with exaggerated and prolonged thyrotropin response to protirelin. We believe that this aberrant response may represent a state of compensated hypothyroidism in these children. Whether this abnormal thyrotropin response represents an earlier, more sensitive indicator for thyroidal illness than the progressive fall in T_3 and T_4 levels seen in the patients of LoPresti et al remains to be determined.

Although failure to thrive and growth disturbances characterize many pediatric patients infected with HIV, we could find no single endocrine abnormality that could be directly responsible for this. Two intriguing abnormalities were noted. The first is that of depressed somatomedin C levels in the setting of normal growth hormone secretion after pharmacologic stimulation. This may represent a state of resistance or insensitivity to the peripheral actions of growth hormone. However, it is also possibly a reflection of a chronic illness. Subtle degrees of malnutrition that we were not able to pick up with one clinical and laboratory assessment of nutritional status also may have lowered somatomedin C concentrations.[27] The second, perhaps more important, finding is a state of compensated hypothyroidism in a subset of subjects that demonstrated a trend toward slower growth velocities and shorter statures. The importance of these findings has yet to be determined, but it is conceivable that if alterations of thyroid regulation contribute to failure to thrive in some HIV-infected pediatric patients, this may represent a potentially correctable defect.

This study was supported by grants T32-HD07053-13 and UOAI

20671 from the National Institutes of Health, Bethesda, Md.

We gratefully acknowledge Hasoon Lee, MD, and Sara Paterson, RN, for their assistance in enrolling participants in this study. Ken Fishman aided in statistical analysis.

References

1. Guarda LA, Luna MA, Smith JL Jr, Mansell PWA, Gyorkey F, Roca AN. Acquired immuno deficiency syndrome: postmortem findings. *Am J Clin Pathol.* 1984;81:549-557.

2. Tapper ML, Rotterdam HZ, Lerner CW, Al'Khafaji K, Seitzman PA. Adrenal necrosis in the acquired immunodeficiency syndrome. *Ann Intern Med.* 1984;100:239-241.

3. Glasgow BJ, Steinsapir KD, Anders K, Layfield LJ. Adrenal pathology in the acquired immune deficiency syndrome. *Am J Clin Pathol.* 1985;84:594-597.

4. Ferreiro J, Vinters HV. Pathology of the pituitary gland with the acquired immune deficiency syndrome (AIDS). *Pathology.* 1988;20:211-215.

5. Membreno L, Irony I, Dere W, Klein R, Biglieri EG, Cobb E. Adrenocortical function in acquired immunodeficiency syndrome. *J Clin Endocrinol Metab.* 1987;65:482-487.

6. Dobs AS, Dempsey MA, Ladenson PW, Polk BF. Endocrine disorders in men infected with human immunodeficiency virus. *Am J Med.* 1988;84:611-616.

7. Aaron DC. Endocrine complications of the acquired immunodeficiency syndrome. *Arch Intern Med.* 1988;149:330-333.

8. LoPresti JS, Fried JC, Spencer CA, Nicoloff JT. Unique alterations of thyroid hormone indices in the acquired immunodeficiency syndrome (AIDS). *Ann Intern Med.* 1989;110:970-975.

9. Rubinstein A. Pediatric AIDS. *Curr Probl Pediatr.* 1986;16:384.

10. Centers for Disease Control. Classification for human immunodeficiency virus (HIV): infection in children under thirteen years of age. *MMWR.* 1987;36:225, 235.

11. Utiger RD. Tests of thyroregulatory mechanisms. In: Ingar SH, Braverman LE, eds. *Werner's The Thyroid.* 5th ed. Philadelphia, Pa: JB Lippincott; 1986:511-523.

12. Bricaire F, Marche C, Zoubi D, Regnier B, Saimot AG. Adrenocortical lesions and AIDS. *Lancet.* 1988;1:881.

13. Saimot AG, Marche C, Mayorga R, et al. Pituitary gland involvement in AIDS: a 57 case pathological study. In: Proceedings of the Third International Conference on AIDS; June 1987; Washington, DC. Abstract 137.

14. Kruth PH, Katz JF. Kaposi's sarcoma involving the thyroid in a patient with AIDS. *Clin Nucl Med.* 1987;12:84-89.

15. Frank JS, Livolsi VA, Connor AM. Cytomegalovirus infection of the thyroid in immunocompromised adults. *Yale J Biol Med.* 1987;60:1-8.

16. Greene LW, Cole W, Greene JB, et al. Adrenal insufficiency as a complication of the acquired immunodeficiency syndrome. *Ann Intern Med.* 1984;101:497-498.

17. Guenthner BE, Rabinowe SL, Van Neil A, Naftilan A, Dluhy RG. Primary Addison's disease in a patient with the acquired immunodeficiency syndrome. *Ann Intern Med.* 1984;100:847-848.

18. Kalin MF, Pretsky L, Seres DS, Zumoff B. Hyporeninemic hypoaldosteronism associated with the acquired immune deficiency syndrome. *Ann J Med.* 1987;82:1035-1038.

19. Mulhall BP, Fieldhouse S, Deam D. Adrenocortical lesions and HIV infection. *Lancet.* 1988;1:1345.

20. Verges B, Chavanet P, Kisterman JP, et al. Adrenocortical lesions and HIV infection. *Lancet.* 1988;1:1345.

21. Milligan SA, Katz MS, Craven PC, Strandberg DA, Russell LJ, Becker RA. Toxoplasmosis presenting as panhypopituitarism in a patient with the acquired immune deficiency syndrome. *Am J Med.* 1984;77:760-764.

22. Miller JD, Zaia JA. Isolated growth hormone deficiency in association with human immunodeficiency virus (HIV) infection. *Pediatr Res.* 1987;21:25A.

23. Rappaport R, McSherry G, Connor E, et al. Growth and hormonal parameters in symptomatic human immunodeficiency virus (HIV) infected children. *Pediatr Res.* 1989;25:187A.

24. Goodinson SM, Dickerson JW. Assessment of nutritional status. In: Dickerson JW, Lee HA, eds. *Nutrition in the Clinical Management of Disease.* Baltimore, Md: Edward Arnold Publishers Ltd; 1988:468-469.

25. Kaufman FR, Gomperts ED. Growth failure in boys with hemophilia and HIV infection. *Am J Pediatr Hematol Oncol.* 1989;11:292-294.

26. Welch K, Finkbeiner W, Alpers CE, et al. Autopsy findings in the acquired immunodeficiency syndrome. *JAMA.* 1984;252:1152-1159.

27. Clemmons DR, Klibanski A, Underwood LE, et al. Reduction of immunoreactive somatomedin-C during fasting in humans. *J Clin Endocrinol Metab.* 1981;53:1247-1250.

REFERENCE 1. Schuckit MA. *Drug and Alcohol Abuse. A Clinical Guide to Diagnosis and Treatment.* New York, NY: Plenum Medical Book Company; 1979: 25, 71-73.

Radiological Case of the Month

Michele K. Holloway, MD; Suman Wason, MD, MBA; J. Paul Willging, MD; Charles M. Myer III, MD (Contributors); *Beverly P. Wood, MD* (Section Editor)

A 5-year-old girl presented to the emergency department with a history of shortness of breath and coughing. Although she had been coughing for several weeks, there was an abrupt change in character and the cough became more "croupy" on the night of her presentation to the hospital. The patient complained of a "scratchy" sensation in her throat. No fever was reported.

On physical examination, the patient's vital signs were as follows: temperature, 37.2°C; pulse, 150 beats per minute; respiratory rate, 26 per minute; and blood pressure, 120/65 mm Hg. She was a well-developed child who was alert and cooperative. She was not in respiratory distress, but had a dry, croupy cough and mild inspiratory and expiratory stridor, and constantly attempted to clear her throat. The remainder of the examination findings were normal. A pulse oximeter reading showed 95% to 100% oxygen saturation in room air. Chest radiographic findings were normal.

A diagnosis of foreign body aspiration or foreign body lodged within the pharynx was entertained, although the patient denied any foreign body ingestion. A lateral neck roentgenogram was obtained (Fig 1), and reportedly demonstrated a calcified foreign body at the level of the hypopharynx. An otolaryngologist was consulted to remove the foreign body.

Accepted for publication March 12, 1990.

From the Emergency Department (Drs Holloway and Wason) and the Department of Otolaryngology and Maxillofacial Surgery (Drs Willging and Myer), Children's Hospital Medical Center, University of Cincinnati, Ohio.

Reprint requests to the Department of Radiology, Childrens Hospital of Los Angeles, 4650 Sunset Blvd, Los Angeles, CA 90027 (Dr Wood).

Figure 1.

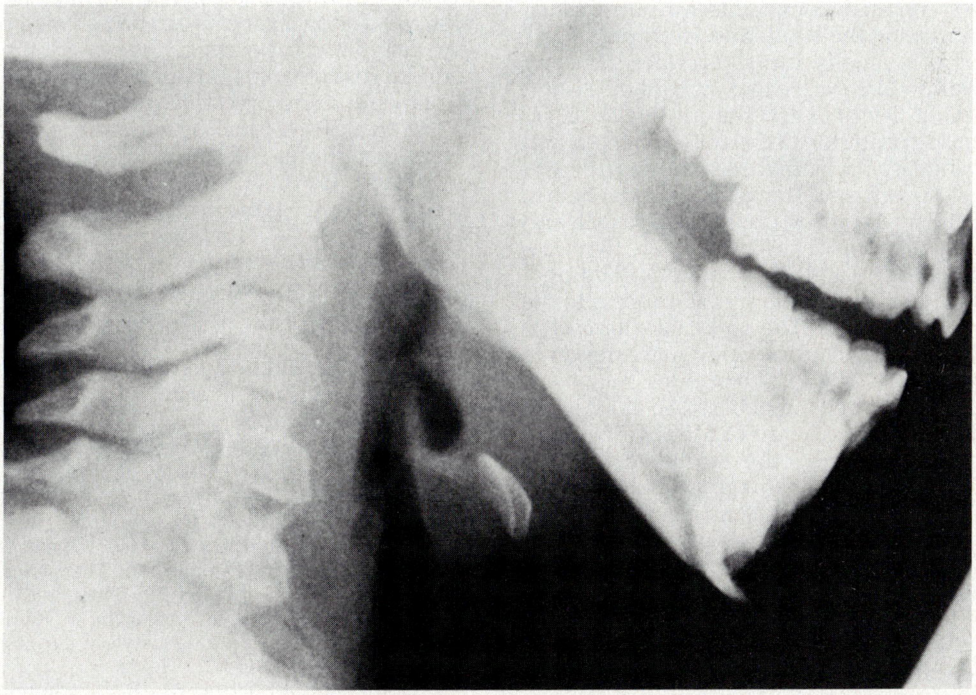

Denouement and Discussion

A Pediatric Case of Eagle's Syndrome

Fig 1.—*Lateral neck roentgenogram showing a calcification extending from C-1 to the angle of the mandible.*

Fig 2.—*Diagram demonstrates the stylomandibular, stylohyoid ligament complex. A indicates stylomandibular ligament; and B, stylohyoid ligament.*

On review of the radiographs, we identified the "foreign body" as a calcified stylomandibular ligament. The scratchy sensation and continual clearing of the throat were symptoms associated with this calcified ligament. The patient was reassured and no therapy was administered. Incidental sinus radiograms were obtained and showed bilateral maxillary sinus opacification. The patient was given a diagnosis of chronic sinusitis and symptomatic calcified stylomandibular ligament; she was discharged while receiving amoxicillin treatment.

Eagle's syndrome is defined as the symptomatic mineralization of the stylohyoid-stylomandibular ligament complex (MSSLC).[1] The variations of the styloid process and its adjoining ligaments have been of interest to anatomists for 300 years, most recently in relation to the advent of diagnostic radiology.

Eagle reported more than 200 cases in the 1930s and 1940s and documented symptoms associated with anomalies of the styloid process. Although many patients are asymptomatic, the symptoms associated with MSSLC are related to the hypopharynx. These include dysphagia (80%), pharyngeal foreign body sensation (55%), and constant aching in the throat (40%).[2] Less common complaints include otalgia, headache, pain on turning the head, and facial pain.[3]

The styloid process is usually a small, slender, tapering projection of the temporal bone located in front of the stylomastoid foramen. It lies between the internal and external carotid arteries, posterior to the tonsillar fossa and lateral to the pharyngeal wall, with three muscles (the stylopharyngeus, stylohyoid, and styloglossus) attached to it. These are supplied by the glossopharyngeal, facial, and hypoglossal nerves, respectively. At the apex, two ligaments are inserted into the styloid. The stylohyoid ligament extends from the far end of the styloid process to the lesser cornu of the hyoid bone. The stylomandibular ligament is inserted at the angle of the apex and extends to the angle of the mandible (Fig 2).[2-5]

A radiographic survey of 4200 men aged 18 to 22 years demonstrated only a 1.4% incidence of MSSLC. None of the patients was symptomatic. In other studies, 8% to 28% of patients with MSSLC have been symptomatic. Clinically, the syndrome is usually not seen prior to age 30 years.[3] In a review of the literature by Gossman and Tarsitano,[3] only one patient younger than 30 years was found to be symptomatic. The anomaly is present more frequently in the 40- to 80-year age range, with symptoms developing after the fourth decade.[6] The etiology of the mineralization is unknown. There is no significant sex predilection in the occurrence of MSSLC[3]; however, symptoms are more common among women.[4]

The radiographic diagnosis of the MSSLC is best made with a temporomandibular joint panoramic radiograph and frontal and lateral projections of the neck to visualize the anatomy in three planes. The anomaly is bilateral and the elongated styloid process can be palpated by inserting a finger orally along the occlusal line posterior to the region of the tonsillar fossa. Pain is experienced as the elongated process is palpated. Another test is to administer regional anesthesia in the area of the tonsillar fossa for relief of symptoms.[3]

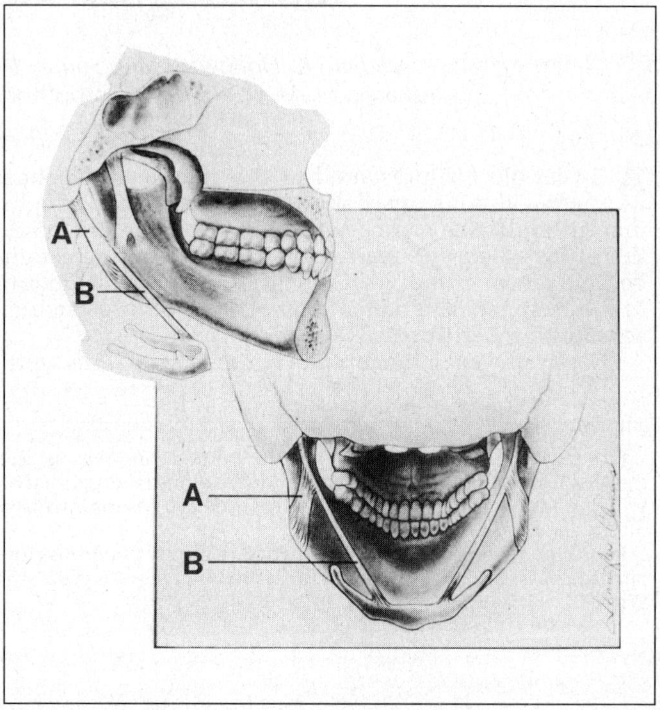

Figure 2.

The differential diagnosis of Eagle's syndrome includes impacted third molars; migrainous neuralgias; trigeminal, vagoglossal, or geniculate neuralgias; temporomandibular joint abnormalities; and psychosomatic disease.[1]

Treatment in severely symptomatic patients is surgical excision of the styloid process. Most patients require only reassurance and symptomatic treatment. Calcification of the styloid process is not an uncommon occurrence and physicians should be aware of this entity when entertaining the diagnosis of an atypical pharyngeal foreign body.

References

1. Correll RW, Wescott WB. Eagle's syndrome diagnosed after history of headache, dysphagia, otalgia, and limited neck movement. *J Am Dent Assoc.* 1982;104:491-492.
2. Lavine MH, Stoopack JC, Jerrold TL. Calcification of the stylohyoid ligament. *Oral Surg Oral Med Oral Pathol.* 1968;25:55-58.
3. Gossman JR Jr, Tarsitano JJ. The styloid-stylohyoid syndrome. *J Oral Surg.* 1977;35:555-560.
4. Keur JJ, Campbell JP, McCarthy JF, Ralph WJ. The clinical significance of the elongated styloid process. *Oral Surg Oral Med Oral Pathol.* 1986;61:399-404.
5. Goldstein GR, Scopp IW. Radiographic interpretation of calcified stylomandibular and stylohyoid ligaments. *J Prosthet Dent.* 1973;30:330-334.
6. Correll RW, Jensen JL, Taylor JB, Rhyne RR. Mineralization of the stylohoid-stylomandibular ligament complex: a radiographic incidence study. *Oral Surg.* 1979;48:286-291.

SPECIAL FEATURE

Picture of the Month

Diane E. Friedman, MEd; Richard J. Pines, DO; Matthew Shelley, MD; Pamela Fisher, MD; G. Michael Silberbach, MD (Contributors); *Murray Feingold, MD* (Section Editor)

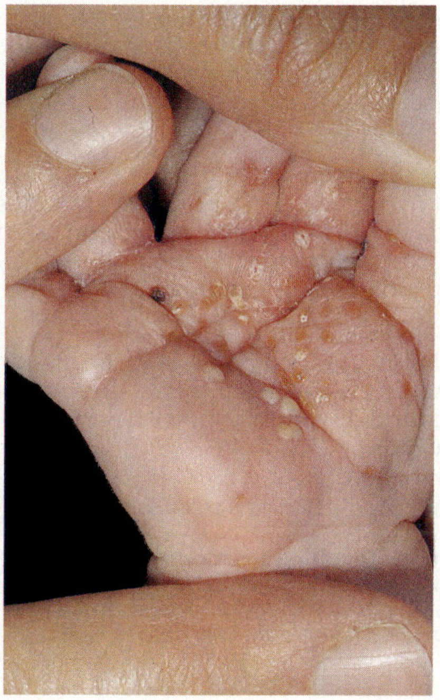

Figure 1.

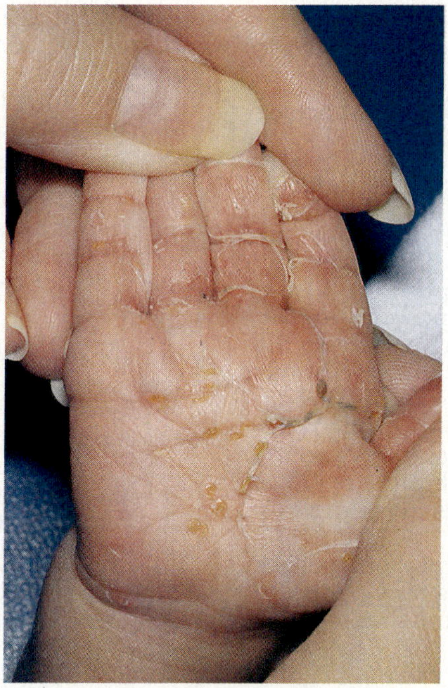

Figure 2.

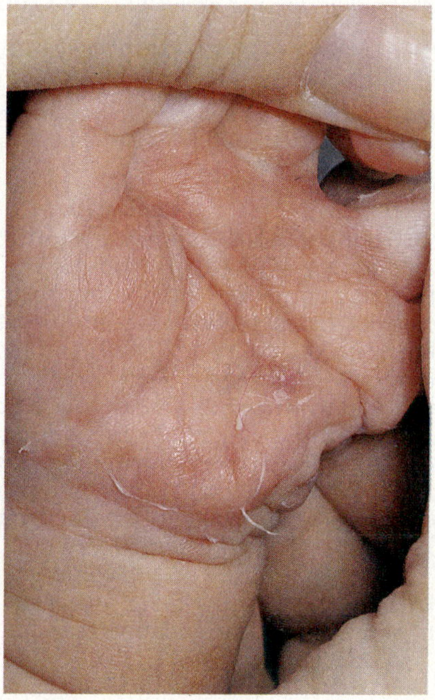

Figure 3.

Figure 4.

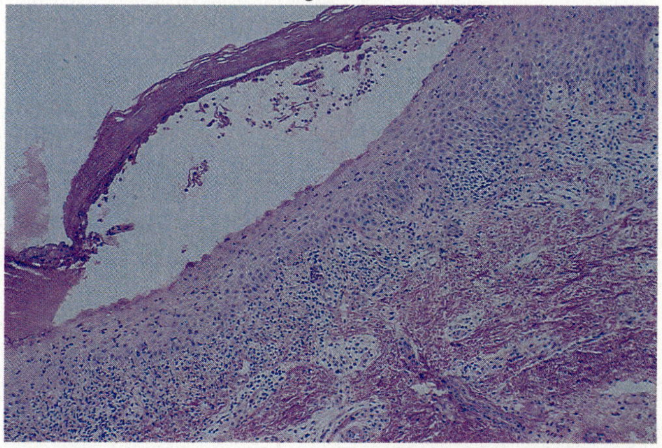

Accepted for publication November 3, 1990.

Contributed from the Department of Pediatrics, Oregon Health Sciences University, Portland.

Reprint requests to the National Birth Defects Center, Franciscan Children's Hospital, 30 Warren St, Brighton, MA 02135 (Dr Feingold).

The Editors welcome contributions to Picture of the Month and Radiological Case of the Month. Those who wish to contribute should send their manuscripts to Dr Feingold (Picture of the Month), National Birth Defects Center, Kennedy Memorial Hospital, 30 Warren St, Brighton, MA 02135, or Dr Wood (Radiological Case of the Month), Department of Radiology, Childrens Hospital of Los Angeles, 4650 Sunset Blvd, Los Angeles, CA 90027. Articles and photographs accepted for publication will bear the contributor's name. There is no charge for reproduction and printing of color illustrations.

Denouement and Discussion

Acropustulosis of Infancy

Fig 1.—*Hand at presentation showing circumscribed, intensely pruritic, pustular dermatitis.*

Fig 2.—*Hand 1 week after presentation showing resolving lesions with peeling skin and no pustules.*

Fig 3.—*Hand 2 weeks after presentation, with minimal peeling of the skin.*

Fig 4.—*Photomicrograph of biopsy specimen of pustule showing subcorneal accumulation of neutrophils.*

Manifestations

Acropustulosis of infancy is an uncommon but distinctive dermatosis often mistaken for pustular impetigo. The unusual cutaneous distribution is the principle distinguishing characteristic. Sterile, pruritic pustules appear mainly on the palms and soles and less frequently on the dorsum of the hands, feet, wrists, and ankles. Lesions evolve from pinpoint-sized erythematous papules that enlarge to form well-circumscribed pustules. Eruptions appear to be more severe during the summer. Onset occurs usually between ages 2 and 10 months, but the rash has been observed in newborns. Recurrences in children up to age 2 years have been reported.

Diagnosis is based on the clinical presentation and lack of response to antibiotic or antifungal therapy. Cultures of the pustules are invariably sterile unless associated with secondary infection. Histologic examination of the lesion demonstrates a circumscribed, subcorneal pustule filled with polymorphonuclear leukocytes. The floor of the pustule consists of compact keratin and the base has a compressed atrophic malpighian layer. The papillary dermis shows slight edema.

The differential diagnosis of acropustulosis of infancy includes dyshidrotic eczema, pustular psoriasis, toxic erythema of the newborn, transient neonatal pustular melanosis, infantile scabies, subcorneal pustular dermatosis, and impetigo.

Genetics

The cause is unknown. A genetic predisposition has been postulated since most cases occur in black or Asian children. Unlike other types of aseptic dermatosis, a family history of atopy or psoriasis is uncommon.

Treatment

Acropustulosis of infancy is self-limited, with no known adverse sequelae. Therapy is directed toward relieving the symptoms of pruritus and discomfort and preventing secondary bacterial infection.

References

1. Kahn G, Rywlin AM. Acropustulosis of infancy. *Arch Dermatol.* 1979;115:831-833.
2. Jarratt M, Ramsdell W. Infantile acropustulosis. *Arch Dermatol.* 1979;115:834-836.
3. Newton JA, Salisbury J, Marsden A, McGibbon DH. Acropustulosis of infancy. *Br J Dermatol.* 1986;115:735-739.

Ambulatory Pediatric Association

Program and Abstracts

31st Annual Meeting
April 29–May 3, 1991
Riverside Hilton
New Orleans, La

All of the material received from the Ambulatory Pediatric Association, including the abstracts, has been printed as received without copyediting by the staff at AJDC *or the AMA. The AMA,* AJDC, *and the Editor are not responsible for any errors in content, style, grammar, or spelling.*

APA Application for Membership

Information for Prospective Members

The objectives of the Ambulatory Pediatric Association are to improve the teaching of general pediatrics, to improve research in general pediatrics, to improve patient services in general pediatrics, and to affect public and governmental opinion regarding issues vital to teaching and research in general pediatrics. Applications for membership will be considered from members of the health care professions involved in teaching and patient care or research in general pediatrics.

Application forms are obtained from the Executive Secretary's Office:

Executive Secretary
Ambulatory Pediatric Association
6728 Old McLean Village Dr
McLean, VA 22101
(703) 556-9222

Future Annual Meetings

1992—*May 4-8, Baltimore Convention Center, Baltimore, Md*
1993—*May 3-7, Sheraton Hotel, Washington, DC*
1994—*May 2-5, Seattle Convention Center, Seattle, Wash*
1995—*May 8-12, San Diego, Calif*
1996—*May 6-10, Washington, DC*

APA PROGRAM SCHEDULE

Sunday, April 28

Time	Event	Room
5 PM-10 PM	APA Board of Directors Meeting	Oak Alley

Monday, April 29

Time	Event	Room
8 AM-NOON	*APA Board of Directors Meeting*	Melrose
3:30 PM-7 PM	*Poster Session APA/APS/SPR (p 373)*	South Hall Rivergate Convention Center
7 PM-8 PM	*Opening Reception APA/APS/SPR*	South Hall Rivergate Convention Center

Tuesday, April 30

Time	Event	Room
7:30 AM-9 AM	*Past Officers Breakfast*	Belle Chasse
	APA Special Interest Groups	
8 AM-NOON	Clerkship Directors	Marlborough Suite
	Emergency Medicine	Versailles
9 AM-NOON	*APA Special Interest Groups*	
	Women in Medicine	Cambridge
	International Health	Grand Salon Section 3
	Residency Program Directors	Prince of Wales
	Serving the Underserved	Grand Salon Section 6
	APA Workshops 1-10 (p 372)	
	Workshop 1	Oak Alley
	Workshop 2	Newberry
	Workshop 3	Eglington & Winton
	Workshop 4	Norwich
	Workshop 5	Durham
	Workshop 6	Jasperwood
	Workshop 7	Burgundy
	Workshop 8	Magnolia
	Workshop 9	Chequers
	Workshop 10	Grand Salon Section 4
NOON-2 PM	*APA Regional Chairs Luncheon*	Trafalgar
	APA SIG Chairs Luncheon	Ascot
2:40 PM-3 PM	*St. Geme Award*	Grand Ballrooms A&B
3 PM-6:30 PM	*APA/APS/SPR Joint Topic Sessions (p 374)*	
	Adolescent Medicine	Grand Ballroom C
	Behavioral Pediatrics	Grand Salon D
	Epidemiology & Preventive Pediatrics	Grand Salon C
	General Pediatrics & Pediatric Education	Grand Ballroom D
6:30 PM-8:30 PM	*APA Committees*	
	Child Health Care Delivery	Newberry
	Research	Norwich
	Education	Durham
	Public Policy	Ascot
	Communications	Warwick

Wednesday, May 1

Time	Event	Room
7:30 AM-9 AM	*APA Regional Breakfast Meetings*	
	Region I	Durham
	Region II	Elmwood
	Region III	Cambridge
	Region IV	Norwich
	Region V	Magnolia
	Region VI	Newberry
	Region VII	Prince of Wales
	Region VIII	Ascot
	Region IX	Eglington & Winton
	Region X	Chequers
9 AM-NOON	*APA Topic Plenary Session (p 377)*	
	Clinical Issues	Grand Ballroom C
	Developmental & Behavioral Pediatrics	Grand Salon A
	Emergency Medicine & Child Abuse	Grand Salon B
	General Pediatrics	Grand Salon C
	Prevention & Epidemiology	Grand Salon D

APA Program Schedule

Time	Event	Room
1:30 PM-4:30 PM	*APA Workshops 11-20 (p 372)*	
	Workshop 11	Jasperwood
	Workshop 12	Cambridge
	Workshop 13	Eglington & Winton
	Workshop 14	Newberry
	Workshop 15	Ascot
	Workshop 16	Norwich
	Workshop 17	Burgundy
	Workshop 18	Durham
	Workshop 19	Elmwood
	Workshop 20	Trafalgar
	APA Special Interest Groups	
	Adolescent Medicine	Rosedown
	AIDS	Chequers
	Behavioral Pediatrics	Magnolia
	Child Abuse	Prince of Wales
	Injury Control	Oak Alley
	Primary Care	Melrose
4:45 PM-6:45 PM	*APA Awards & Business Meeting*	Grand Salon C
	APA Research Award	
	APA Teaching Award	
	APA Business Meeting	
8:30 PM-10 PM	*APA Debate*	Grand Salon A

Thursday, May 2

Time	Event	Room
8 AM-NOON	*APA General Plenary Session (p 379)*	Grand Salon D
	Distinguished Career Award	
	President's Address	
1:30 PM-4:30 PM	*APA Workshops 21-30 (p 373)*	
	Workshop 21	Jasperwood
	Workshop 22	Ascot
	Workshop 23	Newberry
	Workshop 24	Durham
	Workshop 25	Magnolia
	Workshop 26	Cambridge
	Workshop 27	Trafalgar
	Workshop 28	Chequers
	Workshop 29	Eglington & Winton
	Workshop 30	Prince of Wales
	APA Special Interest Groups	
	Chronic Illness	Elmwood
	Continuity Clinic	Rosedown
	Day Care	Melrose
	Homeless Children	Oak Alley
	Nutrition	Norwich
5:15 PM-6 PM	*APA Armstrong Award*	Grand Ballroom C
6 PM-7 PM	*APA Reception*	Melrose

Friday, May 3

Time	Event	Room
8 AM-2 PM	APA Board of Directors Meeting	Oak Alley

Registration Hours

Sunday, April 28	NOON-5 PM
Monday, April 29	8 AM-8 PM
Tuesday, April 30	7 AM-8 PM
Wednesday, May 1	7 AM-6 PM
Thursday, May 2	7:30 AM-5 PM
Friday, May 3	8 AM-NOON

Workshop Registration

Tuesday, April 30	7:15 AM-6 PM
Wednesday, May 1	7:15 AM-5:30 PM
Thursday, May 2	7:15 AM-12:30 PM

As an organization accredited for continuing medical education, the America Academy of Pediatrics designates this continuing medical activity as meeting the criteria for 43.5 credit hours in category 1 of the Physician's Recognition Award of the American Medical Association. To those currently enrolled in the American Academy of Pediatrics PREP program, this course is eligible for 43.5 PREP credits.

The California State Board of Registered Nursing has approved this program for 23 Continuing Education Credits for Registered Nurses. Certificates will be available at the APA registration desk.

Officers

President	*Carol Berkowitz, MD,* Torrance, Calif
President-Elect	*Kathleen G. Nelson, MD,* Birmingham, Ala
Secretary-Treasurer	*Thomas G. DeWitt, MD,* Worcester, Mass
Immediate Past President	*Paul McCarthy, MD,* New Haven, Conn
Newsletter Editor	*John M. Pascoe, MD, MPH,* Madison, Wis

Board of Directors

Ruth T. Gross, MD, Stanford, Calif
John M. Leventhal, MD, New Haven, Conn
Stephen Ludwig, MD, Philadelphia, Pa
Lucy Osborn, MD, Salt Lake City, Utah
Robert H. Pantell, MD, San Francisco, Calif
Modena E. H. Wilson, MD, MPH, Baltimore, Md

Past Presidents

1961-1962 *Richard W. Olmsted*
1962-1963 *Morris Green*
1963-1964 *Robert J. Haggerty*
1964-1965 *Frederic M. Blodgett*
1965-1966 *Donal Dunphy*
1966-1967 *Loren G. MacKinney*
1967-1968 *Lewis M. Fraad*
1968-1969 *Hugo Dunlap Smith*
1969-1970 *Joel J. Alpert*
1970-1971 *John H. Kennell*
1971-1972 *Donald Fink*
1972-1973 *Ray E. Helfer*
1973-1974 *Katherine S. Lobach*
1974-1975 *Evan Charney*
1975-1976 *Frederick North, Jr.*
1976-1977 *Margaret C. Heagarty*
1977-1978 *Robert Hoekelman*
1978-1979 *George Comerci*
1979-1980 *Ivan Barry Pless*
1980-1981 *Barbara Starfield*
1981-1982 *Alvin Novack*
1982-1983 *Philip Nader*
1983-1984 *Fredric D. Burg*
1984-1985 *Abraham B. Bergman*
1985-1986 *Catherine DeAngelis*
1986-1987 *Jay E. Berkelhamer*
1987-1988 *Ruth E. K. Stein*
1988-1989 *Steven P. Shelov*
1989-1990 *Paul McCarthy*

Regional Chairs

I. *William G. Bithoney, MD,* West Roxbury, Mass
II. *Alan B. Bernstein, MD,* Brooklyn, NY
Mary Ann LoFrumento, MD, Morristown, NJ
III. *Kenneth M. McConnochie, MD,* Rochester, NY
IV. *Gregory Hayden, MD,* Charlottesville, Va
V. *John Chessare, MD, MPH,* Toledo, Ohio
Daniel Coury, MD, Columbus, Ohio
VI. *Timothy Russell Schum, MD,* Milwaukee, Wis
Patricia S. Simmons, MD, Rochester, Minn
VII. *Pamela Wood, MD,* San Antonio, Tex
VIII. *Joseph Pesek, MD,* Jacksonville, Fla
IX. *Sandra L. Elvik, MS, CPNP,* Torrance, Calif
Stanley Howard Inkelis, MD, Los Angeles, Calif
X. *Kathi Kemper, MD,* Seattle, Wash

Past Secretary-Treasurers

1961-1963 Frederic M. Blodgett
1963-1966 Hugo Dunlap Smith
1966-1969 Abraham B. Bergman
1969-1972 Katherine S. Lobach
1972-1974 Elizabeth S. Hillman
1974-1977 George Comerci
1977-1980 Fredric D. Burg
1980-1983 Barbara Durand
1983-1986 Marie McCormick
1986-1989 Kathleen Nelson

APA Teaching Award

The purpose of this award is to foster interest in the teaching of ambulatory pediatrics by giving national recognition to an outstanding ambulatory pediatric program. Programs must demonstrate excellence in educational teaching methods, acceptance by students and/or residents, acceptance by the community and the institution, innovations and adaptability, or outstanding quality of the individuals trained in the program. Emphasis is placed on the award being given to *an* outstanding *program*.

1972 University of Arizona
College of Medicine
Department of Pediatrics
Division of Ambulatory Pediatrics
Tucson

1976 University of Chicago
Pritzker School of Medicine
Wyler Children's Hospital
Division of Ambulatory Pediatrics

1977 University of Vermont
College of Medicine
Department of Pediatrics
Division of Ambulatory Pediatrics
Burlington, Vt

1978 Children's Hospital of Philadelphia
Division of Ambulatory Services
Resident Group Practice

1980 Primary Care Training Program
Department of Pediatrics
University of Arizona
College of Medicine
Tucson

1981 Sinai Hospital of Baltimore
Pediatric Residency Training Program

1982 Child Health Associate Program
University of Colorado
Health Sciences Center
Denver

1984 University of North Carolina—Chapel Hill
Department of Pediatrics
Community Outreach Training Program

1986 Pediatric Practice Model
University of Oklahoma College of Medicine
Oklahoma City

1987 Chronic Illness Teaching Program
Department of Pediatrics and
Human Development
Michigan State University
East Lansing

1988 Emergency Room Teaching Program
Children's Hospital of Philadelphia (Pa)
and
Behavioral and Developmental
Pediatric Fellowship Program
Department of Pediatrics
Ohio State University
Columbus

1989 Primary Care Training Program
University of California—
San Diego Department of Pediatrics
Division of General Pediatrics

1990 Behavioral Science Training Program
University of California—San Francisco

1991 University of Utah Pediatric Residency Program
University of Utah Center for Health Sciences
and the
Primary Children's Medical Center
and
Third Year Pediatric Clerkship (MS III)
Department of Pediatrics
F. Edward Hebert School of Medicine
Uniformed Services University of the
Health Sciences

APA RESEARCH AWARD

The APA Research Award acknowledges the contribution of an individual in advancing pediatric knowledge through excellence in research. Research excellence is characterized by originality, creativity, and methodological soundness. The findings should contribute significantly to the general health of children in such areas as understanding mechanisms of health and disease, methods of education, and innovative ways of providing children's services.

1990 ***Barbara Starfield***

1991 ***Ivan Barry Pless***

APA DISTINGUISHED CAREER AWARD

The APA Distinguished Career Award recognizes members of the Association who have fostered the goals of the APA throughout their careers. They have distinguished themselves in the promotion of improved patient care, teaching, and research in ambulatory pediatrics.

1991 ***Barbara M. Korsch***

The George Armstrong Lectures

George Armstrong, an English physician of the 18th century, established the first dispensary for children in London, England, in 1769. There he served with great devotion and taught others the care of sick children. He is honored as one of the fathers of modern pediatrics, and those who deliver this lecture are also honored as outstanding teachers and contributors to our knowledge of the care of children.
The lecture is sponsored by Ross Laboratories, Columbus, Ohio.

1967 George A. Silver
1968 Allan M. Butler
1969 Robert H. Haggerty
1970 Julius B. Richmond
1971 Morris Green
1972 Henry K. Silver
1973 Barbara M. Korsch
1974 Lewis Fraad
1975 C. Henry Kempe
1976 Abraham B. Bergman
Waldo Nelson
1977 Wilbur J. Cohen
1978 Richard W. Olmsted
1979 John H. Kennell
(Children's Defense Fund)
1980 OXFAM (Tim Lusty)
1981 Benjamin Spock
1982 Evan Charney
1983 Barbara Starfield
1984 Victor Vaughan
1985 Gerold L. Schiebler
1986 Marian Wright Edelman
1987 Robert A. Hoekelman
1988 Ivan Barry Pless
1989 Joel J. Alpert
1990 Catherine DeAngelis
1991 Paul L. McCarthy

APA Workshops and Special Interest Groups

Tuesday, April 30, 1991
9 AM-NOON

1. **Federal Funding for Health Services Research in Primary Care** *Oak Alley*
   Leaders: *P. A. Nutting and B. A. White*
2. **Evaluation Research: The Impossible Made Easy** *Newberry*
   Leaders: *L. J. Bauman and R. E. K. Stein*
3. **Logistic Regression: A Guide for the Slightly Perplexed** *Eglington & Winton*
   Leaders: *P. Margolis and S. Goodman*
4. **Sex Education in Adolescents with Chronic Diseases and Disabilities** *Norwich*
   Leaders: *B. A. Cromer, S. J. Rost, and M. J. Gerhardstein*
5. **Foster Children—Meeting Their Health Care Needs** *Durham*
   Leaders: *R. Chernoff, H. Dubowitz, D. Chadwick, M. Simms, and N. Kaufman*
6. **Pediatricians Facilitation of Healthy Sexual Development With Families** *Jasperwood*
   Leaders: *C. A. Croft and M. C. Sorrentino*
7. **Primate Parallels: Mothers, Infants and Love** *Burgundy*
   Leader: *R. E. Helfer*
8. **"Please Don't Die on My Shift"—Helping the Pediatrician Deal With Patient Death** *Magnolia*
   Leaders: *D. J. Timmel and D. J. Schonfeld*
9. **Children and Venipuncture: Coping Skills for Professionals and Patients** *Chequers*
   Leaders: *M.H. Young, S. Franklin, N. Powers, and D. Moiles*
10. **Society for Behavioral Pediatrics Workshop: Child Development Projects: Collaboration Between Educators and Pediatricians** *Grand Salon Section 4*
    Leaders: *B. Zuckerman, M. Kaplan-Sanoff, R. Needlman, and K. Bresnahan*

Special Interest Groups

Clerkship Directors (8 AM-NOON) *Marlborough Suite*
Emergency Medicine (8 AM-NOON) *Versailles*
Women in Medicine *Cambridge*
International Health *Grand Salon Section 3*
Residency Program Directors *Prince of Wales*
Serving the Underserved *Grand Salon Section 6*

Wednesday, May 1, 1990
1:30 PM-4:30 PM

11. **New Concepts in the Screening, Management, and Neurotoxicity of Childhood Lead Poisoning** *Jasperwood*
    Leaders: *J. W. Graef, M. Shannon, and D. Bellinger*
12. **Schools and Day Care Centers: Innovative Settings for Residency Training** *Cambridge*
    Leaders: *E. C. Allen, L. S. Grossman, and J. C. Joost*
13. **Community-Based Continuity Clinic Programs: Practical Approaches to Implementation** *Eglington & Winton*
    Leaders: *L. M. Osborn, J. R. Sargent, S. D. Williams, T. G. DeWitt, and K. B. Roberts*
14. **Child Development, Pain, and Mental Imagery** *Newberry*
    Leaders: *R. Solomon and C. Saylor*
15. **Preparing Interns for Residency: A "Teaching and Leadership" Seminar** *Ascot*
    Leaders: *J. Anderson, C. Chantry, R. Kamei, and K. Overby*
16. **Stayin' Alive in Pediatric Emergency Medicine** *Norwich*
    Leaders: *S. Selbst, F. Henretig, S. Ludwig, K. Shaw, and C. McAneney*
17. **Quality Assurance in the Emergency Department** *Burgundy*
    Leaders: *F. Oberklaid and F. Jarman*
18. **Problem-Based Learning in Pediatrics** *Durham*
    Leaders: *F. A. McCurdy, J. O. Lopreiato, C. B. White, and B. A. DeFrancesco*
19. **Resuscitating Your Continuity Clinic** *Elmwood*
    Leaders: *J. E. Drutz, D. Kittredge, D. C. Hurley, C. R. Reed, R. M. Rutstein, R. C. Baker, L. R. First, J. N. Middlekamp, and M. E. H. Wilson*
20. **An Academic Seminar: Beyond Epidemiology and Biostatistics** *Trafalgar*
    Leaders: *H. Bauchner, J. Howland, and R. Needlman*

Special Interest Groups

Adolescent Medicine *Rosedown*
AIDS *Chequers*
Behavioral Pediatrics *Magnolia*
Child Abuse *Prince of Wales*
Injury Control *Oak Alley*
Primary Care *Melrose*

APA Workshops and Special Interest Groups

Thursday, May 2, 1991
1:30 PM-4:30 PM

21. **Anatomy and Physiology of Successful Residency Educational Programs: What We Can Learn and Apply Back Home** *Jasperwood*
Leaders: *J. M. Devries and L. Osborn*

22. **How to Write an Abstract** *Ascot*
Leaders: *K. J. Kemper and F. P. Rivara*

23. **Sample Size Estimation for Clinical Research** *Newberry*
Leader: *T. B. Newman*

24. **The Medical Interview and Clinical Problem Solving as an Educational Orientation for Medical Students and House Officers** *Durham*
Leaders: *A. P. Scheiner and B. Siegel*

25. **Reinterpreting Disability: Origins and Consequences of the Supreme Court SSI Decision** *Magnolia*
Leaders: *J. M. Perrin, R. E. K. Stein, and S. Davis*

26. **Integration of International Child Health Training into Undergraduate and Graduate Pediatric Programs** *Cambridge*
Leaders: *A. Brann, B. Duncan, J. Ey, J. Goldhagen, R. Hill, and R. Pust*

27. **Teaching Residents the Fundamentals of the Sexual Abuse Evaluation Towards a Comprehensive Curriculum** *Trafalgar*
Leaders: *A. Giardino, C. Christian, T. Seidl, W. Schwartz, and S. Ludwig.*

28. **Use of Computer Simulations to Expand the Teaching of General Pediatrics** *Chequers*
Leader: *W. Schwartz*

29. **Wound Management for the Pediatrician: Abrasions to Z-Plasty** *Eglington & Winton*
Leaders: *L. S. Fitzmaurice, J. F. Knapp, and T. M. Barnett*

30. **Law and Order in the Emergency Department—Avoiding Hill Street Blues** *Prince of Wales*
Leaders: *S. Selbst, S. Ludwig, J. Loiselle, and C. Barcliff*

Special Interest Groups

Chronic Illness	*Elmwood*
Continuity Clinic	*Rosedown*
Day Care	*Melrose*
Homeless Children	*Oak Alley*
Nutrition	*Norwich*

General Poster Session

Monday, April 29, 1991
3:30 PM-7 PM
South Hall and Rivergate Convention Center

147 **Direct Bilirubin Measurements in Jaundiced Term Newborns: A Waste of Blood and Money?** *T. B. Newman, S. Hope, and D. K. Stevenson. General Pediatrics and Epidemiology, University of California, San Francisco, and Stanford University, San Francisco.*

148 **Home Phototherapy—Use and Attitudes Among Community Pediatricians.** *S. B. Meropol, A. A. Luberti, A. R. DeJong, and J. C. Weiss. Department of Pediatrics, Jefferson Medical College, Philadelphia, Pa.*

149 **The Health Status of Children Placed with Relatives.** *H. Dubowitz, S. Feigelman, S. Zuravin, V. Tepper, R. Lichenstein, and N. Davidson. Department of Pediatrics, University of Maryland Medical School, Baltimore.*

150 **Foster Children: Predictors of Developmental Problems on Baseline Health Assessment.** *S. M. Horwitz and M. D. Simms. Yale University, Department of Epidemiology and Public Health, New Haven, Conn, and Foster Care Clinic, St Mary's Hospital, Waterbury, Conn.*

151 **Measurement of Gestational Cocaine Exposure.** *C. M. Callahan, T. M. Grant, P. Phipps, G. D. Clark, A. H. Novack, A. P. Streissguth, and V. A. Raisys. University of Washington, Seattle.*

152 **Effects of Head Start on Children with Lead Poisoning.** *B. Howard and E. Charney. Department of Pediatrics, Duke University Medical Center, Durham, NC, and Department of Pediatrics, University of Massachusetts Medical Center, Worcester.*

153 **Elevated Lead (Pb) Levels in Abused Children.** *W. Bithoney, W. Barbaresi, A. Vandeven, and A. Ryan. Children's Hospital, Department of Medicine, Boston, Mass.*

154 **Getting Away with Murder? A Study of Unintentional Child Shootings.** *J. T. Maurer, M. J. Barthel, and R. R. Tanz. Department of Pediatrics, Children's Memorial Hospital, Northwestern University Medical School, Chicago, Ill.*

155 **Patterns of Causation for Intentional Injury in a Population Based Study of Urban Children.** *L. L. Davidson, M. S. Durkin, P. O'Connor, B. Barlow and M. C. Heagarty. Departments of Pediatrics, Pediatric Surgery, and Public Health, Columbia University, New York, NY, and Russell Sage College, Troy, NY.*

156 **Physician Decisions to Report and Label Suspected Child Maltreatment.** *L. S. Wissow, M. E. H. Wilson, and G. L. Zellman. Department of Pediatrics, Johns Hopkins University School of Medicine, Baltimore, Md, and The Rand Corporation, Santa Monica, Calif.*

157 **Sexual Abuse by Father-Figures: A Comparison of Natural Fathers, Stepfathers, and Mothers' Paramours.** *A. R. DeJong. Department of Pediatrics, Jefferson Medical College of Thomas Jefferson University, Philadelphia, Pa.*

158 **An Association Between Sexual Abuse and Early Adolescent Pregnancy.** *J. E. Cox, L. Coyne, and W. G. Bithoney. Department of Pediatrics, Harvard Medical School and Children's Hospital, Boston, Mass.*

159 **Utilization of Prenatal Care by Adolescents: Who Starts When?** *M. C. Pew, J. M. Leventhal, and S. M. Horwitz. Department of Pediatrics, Yale University School of Medicine, New Haven, Conn.*

160 **Adolescent AIDS Education in a Pediatric Emergency Department.** *A. J. Behrman, K. N. Shaw, and F. S. Shofer. Departments of Internal Medicine and Pediatrics, University of Pennsylvania School of Medicine, Philadelphia.*

161 **Clinical Utility of *Chlamydia Trachomatis* Diagnostic Techniques in Adolescent Women.** *F. M. Biro, S. F. Reising, and J. A. Doughman. Department of Pediatrics, Children's Hospital Medical Center, University of Cincinnati (Ohio).*

162 **Peer Screeners to Identify Substance Abuse in Pregnant Teens.** *S. Barnett, D. P. McCormick, G. Wilkinson, and A. Berensen. Departments of Pediatrics, Preventive Medicine/Community Health and Obstetrics, University of Texas Medical Branch, Galveston.*

163 **PID: Evaluation and Treatment in a Pediatric vs Adult Emergency Department.** *J. M. Lavelle, I. Reyes, and K. N. Shaw. Department of Pediatrics, University of Pennsylvania School of Medicine, The Children's Hospital of Philadelphia, and the Hospital of the University of Pennsylvania, Philadelphia.*

164 **Prior Advice Seeking and Appropriate Use of a Pediatric Emergency Room.** *T. F. Oberlander, I. B. Pless, G. E. Dougherty, and D. McGillivray. Department of Pediatrics, McGill University, Montreal, Quebec.*

165 **Prehospital IV Placement in Children.** *K. A. Grisanti and D. M. Jaffe. Department of Pediatrics, Hospital for Sick Children, University of Toronto (Ontario).*

166 **Responses of Children, Parents, and Nurses to Tympanic Thermometry in the Pediatric Office.** *D. T. Alexander and B. A. Kelly. Department of Pediatrics, University of Pennsylvania School of Medicine, Philadelphia, and Children's Hospital of Philadelphia.*

167 **Effect of Personalized Letter Reminders on Preventive Appointment Show Rates and Vaccination Status.** *J. R. Campbell, P. G. Szilagyi, L. E. Rodewald, C. B. Doane, and K. J. Roghmann. Department of Pediatrics, University of Rochester (NY), Strong Memorial Hospital, Rochester.*

168 **Metal Detectors—An Alternative Approach to the Evaluation of Coin Ingestions in Children?** *S. P. Ros and F. Cetta. Pediatrics, Loyola University Medical Center, Maywood, Ill.*

169 **Efficacy of Cough Suppressants in Treating Nighttime Cough in Children.** *J. A. Taylor, A. H. Novack, J. R. Almquist, and J. E. Rogers. Department of Pediatrics, University of Washington, Seattle, and Carolinas Medical Center, Charlotte, NC.*

170 **Milder Symptoms Occur in Recurrent Episodes of Streptococcal Infection.** *K. A. Woodin, L. H. Lee, and M. E. Pichichero. Department of Pediatrics, University of Rochester, (NY).*

171 **Strategies for Diagnosis (Dx) and Treatment of Febrile Infants: Clinical and Cost-Effectiveness.** *T. A. Lieu, M. N. Baskin, J. S. Schwartz, and G. R. Fleisher. Department of Pediatrics, University of Pennsylvania, Philadelphia.*

172 **Blood Culture in the Outpatient Setting: What is the Optimum Number & Method?** *K. J. DiPasquale, G. G. Gaar, and A. B. Anderson. The Emergency Associates for Medicine, The Tampa (Fla) General Hospital.*

173 **Diagnostic Test Ordering in the Evaluation of Febrile Children: The Role of Physician and Environmental Factors.** *D. L. McGillivray, R. Roberts-Brauer, and M. S. Kramer. Departments of Pediatrics and Epidemiology and Biostatistics, McGill University, Montreal, Quebec.*

174 **Management of Febrile Infants by Practicing Pediatricians.** *D. Bergman, R. Pantell, S. Brotherton, and the PROS Network of the AAP. Department of Pediatrics, University of California, San Francisco.*

175 **The Value of Early Treatment for the Prevention of Lyme Disease.** *F. Agre and R. M. Schwartz. Department of Pediatrics, College of Physicians and Surgeons, Columbia University, New York, NY.*

176 **Adaptive Behavior in Subgroups of Children with Attention Deficit Disorder and Hyperactivity Disorder (ADHD).** *N. J. Roizen, T. A. Blondis, and M. Stein. Department of Pediatrics, University of Chicago (Ill) Pritzker School of Medicine, Wyler Children's Hospital, Chicago.*

177 **Who Provides Health Care to the Children of Physicians?** *L. Dusdieker, J. Murph, C. Dungy, and W. Murph. Department of Pediatrics, University of Iowa Hospitals and Clinics, Iowa City.*

178 **Vulnerable Infants and Doctor-Shopping: Common Psychosocial Determinants?** *A. Okun and R. E. K. Stein. Department of Pediatrics, Albert Einstein College of Medicine, Division of Ambulatory Pediatrics, Bronx (NY) Municipal Hospital Center.*

179 **Agreement of the Mother's and Physician's Perception of the Child's Health Status Correlates with Clinic and Emergency Room Use.** *M. Irigoyen and M. Goldstein. Department of Pediatrics, Babies Hospital and Columbia University, New York, NY.*

180 **Parenting Stress in Families of Urban Third Graders.** *L. S. Grossman, M. M. Kappelman, and R. G. Chernoff. Department of Pediatrics, University of Maryland School of Medicine, Baltimore.*

181 **Maternal Emotional Response to Low Birthweight vs Healthy Infants: Role of Social Support.** *S. J. Hershman, H. T. Ireys, and E. J. Silver. Pediatrics, Albert Einstein College of Medicine, Preventive Intervention Research Center, Bronx, NY.*

182 **Third Trimester Maternal Psychosocial Factors and Home Stimulation for Four Month Old Infants: A Prospective Study.** *J. M. Pascoe and J. French. Department of Pediatrics, University of Wisconsin, Madison, and Department of Human Ecology, Michigan State University, East Lansing.*

183 **The Prevalence of Behavioral and Psychosocial Problems in Pediatric Practices.** *P. J. Leaf, S. M. Horwitz, J. M. Leventhal, and K. N. Speechley. Department of Epidemiology and Public Health, Yale University School of Medicine, New Haven, Conn.*

184 **The Relationship Between Maternal Self-Reported Health Status and Maternal Report of Children's Health Status Among Hispanics.** *F. Mendoza, G. Takata, K. Baisden, L. Herrera, and R. Mortorell. Department of Pediatrics and Food Research Institute, Stanford (Calif) University.*

185 **Life Change Events, Disease Course, ESR, and CPR in Patients with Juvenile Arthritis.** *D. M. Siegel, J. Baum, and S. P. Ellis. Department of Pediatrics, University of Rochester (NY) School of Medicine and Dentistry.*

186 **The Preceptor Report Form: An Assessment Tool for Use in Evaluating Residents in Ambulatory Pediatric Settings.** *J. K. Davis and B. Hermosa. Department of Pediatrics, New York (NY) Medical College and Lincoln Medical and Mental Health Center, Bronx, NY.*

187 **The Care Giving Role: Influences of Residents' Background Characteristics.** *M. E. Zondorak-Perez and R. E. K. Stein. Department of Pediatrics, Albert Einstein College of Medicine, Division of Ambulatory Pediatrics, Bronx (NY) Municipal Hospital Center.*

188 **Medicaid During the Reagan Years: Federal and State Reforms.** *J. D. C. Cartland. Department of Research, American Academy of Pediatrics, Elk Grove Village, Ill.*

189 **Linking Medicaid and Special Education in a Rural State.** *C. Field, R. Kirby, and T. Nosal. Department of Pediatrics, University of Arkansas for Medical Sciences, Little Rock.*

Joint Topic Sessions

With American Pediatric Society and Society for Pediatric Research

Tuesday, April 30, 1991
3 PM-6:30 PM

ADOLESCENT MEDICINE

Grand Ballroom C

Moderators: *Robert H. DuRant, PhD, Martin Fisher, MD, and Elizabeth R. McAnarney, MD*

3:00 ***Gender Differences in Establishing Causal Paths for Self Esteem.** *S. K. Steinmetz and D. P. Orr. Departments of Sociology and Pediatrics, Indiana University, Indianapolis.*

3:15 ***Late Pubertal Maturation is Associated with Less Behavioral Risk.** *D. P. Orr, M. Beiter, J. Ryser, and G. M. Ingersoll. Department of Pediatrics, Indiana University School of Medicine, Indianapolis.*

3:30 ***Street Youth: A Heterogeneous Population.** *N. E. MacDonald, S. I. Davidson, B. Ferguson, G. Wells, W. A. Fisher,*

D. Tate, W. Warren, J. A. Doherty, and W. R. Bowie. CYAS Research Group, Children's Hospital of Eastern Ontario, Ottawa.

3:45 **Access to Handguns Among Urban Adolescents.** *C. M. Callahan and F. P. Rivara. Department of Pediatrics, University of Washington, and Harborview Injury Prevention and Research Center, Seattle.*

4:00 ***HIV Seroprevalence Rates in Sexually Active Adolescent Members of a Health Maintenance Organization.** *A. Tipton, S. Black, and L. Hurley. Department of Pediatrics, Kaiser Permanente Medical Center, Oakland, Calif.*

4:15 ***The Impact of AIDS on a Population of Urban Adolescents: Implications for Intervention.** *K. J. Overby and S. M. Kegeles. Departments of Pediatrics and Medicine, University of California, San Francisco.*

4:30 **Risk Factors for Repeat Adolescent Childbirth.** *L. B. Heery, M. J. Werner, and R. M. Brayden. Department of Pediatrics, Division of Community Pediatrics, Vanderbilt University, Nashville, Tenn.*

4:45 **Predictors of Depression and Substance Abuse in Adolescent Offspring of Former Teenage Mothers.** *S. M. Horwitz, L. V. Klerman, and J. F. Jekel. Department of Epidemiology and Public Health, Yale University School of Medicine, New Haven, Conn.*

5:00 ***Rurality and Patterns of Early Adolescent Alcohol Use.** *K. J. Kelleher, V. Rickert, B. Hardin, and S. Pope. University of Arkansas for Medical Sciences and Department of Pediatrics, Arkansas Children's Hospital, Little Rock.*

5:15 ***Patterns of Smokeless Tobacco Use by Early Adolescents.** *V. I. Rickert, A. A. Gottlieb, S. K. Pope, and B. H. Hardin. University of Arkansas for Medical Sciences and Department of Pediatrics, Arkansas Children's Hospital, Little Rock.*

5:30 ***The Virginal Male Adolescent: Differences in Attitudes and Knowledge?** *K. A. Woodward, L. J. D'Angelo, P. R. Getson, and C. O. Brasseux. Children's National Medical Center, Washington, DC.*

5:45 ***Factors Associated with High School Students' Attrition from Organized Sports.** *R. H. DuRant, R. A. Pendergrast, J. Donner, C. Seymore, and G. L. Gaillard. Department of Pediatrics, Medical College of Georgia, Augusta, Ga.*

6:00 **Evaluation of Sexual Behavior in Sports Preparticipation Examination.** *B. J. Foch, M. K. Oh, C. H. Hong, B. C. Cotton, B. C. Brown, and R. A. Feinstein. Department of Pediatrics, University of Alabama, Birmingham.*

6:15 ***Mental Health Effects of a Social Skills Intervention for Adolescents with Chronic Illness.** *S. M. Coupey, L. J. Bauman, J. L. Lauby, C. R. Koeber, and R. E. K. Stein. PreventiveIntervention Research Center, Department of Pediatrics, Albert Einstein College of Medicine, Bronx, NY.*

BEHAVIORAL PEDIATRICS

Grand Salon D

Moderators: *Daniel Coury, MD, Morris Green, MD, and Sheridan Phillips, PhD*

3:00 **The Cry of Colic Facies.** *R. G. Barr, A. Rotman, J. Yaremko, D. Leduc, T. E. Francoeur, and B. Katchan. Department of Pediatrics, McGill University, and Montreal Children's Hospital, Montreal, Quebec.*

3:15 ***Infant Cry Analysis Predicts Developmental Outcome in Term and Preterm Infants.** *B. Lester, C. F. Z. Boukydis, M. Corwin, C. Sepkoski, M. Peucker, and H. Golub. Brown University Bradley, and Women and Infants' Hospital, Boston (Mass) University and Cry Research, Inc.*

3:30 ***Predictor of Failure to Thrive in Low Birth Weight Infants.** *K. J. Kelleher, P. Casey, R. Bradley, M. Swanson, L. Whiteside, S. Pope, and K. Barrett. Infant Health and Development Program, Department of Pediatrics, University of Arkansas Medical Sciences, Little Rock.*

3:45 ***Patterns of Affect Expression in Infants with Nonorganic Failure to Thrive Syndrome (NFTT).** *D. K. Wilcox, H. Bauchner, and D. Frank. Division of Developmental and Behavioral Pediatrics, Boston (Mass) City Hospital, Boston University School of Medicine.*

4:00 ***Early Temperament and Cardiac Responses of Preterm (PT) Infants with Bronchopulmonary Dysplasia (BPD).** *C. G. Coll, B. M. Lester, M. Peucker, C. F. Z. Boukydis, and B. R. Vohr. Brown University, Women and Infants Hospital, Providence, RI.*

4:15 **Reducing Low Birthweight, Depression, and Stress Through Social Support in Pregnancy.** *A. W. Cross, K. J. Welshimer, E. Jackson, and J. Chapman. Center for Health Promotion Disease Prevention, University of North Carolina, Chapel Hill.*

4:30 ***Effects of Theophylline on Behavior in Children with Chronic Asthma.** *N. F. Slater, M. Green, H. Eigen, S. Hui, and H.G. Taylor. Indiana University School of Medicine, Departments of Pediatrics and Biostatistics, Indianapolis, and Case Western Reserve University, Cleveland, Ohio.*

4:45 **Evaluating a Parent Support Program for Mothers of Chronically Ill Children.** *H. T. Ireys, E. J. Silver, R. E. K. Stein, K. Bencivenga, and C. Koeber. Pediatrics, Albert Einstein College of Medicine, Preventive Intervention Research Center, Bronx, NY.*

5:00 ***Hypnoanalgesia in Sickle Cell Anemia.** *C. J. Erickson. Department of Pediatrics, Babies Hospital, Columbia University College of Physicians and Surgeons, New York, NY.*

5:15 ***Immunologic Changes Occurring at Kindergarten Entry Predict Respiratory Illnesses Following the Loma Prieta Earthquake.** *W. T. Boyce, E. A. Chesterman, D. Wara, F. Cohen, S. Folkman, and N. Martin. Department of Pediatrics, University of California, San Francisco.*

5:30 ***Rapid Calming Effect of Intraoral Sucrose in Crying Newborns.** *R. G. Barr, V. Quek, S. Young, and T. Oberlander. Departments of Pediatrics and Psychiatry, McGill University, Montreal, Quebec, and Montreal Children's Hospital.*

5:45 **Can the Reliability of Mothers' Clinical Judgments be Predicted?** *P. McCarthy, D. Cicchetti, S. Sznajderman, B. Forsyth, M. Baron, H. Fink, N. Czarkowski, B. Bauchner, and K. Lustman-Findling. Department of Pediatrics, Yale University School of Medicine, New Haven, Conn.*

6:00 **Cognitive Dysfunction in Children with Post-Meningitic Deafness.** *D. Kelly, B. Kelly, M. Jones, S. Verhulst and S. Bell.*

6:15 ***The Preschool Rapid Screen.** *M. L. Suchoff, M. H. Lifschitz, G. S. Wilson, N. LaFevers, and W. D. Williamson. Department of Pediatrics, Baylor College of Medicine, Texas Children's Hospital, Houston.*

EPIDEMIOLOGY AND PREVENTIVE PEDIATRICS

Grand Salon C

Moderators: *Robert Haggerty, MD, Nigel Paneth, MD, MPH, and Steven Shelov, MD*

3:00 **Firearms: Family Attitudes and Household Safety Practices.** *C. C. Wiley and R. Casey. Division of General Pediatrics, Children's Hospital of Philadelphia (Pa).*

3:15 **Previous Injury as a Risk Factor for Youth Suicide.** *D. C. Grossman, R. W. Soderberg, and F. P. Rivara. Department of Pediatrics, University of Washington, Harborview Injury Prevention Center, Seattle.*

*Abstract was published in the Program Issue of the American Pediatric Society and the Society for *Pediatric Research*, Pediatric Research, April 1991.

3:30 ***Parental Alcohol Consumption and Children's Injuries: Evidence from the 1988 National Health Interview Survey (NHIS).** *P. E. Bijur and M. Kurzon. Albert Einstein College of Medicine, Department of Pediatrics, Bronx, NY.*

3:45 ***Increased Susceptibility of Infants to Red Measles (Rubeola) in a Well Vaccinated Society.** *D. W. Spady, H. F. Pabst, R. Marusyk, L. Chui, and M. Carson. Departments* of Pediatrics and Medical Microbiology and Infectious Diseases, University of Alberta, Edmonton

4:00 ***Measles Antibody in Baltimore Children.** *J. C. King, S. Feigelman, E. M. Hirshorn, C. L. Luna, C. A. Loffredo, and R. Lichenstein. Department of Pediatrics, University of Maryland, University of Maryland Hospital, Baltimore.*

4:15 ***Waning Immunity and Mild Measles in School-Aged Children Who Received Measles Vaccine Before 1979.** *M. B. Edmonson, J. L. Berg, and J. P. Davis. University of Wisconsin, Department of Pediatrics, and Wisconsin Division of Health, Madison.*

4:30 ***Risk Factors for Invasive Haemophilus Influenza Type b Disease in Victoria, Australia.** *D. Clements, I. Guise, and G. Gilbert. Department of Pediatrics, Duke University Medicine Center, Durham, NC, and Department of Microbiology and Infectious Diseases, Royal Children's Hospital (RCH), Melbourne, Australia.*

4:45 ***Validation of the Case-Control Method of Assessing A Vaccine's Efficacy.** *E. D. Shapiro. Yale School of Medicine, New Haven, Conn.*

5:00 ***Cigarette Smoking and Sudden Infant Death Syndrome (SIDS): No Dose Response in Data From the United States.** *H. J. Hoffman, M. Malloy, and D. Peterson. Prevention Research, NICHD, NIH, Bethesda, Md, and School of Public Health, University of Washington, Seattle.*

5:15 ***Maternal Substance Use and Sudden Infant Death Syndrome (SIDS) in Offspring.** *S. R. Kandall, K. Damus, J. J. Gaines, and L. Habel. Mt Sinai School of Medicine, Department of Pediatrics, Beth Israel Medicine Center; New York City Department of Health; Medical and Health Research Association of New York City, Inc, New York.*

5:30 ***Paternal and Maternal Birth Weights and Subsequent Pregnancy Outcome.** *M. A. Klebanoff. NICHD, NIH, Bethesda, Md.*

5:45 ***Cumulative Incidence of Atopic Disorders in High Risk Infants Fed Whey Hydrolysate, Soy, and Conventional Cow Milk Formulas.** *R. K. Chandra and A. Hamed. Memorial University of Newfoundland, Janeway Child Health Centre, St John's, Newfoundland.*

6:00 **Effects of Screening Children for High Cholesterol.** *C. M. Lannon and J. A. Earp. Department of Pediatrics, School of Medicine, and Department of Health Education and Health Behavior, School of Public Health, University of North Carolina, Chapel Hill.*

6:15 **Access to Care for Poor and Nonpoor Children: Separate and Unequal?** *R. F. St Peter and P. W. Newacheck. Robert Wood Johnson Clinical Scholars Program, Department of Pediatrics and Institute for Health Policy Studies, University of California, San Francisco.*

*Abstract was published in the Program Issue of the American Pediatric Society and the Society for *Pediatric Research*, Pediatric Research, April 1991.

GENERAL PEDIATRICS AND PEDIATRIC EDUCATION

Grand Ballroom D

Moderators: *Frederick H. Lovejoy, Jr, MD, Lucy Osborn, MD, and Michael Weitzman, MD*

3:00 ***Office Diagnosis of Neonatal Chlamydial Conjunctivitis: Use of Kodak Surecell®.** *M. R. Hammerschlag, M. Gelling, P. Roblin, W. Dumornay, and M. Worku. Department of Pediatrics, SUNY Health Science Center at Brooklyn (NY).*

3:15 ***Missed Opportunities for Vaccinations in Pediatric Practices and the Effect on Vaccination Status.** *P. G. Szilagyi, L. E. Rodewald, S. G. Humiston, R. F. Raubertas, K. J. Roghmann, and C. B. Hall. Department of Pediatrics, University of Rochester (NY) School of Medicine and Dentistry.*

3:30 ***Prevalence of Urinary Tract Infection (UTI) in Febrile Infants.** *A. Hoberman, H. Chao, D. M. Keller, R. Hickey, H.M . Davis, and D. Ellis. University of Pittsburgh (Pa), Children's Hospital of Pittsburgh, Department of Pediatrics.*

3:45 ***Outbreaks of Human Enteric Adenovirus Types 40 and 41 in Houston Day Care Centers (DCC).** *R. Van, M. L. O'Ryan, D. O. Matson, L. Jackson, and L.K. Pickering. University of Texas Medical School at Houston and Baylor College of Medicine, Houston.*

4:00 ***Toxic Changes in Neutrophils as a Test for Kawasaki Syndrome (KS).** *P. C. Rowe, A. Quinlan, and B. K. Luke. Departments of Pediatrics and Epidemiology, University of Ottawa School of Medicine, Children's Hospital of Eastern Ontario, Ottawa.*

4:15 **Has the Eighty Hour Week Lessened Stress Levels in PL-1 Residents?** *J. E. Berkelhamer and N. H. Pliskin. Departments of Pediatrics and Psychiatry, Wyler Children's Hospital, University of Chicago (Ill) Pritzker School of Medicine.*

4:30 **Diagnostic Trends in a Pediatric Primary Care Clinic.** *C. Calderon, G. Gonzalez, and M. Valcarcel. Pediatric Department, University of Puerto Rico Ciencias Medicas, San Juan, Puerto Rico.*

4:45 **Comparison of Interviewing Skills of Fourth Year Medical Students with Their Individual Performance as Second Year Medical Students.** *R.D.OlsenandB.Anderson. Department of Pediatrics, Mayo Clinic, Rochester, Minn.*

5:00 **Reduction of Morbidity in Asthmatic Children Given a Spacer Device.** *S. J. Cunningham and E. F. Crain. Department of Pediatrics, Albert Einstein College of Medicine, Division of Pediatric Ambulatory Care, Bronx (NY) Municipal Hospital Center.*

5:15 ***Conductive Hearing Loss at Age 4 Years in Children Who Were <32 Weeks of Gestational Age.** *S. J. Gross. Department of Pediatrics, SUNY Health Science Center, Syracuse, NY.*

5:30 ***Appropriateness of Hospitalization in a Canadian Pediatric Hospital.** *J. E. Gloor, N. Kissoon, and G. I. Joubert. Children's Hospital of Western Ontario, Victoria Hospital, London, Ontario.*

5:45 ***Erythrocyte Protoporphyrin (EP) in Screening for Lead Poisoning at Blood Lead Levels Below 25 mcg/dl.** *S. Rajkumar and V. Rajagopal. SUNY Health Science Center at Brooklyn, Brooklyn, NY.*

6:00 ***A Change in Dietary Fat Composition Improves Serum Cholesterol Values in 7 to 13 Month Old Infants.** *H. Kovanen, E. Jokinen, A. Myyrinmaa, P. Salo, T. Ronnemaa, J. Viikari, I. Valimaki, and O. Simell. Cardiorespiratory Research Unit and Departments of Medicine and Pediatrics, University of Turku, and Rehabilitation Research Center of the Social Insurance Institution, Turku, Finland.*

6:15 **An Assessment of Nutritional Status in Homeless Children.** *J. H. Gould, T. L. Pelham, and J. C. Weiss. Department of Pediatrics, Jefferson Medical College, Philadelphia, Pa.*

Wednesday, May 1, 1991
9 AM-NOON

CLINICAL ISSUES

Grand Ballroom C

Moderators: Paul McCarthy, MD, and Robert Pantell, MD

9:00 **Double-blind, Cross-over Trial of Psyllium Fiber in Hypercholesterolemic Children.** *B. A. Dennison. Department of Pediatrics, Cornell University Medical College and The Rogosin Institute, New York, NY.*

9:15 **Bacteriology of Acute Otitis Media (AOM): A New Perspective.** *M. A. DelBeccaro, P. M. Mendelman, A. F. Inglis, M. A. Richardson, and C. Clausen. Departments of Pediatrics and Otolaryngology, University of Washington, Seattle.*

9:30 **Brush Culture Method for Diagnosing Tinea Capitis.** *T. W. Hubbard and J. M. de Triquet. Department of Pediatrics, Eastern Virginia Medical School, Norfolk.*

9:45 **Utility of Oxygen Saturation in Evaluating the Response to Treatment in Wheezing Infants.** *A. J. Alario, W. J. Lewander, P. H. Dennehy, R. Seifer, and A. L. Mansell. Department of Pediatrics, Rhode Island Hospital, Providence.*

10:00 **Initial Weight Loss and Return to Birth Weight Criteria for Breast-Fed Infants: Challenging the "Rules of Thumb."** *S. DeMarzo, J. Seacat, and M. Neifert. Lactation Program, Presbyterian/Saint Luke's Medical Center, Denver, Colo.*

10:15 **Appropriateness of Admissions to a Canadian Children's Hospital.** *K. R. Kowaleski and M. Li. Division of Emergency Medicine, Department of Pediatrics, Children's Hospital of Eastern Ontario, Ottawa.*

10:30 **Parental Time and Expenses for Diabetes Care.** *G. E. Dougherty, A. Schiffrin, and L. Ball. Departments of Pediatrics and Epidemiology and Biostatistics, McGill University, Montreal, Quebec.*

10:45 **Simethicone in the Treatment of Infant Colic.** *T. J. Metcalf, T. G. Irons, L. D. Sher, and P. C. Young. Willow Creek Pediatrics, Salt Lake City, East Carolina University, Greenville; Pennisula Allergy and Pediatrics, Rolling Mills Estate, Calif; and University of Vermont, Burlington.*

11:00 **Tympanic Membrane Thermometers: Caveat Emptor.** *M. Nypaver, E. Zieserl, B. Nachtsheim, and A. T. Davis. Department of General and Emergency Pediatrics, Children's Memorial Hospital, Chicago, Ill.*

11:15 **Over-the-Counter (OTC) Medication Use in Children with Colds—A Critical Appraisal.** *M. B. H. Smith and W. Feldman. Department of Pediatrics, University of Ottawa, Ontario.*

11:30 **Intermittent Versus Continuous Amoxicillin Prophylaxis for Infants and Children with Recurrent Otitis Media With Effusion.** *S. Berman, R. Nuss, R. Roark, C. Huber-Navin, K. Grose, and M. Herrera. Department of Pediatrics, University of Colorado Health Sciences Center, Denver.*

11:45 **Duration of Positive Streptococcal Throat Cultures After Initiation of Antibiotics.** *L. W. Snellman, H. J. Stang, J. M. Stang, D. R. Johnson, and E. L. Kaplan. Departments of Pediatrics, Group Health Inc, and University of Minnesota, White Bear Lake.*

DEVELOPMENTAL AND BEHAVIORAL PEDIATRICS

Grand Salon A

Moderators: John Pascoe, MD, MPH, and Modena Wilson, MD, MPH

9:00 **School Outcomes of Children with Asthma.** *M. G. Fowler, R. Garg, and M. G. Davenport. Office of Analysis, National Center for Health Statistics, Hyattsville, Md, and Clinical Trials Branch, National Health, Lung, and Blood Institute.*

9:15 **Homage to a Clinical Observation: Empirical Support for Wessel's Definition of "Colic."** *R. G. Barr, A. Rotman, J. Yaremko, D. Leduc, T. E. Francoeur, J. Desilets, and R. DuBerger. Department of Pediatrics, McGill University and Montreal (Quebec) Children's Hospital, Montreal.*

9:30 **Preventing Disruptive Night Waking in Infancy: An Effective Primary Care Intervention.** *R. Adair, H. Bauchner, B. Philipp, S. Levenson, and B. Zuckerman. Department of Pediatrics, Boston (Mass) City Hospital, Boston University School of Medicine.*

9:45 **Identifying Sources of Discrepancy Between Pediatricians' Diagnoses and the Child Behavior Checklist.** *S. M. Horwitz, P. J. Leaf, J. M. Leventhal, B. W. C. Forsyth, and K. N. Speechley. Departments of Epidemiology and Public Health and Pediatrics, Yale University School of Medicine, New Haven, Conn.*

10:00 **Understanding the Development of Failure to Thrive in a Low Birth Weight, Preterm Cohort: A Prospective Study to Age Three.** *P. H. Casey, K. Kelleher, R. H. Bradley, M. Swanson, L. Whiteside, S. Pope, and K. Barrett. Department of Pediatrics, University of Arkansas for Medical Sciences, Little Rock.*

10:15 **The Mental Health of Children Placed With Relatives.** *H. Dubowitz, V. Tepper, S. Zuravin, and S. Feigelman. Department of Pediatrics, University of Maryland Medical School, Baltimore.*

10:30 **Child Rearing Practices and Nursing Caries.** *J. R. Serwint, R. Mungo, V. Negrete, M. Guzman, and B. M. Korsch. Departments of Pediatrics and Pediatric Dentistry, University of Southern California School of Medicine and Children's Hospital of Los Angeles.*

10:45 **Detecting Family Violence in the Context of Pediatric Continuity Care.** *L. S. Wissow, M. E. H. Wilson, and D. Roter. Johns Hopkins Medical Institutions, Baltimore, Md.*

11:00 **Depression and Role Satisfaction in Mothers of Toddlers.** *A. L. Olson and L. A. DiBrigida. Department of Maternal and Child Health, Dartmouth Medical School, Hanover, NH.*

11:15 **Maternal Attitudes as Predictors of Infant Feeding Decisions.** *C. I. Dungy, J. Christensen-Szalanski, M. Losch, and D. Russell. Department of Pediatrics, The University of Iowa, Iowa City.*

11:30 **The Feasibility and Utility of Psychosocial Screening in a Pediatric Clinic.** *K. J. Kemper. Department of Pediatrics, University of Washington, and Harborview Medical Center, Seattle.*

11:45 **Developmental Delay Among Homeless Children.** *B. P. Dreyer, C. D. Courtlandt, A. H. Fierman, A. Arbel, G. Bencincasa, C. Squittieri, L. Palevsky, and N. Mann. Department of Pediatrics, New York (NY) University School of Medicine, NY.*

EMERGENCY MEDICINE AND CHILD ABUSE

Grand Salon B

Moderators: John Leventhal, MD, and Stephen Ludwig, MD

9:00 **The Failure of Tympanic Thermometry to Detect Fever Accurately in a Pediatric Emergency Department (PED).** *C. Garabedian, R. Vinci, D. Dwyer, and H. Bauchner. Division of Pediatric Emergency Medicine, Department of Pediatrics, Boston (Mass) University School of Medicine, and Boston City Hospital.*

9:15 **Refinement of the Child Vulnerability Scale.** *B. W. C. Forsyth, P. J. Leaf, S. M. Horwitz, and J. M. Leventhal. Departments of Pediatrics and Epidemiology and Public Health, Yale University School of Medicine, New Haven, Conn.*

9:30 **Cocaine-Exposed Newborns in an Inner-City Community Hospital.** *A. Theodorou, T. Holtrop, J. Marshall, K. Meert, and A. Sarnaik. Children's Hospital of Michigan, Wayne State University, and Samaritan Health Center, Detroit, Mich.*

9:45 **Pediatric Emergency Medicine—State of the Art.** *D. J. Isaacman, R. B. Karasic, and H. W. Davis. Department of Pediatrics, University of Pittsburgh (Pa) School of Medicine.*

10:00 **Defervescence as a Guide to Resolution of Bacteremia** in Ambulatory Children. *F. Agre and L. R. Prieto. Department of Pediatrics, College of Physicians and Surgeons, Columbia University, New York, NY.*

10:15 **Positive Effect of an Educational Intervention on Compliance With Universal Precautions in a Pediatric Emergency Department.** *L. R. Friedland, M. Joffe, and J. F. Wiley, II. Emergency Medicine, Section of General Pediatrics, St Christopher's Hospital for Children, Philadelphia, Pa.*

10:30 **Historical Correlates to Anogenital Trauma in 1,150 Suspected Child Sexual Abuse Victims.** *D. L. Kerns and M. L. Ritter. Department of Pediatrics, Santa Clara Valley Medical Center, San Jose, Calif.*

10:45 **Screening for Cocaine Intoxication in Children with Unexplained Seizures in the Emergency Department.** *S. E. Krug, R. D. Marble, D. L. Lubitz, and T. J. Long. Department of Pediatrics, Case Western Reserve University School of Medicine, Cleveland, Ohio.*

11:00 **The Value of Chest Radiographs in the Evaluation of Febrile Infants Less Than Two Years Old.** *J. A. Taylor, S. Roncevich, E. Kouri, C. Talarico, and R. Schneider. Departments of Pediatrics, Radiology, and Emergency Medicine, Carolinas Medical Center, Charlotte, NC.*

11:15 **A New Instrument to Improve the Ability of Non-Experts to Identify Infants at Risk of Subsequent Child Abuse or Neglect.** *D. H. K. Ihnat, J. M. Leventhal, D. V. Cicchetti, D. R. Wasserman, and J. P. Hamilton. Department of Pediatrics, Yale University School of Medicine, New Haven, Conn, and Yale-New Haven Hospital.*

11:30 **Maltreatment of Children Born to Cocaine Dependent Mothers.** *D. R. Wasserman and J. M. Leventhal. Department of Pediatrics, Yale University School of Medicine, New Haven, Conn.*

11:45 **Are Interdisciplinary Evaluations of Alleged Sexual Abuse Cases Necessary?** *P. K. Jaudes and M. Martone. La Rabida Children's Hospital and Department of Pediatrics, University of Chicago (Ill) Pritzker School of Medicine.*

GENERAL PEDIATRICS

Grand Salon C

Moderators: Thomas G. DeWitt, MD, and Ruth T. Gross, MD

9:00 **Doctorhoppers: Myth or Reality?** *C. Gosselink, D. Brazdziunas, E. Ekwo, A. Kresheck, and M. Lehmann. Department of Pediatrics, University of Chicago (Ill)/La Rabida Children's Hospital and Research Center.*

9:15 **What Factors Predict School Absence in Children with Chronic Medical Conditions? A Controlled Population Based Study.** *F. C. Jarman and M. C. Starr. Department of Pediatrics, University of Massachusetts Medical Center, Worcester.*

9:30 **Comparison of Two Methods of Assessing Appropriateness of Admission.** *K. R. Kowaleski, P. Griffin, and M. Li. Department of Pediatrics, Children's Hospital of Eastern Ontario, Ottawa.*

9:45 **Validity, Bias, and "Overcall" in Interpreting Chest Radiographs in Young Febrile Children.** *M. S. Kramer, R. Roberts-Brauer, and R. Williams. Departments of Pediatrics and Epidemiology and Biostatistics, McGill University, Montreal, Quebec.*

10:00 **An Analysis of Mental Health Service Utilization by Children in Foster Care in California.** *N. Halfon, G. Berkowitz, and L. Klee. Center for the Vulnerable Child, Children's Hospital Oakland, Calif.*

10:15 **The Relation of Family Mobility to Children's Emotional and School Functioning.** *G. A. Simpson and M. G. Fowler. National Center for Health Statistics, Hyattsville, Md.*

10:30 **Biofeedback: Initial Success in Treating Recurrent Abdominal Pain.** *A. J. Rosenberg, and T. Whitehead. Department of Pediatrics, University of Kansas Medical Center, Kansas City.*

10:45 **Are School-Based Clinics Serving the High-Risk Student?** *J. W. Stout and C. R. Anderman. Departments of Pediatrics and Epidemiology, University of Washington, Seattle.*

11:00 **A Clinic-Based Intervention to Promote Literacy.** *R. D. Needlman, L. E. Fried, and B. S. Zuckerman. Division of Developmental and Behavioral Pediatrics, Boston (Mass) City Hospital.*

11:15 **A Critical Appraisal of the Quality of Pediatric Journal Articles that Evaluate Diagnostic Tests.** *A. S. Bates, P. X. Margolis, and A. E. Evans. Departments of Pediatrics and Medicine, University of North Carolina, Chapel Hill, and Indiana University, Indianapolis.*

11:30 **Educational Effectiveness of a Lead Poisoning Video.** *S. Melman, S. Schorr, R.Lempert,and M. Polansky. Department of Pediatrics, Hahnemann University Hospital, Philadelphia, Pa.*

11:45 **Impact of Shorter Working Hours on Pediatric Housestaff Training.** *A. Willenborg, S. Shelov,and D.Neuspiel. Department of Pediatrics, Albert Einstein College of Medicine, Bronx, NY.*

PREVENTION AND EPIDEMIOLOGY

Grand Salon D

Moderators: Katherine K. Christoffel, MD, MPH, and Sandra Elvik, MSN, CPNP

9:00 **Immunization Opportunities Missed Among Urban Poor Children.** *K. M. McConnochie and K. J. Roghmann. Department of Pediatrics, Rochester (NY) General Hospital, University of Rochester.*

9:15 **Predictors of Parental Injury Prevention Behavior.** *D. F. Schwarz, C. B. Forrest, J. A. Grisso, C. G. Miles, and V. M. Wolfson. Department of Pediatrics and Clinical Epidemiology Unit, University of Pennsylvania School of Medicine, Philadelphia.*

9:30 **The Functional Impact of Asthma.** *J. M. Perrin, M. L. Weitzman, and S. L. Gortmaker. Children's Service, Massachusetts General Hospital, Boston; Harvard School of Public Health, Boston; and University of Rochester (NY) School of Medicine.*

9:45 **Avoidable Pediatric Hospital Use: A Comparison of Admitting Physician Judgement With Utilization Review.** *J. L. Soulen, A. K. Duggan, and C. DeAngelis. Department of Pediatrics, Johns Hopkins University, Baltimore (Md).*

10:00 **Lead Intoxication in Early Infancy.** *M. W. Shannon and J. W. Graef. Department of Pediatrics, Harvard Medical School, Department of Medicine, Children's Hospital, Boston, Mass.*

10:15 **Children's Household Exposure to Guns.** *Y. D. Senturia, A. M. Teuscher, and K. K. Christoffel. Pediatric Practice Research Group, Children's Memorial Hospital, Chicago, Ill.*

10:30 **Finding the Missing Data—A Statewide System for Injury Surveillance in the Pediatric Office Setting.** *J. K. Sanders, E. R. Waring, and J. R. Zanga. Division of General Pediatrics and Emergency Care, Children's Medical Center, Medical College of Virginia/Virginia Commonwealth University, Richmond.*

10:45 **Management of Childhood Lead Poisoning: A Survey.** *D. Glotzer and H. Bauchner. Department of Pediatrics, Boston (Mass) University School of Medicine and Boston City Hospital.*

11:00 **Who Needs the Lead (Pb) Mobilization Test (LMT)? Blood Pb as the Sole Determinant of Need for Treatment.** *M. E. Markowitz and J. F. Rosen. Department of Pediatrics, Albert Einstein College of Medicine and Montefiore Medical Center, Bronx, NY.*

11:15 **Can We Influence Parents Whose Preschooler Has Been Recently Poisoned to Take Preventive Precautions?** *A. D. Woolf, A. Saperstein, and S. Forjuoh. Department of Pediatrics, Harvard Medical School, Boston; Division of General Pediatrics, Children's Hospital, Boston; and Massachusetts Poison Control System, Boston.*

11:30 **Gender Difference in Health Care Utilization by Children Away from Parental Influence.** *M. C. J. Rudolf and A. J. Alario. Department of Pediatrics, Rhode Island Hospital, Brown University, Providence.*

11:45 **Barriers to Influenza Vaccination in Children with Asthma.** *P. G. Szilagyi, L. E. Rodewald, J. Savageau, L. M. Yoos, and C. B. Doane. Department of Pediatrics, University of Rochester (NY) School of Medicine and Dentistry.*

APA Debate

Wednesday, May 1, 1991
8:30 PM-10 PM
Grand Salon A

Resolved: That professional societies should accept financial contributions from commercial enterprises.

Moderator: *Kathleen Nelson, MD, APA President Elect; Professor of Pediatrics; and Director, Division of General Pediatrics, Children's Hospital, Birmingham, Ala.*

Pro Resolution: Larry Shapiro, MD, Professor of Pediatrics and Biological Chemistry, Harbor UCLA Medical Center, Torrance, Calif, and Carol Berkowitz, MD, APA President; Professor, Clinical Pediatrics, UCLA School of Medicine; and Acting Chair, Department of Pediatrics, Harbor UCLA Medical Center, Torrance, Calif

Con Resolution: Catherine De Angelis, MD, Associate Dean for Academic Affairs and Professor of Pediatrics, Johns Hopkins Medical Institute, Baltimore, Md, and Steven P. Shelov, MD, Director, Pediatric Education, Albert Einstein College of Medicine, Montefiore Medical Center, Bronx, NY

General Plenary Session

Thursday, May 2, 1991
8 AM-NOON
Grand Salon D

Moderator: Kathleen G. Nelson, MD

8:00 **Managed Care for New York Medicaid Children: Cost Analysis of Referred Services.** *T. D. Sullivan. Department of Pediatrics, SUNY at Buffalo (NY), The Children's Hospital of Buffalo.*

8:15 **The Efficacy of Non-Invasive In-Hospital and Outpatient Management of Febrile Infants: A Four Year Experience.** *M. D. Baker, L. M. Bell, and J. R. Avner. Divisions of General Pediatrics, Emergency Medicine, and Infectious Diseases, The Children's Hospital of Philadelphia (Pa).*

8:30 **Increased Growth Velocities in Children Living in Shelters.** *C. D. Courtlandt, A. H. Fierman, B. P. Dreyer, K. Hick, D. Arnold, E. Keating, and N. Mann. Department of Pediatrics, New York (NY) University School of Medicine.*

8:45 **The Prediction of Preschool Behavior Problems from Temperament and Other Variables in Infancy.** *F. Oberklaid, A. Sanson, R. Redlow, and M. Prior. Department of Ambulatory Pediatrics, Royal Children's Hospital, Victoria, Australia.*

9:00 **Vaccine Storage Errors in Pediatric Practice: The Tip of an Iceberg?** *D. M. Bishai, S. Bhatt, L. T. Miller, and G. F. Hayden. Department of Pediatrics, Cedars-Sinai Medical Center, Los Angeles, Calif, and University of Virginia Health Sciences Center, Charlottesville.*

9:15 **Use of the Fentanyl Lollipop for Analgesia During Painful Procedures in Children.** *N. L. Schechter, S. J. Weisman, M. Rosenblum, P. L. Conard, B. Bernstein, C. Bartolotta, C. San Antonio, B. Shapiro, and D. Cohen. Departments of Pediatrics and Anesthesia, University of Connecticut Health Center, Farmington; St Francis Hospital and Medical Center, Hartford, Conn; and Children's Hospital at Philadelphia (Pa).*

9:30 **DISTINGUISHED CAREER AWARD**

INTERMISSION

10:00 **PRESIDENT'S ADDRESS**

10:30 **The CBC Revisited: A Bayesian Reappraisal.** *M. S. Kramer, S. M. Tange, E. G. Mills, and M. L. Bernstein. Departments of Pediatrics and of Epidemiology and Biostatistics, McGill University Faculty of Medicine, Montreal, Quebec.*

10:45 **Clinical Risk Index for Bacterial Meningitis Among Febrile Children.** *R. Lembo, D. Krowchuk, and P. McCarthy. Department of Pediatrics, Yale University, New Haven, Conn, and Department of Pediatrics, Case-Western Reserve University at MetroHealth Medical Center, Cleveland, Ohio.*

11:00 **Randomized Trial of Laxatives in the Treatment of Encopresis.** *T. Nolan, G. Debelle, F. Oberklaid, and C. Coffey. Department of Pediatrics and Ambulatory Pediatrics, University of Melbourne, Royal Children's Hospital, Melbourne, Australia.*

11:15 **Maternal Emotional State and Infant Behavior: Are They Related?** *A. R. Miller and R. G. Barr. Department of Pediatrics, Montreal (Quebec) Children's Hospital.*

11:30 **Perinatal Injuries: Why Families File Suit.** *G. B. Hickson, E. W. Clayton, P. B. Githens, and F. A. Sloan. Vanderbilt Institute for Public Policy Studies, Health Policy Center, Vanderbilt University, Nashville, Tenn.*

11:45 **Maltreatment of Young Children Born to Teenage Mothers: A Comparison Between the Late 1960's and the Early 1980's.** *C. S. Rude, J. M. Leventhal, S. M. Horwitz, and D. M. Stier. Departments of Pediatrics, Epidemiology, and Public Health, Yale University School of Medicine, New Haven, Conn.*

Annual Meeting
The American Pediatric Society and The Society For Pediatric Research

New Orleans Hilton Riverside & Towers
and Rivergate Convention Center

Monday, April 29	Tuesday, April 30	Wednesday, May 1	Thursday, May 2
	7:45 AM-10:15 AM Poster Session II*, Poster Symposia, Nos. 7-12 **7:45 AM-11 AM** APS/SPR/APA Commercial Exhibits	**8 AM-9:30 AM** SPR Plenary Session; SPR Presidential Address; Young Investigator Award; Richard D. Rowe Award; Medical Student, House Officer, and Fellow Awards	**8 AM-11:30 AM** Subspecialty Platform Sessions III
	10:30 AM-1 PM APS Plenary Session; APS Presidential Address; APS Presidential State-of-the-Art Symposium, *Maternal & Child Health: Global Perspectives*	**9:30 AM-12:30 PM** Poster Session III* **9:30 AM-1:30 PM** APS/SPR/APA Commercial Exhibits **10 AM-12:30 PM** Poster Symposia, Nos. 13-18 **12:30 PM-1:45 PM** APS Business Meeting	**11:30 AM-12:45 PM** SPR Business Meeting
3:30 PM-7 PM Poster Session I* **3:30 PM-8 PM** APS/SPR/APA Commercial Exhibits **4:30 PM-7 PM** Poster Symposia, Nos. 1-6 **7 PM-8 PM** APS/SPR Opening Reception	**2 PM-3 PM** APS Howland Award, Joseph W St Geme, Jr, Leadership Award **3 PM-6:30 PM** Subspecialty Platform Sessions I and concurrent Joint APS/SPR/APA Subspecialty Platform Sessions	**2 PM-4:30 PM** SPR Presidential State-of-the-Art Symposium, *The Medical Social Crisis in Child Health* **2 PM-5:30 PM** Subspecialty Platform Sessions II	**1:30 PM-5 PM** Subspecialty Platform Sessions IV

*Please see poster session schedule for author attendance times.

Society For Pediatric Research 1991 — Subspecialty Platform Session Schedule

TUESDAY, APRIL 30, 3:00 PM—6:30 PM

Adolescent Medicine *(Grand Ballroom C)*
Behavioral Pediatrics *(Grand Salon D)*
Developmental Pharmacology I *(Belle Chasse)*
Epidemiology and Preventative Pediatrics *(Grand Salon C)*
General Pediatrics & Pediatric Education *(Grand Ballroom D)*
Hematology & Oncology I *(Napoleon)*
Immunology I *(Versailles)*
Infectious Diseases I *(Grand Salon B)*
Metabolism & Diabetes I *(Grand Salon A)*
Neonatology I *(Grand Ballroom A/B)*
Nephrology I *(Marlborough Suite)*

WEDNESDAY, MAY 1, 2:00 PM—5:30 PM

Gastroenterology/Nutrition I *(Grand Salon A)*
Genetics I *(Grand Salon B)*
Metabolism & Diabetes II *(Grand Salon D)*
Neonatal Cardiology *(Belle Chasse)*
Neonatal Epidemiology & Follow Up *(Versailles)*
Neonatal Immunology & Hematology *(Napoleon)*
Nephrology II *(Marlborough Suite)*
Pulmonology I *(Grand Ballroom C)*

THURSDAY, MAY 2, 8:00 AM—11:30 AM

Cardiology I *(Napoleon)*
Developmental Biology I *(Versailles)*
Endocrinology I *(Grand Ballroom D)*
Genetics II *(Grand Salon C)*
Gastroenterology/Nutrition II *(Grand Salon A)*
Neurology *(Marlborough Suite)*
Infectious Diseases II *(Grand Salon B)*
Neonatology II *(Grand Ballroom A/B)*
Pulmonology II *(Grand Ballroom C)*

THURSDAY, MAY 2, 1:30 PM—5 PM

Cardiology II *(Napoleon)*
Critical Care *(Grand Salon A)*
Developmental Biology II *(Versailles)*
Developmental Pharmacology II *(Belle Chasse)*
Dysmorphology and Teratology *(Marlborough Suite)*
Endocrinology II *(Grand Ballroom D)*
Immunology II *(Grand Salon D)*
Neonatal Infectious Diseases *(Grand Salon C)*
Neonatal Nutrition & Metabolism *(Grand Ballroom C)*
Neonatal Pulmonology *(Grand Ballroom A/B)*
Hematology and Oncology II *(Grand Salon B)*

1991 APS/SPR/APA Exhibitors

EXHIBITING COMPANY	CITY, STATE	BOOTH NUMBER
Air-Shields Vickers	Hatoboro, Pa	302, 304, 401, 403
Airborne Life Support Systems	Austin, Tex	419
Allied Healthcare Products, Inc.	St. Louis, Mo	514
Ameda/Egdell	Cary, Ind	102
American Journal of Diseases of Children	New Orleans, La, and Chicago, Ill	707
Appleton & Lang	East Norwalk, Conn	203
Applied Biometrics, Inc.	Eden Prairie, Minn	519
Baby's Benefit, Inc.	Colorado Springs, Co	404
Baxter Hyland Division	Glendale, Calif	418
Bear Medical Systems, Inc.	Riverside, Calif	207
Bunnell Incorporated	Salt Lake City, Utah	717, 719
Burroughs Wellcome Company	Research Triangle Park, NC	610, 612, 709, 711
Carnation Nutritional Products	Washington, DC	319
CNS, Inc.	Eden Prairie, Minn	609
Contemporary Pediatrics	Montvale, NJ	211
Corometrics Medical Systems, Inc.	Wallingford, Conn	414, 416
Davol, Inc.	Cranston, RI	209
DeVILBISS Health Care, Inc.	Somerset, Pa	611
Eli Lilly Company	Indianapolis, Ind	606, 608
Encyclopaedia Britannica, Inc.	Chicago, Ill	505
Endocrine Sciences	Calabasas, Calif	405
Fiberoptic Medical Products, Inc.	Allentown, Pa	507
Flexco Medical Instruments AG	Hendon, London, United Kingdom	513
Fujisawa Pharmaceuticals Inc.	Deerfield, Ill	110
Genentech, Inc.	South San Francisco, Calif	410, 412

EXHIBITING COMPANY	CITY, STATE	BOOTH NUMBER
Gerber Products Company	Fremont, Mich	508
Hemocue, Inc.	Mission Viej, Calif	502
Hewlett-Packard Company	Waltham, Mass	213, 215
Hologic, Inc.	Waltham, Mass	618, 620
ICN Pharmaceuticals	Costa Mesa, Calif	617, 619
Infrasonics, Inc.	San Diego, Calif	703
Infusaid, Inc.	Norwood, Mass	206
Intelligent Medical Systems	Carlsbad, Calif	104
International Technidyne Corporation	Edison, NJ	518
J.B. Lippincott Company	Philadelphia, Pa	307
John Wiley & Sons, Inc.	New York, NY	713
La Leche League International	Franklin Park, Ill	420
Lederle Laboratories	Wayne, NJ	614
Mallinckrodt Medical, Inc.	St. Louis, Mo	503
Marquette Electronics	Milwaukee, Wis	317
Mead Johnson Nutritionals	Evansville, Ind	306, 308
MED MARK, Inc.	Olathe, Kan	517
MEDELA, Inc.	Crystal Lake, Ill	520
Medfusion, Inc.	Duluth, Ga	201
Medical Associated Services, Inc.	Hatfield, Pa	615
Medical Data Systems	Wayne, Pa	406, 408
Medical Research Center	New York, NY	512
Merck, Sharp, & Dohme	West Point, Pa	705
Mosby-Year Book, Inc.	St. Louis, Mo	218
N.I.C.H.D.	Bethesda, Md	511
National Center for Health Statistics	Hyattsville, Md	112
Natus Medical Inc.	Foster City, Calif	407
Neonatal Intensive Care	Santa Monica, Calif	305
Nichols Institute	San Juan Capistrano, Calif	118
Non-Invasive Monitoring System, Inc.	Miami, Fla	504
NTI/White River	Laguna Hills, Calif	120
Nurticia-Loma Linda Foods	Riverside, Calif	318
Ohmeda	Madison, Wis	602, 604
Physicians Engineered Products	Park Rapids, Minn	320
Plenum Publishing Corporation	New York, NY	605
Preemicare Corporation	Houston, Tex	106, 108
Promedica, Inc.	Burlingame, Calif	616
Ross Laboratories	Columbus, Ohio	402
Sandoz Pharmaceuticals Corp.	East Hanover, NJ	301, 303
Scale Tronix, Inc.	White Plains, NY	613
Schering-Plough Corporation	Kenilworth, NJ	603
Sechrist Industries	Anaheim, Calif	607
Serono Laboratories, Inc.	Norwell, Mass	202
Sigma Tau Pharmaceuticals	New York, NY	506
SmithKline Beecham Pharmaceuticals	Philadelphia, Pa	205, 208
Social Security Administration	Baltimore, Md	515
SpaceLabs, Inc.	Redmond, Wash	217
Springer-Verlag NY Publishers	New York, NY	501
The Langer Biomechanics Group, Inc.	Deer Park, NY	715
Thermoscan, Inc.	San Diego, Calif	417
W.B. Saunders Company	Philadelphia, Pa	601
Western Reserve Care Systems	Youngstown, Ohio	509
Williams & Wilkins	Baltimore, Md	510
Wyeth Pediatrics	Philadelphia, Pa	701
Zila Pharmaceuticals, Inc.	Phoenix, Ariz	114

Annual Meeting of the Ambulatory Pediatric Association

GENERAL POSTER SESSION
Monday, April 29, 3:30 PM-7 PM

Poster No. 147
Direct Bilirubin Measurements in Jaundiced Term Newborns: A Waste of Blood and Money?

T. B. Newman, S. Hope, and D. K. Stevenson

General Pediatrics and Epidemiology,
University of California, San Francisco,
and Stanford (Calif) University

Most authorities recommend measurement of direct bilirubin as an initial step in the evaluation of jaundiced newborns. However, true conjugated hyperbilirubinemia is rare, and measurements of direct bilirubin are often inaccurate, suggesting that the predictive value of a high direct bilirubin value might be low. To investigate this possibility, we used a computerized database and medical records to review the outcome of 5255 measurements of direct bilirubin on 2877 term newborns in two hospitals. Test ordering frequency and results varied markedly between the two institutions: direct bilirubins were ordered about 10 times more often at the University of California, San Francisco than at Stanford, and the reported results were more than twice as high. One hundred forty-nine babies had maximum direct bilirubin values in the top 5% for their hospital of birth. In most, the high direct bilirubin remained unexplained (52%) or was due to laboratory error (21%). Forty infants (27%) had possibly associated conditions. These conditions were identified as a result of elevation of direct bilirubin in only four, all of whom had minor laboratory abnormalities which resolved spontaneously. Thus, none of the 5255 measurements of direct bilirubin in this study was clearly useful. Because of the low yield of unsuspected treatable pathology and very poor specificity, measurement of direct bilirubin is a poor screening test. More selective ordering of direct bilirubin tests could lead to considerable cost savings without an adverse effect on health.

Poster No. 148
Home Phototherapy—Use and Attitudes Among Community Pediatricians

S. B. Meropol, A. A. Luberti, A. R. De Jong, and J. C. Weiss

Department of Pediatrics,
Jefferson Medical College, Philadelphia, Pa

Despite almost 20 years of published experience with the use of home phototherapy (HP) for the treatment of neonatal unconjugated hyperbilirubinemia, many pediatricians still admit such patients to the hospital. This study investigates the fears and experiences of pediatricians related to the use of HP.

A questionnaire was sent to 139 pediatric practices in the Philadelphia area. Of the 93 responders, (67% response rate), only 30 (32%) had used HP. Similarly, of the 10 non-responders who were contacted by telephone, only 30% had used HP.

Twenty-two users (81%) had less than a 10% failure rate with HP. Twenty-four users (89%) stated that more than 75% of parents were satisfied with HP. While 25 (41%) of the non-users had worries about parental non-compliance with eyeshields and with phototherapy itself, only 1 (4%) of the users actually had major problems in each of these areas. Although 23 (38%) of the non-users reported a fear of medico-legal consequences as a reason for non-use, none of the practitioners using HP had ever been threatened with a potential lawsuit stemming from its use. Eighteen (30%) of the non-users feared overheating and dehydration, but none of the users experienced major difficulties with these problems.

Some of the perceived fears of non-users actually were confirmed as major problems by the users: parental anxiety (non-users 28% vs. users 24%); and difficulty obtaining home blood testing (non-users 26% vs. users 17%). Also, 17% of the users experienced major difficulties with insurance reimbursement.

This study reveals that the use of home phototherapy is still limited in this region despite favorable reviews in the literature and positive experiences of local practitioners. There is a substantial discordance between the disadvantages of HP feared by non-users and the problems actually experienced by those who utilize this home treatment. Providing education and better ancillary support services supports may allow more practitioners to feel comfortable using this method of treatment.

No. 149
The Health Status of Children Placed With Relatives

H. Dubowitz, S. Feigelman, S. Zuravin, V. Tepper, R. Lichenstein, and N. Davidson

Department of Pediatrics,
University of Maryland Medical School, Baltimore

Placement with relatives is generally the first option of public agencies seeking substitute care for children, mostly due to child abuse or neglect. This is the first evaluation of the health care, prevalence of chronic health problems, and need for further treatment of children placed in this type of foster care.

METHOD: Subjects were *all* 524 children living in relative placements in Baltimore in April 1989. Data were gathered from medical records, mailed questionnaires to health care providers, parents, relative caretakers, caseworkers and the adolescents, and by a history and physical exam.

RESULTS: Primary care was clearly received by about 25% of the children, with uncertainty accounting for another 66% of the children. About 50% were adequately immunized; most of the remainder had uncertain status. Over 40% of the children had not seen a dentist in the prior year. The salient medical findings included poor vision (10%), poor hearing (eg, 9% of 6-11 year olds), failure to thrive (10% of 0-5 year olds), obesity (20% of teens), dental caries (22%) and asthma (18%). Only 10% of the children had no medical problem; 52% had 1-2 problems and the remainder had >2 diagnoses. Many of the problems had not been previously identified, evaluated or treated. Over half the children had ≥1 health problem that definitely needed follow-up.

Few background variables predicted the number of health problems. However, children with more health problems were more likely to have a caretaker who made frequent contact with the caseworker ($p=.04$), was unemployed ($p=.004$), and who received more services ($p=.009$). Children who were older at placement ($p=.001$), and had less educated caretakers ($p=.04$) who were noncompliant with keeping appointments ($p=.04$) had a greater number of *untreated* health problems.

IMPLICATIONS: Children placed with relatives appear to have substantial health care needs. However, their problems are similar to those of poor and other foster children. Nevertheless, greater responsivity to their needs by families, health professionals and the social service system is indicated.

Poster No. 150
Foster Children: Predictors of Developmental Problems on Baseline Health Assessment

S. M. Horwitz and M. D. Simms

Department of Epidemiology and Public Health,
Yale University, New Haven, Conn, and
Foster Care Clinic, St Mary's Hospital, Waterbury, Conn

We know little about the rate or predictors of developmental problems for children entering foster care. We investigated these issues in a cohort of 272 children who received a unique baseline medical/developmental assessment in the Foster Care Clinic (FCC), St. Mary's Hospital, Waterbury, CT, from 6/85 to 12/89. Children ranged in age from 1 mo. to 7.8 yrs. at initial assessment, 57% were male, 39% were caucasian, 31% African-American, 20% Hispanic, and had been in foster care an average of 7 months at assessment. Reasons for placement included 15% abuse, 49% neglect, and 36% at risk for abuse/neglect. Significant growth stunting was noted in 19.5% and wasting in 8.4%. Children were assessed with the Battelle Developmental Inventory (BDI). Fifty-three percent ($N=144$) of children scored $\leq$10th% in at least one area of development, with 39% ($N=106$) of children impaired in $\geq$2 areas.

Factors related to developmental problems included: older age (>1 year) at first foster placement ($RR=1.8$, $p=.01$); placement for abuse/neglect rather than "at risk" status ($RR=1.6$, $p=.02$); and less time in foster care prior to the assessment ($RR=2.0$, $p=.000$). Using these three variables, we constructed 2 risk categories: in the high risk category, 87% (39/45) had $\geq$2 developmental problems; in the moderate risk category, 32% (56/176) had multiple developmental problems. High risk children were: older at entry into care, placed for abuse/neglect, and had been in care <3 months at baseline assessment.

We conclude that many children entering foster care have developmental problems and that problems are highly prevalent in a particular subgroup of children. Given the importance of early intervention, it is critical that all children entering substitute care receive a complete evaluation and, further, that particular attention be paid to older children who are placed for abuse/neglect.

Poster No. 151
Measurement of Gestational Cocaine Exposure

C. M. Callahan, T. M. Grant, P. Phipps, G. D. Clark, A. H. Novack, A. P. Streissguth, and V. A. Raisys

University of Washington, Seattle

Studies of fetal cocaine exposure have challenged the validity of maternal drug history and recommended analysis of infant biologic specimens. We studied the relationships between history of maternal drug use, radioimmunoassay (RIA) of trimester specific segments of maternal hair, meconium, newborn urine and hair. We hypothesized that meconium and newborn hair would prove most sensitive.

We studied 60 postpartum women who delivered a live newborn between 11/89 and 12/90. Subjects were eligible if they completed an anonymous questionnaire and a confidential interview. Meconium was analyzed by fluorescence polarization immunoassay and gas chromatography/mass spectrometry (GCMS).

Maternal history for cocaine use and RIA of maternal hair correlated (kappa statistic = 0.95). The sensitivities of newborn biologic specimens were assessed by McNemars Test for Correlated Proportions-Exact Method. Multiple regression analysis was used to evaluate the relationship between the quantity of cocaine found in the newborn hair with the amount detected in the trimester specific maternal hair segments.

RIA of newborn hair and GCMS of meconium were more sensitive than immunoassay of urine ($P< 0.05$).

The quantity of benzoylecgonine found in the newborn hair correlated best with that detected in the segment of maternal hair representing the third trimester ($R=0.66$, 95% C.I. $0.48<R<0.79$).

Analysis of either newborn hair by RIA or meconium by GCMS are more sensitive than immunoassay of urine in determining gestational cocaine exposure. Drugs detected in newborn hair correlate with the maternal pattern of use during the third trimester.

Immunoassay of urine to detect gestational cocaine exposure is not sensitive. Newborn hair or meconium is more sensitive and can detect most third trimester fetal cocaine exposure.

Poster No. 152
Effects of Head Start on Children With Lead Poisoning

B. Howard and E. Charney

Department of Pediatrics,
Duke University Medical Center, Durham, NC,
and Department of Pediatrics,
University of Massachusetts Medical Center, Worcester

Children with lead poisoning are at high risk for poor developmental outcome from the CNS toxicity of lead and also from poor nutrition including Fe deficiency and suboptimal parenting. We attempted to improve their outcome with a combined program: a small group Head Start class 5½ days/week plus parenting-nutrition sessions for their mothers. A prior pilot study demonstrated developmental gains in the children and suggested that the parent group program was key to its success. This study involved 36 low-income black children 30-54 months with Class II/III lead poisoning (PbB 25-50 ug/dl) and their mothers, enrolled in both child and parent groups for one school year; 31 matched controls attended regular Head Start with no parent groups. After one year there were no between group differences. However, both groups had significant verbal IQ gains (3.3) and improved HOME environment scores (4.0). HOME scores improved whether or not the mothers attended the parenting sessions. Drops in PbB (3.2 ug/dl) and FEP (6.6 ug/dl) were significant and comparable in both groups. IQ correlated negatively with PbB but also with maternal depression (CES-D), # of social problems and negative parenting attitudes (PSI). Behavior problems (CBCL) correlated with social factors (CES-D, PSI, HOME, # social problems, life stress) and iron deficiency but not with PbB (all $p<.05$). This study indicates that gains in Head Start may relate to its effect on parents, not well studied previously. The study also suggests that the neurobehavioral effects attributed to lead are also significantly related to family dysfunction and iron deficiency. We conclude that lead poisoned children can particularly benefit from Head Start with its effects on both parent and child.

Poster No. 153
Elevated Lead (Pb) Levels in Abused Children

W. Bithoney, W. Barbaresi, A. Vandeven, and A. Ryan

Department of Medicine,
Children's Hospital, Boston, Mass

To test our hypothesis that abused children are at increased risk for lead (Pb) poisoning we measured whole blood Pb levels in 95 children who had reports of physical abuse made by clinicians in our primary care clinic (PCC) and a comparison group of 95 children from the PCC without symptoms of abuse. All parents completed a demographic and housing questionnaire. Comparison subjects were matched to cases on age, race, SES and housing type. All cases were identified prospectively over a 48 month period. Cases were ascertained in all seasons.

During the study periods 74% of eligible case children had lead levels determined. Abused children had Pb levels of 17± 4.25 μgm/dl SEM. Comparison subjects Pb was 11±3.82, p<.001 by paired t-test. Abused children were more frequently anemic, a possible Pb effect, had higher FEP levels, p<.001, and had significantly more peeling paint in their homes, p<.04. 19% of abused children had Pb levels so high as to require chelation while only 4% of comparison subjects had Pb levels this high. Many authors have suggested that lead levels formerly thought to be inconsequential are toxic. Clinicians caring for abused children must attend to a broad range of concerns, thus, all abused children, known to be epidemiologically at risk for Pb elevation, should have Pb levels drawn. Correction of iron deficiency and elevated Pb may result in improved developmental outcome in these children.

Poster No. 154
Getting Away With Murder?: A Study of Unintentional Child Shootings

J. T. Maurer, M. J. Barthel, and R. R. Tanz

Department of Pediatrics, Children's Memorial Hospital, Northwestern University Medical School, Chicago, Ill

Is anyone held accountable when children are shot unintentionally, i.e. without intent for anyone to be injured, or are such shootings considered just the cost of gun ownership in our society?

Using a database of children <17 years old treated at our hospital for gun injuries from 1980-1990, we identified children shot unintentionally. Police data available since 1984 were then linked to medical and court records to determine the identity of the shooter, the weapon used, the legal charges filed and the legal outcome in each case. Police officers were interviewed whenever possible. Involvement of child protective services (CPS) was determined. From 1/84-3/90, 19/78 (24%) children were shot unintentionally. 13/19 (68%) shootings involved handguns. 4/19 (21%) victims died, 7 (37%) suffered neurologic impairment. Most victims were male (68%) and nonwhite (53%). 11 (58%) victims were <10 years old. Shooters were older: 15 (79%) ≥10 years old; 18/19 were male. 95% of the gun owners were related to the victim or the shooter. At least 11 state and local laws covered the shootings. Police interviewed were ambivalent about filing charges in these cases. Charges were filed against the shooter in 4/19 (21%) cases; 2 were convicted. Gun owners were charged in 8 (42%) cases; 3 were convicted. Fines totalled $150 and no one was imprisoned. Hospital social services became involved in 10 cases; 5 were reported to state CPS with 1 finding of neglect.

CONCLUSIONS: 1) Handguns were the predominant weapon used in these unintentional shootings; 2) Shooters and gun owners were rarely held accountable for the injuries caused; 3) The state child protection agency was rarely involved; 4) Making gun owners and shooters responsible for unintentional shootings of children will require a shift in attitudes throughout our society.

Poster No. 155
Patterns of Causation for Intentional Injury in a Population Based Study of Urban Children

L. L. Davidson, M. S. Durkin, P. O'Connor, B. Barlow, and M.C. Heagarty

Departments of Pediatrics, Pediatric Surgery, and Public Health, Columbia University, New York, NY, and Russell Sage College, Troy, NY

Although the proportion of intentional injuries causing death to urban children is rising, little is known of the pattern of injury causation which does not result in death. The denominator in this epidemiological study of injuries was an urban population of 91,000 children under 17. The numerator was drawn from three sources covering a five year period: the medical records of the two primary hospitals serving the area and the deaths certificates from the Department of Health. This represents 100% of the deaths and a sample of 77% of the hospitalizations.

Of the 2752 injuries causing hospitalization or death, almost 9% were intentional. Of the 76 deaths to children, 34% were intentional. This varied by age in a J shaped distribution rising sharply in adolescence: 4% of the 841 injuries to 1-4 year olds were intentional, while 12% of the 685 to 10-14 year olds and 25% of the 353 to 15 and 16 year olds were intentional assaults. The patterns of specific causes were also related to the age of the children.

Proportion of Intentional Injuries Due to Specific Causes

Causes(%):	Striking	Falls	Drown	Burns	Guns	Pierce	Ingest	Undetermined*
Age Groups(N)**								
<1 yr(17)	35	18	6	6	0	0	0	35
1-4 yr(30)	27	3	0	17	7	0	7	37
5-9 yr(38)	68	3	0	3	13	3	0	3
10-14 yr(83)	52	5	0	0	16	22	0	5
15-16 yr(88)	36	4	0	0	32	25	0	1

*This category includes what seemed to be primarily striking injuries, but the history was not clear enough to assign an E-code

**N = number of intentional injuries

What can be concluded is that drowning, ingestions and burns are primarily found as intentional injuries only in the younger age groups while gun shot wounds and stab/piercing injuries occur with increasing frequency in the older age groups. Given that the underdetermined category seem to be primarily striking injuries, striking as a cause of intentional injury occurs across the age range.

Poster No. 156
Physician Decisions to Report and Label Suspected Child Maltreatment

L. S. Wissow, M. E. H. Wilson, and G. L. Zellman

Department of Pediatrics, Johns Hopkins University School of Medicine, Baltimore, Md, and The Rand Corp, Santa Monica, Calif

Despite legal requirements many physicians do not report all cases in which they suspect maltreatment. This study examined how differences in specialty, attitudes, and experience influence the decisions of primary care physicians to make reports and label cases as abuse or neglect. Subjects were a random sample of Maryland pediatricians, family practitioners, and emergency physicians (n=727). Mailed questionnaires asked for anonymous responses to vignettes of 3 cases of injury said to be related to a small child's accidental household fall. Variations in the cases allowed separate measurement of the effects of caretaker identity (mother or stepfather) and injury type (head contusion, skull or femur fracture). For each case physicians were asked if they would report suspected maltreatment and if the report would be for abuse or neglect. They were also asked for opinions on 8 statements about the impact of reporting (the chance of resolving the problem alone, the risk of losing the family, etc.). There were 351 questionnaires returned (48%); differences in response rate by specialty and rural/urban residence were considered in the calculation of results, as were variations in the vignettes' portrayal of injury severity and caretaker.

The specialties differed in practice setting, prior experience with maltreatment, and attitudes about the effects of reporting. Family practitioners were most likely to be working in direct contact, continuity settings. They were least likely to have ever reported child abuse (76% vs. more than 90% for pediatricians and emergency physicians). Emergency physicians were most likely to support prompt reporting; family practitioners tended to endorse a more cautious approach. Attitudes about reporting were more important determinants of intention to report the study vignettes than was specialty. On average, less cautious physicians were 40% more likely to say they would report study cases than were physicians who were more cautious. Physicians endorsing a cautious approach to reporting were more likely to label the cases they intended to report as neglect rather than abuse. We conclude that differences in physician attitudes about reporting may contribute to inconsistencies in the application of reporting laws and the responses of agencies whose actions vary by the type of report received.

Poster No. 157
Sexual Abuse by Father-Figures: A Comparison of Natural Fathers, Stepfathers, and Mothers' Paramours

A. R. De Jong

Department of Pediatrics, Jefferson Medical College of Thomas Jefferson University, Philadelphia, Pa

Sexually abused children often name father-figures as abusers. Although increased abuse risk has been suggested within stepfamilies, little has been written comparing abuse by stepfathers (SF), natural fathers (NF), and mothers' paramours (MP). The purpose of this study was to compare specific features of the abuse and the childrens' responses to abuse by NF, SF, and MP.

All victims under age 15 years seen at a sexual assault center were included in the descriptive data and behavioral assessments were obtained on all keeping followup appointments. Father-figures were abusers in 308 cases (NF=128, SF=65, MP=115), representing 23.3% of all child victims. No significant variation was found among the three father-figure groups with respect to the victims' age or gender, type of sexual contact, presence of physical trauma, whether violence was involved, whether followup appointments were kept, or the frequency of phobias, sleep problems, regression, somatic complaints or behavior changes in their victims. (Chi square, $p>.05$)

Stepwise regression analysis was performed using the abuser group as the dependent variable. The analysis included 14 sociodemographic variables, abuse descriptors, and childrens' responses which were significant or approached significance. Only four variables were predictors of the abuser group: duration of abuse ($p<.01$, $R^2 = .068$), child expressed anger ($p<.01$, $R^2 = .101$), race ($p<.01$, $R^2 = .145$), and child expressed guilt ($p<.01$, $R^2 = .175$). NF often abused children for >1 year (34%). Victims verbalized more guilt (19%) and less anger (27%). SF also often abused children for >1 year (42%). Victims verbalized average guilt (12%), but more anger (45%). MP rarely abused victims for >1 year (8%), and abuse was more often disclosed after a single episode than NF or SF abuse (32% vs 18%). Their victims rarely expressed guilt (0%), but frequently expressed anger (47%). A higher percentage of NF abusers were white (NF=41%, SF=18%, MP=15%).

Despite many similarities in specific features of abuse by NF, SF, and MP, significant differences in abuse dynamics are reflected in the victims' responses and expressed feelings.

Poster No. 158
An Association Between Sexual Abuse and Early Adolescent Pregnancy

J. E. Cox, L. Coyne, and W. G. Bithoney

Department of Pediatrics, Harvard Medical School, and Childrens Hospital, Boston, Mass

We examined the hypothesis that a history of sexual abuse predisposes adolescents to early parenthood. The medical records, which included detailed interviews, of 147 inner-city, welfare dependent adolescent mothers, aged 13-17 years, followed in a hospital based teen tot clinic were examined for history of sexual abuse and age of first pregnancy. The population was 76% black, 22% hispanic, and 2% white. 28 (19.3%) of young mothers had history of sexual abuse prior to their first pregnancy. 16 of the 34 perpetrators (47.1%) were family members. Only 8/34 episodes (23.5%) were immediately disclosed with 9 (26.5%) revealed more than one year later. Of the 28 mothers with history of sexual abuse, 19 were abused prior to age 12 (67.8%) and 9 (32.2%) after age 12 with an average age of first abuse of 9.7 years. 9/19 (47.4%) of the episodes prior to age 12 years involved intercourse compared to 7/9 (77.8%) of episodes after age 12 years ($p<0.05$). 11 of the 28 mothers with history of sexual abuse received psychotherapy.

These 28 teen mothers were compared to the 119 teen mothers without past history of sexual abuse. The mothers with history of sexual abuse were younger at first pregnancy with a mean age of 15.0 ± 1.4 years than those without history of sexual abuse who first became pregnant at 16.3 ± 1.3 years ($p<0.005$). Mothers with history of sexual abuse were more likely to have been in foster care, 14/28 (50%) vs. 23/119 (19.3%), ($p<0.005$), and to have used illicit drugs, 7/28 (25%) vs. 10/119 (8.4%), ($p<0.01$). Since our study was based on a record review, it probably underestimates the extent of sexual abuse in our population. However, our study demonstrates that history of sexual abuse is common in adolescent mothers. More importantly, adolescents with a history of sexual abuse become parents at an earlier age than do adolescents without a prior history of sexual abuse. Further studies are needed to examine both the background of sexual abuse in our population and the sequelae of sexual abuse.

Poster No. 159
Utilization of Prenatal Care by Adolescents: Who Starts When?

M. C. Pew, J. M. Leventhal, and S. M. Horwitz

Department of Pediatrics,
Yale University School of Medicine, New Haven, Conn

Early prenatal care has been associated with better outcomes for teenage mothers and their children, yet only half of teenage mothers begin care early. The purpose of this study was to assess whether adolescents delay because of 1) limited access to care or 2) characteristics of the teens themselves. We surveyed 57 primigravida women ≤ 18 yrs. of age (mean age: 16 yrs.), who sought care in a hospital-based program for inner-city young mothers from 1/90-8/90. With a semi-structured interview and review of the medical records, we collected information about barriers to care and personal and social details. Teens who enrolled early (in the first trimester) were compared to late enrollees.

Thirty of the 57 teens (53%) enrolled early, and 27 (47%) enrolled late. There were no differences between early vs. late enrollees in age, race, grade in school, method of payment, waiting time for the appointment or transportation time to the clinic. In contrast, the early enrollees were more likely to have a telephone (97% vs. 74%; $p<.002$), and to seek other medical care before pregnancy (50% vs. 18%; $p<.02$). While both groups suspected pregnancy early, the early enrollees shared the news sooner (1.9 mo.vs. 2.9 mo.; $p<.002$), were more likely to tell only family at first (27% vs. 0%; $p<.005$), and less likely to plan to move after delivery (20% vs. 48%; $p<.03$). Depression was twice as frequent among late enrollees (52% vs. 26%; $p=.05$).

In summary, young teenagers who began prenatal care late had the same access to care as those who began early, but their socioeconomic status, health behaviors, reliance on family and prevalence of depression were different. We conclude that the tendency to delay prenatal care accompanies important risk factors for a poor outcome of pregnancy, such as extreme poverty and depression. Improving the outcomes of teenage pregnancies will require more than increasing access to prenatal care.

Poster No. 160
Adolescent Aids Education in a Pediatric Emergency Department

A. J. Behrman, K. N. Shaw, and F. S. Shofer

Departments of Internal Medicine and Pediatrics,
University of Pennsylvania School of Medicine,
Philadelphia

Two-hundred and seventy-eight subjects aged 12-25 from an inner-city pediatric emergency department (ED) serving a minority population were surveyed for AIDS-related knowledge, attitudes, and risk behavior as they waited for care for themselves or their children. Subjects completed a 61-question survey followed by a short videotape or no educational intervention. Both groups were re-interviewed by telephone at 1-2 weeks. There were no significant differences between the groups for age, gender, parental status, baseline knowledge or follow-up rates. Twenty-nine percent admitted risk factors for HIV infection.

Analysis showed that over 90% knew HIV transmission could occur via sex, intravenous drug abuse (IVDA), contaminated blood products, and perinatal transmission. However, there were striking deficiencies in baseline knowledge. For example, many believed that AIDS was transmitted via toilets (26%), eating utensils (39%), coughing (29%), blood donation (28%), and mosquitos (54%); blood transfusion was considered a high risk by 54%. A high percentage did not know that AIDS could be acquired from anal sex (26%), oral sex (40%), or sex with a healthy IVDA (21%); nor that other sexually transmitted diseases (STDs) increased the risk of HIV infection (75%). Seventy percent did not know AIDS is increasing among black women. Only 56% remembered ever hearing about AIDS in school (despite a well established K-12 public school AIDS program). There were no differences in baseline knowledge scores with respect to age, gender, or admitted risk behavior. Follow-up knowledge scores were better overall for the intervention group than the controls ($p<0.05$). Specifically, scores were significantly improved in the intervention group with respect to the risk of anal sex, oral sex, and coexisting STDs; the increase in AIDS among black women; and knowing where to get further information.

High risk adolescents and young adults seeking non-acute care in inner city EDs may lack access to other sources of AIDS education. The ED waiting room can be a site for effective educational intervention.

Poster No. 161
Clinical Utility of Chlamydia Trachomatis Diagnostic Techniques in Adolescent Women

F. M. Biro, S. F. Reising, and J. A. Doughman

Department of Pediatrics,
Children's Hospital Medical Center,
University of Cincinnati, Ohio

To evaluate the clinical utility of various diagnostic tests, 2 enzyme immunoassays (Abbott Chlamydiazyme (CZM), Syva Microtrak (MT), and a non-isotopic DNA probe (Gen-Probe Pace II (GPP) were compared to cell culture (with monoclonal antibody confirmation) for the diagnosis of endocervical *Chlamydia trachomatis* infection. There were 479 consecutive patients enrolled, of whom 473 had complete data collection. The order of sample collection was randomized. Patients were stratified according to whether they were asymptomatic (N=206), symptomatic (defined by patient's symptoms of dysuria, discharge, burning, or abdominal pain) (N=219), or test of cure (N=48). Discrepant analysis was performed when culture was negative and nonculture technique was positive. The patient was considered to have *C. trachomatis* if culture was positive, or if 2 or more alternate techniques were positive. Overall prevalence of *C. trachomatis* was 11.7% in the asymptomatic, 23.2% in the symptomatic, and 6.2% in the test of cure group. Because there were few positive Chlamydia results in the test of cure group (4 of 48), no further analyses were performed. Sensitivity (SENS), specificity (SPEC), positive predictive value (PPV), and negative predictive value (NPV) were calculated for both symptomatic and asymptomatic groups. Pending discrepant analysis for GPP, the following results were obtained:

	Symptomatic				Asymptomatic			
	SENS	SPEC	PPV	NPV	SENS	SPEC	PPV	NPV
Culture	72.5	100	100	92.3	79.2	100	100	97.3
CZM	72.5	100	100	92.3	50.0	100	100	93.8
MT	86.3	98.8	95.7	96.0	79.2	98.9	90.5	97.3
GPP	70.6	95.8	83.7	91.4	70.8	95.6	68.0	96.1

Clinical presentation should influence the choice of test(s) for a specific patient.

Poster No. 162
Peer Screeners to Identify Substance Abuse in Pregnant Teens

S. Barnett, D.P. McCormick, G. Wilkinson, and A. Berensen

Departments of Pediatrics,
Preventive Medicine/Community Health, and Obstetrics,
University of Texas Medical Branch at Galveston

Despite the growing recognition of disastrous outcomes in pregnant adolescents using drugs and alcohol, the early diagnosis of this problem remains elusive. In a meta analysis of prevention studies Tobler reported improved results using peer-oriented drug prevention programs.

We compared two methods of screening adolescents for drug use. First, a peer screener (PS), a 16 year old Hispanic female, used a structured interview beginning with innocuous questions and progressing to queries regarding substance use in pregnant/post partum teens. Second, during a routine prenatal exam, obstetrical practitioners (OBP), female physicians' assistants with 5-9 years of experience, queried pregnant teens about cigarette, alcohol, and drug use. IRB approved oral assent obtained by the PS; confidentiality was maintained. Results are:

No. of Patients	Peer Screeners n=69 % #	OB Practitioners n=41 % #	Relative Risk
Any Substance Use	65.0(45)	27.0(11)	2.41
Smoking	18.7(13)	19.5(8)	0.96
Alcohol	33.2(23)	12.2(5)	2.72
Drugs	37.7(26)	19.4(8)	1.94

The two groups were similar in age, race, and socio-economic mix. The PS was 2.41 times more likely to identify a history of positive substance use than the OBP. Similar findings occurred in identifying alcohol (2.72) and drug (1.94) use but not tobacco use (0.96).

A peer screener may be more likely to identify substance use in pregnant teens. Controlled studies to evaluate these findings are planned to determine whether peers on clinical health teams could improve diagnosis of substance use in pregnant adolescents.

Poster No. 163
PID: Evaluation and Treatment in a Pediatric vs Adult Emergency Department

J. M. Lavelle, I. Reyes, and K. N. Shaw

Department of Pediatrics, University of Pennsylvania
School of Medicine, Philadelphia;
The Children's Hospital of Philadelphia;
and The Hospital of the University of Pennsylvania,
Philadelphia

A one year retrospective study of 399 adolescent females who presented to an adult (194) or pediatric (205) emergency department and evaluated for PID was conducted. Race, socioeconomic status, presenting complaints, rate of positive GC cultures, severity of illness as determined by objective clinical and laboratory criteria, and treatment rate at first visit were similar at both institutions. Although charts from both institutions lacked important documentation, information was more likely to be lacking from the pediatric charts; gravity was not recorded in 86% as compared to 18% at the adult ED, and results of pregnancy testing were unknown in 24 pediatric ED patients vs. 7 adult ED patients. At both institutions RPR results were unknown in 30% of cases, of those done, 12% were reactive. Ultrasounds were done in 22% pediatric patients vs. 4% adult patients with similar rates of positive results.

Adolescents diagnosed with PID were more likely to be admitted if they presented to a pediatric ED, [odds 2.5 (95% CI: 1.3-5), $p<0.005$] even when physical exam findings were absent; 18% had no cervical motion tenderness, 20% had no adnexal tenderness, and 43% had no lower abdominal tenderness. However, no patient was admitted to the adult hospital without these findings. When only patients who met objective criteria for PID were compared, the adolescent at the pediatric hospital was still more likely to be admitted, [odds 4.4 (95% CI: 1.8-11), $p<0.001$], especially those under 16 years of age ($p<0.02$).

Many adolescent patients are seeking care for PID in pediatric settings, therefore education and standard of care need to be improved. These data are also reflective of conflicting policies regarding hospitalization of young females for PID.

Poster No. 164
Prior Advice Seeking and Increased Appropriate Use of a Paediatric Emergency Room

T. F. Oberlander, I. B. Pless, G. E. Dougherty, and D. McGillivray

Department of Pediatrics,
McGill University, Montreal, Quebec

Seeking advice prior to an unscheduled visit to a pediatric emergency room (PER) may influence the appropriate use of this setting for minor illnesses. To address this issue a questionnaire was given to parents of children 0-18 years ($n=489$) visiting a PER, asking whether they had sought advice from family, friends, or a physician and about factors possibly related to the decision to seek care. Appropriateness was rated, blind to discharge diagnosis, by two pediatricians using an established algorithm incorporating child's age, time of visit, clinical state and problem at presentation. Substantial agreement was found between these pediatricians (Kappa = .71). The response rate was 50% and non-responders did not differ significantly with respect to age, sex, time of visit and appropriateness rating. Overall, 34% of visits were appropriate.

Bivariate analysis showed appropriateness was significantly related to advice seeking, having a regular physician, two or more children, older parents and the absence of prior treatment ($p<.05$); it was not related to sex, time since last physician visit or level of parents' education ($p>.05$).

A logistic regression model with appropriateness (Yes/No) as outcome showed appropriate visits occurred significantly more often when a parent spoke to both a physician and non-physician prior to visiting the PER, than when only one of these individuals was consulted, or when no advice was sought (Odds Ratio [OR] 2.7, 95% confidence interval [CI] 1.4-5.3). [Talking to a physician alone, OR 1.7, CI 1.0-2.8; talking to a non-physician alone, OR 1.6, CI .9-2.9]. The model also showed that having a regular physician and two or more children contributed significantly (OR 2.2, CI 1.1-4.3; OR 2.1, CI 1.3-3.1, respectively).

These findings suggest that appropriate use of a PER is positively influenced by prior advice seeking, especially with a physician and family member, having a regular physician and a parent's past child care experience.

Poster No. 165
Prehospital IV Placement in Children

K. A. Grisanti and D. M. Jaffe

Department of Pediatrics, Hospital for Sick Children, University of Toronto (Ontario)

Sick and injured children present unique challenges in diagnosis, psychosocial care, and successful accomplishment of essential procedures to prehospital care providers. Our purpose was to examine the ability of a unified metropolitan paramedic system with no intraosseous protocol to provide intravenous (IV) access when indicated. All paramedic transports involving children in metropolitan Toronto from January, 1988 through October, 1990 were reviewed. Indications for IV access, rates of successful placement, and time to achieve access were determined. Age related failure rates were compared using the chi-square statistic and time to achieve IV access using the t-test.

There were 477 children < 19 years, comprising 4.7% of all paramedic transports. The mean age was 9.0 years. 40% were < 6 years, and 61% were male. The paramedic diagnoses were: trauma (31%); seizures (27%); asthma (13%); cardiac arrest (5%); and respiratory distress (5%). Condition during transport included 34% with decreased level of consciousness, 9% with seizures, and 8% with vital signs absent (VSA).

IV attempts were made in 277 children (58%). IV placement was obtained in 236 (85% of patients attempted). The mean time from arrival on scene to IV placement was 9.8 minutes (range 1-45 minutes). Our strict criteria for IV placement were: cardiac arrest, shock, extensive burns, major trauma, and intubation. Of the 152 children who met criteria, 29% failed to receive an IV. IV placement was not attempted or unsuccessful in 47% of children < 6 years meeting criteria, as compared to 22% in children ≥ 6 years ($p = .003$). Non-trauma patients accounted for most of the age related difference. Of children < 6 years with VSA, the failure rate was 63% but only 23% in children ≥ 6 years ($p = .026$). Time to achieve successful access did not differ among age groups.

We conclude that skilled paramedics are unable to achieve IV access when indicated in a significant proportion of children especially those < 6 years of age. Intraosseous access may provide a useful alternative.

Poster No. 166
Responses of Children, Parents, and Nurses to Tympanic Thermometry in the Pediatric Office

D. T. Alexander and B. A. Kelly

Department of Pediatrics,
University of Pennsylvania
School of Medicine, Philadelphia,
and Children's Hospital of Philadelphia

This study was designed to assess children's behavioral responses to tympanic thermometry. In addition, parents' and nurses' impressions of this new technology were evaluated. Infrared tympanic thermometry eliminates the risks associated with traditional methods of temperature taking including mucus membrane contact and glass breakage. Temperature taking by this method is rapid taking only one second. 224 patients were enrolled from three private pediatric practices in suburban Philadelphia during regular office hours. Patients were alternately assigned to have their temperature taken with either a tympanic thermometer or with a rectal or oral thermometer depending on the patient's age. Parents and nurses were then asked to fill out a short questionnaire to describe their observations of the child's behavior during temperature taking and to describe their own feelings about the temperature taking method used. Parents were also asked to assess their usual method of temperature taking at home and their child's usual behavioral response at home.

Tympanic thermometry was rated higher by both parents and nurses for speed, ease, cleanliness, and safety. These differences were statistically significant. Parents and nurses were more confident in the accuracy of traditional temperature taking methods. Children whose temperatures were taken rectally were more likely to be observed by both parents ($p=.02$) and nurses ($p=.01$) to have a negative behavioral reaction to the procedure than children whose temperatures were taken by tympanic thermometry. There was no difference observed between the behavioral responses of children who had temperatures taken orally and those who had tympanic thermometry.

Our data show that the benefits of tympanic thermometry are appreciated by both parents and nursing professionals. Temperature taking can be particularly upsetting for the younger child. The data from this study clearly suggest that young children prefer tympanic thermometry to rectal temperature taking.

Poster No. 167
Effect of Personalized Letter Reminders on Preventive Appointment Show Rates and Vaccination Status

J. R. Campbell, P. G. Szilagyi, L. E. Rodewald, C. B. Doane, and K. J. Roghmann

Department of Pediatrics, University of Rochester (NY), Strong Memorial Hospital

Postcard reminders specifying the time of preventive health care (PHC) visits improve show rates in primary care settings. Few studies have evaluated personalized letter reminders that specify the content of an upcoming PHC visit (e.g., immunizations, anticipatory guidance). While personalized reminders are costly to create, they can inform parents of the benefits of an upcoming PHC visit. We studied the effect of personalized letter reminders (L), generic postcard reminders (P) or no reminders (control; C) on PHC visits of infants enrolled at a teaching hospital pediatric continuity clinic.

In this prospective clinical trial, newborns (N=295) were randomized to one of the three study groups and followed for 13 months. The clinic staff were blind to group allocation. For every PHC visit the investigators sent either postcards to the P group or letters specific to the particular PHC visit to the L group.

There were no differences in demographic features among the groups (Table). The show rates for the L and P groups were not different from each other, and were significantly higher than the show rate for the control group. The L and P groups had fewer appointments scheduled per patient, but the number of kept appointments per patient was the same for all groups. The mean age of completion of the primary DPT series was the same for the 3 groups.

We conclude that (1) costly personalized letter reminders, while providing more information to parents, are no more effective than inexpensive postcard reminders in this setting, (2) vaccination status is not improved by either type of reminder in a setting having high immunization rates for infants, and (3) letter and postcard reminders improve clinic efficiency by decreasing the number of unused, scheduled appointments.

	Percent Medicaid[2]	2-Factor Hollingshead[3]	PHC SR[4]	# Sched Visits	# Kept Visits	Age at 3rd DPT
Letter[1]	89	57	73.1%*	5.9*	4.2	7.6 mo.
Postcard[1]	78	55	74.4%*	6.0*	4.3	7.0 mo.
Control	83	58	67.6%	6.7	4.3	7.6 mo.

[1] Group compared with control group (t-test) * $P < 0.05$ [2] Chi-square among all groups = 3.87, P = 0.2 [3] Hollingshead score, based on head of household occupation and education [4] Show rate (SR)

Poster No. 168
Metal Detectors—An Alternative Approach to the Evaluation of Coin Ingestions in Children?

S. P. Ros and F. Cetta

Pediatrics, Loyola University Medical Center, Maywood, Ill

Foreign body ingestions constitute a common problem in pediatric emergency medicine. Recent data indicate that, despite current recommendations, most children who ingest coins do not undergo radiologic evaluation. The purpose of this study was to determine the accuracy of a metal detector in localizing coins in a model simulating coin ingestions in children. The distance between the anterior chest wall (ACW) and the esophagus was measured on seventeen chest computed tomograms obtained on children between the ages of three months and six years. Subsequently, a diameter equal to the mean ACW to lower esophageal sphincter measurement was marked across the investigator's forearm. A second investigator then attempted to detect the presence of the coin through the forearm by using a Super Scanner (Garrett Security Systems Inc, Texas) metal detector. The study was conducted in a blinded manner and consisted of fifty attempts equally divided between pennies, nickels, dimes, quarters and controls (no coin). The accuracy of the metal detector in identifying the presence or absence of coins in our model was 100%. We conclude that the metal detector evaluated by us is highly accurate in identifying coins through human tissues and it should become a valuable and practical tool in the evaluation of children following a coin ingestion.

Poster No. 169
Efficacy of Cough Suppressants in Treating Nighttime Cough in Children

J. A. Taylor, A. H. Novack, J. R. Almquist, and J. E. Rogers

Department of Pediatrics,
University of Washington, Seattle,
and Carolinas Medical Center, Charlotte, NC

Data are not available on the efficacy of cough suppressants in pediatrics patients with acute cough. To test our hypothesis that guaifenesin with codeine (C) or with dextromethorphan (DM) are effective in alleviating the symptoms of nighttime cough a double-blinded, placebo-controlled study was conducted. Children 18 months-12 years old with significant nighttime cough were recruited from private pediatric practices. Parents responded to a questionnaire describing the severity of 3 symptoms (amount of coughing, loss of sleep, and post-tussive emesis) on the previous night for use as baseline data for each patient. The child was then randomized to receive C, DM or placebo (PL) at bedtime for 3 consecutive days with completion of an identical questionnaire rating the symptoms each night. Answers were transformed to an ordinal scale for analysis. A successful therapeutic intervention was defined as a reduction of at least 2 points in cough score on any day of the study from cough score at baseline (range 0-4 for each day). A composite symptom score was computed for each day (range 0-10); reduction in symptom score was calculated by subtracting symptom score for any day of study from symptom score at baseline. Of 49 eligible children 13 received PL, 19 DM, and 17 C. On entry mean cough and symptom scores were similar for each group ($P > 0.2$). Percent of patients with a successful therapeutic intervention, and mean reduction in symptom score for each drug for each day are summarized below.

	% of Patients With Successful Therapy			Mean Reduction in Symptom Score		
	day 1	day 2	day 3	day 1	day 2	day 3
PL	46.2	46.2	76.9	2.67	3.62	4.69
DM	57.9	47.4	63.2	2.95	3.28	4.13
C	29.4	64.7	82.4	1.76	2.47	3.85

For every comparison between study drugs the P value was > 0.05; the smallest P value was 0.10 comparing reduction in symptom score on day 1 between DM and C. We conclude that there is little difference between PL, DM and C. Cough suppressants are not indicated for treatment of nighttime cough in children.

Poster No. 170
Milder Symptoms Occur in Recurrent Episodes of Streptococcal Infection

K. A. Woodin, L. H. Lee, and M. E. Pichichero

Department of Pediatrics, University of Rochester, NY

We hypothesized that Group A streptococcal (GABHS) recurrences with homologous serotypes present with milder symptoms than those encountered on initial infection.

Data collected prospectively as part of a multi-centered, randomized antibiotic efficacy trial performed during 1981-1983 was re-evaluated to answer this question. Patients were routinely evaluated at 4-6 days, 18-21 days and 32-35 days following the start of treatment or if they were symptomatic. All casebooks were reviewed and patients with second infections in which M typing or T agglutination data and anti-streptolysin O and anti-DNAase serology was available were evaluated. Recurrences were defined as the presence of the same serotype on follow-up culture with evidence of antibody rise. Charts from all eligible patients were abstracted for signs and symptoms of GABHS infection. The data was analysed with the Student t test and chi-square analysis; each recurrent infection was compared with the initial infection.

Seventy (24%) of the 295 patients had a second episode of GABHS infection during the study period. Twenty-eight recurrences were identified; they occurred a mean of 23 days following the initial infection (median 21 days). These patients showed significant differences between their two infections for symptoms of sore throat, headache, chills ($p<.001$), and signs of fever ($p=.003$), pharyngeal erythema ($p<.001$), exudate ($p=.007$), palatal petechiae ($p=.01$), and ≥2+ adenitis ($p=.004$). However, earache, upper respiratory tract symptoms, stomache, tonsillar enlargement, and scarletina were similar on both occasions.

Milder symptoms occur with recurrent homologous GABHS infections compared with the initial infection. These findings are relevant since patients with milder symptoms may be less likely to seek physician attention.

Poster No. 171
Strategies for Diagnosis (Dx) and Treatment of Febrile Infants: Clinical and Cost-effectiveness

T. A. Lieu, M. N. Baskin, J. S. Schwartz, and G. R. Fleisher

Department of Pediatrics,
University of Pennsylvania, Philadelphia

Fever in infants may signify serious bacterial infection. We conducted a clinical and cost-effectiveness analysis for Dx and Rx of infants 29-89 days with T≥38.0 C. The baseline analysis used data on 503 pts in a study of intramuscular ceftriaxone (IM cef) and estimates from the literature to evaluate 6 strategies: (1) No Dx, No Rx; (2) Lumbar puncture (LP) with CSF, blood (Bcx), and urine (Urcx) cultures, white blood count (WBC) and urinalysis (UA), + intravenous antibiotics (IV abx) for all pts; (3) LP + IM cef for all pts with nl LPs; (4) Bcx & Urcx with WBC and UA; (5) WBC & UA; (6) Judgment. In strategies 4, 5, and 6, pts judged at high risk had Rx with IV abx; low-risk pts were observed as outpts without abx. For a hypothetical cohort of 100,000 febrile infants, the results are:

	# of Deaths or major sequelae	# (%) of sequelae prevented	# of abx compls/ sequelae prevented	Avg cost/ pt	Cost/death or sequelae prevented
LP + IV abx	244	747 (75)	34	$2038	$272,600
LP + IM cef	248	743 (75)	23	528	71,000
Bcx & Urcx	398	594 (60)	14	846	142,500
WBC & UA	468	523 (58)	16	841	160,800
Judgment	692	299 (30)	30	823	275,300
No Dx, No Rx	991	0 (00)	NA	247	NA

Sensitivity analyses show that the choice of strategy depends greatly on the effectiveness of im cef and the sensitivity of the WBC & UA. WBC & UA prevents more sequelae than LP + IM cef only when IM cef is assumed to be less than 53% effective. We conclude that: (1) strategies which combine LP and abx for all pts prevent the most sequelae; (2) LP + IM cef has equal clinical and superior cost-effectiveness compared with LP + IV abx; (3) strategies which use WBC & UA or clinical judgment do not surpass strategies which use LP + abx even when test sensitivity is very high.

Poster No. 172
Blood Cultures in the Outpatient Setting: What Is the Optimum Number & Method?

K. J. DiPasquale, G. G. Gaar, and A. B. Anderson

The Emergency Associates for Medicine,
The Tampa (Fla) General Hospital

Obtaining blood cultures (BC's) in young children to rule out bacteremia without contaminating the specimen has always been a challenge in the outpatient setting. Pediatricians traditionally obtain one BC while in the adult population multiple cultures are routinely obtained. The optimum number of cultures and method of collection for pediatric patients remain to be determined. This study was designed to analyze 1) the sensitivity of one versus two BC's and 2) the difference in contamination rates between collection methods.

In this prospective clinical study, all patients 0-18 years of age who met predetermined criteria to have a BC drawn were eligible. 408 patients were enrolled from August to November, 1990, representing 6.6% of total patient visits to the Pediatric Emergency Care Center at Tampa General Hospital. Two sets of BC's were obtained from each patient using a standard protocol employing aseptic technique. The first set was collected through a newly inserted IV catheter. The second set was collected at a separate venipuncture site using a butterfly or straight needle exclusively for collection of the BC specimen. A minimum blood volume of 0.5 ml was obtained for each bottle. Cultures were separated by an interval of at least 10 minutes. A standard data collection sheet was completed on each patient. All cultures were processed in the clinical microbiology lab. Followup was done by chart review and or telephone contact. Data analysis was done using the sign test.

To date, true pathogens were identified in 11/408 (2.7%) BC's. All 11 pathogens were identified in the first set of BC's, while only 8/11 (73%) cultures were also positive in the second set. Analysis of contaminants shows that 38/408 (9.3%) of the first specimen were contaminated versus 7/408 (1.7%) from the second specimen ($p < .01$).

At the present time our data do not allow us to draw a statistical conclusion concerning the necessity of more than one BC. Further data from this ongoing study will be presented at the time of the meetings. It is clear that obtaining BC's through newly inserted IV catheters significantly increases the risk of contamination ($p < .01$). The ideal method for obtaining BC's appears to be phlebotomy for the sole purpose of obtaining a specimen for culture.

Poster No. 173
Diagnostic Test Ordering in the Evaluation of Febrile Children: the Role of Physician and Environmental Factors

D. L. McGillivray, R. Roberts-Brauer, and M. S. Kramer

Departments of Pediatrics and Epidemiology
and Biostatistics, McGill University, Montreal, Quebec

Patient factors such as age, temperature, duration of illness, and "toxicity" are known to affect physicians' use of diagnostic tests in febrile children. Our objective was to assess the independent effects of physician (gender, practice type, and experience of attending staff; presence and level of trainees) and environmental (pre- or post-July 1, patient load, time of day, day of week, referral status) factors on ordering a complete blood count, blood culture, BUN, urinalysis, urine culture, throat culture, chest x-ray, and lumbar puncture. We prospectively studied 6,191 consecutive visits by nonadmitted febrile (rectal T ≥38.0°C) children <18 years of age to a children's hospital emergency department from March 1989 to November 1989. Multiple logistic regression analysis was used to control for the mutually confounding effects of patient, physician, and environmental factors and to assess attending staff-trainee interactions (effect modification).

One or more diagnostic tests were ordered in 39.6% of the visits. Patients evaluated by hospital-based subspecialists were more likely to receive tests than those evaluated by community-based physicians [e.g., odds ratio (OR) for complete blood count = 1.28 (95% confidence interval = 1.12-1.46)]. Children seen by physicians with >10 years experience were significantly less likely to receive tests than those seen by their more junior colleagues, but this effect was modified substantially by trainee presence and level. For example, when no trainee was involved, care by experienced physicians had an OR (relative to care by those with <5 years experience) of 0.51 (0.38-0.68) for ordering a chest x-ray. Involvement by a junior trainee (medical student, intern, or first-year resident), however, increased the OR to 0.79 (0.59-

1.07), while involvement by a senior resident increased the OR to 0.96 (0.72-1.29). For all tests except the throat culture, patients seen on or after July 1 were significantly more likely to be tested [e.g., OR = 1.36 (1.16-1.58) for blood culture]. These attending staff, trainee, and seasonal effects on test ordering have important implications for febrile children and their families, clinical training and supervision, and health care costs.

Poster No. 174
Management of Febrile Infants by Practicing Pediatricians

D. Bergman, R. Pantell, S. Brotherton, and the PROS Network of the AAP

Department of Pediatrics,
University of California, San Francisco

The optimal management of febrile infants remains elusive. Because of the low incidence of serious illness (bacterial meningitis and sepsis) for which errors in clinical judgment are of considerable consequence, adequate sample sizes of febrile infants have not been achieved making studies of clinical predictors unconvincing.

The Pediatric Research in Office Settings (PROS) Network of the American Academy of Pediatrics has completed two separate two month pilot studies (n = 200, n = 120) of febrile (>38.0°C) infants (<2 months). Two hundred and thirty-eight physicians in 91 practices from 33 states provided prospective observational data on their diagnostic and management approaches to febrile infants seen in their offices. This group of infants were predominantly white (82.2%) and only 15.7% received Medicaid or were without insurance. Sixty-nine percent of infants did not appear ill and 10% had no further laboratory evaluation. Screening laboratory tests were commonly performed with 90% obtaining WBC, 77% blood cultures, 74% urinalysis, 69% urine culture and 64% lumbar puncture. Twenty one percent of infants did not receive antibiotics and 34% of infants were sent home. Of those infants hospitalized 52% had a specific illness diagnosed or suspected, while 48% were hospitalized as part of the physicians' routine management. The incidence of bacterial meningitis (1%) and sepsis (3%) in these studies from office practice are similar to reports from hospital-based series, and too small to make meaningful statements about the accuracy of clinical predictors. Also clinically noteworthy was urinary tract infection being diagnosed in 8% of the total sample (11% of infants with urinalysis).

In conclusion, this study documents the considerable variation in diagnostic and management approaches to febrile infants by a large national sample of practicing pediatricians. This practice variability and the capacity of a nationwide collaborative network provides an opportunity to complete the large scale (n>3000) outcome study required to determine the accuracy of different clinical strategies in detecting serious illness.

Poster No. 175
The Value of Early Treatment for the Prevention of Lyme Disease

F. Agre and R. M. Schwartz

Department of Pediatrics,
College of Physicians and Surgeons,
Columbia University, New York, NY

Over a three year period 179 patients were enrolled in a double blind, placebo controlled early treatment program for the prevention of Lyme disease. Enrollment criteria were that the patient be age 3 to 19 years of age and that the deer tick bite occurred no more than three days prior to treatment. The tick was brought to the physician for identification or identified by the family after looking at preserved specimens or pictures. Acute and six week convalescent blood samples were drawn for Lyme titer rise. Serological testing was done by I.F.A. 89 patients were randomized to treatment with penicillin or tetracycline, 250 mgm Q.I.D. for 10 days and 90 patients to placebo. Of four patients with weekly positive titer rise, one patient had clinical Lyme disease that received placebo. Of the remaining 3 patients with weekly positive titer rise, all of whom received a placebo, 1 had a Flu-like illness and 2 had no symptoms. No patients receiving an antibiotic had a significant titer rise. In a two and half year follow-up, no patient developed stage 2 or 3 Lyme disease. We conclude that because of the low incidence of Lyme disease in children bitten by a deer tick early prophylactic treatment is not warranted.

Poster No. 176
Adaptive Behavior in Subgroups of Children With Attention Deficit Disorder and Hyperactivity Disorder (ADHD)

N. J. Roizen, T. A. Blondis, and M. Stein

Department of Pediatrics,
University of Chicago (Ill)
Pritzker School of Medicine,
and Wyler Children's Hospital, Chicago

Children with ADHD often have impaired social competence. To better describe and quantitate this, the scores on the Vineland Adaptive Behavioral Scales (1984) (Vineland) which measure personal and social sufficiency were compared to Wechsler Intelligence Scale for Children-Revised (WISC-R) scores in children with ADHD. The subjects consisted of 74 children diagnosed in the multidisciplinary Hyperactivity and Learning Problem Clinic as having ADHD based on a combination of history, clinical observation, and standardized IQ tests, achievement tests, and behavior rating scales. The children with ADHD were separated into 3 subgroups: ADHD (n = 31), ADHD plus a learning disorder (LDADHD, n = 21), and ADHD plus oppositional defiant disorder. (ODDADHD, n = 22). The following was found:

	ADHD	LDADHD	ODDADHD
WISC-R Verbal IQ	99.0(SD±19.0)	98.4(SD±14.7)	99.6(SD±15.3)
WISC-R Performance IQ	97.9(SD±15.5)	96.8(SD±20.9)	100.7(SD±13.7)
WISC-R Full Scale IQ	97.8(SD±16.0)	97.0(SD±17.9)	100.4(SD±14.1)
Vineland Communication SS	82.0(SD±12.8)	70.7(SD±13.3)	71.3(SD±14.3)
Vineland Socialization SS	87.7(SD±17.2)	84.0(SD±17.9)	72.0(SD±14.3)
Vineland 3 Factor SS	79.7(SD±12.9)	73.1(SD±14.2)	68.6(SD±11.9)

Results indicated significant discrepancies between IQ and Vineland functions for all subgroups ($p \leq 0.04$). When all subgroups are combined and comparisons between WISC-R and Vineland scores are made the results show dramatic significance ($F = 136$, $p \leq 0.00001$). This study demonstrates that ADHD children with average intelligence show major adaptive dysfunction which is greater if the ADHD is associated with LD or ODD.

Poster No. 177
Who Provides Health Care to the Children of Physicians?

L. Dusdieker, J. Murph, C. Dungy, and W. Murph

Department of Pediatrics, University of Iowa
Hospitals and Clinics, Iowa City

To define health care interventions performed by physicians for their own children, a Likert scale questionnaire was sent to 701 physicians (residents, fellows and faculty) at a large midwestern teaching hospital. Of the 492 respondents 353 were parents of children ≤ 18 yrs of age. The father was identified as the parent physician (PP) in 78% of cases, the mother in 5% and both mother and father in 16%. A non-family physician was listed as the child's MD by 96% of the respondents. The majority of PP reported treating their afebrile child for acute illnesses such as vomiting, diarrhea, colds, etc. In this situation, 36% of PP rarely or never contacted the child's primary doctor. However, if the ill child was febrile (⩾38.5°C), 55% of PP rarely or never treated without consultation. Only 47% of PP always performed a physical exam of the ill child prior to treatment. Physicians were most likely to auscultate the chest of a child with a cough or examine the tympanic membranes of a child with ear pain and least likely to obtain a clean catch urine in a child with dysuria or a throat swab from a child complaining of a sore throat. 62% of PP never performed routine physical examinations of their children. Likewise, 54% of PP did not complete school/sports participation forms. Prescription medications were prescribed for children by 65% of PP. However, only half of the respondents considered the physical exam in their decision to use antibiotics. For children treated with antibiotics, 42% of parents rarely or never notified the child's MD so the event could be recorded in the child's health record. Also, 29% of PP self-referred their children to a specialist without consulting the child's MD. Analyses of treatment by the PP were performed comparing level of physician training, physician sex and primary care (pediatrics, internal medicine, family practice, emergency room) vs all other specialties. Primary care physicians consulted the child's MD for advice less often when their child was febrile ($p = 0.001$) and other physicians completed school/sports forms more frequently ($p = 0.04$). Physicians gave a variety of reasons for treating their own children with convenience listed as most important for 72% of PP and confidence in their own diagnostic and treatment skills as most important for 21% of respondents.

Poster No. 178
Vulnerable Infants and Doctor-Shopping: Common Psychosocial Determinants?

A. Okun and R. E. K. Stein

Department of Pediatrics,
Albert Einstein College of Medicine, Bronx, NY,
and Division of Ambulatory Pediatrics,
Bronx Municipal Hospital Center

Mothers who view their children as "vulnerable" may use medical services erratically, seek care from different doctors, or make emergency room (ER) or other unscheduled visits with seemingly minor complaints. Similar use patterns are associated with maternal psychological distress and, in adult services, with the need for social support. We hypothesized that postpartum women who reported greater levels of psychological distress and inadequate social support would view their infants as more vulnerable and display inconsistent patterns of pediatric medical care use.

Postpartum mothers of infants in the well-baby nursery of an urban, municipal hospital were interviewed and given Ilfeld's Psychiatric Symptom Index and five original questions about the quality of anticipated social support. Telephone interviews were conducted 3-4 months later to obtain details of the infants' medical encounters and administer Kemperer and Forsythe's Vulnerable Child Scale.

169 subjects were enrolled, and 121 (72%) were reached for follow-up. Mothers who perceived their 3-4 month-old infants as more vulnerable had greater levels of postpartum psychological distress ($r = .26$, $p < .01$) and had anticipated being subjected to more frequent demeaning remarks or worrisome advice ($r = .33$, $p < .001$). 30 (25%) mothers visited more than one doctor for a regular check-up, 59 (49%) made unscheduled walk-in visits, and 37 (30%) made ER visits, 6 with minor complaints. A trend toward higher levels of postpartum psychological distress existed among those who made ER visits with minor complaints. Psychological and social variables bore no other associations with specific medical care use patterns.

These findings support the hypothesis that certain social and psychological factors contribute to the development of a mother's perception of her infant as vulnerable. Further research is needed to determine if these in turn lead to different patterns of medical care use later in childhood.

Poster No. 179
Agreement of the Mother's and Physician's Perception of the Child's Health Status Correlates With Clinic and Emergency Room Use

M. Irigoyen and M. Goldstein

Department of Pediatrics, Babies Hospital,
and Columbia University, New York, NY

It has been alleged that many emergency room (ER) visits are trivial and primarily due to maternal concern. This study examines how mother's and physician's agreement on the child's health status correlates with ER and clinic use.

We surveyed 600 mother-physician pairs at the time of a scheduled visit at a pediatric clinic. The patient population was minority (70% Hispanic, 30% Black) and poor (82% welfare). Mothers and physicians were each asked to separately rate the child' health status: 1) how is the overall health of the child?, 2) does the child have a specific health problems?, 3) does the child get sick easily?, and 4) how worried are you about the child's health? On the basis of these ratings, children were categorized into one of three groups for each measure of health: mother and physician agree the child's health is poor, mother and physician disagree, and mother and physician agree the child's health is good. For each of the four measures of health status, when the mother and the physicians agreed that the child's health was poor, there was higher ER and clinic visits. Conversely, when they agreed that the health was good, there was lower ER and clinic visits. When the mother and the physicians disagreed, the number visits to ER and clinic was intermediate. (Sick easily for clinic and ER visits $p<0.05$, worry for clinic $p<0.001$, health problems for clinic $p<0.05$).

In conclusion, in this inner city population, the agreement and disagreement in the perceptions of children's health status by mothers and pediatricians correlated with visits to pediatric health services. This study provides evidence that the increased number of visits made by some children is warranted by their poor health and is associated with physician as well as maternal concerns for their health.

Poster No. 180
Parenting Stress in Families of Urban Third Graders

L. S. Grossman, M. M. Kappelman, and R. G. Chernoff

Department of Pediatrics,
University of Maryland School of Medicine, Baltimore

Pediatricians have been well trained in counseling parents of infants and toddlers regarding parenting. Substantially less attention is paid to counseling parents of school age children. This study was designed to identify the stressful areas in parenting for inner city families of elementary age children.

Parents of 146 randomly selected 3rd grade children were invited to complete the Parenting Stress Index (PSI). The female caretakers (96) or fathers (2) came in for 98 children (67% participation). Participants and non-participants were identical in race, sex, and achievement test results. The schools supplied demographic and school function information.

Study families did not differ significantly from the more middle class normative sample on PSI Total Stress, Parent Domain, or Life Stress scores using 95% confidence intervals. Study families did have significantly higher scores on the Child Domain portion of the PSI ($p<.02$). On subscales, parents of this urban sample felt their children were less acceptable ($p<.01$), more demanding ($p<.05$), moodier ($p<.01$), and less likely to reinforce them in their role as parents ($p<.001$) than norms. Parent subscales were similar to norms except these parents felt less depressed ($p<.02$), less attached to their children ($p<.05$), and less restricted in their lives ($p<.01$). There were no significant differences in responses based on child's sex or race. Parents whose children were performing poorly in school (achievement tests below grade level or enrollment in special education) were more likely to report parenting stress (parent domain, $p<.04$; child domain, $p<.001$) than those doing well.

This study suggests that there are areas in which parents of school age children could benefit from counseling. These include teaching about "normal" behavior, helping parents see the positive features of their child, and assisting parents to help their child be successful in school.

Poster No. 181
Maternal Emotional Response to Low Birthweight vs Healthy Infants: Role Of Social Support

S. J. Hershman, H. T. Ireys, and E. J. Silver

Pediatrics/Albert Einstein College of Medicine,
Preventive Intervention Research Center, Bronx, NY

Despite previous work, the relationship between social support and the mental health of mothers of low birthweight (LBW) infants remains poorly understood. This study investigated how mothers' psychological responses to the birth of full-term or premature infants were influenced by the need for the availability of social support. 22 mothers of LBW infants and a comparison group of 27 mothers of full-term healthy (FTH) infants were interviewed in person within 48 hours after birth and by telephone about 4 weeks later. The sample consisted of black, Hispanic, and white mothers from mid to low SES. Mental health was measured by the Psychiatric Symptom Index (PSI); social support variables were derived from 13 structured items related to need for and availability of support.

At T1, mothers in both groups had moderate to high psychiatric symptoms. Both groups decreased symptoms at T2 but mothers of the FTH infants decreased much more in total PSI scores ($M=18.7$ at T1, 7.0 at T2) in comparison to mothers of LBW infants ($M=20.6$ at T1, 11.7 at T2). Mothers of the FTH infants scored lower at T2 than mothers of LBW infants on the PSI anxiety subscale (4.2 vs 10.2, $p<.05$) and on the depression subscale (8.8 vs 15.5, $p<.10$). The mean number of support items needed by mothers in both groups was similar at T1 (FTH = 6.2, LBW = 5.9) and did not change at T2. In both groups, the need for social support was modestly correlated with PSI total scores at T1 ($r=.22$, FTH; .31, LBW) and more strongly associated at T2 ($r=.52$, FTH; .61, LBW; $p<.01$). The mean number of items related to availability of support was also similar in both groups at T1 (FTH = 12.4, LBW = 12.3) and did not change at T2. Availability of support was inversely related to PSI total scores in the mothers of LBW infants at both T1 ($r=-.47$, $p<.05$) and T2 ($r=-.50$, $p<.05$), but was unrelated at either time in mothers of FTH infants.

It appears that (1) the need for support is similar in both groups over time, with greater need associated with poorer mental health and (2) for mothers of LBW infants only, less available support is associated with more psychiatric symptoms.

Poster No. 182
Third Trimester Maternal Psychosocial Factors and Home Stimulation for 4 Month Old Infants: A Prospective Study

J. M. Pascoe and J. French

Department of Pediatrics,
University of Wisconsin, Madison, and
Department of Human Ecology,
Michigan State University, East Lansing

PURPOSE: To examine the association between primiparous mothers' prenatal psychosocial factors and the amount of home stimulation provided to their 4 month old infants.

METHOD: A group of primiparous mothers ($N=60$) from community-based public and private prenatal clinics were studied during the third trimester and about 4 months after delivery to identify antecedents of higher levels of home stimulation during the first few post-partum months. All mothers in this study vaginally delivered normal newborns. The following variables were assessed at a third trimester prenatal visit: maternal demographic characteristics, social support (Maternal Social Support Index), maternal depressive symptoms (Center for Epidemiologic Depression Scale), as well as satisfaction with the male support figure (Dyadic Adjustment Scale). Home stimulation was measured 4 months after delivery during a home visit using Caldwell's Home Observation for Measurement of the Environment. Data analysis included descriptive statistics, zero-order correlations, and hierarchical regression.

RESULTS: Age range was 14-35 years (median = 20 years), 78% had at least a high school education, 48.9% were single, never married, 76.1% were white. Third trimester social support ($r=.27$, $p=0.009$) and satisfaction with the male support figure ($r=.45$, $p=0.0001$) both had significant, positive correlations with home stimulation at 4 months. Maternal depressive symptoms were inversely, but not significantly, correlated with home stimulation ($r=-.12$, $p=0.26$). Using hierarchical regression, social support and satisfaction with the male support figure continued to explain a significant amount of variance in home stimulation after maternal age, education and socioeconomic status (Hollingshead) were included in the model (Total $R^2=.47$, $p=0.0001$).

CONCLUSION: Mothers' prenatal social environments are associated with their abilities to provide their infants with stimulating home environments. Subsequent research should investigate cost-effective interventions designed to support mothers as they strive to provide stimulating environments for their infants.

Poster No. 183
The Prevalence of Behavioral and Psychosocial Problems in Pediatric Practices

P. J. Leaf, S. M. Horwitz, J. M. Leventhal, and K. N. Speechley

Department of Epidemiology & Public Health,
Yale University School of Medicine,
New Haven, Conn

The prevalence and age specific patterns of psychosocial (PS) problems in pediatric practices has been the subject of considerable debate. We investigated rates and patterns of PS problems as part of a study of the detection of these problems by pediatric clinicians. We administered the Child Behavior Checklist to adults accompanying 1886 consecutive children ages 4-8 seen in the 19 different pediatric practices in South-Central Connecticut. Settings included pre-paid group practices, health centers, and solo and group practices.

Overall 17% of all the children seen, 13% of children ages 4-5 and 21% of children 6-8 years of age scored above the standard cut-point for the CBCL. Girls and boys had similar rates of problems in both the younger (13% vs. 14%) and older (22% vs 21%) age groups. Age related differences were least for the internalizing problems, 5% for children 4-5 years old vs. 6% for children 6-8 years old. Externalizing problems were more common in the older than younger children (6% vs. 3%).

There was some variation by age and sex in the specific CBCL sub-scales with the schizoid scale showing the highest rate of problems for boys ages 6-8 (10%) and the aggressive scale producing the highest rates of problems for boys 4-5. Over 10% of the girls ages 6-8 scored above the standard cut-point for the depressed sub-scale and hyperactivity was the most common problem for girls 4-5. These findings confirm that a significant number of children seen by pediatricians have disorders similar in nature and severity to those treated in child guidance clinics. Further, they show that even within a narrow age range, there are major differences in the patterns of PS symptoms.

Poster No. 184
The Relationship Between Maternal Self-Reporting Health Status and Maternal Report of Children's Health Status Among Hispanics

F. Mendoza, G. Takata, K. Baisden, L. Herrera, and R. Martorell

Department of Pediatrics and the Food Research Institute, Stanford (Calif) University

The percent of Mexican-American and mainland Puerto Rican mothers who perceive their children to be in poor health, 18.0% and 19.3% respectively, is significantly higher than the rates reported by non-Hispanic mothers. This study examined the hypothesis that these higher rates were associated with mothers' perception of their own health status. Data from the Hispanic Health and Nutrition Examination Survey were used to identify 1,183 Mexican-American and 332 mainland Puerto Rican mother-child pairs. Mothers reported on the perceived health status of their children (6 months to 12 years) and of themselves. Poor health status was reported by 32.4% of Mexican-American mothers and 38.9% of Puerto Rican mothers. These prevalences were affected by the mother's socioeconomic status ($p<.01$), educational level ($p<.001$), and the presence of a chronic illness ($p<.001$). In addition, for Puerto Rican mothers, marital status was also a significant determinant of perceived poor health status ($p<.01$), while acculturation was a determinant for Mexican-American mothers ($p<.001$). Bivariate analysis showed that mothers' perception of their own health status significantly influenced their perception of their children's health status ($p<.001$) for both groups. However, logistic regression indicated that this was true only for Mexican-Americans after other sociodemographic variables were considered. These findings will be important in assessing the reported health care needs of Hispanic children.

Poster No. 185
Life Change Events, Disease Course, ESR, and CRP in Patients With Juvenile Arthritis

D. M. Siegel, J. Baum, and S. P. Ellis

Department of Pediatrics,
University of Rochester (NY)
School of Medicine and Dentistry

The relationship between stressful life events and the course of many childhood chronic illnesses remains unclear. We conducted a study to test the hypothesis that life change events are associated with the course of juvenile arthritis (JA). Forty-two children, ages 2-20 years (mean age 10.1 years) attending the rheumatology clinic for a scheduled appointment were consecutively enrolled and followed for 6 months at 3 month intervals (total of 3 visits). Data gathered at each visit included: Coddington Life Events Scale, count of involved joints at time of visit, parent and patient assessments of status over the preceeding 3 months (much worse, worse, same, better, much better), ESR and CRP. Data Analysis utilized Chi Square and Pearson Correlation.

All subjects experienced at least 1 change in disease status (increase or decrease in the number of involved joints) over the 6 month period. Whereas life events scores (LES) did not correlate with the number of involved joints at the previous, same, or next visit, parent's global assessment of the child's arthritis status was correlated with LES at the same visit (Chi square = 5.98, df = 2, $p = .05$). LES did not correlate with ESR or CRP at the same visit, LES from visits I and II were correlated with ESR (but not CRP) at visits II and III, respectively ($R^2 = .401$, $p = .006$).

These data suggest that stressful life events are not associated with the course of JA as measured by clinically apparent changes in the number of inflamed joints, but they may influence the degree of inflammation as assessed by some laboratory measures. In addition, stress as measured by Coddington's scale, appears to be associated with parents' perception of their child's disease course.

Poster No. 186
The Preceptor Report Form: An Assessment Tool for Use in Evaluating Residents in Ambulatory Pediatric Settings

J. K. Davis and B. Hermosa

Department of Pediatrics, New York Medical College, Lincoln Medical and Mental Health Center, Bronx

Rating scales are widely used to assess on-the-job performance in medical education. We developed a 15-item scale for use by preceptors to assess clinical competence, interpersonal behavior, and personal responsibility of housestaff in the ambulatory pediatrics setting. This study was to determine if each of these dimensions could be reliably assessed. Thirty-six residents received ratings for the first quarter of 1990-1991 from each of two team preceptors. A principal axis factor analysis with varimax rotation yielded only two factors: interpersonal behavior (makes certain parent and patient know his/her name, communicates pleasure in seeing them, demonstrates sensitivity to feelings, etc.) and clinical competence (shows good clinical judgement, is able to formulate a sound diagnostic hypothesis, is accurate and thorough in maintaining charts, etc.). Internal consistency reliabilities were quite high (alpha = 0.90 and alpha = 0.97). Interrater agreement was significant ($r = 0.35$, $P < .05$ and $r = 0.44$, $p < .01$). Contrary to expectation clinical competence scores did not show significant correlation with American Board of Pediatrics Intraining Exam (ITE) scores. It is concluded that preceptors can reliably assess two dimensions of resident performance early in the academic year. Interrater agreement is expected to improve as the year progresses. With this increased precision of ratings, correlation between clinical competence and ITE scores should also improve. A mid-year replication is in progress.

Poster No. 187
The Care Giving Role: Influences of Residents' Background Characteristics

M. E. Zondorak-Perez and R. E. K. Stein

Department of Pediatrics,
Albert Einstein College of Medicine,
Division of Ambulatory Pediatrics,
Bronx (NY) Municipal Hospital Center

Little is known how background characteristics affect attitudes towards the care giving role among pediatric trainees. As part of a larger study about resident characteristics and continuity in a primary care setting, we developed a 21-item scale to measure positive care giving attitudes and related self-reported behaviors. It has high internal reliability (Cronbach's $\alpha = 0.82$) as does a 7-item psychosocial subscale ($\alpha = 0.80$). 53 of 56 residents (including 45 pediatric and 8 triple board residents: pediatrics, psychiatry, and child psychiatry) caring for patients in a large municipal university affiliated pediatric primary care clinic completed a self-administered demographic questionnaire and the scale.

There were no significant differences on total scale score or psychosocial subscale by race, marital status, number of children, educational loans, sibling number, training level, or foreign vs US medical school training. However, total scale scores were significantly higher ($p<.05$) for women, and residents with work experiences with children, additional graduate degrees or programs, or plans to work in a socio-economically depressed area. Scale scores did not differ by self-perceived adequacy of preresidency preparation for interviewing, emotional support from colleagues, or perceived ability to get needed information by interviewing. Total scale scores did differ significantly ($p<.05$) by previous job experience involving interviewing, medical school interview training, and perceived emotional support from noncolleagues. Pediatric residents scored significantly lower on the total scale ($p = .003$) than triple-board residents.

The higher scale scores among residents who have reported additional interviewing experiences, graduate training, or employment experiences with children raise important educational issues in the training of pediatric residents. Further study is needed to investigate the possibilities of affecting care giving attitudes with strategic supplemental training opportunities.

Poster No. 188
Medicaid During the Reagan Years: Federal and State Reforms

J. D. C. Cartland

Department of Research,
American Academy of Pediatrics, Elk Grove Village, Ill

As states gain more and more control over health and welfare policy, it becomes increasingly important for child health advocates to gauge whether state governments are more or less likely than the federal government to take a conservative approach to setting policy that affects children's health.

Many researchers have examined whether states have the capacity or the will to establish generous welfare policy independently of the federal government. This study analyzes the effect of federal and state Medicaid policy changes, state economic and state social conditions on state Medicaid and AFDC eligibility policy output during the Reagan years.

States' AFDC need standards are examined for the years 1978 through 1983, during which time the need standard was reduced by the states from an average of 60% of states' per capita income to 45%. Medicaid eligibility thresholds for first-time pregnant women are examined for the years 1983 through 1988, when the eligibility threshold increased from 54% of states' per capita income to 72%.

Pooled regression is used to analyze states cross-sectionally as well as longitudinally. When controlling for the unemployment rate, age distribution, region, and various Medicaid program characteristics, the multivariate analyses indicate that, while states may not require federal mandates to increase the generosity of their Medicaid programs, they do require a federal commitment to share the costs of these programs in order to expand them. The findings show that without evidence of a federal commitment, states are likely to compete with each other for lower welfare loads by reducing the generosity of their Medicaid programs.

These findings indicate that child health advocates will be most effective if they attempt to influence both state and federal governments for more generous child health policy in the coming years.

Poster No. 189
Linking Medicaid and Special Education in a Rural State

C. Field, R. Kirby, and T. Nosal

Department of Pediatrics,
University of Arkansas
for Medical Sciences, Little Rock

P.L. 100-360 (1988) for the first time allowed Medicaid (MA) reimbursement of medically related special education (SE) services, but has resulted in limited participation by schools. We describe the successful implementation of an assistance program by a university Department of Pediatrics to public schools using MA. In Arkansas for 1989-90, the mean percent eligible for MA across school districts was 6.6%. The average SE enrollment was 11.0%. The mean percent of SE pupils with speech and language as the primary handicapping condition was 19.4%, the single most common served group.

The professional/technical services for the College of Medicine were made available to schools to assist in obtaining provider status, billing and tracking MA claims for SE services, as well as implementing OBRA 1989 and 1990 changes in MA, especially EPSDT. In the first year, 46 school districts and 8 of 16 3-5 year-old P.L. 99-457 preschool programs in Arkansas began participating as MA providers accessing MA through the Department of Pediatrics. In one district, 19.2% of MA eligibles were in SE programs; MA paid $196/pupil/yr. Participating districts have enrollments ranging from 236 to 6,412 (mean = 1,351), and would have had difficulty billing MA for SE services without assistance and support.

MA funds for SE are not being utilized. Twelve states participated in 1989-90 (four on a pilot basis only), with 22 states projected for 1990-1991 (eight as pilots). Districts this project assisted are rural and small, unfamiliar with MA billing and procedures. P.L. 99-457 funds are payor of last resort; thus MA is vital to the support of early intervention services. This project allows rural schools with limited resources efficient access to MA for SE. Physicians can provide MA expertise to schools as the relationship between the MA and SE entitlement programs evolves. This improves services to children at risk from both low income and educational handicaps.

JOINT TOPIC SESSIONS
Tuesday, April 30, 3 PM-6:30 PM
ADOLESCENT MEDICINE

Access to Handguns Among Urban Adolescents

C. M. Callahan and F. P. Rivara

Department of Pediatrics,
University of Washington, Seattle,
and Harborview Injury Prevention and
Research Center, Seattle

Although mortality of urban adolescents due to firearms has risen sharply in recent years, little data are available on adolescents' access to or ownership of handguns, nor are there reliable data on the relationship of access or ownership to demographic characteristics. This study attempted to determine the access or ownership of firearms by urban adolescents. In addition, we hypothesize that access/ownership would be positively related to deviant behavior and inversely related to socioeconomic status.

Data were gathered through a voluntary anonymous questionnaire, administered to third-year students (N = 491) at two Seattle public high schools during non-elective class time (84% responded, 13% were absent and 3% refused to participate).

Respondents were judged to have easy access to a handgun if they reported ownership or they believed they could acquire a handgun within a few days. A handgun was considered inaccessible for those reporting that acquisition would be difficult or their need for a handgun was unlikely.

Half of the sample was male. Of the males, 6.8% reported carrying a handgun to school. Thirty-five percent reported easy access, and of these, 10% reported having fired the handgun at another person. Easy access to handguns was positively related to gang membership (OR 9.1, C.I. 3.1, 31.3), expulsion from school (OR 4.2, C.I. 2.2, 7.8), crimes against persons (OR 5.0, C.I. 2.7, 9.6) and crimes against property (OR 7.7, C.I. 4.6, 12.6).

The availability and use of handguns by high school juniors is common and for some students handguns are integrated with other risk-taking behaviors.

Risk Factors for Repeat Adolescent Childbirth

L. B. Heery, M. J. Werner, and R. M. Brayden

Department of Pediatrics,
Division of Community Pediatrics,
Vanderbilt University, Nashville, Tenn

Repeat childbirth to an adolescent mother may exacerbate the adverse social, educational, and economic consequences of adolescent parenthood. To identify risk factors for rapid repeat delivery, we evaluated data collected during initial pregnancy on 186 low socioeconomic nulliparous adolescents enrolled in an observational cohort study. Subjects were randomized either to routine care or to an invervention clinic offering comprehensive medical care and psychosocial support from entry into prenatal care until the child's second birthday. Subjects were 13-18 years old (mean = 16.3 years, SD = 1.3), 44% black, 56% white, and 24% married. State vital statistics records searched for 3 years following the initial delivery revealed repeat delivery rates of 19.4% at 2 years, and 31.5% at 3 years after first delivery. Repeat delivery at 2 or 3 years was not associated with marital status; however, black race and younger maternal age were associated at 3 years ($p<.04$ and $<.03$ respectively). Fewer years of education was associated with repeat delivery at both 2 ($p<.01$) and 3 ($p<.001$) years. Later entry into prenatal care for the initial pregnancy was associated with repeat at 2 years ($p<.04$), and approached significance at 3 years ($p=.06$). Seventy-eight subjects were administered the Tennessee Self Concept Scale. As a group, their mean self-concept score did not differ from the normative population; however, repeaters had significantly lower self-concepts than non-repeaters at 2 ($p<.02$) and 3 years ($p<.03$). Enrollment in the intervention clinic had no significant effect on the rate of repeat delivery. Addressing educational and self-concept issues with pregnant adolescents may help reduce repeat deliveries; whereas, comprehensive prenatal and child care alone does not appear to be effective.

Predictors of Depression and Substance Abuse in Adolescent Offspring of Former Teenage Mothers

S. M. Horwitz, L. V. Klerman, and J. F. Jekel

Department of Epidemiology and Public Health,
Yale University School of Medicine,
New Haven, Conn

Children born to teenage mothers are reported to have more behavioral and emotional problems than children born to older mothers. Most of the evidence concerns preadolescent children, and virtually nothing is known about the psychiatric morbidity of these children as they pass through adolescence. We examined the rates and predictors of two important mental health outcomes, major depression and substance abuse in adolescents born to 154 (13-18 yr.) black primiparas enrolled in an early (1967-69) program for school-age mothers. We located 128/149 living mothers (86%) and interviewed 121 (95%). Of the adolescents born to these women, 2 could not be interviewed, 2 refused, 6 were not located, and 111 were interviewed (92%).

Of these 111 adolescents, the mean age was 18, 42% were females, 83% had completed or were in high school, 62% lived with their mothers, and 74% were employed. Four females (8.5%) and 1 male (1.6%) met DSMIII criteria for major depression (MD). Seven males (16.3%) met criteria for substance abuse (SA). Predictors of SA and MD were similar for mothers' 20-year success ($RR=4.5$, 11.0 respectively) and low fertility ($RR=3.7$, 11.0). The predictors differed for gender (female sex, $RR=4$ for MD; male sex, $RR=11.5$ for SA), contact with grandmothers ($RR=3.7$ for SA only), and divorce ($RR=12.2$ for SA only). Because SA and MD had two common predictors and the outcomes were rare, we constructed risk categories with the two outcomes merged.

Using these variables (with the exception of gender), we constructed (4) risk categories with increasing probability of developing SA or MD: 1=3% (2/73), 2=13% (3/24), 3=38% (3/8); 4=80% (4/5). Low risk offspring had mothers who were unsuccessful in the 1967-69 program regardless of other variables. The highest risk adolescents had low contact with their grandmothers, and had mothers who were: 1) successful in the 1967-69 program; 2) divorced; and 3) had few children.

We concluded that these adolescents have considerable psychiatric morbidity and that losses of important emotional relationships are strongly related to this morbidity.

Evaluation of Sexual Behavior in Sports Preparticipation Examination

B. J. Foch, M. K. Oh, C. H. Hong, B. C. Cotton, B. C. Brown, and R. A. Feinstein

Department of Pediatrics,
University of Alabama at Birmingham

Adolescent males infrequently utilize the health care system. One reason they do seek medical care is for the sports preparticipation evaluation (PPE). The purpose of this study was to determine the feasibility of taking sexual history during PPE, and usefulness of such information in health care delivery. The subjects consisted of 657 males (mean age 16.6 yrs; 12-20 in range) seen during one week of station-oriented PPE at the Adolescent clinic of UAB. 370 (56.3%) were black, 233 (35.5%) white, and 54 (8.2%) of unknown race. 148 (22.5%) were under 15 years of age. Each subject was asked about his sexual experience (history of intercourse; age at first sex; number of lifetime sex partners; condom use in past 4 months, always, sometimes, never; and history of STD) in the Abdomen-Genital station.

Sixty-two percent (407/657) were sexually experienced. Mean age of this group was 16.0 ± 1.1 yrs (compared with 14.8 yrs, of those who never had sex), age at first sex 13.3 ± 1.9 yrs and number of lifetime sex partners 5.5 ± 6.2. 84% of blacks and 34% of whites were sexually experienced. Blacks tended to start intercourse at a younger age (13.0 ± 1.9 vs 14.4 ± 1.7, $p=.0001$) and have more sex partners (6.1 ± 6.3 vs. 3.6 ± 6.0, $p=.001$). Only 15% reported a consistent condom use. Condom use was significantly less prevalent among blacks ($p=.002$). 50% of sexually active blacks and 38% of whites had "never" used condoms, 11% of blacks and 21% of whites used "always" and the rest "sometimes". A history of an STD was reported by 4% of whites and blacks.

Prevalent high risk sexual behaviors (early age of sexual intercourse, multiple sex partners, and inadequate condom use) we found among Jr. and Sr. high school athletes in this study indicate sexual history and counseling may be an efficient health care delivery measure during PPE to an otherwise inaccessible population. We concluded sexual history taking was a feasible and useful adjunct to the PPE.

BEHAVIORAL PEDIATRICS

The Cry of Colic Facies

R. G. Barr, A. Rotman, J. Yaremko, D. Leduc, T. E. Francoeur, and B. Katchan

Department of Pediatrics,
McGill University, Montreal, Quebec,
and Montreal Children's Hospital

Pain or pain facies is reported as a criterion in 25% of published descriptions of colic. To determine empirically if the crying facies of infants with colic differs from normals, crying bouts of 38 infants whose mothers considered crying a problem ("colic") and 38 age, sex, parity and ethnicity pair-matched controls were videotaped at home for 10 min. before and after an evening feed. Recording was completed when 2 mins. of crying occurred. On the basis of 7-day pre-validated maternal diaries, "colic" infants were sub-defined as *Wessel's Colic* if cry and fuss duration was ≥3 hrs/day for ≥3 days/wk or as *Non-Wessel's Colic* if not. Using the Neonatal Facial Coding System (Gruneau & Craig 1987), tapes were scored without sound and blind to identity, group, and prandial state. Rates of occurrence/120 seconds were determined for 7 facial actions (brow bulge [BB], eye squeeze [ES], nasolabial furrow [NLF], open lips [OL], vertical mouth stretch, horizontal mouth stretch, taut tongue), plus Total Facial Activity (TFA) and "pain concatenation" (simultaneous presence of BB, ES, NLF, OL). Interobserver reliability (kappa) averaged .83 for all measures (range .57 to 1.0). Groups were compared by ANOVA with post hoc Tukey tests.

After feeding, there were no significant differences on any measure. Before feeding, however, Wessel's Colic infants differed from *both* Non-Wessel's Colic and Controls on Total Facial Activity (mean ± SD: 78 ± 7 vs. 63 ± 14 and 68 ± 11 respectively; $F[2,56]=5.1$, $P=.01$) and almost on pain concatenation (106 ± 14 vs. 83 ± 30 and 89 ± 24; $F=2.9$, $P=.07$). The same pattern occurred specifically for brow bulge (118 ± 3.2 vs. 99 ± 22 and 109 ± 15; $F=4.1$, $P=.02$), taut tongue (73 ± 30 vs. 43 ± 34 and 44 ± 33; $F=3.3$, $P=.05$) and, probably, nasolabial fold (108 ± 14 vs. 85 ± 29 and 94 ± 25; $F=2.8$, $P=.07$).

CONCLUSIONS: Under some conditions, the crying facies of infants meeting Wessel's criteria differs from that of both non-Wessel colic and normal infants. This includes a facial expression often seen with pain stimuli, which may reflect differences in the infants and/or stimulate parental concern.

Reducing Low Birthweight, Depression, and Stress Through Social Support in Pregnancy

A. W. Cross, K. J. Welshimer, E. Jackson, and J. Chapman

Center for Health Promotion and Disease Prevention, University of North Carolina at Chapel Hill

Accumulating evidence suggests that stress and social isolation can have a negative impact on pregnancies. The Helping Mothers Program was created in 2 rural counties to reduce low birthweight. Through this program, volunteers were recruited among women already perceived as natural helpers. Training served to enhance the volunteers' helping skills, while providing greater information on the prevention of problems in pregnancy. Volunteers were then paired with pregnant women at risk for low birthweight. The volunteers met regularly with the mothers throughout pregnancy offering friendship, support and assistance.

The frequency and nature of the interactions between mother and volunteer varied greatly among the 116 mother-volunteer pairs. Seventy mothers were interviewed extensively early and late in pregnancy. Mothers experienced a 19% reduction in stress ($p=0.007$) and 13% reduction in depression ($p=0.0001$) over the course of participation, which was significantly associated with the number of contacts between mother and volunteer. All 116 program mothers were compared with 3 control groups matched for age, race, parity and education. The first was from the same counties prior to the time of the program. The other 2 were from a demographically similar county prior to and concurrent with the program. In the program counties, the low birthweight rate was 6% among the retrospective control group and remained 6% among program participants. In the comparison county, the low birthweight rate was 7.8% prior to the program and rose to 13.8% at the time of the program which was significantly worse ($p=0.03$) than the program mothers. For prenatal care, program participants received more prenatal care than mothers in all 3 control groups with that difference being statistically significant when compared with the same county retrospective group ($p=0.001$).

We conclude that a volunteer social support program in pregnancy can be associated with reduced stress and depression, fewer low birthweight babies and improved prenatal care.

Evaluating A Parent Support Program For Mothers Of Chronically Ill Children

H. T. Ireys, E. J. Silver, R. E. K. Stein, K. Bencivenga, and C. Koeber

Pediatrics, Albert Einstein College of Medicine, Preventive Intervention Research Center, Bronx, NY

In view of increased mental health risks for children with serious on-going health conditions and for their parents, many pediatric services have sponsored parent support programs. Few such programs, however, have been evaluated in terms of their impact on parental mental health or child behavior. We postulate that such programs will have a long-term positive effect on maternal mental health by initially enhancing aspects of parental competence and efficacy. We are conducting a randomized controlled trial of a parent support program for mothers of children aged 5-9 years who have serious on-going health conditions. The Parent-to-Parent Network (PTPN) includes three women from the community who have themselves raised children with serious ongoing health problems. PTPN staff provide information, affirmation of the mothers' skills, and emotional support to mothers through bi-weekly phone calls and regular face-to-face contacts for 1 year. Mothers in the study are primarily of minority background and have low to middle income. We have used the Rosenberg Self-Esteem scale (RSE), Sense of Competence subscale of the Abidin Parenting Stress Index (PSI) and the Ilfeld Self-Efficacy scale (ISE) to measure mothers' self-esteem, sense of parenting competence, and self-efficacy, respectively.

In paired t-tests comparing baseline (T1) and 6 month scores (T2), mothers in the intervention group ($N=64$) had improved self-efficacy ($t=3.89$; $p<.01$) and improved self esteem ($t=3.49$; $p<.01$). Mothers in the control group ($N=31$) did not change significantly on either measure. The control group showed increased parenting stress from T1 to T2 ($t=2.45$; $p<.05$), but scores of intervention mothers did not change significantly. These results suggest that the PTPN is achieving its initial goals of increasing mothers' feelings of self-worth and control over life experiences and also prevents deterioration in mothers' sense of parenting competence. More work is needed to determine long-term mental health effects of parent support programs for mothers of children with chronic health conditions.

Can the Reliability of Mothers' Clinical Judgments be Predicted?

P. McCarthy, D. Cicchetti, S. Sznajderman, B. Forsyth, M. Baron, H. Fink, N. Czarkowski, B. Bauchner, and K. Lustman-Findling

Department of Pediatrics, Yale University School of Medicine, New Haven, Conn

The purpose of this study was to identify descriptive data gathered at the two week well child visit which would predict the reliability of mother's clinical judgments during their children's subsequent acute illnesses. It was a pre-existing hypothesis that mothers who a) demographically, were younger, unmarried, on welfare, resided in the inner city, had less education, who b) clinically had fewer previous children, less adult support, previous children with serious illnesses, and who c) psychosocially, had concerns about the pregnancy outcome, higher Spielberger State-Trait Anxiety scores and higher Maternal Anxiety About the Baby Scores would be more unreliable. The study was a randomized trial of the Acute Illness Observation Scales (AIOS); 369 mothers participated, 183 in the Intervention Group, and 186 in the Control Group. There were 704 acute illnesses judged simultaneously and independently by mothers and pediatricians in the 33 months of study. Intervention Group mothers used the AIOS; Control Group mothers a 3 point global assessment scale.

Pearson r correlations were performed between the independent variables, taken singly and in all possible combinations, and the dependent variable, reliability of mothers' judgments as measured by weighted kappa (Kw). Group assignment was entered as an independent variable. Analyses were performed separately for all first, second, and third acute illness visits to control for any "practice effect" (Analysis I). To control for consistency of observers, the first, second, and third visits of mothers with three visits were also analyzed (Analysis II).

Results indicate that, depending on the visit number, adverse demographic, clinical and psychosocial characteristics did correlate with poorer reliability independent of group assignment. The correlations ranged from small (Analysis I, first visit, multiple variable $r^2=3\%$) to large (Analysis II, second visit, multiple variable $r^2=28\%$). Controlling for both visit number *and* consistency of observers versus visit number alone (Analysis II versus Analysis I) increased multivariate correlations to Kw. Except for one variable, number of previous children, correlations were in the hypothesized direction. The results support the untoward impact that adverse demographic, clinical, and psychosocial factors have on mothers' clinical judgment. These data may assist pediatricians in identifying parents who might benefit from more intensive teaching and support about acute illness episodes in their children.

Cognitive Dysfunction in Children With Post-Meningitic Deafness

D. Kelly, B. Kelly, M. Jones, S. Verhulst, and S. Bell

Department of Pediatrics, Southern Illinois University School of Medicine, Springfield, and Illinois School for the Deaf, Jacksonville

The long term sequelae of bacterial meningitis, including subtle neuropsychologic dysfunction, are not clearly delineated. While hearing loss is the most frequent neurologic complication, it has been suggested that this reflects damage to the inner ear or eighth nerve specifically, without central nervous system involvement. This study utilized a wide range of measurements including computerized neuropsychologic tests to compare the function of children with deafness secondary to bacterial meningitis with hereditarily deaf peers.

Twenty-four prelingually profoundly deaf students (16 males, 8 females) at a residential school for the deaf were studied. Eleven had post-meningitic deafness (mean age 13.2 yrs., mean age of infection 9.8 months). Controls were 13 children with hereditary deafness (mean age 13.8 yrs.). All subjects were of normal intelligence with no other physical handicaps. Measures included medical and neurologic evaluation, IQ and academic achievement testing, behavioral ratings by parents, teachers and dormitory supervisors (Child Behavior Checklist, ACTeRS and ANSER questionnaires), neurodevelopmental testing and computerized testing (visual attention and memory scanning tasks using the MEL system).

Study groups did not differ significantly with regard to medical complications, standard neurologic findings, WISC-R Performance IQ or behavioral measures. However, significant differences were seen on academic and computer tests with the post-meningitic students performing less well on the Stanford Achievement Tests (Math: $t = 2.76$, $p = .014$); reaction-time on the visual attention test ($t = 2.13$, $p = .045$); and accuracy of responses on memory scanning task ($t = 2.87$, $p = .009$). The accuracy measure correlated significantly with achievement scores.

Thus, while general psychologic and neurologic assessment did not reveal differences, more precise measures of cognitive processing efficiency did show dysfunction in students with post-meningitic deafness which was also reflected in their academic achievement. These findings suggest that nervous system damage in children with post-meningitic deafness is not isolated to the eighth nerve.

EPIDEMIOLOGY AND PREVENTIVE PEDIATRICS

Firearms: Family Attitudes and Household Safety Practices

C. C. Wiley and R. Casey

Division of General Pediatrics, Children's Hospital of Philadelphia, Pa

This prospective study was conducted to examine firearm safety practices, experience with shootings, and attitudes concerning firearms. We interviewed 208 children (ages 5-12 years) and surveyed 242 parents (92% mothers) from a pediatric clinic and a private group practice. Boys and girls were equally represented. Payment for health care was 51% medical assistance (MA) and 49% private insurance (PI). The MA and PI groups differed by employment (44% vs 84%), college education (30% vs 85%), single parent families (74% vs 16%), race (93% black vs 34% black) and mean maternal age (31.5 vs 37.4 years).

Gun ownership was reported by 10% of parents. The majority of guns were potentially accessible, 36% were not always locked and 18% were sometimes or always kept loaded. Only 3% of parents discussed gun safety with a pediatrician. MA parents were less likely to be in favor of gun control (56% vs 89%, $p < .001$).

Parents underreported their children's toy gun play (44% parents vs 81% children, $p < .001$) and pretend gun play (33% parents vs 53% children, $p < .05$). More boys reported toy gun play but many girls also played with toy guns (93% vs 70%, $p < .001$).

Personal knowledge of shootings was common among children (24%). MA children more often reported shootings of family members or friends (37% MA vs 11% PI, $p < .001$) and were more likely than PI children to have witnessed a shooting (12% MA vs 2% PI, $p < .01$).

Few children felt it was appropriate to shoot animals (27%) or people (6%). Four percent thought they might ever shoot someone. One third of children thought about being shot themselves. Of note, despite the MA children's greater exposure to shooting, all children's attitudes about guns were similar and did not differ by method of payment, income, level of maternal education, site of health care or sex.

We conclude that parents owning guns describe unsafe storage of guns and very few parents report having had anticipatory guidance concerning gun safety. Many children have personal experience with firearm-related violence and think about being shot themselves. Children are similar in their gun play and attitudes about gun use despite disparate socioeconomic backgrounds and exposure to violence.

Previous Injury As A Risk Factor for Youth Suicide

D. C. Grossman, R. W. Soderberg, and F. P. Rivara

Department of Pediatrics, Harborview Injury Prevention Center, University of Washington, Seattle

While suicide attempts are known to be risk factors for later suicide completion, it is unclear whether other injuries are also associated with increased risk of later suicide. It has been widely hypothesized that other intentional or unintentional injuries represent suicide attempts in disguise.

We conducted a population based case-control study to answer the following question: What is the risk of death by suicide for persons ages 10-35 with a past history of hospital admission for a previous suicide attempt, or other intentional and unintentional injuries? We hypothesized that a past hospital admission for both intentional and unintentional injury would be significant risk factors for eventual suicide.

Cases were all Washington State residents ages 10-35 whose death certificate indicated suicide as the cause of death during 1987-89. Controls were a sample of licensed drivers in Washington State matched by age, sex, race and zip code. Exposure to previous injury was ascertained by linking cases and controls to a statewide hospital database (CHARS) of all civilian hospital admissions over the same time period. Using the ICD-9 E-codes, hospitalizations were classified as related to suicide attempts (SA), unintentional injury (UI), and other intentional injury of intentional or undetermined intent (II).

Of the 838 cases, 81% were male. Eighteen percent of the cases and 4% of the controls had a record of a hospital admission in the CHARS database during the exposure period. Among cases, there were 9 persons with a past admission for *UI*, 29 with a past *SA*, and 9 with a past *II*. In contrast, the controls only had 14 *UI* (3.0%), 3 *SA* (3.0%) and 5 admissions for *II*. Compared to controls, cases were more likely to be exposed to hospitalizations for suicide attempts (OR = 48, 95% CI = 14-198), unintentional injury (OR = 3.1, 95% CI = 1.3-6.9), and injuries of intentional or undetermined intention (OR = 9.0, 95% CI = 3-31).

We conclude that, compared to controls, adolescent and young adult suicide victims have a small but significant history of both intentional and unintentional injuries resulting in a hospitalization prior to their death. These findings support the hypothesis that the increased rate of injury in this population may represent additional suicide attempts.

Effects of Screening Children for High Cholesterol

C. M. Lannon and J. A. Earp

Department of Pediatrics, School of Medicine,
and Department of Health,
Education, and Health Behavior,
School of Public Health,
University of North Carolina, Chapel Hill

Many pediatricians are enthusiastically instituting cholesterol screening despite controversy about the long-term implications of an elevated cholesterol level in children. The American Academy of Pediatrics (AAP), concerned that screening may lead to mislabeling and overly restrictive diets, stresses laboratory confirmation and nutritional follow-up for children with elevated cholesterols. We studied parents' behavior and attitudes toward screening children for high cholesterol.

During an eight-week period in summer of 1989 all children between the ages of 2 to 15 years seen for well-child examinations at a community pediatric group practice were offered cholesterol screening by fingerstick method. Most parents were well-educated and white.

Of 440 children screened, 134 (30%) had cholesterol levels above the recommended cutpoint of 175 mg/dl (75th percentile). Parents were notified of results and encouraged to comply with AAP guidelines. Only sixty-four children returned for follow-up; hypercholesterolemia was confirmed in 97% of children with screening values > 199 mg/dl (95th percentile) and in 76% with values between 175 and 199 mg/dl. Parents of the children with high screening levels who did not return for lipid panels (N = 70) were interviewed by telephone; 86% responded. Reasons for non-compliance included "not sure test machine was accurate" (67%); "child too traumatized by fingerstick" (47%); and "will try low-cholesterol diet before recheck" (40%). A third of these parents (N = 20) felt that confirmation of an elevated cholesterol "would make the child worry too much." Only 29 of 101 parents of children with high screening levels (29%) talked with a dietician. In a follow-up of this cohort, we will evaluate whether identifying children as hypercholesterolemic has affected parents' health perceptions of their children (labeling) and family habits.

In this middle-class, well-educated population, a large proportion of children had elevated screening cholesterols, but few complied with AAP guidelines. As a result, many children may be mislabeled as hypercholesterolemic and may not benefit from screening.

Access to Care for Poor and Nonpoor Children: Separate and Unequal?

R. F. St. Peter and P. W. Newacheck

Robert Wood Johnson Clinical Scholars Program,
Department of Pediatrics
and Institute for Health Policy Studies,
University of California, San Francisco

Access to care for poor children has improved since the implementation of Medicaid. Recent legislation expanding Medicaid eligibility will significantly increase the number of children covered by this program. We examined how coverage by Medicaid affects the use, location, and continuity of care for poor children. The findings reported are from data in the 1988 National Health Interview Survey, which contains information on 17,110 children under 18 years of age.

Poor children with Medicaid were more likely than uninsured poor children to have a regular source of care (93% v 76%, $p<0.001$) and to receive routine care within an appropriate time interval (85% v 66%, $p<0.001$). However, poor children with Medicaid were less likely than nonpoor children to identify a doctor's office as their regular source of care (57% v 82%, $p<0.001$), and more likely to identify a hospital clinic (12% v 3%, $p<0.001$) or neighborhood health center (15% v 3%, $p<0.001$). Those children receiving routine care at a neighborhood health center rather than a doctor's office were 12 times more likely to receive sick care at a different location than where they receive routine care (37% v 3%, $p<0.001$). Such children were also 5 times more likely to identify an emergency room as their regular source of sick care.

While Medicaid does improve access to care for poor children, it does not ensure that they have access to the same locations and continuity of care as nonpoor children. Future legislation designed to improve access to care for poor children should also address the separateness and inequality of care to which these children gain access.

GENERAL PEDIATRICS AND PEDIATRIC EDUCATION

Has the Eighty Hour Work Week Lessened Stress Levels in PL-1 Residents?

J. E. Berkelhamer and N. H. Pliskin

Departments of Pediatrics and Psychiatry,
Wyler Children's Hospital,
University of Chicago (Ill)
Pritzker School of Medicine

We investigated whether implementation of the Association of American Medical Colleges recommendations on work hours lessened stress levels in first year pediatric residents. The Holmes and Rahe Social Readjustment Rating Scale (HRSRRS) and the Farguhar Stress Questionnaire (FSQ) were administered to two groups of PL-1 residents (1988 and 1990) and results were compared. After July 1, 1990 rotations have averaged no more than 80 hours of work per week; residents are relieved of duties one 24 hour period per week and when displaying signs of fatigue.

23 of 24 1988 participants and 17 of 19 1990 participants returned completed HRSRRS forms. The mean scores were 296 (sd = 121) and 272 (sd = 129) respectively, both well into the "moderate" crisis range defined by the test instrument (200 to 299). The mean scores showed no significant difference using the t test for independent samples. The number of positive responses to those most frequently cited items did not differ significantly between the 1988 and 1990 groups (Chi square = ns). Using weighted HRSRRS point values (pv), the most contributory factors to overall stress levels in both groups were change in responsibilities at work (pv = 24), change in financial state (pv = 22), change in work hours or conditions (pv = 18), end of school (pv = 18), change in living conditions (pv = 16), change in residence (pv = 13), and change in sleeping habits (pv = 12).

All 1988 (n = 24) and all 1990 (n = 19) residents returned completed FSQ scores. The mean scores were 7.7 (sd = 3.8) and 7.3 (sd = 3.0) respectively, both within the "average" stress range of 6 to 9 points defined in the test instrument. The mean scores showed no significant difference using the t tests for independent samples. The FSQ scores demonstrated that both resident groups were in the average range in terms of symptomatology due to stress, suggesting that both groups were coping well considering the stressful demands of residency training.

The results of this study do not support the contention that the eighty hour work week alone will lessen resident stress.

Diagnostic Trends in a Pediatric Primary Care Clinic

C. Calderon, G. Gonzalez, and M. Valcarcel

Pediatric Department, University of Puerto Rico,
Recinto Ciencias Medicas, San Juan

A major goal of General Training Programs is to teach trainees to diagnose and manage the common pediatric morbidity. Many programs have increased the ambulatory experience, providing exposure to the changing morbidity pattern, including the management of psychosocial and psychosomatic conditions. Since 1979 a model General Pediatric clinic has been operational in Cataño, Puerto Rico, serving as a clinical training site with emphasis on ambulatory, preventive, and biopsychosocial aspects of pediatric care. A retrospective and descriptive study was done with the purpose to identify the diagnoses to which the trainees have been exposed in this population and changes in the patterns of these diagnoses. Data collected included: number of patient-doctor contacts, type of patient visit, patient age, frequency of diagnoses, and patient absenteeism. A patient-doctor contact was defined as that occurring during a first visit to clinic, follow up, or urgent care visit. Diagnostic patterns were compared between each year. A total of 66,054 patient-doctor contacts occurred in nine years, 79% for scheduled health care visits and 20% for urgent care. The main diagnoses were: healthy child or adolescent (HV), well baby (WB), upper respiratory tract infection (URTI), skin condition (SC), bronchial asthma (BA), acute gastroenteritis (AGE), otitis media (OM), anemia (A), incomplete immunization (II), psychosocial condition (PS), nutritional and/or linear growth problems (N), psychosomatic condition (PC), parasites (P), pneumonia (PN), and others. There was a significant decrease ($p<.005$) in the diagnosis of infectious diseases (URTI, AGE, P, PN), comparing 1979 to 1989. There was a significant increase ($p<.005$) in the proportion of patients with the diagnoses of WB and HV, (two most common diagnoses of 1989). This data supports the curricular goal of exposing the trainees to diagnosis and management of common pediatric morbidity.

Comparison of Interviewing Skills of Fourth Year Medical Students With Their Individual Performance as Second Year Medical Students

R. D. Olsen and B. Anderson

Department of Pediatrics,
Mayo Clinic, Rochester, Minn

There are many articles in the pediatric literature on doctor-patient communications and its effect on parents, but little has been written on the development of interviewing skills in medical students. This study was designed to assess and compare interviewing skills of medical students as they progress from their second to fourth year.

In this longitudinal study a class of 33 students completed videotaped interviews with a simulated parent who had been trained to portray the mother of a child with chronic illness (during their second year and fourth year of medical school). The evaluation process involved: 1) measurement of historical content using a checklist of specific facts; and 2) evaluation of the interview process based on a rating instrument which was subdivided into the following sections: organization, questioning skills, rapport, and closure. Observations were made by pediatric parent-instructors who had been trained to analyze the interaction and had obtained 90% interobserver reliability. During the testing in the fourth year, parent-instructors were blinded to any previous data.

Results: There was generalized improvement in the questioning skills between the second and fourth year ($p = .02$ sign rank). There was no improvement in skills related to rapport-building, which included items such as empathy, support, and nonverbal messages. In fact, there was a downward trend in the rapport-building skills; 9% failed in the second year vs. 18% in the fourth year, and 36% scored skillful in the second year vs. 11% in the fourth year ($.05 < p < .10$, sign rank). There was no significant change in ability to obtain historical information. During the post interview feedback session between the parent-instructor and fourth year medical students, it became evident that as the students progressed through medical school they based their interviewing skills more and more on performance and expectations of the role models—the residents and faculty. They felt their role models were fact-oriented. They did not feel encouraged by the faculty to improve rapport-building skills, nor was this routinely assessed.

Reduction of Morbidity in Asthmatic Children Given a Spacer Device

S. J. Cunningham and E. F. Crain

Department of Pediatrics, Albert Einstein College of Medicine,
Division of Pediatric Ambulatory Care,
Bronx (NY) Municipal Hospital Center

Spacer devices have made inhaled medication available to young children with asthma. However, their effectiveness is unsubstantiated in settings where ongoing reinforcement is unavailable. We hypothesized that providing a spacer device and a single, brief demonstration regarding its proper use would result in earlier resolution of asthma symptoms, improved school attendance and decreased frequency of unscheduled medical visits for asthma among children receiving noncontinuous care in an urban emergency room (ER).

Children between the ages of 3 through 10 years, who presented to the ER for the treatment of asthma, were randomly assigned to receive either: 1) a spacer device plus inhaled beta agonist or, 2) oral or inhaled beta agonist without a spacer device. Subjects in both groups received other medications at the discretion of the evaluating physician. A questionnaire assessing the child's asthma history was administered to the parent at the time of ER discharge. In follow-up telephone interviews at 1 week, and at 2 and 4 months, parents reported days of wheeze and cough, missed school days and unscheduled medical visits related to asthma.

Ninety-eight patients were enrolled. Eighty-four patients (86%) completed the study. Seven patients from each group were lost to follow-up. The groups did not differ in age, ethnicity, age at onset or baseline severity of asthma. At 1 week there were no significant differences in reported days of cough or wheeze or days missed from school. At the 2 and 4 month follow-up, patients given the spacer device had experienced significantly earlier resolution of cough (4.7 and 2.6 days vs. 11.3 and 6.8 days, $p<.01$) and wheeze (2.3 and 0.4 days vs. 7 and 3.6 days, $p<.001$), and had missed fewer school days because of their asthma (1.2 and 2.5 days vs. 6.7 and 5.7, $p<0.03$). Unscheduled medical visits were reported at similar, low frequencies in both groups.

We conclude that introducing a spacer device to patients in a busy, urban ER is an effective and efficient intervention that improves the functioning of asthmatic children.

An Assessment of Nutritional Status in Homeless Children

J. H. Gould, T. L. Pelham, and J. C. Weiss

Department of Pediatrics,
Jefferson Medical College,
Philadelphia, Pa

The association between poverty and poor health and nutrition is well known. However, to date there has been no comprehensive nutritional assessment of the pediatric homeless population. The purpose of this study is to determine the nutritional status of children living in homeless shelters.

Dietary history, anthropomorphic measurements, and blood studies were obtained from 102 children, ages 0.5 yrs. to 5.6 yrs. (mean = 2.7 yrs.), living in four Philadelphia area homeless shelters. The duration of homelessness averaged 16.5 ± 13.8 wks. Although all of the children were eligible for WIC, only 48 children had been enrolled in the past twelve months. For children greater than one year of age, the primary source of nutrition was meals provided by the shelters.

Anemia (Hgb $<$ 2 SD below mean for age) was found in 23% of children. Iron deficiency (serum ferritin $\leq$ 15ng/ml) was seen in only 5% of anemic children and 4% overall.

Weight for age measurements did not differ significantly from expected NCHC standard norms, and the tricep skinfold measurements were also normal, suggesting adequate caloric intake.

In contrast, 33% of the children had heights below the tenth percentile for age, and 32% had mid-arm muscle area (MAMA) below the tenth percentile, indicating chronic protein malnutrition. Retinol binding protein (RBP), a blood test that measures acute protein malnutrition, was abnormal in 53% of the children. Of the children with MAMA and height above the twenty-fifth percentile, 45% and 53% respectively had abnormally low RBP. Thus, the RBP was able to identify protein malnutrition that would not have been detected by anthropometry alone.

In summary, this study demonstrates that anemia and both acute and chronic protein malnutrition are common in homeless children. These nutritional findings, which did not show statistical correlation with duration of homelessness, WIC enrollment, or percentage of meals provided by the shelter, may be associated with other aspects of homelessness and will require further investigation.

APA TOPIC PLENARY SESSION
Wednesday, May 1, 9 AM-NOON
CLINICAL ISSUES

Double-blind, Cross-over Trial of Psyllium Fiber in Hypercholesterolemic Children

B. A. Dennison

Department of Pediatrics, Cornell University Medical College, and the Rogosin Institute, New York, NY

Water-soluble fiber has been shown to have a cholesterol lowering effect in adults. A randomized, double-blind, placebo-controlled, cross-over trial was designed to test the efficacy of psyllium fiber in lowering elevated LDL-cholesterol (LDL-C) levels in children (5-18 years). Subjects with LDL-C levels $\geqslant$ 2.84 mmol/L (110 mg/dL), despite $\geqslant$ 3 months of a low fat, low saturated fat, low cholesterol diet were enrolled. Two ready-to-eat cereals, with psyllium fiber (6 g per day) and without, were prescribed for 4-5 weeks each, with an intervening 2 week washout phase. Reported compliance rates exceeded 90% in the 20 subjects completing the study. Mean initial total cholesterol (TC), LDL-C, HDL-C, and triglyceride (TG) values were: 5.23, 3.60, 1.18, and 2.22 mmol/L, respectively. Comparison of the mean changes (from baseline) in lipid values following the two periods of cereal consumption revealed no statistically or clinically significant differences in TC, LDL-C, or HDL-C values. Triglyceride levels, however, increased significantly (0.68 mmol/L (26 mg/dL), $p < 0.05$) after the control cereal, compared to the psyllium cereal. No significant differences were noted in the children's dietary intake (assessed by 7-day diet records) during the two study periods. Growth parameters (height, weight, skinfold thicknesses), vitamin (folic acid, Vitamin A, D, and E), and mineral (iron, zinc, and calcium) levels were not affected. In this study, psyllium fiber had no additional TC or LDL-C lowering effect in children who were following low fat, low cholesterol diets.

Bacteriology of Acute Otitis Media (AOM): A New Perspective

M. A. DelBeccaro, P. M. Mendelman, A. F. Inglis, M. A. Richardson, and C. Clausen

Departments of Pediatrics and Otolaryngology, University of Washington, Seattle

Previous studies have reported 20% to 50% of middle ear cultures from patients with AOM are sterile. We describe our isolation of bacterial pathogens from patients with AOM.

Children were recruited from the Emergency Room, during Otolaryngology Clinic hours, as part of a multicenter single blind study comparing oral antibiotics in the treatment of AOM. Eligibility required symptoms $\leqslant$ 7 days duration, an erythematous or bulging tympanic membrane (TM), and no antibiotics in the last 5 days. Surface cultures of the TM, and an aspirate of middle ear fluid (MEF) were taken immediately to the microbiology lab and cultured aerobically. MEF specimens were also cultured anaerobically. If there was no growth on the primary plates a blind subculture of the Tryptic Soy Yeast broth was performed at 48 hours. A positive culture was considered to be a pathogen if it was isolated only from the MEF. If a child had recurrent otitis within 30 days a repeat tympanocentesis was performed.

Forty-one patients between the ages of 6 months and 15 years were enrolled; 27 (66%) were female, 33 (80%) white, and 14 (34%) had health insurance. Thirty-eight (93%) of the 41 patients yielded the following 43 pathogens from their MEF: *S. pneumoniae* 19 (44%); *M. catarrhalis* 11 (26%); *H. influenzae* 9 (21%); others 4 (9%). Ten (91%) of the *M. catarrhalis* and 3 (33%) of the *H. influenzae* strains produced the β-lactamase enzyme. Four patients had $>$ 1 pathogen in their MEF. No growth was observed on the primary plates of 7 (18%) of the 38 positive cultures, but grew from the broth subcultures. Ten (24%) patients had a recurrence, all 10 (100%) were culture positive on repeat tympanocentesis, and 7 (70%) of the 10 had different organisms.

CONCLUSIONS: 1) Bacterial pathogens are recoverable in $>$ 90% of AOM if specimens are promptly cultured and if broth subcultures are used; 2) recurrent infections often are due to new organisms.

Brush Culture Method for Diagnosing Tinea Capitis

T. W. Hubbard and J. M. de Triquet

Department of Pediatrics, Eastern Virginia Medical School, Norfolk

Tinea capitis (TC) is a common dermatophytosis in childhood. Documenting fungal infection is prudent before starting systemic antifungal agents, but culture methods involving scraping and pulling hairs are time-consuming and cumbersome. A quicker, less painful method for diagnosing TC was tested.

During March to October 1990, 70 children (mean age 5.1 years, range 8 months - 11 years) presenting to the Children's Hospital of The King's Daughters (CHKD) with symptoms suggesting tinea capitis (e.g. alopecia, scaling) were cultured using both the traditional method (TM) and an experimental brush culture method (BCM). First, in the BCM a small, sterile brush (Reach juvenile toothbrush) was gently rubbed over the affected areas; the brush fibers then were gently depressed into the surface of the dermatophyte test medium: ACU-DTM (Acuderm) agar slant, and then discarded. The TM was then used, scraping scale if present and removing hairs from the same lesions, embedding them on another ACU-DTM. The slants were read daily. No color change in 21 days signified a negative result. Positive cultures were subcultured to identify the dermatophyte. There was no significant difference between methods in detecting disease or lack thereof; culture results agreed in 64 patients; in 5 cases BCM was positive, TM negative; in 1 case TM was positive, BCM negative (Wilcoxon, $p > .4$). Of the 51 paired positive cultures, BCM samples turned positive before TM in 39, and later than TM in 12 (9.6 days (BCM) vs. 10.6 days (TM); $p < .01$, T-test). *Trichophyton tonsurans* was the dermatophyte in all cases of TC.

BCM is a reliable, painless, and simpler alternative to TM in culturing a scalp for fungal disease. BCM produces positive results significantly faster and is a more sensitive method than TM in detecting TC.

Utility of Oxygen Saturation in Evaluating the Response to Treatment in Wheezing Infants

A. J. Alario, W. J. Lewander, P. H. Dennehy, R. Seifer, and A. L. Mansell

Department of Pediatrics, Rhode Island Hospital, Providence

To determine the utility of oxygen saturation measurements in acutely wheezing children, we evaluated 74 full term, previously well infants (mean age 10.1 months) presenting as outpatients with acute wheezing. As participants in a double-blind, randomized, placebo controlled trial infants received nebulized metaproterenol sulfate, as an initial treatment or after a control treatment with normal saline. At baseline and 20 minutes after each treatment a clinical assessment was made which included respiratory rate (RR), and a standardized respiratory distress index (RDI) based on 3 key variables: wheezing, retractions, and flaring. To keep the clinical assessors blinded, oxygen saturations (measured by pulse oximetry) were recorded by a research assistant. Oxygen saturations before and after medication were compared in a post-hoc analysis with the clinical response to treatment defined as *both* a decrease in RR of ≥20% *and* an improvement in RDI score of ≥50% compared to premedication values.

At baseline, the mean (±SEM) oxygen saturation for the entire sample was 94.1±.3% (vs. 97.7±.3% from a sample of healthy controls, P≤.01). Forty-two percent (31/74) of the infants were classified as responding to metaproterenol. No significant difference in oxygen saturation was observed with treatment: pre = 94.6±.5% vs. post = 95.5±6%, with a mean difference per patient of 0.86%, (CI_{95} = −.34 to 2.06%, P = .15). Forty-six percent of responders showed no change (25%) or a decrease (21%) in oxygen saturation following medication. Likewise, 23% of nonresponders showed no change in oxygen saturation and 27% a decrease. These data suggest that although oxygen saturation measurements may indicate hypoxemia in an acutely wheezing infant, change in saturation may not be a useful determinant of the clinical response to bronchodilators. The deterioration in oxygen saturation with treatment in some infants may be due to vasodilation of under-ventilated areas of the lung, resulting in a decrease in measured oxygen saturation.

Initial Weight Loss and Return to Birth Weight Criteria for Breast-fed Infants: Challenging the 'Rules of Thumb'

S. DeMarzo, J. Seacat, and M. Neifert

Lactation Program, Presbyterian/Saint Luke's Medical Center, Denver, Colo

Weight loss up to 10% of birth weight and return to birth weight by 2-3 weeks are commonly cited clinical criteria for acceptable initiation of breast-feeding. To explore these criteria, patterns of initial weight loss and return to birth weight were examined among 264 healthy, term, breast-fed infants. Primiparous mothers in a convenience sub-sample from a prospective study maintained infant feeding and elimination diaries during the first 2 weeks postpartum. Mothers received breast-feeding guidance and support. Infants were weighed naked twice during the 1st 2 weeks using the Sartorius integrating balance, and % weight change from birth weight was calculated. Milk ingestion was measured by change in infant weight before and after a feeding and milk yield was calculated in cc/hr since the infant last nursed.

Data were analyzed using SPSS/PC. Percent infant weight change from birth weight at the 1st visit (mean age = 5d) ranged from −14.3 to +15.3 (mean −1.79, median −1.80, S.D. 4.24). Weight loss exceeded 7% in 8.7% of infants. Among 236 exclusively breast-fed infants who were seen at a 2nd visit (mean age = 10d), 88.7% were above their birth weight. Pearson Product Moment Correlations were performed to ascertain the strength of association between % infant weight loss and selected infant feeding, elimination and milk intake variables. The timing of the first yellow "milk" stool was negatively correlated with % infant weight loss at the 1st visit (r = −.30, p = .000). A moderate correlation was found between % infant weight loss and total breast-milk intake measured at a feeding (r = .50, p = .000), as well as maternal milk yield calculated in cc/hr (r = .48, p = .000). Multiple regression analysis was performed to determine predictors of % weight loss at the 1st visit. Significant predictors were birth weight and maternal milk yield. The resultant equation (F [9,128] 8.07, P = 0.0000) accounted for 36% of the explained variance.

These findings suggest that, with conscientious breast-feeding management, few infants lose >7% of birth weight or fail to regain their birth weight by 2 weeks. Thus, emphasizing the extremes in breast-feeding "rules of thumb" may not be appropriate. Further studies are warranted to establish definitive criteria to assess the onset of breast-feeding.

Appropriateness of Admissions to a Canadian Children's Hospital

K. R. Kowaleski and M. Li

Division of Emergency Medicine, Department of Paediatrics, Children's Hospital of Eastern Ontario, Ottawa

Universal health care coverage may result in meaningful differences in hospital utilization between the U.S. and Canada. We analyzed the rate of inappropriate admission (RIA) to CHEO through the use of the Pediatric Appropriateness Evaluation Protocol (PAEP), a set of objective, diagnosis-independent criteria. We also examined variables that may have influenced this rate. The extent to which potential admissions that would have qualified as appropriate were diverted to the emergency room (ER) holding unit (HU) was also determined.

All non-psychiatric admissions every 12th day in 1989 was retrospectively reviewed. The primary rater was a medical student; a pediatric fellow also reviewed half the charts. The criteria are brief and straightforward; we believed a relatively inexperienced individual could use them reliably. The fellow's results were used to determine interrater reliability.

786 admissions were reviewed, 380 by both raters. 60.1% were male; median age was 4y. Classification by source was: 46.8% ER, 33.5% elective (L), 16.0% urgent (U) and 3.7% neonatal (N). 53.6% were admitted to a medical service, 46.4% surgical.

Overall RIA was 21.3%; however, RIA varied substantially depending on source: N 3.4%, ER 7.1%, U 33.3%, L 37.3% (p<.001). Sex (males 18.7%, females 25.2%; p<.05) was the only other variable demonstrating significant effect on overall results. Age, stay <1 day, day of week, season of year did not. For ER admissions, physician (full-time ER 2.4% vs. other 13.9%), medical (4.8%) vs. surgical (11.8%), and distance from home (<20mi 5.5%, >20mi 13.3%) were of significance (p<.05).

The most common reason for inappropriateness for L was premature admission; for U and ER, inpatient care unnecessary for tests/treatment given. 107 patients admitted to HU met appropriateness criteria. Between raters, general agreement was 93.4%, kappa = 0.82, demonstrating high interrater reliability.

RIA at CHEO compares well with that of U.S. pediatric hospitals reported in the literature. We found ER RIA to be especially low. Overall RIA could be lowered by better timing of L admissions and/or having U admissions screened in the ER.

Parental Time and Expenses for Diabetes Care

G. E. Dougherty, A. Schiffrin, and L. Ball

Departments of Pediatrics and Epidemiology and Biostatistics, McGill University, Montreal, Quebec

Parental time and out of pocket expenditure in the first month after diagnosis of childhood type I diabetes mellitus were measured as part of a randomized trial of traditional (T) versus comprehensive ambulatory care (CAC). Patients in the CAC group were discharged after stabilization of acute metabolic complications (0-5 days) and teaching and insulin adjustment were accomplished at home by a visiting nurse practitioner. Patients in the traditional group were admitted for 2 to 8 days to titrate insulin requirements, complete a formal educational program and allow for adjustment in the family.

The families' out of pocket expenses, parental time devoted to diabetes and time lost from work in the first month were collected via a telephone administered questionnaire supplemented by direct interview.

Mean total parental time expenditure was 144.6 hrs for the traditional group (N = 15), and 101.9 hrs for CAC parents (N = 18), (T = 2.07 P = .047). The main differences occurred in the first 11 days when "T" parents spent a mean of 115.8 hrs at the hospital or providing direct care vs 74.9 hrs for CAC parents (T = 2.40, P = .023). Time lost from work did not differ significantly and was 28.9 hrs vs 27.0 hrs, for T vs CAC.

Total out of pocket expenses for transportation, meals, child care, medical supplies and miscellaneous expenses were $350.68 vs $317.42 with the difference mainly due to transportation, meals and child care, T vs CAC, \$123.76 vs \$71.03 ($T=2.32$, $P=.027$).

Short term medical outcomes did not differ significantly in the two groups. HbA1c's at 3 months were 5.40 vs 5.76% for T vs CAC.

Traditional care occupied more parental time and was more costly to families than comprehensive ambulatory care.

Simethicone in the Treatment of Infant Colic

T. J. Metcalf, T. G. Irons, L. D. Sher, and P. C. Young

Willow Creek Pediatrics, Salt Lake City, Utah;
East Carolina University, Greenville, NC;
Pennisula Allergy and Pediatrics,
Rolling Hills Estates, Calif;
and University of Vermont, Burlington

Simethicone, an antiflatulent, has been used by parents in the treatment of infantile colic for a number of years, on the advice of pediatricians, friends, or relatives. The authors designed a multicenter, randomized, double-blind, placebo-controlled, crossover trial to test the efficacy of Simethicone in infants with symptoms of colic, using a commonly accepted definition of the disorder. Eighty-three infants from three centers formed the data base. Each infant was randomly assigned to receive either simethicone or placebo for a one week treatment period followed by the opposite agent for a second treatment period. A total of 166 treatment periods were evaluated in 83 infants. Fifty-three percent of the treatment periods resulted in improvement compared to baseline; in 22% symptoms worsened, and in 24% no change was noted. The likelihood that an infant would improve, stay the same, or worsen during a treatment period was the same whether the infant was receiving simethicone or placebo (no significant difference by ANOVA). No difference could be shown even when infants with "gas-related symptoms" (by parental report) were evaluated as a group. We conclude that simethicone is no more effective than placebo in the treatment of infantile colic.

Tympanic Membrane Thermometers: Caveat Emptor

M. Nypaver, E. Zieserl, B. Nachtsheim, and A. T. Davis

Department of General and Emergency Pediatrics,
Children's Memorial Hospital, Chicago, Ill

Temperature (temp) measurement is integral to the evaluation of pediatric patients visiting the emergency department (ED). Glass and electronic thermometers are slow, cumbersome and uncomfortable for children. If reliable, the Tympanic Membrane Thermometer (TMT) offers a rapid, noninvasive alternative to the problem of temp measurement in children. Results of previous studies with the TMT are contradictory due to study design flaws. We hypothesized that the TMT yields a reliable measure of temp in children. In this prospective, comparative study we sought to: 1) determine the reliability of the Firstemp TMT to detect fever compared to our current standard, the IVAC digital thermometer, and 2) to determine if reliability was affected by patient age or range of temp. 1959 children of all ages were enrolled from the Children's Memorial Hospital ED during 2 months in 1990. Bilateral TMT temps were taken in all patients (pts) in addition to oral (ORL)-IVAC and/or rectal (REC)-IVAC temps depending on age and ability to cooperate. All temps were taken by ED nursing staff. Findings of cerumen, otitis media, perforation, myringotomy tubes, and foreign bodies were noted. Fever was defined as IVAC temp $\geqslant 38.5°C$.

RESULTS: 1040 pts had ORL-IVAC temps, 939 pts had REC-IVAC temps and 23 pts had both. Mean difference (diff) between right and left ears $= 0.005°C \pm 0.45°C$, ($r=.88$). For febrile children, mean diff between TMT and REC-IVAC $= -0.35°C \pm 0.47°C$ ($r=.87$); between TMT and ORL-IVAC $= -0.13°C \pm 0.54°C$ ($r=.79$). Although correlation was good, 28% of children with fever had normal TMT temps. The TMT underestimated IVAC temps more in febrile pts than nonfebrile pts (mean diff $=0.44°C$ vs. $0.31°C$, $p<.001$, t-test) regardless of age.

CONCLUSIONS: The Firstemp TMT is not a reliable indicator of fever in children due to its imprecision and significant variability; it missed almost 30% of children with fever and performed worse at higher temperatures. Age did not contribute to TMT performance. The Firstemp TMT should not replace electronic digital thermometers.

Over-the-Counter (O.T.C.) Medication Use in Children With Colds—a Critical Appraisal

M. B. H. Smith and W. Feldman

Department of Pediatrics,
University of Ottawa (Ontario)

Previous review articles on the use of OTC cough and cold medications in children have been inconclusive. Despite the lack of firm evidence supporting their use, these substances are present in most homes and continue to be a common cause of accidental ingestion in young children. In order to demonstrate a greater good than harm, these products must be shown to be effective for the symptomatic relief of the common cold in children. Our objective was to critically evaluate the medical literature to determine what medications have been shown to be effective in controlled trials and particularly their evaluation in children.

All relevant citations from January 1950 to November 1990 were categorized into six groups and given a scientific validity score based on the representativeness of the subjects, treatment design and objectivity of outcome measures. Those articles scoring over 70% were included in the final synthesis. 50 studies were analyzed in detail. Interrater reliability was good (weighted Kappa = .80).

No. of studies and mean scientific validity score (%)	Supporting Use	Not Supporting Use
Adult Studies		
Antihistamines	3 (79)	6 (83)
Decongestants	4 (77)	1 (70)
Antitussives	-	-
Expectorants	-	1 (77)
Anticholinergics	1 (100)	1 (92)
Combinations	6 (85)	1 (92)
Child Studies		
(Age > 5 Years)	1 (85)	1 (77)

We conclude that some OTC cold medications have been demonstrated to reduce the symptoms of the common cold in adults including smokers. Only 2 studies involved children (5 - 12 years) and their results were diametrically opposed. No controlled trials have been done in children under 5 years. Since this is the age group most likely to use or ingest excessive amounts, these products should be considered experimental for young children.

Intermittent Versus Continuous Amoxicillin Prophylaxis for Infants and Children With Recurrent Otitis Media With Effusion

S. Berman, R. Nuss, R. Roark, C. Huber-Navin, K. Grose, and M. Herrera

Department of Pediatrics, University of Colorado
Health Sciences Center, Denver

The efficacy of continuous (C) amoxicillin prophylaxis was compared to intermittent (I) prophylaxis with cold symptoms in a randomized single blinded prospective clinical trial. Eighty-four patients (31 infants and 53 children) who experienced three episodes of otitis media with effusion (OME) in the 6 months preceding entry into the study were randomized to I amoxicillin and 89 patients (38 infants and 51 children) to C amoxicillin. For infants less than 12 months of age, the overall OME incidence rate per 120 days at risk was 1.18 for I amoxicillin versus 1.25 for C amoxicillin. C amoxicillin was associated with a lower OME incidence rate for infants enrolled during the winter months while I amoxicillin had a lower incidence rate for infants enrolled during the remaining months. For children 1 year of age or older, the overall incidence rate per 120 days at risk was 0.70 for I versus 0.43 for C amoxicillin. During winter months the incidence of OME for children on I amoxicillin was 3.5 times higher than the rate for children on continuous amoxicillin (0.80 versus 0.23).

	Intermittent Amoxicillin			Continuous Amoxicillin		
	Entered During			Entered During		
	All Year	Winter	Non-Winter	All Year	Winter	Non-Winter
Total Patients	84	37	47	89	35	54
Infants <12 mos.	31	16	15	38	10	28
Children >12 mos.	53	21	32	51	25	26
Incidence Rate						
Total Patients	0.87	1.10	0.70	0.74	0.46	0.97
Infants <12 mos.	1.18	1.52	0.85	1.25	1.15	1.30
Children >12 mos.	0.70	0.80	0.64	0.43	0.23	0.68

The results support treating infants and children with continuous antibiotic prophylaxis during winter months and with intermittent prophylaxis at other times.

Duration of Positive Streptococcal Throat Cultures After Initiation of Antibiotics

L. W. Snellman, H. J. Stang, J. M. Stang, D. R. Johnson, and E. L. Kaplan

Departments of Pediatrics, Group Health, Inc, and
University of Minnesota,
White Bear Lake and Minneapolis

Recommendations differ concerning when, after initiating antibiotics, a patient with group A streptococcal (GAS) pharyngitis may return to school with diminished risk of transmission. We are aware of no prospectively collected data which completely address this issue. This study was undertaken to determine the period of contagiousness as manifested by positive throat culture.

Children (4-18 years) with pharyngitis associated with the presence of GAS were enrolled. They received either oral penicillin V (OP), oral erythromycin estolate (OE), or intramuscular benzathine penicillin G (BPG). During three home visits in the 24 hours following initiation of antibiotic therapy, additional throat cultures were obtained and clinical signs and symptoms were recorded. Serum samples were obtained at enrollment and at 4 weeks for anti-streptolysin O (ASO) and anti-DNAse B titers.

Of 47 children enrolled, 39 (83%) became culture negative within 24 hours. For these 39 patients, the mean time to first negative culture was 17.6 hours. Neither time to conversion to negative nor positivity of any single culture could be predicted by clinical signs or symptoms. There was no difference in mean time to first negative culture between the OP and BPG groups. However, 75% of patients who failed to convert to negative within the first 24 hours were in the OE group (OP: 1/17 [5.9%]; BPG: 1/15 [6.7%]; OE: 6/15 [40%]). There was also no difference in either time to conversion to negative or the positivity of culture at 24 hours between those who had a rise in ASO and/or anti-DNAse B titers and those who did not.

These data suggest that children with GAS pharyngitis treated with penicillin have reduced communicability and may usually return to school after 24 hours of therapy. These data further suggest that erythromycin may be less effective.

DEVELOPMENTAL AND BEHAVIORAL PEDIATRICS

School Outcomes of Children With Asthma

M. G. Fowler, R. Garg, and M.G. Davenport

Office of Analysis, National Center for
Health Statistics,
Hyattsville, Md, and
Clinical Trials Branch,
National Heart, Lung, and Blood Institute, Bethesda, Md

Children with asthma are at increased risk for school problems. Data from the 1988 U.S. National Health Interview Survey on Child Health, a representative national cross-sectional survey, were used to determine national estimates of school outcomes for children reported to have asthma (CWA) compared to children without current conditions (CWNOCC). Among the 10,362 survey children in school grades 1-12, families reported that 536 (5%) had had asthma in the previous 12 months; prevalence varied little by demographic factors although blacks had slightly higher rates than nonblacks.

Regarding school outcomes, mean days absent were 7.5 days for CWA versus 2.5 days for the CWNOCC group; twenty percent of CWA missed 11 or more school days in the previous 12 months versus only 2.5% for CWNOCC. Seventeen percent of CWA had ever repeated a grade compared to 15% of CWNOCC, and 9% CWA were reported to have learning disabilities compared to 5% of CWNOCC. Thirty percent of CWA were reported to have some activity limitation, compared to only 2% of CWNOCC. Using logistic regression to control for demographic factors, CWA had similar (OR = 1.3) risk of grade failure but 1.7 times the risk of learning disability compared to children without chronic conditions. For CWA, activity limitation was an important predictor of school outcomes: those children with activity limitations were 2.5 times as likely to repeat a grade, and 5 times as likely to have a learning disability, compared to CWA without limitations. Likewise, CWA with activity limitations averaged 11 days absent versus 7 days for those with no limitations. These national data underscore the importance of evaluating children with asthma for special academic needs and also suggest that optimal treatment to reduce activity limitations among asthmatic children may facilitate their school functioning.

Homage to a Clinical Observation: Empirical Support for Wessel's Definition of 'Colic'

R. G. Barr, A. Rotman, J. Yaremko, D. Leduc, T. E. Francoeur, J. Desilets, and R. DuBerger

Department of Pediatrics, McGill University,
Montreal, Quebec, and
Montreal Children's Hospital

To provide the first controlled empirical description of the clinical features of colic, 38 infants whose mothers considered crying a problem ("colic") and 38 age, sex, parity and ethnicity pair-matched controls were observed at home 10 min. before and after an evening feed and by mothers for 7 days with pre-validated diaries. Measures included (1) duration and frequency of cry and fuss (C/F), (2) crying after feed, (3) distention (fat free abdominal girth), (4) temperament ratings, and (5) 8 parent ratings of cry quality. Following Wessel (1954), each "colic" infant was classified by number of days/wk of C/F duration ⩾3 hrs/day. The distribution showed 2 peaks at 0 and 3 days/wk. Colic infants with C/F ⩾3 hrs/day for ⩾3 days/wk were called *Wessel's* Colic (WC), the others *Non-Wessel's* Colic (NWC). Groups were compared by ANOVA (post hoc Tukey) or χ^2 analyses.

Neither crying after feed nor distention differed between groups. WC infants cried over twice as long as *both* NWC and Controls (4.1 vs. 1.7 and 1.7 hrs/day; F [2,70] = 37.1, P<.001) but there was no difference in frequency (7.8 vs. 5.7 vs. 7 bouts/day; F=1.4, P=.25). The same pattern occurred with Temperament: WC were significantly more negative than NWC and Controls (−5.2 vs. −0.7 and 1.3: F[2,65]=7.8, P=.001). In contrast, there was no difference before or after feeds on 7 of 8 cry ratings except on the "sickness" rating. It *increased* after feeds for *both* WC *and* NWC infants (3.8 and 3.2) compared to cries before feed (2.3 and 1.9, respectively) and controls (1.8 before and 1.7 after feed: group × feed F[2,45]=3.5, P=.04).

CONCLUSION: In infants presenting with problem crying, there are probably 2 groups: (1) "Wessel's" colic with longer cry duration and negative temperament, and (2) "non-Wessel's" colic with cry duration and temperament similar to controls. Cry is equally likely after feeding in all infants and quality is similar. However, if seen as indicating "sickness," crying may be a complaint in both groups.

Preventing Disruptive Night Waking In Infancy: An Effective Primary Care Intervention

R. Adair, H. Bauchner, B. Philipp, S. Levenson, and B. Zuckerman

Department of Pediatrics,
Boston (Mass) City Hospital,
Boston University School of Medicine

Approximately 25% of young infants wake at night. The purpose of this study was to implement and evaluate a brief intervention to prevent disruptive night waking. Parents were enrolled as they sought care at the Lahey Medical Center, Burlington, MA. The control group was enrolled at the 9 month visit, the intervention group at the 4 month visit. For the intervention parents: (1) were advised to place their infants partially awake in the crib at bedtime starting at 4 months, and (2) completed a daily routine chart prior to the 6 month visit then reviewed it with the MD. Parents in both groups completed an outcome questionnaire when their children were 9 months old. All contacts addressed feeding and sleeping in order to obscure the purpose of the study.

128 of 172 (74%) invited infant-parent pairs comprised the control group and 164 of 222 (74%) the intervention group. The majority of families were white (97%), well-educated (66% parents college graduates) and financially secure (83% yearly income > $30,000). The groups were also similar with regards to infant age, gender, number of siblings; parental age, marital status; and factors shown to be related to night waking: current breast feeding, thumb/pacifier sucking and maternal isolation.

Infants in the intervention group averaged 2.5 wakings/week versus 3.9 in the control group (p=.02), a 36% reduction. Frequent night waking (> 7 wakings/week) occurred in 14% of intervention infants versus 27% of control infants (p=.01), a 48% reduction. We conclude that with this intervention pediatricians can help parents prevent disruptive night waking in young infants.

Identifying Sources of Discrepancy Between Pediatricians' Diagnoses and the Child Behavior Checklist

S. M. Horwitz, P. J. Leaf, J. M. Leventhal, B. W. C. Forsyth, and K. N. Speechley

Departments of Epidemiology and
Public Health and Pediatrics,
Yale University School of Medicine,
New Haven, Conn

Previous research indicates that when pediatricians' diagnoses of psychosocial (PS) problems are compared to those from a structured assessment tool such as the Child Behavior Checklist (CBCL), there is little agreement on which children have PS problems. The purpose of this study was to measure disagreement between the CBCL and clinicians and identify sources of conflict. We hypothesized that issues such as clinician's knowledge of a child, type of visit, and differences in diagnostic thresholds between clinicians and the CBCL may account for the discrepancies. We investigated this in a random sample of 19 out of 23 (83%) pediatric practices in New Haven, CT. We collected PS information from physicians using a 12-category checklist based on a WHO-sponsored primary care classification system.

Of the 2006 children 4-8 years visiting these practices, 1886 children and their families (91%) participated. At entry, 52% were 4-5 years, 50% were male, 80% were white, and 59% were visiting for acute care.

Pediatricians identified 515 children (27%) with ≥1 PS problems, while the CBCL identified 322 children (17%). Overall, pediatricians and the CBCL disagreed on 29% of the children. When we examined disagreement for that group of children in which the hypothesized methodological problems had been corrected [i.e., for well-child or follow-up visits to the usual clinician who knew the child well (N=485)], the disagreement rate was similar (36%). Within the 485 children, we next examined the reasons for these discrepancies. In 83/155 children (54%) where the pediatrician but not the CBCL indicated a PS problem, children had CBCL scores of 50 or more, indicating many problem behaviors. These CBCL scores were not high enough to meet the diagnostic cutoff. In children with CBCL scores less than 50 (N=72), pediatricians and the CBCL identified the same problem in 34 children (47%). Of the 25 cases where the CBCL but not the physician indicated a problem, 7 (28%) had a past problem indicated by the clinician.

We conclude that previously reported discrepancies are largely due to differences in diagnostic thresholds between clinicians and the CBCL.

Understanding the Development of Failure to Thrive in a Low Birth Weight, Preterm Cohort: A Prospective Study to Age Three

P. H. Casey, K. Kelleher, R. H. Bradley, M. Swanson, L. Whiteside, S. Pope, and K. Barrett

Department of Pediatrics, University of Arkansas
for Medical Sciences, Little Rock

The development of Failure to Thrive (FTT) was assessed in a prospective study of low birth weight (LBW) preterm (PT) infants to avoid methodologic problems of previous retrospective research. 985 infants (birth weight ≤2500 gm, gestation age ≤37 wks) were recruited in the nursery in a 8 site collaborative research program. All infants received routine follow up care at standard intervals, and a broad range of infant, parent, and environmental data were collected in the nursery and at 40 wks, 4, 8, 12, 18, 24, 30, and 36 mos gestation corrected age (GCA). Clinicians were instructed to utilize a standard definition using growth data; in addition, a computer model was employed to assess normal interval growth. One hundred fifty six (156) infants met both criteria by 36 mos and were considered FTT. 144 infants were excluded as they met only 1 criteria. Bivariate analyses compared all independent variables collected from 40 wks to 30 mos GCA between 156 FTT and 685 non-FTT infants. Of all the maternal and environmental variables, only the 12 mos household density and the quality of home environment as measured by the total HOME Inventory and its Responsivity, Play Materials, and Involvement subscales differentiated the groups (p≤.01). FTT infants were rated lower by their mothers on the 12 and 24 mos Health Rating Scale (p<.001), had more chronic conditions at 12 and 24 mos (p<.001), and were more likely to be judged suspect or abnormal on the neurologic examination at all clinical visits (p<.01). The FTT infants scored lower on the Bayley MDI and PDI at 12 and 24 mos GCA (p<.002). There were no differences in neonatal health, infant temperament, family stress, support, SES, or maternal mental health, knowledge, or I.Q.

In this large cohort of LBW, PT infants followed longitudinally, several medical characteristics of the child, along with the quality of their home environments, differentiated the group of children with FTT from those without FTT. These results should assist in the development of identification and intervention strategies regarding FTT in LBW, PT infants.

The Mental Health of Children Placed With Relatives

H. Dubowitz, V. Tepper, S. Zuravin, and S. Feigelman

Department of Pediatrics,
University of Maryland Medical School, Baltimore

Placement with relatives is generally the first option of public agencies seeking substitute care for children, mostly due to child abuse or neglect. This is the first evaluation of the prevalence and treatment status of mental health problems of children in this type of foster care.

METHOD: Subjects were *all* 524 children living in relative placements in Baltimore in April, 1989. Data were gathered from medical records, mailed questionnaires to health care providers, parents, relative caretakers, caseworkers and the adolescents, and a clinical assessment involving standardized measures and interviews.

RESULTS: Only 58% of the children aged 0-5 years passed the Battelle developmental screening test. The median percentiles on a test of cognitive functioning were far below normal for the older children. Forty-six percent of the children had clinically significant behavior problems on the Achenbach CBCL; 32% were depressed. Only 27% of the children, mostly in the 0-5 age group, had no mental health diagnosis. Fifty-eight percent had 1-2 problems and the remainder had >2. Many of these problems had not been identified or were not being addressed and 38% of the children clearly needed follow-up.

Increased mental health problems were associated with older age at placement ($p=.001$), increased duration of placement ($p=.001$), older current age ($p=.001$), and male gender ($p=.0001$). Increased problems were also associated with previous abuse ($p=.01$), the caretaker having made more contact with the caseworker ($p=.01$) and receiving more services ($p=.003$). Children with increased problems were more likely to be placed with older relatives ($p=.01$), in homes with more children ($p=.01$), and viewed by the relative as "difficult".

IMPLICATIONS: Children placed with relatives appear to have substantial mental health problems, many of which are not being addressed. Their problems are similar to those of other foster children, but appear to be greater than those of poor children and the population in general. Families, health professionals, and the child welfare system should address these needs.

Child Rearing Practices and Nursing Caries

J. R. Serwint, R. Mungo, V. Negrete, M. E. Guzman, and B. M. Korsch

Departments of Pediatrics
and Pediatric Dentistry,
University of Southern California
School of Medicine, Los Angeles,
and Children's Hospital of Los Angeles

In the dental literature, nursing caries are attributed to factors such as bottle feeding past 12 months of age, night time bottles and parental inability to say no to their children. We conducted a cross-sectional study in a pediatric residents' clinic to determine which factors may be predictive of nursing caries.

Caregivers of children aged 18 to 36 months were interviewed to determine feeding practices, dental health behavior, limit setting and sleep issues after which the children's teeth were examined. Of 110 children enrolled, 22 (20%) were found to have nursing caries.

Children with caries were older, and compared to children without caries, were more likely to have younger siblings, 69% vs. 35% ($p = .03$), lower maternal educational level, 8.6 vs. 11.2 years ($p = .02$), and mothers with 8 or more cavities, 55% vs. 19% ($p = .002$). At the time of the interview, 50% of those who had caries and 72% of those who did not were still taking the bottle (p = ns).

More infants in the caries group had been breast fed, 77% vs. 46% ($p = .02$), although length of breast feeding was similar, 5.3 vs. 6.3 months. Fewer children with caries drank tap water, 27% vs. 54 % ($p = .05$); there were no differences in topical fluoride use, tooth brushing practices or visits to the dentist.

Ninety-five percent of children with caries and 97% without had taken bottles while sleeping. There were no differences in number of daytime or night time bottles, or use of a pacifier or security object. There were also no differences reported in night waking, cosleeping, or parental report of difficulty in saying no to the child or difficulty disciplining the child. However, children with caries were more likely to specifically wake for a bottle at night, 64% vs. 36% ($p = .05$), and their mothers were more likely to feel that the bottle helped motivate the child to do things, 58% vs. 23% ($p = .02$).

These data fail to substantiate a straightforward relationship between child rearing practices and nursing caries and suggest that well designed prospective studies are needed to clarify the etiology of early caries.

Detecting Family Violence in the Context of Pediatric Continuity Care

L. S. Wissow, M. E. H. Wilson, and D. Roter

Johns Hopkins Medical Institutions, Baltimore, Md

Family violence is a common but frequently undisclosed contributor to problems with child behavior and development. We compared 3 methods of detecting family violence in the context of pediatric continuity clinic visits: 1) prior to a scheduled visit with their child's pediatrician mothers completed an adaptation of the Conflict Tactics Scale (CTS) (Straus, 1979), a measure of violent behavior among any members of the child's family; 2) the visit was audiotaped and coded by a research assistant who documented disclosures of corporal punishment, which often occurs in conjunction with violence among other family members; 3) at the end of the visit the physician, without knowledge of the mother's response to the CTS, rated the chance that there might be a problem with interpersonal violence in the family. The study took place in an inner city hospital's residents' continuity clinic. Fifty-seven mothers were systematically enrolled, representing visits to 19 PGY2 and PGY3 pediatric residents.

Nearly half (26/57) of the mothers gave positive responses to the CTS (answered "at least once or twice in the past year" to one or more of the last five items, including "kicked, bit or hit with a fist" through use of a weapon). During 15 of the 57 visits (26%) there was an explicit disclosure of corporal punishment. These 15 disclosures included labeling the child as "bad" or a cause of extreme parental distress (4), mentioning the threat of a beating as a means of controlling the child (2), and either describing a specific beating or striking the child in the exam room (6). Eight of the 15 disclosures were initiated by the mother, with the remainder coming in response to physician questions about behavior or discipline. Physicians rated 53 of the 57 families as having little or no chance of experiencing a problem with interpersonal violence, including 13 of the 15 families that had disclosed or demonstrated corporal punishment during the preceding visit. Neither disclosure of corporal punishment nor physician prediction was a sensitive or specific predictor of a mother's response to the CTS. We conclude that instruments such as the CTS are important parts of the effort to help physicians become aware of the broader range of intrafamilial violence experienced by children.

Depression and Role Satisfaction in Mothers of Toddlers

A. L. Olson and L. A. DiBrigida

Department of Maternal and Child Health,
Dartmouth Medical School, Hanover, NH

Maternal depression is an important problem for pediatricians caring for toddlers since it can affect children's behavior and development. Work can affect the mental health of mothers in a positive or negative manner. Mothers may find themselves against their wishes in a position of working or staying at home which may influence their mental health. Pediatricians have frequent contact with mothers during the toddler year. We gathered data on the prevalence of depression and its association with employment. We hypothesized that mothers who are satisfied with their current role, whether at home, or employed, will have less depression than mothers who are not.

To test this hypothesis we conducted a cross-sectional practice based survey of maternal self reported symptoms of depression with 234 mothers of toddlers (12-24 mon.) at well child visits in two community pediatric practices from the Dartmouth-Hitchcock Pediatric Practices Collaborative Research Group. Depression was assessed with a 20 item depression screening inventory, developed by Barrett, Oxman and Gerber and based on the Hopkins Symptom Checklist-90 for use in primary care practice. It allows one to assess 3 levels of depressive symptomatology (depressive mood, syndrome or disorder) with cut off levels on a scale of 0 to 60 of ⩾9, ⩾14 and ⩾19. It also allows a mean depression score to be calculated. Data was obtained on parents' socioeconomic status, hours worked, and whether the mother was satisfied with her current role of being at home or employed.

Depressive symptoms were present to some degree in 52% overall. This included depressive mood only in 10%, depressive syndrome in 25%, and depressive disorder in 17%. Mean scores for depression were somewhat better for working than nonworking mothers (11.3 work vs 13.2 home, t-test, p = .02) but the 42 mothers who were disatisfied with their current roles had much higher depression scores (20.5 dissatisf. vs 10.3 satisf., t-test, p = .002). The association of satisfaction and depression with maternal education or employment, parental SES, parity and maternal age were also examined.

These results indicate that the majority of mothers of toddlers in a pediatric practice were depressed to some extent. Role satisfaction was more important than employment status in depressive symptoms. We need to give more careful attention to these issues during toddler visits.

Maternal Attitudes As Predictors of Infant Feeding Decisions

C. I. Dungy, J. Christensen-Szalanski, M. Losch, and D. Russell

Department of Pediatrics,
The University of Iowa, Iowa City

The rate of breast feeding among women in the United States has been declining since 1982. In order to develop intervention strategies to reverse the downward trend it is important to determine the factors influencing maternal infant feeding decisions. Most previous studies have evaluated various socio-demographic characteristics to predict infant feeding behavior. The present study reports an easily constructed attitude profile that is closely correlated with maternal infant feeding behavior. 219 women were interviewed within 48 hours of birth to determine those factors most closely associated with the infant feeding decision. Socio-demographic characteristics including age, ethnicity, education, family income and parity were obtained for each respondent. In addition, maternal attitudes concerning infant feeding were assessed through the use of a multi-attribute utility (MAU) scale composed of ten topic areas. Five topic areas (nutrition, cost, maternal appearance, pleasure and well-being) addressed selected aspects of breast milk and infant formula (product dimension). The remaining 5 areas (parental role, physical closeness, infant intake, feeding ease and night feeding) focused on breast feeding and bottle feeding (process dimension). A discriminant function analysis using socio-demographic variables previously shown to be correlated with maternal feeding decisions was only marginally able to discriminate breast feeding from bottle feeding women (kappa = .30). However, a discriminant function analysis based on the MAU was able to identify correctly nearly all mothers' infant feeding choices (kappa = .90). Thus, the attitude profile was significantly better ($p < .001$) in predicting feeding choices than were socio-demographic characteristics. The results indicate that the MAU provides easily obtained information useful in predicting maternal infant feeding decisions.

The Feasibility and Utility of Psychosocial Screening in a Pediatric Clinic

K. J. Kemper

Department of Pediatrics,
University of Washington,
and Harborview Medical Center, Seattle

Screening for psychosocial risk factors which affect parenting has been limited by lack of a structured approach. The purpose of this study was to assess the feasibility and utility of a self-administered questionnaire in screening for risk factors for poor parenting; eg. substance abuse, history of parental abuse as a child, depression, self-esteem and social support. Questionnaires were offered to mothers bringing their children for routine care at an urban pediatric clinic from April 15-June 15, 1990. In addition to routine medical history, the questionnaire included standard screening questionnaires on psychosocial conditions, eg. Cyr's two-item screening test for alcoholism, Rosenberg's Self-Esteem questionnaire, and the Screening Instrument for Depression. Charts were reviewed for 114 children whose mothers completed part or all of the questionnaire and 117 randomly selected children whose mothers had not. Mothers who filled out questionnaires were similar to mothers who did not in terms of maternal age (x = 25 years) and education (x = 11.5 years), payor status (Medicaid = 70%) and the frequency with which psychosocial problems were noted on the chart (eg. drug problem in the home in 24% vs. 22%). For those who returned questionnaires, the response rate, even for sensitive questions was high (eg. household income, 85%; maternal drug use, 97%; and domestic violence, 89%). Overall, the questionnaire identified significantly more children with one or more of the risk factors for poor parenting than the chart did (64/114, 56% vs. 43/117, 37%, P = 0.005). For example, parental history of abuse as a child was noted on 41 questionnaires vs. 3 charts (P<0.001). Self-administered questionnaires addressing psychosocial risk factors are feasible, yield important information for family health and parenting, and should be considered as part of routine intake procedures in pediatric clinics, especially those serving high-risk populations.

Developmental Delay Among Homeless Children

B. P. Dreyer, C. D. Courtlandt, A. H. Fierman, M. Arbel, G. Benincasa, C. Squittieri, L. Palevsky, and N. Mann

Department of Pediatrics,
New York (NY) University School of Medicine

To determine whether young homeless children are at risk for developmental delays, we studied children residing in a shelter for single homeless mothers and their children. Medical, social, and family histories were obtained, and the Revised Gesell Developmental Examination and the Denver Developmental Screening Test (DDST) were administered to all children 15-30 months of age with no known developmental problems (N = 25). Each item on the Gesell was scored by two observers. Developmental ages were determined by a third researcher blinded to the age, sex, race, and performance of the child. All families were Hollingshead SES Group V, medicaid eligible, and receiving AFDC benefits. 20 (80%) mothers failed to complete high school. 16 (64%) fathers were arrested for a violent or drug-related crime. Only 3 mothers admitted to drug use.

The mean (±SE) developmental quotients (DQ) on the sections of the Gesell were as follows: adaptive 77.6 (1.6); fine motor 79.4 (1.9); language 77.1 (1.8); gross motor 95.9 (2.2); personal-social 93.5 (2.4). Mean DQs for the homeless children were compared with those of the 15-36 month-old subset of the 1980 Gesell sample with a maternal education level of high school or less. Homeless children scored significantly lower on all sections (adaptive, fine motor, language p<.001; gross motor p<.05; personal-social

$p<.01$). 10/25 (40%) homeless children failed the Gesell. An additional 11/25 (44%) scored in the questionably abnormal range. After controlling for sex, race, birth weight, gestational age, birth order, child's current age, chronic/ recurrent illness, maternal age and educational level, family size, and paternal arrest, a duration of homelessness of greater than four months was significantly associated with lower scores on the Gesell adaptive, language, and fine motor schedules ($p<.05$). All children passed the DDST; one child had a questionable result.

We conclude that young homeless children exhibit significant which may influence their mental health. Pediatricians have fre-delays in development. Longer duration of homelessness was associated with more extreme delays. The DDST was insensitive in identifying these delays. Effective developmental evaluation and intervention programs are indicated for young children residing in homeless shelters.

EMERGENCY MEDICINE AND CHILD ABUSE

The Failure of Tympanic Thermometry to Detect Fever Accurately in a Pediatric Emergency Department (PED)

C. Garabedian, R. Vinci, D. Dwyer, and H. Bauchner

Division of Pediatric Emergency Medicine,
Department of Pediatrics,
Boston (Mass) University School of Medicine
and Boston City Hospital

The presence of fever is an important finding in the evaluation of the pediatric patient. Tympanic thermometry (TT) is a new technique that assesses body temperature by measuring infrared radiation from the tympanic membrane. The purpose of this report is to assess the accuracy of TT in the PED.

Following an inservice program, nurses performed both TT and rectal or oral temperatures in 845 consecutive patients who presented to the PED. The majority were male (53%) and black (65%). We identified a discrepancy between TT and rectal temperature in 6% (15 of 239) of children < two years of age. Using temperature ≥ 100.4°F in children ≤ 3 months of age as the clinical marker of serious illness, 1 of 57 children was afebrile by rectal temperature, but had a temperature by TT. Using temperature ≥ 102°F in children between 3 and 24 months of age as a clinical marker of serious illness, 14 of 209 children may have had their clinical management changed if TT alone was used, with 7 potentially having additional studies (such as a CBC and blood culture) and 7 potentially less studies. We found no discrepancies between TT and rectal temperatures, when rectal temperatures were ≤ 100°F (N = 126) in children between 3 and 24 months of age.

We conclude (1) TT is not accurate in assessing febrile children, and that in a substantial number of patients, clinical management may be different if TT alone is used to assess temperature, and (2) when TT indicates, in children between 3 and 24 months of age, that the temperature is ≤ 100°F no rectal temperature is necessary.

Refinement of the Child Vulnerability Scale

B. W. C. Forsyth, P. J. Leaf, S. M. Horwitz, and J. M. Leventhal

Departments of Pediatrics and
Epidemiology and Public Health,
Yale University School of Medicine,
New Haven, Conn

Parents' perceptions of their child's vulnerability can affect both their child's psychological development and use of health care. The Child Vulnerability Scale (CVS) has previously been used to demonstrate factors associated with increased perceptions of vulnerability. To date, there has been no validation of the CVS.

By definition, two major factors contribute to perceptions of vulnerability: prior fears that a child might die; and the presence of severe medical illness. In this research, association with these two factors is used to refine the CVS.

Children, ages 4-8 yrs, were enrolled in a community-based study and 1095 mothers completed interviews which included the 12-item CVS and questions about the two factors. Mothers of 226 children (21%) reported that they had feared their child might die (factor A) and 45 children had a severe medical illness (factor B).

Four items were deleted from the CVS because item scores were not significantly different for subjects with and without the two factors. Changes were made in the scoring of the new 8-item scale and comparisons made between new and old scales. Using the new scale, 22.1% of children with factor A were categorized as vulnerable vs. 7.5% without factor A (Risk ratio 2.9, $P<.001$); 37.8% of those with factor B were vulnerable vs. 3.1% without factor B (RR 12.1, $P<001$). Using the old 12-item scale the RRs for these two comparisons were only 2.0 and 5.4 respectively. Using the new scale, only 1.9% of those without either factor were categorized as vulnerable. By comparison, 13.3% of those with factor A alone (RR 6.9), 33.3% of those with factor B alone (RR 17.2) and 42.8% of those with both A and B (RR 22.1) were categorized as vulnerable. Further analyses using the new scale confirmed previously reported associations with vulnerability.

Cocaine-Exposed Newborns in an Inner-city Community Hospital

A. Theodorou, T. Holtrop, J. Marshall, K. Meert, and A. Sarnaik

Children's Hospital of Michigan,
Wayne State University, and
Samaritan Health Center, Detroit

The prevalence of newborn cocaine-exposure has been estimated at 15% at inner city, tertiary care centers based on urine drug screens. We believe the problem is not limited to large medical centers, and initiated this study to evaluate the problem in a community hospital. We reviewed all the deliveries in 1987 (n = 1131) and identified 105 (9.3%) newborns with in-utero drug-exposure, the diagnosis made by urine drug screen and/or maternal history. Of these, 87 were exposed to cocaine either as the only drug or in combination with other drugs. Those exposed to cocaine alone (n = 73) were compared to a randomly selected group of non-drug-exposed infants born during the same time (n = 140). Dependent variables recorded include birthweight, Apgar score, presence of meconium staining, type of delivery, prematurity (<37 weeks), symptoms of tremors or irritability. The cocaine-exposed infants demonstrated lower birth weight (controlled for smoking), higher incidence of meconium staining, increased tremors and irritability, and a greater number of home deliveries (table).

	Birth Wt (grams)	Meconium Stained	Home Delivery	Tremors	Irritability
Cocaine	2677±439	30%	15%	51%	37%
Control	3024±564	11%	3%	16%	6%
p value	<.005	<.005	<.005	<.0005	<.0005

No significant differences were observed in the incidence of prematurity, c-section, or Apgar scores. Twenty-six (36%) of the cocaine-exposed infants had no observable symptoms. There were two deaths in the drug-exposed group. One infant died of SIDS at 4 mos. of age and another from an acute ingestion of cocaine at 5 mos.

We conclude that intra-uterine cocaine-exposure is a problem that can exist in a community hospital. The neonatal characteristics that we identified are consistant with the physiologic effects of cocaine on the fetus, placenta and uterus. Since a large number of cocaine-exposed newborns may remain asymptomatic, we recommend routine drug screening in high risk areas.

Pediatric Emergency Medicine—State of the Art

D. J. Isaacman, R. B. Karasic, and H. W. Davis

Department of Pediatrics,
University of Pittsburgh (Pa) School of Medicine

To assess the current practice of pediatric emergency care in the US, a questionnaire was mailed to the directors of all 240 emergency departments (EDs) affiliated with pediatric residency training programs in the US. One hundred fifty-three (63.8%) programs returned completed surveys, which comprised 32 questions highlighting staffing patterns, ancillary services, clinical issues, and resident education. Selected data are presented.

The mean annual ED census was 39,376; 6.5% of visits were categorized as critical, 22.3% urgent, and 71.2% non-urgent. Eleven percent of patients were admitted to the hospital. During peak periods, non-urgent patients waited an average of 1.5 hours to be seen by a physician.

Twenty-two percent of programs provided 24 hour on-site coverage by a pediatric attending or fellow. Of the remaining programs, the average daily on-site pediatric attending coverage was 8.3 ± 6.1 hours. Seventeen percent of programs utilized physician assistants or nurse practitioners in the ED. During the first, second, and third years, pediatric residents spent 4.8, 5.4 and 3.8 weeks in the ED, respectively.

The majority (88.1%) of EDs handled all levels of pediatric trauma, had dedicated trauma teams (71.2%), employed social workers specifically assigned to the ED (62.9%), and had child abuse teams (69.9%). Ninety-two percent of EDs had radio communications with pre-hospital care vehicles and 69.9% provided medical command for incoming pediatric patients.

Fifty-three percent of programs had a mechanism for ensuring telephone follow-up of worrisome patients, and 69.6% utilized a system for ensuring feedback to the referring physician. Ninety-four percent of programs had a system in place for contacting patients with positive cultures; in most cases this function was handled by physicians. Seventy-five percent of programs provided medical advice over the telephone.

These data highlight current practice patterns in EDs associated with pediatric training programs and may assist in the development of practice standards for pediatric emergency care.

Defervescence As a Guide to Resolution of Bacteremia in Ambulatory Children

F. Agre and L. R. Prieto

Department of Pediatrics,
College of Physicians and Surgeons,
Columbia University, New York, NY

We wanted to determine whether presence or absence of fever correlated with persistence or resolution of bactermia in children. Bacteremic children between the ages of 1 month and 19 years were eligible for study. Every patient with a positive blood culture was recalled for evaluation and reculturing by a physician. From 1986 to 1990, 95 bacteremic children were identified, 92 of whom made return visits. Medical records were retrievable for 84 of the 92, and these form the study group. 79/84 children were previously healthy. 70/84 were in the age range of 2 to 24 months. 9 pathogenic organisms were isolated, of which the three most common ones were *Streptococcus pneumoniae* (69%), *Salmonella enteritidis* (15%), and *Haemophilus influenzae* (5%).

5/84 patients had persistently positive blood cultures and were febrile (T>38° C) at the time of the return visit. 79/84 patients had negative repeat blood cultures at the time of the return visit. Of these, 20/79 were febrile and 59/79 were not. No afebrile patient was persistently bacteremic. Using Fisher's exact test a statistically significant difference was found between the persistently and resolved bacteremic patients with regards to fever ($p=0.002$). 2/5 persistently bacteremic patients were prescribed antibiotics at the first visit and 3/5 were not. 58/79 resolved bacteremic patients were prescribed antibiotics at the first visit and 21/79 were not.

We conclude that the majority of ambulatory bacteremic patients have resolution of their bacteremia whether they are treated with antibiotics or not. The presence of fever was not necessarily indicative of persistent bacteremia. However, the absence of fever was consistently indicative of resolved bacteremia.

Positive Effect of an Educational Intervention on Compliance With Universal Precautions in a Pediatric Emergency Department

L. R. Friedland, M. Joffe, and J. F. Wiley II

Emergency Medicine, Section of General Pediatrics,
St Christopher's Hospital for Children,
Philadelphia, Pa

We prospectively studied compliance with universal precautions by nurses and residents in our pediatric emergency department (ED), and then investigated the effect of an intensive educational intervention (lectures, written materials, posters) which stressed the need for universal precautions in the ED. The cohort was observed without their knowledge in a time-series study design. We monitored glove use during venipuncture/IV placement, and face visor use during wound irrigation, pre and post intervention phases. Pre intervention phase the RN's wore gloves 13/51 times (25%), and over a 4 week period post intervention phase they wore gloves 65/70 (93%) ($p<.001$; RR = 3.6, CI 2.3-5.8). The RN's were observed for another 3 weeks and their continued compliance was 50/56 (89%). The compliance by the RN's 5-7 weeks post intervention phase (89%) was not statistically different compared with 1-4 weeks post intervention phase (93%) ($p=0.5$, RR = 0.9, CI 0.8-1.1). The MD's pre intervention phase wore gloves 9/51 (18%) vs. 55/59 (93%) over a 4 week period post intervention phase ($p<.001$; RR = 5.3, CI 2.9-9.6). The entire cohort's success rate on the first attempt at vascular access while wearing gloves was 141/192 (73%) vs. 63/95 (66%) without gloves ($p=0.27$; RR = 1.1, CI 0.9-1.3). The MD's wore a face visor 0/21 times pre intervention phase vs. 5/14 post intervention phase ($p<.001$). We conclude: (1) intensive educational intervention dramatically improves compliance with universal precautions by RN's and MD's in the ED; (2) this improvement did not extinguish among RN's over a 7 week period post intervention; (3) glove use did not interfere with the proficient performance of vascular access procedures; (4) longer term follow-up data is being collected to better plan for continuing education.

Historical Correlates to Anogenital Trauma in 1,150 Suspected Child Sexual Abuse Victims

D. L. Kerns and M. L. Ritter

Department of Pediatrics,
Santa Clara Valley Medical Center, San Jose, Calif

Between July 1985 and January 1990 comprehensive medical evaluations were performed on 1,150 children and adolescents who were suspected to be victims of sexual abuse. These evaluations included the collection of demographic, historical and behavioral data, and physical examinations including colposcopic photography. A computerized data base was developed for the detailed analysis of these cases. By virtue of anogenital physical findings, the cases were diagnostically classified into five categories: (1) Benign (57.22%), (2) Benign with Reservations (11.39%), (3) Uncertain (4.7%), (4) Suggestive of Trauma (10.09%), and (5) Trauma (16.35%). For purposes of analysis, "Uncertain" cases were dropped, categories (1) and (2) were combined as the "Benign Cluster" (68.61%), and categories (4) and (5) were combined as the "Trauma Cluster" (26.17%). Chi-Square analysis was used to determine the association of a variety of historical variables to the physical finding of anogenital trauma (i.e. categorization in the "Trauma Cluster").

Females were nearly twice as likely as males to have trauma (28.82% vs. 15.81%; $p<0.001$). In females, positive associations to trauma included age greater than 3 years ($p<0.001$), separation from biologic parents ($p<0.01$), acute (vs. elective) visits ($p<0.05$), penile contact ($p<0.001$), penetration ($p<0.001$), pain ($p<0.001$), bleeding ($p<0.001$), ejaculation ($p<0.01$), urinary tract infection ($p<0.01$), and aggression ($p<0.05$). In males, positive associations to trauma included penile contact ($p<0.01$), penetration ($p<0.01$), and feeding disorder ($p<0.05$). Among historical variables not positively associated with trauma were ethnicity, confessions, number of perpetrators, number of episodes, depression/suicide, regression, sexualization, school disturbance and sleep disorder.

Screening for Cocaine Intoxication In Children With Unexplained Seizures in the Emergency Department

S. E. Krug, R. D. Marble, D. L. Lubitz, and T. J. Long

Department of Pediatrics,
Case Western Reserve University School of Medicine,
Cleveland, Ohio

Recent literature has demonstrated a significant incidence of cocaine exposure and intoxication in pediatric populations and suggests an increased susceptibility for cocaine induced convulsions in children. Children presenting for emergency care with an unexplained convulsion may, therefore, represent a population at risk for cocaine intoxication.

All children between the ages of 0 and 16 years presenting to an urban university hospital emergency department (ED) with a history of a convulsion within the preceding 12 hours were considered for study enrollment. Children with a known history of epilepsy or prior seizures, an identifiable traumatic, metabolic or infectious precipitant, or a presentation consistent with a simple febrile seizure were excluded.

As part of their ED evaluation, all enrolled children had blood and urine samples collected for toxicology screening. The presence of the cocaine metabolite benzoylecgonine, was determined via the EMIT® urine assay. All ED visits for the period of the study were reviewed to determine completeness of patient enrollment.

Over a period of one year, 66 children were enrolled, representing 80% of all potential enrollees. 30 of these enrolled patients were then excluded based upon subsequent identification of a cause of their seizure including trauma (5), metabolic (6), infection (7), epilepsy (4) and simple febrile convulsion (8). None of these children had a positive toxicology screen. Of the remaining 36 patients, 4 (11%) had a positive urine toxicology screen for cocaine. Subsequent history confirmed either an intentional (ages 14 & 15 years) or accidental ingestion (ages 14 and 32 months) in all 4 children.

The data from the study suggests that children presenting to an urban ED with an unexplained convulsion represent a group at risk for cocaine intoxication and warrant consideration for toxicology screening.

The Value of Chest Radiographs in the Evaluation of Febrile Infants Less Than Two Years Old

J. A. Taylor, S. Roncevich, E. Kouri, C. Talarico, and R. Schneider

Departments of Pediatrics, Radiology,
and Emergency Medicine,
Carolinas Medical Center, Charlotte, NC

In the evaluation of febrile infants less than 2 years old chest radiographs (CXR) are frequently obtained even in the presence of a normal chest examination. We postulated that if every component of a systematic lung exam in a febrile infant were normal the yield of a CXR would be low. Between December, 1989, and July, 1990, examining physicians in the Emergency Department of a large urban teaching hospital completed a study questionnaire on febrile infants < 2 in whom a CXR was obtained. The presence or absence of the following respiratory signs was recorded: rales, grunting, retractions, nasal flaring, and asymmetry of breath sounds. The child's temperature, age, and resting respiratory rate were also recorded. Tachypnea was defined as a respiratory rate of > 50 in infants 0-6 months old, > 45 for infants 7-12 months old, and > 40 in those 13-24 months old. If all signs were absent the exam was considered negative; if one or more signs were present the exam was positive. CXR were independently classified as pneumonia, no pneumonia or indeterminate by 2 radiologists unaware of the child's clinical condition. Agreement between radiologists was 74% (Kappa = .53). For the analysis CXR were considered positive only if classified as pneumonia by both radiologists.

One hundred thirty-one infants were enrolled: radiologic evidence of pneumonia was found in 32 (24.4%), and no evidence of pneumonia was found in 89 (67.9%); in 10 children (7.6%) the CXR was classified as indeterminate. Although patients with radiographic evidence of pneumonia were more likely to demonstrate positive physical findings than those with negative CXR (20/32 vs. 35/89, P = .04), more than a third of our infants (12/32) with positive radiographs had no findings suggestive of lower respiratory tract infection. Thus our bias was not supported by the findings of this study. An appreciable number of febrile infants 0-2 years old with pneumonia have a normal physical examination of the lungs.

A New Instrument to Improve the Ability of Non-Experts to Identify Infants at Risk of Subsequent Child Abuse or Neglect

D. H. K. Ihnat, J. M. Leventhal, D. V. Cicchetti, D. R. Wasserman, and J. P. Hamilton

Department of Pediatrics,
Yale University School of Medicine, New Haven, Conn,
and Yale–New Haven Hospital

Prior studies have indicated that clinicians can identify some newborns who are at high risk of subsequent child abuse or neglect. To provide a standardized approach to the assessment of risk during the post-partum period, we developed a clinical rating scale and compared the assessments of clinicians who use this scale with those of child abuse experts.

The clinical rating scale (CRS) consisted of 22 risk factors, including items about the mother (e.g. use of drugs), father, past care of children, family, pregnancy, and the mother's in-hospital behaviors. Each item was scored on a 4-point ordinal scale, in which 1 represented no risk, 2 low, 3 moderate, and 4 high risk. For each item, a clear example was given for each level of risk. The score was the sum of those items rated ≥ 2; a total score of ≥ 9 was labeled High Risk.

Pairs of experts in the field of child abuse rated the risk statuses of 32 newborns born to inner city mothers. After jointly interviewing a mother on the postpartum ward, each expert used unstructured clinical judgment to provide an overall assessment of the newborn's risk status, as either high or low risk. The nurses and pediatric residents caring for these same families served as non-expert clinicians and independently assigned risk using the CRS.

The experts' overall assessment, which had an agreement (P_o) of 91% and a kappa of 0.80, served as the gold standard of prediction. Of the 32 assessments, 44% were considered high risk by these experts. Compared to the assessments of the experts, the nurses' CRS's had a sensitivity of 64% and a specificity of 78%, and the pediatricians' CRS's had a sensitivity of 63% and a specificity of 92%.

We conclude that experts agree with each other in their overall evaluations and that using the CRS, non-experts have fair sensitivity and good specificity. The CRS should help clinicians caring for newborns assess the risk of subsequent abuse or neglect and thus focus scarce resources on those at highest risk.

Maltreatment of Children Born to Cocaine Dependent Mothers

D. R. Wasserman and J. M. Leventhal

Department of Pediatrics,
Yale University School of Medicine, New Haven, Conn

Much of the recent rise in national reporting of child abuse and neglect has been attributed to parental substance abuse, particularly the use of cocaine, yet there are no systematic studies that have examined this association. The purpose of this ongoing study is to investigate the relationship between maternal cocaine dependency and child maltreatment in a cohort of young children.

We have identified 43 infants, born between 10/88 and 7/89, whose mothers were identified as regular users of cocaine during pregnancy based on history and the results of urine toxicology screens. These "exposed" infants were matched to a comparison group of 43 "unexposed" infants whose mothers did not use cocaine during pregnancy. Matching was on the basis of birthdate, race, method of payment for the hospitalization, and marital status of the mother. Through a review of medical records, we determined the occurrence of maltreatment (physical abuse, sexual abuse, or neglect), as well as placements in foster care or with a substitute caretaker. To identify episodes of maltreatment, a reviewer who was unaware of the group status categorized each injury as due to abuse, neglect, household violence, or an accident.

During the first 18 months of life, maltreatment occurred in 23% of the "exposed" vs. 2% of the "unexposed" groups (RR=9.6, 95% C.I.: 1.2-78.6). Physical abuse occurred in 9% of the "exposed" vs. 2% of the "unexposed" groups (RR=4.7, 95% C.I.: 0.4-35.6), while neglect occurred in 12% vs 0% ($P<.05$). Changes in placement occurred in 23% of the "exposed" vs. 2% of the "unexposed" groups (RR=9.6, 95% C.I.: 1.2-78.6). Of the 10 placements, only 2 were directly linked to an episode of maltreatment: 3 occurred while their mothers were in residential drug treatment programs and 3 after the mother deserted the children to the care of a relative.

Children identified during the neonatal period as regularly "exposed" to cocaine *in utero* are at a substantially increased risk both of maltreatment and of changes in the primary caretaker during the first 18 months of life. Further studies are necessary to determine whether intensive interventions can prevent these parenting failures.

Are Interdisciplinary Evaluations of Alleged Sexual Abuse Cases Necessary?

P. K. Jaudes and M. Martone

La Rabida Children's Hospital, Chicago, Ill, and Department of Pediatrics, University of Chicago Pritzker School of Medicine

Alleged sexually abused children often go through grueling interrogations to relate to adults their experiences and even then, most are not viewed as reliable sources of information. The Victim Sensitive Interview Program (VSIP) was initiated to decrease the number of interviews for which a child who allegedly had been sexually abused had to endure. The program brought together the disciplines involved in the evaluation of these cases: hospital based medical social worker and pediatrician, state child protective agency worker, police youth officer, and assistant state's attorney. This team established a protocol for an investigative interview to be conducted by a team member.

We compared by t-test analysis preVSIP sexual abuse evaluations from 1985 to 1986 (38) with VSIP evaluations (224) from 1987 to 1988. There was no significant difference between the two groups in relation to gender or age of victim, physical symptoms, sexually transmitted diseases present, age of perpetrator, or length of stay in hospital. There were significant differences between the two groups in (1) number of interviews ($p<0.003$), 11% preVSIP versus 80% VSIP receiving only one interview, (2) indicated cases of sexual abuse ($p<0.006$), 68% preVSIP versus 85% VSIP, (3) identification of the perpetrator ($p<0.026$), 70% preVSIP versus 85% VSIP, and (4) charges pressed ($p<0.029$), 32% preVSIP versus 55% VSIP.

To assess if police evaluations of child sexual abuse cases were similar, we compared VSIP cases (224) to cases (235) for the same years in a designated police area that did not have an interdisciplinary program. Significant differences were found for identification of the perpetrator ($p<0.000$), 85% VSIP versus 37% Police and charges pressed ($p<0.018$), 55% VSIP versus 40% Police. There were no difference in gender of the victim but the children interviewed by the police were slightly younger (6.7 years compared to 7.3 years of those in VSIP).

From this study, interdisciplinary evaluations of alleged sexually abused children not only decreased the number of interviews a child must undergo but also increased the likelihood of indicated cases, identification of the perpetrator, and charges being pressed. We strongly recommend formation of interdisciplinary teams to assess allegedly sexually abused children.

GENERAL PEDIATRICS

Doctorhoppers: Myth or Reality?

C. Gosselink, D. Brazdziunas, E. Ekwo, A. Kresheck, and M. Lehmann

Department of Pediatrics, University of Chicago (Ill)/ La Rabida Children's Hospital and Research Center

ER pediatricians frequently claim that one of the reasons for congested emergency services is that caregivers (CGs), unconvinced that their children's symptoms are being correctly diagnosed or treated, go from doctor to doctor for the same presenting complaint. "Doctorhoppers" (DHs), as these CGs are commonly called, are perceived as unnecessarily overburdening ER services when they should return to their child's primary care provider to seek reassurance or better understanding about their child's condition. To examine whether DHs really do exist, a sample of CGs of children visiting an inner-city ER during a 2-month period were surveyed by trained interviewers regarding sociodemographics, health care use, and medical history. CGs were asked how many times in the past 2 weeks they had taken their child to another doctor, clinic, or ER for the same presenting complaints.

116 (16.5%) of the 704 CGs acknowledged having taken their child to another doctor in the last 2 weeks for the same presenting complaints. 72.4% had only gone to one other doctor, although 32 (27.6%) had seen ≥2 for the same symptoms. 47 (40.5%) of the CGs had received written instructions from the other doctor and all claimed they were able to understand this information. However, reasons given for not returning to the other doctor included wanting a 2nd opinion (28.7%), the doctor's office being closed (20.9%), and not trusting the other doctor (13.9%).

Multiple logistic regression was performed to compare DHs with the other 588 sampled CGs (NonDHs) and odds ratios (OR) were calculated. DHs were significantly more likely than NonDHs to be single (OR=3.1), to have been aware of their child's symptoms for more than 24 hours (OR=2.7), to state they would go to another doctor if their child did not seem to be getting better (OR=1.9), and required >15 minutes to get to the ER (OR=1.8). However, they were significantly less likely than nonDHs to mention convenience of ER location (OR=.30), be up to date on their child's shots (OR=.37), or to be familiar with the study ER (OR=.62).

We conclude that DHs do indeed exist. However, we believe DHs are comprised of highly-motivated CGs who appear to be concerned about their children's welfare. We suggest that better CG-doctor relations and education could encourage CGs to return to the child's primary care physician and may improve immunization status. This would be better for the child and could help reduce ER overcrowding.

What Factors Predict School Absence in Children With Chronic Medical Conditions?: A Controlled Population Based Study

F. C. Jarman and M. C. Starr

Department of Pediatrics, University of Massachusetts Medical Centre, Worcester

Excessive school absence has been identified as the single most important administrative problem facing educators in the United States. School absence may be associated with poor achievement, psychosocial problems, and early school drop-out. Children with chronic medical conditions are known to be at high risk for school absence, although the specific determinants and correlates of absence in a community-representative sample of chronically ill and well children remain to be further clarified.

We prospectively surveyed parents of all 1601 fourth grade students attending the 41 public elementary schools in Worcester using a standardized health screening instrument. Of the 1168 (73%) children who participated in the study, 306 (26%) had chronic medical conditions, and these children were individually paired with healthy classroom controls matched for age, sex, race, and sociodemographic characteristics. Cases and controls were then compared on standardized measures of behavior, academic performance, perceived self competence, health locus of control, and number of days absent over the preceding school year. The predictors of school absence were also examined.

Children with chronic medical conditions were absent an average of 10.0 days over the preceding school year, compared to 8.2 days for healthy controls ($p<.006$). In both groups, univariate analysis revealed school absence to be significantly associated with non-white race ($p<.001$), lower socioeconomic status ($p<.001$), and parent perceptions of their children being less well ($p<.001$). In chronically ill children but not healthy controls school absence was significantly correlated with female sex ($p<.001$), greater physical limitations ($p<.001$), and lower academic aptitude ($p<.01$) and achievement ($p<.001$). School absence was not related to the child's diagnosis, whether or not the child received special education services, parent or teacher rated child behavior problems, child health locus of control, or child self-perceptions ($p>.05$). Multiple regression analysis identified family socioeconomic status and degree of physical limitation as the only independent predictors of school absence in chronically ill children; these variables explained 16% of the total variance. For healthy controls, parent perception of child health status was the only independent predictor of school absence identified, accounting for 10% of the total variance.

We conclude that school absence has different correlates in chronically ill compared to healthy children, despite only a 2 day per year attendance discrepancy between the two groups. Children with chronic medical conditions appear to be more vulnerable to the effects of time off school than their healthy peers.

Comparison of Two Methods of Assessing Appropriateness of Admission

K. R. Kowaleski, P. Griffin, and M. Li

Department of Paediatrics,
Children's Hospital of Eastern Ontario, Ottawa

Interest in limiting unnecessary expenditures in inpatient hospital care has stimulated the development of a number of methods for assessing appropriateness of hospital admission. We compared two, the Intensity-Service-Discharge-Appropriateness (ISDA) criteria and the Pediatric Appropriateness Evaluation Protocol (PAEP). Each consists of explicit, objective, diagnosis-independent criteria that are designed to require minimal subjective judgment. However, they differ in many respects in their composition and application.

All non-psychiatric admissions to CHEO every 12th day in 1989 were retrospectively reviewed. Three raters reviewed each record: the first used PAEP, the second ISDA; their results were used in the comparison of the two methods. The third rater alternated the two to determine interrater reliability with each.

778 of a possible 786 records were assessed. Overall rate of inappropriate admission (RIA) was similar: PAEP=21.3%, ISDA=21.0%. However, general agreement (GA) was only 77.5%, kappa(k)=0.33, and there were significant differences when admissions were examined by source:

	PAEP(RIA)	ISDA(RIA)	
Emergent (E)	7.1%	20.6%	$p<.001$
Elective (L)*	81.7%	17.5%	$p<.001$
Urgent (U)	32.8%	53.6%	$p<.01$
Neonatal (N)	3.6%	0.0%	N.S.

*excludes short stay surgery

A few major differences in PAEP and ISDA accounted for these discrepancies. PAEP requires elective procedures be done on the day of admission; ISDA does not. E and U admissions must meet two different ISDA criteria (severity of illness, intensity of service), but only one PAEP criterion.

Interrater reliability with PAEP showed GA of 93.4%, k=0.82; with ISDA, GA=89.0%, k=0.71; the difference in the two kappas was significant at $p<.05$. Considering only E and U admissions, the two kappas were similar: PAEP, k=0.70; ISDA, k=0.67.

PAEP, being brief, was easily committed to memory and could be applied more quickly than ISDA, which consists of many pages of criteria. Nevertheless, the two showed similar interrater reliability in assessing E and U admissions. Although overall RIA is similar with each, PAEP and ISDA exhibited frequent disagreement in individual patients.

Validity, Bias, and 'Overcall' in Interpreting Chest Radiographs in Young Febrile Children

M. S. Kramer, R. Roberts-Brauer, and R. Williams

Departments of Pediatrics
and of Epidemiology
and Biostatistics,
McGill University, Montreal, Quebec

Few studies have examined the diagnostic validity of the examining physician's interpretation of chest radiographs in young febrile children, and none (to our knowledge) the extent to which the "official" (i.e., the radiologist's) reading may be biased by access to the examining physician's reading and to other clinical information. We studied 229 consecutive chest radiographs obtained in febrile, nonasthmatic children 3 to 24 months of age who presented to a children's hospital emergency department between March 1989 and August 1990. We compared the readings by the examining staff pediatrician, the subsequent (usually next day) official pediatric radiologist's reading, and a "blind" reading by a pediatric radiologist. The official radiologist had access to the examining pediatrician's readings and the clinical information provided on the x-ray requisition. The blind radiologist knew only that each child was 3 to 24 months of age and febrile; he was asked to judge the presence or absence of pneumonia.

Of the 229 total radiographs, the examining pediatrician interpreted 53 (23%) as demonstrating pneumonia, a significantly ($P<.01$ by McNemar χ-test) lower number (72, or 31%) than the official radiologist but similar to that of the blind radiologist (47, or 21%). The positive predictive value (PPV) of the examining pediatrician's reading was significantly ($P<.001$) lower when based on the blind radiologist as gold standard (.34) than when based on the official radiologist (.70). When the analysis was restricted to children without suggestive clinical signs of pneumonia, PPV decreased when based on the blind reading (.19) but not when based on the official reading (.80). Agreement between the official and blind radiologists' readings was barely better than could be explained by chance [($\kappa=.15$ (95% confidence interval=.05-.25)].

These results indicate that official interpretations systematically "overcall" pneumonia, particularly in cases without suggestive clinical findings, and appear to be influenced (biased) by the examining physician's reading. Since these tendencies can lead to unnecessary antibiotic treatment and hospital admission, strategies to reduce them should receive high priority.

An Analysis of Mental Health Service Utilization by Children in Foster Care in California

N. Halfon, G. Berkowitz, and L. Klee

Center for the Vulnerable Child,
Children's Hospital, Oakland, Calif

An examination of Medi-Cal paid claims was undertaken to assess the utilization of mental health services by children in California's foster care system. Using unduplicated counts of service use and diagnoses, it was determined that children in foster care account for 41% of all users of mental health services even though they represent less than 4% of Medi-Cal eligibles. When partitioned into specific service categories, children in foster care account for 53% of all psychologist visits, 47% of psychiatry visits, 43% of Short Doyle/Medi-Cal inpatient hospitalization in public hospitals, and 27% of inpatient psychiatric hospitalizations. Expenditure for services paralleled utilization frequency. When compared to the non-foster care Medi-Cal eligible child population, children in foster care have 10 - 20 times the rate of utilization per eligible for selected services. For children in foster care 75% of all diagnoses for billed services were accounted for by four diagnoses: adjustment disorders (28.6%); conduct disorders (20.5%); anxiety disorders (13.8%); and emotional disorders (11.9%), with clear age related differences in the distribution of diagnoses. This study raised several questions about the natural histories of mental health disorders of children in foster care, the availability of appropriate services as well as questions about the need for early intervention and preventive mental health services.

The Relation of Family Mobility to Children's Emotional and School Functioning

G. A. Simpson and M. G. Fowler

National Center for Health Statistics, Hyattsville, Md

The impact of multiple family moves on childrens' emotional and school adaptation have not been well delineated. To address this issue, we utilized data from the 1988 National Health Interview Survey on Child Health (NHIS-CH), a cross-sectional survey which included a representative national sample of 10,362 school aged children in grades 1 through 12.

We found that 39 percent of children aged 6 to 17 had moved three or more times in their lifetime—42 percent of Hispanic children, 39 percent of whites, and 34 percent of black children. Among children living below the poverty level, 48 percent had moved multiple times versus 37 percent of children at or above the poverty level. Likewise, 53 percent of children on Medicaid had moved three or more times compared to only 36 percent of children with private health insurance. In addition, 51 percent of children in one parent families moved three or more times, while only 35 percent of children in two parent families moved that often. Using multiple logistic regression to control for demographic variables, children who moved three or more times were 2.4 times as likely to have had emotional problems, 2.2 times as likely to have received psychological help, 1.7 times as likely to have repeated a grade, and to have been suspended or expelled from school compared to children who had never moved. Likewise, using multiple linear regression, the adjusted mean score on the Behavior Problem Index for children who had moved three or more times was significantly higher than for children who had never moved, 6.8 versus 5.5. These findings confirm that children who move multiple times are at high risk for emotional and school problems.

Biofeedback: Initial Success in Treating Recurrent Abdominal Pain

A. J. Rosenberg and T. Whitehead

Department of Pediatrics, University of Kansas Medical Center, Kansas City

Recurrent abdominal pain (RAP) is reported in 16% of school age children. A study using progressive relaxation with biofeedback in children with RAP was initiated at the University of Kansas Medical Center. RAP is defined as a minimum of three occurrences of significant abdominal pain within at least a three month period interfering with normal activity. Sixteen children, 13 girls and 3 boys with an average age of 10 years (6-14 years) met the criteria for RAP. The frequency of abdominal pain averaged 13 episodes per week per child. RAP children were randomized into two groups. The Treatment Group (Group I) consisted of 8 girls, average age 10 years with an average of 15 episodes of pain per week, and the Control Group (Group II) 8 children, 3 boys and 5 girls, average age 11 years, averaging 11 episodes of pain per week. All children were evaluated for frequency and severity of pain by self report at entry and after the six week period. The biofeedback treatment group was taught progressive relaxation while being continuously monitored for skin temperature and EMG, which were converted to digital pulse and displayed to the subject as light and sound on a BMI SRI PRO series model 421 biofeedback instrument. Subjects attended six weekly relaxation - biofeedback sessions. Subjects were given a relaxation tape with which to practice at home between sessions. After six weeks, Group I children had a reduction of abdominal pain to an average of less than one episode per week. This was statistically significant in the relief of abdominal pain in the treatment group at alpha level .05, using the t test of paired samples. Five of the biofeedback children (63%) reported complete absence of abdominal pain. Although the frequency of abdominal pain in the Group II fell to an average of five episodes of pain per week, this was not statistically significant. This demonstrates the Hawthorn effect in the control group of symptom reduction as a result of participating in a study. Biofeedback training had a significant effect on reduction of abdominal pain over the six weeks of training sessions. This treatment method may have a significant impact on reducing recurrent abdominal pain in children and its sequelae in adults.

Are School-Based Clinics Serving the High-Risk Student?

J. W. Stout and C. R. Anderman

Departments of Pediatrics and Epidemiology, University of Washington, Seattle

Oregon's school-based clinics offer comprehensive primary care, including services designed to alter risk-taking behavior. However, it is not clear whether the students who utilize these services are in fact those at increased risk. The purpose of this study is to examine whether these clinics are reaching the population engaging in various kinds of risk-taking behavior, such as substance use and unprotected sex. Data concerning clinic utilization and risk-taking behavior were collected with an 88-item adolescent health survey, administered in the fall of 1990 to students in four Oregon high schools where school-based clinics have been operating for at least three years. In addition to treatment of acute illness and injury, these clinics provide counseling and care for reproductive health which may include prescribing (but not dispensing) contraceptives, and counseling or referral for substance use and mental health problems. Of the 2530 students who completed the survey, 50% reported ever using the clinic. In the area of substance use, students using clinic services were significantly more likely to engage in binge drinking (27% vs. 15%, $p<.01$), regular cigarette smoking (19% vs. 11%, $p<.01$), or marijuana smoking (28% vs. 16%, $p<.01$) than those who do not use clinic services. Regarding reproductive health, clinic utilizers were significantly more likely to be currently sexually active than non-utilizers (35% vs. 19%, $p<.01$). In the area of mental health, students who use the clinic were significantly more likely to be suicidal than non-utilizers (20% vs. 13%, $p<.01$). In conclusion, students who utilize clinic services are more likely to engage in risk-taking behavior than those who do not utilize these services. Subsequent analyses will determine whether risk-taking behaviors are addressed during clinic visits, and further characterize all students engaging in these risk-taking behaviors.

A Clinic-Based Intervention to Promote Literacy

R. D. Needlman, L. E. Fried, and B. S. Zuckerman

Division of Developmental and Behavioral Pediatrics, Boston (Mass) City Hospital

Educational research has shown that exposure to story books is an especially potent stimulus to preschool language development and the acquisition of literacy. To encourage book use among children at risk, we developed and evaluated a primary care clinic-based program which included (1) volunteers who read aloud to children in the waiting room, modeling book use for parents; (2) individualized guidance on book use by pediatricians; and (3) distribution of developmentally and culturally appropriate books to children age 6 months through 5 years at each clinic visit. To assess program effectiveness, 79 parents were interviewed in the waiting room several months after the program began. Thirty-nine percent of the parents received AFDC, 40% were single, 49% were Black, and 3% were White. In order to minimize misreporting, parents were asked to provide a 24-hour recall of everything they did with their child, modelled after a 24-hour diet recall, and to state their child's three favorite activities. After controlling for possible confounders, parents who had received one or more books were four times more likely to report looking at books with their children in the last 24 hours, or that looking at books was a favorite activity (adjusted odds ratio = 4.05, P = .028). This association was strongest among parents receiving AFDC (odds ratio = 7.8, P = .001). This preliminary study suggests that pediatricians can play a role in enriching children's early literacy environments, especially for children at high risk for school failure.

A Critical Appraisal of the Quality of Pediatric Journal Articles That Evaluate Diagnostic Tests

A. Bates, P. X. Margolis, and A. E. Evans

Departments of Pediatrics and Medicine,
University of North Carolina, Chapel Hill, and
Indiana University, Indianapolis

Studies reported in peer-reviewed journals play a major role in disseminating information about the value of diagnostic tests and therefore may affect the quality of patient care. We conducted a systematic critical appraisal of the quality of pediatric journal articles that evaluate diagnostic tests.

We identified all studies of diagnostic tests published in three major pediatric journals over a three year period. Articles were included if they evaluated a test for clinical use in diagnosis, presented original data, and used human subjects. We used 28 criteria to evaluate the following 5 areas of study quality: adequacy of the patient sample, application of diagnostic test, application of gold standard, reporting of results, and discussion of potential utility.

Forty-two articles met our inclusion criteria. Half had serious methodologic short-comings. Of these serious problems, 80% were a result of uneven application of the gold standard; either eligible patients were excluded from analysis because the gold standard had not been applied, or patients with positive diagnostic test results were more likely to have had a definitive work-up compared to those who tested negative. The remaining 20% used a study sample with unusually prevalent or severe disease. An average of 10 of the remaining 26 criteria were not satisfied (range 3 to 20). Most involved failing to report information: the precision of test characteristics, (94%), uninterpretable test results, (86%), technical or observer variability, (83%), and the accuracy of the gold standard, (75%).

A striking number of the pediatric journal articles evaluating diagnostic tests may be so seriously flawed that their results are of questionable validity. These findings suggest that information about methodologic standards for conducting, evaluating, and reporting studies of diagnostic tests should be more widely disseminated. Journal editors and reviewers might also benefit from more structured approaches to assessing studies of diagnostic tests.

Educational Effectiveness of a Lead Poisoning Video

S. Melman, M. Schorr, R. Lempert, M. Polansky

Department of Pediatrics,
Hahnemann University Hospital, Philadelphia, Pa

Lead poisoning is a serious pediatric health threat, which often causes impaired learning and behavioral disturbances. In Philadelphia, over 30% of children <5 years of age are estimated to have lead levels >0.70 μmol/L, yet only 13% of high-risk children were screened in 1989. We developed a ten-minute educational video to teach parents lead poisoning prevention and the importance of screening. The video includes scenes of children playing among peeling paint and dust, inspectors checking homes for lead paint content, and a child being screened for lead poisoning. The purpose of this study was to test the educational effectiveness of this video.

50 English-speaking parents from our inner-city pediatric clinic were randomly assigned to view either the lead video or a commercially available general safety video. Both groups took pre and post-tests to measure their lead poisoning knowledge.

The lead and control groups were comparable in terms of age (31.3 ± 7.0 S.D. vs. 31.5 ± 8.6), gender (proportion of females 0.63 ± 0.48 vs. 0.83 ± 0.38), highest grade level attained (11.8 ± 0.9 vs. 11.8 ± 1.8), insurance (proportion of private 0.42 ± 0.49 vs. 0.26 ± 0.44), and baseline score (9.6 ± 0.4 vs. 10.6 ± 0.4).

The mean increase in score for the lead-video group was 33.0% (SE = 6.3%) in comparison to an 1.5% decrease (SE = 3.0%) for the control group (p < .001). Even after controlling for baseline score, age, sex, educational level, and insurance coverage, a multiple regression confirmed a strongly significant improvement in the lead video group.

The results indicate that this brief educational intervention was effective in significantly increasing short-term lead poisoning knowledge in an inner-city clinic parent population. A six-month follow-up study is planned to test retention. By successfully educating parents about the seriousness of lead poisoning, we will encourage their efforts towards prevention and early detection.

Impact of Shorter Working Hours on Pediatric Housestaff Training

A. Willenborg, S. Shelov, and D. Neuspiel

Department of Pediatrics,
Albert Einstein College of Medicine, Bronx, NY

Residency training has traditionally involved extended hours and long work weeks. In July 1989 New York State implemented strict limitations on resident working hours. In order to monitor the effects of these changes on patient care, resident education, and the personal lives of pediatric housestaff, we initiated a longitudinal study in the spring 1989. Pediatric residents from 30 New York State(NY), and 14 Chicago and Los Angeles where no such changes were instituted (CHI/LA) programs were asked to complete a questionnaire both prior to the onset of limitations (Spring 1989) and one year later, including information concerning demographic data, patient care, education, supervision, and personal issues. In 1989, 533 residents from 22 NY and 10 CHI/LA programs completed questionnaires: in 1980, 439 residents from 16 NY and 8 CHI/LA programs participated. Mean maximum consecutive work hours were reported as:

	1989			1990		
	NY	CHI/LA	P	NY	CHI/LA	P
Inpatient (S.D.)	34(6)	35(3)	.05	30(5)	36(4)	<.0005
Outpatient (S.D.)	17(10)	20(10)	.03	15(8)	20(10)	<.0005

NY residents reported more sleep while on inpatient rotations, greater time with their spouse or significant other, and increased time for social life and personal needs compared with CHI/LA residents in 1990 (all p<.005), but no in 1989 (all NS). However, NY residents spent more time than CHI/LA residents performing non-physician tasks and participating in sign-out rounds in both years (p<.005).

It appears that the limitation of work hours has improved the quality of life for NY pediatric residents. However, NY residents continue to spend more time doing non-physician tasks and in sign-out rounds. The effects of shorter working hours on education, patient care, and supervision were also examined any analyses of these differences also will be presented.

PREVENTION AND EPIDEMIOLOGY

Immunization Opportunities Missed Among Urban Poor Children

K. M. McConnochie and K. J. Roghmann

Department of Pediatrics,
Rochester (NY) General Hospital, University of Rochester

Low immunization (IZ) rates among United States preschool-age children suggest a need for altered vaccination practices. Computer IZ and encounter records as well as traditional medical records were reviewed to ascertain IZ rates and missed opportunities (MOs) for vaccine administration among 540 children. Subjects included all preschool children over 30 months of age who were active for at least 6 months in an urban, hospital-based primary care practice serving lower SES families (74% Medicaid-covered visits). Subjects averaged 17 visits over their first three years. Despite such frequent contacts, the point prevalence at abstraction (mean age 4.4 yrs) for lack of one or more recommended IZs was 29%; 8% lacked MMR, 20% lacked Hib, 9% lacked two or more DPT, and 5% lacked two or more OPV. Many more (79%) experienced at least one period of undervaccination at any time during their first 36 months.

Any visit when IZs were due but not given was counted as MO; if multiple IZs were due, multiple MOs were counted. For the 79% of children with a period of undervaccination, there were an average of 7.3 missed opportunities per child. Although over half of MOs occurred during an acute illness, 28%, 11% and 4% occurred at well child visits, follow-up visits and chronic illness visits, respectively. Eighteen percent of MOs occurred at Emergency Department visits where IZ records were not readily available. Had opportunities not been missed, the average undervaccination period would have been reduced by 4.8, 4.7, 4.4 and 5.3 months for DPT, OPV, MMR and Hib.

Thoughtful evaluation of IZ contraindications at acute visits, readily available IZ records, and better use of IZ opportunities at non-acute visits would reduce undervaccination risks substantially.

Predictors of Parental Injury Prevention Behavior

D. F. Schwarz, C. B. Forrest, J. A. Grisso, C. G. Miles, and V. M. Wolfson

Department of Pediatrics
and Clinical Epidemiology Unit, University of Pennsylvania
School of Medicine, Philadelphia

Effective injury prevention strategies need to target those who are least likely to change their behavior. We evaluated parental injury prevention behavior that occurred as a result of a fall in children under 2 years. Using structured interviews, we assessed families of 123 consecutive children evaluated in 11 emergency rooms involved in an ongoing injury surveillance program. We theorized that pre-fall injury prevention behavior, circumstances of the fall, and demographics of the child and family could be used to describe families as those who made changes (CH) and others who did not change (NCH) their injury prevention behavior.

We found significant differences in injury circumstances between CH and NCH groups. For example, CH infants were more likely to have sustained falls from heights >36 inches ($p<.01$) and in settings where home modifications could occur (indoors v. outdoors, $p<.01$, and on indoor v. outdoor stairwells, p.<001). Of falls from beds, 89% were associated with CHs ($p<.05$). CHs were more common in children learning to walk than in those already walking ($p<.05$); and in keeping with this finding, anterior head injuries were more common in CHs than posterior head trauma ($p<.05$). Fallers 18-24 months were more likely NCHs ($p<.01$). Of falls involving girls 78% were CHs ($p<.10$). Maternal perception of the injury as severe ($p<.05$) and high levels of stress ($p<.05$) were associated with CHs; surprisingly, pre-fall injury prevention behavior, household composition, caregiver age, socioeconomic status and social support had no effect on injury prevention behavior.

We conclude that specific patient characteristics and circumstances of the fall can be identified as important predictors of injury prevention behavior. Strategies to prevent injuries due to falls should focus on these factors in order to target groups in need of additional intervention.

The Functional Impact of Asthma

J. M. Perrin, M. L. Weitzman, and S. L. Gortmaker

Children's Service, Massachusetts General Hospital,
and Harvard School of Public Health, Boston;
University of Rochester (NY) School of Medicine

Asthma and other chronic health conditions affect the functioning of children, as measured by days spent in bed or hospital and by school absence. We used the 1988 Child Health Supplement (CHS) to the National Health Interview Survey to examine the extent of asthma-related functional disability in this nationally representative random household survey. The 1988 CHS provides data about health status, utilization, functional impact, and psychological status for 17,110 children. All analyses were performed by linear regression, controlling for age and maternal education.

Children with asthma spent more than twice as many days in bed for illness (7.56 vs 3.01, $p<0.001$), had four times more hospital days (1.08 vs 0.23; $p<0.0001$), lost more days of school (7.82 vs 3.90; $p<0.0001$), and had higher scores on a behavior problems index ($p<0.01$) than children without asthma. Boys with asthma missed more days of school than did girls ($p<0.05$). Among those with asthma, black children experienced no significant differences in bed or hospital days or school absence, although they were reported by their parents as being in poorer health ($p<0.004$) and had fewer doctor visits (4.63 vs 7.05, $p<0.02$) than did white children with asthma. Lower maternal education was independently associated with increased home and hospital bed days and school absence and decreased reported general health status.

These findings indicate that asthma has a significant effect on children's participation in usual daily activities. Black children with asthma, despite apparently similar functional impact of asthma, appear to use medical services less than do white children with asthma.

Avoidable Pediatric Hospital Use: A Comparison of Admitting Physician Judgment With Utilization Review

J. L. Soulen, A. K. Duggan, and C. DeAngelis

Department of Pediatrics,
Johns Hopkins University, Baltimore, Md

Current mechanisms for identifying avoidable hospital use, such as Utilization Review (UR), rely on the opinion of persons other than those caring for the patient. The agreement between hospital use ruled unjustified by UR and use judged avoidable by admitting physicians is unknown. This study determined 1) the proportion of acute, medical admissions to an urban teaching hospital which the admitting physician considered potentially avoidable; 2) specific services that would have helped prevent avoidable admissions; 3) social factors influencing decisions to admit; and 4) the agreement between physician judgment and UR in identifying avoidable hospital use.

A random sample ($n=600$) of acute medical admissions from March to October, 1990 was chosen. Questionnaires were completed by 96 admitting physicians, with 90% completed within 3 days of admission. Responses were compared with hospital UR data.

Admitting physicians judged 166 of 600 admissions (27.7%) as potentially avoidable had specific services been available and accessible. Services most frequently desired were a 24 hour short stay unit (23.0% of all admissions), an outpatient discharge coordinator to arrange known services (7.5%), and home nursing services (4.8%). UR identified only two (1.2%) of these 166 admissions as medically unjustified. Social context contributed to 88 of 600 admissions (14.7%). The major social factors were not trusting the family (39/88 = 44%), family overwhelmed (41%), and not knowing the family well (18%). Thirty eight (6.3%) of 600 would not have been admitted if not for social factors. UR identified only one (2.6%) of these 38 admissions as medically unjustified. Physicians identified services that might have helped prevent admission for 30 of these 38. Of the 434 admissions which physicians judged unavoidable, UR identified none as medically unjustified.

We conclude that 1) admitting physicians identified a large number of avoidable admissions which were not identified by UR, and 2) Utilization Review did not identify admissions as unjustified when admission was needed. Policy implications will be discussed.

Lead Intoxication in Early Infancy

M. W. Shannon and J. W. Graef

Department of Pediatrics,
Harvard Medical School,
and Department of Medicine,
Children's Hospital, Boston, Mass

The traditional view of childhood plumbism is that it is a disease of ambulatory toddlers who live in dilapidated housing and ingest lead-based paint chips or dust. However, this belief potentially serves both to discourage testing of young infants and, if lead poisoning is discovered, to divert practitioners from obtaining information on all potential lead sources. We reviewed our 4 year experience in the management of infants who developed plumbism in the first year of life in order to characterize this younger age group. This study was undertaken in a Lead/Toxicology referral program within the state of MA, whose comprehensive lead laws include extensive (and, recently, mandatory) screening of all children beginning by age 1 year. Over the 4 years, of 370 new patients enrolled in our clinic, 49 (13%) were ≤ 1 year. Mean age was 10 months (range 1-12 months). Six patients < 9 months were detected through select rather than routine screening. Mean peak whole blood lead level was 1.87 umol/L (range 1.01-3.02 umol/L) while mean peak zinc protoporphyrin was 1.20 umol/L. Twenty-two patients (45%) had a hemoglobin < 114 g/L. No infants had clinical signs of lead intoxication. Only 12 patients (25%) had parents who were welfare dependent. Sixty-three percent were non-ambulatory at the time lead poisoning was diagnosed; 34% had a history of pica. Likely sources of lead poisoning included household renovation (n = 20), ingestion of lead-based paint (n = 8), formula preparation with lead-contaminated water (n = 9), indeterminate (n = 7) and congenital (n = 1). The 9 cases of plumbism from formula preparation (7 of which were confirmed by water analysis and review of preparation practices) were unexpected and occurred after either: 1) use of first draw morning water to reconstitute a days supply of formula, 2) boiling tap water before reconstituting formula, thereby increasing its lead concentration or 3) inadvertently boiling water in lead-containing vessels.

From these data we conclude: 1) lead intoxication occurs at significant frequency in young, non-ambulatory infants, 2) pica is a less frequent cause of plumbism in this age group, 3) unsafe formula preparation practices may expose infants to lead throughout the first year of life and 4) lead screening of all infants, regardless of socioeconomic status should begin by age 1 year if not before.

Children's Household Exposure to Guns

Y. D. Senturia, A. M. Teuscher, and K. K. Christoffel

Pediatric Practice Research Group,
Children's Memorial Hospital, Chicago, Ill

OBJECTIVES: To determine what proportion of households with children who go to pediatricians contains firearms, the types owned, purposes for which they are kept, condition in which they are stored, and the social correlates of each.

METHODS: In-office completion of a short questionnaire by parents of all children attending 20 participating pediatric offices during 1 week study period.

RESULTS: 1608 questionnaires completed in the first 11 offices have been analyzed. The % of respondents reporting any gun ownership (GO) varied independently by practice (mean: 29%; range: 6-53%; P<.00001) and by area of residence (urban (U): 20%, suburban (S): 31%, rural (R): 57%; P<.00001). Homes with males >17 years were more likely to own guns (P<.0001. U: P = .0015; S: P = .13; R: P = .02). As the number of children <5 years increased, GO decreased (P<.06).

Type of firearm owned varied by area:

	Urban	Suburban	Rural	
Rifle (RIF)	12%	20%	47%	P<.0001
Handgun (HG)	9%	11%	23%	P<.0001

RIF were usually kept for recreation (72%); HG for self-protection (50%) or recreation (54%). The majority of firearms were stored in the bedroom (52%). HG were more often kept locked (LK) 51% and loaded (LD) 24% than RIF (LK, 38%: P<.01; LD, 3%: P<.0001). HG were more often reported loaded and not locked than RIF (5.3% vs 1.3%: P<.01).

CONCLUSIONS: (1) GO is more common in rural areas and in homes without preschool children. (2) GO is more common in homes with adult males. (3) Anticipatory safety guidance regarding children and guns must be tailored to patterns of actual gun ownership, which vary from area to area and practice to practice.

Finding the Missing Data—a Statewide System for Injury Surveillance in the Pediatric Office Setting

J. K. Sanders, E. R. Waring, and J. R. Zanga

Division of General Pediatrics and Emergency Care,
Children's Medical Center, Richmond, Va

Injury is the leading cause of death among children ages 0-19 in the United States. In 1985, over 20,000 children and adolescents died in the United States due to injuries. Mortality statistics alone do not accurately reflect the extent of the injury problem. Indeed, deaths due to injury are just the tip of the iceberg. Nonfatal injury statistics further illuminate the injury problem. A study in Massachusetts estimated that for every injury related death, there are 45 injuries requiring hospital admission and 1,300 injuries requiring emergency department treatment. Because nonfatal injury statistics are generally derived from hospital discharge data, they still do not fully depict the extent of the problem. It is the investigator's belief that a large number of childhood injuries are being seen and treated in the physician's office setting and are not being captured by routine injury surveillance. Therefore, a childhood injury surveillance system has been developed in Virginia to track the incidence of childhood injuries not requiring admission to the hospital system. The objectives are to collect data that will add to our ability to determine injury trends and to develop injury prevention strategies based on trends revealed by the surveillance data.

Sixty private pediatricians, representing virtually every geographic region in the state, have agreed to record information on a monthly basis, using a specially designed instrument, about children seen and treated in their practices for injuries. Monthly physician return rates average 75%. Categories of data collection include patient age, sex, race, family income, agent of injury, location of injury, cause of injury, pathology and severity.

Eight months of data indicate that 2,232 injured children have been treated in the office. Falls, collision with objects and collision with persons head the list of causes. While most injuries are mild, 34% are moderate to severe. Data analysis highlights the gaps in hospital based injury surveillance.

We conclude that injury surveillance data from pediatricians' offices significantly adds to our knowledge of injury epidemiology.

Management of Childhood Lead Poisoning: A Survey

D. Glotzer and H. Bauchner

Department of Pediatrics,
Boston (Mass) University School of Medicine,
and Boston City Hospital

Published recommendations (1985) for the management of childhood lead (Pb) poisoning suggest the use of EDTA provocation testing and chelation as the mainstay of treatment for blood Pb (BPb) levels between 25 and 55 μg/dL. Since 1985 evidence has accumulated indicating that: 1) levels of BPb < 25 μg/dL are detrimental to cognitive development; 2) EDTA provocation testing may result in potentially harmful shifts in the body Pb burden; and, 3) oral agents such as penicillamine (PCA) and DMSA are effective in reducing elevated Pb levels. To determine how this evidence impacts on the management of childhood Pb poisoning we surveyed the Pb poisoning clinics of pediatric departments in the cities estimated by the U.S. Public Health Service to have the largest number of children affected by Pb poisoning.

21 of 43 (49%) surveys were completed. Respondents indicated that the lowest BPb level for which they would use a chelating agent to reduce the Pb burden was: ≥ 40 μg/dL (24%), 35 μg/dL (5%), 30 μg/dL (24%) and 25 μg/dL (48%). For the following BPb levels respondents indicated their initial recommended management of an asymptomatic child with BPb elevation would be:

	25-29 μg/dL	30-34 μg/dL	35-39 μg/dL	40-44 μg/dL	45-49 μg/dL	50-55 μg/dL
No chelation	40%	25%	20%	5%	5%	0%
EDTA if Prov+	40%	45%	55%	50%	40%	20%
EDTA chelation	5%	5%	5%	40%	50%	75%
PCA	10%	20%	15%	5%	5%	5%
DMSA	5%	5%	5%	0%	0%	0%

For a child with a negative EDTA provocation test, with the following BPb levels, the percent of respondents recommending the use of any chelation therapy is as follows: 25-29 μg/dL (12%), 30-34 μg/dL (25%), 35-39 μg/dL (25%), 40-44 μg/dL (31%), 45-49 μg/dL (50%) and 50-55 μg/dL (62%).

The results of this survey indicate that: (1) The majority of children with elevated BPb burdens are managed using EDTA. Only a small minority of Pb clinics currently use oral chelating agents; (2) The EDTA provocation test continues to be widely used, and the majority of children with BPb 25-40 μg/dL with negative provocation tests do not receive chelation therapy; (3) No common approach for the treatment of Pb toxicity appears to exist; and, (4) In the majority of pediatric centers current management of BPb elevation does not appear to reflect new information regarding the effects and treatment of Pb poisoning.

Who Needs The Lead (Pb) Mobilization Test (LMT)? Blood Pb As the Sole Determinant of Need for Treatment

M. E. Markowitz and J. F. Rosen

Department of Pediatrics,
Albert Einstein College of Medicine,
and Montefiore Medical Center, Bronx, NY

The Centers for Disease Control have recommended that the evaluation of children with moderate Pb poisoning (blood Pb ≥25 and ≤55 ug/dl and erythrocyte protoporphyrin ≥35 ug/dl*) include the LMT to determine which children will respond to a course of chelation therapy with an enhanced Pb diuresis. However, few medical centers are equipped to perform this test in either its 24 hour in-hospital or 8 hour out-patient forms. As a result, many children with moderate Pb poisoning may not be receiving optimal therapy. To determine if selection criteria for chelation treatment could be simplified, we analyzed the relationship between blood Pb and LMT outcomes in 179 previously untreated children with moderate Pb poisoning. After a blood sample for repeat Pb measurement was obtained, each child received a 500 mg/m^2 dose of $CaNa_2EDTA$, i.m., followed by an 8 hour urine collection for urinary Pb determination. The correlation between blood Pb and the ratio of urinary Pb to dose of EDTA (uPb^r) was .6399, p <.001. Of 28 children with blood Pb levels >40 ug/dl 23 had uPb^r ≥.70, indicating a likely benefit from chelation with $CaNa_2EDTA$. Of 22 children with blood Pb levels <25 ug/dl on the day of the LMT, none had a uPb^r ≥.70. We conclude that in circumstances where the LMT cannot be performed, children with blood Pb concentrations >40 be chelated empirically because of the likelihood of responding to $CaNa_2EDTA$ (82%). Previously untreated children with blood Pb levels <25 need not undergo a LMT.

*(Pb μg/dL)/20.7 = Pb μmol/L; (EP μg/dL)/56.3 = EP μmol/L

Can We Influence Parents Whose Preschooler Has Been Recently Poisoned to Take Preventive Precautions?

A. D. Woolf, A. Saperstein, and S. Forjuoh

Department of Pediatrics,
Harvard Medical School, Boston, Mass;
Division of General Pediatrics,
Children's Hospital, Boston;
and Massachusetts Poison Control System

Among the 960,000 poisonings of children under 6 yo recorded by US poison centers annually, up to 20% will have a repeat poisoning episode before they turn 6 years old. We investigated the prevention practices of families whose preschool child had experienced a recent poisoning incident. Of 906 families queried, 336 (38%) did not have syrup of ipecac on hand one week after the poisoning incident. The families without ipecac were randomly assigned to receive (E1; N = 169) or not receive (C1; N = 167) a mailed intervention from the poison center. The intervention consisted of telephone stickers with the poison center's number, a slide cabinet lock, a coupon for $1 off the purchase price of ipecac, pamphlets on poisoning prevention, a 9-step checklist for poison-proofing the home, and a cover letter. The unit cost of the intervention packet was $2.87 (includes coupon redemption and postage). All families received a structured telephone interview 3 months after the intervention. Over 90% of enrolled families completed the follow-up. The groups were demographically comparable; these families were predominately white, middle class, and well educated. E1 families were more likely to have a poison control sticker than C1 families (78% vs 39%; $\chi^2 = 60.92$; p<0.0001) and were more likely to have in use at least one slide lock on their home cabinets (59% vs 40%; $\chi^2 = 10.8$; p<0.001). However E1 families, who had received a coupon for ipecac, were no more likely to have ipecac on hand 3 months later than those who had not (57% vs 52%; p = ns). There were no differences between groups in their implementation of other advice offered in the "9 steps." We conclude that, even after a preschooler's poisoning, parents are often not motivated to undertake poisoning prevention strategies on their own. A mailed intervention can be effective if it removes barriers to compliance with poisoning prevention advice.

Gender Difference in Health Care Utilization By Children Away From Parental Influence

M. C. J. Rudolf and A. J. Alario

Department of Pediatrics, Rhode Island Hospital,
Brown University, Providence

The increased morbidity and use of health services by women is usually explained by social and biological differences in adult life. In order to explore gender differences in the pediatric age group, infirmary utilization was studied at a residential summer camp where parental influence is at a minimum. Campers were classified according to frequency and necessity of infirmary visits. These were graded by infirmary staff, blind to the study purpose as major, minor or trivial (agreement among investigators = 88%, weighted kappa 0.63, P<0.001).

398 campers aged 8-18 years (F:M ratio 1.1:1) made 498 visits (1.5 visits/girl vs 1.0/boy, $P<0.005$). 237 campers used the infirmary of whom 142 were girls ($P<0.01$). No gender difference was seen in those visiting for major medical problems, e.g febrile illness (5% of all girls vs 4% of boys) or in those admitted (15% of girls vs 13% of boys). However a difference was seen in those visiting for minor and trivial purposes (63% of girls vs 48% of boys, $P<0.05$) and particularly in those making multiple (3+) visits for minor/trivial problems (21% of girls vs 11% of boys, $P<0.02$). There was no correlation between age and frequency of visits. Gender differences were particularly evident in those visiting for minor musculoskeletal trauma (F:M ratio 1.6:1, $P<0.05$) and skin trauma (1.9:1, $P<0.01$). Girls were no more likely than boys to involve a counselor in the decision to visit, (49% vs 43%) nor more likely to receive treatment for trivial visits (33% vs 30%) suggesting that staff were not favoring girls and encouraging return visits.

Although obvious morbidity was no different in campers, girls used the infirmary more than boys in a manner similar to that reported for adult health behavior. This suggests that gender differences occur earlier than suspected and are not simply related to adult social roles.

Barriers to Influenza Vaccination in Children with Asthma

P. G. Szilagyi, L. E. Rodewald, J. Savageau, L. M. Yoos, and C. B. Doane

Department of Pediatrics, University of Rochester (NY) School of Medicine and Dentistry

The AAP recommends influenza vaccination for children with moderate or severe asthma, yet few such vaccinations are provided annually. There may be several barriers to vaccination. Many providers lack a computerized database that can identify children with asthma for annual vaccination. Patient barriers may include (1) health beliefs about asthma and influenza vaccination and (2) "control" beliefs about whether their behaviors affect health status. This study examined both provider and patient barriers at a pediatric continuity clinic in an urban teaching hospital.

A computerized database identified 124 children who had a significant asthma attack within the prior year. Patients were randomly assigned to either a study group ($N=63$), who were sent a personalized letter reminder about the need for an influenza vaccination, or to a control group ($N=61$), who received no reminder. Study group mothers were interviewed 2 months after the letter was sent so that potential factors predicting compliance with influenza vaccination could be assessed. Questions included (1) the four major dimensions of the Health Belief Model and (2) the Multidimensional Health Locus of Control Scale (MHLC).

Eighteen study group patients (29%) and only four control patients (7%) received an influenza vaccination [$\chi^2=10.3$; df=1; $p<0.01$]. Forty-three study group mothers were interviewed; 14 (33%) of interviewed mothers had complied with influenza vaccination recommendations. The 20 patients not interviewed had a similar vaccination rate, but could not be reached because of lack of phones, clinic visits or current addresses. Two measures correlated with vaccination compliance: high levels of parental worry about asthma, which increased compliance (odds ratio = 23.3, $p<0.01$) and high levels of parental worry about vaccine side effects, which decreased compliance (odds ratio = 0.087, $p=0.025$). Variables not predicting compliance included: socioeconomic status, asthma severity, perceived influenza susceptibility or vaccination benefits, physical barriers to care (e.g., transportation), or results of the three MHLC instrument subscales (Internal, Powerful Others, Chance).

We conclude that (1) a computerized database is useful in recalling children with asthma for influenza vaccination; (2) although reminders increase compliance, only a subset of parents will respond to personalized letter reminders; (3) parental worry is an important intervening variable affecting compliance; and (4) assessment of parental worry may allow physicians to tailor parental education to increase influenza vaccination rates.

GENERAL PLENARY SESSION
Thursday, May 2, 8 AM-NOON

Managed Care for New York Medicaid Children: Cost Analysis of Referred Services

T. D. Sullivan

Department of Pediatrics, SUNY at Buffalo (NY), and The Children's Hospital of Buffalo

The Children's Medicaid Program (CMP) is a State and County sponsored ongoing (5/1/87-4/30/91) demonstration project in prepaid, capitated, case-managed care for Erie Co. N.Y. Medicaid children. A cost analysis for the first 24 months presented at the 1990 APA Annual Meeting showed a decrease in overall costs despite an increase in primary care costs. The object of this study was to see if this trend has continued through 36 months and to more closely analyze referred services costs.

CMP pediatricians received a monthly fee (ranging from $8.34 to 42.47 and varying by age and sex) to provide primary care to a group of Medicaid eligible children. Most referred services with some exceptions (ER, dental) required pediatrician approval. CMP costs were compared to costs for a similar comparison group (CG) of Erie Co. Medicaid children using data from New York's computerized payment system. Participation was measured in eligible months (EM). One child in the program for 1 month equalled 1 EM. At 24 months there were 13,861 CMP EM's and 996,024 CG EM's. By 36 months EM's had more than doubled to 28,135 while CG EM's had risen to 1,515,045.

Primary care costs per EM continued to be higher for CMP children compared to the CG ($12.31 vs. $9.14, $p<.001$) although the gap has narrowed ($14.91 vs. $8.94, $p<.001$). Referred services costs per EM were much higher for the CG as follows:

	CMP	CG	p Value
Inpatient Hospital	$ 4.74	$ 9.46	<.001
Specialty MD/Clinic	2.89	7.47	<.001
Emergency Room	2.75	4.62	<.001
Pharmacy	.61	2.49	<.001
Lab/Radiology	.58	.44	<.01
Other	.15	1.06	<.001
Total	11.72	25.54	<.001

Money invested in a sound primary care system pays dividends later in decreased costs for referred services.

The Efficacy of Non-Invasive In-Hospital and Outpatient Management of Febrile Infants: A Four Year Experience

M. D. Baker, L. M. Bell, and J. R. Avner

Divisions of General Pediatrics, Emergency Medicine, and Infectious Diseases,
The Children's Hospital of Philadelphia (Pa)

Since 1987, we have prospectively studied the safety and cost-effectiveness of non-invasive in-hospital and outpatient management of well-appearing febrile infants. Four hundred twenty-five infants 29-56 days old with rectal temperatures in excess of 38.2°C presenting to the CHOP Emergency Department were enrolled. Following a complete history, physical examination, and sepsis work-up, each child was assigned to one of three groups. In hospital controls (IHC, $N=250$), were those children with either laboratory or clinical parameters suggestive of serious infection. The remaining 175 well-appearing infants with normal laboratory parameters were randomly selected for either in-hospital observation without treatment (IHO, $N=92$), or outpatient observation without treatment (OPO, $N=83$), but with repeat physical examinations at 24 and 48 hours. Serious illness (SI) occurred in 116

(27.3%) of 425 infants. SI included: meningitis, sepsis, UTI, pneumonia, cellulitis, and bacterial gastroenteritis. One hundred fifteen of 116 children with SI were identified by our admission criteria (sensitivity = 99.1% [95% CI = 95.3% - 100%]). The negative predictive value was 99.4% (95% CI = 97.0-100%). One child, in the IHO group, subsequently was diagnosed with ectodermal dysplasia and had persistently positive blood cultures. Compared to IHC, substantial savings were realized in both IHO and OPO groups. Average medical charges were: $5,653 (IHC), $2,947 (IHO), and $716 (OPO). Our data indicate that using strict selection criteria, it is possible to safely and cost-effectively manage febrile one-two month old infants without initial antibiotic treatment in either the in-hospital or outpatient setting. Furthermore, outpatient management results in significant savings in patient charges.

Increased Growth Velocities in Children Living in Shelters

C. D. Courtlandt, A. H. Fierman, B. P. Dreyer, K. Hick, D. Arnold, E. Keating, and N. Mann

Department of Pediatrics,
New York (NY) University School of Medicine

We have previously demonstrated in a cross sectional study that homeless children have linear growth delays when compared with national standards and domiciled poor children. In this study, we examined the growth over time of children living in a NYC homeless shelter with an on-site medical clinic and nutrition supplementation programs. We collected height data, age, sex, and ethnicity from the records of all children between two and eight years of age who had routine physicals on two occasions, six to eighteen months apart (N=69). All were Medicaid eligible. Height z-scores were determined using the CDC Anthropometric Software Package. Height velocity z-scores were determined using the Genentech Growth Calculator™, which corrects the z-score for growth intervals of less than one year. Both programs define z-scores according to the National Center for Health Statistics (NCHS) standards.

Height velocity z-scores were significantly skewed toward higher values when compared with the expected NCHS distribution (chi-square goodness of fit, <.0001). The median height velocity z-score was +1.0, with 25/69 (36%) children having height velocities >2 SD above the mean. After controlling for age, sex, ethnicity, growth time interval, and season, there was a significant negative correlation between the initial height z-score and the height velocity z-scores (semipartial r = −.27; p=.02). Children with the lowest initial height z-scores thus had the highest growth velocities; however, even those with normal to high initial height z-scores had elevated height velocities (see Table).

	Height z-score				
	<−2	−2 to −1	−1 to +1	>+1	Total
Height velocity z-score (mean)	+4.07	+2.02	+0.89	+0.97	+1.36
N	6	11	40	12	69

Homeless children, especially those with the lowest initial height z-scores, exhibited catch-up growth while in the shelter system. This may be due to improved access to WIC and other supplemental food programs in shelters, and supports the need for on-site nutrition programs in homeless shelters.

The Prediction of Preschool Behaviour Problems From Temperament and Other Variables in Infancy

F. Oberklaid, A. Sanson, R. Pedlow, and M. Prior

Department of Ambulatory Paediatrics,
Royal Children's Hospital, Parkville, Victoria, Australia

Difficult temperament in infancy has consistently been shown to be associated with concurrent behavioural problems (BPs) such as excessive crying, sleep difficulties and colic. However conflicting results of previous studies have resulted in uncertainty about the relationship between difficult temperament in infancy and reported problem behaviours later in childhood. In this study we utilised data from a large, representative community cohort (Total N studied = 1583) to determine if we could predict difficult preschool behaviour problems (at age 4-5 years) from difficult temperament and other variables in infancy.

In addition to global ratings of their infant's temperament (MOR), mothers completed the Revised Infant Temperament Questionnaire (RITQ) (Carey & McDevitt), a 4 point rating scale of infant behaviour problems (BPs)—excessive crying, sleep problems and colic—and provided sociodemographic data, and maternal and child health nurses globally rated the infant's temperament on a 5 point scale (NOR). Preschool behaviour problems were defined as a score greater than 1 SD above the mean on the Preschool Behaviour Questionnaire (Behar & Stringfield).

Maternal ratings of difficult temperament on the RITQ predicted only 17.5% (NS) of those with preschool behaviour problems, a percentage not significantly greater than the 14% of the total sample rated as having problems. There was some improvement in prediction when difficult temperament was added to other variables such as male sex (28%, p<.05), and low socioeconomic status (24%, p<.001). However MOR was a more powerful predictor of preschool behaviour problems, both alone (26.0%, p<.005) and in combination with other variables such as perinatal stress (36.8%, p<.01), male sex (29.5%, p<.005), non-Australian parent (29.4%, p<.05). Similarly maternal reports of infant BPs was a more powerful predictor of preschool behaviour problems both alone (21.8%, p<.001) and in combination with male sex (24.6%, p<.001), low socioeconomic status (26.1%, p<.001), non-Australian parent (21.8%, p<.01), and NOR (21.9%, p<.05). The best consistent predictor of later problems was the combination of MOR and BPs (27.0%, p<.001) and especially when combined with other infant variables such as perinatal stress (35.3%,m p<.05), male sex (31.5%, p<.001), and non-Australian parent (30.0%, p<.05).

We conclude that difficult temperament in infancy, as traditionally conceptualised and measured on the RITQ, is not on its own significantly associated with behaviour problems at 4-5 years of age. Of far greater importance for clinicians is the significant relationship between preschool behaviour problems and maternal *perceptions* of difficult temperament and behaviour in infancy. Discrepancies between detailed ratings and global perceptions of temperament in infancy may indicate stresses in the parent-child relationship which are ultimately more predictive of problems than difficult temperament *per se*.

Vaccine Storage Errors in Pediatric Practice: The Tip of an Iceberg?

D. M. Bishai, S. Bhatt, L. T. Miller, and G. F. Hayden

Department of Pediatrics,
Cedars-Sinai Medical Center, Los Angeles, Calif,
and University of Virginia Health Sciences Center,
Charlottesville

Recent increases in measles and mumps activity and the occurrence of illness among vaccinees have prompted questions about the adequacy of vaccine handling in pediatric practice. To evaluate this potential problem, we visited 46 pediatric offices (selected randomly from a list of practitioners affiliated with a metropolitan hospital), 3 hospital-based clinics, and 1 community clinic. A questionnaire was administered to the person in each office taking primary responsibility for the care of vaccines (the vaccine coordinator or VC), and each vaccine refrigerator was inspected according to a standard protocol.

The VC was neither a physician nor a nurse in 23 (46%) offices; a written description of his vaccine-related duties was infrequently available (12 offices or 24%). Only 8 (16%) VCs could cite appropriate storage temperatures for vaccines. Nine (18%) VCs were unaware that heat can harm certain vaccines, and 18 (36%) did not know that freezing can likewise be harmful. A thermometer was kept in the refrigerator in only 18 (36%) offices; the temperature was checked at least weekly in only 10 (20%) offices. On inspection, the temperature was inappropriately high (>8 deg.C) in 11 (22%) refrigerators. More than half of the refrigerators contained one or more of: outdated vaccine (62%); >1 opened vial of the same type of vaccine (52%); an opened vial which had not been dated (70%); and food or drink (62%). Vaccines were often observed on the door shelf (46%) and outside the refrigerator in uninsulated trays (16%).

Errors in vaccine handling were encountered at an alarmingly high frequency. Pediatricians should follow the guidelines for optimal vaccine storage to minimize the potential for vaccine failure among their patients.

Use of the Fentanyl Lollipop for Analgesia During Painful Procedures in Children

N. L. Schechter, S. J. Weisman, M. Rosenblum, P. L. Conard, B. Bernstein, C. Bartolotta, C. San Antonio, B. Shapiro, D. Cohen

Departments of Pediatrics and Anesthesia,
University of Connecticut Health Center, Farmington;
St Francis Hospital and Medical Center, Hartford, Conn;
and Children's Hospital at Philadelphia (Pa)

For many children with chronic illness, the painful procedures associated with their disease are worse then the disease itself. To address the need for rapidly-acting, safe oral analgesia and sedation for children undergoing painful diagnostic and therapeutic procedures, we examined the efficacy of oral transmucosal fentanyl citrate (OTFC) commonly known as the fentanyl lollipop in a double-blind, placebo-controlled randomized clinical trial. This preparation which is absorbed through the buccal mucosa offers a more rapid onset of action than oral medications and avoids the discomfort of intravenous cannulation or intramuscular injection.

Fifty-eight children with cancer (aged 3-17 years) scheduled for bone marrow aspiration, lumbar puncture, or central venous line removal were randomized to receive either a placebo lollipop or OTFC (17.5 mcg/kg). Children were instructed to suck on the lollipop until it was finished. The procedure was performed approximately 20 minutes later. One hour after the procedure was completed, the nurse, all children over 8, and the parent were asked to rate the pain associated with the procedure using 1-10 visual analogue scale. Children 3-7 years used the Oucher yielding a 1-6 score on both scales, 1 represents no pain.

RESULTS:	Mean Pain Rating		
	Placebo	OTFC	P
Nurse	4.1±2.0	2.8±2.0	0.01
Children (3-7)	4.1±1.7	2.5±1.6	0.01
(over 8)	4.7±2.5	2.1±1.9	0.007
Parent	5.3±2.7	3.2±2.2	0.003

As is evident, OTFC afforded significant reductions in discomfort as assessed by the nurse, child, and parent. Side effects were frequent but not disabling and included itching (60%) and nausea and/or vomiting (30%). One child experienced oxygen desaturation but remained alert and required only stimulation.

IMPLICATIONS: This study suggests that OTFC offers the rapid onset of safe analgesia via a pleasant route. It may well have applicability to other settings such as emergency departments. It offers an excellent analgesic alternative for children who require painful procedures.

The CBC Revisited: A Bayesian Reappraisal

M. S. Kramer, S. M. Tange, E. G. Mills, and M. L. Bernstein

Departments of Pediatrics and of
Epidemiology and Biostatistics, McGill University
Faculty of Medicine, Montreal, Quebec

Previous studies of the value of the CBC in distinguishing viral from bacterial infection in young febrile children have failed to exclude children with clinically evident bacterial infection and thus have inflated the positive predictive value of the test for occult focal infection. We prospectively studied 2844 children 3 to 24 months of age who presented to a children's hospital emergency department between March 1989 and August 1990 with fever (≥38.0°C) of acute (≤4 days) onset but no evident bacterial focus of infection, 541 (19%) of whom received a CBC. We also carried out an 8-year retrospective analysis to provide data (prior probabilities, CBC results) on rare occult bacterial infections (meningitis, osteomyelitis, septic arthritis, and enteritis).

Prior probabilities for the four most common diagnostic categories were: viral, .932; UTI (≥10^4 organisms/ml), .060; pneumonia (based on "blind" reading by a pediatric radiologist), .008; and bacterial meningitis, .00005. The likelihood of WBC ≥15,000/mm^3 was 30, 60, 57, and 50% for viral, UTI, pneumonia, and meningitis, respectively, yielding significantly (P<.001) elevated likelihood ratios (LR's) (relative to viral) of 1.98, 1.89, and 1.65 for the three occult infections. Among children with high WBC, neither total polymorphonuclear count ≥10,000/mm^3 nor band count ≥500/mm^3 was associated with significantly elevated LR's for any of the three occult infections, a finding confirmed by multiple logistic regression analysis. Based on the prior probabilities and likelihoods of WBC ≥15,000/mm^3 for each diagnosis, the revised (posterior) probabilities were: viral, .874; UTI, .112; pneumonia, .014; and meningitis, .00008. Thus a high WBC count approximately doubles the overall probability of occult focal bacterial infection; even then, however, a viral diagnosis remains far more likely. The increase in probability given a high WBC count is clinically important only for UTI, for which an equally sensitive and far more specific test (i.e., the urinalysis) is readily available. These results seriously undermine the diagnostic value of the CBC in the young febrile child.

Clinical Risk Index for Bacterial Meningitis Among Febrile Children

R. Lembo, D. Krowchuk, and P. McCarthy

Department of Pediatrics,
Yale University, New Haven, Conn, and
Department of Pediatrics, Case-Western Reserve University
at MetroHealth Medical Center, Cleveland, Ohio

We have previously reported a multivariate model to assess risk of bacterial meningitis (BM) among febrile children. To translate this model into a clinical instrument suitable for risk assessment, we derived a weighted numerical index based on 3 predictor variables (meningeal signs [MS], physician impression of toxicity [TOX], and the ratio of immature-to-total neutrophils [ITR] in peripheral blood) from a sample of 223 children (median age: 3 months; prevalence of BM: 20%) and then validated its diagnostic efficacy in an independent sample of 171 consecutive children (median age: 3 months; prevalence of BM: 3%) undergoing a lumbar puncture as part of an evaluation of fever.

Predictor variables were identified by logistic regression analysis. MS were considered as a binary variable (any present = 1/all absent = 0). TOX was quantified retrospectively by a naive rater based on 3 clinical items (level of consciousness, color, hydration) and considered as an ordinal score (range: 0 [non-toxic] to 15 [highly toxic]. The ITR was considered as a decimal value (range: 0.0 to 1.0). The weights represented the exponentiated beta coefficients derived from the logistic regression equation. The risk index was computed as the sum of the products of the weight times the value for each variable (numerical range: 0 to 117 points).

Subjects with BM in the derivation and validation samples had a significantly (p<0.01) higher median index (55.2 and 65.3 points) then did children without BM (16.6 and 10.6). The ability of the index to differentiate subjects with and without BM, as assessed by the area (c) under the receiver operating characteristic curve, was high in both samples (c = 0.86 and 0.99; perfect differentiation: c = 1.0). At a threshold value of 21 points, the index's sensitivity, specificity and predictive accuracy for BM were 0.91, 0.61, and 0.37 in the derivation sample, and 1.00, 0.70, and 0.09 in the validation sample. Raising the threshold value incrementally to 50 points maintained sensitivity at 1.0 but increased specificity to 0.96 and predictive accuracy to 0.42 in the validation sample.

We conclude that this numerical index based on data readily accessible in the acute care setting and easily computed with a hand-held calculator is of value to clinicians for objectively assessing risk of BM in febrile children.

Randomized Trial of Laxatives in the Treatment of Encopresis

T. Nolan, G. Debelle, F. Oberklaid, and C. Coffey

Department of Paediatrics and Ambulatory Paediatrics, University of Melbourne, Royal Children's Hospital, Victoria, Australia

Management of encopresis involves the use of laxative medication and behavior modification aimed at promoting toileting regularity. There has never been an adequate controlled evaluation of the additional benefit conferred by laxatives. A total of 169 children with encopresis and radiographic evidence of stool accumulation were randomized to either multimodal therapy (MM—laxatives plus behavior modification; n = 83), or to behaviour modification alone (BM; n = 86). Treatment failure was defined as failure to achieve substantial progress towards remission by at least 6 weeks from study entry (BM group). This occurred in 32 cases (37%). These subjects were deemed to have reached a study end-point at the time treatment failure was declared. Mean follow-up was 55.1 (sd 26.96) months for the MM group, and 56.7 (sd 31.97) months for the BM group. Remission and improvement rates at follow-up were—n(%):

	Remission			Remission/Partial Remission		
Group	3mo	6mo	12mo	3mo	6mo	12mo
MM (n = 83)	32 (39)	41 (49)	42 (51)	39 (47)	50 (60)	52 (63)
BM (n = 86)	18 (21)	26 (30)	31 (36)	21 (24)	31 (36)	37 (43)
P-value	0.019	0.017	0.079	0.004	0.003	0.016

The MM group came into remission significantly sooner than the BM group, and the difference in the Kaplan-Meier remission curves was most striking in the first 30 weeks of follow-up (p = .012). Separate hazard functions were modelled for follow-up prior to and subsequent to 26 weeks (phase I & II). After covariate adjustment, the phase I hazard ratio was 1.91 (MM/BM, 95% ci 1.18, 3.09; p = .008). However, the hazard ratio was not significantly different for phase II (1.02, 95% ci 0.46, 2.26; p = .95). There were nearly identical patterns of compliance with toileting in both treatment groups, although about 1 in 8 children overall did not comply with the sitting program. The BM group children who complied poorly (n = 11) did significantly worse than all others overall (p = .016). After removal of the poor compliers in both treatment groups from the dataset (n = 24), there was no significant difference between BM and MM groups in phase I (hazard ratio 1.49, 95% ci 0.90, 2.47; p = .12) or in phase II (hazard ratio 0.73, 95% ci 0.32, 1.70; p = .46). More multimodal therapy subjects experienced at least 1 relapse (33/55, 51%) than did BM group patients (17/46, 37%), but the 14% difference was not statistically significant (p = .21, 95% ci on difference −5%, 33%). Only 1 BM subject had more than 1 relapse, compared to 6 MM subjects. These results demonstrate a clear advantage overall for the use of laxative medication, but also show that compliant patients may just as successfully be managed without medication.

Maternal Emotional State and Infant Behaviour: Are They Related?

A. R. Miller and R. G. Barr

Department of Pediatrics, Montreal (Quebec) Children's Hospital

Laboratory studies have demonstrated a relationship between clinical maternal depression and infant behaviour. To determine if emotional distress in otherwise-healthy first-time mothers is related to infant crying, 88 mother-infant pairs were studied prospectively in their homes. At 35 weeks gestation and 6 weeks postpartum, mothers completed the General Health Questionnaire 30 (GHQ), a measure of non-psychotic emotional perturbation, plus Pitt's Pre/Postpartum Anxiety-Depression Scale and Spielberger's State Anxiety Inventory. These measures were highly intercorrelated (r's .68 to .82) so GHQ was used as the primary measure. Infant cry and fuss duration (C/F-dur; hours/day) and frequency (C/F-freq; bouts/day) were obtained from a validated diary kept by mothers for the infant's sixth week. Diary "quality", scored for detail, clarity, completeness and flaws by a rater unaware of maternal emotional state, was not related to pre- or postpartum emotions (both r's <.08, p's >.5).

RESULTS: *Prenatal* GHQ was not associated with infant C/F parameters (both r's <.07, p's >.5). In contrast, *postnatal* GHQ was associated with C/F-freq (r = .28, p <.01) and especially C/F-dur (r = .45, p<.001). Postpartum GHQ retained importance in multiple regression models incorporating significant covariates (mother's age, infant birthweight, feeding type, one parent in home, etc), accounting for 8% of variance in C/F-freq [F(4,83) = 6.2, p<.001] and 31% of C/F-dur [F(3,84 = 16.9, p<.001]. *Changes* in maternal distress from pre- to postpartum periods were examined. Infants of mothers whose scores increased on at least 2 of the 3 measures cried more (2.9 ± 1.4 hrs/day; n = 24) than those whose scores decreased (2.1 ± .9 hrs/day; n = 50) or did not change (2.2 ± 1.1 hrs/day; n = 14)[F(2,85) = 5.6, p = .005].

CONCLUSIONS: Though unrelated to prenatal emotions, crying in 6 wk-olds is related to concurrent maternal emotional distress and changes in emotional state, independent of background influences and quality of maternal diary records. Causal interpretations of this relationship must, however, remain speculative.

Perinatal Injuries: Why Families File Suit

G. B. Hickson, E. W. Clayton, P. B. Githens, and F. A. Sloan

Vanderbilt Institute for Public Policy Studies, Health Policy Center, Vanderbilt University, Nashville, Tenn

It is assumed that following perinatal injuries, families need money to provide care for their children and therefore file suit. Yet, it is likely that reasons for filing may be more complex. To examine this possibility, Florida families (n = 169) identified from a random sampling of closed claims filed between 1978 and 1989, were asked to participate in a one hour interview and provide written consent for release of pertinent medical records to investigators; 127 (75%) agreed. Families offered 179 responses to the question, "Why did you file suit?". These responses were categorized by two independent reviewers who achieved 91% agreement for category assignments. Reasons for filing included: advised to sue by influential others (32% of families), believed a cover-up existed (24%), needed money (23%), child had no future (23%), wanted to find out what happened (20%), and revenge (19%). Reasons for suit were evaluated with respect to potential discriminant variables (family characteristics, medical experiences). Predictors for "advised to sue" included being told by a medical professional that care offered had caused injury (F = 13.9, p<.01) before the family recognized that a problem existed (F = 7.9, p<.01). Predictors for "belief in cover-up" included the perception that a physician tried to mislead (F = 18.3, p<.01), failed to mention the existence of a long term problem (F = 7.6, p<.01) and offer NICU care (F = 6.5, p<.01). "Needed money" was predicted by knowing before birth there might be a problem (F = 5.7, p<.02) and previous contact with a lawyer (F = 4.9, p<.03). "Needed information" was predicted by the perception that an M.D. was unwilling to talk (F = 16.4, p<.01), while the desire for "revenge" was predicted by a child's death (F = 15.0, p<.01), belief that an M.D. would not listen (F = 7.4, p<.01), and overhearing a medical conversation (F = 3.28, p<.07).

Families express reasons for suit other than simply the need for dollars. A no-fault system might meet monetary needs, but would not necessarily provide families with information and a public forum to express distress, frustration and anger with the medical profession.

Maltreatment of Young Children Born to Teenage Mothers: A Comparison Between the Late 1960's and the Early 1980's

C. S. Rude, J. M. Leventhal, S. M. Horwitz, and D. M. Stier

Departments of Pediatrics and Epidemiology and Public Health, Yale University School of Medicine, New Haven, Conn

Despite a marked increase in reported cases of child maltreatment, controversy exists about whether this represents an actual increase in child maltreatment or simply increased reporting. To examine this question, we studied two cohorts of children born at Yale-New Haven Hospital (YNHH) to Black mothers who were <19 years old at the time of delivery. One cohort was enrolled from 9/67-6/69 (N = 148) and the other from 10/79-12/81 (N = 159). Information about each child's first five years of life was obtained from medical records at YNHH and at the three other major health care facilities providing care to these children. Two pediatricians independently rated each reported injury as accident, maltreatment (abuse, sexual abuse, or neglect), or insufficient information using predefined criteria. Disagreements between reviewers were resolved by consensus.

There were no statistically significant differences between the two cohorts ('60's vs. '80's) in terms of maternal age (mean = 16.6 years for both groups), male gender (56% vs. 55%), low birthweight (10% vs. 11%), prematurity (11% vs. 5.6%, $p = 0.11$), 5 minute Apgars <8 (8.3% vs. 5.9%, $p = 0.42$) and neonatal complications (11.5% vs. 18.2%, $p = 0.10$). There was, however, a lower rate of Title 19 enrollment in the earlier group (88% vs. 95%, $p < 0.05$). The mean number of injuries per case in the two cohorts was similar (1.59 vs. 1.65), as was the percentage of cases with ≥1 accidents (49.3% vs. 59.7%, $p = 0.07$). There was no significant difference in the percentage of cases with maltreatment between the two cohorts (14.9% vs. 10.7%, $p = 0.27$). In the earlier cohort, there was a significantly greater percentage of cases with insufficient information recorded in the chart about certain events (17.6% vs. 5.0%, $p < 0.005$).

These results indicate that when the events of the two cohorts are examined using the same criteria, there is no difference in the rates of maltreatment in children in teenage mothers from the 1960's to the 1980's. We suggest that the marked increase in reporting is likely due to better recognition rather than to true changes in the frequency of maltreatment over time.

Author Index to APA Abstracts

Adair, R. 405
Agre, F. 391, 409
Alario, A.J. 401, 417
Alexander, D.T. 388
Almquist, J.R. 389
Anderman, C.R. 413
Anderson, A.B. 390
Anderson, B. 400
Arbel, A. 407
Arnold, D. 419
Avner, J.R. 416
Baisden, K. 394
Baker, M.D. 418
Ball, L. 402
Barbaresi, W. 384
Barlow, B. 385
Barnett, S. 387
Baron, M. 397
Barr, R.G. 396, 404, 421
Barrett, K. 405
Barthel, M.J. 385
Bartolotta, C. 420
Baskin, M.N. 390
Bates, A.S. 414
Bauchner, B. 397
Bauchner, H. 405, 408, 417
Baum, J. 394
Behrman, A.J. 386
Bell, L.M. 418
Bell, S. 398
Bencivenga, K. 397
Benincasa, G. 407
Berensen, A. 387
Bergman, A.B. 391
Bergman, D. 391
Berkelhamer, J.E. 399
Berkowitz, G. 412
Berman, S. 403
Bernstein, B. 420
Bernstein, M.L. 420
Bhatt, S. 419
Biro, F.M. 387
Bishai, D.M. 419
Bithoney, W.G. 384, 386
Blondis, T.A. 391
Bradley, R.H. 405
Brayden, R.M. 395
Brazdziunas, D. 411
Brotherton, S. 391
Brown, B.C. 396
Calderon, C. 399
Callahan, C.M. 384, 395
Campbell, J.R. 389
Cartland, J.D.C. 395
Casey, P.H. 405
Casey, R. 398
Cetta, F. 389
Chapman, J. 397
Charney, E. 384
Chernoff, R.G. 392
Christensen-Szalanski, J. 407
Christoffel, K.K. 416
Cicchetti, D. 397, 410
Cicchetti, D.V. 410
Clark, G.D. 384
Clausen, C. 401
Clayton, E.W. 421
Coffey, C. 421
Cohen, D. 420
Conard, P.L. 420
Cotton, B.C. 396
Courtlandt, C.D. 407, 419
Cox, J.E. 386
Coyne, L. 386
Crain, E.F. 400
Cross, A.W. 397
Cunningham, S.J. 400
Czarkowski, N. 397
Davenport, M.G. 404
Davidson, L.L. 385
Davidson, N. 383
Davis, A.T. 403
Davis, H.W. 409
Davis, J.K. 394
De Jong, A.R. 383, 386
de Triquet, J.M. 401
DeAngelis, C. 415
Debelle, G. 421
DelBeccaro, M.A. 400
DeMarzo, S. 402
Dennehy, P.H. 401
Dennison, B.A. 401
Desilets, J. 404
DiBrigida, L.A. 406
DiPasquale, K.J. 390
Doane, C.B. 389, 418
Dougherty, G.E. 388, 402
Doughman, J.A. 387
Dreyer, B.P. 407, 419
DuBerger, R. 404
Dubowitz, H. 383, 406
Duggan, A.K. 415
Dungy, C. 391, 407
Durkin, M.S. 385
Dusdieker, L. 391
Dwyer, D. 408
Earp, J.A. 399
Ekwo, E. 411
Ellis, S.P. 394
Evans, A.E. 414
Feigelman, S. 383, 406
Feinstein, R.A. 396
Feldman, W. 403
Field, C. 395
Fierman, A.H. 407, 419
Fink, H. 397
Fleisher, G.R. 390
Foch, B.J. 396
Forjuoh, S. 417
Forrest, C.B. 415
Forsyth, B.W.C. 397, 405, 408
Fowler, M.G. 404, 413
Francoeur, T.E. 396, 404
French, J. 393
Fried, L.E. 413
Friedland, L.R. 409
Gaar, G.G. 390
Garabedian, C. 408
Garg, R. 404
Githens, P.B. 421
Glotzer, D. 417
Goldstein, M. 392
Gonzalez, G. 399
Gortmaker, S.L. 415
Gosselink, C. 411
Gould, J.H. 400
Graef, J.W. 416
Grant, T.M. 384
Griffin, P. 412
Grisanti, K.A. 388
Grisso, J.A. 415
Grose, K. 403
Grossman, D.C. 398
Grossman, L.S. 392
Guzman, M. 406
Halfon, N. 412
Hamilton, J.P. 410
Hayden, G.F. 419
Heagarty, M.C. 385
Heery, L.B. 395
Hermosa, B. 394
Herrera, L. 394
Herrera, M. 403
Hershman, S.J. 393
Hick, K. 419
Hickson, G.B. 421
Holtrop, T. 408
Hong, C.H. 396
Hope, S. 383
Horwitz, S.M. 384, 386, 393, 396, 405, 408, 422
Howard, B. 384
Hubbard, T.W. 401
Huber-Navin, C. 403
Ihnat, D.H.K. 410
Inglis, A.F. 401
Ireys, H.T. 393, 397
Irigoyen, M. 392
Irons, T.G. 403
Isaacman, D.J. 409
Jackson, E. 397
Jaffe, D.M. 388
Jarman, F.C. 411
Jaudes, P.K. 411
Jekel, J.F. 396
Joffe, M. 409
Johnson, D.R. 404
Jones, M. 398
Kaplan, E.L. 404
Kappelman, M.M. 392
Karasic, R.B. 409
Katchan, B. 396
Keating, E. 419
Kelleher, K. 405
Kelly, B. 398
Kelly, B.A. 388
Kelly, D. 398
Kemper, K.J. 407
Kerns, D.L. 409
Kirby, R. 395
Klee, L. 412
Klerman, L.V. 396
Koeber, C. 397
Korsch, B.M. 406
Kouri, E. 410
Kowaleski, K.R. 402, 412
Kramer, M.S. 390, 412, 420
Kresheck, A. 411
Krowchuk, D. 420
Krug, S.E. 410
Lannon, C.M. 399
Lavelle, J.M. 387
Leaf, P.J. 393, 405, 408
Leduc, D. 396, 404
Lee, L.H. 389
Lehmann, M. 411
Lembo, R. 420
Lempert, R. 414
Levenson, S. 405
Leventhal, J.M. 386, 393, 405, 408, 410, 422
Lewander, W.J. 401
Li, M. 402, 412
Lichenstein, R. 383
Lieu, T.A. 390
Long, T.J. 410
Losch, M. 407
Luberti, A.A. 383
Lubitz, D.L. 410
Lustman-Findling, K. 397
Mann, N. 407, 419
Mansell, A.L. 401
Marble, R.D. 410
Margolis, P.X. 414
Markowitz, M.E. 417
Marshall, J. 408
Martone, M. 411
Martorell, R. 394
Maurer, J.T. 385
McCarthy, P. 397, 420
McConnochie, K.M. 415
McCormick, D.P. 387
McGillivray, D. 388, 390
Meert, K. 408
Melman, S. 414
Mendelman, P.M. 401
Mendoza, F. 394
Meropol, S.B. 383
Metcalf, T.J. 403
Miles, C.G. 415
Miller, A.R. 421
Miller, L.T. 419
Mills, E.G. 420
Mungo, R. 406
Murph, J. 391
Murph, W. 391
Nachtsheim, B. 403
Needlman, R.D. 413
Negrete, V. 406
Neifert, M. 402
Neuspiel, D. 414
Newacheck, P.W. 399
Newman, T.B. 383
Nolan, T. 421
Nosal, T. 395
Novack, A.H. 384, 389
Nuss, R. 403
Nypaver, M. 403
O'Connor, P. 385
Oberklaid, F. 419, 421
Oberlander, T.F. 388
Oh, M.K. 396
Okun, A. 392
Olsen, R.D. 400
Olson, A.L. 406
Palevsky, L. 407
Pantell, R. 391
Pascoe, J.M. 393
Pedlow, R. 419
Pelham, T.L. 400
Perrin, J.M. 415
Pew, M.C. 386
Philipp, B. 405
Phipps, P. 384
Pichichero, M.E. 389
Pless, I.B. 388
Pliskin, N.H. 399
Polansky, M. 414
Pope, S. 405
Prieto, L.R. 409
Prior, M. 419
Raisys, V.A. 384
Reising, S.F. 387
Reyes, I. 387
Richardson, M.A. 401
Ritter, M.L. 409
Rivara, F.P. 395, 398
Roark, R. 403
Roberts-Brauer, R. 390, 412
Rodewald, L.E. 389, 418
Rogers, J.E. 389
Roghmann, K.J. 389, 415
Roizen, N.J. 391
Roncevich, S. 410
Ros, S.P. 389
Rosen, J.F. 417
Rosenberg, A.J. 413
Rosenblum, M. 420
Roter, D. 406
Rotman, A. 396, 404
Rude, C.S. 422
Rudolf, M.C.J. 417
Russell, D. 407
Ryan, A. 384
San Antonio, C. 420
Sanders, J.K. 416
Sanson, A. 419
Saperstein, A. 417
Sarnaik, A. 408
Savageau, J. 418
Schechter, N.L. 420
Schiffrin, A. 402
Schneider, R. 410
Schorr, S. 414
Schwartz, J.S. 390
Schwartz, R.M. 391
Schwarz, D.F. 415
Seacat, J. 402
Seifer, R. 401
Senturia, Y.D. 416
Serwint, J.R. 406
Shannon, M.W. 416
Shapiro, B. 420
Shaw, K.N. 386, 387
Shelov, S. 414
Sher, L.D. 403
Shofer, F.S. 386
Siegel, D.M. 394
Silver, E.J. 393, 397
Simms, M.D. 384
Simpson, G.A. 413
Sloan, F.A. 421
Smith, M.B.H. 403
Snellman, L.W. 404
Soderberg, R.W. 398
Soulen, J.L. 415
Speechley, K.N. 393, 405
Squittieri, C. 407
St Peter, R.F. 399
Stang, H.J. 404
Stang, J.M. 404
Starr, M.C. 411
Stein, M. 391
Stein, R.E.K. 392, 394, 397
Stevenson, D.K. 383
Stier, D.M. 422
Stout, J.W. 413
Streissguth, A.P. 384
Sullivan, T.D. 418
Swanson, M. 405
Szilagyi, P.G. 389, 418
Sznajderman, S. 397
Takata, G. 394
Talarico, C. 410
Tange, S.M. 420
Tanz, R.R. 385
Taylor, J.A. 389, 410
Tepper, V. 383, 406
Teuscher, A.M. 416
Theodorou, A. 408
Valcarcel, M. 399
Vandeven, A. 384
Verhulst, S. 398
Vinci, R. 408
Waring, E.R. 416
Wasserman, D.R. 410
Weisman, S.J. 420
Weiss, J.C. 383, 400
Weitzman, M.L. 415
Welshimer, K.J. 397
Werner, M.J. 395
Whitehead, T. 413
Whiteside, L. 405
Wiley, C.C. 398
Wiley, II, J.F. 409
Wilkinson, G. 387
Willenborg, A. 414
Williams, R. 412
Wilson, M.E.H. 385, 406
Wissow, L.S. 385, 406
Wolfson, V.M. 415
Woodin, K.A. 389
Woolf, A.D. 417
Yaremko, J. 396, 404
Yoos, L.M. 418
Young, P.C. 403
Zanga, J.R. 416
Zellman, G.L. 385
Zieserl, E. 403
Zondorak-Perez, M.E. 394
Zuckerman, B.S. 405, 413
Zuravin, S. 383, 406

INSTRUCTIONS FOR AUTHORS

General Information.—Please send manuscripts and correspondence to the Editor, Vincent A. Fulginiti, MD, *AJDC*, Dean's Office, Tulane University School of Medicine, 1430 Tulane Ave, New Orleans, LA 70112. *AJDC no longer returns nonaccepted manuscripts. Original artwork and photographs will be returned.* Manuscripts are considered with the understanding that they have not been published previously and are not under consideration by another publication.

Type of Manuscripts Suitable for Submission

Original Articles.—New observations that have not been submitted or published elsewhere.

Pediatric Forum.—A mixture of brief, peer-reviewed observations or investigations *and* letters to the editor and other short commentaries.

From Research to Relevance.—Significant research that has a high probability of being translated into clinical usefulness.

Educational Intervention.—Information concerning any educational efforts in the broad field of pediatrics.

Pediatric Legal Medicine.—A forum for discussion of broad issues relating to children and the law in today's environment.

Pediatric Perspectives.—Current information on clinical and scientific pediatric medical advances and analyses of current controversies in pediatrics.

Sports Medicine.—Current information relating to the medical needs of young athletes, as well as current concepts in the prevention, diagnosis, and treatment of sports-related illnesses and injuries.

Picture of the Month.—Submissions should be sent directly to Walter W. Tunnessen, Jr, MD, Children's Hospital of Philadelphia, Room 2143, 34th and Civic Center Blvd, Philadelphia, PA 19104.

Radiological Case of the Month.—Submissions should be sent directly to Beverly P. Wood, MD, Childrens Hospital of Los Angeles, Department of Radiology, 4650 Sunset Blvd, Los Angeles, CA 90054-0700.

AJDC Archives.—Occasional revivals of classic *AJDC* articles with contemporary commentary.

Pediatric Reviews.—Timely, comprehensive, well-referenced topics.

Conforming with all of the steps listed below will facilitate the editorial processing of your manuscript.

Step 1.—*Cover Letter.*—All manuscripts must be accompanied on submission by a cover letter giving the name, address, affiliation, and telephone and fax number of the corresponding author. The letter must include ALL of the following statements SIGNED BY ALL AUTHORS (ORIGINAL SIGNATURES):

1. Authorship Responsibility.—"I certify that I have participated sufficiently in the conception and design of this work and the analysis of the data (when applicable), as well as the writing of the manuscript, to take public responsibility for it. I believe the manuscript represents valid work. I have reviewed the final version of the manuscript and approve it for publication. Neither this manuscript nor one with substantially similar content under my authorship has been published or is being considered for publication elsewhere, except as described in an attachment. Furthermore, I attest that I shall produce the data upon which the manuscript is based for examination by the editors or their assignees if requested."

2. Financial Disclosure.—"I certify that affiliations (if any) with or involvement in any organization or entity with a direct financial interest in the subject matter or materials discussed in the manuscript (eg, employment, consultancies, stock ownership, honoraria, expert testimony) are disclosed below."

Research or project support should be listed in an acknowledgment.

3a. Copyright Transfer.—"In consideration of the action of the American Medical Association (AMA) in reviewing and editing this submission, the author(s) undersigned hereby transfer(s), assign(s), or otherwise convey(s) all copyright ownership to the AMA in the event that such work is published by the AMA."

3b. Federal Employment.—"I was an employee of the US federal government when this work was investigated and prepared for publication; therefore, it is not protected by the Copyright Act and there is no copyright of which the ownership can be transferred."

Editing.—Accepted manuscripts are copy edited according to AMA style and returned to the author for approval. Authors are responsible for all statements made in their work, including changes made by the copy editor and authorized by the corresponding author.

All accepted manuscripts become the permanent property of the AMA and may not be published elsewhere without written permission from both the author(s) and the AMA. After publication, certain articles may appear in translation in the foreign-language editions of *AJDC*. The corresponding author will receive typeset pages for approval. Forms for ordering reprints are included with the typeset pages. Reprints are shipped 6 to 8 weeks after publication.

Step 2.—*Manuscript Format.*—All articles submitted should have the following features:

1. Four copies of the manuscript should be submitted; three are for transmission to referees and one is retained in the editorial office. We prefer an original and three copies.
2. Manuscripts should be typed in double-spaced format throughout, including title page, abstracts, text, acknowledgments, references, legends for illustrations, and tables. Please number pages. *Do not use justified right margins.*
3. Title should be no more than 75 characters.
4. Authors should be limited to six, all of whom have contributed to the study and manuscript preparation, are familiar with its substance, and are able to defend its conclusions.
5. The title page should give full names, degrees, and academic affiliations of all authors, address for requests of reprints, and, if the manuscript was presented at a meeting, the organization, place, and exact date on which it was read.
6. Writing style should conform to proper English usage and syntax; consult the *American Medical Association Manual of Style,* available from Williams & Wilkins, 428 E Preston St, Baltimore, MD 21202.
7. Abstract should be limited to 135 words or less.
8. Each table should be typed, with a title, on a separate sheet of paper, with each line, including headings, *double-spaced.* Continuations should be on a second sheet with all headings repeated.
9. Use Système International (SI) measurements throughout the manuscript.
10. Illustrations should be high-contrast, glossy prints, in quadruplicate, in a proportion of 5x7 in. Figure number, name of first author, and arrow indicating "top" should be typed on a gummed *label* and affixed on the back of each illustration. *Do not write directly on the print.*

Full-color illustrations should be submitted as 35-mm, positive color transparencies, mounted in cardboard, and carefully packaged. Fee is $400 for up to six square-finished color illustrations that fit on one page. A letter of intent to pay the fee must accompany submission.

All photographs in which there is a possibility of patient identification should be accompanied by a signed statement of consent from both parents (or guardians). Covering eyes to mask identity is not sufficient.

11. References should be listed in order of their appearance in the text, typed double-spaced, and in AMA format. Please follow the exact order of information and punctuation in the examples below. Note: List all authors and/or editors up to six; if more than six, list the first three and "et al."

Journal articles: Bier DM, Fulginiti VA, Garfunkel JM, et al. Duplicate publication and related problems. *AJDC.* 1990;144:1293-1294.

Books: Naeye RL. How and when does antenatal hypoxia damage fetal brains? In: Kubli F, Patel N, Schmidt W, Linderkamp O, eds. *Perinatal Events and Brain Damage in Surviving Children.* New York, NY: Springer Verlag NY Inc; 1988:83-91.

Unpublished data, personal communications, or manuscripts "in preparation" or "submitted" should not be included in the list of references. Such material, if essential, may be incorporated in the body of the article.

Authors are responsible for the accuracy of the references.

12. Investigations involving human subjects require a specific statement in the "Methods" section that an appropriate institutional review board approved the project and/or that informed consent was obtained from both legal guardians and/or child, if appropriate.
13. Illustrations and tables from other publications should be suitably acknowledged, with written permission from *publisher* and *author.* Brief acknowledgments to specific contributors directly involved in the content of the manuscript may be placed at the end of the text, before the references.

Patient Reports: Reports of patient descriptions that do not contain sufficient new information are discouraged; normally, these will be returned without review. If new information is provided, such manuscripts will be submitted for critical review and may be published as a full original article or as a brief report in the Pediatric Forum.

1991 Annual Meeting

The annual meeting of The American Pediatric Society, The Society for Pediatric Research, and The Ambulatory Pediatric Association will be held April 29 through May 2, 1991, at the New Orleans (La) Hilton and Rivergate Convention Center. For further information, contact the APS/SPR Association Headquarters, 2650 Yale Blvd SE, Suite 104, Albuquerque, NM 87106; (505) 764-9099; FAX (505) 842-8227; or the Ambulatory Pediatric Association, 6728 Old McLean Village, McLean, VA 22101; (703) 556-9222.

Diphtheria and Tetanus Toxoids and Pertussis Vaccine Litigation

Sir.—Orenstein's letter,[1] published in the May 1990 issue of *AJDC*, points out what is naive and bad in current thinking concerning litigation over the diphtheria and tetanus toxoids and pertussis vaccines. The National Vaccine Injury Compensation Program, effective October 1, 1988, was the most naive, if not the most stupid attempt at controlling a segment of our legal system that needs to be controlled. Intended to offer a good method of avoiding costly legal battles, it did just the opposite. Lawyers now have two recourses to sue. They can always sue if the National Vaccine Injury Compensation Program is not to their liking.

For the private sector, the program did nothing but increase our cost of the vaccine to approximately $17 per dose (not the $7.96 the government pays).

Numerous studies have indicated that the vaccine itself had nothing to do with the "brain damage" reported by attorneys and parents. Because the availability of these vaccines is in the public interest, the government and the infectious disease "moguls" should take a firm stand supporting the safety of these vaccines. Those who claim a child was damaged by the vaccine should show that similar outbreaks occurred among recipients of the same "batch" of vaccine. If this is not proven, and other malpractice is not shown, no million-dollar settlements should be made. At most, I advocate providing facilities and funds to care for the affected children on an ongoing basis. Without these requirements of proof, we will be "overcharging" continually for essential vaccines. The legal profession has caused this excessive expense. There is no medical justification to it, and as soon as the truth is told, maybe an end to this problem will be achieved. Crossing our fingers or eating garlic will not keep the vampires from their litigation. We need a wooden stake!

Howard Lokietz, MD
Arcadia Medical Arts Bldg
624 W Duarte Rd, Suite 104
Arcadia, CA 91006

1. Orenstein WA. DTP vaccine litigation, 1988. *AJDC.* 1990;144:517.

In Reply.—The author did not wish to respond. I have a great deal of interest in this area, however, and thought that a response to Dr Lokietz' letter was important.

I do not agree with his assessment of the National Vaccine Compensation Program and its implementation. Having participated in the defense of physicians and others in vaccine-related litigation, I can attest to the harm that the tort-system handling of these claims has for everyone concerned. In my view, substitution of the compensation method for adjudicating claims of vaccine-induced injuries is a far better method than the adversarial legal method.

Initially, an agreement on what would be included in the Vaccine Injury Table,[1] which is the source for determining the applicability of a given claim, was the only way that the system could work. That the table will need refinement in the future is clear. That not everyone accepts "brain damage" as a consequence of pertussis vaccine is also clear, as my recent editorial points out.[2] Some insist that such an association is causal and true. A national debate that could alter the entries in the Vaccine Injury Table is now under way. This is an evolutionary process, and time to effect change is to be expected, since the scientific establishment has long considered central nervous system damage a rare consequence of administration of pertussis vaccine. To overturn that viewpoint simply by declaring it not to be so is naive.

One of the problems with the democratic system is that change is cumbersome and requires extensive negotiation, persuasion, examination of facts and myths, and sorting of fact from myth, with ultimate resolution, often with compromises. On the other hand, I know of no other system that works as well as the democratic one, so I will continue to work within it, doing my part to effect change, when change is indicated.

Vincent A. Fulginiti, MD
Editor, *AJDC*

1. Committee on Infectious Diseases, American Academy of Pediatrics. *1988 Red Book.* Elk Grove Village, Ill: American Academy of Pediatrics; 1988:531-534.
2. Fulginiti VA. A pertussis vaccine myth dies. *AJDC.* 1990;144:860-861.

Antibody Response to MMR Vaccination in Children Who Received IVIG as Neonates

Sir.—The administration of intravenous immunoglobulin (IVIG) to

This department of *AJDC* is reserved for comment, criticism, observation, and discussion of issues of current concern and importance for children's health. The Editor encourages our readers to express themselves on a variety of topics and issues. Further, we encourage the submission of unique and brief clinical and scientific observations that do not fulfill the criteria for original articles.

Gestational Age (GA), Birth Weight (BW), No. of Intravenous Immunoglobulin (IVIG) Infusions, and Total IVIG Dose Given to Five Infants Later Studied for IgG Antibody Response to Measles, Mumps, Rubella (MMR) Vaccination

GA, wk	BW, g	No. of IVIG Infusions	Total IVIG Dose, g	Rubeola IgG*	Mumps IgG*	Rubella IgG*
27	535	5	5.9	0.43	2.93	4.14
26	890	3	5.4	0.40	4.81	3.54
28	1150	3	5.4	0.41	1.85	3.88
31	1000	3	3.9	0.62	1.67	5.01
30	1500	1	1.6	0.44	4.00	3.45

*Reference ranges (enzyme immunoassay units) for IgG response to MMR are as follows: rubeola, >0.16; mumps, >0.9; and rubella, >1.5. They represent the means + 3 SDs for 150 normal people, as stated by the manufacturers of the enzyme immunoassay kits used (rubeola and mumps from Whittaker Bioproducts Inc, Walkersville, Md; rubella from Pharmacia Diagnostics Inc, Fairfield, NY).

neonates has few or no acute short-term effects,[1] but less is known about the subsequent effect on humoral immune function. We studied the response to measles, mumps, rubella (MMR) vaccination in five children who received multiple infusions of IVIG during the neonatal period.

We obtained serum from five children who had participated in a study of IVIG pharmakokinetics in infants of 32 weeks' gestation or less weighing 1500 g or less in the Cedars-Sinai Neonatal Intensive Care Unit, Los Angeles, Calif.[2] The Table shows the gestational age and birth weight of each infant, the number of IVIG infusions, and total IVIG dose. These infants were subsequently vaccinated against rubeola, mumps, and rubella at 15 months of age. Serum samples were obtained 2 months after vaccination. The Table also shows the IgG response to MMR vaccination with reference ranges. Following vaccination, normal amounts of IgG antibodies were found in all children. There was no evidence of recent immunologic response to rubeola, mumps, or rubella as manifested by the absence of specific IgM antibodies to these viruses.

Our data indicate a normal response to MMR vaccination 15 months after IVIG infusion. Results of another study of 19 infants weighing less than 1500 g at birth who received one 1-g dose of IVIG for prophylaxis against acquired cytomegalovirus infection confirm the normal antibody response to MMR.[3] Our five infants received repeated doses of IVIG during hospitalization necessary to maintain protective IgG levels. Thus, the response to MMR appears to remain intact following larger IVIG doses. Our results are encouraging because the use of IVIG is increasing in both investigations and in the community.

Jeanne W. Ruderman, MD
Division of Neonatology
Ahmanson Department of Pediatrics
Cedars-Sinai Medical Center
Los Angeles, CA 90048
Noori Barka, PhD
James B. Peter, MD, PhD
Specialty Laboratories Inc
Santa Monica, CA 90404
E. Richard Stiehm, MD
Division of Immunology
Department of Pediatrics
UCLA School of Medicine
Los Angeles, CA 90024

1. Christensen RD, Hardman T, Thornton J, Hill HR. A randomized, double-blind, placebo-controlled investigation on the safety of intravenous immune globulin administration to preterm neonates. *J Perinatol.* 1989;9:126-130.

2. Ruderman JW, Peter JB, Gall RC, Stewart ME, Pomerance JJ, Stiehm ER. Prevention of hypogammaglobulinemia of prematurity with intravenous immune globulin. *J Perinatol.* 1990;10:150-155.

3. Berzen A, Whyte H, Chabot J, Roifman C. Treatment with gammaglobulin in newborns does not affect subsequent humoral immune function? *Pediatr Res.* 1990;27:262. Abstract.

Vaccine Myth and Physician Handouts

Sir.—I read with interest the editorials by Cherry[1] in the March 23/30 1990 issue of *JAMA* and by Fulginiti[2] in the August 1990 issue of *AJDC* and am concerned about an issue neither physician addressed, namely, the handouts from the Centers for Disease Control that pediatricians have been strongly encouraged to give to our patients. These handouts hardly help to dispel the myth of the connection between diphtheria-pertussis-tetanus vaccine and encephalopathy.

These pamphlets not only tell parents that there is a connection, but give the approximate odds of encephalitis and permanent brain damage occurring. We have distributed these pamphlets not only to protect ourselves from the liability of failing to properly inform parents, but also to educate them about these possible problems associated with the vaccine. Now we are told the problem is all a myth. Thus, we are handing out pamphlets with misinformation. Should we continue to distribute these pamphlets and further spread the myth, or should we stop, thus leading to possible serious liability problems?

Thomas P. Lynch, MD
DuPage Pediatrics Ltd
805 Plainfield Rd
Darien, IL 60559

1. Cherry JD. 'Pertussis vaccine encephalopathy': it is time to recognize it as the myth that it is. *JAMA.* 1990;263:1679-1680.

2. Fulginiti VA. A pertussis vaccine myth dies. *AJDC.* 1990;144:860-861.

In Reply.—Dr Lynch raises an important point in regard to the diphtheria-pertussis-tetanus "Important Information" forms currently being distributed by the Centers for Disease Control.

As noted in the 1988 *Report of the Committee of Infectious Diseases* of the American Academy of Pediatrics, "The National Childhood Vaccine Injury Act (PL99-660; Amended by PL100-203), which became effective in 1988 includes requirements for detailed notification of patients/parents about vaccine benefits and risks in both the private and public sectors. This legislation requires development and distribution of standardized benefits/risk statements when administering vaccines for which vaccine injury compensation is available. These statements are in preparation and physicians will be notified by the federal government when their use becomes mandatory." The Centers for Disease Control has been working on the new forms (*which will be mandatory*), and draft editions have been reviewed by many people. At present, members of the Vaccine Commission and members of the parents group (Dissatisfied Parents Together) have strenuously objected to attempts to make the new forms reflect the level of information we currently have. I do not know when new, more appropriate forms will be available.

What to do in the interim, the question posed by Dr Lynch, is intriguing. It clearly is dishonest to use the present forms. However, there is no easy alternative. One possibility would be to continue to use the present forms but to tell parents that the risk of neurologic illness and death resulting from diphtheria-pertussis-tetanus immunization is grossly exaggerated on the forms. If this is done, it would be wise to indicate on the form and in the medical record what information the parents were given.

James D. Cherry, MD
Department of Pediatrics
Division of Infectious Diseases
UCLA School of Medicine
10833 LeConte Ave
22-442-MDCC
Los Angeles, CA 90024-1752

In Reply.—Dr Lynch outlines a problem in using the current generation of "Important Information" documents prepared by the Centers for Disease Control, and in wide use among pediatricians, and the need for a new generation of such statements. As Dr Cherry indicates in his response, we are not yet there. The new set of informational pamphlets for patients and physicians has been in preparation for some time now. The issues are controversial and have caused delays in the preparation and ultimate distribution of these newer statements.

Major controversy stems from the emphasis to be given to adverse effects of vaccines vs adverse outcomes of disease and benefits of vaccine. Most physicians, including me, believe that the data clearly support an overwhelming degree of benefit of the vaccine compared with the risk. However, a number of individual laypersons, groups of laypersons, and some physicians believe that the public is ill informed about the risks of vaccines. These persons wish to place greater emphasis on the potential adverse events, to "enlighten" the public. Unfortunately, this dispute has led to disruption of an orderly process in preparing these materials.

For example, if a vaccine can cause one death in tens of millions of doses, should that fact be trumpeted? Some persons feel that the only correct way to inform the public is by having a black box surround such data on the face sheet of any document that "informs." Obviously, many of us believe this is extreme, inaccurate, and misleading. We believe that such misrepresentation of the risk/benefit ratio would lead to disenchantment with the vaccine. Advocates of such methods fail to take into account the much larger number of deaths that would occur among those who are not vaccinated, and fight against emphasizing such data. In one debate in which I was involved, the phrase "vaccines are safe and effective, but not perfectly safe nor perfectly effective" drew considerable opposition. To me, and others, the phrase concisely sums up the issue, but to opponents of the vaccine, it is believed to deliver a message that is too optimistic and fails to warn adequately.

The debate will continue until statements can be prepared that satisfy neither party completely, but do what both parties basically want it to do. Multiply this type of discussion/debate times 100 and one begins to see the difficulty in preparing reasonable statements.

Adding fuel to such debate is the emergence of new knowledge. The issue of brain damage alleged to accompany pertussis vaccine administration is a case in point. Dr Cherry and I have attempted to point out that such causal association is a "myth," perpetuated by inaccurate reports and scientific uncertainty in the past. We have called for an end to the myth, but simply stating that position does not make it happen. Dr Lynch and his colleagues will hear a great deal more on this issue as the various advisory committees consider the scientific data, reach their own conclusions, and make recommendations. This is a time-consuming process, which means that we will not see the type of documents that Dr Lynch seeks in the near future.

Vincent A. Fulginiti, MD
Editor, *AJDC*
Dean's Office, Room 1529
Tulane University School of Medicine
1430 Tulane Ave
New Orleans, LA 70112

Exhibitor "Giveaways": A Curmudgeon's View

Sir.—I attended the Fall meeting of the American Academy of Pediatrics in Chicago last year. Everybody seemed to love the trinkets, snacks, pens, flashlights, and other paraphernalia given away by convention exhibitors. As I watched the escalators to the exhibit hall, participants descended with only their programs in hand; but on the way up, many carried shopping bags bulging with "goodies." As listed below, most of the giveaways did not bear the slightest relationship to the products being promoted, but who cared? They were free!

Exhibitor's Product	Giveaway Item
Steroid cream	Book underliner
Immunoglobulin	Writing pen
Allergy medication	Instant photo
Fever control medication	Windbreaker
Sore throat spray	Coffee mug
Skin cleansing products	Rubber bath toy
Laxative	Doughnuts
Digestive enzyme	T-shirt
Sun cream	Beach ball
Pain reliever	Coffee mug
Skin ointment	Travel contest

We all know that you do not get something for nothing. The cost of these promotion items—one part of the pharmaceutical industry's multi–billion-dollar advertising expenses—are eventually absorbed by consumers, the children and families we serve. In 1988, there were 16 pharmaceutical companies listed in the Fortune 500 group of the largest industrial corporations in the United States. Their combined sales of over $61 *billion* resulted in reported profits of nearly $8.3 billion. Fifteen of the companies had higher profits as a percent of sales than General Motors (*Fortune Magazine*. April 24, 1989:354-399)!

The other price of giveaways is a more subtle one, difficult to quantify, but arguably as real. Giveaways have the potential to cloud the objective evaluation of products by physicians.[1] At the American Academy of Pediatrics meeting, an exhibitor promoting a prescription-only topical steroid enticed pediatricians to the booth by giving away book underliners and magnifying lenses. After accepting such "gifts," people are much more likely to courteously listen to the sales pitch. They are also less likely to ask pointed questions, such as, Is this steroid any more effective [probably not] or more costly [almost certainly] than plain hydrocortisone?

I think giveaways should be abolished from professional meetings. As listed below in the tabulation of starting salaries, physicians are among the highest-earning individuals in the United States.[2,3]

Occupation	Income, $
Physicians	85 630
Dentists	40 190
Lawyers	32 757
Registered nurses	23 443
Computer programmers	22 531
Accountants	22 198
Typists	13 538
Minimum-wage earners ($3.35/h)	6968

They would not suffer any severe effects if deprived of free coffee mugs, writing pens, or book underliners. Instead of snapping instant photographs or offering free pens, let exhibitors use their marketing dollars to describe and demonstrate products, provide and discuss scientific studies (perhaps we can see some of the "data on file" that are often cited in drug advertisements), and answer probing questions about cost, toxicity, and relative effectiveness of alternate therapies. For the pediatrician who wants objective information about a medication or therapy, there is *The Medical Letter on Drugs and Therapeutics*, a nonprofit publication that does not accept drug company advertising. The giveaway ban should include product samples. If physicians want samples, they can have them mailed to their offices. This approach would be much less wasteful, and much safer for physicians' children, who need not have access to drugs brought home from medical meetings.

Of course, there is no guarantee that companies will pass on to consumers whatever savings are realized by a ban on giveaways. Even if the cost burden on families does not become lighter, at least our carry-on luggage—and our consciences—will be.

Lawrence R. Berger, MD, MPH
Lovelace Medical Foundation
2441 Ridgecrest SE
Albuquerque, NM 87108

1. Chren MM, Landefled S, Murray TH. Doctors, drug companies, and gifts. *JAMA*. 1989;262:3448-3451.
2. Average starting salary, by degree, 1988. In: *The World Almanac and Book of Facts 1989*. New York, NY: Newspaper Enterprise Association Inc; 1988:158-159.
3. *National Survey of Professional, Administrative, Technical and Clerical Pay: Private Non-Service Industries, March, 1988*. Washington, DC: US Dept of Labor, Bureau of Labor Statistics; 1988:12-14.

New York State Health Code 405 Update

Sir.—We appreciate Bedrick's editorial comments in the August issue of *AJDC*.[1] We would like to update our experience in more recent schedule revisions. The ultimate outcome measures of the schedule must be the quality of both patient care and resident learning. One must recall that, when night call was changed by a quantum leap from every second night to every third night for interns, studies of that modification were nonexistent. Thus, we are charting new waters. We plan to carefully monitor the quality of medical care with measures addressed by the hospital and Pediatric Department quality assurance protocols. Also, board scores will be closely scrutinized and each resident's yearly improvement compared with the individual resident improvement before the "405" schedule was started.

The only objective data to be reported thus far is the observations by the faculty that (1) the residents are more alert and awake than they were in the old system, and (2) continuity has improved compared with prior schedules. It is interesting to note that we are matching for the same number of residents that we did prior to the "405" regulations. Our straight pediatric postgraduate level 1 roster has been as follows: 51 in 1987-1988; 49 in 1988-1989; 52 in 1989-1990; and 49 in 1990-1991.

While the actual total number of house staff members has remained stable, there has been a small adjustment in service commitment and a reassignment of duties internally to accomplish our overall objective.

In addition to the above, the schedule has been changed to accommodate a "night float"/floor resident team and also a "day float" senior resident. Acceptance of these new revisions has been positively received by the house staff. It does seem that there is a realistic way to make resident working hours more reasonable and humane while maintaining a high-quality learning experience and providing high-quality patient care.

Gerald E. Daigler, MD
Robert C. Welliver, MD
F. Bruder Stapleton, MD
219 Bryant St
Buffalo, NY 14222

1. Bedrick AD. The eighty-hour workweek: residency friend or foe? *AJDC*. 1990;144:857.

Complex Problem: Complex Solutions

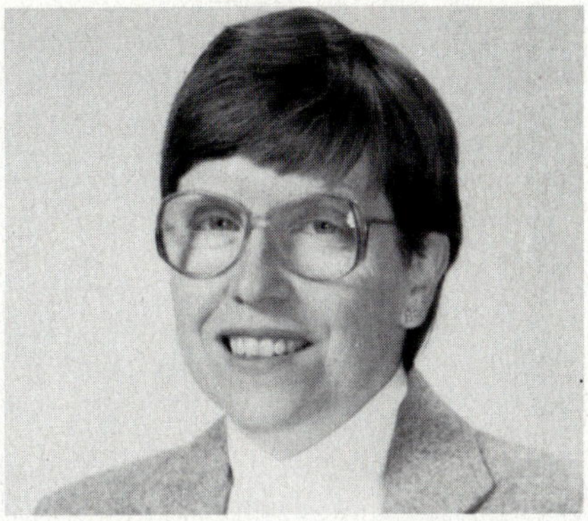

Elizabeth McAnarney, MD

"Lissa" continues to be a valuable addition to our editorial board. Her respected position within adolescent medicine has assisted us in the review of manuscripts, in ideas concerning features for* AJDC *involving adolescent issues, and in encouraging authors to submit their work to us for consideration.Currently, Lissa serves as associate chair of Academic Affairs in the Department of Pediatrics at the University of Rochester (NY) Medical Center and continues to head a vigorous Division of Adolescent Medicine as well. She serves as chair of the department's Promotion and Tenure Committee.

In 1990, Lissa received the Job Lewis Smith Award of the Section of Community Pediatrics, American Academy of Pediatrics, for her work in adolescent health. She also received a Distinguished Service Award from the American Medical Association at the National Congress on Youth in 1990.

Lissa is a much sought-after lecturer and most recently delivered talks at the University of Cincinnati, Ohio, and St Louis (Mo) University. She also continues her roles as mentor to fellows and as researcher; she published seven reports in 1990.

Lissa remains enthusiastic and of great help to* AJDC. *Her commentary on the complex problems of adolescent pregnancy below offers some principles to serve this troubled group.

The challenge of adolescent pregnancy has evoked responses from many sectors: society at large, religious groups, educators, health care professionals, parents, and adolescents themselves. We have every reason to engage in this dialogue, for adolescent pregnancy is one of our greatest challenges. As pediatricians, we are concerned about the health of adolescents and their children.

Adolescent pregnancy is a complex sociocultural and biologic condition. Attitudes about sexuality, sexual activity, pregnancy, contraception, and abortion are all rooted in the cultures and subcultures of our pluralistic society. The biologic capacity to reproduce is one of the hallmarks of adolescence and, for many young people, provides opportunities to fulfill lives that previously have had few accomplishments. To be close to another person (if only transiently), to attempt to prove one's femininity or masculinity by becoming pregnant or impregnating another, and/or to become a parent with new status are powerful motivators for some young people.

There may be few reasons for some young people to plan ahead, either by delaying sexual activity or, if sexually active, delaying pregnancy by using effective contraception. Adolescents, as they have in the past, will continue to become pregnant. Assuming, therefore, that adolescent pregnancy is an ongoing problem, we might ask a question similar to that asked by former New York City Mayor Edward Koch: How are they (adolescents and their children) doing? The answer to that question might be, "not too bad, but not too good."

The "not too bad" part reflects those successful prenatal interdisciplinary adolescent maternity projects that have resulted in improved short-term (ie, obstetric, neonatal, and psychosocial) outcomes as shown in several studies.[1,2] There have also been long-term, promising outcome data for the majority of mothers who were cared for in an adolescent maternity project in the late 1960s and were followed up 17 years later. The majority of these mothers had finished their educations, were not receiving public assistance, and were working at the time of follow-up.

The "not too good" part comes from data indicating distressing long-term outcomes for the children of these adolescent mothers, who themselves did so well. These children, as adolescents, had distressingly poor outcomes, eg, school failure, early sexual activity, and adolescent pregnancy.[3] In addition, the United States still has the highest adolescent pregnancy, birth, and abortion rates compared with those of other industrialized countries (the rate is expressed as the number of pregnancies per 1000 women in that age group). The following data compare the United States and the Netherlands: pregnancy rate, 109.9 vs 15.0, respectively; birth rate, 51.7 vs 7.7, respectively; and abortion rate 43.5 vs 5.3, respectively.[4]

Overall, these data, which are far from complete, indicate the complex nature of adolescent pregnancy and outcome. The solutions to adolescent pregnancy are complex; we should not promise simple panaceas for this challenging sociocultural-biologic phenomenon. Merely dedicating more financial resources to "solving" adolescent pregnancy is not the only strategy. If we articulate clear, nonjudgmental basic principles *and* follow them, adolescents and society will be well served. These basic principles might include the following:

1. It is better to delay sexual activity during early and middle adolescence and to avoid pregnancy. This principle could be supported by modeling dignity and respect between the sexes, demonstrating responsible sexual behavior, and providing decreased media attention to irresponsible sexual activity.
2. If young people become sexually active, they need to consider the consequences, not only to themselves, but also to their potential offspring and to society. Some may believe that most adolescents do not have the capacity to consider consequences meaningfully; some obviously will not be able to. Nevertheless, we must reinforce this basic principle by educating our young people in their families, schools, and health care settings about responsible sexuality. Parenthetically, we need better contraceptive methods that are independent of adolescents' behavior.
3. If a young person becomes pregnant and decides to keep her infant, she must enter prenatal care early and continue with it to optimize her outcome as well as her infant's. Other goals include returning to school to finish her education and securing the best child care possible to make sure the children have the best chance of achieving healthy futures.

If we follow these principles and perhaps others, we shall have served society and its young people honestly and consistently.

References

1. Felice EM, Granados JL, Ances IG, Hebel R, Roeder LM, Heald FP. The young pregnant teenager: impact of comprehensive prenatal care. *J Adolesc Health Care.* 1981;1:193-197.

2. McAnarney ER, Roghmann KJ, Charney E, et al. Obstetric, neonatal, and psychosocial outcome of pregnant adolescents. *Pediatrics.* 1978;61:199-205.

3. Furstenberg FF, Brooks-Gunn J, Morgan SP. Adolescent mothers and their children in later life. *Fam Plann Perspect.* 1987;19:142-152.

4. Jones EF, Forrest JD, Goldman N, et al. Teenage pregnancy in developed countries. *Fam Plann Perspect.* 1985;17:53-63.

Acquired Immunodeficiency Syndrome and Adolescents

Knowledge, Attitudes, and Behaviors of Runaway and Homeless Youths

Susan Tucker Sugerman, MD, MPH; Albert C. Hergenroeder, MD; Mariam R. Chacko, MD; Guy S. Parcel, PhD

• *Objective*: To describe the knowledge, attitudes, and behaviors of runaway and homeless youths regarding infection with the human immunodeficiency virus (HIV).
***Design*: Cross-sectional, descriptive.**
***Setting*: A crisis shelter for runaway and homeless youths.**
***Participants*: One hundred one residents, aged 13 to 20 years, of a shelter for homeless and runaway youths in Houston, Tex.**
***Intervention*: None.**
***Measurements/Main Results:* A self-administered questionnaire was used to examine the knowledge, attitudes, and behaviors of these youths regarding infection with HIV. Nearly one fourth had injected illegal drugs; one fifth had shared needles for other purposes. Sixteen percent had had anal intercourse, 19% had engaged in prostitution, and 67% of all subjects reported having four or more sexual partners. One fifth reported that they always use condoms. While quite knowledgeable about means of transmission, they held prevalent misconceptions about casual contact and risk reduction. Youths perceive few barriers to condom use, have fairly high intentions to practice preventive behavior, and have high self-efficacy to do so. Most believe they are at little or no risk for acquiring HIV. These findings support the need for medical, educational, and social service programs to reduce the risk of HIV among these youths.**
***Conclusion*: Runaway and homeless youths practice behaviors that place them at high risk for acquisition of HIV infection. Risk reduction is imperative and will require programs that address the educational, psychological, social, and medical needs of these youths.**
***(AJDC.* 1991;145:431-436)**

The adolescent population in the United States represents a potential high-risk group for acquiring the human immunodeficiency virus (HIV) and subsequently suffering acquired immunodeficiency syndrome (AIDS) because of sexual activity and experimentation with illegal drugs. Although persons aged 13 to 19 years account for less than 1% of all cases of AIDS in this country, young adults between the ages of 20 and 29 years represent 20% of all reported cases.[1] As the median interval between infection and onset of AIDS is nearly 10 years,[2] it is likely that many of these young adults with AIDS acquired the infection during their teenage years.

Information available on the seroprevalence of antibodies to HIV in adolescents is limited. Studies of groups of youths and young adults have shown seropositivity rates of 0.34% among 1 141 164 teenaged youths (younger than 20 years) applying for military service,[3] 0.41% among 84 089 Job Corps entrants, and 0.2% among 12 000 college students.[4,5] Ten (0.32%) of 3124 patients tested positive for HIV antibodies at an ambulatory clinic and emergency facility for adolescents in an urban center.[6]

Seroprevalence rates among homeless and runaway youths are remarkably higher. A shelter for such youths in New York, NY, reported that nearly 7% (74/1111) of its residents tested positive for HIV antibodies.[7] A Vancouver (British Columbia) study of HIV in the homeless reported a seroprevalence of 5.4% among 92 street youths aged 14 to 19 years.[8] A shelter for homeless and runaway youths in Houston, Tex, reported that 2.1% of 864 individuals tested between October 1988 and September 1989 showed evidence of HIV antibodies (L. F. Novick, MD, PhD, written communication, December 6, 1989). Similarly, serum testing of street youths using intravenous drugs in Houston revealed a positivity rate of 2% (M. L. Williams, PhD, written communication, March 22, 1990).

While many published studies address the knowledge, attitudes, and behaviors of the general adolescent population regarding HIV infection,[9] little is known about homeless adolescents. The few investigators examining risk behaviors of homeless and runaway youths have shown high rates of heterosexual and homosexual behavioPMR,[8,10,11] as well as prevalent anal intercourse,[8] prostitution, and drug abuse.[8,11,12] Many runaway and homeless youths have been abused sexually, suggesting another potential source of infection for these teenagers.[8,11,13]

To develop appropriate medical, educational, and social services to reduce the transmission of HIV among homeless and runaway youths, a better understanding is needed of the behavioral and psychosocial factors that

Accepted for publication September 4, 1990.
From the Univeristy of Texas School of Public Health (Dr Sugerman) and the Center for Health Promotion Research and Development (Dr Parcel), University of Texas School of Public Health, Houston; and the Sections of Adolescent Medicine (Drs Hergenroeder and Chacko) and Academic Ambulatory Pediatrics (Dr Chacko), Department of Pediatrics, Baylor College of Medicine, Houston, Tex. Dr Sugerman is currently with University of Cincinnati (Ohio) Children's Hospital Medical Center.
Reprints not available.

Table 1.—Demographic Characteristics of 101 Runaway and Homeless Youths at Shelter Facility in Houston, Tex, 1990

Characteristic	No. (%)
Sex	
F	38 (37.6)
M	63 (62.4)
Age, y	
13-14	6 (5.9)
15-16	19 (18.8)
17-18	37 (36.6)
19 or older	39 (38.6)
Race/ethnicity	
Black	29 (28.7)
White	52 (51.4)
Hispanic	12 (11.9)
Other	8 (8.0)

place this population at risk. This study examines the behaviors, knowledge, and attitudes regarding HIV and AIDS among adolescents recruited from a shelter for homeless and runaway youths in Houston.

SUBJECTS AND METHODS

Selection of Participants

This study was approved by the Committee for the Protection of Human Subjects at the University of Texas Health Science Center and the Institutional Review Board of Baylor College of Medicine, Houston.

Subjects were residents, aged 13 through 20 years, of a shelter for homeless and runaway youths who were invited to complete an anonymous, self-administered questionnaire at the shelter's clinic facility. Residents coming to the shelter clinic for any reason were invited to participate; youths in the residential buildings were invited to come to the clinic as their schedules permitted.

Verbal consent was obtained from the subjects after explaining the purpose of the study, stressing that no coding devices would be used, that names would not be recorded, and that participation was strictly voluntary. Each subject completed the questionnaire in a private room and returned it in a sealed envelope to a locked box. The principal investigator then met with each subject to answer any questions and provided them with educational pamphlets and information about HIV/AIDS counseling and testing resources.

Survey Instrument

The survey questionnaire was adapted with minor revisions from the Student Health Risk Survey by K. Basen-Engquist, PhD, and G.S.P. (written communication, November 13, 1989), which was designed to investigate knowledge, attitudes, behaviors, and various other cognitive variables regarding HIV and AIDS among high school students. To measure specific behavioral and psychosocial constructs, the questionnaire was divided into several scales made up of items specific to that variable. These scales could then be used to examine the relationships between variables associated with risk behaviors for HIV infection. Four behavior scales measured sexual activity (three questions), anal intercourse (two questions), prostitution (three questions), and needle use or exchange activities (five questions). An additional question addressed frequency of condom use. Twenty-three items determined a scale of factual knowledge regarding AIDS. Individual items addressed sources of information and testing resources. Cognitive variables derived from the Health Belief Model,[14] Theory of Reasoned Action,[15] and Social Learning Theory[16] were employed to examine perceived barriers to condom use (six questions), perceived susceptibility to HIV (two questions),[14] personal beliefs and social norms regarding sexual activity and condom use (three questions each), behavioral intentions to enact preventive behaviors (four questions),[15] and self-efficacy to perform preventive behaviors (13 questions).[16]

Table 2.—Risk Behaviors for HIV Infection Among 101 Runaway and Homeless Youths at Shelter Facility in Houston, Tex, 1990

Behavior (No. Responding)	No. (%)
Sexual activity	
No. of sexual partners	
Ever (100)	
0	4 (4.0)
1	19 (19.0)
2-3	10 (10.0)
4 or more	67 (67.0)
Last year (97)	
0	13 (13.4)
1	25 (25.8)
2-3	22 (22.7)
4 or more	37 (38.1)
Age at first intercourse, y (100)	
Virgin	4 (4.0)
12 or younger	38 (38.0)
13-15	41 (41.0)
16-17	15 (15.0)
18 or older	2 (2.0)
Frequency of condom use (99)	
Virgin	4 (4.0)
Always	20 (20.2)
Sometimes	42 (42.4)
Rarely or never	33 (33.3)
Anal intercourse (98)	
Ever	16 (16.3)
Last year	15 (15.3)
Prostitution (100)	19 (19.0)
Sexual preference (males; 61)	
Virgin	1 (1.6)
Heterosexual	49 (80.3)
Homosexual	7 (11.5)
Bisexual	4 (6.6)
Needle use	
Ever injected drugs (99)	24 (24.2)
Injected in last year (98)	14 (14.3)
Shared needles for drugs (100)	12 (12.0)
Shared needles last year (100)	11 (11.0)
Shared for blood brothers, tattooing, piercing ears (100)	21 (21.0)

Another scale involved anxiety regarding interacting with persons with AIDS.

Data Analysis

Data were collected during a 3-week period ending in February 1990. Subjects' responses were entered into dBASE III PLUS[17] and subsequently analyzed using the Statistical Package for the Social Sciences (SPSS).[18] Items were examined individually and by scales where appropriate. Descriptive analysis was performed using all responses, with percentages reported excluding missing values. For χ^2 tests of independence of items, missing values were excluded pairwise. For the purpose of scale analyses, four cases were deleted because subjects left more than 20% of the questionnaire unanswered, and all scale items were counted as missing if subjects left more than 20% of that scale unanswered. Student's t tests for independence of means excluded missing values pairwise. Pearson's correlation coefficient was used to determine correlation between scale scores.

RESULTS

Of 110 residents invited, 101 agreed to participate (92% response rate), representing 46% of the 221 youths residing at the shelter at any time during the study period. One individual was excluded owing to inability to speak or understand English. Subject characteristics are reported in Table 1.

Table 3.—Scale and Reliability Scores Measuring Behavior and Cognitive Variables for 97 Runaway and Homeless Youths at Shelter Facility in Houston, Tex, 1990*

Variable (No. Responding)	Range	Mean ± SE	Cronbach's α
Sexual activity: first intercourse, No. of partners in lifetime, past year (95)	0-12	8.55 ± 0.328	.738
Anal intercourse: lifetime or past year (95)	0-2	0.305 ± 0.070	.887
Prostitution for money, drugs, place to stay (97)	0-3	0.402 ± 0.092	.862
Needle use: IV drugs or needle sharing (95)	0-5	0.853 ± 0.150	.838
Knowledge (97)	0-23	17.0 ± 0.478	.864
Personal beliefs supporting intercourse with boyfriend or girlfriend, multiple partners, sex without condoms (96)	0-12	4.65 ± 0.242	.354
Social norms supporting intercourse with boyfriend or girlfriend, multiple partners, sex without condoms (96)	0-12	6.76 ± 0.282	.517
Behavioral intentions regarding preventive behaviors (92)	0-16	9.42 ± 0.339	.626
Perceived barriers to condom use (95)	0-24	7.23 ± 0.545	.654
Perceived susceptibility to HIV (92)	0-6	2.28 ± 0.193	.835
Self-efficacy to enact preventive behaviors (86)	0-39	30.2 ± 0.773	.889
Anxiety about interacting with persons with AIDS (97)	0-12	2.87 ± 0.278	.710

*Four respondents were deleted owing to greater than 20% missing responses. IV indicates intravenous; HIV, human immunodeficiency virus, and AIDS, acquired immunodeficiency syndrome.

Risk behaviors are reported in Table 2. Scale and reliability scores measuring behavior and cognitive variables and reliabilities are reported in Table 3.

Risk Behaviors for HIV Infection and AIDS

It is evident from Table 2 that many youths are involved in high-risk behavior for acquisition of HIV infection. Based on scale scores for risk behaviors, those who had ever injected drugs or had recently shared needles for injecting drugs were more likely to have been involved in a sexual exchange for money, drugs, or a place to stay ($F=4.94$, $P<.01$; $F=3.14$, $P=.04$); likewise, those trading sex for money, drugs, or a place to stay scored higher on a scale for needle use ($F=1.73$, $P<.01$; $F=1.97$, $P<.01$; and $F=1.6$, $P<.01$). Those who reported being forced to have sexual intercourse scored higher on scales for prostitution ($F=1.69$, $P=.05$) and anal intercourse ($F=4.34$, $P<.01$).

Knowledge

On 23 questions testing knowledge regarding HIV and AIDS, subjects scored a mean of 75% correct responses. At least 86% correctly identified having sex without a condom, sharing needles or syringes, and pregnancy as means of transmitting HIV. Most subjects (72%) knew that AIDS is not transmitted by having a blood test; however, only 49% knew that it is not transmitted by donating blood, and only 31% responded that almost all transfusions are now safe. The subjects answered questions correctly about whether casual contact transmits HIV at least 85% of the time, with some exceptions: few knew that mosquitoes (47%), public toilets (69%), and coughs or sneezes (69%) do not pose risks for HIV transmission. More than one third believed they could reduce their risk by washing or urinating after sex (39% and 37%, respectively) or by making sure a sexual partner looks healthy (38%). Most knew that one cannot tell by appearances if someone has AIDS (68%), that people other than homosexual men can get the disease (84%), and that there is no cure for AIDS (78%).

Attitudes and Cognitive Variables

Regarding condom use, few had religious or moral objections to using condoms (15%) or believed that condoms make sex seem dirty (16%), and only 16% believed that using a condom to prevent AIDS is embarrassing. Twenty-six percent believed it can be important not to use a condom to show love and trust for someone, and 55% believed that condoms make sex seem planned. The majority (87%) believed that condoms probably or definitely should be used if a person is sexually active; however, only 58% believed that their peers shared this belief.

Ninety-two percent reported knowing where to get condoms. They felt certain they could get a condom if they wanted one (90%), could have it with them when they needed it (76%), and could get their partner to agree to use the condom (74%). Similarly, 74% felt confident that they could refuse sexual intercourse if their partner refused to use a condom. Less than half (32%) of those feeling confident about having a condom with them when they needed it reported actually using them always or sometimes ($\chi^2=13.76$, $P<.01$), and only 44% of those feeling confident about getting their partner to agree to use condoms reported using condoms always or sometimes ($\chi^2=5.85$, $P=.02$).

Results regarding beliefs about sexual activity indicated that 76% believed sex with a steady boyfriend or girlfriend was appropriate, and 74% believed that their peers believed the same. Of note, only 18% personally believed sex with multiple partners was appropriate, whereas 54% believed that their peers held this view.

Overall, 29% reported being worried about getting AIDS, although more female respondents (46%) reported being worried than male respondents (19%). Those who reported being worried were more likely to respond that someone had tried to force them to have sex against their will (68%) than those who were not worried (36%). More female (68%) than male respondents (28%) reported someone attempting to force them to have sex when they did not want to.

Regarding their perceived risk of getting HIV or AIDS, only 9% of the subjects viewed themselves as being at high risk for acquiring HIV; 19% believed they were at medium risk. Thirty-five percent reported themselves at low risk, and 36% believed they were at no risk at all. When asked about their risk at some future time (age 21 years), the numbers of those who predicted themselves to be at high, medium, and low risk increased to 17%, 18%, and 38%, respectively; 28% predicted that they would be at no risk in the future. Among those who predicted themselves to be at high risk for HIV infection in the future, only 29% reported using condoms always or sometimes.

Regarding their intentions to practice preventive behaviors to protect themselves from HIV infection and AIDS, 31% responded that they would abstain from sex, 22% were not sure, and 48% probably or definitely would not refrain from sex. Sixty-eight percent said they would talk with their partners about HIV and AIDS before deciding whether or not to have intercourse; 85% felt confident they could do this. Fifty-two percent said they would always, and 24% said they would sometimes discuss using condoms with their partners before deciding whether or not to have sex; 88% felt sure they could do the same. Fifty-one percent intended always to use condoms when having sex, and 27% intended to use them sometimes. Female respondents were more likely than male respondents to intend to practice preventive behaviors ($F=1.16$, $P=.01$).

On the whole, subjects felt little anxiety about interacting with persons with AIDS. Only 4% said they would stop being friends with someone with AIDS; 7% said they would be afraid to hug a friend who had AIDS. Few believed persons with AIDS should be kept away from others or would mind being in the same room as someone with AIDS (8% and 9%, respectively). More were worried about catching AIDS in a public restroom (35%) and reported they would be afraid to kiss a boyfriend or girlfriend who had AIDS (31%).

While more subjects reported having talked with a friend (81%) than an adult (60%) about HIV and AIDS, most believed they knew where to get information about AIDS (71%) and how to avoid acquiring HIV (93%). Two thirds (67%) reported knowing where to get tested for antibodies to HIV.

Correlations of Scale Score

Scale analysis showed a significant positive correlation between prostitution and needle use ($r=.316$, $P<.01$). Anal intercourse was weakly correlated with needle use as well ($r=.214$, $P=.04$). Increased sexual activity was weakly correlated with prostitution ($r=.198$, $P=.05$) and with decreased intention to practice preventive behavior ($r=-.354$, $P=.001$). Prostitution was inversely correlated with intention to practice preventive behaviors ($r=-.227$, $P=.03$). Increased social anxiety about interacting with persons with AIDS was correlated with increased barriers to using condoms ($r=.441$, $P<.001$). While behavior was not associated significantly with knowledge, increased knowledge was correlated with decreased anxiety about interacting with persons with AIDS ($r=-.409$, $P<.001$) and with decreased barriers to condom use ($r=-.531$, $P<.001$). Increased self-efficacy to enact preventive behavior was found to be correlated with decreased anxiety ($r=-.307$, $P<.01$), decreased barriers to condom use ($r=-.426$, $P<.001$), and decreased perceived susceptibility to AIDS ($r=-.243$, $P=.03$).

COMMENT

This study confirms that homeless and runaway youths engage in behavior putting them at increased risk for acquiring HIV infection. The rate of intravenous drug abuse, rate of needle sharing among drug users, number of sexual partners, and rate of prostitution reported herein compare with results in other studies of runaways, street youths, and crack users.[6,8,11,12,19] The rate of intravenous drug abuse, however, is much higher than that of American high school students, reported to be between 1%[20] and 6.3%.[21] It is difficult to make an exact comparison of the number of sexual partners reported in this study with numbers in college and high school studies, as investigators report the number of partners according to varying parameters.[21,22]

Reported rates of anal intercourse in this study must be interpreted with caution, as several subjects inquired about the meaning of the term "anal intercourse." It may be that others also were unclear about its meaning and did not ask. Noting this, the rate of anal intercourse found in the study sample is similar to rates reported for inner-city black and Hispanic youths, other homeless youths, and black college students[8,23-25] and higher than reported for college women (9%).[22]

While many of the subjects are at high risk for acquiring HIV, participants perceive themselves to be at less risk than adolescents surveyed in other studies. Fewer than 10% of the subjects in this study view themselves at high risk now, and 17% believe they will be at high risk in the future. The reason for the perception of low risk is unclear, but one may speculate that survival on the street gives these youths a false sense of security and perceived invulnerability.

These youths are knowledgeable about high-risk behavior for the transmission of HIV but understand less about the low risk of casual contact and about blood products. These results are similar to those of other adolescent HIV/AIDS knowledge surveys.[21,25-29] The misunderstandings about oral contraceptives, washing after sexual intercourse, urinating after sexual intercourse, and choosing partners who look healthy indicate that myths about reducing risk of acquiring HIV infection persist despite high levels of factual knowledge regarding other aspects of HIV and AIDS. The media and medical communities should work together to reinforce the facts and dispel the myths.

This study found no relationship between knowledge and behavior but did find significant relationships between increased knowledge and decreased perceived barriers to condom use and between increased knowledge and decreased social anxiety about interacting with persons with AIDS. The latter two findings are encouraging and suggest that knowledge may be associated with more favorable beliefs and behaviors. The low anxiety about interacting with people with AIDS may have been influenced by the presence of an HIV-infected individual residing at the shelter shortly before the study period. This person was open about the diagnosis, which led to much discussion about HIV and AIDS among the residents.

The number of youths in this study who always or sometimes use condoms is similar to numbers reported in other studies on homeless and runaway youths,[8] Massachusetts teenagers,[26] and males at an urban health center.[30] It seems that these youths know the value of condoms in preventing the spread of AIDS, know where to get them, and feel comfortable using them when they need to. This information suggests that lack of information about condoms or access to them may not be the primary cause of their actual failure to use condoms. Rather, it may be related to the decision to use condoms at the time of intercourse. Counseling on how to use the condom during moments of sexual intimacy may improve condom use.

Significant discrepancies were noted between subject's personal beliefs about sexual behavior and their perceptions of their peers' beliefs about sexual behavior and condom use. This information suggests that perceived peer opinion may be more influential than personal beliefs in determining behavior for these adolescents. Weinstein's[31] theory of optimistic bias may also partly explain the discrepancy between perceived peer beliefs and personal beliefs. He observed that college students consistently believed that their actions, life-styles, and personalities were more advantageous than those of their peers and were capable of keeping their thoughts about their own behavior and their vulnerability in quite separate mental compartments. Educational efforts should therefore take into consideration the perceived norms for behavior and strategies used to develop norms more consistent with lower-risk behavior. In addition, educational efforts need strongly to emphasize the link between behavior and susceptibility, stressing that youths who engage in high-risk behavior need to see themselves as the ones most likely to suffer harm.

Scale analysis proved useful in determining associations and correlations among factors that may contribute to the risk status of these youths. Of particular note, subjects scored high on the scale for self-efficacy to enact preventive behavior, a finding that contrasts sharply with their reported behaviors. It is paradoxical also that those who are least confident both of their ability to have condoms when necessary and to get partners to use condoms actually reported using them more often than those who are more confident. One could hypothesize that their reported self-efficacy to enact preventive behavior is a reflection of their highly developed survival skills as runaways.

Study Limitations

Because subjects were not recruited using random probability techniques, results may be subject to bias. Youths with full-time day jobs or those attending school participated in the study before or after these other commitments but may have been underrepresented. While closely representative of gender and age distributions noted among shelter residents in 1989, this sample may be disproportionately overrepresented by whites (51.5% in this study vs 32.8% in 1989) and underrepresented by blacks (28.7% in this study vs 45.3% in 1989).[32]

The self-reporting of risk behaviors, which could not be independently verified, represents a potential source of bias in this and any study investigating behavior associated with acquisition of HIV. However, all efforts were made to provide confidentiality and anonymity to encourage subjects to represent their behaviors accurately.

Conclusion

This study describes a population whose knowledge and attitudes are inconsistent with their high-risk behaviors. Programs are needed to help these youths develop more realistic perceptions of their susceptibility. Also, more research is needed regarding the factors that contribute to condom use at the time of intercourse and on how behavioral intentions translate into actions. The relative impact on behavior of social norms vs personal beliefs deserves further investigation. The relationship of self-efficacy to behavior warrants more study as well.

As suggested by their prevalent risk behaviors and substantiated by seroprevalence studies, homeless and runaway youths are vulnerable to acquiring HIV infection. Efforts aimed at protecting these youths from HIV should also help slow the spread of the disease generally, as intervention may be more efficiently directed toward a smaller subgroup with known risks than toward a larger population with fewer risks. Unfortunately, homeless and runaway youths may be among the most difficult to access, as their life-styles cause them to be disfranchised from conventional medical and social services. Public health efforts to stop the spread of the disease among them should take advantage of and expand on existing resources that reach these youths, including shelter facilities, street outreach programs, food pantries, community health clinics, and other social service agencies. Furthermore, serious efforts should be directed toward understanding the determinants of their homelessness, such as dysfunctional family situations, home sexual abuse, poverty, and poor education. Taking steps to alleviate these conditions should help prevent these youths from adopting the behaviors that place them at risk for acquiring HIV infection.

We are indebted to Hardy Loe, Jr, MD, MPH, and Karen Basen-Engquist, PhD, for their roles in making this study possible, and to Ronald Lorimer, PhD, for his assistance with data analysis. We are grateful to Lin Holliday, RN, Doris Walker, RN, and Margaret Gonzalez of Covenant House, Houston, for their support and cooperation in conducting this study, as well as to Karen Griffin and Norma Womack of Texas Children's Hospital, Houston, for their administrative assistance. Special thanks for his valuable suggestions and editorial skills are due to Robert W. Sugerman, MD.

References

1. Centers for Disease Control. AIDS cases by sex, age at diagnosis, and race/ethnicity, reported through January 1990, United States. *HIV/AIDS Surveil.* Washington, DC: US Dept of Health and Human Services. February 1990:1-18.

2. Bacchetti P, Moss AR. Incubation period of AIDS in San Francisco. *Nature.* 1989;338:251-253.

3. Burke DS, Brundage JF, Goldenbaum M, et al. Human immunodeficiency virus infections in teenagers: seroprevalence among applicants for US military service. *JAMA.* 1990;263:2074-2077.

4. Centers for Disease Control. AIDS and human immunodeficiency virus infection in the United States: 1988 update. *MMWR.* 1989;38(suppl 4):1-38.

5. Dondero TJ Jr, Pappaioanou M, Curran JW. Monitoring the levels and trends of HIV infection: the Public Health Service's HIV surveillance program. *Public Health Rep.* 1988;103:213-220.

6. D'Angelo LJ, Getson P, David C, Luban N, Gayle H. Seroprevalence of HIV infection in urban adolescents. *Pediatr Res.* 1989;25:4A. Abstract.

7. Stricof RL, Novick LF, Kennedy JT, Weisfuse IB. Seroprevalence of antibodies to human immunodeficiency virus I in a facility for runaway or homeless adolescents in New York City. Presented at the annual meeting of the American Public Health Association; November 14, 1988; Boston, Mass.

8. Radford JL, King AJC, Warren WK. *Street Youth and AIDS.* Ottawa, Ontario; Social Program Evaluation Group, Queen's University at Kingston; 1989. Federal Centre for AIDS, Health Protection Branch, Health and Welfare Canada.

9. Hein K. AIDS in adolescence: exploring the challenge. *J Adolesc Health Care.* 1989;10:10S-35S.

10. Council on Scientific Affairs. Health care needs of homeless and runaway youths. *JAMA.* 1989;262:1358-1361.

11. Yates GL, MacKenzie R, Pennbridge J, Cohen E. A risk profile comparison of runaway and non-runaway youth. *Am J Public Health.* 1988;78:820-821.

12. Goldman B. Health of Toronto's street kids disturbing, study reveals. *Can Med Assoc J.* 1988;138:1041-1043.
13. Swartz J. Runaways often sexually abused: symposium. *Can Med Assoc J.* 1986;134:944-948.
14. Janz NK, Becker MH. The Health Belief Model: a decade later. *Health Educ Q.* 1984;11:1-47.
15. Azjen I, Fishbein M. *Understanding Attitudes and Predicting Social Behavior.* Englewood Cliffs, NJ: Prentice-Hall International Inc; 1980.
16. Bandura A. *Social Foundations of Thought and Action: A Social Cognitive Theory.* Englewood Cliffs, NJ: Prentice-Hall International Inc; 1986.
17. dBASE III PLUS. Torrance, Calif: Ashton-Tate; 1986.
18. SPSS/PC+ V2.0. Chicago, Ill: SPSS, Inc; 1988.
19. Fullilove RE, Fullilove MT, Bowser BP, Gross SA. Risk of sexually transmitted disease among black adolescent crack users in Oakland and San Francisco, Calif. *JAMA.* 1990;263:851-855.
20. Kandel DB, Logan JA. Patterns of drug use from adolescence to young adulthood, I: periods of risk for initiation, continued use, and discontinuation. *Am J Public Health.* 1984;74:660-666.
21. Centers for Disease Control. HIV-related beliefs, knowledge, and behaviors among high school students. *MMWR.* 1988;37:717-721.
22. DeBuono BA, Zinner SH, Daamen M, McCormack WM. Sexual behavior of college women in 1975, 1986, and 1989. *N Engl J Med.* 1990;322:821-825.
23. Jaffe LR, Seehaus M, Wagner C, Leadbeater BJ. Anal intercourse and knowledge of acquired immunodeficiency syndrome among minority-group female adolescents. *J Pediatr.* 1988;112:1005-1007.
24. Thomas SB, Gilliam AG, Iwrey CG. Knowledge about AIDS and reported risk behaviors among black college students. *J Am Coll Health.* 1989;38:61-66.
25. You know about safe sex, but are you using condoms? *AIDS Alert.* 1990;5:21-40.
26. Hingson R, Strunin L, Berlin B. Acquired immunodeficiency syndrome transmission: changes in knowledge and behaviors among teenagers, Massachusetts statewide surveys, 1986 to 1988. *Pediatrics.* 1990;85:24-29.
27. DiClemente RJ, Zorn J, Temoshok L. Adolescents and AIDS: a survey of knowledge, attitudes and beliefs about AIDS in San Francisco. *Am J Public Health.* 1986;76:1443-1445.
28. Goodman E, Cohall AT. Acquired immunodeficiency syndrome and adolescents: knowledge, attitudes, beliefs, and behaviors in a New York City adolescent minority population. *Pediatrics.* 1989;84:36-42.
29. Seltzer VL, Rabin J, Benjamin F. Teenagers' awareness of the acquired immunodeficiency syndrome and the impact on their sexual behavior. *Obstet Gynecol.* 1989;74:55-58.
30. Glasser M, Dennis J, Orthoefer J, Carter S, Hollander E. Characteristics of males at a public health department contraceptive service. *J Adolesc Health Care.* 1989;10:115-118.
31. Weinstein ND. Why it won't happen to me: perceptions of risk factors and susceptibility. *Health Psychol.* 1984;3:431-457.
32. Hustoft K. *A Descriptive Cross-sectional Study of Runaways and Homeless Adolescents, 10 to 21 Entering Covenant House Texas, a Shelter for Homeless Children in Houston, Texas.* Houston, Tex: University of Texas School of Public Health; 1989. Thesis.

In Other AMA Journals

ARCHIVES OF GENERAL PSYCHIATRY

Traumatic Events and Posttraumatic Stress Disorder in an Urban Population of Young Adults

Naomi Breslau, PhD; Glenn C. Davis, MD; Patricia Andreski, MA; Edward Peterson, PhD
(*Arch Gen Psychiatry.* 1991;48:216-222)

ARCHIVES OF NEUROLOGY

Seizure Disorders in Down Syndrome

Siegfried M. Pueschel, MD, PhD, MPH; Sydney Louis, MD; Pamela McKnight, MD
(*Arch Neurol.* 1991;48:318-320)

Arthur Conan Doyle, Joseph Bell, and Sherlock Holmes: A Neurologic Connection

Barbara F. Estmoreland, MD, Jack D. Key, MS
(*Arch Neurol.* 1991;48:325-329)

ARCHIVES OF PATHOLOGY & LABORATORY MEDICINE

Extramedullary Hematopoiesis in the Liver in Sudden Infant Death Syndrome

Enid F. Gilbert-Barness, MD; Katherine Kenison; Gary Giulian; Sunita Chandra, MBBS
(*Arch Pathol Lab Med.* 1991;115:226-229)

The Ectopic Ovary: A Case Report and Review of the Literature

Mary F. Lachman, MD, Martin M. Berman, MD
(*Arch Pathol Lab Med.* 1991;115:233-235)

The Role of the United Network for Organ Sharing and Designated Organ Procurement Organizations in Organ Retrieval for Transplantation

James S. Wolf, MD
(*Arch Pathol Lab Med.* 1991;115:246-249)

The Total Iron-Binding Capacity in Iron Poisoning

Is It Useful?

Milton Tenenbein, MD, FRCPC, FAAP, Randall W. Yatscoff, PhD, FCACB

• **Traditionally, a serum iron concentration in excess of the total iron-binding capacity (TIBC) is considered as an indication for deferoxamine therapy in acute iron poisoning. We observed a reversible elevation of the TIBC in patients with iron poisoning that coincided with their acute hyperferremia and have hypothesized that this is a laboratory aberration. We tested this hypothesis in vitro and found that the addition of iron to test serum samples produced a related increase in the TIBC, and alteration of the assay by providing additional adsorbent prevented this occurrence. We also evaluated the reproducibility of the TIBC as performed by 500 laboratories on 10 different reference samples. The mean coefficient of variation was 16%, which was unsatisfactory. We concluded that the TIBC should not be used in the decision for the initiation of deferoxamine therapy in acute iron poisoning. Furthermore, high TIBC values that are occasionally seen in patients with iron poisoning should not be considered as providing a protective effect.**

(*AJDC.* 1991;145:437-439)

A serum iron concentration greater than the total iron-binding capacity (TIBC) is often cited as a criterion for the initiation of deferoxamine therapy in patients with iron poisoning.[1] This recommendation is attractive because it assumes that the binding of iron to plasma proteins prevents toxic damage. Our review of the literature could not find data that support this practice; however, we did find that this recommendation coincides with the commercial availability of deferoxamine.[2] We have observed several patients with iron poisoning with TIBC determinations that are above the reference range and that return to normal with a fall in the serum iron concentration (Table). An unusual TIBC in a patient with hyperferremia has been documented by others.[3] We designed the following experiments to test the hypothesis that this elevation of the TIBC is a laboratory aberration and not a true event.

Accepted for publication November 27, 1990.

From the Departments of Pediatrics (Dr Tenenbein), Medicine (Drs Tenenbein and Yatscoff), and Clinical Chemistry (Dr Yatscoff), University of Manitoba, Winnipeg, and The Manitoba Poison Control Centre, Winnipeg (Dr Tenenbein).

Presented at the annual scientific meeting of the American Academy of Clinical Toxicology, Atlanta, Ga, October 12, 1989.

Reprint requests to Children's Hospital, 840 Sherbook St, Winnipeg, Manitoba, Canada R3A 1S1 (Dr Tenenbein).

MATERIALS AND METHODS

An automated analyzer (Du Pont aca, Du Pont Inc, Wilmington, Del) was used for the serum iron and TIBC measurements. The manufacturer's method for measuring serum iron was followed, and the magnesium carbonate method of Ramsay[4] (100 mg of magnesium carbonate) was used for measuring the TIBC (Fig 1, top). Tests were done in the hospital service laboratory that participated in the Wellcome General Clinical Chemistry Quality Assessment Program (Wellcome Diagnostics, Division of the Wellcome Foundation, London, England).

Four experiments were performed as follows: (1) Test serum samples were spiked with iron to final measured concentrations of 52 to 1560 μmol/L (286 to 8560 μg/dL), and TIBCs were quantified. (2) Test serum samples were spiked with iron as ferrioxamine to final calculated concentrations of 0 to 1000 μmol/L, and TIBCs were quantified to determine if ferrioxamine interfered with the measurement of the TIBC. (3) Two pools of test serum samples were spiked with 10 and 100 μmol/L (55 and 550 μg/dL) of iron. To each, serial dilutions of deferoxamine mesylate were added in concentrations of 0 to 500 μmol/L, and TIBCs were quantified to determine if deferoxamine interfered with this assay. (4) Experiment 1 was repeated with twice the amount of magnesium carbonate. Pooled human serum obtained from the Canadian Red Cross Blood Bank, Winnipeg, Manitoba, were used throughout. Deferoxamine was obtained from a manufacturer (Ciba-Geigy Canada, Mississauga, Ontario), and ferrioxamine was prepared in house by combining equimolar amounts of stock iron with deferoxamine. The concentration of ferrioxamine was confirmed by its absorbability at 435 nm, ie, its absorption maximum. All experiments were done in triplicate, and mean results are presented.

We also assessed the interlaboratory reproducibility of the TIBC measurement under conditions of normoferremia. We chose the results for 10 random samples from 500 laboratories that submitted values for the TIBC to the Wellcome General Clinical Chemistry Quality Assessment Program. We calculated the mean coefficients of variation of the TIBC determinations for each of the 10 submitted specimens performed by these laboratories.

RESULTS

The results of experiments 1, 2, and 4 are shown in Fig 2. For illustrative purposes, we have only included iron concentrations of 0 to 600 μmol/L (0 to 3300 μg/dL). The trends continue to be unchanged beyond this range, and the clinically relevant concentrations are included within it. The TIBC began to rise when the serum iron concentration exceeded 72 μmol/L (396 μg/dL) and consistently rose in a nonproportional fashion. This was not observed with the addition of iron as ferrioxamine (experiment 2) or with the addition of deferoxamine to serum samples that were previously spiked with iron (experiment 3). The

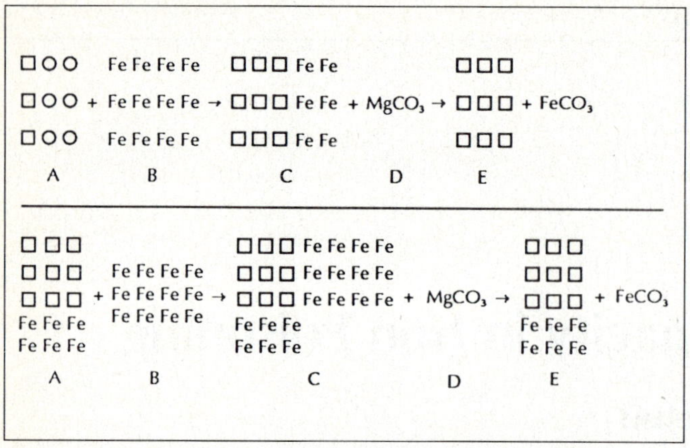

Fig 1.—*Top, Measurement of the total iron-binding capacity in the normal patient. To the patient's serum (A), a standard amount of exogenous iron (B) is added. This occupies all of the binding sites and produces a mild excess of unbound iron (C). To this, a standard amount of magnesium carbonate ($MgCO_3$) (D) is added that forms complexes with the unbound iron (E). After centrifugation, the iron in the supernatant is measured, that is the total iron-binding capacity. Bottom, Measurement of the total iron-binding capacity in the patient with iron poisoning. In this situation, the binding sites are totally saturated, and exogenous iron is present (A). Addition of the standard amount of excess iron (B) creates a situation of massive unbound iron (C). This exogenous iron, along with the ingested iron, overwhelms the capacity for complexation by the routine amount of $MgCO_3$. Because centrifugation only removes the iron carbonate complexes, the subsequent iron assay measures both the bound and free iron (E), thus overestimating the total iron-binding capacity. Squares indicate bound iron; circles, binding sites; Fe, free iron; and $FeCO_3$, iron carbonate.*

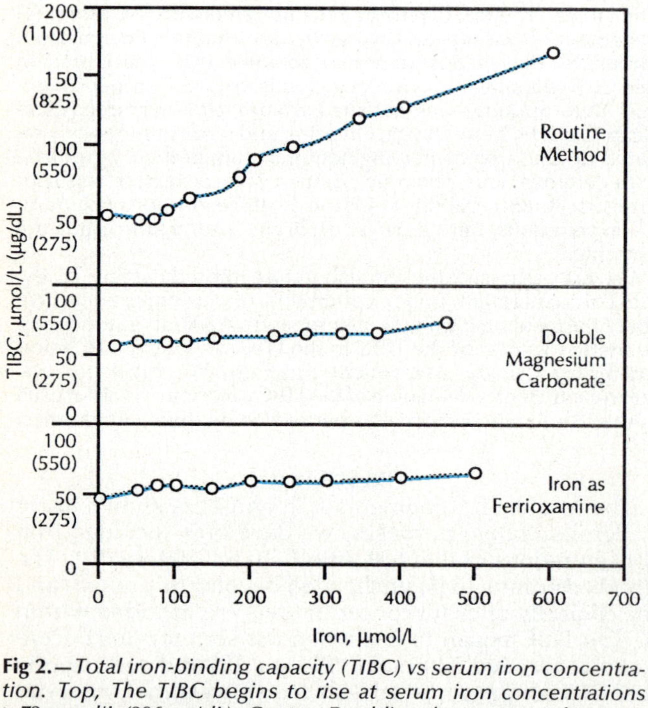

Fig 2.—*Total iron-binding capacity (TIBC) vs serum iron concentration. Top, The TIBC begins to rise at serum iron concentrations >72 µmol/L (396 µg/dL). Center, Doubling the amount of magnesium carbonate largely ablates this observation. Bottom, Iron as ferrioxamine does not affect the TIBC.*

Serum Iron Concentrations and TIBCs in Four Patients With Iron Overdose*

Patient	Hours After Overdose	Serum Iron Concentration, µmol/L (µg/dL)	TIBC, µmol/L (µg/dL)
1	5	1631 (8970)	560 (3080)
	8	958 (5270)	244 (1344)
	24	44 (244)	47 (256)
2†	2	108 (594)	114 (627)
	7	76 (418)	90 (495)
	8	57 (314)	87 (479)
3	3	83 (457)	81 (446)
	7	72 (396)	69 (380)
	15	42 (231)	63 (347)
4	3	95 (523)	87 (479)
	6	540 (2970)	159 (875)
	10	281 (1546)	123 (677)
	26	44 (242)	57 (314)
Normal range	. . .	8-24 (44-132)	45-72 (250-400)

*TIBCs indicates total iron-binding capacities.
†This patient was treated with deferoxamine, and she produced orange urine, indicating the presence of ferrioxamine.

addition of twice the amount of magnesium carbonate (experiment 4) largely ablated the increase of the TIBC. However, minor increases of approximately 30% to 40% were still observed when the serum iron concentration was greater than 225 µmol/L (1238 µg/dL).

Our evaluation of the results of the 10 random samples from the Wellcome General Clinical Chemistry Quality Assessment Program found coefficients of variation that ranged from 11.8% to 21.4%, with a mean of 16%. For a TIBC of 60 µmol/L (325 µg/dL), this represented a 95% confidence interval of 41 to 79 µmol/L (221 to 429 µg/dL), which is clearly too broad a range to be acceptable as a criterion for initiation of deferoxamine therapy.

COMMENT

Unreliability of the TIBC has previously been mentioned,[3] and we have found other examples of abnormally elevated TIBC values, albeit uncommented on, in published series of patients with iron poisoning. In one study, there were five patients with TIBC determinations greater than 90 µmol/L (495 µg/dL), with the highest being 212 µmol/L (1168 µg/dL),[5] while another study had seven such patients, with the highest TIBC determination being 169 µmol/L (930 µg/dL).[6] An ion exchange resin rather than the magnesium carbonate method was used in the latter study.[6] Although these reagents differ, they both serve as adsorbents for the excess iron; thus, the principle of the assays is identical. The upper limit of normal was not stated in these studies, but in our laboratory, it is 72 µmol/L (400 µg/dL). In addition to the hyperferremia of acute iron overdose, a TIBC elevation as high as 273 µmol/L (1500 µg/dL) has been observed after the therapeutic administration of iron dextran.[7] These data complement our observation (Table).

We believe we have proved our hypothesis that the increase of the TIBC in iron poisoning is a laboratory aberration because we have replicated this finding in vitro, and we have prevented its occurrence by altering the laboratory procedure (experiment 4).

Examination of the principles of TIBC determination, as depicted in Fig 1, helps to provide an explanation for this phenomenon. Another source for error is that the adsorbed iron is not always centrifuged out from the supernatant.[8] Reliability could be improved by modifying the assay or using a different one altogether. The obvious modification is to increase the amount of added magnesium carbonate. However, the actual amount needed is dependent on prior knowledge of the serum iron concentration, and the use of variable amounts of magnesium carbonate creates a greater potential for error. Also, these determinations would then have to be consecutive rather than concurrent, which lengthens the turnaround time for a test that is required on an emergent basis. A further complicating factor is that the amount of magnesium carbonate required is also dependent on its adsorptive properties, which can vary from one preparation to another.[4]

Total iron-binding capacity methods, based on other analytical principles, have been reported. Some used ion exchange resins or hemoglobin-coated charcoal rather than magnesium carbonate,[9] while others used alumina columns.[8] However, because the principle is the same, abnormal TIBC determinations could result and indeed have been observed.[6] In one comparison study, the magnesium carbonate method was preferred.[9]

The immunochemical methods for measuring the TIBC actually measure transferrin that is then considered as the TIBC.[10] This is reasonable in patients with normal or near-normal iron status[10] but may not be so with the acute hyperferremia of iron overdose. In this situation, other plasma constituents could contribute to the TIBC. For example, complexation of iron with other plasma proteins and organic ligands is known to occur in chronic hyperferremia.[11] For most laboratories, the equipment required for an immunochemical TIBC method is costly, and the technical expertise for its determination is high.[10] Of greater importance is that its turnaround time is unsuitable for this clinical situation.

The principle that the patient with an iron overdose is at risk when the serum iron concentration exceeds the TIBC is intuitively attractive. However, it ignores other defense mechanisms, such as rapid hepatic uptake of iron with subsequent storage of ferritin. This relationship has not been validated and has been questioned,[3] and recent clinical data cast doubt on its existence.[12] The Fischer test was developed as an immediate screen for serum iron in excess of the TIBC during an era of unavailability of rapid iron and TIBC determinations,[2,6] but it was not validated with outcome criteria.

A high TIBC, occasionally seen in iron poisoning, should not be considered as providing a protective effect. Patient 2 (Table) in this report had chelatable iron as demonstrated by her orange urine during deferoxamine therapy despite having a serum iron concentration less than her TIBC.

Being nonautomated, the TIBC is labor intensive and prolongs the turnaround time. It can be unreliable during acute hyperferremia, and we have demonstrated that the interlaboratory reproducibility of the TIBC under conditions of normoferremia is unsatisfactory. Furthermore, the relationship between exceeding the TIBC by the serum iron concentration and clinical iron toxicity has never been shown, to our knowledge, and has been questioned.[12] Thus, we conclude that the TIBC should not be used in the decision for the initiation of deferoxamine therapy in patients with acute iron poisoning. Appropriate indications are clinical criteria, an absolute serum iron concentration, or a positive chelation challenge test.[1]

This study was supported in part by The Children's Hospital of Winnipeg (Manitoba) Research Foundation.

References

1. Ellenhorn MJ, Barceloux DG. Iron. In: Ellenhorn MJ, Barceloux DG, eds. *Medical Toxicology: Diagnosis and Treatment of Human Poisoning*. New York, NY: Elsevier Science Publishing Co Inc; 1988:1023-1030.
2. Fischer DS. A method for the rapid detection of acute iron toxicity. *Clin Chem.* 1967;13:6-11.
3. Banner WJ Jr, Tong TG. Iron poisoning. *Pediatr Clin North Am.* 1986;33:393-409.
4. Ramsay WNM. The determination of the total iron binding capacity of the serum. *Clin Chim Acta.* 1957;2:221-226.
5. Greenblatt DJ, Allen MD, Koch-Weser J. Accidental iron poisoning in childhood: six cases including one fatality. *Clin Pediatr (Phila).* 1976;15:835-838.
6. Fischer DS, Parkman R, Finch SC. Acute iron poisoning in children: the problem of appropriate therapy. *JAMA.* 1971;218:1179-1184.
7. Markowitz H, Fairbanks VF. Transferrin assay and total-iron binding capacity. *Mayo Clin Proc.* 1983;58:827-828.
8. Starr RT. Use of an alumina column in estimating total iron-binding capacity. *Clin Chem.* 1980;26:156-158.
9. Cook JD. An evaluation of adsorption methods for measurement of plasma iron-binding capacity. *J Lab Clin Med.* 1970;76:497-506.
10. Buffone GJ, Lewis SA, Iosefsohn M, Hicks JM. Chemical and immunochemical measurement of total iron-binding capacity compared. *Clin Chem.* 1978;24:1788-1791.
11. Hershko C, Peto TEA. Non-transferrin plasma iron. *Br J Haematol.* 1987;66:149-151.
12. Chyka PA, Brady AY. Elevated ratio of serum iron concentration to total binding capacity in the assessment of systemic iron poisoning. *Vet Hum Toxicol.* 1989;31:343.

Improving the Use of Early Follow-up Care After Emergency Department Visits

A Randomized Trial

Eliot W. Nelson, MD; Susan Van Cleve, RN, MSN, PNP; Martha K. Swartz, RN, MSN, PNP; William Kessen, PhD; Paul L. McCarthy, MD

• ***Objective:*** **To test the hypothesis that the appropriateness of parents' use of early follow-up care after emergency department (ED) visits can be improved by postvisit support from a nurse practitioner.**
Design: **Randomized controlled trial, single blinded.**
Setting: **Urban university hospital ED linked to hospital's primary care center.**
Participants: **Parents of 190 children younger than 8 years who sought care in the ED for acute illnesses and who were treated as outpatients with primary care center follow-up at the discretion of ED clinicians.**
Intervention: **Parents in the experimental group were called by a nurse practitioner who offered both individualized guidance regarding follow-up and access to a nurse practitioner for further help as needed. The control group received "usual" follow-up advice during ED visits.**
Measurements/Main Results: **In the week after the ED visits, parents in the experimental group, compared with parents in the control group, were more compliant with instructions regarding follow-up (79% vs 61%), less apt to miss appointments (15% vs 31%), and less apt to "shop" elsewhere for care (2% vs 9%). Appropriateness of follow-up was assessed in "blinded" fashion using preestablished guidelines. Inappropriate use of follow-up care was significantly reduced among experimental group subjects (10% vs 20%).**
Conclusion: **The nurse practitioner's intervention improved parents' use of follow-up care in our sample. Overall care for episodic ED users might be improved by similar interventions.**

(AJDC. **1991;145:440-444)**

Parents who bring their children to emergency departments (EDs) for acute illnesses frequently have problems with follow-up. Most EDs are poorly suited to provide continuity of care, and ED clinicians are inconsistent in providing plans for follow-up.[1] However, even when follow-up *is* available, parents often fail to make appropriate use of it.[2-6]

Inappropriate parental use of follow-up care can be most worrisome in the first days after ED visits, when the child is most likely to remain ill. "Inappropriate" use can occur in various forms, such as missed appointments, revisits to the same or another ED for nonurgent problems, failure to follow specific instructions or contingency plans, or failure to use the telephone to obtain information, test results, or further guidance. Any of these forms can raise the costs of care or adversely affect the child's health. A review of records from our hospital indicated that inappropriate follow-up occurred in 20% to 25% of cases in the week after visits to our pediatric ED for acute problems.

In this study, we conducted a randomized trial to test the effectiveness of an intervention to improve patterns of parental use of early follow-up care in an urban ED setting. We hypothesized that telephone support, given by pediatric nurse practitioners (NPs) to parents within 1 day after visits to the ED for their childrens' acute illnesses, could improve the appropriateness of the parents' use of follow-up care. Our study design allowed us to consider a variety of forms of use in the follow-up period, so that we could ascertain inappropriate overuse as well as underuse of such care.

METHODS

Setting

The study was based at the Yale-New Haven (Conn) Hospital. Patients who receive primary health care at this hospital are predominantly black or Hispanic, poor, and receiving state assistance. The Pediatric ED is open 24 hours daily for emergencies or unscheduled visits. A Primary Care Center (PCC), located across the street, provides routine scheduled medical care for patients during daytime hours on weekdays. The PCC patients who need follow-up care after ED visits are generally expected to receive this care at the PCC, which can offer better continuity of care than can the ED.

Study Design

The study protocol was approved by the Yale University Human Investigations Committee. All subjects gave oral consent to participate. The protocol permitted us not to inform participants of the randomized trial we were conducting (so as to minimize

Accepted for publication September 4, 1990.
From the Departments of Pediatrics, Yale University School of Medicine (Drs Nelson and McCarthy), the School of Nursing (Mss Van Cleve and Swartz), and the Department of Psychology, Yale University (Dr Kessen), New Haven, Conn. Dr Nelson is now with the Division of General Pediatrics and Primary Care, University of Vermont Medical Center, Burlington. Read in part at the meeting of the Western Society for Pediatric Research, Carmel, Calif, February 9, 1989.
Reprints not available.

the "Hawthorne effect"[7]). Instead, we told subjects initially that we were conducting a survey of parent ED users, now and later over the phone, to try to learn ways of improving pediatric ED care.

Potential subjects were identified on arrival at the ED. Each child was younger than 8 years, was accompanied by a parent or usual caretaker, was free of active chronic illness, and presented with a chief complaint suggesting an acute infectious or allergic condition. Children remained eligible for the trial only if they were treated as outpatients. Further eligibility criteria required parents to be English speaking, to have access to a telephone in their home or nearby, and to identify the hospital's PCC as their chosen source for primary care for their children.

Subjects were enrolled during visits to the ED, and pretrial ("survey") data were collected uniformly. Those patients randomized to the experimental group received the telephone intervention per protocol after ED discharge, while those in the control group received usual care with respect to follow-up (see detailed descriptions below). Approximately 8 days later, outcome data were collected regarding any type or pattern of use of follow-up care over the interval, and the "appropriateness" of the use was assessed for each case.

Pretrial Baseline Data

Collection of baseline data allowed us to compare the trial groups for similarity. Methods included a standardized interview of the parent both before and after the child was seen for care, a questionnaire completed by the ED physician after ED discharge, and a review of each patient's hospital chart and ED record for the visit. We focused on factors that might influence parents' use of follow-up care, such as demographic and socioeconomic traits, previous use of health care for the child, clinical features of the ED visit, and both parents' and physicians' perceptions of the visit, including how sick the child seemed and how satisfied the parents were with the care given. When questions called for opinions or subjective assessments, either "yes/no" or Likert-format scales were used.

Trial and Intervention

Random assignment to the experimental or control group was predetermined according to study identification number with use of a random number table and a balanced block-randomization scheme. To avoid contamination of the control group and to protect the "blinded" status of the principal investigator (PI) with respect to trial-group assignment, all parents were handed a sealed envelope on leaving the ED that contained written information about the survey in which they had participated. For the experimental group parents, however, these envelopes also contained a message, saying that they would be contacted soon by telephone by an NP, and a printed yellow card, giving the names of the two NPs and a 24-hour telephone access number for reaching an NP in case of need during the child's illness.

An NP called each parent in the experimental group 6 to 18 hours after discharge from the ED. She offered further explanation about the child's diagnosis and treatment, reinforced follow-up instructions, both for specific appointments and contingency plans, and offered round-the-clock access to herself or the other NP by telephone (via the number on the yellow card) if needed. The protocol allowed her to answer questions or offer clinical assistance over the phone herself if it seemed warranted. However, she emphasized the advantages of continuity of care with the child's usual primary care provider and offered to facilitate communication with that provider if the parent wanted help.

Parents in the control group received no additional contact from the investigators until outcome interviews; thus, they received "usual care" with respect to follow-up. In usual care, plans and instructions for follow-up were at the discretion of the individual ED clinician and were communicated simply by the physician and/or nurse who discharged the child. There was no guarantee of further access to or contact with any physician or nurse already familiar with the child's case.

Outcome Data and Assessments

Prior to collection of outcome data, we developed a set of criteria for assessing the overall appropriateness of parents' use of follow-up care for their children. These preestablished criteria favored continuity and economy of care; examples of "appropriate" use included keeping appointments, following instructions regarding reuse of care, using the PCC rather than the ED for nonurgent care, and using the telephone prior to or instead of coming to the hospital for an unscheduled visit. The criteria were flexible in allowing parents to call to reschedule or cancel appointments if the need for care changed; thus, compliance with the original follow-up plan was not absolutely required for use of care to be deemed appropriate. In addition, because all subjects had identified our hospital as their choice for the child's primary care, we considered the seeking of care elsewhere ("outside care") during the follow-up period to be inappropriate.

Outcome data were collected by the PI, who remained blinded to the subject's trial group, approximately 8 days after the initial ED visit. Initially, he reviewed clinic and ED logs, both at Yale-New Haven Hospital and at the city's only other major hospital, to ascertain appointment keeping and use of care in those locations over the interval. He then telephoned each parent to conduct a standardized interview to gather detailed information on the course of the child's illness subsequent to the initial visit, the use of any follow-up care for the child, and the parents' reasons for such use.

This final interview was designed to minimize the risk of unblinding the PI regarding trial-group assignment, with questions focusing simply on how the parents felt about the child's condition and whether they had sought any care during the week. The format allowed the PI to apply the preestablished criteria directly in rating the overall appropriateness of parental use of follow-up care. The rating was then made along a four-point balanced scale (appropriate or probably appropriate vs probably inappropriate or inappropriate), giving consideration both to medical records and parents' information so that needs of individual patients were taken into account.

Validation of Outcome Assessments

To obtain an independent validation of the PI's ratings of overall appropriateness, we submitted 36 case abstracts, including many "hard-to-rate" ones, with our preestablished guidelines, to six outside "judges" experienced in urban pediatric ED care. When the ratings of these judges were pooled, agreement between their ratings and those of the PI was 94%. Agreement between individual judges' ratings and those of the PI ranged from 72% to 94%; corresponding κs were .44, .61, .67, .67, .88, and .88.

Data Analysis

Differences between trial groups with respect to both baseline variables and outcomes were evaluated principally using the χ^2 test, with Yates' continuity correction where appropriate. An α of .05 was considered significant for outcomes of the trial.

RESULTS

Characteristics of Sample: Pretrial Variables

From August 1984 to March 1985, we enrolled 190 subjects in the study. The balanced randomization scheme resulted in equal numbers of subjects initially in each trial group. Four of the subjects in the experimental group and two in the control group could not be reached for outcome interviews. Thus, the final sample available for analysis consisted of 184 subjects, 91 in the experimental group and 93 in the control group.

Some of the key demographic characteristics of the 184 subjects and clinical features of their initial ED visits are shown in Tables 1 and 2. The trial groups were highly similar in these characteristics and most others assessed at baseline. However, as shown, the groups did differ with respect to a few of the important baseline variables, including parents' educational level, the degree of fever in the children, the recorded primary diagnoses for the children, and the specific forms of treatment prescribed. (Although these differences may have arisen by chance considering the multiple comparisons involved, we did stratify the sample with respect to each of these variables

Table 1.—Demographic Characteristics of Sample (n=184)	
Characteristic	**%**
Children (median age, 27 mo)	
Gender, % M	48
Race, % black	77
Parents	
Single	86
Education, % completed 12th grade	62*
Unemployed	74
Receiving state assistance	80

*Experimental vs control, 54% vs 71%, respectively ($P<.05$).

Table 2.—Clinical Features of Emergency Department Visits (n=184)	
Feature	**%**
Chief complaints	
Fever	47
Respiratory/earache	23
Vomiting or diarrhea	7
Rash	13
Other	10
Recorded temperature, °C	
<38	55
38 to <39	17
39 or higher	21*
Not measured	7
Laboratory tests done, % of patients	33
Recorded primary diagnoses	
Viral infection	45
Bacterial infection/otitis	37†
Candida or unspecified rash	11
Other	7
Primary treatment prescribed	
None or supportive only	22
Antibiotic	46‡
Drug(s) other than antibiotics	32

*Experimental vs control, 14% vs 27%, respectively ($P<.05$).
†Experimental vs control, 51% vs 25%, respectively ($P<.001$).
‡Experimental vs control, 57% vs 35%, respectively ($P<.01$).

Table 3.—Plans for Use of Follow-up Care During Week After Emergency Department Visit	
Type of Plan	**Proportion of Subjects, % (n=184)**
None	17
Contingency ("prn") only*	42
Definite appointment	20
Other definite instructions	12
More than one type of definite plan	7
Other/unclear	2

*prn indicates as occasion requires.

to look for any impact on the trial. Importantly, this stratification revealed that the differences did not affect the outcome of the trial.)

With regard to previous use of care for the child, although 89% of the parents had already sought well-child care in the PCC (and more than 90% of these expressed satisfaction with that care), only 15% had sought care for an episode of acute illness in the child at the PCC. By contrast, 77% of the parents had previously sought care in the ED for acute illness in the child, including 28% who had sought such care at least twice in the preceding 6 months. Thus, the sample reflected a clear previous parental predilection for ED use for illness in their children.

Table 3 shows the types of follow-up plans established by the ED clinicians for further care within the first week after the visit. The majority of patients were not believed to require any definite short-term use of follow-up care, although many were given contingency instructions (eg, to call the physician if the child's condition worsened). Definite appointments and/or instructions regarding the use of follow-up care (eg, absolutely to call the physician for test results or to discuss the need for further care) were given in 39% of the cases. There were no significant differences between the trial groups with regard to follow-up plans.

Parents and physicians independently rated the seriousness of the childrens' sicknesses along a five-point scale (dangerously, very, moderately, mildly, or hardly sick). Parents rated their children as moderately, very, or dangerously sick in 57% of cases, whereas physicians rated only 17% of the children as moderately sick or sicker. Perhaps accordingly, physicians classified a majority (56%) of these initial ED visits as inappropriate. Parents generally expressed satisfaction with the visits (48% "highly" and 43% "somewhat" satisfied), as well as with the instructions given them (84% felt these were "very clear").

The Intervention and Outcomes of the Trial

The NP's intervention consisted of only a single telephone call in 78 (86%) of the experimental group cases. For the majority of these calls, the total time required of the NP was less than 5 minutes. The total time spent by NPs in phone contact with parents exceeded 15 minutes for only 8% of these parents, and only five of the parents made use of the NP's availability by phone. The NPs were unable ever to reach three of the parents by phone. These parents were nevertheless considered in the experimental group for analysis because they had received the initial part of the intervention.

During the first week after the initial ED visit, the majority of subjects in this study made no use of follow-up care. In most of these cases, it was not necessary because the child's illness improved or resolved and no specific appointment or instructions for further care had been given. In such cases, the "use of follow-up care" was assessed as appropriate. Similarly, among the 71 patients for whom definite plans for follow-up had been established for the 1-week interval, most parents appropriately kept appointments and/or followed specific instructions.

However, several types of use of follow-up care occurred that were assessed as inappropriate, and in this respect the trial groups showed differences (Table 4). Parents in the experimental group who were given definite appointments and/or instructions for follow-up were much more likely to comply with these than were parents in the control group. Moreover, parents in the experimental group were much less likely to make use of outside care. Unnecessary revisits to the ED were unusual, but they occurred with equal frequency in the two groups. (It should be noted that more than one type of inappropriate use occurred in some cases.)

The ratings of overall use of follow-up care for each patient showed that inappropriate or probably inappropriate use occurred with significantly greater frequency in the control group than in the experimental group (20.4% vs

Table 4.—Results of Trial

Types of Inappropriate Use of Follow-up Care	Frequency Within Groups (%)	
	Experimental	Control
Missed appointments (among those given appointments)	3/20 (15)	8/26 (31)
Failure to follow instructions (among those given them)	3/14 (21)	7/18 (39)
Use of outside care (among all subjects)	2/91 (2)	8/93 (9)
Unnecessary revisits to emergency department (among all subjects)	2/91 (2)	2/93 (2)

Table 5.—Results of Trial

Ratings of Overall Appropriateness of Use of Follow-up Care	Frequency (%) of Ratings Within Trial Groups*	
	Experimental	Control
Appropriate or probably appropriate	82/91 (90.1)	74/93 (79.6)
Inappropriate or probably inappropriate	9/91 (9.9)	19/93 (20.4)

*$\chi^2=3.96$; $P<.05$.

9.9% [Table 5]). Thus, the NP's intervention reduced the frequency of such inappropriate use of follow-up care by half.

Finally, we performed exploratory analyses to find those subgroups, identified at baseline, that were most responsive to the intervention. Inappropriate use of follow-up care was most significantly reduced for experimental group subjects, compared with controls, within three subgroups as follows: parents whose children were younger than 18 months (n=69; 3% vs 29%, $P<.01$); subjects with neither parent employed (n=136; 7% vs 24%, $P<.01$); and parents who perceived their children as at least "moderately" sick at the initial visit (n=105; 6% vs 24%, $P<.02$). Because these analyses required multiple comparisons,[8] we can only consider their results as suggestive.

COMMENT

Provision of follow-up care, including a return of patients to their primary care delivery system, is an important aspect of ED care[9] that frequently fails to receive sufficient attention, perhaps because ED physicians are often confronted with patients who fail to comply with follow-up arrangements. Lack of good follow-up contributes to the inappropriateness of episodic ED use, which in turn is associated with high rates of hospitalization, high costs of care, and poor continuity of care.[10-12]

Weitzman et al[5] observed in 1980 that follow-up care for children after ED or "urgent-care" clinic visits had not been well-studied. Past efforts to improve follow-up and overall use of care among such children have included mailed reminders,[13] telephone reminders,[6] and increased availability of comprehensive and continuous care.[11] The interventions studied have not provided individualized or specific support to parents, and the studies have generally focused on long-term use[12,14] and/or on appointment keeping as the sole outcome. To our knowledge, no previous study has examined all forms of parental reutilization of care (instead of only appointment keeping) within specific episodes of illness, even though authors have suggested that such reutilization should be especially amenable to influence.[15]

The design of our intervention was based in part on the work of Korsch et al,[16] who showed that both improved compliance and increased parent satisfaction were associated with better physician-parent communication in an urban hospital outpatient and ED setting. Because many ED visits are considered inappropriate by physicians[17] (a finding replicated by our study), we believed that discussion of follow-up plans might often be relatively neglected. We thus hoped that even a modest amount of additional supportive communication would improve patterns of follow-up.

Within the early follow-up period on which we focused, our intervention was successful in improving parents' reuse of care. Specifically, it increased short-term compliance with both appointments and instructions, and it also reduced the frequency of "shopping" elsewhere for care for the same problem.

Our results complement and extend the findings of Korsch et al[16] by showing that an intervention consisting of increased supportive communication can improve parental use of health care in a similar setting. On the other hand, the fact that inappropriate use of follow-up care occurred among almost 10% of our experimental group subjects underscores the challenge facing any such effort.

The clinical significance of the improvements in follow-up that we observed may have been relatively minor in some of these cases, but the *potential* importance for individual cases was illustrated vividly by the experience of one noncompliant subject (from the control group) in our study:

A 22-month-old girl had a 3-day history of fever, cold, and vomiting. The mother reported she had been playful at home. In the ED her rectal temperature was 40.5°C, and examination revealed no focal source of infection. A blood sample was taken for culture. A diagnosis of "probable viral syndrome" was made; treatment included acetaminophen and a decongestant. A follow-up appointment for the next day with the child's physician at the PCC was arranged; the mother was also told to return sooner if the child's condition worsened.

The mother failed to appear for the PCC appointment. However, a day later she brought the child back to the ED; the child was then found to have pneumonia with a pleural effusion and was admitted to the hospital.

Although our experience with seriously ill febrile children was not extensive enough in this study to allow statistically significant conclusions, our results suggest that an intervention such as ours will increase the likelihood of appropriate follow-up for some of these most worrisome patients and might in turn decrease morbidity for some of them.

A major cause of inappropriate follow-up may be that parents do not clearly understand options for care or feel that they have access to appropriate forms of care. The NPs in our study were able to offer guidance, using clinical judgment and their training[18] where necessary, to help parents make appropriate decisions. The study design allowed us to examine the intervention of extra supportive communication in a controlled fashion *apart* from usual care; we recognize that other clinicians, including physicians themselves, might provide equally effective extra support. While a "follow-up clerk" or secretary has sufficed in projects designed simply to increase appointment keeping,[6,19] such an individual might lack clinical skills needed to help parents with unforeseen questions regarding follow-up.

It is difficult to predict financial costs and benefits of such an intervention based on a trial of our size. However, our intervention required little time and only a single call in most cases; and we would expect that a 50% reduction in inappropriate use of follow-up care would improve cost-effectiveness as well as quality of care. Moreover, our exploratory analyses suggest that similar interventions might be aimed more efficiently at certain "target" parents most likely to respond (eg, those who are unemployed or whose children are younger than 18 months).

Lack of existing criteria for evaluating appropriateness of follow-up made it necessary for us to develop our own criteria. It was striking that the ratings of the outside judges, who considered many of the most difficult-to-rate cases, showed substantial agreement with those of the PI. This suggests that similar criteria might be useful in other settings or in efforts to evaluate the quality of follow-up care.

In summary, we have shown that a supportive telephone call, made to parents within a day of visits to our ED for their childrens' acute illnesses, improved use of follow-up care for those illnesses. We believe that interventions such as this one can improve the overall provision of health care to poor urban children whose parents frequently seek attention for acute illnesses in EDs. Such efforts must continue to emphasize the importance of supportive communication and access to continuity of care. We believe they can be performed efficiently and can potentially decrease costs by decreasing overuse of unnecessary care. For disadvantaged children whose parents might have related poorly to health care systems in the past, such direct interventions may be the most effective way of influencing parental behavior to achieve improved use of care in the future.

This research was supported by a Robert Wood Johnson Foundation General Pediatric Academic Development Award.

The following gave advice on study design and analysis: James Jekel, MD; John Leventhal, MD; Eugene D. Shapiro, MD; Brian Forsyth, MD; and Sally Horwitz, PhD. The following judged the case abstracts: Allison Anderson, MD; Anthony Haftel, MD; Dee Hodge, MD; Stanley Inkelis, MD; John O'Shea, MD; and Bobbie Phillips, MD. The Yale Pediatric house staff and Yale-New Haven Hospital Pediatric Emergency Department Nursing Staff provided cooperation and support; and Barbara M. Korsch, MD, gave critical review of the manuscript.

References

1. DeAngelis C, Fosarelli P. Assignment of follow-up appointments from an emergency room by pediatric residents. *AJDC.* 1985;139:341-342.

2. Fink D, Malloy MJ, Cohen M, Greycloud MA, Martin F. Effective patient care in the pediatric ambulatory setting: a study of the acute care clinic. *Pediatrics.* 1969;43:927-935.

3. Spivak HR, Levy JC, Bonanno RA, Cracknell M. Patient and provider factors associated with selected measures of quality of care. *Pediatrics.* 1980;65:307-313.

4. Scherzer LN, Druckman R, Alpert JJ. Care-seeking patterns of families using a municipal hospital emergency room. *Med Care.* 1980;18:289-296.

5. Weitzman M, Moomaw MS, Messenger KP. An after-hours pediatric walk-in clinic for an entire urban community: utilization and effectiveness of follow-up care. *Pediatrics.* 1980;65:964-970.

6. Casey R, Rosen B, Glowasky A, Ludwig S. An intervention to improve follow-up of patients with otitis media. *Clin Pediatr.* 1985;24:149-152.

7. Franke RH, Kaul JD. The Hawthorne experiments: first statistical interpretation. *Am Sociol Rev.* 1978;43:523-643.

8. Pocock SJ, Hughes MD, Lee RJ. Statistical problems in the reporting of clinical trials: a survey of three medical journals. *N Engl J Med.* 1987;317:426-432.

9. Jacobsen S. Why is primary care secondary to emergency medicine? *Ann Emerg Med.* 1986;15:969-970.

10. Halperin R, Meyers AR, Alpert JJ. Utilization of pediatric emergency services: a critical review. *Pediatr Clin North Am.* 1979;26:747-757.

11. Starfield B, Simborg DW, Horn SD, Yourtee SA. Continuity and coordination in primary care: their achievement and utility. *Med Care.* 1976;14:625-636.

12. Alpert JJ, Robertson LS, Kosa J, Heagarty MC, Haggerty RJ. Delivery of health care for children: report of an experiment. *Pediatrics.* 1976;57:917-930.

13. O'Shea JS, Collins EW, Pezzullo JC. An attempt to influence health care visits of frequent hospital emergency facility users. *Clin Pediatr.* 1984;23:559-562.

14. Straus JH, Orr ST, Charney E. Referrals from an emergency room to primary care practices at an urban hospital. *Am J Public Health.* 1983;73:57-61.

15. Horwitz SM. *The Impact of Social Stressors and Social Networks on Medical Care Utilization in a Pediatric Population.* New Haven, Conn: Yale University; 1984. Unpublished doctoral dissertation.

16. Korsch BM, Gozzi EK, Francis V. Gaps in doctor-patient communication. *Pediatrics.* 1968;42:855-871.

17. Kahn L, Anderson M, Perkhoff GT. Patients' perceptions and uses of a pediatric emergency room. *Soc Sci Med.* 1973;7:155-160.

18. Breslau N. The contribution of pediatric nurse practitioners to child health care. *Adv Pediatr.* 1982;29:387-405.

19. Fletcher SW, Appel FA, Bourgois M. Improving emergency-room patient follow-up in a metropolitan teaching hospital: effects of a follow-up clerk. *N Engl J Med.* 1974;291:385-388.

Influenza Vaccination in the Prevention of Acute Otitis Media in Children

Terho Heikkinen, MD; Olli Ruuskanen, MD; Matti Waris, MSc; Thedi Ziegler, PhD; Mikko Arola, MD; Pekka Halonen, MD

• We studied a new approach to the prevention of acute otitis media through the administration of influenza vaccine to 187 day-care center children aged 1 to 3 years before the influenza A epidemic of 1988-1989. The control group consisted of 187 unvaccinated children of similar age and background. During the 6-week study period, influenza A infection was diagnosed in five (3%) of 187 vaccinees and in 29 (16%) of 187 controls. Acute otitis media developed in three (60%) of five vaccinees with an influenza A infection compared with 18 (67%) of 27 controls (excluded were two children with a double viral infection). The incidence of acute otitis media associated with influenza A was reduced by 83% in the vaccinees. The total number of children with acute otitis media in the vaccine group was 35, compared with 55 in the control group, disclosing a 36% reduction among the vaccinees. We conclude that influenza vaccination decreases the incidence of acute otitis media in children during an influenza A epidemic, suggesting also that other vaccines against respiratory viruses may be an effective way to reduce the incidence of acute otitis media.

(*AJDC.* 1991;145:445-448)

Otitis media in children is a major health care problem, not only because of the distress it causes to the child and his or her family but also because of the substantial economic burden to the health care system.[1] According to Teele et al,[2] more than 60% of children in the United States have had at least one attack of acute otitis media (AOM) by their first birthday and more than 80% have had an attack by 3 years of age. Similar findings have been reported in Finland.[3] Obviously, it is of utmost importance to find a way to prevent otitis media in children. In most cases, AOM is a bacterial infection. A great deal of research has been conducted in an attempt to develop a bacterial vaccine for otitis media.[4] The results of extensive vaccine trials against the most common causative agent, *Streptococcus pneumoniae,* have not so far been very satisfying.[5-8]

Clinical evidence has shown that in most cases AOM is preceded by a respiratory viral infection.[9] A simultaneous viral infection has been documented in 26% to 42% of patients with AOM.[10-14] The greatest risk for the development of AOM lies in infections caused by respiratory syncytial viruses (RSVs), rhinoviruses, influenza A viruses, or adenoviruses.[11,14,15]

Our study was based on the hypothesis that prevention of the preceding respiratory viral infection would decrease the incidence of AOM. We decided to concentrate on the influenza A virus infection because an available vaccine has been shown to be safe and effective, even in young children,[16] and also because AOM is a common complication of influenza A infection.[15] The attack rate for influenza in children is, moreover, usually high (30% to 60%),[17] epidemics are of short duration, and there is a rapid and sensitive immunoassay available for the direct detection of influenza virus antigens in nasopharyngeal aspirates.[18]

SUBJECTS AND METHODS

Subjects

In October 1988, of a total of 26 day-care centers serving 831 healthy children in Turku, Finland, all 291 children from 11 randomly selected day-care centers were invited to be vaccinated against influenza; the enrollment of children known to be allergic to eggs was discouraged. Informed consent was obtained from the parents of 207 children (71%); 14 children were vaccinated only once or not at all because of either acute infection or absence from day care at the time of vaccination. A total of 193 children (66% of the original total; range, 33% to 83% per center) were vaccinated twice, as recommended. Six children were excluded from the analysis because they left day care before the study began. The final vaccine group consisted of 187 children.

An unvaccinated control group was formed by inviting all 273 children from eight other randomly selected day-care centers in Turku to participate. Informed consent was obtained from the parents of 188 children (69% of the total; range, 56% to 82% per center). One child was excluded from the analysis because of absence from day care during the study period. The final number of children in the control group was 187.

Data on the families and children's previous infections were assembled from a questionnaire completed by the parents (Table 1). The mean age of the children was 2.2 years in both groups. Most of the children were otitis prone: 128 (68%) of 187 children in the vaccine group and 118 (63%) of 187 children in the control group had a history of at least two attacks of AOM. The average number of previous attacks of AOM in the vaccine group was 4.5 (range, 0 through 30) compared with 4.2 (range, 0 to 25) in the control group. No significant differences were noted between the groups regarding the number of siblings, smoking in the household, or earlier adenoidectomy or placement of tympanostomy tubes.

Accepted for publication October 8, 1990.

From the Department of Pediatrics (Drs Heikkinen, Ruuskanen, and Arola) and Virology (Drs Ziegler and Halonen and Mr Waris), University of Turku (Finland).

Presented in part at the Conference on the Eustachian Tube and Middle Ear Diseases, Geneva, Switzerland, October 29, 1989.

Reprint requests to the Department of Pediatrics, Turku University Hospital, SF-20520 Turku, Finland (Dr Heikkinen).

Table 1.—Characteristics of the Study Groups*

Variable	Vaccinees	Controls
Total No. of children	187	187
Male (%)	92 (49)	103 (55)
Mean age, y (range)	2.2 (0.9-3.5)	2.2 (0.6-4.2)
<1	1	5
1-<2	76	65
2-<3	67	76
≥3	43	41
No. of siblings (range)	0.6 (0-3)	0.6 (0-3)
Smoking in the household (%)	30 (16)	42 (22)
No. of previous attacks of AOM (range)	4.5 (0-30)	4.2 (0-25)
No. of children with ≥2 episodes of AOM (%)	128 (68)	118 (63)
Adenoidectomy (%)	40 (21)	47 (25)
Tympanostomy tubes (%)	35 (19)	35 (19)

*AOM indicates acute otitis media.

Table 2.—Results of Viral Antigen Detection in Nasopharyngeal Aspirates and the Corresponding Numbers of Cases With AOM in the Study Groups*

	Vaccinees (n=187)		Controls (n=187)	
Virus	No.	AOM	No.	AOM
Influenza A	5	3	27	18
Influenza A and adenovirus	0	0	1	1
Influenza A and RSV	0	0	1	0
RSV	1	1	9	5
Adenovirus	5	2	4	1
Parainfluenza type 3	7	5	0	0
Parainfluenza type 1	1	0	0	0
Virus detected	19	11	42	25
No virus detected	79	25	65	31
No specimen available	7	0	7	4
Total No. of respiratory tract infections or episodes of AOM	105	36	114	60

*AOM indicates acute otitis media; RSV, respiratory syncytial virus.

The study protocol was approved by the Ethical Committee of Turku University Hospital.

Vaccination

The vaccinations were administered between November 17 and December 15, 1988, with a trivalent subvirion influenza virus vaccine (Fluzone, Connaught Laboratories Inc, Swiftwater, Pa) containing the three prototype strains recommended for the season (influenza A/Taiwan/1/86[H1N1], influenza A/Sichuan/2/87[H3N2], and influenza B/Victoria/2/87). Two doses of 0.25 mL were injected into the deltoid muscle, with a 3-week interval between the injections. No serious adverse reactions were reported.

Study Period

From the beginning of November 1988, an intensive screening of influenza virus activity in the community was conducted, with the use of rapid viral antigen detection in nasopharyngeal aspirates of febrile children seen both in private practice and at the University Hospital in Turku. Before commencement of the study, 340 specimens were tested.

The first case of influenza A to be diagnosed in Turku was found on December 2, 1988. The study commenced on December 19, after 11 influenza A infections had been diagnosed in children in the city, and it was discontinued on January 26, 1989, at 1 week after the last recorded case of influenza A in the study population. The first case of influenza A among the children enrolled in this study was diagnosed on December 19. During the epidemic, both H1N1 and H3N2 strains of influenza were circulating, the latter being predominant in Turku.

During the 6-week study period, the parents of all 374 children were asked to bring their children to the study office whenever fever or signs of a respiratory tract infection appeared. No charge was made for these visits. The parents were not asked by the study physicians (T.H., M.A., and O.R.) whether the child had been vaccinated, which means that in most cases the investigator did not know to which group the child belonged. During each episode of infection, a nasopharyngeal mucus specimen was aspirated for rapid viral antigen detection. In 14 cases, however, it proved impossible to obtain the specimen (seven cases in each group). Children without AOM at the first examination were reexamined 1 week later, unless symptoms of AOM developed in the meantime. The diagnosis of AOM was based on signs and symptoms of acute infection, together with the presence of middle-ear fluid detected by pneumatic otoscopy or purulent discharge from a tympanostomy tube.

Viral Diagnosis

Nasopharyngeal secretions were aspirated through the nostrils with use of a disposable mucus extractor (Vygon, Laboratoires Pharmaceutiques, Ecouen, France). The specimens were transported at room temperature to the laboratory, where they were processed the following day. Viral antigens in the aspirates were detected by one-incubation, monoclonal time-resolved fluoroimmunoassay for influenza A and B viruses; parainfluenza types 1, 2 and 3 viruses; RSV; and the group-reacting hexon antigen of adenoviruses.[19-22] The reliability of time-resolved fluoroimmunoassay with the use of monoclonal antibodies for the detection of influenza virus antigens has been established.[18]

Statistical Analysis

Significance testing was performed by means of the standard χ^2 test. Confidence intervals were calculated at the 95% level of confidence.

RESULTS

During the study period, 105 respiratory tract infections were recorded in the 187 vaccinees, compared with 114 in the 187 controls; in each group, 14 children each had two episodes of infection. Acute otitis media was diagnosed in 36 (34%) of the 105 cases in the vaccine group, compared with 60 (53%) of the 114 children in the control group. One child in the vaccine group and five in the control group had two consecutive attacks of AOM, the numbers of children with AOM during the study thus being 35 and 55, respectively ($P<.02$).

A total of 205 nasopharyngeal aspirates were obtained from the children, with viral antigen being detected in 61 cases (30%). Viral findings and the corresponding numbers of cases of AOM are presented in Table 2. Influenza A was diagnosed in five (3%) of the 187 vaccinees (confidence interval, 1% to 5%), three (60%) of whom also had AOM. In the control group, influenza A was diagnosed in 29 (16%) of the 187 children (confidence interval, 11% to 21%; relative risk, 5.8; $P<.0001$). The protective efficacy of the vaccination against influenza A was 83% (five vs 29). Two controls had both influenza A and another viral infection simultaneously, one with adenovirus and the other with RSV. Not including these two children, AOM developed in 18 (67%) of 27 controls with influenza A. The decrease in the incidence of AOM associated with influenza A in the vaccine group was 83% (three vs 18; $P<.001$).

Influenza A was detected in the participants of four (of 11) day-care centers in the vaccine group compared with six (of eight) day-care centers in the control group. Other viruses detected in the children studied were adenovirus, RSV, and parainfluenza types 1 and 3 viruses.

COMMENT

We studied a new approach to the prevention of AOM through prevention of the respiratory viral infection that usually precedes it. The results of our study suggest that this may be a successful way to prevent AOM when an effective vaccine against a specific predisposing virus is available. In our study, the efficacy of the vaccination against influenza A was 83%, with a consequent 83% decrease in the incidence of AOM associated with influenza A infection in the vaccinees. Obviously, the most important result of our study is, however, the clear-cut 36% reduction in the overall morbidity due to AOM in the vaccine group, although the attack rate for influenza A in the control group was only 16% and several other respiratory viruses were present in the community.

Streptococcus pneumoniae is the most common causative agent in AOM, and several pneumococcal vaccine trials to prevent AOM have been reported.[5-8] Immunization with a polyvalent pneumococcal polysaccharide vaccine reduces the number of episodes of AOM caused by the serotypes contained in the vaccine when there is a good antibody response in the children. The immunogenicity of some of the serotypes commonly associated with AOM, however, is poor, especially in children younger than 2 years, and the trials have therefore failed to show any convincing reduction in the total number of cases of AOM. The conjugated pneumococcal vaccines that have recently been developed may prove more effective in the prevention of AOM in young children.[23]

Our findings are in accordance with earlier evidence of a clear connection between respiratory viral infections and AOM.[11,15,24] In a 14-year longitudinal study, Henderson et al[11] showed that respiratory viral infections conferred a greater risk of AOM than did colonization of the nasopharynx with *S pneumoniae*. Not all respiratory viruses predispose equally to AOM, but it appears that the principal culprits are RSV, rhinovirus, influenza A virus, and adenovirus.[11,14,15] In particular, influenza A and RSV cause major epidemics. If children could be protected from these viruses, there would be a considerable decrease in the incidence of AOM. A fusion-protein vaccine against RSV has recently been developed, and this has been shown to be safe in toddlers.[25] Further clinical trials will be needed to determine its efficacy in the prevention of RSV infection and RSV-associated otitis media.

Acute otitis media was diagnosed in 67% of the unvaccinated children who had an influenza A virus infection. In an earlier study of hospitalized children with influenza A, 35% appeared to have AOM.[15] The difference can most probably be explained by the fact that our study concerned children from day-care centers, most of whom were otitis prone and also younger than those studied earlier.

Influenza vaccination is currently recommended for high-risk children and those in close contact with them, although other children (for example, those in day care) are also thought to benefit from the vaccination.[26] Because children at school and in day-care centers are the main disseminators of viruses during epidemics, there has been discussion as to whether all children should be regularly vaccinated against influenza.[17] To achieve this, however, would not be easy. First, it is necessary to administer the vaccine annually, and two doses must be given in the first instance. Then, there is the question of the continual antigenic variation of influenza viruses and the resulting fluctuation in the efficacy of the vaccine. Our findings nevertheless support the view that children in day care, especially those suffering from recurrent otitis media, would greatly benefit from influenza vaccination. As an alternative to vaccination, the antiviral agent rimantadine hydrochloride could be used to prevent influenza A infection.[27]

Ours was not a double-blind, placebo-controlled study, but this was largely offset by the fact that the parents were not asked whether their child had been vaccinated. In most cases, therefore, the investigator did not know to which group the child belonged; nor were the viral results available when AOM was diagnosed. There was, nevertheless, a similar incidence of AOM in children with different respiratory virus infections in the two groups. It could be argued that because the assignment of children to the groups was based on randomization of the day-care centers, not individual children, a possible clustering of influenza A around a limited number of day-care centers might invalidate the study. Influenza A was diagnosed in participating children from four of 11 day-care centers in the vaccine group compared with six of eight day-care centers in the control group. The smaller incidence of influenza in the vaccinees (3%) compared with the controls (16%) is most likely a result of the protective effect of the vaccine, but lesser exposure to influenza A virus is also possible. It must be emphasized, however, that the actual exposure to influenza A in both groups was in all probability greater than recorded, because about one third of children in each day-care center were not enrolled in the study; consequently, their possible morbidity due to influenza could not be demonstrated.

In conclusion, our findings suggest that influenza vaccination considerably decreases the incidence of AOM in children during an epidemic of influenza A. It therefore seems possible that other vaccines against respiratory viruses may also be an effective way to reduce the incidence of AOM.

This work was supported by grants from the Foundation of Päivikki and Sakari Sohlberg, the Research Foundation of Hoechst Fennica, the Research Society for the Study of Viral Diseases, the Foundation of Wilho Kyttä, Finland, and the city of Turku. The vaccines were supplied by the National Public Health Institute of Finland.

We thank Reijo Pyhälä, PhD, for identification of influenza viruses, Riikka Yli-Kerttula, RN, for vaccine administration, and Merja Kleme for virus antigen detections.

References

1. Stool SE, Field MJ. The impact of otitis media. *Pediatr Infect Dis J.* 1989;8(suppl):S11-S14.

2. Teele DW, Klein JO, Rosner B, and the Greater Boston Otitis Media Study Group. Epidemiology of otitis media during the first seven years of life in children in Greater Boston: a prospective cohort study. *J Infect Dis.* 1989;160:83-94.

3. Pukander J, Luotonen J, Sipilä M, Timonen M, Karma P. Incidence of acute otitis media. *Acta Otolaryngol (Stockh).* 1982;93:447-453.

4. Nelson JD, Scheetz MD, eds. Proceedings of a workshop on vaccines for otitis media. *Pediatr Infect Dis J.* 1989;8(suppl):S1-S97.

5. Mäkelä PH, Leinonen M, Pukander J, Karma P. A study of the pneumococcal vaccine in prevention of clinically acute attacks of recurrent otitis media. *Rev Infect Dis.* 1981;3(suppl):S124-S130.

6. Teele DW, Klein JO, and the Greater Boston Collaborative Otitis Media Study Group. Use of pneumococcal vaccine for prevention of recurrent acute otitis media in infants in Boston. *Rev Infect Dis.* 1981;3(suppl):S113-S118.

7. Sloyer JL Jr, Ploussard JH, Howie VM. Efficacy of pneumococcal polysaccharide vaccine in preventing acute otitis media in infants in Huntsville, Alabama. *Rev Infect Dis.* 1981;3(suppl):S119-S123.

8. Karma P, Pukander J, Sipilä M, et al. Prevention of otitis media in children by pneumococcal vaccination. *Am J Otolaryngol.* 1985;6:173-184.

9. Kovatch AL, Wald ER, Michaels RH, Blatter MM, Reisinger KS, Wucher FP. Clinical profile of children with acute otitis media caused by *Branhamella catarrhalis.* In: Lim DJ, Bluestone CD, Klein JO, Nelson JD, eds. *Recent Advances in Otitis Media With Effusion.* Philadelphia, Pa: BC Decker Inc; 1984:111-114.

10. Klein BS, Dollete FR, Yolken RH. The role of respiratory syncytial virus and other viral pathogens in acute otitis media. *J Pediatr.* 1982;101:16-20.

11. Henderson FW, Collier AM, Sanyal MA, et al. A longitudinal study of respiratory viruses and bacteria in the etiology of acute otitis media with effusion. *N Engl J Med.* 1982;306:1377-1383.

12. Sarkkinen H, Ruuskanen O, Meurman O, Puhakka H, Virolainen E, Eskola J. Identification of respiratory virus antigens in middle ear fluids of children with acute otitis media. *J Infect Dis.* 1985;151:444-448.

13. Chonmaitree T, Howie VM, Truant AL. Presence of respiratory viruses in middle ear fluids and nasal wash specimens from children with acute otitis media. *Pediatrics.* 1986;77:698-702.

14. Arola M, Ziegler T, Ruuskanen O, Mertsola J, Näntö-Salonen K, Halonen P. Rhinovirus in acute otitis media. *J Pediatr.* 1988;113:693-695.

15. Ruuskanen O, Arola M, Putto-Laurila A, et al. Acute otitis media and respiratory virus infections. *Pediatr Infect Dis J.* 1989;8:94-99.

16. Boyer KM, Cherry JD, Wright PF, et al. Clinical reactions and serologic responses in healthy children aged 6 to 35 months after two-dose regimens of inactivated A/New Jersey/76 influenza virus vaccines. *J Infect Dis.* 1977;136(suppl):S579-S583.

17. Glezen WP. Consideration of the risk of influenza in children and indications for prophylaxis. *Rev Infect Dis.* 1980;2:408-420.

18. Walls HH, Johansson KH, Harmon MW, Halonen PE, Kendal AP. Time-resolved fluoroimmunoassay with monoclonal antibodies for rapid diagnosis of influenza infections. *J Clin Microbiol.* 1986;24:907-912.

19. Nikkari S, Halonen P, Kharitonenkov I, et al. One-incubation time-resolved fluoroimmunoassay based on monoclonal antibodies in detection of influenza A and B viruses directly in clinical specimens. *J Virol Methods.* 1989;23:29-40.

20. Hierholzer JC, Bingham PG, Coombs RA, Johansson KH, Anderson LJ, Halonen PE. Comparison of monoclonal antibody time-resolved fluoroimmunoassay with monoclonal antibody capture-biotinylated detector enzyme immunoassay for respiratory syncytial virus and parainfluenza virus antigen detection. *J Clin Microbiol.* 1989;27:1243-1249.

21. Waris M, Halonen P, Ziegler T, Nikkari S, Obert G. Time-resolved fluoroimmunoassay compared with virus isolation for rapid detection of respiratory syncytial virus in nasopharyngeal aspirates. *J Clin Microbiol.* 1988;26:2581-2585.

22. Hierholzer JC, Johansson KH, Anderson LJ, Tsou CJ, Halonen PE. Comparison of monoclonal time-resolved fluoroimmunoassay with monoclonal capture-biotinylated detector enzyme immunoassay for adenovirus antigen detection. *J Clin Microbiol.* 1987;25:1662-1667.

23. Anderson P, Betts R. Human adult immunogenicity of protein-coupled pneumococcal capsular antigens of serotypes prevalent in otitis media. *Pediatr Infect Dis J.* 1989;8(suppl):S50-S53.

24. Sanyal MA, Henderson FW, Stempel EC, Collier AM, Denny FW. Effect of upper respiratory tract infection on eustachian tube ventilatory function in the preschool child. *J Pediatr.* 1980;97:11-15.

25. Lewin EB, Hildreth SW, Hogerman DA, Oren J, Paradiso PR, Smith DH. Evaluation of subunit vaccine for RSV in toddlers: acute and long-term clinical safety. In: Program and abstracts of the 29th Interscience Conference on Antimicrobial Agents and Chemotherapy; September 19, 1989; Houston, Tex. Washington, DC: American Society for Microbiology; 1989. Abstract.

26. Peter G, Hall CB, Lepow ML, Phillips CF, eds. Influenza. In: *Report of the Committee on Infectious Diseases: The 1988 Red Book.* 21st ed. Elk Grove, Ill: American Academy of Pediatrics; 1988:243-251.

27. Clover RD, Crawford SA, Abell TD, Ramsey CN, Glezen WP, Cough RB. Effectiveness of rimantadine prophylaxis of children within families. *AJDC.* 1986;140:706-709.

In Other AMA Journals

ARCHIVES OF INTERNAL MEDICINE

Bad News: Delivery, Dialogue, and Dilemma

Timothy E. Quill, MD,
Penelope Townsend, RN, BSN
(*Arch Intern Med.* 1991;151:478-484)

The Association of Allergen Skin Test Reactivity and Respiratory Disease Among Whites in the US Population: Data From the Second National Health and Nutrition Examination Survey, 1976 to 1980

Peter J. Gergen, MD, MPH,
Paul C. Turkeltaub, MD
(*Arch Intern Med.* 1991;151:487-492)

Sharing of Information by Students in an Objective Structured Clinical Examination

Paul J. Rutala, MD; Donald B. Witzke, PhD; Elizabeth O. Leko, MPA; John V. Fulginiti, MA; Preston J. Taylor, MD
(*Arch Intern Med.* 1991;151:541-544)

Physicians' Effectiveness in Assessing Risk for Human Immunodeficiency Virus Infection

Kristi J. Ferguson, PhD; Jack T. Stapleton, MD; Charles M. Helms, MD, PhD
(*Arch Intern Med.* 1991;151:561-564)

Discussing Life-Sustaining Treatment: A Teaching Program for Residents

Geoffrey H. Gordon, MD, Susan W. Tolle, MD
(*Arch Intern Med.* 1991;151:567-570)

The Pediatric Program Director

An Analysis of the Role and Its Problems

Jeffrey C. Weiss, MD; Robert A. Doughty, MD; Richard Lampe, MD

• A questionnaire designed to elicit information about the work environment, knowledge, and stresses of pediatric residency program directors was mailed to the 235 member programs of the Association of Pediatric Program Directors (APPD). At the time that the 187 respondents (80% return rate) assumed responsibility for their training programs, many rated their knowledge of various aspects of residency program administration as "poor." The respondents indicated that a lack of time, the pressures of too many other academic responsibilities, and a fear of not "filling" all positions in the National Intern Matching Program created much personal stress. Most program directors felt that educational conferences designed to teach educational methods, and administrative skills, and provide technical information knowledge necessary for residency program supervision would be beneficial.

(*AJDC*. 1991;145:449-452)

In April 1989, a workshop entitled "Stress and Burnout in Residency Program Directors" was held as part of the Sixth Annual Pediatric Chief Residents and Program Directors Conference at the Alfred I. duPont Institute in Wilmington, Del. The participants identified and discussed numerous problems related to fulfilling the role of a residency training program supervisor. As an outgrowth of the workshop, the present study was designed to collect demographic information about those pediatricians serving as program directors, to identify areas that program directors believed created major job stress, and to determine the skills or areas of learning in which the directors believed they had been inadequately prepared by their educational experience.

METHODS

A 75-item, four-page questionnaire was mailed to the 245 member programs of the APPD. Ten programs were identified as having closed or merged. Of the remaining 235 programs, 187 (80%) returned the completed form.

The questionnaire contained items designed to elicit information about the individuals who were program directors and about their experience, job description, time allotments, budget, and support staff. For 12 job-related areas, the program directors were asked to respond to the question, "How would you rate your knowledge (excellent, good, fair or poor) at the time you initially became program director?" The directors were also asked to indicate on a five-point Likert scale, "How much personal aggravation and stress does each of the following [23] items create for you?" The questionnaire stated specifically, "We want to know what bothers you the most, not necessarily what takes up most of your time!"

A high score of "4" or "5" indicated that the item represented a major problem and created a good deal of stress for the program director. Low numbers signified that the item was not a problem. Finally, the respondents were asked to indicate whether they believed an extended educational conference for program directors would be of value, and, if so, which of three topic areas (basic educational methods, administrative skills, or technical information for program directors) would be most beneficial. All responses were statistically analyzed using a microcomputer (Apple Macintosh SE, Apple Computer, Cupertino, Calif) and statistical software (Statview, Brainpower Inc, Calabasas, Calif).

RESULTS

Program Director Demographic Data

The sample consisted of 145 men (78%) and 37 women (20%); five anonymous program directors did not indicate their gender. The respondents' mean (±SD) age was 48±8.8 years, with an observed age range of 32 to 68 years (Table 1). Fifty-one percent of the respondents had achieved the rank of professor, 26% were associate professors, and 22% were assistant professors. Thirty-nine percent functioned as department chairperson as well as program director. Table 2 shows the distribution of specialty training among program directors. The number of

Accepted for publication November 1, 1990.

From the Departments of Pediatrics, Jefferson Medical College, Philadelphia, Pa (Dr Weiss); Alfred I. duPont Institute, Wilmington, Del (Dr Doughty); Walter Reed Army Hospital, Washington, DC (Dr Lampe); and the Association of Pediatric Program Directors.

Reprint requests to the Department of Pediatrics, Jefferson Medical College, 1025 Walnut St, Philadelphia, PA 19107 (Dr Weiss).

Purpose.—*This department is intended to share information concerning educational efforts in the broad field of pediatrics. We welcome studies on the following topics: undergraduate and graduate education in medicine and allied health occupations; continuing education of health professionals; education of patients and families; and health education for the general public, the community, and organizations that contribute to the promotion and improvement of the health of children.*

Editorial Comment.—*Did you feel that your residency training program director was well prepared and had adequate time for the task? If you said yes, this survey indicates that many directors feel differently. See what you think about the suggestions for improvement.*—H.D.A.

Table 1.—Age Distribution of Program Directors

Age, y	No. (%) of Directors (n=176)*
25-34	10 (6)
35-44	54 (31)
45-54	71 (40)
55-64	34 (19)
≥65	7 (4)

*Eleven directors did not answer this question.

Table 2.—Distribution of Specialty Training

Specialty	No. (%) of Directors
General pediatrics	60 (32)
Neonatology	27 (14)
Infectious disease	22 (12)
Endocrinology	14 (7)
Nephrology	12 (6)
Hematology	12 (6)
Cardiology	10 (5)
Other (miscellaneous)	30 (16)

Table 3.—Program Director Job Longevity*

No. of Years as Program Director	No. (%) of Respondents (n=186)	No. (%) of Predecessors (n=148)
≤3	69 (37)	54 (36)
4-6	49 (26)	45 (30)
7-9	21 (11)	14 (9)
≥10	47 (25)	35 (24)

*The numbers do not total 187 because one director did not indicate his job longevity and 39 were either directing new programs or were unaware of their predecessor's job longevity.

Table 4.—Support Staff

Position	No. of Support Staff (% of Directors)
Secretary	167 (89)
Administrative assistant	56 (30)
Education specialist (PhD)	21 (11)
Associate director (MD)	72 (39)
Chief resident (postgraduate level 4)	63 (34)

Table 5.—Knowledge Level On Becoming Program Director*

	Knowledge Level, No. (%) of Directors			
Knowledge Area	Poor	Fair	Good	Excellent
Curriculum design	22 (12)	56 (30)	85 (46)	22 (12)
Evaluation methods	19 (10)	72 (39)	72 (39)	23 (12)
"Match" process	13 (7)	51 (28)	77 (42)	42 (23)
Recruiting methods	20 (11)	62 (33)	80 (43)	24 (13)
RRC requirements	33 (18)	66 (36)	60 (33)	24 (13)
Board certification	16 (9)	44 (24)	86 (46)	39 (21)
Resident stress issues	14 (8)	56 (30)	96 (51)	19 (10)
Dealing with difficult and impaired residents	30 (16)	69 (37)	70 (38)	17 (9)
Conflict resolution	21 (11)	56 (30)	87 (47)	22 (12)
Fiscal issues/budgets	58 (31)	56 (30)	54 (29)	18 (10)
Maternity leave policies	53 (29)	62 (34)	62 (34)	8 (4)
Time management	24 (13)	67 (36)	73 (39)	21 (11)

*RRC indicates Residency Review Committee. The numbers in each knowledge area do not all total 187 because some directors did not answer each question.

years that the program director had served to date is shown in Table 3, along with information about job longevity of the program's prior director. These data clearly demonstrate the rapid turnover in the position of residency program director. Those program directors who were not departmental chairpersons served for significantly shorter periods than those who were also departmental chairpersons (5.4 years vs 9.3 years; $t=3.77$; $P=.0002$).

Working Situation of Program Directors

Only 28% of the respondents indicated that they had any type of formal job description and only 13% had been allotted a specific number of hours or percentage of time to accomplish their duties as program director. Fifty-one percent had a formal budget for the residency program, but the chairperson was in control of the budget in 60% of the programs with nonchairperson directors. On average, the program directors devoted 27% of their time to residency administrative activities, 21% to other administrative activities, 23% to direct patient care, 22% to teaching, and only 7% to research activities. Table 4 shows the percentage of directors who had the help of various support staff in the operation of their residency programs. In response to the question, "When you were appointed program director, did you receive a significant raise or increase in fringe benefits?" 73% of the directors answered "No."

Initial Knowledge Needed for Job Performance

Table 5 shows, for each of 12 content areas, how the respondents rated their knowledge at the time they assumed the role of program director. A large percentage of the program directors indicated weak initial knowledge in almost all of the educational, technical, and administrative aspects of their job.

Problems Faced by Program Directors

Table 6 indicates the amount of stress that each of 23 tasks or problems reportedly caused for program directors. The first column shows the mean Likert scale scores and the second column indicates the percentage of directors who gave the item a score of "4" or "5," indicating that the item was a major problem for them. No strong correlations were found when the scores on these items were analyzed with respect to program director age, gender, or job longevity.

Table 6.—Problems for Program Directors

Problem Area*	Mean Likert Scale Score	Major Problem (Score of 4 or 5), % of Directors
Lack of time	3.49	56
Too many other practice or academic responsibilities	3.40	52
Fear of not "filling" in the match	3.38	52
Completing questionnaires	3.32	44
Recruiting and interviewing	3.15	40
Counseling residents with problems	3.11	41
ACGME accreditation	3.11	39
Rescheduling (eg, illness, pregnancy)	3.09	41
Resident working-hour limitations	3.02	37
RRC requirement changes	3.02	35
Lack of adequate support staff	3.01	37
Dealing with hospital administration	2.97	33
Lack of time allotted for program administration	2.85	35
Being a buffer for resident-faculty conflict	2.83	29
Curriculum (need for improvement)	2.74	27
Lack of budget or financial control	2.73	26
Scheduling (eg, block, night)	2.72	30
National funding policies for Graduate Medical Education	2.72	28
Evaluating residents and giving feedback	2.72	24
Lack of clarity of responsibilities	2.38	21
Lack of faculty support	2.29	19
Patient complaints about residents	1.89	5
Lack of chairperson support	1.62	9

*ACGME indicates the Accreditation Council on Graduate Medical Education; and RRC, Residency Review Committee.

Attitudes About an Extended Conference for Program Directors

Eighty-six percent of the directors said that an educational conference to teach them the skills and provide the information needed to be an effective program director would have been valuable when they assumed their jobs. Seventy-five percent indicated that they would still find such a conference useful and almost all (88%) in that group were willing to attend a seminar lasting at least 2 days. Forty-five percent of all directors chose basic educational methods as their first choice of topics for this proposed seminar; examples of methods included curriculum design, formulation of learning objectives, evaluation and feedback methods, and methods to improve conferences. Thirty-six percent wanted to develop administrative skills, such as directing the budgetary process, leadership and motivational techniques, conflict management, and methods to deal with problem residents. The primary choice of 19% of the program directors was technical information, which included the residency program accreditation process, Residency Review Committee requirements, the certification process of the American Board of Pediatrics, and technical aspects of the National Intern Matching Program.

COMMENT

The job of a residency program director is complex and requires special knowledge and skills. The director is expected to be teacher, evaluator, employer, career counselor, scheduler, advisor, arbitrator, and administrator. He or she must have a working knowledge of the laws, rules, and regulations of the many agencies that are responsible for the accreditation of training programs and the licensing and certification of physicians. The program director is responsible for obtaining highly competent trainees for the program, providing them with a good curriculum, measuring and providing feedback about their progress, and identifying and dealing with those trainees who are impaired or otherwise having difficulty.

When dismissal of a resident is being considered, the program director must follow "due process" requirements so that legal action against the program can be avoided. The director is often called on to help create and revise schedules, to ensure that residents are providing competent medical care, to arbitrate disputes between faculty members and residents, to eliminate stress, and to "keep everyone happy." The program director in an academic center must also meet committee responsibilities, write scientific papers and grants, teach medical students, and provide direct patient care. He or she must also write letters of recommendation, sign loan deferment forms, and fill out questionnaires. This diversity of roles must be accomplished within an environment of limited resources, time constraints, and little formal training.

For decades, industry has invested significant resources to train middle and senior management staff and to promote their personal growth and retention. It is only in recent years that the managerial role of physicians has gained attention. The American College of Physician Executives, established in 1989, serves as a forum for research, training, and group discussion relating to skills applicable to physicians in senior management roles.[1] Several medical specialties sponsor periodic orientation and training events for new chairpersons. Management skill training activities for chief residents have recently emerged.[2] To date, however, little attention has been paid to developing effective management skills in the critical "middle manager" role of residency program director.

The issue of stress during residency training has received much attention in recent years. Among the many stressors that have been identified by house officers are a lack of faculty support, a poor learning environment, and an insufficient number of good role models.[3-6] It is not easy for a program director to provide support to others and to create a good learning environment if he or she feels time pressures. As Pfifferling[7] pointed out, "harried, overworked, time-juggling attendings" are not particularly good role models for residents. It certainly seems plausible that the stress felt by program directors contributes to the development of resident stress.

The Pediatric Special Requirements of the Accreditation Council on Graduate Medical Education[8] state that the program director "must be capable of administering the program in an effective manner and be competent in the care of pediatric patients. He/she should have demonstrated ability as a teacher and be knowledgeable in the related basic sciences and in research methodology. The director should be certified by the American Board of Pediatrics or should possess suitable equivalent qualifications."

Our results document the perceived needs of program directors for organized training in specific content areas, such as curriculum design, budgetary processes, and Residency Review Committee requirements, as well as in such areas as motivational techniques, skills of conflict management, and evaluating residents and giving them feedback. Such courses exist for other physician managers and it seems both feasible and reasonable that they be developed for residency program directors. Continuity is an important factor in the leadership of residency training, according to the Accreditation Council on Graduate Medical Education.[8] A program director management training program might lessen the rate of turnover of program directors and promote growth of continuity and expertise in this role, with attendant improvement in the quality of residency training.

References

1. Betson C, Pedrojz A. Physician managers: a description of their job in hospital. *Hosp Health Serv Admin*. 1989;34:353-369.
2. Whitman N. A management skills workshop for chief residents. *J Med Educ*. 1988;63:442-446.
3. Resident Services Committee, Association of Program Directors in Internal Medicine. Stress and impairment during residency training: strategies for reduction, identification and management. *Ann Intern Med*. 1988;109:154-161.
4. Green M. Individual and group support systems: a residency adaptation program. In: Hoekelman RA, ed. *Stress in Pediatric House Staff Training*. Columbus, Ohio: Ross Laboratories; 1986:146-156.
5. McCue JD. The distress of internship: causes and prevention. *N Engl J Med*. 1985;312:449-452.
6. Hoekelman RA. Stress experienced during pediatric residency training: its causes, consequences, recognition and solutions. *AJDC*. 1989;143:177-182.
7. Pfifferling JH. Stress in residency training: an anthropological perspective. In: Hoekelman RA, ed. *Stress in Pediatric House Staff Training*. Columbus, Ohio: Ross Laboratories; 1986:2-13.
8. Special requirements for programs in pediatrics. In: *1989-90 Directory of Graduate Medical Education Programs*. Chicago, Ill: American Medical Association; 1989:87.

In Other AMA Journals

ARCHIVES OF OTOLARYNGOLOGY—HEAD & NECK SURGERY

Reconstruction of Pediatric Larynx and Upper Trachea With the Sternohyoid Rotary Door Flap

Isaac Eliachar, MD, FRCS,
Harvey M. Tucker, MD, FRCS
(*Arch Otolaryngol Head Neck Surg*. 1991;117:316-320)

Noncongenital Hereditary Hearing Loss in Children: Prospective Documentation

Jane R. Madell, PhD, Nancy Sculerati, MD
(*Arch Otolaryngol Head Neck Surg*. 1991;117:332-335)

ARCHIVES OF DERMATOLOGY

An Observational Study of Isotretinoin Recipients Treated for Acne in a Health Maintenance Organization

Newell E. McElwee, PharmD, MSPH;
Mary Catherine Schumacher, MD, MSPH;
Sylvia C. Johnson, MD; Thomas W. Weir, MD;
Steven L. Greene, MD; Marvin J. Scotvold, MD;
Judith R. Hunter; Barbara J. Dinan, RN;
Hershel Jick, MD
(*Arch Dermatol*. 1991;127:341-346)

Nasal Midline Masses in Infants and Children: Dermoids, Encephaloceles, and Gliomas

Amy S. Paller, MD; Jay M. Pensler, MD;
Tadanori Tomita, MD
(*Arch Dermatol*. 1991;127:362-366)

Mineral Metabolism and Calcitriol Therapy in Idiopathic Juvenile Osteoporosis

Giuseppe Saggese, MD; Silvano Bertelloni, MD; Giampiero I. Baroncelli, MD; Giuseppe Perri, MD; Andrea Calderazzi, MD

• Idiopathic juvenile osteoporosis is a rare cause of osteoporosis during childhood. We examined four children (three boys and one girl, ranging in age from 2.3 to 12.6 years) with idiopathic juvenile osteoporosis. All of these patients had normal serum calcium, ionized calcium, phosphate, magnesium, 25-hydroxyvitamin D, intact parathyroid hormone, and total and extractable calcitonin levels. 1,25-Dihydroxyvitamin D values were low in three patients and slightly decreased in one. Three children were treated with calcitriol (1,25 - dihydroxycholecalciferol) (0.50 μg/d in two and 0.25 μg/d in the other). The fourth patient was not treated because of parental refusal. Therapy reduced the fracture rate. Follow-up at 6 and 12 months showed a significant increase in bone mineralization, which reached normal values in two children after 12 months of treatment. No side effects of calcitriol therapy were observed. The untreated patient did not show an improvement of bone mineralization in the same time.
***(AJDC*. 1991;145:457-462)**

Idiopathic juvenile osteoporosis (IJO) is a rare form of bone demineralization during childhood.[1] The diagnosis is difficult since symptoms are not specific; it is based on the exclusion of known causes of osteoporosis in childhood, mainly the mild forms of osteogenesis imperfecta.[1] Typical features are fractures of the long bones and of the vertebrae, bone pain, difficulty in walking, and variable time to spontaneous recovery of bone mineralization, generally within 3 to 4 years.[2-4] In most patients, the onset of disease is just before puberty.[3,4] Kooh et al[5] and Exner et al[6] described some cases in which symptoms became evident before the age of 5 years. These periods of life, ie, the early years and peripuberty, are characterized by a high height velocity,[7] and it is likely that IJO requires rapid growth to be manifest clinically.

The pathogenesis of IJO is unknown.[2] A negative calcium balance, detected in some[3,8,9] but not in all patients,[10] is the main metabolic abnormality observed. Marder and coworkers[11] found low 1,25-dihydroxyvitamin D [$1,25(OH)_2D$] levels in one patient, while Leroy et al[12] found high $1,25(OH)_2D$ concentrations associated with low levels of 25-hydroxyvitamin D (25-OH-D) and 24,25-dihydroxyvitamin D in the girl they observed. Recently, Jackson et al[13] suggested a possible calcitonin deficiency in some cases.

Therapeutic trials with vitamin D, calcium supplements, calcitonin, and anabolic steroids failed to modify the natural course of IJO.[3,13] Marder et al[11] found that calcitriol (1,25-dihydroxycholecalciferol) was effective, even if the same group did not confirm this finding in another patient.[13]

Since the pathogenesis of IJO has been related to an impaired secretion of $1,25(OH)_2D$[11] or calcitonin,[13] we studied serum basal and stimulated levels of $1,25(OH)_2D$ and calcitonin to clarify the relationships between these hormones and IJO. In this study, we evaluated both total plasma calcitonin (tCT) and extractable calcitonin (exCT) levels, since it has been demonstrated that the exCT measurement reflects more accurately the biologically relevant plasma monomeric calcitonin level than the tCT assay does.[14] Moreover, we report bone mineralization, assessed by single photon absorptiometry (SPA), at diagnosis and during 3 years of follow-up. In the first year of follow-up, three patients received calcitriol therapy; the fourth was not treated because of parental refusal.

SUBJECTS AND METHODS

Patients

We examined three boys and one girl with IJO (Table 1). Symptoms were bone pain, recurrent fractures at the methaphyses of long bones in all but one (patient 2), and difficulty in walking. In none of the patients was there any history of nausea, vomiting, recurrent diarrhea, steatorrhea, immobilization, bleeding tendency, familial osteogenesis imperfecta, or other metabolic bone disease. A detailed evaluation of diet showed an adequate intake of energy, protein, calcium, and phosphate. Roentgenographic films showed diffuse osteoporosis in the three boys only. No signs of rickets, ossa suturarum, or abnormalities of the lamina dura were present. More clinical details of these patients at diagnosis were reported elsewhere.[15]

Study Protocol

All subjects were studied in the supine position after an overnight fast; blood samples were taken from an antecubital vein through an indwelling catheter between 8 and 9 AM for the determination of calcium, phosphate, magnesium, alkaline phosphatase, osteocalcin (the major noncollagenous bone protein secreted by osteoblasts),[16] intact parathyroid hormone (PTH), tCT, exCT, 25-OH-D, and $1,25(OH)_2D$ levels in basal condition. After

Accepted for publication August 23, 1990.
From the Vitamin D Laboratory and Calcium Research Center, Endocrine Unit, Department of Pediatrics (Drs Saggese, Bertelloni, and Baroncelli), and Institute of Radiology (Drs Perri and Calderazzi), University of Pisa, Italy.
Reprint requests to Vitamin D Laboratory and Calcium Research Center, Endocrine Unit, Department of Pediatrics, University of Pisa, Via Roma, 35, 56100 Pisa, Italy (Dr Saggese).

Table 1.—Clinical and Radiological Findings

	Patient No.			
	1	2	3	4
Age, y/sex	12.1/M	2.0/M	12.6/F	9.0/M
Symptom onset, age, y	9.5	1.3	10.5	2.1
Height, cm	148	91	148	126
Height percentile*	50	75	10-25	10-25
Weight, kg	44	14	40	25
Weight percentile*	75-90	50	25	25
Pubertal stage*	G1Ph1	G1Ph1	B2Ph1	G1Ph1
Bone age, y†	12.0	1.7	10.0	9.0
Family history	No	No	No	No
Bone pain	Diffuse	Knee, foot	Diffuse	Legs, spine
Walking difficulty	Yes	No	Yes	No
Loss of height	No	No	Yes	Yes
Backache	No	Yes	No	Yes
Pigeon chest	No	Yes	No	No
Fractures	Legs, arms	No	Hands, knees, long bones	Vertebrae, long bones
Fracture rate, No./y	6	...	8	9
Osteoporosis (roentgenography)	Skull, sella, long bones	Widespread	No	Vertebrae, carpal and long bones

*Tanner and Whitehouse standards.[7] G, Ph, and B (pubertal stage) indicate genitalia, pubic hair, and breast.
†Gruelich and Pyle[35] method.

clotting, the serum was separated by centrifugation and the samples were aliquoted and stored in the dark at −20°C until assayed. Measurement of ionized calcium was performed on blood samples collected in anaerobic tubes that had been completely filled; after centrifugation, the serum was analyzed within 1 hour. The calcitonin levels were also measured after calcium infusion; 50 mL of isotonic saline containing calcium gluconate (2 mg of elemental calcium per kilogram of body weight) was infused intravenously during a 5-minute period.[14] Blood samples for the measurement of ionized calcium, tCT, and exCT were obtained before infusion and at 5 and 10 minutes after the beginning of the infusion. Blood for ionized calcium determination was obtained from a site distant from that of the calcium infusion. No adverse effects were observed.

A dynamic evaluation of PTH and 1,25$(OH)_2$D levels, using low-calcium diet as previously described,[17] was started 1 day later. Briefly, serum for measuring ionized calcium, intact PTH, and 1,25$(OH)_2$D was obtained; during the following 3 days, the patients assumed a low-calcium diet, providing a calcium intake of 2 mg/kg per day or less. The diet was formulated with common foods on the basis of the standard tables of foods and their mineral contents; it is effective in increasing PTH and 1,25$(OH)_2$D serum levels in normal children.[17] The diet satisfied the requirements of magnesium and phosphate; energy intakes were appropriate for age and weight. The children were studied as outpatients, and the parents were provided with quantitative daily diet instructions. The parents recorded the exact weight of eaten foods, and the daily diary diet was reviewed by one of us (S.B.). At the end of the 3-day diet, ionized calcium, intact PTH, and 1,25$(OH)_2$D levels were reevaluated.

Subsequently, patients 3 and 4 were treated with 0.50 μg/d of calcitriol in two divided doses; patient 2 received 0.25 μg of calcitriol once a day. Doses were calculated on the basis of a minimal daily 1,25$(OH)_2$D production rate[18] given that endogenous production was present. Child 1 was not treated because the parents did not consent.

Side effects of calcitriol in the treated children were monitored measuring serum ionized calcium and urinary calcium–urinary creatinine ratio every 3 months.

Informed consent was obtained from both parents of each child. The study was approved by the Committee for Investigations in Children of our department; one child's parents did not consent to treatment.

Methods

Serum levels of calcium (normal range, 2.1 to 2.7 mmol/L), phosphate (1.2 to 2.0 mmol/L), magnesium (0.8 to 1.3 mmol/L), alkaline phosphatase (86 to 645 U/L), glucose (4.0 to 6.4 mmol/L), creatinine (<0.88 μmol/L), alanine aminotransferase (<40 U/L), and aspartate aminotransferase (<40 U/L) were assessed by an automatic analyzer (model Chem-1 System, Technicon Instruments Co, Tarrytown, NY). The serum ionized calcium level was measured by a selective electrode (ORION SS-20, Cambridge, Mass) at 37°C and corrected for pH at 7.4 (normal level, 1.1 to 1.3 mmol/L; N = 57 healthy children). Levels of cortisol (normal value at 8 AM, 138.0 to 691.0 nmol/L; at midnight, 55 to 113 nmol/L), total thyroxine (normal level, 51.0 to 154.0 nmol/L), total triiodothyronine (normal level, 1.2 to 3.1 nmol/L), and thyrotropin (normal level, 0.6 to 6.3 mU/L) were detected by commercially available radioimmunoassays (RIAs) (Biodata, Milan, Italy).

The osteocalcin level was assayed by RIA using a commercially available kit (Osteocalcin, INCSTAR Co, Stillwater, Minn). Sensitivity was 0.2 ng/mL; interassay and intra-assay variations were 8.9% and 6.3%, respectively. Our normal values were as follows: 12.2±5.5 ng/mL for 1- to 9-year-olds; 20.8±8.5 ng/mL for 9- to 14-year-olds; and 7.3±3.4 ng/mL for 14- to 18-year-olds.[18]

Parathyroid hormone levels were measured by a two-site immunoradiometric assay for the biologically intact 1-84 amino acid chain of the hormone based on two different goat polyclonal antibodies specific for well-defined regions of the molecule (Allegro Intact PTH, Nichols Institute Diagnostics, San Juan Capistrano, Calif). Sensitivity of the method was 1 ng/L; interassay and intra-assay variations were 5.5% and 4.1%, respectively. Normal values in our laboratory were 31.2±10.8 ng/L, with no significant variations between ages.[19]

Total calcitonin levels were measured in whole serum by an RIA method based on a highly sensitive and specific antiserum capable of detecting hormone levels as low as 3 ng/L (Calcitonin, Nichols Institute Diagnostics). Sequential analysis with delayed tracer addition is employed to maximize assay sensitivity. The calcitonin standard is calibrated against the World Health Organization calcitonin preparation (code 70/234 human, synthetic), National Institute for Biological Standards and Controls, London, England. Interassay and intra-assay variations were 8.9% and 6.7%, respectively; our normal values were 25.0±15.0 ng/L.[20] Levels of exCT were evaluated by the same RIA after an extraction-concentration step performed by a slight modification of the Body and Heath[14] method. Briefly, 3 mL of serum was applied to prewashed (5 mL of distilled water minicolumns (Silica Sep-pak, Waters Associates, Milford, Mass); the cartridges were washed with acetic acid in water (4:96, vol/vol), and exCT was eluted with 3 mL of methanol in water (70:30, vol/vol). The sample was dried, redissolved in assay buffer, and measured by calcitonin RIA. An internal standard was employed to calculate the recovery of exCT after the extraction-concentration procedure. Normal values were 6.0±3.0 ng/L.[20]

Levels of 25-OH-D and 1,25$(OH)_2$D were measured by a competitive protein-binding assay after high-performance liquid chromatography purification, as previously described,[21] with minor modifications. In the 1,25$(OH)_2$D assay, we employed calf thymus receptor instead of chick intestinal receptor, because the

Table 2.—Mineralometric and Biochemical Data at Diagnosis*

	Patient No.			
	1	2	3	4
BMC, %	−23.0	−18.5	−14.0	−33.4
BMC/BW, %	−21.0	−17.6	−15.3	−40.2
Red blood cells, $\times 10^{12}$/L	4.9	4.3	4.5	4.7
White blood cells, $\times 10^{9}$/L	7.0	6.4	5.8	6.9
Platelets, $\times 10^{9}$/L	210	179	156	230
Bone marrow	N	N	N	N
Glucose, mmol/L	4.5	4.3	5.0	4.0
Creatinine, μmol/L	61.7	71.0	44.2	76.9
AST, U/L	12	17	25	15
ALT, U/L	8	23	15	7
Calcium, mmol/L	2.45	2.65	2.40	2.50
Ionized calcium, mmol/L	1.17	1.16	1.13	1.22
Phosphate, mmol/L	1.22	1.42	1.25	1.69
Magnesium, mmol/L	1.22	1.06	0.91	1.06
Alkaline phosphatase, U/L	280	450	330	340
Osteocalcin, ng/mL	19.2	15.3	7.2	14.3
T_3, nmol/L	2.7	2.9	2.5	2.7
T_4, nmol/L	79.4	140.1	115.5	107.5
TSH, mU/L	2.0	3.5	2.1	2.7
Cortisol (8 AM), nmol/L	496.2	579.6	538.2	452.6
Cortisol (midnight), nmol/L	183.2	138.0	63.5	129.7
Intact PTH, ng/L	24.0	32.2	25.0	42.0
tCT, ng/L	19.5	28.0	39.0	18.6
exCT, ng/L	5.8	7.9	4.5	6.0
25-OH-D, nmol/L	102.7	88.5	76.0	85.0
$1,25(OH)_2D$, pmol/L	94.1	170.4	84.2	36.9
Karyotype	46,XY	46,XY	46,XX	46,XY

*BMC indicates bone mineral content; BW, bone width; N, normal; AST, aspartate aminotransferase; ALT, alanine aminotransferase; T_3, triiodothyronine; T_4, thyroxine; TSH, thyrotropin; PTH, parathyroid hormone; tCT, total plasma calcitonin; exCT, extractable calcitonin; 25-OH-D, 25-hydroxyvitamin D; and $1,25(OH)_2D$, 1,25-dihydroxyvitamin D.

former shows higher sensitivity and specificity for $1,25(OH)_2D$.[22] The method was improved with a disequilibrium procedure using delayed tracer addition to test tubes to increase sensitivity. Each metabolite was measured in duplicate against a reference standard. Interassay and intra-assay variations and sensitivity were, respectively, 4.0%, 3.1%, and 1.3 nmol/L for 25-OH-D and 4.3%, 3.6%, and 5.0 pmol/L for $1,25(OH)_2D$. Our normal values for age are as follows: for 25-OH-D, 97.0±24.2 nmol/L for ages 1 month to 2.0 years; 83.0±12.0 nmol/L for ages 2.1 to 10.7 years; and 86.7±16.5 nmol/L for ages 11.0 to 17.0 years; for $1,25(OH)_2D$, 208.0±20.0 pmol/L for ages 1 month to 2.0 years; 92.0±17.5 pmol/L for ages 2.1 to 10.7 years; and 179.0±17.0 pmol/L for ages 11.0 to 17.0 years.[21]

Bone mineral analysis was performed by SPA (model 2783, Norland Corporation, Atkinson, Wis) at the distal third of the nondominant radius. Bone mineral content (BMC) (grams per centimeter) and BMC/bone width (BMC/BW) (grams per square centimeter) of each subject represented the mean of two scans. The results were calculated as percentage means of BMC and BMC/BW values in respect to the values expected for sex- and age-matched normal subjects (2-year age groups).[23] The method has a coefficient of variation of 2% or lower.

Table 3.—Dynamic Evaluation of tCT, exCT, PTH, and $1,25(OH)_2D$*

Stimulus	Levels			
	IV Calcium (2 mg/kg)			
	Patients (n=4)		Controls (n=10)	
	0 min	10 min	0 min	10 min
Ionized calcium, mmol/L	1.15± 0.03	1.34± 0.06†	1.17± 0.05	1.39± 0.09‡
tCT, ng/L	26.3± 8.2	57.7± 14.5§	28.4± 15.5	65.7± 28.9†
exCT, ng/L	6.0± 1.2	24.8± 5.6†	5.2± 2.3	22.2± 10.1‡
	Low-Calcium Diet			
	Patients (n=4)		Controls (n=13)	
	Day 1	Day 3	Day 1	Day 3
Ionized calcium, mmol/L	1.15± 0.02	1.05± 0.03§	1.20± 0.05	1.1± 0.04‡
Intact PTH, ng/L	28.4± 6.0	45.1± 7.5‖	32.0± 11.2	52.1± 15.5†
$1,25(OH)_2D$, pmol/L	90.0± 32.6	103.7± 25.7	110.9± 9.4	168.5± 13.2‡

*tCT indicates total plasma calcitonin; exCT, extractable calcitonin; PTH, parathyroid hormone; $1,25(OH)_2D$, 1,25-dihydroxyvitamin D; and IV, intravenous. Control values for IV calcium[20] and low-calcium diet[17] were selected from previous data obtained in healthy children matched for age, sex, and vitamin D status in respect to patients.
†$P<.01$ vs 0 minutes or day 1.
‡$P<.001$ vs 0 minutes or day 1.
§$P<.02$ vs 0 minutes or day 1.
‖$P<.05$ vs day 1.

RESULTS

Mineralometric and Biochemical Data at Diagnosis

Bone mineralization and biochemical data at diagnosis are reported in Table 2. Bone mineral analysis showed a reduction of both BMC and BMC/BW in patients with IJO in respect to our age- and sex-matched normal values.

Levels of calcium, ionized calcium, phosphate, magnesium, alkaline phosphatase, glucose, creatinine, alanine aminotransferase, aspartate aminotransferase, cortisol (basal and circadian rhythm), triiodothyronine, thyroxine, and thyrotropin were in the normal range; the level of osteocalcin was low in patient 3 and normal in the others. The concentration of $1,25(OH)_2D$ was reduced in three subjects (patients 1, 3, and 4) and slightly decreased in the last one (patient 2); the other examined measures were in the normal range (Table 2).

The calcium stimulation test showed a normal secretory reserve of tCT and exCT (Table 3). While receiving a low-calcium diet, the patients' ionized calcium values fell and intact PTH levels rose, as in healthy subjects, but $1,25(OH)_2D$ concentrations did not increase (Table 3).

Follow-up

Calcitriol administration in the treated patients reduced the frequency of fractures and resulted in improvement of the clinical symptoms, which disappeared within 5 to 9 months. During the first month of treatment, patients remained in their homes to minimize the opportunity for trauma, and no fractures occurred. In the following 6 months, two adjunctive fractures were experienced by patient 4 (one from major trauma in a bicycle accident, the second from intensive physical activity) and one by patient

Table 4.—Bone Mineral Data During Follow-up*

Bone Loss, mo	Patient No. 1	2	3	4
6				
BMC	−27.0	−9.3	−5.2	−18.0
BMC/BW	−25.1	−7.4	−15.1	−24.2
12				
BMC	−22.5	−2.4	N	−7.5
BMC/BW	−18.7	N	−4.1	−10.5
18				
BMC	−23.0	+3.7	N	...
BMC/BW	−27.8	+4.0	N	...
24				
BMC	−20.2	+5.0	N	...
BMC/BW	−18.7	N	+4.5	...
30				
BMC	−13.3	−5.2	N	...
BMC/BW	−16.6	N	+6.7	...
36				
BMC	...	+5.1	N	...
BMC/BW	...	+6.2	N	...

*BMC indicates bone mineral content; BW, bone width; and N, normal. Values are percent. Patient 1 stopped follow-up after 30 months; patient 4 discontinued therapy and follow-up after 12 months.

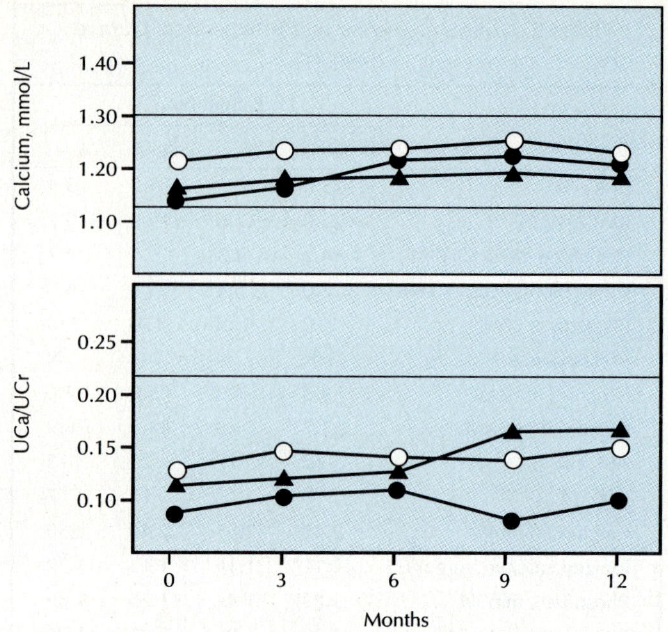

Serum ionized calcium levels and urinary calcium excretion (urinary calcium–urinary creatinine ratio [UCa/UCr]) in the three patients with idiopathic juvenile osteoporosis during calcitriol treatment. Open circles indicate patient 2; solid circles, patient 3; and triangles, patient 4.

3 (traumatic metacarpal fracture). Additional fractures did not occur for the remaining period of observation. After 6 months of treatment, BMC and BMC/BW increased in all treated subjects (Table 4). After 1 year of therapy, bone mineralization reached normal values in patients 2 and 3; patient 4 also showed a clear improvement of BMC and BMC/BW. After this control period, patient 4 discontinued care, and no other data are available. In the other two treated children (patients 2 and 3), BMC and BMC/BW increased in the subsequent 2 years according to age-related increments (Table 4), and no other fractures were experienced by these patients.

No side effects of calcitriol therapy were observed. The serum ionized calcium level and urinary calcium–urinary creatinine ratio remained in the normal range in the three patients during treatment (Figure).

The untreated boy (patient 1) showed a slow increment of mineralization with no improvement at 1 year of follow-up and with only a slight increase of bone mineralization 30 months after the initial evaluation (Table 4). During this period, fractures occurred with the same rate as before the initial evaluation (3 to 5 fractures per year).

COMMENT

Diagnosis of IJO in our patients was made by the presence of typical skeletal involvement and by ruling out the other known causes of osteoporosis in childhood on the basis of history, physical examination, and laboratory data.[2-4] Our patients showed neither the typical features of osteogenesis imperfecta (blue sclerae, lax ligaments, dental abnormalities, family history, deafness, skull abnormalities), the main differential diagnosis,[1] nor the signs or symptoms of thyrotoxicosis, Cushing's syndrome, defects in secretory activity of parathyroid glands, diabetes, connective tissue disorders, chronic rheumatic diseases, hematological malignant neoplasm, malabsorption syndromes, or chromosomal disorders. Vitamin D deficiency was ruled out by history of sufficient solar exposure and normal serum 25-OH-D levels, the best index of individual vitamin D status.[24] Dietetic deprivation was excluded by patient history, which showed adequate calcium and phosphate intake. Moreover, skeletal fractures, occurring mainly at metaphyseal sites, are pathognomonic of IJO.[3,4,25-27]

Bone demineralization is the constant finding in all described cases of IJO.[1,2] Radiological evidence of osteoporosis was present in only three of our children; in one (patient 3), bone loss was evident only when assessed by SPA, suggesting that in cases of children with a history evoking IJO but with normal roentgenograms, a more sensitive evaluation of skeletal mineral content is required. Furthermore, SPA may allow a more accurate follow-up of bone mineralization if some kind of treatment is employed. The lack of fractures, first reported by Lapatsanis et al[9] in patients with IJO, was found by us in one boy (patient 2).

The pathogenesis of IJO is largely unknown.[2] The disease shows a fairly uniform age at presentation around the pubertal growth spurt, with spontaneous recovery after 3 to 5 years.[3,4] Moreover, some instances of childhood osteoporosis of unknown origin have been reported in the first years of life.[5,6] These patients were identical with cases of IJO in regard to symptoms, signs, radiological and biochemical findings, and course of the disease: spontaneous recovery occurred when growth velocity fell after the first 3 to 4 years of life.[5,6] Therefore, the two forms may represent an expression of the same disease,[2,5] in which rapid growth velocity acts as a trigger to make it clinically manifest.

Biochemical data in IJO are characterized by normal levels of calcium, phosphate, and alkaline phosphatase[3-5,8,10] and by a slight increase of urinary total hydroxyproline.[4] The external balance of calcium has been shown to be negative in most affected children,[3,4,8,9] zero in the mild forms, and positive in some other patients.[10] Clinical recovery from the disease is associated with the normalization of calcium balance.[4,9] Parathyroid hormone levels have been measured in the normal range,[4,10-12] as we confirmed in our patients by using an ultrasensitive assay specific for the intact PTH molecule, which allows a complete discrimination of hormone levels in patients with altered parathyroid gland secretion from levels in normal subjects.[28] Marder et al[11] underlined a severe $1,25(OH)_2D$ deficiency in the child they studied and hypothesized that the negative calcium balance could be due to reduced $1,25(OH)_2D$ levels, mostly related to a transient sex steroid deficiency before the onset of puberty. The increase of sex steroid production during puberty[29] would explain the spontaneous improvement in bone mineralization for patients with IJO, and the increase of $1,25(OH)_2D$ values in the patient of Marder et al.[11]

However, the rarity of IJO and its occurrence in some children during the first years of life point out that other factors are involved in the pathogenesis of the disease. Vitamin D deficiency, as suggested by Leroy et al,[12] is ruled out by the evidence of normal 25-OH-D values in our patients, as in others.[11,13] Also, the hypothesis of an increased $1,25(OH)_2D$ catabolism is not supported by the observation that calcitriol treatment in physiological doses is effective and that these low doses increased serum hormone concentrations into the normal range.[11] During the periods of life in which IJO mainly occurs, the $1,25(OH)_2D$ serum levels increase physiologically[30,31] to permit a greater intestinal mineral absorption needed for growth.[30] The low-calcium diet we used to test $1,25(OH)_2D$ production in IJO showed no significant hormone increase over baseline levels, while the same diet enabled determination of a significant $1,25(OH)_2D$ increase in healthy children.[17] In these patients, a partial defect of renal 1α-hydroxylase could be present that is able to maintain $1,25(OH)_2D$ levels in the normal range with usual calcium requirements but is not able to increase hormone levels when calcium needs are stressed, as in ages with higher growth velocity.[30] The relative sex steroid deficiency of prepuberty could cause enhanced bone resorption, as in postmenopausal osteoporosis, depending on bone hypersensitivity to normal PTH levels; thus, normocalcemia and normal PTH levels take place in spite of reduced $1,25(OH)_2D$ levels and negative calcium balance.[11,32]

Recently, Jackson and coworkers[13] described a girl with IJO in whom the $1,25(OH)_2D$ value was elevated and calcitonin was undetectable; the levels of these components returned to normal when the IJO resolved. The authors suggested that calcitonin deficiency may have a causative role in the pathogenesis of the disease. In our patients, both basal and calcium-stimulated tCT and exCT values, the latter being more representative of biologically active hormone,[14] were normal. These findings do not support the hypothesis of impaired calcitonin secretion in IJO, at least in our series. In this regard, it is of interest that calcitonin therapy administered to a girl described by Jackson et al[13] improved neither bone mineralization nor fracture rates. Furthermore, the possibility that a derangement of calcitonin secretion is involved in bone demineralization seems to be ruled out by the evidence that subjects with prolonged whole calcitonin deficiency did not have increased bone loss as compared with appropriate controls. Conversely, calcitonin excess did not cause increased bone mass.[33] Moreover, reduced bone mineralization did not develop in hypothyroid children with calcitonin deficiency from congenital thyroid agenesia in comparison with controls.[34]

In conclusion, our data support the evidence of decreased $1,25(OH)_2D$ serum levels in some patients with IJO. Calcitriol treatment seems to be effective in these subjects; however, since IJO is a disease that remits spontaneously, further study of treated patients will be required to draw definitive conclusions.

References

1. Dent CE. Osteoporosis in childhood. *Postgrad Med J.* 1977;53:450-456.
2. Smith R. Idiopathic juvenile osteoporosis. *AJDC.* 1979;133:889-891.
3. Teotia M, Teotia SPS, Singh RK. Idiopathic juvenile osteoporosis. *AJDC.* 1979;133:894-900.
4. Jowsey J, Johnson KA. Juvenile osteoporosis: bone findings in seven patients. *J Pediatr.* 1972;81:511-517.
5. Kooh SW, Cumming WA, Fraser D, Fraser A. Transient childhood osteoporosis of unknown cause. In: Frame B, Parfit AM, Duncan H, eds. *Clinical Aspect of Bone Disease.* Princeton, NJ: Excerpta Medica; 1973:329-332.
6. Exner GU, Prader A, Elsasser U, Anlinker M. Idiopathic osteoporosis in a three-year old girl: follow-up over a period of 6 years by computed tomography bone densitometry. *Helv Paediatr Acta.* 1984;39:517-529.
7. Tanner JM, Whitehouse RH. Clinical longitudinal standards for height, weight, height velocity, weight velocity, and stages of puberty. *Arch Dis Child.* 1976;51:170-181.
8. Dent CE, Friedman M. Idiopathic juvenile osteoporosis. *Q J Med.* 1965;34:177-210.
9. Lapatsanis P, Kavadias A, Vretos K. Juvenile osteoporosis. *Arch Dis Child.* 1971;47:66-71.
10. Lachmann D, Willvonsender R, Hofer R. A case report of idiopathic juvenile osteoporosis with particular reference 47-calcium absorption. *Eur J Pediatr.* 1977;125:265-273.
11. Marder HK, Tsang RC, Hug G, Crawford AC. Calcitriol deficiency in idiopathic juvenile osteoporosis. *AJDC.* 1982;136:914-917.
12. Leroy D, Garabedian M, Guillozo H, Bourdeau A, Sauvegrain J, Balsan S. Evolution des concentrations seriques en metabolites de la vitamine D (25-OH-D, $24,25(OH)_2D$, $1,25(OH)_2D$) dans un case d'osteoporose juvenile idiopathique. *Arch Fr Pediatr.* 1981;38:165-170.
13. Jackson EC, Strife F, Tsang RC, Marder HK. Effect of calcitonin replacement therapy in idiopathic juvenile osteoporosis. *AJDC.* 1988;142:1237-1239.
14. Body JJ, Heath H III. Estimates of circulating monomeric calcitonin: physiological studies in normal and thyroidectomized man. *J Clin Endocrinol Metab.* 1983;57:897-902.
15. Perri G, Saggese G, Bertelloni S, Saggese G, Bertelloni S, Baroncelli GI. Idiopathic juvenile osteoporosis. *Radiol Med.* 1987;74:399-403.
16. Saggese G, Bertelloni S, Baroncelli GI, Buggiani B. Osteocalcin values in childhood: relationship with bone mineralization and with 1,25-dihydroxyvitamin D variations. *Riv Ital Pediatr.* 1989;15:109-112.
17. Saggese G, Bertelloni S, Baroncelli GI, Buggiani B. A simple and reliable stimulatory test for 1,25-dihydroxyvitamin D in childhood. *Horm Metab.* 1987;1:29-35.
18. Portale AA, Halloran BP, Murphy MM, Morris RC Jr. Oral intake of phosphorus can determine the serum concentrations of 1,25-dihydroxyvitamin D by determining its production rate in humans. *J Clin Invest.* 1986;77:7-12.
19. Saggese G, Baroncelli GI, Bertelloni S. Two-site immunoradiometric assay of intact parathyroid hormone in children: methodological aspects. *G Ital Chim Clin.* 1989;14:123-129.
20. Saggese G, Bertelloni S, Baroncelli GI, Buggiani B, Papini A. Calcitonin secretion in osteoporosis of Turner's syndrome. *Riv Ital Pediatr.* 1988;14:674-678.
21. Saggese G, Bertelloni S, Baroncelli GI. Radioreceptor assay of vitamin D metabolites after high performance liquid chromatography using ultraphine stationary phases. *G Ital Chim Clin.* 1986;11:177-182.
22. Reinhardt TA, Horst RL, Littledike ET. 1,25-Dihydroxyvitamin D receptor in bovine thymus gland. *Biochem Biophys Res Commun.* 1982;106:1012-1015.
23. Saggese G, Federico G, Ghirri P, Cipriani J, Bertelloni S, Baroncelli GI. Bone mineral content in pediatrics: normal values between 2 and 19 years: first Italian data. *Minerva Pediatrica.* 1986;38:545-551.

24. Holick MF. Vitamin D requirements for the elderly. *Clin Nutr.* 1986;5:121-127.
25. Houang MTW, Brenton DP, Renton P, Shaw DG. Idiopathic juvenile osteoporosis. *Skeletal Radiol.* 1978;3:17-23.
26. Gooding CA, Ball JH. Idiopathic juvenile osteoporosis. *Radiology.* 1969;93:1349-1351.
27. Sauvegrain J, Leroy D, Finidori G, Kalifa G. Osteoporose juvenile idiopathique. *J Radiol.* 1979;60:821-824.
28. Pandian MR, Potts JT, Lavigne JR, Segre GV, Carlton EI, Sherrard DJ. *Immunoradiometric Assay for Intact PTH: A New Generation of PTH Assay for Assessment of Parathyroid Function.* San Juan Capistrano, Calif: Nichols Institute; 1988.
29. Sizonenko P. Endocrinology in preadolescents and in adolescents. *AJDC.* 1978;132:704-711.
30. Chesney RW, Rosen JF, Hamstra AJ, De Luca HF. Serum 1,25-dihydroxyvitamin D levels in normal children and in vitamin D disorders. *AJDC.* 1980;134:135-139.
31. Aksnes L, Aarskog D. Plasma concentrations of vitamin D metabolites in puberty: effect of sexual maturation and implication for growth. *J Clin Endocrinol Metab.* 1982;55:94-99.
32. Riggs BL. Vitamin D and involutional osteoporosis. In: Kumar R, ed. *Vitamin D: Basic and Clinical Aspects.* Boston, Mass: Martinus Nijhoff Publishers; 1984:559-597.
33. Hurley DL, Tiegs RD, Wahner HW, Heath H III. Axial and appendicular bone mineral density in patients with long-term deficiency or excess of calcitonin. *N Engl J Med.* 1987;317:537-541.
34. Kruse K, Suss A, Busse M, Kract U. Monomeric serum calcitonin and bone turnover during anticonvulsant treatment and in congenital hypothyroidism. *J Pediatr.* 1987;111:57-63.
35. Greulich WW, Pyle SI. *Radiographic Atlas of Skeletal Development of the Hand and Wrist.* Stanford, Calif: Stanford University Press; 1959.

BOOK REVIEW

Current Concepts in Childhood Spinal Muscular Atrophy

Edited by L. Merlini, C. Granata, and V. Dubowitz, 226 pp, $89.30, New York, NY, Springer-Verlag NY Inc, 1989.

There has been a surge of interest in neuromuscular disease in the past 2 years, sparked primarily by major genetic discoveries. While initial attention focused appropriately on Duchenne muscular dystrophy, the momentum has now swung to the spinal muscular atrophies, which, the authors note, are equally frequent and no less important in childhood because of their severe handicaps and disabilities. This book covers the clinical picture, research strategies, pathogenesis, genetics, natural history, rehabilitative care, and other clinical management problems. New avenues of therapy are discussed, including attention to nutrition, respiratory care, physical and occupational therapy, and psychological management. Gloria Eng, long a pioneer in the treatment of children with this disorder, notes that the terminal course may be particularly difficult: "Every parent reacts differently when the baby has a protracted course and begins to die. At that point everyone is worn out, including the physician." "No code" status, preference of the child dying at home, and hospice care are discussed. This book provides an important update and new optimism in our understanding of the basic neurobiologic characteristics of this previously fatal disorder, along with important new avenues of treatment and hope for the future as the basic genetic origin unravels even further.

Peggy C. Ferry, MD
Section of Child Neurology
Department of Pediatrics
University of Arizona
College of Medicine
Tucson, AZ 85724

Evaluation of Bayesian Forecasting for Individualized Gentamicin Dosage in Infants Weighing 1000 g or Less

Kei Lui, MBBS, FRACP; Scott M. Bryson, MSc Pharm; Danica B. Irwin, BSc Pharm; Simon Costello, MBBS, FRACP

• We evaluated the use of Bayesian forecasting for gentamicin therapy in outborn infants weighing 1000 g or less irrespective of postnatal age. Dosages were individualized using a computer program, guided by early serum gentamicin assays after a loading dose and a database of population kinetics. Steady-state gentamicin levels achieved were compared with those from a regimen based on guidelines. A total of 26 gentamicin courses were individualized in 19 infants of 22 to 33 weeks' gestation, weighing 500 to 1000 g at 1 to 41 days of age. All steady-state trough levels were between 1 and 2.4 mg/L; peak levels were between 4.4 and 9.3 mg/L. The 95% confidence intervals were in almost identical ranges. The prevalence of toxic and suboptimal trough levels was less when compared with that of 23 gentamicin courses based on guidelines in 17 control infants. We conclude that early individualized gentamicin dosage over a range of postnatal age is a practical alternative and serum level distributions appear superior.

(*AJDC.* 1991;145:463-467)

Gentamicin is an aminoglycoside frequently used in the management of neonatal sepsis. Appropriate dosage is desirable to provide adequate treatment and to avoid drug-related toxic reactions. Low-gestation infants have a high percentage of body water and, thus, a large volume of distribution in gentamicin disposition.[1] They may require large initial doses to achieve therapeutic serum peak concentrations.[2,3] Glomerular filtration rate is the main determinant of gentamicin plasma clearance and half-life. Although there exists a significant difference in half-life among infants of different gestations, the range is considerably wider in low-gestation infants.[1,2] This may relate to the wide differences in glomerular filtration rate in infants of similar gestation.[4,5] Furthermore, sick preterm infants often have reduced gentamicin clearance.[6] Owing to the combined effects of intrarenal drug accumulation, developmental acquisition of renal competence, and the influences of disease states, there is a need for an individualized regimen in these infants.[6,7]

In this study, we report the experience of an individualized gentamicin sulfate regimen using the Bayesian forecasting in outborn infants weighing 1000 g or less. The performance in achieving steady-state serum levels within acceptable ranges was compared with the performance from a comparable group where dosages were based on guidelines.

PATIENTS AND METHODS

During a 5-month period in our outborn neonatal intensive care unit, all infants were candidates for the study if they weighed 1000 g or less when gentamicin therapy was started. Infants who had received repeated doses from other nurseries were excluded. In each study, we individualized gentamicin therapy within 24 hours of a loading dose.

All infants who received gentamicin courses based on our unit guidelines over the immediate preceding 5 months were selected for comparison. Infants younger than 7 days receive 3.5 mg/kg every 24 hours, and infants 7 days or older may receive 2.5 mg/kg every 12 or 8 hours. There is allowance for modest alteration by the house staff when renal immaturity or impairment is suspected. The clinical profiles of the two infant groups at the start of gentamicin therapy were compared. Medications or illnesses that could alter renal clearance or volume of distribution in gentamicin kinetics were documented.

Gentamicin Loading Dose and Assays for Bayesian Forecasting

Gentamicin was given intravenously as a slow bolus over 3 to 5 minutes. Following a 3.5-mg/kg loading dose of gentamicin sulfate, two serum gentamicin concentrations 6 to 11 hours apart obtained by heel prick or arterial sampling were assayed (EMIT, Syva Diagnostics, Palo Alto, Calif). The first sample was collected between 1 and 2 hours after the loading dose. In infants who had received intravenous volume expansion, blood samples were taken at least 1 hour after infusion. Infants older than 7 days were given a second dose of gentamicin sulfate (2.5 mg/kg) 12 hours after the loading dose if results of assays were not immediately available.

Bayesian Forecasting

Forecasting was performed using a computer method established in the Department of Pharmacy. The program was adopted from an adult program,[8] and the population kinetic data used were mainly derived from the previously published Glasgow cohort of preterm and term infants (gestation, 26 to 39 weeks; age, 2 to 120 days old).[9] Pharmacokinetics were described by a simplified one-compartment open model and elimination was of first-order (exponential) kinetics.

Accepted for publication September 27, 1990.

From the Departments of Pediatrics (Drs Lui and Costello) and Pharmacy (Mr Bryson and Ms Irwin), Hospital For Sick Children, Toronto, Ontario. Dr Lui is now with the Westmead Hospital, Westmead, New South Wales, Australia.

Reprint requests to Neonatal Intensive Care Unit, Department of Pediatrics, Westmead Hospital, Westmead, New South Wales, Australia 2145 (Dr Lui).

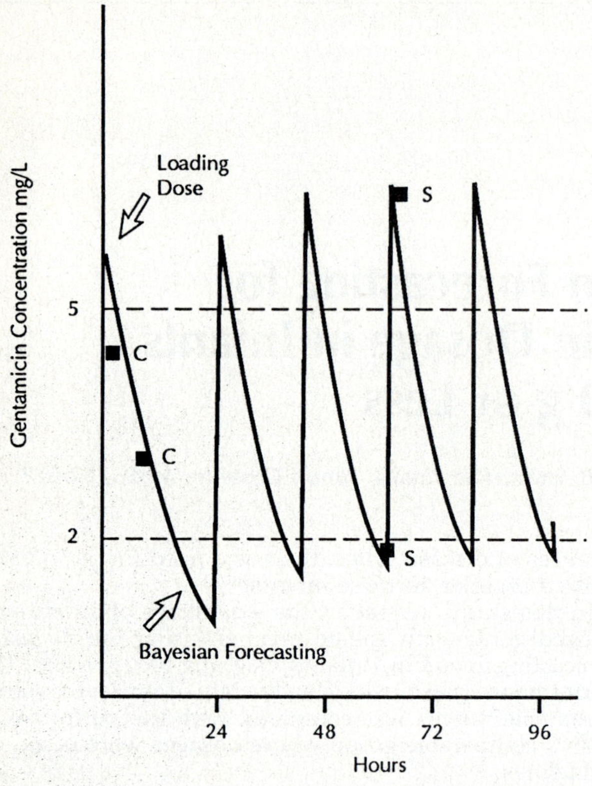

Fig 1.—*Example of Bayesian forecasting in a 27-weeks' gestation, 900-g infant who was started on gentamicin therapy on day 1. An individualized dosage of 2.6 mg (2.9 mg/kg) every 18 hours resulted in steady-state trough and peak concentrations of 1.8 mg/L and 6.7 mg/L. Computer-fitted line of gentamicin concentration is based on the Bayesian kinetic estimates in Table 1. Assayed gentamicin concentrations are also plotted for illustration. C indicates concentrations used for Bayesian forecasting; S, the measured steady-state concentrations of the implemented dosage.*

The method used population-derived kinetics as the starting point. Using three simple patient variables—gestational age, postnatal age, and current weight—the program retrieved a set of normally distributed kinetic estimates of similar clinical characteristics based on all available data from the infant population. These estimates allowed the calculation of theoretical (expected) gentamicin concentrations at any specific time (see example in Fig 1 and Table 1; this initial step is highlighted as boxed area in Table 1). Assessing the differences between the gentamicin assay results and the expected concentrations to reflect interindividual variations, the kinetic factors were adjusted by a weighting function based on the Theory of Maximum Likelihood.[10] From this most probable (Bayesian) kinetics, the steady-state levels of a given dosage were predicted. Predicted trough and peak (1 hour after dose) levels of the recommended or "optimized" dosage were targeted in the range of 1 to 2 mg/L and 5 to 7 mg/L, respectively. Dose intervals were limited to 12, 18, 24, 30, or 36 hours to make the repeated administrations practical to the nursing staff.

In infants weighing 1000 g or less at a later age when gentamicin therapy was restarted, complete forecasting procedures, including the loading doses, were carried out. With considerable changes in age and body weight, independent sets of population kinetics were retrieved for individualization.

Evaluation

To evaluate performance of the forecasting, we examined the following: (1) the 95% confidence intervals of trough and peak steady-state levels compared with the accepted ranges of gentamicin levels; (2) differences in the prevalence of "toxic" and "suboptimal" steady-state levels compared with those in the control infants; and (3) differences between predicted and measured steady-state levels, denoted as prediction bias. In both infant groups, trough and peak gentamicin levels were routinely measured around the third maintenance dose to reflect steady-state concentrations. In our unit, trough levels between 1 and 2 mg/L[11] and peak levels between 5 and 10 mg/L[12] are denoted as optimal. We regard levels above 2.5 mg/L as toxic where dosage adjustments are mandatory consistent with the standard policy of our unit.[13] Peak levels above 4 mg/L could be accepted as therapeutic.[11]

Table 1.—Population and Bayesian Kinetics and Steady-State Level Predictions*

Concentration Measurements			
Dose Interval	Time From Last Dose, h	Measured Concentration, mg/L	Expected Concentration (Population)
1	2.00	4.5	5.3
1	9.00	3.1	3.1
Parameter Estimates		**Bayesian, Mean ± SD**	**Population Mean ± SD**
Clearance		0.039 ± 0.005	0.036 ± 0.018 L/h
Volume of distribution		0.0498 ± 0.061	0.0414 ± 0.083 L
Eliminated rate constant		0.078/h	
Eliminated half-life		8.8 h	
Dose Recommendation			
Dose,		2.6 mg	
Dose interval,		18 h	
Estimated Steady-State Concentration With Recommended Dosage, mg/L			
Concentration			
Minimum,		1.7	
Maximum		6.9	
At 1 h,		6.4	
Average,		3.7	

*The population estimates (the initial step in Bayesian forecasting) are highlighted as the boxed area. See text for details.

RESULTS AND ANALYSIS

Patients

A total of 30 gentamicin dosage individualizations were performed in 23 infants weighing 1000 g or less. Four studies in four infants were excluded because gentamicin therapy was stopped or death occurred before steady state was reached. The remaining 19 infants, 11 girls and eight boys, were of (mean±SD) 25±2 weeks' gestation (range, 22 to 33 weeks' gestation), and weighed 500 to 1000 g at birth. Among the 26 studies, 13 were entered on day 1, one was entered on day 6, and the remaining 12 were entered between 9 and 41 days of age (including seven repeated studies at a later day).

In the preceding 5 months, 17 infants received 23 completed gentamicin courses from our routine guidelines. Their gestational age was 25±2 weeks (range, 23 to 29 weeks), and birth weight was from 630 to 1000 g. Among the 23 gentamicin courses, 12 were started on day 1, two were started on days 5 and 6, and the remaining nine were started between days 8 and 36 (including six repeated gentamicin courses). The clinical profiles and dosages for the two groups are summarized in Table 2. Almost all infants were receiving ventilatory assistance when treatment with gentamicin was started. The indication for gentamicin, the renal function, exposure to nephrotoxic medications, and concurrent illnesses were similar.

Gentamicin Dosage

The gentamicin dose was similar between the two groups (Table 2). Dose interval of regimens guided by the

Table 2.—Summary of Clinical Profiles of Infants and Gentamicin Dosages for the Two Regimens

	Bayesian Forecasting	Standard Guideline
No. of studies	26	23
Clinical profile		
Postnatal age, d		
<7	14	14
>7	12	9
Range	1-41	1-36
Postconceptional age, wk		
Mean ± SD	26 ± 2	26 ± 1
Body weight, g		
Mean ± SD	811 ± 150	792 ± 135
Range	500-1000	630-1000
Indications		
Sepsis		
Proved	3	4
Suspected	20	17
Necrotizing enterocolitis	2	2
Need for ventilation	25	23
Nephrotoxic drugs		
Indomethacin	2	0
Vancomycin hydrochloride	3	3
Amphotericin B	0	1
Oliguria <1 mL/kg/h	1	1
Serum creatinine, µmol/L		
Mean ± SD	74 ± 32	69 ± 17
Range	42-159	44-102
Illnesses predispose to abnormal fluid accumulation		
Patent ductus arteriosus	8	5
Hydrocephalus	1	1
Gentamicin dosage		
Postnatal age <7 d		
Dose/kg, mg		
Mean ± SD	3.4 ± 0.4	3.1 ± 0.3
Range	2.7-4.2	2.5-3.5
Dose interval, h		
Mean ± SD	25 ± 7	24 ± 6
Range	12-36	12-36
Postnatal age ≥7 d		
Dose/kg, mg		
Mean ± SD	3.1 ± 0.3	2.8 ± 0.5
Range	2.9 ± 3.5	2.2-3.9
Dose interval, h		
Mean ± SD	15 ± 5	20 ± 12
Range	18-24	8-36

Bayesian forecasting ranged from 18 to 36 hours for infants younger than 7 days, and from 12 to 24 hours for postnatal age older than 7 days. In the gentamicin courses based on guidelines, dose intervals were increased by the house staff in seven instances because of clinical evidence of preexisting renal impairment or in older immature infants who had high trough levels during previous gentamicin courses. In two infants younger than 7 days who were born at 29 and 28 weeks' gestation, dose intervals were decreased to 12 and 18 hours accompanied with decreased doses per kilogram.

Steady-State Gentamicin Levels

The initial forecasting in the 19 study infants resulted in steady-state trough concentrations between 1 and 2.4 mg/L; their peak levels were between 4.7 and 9.3 mg/L. In the seven repeated studies, the trough and peak levels ranged from 1.0 to 2.3 mg/L and from 4.4 to 7.8 mg/L, respectively. The overall 95% confidence interval for trough levels was between 0.9 and 2.5 mg/L (acceptable range, 1 to 2.5 mg/L) and that of peak levels was between 4 and 9.5 mg/L (acceptable range, 4 to 10 mg/L).

In the group in which standard guidelines were used, three of 17 initial trough levels were above 2.5 mg/L (between 2.8 and 3.2 mg/L) and two were below 1 mg/L. Among the six repeated gentamicin courses, two trough levels were above 2.5 mg/L (3.4 and 3.6 mg/L) and two were less than 1 mmol/L. All 23 peak gentamicin levels, except one (3.0 mg/L), were between 5 and 9.2 mg/L. The overall 95% confidence interval for trough level was between 0.0 and 3.5 mg/L, and it was between 4 and 10 mg/L for the peak level. While the mean trough levels of the two regimens were similar, trough levels guided by Bayesian forecasting had a smaller scatter in distribution (F ratio 4.0, $P<.01$). Results are summarized in Fig 2.

Using greater than 2.5 mg/L and less than 1 mg/L as our criteria of toxic and suboptimal trough levels, prevalence of these concentrations was significantly less in regimens guided by the Bayesian forecasting (0/26 vs 5/23, $P<.01$; 0/26 vs 4/23, $P<.01$, respectively, Fisher's Exact Test). For the peak levels, we found no significant difference between the two regimens, and almost all were within acceptable range.

We found the Bayesian forecasting had a tendency to underestimate the trough and peak steady-state levels. The mean prediction bias for trough levels (predicted steady-state levels—measured levels) was −0.3 mg/L, and the mean prediction bias for peak levels was −0.4 mg/L. Results are summarized in Table 3. The prediction bias of studies entered within the first 7 days of life was considerably smaller than those studied at a later postnatal age.

COMMENT

Adequate therapy with aminoglycosides requires serum concentrations to be maintained within certain limits. Difficulties arise in patients with impaired renal function in whom serum levels decline slowly. Variable doses or variable dose frequency regimens as an adjunct to guidelines[14,15] have been suggested. However, prolonged periods of low serum levels could invite the possibility of undertreatment.[16] McCracken and Nelson[11] suggested a peak concentration of 4 to 8 mg/L and trough levels of 1 to 2 mg/L as desirable ranges for safe and effective therapy in newborn infants with impaired renal function.

In older children and adults, tables, nomograms, and computer programs based on patient variables such as weight, height, sex, and serum creatinine concentration are available to aid in aminoglycoside administration. However, assessment of renal function within the first 24 hours of life could be difficult in clinical practice. Serum creatinine concentration during this period is a reflection of the maternal renal function, while serum creatinine concentration on days 2 to 3 is a reasonable index of glomerular filtration rate in very-low-birth-weight infants.[2] Furthermore, the degree of asphyxial insult at birth is difficult to ascertain. The usefulness of Apgar scores as an indication of asphyxia in premature infants has been seriously questioned.[17]

The pharmacokinetic advantage of the Bayesian forecasting for aminoglycoside therapy has been documented

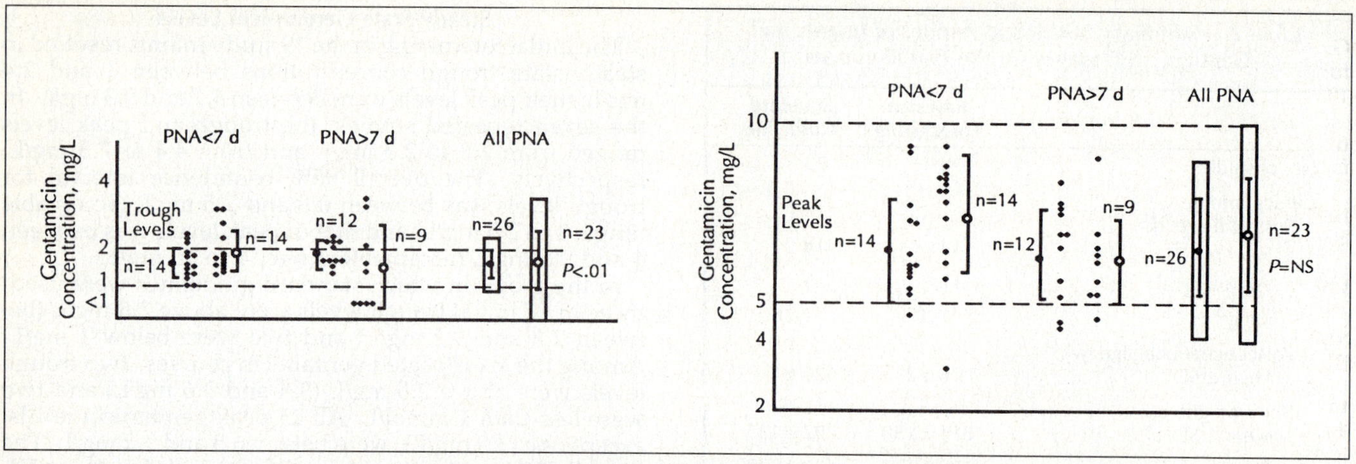

Fig 2.—*Comparison of steady-state gentamicin levels according to postnatal age (PNA) between regimens by Bayesian method and by guidelines. NS indicates not significant. Left, Trough levels. Right, Peak levels. Means and SDs are shown in closed circles for the Bayesian forecasting and in open circles for guidelines for each comparison. The 95% confidence intervals are shown in boxes.*

Table 3.—Prediction Bias of the Bayesian Forecasting Showing a Consistent Tendency of Underestimation of Steady-State Levels*

	n	Mean Predicted Gentamicin Concentration, mg/L, (Range)	Mean Prediction Bias (Predicted-Measured), mg/L, (Range)
Trough			
PNA <7 d	14	1.5 (0.8-2.1)	−0.1 (−0.9-0.5)
PNA ≥7 d	12	1.4 (0.9-1.7)	−0.5†(−1.4-0.7)
All	26	1.4 (0.8-2.1)	−0.3 (−1.4-0.7)
Peak			
PNA <7 d	14	6.1 (5.1-7.2)	−0.1 (−2.6-1.4)
PNA ≥7 d	12	5.7 (4.4-7.1)	−0.7 (−2.2-1.3)
All	26	6.1 (4.4-7.2)	−0.4 (−2.6-1.4)

*Mean and range are shown. PNA indicates postnatal age.

†Significant difference between prediction bias of trough levels at PNA <7 days and ≥7 days, Student's *t* test.

in children and adults[18-21] and in patients in the intensive care unit who exhibit considerable interindividual variations of drug disposition.[22] In reality, laboratory variations are inherent in the assay of gentamicin concentrations. This may result in errors of exponential magnitude if concentrations alone are used for kinetic extrapolations. We used three simple variables—gestation, postnatal age, and body weight—and two serum concentrations for kinetic adjustment. Bayesian theorem in this setting has the advantage that data input errors cannot easily result in misinterpretation. Therapy can be individualized from the outset and kinetics can be adjusted for the expected postnatal renal maturation. In our outborn infants weighing 1000 g or less, we achieved steady-state trough and peak levels ranging from 1 to 2.4 mg/L and from 4.4 to 9.3 mg/L, respectively. Moreover, their 95% confidence intervals were within our preset acceptable ranges.

Studies suggested the volumes of distribution were relatively consistent for infants over a small range of body weight.[2,3] When a similar total dose per body weight was used in both regimens, we were not surprised to find no significant difference in their steady-state peak levels. However, there was less variation in the trough levels from a Bayesian forecasting regimen resulting in a lower prevalence of toxic or suboptimal levels.

Seven study infants were recommenced on a regimen of gentamicin therapy at a later age. The steady-state levels appeared superior to the six repeated gentamicin courses in the control infants. Results suggest individualizing each course of gentamicin therapy to be beneficial. A guideline regimen influenced by a "previous experience" in the infant may also lead to underestimation or overestimation of the infant's renal competence.

In the first few days of life, body fluid composition and renal blood flow change considerably. Despite these, Bayesian forecasting performed well in the early postnatal ages. We suspect its performance at the older postnatal ages may improve with increased size of the population kinetic database.

Premature animals[23,24] were thought to be somewhat protected from aminoglycoside-induced nephrotoxic reactions. Recently, increasing concern has been expressed against its apparent safety.[13,25] Furthermore, optimal therapy may not only be important for infants with impaired renal function but also for infants with normal renal function. These infants may receive inadequate dosages. While the clearance of aminoglycosides is considerably decreased in this specific study population, it provides ample time for the use of Bayesian forecasting in clinical practice.

CONCLUSION

We found Bayesian forecasting for gentamicin therapy to be a practical alternative. It compared favorably with dosage based on guidelines in infants weighing 1000 g or less over a range of postnatal age, and this may potentially minimize suboptimal gentamicin treatment and dose-related toxic reactions. Serum drug level was the only factor evaluated; further studies examining clinical toxic reactions would be desirable.

Andrew W. Kelman, PhD, of Clydesoft Scientific Software provided support with the computer programming. The computer program for the Bayesian forecasting may be obtained from Mr Bryson, assistant director, Clinical Research Education Program, Department of Pharmacy, British Columbia Children's Hospital, Vancouver, or Dr A. W. Kelman, Clydesoft Scientific Software, 78 Meadows Ave, Larkmall, Lanankshire, Scotland ML9 2JG.

References

1. Miranda JC, Schimmel MM, James LS, Spinelli W, Rosen TS. Gentamicin kinetics in the neonate. *Pediatr Pharmacol.* 1985;5:57-61.

2. Landers S, Berry PL, Kearns GL, Kaplan SL, Rudolph AJ. Gentamicin deposition and effect on development of renal function in the very low birth weight infant. *Dev Pharmacol Ther.* 1984;7:285-302.
3. Koren G, Leeder S, Harding E, Jacques D, MacLeod S. Optimization of gentamicin therapy in very low birth weight infants. *Pediatr Pharmacol.* 1985;5:79-87.
4. Leake RD, Trygstad CW. Glomerular filtration rate during the period of adaption to extrauterine life. *Pediatr Res.* 1977;11:959-962.
5. Arant B. Developmental pattern of renal functional maturation in the human neonate. *J Pediatr.* 1978;92:705-712.
6. Friedman CA, Parks BR, Rawson JE. Gentamicin deposition in asphyxiated newborns: relationship to mean arterial blood pressure and urine output. *Pediatr Pharmacol.* 1982;2:189-192.
7. Assael BM, Gianni V, Marini A, Peneff P, Sereni F. Gentamicin dosage in preterm and term neonates. *Arch Dis Child.* 1977;52:883-886.
8. Kelman AW, Whiting B, Bryson SM. OPT: a package of computer programs for parameter optimisation in clinical pharmacokinetics. *Br J Clin Pharmacol.* 1982;14:247-256.
9. Kelman AW, Thomson AH, Whiting B, et al. Estimation of gentamicin clearance and volume of distribution in neonates and young infants. *Br J Clin Pharmacol.* 1984;18:685-692.
10. Sheiner LB, Beal SL, Rosenberg B, Marathe VV. Forecasting individual pharmacokinetics. *Clin Pharmacol Ther.* 1979;26:294-305.
11. McCracken GH, Nelson JD. Clinical application of laboratory test. In: *Antimicrobial Therapy for Newborns.* New York, NY: Grune & Stratton; 1977:73-80.
12. Moore RD, Smith CR, Leitman PS. The association of aminoglycoside plasma levels with mortality in patients with gram-negative bacteremia. *J Infect Dis.* 1984;149:443-448.
13. Rajchogot P, Prober CG, Soldin S, et al. Aminoglycoside-related nephrotoxicity in the premature newborn. *Clin Pharmacol Ther.* 1984;35:394-401.
14. Schumacher GE. Pharmacokinetic analysis of gentamicin dosage regimens recommended for renal impairment. *J Clin Pharmcol.* 1975;15:656-665.
15. Goodman EL, Van Gelder J, Holmes R, et al. Prospective comparative study of variable dosage and variable frequency regimens for administration of gentamicin. *Antimicrob Agents Chemother.* 1975;8:434-438.
16. Barza M, Lauermann M. Why monitor serum levels of gentamicin? In: Gibaldi M, Prescott L, eds. *Handbook of Clinical Pharmacokinetics.* Sydney, NSW: ADIS Health Science Press; 1983:164-174.
17. Sykes GS, Molloy PM, Johnson P, et al. Do Apgar scores indicate asphyxia? *Lancet.* 1982;1:494-496.
18. Bachmann K, Pongsin V, Forney R, Gronau G. Experience with a computer-based technique for estimating pharmacokinetic constants from limited data. *Ther Drug Monit.* 1985;7:258-264.
19. Bachmann GE, Barr JT. Bayesian approaches in pharmacokinetic decision making. *Clin Pharm.* 1985;3:525-530.
20. Burton ME, Brater C, Chen PS, Day RB, Huber PJ, Vasko MR. A Bayesian feedback method of aminoglycoside dosing. *Clin Pharmacol Ther.* 1985;37:349-357.
21. Zantvoort FA, Wagenvoort JH, Derkx FH, Michel MF. Evaluation of a microcomputer program (OPT) for parameter optimization in clinical pharmacokinetics: gentamicin and tobramycin. *Br J Clin Pharmacol.* 1987;24:511-518.
22. Rodvold KA, Pryka RD, Kuehl PG, et al. Bayesian forcasting of serum gentamicin concentration in intensive care patients. *Clin Pharmacokinet.* 1990;18:409-418.
23. Provoost AP, Adejuyigbe O, Wolff ED. Nephrotoxicity of aminoglycosides in young and adult rats. *Pediatr Res.* 1985;19:1191-1196.
24. Cowan RH, Jukkola AF, Arant BS Jr. Pathophysiological evidence of gentamicin nephrotoxicity in neonatal puppies. *Pediatr Res.* 1980;14:1204-1207.
25. Aldeman RD, Wirth F, Rubio T. A controlled study of nephrotoxicity of mezlocillin and gentamicin plus ampicillin in the neonate. *J Pediatr.* 1987;111:888-893.

In Other AMA Journals

ARCHIVES OF DERMATOLOGY

Childhood Bullous Pemphigoid:Clinical and Immunologic Features, Treatment, and Prognosis

Albert J. Nemeth, MD; Alan D. Klein, MD; Edwin W. Gould, MD; Lawrence A. Schachner, MD
(*Arch Dermatol.* 1991;127:387-390)

Cytomegalovirus Diaper Dermatitis

Diane M. Thiboutot, MD; Avril Beckford, MD; Christopher R. Mart, MD; Mack Sexton, MD; Mary E. Maloney, MD
(*Arch Dermatol.* 1991;127:396-398)

ARCHIVES OF SURGERY

The Town-Gown Syndrome: An Ancient Disease, as Yet Uncured

Robert J. Baker, MD
(*Arch Surg.* 1991;126:287-288)

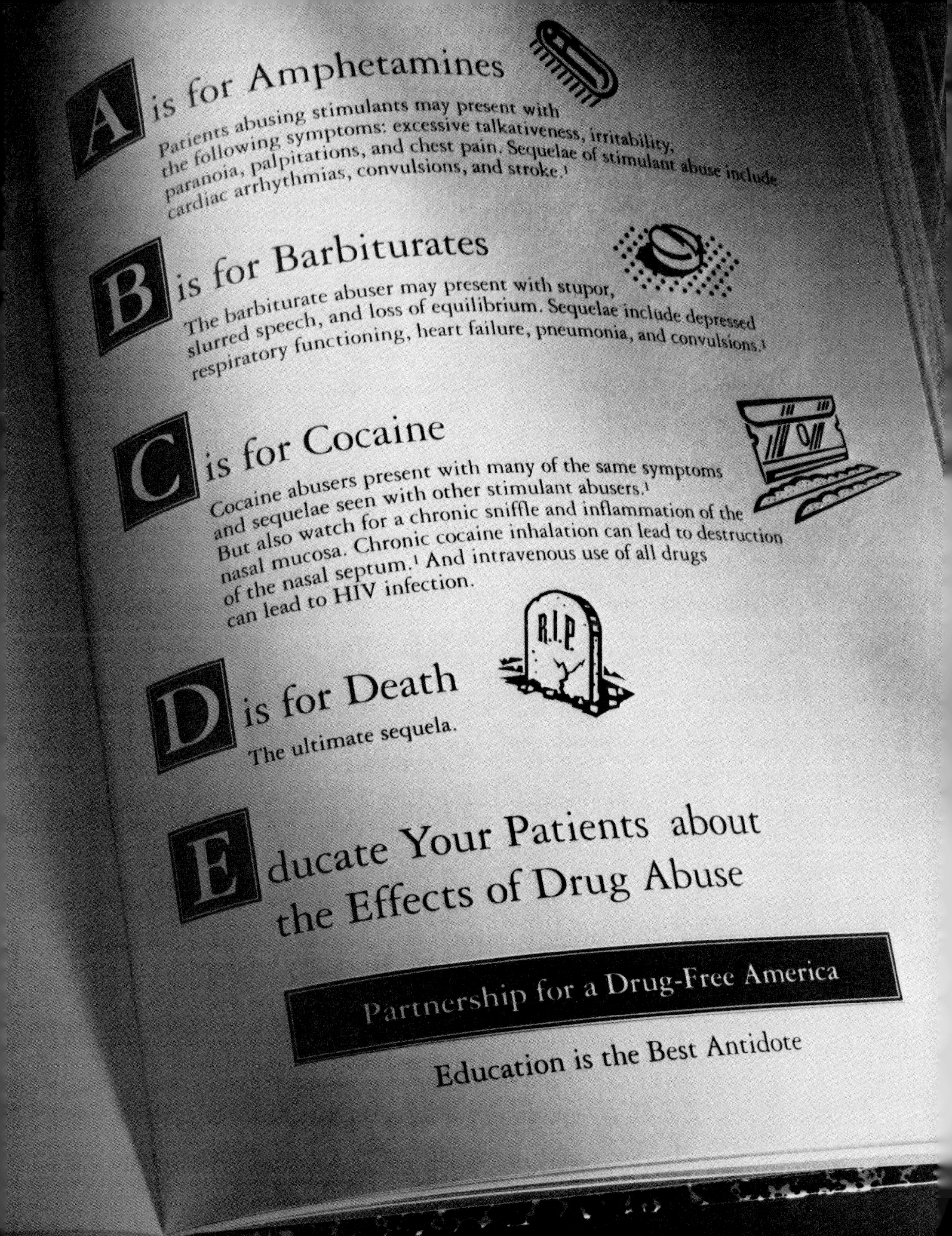
A is for Amphetamines
Patients abusing stimulants may present with the following symptoms: excessive talkativeness, irritability, paranoia, palpitations, and chest pain. Sequelae of stimulant abuse include cardiac arrhythmias, convulsions, and stroke.[1]
B is for Barbiturates
The barbiturate abuser may present with stupor, slurred speech, and loss of equilibrium. Sequelae include depressed respiratory functioning, heart failure, pneumonia, and convulsions.[1]
C is for Cocaine
Cocaine abusers present with many of the same symptoms and sequelae seen with other stimulant abusers.[1] But also watch for a chronic sniffle and inflammation of the nasal mucosa. Chronic cocaine inhalation can lead to destruction of the nasal septum.[1] And intravenous use of all drugs can lead to HIV infection.
R.I.P.
D is for Death
The ultimate sequela.
Educate Your Patients about the Effects of Drug Abuse
Partnership for a Drug-Free America
Education is the Best Antidote

SPECIAL FEATURE

Radiological Case of the Month

Janice W. Allison, MD; Carol A. Stephenson, MD; Teresita L. Angtuaco, MD; Charles M. Glasier, MD (Contributors); *Beverly P. Wood, MD* (Section Editor)

A fetal cardiac abnormality was detected in a prenatal ultrasound examination of a 31-year-old woman. No family history of genetic syndromes or congenital heart disease was elicited, and she had two normal children. The infant, delivered by spontaneous vaginal delivery at 36 weeks' gestation, developed respiratory distress shortly after birth and was intubated.

Physical examination revealed afebrile, cyanotic female infant with tachycardia (heart rate, 116 to 152 beats per minute) and tachypnea (48 to 76 breaths per minute).

Accepted for publication January 23, 1991.

Contributed from the Departments of Radiology, University of Arkansas for Medical Sciences (Drs Allison and Angtuaco) and Arkansas Children's Hospital (Drs Stephenson and Glasier), Little Rock.

Reprint requests to Department of Radiology, Childrens Hospital of Los Angeles, 4650 Sunset Blvd, Los Angeles, CA 90027 (Dr Wood).

Hypopigmented macules were present on her back and buttocks. The liver was palpable 3 cm below the costal margin.

An electrocardiogram revealed Wolff-Parkinson-White complex, biventricular hypertrophy, and atrial enlargement. Laboratory values were unremarkable except for hypoxia. A chest roentgenogram (Fig 1), echocardiogram, cardiac magnetic resonance imaging (MRI) (Fig 2), and cranial computed tomography (CT) (Fig 3) and MRI (Fig 4) were performed during diagnostic workup.

The infant's congestive heart failure was treated and she no longer required assisted ventilation by 3 days of age. On the sixth day, respiratory distress returned and the infant became cyanotic with feedings. She died of cardiac failure on the eighth day.

Figure 1.

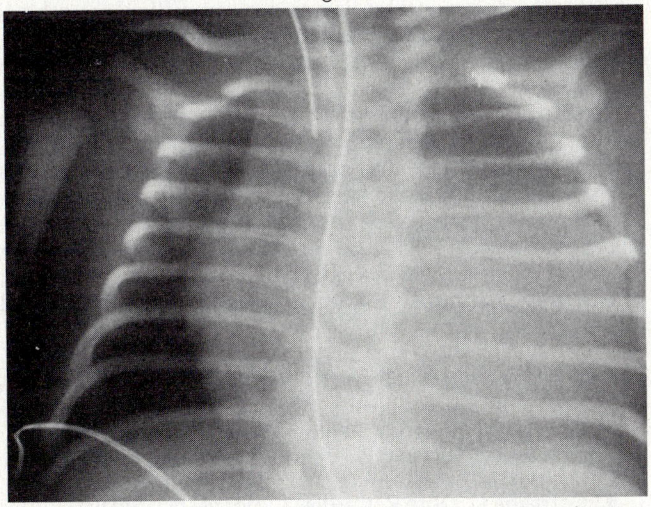

Figure 2.

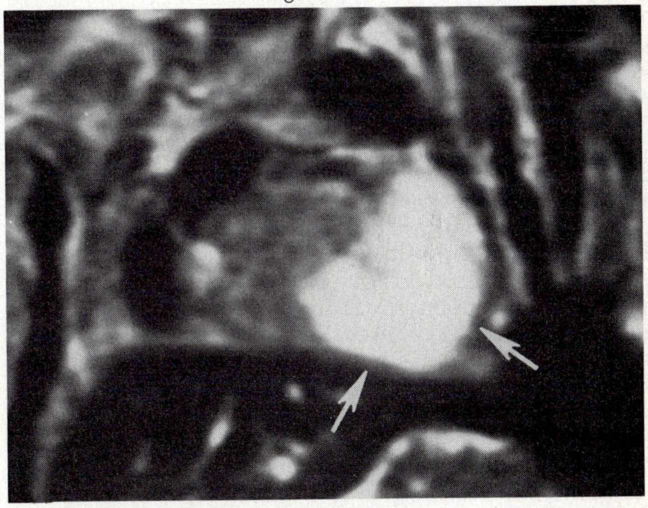

Figure 3.

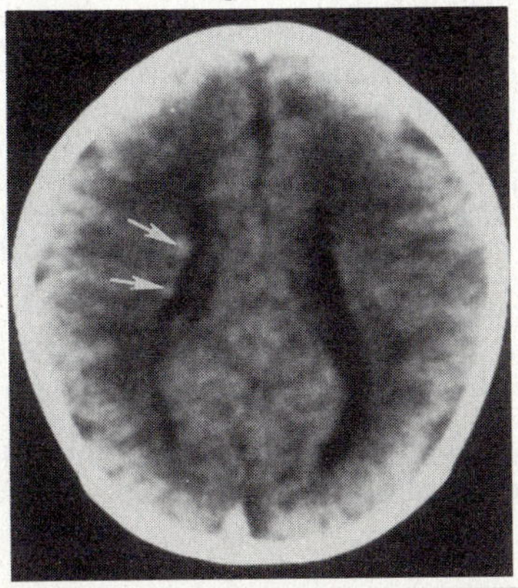

Figure 4.

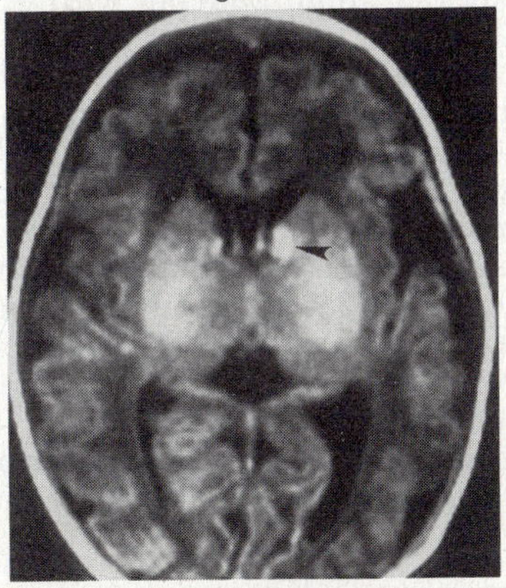

Denouement and Discussion

Tuberous Sclerosis With Myocardial and Central Nervous System Involvement at Birth

Fig 1.—*Anteroposterior chest roentgenogram reveals massive cardiomegaly.*

Fig 2.—*T1-weighted coronal magnetic resonance imaging of the chest shows a high-signal-intensity mass in the ventricular wall (arrows).*

Fig 3.—*Computed tomography of the head reveals high-density periventricular nodules (arrows).*

Fig 4.—*Axial inversion-recovery magnetic resonance imaging of the brain reveals a high-signal-intensity periventricular nodule (arrowhead). uberous sclerosis (TS) is a neurocutaneous dysplasia with clinical manifestations resulting from hamartomatous malformations of the skin, brain, heart, and kidneys. Inheritance is autosomal dominant with variable penetrance or spontaneous mutation.[1] The classic clinical triad is mental retardation, skin lesions (adenoma sebaceum or ash leaf macules), and seizures.*

This infant presented with cardiomegaly and congestive heart failure. The echocardiogram disclosed a pericardial effusion, a ventricular mass, and echogenic septal masses. Cardiac magnetic resonance imaging (MRI) and autopsy revealed multiple rhabdomyomas in the myocardium with distortion of the chambers. The largest tumor was within the septum and measured 3.2×3.3 cm at autopsy. Go et al[2] compared the diagnostic advantages of gated cardiac MRI with two-dimensional echocardiography in the diagnosis and characterization of intracardiac tumors in adult patients and concluded that the tumor size, shape, and surface characteristics were most specifically delineated by MRI.

In infants, 60% of primary cardiac tumors are rhabdomyomas, most commonly found in the ventricular walls, and multiple in 90% of cases. Fifty percent of infants with cardiac rhabdomyomas have TS. Seventy percent of patients with multiple rhabdomyomas die within the first year of life, and 92% die by the fifth year without surgical treatment.[3]

The most common renal abnormality associated with TS is angiomyolipoma, seen in 40% to 50% of patients. Cystic renal changes are less commonly seen in TS. Abdominal ultrasound study is indicated in all patients with TS to identify these abnormalities.

The typical cranial findings of TS include calcified periventricular subependymal nodules and low-attenuation areas (on computed tomography [CT]) in the cortex and subcortical white matter. These correspond to parenchymal hamartomas (tubers). Cortical tubers are usually found at the gray-white matter interface and may also be calcified.[4] The abnormalities noted on this infant's cranial CT were subependymal nodules (Fig 3). Sugita et al[5] described two infants with TS with intracranial calcifications detected with CT within 1 week of birth. The subependymal nodules may later transform into astrocytomas. If these occur at the foramen of Monro, they cause ventricular obstruction.[4] Astrocytomas are enhanced by intravenous contrast injection, whereas subependymal and cortical tubers are not. Therefore, routine contrast enhancement is indicated in evaluating patients with TS with CT or MRI.

The cranial MRI findings of TS include multiple cortical and subcortical regions of high signal intensity on T2-weighted images corresponding to the hypodense areas seen on CT; subependymal nodules of intermediate signal intensity on all pulse sequences; and distortion of the cortical architecture.[6] Large calcifications are seen as absent signal. Small or large calcifications are better identified with CT.[7] Subependymal nodules are demonstrated on inversion-recovery or T1-weighted images.[8] This infant's cranial MRI features were typical for TS. Subependymal nodules showed high signal intensity on inversion-recovery images and signal dropout on T2-weighted images due to calcification. Multiple areas of cortical high signal intensity were identified on the T2-weighted images.

Magnetic resonance imaging is more sensitive than CT for the detection of cerebral change in TS. Both MRI and CT are important in the early detection of TS before the clinical signs are manifested.[5] Roach et al[1] noted a correlation between the number of cortical tubers on MRI and the clinical severity of the disease as manifested by more severe developmental delay and more difficulty with seizure control. Direct correlation between the abnormalities on CT and the clinical severity of disease has not been shown.

In this infant, cranial MRI and CT were instrumental in confirming the diagnosis of TS, already suggested by the presence of multiple myocardial tumors and skin lesions. Cardiac MRI depicted extensive rhabdomyomas and ventricular distortion. These studies assisted in reaching a decision to provide palliative care because of the poor prognosis for extensive myocardial lesions. Autopsy confirmed the presence of multiple cardiac rhabdomyomas and multiple cerebral hamartomas.

References

1. Roach ES, Williams DP, Laster DW. Magnetic resonance imaging in tuberous sclerosis. *Arch Neurol.* 1987;44:301-303.
2. Go RT, O'Donnell JK, Underwood DA, et al. Comparison of gated cardiac MRI and 2D echocardiography of intracardiac neoplasms. *AJR Am J Roentgenol.* 1985;145:21-25.
3. Cornalba G, Dore R. Cardiac tumor associated with tuberous sclerosis: CT diagnosis. *J Comput Assist Tomogr.* 1985;9:809-811.
4. Altman NR, Purser RK, Donovan Post MJ. Tuberous sclerosis: characteristics at CT and MR imaging. *Radiology.* 1988;167:527-532.
5. Sugita K, Itoh K, Takeuchi Y, et al. Tuberous sclerosis: report of two cases studied by computer-assisted cranial tomography within one week after birth. *Brain Dev.* 1985;7:438-443.
6. McMurdo SK Jr, Moore SG, Brant-Zawadzki M, et al. MR imaging of intracranial tuberous sclerosis. *AJR Am J Roentgenol.* 1987;148:791-796.
7. Nixon JR, Houser OW, Gomez MR, Okazaki H. Cerebral tuberous sclerosis: MR imaging. *Radiology.* 1989;170:869-873.
8. Inoue Y, Nakajima S, Fukuda T, et al. Magnetic resonance images of tuberous sclerosis: further observations and clinical correlations. *Neuroradiology.* 1988;30:379-384.

Picture of the Month

Zvi Laron, MD; Beatrice Klinger, MD; Michael Grunebaum, MD (Contributors);
Murray Feingold, MD (Editor for This Case); *Walter W. Tunnessen, MD* (Section Editor)

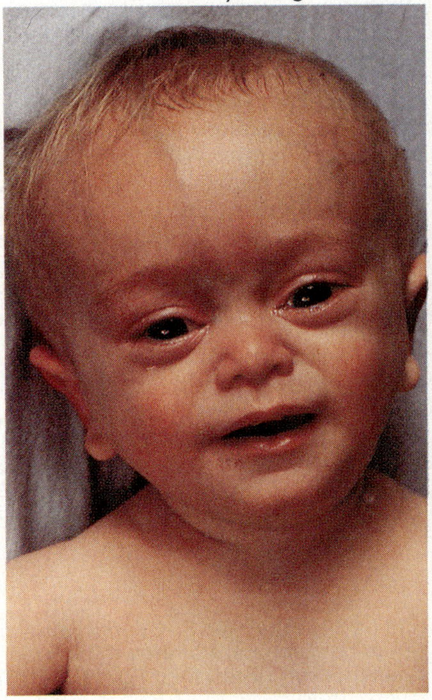

Figure 1.

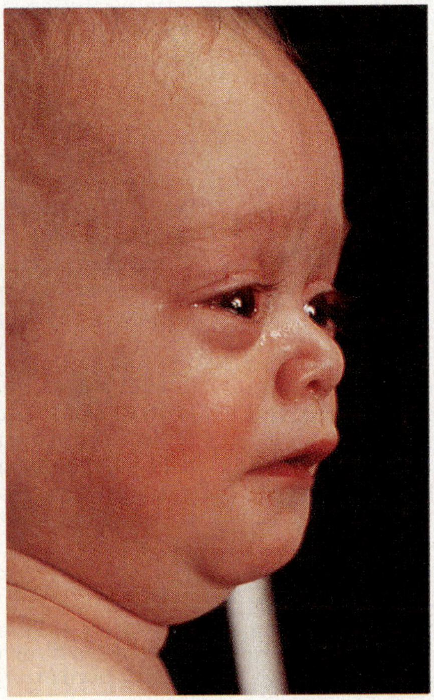

Figure 2.

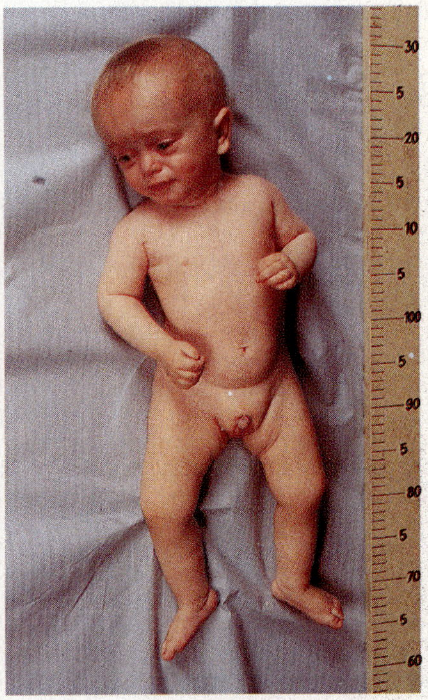

Figure 3.

Figure 4.

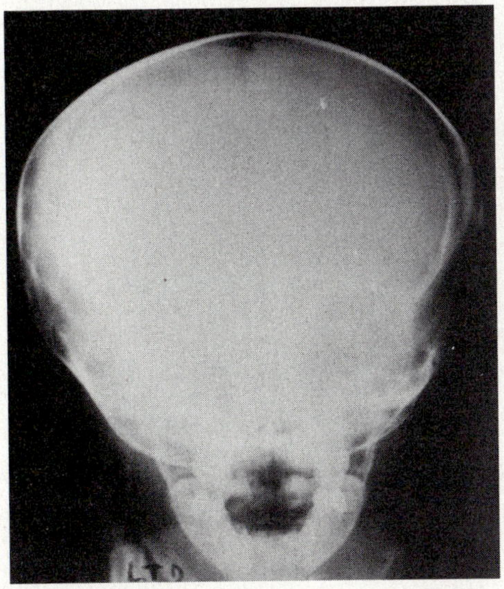

Figure 5.

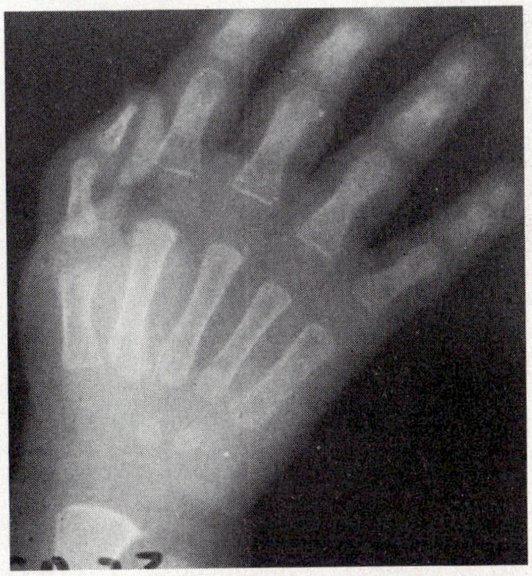

Accepted for publication December 12, 1990.

Contributed from the Institute of Pediatric and Adolescent Endocrinology (Drs Laron and Klinger) and Department of Pediatric Roentgenology (Dr Grunebaum), Beilinson Medical Center, Petah Tikva and Sackler Faculty of Medicine, Tel Aviv (Israel) University.

Reprint requests to National Birth Defects Center, Franciscan Children's Hospital, 30 Warren St, Brighton, MA 02135 (Dr Feingold).

The Editors welcome contributions to Picture of the Month and Radiological Case of the Month. Those who wish to contribute should send their manuscripts to Dr Tunnessen (Picture of the Month), The Children's Hospital of Philadelphia, 34th Street and Civic Center Blvd, Philadelphia, PA 19104, or Dr Wood (Radiological Case of the Month), Department of Radiology, Childrens Hospital of Los Angeles, 4650 Sunset Blvd, Los Angeles, CA 90027. Articles and photographs accepted for publication will bear the contributor's name. There is no charge for reproduction and printing of color illustrations.

Denouement and Discussion

Laron-Type Dwarfism

Figs 1 and 2.— *3 1/2-year-old boy with Laron-type dwarfism with sparse hair, frontal bossing, prominent veins, saddle nose, micrognathia, and small facial bones.*

Fig 3.—*Obesity and micropenis.*

Fig 4.—*Underdevelopment of facial bones and small bicondylar diameter.*

Fig 5.—*Marked retardation in skeletal maturation.*

Manifestations

Laron-type dwarfism is characterized by marked growth retardation, acromicria (small hands, feet, and chin), obesity, and micropenis. Craniofacial abnormalities include a protruding forehead, saddle nose, and an increased biparietal-bicondylar ratio, all caused by marked underdevelopment of the facial bones. Head circumference is decreased, skeletal maturation is markedly retarded, the bones are very thin, and there is an increased incidence of minor skeletal abnormalities such as slipped femoral epiphyses and Legg-Calve-Perthes disease. The obesity is generalized and there is underdevelopment of muscle mass. Genitalia and gonads are small, and puberty is delayed but ultimately attained. Final height ranges between 110 and 138 cm. Afflicted children have a typically high-pitched voice and are clinically indistinguishable from patients with growth hormone deficiency.

Biochemical abnormalities are characterized by hypoglycemia, often symptomatic at an early age, high circulating levels of growth hormone, and low serum insulinlike growth factor levels that do not rise with the administration of exogenous human growth hormone. There is resistance to growth hormone due to a defect in growth hormone receptors.

Genetics

Laron-type dwarfism is a hereditary disease occurring mainly in children of Jewish, Oriental, Arab, Spanish, Portuguese, and Italian descent. However, patients have been diagnosed in white, Japanese, and Eskimo populations. Because the extracellular part of the growth hormone receptor is identical to the circulating growth hormone–binding protein, it is possible to diagnose homozygous patients and identify heterozygote carriers.

Treatment

The recent recombinant biosynthesis of insulinlike growth factor 1 has resulted in therapeutic trials aimed at replacing the hormone that the body cannot generate. Nutritional counseling is also needed to prevent hypoglycemia and progressive obesity. Continuous psychosocial counseling of the parents and patients may be indicated.

References

1. Laron Z, Pertzelan A, Mannheimer S. Genetic pituitary dwarfism with high serum concentration of growth hormone: a new inborn error of metabolism? *Israel J Med Sci.* 1966;2:152-155.

2. Laron Z, Klinger B, Erster B, Anin S. Effects of acute administration of insulin like growth factor I in patients with Laron type dwarfism. *Lancet.* 1988;2:1170-1172.

3. Laron Z, Klinger B, Erster B, Silbergeld A. Serum GH binding protein deficiency activity identifies the heterozygous carriers for Laron type dwarfism. *Acta Endocrinol.* 1989;121:603-608.

Far From the Ideal

The Plight of Poor Children in the United States

The child on the cover of this month's issue of *AJDC* was visualized as an ideal by an unknown painter in colonial times. The child is beautiful, well nourished, placid, and obviously well cared for. This is the ideal that many think of when asked to picture our aspirations for our children. Unfortunately, in the United States today, we fall far short of providing that ideal for millions of infants, children, adolescents, and young adults. This issue of *AJDC* is devoted to exploring the dimensions of and reasons for the problems as well as offering potential corrective actions that might be applied to the plight of our underserved or unserved youth. We embarked on this issue as part of the family of American Medical Association journals' efforts to highlight what has become a national disgrace: 47 000 000 or more individuals are neglected at a time when many in the United States enjoy the highest level of health in the history of humanity. We hope that our readers will learn of this awful circumstance and, to the extent possible, take action locally, regionally, and nationally to effect some of our authors' remedial suggestions.

We embarked on the development of this issue by inviting commentaries from individual leaders in pediatrics, from spokespersons for our professional societies, and from directors of our major foundations and organizations that offer support and funding for programs that benefit children. We may not have invited all who could participate to do so, and some of those invited did not respond. However, a cross section of individuals did respond and covered all of the issues one might think of when considering the extent of the problems. We thank those who did so and offer our readers their comments.

We also received unsolicited manuscripts whose themes were consistent with the major intent of this issue of the journal. We have included those that seemed pertinent in our "Pediatric Forum" and "Original Article" departments. They form a unified whole with the solicited articles.

To highlight some of the generic issues common to many of the thematic articles in this issue, I offer the following observations:

1. The dimension of the problem is enormous. More than 37 million children live in poverty, an additional 10 million have no health insurance, and an unknown number have inadequate health care. Many of these children receive no care at all or only urgent care, in fragmented fashion, often for late-stage or even end-stage disease. For most of this population, preventive services are nonexistent or inaccessible because of poverty, lack of knowledge, or failure of insurance programs to cover preventive services. The legacy of this neglect will be felt for many generations to come if we do not take urgent and emphatic action. We will have a host of unhealthy adults and lose significant numbers of otherwise contributing members of society. We also will lose the diversity of ethnicity that is desirable in our leadership ranks in all areas of society.

2. The reasons for the lack of medical care are legion; the most often cited in the reports in this issue are financial. Our national economic plight, with high national debt, diversion of funds from social programs to other areas of the budget, redistribution of federal support to states and cities (which cannot supply the redistributed services because of their own economic difficulties), and now, the added potential cost of the conflict in the Persian Gulf area, has resulted in inadequate resources for health-related programs. Non–health care social programs suffer from the same maldistribution of resources. As a result, poverty increases, homelessness skyrockets, and the causes of ill health multiply.

Apart from financial considerations, which are a major part of the problem, societal issues combine to deny adequate health care. For reasons that are unclear, children lack a voice in the halls of power, especially compared with other segments of our population, such as the elderly. Society voices the bland sentiment that children are our "most valuable resource" but does not protest when we do not ensure that this most valuable resource has an opportunity for a healthy life. In recent years, the American Academy of Pediatrics has become a voice heard in Congress and in other settings as an advocate for children and their needs. However, this is a relatively recent phenomenon and has not yet reached the magnitude of advocacy for the elderly. Strain's contribution[1] in this issue outlines the approach taken by the academy to influence adequate health planning for our youth.

Children whose parents have habits that result in congenital drug addiction and/or congenital infection with human immunodeficiency or hepatitis viruses receive a legacy over which they have no control. They are innocent victims of society's inability or lack of commitment to deal with these problems of their parents. Several contributors to this issue focus on the resulting ill health attendant on such neglect.

Another contributing factor is what I term the *disease of the month* mentality prevalent in allocating money to health programs. Many governmental and private programs are funded to satisfy the demands of potent advocacy groups for specific diseases. In other instances, a powerful individual, sometimes for personal reasons, supports a specific disease program. Added to this set of factors is advocacy by specific professional societies, each with its own agenda. Although this kind of advocacy, and subsequent funding, results in good care for some segments of the population, such specialized program development often substitutes for a more coherent, more widely applicable medical or preventive care program that could offer greater benefit for a larger proportion of our population. Cleveland[2] elaborates on this theme in his discussion of the "patchwork" vs "quilt" approach to health care.

Society also has neglected our adolescents, whose rising pregnancy rate results in increased prematurity, inadequate parenting, and reinforcement of poverty, ill health, and dangerous life-styles. A number of our authors have highlighted this critical area.

Members of society "bill and coo" over the infant born to parents in good financial condition, but ignore the minority infant in the intensive care unit who struggles first to exist and then to remain functionally intact. Members of society bemoan our high neonatal and infant mortality rates compared with other developed societies but do little to advocate for the resources that are needed to prevent prematurity and manage conditions leading to excessive morbidity and mortality. Commentators in this issue highlight the toll resulting from such inattention to this critical period in life.

3. Potential corrective actions are outlined for each of the areas covered by the articles in this issue. Some are relatively simple to accomplish, requiring some rededication of effort but little extra funding. Others will require considerable funding and a change in our national priorities. However, most readers reach the overwhelming conclusion that we need a fundamental change in our national commitment. We need to behave as if children are really our most valuable resource and our future. Therefore, mothers must be afforded healthy pregnancies so newborns will be healthy and born at term, and children must be freed from preventable childhood diseases. They must enjoy normal growth and development and receive an effective education, which should include knowledge and skills needed to understand health and to effect behavioral changes that lead to prevention and avoidance of disease. Parents and children must also learn how to gain early and effective access to the health care system.

Rather than be discouraged by the scope of the problem, we suggest that readers use the data and recommendations in this issue to take action in individual practices, professional societies, medical schools, residency programs, and communities to become advocates for change at all levels of government. We need to take such actions now, not later. We can solve these problems with a unified will, but it will take a society that is willing to move itself from complacency to a new position of concern and action. We at *AJDC* believe we have taken a first step by presenting the articles in this issue; each of you can now take the necessary steps in the immediate future.

Vincent A. Fulginiti, MD
Editor, *AJDC*
Dean's Office
Tulane University School of Medicine
1430 Tulane Ave
New Orleans, LA 70112

References

1. Strain JE. The American Academy of Pediatrics response to the growing health needs of children. *AJDC.* 1991;145:536-539.

2. Cleveland WW. Redoing the health care quilt: patches or whole cloth? *AJDC.* 1991;145:499-504.

Youth Alienation as an Emerging Pediatric Health Care Issue

Many young people have withdrawn or are separated from the values of their society or family. These are our alienated youth. The number of adolescents without a defined role in modern society is growing.[1] The inability of children to find a meaningful and productive place in American society both contributes to and stems from the "new morbidities of youth," including early sexual activity, drug abuse, school failure, family violence, and the like. A dearth of descriptive information exists on this growing population of alienated adolescents, which includes runaways, teenaged prostitutes, street youth, school dropouts, and delinquents, to name but a few.[2] The problem of alienation during adolescence, which began to be of major sociological concern in the 1960s, today constitutes an emergent area of study for health care professionals.

These young people, because of forced or adopted destructive life-styles, are exposed more than most youth to both physical and emotional illness and to the untoward consequences of early sexual activity, such as pregnancy and exposure to sexually transmitted diseases, including acquired immunodeficiency syndrome.[3] For example, more than half of all homeless adolescent girls become pregnant while on the streets.[4] Likewise, those who live in inner cities and come from the underclass often migrate to environments where violence and bodily injury occur frequently and gang affiliation becomes inevitable. Opportunities therefore to reclaim these "wayward" youth become more difficult if the pattern of alienation is not recognized early.

While the largest group of alienated young people are of ethnic minority backgrounds, generally from the lower socioeconomic strata, their values and attitudes often remain similar to those of their families and culture.[5] Equally alarming is the increasing number of alienated youth who come from middle-class America: runaways, street youth, punk rockers, delinquents, and school dropouts. Many of these youth are in conflict with their families and middle-class institutions because of a rejection of parental values or an attraction to subcultures that are perceived as more akin to themselves and supportive than their families, schools, or everyday peers. Few of these young people are running away from unfortunate or abusive home lives. Yet another group, the so-called throwaway kids, are asked by their families to leave at a young age. Many of these young people are depressed, have limited educations, and are unemployable; thus, they are unlikely to become productive citizens.

The number of alienated youth in America is large. By conservative estimates, more than 1 million youth run away from home each year.[6] Nationwide, more than 25% of all high school students drop out.[7] More than ½ million adolescents are incarcerated in secure facilities each year.[8] Estimates of the number of homeless teenagers on the street are rough at best. It is impossible to obtain accurate data for these large groups, in part because they do not congregate and many return home and to the streets in an unpredictable fashion. At a very young age these adolescents begin having difficulties fitting in, and the likelihood is high that as young adults they will have even more difficulty becoming independent, productive members of society.

Alienated youth are frequently outside the health care system and tend to remain there unless efforts are made to identify them and develop health services that are acceptable to them. The adoption of destructive life-styles by many of these youth contributes heavily to physical and psychological morbidity and to an alarmingly high mortality rate. Because health care is one of the more acceptable areas of interaction with these adolescents, some members of the health care community have been remarkably creative in their outreach and development of health services. A few model adolescent and young adult "street clinics" offer free, comprehensive health care services to this population. Those clinics that are affiliated with medical schools and specifically adolescent medicine provide many opportunities for pediatricians in training or in practice to be involved.

Even when the pediatrician is not involved in the regular care of homeless and alienated adolescents, motivated clinicians are aware of specialized resources in the community for this group. These resources include shelter services, free or easy-access adolescent clinics, counseling or support groups for gay and lesbian youth, adolescent chemical dependency treatment programs, and alternative schools. However, few cities have successfully developed comprehensive service programs and many of these components of care may not be available, or homeless and "emancipated" minors may not be eligible. Job training programs for runaways, juveniles involved in prostitution, and older street youth are becoming more prevalent in cities, but often cannot meet the great demand for services.[9]

Perhaps even more important is the pediatrician's advocacy role in promoting healthier outcomes before the alienation process progresses in adolescence. Pediatricians frequently see children who are beginning to have problems associated with alienation. Alienation is often preceded by childhood emotional trauma and ongoing stress. Repeated stress-related illness, school absences, new behaviors stemming from depression, irritability, or anxiety may ultimately escalate into a situation during early adolescence that makes reconciliation between children and parents more difficult.

The pediatrician should take every opportunity during the earlier years to explore family relationship concerns and problem behaviors with children and parents. For older children and younger adolescents, the general psychosocial history should be discussed with the young person in a confidential setting. The degree to which the young person has begun to separate himself or herself from activities normal for his or her age should be assessed. Family relationships, leisure activities, the patient's association with a deviant peer group, school attendance and performance, alcohol and drug experience, sexual behaviors and concerns about sexual identity, and symptoms of depression and withdrawal are important areas to explore. Alienated youth have usually encountered problems in most of these areas.

Early intervention and referral, orchestrated by a caring pediatrician who recognizes the early signs of alienation, who has developed empathy for the experience of these young people and their families, and who knows community resources can be of great help in averting future adoption of destructive behaviors and lifestyles.

While physicians as individual practitioners have a responsibility for providing anticipatory guidance to families and caring for these youth in clinical settings, a great deal more regional and national attention should be given to this large portion of American youth. Physicians can take an active role in developing community resources to meet the needs of alienated youth. They can volunteer to serve on agency boards, committees, and groups to provide the expertise and understanding of a physician who is familiar with these youth and their health issues. The health perspective is important. We are at great risk of losing through apathy, illness, injury, and death many children who have a great deal more potential for productive adult lives than we often recognize.

James A. Farrow, MD
Division of Adolescent Medicine
University of Washington
WJ-10
Seattle, WA 98105

References

1. Nightingale EO, Wolverton L. *Adolescent Rolelessness in Modern Society.* New York, NY: Carnegie Corporation of New York; 1988.
2. Resnick MD, Hibbard R. Chronic physical and social conditions of youth. Presented at the National Invitational Conference on Health Futures of Adolescents; April 2-5, 1986; Daytona Beach, Fla.
3. Kusserow RP. *HIV Infection Among Street Youth.* Washington, DC: Office of Inspector General; 1990. US Department of Health and Human Services publication OEI-01-90-00500.
4. Deisher RW, Farrow JA, Hope K, Litchfield C. The pregnant adolescent prostitute. *AJDC.* 1989;143:1162-1165.
5. Deisher RW, Farrow JA. Recognizing and dealing with alienated youth in clinical practice. *Pediatr Ann.* 1986;15:759-763.
6. National Network of Runaway and Youth Services. *AIDS Education: Programs for Out-of-School Youth Slowly Evolving.* Washington, DC: US General Accounting Office; May 1990. HRD-90-111.
7. Commission on Work, Family and Citizenship. *The Forgotten Half: Pathways to Success for America's Youth and Young Families.* New York, NY: William T. Grant Foundation; 1988.
8. Stone D. Juvenile crime rate: myth vs reality. *Youth Law News.* 1982;2:1-2.
9. Deisher RW. Our alienated youth. Presented at the National Invitational Conference on Health Futures of Adolescents; April 2-5, 1986; Daytona Beach, Fla.

New Initiatives in Adolescent Health Promotion

Sir.—Health issues facing adolescents have changed dramatically over the last several decades.[1] Twenty years ago, adolescent morbidity and mortality were associated predominantly with natural causes. Adolescents today, however, are endangered predominantly by their own behaviors. Drinking, tobacco and drug use, pregnancy, sexually transmitted diseases, and injuries take a major toll on youth and place them at risk of developing disease as adults. Because these health risks do not lend themselves to traditional models of medical intervention, greater emphasis is needed on prevention as a way to improve the health and well-being of adolescents.

The process of identifying and implementing a broad prevention strategy has gained momentum with the recent release of two documents by the US Public Health Service (PHS):— *Healthy People 2000: The National Health Promotion and Disease Prevention Objectives*[2] and *the Guide to Clinical Preventive Services*.[3] Unfortunately, pediatricians and other health care professionals treating adolescents have been relatively quiet in the national dialogue stimulated by these documents. Because the information contained in these two reports can, however, affect the provision of health care to adolescents, they are worth reviewing.

Healthy People 2000 was developed to focus ". . . a national strategy for significantly improving the health of the Nation over the coming decade."[2] The initiative promotes three broad health goals: "(1) increase the span of healthy life for Americans; (2) reduce health disparities among Americans; and (3) achieve access to preventive services for all Americans." To meet these goals, the PHS defined 22 areas for special emphasis. Eight relate to health promotion topics (eg, physical activity and fitness, mental health, and mental disorders), five involve health protection topics (eg, unintentional injuries and oral health), eight involve preventive services for targeted issues (eg, sexually transmitted disease and maternal and child health), and one relates to surveillance and data systems. Except for surveillance and data systems, each area includes health status,risk reduction, and service and protection objectives. Of the almost 300 national health objectives in the document, 45 target adolescents directly, and approximately 51 affect adolescents as part of the broader population. An introductory section of the document delineates the predominant health problems experienced by various age groups (including adolescents) and by special populations, such as people with low income, minorities, and the disabled.

The *Guide to Clinical Preventive Services*, the final report of the US Preventive Services Task Force,[3] describes 169 clinical screening, counseling, and immunization practices recommended for treatment or therapy of 60 target conditions. The procedures are grouped by patient age, including preadolescents (aged 8 to 12 years), young adolescents (aged 13 to 17 years), and older adolescents (aged 18 to 24 years). Only those conditions for which effective preventive intervention procedures exist or that cause a high "burden of suffering" were addressed in the report. Most of the conditions relating to adolescents qualified for inclusion in the latter category.

For at least four reasons, these two documents are important to those who work to improve the health of adolescents. First, they direct the debate on improving adolescent health to developing and implementing more effective preventive strategies. Most adolescent preventive interventions now are provided by schools, churches, youth organizations, or media campaigns. Not only do the PHS documents promote these methods of intervention, but they also renew interest in how physicians and other health care providers can provide effective preventive services in the office. Second, these documents present a framework for actions that can be taken by both the private and public health sectors. They provide impetus for the development of new strategies for physicians and health professionals who work in both traditional (eg, hospitals and private, community, and public health clinics) and nontraditional (eg, school clinics, correctional institutions, and drop-in centers) settings. Third, *Healthy People 2000* provides a structure for focusing human and financial resources. States, communities, and health organizations can use it to determine health priorities for their populations. With clearly defined objectives, organizations and health care professionals can better coordinate their efforts, producing a more efficient and comprehensive preventive health strategy. As called for in the recent report from the National Commission on the Role of the School and the Community in Promoting Adolescent Health,[4] better access to appropriate, comprehensive, coordinated, and confidential health services is necessary to solve the complex array of adolescent health problems. Providing such services will require cooperation and focused efforts from all segments of the health care community. Fourth, the PHS documents set goals that provide opportunities that allow for research on the effectiveness of various prevention strategies. As preventive interventions are developed and implemented, a rigorous agenda for evaluation of research must be followed to determine how best to use scarce health care funds.

Neither the national health objectives nor the *Guide to Clinical Preventive Services* has received universal approval. The public health care community is concerned that the national health objectives ". . . have no implementation plan, they overemphasize individual responsibility, and they abrogate governmental responsibility."[5] Critics also state that preventive health goals cannot be achieved without additional federal funding and that the multifunded nature of the US health care system precludes effective implementation.[6] The professional pediatric community has criticized the *Guide* because it recommends a specified frequency of preventive health visits for adults while leaving the frequency of such visits by adolescents and children to the discretion of the provider.[7] Other concerns are that the recommendations do not include all pediatric preventive health practices and that they tend to overemphasize change in existing behavior rather than focusing on anticipatory guidance as a way to prevent the onset of health-compromising behavior. In general, the *Guide* fails to recognize many of the risks that endanger adolescents specifically and the opportunity for promoting healthy behaviors during this developmental period. Although the *Guide* clearly "shortchanges" children and youth, it and *Healthy People 2000* together provide health professionals, administrators, and the federal government a structure on which to build sound preventive health strategies for adolescents.

It is important that advocates of adolescent health work to ensure that the interests of adolescents are well represented as the nation begins to implement broad intervention strategies for preventive health. Because adolescents and children are not empowered politically, adolescent health concerns easily may be overshadowed by concerns of other populations.

Various organizations have been funded by the PHS to promote the national health objectives as they relate to special populations or settings, such as Hispanics, blacks, schools, and hospitals. As part of these efforts, the American Medical Association received funds to be used in the dissemination of information related to adolescents. For information on this initiative for adolescents, write to the Department of Adolescent Health, AMA, 515 N State St, Chicago, IL 60610. For general information, write to the Office of Disease Prevention and Health Promotion, Department of Health and Human Services, Washington, DC 20201.

Arthur B. Elster, MD
Department of Adolescent Health
American Medical Association
515 N State St
Chicago, IL 60610

1. Gans JE, Blyth DA, Elster AB, Gaveras LL. *America's Adolescents: How Healthy Are They?* Chicago, Ill: American Medical Association; 1990.
2. *Healthy People 2000: National Health Promotion and Disease Prevention Objectives*. Washington, DC: Department of Health and Human Services; 1990. US Public Health Service publication 017-001-00474-0.
3. US Preventive Services Task Force. *Guide to Clinical Preventive Services*. Baltimore, Md: Williams & Wilkins; 1989.
4. National Commission on the Role of the School and the Community in Promoting Adolescent Health. *Code Blue: Uniting for Healthier Youth. Chicago, Ill: American Medical Association; 1990.*
5. *Nation's Health: Year 2000 Objectives Are Important, But Imperfect Guide*. Washington, DC: American Public Health Association; 1990.
6. *Media Information Alert*. Washington, DC: Advocacy Institute; November 14, 1990.
7. *AAP News: From the President*. Elk Grove Village, Ill: American Academy of Pediatrics; February 1990.

Redoing the Health Care Quilt

Patches or Whole Cloth?

William W. Cleveland, MD

The current health care system of the United States, like a quilt that is tattered and full of holes, badly needs attention. The question is whether we should repair it with patches or replace it with a new quilt of whole cloth. That the system needs fixing is evident; the deficiencies have been described by abundant commentaries. The major deficiencies include those cited below.

The Uninsured.—An estimated 37 million people in the United States do not have health insurance. Of these, about 12 million are children; another major segment comprises pregnant women. These numbers are estimated to have increased approximately 30% in the last decade. This reflects lack of employee coverage, particularly in small businesses, and a high rate of job turnover. It also reflects an inadequate Medicaid program that varies by state but that generally leaves a significant fraction of indigent families uncovered. The problem of uninsured children has been extensively reviewed by Oberg.[1]

Expanding Health Care Costs and an Apparent Lack of Efficiency.—If infant mortality rate is an acceptable indicator of maternal and child health, the comparison of rates in the United States with those of other nations relative to expenditure provides a discouraging picture indeed (Fig 1).[2] Our per capita medical expenditure is the highest in the world, but we rank 21st in infant mortality rates. When infant mortality rates are compared in terms of percentage of gross national product spent on health care, the result is the same (Fig 2). One factor to be considered is whether the US government is spending its money in the right places. For example, if infant mortality rates among developed nations are compared with the percentage of health care dollars spent for public health, our position is reversed—the United States spends the lowest percentage for public health and is still 21st in mortality rate (Fig 3).

A Burdensome Bureaucracy.—Costs of administering US health care programs are staggering. Of the approximately 11.5% of the gross national product expended, an estimated 2.6% funds the bureaucracy. For the physician, penetrating the administrative barriers of either governmental agencies or insurance companies to render service charges is a familiar problem. For the patient, dealing with these groups is perhaps even more difficult. The bureaucracy of health care appears to be in a state of chronic and self-sustained hyperplasia.

An Inadequate Medicaid Program.—This system is federally mandated but managed through varying policies by the states. These variances include the standards for inclusion in the program, the scope of benefits provided, the amount of public funds allocated, and rates of provider reimbursement. Financial criteria for eligibility vary widely, but in most states a significant portion of the indigent population of children and pregnant women is not covered. For persons eligible, the mechanisms for registration are often cumbersome and patients with limited social resources may not be able to gain access to the system. A further deficiency is that payment to providers may be so low as to offer no incentive to render services. In some states, payments for preventive care, including well-child visits, are so low that they do not cover physicians' overhead, much less reimburse them for professional services.

A Troubled Health Insurance Industry.—More than 1500 health plans in this country compete for coverage in an entrepreneurial system. Each maintains its separate administration; each has its own policies as to eligibility and coverage and each is a for-profit operation. Providers must deal with a variety of provisions and regulations that significantly contribute to costs of delivering care. Insurance companies also must spend large amounts of money on administrative costs—approximately 12% of premiums.

Lack of Emphasis on Prevention.—The insurance industry does not embrace preventive medicine as its goal. Pediatricians in Florida were able to promote legislation mandating well-child care provision by insurers; this was accomplished with great travail and with much resistance by the industry. As previously noted, an inordinately low percentage of our health care funds goes to public health agencies. Medicaid struggles to provide treatment of illness with incomplete success, and little is left for preventive care.

Litigious Factors Expanding Costs.—Physicians who practice in areas where malpractice suits flourish and attorneys become rich cannot help but be influenced by this threat in making clinical decisions. The remote chance that a child not growing well has a hypothalmic lesion not clinically evident provokes the performance of magnetic resonance imaging, which currently costs $1200. (Why this procedure should cost $1200 or growth hormone should cost $50/mg is also of interest, but that is the subject of

Accepted for publication January 11, 1991.

From the Department of Pediatrics, School of Medicine, University of Miami (Fla).

Reprint requests to Department of Pediatrics, PO Box 016980 (R 131), Miami, FL 33101 (Dr Cleveland).

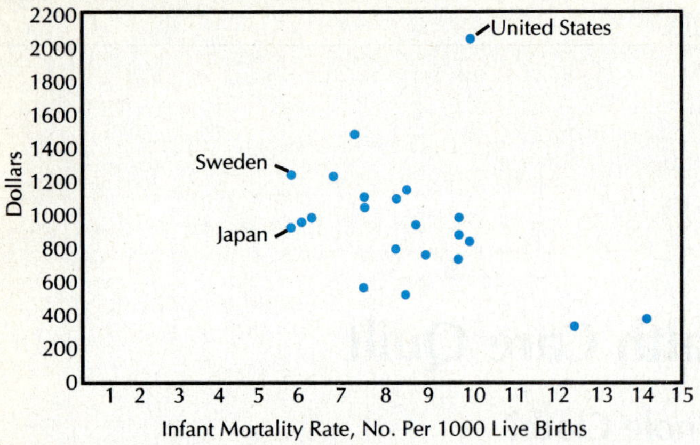

Fig 1.—*Per capita health expenditures and infant mortality rates in 1987.*

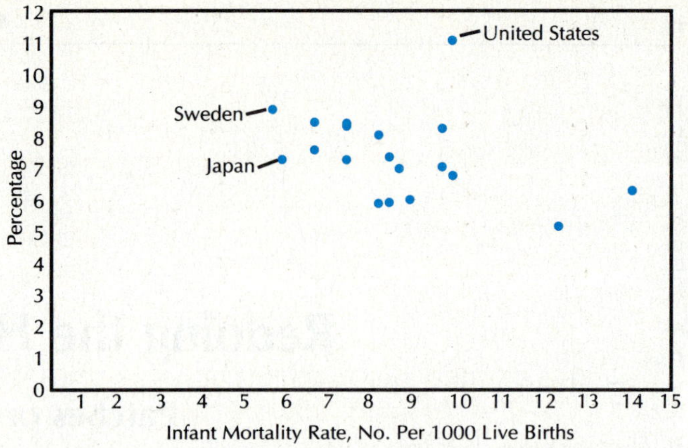

Fig 2.—*Infant mortality rates and public health expenditures as percentages of all health expenditures in 1987.*

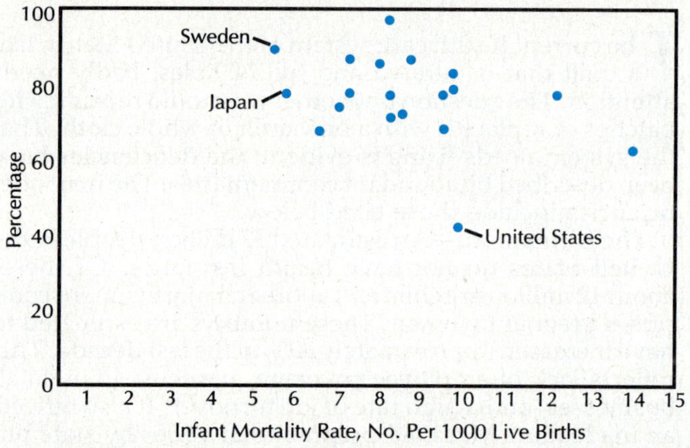

Fig 3.—*Infant mortality rates and health expenditures as percentages of gross national product in 1987.*

another essay.) And so it goes—the expansion of these ultraconservative decisions contributes to health care costs, to say nothing of its contribution to the costs of malpractice insurance. The many holes in the ragged quilt are evident. All agree that repairs are urgently needed. The question remains as to the best approach. Many alternatives have been proposed—patches and new quilts of whole cloth.

THE PATCHES

Various proposals have been made at several levels to patch the holes. The essential features of some of these are summarized below. The review is intended to be illustrative but not all-inclusive.

Medicaid Expansion and Reform.—This is a part of several proposals listed below, but has been specifically addressed by the Health Policy Agenda for the American People.[3,4] Eight major reforms were recommended by the Ad Hoc Committee on Medicaid and are as follows:

1. The Medicaid program should be governed by national standards and goals.

2. The categorical link of Medicaid eligibility to public cash assistance (welfare) programs should be broken; income eligibility for the program should be set at no less than the federal poverty level.

3. All states should be mandated to adopt a Medically Needy program with "spend down" eligibility provisions. Asset testing should be an acceptable eligibility requirement only through the Medically Needy provisions. "Medically needy" persons are those whose incomes exceed the Medicaid eligibility level but who have been impoverished by catastrophic medical bills.

4. A standard benefit package should be provided by each state and federally mandated. It should include physician services, inpatient and outpatient hospital services, laboratory and roentgenogram services, prescription drugs, institutional care for the elderly and the physically or mentally disabled, dental services, early and periodic health screenings, diagnostic and treatment services, family planning services, home health and personal care services, and other medically necessary professional services.

5. Medicaid expansion should include measures to promote cost-effective provision of services.

6. Medicaid expansion should include policies and incentives to encourage broader health care provider participation.

7. A greater burden of the fiscal impact of eligibility expansion should be borne by the federal government, and the federal formula governing reimbursement to states should be revised to correct for tax-burden inequities.

8. Long-term care services should be continued under Medicaid or through a structurally improved program.

Basic Health for All Americans Act.—Proposed by Kennedy[5] in 1987, the act recommends major expansion of employer coverage for health care and mandates a minimum level of health benefits to be provided, including hospital and physician care, preventive testing, prenatal testing, and well-baby care.

Universal Maternal and Child Health Program.—Proposed by Oberg,[1] this would ensure universal and equitable access to health services by pregnant women and children independent of age, income, family composition, or employment. Coverage would be provided for preventive as well as acute and catastrophic services.

Recommendations of the Pepper Commission.—The commission's recommendations[6,7] include insurance reforms by which income-based cost sharing of premiums by employers and a public plan guaranteeing health care coverage for all workers would be implemented. Ultimately, this plan would provide coverage for all children. Insurance reforms would include coverage of primary and preventive care, elimination of exclusions because of preexisting conditions, and elimination of coinsurance payments by consumers for prenatal and well-child care. The commission also recommended Medicaid reforms (including physician reimbursement for obstetric and pediatric care), ultimate replacement of Medicaid with a new federal program expanding access and payment according to Medicare rules, a quality assurance strategy that would include reform of the medical malpractice system, and cost containment measures.

American Academy of Pediatrics National Child Health Policy.—This policy[8] includes health care coverage for all children and adolescents through age 21 years and mandates employer-based coverage or coverage by private insurance companies contracted by the state. The policy also calls for state health care funding (including funding of Medicaid expenditures), state and federal insurance premiums, an employer payroll tax for those employers who choose not to cover pregnant women and children, and methods of ensuring adequate provider reimbursement.

HR 4280 Health Insurance for Children and Mothers Act of 1990.—This act[9] requires health insurance for pregnant women and children, mandates comprehensive benefits, calls for elimination of financial barriers to health care (development of a one-tier health care system), recommends that Medicaid dollars be refocused in a more efficient and effective program, emphasizes preventive services (including immunizations, and prenatal and well-child care), and directs that payroll tax be increased to match current Medicare tax paid by employer and employees.

A Consumer Choice Health Plan for Universal Health Insurance.—The proposal[10] states that "To remedy the deprivation, we propose that everyone not covered by Medicare, Medicaid, or some other public program be enabled to buy affordable coverage, either through their employers or through a 'public sponsor.' To attack the excess, we propose a strategy of managed competition in which collective agents, called sponsors, such as the Health Care Financing Administration and large employers, contract with competing health plans and manage a process of informed cost-conscious consumer choice that requires providers who deliver high-quality care economically."

State Programs.—These programs include Massachusetts legislation designed "to make health security available to all citizens of the Commonwealth and to improve hospital financing." This legislation would create a Department of Medical Security that contracts with health plans to make coverage available to small businesses and unsponsored individuals. It proposes a tax on all employers of five or more workers.[11] The New York State Department of Health has developed a program called Universal New York Health Care, or UNY-CARE.[12] It would retain existing payers, including employer-based insurance coverage, but would combine them in a one-payer framework. This one payer would be the only resource for most services and would negotiate reimbursement rates, hopefully to exercise some cost controls.

Rationing Health Services.—Oregon legislation proposes altering Medicaid coverage to provide services based on a "net benefit" concept.[13] This involves prioritizing medical services on the basis of cost and benefit to the overall public. A list of such priorities has been generated. Different priorities have been established for different age groups. High priorities are given to family planning, prenatal care (including nutritional care), childhood immunizations, labor and delivery services, and the treatment of acute illness. Low-priority items include infertility services, plastic surgery, routine dental care for adults, and most transplantations. These priorities are established by a Health Services Commission consisting of five physicians, a public health nurse, a social worker, and four consumers. The basic principle is expansion of numbers served by restriction of services provided. Thus far it proposes rationing services only to those served by Medicaid.

Rationing Medical Progress.—Callahan[14] describes his proposal as follows: "In any case, we must be prepared to ration medical progress and in particular to forego potentially beneficial advances in the application and development of new techniques. I am not proposing a diminution of efforts to extend our store of theoretical biologic and medical knowledge. A strong commitment to basic biomedical research remains an attractive and desirable goal. That commitment is not incompatible, however, with several insistent requirements: (1) that clinical applications be subjected to stringent technological assessments before dissemination; (2) that the social and economic standards for the assessment be biased toward restrictiveness ('straight is the gate and narrow the way' might be a pertinent maxim here); and (3) that it is understood and accepted that some, perhaps many, beneficial applications will have to be passed over on grounds of cost and other, more pressing social priorities."

Rationing Health Care According to Age.—Levensky[15] summarized these proposals as follows: "Why is it acceptable to propose limits on health care for the elderly, in contrast to the obvious unacceptibility of such a proposal applied to other groups and classes of citizens? A number of philosophers and medical ethicists, prominent among them Callahan, Daniels, and Veatch, have published carefully formulated arguments favoring the use of age as a criterion for rationing health care. Although the details of their various arguments differ, the essential philosophical underpinnings are quite similar. They argue that limits on health care for the elderly are justifiable because each citizen, throughout a lifetime, would benefit if funds now used to extend life at its end were redirected to earlier stages of life. They envision the national health care budget equitably distributed among all citizens. Each person would be entitled to a fair share of national health care expenditures as a personal lifetime 'health care budget.' "

THE QUILTS

The Canadian Health Care System

Much discussion of adopting a variant of the Canadian system has been heard.[16] In Canada, one national health program is administered by the provinces, and universal coverage for all citizens is provided regardless of age, health status, or financial means.

All medical costs, with no copayments or deductibles and including costs of long-term stays in health care facilities, are covered. Services include care by physicians in offices, in hospitals, and at home. Also covered are diagnosis and treatment of illness and injury (including and drugs prenatal and postnatal obstetrical care); laboratory, radiologic, and other ancillary services; radiotherapy; and home dialysis. Most of the provinces also provide land and air ambulance services. Private or semiprivate hospital accommodations are not covered by the plan but may be financed through commercial insurers with premiums paid by employers. (These plans may not, however, offer benefits provided by the provincial plans.)

Payments to providers include fee-for-service reimbursement of physicians according to a schedule negotiated between organized medicine and provincial government. Some provinces have capitation systems. Patients can choose any physician. Extra billing by physicians is barred. Hospitals are paid an annual global sum for provision of services, which is similarly negotiated. In Canada, centralized government controls are exercised over major forms of technology and capital spending, with an effort to regionalize highly technologic services. The system is financed by payment of premiums by employers and individuals. Funding is also provided by the provincial and federal governments through general revenues. Participants older than age 65 years pay no premiums; individuals or families lacking resources to pay also are not charged.

Comprehensive Health Care for All Americans Act (the Claude Pepper Comprehensive Health Care Act)

This comprehensive plan includes many features of the Canadian system.[17] Its principal elements are as follows:

Eligibility.—All residents of the United States who are citizens, nationals, or lawful resident aliens may enroll. The enrollee may choose among qualified health plans as approved by the state of residency.

Administration.—The act would establish a National Comprehensive Health Care (CHC) Board to which each state would submit a plan for its CHC program. To be approved, the state plan must provide for (among other things): adequate financing, freedom of choice among qualified health plans by enrollees, effective cost containment measures, adequate administration (including establishment of a public advisory boards), responsive quality control mechanisms, and organization of a state commission to reduce excess hospital beds. The National CHC Board would establish a commission to provide advice regarding technology development and effectiveness and to recommend such technologies for inclusion as covered health services. Each state CHC program would approve qualified health plans for inclusion based on defined criteria. The number might be limited, except for health maintenance organizations.

Financing.—The federal CHC program would make a per capita contribution to each state annually according to defined criteria for support of the state plan. The state CHC program would generate funds from general revenues, earmarked taxes, sales taxes, employer and employee health insurance premiums, and cost sharing. Services for low-income groups, pregnant women, and well-child care might be exempt from premiums or cost sharing.

Reimbursement.—The CHC program would include payment of institutions according to a biennial budget plan and to physicians according to payment schedules negotiated with medical organizations and based on a national relative value scale. Alternate methods such as capitation, annual salary, and hourly payments might be approved with some restrictions.

Benefits.—The plan provides very broad coverage, including physicians' and other professional medical services, inpatient and outpatient hospital care, diagnostic and screening tests, prenatal and well-baby care, mental health services, long-term care, and hospice services. Preventive services would include basic immunizations, prenatal and postnatal care, well-child care (including periodic physical examinations and hearing and vision screening until age 23 years), Papanicolaou smears, and mammographic examinations. This legislation also proposes extensive programs for long-term and geriatric care and authorization for support of research of acquired immunodeficiency syndrome, hypertension, sickle cell anemia, infant mortality, and breast cancer.

Mediplan

This proposal mandates a broad health care program[18] by which all US residents would be enrolled and issued a Mediplan card entitling them to care. Subsequently, residents would be enrolled at birth. Children, pregnant women, and low-income groups particularly are identified to receive services. Benefits would include those provided currently by Medicare and special preventive health services for women and children (including well-child care and pregnancy-related services). Providers would be paid according to a resource-based relative value scale. Physicians would be required to accept a Mediplan rate and charge no additional fees. Mediplan includes a global obstetrical fee and a bonus for prenatal care. Children, pregnant women, and low-income groups would be exempt from the $500 annual deductible. Financing of Mediplan would be generated from income tax, employer contributions, and income-related employer premiums. Deductibles, copayments, and co-insurance would be limited to $2500 per year.

A National Health Program for the United States: A Physician's Proposal

Himmelstein et al[19] and Woolhandler and Himmelstein,[20] along with the Writing Committee of the Working Group on Program Design representing Physicians for a National Health Program, describe a comprehensive health plan by which everyone would be covered by one public plan and all alternative insurance coverage, copayments, and deductibles would be eliminated. All medical services, including those to treat acute problems and problems requiring long-term and rehabilitative care, would be covered. Prevention and public health programs would be covered, as would dental services and occupational therapy. A lump-sum budget would be negotiated annually with hospitals for patient services. Improvements, expansion, and major capital services would be funded by independent appropriations. Three options would be available: fee-for-service, salaried positions in institutions receiving global budgets, and per capita payments to group practices or health maintenance organizations. Fee schedules would be negotiated by a medical organization, and extra billing would be limited to uncovered services such as cosmetic surgery. All funding sources currently used would continue during a transitional period (including insurance premiums, Medicaid, Medicare, and employer contributions), but all would flow through a single payer, the national health plan. Private health insurance would be phased out over 3 years, and general tax revenues would be developed based on income or some other progressive tax.

COMMENT

Most would agree that our health care system needs urgent attention. There are obviously many options. The continuing flow of thoughtful commentaries on the problem in our medical journals[21-34] reflects the intense interest of health care professionals. Various polls have demonstrated that Americans favor a major overhaul of the health care system, but their dissatisfaction has apparently not reached a level sufficient to bring pressure on politicians, which is ultimately needed if change is to occur. In contrast, powerful elements in the health care industry exert major influence in determining changes or lack thereof. As Levey and Hill[21] put it: "The voices now raised to support national health care will not produce universal health insurance soon . . . . Americans lack a necessary level of discontent with our health care system, agreement on a widely endorsed program of universal health insurance, and the political stamina to drive legislation through Congress." However, perhaps enlightened leadership in the medical community can stimulate the necessary action in both lay and professional circles. Relman,[22] in a valuable discussion of the subject, reviews the options and concludes: "In my view, nothing short of a comprehensive plan which includes improved technology assessments and malpractice reform as well as other reforms of medical practice is likely to achieve the goals of universal access, cost containment and preservation of quality that everyone seems to want. . . . Now is the time for our profession to make common cause with government and with the major private payers in seeking solutions to a pressing social problem that is not going to solve itself."

If political and other realities limit us to patches, even if in the process of shopping for a new quilt, then we should get on with it. The most practical of these is modification of the Medicaid program: extended coverage for indigent children and pregnant women; increased benefits provided, with emphasis on preventive care; and payments to providers that are adequate to attract their services. These changes can be relatively simply made by federal and state governments. This is an urgently needed first step that can be taken while plans for broader coverage are being developed. Medicaid expansion in one or another form is part of several broader recommendations, including the legislation proposed by Stark,[8] the American Academy of Pediatrics,[9] and, at least temporarily, the Pepper Commission.[5,6] If we pursue patchwork remedies, these broader proposals should be evaluated as to overall benefit and political reality.

A modification of the Medicaid patch proposed by the state of Oregon would ration services based on net benefit. (This is in contrast to our present system of rationing care by limiting populations served.) This proposal has generated much and varied reaction.[13,23,24] Variations on this idea causing even more violent reactions have included Callahan's proposal[14] to ration new technology and a scheme to ration services based on age, restricting access to some benefits by the elderly. The Canadian system controls provision of some services by having the health plan approve implementation of new technology in clinical practice and by controlling capital expenditures by institutions. The chances of implementing any of these proposals seem slim.[24]

If we are to consider a new quilt, how should it be sewn? The Canadian system has been much discussed[25-28] and has many advantages: universal coverage under one plan; coverage of all reasonable benefits; one system of management that simplifies procedures for patients, physicians, and hospitals; free choice of physicians; emphasis on the role of the primary care practitioner; regulated application of new technology that encourages regionalization; controlled capital expenditures; fee-for-service physician reimbursement; and controlled hospital costs through development of an annual, realistically-negotiated budget. Studies comparing the Canadian and American health care systems[27,28] have emphasized reduced administrative costs in Canada, costs that contribute to premiums for patients and to overhead for physicians in the United States. The cost of health care in the United States is approximately 11% of the gross national product, while in Canada it is approximately 8%, despite the latter's broader coverage. The difference has been attributed largely to our higher administrative costs, higher payments to physicians, and hospital costs. Concerns about the Canadian system include its larger role of government and the potential of increased regulation, yet there is apparently more regulation of clinical practice in this country than in Canada. Evans et al[28] point out that "In the United States corporate competitors or employers may turn out to be more ruthless than public regulators." Another concern, not so regularly expressed, is the impact on physician's incomes. A comparison of fee costs in 1985[27] revealed the following ratios for some services.

Service	Fee Ratio, United States to Canada
Surgery	3.21:1
Anesthesiology	3.73:1
Radiology	3.50:1
Office visit	1.56:1
Hospital visit	4.77:1

A comparison of net physician incomes (US physicians vs Canadian physicians) produced a ratio of 1.35:1, and, according to one report, after adjustment for costs of resources (including liability insurance) the ratio became 1.30:1.[16] In 1984, the mean net income of physicians (before taxes) in Ontario was $160 000 per year for specialists and approximately $112 000 for general practitioners. Another report[27] lists net income for office-based physicians in Canada in 1985 as $73 607, compared with $112 109 in the United States. Interestingly, this report states that payments to physicians (before income taxes) represent 52% of the gross income in the United States and 66% in Canada.

The United States needs a health care system that will provide access to coverage by all citizens. It must provide services of broad scope and high quality, and it must do so with emphasis on measures for cost containment and preventive health. The evidence seems compelling that this can be done only by the institution of a new system. As Iglehart[25] puts it, "Muddling through, as we are now doing, is not a prescription for the ages, nor is it a policy that allows the United States to stand tall." Of the options, a variant of the Canadian system appears most attractive. The program described by Himmelstein et al[19,20] embraces many of the desirable features and would be a new, first-class quilt, but quilts imply bedfellows, and it is desirable, almost essential, that bedfellows be compatible. There are a number of large fellows in the bed, including the health insurance industry, hospitals, employers, government, politicians, and the public. The chances of compatibility under a new quilt seem remote, particularly when some bedfellows may get kicked out of bed. Nevertheless, it is imperative that we keep trying and that the medical profession lead the efforts to ultimately find a new quilt rather than to continue patching the old one.

References

1. Oberg CN. Medically uninsured children in the United States: a challenge to public policy. *Pediatrics.* 1990;85:824-832.
2. Wegman ME. Annual summary of vital statistics. *Pediatrics.* 1989;84:943-956.
3. Boyle JD. Health policy agenda for the American people. *JAMA.* 1987;257:1199-1210.
4. Tallon JR. A health policy agenda proposal for including the poor. *JAMA.* 1989;261:1044.
5. Basic Health for All Americans Act of 1987. S768.
6. Rockefeller JD. Access to Health Care and Long Term Care for all Americans: Preliminary Recommendations to the 101st Congress by the Pepper Commission. March 2, 1990.
7. Rockefeller JD. The Pepper Commission report on comprehensive health care. *N Engl J Med.* 1990;323:1005-1007.
8. Health Insurance for Children and Mothers Act of 1990. HR 4280.
9. Harvey B. Toward a national child health policy. *JAMA.* 1990;264:252-253.

10. Enthoven A, Kronick R. A consumer-choice health plan for the 1990s: universal health insurance IHA system designed to promote quality and economy. *N Engl J Med.* 1989;320:29-37, 94-101.

11. Sager A, Hiam P, Socolar D. *Promise and Performance: First Monitoring Report on 'An Act to Make Health Security Available to All Citizens of the Commonwealth and to Improve Hospital Financing.'* Boston, Mass: Boston University School of Public Health; 1989.

12. Beauchamp DE, Rouse RL. Universal New York health care: a single payer strategy linking cost control and universal access. *N Engl J Med.* 1990;323:640-644.

13. Relman AS. Is rationing inevitable? *N Engl J Med.* 1990;322:1809-1810.

14. Callahan D. Rationing medical progress: the way to affordable health care. *N Engl J Med.* 1990;322:1810-1813.

15. Levensky NG. Age as a criterion for rationing health care. *N Engl J Med.* 1990;322:1813-1815.

16. Iglehart JK. Canada's health care system. *N Engl J Med.* 1986;315:202-208, 778-784, 1623-1628.

17. The Comprehensive Health Care for All Americans Act of 1990. HR 4253.

18. Mediplan Act of 1990. HR 5300.

19. Himmelstein DU, Woolhandler S, The Writing Committee of the Working Group on Program Design. A national health program for the United States: a physician's proposal. *N Engl J Med.* 1989;320:102-108.

20. Woolhandler S, Himmelstein DU. A national health program: northern light at the end of the tunnel. *JAMA.* 1989;262:2136-2137.

21. Levey S, Hill J. National health insurance: the triumph of equivocation. *N Engl J Med.* 1989;321:1750-1753.

22. Relman AS. Universal health insurance: its time has come. *N Engl J Med.* 1989;320:117-118.

23. Russell LB. Some of the tough decisions required by a national health plan. *Science.* 1989;246:892-896.

24. Relman AS. The trouble with rationing. *N Engl J Med.* 1990;323:911-913.

25. Iglehart JK. The United States looks at Canadian Health Care. *N Engl J Med.* 1989;321:1767-1772.

26. Linton AL. The Canadian health care system: a Canadian physician's perspective. *N Engl J Med.* 1990;322:197-199.

27. Fuchs VR, Hahn JS. How does Canada do it?: a comparison of expenditures for physician's services in the United States and Canada. *N Engl J Med.* 1990;323:884-890.

28. Evans RG, Lomas J, Rarer ML, et al. Controlling health expenditures: the Canadian reality. *N Engl J Med.* 1989;320:571-577.

29. Ginzberg E. Health care reform: why so slow? *N Engl J Med.* 1990;322:1464-1465.

30. Schorr AL. Job turnover: a problem with employer-based health care. *N Engl J Med.* 1990;323:543-545.

31. Shortell SM, McNerney WJ. Criteria and guidelines for reforming the health care system. *N Engl J Med.* 1990;322:463-466.

32. Kinzer DM. Universal entitlement to health care: can we get there from here? *N Engl J Med.* 1990;322:467-470.

33. Relman AS. Reforming the health care system. *N Engl J Med.* 1990;323:991-992.

34. Newachek PW. Improving access to health care for children, youth and pregnant women. *Pediatrics.* 1990;86:626-635.

A Regional Pediatric Approach to the Epidemic of Social Ills Within Our Cities

Waldo E. Nelson, MD

'Twas midsummer 1990, I received a letter from Vince Fulginiti:

> In May 1991, each of the AMA family of journals will devote all or most of their issues to articles that report individual and professional societies' ideas and suggestions for improving health care to the poor and underserved in this country. *AJDC* will focus on infants, children, adolescents, and young adults . . . who are not receiving it [health care] currently, or who are poorly served by our present system. . . . This would be an excellent opportunity . . . for you to [record] your concept of the academic health center/community relationships . . . [for the health care of] the underserved and unserved . . . ."

Vince (my one-time student, now colleague, and from the beginning, my teacher) is correct in his implication that an overriding concern of mine is that the state of our national health care is not nearly as good as it could be. The most serious deficits are evident in the health care available for the poor and are, to a great extent, concentrated in our large metropolitan areas. The issue at hand for the medical community appears to be not only the search for ways to improve the quality of health care, but also for an adequate distribution of it and the means to pay for it. This is not a new concept. My own recognition of these inadequacies goes back to the mid 1920s.

No attempt will be made here to review the many aspects of this multifaceted subject. Rather, I venture to suggest an initiative for medical care of the underprivileged that may have some potential to be effective now, and even to provide some serendipitous dividends for the future.

I am convinced that more is likely to be gained at the local level within an area or region that functions as a natural medical service unit rather than by a limited national program. In recent years there have been several national programs designed to provide care for the socioeconomically deprived, especially within the inner cities. At best they were of limited value and were relatively expensive.

The medical unit in this concept is a regional area with complete primary, secondary, and tertiary medical services for its inhabitants. In general, they are not demarcated by state or other political boundaries, but have been determined by growth and developmental factors within and around urban centers and extend into the surrounding rural areas. Primary services are those available through physicians in private practice, in particular, pediatricians, internists, family practitioners, and pediatric nurse practitioners, and through their respective counterparts in the community and tertiary hospitals.[1]

The regional medical unit will contain a number of neighborhood hospitals (secondary), and at least one tertiary (usually associated with a medical school) hospital. In most large metropolitan areas there are usually two or more medical schools. Each hospital will naturally have its own coterie of practicing physicians who preferentially refer their patients who need specialized care. Hospitals that have attained particular competence in a certain highly specialized clinical field should expect preferential referrals to them from the primary physician whose principal affiliation is with another tertiary hospital and even from the clinical staffs of other academic hospitals. If such an objective policy were adhered to, it would represent a major step toward high-quality care in that regional medical unit.

For such a utopia to come into existence, not only goodwill but free and open communication among the physicians within that region will be required. Furthermore, it will necessitate elimination of competitive advertising by hospitals, health maintenance organizations, and individual physicians. To be sure, such activity is not only condoned by the federal government, it is even encouraged, and so far as I am aware, it is not objected to by AMA-related societies. It can only be destructive in some of its current forms. Information about services available in the various hospitals, health maintenance organizations, and other medical service units is essential for the primary physician and for the lay public, but inflammatory advertising that is unjustly self-serving should be abolished.

What I speak for is simply a realistic bonding between practicing physicians and those in academia in accepting responsibility for the quality of medical care within and "beyond their office walls," ie, within their respective region. I tend to designate those physicians who are primarily in private practice as "The Town" and those who are solely or mainly in academic activities as "The Gown."[2] It is the close integration of these physicians within a given region that is so essential in determining the ways and means to meet the medical needs of the underserved.

Those of us in the medical field should sense our personal responsibility not only for the quality of medical care in our respective roles, but also for the quality of health care within our community.[1] For example, activities centered more or less in the Philadelphia Pediatric Society,

Accepted for publication December 27, 1990.
From the Department of Pediatrics, Temple University School of Medicine at St Christopher's Hospital for Children, Philadelphia, Pa.
Reprint requests to CME office, St Christopher's Hospital for Children, Erie Ave at Front St, Philadelphia, PA 19134-1095 (Dr Nelson).

concerning the epidemic proportions of socioeconomic health problems among children and youth in our area, led to the formation of a task force under the leadership of William N. Mebane, MD, Director of the Family Practice Residency Program at the Chestnut Hill (Pa) Hospital. It was thought that this group could bring together those in the Gown sector (medical school hospitals) who were currently involved in pediatric activities in public schools and in shelters for the homeless with members of the Town sector who might be interested in sharing in this work. Both resident physicians and medical students are becoming involved in these activities.

Recently, the Philadelphia Pediatric Society circulated a questionnaire among its membership to identify additional Town and Gown physicians who might be interested in joining in this work. To date, there have been some 120 favorable replies. It will be of considerable interest to see what eventually evolves from these activities.

One of the recent encouraging outcomes has been the "spontaneous creation" by the resident physicians from one of the hospitals of a volunteer group of their own to provide medical services at an evening clinic in one of the shelters, an activity that does not interfere with their hospital program. I visited an evening clinic recently. It was a busy sight that included mothers, some fathers, infants and children, doctors, a nurse, and two social workers. It was truly a rewarding experience. Had one not known, one would not have surmised the variety of medical problems that were represented.

A necessary step will be the funding of this local effort. At the moment it is expected that the salaried members of the pediatric departments will continue receiving their current support, and it is hoped that, at least for the foreseeable future, the private physicians from the Town will "gain most," if they serve on a volunteer basis. In days past, when the Town was so essential in sharing in the clinical teaching load of pediatric departments, most of them served without pay. To this day, I have not found more loyal members of the two departments I was privileged to serve in my active days than those whose participation was on a volunteer basis. However, there will be a need for additional money. More can be expected from a number of sources—local governments, foundations, corporations, labor unions, and private individuals.

Separate from our considerations in support of a regional approach to the solution of community health problems is the necessity to devise a new national health insurance program that will include all persons on as nearly an equitable basis as possible. The time is past when we should expect anything less. It is estimated that 30 to 40 million of our children who are mainly in the lowest socioeconomic grouping are either uninsured or underinsured. To include them in a revised program will likely necessitate reduction in the payments to some of those in the older age group. There will be opposition, and the lobby for this group is not impotent. I am in this age group, and I am comfortable in saying that there are a number of us who could do with less in "third party payments" for care in our terminal years even if it is not the most pleasant of possibilities. The uninsured children must also be served. They have years of growth and development and of contribution to mankind ahead of them.

A national commission made up of competent, objective, and socially minded citizens should be formulated to develop such a program, and soon!

So, my concept of a common goal for those who are committed to the search for excellence in the provision of health care is simply that in each successive period, the medical care for each person, in health and in disease, will come to approximate the potentials of the moment; that such high-quality health care will be available to all those who want and can profit from it; that the lay person will recognize that he or she must come to appreciate "good care" and be responsible for cooperating with it and for maintaining a healthy pattern of living; and that the legal profession will share in attempts to develop a truly objective and ethical climate in the region.

Within our own time, what can be done by the medical profession and, especially, by the pediatric segment of it, to develop a workable plan to meet the above-mentioned goals?

1. Town and Gown will join together in determination to see "that their (invisible) walls shall come tumbling down," a true bonding.[2] Their constant priority will be to assume joint responsibility for the general health of the community in conjunction with their public health departments, including those of the school systems.

2. Town will have access to and make use of Gown's personnel and facilities, when indicated, in the treatment of their acutely ill patients as well as in the study and treatment of chronically ill ones, often on a continuing basis.

3. Gown will tap the Town segment for bolstering its teaching programs in inpatient and outpatient divisions. Some of our best teachers are among the Town personnel and some of our best clinicians among the Gown segment.[1]

4. Town and Gown will participate in efforts to devise a health insurance program available to all citizens, and everyone, including professionals and laity, will cooperate in efforts to make its operation fiscally sound.

Important as the medical aspects are, the social, educational, and economic deficits present as great or greater challenges in planning a total community program. These deficits are manifested by the lack of personal motivation among school-age children, the number of school dropouts, the failure to take advantage of work opportunities, teenage pregnancies, and other deviations that often result in anger against society, not only leading to lives of crime but to loss of potentially productive careers.

The issue at hand is patently a moral one that will not go away except by appropriate mass determination and action. It is my contention that the desired goal of giving each child the opportunities that could lead to readiness for responsible adulthood is most likely to be attained by local efforts within multiple communities.

Those of us in the health field constitute one channel of support. Within the confines of our communities, we can, in conjunction with other disciplines, the family, education, business, law and, not the least, the church, find ways to reactivate the spirit and determination to make this country truly a land of equality in freedom and in opportunity for the child to find a fulfilling role in society.

References

1. Nelson WE. Regionalization of pediatric activities: a challenge for Town and Gown. 30th Anniversary, The Ambulatory Pediatric Association - Its History and The Collection of the George Armstrong Lectureships (1960-1990).

2. Nelson WE. And the walls come tumbling down: a tribute to Lee Forrest Hill. *J Pediatr.* 1976;89:1-2.

Poverty and the Health of American Children

Implications for Academic Pediatrics

Richard B. Johnston, Jr, MD

The headline of a recent editorial in the *Philadelphia Inquirer* posed a loaded question: "How is it that we have such great hospitals—and such poor public health?" (August 22, 1989:14-A).

The reference point was Philadelphia in which "high-tech progress and abysmal public health performance . . . coexist too comfortably." Instead of just "cranking out specialists," the editorial said, "academic medicine ought to be taking stock of its broader mission—preventing sickness, making care more easily available and figuring ways to improve the state of public health." The present focus of medical schools has led to sophisticated methods of treatment but

> has left too much undone, too many unserved, in a nation with the resources and imagination to make life healthier, even for the poorest, most vulnerable of its people. . . . On matters of public health, academic medicine has been embarrassingly slow to show leadership. . . . Doctors have won heroic fights to save babies. But when it has come to shaping strategies to save generations, their record is skimpier. Medicine has been reactive, repairing the damage *after* it has been done.

The editorial was indeed provocative. The responses from the academic medicine and public health communities correctly emphasized the unfair implication that medical schools and their hospitals can be blamed for the serious health issues that affect the city. Little was said, however, in response to the editorial's basic question: What are medical school people doing to correct these health problems that affect so many humans so profoundly? The fact that the editorial's fundamental question also should have been addressed to our political leaders at a local and national level is frustrating. That so many of the city's (and the country's) people do not receive even basic medical care cannot reasonably be blamed on academic medical centers. In fact, these centers bear much of the burden of this society's failure in public health, because they spend a great deal of largely nonreimbursed time, emotion, and expertise dealing with its consequences. This underreimbursed effort, as important as it may be, makes it harder for academic medicine to accomplish its special mission of education and research.

Nevertheless, the validity of the challenge remains, and it is hard to escape the conclusion that we have a responsibility in academic pediatrics to respond somehow to these issues as they relate to children. Those children who have reduced access to preventive medical care suffer the most illness. Poor children have significantly higher rates of a variety of health-related problems, from infant mortality and traumatic death to prematurity (and consequently its related disabilities), failure to thrive, iron deficiency anemia, lead poisoning, perforated appendix, sick days out of school, and hearing loss.[1] The physical, intellectual, and emotional sequelae of these largely preventable conditions can only decrease the chances that these children will work their way out of poverty as adults.

If academic pediatrics has a responsibility to respond to this tragic situation, what should we do? What about staffing clinics in underserved areas? Editors of the American Medical Association and the American Bar Association journals have advocated giving 1 week per year for pro bono service, reminding us of an historic element of professionalism that may have faded in recent years.[2] Certainly, this sort of service can make a major difference in the lives of the children actually treated, and it can be rewarding for the physician. However, to suggest that academic personnel should necessarily contribute even more free medical care, with even further dilution of their academic efforts, seems, in the long run, unwise. Academic departments have special opportunities and faculty with special expertise. These offer the potential to go beyond the immediate problems toward more fundamental solutions with more lasting benefits.

Education is obviously the special province of the academic institution, but what should we teach? The problems are overwhelming, and we have little to offer in the way of solutions; perhaps this is what our students and residents should learn first. It is a widely held tenet of education that the student learns better when knowledge is gained by his or her own initiative and best of all when he or she is truly involved. Involvement in this case necessitates exposure to the societal failures that are related so closely to the poor health of many Americans. This means that students and residents must leave the medical school and hospital and go out into the community where they can see first-hand the consequences of weak education systems, insufficient job training, inadequate low-income housing, the high costs of medical care, and the downward, grinding spiral of poverty. Endorsement

Accepted for publication January 22, 1991.

From the Department of Pediatrics, University of Pennsylvania School of Medicine and The Children's Hospital of Philadelphia.

Reprint requests to the Department of Pediatrics, University of Pennsylvania School of Medicine, The Children's Hospital of Philadelphia, 34th Street and Civic Center Boulevard, Philadelphia, PA 19104 (Dr Johnston).

and collaboration of community leaders are prerequisites. The format might be health promotion and provision of medical care (with faculty) at housing projects, schools, shelters, and clinics within an underserved community, but these activities should be part of an educational program with defined educational goals.

For example, with guidance from pediatric faculty, residents and medical students in Philadelphia have taught health care in inner-city biology classes, conducted perinatal clinics in housing projects, made home visits to adolescent mothers, and assumed responsibility for pediatric care in shelters for homeless or battered women. Participating residents carry a beeper that allows them to offer 24-hour coverage. Teams comprising a resident and one or two medical or nursing students make shelter calls weekly and conduct health fairs at 4- to 6-week intervals to immunize, screen for disease, and educate mothers.

What have the students and residents learned from these experiences? Most respond first that they have gained a "gut feeling" for the broad needs of the mothers and children. The complexity of poverty and the plight of real people elicit frustration, anger, and sadness. A second lesson has been that health is not a survival issue for poor people. When food, clothes, and shelter cannot be assured, baby shots or even treatment for infection or anemia become minor concerns; poor compliance is understood differently. Third, these residents and students have learned the serious handicap imposed by the lack of a record system to track children who have no consistent source of care, no consistent financial aid, and sometimes no consistent parent or caregiver. Three additional lessons have probably been the most important: (1) Most residents report a new recognition of their own limitations in addressing the enormity of the need. (2) Most residents clearly realize that throwing even larger numbers of medical personnel at this problem in efforts like theirs will not make it go away. (3) Finally, often to their surprise, the residents identify a clear need for *research*—research on fundamental causes, on what really works, and even on whether their own efforts have made a lasting impact.

Projects like these, established for the purpose of service and education, may be very important to many individual children, but they do not represent a solution to the fundamental problems; however, they can function as an important means toward that end. Projects like these could serve to recruit the next generation of researchers, teachers, and policymakers, better prepared as a group than their predecessors to formulate meaningful and answerable research questions, to emphasize the importance of disease prevention, and to create public health policies that will work. At the very least, participants will be unlikely to underestimate the magnitude of the problem, and some will become informed and intelligent advocates for change.

How can academic pediatrics work most effectively to achieve fundamental, broad-based solutions? A major part of the answer must lie with research, obviously an essential function of the academic medical center. Basic biomedical research has made tremendous contributions to public health and also, incidentally, to reduced expenditures for the treatment of many diseases.[3] However, there has been too little research conducted regarding possible solutions to the health problems of the poor in America, and an estimated one fifth of our nation's children fall into that socioeconomic class.[4] The critical peer-review system that controls expenditure of public research funds should endorse with enthusiasm good scientific investigation into health promotion and disease prevention. What questions could be more substantial in pediatrics than those related to the reduction of problems such as adolescent pregnancy, premature delivery, adolescent suicide, and accidental deaths?

Research is needed regarding methods to provide care to poor children in our cities and remote rural areas. How can we be more accessible to these children? How can we finance systems to provide this care? How can we reduce medical expenditures in other areas and release funds to meet the need for basic care for poor children? How can we maintain a medical record that will be easily accessible to any pediatrician?

Research into outcomes is needed. Which programs work, and which programs are worth the money and effort? For example, can improved education and counseling reduce prematurity? The fundamental question is whether preventive medicine is cost-effective. Common sense and a quick review of hospital costs suggest that it is, and experience with programs for prenatal care, immunizations, and supplemental food for women, infants, and children (WIC program) support this view.[5,6] However, the content of medical school and residency curricula and the behavior of organized medicine, hospitals, government agencies, and insurance companies reflect little support for such a concept. In their defense, too little scientifically based research has been done in this area to prove that the principle of cost-effective prevention is broadly applicable.

Consider, for example, extracorporeal membrane oxygenation (ECMO) and the problem of nonreimbursed costs for long-term care in nurseries. It is hard to believe that ECMO, employed to save selected neonates, is more cost-effective (much less more humane) than adding equivalent nursing and support personnel to try to prevent unwanted adolescent pregnancy, to help carry pregnancies to term, or to make routine home nurse visits after delivery, which is the standard of care in Britain. Yet more and more hospitals are establishing ECMO programs but not programs to prevent prematurity in the communities they serve. Research is needed.

Research such as that which might compare cost-effectiveness and outcomes of ECMO and preventive care is extremely difficult to conduct, however. Few academic pediatricians have yet had sufficient knowledge, funding, or whatever it takes to try. Although foundations have provided some financial support for such research, too little public money has been available for this purpose compared with the human need, the critical importance of healthy children to the country's future, and the reasonable possibility that research might lead to a reduction in health care costs. The Medical Treatment Effectiveness Program, established in 1989 under the Agency for Health Care Policy and Research, US Public Health Service, may begin to correct this serious deficiency. This program supports research into fundamental issues of health services, such as which treatments actually work best and which are cost-effective. (Inquiries may be addressed to the Agency for Health Care Policy and Research, 18-12 Parklawn Bldg, Rockville, MD 20857.)

Although experimental proof of cost-effectiveness and clinical efficacy is necessary to effect fundamental, broad-based change, provision of the data will not guarantee implementation. Federal and state governments have only recently appropriated enough money to support approximately 60% of those eligible for the women, infants, and children (WIC) supplemental food program, fewer than one sixth of those eligible for Head Start, and about half those who need remedial education, and these programs have been proved to be effective.[7] Expenditures for defense, in the meantime, have far exceeded those for all children's programs combined. Not many pediatricians, either academic or practicing, have had the fortitude to take on the shameful, short-sighted governmental policies that ignore the critical needs of so many of our children. Fortunately, a few have done so, and our professional organizations have begun to guide us toward more effective participation in the area of public policy. Pediatricians are uniquely and eminently qualified to participate effectively by testifying or writing about and by lobbying for legislation related to children.[8] Considering the critical importance of directing public support toward children, serious efforts to accomplish this should be recognized as legitimate academic endeavor, worthy of endorsement by the departmental and medical school promotions committees.

The devastating effect of poverty on the health of so many American children has created opportunities that are as intellectually demanding, emotionally fulfilling, and immediately important as any available in academic pediatrics. The laboratory becomes the community of which the medical school is a part. Which faculty should participate? Not all of them, as the poor are not our only responsibility, but more is needed than we have offered so far, especially with regard to research. No group understands the needs of children better or cares more deeply than do pediatricians. The longer we wait for others to solve the problem, the longer the preventable suffering will continue, the greater the number of children who will sustain permanent injury, and the more profound will be the losses to their future and to ours. Academic pediatrics has a responsibility to use its special talents to address these problems. Those faculty who accept the challenge deserve our highest respect and support.

I thank Donald Schwartz, MD, Kenneth R. Ginsburg, MD, Robert E. Merrill, MD, and Waldo E. Nelson, MD, for inspiration and guidance and Charles L. Johnston and Margi Ide for critical review.

References

1. Wise PH, Meyers A. Poverty and child health. *Pediatr Clin North Am.* 1988;35:1169-1186.
2. Lundberg GD, Bodine L. Fifty hours for the poor. *JAMA.* 1989;262:3045.
3. Schroeder SA, Zones JS, Showstack JA. Academic medicine as a public trust. *JAMA.* 1989;262:803-812.
4. Bane MJ, Ellwood DT. One fifth of the nation's children: why are they poor? *Science.* 1989;245:1047-1053.
5. Dutton DB. Social class, health, and illness. In: Aiken LH, Mechanic D, eds. *Applications of Social Science to Clinical Medicine and Health Policy.* New Brunswick, NJ: Rutgers University Press; 1986:31-62.
6. Committee to Study the Prevention of Low Birthweight, Division of Health Promotion and Disease Prevention, Institute of Medicine. Preventing low birthweight: summary. Washington, DC: National Academy Press; 1985.
7. *Children 1990: A Report Card, Briefing Book, and Action Primer.* Washington, DC: Children's Defense Fund; 1990:11-12.
8. Berger LR. The pediatrician's role in child advocacy. *Adv Pediatr.* 1982;29:273-291.

Improving Health Care Provision to Neonates in the United States

Mildred T. Stahlman, MD

Any discussion concerning the possible approaches toward improving health care provision to neonates naturally encompasses the improvement of health care provision to their mothers, both before and after delivery. In a larger sense, it encompasses solving the deficiencies in health care provision to the entire population, as babies and their mothers are only two of the overlapping circles in this large Venn diagram.

Thirty-seven million Americans are without health insurance, and therefore frequently without access to necessary care. Simultaneously, we devote a larger portion of our gross domestic product to health care than any other industrialized country, yet we rank 15th in male life expectancy, seventh in female life expectancy, and 19th in infant mortality. There is a national realization, by politicians and the public alike, that health care costs are not only excessively high, but that health care resources are unwisely and inequitably distributed.[1]

A change in perception of the problem is necessary before a solution can be found. We must learn that health, both mental and physical, is a by-product of a national standard of living, which includes adequate housing and nutrition, a meaningful job with reasonable pay scale, a good (we hope excellent) public educational system, and a national economy that does not fluctuate extremely with changes in political leadership. Second, we must admit that despite our high national expenditure on health care, we are unwilling to pay, as a national priority, for equal access and basic care for all, including those who cannot pay.

In days of increasingly restricted federal and state budgets and skyrocketing medical costs, the inevitable questions arise about the direction we should choose (assuming we still have a choice): should we limit our expenditures for tertiary care medicine and opt for better-supported preventive medicine for the majority of patients, or should we continue to support, without regard to the cost-benefit ratio, each new and exciting technological advance, which may be lifesaving for the few who need it but extremely costly for the patient, third-party carriers, and society in general? Nobody wants to make these hard choices, but clearly the time is rapidly coming when someone must. If the medical profession does not choose to participate in this debate, health care planners and politicians will dictate their decisions to us.

Accepted for publication November 12, 1990.

From the Department of Pediatrics, Vanderbilt University School of Medicine, Nashville, Tenn.

Reprint requests to the Department of Pediatrics, Vanderbilt University School of Medicine, Nashville, TN 37232-2370 (Dr Stahlman).

I propose that both approaches are desirable, necessary, and, to some extent, affordable if we set our priorities straight. Preventive measures have long-term benefits, with no exciting publicity or dramatic breakthroughs, but, in the long run, they save more lives and prove to be more cost effective than crisis medicine. They require, in a country such as ours with such a wide diversity of health care provisions and patient acceptance, a hard sell from kindergarten onward. It is too late to try to change health patterns in high school, and well nigh impossible in adults with their fixed life-styles. This is especially true in the medically underserved since they are trapped in an environment in which changes in life-style to improve health may be totally unrealistic.

Easily learning new ideas is one of the characteristics of the very young, and the focus on good health patterns must begin then. Successful approaches elsewhere have been to assign each child to the equivalent of a public health nurse, who then knows each child's health problems sequentially and sees to it that parents take advantage of available facilities.

This begins with immunizations and well child care, not with the first major illness. Public television programs are used to promote preventive medicine, often called "social medicine," as the society takes responsibility for its organization and cost. If preventive medicine is begun early in life, a generation of essentially healthy young adults can grow up and, with good health care availability and accessibility ingrained in them, pregnant women can care for themselves and their fetuses from conception onward. This will not be an easy concept to sell, either to the Congress or to neonatal intensive care unit (NICU) physicians, but in the long run it will be seen as a necessity.

If we are to change health care provision to mothers and babies, we must first change their lives. We must educate them to consider health as a goal rather than to expect society to provide crisis care that might have been avoided. One of our major problems is the many medical and social consequences of teenage pregnancy. Unless we can reverse this social trend, high-risk pregnancies and very expensive, very-low-birth-weight infants will continue to consume an inordinate amount of our dwindling health care dollars.

How do we decrease the incidence of teenage pregnancies? First, we must admit the truth about the sexual mores of the young. Ever since the introduction of the birth control pill in the early 1960s and the sexual revolution that followed, sexual activity, much of it casual, has been increasing among our teenage population. Unfortunately, we have failed to encourage the use of responsible and effective contraception, and unwanted and high-risk pregnancies and infants have been the consequences of this failure.

Another social result has been the 1½ million abortions performed each year in this country. Until parents, schools, churches, and society in general become realistic about their children's sexual mores and either educate them to different social mores or provide them with the knowledge and means to prevent unwanted pregnancy, abortions, high-risk pregnancies, and low-birth-weight infants will continue to be the result. This lack of responsibility on the part of parents, schools, communities, politicians, and teenagers themselves presents appalling consequences to those whose responsibility it is to provide medical and social care for the tragic outcomes of these failures. We cannot change social mores overnight, but we must begin by telling it like it is. The specter of acquired immunodeficiency syndrome has begun to have an impact on so-called safe sex, but it is ironic that a social good—the prevention of teenage pregnancy—may be a consequence of fear of an international plague!

One of the most pressing current ethical questions in NICUs is that of resuscitating infants of borderline viability. Some would even put it in financial terms. It is an excellent example of expending a large amount of health care resources on a small number of infants who can questionably benefit from them. Should we continue to resuscitate infants born before 25 weeks' gestation and/or whose birth weight is below 500 g? There are those who would put the question at even more mature limits. In contrast to this are some societies in which health care is a priority and prenatal care is provided to all pregnant women early in gestation; in these countries (eg, Sweden), ultrasonography is routinely performed by 16 weeks' gestation and correct dating of almost all pregnancies can be done.

In this country, especially among teenagers, the medically underserved, and the poor, accurate estimation of gestational age is often impossible. Likewise, intrauterine estimates of birth weight are very likely to be overestimates. We then are faced with the terrible decision in the delivery room in cases of fetuses of borderline weight. These infants are almost always in need of some sort of resuscitation, and delay in doing so may affect outcome adversely in very important ways. The decision is frequently the responsibility of a young house officer serving time in a neonatal intensive care unit who may not be prepared by experience or ethical considerations to make such important decisions.

One of our best perinatal centers has taken the position of using constant positive airway pressure (CPAP) and oxygen in the delivery room if needed, and delaying assisted ventilation in most cases of borderline viability until the infant can be carefully assessed with regard to maturity and chances of survivability. If the decision is made to continue the most intensive care, nothing reasonable is withheld until the infant is clearly unsalvageable. If, however, the infant is judged too immature to survive after weighing and careful examination, including functional estimates of maturation, no additional intensive care procedures are carried out. This is a hard line to draw, but some guidelines need to be agreed on since the need to discontinue intensive care, once begun, can be a difficult dilemma to face. We know, based on anatomic and functional evidence, that there is a level of maturation necessary for successful extrauterine life, even when all current technologies are available. Perhaps now is the time for consensus on withholding extraordinary means of life support to the extremely immature but live-born fetus.

The development of regional high-risk perinatal and neonatal care networks during the 1970s was one of the most important concepts leading to improved health care provision to newborns and mothers. It was medically sound and fiscally responsible, as it served to provide the most highly skilled individuals with the most sophisticated (and expensive) technology for high-risk patient care. Most regional centers have had an important educational component, serving to raise the regional hospitals' level of expertise to be commensurate with their facilities and personnel. This system has proved to be cost effective and has been associated with a dramatic lowering of perinatal mortality and morbidity, the byproduct of which has been the survival of infants with lower and lower birth weights.

A new move, called deregionalization by some, has developed in recent years, brought about by an overabundant number of trainees flocking into an exciting new field, the realization by hospital administrators that newborn intensive care *can* be profitable for the hospital, and the willingness of third-party payers to pay both hospitals and physicians for high-risk care. Private hospitals have chosen to leave the network and rely on their own facilities and personnel for this highly visible service. The consequence, in many instances, is the skimming off of paying and insured patients, leaving the regional center, usually a university teaching hospital, to care for the uninsured, the poor, and the highest-risk and most costly patients, socially and medically. No reversal of this trend is foreseeable, and I believe that catastrophic health insurance and some method of limiting the enormous profits from high technology and high-risk care will be the ultimate solution.

When I worked briefly as a cardiologist, I said that I was interested in cardiac success, not cardiac failure. We must be more interested in successful pregnancy outcome than pregnancy failure. Our NICUs are filled with these failures and we tend to focus on them as the exciting problems. However, this excitement generates new ideas and new approaches to patient care, and neonatal/perinatal research has been responsible during the last 30 years for the dramatic changes in survival of the high-risk and very-low-birth-weight newborn. We should not abandon newborn intensive care, but should try to limit our use of technology in place of careful clinical medicine.

Above all, NICUs should be the breeding grounds for bright young investigators who will make the breakthroughs and solve the clinical problems, with basic research followed by carefully designed clinical trials. An interesting suggestion has been made that in times of severe fiscal restraints, such as now, a fixed percentage of the entitlement programs should be set aside for research, much as industry sets aside a fixed percentage of costs for research and development (R. B. Cotton, MD, oral communication, October 1990). Without continuous research, and without a continuous cadre of bright young investigators entering neonatology, we will find ourselves frozen in time with no innovations in patient care in the near future. The by-product of exciting new ideas makes much of the pain, frustration, and cost of intensive care worthwhile.

I am not a medical economist. I was not educated to be one, and the idea of matching the quality of patient care with dollars is abhorrent to me. However, it does not take a financial genius to see the enormous profits that the practice of medicine, the hospitalization of the sick, and the provision of technology and medication can provide to their respective areas of the health care provision system. It has been said that this is the "me" generation, and many physicians have joined those who rank patients' interests below those of first, themselves, the care providers; second, the hospital or academic institution; and finally, third parties (ie, insurance companies, the government, and employers). This attitude is unfortunately becoming increasingly prevalent in maternal and newborn high-risk care.

Third-party reimbursement engendered by procedures and action rather than by thoughtful and responsible inaction has become the norm. The insistence on shorter hours for medical personnel, less personal responsibility, and more consultations, as well as the reliance on technology, the pressures of hospital administrators to fill beds with paying patients, and the enormous markup on pharmaceutical and disposable products, all contribute to enormous patient charges, to less personal satisfaction on the part of care providers, and to more malpractice suits stemming from failures in communication. The result is now the real threat of rationing high-risk (high-cost) care and the development of a two-tiered system of health care provision.

One tier would provide basic, less costly care for the poor and uninsured, and a second tier would provide specialized, more costly care, including all the new technological advances, for the insured and those who can pay. The use of technology has been shown to be directly related to reimbursement for its use.[2] The only redeeming feature of such a two-tiered system besides the expense might be the reemergence of physicians in the first tier who rely on their own skills rather than those of others or on machines and tests. The downside, of course, would be the enormous inequity of accessibility to needed expertise and technology in complicated cases that are unreimbursable.

This two-tiered system is not the answer to the lack of universal health care insurance, and catastrophic health insurance is an imperative. Nowhere is this more apparent than in newborn intensive care. A realistic reassessment of physicians' fees and hospital reimbursement coupled with the need to accept patients on the basis of medical need might even start a trend toward lower charges!

Some corporate participants in the health care provision system, such as for-profit hospitals, pharmaceutical houses, and high-technology equipment manufacturers, and a small percentage of physicians have always been considered to be motivated, at least in part, by greed. Until recently, these were considered the few bad apples in the barrel to be identified and avoided. However, the public's perception has shifted and polls now show that physicians are no longer esteemed above other members of society. Many physicians are considered to not care about their patients' welfare, and medical negligence is the common complaint leading to malpractice litigation.

Communication has broken down between physician and patient, and we have lost our youthful idealism. We, as physicians, are seen as part of the problem of maldistribution of adequate health care, rather than as part of its solution. Darwin taught us that we must change or our species would disappear. Before it is too late, physician, heal thyself.

References

1. Priester R. *Overview on Distributing Limited Health Care Resources. Biomedical Ethics Reading Packet No. 5.* Minneapolis, Minn: Center for Biomedical Ethics, University of Minnesota Health Center; December 1988:1-13.

2. Evans RW. Health care technology and the inevitability of resource allocation and rationing decisions, part I. *JAMA.* 1983;249:2047-2053.

Child Abuse and Neglect: Critical First Steps in Response to a National Emergency

The Report of the US Advisory Board on Child Abuse and Neglect

Richard D. Krugman, MD

In June 1990, the US Advisory Board on Child Abuse and Neglect presented its first report to the Secretary of the Department of Health and Human Services and Congress. The board had studied the status of the child protection system (broadly defined as the *system,* not just the child protective services (CPS) agencies involved in the multidisciplinary recognition, intervention, treatment, and prevention of child abuse and neglect). The board was established under provisions of public law 100-294, and the 1988 Amendments to the Child Abuse Prevention and Treatment Act. The mission of the board is to evaluate the nation's efforts to accomplish the purposes of the Act and to make recommendations on ways in which those efforts can be improved.

The board concluded that child abuse and neglect in the United States now represents a national emergency. This conclusion is based on three findings: (1) each year, hundreds of thousands of children are being starved and abandoned, burned and severely beaten, raped and sodomized, berated and belittled; (2) the system created by the nation to respond to child abuse and neglect is failing; and (3) the United States spends billions of dollars on programs that deal with the results of the nation's failure to prevent and treat child abuse and neglect.

The board believes that the extent of the emergency is so compelling that it dictates an immediate response and has recommended 31 critical first steps that will provide a framework for a decade of review and reconstruction of policies and programs that have exacerbated the emergency. These 31 critical first steps, if implemented, will only control the emergency. Once it is brought under control, the board believes that the nation should commit itself to achieving an equally important goal: the replacement of the existing child protection system with a new, national, child-centered, neighborhood-based, child protection strategy. The Board's 31 recommendations (numbered in parentheses below) are organized into the following eight areas.

Accepted for publication January 23, 1991.

From the Department of Pediatrics University of Colorado School of Medicine, Denver, and the C. Henry Kempe National Center for the Prevention of Child Abuse and Neglect, Denver.

Reprint reprints to C. Henry Kempe National Center for the Prevention of Child Abuse and Neglect, 1205 Oneida St, Denver, CO 80220 (Dr Krugman).

RECOGNIZING THE NATIONAL EMERGENCY

Each citizen (recommendation 1), each elected official (recommendation 2), and each legislative body (recommendation 3) is called on to recognize the extent of the problem in our society and take personal responsibility to join with others to resolve this emergency.

PROVIDING LEADERSHIP

The president (recommendation 4), the governors of the several states (recommendation 5), the county executives, and mayors (recommendation 6) are called on to become visible and effective leaders within their jurisdiction in renewed child protection efforts. Legislative bodies at all levels are urged to support these efforts by providing funding for the initiatives developed. The rebuilding of our family-support infrastructure is as important as our willingness to rebuild our banking system (recommendation 7). Scientific societies and professional organizations are urged to respond to the emergency by making the issue a priority, stimulating research, and providing guidance to their members (recommendation 8).

COORDINATING EFFORTS

The secretary is called on to work with the governors of the states to eliminate barriers that stand in the way of providing coordinated community services related to the protection of children (recommendation 9), to work with the director of the Office of National Drug Control Policy in the White House to assure coordination of efforts to control substance abuse and child abuse (recommendation 10), and to coordinate with the attorney general to address the issue of fatal child abuse and neglect (recommendation 11).

GENERATING KNOWLEDGE

This area has four recommendations shaped by the board's conviction that good policy begins with good facts. The secretary is asked to establish a federal data collection system that reflects not only social service dimensions of the problem, but the public health, mental health, and legal/judicial dimensions as well (recommendation 12). The secretary is also asked to launch major coordinated initiatives to promote the systematic conduct of research related to abuse and neglect (recommendation 13), to coordinate knowledge about what does and does not work in the child protection system (recommendation 14), and to increase the number and professional qualifications of researchers in child abuse and neglect (recommendation 15).

DIFFUSING KNOWLEDGE

The secretary is asked to ensure that practitioners, policy makers, and the general public have ready and continuous access to information through the establishment of a permanent governmental unit (recommendation 16). The board also asks journalists, broadcast executives, publishers, as well as individual media outlets to join in a campaign to promote public understanding of the emergency and the most effective ways of addressing it (recommendation 17).

INCREASING HUMAN RESOURCES

These six recommendations are shaped by the board's conviction that the status, qualifications, training, workload, and representiveness of public agency CPS workers are intrinsic to the crisis in the child protection system. The secretary is asked to establish the position of public agency "CPS caseworker" as a professional specialty (recommendation 18), establish minimum educational requirements for the position of a public agency CPS worker (recommendation 19), and ensure that all public agency CPS workers receive adequate preservice and in-service education and training (recommendation 20). The board proposes that the secretary and Congress, with their counterparts at state and county levels, establish acceptable caseload standards for these workers (recommendation 21). State and local social service officials are asked to launch an aggressive campaign for recruitment of CPS workers representative of the racial, ethnic, and cultural composition of the caseload population (recommendation 22). The secretary is also asked to ensure a steady increase in the total number of the nation's professionals in medicine, social work, law, law enforcement, mental health, and education who possess the necessary competence and skill to participate effectively in the protection of children (recommendation 23).

PROVIDING AND IMPROVING PROGRAMS

The secretary is asked to ensure that more resources are allocated to establishing voluntary and nonpunitive access to help. It should become as easy for a person to pick up the telephone and receive help before abusing a child as it is now for a neighbor to report that person after the fact (recommendation 24). The secretary and governors are asked to ensure that efforts to prevent the maltreatment of children are substantially increased. At a minimum, this should involve significant expansion of the availability of home visitation and follow-up services for all families of newborns (recommendation 25). Congress and state and local legislatures are asked to ensure that resources devoted to prevention and to treatment do not come at the expense of each other (recommendation 26). Private sector organizations are encouraged to increase significantly the involvement of their local affiliates and outlet members or employees and child protection efforts (recommendation 27). Congress, the attorney-general, and chief justices are asked to ensure that all state and local courts resolve cases promptly and fairly (recommendation 28). The Secretary of Education and his counterparts at the state and local level are asked to launch a major initiative to establish and strengthen the role of every public and private school in the prevention, identification, and treatment of abuse and neglect (recommendation 29).

PLANNING FOR THE FUTURE

The final two recommendations are shaped by the board's intention to design and propose a new national strategy for the protection of children. The board proposes that Congress direct an appropriate research agency to determine the cost of developing and implementing a comprehensive national program for the prevention and treatment of child abuse and neglect, as well as the projected cost of not developing and implementing such a program (recommendation 30). Finally, the secretary, in concert with the National Governors Association, the US Conference of Mayors, and the National Association of Counties, is asked to develop a model planning process aimed at generating plans for the coordinated comprehensive community-based prevention, identification, and treatment of abuse and neglect with steps taken to ensure that the model process is implemented throughout the nation (recommendation 31).

In presenting these recommendations to the nation, the board has attempted to provide direction, vision, and leadership and expects that its recommendations will serve as the impetus for much needed action to address the national emergency. What does this mean for pediatricians, and why should we care?

Throughout the United States, many pediatricians are faced with a major dilemma; they are knowledgeable about statutes that require them to report all cases of suspected abuse and neglect and yet, in many communities, they observe that their reports are received but inadequately acted on. The child protection system in the United States is fragmented, under-funded, overworked, episodic, and unable to generate any information that would let us know that children are, in fact, being protected. Some physicians have deliberately followed a pattern of civil disobedience and do not report child abuse because of their belief that above all they should "do no harm." In my view, such an approach leaves physicians, and more importantly children, at serious risk. The answer is not to capitulate and abandon a child protection system that is in crisis. As the US Advisory Board suggests, it may be necessary to replace our existing system with one that works, but our efforts need to be focused on rebuilding the supportive infrastructure for families that has been lost in this country (ie, the prevention and treatment arms of the system) without abandoning our recognition and investigation arm. All over the United States, CPS agencies are refusing to open more and more cases so that they will have fewer and fewer with which to deal.

In Colorado, a bill is currently pending in the legislature that would raise the requirements necessary to "prove" a case of abuse from "credible evidence" to "the preponderance of the evidence." The bill will also remove the requirement that home visits be done on all reports, and finally will put in statute that CPS agencies need no longer be involved when children are abused outside the family. This is already happening in practice, but if it becomes the norm nationally to reset in statute those things that we *are* doing instead of those things that we *should* be doing, it is clear that we will continue to erode our ability to protect children. Such statutes are the single best milestones of the decline of a society's moral values.

If children are to be protected and death rates are to decline, we must do more about prevention. Throughout the country, efforts are being made to develop "family preservation programs." These programs, described over 20 years ago by Kempe and colleagues[1] have been rediscovered. They provide intensive 4- to 8-week treatment to families to help them out of crises, and have the advantage of leaving children in the home. They are clearly cost effective in that they reduce the need for foster care, but an 8-week fix for after-the-fact abuse is treatment, not prevention, and may be insufficient for long-term success.

It is time for pediatricians in this country to recognize that our long experiment in making the departments of social services in the country responsible for the protection of children has failed. It is not their fault. Beset by budget cuts, caught in a web of legal expectations that they could not possibly fulfill, public child welfare agencies, public health nursing, and mental health agencies simply cannot do what they should be doing. These three critical components of the supportive infrastructure that used to care for families have literally disappeared. The role of child welfare is now primarily income maintenance and investigation of abuse reports. Public health nursing is now primarily fee for service home health care nursing. The mental health system is completely clogged with the long-term, deinstitutionalized, severely mentally ill. It is no longer possible in this country for a family who needs help *before* they abuse their child to get that help by calling any of these three agencies. Further, the approach of these agencies is episodic: none has continuity of care as a principle. It is increasingly difficult in our competitive, prepaid health care environment to provide the continuity of care that these families desperately need, but it is my view that only the health system has the opportunity to save children from the failures of our child protection system.

There are several recommendations within the Advisory Board Report that would form the basis of what pediatricians can do. We need to recognize that this *is* an emergency! We can provide leadership through our professional societies to ensure that the problems of abuse and neglect will be dealt with as a priority during the coming decade (not *the* priority, but one of the priorities that we must pay attention to during this decade). We desperately need more physicians and child health professionals to work in both the clinical and research areas of abuse and neglect. We need to take responsibility for prevention. The work by Gray et al,[2] Olds et al,[3] Helfer,[4] and others has shown that we have the technology to be able to prevent the physical abuse of children. *Not* implementing what we know is tantamount to the withholding of poliovirus vaccine from children when an epidemic is poised to strike.

Pediatricians, through their contact with families, can make a difference. They can develop home visitation systems out of their offices, multispecialty groups, or hospitals that will provide support to new families in their community. Ultimately, if we make it as easy for a family to pick up the telephone and get help *before* they abuse their child as it is now for their neighbors to report them after the abuse has occurred, we will have taken a major step in preventing the abuse and neglect of our children. The Advisory Board's recommendations make it clear that this is no easy task. A future report will outline a new, coordinated, comprehensive, child-centered neighborhood-based child protection system. Pediatricians need to be part of that system so that we can avoid spending millions of dollars on the technology that allows babies born at 28 weeks' gestation to leave the hospital only to go home to an environment in which they are violently shaken or killed within weeks or months of their discharge, or stand by helplessly while millions more go to build prisons that will house the abused children of the 1970s and 1980s who are the failures of our present child protection system.

References

1. Kempe CH, Helfer RE, eds. *Helping the Battered Child and His Family*. Philadelphia, Pa: JB Lippincott; 1972.
2. Gray JD, Cutler CA, Dean JG, Kempe CH. Prediction and prevention of child abuse and neglect. *J Soc Issues*. 1984;35:127.
3. Olds D, Chamberlin R, Henderson C. The prevention of child abuse and neglect: a randomized trial of nurse home visitation. *Pediatrics*. 1986;78:65.
4. Helfer RE. A review of the literature on the prevention of child abuse and neglect. *Child Abuse Negl*. 1982;251:6

Correction

Transposed Wording.

In the article entitled "Lipoprotein Profiles in Hypercholesterolemic Children," published in the February 1991 issue of *AJDC* (1991;145:147-150), an error was made in the "Results" section. On page 148, in the sixth line of the first full paragraph in the left column, triglyceride levels should have read "lower than 1.3 mmol/L" and two lines below, triglyceride levels should have read "higher than 1.3 mmol/L."

Children in and of the Streets

Health, Social Policy, and the Homeless Young

James D. Wright, PhD

The nature of homelessness in the United States was transformed dramatically in the 1980s. Once dominated by older, largely white, broken-down, alcohol-abusive men, today's homeless population contains a sizable fraction of women and children.[1,2] Indeed, women, children, and youth now comprise perhaps three eighths of the total.[3] What are the effects of homelessness on the health and well-being of children? How do these effects compare with those of simply being poor? What are the likely long-term consequences of these effects on the ability of homeless children to mature normally and to achieve productive, independent adult lives? Scholars have been researching these and a range of related questions for the past 10 years, and the results are not encouraging.

That homelessness and extreme destitution exist at all in a society so affluent as ours is shocking. That increasing numbers of the homeless are women, children, and youth—groups that society has traditionally obliged itself to protect—further offends one's sensibilities. It is easy enough (too easy, perhaps) to be indifferent to the plight of Skid Row drunks, but indifference to the circumstances of homeless women and their children requires an unmistakable coldness of heart.

There are many good reasons for the pediatric community to be concerned about the health status of homeless children and youth. Poor physical health and especially chronic physical illness contribute to the cycle of poverty, whereby sick, homeless children of today become the unemployable, destitute, and homeless adults of tomorrow. Recurring health problems of even minimal severity disrupt school attendance and interfere with studying and homework activities. Chronically poor health or physical disabilities will interfere with, if not preclude, normal labor force participation and, with it, the ability to lead an independent adult existence. Thus, poor health is one mechanism by which homelessness reproduces itself in subsequent generations.

Every aspect of a homeless existence compromises physical health to some degree or at least complicates the provision of adequate health services; this is true of both children and adults. Life without shelter corrodes physical well-being in 1000 different ways, most of them too obvious to belabor here. Much that ails children requires little more than a day or two at home in bed—but what if you have neither home nor bed? Nothing is quite so therapeutic to an ailing child as the tender, loving care of a parent. But homelessness is a mean existence in which tenderness, love, and care are often in short supply. Further compounding the difficulties are an often inadequate diet, uncertain sleeping location, limited facilities for daily hygiene, exposure to the elements and to the social environment of the streets, extended periods on one's feet, an absence of support networks to draw on in times of illness, extreme poverty, and on through a long list.[4-8]

Among homeless children and youth in particular, there are additional complications. The shelters for women and children may well present optimal conditions for transmitting the infectious and communicable diseases of childhood.[9] A second problem is that immunization protocols are frequently found to be incomplete or nonexistent[10]; a third is the possibility of widespread physical and sexual abuse. Among homeless teens already out on their own, rates of pregnancy, sexually transmitted diseases, and alcohol and drug abuse and the associated health problems are all inordinately high.[11,12]

Many of the health and nutritional problems of homeless children and youth stem from the extreme poverty of their parents. (The notion that most, many, or even a sizable number of the homeless are "homeless by choice" has been thoroughly discredited by the research of the past decade.[13]) The evident role of poverty in creating homelessness also implies that the recent increases in the numbers of homeless women (and therefore homeless children) are a consequence of the so-called feminization of poverty about which much has recently been written.[14-16] In 1984, approximately two thirds of the nation's poor adults were women[14]; this proportion is increasing. As a consequence, the poverty rate among American children is about twice that of adults. Four of 10 poor people in the United States today are children.[17]

Poverty is a well-known "risk factor" for poor health among children and certainly contributes to the poor health of homeless children. Poverty is strongly correlated with infant mortality in every study that has inquired into the matter, and is also associated with a range of morbidities as well. Homeless children, being poor, must suffer the health consequences of their poverty as well as those resulting from their unsettled living conditions.

Although the effects of poverty on infant mortality are

Accepted for publication December 5, 1990.

From the Department of Sociology, Tulane University, New Orleans, La.

Reprint requests to Department of Sociology, Tulane University, New Orleans, LA 70118 (Dr Wright).

well documented, no study has yet examined the rate of infant mortality among the homeless poor. Among homeless adults, mortality is exceptionally high[8,18]; indeed, the average age at death for various samples of the homeless is reported to be in the range of 50 to 55 years. It is, therefore, a safe bet that homeless infants also die prematurely at a rate substantially higher than average, although, as indicated, this point has yet to be researched.

One mechanism that links poverty to poor health is inadequate nutrition—a problem for poor children in general and the homeless poor in particular. Specific studies of dietary intake or nutritional deficiency disorders among homeless persons, whether child or adult, are relatively rare. Winick[19] has noted that the menu used by the city of New York in its shelters for homeless persons supplies at least one third of the daily requirements for all known nutrients, and is to that extent "sufficient." These diets, however, are typically high in cholesterol, fat, sugar, salt, and starch, so while they may well offer adequate caloric intake, they are far short of optimal. As for the nutrition of those homeless who do not avail themselves of shelters and soup kitchens and who eat mainly what they can scavenge from street sources, nothing further need be said.

A few studies have inquired into the prevalence of nutritional deficiency disorders among homeless children; as would be expected, the rates are high. I[11] reported that 2.2% of homeless children who received care during the first year of the National Health Care for the Homeless program were diagnosed as anemic; this is twice the rate for "normal" children seen in ambulatory pediatric clinics nationwide.[20] An additional 1.6% of the homeless children had nutritional deficiency disorders other than anemia (most of them vitamin deficiency disorders); among children in general, such deficiencies are practically nonexistent (Wright,[11] Table 1). About 2% of the homeless children studied by Miller and Lin[20] were diagnosed as having "growth problems," possibly secondary to dietary insufficiencies, similar to the results reported by Alperstein et al.[10]

General morbidity among homeless children appears to be much more widespread than among children in general or among poor children in particular. Miller and Lin[20] studied 158 homeless children in Seattle, Wash, and reported that "although the majority of the children were considered to be in good or excellent health, the proportion whose health was described as 'fair' or 'poor' was four times higher than in the general US pediatric population."[20(pp671-672)] This study also found a high prevalence of abnormal anthropometry and immunization delays within this population. Homeless children appear to overutilize emergency department services, underutilize preventive health services, and have far fewer dental visits than the general pediatric population. Similar results for homeless children in Boston have been reported by Bassuk et al,[21] and for homeless children in New York by Alperstein et al.[10]

I[11] compared the health problems of homeless children seen in the National Health Care for the Homeless program with those of children included in the National Ambulatory Medical Care Survey. Nearly all disorders are more common among the homeless group. About 7% of the homeless children were found to have scabies and lice infestations, for example, compared with 0.2% of the National Ambulatory Medical Care Survey children; upper respiratory infections were about twice as common, skin disorders four times as common, poor dentition 10 times as common, etc. Homeless children were also more likely than normal children to suffer from chronic physical disorders. Similar patterns were observed among homeless teenagers as well.[12]

Mental health problems of homeless children have been studied in depth by Bassuk et al[21] and Bassuk and Rubin.[22] Depression, developmental delays of varying severity, anxiety, and learning difficulties are reported to be distressingly common. Psychiatric morbidity is also widespread among homeless adults.[23,24]

The general configuration of illness among homeless children is similar to that of children in general. That is to say, the health problems faced by homeless children are not exotic or unusual; they are, rather, the same health problems that all children face. In all studies, by far the most common disorders observed among homeless children are minor upper respiratory infections, followed by minor skin ailments, ear disorders (mostly otitis media), then gastrointestinal problems, trauma, eye disorders, and lice infestations. In most cases, differences in the rates of disorder between homeless boys and girls are reported to be minor.

Differences between homeless children and children in general, in contrast, are often large and in some cases dramatically large. Although the general pattern of illness among homeless children is not atypical of children's illnesses in general, the comparative rates of occurrence are often inordinately elevated.

Children, clearly, are not immune to the deleterious effects of homelessness on physical health. That many of these children are over age 5 years and therefore required to attend school, where their illnesses can then circulate to other children, is an additional point of concern.

It is important to stress here that the best available studies of the effects of poverty on child health report relatively slight differences in the *prevalence* of most disorders between poor and nonpoor children, whether chronic or acute.[25,26] The larger differences are found in the ensuing *consequences* of disease. Differentials on the order of those reported in the studies of homelessness and child health are not to be found anywhere in the published literature on poverty and child health. The evidently disproportionate rate of illness observed among homeless children, in short, is not just a consequence of their impoverished circumstances. Homelessness is an independent and quite consequential risk factor in its own right.

The life chances of homeless children are obviously not bright to begin with. They are saddled first with the burdens of poverty and then with the unique burdens of not having a safe, stable place to live. The effects of homelessness on school performance and intellectual development are now well-known,[22] as are the effects on various physical disorders, both acute and chronic. Among the many good reasons to "do something" about homelessness is that homelessness makes people ill.

These days, the people being made ill by homelessness are increasingly children and youth, who comprise a tenth or more of the total homeless population. To be a poor child is one thing, but to be poor *and* homeless is a thing apart. It is hard to imagine a social environment less conducive to health or normal maturation and development.

Pediatricians at the New York City Children's Health Project have identified what they call the "homeless child syndrome," which comprises "poverty related health problems, immunization delays, untreated or undertreated acute and chronic illnesses, unrecognized disorders, school, behavioral, and psychological problems, child abuse and neglect."[27] It is not true that all homeless children exhibit all aspects of this syndrome. However, most homeless children do exhibit one or more of these problems and disorders; at the very least, they are more commonly observed among homeless children than among children in general or even those at the poverty level.

Knowing how and to what extent homelessness affects the health of children does not in itself tell us what needs to be done. Most of what has been done to date is along the lines of amelioration. There is an evident need to continue such programs: aggressive screening of homeless children for health disorders and proper treatment and health care once problems have been identified. But here, as in many other areas of public health, the only long-term solutions are to be found in prevention. We will avoid the negative consequences of homelessness on the health of children only when we find a way to prevent children from being homeless in the first place.

Sad to say, this obvious truth is much easier to state than to act on. Homelessness is a complex problem rooted in recent trends in the political economy of the nation.[13] A rising poverty rate coupled with a serious and ongoing decline in available low-income housing has served to price an increasingly large segment of the urban poverty population out of the private housing market.[28] Inflation has reduced the purchasing power of Aid to Families with Dependent Children and other welfare programs to the point where the welfare-dependent can no longer maintain stable residences with their monthly payments.[2] In the absence of other sources of support, mothers with children dependent on Aid to Families with Dependent Children find themselves virtually consigned to homelessness in all but the most generous states, unless they are also among those fortunate enough to receive a federal Section Eight housing voucher.

An aggressive, broad-scale federal assault on homelessness in all its various manifestations would easily add several tens of billions of dollars to the annual federal expenditure on housing, health, and human services.[29] No one who has followed the Washington, DC, scene closely for the past few years would consider this the least bit likely anytime in the coming decade. The prospects for community-based local programs are scarcely brighter, since most of the cities and states face budget problems every bit as serious as the federal problem. That would seem to leave the private sector as the most promising source for new programs, but the limit may well have been reached here as well. In fact, approximately three quarters of the total national expenditure for assistance to the homeless already comes from the private sector, principally the churches, and one is entitled to wonder just how much wattage can be cranked from the "thousand points of light." Thus, for the foreseeable future, we will have to content ourselves with programs of amelioration such as those embodied in the Stewart B. McKinney Homeless Assistance Act, knowing full well that such measures do not and cannot provide any final solutions to this problem.

The large number of children now being seen on the streets and in the shelters and other facilities providing services to homeless people means that the homelessness of the 21st century is already being created today. As this is being written, the lives and futures of many tens of thousands of children around the nation are being destroyed by forces over which they have no control. The Children's Defense Fund estimates that "more children die each year from poverty-related causes than traffic fatalities and suicides combined,"[30] and while this is probably an exaggeration, it is nonetheless an exaggeration that makes a point. It is useful, if troubling, to ask, What does the very existence of homeless children say about us as a nation? What image does this present to the world?

In February 1987, I appeared at hearings before the House Select Committee on Children, Youth, and Families to testify to the effects of homelessness on the physical health of children. Among the several witnesses present at the hearings was a lovely 12-year-old Hispanic girl living with her mother and three siblings at one of the large welfare hotels in midtown Manhattan. In the course of her testimony, this young woman remarked, "If I could have anything that I could want, I wish that we could have our own apartment in a nice clean building and a place that I could go outside to play in that is safe. I want that most of all for me and my family." A clean place to live and a safe place to play do not seem like too much to ask. These are not the rapacious demands of some welfare-dependent drug addict, but the plaintive wishes of a young child to have those things that normal children have. As the hearings closed, the thought occurred to me, What kind of world is this, where such simple things can only be a dream to some children? As a kind and generous nation, are we truly prepared to let this continue?

This report has been adapted from a previously published study by Dr Wright.[31]

References

1. Lam J. *Homeless Women in America: Their Social and Health Characteristics*. Amherst, Mass: University of Massachusetts; 1987. Thesis.
2. Rossi PH. *Without Shelter: Homelessness in the 1990s*. New York, NY: Priority Press; 1989.
3. Wright JD. The worthy and unworthy homeless. *Society*. 1988;25:64-69.
4. Brickner PW, Scharer LK, Conanan B, Elvy A, Savarese M, eds. *Health Care of Homeless People*. New York, NY: Springer-Verlag NY Inc; 1985.
5. Brickner PW, Scharer LK, Conanan BA, Savarese M, Scanlan BC, eds. *Under the Safety Net: The Health and Social Welfare of the Homeless in the United States*. New York, NY: WW Norton; 1990.
6. Institute of Medicine. *Homelessness, Health and Human Needs*. Washington, DC: National Academy Press; 1988.
7. Wright JD, Brickner PW. The health status of the homeless: diverse people, diverse problems, diverse needs. Presented at the annual meeting of the American Public Health Association; November 15, 1985; Washington, DC.
8. Wright JD, Weber E. *Homelessness and Health*. New York, NY: McGraw-Hill International Book Co; 1987.
9. Gross TP, Rosenberg ML. Shelters for battered women and their children: an under-recognized source of communicable disease transmission. *Am J Public Health*. 1987;77:1198-1201.
10. Alperstein G, Rappaport C, Flanigan J. Health problems of homeless children in New York City. *Am J Public Health*. 1988;78:1232-1233.
11. Wright JD. Homelessness is not healthy for children and other living things. *Child and Youth Services*. 1990;14:65-88.
12. Yates G, MacKenzie R, Pennbridge J, Cohen E. A risk profile comparison of runaway and non-runaway youth. *Am J Public Health*. 1988;78:820-821.
13. Wright JD. *Address Unknown: Homelessness in Contemporary America*. Hawthorne, NY: Aldine de Gruyter; 1989.
14. Sidel R. *Women and Children Last: The Plight of Poor Women in Affluent America*. New York, NY: Viking Penguin; 1986.
15. Ehrenreich B, Piven F. The feminization of poverty. *Dissent*. 1984;31:162-170.
16. Duncan G. *Years of Poverty, Years of Plenty*. Ann Arbor, Mich: Institute for Social Research Press; 1984.
17. US Department of Commerce. *Money Income and Poverty Status in the United States*. Washington, DC: Bureau of the Census, Current Population Reports; 1987. Consumer Income Series P-60, Number 161.
18. Alstrom CH, Lindelius R, Salum I. Mortality among home-

less men. *Br J Addict.* 1975;70:245-252.
19. Winick M. Nutritional and vitamin deficiency states. In: Brickner PW, Scharer LK, Conanan BA, Savarese M, Scanlan BC, eds. *Health Care of Homeless People.* New York, NY: Springer-Verlag NY Inc; 1985;8:103-108.
20. Miller D, Lin E. Children in sheltered homeless families: reported health status and use of health services. *Pediatrics.* 1988;81:668-673.
21. Bassuk E, Rubin L, Lauriat A. Characteristics of sheltered homeless families. *Am J Public Health.* 1986;76:1097-1101.
22. Bassuk E, Rubin L. Homeless children: a neglected population. *Am J Orthopsychiatry.* 1987;57:279-286.
23. Bassuk E. The homeless problem. *Sci Am.* 1984;251:40-45.
24. Wright JD. The mentally ill homeless: what is myth and what is fact? *Soc Problems.* 1988;35:182-191.
25. Egbuono L, Starfield B. Child health and social status. *Pediatrics.* 1982;69:550-557.
26. Newacheck P, Starfield B. Morbidity and use of ambulatory care services among poor and nonpoor children. *Am J Public Health.* 1988;78:927-933.
27. Today's Child. 1988. "The homeless child syndrome." *Today's Child.* 1988;2:4.
28. Rubin B, Wright JD, Devine JA. Unhousing the urban poor: the Reagan legacy. *J Sociol Soc Welfare.* In press.
29. Wright JD. Science, passion and polemics. *Society.* 1989;26:21-23.
30. Oberg C. Pediatrics and poverty. *Pediatrics.* 1987;79:567-568.
31. Wright JD. Poverty, homelessness, health, nutrition, and children. In: Kryder-Coe J, Salamon L, Molnar J, eds. *Homeless Children and Youth: A New American Dilemma.* New Brunswick, NJ: Trans-action Books; 1990.

A Survey of the Health of Homeless Children in Philadelphia Shelters

Ruth M. Parker, MD; Leslie A. Rescorla, PhD; Jonathan A. Finkelstein, MD; Nathaniel Barnes, MD; John H. Holmes, MS; Paul D. Stolley, MD, MPH

• We conducted a random-sample survey of homeless children and their mothers residing in Philadelphia (Pa) shelters. One hundred forty-six families were included in the final sample, resulting in an 80% response rate. The aims of the survey were to characterize the child's current and past health status, to determine access to and use of medical services, and to determine the serum erythrocyte protoporphyrin levels and tuberculin skin test status of the children. In addition, psychological tests were administered to both child and parent to assess developmental level and psychological problems. Finally, detailed questions were asked concerning the reasons for the homeless condition. The important reasons for homelessness cited in the survey included physical abuse, substance abuse, disagreements with landlords, and poor living conditions. The children's health problems included a high incidence of reported accidents and injuries, burns, and lead toxicity; the parents suffered from depression, physical abuse, and substance abuse. School-aged children tended to have low scores on tests of expressive vocabulary and word decoding, and preschoolers seemed to be below age expectations in receptive vocabulary and visual motor skills. The findings of this study suggest that homeless children tend to score poorly on developmental and psychological tests and tend to sustain serious burns and accidents. Policy implications of the survey include suggestions for health screening, rehabilitation, and education.

(*AJDC*. 1991;145:520-526)

Several studies have described the health problems of homeless persons. The health of homeless families and their children is less well defined, but a few studies examining the health status of homeless children are available. Bassuck et al[1] studied 80 families and their 151 children living in 14 Massachusetts shelters in 1985 and reported that about half of the children had developmental lags as assessed by the *Denver Developmental Screening Test*. They also reported a high frequency of learning disabilities, depression, and anxiety. Alperstein et al[2] reviewed clinic records of 256 homeless children younger than age 5 years who attended a primary care clinic in New York, NY. Higher rates of hospitalization, higher serum lead levels, delayed immunization, and increased reports of child abuse were found compared with a population of children of the same age and socioeconomic status who lived at home but attended the same clinic.

A 1986 probability sample of homeless families in King County, Washington, described 82 families with 158 children younger than age 17 years. Thirteen percent of these parents reported their children's health as "fair" or "poor." Compared with the general US population, this sample of homeless persons had a higher rate of emergency department use, and a higher proportion had no health insurance (35% vs 12.5% for the general US population). The population studied was 27% white, 44% black, 8% Hispanic, 6% native American, and 15% mixed. Approximately one third of the children were obese, scoring above the 95th percentile in weight for height measurements.[3]

Comparing 98 children younger than age 12 years residing in New York City welfare hotels with 253 domiciled poor children, Acker et al[4] found an increased rate of iron deficiency among the homeless children.

The *Health Care for the Homeless Project*[5] listed the most common reasons homeless children were brought by their parents to see health care workers: respiratory infection, minor skin problems, ear problems, gastrointestinal complaints, trauma, eye problems, and lice infestations.

PHILADELPHIA SHELTER SYSTEM FOR HOMELESS FAMILIES

Estimates of the composition of the homeless population in Philadelphia were derived from a project directed by the Philadelphia Health Management Corporation, and the 1985 estimates portray a total homeless population in Philadelphia of 10 000 to 13 000 people.[6] At the time of the study, an estimated 2500 to 5000 homeless children lived in Philadelphia, a majority of whom were thought to be younger than age 5 years.

The city shelter network included the one city-owned facility and 22 other privately owned shelters under contract with the city. On presentation to the city authorities, an appropriate space was usually located and the family

Accepted for publication January 30, 1991.

From the Department of Medicine, Emory University School of Medicine, Atlanta, Ga (Dr Parker); the Department of Human Development, Bryn Mawr (Pa) College (Dr Rescorla); the Department of Pediatrics, Children's Hospital, Boston, Mass (Dr Finkelstein); the Department of Urology, Duke University Medical Center, Durham, NC (Dr Barnes); and the Clinical Epidemiology Unit, Section of General Internal Medicine, Department of Medicine, University of Pennsylvania School of Medicine, Philadelphia (Mr Holmes and Dr Stolley).

Reprint requests to Emory University School of Medicine, Department of Medicine, 69 Butler St SE, Atlanta, GA 30345 (Dr Parker).

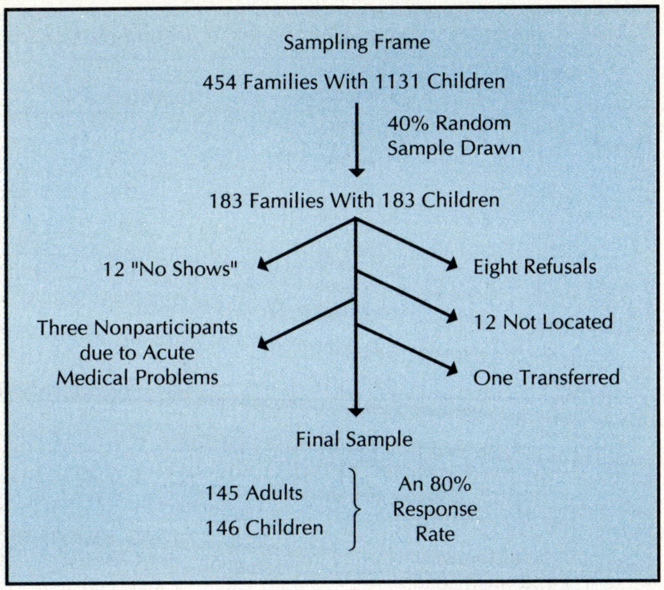

Diagrammatic representation of sample and final response rate.

was placed within a few hours; however, if an appropriate unit could not be found, the family was housed in a large gymnasiumlike room at the city-owned facility, which accommodated as many as 75 families.

All of the 22 shelter buildings in our sample were structures converted from former uses, ie, a car dealership, a retirement home, an orphanage, a funeral home, and a school. The capacity of the shelters and the actual living arrangements for families varied greatly, with from one to six families housed in one room. Few cribs were available and only one shelter had an isolation room for persons with communicable diseases. All of the shelters housed single women with dependent children, and four of the shelters also housed single women without children. One shelter housed a large proportion of troubled girls placed there for supervision and guardianship.

Most shelters referred their clients to local neighborhood clinics or hospitals for medical assistance. One shelter had a nurse and an infirmary, and another shelter employed the services of a visiting nurse practitioner organization. All shelters had paid staff, including nighttime staff. Three privately owned shelters were managed by formerly homeless women who resided there.

AIMS AND OBJECTIVES

When we planned our study in September 1987, there was little published information concerning the health status of homeless families, and much of what was available had not been obtained using random sampling methods. We therefore designed a survey of homeless families residing in shelters in Philadelphia to obtain descriptive information that would be helpful in health planning and in identifying specific problems and unmet health needs. In surveying randomly selected homeless families in Philadelphia shelters to describe their health status and other characteristics, we targeted seven main areas: (1) the child's health, including general health perceptions, medical history, and recent illnesses; (2) access to health services for children; (3) social, economic, and demographic features of the family, such as family structure, income, work history, and school performance; (4) parental health history, which focused on drug and alcohol use, chronic illnesses, and childbearing history; (5) visual screening of the children; (6) laboratory investigation of the children using a tine test for tuberculosis and determination of erythrocyte protoporphyrin (EP) levels; and (7) developmental and psychological screening of the children using tests appropriate to their ages. By obtaining such information we hoped to better understand how resources can be best allocated to the homeless population.

SUBJECTS AND METHODS

Defining the Population and the Sampling Method

After receiving permission from the Philadelphia government to conduct the study, we obtained information regarding the number, type, and location of all shelters with which the city contracts. We excluded homeless families residing at noncontracting shelters since there was no available list of all such facilities and they housed only a small proportion of the city's homeless families. We contacted each of the 21 privately owned shelters and the one city-owned facility to request their participation in our study and to ascertain their current occupancy. Two shelters, each housing about 20 families, refused to participate; seven shelters had only one to eight families present and were excluded from our sampling frame due to their small size. Because homeless families were randomly assigned to shelters regardless of shelter size, the exclusion of these nonparticipating shelters was unlikely to have biased our sample. The remaining 13 shelters agreed to participate. We conducted on-site visits to interview shelter directors and conduct the survey.

Our research team spent prearranged days at each shelter conducting the survey. Each shelter maintained a roster of resident families. Using a table of random numbers, we selected from 28% to 49% of the families present at each shelter for study. The family was contacted at least twice to set up an appointment. Next, we randomly selected one child, aged 12 years or younger, from each family and invited this child to participate in the study. There were 454 families, with 1131 children, in the 13 shelters during our census. One hundred eighty-three families, with one randomly selected child per family, were selected for study. One hundred forty-six families enrolled in the study. There were 37 nonrespondents, including eight who refused to participate, 12 who did not show up for interviews, 12 who could not be located to request participation on at least two attempts, three who could not participate due to acute medical problems (ie, premature labor for one woman and bleeding during pregnancy for two women), one who was transferred to another shelter before her scheduled appointment, and one who was inebriated on the two occasions we arranged for the interview. The mother's responses in this latter case were not included in our analysis, but those of her child were included.

The study included information on 145 families and 146 children (Figure). Psychometric data were requested only for the 98 children aged 2 years and older. Following completion of this study of homeless children, we were able to collect psychometric data on a small sample of inner-city–domiciled children in Philadelphia. These comparative data are reported elsewhere.[7]

Parents signed informed consent forms, and an oral interview was conducted lasting 45 minutes. The survey questionnaire targeted four main areas: (1) demographic and socioeconomic characteristics, including family structure, a calendar of homelessness (a chronological list of all places the family resided in the previous 5 years), and use of social services; (2) access to medical care; (3) the child's health history, including perceptions of general health, functional status, chronic medical conditions, hospitalizations, immunization status, and school performance; and (4) parental health history, including chronic and recent acute illnesses, history of smoking, and alcohol and drug use.

Adult subjects completed the Peabody Picture Vocabulary Test-Revised (PPVT-R), Beck Depression Inventory (BDI), and an age-appropriate Achenbach Child Behavior Checklist (CBCL). Simultaneously, the children completed a battery of age-appropriate psychological and developmental tests, listed and described below.

Tests Administered

Wechsler Intelligence Scale for Children-Revised (WISC-R) Vocabulary.—The best predictor of WISC-R IQ, this subtest involves asking the child to give definitions for a list of vocabulary

Table 1.—Highest Level of Education Achieved by Homeless Mothers (N=145)	
Education Level	No. (%) of Mothers
<12 years of school	72 (50)
<12 years and vocational school	2 (1)
High school equivalence degree	5 (3)
High school graduate	38 (26)
High school graduate and vocational school	18 (12)
Some college	10 (7)
College graduate	0

Table 2.—Parity of Homeless Mothers (N=145)		
No. of Children	No. (%) of Mothers	Cumulative %
1	22 (15)	15
2	35 (24)	39
3	44 (30)	69
4	20 (14)	83
5	9 (6)	89
6	8 (6)	95
7	2 (1)	96
8	3 (2)	98
9	2 (1)	99

Table 3.—Maternal Age at Delivery of First Child (N=145)		
Maternal Age, y	No. (%) of Mothers	Cumulative %
13	1 (1)	1
14	6 (4)	5
15	13 (9)	14
16	21 (14)	28
17	20 (14)	42
18	25 (17)	59
19	14 (10)	69
20	14 (10)	79
≥21	31 (21)	100

Table 4.—Incidence of Illness Among Homeless Children During Previous 4 Weeks (N=145)	
Type of Illness	No. (%) of Children
Gastrointestinal	54 (37)
Cough with fever	35 (24)
Ear infection	29 (20)
Conjunctivitis	25 (17)
Other	2 (1)

words. The test was given to children aged 6 to 12 years to measure verbal ability.

WISC-R Block Design.—The child assembles geometric blocks to duplicate a model under a time limit. Block Design is the subtest correlating most highly with WISC-R Performance Scale IQ, and was given to children aged 6 to 12 years.

Wide Range Achievement Test–Revised (WRAT-R) Reading.—On this subtest, the children aged 6 to 12 years were asked to read a list of words. Children who could not read were asked to match and identify letters of the alphabet.

House-Tree-Person (HTP).—The child is asked to draw a picture of a house, a tree, and a person and then to answer a few questions about each drawing. The drawing of a person was scored by certified school psychologists using the Goodenough-Harris developmental system.

Stanford-Binet Intelligence Scale: Fourth Edition (IV) Vocabulary.—This subtest assesses a child's ability to label pictures and give word definitions for common words. The vocabulary subtest is the best predictor of overall Stanford-Binet IV Test Composite Score (IQ) and was given to children aged 2 to 5 years.

PPVT-R.—This test was given to children aged 3 to 5 years to assess their receptive vocabulary by asking them to point to one of four pictures on a page that depicts the stimulus word.

Beery Visual-Motor Integration (VMI).—The Beery VMI Test involves copying a series of simple geometric forms (eg, line, circle, and cross) and was given to children aged 3 to 5 years.

Yale Cubes.—Children aged 2 to 5 years were asked to copy a series of cube formations (ie, tower, bridge, house, and steps). This task was drawn from the Gesell Preschool Screening Test and the Yale Developmental Schedules.

Yale Drawings.—Two-year-old children were asked to copy a set of geometric forms (ie, vertical line, horizontal line, cross, and circle).

CBCL.—Mothers of all the children completed the CBCL. This involved reading a list of 118 behavioral symptoms and indicating for each one whether it was "untrue," "somewhat true," or "very true" of her child. The scores for "Total Problems," "Externalizing," and "Internalizing" were calculated for each child.

BDI.—A questionnaire for adults (mothers in this study) was administered that measures the presence and degree of "depression" or depressive affect.

Three Wishes.—Each child was asked to tell three things he or she would wish for if wishes could come true.

Children older than age 6 years had their vision screened using the Richmond Kindergarten Test Chart.

Parents gave separate informed consent for laboratory testing of their children. These tests included a tine test placed on the right forearm by a standard procedure (read by an interviewer 48 to 72 hours later) and a determination of the EP level from a finger stick sample of blood to assess lead exposure. The EP level was determined by the City of Philadelphia Health Department Laboratory. Values greater than 0.62 μmol/L were considered abnormal, and a follow-up determination of serum levels was requested. Parents were notified of abnormal EP levels and instructed on the proper follow-up procedures.

RESULTS

Population Studied

Adults.—One hundred forty-five adults completed our interview and examination. One hundred thirty-one subjects (90%) were black, 11 (8%) were white, and three (2%) were white or Hispanic. Fifteen percent stated that they were currently married and 46% were "never married"; the remainder said they were divorced or separated. Half of these 145 adult respondents had not completed high school; 10 (7%) of the participants in the study stated that they had completed at least 1 year of college (Table 1).

Concerning parity, 44 (30%) of the 145 respondents reported that they had three or more living children, and two individuals (1%) reported that they had nine children (Table 2). Eighty six (59%) of the respondents had delivered their first child by age 18 years (Table 3). One-hundred forty (97%) of the 145 mothers stated that they were not working; only five (3%) were currently engaged in some part-time work.

Although the mean length of stay in the current shelter was 12.7 weeks, the range was wide (<1 week to 82 weeks), and the mean length of homelessness was 19.3 weeks. Families had resided in a mean of 3.2 places (range, one to 20 places) in the previous 12 months, and in the previous 5 years had moved a mean of 4.7 times (range, one to 22 times). In the previous year, 14 (10%) owned their

Table 5.—Incidence of Major Accidents, Injuries, or Medical Conditions Over the Lifetime of Homeless Children (N=145)

Condition	No. (%) of Children
Burn with scar formation	20 (14)
Lead poisoning	16 (11)
Poison/pill ingestion	10 (7)
Fracture	9 (6)
Unconsciousness	9 (6)
Seizure	6 (4)

Table 6.—Reasons for the Hospitalization of Homeless Children in the Previous Year (N=145)

Reason for Hospitalization	No. (%) of Children Hospitalized
Injury	12 (8)
Other illness	12 (8)
Asthma	7 (5)
Dehydration	6 (4)
Seizure disorder	4 (3)
Respiratory infection	3 (2)
Other infection	3 (2)

Table 7.— Chronic Illnesses of Homeless Mothers Requiring Regular Medical Care (N=145)

Illness	No. (%) of Mothers
Hypertension	13 (9)
Renal disease	6 (4)
Cardiovascular disorder	5 (3)
Diabetes mellitus	4 (3)
Cancer	3 (2)
Physical disability	6 (4)
Other	23 (16)

Table 8.— Drug Use Reported by Homeless Mothers in the Previous Year (N=145)

Type of Drug	No. (%) of Mothers
Marijuana	61 (42)
Cocaine ("crack")	32 (22)
Amphetamines	4 (3)
Polychlorinated biphenyl	4 (3)
None	44 (30)

own homes, 112 (77%) rented their own apartments, 72 (50%) lived with their mothers, 78 (54%) "doubled up" or shared housing, and 10 (7%) lived on the streets, in abandoned buildings, or in cars. (This total is greater than 100% because more than one living arrangement was possible during the year.)

When asked about their *primary* reason for homelessness, 36 (25%) cited poor living conditions at a previous residence; 33 (23%) were evicted; 29 (20%) had disagreements with their landlord, other tenants, or family members; 15 (10%) attributed their homelessness to a lack of money or loss of a job; 10 (7%) had experienced a disaster (eg, fire or flood); seven (5%) cited abuse, and four (3%) cited divorce or separaton.

Findings Concerning General Health and Use of Services

When queried about their child's health, 55 (38%) of the respondents believed it was "excellent"; 39 (27%), "very good"; 29 (20%), "good"; 19 (13%), "fair"; and only three (2%) thought that their child's health was "poor." This favorable assessment of their children's health was restated when the parents were asked to compare the health of their child with that of other children; very few stated that their child's health was worse than that of most other children. Furthermore, only nine (6%) of 145 parents said that their child had a condition that interfered with usual activities.

When mothers were asked about recent health problems their child had encountered in the previous 4 weeks, gastroenteritis, otitis, cough, and conjunctivitis were the conditions most frequently mentioned (Table 4). Twenty-nine (20%) of the 145 respondents for these questions reported that their child had been seen in an emergency department during the past year as a result of an injury or fall, and nine (6%) of these children had sustained a fracture; nine children (6%) were reported "knocked unconscious" because of trauma during the previous year. Twenty (14%) of the 145 children had received burns during the previous year severe enough to have scarred; 10 children (7%) had swallowed a poison or medicine and required emergency treatment (Table 5).

Seventeen of the children (12%) had been hospitalized during the previous year; the major reasons for hospitalization included injury, seizures, dehydration, asthma, and other respiratory infections (Table 6).

The mothers of the homeless children were asked about the antenatal care they received when pregnant with the child in question: only four (4%) of the 104 mothers who answered this question reported receiving no care at all, and most of the other respondents reported first receiving care during their first trimester. Fourteen (13%) said that their care began during the fifth month of pregnancy or later.

By and large, parents seemed to have found some sort of medical care for themselves and their child; however, 23 (19%) of 124 respondents could not identify a place to which they could go for care. Fifty-five (44%) used the hospital emergency department or clinics for care, 53 (43%) went to a community clinic, 12 (10%) went to a private physician's office, and only four (3%) visited a health maintenance organization.

Dental care was harder to evaluate since many of the children were aged 3 years or younger, an age group that usually does not receive regular dental care.

Findings of Physical and Laboratory Examinations

Tine tests to screen for tuberculosis were placed on 92 children. Interviewers read the results between 48 and 72 hours later and found six positive findings (7%) from 0 to 5 mm, one positive finding (1%) from 6 to 10 mm, and 69 negative findings (75%). We were unable to locate 16 children (17%) for the test reading. Finger-stick blood samples for EP determination by extraction were obtained from 96 children, but 20 samples were not processed because of clotting or insufficient quantity. Nine (12%) of the remaining 76 samples had abnormal values (>35 μg/dL).

Visual acuity of children older than age 6 years was checked using the Richmond Kindergarten Test Chart. Ten (26%) of the 39 children tested failed to identify pictures at a distance of 600 cm with visual acuity better than 20/40.

Table 9.—Descriptive Statistics for Psychometric Measures

Measure*	Age Range, y	Domain	Normative	Mean (SD) School-Aged (6-12 y) (n=43)	Preschool (Aged 3-5 y) (n=40)	Toddlers (Aged 2 y) (n=15)	Mothers (n=145)
WISC-R Vocabulary	6-12	Verbal ability	10 (3)	6.67 (2.92)	...	...	...
WISC-R Block Design	6-12	Nonverbal problem solving	10 (3)	7.72 (3.33)	...	...	...
WRAT-R Reading	6-12	Reading, decoding	100 (15)	80.88 (20.81)	...	...	...
Draw-A-Person	3-12	Visual-motor skill	100 (15)	85.50 (16.22)	79.96 (13.12)	...	...
Binet IV Vocabulary	2-5	Verbal ability	50 (8)	...	41.44 (4.25)	45.27 (2.97)	...
PPVT-R	3-5, Mothers	Receptive vocabulary	100 (15)	...	67.84 (13.89)	...	71.99 (14.48)
Beery VMI	3-5	Visual-motor skill	100†	...	82.46 (9.06)	...	...
Yale Cubes	2-5	Nonverbal problem solving	100†	...	85.41 (21.43)	87.13 (11.72)	...
Yale Drawings	2	Visual motor skill	100†	...	...	88.67 (32.28)	...
CBCL Internalizing	2-12	Emotional problems	50 (10)	57.02 (9.11)	59.05 (11.61)	47.00 (6.98)	...
CBCL Externalizing	2-12	Behavior problems	50 (10)	57.68 (11.49)	55.05 (9.56)	45.13 (7.90)	...
CBCL Total Problems	2-12	Overall problems	50 (10)	57.92 (10.42)	59.87 (11.08)	44.73 (8.06)	...
Beck Depression Inventory	Mothers	Depression	...	...	...	...	13.26 (10.28)

*WISC-R indicates Wechsler Intelligence Scale for Children-Revised; WRAT-R, Wide Range Achievement Test–Revised; PPVT-R, Peabody Picture Vocabulary Test–Revised; Beery VMI, Beery Visual-Motor Integration; and CBCL, Child Behavior Checklist.
†Quotients produced by dividing mental age by chronological age.

Health of Parents

The reported health status of the mothers is summarized in Table 7. Seventeen (12%) of the 138 respondents stated that they were pregnant at the time of the interview. Ninety-nine (68%) of 145 mothers rated their own health as "good" or better, but specific health problems were cited by many women. Six (4%) of 145 respondents reported physical disabilities that interfered with their daily activities, and 13 (9%) reported that they had hypertension. Twenty-one respondents (14%) reported having been hospitalized in the previous year for a reason other than childbirth. While most respondents felt their health was "adequate," a significant number had conditions that required short- or long-term medical care, and this may have contributed to their difficulties in finding employment, housing, and child care.

The incidence of emotional difficulties severe enough to cause the mother to consult a psychiatrist, counselor, or therapist in the preceding 6 months was 14% (20 respondents), and seven mothers (5%) reported having been hospitalized at some time in their lives specifically for mental illness.

The prevalence of *reported* alcohol use was surprisingly low, with 102 (70%) of the 145 women stating that they consumed less than one alcoholic drink per day, and only four (3%) stating that their alcohol use had contributed, even slightly, to their present circumstances. Seventeen (12%) reported that alcohol use by others in their household was "a big part" or "the main cause" of their present problems. Thirteen women (9%) reported that their own drug use was "a big part" or "the main cause" of their present problems; 26 (18%) reported that drug use by others had created a significant problem for them. Table 8 shows the number of respondents who used specific drugs during the previous year.

Finally, thirty-one women (21%) reported having been battered or physically abused in the preceding 12 months, while only four (3%) reported that their children had been physically abused in the preceding year.

The estimates of the incidence and prevalence of these health and substance use problems may be falsely low because of underreporting. It is possible, for instance, that the clients perceived that admitting to some of these problems might cause them to be forced out of the shelter, despite our guarantees of confidentiality.

These women appeared to have the range of health problems found in the general population of women in this age group. However, the number who became pregnant as teenagers, who had been recently battered, and who cited drugs as a major cause of their difficulties was impressive, although we have no control group with which to compare the data.

Psychometric Data on School-Aged Children

Descriptive statistics for the psychometric data for the 6- to 12-year-old children appear in Table 9. These 43 children scored significantly below average in WISC-R Vocabulary and Block Design tests. However, these scores were within the range of scores obtained by black children whose parents are in the lowest occupational category of the WISC-R standardization sample.[8]

The mean score for this group of children aged 6 to 12 years on the Goodenough-Harris scoring of Draw-A-Person (DAP) was 85.5, indicating performance about one SD below average. Only 28% of the children scored in the average range or higher on the human figure drawing.

The mean score on the reading subtest of the WRAT-R for these 43 children was 80.9, or more than one SD below the mean for the standardization sample. Only one third of the children were reading at age level. This is consistent with the fact that only 25 (63%) of 40 children were in the correct grade for their age. However, it is somewhat inconsistent with the mothers' reports that 19 (48%) of 40 children had "good" or "excellent" performance in school, 11 (28%) had "average performance," and only 10 (25%) performed "below average" or were not attending school. School information was not obtained for three of the 43 school-aged children.

Absence from school was a major problem for these homeless children: 12 (30%) of 40 had missed 10 or more days of school in the past 2 months and another eight (20%) had missed between 5 and 9 days.

Psychometric Data on Preschool Children

Table 9 presents the scores on the Binet IV Vocabulary subtest, which measures expressive vocabulary performance. These 40 homeless preschool children scored about 1 SD below the mean for the general population. The children performed even more poorly in the PPVT-R, the test of receptive vocabulary; their mean score of 67.8 was more than two SDs below the mean for the general population. This was comparable with the performance of their mothers, who obtained a mean PPVT-R score of 72.0, indicating extremely poor receptive vocabulary skills.

The 40 preschool children scored below age level on the Yale Cubes, with a mean score of 85.6. These preschool children obtained a mean score of 82.5 on the VMI, indicating below-average performance on design copying. Visual motor immaturity was also shown on the DAP test, in which the mean score (based on the Goodenough-Harris norms) was 79.7; however, only 26 (65%) of 40 of the 3- to 5-year-olds were able to draw anything even "scorable" on the DAP.

Psychometric Data on 2-Year-Old Children

Few 2-year-olds were tested; their mean score on the Binet IV Vocabulary was 45.3, which is within one SD of the population mean. These 2-year-olds performed somewhat below age level on the Yale Cubes, with a mean score of 87.1. Their visual-motor skills were examined with the Yale drawings. Based on a ratio score using developmental age, these children scored slightly below average for their ages (88.7).

Behavioral-Emotional Adjustment of All Age Groups

The mother of each child aged 2 years and older completed the CBCL. Research has demonstrated that differences by social and economic group are minimal on this measure.[9] Maternal reports on the CBCL for school-aged and preschool children yielded mean scores close to the population mean; CBCL scores for the 2-year-olds were slightly below the mean (Table 9). Four (9%) of the 43 older children had scores above 70, or in the "clinical range," while seven children had scores between 65 and 70 for "Total Problems." Eight (20%) of 40 preschoolers had "Total Problems" scores in the "clinical range." No 2-year-olds were reported to score in the "clinical range" for "Total Problems," "Internalizing," or "Externalizing." On average, they did not show more emotional or behavioral symptoms than 2-year-olds in the CBCL standardization sample.[10]

These 145 homeless mothers reported substantial depression, according to the Beck Depression Inventory.[11] Although 69 (48%) scored in the normal range, 38 (26%) scored in the mild-to-moderate range, and 38 (26%) scored in the moderate-to-severe range of depression.

Clinical Measures: Three Wishes and HTP Drawings

The school-aged children showed a strong tendency to wish for major changes in their life situation, indicating an intense awareness of their plight as homeless poor people. Thirteen (48%) of the 27 older boys and eight (50%) of the 16 older girls made at least one wish to be out of the shelter or to have a new house. Fourteen (33%) of the 43 older boys and girls wished for money. Four (25%) of the 16 older girls wished for the family to be together and healthy, and 10 (37%) of the 27 boys wished for a car. In contrast, only 11 (28%) of the 40 younger children wished for these major life-style changes affecting the family. Rather, preschoolers showed a strong tendency to wish for more immediate personal pleasures: 11 (85%) of the 13 younger boys and 12 (44%) of the 27 younger girls wished for toys. Only younger children used their wishes for miscellaneous or minor objects. Thirty one percent of older girls (five girls) and younger boys (four boys) wished for fulfillment of "dreams," such as to be a princess, to be a flower, to visit Disney World, to be a "man," or to "do anything I want."

The older children's drawings of houses were remarkable as expressions of their wish for a comfortable and well-appointed home. Embellishments such as curtains, flower pots, "welcome" signs, and decorative details were common. The children's comments explicitly and poignantly expressed their unhappiness at being homeless and their desire for an inviting house in which to live.

COMMENT

This 1988 survey of homeless families residing in Philadelphia shelters revealed some results that were expected and some that were surprising. Unlike many previous studies of this population, selection of participants was random and should therefore be representative of Philadelphia's homeless population at that time. Because this was a field study, the conditions of data collection were suboptimal. There was often no appropriate area to interview parents or test children. Technical problems (20 of 96 blood specimens clotted before reaching the laboratory) and probable underreporting, especially on issues of drug use and physical abuse, may have hampered data interpretation. A comprehensive assessment of causes and consequences of homelessness would require comparative sampling, which was beyond the scope of this project. Thus, our analysis was limited to descriptive statistics.

The homeless parents interviewed most commonly cited poor living conditions, eviction, or disagreement with a landlord as their primary reasons for homelessness. Thirty-nine (27%) described illegal drug use by themselves or other household members as a major contributor to their current problems. Our overall impression was that the majority of these families lived in marginal situations (ie, doubled up, overcrowded, and/or unsafe), until some recent event (ie, argument, abuse, drug problem, pregnancy, or birth of a baby) forced them to leave. Many families described "choosing" to enter the shelter system as a better alternative than their current housing arrangements.

The children's reported health problems were those most prevalent at this socioeconomic level. Injuries and accidents were commonly reported, as were communicable diseases, such as gastroenteritis and upper respiratory infections. Nine (12%) of 76 children had abnormally high free EP levels. We do not know what proportion of these results represents lead intoxication or anemia from iron deficiency or other causes. However, parents reported that 16 (11%) of 145 children had been diagnosed as having lead poisoning in the previous year.

Despite the health problems described by parents, most believed that their children were in good or excellent health. Although most families could identify a source of care, almost half named a hospital emergency department or clinic rather than local health centers or individual practitioners.

The homeless mothers had a high degree of parity and, on average, had delivered their first children while teenagers. Their level of schooling was low and they performed poorly on a test of receptive vocabulary. They tended to suffer from depression, and many reported being abused by husbands or male companions. In addition to self-reported emotional difficulties requiring recent hospitalization, many mothers reported significant chronic medical problems.

The children had poor school attendance records and scored poorly on intelligence tests and receptive vocabulary tests, as well as having impaired ability to perform visual-motor skills. The older children expressed yearnings for a stable family structure, a desire to leave the shelter, and hope to have a home.

The problems of the homeless are protean and complex, just as the causes are multifactorial. The shelter system, created to supply emergency and temporary housing, is often the residence for homeless persons for prolonged periods. The health of the resident mothers was characterized by depression and multiparity as well as the presence of serious psychiatric and medical illnesses for some. The resident children tended to suffer serious injuries, such as burns, and many may have had anemia and/or high blood lead levels. The children scored poorly on developmental and psychological tests.

Some of the problems of homeless persons living in shelters that need to be addressed include lead toxicity, anemia, and accidents of children, as well as substance abuse and physical abuse of mothers. The psychological and developmental needs of homeless children may require special programs if these deficits are to be overcome.

This work was supported by a grant from the University of Pennsylvania Research Foundation, the United Way, the Manealoff Foundation, and the Robert Wood Johnson Clinical Scholars Program.

Drs Barnes and Finkelstein were Charles A. Dana Foundation Scholars at the time of this study, and Dr Parker was a Robert Wood Johnson Clinical Scholar at the University of Pennsylvania School of Medicine, Philadelphia.

References

1. Bassuck EL, Rubin L, Lauriat AS. Characteristics of sheltered homeless families. *Am J Public Health*. 1986;76:1097-1101.
2. Alperstein G, Rappaport C, Flanigan JM. Health problems of homeless children in New York City. *Am J Public Health*. 1988;78:1232-1233.
3. Miller DS, Lin E. Children in sheltered homeless families: reported health status and use of health services. *Pediatrics*. 1988;81:668-673.
4. Acker PJ, Fierman AH, Dreyer BP. An assessment of parameters of health care and nutrition in homeless children. *AJDC*. 1987;141:388.
5. Wright JD, Weber E. *Homelessness and Health*. Washington, DC: McGraw Hill International Book Co; 1987:112.
6. *Homelessness in Philadelphia: People, Needs, Services*. Philadelphia, Pa: Philadelphia Health Management Corporation; 1985.
7. Rescorla L, Parker R, Stolley PD. Ability, achievement and adjustment in homeless children. *Am J Orthopsychiatry*. In press.
8. Kaufman AS, Doppelt JE. Analysis of WISC-R standardization data in terms of the stratification variables. *Child Dev*. 1976;47:165-171.
9. Achenbach TM, Edelbrock CS. Behavioral problems and competencies reported by parents of normal and disturbed children aged four through sixteen. *Monogr Soc Res Child Dev*. 1981;46.
10. Achenbach T, Edelbrock CS, Howell C. Empirically-based assessment of the behavioral/emotional problems of 2-3-year-old children. *J Abnorm Child Psychol*. 1987;15:629-650.
11. Beck AT. *Depression: Causes and Treatment*. Philadelphia, Pa: University of Pennsylvania Press; 1987.

Pediatric Acquired Immunodeficiency Syndrome, Poverty, and National Priorities

Margaret C. Heagarty, MD

Human immunodeficiency virus (HIV) infection or acquired immunodeficiency syndrome (AIDS), as found in children, represents a microcosm of the problems and failures of this nation's health care system for the poor.

EPIDEMIOLOGY

When Oleske et al[1] and Rubenstein et al[2] first described the disease in children, it was not evident that AIDS was to become a disease found predominantly in poor children of minority status. But in the years since those first reports appeared, epidemiologic studies have demonstrated that AIDS in children is largely acquired through perinatal transmission from HIV-infected mothers who are or have been involved in intravenous drug use or who have had intercourse with someone involved in the drug culture. About 15% of children with AIDS are hemophiliacs or others who were infected by contaminated blood products before the advent of the national universal HIV blood screening program. Presumably, the number of transfusion-related cases will decrease with time.

To date, children with AIDS have been found in most urban areas of the country, but the disease continues to cluster in three distinct geographic areas: low-income areas of New York City, Northern New Jersey, and Miami, Fla. Those who live in these disadvantaged communities are of either African American or Hispanic origin; 53.4% of children with AIDS are from New York, New Jersey, or Florida, and 77.5% are of either Hispanic or African American ethnicity.[3] Since many are children of intravenous drug–using parents, some of whom have AIDS themselves, they and their parents live on the fringes of their disadvantaged communities, often isolated from their larger families or from other social supports that might be more easily mobilized for other, more advantaged groups with such a serious, lethal disease. In short, most children with AIDS and their families come largely from the most socially disorganized, economically deprived segments of our society.

PROGNOSIS

During the recent past, the prognosis for children with AIDS has improved for two reasons. First, pediatricians in areas in which the disease is prevalent have become more experienced in its early diagnosis and in the use of vigorous antibiotic therapy for bacterial infections to which these children are particularly prone. Second, research and development of scientific antiviral therapy for children, which, at times, has seemed too slow and too little, has finally become available in most areas in which significant numbers of children with the disease are found. While much more research is required before we fully understand AIDS and therefore its medical treatment, by now, some 10 years into the AIDS epidemic, the prognosis for children with AIDS has improved. Nevertheless, these children and their families face a complicated, chronic disease with a very guarded prognosis.

MEDICAL CARE SYSTEM

Because these children and their families are poor, they must also face a system that at times seems designed to impede rather than facilitate the provision of medical care. During the past 40 or more years, local and federal governments have developed a series of social and financial supports for the poor. However, the statutory and regulatory requirements of these programs are so complex, dysfunctional, fragmented, and disorganized that professionals providing care for these families often spend as much or more time dealing with a variety of local, state, and federal governmental bureaucracies as they do providing direct medical care or social support. In our zeal to make absolutely certain that no rascals or scoundrels get something to which we judge they are not entitled, we have constructed paper edifices and barriers that no one could easily master. We wonder why the most socially disorganized and disadvantaged members of our communities have trouble "getting on Medicaid" or registering for this or that social program. Indeed, we sometimes blame them, call them unmotivated, noncompliant, or worse. Since I have an acute anxiety attack when facing a Bureau of Motor Vehicles for a driver's license, I suspect that I, and probably most of us, would decompensate entirely if we had AIDS and had to try to qualify for Medicaid or Social Security benefits.

Finally, more than half the cases of AIDS reported to the Centers for Disease Control, Atlanta, Ga, have come from only 15 cities in this nation. Because our major urban disadvantaged communities contain large numbers of intravenous drug users and because HIV is transmitted via the shared needles of intravenous drug users, the prevalence of HIV infection in these communities is very high. This increased prevalence of the infection has led to rapid

Accepted for publication January 3, 1991.

From the Department of Pediatrics, Harlem Hospital Center, and the College of Physicians and Surgeons of Columbia University, New York, NY.

Reprint requests to Harlem Hospital Center, Department of Pediatrics, 506 Lenox Ave, New York, NY 10037 (Dr Heagarty).

spread, not only among the intravenous drug–using population, but also by heterosexual contact among adults who do not use drugs. It is not uncommon to make the diagnosis of AIDS in a child of a woman who is not a drug user and who is completely unaware that she has acquired the HIV infection from an infected sexual partner.

Because AIDS in children is a disease of the urban poor, the public general hospitals in our major cities provide much, if not most, of their medical care. In the best of times, these city or county hospitals are underfinanced, embattled medical care institutions of last resort. Historically, they have survived in a financial hand-to-mouth existence, relying on funds from local governments to subsidize the cost of care for the medically indigent. Unfortunately, these same cities are also besieged by the current drug epidemic so that these institutions must deal not only with the increased burden of AIDS, but also with the morbidity and mortality associated with crack/cocaine.

While their public health institutions are struggling to cope with these serious problems, these municipalities, particularly those in the Northeast, also face serious economic problems. Despite the increased needs associated with AIDS and the drug epidemic in these cities, medical and social care systems for the poor must cope with fixed or declining resources. This serious lack of resources imperils the care not only for children with AIDS, but for all who must rely on these systems for medical care.

EFFECT ON THE FAMILY

Any serious, chronic disease obviously affects the function of the entire family, including adults and siblings, as well as the ill child. But AIDS is even more catastrophic for families. Because most children have been infected by their mothers during pregnancy, the family must deal not only with the disease in the child, but also in the mother and often in the father. While the problems of children with AIDS have been widely publicized in the lay press, the fact that virtually all their mothers are infected and thus at risk for developing the disease has not been equally appreciated. However, estimates from the New York City Department of Health suggest that in that city alone, some 40 000 children may be orphaned by AIDS during the next decade (Pauline Thomas, MD, director of AIDS and HIV Surveillance, oral communication, September 1990). Finally, despite considerable efforts at public and professional education, the fear of AIDS with the resulting discrimination makes the care and support of these unfortunate children and their families even more problematic.

A CALL TO ACTION

The story of AIDS in children mirrors our lack of concern for the poor children of this nation. In our current national obsession with budget deficits, the needs of constituencies with political power, and foreign policy issues, the care and welfare of the nation's children do not seem to have a high priority in the national agenda. While our political rhetoric may deny such an assertion, actions speak louder than words. The reality is that we are unwilling to provide the resources necessary to provide medical care to children with AIDS, to provide medical care to all poor children, or even to provide them with adequate housing or education.

To solve the problems of children with AIDS and indeed of all poor children, we must develop a simple method of financing medical care for the poor. For large numbers of families and children to have no access to medical care because of a lack of financial resources is simply unacceptable. Over the years, any number of proposals to remove the financial barriers to health care have been debated. A detailed analysis of these proposals is beyond the scope of this essay, but one thing is clear: any remedy to this problem must have much simpler administrative procedures than does our current highly bureaucratic Medicaid system. While money is a necessity, it is not sufficient for the humane care of these children and their families who represent some of the most socially isolated and bereft of our society. We must develop social support, housing, and respite systems that afford them the compassion and care that any of us would need in the face of such a devastating illness.

A nation that neglects its children places itself in greater danger than any foreign power could possibly muster. The clich´e is true: children are the future of the country. If we do not begin to attend to the needs of children with AIDS, indeed all children in poverty, the final judgment of history will surely be very harsh indeed.

References

1. Oleske J, Minnefor A, Cooper R Jr, et al. Immunodeficiency syndrome in children. *JAMA.* 1983;249:2345-2349.
2. Rubenstein A, Sicklick M, Gupta A, et al. Acquired immunodeficiency with reversed T4/T8 ratios in infants born to promiscuous and drug addicted mothers. *JAMA.* 1983;249:2350-2356.
3. Centers for Disease Control. *HIV/AIDS Surveillance Report.* Atlanta, Ga: Centers for Disease Control; September 1990:1-18.

Pediatric Human Immunodeficiency Virus Infection and the Acquired Immunodeficiency Syndrome

A Health Care Crisis of Children and Families

Russell B. Van Dyke, MD

• The number of children infected with the human immunodeficiency virus (HIV) is rapidly increasing. Most infected children acquire their infection by vertical transmission from an infected mother, and this increase in the number of infected children reflects a similar increase in the number of infected women. Many features of HIV infection in children differ from those in adults, and it is important for the physician to be familiar with the varied presentations of pediatric HIV infection. Transmission of HIV during adolescence, by sexual contact and illicit drug use, is also a growing problem, accounting for most cases of acquired immunodeficiency syndrome (AIDS) seen in young adults in their 20's. The HIV-infected child represents only one member of a family affected by the HIV virus; frequently, multiple other members of the family are infected as well. These families are predominantly underpriviledged, coming from inner city minority populations with limited access to medical care and social service support. Pediatric AIDS is a preventable disease, by the prevention of HIV infection in women. In short term, it is likely that education will have the greatest impact on altering the course of the AIDS epidemic. Most infected children are cared for in a limited number of public inner city hospitals, and the ability of these hospitals to continue to provide adequate care will be threatened by the rising number of cases. A multidisciplinary approach to providing care for these children and their families is essential, with the primary care physician coordinating this effort. Rapid advances in the treatment of HIV and its associated opportunistic diseases raise difficult questions concerning the access of women, including pregnant women, and children to clinical trials of investigational agents. The commitment of individual health care workers and an increased level of financial support will be necessary to provide the care that these children and their families require and deserve.

(*AJDC.* 1991;145:529-532)

The acquired immunodeficiency syndrome (AIDS) was first recognized in the United States in 1981 as a disease occurring in homosexual men. However, as the epidemic evolved, the disease appeared in other groups, including hemophiliacs, intravenous drug users, women, and children. Currently, children less than 13 years of age comprise 1.8% of all cases of AIDS in the United States; by the end of 1991, it is estimated that there will be approximately 3000 pediatric AIDS cases in the United States. Most cases of AIDS in children result from the vertical transmission of human immunodeficiency virus (HIV) from an infected mother to her child, and the rising number of pediatric AIDS cases reflects a parallel rise in the number of HIV-infected women. Between 20% and 40% of infants born to an HIV-infected mother become infected themselves.[1-3] Factors that influence the transmission rate are not clearly defined, but maternal antibodies directed against specific portions of HIV surface glycoproteins appear to be an important factor in protecting the infant from infection.[4-6]

The proportion of AIDS cases in the United States that occur in women has been rising steadily since the onset of the epidemic and currently stands at 11% of all reported cases. Between 1988 and 1989, the number of cases in women increased by 29%, while the number in men rose by only 18%.[7] Approximately one half of women with AIDS acquired their infection through parenteral drug use, while one third acquired their infection through heterosexual transmission. Most HIV-infected women are of childbearing age. The proportion of AIDS cases in the United States due to heterosexual transmission increased from 0.9% in 1983 to 6% in 1990, with this rise expected to continue. This emphasizes that HIV is fundamentally a sexually transmitted disease, spread by both heterosexual and homosexual contact. Heterosexual transmission is the principal route of transmission of HIV in many developing countries and is playing an increasingly important role in the United States.

Although many of the clinical features of HIV infection are similar in adults and children, some are unique to children.[8] The typical clinical presentation of pediatric AIDS includes growth failure, developmental delay, hepatosplenomegaly, diffuse lymphadenopathy, recurrent bacterial infections, and chronic *Candida* infections. However, in many children the infection presents in an atypical fashion, manifesting isolated features of the disease, such as thrombocytopenia, pneumonia, parotitis, diarrhea, recurrent infections, failure to thrive, or loss of developmental milestones. Involvement of the central nervous system is a particularly important problem in children with HIV

Accepted for publication January 28, 1991.
From the Section of Pediatric Infectious Diseases, Department of Pediatrics, Tulane University School of Medicine, New Orleans, La.
Reprints not available.

infection. Since children have not yet reached physical and developmental maturity, early features of HIV infection include poor growth and loss of mental and motor milestones. The immunologic immaturity and naïveté of children makes them prone to recurrent infections with common bacterial pathogens.

Infection with HIV must now be considered when a broad range of common and uncommon clinical syndromes are seen in children. Testing for HIV should be performed as part of the diagnostic evaluation of these children, whether or not risk factors for HIV infection are present. Consequently, the clinician must understand the difficulties in establishing HIV infection in children, particularly in those less than 15 months of age, in whom maternal antibody can result in a falsely positive HIV antibody test.[9] The results of HIV testing must be kept confidential. I believe that parents should be informed whenever HIV testing is performed on their child, but informed consent is usually not required unless mandated locally. Concerns about confidentiality should not prevent a child from being examined for HIV infection when appropriate.

Infection with HIV in the adolescent is a problem that deserves special attention. Currently, only 3.8% of AIDS cases in the United States occur in individuals between 13 and 19 years of age. However, the proportion of cases in this age group due to heterosexual transmission has increased substantially in recent years and currently stands at 23% for male patients and 44% for female patients.[10] Females currently make up 20% of adolescents with AIDS, in contrast to only 9% of adults with AIDS, further pointing out that heterosexual transmission plays a major role in the spread of HIV during adolescence.

Furthermore, these figures underestimate the importance of HIV *transmission* during adolescence. Currently, 20% of all cases of AIDS occur in young adults between 20 and 29 years of age. Since the median incubation period of AIDS in adults is between 8 and 10 years, the majority of individuals who develop AIDS in their 20's acquired their HIV infection during adolescence. The growing problem of HIV transmission during adolescence requires a response directed toward prevention of infection. This is particularly important in light of the increasing proportion of adolescents who are sexually active. At the present time in the United States, 32% of 16-year-old girls and 70% of 18-year-old women engage in premarital sexual activity.[11] There are several reasons why adolescents are at increased risk of HIV infection: they have a greater risk of other sexually transmitted diseases than older persons, they are less likely to use barrier methods of contraception, and they frequently have multiple sexual partners.[12] However, adolescents are receptive to being taught about AIDS; Steiner et al[13] demonstrated an excellent level of knowledge about this disease among a group of adolescents in Wisconsin. One hopes that these young adults will apply this knowledge to their own behavior.

Pediatric AIDS is not only a disease of the child; it is a disease of the whole family unit. Eighty percent of children with AIDS, and nearly all seropositive infants, have a mother who is HIV infected. Frequently, the mother's sexual partner is infected, and other children in the family may be infected as well. A disproportionate number of children with AIDS belong to minority groups; 53% are black and 23% Hispanic. Most cases occur in inner-city populations, which suffer from poverty, racism, illicit drug use, inadequate housing, poor access to medical care, and a nonintact family unit. As the HIV infection progresses in the child's parents, they are unable to care adequately for themselves and their child, and it falls on the extended family or the community to provide this care. These children are very difficult to place in foster care and hospice care. Not surprisingly, then, the hospital often provides this care, resulting in a large number of hospitalized "boarder babies" in regions with a large number of pediatric AIDS cases. At Harlem Hospital (New York, NY), more than 20% of hospitalizations of children with AIDS resulted from social problems rather than medical needs. The mean length of stay for these boarder babies was 339 days, as opposed to 89 days for children cared for at home.[14] The cost of this care is great; in that report from 1988, the authors estimated the mean lifetime hospital cost for a child with AIDS to be greater than $90 000. The increased use of outpatient services and foster care substantially reduces unnecessary hospitalizations among these children.[15]

Pediatric AIDS has its greatest impact on those minority groups that have the poorest access to medical care and are least likely to benefit from advances being made in the prevention and treatment of this disease. Indeed, more than any other disease, pediatric AIDS highlights the deficiencies in the health care system that exists in the United States today. Our efforts at delivering health care to these disadvantaged children have not been completely successful. For example, less than two thirds of nonwhite children in the United States are up to date in their immunizations at 2 years of age.[16] It can only be hoped that we will be more successful at delivering preventive and therapeutic care to HIV-infected children.

The rising number of children with AIDS will impact all areas of health care and rapidly overwhelm those areas where cases are concentrated. Infection with HIV is currently the ninth leading cause of death among children aged 1 to 4 years in the United States. By the end of 1991, it is anticipated that children with AIDS will occupy 10% of all pediatric hospital beds in the United States.[17] Most of these children will not have private health insurance, and their medical care will be funded by such public sources as the Medicaid program. Of the children in our pediatric HIV clinic, approximately 90% qualify for Medicaid through the Aid to Families With Dependent Children program. An additional 5% qualify through participation in the Supplemental Security Income program, which is available only to those children who carry an AIDS diagnosis. The remaining 5% of children have other sources of insurance or do not qualify for Medicaid. Unfortunately, each state administers its own Medicaid program, and states have differing eligibility criteria and benefits. In many states, the level of reimbursement is too low to meet adequately the needs of the child. In addition, home nursing care, ambulatory care, foster care, hospice care, and social service support may not be available or have limited benefits in some states. Finally, many health care providers do not accept Medicaid patients, further limiting access of these children to medical care.

The impact of pediatric AIDS on the practice of pediatrics and the training of young pediatricians needs to be addressed. All pediatric subspecialists will need to develop expertise in the problems of HIV-infected children. However, in most instances, the pediatrician or family practitioner will provide primary care for these children. In the ideal situation, the primary care physician will work with a team of specialists, including pediatric subspecialists, nurses, social workers, nutritionists, and developmentalists. The assessment and treatment of HIV-infected children must become part of the curriculum of all pediatric and family practice training programs. It is hoped that the increasing number of HIV-infected children will not be seen as a deterrent to those entering the field of pediatrics, but rather as a challenge to those committed to the health of children and their families.

A major concern raised by those caring for HIV-infected children has been a delay in access to new forms of treatment. Children have traditionally been excluded from clinical trials involving new medications until efficacy has been demonstrated in adults. The intent of this is to protect the child from possible adverse effects of a new medication until efficacy is established and the profile of adverse reactions is known. Unfortunately, it also delays the initiation of clinical trials in children and ultimately the availability of effective new forms of therapy. For instance, zidovudine was not available to children until clinical trials in adults were completed. The AIDS Clinical Trials Group, a collaborative group of AIDS researchers funded by the National Institutes of Health, has an active group of pediatric investigators responsible for designing and conducting clinical trials in HIV-infected children. This group has been very vocal in this concern, and children and women are currently benefiting from early involvement in the evaluation of promising new agents.

A question that arises in designing treatment protocols for children is whether results obtained in adult trials should be applied to children. An example is the recent demonstration that the early administration of corticosteroids increases survival in adults with *Pneumocystis carinii* pneumonia.[18] There is reason to suspect that pediatric *P carinii* pneumonia may respond differently than adult disease, because it represents primary infection rather than reactivation disease. The pediatric members of the AIDS Clinical Trials Group are currently considering whether a similar trial should be conducted in children.

What should the response of the medical community be to the growing problem of HIV-infected children? In the short term, the most successful response to the AIDS epidemic will be in the area of prevention. Pediatric AIDS *is* a preventable disease—by the prevention of HIV infection in women of childbearing age. To protect themselves, all young adults must understand, before they become sexually active, that HIV is a sexually transmitted disease. They need access to counseling about HIV and other sexually transmitted diseases, and they need to know how to protect themselves from infection, including the use of condoms. In addition, they need to understand the risk of parenteral drug use. Information about HIV transmission and AIDS must be taught to all children while they are in middle or junior high school. Finally, women need greater access to HIV testing so that pregnancy prevention and termination can be considered by those who are infected. Guidelines for HIV testing of pregnant women have been published.[17]

The development of new forms of treatment for HIV and the opportunistic diseases associated with AIDS must be of the highest priority. It is gratifying that the AIDS Clinical Trials Group has recently identified pediatrics as a major area of emphasis, and funds have been made available for additional sites to conduct pediatric studies. Both clinical research and basic research in the field of AIDS deserve additional support.

It is currently unknown whether HIV infection can be prevented in the child born to an infected mother. We are hindered by a lack of understanding of two key points: when during gestation and delivery the child becomes infected, and why only one of three infants born to an infected mother becomes infected. The AIDS Clinical Trials Group is initiating a study to determine whether the administration of zidovudine during the second and third trimesters of pregnancy, and continued in the infant for 6 weeks after delivery, will interrupt perinatal transmission. Other strategies for the prevention of perinatal transmission being considered include passive and active immunization of the woman before delivery and the prevention of infection in the child after delivery by the administration of such agents as recombinant CD4, which blocks infection from being established. We clearly need to learn much more about the mechanism and immunology of perinatal HIV infection.

Because of the complex medical and social needs of HIV-infected children and their families, a multidisciplinary team approach to providing care is necessary. In our Pediatric HIV Clinic at Charity Hospital of New Orleans (La), primary ongoing care is provided by general pediatricians with an interest in HIV disease, supported by pediatric subspecialists in infectious diseases, hematology, neurology, and other subspecialties. Adolescents infected with HIV are cared for by an adolescent medicine physician in the pediatrics clinic. We are currently developing a combined mother-child clinic to allow HIV-infected mothers and their infants to be seen at the same clinic visit. This takes advantage of our observation that HIV-infected women are much more compliant with their child's care than with their own care. A case manager/social worker is assigned to each family to assist with financial arrangements, transportation to and from the clinic, home health care, and referrals to other health care agencies. Finally, a pediatric therapist and clinical psychologist assist in neurodevelopmental evaluations and provide physical therapy.

This multidisciplinary approach to providing care is expensive and requires the commitment of a large group of health care professionals. Funds must be made available to support these programs, and personnel must be trained to provide the care. Developed countries, such as the United States, have the resources to deliver this care; it remains to be seen whether we have the wisdom to insist that it be done.

References

1. The European Collaborative Study. Mother-to-child transmission of HIV infection. *Lancet.* 1988;2:1039-1043.
2. Blanche S, Rouzioux C, Moscato MG, et al. A prospective study of infants born to women seropositive for human immunodeficiency virus type 1. *N Engl J Med.* 1989;320:1643-1648.
3. Willoughby A, Mendez H, Goedert J, et al. Natural history of infants born to HIV-positive women. Program and abstract of the Fifth International Conference on AIDS; June 4-9, 1989; Montreal, Quebec. Abstract MBO 2.
4. Davish Y, Calvelli TA, Wood DG, et al. Vertical transmission of human immunodeficiency virus is correlated with the absence of high-affinity/avidity maternal antibodies to the gp120 principal neutralizing domain. *Proc Natl Acad Sci U S A.* 1990;87:3445-3449.
5. Rossi P, Moschese V, Broliden PA, et al. Presence of maternal antibodies to human immunodeficiency virus 1 envelope glycoprotein gp120 epitopes correlates with the uninfected status of children born to seropositive mothers. *Proc Natl Acad Sci U S A.* 1989;86:8055-8058.
6. Goedert JJ, Mendez H, Drummond JE, et al. Mother-to-infant transmission of human immunodeficiency virus type 1: association with prematurity or low anti-gp 120. *Lancet.* 1989;2:1351-1355.
7. Centers for Disease Control. AIDS in women—United States. *MMWR.* 1990;39:845-846.
8. Falloon J, Eddy J, Wiener L, Pizzo PA. Human immunodeficiency virus infection in children. *J Pediatr.* 1989;114:1-30.
9. Husson RN, Comeau AN, Hoff R. Diagnosis of human immunodeficiency virus infection in infants and children. *Pediatrics.* 1990;86:1-10.

Centers for Disease Control. *HIV/AIDS Surveillance Re-* ... 1. Atlanta, Ga: Centers for Disease Control; November ... 1-18.
11. Centers for Disease Control. Premarital sexual experience among adolescent women—United States 1970-1988. *MMWR.* 1991;39:929-932.
12. Cates W Jr. The epidemiology and control of sexually transmitted diseases in adolescents. *Adolesc Med.* 1990;1:409-427.
13. Steiner JD, Sorokin G, Schiedermayer DL, Van Susteren TJ. Are adolescents getting smarter about acquired immunodeficiency syndrome? *AJDC.* 1990;144:302-306.
14. Hegarty JD, Abrams EJ, Hutchinson VE, et al. The medical care costs of human immunodeficiency virus–infected children in Harlem. *JAMA.* 1988;260:1901-1905.
15. Kemper K, Forsyth B. Medically unnecessary hospital use in children seropositive for human immunodeficiency virus. *JAMA.* 1988;260:1906-1909.
16. Centers for Disease Control. *U.S. Immunization Survey.* Atlanta, Ga: Centers for Disease Control; 1986.
17. Working Group on HIV Testing of Pregnant Women and Newborns. HIV infection, pregnant women, and newborns: a policy proposal for information and testing. *JAMA.* 1990;264:2416-2420.
18. Bozzette SA, Stattler FR, Chiu J, et al. A controlled trial of early adjunctive treatment with corticosteroids for *Pneumocystis carinii pneumonia in the acquired immunodeficiency syndrome. N Engl J Med.* 1990;323:1451-1457.

In Other AMA Journals

ARCHIVES OF OTOLARYNGOLOGY—HEAD & NECK SURGERY

Pediatric Sinusitis: The Role of Endoscopic Sinus Surgery in Cystic Fibrosis and Other Forms of Sinonasal Disease

J. Kevin Duplechain, MD;
John A. White, MD;
Robert H. Miller, MD
(*Arch Otolaryngol Head Neck Surg.* 1991;117:422-426)

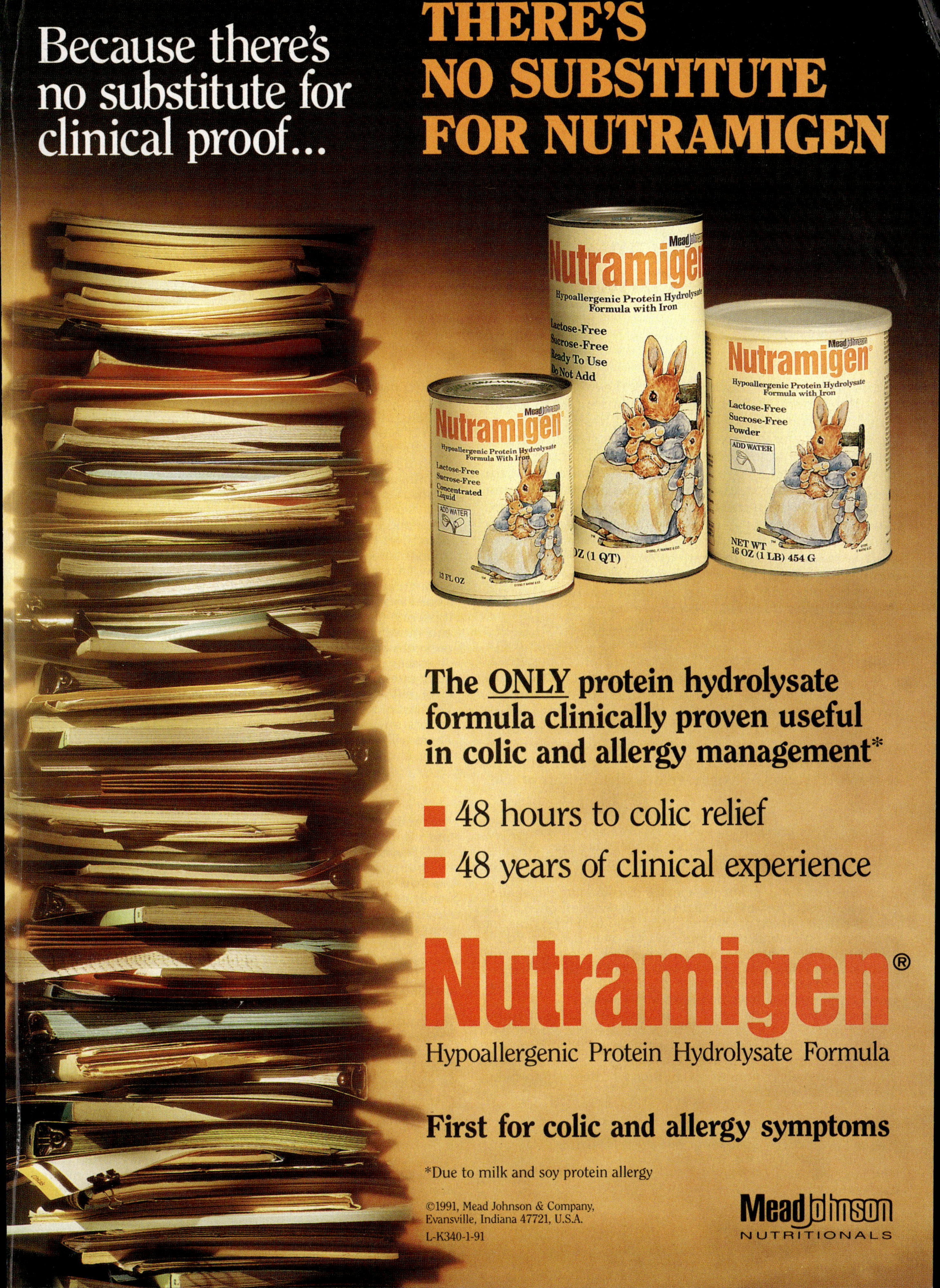
Because there's no substitute for clinical proof...
THERE'S NO SUBSTITUTE FOR NUTRAMIGEN
Nutramigen
Hypoallergenic Protein Hydrolysate Formula with Iron
Lactose-Free
Sucrose-Free
Powder
ADD WATER
NET WT 16 OZ (1 LB) 454 G
The ONLY protein hydrolysate formula clinically proven useful in colic and allergy management*
48 hours to colic relief
48 years of clinical experience
Nutramigen®
Hypoallergenic Protein Hydrolysate Formula
First for colic and allergy symptoms
*Due to milk and soy protein allergy
©1991, Mead Johnson & Company, Evansville, Indiana 47721, U.S.A.
L-K340-1-91
Mead Johnson
NUTRITIONALS

The American Academy of Pediatrics Response to the Growing Health Needs of Children

James E. Strain, MD

At its planning meeting in May 1988, the executive board of the American Academy of Pediatrics (AAP) established the promotion of access to child health care as its top priority. Later in the year, the following resolution was passed at the chapter president's forum: "That the Academy develop and support legislation to assure a health program that guarantees all children and pregnant women access to a comprehensive (basic) package of health care benefits that treats all children and pregnant women equally, and that the Academy work with legislators to draft a model program that, to the extent practicable, maintains parental control of health care decisions, preserves the physician's primary obligation to his or her patient, and effectively utilizes private insurers."

In October 1988, the executive board approved a universal access-to-care proposal consisting of three components: (1) the introduction of federal legislation that guarantees financial access to medical care for all children and pregnant women; (2) the establishment of community-based health projects that meet the special needs of children at the local level; and (3) the introduction of a public relations program that increases public awareness of the importance of child health issues. The three components of the AAP access initiative are described in this article.

FEDERAL LEGISLATION

In 1987, approximately 10 million children aged 0 through 21 years were without health insurance for the entire year. Another 10 million were uninsured for part of the year.[1] Employers faced with escalating insurance costs are increasing employees' share of premium costs for dependents, thereby discouraging dependent coverage.[2] In addition, plans that do cover dependents often fail to meet the health needs of children. Most child health services are provided in an ambulatory setting and are often not covered by health insurance. Traditional insurance has been designed to cover hospital care. While this type of coverage is important for the occasional child with a catastrophic or long-term illness, the vast majority of children will have no need for this service.

Some children are classified as uninsurable because of a preexisting condition. Children with congenital defects, chronic diseases, or other disabling conditions are often excluded from coverage, particularly when a parent changes jobs. Insurance companies are reluctant to accept children who may require more than the usual amount of care.

Accepted for publication January 3, 1991.

From the American Academy of Pediatrics, Elk Grove Village, Ill.
Reprint requests to the American Academy of Pediatrics, 141 Northwest Point Blvd, PO Box 927, Elk Grove Village, IL 60009-0927 (Dr Strain).

More than one in five children in this nation live in poverty.[3] About half of the poor children are receiving Medicaid benefits.[4] Although 52% of those eligible for Medicaid are children, less than 20% of Medicaid dollars are spent for their care.[4] Thus, in both the private and public sectors, there are significant gaps in the health insurance coverage for children.

Uninsured children utilize physician services less often than do insured children,[5,6] particularly preventive health services.[6] Delays in treatment often add to the cost of care and reduce the likelihood of a successful outcome.

To meet the needs of all children, including the uninsured, underinsured, and uninsurable, the AAP has developed a proposal that guarantees financial access to care for all children through age 21 years and all pregnant women. This plan is designed to be the least disruptive of the present health care system. It is a one-tiered system in which children insured in the private and public sectors have equal benefits. These benefits include preventive health services, the treatment of acute and chronic illnesses, and the management of disabling conditions that require care coordination. Standards of care will be set at the federal level, but administration of the program will be left to the states. The cost of the program will be borne by the public and private sectors, and families that can afford to pay will share in the costs. There will be a fair and equitable payment for services rendered and a simplified billing system.

THE AAP PLAN

Benefits

Benefits include preventive health care, primary medical care, and extended care requiring coordination of services.

1. Preventive health care includes the following: (*a*) office visits, immunizations, and laboratory services as recommended by the AAP in its periodicity schedule; (*b*) maternity services; (*c*) family planning services; (*d*) care of the newborn, including physician attendance at high-risk deliveries; (*e*) child abuse and neglect assessment; and (*f*) preventive dental care. Because of the importance of preventive health care, there will be no copayments or deductibles for anyone receiving these services.

2. Primary medical care includes the following: (*a*) hospital care; (*b*) physician services for acute and chronic conditions; (*c*) laboratory and other diagnostic services; (*d*) acute dental care; (*e*) medical and surgical supplies; (*f*) corrective eyeglasses and lenses; (*g*) hearing aids; (*h*) medical equipment; and (*i*) prescription drugs, including nutritional supplements. For families below 133% of the poverty level, no coinsurance or deductibles will be required for these services. For those above 200% of the poverty level, there will be a $200 annual deductible per family and a 20% copayment. A sliding scale will be used for families between 133% and 200% of the poverty level.

3. Extended medical care requiring care coordination includes the following: (*a*) care coordination for chronically ill and other "at risk" children; (*b*) orthodontia; (*c*) treatment of developmental and learning disabilities; (*d*) substance abuse services; (*e*) speech

therapy; (*f*) occupational therapy; (*g*) physical therapy; (*h*) hospice care; (*i*) respite care; (*j*) recuperative stays in long-term care facilities; and (*k*) nutritional assessment and counseling. For those above 200% of the poverty level, there will be a maximum coinsurance of 30% for these services. No copayments or deductibles will be required of families with incomes below 133% of poverty. A sliding scale will be used for families between 133% and 200% of poverty. There will be an out-of-pocket cap of 10% of family income or $1000 per year for an individual and $3000 per family, whichever is less, for all services provided under the plan.

To the extent possible, insurance mechanisms will be used to fund benefits included in the AAP proposal. However, direct state or federal funding will be required for some services. Services for children with special health care needs and primary care services where none are locally available are among those that may need direct funding. The state Title V maternal and child health agencies will continue to play an important role in monitoring care and providing services not covered by insurance.

Financing

Funding for this plan will come from private and public sources. In the private sector, employers will be required to provide the mandated benefit package for children and pregnant women or pay a 3.17% employee payroll tax based on 1990 calculations. The shared cost of dependent coverage cannot be a greater percentage of the total premium than the shared cost of the employee coverage and cannot exceed 25% of the total premium.

In the public sector, a fund will be established at the state level to purchase insurance for families not covered by employer insurance. It will have several income streams. The tax imposed on employers who elect not to provide coverage for dependents of their employees or whose benefit package fails to meet mandated benefit standards will be one source of funding. Federal and state Medicaid funds currently being used to provide medical services for children and pregnant women will be another source. Finally, premiums paid by families not covered by employer insurance will be added to the fund. If the family income is above 200% of the poverty level, an annual premium of $458 will be paid per family. No premium payments will be required for those families below 133% of the poverty level, and a sliding scale will be used to determine the premium costs for families falling between 133% and 200% of the poverty level.

Multiple private insurers will bid on the state contracts just as they do in the private sector. The benefit package must be the same for employer insurance and for the state-administered fund. In the required package, insurers will be allowed some flexibility in the scope and duration of benefits and in the amount of cost sharing, provided the plan is actuarially equivalent.

Administration

The federal government will mandate a benefit package. The Secretary of the US Department of Health and Human Services will have the authority to establish boundaries within which the states must function.

The actual administration of the program will be at the state level. States will establish policies that control marketing of insurance and will develop and maintain the system. They will monitor the health status of children and pregnant women and will collect data on unmet needs. They will be responsible for regulating fiscal intermediaries and for developing performance standards for insurers.

COMMENT

The AAP plan replaces the children's and pregnant women's portions of Medicaid. Medicaid has perpetuated a two-tiered system of care in which eligibility, benefits, and reimbursement limited by lack of funds, vary from state to state. Physician participation in Medicaid has declined in recent years.[6] Billing procedures have become burdensome.

The plan proposed by the AAP provides a uniform package of benefits for all children and pregnant women. It is an insurance-based program with private insurers bidding for contracts in the public and private sectors. It provides for cost sharing of premiums, copayments, and deductibles based on the ability to pay. It underwrites the cost of care for the poor.

The AAP's proposal will increase the total cost of health services for children and pregnant women from the 1990 level of $98.8 billion to $111.4 billion, an increase of approximately $12 billion. Compared with the total cost of medical care in the United States, which was $650 billion in 1990,[7] the added cost of providing health care for all children and pregnant women is relatively low.

The AAP intends to introduce legislation in the 1991 session of Congress that incorporates the principles enunciated in the plan. Because of the widespread dissatisfaction with the current methods of financing health care, it is likely that many new health care financing proposals will be considered by the 102nd Congress. The AAP plan is the only one that specifically addresses the care of children and pregnant women. The AAP supports guaranteed financial access to care for all United States citizens, but we believe that if an incremental approach is necessary, the first step should be coverage for children and pregnant women. The value of preventive care and early intervention for children and pregnant women, the relatively low cost, and the large number of women and children living in poverty are strong arguments for making children and pregnant women our top priority.

Community-Based Programs

While providing health insurance for all children and pregnant women is an important first step in guaranteeing access to medical care, it is clearly not the total solution to the mounting health problems of the young. Poverty and its social consequences account for much of the morbidity in our nation's children. Until mothers and children live in a safe environment and have sufficient food and adequate housing, the availability of medical care will have limited impact on the health of our children.

These societal problems are beyond the scope of activity of the AAP; however, we should be able to address many nonfinancial barriers to health care. For example, there are inadequate numbers of health professionals to deliver care in some parts of the country, particularly in rural and inner-city areas. Transportation to and from the sources of care can be difficult when medical care is not readily accessible. The process of enrollment in the Medicaid program is often difficult and demeaning. Many of the Medicaid registration requirements appear to be designed to keep children out of the program rather than bring them in.

In addition, cultural differences sometimes make it difficult for families to use traditional health care services. They often feel ill-at-ease in physicians' offices or in emergency centers. Reliance on folklore medicine is common among some ethnic groups.

The AAP believes that many of these problems can be solved at the local level. Communities understand the health needs of their children and, given the necessary resources, are able to develop programs that meet those needs.

To assist communities in this effort, the AAP initiated two community-based programs. The first, "The Healthy Tomorrows Partnership For Children," is a program funded by the federal Maternal and Child Health Bureau and jointly administered with the AAP. The program is designed to fund community-based projects in areas where access to care is limited and child health needs are not being met. A funded program receives $50 000 each year for 5 years provided that annual matching funds of $100 000 are obtained from local sources. An additional requirement is the participation of the local pediatric community and the state Maternal and Child Health Agency.

In 1989, 113 grant applications were submitted. Ten were selected by a panel of experts appointed by the AAP and Maternal and Child Health Bureau. Among the projects selected were the Family Care Center Health Project in Lexington, Ky; the Healthy Start Children's Clinic in Fort Collins, Colo; the Parent-Pediatric Partnership in Honolulu, Hawaii; and Project Caring in Pittsburgh, Pa. Site visits were carried out by members of the AAP Project Advisory Committee and each of the 10 programs has been approved for continued funding for a second year.

The program was continued in 1990 with the selection of 10 additional projects, all created to meet the special needs of children in local communities. These include the Jackson County Prenatal Clinic in Jackson, Mich; the First Steps Primary Program in Baton Rouge, La; and the Rural Partnership For Children in Omaha, Neb.

The second AAP community-based effort is the Healthy Children program, originally conceived and directed by Philip Porter, MD, and funded by the Robert Wood Johnson Foundation. Dr Porter has had great success during the past 20 years in helping communities recognize their child health needs and sharing with them the experiences of other communities. He has accomplished this by providing consultants from other successful programs and advising on new and innovative ways to secure local funding. Among the programs developed with the assistance of Dr Porter are a school-based primary care program, a program for social enrichment and primary care of preschool children, a pregnancy prevention program, a comprehensive primary care program for mothers and children, and a program for the care of handicapped children in rural America.

Healthy Children has demonstrated that a broad base of community leadership is needed to successfully introduce a health care program at the community level. Public health officials, school administrators, political leaders, nurses, child advocates, church leaders, and pediatricians all bring special skills and experience to the programs. All can play a significant role in meeting the needs of children in their communities.

During the past 2 years, as a result of funding from the Robert Wood Johnson Foundation, the Healthy Children concepts have been incorporated into an AAP program to assist local communities in their planning efforts. The program does not make grants, but provides technical assistance and advice under the direction of Dr Porter. Forty thousand pediatricians have learned about the program through direct mailings from the AAP. Using the existing network of state AAP chapters, pediatricians with a special interest in community-based activities have been identified and have agreed to serve as state facilitators.

In August 1990, these facilitators met in Chicago, Ill, to discuss their programs and share information. This very successful conference laid the groundwork for future development of community-based programs throughout the country. In addition, lessons learned from these programs can contribute to a better understanding of child health needs and to the establishment of an effective national child health policy.

Public Awareness Program

The third component of the AAP access initiative is the public awareness program. The public must become convinced of the importance of child health to the future of the nation. We must assume responsibility for the health of all of our children—rich and poor, black and white, disabled and healthy. This will require a commitment on the part of the public and, ultimately, state and federal legislators to put children's issues first. The AAP expects to accomplish this with the public awareness program.

Health professionals have an important role to play in keeping children healthy and in treating their illnesses. However, other factors are equally important. A polluted environment can have serious health consequences. Lead and toxic chemicals can have damaging effects on children.[8,9] Certain activities related to life-styles, such as substance abuse and risk-taking behaviors, have an immediate impact on health. Inappropriate diets, sedentary behavior, and tobacco use can also have long-term consequences.

There is a definite relation between health and education. An unhealthy child will not do well in school. In 1988, there were 4 300 000 children and young adults aged 14 to 24 years who did not attend school regularly and/or had not completed 12th grade or received a general equivalency degree.[10] Many children who do graduate are functionally illiterate. These are alarming statistics in a nation that is being forced to compete in the world market. Children's health and education go hand in hand and must be our nation's highest priorities.

These messages will be taken to the public with the assistance of a national public relations firm. Marketing a product is difficult and expensive. Marketing an idea is even more challenging. The AAP intends to seek industry support for programs that highlight solutions to the problems of children. We believe industry is interested, not only from a humanistic point of view, but also out of concern for the health and education of our nation's future work force. Contributions from foundations and individuals will also be solicited to support the public awareness program.

The AAP also recognizes that there are other groups with an interest in promoting child health. We intend to work with these organizations to enhance their activities and to broaden their scope of influence.

The specific objectives of the public awareness program are (1) to convince business leaders, legislators, and the public at large of the importance of child health and the long-term benefits of improving the health of our nation's children, and (2) to generate public support for improving access to care for children and pregnant women by defining the barriers to care and the means of overcoming those barriers.

The AAP is under no illusion that changing public opinion or creating a ground swell of public support for children's health issues will be easily accomplished, but over a period of time, we believe an informed and aroused public will demand that children's issues be given a higher priority on the legislative agenda.

The AAP invites the support and participation of all pediatric organizations and other child advocates in these important child health initiatives.

References

1. Short P. *Estimates of the Uninsured Population, Calendar Year 1987.* Rockville, Md: US Public Health Service; 1990. US Dept of Health and Human Services publication (PHS) 90-3469.

2. Congressional Research Service. *Health Insurance and the Uninsured: Background Data and Analysis.* Washington, DC: US Government Printing Office; 1988.

3. Plotnick RD. Directions for reducing child poverty. *Social Work.* 1989;34:523-530.

4. Office of Maternal and Child Health. *Child Health USA 1989*. Washington, DC: US Government Printing Office; 1989.
5. Rosenbach ML. The impact of Medicaid on physician use by low-income children. *Am J Public Health*. 1989;79:1220-1226.
6. Bloom B. *Health Insurance and Medical Care: Health of Our Nation's Children, United States, 1988*. Hyattsville, Md: National Center for Health Statistics; 1990.
7. Yudkowsky BK, Cartland JDC, Flint S. Pediatrician participation in Medicaid 1978-1989. *Pediatrics*. 1990;85:567-577.
8. American Academy of Pediatrics, Committee on Environmental Hazards and Committee on Accident and Poison Prevention. Childhood lead poisoning. *Pediatrics*. 1989;83:799-800.
9. American Academy of Pediatrics, Committee on Environmental Hazards. Pesticide residue in the diet of children. *AAP News*. 1989;5:10.
10. Statistical Abstract of the United States. *The National Data Book*. 110th ed. US Department of Commerce, Bureau of the Census; 1990.

BOOK REVIEW

Seizures and Epilepsy in Childhood: A Guide for Parents

By John M. Freeman, Eileen P. G. Vining, and Diana J. Pillas, 287 pp, $18.95, Baltimore, Md, Johns Hopkins University Press, 1990.

Good books for parents of children with seizures are hard to come by. This new volume fills a much-needed gap. Written by two pediatric neurologists and a clinic coordinator–counselor from the Pediatric Epilepsy Center at The Johns Hopkins Medical Institutions (Baltimore, Md), the book addresses both the medical facts about seizure disorders and the fears and concerns of parents.

The book is divided into five parts: why seizures occur; diagnosing and treating seizures and epilepsy; treating seizures and epilepsy; coping with epilepsy; and living with epilepsy. Using clinical examples, tables, and illustrations, the areas are clearly and matter-of-factly reviewed. The "new" and "old" systems of classification of epilepsy are included, as well as simplified neuroanatomy and sample electroencephalograms. Because I agree strongly, I was delighted to see the authors state, "It is not necessary to do a CT or MRI scan on every child who has had a first seizure" (page 103). Discussion of therapy is simple but thorough, as are the chapters on school, driving, participation in sports, insurance, and support organizations such as the Epilepsy Foundation of America.

Toward the end of the book, the authors state, "There are no references in this book because the information about epilepsy is changing and evolving. Parents are encouraged to contact the Epilepsy Foundation of America for further information." This seems like a bit of a shortcut; other references could have been included for completeness. Finally, an excellent glossary is included at the end for parents bewildered by the terminology of epilepsy and seizures.

Peggy C. Ferry, MD
Section of Child Neurology
Department of Pediatrics
University of Arizona
College of Medicine
1501 N Campbell
Tucson, AZ 85724

The Growing Neglect of American Children

Harold M. Maurer, MD

America is not doing enough to meet the health care needs of poor children. Unless we face up to this growing neglect, our nation's future is in doubt. Although we frequently hear that "children are our greatest national resource," we see little evidence to indicate that our policy makers believe it or are willing to act to prevent the terrible waste in human resources as a result of poverty. The money spent on health care for the elderly in America is 15 times that spent on health care for children.[1] Although children represent 50% of the Medicaid population, they receive less than 20% of the money spent for health services.[1] Furthermore, Medicaid reimbursement for health services for children is so low that few physicians in private practice can afford to see Medicaid patients.

The facts regarding impoverished children are staggering. They are cause for concern regarding the values and priorities of our nation. The data speak for themselves.

1. Thirty-seven million American children live in poverty, 9 to 12 million have no health insurance, and millions of others have less than adequate health insurance.[2] Children are the poorest group in society.
2. One in four to six pregnant women lacks health insurance for maternity care, and one in four does not receive prenatal care during the first trimester.[2]
3. The infant mortality rate is higher in America than in some third-world countries. In 1989, there were 9.7 deaths per 1000 live births; it was twice that for blacks.[3]
4. Nearly 5000 low-birth-weight babies are born every week in America.[1] Low birth weight, which, in many instances, is preventable through improved prenatal care for the mother, places these babies at high risk for serious illness and handicapping condi-tions.[1]
5. Each year, as many as 1 million teenagers become pregnant, and 18% of newborn infants in some city hospitals are victims of transplacental exposure to alcohol, crack, and other hard drugs (*The New York Times Magazine.* September 9, 1990:41).
6. One third of poor children are not immunized by the second year of life against measles, mumps, and rubella.[2] Ten percent of children younger than 4 years have not seen a physician in a year.[2] Poor children tend to be taken episodically to costly city or county hospital emergency departments for care, often late in the course of an illness. Because poor children lack a "medical home," they often do not receive continuing care, anticipatory guidance, or counseling, which could eliminate preventable health problems.

America must come to grips with these devastating but correctable problems. We have the knowledge to prevent illness, promote health, and save lives. We must provide access to health and social services for all pregnant women and children through the provision of universal health insurance. The plan proposed by the American Academy of Pediatrics meets this objective, and this plan or an equivalent one should be enacted into law. In addition, we must provide a "medical home" for every pregnant woman and child so that primary health and continuity of care can be provided to promote health. Widening medical coverage alone to cover more pregnant women may not be the answer. Women must be able to enroll before they become pregnant, or else they may become pregnant months before they sign up. The application process also needs to be accelerated and health care should be provided during the processing of the application. We should support all programs, agencies, policies, and strategies that guarantee the full spectrum of health care services for these underserved.

Expanding access to health care will also affect health manpower needs. More primary care physicians will be required to care for the population of pregnant women and children who are currently underserved, or whose needs are not being met. Resident physician education should include a curriculum segment that deals with the specific health care needs of the poor.[4] Moreover, incentives such as loan forgiveness should be created to attract residents to pursue careers in serving the poor.

During the next century, we can expect considerable change in the demographics of our nation. The current migration of people throughout the world is greater than ever before. The distinction between minority and majority groups will fade. In the next century minority groups will become the majority of the population in the United States. It is essential that we recognize this changing environment and begin to provide access to health care for poor women who do not receive prenatal care and for poor children in our society. We must ensure that every child has the opportunity to grow up healthy, gain an education, and become economically productive.

Accepted for publication January 22, 1991.

From the Association of Medical School Pediatric Department Chairmen Inc, Salt Lake City, Utah, and the Department of Pediatrics, Children's Medical Center, Medical College of Virginia, Virginia Commonwealth University, Richmond.

Reprint requests to the Department of Pediatrics, Children's Medical Center, Medical College of Virginia, Virginia Commonwealth University, Richmond, VA 23298 (Dr Maurer).

The following are the members of the Executive Committee of the Association of Medical School Pediatric Department Chairmen Inc: Robert P. Kelch, MD, president; Ralph Feigin, MD, president-elect; Michael A. Simmons, MD, secretary-treasurer; George W. Brumley,

MD; Robert A. Hoekelman, MD; Harold M. Maurer, MD; Donald N. Mederis, Jr, MD; Alfred E. Michael, MD; Carol F. Phillips, MD; Irving Schulman, MD; James A. Stockman III, MD.

References

1. *Myth vs Reality Fact Sheet.* Washington DC: American Academy of Pediatrics Department of Government Liaison. 1990.
2. *A Promise to Keep: A Conference on Cross-National Comparisons of Child Health.* Sponsored by the American Academy of Pediatrics. March 17-19, 1990.
3. Saving infants lives. *Faulkner & Gray's Medicine and Health.* 1990;44:36.
4. *Educating Pediatric Residents to Provide Health Care to Underserved Children.* McLean, Va: Ambulatory Pediatric Association; 1990.

BOOK REVIEW

Difficult Diagnosis in Pediatrics

Edited by J. A. Stockman III, 464 pp, $45, Philadelphia, Pa, WB Saunders Co, 1990.

Books for the general physician who encounters children with difficult diagnoses and management problems are few, but in great demand. The major pediatric textbooks emphasize individual diseases rather than problems of diagnosis and management. This book attempts to fill that void.

The book is divided into two sections. We are told that the first section deals with approaches to evaluations of common problems and that the second section deals with specific disease entities that are difficult to diagnose or to distinguish from similar disorders. I was confused by exactly how each chapter was chosen for one section vs the other, and, therefore, this division into two sections did not help organize the book for me. Nevertheless, each chapter easily stands by itself. The book discusses a broad spectrum of disease categories, but as Stockman warns in his introduction, the list can hardly be comprehensive.

While reading each chapter, it seemed I was sitting at grand rounds listening to the author. Included in the discussion is the pathophysiology of the disease and a thorough differential diagnosis of the problem. The biochemical, radiologic, and other techniques available to evaluate each problem are then described. The chapters are stimulating and often information-packed.

The topics are usually presented with a subspecialty orientation. The bulk of each chapter is not devoted to the most likely diagnosis to be encountered by the generalist but instead focuses on the most difficult disorders for subspecialists to distinguish and diagnose. A good example of this is in the chapter on hyperbilirubinemia. Physiologic and breast milk jaundice are discussed only briefly. Most of the discussion centers on intrahepatic and extrahepatic causes of cholestatic jaundice. The choice of topics also reflects a subspecialty bias. Poor glucose control, chronic interstitial pneumonia, unexplained acidosis, and acute hepatic failure thankfully are only occasionally encountered by most generalists, but are more typical of problems faced by the subspecialist.

There are a few excellent chapters on problems that generalists encounter more frequently. Chapters entitled "Innocent Murmurs," the "Nonsleeping Child," and "Growing Pains" discuss the initial outpatient evaluation and suggest when a more in-depth evaluation will be needed and the optimal time at which the input of a subspecialist will be helpful. The chapter on failure to thrive is one of the best I have read. It minimizes the importance of laboratory screening tests and includes a well-developed discussion of the importance of psychosocial issues in the work-up. Those chapters turned out to be my favorites, but perhaps they give the book too broad an audience.

Busy practitioners will be disappointed if they purchase this book only for quick guidance to the evaluation of a variety of symptoms or problems. While controversies in management and therapeutics are discussed, the discussion focuses on subspecialty procedures. The view presented is that general pediatricians should continue to have input in determining if and when procedures such as skin biopsies, bronchoscopies, or D-xylose absorption tests should be performed, although they rarely perform and/or interpret these evaluations by themselves. This book is not meant to replace the subspecialist.

All general pediatricians undoubtedly will encounter many patients who defy diagnosis and and whose conditions require subspecialty consultation. To manage these patients, the general pediatrician must be able to work with other physicians and coordinate the care of patients with difficult problems. This is a difficult but vital job that requires a tremendous breadth of knowledge to perform well. Books like this are in demand by all physicians who seek to broaden their knowledge and understand the approaches used by specialists. The medical student and pediatric resident working at a referral center, who will see every day the problems discussed in this book, especially will find this book ideal.

Robert Kamei, MD
San Francisco, Calif

The Challenge of Care for the Poor Child

The Research Agenda

Steve Kohl, MD

The Society for Pediatric Research is a diverse group of scientists bonded by the common interest in research dealing with problems of children. Many of the society's members have very strong feelings regarding the social and political problems of health care for the poor and, in particular, health care for poor children. Nevertheless, it is not in the usual scope of our organization to comment as a group on these problems or even to claim particular expertise in this area. Indeed, other segments of the pediatric community have been asked to address these issues, and their efforts can be found in this issue.

As a research-oriented organization, the Society for Pediatric Research can make cogent comments and suggestions concerning the role of investigation in this problem area. In this regard, one must view research in its broadest sense; that is, research on the molecular level at one end to research on the societal level at the other end. There is a clear and pressing role for research methods in identifying the problems facing the poor and in arriving at rational solutions to them on all levels.

To enumerate many of the health problems particularly facing poor children in this country would surely be redundant. I will outline only a few that are of markedly increased incidence in poor children, take a deadly toll, and are obviously amenable to investigation. These include prematurity, perinatal infections (including acquired immunodeficiency syndrome), substance abuse effect on the fetus and infant, infectious diseases of early childhood (notably gastrointestinal and respiratory infections, meningitis, and measles), child abuse, trauma, homicide and suicide, teenage pregnancy, and school failure. The impact of these maladies converts potentially valuable and productive members of society into long-term financial liabilities as well as poignant catastrophes.

Each of these problems can be, and indeed must be, attacked from the research level to find a cogent solution. As an infectious disease expert, I think it is reasonable to use *Haemophilus influenzae* meningitis as an example. This is the most common type of bacterial meningitis in the young child, resulting in considerable sequelae. The incidence of this illness is markedly increased in the poor child.[1,2] The particular epidemiology of various organisms and host interactions can be discerned to determine the reasons for the increased incidence. The relationships of family crowding, day-care center care, and breast-feeding to the increased incidence of meningitis in poor children are being elucidated.[1,2]

The definition of the basic immune response on the molecular level, with particular attention given to possible immune defects in special population groups to the etiologic pathogens,[3] have spurred rational development of vaccines (as we are now seeing with conjugate polysaccharide vaccines). These are active areas of research bearing directly on this particular problem of health care for poor children. Finally, it is critical that research be conducted into systems of health care provision on a societal level that will facilitate reliable access for the poor child to the fruits of the health care system, in this case vaccine provision.

This type of investigation is not as "sexy" as dissection of molecular mechanisms, but in the broad sense is every bit as valid a research question. In this area, as in all other areas, the research must be scientifically rigorous and creative, with a mechanistic, not purely descriptive, approach. Without such research, society would deprive the most financially and health-deficient members of our population of the benefits of the more basic research advances. I have used the specific example of *H influenzae* meningitis, but equally cogent and perhaps more dramatic cases can be made for any of the problems outlined above. While some are less basic (eg, the behavioral problems) than others (eg, acquired immunodeficiency syndrome and infectious diseases), in all there is a complex and as yet poorly understood blend of basic biologic and sociopolitical issues.

Identification of the problems is the first step in finding possible solutions. To arrive at accurate solutions requires research. Again, this must include research in the broadest sense, from the molecular to the societal arena. One promising new approach is the recently established Child Health Research Centers program within the National Institute for Child Health and Human De-velopment. Seven centers were established in 1990 with the expectation of creating "centers of excellence" in a specific subject area, with considerable flexibility provided to promote the development of new pediatric investigators. Unfortunately, with the exception of this new initiative, research in general, and research into child health issues in particular, remains among the lower priorities in this country. With

Accepted for publication November 30, 1990.

From the Division of Pediatric Infectious Diseases, University of California, San Francisco, and San Francisco General Hospital.

Reprint requests to San Francisco General Hospital, 1001 Potrero, 6E9 San Francisco, CA 94110 (Dr Kohl).

the current financial situation, there has been a progressive decline in newly funded research grants and a reduction in funding to established grants. The percentage of funded NIH grants has dropped from 62% in 1974 to an estimated 22% to 24% in 1990.[4-7] I would like to offer a list of possible solutions to these problems:

1. A basic shift in national priorities to acknowledge that the main threat to our security comes from profound internal societal problems, not external military challenges.
2. A fundamental restructuring of budgetary goals to acknowledge the change in national priorities; health care research would be placed closer to the top of the list along with other social and domestic programs.
3. Acknowledgment that problems of the poor child and child health in particular, if not addressed, will lead to crippling problems in society as the demand for productive and increasingly skilled workers accelerates.
4. With this acknowledgment, increased funding of all areas of child health problems becomes vital.
5. Recognition that funding of scientifically rigorous, creative, and mechanistic research into broad societal problems is as valid as research into molecular mechanisms.
6. Similarly, increased awareness in the pediatric academic world, including our medical school departments and research organizations, of the breadth of research, with rewards for the societal-oriented researcher being similar to those for the molecular scientist.
7. Creation of a cadre of pediatric scientists rigorously trained in the social sciences (eg, sociology, economics, and epidemiology) to enable them to contribute to the solution of the broad arena of medicosocial problems of the poor child through research.
8. A rational, long-term plan for stable national funding mechanisms to maintain the fragile research infrastructure, to provide a level of confidence in the research community, and to ensure a continuity of research and training of entry-level researchers.
9. Increased funding for the Child Health Research Centers to allow the opening of more than the initial seven funded centers.
10. Broadening the scope of Child Health Research Centers to include training and research on every level into the problems that affect children, and enhanced coordination of molecular and societal research efforts.
11. Enhanced cooperation among the public sectors of funding and the private sectors, including foundations and industry, regarding child health problems.

The problems we face in child health care, and child health care of the poor in particular, are immense. Nevertheless, they are every bit as amenable to solution as those involving Middle East oil or the savings and loan institutions. Indeed, health care problems will erode this nation's security as surely as will the more publicized national and international problems. The most efficient solutions to the problems of child health involve the traditional research methods focused on a broad plane. Once a reliable database is established and interventional techniques are validated, the solutions themselves can be instituted. Some believe that a conflict exists between research and health care for the poor, since each requires scarce resources. It is my contention that this nation is wealthy enough to fund both adequately once we reorder our priorities. Indeed, it will be the poor, so disproportionately burdened by ill health, who will benefit the most from the fruits of all research advances.

The theme of the 1991 Society for Pediatric Research's Presidential State of the Art Symposium (occurring at our annual meeting in May in New Orleans, La) is entitled "The Medical-Social Crisis in Child Health." The main areas discussed will include an overview of the vulnerable child, pediatric acquired immunodeficiency syndrome, substance abuse, and health care access for children. Thus, the research societies are acknowledging and beginning to come to grips with these issues. It will be up to the nation to further use the tools of pediatric research to aid in the solution of these problems.

I would like to thank the following people for their reviews and helpful comments: Larry J. Shapiro, MD, president-elect of the Society for Pediatric Research, Department of Pediatrics, UCLA School of Medicine, Los Angeles, Calif; Thomas N. Hansen, MD, secretary-treasurer of the Society for Pediatric Research, Baylor College of Medicine, Houston, Tex; Moses Grossman, MD, University of California Medical School and San Francisco General Hospital; Richard E. Behrman, MD, Stanford (Calif) University and the Center for the Future of Children, David and Lucille Packard Foundation, Los Altos, Calif; and Myron Genel, MD, Yale University, New Haven, Conn, chairman of the Public Policy Council.

References

1. Cochi SL, Fleming DW, Hightower AW, et al. Primary invasive *Haemophilus influenzae* type b disease: a population-based assessment of risk factors. *J Pediatr.* 1986;108:887-896.
2. Wilfert CM. Epidemiology of *Haemophilus influenzae* type b infection. *Pediatrics.* 1990;85:631-635.
3. Granoff DM, Sheetz K, Pandey JP, et al. Host and bacterial factors associated with *Haemophilus influenzae* type b disease in Minnesota children vaccinated with type b polysaccharide vaccine. *J Infect Dis.* 1989;159:908-916.
4. Cassman M. Issues behind the drop in the NIH award rate. *ASM News.* 1990;56:465-469.
5. Institute of Medicine. *1990 Funding Health Sciences Research: A Strategy to Restore Balance.* Washington, DC: National Academy of Sciences; 1990.
6. Kennedy DE. The rising cost of NIH-funded biomedical research? *Acad Med.* 1990;65:63-73.
7. Kelley DM. NIH Funding for biomedical research, 1990: perceptions and reality. *Endocrinology.* 1990;126:2233-2236.

Serving the Underserved

Impact on Resident Education

Carol D. Berkowitz, MD

Numerous obstacles stand in the way of universal access to health care.[1,2] Some of these barriers are political, and influencing them is more problematic, slow, and subject to the climate of the time. Other aspects may be addressed by increasing the pool of physicians aware of and involved in the issues of serving the underserved.

The Ambulatory Pediatric Association (APA), under the leadership of Paul McCarthy, MD, began addressing the issue of serving the underserved in March 1990. A conference, cosponsored by the APA and the Bureau of Maternal and Child Health, was convened. Participants in the conference included nurses, social workers, and physicians, many of whom were chief residents in their respective training programs. These individuals were representative of different regions in our nation and cared for different populations within these regions. Participants were asked to address one aspect of the impact of underserved children on resident education.[3] The proceedings of this conference have been published and distributed.[4] The reasons for this focus on education were multiple. It is readily apparent that the underserved represent a diverse group, including a large portion of financially disadvantaged and/or geographically isolated children (rural and migrant workers). Care of these children, particularly the economically restricted, often falls into the bailiwick of pediatricians in training. By properly preparing these (and all) residents, not only may health care be improved for the children, but commitment and advocacy by the house staff may be encouraged. How will this be achieved? The purpose of this article is to outline the means to accomplish this end.

The APA took on as a project the development of a strategic plan regarding residency education. This plan has both short- and long-term objectives. The major short-term objective is the development of a core curriculum of fundamental knowledge, of necessary skills, and of unique techniques for resident education. Methods for curriculum implementation will also be defined.

The first curriculum category concerns what can broadly be referred to as clinical issues. First, the house officer needs to be able to identify the underserved individual and recognize the numerous barriers (ie, financial, governmental, geographic, institutional, or personal) to health care. The second clinical issue addresses the *specific* health problems of the underserved and educates individuals about diseases unique to or at higher incidence among certain populations. An example of this would be recognizing and being prepared to treat conditions such as tuberculosis, child abuse and neglect, and dental caries among migrant farm workers and their children.[5]

A third clinical issue involves the teaching of the interpersonal aspects of care, focusing on psychosocial issues and interviewing skills. The means to teach these to house officers have been eloquently addressed by Julia Hamilton, MSW, CISW, a social worker from Yale–New Haven (Conn) Medical Center.[6] Ms Hamilton teaches about the "five C" model of intervention. These five stages include caring, confrontation, creativity, culture, and closure. The stages are consecutive and developmental, and require mastery of one before proceeding to the next. They are practical and readily learned by house officers. Caring means demonstrating to the patient (by touching or through statements) that one cares. Confrontation involves open discussions with patients about their goals and expectations from the health care system. Creativity includes role modeling or reframing things for patients and their parents. Culture means being sensitive not just to ethnic differences, but to the culture of poverty. Last, closure means letting go, and allowing the family to solve its problems on its own. The goal of Ms Hamilton's five C model is to nurture the unnurtured. Intimately integrated in the clinical issues is teaching the house staff to identify strengths in families and children and to utilize these strengths while providing health care. These families can often benefit from a family systems approach.[7]

In addition to teaching the resident about clinical issues, the curriculum must also include community or environmental issues. First, one must address ecology, the relationship of the child to his or her environment, family, and the social systems that regulate his or her life. One must be knowledgeable about public laws, such as 94-142, that affect the care of children. Likewise, the physician must know about available categorical programs, such as the Special Supplemental Food Program for Women, Infants, and Children; Aid to Families With Dependent Children; and Medicaid, and help patients achieve access to these programs.[8] The issues of advocacy, ethics, and the legislative process should be addressed in a formal way. Didactic sessions, as well as opportunities to become in-

Accepted for publication November 19, 1990.
From the Ambulatory Pediatric Association, McLean, Va, and the Department of Pediatrics, UCLA School of Medicine.

Reprint requests to Department of Pediatrics, Harbor/UCLA Medical Center, 1000 W Carson St, BIN 437, Torrance, CA 90509 (Dr Berkowitz).

volved in organizations geared to muster change, should be offered.

The house officer needs to be taught about the organization of health care systems. Included in this is formal instruction on practice management.[9] Residents should be given career counseling. The realities of reimbursement should be taught. Residents should be encouraged (inspired) to assume some responsibility for the health care of individuals whose major barrier is a financial one. Instruction about health care access and barriers, both financial and otherwise, should be given.

How many training programs already address these issues, and what methods are available to teaching house staff about serving the underserved? The APA is developing a questionnaire to assess the extent of such programs. It is hoped that programs with an established curriculum will make their curriculum available to others.

There are key methods in teaching residents to care for the underserved. First, institutions may develop rosters of faculty mentors, individuals who are knowledgeable about the issues of the underserved, who care for the underserved, and who are role models for young physicians. Such faculty members are often the ones who are overworked and overutilized. They often do not have time to do what they do, much less take on additional tasks as mentors. However, academic acknowledgment for their contribution would validate the importance of their role. Didactic lectures are another forum in which to teach about serving the underserved. These may be included in continuing care conferences. The continuing care clinic, for many house officers, is an excellent setting in which to recognize psychosocial and medical concerns of underserved children.[10] The five C model of intervention could be incorporated in this setting.[6] Block rotations could be developed, particularly in specific underserved communities. Institutions could develop "exchange" programs to allow for greater exposure of house staff to different underserved populations. Examples of such block rotations would include the homeless, migrant children, inner-city health care, etc. Built into these rotations, or as a separate part of the training experience, would be structured extramural experiences such as home visits, or visits to the welfare office. Such experiences are meant to help the house officer understand and empathize with the day-today struggle many of the underserved face.

The educational experience of working on a multidisciplinary team cannot be overstated. The purpose of such exposure is to increase the skills of the house officer through contact with individuals with greater expertise in areas such as interviewing.[11] The use of timely feedback using tools such as videotaping is also important to the teaching of communication skills.[12]

The appropriate timing of this instruction is also important. It is critical to use the orientation process to teach the house staff about the demographics of the people for whom they are caring. Likewise, a separate house staff retreat, away from the hectic hospital setting, is to be encouraged as a means to reinspire house staff and focus on these issues. The idealism of the medical student is lost (or put on the back burner) after graduation by the new demands and responsibilities of being a house officer.[13]

In addition to working toward developing a curriculum, organizations such as the APA should work to affect public policy to encourage resident education in the area of underserved children. For example, state and federal programs that would fund initiatives in resident education regarding the underserved should be encouraged. Inclusion of instruction on caring for the underserved should be a priority in all federally funded primary care programs. Primary-care fellowships with a focus on the underserved should be developed.

Likewise, financial issues related to the underserved should be addressed. Physicians need to be encouraged to join organizations that actively lobby for universal access to health care regardless of financial status. Physicians, individually and as members of organizations, should then be encouraged to support agencies (eg, the Health Resources and Services Administration and the Bureau of Maternal and Child Health) that focus on the underserved and support health policies that provide full funding or primary-care services and a full spectrum of care for the underserved. Loan forgiveness for those pursuing careers in serving the underserved should be encouraged.

The APA as an organization is firmly committed to the issue of serving the underserved. To date, the organization has held a conference exploring this issue and the impact that underserved children have on residency education. The APA has chosen to focus on teaching house staff about underserved children as one approach to combating the problem. It is both hoped and anticipated that better training of house officers will result in a pool of physicians who are not only more knowledgeable about health care issues of the underserved, but also more willing to care for such children, and serve as advocates and forces for change.

References

1. Hubbell A, Waitzkin H, Mishra SI, Dombrink J. Evaluating health care needs of the poor: a community-oriented approach. *Am J Med.* 1989;87:127-131.
2. Schmidt DD. The challenge of caring for the underserved. *Fam Med.* 1989;21:257-260.
3. Lurie N, Yergan J. Teaching residents to care for vulnerable populations in the outpatient setting. *J Gen Intern Med.* 1989;5(suppl):526.
4. *Educating Pediatric Residents to Provide Health Care to Underserved Children.* McLean, Va: Ambulatory Pediatric Association; 1990.
5. Markello J. Children of migrant farm workers living in rural poverty. In: *Educating Pediatric Residents to Provide Health Care to Underserved Children.* Alexandria, Va: Ambulatory Pediatric Association; 1990:63-69.
6. Hamilton J. The process of helping residents learn how to nurture the unnurtured. In: *Educating Pediatric Residents to Provide Health Care to Underserved Children.* Alexandria, Va: Ambulatory Pediatric Association; 1990:11-15.
7. Allmond BW Jr, Buckman W, Gofman HF. *The Family Is the Patient: An Approach to Behavioral Pediatrics for the Clinician.* St Louis, Mo: CV Mosby Co; 1979.
8. Modena W. Serving the underserved: public policy issues. In: *Educating Pediatric Residents to Provide Health Care to Underserved Children.* Alexandria, Va: Ambulatory Pediatric Association; 1990:29-34.
9. Berkelhamer JE. The organization of practice for underserved children: implications for resident education. In: *Educating Pediatric Residents to Provide Health Care to Underserved Children.* Alexandria, Va: Ambulatory Pediatric Association; 1990:29-34.
10. Hodge RH. The method for assuring continuity of care in residency training experience. *J Med Educ.* 1977;52:739-744.
11. Berkowitz C. Comprehensive pediatric management of failure to thrive: an interdisciplinary approach. In: Drotar D, ed. *New Directions in Failure to Thrive.* New York, NY: Plenum Press; 1985.
12. Menahem S. Interviewing and examination skills in pediatric medicine: videotape analysis of student and consultant performance. *J R Soc Med.* 1987;80:138-142.
13. Thomas CB. What becomes of medical students: the dark side. *Johns Hopkins Med J.* 1976;139:185-195.

The Challenge of Care for the Poor and Underserved in the United States

An American College of Obstetricians and Gynecologists Perspective on Access to Care for Underserved Women

Ezra C. Davidson, Jr, MD; Charles E. Gibbs, MD; Janet Chapin, MPH

● Access to pregnancy-related care for women and their infants and to reproductive health services for adolescents are significant concerns to the American College of Obstetricians and Gynecologists (ACOG). Adolescent and young adult women are among those most likely to be uninsured and lack access to health care services. Adolescent pregnancy, low-birth weight, and infant mortality remain major national burdens. The ACOG has taken the position that quality health care should be accessible to all women. The ACOG recommendations regarding health services for adolescents and the ACOG Committee on Health Care for Underserved Women's statement of principles regarding universal access for pregnancy-related care, which includes the basic scope of benefits, the characteristics of the providers, and the organization of services are described.

(*AJDC*. 1991;145:546-549)

In 1988, more than 794 000 women did not receive prenatal care in the first trimester of pregnancy.[1] Every year, more than 10% of all 15- to 19-year-old women become pregnant.[2] Access to care for underserved women—in particular, pregnancy-related care for women and their infants and reproductive health services for adolescents—is a significant concern to the American College of Obstetricians and Gynecologists (ACOG). More than 30 reports and policy recommendations have been published in the past 5 years alone on the subjects of infant mortality and access to pregnancy-related services.[3] Reports on adolescent pregnancy have multiplied, reflecting the concerns about pregnancies in this age group. Although some responses to the recommendations have been forthcoming at the state and federal levels, much more is needed before we will see significant improvements in health status. The time for study is past. Although we always need current data, it is time now to move forward to implement many of these recommendations.

Accepted for publication January 24, 1991.

From the American College of Obstetricians and Gynecologists, Washington, DC.

Reprint requests to American College of Obstetricians and Gynecologists, 409 12th St SW, Washington, DC 20024-2188 (Ms Chapin).

THE PROBLEMS

Lack of health insurance decreases the likelihood that a woman will receive appropriate health care.[4] In 1985, of the women of reproductive age, 26% did not have insurance to cover maternity care, and 15% of the 3.7 million births in that year were to women with no health insurance coverage.[5]

One measure of access is entry into prenatal care. In 1988, for the nation as a whole, 24% of the women who gave birth did not receive prenatal care in the first trimester of pregnancy, and 6% received little or no care at all before delivery. For black women, the situation was worse; 40% did not receive care in the first trimester, and 11% received little or no care during pregnancy.[1]

Access to prenatal care is a major factor associated with low birth weight and infant mortality.[6] The personal and public costs of the stubbornly high percentage of low-birth-weight infants remain a national burden. The Office of Technology Assessment has estimated that a single low-birth-weight infant incurs between $12 000 to $40 000 in short-term hospital costs.[7] Handicapping conditions occur in approximately 5% to 16% of the low-birth-weight infants treated in today's neonatal intensive care units.[7] Long-term domiciliary and education costs for these disabled children are estimated at $6000 to $37 000 per year.[8]

In addition, adolescents and young adults are among the groups more likely to be uninsured for health care services. As of 1984, about one in every seven adolescents, approximately 4.5 million adolescents aged 10 to 18 years, had no health insurance coverage. Black adolescents were 63% more likely than white adolescents to be uninsured. Hispanic adolescents were nearly three times as likely as non-Hispanic whites to be uninsured. Adolescents living in families earning less than the federal poverty standard were three times more likely than their nonpoor counterparts to be uninsured.[9]

More than 6 million young adults, 26% of those 19 to 24 years old, were uninsured in 1984. Hispanic, black, poor and near poor, unemployed, and high school dropouts were among those young adults most likely to be without insurance. Three fourths of white young adults 19 to 24 years of age had private insurance compared with only half of blacks of the same age. More than 40% of Hispanics had no insurance, twice the rate of non-Hispanic whites.[9] One of the most troubling issues in adolescent health care is adolescent pregnancy. More than 1 million adolescents become pregnant every year in the United States.[2] The birth rate for teens aged 15 to 17 years rose in 1988 for the first time in a decade, to 33.8 births per 1000 women aged 15 to 17 years.[1] Compared with the rate in other developed countries, the pregnancy rate among American teenagers is among the highest in the world. It is twice the rate in England, Wales, and Canada, three times that in Sweden, and more than six times the rate in the Netherlands.[2]

ACOG RECOMMENDATIONS

Since 1971, ACOG has taken the position that quality health care should be accessible to all women.[10] This position was reaffirmed in a policy statement adopted in July 1988.[11] Since 1985, through its Committee on Health Care for Underserved Women, ACOG has addressed various components of the problems related to access to care. The ACOG also has a long-standing interest in the development of adequate, comprehensive, and high-quality health services for adolescents, with special reference to reproductive health services. Since 1964, ACOG has organized initiatives in the area of adolescent health. Over the years, more than 10 policy statements, as well as numerous other reports and committee statements regarding adolescent health, have been issued. In 1985, ACOG began a public education program that broke network television barriers that prevented the provision of good, reliable information on unintended pregnancy to the American public.

SERVICES FOR ADOLESCENTS

The ACOG holds the position that health services for adolescents must be broad in scope and must be provided in the context of adequate education, social services, and family support. Health education that includes education regarding sexuality and reproduction, beginning early in a child's life, is a cornerstone of effective reproductive health services.

Moreover, contraception and family planning services must be available and accessible for all women, regardless of age, whose sexual behavior exposes them to the risk of unintended pregnancy. Contraceptive services should be offered, whenever possible, in a general health care setting that includes counseling regarding psychosocial considerations and sexually transmitted diseases. Much more outreach and publicity should be undertaken to inform sexually active adolescents about the importance and safety of contraceptive use, as well as to assist them in locating and accessing services. The ACOG has called for responsible advertising of prescription and over-the-counter contraceptives and has indicated that it would be willing to work with publishers and broadcasters to make sure the advertising claims were accurate and scientifically verifiable.[12]

The ACOG endorses the programs, including those located in schools, that provide reproductive health services in areas where such services are not available and where such services have the support and input of parents and communities. These programs appear to be most effective when they are offered within a system of comprehensive health care services. One aim of such programs should be to encourage sexually responsible behavior that is both nondestructive and nonexploitive. The ACOG also supports the recommendations of the National Academy of Science's report *Risking the Future: Adolescent Sexuality, Pregnancy and Childbearing,* including the need to mainta the availability of adoption and abortion as needed optior for adolescents.[13]

The issue of confidentiality has been identified by both providers and young people as having a significant impact on access to health care. This is particularly true for reproductive health services. Health professionals have an ethical obligation to provide the best possible care and counseling in response to the needs of their adolescent patients. This obligation includes reasonable efforts to encourage the adolescent to involve her or his parents in health care decisions. The support of parents can, in many instances, increase the potential for resolving the adolescent's problems on a continuing basis. The restrictive laws and regulations affecting confidentiality found in many jurisdictions are often impediments to care and need to be revised as a matter of public policy. The ACOG, in collaboration with the American Academy of Family Physicians, the American Academy of Pediatrics, NAACOG—the Organization of Obstetric, Gynecologic and Neonatal Nurses, and the National Medical Association, has developed a policy statement on confidentiality, since such assurances are essential to serve adolescents effectively. This policy statement sets forth the obligation of the providers of adolescent health care to protect confidentiality, as well as suggesting methods for clarifying the relationship to the adolescent and her or his parents.[14]

IMPROVING ACCESS TO PREGNANCY-RELATED CARE FOR UNDERSERVED WOMEN

Although access to all health services is important for women of all ages, among the most critical needs is access to pregnancy-related care. The ACOG Committee on Health Care for Underserved Women has developed a statement of principles regarding universal access for pregnancy-related care and the necessary characteristics of any legislation or plan that would provide such care.

The ACOG is aware of the importance of controlling costs, and this statement of principles regarding universal access should not be seen as a call for unrestrained spending. To the contrary, the college believes that comprehensive pregnancy-related care, appropriate to the various needs of each patient, is worth the initial costs and will contribute importantly to cost containment. For example, a good system of care will facilitate rapid and accurate evaluation of the effectiveness and the role of new technologies and therefore is likely to prevent unnecessary, expensive services. Administering authorities and financing plans for universal access need to be specified, but these issues are beyond the scope of the current development of the ACOG statement of principles.

Universal Access

Access to the full range of pregnancy-related services (see the list below) should be provided for all women and infants who live in the United States. It is important to note that these principles do not call for all women and infants to be covered under a single program, but there must be certain characteristics common to all coverage. Minimum benefits for all coverage and the eligibility requirements for any publicly funded and operated program should be established across the nation. Care must be organized and delivered in a manner appropriate for, and acceptable to, the pregnant woman and her family. Current public and private resources should be used whenever possible. Any unded and operated health services must be kept separate, administratively and financially, from assistance/welfare programs.

Scope of Services in Maternal and Infant Care

The ACOG Committee on Health Care for Underserved Women has established the following list of basic elements of care to which it is particularly important to ensure accessibility. Pregnancy-related care must be understood as broad in scope and variable in intensity and complexity. To the degree that an element is needed but missing or inadequate, the care is deficient. Additional emphasis should be placed on prevention and early intervention in all services, and all services should be coordinated and linked.

Planning pregnancy, and the prevention of those pregnancies that are unplanned, is an important strategy to improve maternal and infant health. All women in the United States should have access to family planning and contraceptive services.

Additionally, ACOG actively supports individual choice in regard to abortion as a necessary and safe option for all women. This position is based on the belief that decisions concerning abortion are so bound in ethical, moral, and religious complexities, as well as other personal considerations, that they are best left to a woman in consultation with her physician. The ACOG believes that continued availability of safe, legal abortion services is essential to maternal health.

A prepregnancy-related health examination is important to identify behavioral and medical factors that require modification before pregnancy to improve outcome, such as control of diabetes or smoking cessation, and should be available to all women. This evaluation is not meant to include infertility services. Additionally, early pregnancy diagnosis facilitates appropriate and timely prenatal care and should be available.

Prenatal, pregnancy-related services should be based on risk assessment with an appropriate response and include care for new or preexisting conditions that affect the pregnancy, fetal evaluation, health and childbirth education, nutritional support and counseling, substance abuse counseling and treatment, and linkage of prenatal care and delivery.

Labor and delivery should be provided in an optimal, risk-appropriate environment, as should neonatal care appropriate to the needs of the infant. Postpartum evaluation and services, including family planning and postpartum sterilization, and infant follow-up for at least 1 year should be provided after delivery. Social services support as needed should be provided throughout the pregnancy and follow-up period.

Provider Characteristics

Providers of pregnancy-related services include health care professionals and such institutions as laboratories, hospitals, health departments, and community and migrant health centers. All providers should be licensed or certified when license is not required in their jurisdiction and subject to a quality review process involving peer review. There must be a sufficient number of providers, and they must be of the appropriate disciplines required to render all of the necessary services. The relationships between the primary and referral levels of care, and between the various disciplines involved in care, should be clearly defined in contractual documents between providers. Such agreements tend to clarify both responsibility and authority and also describe the extent to which any provider should commit resources. These contracts should contain cancellation clauses and should be renegotiated at regular intervals.

Organization of Services

Maternal and infant health services may be delivered by both private and publicly funded and operated services. There are, however, certain characteristics that are important for all components. The focus of care should be health-outcome oriented. However, outreach (recruitment) for both patients and providers should be supported financially, and undergraduate, graduate, and continuing education should be supported to provide an ongoing supply of qualified providers. Additionally, research designed to improve patient care should be identified and a suitable environment for investigation encouraged.

The organization and methods used to deliver services should be efficient and cost-effective and responsive to patient needs. Both the management and clinical components of the programs should be evaluated by means of outcome and process objectives, and these evaluation results should be used in decision making. All types of qualified health care professionals and other providers should be used, and incentives must be available to encourage the provision of services in geographic areas that are difficult to serve.

Certain administrative characteristics are important for any private or public organization or agency that pays for health services. There must be a simple, responsive, and prompt paper and reimbursement flow for patients and providers. Easy access to decision makers and clerical-level workers is essential for both patients and providers. Furthermore, reliable, sufficient, and consistent funding mechanisms must be present.

Additional characteristics apply specifically to those that are publicly funded and operated. The administrating agency should have a simple table of organization with clear lines of responsibility. Clinical expertise should be present within the senior management, with assurance of both professional and consumer input at the governance level. Where or when it is necessary to restrict the breadth or depth of the services to be supported or provided, the selection of the services included or excluded should be determined by a group including both health care professionals and lay persons. The particulars of reimbursement, quality assurance, and utilization review should be specified through a negotiated contract between the provider and the administrating authority. Health services should be completely separate from welfare services, in attitude and approach.

CONCLUSION: FUTURE ACTIONS

The ACOG will continue its organizational focus on these issues through two permanently established committees of its executive board. In 1990, a specific goal of advocacy for access to prenatal care for all women was articulated by the ACOG. A significant portion of ACOG's government relations activity focuses on improving access to quality health care. The college believes that this nation has a moral obligation to ensure health care for women and children at the most vulnerable time in their lives. Furthermore, providing effective maternal and infant care is cost-effective for our society as a whole.

Public education must continue to focus on the consequences that will result if we fail to improve the system of health care for pregnant women and infants in this country. The ACOG intends to educate its fellows about how to improve systems of health care and access to care and to solicit their involvement, in conjunction with government and other policy makers, in actively working toward these solutions.

Perhaps one of our most important activities is the recently established National Fetal and Infant Mortality Review Program. With grant support from the Maternal and Child Health Bureau, we have brought together many organizations to provide guidance and assistance to communities to identify the specific causes of fetal and infant mortality in their areas and to develop solutions targeted to those specific problems.

Several other aspects of this nation's health care delivery system must be repaired if access to care for the poor and the uninsured is to be guaranteed.

The problems regarding professional liability must be ameliorated by ensuring care for affected infants and support for their families. To promote self-discipline in the profession, there must be protection for those who participate in peer review and sanctioning activities.

In addition, difficulties surrounding referrals, transfers of high-risk patients, and the provision of consultation must be resolved in ways that both protect patients and allow physicians to provide appropriate levels of care for higher-risk patients. Furthermore, reimbursement and compensation for nurses, technical workers, and hospitals must be enhanced.

It is clear that public hospitals and health departments, which constitute only a portion of the current system, can no longer be expected to bear the major burden of providing care for the poor and uninsured without a greatly increased level of support.

It is naive to assume that one organization or group of organizations alone, such as organized medicine, no matter how well intentioned, can solve the problems of access to care. What is needed in this country, as in other countries, is leadership and the social will to make sure that universal access to care becomes a reality.

A history of ACOG activities in adolescent health care and a summary of all ACOG policies regarding adolescent health are available from the Resource Center of the American College of Obstetricians and Gynecologists, 409 12th St SW, Washington, DC 20024-2188.

References

1. National Center for Health Statistics. Advance report of final natality statistics, 1988. *Monthly Vital Stat Rep.* 1990;39(4; suppl):1-48.

2. Henshaw SK, Kenney AH, Somberg D, Van Vort J. *Teenage Pregnancy in the United States: The Scope of the Problem and State Responses.* New York, NY: Alan Guttmacher Institute; 1989.

3. Healthy mothers, healthy babies: recent policy recommendations. In: *Supplement to a Compendium of Program Ideas for Serving Low Income Women.* Washington, DC: US Dept of Health and Human Services, Public Health Service, Health Resources and Services Administration, Maternal and Child Health Bureau; January 1990:1-4.

4. *Medicaid Recipients and Uninsured Women Obtain Insufficient Care.* Washington, DC: United States General Accounting Office; September 1987.

5. *Blessed Events and the Bottom Line: Financing Maternity Care in the United States.* New York, NY: Alan Guttmacher Institute; 1987.

6. Brown S, ed. *Preventing Low Birthweight.* Washington, DC: National Academy Press; 1985.

7. *Neonatal Intensive Care for Low Birthweight Infants: Costs and Effectiveness, Health Technology Case Study 38.* Washington, DC: Congress of the United States, Office of Technology Assessment; December 1987.

8. *Healthy Children: Investing in the Future.* Washington, DC: Congress of the United States, Office of Technology Assessment; February 1988. OTA-H-345.

9. Newacheck PW, McManus MA, Brindis C. Financing health care for adolescents: problems, prospects, and proposals. *J Adolesc Health Care.* 1990;11:398-403.

10. American College of Obstetricians and Gynecologists. National health care for women. *Obstet Gynecol.* 1972;39:603-608.

11. *Access to Women's Health Care: ACOG Policy Statement.* Washington, DC: American College of Obstetricians and Gynecologists; 1988.

12. *Contraceptive Advertising: ACOG Policy Statement.* Washington, DC: American College of Obstetricians and Gynecologists; 1987.

13. Hayes C, ed. *Risking the Future: Adolescent Sexuality, Pregnancy and Childbearing.* Washington, DC: National Academy Press; 1987.

14. *Confidentiality in Adolescent Health Care: ACOG Policy Statement.* Washington, DC: American College of Obstetricians and Gynecologists; 1988.

Poverty and Cardiac Disease in Children

Hugh D. Allen, MD; Kathryn A. Taubert, PhD; Richard J. Deckelbaum, MD; David Driscoll, MD; Ann Dunnigan, MD; Samuel S. Gidding, MD; Paul Herndon, MD; Rae-Ellen W. Kavey, MD; Charles Mullins, MD; A. Rebecca Snider, MD; William B. Strong, MD; Reginald Washington, MD

Almost 80 million children live in the United States. At least eight of every 1000 infants born each year have congenital heart defects.[1] When mortality and spontaneous defect improvement are factored into live birth data, Roberts and Cretin[2] estimated that by 1995 there will be 300 000 children under the age of 21 years with congenital heart disease; 38% will have had one or more surgical procedures. Other children will develop acquired heart disease, such as cardiomyopathies, rheumatic fever, acquired immunodeficiency syndrome with its myocarditis, Kawasaki disease, and arrhythmias. The projected incidence estimate for supraventricular tachycardia alone is between one and four per 1000.[3] Familial hypercholesterolemia will affect the future of an unknown but probably large number of children. Therefore, at least one-half million children in the United States have some form of cardiac problem.

One quarter to one third[4,5] of the more than 4 million infants born each year[6] are born into poverty. Therefore, approximately 150 000 to 200 000 children have the problems of both being poor and having heart disease. Considering the birth rate and incidence of heart disease, 8000 to 10 000 infants with heart problems will be added to this population each year. The impact of illegal immigrants on the overall population figure is unknown. Additionally, the assignment of the term *poverty* for a family of four at $12 675 is probably unrealistic; according to the National Center for Health Statistics, many families will still live in poverty even at a breakpoint of $20 000.[7] Some families with incomes greater than $20 000 live in a notch group between poverty and affordability. These groups will further inflate the numbers of poor children with heart problems.

Nearly every child who has been diagnosed as having a heart problem will require some follow-up care. In the Baltimore-Washington Infant Study, for example, among all patients with heart disease diagnosed during the 1st year of life, more than 80% required ongoing pediatric cardiology visits. Furthermore, about 50% required invasive diagnostic procedures and approximately 40% needed cardiac surgery (C. Ferencz, MD, MPH, Principal Investigator, Baltimore-Washington Infant Study, unpublished data, 1981-1987). Regardless of ability to pay, affected children require access to the pediatric cardiac health care system.

Accepted for publication November 19, 1990.

From the Committee on Congenital Cardiac Defects, the Committee on Atherosclerosis and Hypertension in Childhood, and the Committee on Rheumatic Fever, Endocarditis, and Kawasaki Disease of the Council on Cardiovascular Disease in the Young of the American Heart Association, Dallas, Tex.

Reprint requests to Office of Scientific Affairs, American Heart Association, 7320 Greenville Ave, Dallas, TX 75231 (Dr Taubert).

UNIQUENESS OF THE POVERTY POPULATION

Pregnant women who live in poverty have less prenatal care than affluent patients. This creates a problem for certain fetal conditions that must be detected in enough time to institute treatment that will allow fetal salvage. For example, fetal echocardiography permits the diagnosis of supraventricular tachycardia in hydropic fetuses. These can be successfully treated by administration of antiarrhythmic drugs to the mother. Otherwise the fetus could die. Detection and careful control of the diabetic mother results in less frequent occurrence of diabetic cardiomyopathy in the newborn. Maternal drug abuse and acquired immunodeficiency syndrome are both associated with poverty and with newborn cardiac disorders.[8-10]

The poor have greater exposure to certain environmental risk factors, such as lead, solvents, traffic and factory emissions, and pesticides.[11,12] They can be exposed to these atmospheric teratogens both at home and in the workplace.

The poor have a higher illiteracy rate, often have large families, and often experience difficulty accessing (or paying for) transportation to cardiac care for their children. This is especially the situation for the rural poor. The quality of the system accessed can be variable. All these factors contribute to fewer postnatal visits where early detection of cardiovascular disorders can make a significant difference in the survival rate of children who have potentially treatable lesions that are lethal if not detected and treated.

Subsequent problems of infants and older children with heart disease include availability of and receiving immunizations, proper nutrition, and ability to comply with ongoing treatment plans, including filling prescriptions. If the child with a significant cardiac defect becomes infected with, for example, pertussis, that superimposed disease could prove fatal in the already compromised patient. Children with cyanotic heart disease, those with congestive heart failure, and those being prepared for operation or who have had an operation require proper nutrition to maintain growth and to keep up with increased energy intake demands imposed by their condition. The child may receive an initial prescription provided by a cardiologist; however, access to a pharmacy or ability to afford the sometimes very expensive drugs necessary to control the child's condition may prevent the parent from providing that medication on an ongoing basis. Compliance with administration of the medication is sometimes compromised by problems as simple as the parent's inability to read and understand the directions printed on the label.

Older children in the poverty level have more risk factors for cardiovascular disease as adults than do the affluent. These include at least hypertension, smoking, and diet. With their known increased exposure to drug abuse, they have a greater risk of endocarditis, of acquired immunodeficiency syndrome with its myocarditis, and of their own offspring having congenital heart disease, such as that encountered with exposure to cocaine and alcohol. Rheumatic fever has always been primarily considered a disease of the poor, and studies from the 1970s and 1980s continue to show this pattern.[13-15] Recent data show that rheumatic fever attacks are still being reported in all areas of the country.[16] Other published focal experiences have shown that numbers of cases of acute rheumatic fever are increasing at least in these areas, which may or may not portend a national phenomenon.[17-21] Compliance with ongoing prophylactic measures for prevention of secondary attacks of rheumatic fever is compromised by poverty, access to medication, and understanding of the disease process.

COVERAGE PATTERNS

Crippled Children's Services or Medicaid coverage is available to many poor children with heart disease. For those who can afford it, insurance is available but may not be granted to those with preexisting conditions. With rising costs of health insurance, insurance may not be affordable to those just above the poverty level no matter whether the condition is covered or not. Certain groups have unique problems. These include the young adult over 21 years of age who previously had Crippled Children's Services coverage but no longer qualifies because of age. Another is the young adult who leaves college and/or reaches the age of 23 years and is no longer eligible for parental private health insurance coverage. If these patients are faced with the need for a major intervention, such as cardiac surgery, their lack of coverage, no matter what profession they have entered, may move them into poverty. This group was much smaller in the past because many of these children did not survive into adulthood. However, surgical and medical advances have improved the survival and quality of life for these young adult cardiac patients, and many more will enter adulthood during the next decades.

A notch group of those parents who do not qualify for public assistance yet cannot afford private insurance can be similarly devastated by an expensive interventional procedure that is considered necessary for treating their child's cardiac condition. This sometimes presents the dilemma of either entering poverty or not treating the heart problem.

Only 53% of the children below the poverty line are covered by Medicaid for reasons of either not qualifying, not applying, or not understanding the application.[22] Most states limit children's Medicaid eligibility level, some to a level as low as 14% of the poverty line.[23] Particularly affecting the cardiac patient is that several states limit the number of hospital days covered and/or the number of physician visits allowed.[24]

Since the introduction of the "War on Poverty" 25 years ago and the birth of Medicare/Medicaid, a dramatic but not yet adequate reduction in the percentage of the elderly classified as "poor" (28.5% in 1966 to 12.4% in 1986) has been achieved.[23] During the same time span, children have formed the majority of the poverty population (the so-called new poor) and also represent the segment with the least insurance coverage.[23,25] Over 4 million children uninsured and living in poverty are not eligible for Medicaid.[26] The popular press has also recently discussed this problem. *Time* magazine reported that between 1978 and 1987, spending on programs for the elderly rose 52% while spending on children dropped 4% (October 8, 1990:41-48). It is apparent, therefore, that children have much less vocal representation and impact at the voting booth.

Children of the homeless, the migrant worker, and the illegal immigrant may have greater problems than those who have permanent shelter. These include less coverage because of their transience, variations in state Medicaid coverage, language difficulties, problems understanding the application process, and fear of discovery of their immigrant status.[4]

UTILIZATION OF THE SYSTEM

Some pediatric cardiology systems are not user friendly and can be confusing and intimidating, especially for poor patients. Difficulties can include transportation to the facility, parking or finding the right bus line, finding someone to stay with the other children at home, and coping with an inpatient environment where the child's illness already imposes confusion and anxiety. Many of these parents cannot afford food or housing for themselves during their child's inpatient stay. Furthermore, they may have no resources for the care of the children who remain at home.

Outpatient costs may be affordable for such situations as a physician visit but not for expensive testing, such as Doppler echocardiography or magnetic resonance imaging. All of these factors tend to discourage the parents from keeping return appointments, refilling prescriptions, or dealing with their child's ongoing cardiac health care needs.

There are up to 3 million homeless people in the United States. Depending on the geographic location, one third to three quarters are children.[27,28] Characteristics of this population include less use of the health care system, as eating is a higher priority; episodic usage of acute facilities when problems arise; and less follow-up care because of their mobility and difficulty in accessing a consistent system. Similarly, children of migrant workers, whether having immigrated illegally or not, do not have access to ongoing health care. Such parents do not always have a clear understanding of their child's cardiac condition, do not remember the name of their last provider, and move from community to community without carrying adequate documentation of their child's condition. This, in addition to lack of continuity of care in one location, complicates the situation for their child with a cardiac condition. Additionally, cultural differences, language difficulty, and fear of being detected as an illegal immigrant often delay or inhibit proper cardiac health care to this group. Certain hospitals, because of economic pressures, deny admission or care to these children unless an absolute and dire emergency is detected. They then force early discharge after the child's condition has been stabilized, but not necessarily when maximum benefit has been achieved.

Guidelines and handout materials are often written for those who have attained a fairly high educational level. For example, nutritional advice is sometimes aimed at the affluent but does not take into account foodstuffs available to the poor, who must be careful of every dollar spent at the supermarket.

Atherosclerotic risk factor prevention is likewise directed toward the affluent. Such physical activities as swimming or tennis almost categorically exclude the poor, who do not have access to such sports facilities. Tobacco advertising is characteristically directed at the poor. Risk factor education and implementation may be available only through the schools, but many inner-city or rural schools cannot afford to provide nutritional programs, hypertension screening, or physical education programs aimed toward improved fitness.

RESPONSE OF THE PRESENT SYSTEM

Pediatric cardiologists currently respond to these problems by availability, especially for emergencies on a 24-hour basis, writing off bills, and providing free care both in outpatient clinics and as inpatient teaching attending physicians. Some offer flexible office hours and scheduling to meet the time constraints of working families. Many provide free or less expensive care at outlying clinics throughout their state, which are usually sponsored by Crippled Children's Services or the Bureau of Maternal and Child Health. These take the physician to the patient and often offer care that would otherwise be unavailable. Many pediatric cardiologists also provide education and exert political influence directly or through such organizations as the American Heart Association, American Academy of Pediatrics, and the American College of Cardiology. For example, the American Heart Association Schoolsite Program has presented heart health education to more than 7 million US schoolchildren.

Most pediatric cardiology programs directly include social workers and nurse clinicians as members of the cardiac health care team. A few programs have access to patient ombudsmen and translators. Many hospitals allow rooming in and recognize and help with the other individual needs of parents.

Certain private and charitable organizations offer support for these patients. Some of these include the Variety Club, Ronald McDonald housing programs, Children's Heart Fund, Make-A-Wish Foundation, and the businessman's Wings of Hope program, which uses unoccupied corporate jet seats to allow transportation between the child's home and a cardiac center.

CONCLUSIONS AND RECOMMENDATIONS FOR THE FUTURE

Physicians who provide prenatal, perinatal, and pediatric cardiac care must increase collaborative efforts that will lend insight into identification and care of the at-risk poverty mother at a level equivalent to that offered the affluent. Ways must be found to identify and treat the at-risk pregnant woman. Strategies should be directed toward adequate nutrition, maternal diabetes detection and treatment, substance abuse prevention (including smoking), the effects of maternal age, and the influence of multiple pregnancies. Similarly, research support and activities should evaluate reasons for inadequate follow-up of poor children who have cardiac disease. This could include evaluation of problems with transportation, system access, finances, and disease understanding.

The number of pediatric cardiologists in the United States is limited. To provide the time for provision of equal and adequate care, more must be trained, and that training must be supported. Present resources should be used more discriminantly. For example, pediatric specialists (pediatricians) should be able to examine patients with chest pain and innocent murmurs and provide follow-up for patients with less significant cardiac problems, such as small ventricular septal defects, mild pulmonary stenosis, and the like. This can be accomplished by their gaining greater confidence through continuing education and experience. The medicolegal climate that currently drives pediatric specialists to refer and not to manage such conditions must be modified so that fear of inappropriate litigation is not a factor behind these actions. Likewise, patient attitudes must be modified to accept the pediatric specialist as a consultant and provider for such cases. Ancillary health personnel should be used to greater advantage for patient education, handling minor problems, writing to schools and insurance companies, and handling other paperwork that absorbs much of the pediatric cardiologist's time.

All pediatric cardiac care providers should be sensitive to the problems of the poor. Their practices should be near mass transportation. They should track their patients' follow-up appointments and treatments to assure compliance. This may be accomplished through development of computer databases that are simple enough to be used even by those of us who are not "computer literate." Printed materials and patient teaching materials should be written to the reading level and in the language understood by the patient's parent. When programs are developed that include general population strategies, such as hypertension education and treatment, those materials and programs must be critiqued by the group for whom their use is intended, and those critiques must receive an acceptable response before implementation.

Preventive programs should be coordinated through the school system. After-school care could be provided by parents and siblings from the same population, offering employment opportunities to them that would otherwise not be available. Physical activity programs should include all children without creating embarrassment for any child, even the clumsiest. Exercise should be viewed as fun, and lifelong sport activities should be taught instead of sports in which only a few will achieve success. Not every child will ultimately be a professional athlete. Cafeteria meal planning should address heart-healthy eating habits, and poor children should eat two meals per day at the school site. Cities should provide funding for health clinics based at the school. With these school health clinics, health promotion, not just disease diagnosis, should be emphasized. Children should receive anti-smoking education that is proved to be effective, and tobacco usage advertising directed toward children and the disadvantaged should be outlawed. Other community resources, such as churches and community centers, should be included in development of cardiovascular and other health strategies that will help the poor.

There must be universal access of adequate care to the child with cardiac disease no matter what the socioeconomic status. Medicaid and Crippled Children's Services eligibility and coverage must be improved. Care of those over age 21 years who had heart problems as children must receive continued funding similar to that provided to patients with cystic fibrosis or hemophilia. Private insurance carriers may wish to consider strategies to cover this group, which might include making a general insurance pool available to all with cardiac disease. If no private solution to the problem is forthcoming, a national health insurance alternative may be the only answer.

These children do not have a voice in politics. The effects of that lack are apparent as their general support has declined despite increases in other segments of the population. These children must be treated fairly, and it is up to us as their providers to be an effective political voice that will be heard on their behalf.

References

1. Clark EB, Takao A. Overview: a focus for research in cardiovascular development. In: Clark EB, Takao A, eds. *Development Cardiology: Morphogenesis and Function.* Mount Kisco, NY: Futura Publishing Co Inc; 1990:3.
2. Roberts NK, Cretin S. The changing face of congenital heart disease: a method for predicting the influence of cardiac surgery upon the prevalence and spectrum of congenital heart disease. *Med Care.* 1980;18:930-939.
3. Ludomirsky A, Garson A Jr. Supraventricular tachycardia. In: Garson A Jr, Bricker JT, McNamara DG, eds. *The Science and Practice of Pediatric Cardiology.* Philadelphia, Pa: Lea & Febiger; 1990:1809.
4. Children's Defense Fund. Testimony of the Children's Defense Fund Before the House Energy and Commerce Committee Subcommittee on Health and the Environment; September 10, 1990; Washington, DC.
5. Sealing PA. *Profile of Child Health in the United States.* Alexandria, Va: National Association of Children's Hospitals and Related Institutions; 1989.
6. National Center for Health Statistics. *Monthly Vital Statistics Report.* Washington, DC: US Dept of Health and Human Services; 1990;39(6):1.
7. Ries P. Americans assess their health: United States, 1987. *Vital Health Stat 10.* 1990; No.174:10.
8. Johnson SF, McCarter RJ, Ferencz C. Changes in alcohol, cigarette, and recreational drug use during pregnancy: implications for intervention. *Am J Epidemiol.* 1987;126:695-702.
9. Curran JW, Jaffe HW, Hardy AM, Morgan WM, Selik RM, Dondero TJ. Epidemiology of HIV infection and AIDS in the United States. *Science.* 1988;239:610-616.
10. Little BB, Snell LM, Klein VR, Gilstrap LC III. Cocaine abuse during pregnancy: maternal and fetal implications. *Obstet Gynecol.* 1989;73:157-160.
11. Correa A, Loffredo C, Ferencz C, Wilson PD. Lead and solvent exposure during pregnancy: possible risk of cardiovascular malformations (CVM). *Teratology.* 1990;41:545.
12. Ferencz C, Neill CA, Brenner JI, Perry LW, Martin GR. Ventricular septal defect in infants: an eight-year population-based study. *Am J Cardiol.* 1990;66:524.
13. Griffiths SP, Gersony WM. Acute rheumatic fever in New York City (1969 to 1988): a comparative study of two decades. *J Pediatr.* 1990;116:882-887.
14. Land MA, Bisno AL. Acute rheumatic fever: a vanishing disease in suburbia. *JAMA.* 1983;249:895-898.
15. Bisno AL, Ferguson GW, Shultz JM. Epidemiology of acute rheumatic fever in Miami, Florida, USA, 1984-1988. XI Lancefield Symposium on Streptococci and Streptoccal Diseases; September 10-14, 1990; Siena,Italy. Abstract L37.
16. Taubert KA, Rowley AH, Shulman ST. A U.S. nationwide survey of Kawasaki disease (KD) and acute rheumatic fever (ARF). *J Pediatrics.* In press.
17. Veasy LG, Wiedmeier SE, Orsmond GS, et al. Resurgence of acute rheumatic fever in the intermountain area of the United States. *N Engl J Med.* 1986;316:421-427.
18. Congeni B, Rizzo C, Congeni J, Sreenivasan VV. Outbreak of acute rheumatic fever in northeast Ohio. *J Pediatr.* 1987;111:176-179.
19. Wald ER, Dashefsky B, Feidt C, Chiponis D, Byers C. Acute rheumatic fever in western Pennsylvania and the tristate area. *Pediatrics.* 1987;80:371-374.
20. Hosier DM, Craenen JM, Teske DW, Wheller JJ. Resurgence of acute rheumatic fever. *AJDC.* 1987;141:730-733.
21. Westlake RM, Graham TP, Edwards KM. An outbreak of acute rheumatic fever in Tennessee. *Pediatr Infect Dis J.* 1990;9:97-100.
22. Newacheck PW. Improving access to health care for children, youth, and pregnant women. *Pediatrics.* 1990;86:626-635.
23. Steinhardt BJ, DeCuypere M. *Assuring Children's Access to Health Care: Fixing the Medicaid Safety Net.* Alexandria, Va: National Association of Children's Hospitals and Related Institutions; 1989.
24. *Medicaid Source Book: Background Data and Analysis.* Washington, DC: Congressional Research Service; November 1988.
25. Oberg CN. Medically uninsured children in the United States: a challenge to public policy. *Pediatrics.* 1990;85:824-833.
26. Waxman HA. Kids and Medicaid: progress but continuing problems. *Am J Public Health.* 1989;79:1217-1218.
27. Hu DJ, Covell RM, Morgan J, Arcia J. Health care needs for the children of the recently homeless. *J Community Health.* 1989;14:1-8.
28. Committee on Community Health Services. Health needs of homeless children. *Pediatrics.* 1988;82:938-940.

In Other AMA Journals

ARCHIVES OF INTERNAL MEDICINE

Change in Cholesterol Awareness and Action: Results From National Physician and Public Surveys

Beth Schucker, MA; Janet T. Wittes, PhD;
Nancy C. Santanello, MD, MS;
Stephen J. Weber, PhD; Daniel McGoldrick;
Karen Donato, MS, RD; Alan Levy, PhD;
Basil M. Rifkind, MD, FRCP
(*Arch Intern Med.* 1991;151:666-673)

Health Effects of Radon Exposure: Report of the Council on Scientific Affairs, American Medical Association

American Medical Association Council on Scientific Affairs
(*Arch Intern Med.* 1991;151:674-677)

The Challenge of Caring for Indigent Children With Rheumatologic Diseases

Michael L. Miller, MD, Patience H. White, MD

● Poverty and lack of insurance prevent complete access to tertiary care for many children with rheumatologic diseases. Long-term solutions to provide community based support for local teams and other services are needed. Physicians need to work with colleagues in health care systems and government to make the health care system fully available to all families. Medical schools can act as catalysts in helping government agencies redefine policies to support outreach and other health care programs for the indigent. Governmental agencies must collaborate with insurance companies to change policies so as to cover all aspects of service, including those provided by arthritis health professionals. With coordinated effort, the goal of adequate services to indigent children with rheumatologic and other chronic illnesses can become reality.

(*AJDC*. 1991;145:554-558)

Poverty amplifies problems that rheumatologic diseases impose on children and their families. Providing adequate care becomes a challenge for society no less than for physicians and other health care professionals. For the many indigent children with these diseases who do not receive continuing primary care, access to pediatric rheumatology centers becomes difficult. Those who do get to pediatric rheumatology centers often have difficulty in getting prescribed services, such as physical therapy. As a result, potentially reversible problems, such as joint contractures, may last well into adulthood; persisting disability can interfere with the ability to work. This article will examine problems with access to and delivery of care for impoverished children with rheumatologic diseases. We will suggest some approaches health care professionals can take in dealing with these problems.

PROBLEMS IN ACCESSING CARE

Poverty and lack of insurance prevent access to tertiary care for many children with rheumatologic and musculoskeletal diseases. Among youths aged 19 to 24 years, these illnesses account for more than half of chronic disabilities in this country; 20% of affected children are uninsured.[1] For the uninsured, the Medicaid program has yet to live up to its promise. Although it increased access to ambulatory services for children of lower socioeconomic status, Medicaid has covered less than half of children from low-income groups during the past decade.[2] This may explain why indigent children with health problems do not visit physicians as often as those from higher socioeconomic groups.[3,4] Because their parents cannot afford it, many indigent children with chronic diseases do not receive continuing primary care.[5] Thus, impoverished children with arthritis often cannot get longitudinal monitoring of their illness. The result can be delayed diagnosis and later referral to pediatric rheumatology centers, which can affect prognosis.

Even when Medicaid or insurance companies cover rheumatologic illnesses, many children cannot get the coordinated services they need for optimal care. Federal and state governmental agencies do not pay for all the necessary care. Those indigent families with some form of health insurance are usually underinsured because their employers offer benefits programs that do not provide full coverage. As health care costs increase, coverage becomes even more restricted. Reimbursement for physical and occupational therapy, nutritional counseling, and orthotic devices is either insufficient or, in some cases, nonexistent. Families with marginal incomes often cannot afford to pay for uncovered services.[5]

Decreased access to care for indigent children with chronic rheumatologic diseases causes serious consequences. Families experience fragmentation of services: they may need to choose between paying for primary preventative care locally or for transportation to and care at tertiary care centers. Decreased services can lead to uncorrected disability that worsens over time. Community-based services could provide some of these services if they were more complete. Respite programs offering parents help with affected children and their siblings are only partially funded.

Impoverished children with arthritis face additional problems when they enter the adult world. Young adults may lose funding for medical care because of age limits set by state agencies. Those on the lower end of the socioeconomic scale tend to have lower educational achievements. In adults with rheumatoid arthritis, low educational levels correlate with worse prognosis[6]; the resulting disabilities make getting work more difficult. Available jobs often do not offer adequate health insurance, perpetuating the cycle of decreased access to health care.

Accepted for publication December 27, 1990.

From the Department of Pediatrics, University of Texas Health Science Center, San Antonio (Dr Miller); and the Department of Pediatrics, Children's National Medical Center, George Washington University, Washington, DC (Dr White).

Reprint requests to Department of Pediatrics, UTHSC, 7703 Floyd Curl Dr, San Antonio, TX 78284 (Dr Miller).

Thus, indigent young adults who are poorly educated may have the most severe disease and the last access to health care.

SERVICES THAT ARE NEEDED FOR OPTIMAL CARE

For children who regularly visit pediatric rheumatology centers, prognosis depends on the nature of their illness and the availability of medical services. The three most common rheumatologic illnesses of childhood are juvenile rheumatoid arthritis (JRA), systemic lupus erythematosus, and dermatomyositis.[7] Juvenile rheumatoid arthritis is not rare; in the United States, it is estimated to affect more than 10 children per 100 000.[8] Juvenile rheumatoid arthritis is classified into systemic, pauciarticular, and polyarticular types, based on clinical presentation, including number of joints affected, and course. Patients with JRA need close monitoring of their anti-inflammatory medications. They also need close follow-up by ophthalmologists, physical and occupational therapists, and other health care professionals. Lupus, an autoimmune disease of unknown etiology, can present at any age, but most pediatric cases occur in adolescent girls. Services needed depend on complications, which include chronic renal disease, pleuritis, pericarditis, and arthritis.

Patients with systemic lupus erythematosus often require chemotherapeutic agents, necessitating regular hospitalization and outpatient follow-up. Dermatomyositis, an inflammatory disease of skin and muscle, requires intensive physical therapy and anti-inflammatory or immunosuppressive medication. Most pediatric rheumatologic patients survive into adulthood. Because their illnesses often remain active, they need complex transition services. These include identifying primary care physicians familiar with their type of illness, training in job readiness skills, and sex counseling (as many are at risk for teenage pregnancy).

No matter what their socioeconomic status, children with rheumatologic illnesses and their families need help in using disparate resources scattered throughout the community. This is often best done in a planning process called "case management" by pediatric rheumatology teams. The coordinating team often includes parent representatives, physicians, nurses, social workers, and physical and occupational therapists. Team members also use their individual skills to provide coordinated care in a single setting. For instance, children and their families need to comprehend clearly the nature of their illness. Nurses help families to understand further the information communicated by other health care professionals. Families can then select from the many materials (including videotapes, pamphlets, and coloring books) now available on JRA and other rheumatologic diseases. Nurses are often the first to help families decide whether a visit to the primary physician or subspecialist is needed. In this sense, pediatric rheumatology nurses perform triage as important as that provided in emergency departments for patients with acute problems.

Indigent families need help in using resources effectively. They often do not know where to find local community services; they may not understand the bureaucratic processes required to maintain eligibility for aid. Social workers on pediatric rheumatology teams help families in a variety of ways, such as helping them get emergency funds to purchase food or obtain, complete, and follow up on application forms for state and federal aid. Since parents of children with chronic illnesses are more likely to divorce, social workers provide counseling for families in distress. Social workers identify and arrange intervention for children at risk for medical or physical neglect. These important services are seldom reimbursed. Yet social workers obtain clinical revenues from state and federal sources for medical care that would otherwise be unavailable.

Many children with JRA and other rheumatologic illnesses need to improve their independence by increasing joint mobility and muscle strength, obtaining adaptive aids for daily living, and learning coping skills to minimize pain. Physical therapists can help by recommending exercise programs for home and school. When joint flexion contractures develop in patients with JRA, occupational therapists can make some of the necessary splints. They also work with patients to improve activities of daily living. Occupational therapists work with school personnel to adjust schedules, giving appropriate periods for rest or for walking between classes. They monitor other changes in the school environment that will improve the student's ability to function.

Some patients with JRA have growth abnormalities,[9-11] become anorectic,[12] or are at risk for becoming malnourished.[13] These problems are exacerbated by the difficulty many poor families have in affording sufficient food to feed their children.[14,15] Dieticians on pediatric rheumatology teams document food intake and identify for the social worker which families need aid for nutritional supplements. They counsel families on how to prepare a balanced diet on a limited income.

Career maturity is often delayed in adolescents with rheumatologic diseases, compared with their nondisabled peers. It is most severe in those teenagers whose disease onset was in early adolescence.[16] In most of the United States, current services are inadequate to handle this group of chronically ill and disabled adolescents. For example, a recent Harris poll found that between 50% and 75% of young adults with disabilities are jobless; 67% of those who were unemployed wanted to work.[17] However, the Federal Vocational Rehabilitation System only provides services to young adults over 18 years old in many states. Earlier delivery of vocational programs might help children with rheumatologic diseases make a better transition from school to work. The widespread absence of this type of program typifies some of the problems that exist in delivering services.

PROBLEMS IN DELIVERING SERVICES

Delivering services to indigent children with rheumatologic diseases is difficult. Parents may be unable to take children for physical or occupational therapy if they lack funds for transportation. Delays in insurance reimbursement sometimes prevent families ineligible for assistance from buying medications. Inadequate funding for services makes it difficult for some medical centers to recruit and keep arthritis health care professionals.

School districts in poverty-stricken areas do not always provide special education services mandated by the federal Public Law No. 94-142 (Education for All Handicapped Act, 20 USC, §1401 (1). (15)) for children with "other health impairments," including JRA.[18] Low budgets may prevent administrators from providing school facilities that have adequate access for the physically handicapped. To be able to sit in the classroom and write their assignments, some students with severe arthritis need range of motion and stretching exercises in school. However, many poor school districts cannot offer competitive salaries or fees to recruit physical therapists, even when state funds are available for therapy sessions. Children with arthritis in these districts may suffer increasing pain, weakness, or joint contractures. As a result, they miss more days of school; when in school, they have difficulty in concentrating.[19,20]

In many states throughout the country, agencies that administer the Chronically Ill and Disabled Children's Services programs encounter fiscal constraints in caring for indigent children. To meet budgets passed by cost-conscious state legislatures, these agencies sometimes must set limits on reimbursement that interfere with care for chronic illness. Limits to the number of hospital days reimbursable for rehabilitation deny some impoverished children with severe arthritis and dermatomyositis the intensive inpatient physical and occupational therapy needed for optimal recovery. Agencies in some states must also restrict the coverable diagnoses or complications to meet budgets; for instance, only musculoskeletal complications of systemic lupus erythematosus may be covered. States do not always cover costs for necessary services provided by team members. Social work services, for example, are rarely covered. Nutritional counseling for poor children may not be available in states that do not offer reimbursement. Another example of limited service for children with arthritis concerns splinting, often necessary to restore function to contracted joints. When budget crises affect state medical programs, state agencies are forced to delay reimbursements to vendors, who in turn may not honor orthotic prescriptions. Ironically, the result may be a nonbiologic seasonal variation in the duration of joint contractures, in which increases occur at the end of the state's fiscal year.

State funding problems have also affected some outreach programs, in which pediatric rheumatologists visit outlying areas. They work with locally based health care teams, which may also care for children with other chronic illnesses. The federal or private grants that start these programs are usually temporary; when support ends, local funding may not always be sufficient to maintain all the local team members. Long-term solutions to provide community-based support for local teams and other services are needed.

POSSIBLE APPROACHES

Physicians and other health care professionals have been making progress on the problems described above. Much work remains to be done by people at all levels of the health care system. Parents, community organizations, primary care physicians, pediatric rheumatologists and their teams, and medical schools all have their role to play. With coordinated effort, the goal of adequate services to indigent children with rheumatologic and other chronic illnesses can become reality.

Parents are their children's best advocates when they understand some fundamental issues about health care. Specifically, impoverished children with rheumatologic diseases will only receive services for which society is willing to pay. Enhancing those existing services that are suboptimal will require advocacy. Therefore, parents must form new coalitions with health care professionals, community agencies, and foundations in being strong advocates for government-supported services for all indigent children with chronic illnesses.

The American Juvenile Arthritis Organization (AJAO), part of the Arthritis Foundation, provides parents a forum for advocacy, education, and support. Both parents and professionals belong to and help operate AJAO. A quarterly newsletter provides information on care and research of JRA and related illnesses. Local chapters conduct camps and other activities. An excellent compendium of information about JRA is available through the Arthritis Foundation.[21]

The Arthritis Foundation is interested in new ways in which parents can get better care for their children with rheumatologic diseases. For instance, the AJAO will be starting a new program to involve parents in regionalization of services. Regionalization is described by Perrin and Ireys[5] as the establishment of regionwide standards of referral, evaluation, and care of children with chronic illnesses. The authors discuss the utility of a database that identifies medical and nonmedical resources, and they recommend a plan for regional care that includes referral mechanisms and community education.

To establish its program fostering regionalization, the Arthritis Foundation collaborated with Daniel Lovell, MD, MPH, University of Cincinnati, Ohio, in obtaining federal support from the Maternal and Child Health Bureau of the US Department of Health and Human Services. The Arthritis Foundation is establishing the National Resource Center for Childhood Rheumatic Diseases (NRCCRD). The NRCCRD will train parents to participate in support groups, become advocates for improved services, and give feedback concerning programs to health care professionals. Local Arthritis Foundation chapters will train parent-professional teams, which will in turn train parents in pediatric rheumatology centers. Indigent families can receive training directly from these teams. The NRCCRD may serve as a model for involving indigent parents of children with many other chronic illnesses in the regionalization of health care delivery.

Community organizations need to petition state legislatures and the federal government to fund services at adequate levels for children with rheumatologic and other chronic diseases. Many organizations are currently advocating improvements in health care coverage for children with chronic illnesses, including rheumatic disease. The American Academy of Pediatrics (AAP) has proposed a comprehensive health insurance plan.[22] The AAP is also collaborating with the Maternal and Child Health Bureau in developing strategies for improving community-based access to care.

Health services research has documented the need for services; communities can help investigators get funding for further research through fund-raising and legislative advocacy. Some local health departments have been successful in convincing public health degree candidates to conduct research on delivery of health care as part of their training. Local organizations can also learn more about these issues and meet some service needs by offering to place volunteers in outreach clinics for children with rheumatologic and other chronic illnesses.

Pediatricians and other primary care physicians provide critical help for indigent children with chronic rheumatologic illnesses by following up these children along with subspecialty health care teams. In clinics serving indigent areas, primary care physicians are the first to identify problems worsened by poverty. Close communication between primary care physicians and pediatric rheumatology teams allows the teams to identify which children need help with noncompliance and school problems. Primary care physicians also work closely with pediatric rheumatology teams in coordinating provision of local services for families, thus helping to reduce fragmentation.

If primary care physicians and other health care professionals need more information about pediatric rheumatologic illnesses, information is available through local continuing medical education and AAP education programs. The Arthritis Foundation and the American College of Rheumatology also provide educational materials. In addition, programs are available where health care professionals can rotate through pediatric rheumatology services. Informed health care professionals can work more closely with community groups, local schools, and subspecialty health care teams. Using limited resources, they can make the best choices possible in upgrading local health care delivery.

Members of pediatric rheumatology teams help provide comprehensive service to indigent children with rheumatologic illnesses, as mentioned above. In the future, the increased use of questionnaires will help pediatric rheumatology team members evaluate and monitor the progress of children with JRA and related diseases. A school questionnaire assesses the physical problems confronting children in school and suggests solutions to these problems.[18] The Family Environment Scale measures the ability of families to cope with emotional issues.[23] Myones et al[24] have used it to study families of patients with JRA. Dieticians use 24-hour recall questionnaires and diet diaries. Monitoring the functional disability caused by JRA can help pediatric rheumatology teams identify patients in need of rapid services. Lovell et al[25] recently developed and validated a pediatric version of the Health Assessment Questionnaire used in adults with arthritis.[26] Indigent children will benefit greatly; the Lovell et al instrument can monitor the ability of intervention to improve function in situations where many complex underlying factors may contribute to impairment.

Outreach programs are an important indicator of how carefully different professionals must work together. As mentioned, government or foundation sources of initial funds will not always provide continuing support. The survival of outreach programs therefore requires that local medical and nonmedical organizations arrange for continuing financial support through foundations, fundraising, and advocacy through state legislatures. During the planning stages for new outreach programs, local organizations, state agencies, and medical schools need to discuss how they can best make the transition from temporary to permanent sources of funding without interrupting services.

Medical schools can act as catalysts in helping government agencies redefine policies to support outreach and other health care programs for the indigent. For example, the University of Texas, San Antonio, has begun a program for working with state health agencies in delivering care to the poor of all ages in the Rio Grande Valley. In this program, called the University of Texas System Valley/Border Health Services Task Force, university health care professionals and administrators meet with local and state counterparts in designing delivery systems that conserve fiscal and professional resources. The collaboration between university, state government, and local health departments is critical in linking primary and specialty health care in south Texas.

Children's hospitals can establish programs for adolescents with chronic illnesses that help them prepare for employment. At the Children's National Medical Center in Washington, DC, the Adolescent Employment Readiness Center offers career and academic counseling to individual teenagers. A newsletter informs adolescents and their families about career awareness and other workshops. The center also holds seminars for schools, community groups, and employers.

Economic conditions in the immediate future may require a decrease in budgets for the care of children with rheumatologic diseases. The approaches mentioned will be feasible only if financial planning is at the core of planning coordinated programs. For instance, some children's hospitals cannot afford dedicated pediatric rheumatology teams. They may be able to establish teams caring for children with related problems, such as musculoskeletal teams for children with rheumatologic and orthopedic problems. Health care teams can use computer programs to produce more efficient schedules by tracking time required to deliver services. Administrators may be able to help teams set up fiscal models. Such models could determine the most cost-effective use of community resources by families as well as by the teams.

Eliminating rheumatologic diseases through cures generated by basic research is the ultimate solution to problems worsened by poverty. Research establishing a vaccine resulted in eliminating polio as a major health problem. Similarly, etiologies and better treatment will probably be determined by studies of transgenic mice. However, the best therapy is only as good as the ability to make it uniformly available. Governmental agencies must collaborate with insurance companies to change policies so as to cover all aspects of service, including those provided by arthritis health care professionals. Physicians need to work with colleagues in health care systems, government, and the Arthritis Foundation to make the health care system fully available to all families. Educating the public about chronic illnesses in childhood will be necessary to reach this goal. Only then will children with rheumatic diseases, irrespective of their socioeconomic status, get the primary and coordinated subspecialty care they deserve.

We greatly appreciate comments on the manuscript provided by John A. Mangos, MD, and Victor German, MD, PhD.

References

1. McManus MA, Newacheck PW, Greaney AM. Young adults with special health care needs: prevalence, severity, and access to health services. *Pediatrics.* 1990;86:674-682.

2. Newacheck PW, Halfon N. Access to ambulatory care services for economically disadvantaged children. *Pediatrics.* 1986;78:813-819.

3. Kleinman JC, Gold M, Makuc D. Use of ambulatory medical care by the poor: another look at equity. *Med Care.* 1981;19:1011-1029.

4. Newacheck PW, Starfield B. Morbidity and use of ambulatory care services among poor and nonpoor children. *Am J Public Health.* 1988;78:927-933.

5. Perrin JM, Ireys HT. The organization of services for chronically ill children and their families. *Pediatr Clin North Am.* 1984;31:235-257.

6. Callahan LF, Pincus T. Formal education level as a significant marker of clinical status in rheumatoid arthritis. *Arthritis Rheum.* 1988;31:1346-1357.

7. Cassidy JT, ed. *Textbook of Pediatric Rheumatology.* New York, NY: John Wiley & Sons Inc; 1982.

8. Towner SR, Michet CJ Jr, O'Fallon WM, Nelson AM. The epidemiology of juvenile arthritis in Rochester, Minnesota. *Arthritis Rheum.* 1983;26:1208-1213.

9. Lovell DJ, White PH. Growth and nutrition in juvenile rheumatoid arthritis. In: Woo P, ed. *Pediatric Rheumatology Update.* New York, NY: Oxford University Press Inc; 1990:47-56.

10. White PH. Growth abnormalities in children with juvenile arthritis. *Clin Orthop.* 1990;259:46-50.

11. Bacon MC, White PH, Raiten DJ, et al. Nutritional status and growth in juvenile rheumatoid arthritis. *Semin Arthritis Rheum.* 1990;20:97-106.

12. Miller ML, Chacko JA, Young EA. Dietary deficiencies in

children with juvenile rheumatoid arthritis. *Arthritis Care Res.* 1989;2:22-24.

13. Henderson CJ, Lovell DJ. Assessment of protein-energy malnutrition in children and adolescents with juvenile rheumatoid arthritis. *Arthritis Care Res.* 1989;2:108-113.

14. Karp RJ. Undernutrition and the cycle of poverty. *Pediatr Ann.* 1990;19:268-271, 274-275.

15. Karp RJ. The social context of malnutrition in childhood. *Bull N Y Acad Med.* 1989;65:1026-1031.

16. White PH, Gussak D, Hixson D. Career maturity of adolescents with juvenile rheumatoid arthritis (JRA) compared to other chronically ill adolescents. *Arthritis Rheum.* 1989;32S:29.

17. Rosch D, Phelps A. Secondary special education and transition from school to work: a national priority. *Except Child.* 1987;53:487-491.

18. Spencer CH, Zanga J, Passo M, Walker D. The child with arthritis in the school setting. *Pediatr Clin North Am.* 1986; 33:1251-1264.

19. Stoff E, Bacon MC, White PH. The effects of fatigue, distractibility, and absenteeism on school achievement in children with rheumatologic diseases. *Arthritis Care Res.* 1989;2:49-53.

20. Lovell D, Arthreya B, Emery H, et al. School attendance patterns, special services, and special needs in pediatric patients with rheumatoid diseases: results of a multicenter study. *Arthritis Care Res.* In press.

21. Kovalesky A, Boutaugh M, Erlandson D, et al. *Juvenile Rheumatoid Arthritis: A Health Professional's Guide to Teaching Children and Patients.* Atlanta, Ga: Arthritis Foundation; 1987.

22. Harvey B. A proposal to provide health insurance to all children and all pregnant women. *N Engl J Med.* 1990;323:1216-1220.

23. Moos RH, Moos BS. *Family Environment Scale Manual.* Palo Alto, Calif: Consulting Psychologists Press; 1981.

24. Myones BL, Williams GF, Billings A, Miller III JJ. Social environment in families of children with juvenile arthritis. *Arthritis Care Res.* 1988;1:17-22.

25. Lovell DJ, Howe S, Shear E, et al. Development of a disability measurement tool for juvenile rheumatoid arthritis: the Juvenile Arthritis Functional Assessment Scale. *Arthritis Rheum.* 1989;32:1390-1395.

26. Fries JF, Spitz P, Kraines RG, Holman HR. Measurement of patient outcome in arthritis. *Arthritis Rheum.* 1980;23:137-145.

What Will It Take to Fully Protect All American Children With Vaccines?

Alan R. Hinman, MD, MPH

• Although 95% of children have had a full course of vaccines by the time they enter school, immunization levels among poor inner-city preschoolers may be substantially lower. Among the factors responsible for the disparity are the lack of a uniform data system to identify children who need vaccine; missed opportunities to offer immunizations; overinterpretation of contraindications; and administrative barriers to immunization. Remedies lie in a multifaceted approach: a tracking system that will prompt a reminder and then sound an alarm when an immunization is overdue; means of informing parents, probably best accomplished by an outreach worker of the same racial or ethnic background as the parent; removal of administrative barriers and increased access to services; incentives, either positive or negative, to raise the priority of immunizations; and more education for health care providers to ensure that they understand contraindications and do not miss opportunities to offer vaccines. Other possibilities are "express lane" services to immunize all children who come to a health care provider and the delivery of immunizations in child care settings and in programs such as Women, Infants, and Children, and Aid to Families With Dependent Children.

(*AJDC.* 1991;145:559-562)

Recent newspaper and journal articles headline the continuing occurrence of measles outbreaks in this country and report that a high proportion of young children are unvaccinated. At the same time, the Centers for Disease Control, Atlanta, Ga, describes immunization levels in school-age children as being at an all-time high, with more than 95% of students having records documenting receipt of a full course of vaccines. In this article, I assert that both of these seemingly contradictory statements are true, attempt to describe some of the factors responsible for the present situation, and consider possible remedies.

BACKGROUND

Current recommendations call for a child to receive eight different vaccines or toxoids (many in combination form and all requiring more than one dose) in a total of five visits for immunization between birth and school entry. The basic immunization schedule of the US Public Health Service's Immunization Practices Advisory Committee is summarized in Table 1.[1] Two discrepancies between this committee's recommendations and those of the American Academy of Pediatrics Committee on Infectious Diseases (the "Red Book" Committee)[2] are that the Red Book Committee recommends two immunization visits during the second year of life (at 15 months for measles, mumps, and rubella [MMR] and *Haemophilus* b conjugate vaccines and at 18 months for diphtheria and tetanus toxoids and pertussis vaccine [DTP] and oral polio vaccine [OPV]) and also recommends that the second dose of MMR vaccine be given at approximately 12 years of age, rather than at 5 to 6 years of age, along with DTP and OPV. Thus, a child being immunized according to the Red Book schedule would have six immunization visits before school entry (and a seventh later).

Half of US children are immunized by private physicians (commonly pediatricians) as part of overall well-child preventive care. Their parents either pay for this service or have it paid for by third-party reimbursement mechanisms. The current private-sector price for the vaccines each child should receive totals $198.55; with an estimated cost per physician visit of $15, the total for full immunization would be $303.55, following the Red Book schedule.

The other half of US children receive immunizations in the public sector, often as a specific, categorical service independent of other preventive care services. Their parents do not pay for the vaccine received (which at current public-sector prices totals $92.53) but may pay a small fee for administration. These children are likely to be members of racial or ethnic minorities and to be socioeconomically disadvantaged.

Since passage of the Vaccination Assistance Act of 1962, a federal grant program, administered by the Centers for Disease Control, has provided financial and technical assistance to supplement state and local health department efforts to provide the public sector immunizations. Grant funds typically provide half of the public-sector vaccines (approximately one quarter of the national total). The level of funding for this program has increased dramatically in the past 14 years (Figure), from a low of $5 million in fiscal year 1976 to the fiscal year 1991 appropriation of $185 million. The striking increases are largely a reflection of the dramatic increases in vaccine prices and the introduction of new vaccines. As shown by the nonvaccine grant dollars in the Figure, funding for program operations (surveillance of disease and adverse events, coordination, assessment of immunization coverage, evaluation, education, etc) has not increased significantly. Grant funds have not paid for actual administration of vaccine; this typically comes from

Accepted for publication December 27, 1990.

From the Center for Prevention Services, Centers for Disease Control, Atlanta, Ga.

Reprints not available.

Table 1.—Routine Immunization Schedule*	
Age, mo	Vaccines
2	DTP, OPV, HbCV
4	DTP, OPV, HbCV
6	DTP, HbCV
15	MMR, HbCV, DTP, OPV
School entry (4-6 y)	DTP, OPV, MMR

*Based on recommendations of the Immunization Practices Advisory Committee. DTP indicates diphtheria and tetanus toxoids and pertussis vaccine; OPV, oral polio vaccine; HbCV, *Haemophilus* b conjugate vaccine (the dose at 6 months of age may not be required, depending on which vaccine is used); and MMR, measles, mumps, and rubella vaccine.

Table 2.—Immunization Levels United States, 1989-1990 School Year				
	Weighted Average, %			
Vaccine	Head Start	Day Care	K-1	K-12
DTP	97	95	98	98
Polio	97	95	98	98
Measles	95	95	97	98
Rubella	94	95	97	98
Mumps	97	95	98	98

*Provisional. K-1 and K-12 indicate kindergarten through first and 12th grades; DTP, diphtheria and tetanus toxoids and pertussis vaccine.

local or state health department funds, although some funds from the Federal Prevention Services Block Grant, Maternal and Child Health Block Grant, or Medicaid may also be used.

Because of the existence and enforcement of laws requiring immunization before school entry in all 50 states, there is a mechanism for ascertaining with confidence the immunization levels of 5- to 6-year-old children. For the 1989-1990 school year, more than 97% of such children had documentary evidence of having received a full course each of DTP, MMR, and OPV (Table 2), with little variation around the country. Levels nearly as high are reported from Head Start and other licensed day-care centers, where the school immunization requirements also apply. By contrast, there is no single nationwide mechanism for monitoring immunization levels in infants and young children and no mechanism for requiring immunizations. In the past, the US Immunization Survey carried out by the Bureau of the Census[3] was used, but it was discontinued in 1985 because of concerns about accuracy and budgetary restrictions. It is estimated that, nationwide, 70% to 80% of children have received a full series of individual immunizations by the time of their second birthday (a convenient measuring point), although the proportion who have received the full course of all immunizations is doubtless lower. However, there is marked variation around the country. In particular, immunization levels among poor inner-city children may be substantially lower. A survey in early 1990 of kindergarten and first-grade public school students in eight inner-city areas (Boston, Mass; Bronx, NY; Cleveland, Ohio; Houston, Tex; Jersey City, NJ; Phoenix, Ariz; Pittsburgh, Pa; and Seattle, Wash) revealed that, although more than 95% had received measles vaccine by the time of school entry, only 51% to 81% (depending on the city) had received the vaccine before their second birthday (median, 68%).[4] Some had been vaccinated only shortly before entering school to comply with school immunization requirements and thus had been at risk of disease for several years.

Those who are not immunized on time are likely to be members of racial and ethnic minorities and to be socioeconomically disadvantaged. A recent investigation in Chicago, Ill, demonstrated that only 50% of the students enrolled in predominantly black and Hispanic schools had been immunized against measles by their second birthday, compared with 80% of students in predominantly white schools.[5] In predominantly black or Hispanic schools 25% to 30% of the students had been vaccinated shortly before school entry, presumably to meet school entry criteria. An inverse correlation was noted between immunization coverage by the age of 2 years and the incidence of measles in preschoolers.

The striking disparity between the extraordinary success in assuring immunization in school-age children and the unacceptable levels seen in inner-city (and in some nonurban area) preschoolers demonstrates two important facts. First, the high immunization levels in schoolchildren indicate that parents want to have (or at least do not mind having) their children immunized. Immunization ranks with motherhood and apple pie as a value for most Americans. Aggressive enforcement of the school immunization requirements, which began in the late 1970s, did not meet widespread opposition. Indeed, in Los Angeles, Calif, and New York, NY, to cite two examples, although thousands of children were denied entry to school (or were sent home) because of a lack of evidence of immunization, most returned to school within 1 or 2 days, either having found their immunization records or having been immunized.

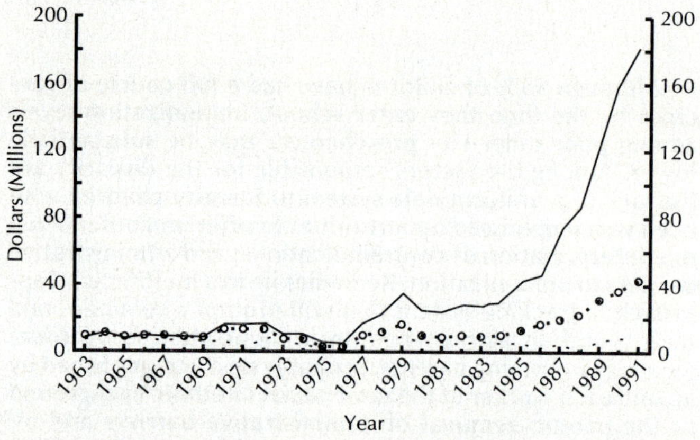

Immunization grant dollars, 1963 to 1991, including supplemental funding in 1970, 1974, 1977, 1979, and 1982; grant dollars at current value (solid line), grant dollars adjusted at the 1964 purchasing power base (broken line with circles), and nonvaccine grant dollars adjusted to the 1963 purchasing power base (broken line).

Second, the private and public "system" to deliver immunizations in the United States has the capacity to serve all children (because it ultimately does so) and that the costs of immunization in either the private or the public sector do not pose insurmountable barriers (again, because almost every child ultimately is immunized). This is not to say that the costs of immunization are unimportant; any parent would find the $59.01 (private sector) vaccine cost of the 15- to 18-month immunization with DTP, OPV, MMR, and *Haemophilus* b conjugate vaccine daunting. In fact, postponing this expenditure may contribute to the delayed receipt of vaccines. However, in the final analysis, some way is found to meet these costs.

FACTORS RESPONSIBLE

Given a willing populace and a system capable of meeting the need, why is it that we are in such trouble? Here the analysis gets softer with difficulty in documentation and in assigning weights. At least three factors seem to be involved.

Inattention by the Provider

This is a problem both in the private and the public sectors. Even though all births are registered with vital statistics authorities and more than 98% of children in this country are born in hospitals, no uniform data system keeps track of all children and identifies those in need of a dose of vaccine at a particular time. Individual physician offices may have reminder systems, but surveys of private physician records have demonstrated that 10% to 30% (or more) of their patients are not up-to-date for immunizations.[6] In the public sector, some health departments have automated systems that track individual children, identify those in need of immunizations, and may even generate mailed reminders. A few may employ outreach workers who go into the community and talk with parents about the need for immunization. In the majority of both private and public providers, however, it seems that no comprehensive system exists to identify and notify individuals who need immunization or to assess overall immunization levels in their client populations. Thus, appropriate immunization may depend on a highly motivated parent or a provider who views immunization as a priority.

Another problem arises when the provider does not review immunization status and offer needed immunizations when a child is seen for whatever reason. Each contact with the health care system should include review of immunization status and provision of needed immunizations. Other factors include excessive interpretation of contraindications to vaccination and failure to administer all indicated vaccines at a single visit. A recent review of records at a public health department child health clinic in Los Angeles revealed that only two thirds of the children received MMR vaccine on their first visit after becoming eligible (K. M. Farizo, MD, P. A. Stehr-Green, DrPH, L. E. Markowitz, MD, and P. A. Patriarca, MD, unpublished data, August 1988). None of the "missed opportunities" arose from a valid reason for withholding the vaccine.

Competing Priorities

Simply put, modern parents have many things on their minds. Many children are being raised by single parents who have jobs that do not pay well and that do not provide many benefits. In addition, other children in the home may have other problems. Thus, priorities may focus on more immediate needs, such as food, shelter, clothing, or acute medical care. "Nonurgent" issues, such as immunization of a well child, simply do not reach the threshold for action.

Another indication that immunization may not achieve high priority comes from a consideration of where (and with whom) children are during the day. Sixty percent of children younger than 5 years are in a child-care setting (including 50% of those younger than 2 years, who are most in need of immunization).[7] Of these, 31% are in a group-care setting (eg, nursery, preschool, or day-care center) where state immunization requirements may ensure immunization. As noted earlier, immunization levels in these settings are generally high. However, more than two thirds of these children (and more than 85% of those younger than 2 years) are being cared for in another setting, such as a home. Bringing these children to immunization clinics (or bringing immunization services to them) may be difficult.

Barriers to Immunization

Barriers may be as seemingly trivial as the requirement in some health department clinics that immunizations be given only by appointment rather than on a walk-in basis, or they may be more apparent, such as limited clinic hours, no evening or weekend clinics, or insufficient staff. A recent survey of state health department immunization projects revealed that 50% had such barriers.[8]

It is important that parents understand all of the benefits and risks of immunizations, and considerable effort (and legislation) has gone into trying to ensure this.[9] However, the "Vaccine Information Pamphlets" that are being developed and are required for use with all vaccines may themselves pose a barrier. Despite considerable work, they are written at an eighth-grade reading comprehension level and average 2000 words each. Given that many adults read fewer than 100 words per minute and that there will be three forms to be read at the 15-month visit (DTP, polio, and MMR), it seems likely that the process itself might be a disincentive to parents, not to mention creating an office traffic problem and tying up office staff, whose time may not be adequately reimbursed by third-party payers.

Another potential barrier is less obvious and also results from good intentions: the desire to provide comprehensive care. This may be manifested by a requirement that a child have a complete well-child appraisal before receiving vaccines. Because many health care providers (particularly in the public sector) are overextended, children must wait weeks to months for these appraisals. Meanwhile, they remain susceptible to vaccine-preventable diseases (and, in fact, may be exposed to such diseases when they visit the health care provider). This recalls Voltaire's maxim that "the best is the enemy of the good."[10]

Financial barriers may also exist. More than 15% of preschoolers are covered neither by health insurance nor Medicaid and almost 10% have no regular source of care.[11] If free public services are not readily available, these children may lose out. In addition, reimbursement mechanisms may cover acute curative care but not preventive services such as immunizations; only 45% of employment-based conventional health insurance plans covered basic childhood immunizations in a recent survey.[12]

POSSIBLE REMEDIES

The easiest recommendation is to say, "Put more resources into immunization programs." Although I agree that more resources will be required, it seems clear that money alone is not the answer.

Some have proposed that the government should provide all recommended childhood vaccines as an entitlement for all children.[13] As a lifelong advocate of immunization, I find it difficult to argue that this would be inappropriate. However, further reflection suggests that this would not solve the problem. The government (federal, state, or local) provides vaccines for socioeconomically disadvantaged children. Consequently, additional government expenditures for vaccines would essentially subsidize vaccination for the middle class and well-to-do, who seem to be getting immunized on schedule. Nevertheless, arguments have been made that free services should be provided for all, not just for the poor, so as not to establish a "two-tier" or "second-class" category of care for the disadvantaged. Another reason, given increasing vaccine costs and the increasing number of vaccines, would be to prevent diversion of private-sector patients to the public sector (where vaccines are free), thus preventing further fragmentation of care. In any event, continued government support for all recommended vaccines for socioeconomically disadvantaged children is essential.

More likely remedies flow from the factors mentioned in the preceding section. First, information systems must be developed and put into practice to (1) track the immunization status of each child, (2) prompt a reminder of needed immunizations coming up, and (3) sound an alarm when a child is overdue. Possibly even more important, such information systems would allow health care providers to assess how well they are doing in protecting their clientele. The suboptimal immunization levels found on record reviews are usually a surprise to the provider and commonly result in remedial action.

Second, effective means must be developed to get the word to the child's parents. In many areas, mail or telephone may suffice, but in many poorer areas, parents may be marginally literate, distrust official mail, or have no telephone. Direct contact by an outreach worker seems most likely to be successful in these circumstances, particularly if the outreach worker is of the same racial or ethnic background as the parent. However, additional resources would be required to fund such labor-intensive activities.

Third, some mechanism must be found to raise the priority of immunization. Mechanisms that come to mind are incentives, either positive or negative. A positive incentive might include payment (either monetary or in kind) to the parent when the child is immunized. A negative incentive might be the threat of denial of services or support if the child is not immunized. A large proportion of the children most likely to be behind schedule are enrolled in some type of public-assistance program. In four large, inner-city measles outbreaks recently investigated, it was found that of the nonimmunized children with measles who were old enough to have been vaccinated, as many as 86% were enrolled in the Aid to Families With Dependent Children program and up to 61% were enrolled in the Special Supplemental Food Program for Women, Infants, and Children.[14] Perhaps it would be possible to require age-appropriate immunization as a condition for continued participation (not initial enrollment) in these programs. Although there is justifiable concern that this might result in needy children being denied services, it seems likely that the experience encountered when first enforcing school immunization requirements would be repeated and no, or only temporary, withdrawal of benefits would occur. Additionally, such a process would also ensure that children were gotten into the health care system where they could receive other important services.

Increased efforts to promote or "market" immunizations are needed to raise the priority of immunizations.

Efforts to reduce barriers are also needed. Administrative procedures must be reviewed to ensure that they do not impede immunization. In addition, clinic services need to be increased, in terms of their overall capacity, their location, and the times at which they are offered. This strengthening of the public health "infrastructure" has historically been primarily a local and state activity, with federal involvement playing a minor role. A recent Institute of Medicine study has described the public health system in this country as being "in disarray," not just in terms of immunizations but with regard to the entire public health mandate. A societal commitment is necessary to ensure that the public sector is capable of providing needed services, and this will require increased public-sector resources from all levels.

More education is needed for health care providers to ensure that they realize the importance of immunizations, understand true and false contraindications, and eliminate missed opportunities for immunizations. Professional societies can play a leading role in this aspect.

It is not at all clear how we can reconcile the need to ensure informed participation with the fact of extensive, and often conflicting, information about the benefits and risks of particular vaccines. It is clear, however, that the days have gone of the "MDeity" deciding unilaterally what is best for the patient.

Reducing the barriers relating to the desire for comprehensive care may be difficult but should not be impossible. Even while scheduling children for future comprehensive evaluations, it should be possible to establish "express lane" immunization services to immunize all children who come to a health care provider. Leadership from professional societies will be essential to bring about this change in orientation. Immunizations should also be brought to children in child-care settings and in programs such as the Women, Infants, and Children program and Aid to Families With Dependent Children. Given the overburdened facilities of the Women, Infants, and Children program and Aid to Families with Dependent Children, the provision of immunization on site will require increased resources.

COMMENT

Although we have much to be proud of in the way we are protecting our children with immunizations, significant problems remain. No single "magic bullet" is apparent that would remove all the problems. A multifaceted approach is needed to reduce the problems already identified, and research is needed to define the factors involved in immunization and nonimmunization and to develop more effective interventions. Immunizations are among the most precious health gifts we can give our children; we must find the ways to ensure full and equitable distribution of these gifts.

References

1. Centers for Disease Control. General recommendations on immunization. *MMWR.* 1989;38:205-214, 219-227.
2. American Academy of Pediatrics, Committee on Infectious Diseases. Measles. *Pediatrics.* 1989;84:1110-1113.
3. Orenstein WA, Bernier RH. Surveillance. *Pediatr Clin North Am.* 1990;37:709-734.
4. Centers for Disease Control. Measles vaccination levels among preschool-aged children in 8 selected cities, United States. *MMWR.* 1991;40:36-39.
5. Centers for Disease Control. Update: measles outbreak—Chicago, 1989. *MMWR.* 1990:39:317-319, 325-326.
6. Ector WL. Immunization levels of children in private practice. In: Proceedings of the 15th Immunization Conference of the Centers for Disease Control; March 10-13, 1980; Denver, Colo; pp 70-72.
7. Dawson DA, Cain VS. Child care arrangements: health of our nation's children, United States, 1988. Advance data No. 187. Hyattsville, Md; National Center for Health Statistics; 1990.
8. Orenstein WA, Atkinson W, Mason D, Bernier RH. Barriers to vaccination of preschool children. *J Health Care Poor Underserved.* 1990;1:315-329.
9. Bruce R. Status and use of vaccine information pamphlets. In: Proceedings of the 24th National Immunization Conference of the Centers for Disease Control; May 21-25, 1990; Orlando, Fla; pp 99-100.
10. Arouet FM (Voltaire). *Dictionnaire Philosophique.* 1764.
11. Bloom B. Health insurance and medical care: health of our nation's children, United States, 1988. Advance data No. 188. Hyattsville, Md: National Center for Health Statistics; 1990.
12. *Health Insurance Association of America Survey 1989.* Washington, DC: Health Insurance Association of America; 1989.
13. American Academy of Pediatrics. Cross-national comparisons of child health. *Pediatrics.* In press.
14. Hutchins SS. Access of preschool-aged children to health care services and federal assistance programs. In: Proceedings of the 24th National Immunization Conference of the Centers for Disease Control; May 21-25, 1990; Orlando, Fla; pp 87-92.

Improving Health Care for Underserved Infants, Children, and Adolescents

The Robert Wood Johnson Foundation's Experience

Michael P. Beachler

Improving the health care of this nation's infants, children, and adolescents has been a priority of The Robert Wood Johnson Foundation since its inception as a national philanthropy in 1972. The foundation has awarded grants totaling almost $243 million, approximately 22% of the foundation's overall grant-making to date, to programs whose aim is to improve the health of infants, children, and adolescents.

The foundation has used three major strategies in its child health efforts: service demonstrations to develop and test new models of care, research to improve the knowledge base and assess the efficacy of its service demonstrations, and training to better prepare health care providers to address common child health problems. Given the foundation's mission to improve the health care system, and particularly its long-standing interest in improving access to care, more than two thirds of its child health funding has supported service projects targeting underserved children.

The foundation's primary objective in its early years (1972 to 1980) was to increase access to personal health services. In light of the nation's high infant mortality rate, which accounted for 70% of all deaths among children under age 15 years, many of the foundation's early child health efforts emphasized improving access to perinatal care.

In the early 1980s, the foundation announced a broader agenda, one that went beyond improving access to include support of programs to help people maintain or regain maximum attainable function and to make health care arrangements more effective and affordable.

The development of its most recent child health efforts has been influenced by major changes in the organization and financing of child health services and by the changing nature of child health problems.

A CHANGING HEALTH CARE ENVIRONMENT FOR CHILDREN

With the foundation's earliest child health efforts, it was presumed that once a program was successfully implemented the health system would have sufficient resources to sustain it beyond the grant period and to replicate it more broadly. This expectation may have been appropriate in the 1970s when federal financing for child health programs was increasing, but by the early 1980s, an era of fiscal retrenchment, it was no longer realistic.

In the late 1970s, the number of children without health insurance was increasing, yet in the early 1980s public financing for child health services was cut back. From 1977 to 1985, the proportion of children younger than age 18 years without public or private health insurance increased from 17.6% to 23.4%.[1,2] Today, more than one third of the uninsured are children.

Economic changes have had a major influence on the decrease in private insurance coverage for children. For some, parents' manufacturing jobs, and accompanying health insurance, have been lost, to be replaced with service-sector jobs less likely to provide health insurance benefits. The growth of single-parent households and a reduction in the share of group health premiums paid by employers have also contributed to the decrease in private coverage.[3] Regarding public insurance, changes in Medicaid eligibility requirements reduced the proportion of low-income Americans covered from 63% in 1975 to 46% in 1983.[4] From 1978 to 1984, Medicaid expenditures (measured in constant dollars) declined 13%, and federal funding for three important sources of primary health care for poor women and children—maternal and child health services, community health centers, and health centers for migrants—declined 32%.[5]

During this period, a shift in responsibility for child health policy from the federal to the state level occurred under the Reagan administration's "New Federalism" policy. States now had primary administrative responsibility for several key child health programs, such as the Maternal and Child Health; Prevention; and Alcohol, Drug Abuse, and Mental Health block grant programs. Accompanying federal funding cuts pressured state governments to increase their support of these services. Federal Medicaid policy also started to allow states greater flexibility concerning the range of child health services they could cover and greater discretion as to who was eligible for services. In the last 5 years, Congress passed legislation allowing states to increase covered services and to provide Medicaid coverage to mothers and children without having to increase welfare payments.

Accepted for publication December 21, 1990.

From The Robert Wood Johnson Foundation, Princeton, NJ.

The views expressed in this article are those of the author, and no official endorsement by The Robert Wood Johnson Foundation is intended or should be inferred.

Reprint requests to The Robert Wood Johnson Foundation, PO Box 2316, Princeton, NJ 08543-2316 (Mr Beachler).

While these policy changes unfolded, the changing health problems of America's children presented significant new challenges. The premature infant of the early 1970s may have required admission to a state-of-the-art neonatal intensive care unit; by contrast, today's cocaine-addicted premature infant—in addition to neonatal intensive care—may require detoxification, foster care, and many other health and social services involving many agencies, institutions, and funding sources. The mother also requires drug treatment and help coping with an at-risk newborn. In a child health system that is fragmented and funded through a bewildering array of separate categorical programs at the federal, state, and local levels, ensuring that a child with multiple health problems obtains needed services becomes extremely difficult.

These changes in public policy, children's needs, and what are considered health-related problems have resulted in a broader focus for the foundation's programs in this area, which now concentrate on helping the child health system be more responsive to children's health needs.

SELECTED CHILD HEALTH EFFORTS

This evolution in the foundation's programs can be illustrated through brief descriptions of several of its major maternal and infant care programs. The first major initiative in this area was the Perinatal Program, an eight-site demonstration program, implemented between 1975 and 1980, designed to demonstrate the feasibility of regionalized perinatal services and to measure their impact on infant mortality and morbidity. Through this program, major medical centers worked with community hospitals to establish common perinatal risk assessment systems, maternal and neonatal transport systems, consultation and outreach education programs, and management information systems to track care. An independent evaluation of the program found that neonatal mortality rates declined by an average of 20% at the eight sites. At the same time, there was no increase in the number or proportion of infants with serious physical or developmental handicaps at age 1 year.[6] The concept of regionalizing perinatal care has taken hold strongly in most parts of the country, yet, key elements of this system—common records, training, and outreach—are not widely adopted. In fact, even former grantees have had difficulty sustaining these components of a regional system.[7]

The Rural Infant Care Program (1980 to 1985) extended this regionalized approach to isolated rural areas that had extremely high infant mortality rates. This effort supplemented the federal government's Improved Perinatal Outcomes and Improved Child Health programs. The Rural Infant Care Program mobilized 10 medical schools to provide technical support to providers in outlying communities. It also included aggressive efforts by nurses and lay outreach workers to encourage high-risk mothers to obtain prenatal care early in their pregnancies. The evaluators of the program found significantly greater reductions in infant mortality in most of the program sites compared with other rural counties in their states without this program. They also found that a significantly larger proportion of low-birth-weight deliveries in the area served were taking place in medical centers.[8] Almost all of the sites have maintained some identifiable elements of the program, although the project's interventions have not been widely implemented in other sites in these states.

By the mid-1980s, the foundation's focus had shifted. The intent of Healthy Futures: A Program to Improve Maternal and Infant Care in the South (1988 to 1992) is not to demonstrate the effectiveness of new models of care, but to encourage states and communities to incorporate what has already been learned from past demonstrations into their permanent systems of care. In contrast to the two earlier programs, in which the grantees were academic medical centers, the grantees in the Healthy Futures program are the state health departments in five southern states and Puerto Rico. (Another six sites are funded through the federal government's Healthy Generations Program, which resembles and has worked closely with the Healthy Futures program.) This $7.2-million program emphasizes promotion of regionalized systems and prenatal care outreach, improved coordination between the state's maternal and child health and Medicaid agencies, better financing for the state's perinatal care service system, and increased cooperation between public officials and private providers.

The grantees in this program have made considerable progress during the first 2 years of foundation support. For example, several states have actively promoted the adoption of uniform prenatal risk assessment tools and have improved financing (eg, expanded Medicaid eligibility, reimbursement, and perinatal service coverage).

Another example of a program developed with this broader focus is the Mental Health Services Program for Youth (1989 to 1994). Here, too, the grantees are state agencies. In this eight-site, $20.4-million program, the foundation seeks to demonstrate that through a collaborative effort between states and local communities, services for children and youth with serious mental illnesses can be organized and delivered far more effectively. Mental health, child welfare, juvenile justice, and special education agencies at the community and state levels are responsible for improving the financing and coordination of services. They also are charged with developing a continuum of mental health and supportive services to maintain seriously mentally ill children in the most appropriate settings. During the 1-year development phase of the program, each of the sites made statewide financing changes that will increase the availability of home- and community-based services.

The importance of multiple agencies and community leaders in making the child health system more responsive is also illustrated by the School-Based Adolescent Health Care Program (1987 to 1993). This 18-site, $14.5 million program is a collaborative effort involving schools, health care providers (such as hospitals or community health centers), and the community (through a formal community advisory committee). The program provides start-up support for school-based health centers that offer a comprehensive range of services in public secondary schools. The partnership between the schools and the community health providers has helped the sites secure third-party reimbursement of clinical services. In the 1989 to 1990 school year, reports Julia Lear, PhD, program codirector, more than 15 200 students received health services in the 23 schools involved, and more than 58 000 patient visits were made (oral communication, November 1990).

The foundation's most recent multi-site child health effort is a 3-year pilot test of the feasibility of restructuring publicly funded health services for children with a special emphasis on how these services are financed and delivered. It is intended to help communities simplify the complex web of categorical programs that fund services for children with many health needs and to make these services more accessible. The hoped-for result is a system more responsive to the needs of the individual child.

SINGLE-SITE PROJECTS

In addition to these demonstration programs, the foundation also supports many single-site projects funded in response to unsolicited proposals. Some of these projects also are aimed at improving children's health by making the health and social service systems more responsive.

Harlem Hospital, New York, NY, for example, has developed an injury prevention program (1988 to 1992) that mobilizes coalitions of parents and community leaders to work with representatives from the city departments of education, parks and recreation, and transportation. During the last 2 years, substantial improvements have been made in the maintenance and supervision of equipment at 28 playgrounds, and a recent hospital survey indicates that window-guard use in apartments has increased from 50% to 80% during the last few years. The hospital's childhood injury–related admissions declined by 14% from 1988 to 1989—the first recorded reduction since 1975. During the next 2 years, the injury prevention program will continue to expand the playground and window safety projects and will develop programs targeted at adolescents.

In another urban project targeting underserved children, Montefiore Medical Center, New York, NY, has developed a lead poisoning prevention and treatment program (1988 to 1992) in The Bronx that combines new services and creative financing and involves city and state social service, health, and housing agencies. The project includes community-based mobile screening and a full range of treatment. Two new services—outpatient chelation and transitional housing—will complement Montefiore's existing inpatient chelation, nutritional counseling, and after-care services. The project has already secured financing for some transitional housing from city and state housing agencies and will work with housing and Medicaid agencies to increase this capacity and secure permanent financing for the mobile screening and outpatient chelation services.

In a rural project (1988 to 1990) funded by The Robert Wood Johnson Foundation, the Freedom from Hunger Foundation is working with the Mississippi Cooperative Extension Service and the state health department to reduce nutrition-related health problems among children in the Mississippi Delta. The project is designed to integrate the nutrition education efforts of the Extension Service–administered Expanded Food and Nutrition Service Program and the state-administered Supplemental Food Program for Women, Infants, and Children (WIC). Program coordinators are training Cooperative Extension Service staff in six counties and revising policies and procedures to facilitate better coordination of the two agencies' efforts.

CHILD HEALTH RESEARCH EFFORTS

The Robert Wood Johnson Foundation's child health demonstration programs have raised many important research questions. For example, the success of the regional Perinatal Program in improving the survival of low-birth-weight infants raised the critical question of what, if anything, can be done to improve long-term health and developmental outcomes of low-birth-weight infants. In response, the foundation designed the Infant Health and Development Program (1983 to 1990), the largest randomized clinical trial of intensive early childhood interventions for low-birth-weight infants. The study principally was underwritten by the foundation with additional support from the federal government, The Pew Charitable Trusts, and Stanford (Calif) University's Center for the Study of Families, Children, and Youth. Eight cities were involved in the program: Boston, Mass; Dallas, Tex; Little Rock, Ark; Miami, Fla; New Haven, Conn; New York, NY; Philadelphia, Pa; and Seattle, Wash. The 985 children in the study sample were randomly assigned to one of two groups: children in the intervention group received home visits and were enrolled in special child development centers, with support groups for parents; children in the intervention and follow-up groups received high-quality pediatric follow-up care. The study found that children in the intervention group had significantly higher mean IQ scores and fewer maternally reported behavior problems than children in the control group. The study also provided conclusive evidence that high-quality group day care can be both safe and beneficial to low-birth-weight infants, despite their increased vulnerability to illness and their special developmental needs.[9]

Another foundation-supported child health research effort (1979 to 1983), conducted by the University of Rochester (NY) School of Medicine, assessed the effectiveness of a nurse home-visitor program for pregnant women and their infants in rural Chemung County, New York. Additional support for this project came from the W. T. Grant and Ford Foundations and the federal government. The study found that children whose families received home visits tended to have better language and fine motor skills, less use of emergency room and hospital services, and lower rates of child abuse than did children in families that did not receive these services. Home-visited mothers had fewer additional pregnancies and therapeutic abortions, were more likely to return to work, and used fewer welfare services.[10] The positive findings of this randomized controlled trial have led to a second study (1988 to 1994) to test whether the model could be replicated in an urban setting (Memphis, Tenn), again supported by multiple funding agencies, including The Robert Wood Johnson Foundation, the federal government, The Pew Charitable Trusts, the Carnegie Corporation of New York, and the W. T. Grant Foundation.

CONTINUATION AND REPLICATION

The foundation faces a continuing challenge in helping grantees identify sources of ongoing support for program services following grant expiration. Identifying such funding sources also has significant implications for whether foundation-supported programs can be replicated more broadly.

To help grantees address these issues, the foundation encourages the early involvement of potential long-term funders, sometimes through the use of declining-balance budgeting (by which foundation funds decrease over time) and matching funds requirements. In addition, several of the foundation's recent child health programs, such as the Mental Health Services for Youth Program and the Child Health Initiative, are specifically designed to encourage agencies to redeploy existing funds to maximize their impact.

Clearly, meeting the needs of underserved children and youth will remain a major and important challenge for families, the health care system, and this country. Factors such as poverty, homelessness, and family dysfunction make it difficult to address adequately the health care needs of children with complex problems, such as acquired immunodeficiency syndrome, substance abuse, and mental illnesses. For the foreseeable future, multiple organizations and constituencies, from both the health and other child-serving sectors, must be engaged in efforts to develop a comprehensive response to children's needs.

I would like to acknowledge the thoughtful contributions of my colleagues, Ruby P. Hearn, PhD, Paul Jellinek, PhD, Richard Reynolds, MD, and Steven Schroeder, MD.

References

1. *1977 National Health Care Expenditures Survey.* Washington, DC: US Dept of Health and Human Services; 1980:6. Publication (PHS) 85-3377.
2. *1987 National Medical Expenditures Survey.* Washington, DC: US Dept of Health and Human Services; 1990:6. Publication (PHS) 90-3469.
3. Chollet D. *The Changing Pattern of Health Insurance Coverage Among Non-Elderly Families* [oral presentation]. Washington, DC: US House of Representatives Select Committee on Children, Youth and Families; July 1, 1987.
4. Blendon R, Aiken L, Freeman H, Kirkman-Liff B, Murphy T. Uncompensated care by public hospitals or public insurance for the poor: does it make a difference? *N Engl J Med.* 1986;314:1160-1163.
5. *Healthy Children: Investing in the Future.* Washington, DC: Office of Technology Assessment; 1988:5-6.
6. McCormick MC, Shapiro S, and Starfield BH. The regionalization of perinatal services: summary of the evaluation of a national demonstration program. *JAMA.* 1985;253:799-804.
7. *The Robert Wood Johnson Foundation Special Report: The Perinatal Program: What Has Been Learned?* Princeton, NJ: The Robert Wood Johnson Foundation; 1985:8.
8. *The Robert Wood Johnson Foundation Special Report: The Rural Infant Care Program.* Princeton, NJ: The Robert Wood Johnson Foundation; 1986:6.
9. Gross R, Spiker D, Contstantine NA, et al. Enhancing the outcomes of low-birth-weight, premature infants: a multisite randomized trial. *JAMA.* 1990;263:3035-3042.
10. Olds DL, Henderson CR Jr, Tutelbaum R, Chamberlin R. Improving the delivery of prenatal care and outcomes of pregnancy: a randomized trial of nurse home visitation. *Pediatrics.* 1986;86:16-28.

In Other AMA Journals

ARCHIVES OF INTERNAL MEDICINE

What Should We Do About HIV-Positive Health Professionals?

David M. Price, PhD
(*Arch Intern Med.* 1991;151:658-659)

The HIV-Infected Health Care Professional: Public Policy, Discrimination, and Patient Safety

Larry Gostin
(*Arch Intern Med.* 1991;151:663-665)

Care of the Poor and Underserved in America

Older Adolescents: A Group at Special Risk

Robert J. Haggerty, MD

Jeff, a 19-year-old who dropped out of school after tenth grade, has lived "emancipated" for the past 3 years on his own in New York, and survived for a time as a male prostitute. At a community health center he was recently discovered to have AIDS. When his disease progressed far enough to require hospitalization, it was found that he was ineligible for Medicaid without a prior assessment of whether his parents' health insurance covered him. But he did not want his parents to know that he had AIDS. While this may be seen as a problem with Jeff's pride, the fact that there is not presumptive eligibility for Medicaid, as there is for pregnancy, is a failure of our health system. This catch-22 situation is extreme, to be sure, but Jeff is one example of a group of poor and underserved children often forgotten by pediatricians and, indeed, by society: young people roughly 16 to 24 years of age who drop out of high school or do not go on to any further education.

The William T. Grant Commission on "Youth and America's Future"[1] labeled this group "the forgotten half." There are many other groups of children who are poor and underserved in America. Other authors in this issue address these. Older adolescents and youth are often forgotten by pediatricians and society.

Why are the forgotten half a problem today? In past decades, the majority of young people did not graduate from high school, and certainly not from college. Why are they now part of the growing population of poor and underserved young people? Because the world, especially the United States, has changed. The job opportunities for today's young workers who begin their careers with only a high school diploma or less are far more constrained than they were 15 or 20 years ago. Jobs in manufacturing that offer pay sufficient to raise a family are far less available for this group than they were 20 years ago. Unemployment for this age and educational group is high, irrespective of race, but especially for black and other minority youth. And even those with jobs have had a steep decline in income. The mean earnings of young male workers (from 20 to 24 years of age) dropped from $12 166 in 1973 to $9027 in 1984 (and the figures are probably even lower today). For those young men who are trying to head a family, the decline in earnings is striking (Fig 1, Table 1). If the family is headed by a woman or belongs to a minority group (or both), the decline in income is even greater. Between 1967 and 1986 the poverty rate among young families has doubled (Fig 2, Table 2).

The changing economy, which calls for workers in high-skill jobs rather than manual jobs, has led to a sharp increase in a new poor and underserved group.

CONSEQUENCES OF A POOR JOB MARKET

We usually do not think of the health and related problems that result from poor jobs, but they are many. Because unemployed men, or even those with full-time but dead-end jobs at minimum wage, cannot support families, young women are quite understandably reluctant to marry them. Yet given current sexual practices, they have their children. Unwed teen pregnancy can be a consequence of poor jobs. High school graduates earn more than non–high school graduates, and are more likely to be married (Fig 3). Lack of coverage by health insurance is a major problem for this age group, especially for those with low-paying and part-time jobs that traditionally offer little employee health insurance. However, these young people, when employed, earn slightly above the Medicaid eligibility level. They are in limbo regarding health insurance. One major finding of several research groups is the large number of fully employed young men who earn too little to support a family, have no health insurance, and have a high risk of health problems.

While this presents a bleak picture, we should not blame the victim. A particularly revealing finding of the W. T. Grant Foundation's Commission is that the vast majority of youth are trying to get jobs, trying to "make it" (82% of the 20- to 24-year-olds are in the work force). It is not that we have a generation of lazy workers. Young people today seem little different from those of the past. Interviews with hundreds of inner-city and rural young people in the forgotten half study demonstrate that they have the same aspirations and willingness to work as those who go on to college, but our current economy has far fewer places for such youth, and the health consequences are great.

Certainly not all cases of substance abuse, teen pregnancy, sexually transmitted diseases, acquired immunodeficiency syndrome, and low-birth-weight babies come from this group, but for a variety of reasons the risk of all of these problems is greater among the forgotten half. In addition, these problems often cluster together in the same individuals, thus geometrically compounding the problem. The medical system has greater difficulty dealing

Accepted for publication November 19, 1990.
From the William T. Grant Foundation, New York, NY.
Reprint requests to the William T. Grant Foundation, 515 Madison Ave, New York, NY 10022-5403 (Dr Haggerty).

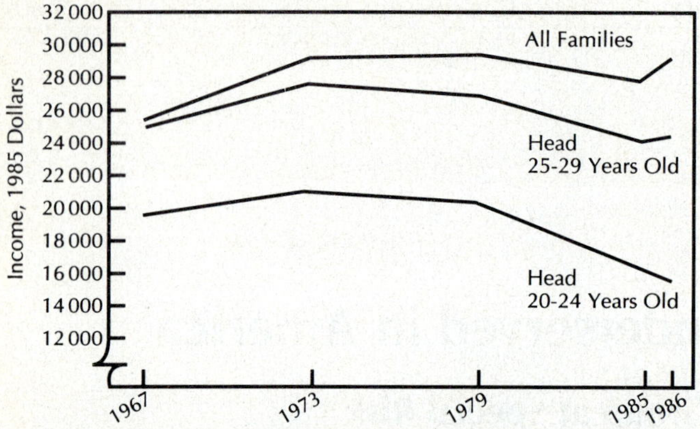

Fig 1.—*Incomes in 1985 dollars of all families and those families with heads aged between 20 and 24 years and between 25 and 29 years for the period 1967 to 1986.*

Table 1.—Trends in Real Median Incomes of Families, 1967-1986, by Age of Family Head (in 1985 Dollars)

Year	All Families	Age of Family Head, y 25-29	20-24
1967	25 560	25 132	19 654
1973	29 175	27 551	20 821
1979	29 028	26 676	20 025
1985	27 735	24 000	16 000
1986	28 898	24 400	15 107
% change			
1967-1973	+14.1	+9.6	+5.9
1973-1986	−1.0	−11.4	−27.4

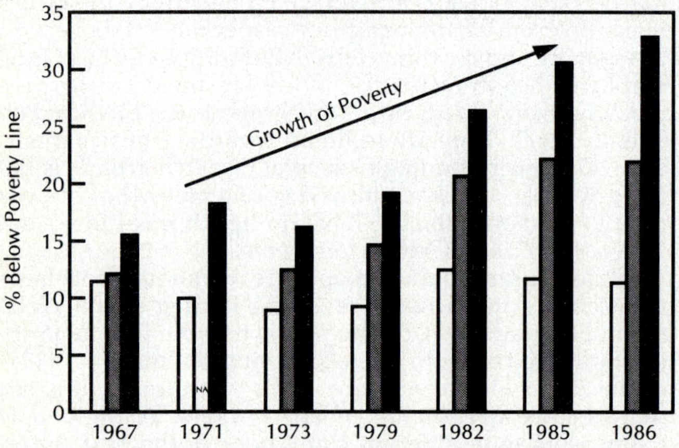

Fig 2.—*Growth of poverty in all families (open bars) and families with heads aged less than 30 years (shaded bars) and less than 25 years (solid bars) for the years 1967, 1971, 1973, 1979, 1982, 1985, and 1986. NA indicates not available.*

with these problems in people from this group, since they have so many associated social problems.

WHY SHOULD PEDIATRICIANS BE CONCERNED?

Young people 16 to 24 years of age have not traditionally been the responsibility of pediatricians. Why should we now focus on this group? I believe that pediatricians should become more involved at least with the health care

Table 2.—Primary Families With Income Below the Poverty Line, by Age of Family Head, 1967-1986 (in Percentages)*

Year	All Families	Age of Family Head, y <30	<25
1967	11.4	12.1	15.3
1971	10.0	NA	18.0
1973	8.8	12.3	15.8
1979	9.1	14.5	19.1
1982	12.2	20.6	26.1
1985	11.4	21.8	30.2
1986	10.9	21.6	32.6

*NA indicates not available.

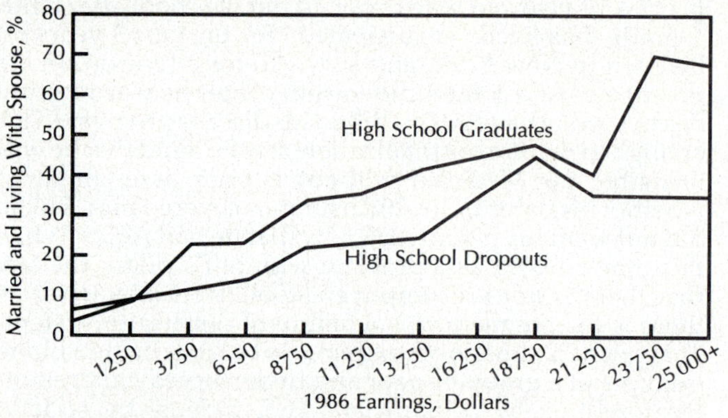

Fig 3.—*Proportion of 20- to 24-year-old men who were married and living with their spouses by 1986 annual earnings and by educational subgroup (March 1987).*

of this group, and if they do, they will of necessity become involved as advocates for change in the socioeconomic and educational aspects of these young people's lives. Without such involvement, medical care by itself will be of only moderate benefit.

First, few other medical specialties are dealing with this age group, in part because of their lack of health insurance. Among all young people, health coverage is poor, but blacks, Hispanics, and other minorities are even less likely to have health insurance than other American youth. In 1984, 21.4% of 16- to 24-year-olds nationwide (7.4 million young people) had no health insurance, compared with 13.3% of all the civilian population.

Second, the diseases young people have are similar to those of younger children rather than being the degenerative diseases of older people that constitute such a large part of internal medical practice. Pediatricians are likely to be very competent in dealing with these health problems.

Third, no other medical specialty really specializes in all of the many interrelated problems of this age group, such as substance abuse, sexually transmitted diseases, infections, and closely related social problems. True, these problems require skills in social pediatrics, but many pediatricians are well versed in these skills. Pediatricians have generally been more involved in social action than many medical specialists.

Fourth, the field of chronic illness in this age group, while small, is especially pertinent for pediatricians. Many children with chronic childhood illnesses, such as asthma, cystic fibrosis, hemophilia, and rheumatoid arthritis, now live into their twenties. If they have been under pediatric care earlier, it makes little sense to transfer their care to another specialty when they are 16 or 18 or 20 years old, since their medical care is very similar to what it was when they were 10 years old.

Finally, we now recognize that considerable development, especially psychological, is still going on while young people are in their early twenties. Few young people take on permanently the major tasks of adulthood—family, permanent career, and citizen participation—in their early twenties. Most, especially middle-class children, try out a number of possibilities in their twenties before settling in. One of the problems of disadvantaged youth is the difficulty they have in getting second and third chances. Since understanding development is one of the pediatrician's main skills, it makes sense for us to add to our knowledge and skill to provide health care for a group of young people undergoing rapid social and emotional development in their late teens and early twenties.

WHAT CAN PEDIATRICIANS DO FOR THIS GROUP OF POOR AND UNDERSERVED CHILDREN?

At first glance, one can legitimately question whether pediatricians can do much for the forgotten half, since so many of their problems lie in the changed economic sphere. It is true that without change in job opportunities other services are going to be less than adequate. Pediatricians need to advocate promising programs in the job area, such as better vocational education programs, apprenticeship (school-job linkage) programs, educational reform that produces schools that encourage an individual's strengths and foster success, and enhanced job training partnership programs. Most of these require national initiatives and policy changes, and we can at best be supportive.

There are a number of initiatives at the local level that pediatricians can take to meet the needs of this group of poor and underserved youth. Closest to home would be to foster comprehensive service programs. Most such youth need a combination of social services, remedial education, and rehabilitation, together with medical care. Sometimes this can be organized in a group practice setting. More often the pediatrician will have to go where the young people are—the school, workplace, church, or community service center. The need for age-appropriate comprehensive services rather than any one of these services in isolation is very great. We can work toward that goal in every community.

Strengthening of families is another very important task. We often think that this age group is totally emancipated, but most still maintain contact with their parents; indeed, many remain in the parental home. Many of the young people interviewed by the W. T. Grant Foundation Commission expressed the wish to have more contact with parents and adults. Parent education programs, enhancement of parent participation in schools, involvement of parents in health programs, mentoring programs for youth, and efforts by parents, teachers, and employers to plan reasonable part-time work schedules can be done at a local level. Communities must tap the youthful energy and idealism of youth. Many youths volunteer their time to rebuild communities. Such volunteer programs have demonstrated useful ways to capture this energy of young people. For the poor, however, all of this activity cannot be voluntary. Such young people must be paid, or else they will turn to activities, legal or illegal, that yield some income. Many of the successful "volunteer" corps programs provide incentives for further education by providing an amount (usually around $5000) for each year completed toward further education. Many high school systems are now requiring a certain amount of community service as a requirement for graduation. Such service utilizes the idealism of the young, brings them in contact with adults, and gives them a true sense of value to society. One group in New York City provided an opportunity for young people to read to elderly people in nursing homes. Teachers have noticed that these young people, who could not sit still in school, became very patient and invested in their relationships with the old people. This also gave the young people a real sense of accomplishment. Every community can organize some youth activities such as these.

COMMENT

Young people in late adolescence and young adulthood, roughly 16 to 24 years of age, are a neglected group of children in our society. They are neglected by schools, health services, and employers. If they have not graduated from high school or do not go on to higher education, their future today in America is limited. They are the forgotten half. While most are energetic and ambitious, without adequate jobs to support a family, they are at increased risk of becoming single parents, engaging in substance abuse, contracting diseases, and exhibiting problem behaviors. Even those who go on to higher education often go through a period of testing alternatives in intimate social relations, jobs, and citizen roles.

A number of solutions are possible for the problems of this age group, but they require attention to programs that combine education reform, job opportunities, integrated comprehensive services, meaningful community roles, and contact with adults. Pediatricians have an important role as part of the team caring for youth, but they must also be willing to work with other disciplines in comprehensive programs and as advocates for this age group.

We may not be able to solve Jeff's problem by ourselves, but with more of the comprehensive community approaches I have outlined, we should be able to prevent many young people from reaching his state. Prevention has always been the pediatrician's main job. Now it requires social change as well as immunizations.

Some will ask, How can we convince the public of the need? People accuse me of being a congenital optimist, but I see more opportunity now than in the past 10 years. Businesses are concerned that there will not be enough skilled workers in the future. Schools are being reformed. Links between school and work are being developed. The task will not be easy, but pediatricians must add their prestige to these efforts, and join the growing chorus of those who are coming together in coalitions to make the lives of the forgotten half more healthy and effective. In so doing, they will improve the competitiveness of America in the future.

Reference

1. The William T. Grant Foundation Commission on Work, Family and Citizenship. *The Forgotten Half: Pathways to Success for America's Youth and Young Families.* Washington, DC: The William T. Grant Foundation; 1988.

Health Care for Pregnant Women and Young Children

Richard E. Behrman, MD, Carol S. Larson, JD

Inadequacy of family resources to purchase health care is the major reason poor, near-poor, and underserved children and youth do not obtain needed preventive, acute, and chronic health care services.[1] Other factors also can significantly limit access to health service, such as distance to facilities, availability of health providers, barriers in the organization and function of the health care system, and the attitudes and behaviors of patients.[2,3] However, inadequacy of resources to purchase medical care is the central problem. The child population whose families are unable to afford medical insurance coverage now includes 27 to 28 million infants, children, and youth who are uninsured, partially insured, or enrolled in Medicaid. The number of pregnant women who cannot afford care must also be considered when addressing the health care needs of children. Twenty-seven percent of women between ages 20 and 24 years are without private health insurance, as are 22% of teenage girls and women between ages 15 and 19 years.[3]

It is time for this country to meet the health care needs of its pregnant women and children. A strengthened partnership between the private and public sectors can meet these needs through a uniform, comprehensive, and federally initiated plan. As the debate proceeds over major restructuring of the health care system, comparatively minor changes to the current system can be made today to care for our youngest and most vulnerable population. These changes could apply immediately to pregnant women and all young children or could be phased in by birth cohorts. In the long run, the costs of providing this health care will be low compared with the health and social costs that follow in adulthood from lack of health care during early childhood.

BACKGROUND

The opportunity for many of our nation's children to fulfill their potentials as productive citizens is being severely compromised even before they reach school age. A child's capacity to thrive in later years is limited by health and developmental problems ignored in early life during the especially critical period from conception through age 5 years. This is also the period of life for which the evidence of the beneficial effects of appropriate health and developmental interventions is strongest. At any time, this most vulnerable population totals about 26 million individuals, consisting of approximately 22 million children aged 5 years or younger and 4 million pregnant women. An estimated 23% of this population are below the poverty line[4] and particularly likely to fall into a health care gap, ie, are likely not to receive important health and related services between conception and delivery (eg, prenatal care and treatment of substance abuse) and between birth and entering public programs (eg, Head Start, child care, or school, which can provide such services as immunization and screening for disabilities).[5,6]

The families of children without disabilities or illness can often bridge any gaps financially to see that their children receive the care they need. Many families cannot afford the health services their children require, however, and are ineligible for Medicaid and other programs.[3] Indeed, given the widely varying eligibility standards of Medicaid among the states, whether poor children are covered has more to do with where they live than what they need. Even families with children covered either by Medicaid or private insurance can experience tragic gaps in health care. Both public and private benefit packages are limited in coverage, and an increasing number of barriers make it more difficult to maintain coverage and obtain access to services.

Myriad proposals have emerged in recent years to reform the health system for people of all ages. Some build on the current structure; others urge a complete overhaul. They use, in different combinations, diverse strategies such as a single-payer system, managed care, and employer-mandated coverage.

The debate over health care provision in this country is not likely to be resolved quickly. Indeed, a new health care system may most likely evolve from lessons learned from relatively incremental change. If so, that change should start with pregnant women and young children. As the recent congressional expansions of Medicaid attest, there is consensus that the health needs of this population should receive high priority.

The American Academy of Pediatrics (AAP) has proposed a plan that would build on the current system to better meet the health care needs of pregnant women and children.[7] The following proposal contains many of the components of that plan and a few additional provisions: to allow a phase-in that targets young children first, to establish health providers in underserved areas, to establish a national insurance commission, to create a public/private council for citizen participation in the monitoring of health care provision, and to provide ongoing outcome measures of effectiveness.

Accepted for publication November 19, 1990.

From the Center for the Future of Children, the David and Lucile Packard Foundation, Los Altos, California.

Reprint requests to the Center for the Future of Children, the David and Lucile Packard Foundation, Los Altos, CA 94022 (Dr Behrman).

PROPOSAL

We propose a targeted national health care program that could be phased in incrementally over 6 years by enrolling all pregnant women and newborns each year by birth cohorts. In addition to requiring lower initial outlays, this approach would also provide an opportunity to implement a new public/private health insurance partnership program without significantly disrupting the existing complex of health care providers, payers, and employers. Furthermore, the program could be implemented on a controlled, small scale that would make it possible to troubleshoot unforeseen problems during the phase-in. This approach also takes a first step in addressing the larger health insurance problem in this country without incurring the enormous financial obligation inherent in the more global solutions that have been proposed.

The major points in this proposal are as follows:

1. All pregnant women and young children would be covered by private health insurance (indemnity or managed care) purchased through either public or private funds and consisting of a basic benefit package (including preventive health and screening programs, ambulatory and hospital care, and related social services). The health benefit package would be developed with reference to the AAP benefit list and current provisions of the Medicaid and Early Periodic Screening, Diagnosis, and Treatment program.[7]

2. All private health insurance policies and contracts would be required to include this benefit package, and a special payroll tax would be levied on employers who did not offer insurance. For children whose parents cannot afford a policy and do not receive coverage from an employer, coverage would be purchased and premiums paid through a combination of income-graduated, family payments; public funds financed by the payroll tax on employers and employees; and allocations from federal and state budgets. Payments from the latter sources might be indexed to the proportion of children under age 6 years in the state. Premiums for insurance purchased by the public fund would be negotiated with consideration of the cost of purchasing the health benefits in the marketplace and of variations in health care costs.

3. Many of the health and related services that would be required under this proposed children's health plan are currently provided for some children through a variety of federal and state programs, and these program funds would be transferred and consolidated to fund this plan. This would likely include transfers from federal programs such as Medicaid; Title V of the Social Security Act; the Supplemental Food Program for Women, Infants, and Children; and immunization grants.

4. The existing provider health provision systems would be used. The Public Health Service would be expanded and authorized to provide care in areas where numbers of health professionals are inadequate. This public program would include a voluntary program by private physicians, perhaps with subsidized professional insurance coverage or other provisions to attract these health providers. Recruitment of young physicians to the Public Health Service might also be facilitated by an educational loan forgiveness program in exchange for service.

5. Reimbursements to providers would be based on diagnosis related groups and a professional relative value system schedule developed for this population.

6. A Federal Child Health Insurance Commission would be created to establish standards and the basic benefit package, to coordinate states and their insurance commissions, and to oversee the insurance broker function and negotiation and payment of premiums. State agencies would be identified as the agents for disbursement of public funds.

7. A Council for Children's Health and Related Social Services would be established with broad representation from private and public sectors, including appropriate professionals. This council would be a national umbrella organization to advise and monitor the health delivery system. The council would have state and local units, creating a federation of local volunteer and public agencies throughout the country to assist in monitoring and coordinating outreach and volunteer efforts in health care.

The national council would be responsible for making recommendations about the basic benefit package to the federal and state insurance commissions and for monitoring the implementation of these recommendations. Its recommendations would also inform the premium negotiations.

The national council, in cooperation with the Department of Health and Human Services and state departments of health and education, would also annually review and report on the status of this insured population based on available selected health outcome measures, such as the proportion of women receiving late or no prenatal care, infant mortality, immunization rates, hospital use by children, and primary school absenteeism and performance.[8,9] This would be an important element in evaluating effectiveness of the services provided under this program and in making recommendations for change in benefits, payments, or other services.

The state and local affiliates of the council would assist in oversight and coordination of services, community innovation, and problem solving. "Lead organizations" would be selected at the state and local levels from among the private and public organizations concerned with child health and welfare. These lead organizations would be responsible for working with families, providers, and various local voluntary and public agencies to ensure that each pregnant woman and young child obtains needed high-quality services. These groups would also regularly report to the council on provider and insurance carrier performance. These reports would be incorporated into the council's recommendations to the insurance commission.

COSTS AND ADMINISTRATION

The AAP estimates that its plan to insure pregnant women and children aged 18 years and younger would increase the $98.8 billion currently spent on this population annually to $111.4 billion.[7] This more modest plan focusing on the youngest children would cost significantly less. Because of its incremental approach and the relatively small population covered, it would facilitate the field-testing of the new administrative structures and the private-public partnership in program implementation. Thus, unanticipated problems could be better dealt with than might otherwise be possible. It would cause minimal disruption in the insurance industry and various provider systems.

CONCLUSION

Initiating change in the current system would be less costly than maintaining the status quo. Failing to provide preventive health and early treatment services results in larger direct and indirect costs to society than providing services early in life. In addition, the costs of such a program are probably lower than one might assume because most members of this population are healthy. The costs of providing health services for all children and pregnant women account for a relatively small portion of total national health care expenditures.

To address the health needs of this overlooked group in a cost-efficient way, we need to elicit significant efforts from local private and public sectors and from the federal government. All share in the potential benefits when these children succeed in becoming productive citizens.

Failure to address the health needs of today's children is having insidious consequences for our society, causing uncertainty and suffering for our families and compromising our future productivity and competitiveness.[6,9] Our future will be mortgaged to a much greater extent by this negligence than by failure to reduce the federal budget deficit. The proposed program would start to address this problem by focusing on pregnant women and young children, those whose health needs are not only great, but also will have consequences for the well-being of this country for decades to come.

References

1. Oberg CN. Medically uninsured children in the United States: a challenge to public policy. *Pediatrics*. 1990;85:824-833.

2. Children's Defense Fund. *The Health of America's Children: Maternal and Child Health Data Book*. Washington, DC: Children's Defense Fund; 1989.

3. Erdman K, Wolfe SM. *Poor Health Care for Poor Americans: A Ranking of State Medicaid Programs*. Washington, DC: Public Citizen Health Research Group; 1988.

4. National Center for Children in Poverty. *Five Million Children: A Statistical Profile of Our Poorest Young Citizens*. New York, NY: Columbia University; 1990.

5. National Commission on Children. *Reference Book*. Washington, DC: National Commission on Children; 1989.

6. Wise PH, Meyers A. Poverty and child health. *Pediatr Clin North Am*. 1988;35:1169-1186.

7. Harvey B. A proposal to provide health insurance to all children and all pregnant women. *N Engl J Med*. 1990;323:1216-1220.

8. US Office of Technology Assessment. *Healthy Children: Investing in the Future*. Washington, DC: US Government Printing Office; 1988.

9. US Public Health Service. *Healthy People 2000*. Washington, DC: US Dept of Health and Human Services; 1990.

Children's Services in an Era of Budget Deficits

Barbara B. Blum, Susan Blank

It is virtually impossible to address the issue of how to improve the care of the nation's poor children without confronting the question of the resources society is willing to spend on those children. As a first step in examining that question, I suggest we visualize an increasingly common sight in contemporary hospitals: a premature, low-birth-weight infant, born with medical complications and hooked up to a life-support system. The baby's mother is penniless; the hospital, or, in other words, society at large will spend thousands of dollars to give the infant all the medical assistance he or she needs to breathe and eat and develop.

What the scenario tells us is that in this instance, society has concluded that almost no amount of money is too much to spend to save the life of a child. The statement is a powerful one. Granted, the work of the neonatal care unit reflects society's stake in preserving any human life, but it is fair to say that commitment assumes a special force and urgency when its subject is a *young* life. The resources we devote to premature infants born into poverty suggest that we honor the potential to develop and grow in any child, however frail or disadvantaged.

But that commitment to children has its limits. If we pursued it to its logical conclusion, we would not live in a society that cares for the baby until he or she can leave the neonatal unit and then allows the infant to go home to an apartment infested with rats. When the infant reaches school age, we could not be satisfied to let the child begin an education in a badly overcrowded and dilapidated building where it takes years to fix a leaky roof. We would also not be able to live with the fact that the emergency department will be that child's only source of health care.

Clearly, almost no one actively endorses such a level of risk to children's health and development, yet childhood deprivation persists and worsens. One reason is the isolation of poor children. Despite growing attention to childhood poverty in the United States, many low-income children live in neighborhoods separated from a mainstream society that reads about them in newspapers but does not personally witness their plight.

Another reason for the neglect of children is the racism and classism that pervade a supposedly egalitarian society. Racism and classism make it easier to ignore children in poor neighborhoods; indeed, racism and classism may even make it more attractive to care for babies in the highly technological professionalized neonatal environment than in the communities to which they return.

However, efforts to make poor children more visible to the public at large will be of little consequence unless underlying questions about resources can be answered. Growing state and federal budget deficits confront children's advocates with a seemingly open-and-shut objection to greater investments in services. Children do have unmet needs, concede the budget cutters, but there is simply no more money. Government, they contend, is in much the same position as a poor family that needs every penny to make it through the week. When short-term budgets are tight, long-term prevention gets defined as a luxury.

For the family, pinched resources manifest themselves as hesitating to take a child to the doctor until an illness grows sufficiently serious to require treatment in the emergency department. For society, budget constraints mean spending more on shelters and welfare hotels after people become homeless than on raising the public assistance allowance, or they mean providing expensive neonatal care to some women because prenatal care is not universally available. Just as the family scrapes enough together to buy a used car, but has nothing left for its upkeep, so society funds the popular Head Start program but dissipates its gains by failing to provide the high-quality education that would reinforce the enriched early childhood experience. Scarce resources must be reserved for averting or alleviating crises; prevention and long-term maintenance are worthy but unattainable luxuries. These principles, argue supporters of fiscal austerity, are as true for government as they are for families.

However persuasive, the analogy is flawed. A wealthy society with its government in budget straits is not the same as a family in budget straits. The government simply has more choices. To pay for better services to meet children's basic needs, this wealthy nation can raise taxes. Used for better prenatal care or drug treatment for pregnant addicts or decent housing allowances, the resources would be money well spent.

At this juncture, however, another set of objections to investing in services must be confronted. There are two meanings to the phrase "money well spent," and we have thus far focused only on the first, the sense that resources will be used for worthwhile ends. When the services are better health care, housing, and early childhood education, their value is easy to defend. It is the second meaning of "money well spent," the concept of *money used efficiently*, that raises more difficult questions.

The source of the difficulty is that as currently structured, our human services system does waste resources.

Accepted for publication November 30, 1990.
From the Foundation for Child Development, New York, NY.
Reprint requests to the Foundation for Child Development, 345 E 46th St, New York, NY 10017-3562 (Ms Blum).

To a degree, the problem is the one already discussed: the overemphasis on costly crisis intervention at the expense of prevention. However, the crisis mode is not the only source of inefficiency. Another is the lack of accountability for public funds spent on human services. The problem is familiar. A program is launched, funds are allocated, and, once established, the program continues to receive support year after year. The principal measure of the program's performance is whether it follows certain procedures. Too little effort is made to find out whether the program is making a difference for children and families. As the public sees it, tax dollars disappear into a void.

In fact, considerable progress has been made on this front, and to a certain extent public perceptions have not caught up with what has been accomplished. We must recognize that this country is the beneficiary of more than a decade of large-scale experimental research efforts that have used controlled studies to measure the effects of various programs. Even when it is impossible to conduct sophisticated treatment/control group studies, as is the case with most programs, officials recognize more and more the value of regularly examining indicators on families at risk. In the absence of controlled studies, it is of course impossible to know precisely how much change can be attributed to particular interventions and how much to external factors. Nevertheless, as new programs are tried, indicators do offer practitioners, policymakers, and the public a general sense of whether initiatives are moving in the right direction.

One of the many examples of this new interest in program accountability comes from the Council of Governors' Policy Advisors (formerly the Council of State Policy and Planning Agencies), an affiliate of the National Governors' Association, which, in the summer of 1990, completed what it calls a Policy Academy on children and families at risk. The academies are intensive technical assistance conferences for teams of top state officials who meet to develop a plan for solving complex policy problems. The teams taking part in the recent academy series on children and families devoted a great deal of time to the issue of how to gauge the success of the plans they developed by examining changes in specific indicators, such as rates of low-birth-weight infants or of teen pregnancy. We need to infuse much more of the planning associated with human services with this approach, which moves beyond mechanistic, procedural measures of how a program functions to a more probing assessment of whether it seems to be effecting change.

Another, still more fundamental source of inefficiency in the way money is spent to help families is the very structure of the country's health and human services systems. These systems are both overly centralized and fragmented. Multiple agencies with multiple funding streams are charged with specialized responsibilities for serving the same families. These families are neither equipped nor inclined to sort through their life problems and fit them into boxes constructed by government. Consequently, they often do not know which agency they should approach for help. When they do locate the right system, they often discover that services are offered only at central, inconvenient locations.

Families pay a high price in frustration and discouragement when they try to negotiate the service maze. Society pays a high price when the maze keeps multiproblem families from getting access to the help they need, thereby allowing their problems to worsen. Government wastes precious resources in duplicative intake processes and reporting requirements and in the time and energy spent piecing together funds from different sources to support single programs.

How should the system function? There are a variety of ways to conceptualize what reform would look like. Many of us who are familiar with social services in New York City like to point to an exemplary program, the Center for Family Life in the low-income community of Sunset Park, Brooklyn, to illustrate what could be done. The center, which is supported by a mixture of private and public funding sources, is open to any family in the neighborhood with children. Through the center, families have access to a rich array of services, including a therapeutic nursery program, job search assistance, parenting education, and many others.

Regardless of the reason why someone first walks through the center's door, staff members are always alert to other kinds of help that that person *and* his or her family may need. While a child may enroll in the center's after-school program, the mother may later avail herself of its counseling services, turn to its employment program for help in finding a job, and, as she comes to feel at home, bring her whole family to its community dinners. The center client, say its staff, is typically not an individual, but the entire family. Every effort is made to avoid artificial distinctions between, for example, "child welfare families," "substance abusing families," and "families receiving public assistance." Instead, the criterion for service is, What help does the family need to function well?

Around the country are hundreds of local programs that share the center's vision of holistic services. They operate with many different funding sources, from many different bases, serving many kinds of families and communities. However, the efforts of these innovative community-based programs are overshadowed by the large public bureaucracies that poor families must typically turn to for assistance. The question is, can these bureaucracies possibly be reconfigured so that the maze becomes a neighborhood center? The center would be friendly and convenient, its mode of operation would be to keep a limited number of staff members closely and continuously involved with one family, and, finally, it would give the family easy access to many different kinds of key services, such as income and housing assistance, preventive health care and child welfare programs, employment and training initiatives, and drug treatment programs.

In New York City, where children's advocates have repeatedly called for integration and decentralization of publicly funded services for poor families, there is now some ground for optimism. A project called Agenda for Children Tomorrow (ACT), which was privately initiated but is now supported in part by the mayor's office, is beginning to map service needs and usage patterns in 10 of the city's poorest neighborhoods. The mapping is the first step in a plan to build a neighborhood-based service system in these districts and eventually throughout the city. It will take time, patience, skill, political commitment, and a generous portion of good luck to create coordinated community services in New York City. However, those of us who have been involved with ACT are gratified that at last a systematic effort to realize the vision is under way.

Local reform efforts like ACT, however, cannot proceed in a vacuum. Initiatives to reconfigure services at the community level are much more likely to succeed if they enjoy a supportive policy environment at the state and national levels. Unfortunately, the federal environment often chills and constricts, rather than nurtures, state and local experimentation. As with almost all generalizations, this one demands qualifications. First, most federal officials want to foster flexibility. However, legislative and institutional practices frequently obstruct that good impulse. Second, some developments of the 1980s, including, for example, the use of block grants or the new latitude given to states to create their own welfare-to-work programs, did favor service coordination. Too often, however, the freedom given to states and localities by the federal government was undercut by funding cuts and freezes. More importantly, despite block grants and special programs that encourage coordination, state and local officials are still met at every turn with federal policies that encourage them to think categorically rather than holistically. We need to look no further than the Congressional committee structure for an example of this problem.

Congressional staffers, when approached with ideas for new federal initiatives that crosscut conventional program areas, typically acknowledge that the House and Senate committee structures are hurdles that must be surmounted if more integrated programs are to be authorized. Because Congress should serve as an aid, not an obstacle, to decategorization, careful thought is needed about how to rationalize the way the committees do business.

At best, however, improvements will be very gradual. Thus, we must also consider if there are ways to give states more immediate relief from the constraints of federal policies. One answer may be to modify the assumptions that underlie decisions about whether to grant states waivers for federal regulations on programs for children and families—to presume that states should be permitted flexibility in following the rules established for categorical funding unless there is good evidence to the contrary.

A starting point for this more short-term reform might be to look into the work of a panel that until recently was known as the Low Income Opportunity Control Board. Established in 1987 under the White House Office of Policy Development, the panel has been renamed the Economic Empowerment Task Force and will operate under the direction of Housing Secretary Jack Kemp. The task force is an unusual federal entity in that it brings together assistant secretaries from the wide range of departments that oversee social welfare programs. Its mission is to examine ideas for state-sponsored demonstrations—programs established for the purposes of evaluation—and a key element of that work is to review state requests for waivers to conduct them. With representatives from all the agencies from which a state would be likely to need waivers, the board offers a shortcut to states that would otherwise need to apply to multiple agencies to launch a complex demonstration.

The board's new name and leadership suggest there is probably federal interest in broadening its authority to take advantage of its unusually wide-ranging representation. There are several good possibilities for such an expansion. Perhaps the task force could become more proactive in encouraging states to undertake demonstrations. Also, rather than confining itself to demonstrations, the task force could also simplify the waiver process when states wish to apply for experiments that involve administrative, nonresearch activities. In addition, the rule now followed by the task force that waivers will be approved only for demonstrations that are revenue neutral should be modified. Because this stipulation ignores the start-up costs associated with almost all demonstration programs, it places unnecessary restraints on experimentation.

Expanding the functions of the task force is one possible route that the federal government could take to make it easier for states to innovate; there are clearly many others that would likewise offer states greater flexibility in the use of funds, leaving them in a stronger position to support locally based, coordinated services.

States, however, do not inherit all their problems in this area; some are indigenous. Like the federal government, states have legislative committees that carve the needs of high-risk families into pieces that are difficult to fit together. Similarly, states have their own centralized bureaucracies that take too many decisions out of the hands of communities.

There are, however, signs of change. In many ways, states are now exploring possibilities for restructuring. For example, the American Public Welfare Association has formed a commission of top state welfare and child welfare officials to recommend reforms in the child welfare system, and that group strongly supports the creation of a more integrated service system for children and families. Efforts to build integrated family services are already under way in Iowa and in states taking part in a special child welfare initiative sponsored by the Annie E. Casey Foundation.

In addition to the federal and state policy environments, a third sector of our society, the professional community, must change if more efficient and helpful local service systems are to be developed. The challenge to professionals has two dimensions, each reflecting one of the two structural problems in contemporary health and human services systems discussed earlier: their fragmentation and overcentralization.

First, to heal the system's fragmentation, the psychologist, child welfare worker, nurse, and many other professionals must be willing to move outside the confines of their own disciplines. The social worker cannot become a public health specialist, but perhaps he or she can become more attuned to the way the public health specialist views families and their needs. The employment specialist need not be a child welfare worker, but perhaps he or she should become more conversant in the language that child welfare workers speak.

Second, to decentralize systems and make them more accessible to clients, professionals must be willing to hand some of the control they now exercise over to local leaders and, ultimately, to families. Families must have a choice in the way services are designed, provided, and prioritized. If they say they prefer family day care to center-based programs, if they believe the neighborhood needs drug treatment more than recreational services, and if they conclude that a single mothers' group established for parenting education purposes should focus less on child-rearing and more on how to find a job, then professionals should listen.

In fact, many professionals are beginning to collaborate across disciplines and shape programs in response to what families themselves say they need. In some cases, these professionals have the wholehearted backing of their agencies, but, overall, more top-down institutional support is needed for this kind of innovation.

In addition, workers must be *trained* to function in a more multidisciplinary system. On-the-job innovation is heartening, but many of the fresh approaches now being taken by health and human service professionals ought to become the standard practice taught to students before they begin their careers. Equally important is orienting current workers to the challenges and demands of coordinated and locally based service provision.

Because there is a tendency to oversell every solution to poverty problems in this country, we should be well aware that, however desirable, a more coordinated and decentralized service system is no panacea. First, while coordination should save precious resources, it will also require new investments in the short run. Changing service systems requires planning, training, and consulting, and none of these activities is without its price tag.

Second, and even more critical, is the fact that clustering services and even clustering them in neighborhoods is likely to be a necessary but insufficient step to bring about the full measure of systemic change that should occur. Services can be integrated, but if they are of poor quality or if there are simply not enough of them, little has been gained.

On the other hand, the potential benefits of coordination are undervalued if there is an assumption that the *way* in which services are provided has little or nothing to do with their *substance*. In fact, the kind of reconfiguration discussed here could improve the quality and possibly even the quantity of family interventions. Convenient, accessible services provided by workers who think about the needs of the entire family constellation would axiomatically be better services. As to the question of supply, if integration reforms created systems that made more sense to workers and families than do current arrangements, the improved morale could, in turn, help to convince the public to invest the dollars needed to create a decent supply of services for children at risk.

Perhaps it is idealistic to expect that the country can create a new and vital service system during the next 10 to 20 years, but there are times when idealism is the only appropriate response to reality. In 1991, when large numbers of children are vulnerable to poverty, homelessness, ill health, and developmental disabilities, it is time, if not past time, for bold and creative systemic change.

In Other AMA Journals

ARCHIVES OF NEUROLOGY

Corpus Callosotomy for Intractable Seizures in the Pediatric Age Group

Richard E. Nordgren, MD; Alexander G. Reeves, MD; Adele C. Viguera; David W. Roberts, MD (*Arch Neurol*. 1991;48:364-372)

The Caring Program for Children

The Michigan Experience

Marianne Udow, MHSA; Vernon K. Smith, PhD; Margaret H. Mason, MHSA

• **Public-private partnerships may offer the best opportunity in the near-term for addressing the problem of the uninsured. In Michigan, a broad spectrum of groups has studied the issue of the uninsured and, despite the diversity of the groups, arrived at a consensus that providing coverage to uninsured children is an urgent priority. The Caring Program for Children, a private program initiated by Blue Cross of Western Pennsylvania to provide primary and preventive health care coverage to children in low-income, uninsured families, gained support from the Michigan legislature and advocacy and provider groups as a means to address the problem. Blue Cross Blue Shield of Michigan and the Michigan Department of Social Services joined to expand the Caring Program for Children from a private program to a public-private venture funded by federal and state funds and private donations that has the potential to provide coverage to more than 12 000 children. The Michigan experience may be instructive to other states attempting to devise immediate local solutions to the problem of the uninsured.**

(*AJDC.* 1991;145:579-580)

Health care financing and delivery mechanisms used in other industrialized nations have been suggested by many as models for reform of the American health care system. Given the pluralistic nature of American politics, however, it is unlikely that approaches used by other countries can be successfully duplicated in this country. At least in the near term, reforms that build on the current system rather than necessitating radical restructuring of existing mechanisms are most likely to garner sufficient support to be implemented. We describe one approach to building on the current financing and delivery mechanisms to address issues of access to care. Implications for broader applicability are also considered.

The Caring Program for Children (CPC) is a well-established private program offering health benefits to uninsured children who meet eligibility criteria. The program was initiated by Blue Cross of Western Pennsylvania and implemented in 11 additional Blue Cross and Blue Shield plans throughout the country. While the programs have provided health benefit coverage to some children who are not eligible for other private or public programs and whose families cannot afford private insurance, as a private effort the programs have had relatively modest impacts on the problem of uninsured children. In Michigan, the Department of Social Services (DSS) and Blue Cross and Blue Shield of Michigan (BCBSM) have worked together to expand the CPC into a public-private partnership plan. This effort will be a laboratory to test the effectiveness of combining federal, state, and private funding to offer health benefits through a private delivery and administrative mechanism.

Accepted for publication February 5, 1991.

From Blue Cross and Blue Shield of Michigan, Detroit (Mss Udow and Mason) and the Michigan Department of Social Services, Lansing (Dr Smith).

Reprint requests to Blue Cross Blue Shield of Michigan, 600 Lafayette E, J218, Detroit MI 48226 (Ms Mason).

BACKGROUND

Across the United States over the last half decade, key state and local policymakers have become involved in efforts to identify the number of uninsured Americans and to devise local strategies to address the problem. Some states have initiated programs ranging from universal access models and mandated employer-based health coverage to initiatives that target specific population groups.

There is no "silver bullet" approach toward which policymakers automatically migrate as each state grapples with the need to strike a balance between cost and coverage. Common to all the states' efforts, however, is that diverse groups and coalitions have developed consensus on the urgency of the local situation and that the solutions reflect the unique circumstances and conditions each locality. The recent Michigan experience illustrates how coalitions can develop to create a policy environment conducive to implementation of programs that address health care for the uninsured.

In the middle to late 1980s, the increasing priority given to health care of the uninsured in Michigan was reflected in the creation of task forces, commissions, and work groups by provider, advocate, and health policy organizations. In Michigan, this included The Greater Detroit Area Health Council, the Michigan Hospital Association, the Michigan State Medical Society, the Michigan Protection and Advocacy Service, and the Michigan League for Human Services. Remarkably, given the diversity of the groups examining the issue, a sense of urgency about the creation of programs to provide health care for children was common among all groups. The findings that one third, or about 300 000, of the uninsured in Michigan are children—most of them in families of the "working poor"—and that uninsured children in need of medical care do face severe obstacles to obtaining care, generated consensus that any strategy should include as its first priority a focus on children. All who studied this issue concluded that neither private nor public approaches alone will solve this problem, but that a combination of public and private approaches will be necessary.

For example, based on the findings of the Governor's Task Force on Access to Health Care, a broadly representative, 40-member body, "Healthy Start" was proposed as an expansion of Medicaid to provide health care coverage to children up to age 18 years in families with incomes of up to 200% of the federal poverty level. At the same time, BCBSM announced plans to implement the CPC, to be financed by private donations. The DSS and BCBSM began discussing ways to work together to ensure that the programs would be complementary.

Meanwhile, two legislative committees were examining the issue of the uninsured. The House Republican Task Force on Affordable Health Care for the Uninsured included in its final report,[1] issued in July 1990, eight recommendations largely focused on making health insurance more affordable to small-business owners. Notably, the primary recommendation was that legislation should be enacted to allow BCBSM to implement the CPC. The House Democratic Commission on Families identified health care as one of the key issues affecting the strength of families and urged in its September 1990 report[2] that priority be given to the adoption of statutory changes necessary to implement the CPC.

Owing to other budget priorities, Healthy Start was not enacted by the 1990 state legislature. The DSS and BCBSM then joined forces and secured a 3-year, $6.6 million matching grant from the Health Care Financing Administration to supplement private and state funds for the CPC. Underlying the grant proposal was the premise that through public-private partnerships programs such as the CPC are greatly enhanced—use of public funds allows the Michigan CPC to provide coverage to more children and broaden benefit coverage, while use of private sector delivery mechanisms offers access to more providers. The federal grant allowed the CPC to expand coverage to include prescription drugs, and the program has the potential to provide coverage to more than 12 000 children.

PROGRAM DESIGN

The CPC is designed to provide the highest priority services to the population group with the greatest need for health care services.

Administrative Structure

Blue Cross and Blue Shield of Michigan provides free administrative services, and the DSS administers the funds and assists with outreach and coordination with government programs. To ensure broad community involvement in the program, an advisory committee composed of 30 representatives from business, labor, religious organizations, the health care providers, parents, and state government provides fund-raising, outreach support, and general oversight of the CPC.

Target Population

The CPC provides primary health care coverage to children aged 18 years and younger whose household incomes are at or below 185% of the federal poverty level and who are not eligible for Medicaid or other sponsored health coverage. Under the terms of the Health Care Financing Administration grant, priority for coverage is given to children of employed former welfare recipients. All eligible children in a family are required to enroll simultaneously to provide a mixed risk pool of sick and well children. Enrollees are recertified annually.

Benefits

Benefits under the CPC are aimed at providing the basic preventive and primary health care coverage children need to avoid chronic illness and permanent disability. Because children are hospitalized less often than adults, and to provide coverage for as many children as possible, inpatient care is not covered under the program. Benefits of CPC include preventive care (including well-child care and immunizations), office visits to physicians, outpatient and office diagnostic and therapeutic laboratory and radiology services, outpatient and office surgery and anesthesia, outpatient and office accident medical emergency care, outpatient substance abuse services, and prescription drugs. These are covered in full, with no deductibles or copayments.

Provider Arrangements

All BCBSM participating physicians and BCBSM Participating Provider Organization pharmacies are eligible for reimbursement through the CPC. A number of pediatricians, family practitioners, and other providers are participating with BCBSM especially for the CPC.

Funding

The CPC is supported by private funds raised by BCBSM and state funds, which are matched by a special grant from the federal government. Private contributions to the program are tax deductible.

IMPLICATIONS

While the Michigan CPC is only a relatively small step toward providing health benefit coverage to the uninsured, it can have profound lessons for a more comprehensive solution. First, the program is easily duplicated in other states. Second, existing structures necessary to implement the program are for the most part already in place so that implementation can occur relatively quickly. Finally, the program builds widespread coalition support. Indeed, the strength of this effort has been the broad base of interest from providers and consumers of health care as well as from private health benefit carriers, financiers, regulators, and legislators. The depth of this support, including the willingness to commit to this effort on a long-term basis, will be key to the general applicability of this kind of an approach.

In the long term, more radical restructuring of our mechanisms to finance health care may be necessary to ensure access to health care for all. It does not appear, however, that this country is yet ready for such a major change in health policy. In that context, much can be learned from the several efforts under way across the country that use public-private partnerships to deliver health care services to segments of the uninsured populations. Programs that can be implemented now and that maximize funding and administrative capabilities from all sources, such as the Michigan CPC, are likely to have much more immediate impacts on delivering needed care to the uninsured.

References

1. House Republican Policy Committee. *Recommendations of the House Republican Task Force on Affordable Health Care for the Uninsured.* July 1990.

2. The House Majority Commission on Families. *Interim Report.* September 1989.

Comments on Life After Residency

Sir.—I read the editorial by Boyce[1] in the August 1990 issue of *AJDC* and believe it discusses a subject that should be of great interest to everyone. Dr Boyce is a thoughtful and kind individual who has given the reader his "highly personal" view on this subject. While personal views are sometimes insightful and creative, they may also fail to note that there may be extensive literature on the subject.

Twenty-five years ago, I began what has evolved into an annual lecture to freshmen medical students at Jefferson Medical College, Philadelphia, Pa, entitled "Medicine, An Excuse From Living."[2] It was published in 1978 and reprinted in 1990.[3] Before and since the 1978 publication, many articles have been published dealing with this subject. The publications are not all in agreement and they do not reflect the same level of scholarship or insight.

Dr Boyce discusses five criteria or assumptions that he believes "guide our collective approach" to setting priorities and making key decisions. Some might refer to these concepts as dogma or truisms: (1) "The development of meaningful personal relationships (such as one's marriage) can and often must be postponed until certain professional goals are attained." (2) "Medicine must be the physician's highest priority (with the corollary that the more time devoted to medicine, the greater the rewards)." (3) "The single objective in setting priorities is to establish a balance between work life and home life." (4) "In most issues of competing demands on time, efficiency is the solution." (5) "Lack of time with children can be balanced by spending 'quality time.'" Dr Boyce's comments about these criteria are sensitive and thoughtful, but they are of little assistance to the individual who wishes to prevent personal or professional tragedies. His approach is a positive one but he does not address the reasons why individuals may ignore their professional or personal responsibilities or why relationships between spouses or children and parents may fail to mature.

He also fails to commit himself with regard to the problem of postponing personal responsibilities. He vacillates between the importance of professional and personal responsibilities and says "Perhaps the solution lies instead in a dialectic that simultaneously embraces a deep-seated commitment to both professional and personal life. . . . There is a sense in which the building of a 'creative tension' between one's public and private lives results in greater contentment and well-being than a unifocal dedication to either." I find these concepts difficult to translate into specific behaviors that will assist one in establishing priorities or preventing personal or professional tragedies. His discussion of the establishment of priorities is even further removed from practical application since it is "derived from a context of true spirituality." I believe there are more understandable concepts to assist individuals in establishing priorities.

I *do* agree that the concept of quality time with children is a myth. However, I do not believe that "moments of joy and extraordinary closeness" are the basis for successful parent-child relationships and child rearing. The basis of success is the degree to which you can make that child feel special, loved, and respected. This will come only when the child knows he or she is one of your high priorities.

This subject matter has been developed into a course at Jefferson Medical College called "Personal Problems of Physicians," a 20-hour elective for second-year medical students. With regard to the competition between one's professional and personal lives, the following are some of the concepts discussed in that curriculum.

1. A percentage of marriage partners will have serious psychiatric disorders or personality problems. Rational principles for building and strengthening interpersonal relationships may not be successful with these partners. Recognition of the seriousness of the situation is the first step to possible resolution of problems.

2. One cannot treat all interpersonal relationships identically. Individuals come into a marriage with varied backgrounds and expectations. Therefore, preventive measures have to focus on the areas of greatest deficiencies in coping skills and on unrealistic expectations.

3. The most serious barrier to the development of mature and loving relationships between healthy spouses is a discrepancy in expectations and an unwillingness to discuss these differences and resolve them.

4. "Becoming a good doctor is, relatively speaking, an egocentric although respectable goal and that the most difficult and most important accomplishments in life are the development of giving relationships with other human beings, be they spouse, parents, children or friends."[2]

5. "When things go wrong at the interpersonal level the anguish and heartache are measurably greater than you will ever experience from disappointment in your profession."[2]

6. Physicians may learn, or be trained by their loved ones, that their medical responsibilities *can* be used to defer other responsibilities, whenever and wherever they choose, because families can easily be intimidated by the accusation that they are taking their spouse or parent away from a sick or dying patient.

7. While time management and organizational skills may be important in determining whether one is successful in his or her personal or professional life, they are secondary to commitment. It is much easier to be committed to the portion of your life that is filled with numerous short-term rewards. External recognition for developing mature and giving interpersonal relationships is meager

and long-term. The psychological basis of commitment has to be brought to consciousness. The saving grace is that commitment can be taught to the uncommitted.

These are just a few of the points we discuss in our elective course. The important point is that this is an extensive subject matter that has to be introduced to help physicians prepare for their personal and professional lives. As pediatricians, we believe in preventive medicine and, therefore, it is appropriate for this subject matter to be part of medical school education. It may prevent some family tragedies.

I am further indebted to Dr Boyce for one clever innovation. He says he has 18 years of parenting experience. I do not know whether he has 6-year-old triplets or 11- and 7-year-old children. But this innovative way of expressing parental experience permits my wife and me to now claim 317 years of parenting and grandparenting experience!

Robert L. Brent, MD, PhD
Department of Pediatrics
Jefferson Medical College
Philadelphia, PA 19102

1. Boyce WT. Life after residency: setting priorities in pediatric professional life. *AJDC.* 1990;144:858-860.
2. Brent RL, Brent LH. Medicine, an excuse from living. *Resident Staff Phys.* 1978;24:61-65.
3. Garfield E. Science and emotion are compatible: a tribute to Robert and Lillian Brent. *Curr Contents Clin Med.* 1990;18:2-10.

How Much Iron Is Enough?

Sir.—I write to take issue with the commentary by Finberg[1] in the November 1990 issue of *AJDC.* I do not agree that all infant formulas should have added iron. I say this for two reasons.

First, Finberg seems to assume that iron-fortified formula is the only source of iron for the infant and small child. All the cereals that I (and many others) have our patients start taking at age 2 months are now fortified. Meats are recommended by many of us at 4 months or even earlier. Many foods such as beans, nuts, and raisins have a high iron content. Most bread, macaroni, and spaghetti products are now iron fortified. So infants and toddlers get enough iron without fortifying their formulas.

Second, based on my experience, I disagree that extra iron gives no problems to a baby. Take an infant at 1, 2, or 3 months of age, as I have, who has been on a low-iron formula. Offer the mother three to four cans of an iron-enriched formula and ask her if she can see the difference. I have found many mothers who said "Iron gave gas and cramps; I had the same trouble when I had to take extra iron during my pregnancy!"

If what you advocate were true, I should have hundreds of anemic children in my practice—and I do not! My only rare patients with anemia are ones whose mothers keep on the bottle for over a year and take milk at the expense of a normal diet.

William B. Rogers, MD
1935 Second St
Cuyahoga Falls, OH 44221

1. Finberg L. Remembrance and loose ends of controversies past. *AJDC.* 1990;144:1188.

In Reply.—I am particularly pleased to respond to Dr Rogers' letter because he raises issues that are important and to which I believe there are completely satisfactory answers.

First, consider the issue of iron sources for most infants. Remember that we are here recommending a population approach that is appropriate as long as there is no harm and no excessive cost. The fortunate infants under Dr Rogers' care do not typify the population and most of them undoubtedly have done well with their iron nutrition. Many American infants are not offered fortified solid foods early on, and 10 or 15 years ago, this group had a very high incidence of iron deficiency. Some of those taking "low-iron" formulas still do. An analogy would be to oppose adding vitamin D to milk because many infants have enough sun exposure to avoid rickets.

Second, Dr Rogers raises the issue of symptoms experienced by infants taking iron-fortified milk. Objective studies[1] have shown that the symptoms are not related to the iron and occur no matter what feeding change is made and for the same number of infants. Thus, the symptom argument does not stand up under scrutiny.

Third, Dr Rogers states that he does not have "hundreds of anemic children" in his practice. I am sure he is correct; however, I believe that if he recommended fortified formula the overall prevalence of iron adequacy would be even better.

Anemia is only one ill effect of iron deficiency. We can only know if Dr Rogers or others with similar situations have such indexes as transferrin saturation, ferritin levels, and body storage iron. Iron contributes to cellular function, probably to growth and possibly to both intelligence and resistance to infection, the last having some exceptions of importance. More important in this context, though, are the inner city and rural poor whose need for iron is more crucial.

Finally, no harm is done and the cost of this low but very useful amount of iron fortification is negligible. I thank Dr Rogers for writing and allowing for greater explication.

Laurence Finberg, MD
450 Clarkson Ave, Box 49
Brooklyn, NY 11203

1. Nelson SE, Ziegler EE, Copland AM, Edwards BB, Foman SJ. Lack of adverse reactions to iron fortified formula. *Pediatrics.* 1988;87:360-364.

Acute Glossitis and Bacteremia Caused by *Streptococcus pneumoniae:* Case Report and Review

Sir.—Acute bacterial glossitis is a rare but extremely serious entity. To date, only a handful of case reports have appeared in the literature. A variety of causative organisms have been identified, including three cases of acute glossitis resulting from *Haemophilus influenzae* type B,[1-3] two cases of suppurative glossitis from *Pseudomonas* species and hemolytic streptococci,[4] and one case of glossitis associated with *Trichomonas* species.[5] We report the first case, to our knowledge, of acute glossitis and associated bacteremia caused by *Streptococcus pneumoniae* to recognize this organism's role in this disease.

Patient Report.—A 28-month-old, previously healthy white boy presented to the clinic with a 1-day history of fever, cold symptoms, and mild crankiness. He refused any oral intake during the morning of his presentation. His mother noted rapidly progressive swelling of the tongue during the 3 hours prior to the office visit. No history of tongue trauma, toxin ingestion, or allergies was elicited. The patient's temperature was 39.6°C. The physical examination revealed a mildly

Reported Cases of Infectious Glossitis

Source, y	Patient Age	Causative Organism	Comment
Chandra and Prakash,[4] 1965	5 y 6 y	*Pseudomonas* species hemolytic streptococci	Suppurative parenchymatous glossitis requiring incision and drainage of residual abscesses (both cases)
Granoff and Nankervis,[1] 1976	14 mo	*Haemophilus influenzae* type B	Diffuse swelling of tongue and uvula; resembled angioneurotic edema
Edwards and Reynolds,[2] 1978	20 mo	*H influenzae* type B	Associated bacteremia; tongue excoriation present
San Joaquin et al,[3] 1980	4 y	*H influenzae* type B	Associated bacteremia
Brenner and Simon,[5] 1984	29 y	*Trichomonas* species	Communicated by orogenital sexual contact
Present report	28 mo	*Streptococcus pneumoniae*	Associated bacteremia

distressed boy with an enlarged, edematous, and erythematous tongue protruding slightly from his mouth. Involvement was greatest at the anterior aspect of the tongue. No evidence of laceration or trauma was observed. Phonation was normal and there was no evidence of stridor, dyspnea, or airway compromise. An otolaryngologist evaluated the child on his admission to the local hospital; there, the working diagnosis of tongue cellulitis was made. Blood cultures were obtained, and the child was given a dose of intravenous ceftriaxone sodium and was transferred to the Johns Hopkins Pediatric Intensive Care Unit, Baltimore, Md, for further treatment.

On his arrival at the unit, the child's temperature was 38.5°C and his respiratory rate was 20 to 30 per minute; profound drooling was observed. The anterior aspect of his tongue was diffusely enlarged, thickened, and erythematous. A few scattered vesicular lesions were noted on the tongue's ventral aspect. The patient's neck was supple, with marked bilateral, anterior cervical lymphadenopathy and left-sided posterior cervical lymphadenopathy. No cough, stridor, wheeze, or hoarseness was noted. Pulse oximetry demonstrated oxygen saturation of 97% to 100% in room air. Lateral neck roentgenograms showed a normal airway, pharynx, and epiglottis. The patient's white blood cell count was 24.7×10^9/L, with 0.47 neutrophils, 0.17 band forms, 0.21 lymphocytes, and 0.13 monocytes. Repeated blood culture, throat culture for group-A streptococci, and viral culture of the vesicular lesions were performed, the results of which were all negative, as were the results of an *H influenzae* type B latex agglutination assay of urine. The C1 esterase inhibitor level was normal.

On admission to the intensive care unit, the child's antibiotic therapy was changed to intravenous penicillin G potassium (250 000 U/kg per day) and cefuroxime sodium (150 mg/kg per day). He promptly defervesced, becoming afebrile within 12 hours after the onset of symptoms, and showed a rapid decrease in tongue swelling during the 24 hours following presentation. No subsequent complications were encountered. The original blood culture (obtained before antibiotics were administered) was positive for *S pneumoniae* after 24 hours. The child was discharged the following day.

Comment. — Few epidemiologic data are available on acute infectious glossitis (Table). Indeed, the available literature consists only of scattered case reports. Of those cases, the most common pathogen responsible for the infection is *H influenzae* type B. The authors' descriptions indicate that these cases were cellulitic and not pyogenic in nature. By contrast, Chandra and Prakash[4] described two instances in children of suppurative parenchymatous glossitis, resulting in abscess formation requiring incision and drainage; *Pseudomonas* species and hemolytic streptococci were the identified causative organisms in these cases. Finally, Brenner and Simon[5] reported *Trichomonas* species as the causative agent in a case of acute glossitis with prominent white plaques appearing in a 29-year-old man with a history of orogenital contact with a new sexual partner within the week before symptom onset.

To our knowledge, no other cases of pneumococcal glossitis have been reported. Clinically, our patient resembled the patient described by San Joaquin et al.[3] There was no obvious source of entry (tongue or mucosal or skin lesion) in either patient, and tongue swelling progressed rapidly. Because life-threatening respiratory impairment can develop rapidly in such cases, early recognition and prompt treatment are imperative. Treatment decisions in cases of acute glossitis should take into consideration *S pneumoniae* as a possible causative agent.

Jeffrey J. Stoddard, MD
Department of Pediatrics

Jayant K. Deshpande, MD
Department of Pediatrics
Department of Anesthesiology/Critical Care Medicine
Johns Hopkins Medical Institutions
600 N Wolfe St
Baltimore, MD 21205

1. Granoff DM, Nankervis GA. Cellulitis due to *Haemophilus influenzae* type B: antigenemia and antibody responses. *AJDC.* 1976;130:1211-1214.

2. Edwards MS, Reynolds GES. Acute glossitis due to *Hemophilus influenzae* type B. *J Pediatr.* 1978;93:532-533.

3. San Joaquin VH, Granum M, Surpure JS, Srouji ES. Acute glossitis and septicemia owing to *Haemophilus influenzae* type B. *AJDC.* 1980;134:91.

4. Chandra T, Prakash A. Suppurative parenchymatous glossitis. *Br J Surg.* 1965;52:234-235.

5. Brenner BE, Simon RR. Glossitis and dysgeusia. *Am J Emerg Med.* 1984;2:147.

Puncture Wound–Induced *Achromobacter xylosoxidans* Osteomyelitis of the Foot

Sir.—*Achromobacter xylosoxidans* is a gram-negative bacteria, found in the vertebrate intestinal tract and isolated from aqueous environments. The majority of infections caused by *A xylosoxidans* are either nosocomially acquired or involve immunocompromised hosts, but sporadic community-acquired infections in presumed normal patients have been described.[1]

Osteomyelitis of the foot following puncture wounds through sneakers is most often associated with *Pseudomonas aeruginosa* or other *Pseudomonas* species.[2-4] We describe a child with community-acquired *A xylosoxidans* osteomyelitis of the foot that resulted from a puncture wound.

Patient Report.—A previously healthy 11-year-old boy stepped on two nails 2.5

weeks before seeking care. The nails penetrated his tennis shoe to a presumed depth of about 2 inches. Immediately after the injury, the foot was soaked in hydrogen peroxide and alcohol. The wounds initially appeared to be healing well without evidence of drainage, pain, or swelling. In the week before admission the child complained of progressive, severe left foot pain. Several days before admission, swelling and a bluish discoloration of the sole of his foot just distal to one of the puncture wounds was noted.

On admission, the following were noted: temperature of 37.4°C and two puncture wounds on the plantar surface of his left foot, one of which was tender; the remainder of his physical examination was unremarkable. The peripheral white blood cell count was 11.1×10^9/L with 0.43 polymorphonuclear cells, 0.53 lymphocytes, and 0.04 monocytes. Wintrobe erythrocyte sedimentation rate was 12 mm/h. Roentgenography of the foot showed a lucency in the metaphysis of the left fifth metatarsal with associated soft-tissue swelling.

Blood cultures were obtained and therapy with intravenous ticarcillin disodium–clavulanate potassium (200 mg/kg per day) and gentamicin (7.5 mg/kg per day) therapy was begun; the child underwent surgical exploration of the wound within 24 hours. The fifth digital flexor tendon was necrotic; there was a lytic lesion in the fifth metatarsal that had broken through the plantar cortex. The bone was curetted, irrigated, and externally drained. Aerobic culture of the wound yielded coagulase-negative staphylococci. An oxidase-positive, gram-negative rod, subsequently identified as *A xylosoxidans*, was isolated from the bone specimen. This organism was resistant to gentamicin, tobramycin sulfate, and amikacin sulfate and sensitive to ticarcillin, trimethoprim-sulfamethoxazole, ticarcillin-clavulanic acid, and ceftazidime sodium. The child remained afebrile throughout his hospitalization. His foot swelling resolved by the fifth hospital day. Fourteen days after surgery, the erythrocyte sedimentation rate was 22 mm/h. He received ticarcillin-clavulanic acid and gentamicin after surgery for a total of 14 days and was discharged receiving oral trimethoprim-sulfamethoxazole therapy (16 mg/kg per day). At follow-up examination 2.5 months after surgery he was completely asymptomatic; roentgenographs showed periosteal reaction around the metaphysis of the fifth metatarsal.

Comment.—Achromobacter xylosoxidans is an aerobic gram-negative rod whose taxonomy remains in dispute. It is also known as *Alcaligenes dentrificans* subspecies *xylosoxidans* or *Achromobacter xylosoxidans* subspecies *xylosoxidans* and is listed in *Index Medicus* under *Alcaligenes*.[5] The organism has been recovered from a number of human sources including ear discharge; pleural and peritoneal fluid; urine; feces; cerebrospinal fluid; swabs of the eyes, ears, and pharynx; blood; prosthetic heart valves[1]; and bone.[6] It has also been isolated from numerous aqueous sources, including disinfectants commonly employed in hospitals.[1] Osteomyelitis due to *A xylosoxidans* is rare. To our knowledge, only one other case of *A xylosoxidans* osteomyelitis, in a patient with a fractured tibia, has been reported.[6]

Osteomyelitis of the foot following puncture wounds is usually caused by *P aeruginosa*, although infections with *Pseudomonas stutzeri* and *Pseudomonas maltophilia* have been described.[3,4] Our patient displayed the characteristics usually associated with *P aeruginosa*–induced osteomyelitis, including delayed symptomatology after puncture, lack of fever or systemic symptoms, and a normal white blood cell count. However, his erythrocyte sedimentation rate did not become elevated until 10 days after surgery.[7]

The most active antimicrobial agents against *A xylosoxidans* and nonaeruginosa *Pseudomonas* isolates appear to be the third-generation cephalosporins and trimethoprim-sulfamethoxazole. They are usually resistant to aminoglycosides and are variably susceptible to antipseudomonal penicillins.[8] Initial treatment of *P aeruginosa* osteomyelitis has generally included an aminoglycoside and antipseudomonal penicillin or a cephalosporin.[9] This may be inadequate therapy for *A xylosoxidans* infections and may lead to progression of disease or prolonged hospitalization. The duration of therapy of *A xylosoxidans* osteomyelitis of the foot awaits further definition.

As in our patient, it has been repeatedly demonstrated that sinus tract cultures do not reliably predict the causative agent of underlying acute or chronic osteomyelitis.[6,10] Bone cultures thus remain essential to determine antimicrobial therapy.

David M. Hoddy, MD
Department of Pediatrics
St Louis University School of Medicine
St Louis, MO 63104

Leslie L. Barton, MD
Department of Pediatrics
University of Arizona Health Sciences Center
Tucson, AZ 85724

1. Mandell WF, Garvey GJ, Neu HC. *Achromobacter xylosoxidans* bacteremia. *Rev Infect Dis.* 1987;9:1001-1005.
2. Fisher MC, Goldsmith JF, Gilligan PH. Sneakers as a source of *Pseudomonas aeruginosa* in children with osteomyelitis following puncture wounds. *J Pediatr.* 1985;106:607-609.
3. Rowley AH, Dias LD, Chadwick EG, Shulman ST. *Pseudomonas stutzeri*: an unusual case of calcaneal *Pseudomonas* osteomyelitis. *Pediatr Infect Dis J.* 1987;6:296-297.
4. Baltimore RS, Jenson HB. Puncture wound osteochondritis caused by *Pseudomonas maltophilia. Pediatr Infect Dis J.* 1990;9:143-144.
5. Kiredjian M, Holmes B, Kersters K, Guilvout I, DeLey J. *Alcaligenes piechaudii:* a new species from human clinical specimens and the environment. *Int J Syst Bacteriol.* 1986;36:282-287.
6. Dubey L, Krasinski K, Hernanz-Schulman M. Osteomyelitis secondary to trauma or infected contiguous soft tissue. *Pediatr Infect Dis J.* 1988;7:26-34.
7. Jacobs RF, McCarthy RE, Elser JM. *Pseudomonas* osteochondritis complicating puncture wounds of the foot in children: a 10 year evaluation. *J Infect Dis.* 1989;160:657-661.
8. Schoch PE, Cunha BA. Nosocomial *Achromobacter xylosoxidans* infections. *Infect Control Hosp Epidemiol.* 1988;9:84-87.
9. Joseph WS, LeFrock JL. Infections complicating puncture wounds of the foot. *J Foot Surg.* 1987;26:S30-S33.
10. Mackowiak PA, Jones SR, Smith JW. Diagnostic value of sinus-tract cultures in chronic osteomyelitis. *JAMA.* 1978;239:2772-2775.

Condylomata Acuminata: Still Usually a Sexually Transmitted Disease in Children

Sir.—A number of points about the recent article by Boyd[1] on human papillomavirus (HPV) genital infections in children need to be made so that pediatricians and other concerned professionals, such as Family Court judges, are not confused or misled by this attempt at a "meta-analysis" of previous case reports.

First, as Disraeli once noted, "There are lies, there are damned lies, and there are statistics!" I have a very basic quarrel with Boyd's statistical analysis because he analyzes all cases together. One major question—how often condylomata acuminata are representative of sexual transmission, ie, sexual abuse in children—does not lend itself to this "lumping" of data.

To answer this important question, one must exclude children younger than age 1.5 years, since most of these cases are due to vertical transmission at or even before birth. One must also exclude teenagers, who may be having consensual sexual relations, and at any rate can give a clear history so that the mode of transmission is much less often an issue. When the denominator in Table 2[1] is thus revised, we have a sexual abuse reporting rate of 43% of the relevant cases of condylomata acuminata, a rate that is compatible with previous reports,[2] and not the very low and misleading 28% that Boyd reports.

Furthermore, the fact that a sexual mode of transmission cannot be clearly established in no way means that sexual transmission of wart virus did not occur! Children younger than age 7 years who are evaluated for sexual abuse often give unreliable histories due to fear, immaturity, or inadequate language. Boys are the worst at reporting and seldom reveal abuse at ages younger than 16 years,[3] even when confronted with incontrovertible evidence. For example, I reported a case of a 10-year-old boy with perirectal condyloma lata—proven syphilis—who refused to acknowledge what had happened to him despite our best efforts.[4]

Finally, I must take issue with Boyd's Table 3.[1] I can find no evidence from good, original sources to support the idea that HPV types 1 through 4 or 10 cause condylomata acuminata genital warts. No author or investigator I have known in the past 6 years has ever detected DNA from these subtypes in any clinical specimens from perineal or rectal area condylomata acuminata, in either adults or children. If Boyd knows of such data, I would appreciate references to *primary sources* that he believes are authoritative and use good methods. I previously pointed out[5,6] possible methodologic errors in an often-quoted 1980 study.[7] This report, which I once quoted in a review[8] before realizing its flaws, exemplifies why reliance on critically and meticulously reviewed original reports is essential when developing references in this extremely difficult and potentially controversial field of investigation.

Therefore, I must emphasize that Boyd's analysis should be viewed with skepticism if he intends us to conclude that nonsexual transmission of HPV takes place with any degree of commonness. It clearly can happen,[9] but under very circumscribed clinical circumstances.[5,6] I stick strongly to my position (also taken by other experts[10]) that there is only rare evidence of nonsexual transmission of condylomata acuminata–type warts.[5,6,8] I have previously suggested a clinical scheme for determining whether warts in the rectoperineal area in children are probably sexually transmitted and should be reported for investigation.[6]

John M. Goldenring, MD, MPH
245 Terracina Blvd, No. 202
Redlands, CA 92373

1. Boyd AS. Condylomata acuminata in the pediatric population. *AJDC.* 1990;144:817-824.

2. Schachner L, Hankin DE. Assessing child abuse in childhood condyloma acuminata. *J Am Acad Dermatol.* 1985;12:157-160.

3. Johnson RL, Shrier DK. Sexual victimization of boys. *J Adolesc Health Care.* 1985;6:372-376.

4. Goldenring J. Secondary syphilis in a prepubertal child: differentiating condylomata lata from condylomata acuminata. *NY State J Med.* 1989;89:180-181.

5. Goldenring JM. Condylomata acuminata in the evaluation of child sexual abuse. *Arch Dermatol.* 1987;123:1265-1266.

6. Goldenring JM. Warts and diagnosis of sexual abuse. *Lancet.* 1987;2:1018-1019.

7. Kryzek RA, Watts SL, Anderson DL, et al. Anogenital warts contain several distinct species of human papilloma virus. *J Virol.* 1980;36:236-244.

8. Neinstein LS, Goldenring J, Carpenter S. Non-sexual transmission of sexually transmitted diseases: an infrequent occurrence. *Pediatrics.* 1984;74:67-76.

9. Rock B, Naghasfar Z, Barnett N, et al. Genital papilloma virus in children. *Arch Dermatol.* 1986;22:1129-1132.

10. Verdich JH. Venereal diseases in children and sexual abuse. *Ugeskr Laeger.* 1989;151:555-557.

In Reply.—I would like to thank Dr Goldenring for his careful analysis of my article. Although I am unsure of the exact meaning of "meta-analysis" in this context, I can assure him that, like most retrospective analyses of the literature, this project was undertaken with the desire to better define the picture, not muddy the waters. It was never my intent to assess the problem with a statistical analysis; otherwise, inferences would have been made from them. These figures are simply a compilation of what is present in the literature.

Goldenring seems to intimate that the percentage of children who acquire venereal warts from molestation is much higher, an opinion not held by all experts and for which significant evidence to the contrary now exists.[1,2] Cohen et al[1] evaluated 73 children with anogenital warts and concluded that fewer than 10% had been sexually abused. Likewise, Obalek and coworkers[2] recently reported that of 32 children with condylomata acuminata, only one (3%) was suspected of having been molested. It appears that the 28% figure cited in my article may be more accurate than Goldenring acknowledges.

Eliminating children younger than age 1.5 years and teenagers will certainly lessen the pool of patients to analyze, but it may also exclude some patients. Most, but not all, children younger than 18 months probably do indeed acquire their lesions by vertical transmission.[3-5] Goldenring's statement, ". . . the fact that a sexual mode of transmission cannot be clearly established in no way means that sexual transmission of wart virus did not occur!" should be taken *prima facia*. The 37% of the cited cases in which the infection was acquired by unknown means are simply that, cases in which the authors failed to discover a means of infection.

Finally, Goldenring takes issue with Table 3 in which HPV types 1, 2, 6, 10, 11, 16, and 18 are cited as being associated with anogenital warts. The types he questions the most, 1, 2, and 10, were cited by a group of investigators[6] who included those types on a table in their article. On more careful inspection of their references, I was unable to find documentation for the discovery of condylomata acuminata with these HPV types. However, the authors of the two previously cited reports,[1,2] as well as our clinic, have found "nonclassical" HPV types, *including* type 2, in cases of pediatric venereal warts. Those who also "stick strongly" to Golden-ring's position that ". . . there is only rare evidence of nonsexual transmission . . ." for anogenital warts may want to reexamine their views in light of the recent evidence to the contrary.

ALAN S. BOYD, MD
Department of Dermatology
Texas Tech University
Health Sciences Center
Lubbock, TX 79430

1. Cohen BA, Honig P, Androphy E. Anogenital warts in children. *Arch Dermatol.* 1990;126:1575-1580.
2. Obalek S, Jablonska S, Favre M, Walczak L, Orth G. Condylomata acuminata in children: frequent association with human papillomaviruses responsible for cutaneous warts. *J Am Acad Dermatol.* 1990;23:205-213.
3. Herman-Giddens ME, Gutman LT, Berson NL. Association of coexisting vaginal infections and multiple abusers in female children with genital warts. *Sex Transm Dis.* 1988;15:63-67.
4. McCoy CR, Applebaum H, Besser AS. Condyloma acuminata: an unusual presentation of child abuse. *J Pediatr Surg.* 1982;17:505-507.
5. Sadan O, Koller AB, Adno A, Peale PG. Massive vulval condylomata acuminata in a 10-month-old child with suspected sexual abuse: case report. *Br J Obstet Gynaecol.* 1985;92:1201-1203.
6. Silva PD, Micha JP, Silva DG. Management of condyloma acuminatum. *J Am Acad Dermatol.* 1985;13:457-463.

Lead Poisoning in Children With Developmental Disabilities

Sir.—We were pleased to read the article by Friedman and Weinberger[1] in the September 1990 issue of *AJDC* regarding the screening, diagnosis, and treatment of children with lead poisoning. We describe a child with mental retardation whose pica behavior led to lead poisoning.

Patient Description.—An 8-year-old boy with previously diagnosed infantile autism and mental retardation underwent interdisciplinary team evaluation. The medical history incorporated questions regarding stereotypic behaviors, specifically pica. With confirmation of pica, a lead level of 3.13 μmol/L and an erythrocyte protoporphyrin level of 364 μg/dL were measured. Lead-based paint was discovered in the home of the boy's grandparents. He received chelation treatment with intramuscular calcium disodium ethylenediaminetetraacetic acid (EDTA) and oral penicillamine on an outpatient basis. His lead level dropped to 1.45 μmol/L. Repeated developmental testing 4 years later showed performance at the 8-month level in language skills and at the 2- to 3-year level in other skills. The patient's lead level at that time was 2.41 μmol/L, with an erythrocyte protoporphyrin level of 90 μg/dL. Pica behavior was still present.

What Can We Learn From This Patient?—Children and adults with developmental disabilities including autism and mental retardation, regardless of cause, can display behaviors inappropriate to their chronologic ages. These behaviors can be stereotypic or can result from associated medical problems such as iron deficiency. Other features of developmental disorders, such as overactivity and cognitive and motor abnormalities, can obscure the clinical signs of lead poisoning. The prevalence of pica behavior in groups of persons with severe and profound retardation ranges between 5% and 15%.[2,3]

Physicians, family members, and others involved in the care of persons with developmental disabilities should not fail to consider the presence of pica behavior in such individuals. Lead poisoning and other associated problems, such as parasitic infection and foreign body ingestion, are potential causes of additional disabilities that are reversible.

STEPHEN B. SULKES, MD
University Affiliated Program
for Developmental
Disabilities
University of Rochester
Medical Center
Rochester, NY 14642
DENNIS W. O'CONNOR, MD
Keuka Family Practice
Associates
Bath, NY 14810

1. Friedman JA, Weinberger HL. Six children with lead poisoning. *AJDC.* 1990;144:1039-1044.
2. McAlpine C, Singh NN. Pica in institutionalized mentally retarded persons. *J Ment Defic Res.* 1986;30:171-178.
3. Sachdev A, McNiff C. Pica. In: Rubin IL, Crocker AC, eds. *Developmental Disabilities: Delivery of Medical Care for Children and Adults.* Philadelphia, Pa: Lea & Febiger; 1989:361-366.

Neurodevelopmental Outcome of Offspring of the Diabetic Mother: Need for Further Research

Sir.—The improved care of diabetic women prior to conception and during pregnancy has significantly decreased the incidence of mortality, morbidity, and congenital anomalies in the infants of these diabetic mothers.[1-3] However, postnatal complications still occur more frequently among these infants than among infants of nondiabetic mothers.[4-8] The significance of these complications for the developing child of the diabetic mother must be established to determine whether the complications at birth predispose these children to later neurodevelopmental dysfunction.

An analysis of the results of follow-up studies of children whose mothers had diabetes during pregnancy should address this issue. Results of five major follow-up studies have been published between 1977 and 1988.[9-13] However, the results have often been contradictory and limited by methodologic flaws. For example, only two of the studies employed control groups.[12,13] In all the studies, sample sizes were relatively small (73 to 174 children) and attrition rates were high (15% to 42%). The high mortality rates (ranging from 7% to 14%) combined with the relatively high attrition rates make inferences based on the findings problematic, since only 58% to 85% of the cohorts were actually evaluated.

The variability of the study designs further confounds comparisons between studies. The instruments used to evaluate outcome included standardized intelligence tests,[9,10] a developmental screening device,[13] and behavioral questionnaires.[11,12] Conclusions based on the data collected were often inconsistent and contradictory. For example, Stehbens et al[9] found impaired intellectual functioning among 5-year-old children of diabetic mothers who were small for gestational age or whose mother's pregnancy was complicated by acetonuria. On the other hand, Persson and Gentz[11] found no relationship between maternal acetonuria and intelligence. Cummins and Norrish[10] reported a normal distribution of intellectual functioning among children of diabetic mothers. Petersen et al[13] determined a relationship between early intrauterine growth delay and lowered developmental scores among children of diabetic mothers.

Similar contradictory results were reported in studies focusing on behavioral data. Persson and Gentz[11] determined that diabetic mothers under high stress reported more behavioral problems among their children. Hadden et al[12] found no differences between the emotional or academic status of children of diabetic mothers and a matched group of children of nondiabetic mothers.

To our knowledge, no one study has comprehensively evaluated neurologic, intellectual, and behavioral outcomes of children of diabetic mothers with a sufficiently large population and a matched control group. Explicit data on maternal pregnancy and newborn outcome, appropriate control groups, large sample size, and a broad range of tests of neurologic, intellectual, and behavioral functioning at school ages are needed to attempt any attribution to the diabetic pregnancy per se. It is yet unclear whether the influence of the diabetic state in pregnancy produces subtle developmental dysfunctions. This can only be detected through a thorough evaluation of the child in a wide range of areas. If it is determined that the child of the diabetic mother is at greater risk for subtle dysfunctions, this child must be followed up closely from birth. Early detection is critical so that remedial programs can be developed and implemented to prevent the predisposition from becoming a precursor for major developmental and learning handicaps.

Esther Goldstein, PhD
Department of Education
Center for Child Development
Basil Porter, MBBCh
Aharon Galil, MD
Center for Child Development
Soroka University Hospital
Ben Gurion
University of the Negev
PO Box 151
Beer Sheva, Israel 84110

1. Fleischman AR, Finberg L. The infant of the diabetic mother and diabetes in infancy. In: Ellenberg M, Rifkin H, eds. *Diabetes Mellitus*. 3rd ed. New York, NY: Medical Examination Publishing Co; 1983:715-725.
2. Schwartz R. The infant of the diabetic mother. In: Davidson JK, ed. *Clinical Diabetes Mellitus*. New York, NY: Thieme-Stratton Inc; 1986:496-504.
3. Damm P, Molsted-Pedersen L. Significant decrease in congenital malformation in newborn infants of an unselected population of diabetic women. *Am J Obstet Gynecol*. 1989;161:1163-1167.
4. Fraser D, Weitzman S. Diabetes in pregnancy and the newborns of diabetic mothers. In: *Epidemiology in Diabetes*. Beer Sheva, Israel: Israeli National Council for Research and Development; 1989.
5. Drexel H, Bichler A, Sailer S, et al. Prevention of perinatal morbidity by tight metabolic control in gestational diabetes mellitus. *Diabetes Care*. 1988; 11:761-768.
6. Lowy C, Beard RW, Goldschmidt J. Congenital malformations in babies of diabetic mothers. *Diabetes Med*. 1986; 3:458-462.
7. Raymond CA. Combing diabetes' teratogenic 'suspect list.' *JAMA*. 1988; 259:333.
8. Cousins L. Congenital anomalies among infants of diabetic mothers. *Am J Obstet Gynecol*. 1983;147:333-338.
9. Stehbens JA, Baker GL, Kitchell M. Outcome at ages 1, 3, and 5 years of children born to diabetic women. *Am J Obstet Gynecol*. 1977;127:408-413.
10. Cummins M, Norrish M. Follow-up of children of diabetic mothers. *Arch Dis Child*. 1980;55:259-264.
11. Persson B, Gentz J. Follow-up of children of insulin dependent and gestational diabetic mothers. *Acta Paediatr Scand*. 1984;73:349-358.
12. Hadden DR, Byrne E, Trotter I, Harley JMG, McClure G, McAuley RR. Physical and psychological health of children of type 1 (insulin-dependent) diabetic mothers. *Diabetologica*. 1984; 26:250-254.
13. Petersen MB, Pedersen SA, Greisen G, Pedersen JF, Molsted-Pedersen L. Early growth delay in diabetic pregnancy: relation to psychomotor development at age 4. *Br Med J*. 1988;296:598-600.

Albuterol Inhalations in Acute Chest Syndrome

Sir.—Recently we treated a 12-year-old boy with sickle cell anemia and acute chest syndrome (ACS) who had decreased air entry in the same way an asthmatic patient does. This prompted us to treat him with nebulized albuterol, which improved his dyspnea and aeration. Finding no reports of β_2 agonist use in acute chest syndrome we performed the following preliminary study to determine if albuterol inhalation therapy could be a useful adjunct in the treatment of ACS in sickle cell anemia.

Patient Reports.—Four patients, including the aforementioned one, all with ACS and sickle cell anemia, were evaluated. None had a personal or family history of asthma or wheezing. Each was at least 8 years old, enabling use of the Wright peak flow meter. Initially each patient had chest pain, difficulty breathing, decreased breath sounds and/or crackles on chest auscultation, and roentgenographic evidence of an acute pulmonary infiltrate. Each was thus diagnosed as having ACS.

The four patients received conventional treatment for ACS, including oxygen, intravenous fluids, antibiotics, and in two cases, exchange transfusions. Each child also received 0.02-mL/kg albuterol sulfate (5 g/L) via 15-minute nebulization. Peak expiratory flow rate was measured before and after each albuterol treatment. Two or three measurements were taken before and after inhalation, thus making improved technique an unlikely cause of peak flow increase. A 15% increase in peak flow was considered a significant positive response.

All four patients in this survey had positive responses. Their improvement was greater earlier in the course of their illness, and lessened as their signs and symptoms of pulmonary disease diminished. The Table shows the maximum increase in peak flow for each patient following albuterol inhalation. Each child tolerated the therapy without ill effects, and no child failed to respond positively to the treatment.

Repeated peak flow determinations before and after bronchodilator treatments were performed at follow-up visits in all four children at least 8 weeks after recovery from ACS. All showed no significant (less than 15%) peak flow increase after nebulization. This, plus the lack of wheezing or asthma history discounts preexisting reactive airway disease as a basis for the response to albuterol.

Comment.—Based on these preliminary findings, a double-blind placebo-controlled study is needed to evaluate the potential role of al-

Maximum Peak Flow Increase After Albuterol Treatment

Patient No.	Pretreatment Peak, L/min	Posttreatment Peak, L/min	% Increase
1	85	170	100
2	50	95	90
3	230	300	30
4	50	150	200

buterol in the treatment of acute chest syndrome.

EDWARD HANDELSMAN, MD
Department of Pediatrics
Schneider Children's Hospital
Long Island Jewish Medical Center
New Hyde Park, NY 11042
DEBRA VOULALAS, MD
Children's Seashore House
Children's Hospital of Philadelphia
Philadelphia, Pa

Penile Vasculitis With Impending Necrosis Treated With Prostaglandin E_1 Infusion

Sir.—Prostaglandin E_1 (PGE_1) infusions have been used in the treatment of occlusive vascular diseases since 1973, when Carlson and Eriksson[1] described subjective improvement in three of four patients with peripheral atherosclerotic vascular disease and ischemic rest pain given PGE_1 by femoral artery infusion. Since that time, PGE_1 has been reported to be effective in Raynaud's syndrome, peripheral vascular occlusive disease, and Kawasaki's disease.[2-4] We report the dramatic clinical reversal of severe, apparently immune complex–mediated vasculitis of the penis following the use of intravenous PGE_1 in an 8-year-old boy.

Patient Report.—An 8-year-old black boy presented to the UCLA Medical Center in 1981 with a 1-day history of severe pain and swelling of his penile shaft. He had no other somatic complaints, gave no history of recent febrile illness, and was able to void without difficulty on admission.

The patient had a complex medical history, including hereditary spherocytosis, tetralogy of Fallot with surgical correction at age 5 years, and intermittent bloody diarrhea of unclear origin that began at age 2 years. In addition, he had multiple episodes of peripheral vasculitis leading to the partial or complete amputation of several digits on his hands and feet. An exhaustive effort had been made to elucidate the origin of the vascular disease, and the only consistent finding had been a rise in the level of circulating immune complexes at the onset of symptoms, and a fall with their resolution. Unfortunately, no pathologic information from the previously amputated digits was available, and although an attempt had been made to perform a biopsy on an artery, it was unsuccessful.

On earlier occasions a variety of therapeutic interventions had been used, including dextran-40, aspirin, dipyridamole (Persantine), intra-arterial reserpine, corticosteroids, and plasmapheresis. There had been a modest response to corticosteroid therapy in conjunction with plasmapheresis, but each episode had led to some degree of amputation.

Physical examination revealed an afebrile, thin, black child whose penis was markedly swollen, although not erect, with marked ecchymosis of the entire shaft and moderate tenderness. The foreskin was edematous and phymotic. His testes were descended bilaterally, and he had a normal scrotal sac. A 3 × 4-cm ecchymotic area was noted over the lateral malleolus of the left leg. Results of admission laboratory studies were essentially normal with the exception of increased immune complexes at a level of 730 mg/L (normal, up to 310 mg/L) by polyethylene glycol precipitation.

Because of concern over the possibility of necrosis with amputation of the penis, PGE_1 was administered in an emergency investigational new drug protocol beginning approximately 2 hours after admission. In addition, due to a modest previous response to steroids, hydrocortisone (500 mg, intravenous bolus) was administered on day 1 of his PGE_1 infusion, and continued as prednisone (20 mg by mouth) once daily for the next 3 days.

The patient started receiving a continuous intravenous PGE_1 infusion (0.5 mg per 200 mL of 5% dextrose solution) at a rate of 0.007 μg/kg per minute, and this was increased over the next 5 hours to a rate of 0.02 μg/kg per minute. The patient received a total dose of 2296 μg or 112 μg/kg over 92 hours, without any discernible side effects. Four hours after beginning the infusion, the patient noted a marked decrease in pain and an associated slight decrease in penile swelling. By day 2 the swelling was notably reduced, and by day 3 the swelling had completely resolved. By the time the PGE_1 infusion was completed on day 4, the ecchymosis of the penile shaft, and over the left lateral malleolus had disappeared, and the patient had entirely normal genital urinary examination results. At this point the level of circulating immune complexes was 350 mg/L. He made a complete and uneventful recovery and has not suffered from symptomatic vasculitis in the last 9 years.

Comment.—PGE_1 affects platelet aggregation and peripheral vascular tone, and has been used in the treatment of both Raynaud's syndrome and peripheral vascular disease, with dramatic benefits in some but not all patients. Recently, PGE_1 has been used to improve renal blood flow after kidney transplantation (Allen Wilkinson, MD, personal communication, March 1990), and to decrease pulmonary vascular resistance after heart transplantation.[5] A recent case report describes a striking reversal of peripheral ischemia of the hands of an infant with Kawasaki's disease.

We noted dramatic improvement in our patient within 4 hours after PGE_1 infusion was started, and a full recovery 4 days later. This response may well have been due to vasodilation and/or inhibition of platelet aggregation. However, work by McLeish et al[6] and others has demonstrated that PGE_1 infusion leads to a reduction in immune complex deposition and in the synthesis of the specific antibody responsible for this deposition in a murine model for immune complex– mediated glomerular nephritis. Although only a speculation, PGE_1 may have had an immune-modulating effect in this patient as well, outlasting its temporary effect on platelet aggregation, and vascular tone. Prostaglandin E_1 is currently only licensed for use in maintaining the patency of the ductus arteriosus in congenital heart disease. Although its value is unproven, we suggest that PGE_1 treatment may be of benefit in selected patients with vascular disease unresponsive to other therapies.

ANTHONY A. HORNER, MD
KAREN DUNN, MD
E. RICHARD STIEHM, MD
UCLA Medical Center
Los Angeles, CA 90024

1. Carlson LA, Eriksson I. Femoral-artery infusion of prostaglandin E_1 in severe peripheral vascular disease. *Lancet.* 1973;1:155-156.
2. Kyle V, Parr G, Salisbury R, Page TP, Hazleman B. Prostaglandin E_1 vasospastic disease and thermography. *Ann Rheum Dis.* 1985;44:73-78.
3. Trubestein G, Diehm C, Gruss JD, Horsch S. Prostaglandin E_1 in chronic arterial disease: a multicenter study. *Vasa.* 1987;17(suppl):39-43.
4. Wilstphalen MA, McGrath A, Kelly W, Moore FJ, Ziegler JB. Kawasaki disease with severe peripheral ischemia: treatment with prostaglandin E_1 infusion. *J Pediatr.* 1988;112:431-433.
5. Armitage JM, Hardesty RL, Griffith BP. Prostaglandin E_1: an effective treatment of right heart failure after orthotopic heart transplantation. *J Heart Transplant.* 1987;6:348-351.
6. McLeish ER, Stelzer GT, Eades DS, Cohen R, Wallace JH. Serial changes in humoral and cellular immunity induced by prostaglandin E_1 treatment of murine immune complex gromerulonephritis. *J Lab Clin Med.* 1985;106:517-523.

THE EDITORIAL BOARD SPEAKS...

Losing Time

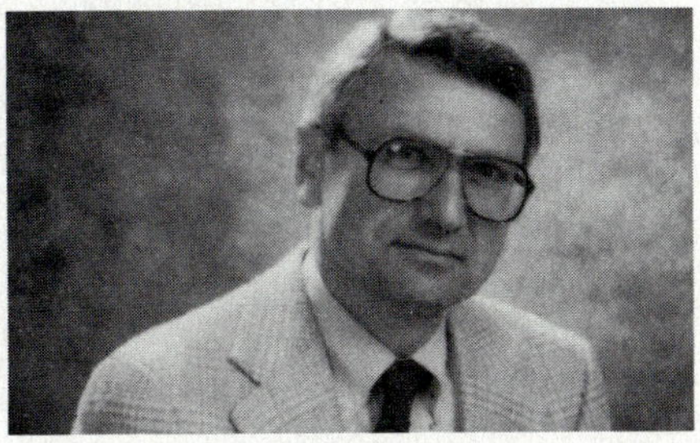

Albert W. Pruitt, MD

"Al" has been the mainstay of the editorial board for pharmacologic and toxicologic information. Despite his heavy academic and administrative load, Al has actively reviewed for us and has participated in all phases of the board's activities.

Most recently, he participated in the Advanced Management Program of the Harvard Graduate School of Business in Boston, Mass. He also participated in the Program in Clinical Effectiveness of the Harvard School of Public Health, covering such areas as biostatistics, epidemiology, and health policy and management. These experiences served to broaden his administrative experience and skills.

He remains the Ellington Charles Hawes Professor and Chairman of the Department of Pediatrics, Medical College of Georgia, positions he has held for more than 10 years. He also served as interim dean of the School of Medicine of the Medical College of Georgia from 1985 to 1986, and again in 1988. His professional activities have included the following: chairmanship of the Committee on Substance Abuse of the American Academy of Pediatrics (1990 to present); member of the Physician Task Force, National Training Systems, Office for Substance Abuse Prevention (1990 to present); member of the Pediatric and Adolescent Medicine Committee of the National Council of Juvenile and Family Court Judges (1990 to present); member of the Steering Committee of the Georgia General Assembly's Conference on Children of Cocaine and Substance Abuse (1990); and member of the National Advisory Council on Maternal, Infant and Fetal Nutrition of the US Department of Agriculture (1990 to present).

After his release from prison, "Johnny" learned quickly that no one would hire him if he admitted to his record, so he stopped letting prospective employers know of it and got a job repairing engines. For a few months, he worked successfully and contentedly. When the boss found out about the prison record, he promptly fired young Johnny. There was no one to whom Johnny could turn for counsel, advice, or help of any kind. Whatever help Johnny was entitled to along those lines he had already received while "behind the fence." Sooner, rather than later, Johnny was once again back there.

This little story, with its accompanying emotion and attempt at justification, is one I know to be true; I am acquainted with Johnny. However, it is also a generic tale of young men, boys really, who do time early in their lives. We all acknowledge the need to identify those youngsters who are at risk of becoming Johnny, but judging from their health status at the time of arrest, most have not been in our offices. The prison population of incarcerated youth is increasing rapidly and sharply in almost every state, largely due to drug-related crimes. Many factors contribute to the growing number of "Johnnies" today, young men who are incarcerated at an early age and therefore often released at an age at which they should have several decades of productivity left. How hollow is that prospect in reality? For many, release from prison is really only an intermission in a life that, after the first incarceration, is almost certain to be spent largely in prison. The mere fact of having "done" time is almost a curse that means the experience will be repeated, in many cases, many times.

One view, of course, is to say that these young men deserve what they get and get what they deserve. There is at least some truth to this. They have broken the law and have committed acts that are dangerous and destructive to other people and to the fabric of society. However, I have made two observations that I would like to share: the first is about what some of these young men are like, and the second is about what exactly the punishment may amount to.

For the past few years, I have been permitted to get to know a large number of young men and older men in a nearby state prison. Being with both age groups is important because meeting "John," who was "Johnny" decades ago, only intensifies my concern about what time holds for incarcerated youth. One can be certain that John's story is known by every Johnny, and those stories do not help.

So what is this Johnny like? Who are these young guys so probably "sentenced to life" just because they are doing time? The thing that I found truly shocking initially, and that continues to astonish me every time I face it, is that these young men are so utterly familiar to me. They are by no means a different breed. They are neither especially vicious nor especially hotheaded. They are neither particularly unwise nor particularly cunning. They are no more open or more closed than the house officers with whom I work.

The one thing that sets these young men apart from those on the outside is how scared they are. They are scared about what has happened to them, about what it all means, and about who they themselves are becoming as they look at John. They are scared about the short term, and very tense and frightened about what will happen "when I get out."

Their anxiety about the future is all too well founded and relates to my second observation. Despite all the attempts to make the time in prison in some way productive and corrective through education, job training, personal rehabilitation, health care, and so forth, there is no room for many of these young men when they come out. Very often there is no room in their families, who are disgraced and disgusted by them; there is no room in the work force, in which they are regarded as poor risks, undeserving of help, or deserving of further punishment. Most of all, however, there is no room for these young men in our society's collective heart, so filled are we with fear of them. Unless we can somehow change that feeling, these men are condemned to a life of "losing time."

EDITORIAL

Parental Alcoholism

A Neglected Pediatric Responsibility

Despite the high prevalence of parental alcoholism and its many serious consequences, pediatricians have little awareness of the drinking problems in the families of the patients they treat.

The article by Duggan et al[1] in this issue of *AJDC* speaks for itself. My comments only underscore the points these authors have made so well. Particularly important is the question "Why?" Why do pediatricians do such a poor job of recognizing alcohol problems? Implicit in the article and my comments is a plea; a plea to do a better job.

See also p 613.

The findings of Duggan et al should come as no surprise. Fewer than half of US medical schools provide any formal instruction in alcohol or drug treatment.[2] The findings highlight the sorry state of physician interest in and involvement with the major health problems associated with alcohol use.

When the families of 147 pediatric inpatients aged 10 years and older were interviewed, 22 families (15%) screened positive for alcoholism. Only one of the 22 families had been identified by an attending pediatrician. The pediatric house staff had identified no one. Other departments at the same institution did considerably better. Psychiatric attending physicians correctly identified 65% of alcoholic family members, and psychiatric house staff, 66%. For medicine, the rates were 35% and 52%, and for surgery they were 35% and 20%, respectively. Only obstetricians approached the low pediatric rates.

Why is this? Is it because of a lack of knowledge, or is it because of a feeling that parental drinking is none of the pediatrician's business? Do physicians feel uncomfortable about what may be perceived to be an issue that is too personal to discuss? The answer is probably some combination of all of the above.

Biomedical research advances have fueled a tremendous expansion of our clinically relevant knowledge base. Because so much worthwhile information has been generated, subjects must fight for inclusion in the course of medical studies.

How much do we really need to know? Most of the information necessary to recognize and intervene with families troubled by alcoholism is not hard to come by. Nor does it require a great deal of curriculum time. It might, however, require the recruitment and training of qualified instructors. Harder to accomplish is the instillation of a sense that alcohol abuse and alcoholism are medical problems that physicians should become involved with. At a minimum we should know the following: (1) Many parents are alcohol abusers and alcoholics. (2) Parental alcoholism may have many serious consequences for children. (3) Screening for parental alcoholism is easy and quick. (4) Intervention can make a difference. (5) Physicians need to know how to overcome feelings of discomfort in dealing with alcoholic parents.

Many Parents Are Alcohol Abusers and Alcoholics

The 15% prevalence rate of alcoholism found by Duggan et al[1] agrees with national estimates of 13.5% lifetime prevalence rates of alcohol abuse and alcoholism in the general population.[3] It also agrees with the estimates that one in eight American children has alcoholic parents.[4]

Parental Alcohol Abuse and Alcoholism Can Have Many Serious Consequences for Children

These consequences include highway deaths, child abuse, fetal alcohol syndrome, and an increased incidence of alcoholism and other drinking problems in children of alcoholics. Consequences also include dysfunctional family life that may be chaotic, nonsupportive, and abusive.[5] Pediatricians generally do know these things, but for reasons that are far from clear do not usually become involved.

Perhaps the most obvious consequence of parental drinking is death on the highway. Each year more than 40 000 Americans die in traffic accidents. More than 8000 of these deaths are in the pediatric age range. Estimates are that drunken driving accounts for more than 60% of these fatalities. Hundreds of thousands more suffer serious injuries because of automobile accidents.[6]

Another major consequence of parental drinking is child abuse. Pediatricians, who are such strong advocates of child protection and child abuse regulations, have not as a rule made the link between parental drinking and child abuse; however, there is a link. A significant number of child abusers are alcohol abusers as well.[7] Whether it be physical abuse, incest, neglect, abandonment, or emotional abuse, child abuse is an important pediatric issue.

Pediatricians are familiar with fetal alcohol syndrome and know that it is caused by maternal drinking. Failure to obtain an adequate family history, however, robs the pediatrician of the opportunity to detect maternal alcohol abuse and to initiate action to prevent problems in unborn children. The fact that obstetricians do such a poor job of recognizing alcoholism makes pediatrician involvement even more important.

Still another problem is that children of alcoholics are at increased risk of becoming problem drinkers themselves. Genetic and environmental factors may both play a role.[8] The road to adult alcoholism usually begins in adolescence when abuse can be particularly disastrous. The three leading causes of death in the 15- to 24-year-old age range are accidents, suicide, and homicide. All three are frequently associated with the abuse of alcohol.

Alcohol abuse in adolescence does more than kill. There may be learning problems, emotional problems, and delayed, inadequate, or abnormal development of relationships with family, friends, and dating partners.[5]

Screening for Alcoholism Is Easy and Quick

Families generally do a good job of hiding their alcohol problems. Pediatricians must make a conscious effort to identify these problems or they will be missed. Fortunately, there are readily available screening tests that are easy and quick to administer. It should not take more than 10 minutes to complete the short version of the Michigan Alcohol Screening Test and the CAGE, used by Duggan et al.[1]

Intervention Can Make a Difference

If physicians do not believe anything can be done for the child of an alcoholic or for the drinking parent, then there is little therapeutic reason for obtaining a history except to explain current problems or to predict future problems. If we know that alcoholics can be treated and do recover, we will realize that medical histories are essential. Pediatricians should know which treatment methods work and how to use locally available resources.

Treatment of adult alcoholics has a 50-year history of success. That success began far outside the medical mainstream. Two alcoholics, one of them a physician, formed a fellowship of alcoholics that we know today as Alcoholics Anonymous. Medical acceptance of the principles of Alcoholics Anonymous was late in coming, but today few alcohol treatment programs do not include at least some of its principles. Many are based almost entirely on Alcoholics Anonymous.

How to Overcome Feelings of Discomfort in Dealing With Alcoholic Parents

A 1988 survey of pediatric faculty and house staff revealed that 33% of the faculty and 25% of the house staff felt little or no responsibility for referring patients' family members with alcohol problems.[9] Why is this?

Perhaps it is that pediatricians feel uncomfortable asking people about their drinking habits. Should they? There is precedent for asking questions in potentially sensitive personal areas. For example, few physicians feel any discomfort asking people about their bowel habits. Even once taboo questions about sexual practice are becoming accepted as part of what a physician is expected to ask. Questions about the use of alcohol and other drugs are more than appropriate.

Perhaps it is the fear of confrontation. It is not easy to suggest that someone has a drinking problem. Denial is to be expected and anger is common. However, with training and practice, intervention can be successful.[10] For those who are untrained, referral is appropriate. Few communities do not have someone skilled at intervention.

Putting it all together means knowing that there is a problem and learning how to manage that problem. Even if no intervention is planned, knowledge of alcoholism is an important component of understanding family dynamics. The article by Duggan et al[1] lays the groundwork. Now, it is up to those who take responsibility for children's health to act responsibly.

Donald Ian Macdonald, MD
Employee Health Programs
6550 Rock Spring Plaza
Suite 280
Bethesda, MD 20817

References

1. Duggan AK, Adger H, McDonald EM, et al. Detection of alcoholism in hospitalized children and their families. *AJDC.* 1991;145:610-611.

2. Adger H, McDonald EM, DeAngelis C. Substance abuse education in pediatrics. *Pediatrics.* 1990;86:555-560.

3. Regier DA, Boyd JH, Burke JD, et al. One month prevalence of mental disorders in the United States based on five epidemiologic catchment area sites. *Arch Gen Psychiatry.* 1988;45:977-986.

4. Russell M, Henderson C, Blume SB. *Children of Alcoholics: A Review of the Literature.* New York, NY: Children of Alcoholics Foundation; 1984.

5. Macdonald DI, Blume SB. Children of alcoholics. *AJDC.* 1986;140:750-754.

6. Fatal Accident Reporting System. *Computerized Data Base of US Fatal Motor Crashes.* Washington, DC: US Dept of Transportation; 1987.

7. Bland R, Orn H. Family violence and psychiatric disorder. *Can J Psychiatry.* 1986;31:129-137.

8. Cloninger CR, Bohman M, Siguardsson S. Inheritance of alcohol abuse. *Arch Gen Psychiatry.* 1981;38:861-868.

9. Adger H, McDonald EM, Duggan AK. Evaluation of a pediatric substance abuse curriculum. Presented at the annual meeting of the Association for Medical Education and Research in Substance Abuse; November 1989; Washington, DC.

10. Johnson Institute. *How to Use Intervention in Your Professional Practice.* Minneapolis, Minn: Johnson Institute Books, Professional Series; 1987.

Detection of Alcoholism in Hospitalized Children and Their Families

Anne K. Duggan, ScD; Hoover Adger, Jr, MD, MPH; Eileen M. McDonald;
Emma J. Stokes, PhD; Richard Moore, MD, MHS

• The study sought to measure provider recognition of family alcohol-related problems among hospitalized children and to identify characteristics distinguishing "positive" families. The study sample (N = 147) was drawn from admissions to the general pediatric medical service of a metropolitan teaching hospital. Positivity was assessed through parent and patient interviews that included standard alcohol abuse screening instruments. Provider recognition was assessed through record review and physician interview. Of the 22 families screened positive, only one was so identified by the child's attending or resident physician. Positive and "negative" families were similar in most respects, although parents in positive families were more likely to report stress and sleeping problems and adolescents were more likely to report being troubled by a parent's drinking. The similarity of positive and negative families and the low pediatrician recognition rate suggest that alcohol problems are likely to go unnoticed without a conscious screening effort.

(*AJDC.* 1991;145:613-617)

The importance of substance abuse as a pediatric health care problem stems from its high prevalence among patients and their families, its unfavorable and serious consequences, and the effectiveness of timely recognition and treatment. More than 15 million Americans are estimated to meet the *Diagnostic and Statistical Manual of Mental Disorders, Third Edition,* criteria for alcohol abuse or dependence,[1] and about one in eight American children has a parent with a past or present drinking problem.[2]

For editorial comment see p 609.

Adverse consequences of this disease extend beyond the alcoholic to his or her family. For children in an alcoholic household, home life is chaotic and emotionally unsupportive.[3] In the short run, such an environment erodes the child's physical and emotional well-being.[4] In homes where alcoholism remains undetected and untreated, consequences extending to adulthood include low self-esteem, inability to trust, difficulty in expressing anger appropriately, and a distorted sense of the extent and limits of one's responsibilities.[5]

Adult substance abuse often begins in adolescence. Among high school seniors nationally, use in the past month was reported by 64% for alcohol and 18% for marijuana.[6] Substance abuse can adversely affect the adolescent's physical, mental, and emotional health. Alcohol use is related to 40% of accidental deaths, 30% of homicides, and 20% of suicides among adolescents.[7] Cognitive and psychosocial consequences include developmental lag, amotivational syndrome, escapism, egocentrism, self-deprecation, and alienation.[8]

Pediatricians are in a unique position to identify and respond to substance abuse among patients and their families. Even so, because substance abuse is given low priority in pediatric medical education, pediatricians are ill equipped to identify and respond to substance abuse in patients and their families.[9] Potential barriers to detection and response are varied, and they relate to the individual provider, his or her medical training, and characteristics of the disease. The pediatrician may not perceive his or her role as extending to the patient's family. Medical training in all but the end stages of the disease of alcoholism and drug addiction may be inadequate. The provider may be unaware of available treatment resources or may question the effectiveness of treatment. Even those who are motivated and knowledgeable may lack the interviewing skills necessary to break through patient and family denial of alcoholism and other drug dependence.

As part of a larger institutional effort to develop a comprehensive approach to drug and alcohol education, a baseline survey of the prevalence and provider recognition of alcoholism among hospital inpatients was conducted. An earlier article describes the methods and findings for the departments of internal medicine, obstetrics and gynecology, surgery, and psychiatry.[10] This article focuses on the department of pediatrics, for which the survey assessed alcohol abuse prevalence and provider recognition not only among patients but also among their parents and other primary caregivers. Families screened "positive" are compared with those screened "negative" in terms of demographic, health, and behavioral characteristics.

PATIENTS AND METHODS

The study population was defined as children and adolescents admitted to the general pediatric medical service of The Johns

Accepted for publication December 13, 1990.

From the Departments of Pediatrics (Drs Duggan and Adger and Ms McDonald) and Medicine (Dr Moore), and the Blades Center for Clinical Practice and Research in Alcoholism (Dr Stokes), The Johns Hopkins University School of Medicine,Baltimore, Md.

Reprint requests to Department of Pediatrics, Park 307, The Johns Hopkins Hospital, 600 N Wolfe St, Baltimore, MD 21205 (Dr Adger).

Hopkins Children's Center, Baltimore, Md. The study sample was drawn from all such hospital admissions from August 1987 to November 1987. Signed informed consent was obtained for participating parents and children aged 10 years or older. As mandated by the institutional review board, patients judged by the unit nurse as too sick to be interviewed and those with a new diagnosis of cancer were excluded.

Prevalence data were collected by trained interviewers through structured interviews with the parent and with patients older than 9 years. Priority was given to interviewing the mother but, where this was impossible, the father or grandmother was interviewed. Data on provider recognition of substance abuse problems were collected through record review and through interviews with the house officer and attending physician for each family that screened positive and for a sample of those who had screened negative on parent or child interview.

The parent interview solicited information on family demographics, parent health status, and health-related behaviors. When the child was younger than 10 years, the parent interview included the Child Behavior Checklist[11] to measure parent-reported behavior.

The parent's use of alcohol was assessed in terms of quantity-frequency and by responses to the brief version of the Michigan Alcohol Screening Test (Brief MAST)[12,13] and the CAGE (which is explained below).[14] Alcohol use by the child's other parent, including both a surrogate parent living in the home and a biological father whether in or out of the child's home, was also ascertained. This was accomplished by administering the Brief MAST and CAGE to the participating parent as a proxy respondent for the other parent.[15]

The Brief MAST is a set of 10 questions concerning alcohol use and associated consequences. The questions are weighted, and a score is derived as the weighted sum of answers suggestive of alcohol-related problems. The CAGE is a screening framework whose name is derived from the first letters of four areas of questioning about the subject's or another's drinking: *C*oncern over alcohol use, *A*nnoyance with another's suggestion to alter use, *G*uilt over behavior while intoxicated, and need for an *E*ye-opener drink to start the day. The CAGE score is the number of these four areas in which the subject replies in the affirmative.

The interview for older children and adolescents included questions on family composition, the child's health care utilization and health habits, indicators of health status, and use of cigarettes and alcohol and other drugs. Alcohol use was measured in terms of quantity-frequency, the Adolescent Alcohol Involvement Scale (AAIS),[16] and the CAGE. The adolescent's reasons for drinking were measured by the Perceived Benefits of Drinking Scale.[17] Experience with each of several classes of drugs was measured as never used/nonregular use/regular use. Finally, the adolescent was asked whether he or she had ever been troubled by the drinking of a parent or caregiver.[18]

A Brief MAST score of 6 or greater was considered positive for alcoholism; two or more affirmative responses to the four CAGE items was also considered positive. For the AAIS scale, a score of 42 or greater indicated positivity. A family was considered positive for alcohol abuse if the Brief MAST or CAGE score for a biological parent or surrogate parent in the household was positive or if the CAGE or AAIS score was positive for an adolescent patient.

For all families who screened positive and a random 15% sample of those who screened negative for alcohol abuse, data on provider recognition of and response to alcoholism were collected through record review and interviews with the resident and attending physicians. Documented assessment of substance use by both the patient and family was determined through record review. The provider interviews determined whether the provider had identified substance use in the patient or a family member, the means of identification, and the treatment given. The statistical significance of differences between positive and negative families was assessed using Student's t test and χ^2.

RESULTS

There were 246 general pediatric medical admissions to the hospital during the study period. Of these, 19 children (8%) were judged by the unit nurse to be too sick to participate in the study. Of the remaining 227 children, 27 parents (12%) refused participation, and no parent or caregiver was available for interview in 53 instances (23%). Parents of 147 children (65%) agreed to participate in the study. Of the 147 admitted children in participating families, 82 were 10 years or older. Of these, 59 (72%) were interviewed, nine (11%) were unavailable for interview during times of interviewer coverage, and 14 (17%) refused to be interviewed.

In 22 (15%) of the 147 participating families, either a parent or child was determined to be positive for alcoholism. Screen-positive family members included four primary female caretakers, eight biological or surrogate fathers inside the household, nine biological fathers living outside the household, and one adolescent patient. In 15 of the 22 positive households, the patient was aged 10 years or older, and in seven positive households the patient was younger than 10 years.

Provider recognition of alcoholism was poor. Of the 22 families screened positive by parent or adolescent interview, only one was identified as such by the attending physician; none were identified by house officers. Two of the families screened negative in the study were identified as having a family history of alcoholism by the resident or attending physician.

Table 1.—Comparison of Parents by Household Screening Status

		Household Screening Status, %		
Characteristics of Parent Interviewed	Total, % (n=147)	Positive (n=22)	Negative (n=125)	*P*
Age, y*	35.7±6.2	36.0±5.1	35.7±6.6	.83
Sex, F	99	100	98	1.00
Race, W	76	73	77	.89
Employed	59	68	57	.44
Income <$20 000	30	46	27	.15
Education				.87
<High school	15	18	15	...
High school and some college	62	64	62	...
≥College graduate	22	18	23	...
Gets adequate sleep seldom or never	25	41	22	.11
Has insomnia usually/always	17	32	14	.07
Has had stress frequently/constantly in past year	36	54	30	.04
Depressed for period of >2 wk in past year	28	41	26	.25
Perceives own health as				.34
Excellent	32	18	34	...
Good	54	64	52	...
Fair or poor	15	18	14	...
Smokes	43	54	41	.33
Perceives patient's health as				.06
Excellent	30	27	30	...
Good	48	32	51	...
Fair or poor	22	41	19	...

*Values are means ± SDs.

Table 2.—Comparison of Adolescents by Household Screening Status

Adolescent Characteristics	Total, % (n=59)	Household Screening Status, % Positive (n=10)	Negative (n=49)	P
Age, y*	14.6±2.7	14.6±2.4	14.6±2.8	.99
Race, B	22	20	23	1.00
Sex, M	49	60	47	.68
Sees dentist annually	75	80	74	.97
Has annual medical checkup	61	50	63	.67
Eats balanced meals daily	76	78	76	1.00
Exercises ≥3 times weekly	66	60	67	.94
Gets adequate sleep seldom/never	20	30	18	.69
Has insomnia most every night	15	20	14	1.00
Depressed for a period of ≥2 wk in past year	39	50	37	.69
Has headaches, stomachaches, or other recurrent problems	75	80	74	.97
Discusses problems with no one	16	10	17	.96
Not active in extracurricular activities	50	30	54	.30
Has been troubled by a parent's drinking	5	23	2	<.001
Has used drugs	5	20	2	.07
Does drink alcohol	8	10	8	1.00

*Values are means±SDs.

Positive and negative families were similar for most of the demographic parent characteristics examined (Table 1). The interviewed parents were 36 years old on average, almost all were female, and three quarters were white. About three fifths of the interviewed parents were employed. Differences in household income approached significance ($P=.15$); 46% of those in positive households as compared with 27% of those in negative households reported an income of less than $20 000. Parents did not differ in terms of educational status, with less than a fifth in each group lacking a high school diploma.

Parents in positive households were less likely to report routinely getting adequate sleep ($P=.11$), and they were more likely to report frequent insomnia ($P=.07$) and frequent or constant stress in the past year ($P=.04$). Group differences in the proportion reporting depression for more than 2 weeks were similar but less pronounced (positive households 41% vs negative households 26%, $P=.25$). Positivity was not related to parent smoking or to the parent's perception of his or her own health status. Parents in positive households were more likely to characterize their child's health as only fair or poor (41% vs 19%, $P=.06$).

Among adolescent patients, household positivity for alcoholism was not related to patient age (mean, 14.6 years), race (22% black), or sex (49% male) (Table 2). Most adolescents in both positive and negative households reported good health practices: 61% of the adolescents had annual medical checkups; 75% had annual dental checkups; 76% ate balanced meals daily; and 66% exercised at least three times weekly.

Table 3.—Differences in Child Behavior* by Household Screening Status

Child Behavior Score	Household Positive (n=7)	Negative† (n=14)	P
Activity	35.1	47.3	.14
Social	43.5	44.6	.79
T			
Sum	51.4	52.5	.83
Internal	55.4	51.1	.35
External	46.9	50.2	.52

*As measured by parental report using the Achenbach Child Behavior Checklist.[11]

†Each subject younger than 10 years old in positive households was matched on age, sex, and race with two controls from negative households.

The likelihood of health-related problems did not differ significantly between adolescents in positive and negative families. Sleep problems were fairly common: 20% seldom or never got adequate sleep; 15% indicated they had insomnia most nights. Two-fifths reported feeling depressed 2 weeks or more in the past year. Headaches, stomachaches, or other recurrent problems were the norm and were reported by 75% of the adolescents. About one in six adolescents reported having no one with whom to discuss problems. Half of the adolescents were not involved in extracurricular activities at school.

The groups differed markedly in their reaction to parental drinking. Those in positive households were much more likely to indicate they had been troubled, scared, or angry because of a parent's drinking (23% in positive households vs 2% in negative households, $P<.001$).

Group differences in reported prior use of drugs approached significance (20% of those in positive households vs 2% in negative, $P=.07$). The three patients with prior drug use all reported using marijuana. In addition, the adolescent who screened positive for alcohol use also reported having used amphetamines and lysergic acid diethylanmide.

Five adolescents (8%) reported current alcohol use. One adolescent screened positive on the CAGE, although not on the AAIS, where scores ranged from 24 to 41. When queried about the perceived benefits of drinking, one of the five adolescents reported that drinking helped him be friendly, and two adolescents, including the adolescent who screened positive, reported it helped them relax. None of the five adolescents reported drinking as a means to help forget problems, feel good about oneself, or be friends with others who drink.

Table 3 summarizes parental assessment of behavior for patients younger than 10 years by household positivity. Each of the seven children from positive households was matched by age and sex with two controls from negative households. Children in positive and negative households did not differ significantly on any behavior subscore and had behavior scores within group norms.

COMMENT

The 15% prevalence rate of positive screens for alcoholism in hospitalized pediatric patients and their parents was consistent with national estimates of the lifetime prevalence of alcoholism and alcohol abuse (11.5% to 15.7%)[19] and somewhat lower than rates found for adult inpatients in most other departments of our institution: psychiatry (30%); medicine (25%); surgery (23%); neurology (19%); and obstetrics-gynecology (12.5%).

There are several reasons to suspect that the 15% prevalence rate is conservative. First, anecdotal evidence suggested that positive families were more likely to decline study participation. Many families were known to nursing staff from prior hospitalizations. At least a few parents who refused to be interviewed or who judged their child too sick to participate were believed by nursing staff to be from alcohol-dependent families. Second, parent interviewing was limited to the inpatient setting. To the extent that family alcoholism negatively influenced hospital visiting, parents in positive households were less likely to be recruited for participation. Third, insofar as alcoholism was viewed by parents as socially unacceptable behavior, there was motivation for underreporting by those interviewed. A final reason pertains to the interviewed parent's role as proxy respondent for the Brief MAST and CAGE items relating to the other parent. To the extent that the interviewed parent could not or would not answer items, the likelihood of a positive screen for the other parent was decreased.

Screen positivity for alcoholism was not a problem limited to any particular patient subgroup. Both parents and patients in positive and negative families were similar in most respects. Parents in positive households were more likely to suffer from stress and sleep problems, and adolescents were more likely to be troubled by a parent's drinking. Given the small sample sizes, only substantial group differences could attain statistical significance. From the perspective of teaching pediatricians how to identify families with alcohol-related problems, the similarities between positive and negative families are perhaps more important. The similarities demonstrate the lack of sensitivity of typical substance abuse stereotypes—unemployment, low income, lack of education—as a way of identifying families with problems.

Provider recognition of families who screened positive was low. Only one of the positive families was identified as such by the physician. In this family, both parents had a positive history, the child had been removed from home for a time, one parent had been in treatment in the past, and the provider reported not knowing the parents' current state of recovery. The adolescent patient who screened positive for alcohol use also reported past use of marijuana, amphetamines, and lysergic acid diethylamide. This patient was not recognized as positive by either the attending or resident physician.

Provider recognition rates were substantially lower in pediatrics than in most other departments. Only one (5%) of the positive families was so identified by a pediatric attending physician as compared with 27% of positive cases detected by attending physicians in neurology and in surgery, 35% in medicine, and 65% in psychiatry. While pediatric house officers detected none of the screen-positive families, house staff recognition rates in other departments were 20% in surgery, 46% in neurology, 52% in medicine, and 66% in psychiatry. As in pediatrics, attending physicians in obstetrics-gynecology recognized only 7% of positive cases and house officers recognized none.

No doubt the pediatric recognition rate was lower because positivity was defined to include parents as well as patients and because many pediatricians did not view their role as extending to family members. This attitude was demonstrated in a 1988 survey of our pediatric faculty and house staff.[20] Faculty were twice as likely to feel little or no responsibility for substance abuse referral of patient family members as compared with adolescent patients (33% vs 15%). This trend was even more pronounced for house staff, of whom 25% and 3% reported feeling little or no responsibility for referral of patient family members as compared with adolescent patients.

The low provider recognition rate of this study is congruent with reported practice behavior. In the 1988 survey cited above, 62% of faculty and house staff reported taking a personal alcohol/drug use history from most or all of their adolescent patients. However, only 34% reported taking a family substance abuse history for their pediatric patients.

Some may question whether it is appropriate to expect physicians providing inpatient care to identify patient and family alcohol problems. Certainly, a family history of alcohol and drug abuse is more likely than many other aspects of history to affect a patient's immediate and follow-up treatment. Family problems with alcohol and other drugs can jeopardize a parent's ability to carry out necessary therapeutic regimens. A thorough history, including family and social histories, is required for all patients admitted to the hospital. We believe personal and family histories for substance abuse are just as important as a history for hypertension, cancer, or diabetes mellitus.

The generalizability of findings is limited by study of an inpatient population rather than a primary care setting. The inpatient setting was chosen because it was suspected to have the lowest provider recognition rate and the greatest provider resistance to patient and family substance abuse screening. Certainly, replication of this study in primary care settings serving both general populations and children with chronic conditions would provide much needed information on the prevalence and pediatrician identification and management of family substance abuse problems.

CONCLUSION

This study was undertaken to assess the prevalence of patient and family positivity for alcoholism in an inpatient pediatric setting and to describe provider behavior in dealing with identified families. We found that family alcoholism was distributed in this population as it is distributed more generally, across all socioeconomic and demographic strata. We conclude from this that if alcohol-dependent families of pediatric patients are to be identified, all families must be screened.

We also found that pediatricians in our setting failed to recognize most alcohol-dependent families. We conclude from this that in many instances, family alcoholism is not likely to be a blatant problem, but rather one whose identification requires a deliberate and skilled screening effort. If pediatricians are to make family screening for substance abuse a routine part of care, they must learn how to screen and they must be convinced of the importance of doing so. Macdonald and Blume[3] have well described the importance of family screening and have suggested the utility of the CAGE framework as a means for detecting alcohol abuse.

What might pediatricians do with increased awareness of parental drinking problems? It is important for the pediatrician to remember that a positive screen does not make a diagnosis. As Macdonald and Blume[3] point out, a diagnosis of alcoholism is often difficult for a parent to accept. A diagnosis that is reached too hastily and without a complete and thorough assessment may sever the physician-family relationship rather than strengthen it. The pediatrician should advocate further exploration into the area, either with himself or herself or with an assessment specialist. It is important for the pediatrician to express his or her concern for the parent and child and the belief that alcoholism is not a moral weakness but a treatable disease. In addition, the pediatrician can play an important role in educating the family and can help the parent to explore the links between parental drinking and family dysfunction. The pediatrician can offer the parent referral to a substance abuse counselor or support group as a means for learning more about whether there is a problem with family alcoholism, and if so, how to deal with it. In this spirit, the parent is more likely to interpret the pediatrician's actions as genuine concern and to respond in a positive manner.

In our institution, the results of this study and related research are being used to help motivate pediatricians to incorporate substance abuse identification and initial management in their practice. Essential aspects of this effort include the teaching of clinical screening skills, including the CAGE framework, reinforcing the role of the physician in early detection and minimal interventions, and disseminating information on the availability of institutional and community treatment resources. Our experience suggests that assessing prevalence and practice is a useful first step for improving physician recognition and response to substance abuse.

This investigation was supported by a grant from the Pew Memorial Trust, Philadelphia, Pa.

References

1. Williams GD, Grant BF, Harford TC, Noble J. Population projections using *DSM-III* criteria: alcohol abuse and dependence, 1990-2000. *Alcohol Health Res World*. 1989;13:366-370.
2. Russell M, Henderson C, Blume SB. *Children of Alcoholics: A Review of the Literature*. New York, NY: Children of Alcoholics Foundation; 1984.
3. Macdonald DI, Blume SB. Children of alcoholics. *AJDC*. 1986;140:750-754.
4. Harrigan JA. Children of alcoholics. *Am Fam Physician*. 1987;35:139-144.
5. Reich W, Early F, Powell J. A comparison of the home and social environments of children of alcoholic and non-alcoholic parents. *Br J Addict*. 1988;83:831-839.
6. Johnston LD, O'Malley PM, Bachman JG. *Drug Use, Drinking and Smoking: National Survey Results from High School, College, and Young Adult Populations, 1975-1988*. Washington, DC: National Institute on Drug Abuse; 1989. US Dept of Health and Human Services publication (ADM) 89-1638.
7. Schonberg SK, ed. *Substance Abuse: A Guide for Health Professionals*. Elk Grove Village, Ill: American Academy of Pediatrics; 1988.
8. Baumrind D, Moselle KA. A developmental perspective on adolescent drug abuse. *Adv Alcohol Subst Abuse*. 1985;4:41-66.
9. Adger H, McDonald EM, DeAngelis C. Substance abuse education in pediatrics. *Pediatrics*. 1990;86:555-560.
10. Moore RD, Bone LR, Geller G, Mamon JA, Stokes EJ, Levine DM. Prevalence, detection and treatment of alcoholism in hospitalized patients. *JAMA*. 1989;261:403-407.
11. Achenbach TM, Edelbrock C. *Manual for the Child Behavior: A Checklist and Revised Child Behavior Profile*. Burlington, Vt: Department of Psychology, University of Vermont; 1983.
12. Selzer M. The Michigan Alcoholism Screening Test: the quest for a new diagnostic instrument. *Am J Psychiatry*. 1971;127:1653-1658.
13. Pokorny AD, Miller BA, Kaplan HB. The Brief MAST: a shortened version of the Michigan Alcoholism Screening Test. *Am J Psychiatry*. 1972;129:342-345.
14. Ewing J, Mayfield D. CAGE. *Am J Psychiatry*. 1974;131:1121-1122.
15. Davis LJ, Morse RM. Patient-spouse agreement in the drinking behaviors of alcoholics. *Mayo Clin Proc*. 1987;62:689-694.
16. Mayer J, Filstead WJ. The adolescent alcohol involvement scale: an instrument for measuring adolescents' use and misuse of alcohol. *J Stud Alcohol*. 1979;40:291-299.
17. Petchers MK, Singer MI. Perceived-benefit-of-drinking scale: approach to screening for adolescent alcohol abuse. *Pediatrics*. 1987;110:977-981.
18. Biek JE. Screening test for identifying adolescents adversely affected by a parental drinking problem. *J Adolesc Health Care*. 1981;2:107-113.
19. Niven RG. Alcoholism—a problem in perspective. *JAMA*. 1984;252:1912-1914.
20. Adger H, McDonald EM, Duggan AK. Evaluation of a pediatric substance abuse curriculum. Presented at the annual meeting of the Association for Medical Education and Research in Substance Abuse; November 8, 1989; Washington, DC.

In Other AMA Journals

ARCHIVES OF OTOLARYNGOLOGY—HEAD & NECK SURGERY

Balloon Dilatation of Esophageal Strictures in Children

Charles M. Myer III, MD; William S. Ball Jr, MD; George S. Bissett III, MD
(*Arch Otolaryngol Head Neck Surg*. 1991;117:529-532)

The Causes of Hospital-Treated Acute Lower Respiratory Tract Infection in Children

Hanna Nohynek, MD; Juhani Eskola, MD; Eija Laine, MD; Pekka Halonen, MD; Petri Ruutu, MD; Pekka Saikku, MD; Marjaana Kleemola, MD; Maija Leinonen, PhD

• **Objective:** To determine the etiologic agents in children with acute lower respiratory infection.

Design: A survey of a series of patients.

Setting: General pediatric hospital serving an urban population with and without referrals in Helsinki, Finland.

Participants: 135 Finnish children aged 2 months to 15 years (mean, 1.75 years), with clinically defined acute lower respiratory infection (with difficulty of breathing), or found to have fever and a pneumonic infiltrate on chest roentgenogram.

Selection Procedures: Consecutive sample on voluntary basis.

Interventions: None.

Main Results: Of 121 children with adequate samples, an etiologic diagnosis could be established in 84 (70%): 30 (25%) had bacterial, 30 (25%) viral, and 24 (20%) mixed infections. Antibody assays alone identified the agent in 91% of positive cases.

Conclusions: Bacterial infections are common but generally underestimated in acute lower respiratory infection; serologic methods add significantly to their detection.

(*AJDC.* 1991;145:618-622)

Acute lower respiratory tract infection (ALRI), ie, pneumonia and bronchiolitis, is a major cause of morbidity among children worldwide.[1] In addition, these diseases cause significant mortality in the developing countries.[1-3] The causes of ALRI are still partly unknown, primarily because of difficulties in obtaining adequate samples and lack of reliable diagnostic methods.[4,5] This is a major shortcoming, since knowledge of the etiologic agents of ALRI in different patient populations would be of crucial importance for both development of vaccines and recommendations regarding treatment.

We report here a study of 121 urban Finnish children hospitalized because of clinically defined ALRI. We used both conventional microbiological methods and a broad range of serologic methods, including bacterial antibody assays and detection of viral and bacterial antigens and nucleic acid, which allowed us to find the presumptive cause of ALRI in 70% of the patients.

Accepted for publication July 2, 1990.

From the National Public Health Institute, Helsinki, Finland (Drs Nohynek, Eskola, Kleemola, and Leinonen); Aurora Hospital, Helsinki (Drs Eskola and Laine); Second Department of Medicine, Helsinki University Central Hospital (Dr Ruutu); and the Departments of Virology, Universities of Helsinki (Dr Saikku) and Turku (Finland) (Dr Halonen).

Reprint requests to National Public Health Institute, Mannerheimintie 166, SF-00300 Helsinki, Finland (Dr Eskola).

PATIENTS AND METHODS

The study was carried out from December 1987 to November 1988 in Aurora Hospital, Helsinki, Finland, with the permission of its Ethics Committee. The hospital serves an urban population with and without referrals. Informed consent was obtained from the parents in each case.

Patients

All children aged 15 years or younger hospitalized for respiratory infection were enrolled in the study if they fulfilled the following criteria judged by the pediatrician on duty: symptoms of acute respiratory infection lasting 7 days or less, together with difficulty of breathing defined as chest indrawing or respiratory rate of more than 40/min for infants or more than 30/min for those older than 1 year. In addition, children hospitalized for other reasons but found to have fever (≥38°C) and a pneumonic infiltrate on chest roentgenogram were included in the study.

Specimens

Nasopharyngeal aspirates (NPAs) of respiratory secretions and urine were collected on admission. Blood was collected on admission, on days 3 and 5, and during convalescent checkup examination (day 36 on the average; range, 14 to 96 days).

Blood Culture

One to five milliliters of venous blood taken on admission was cultured using standard techniques (Bactec NR 660, Becton Dickinson Diagnostics Instruments Systems, Towson, Md).

Bacterial Antigen Detection

The urine samples were tested for capsular polysaccharide of *Haemophilus influenzae* type b and for pneumococcal polysaccharides of the most common serotypes reported in Finnish children (types 4-9, 11, 14, 15, 19, and 23) (M.L., unpublished observations, 1988) by type-specific latex reagents made from monospecific antiserum (for *H influenzae* type b: burro 46, provided by John B. Robbins, MD, National Institutes of Health, Bethesda, Md; for *Streptococcus pneumoniae* serotypes: Statens Seruminstitut, Copenhagen, Denmark) as described.[6] The serum samples obtained on admission were tested with a commercial latex agglutination test (Bactigen, Wampole Laboratories, Cranbury, NJ) for pneumococcal capsular polysaccharide antigens.

Mycoplasmal RNA Hybridization

Homogenized NPA was used for detection of nucleic acid of *Mycoplasma pneumoniae* by RNA hybridization as specified by the producer of the kit (Gen-Probe Rapid Diagnostic System, San Diego, Calif).

Table 1.—Methods Used to Measure Antibodies to the Common Respiratory Pathogens Studied*

Agent	Antigen Used	Antibody Class	Method	Significant Response	Source, y
S pneumoniae	Pneumolysin	IgG	EIA	2-fold† increase in titer	Jalonen et al,[11] 1989
H influenzae	Whole cell‡	IgG, IgA	EIA	3-fold† increase in titer	Leinonen et al,[12] 1981
M catarrhalis	Whole cell‡	IgG, IgA	EIA	3-fold† increase in titer	Leinonen et al,[12] 1981
M pneumoniae	Whole cell§	IgG, IgM	EIA	3-fold increase in titer	Kleemola et al,[13] 1990
C pneumoniae, C psittaci, C trachomatis	Type-specific elementary bodies‖	IgG, IgM	mIF	4-fold increase in titer or presence of IgM	Wang et al,[14] 1970
Respiratory syncytial virus	Cell-lysed viruses	IgG	EIA	4-fold increase in titer	Meurman et al,[15] 1984
Influenza A or B	AFP	IgG	EIA	3-fold increase in unit value	Koskinen et al,[16] 1987
Parainfluenza types 1, 2, or 3	1, AFP; 2, 3, CL	IgG	EIA	3-fold increase in unit value	Vuorinen et al,[17] 1989
Adenovirus	Group-reacting hexon	IgG	EIA	3-fold increase in unit value	Meurman et al,[18] 1983

*EIA indicates enzyme immunoassay; mIF, microimmunofluorescence; and AFP, allantoic fluid-pelleted viruses. Full expansion of names of agents appears in the text.
†Based on measurements of antibodies in paired serum samples from 158 healthy children (M.L., unpublished observations).
‡Whole bacterial cell suspension of 10 different strains.
§*Mycoplasma pneumoniae* organisms lysed by 2% sodium dodecylsulfate.
‖Following elementary bodies were used: *C trachomatis,* A, C-H-I-J, K-G-F, B-D-E; *C pneumoniae,* AR-39; and *C psittaci,* V-394.

Viral Antigen Detection

Sonicated NPA diluted 1:5 in assay buffer was used for detection of respiratory syncytial virus (RSV), group-reacting hexon antigen of adenoviruses, influenza A and B, and parainfluenza types 1, 2, and 3 antigens by one-incubation time-resolved fluoroimmunoassay based on immunoreagents prepared from monoclonal antibodies.[7-10]

Antibody Assays

The methods and diagnostic criteria used in antibody assays are listed in Table 1.[11-18] Serum samples were tested for antibodies to *S pneumoniae, H influenzae, Moraxella (Branhamella) catarrhalis, M pneumoniae, Chlamydia trachomatis, Chlamydia psittaci,* and *Chlamydia pneumoniae,* and for antibodies to RSV and adenovirus, influenza A and B, and parainfluenza types 1, 2, and 3.

Criteria for Etiology

The infection was considered bacterial if at least one of the following criteria was fulfilled: a positive blood culture, a significant bacterial antibody response, or positive antigen detection in serum or urine. For *M pneumoniae,* a positive RNA hybridization test result in NPA was also considered indicative of infection. Viral infection was defined as a positive antigen finding in NPA or a significant antibody response. Mixed infection was defined as a concomitant finding of a bacterial and viral agent. If two or more bacterial or viral agents were found, the infection was considered to be a bacterial or viral coinfection, respectively.

Statistical Methods

The χ^2 test with Yates' correction or Fisher's Exact Test, when appropriate, were used to test the differences in distributions of the etiologic agents. The Wilcoxon rank sum test was used to analyze the differences in clinical and laboratory variables indicative of infection.

RESULTS

A total of 135 patients were enrolled during the 1-year study period. Fourteen patients lacked paired serum samples and were excluded from the etiologic part of the study; they did not differ from the rest of the patients in age, clinical signs and symptoms or laboratory indexes, erythrocyte sedimentation rate, white blood cell count, and C-reactive protein level.

Table 2.—Comparison of Assays Detecting Microbial Antigen (or RNA) With Those Detecting the Antibody Response

	Combination of Findings*			
Pathogen†	Ab+/Ag−	Ab+/Ag+	Ab−/Ag+	Total
S pneumoniae	15	0	4‡	**19**
H influenzae type b	0	1	1	**2**
M pneumoniae	4	4	3	**11**
Respiratory syncytial virus	12	19	3	**34**
Adenovirus	11	4	1	**16**
Parainfluenza 1, 2, or 3	7	1	0	**8**
Influenza A or B	2	2	0	**4**
Total	**51**	**31**	**12**	**94**

*Ab indicates significant antibody response; Ag, antigen or RNA (for *M pneumoniae*) detection; plus sign, positive finding; and minus sign, negative finding.
†Full expansion of names of pathogens appears in the text.
‡One case with a positive blood culture.

The median age of the remaining 121 children was 1.75 years (range, 4 months to 15 years). Fifty-nine percent were male and 41% female. The majority (n = 108) were enrolled on the basis of clinical criteria of ALRI, and 13 on the basis of fever and chest roentgenographic findings. Of the 108 patients enrolled on clinical criteria, a pneumonic infiltrate was found in 80%. Acute otitis media, defined as

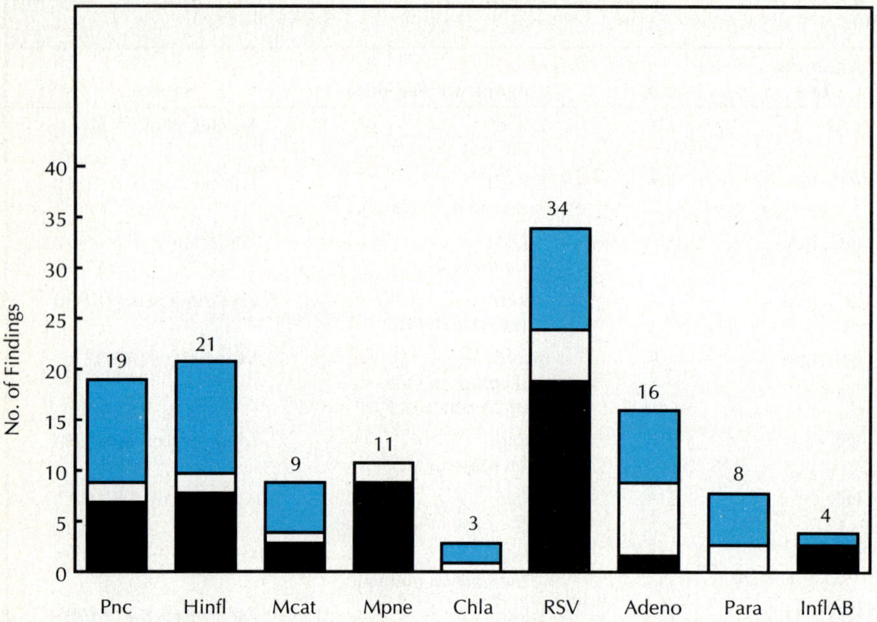

Fig 1.—*The presumptive etiologic findings in 121 children with acute lower respiratory infection based on blood culture, measurement of antibodies, and detection of antigen or RNA. Pnc indicates* Streptococcus pneumoniae; *Hinfl,* Haemophilus influenzae; *Mcat,* Moraxella catarrhalis; *Mpne,* Mycoplasma pneumoniae; *Chla,* Chlamydia *species; RSV, respiratory syncytial virus; Adeno, adenovirus; Para, parainfluenza viruses types 1, 2, and 3; and InflAB, influenza A and B viruses. Closed bars represent a single finding; open bars, two or more bacterial findings together, or two or more viral findings together; and tinted bars, one or more bacterial with one or more viral findings.*

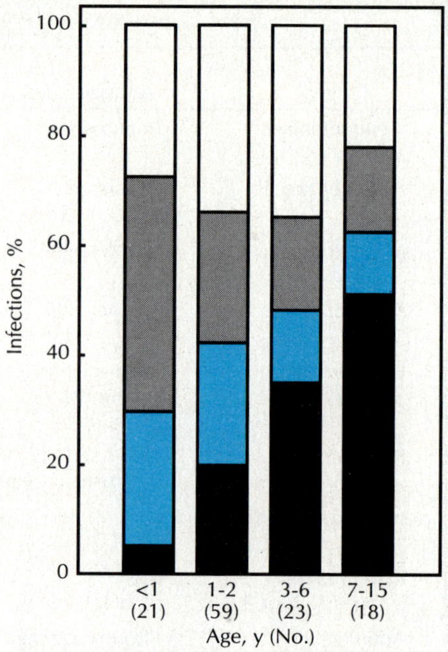

Fig 2.—*Percentages of bacterial (closed bars), mixed (tinted bars), viral (shaded bars), and unknown (open bars) etiologic agents of acute lower respiratory infection in different age groups among 121 children.*

detection of an immobile and inflamed tympanic membrane by pneumatic otoscopy or purulent secretion by myringotomy, was found in 15 of the 96 patients in whom the status of the middle ear was recorded. All children received antimicrobial therapy. The majority of the patients were treated parenterally with procaine penicillin G for 3 to 5 days; 11 patients received other antimicrobial agents (sodium cefuroxime, cefaclor, erythromycin ethylsuccinate, or ampicillin sodium). There were no deaths. All patients recovered without major complications.

Etiologic Diagnosis

Presumptive evidence for the etiologic characteristics of ALRI was detected in 84 (69%) of the 121 patients. Thirty (25%) episodes were found to be associated with a bacterial and 30 (25%) with a viral agent; in 24 (20%), a mixed infection was diagnosed. The methods by which the different etiologic agents were detected are shown in Table 2. Antibody assays alone would have identified the agent in 91% of the positive episodes; antigen detection was less sensitive for most of the microbes (*H influenzae* type b being an exception). Hybridization of RNA identified *M pneumoniae* as often as did antibody assays. The presence of acute otitis media did not increase the etiologic yield; acute otitis media was not associated with any specific etiologic agent or group, or with any one method to implicate the etiologic agent. The finding of a pneumonic infiltrate on chest roentgenogram also did not influence the distribution of causative agents.

Bacterial Agents

Among the bacterial agents (Fig 1), *H influenzae* and *S pneumoniae* were the most common findings, in 17% and 16% of all patients, respectively. *Moraxella catarrhalis* was found in 7% and *M pneumoniae* in 9% of the cases. *Chlamydia* species were found in three patients: *C trachomatis* in two and *C pneumoniae* in one; no *C psittaci* were found. In five patients, two bacterial agents were identified: *S pneumoniae* together with *M pneumoniae* and *H influenzae; H influenzae* with *M pneumoniae* or *M catarrhalis;* and *M catarrhalis* with *C trachomatis.*

Viral Agents

Of the viral agents (Fig 1), RSV was the most common finding, seen in 28% of the patients. The majority of the RSV cases (32 of 34) occurred during a local epidemic in the beginning of the study (December to January). No other seasonal variation was seen among the viral or bacterial agents. The rest of the viral findings were adenovirus in 13%, influenza A or B in 3%, and parainfluenza type 1, 2, or 3 in 7% of the cases. Eight patients had a viral coinfection: RSV together with adenovirus or parainfluenza 1 and 3, and adenovirus with parainfluenza 1 and 3.

Mixed Causes

All bacterial agents except *M pneumoniae* were found with a concomitant viral agent in some patients. Among the viruses, all but influenza B and parainfluenza type 2 were found in association with a concomitant bacterial agent. There was no specific association between a certain bacterium and a certain virus. The proportions of mixed findings among the different agents are shown in Fig 1.

Etiologic Characteristics and Age

The relationship between the different etiologic groups and the age of the patient is shown in Fig 2. The proportion of bacterial ALRI steadily increased with age, whereas the proportion of mixed and pure viral ALRI decreased. *Streptococcus pneumoniae* was seen in all ages and *M pneumoniae* in all ages except for infants; the proportional roles of both

Table 3.—The Relation Between the Age of the Patient and the Etiologic Agent*

Etiologic Agent	No. (%) of Findings by Age Group, y <2 (n=66)	≥2 (n=55)	P
S pneumoniae	6 (9)	13 (24)	<.03
H influenzae	13 (19)	8 (14)	NS
B catarrhalis	5 (7)	4 (7)	NS
M pneumoniae	2 (3)	9 (16)	<.01
Chlamydiae	2 (3)	1 (2)	NS
Respiratory syncytial virus	26 (38)	8 (14)	<.003
Adenovirus	12 (17)	4 (7)	NS
Parainfluenza	3 (4)	5 (9)	NS
Influenza A or B	0 (0)	4 (7)	NS
Total	**69**	**56**	...
No findings	20	17	...

*NS indicates not significant. Full expansion of names of agents appears in the text.

increased with age (Table 3). Respiratory syncytial virus, adenovirus, and *H influenzae* were more common in the younger children; the difference was statistically significant ($P<.003$) for RSV only.

COMMENT

Several problems are faced in establishing the etiologic diagnosis of bacterial ALRI. Blood culture, the "gold standard" of diagnosis, is specific, but insensitive in children with bacterial ALRIs of which less than 10% are bacteremic.[19,20] Invasive methods such as transtracheal aspiration, bronchoalveolar lavage, and lung puncture can seldom be considered justified in pediatric practice, and nasopharyngeal samples provide little etiologic information because of high carriage rates of the potential bacterial pathogens.[21,22] Methods to detect antigens in serum and urine are available, but both their specificity and sensitivity have, until recently, been unsatisfactory.[5,6,20]

Demonstration of a serum antibody response is a well-established indication of viral infection. Antibody assays to detect *S pneumoniae*, nontypable *H influenzae*, and *M catarrhalis* have recently been used in several studies of adult pneumonia,[23,24] demonstrating that bacteria play a significant etiologic role. These new enzyme immunoassays have also been validated in children as follows: when paired serum samples from 158 healthy children less than 14 years old (range, 3 months to 13 years) were studied, no significant responses were found to *M catarrhalis*, and responses to *H influenzae* were seen in less than 4% of the children (M.L., unpublished observations, 1989). So far only a few studies have applied these methods to children with ALRI.[25,26] In accordance with the findings in adult patients, these studies have found a larger involvement of the bacterial pathogens than previously estimated in ALRI of children.

An etiologic diagnosis would have been identified in 45% of the cases, and viruses would have appeared dominant in the etiology of ALRI, had we relied on generally used microbiological methods alone. The use of bacterial antibody assays and antigen detection in addition to conventional methods enabled us to find presumptive evidence for the causes of ALRI in 70% of the patients.

The distribution of the bacterial pathogens corresponded to expectation with the exception of the frequently nontypable *H influenzae*. In children less than 3 years of age, *H influenzae* was a more common bacterial agent than *S pneumoniae*, a finding that, to our knowledge, has not been reported previously from the industrialized world. *Moraxella catarrhalis* was also mainly implicated in children less than 3 years of age and in mixed infections. Although both nontypable *H influenzae* and *M catarrhalis* are common findings in acute otitis media[27,28] and have been also reported in pneumonia in children,[4] their role in the pathogenesis of ALRI is still unclear.

The present study began in December 1987 during a major RSV epidemic. The RSV was by far the most common viral finding in this study, and the majority of them occurred in children younger than 3 years. Adenovirus was the next most common viral finding, outnumbering parainfluenza viruses; it was seen mainly in the same age group as RSV.

In this study, the younger children had few bacterial findings; by contrast, the older children had few viral findings. Several factors probably contribute to these differences. The clinical picture of ALRI in the older children may have been severe enough to require hospitalization only if there was bacterial involvement, whereas in the younger children, ALRI, regardless of etiologic characteristics, may have caused symptoms requiring hospital treatment. Viral epidemics, like the RSV epidemic during this study period, usually affect the youngest children, while the older ones, in whom immunity is already developed, are spared.

The etiologic causes remained unknown in 30% of the children despite a broad range of methods used. There are many possible reasons for this. First, the immaturity of the child's immune system may have led to lack of a measurable seroresponse. Second, antibiotic treatment might have been started in such an early phase of the illness that the immune system did not have enough time to respond to detectable limits[29]; this would reduce the detection of both bacterial and mixed, but not viral, infection. Finally, there might have been etiologic agents we did not search for, such as *Staphylococcus aureus*, *Bordetella pertussis*, cytomegalovirus, coronavirus, and, probably most important, rhinoviruses.[30]

This work was supported by the Academy of Finland (Drs Eskola and Ruutu).

We thank Professor P. Helena Mäkelä, MD, PhD, for discussions and critical reading of the article. We also thank the staff of Aurora Hospital, Helsinki, Finland, Raili Kalliokoski, RN, and Panu Rekola, MSc, for their assistance.

References

1. Bulla A, Hitze KL. Acute respiratory infections: a review. *Bull WHO.* 1978;56:481-498.

2. Berman S, McIntosh K. Selective primary health care: strategies for control of disease in the developing world, XXI: acute respiratory infections. *Rev Infect Dis.* 1985;7:674-691.

3. Leowski J. Mortality from acute respiratory infections in children under five years of age: global estimates. *World Health Stat Q.* 1986;39:138-144.

4. Shann F. Etiology of severe pneumonia in children in developing countries. *Pediatr Infect Dis J.* 1986;5:247-252.

5. Isaacs D. Problems in determining the etiology of community-acquired childhood pneumonia. *Pediatr Infect Dis J.* 1989;8:143-148.

6. O'Neill KP, Lloyd-Evans N, Campbell H, Forgie IM, Sabally S, Greenwood BM. Latex agglutination test for diagnosing pneumococcal pneumonia in children in developing countries. *BMJ.* 1989;298:1061-1064.

7. Halonen P, Obert G, Hierholzer JC. Direct detection of viral antigens in respiratory infections by immunoassays: a four year experience and new development. In: de la Maza LM, Peterson EM, eds. *Medical Virology IV.* Hillsdale, NJ: Lawrence Erlbaum Associates Publishers; 1985:65-85.

8. Walls HH, Johansson KH, Harmon MW, Halonen PE, Kendal AP. Time-resolved fluoroimmunoassay with monoclonal antibodies for rapid diagnosis of influenza infections. *J Clin Microbiol.* 1986;24:907-912.

9. Hierholzer JC, Johansson KH, Anderson LJ, Tsou CJ, Halonen PE. Comparison of monoclonal time-resolved fluoroimmunoassay with monoclonal capture-biotinylated detector enzyme immunoassay for adenovirus antigen detection. *J Clin Microbiol.* 1987;25:1662-1667.

10. Hierholzer JC, Bigham PG, Coombs RA, Johansson KH, Anderson LJ, Halonen PE. Comparison of monoclonal antibody time-resolved fluoroimmunoassay with monoclonal antibody capture-biotinylated detector enzyme immunoassay for respiratory syncytial virus and parainfluenza virus antigen detection. *J Clin Microbiol.* 1989;27:1243-1249.

11. Jalonen E, Paton JC, Koskela M, Kerttula Y, Leinonen M. Measurement of antibody responses to pneumolysin: a promising method for the presumptive etiological diagnosis of pneumococcal pneumonia. *J Infect.* 1989;19:127-134.

12. Leinonen M, Luotonen J, Herva E, Valkonen K, Mäkelä PH. Preliminary serologic evidence for a pathogenic role of *Branhamella catarrhalis. J Infect Dis.* 1981;144:570-574.

13. Kleemola M, Karjalainen JE, Räty RKH. Rapid diagnosis of *Mycoplasma pneumoniae* infection: clinical evaluation of a commercial probe test. *J Infect Dis.* 1990;162:70-75.

14. Wang SP, Grayston JT. Immunologic relationship between genital TRIC, lymphogranuloma venereum, and related organisms in a new microtiter indirect immunofluorescence test. *Am J Ophthalmol.* 1970;70:367-374.

15. Meurman O, Ruuskanen O, Sarkkinen H, Hänninen P, Halonen P. Immunoglobulin class-qi specific antibody response in respiratory syncytial virus infection measured by enzyme immunoassay. *J Med Virol.* 1984;14:67-72.

16. Koskinen P, Vuorinen T, Merman O. Influenza A and B virus IgG and IgM serology by enzyme immunoassays. *Epidemiol Infect.* 1987;99:55-64.

17. Vuorinen T, Meurman O. Enzyme immunoassays for detection of IgG and IgM antibodies to parainfluenza types 1, 2 and 3. *J Virol Methods.* 1989;23:63-70.

18. Meurman O, Ruuskanen O, Sarkkinen H. Immunoassay diagnosis of adenovirus infections in children. *J Clin Microbiol.* 1983;18:1190-1195.

19. Teele DW, Pelton SI, Grant MJA. Bacteremia in febrile children under 2 years of age: results of cultures of blood of 600 consecutive children seen in a "walk-in" clinic. *J Pediatr.* 1985;18:1190-1195.

20. Ramsey BW, Marcuse EK, Foy HM, et al. Use of bacterial antigen detection in the diagnosis of pediatric lower respiratory tract infections. *Pediatrics.* 1986;78:1-9.

21. Loda FA, Collier AM, Glezen WP, Strangert K, Clyde WA, Denny FW. Occurrence of *Diplococcus pneumoniae* in the upper respiratory tract of children. *J Pediatr.* 1975;87:1087-1093.

22. Trottier S, Stenberg K, Svanborg-Eden C. Turnover of nontypable *Haemophilus influenzae* in the nasopharynges of healthy children. *J Clin Microbiol.* 1989;27:1275-1279.

23. Kerttula Y, Leinonen M, Koskela M, Mäkelä PH. The etiology of pneumonia: application of bacterial serology and basic laboratory methods. *J Infect.* 1987;14:21-30.

24. Lehtomäki K, Leinonen M, Takala A, Hovi T, Herva E, Koskela M. Etiological diagnosis of pneumonia in military recruits by combining bacterial culture and serological methods. *Eur J Clin Microbiol Infect Dis.* 1988;7:348-354.

25. Korppi M, Leinonen M, Mäkelä PH, Launiala K. Bacterial coinfection in children hospitalized with respiratory syncytial virus infections. *Pediatr Infect Dis J.* 1989;8:687-692.

26. Claesson BA, Trollfors B, Brolin I, et al. Etiology of community-acquired pneumonia in children based on antibody responses to bacterial and viral antigens. *Pediatr Infect Dis J.* 1989;8:856-861.

27. Schneerson R, Robbins JB, Parke JC. Studies on *Haemophilus influenzae* isolated from otitis media. In: Sell SH, Karzon DT, eds. *Haemophilus Influenzae.* Nashville, Tenn: Vanderbilt University Press; 1973:13-20.

28. Shurin PA, Marchant CD, Kim CH, et al. Emergence of beta-lactamase-producing strains of *Branhamella catarrhalis* as important agents of acute otitis media. *Pediatr Infect Dis J.* 1983;2:34-38.

29. Pichichero ME, Disney FA, Talpey WB, et al. Adverse and beneficial effects of immediate treatment of group A beta-hemolytic streptococcal pharyngitis with penicillin. *Pediatr Infect Dis J.* 1987;6:635-643.

30. Paisley JW, Lauer BA, McIntosh K, Glode MP, Schachter J, Rumack C. Pathogens associated with acute lower respiratory tract infection in young children. *Pediatr Infect Dis J.* 1984;3:14-19.

In Other AMA Journals

ARCHIVES OF OTOLARYNGOLOGY—HEAD & NECK SURGERY

Mandibular Fractures in the Pediatric Patient

Michael B. Siegel MD; Ralph F. Wetmore, MD; William P. Potsic, MD; Steven D. Handler, MD; Lawrence W. C. Tom, MD
(*Arch Otolaryngol Head Neck Surg.* 1991;117:533-536)

Periorbital Hematoma Secondary to Sinusitis in a Child

George H. Zalzal, MD
(*Arch Otolaryngol Head Neck Surg.* 1991;117:557-559)

Influenza Type A and B Infections in Hospitalized Pediatric Patients

Who Should Be Immunized?

Janet R. Serwint, MD; Ross M. Miller, MD; Barbara M. Korsch, MD

• Medical records of 99 hospitalized pediatric patients whose respiratory viral cultures yielded influenza type A or B during the winter of 1988/1989 were reviewed. We compared the records of patients considered to be at high risk (n = 43) with those of patients considered to be at low risk (n = 56) to determine differences in morbidity and mortality and if vaccination was warranted. Sixty-six percent of high-risk patients had chronic pulmonary disease. Forty-four percent of the high-risk and 11% of the low-risk patients were hospitalized for 14 or more days. Nosocomial influenza infections were identified in 14% of the high-risk and 4% of the low-risk patients. Four of the high-risk patients and only one of the low-risk patients were intubated. Of the three deaths, two occurred in the high-risk group. None of the high-risk patients who experienced significant morbidity had been immunized. We need to immunize high-risk patients, particularly high-risk pulmonary patients.
(*AJDC*. 1991;145:623-626)

According to the recommendations of the Committee on Infectious Diseases in Children,[1,2] children aged 6 months or older in the following high-risk groups should be immunized against influenza: (1) chronic pulmonary disease; (2) hemodynamically significant cardiac disease; (3) patients receiving immunosuppressive therapy; (4) sickle cell disease and other hemoglobinopathies; (5) chronic renal and metabolic diseases; (6) diabetes; (7) symptomatic human immunodeficiency virus infections; and (8) patients receiving long-term aspirin therapy.

Despite these recommendations, only 1% to 7% of high-risk children for whom the vaccine is recommended receive the vaccine.[3] Reasons for such a low rate of immunization may include the following[3]: (1) influenza is not thought to be associated with significant morbidity or mortality in children; and (2) there is uncertainty about which children aged 6 months or older with high-risk conditions really need the vaccine.

Some of this uncertainty may be justified because vaccine recommendations for children are inferred from risk data in adults. Few investigators have studied children considered to be at high risk.[4-8]

Several studies, including those by Brocklebank et al,[9] Liou et al,[10] and Mullooly et al,[11] have examined influenza infections in hospitalized children, but their definitions of high risk and underlying disease were varied and rather broad. Few studies have compared the sequelae from influenza in high-risk patients, as defined by the Committee of Infectious Diseases, with the sequelae in low-risk patients[12,13] or determined which high-risk patients are most affected by influenza and, thus, would benefit most from immunization.

The purpose of this study was to determine how much morbidity from influenza occurred in high-risk groups for whom the influenza vaccine is recommended compared with low-risk groups, and to determine whether certain high-risk groups are at greater risk for influenza sequelae than other high-risk groups. We hypothesized that high-risk children experience more significant morbidity than low-risk children and that certain high-risk groups are at greater risk of influenza morbidity than other high-risk groups.

MATERIALS AND METHODS

We retrospectively reviewed microbiology records to identify all hospitalized patients from December 1988 through March 1989 with positive influenza A or B respiratory viral cultures. A viral respiratory culture was done on patients hospitalized with a respiratory illness suspected to be of viral cause. The primary reason for obtaining the culture was to diagnose respiratory syncytial virus and to place these patients in contact isolation to avoid nosocomial transmission.

The medical records of these patients were reviewed to identify those who met high-risk criteria. Influenza immunization status was determined by examining hospital charts, influenza immunization lists from subspecialty and primary care clinics, and, when in doubt, contacting the primary care provider. The patients were categorized into high-risk and low-risk groups according to the Committee on Infectious Diseases criteria[1] and were then compared for age at hospitalization and type of influenza yielded. The cutoff age of 6 months was selected for analysis since this is the age at which influenza immunization is recommended. Morbidity from influenza, as measured by length of hospitalization, incidence of intubation, and mortality, was also

Accepted for publication August 20, 1990.
From the Division of General Pediatrics, Department of Pediatrics, Childrens Hospital of Los Angeles, Calif, and the University of Southern California School of Medicine, Los Angeles. Dr Serwint is now with the Division of General Pediatrics, The Johns Hopkins Hospital, Baltimore, Md.
Presented in part at the Annual Meeting of the Western Society for Pediatric Research, Carmel, Calif, February 8, 1990.
Reprints are not available.

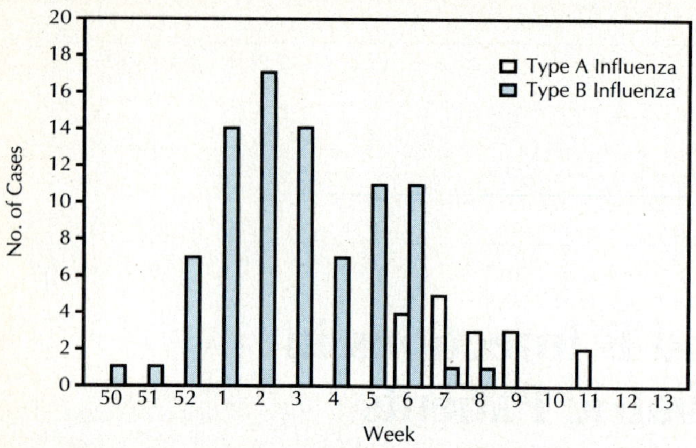

Type of influenza yielded by week.

measured and compared between groups. We identified cases of influenza acquired in nosocomial fashion during hospitalization as another component of morbidity. The high-risk group outcome variables were then divided into subgroups by disease, such as pulmonary and cardiac, to determine if certain high-risk patients experienced more morbidity.

The data were analyzed using χ^2 analysis or Fisher's Exact Test when appropriate.

Specimens from nasopharyngeal swab, endotracheal tube, and tracheostomy suction were first inoculated onto MRC-5 cells (fetal lung tissue), rhesus monkey kidney tissue cells, human foreskin fibroblasts, Hep-2 cells, and A-549 cells (human lung carcinoma). These cells were inoculated at 34°C and observed for cytopathic effect every 3 to 4 days for 2 weeks. Rhesus monkey kidney tissue cell tubes were hemadsorbed with 0.2 mL of 0.5% guinea pig blood cells at 4°C during the first 14 days. Hemadsorption-positive cultures were further evaluated using immunofluorescence staining for influenza A or B virus.

RESULTS

Of 790 viral respiratory cultures obtained from hospitalized patients from December 1988 through March 1989, 112 (14%) were positive for influenza in 99 patients. The hospital records of those 99 patients were reviewed. Their ages ranged from 14 days to 19 years; 53% were male. Of those 99 patients, 43 met the criteria for high risk. In 37 of these high-risk patients and 54 of the low-risk patients, viral cultures were obtained at or shortly after admission. The remaining six high-risk and two low-risk patients were asymptomatic for respiratory symptoms at the time of admission, but cultures for them were obtained 7 or more days after admission when they became symptomatic.

In comparing high-risk and low-risk patients by age, 38 (88%) of the high-risk patients and 21 (38%) of the low-risk patients were aged 6 months or older. This difference was significant at $P<.001$. There was no difference between the high-risk and low-risk groups in type of influenza yielded. Cultures yielded type B influenza more often in both groups (82% of high-risk patients and 80% of low-risk patients). The viral culture from one patient in each group yielded types A and B concomitantly, while the viral culture from an additional high-risk patient yielded influenza B during her first hospitalization and then type A during a second hospitalization, 2½ months later.

We noted that there was an apparent interseasonal distribution in the types of influenza yielded. From December 16 through February 10, cultures yielded only influenza type B except for one case of A in late January. From February 10 through March 15, cultures yielded both types A and B (Figure). The distribution of the high-risk patients by diagnosis according to the criteria established by the

Table 1.—Comparison of High-Risk Patients (n=43) by Diagnosis, Age, and Immunization Status

Diagnosis	Age, mo <6	Age, mo ≥6	No. of Patients Immunized
Pulmonary disease	3	25	4
Cardiac disease	2	3	0
Hemoglobinopathy	0	3	0
Immunosuppression	0	3	0
Immunodeficiency	0	2	0
Renal disease	0	2	0
Total (%) of Patients	**5** (12)	**38** (88)	**4** (11)

Table 2.—Comparison of Morbidity From Influenza Infections Between High- and Low-Risk Patients

Type of Morbidity	No. (%) of Patients: High-Risk (n=43)	No. (%) of Patients: Low-Risk (n=56)	*P*
Hospitalization ≥14 d	19 (44)	6 (11)	.001
Nosocomial influenza infection	6 (14)	2 (4)	.05*
Intubation	4 (9)	1 (2)	.10*
Death	2 (5)	1 (2)	.32*

*Fisher's Exact Test.

Committee of Infectious Diseases is shown in Table 1. The large majority of these patients had pulmonary disease, including patients with asthma, bronchopulmonary dysplasia, congenital emphysema, restrictive lung disease, or chronic aspiration. The other high-risk categories were less well represented in the sample. No patients with diabetes or those receiving long-term aspirin therapy were hospitalized or had culture-positive influenza.

Of the 38 high-risk patients aged 6 months or older who were eligible for immunization, only four (11%) had been appropriately immunized with influenza vaccine. All four of these immunized patients had underlying pulmonary disease. None of the high-risk patients received amantadine as prophylaxis or treatment. Examining morbidity based on the length of hospitalization, 19 patients (44%) in the high-risk group were hospitalized for 14 days or more compared with six patients (11%) in the low-risk group. This difference was significant at $P<.001$. When the length of hospitalization for patients with nosocomial influenza infections was excluded, this difference still remained significant at $P<.001$ (Table 2).

Nosocomial or hospital-acquired influenza infections were defined as influenza infections in patients who did not have respiratory symptoms at the time of admission but who developed symptoms and had a positive influenza culture 7 or more days after they were admitted to the hospital. Six patients in the high-risk group (14%) had nosocomial influenza infections compared with two patients (4%) in the low-risk group. ($P=.05$ by Fisher's Exact Test; Table 2).

Of the six high-risk patients with nosocomial infections, three had underlying pulmonary disease, two were immunosuppressed, and one had cardiac disease. Of the four high-risk patients who were eligible by age for immunization, none had received the influenza vaccine. There did not appear to be any differences in the rate of nosocomial acquisition between influenza type A and B. The mean length of hospital stay at the time cultures were obtained in these patients was 58 days.

Morbidity in these patients was also assessed in terms of the need for intubation directly related to their influenza infection. Four patients (9%) in the high-risk group compared with only one patient (2%) in the low-risk group required intubation. All four of the high-risk patients who were intubated had underlying pulmonary disease. None of the patients who were eligible by age had been immunized with influenza vaccine. Two home ventilator–dependent patients who required hospitalization in the intensive care unit because of increasing ventilatory settings due to influenza infections were not included in this analysis.

Mortality in the cohort was also assessed. Three patients died, resulting in a mortality rate of 3%. Two of these patients met the criteria for the high-risk group. The first patient was a 3-month-old infant with atrioventricular canal who died after 10 days of an influenza B infection. The second patient was a 12-year-old child with restrictive lung disease, juvenile dermatomyositis, and calcinosis universalis. She became infected with influenza A via nosocomial spread after being in the hospital for 175 days and died 7 days later. She had not been immunized with the influenza vaccine.

In summarizing the morbidity from influenza in high-risk, vaccine-eligible patients (aged 6 months or older), there were more patients with pulmonary disease (66%) than other high-risk conditions. These patients also had a longer mean length of hospital stay (20 days) than the other high-risk patients, including those with immunodeficiency (mean stay, 15 days), cardiac disease (mean stay, 13 days), renal disease (mean stay, 11 days), and hemoglobinopathy and immunosuppression (mean stay, 8 days each). There were three intubations and one death within the pulmonary group and none in the other high-risk groups in this age range.

Significant morbidity occurred in the high-risk patients younger than 6 months. Of three pulmonary patients, one acquired influenza via nosocomial spread and a second patient required intubation. Of the two cardiac patients, one acquired a nosocomial influenza infection and the second patient died secondary to influenza. Of the five high-risk patients younger than 6 months, four (80%) experienced significant morbidity from influenza.

COMMENT

Our data show that high-risk patients experienced more morbidity from influenza infections than low-risk patients when length of hospitalization and nosocomial influenza infections were considered. Since this was a retrospective study, it was difficult to determine what portions of the hospitalizations were due solely to influenza infections and their sequelae. This statistical difference in length of hospitalization persisted even when the length of hospitalization for patients with nosocomial-acquired influenza was excluded.

The nosocomial acquisition of influenza infections in high-risk patients is undoubtedly related to prolonged hospitalization and exposure to other patients and health care workers with respiratory viral infections. This has important ramifications concerning isolation and immunization policies. Although we cannot draw any conclusions concerning isolation techniques from our study, it does point out that nosocomial spread does occur and has serious consequences. Current recommendations include immunization for health care providers who treat high-risk patients. We do not have data to document health care workers' immunization rates at our institution, but this may remain another way in which nosocomial spread can be minimized. The fact that two of the nosocomial infections occurred in infants younger than 6 months for whom immunization is not recommended suggests that immunization of health care personnel may be essential.

Our sample was too small to compare differences between the high-risk and low-risk patients for the number of intubations and deaths. However, the mortality rate of 3% in our study is consistent with the rates of 1% to 4% found in other studies. Interestingly, cultures yielded both influenza A and B that year, with type B more predominant in our cohort. Although it has been suggested in the literature that type A disease results in more serious morbidity than type B,[14] we did not find this to be the case. Type B disease resulted in four of six nosocomial infections, five of five intubations, and two of three deaths. Influenza A is thought to lead to more morbidity because of its association with antigenic shift. Since no major shifts have occurred in the last few years, we did not expect to note a difference in our cohort. Also, Reye's syndrome has been shown to correlate with cases of influenza B infection.[15,16] There were no cases of Reye's syndrome in our cohort.

It is worth noting that cultures from four immunized patients yielded influenza. Although we did not have the influenza subtypes cultured from these four individuals, the circulating subtypes in the community did match those present in the vaccine that year.[17] The four patients constituted too small a sample for statistical significance to be determined. However, their mean hospital stay was only 8 days, which was much shorter than the 20 days for the remainder of the pulmonary patients. None of the four patients acquired nosocomial influenza infections and none required intubation or died. Although the efficacy of the vaccine is thought to be 70% to 80%, it may be that the disease course is modified secondary to receipt of the vaccine.

The majority of the high-risk patients admitted to the hospital had pulmonary disease, although there were several patients in other high-risk groups. These data may have been biased if more pulmonary patients than other high-risk patients were followed up by physicians who admit to our hospital, but we have no reason to suspect this. Also, the criteria for admission of patients with pulmonary conditions might be less stringent than for other patients. However, since many patients with acute problems are admitted through the emergency department, we would not expect the criteria to depend on subspecialist bias. In addition, other studies[8-10] have shown pulmonary patients to constitute a large proportion of the high-risk patients hospitalized.

We were impressed by the fact that of the five high-risk patients younger than 6 months, one required intubation and a second died. At present, these patients are not eligible for the influenza vaccine. Perhaps further research will lead to the development of a vaccine that can be used in younger children. The only other ways to minimize morbidity in these young high-risk patients is by immunization of caretakers, family members, and hospital personnel.

We need to immunize all high-risk patients; in particular, high-risk pulmonary patients. Immunization should be considered in all high-risk hospitalized patients. Since hospitalized patients are a captive audience and the vaccine is an inactivated viral vaccine, it may be appropriate to immunize patients once their acute symptoms have resolved. Immunization of family members and health care workers needs to be encouraged.

More studies are needed to determine which high-risk children need to be immunized, to develop an effective vaccine in younger infants, and to determine the impact of nosocomial spread and isolation techniques in influenza.

The authors thank Vida Negrete for her input in this project and Linda Leahy for her secretarial assistance.

References

1. American Academy of Pediatrics. *Influenza Infection in the Report of the Committee on Infectious Diseases.* Elk Grove Village, Ill: American Academy of Pediatrics; 1988:243-251.
2. Immunization Practices Advisory Committee. Prevention and control of influenza. *MMWR.* 1988;37:361-373.
3. Hall CB. Influenza: a shot or not? *Pediatrics.* 1987;79:564-566.
4. Glezen WP, Couch RB. Interpandemic influenza in the Houston area. *N Engl J Med.* 1978;298:587-592.
5. Wright PF, Ross KB, Thompson J, Karzon DT. Influenza A infections in young children. *N Engl J Med.* 1977;296:829-834.
6. Glezen WP. The pediatrician's role in influenza control. *Pediatr Infect Dis.* 1986;5:615-618.
7. Glezen WP. Serious morbidity and mortality associated with influenza epidemics. *Epidemiol Rev.* 1982;4:25-44.
8. Glezen WP. Consideration of the risk of influenza in children and indications for prophylaxis. *Rev Infect Dis.* 1980;2:408-420.
9. Brocklebank JT, Court SMD, McQuillin J, Gardner PS. Influenza A infection in children. *Lancet.* 1972;2:497-500.
10. Liou YS, Barbour SD, Bell LM, Plokin SA. Children hospitalized with influenza B infection. *Pediatr Infect Dis J.* 1987;6:541-543.
11. Mullooly JP, Barker WH. Impact of type A influenza on children: a retrospective study. *Am J Public Health.* 1982;72:1008-1016.
12. Kempe A, Hall CB, Macdonald NE, et al. Influenza in children with cancer. *J Pediatr.* 1989;115:33-39.
13. Glezen WP, Decker M, Perrotta DM. Survey of underlying conditions of persons hospitalized with acute respiratory disease during influenza epidemics in Houston 1978-1981. *Am Rev Respir Dis.* 1987;136:550-555.
14. Kendal AP. Epidemiologic implications of changes in the influenza virus genome. *Am J Med.* 1987;82(suppl 6A):4-14.
15. Corey L, Rubin RJ, Hatwick MNW, Noble GR, Cassidy E. A nationwide outbreak of Reye's syndrome: its epidemiologic relationship to influenza B. *Am J Med.* 1976;61:615-625.
16. Reynolds DW, Riley HD, LaFont DS, Vorse H, Stout C, Carpenter RL. An outbreak of Reye's syndrome associated with influenza B. *J Pediatr.* 1972;80:429-432.
17. Immunization Practices Advisory Committee. Prevention and control of influenza: recommendations of the Immunization Practices Advisory Committee. *MMWR.* 1988;37:361-373.

In Other AMA Journals

ARCHIVES OF INTERNAL MEDICINE

The Cruzan Decision and Medical Practice

David C. Thomasma, PhD
(*Arch Intern Med.* 1991;151:853-854)

Persistant Vegetative State: Where Do We Go From Here?

Joseph S. Alpert, MD
(*Arch Intern Med.* 1991;151:855-856)

Insuring the Uninsured Is Not Enough

James E. Dalen, MD, Jose Santiago, MD
(*Arch Intern Med.* 1991;151:857-859)

Overcoming the Prejudice Against Establishing a National Health Care System

Richard J. Botelho, MD
(*Arch Intern Med.* 1991;151:853-869)

What Does Cruzan Mean to the Practicing Physician?

Bruce David White, DO, JD; Mark Siegler, MD;
Peter A. Singer, MD, MPH; Kenneth V. Iserson, MD, MBA
(*Arch Intern Med.* 1991;151:925-928)

Pediatric Cardiac Rehabilitation

Ian C. Balfour, MBBS; Ami M. Drimmer, PhD; Soraya Nouri, MBBS; D. Glenn Pennington, MD; Carol L. Hemkens, RN; Linda L. Harvey, RN

• Sixteen patients participated in a Pediatric/Young Adult Cardiac Rehabilitation Program that included exercise training, education about cardiovascular diseases, dietary counseling, and counseling on stress management. Seven patients completed the program, and complete data were available on six. The subjects demonstrated significant changes in their hemodynamics and exercise tolerance after completing the program. Resting blood pressure decreased by 7%, from 119±12 to 111±10 mm Hg; peak oxygen consumption increased by 20%, from 31.9±4.3 mL/kg of body weight per minute to 38.4±6.0 mL/kg of body weight per minute; and exercise treadmill time increased by 21%, from 8.5±1.4 to 10.3±1.0 minutes. No complications occurred during exercise training or testing. Supervised exercise training at moderate intensity is safe and produces significant and beneficial changes in hemodynamics and exercise time in children with cardiac disease.

(*AJDC*. 1991;145:627-630)

Cardiac Rehabilitation Programs (CRPs) are recognized as valuable for the treatment of adults with cardiac disease.[1] Recently, similar programs have been developed for children.[2,3] The CRP at Cardinal Glennon Children's Hospital/St Louis (Mo) University Medical Center was developed for children and young adults with congenital or acquired cardiac disease, children with increased risk of developing coronary disease, and chronically ill children who might benefit from exercise training. The goals of the program are similar to those of the American College of Cardiology[4]: (1) to help individuals attain optimal physiologic and psychologic function; (2) to reverse the adverse physiologic effects of deconditioning that result from an overprotected, sedentary lifestyle; (3) to encourage the patient and family through education to adopt a life-style that may reduce the risk of coronary heart disease and hypertensive cardiovascular disease, including avoiding smoking, controlling blood pressure and diabetes mellitus, and decreasing emotional stress, and to educate the patient and family about cardiovascular disease and the importance of a program of suitable and regular physical activity; (4) to reduce the emotional disorders that often accompany serious and chronic health disorders; and (5) to reduce the cost of health care by diminishing physical and psychological disability and the need for medical treatment.

Accepted for publication January 3, 1991.

From the Departments of Pediatrics/Adolescent Medicine (Drs Balfour and Nouri and Ms Harvey) and Surgery (Dr Pennington) and the Cardiovascular Fitness and Rehabilitation Center (Dr Drimmer and Ms Hemkens), St Louis (Mo) University Medical Center.

Reprint requests to St Louis University Medical Center, Department of Pediatrics/Adolescent Medicine, 1465 S Grand Blvd, St Louis, MO 63104 (Dr Balfour).

PATIENTS AND METHODS

The CRP at Cardinal Glennon Children's Hospital/St Louis University Medical Center is a 3-month program that combines exercise training, dietary counseling, counseling on stress management, and education concerning cardiovascular physiology and congenital and acquired cardiovascular diseases. Family members are encouraged to participate in the program, particularly in the educational sessions. Most participants were referred to this facility from the Cardiology Clinic at Cardinal Glennon Children's Hospital, but patients also were referred from other clinics (eg, the Renal Clinic). Before entering the program, patients were encouraged to set reasonable goals: improved fitness, weight loss, etc. Informed consent was obtained from the participants' parents. Each patient was evaluated by a pediatric cardiologist. An electrocardiogram and chest roentgenogram were obtained in each case. When indicated, patients also underwent Holter monitoring and echocardiography as part of their preparticipation evaluations. All patients underwent a graded maximal exercise treadmill test (Bruce protocol)[5] to evaluate their exercise tolerance and cardiovascular fitness. During the exercise test, the patient's time on the treadmill, heart rate, blood pressure, and electrocardiographic results were recorded. Metabolic parameters, oxygen consumption ($\dot{V}O_2$), and carbon dioxide production ($\dot{V}CO_2$) also were measured using a metabolic cart (Beckman Instruments Inc, Anaheim Calif). Metabolic measurements were obtained at 15-second intervals during the exer cise test. The highest measured $\dot{V}O_2$ after the patient has reached anaerobic threshold is the patient's peak $\dot{V}O_2$. Anaerobic threshold was regarded as the point at which the $\dot{V}CO_2$-$\dot{V}O_2$ ratio reached or exceeded 1.0 and a sharp rise in the $\dot{V}CO_2$-$\dot{V}O_2$ curve occurred when this ratio was plotted against time. Using the data from the exercise test, an exercise program was prescribed for each patient. The exercise programs were individualized to meet the abilities, needs, and goals of each patient. The program emphasized dynamic exercise (eg, walking and riding a stationary bicycle). Patients were encouraged to exercise strenuously enough to increase and maintain heart rates of 70% or more of their maximal heart rates. Supervised exercise sessions were held 3 days per week, and patients were encouraged to exercise at home on 1 or 2 additional days. The sessions lasted 30 to 40 minutes and were supervised by exercise trainers who were registered nurses, an exercise physiologist, and a physician. The initial and final 10 minutes of each exercise session were used as "warm-up" and "cool-down" periods during which stretching exercises were done. Patients at risk of developing dysrhythmias were screened with telemetry and Holter monitoring during their first three sessions. Patients were taught to monitor their responses to exercise by counting their pulse rates and to monitor exercise intensity using Borg's scale of perceived exertion.[6] Initially, the program was structured to last 6 months, with 56 sessions. Subsequently,

Table 1.—Data of Patients Who Did Not Complete the Cardiac Rehabilitation Program

Patient No.	Diagnosis*	Age, y	Reason for Not Completing Program
1	DC, obesity	16.3	Insufficient interest
2	Mild AS, obesity	12.8	Insufficient interest
3	TOF (repaired)	7.8	Insufficient interest
4	IHSS, obesity	18.6	No transportation
5	Hypertension	14.2	No transportation
6	AVR	10.6	Torsion of testes
7	VSD	14.4	Sprained ankle
8	VSD	7.3	Travel
9	MVP	16.1	Family problems
10	Fontan	9.9	Completed program (follow-up test not suitable for analysis)

*DC indicates dilated cardiomyopathy; AS, aortic stenosis; TOF, tetralogy of Fallot; IHSS, idiopathic hypertrophic subaortic stenosis; AVR, aortic valve replacement; USD, ventricular septal defect; MVP, mitral valve prolapse; and Fontan, Fontan procedure for tricuspid atresia.

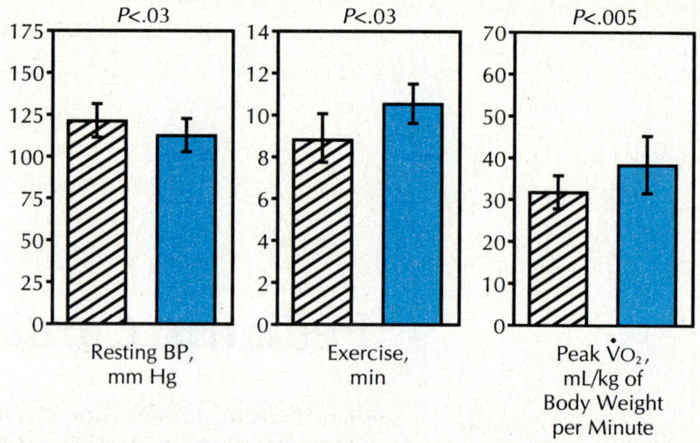

Patients' mean resting systolic blood pressure (BP), exercise time, and peak oxygen consumption ($\dot{V}O_2$) before (hatched bars) and after (solid bars) rehabilitation exercise tests. Vertical lines intersecting the bars indicate SD.

it was shortened to 3 months and 36 sessions to improve patient compliance. The exercise test and metabolic measurements were repeated at the end of the program. Seven patients completed the CRP, and six underwent satisfactory preparticipation and postparticipation evaluations.

Dietary intervention was an important aspect of the program. On entry, each participant was directed to keep a 3-day food log. This was reviewed by a dietitian, and the patient and family were advised on making dietary changes when necessary to reduce cardiovascular risk factors, control weight gain, or promote weight loss. Parents and patients also were evaluated by a psychologist and instructed in stress management through relaxation and biofeedback techniques.

The preparticipation and postparticipation test data were compared using the Student's paired t test.

RESULTS

Sixteen patients were enrolled in the program. Their diagnoses are listed in Tables 1 and 2. All patients were ignorant about appropriate exercise and anxious about exercise. Complete data from preparticipation and postparticipation exercise tests were available on six patients, aged 13.5 to 19.8 years (mean, 17.3±2.8 years), who completed an average of 29 sessions. One patient completed the program, but results of his follow-up exercise test were unsuitable for analysis because it was a submaximal test. Nine patients either did not complete the program or completed the program but did not undergo follow-up tests. These latter patients took part in an average of 18 sessions. There were many reasons for patients not completing the program (Table 1). Of the six patients who completed the program and had satisfactory preparticipation and postparticipation tests, three had undergone successful repair of congenital heart defects, and three had not undergone cardiac surgery (Table 2). The preparticipation and postparticipation evaluations of these patients are shown in Table 2 and the Figure. No significant differences were observed in the subjects' mean resting heart rates, mean peak heart rates, or mean peak blood pressures when their prerehabilitation and postrehabilitation exercise test results were compared. The subjects' resting systolic blood pressures decreased (as measured by a sphygmomanometer) after training. As a group, the patients significantly improved in exercise time and peak $\dot{V}O_2$ (Figure). One patient did not improve in these parameters. This patient had been a very active adolescent boy when he developed sudden-onset severe chest pain and electrocardiographic changes suggestive of an anteriorseptal myocardial infarct. He was thought to have had myocarditis. Results of a cardiac muscle biopsy were normal, and he eventually recovered completely. This patient did not have structural cardiac disease and probably did not exercise strenuously enough to improve his conditioning level.

COMMENT

Physical activity (play or recreational sports) is important for the normal development and general well-being of children[7,8] and may help prevent coronary heart disease.[9] Many children with heart disease remain sedentary even after successful repair of congenital defects or recovery from acquired diseases such as myocarditis. Because the activity of these children may have been restricted for many years, they and their families may be apprehensive about their participation in normal physical activity. The psychological adjustment a child makes to a chronic disease is primarily determined by parental anxiety and pampering rather than by the severity of the illness.[7,8] By participating in a rehabilitation program that includes education, the child and the family are shown exercises that are safe, ways of monitoring the severity of exercise, and ways of measuring the body's response to exercise. Thus, the undue anxiety of the family may be alleviated, and the child's illness viewed in a more pragmatic manner. Rehabilitation that includes exercise training may also improve exercise tolerance and cardiovascular function[10,11] and reduce risk factors for coronary heart disease.[9] Mathews et al[2] demonstrated that exercise training by four pediatric cardiac patients increased maximal oxygen consumption and decreased total serum cholesterol levels. The patients' and their mothers' psychologic outlooks in terms of fear of death and apprehension about exercise improved. Bradley et al[3] also have reported increased $\dot{V}O_2$, treadmill time, and peak systolic blood pressure after exercise training by patients who had undergone repair of tetralogy of Fallot and transposition of the great arteries.

Normal subjects exhibit many physiologic changes after training, such as increased exercise time and peak $\dot{V}O_2$, which are due in part to an increase in maximal cardiac output.[11-13] Because maximal heart rate does not change

Table 2.—Data of Patients Who Completed the Cardiac Rehabilitation Program*

			Before Program			After Program		
Patient No.	Diagnosis	Age, y	Resting SBP, mm Hg	Peak $\dot{V}O_2$, mL/kg of Body Weight per Minute	ETT, min	Resting SBP, mm Hg	Peak $\dot{V}O_2$, mL/kg of Body Weight per Minute	ETT, min
11	Fontan	19.8	128	28.7	7.75	125	30.5	9.28
12	Mild AS, obesity	14.3	110	32.6	8.13	100	44.1	10.37
13	PVCs, obesity	13.5	98	31.6	7.13	100	36.0	9.22
14	PS	18.3	120	25.9	7.18	113	32.5	9.80
15	Myocarditis (resolved)	18.2	127	38.5	11.10	108	39.1	11.10
16	AVR	18.9	128	33.8	8.50	120	48.4	11.40

*SBP indicates systolic blood pressure; $\dot{V}O_2$, oxygen consumption; ETT, exercise treadmill time; Fontan, Fontan procedure for tricuspid atresia; AS, aortic stenosis; PVCs, premature ventricular contractions; PS, pulmonary stenosis; and AVR, aortic valve replacement.

with training and cardiac output equals heart rate multiplied by stroke volume, stroke volume must increase to change cardiac output. An increase in myocardial contractility would explain the increased stroke volume, but this has not been proven.[12,13] Patients with congenital heart disease, even those who have undergone repair for the condition, may not be capable of responding as normal subjects would, although they demonstrate similar physiologic changes. For example, a study[14] of patients who underwent the Fontan procedure for tricuspid atresia showed that those patients in whom the right ventricle was incorporated as part of the repair (right atrium to ventricle to pulmonary artery anastomosis) were not able to increase their stroke volumes during exercise as well as those patients who had direct anastomoses from right atrium to pulmonary artery. The participants in our study improved their exercise times and peak $\dot{V}O_2$ and sustained decreases in their resting systolic blood pressures. A decrease in peripheral resistance (afterload), resulting in a decrease in the work of the left ventricle, is another physiologic change observed in normal subjects that may lead to increased stroke volume.[10,11] As a group, our patients demonstrated lower resting systolic blood pressures after training, indicating a reduction in peripheral resistance. This could have been the result of lower catecholamine levels. Studies in adult patients[15,16] have shown that training lowers the levels of these hormones at rest and during exercise. Peripheral resistance may also decrease because of the development of new capillaries in the trained skeletal muscle, which increases the total cross-sectional area of the vascular bed, a phenomenon previously demonstrated in animal studies.[10] Whatever the mechanism, training may produce physiologic changes that increase maximal cardiac output. This allows more oxygen to be taken up from the lungs for delivery to the exercising muscles. Additionally, the skeletal muscles may undergo changes such as an increase in the number of mitochondriae and the level of metabolic enzymes. Such changes improve the aerobic capacity and endurance of the trained muscle by causing more oxygen to be extracted from the blood.[10] With more oxygen available during exercise, exercise time and peak $\dot{V}O_2$ increase.

Hagberg et al[17] and others[18,19] have demonstrated the antihypertensive effect of exercise. Therefore, in addition to a beneficial effect on cardiac performance, exercise training may lower risk factors such as hypertension that contribute to the development of atherosclerotic disease. The resting heart rates of our patients did not decrease. A reduction in resting heart rate is usually observed in normal subjects after training.[11,12] Perhaps the exercise program was not long enough or intense enough to induce changes in heart rate, or these patients, in association with structural heart disease, had sinus node dysfunction.

The program's success in achieving physiologic changes in patients was limited by the relatively large number of patients who did not complete the protocol. Two patients developed coincidental medical illnesses unrelated to their cardiac conditions or to the CRP exercises (one patient developed testicular torsion and another sprained her ankle while at school), so their absences were unavoidable. The remaining patients who did not complete the program cited many preventing factors, including family problems, an out-of-state visit to a noncustodial parent, transportation problems, and lack of interest. We have made some changes in the program to improve compliance. Its duration has been shortened from 6 to 3 months. We encourage parents to participate in the exercise classes whenever possible (after obtaining appropriate medical clearance). The number of educational sessions has been increased to improve parental participation. Future programs will be held in fall only, rather than year-round. This may prevent conflicts with summer vacation plans and the difficulty in transportation during the winter. Another problem is the cost of maintaining the staff and facilities necessary for the program. We limited the cost by sharing the facilities and staff with an Adult Cardiac Rehabilitation Program, and if at any time fewer than five patients were enrolled, the pediatric exercise sessions were combined with those of the adult cardiac patients.

The authors thank Marilyn Arnold, RN, BSN; Diane Dubois, RN, MSN; Dave Friederich, MS, PE; Mary Lavin, RD; Martha Manley, RN, MSN, and Pam Zook, RN.

References

1. O'Connor GT, Buring JE, Yusuf S, et al. An overview of randomized trials of rehabilitation with exercise after myocardial infarction. *Circulation.* 1989;80:234-244.

2. Matthews RA, Nixon PA, Stephenson RJ, et al. An exercise program for pediatric patients with congenital heart disease. *J Cardiac Rehabil.* 1983;3:467-475.

3. Bradley LM, Galioto FM, Vaccaro P, Hansen DA, Vaccaro J. Effect of intense aerobic training on exercise performance in children after surgical repair of tetralogy of Fallot or complete transposition of the great arteries. *Am J Cardiol.* 1985;56:816-818.

4. Parmley WW. President's page: position report on cardiac rehabilitation (recommendations of the American College of Cardiology). *J Am Coll Cardiol.* 1986;7:451-452.

5. Wasserman K, Hansen JE, Sue DL, Whipp BJ. *Principles of Exercise Testing and Interpretation.* Philadelphia, Pa: Lea & Febiger; 1987:58-71.

6. Goforth D, James F. Exercise training in noncoronary heart

disease. *Cardiovasc Clin*. 1985;15(2):243-253.
7. Linde LM. The psychiatric aspects of congenital heart disease. *Psychiatr Clin North Am*. 1982;5:399-406.
8. Strunk RC, Mrazek DA, Fukuhara JT, Masterson J, Ludwick SK, LaBrecque JF. Cardiovascular fitness in children with asthma correlates with psychologic functioning of the child. *Pediatrics*. 1989;84:460-464.
9. Hartley HL. The role of exercise in the primary and secondary prevention of atherosclerotic coronary artery disease. In: Wenger NK, ed. *Exercise and the Heart*. Philadelphia, Pa: FA Davis Co Publishers; 1985:1-8.
10. Holloszy JO, Coyle EF. Adaptations of skeletal muscle to endurance exercise and their metabolic consequences. *J Appl Physiol Respir Environ Exerc Physiol*. 1984;56:831-838.
11. Blomquist CG, Saltin B. Cardiovascular adaptations to physical training. *Annu Rev Physiol*. 1983;45:169-189.
12. Hammond HK, Froelicher VF. The physiologic sequelae of chronic dynamic exercise. *Med Clin North Am*. 1985;69:21-39.
13. Schaible TF, Scheuer J. Cardiac adaptations to chronic exercise. *Prog Cardiovasc Dis*. 1985;27:297-324.
14. Gewillig MH, Lundstrom VR, Bull C, Wyse RK, Deanfield JE. Exercise responses in patients with congenital heart disease after Fontan repair: patterns and determinants of performance. *J Am Coll Cardiol*. 1990;15:1424-1432.
15. Cooksey JD, Reilly P, Brown S, Bomze H, Cryer PE. Exercise training and plasma catecholamines in patients with ischemic heart disease. *Am J Cardiol*. 1978;42:372-376.
16. Nelson L, Esler MD, Jennings GL, Korner PI. The effect of changing levels of physical activity on blood-pressure and hemodynamics in essential hypertension. *Lancet*. 1986;2:473-476.
17. Hagberg JM, Goldring D, Ehsani AA, et al. Effect of exercise training on the blood pressure and hemodynamic features of hypertensive adolescents. *Am J Cardiol*. 1983;52:763-768.
18. Choquette G, Ferguson RJ. Blood pressure reduction in 'borderline' hypertensives following physical training. *Can Med Assoc J*. 1973;108:699-703.
19. Drimmer AM, Hibbert A, Arnold M. Exercise effect on long term control of mild hypertension. *J Cardiopulmonary Rehabil*. 1989;10:404. Abstract.

In Other AMA Journals

JAMA

Clinical and Laboratory Correlates of *Pneumocystis carinii* Pneumonia in Children Infected With HIV

E. Connor; M. Bagarazzi; G. McSherry; B. Holland;
M. Boland; T. Denny; J. Oleske
(*JAMA*. 1991;265:1693)

CD4 T-Lymphocyte Counts and *Pneumocystis carinii* Pneumonia in Pediatric HIV Infection

A. Kovacs; T. Frederick; J. Church;
A. Eller; M. Oxtoby; L. Mascola
(*JAMA*. 1991;265:1698)

Prevalence of HIV Infection in Childbearing Women in the United States

M. Gwinn; M. Pappaioanou; J. R. George; W. H. Hannon;
S. C. Wasser; M. A. Redus; R. Hoff; G. F. Grady;
A. Willoughby; A. C. Novello; L. P. Petersen;
T. J. Dondero, Jr; J. W. Curran
(*JAMA*. 1991;265:1704)

Trends of HIV Seroconversion Among Young Adults in the US Army, 1985 to 1989

J. G. McNeil; J. F. Brundage; L. I. Gradner; Z. F. Wann;
P. O. Renzullo; R. R. Redfield; D. S. Burke;
R. N. Miller; US Army Retrovirus Research Group
(*JAMA*. 1991;265:1709)

Opinion Leaders vs Audit and Feedback to Implement Practice Guidelines: Delivery After Previous Cesarean Section

J. Lomas; M. Enkin; G. M. Anderson;
W. J. Hannah; E. Vayda; J. Singer
(*JAMA*. 1991;265:2202)

Dietary Calcium and Bone Mineral Status of Children and Adolescents

Gary M. Chan, MD

• **We studied 164 healthy, white children aged 2 to 16 years; there were 88 boys and 76 girls. By the method of single photon absorptiometry, we found that age, height, and weight correlated positively with bone mineral content of the radius bone. In the children's diet, most of those aged 2 to 11 years met the recommended dietary allowance (800 mg daily) for calcium. Children older than 11 years had low dietary calcium intake; only 15% met the recommended dietary allowance for calcium (1200 mg daily). Dietary calcium intake was associated with bone mineral status. Children ingesting more than 1000 mg of calcium daily had higher bone mineral content than those ingesting less. Almost all serum determinations of calcium, phosphate, magnesium, alkaline phosphatase, parathyroid hormone, 25-hydroxyvitamin D, and 1,25-dihydroxyvitamin D were within normal limits and had no correlation with children's bone mineral status.**

(*AJDC.* 1991;145:631-634)

Calcium is the most abundant mineral in the human body. Ninety-nine percent of the body's calcium is found in the bones and teeth. It is an essential nutrient for growth during infancy and childhood.[1] Skeletal growth and development may be the most important concern in nutrition for children. From birth to age 20 years, the bones are in a phase of active growth. Peak bone mass is achieved between ages 12 and 40 years.[2]

There are little data on the role of calcium nutrition in bone status in children during this crucial period. Children need to receive sufficient calcium for building bone mass. The purpose of this study was to investigate the nutritional and biochemical factors that may affect children's bone mineral status.

SUBJECTS AND METHODS

Subjects

All children were recruited from the author's private pediatric clinic and local schools. The subjects were healthy, white, and free of any medications that may affect calcium metabolism. None of the children reported smoking or consuming alcohol. Children aged 2 to 16 years were eligible for the study. All children were within the 10th and 90th percentiles for weight and height, respectively, recommended by the National Center for Health Statistics.[3] This study was approved by our institutional review board. Informed consent was obtained from the children's parents and assent of the older children.

Experimental Design

Each child was seen twice during a 3-month period. At each visit, routine weight and height were recorded. A 2-day dietary history (home diet diary) was taken 3 days prior to the office visit. Each child's history was checked by a dietitian and verified by the parents. Food brands and amounts were recorded. All dietary records were coded and checked by our dietitian, who was blinded to the study's results. These records were then evaluated by a dietary computer program (Nutripractor, San Diego, Calif). All dietary and anthropometric values obtained at each visit were averaged and used in the final analyses.

Blood was drawn once during the study by venipuncture for measurements of serum concentrations of calcium, phosphate, magnesium, alkaline phosphatase, parathyroid hormone, 1,25-dihydroxyvitamin D, and 25-hydroxyvitamin D. All blood samples were drawn in the afternoon between 1 and 4 PM after the bone mineral analysis. The methods for analysis of calcium, phosphate, magnesium, alkaline phosphatase, 1,25 dihydroxyvitamin D, and 25-hydroxyvitamin D have been described previously.[4] Our children's normal range for 1,25-dihydroxyvitamin D was from 34 to 220 pmol/L. The parathyroid hormone assay (Nichols Institute Diagnostic, San Pedro, Calif) uses the goat antisera that recognize primarily the C-terminal of the molecule. Our normal parathyroid hormone range was 6 to 32 pmol/L.

Bone mineral status was determined for all subjects by the method of photon absorptiometry using the Lunar bone mineral analyzer (Lunar Corp, Madison, Wis). The analyzer consists of a scanner module containing a narrow collimated scintillation detector and an iodine 125 radionuclide source. As the scanner moves across the bone to be measured, the scintillation detector counts the attenuated counts, and the absorbance of the photons is proportional to the bone mineral content (BMC) in grams per linear centimeter. The bone width is also measured, as it is proportional to the length of the scan path over the bone. The nondominant radius was measured at the midshaft (distal third) site. The bone was measured once during the study. In adults and infants, this method correlates very highly with the ash weight of the bone,[5] and has been correlated with total body calcium ($r = .85$).[6] In our laboratory, the day-to-day error rate in infants and adults is 2.5%.

Statistical Analysis

All statistical analyses were performed with a commercially available computer program (Statworks, Philadelphia, Pa). Standard t tests and analysis of variance were used for comparison between groups. The correlations between variables were analyzed with regression analysis. Multivariate analyses were performed when two or more independent variables influenced BMC. To compare bone mineral data at different ages, the children's ages were arbitrarily divided into five age categories, and

Accepted for publication January 11, 1991.
From the Department of Pediatrics, University of Utah Medical Center, Salt Lake City.

Reprint requests to Department of Pediatrics, 2A210, University of Utah Medical Center, Salt Lake City, UT 84132 (Dr Chan).

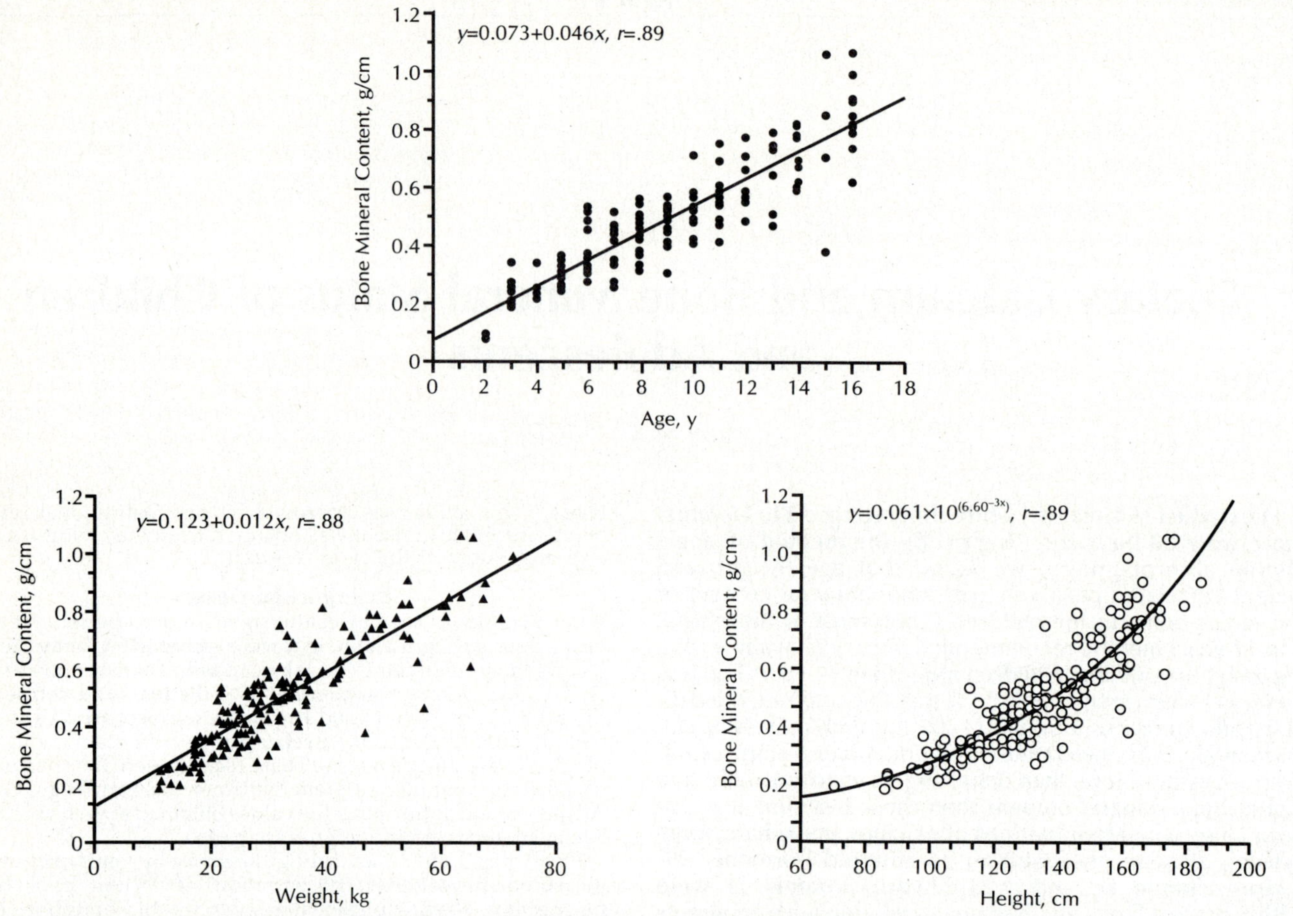

Fig 1.—*Relation of weight, height, and age to bone mineral content in 164 children. Correlation was significant for all three variables.*

Table 1.—Children's Daily Dietary Intakes

	Mean (±SD) Intakes					
Age, y	**Total Energy, kJ**	**Protein, g**	**Calcium, mg**	**Phosphate, mg**	**Sodium, mg**	**Magnesium, mg**
2-5	316.9±0.23	56±21	1126±566	1181±510	2006±786	255±265
6-8	350±75	61±16	1075±368	1206±389	2176±930	213±165
9-11	364.3±0.23	65±21	966±361	1154±371	2294±856	180±63
12-14	445.7±140.7	72±18	1179±485	1307±418	2165±801	208±61
15-16	394.0±168.8	64±28	925±524	1121±496	2054±936	178±80

a *z* score or standard normal variate was determined for each BMC value within each age category. The *z* score is a measure of the deviation from the expected population mean.

RESULTS

Description of Subjects

Eighty-eight boys and 76 girls aged 2 to 16 years completed the study. No drugs, tobacco, or alcohol were reported to be taken by our subjects. The mean age (±SD) of our children was 9.1±3.6 years.

Relation of Age, Weight, Height, and Sex to Bone Mineral Status

Age, weight, and height correlated with bone mineral status ($r = .88$ to $.89$; $P < .01$; Fig 1). The exponential equation improved the fit of the height data over the linear equation from $r = .86$ to $r = .89$. Boys had a higher BMC status than girls, their mean *z* score being 0.106 and the girls' mean *z* score being −0.123 ($P < .001$). After controlling for weight, there were no differences between bone mineral status of boys vs girls as determined by their *z* scores.

Relation of Diet to Bone Mineral Status

Children's dietary intakes are shown in Table 1. There was no difference between the two diet histories, and no association between dietary intakes and ages of the subjects. A majority of children (70%) younger than 11 years were consuming at least the recommended dietary allowance for calcium, 800 mg daily. However, 63% of children older than 11 years were not consuming the recommended dietary allowance for calcium, 1200 mg daily. Girls older than 11 years had a mean daily dietary calcium intake of 750±450 mg; only 15% of the girls and 53% of the boys met the recommended dietary allowance for calcium. The differences in calcium intake between girls and boys older

Table 2.—Children's Mean Serum Values and Ranges*							
Age, y	Total Calcium, mmol/L	Phosphate, mmol/L	Magnesium, mmol/L	Alkaline Phosphate, IU/L	25-OH D, mmol/L	1,25 $(OH)_2D$, pmol/L	PTH, pmol/L
2-5	2.4(2.2-2.7)	1.6(1.2-2.0)	1.1(0.9-1.4)	123(60-220)	82(55-110)	136(61-238)	6(3-9)
6-8	2.3(1.7-2.8)	1.7(0.8-3.6)	1.2(0.9-1.4)	91(33-277)	65(40-102)	117(34-243)	9(3-18)
9-11	2.3(1.6-2.8)	1.7(0.7-2.6)	1.1(0.8-1.2)	100(33-222)	68(32-112)	112(46-294)	7(2-18)
12-14	2.3(1.6-2.7)	1.5(0.9-2.6)	1.1(0.8-1.2)	12(50-191)	62(8-110)	122(44-199)	9(2-18)
15-16	2.3(1.6-2.7)	1.3(0.5-1.8)	1.1(0.8-1.5)	63(21-155)	72(35-138)	122(68-275)	9(2-22)
Normal range	2.2-2.7	1.1-1.7	0.6-1.2	47-112	25-150	34-792	6-32

*25-OH D indicates 25-hydroxyvitamin D; 1,25 $(OH)_2D$, 1,25-dihydroxyvitamin D; and PTH, parathyroid hormone. Values in parentheses represent ranges.

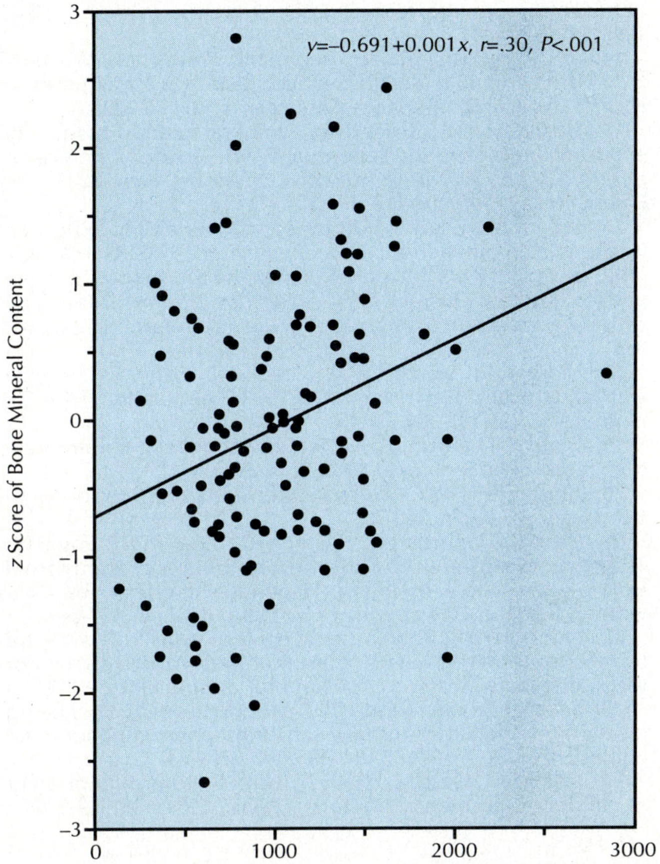

Fig 2.—*z Score of bone mineral content and daily calcium intakes in children. A z score of zero or the average bone mineral content corresponded to a dietary calcium intake of 1000 mg daily.*

than 11 years was not significant ($P<.13$). In children older than 11 years, the *z* score of the girls' BMCs was not lower than that of boys' BMCs. Of all the nutrients analyzed, only dietary calcium, phosphate, and protein intakes were associated with the *z* scores of the bone mineral data. All three variables were highly associated with each other. The multiple correlation coefficient of the *z* score on dietary calcium, phosphate, and protein intakes was .277 ($P=.02$). However, by multivariate analyses, only dietary calcium intake was related to the children's bone mineral status (partial correlation coefficient, .18, $P<.05$) after adjusting for phosphate and protein intakes. By regression analysis, a dietary calcium intake of 1000 mg corresponded to a *z* score of zero or the average BMC (Fig 2).

Children consuming at least 1000 mg of calcium daily had a higher BMC than those consuming less. The *z* score of children ingesting less than 1000 mg of calcium daily was -0.30 ± 1.03 compared with 0.21 ± 0.91 for children ingesting more than 1000 mg of calcium daily ($P=.001$ by *t* test). The difference between these two groups represents 0.51 *z* units or 0.51 SDs from the mean BMC of each group.

Relationship of Biochemical Values to Bone Mineral Status

Serum values of calcium, phosphate, magnesium, alkaline phosphatase, and vitamin D did not correlate with bone mineral status. Almost all (>90%) serum values were within the normal range (Table 2).

COMMENT

In this study, we have demonstrated that children's bone mineral status was associated with age, weight, height, and dietary calcium intake. Other investigators have shown that BMC is associated with age, weight, and height in children aged 4 to 16 years.[7]

Other factors reported to affect skeletal mass are race and genetics. Some studies have shown that young black children have higher skeletal mass than white children by roentgenographic films and other morphological indexes.[8,9] Because all our subjects were white, we could not evaluate the effect of race on children's bone status. Other ethnic populations may differ from our population. Adult studies on osteoporosis have shown a familial resemblance in bone mass.[10,11]

In our study of children aged 2 to 16 years, BMC increases exponentially with age, weight, and height. Bone mass should normally increase as the child grows. From birth to age 20 years, the skeleton is in an active phase of growth. Peak bone mass is determined in these early years.[2] There were no differences in bone mineral status between boys and girls in our study after controlling for weight. Other researchers in Wisconsin and Ohio have reported a lower bone mineral status in girls.[12,13] In adults, the influence of sex hormones may play a bigger part in the difference of bone mass between men and women.[14]

Dietary intakes of calcium, phosphate, vitamin D, protein, and copper are important nutrients in bone mineralization.[1,2,15] In the present study, only dietary calcium intake appears to contribute to bone mineral status in children. The limited sample size may have affected the detection of other nutrients in children's diet contributing to bone mineralization. Dietary histories generally produce higher estimates of group mean intakes than weighed food records.[16] However, calcium, phosphorus, and protein determinations from dietary histories have shown minor daily variations compared with food records.[17] In the present study, children ingesting more than 1000 mg of calcium daily had higher BMC than those ingesting less. The dietary calcium intake of our children younger than 11 years old was better than that of those who were older. Children, especially adolescent girls older than 11 years, had low calcium intakes. This low calcium intake in school-age children has been reported by others.[18,19] Dairy consumption, which is our major source of calcium, has continued to decline in the United States with the substitution of soft drinks. Some studies in children and adults have shown a relation between dietary intakes of milk and calcium and bone mineral status.[20-22] Increased milk consumption in childhood and adolescence may prevent low postmenopausal bone density.[23]

In children, it may be important to achieve optimal bone mass. There is preliminary evidence to suggest that sufficient intake of calcium and phosphate increases the mineral content in children's bones and might decrease the risk of accidental fractures.[24] Supplemental dietary calcium has also been shown to prevent bone loss during lactation in adolescents.[4] Low peak bone mass rather than excessive loss of bone also may be the major contributor to osteoporosis. Our study has shown that the majority of older children's diets are low in calcium intake, and this low calcium intake may affect their bone mineral status.

This study was supported in part by the National Dairy Council, Rosemont, Ill.

References

1. Avioli LV. Calcium and phosphorus. In: Shels ME, Young VR, eds. *Modern Nutrition in Health and Disease*. 7th ed. Philadelphia, Pa: Lea & Febiger; 1988:142-158.
2. Heaney RP, Gallagher JC, Johnston CC, Neer R, Parfitt AM, Whedon GD. Calcium nutrition and bone health in the elderly. *Am J Clin Nutr.* 1982;36(suppl):986-1013.
3. Hamill PVV, Drizd TA, Johnson CL, Reed RB, Roche AF, Moore WM. Physical growth: national center for health statistics percentiles. *Am J Clin Nutr.* 1979;32:607-629.
4. Chan GM, McMurray M, Westover K, Engelbert-Fenton K, Thomas MR. Effects of increased dietary calcium intake upon the calcium and bone mineral status of lactating adolescent and adult women. *Am J Clin Nutr.* 1987;46:319-323.
5. Cameron JR, Mazess RB, Sorensen JA. Precision and accuracy of bone mineral determination by direct photon absorptiometry. *Invest Radiol.* 1968;3:141-150.
6. Manzke E, Chestnut CH III, Wergedal JE, Baylink DJ, Nelp WB. Relationship between local and total bone mass in osteoporosis. *Metabolism.* 1975;24:605-615.
7. Landin L, Nilsson BE. Forearm bone mineral content in children: normative data. *Acta Paediatr Scand.* 1981;70:919-923.
8. Trotter M, Broman GE, Peterson PR. Densities of bones of white and negro skeletons. *J Bone Joint Surg Am.* 1960;42:50-58.
9. Garn SM. The phenomenon of bone formation and bone loss. In: DeLuca HF, Frost HM, Jee WSS, Johnston CC, Parfitt AM, eds. *Osteoporosis: Recent Advances in Pathogenesis and Treatment.* Baltimore, Md: University Park Press; 1980:1-18.
10. Lutz J. Bone mineral, serum calcium, and dietary intakes of mother/daughter pairs. *Am J Clin Nutr.* 1986;44:99-106.
11. Seeman E, Hopper JL, Bach L, et al. Reduced bone mass in daughters of women with osteoporosis. *N Engl J Med.* 1989;320:554-558.
12. Mazess RB, Cameron VR. Growth of bone in school children: comparison of radiographic and photon absorptiometry. *Growth.* 1972;36:77-92.
13. Specker BL, Brazerol W, Tsang RC, Levin R, Searcy J, Steichen J. Bone mineral content in children 1 to 6 years of age: detectable sex differences after 4 years of age. *AJDC.* 1987;141:343-344.
14. *Osteoporosis: Cause, Treatment, Prevention.* Washington, DC: US Public Health Service; 1986. US Department of Health and Human Services publication NIH 86-2226.
15. Chan GM. Calcium and bone mineral status in infants' and children's nutrition. In: Lebenthal E, ed. *Textbook on Gastroenterology and Nutrition in Early Childhood.* New York, NY: Raven Press; 1989:403-413.
16. St Jeor ST, Guthrie HA, Jones MB. Variability in nutrient intake in a 28-day period. *J Am Diet Assoc.* 1983;83:144-146.
17. Mahalko JR, Johnson LK, Gallagher SK, Milne DB. Comparison of dietary histories and seven-day food records in a nutritional assessment of older adults. *Am J Clin Nutr.* 1985;42:542-553.
18. Morgan KJ, Stampley GL, Zabek ME, Fisher DR. Magnesium and calcium dietary intakes of the US population. *J Am Coll Nutr.* 1985;4(2):195-206.
19. Evans MD, Cronin FJ. Diets of school-age children and teenagers. *Fam Econ Rev.* 1986;3:14-21.
20. Amschler DH. Calcium intake: a lifelong proposition. *J Sch Health.* 1985;55:360-363.
21. Yano K, Heilbrun LK, Wasnich RD, Hankin JH, Vogel JM. The relationship between diet and bone mineral content of multiple skeletal sites in elderly Japanese-American men and women living in Hawaii. *Am J Clin Nutr.* 1985;42:877-888.
22. Lindergard B. Bone mineral content measured with photon absorptiometry: a methodological study carried out on normal individuals. *Scand J Urol Nephrol Suppl.* 1981;59:1-37.
23. Sandler RB, Slemenda CW, LaPorte RE, et al. Post menopausal bone density and milk consumption in childhood and adolescence. *Am J Clin Nutr.* 1985;42:270-274.
24. Chan GM, Hess M, Hollis J, Book LS. Bone mineral status in childhood accidental fractures. *AJDC.* 1984;138:569-570.

Chief Resident Training

Developing Leadership Skills for Future Medical Leaders

Robert A. Doughty, MD, PhD; Patricia D. Williams, MD; Charles N. Seashore, PhD

• Most future medical leaders receive little or no formal exposure to management and leadership training activities. Industry invests considerable resources in such training for middle and senior level managers. With the increasing complexity of health care delivery systems and the increased involvement of diverse teams of individuals in the care of patients, it was believed that a training activity designed to enhance participant human interaction skills and teach about group behavior and team management might be valuable to pediatric chief residents. This article describes a 3-day workshop designed to develop such leadership skills. It has been conducted for 3 years with 117 participants. Results of end-of-course and 6-month follow-up evaluations show that participants enjoyed the training experience and believed it was valuable in helping them fulfill their leadership role as chief resident.

(*AJDC.* 1991;145:639-642)

In recent years, medical educators have increasingly discussed the importance of incorporating human relations skills into medical school curricula and residency training programs.[1-6] At least three issues have contributed to this trend. First, the effects of stress on the emotional well-being of medical students and residents are now recognized as having a potential adverse effect on learning and patient care and, furthermore, may contribute to later physician impairment.[3,4,7] Second, health care consumers are demanding that physicians have effective interpersonal skills.[8-11] Finally, although the traditional model of health care has been a pyramid with the physician as decision-maker issuing orders from the top to those below, health care increasingly involves teamwork among a variety of individuals with differing skills and perspectives.[2,11,12]

Thus, facility in negotiating relationships with many diverse individuals in various group settings promotes optimal learning during medical training and good patient care. Traditionally, however, medical schools and residency programs have done little to address this area of expertise.[13]

The field of organization development grew out of theory and research on the application of behavioral science to work groups and other organizations. In many organizations outside of health care, workshops led by trained facilitators are used to teach executives and managers the principles and practice of effective leadership and teamwork.[14] The successful adaptation of this concept to the "work group" of first-year pediatric residents at a residency program has been described elsewhere.[15]

In this article we describe a leadership training program designed to teach pediatric chief residents skills involving human interaction and the management of teams. Chief residents were targeted for several reasons: first, their role typically requires management skills in which they have little or no experience[13]; second, they serve as teachers and role models for other residents and medical students[2,3,11]; and third, many chief residents subsequently hold important leadership positions in medical education—as attending physicians, program directors, and department chiefs and in such roles, they could foster further training in these areas of leadership skills.

DESCRIPTION

The Pediatric Chief Resident Training Program is a structured, 3-day experiential workshop conducted at sites on the East and West coasts. Content and process are based on organization development techniques and human interaction training methods.[16]

Accepted for publication October 1, 1990.

From the Alfred I. duPont Institute, Wilmington, Del, and Jefferson Medical College, Philadelphia, Pa (Drs Doughty and Williams). Dr Seashore is a private consultant.

Reprint requests to Alfred I. duPont Institute, PO Box 269, Wilmington, DE 19899 (Dr Doughty).

Department Editors.—*Hugh D. Allen, MD, Columbus, Ohio; Fredric Burg, MD, Philadelphia, Pa; Harold Levine, MPA, Galveston, Tex; Barbara Starfield, MD, Baltimore, Md; Larrie W. Greenberg, MD, Washington, DC*

Purpose.—*This department is intended to share information concerning educational efforts in the broad field of pediatrics. We welcome studies on the following topics: undergraduate and graduate education in medicine and allied health occupations; continuing education of health professionals; education of patients and families; and health education for the general public, the community, and organizations that contribute to the promotion and improvement of the health of children.*

Editorial Comment.—*We select our brightest and best to be chief residents, but this new role may require more than handing them a beeper. This article describes a training program designed to teach them how to handle the problems that they may encounter in a management and leadership role.*—H.D.A.

Table 1.—Typical Agenda for Pediatric Chief Resident Training Program		
	Time	**Activity**
Day 1		
	8:30-10:30 AM	Introduction and review of agenda; the role of chief resident
	10:30-12:30 PM	Leadership roles and group functioning
	12:30-1:30 PM	Lunch
	1:30-5 PM	Group process exercise: residency program design
	5-5:30 PM	Midcourse evaluation
Day 2		
	8-10 AM	Personal leadership skills and styles
	10-12:30 PM	Dealing with conflict
	12-1:30 PM	Lunch
	1:30-3 PM	Dealing with conflict (continued)
	3-5:30 PM	Effective feedback
	5:30-7 PM	Dinner
	7-8:30 PM	Stress management; managing the boundary between work and home life
Day 3		
	8-12 PM	Working with hospital administration
	12-1 PM	Lunch
	1-3:30 PM	Hollow square simulation
	3:30-4:30 PM	Review of workshop learnings and applications; reentry to work environment; closure
	4:30-5:30 PM	Written evaluation

The program is offered in the spring to any newly appointed pediatric chief resident who has recently assumed or, in most cases, is about to assume the responsibilities of the position. To date, the program has had 117 participants representing 50 different institutions.

The object of the workshop is to train medicine's future leaders in leadership skills involving human interaction and the management of teams. The basic workshop schedule is given in Table 1. Each workshop's design is modified based on written and verbal feedback obtained during and after the program.

Although the content of each workshop varies depending on group interests and concerns and feedback from previous workshops, a typical session begins with an initial exercise in which participants share ideas and concerns about their new role; this promotes the feeling of the workshop as a "safe" place in which experiences and concerns can be revealed and discussed. Participants thus learn early that sharing in the group fosters mutual learning and support because of the commonality of their experiences and the unique perspectives of each individual.

After the opening exercise, operating norms are suggested and agreed to by all participants. In particular, confidentiality is established as a norm, allowing for open participation and discussion of sensitive topics (eg, personal feelings of incompetence or perceived negative aspects of a particular residency program). Basic theories of group development and experiential learning are introduced with suggestions on how to maximize the educational benefits of the workshop. Next, a session on the dynamics of group function initiates an exploration of general forces that operate in the development and functioning of working groups and applications of this learning to various work groups encountered in the residency setting. The large group is divided into smaller groups that each design a program addressing an area of residency training that participants have identified as problematic, such as resident orientation or resident evaluation systems. Observers note the interpersonal dynamics involved as the groups work to complete their tasks. The exercise affords an opportunity to learn more about the roles individuals take in groups and how those roles can contribute to or detract from effective teamwork as well as provide concrete ideas for implementing changes in each individual's residency program.

The first day concludes with a midcourse evaluation. This session serves two purposes. First, it provides the facilitators with valuable information on whether they need to modify the agenda. Second, it models a technique for giving and receiving feedback that is developed in more depth the next day.

The second morning begins with distribution of individual results on the Myers-Briggs Type Indicator, a self-administered personality instrument that measures an individual's preferences for various styles of perception and decision-making.[17] This is followed by exercises designed to enhance understanding of different style preferences and their effect on professional life.

The theme of appreciating and learning from differences is developed further through administration of the Thomas-Kilmann Conflict Mode Instrument,[18] a self-administered and scored instrument that indicates an individual's preferred styles of managing conflict. Discussion of results is typically followed by a role-playing exercise. The large group is divided into three smaller groups. Each group reconstructs the scenario of a typical conflict situation between a resident and another individual, such as an attending, nurse, parent, or patient. After the three groups reconvene, one group describes its scenario. Residents from the other groups volunteer to act out the scenario. In the ensuing role plays, participants practice a variety of responses to difficult interactions and learn about the advantages and disadvantages of their usual styles.

The afternoon of the second day typically focuses on how to give and receive feedback regarding work performance. Although residents are eager to receive this information from colleagues and supervisors, they are generally unfamiliar with the behaviors required to obtain and give feedback that is nonjudgmental, effective in contributing to improvement in professional skills, and relationship enhancing.

After dinner, the evening is usually devoted to discussion, often in small interest groups, of the stresses of residency training. Typical areas of interest have included the boundary between work and home life, and the different stressors experienced by various groups, such as married and unmarried residents and men and women. The intimacy of the smaller groups followed by sharing in the larger group combine to make this segment uniquely rich in increasing understanding and support for each other.

The morning of the third day is spent on how to work effectively with hospital administration. Small groups again devise role plays addressing significant issues they wish to present to a hospital administrator. An actual hospital administrator serves as a facilitator in enacting role plays with the residents. Discussion focuses on effective negotiating styles, responses to authority, and socialization differences between physicians and administrators that affect their interactions.

On the last afternoon, chief residents participate in the Hollow Square Exercise.[19] In this "game," small groups are assigned roles and given a complex task to complete in competition with each other within a limited time. Observers note the effective and ineffective individual and group behaviors demonstrated as participants attempt to "win" by completing the task. A variety of constructive and detrimental behaviors emerge under these conditions. This provides an excellent opportunity for the group members to examine their personal contributions to effective and ineffective leadership and group behavior.

The final part of the afternoon is given to a review of the workshop experience, further discussion of "back-home" applications, and preparation for reentry into the residency environment. Attention is given to ensure that the experiences of the workshop are integrated into the residents' further professional development rather than left behind as 3 days isolated from the rest of their training. One technique, for example, is to have participants complete individual time capsules in which they list key learnings from the workshop. The learnings are then reinforced the following September when the facilitators mail back the time capsules. The workshop ends with the completion of written evaluation forms.

Table 2.—Mean Ratings of Chief Resident Training Program*

	1988 n=23	1989 n=47	1990 n=47
Introduction to conference: Johari window	7.4	6.6	8.2
Ice-breaker communication process	8.2	7.2	9.1
Task-process leadership instrument and discussion	7.4	7.3	8.7
Group process	8.4	8.0	8.1
Giving and receiving feedback	7.7	8.1	7.9
Hollow square exercise	7.6	7.2	9.3
Myers-Briggs type indicator	9.3	9.3	9.8
Conflict management skills	8.9	8.1	8.9
Conflict resolution process	9.2	7.6	9.1
Stress and stress management	7.0	6.0	N/A
Personal feedback process	9.2	7.3	N/A
Working with hospital administrators	8.3	7.1	9.1
Time capsule	8.4	7.1	9.3
Chief resident/program director role analysis	7.4	N/A	N/A
Mean ratings of all aspects	8.2	7.6	8.9

*Specific aspects of the course were rated on a 10-point scale (1, poor/useless; 10, excellent/useful); n indicates number of chief resident participants; and N/A, not offered in this workshop.

RESULTS

It is difficult to measure objectively the success of this workshop in training participants in leadership skills that improve their effectiveness as chief residents. First, it is difficult to quantify noncognitive learning and its contribution to performance of the chief resident's duties. Second, the duties vary from program to program and include such complex skills as giving feedback to other residents and managing conflicts involving house staff. It might be possible to compare data from residency programs that have sent a chief resident to the workshop with those that have not participated in the workshop or even to assign chief residents to experimental and control groups; but the multiple ways in which programs differ would preclude any significant conclusions about the effectiveness of the workshop alone as an intervention.

Nevertheless, despite the lack of quantifiable data from carefully controlled studies, there are several indicators that the course is valuable to participating chief residents and their residency programs. First, enrollment doubled from the first to the second year of the program. Also, more than two thirds of residency programs where a chief resident attends the workshop send a chief resident in subsequent years. This suggests that workshop attendance is seen as worth the investment in time and financial resources.

Ratings by the chief residents themselves on the end-of-workshop evaluation forms are presented in Table 2. They were asked to rate specific aspects of the course on a scale from 1 to 10, with 1 representing "poor/useless" and 10 representing "excellent/useful." The mean ratings given were 8.2 for the 1988 course, 7.6 for the 1989 course, and 8.9 for the 1990 course, for an overall weighted average rating of 8.2. When asked: "Do you believe this conference would be useful to other chief residents?" 97% of the respondents said yes, and most added comments such as: "Absolutely," "Every chief resident should attend," and "More than useful, it should be mandatory."

Twenty chief resident participants among the 67 attendees in 1988 and 1989 responded to a 6-month follow-up questionnaire asking them to comment on their experience as chief resident, those aspects of the course that have proved most useful, and any areas they think should be included or expanded on. Behaviors that individual respondents perceived to have been significantly modified as a result of the course included the following: insight into differences in personality types; improved ability to manage conflict; greater awareness of their personal strengths and weaknesses in leadership situations; greater ability to appreciate the perspectives of others; and improved ability to give negative feedback.

Finally, the questionnaire asked: "Any other comments about the course, questions, suggestions, etc." Ten of the 14 people who responded to that request specifically praised the course again, with comments such as the following: "I...feel that it was an invaluable experience and one which I will never forget," and "I have encouraged our future chief residents to go wholeheartedly."

COMMENT

The 1980s saw the development of a number of new initiatives to address the training of physicians in interpersonal skills—from courses on interviewing skills,[20-22] to Balint-type discussion groups,[23] to psychosocial support groups for medical students and resident physicians,[1,24] to resident retreats.[15] The Chief Resident Leadership Training Program addresses such training by applying theories and techniques from the field of organization development and management training to a group of individuals who are or who shortly will be in leadership roles in medicine and who will likely be in leadership roles in the future.

While other initiatives are designed to enhance physicians' interpersonal skills by broadening physicians' perspectives on the role of medicine in society,[25] minimizing the effects of stress during medical training,[15,25] improving communication with patients,[20-22] or teaching skills specific to middle managers,[26] this Chief Resident Training Program addresses another important aspect of current medical training and practice: awareness of personal leadership traits and the critical importance of teamwork—with fellow physicians, hospital administrators, other health care workers, and patients. Group interaction skills can be expected to have value in a myriad of other groups of which physicians are members. These groups include departments, committees, specialty groups, and others. Indeed, never before have physicians found themselves practicing in relation to so many different individuals and organizations, with all the attendant opportunities for collaboration and conflict.[2,11-13,27]

Judging from the evaluation forms and comments of workshop participants, this program successfully addresses the leadership training of residents making the transition to chief resident. Optimally, one would like a well-designed study demonstrating a positive effect on residency programs due to the improved efficiency, effectiveness, and job satisfaction of Chief Residents who have attended the workshop. However, such a study is difficult, perhaps impossible, to design. Yet there is no question that, subjectively, participants benefit from the course.

The importance of the leader in setting group norms and modeling behaviors has been well documented outside the field of medicine.[14,28,29] Presumably, similar principles apply to medical education: the benefits of having well-trained leaders in the role of pediatric chief resident are expected to "trickle down" to residents and medical students and affect their medical education process. Yet it is important that this course be placed in the context of overall organizational change.[3,11,30] It is hoped, therefore, that similar training programs can be developed for residents in other specialties, program directors, department chiefs, and others in significant leadership roles in medicine.

As medical education enters the next decade, a number of new strategies for training the physicians of the future are likely to unfold, of which the Pediatric Chief Resident Training Program is one. Training in the skills of human interaction, effective leadership, and teamwork may have a positive effect on the actual process of medical education and on ultimate satisfaction with the effectiveness of clinical practice as well.

References

1. Kahn G, Cohen B, Jason H. Teaching interpersonal skills in family practice: results of a national survey. *J Fam Pract.* 1979;8:309-316.
2. Subcommittee on Evaluation of Humanistic Qualities in the Internist. American Board of Internal Medicine evaluation of humanistic qualities in the internist. *Ann Intern Med.* 1983;99:720-724.
3. Resident Services Committee, Association of Program Directors in Internal Medicine. Stress and impairment during residency training: strategies for reduction, identification, and management. *Ann Intern Med.* 1988;109:154-161.
4. Lemkau JP, Purdy RR, Rafferty JP, Rudisill JR. Correlates of burnout among family practice residents. *J Med Educ.* 1988;63:682-691.
5. Colford JM Jr, McPhee SJ. The raveled sleeve of care: managing the stresses of residency training. *JAMA.* 1989;261:889-893.
6. Hoekelman RA. Stress experienced during pediatric residency training: its causes, consequences, recognition, and solutions. *AJDC.* 1989;143:177-180.
7. McCue JD. The distress of internship: causes and prevention. *N Engl J Med.* 1985;312:449-452.
8. Matthews DA, Sledge WH, Lieberman PB. Evaluation of intern performance by medical inpatients. *Am J Med.* 1987;83:938-944.
9. Falvo D, Tippy P. Communicating information to patients: patient satisfaction and adherence as associated with resident skill. *J Fam Pract.* 1988;26:643-647.
10. Nelson AR. Humanism and the art of medicine. *JAMA.* 1989;262:1228-1230.
11. Tosteson DC. New pathways in general medical education. *N Engl J Med.* 1990;322:234-238.
12. Stein LI, Watts DT, Howell T. The doctor-nurse game revisited. *N Engl J Med.* 1990;322:546-549.
13. Colenda CC III. The psychiatric chief resident as information manager. *J Med Educ.* 1986;61:666-673.
14. Dyer WG. *Team Building: Issues and Alternatives.* Reading, Mass: Addison-Wesley; 1987.
15. Doughty RA, Krantz J. Teaching fundamentals in group and interpersonal relations: an intervention designed to enhance resident learning and productivity and the quality of work life. *AJDC.* 1985;139:1206-1210.
16. Porter L, Mohr B, eds. *Reading Book for Human Relations Training.* Arlington, Va: National Training Laboratory Institute; 1982.
17. Myers IB, McCaulley MH. *Manual: A Guide to the Development and Use of the Myers-Briggs Type Indicator.* Palo Alto, Calif: Consulting Psychologist Press; 1985.
18. Thomas KW, Kilmann RH. *Thomas-Kilmann Conflict Mode Instrument.* Tuxedo, NY: Xicom Inc; 1974.
19. Shedlin A, Schmidt, WH. Hollow square: a communications experiment. In: Pfeiffer JW, Jones JE, eds. *A Handbook of Structured Experiences for Human Relations Training.* San Diego, Calif: University Associates; 1974;2:32-35.
20. Bertakis KD. The communication of information from physician to patient: a method for increasing patient retention and satisfaction. *J Fam Prac.* 1977;5:217-222.
21. Monahan DJ, Grover PL, Kavey RE, Greenwald JL, Jacobsen EC, Weinberger HL. Evaluation of a communication skills course for second-year medical students. *J Med Educ.* 1988;63:372-378.
22. Mason JL, Barkley SE, Kappelman MM, Carter DE, Beachy WV. Evaluation of a self-instructional method for improving doctor-patient communication. *J Med Educ.* 1988;63:629-635.
23. Pomeroy DP. Balint groups and difficult physician-patient relationships. *J Fam Pract.* 1989;29:16-17.
24. Siegel B, Donnelly JC. Enriching personal and professional development: the experience of a support group for interns. *J Med Educ.* 1978;53:908-914.
25. Blurton RR, Mazzaferri EL. Assessment of interpersonal skills and humanistic qualities in medical residents. *J Med Educ.* 1985;60:648-650.
26. Whitman N. A management skills workshop for chief residents. *J Med Educ.* 1988;63:442-446.
27. Relman AS. The new medical-industrial complex. *N Engl J Med.* 1980;303:963-970.
28. Peters TJ, Waterman RH Jr. *In Search of Excellence.* New York, NY: Harper & Row Publishers Inc; 1982.
29. Bradford DL, Cohen AR. *Managing for Excellence.* New York, NY: John Wiley & Sons Inc; 1984.
30. Giardino AP, Giardino ER. Resident stress. *AJDC.* 1989;143:1129-1130.

Percentile Curves for Various Hematologic Measurements at Birth in Arab Preterm Babies of Different Gestational Ages

Khalid N. Haque, FRCP, DCH, Hassan M. Bahakim, MD

• Percentile curves were calculated for hemoglobin; hematocrit; total red and white blood cell counts; mean corpuscular volume; mean corpuscular hemoglobin; mean corpuscular hemoglobin concentration; and platelet, neutrophil, band cell, lymphocyte, monocyte, basophil, and eosinophil counts in preterm babies of 24 through 36 weeks' gestation. The curves were derived from mainly Saudi Arabian preterm babies who were born in Riyadh, which is just above sea level. Babies born to mothers with hematologic problems or babies who themselves had any evidence of hematologic disorder, blood loss, or disorders that affect hematologic values, eg, asphyxia, were excluded from the reference population. Six hundred two newborns were included in the study; however, after exclusions, the final reference population was 550. A minimum of 50 babies were studied for each gestational age except for gestations of 24 and 25 weeks. For these two gestations, 27 and 21 babies were studied, respectively. The percentile curves should be useful as a guide to the normal range of these variables in babies, particularly those of Arab origin.

(*AJDC*. 1991;145:645-649)

Although information concerning the normal values for various hematologic variables is abundant,[1-5] to our knowledge, very few studies have related these values to gestational age in premature babies.[5] This age group is of interest because values for most hematological variables undergo changes with gestational age. Moreover, extrapolation of normal limits available for children and infants may result in marked underestimation or overestimation.[6]

With increasing survival of smaller and smaller babies of shorter and shorter gestational age,[7,8] it has become important to establish normal hematologic values for these tiny babies. We report herein various hematologic variables in babies with gestational ages of 24 through 36 weeks.

Accepted for publication September 4, 1990.

From the Department of Pediatrics, College of Medicine, Riyadh, Saudi Arabia. Dr Haque is now with Chase Farm Hospital, Enfield, England.

Reprint requests to Department of Paediatrics, Chase Farm Hospital, The Ridgeway, Enfield EN2 8JL, England (Dr Haque).

PATIENTS AND METHODS

The study was conducted over a 6-year period from 1983 to 1989. During this period all babies born between 24 and 36 weeks' gestation were admitted to the Neonatal Intensive Care Unit (NICU) at King Khalid University Hospital, Riyadh, Saudi Arabia.

Gestational age was assessed by a combination of maternal dates, antenatal ultrasound examination, and postnatal gestational assessment done within 24 hours after birth using the Ballard[9] scoring system. Where there was a difference of more than 2 weeks between maternal dates and gestational assessment, the latter value was used. Babies were enrolled into the study if they were admitted to NICU with a gestational age of 24 through 36 weeks and if they and their mothers had no evidence of hematologic disorder, eg, antepartum hemorrhage, thrombocytopenia, or bleeding disorder. Babies who had conditions that could affect the hematologic[6] variables, eg, asphyxia, were also excluded from the study.

Every baby enrolled in the study had a 1-mL venous blood sample taken into an ethylenediaminetetraacetic acid tube for analysis of hematologic variables. The analysis was done on an automated blood cell counter (Coulter Counter S plus IV, Coulter Corp, Hialeah, Fla). Blood samples were taken between 4 and 6 hours after birth and differential cell count was done manually. No blood sample was drawn from either an umbilical vein or artery catheter.

During the period of study (October 1983 to October 1989) a total of 2050 babies were admitted to the NICU. Of those, 602 were eligible for enrollment into the study according to the criteria described above. Fifty-two babies were excluded later after developing disorders that would have affected their hematologic variables; a total of 550 babies were studied. All values thus obtained were analyzed on a personal computer (IBM, North Harbour, Portsmouth, England) using software from Statistical Analysis System (SAS Institute, Cary, NC). Scattergrams and percentile lines were also drawn using this program. To smooth out the curves a Harvard Graphics software program (Harvard Graphics Software Publishing Corp, Bracknell, England) also was used.

RESULTS

To make optimal use of our results we developed percentile grids for the following hematologic variables: hemoglobin and hematocrit; red blood cell count; white blood cell count; and platelet, neutrophil, band cell, lymphocyte, eosinophil, basophil, and monocyte count. These are presented in Figs 1 through 11. Although other percentile lines were also derived, for clarity of presentation only the 5th, 50th, and 95th percentiles are shown in the Figures. The absolute values for mean corpuscular

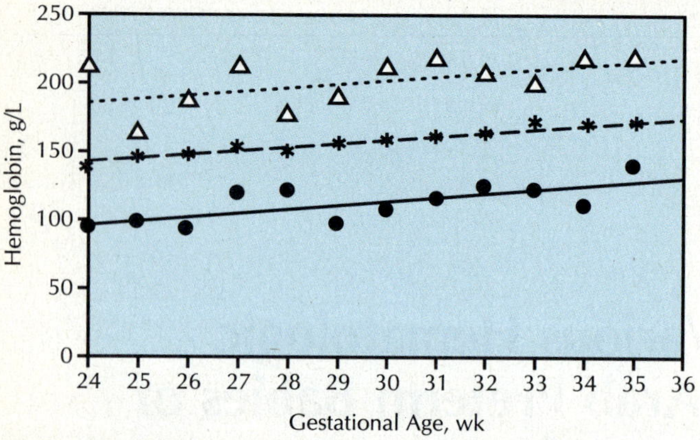

Fig 1.—*Hemoglobin percentiles in preterm babies. Solid line represents 5th percentile; dashed line, 50th percentile; and dotted line, 95th percentile.*

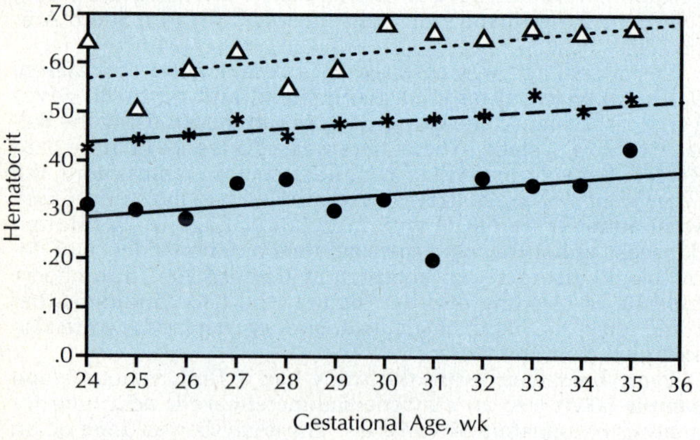

Fig 2.—*Hematocrit percentiles in preterm babies. Solid line represents 5th percentile; dashed line, 50th percentile; and dotted line, 95th percentile.*

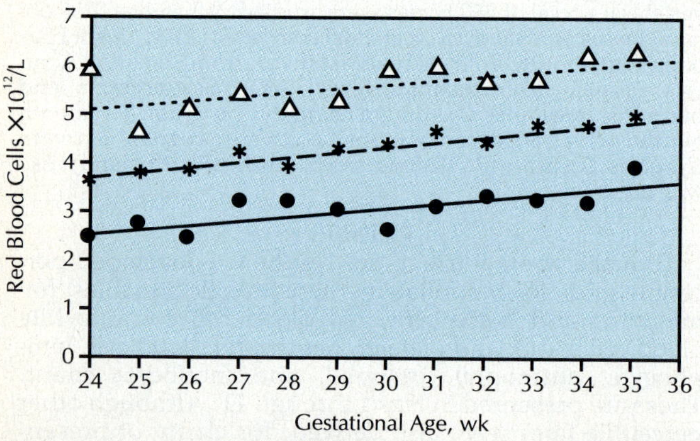

Fig 3.— *Red blood cell percentiles in preterm babies. Solid line represents 5th percentile; dashed line, 50th percentile, and dotted line, 95th percentile.*

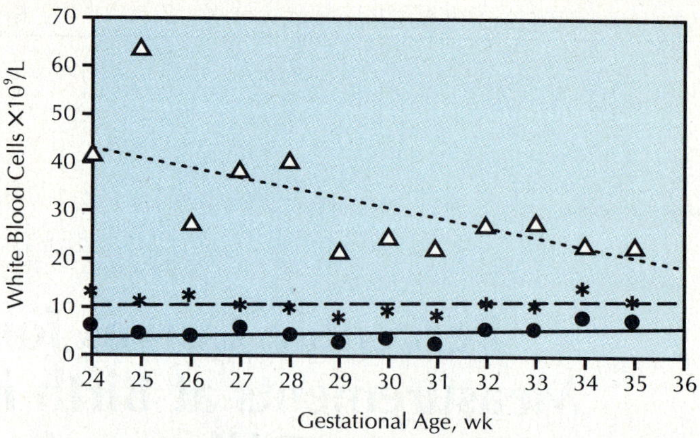

Fig 4.—*White blood cell percentiles in preterm babies. Solid line represents 5th percentile; dashed line, 50th percentile; and dotted line, 95th percentile.*

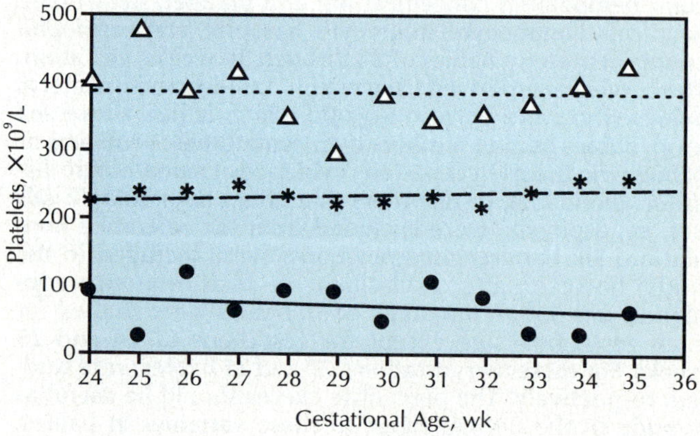

Fig 5.—*Platelet percentiles in preterm babies. Solid line represents 5th percentile; dashed line, 50th percentile; and dotted line, 95th percentile.*

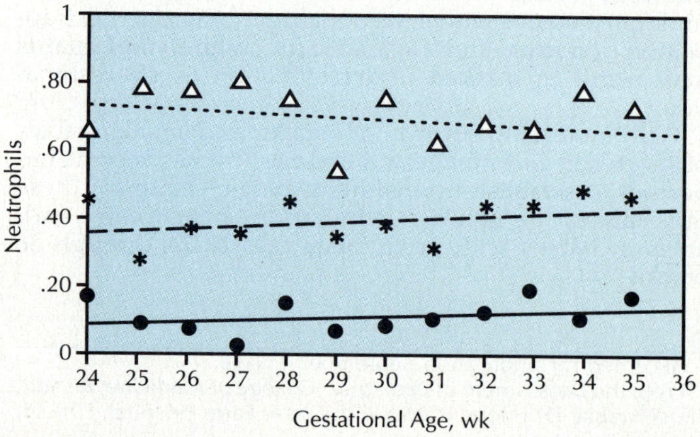

Fig 6.—*Neutrophil percentiles in preterm babies. Solid line represents 5th percentile; dashed line, 50th percentile; and dotted line, 95th percentile.*

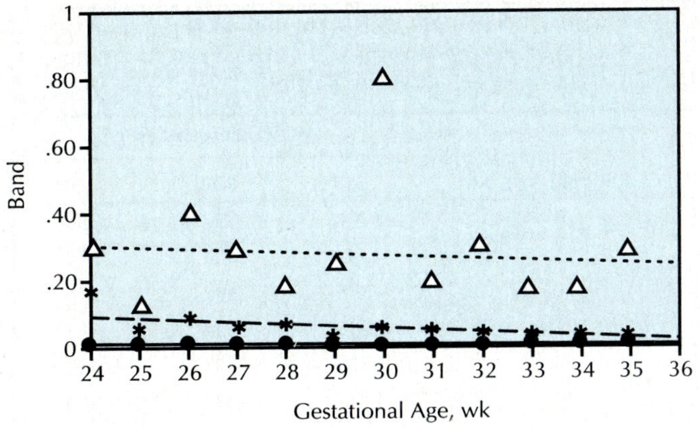

Fig 7.—*Band cell percentiles in preterm babies. Solid line represents 5th percentile; dashed line, 50th percentile; and dotted line, 95th percentile.*

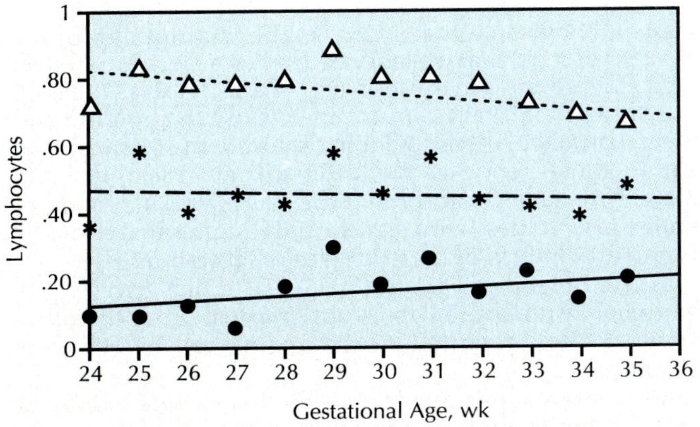

Fig 8.—*Lymphocyte percentiles in preterm babies. Solid line represents 5th percentile; dashed line, 50th percentile; and dotted line, 95th percentile.*

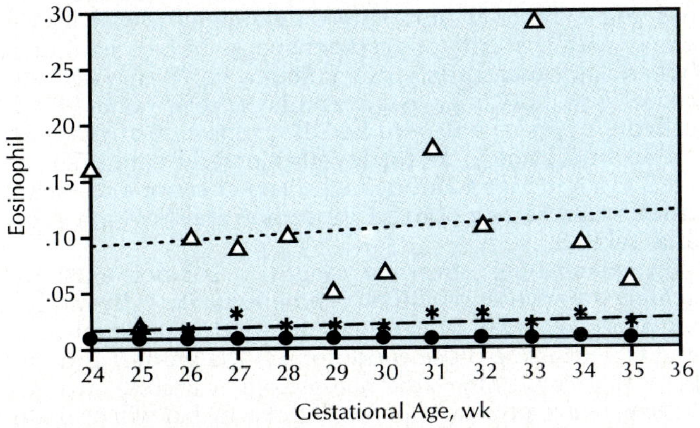

Fig 9.—*Eosinophil percentiles in preterm babies. Solid line represents 5th percentile; dashed line, 50th percentile; and dotted line, 95th percentile.*

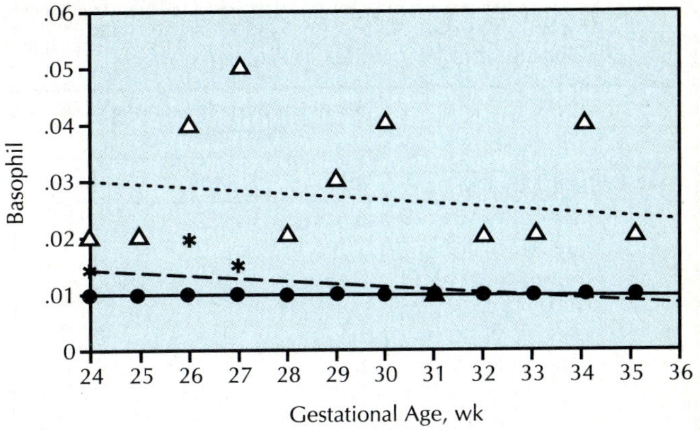

Fig 10.—*Basophil percentiles in preterm babies. Solid line represents 5th percentile; dashed line, 50th percentile; and dotted line, 95th percentile.*

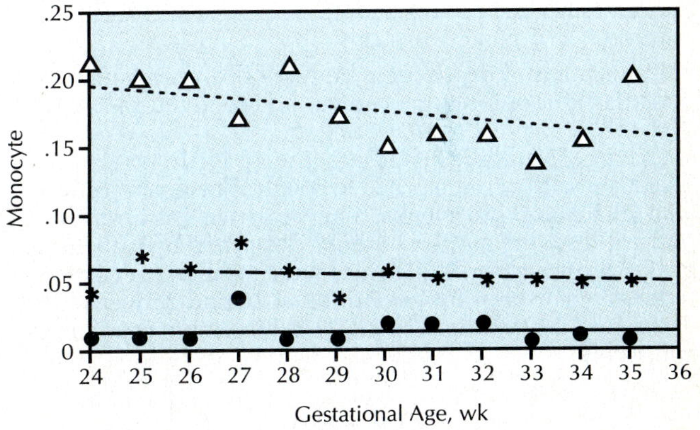

Fig 11.—*Monocyte percentiles in preterm babies. Solid line represents 5th percentile; dashed line, 50th percentile; and dotted line, 95th percentile.*

Table 1.—Absolute Values for Mean Corpuscular Volume Percentile in Preterm Babies

	Mean Corpuscular Volume Percentiles, fL		
Gestational Age, wk	**5th**	**50th**	**95th**
24	81	115.6	128.4
25	102.9	115.5	132.5
26	100.5	114.1	130
27	97.37	110.9	124.5
28	99.9	111.3	128.2
29	94.9	111.3	127
30	87.3	110.9	126.5
31	97	111.3	124
32	97.8	111.2	126.4
33	98.2	109.3	119.8
34	98.3	110.2	124.2
35	95.7	109.8	123.1
36	96.23	109.2	123.9

Table 2.—Absolute Values for Mean Corpuscular Hemoglobin Percentiles in Preterm Babies

Gestational Age, wk	Mean Corpuscular Hemoglobin Percentiles, pg		
	5th	50th	95th
24	26.6	38.5	43.7
25	33.6	38.5	42.2
26	31.12	37.6	42.5
27	31.1	37.6	42.5
28	33.15	37.7	43.62
29	33	37.2	41.2
30	30.7	36.9	41.1
31	32.15	36.1	41.6
32	32.1	37.6	42.7
33	31.5	36.6	39.84
34	31.4	36.8	40
35	33	36.3	41.7
36	32.08	36.3	41.29

Table 3.—Absolute Values for Mean Corpuscular Hemoglobin Concentration (MCHC) Percentiles in Preterm Babies

Gestational Age, wk	MCHC Percentiles, g/L		
	5th	50th	95th
24	306	337	354
25	324	331	346
26	315	331	350
27	313	332	370
28	321	333	352
29	315	332	358
30	318	333	349
31	312	331	348
32	320	337	362
33	312	331	350
34	311	333	348
35	316	334	355
36	321	332	351.6

volume, mean corpuscular hemoglobin, and mean corpuscular hemoglobin concentration are given in Tables 1 through 3.

Of the 550 babies studied, mean birth weight was 1.9800 kg with a range of 480 to 3600 g. The gestational age was 24 through 36 weeks. The birth weight and length percentiles were similar to those described by Lubchenco et al.[10] A minimum of 50 babies were studied for each gestational age except for gestations of 24 and 25 weeks. For these two gestations, 27 and 21 babies were studied, respectively.

COMMENT

For establishing criteria of normality, two approaches are generally used. One commonly used and published in reporting growth standards uses the study by random sample of the total population.[11,12] The disadvantage of this method is that it does not include values of abnormal individuals. Inclusion of such individuals can be misleading if the curves are to be interpreted as representing normal standards.[1] The second method, and the one we chose to use, is to derive the normal data by excluding all subjects with evidence of common abnormalities (influencing variables) that might be expected to bias the data. Although this method has the disadvantage of excluding criteria that may seem arbitrary, it has certain advantages for the derivation of normative hematologic data.[1]

It is difficult to compare our values with earlier published data for the following two reasons: (1) we are not aware of any published data on hematologic values in preterm babies of Arab origin, and (2) previously published data from the Western literature[1,2,12-16] do not relate the values to gestational age. However, from a brief review of the literature,[4,5,13,15,17] it appears that the hematologic variables do not differ significantly between races, and these percentile charts may be applicable to non-Arab races as well. Monroe et al[5] have suggested that gestational age and birth weight do not affect neutrophil counts, but no data are available for other hematologic variables.

Comparison of our values with those published earlier[1,2,5,12-16] indicates that hemoglobin and hematocrit values are significantly higher than those reported by Dallman and Siimes,[1] and contrary to the findings of Monroe et al,[5] we found that gestational age has a significant effect on these two and other values (Figs 1 and 2; Tables 1 and 2).

Although our values of mean corpuscular volume and mean corpuscular hemoglobin (Tables 1 and 2) were similar to those reported by Dallman[13] and Saarinen and Siimes[2] in babies nearer full term, ie, 36 weeks' gestation, both these values were significantly higher in extremely premature babies of 24 to 25 weeks' gestation.

The red blood cell count (Fig 3) was much lower in the extremely premature babies but gradually rose to values similar to those reported in full-term infants[13] by 34 weeks' gestation.

Most interest has focused on the total white blood cell and the neutrophil counts because of their value in the diagnosis of sepsis. A wide range has been described (0.09 to 30 × 10^9/L) with a mean of 18.1 × 10^9/L by Dallman[13] and others.[15] The reason for this wide variation is that maternal conditions, eg, diabetes and hypertension, as well as the baby's condition, eg, asphyxia, respiratory distress syndrome, and hypoglycemia, influence the white blood cell count. In most studies, except for that by Monroe et al,[16] these variables have not been taken into account. We took them into account with our exclusion criteria, and our values (Fig 4; Table 2) show that the range narrows considerably with maturity of gestational age. In fact, of all the hematologic measurements studied by us, the greatest effect of gestational age was seen on the total white blood cell count. We have also studied the proportion of different cells contributing to the total white blood cell count. These are shown in Figs 6 through 11. Platelet count and mean corpuscular hemoglobin concentration are shown in Fig 5 and Table 3.

In establishing reference ranges, a balance must be achieved between sensitivity and specificity.[18] By studying a large number of babies of different gestational ages and by excluding those conditions in the mother and the baby that could affect the hematologic variables, we believe we have produced percentile charts that will provide a guide with 90% confidence of the normal ranges of these variables in healthy Arab babies within these gestational ages.

We thank Erum Shiekh, MD, research assistant, for her valuable help in collecting the data.

References

1. Dallman PR, Siimes MA. Percentile curves for hemoglobin and red cell volume in infancy and childhood. *J Pediatr.* 1979;94:26-31.
2. Saarinen UM, Siimes MA. Developmental changes in red blood cell counts and indices of infants after exclusion of iron deficiency by laboratory criteria and continuous iron supplementation. *J Pediatr.* 1978;92:412-416.
3. Burman D. Hemoglobin levels in normal infants aged 3 to 24 months and the effect of iron. *Arch Dis Child.* 1972;47:261-270.
4. Dallman PR, Barr GD, Allen CM, Shinefield HR. Hemoglobin concentration in white, black, and oriental children: is there a need for separate criteria in screening for anaemia? *Am J Clin Nutr.* 1978;31:337-380.
5. Monroe BL, Weinberg AG, Rosenfeld CR, Browne R. The neonatal blood count in health and disease, I: reference values for neutrophilic cells. *J Pediatr.* 1979;95:89-98.
6. Siimes MA, Saarinen UM. What critical value of transferrin saturation identifies iron deficiency in non-anaemic breast-fed infants? *J Pediatr.* 1977;91:1027.
7. Haque KN. Outcome of low and very low birth weight infants born at King Khalid University Hospital, Riyadh, Saudi Arabia: a case for regionalization. *Ann Saudi Med.* 1986;6:247-251.
8. Haque KN, Bashir OB. Four year perinatal mortality and morbidity at King Khalid University Hospital, Riyadh. *Ann Saudi Med.* 1988;8:190-193.
9. Ballard JL. A simplified assessment of gestational age. *Pediatr Res.* 1977;11:374.
10. Lubchenco LO, Hansman C, Boyd E. Intrauterine growth in length and head circumference as estimated from live births at gestational ages from 26 to 42 weeks. *Pediatrics.* 1966;37:403-408.
11. National Center for Health Statistics. *National Center for Health Statistics Growth Charts: Monthly Vital Statistics Report.* 1976;25(suppl):1120. Document No. HRA 76.
12. National Center for Health Statistics. *National Center for Health Statistics Growth Charts Vital and Health Statistics Series 11.* Rockville, Md: Health Resources Administration, US Government Printing Office; 1976.
13. Dallman PR. In: Rudolf A, ed. *Pediatrics.* 16th ed. East Norwalk, Conn: Appleton & Lange; 1977:1111.
14. Lundstrom U, Siimes MA, Dallman PR. At what age does iron supplementation become necessary in low birth weight infants. *J Pediatr.* 1977;91:872-883.
15. Oski FA, Naiman JL. *Hematological Problems in the Newborn.* 2nd ed. Philadelphia, Pa: WB Saunders Co; 1972:13.
16. Monroe BL, Browne R, Weinberg CR, Rosenfeld CR. Normal leukocyte (WBC) values in neonates. *Pediatr Res.* 1976;10:428.
17. Behrman RE, Vaughan VC. *Nelson Textbook of Paediatrics.* 13th ed. Philadelphia, Pa: WB Saunders Co; 1987;15.1-15.3.
18. Desforges JF, Hollenberg NK, Ingelfinger FJ, et al. What does a healthy control control? *N Engl J Med.* 1977;296:1165-1166.

In Other AMA Journals

ARCHIVES OF NEUROLOGY

Freeze the Ocean

Robert J. Joynt, MD, PhD
(*Arch Neurol.* 1991;48:471)

Caring for the Underserved: Health Insurance Coverage Is Not Enough

Matthew Menken, MD
(*Arch Neurol.* 1991;48:472-475)

Access to Health Care: One Neurologist's Perspective

Michael P. Earnest, MD
(*Arch Neurol.* 1991;48:476-479)

Access to Neurological Care for Minorities

Edgar J. Kenton, MD
(*Arch Neurol.* 1991;48:480-483)

ARCHIVES OF PATHOLOGY & LABORATORY MEDICINE

Passive Inhalation of Free-Base Cocaine ('Crack') Smoke by Infants

Haresh G. Mirchandani, MD; Ila H. Mirchandani, MD;
Fredric Hellman, MD; Rosanne English-Rider;
Samuel Rosen, PhD; Elizabeth Kleinerman, MD
(*Arch Pathol Lab Med.* 1991;115:494-498)

Meconium for Drug Testing

Edward C. Maynard, MD; Louis P. Amoruso, PhD; William Oh, MD

• Samples of meconium from 28 neonates born to women suspected of drug abuse were tested for drugs of abuse (ie, cocaine, morphine, codeine, and marijuana). In each case, testing of urine from the mother, the newborn, or both had been ordered by the attending physician because of suspected maternal drug abuse. Seventeen (61%) of 28 meconium samples tested positive; 28 (60%) of 47 urine samples were positive. Meconium test results were concordant with the results of maternal or newborn urine testing in 24 (86%) of the 28 cases. In three cases, meconium was positive for cocaine when newborn urine was negative; in one case, meconium was negative when maternal urine was positive for cocaine. Compared with the combination of maternal and newborn urine testing, meconium testing had an 82% positive predictive value (14/17) and a 91% negative predictive value (10/11). Collection of meconium is simpler and more reliable than collection of urine, and testing of meconium was easily incorporated into routine procedures at a busy commercial laboratory. Meconium is a useful sample for drug detection in newborns.

(*AJDC.* 1991;145:650-652)

Maternal drug abuse carries considerable risk for injury to the mother and her fetus or neonate.[1,2] The detection and treatment of maternal drug abuse is an area of growing concern to those involved in perinatal care; laboratory tests to detect drugs of abuse are essential to this effort. Maternal self-report is often unreliable for detection of drug abuse[3,4]; even inquiry and testing based on broad indications of possible maternal drug use leave many cases undetected.[5] In addition, social service agencies often request confirmation of perinatal drug abuse by testing of urine from the newborn. However, urine collection in neonates may be difficult or delayed, impairing the ability to screen effectively for fetal drug exposure.[6]

Ostrea and colleagues[7] recently reported on use of meconium as a sample for drug detection in neonates born to drug-dependent mothers. Cocaine, morphine, or cannabinoid was detected in meconium from all 20 neonates tested and in urine from only seven of 19 neonates tested. We report our experience using a modification of the Ostrea et al[8] technique.

Accepted for publication November 5, 1990.

From the Department of Pediatrics, University of Massachusetts Medical School, Worcester (Dr Maynard); Clinical Science Laboratory Inc, Mansfield, Mass (Dr Amoruso); and Department of Pediatrics, Brown University, Providence, RI (Dr Oh).

Read before the New England Perinatal Society, Manchester, Vt, February 24, 1990.

Reprints not available.

SUBJECTS AND METHODS

Meconium was collected during the first 2 days of life from 28 neonates. The meconium was scooped into a specimen cup from the surface of an absorbent diaper to minimize contamination with urine. In each case, the mother was suspected of active drug use by history or symptoms, or had had pregnancy complications associated with drug use (eg, premature rupture of membranes, premature labor, abruptio placentae, intrauterine growth retardation, or poor prenatal care). In each case, testing of urine for drugs had been ordered by the attending physician.

Meconium was refrigerated after collection and tested in a commercial laboratory within 24 hours (Clinical Science Laboratory Inc, Mansfield, Mass). The meconium sample (1 to 2 g) was diluted in 5 mL of normal saline, mixed by vortex for 20 seconds, and allowed to stand refrigerated for a minimum of 15 minutes. After centrifugation at 1200 to 1400*g* for 10 minutes, the supernatant was tested by radioimmunoassay using a commercial kit designed for drug detection in urine (Abuscreen, Roche Diagnostic Systems, Montclair, NJ). Preliminary studies showed no difference in drug detection when meconium was diluted with the acidified buffer supplied with the radioimmunoassay kit or with normal saline (pH 6.3 to 6.7).

Each meconium sample was tested for cocaine and benzoyl ecgonine (a cocaine metabolite), morphine, codeine, and tetrahydrocannabinol. The cutoff for a positive test result was 300 ng/mL for cocaine–benzoyl ecgonine, morphine, and codeine, as recommended by the National Institute on Drug Abuse, Bethesda, Md[9]; in our laboratory, these cutoff values gave no false results when known negative or positive samples of urine or meconium were tested. A positive cutoff of 100 ng/mL was used for tetrahydrocannabinol, because in our laboratory lower cutoff values were found to yield false-positive results in known negative samples of urine and meconium. When the radioactivity in a sample was less than 10% above or below the number of counts per minute in the positive control, the sample was called "borderline negative" or "borderline positive." Two cases with borderline positive results are treated as positive in the data analysis, and one borderline negative result is treated as negative.

Results of the meconium testing were reported only to the principal investigator and not recorded in the patient chart or used for any clinical purpose. The study was approved by the Research and Human Subjects Committee at Women and Infants Hospital, Providence, RI.

Maternal or newborn urine samples were assayed as routine samples in the same commercial laboratory by enzyme immunoassay, thin-layer chromatography, and gas chromatography–mass spectrography.

RESULTS

Drugs of abuse were detected in 17 (61%) of 28 meconium samples and 28 (60%) of 47 urine samples (15 of 21 maternal, 13 of 26 newborn; Table 1). In 21 cases, paired samples of meconium and maternal urine were tested; results were concordant in 19 cases (90%). In 26 cases, paired

Table 1.—Results of Drug Testing*

Patient No.	Meconium	Newborn Urine	Maternal Urine
1	Cocaine	Cocaine	Cocaine
2	Cocaine	Cocaine	Cocaine
3	Cocaine	Cocaine	Cocaine
4	Cocaine	Cocaine	Cocaine
5	Cocaine	Cocaine	Cocaine
6	Cocaine	Cocaine	Cocaine
7	Cocaine	Cocaine	Cocaine
8	Cocaine	Cocaine	Cocaine
9	Cocaine	Cocaine	Cocaine
10	Cocaine	Cocaine	Cocaine
11	Cocaine	Cocaine	Cocaine
12	Cocaine	Cocaine	Cocaine
13	Cocaine, opiates	Cocaine	Cocaine, opiates
14	Cocaine	Negative	Negative
15	Cocaine†	Negative	. . .
16	Cocaine†	Negative	. . .
17	THC	. . .	THC
18	Negative‡	. . .	Cocaine
19	Negative	Negative	Negative
20	Negative	Negative	Negative
21	Negative	Negative	Negative
22	Negative	Negative	Negative
23	Negative	Negative	Negative
24	Negative	Negative	. . .
25	Negative	Negative	. . .
26	Negative	Negative	. . .
27	Negative	Negative	. . .
28	Negative	Negative	. . .

*THC indicates tetrahydrocannabinol. Cocaine includes cocaine metabolites; opiates, morphine and codeine.
†Borderline positive (<10% above positive control value).
‡Borderline negative (<10% below positive control value).

samples of meconium and newborn urine were tested; results were concordant in 22 cases (85%).

Meconium test results were concordant with the combination of maternal and newborn urine testing in 24 (86%) of 28 cases (Table 2). Meconium testing detected the same drugs found in maternal or newborn urine in 14 of 15 cases (sensitivity, 93%; 95% confidence interval [CI], 80% to 100%). Meconium testing was negative in 10 of 13 cases where urine testing was negative (specificity, 77%; CI, 65% to 89%). Meconium testing predicted a positive urine test in 14 of 17 cases (positive predictive value, 82%; CI, 73% to 91%) and predicted a negative urine test in 10 of 11 cases (negative predictive value, 91%; CI, 82% to 100%).

In five cases, part of the meconium sample was frozen at −20°C for 1 month, then retested. Results were identical with the initial testing in every case.

COMMENT

The data presented herein suggest that testing meconium from the newborn compares favorably with testing of maternal or newborn urine as a means of detecting perinatal drug abuse. Certainly, the ideal way to detect maternal drug abuse is by repeated questioning and testing of the mother during and after pregnancy. For practical reasons, however, detection of maternal drug abuse often relies on maternal and newborn urine testing at the time of delivery. While urine testing is not a "gold standard"

Table 2.—Drug Detection in Meconium vs Maternal or Newborn Urine

	Maternal/Newborn Urine	
	Positive*	Negative†
Meconium		
Positive	14	3
Negative	1	10

*One or both positive.
†Both negative, or one negative and one not done.

for identification of perinatal drug abuse, it is appropriate to compare meconium testing with the results of concurrent urine testing when assessing the reliability of this method for drug detection.

Compared with the combination of maternal and newborn urine testing, meconium testing was 93% sensitive, with an 82% positive predictive value. This supports the conclusion of Ostrea et al[7] that testing of meconium is an adequately sensitive method of screening for maternal drug abuse near the time of delivery. Note as well, that the single false-negative meconium result in our series was "borderline negative," or within 10% of the positive control value. In the Ostrea et al series, though, all of the mothers were known to be active drug users, and every newborn had at least one positive meconium sample, so no conclusion about the specificity of meconium testing could be drawn. In our series, meconium testing had a specificity of 77% and negative predictive value of 91% compared with urine testing.

The low specificity of meconium testing in our series reflects three cases in which meconium was positive for cocaine but urine testing was negative. These three cases may represent examples of maternal cocaine use more than 48 hours before the time of delivery. Cocaine is rapidly metabolized and excreted by the kidney and is usually detectable in urine for only 1 to 2 days after use.[10] Urine testing will, therefore, reflect maternal cocaine use only if the most recent use occurred less than 2 days before delivery. Meconium, however, may serve as a repository of drug metabolites excreted in bile and retained in the fetal gut during a period of days to weeks before delivery[7]; further research is needed to evaluate this hypothesis.

An alternative possibility is that the three cases of positive meconium and negative urine represent false-positive results. Any positive screening test must be interpreted in the context of all the information available for a given patient; caution must be exercised before using a screening test to label a patient in a way that might be harmful.[11]

The technique of meconium testing described herein was easily incorporated into routine drug testing procedures in a busy commercial laboratory. The high degree of concordance between the meconium and urine test results supports the use of suspension in saline rather than acid extraction of the meconium sample, at least for detection of cocaine and opiates.

Since the period of this study, meconium testing by the method described herein has been made available as a routine clinical test at another hospital (The Medical Center–Memorial, Worcester, Mass), using the same commercial laboratory. During the first several months, results have supported the findings of this study. In 25 cases, maternal or newborn urine samples have been tested in addition to meconium. Meconium and urine samples were negative in 15 cases and positive for the same drugs in four cases. In one case, meconium and maternal urine tested positive for cocaine, while newborn urine was negative. In five cases, the quantity of newborn urine submitted was insufficient for drug testing; meconium was positive for cocaine in one of these newborns.

Such examples of insufficient urine collection emphasize that a major advantage of meconium is the ease of its collection, which may result in detection of cases of maternal drug abuse that are missed when collection of urine is delayed or unsuccessful. The fact that freezing the sample for up to 1 month did not alter meconium test results also suggests that meconium can be collected and stored for later testing in batch. Meconium testing may thus provide a practical means for assessing the prevalence of perinatal drug abuse in large populations. One such study has been reported, in which both maternal urine and newborn meconium were collected for anonymous drug testing.[12] During a 17-day period, maternal urine was collected during labor at 258 (61%) of 426 deliveries; meconium was collected from 367 (86%) of the newborns, demonstrating significantly greater success in collection of meconium ($P<.001$ by χ^2). The prevalence of perinatal cocaine abuse determined by meconium testing (1.6%) was lower than that estimated by maternal urine testing (3.9%),[13] but not significantly different.

Collection of meconium is simpler and more reliable than collection of urine; testing of meconium for drugs of abuse seems to be both sensitive and specific compared with maternal or newborn urine testing; and meconium testing is easily incorporated into routine procedures at a busy commercial laboratory. Meconium is a useful sample for detection of perinatal drug abuse and may be particularly useful for prevalence surveys in large populations.

References

1. Farrar HC, Kearns GL. Cocaine: clinical pharmacology and toxicology. *J Pediatr.* 1989;115:665-675.
2. Chasnoff IJ. Drug use in pregnancy: parameters of risk. *Pediatr Clin North Am.* 1988;35:1403-1412.
3. Hingson R, Zuckerman B, Amaro H, et al. Maternal marijuana use and neonatal outcome: uncertainty posed by self-reports. *Am J Public Health.* 1986;76:667-669.
4. Zuckerman B, Amaro H, Cabral H. Validity of self-reporting of marijuana and cocaine use among pregnant adolescents. *J Pediatr.* 1989;115:812-815.
5. Maynard EC. Testing for maternal drug abuse: how much is enough? *Pediatrics.* In press.
6. Halstead AC, Godolphin W, Lockitch G, Segal S. Timing of specimen collection is crucial in urine screening of drug dependent mothers and newborns. *Clin Biochem.* 1988;21:59-61.
7. Ostrea EM, Brady MJ, Parks PM, Asencio DC, Naluz A. Drug screening of meconium in infants of drug-dependent mothers: an alternative to urine testing. *J Pediatr.* 1989;115:474-477.
8. Ostrea EM, Parks PM, Brady MJ. Rapid isolation and detection of drugs in meconium in infants of drug-dependent mothers. *Clin Chem.* 1988;34:2372-2373.
9. *Federal Register.* April 11, 1988;53:11970-11989.
10. Barnett G, Hawks R, Resnick R. Cocaine pharmacokinetics in humans. *J Ethnopharmacology.* 1981;3:353-366.
11. American Academy of Pediatrics, Committee on Substance Abuse. Drug-exposed infants. *Pediatrics.* 1990;86:639-642.
12. Griffin JF, Hollinshead WH, Scott HD, Maynard EC, Burke ME. Issues in measuring the prevalence of cocaine use during the perinatal period. Abstract. Presented before the American Public Health Association annual meeting; September 30, 1990; New York, NY.
13. Hollinshead WH, Griffin JF, Scott HD, Burke ME, Coustand DR, Vest TA. Statewide prevalence of illicit drug use by pregnant women—Rhode Island. *MMWR.* 1990;39:225-227.

In Other AMA Journals

ARCHIVES OF OTOLARYNGOLOGY—HEAD & NECK SURGERY

Access to Health Care in the United States

Byron J. Bailey, MD
(*Arch Otolaryngol Head Neck Surg.* 1991;117:481-483)

Indigent Patient Care—Then and Now

Loring W. Pratt, MD
(*Arch Otolaryngol Head Neck Surg.* 1991;117:484-485)

Indigent Care—Now

Neil O. Ward, MD
(*Arch Otolaryngol Head Neck Surg.* 1991;117:486-487)

Access to Care—The Problem of the Uninsured and Underinsured: The View From Washington

Jerome C. Goldstein, MD
(*Arch Otolaryngol Head Neck Surg.* 1991;117:490-492)

Guidelines for Safe Transportation of Children in Wheelchairs

Kathleen M. DiGaudio, RN, MSN, PNP, Michael E. Msall, MD

• Advocacy efforts by health care professionals have prompted state legislative changes mandating the use of car seats and seat belts by children. These initiatives have greatly improved the level of safety in transportation of nonhandicapped children. Despite these positive changes, the transportation needs of nonambulatory children have not been addressed. In addition, implementation of Public Law 99-457 will result in larger numbers of young children with motor impairments requiring transportation to preschool early intervention programs. This study sought to describe how safely children in wheelchairs are transported. Observations of subjects were made as they were transported by their families or agencies at a residential summer camp, a preschool program for children with developmental disabilities, and a school for children with cerebral palsy. A safety score system was developed based on laboratory studies conducted on wheelchair restraint systems. This observation tool described the position of the wheelchair in the vehicle, the occupant restraint system, and the wheelchair restraint system. These structured observations revealed inadequate safety measures. Comparisons of safety scores of subjects transported by families with those transported by agencies were not found to have statistically significant differences. The findings of this study demonstrate a gap between minimal safety standards in wheelchair transportation and actual observed practices. In an effort to promote safe transportation practices of children regardless of their developmental differences, we present guidelines for health care providers for monitoring safe wheelchair practices in family, school, and community settings.

***(AJDC.* 1991;145:653-655)**

Epidemiological data have demonstrated a reduction in the reported incidence of injuries in New Mexico,[1] California,[2] Washington,[3] Michigan,[4] and Tennessee[5] following passage of state child restraint laws. All 50 states had implemented mandatory child restraint laws by 1986. The percentage of restraint use by children tripled between 1974 (20%) and 1984 (60%). It is estimated that 26% of the fatalities that would have occurred in 1984 in children aged 0 to 4 years were prevented.[6]

In 1977, at the University of Michigan Highway Safety Research Institute, Benson and Schneider[7] evaluated the effectiveness of wheelchair restraint devices. This research demonstrated that wheelchairs and restraint systems could be designed to provide effective impact protection for children with disabilities when utilizing the basic safety concepts listed in Table 1. The goal of this study was to provide data that would assess the adherence to these basic safety concepts and to initiate guidelines for the safe transportation of children in wheelchairs.

SUBJECTS AND METHODS

Sample

The target population consisted of 63 nonambulatory subjects between the ages of 2 and 21 years. All subjects were transported in wheelchairs to and from agencies in western New York. Administrators at three sites serving developmentally disabled persons granted permission for data collection with the assurance of anonymity.

Setting

Data were collected at three sites in western New York. Site 1 was a United Cerebral Palsy Association day treatment program. Site 2 was a center for multiply handicapped children aged 2 to 5 years utilizing Association for the Severely Handicapped principles.[8] Site 3 was a summer camp for children with disabilities.

Data Collection

An observation checklist for categorizing and recording specific aspects of the method of transporting the subject in a wheelchair was developed (Table 2).[7] Reliability of the instrument was established by two trained observers in the summer of 1987 at the summer camp. Sidewalk observations of 12 subjects were made as the children boarded or departed the vehicle. Both observers were in 100% agreement on data collected on the 12 subjects. The observer did not interact with the subjects, nor was her purpose known to the subjects or bus personnel. Each safety variable was assigned a point value so a combined "safety score" could be assigned. The presence of minimal essential safety factors equaled a score of 10. The scores ranged from 0 (no safety measures observed) to 10 (essential safety factors observed).

Informal discussions with parents of handicapped subjects and agency personnel provided valuable information on transportation-related injuries, methods of reporting such incidents, and the difficulties encountered by families of handicapped subjects.

Accepted for publication January 24, 1991.

From the School of Nursing (Ms DiGaudio), and the Division of Developmental Disabilities and Rehabilitation, Department of Pediatrics, School of Medicine and Biomedical Science (Dr Msall), State University of New York at Buffalo.

Presented in part as poster exhibits at the 38th Annual American Academy of Cerebral Palsy and Developmental Medicine, Toronto, October 26-29, 1988, and the Annual Meeting of Society of Developmental Pediatrics, Williamsburg, Va, November 18, 1988.

Reprint requests to Children's Hospital of Buffalo, Robert Warner Rehabilitation Center, 936 Delaware Ave, Buffalo, NY 14209 (Dr Msall).

Table 1.—Safety Principles for Wheelchair Restraints*
1. Position of chair: forward or rear facing
2. Occupant restraint system: chest and lap belt system that attaches to side of vehicle
3. Wheelchair restraint system: tie down straps on all four wheels of chair that attach to wheelchair frame and anchor in floor of vehicle

*Modified from Benson and Schneider.[7]

Table 2.—Observation Checklist	Score	
Category (Points)	2	0
Position of chair (2)	Backward Front facing	Side facing
Restraint belts (4)	Lap belt/buckle Chest or shoulder strap	Velcro None
Wheel restraints (4)	Tie-down strap Front Rear	Locking bar Front Rear

Table 3.—Safety Scores by Transporters*	Score		
	<2	4	6
Agency (n=50)	76	22	2
Parent (n=13)	92.3	7.7	0

*Values are percentages. Maximum score observed was 6; mean was 1.10.

Table 4.—Safety Principles	
Principle	No. (%)
1. Position of wheelchair	
Forward facing	11 (17.5)
Rear facing	0 (0)
2. Child restraint system	
Shoulder belts	0 (0)
Buckle lap belts	11 (17.5)
3. Wheelchair restraints	
Four tie-down straps	3 (4.8)

Statistical Analysis

Descriptive data analysis was performed by measurements of central tendency. Safety scores of the three agencies were analyzed by analysis of variance (ANOVA) using the SPSS-X computer program.[9] The safety of methods of transportation by different agencies was compared using the χ^2 statistic.

RESULTS

Data in Table 3 reveal that the sample of subjects in wheelchairs was not transported safely. The range of safety scores was 0 to 6, with a mean of 1.10. Of the 50 subjects transported by agencies, a safety score of less than 2 was assigned to 38 subjects (76%), a score of 4 to 11 subjects (22%), and a score of 6 to one subject (2%). Thirteen subjects were transported by families, with a safety score of less than 2 in 12 subjects (92%) and a score of 4 in one subject (7.7%).

Table 4 reveals the breakdown of scores by safety principle. The recommended position of forward facing was observed in 11 (17%) of the 63 subjects. None of the subjects observed were transported in a rear-facing position. Similarly, the recommended restraint systems on the wheelchairs were utilized by 11 subjects (17%). Wheelchair restraint systems were safe on only three wheelchairs (4.8%). These alarming statistics confirm that subjects in wheelchairs are not transported safely.

Data were compared to determine if a difference in the level of safety existed among agencies. The mean safety scores of site 1 (1.26), site 2 (1.81), and site 3 (2.0) were analyzed by one-way ANOVA. No significant differences existed ($F=1.139$, $P>.05$).

Cross-tabulation was used to compare the safety scores of subjects transported by families as opposed to agencies. Safety scores were dichotomized into two groups. Group 1 consisted of scores below 3, and group 2 included scores of 3 or more. In group 1, agencies transported 38 subjects and families transported 12 subjects. In group 2, agencies transported 12 subjects and a family transported one subject. Overall, 50 subjects (79.4%) had scores below 3, while 13 (20.6%) had scores of 3 or more.

Discussion with families and agency personnel revealed an absence of documented transportation-related injuries. In addition, no systematic standard reporting mechanism existed if such an event occurred. Last, parents were not aware of the variety of specialized car seats for the disabled or whether their nonambulatory child would be safely restrained by standard seat belts.

COMMENT

Our results demonstrate that subjects with developmental disabilities in wheelchairs are not transported safely. Our results are similar to those of Bull and colleagues,[10] who observed misuse of car seats in 75% of their observations of children without disabilities. Though much of our safety scoring system seems to be commonsensical, ongoing reinforcement of these safety principles required. Safety education should extend beyond parents to educational and developmental professionals serving persons with disabilities.

Car seat laws may have gaps leading to inconsistent protection for children. Legally acceptable exemptions pose significant risks in safe transportation of nondisabled children. For example, in Missouri the legislation applies only to cars registered in the state.[11] Similarly, North Carolina restricts coverage to drivers licensed in that state. In Wyoming, 27% of the children killed in accidents were transported in pickup trucks, which are exempt from legislation.[11]

Our results suggest that exempting children with disabilities from safe transportation guidelines places them at risk for accidents. In addition, children with developmental disabilities in wheelchairs often lack the balance skills or protective responses necessary to avoid injuries during routine swerving, let alone collisions. However, the lack of a standard reporting mechanism for transportation-related injuries of children with disabilities does not allow ongoing collection of data to estimate this risk better. We agree with recent prevention and policy analysis that recommends coding the cause of injury for all hospital discharge or emergency department events to have data for preliminary risk estimates.[12]

Policy Guidelines

In an effort to address the safety needs of all children regardless of motor disabilities, we suggest the following guidelines.

Health Care Professionals as Advocates.—Physicians, nurses, and therapists in schools, agencies serving the disabled, and medical centers have a role in advocating safer transportation practices for children. The initial car seat legislation in Tennessee was the result of advocacy efforts by Robert S. Sanders, MD, a pediatrician.[13] Child advocates can assist handicapped children and their families by increasing awareness of safe transportation practices as well as the means of instituting the needed public awareness.

Health Care Professional–School Collaboration.—Several mechanisms are available to health care professionals to promote optimal safety in transportation of developmentally disabled children in wheelchairs. Physicians, parents, and schools must explicitly specify transportation goals in a child's individual educational plan.[14] School nursing and therapy goals must include an assessment of safety of transportation for children in wheelchairs. School boards should be made aware of medicolegal liabilities that can ensue if injuries result from unsafe transportation practices. Contracts for bus companies can be contingent on provision of safe transportation. Similar medicolegal liabilities exist for bus companies providing services and can be used to promote change.

Uniform Reporting Standards.—Standard incident reports need to be developed for recording transportation-related injuries by agencies and schools. This provides a means of monitoring trends in the incidence of injuries in a standardized fashion. Such standardization would also facilitate data collection for needed ongoing research in this area.

Family Supports.—Decreasing families' burdens in transporting their handicapped children must be emphasized. Wisbeach and Holt[15] had previously described problems that families encounter during routine use of wheelchairs, including folding, lifting, and transferring the chair without the child. Families need to be informed of safety principles in wheelchair transportation when equipment is provided. Financial resources for families must be identified that will aid them in obtaining the safest wheelchairs, the best restraint systems, or both.

Formal Policy Statement by Relevant Professional Organizations.—In the past, policy statements by health care professional organizations such as the American Academy of Pediatrics have greatly influenced public policy in the areas of school bus safety, car seats, and specific services for developmentally disabled children.[16-20] These statements should be expanded to include children in wheelchairs transported in personal and agency vehicles. Such a statement can precipitate the awareness of and the support for critically needed policy changes.

Summary

Both Public Law 94-142 and Public Law 99-457 require greater community and educational services for children with disabilities.[21,22] The recently passed Americans With Disabilities Act of 1989 (Public Law 101-366) also emphasizes greater access to and participation of individuals of all ages with disabilities in the full fabric of community life.[23] A key role for pediatric health care professionals is to stress basic safety principles for children in wheelchairs and to assist families in ensuring safety and alternative mobility. By advocating basic safety practices in transportation, additional disabilities can be prevented and increased participation of the disabled in community and educational settings can occur. This will further expand the partnership among pediatric health care professionals, families, and schools.

This study was supported in part by a grant from the Developmental Disabilities Prevention Program of Western New York (Ms DiGaudio), and by a grant from the New York State Office of Mental Retardation and Developmental Disabilities (Dr Msall).

We thank the United Cerebral Palsy Association, Cheektowaga, NY, Cradle Beach Camp, Angola, NY, and Center for the Handicapped, Cheektowaga, NY, for permission to collect data; Joan Edwards for her support in addressing this issue publicly; the Thesis Committee at the State University of New York at Buffalo School of Nursing for their professional guidance; and Maryann Kihl for her preparation of the manuscript.

References

1. Sewell CM, Hull HF, Fenner J, Graff H, Pine J. Child restraint law effects on motor vehicle accident fatalities and injuries: the New Mexico experience. *Pediatrics.* 1986;786:1079-1084.

2. Guerin D, Mackinnon DP. An assessment of the California child passenger restraint requirement. *Am J Public Health.* 1985;75:142-144.

3. Scherz RG. Restraint systems for the prevention of injury to children in automobile accidents. *Am J Public Health.* 1976;66:451-455.

4. Margolis LH, Wagenaar AC, Liu W. The effects of a mandatory child restraint law on injuries requiring hospitalization. *AJDC.* 1988;142:1099-1103.

5. Decker MD, Dewey MJ, Hutcheson RH, Schaffner W. The use and efficacy of child restraint devices. *JAMA.* 1984;252:2571-2575.

6. *An Evaluation of Child Passenger Safety: The Effectiveness and Benefits of Safety Seats Summary.* Washington, DC: National Highway Traffic Safety Administration; 1986. US Dept of Transportation technical report HS 806 889.

7. Benson J, Schneider L. Improving the crashworthiness of restraints for handicapped children. In: *Society of Automobile Engineers Technical Paper 840528.* Warrendale, Pa: Society of Automobile Engineers; 1984:389-404.

8. Baker D. Severely handicapped: toward an inclusive definition. *Am Assoc Educ Severe/Profound Handicapped Rev.* 1979;4:52-65.

9. Nie NH, Hull CH, Jenkins JG, Steinbrenner K, Bent DH. *SPSS: Statistical Package for the Social Sciences.* New York, NY: McGraw-Hill International Book Co; 1975:181-248.

10. Bull MJ, Bruner Stroup K, Gerhart S. Misuse of car safety seats. *Pediatrics.* 1988;81:98-101.

11. Teret SP, Jones AS, Williams AF, Wells JK. Child restraint laws: an analysis of gaps in coverage. *Am J Public Health.* 1986;76:31-34.

12. Agran P, Castillo D, Winn D. Childhood motor vehicle occupant injuries. *AJDC.* 1990;144:653-662.

13. Christopherson ER. Accident prevention in primary care. *Pediatr Clin North Am.* 1986;33:925-933.

14. American Academy of Pediatrics, Committee on Children With Disabilities. Pediatrician's role in development and implementation of an individual education plan. *Pediatrics.* 1987;80:750-751.

15. Wisbeach A, Holt KS. Children in wheelchairs. *BMJ.* 1980;281:199-201.

16. American Academy of Pediatrics. *Policy Statement on School Bus Safety.* Elk Grove Village, Ill: American Academy of Pediatrics; 1985.

17. American Academy of Pediatrics, Committee on Accident and Poison Prevention. Automatic passenger protection systems. *Pediatrics.* 1984;74:146-147.

18. American Academy of Pediatrics, Committee on Research and Committee on Accident and Poison Prevention. Reducing the toll of injuries in childhood requires support for a focused research effort. *Pediatrics.* 1983;72:736-737.

19. American Academy of Pediatrics, Committee on Children With Disabilities. School-aged children with motor disabilities. *Pediatrics.* 1985;76:648-649.

20. American Academy of Pediatrics, Committee on Children With Disabilities. Provision of related services for children with chronic disabilities. *Pediatrics.* 1985;75:796-797.

21. Education for All Handicapped Children Act of 1975, Pub L No. 94-142, 20 USC § 1401 et seq.

22. Education of the Handicapped Act Amendments of 1986, Pub L No. 99-457, 20 USC § 1419 et seq.

23. Americans With Disabilities Act of 1989, Pub L No. 101-336, 42 USC § 1210 et seq.

Osteochondrodysplasia in Fryns Syndrome

Matthew M. Kershisnik, MD; Catherine M. Craven, MD; A. L. Jung, MD; John C. Carey, MD; A. S. Knisely, MD

• Various skeletal abnormalities have been identified in roentgenograms of persons with Fryns syndrome, but to our knowledge, no histopathologic description of bone or cartilage has been published. We describe disordered endochondral and intramembranous bone formation in a premature female infant with Fryns syndrome. This infant and a full sibling (ie, had same set of parents) with Fryns syndrome in addition exhibited delayed ossification of the basiocciput and of cervical vertebral bodies, also previously undescribed in Fryns syndrome. These findings expand the spectrum of Fryns syndrome to include osteochondrodysplasia.

(*AJDC*. 1991;145:656-660)

Fryns syndrome is a generally fatal autosomal recessive disorder of unknown pathogenesis manifested by a consistent pattern of multiple congenital anomalies such as abnormal facies, diaphragmatic hernia, and distal limb abnormalities, and, more irregularly, by other congenital defects such as axial skeletal abnormalities and malformations of the respiratory, cardiovascular, gastrointestinal, genitourinary, and central nervous systems.[1] Reported defects include cystic dysplasia of the kidneys,[1-4] hypoplastic and abnormally lobulated lungs,[1-4] Dandy-Walker malformation,[2,4,5] Purkinje and granular cell heterotopia,[1,6] agenesis of the corpus callosum,[1,5] and aganglionosis of the colon and ureters.[3] Reported roentgenographic skeletal abnormalities include broad medial ends of the clavicles[1,3]; shortness of long bones, broad ribs, and globularly formed ilium[3]; unusually thin ribs[4]; and abnormal rib-vertebral junctions.[2] To our knowledge, no histopathologic description of bone or cartilage in Fryns syndrome has been published.

We identified, by light microscopy, morphologic abnormalities in rib and humeral physeal osteochondrogenesis in a premature female infant with Fryns syndrome. Delayed ossification of the basiocciput and of cervical vertebral bodies was seen in roentgenograms both of this infant and, on review, of a full sibling (ie, had same set of parents); at autopsy 9 years previously, the sibling was found to have multiple congenital anomalies that on review were compatible with Fryns syndrome. We herein report our observations, which expand the spectrum of Fryns syndrome to include osteochondrodysplasia with delayed cervical vertebral body and basioccipital ossification.

Accepted for publication January 4, 1991.

From the Departments of Pathology (Drs Kershisnik, Craven, and Knisely) and Pediatrics (Drs Jung and Carey), University of Utah Medical Center, Salt Lake City.

Presented in part at the interim meeting of the Society for Pediatric Pathology, Oklahoma City, Okla, October 20-21, 1990.

Reprint requests to Department of Pathology, University of Utah Medical Center, 50 N Medical Dr, Salt Lake City, UT 84132 (Dr Knisely).

PATIENT REPORT

A 1200-g female infant was delivered by cesarean section prematurely at 27 weeks' gestation following acute maternal vaginal hemorrhage secondary to placenta previa. The pregnancy had been complicated by polyhydramnios, which was identified during preoperative ultrasonography.

The family history included parental consanguinity (parents are third cousins once removed [Fig 1]). A female full sibling died of multiple congenital abnormalities 9 years earlier; no syndromic diagnosis was assigned clinically or at autopsy. Two male full siblings are phenotypically normal.

Apgar scores were 0, 5, and 7 at 1, 5, and 10 minutes, respectively. Crown to heel length was 41.5 cm, and occipitofrontal circumference was 24.0 cm. The infant was intubated and surfactant was administered. Craniofacial dysmorphism was present with narrow skull, hypertelorism, lower canthal folds, upturned nose, and broad mouth (Fig 2). The nipples were widely spaced. The cartilaginous portions of the inferior ribs were abnormally pliable. The thumbs were broad and digitalized. The distal phalanges were short, and the nails were hypoplastic (Fig 3). Flexion contractures were present at all distal interphalangeal joints. A right calcaneovalgus deformity was present. M-mode ultrasonic examination of the infant's heart revealed double outlet right ventricle with subaortic ventricular septal defect, thickened mitral valve, thickened pulmonary valve with abnormal motion, and patent ductus arteriosus with bidirectional flow. Abdominal and cranial ultrasonic examinations were normal. The placenta, membranes, and cord (three vessels) were grossly unremarkable. Fryns syndrome was diagnosed clinically. Severe hypoxemia and bradycardia led to death at 12 hours.

Cultured peripheral blood lymphocytes showed a normal 46,XX Giemsa-banded karyotype. Fascial fibroblasts from the infant (NIGMS GM 10879) and peripheral-blood lymphocytes from the parents (NIGMS GM 10930 [mother], NIGMS GM 10931 [father]) were cultured and banked (NIGMS Mutant Cell Repository, Coriell Institute for Medical Research, Camden, NJ).

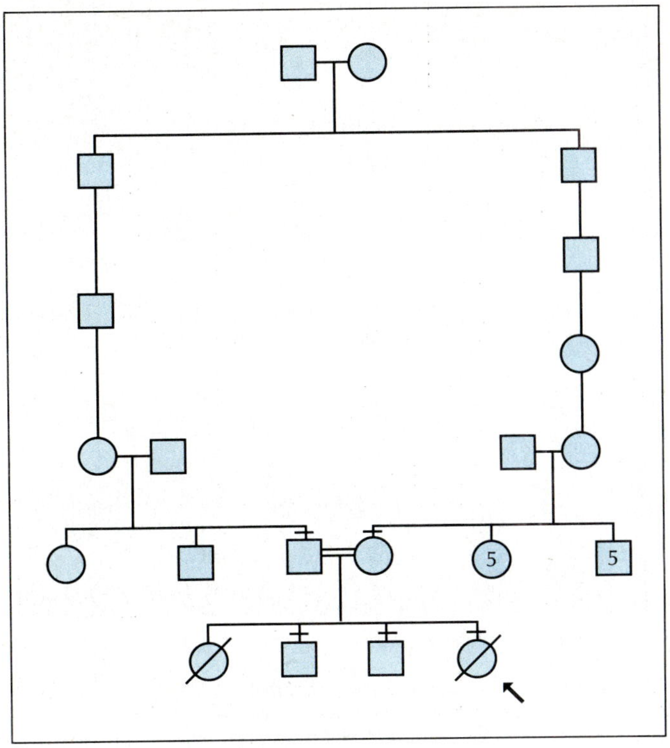

Fig 1.—*Family tree of kindred reported. Arrow indicates proposita; parents are third cousins once removed.*

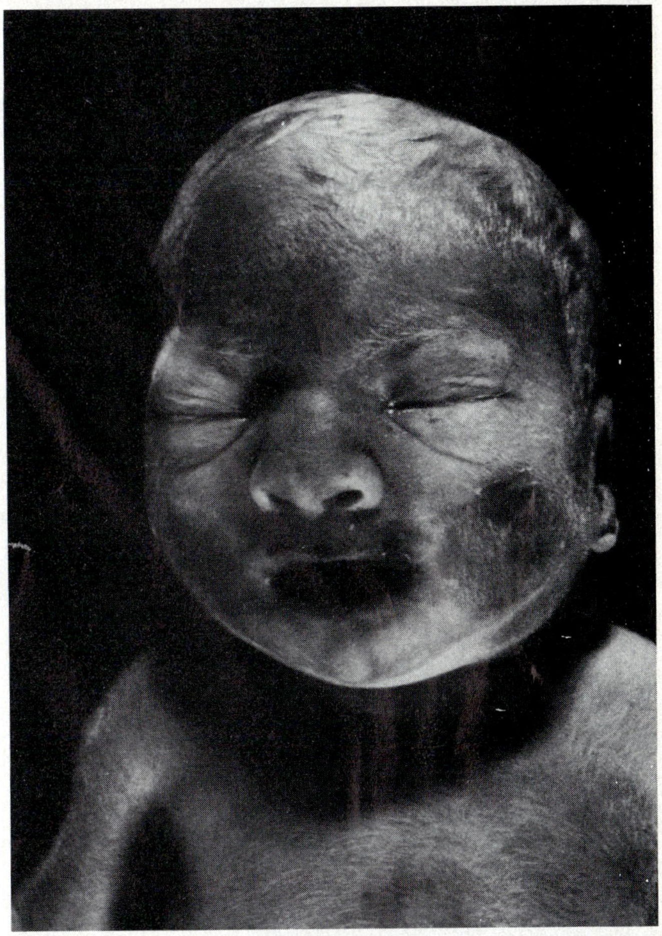

Fig 2.—*Face of younger sibling with Fryns syndrome. There is hypertelorism, the nasal tip is upturned, and the mouth is broad.*

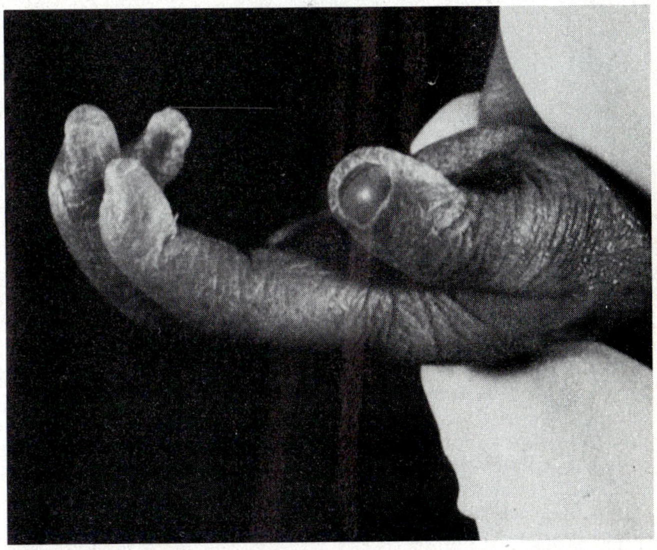

Fig 3.—*Hand of younger sibling with Fryns syndrome. There are flexion contractures of the distal interphalangeal joints. The distal phalanges are hypoplastic.*

At autopsy, external examination confirmed the antemortem findings. No disproportionate shortening of the extremities was noted. Asymmetric toe-heel lengths were 4.9 and 5.2 cm (expected,[7] 4.7 to 5.7 cm), and bilateral ulnar deviation of the hands at the radiocarpal joints was also noted. The inner canthal distance was 2.1 cm (expected,[7] 1.3 to 1.8 cm). The intercommissural distance was 2.9 cm (expected,[7] 1.6 to 2.2 cm). Postmortem roentgenograms showed broadening of the medial ends of the clavicles and delayed ossification of cervical vertebral bodies and basiocciput (Fig 4, top and bottom).

On internal examination, a 1.3×1.0-cm left posterolateral membranomuscular diaphragmatic defect was found, with displacement of the spleen into the left thoracic cavity. Clear ascitic fluid (20 mL) and bilateral pleural effusions (8 mL total) were present. The lungs were hypoplastic (combined weight, 11.8 g; expected,[7] 27.0±7.0 g [mean±2 SDs]) with failure of fissure formation between upper and middle lobes of the right lung. Cardiovascular findings included a persistent left superior vena cava with cardiomegaly (13.2 g; expected,[7] 9±5 g), a 0.2×0.3-cm membranomuscular ventricular septal defect, an abnormally thickened pulmonic valve cusp, agenesis of the nonseptal mitral papillary muscle, and a patent ductus arteriosus. Hepatosplenomegaly was present (liver and spleen weights, 101.5 and 6.0 g, respectively; expected,[7] 60±16 and 3±3 g, respectively). The genitourinary tract was normal with the exception of a uterus bicornis unicollis. The cerebrum, cerebellum, brain stem, and spinal cord were small but externally normal (brain weight, 100 g; expected, 180±53 g[7]). The cervical spine and cord were removed en bloc and serially transversely sectioned at levels inclusive of C-2 through C-6, corresponding to the innervation of the upper extremities; the cord and the brachial plexuses were grossly normal.

On microscopy, bilateral acute pneumonia with hyaline membrane disease was present. The hepatic sinusoids and splenic red pulp were congested. The glomeruli and renal tubules were normal. Myenteric neural elements were present in the colon. An ectopic focus of poorly organized Purkinje and granular cells within inferior cerebellar white-matter tracts was identified. All other organs were

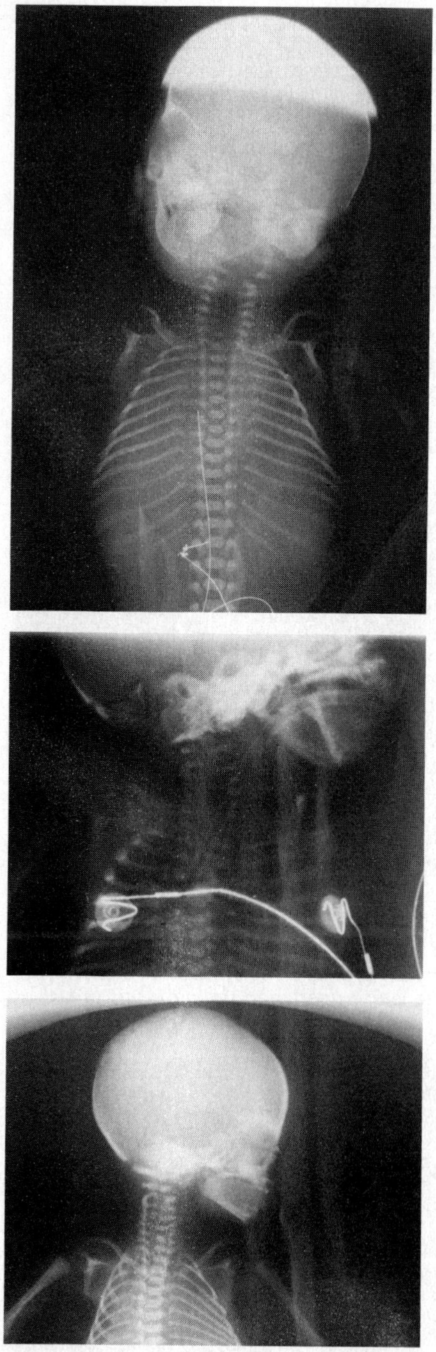

Fig 4.—*Top, Roentgenogram of younger sibling with Fryns syndrome (gestational age, 27 weeks). The medial aspects of the clavicles are broadened, and the basiocciput and the bodies of the first through sixth cervical vertebrae are not mineralized. Center, Roentgenogram of older sibling with Fryns syndrome (gestational age, 28 weeks). The medial ends of the clavicles are broadened, and the basiocciput and the cervical vertebral bodies are not mineralized. Bottom, Roentgenogram of infant without Fryns syndrome (gestational age, 25 weeks). The medial ends of the clavicles are slender. The basiocciput and the cervical vertebrae are clearly mineralized.*

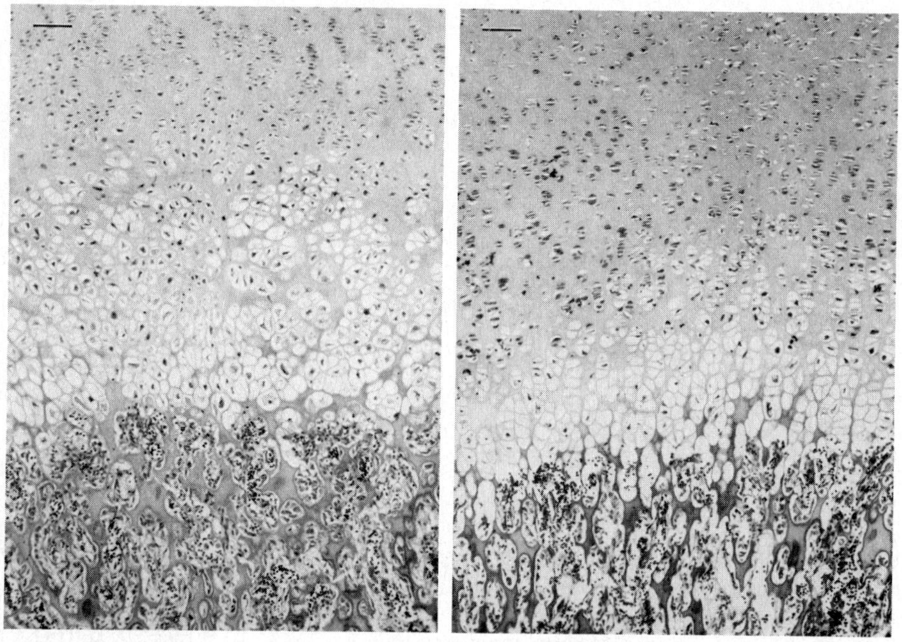

Fig 5.—*Left, Center of proximal humeral physeal plate of younger sibling with Fryns syndrome. Chondrocyte columnarization in the zones of proliferation and hypertrophy are markedly disorganized (hematoxylin-eosin, original magnification ×100; bar=100 μm). Right, Center of proximal humeral physeal plate of age-matched comparison infant without osteochondrodysplasia. Compare with Fig 5, left (hematoxylin-eosin, original magnification ×100; bar=100 μm).*

Fig 6.—*Left, Margin of proximal humeral physis of younger sibling with Fryns syndrome. Metaphyseal trabeculae are coarse and thickened. Subperiosteal bone is discontinuous and the periosteum is thickened (arrow) (hematoxylin-eosin, original magnification ×100; bar=200 μm). Right, Margin of proximal humeral physis of age-matched control infant without osteochondrodysplasia. Trabeculae are slender; subperiosteal bone is delicate and continuous (arrow) (hematoxylin-eosin, original magnification ×50; bar=200 μm).*

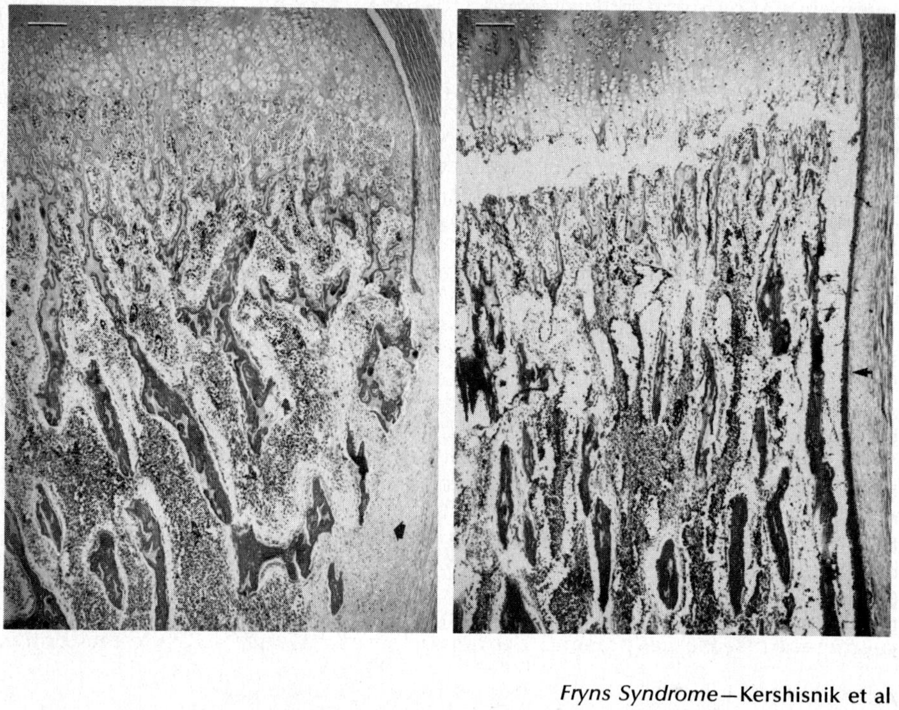

unremarkable microscopically with the exceptions of the cervical vertebral, anterior costal, and proximal humeral physes (see below). The diagnosis of Fryns syndrome was supported by the characteristic dysmorphic features, diaphragmatic hernia, and cardiovascular, pulmonary, and genitourinary system abnormalities.

Patient Report of Sibling

Clinical, roentgenographic, and autopsy records, including glass slides, for the deceased full sibling were reviewed. The infant, an 1190-g girl, was prematurely born (28 weeks' gestation) and died 5.5 hours after delivery. A Giemsa-banded karyotype was 46,XX. External abnormalities included an abnormal face with suborbital creases, micrognathia, low-set ears, and mild neck webbing; bilateral clinodactyly and flexion contractures of distal interphalangeal joints of hands with deep palmar creases; bilateral flexion contractures of knees; bilateral club feet; and omphalocele. Internal abnormalities included a ventricular septal defect; incomplete rotation of the bowel with infrahepatic cecum; agenesis of the corpus callosum; and Dandy-Walker malformation. Diaphragmatic hernia was not seen. Broadening of the medial clavicles and delayed cervical vertebral body and basioccipital ossification were identified on review of antemortem roentgenograms (Fig 4, center and bottom). Bone and cartilage had not been sampled for histologic examination; abnormalities were not identified in other tissues by microscopy. The diagnosis of Fryns syndrome was retrospectively assigned.

Bone Histologic Features

Longitudinal sections of proximal humeral and anterior costal physes of the younger sibling and age-matched controls without apparent osteochondrodysplasia were stained with the following: hematoxylin-eosin; periodic acid–Schiff with and without diastase digestion; Masson's trichrome; toluidine blue O; and alcian blue at a pH of 1.8, with and without hyaluronidase digestion, using conventional techniques.[8] In hematoxylin-eosin–stained sections, the Fryns cartilage, by comparison with that of the age-matched controls, contained poorly oriented columns of chondrocytes and strands of matrix in physeal zones 1 and 2 (zones of hypertrophy and proliferation, respectively). Columns of chondrocytes were crowded and irregularly shaped (Fig 5, left). In age-matched controls, chondrocyte columnarization and strands of matrix in zones 1 and 2 were longitudinally oriented and organized (Fig 5, right).[9,10]

The central bony trabeculae of the Fryns metaphysis were coarse and thickened, and they generally lacked longitudinal orientation (Fig 6, left). The control metaphyses were strikingly different. They contained delicate, thin, homogeneous, generally longitudinally oriented bony trabeculae (Fig 6, right).

The metaphyseal periosteum of the infant with Fryns syndrome was abnormally thickened. The subperiosteal bone was coarse and discontinuous; it did not extend to zone 1 at the lateral margins (Fig 6, left). Similar morphologic changes were identified in sections of cervical vertebral laminae of the infant with Fryns syndrome. In contrast, a distinctly continuous subperiosteal rim of bone extending to zone 1 at the lateral margins was present in the control metaphyses; the periosteum was thinner and did not envelop subperiosteal islands of trabecular bone (Fig 6, right). No histochemical differences between sections from the infant with Fryns syndrome and comparison sections were seen using special stains.

COMMENT

Fryns syndrome is an autosomal recessive disorder characterized by craniofacial anomalies, diaphragmatic hernia, and distal digital hypoplasia.[1,3,4,11] Relatively common conditions that may be confused with Fryns syndrome include trisomy 18 (Edwards' syndrome) and Robert's syndrome. Limb abnormalities readily distinguish Fryns syndrome from these syndromes. Patients with Edwards' syndrome show hypoplasia of the hallux and nails; patients with Robert's syndrome show phocomelia.[12] Neither syndrome manifests diffuse distal digital hypoplasia, which is characteristic of Fryns syndrome. Several other syndromes[12,13] also possess some of the anomalies seen in Fryns syndrome; however, each of these syndromic malformation patterns is different from that seen in Fryns syndrome.

The two patients we describe bring the total number of reported cases of Fryns syndrome to 35. They represent the fourth and fifth cases involving parental consanguinity,[6,11,14] the 10th instance of familial recurrence,[1-4,14,15] and the 25th and 26th confirmed cases of patients with normal karyotypes.[1,5] (Tandem duplication and ring chromosome abnormalities have been recently reported in patients with some features of Fryns syndrome[16,17] who are not considered cases of Fryns syndrome in this article.) The older sibling represents the fourth case of a patient with Dandy-Walker malformation[2,4,5] and the third case of a patient with callosal agenesis.[1,5]

Previously identified roentgenographic abnormalities in patients with Fryns syndrome include the following: bifid manubrial ossification centers[1]; broad medial ends of the clavicles; shortness of the long bones, broad ribs, and globularly formed ilium[3,6]; unusually thin ribs[4]; and abnormal rib-vertebral junctions.[2] Both infants described here had broadened medial ends of the clavicles and delayed cervical vertebral body and basioccipital ossification; their skeletons were otherwise grossly and roentgenographically unremarkable. The observed skeletal abnormalities are presumed manifestations of the genetic defect(s). These findings, in conjunction with previous case reports, suggest partial expression of a short limb dwarfism.[3]

Histologic sections of bone from the youngest sibling showed disordered endochondral and intramembranous bone formation. Chondrocyte columnarization was disorganized, metaphyseal bone was irregular and coarse, metaphyseal periosteum was thickened, and subperiosteal intramembranous bone formation was discontinuous. The observed histopathologic abnormalities in endochondral and intramembranous bone formation were most striking in the proximal humeral physis. The anterior costal physis showed similar histopathologic changes; however, the changes were more subtle than those seen in the proximal humeral physis. Disordered intramembranous (subperiosteal) ossification is characteristic of some osteochondrodysplasias (fibrochondrogenesis, thanatophoric dysplasia[18]) and has been reported in oto-palato-digital syndrome, type II.[19] While abnormalities in endochondral ossification have been identified at autopsy in 60% of infants of less than 32 weeks' gestation,[20] these have not been associated with frank skeletal malformation or heritable syndromic disease, but rather with intrauterine growth retardation. Neither sibling was small for gestational age. Accordingly, our findings indicate osteochondrodysplasia rather than nonspecific intrauterine growth retardation.

On microscopic review of sections of an anterior costal physis from an infant with Fryns syndrome whose case had been reported previously,[1] we found no abnormalities. This suggests that osteochondrodysplasia may not be a consistent finding in Fryns syndrome or that histopathologic changes may be better appreciated in the appendicular skeleton (proximal humeral physes). Future investigations of patients with Fryns syndrome should include histologic examination of bony physes[8] obtained either at autopsy or at diaphragmatic herniorrhaphy.

Many new and superficially unrelated abnormalities have been described in patients with Fryns syndrome[1-5,11,15-17,21,22] since its initial recognition.[13] This report adds osteochondrodysplasia to the spectrum of associated defects, suggesting that the responsible gene affects skeletal development as well as body wall, cardiovascular, genitourinary, and central nervous system organogenesis. Our studies of these two siblings provide new roentgenographic (delayed basiocciput and cervical vertebral body ossification) and histopathologic evidence of osteochondrodysplasia as a feature of Fryns syndrome.

C. Richard Nixon, MD, Department of Medical Imagery at Primary Children's Medical Center, Salt Lake City, Utah, assisted in interpreting the roentgenograms; Kurt Benirschke, MD, Department of Pathology, University of California at San Diego, provided access to sections of rib from the infant with Fryns syndrome whose case was previously reported; and Susan L. Wall, MT(ASCP), and her staff provided technical assistance.

References

1. Cunniff C, Jones KL, Saal HM, Stern HJ. Fryns syndrome: an autosomal recessive disorder associated with craniofacial anomalies, diaphragmatic hernia, and distal digital hypoplasia. *Pediatrics.* 1990;85:499-504.

2. Lubinsky M, Severn C, Rapoport JM. Fryns syndrome: a new variable multiple congenital anomaly (MCA) syndrome. *Am J Med Genet.* 1983;14:461-466.

3. Bamforth JS, Leonard CO, Chodirker BN, et al. Congenital diaphragmatic hernia, coarse facies, and acral hypoplasia: Fryns syndrome. *Am J Med Genet.* 1989;32:93-99.

4. Moerman P, Fryns JP, Vandenberghe K, Devlieger H, Lauweryns JM. The syndrome of diaphragmatic hernia, abnormal face and distal limb anomalies (Fryns syndrome). *Am J Med Genet.* 1988;31:805-814.

5. Aymé S, Julian C, Gambarelli D, et al. Fryns syndrome: report on 8 new cases. *Clin Genet.* 1989;35:191-201.

6. Schwyzer U, Briner J, Schinzel A. Fryns syndrome in a girl born to consanguineous parents. *Acta Paediatr Scand.* 1987;76:167-171.

7. Hall JG, Froster-Iskenius UG, Allanson JE, eds. *Handbook of Normal Physical Measurements.* New York, NY: Oxford University Press Inc; 1989:27,64,84,139,193,435.

8. Yang SS, Kitchen E, Gilbert EF, Rimoin DL. Histopathologic examination in osteochondrodysplasia. *Arch Pathol Lab Med.* 1984;110:10-12.

9. Rimoin DL, Hollister DW, Lachman RS, et al. Histologic studies in the chondrodystrophies. In: Bergsma D, ed. *Skeletal Dysplasia: Papers Presented at the Johns Hopkins Hospital.* New York, NY: American Elsevier Publishing Co, Inc, for The National Foundation-March of Dimes; 1974;10:274-295. Birth Defects: Original Articles Series.

10. Di Fiore MSH, ed. *Atlas of Human Histology.* 3rd ed. Philadelphia, Pa: Lea & Febiger; 1967:36-49.

11. Meinecke P, Fryns JP. The Fryns syndrome: diaphragmatic defects, craniofacial dysmorphism, and distal digital hypoplasia. *Clin Genet.* 1985;28:516-520.

12. Jones KL, ed. *Smith's Recognizable Patterns of Human Malformations.* 4th ed. Philadelphia, Pa: WB Saunders Co; 1988:16-19,256,257.

13. Fryns JP, Moerman F, Goddeeris P, Bossuyt C, Van den Berghe H. A new lethal syndrome with cloudy corneae, diaphragmatic defects and distal limb deformities. *Hum Genet.* 1979;50:65-70.

14. Fitch N, Srolovitz H, Robitaille Y, Guttman F. Absent left hemidiaphragm, arhinencephaly, and cardiac malformations. *J Med Genet.* 1978;15:399-401.

15. Samueloff AS, Navot D, Birkenfeld A, Schenker JG. Fryns syndrome: a predictable, lethal pattern of multiple congenital anomalies. *Am J Obstet Gynecol.* 1983;156:86-88.

16. de Jong G, de Rossouw RA, Retief AE. Ring chromosome 15 in a patient with Fryns syndrome. *J Med Genet.* 1989;26:469-470.

17. Clark RD, Fenner-Gonzales M. Apparent Fryns syndrome in a boy with a tandem duplication of 1q24-31.2. *Am J Med Genet.* 1989;34:422-426.

18. Gilbert EF, Yang SS, Langer L, Opitz JM, Roskamp JO, Heidelberger KP. Pathologic changes of osteochondrodysplasia in infancy: a review. *Pathol Ann.* 1987;22(pt 2):283-345.

19. Ogata T, Matsuo N, Nishimura G, Hajikano H. Oto-palato-digital syndrome, type II: evidence for defective intramembranous ossification. *Am J Med Genet.* 1990;36:226-231.

20. Emery JL, Kalpaktsoglou PK. The costochondral junction during later stages of intrauterine life, and abnormal growth patterns found in association with perinatal death. *Arch Dis Child.* 1967;42:1-13.

21. Fryns JP. Fryns syndrome: a variable MCA syndrome with diaphragmatic defects, coarse face, and distal limb hypoplasia. *J Med Genet.* 1987;24:271-274.

22. Young ID, Simpson K, Winter RM. A case of Fryns syndrome. *J Med Genet.* 1986;23:82-88.

Autosomal Recessive Lethal Infantile Cytochrome C Oxidase Deficiency

Gideon Eshel, MD; Eliezer Lahat, MD; Kalman Fried, MD, PhD; Josef Barr, MD; Varda Barash, MD; Alisa Gutman, MD; Salvatore DiMauro, MD; Mordechei Aladjem, MD

• Three bedouin children with mitochondrial myopathy due to cytochrome c oxidase deficiency presented with progressive muscle weakness, failure to thrive, proximal renal tubular acidosis, and lactic acidemia leading to death. Two died by age 5 months and one by age 16 months. Cytochrome c oxidase was markedly reduced in skeletal muscle extracts of all three. Three other children of the same family with most probably the same metabolic aberration are also described. We suggest an autosomal recessive inheritance for this lethal mitochondrial myopathy.

(*AJDC.* 1991;145:661-664)

Biochemical abnormalities of mitochondria may affect lipid or pyruvate metabolism, the respiratory chain, or the coupling of respiration and phosphorylation.[1] The concept of mitochondrial myopathy was introduced by Luft et al[2] in 1962 and was based on morphological and biochemical abnormalities of muscle mitochondria in a patient whose clinical manifestations could be explained by the mitochondrial dysfunction. In the past decade, clinical and biochemical investigations have led to the identification of several specific errors of mitochondrial metabolism and the current classification of mitochondrial myopathies based on primary biochemical defects.[1] A defect of the respiratory chain affecting cytochrome *c* oxidase (COX) was described in a baby with generalized weakness from birth, severe lactic acidosis, and a renal disorder similar to de Toni-Fanconi-Debré syndrome. The child died of respiratory failure at age 13 weeks.[3] Since this original description, 10 patients with the same clinical and biochemical syndrome have been reported.[4-9] Most of the patients died before age 4 months. In their families, autosomal recessive inheritance appeared likely because twin sisters of one patient[3] and the brother of another[6] died in infancy with similar symptoms, and two patients were siblings.[7]

We describe a bedouin family with three children who had COX deficiency and three who presented with clinical and laboratory findings highly suggestive of the deficiency. This highly inbred family is large enough to provide conclusive evidence of an autosomal recessive mode of inheritance for this disorder.

Accepted for publication July 9, 1990.

From the Pediatric Division (Drs Eshel, Lahat, Barr, and Aladjem) and Department of Genetics (Dr Fried), Assaf Harofeh Medical Center, Sackler School of Medicine, Tel Aviv, Israel; the Department of Clinical Biochemistry, Hadassah Medical Center, Jerusalem, Israel (Drs Barash and Gutman); and the Center for Muscular Dystrophy and Related Diseases, Columbia University, New York, NY (Dr DiMauro).

Reprint requests to Assaf Harofeh Medical Center, Zerifin 70300, Israel (Dr Eshel).

PATIENT REPORTS

The father of four of these children was polygamous and married to two first cousins and to an unrelated woman, all of whom were healthy. The family pedigree is presented in Fig 1.

Patient III-7 (Proband).—A 5-month-old boy was admitted with respiratory distress and hypothermia. He had been delivered after a full-term, uneventful pregnancy. Birth weight was 2100 g. Prior to hospitalization, several episodes of diarrhea and vomiting were noted. Feeding problems started immediately after birth. On admission, he weighed 2170 g, was severely dehydrated and floppy, and had a weak cry. Rectal temperature was 34°C, and respiratory rate was 60 beats per minute. Tendon reflexes were decreased symmetrically. Chest roentgenograms were normal. Measurements of arterial blood gases showed partially compensated metabolic acidosis with pH 7.30, a P_{CO_2} level of 19 mm Hg, P_{O_2} level of 70 mm Hg, and base excess level of −13 mmol/L. Additional levels were as follows: serum lactate, 4.0 mmol/L (normal, <2.0 mmol/L); serum pyruvate, 148 μmol/L (normal, <114 μmol/L); blood ammonia, 44 μmol/L (normal, 47 to 64 μmol/L); and plasma glucose, 4.8 mmol/L (normal, 3.85 to 6.05 mmol/L). No organic acids were found in the urine. On urinalysis, proteinuria was +3, glycosuria was +3, and generalized aminoaciduria was present. An electroencephalogram showed generalized diffuse slowing of the background activity, and a brain sonogram was normal. The child died 10 days after admission. A detailed autopsy was not performed, and only a skeletal muscle specimen was obtained from the vastus lateralis. The biochemical analysis of mitochondrial enzymes was performed by methods described elsewhere previously.[8] The results are presented in Table 1.

Patient III-10.—A 5-month-old girl presented with severe failure to thrive and had the following test values: serum lactate,

Fig 1.—*Family pedigree. Circles indicate females, and squares, males. The black squares and circles represent the clinically affected patients who are deceased. The arrow indicates the proband.*

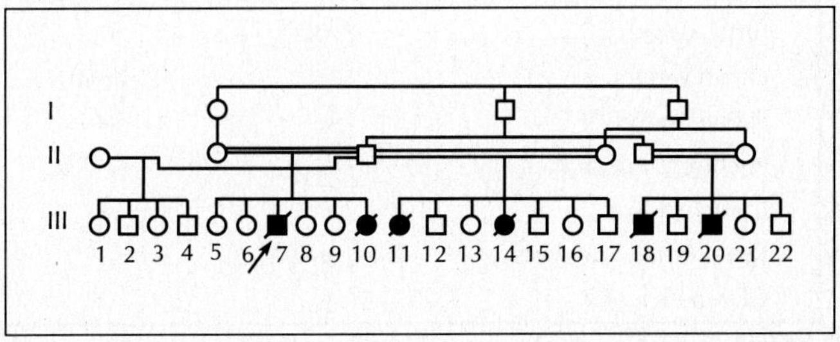

3.7 mmol/L; serum pyruvate, 136 µmol/L; blood ammonia, 56 µmol/L. She died of respiratory failure. Results of biochemical analysis of a muscle biopsy specimen obtained shortly before her death are shown in Table 1.

Patient III-20.—A 2-month-old boy was admitted because of prolonged diarrhea. He had been delivered after an uneventful pregnancy and weighed 3220 g. On admission, he weighed 3000 g; except for marked dehydration, results of physical examination were unremarkable. Laboratory examinations revealed metabolic acidosis with pH 7.27, $Paco_2$ level of 24.8 mm Hg, Pao_2 level of 65 mm Hg, and base excess level of −13 mmol/L. Test results included the following values: serum phosphate, 1.2 mmol/L; calcium, 2.24 mmol/L; serum lactate, 6.2 mmol/L; serum pyruvate, 132 µmol/L; blood ammonia, 62 µmol/L; and plasma glucose, 5.1 mmol/L. No organic acids were found in the urine, and serum carnitine levels were within normal limits. Urinalysis showed proteinuria, phosphaturia, glycosuria, and generalized aminoaciduria. Stool cultures were positive for *Salmonella*. The metabolic acidosis persisted, and oral treatment with bicarbonate, calcium lactate, and phosphate was begun. Starting at age 3 months, progressive diffuse hypotonia, gradual decrease in deep tendon reflexes, and increasing opsoclonus (involuntary eye movements) were noted. Electroencephalography revealed diffuse slowing of the background activity. Computed tomography showed diffuse cortical atrophy. The infant was readmitted several times following repeated episodes of bacterial infections until his death at age 16 months. Immunologic screening tests were normal. Muscle, heart, and brain tissue were obtained after death for biochemical analysis. The results of analysis for mitochondrial enzymes are presented in Table 1.

Patients III-11, III-14 and III-18.—Three additional siblings and half-siblings of patients III-7, III-10, and III-20 presented at ages of 1, 4, and 5 months with severe failure to thrive and progressive hypotonia. Clinical and biochemical findings were very similar to those observed in patients III-7, III-10, and III-20 (Tables 2 and 3). Proximal tubular dysfunction was diagnosed after laboratory findings disclosed proteinuria, glycosuria, and generalized aminoaciduria. Computed tomography of patient III-14 showed diffuse cortical atrophy (Fig 2). The three children died at ages 6, 15, and 23 months. Cytochrome *c* oxidase activity in tissues was not examined.

COMMENT

The mitochondrial respiratory chain is divided into four functional units or complexes, each composed of several

Table 1.—Mitochondrial Enzymes in Skeletal Muscles of Three Patients and in the Brain and Heart of Case III-20*

Tissue Type and Patient No.	COX	Succinate	NADH Cytochrome C Reductase	Succinate DH	NADH DH	CS
Muscle						
III-7	0.231	0.513	0.970	0.60	20.64	4.27
III-10	0.000	0.605	1.400	1.44	25.00	8.42
III-20	0.108	0.378	0.270	0.63	24.03	3.90
Controls (No.)	2.80±0.52 (71)	0.70±0.228 (68)	1.020±0.377 (78)	1.00±0.526 (78)	35.48±7.07 (76)	9.88±2.55 (73)
Brain						
III-20	0.486	0.432	0.217	0.406	12.10	6.176
Controls (No.)	0.517±0.168 (13)	0.336±0.228 (12)	0.640±0.240 (9)	1.920±0.500 (8)	9.29±2.54 (21)	6.05±1.77 (21)
Heart						
III-20	3.45	4.41	0.649	3.67	79.03	34.56
Controls (No.)	4.63±1.59 (10)	1.70±0.44 (9)	3.10±1.45 (7)	1.78±0.55 (7)	69.66±11.4 (7)	35.68±14.2 (7)

*All assays were carried out on crude extracts. COX indicates cytochrome *c* oxidase; NADH, rotenone-sensistive reduced nicotinamide-adenine dinucleotide; DH, dehydrogenase; and CS, citrate synthase. Enzyme values are in micromoles of substrate per minute per gram of tissue. Control values are means±SEMs.

Table 2.—Clinical and Biochemical Data of the Six Patients*

	Patient III-7	Patient III-10	Patient III-11	Patient III-14	Patient III-18	Patient III-20
Date of birth	12/21/83	5/20/81	1/16/77	7/22/80	10/10/80	5/23/83
Sex	M	F	F	F	M	M
Age at admission, mo	1	1	5	1	4	2
Age at death, mo	5	5	15	23	6	16
Birth weight, g	2100	2000	2500	3000	3500	3220
Death weight, g	2170	2650	4100	4600	4720	4610
Failure to thrive	+	+	+	+	+	+
Recurrent infections	+	−	+	−	+	+
Lactic acidosis	+	+	+	+	+	+
Renal tubular acidosis	+	+	+	+	+	+
COX deficiency	+	+	ND	ND	ND	+

*COX indicates cytochrome *c* oxidase, and ND, not done.

proteins that are embedded in the inner mitochondrial membrane. Complex IV (COX) is composed of 13 polypeptides. Subunits I, II, and III are transcribed by mitochondrial DNA, while the remaining 10 are encoded by nuclear DNA. Genetic errors affecting the nuclear-coded subunits may impair the assembly of the whole complex in muscle or other tissues and cause different clinical syndromes.[1,10]

Table 4 summarizes a tentative clinical classification of COX deficiency based on differential tissue involvement.[10]

Sixteen patients have been reported to have lethal in-

Table 3.—Neurologic Manifestations*

	Patient III-7	Patient III-10	Patient III-11	Patient III-14	Patient III-18	Patient III-20
Hypotonia	+	+	+	+	+	+
Psychomotor retardation	+	+	+	+	+	+
Convulsions	−	−	−	+	−	−
Opsoclonus	−	−	−	−	+	+
Optic atrophy	−	−	+	−	−	−
Abnormal EEG	+	+	+	+	ND	+
Abnormal CT	ND	+	ND	+	ND	+

*EEG indicates electroencephalogram; CT, computed tomogram; and ND, not done.

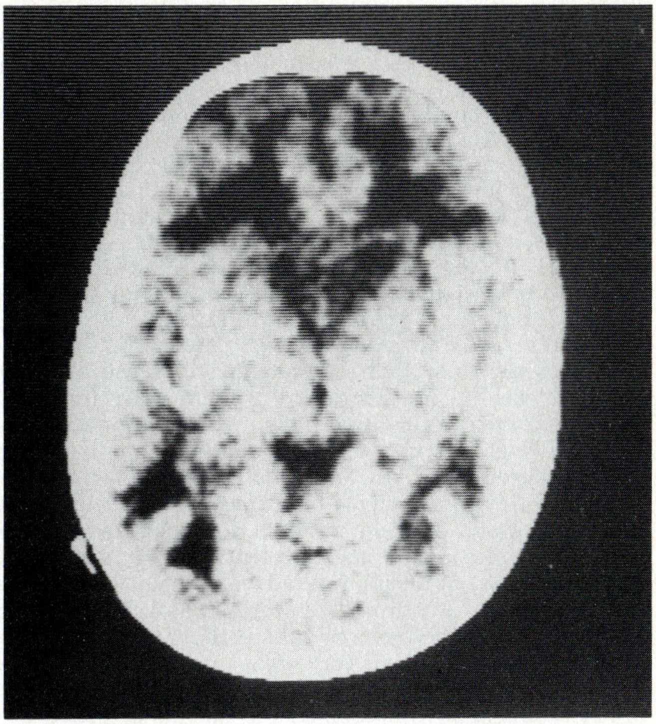

Fig 2.—*A computed tomogram of patient III-14 shows diffuse cortical atrophy with enlargement of the ventricular system.*

Table 4.—Cytochrome Oxidase Deficiency: Clinical and Laboratory Features

Clinical Syndromes	Reference No.	Myopathy	CNS Involvement*	Generalized Weakness	Hypotonia	Hyporeflexia	Respiratory Failure	Renal Tubular Acidosis	Cardiopathy	Liver Involvement	Lactic Acidosis
Syndromes dominated by muscle involvement											
Fatal infantile myopathy	7, 8, 11, 12	+	−	+	+	+	+	−	−	−	+
Fatal infantile myopathy and renal dysfunction	3-6, 13-15	+	+	+	+	+	+	+	−	−	+
Myopathy and cardiopathy	16-18	+	−	+	−	−	+	−	+	+	+
Myopathy and liver disease in second cousins	19	+	−	+	+	+	−	−	−	−	+
Benign infantile mitochondrial myopathy	20-21	+	−	+, reversible	+	+	−	−	−	−	+
Syndromes dominated by brain involvement											
Subacute necrotizing encephalomyelopathy (Leigh syndrome)	22-25	+	+	+	+	+	+	−	−	+	+
Progressive sclerosing poliodystrophy of children (Alper's disease)	26	−	+	−	−	−	+	−	−	+	−
Trichopol iodystrophy (Menkes' disease)	27	+	+	+	+	+	+	−	−	+	+

*CNS indicates central nervous system.

fantile myopathy.[3-9,11-18] Manifestations included generalized weakness, lactic acidosis, and de Toni-Fanconi-Debré syndrome. We add six patients with similar clinical and biochemical findings, three of whom had proven COX deficiency. This family enlarges our understanding of the spectrum of the natural history of COX deficiency. Our patients are different from those previously described in their longer survival and heterogeneous neurologic manifestations. Most of the other described patients died before age 4 months. All our patients survived for at least 5 months, the longest survival being 23 months.

In addition to generalized weakness, hypotonia, and hyporeflexia already reported in previous cases, our patients presented a variety of neurologic abnormalities, including severe psychomotor retardation in all affected children, seizure (one patient), optic atrophy (one patient), and opsoclonus (two patients). Electroencephalograms of five patients were abnormal, showing irregular slow background activity and irritative features in the patient with seizure activity. Computed tomography of the brain performed on three patients demonstrated diffuse cortical atrophy with enlarged ventricular systems. The possibility that our patients had variants of COX deficiency and Leigh syndrome[22-25] seems to us unlikely, since COX activity in the brain of patient III-20 was normal.

Autosomal recessive inheritance appeared likely in the families described previously in the literature. The large affected sibships in this highly inbred family prove the autosomal recessive mode of transmission.

References

1. DiMauro S, Bonilla E, Zeviani M, Nakagawa M, DeVivo DC. Mitochondrial myopathies. *Ann Neurol.* 1985;17:521-538.
2. Luft R, Ikkos D, Palmieri G, et al. A case of severe hypermetabolism of nonthyroid origin with a defect in the maintenance of mitochondrial respiratory control: a correlated clinical, biochemical and morphological study. *J Clin Invest.* 1962;41:1776-1804.
3. Van Biervliet JPGM, Bruinvis LK, Ketting D, et al. Hereditary mitochondrial myopathy with lactic acidemia, a de Toni-Fanconi-Debré syndrome, and a defective respiratory chain involuntary striated muscles. *Pediatr Res.* 1977;11:1088-1092.
4. DiMauro S, Mendell JR, Sahenk Z, Bachman A, Scarpa RM, Scofield C. Fatal infantile mitochondrial myopathy and renal dysfunction due to cytochrome-c-oxidase deficiency. *Neurology.* 1980;30:795-804.
5. Heiman-Patterson TD, Bonilla E, DiMauro S, Foreman J, Schotland DL. Cytochrome-c-oxidase deficiency in a floppy infant. *Neurology.* 1982;32:898-900.
6. Minchom PE, Dormer RL, Hughes IA, et al. Fatal infantile mitochondrial myopathy due to cytochrome *c* oxidase deficiency. *J Neurol Sci.* 1983;60:453-463.
7. Muller-Hocker J, Pongratz D, Deufel TH, Trijbels W, Endres G. Fatal lipid storage myopathy with deficiency of cytochrome-c-oxidase and carnitine. *Virchow's Arch A.* 1983; 399:11-23.
8. Zeviani M, Nonaka I, Bonilla E, et al. Fatal infantile mitochondrial myopathy and renal dysfunction caused by cytochrome *c* oxidase deficiency: immunological studies in a new patient. *Ann Neurol.* 1985;17:414-417.
9. Oldfors A, Solmmerland H, Holme E, Tulinius M, Kristiansson B. Cytochrome-c-oxidase deficiency in infancy. *Acta Neuropathol (Berl).* 1989;77:267-275.
10. DiMauro S, Zeviani M, Servidei S, et al. Cytochrome oxidase deficiency: clinical and biochemical heterogeneity. *Ann N Y Acad Sci.* 1987;484:19-32.
11. Trijbel F, Sengers R, Monnens L, Janssen A, Willem H, ter Laak H. A patient with lactic acidemia and cytochrome oxidase deficiency. *J Inherited Metab Dis.* 1983;6(suppl 2):127-128.
12. Bresolin N, Shanske S, Miller RH, et al. Fatal infantile cytochrome *c* oxidase deficiency: decrease of immunologically detectable enzyme in muscle. *Neurology.* 1985;35:802-812.
13. DiMauro S, Zeviani M, Bonilla E, et al. Cytochrome *c* oxidase deficiency. *Biochem Soc Trans.* 1985;13:651-653.
14. Kuhn-Nentwig L, Kadenbach B. Isolation and properties of cytochrome *c* oxidase from rat liver and quantification of immunological differences between isozymes from various rat tissues with subunit-specific antisera. *Eur J Biochem.* 1985;149:147-158.
15. Capaldi RA, Malatesta F, Darley-Usmar VM. Structure of cytochrome *c* oxidase. *Biochim Biophys Acta.* 1983;726:135-148.
16. Rimoldi M, Bottacchi E, Rossi L, Cornelio F, Uziel S, DiDonato S. Cytochrome *c* oxidase deficiency in muscles of a floppy infant without mitochondrial myopathy. *J Neurol.* 1982;227:201-207.
17. Sengers R, Trijbel F, Bakkeren JAJM, et al. Deficiency of cytochromes *b* and aa_3 in muscle from a floppy infant with cytochrome oxidase deficiency. *Eur J Pediatr.* 1984;141:178-180.
18. Zeviani M, Van Dyke DH, Servidei S, et al. Myopathy and fatal cardiopathy due to cytochrome *c* oxidase deficiency. *Arch Neurol.* 1986;43:1198-1202.
19. Boustany RN, Aprille JR, Halperin J, Levy H, DeLong GR. Mitochondrial cytochrome deficiency presenting as a myopathy with hypotonia, external ophthalmoplegia and lactic acidosis in an infant and as fetal hepatopathy in a second cousin. *Ann Neurol.* 1983;14:462-470.
20. DiMauro S, Nicholson JF, Hays AP, et al. Benign infantile mitochondrial myopathy due to reversible cytochrome *c* oxidase deficiency. *Ann Neurol.* 1983;14:226-234.
21. Zeviani M, Peterson P, Servidei S, Bonilla E, DiMauro S. Benign reversible muscle cytochrome *c* oxidase deficiency: a second case. *Neurology.* 1987;37:64-67.
22. DiMauro S, Servidei S, Zeviani M, et al. Cytochrome *c* oxidase deficiency in Leigh syndrome. *Ann Neurol.* 1987;22:498-506.
23. Miyabayashi S, Narisawa K, Tada K, Sakai K, Kobayashi K, Kobayashi Y. Two siblings with cytochrome *c* oxidase deficiency. *J Inherited Metab Dis.* 1983;6:121-122.
24. Hoganson GE, Paulson DJ, Chun R, Sufit RL, Shug AL. Deficiency of muscle cytochrome *c* oxidase in Leigh's disease. *Pediatr Res.* 1984;18:22A. Abstract.
25. Servidei S, Zeviani M, DiMauro S, et al. Cytochrome oxidase deficiency in Leigh's syndrome. *Ann Neurol.* 1986;20:400. Abstract.
26. Prick MJJ, Gabreels FJM, Trijbels JMF, et al. Progressive poliodystrophy (Alper's disease) with a defect in cytochrome *aa*, in muscle: a report of two unrelated patients. *Clin Neurol Neurosurg.* 1983;85:57-70.
27. French JH, Sherard ES, Lubell H, Brotz M, Moore CL. Trichopoliodystrophy, I: report of a case and biochemical studies. *Arch Neurol.* 1972;26:229-244.

Tracking of Elevated Blood Pressure Values in Adolescent Athletes at 1-Year Follow-up

Jeffrey L. Tanji, MD

• Resting blood pressures were measured in 467 adolescents during preparticipation physical examinations for high school sports. Fifty-seven of the athletes (12.2%) had significantly elevated blood pressures. Forty-three (79.6%) of 54 subjects demonstrated significantly and persistently elevated blood pressures at 1-year follow-up. A family history of hypertension was positively associated with elevated blood pressures in 46 (80.7%) of 57 subjects compared with controls (23/410 [5.6%]). Consistent with previous studies, subjects with elevated blood pressures had a greater body weight (94.5±25.7 kg) compared with normotensive subjects (75.2±14.0 kg). Subjects with elevated blood pressures engaged in heavy resistance weight training (three times a week or more) more often (41/57 [71.9%]) than normotensive subjects (65/410 [15.8%]). These data support the idea that blood pressures measured during routine preparticipation physical examinations for high school sports are a useful tool in screening for elevated blood pressure in adolescents.

(*AJDC.* 1991;145:665-667)

Hypertension is a widespread condition affecting an estimated 58 million adults in the United States.[1] It is a proved risk factor for cardiovascular morbidity and mortality[2] and contributes to the leading cause of death in the adult American population.[3] Often, the diagnosis of hypertension is not made until the third or fourth decade of life, despite the hypothesis that borderline hypertension may exist before this for a long time. One of the obstacles in the early diagnosis of hypertension is the concept that many young adults, specifically adolescents, do not present as often for medical care compared with other age groups. An estimated 25 million adolescents participate regularly in organized sports.[4] Thirty-five states require an annual physician's examination before participating in organized sports at the high school and junior high school levels.[5] It is the hypothesis of this article that elevated blood pressures taken during the preparticipation sports physical examination correlate with elevated blood pressures at 1-year follow-up. This screening examination, therefore, may be useful in identifying a cohort at risk for the development of hypertension at a later date. Corollary findings from the project will ascertain if an association exists between elevated blood pressure and increased body weight and if an association exists between elevated blood pressure and regular weight training.

Longitudinal studies of children with blood pressures above the 95th percentile for age have revealed consistent tracking of elevated blood pressure, particularly in adolescent and obese subjects.[6] Previous studies have indicated that the single best correlate of elevated blood pressure is body mass.[6] The report of the Second Task Force on Blood Pressure Control in Children[7] has categorized significant hypertension as blood pressure persistently equal to or greater than the 95th percentile for age (≥142 mm Hg systolic and ≥92 mm Hg diastolic, group aged 16 to 18 years) and severe hypertension as blood pressure equal to or greater than the 99th percentile for age (≥150 mm Hg systolic and ≥98 mm Hg diastolic, group aged 16 to 18 years).

SUBJECTS AND METHODS

Subjects were 467 male and female adolescents (aged 15 to 19 years) who were enrolled in high school and required preparticipation physical examinations before their sports season. Included were all subjects who underwent screening examinations

Department Editors.—*William B. Strong, MD, Augusta, Ga; Carl L. Stanitski, MD, Pittsburgh, Pa; Ronald E. Smith, PhD; Seattle, Wash; Jack H. Wilmore, PhD, Austin, Tex*

Purpose.—*This section provides current information related to the medical needs of young athletes, as pertinent to counseling young athletes and their parents regarding sports participation and practices contributing to the health maintenance of the athlete, as well as current concepts in the prevention, diagnosis, and treatment of sports-related illnesses and injuries.*

Editorial Comment.—*This prospective study of blood pressure assessment of adolescent athletes addresses a common problem. It demonstrates the importance of medical follow-up and more aggressive evaluation of the youngster with elevated blood pressure. Family history, body size, the type of strength training in which the athlete participates, and the use of anabolic steroids are issues that need to be addressed.*—*W.B.S.*

Accepted for publication October 29, 1990.

From the Department of Family Practice, University of California, Davis Medical Center, Sacramento.

Reprint requests to Department of Family Practice, University of California, Davis Medical Center, 2221 Stockton Blvd, Sacramento, CA 95817 (Dr Tanji).

from seven Sacramento (Calif) metropolitan high schools. Excluded were subjects who were absent on the days of the examination and students enrolled in their senior year of high school (for the purpose of tracking blood pressure more easily at 1-year follow-up). To decrease the possibility of selection bias, profiling of blood pressures was done for the excluded group (n = 113). No differences were noted compared with the study population.

All subjects underwent a screening history and physical examination, which was performed by five physician examiners according to a nationally published format.[4] The history included questions regarding current health status; symptoms; previous level of competition; and medical history, including trauma, surgeries, fractures, sprains, medications, allergies, and habits (ie, smoking, alcohol, recreational drugs). Specifically, a history of hypertension in first-degree relatives, history of loss of consciousness, palpitations, family history of heart disease or hypertension, and a cardiovascular review of systems were documented. The validity of the reported findings was strengthened by having a history questionnaire distributed 1 week before the examination for parental review and input. A history of weight training was elicited retrospectively by self-report from the participants; this was validated through the athletic coaching staffs by written survey.

The physical examination adhered to previously published standards[4] and included blood pressure determination using a manual sphygmomanometer according to American Heart Association criteria.[8] Cuff size selection, however, was not based on American Heart Association criteria for adults; rather, it was chosen using criteria for children and adolescents according to the Second Task Force on Blood Pressure Control in Children.[7] A cardiovascular examination, including auscultation of the heart and palpation of peripheral pulses, was included.

All findings were recorded using a standardized format,[4] which included the name of the subject's physician, home telephone number, sports, and high school. Criteria for an elevated blood pressure response were derived from the Report of the Second Task Force on Blood Pressure Control in Children[7] and used a blood pressure of 142 mm Hg or greater systolic or 92 mm Hg or greater diastolic as significant. All subjects with significant elevation in blood pressure according to these criteria were reported to the coach and school nurse after the examination for follow-up blood pressure checks within 3 months.

One year after the initial examination, 436 of the initial cohort of 467 (31 subjects were unavailable for follow-up) were examined again for their annual sports preparticipation physical examination. The same procedures as described previously were performed.

Statistical analysis was performed using a mean±SD value from the mean for descriptive data. A correlation coefficient analysis was used to analyze the relationship of elevated blood pressure between the two examinations. Student's paired *t* test was used to analyze differences between hypertensive and normal subjects. A χ^2 test was used to analyze categorical differences.

RESULTS

The study population consisted of 359 male and 108 female adolescents (mean age, 16.2±2.2 years; range, 15 to 19 years) who were enrolled in high school and participating in a school-organized sports team. The group included 289 white (61.9%), 73 black (15.6%), 59 Hispanic (12.6%), and 46 Asian (9.9%) subjects; this racial distribution was representative of the demographic characteristics of the seven high schools.

As might be expected, the study population was a generally healthy group, with the only prior hospitalizations being for orthopedic trauma (12 [2.6%]) and asthma exacerbation (two [0.4%]). Twenty (4.3%) of the cohort of 467 reported a history of an elevated blood pressure; none reported a history of using an antihypertensive medication or illnesses or complications as a result of elevated blood pressure.

At the initial evaluation, 57 of the subjects (12.2%) had significantly elevated (≥142 mm Hg systolic, ≥92 mm Hg diastolic) blood pressures according to the stated criteria.[7] Forty-eight (13.4%) of 359 men and nine (8.3%) of 108 women met these criteria. A family history of hypertension by self-report was present in 46 (80.7%) of the 57 subjects with significantly elevated blood pressures as opposed to 23 (5.6%) of 410 normal subjects. Subjects with elevated blood pressures had a greater body weight (94.5±25.7 kg) than normal subjects (75.2±14.0 kg; $P<.05$). Subjects with elevated blood pressures engaged in heavy resistance training (defined as three times a week or more), 41 (71.9%) of 57 to a greater frequency than normotensive subjects (65/410 [15.8%]; $P<.5$). Subjects with an elevated blood pressure did not demonstrate racially related patterns, as 31 (10.7%) of 289 white, nine (12.3%) of 73 black, eight (13.6%) of 59 Hispanic, and nine (19.6%) of 46 Asian subjects met the criteria for a significantly elevated blood pressure.

Blood Pressures of 436 High School Athletes at Initial Examination and Follow-up

Blood Pressure	Initial Examination	1-y Follow-up	*r* Value Systolic	*r* Value Diastolic
Normal	382	368	.77	.79
Elevated	54	43	.72	.74

At 1-year follow-up, of the original cohort of 467, 31 (6.6%) were unavailable for follow-up, leaving a group of 436, who were tracked longitudinally for the 1-year study. Three (9.7%) of the 31 subjects unavailable for follow-up met the criteria for a significantly elevated blood pressure. The group unavailable for follow-up did not differ significantly in blood pressure compared with the original study population. Of the group of 436 tracked at 1-year follow-up, 48 (11.0%) demonstrated a significantly elevated blood pressure. Forty-three (79.6%) of 54 subjects with an elevated blood pressure at the initial examination demonstrated a persistently elevated blood pressure at 1-year follow-up.

Three hundred eighty-two subjects of the group of 436 tracked at 1-year follow-up initially had a normal blood pressure. At 1-year follow-up, 368 (96.3%) of the 382 continued to have a normal blood pressure, and the remaining 14 (3.7%) manifested a significantly elevated blood pressure not noted on the initial screening. Eleven (20.4%) of the cohort of 54 had a significantly elevated blood pressure at the initial screening examination and had a normal blood pressure at 1-year follow-up (Table). For both systolic and diastolic pressures in subjects with normal and elevated blood pressures, all *r* values were greater than .7.

COMMENT

These data support the hypothesis that elevated blood pressures according to the Second Task Force on Blood Pressure Control in Children criteria[7] taken as a part of a routine preparticipation sports examination are positively related to persistently elevated blood pressures at 1-year follow-up. These findings reinforce the concept that stratification of blood pressures in relation to peer groups begins before adulthood.[6] A normal blood pressure at initial evaluation is correlated with normal blood pressures at 1-year follow-up.

The implications of this study are to validate the significance of elevated blood pressures during routine screening of the 25 million adolescents who participate in annual school sports competition. Closer observation of the elevated blood pressures by follow-up has been recommended previously.[7] These findings support such recommendations. Earlier detection of patients at risk for hypertension would theoretically imply that earlier evaluation and intervention and improved control of blood pressure could occur. The Joint National Committee on the Detection, Evaluation, and Treatment of Hypertension proposes clear guidelines to follow and treat such patients.[3]

A 3-month follow-up evaluation after an initially elevated blood pressure for mild or borderline hypertension is the currently recommended standard of care. A clinically relevant question that arises after the detection of an elevated blood pressure according to the task force criteria[7] is whether a young athlete should continue to participate in his or her chosen sport. The American Academy of Pediatrics has published specific guidelines for this decision,[9] and the recommendations have been discussed and supported in the literature.[10] Generally, an athlete with no symptoms or end-organ damage in the presence of significantly elevated blood pressure may be allowed to compete in sports as long as blood pressure is carefully tracked.

Limitations of this study include the use of the standard manual sphygmomanometer, which could account for observer bias and errors in measurement of blood pressure. The rationale for using such a device is that in practice, such devices are used routinely to determine blood pressures and constitute the standard for measurement. Observer bias was minimized by "blinding" the observer as to the result of the previous blood pressure measurement, and all subjects were randomized to be examined by a group of five examiners.

One can be critical of the fact that in this prospective, longitudinal cohort study, 6.6% of the subjects were unavailable for follow-up. Attrition was minimized by initially excluding senior students from the cohort, although data were collected in this group to demonstrate no difference between this group and the study population. We believe that 6.6% attrition is a reasonable figure in light of the general issue of high school attendance as well as migration away from school. Within the group unavailable for follow-up, no variance in blood pressures were noted between that group and the study population.

Selection bias is a valid issue in this study. The fact that the study population represents high school athletes probably selects for a more active, fit, and healthier group than a typical adolescent population. The practical avenue of the preparticipation sports physical examination facilitated data collection for this cohort. Realistically, this screening examination in many cases may very well be the only contact that a healthy adolescent has with the health care delivery system. The issue of cuff size leading to falsely elevated blood pressures in subjects with greater body mass was addressed by using the criteria from the Second Task Force on Blood Pressure in Children as the method for determining appropriate cuff size for subjects.[7]

Strengths of the study include the large study population (N = 467), the low percentage of attrition in the study group (6.6%), the detail of information gathered in the history and physical examination, and the fact that this was a longitudinal, prospective cohort study.

A confounding variable that merits discussion is the possibility that elevated blood pressures in adolescents with increased body weight who engage in weight training may be associated with the illicit use of anabolic steroids.[11] The prevalence of anabolic steroid use has been estimated to be as low as 6%[12] and as high as 10%[13] among high school and college athletes. An experimental study to analyze the effect of anabolic steroid use on blood pressure is not ethically viable at this point, and retrospective self-report studies are flawed by the possible issue of underreporting of illegal drug use. It is stimulating to note the relationship between elevated blood pressures in larger athletes who weight train, but it is by no means valid to conclude that a relationship with anabolic steroid use may exist.

Further studies would point to continued follow-up of this cohort in a prospective, longitudinal study to determine when the diagnosis of hypertension is made. This sort of study sets the stage for interventional trials with closer follow-up and perhaps the earlier use of nonpharmacologic therapy for this population.

Randy Armstrong, MD, Pat Browning, MD, Belinda Murphy, DO, Terry Wrobel, DO, and Don Yokoyama, MD, provided support in data collection, and Barbara Claire prepared the manuscript.

References

1. American Heart Association. *Heart Facts.* Dallas, Tex: American Heart Association; 1988.

2. Kannel WB, Doyle JT, Ostfeld AM, et al. The Framingham Study. *Circulation.* 1984;70:157A-162A.

3. Joint National Committee on Detection, Evaluation, and Treatment of High Blood Pressure. The 1988 Report of the Joint National Committee on Detection, Evaluation, and Treatment of High Blood Pressure. *Arch Intern Med.* 1988;148:1023-1038.

4. Tanji JL. Sports safety. In: Hudson TW, ed. *Clinical Preventive Medicine.* Boston, Mass: Little Brown & Co Inc; 1988:251-259.

5. Smilkstein G. Health evaluation of high school athletes. *Phys Sports Med.* 1981;9:73-81.

6. Lieberman E. Hypertension in childhood and adolescence. In: Kaplan NM, ed. *Clinical Hypertension.* Baltimore, Md: Williams & Wilkins; 1986:447-472.

7. Second Task Force on Blood Pressure Control in Children. Report of the Second Task Force on Blood Pressure Control in Children: 1987. *Pediatrics.* 1987;79:1-25.

8. American Heart Association. *Recommendations for Human Blood Pressure Determinations by Sphygmomanometers.* Dallas, Tex: American Heart Association; 1980.

9. American Academy of Pediatrics, Committee on Sports Medicine. Recommendations for participation in competitive sports. *Pediatrics.* 1988;81:737-739.

10. Tanji JL. The preparticipation physical examination for sports: an update for 1990. *Am Fam Physician.* 1990;42:397-402.

11. National Task Force on Anabolic/Androgenic Steroids. *Report of the National Consensus Meeting on Anabolic/Androgenic Steroids.* Los Angeles, Calif: US Olympic Committee; 1989.

12. Buckley WE, Yesalis CE, Friedl KE, et al. Estimated prevalence of anabolic steroid use among high school seniors. *JAMA.* 1988;260:3441-3445.

13. Shroyer J. Getting tough on anabolic steroids. *Phys Sports Med.* 1990;18:106-118.

Escherichia coli Bacteremia in Children

A Review of 91 Cases in 10 Years

William A. Bonadio, MD; Douglas S. Smith, MD; Elisabeth Madagame, MD; Jane Machi, MD; Narendra Kini, MD

• We reviewed 91 cases of pediatric *Escherichia coli* bacteremia during a 10-year period. Thirty one patients were afebrile; a significantly greater proportion of these patients were aged less than 1 month, had ampicillin-resistant *E coli* isolates, or had persistent bacteremia 24 hours after initiating antibiotic therapy. Infection was community acquired in 65 cases; associated urinary tract infection was six times more common in this setting than in nosocomially acquired infections. In 85 cases at least 1 underlying medical condition/focus of infection was identified at the time the positive blood culture was obtained, the most common were immune deficiency states (38 cases), urinary tract infection (29 cases), and lesions of the gastrointestinal tract (27 cases). Polymicrobial bacteremia occurred in five cases. Twelve patients died; significantly associated with death were hypotension requiring pressor therapy, presence of a central venous catheter, and neutropenia.

(*AJDC*. 1991;145:671-674)

Escherichia coli is a gram-negative bacterium of the family Enterobacteriaceae, which has been shown to be a common cause of gram-negative sepsis in adults,[1,2] in children with underlying malignant neoplasms,[3,4] and in pediatric nosocomial infection.[3] *Escherichia coli* bacteremia in children is a potentially serious infection, as evidenced by the 60% associated mortality reported in one study.[3]

Information regarding pediatric *E coli* bacteremia is limited; most studies related to this infection have either examined specific patient populations[1,5] or described associated clinical characteristics within the larger context of gram-negative bacteremia.[2,3] We conducted a computer-assisted medical literature search of the past 20 years and were not able to identify a study that specifically described a large series of children with *E coli* bacteremia.

The purpose of this study was to delineate the clinical characteristics and outcomes of a large series of children with *E coli* bacteremia.

PATIENTS AND METHODS

We reviewed the results of consecutive blood cultures at Children's Hospital of Wisconsin, Milwaukee, from 1980 to 1990. Identified were instances in which the isolate was *E coli*. Microbiologic identification of these organisms was performed by standard methods.[6] Routine in vitro testing for susceptibility of isolates to a standard panel of antibiotics (which included ampicillin and gentamicin in all cases) was performed by means of the Kirby-Bauer disk method.[7] The medical records of all patients were reviewed, and all contained the following information: patient age/race/sex; underlying medical condition; current medications; symptoms; vital signs, physical findings, and results of laboratory tests performed at the time the positive blood culture was obtained; culture and sensitivity results; treatment received; subsequent clinical course; and outcome.

Fever was considered to have occurred when the body temperature was greater than 38.0°C during the 24-hour period of hospitalization before the original positive blood culture was obtained. Infection that occurred after 72 hours of hospitalization was considered nosocomially acquired. *Escherichia coli* bacteremia occurred when the organism was (1) the sole isolate from a single blood sample (both culture media) collected from a peripheral vein or artery when associated with an acute illness or (2) an isolate in two or more separate blood cultures when associated with another organism. Patients with *E coli* and a different organism isolated from a single blood culture were excluded from study unless these bacteriologic findings were confirmed by a subsequent blood culture (then consistent with polymicrobial bacteremia). Blood cultures positive for *E coli* obtained through a central venous or arterial catheter were considered consistent with bacteremia only if corroborated by an additional positive blood culture obtained from a peripheral vessel. Preceding antibiotic therapy was administered when a patient received parenteral antibiotics within 72 hours before the the initial positive blood culture was obtained. Persistent bacteremia occurred when *E coli* was isolated in two or more separate blood cultures obtained at least 24 hours apart. Neutropenia occurred when the peripheral absolute neutrophil count was less than 1.0×10^9/L. Death was associated with *E coli* bacteremia if it occurred while patients received treatment for this infection, unless clear clinical and pathologic data suggested otherwise.

The 11 variables analyzed included the following: mortality, presence of fever, presence of urinary tract infection, nosocomially acquired infection, hypotension requiring pressor therapy, presence of a central venous catheter, persistent bacteremia, isolate sensitivity to ampicillin, patient receiving care in an intensive care unit, preceding antibiotic therapy, and patient age less than 1 month. We chose the outcome variables to address the clinical questions of interest; they included mortality and presence of fever. Univariate analysis comparing these variables with all other variables was performed by means of χ^2 or Fisher's Exact Test where appropriate (the significant variables are given in Table 1). Many of these variables were not independent of one another. Spearman's correlation coefficients were determined along with *P* values for each correlation. Significant correlations

Accepted for publication January 25, 1991.
From the Medical College of Wisconsin, Children's Hospital of Wisconsin, Milwaukee.

Reprint requests to 1240 Pioneer Trail, Waukesha, WI 53186 (Dr Bonadio).

Table 1.—Univariate Analysis*

Significant Variable	*P*
Mortality	
Hypotension requiring pressor therapy	.0015
Neutropenia	.016
Persistent bacteremia	.024
Presence of central venous catheter	.029
Nosocomial infection	.34
Preceding antibiotic therapy	.35
Fever	
Age<1 mo	.001
Ampicillin-resistant isolate	.001
Persistent bacteremia	.0039
Hypotension requiring pressor therapy	.012

*By χ^2 or Fisher's Exact Tests.

Table 2.—Spearman's Correlation Coefficients

Variables	Coefficient	*P*
Preceding antibiotic therapy/ nosocomial infection	.51168	.0001
Neutropenia/persistent bacteremia	.33819	.0010
Preceding antibiotic therapy/ persistent bacteremia	.30085	.0038
Preceding antibiotic therapy/ neutropenia	.22421	.0326
Central venous catheter/ nosocomial infection	.22404	.0328
Hypotension requiring pressor therapy/ age <1 mo	.21463	.0411

Table 3.—Stepwise Logistic Regression

Significant Variable	Odds Ratio	95% Confidence Interval
Mortality		
Hypotension requiring pressor therapy	14.45	2.80,74.44
Central venous catheter	14.89	1.70,130.64
Neutropenia	5.57	1.15,26.92
Fever		
Ampicillin-resistant isolate	9.17	2.61,32.17
Age <1 mo	0.10	0.029,0.35
Persistent bacteremia	14.64	2.15,99.56

among those variables significant in the univariate analysis are given in Table 2. Stepwise logistic regression analysis was then performed to control for this confounding; this analysis allows identification of variables that are independently significant after the effects of all others are controlled. These variables are given in Table 3 along with their odds ratios and 95% confidence intervals derived from the logistic coefficients and SEs.

RESULTS

During the study period, 4685 blood cultures were positive for bacterial isolates in 84 331 hospitalized patients. *Escherichia coli* accounted for 101 isolates (2%); 10 cases were eliminated from study because only a single positive blood culture yielded both *E coli* and at least one other organism.

There were 91 cases that met the study criteria for *E coli* bacteremia; their clinical characteristics are given in Table 4. The distribution of cases by season was 27 in spring (April through June), 29 in summer (July through September), 13 in autumn (October through December), and 22 in winter (January through March). All patients who survived at least 24 hours after the original positive blood culture was obtained had one or more additional blood culture performed. After the original positive blood culture was obtained and antibiotic therapy to which the organism exhibited in vitro sensitivity was initiated, 10 patients had persistent *E coli* bacteremia. The other isolates associated with the five cases of *E coli* polymicrobial bacteremia were *Enterobacter cloacae* (two cases), enterococcus, *Klebsiella pneumoniae*, and *Acinetobacter anitratus*; all five patients had persistent *E coli* bacteremia after antibiotic therapy to which the organism exhibited in vitro sensitivity was initiated, and one of these patients died. *Escherichia coli* isolates were sensitive to an aminoglycoside in all instances and to ampicillin in 62 instances; 29 isolates were resistant to ampicillin. Other sources of *E coli* isolates were urine (29 patients; 14 were aged <2 months and 27 had community-acquired infection), cerebrospinal fluid (eight patients; six were aged <1 month, four of whom were afebrile), indwelling central venous catheter (six patients), peritoneal fluid (seven patients), and abscess drainage (three patients).

Table 4.—Clinical Characteristics of Patients With *Escherichia coli* Bacteremia

Variable	No. of Patients
Patient age	
0-1 mo	33
1-2 mo	6
2-12 mo	18
1-5 y	10
5-10 y	4
10-18 y	20
Sex	
M	44
F	47
Race	
W	64
B	21
Hispanic	6
Abnormal clinical findings when positive blood culture obtained*	
Ill/toxic appearance	84
Fever	58
Respiratory rate >60/min	25
Heart rate >180 beats/min	24
Hypotension requiring pressor therapy	13†
Disseminated intravascular coagulation	10
Apnea	8
Nosocomial infection	26‡

*At least one finding was exhibited by each of the 91 patients.
†Seven aged less than 1 month.
‡Thirteen aged less than 12 months and eight aged 10 to 18 years.

The 117 underlying conditions/foci of infection identified at the time the original positive blood culture was obtained are given in Table 5. Of 20 patients aged 10 to 18 years, 15 had an immune deficiency, whereas five of 57 patients less than 12 months of age had a similar condition

Table 5.—Underlying Conditions/Foci of Infection Identified When the Original Positive Blood Culture for *Escherichia coli* Was Obtained

Condition/Foci of Infection	No. of Patients
Immune deficiency	
Neutropenia	19
Malignant neoplasm/received chemotherapy within 2 wk of presentation	17
Sickle cell disease	2
Urinary tract infection	29
Gastrointestinal tract lesion	
Gastroenteritis	7
Perforated bowel/peritonitis	7
Typhlitis	5
Hepatic failure/ascites	3
Cholangitis	2
Intra-abdominal abscess	1
Necrotizing enterocolitis	1
Bowel obstruction	1
Bacterial meningitis	8
Central venous catheter	5
Pneumonia*	5
Cutaneous lesion	
Cellulitis	2
Abscess	2
Osteomyelitis	1
None identified	6

*Roentgenographic presence of pulmonary infiltrate per pediatric radiologist.

identified. The clinical characteristics of patients with underlying malignant neoplasms and *E coli* bacteremia are given in Table 6.

COMMENT

In our series, the isolation of *E coli* by blood culture was rarely classified as a contaminant, as 90% of instances fulfilled the criteria for clinical sepsis. The frequency of this infection was one per 1000 hospitalized patients and did not exhibit a distinct seasonal distribution. The majority of patients with *E coli* bacteremia were young; two thirds were younger than than 12 months, and one third were younger than 1 month. At the time the original positive blood culture was obtained, patients were febrile in only 64% of cases and required pressor therapy for hypotension in 14% of cases; both rates are lower than those previously documented in a series[3] of children with gram-negative sepsis, in which 91% had fever and 25% had septic shock.

Certain distinctions were noted in the clinical characteristics of children with *E coli* bacteremia related to patient age. Most patients younger than 12 months experienced community-acquired infection (78%) and had no associated immune deficiency identified (91%). By contrast, the majority of patients aged 10 to 18 years had an associated underlying immune deficiency (75%), and nearly one half had nosocomially acquired infection. Very young infants were a distinct subgroup with regard to clinical characteristics and outcome. Compared with those older than 1 month, neonates were significantly more likely to present without fever; specifically, four of six neonates with *E coli* meningitis had an afebrile presentation. *Escherichia coli* sepsis could be a particularly fulminant process in neonates, as evidenced by the fact that these patients accounted for over one half of all instances of hypotension requiring pressor therapy.

Table 6.—Clinical Characteristics of 17 Children With Malignant Neoplasms and *Escherichia coli* Bacteremia

Characteristic	No. (%)
Received chemotherapy within 2 wk of presentation	17 (100)
Neutropenia	15 (88)
Aged 10-18 y	13 (76)
Fever	13 (76)
Ampicillin-resistant isolate	10 (60)
Identified portal of infection	8 (47)
Nosocomially acquired infection	6 (35)
Death	5 (29)
Persistent bacteremia	4 (24)
Antibiotic therapy being received when positive blood culture obtained	3 (17)
Hypotension requiring pressor therapy	2 (11)
Polymicrobial bacteremia	1 (6)

Escherichia coli bacteremia was nosocomially acquired in 29% of cases, much lower than the 76% rate of nosocomially acquired pediatric *E coli* bacteremia described by DuPont and Spink.[3] Underlying medical conditions or foci of infection were identified in 90% of cases of pediatric *E coli* bacteremia at the time the original positive blood culture was obtained, which is greater than the 60% rate previously reported.[3] The most frequent were immune deficiencies, urinary tract infections, and lesions of the gastrointestinal tract. In accord with this trend were the findings by DuPont and Spink[3] that underlying malignant neoplasm (with administration of immunosuppressive agents) was the most common chronic disorder associated with pediatric gram-negative sepsis and that the two most commonly identified portals of infection associated with pediatric *E coli* sepsis were the genitourinary and gastrointestinal tracts. A previous series of another cause of pediatric gram-negative bacteremia (*K pneumoniae*[8]) showed a common association with both underlying gastrointestinal tract lesions and immune deficiencies; yet, by comparison with *E coli* bacteremia, sepsis due to this other pathogen was rarely associated (5%) with urinary tract infection. *Escherichia coli* urosepsis was common in young infants, being documented in one third of all patients aged less than 2 months with *E coli* bacteremia.

Escherichia coli has been shown to be one of the most common causes of bacteremia experienced by patients with underlying malignant neoplasms.[4,9] In our series, this pathogen was especially prevalent in children with hematologic malignant neoplasms who received chemotherapy within 2 weeks of the bacteremic episode. The majority of patients with malignant neoplasms were older (76% were aged 10 to 18 years); although the majority of isolates were ampicillin resistant (60%), only one third of infections were nosocomially acquired, and only 17% of patients had been receiving antibiotic therapy at the time the original positive blood culture was obtained. Compared with a previous series of adults with malignant neoplasms and *E coli* sepsis,[9] we found comparable rates of children with persistent bacteremia (24% vs 25%, respectively), fever (96% vs 76%), and an identified portal of infection (51% vs 47%). By contrast with the same series,[10] we found a higher rate of associated neutropenia (52% vs 88%, respectively) and only one half the rate of hypotension requiring pressor therapy. The mortality in our group with underlying malignant neoplasms and *E coli* sepsis was 29%, which was lower than both the 40% mortality for sepsis (all causes) associated with childhood malignant neoplasms[4] and the 73% mortality for gram-negative sepsis in children with malignant neoplasms receiving immunosuppressive therapy.[3]

Certain clinical features were predictive of the outcome of children with *E coli* bacteremia. Patients who were afebrile when the positive blood culture was obtained were more likely to experience a complicated clinical course; compared with those manifesting fever, they experienced significantly greater rates of both persistent bacteremia despite the administration of antibiotics to which the isolate exhibited in vitro sensitivity and ampicillin-resistant isolates. Afebrile presentation is perhaps an index of inadequate host response to *E coli* bacteremia, in that it was significantly associated with the individual variables of neutropenia and persistent bacteremia. Despite this, we did not find a significant difference in mortality between children with and without fever on presentation, which contrasts with the findings of a previous study of adults with *E coli* bacteremia[10] that also compared like presentations. Finally, polymicrobial bacteremia in which *E coli* was a constituent was rare, occurring in only 5% of cases; the mortality observed in this group was not significantly different from that associated with monomicrobial *E coli* bacteremia (although the sample examined was small).

The overall mortality associated with pediatric *E coli* bacteremia was 12%, which is much lower than the 60% mortality reported by DuPont and Spink.[3] The three independent clinical characteristics significantly associated with death were hypotension requiring pressor therapy, presence of a central venous catheter, and neutropenia at the time the original positive blood culture was obtained. A significantly greater mortality was demonstrated in adults with *E coli* sepsis who experienced shock,[3,10] yet the significantly greater mortality in neutropenic than nonneutropenic children with *E coli* bacteremia contrasts with the findings of two previous series of adults with *E coli* bacteremia.[3,10]

References

1. Gardener P, Carles DG. Infections acquired in a pediatric hospital. *J Pediatr.* 1972;81:1205-1210.
2. Kreger BE, Craven DE, Carling PC, McCabe WR. Gram-negative bacteremia, III: reassessment of etiology, epidemiology and ecology in 612 patients. *Am J Med.* 1980;68:332-343.
3. DuPont HL, Spink WW. Infections due to gram-negative organisms: an analysis of 860 patients with bacteremia at the University of Minnesota Medical Center, 1958-1966. *Medicine.* 1969;48:307-322.
4. Miser JS, Miser AW, Bleyer WA, Chard RL. Septicemia in childhood malignancy: analysis of 101 consecutive episodes. *Clin Pediatr.* 1981;20:320-323.
5. Shapiro ED, Wald ER, Spiegelman KN. Broviac catheter–related bacteremia in oncology patients. *AJDC.* 1982;136:679-681.
6. Lynnette EH, Spaulding EH, Truant J, eds. *Manual of Clinical Microbiology.* 2nd ed. Washington, DC: American Society for Microbiology; 1974:74-82.
7. Bauer AW, Kirby WM, Sherris JC, et al. Antibiotic susceptibility testing by a standard single disk method. *Am J Clin Pathol.* 1966;45:493-496.
8. Bonadio WA. *Klebsiella pneumoniae* bacteremia in children: a 12-year experience. *AJDC.* 1989;143:178-181.
9. Bodey GP, Elting L, Kassamali H, Lim BP. *Escherichia coli* bacteremia in cancer patients. *Am J Med.* 1986;81:85-95.
10. Kreger BE, Craven DE, McCabe WR. Gram-negative bacteremia, IV: re-evaluation of clinical features and treatment in 612 patients. *Am J Med.* 1980;68:344-355.

In Other AMA Journals

ARCHIVES OF SURGERY

Surgical Care for the Uninsured and Underinsured

Claude H. Organ, Jr, MD
(*Arch Surg.* 1991;126:549-550)

The Underinsured and the Uninsured

Maria D. Allo, MD
(*Arch Surg.* 1991;126:551)

Inflammatory Pseudotumor in Childhood: A Diagnostic and Therapeutic Dilemma

Enrique Freud, MD; Ron Bilik, MD, MS; Isaac Yaniv, MD;
Gadi Horev, MD; David Cohen, MD;
Marc Mimouni, MD; Michael Zer, MD
(*Arch Surg.* 1991;126:653-655)

Factors Associated With Umbilical Catheter-Related Sepsis in Neonates

Susan Landers, MD; Alicia A. Moise, MD; J. Kennard Fraley, MPH; E. O'Brian Smith, PhD; Carol J. Baker, MD

• To determine factors associated with risk for umbilical catheter-related sepsis, we studied neonates with one or more catheters in place for more than 3 days. Among 225 infants with 357 umbilical catheters, catheter-related sepsis occurred in 14 infants (6%). Catheter-related sepsis occurred in 5% of infants with umbilical arterial catheters and in 3% of infants with umbilical venous catheters. Staphylococcal species accounted for 71% of cases of catheter-related sepsis. Multiple logistic regression analysis revealed that very low birth weight and longer duration of antibiotic therapy were significantly associated with risk for umbilical arterial catheter-related sepsis. Increased risk for umbilical venous catheter-related sepsis was best predicted by the simultaneous occurrence of higher birth weight and infusion of hyperalimentation solution. Catheter duration correlated with duration of antibiotic therapy and with infusion of hyperalimentation solution for both types of catheters; however, in the multivariable analysis, duration of catheterization was not found to be a significant independent predictor of risk for catheter-related sepsis for either type of catheter.
(*AJDC.* 1991;145:675-680)

Umbilical arterial catheters (UACs) and umbilical venous catheters (UVCs) provide convenient access to sick neonates. However, these catheters are associated with serious infectious complications, such as nosocomial bacteremia or sepsis. The prevalence of umbilical catheter–related sepsis (CRS) among newborns varies from 3% to 16%.[1-4] Umbilical catheter colonization rates have been reported to be as high as 60%.[4-6]

Because little is known about the factors influencing CRS associated with umbilical catheters, especially in the extremely preterm infant, we sought to determine these risk factors in our neonatal intensive care unit (NICU). We evaluated numerous clinical variables in an effort to identify predictors of CRS and potentially to establish methods for the prevention of CRS in neonates.

SUBJECTS AND METHODS

Subjects

All neonates admitted to the NICU from March 1, 1984, to March 31, 1985, who required umbilical artery and/or venous catheterization for more than 72 hours were studied. Physicians caring for the infants determined the need for catheterization. Most UACs were inserted for blood gas monitoring in neonates with respiratory distress or premature neonates. Most UVCs were placed for administration of fluids and medications to very-low-birth-weight (VLBW) infants (ie, those weighing <1500 g at birth).

Accepted for publication February 8, 1991.

From the Department of Pediatrics, Baylor College of Medicine and Jefferson Davis Hospital, Houston, Tex.

Reprint requests to the Department of Pediatrics, Baylor College of Medicine, One Baylor Plaza, Houston, TX 77030 (Dr Landers).

Catheter Insertion and Maintenance

Physicians working in the NICU used uniform technique for catheter insertion and maintenance and routinely obtained catheter surveillance cultures, as recommended by the hospital infection control committee.

The umbilicus was disinfected with povidone-iodine solution, excess solution was removed from the skin, and each catheter was inserted with use of sterile technique and secured with sterile suture and tape. Polyvinyl chloride catheters (Argyle Umbilical Vessel Catheter, Sherwood Medical, St Louis, Mo) were used exclusively. The UACs were placed with the tip at the third or fourth lumbar vertebral interspace, and the UVCs were placed in the inferior vena cava at the level of the diaphragm or in the umbilical vein below the liver. Catheter position was confirmed roentgenographically, and improperly positioned catheters were repositioned. The umbilicus remained uncovered, and povidone-iodine solution was applied every 4 hours. All catheter infusates and connecting tubes were changed daily.

Antimicrobial prophylaxis was not given for catheterization. Instead, antibiotics were administered when infection was suspected clinically. Antibiotic therapy included ampicillin and gentamicin for infections acquired before 3 days of life and vancomycin and amikacin with or without ampicillin, ticarcillin, or clindamycin for infections of later onset.

Catheters were infused with 5% or 10% dextrose solution, normal saline solution, or hyperalimentation solution. Each solution contained 1 U of heparin sodium per milliliter. Central strength hyperalimentation fluid contained 20% dextrose, and peripheral strength hyperalimentation fluid contained 12.5% or less. All catheters were infused continuously, except when flushed with heparinized saline after withdrawal of blood samples. Entries into all umbilical catheters were kept at a minimum; however, catheters were used for blood sampling and administration of medications (eg, antibiotics, sodium bicarbonate, and calcium gluceptate) and blood products.

Catheters remaining in place for longer than 7 days were maintained predominantly for infusion of hyperalimentation solutions. Only peripheral strength solutions were infused through UACs. Umbilical venous catheters infusing central strength hyperalimentation solution into the right atrium were entered only for daily solution changes.

Catheter Surveillance Cultures

Weekly surveillance blood cultures were obtained from infants whose catheters were maintained for longer than 7 days. The stopcock was disinfected with povidone-iodine solution, and

Table 1.—Cross-Tabulation of Catheter Status and Culture Data*

	Infants With UAC				
	• UAC Cultured	• UAC Not Cultured	No UAC	Total No. of Infants Cultured	Total No. of Infants
Infants with UVC					
• UVC cultured	108†‡	24†	12	144	179
• UVC not cultured	35‡	. . .	. . .	. . .	
No UVC	46	. . .	. . .	. . .	
Total No. of Infants Cultured	189	. . .	. . .	. . .	. . .
Total No. of infants	213		. . .		225

*UAC indicates umbilical arterial catheter; UVC, umbilical venous catheter.

†Infants with UVC cultured and a simultaneous UAC: 108+24=132.

‡Infants with UAC cultured and a simultaneous UVC: 108+35=143. Infants with both a UAC and UVC: 108+24+35=167.

1 mL of blood was withdrawn through the catheter and placed in thioglycollate broth. When any surveillance catheter culture was positive, a blood culture was obtained from a peripheral vessel within 24 to 48 hours. The catheter was maintained only if the infant remained asymptomatic and the subsequent peripheral blood culture was sterile. Catheters were maintained in infants treated for early-onset sepsis (sepsis occurring during the first 3 days of life) who had negative blood cultures following therapy and in whom the catheter was necessary for care.

Catheters were removed when (1) an infant with a positive surveillance culture either manifested clinical signs of sepsis or had a confirmatory positive peripheral blood culture, (2) the catheter was no longer needed for care, or (3) a noninfectious complication of catheterization occurred. When a catheter was removed, the tip was cut off with sterile scissors and placed in thioglycollate broth. All surveillance cultures were processed by standard bacteriologic methods for identification of isolates and their antimicrobial susceptibility.

Definitions

A "culture-negative" infant was one in whom all surveillance blood and catheter tip cultures were sterile and who remained asymptomatic. A "colonized infant" was an infant with a positive surveillance catheter blood culture or catheter tip culture, who also had a sterile peripheral blood culture and who was not clinically ill.[7,8] An infant was diagnosed as having CRS when the infant was clinically ill with no other obvious source for bacteremia and had either a positive blood culture obtained through the catheter and a peripheral blood culture positive for the same organism[7,9,10] or had cultures of the catheter tip and the peripheral blood positive for the same organism.[8,11]

Clinical Variables

We recorded birth weight, number and duration of catheterization(s), simultaneous UAC and UVC placement, predominant catheter infusate, type and duration of antimicrobial therapy, and all noninfectious complications for each infant. For infants with multiple catheters, the sum of days duration for each catheter was considered the total duration of catheterization. If more than one infusate was used, the solution that was infused for the longest time was analyzed. Only antibiotics administered before final catheter removal or before onset of documented CRS were analyzed. Noninfectious, thrombotic, or vasospastic catheter-related events consisted of any occurrence of dampened blood pressure wave form, clotted catheter, pale or cyanotic "catheter toes," decreased pulses, or altered perfusion distal to the catheter for which a catheter was removed or replaced.

Statistical Methods

All data are expressed as mean and SD or as percentages and their 95% confidence intervals (CIs). Potential factors associated with CRS were analyzed for UACs and UVCs separately. Categorical variables were analyzed by χ^2, and continuous variables were analyzed by t test.

To determine the independent contribution of each variable and which variable(s) best predicted CRS, multiple logistic regression analysis was performed. The multivariable analysis adjusted for possible correlations between variables and served to overcome the inflation in type I error associated with repeated univariate significance testing. The occurence of CRS was the dependent variable and was regressed on all other independent variables. The data from infants with UACs were analyzed separately from data from infants with UVCs. Simultaneous UAC and UVC catheterization was included as one of the variables, so that for each infant the presence of both types of catheters was analyzed as a confounding variable.

RESULTS

Frequency of CRS and Demographic Data

Two hundred twenty-five infants had one or more catheters in place for longer than 72 hours. Their mean birth weight was 1560 g (SD, 865 g), with a range of 620 to 4700 g. Twenty-three percent weighed less than 1000 g, 50% weighed 1001 to 1500 g, 9% weighed 1501 to 2000 g, and 18% weighed more than 2001 g. Their mean gestational age was 31.3 weeks (SD, 4.1 weeks).

Fourteen infants developed CRS (14/225 [6%]). Ten had CRS associated with a UAC and four had CRS associated with a UVC. Thirty-nine percent of infants (87/225) were colonized, and 55% (124/225) had sterile surveillance cultures.

Overall, the infants had 1.6 (SD, 0.8) catheters each, with a range of one to six catheters. Twenty percent (46/225) of infants had a UAC only, 75% (167/225) had both a UAC and a UVC, and 5% (12/225) had a UVC only. Culture data were available for analysis from 189 of the 213 infants with UACs and from 144 of the 179 infants with UVCs. Table 1 presents a cross-tabulation of the infants' catheter status and available catheter culture data. To describe the prevalence of CRS and to determine risk factors for CRS, the multivariable analysis examined only data from those infants with catheters and available culture data. The multivariable analysis examined data from infants (cultured) for each catheter type separately (UAC and UVC) and accounted for simultaneous UAC and UVC catheterization as a confounding variable within the analysis. Repeated analysis of the same infants did not occur, except for those infants who had simultaneous UAC and UVC catheterization and culture data available for each catheter type. At the time of diagnosis of CRS, exact catheter status was known for each of the 10 infants with UAC-related CRS and each of the four infants with UVC-related CRS, and their catheter status did not change during either analysis.

The prevalence of CRS among infants with UACs was 5% (10/189) and among those with UVCs was 3% (4/144). Catheter colonization was noted more often among infants with UACs (76/189 [40%]) than UVCs (32/144 [22%]) ($P<.002$). Colonization of either catheter type occurred more often among infants who weighed more than 1500 g at birth (31/61 [51%]) than among VLBW neonates (56/164 [34%]) ($P<.03$).

Simultaneous UAC and UVC catheterization was common. Seventy-five percent of infants had both a UAC and a UVC in place at some time. However, the majority of

Table 2.—Variables Assessed as Potential Risk Factors for UAC-Related CRS*

Risk Factor	UAC-Related CRS	No CRS	Univariate Significance	Multivariate Significance
Catheter duration, d	16.9 (8.9)	10.7 (7.0)	$P=.059$	NS
Birth weight, g [range]	959 (221) [620-1270]	1609 (874) [660-4700]	$P<.001$	$P<.02$
VLBW infants	10/10 (100)	127/179 (71)	. . .	. . .
Antibiotic therapy, d	9.7 (4.5)	5.0 (3.6)	$P<.01$	$P<.02$
Antibiotics at catheter removal	7/10 (70) [34-94]	40/179 (22) [16-29]	$P<.001$	$P<.02$
Hyperalimentation infusate	7/10 (70) [34-94]	47/179 (26) [19-33]	$P<.01$	NS
Vascular complication	6/10 (60) [25-88]	44/179 (25) [19-32]	$P<.05$	NS
Total No. of catheters per infant	2.5 (1.1)	2.1 (0.8)	NS	NS
Simultaneous UAC and UVC catheterization	8/10 (80) [42-98]	135/179 (75) [68-82]	NS	NS

*UAC indicates umbilical arterial catheter; CRS, catheter-related sepsis; VLBW, very-low-birth-weight; NS, not significant ($P>.05$); and UVC, umbilical venous catheter. Data are mean (SD) or number/total number (percent); values in brackets are 95% confidence interval, unless otherwise stated.
†Univariate analysis by t test for continuous variables, and χ^2 test for categorical variables.

infants who developed CRS had only one type of catheter in place when CRS was diagnosed; the other catheter had been removed days previously. Among the 10 infants with UAC-related CRS, two had a UAC alone and eight had both a UAC and a UVC at some time. Six of these eight infants with UAC-related CRS had a UVC simultaneously, but had both catheters cultured so that it was possible to ascertain which catheter had caused the CRS, or their UVC had been removed days earlier with negative surveillance cultures at that time. In the other two infants with UAC-related CRS, the UVC had been removed more than 4 days previously, although it was not cultured. Similarly, among the four infants with UVC-related CRS, one infant had a UVC alone; the other three infants had both UAC and UVC cultured at the time of diagnosis of UVC-related CRS (two of the three) or their UAC had been removed days earlier. So, for each case of CRS, despite simultaneous UAC and UVC catheterization, adequate culture data were available or the other catheter had been removed days previously, permitting accurate assessment of catheter status and diagnosis of CRS.

Sixty-five percent of catheters were removed electively (the catheter was no longer needed for care). Twenty-two percent were removed because of a noninfectious, vascular complication. Thirteen percent fell out accidentally or were removed for other reasons, such as necrotizing enterocolitis. Culture-proven early-onset sepsis was not an indication for catheter removal.

Causative Agents

Staphylococci were the most common isolates from infants with colonized catheters (80%) and from those who developed CRS (10/14 [71%]). Coagulase-negative staphylococci were the most frequent cause of CRS (6/14 [43%]). *Staphylococcus aureus* (4/14 [28%]) and gram-negative bacilli (3/14 [21%]) accounted for the majority of the other cases of CRS. One case of CRS was due to *Candida* species. During the period of study, 67% of coagulase-negative staphylococcal isolates from all neonatal blood and cerebrospinal fluid cultures were resistant to methicillin, while 100% of isolates causing CRS were methicillin resistant ($P<.02$).

Surveillance Cultures

Eighty-two surveillance blood cultures were drawn through catheters remaining in place for longer than 7 days. Sixteen cultures were positive, six of which accurately identified CRS. The sensitivity and specificity of this surveillance method were 67% (95% CI, 30% to 92%) and 86% (95% CI, 75% to 94%), respectively. The positive predictive value calculated for catheter blood cultures was 37% (95% CI, 14% to 65%).[12]

There were 121 positive catheter tip cultures among the 351 tip cultures obtained. Only 12 of the positive tip cultures accurately identified CRS. For the diagnosis of CRS, this method of surveillance had a sensitivity of 92% (95% CI, 63% to 99%) and a specificity of 68% (95% CI, 63% to 72%). A very low positive predictive value of 10% (95% CI, 5% to 17%) was found for catheter tip cultures.[12]

Analysis of Risk Factors for UAC-Related CRS

Table 2 summarizes the factors evaluated by both univariate and multiple logistic regression analyses. The multivariable analysis revealed that VLBW was the best predictor of risk for CRS in infants with UACs ($P<.02$). Duration of antibiotic therapy and antibiotic therapy at catheter removal were also significant, although interchangeable, in their ability to predict risk for CRS ($P<.02$). The odds of an infant developing CRS if he or she had received antibiotics at the time of UAC removal were 6.2 times that if he or she had not. The odds of developing CRS were 1.2 times greater for each day of antibiotic administration.

Prolonged UAC catheterization was not found to be significant as an independent risk factor for CRS after birth weight and antibiotic therapy were introduced into the multivariable analysis. Duration of UAC correlated with both duration of antibiotic therapy ($r=.651$, $P<.001$) and with use of hyperalimentation solution ($r=.616$). Similarly, infusion of hyperalimentation solution through a UAC was not significant as an independent risk factor for CRS after adjusting for other variables. Although birth weight correlated inversely with the total number of catheters ($r=-.264$, $P<.001$), neither simultaneous UVC catheterization nor multiple UAC catheterizations was significant as an independent risk factor for CRS in the multivariable analysis.

Table 3 summarizes the relationship between several of the independent variables that were correlated. Umbilical arterial catheters infused with hyperalimentation fluid

Table 3.—Relationships Between Selected Risk Factors*

	Hyperalimentation Solution	No Hyperalimentation Solution	Univariate Significance†
Variables for UAC-related CRS			
Birth weight, g	1206 (654)	1722 (895)	$P<.001$
Antibiotic duration, d	7.4 (4.5)	4.4 (3.1)	$P<.001$
Catheter duration, d	18.0 (7.6)	8.2 (4.7)	$P<.001$
Variables for UVC-related CRS			
Birth weight, g	1858 (1248)	1262 (513)	$P<.02$
Antibiotic duration, d	6.6 (4.9)	4.3 (2.2)	$P<.02$
Catheter duration, d	12.5 (5.4)	6.8 (2.1)	$P<.001$

*Data are mean (SD). UAC indicates umbilical arterial catheters; CRS, catheter-related sepsis; and UVC, umbilical venous catheters.
†Univariate analysis by two-sample *t* test.

were maintained longer than those that infused other solutions. In addition, smaller infants tended to have hyperalimentation fluid infused through their UACs. These correlations probably explain why UAC infusion with hyperalimentation fluid was associated significantly with CRS in the univariate but not in the multivariable analysis.

Because duration of antibiotic therapy was a significant predictor of risk for UAC-related CRS, we examined why infants with UACs received prolonged antibiotic therapy. Among infants with UACs, 12% (23/189) received antibiotic therapy for more than 10 days. Culture-proven early-onset sepsis was the indication in 26% (6/23) of cases. Clinical suspicion of sepsis (without positive cultures) or nosocomial pneumonia were indications in 74% (17/23) of cases.

Analysis of Risk Factors for UVC-Related CRS

Factors evaluated by both univariate analysis and multiple logistic regression analysis are summarized in Table 4. The multivariable analysis revealed that overall risk of UVC-related CRS was greatest for infants with higher birth weight ($P<.05$). In addition, the presence of two factors interacting—birth weight and infusion of hyperalimentation solution—was significant as a predictor of risk for UVC-related CRS ($P<.05$).

Duration of UVC catheterization was not a significant independent predictor of risk for CRS after antibiotic therapy and hyperalimentation fluid were accounted for in the multivariable analysis. Risk for UVC-related CRS was not influenced significantly by duration of antibiotic therapy, multiple or simultaneous catheterizations, or the occurrence of vascular complications.

Table 3 illustrates that UVC infusion with hyperalimentation fluid correlated with birth weight and with catheter duration ($r=.321$ and $r=.607$ [$P<.001$], respectively). Larger infants tended to have UVCs infused with hyperalimentation fluid. Infants with hyperalimentation fluid infusing through their UVCs were catheterized longer than those who had other solutions infused.

COMMENT

Few data are available concerning CRS or bacteremia associated with umbilical catheters,[1-5] especially for VLBW neonates who require catheters for more than a few days. In our study, CRS occurred in 6% of infants who required catheterization for more than 3 days. As expected, the majority of these were VLBW infants. Utilizing a similar definition of CRS, Bard et al[2] reported a frequency of 3%, but most of the 75 infants in their study had catheters in place for less than 4 days and weighed more than 1500 g. In our study, infants tended to develop CRS from UACs slightly more frequently (5%) than from UVCs (3%), but this difference was not statistically significant. Similarly, Hall and Rhodes[3] analyzed CRS by umbilical vessel site and found a frequency of UAC-related CRS of 16% and a frequency of UVC-related CRS of 11%.

As with catheter-related infections in older patients, the most common causative agents for umbilical CRS in neonates were staphylococci. Coagulase-negative staphylococci were the most frequent isolates, and all were resistant to methicillin but susceptible to vancomycin. Coagulase-negative staphylococci frequently cause nosocomial sepsis in VLBW neonates, and most strains are resistant to methicillin.[9,13,14] In adults with central venous catheters, *Staphylococcus epidermidis* is the most frequent organism colonizing catheters and causing CRS.[8,15] The virulence properties of certain strains, their antibiotic resistance patterns, and the immature immunologic status of neonates all account for their prevalence in causing CRS.[9,16] Properties of the umbilical catheter itself may be influential, as slime-producing coagulase-negative staphylococci preferentially adhere to surface irregularities of the polyvinyl chloride catheter and account for a majority of CRS isolates.[17,18] Other cases of CRS in our study were due to *S aureus*, gram-negative bacilli, and *Candida* species, agents commonly causing CRS in adults.[8]

A major finding in our study was that risk for CRS from UACs was related to both VLBW and longer duration of antibiotic therapy. Other reports have documented the higher risk for nosocomial sepsis among VLBW infants.[14,19,20] However, the influence of prolonged antibiotic therapy on the risk for CRS has not been described, to our knowledge. Prolonged antibiotic therapy may increase the risk for CRS by increasing the prevalence of resistant organisms, or it may be a marker for overall severity of illness and susceptibility to infection. Bard et al[2] noted that prophylactic antibiotics given for umbilical catheterization decreased catheter colonization but did not prevent CRS. In our study, prolonged administration of broad-spectrum antibiotic therapy was associated with increased risk for CRS predominantly among VLBW infants treated for multiple episodes of presumed sepsis or nosocomial pneumonia.

For infants with UVCs, the occurrence of two factors interacting—higher birth weight and infusion of hyperalimentation fluid—influenced risk for CRS. This is in agreement with the report of Munson et al[13] that UVCs and central venous catheters infusing hyperalimentation fluid often led to coagulase-negative staphylococcal sepsis in neonates. Every infant in our study who developed UVC-related CRS had central strength hyperalimentation

Table 4.—Variables Assessed as Potential Risk Factors for UVC-Related CRS*

Risk Factor	UVC-Related CRS	No CRS	Univariate Significance†	Multivariate Significance
Catheter duration, d	11.8 (3.6)	8.1 (3.9)	NS	NS
Birth weight, g [range]	3530 (1195) [1860-4700]	1342 (691) [620-4050]	$P<.05$	$P<.05$‡
VLBW infants	0/4 (0)	123/140 (88)	...	...
Antibiotic therapy, d	4.0 (6.2)	4.9 (3.1)	NS	NS
Antibiotics at catheter removal	1/4 (25) [0-100]	49/140 (35) [27-43]	NS	NS
Hyperalimentation infusate	4/4 (100) [0-100]	30/140 (21) [14-28]	$P<.001$	$P<.05$‡
Vascular complication	2/4 (50) [0-100]	6/140 (4) [0-7]	$P<.0001$	NS
Total No. of catheters per infants	2.3 (0.5)	2.2 (0.7)	NS	NS
Simultaneous UAC and UVC catheterization	3/4 (75) [0-100]	129/140 (92) [87-97]	NS	NS

*UAC indicates umbilical arterial catheter; CRS, catheter-related sepsis; VLBW, very-low-birth-weight; NS, not significant ($P>.05$); and UVC, umbilical venous catheter. Data are mean (SD) or number/total number (percent); values in brackets are 95% confidence intervals, unless otherwise stated.
†Univariate analysis by t test for continuous variables and χ^2 test for categorical variables.
‡Value represents significance for interaction of birth weight and hyperalimentation fluid.

fluid infusing the catheter. In contrast, the infusion of peripheral strength hyperalimentation fluid through UACs was not a significant risk factor for UAC-related CRS.

We anticipated that longer duration of catheterization would predict risk for CRS. Band and Maki[11] found that both catheter colonization and CRS were related to duration of arterial catheterization, presumably because multiple entries into a catheter increase the risk of infection over time. Similarly, Adam et al[21] reported that longer catheter duration was associated with positive cultures of umbilical catheters. In our study, prolonged catheterization was not an independent risk factor for CRS, most likely because of the correlations that existed between catheter duration, antibiotic therapy, and infusion of hyperalimentation fluid for both catheter types.

Certain variables that we studied (specifically, catheter duration and infusion of hyperalimentation solution) were found to be significant by univariate testing but became insignificant by multivariate testing. This can be explained as a result of interactions and correlations that were found to exist between certain independent variables. This multicollinearity, the finding that some of the predictor variables are highly correlated with each other, is troublesome assessment of the independent significance of prolonged catheterization. When some of the independent variables are highly correlated (such as antibiotic therapy and catheter duration), the multivariable analytic model may retain one variable, such as antibiotic therapy, as a significant risk factor at the cost of diminishing the possible contribution of other variables, such as prolonged catheter duration. If antibiotic therapy had not been introduced into and accounted for in the analysis, then it is possible that prolonged catheter duration might have been a significant independent variable or predictor for CRS.

The best method for detection of catheter colonization has been controversial. Routine cultures of catheter tips at removal may overestimate colonization[21]; as a result, semiquantitative catheter culture techniques have been recommended to enhance specificity.[7,8,10,21] Nevertheless, we performed routine tip cultures and blood cultures obtained through catheters periodically to evaluate each technique's ability to predict CRS. Some catheters determined to be colonized may have been contaminated at the site of blood withdrawal; without semiquantitative cultures or histopathologic examination of catheter tips, our definition of catheter colonization cannot be confirmed.[7] However, our low rate of catheter colonization compared with that previously reported suggests that colonization was not overestimated. The surveillance culture methods correctly predicted CRS in only 10% to 38% of infants subsequently documented to have CRS. However, blood cultures drawn through umbilical catheters may be useful to predict CRS, with the advantage of being performed while the catheter remains in place.

CONCLUSIONS

The benefits from the use of umbilical catheters must be assessed daily and weighed against risk for infection, particularly in VLBW infants. Our results reveal certain factors that significantly influence risk for umbilical CRS. Infusion of hyperalimentation fluid through the UVC places an infant at higher risk for infection. Very low birth weight and prolonged antibiotic therapy increase risk for CRS from UACs. Prolonged catheterization, generally greater than 2 weeks, should be avoided whenever possible.

We do not advocate the widespread use of catheter surveillance cultures. Bloods cultures obtained through catheters, together with peripheral blood cultures, may be of diagnostic benefit in cases where umbilical CRS is clinically suspected.

This work was supported by the United States Department of Agriculture/Agricultural Research Service Childrens Nutrition Research Center, Houston, Tex.

We appreciate the secretarial assistance of Robin Dudley and Jennie Chilson and the help of Joseph Garcia-Prats, MD, Steve Welty, MD, Joan Shook, MD, and Yvonne Barry, MD, and the nurses in the NICU at Jefferson Davis Hospital, Houston, Tex.

References

1. Krauss AN, Caliendo TJ, Kannan MM. Bacteremia in newborn infants following umbilical catheterization. *N Y State J Med.* 1972;72:1136-1137.
2. Bard H, Albert G, Teasdale F, Doray B, Martineau B. Prophylactic antibiotics in chronic umbilical artery catheterization in respiratory distress syndrome. *Arch Dis Child.* 1973;48:630-635.
3. Hall RT, Rhodes PG. Total parenteral alimentation via indwelling umbilical catheters in the newborn period. *Arch Dis Child.* 1976;51:929-934.
4. Balagtas RC, Bell CE, Edwards LD, Levin S. Risk of local and

systemic infections associated with umbilical vein catheterization: a prospective study in 86 newborn patients. *Pediatrics.* 1971;48:359-367.

5. Anagnostakis D, Kamba A, Petrochilouv V, Arseni A, Matsaniotis N. Risk of infection associated with umbilical vein catheterization. *J Pediatr.* 1975;86:759-765.

6. Krauss AN, Caliendo TJ, Kannan MM. Bacteremia in newborn infants following umbilical catheterization. *N Y State J Med.* 1970;77:965-969.

7. Ruderman JW, Morgan MA, Klein AH. Quantitative blood cultures in the diagnosis of sepsis in infants with umbilical and Broviac catheters. *J Pediatr.* 1988;112:748-751.

8. Maki DG, Weise CE, Sarafin HW. A semiquantitative culture method for identifying intravenous-catheter–related infection. *N Engl J Med.* 1977;296:1305-1309.

9. Noel GJ, Edelson PJ. Staphylococcus epidermidis bacteremia in neonates: further observations and the occurrence of focal infection. *Pediatrics.* 1984;74:832-837.

10. Raucher HS, Hyatt AC, Barzilai A, et al. Quantitative blood cultures in the evaluation of septicemia in children with Broviac catheters. *J Pediatr.* 1984;104:29-33.

11. Band JD, Maki DG. Infections caused by arterial catheters used for hemodynamic monitoring. *Am J Med.* 1979;67:735-741.

12. Feinstein AR. Clinical biostatistics, XXXI: on the sensitivity, specificity, and discrimination of diagnostic tests. *Clin Pharmacol Ther.* 1975;17:104-116.

13. Munson DP, Thompson TR, Johnson DE, Rhame FS, Van Drunen N, Ferrieri P. Coagulase-negative staphylococcal septicemia: experience in a newborn intensive care unit. *J Pediatr.* 1982;101:602-605.

14. Starr SE. Antimicrobial therapy of bacterial sepsis in the newborn infant. *J Pediatr.* 1985;106:1043-1048.

15. Sewell CM, Clarridge JE, Young EJ, et al. Clinical significance of coagulase-negative staphylococci. *J Clin Microbiol.* 1982;16:236-239.

16. D'Angio CT, McGowan KL, Baumgart S, St Geme J, Harris MC. Surface colonization with coagulase-negative staphylococci in premature neonates. *J Pediatr.* 1989;114:1029-1034.

17. Peters G, Locci R, Pulverer G. Adherence and growth of coagulase-negative staphylococci on surfaces of intravenous catheters. *J Infect Dis.* 1982;146:479-482.

18. Dunne WM, Nelson DB, Chusid MJ. Epidemiologic markers of pediatric infections caused by coagulase negative staphylococci. *Pediatr Infect Dis J.* 1987;6:1031-1035.

19. LaGamma EF, Drusin LM, Mackles AW, Machalek S, Auld PM. Neonatal infections: an important determinant of late NICU mortality in infants less than 1,000 g at birth. *AJDC.* 1983;137:838-841.

20. Siegel JD, McCracken GH. Sepsis neonatorum. *N Engl J Med.* 1981;304:642-647.

21. Adam R, Edwards LD, Becker CC, Schrom HM. Semiquantitative cultures and routine tip cultures on umbilical catheters. *J Pediatr.* 1982;100:123-126.

A 50-Year Follow-up of Childhood Plumbism

Hypertension, Renal Function, and Hemoglobin Levels Among Survivors

Howard Hu, MD, MPH, ScD

• A group of 192 subjects with well-documented lead poisoning in 1930 to 1942 were identified in this pilot study. Thirty-five of 72 survivors traced to a Boston area address and 22 age-, sex-, race-, and neighborhood-matched controls were recruited into a clinical study. One matched subject with plumbism had grossly abnormal renal function and an elevated blood lead level of an unclear cause. Among the remaining 21 matched pairs, the risk of hypertension was significantly higher in subjects with plumbism (relative risk, 7.0; 95% confidence interval, 1.2 to 42.3). Mean adjusted creatinine clearance rates for subjects with plumbism, however, were significantly higher than those of controls and supranormal in comparison to rates predicted for sex and age. Subjects with plumbism had significantly lower hemoglobin concentrations and hematocrit readings than the controls. Blood lead and serum creatinine levels were low for both groups. These results suggest that survivors of childhood lead poisoning have an increased risk of clinically significant hypertension developing in the setting of supranormal creatinine clearance rates.

(*AJDC.* 1991;145:681-687)

The immediate effects of exposure to high amounts of lead are well known. Intense interest has focused on the long-term effects of lead exposure.[1] Such effects include those caused by continuous exposure to low levels of lead from outside sources as well as the long-term sequelae of lead poisoning.

Pediatric lead exposure continues to be a widespread phenomenon in our society.[2,3] There is growing evidence, moreover, that lead that accumulates in the skeleton is more metabolically active than previously thought[4,5] and may exert multisystemic effects late in life.

Most studies on the long-term effects of pediatric lead exposure have been directed at measuring neuropsychological outcomes. Few have assessed other long-term consequences. High rates of renal disease–associated morbidity and mortality have been reported among adults who had histories of childhood lead poisoning in Queensland, Australia.[6,7] In contrast, investigators in the United States failed to find significant chronic nephropathy among patients studied up to 20 years after childhood lead intoxication.[8-10] To our knowledge, the risk of hypertension without kidney disease or injury to other organ systems has not been closely examined.

In this pilot study, subjects who had well-documented evidence of childhood plumbism in the period 1930 to 1942 were recruited for a detailed investigation of renal, cardiovascular, hematopoietic, and neurobehavioral function. Although small in scale, the investigation had several advantages over previous studies, including the use of strict criteria to define childhood plumbism, the long duration of follow-up, the simultaneous study of a matched control group, and the range of outcomes studied. All research described herein was approved by the Institutional Review Boards of the Brigham and Women's Hospital, Boston Children's Hospital and Medical Center, and the Harvard School of Public Health, Boston, Mass.

SUBJECTS AND METHODS

Defining the Eligible Study Population

The diagnosis of the lead poisoning was based largely on clinical grounds until 1930, when the finding of radiologic evidence of lead's effect was reported in the literature by Vogt[11] of Boston Children's Hospital. This finding is otherwise seen only in patients with rickets, which, in turn, is associated with other characteristic findings (eg, bow deformity of the lower extremities).

This study began with a review of microfilmed medical records of all 322 patients who had been given a diagnosis (primary, secondary, or other) of lead poisoning while at Boston Children's Hospital from 1930 to 1942 and who survived hospitalization. To be eligible for further consideration, a patient needed medical record documentation that fulfilled the following four major criteria based on history, clinical presentation, and radiologic evidence: (1) a definite history of pica for lead-containing material (usually paint) or the use of lead nipple shields; (2) evidence of dense metaphyseal bands ("lead lines") on at least one long bone roentgenogram; (3) clinical evidence of symptoms and signs characteristic of childhood lead intoxication; and (4) the absence of clinical evidence for rickets.

The 192 subjects who remained were divided into three categories based on clinical severity of lead intoxication (Table 1). The classification scheme corresponds to ranges of blood lead concentration that have a small amount of overlap and can serve as approximate indicators of the level of poisoning.[12,13] All subjects for whom race was recorded were white.

Accepted for publication December 11, 1990.

From the Channing Laboratory, Department of Medicine, Brigham and Women's Hospital, Harvard Medical School, and the Occupational Health Program, Departments of Environmental Health and Physiology and Epidemiology, Harvard School of Public Health, Boston, Mass.

Reprint requests to Brigham and Women's Hospital, Department of Medicine, Channing Laboratory, 180 Longwood Ave, Boston, MA 02115 (Dr Hu).

Table 1.—Scoring System for Severity of Childhood Plumbism

Score	Symptoms/Signs	Blood Lead Level at Which Symptoms/Signs Begin, μmol/L
1	Abdominal pain, constipation, vomiting, anorexia, or hyperirritability	2.9-4.8
2	Score 1 symptom(s) plus nerve palsy	4.3-5.8
3	Score 1 symptom(s) plus sign(s) of encephalopathy (somnolence, semistupor, coma, convulsion, or projectile vomiting)	5.8

Tracing of Subjects

Tracing of the 192 eligible subjects was performed using available public records of state and local governments, including birth, marriage, and death certificate records from the state Registry of Vital Records and Statistics, voting lists from state records, drivers license records from the state Registry of Motor Vehicles, and local telephone books. Records of parents and siblings were inspected that provided listings of survivors.

One hundred two eligible subjects were traced to current Massachusetts addresses (Fig 1). Death certificates were obtained on 43 subjects. The 47 remaining subjects (24% of the 192 eligible subjects) were either traced to an out-of-state address or were unavailable for follow-up. As could be expected, dead subjects had a high odds for having had poor Plumbism Severity Scores (2 or 3) in comparison with either all the other eligible subjects (odds ratio [OR], 2.21; 95% confidence interval [CI], 1.04 to 4.67) or survivors who were traced to current Massachusetts addresses (OR, 2.79; 95% CI, 2.14 to 6.30).

Recruitment of Subjects

Of the 102 subjects traced to current Massachusetts addresses, a subgroup of 72 who lived within a 48-km radius of the Ambulatory Clinical Research Center in Boston were targeted for recruitment. Each subject was sent a letter that specifically described the project as a scientific study on "the impact of the environment on health," in which the addressee had been identified as someone who had been "exposed to lead and admitted to Children's Hospital." The evaluation was explained as consisting of a questionnaire, interview, and "simple tests of kidney and neurologic function." Subjects were offered $50 to $75 as compensation for participation, the amount depended on the distance necessary for the subject to travel to participate. Letters were followed by telephone calls to subjects who had not responded.

Thirty-five subjects agreed to participate in the study and followed through on their visit. Fifteen expressed interest in the study but could not schedule a visit to the Ambulatory Clinical Research Center. Seven refused outright to participate in the study. Fourteen did not live at the address listed or did not respond to letters or telephone calls. One subject was found to have died several months prior to the study. Study participants had a low odds (but not statistically significant) of having a Severity Score of 2 or 3 in comparison with all the other nondead subjects (OR, 0.50; 95% CI, 0.18 to 1.34) and the nonparticipating subjects who had been traced to Massachusetts (OR, 0.63; 95% CI, 0.21 to 1.85) or Boston-area addresses (OR, 0.52; 95% CI, 0.15 to 1.72).

Recruitment of Control Subjects

Potential control subjects matched on age (within 2 years), sex, race, and neighborhood (voting precinct) were identified using information derived from town books. Within 4 weeks of evaluating the index case, letters of recruitment were mailed to two potential controls, followed by telephone calls using numbers from telephone book listings. The letter of recruitment specifically described the project as an "approved scientific study on the impact of the environment on health" in which we were focusing on "kidney and nerve function." Subjects were offered $50 to $75 as compensation for participation, the amount depending on the distance necessary for the subject to travel to participate. Failure to respond within 2 weeks or refusal led to successive cycles of recruitment mailing and calling to other potential controls. Subjects were excluded if they had a history of lead intoxication as a child (none did).

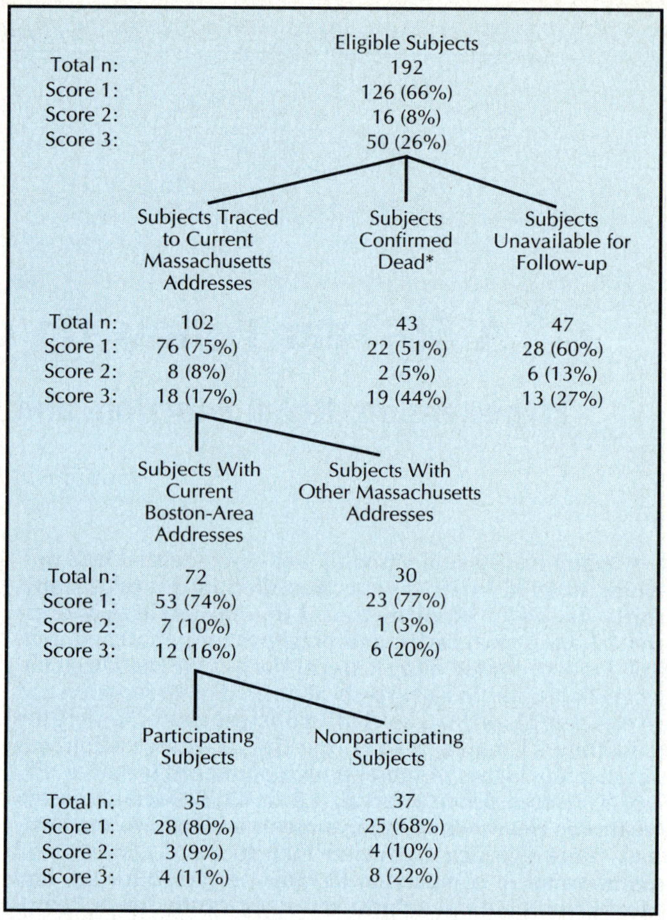

Fig 1.—*Breakdown on tracing, recruitment, and plumbism severity scores. Score 1 indicates abdominal pain, constipation, vomiting, anorexia, or hyperirritability; score 2, score 1 symptom(s) plus nerve palsy; score 3, score 1 symptom(s) plus sign(s) of encephalopathy; and asterisk, death certificate obtained.*

Twenty-two control subjects were recruited in this fashion. Seven were recruited in the first mailing; eight were recruited in the second mailing; one was recruited in the third mailing; four were recruited in the fourth mailing; and two were recruited in the fifth mailing. Exhaustion of the pilot study's funding curtailed further recruitment, and 13 subjects with childhood plumbism were left without matched controls. Unmatched subjects with plumbism tended to live farther away from Boston than the matched subjects with plumbism, which may partially explain the difficulty in recruiting more controls after five mailings.

Evaluation Protocol

Each participant received a package containing a self-administered questionnaire and instructions. The questionnaire elicited information on childhood hospitalizations and illnesses, occupations, hobbies, potentially hazardous exposures, smoking, alcohol ingestion and other drug use, adult hospitalizations, reproductive histories, medications, and chronic diseases (ie, high blood pressure, diabetes, gout, and kidney disease). A subject was classified as receiving antihypertensive medications if taking daily doses of any medication listed by the American Hospital Formulary Service as a hypotensive or diuretic agent, or any β-blocker or calcium channel–blocking agent.

During the visit to the Ambulatory Clinical Research Center, each subject underwent a 3-hour timed urine collection, brief physical examination, a 1½ -hour battery of neuropsychological

Table 2.—Participant Demographics and Severity Scores

	Matched Subjects With Plumbism	Matched Control Subjects	Unmatched Subjects With Plumbism
n	22	22	13
Age, y			
Range	49-60	48-60	47-60
Mean (SD)	54.7+4.0	55.4+4.0	56.7+4.0
Sex M/F	8/14		5/8
Plumbism Severity Score, No.(%)			
1	19 (86)	. . .	9 (69)
2 or 3	3 (14)	. . .	4 (31)
Education, y			
Range	8 -20	8-18	11-18
Mean (SD)	13.5+2.8	14.3+2.9	12.9+1.9
Smoking			
Never	8	7	5
Former	11	12	5
Current	3	3	3
Alcohol Ingestion			
<2 alcoholic drinks per day	19	20	12
≥2 alcoholic drinks per day	3	2	1
Body Mass Index kg/m^2			
Range	21.5-38.3	20.1-40.0	22.4-37.5
Mean (SD)	28.4+5.5	27.7+5.1	28.8+4.6

tests, and phlebotomy. Systolic blood pressure and fifth-phase diastolic blood pressure were measured to the nearest 2 mm Hg, which were taken from the right and left arms while the subject was in the sitting position by a research nurse who was unaware of the subject's classification as lead-exposed or control. A subject's blood pressure was considered elevated if, based on the average of readings from the right and left arm, the systolic blood pressure was greater than 140 mm Hg or the diastolic blood pressure was greater than 90 mm Hg. All subjects with childhood plumbism and their matched controls were given the same evaluation protocol.

Laboratory Tests

The 3-hour timed urine collections underwent standard urinalysis with measurement of creatinine level. Urinary creatinine values were compared with serum creatinine values; creatinine clearance rates were calculated adjusted to a body surface area of 1.73 m^2. Blood specimens were assayed for standard serum chemistry studies, serum urea nitrogen, and creatinine by standard multichannel computerized analysis (Technicon SMAC-2, Technicon, Tarrytown, NY). Complete blood cell counts were performed by an automated cell counter (Coulter, STK-R, Coulter Corp, Hialeah, Fla). Blood specimens that had been collected in metal-free heparinized tubes were assayed for blood lead level using graphite atomic absorption spectroscopy and zinc protoporphyrin level by hematofluorometry (ESA Labs, Bedford, Mass).

Statistical Analyses

Continuous variable data for matched pairs of plumbism and control subjects were plotted; means were compared using paired *t* tests. For each subject, creatinine clearance rate also was compared with the age- and sex-specific expected value generated by the nomogram developed by Rowe et al.[14] Discrete outcomes were compared by analyzing discordant pairs using McNemar's test and calculating relative risks and 95% CIs.[15]

RESULTS

Demographics, Mortality, and Reproductive and Neurobehavioral Outcomes

Matched subjects with plumbism, matched controls, and nonmatched subjects with plumbism were similar

Table 3.—Comparison of Selected Laboratory Values

Factor	Subjects Matched With Plumbism	Matched Control Subjects	*P* Value*	Unmatched Subjects With Plumbism
Blood lead, µmol/L				
Range	0.9-0.53	0.19-0.87		0.19-0.48
Mean (SD)	0.29 (0.11)	0.36 (0.19)	.23	0.30 (0.11)
Zinc protoporphyrin, µg/dL				
Range	6-84	15-79		19-72
Mean (SD)	36.4 (22.8)	32.2 (16.8)	.55	29.8 (16.2)
Serum creatinine, µmol/L				
Range	50-130	60-100		60-130
Mean (SD)	90 (20)	90 (20)	.77	90 (10)
Serum urea nitrogen, mmol/L				
Range	3.6-24.6	3.2-8.6		3.2-16
Mean (SD)	5.9 (1.5)	5.7 (1.1)	.61	6.7 (3.4)
Creatine clearance rate, mL/s per 1.73 m^2				
Range	1.08-2.62	0.78-2.33		0.88-2.97
Mean (SD)	1.88 (0.33)	1.48 (0.48)	.00	1.68 (0.50)
Serum uric acid, µmol/L				
Range	190-460	180-430		170-600
Mean (SD)	330 (80)	320 (70)	.45	360 (120)
Hemoglobin, g/L				
Range	120-152	128-171		122-169
Mean (SD)	138 (11)	147 (12)	.01	145 (15)
Hematocrit				
Range	0.35-0.45	0.39-0.5		0.37-0.5
Mean (SD)	0.41 (0.03)	0.43 (0.32)	.02	0.43 (0.04)
Mean cell volume				
Range	81-99	82-95		80-92
Mean (SD)	86.0(12.9)	86.3(17.8)	.95	84.0(12.8)

*Comparing matched subjects with plumbism with control subjects.

with respect to age, sex ratio, body mass index, years of education, alcohol ingestion, and smoking status (Table 2). A higher proportion of nonmatched subjects with plumbism had high severity scores. All subjects were white.

Hypertension

Among the 22 matched pairs of subjects with plumbism and controls, three (14%) of the controls reported taking daily medications that were classified as antihypertensive, as opposed to nine (41%) of the subjects with plumbism. Each of these controls took a single agent, with two taking β-blockers and one taking a diuretic. Among subjects with plumbism, five were receiving single agents, with two receiving β-blockers, two receiving angiotensin-enzyme inhibitors, and one receiving a diuretic. Three subjects with plumbism were taking two agents, and one was taking a combination of three. There were seven discordant pairs in which the subject with plumbism was taking antihypertensive medications but the control subject was not, compared with one discordant pair in which the subject with plumbism was not taking medications but the control subject was (relative risk, 7.0; 95% CI, 1.2 to 42.3). Of the matched study participants not taking antihypertensive medications, an additional five subjects with plumbism and five controls had elevated blood pressure on physical examination. The ratio of discordant pairs for subjects either taking antihypertensive medications or having elevated blood pressures was also 7:1. Mean systolic blood pressure of subjects with plumbism was higher than that of their matched control subjects (137.4±20.2 vs

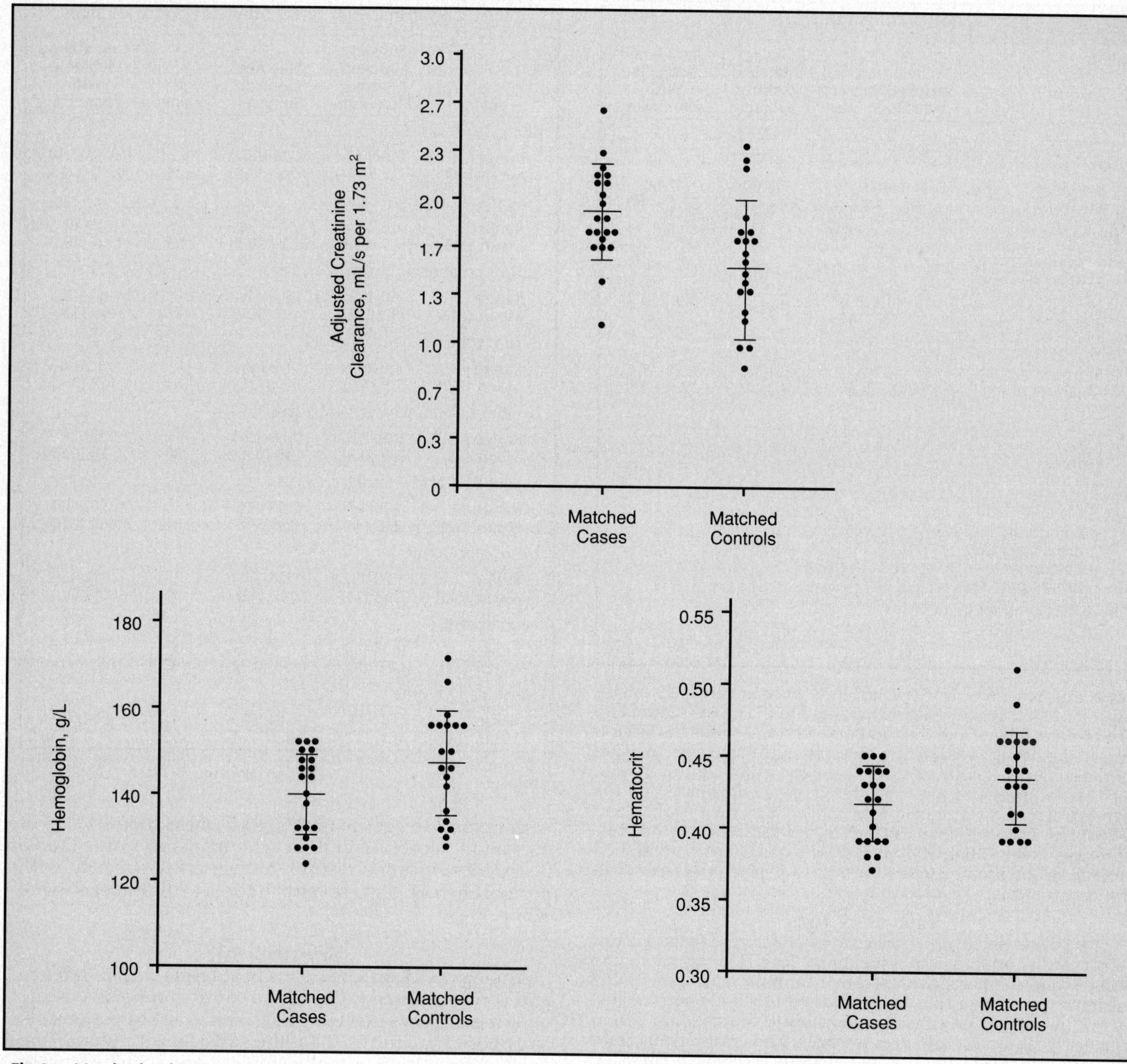

Fig 2.—*Matched subjects with plumbism ("matched cases") vs matched control subjects for selected factors. Bars indicate means with 1 SD.*

132.6±18.9 mm Hg), whereas mean diastolic blood pressure of subjects with plumbism was lower than that of their matched control subject (83.6±9.8 vs 86.4±10.2 mm Hg); however, none of these differences was statistically significant (P=.36 and .32, respectively, by paired t tests).

Seven (54%) of the unmatched subjects with plumbism reported taking medications for hypertension. An additional subject who was not receiving medications had elevated blood pressure.

Renal Function, Blood Lead, and Hematologic Variables

One subject with plumbism had grossly abnormal renal function and hypertension with a serum creatinine value of 390 μmol/L and serum urea nitrogen of 24.6 mmol/L. This subject is discussed further below; she and her matched control were eliminated from the following analyses.

Among the remaining 21 matched pairs, no significant difference was noted between subjects with plumbism and control subjects with respect to mean blood lead level, zinc protoporphyrin, serum creatinine, or mean serum urea nitrogen values (Table 3).

Matched subjects with plumbism had a mean adjusted creatinine clearance rate of 1.88 mL/s per 1.73 m², in comparison to control subjects who had a mean rate of 1.48 mL/s per 1.73 m² (Table 3 and Fig 2). The mean expected age- and sex-adjusted creatinine clearance rate for the matched subjects with plumbism and control subjects was calculated from the data of Rowe et al[14] to be 1.57 mL/s per 1.73 m². Nine (41%) of the matched subjects with plumbism and five (38%) of the unmatched subjects with plumbism had creatinine clearance rates above their individual age- and sex-specific 95th percentile predicted values, compared with four (18%) of the matched controls.

Hemoglobin values and hematocrit readings were found to be significantly lower among subjects with plumbism, both male and female (Table 3 and Fig 2). One subject with plumbism and no control subject had values that were below the lower limit that is considered normal for their sex. (Lower limit for male subjects is as follows: hemoglobin, 131 g/L; hematocrit, 0.4; and lower limit for female subjects is as follows: hemoglobin, 115 g/L; hematocrit, 0.37.) No difference was noted in red blood cell size or shape. No significant difference was noted in other biochemical or hematologic factors.

Subject With Frank Renal Failure

The subject with frank renal failure had a history not notable for renal disease until 1973, when at the age of 40 years, during delivery of her eighth and last child, an elevated serum creatinine value and hypertension were discovered. Renal biopsy specimen demonstrated findings consistent with chronic interstitial nephritis. The subject subsequently has been receiving antihypertensive medications and has had slowly progressive azotemia. On this evaluation, her serum creatinine value was 390 μmol/L, with a serum urea nitrogen level of 24.6 mmol/L and creatinine clearance rate of 0.32 mL/s per 1.73 m^2. Her blood lead and zinc protoporphyrin levels were elevated (1.45 μmol/L and 293 μg/dL, respectively). A detailed environmental and occupational history disclosed no identifiable source of ongoing lead contamination. An early morning sample of tap water revealed no evidence of significant lead contamination.

COMMENT

Previous studies of survivors of childhood plumbism concentrated on adults younger than 35 years. Henderson[7] noted that 20 of 101 survivors of plumbism had blood pressures exceeding 140/90 mm Hg. Tepper[8] commented that only one of the 42 survivors of plumbism whom he studied had a blood pressure exceeding 140/90 mm Hg. Moel et al[10] found that systolic blood pressure was higher in survivors of plumbism than in control siblings, but they attributed this to higher weights among the controls. The finding of an elevated risk for hypertension requiring medications among survivors of plumbism in this study of older adults suggests that a latency period of more than 40 years is necessary before this effect occurs.

Bias in the form of selecting subjects who were more likely to have hypertension is unlikely to account for our finding. Follow-up was successful for 76% of the original cohort. Subjects who were targeted for recruitment were chosen based on geographic proximity to the Ambulatory Clinical Research Center. In the recruitment letter, no mention was made of hypertension as an outcome of interest. Matched subjects with plumbism did not differ from matched controls with respect to smoking, alcohol ingestion, education, and body mass index, which militates against confounding by known hypertension risk factors. Moreover, because participating survivors with plumbism had low severity scores, the risk ratio of 7.0 may actually underestimate the risk of hypertension.

Batuman et al[16] found an association between chelatable lead and hypertension that was confined to patients with evidence of chronic renal failure (serum creatinine concentration >130 μmol/L). Other investigators have reported an association of blood lead levels with elevated blood pressure.[5,17-21] By contrast, the subjects with plumbism in our study had neither elevated serum creatinine concentrations nor elevated blood lead levels. Their increased risk of hypertension suggests that remote exposures can cause hypertension in the absence of clinically significant renal disease and discernible elevations in blood lead levels.

The mechanism by which this occurs may depend on subclinical release of bone lead stores into plasma.[22] Bone is the major reservoir of body lead stores in adults and children,[23,24] with a half-life extending for decades.[25,26] It is accepted that while these deposits are readily exchangeable,[4,5,27-29] they can exist without accompanying elevations in blood lead levels.[18,30-32] Campbell et al[33] recently found that men with long-term subclinical lead exposure had increases in the concentrations of plasma renin activity and plasma aldosterone concentrations. In animal studies, lead exposure has been shown to increase sensitivity of vascular smooth muscle via neurogenic and humoral mediators such as catecholamines.[34-36]

As in previous studies in this country, no evidence was found to support renal dysfunction in survivors of plumbism. On the contrary, adjusted creatinine clearance rates for matched subjects with plumbism were unexpectedly found to be significantly high. A similar finding of supranormal creatinine clearance rates was reported by Odutola et al[37] among patients with mild essential hypertension and has been seen among subjects with newly diagnosed diabetes and young diabetics before the onset of proteinuria.[38] In conjunction with increased *p*-aminohippurate clearance rates observed in some experimental studies of lead poisoned rats[39] and clinical studies of lead-toxic workers,[40] these results suggest that lead may actually increase renal blood flow and/or glomerular filtration rates through a shift in autoregulation, perhaps as an intermediate step in the evolution of eventual renal disease. Alternatively, the elevated creatinine clearance concentration could represent enhanced proximal tubular secretion of creatinine as occurs in sickle cell nephropathy.[41]

The single survivor with plumbism who was found to have frank renal failure hints that this outcome may occur, but at a low incidence. Of additional interest is her elevated blood lead level in the absence of an identifiable occupational or environmental source. This may reflect the additive effects of osteoporosis[42] and renal osteopenia in releasing bone lead stores.

This study also found that matched subjects with plumbism had significantly lower hemoglobin and hematocrit values than controls. Although serum iron, folate, and other factors were not measured, the presence of comparable indexes of red blood cell size and shape argues against confounding by common risk factors for anemia. Only one subject with plumbism was mildly anemic (hematocrit, 0.35; hemoglobin, 120 g/L); none had blood lead levels above 0.72 μmol/L. The lowest blood lead level that carries a risk for anemia has recently been estimated to be 0.96 μmol/L.[43] Therefore, the effect observed may represent a subclinical effect of accumulated bone lead stores on hematopoiesis.

As discussed elsewhere, subjects with plumbism differed from controls in other respects as well. Female subjects with plumbism reported a rate of learning disability among their children that was greater than that for female controls.[44] Subjects of both sexes with plumbism performed the cognitive aspects of neuropsychological tests more poorly than controls.[45]

Clearly, another key aspect of the experience of children poisoned by lead is their mortality. Analysis of the 43 death certificates from this study awaits the completion of tracing for a broader cohort of subjects with plumbism; preliminary results suggest an increased mortality rate from renal disease (N. P. Potter, RN, oral communication, September 10, 1990).

CONCLUSION

A high risk of clinically significant hypertension was found developing among 50-year survivors of childhood plumbism in comparison with an age-, sex-, and neighborhood-matched control group. Survivors with plumbism also had lower hemoglobin and hematocrit values. A single survivor with plumbism had frank renal failure that was suspicious of lead nephropathy. Subjects with plumbism were found to have creatinine clearance rates that were significantly greater than controls. The significance of this finding is unclear.

This research was supported in part by grant ES00002 from the National Institutes for Environmental Health Sciences (NIEHS) Center and NIEHS National Research Service award 2T32 ES07069 at the Harvard School of Public Health and grant RR 02635 from the the National Institute of Health Clinical Research Center at Brigham and Women's Hospital.

Nancy Potter, RN, Dana-Farber Cancer Institute, shared data from her ongoing mortality study; Richard Monson, MD, Stephen Lagakos, ScD, and David Christiana, MD, of the Harvard School of Public Health; John Graef, MD, of Children's Hospital; Burton Rose, MD, and Frank Speizer, MD, of Brigham and Women's Hospital; and Fred Li, MD, of the Dana-Farber Cancer Center, Boston, provided advice. Many research assistants (too numerous to name herein) traced the subjects; Sarah Freeman, Kim Damakosh, and Cynthia Cryan helped recruit the traced subjects; Susan Fisher, RN, helped in examining subjects; and Ilene Brill, Irene Zhao, and Carrie Wager provided computer programming and graphics assistance.

References

1. Landrigan PJ. Toxicity of lead at low dose. *Br J Ind Med.* 1989;46:593-596.

2. Agency for Toxic Substances and Disease Registry. *The Nature and Extent of Lead Poisoning in Children in the United States: A Report to Congress.* Washington, DC: US Dept of Health and Human Services; July 1988. US Dept of Health and Human Services publication 53009/84730.

3. Needleman HL. The persistent threat of lead: a singular opportunity. *Am J Public Health.* 1989;79:643-645.

4. Rabinowitz MB, Wetherill GW, Kopple JD. Lead metabolism in the normal human: stable isotope studies. *Science.* 1973;182:725-727.

5. US Environmental Protection Agency. *Air Quality Criteria for Lead.* Research Triangle Park, NC: Office of Health and Environmental Assessment, Environmental Criteria and Assessment Office: EPA report EPA-600/8-83/028aF-dF. 4v. NTIS, Springfield, Va; PB87-142378; 1986.

6. Nye LJJ. An investigation of the extraordinary incidence of chronic nephritis in young people in Queensland. *Med J Aust.* 1929;2:145-152.

7. Henderson DA. Chronic nephritis in Queensland, Australia. *Aust Ann Med.* 1955;4:163-177.

8. Tepper LB. Renal function subsequent to childhood plumbism. *Arch Environ Health.* 1963;7:76-85.

9. Chisolm JJ, Mellits ED, Barrett MD. Cited by: Goyer RA. Lead and the kidney. *Circ Top Pathol.* 1971;55:147-176.

10. Moel DI, Sachs HK, Cohn RA, Drayton MA. Renal function 9 to 17 years after childhood lead poisoning. *J Pediatr.* 1985;106:729-733.

11. Vogt EC. A roentgen sign of plumbism: the lead line in growing bone. *AJR Am J Roentgenol.* 1930;24:550-553.

12. Gompertz D. Assessment of risk by biological monitoring. *Br J Ind Med.* 1981;38:198-202.

13. Thomas M. Entry on lead. In: Ellenhorn MJ, Barceloux DG, eds. *Medical Toxicology.* New York, NY: Elsevier Science Publishing Co Inc; 1988:1030-1042 .

14. Rowe JW, Andres R, Tobin JD, Norris AH, Shock NW. Age-adjusted standards for creatinine clearance. *Ann Intern Med.* 1976;84:567-569.

15. Schlesselman JJ. *Case-Control Studies.* New York, NY: Oxford University Press Inc; 1982.

16. Batuman V, Landy E, Maesaka JK, Wedeen RP. Contribution of lead to hypertension with renal impairment. *N Engl J Med.* 1983;309:17-21.

17. Harlan WR, Landis JR, Schmouder RL, Goldstein NG, Harlan LC. Blood lead and blood pressure: relationship in the adolescent and adult US population. *JAMA.* 1985;253:530-534.

18. Kirkby H, Gyntelberg F. Blood pressure and other cardiovascular risk factors of long-term exposure to lead. *Scand J Work Environ Health.* 1985;11:15-19.

19. De Kort WL, Verschoor MA, Wibowo AAE, van Hemmen JJ. Occupational exposure to lead and blood pressure: a study of 105 workers. *Am J Ind Med.* 1987;11:145-156.

20. Orssaud G, Claude JR, Moreau T, et al. Blood lead concentration and blood pressure. *BMJ.* 1985;290:244-250.

21. Weiss ST, Munoz A, Stein A, Sparrow D, Speizer FE. The relationship of blood lead to blood pressure in a longitudinal study of working men. *Am J Epidemiol.* 1986;123:800-808.

22. Araki S, Aono H, Fukahori M, Tabuki K. Behavior of lead and zinc in plasma, erythrocytes, and urine and ALAD in erythrocytes following intravenous infusion of CaEDTA in lead workers. *Arch Environ Health.* 1984;39:363-367.

23. Barry PSI. A comparison of concentrations of lead in human tissues. *Br J Ind Med.* 1975;32:119-139.

24. Barry PSI. Concentrations of lead in the tissues of children. *Br J Ind Med.* 1981;38:61-71.

25. Rabinowitz MB, Wetherill GW, Kopple JD. Kinetic analysis of lead metabolism in healthy humans. *J Clin Invest.* 1976;58:260-270.

26. Steenhout A. Kinetics of lead storage in teeth in bones: an epidemiologic approach. *Arch Environ Health.* 1982;37:224-231.

27. Keller CA, Doherty RA. Bone lead mobilization in lactating mice and lead transfer to suckling offspring. *Toxicol Appl Pharmacol.* 1980;55:220-228.

28. Marcus AH. Multicompartment kinetic models for lead, I: bone diffusion models for long-term retention. *Environ Res.* 1985;36:441-458.

29. Rosen JF. Metabolic and cellular effects of lead: a guide to low level lead toxicity in children. In: Mahaffey KR, ed. *Dietary and Environmental Exposure to Lead.* Amsterdam, the Netherlands: Elsevier/North-Holland Biomedical Press; 1985:157-185.

30. Alessio L, Bertazzi PA, Monelli O, Toffoletto F. Curvilinear relationships between blood lead, erythrocyte protoporphyrin and chelatable lead in adults. *Int Arch Environ Health.* 1976;37:84-88.

31. Fascchetti S, Geiss F. *Isotopic Lead Experiment: Status Report.* Brussels-Luxembourg, Belgium: Office for Official Publications of the European Communities; 1982.

32. Rosen JF. The toxicologic importance of lead in bone: the evolution and potential uses of bone lead measurements by x-ray fluorescence to evaluate treatment outcomes in moderately lead toxic children. In: Clarkson TW, Friberg L, Nordberg GF, Sager PR, eds. *Biological Monitoring of Toxic Metals.* New York, NY: Plenum Press; 1988:603-621.

33. Campbell BC, Meredith PA, Scott JJC. Lead exposure and changes in the renin-angiotensin-aldosterone system in man. *Toxicol Lett.* 1985;25:25-32.

34. Iannaccone A, Carmignani M, Boscolo P. Neurogenic and humoral mechanisms in arterial hypertension of chronically lead-exposed rats. *Med Lav.* 1981;1:13-21.

35. Carmignani M, Boscolo P, Galli G, Iannaccone A, Porcelli F. Effects of chronic exposure to cadmium and/or lead on some neurohumoral mechanisms regulating cardiovascular function in the rat. *Int Conference Heavy Metals Environ.* 1983;1:557-560.

36. Baksi SN, Hughes MJ. Effects of chronic lead ingestion by the weaning rat on adrenal catecholamine levels. *J Auton Nerv Syst.* 1983;8:287-289.

37. Odutola TA, Ositelu SB, D'Almeida EA, Okeiyi JC. Supranormal creatinine clearance in black mild hypertensive patients in Nigeria. *J Hum Hypertens.* 1988;2:133-139.

38. Mogensen CE, Osterby R, Gundersen HJG. Early functional and morphologic vascular renal consequences of the diabetic state. *Diabetologia.* 1979;17:71-76.
39. Pardoe AU. Renal function in lead poisoning. *Br J Pharmacol.* 1952;7:349-357.
40. Cramer K, Goyer RA, Jagenburg R, Wilson MH. Renal ultrastructure, renal function, and parameters of lead toxicity in workers with different periods of lead exposure. *Br J Ind Med.* 1974;31:113-127.
41. DeJong PE, van Eps LWS. Sickle cell nephropathy. *Kidney Int.* 1985;27:711-717.
42. Silbergeld EK, Schwartz J, Mahaffey K. Lead and osteoporosis: mobilization of lead from bone in postmenopausal women. *Environ Res.* 1988;47:79-94.
43. Schwartz J, Landrigan PJ, Baker EL, Orenstein WA, Lindern IH. Lead-induced anemia: dose-response relationships and evidence for a theshold. *Am J Public Health.* 1990;80:165-168.
44. Hu H, Potter N. A fifty-year follow-up of the long-term consequences of childhood plumbism: knowledge of diagnosis and reproductive history among survivors. *Arch Environ Health.* In press.
45. White R, Gendzler RD, Proctor S, Hu H, Potter N. A fifty-year follow-up of the long-term consequences of childhood plumbism: neurobehavior among survivors. *Arch Environ Health.* In press.

In Other AMA Journals

JAMA

Health Care Use Among Young Children in Day Care

M. C. McCormick; J. Brooks-Gunn; S. Shapiro;
A. A. Benasich; G. Bloac; R. T. Gross
(*JAMA.* 1991;265:2212)

Setting Health Care Priorities in Oregon

D. C. Hadorn
(*JAMA.* 1991;265:2218)

Is The Oregon Rationing Plan Fair?

N. Daniels
(*JAMA.* 1991;265:2232)

Resident Physician Substance Use in the United States

P. H. Hughes; S. E. Conard; D. C. Baldwin, Jr;
C. L. Storr; D. V. Sheehan
(*JAMA.* 1991;265:2069)

Substance Use Among Senior Medical Students

D. C. Baldwin, Jr; P. H. Hughes; S. E. Conard;
C. L. Storr; D. V. Sheehan
(*JAMA.* 1991;265:2074)

Do House Officers Learn From Their Mistakes?

A. W. Wu; S. Folkman; S. J. McPhee; B. Lo
(*JAMA.* 1991;265:2089)

ARCHIVES OF INTERNAL MEDICINE

Clinical Characteristics of Patients in the Persistent Vegetative State

Donald D. Tresch, MD; Farrol H. Sims, MD; Edmund H. Duthie, MD;
Michael D. Goldstein, PhD; Paul S. Lane, MD
(*Arch Intern Med.* 1991;151:930-932)

Brain and Ocular Abnormalities in Infants With In Utero Exposure to Cocaine and Other Street Drugs

Rodrigo Dominguez, MD; Antonio Aguirre Vila-Coro, MD; John M. Slopis, MD; Timothy P. Bohan, MD, PhD

• We describe 10 infants with developmental delay and congenital cerebral anomalies who were found to have had in utero exposure to vasoactive drugs. Nine infants had ophthalmological abnormalities; these included strabismus, nystagmus, and/or hypoplastic optic discs. Six mothers used cocaine, one used cocaine and heroin, one used only heroin, one used amphetamine, and one used phenylpropanolamine. Each of these cerebral anomalies (agenesis of the corpus callosum, septo-optic dysplasia, schizencephaly, hydranencephaly, congenital hydrocephalus, porencephaly, and cerebral infarctions) can be attributed to insults at different stages of development. There appears to be a relationship between the time of prenatal drug exposure and the type of cerebral anomaly, evoking malformations, disruptions, or fetal strokes. Since many or possibly all of these anomalies are thought to have a vascular origin, it seems appropriate to implicate prenatal exposure to vasoactive drugs.

(*AJDC.* 1991;145:688-695)

In utero exposure to drugs, particularly street drugs, is a social and medical problem of increasing importance. Although the incidence of heroin abuse has remained relatively constant, the abuse of cocaine has increased sharply in the last few years, in part due to the cheap, highly addictive, smokable form called "crack."[1] The use of crack cocaine during pregnancy is apparently now much more prevalent than the use of other street drugs, including heroin. Some studies in the United States have shown that prenatal exposure to cocaine has affected 11% of these surveyed newborns.[2] The percentage of drug-exposed neonates has apparently quadrupled since 1985.[3] There is a low incidence of in utero exposure to other stimulant drugs, such as amphetamine and methamphetamine.[4] The incidence of prenatal exposure to phenylpropanolamine, which is in diet pills and some decongestants, is unknown.

Cocaine use during pregnancy can have a deleterious effect on both the developing fetus and on the outcome of the pregnancy.[5] The human teratogenicity of cocaine is not well known and is still controversial. Even though one study has stated that cocaine does not cause congenital malformations in humans, most other studies have reported cocaine-induced birth defects[6]; these included congenital genitourinary tract malformations,[7,8] encephalocele, microcephaly, limb anomalies, and bony skull defects.[5,9]

Use of cocaine immediately before and during delivery has been reported to cause cerebral infarction,[10,11] necrotizing enterocolitis,[12] decreased cardiac output,[13] and seizures.[11]

Although some are abnormal, the majority of cocaine-exposed newborns show little or no evidence of drug withdrawal injury during the neonatal period.[14] In contrast, many infants with in utero exposure to heroin often have an abnormal nursery course.[15]

We describe a group of 10 infants who were found to have neurological abnormalities and congenital anomalies of the brain. The cerebral lesions found in our patients included early, middle, and late gestational lesions, thereby further expanding the spectrum of cerebral teratogenicity of cocaine into the early part of pregnancy, which includes cerebral malformations.

METHODS

This study was conducted at the University of Texas Medical School, Houston, from 1987 to middle 1990. We studied seven infants (three females and four males) who presented with strabismus before 6 months of age. The last three infants (two males and one female) presented in the newborn period with abnormal findings from a neonatal neurological examination.

All birth records were obtained and reviewed for maternal and gestational age, delivery history, birth weight, Apgar scores, head circumference, and nursery history. Gestational age was based on the results of newborn examination. Pregnancy history, including prenatal drug use, was obtained from the birth records and, for patients 2 and 4 through 7, from an extensive interview with the mother. The findings from a urine drug screening were abnormal in patients 2 and 8. The remaining eight infants did not undergo screening. All infants underwent screening for neonatal infections. This screening included tests for (1) human immunodeficiency virus (Enzyme Immuno Assay, Abbott Laboratories, North Chicago, Ill); (2) TORCH (*t*oxoplasmosis, *o*ther [syphilis, hepatitis, zoster], *r*ubella, *c*ytomegalovirus, and *h*erpes simplex [maternal infections]) infections (Solid Phase Immuno fluorescence, Whittaker Na Bio Products, Walkersville, Md); and (3) syphilis (rapid plasma reagin charcoal agglutination test, Beckton Dickinson, Mountainview, Calif). All infants were examined by both a pediatric ophthalmologist and a pediatric neurologist. In five patients, the brain anomalies were diagnosed with computed tomography only, in two infants with magnetic

Accepted for publication January 4, 1991.

From the Departments of Radiology (Dr Dominguez), Pediatrics (Drs Dominguez, Slopis, and Bohan), Ophthalmology (Dr Aguirre Vila-Coro), Neurology (Drs Slopis and Bohan), and Pharmacology (Dr Bohan), University of Texas Health Science Center, and the Mann Eye Clinic (Dr Aguirre Vila-Coro), Houston.

Reprint requests to Department of Radiology, University of Texas Health Science Center, 6431 Fannin, Room 2.132 MSB, Houston, TX 77030 (Dr Dominguez).

Infant	Gestation, wk	Weight, g	Head, cm	Maternal Age, y	Delivery	Nursery Course	Prenatal Care	In Utero Drug Exposure*
1	40	2810	31.8†	24	Spontaneous delivery	Normal nursery course of 2 d	Some prenatal care	IV cocaine use during first 7 mo
2	27	1070	28	25	Cesarean section for fetal distress	Long course due to prematurity	None	Amphetamine use during most of the pregnancy
3	39	2930	30.5†	28	Precipitous delivery	Normal nursery course of 3 d	Some prenatal care	IV cocaine use during most of the pregnancy
4	40	3068	31.8†	26	Spontaneous delivery after only 2 h of labor	Normal nursery course of 2 d	None	Use of diet pills containing phenylpropanolamine during 6-12 wk
5	38	3350	33	24	Spontaneous delivery	Normal nursery course of 3 d	None	IV heroin use during most of the pregnancy, but no use of cocaine
6	40	4005	31.8†	20	Spontaneous delivery	Normal nursery course of 5 d	Some prenatal care	Crack cocaine use during 1st and 2nd trimester
7	39	3660	36.5	34	Delivery induced due to pregnancy-induced hypertension	R clavicle fracture but otherwise normal nursery course of 2 d	Some prenatal care	IV cocaine and heroin use during 3-8 mo
8	40	2480	32†	24	Precipitous delivery	Complicated by late-onset meningitis	Some prenatal care	Crack cocaine use during most of the pregnancy
9	32	1500	27	35	Spontaneous delivery after premature rupture of membranes	Respiratory distress, seizures, and congenital syphilis that did not involve the brain	None	IV cocaine use throughout pregnancy
10	38	2370	31†	17	Spontaneous delivery	Neonatal seizures	None	In utero cocaine during 1st and 2nd trimester

Table 1.—Pregnancy, Labor, and Delivery History of Infants With In Utero Drug Exposure

*IV indicates intravenous.
†Microcephalic—head circumference more than 2 SDs below the mean for gestational age.

resonance imaging only, and in another infant with neonatal head ultrasound only; two patients were studied with both magnetic resonance imaging and computed tomography.

RESULTS

Prenatal and Perinatal Histories

The pregnancy, labor, and delivery histories of the 10 patients are summarized in Table 1; of the 10 infants, three were adopted. Seven infants were delivered vaginally at full term, and two were premature. One was born by cesarean section due to fetal distress. All infants had normal Apgar scores; seven had a normal nursery course. Six of the 10 infants were microcephalic. All infants had had prenatal exposure to vasoactive drugs, ie, cocaine, heroin, amphetamine, or phenylpropanolamine. For all patients, the drug exposure occurred during at least part of the first trimester, and in four patients, it occurred throughout most of the pregnancy. The mother of patient 4 did not know that she was pregnant when she consumed phenylpropanolamine diet pills during part of the first trimester. The remaining nine mothers were long-term drug addicts, and it was not possible to quantitate accurately their drug intake. All infants had normal karyotypes, and except for patient 9, negative titers for common congenital infections, including human immunodeficiency virus, toxoplasmosis, rubella, cytomegalovirus, syphilis, and herpes simplex. Although patient 9 had congenital syphilis, the results of his cerebrospinal fluid studies were normal, and hence, he did not have neurosyphilis.

In two infants (patients 2 and 8), cocaine was detected in the urine at birth. Patients 1, 2, and 10 had abnormal neurological findings at birth, and their mothers admitted to the use of cocaine during pregnancy. The remaining seven infants were identified later because of their unusual ophthalmological anomalies and were found to have a history significant for drug exposure.

Neurological and Ophthalmological Findings

The neurological and ophthalmological findings are summarized in Table 2. All infants were examined by a pediatric neurologist (T.P.B. or J.M.S.). For some patients, this assessment included a Denver Developmental Assessment and/or a Bayley Neuropsychiatric Assessment of mental and motor performance. All infants had some degree of global developmental delay, that is, a delay in both mental and motor skills. Although the types of abnormalities were similar, the severity varied. Except for the three infants who were examined in the newborn period, distal hypertonicity and some degree of spasticity were consistent features.

Another feature that was found in all patients was truncal ataxia. In the younger infants, this was manifested by poor head control and axillary slippage. Some of the older

Table 2.—Neurologic and Ophthalmologic Findings at Time of Presentation in Infants With In Utero Drug Exposure

Infant/Age, mo	Primary Caretaker*	Neurologic Findings	Ophthalmologic Findings
1/5½	AM	Truncal ataxia, spastic diplegia, L hemiparesis, history of facial seizures, global delay	Intermittent esotropia and hypoplastic optic discs bilaterally
2/Newborn	BM	Motor delay with truncal hypotonia	No apparent strabismus but patient did not have adequate fixation for evaluation, normal funduscopic examination results
3/3	AM	Global delay with truncal ataxia, swallowing difficulties, severe hypertonia with opisthotonic posturing and seizures	Optokinetic nystagmus absent, bilateral disc atrophy with apparent blindness
4/3½	AM	Global delay with truncal ataxia, distal spasticity, hypertonicity, opisthotonic posturing	Incomplete L 3rd nerve palsy with partial ptosis; minimally reactive pupil, exotropia, and vertical nystagmus of the R eye; normal optic discs
5/3	BM	Global delay with truncal ataxia, severe hypertonicity, spasticity, poor head control	Exotropia of 65° with full ductions and versions, subtotal cupping of the L optic disc with spontaneous pulsations of the L central retinal artery
6/6	BM	Global delay with truncal ataxia and distal spasticity, hypertonicity, reduced interactions with environment	Bilateral exotropia of 35° with full ductions and versions
7/4	BM	Global delay, truncal ataxia with distal spasticity and hypertonicity	Variable exotropia of 40-90° with full ductions and versions, fine pendular nystagmus
8/Newborn	BM	Global delay, with seizures	Intermittent esotropia
9/11	BM	Global delay with truncal hypotonia, poor head control, inability to sit, distal hypertonicity	Absent upgaze, poor visual fixation and following, normal funduscopic examination results
10/Newborn	BM	Motor delay with diffuse hypotonia, particularly truncally	Nystagmus with normal fundi

*AM indicates adoptive mother; BM, biologic mother.

infants had achieved head control, but the axillary slippage had not resolved. Patients 1 and 9 were followed up until the 13th and 18th months, respectively, and both had truncal ataxia; this last infant, patient 9, was unable to sit and still had poor head control; and patient 1 had poor sitting posture and was unable to stand without holding on. At 18 months of age, he was about 6 months delayed. Two patients were profoundly delayed. Patient 6 has been bedridden, receiving gastrotomy feedings, and has not achieved any significant developmental milestones. Patient 5 never achieved any developmental milestones and died of pneumonia at 11 months of age. Seizures occurred in five patients; two infants (patients 9 and 10) had transient neonatal seizures, and patient 1 had a single seizure at 6 months of age. Two patients had chronic seizures.

Nine infants had ophthalmological abnormalities. Strabismus was a consistent finding in all infants in whom adequate visual fixation had developed. Adequate visual fixation had not yet developed in infants 2 and 10. Five infants had exotropia, two had esotropia, one had absent upgaze, two had nystagmus, and one had a unilateral third nerve palsy. Two patients were apparently blind. Four patients were followed up for many months, and the eye findings were persistent. By 18 months, patient 1 had some reduction in the angle of the esotropia. The absent upgaze persisted in patient 9; patient 5 died; and patients 6 and 7 had corrective surgery for their strabismus. Three infants also had abnormal optic discs.

Neuroimaging

The anatomical findings of the 10 patients who were under study are described in Table 3 according to the presumed time of insult during pregnancy. These anomalies included midline cerebral malformations (eg, septo-optic dysplasia), errors of neuronal migrations (eg, dysgenesis of the corpus callosum and schizencephaly), disruptions (hydranencephaly, "congenital" hydrocephalus, and porencephaly), or perinatal strokes (Figs 1 through 4). Magnetic resonance imaging, when available, allowed a clearer assessment of the abnormalities due to its inherent properties as follows: better resolution, contrast sensitivity for soft tissues, and multiplanar-imaging capabilities.

Prevalence

Due to the retrospective nature of our study, we could only estimate the prevalence of these cerebral malformations. Two types of estimates were possible: (1) the prevalence of these cerebral malformations in drug-exposed infants and (2) the prevalence of cerebral malformations in infants with drug-induced strabismus. Of the 10 patients described here, five were born at Hermann Hospital, Houston, and one was born at an outlying hospital; they were studied during infancy. The other four infants were born at the new county hospital (Lyndon B. Johnson General, Houston). Three infants were studied in the nursery, and one was studied at 11 months of age. Although the last institution had been open for 16 months, it has only been a University of Texas facility since July 1, 1990. The three newborns in the study were discovered among the

Table 3.—Neuroimaging: Anatomical Findings of the Six Patients Under Study According to the Time of the Vascular Insult During Intrauterine Life*

Infants	Time of Gestational Insult: Trimester	Week	Type of Lesions/Malformations	Radiological Findings(CT and/or MRI)
1 and 2	1st	7	Dysgenesis of the corpus callosum†	Absence of corpus callosum, parallel and widely spaced lateral ventricles, frontal horns narrowed, occipital horns enlarged (colpocephaly), 3rd ventricle in continuity with interhemispheric fissure anteriorly
3	1st	7½	Septo-optic dysplasia with schizencephaly†	Bilateral open-lips schizencephaly with heterotopic gray matter lining lips; both corpus callosum and septum pellucidum are absent
4	1st	7½	Septo-optic dysplasia with schizencephaly†	Bilateral closed-lips schizencephaly at junction of frontal and parietal lobes with thin clefts of subarachnoid space lined by gray matter extending to ventricular margins; septum pellucidum is absent; corpus callosum and optic nerves are hypoplastic
5	2nd	12-24	Encephaloclastic hydranencephaly‡	Replacement of cerebral cortex by CSF-filled sacs with residual occipital lobe and preservation of basal ganglia, cerebellum, and falx
6	2nd	13-14	Porencephaly of 2nd trimester with midline brain anomalies‡	Large porencephalic cavity confluent with R lateral ventricle and replacing most of the R brain mantle, septum pellucidum is absent
7	3rd	28-32	Porencephaly with normal midline structures§	Bilateral wedge-shaped porencephalic cavity at parietal lobes, moderate cerebral atrophy and asymmetrical enlargement of R lateral ventricle
8	3rd	28-32	Porencephaly with normal midline structures§	Microcephaly, mild brain atrophy, noncommunicating hydrocephalus, extensive cerebral infarctions, small bilateral porencephaly
9	3rd	28-32	Porencephaly with partially destroyed normal midline structures§	Noncommunicating hydrocephalus, fenestration of septum pellucidum and thinned-out corpus callosum, large porencephalic cyst at R occipital lobe
10	3rd	36	Bilateral posterior cerebral infarcts§	Diffuse decreased density within cerebral hemispheres affecting mainly deep white matter and most prominently in parieto-occipital watershed areas, mild associated edema with compression of lateral ventricles

*CT indicates computed tomography; MRI, magnetic resonance imaging; and CSF, cerebrospinal fluid.
†Malformation only.
‡Malformation and disruption.
§Encephaloclastic lesion.

2510 infants who were born during these 3 months. Although that hospital does not screen all newborns, limited surveys at that institution suggest that 10% to 15% of the infants have had prenatal exposure to drugs of abuse. We therefore estimate that 250 to 375 of these infants have had prenatal exposure to drugs. We would further estimate that 0.8% to 1.2% of infants with prenatal drug exposure have congenital malformations of the brain. This is probably an underestimation since at that hospital neuroimaging is only done on children with (1) a head of abnormal size or shape or (2) a neurological abnormality, such as a seizure.

Of the 10 infants described here, all but patients 2 and 10 had strabismus. At the time of examination, neither patient had adequate fixation for full evaluation. During the first year covered in this study, our pediatric ophthalmologist (A.A.V.-C.) examined 200 infants with strabismus who were younger than 6 months of age. One hundred ninety-two infants had the much more common condition of infantile congenital esotropia; only eight infants suffered from congenital exotropia, including the four patients who constituted the starting point of our research. The rarity of congenital exotropia[16] and the obvious developmental delay in these four infants led to neuroimaging and neurological evaluation. The findings in these first four patients prompted the remainder of this study.

COMMENT

In the present study, we have reported congenital ocular abnormalities and congenital brain malformations in infants with prenatal exposure to cocaine and/or other vasoactive drugs. Three of these patients had been described previously.[17] Specific cerebral abnormalities that have been associated with maternal cocaine and methamphetamine exposure are perinatal strokes and intracranial hemorrhages, intracerebral cysts,[4,10] exencephaly, bony skull defects, and microcephaly[18] with brain atrophy.[4,5] The strokes and hemorrhage were related to drug exposure during the latter part of the third trimester, and no comment was made about ocular abnormalities. The other anomalies (exencephaly and bony skull defects) would have been related to earlier, probably first-trimester drug exposure.

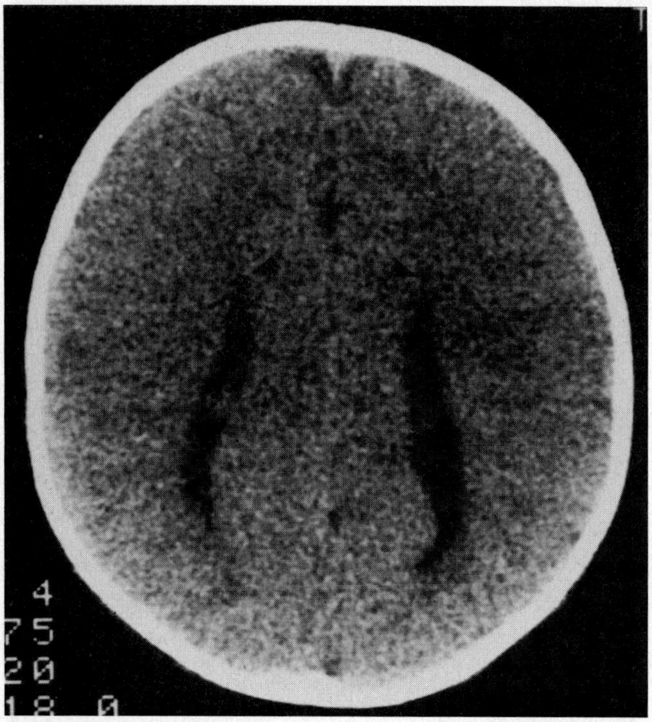

Fig 1.—*Patient 2. Dysgenesis of the corpus callosum. Axial noncontrast-enhanced computed tomographic scan of the brain at the level of the bodies of the lateral ventricles. Note the parallel widely spaced lateral ventricles with narrowing and a characteristic lateral convexity of their frontal horns (due to the formation of the hemilateral bundles of Proust, secondary to the absence of corpus callosum). The fibers that course parallel to the hemispheric fissure indent the medial wall of the lateral ventricles (arrowheads).*

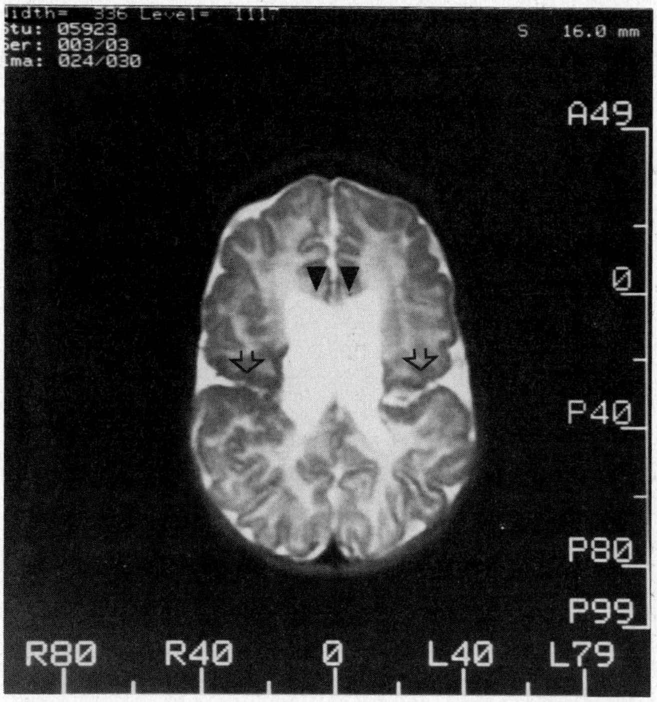

Fig 2.—*Patient 5. Septo-optic dysplasia and schizencephaly. Axial T_2-weighted magnetic resonance imaging of the midbrain at the level of the lateral ventricles. The ventricles communicate freely due to the absence of septum pellucidum; note the shallow anterior and medial margins of the lateral ventricles secondary to the hypoplasia of the corpus callosum (arrowheads). Bilateral closed-lips schizencephaly at the junction of frontal and parietal lobes (open arrows). These thin clefts of the subarachnoid space extend into the ventricular margins. Note, in this magnetic resonance imaging sequence, the dark band of heterotopic gray matter that rims the clefts, as proof of the abnormal neuroblastic migration.*

Other nonneurological effects of prenatal cocaine include spontaneous abortion, abruptio placentae, prematurity, intrauterine growth retardation,[5,9] stillbirth,[18] and neurobehavioral problems.[14] Studies of infants with prenatal exposure to cocaine also reveal a significant incidence of strabismus[19] and congenital microcephaly.[4,5] The lesions that were found in our patients included early, middle, and late gestational lesions, thereby further expanding the spectrum of cerebral teratogenicity of cocaine into the early part of pregnancy.

There have been only a few animal studies of cocaine teratogenicity, and these have produced conflicting results, possibly due to species variability. In CF-1 mice, cocaine produced significant ocular abnormalities, ranging from frequent anophthalmia to lens hypoplasia and microcephaly.[20] In one study of Sprague-Dawley rats, there were significant limb malformations but no anophthalmia.[21] In another study of Long-Evans rats, only one of 360 rat embryos had anophthalmia.[22] The animal studies and human epidemiology seem to indicate that the risk of severe anatomical malformations from cocaine is dose dependent but low.[23] The absence of cerebral malformations in most other studies of cocaine-exposed infants may be due to a combination of the small size (<100 patients) of most studies and the low prevalence (our estimate, 0.8% to 1.2%) of the malformations in drug-exposed infants. In fact, in the one large study, there was a significant incidence of cerebral malformations in cocaine-exposed neonates.[24]

Although some congenital malformations of the brain are associated with strabismus,[25] to our knowledge, there have been no reports that link the prenatal, drug-induced strabismus to cerebral malformations. Strabismus, nystagmus, and ocular torticollis are often found in infants with in utero exposure to heroin, methadone, and/or cocaine, but these abnormalities are often not appreciated until several months of age,[19,26,27] and they have never been correlated with cerebral anomalies. In addition to strabismus, prenatal exposure to cocaine can also cause other ocular abnormalities. These include optic nerve hypoplasia, retinal colobomas, and micro-ophthalmia with retinal dysgenesis.[28]

Similarly, congenital microcephaly is associated with cerebral malformations,[29] but, to our knowledge, there have been no reports that link prenatal, drug-induced microcephaly to cerebral malformations. To date, neurobehavioral problems are the major reported complications of prenatal cocaine exposure.[14]

Cocaine-induced vasoconstriction can occur in all organs, including the placenta,[30] heart,[31] and brain.[32] Cocaine-induced vasoconstriction in the brain can cause strokes and intracranial hemorrhages.[33] Amphetamine and phenylpropanolamine, an anorexic agent that is chemically similar to amphetamine, are both potent vasoconstrictors.[34] Like cocaine, both have also been reported to cause strokes and intracranial hemorrhages.[35] Although less well known, heroin has also been reported to affect cerebral blood flow in humans and cause cerebral anoxia.[36,37] Its actions are presumably mediated via stimulation of endorphinergic systems. Several animal studies also indicate that endorphinergic systems are involved in regulating cerebral blood flow.[38,39]

The congenital anomalies that were present in our patients fall into three categories. In the first category are

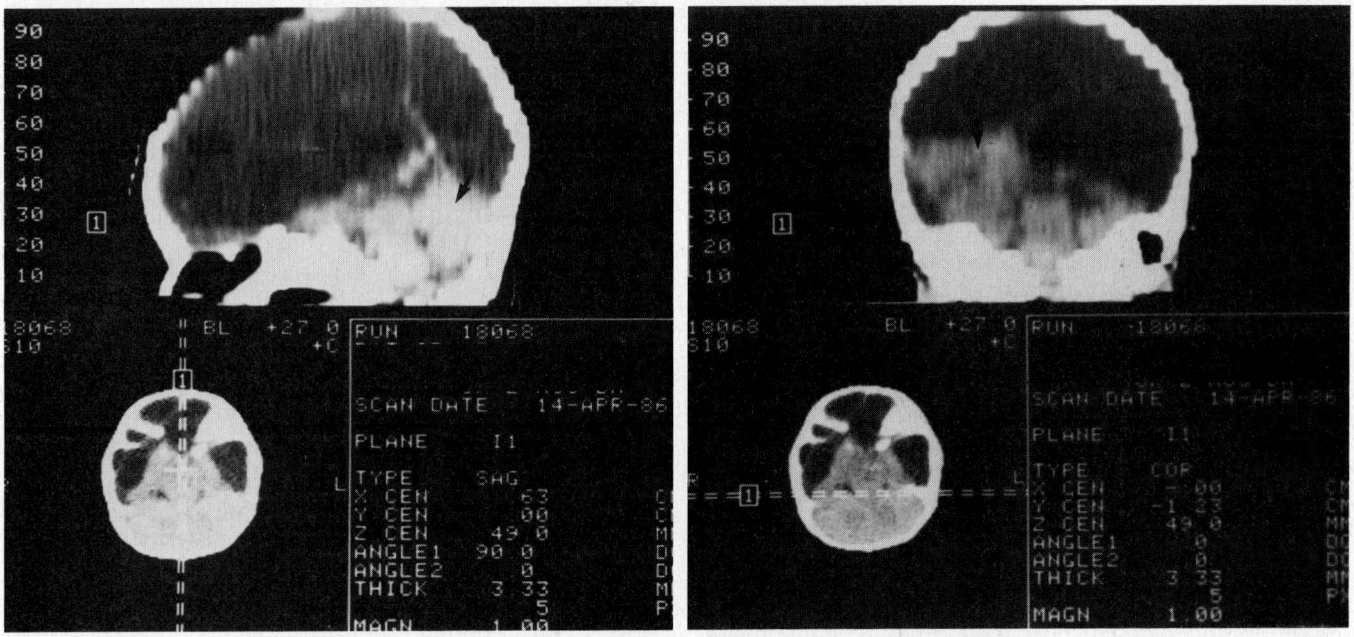

Fig 3.—*Left and right, Patient 7. Hydranencephaly. Midline sagittally reconstructed and coronal noncontrast-enhanced computed tomographic scan planes of the brain reveal incomplete replacement of the cerebral cortex with cerebrospinal fluid–filled sacs. Note the presence of residual occipital cortex and the preservation of the basal ganglia and cerebellum (arrows).*

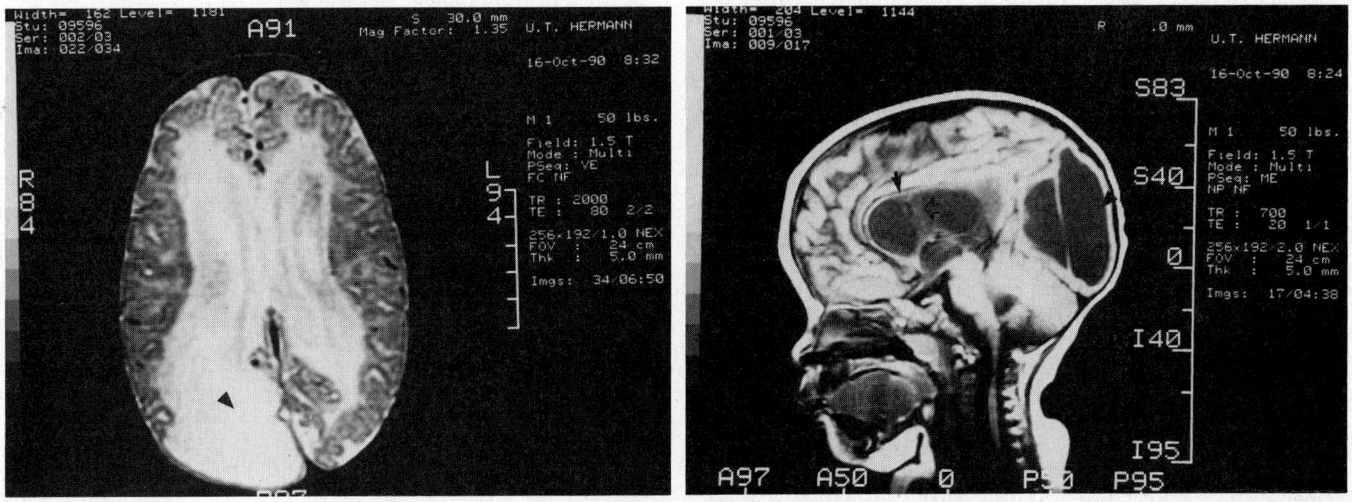

Fig 4.—*Patient 10. Porencephaly. Sagittal (left),* T_1*-weighted and axial (right),* T_2*-weighted magnetic resonance imaging revealing a large porencephalic cyst (arrowhead) at the right occipital lobe illustrated on both the sagittal (left) and axial (right) image. Also note the communicating hydrocephalus. Note the preservation of the midline brain structures, although the ventricular dilatation has thinned out the corpus callosum (arrow on left) and fenestrated the septum pellucidum right (open arrow).*

dysmorphic lesions in which the insult occurred at an early (5 to 7 weeks) stage of embryogenesis. During this time period, ventral induction in the cephalic end of the central nervous system takes place with differentiation of midline brain structures, such as the optic vesicles and retinal ganglion cells; the anterior wall of the diencephalon then forms the commissural plate and septum pellucidum.[40] Our patients' malformations in this category included agenesis of the corpus callosum, septo-optic dysplasia, and schizencephaly (patients 1 through 4). These malformations may be seen alone or in association with each other[41] and/or with hypoplasia of the optic nerves.[42] The results of this and other studies[28,43] support the hypothesis that a hypotensive insult or ischemic event is the cause for this group of anomalies. Although the authors do not make this point, the results of the study by Skarf and Hoyt[42] support linkage of septo-optic dysplasia to a vascular event. They reported the neuroanatomical and neurologic findings in patients with optic nerve hypoplasia. One group in their study consisted of 41 infants with bilateral optic nerve hypoplasia and nystagmus. Three of these 41 patients also had a porencephalic cyst, a lesion that is known to have a vasogenic origin; unless there is one cause for the optic nerve hypoplasia and another for the porencephalic cyst, one has to conclude that, in these three patients, the two lesions had the same, that is, a vascular origin. The vascular origin of septo-optic hypoplasia is also supported by the findings from the recent report of three cocaine-exposed infants with retinal abnormalities, including both optic nerve hypoplasia and retinal dysgenesis; one of the three infants also had a cerebral malformation.[28] Furthermore, three additional patients in the study of Skarf and Hoyt[42] had an encephalocele, a lesion that others have found in infants with prenatal cocaine exposure.[18,24]

Although it is somewhat hypothetical, one could extrapolate from the cocaine-induced anophthalmia report in CF-1 mice[20] to cocaine-induced septo-optic dysplasia in humans. One would hypothesize that septo-optic dysplasia, micro-ophthalmia, and anophthalmia are different points on a continuum, and that an agent that caused anophthamia in one species could cause septo-optic dysplasia in another. This hypothesis is supported by the findings from the recent report of cocaine-exposed infants with optic nerve hypoplasia and micro-ophthalmia.[28]

The second category of lesions are due to an insult that occurs somewhat later in gestation, toward the end of the first trimester, which is a borderline period between late brain malformation and disruptive pathophysiological mechanisms.[44] Lesions in this category include a spectrum of disruptions or destructive anomalies that range from hydranenchephaly to porencephaly and congenital hydrocephalus. In hydranenchephaly (patient 5), there is a nearly complete destruction of the cerebral hemispheres, which are replaced by cerebrospinal fluid–filled sacs.

Porencephaly is understood as a large hemispheric defect that communicates with one of the lateral ventricles. Porencephalic defects that are due to second-trimester insults are located in the territory of the middle cerebral artery, extend across the entire thickness of the cerebral mantle, and are often associated with absence of the septum pellucidum[45] (as in patient 6). In contrast to schizencephaly, porencephalic defects are not lined with gray matter.

In the third category are another type of porencephalic cysts (patients 7 through 9). These do not necessarily involve the entire thickness of the cerebral mantle and are often associated with some degree of homolateral or diffuse cerebral atrophy.[45] The septum pellucidum is usually present. These are also referred to as perinatal strokes.

In some, but not all, of the infants described here, there appeared to be a correlation between the time of prenatal drug exposure and the type of lesion (Tables 1 and 3). Patient 4, who was exposed to phenylpropanolamine during the sixth to 12th weeks, had schizencephaly, a lesion consistent with an early dysmorphic insult. The porencephalic cysts in patient 6 were consistent with an insult during the second but not the third trimester of pregnancy. This patient had exposure to cocaine during the first and second trimesters but not the third trimester. The porencephalic cysts in patients 7 through 9 were consistent with a third-trimester insult, and these patient's mothers consumed cocaine well into the third trimester. Such a correlation is not always possible since many infants are exposed to drugs throughout much of the pregnancy. Additionally, the polydrug abuse that is common in many addicts makes it more difficult to understand the specific effects of maternal street drug consumption. As was the case with three of our patients, these pregnant women often give up their infants for adoption and leave no records of perinatal drug use. Even in infants who are not adopted, the social taboo and the legal complications of admitting drug abuse during pregnancy increase the likelihood of false-negative clinical histories. The presence of congenital strabismus (particularly exotropia), a vascular dysencephaly, and/or congenital microcephaly appear to be an indication to search for a history of prenatal drug exposure. A drug screening with normal results at birth obviously does not exclude significant prenatal drug exposure, and in fact, four of our 10 mothers stopped drug use 1 or more months before delivery. Since cocaine causes vasoconstriction, the presence of either placental or neonatal infarctions in the cerebrum or viscera should also prompt a careful history of prenatal drug exposure.

We would like to thank Phillip Scott, MD, Karen Moreau, MD, Jose Garcia, MD, and Cynthia Castell, MD, for referral of patients. We would also like to thank Adlene Rehfeld for careful preparation of the manuscript.

References

1. Miller JD, Cisin IH. *National Survey on Drug Abuse*: National Institute on Drug Abuse; 1983. US Dept of Health and Human Services, Public Health Service, publication ADM 83-126316.

2. Chasnoff IJ. Drug use and women: establishing a standard of care. *Ann Acad Sci.* 1989;562:208-210.

3. Miller G. Addicted infants and their mothers. *Zero to Three.* 1989;10:20-23.

4. Dixon SD, Bejar R. Echoencephalographic findings in neonates associated with maternal cocaine and methamphetamine use: incidence and clinical correlates. *J Pediatr.* 1989;115:770-778.

5. Hadeed AJ, Siegel SR. Maternal cocaine use during pregnancy: effect of the newborn infant. *Pediatrics.* 1989;84:205-210.

6. Madden JD, Payne TF, Miller S. Maternal cocaine abuse and effect on the newborn. *Pediatrics.* 1986;77:209-211.

7. Chavez GF, Mulinare J, Cordero JF. Maternal cocaine use during early pregnancy as a risk factor for congenital urogenital anomalies. *JAMA.* 1989;262:795-798.

8. Chasnoff IJ, Chisum GM, Kaplan WE. Maternal cocaine use and genitourinary tract malformations. *Teratology.* 1988;37:201-204.

9. Zuckerman B, Frank DA, Hingson R. Effects of maternal marijuana and cocaine use on fetal growth. *N Engl J Med.* 1989;320:762-768.

10. Chasnoff IJ, Bussey ME, Savich R, Stack CM. Perinatal cerebral infarction and maternal cocaine use. *J Pediatr.* 1986;108:456-459.

11. Kramer LD, Locke GE, Ogunyemi A, Nelson L. Neonatal cocaine-related seizures. *J Child Neurol.* 1990;5:60-64.

12. Telsey AM, Dixon S, Merritt TA. Cocaine exposure in a term neonate: necrotizing enterocolitis as a complication. *Clin Pediatr (Phila).* 1988;27:547-550.

13. Van de Bor M, Walter FJ, Ebrahimi M. Decreased cardiac output in infants of mothers who abused cocaine. *Pediatrics.* 1990;85:30-32.

14. Chasnoff IJ, Burns KA, Burns WJ. Cocaine use in pregnancy: perinatal morbidity and mortality. *Neurotoxicol Teratol.* 1987;9:291-293.

15. Zelson C. Acute management of neonatal addiction. *Addict Dis.* 1975;2:159-168.

16. Manley DR. Strabismus. In: Harley RD, ed. *Pediatric Ophthalmology.* 2nd ed. Philadelphia, Pa: WB Saunders Co; 1983;1:237.

17. Dominguez R, Aguirre A. Cerebral dysmorphogenesis in infants of substance abuse mothers. In: Proceedings of the 32nd Annual Meeting of the Society of Pediatric Radiology; April 6-9, 1989; San Antonio, Tex. Page 160.

18. Bingol N, Fuchs M, Diaz V, Stone RK, Gromisch DS. Teratogenicity of cocaine in humans. *J Pediatr.* 1987;110:93-96.

19. Isenberg SJ, Spierer A, Inkelis SH. Ocular signs of cocaine intoxication in neonates. *Am J Ophthalmol.* 1987;103:211-214.

20. Mahalik MP, Gautieri RF, Mann DE. Teratogenic potential of cocaine hydrochloride in CF-1 mice. *J Pharm Sci.* 1980;69:703-706.

21. Webster WS, Brown-Woodman PDC. Cocaine as a cause of congenital malformations of vascular origin: experimental evidence in the rat. *Teratology.* 1990;41:689-697.

22. Church MW, Dintcheff BA, Gessner PK. Dose-dependent consequences of cocaine on pregnancy outcome in the Long-Evans rat. *Neurotoxicol Teratol.* 1988;10:51-58.

23. Brent RL. Relationship between uterine vascular clamping, vascular disruption syndrome, and cocaine teratogenicity.

Teratology. 1990;41:757-760.
24. Mast, J, Carpanzano C, Hier L. Cocaine as a teratogen: a controlled retrospective review. *Ann Neurol.* 1989;26:458-459.
25. Herman DC, Barkley GB, Bullock JD. Ophthalmic finding in hydranencephaly. *J Pediatr Ophthalmol Strabismus.* 1988;25:106-111.
26. Nelson L, Ehrlich S, Calhoun JH, Matteucci T, Finnegan LP. Occurrence of strabismus in infants born to drug-dependent women. *AJDC.* 1987;141:175-178.
27. Chavez CJ, Ostrea EM, Stryker JC, Strauss ME. Ocular abnormalities in infants as sequelae of prenatal drug addiction. *Pediatr Res.* 1979;13:367.
28. Ferriero DM, Dobori JA, Good WV, Golabi M. Retinal defects in cocaine-exposed infants. *Ann Neurol.* 1989;26:458.
29. Jawarski M, Hersh JH, Donat J, Shearer LT, Weisskopf B. Computed tomography of the head in the evaluation of microcephaly. *Pediatrics.* 1986;78:1064-1069.
30. Woods JR, Plessinger MA, Clark KE. Effect of cocaine on uterine blood flow and fetal oxygenation. *JAMA.* 1987;257:957-961.
31. Lange RA, Cigarroa RG, Yancy CW, et al. Cocaine-induced coronary-artery vasoconstriction. *N Engl J Med.* 1989;321:1557-1562.
32. Chokshi SK, Gal D, Whelton JA, Isner JM. Evidence that fetal distress in newborns of cocaine users is due to vascular spasm and may be attenuated by pre-treatment with diltiazem. *Circulation.* 1989;80(suppl 2):II-185. Abstract.
33. Nalls G, Disher A, Daryabagi J, Zant Z, Eisenman J. Subcortical cerebral hemorrhages associated with cocaine abuse: CT and MR findings. *J Comput Assist Tomogr.* 1989;13:1-5.
34. Weiner N. Norepinephrine epinephrine and the sympathomimetic amines. In: Gilman AG, Goodman LS, Gilman A, eds. *The Pharmacological Basis of Therapeutics.* 6th ed. New York, NY: Macmillan Publishing Co Inc; 1980:138-175.
35. Edwards M, Russo L, Harwood-Nuss A. Cerebral infarction with a single oral dose of phenylpropanolamine. *Am J Emerg Med.* 1987;5:163-164.
36. Leeds NE, Malhotra V, Zimmerman RD. The radiology of drug addiction affecting the brain. *Semin Roentgenol.* 1983;18:227-233.
37. Yolkow ND, Valentine A, Kulkarni M. Radiological and neurological changes in the drug abuse patient: a study with MRI. *J Neuroradiol.* 1988;15:288-293.
38. Sandor P, DeJong W, DeWied D. Endorphinergic mechanisms in cerebral blood flow autoregulation. *Brain Res.* 1986;386:122-129.
39. Sandor P, Cox-van Put J, de Jong W, DeWied D. Continuous measurement of cerebral blood volume in rats with the photoelectric technique: effect of morphine and naloxone. *Life Sci.* 1986;39:1657-1665.
40. Byrd SE, Naidich TP. Common congenital brain anomalies, I: imaging in neuroradiology. *Radiol Clin North Am.* 1988;26:755-772.
41. Barkovich A, Norman D. MR imaging of schizencephaly. *AJNR.* 1988;150:1391-1396.
42. Skarf B, Hoyt CS. Optic nerve hypoplasia in children: association with anomalies of the endocrine and CNS. *Arch Ophthalmol.* 1984;102:62-67.
43. Padget DH. The development of the cranial arteries in the human embryo. *Carnegie Inst Contr Embryol.* 1948;32:205-261.
44. Diebler C, Dulac O. Vascular disorders. *Pediatric Neurology and Neuroradiology.* Hydleberg, NY: Springer-Verlag; 1987:185-194.
45. Dekaban A. Large defects in cerebral hemispheres associated with cortical dysgenesis. *J Neuropathol Exp Neurol.* 1965;24:512-530.

In Other AMA Journals

JAMA

Drug Abuse in the United States: Strategies for Prevention

Board of Trustees
(*JAMA.* 1991;265:2102)

Decreased Measles Antibody Response After Measles-Mumps-Rubella Vaccine in Infants With Colds

M. S. Krober; C. E. Stracener; J. W. Bass
(*JAMA.* 1991;265:2095)

Recent Approaches to the Treatment of Sickle Cell Anemia

G. P. Rodgers
(*JAMA.* 1991;265:2097)

Measles Immunization: Recommendation, Challenges, and More Information

G. Peter
(*JAMA.* 1991;265:2111)

A Preliminary Report of Prenatal Cocaine Exposure and Respiratory Distress Syndrome in Premature Infants

Barry Zuckerman, MD; Edward C. Maynard, MD; Howard Cabral, MPH

• A prospective study of maternal drug use during pregnancy and newborn outcomes provided us with an opportunity to assess the relationship between prenatal cocaine use and respiratory distress syndrome among premature infants. Women were consecutively recruited from the prenatal clinics at Boston (Mass) City Hospital between 1984 and 1988 and were interviewed during the prenatal and postpartum period by trained bilingual interviewers. Urine specimens were collected at the time of each interview and were analyzed for marijuana and cocaine metabolites. Following delivery, one of five pediatricians who were "blinded" to the mothers' prenatal and drug history performed a physical examination and abstracted medical information, including the diagnosis of respiratory distress syndrome from the medical record. The study sample consisted of 33 infants born at 34 weeks' or less gestation who were appropriate for gestational age and not exposed to heroin or methadone prenatally. Eight of the mothers of these 33 infants used cocaine prenatally. One (12%) of eight cocaine-exposed infants was diagnosed as having respiratory distress syndrome compared with 13 infants (56%) not exposed to cocaine prenatally. Infants not exposed had an odds ratio of 8.9 (95% confidence interval: 0.9, 83.5) for respiratory distress syndrome compared with infants exposed to cocaine prenatally. When the analysis was controlled for prolonged rupture of membranes, black race, infant gender, or gestational age, the adjusted odds ratio was essentially unchanged. This preliminary observation of a decreased incidence of respiratory distress syndrome among premature infants prenatally exposed to cocaine appears to be biologically plausible and needs to be confirmed in future studies with larger numbers of subjects to control for potentially confounding variables.

(*AJDC.* 1991;145:696-698)

In 1970, it was first noted that premature infants of mothers addicted to heroin have a low rate of respiratory distress syndrome (RDS).[1] During the past 5 years, cocaine has become a much more common drug of abuse, with one study[2] showing that 18% of women receiving prenatal care used cocaine during pregnancy. Published reports show numerous adverse outcomes, including low birth weight, microcephaly, and prematurity, are associated with cocaine use during pregnancy.[2-7]

However, little is known about the relationship between prenatal cocaine use and RDS. It is striking that published reports showing rates of prematurity ranging from 24% to 51% have consistently failed to mention RDS as an adverse neonatal outcome in infants born to mothers using cocaine.[3-5] One retrospective case-control study reported a lower rate of RDS among cocaine-exposed premature infants.[8] As part of a larger study of maternal drug use during pregnancy and newborn outcomes,[2] we investigated the relationship between maternal use of cocaine during pregnancy and RDS among the subsample of premature infants.

Accepted for publication February 11, 1991.

From the Division of Developmental and Behavioral Pediatrics, Department of Pediatrics, Boston (Mass) City Hospital/Boston University School of Medicine (Dr Zuckerman and Mr Cabral), and the Department of Pediatrics, University of Massachusetts Medical School (Dr Maynard), Boston.

Reprint requests to the Division of Developmental and Behavioral Pediatrics, Boston City Hospital, Talbot 214, 818 Harrison Ave, Boston, MA 02118 (Dr Zuckerman).

SUBJECTS AND METHODS

Recruitment of Subjects

Subjects were consecutively recruited at the Women's and Adolescent Prenatal Clinics at Boston (Mass) City Hospital from July 1984 through June 1987. English-speaking and Spanish-speaking women who were willing to give informed consent and who gave birth by December 31, 1987, were eligible to participate in the study. The protocol was approved by the Human Studies Committee of Boston City Hospital. Subjects were protected from the use of data for criminal prosecution by a Writ of Confidentiality under Title 42 of US Code Section 242A. To minimize unavailability for follow-up, participants were paid $10 for each interview.

Assessment of Participants

All participants were interviewed twice, once during the prenatal period and again during the postpartum period, by trained bilingual interviewers. A close-ended, forced-choice interview elicited the timing and frequency of the use of cocaine, marijuana, cigarettes, alcohol, and other illicit psychoactive substances before and during pregnancy. The interviewers were unaware of the results of the infant assessments conducted by the study pediatricians.

Participants were asked to submit urine samples at the time of each interview and were informed that their urine would be assayed for "marijuana and prescription and nonprescription drugs" and that the results would remain confidential and not become part of their clinical record. Urine samples to identify cocaine were obtained from the mother and not the infant during the postpartum period. Women were classified as cocaine users if their urine sample was positive for metabolites of cocaine or if, at either interview, they reported using cocaine during pregnancy. All urine samples were screened for benzoylecgonine, the major metabolite of cocaine, by enzyme-mediated immunoassay

Table 1.—Comparison of Maternal Characteristics Between Women Who Used and Did Not Use Cocaine During Pregnancy (N=33)

	Cocaine Use, %		
	Nonuse (n=25)	Use (n=8)	*P*
Black race	72	75	.62
Cigarette use	36	100	.002
Alcohol use	48	75	.18
Pregnancy-induced hypertension	28	38	.83
Prolonged ROM (>12 h)*	20	50	.12
Abruptio placentae	12	25	.93

*Clinical standard used at Boston (Mass) City Hospital during the study years to indicate increased suspicion for neonatal sepsis. ROM indicates rupture of membranes.

Table 2.—Comparison of Characteristics Between Infants of Mothers Who Used and Did Not Use Cocaine During Pregnancy (N=33)*

	Cocaine Use, %		
	Nonuse (n=25)	Use (n=8)	*P*
Birth weight, g	1554 (730)	1577 (225)	.89
Gestational age, wk	31.1 (2.2)	32.3 (1.1)	.18
Male gender	46	50	.73
Apgar Score at 1 min	5.6 (2.8)	5.5 (2.7)	.90
Apgar score at 5 min	7.0 (2.2)	7.6 (2.0)	.50
RDS	56	13	.03

*Values are mean (SD) or percent. RDS indicates respiratory distress syndrome.

technique (Syva Co, Palo Alto, Calif). When sample volume permitted, presumptive positive samples were confirmed by gas chromatography/mass spectrometry. If specimen volume was insufficient, a second enzyme-mediated immunoassay technique assay performed on a different day was used as a confirmatory test.

Following delivery, one of five pediatricians who were "blinded" to the mothers' prenatal and drug history performed a standard physical examination. Gestational age was determined according to the method of Dubowitz et al.[9] After performing the physical examination, the study pediatrician reviewed the infants' medical records to ascertain the Apgar scores and intrapartum and perinatal complications. The clinical staff of the neonatal intensive care unit diagnosed RDS by clinical symptoms and chest roentgenogram. This information was abstracted from Boston City Hospital's problem-oriented medical record by the study pediatrician. A more complete description of the methods and quality control for urine assays has been published elsewhere.[2]

Statistical Analysis

Bivariate analyses for categorical data were performed with the χ^2 test and Fisher's Exact Test. Means of continuous variables were compared for users and nonusers of cocaine by *t* tests. Unadjusted and adjusted odds ratios and 95% confidence intervals were calculated from logistic regression models[10] assessing the relationship of cocaine use and RDS.

RESULTS

The study sample consisted of 38 infants who were born at 34 weeks' gestation or less. Infants with intrauterine growth retardation (n=1) and opiate (heroin and/or methadone) exposure during pregnancy (n=2) were excluded from the analysis because these conditions are known to be associated with a lower rate of RDS. The research records of two additional infants did not indicate whether RDS was present or absent, leaving a final sample size of 33.

The mean (SD) gestational age of the study sample was 31.4 (2.0) weeks, and mean (SD) birth weight was 1560 (641) g. Forty-five percent of the infants were male. Most of the infants were black (67%), 15% were white, 6% were Hispanic, and 12% were other. Fourteen infants (42%) had RDS. During the years the study was conducted, all mothers with impending delivery between 26 and 36 weeks' gestation received steroids; no infant was treated with surfactant.

Eight of the 33 women used cocaine prenatally. Mothers who used cocaine were similar to those who did not, except that cocaine-using mothers were younger (19.9 [0.8] years vs 26.3 [6.3] years, $P<.001$) and more likely to smoke cigarettes (Table 1). Of the eight cocaine users, three reported using less than once a month, two reported using one to two times a week, and three reported using three or more times a week. Two of the eight cocaine users had a positive urine assay for cocaine metabolites.

The mean birth weight and the mean gestational age of the cocaine-exposed infants were not significantly different from of those of infants not exposed (Table 2). One (12%) of eight cocaine-exposed infants was diagnosed as having RDS compared with 13 infants (56%) not exposed to cocaine prenatally ($P=.03$). Infants not exposed had an odds ratio of 8.9 (95% confidence interval: 0.9, 83.5) for RDS compared with infants exposed to cocaine prenatally. When the analysis was controlled for prolonged rupture of membranes, black race, infant gender, or gestational age, the adjusted odds ratio was essentially unchanged.

COMMENT

Our preliminary investigation suggests that RDS occurs significantly less frequently among premature infants prenatally exposed to cocaine compared with premature infants not so exposed. The findings are similar to those previously reported in a retrospective case-control study, which found RDS in four (25%) of 16 cocaine-exposed infants vs 20 (63%) of 32 controls.[8] To our knowledge, this preliminary report represents the first prospective investigation of prenatal cocaine exposure that has evaluated RDS as an outcome. The relatively small numbers of subjects born at less than 34 weeks' gestation during the 3-year period is in part due to the exclusion of women who did not receive prenatal care; subject recruitment only occurred during prenatal care. While the sample size is small and we do not have information regarding the amount and duration of mechanical ventilation, the strength of our study is that cocaine use was ascertained prospectively both during pregnancy and post partum. The use of both self-report and urine assay is important to identify prenatal cocaine use. In a previous study, had we relied solely on self-report, we would have missed 24% of cocaine users who would have then been misclassified as nonusers.[2] In this study, had we not conducted interviews, we would have missed six of the eight mothers who used cocaine prenatally.

There are several possible mechanisms to explain this observation. Cocaine causes maternal hypertension and decreased uterine blood flow,[11] both of which have been associated with accelerated fetal lung maturation as assessed by amniotic fluid phospholipid analysis.[12] This effect is probably mediated by fetal glucocorticoids that affect surfactant synthesis.[13] Fetal catecholamines may also contribute to accelerated fetal lung maturation by increasing synthesis and secretion of surfactant.[14] Elevated norepinephrine levels among 2-month-old infants[15] and elevated levels of norepinephrine precursors[16] among newborns have been shown in infants born to mothers using cocaine during pregnancy. This increase may be a direct effect of cocaine, which blocks presynaptic reuptake of norepinephrine and epinephrine or a result of adrenal catecholamine release in response to fetal hypoxia secondary to uterine vasoconstriction. Other mechanisms for an effect of cocaine on the developing lung are also possible, as suggested by studies implicating endogenous opioids in fetal lung maturation.[17]

This preliminary observation of a decreased incidence of RDS in cocaine-exposed premature infants appears to be biologically plausible. In fact, data have recently been reported that demonstrate accelerated fetal lung maturation in rabbits following in utero exposure to cocaine.[18] This clinical observation in newborns needs to be confirmed in future studies with an adequate number of subjects to control for other factors known to influence the incidence of RDS, such as intrauterine growth retardation, race, gender, and maternal use of other drugs.

This work was supported in part by grant NIDA-RO1DA03508 from the National Institute of Drug Abuse and grant MCJ-009094 from the Bureau of Health Care Delivery and Assistance, Maternal and Child Health Bureau, Washington, DC.

We thank Jeanne McCarthy for her help in preparing in the manuscript.

References

1. Glass L, Rajegowda BK, Evans HC. Absence of respiratory distress syndrome in premature infants of heroin addicted mothers. *Lancet.* 1971;2:685-686.
2. Zuckerman B, Frank DA, Hingson R, et al. Effects of maternal marijuana and cocaine use on fetal growth. *N Engl J Med.* 1989;320:762-768.
3. MacGregor SN, Keith LG, Chasnoff IJ, et al. Cocaine use during pregnancy: adverse perinatal outcome. *Am J Obstet Gynecol.* 1987;157:686-690.
4. Oro AS, Dixon DS. Perinatal cocaine and methamphetamine exposure: maternal and neonatal correlates. *J Pediatr.* 1987;111:571-578.
5. Cherukuri R, Minkoff H, Feldman J, Parekh A, Glass L. A cohort study of alkaloidal cocaine ('crack') in pregnancy. *Obstet Gynecol.* 1988;72:147-151.
6. Chasnoff IJ, Burns WJ, Schnoll SH, Burns KA. Cocaine use in pregnancy. *N Engl J Med.* 1985;313:666-669.
7. Petitti DB, Coleman C. Cocaine and the risk of low birth weight. *Am J Public Health.* 1990;80:25-28.
8. Maynard EC, Dreyer SA, Oh W. Prenatal cocaine exposure and hyaline membrane disease (HMD). *Pediatr Res.* 1989;25:223A. Abstract.
9. Dubowitz LM, Dubowitz V, Goldberg C. Clinical assessment of gestational age in the newborn infant. *J Pediatr.* 1970;77:1-10.
10. Kleinbaum DG, Kupper LL, Morgenstern H. *Epidemiologic Research.* New York, NY: Van Nostrand Reinhold; 1982.
11. Woods JR Jr, Plessinger MA, Clark KE. Effect of cocaine on uterine blood flow and fetal oxygenation. *JAMA.* 1987;257:957-961.
12. Gluck L, Kulovich MV. Lecithin/sphingomyelin ratios in amniotic fluid in normal and abnormal pregnancy. *Am J Obstet Gynecol.* 1973;115:539-546.
13. Gross I. Regulation of fetal lung maturation: induction and modulation. In: Raivio KO, Hallman N, Kouvalainen K, Valimaki I, eds. *Respiratory Distress Syndrome.* Orlando, Fla: Academic Press Inc; 1984:51-66.
14. Phillippe M. Fetal catecholamines. *Am J Obstet Gynecol.* 1983;146:840-855.
15. Ward SLD, Bautista DB, Buckley S, et al. Circulating catecholamines and adrenoreceptors in infants of cocaine-using mothers. *Ann N Y Acad Sci.* 1989;562:349-351.
16. Mirochnick M, Meyer J, Cole J, Herren T, Zuckerman B. Circulatory catecholamines in cocaine-exposed neonates: a pilot study. *Pediatrics.* In press.
17. Comer CR, Grunstein JS, Mason RJ, Johnston SC, Grunstein MM. Endogenous opioids modulate fetal rabbit lung maturation. *J Appl Physiol.* 1987;62:2141-2146.
18. Kain ZN, Antonio-Santiago MT, Chinoy MR, Marchitelli RN, Scarpelli EM. Fetal rabbit lung maturation following in utero exposure to cocaine. Presented at the American Academy of Pediatrics annual meeting; October 21, 1989; Chicago, Ill.

In Other AMA Journals

ARCHIVES OF GENERAL PSYCHIATRY

On the Care of the Poor and the Uninsured

Boris M. Astrachan, MD, Donald J. Scherl, MD
(*Arch Gen Psychiatry.* 1991;48:481)

ARCHIVES OF DERMATOLOGY

The Dilemma of the Uninsured and Underinsured

Marvin Young, MD
(*Arch Dermatol.* 1991;127:712-713)

Radiological Case of the Month

David Ponder, MD; Gary S. Marshall, MD; Gerard P. Rabalais, MD (Contributors);
Beverly P. Wood, MD (Section Editor)

PATIENT 1.—A previously healthy 2-year-old girl presented with an intermittent low-grade fever, watery diarrhea, malaise, and decreased appetite of 6 weeks' duration. She lived in a rural community on a farm and had a pet dog. The parents confirmed a history of pica. Results of examination revealed a well-developed child with no abnormal physical findings. The lungs were clear on auscultation, the liver was not enlarged, and the optic fundi were normal.

Her white blood cell count was 42.4×10^9/L, with .05 band forms, .13 segmented neutrophils, .29 lymphocytes, .12 monocytes, and .41 eosinophils (the absolute eosinophil count was 17.4×10^9/L). The Westergren erythrocyte sedimentation rate was 87 mm/h, and results of stool examination for ova and parasites were negative. The serum IgG level was greater than 20 g/L, and isoagglutinin titers to A and B blood group antigens were normal. Figure 1 shows the patient's frontal chest radiograph.

PATIENT 2.—A 6-year-old boy presented with a cough, wheezing, fever, and intermittent abdominal pain of 3 months' duration. His family had emigrated from India several years earlier, and he had had a pet dog since arrival in this country. On physical examination, he was an active, well-developed boy with tachypnea, decreased breath sounds on auscultation of the chest, and diffuse expiratory wheezes. The liver was palpated 4 cm below the right costal margin. Results of the remainder of the examination were normal, including results of retinal examination. His white blood cell count was 57.6×10^9/L, with .06 band forms, .06 segmented neutrophils, .15 lymphocytes, .02 monocytes, and .71 eosinophils (the absolute eosinophil count was 40.9×10^9/L). The Westergren erythrocyte sedimentation rate was 108 mm/h, and results of stool examination for ova and parasites were negative. His serum IgG level was 40 g/L, and a serum isoagglutinin titer to blood group B antigen was 1:8192. Figure 2 shows his radiograph.

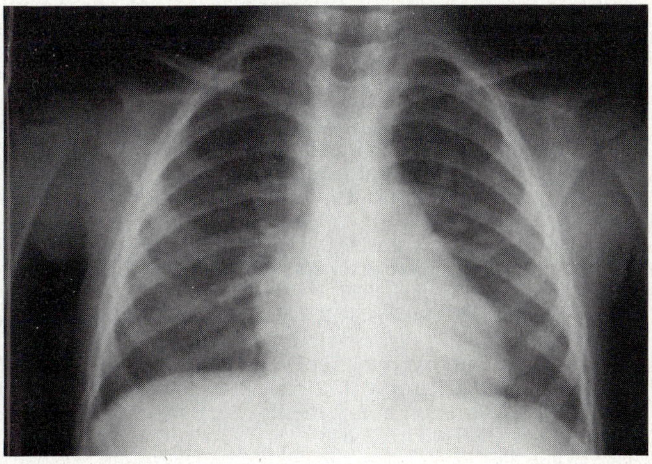

Figure 1.

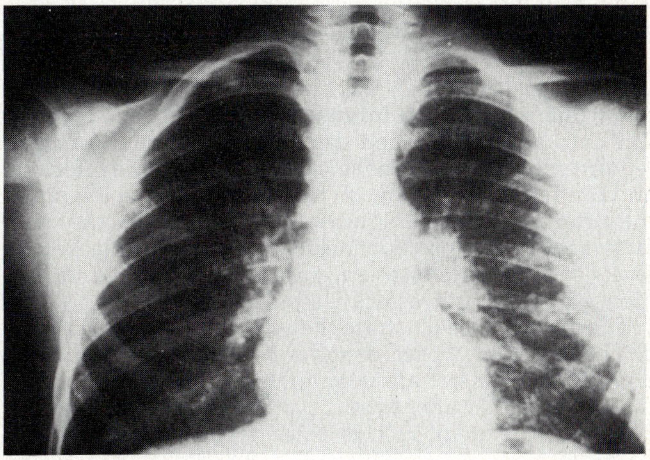

Figure 2.

Accepted for publication March 12, 1990.

From the Department of Pediatrics, University of Louisville (Ky) School of Medicine.

Reprint requests to the Department of Radiology, Childrens Hospital of Los Angeles, 4650 Sunset Blvd, Los Angeles, CA 90027 (Dr Wood).

Denouement and Discussion

Visceral Larva Migrans

Fig 1.—*Case 1. Both lungs have a mild, diffuse interstitial infiltrate. There is no pleural fluid, and the heart and mediastinal structures are normal.*

Fig 2.—*Case 2. Diffuse reticulonodular densities are evenly distributed bilaterally, with hilar adenopathy.*

Visceral larva migrans (VLM), first described in 1952,[1] is an infection of young children. It is characterized by fever, respiratory abnormalities, hepatomegaly, and marked eosinophilia. It is most commonly caused by infection with *Toxocara canis*, a dog ascarid. Infection occurs through ingestion of embryonated eggs in soil.[2] These eggs hatch second-stage larvae in the proximal small bowel that penetrate the intestinal wall and disseminate to the viscera, where they engender intense inflammatory reactions and may become encapsulated in eosinophilic granulomas. The clinical manifestations of VLM infection result from the mechanical effect of migrating larvae and from the vigorous immune response to them. Associated findings of leukocytosis, hypereosinophilia, and hypergammaglobulinemia, illustrated in these two patients, reflect the intensity of this host reaction.

Humans are accidental hosts in the life cycle of these helminths. As such, the helminths' maturation is arrested, and infected humans do not excrete infective eggs. In the most common form of transmission among dogs, puppies are infected in utero by migrating larvae. After birth, the larvae migrate through the lungs into the trachea, posterior pharynx, and gastrointestinal tract. There they mature into adults and shed eggs into the stool. The eggs require prolonged external incubation to become infective and can remain viable in soil for long periods, explaining the strong association between VLM and pica. Other risk factors for *T canis* infection include youth, being black, low levels of parental education, puppy ownership, and residence in the southeastern United States.[3]

These two cases illustrate the variety of manifestations of VLM infection. Fever, cough, wheezing, pallor, and abdominal discomfort are common complaints.[4] Infection can affect the central nervous system and cause seizures. Retinal involvement such as exudative granulomatous lesions is described in VLM-infected older children, who rarely manifest visceral disease. Hepatomegaly is the most common physical finding; rashes and lymphadenopathy can also occur. Rales and/or rhonchi are sometimes present in patients with pulmonary symptoms of VLM infection.

The diagnosis of VLM infection is confirmed by the laboratory findings mentioned above and in elevated levels of isohemagglutinins, as demonstrated in patient 2. The latter results from cross-reactivity between blood group antigens and surface proteins of the parasite. Levels of hepatic transaminase are elevated, as illustrated in both patients. Roentgenographic abnormalities of the lung are evident and include diffuse or patchy alveolar infiltrates, miliary patterns, shifting infiltrates, and chronic interstitial changes.[5] The diagnosis can be confirmed by demonstrating larvae in a liver biopsy specimen or by detecting *Toxocara*-specific antibodies using enzyme-linked immunosorbent assay.[6] This test was performed in patient 1, and results were positive.

Infection with VLM is generally a self-limited condition, but treatment with antilarval chemotherapy or anti-inflammatory agents is indicated in patients experiencing compromised organ function.

References

1. Beaver PC, Snyder CH, Carrera GM, Dent JH, Lafferty JW. Chronic eosinophilia due to visceral larva migrans: report of three cases. *Pediatrics.* 1952;9:7-19.
2. Schantz PM, Glickman LT. Toxocaral visceral larva migrans. *N Engl J Med.* 1978;298:436-439.
3. Worley G, Green JA, Frothingham TE, et al. *Toxocara canis* infection: clinical and epidemiological associations with seropositivity in kindergarten children. *J Infect Dis.* 1984;149:591-597.
4. Huntley CC, Costas MC, Lyerly A. Visceral larva migrans syndrome: clinical characteristics and immunologic studies in 51 patients. *Pediatrics.* 1965;36:523-536.
5. Felman AH, Cohen MD, eds. *Radiology of the Pediatric Chest: Clinical and Pathological Correlations.* New York, NY: McGraw-Hill International Book Co; 1987:332.
6. Cypess RH, Karol MH, Zidian JL, Glickman LT, Gitlin D. Larva-specific antibodies in patients with visceral larva migrans. *J Infect Dis.* 1977;135:633-640.

SPECIAL FEATURE

Picture of the Month

Merlin G. Butler, MD, PhD, Sarah Hassell, MD (Contributors); *Murray Feingold, MD* (Editor for This Case);
Walter W. Tunnessen, Jr, MD (Section Editor)

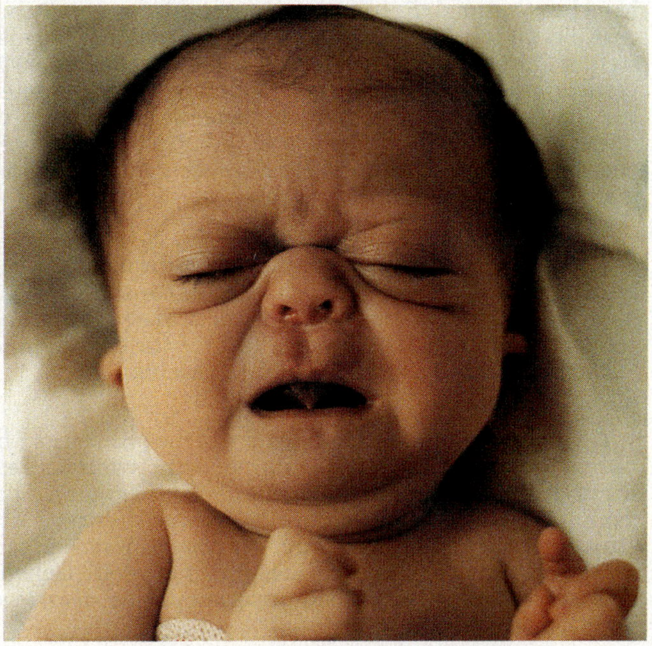

Figure 1.

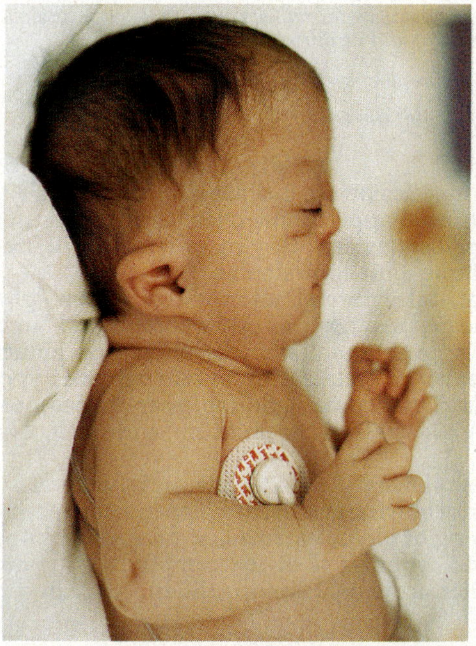

Figure 2.

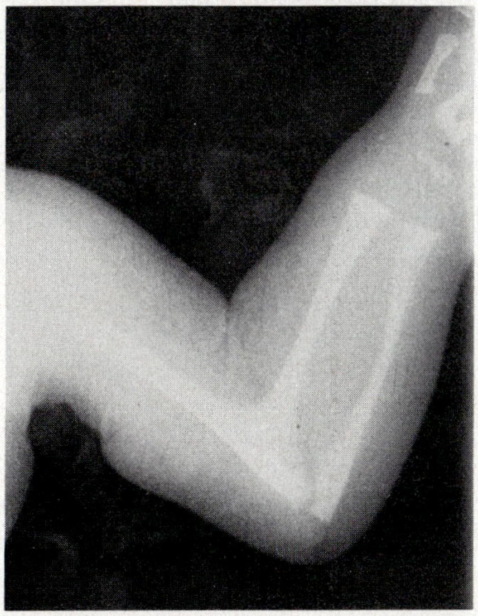

Figure 3.

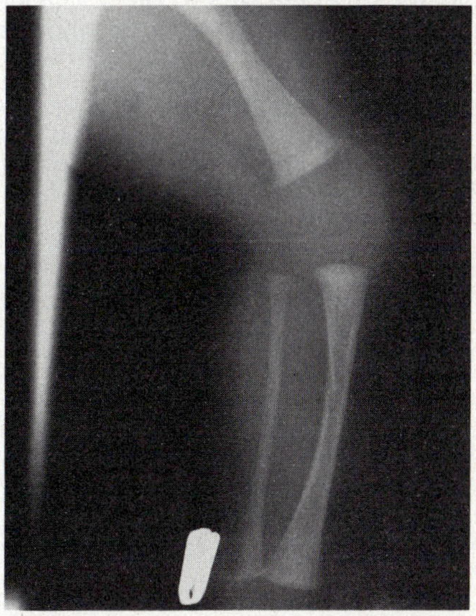

Figure 4.

Accepted for publication December 5, 1990.
Contributed from the Department of Pediatrics, Division of Genetics, Vanderbilt School of Medicine, Nashville, Tenn.
Reprint requests to National Birth Defects Center, Franciscan Children's Hospital, 30 Warren St, Brighton, MA 02135 (Dr Feingold).

Denouement and Discussion

Antley-Bixler Syndrome

Figs 1 and 2.—*3-week-old newborn with brachycephaly; prominent forehead; flat face; low-set, dysplastic ears; flattened nasal bridge; pear-shaped nose; severe, midface hypoplasia; proptosis; flexed position of elbow; and camptodactyly.*

Fig 3.—*Radiohumeral synostosis.*

Fig 4.—*Bowing of the femur.*

Manifestations

Major manifestations include craniosynostosis, a characteristic facial appearance, choanal atresia/stenosis, radiohumeral synostosis, bowing of femurs with fractures, and multiple joint contractures.

Craniofacial abnormalities consist of brachycephaly secondary to craniosynostosis of the coronal and lambdoidal sutures; large anterior fontanelle; and a face characterized by frontal bossing, flat facies, severe midface hypoplasia, proptosis, flattened nasal bridge, pear-shaped nose, choanal stenosis/atresia, long philtrum, and small, dysplastic ears.

Skeletal abnormalities include radiohumeral synostosis, anterior bowing of femurs with neonatal fractures, medial bowing of ulnas, narrow iliac wings, arachnodactyly with distal tapering of digits, camptodactyly, and scoliosis. Other occasional abnormalities are hydrocephalus, atrial septal defects, vaginal atresia, renal defects, multiple hemangiomata, and preauricular tags. Auditory dysfunction may also occur.

In most reported cases, prenatal and postnatal growth have been normal. Respiratory compromise generally occurs secondary to upper-airway obstruction (choanal stenosis/atresia occurs in about one half of affected individuals) and may vary from nasal congestion to apnea leading to death. Some patients have died in infancy of unexplained causes. Patients followed up beyond age 1 year have been ambulatory. Intelligence varies from normal to mild retardation.

Genetics

Antley-Bixler syndrome occurs sporadically, but has been reported in siblings and children of consanguineous parents. Therefore, inheritance is most likely autosomal recessive with a 25% recurrence risk for the condition in subsequent children from the same parents.

Treatment

Treatment consists of management of the orthopedic abnormalities, including the multiple joint contractures, through physical therapy, casting, and/or surgery. Surgery may also be necessary to alleviate upper-airway obstruction and to correct the craniosynostosis. Hearing, cardiac, and renal evaluations are also indicated. Genetic counseling and prenatal diagnosis should be discussed with the family.

References

1. Antley RM, Bixler D. Trapezoidocephaly, midface hypoplasia and cartilage abnormalities with multiple synostoses and skeletal fractures. *Birth Defects Original Articles Series.* 1975;11:397-401.

2. DeLozier CD, Antley RM, Williams R. The syndrome of multisynystotic osteodysgenesis with long-bone fractures. *Am J Med Genet.* 1980;7:391-403.

3. Escobar LF, Bixler D, Sadove M, Bull MJ. Antley-Bixler syndrome from a prognostic perspective: report of a case and review of the literature. *Am J Med Genet.* 1988;29:829-836.

The Editors welcome contributions to Picture of the Month and Radiological Case of the Month. Those who wish to contribute should send their manuscripts to Dr Tunnessen (Picture of the Month)*, The Children's Hospital of Philadelphia, 34th Street and Civic Center Blvd, Philadelphia, PA 19104, or Dr Wood* (Radiological Case of the Month)*, Department of Radiology, Childrens Hospital of Los Angeles, 4650 Sunset Blvd, Los Angeles, CA 90027. Articles and photographs accepted for publication will bear the contributor's name. There is no charge for reproduction and printing of color illustrations.*

THE PEDIATRIC FORUM

More on a Myth

Sir.—I read your very interesting editorial in the August 1990 issue of *AJDC*[1] *on the pertussis vaccine myth and its death.*

I have been practicing pediatrics for 30 years in West Texas and have administered the diphtheria and tetanus toxoid and pertussis vaccine to more children, I am sure, than many physicians in the academic centers. I have probably examined more children than many of the physicians in institutional centers. I have never seen a reaction supporting the findings of encephalopathy that were previously thought to occur in conjunction with diphtheria/pertussis immunizations, particularly pertussis immunizations.

What disturbs me most about your editorial is your discomfort with the fact that there are many unexplained results in medicine leading the "experts" to render opinions that become irrefutable early on, to the degree that they are used by courts of law to hold the practicing physician responsible for injury and therefore financially liable. This is one of the facets that, in my opinion, have led to the high cost of liability. "Cap-and-gowned" experts around the country continue to give their opinions even before evidence is collected on whether a complication is associated with the performance of certain procedures, the application of certain treatments, or the provision of certain medications to patients, thereby creating a situation that is very hard to turn around when an untoward event occurs. It would be certainly more efficacious, safer, and better if the "experts" refrained from making official statements and giving their opinions before having clear evidence to support such definite pronouncements early in the course of any illness.

As a result of the concern for pertussis vaccine and so-called myth of encephalopathy, the fear of God was placed on pediatricians' shoulders. The fear of litigation along with the concomitant rise in the cost of liability and vaccines has put the pediatric community in a position from which it may never recover. In terms of reasonable medical liability insurance coverage fees and affordable immunizations to patients as administered by the private and public pediatric community, I doubt very seriously if, in a free market economy, the price of those vaccines or liability costs will decrease in the face of such a myth. It is so interesting to me that in these United States, myths have such a great degree of control over us that they often explain untoward outcomes more than reality.

Please note also that as a result of the myth, a Vaccine Compensation Act was passed at extreme cost to the providers of care, drug manufacturers, and other entities. It was probably unnecessary in the first place. It appears now that the people who will benefit from the passage of such a law and the creation of such a fund are the managers of the fund and attorneys who, through the process, know how to tap into that fund. I am sure if we now decided that the compensation fund was unnecessary, the money would never be refunded, and even if it were, any savings would not be returned to the people who originally participated in contributing to that fund.

I doubt that my letter will be read with the intent that is meant; I doubt that it will be published; and I also doubt very seriously whether anyone in the academic field and the so-called experts of medicine will get the message.

Jose Roman, Jr, MD
1900 N Oregon, Suite 405
El Paso, TX 79902

1. Fulginiti VA. A pertussis vaccine myth dies. *AJDC*. 1990;144:860-861.

In Reply.—I appreciate Dr Roman's letter in response to my editorial concerning the pertussis vaccine encephalopathy myth. His comments are those of a concerned physician and should be taken seriously. To add further information to the topic he discusses, I refer Dr Roman to my earlier editorial on how standard practice in pediatrics is set.[1]

I do not believe that experts act capriciously. I addressed part of this in my previous editorial, but would like to take this opportunity to expand on those thoughts.

Most experts are dedicated professionals who strive to offer their best opinion in a discipline that does not have all the data it needs but must act on the data available to care for patients. My experience is mostly with recommendations for immunization and infectious diseases practice, so I will draw on that for my examples.

The Academy of Pediatrics Committee on Infectious Diseases (the *"Red Book"* Committee) serves pediatricians by digesting, analyzing, and sorting out the available data on infectious diseases and their prevention and treatment. From this process they develop recommendations for the practitioner by consensus. These are incorporated into the *Red Book* and other statements published by the committee from time to time. The preamble to the latest edition of the *Red Book* states

> Unanswered scientific questions, the complexity of medical practice, new information, and inevitable differences of opinion between experts result in inherent limitations in the *Red Book*. Other committees and experts may not always agree with specific recommendations of the committee and will provide different viewpoints. . . . Inevitably in clinical practice, questions arise which cannot be answered on the basis of currently available data, but in such cases the committee attempts to provide guidelines and information that in conjunction with clinical judgment will facilitate well-reasoned decisions.[2]

This statement, built on earlier versions published in previous editions of the *Red Book*, summarizes my own viewpoint on the issue that Dr Roman raises. The individual practitioner often requests some guidance in areas in which he or she does not have all the available information. Experts and advisory committees attempt to assist by providing the best possible advice. This is precisely what happened with the pertussis vaccine encephalopathy story. As I outlined in my editorial, in the days before we had the data now available, the best analysis was that such an entity existed. It was not irresponsible opinion, it was the best judgment that could be rendered. It was not delivered capriciously or with the intent of harming the practitioner. On the contrary, the opinion was offered to assist the practitioner in avoiding this possible complication by delimiting those children who might be vulnerable (in the form of recommendations for precautions and contraindications for the use of whole-cell pertussis vaccine).

Unfortunately, much of medical expert advice today in all areas of medicine has the same indefinite characteristic. Data are incomplete, significant critical gaps exist, and yet, patients must be treated, vaccines administered, and other forms of treatment provided. Experts, rather than remain silent and indecisive, should offer their opinions. I agree with Dr Roman that the potential consequences of those opinions should be carefully weighed and taken into account, and appropriate qualifications offered. That is precisely what the *Red Book* statement quoted above attempts to do. That society, through the tort system, chooses to act on those opinions cannot be helped. The American Academy of Pediatrics, along with other interested parties, attempted to influence this societal tendency by advocating, assisting in developing, and participating in implementing the Vaccine Injury Compensation Act and Program.

In short, I believe experts need to give their best opinion in areas that are uncertain, and that such opinions indicate the degree of uncertainty and take into consideration potential consequences.

VINCENT A. FULGINITI, MD
Editor, *AJDC*
Tulane University School of Medicine
1430 Tulane Ave
New Orleans, LA 70112

1. Fulginiti VA. Is standard practice in pediatrics 'standard': a potential lesson for experts and practitioner. *AJDC*. 1989;143:529-530.

2. Committee on Infectious Diseases, American Academy of Pediatrics. *Red Book*. Elk Grove Village, Ill: American Academy of Pediatrics; 1988.

The Fallacy of the Hemorrhagic Shock and Encephalopathy Syndrome

Sir.—Chaves-Carballo et al[1] described nine infants with clinical features similar to heatstroke that they diagnosed as hemorrhagic shock and encephalopathy (HSE). An editorial in the same issue focuses on the inconsistencies and perplexities of the mysterious HSE syndrome.[2] During the past 15 years, I recall seeing several fatal cases that were presumptively diagnosed as either HSE or sudden infant death syndrome, but after an investigation of the home, could be diagnosed as heatstroke, exposure to toxic fumes, or both.[3,4] In the cases diagnosed as heatstroke, based on on-site investigations, there was a lack of awareness by some pathologists that exposure of a young infant, like other small mammals, to high environmental temperatures may lead to cardiogenic shock and sudden death.[5]

Chaves-Carballo and coworkers[1] discussed the catastrophic clinical features and sparse laboratory data of HSE but failed to mention anything about the home environment of the young infants who were near death on arrival at the hospital. Similar to a death-scene investigation of infants presumed to have sudden infant death syndrome, questions may be asked concerning presumptive HSE cases. Were the cribs too close to the heat source? Did a defective heating system suddenly and unexpectedly deliver bursts of heat in the early hours during the winter or in the summer during a heat wave? Were the infants prescribed medication that prevented sweating? Was there inadvertent ingestion of cocaine or was the formula contaminated with phencyclidine hydrochloride? Were toxicologic tests, including a search for volatile hydrocarbons, performed on the body fluids before prolonged resuscitative efforts were begun in the hospital?

Standard investigative procedure should be to encourage a thorough evaluation of the home environment from which a previously healthy infant is brought to the hospital and heatstroke is suspected. Information developed from scene investigation may help the physician to confirm a diagnosis of heatstroke and to prevent a similar occurrence. Like the forensic pathologist who may discard the presumptive and exclusionary diagnosis of sudden infant death syndrome for a more obvious cause following a death-scene investigation, the weak and misleading term *HSE* could be eliminated as a legitimate classification by pediatricians after a scene investigation provides evidence of heatstroke. Attempts to pinpoint elusive environmental hazards should be made only by personnel equipped to detect toxic agents in the ambient air and trained to uncover and document other useful information.

Although complete recovery is possible, the consequences of heat shock in infants who survive may include cerebral palsy, epilepsy, and mental retardation. Based on the potential savings in health care costs that could result from eliminating many of the indoor health hazards, an expanded effort is justified to train physicians in environmental medicine, including scene investigation.

MILLARD BASS, DO, MPH, ScD
1 Plaza St
New York, NY 11217

1. Chaves-Carballo E, Montes JE, Nelson WB, Chrenka BA. Hemorrhagic shock and encephalopathy: clinical definition of a catastrophic syndrome in infants. *AJDC*. 1990;144:1079-1082.

2. Corrigan JJ Jr. The 'H' in hemorrhagic shock and encephalopathy syndrome should be 'hyperpyrexia.' *AJDC*. 1990;144:1077.

3. Bass M, Kravath RE, Glass L. Death-scene investigation in sudden infant death. *N Engl J Med*. 1986;315:100-105.

4. Bass M. The fallacy of the simultaneous sudden infant death syndrome in twins. *Am J Forensic Med Pathol*. 1989;10:200-205.

5. Bass M. Sudden infant death syndrome. *N Engl J Med*. 1982;307:891-892.

Hyperpyrexia, Hemorrhagic Shock and Encephalopathy, and Creatinine Phosphokinase

Sir.—In his October 1990 editorial in *AJDC*, Corrigan[1] recommends that the "H" in the syndrome of hemorrhagic shock and encephalopathy (HSE) stand for hyperpyrexia. This is a welcome suggestion to the clinician because it underscores hyperpyrexia as an important clue to the diagnosis of this new syndrome. In February 1985, we were at a loss to explain a difficult patient who showed clinical symptoms of heatstroke. The original description of HSE by Levin et al[2] in 1983 did not view hyperpyrexia as a prominent feature of this disorder. Only two of the 10 patients described had temperatures of 41°C or greater. It was not until a subsequent report[3] emphasized hyperpyrexia that we were alerted to the similarity between our case and those being described in the literature.

Patient Report.—A 3-year-old black girl was well until 11 PM on the evening of admission, when she vomited and had a seizure. The paramedics noted a temperature of 42°C and took her to a local hospital, where a temperature of 41.6°C was recorded and the seizure was stopped with phenobarbital sodium. On arrival at our hospital, the patient was markedly lethargic with occasional seizures. She had sharp disks and no focal neurologic signs. Her blood pressure was 76/40 mm Hg; pulse, 116 beats per minute; respiratory rate, 32/min; and she had normal general examination results. She was treated intravenously with fluids, cefuroxine sodium, gentamycin sulfate, and phenobarbital. Later, fresh frozen plasma, vitamin K, and blood were given. Results of admission laboratory tests showed a hemoglobin level of 123 g/L, white blood cell count of 20×10^9/L (0.87 segmented neutrophils and 0.13 lymphocytes), and a platelet count of 350×10^9/L. The urine had 10 red blood cells per high-powered field. Serum electrolytes were normal with a carbon dioxide content of 15 mmol/L. The serum urea nitrogen was 8.9 mmol/L of urea, creatinine was 123.8 μmol/L, and aspartate aminotransferase was 185 U/L; blood ammonia, sugar, and calcium levels were normal. The cerebrospinal fluid was normal, and computed tomographic scan of the head and chest roentgenogram were normal. Later, her hemoglobin level dropped to 70 g/L and her platelet count was 136×10^9/L. Her aspartate aminotransferase and alanine aminotransferase levels rose to 14 062 U/L and 6297 U/L, respectively, with repeated normal blood ammonia content. The γ-glutamyltranspeptidase level was 61 U/L, bilirubin level was 22.2 μmol/L, and serum protein levels were normal. Liver sonogram was negative. Partial thromboplastin time was 61 seconds (normal, 34 seconds), prothrombin time was 24 seconds (normal, 10.9 seconds), fibrin split products were positive, and the fibrinogen level was more than 4 g/L. The VDRL test had negative results. Serologic test results for hepatitis A and B, amebiasis, Epstein-Barr virus, and toxoplasmosis were negative. She had creatinine phosphokinase (CPK) levels that rose to 13 397 U/L. There was no myoglobinuria. Immunoglobulin levels were normal. Tests for urinary porphyrins, amino acids, and heavy metals had negative results. Results of hypnotic screening were negative. Multiple cultures for bacteria and viruses in the cerebrospinal fluid, blood, stool, and urine were negative. Two electroencephalograms showed diffuse slowing. Repeated cerebrospinal fluid and computed tomographic scans of the head were normal. The patient remained lethargic and febrile (around 39.4°C) for 8 days. She unexpectedly had a recurrence of fever and lethargy (although milder) from day 10 to day 17. Her laboratory values normalized by day 20. She was discharged on day 25, clinically well without neurologic sequelae.

Comment.—Since the original report by Levin et al[2] describing infants who died or had severe neurologic impairment, subsequent reports have enlarged the clinical spectrum of this syndrome. Hyperpyrexia is now frequently described, milder cases have been seen, and older children have been reported. Not every patient has met the criteria suggested by Levin et al and Chaves-Carballo et al[4] to be diagnosed as having HSE. Nonetheless, the cases reported have unmistakable clinical similarities. Their resemblance to heatstroke, noted by several authors, was discussed in Corrigan's editorial.[1] The patient described here had a clinical profile of HSE in association with hyperpyrexia. The hyperpyrexia brought this new syndrome to our attention.

The markedly elevated CPK level (13 397 U/L) in this patient is noteworthy since it is a common finding in heatstroke. In 34 patients with classic heatstroke reported by Tucker et al,[5] for example, CPK elevations were observed in 75% of the cases. There are more than 160 reported cases of HSE, and the CPK levels were not recorded in most of these cases. In a few reports,[4,6-8] markedly elevated CPK levels have been noted. Beaufils and Aujard[6] had seven of seven patients with high CPK levels, and they expressed an interest in knowing these levels in the patients described by Levin et al. It would be interesting to know the CPK levels in all suspected cases of HSE. This information could be helpful in understanding these patients, and in strengthening the connection of heatstroke to the HSE syndrome.

C. Randall Dupee, MD
Department of Pediatrics
Kaiser Los Angeles
Medical Center
4867 Sunset Blvd
Los Angeles, CA 90027

1. Corrigan JJ Jr. The 'H' in hemorrhagic shock and encephalopathy syndrome should be 'hyperpyrexia.' *AJDC.* 1990;144:1077.

2. Levin M, Kay JDS, Gould JD, Hjelm M, Pincott JR, Dinwiddie R. Haemorrhagic shock and encephalopathy: a new syndrome with a high mortality in young children. *Lancet.* 1983;2:64-67.

3. Caspe WB, Nucci AT, Sangho C. Extreme hyperpyrexia in childhood: presentation similar to hemorrhagic shock and encephalopathy. *Clin Pediatr.* 1989;28:76-80.

4. Chaves-Carballo E, Montes JE, Nelson WB, Chrenka BA. Hemorrhagic shock and encephalopathy: clinical definition of a catastrophic syndrome in infants. *AJDC.* 1990;144:1079-1082.

5. Tucker L, Stanford J, Graves B, Swetnam J, Hamburger S, Anwar A. Classic heatstroke: clinical and laboratory assessment. *South Med J.* 1985;78:20-25.

6. Beaufils F, Aujard Y. Haemorrhagic shock and encephalopathy syndrome. *Lancet.* 1983;2:1086.

7. Sofer S, Philip M, Hershkowit J, Bennett H. Hemorrhagic shock and encephalopathy syndrome. *AJDC.* 1986;140:1252-1254.

8. Roth B, Younossi-Hartenstein A, Schroder R, Hornchen H, Heymans L. Haemorrhagic shock-encephalopathy syndrome. *Eur J Pediatr.* 1987;146:83-85.

Hemorrhagic Shock and Encephalopathy: An Entity Similar to Heatstroke

Sir.—We read with interest the article by Chaves-Carballo et al[1] concerning the hemorrhagic shock and encephalopathy (HSE) syndrome. We recently cared for two infants with this entity[2] and we believe that the gastrointestinal tract is the source of this devastating illness. Approximately 74 infants and children with HSE have been described in the literature, most of whom presented with a prodromal illness consisting of vomiting and diarrhea.

The origin of HSE remains unexplained, but the multisystem failure seen in both HSE and heatstroke (HS) may be a final common pathway of an unexplained mediator. The hyperpyrexia may be the result of high metabolic requirements coupled with compensatory vasoconstriction. The shock state leads to increasing splanchnic vasoconstriction (which may actually be worsened by hyperpyrexia) that contributes to the release of these potentially toxic mediators. The vasoconstriction, caused by any combination of hypotension, hyperthermia, or gut ischemia, will allow leakage of endotoxin (lipopolysaccharide [LPS]) from the gastrointestinal tract. Lipopolysaccharide, in turn, may stimulate monokines, such as tumor necrosis factor. Leclere et al[3] described two infants with HSE with elevated tumor necrosis factor levels. Endotoxemia has been noted in heat-stressed animal models[4] and may also play a role in HSE.

The gastrointestinal tract is a reservoir of endotoxin (LPS) and contains 1 mg of LPS per gram of feces.[5] The mucosal barrier of the gut is easily disrupted by trauma, ischemia, hypoxia, hypotension, vasoactive agents, hyperthermia, and viral gastroenteritis.[6] Lipopolysaccaride is usually sequestered by the reticuloendothelial cells (Kupffer cells) in the liver. The liver is very sensitive to heat stress, and autopsies have revealed abnormalities even in the early stages of HS.[7] In patients with HSE the liver may not be able to handle the increased LPS burden. Lipopolysaccharide may alter vascular permeability, impair cell metabolism and oxygen utilization, initiate disseminated intravascular coagulation, and produce hemodynamic changes resulting in hypotension, all of which are seen in both HS and HSE. Tumor necrosis factor has been demonstrated to mediate many of these changes as well. The pathologic features of HS and HSE are very similar, and we feel that cardiovascular failure, either primarily from the hyperthermia or perhaps secondary to the release of endotoxin, is the final pathway of these two entities.

The above discussion has clinical implications in that our patients[2] received fresh frozen plasma, which may have blocked the effects of LPS. Several of the patients described by Chaves-Carballo et al also received fresh frozen plasma, and it would be interesting to review the data of the survivors and see if any received fresh frozen plasma. Animal studies have recently shown that antibodies to LPS improve survival following HS.[8] We need to evaluate more carefully the potential biochemical mediators of both HS and HSE. Levin et al[9] noted elevated trypsin levels in 72% of their patients. These elevations are nonspecific findings and have been noted in hyperdynamic septic shock, adult respiratory distress syndrome, and pancreatitis.[10] Deby-Dupont et al[11] have shown that there is a statistically significant correlation between high trypsin levels and septic phenomena. Many of the biochemical and physiological changes seen in HSE lead us to suspect that it is a "septic-mediated" process. Despite an extensive search, no organism has been implicated to date. It is hoped that the application of specific criteria for a diagnosis of HSE coupled with more extensive research will lead to a better outcome for these children.

Edward E. Conway, Jr, MD
Lewis P. Singer, MD
Albert Einstein College of Medicine
Montefiore Medical Center–Pediatrics
111 E 210 St
Bronx, NY 10467

1. Chaves-Carballo E, Montes JE, Nelson B, Chrenka BA. Hemorrhagic shock and encephalopathy: clinical definition of a catastrophic syndrome in infants. *AJDC.* 1990;144:1079-1082.
2. Conway EE Jr, Varlotta L, Singer LP, Caspe WB. Hemorrhagic shock and encephalopathy: is it really a new entity? *Pediatr Emerg Care.* 1990;6:131-134.
3. Leclere F, Martinot A, Gosset P, Ameisen JC. Cachectin in hemorrhagic shock and encephalopathy syndrome. *J Pediatr.* 1989;115:500-501.
4. Gathiram P, Gaffin SL, Brock-Unte JG, Wells MT. Time course of endotoxemia and cardiovascular changes in heat stressed primates. *Aviat Space Environ Med.* 1987;58:1071-1074.
5. Pinsky MR, Matuschak GM. Multiple systems organ failure: failure of host defense homeostasis. *Crit Care Clin.* 1989;5:199-218.
6. Gaffin SL, Brock-Unte JG, Zanotti A, Wells MT. Hypoxia-induced endotoxemia in primates: role of reticuloendothelial system function and anti-lipopolysaccharide plasma. *Aviat Space Environ Med.* 1986;57:1044-1049.
7. Rubel LR, Ishak KG. The liver in fatal exertional heatstroke. *Liver.* 1983;3:249-260.
8. Gathiram P, Wells MT, Brock-Unte JG, Geffin SL. Antilipopolysaccharide improves survival in primates subjected to heat stroke. *Circ Shock.* 1987;23:157-164.
9. Levin M, Pincott JR, Hjelm M, Taylor F, et al. Hemorrhagic shock encephalopathy: clinical, pathologic, and biochemical features. *J Pediatr.* 1989; 144:194-203.
10. Jocum M, Duswald KM, Neuman S, Witt J, Fritz H. Proteinases and their inhibitors in septicemia: basic concepts and clinical implications. In: Hörl WN, Heidlond A, eds. *International Symposium on Proteases.* New York, NY: Plenum Press; 1983;167:391-422.
11. Deby-Dupont G, Hass M, Pincemaul J, et al. Immunoreactive trypsin in the adult respiratory distress syndrome. *Intensive Care Med.* 1984;16:7.

The 'H' in Hemorrhagic Shock and Encephalopathy Syndrome

Sir.—I agree with the recent editorial by Corrigan[1] that hyperpyrexia is an important, striking element in the so-called hemorrhagic shock and encephalopathy syndrome. My experience with these patients has led me to conclude that the most striking features of this syndrome are the sudden onset of high fever, severe shock, and mental status changes in a previously healthy infant. The shock state is very impressive in that it requires almost unbelievable amounts of volume expanders to reverse it, and occurs suddenly without any loss of extracellular fluid or blood from the body. Presumably this means that the shock is the result of massive third spacing in the gastrointestinal tract and/or massive vasodilatation. Both mechanisms suggest that a toxin is involved. It is my guess that this same, unidentified toxin affects skeletal muscle metabolism in such a way as to cause the hyperpyrexia. I agree with Corrigan[1] that a genetic predisposition (subclinical myopathy) may be required for this toxin to produce the full-blown syndrome.

Whittington et al[2] showed 5 years ago that if these patients were diagnosed early and the shock state reversed rapidly, all the other features of this syndrome were reversible. I have therefore concluded that all the other features of this syndrome are secondary to the shock and/or altered metabolic state of the patient (hyperpyrexia). Certainly, the "hemorrhagic" part of this disease is a minor secondary feature. As Corrigan suggests, this feature is most likely the result of some form of consumptive coagulopathy secondary to shock- and/or toxin-induced damage of the endothelium. Hemorrhage plays no significant role in this syndrome. Even the encephalopathy may be a secondary feature of this syndrome caused by decreased cerebral perfusion or by endogenous toxins produced by the altered metabolic state. It is possible, however, that the toxin causing the syndrome may directly affect the brain and cause the encephalopathic features of this syndrome.

The name given to a syndrome is of great consequence. It may implicitly convey notions about the pathogenesis or pathophysiologic characteristics of the syndrome. As a result of my experience with this syndrome, I wrote more than 5 years ago that "the term 'hemorrhagic shock and encephalopathy syndrome' is misleading, because it may suggest that the shock is secondary to hemorrhage, which is conjecture. We propose that this entity simply be called 'shock and encephalopathy syndrome,' which describes the two main features and does not have implications for pathogenesis."[2] I would not, at this time, disagree with Corrigan's proposal that the syndrome be renamed as the "hyperpyrexia, shock, and encephalopathy syndrome"[1] since hyperpyrexia is probably an important primary feature of this syndrome. I do, however, believe that our article should have been acknowledged in his editorial.

COL John D. Roscelli, MC
Tripler Army Medical Center
Tripler AMC, HI 96859-5000

1. Corrigan JJ Jr. The 'H' in hemorrhagic shock and encephalopathy syndrome should be 'hyperpyrexia.' *AJDC*. 1990;144;1077.

2. Whittington LK, Roscelli JD, Parry WH. Hemorrhagic shock and encephalopathy: further description of a new syndrome. *J Pediatr.* 1985;106:599-602.

Fetal Alcohol Syndrome: Misplaced Emphasis

Sir.—Little et al[1] seem to believe that "better communication" between the obstetric and pediatric staffs would somehow result in better diagnosis and treatment of infants with fetal alcohol syndrome (FAS). They do not seem to consider the dilemma of the pediatric clinician in this situation. The clinician is strictly bound first to do no harm. There has to be substantial benefit to justify telling the mother, "You damaged your child." As far as I can determine, since diagnosis is imprecise and judgmental, the relation between the phenotype and the behavior is highly variable, and specific treatment is nonexistent, there is little value in making the diagnosis of FAS.

What *is* imperative is the sophistication of obstetric services in supporting women during their pregnancies in a way that minimizes consumption of alcohol and other toxic substances and improves nutrition. It is also imperative that pediatricians develop widely available sophisticated services to support these mothers (and fathers) in caring for their children, whatever the degree and cause of their handicaps.

The clinical payoff comes in being sufficiently familiar with one's patients to be able to monitor various dysfunctional situations, including alcohol consumption. Only in the context of providing sufficient support for the family does this diagnosis have a decent chance of being beneficial.

Let us keep our eyes on the prize.

Karl W. Hess, MD, FAAP
3286 Maynard Rd
Cleveland, OH 44122

1. Little BB, Snell LM, Rosenfeld CR, Gilstrap LC III, Gant NF. Failure to recognize fetal alcohol syndrome in newborn infants. *AJDC.* 1990;144:1142-1146.

In Reply.—We thank Dr Hess for commenting on our article. However, we believe that making the diagnosis of FAS is important because these are not simply growth-retarded infants. They are at high risk of having developmental abnormalities, some of which may be ameliorated by appropriate early intervention and occupational therapy. Accurate diagnosis of the syndrome may make a difference because the earlier the diagnosis is made, the sooner intervention and therapy may be implemented. We agree that caring for the mother during and after pregnancy is important. However, FAS may already be induced by the time a woman who drinks heavily realizes she is pregnant because organogenesis is frequently completed when the gravid state is recognized.

Hence, in the prevention of FAS, life-style practices of women of childbearing age are the major issue, not obstetrical services rendered. We also agree that providing "widely available sophisticated services to support" parents is appropriate, but it is obvious that one must target certain services to specific needs. For example, early intervention needs of the mild to moderately mentally retarded child with FAS differ widely from those of a child with a congenital limb amputation.

Children with FAS should certainly be targeted for early intervention, and the earlier the diagnosis is made the greater the potential benefit.

Bert Little, PhD
Larry C. Gilstrap III, MD
Department of Obstetrics and Gynecology
Laura M. Snell, MPH
Department of Family Practice and Community Medicine
Charles R. Rosenfeld, MD
Department of Pediatrics
The University of Texas Southwestern Medical Center at Dallas
5323 Harry Hines Blvd
Dallas, TX 75235-9032

Herpes Zoster Oticus

Sir.—Herpes zoster oticus (HZO) is characterized by varicella zoster virus (VZV) infection of the ear in association with facial nerve palsy. It may result in permanent facial paralysis and denervation more frequently than does idiopathic Bell's palsy.[1] We describe three patients diagnosed with HZO associated with seventh cranial nerve palsy.

Patient Reports.—PATIENT 1.—A 10-year-old boy reported left ear pain for 4 days and progressive left facial weakness for 3 days before hospitalization. Otitis media had been diagnosed, and antimicrobial treatment had been initiated 7 days earlier. He had had chickenpox at age 4 years. Results of physical examination on admission revealed an afebrile child with infranuclear left facial paralysis. The left tympanic membrane was erythematous; vesicles were seen on the annulus of tympanic membrane and on the external auditory canal of the left ear. Intravenous acyclovir (30 mg/kg of body weight per day) was administered in three divided doses for 7 days. Vesicle cultures yielded VZV. The facial weakness partially resolved, and vesicles healed during the 7 days of therapy. Complete recovery ensued.

PATIENT 2.—An 18-year-old woman complained of pain on the left side of her neck for 8 days and weakness on the left side of her face for 7 days. The left side of her neck over the angle of the mandible, the left ear, and the surrounding area anteriorly were tender. The left pinna and external auditory canal were edematous with multiple vesicular lesions. She had a left infranuclear facial nerve weakness. She had had chickenpox at age 5 years. Cultures of the ear lesions yielded neither bacteria nor viruses. She received analgesic therapy, eye care, and acyclovir (22.5 mg/kg of body weight per day), which was administered intravenously for 4 days, followed by oral acyclovir (200 mg) four times a day for 6 days. Complete recovery ensued.

PATIENT 3.—A 9-year-old boy who had undergone cardiac transplantation 10 months earlier and who was receiving immunosuppressive therapy presented with a 2-day history of otalgia. On the day before admission, he developed a painful vesicular rash on his right ear. He had had chickenpox at age 5 years. On admission, he was afebrile and had infranuclear right facial palsy and vesicular lesions scattered over his right ear. Treatment with intravenous acyclovir (30 mg/kg of body weight per day) was initiated. Direct fluorescence antibody stain for VZV (Ortho Diagnostic Systems Inc, Raritan, NJ) and a culture for VZV done before administration of acyclovir were both positive. He rapidly improved, with vesicular crusting and resolution of his facial palsy. After 3 days, therapy was changed to oral acyclovir (200 mg) four times a day for 7 days. At 6 months, the seventh nerve palsy had completely resolved.

Comment.—Facial palsy due to VZV infection is uncommon in children. May et al[2] reported 170 cases of facial palsy in subjects up to age 18 years, of which only four cases (2.4%) were associated with HZO.[2] In 1907, Ramsay-Hunt[3] described a syndrome of herpesvirus infection involving the ear. Four types of HZO have been indentified: HZO without neurologic involvement; HZO with facial palsy; HZO with facial palsy and auditory symptoms; and HZO with facial palsy and both auditory and vestibular symptoms.

The clinical diagnosis of HZO rests on the combined presence of earache, cutaneous vesicles, and inflammation of the pinna, usually with ipsilateral facial weakness. Devriese and Moeskev,[4] in a review of 102 patients with HZO, concluded that (1) in most cases, vesicles and weakness appear at the same time (in 25%, eruptions appear earlier); (2) the external ear has vesicles in 90% of patients; (3) maximal weakness usually occurs within a week; (4) complete paralysis is twice as common as incomplete paralysis; (5) recovery is better when appearance of vesicles precedes complete loss of function; and (6) 10% of patients with complete paralysis, and 66% with incomplete paralysis, recover totally. Clinical diagnosis can be confirmed by either viral culture or fluorescence antibody studies using VZV identification reagent (Fluorescein isothiocyanate–conjugated monoclonal anti-VZV; Ortho Diagnostic Systems Inc) on lesion specimens. Serologic studies are unlikely to be helpful in confirming the diagnosis. When performed, histologic examination of the facial nerve reveals scattered, diffuse, lymphocytic and plasma cell infiltrates and lymphocytic, perilymphatic, perivascular cuffing.[5,6] This is in contrast to the typical edematous neuropathy with an acellular infiltrate seen in idiopathic Bell's palsy.[7] The pathologic changes in facial nerve fibers in HZO are probably secondary to the involvement of Schwann cells by VZV. The observed weakness may result from the inflammatory edema, which results in compression and ischemia of the facial nerve in its course through the narrow canal in the petrous bone.[8]

There are no standard recommendations for the management of HZO. Appropriate supportive therapy, including administration of analgesia and eye care, are indicated for all patients. Corticosteroids have been shown by some investigators to decrease pain during the acute phase, shorten the duration of facial weakness, and possibly decrease postherpetic pain, although the latter claim is controversial.[9] Surgical intervention may be indicated in patients with normal prognostic and stimulation tests of the facial nerve, but with incomplete recovery.[10] Acyclovir has been successfully employed, both orally and parenterally, for the treatment of VZV infections in both normal and immunocompromised hosts.[11-14] While prospective studies are lacking with respect to the specific effectiveness of acyclovir in treating HZO, our data and those of others[15-17] support consideration of its use. Collaborative investigations are necessary before definitive therapeutic recommendations can be made.

MOBEEN H. RATHORE, MD
ALLAN D. FRIEDMAN, MD, MPH
St Louis University
School of Medicine
Cardinal Glennon
Children's Hospital
Division of Infectious Diseases
1465 S Grand Blvd
St Louis, MO 63104

LESLIE L. BARTON, MD
University of Arizona
Health Sciences Center
1501 N Campbell Ave
Tucson, AZ 84724

LISA M. DUNKLE, MD
Bristol-Myers-Squibb
Antiviral Research Division
5 Research Pkwy
Wallingford, CT 06492

The authors would like to thank Diana Duke for her help in the preparation of this manuscript.

1. Adour KK, Swanson PJ. Facial paralysis in 403 consecutive patients. *Trans Am Acad Ophthalmol Otolaryngol.* 1971;75:

1284-1301.
2. May M, Fria TJ, Curtin H. Facial paralysis in children: differential diagnosis. *Otolaryngol Head Neck Surg*. 1981;89:841-848.
3. Ramsay-Hunt J. On herpetic inflammation of the geniculate ganglion: a new syndrome and its complications. *J Nerv Ment Dis*. 1907;34:73-96.
4. Devriese PP, Moeskev WH. The natural history of facial paralysis in herpes zoster. *Clin Otolaryngol*. 1988;13:289-298.
5. Etholm B, Schuknecht HF. Pathological findings and surgical implications in herpes zoster oticus. *Adv Otorhinolaryngol*. 1983;31:184-198.
6. Zajtchuk JT, Matz GJ, Lindsay JR. Temporal bone pathology in herpes oticus. *Ann Otolaryngol*. 1972;81:311-338.
7. McCovern FH. Facial nerve paralysis in herpes oticus. *Va Med Mon*. 1975;102:609-613.
8. Aleksic SN, Budzilovich GN, Lieverman AN. Herpes zoster oticus and facial paralysis (Ramsay-Hunt syndrome). *J Neurosci*. 1973;20:149-159.
9. Elliot FA. Treatment of herpes zoster with high dose prednisone. *Lancet*. 1964;2:610-611.
10. May M, Blumenthal F. Herpes zoster oticus: surgery based upon prognostic indicators and results. *Laryngoscope*. 1982;92:65-67.
11. Peterslund NA, Seyer-Hansen K, Ipsen J, Esmann V, Schonheyder H, Juhl H. Acyclovir in herpes zoster. *Lancet*. 1981;2:827-836.
12. Cobo M. Reduction of the ocular complications of herpes zoster ophthalmicus by oral acyclovir. *Am J Med*. 1988;85:90-93.
13. Peterslund NA, Ipsen VE, Christensen KD, Petersen CM. Oral and intravenous acyclovir are equally effective in herpes zoster. *J Antimicrob Chemother*. 1984;14:185-189.
14. McKendrick MW, McGill JI, White JE, Wood MJ. Oral acyclovir in acute herpes zoster. *BMJ*. 1986;293:1529-1532.
15. Hall SJ, Kerr AG. Acyclovir in herpes zoster oticus. *Lancet*. 1985;1:1103.
16. Ivarsson S, Andreasson L, Ahlfors K. Acyclovir treatment in a case of facial paralysis caused by herpes zoster. *Pediatr Infect Dis J*. 1987;6:84.
17. Stafford FW, Welch AR. The use of acyclovir in Ramsay Hunt syndrome. *J Laryngol Otol*. 1986;100:337-340.

Laparoscopic Cholecystectomy Under Continuous Epidural Anesthesia in Patients With Cystic Fibrosis

Sir.—Patients with cystic fibrosis often develop cholelithiasis. Subsequently, many will suffer from symptoms of their gallstones and develop cholecystitis. Because of the high risks associated with induction of anesthesia in patients whose pulmonary status is compromised, surgery is sometimes delayed or avoided. With the advent of laparoscopic cholecystectomy and anesthetic techniques such as epidural blockade, another option is available that may be safe for many of these patients. I describe a patient whose surgical and anesthetic care was unique.

Patient Report.—An 18-year-old man with cystic fibrosis, severe recurrent pneumonia caused by *Pseudomonas aeruginosa*, and bronchiectasis was admitted to the Baptist Hospital of Miami (Fla) with worsening midepigastric pain, bilious vomiting, belching, and inability to eat. He had a 2- to 3-year history of biliary colic after eating certain foods. An ultrasound examination revealed multiple small gallstones in a contracted gallbladder; the gallbladder was not visualized after 4 hours of radionuclide scanning. His temperature was 102°F. He was emaciated and nonicteric. There were bilateral rales and rhonchi in all lung fields. Results of abdominal examination were unremarkable.

The white blood cell count was 26.7×10^9/L, with 0.75 segmented neutrophils and 0.11 banded neutrophils. This was higher than his usual level of 19×10^9/L to 20×10^9/L. Serum amylase and bilirubin levels were normal. The glutamic oxaloacetic acid transaminase level was 93 U/L (normal range, 7 to 40 U/L), and the alkaline phosphatase level was 257 U/L (normal range, 22 to 125 U/L). A chest roentgenogram showed extensive bilateral changes consistent with cystic fibrosis. A pulmonary function test revealed severe obstructive ventilatory disease. His vital capacity was 1.98 L (51% of the predictive value). Forced expiratory volume in 1 second was 0.76 L (22% of the predictive value), and forced vital capacity was 1.81 L (48% of the predictive value).

Ceftazidime and tobramycin sulfate therapy was begun. Respiratory treatments were strictly enforced, including chest physiotherapy. He also received anhydrous theophylline, ipratropium bromide, and prednisone. Total parental nutrition (with intralipids) was started.

Six days after admission, a laparoscopic cholecystectomy under continuous epidural anesthesia was performed without complication. The umbilicus was infiltrated with 1% lidocaine hydrochloride (Xylocaine) prior to insufflating the abdomen with 2 L of carbon dioxide. A 10-mm trocar was placed in the umbilicus to accommodate the laparoscope, and, visualizing the peritoneal surface of the abdominal cavity, trocars were placed in the anterior axillary line (5 mm), midclavicular line (5 mm), and midepigastrium (10 mm) just beneath the costal margin. The gallbladder was grasped through the 5-mm ports. Dissection, clip application, and electrocauterization were performed through the 10-mm epigastric port. A stone was lodged in the cystic duct, and removal caused a prompt backflow of bile. The common duct was small and normal. The gallbladder was dissected free from the liver bed, and the neck delivered through the umbilical port after placing the laparoscope in the midepigastrium. The gallbladder was decompressed with a small suction instrument and removed intact from the abdomen. The operation lasted 55 minutes. Cholecystitis and cholelithiasis were observed in the removed gallbladder by pathologic description. The patient was transferred to the intensive care unit overnight and was ambulatory in the unit most of the evening. The next morning, he was transferred to a room outside of the intensive care unit, and he was discharged from the hospital 5 days after surgery without complication or exacerbation of his pneumonia.

Comment.—As patients with cystic fibrosis live longer, their risk of developing cholelithiasis increases. Altered bile metabolism, malabsorption of bile acids, abundant mucoproteins, increased bile viscosity, and abnormalities of gallbladder emptying may promote biliary stasis and stone formation.[1] The diagnosis of symptomatic gallstones can be obscured because of the many other causes of abdominal pain in cystic fibrosis. Chronic antibiotic therapy for recurring pneumonia may mask the inflammation of cholecystitis.

The standard treatment for symptomatic cholelithiasis has been removal of the diseased gallbladder under general anesthesia with a subcostal incision. This is associated with the possibility of postoperative chest splinting and worsening pulmonary status. Cholecystectomy using a laparoscope causes lower morbidity and shorter hospital stays.[2] This procedure has been shown to be safe and effective in treating biliary diseases.[3] In addition, use of continuous epidural anesthesia supplementing general endotracheal anesthesia has been reported for relief of postoperative pain in patients with cystic fibrosis.[4]

The procedure is usually performed under general endotracheal anesthesia. I have performed open cholecystectomies under continuous epidural anesthesia in elderly patients and in those patients refusing endotracheal intubation. In a motivated individual, it has not been difficult. Careful preoperative pulmonary function testing was performed almost routinely. The patients undergo surgery in a 30° to 40° sitting position, which is ideal for laparoscopy. This allows the liver to descend and expose the gallbladder. A 7- or 10-mm laparoscope is placed in the umbilicus. Below the costal margin, two 5-mm trocar punctures are made for grasping and manipulating the gallbladder, and a 10-mm trochar is used in the midepigastrium to dissect out and remove the gallbladder. Electrocautery was used in this instance for dissecting the gallbladder from the liver bed, but a laser could also be used. Cholangiograms can be obtained if necessary. Complications are minimal.

Laparoscopic cholecystectomy is a safe and effective treatment for patients with symptomatic gallstones. Patients with cystic fibrosis are at high risk of developing biliary colic and cholecystitis. Additional studies will be necessary to determine the risks and complications of performing this relatively new procedure on this select group of patients. The safety of continuous epidural anesthesia without endotracheal intubation cannot be determined by a single successful patient report, but it may be considered in patients with severe pulmonary disease.

David S. Edelman, MD
Department of Surgery
Baptist Hospital of Miami
8720 N Kendall Dr, #204
Miami, FL 33176

I thank Morton Schwartzmann, MD, for his help in the preparation of this report.

1. Scott W, Block G. Biliary stone disease in adults with cystic fibrosis. *Surgery*. 1989;105:671-673.

2. Reddick E, Olsen D. Laparoscopic laser cholecystectomy. *Surg Endosc.* 1989;3:131-133.

3. Dubois F, Berthelot G, Levard H. Coelioscopic cholecystectomy. *Ann Surg*. 1990;211:60-62.

4. Kang S. Continuous thoracic epidural anesthesia for biliary tract surgery and for postoperative pain relief in a patient with cystic fibrosis. *Anesth Analg.* 1982;61:793-795.

War Souvenir Poisoning

Sir.—We recently had an alarming case of accidental atropine sulfate poisoning in a 4-year-old boy who was brought to the emergency department after injecting himself with 2 mg of atropine from a vacuum-loaded syringe. Why was such an article within reach of a young child? The boy's uncle had recently returned home from military service. He was stationed in Saudi Arabia and issued the syringe to use as an antidote in chemical warfare, ie, in case he suffered symptoms of cholinergic poisoning.

The child was observed for 24 hours after receiving two consecutive doses of activated charcoal.[1] He suffered only minor symptoms of tachycardia, mydriasis, and drying of the mucous membranes, and was released the following day. We were relieved that he had no complications, since, according to reports, people have died of anticholinergic poisoning.[2] In this case, the circumstances of the accident were more alarming than the symptoms. If troops continue to bring home these "souvenirs" to the United States, we will have to warn the families of military personnel about this sort of accident. Since the syringes are vacuum-loaded, a child can simply touch the needle tip of the device to be injected. Poisoning is likely with any curious child who has access to the syringe. We suspect this will not be the only case of atropine poisoning, and we urge other pediatricians to be aware of the possibility.

Elizabeth Secord, MD
Shari Claude, MD
Charles Newton, MD
Staten Island University
Hospital and Department
of Pediatrics
Children's Medical Center
of Brooklyn
450 Clarkson Ave
Brooklyn, NY 11203

1. Fahy P, Arnold P, Curry, SC et al. Serial serum drug concentrations and prolonged anticholinergic toxicity after benztropine (Cogentin) overdose. *Am J Emerg Med.* 1989;7:199-202

2. Sangster B. Dangers of orphenadrine in psychiatric patients. *Lancet.* 1985; 2:280..

Word Choice

Sir.—Wow! Eureka! It's magic! At least that is what Dr Hong says in his article in the September 1990 issue of *AJDC.*[1] He states: ". . . The phenomenological approaches have now been largely [do they have sizes?] abandoned . . ." and ". . . soon to be available through the magic of . . . "

Wow! What a change! Or were the alchemists correct in their hope that magic would create gold?

What a retrogression, really.

Gary M. Gorlick, MD, MPH
Medical Arts Pediatric
Medical Group
6221 Wilshire Blvd
Los Angeles, CA 90048

1. Hong R. Update on the immunodeficiency diseases. *AJDC.* 1990;144:983-992.

In Reply.—Dr Gorlick apparently read my article with care and disagreed with my choice of words. Responding to his confusion, I could have sought refuge in my ethnicity. After all, when one is my age (sixtysomething) and harbors more than one language in his shrinking cerebral cortex, he ought to be entitled to a bit of poetic license. However, that would be a geriatric cop-out, so I consulted my dictionary.

Largely, used as an adverb, means "for the most part; mainly."[1(p715)] Therefore, we can "largely" abandon a procedure without incurring the wrath of Strunk or White or any other protectors of the English language.

Magic, in addition to the common meanings (which include practices of alchemists), is defined as a "mysterious quality of enchantment."[1(p753)] If Dr Gorlick has seen appreciation in the eyes of patients and their families after bringing comfort to their lives, he knows magic. If he has not, he is welcome to come and visit us. Gold from base metals he will not get, but magic he will surely experience.

Richard Hong, MD
Department of Pediatrics
600 Highland Ave
Madison, WI 53792

1. *American Heritage Dictionary.* Boston, Mass: Houghton Mifflin Co; 1982:715, 753.

Saving Money With Home Care

Home care for children dependent on ventilators or other equipment is increasingly common. Until recently, such children remained in acute-care hospitals, using vast amounts of resources, even when they required less-than-acute care. Less than a decade ago, only a few demonstration projects in this country routinely attempted to return ventilator-dependent children to their homes and back into the community.[1] Today, an expanding home-care industry assists many established centers, pediatricians, and specialists in this transfer. The trend toward home care has been stimulated by rising societal expectations, awareness of the needs of the disabled, the increasing number of children rescued from formerly lethal conditions but sustaining disability in the process, and the high cost of inpatient care in acute-care facilities.

See also p 729.

Clearly, the foremost pressure is financial. Third-party payers, both public and private, do not believe they can sustain the high costs of maintaining such children in acute-care hospitals. The drain on hospital resources, once a few such children outlive their insurance coverage, can be devastating. There are two common institutional responses. Institutions faced with unsustainable expenses can devote efforts to shifting the cost to somebody else or to devising a cheaper way to provide quality care. Too many administrators are faithful followers of the first doctrinal response—"let the other guy pay." Meanwhile, others labor to achieve high-quality care in the home.

In this issue of *AJDC*, Fields et al[2] attempt to establish the level of cost-savings available to government agencies that endorse and fund home care for children disabled by respiratory conditions. Their findings make a fascinating and compelling argument. Forget the total costs to society, or the many advantages to the children themselves. Maryland's Medicaid system saved itself almost $80 000 per year per child by fully funding home care for these children. These savings were computed by comparing actual cost with estimates of the cost of care in a skilled-nursing facility. In states where the only option to home care is institutionalization in an acute-care hospital, potential savings are substantially higher.

The other striking finding of this report is the central role of the home nursing expenditure (68% of the total home care cost). Around-the-clock home nursing care for one of the patients described in the report cost Maryland $135 000. While this still reflects a modest savings compared with institutionalization, the long-term success of the home care concept clearly depends on the rational and conservative use of this scarce resource.

Our program at The Children's Hospital of Alabama mandates a transitional period of 2 to 4 weeks in which home nurses are provided for as many hours per day as the patient's life depends on skilled care. While around-the-clock home nursing care during this period is common, some patients may receive considerably fewer hours of skilled care. After a successful transition to the home, the home nursing hours are reduced steadily to a level appropriate to each situation. This "appropriate level" depends largely on the availability and ability of family members to provide nursing care. Respite nursing care is also provided using the same concept. That is, sufficient skilled nursing care must be provided to enable the family to manage the remainder of the patient's care over the long term. Alternative approaches to the problem of providing skilled nursing care deserve further study. The use of nurse-extenders and direct payments to families for the skilled nursing care they provide may enable third-party payers to reduce expenditures for home nursing care, if this can be accomplished without sacrificing safety or quality of care.

A recent article by Quint et al[3] reminds us that the long-term impact of home care is still a subject of study and debate. Moving children from the hospital to the home for 5 to 10 years while we deplete the financial and emotional resources of their families will not benefit society or third-party payers. Establishing rational criteria for the use of home nursing care should be an important subject of future reports in this field because third-party payers will surely scrutinize this expense closely. Nevertheless, the work of Fields et al should help convince Medicaid agencies in other states to adopt waiver programs such as Maryland's.

I do not suggest that the cost-benefit equation is firmly resolved by these recent reports. Further studies of medical outcome, family impact, and psychosocial development are clearly needed. Because most centers are managing only a handful of patients, who have a wide variety of diseases and support requirements, it is difficult to formulate or evaluate generalizable hypotheses. Meticulous attention to the pathophysiologic characteristics of each case has been crucial to our efforts. As more centers report their results with various medical devices and with patients with varying diseases and medical requirements, a clearer view of the role of home care will emerge. Controlled trials are likely to be rare, and skeptical review will be as essential as ever.

Robert A. Schoumacher, MD
Department of Pediatrics
University of Alabama
at Birmingham
Birmingham, AL 35294

1. Burr BH, Guyer B, Todres ID, Abrahams B, Chiodo T. Home care for children on respirators. *N Engl J Med.* 1983;309:1319-1323.
2. Fields AI, Rosenblatt A, Pollack MM, Kaufman J. Home care cost-effectiveness for respiratory technology—dependent children. *AJDC.* 1991; 145:729-733.
3. Quint RD, Chesterman E, Crain LS, Winkleby M, Boyce WT. Home care for ventilatory-dependent children. *AJDC.* 1990;144:1238-1241.

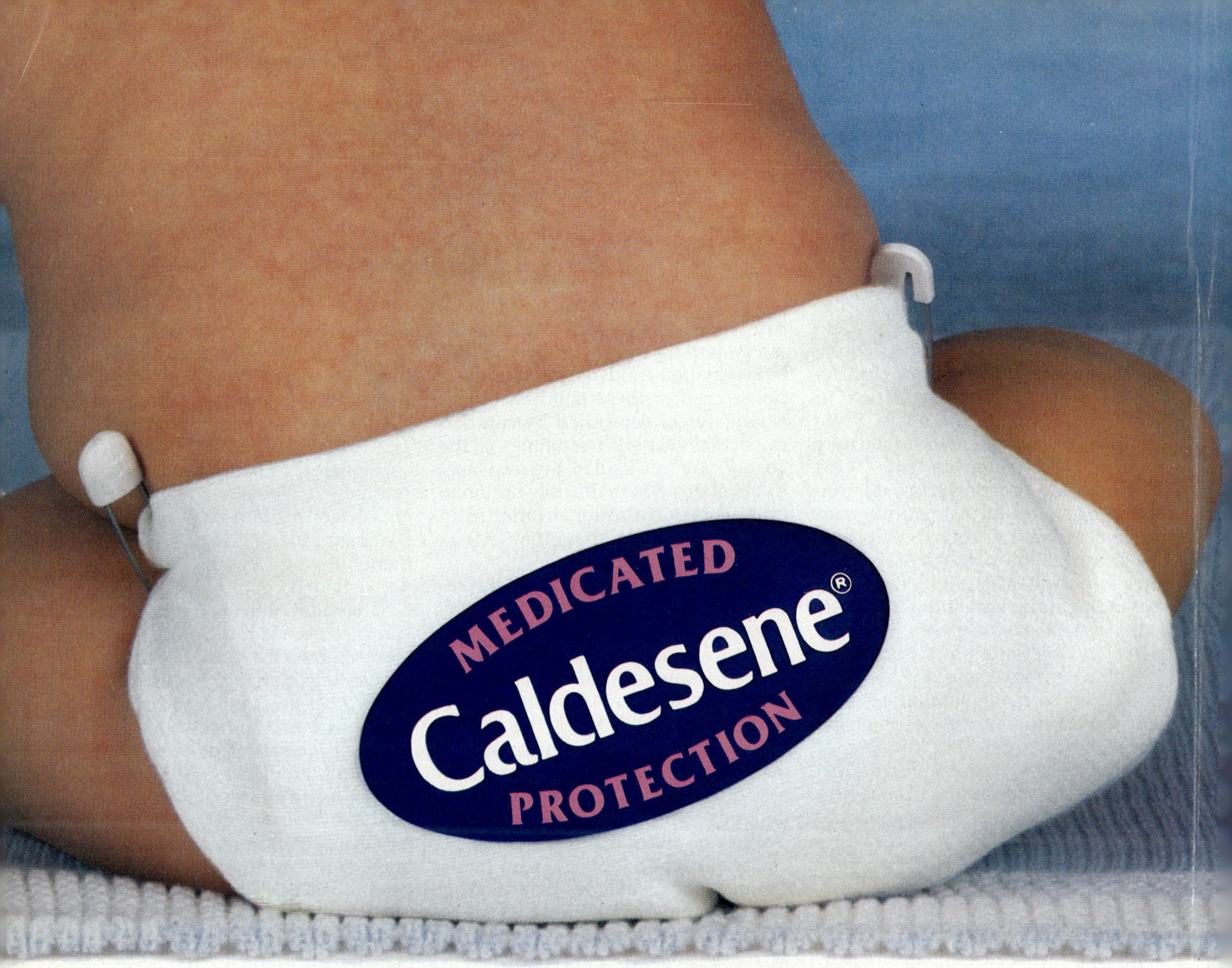

MEDICATED
Caldesene®
PROTECTION

Buddy, Can You Paradigm?

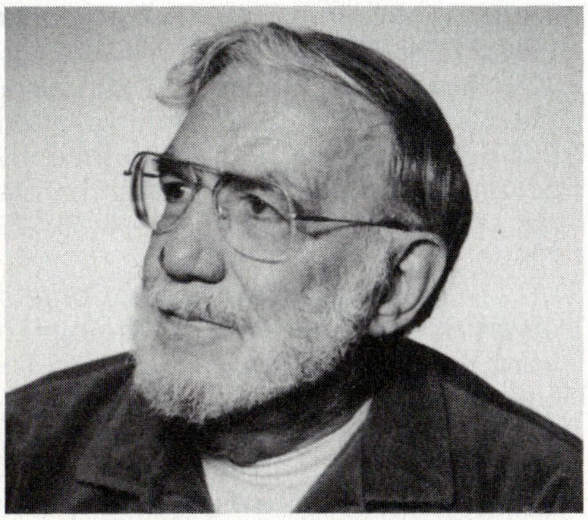

George W. Brown, MD

George is our beloved, self-declared curmudgeon. He is a workhorse for **AJDC**, *holding the record for most manuscripts refereed and for the shortest turnaround time of all of our reviewers. George provides in-depth comments designed to assist authors, whether the decision is to accept or reject the manuscript. Reading his comments is an education for all of us, not the least of whom are the authors. I have received a number of gracious comments concerning his reviews, and not all from authors whose work was accepted.*

George also accompanies his reviews of manuscripts with comments for the editor—these are terse, always humorous, and intended to lighten what he believes is the "burden" of editorship. He comments on my local geography, flora and fauna, the travails of difficult judgments, and sundry other unrelated items. Occasionally, he sends me a cartoon, suitably modified for the editor's lot. In each instance, these "bon mots" bring a smile to me and to those in our editorial group who have the pleasure of reading both his trenchant, on-the-mark reviews and the added fillip. He is not above punning, as the title of this month's contribution clearly illustrates.

George has also contributed scholarly articles to **AJDC** *and other journals on the statistical aspects of research and publication. George also is very persnickety about correct language usage and mathematical expression. He points out small errors that occasionally creep into* **AJDC** *after escaping the eyes of the editors and others. He has even had the audacity to write a letter to the editor of the journal on which he serves as a board member! I guess he does qualify as a curmudgeon, even if it is his own designation, but to all of us at* **AJDC**, *he is a lovable one at that! We are most grateful for his hard work, good sense, and sense of humor. Long live curmudgeons like George.*—**V.A.F.**

Kuhn[1] wrote that a paradigm is the constellation of beliefs, values, standards, and techniques shared by the members of a scientific community. The set of beliefs about classification of disability, impairment, or disease might be called a taxonomic or nosologic paradigm.

"Classification is a basic process man uses for ordering the universe, for simplifying a large amount of information through the placement of objects or events into definable subsets."[2] Blashfield[3] wrote: "Classification is a fundamental process in all sciences. A classification system contains the concepts which are the building blocks for a theory within that science."

On the other hand, in his presidential address to the Society for Behavioral Pediatrics, Levine[4] announced, "We are not invested in any disciplinary diagnostic system or catalog of diagnoses. We are . . . intellectually eclectic and liberated from *a priori* approaches. . . . We need not adhere over time to any fixed set of diagnostic instruments, systems of nosology, or therapeutic algorithms."

The dismissal of formal classification closely followed publication of a report by Barkley[5] reviewing *DSM-III-R* criteria for identifying attention deficit hyperactivity disorder and contrasting *DSM-III-R* criteria to criteria in the draft version of *ICD=10=CM* for identifying hyperkinetic disorders. Barkley et al[6] also reported clinical studies showing that attention deficit disorder with hyperactivity is separable from attention deficit disorder without hyperactivity and that such diagnostic precision must, whenever possible, be included in child development classification systems.

Millon and Klerman[7] edited a monograph in which some authorities defend *DSM-III-R* criteria while several others denounce it. The volume also discusses revisions that may appear in *DSM-IV*. The monograph explores the contempt expressed in some quarters toward "medical" classification schemes. For example, Eysenck[8] describes *DSM-III* as "scientifically disastrous," "antiscientific and irrational," and "empty, atheoretical, and antiexperimental." According to Eysenck, it is the product of "the power structure of contemporary feudal baronetcies."

A valuable contribution of valid classification systems to psychiatry, psychology, or developmental pediatrics would be improved prediction of outcomes of people assigned to particular diagnostic categories. Dawes et al[9] documented that clinical judgments in the diagnosis and prediction of behavior are consistently inferior to actuarial (statistical) judgments about behavior. These authors warned that "Dismissing the scientific evidence or lamenting the lack of available methods will prove much less productive than taking on the needed work."

The "needed work" is the development of a valid classification system along with a set of procedures to produce reliable and valid decisions about behavioral disturbances.

Faust and Ziskin[10] present a devastating account of the poor reliability and validity of behavioral classification systems in legal and forensic environments. They show that classification of antisocial behavior is primitive and that "expert" prediction of violent criminal behavior is about as valid as reading tea leaves or Tarot cards.

Developmental pediatrics is not the private preserve of pediatricians. Child development professionals pride themselves on their interdisciplinary methods; assessments and decisions are made by "teams" of expert participants. It gives us pause to recognize that there does not seem to be anything approaching a consensus in regard to classification of the disorders, the methods of assessment and diagnosis, the role of "theory" in nosology, generally accepted interventions, or prediction of outcomes for children with developmental problems.

Consensus fails both within and across disciplines—consider the needs of educators, language therapists, juvenile justice workers, the courts, and probation officers. Developmental pediatricians, neurologists, psychiatrists, and psychologists should be able to work together. Do they understand each other? Do they use a common language? Do they share paradigms? What about the needs of the geneticist, sociologist, anthropologist, and epidemiologist in this ensemble?

Must we abandon hope for shared theories, models, standards? Where do we begin? Is *DSM-III* a reasonable starting place for building a consensus about classification and diagnosis? Must we throw it out, and begin with a new paradigm? Is the "medical model" obsolete? Should we adopt a doctrine that the "science" of child development can thrive without classification systems? When are we going to agree to "do the needed work"?

References

1. Kuhn TS. *The Structure of Scientific Revolutions.* 2nd ed. Chicago, Ill: University of Chicago Press; 1970.

2. Skinner HA. Construct validation approach to psychiatric classification. In: Millon T, Klerman GL, eds. *Contemporary Directions in Psychopathology Toward the DSM-IV.* New York, NY: The Guilford Press; 1986:307-330.

3. Blashfield RK. Structural approaches to classification. In: Millon T, Klerman GL, eds. *Contemporary Directions in Psychopathology Toward the DSM-IV.* New York, NY: The Guilford Press; 1986:363-380.

4. Levine MD. Presidential address. *J Dev Behav Pediatr.* 1991;12:1-3.

5. Barkley RA. A critique of current diagnostic criteria for attention deficit hyperactivity disorder: clinical and research implications. *J Dev Behav Pediatr.* 1990;11:343-352.

6. Barkley RA, DuPaul GJ, McMurray MB. Comprehensive evaluation of attention deficit disorder with and without hyperactivity as defined by research criteria. *J Consult Clin Psychol.* 1990;58:775-789.

7. Millon T, Klerman GL, eds. *Contemporary Directions in Psychopathology Toward the DSM-IV.* New York, NY: The Guilford Press; 1986.

8. Eysenck HJ. A critique of contemporary classification and diagnosis. In: Millon T, Klerman GL, eds. *Contemporary Directions in Psychopathology Toward the DSM-IV.* New York, NY: The Guilford Press; 1986:73-98.

9. Dawes RM, Faust D, Meehl PE. Clinical versus actuarial judgment. *Science.* 1989;243:1668-1674.

10. Faust D, Ziskin J. The expert witness in psychology and psychiatry. *Science.* 1988;241:31-35.

Home Care Cost-effectiveness for Respiratory Technology–Dependent Children

Alan I. Fields, MD; Alan Rosenblatt, MBA; Murray M. Pollack, MD; Joanne Kaufman, RN, MS

• We evaluated home care costs and the cost-effectiveness of home care vs alternative institutional care for respiratory technology–dependent children in a Medicaid Model Waiver Program. "Cost-savings" was measured as the difference between the established Medicaid reimbursable charges to enact an individualized care plan at a long-term care institution and the actual Medicaid reimbursements for home care. Ten patients—six dependent on mechanical ventilation and four with a tracheostomy who were receiving oxygen—were included in the analysis. The mean (±SD) annual home care costs were \$109 836±\$20 781 for ventilator-dependent children and \$63 650±12 350 for oxygen-dependent patients with a tracheostomy, representing annual savings of approximately \$79 000 per patient and \$83 000 per patient, respectively. The largest portion of home care reimbursements was for nursing care, accounting for 69.0% and 59.0% of the two patient groups. The full program (50 patients) has the potential for a savings of \$4 million per year.

(*AJDC.* 1991;145:729-733)

Home care for technology-dependent children is more cost-effective than institutional care.[1-5] Home care may save up to \$300 000 per year with mean costs of only 50% of institutional costs.[1-5] However, third-party payers frequently will not reimburse fully for the complete range of services required for home care, shifting the financial burden toward the family. Because many families are unable to dedicate the financial and personnel resources necessary for home care, technology-dependent children often remain in short- and long-term care hospitals. In 1981, Congress enacted a law allowing transfer of public funding from hospital care to home care through the creation of a state Medicaid Home and Community-Based Waiver Program.[6] Normally, by statute, the income and resources of parents living in the same household as their child are "deemed" available to the child. The crucial aspect of the Model Waiver Program is the waiving of "deeming of parental income," so that the child's income is the only consideration for financial eligibility. This resulted in the expansion of the Medicaid eligibility criteria to include middle- and upper-income families whose private insurance benefits either reached their maximum or would not reimburse for home care. Unfortunately, few physicians are aware of this program, few states have utilized it to its full extent, and there has been limited analysis of the program's cost-effectiveness.[7]

See also p 725.

Accepted for publication January 24, 1991.

From the Coordinating Center for Home and Community Care Inc, Millersville, Md (Dr Fields, Mr Rosenblatt, and Ms Kaufman); the Department of Critical Care Medicine, Children's National Medical Center, Washington, DC (Drs Fields and Pollack); and the Departments of Anesthesiology and Pediatrics (Drs Fields and Pollack), George Washington University School of Medicine, Washington, DC.

Presented in part at the 18th Annual Society of Critical Care Medicine Educational and Scientific Symposium, New Orleans, La, May 8, 1989.

Reprint requests to the Department of Critical Care Medicine, Children's National Medical Center, 111 Michigan Ave NW, Washington, DC 20010 (Dr Fields).

In 1985, the state of Maryland enacted a Medicaid Home and Community-Based Services Waiver Program for technology-dependent children, including those who are disabled by respiratory conditions and who require long-term mechanical ventilation or a tracheostomy and oxygen. Our purpose was to determine home care costs and the cost-effectiveness of home care vs alternative institutional care for respiratory technology–dependent children in this Medicaid Model Waiver Program.

PATIENTS AND METHODS

Data were collected by the Coordinating Center for Home and Community Care (CCHCC) in Maryland, a not-for-profit consortium of public and private institutions, agencies, and organizations that provided case management for children with respiratory disabilities at home or alternative living facilities. The CCHCC was a subcontractor to the Medicaid Model Waiver Program and was responsible for case management, monitoring the plan of care, and determining the cost-effectiveness of the program for each recipient. The CCHCC was initially funded in 1983 by a 3-year Special Program of Regional and National Significance (SPRANS) grant by the Bureau of Maternal and Child Health. The CCHCC is staffed with administrators, nurse case coordinators, educational coordinators, human service workers, a financial analyst, and a medical director.

All children in this analysis were Medicaid Model Waiver Program recipients who were discharged from short- and long-term care hospitals from April 1985 through June 1987. All patients required either mechanical ventilation or a tracheostomy and oxygen without mechanical ventilation, the need for which remained constant for the first year after hospital discharge, and

Table 1.—Annual Patient Data for Ventilator-Dependent Children

Diagnosis	Age at Discharge	Adjusted AIC*	Home Care Reimbursed†	Savings‡
Osteogenesis imperfecta	10 mo	186	116	70
Traumatic quadriplegia	9 y	210	143	67
Congenital heart disease tracheomalacia	14 mo	190	108	82
Central hypoventilation	4 y	194	80	114
Prune belly, hypoplastic lungs	3 y	200	98	102
Central hypoventilation	2 y	153	113	40
Mean ± SD§	...	188.9±19.5	109.8±20.8	79.1±26.6

*Adjusted alternative institutional care (AIC) costs (in thousands of dollars) are estimates for care at the alternative institution after correction for actual, short-term rehospitalizations.

†Reimbursed home care costs (in thousands of dollars) are actual Medicaid reimbursements, including short-term hospital reimbursements.

‡Savings (in thousands of dollars) is adjusted AIC minus reimbursed home care.

§Means are based on raw data.

all of the first year's Medicaid reimbursable charges for home care were paid in full by July 1988.

To receive the Medicaid Model Waiver Program funding, Maryland State Regulations (COMAR 10.09.27–Home Care for Disabled Children Under a Model Waiver) required patients to be Maryland residents younger than 19 years of age and to meet medical, financial, and cost-effectiveness eligibility requirements.[8] Medical eligibility was determined by a state-sanctioned, peer-review organization based on the primary care physician's assessment of medical conditions and care needs. Medical eligibility criteria specified in the regulations included disabilities requiring technological support. Financial eligibility required that parents apply for medical assistance for the child; only the child's income was considered when eligibility was determined. If the patient was financially and medically eligible, the cost-effectiveness of home care was evaluated. Specific care needs, including the amount of skilled nursing care, were individualized by a separate process (see below).

The cost-effectiveness eligibility was evaluated by comparing the projected costs of home care to the projected costs at an alternative care setting. The alternative care setting was defined as the least costly location capable of meeting the needs as prescribed in an individualized care plan (see below) and included pediatric long-term care facilities and short-term care hospitals. Pediatric long-term care hospitals in this region had in-house physicians 24 hours a day, while skilled nursing care facilities did not have such physician coverage. In this region, skilled nursing care facilities would not accept these children. For all patients in this analysis, the alternative care institutions were pediatric long-term care hospitals.

Annual costs for each patient's care at home or an alternative institutional setting were projected from an individualized care plan developed by a multidisciplinary team. This team consisted of specialty physicians, a primary care physician, parents, a group representing Maryland Medicaid (Children's Medical Services), a CCHCC representative (nurse coordinator), nursing agencies, and vendors. This plan detailed all foreseeable care for the next year, regardless of the medical setting, including nursing care, short-term hospital care, case management, outpatient care, medications, and other items, including durable medical equipment (eg, ventilators and apnea monitors), disposable medical supplies, transportation needs, adaptive equipment, and other therapies, such as occupational, physical, and speech therapies. The primary care physicians estimated the number of short-term care hospital admissions and the projected lengths of stay. For ventilator-dependent children, durable medical equipment and disposable medical supplies were estimated to account for 40% and 33% of the "other" category, respectively. For oxygen-dependent patients with a tracheostomy, these percentages were 29% and 42%, respectively. This care plan considered the patient's home environment and specific parental support needs. For example, the evaluation considered the number of caregivers in the home, the number and health of siblings, and parental employment status (examples are available from the authors on request).

In this analysis, we used standard Medicaid methods to determine projected cost-effectiveness. A financial analyst from CCHCC computed the difference between the established Medicaid reimbursable charges (the Medicaid definition of "costs") at the alternative institution minus the Medicaid reimbursable charges for the same care plan at home. The costs of the projected short-term care hospital admissions were added to both the home care and alternative institutional computed expenses, as per Medicaid requirements. If the estimated costs of alternative institutional care exceeded the estimated costs of home care, the patient met the cost-effectiveness eligibility criteria. All calculations were reviewed by Medicaid before the release of funds.

Once home care was initiated, the multidisciplinary team evaluated the home care plan every 90 days to ensure that medical needs had not changed and that the cost-effectiveness of home care continued. If additional medical expenditures were necessary between the team meetings, they were evaluated by the financial analyst to ensure the continuation of cost-effectiveness before the funds were approved.

Savings by the program ("actual" cost-effectiveness) for the first year were calculated as estimated alternative institutional expenses minus home care reimbursements. Home care costs were calculated with use of actual Medicaid reimbursements and included the cost of case management. Home care nursing rates were reimbursed at $18/h. Alternative institutional costs were estimated with use of Medicaid reimbursement rates (96% of charges) for care at the alternative institution, including ancillary charges. Three of the 10 patients assessed were hospitalized in the least costly alternative institution at the time of discharge, and their Medicaid reimbursements were used to confirm the accuracy of these projections. Because home care costs included reimbursements for short-term hospital care, alternative institutional cost estimates were also adjusted for these expenses, assuming an equal number of days of short-term hospital care for the alternative care institution as for home care. In addition, because nursing costs for home care depend on the number of days of home care, the projected nursing costs were adjusted for the actual number of short-term care rehospitalizations. Data are reported as mean±SD.

RESULTS

Ten patients–six dependent on mechanical ventilation (Table 1) and four with a tracheostomy and receiving oxygen (Table 2)–were included in our analysis. The mean cost of home care for ventilator-dependent children was $109 836±$20 781 per patient for the first year. The estimated cost of alternative institutional care was $188 909±$19 472 per patient, for an estimated annual savings of $79 074±$26 558 per patient. The mean cost of home care for the four oxygen-dependent patients with a

Table 2.—Annual Patient Data for Oxygen-Dependent Children With a Tracheostomy*

Diagnosis	Age at Discharge	Adjusted AIC	Home Care Reimbursed	Savings
Bronchopulmonary dysplasia	1.5 y	118	66	52
Partial trisomy 1, mental retardation with cerebral palsy	10 mo	177	71	106
Congenital heart disease, tracheomalacia	2.5 y	147	46	101
Congenital heart disease, Down syndrome	5 y	146	72	74
Mean ± SD	. . .	146.8±24.0	63.6±12.4	83.2±25.0

*See Table 1 footnotes for additional information.

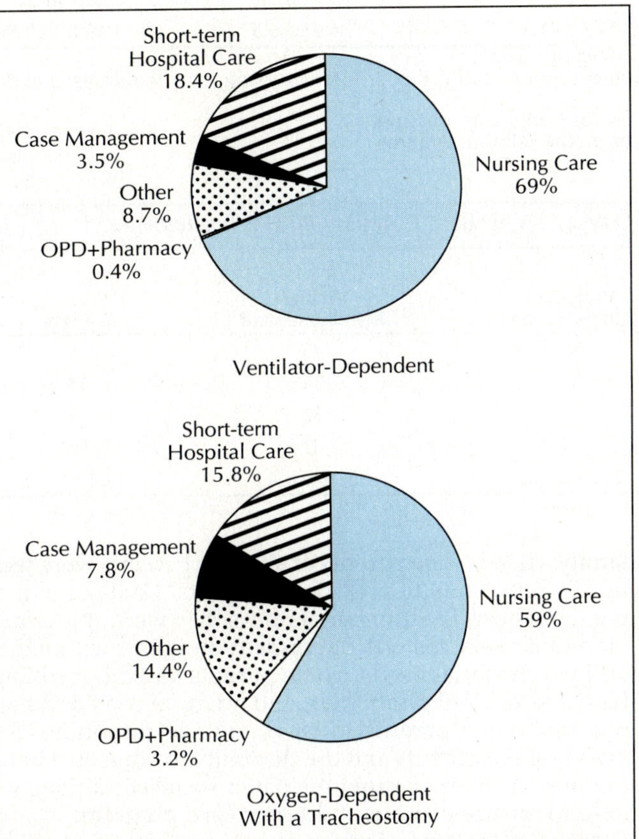

Distribution of annual home care reimbursements for ventilator-dependent and oxygen-dependent children with a tracheostomy in the Medicaid Model Waiver Program. Short-term hospital care includes all reimbursements for rehospitalizations for the first year after discharge; OPD includes physician visits and outpatient hospital charges; and includes other, durable medical equipment, disposable medical supplies, transportation, and occupational, physical, and speech therapies.

tracheostomy was $63 650±$12 350 per patient for the first year, while the estimated cost of alternative institutional care was $146 836±$23 992 per patient, resulting in an estimated annual savings of $83 187±$25 028 per patient.

Components of home care costs for the first year appear in the Figure. For ventilator-dependent patients, nursing care accounted for 69.0% of total costs; short-term hospital care, 18.4%; case management, 3.5%; outpatient costs, 0.3%; and pharmacy, 0.1%; the remaining expenses, including durable medical equipment, disposable medical supplies, occupational and physical therapies, and transportation, accounted for 8.7%. For oxygen-dependent children with a tracheostomy, nursing care accounted for 59.0% of the total costs; short-term hospital care, 15.8%; case management, 7.8%; outpatient care, 2.4%; and pharmacy, 0.8%; the remaining items averaged 14.2%.

Nursing care accounted for more than half of the reimbursements in both groups (Figure). Multidisciplinary team evaluations after the first 90 days at home decreased nursing care for three ventilator-dependent children (Table 3) and one oxygen-dependent child who had a tracheostomy (Table 4), as parents were able to provide more care. Projected nursing requirements did not increase for any child.

The mean reimbursements for nursing care for the first year were substantially lower than were projected from the individualized care plan. Only one patient in each group actually required more nursing care than projected from the initial care plan and quarterly reviews. These increases resulted from the provision of extra nursing care in lieu of rehospitalization for acute illness. The projected cost of home care nursing for ventilator-dependent children was $94 704±$41 381 per patient, while their reimbursements for nursing care were $74 916±$36 508 per patient (Table 3). The difference of $19 788±$21 732 per patient represents 21% of all ordered nursing care that remained unfilled. The projected costs of home care nursing for oxygen-dependent children with a tracheostomy was $51 102±$20 183 per patient, while their reimbursements for nursing care were $37 848±$6397 per patient (Table 4). The difference of $13 254±$17 419 per patient represents 26% of all ordered nursing care that remained unfilled.

COMMENT

Medicaid is the major public funding source for medical services to people with disabilities. Previously, few state Medicaid programs reimbursed for the full range of services needed by technology-dependent children in nonhospital settings. The Omnibus Reconciliation Act of 1981 (Public Law 97-35) expanded eligibility for Medicaid benefits in two major ways. First, it granted eligibility for benefits to finance medical and nonmedical support services and the purchase of equipment to be used in the home, such as mechanical ventilators and skilled nursing care. These services and equipment usually are not covered by Medicaid, frequently requiring Medicaid recipients to remain in a more costly institutional setting. Second, this waiver enables only the child's income to be considered for financial eligibility, expanding the Medicaid eligibility criteria to include middle- and upper-income families whose private insurance benefits either "capped out" or would not reimburse for home care. President Reagan applied this waiver to Katie Beckett, a 5-year-old girl in Iowa, who was ventilator-dependent after contracting encephalitis, to allow Medicaid funding for home care. "Katie Beckett" waivers had to be individually approved by the Health Care Financing Administration (HCFA). In 1982, a Medicaid Home and Community-Based Waiver Program

Table 3.—Annual Home Care Nursing Requirements in Ventilator-Dependent Children

Patient	Nursing Care* Discharge	90 d–1 y	Projected† Reimbursement	Actual Reimbursement‡	Savings§
1	16/7	16/7	103	95	8
2	24/7	24/7	158	135	23
3	24/7	16/7	105	49	56
4	19/5	16/2	43	53	−10
5	16/7	16/7	105	81	24
6	16/7	8/7	54	36	18
Mean ± SD‖	...	...	94.7±41.3	74.9±36.5	19.8±21.7

*Ordered from the individualized care plan. Data are hours per day/days per week.
†Projected reimbursement (in thousands of dollars) are the computed costs to fulfill the ordered nursing care (columns 2 and 3) corrected for actual short-term rehospitalizations.
‡Actual reimbursements (in thousands of dollars) as paid by Medicaid for home care nursing.
§Savings (in thousands of dollars) is projected reimbursements minus actual reimbursements.
‖Means are based on raw data.

Table 4.—Annual Home Care Nursing Requirements in Oxygen-Dependent Children With a Tracheostomy*

Patient	Nursing Care* Discharge	90 d–1 y	Projected Reimbursement	Actual Reimbursement	Savings
1	9/6	9/6	50	45	5
2	16/7	8/5	51	33	18
3	6/5	6/5	27	32	−5
4	12/7	12/7	77	41	36
Mean ± SD	...	...	51.1±20.2	37.8±6.4	13.2±17.4

*See Table 3 footnotes for additional information.

(formerly known as the "Model Waiver") was developed, allowing each state to establish a program for up to 50 blind or disabled children and adults who, in the absence of community services, would require long-term institutional care. The Health Care Financing Administration approved the Medicaid Home and Community-Based Services Waiver Program and expanded the eligible population to include up to 50 technology-dependent children per state, removing the necessity of applying to the Health Care Financing Administration for approval for each child.

The Medicaid Model Waiver Program instituted in Maryland has produced substantial cost savings for the payer. The mean annual home care costs were $109 836 for a ventilator-dependent child and $63 650 for an oxygen-dependent child with a tracheostomy. These home care costs for ventilator-dependent children are comparable with those reported by Frates et al.[2] The estimated annual savings of approximately $79 000 for each ventilator-dependent child and $83 000 for each oxygen-dependent child with a tracheostomy were computed with use of individualized home care plans. Our computations for cost savings may be more reliable than those previously reported, because this Medicaid system reimbursed for almost all (96%) long-term care institutional charges, and care needs were individualized for each child. Other studies compared home care costs with average short-term care hospital costs[3] or simply the minimal daily rate charged by short- or long-term care hospitals.[2,4]

Both medical and social needs are important in determining home care supports. Children with similar technology and care requirements may be discharged with very different amounts of professional caregiver support,[5] because discharge planning attempts to provide for the family's needs. The parents of all these patients were technically competent to provide all required home care nursing. However, the number of hours they were able to provide these services was dependent on their own medical and psychosocial needs. Some parents and other siblings had illnesses and disabilities, and financial considerations required some parents to work outside the home. Frequent reassessments and the flexibility to adjust to changing medical status or unanticipated social conditions will help to ensure a successful home care program.

Actual home care reimbursements for nursing care were considerably less than projected (Tables 3 and 4). For 80% of the patients, the major component of this difference was unutilized nursing care secondary to a lack of available skilled nursing care. For the remaining 20% of patients (one in each group), nursing care reimbursements were greater than projected from their individualized care plan, as these two patients were provided with additional nursing care in lieu of rehospitalization for acute illness. Overall, annual nursing care reimbursements averaged approximately $20 000 per patient less than ordered for ventilator-dependent children and $13 000 per patient less than ordered for oxygen-dependent children with a tracheostomy, equivalent to 21% and 26% of the ordered nursing care hours, respectively. This problem has increased in proportion to the number of children discharged home. Coupled with the existing nursing shortage, maintaining appropriate nurse staffing for children receiving home care may become even more difficult as this patient population continues to increase.

A more complete cost-effectiveness analysis would include other direct and indirect costs, considerations of patient benefits, and quality of outcomes.[9,10] Other costs of home care borne by parents include home remodeling, increased utility charges, lost income from work, transportation, child care, and training of families and personnel. "Out-of-pocket" expenses are a major cause of stress to the family.[11] Items such as lost family leisure time were not considered. Although the lack of inclusion of direct and indirect costs may have resulted in an overestimation of cost savings, several of these additional costs (eg, transportation and child care) could have been a factor if the child was in the alternative institution. In addition, use of the least costly institution (long-term care institutions) as the alternative to home care often underestimated the alternative institutional costs, because long-term care beds for technology-dependent children were frequently unavailable at the time of hospital discharge. Long delays in patient discharges to long-term care institutions in this region were routine. Therefore, many patients would have remained in more costly short-term care facilities for longer periods. With the approximate Medicaid reimbursements of $1000 to $1200 per day for these patients in short-term care hospitals in this region, savings for home care compared with short-term hospital care was approximately $250 000 to $300 000 per year.

The degree to which health services are covered and reimbursed by a state's Medicaid rules affect the setting and the amount of care a technology-dependent child receives. Although these methods could be applied to other states, cost-effectiveness would depend on Medicaid reimbursements for acute care for each individual state. In addition, if Medicaid reimbursements to hospitals for ventilator-dependent children are meager, the financial incentives of resultant savings for a home care program are nonexistent.[12]

In summary, the Medicaid Model Waiver Program is highly cost-effective for the state of Maryland, with approximate mean savings of $79 000 per year for each ventilator-dependent patient and $83 000 per year for each oxygen-dependent patient with a tracheostomy. The full program (50 patients) has the potential to save $4 million per year and allows greater availability of specialized short- and long-term care beds. Although we believe that decisions concerning resource allocations should depend on patients' needs and be proportional to expected benefits, lack of access to financing is a real barrier to appropriate home care. The savings from home care of some individuals also could be used to offset the losses from others, allowing the aggregate costs to remain less costly than alternative institutional care.

This work was supported, in part, by a grant from the US Department of Health and Human Services, Bureau of Maternal and Child Health, through its Special Projects of Regional and National Significance (SPRANS).

References

1. Burr BH, Guyer B, Todres ID, Abrahams B, Chiodo T. Home care for children on respirators. *N Engl J Med.* 1983;309:1319-1323.

2. Frates RC, Splaingard ML, Harrison GM. Outcome of home mechanical ventilation for children. *J Pediatr.* 1985;106:850-856.

3. Goldberg AI, Faure EAM, Vaughn CJ, Snarski R, Seleny FL. Home care for life-supported persons: an approach to program development. *J Pediatr.* 1984;104:785-795.

4. Thilo EH, Comito J, McCulliss D. Home oxygen therapy in the newborn: costs and parental acceptance. *AJDC.* 1987;141:766-768.

5. Eigen H, Zander J. Home mechanical ventilation of pediatric patients: American Thoracic Society. *Am Rev Respir Dis.* 1990;141:258-259.

6. The Omnibus Budget Reconciliation Act of 1981 (OBRA). Pub L No. 97-35, Section 2176, 95 Stat 351.

7. US Congress, Office of Technology Assessment, Health Program. *Technology-Dependent Children: Hospital v Home Care—A Technical Memorandum.* Washington, DC: US Government Printing Office; May 1987. OTA-TM-H-38.

8. COMAR 10.09.27 Home care for disabled children under a Model Waiver. *Maryland Register.* 1985;12:1041-1045.

9. Weinstein MC, Stason WB. Foundations of cost-effectiveness analysis for health and medical practices. *N Engl J Med.* 1977;296:716-721.

10. Doubilet P, Weinstein MC, McNeil BJ. Use and misuse of the term 'cost-effective' in medicine. *N Engl J Med.* 1986;314:253-256.

11. Aday LA, Aitken MJ, Wegener DH. *Pediatric Home Care: Results of a National Evaluation of Programs for Ventilator Assisted Children.* Chicago, Ill: Pluribus Press Inc; 1988.

12. Frates RC, Harrison GM, Splaingard ML. Home care for children on respirators. *N Engl J Med.* 1984;310:1126-1127. Letter.

A Comparative Trial of the Reactogenicity and Immunogenicity of Takeda Acellular Pertussis Vaccine Combined With Tetanus and Diphtheria Toxoids

Outcome in 3- to 8-Month-Old Infants, 9- to 23-Month-Old Infants and Children, and 24- to 30-Month-Old Children

Mikio Kimura, MD; Harumi Kuno-Sakai, MD; Yuji Sato, PhD; Hitoshi Kamiya, MD; Ritsue Nii, MD; Shin Isomura, MD; Kiyoshi Horiuchi, MD; Tatsuo Kato, MD; Masanori Deguchi, MD; Hiroaki Saikusa, MD; Edward A. Mortimer, Jr, MD; James D. Cherry, MD

• The reactogenicity and immunogenicity of the Takeda acellular pertussis vaccine combined with tetanus and diphtheria toxoids were compared in 139 infants aged 3 to 8 months, 60 infants and children aged 9 to 23 months, and 99 children aged 24 to 30 months. Good antibody responses to pertussis toxin (PT), filamentous hemagglutinin (FHA), and agglutinogens occurred in all age groups after both the third and fourth doses. After the fourth (booster) dose, the mean antibody values in initially seronegative infants vaccinated at 3 to 8 months of age were as follows: anti-PT, 67.8 enzyme-linked immunosorbent assay units (EU) per milliliter; anti-FHA, 149.5 EU/mL; the agglutinin titer was 125.6. The values in initially seronegative children vaccinated at 24 to 30 months of age were as follows: anti-PT, 92.9 EU/mL; anti-FHA, 251.7 EU/mL; the agglutinin titer was 275.8. Reactions following immunization were minimal. Except for drowsiness after the first dose in infants, there were no clinically significant differences in reactions between infants and older children. The findings in this study coupled with the recent demonstration of efficacy of this vaccine in 2-year-old children supports the recent Japanese recommendation to lower the age of immunization with acellular pertussis vaccine combined with tetanus and diphtheria toxoids to 3 months.

(*AJDC*. 1991;145:734-741)

Accepted for publication November 12, 1990.

From the Department of Pediatrics, Tokai University School of Medicine, Isehara; Japan (Drs Kimura and Kuno-Sakai), the Department of Pediatrics, Mie National Hospital, Tsu, Japan (Drs Kamiya and Nii), Aichi Prefectural Institute of Public Health, Nagoya, Japan (Dr Isomura), Department of Pediatrics, National Higashi-Tochigi Hospital, Utsunomiya, Japan (Dr Horiuchi), Deguchi Pediatrics Clinic, Omura, Japan (Dr Deguchi), and Saikusa Pediatrics Clinic, Sasebo, Japan (Dr Saikusa), Department of Bacteriology, National Institutes of Health, Tokyo, Japan (Dr Sato); Department of Pediatrics, St Marianna University, Kawasaki, Japan (Dr Kato); Department of Epidemiology and Biostatistics, Case Western Reserve University School of Medicine, Cleveland, Ohio (Dr Mortimer); and Department of Pediatrics, UCLA School of Medicine (Dr Cherry).

Reprint requests to Tokai University School of Medicine, Department of Pediatrics, Isehara, Kanagawa, Japan (Dr Kimura).

In Japan, since the fall of 1981, children have been vaccinated against pertussis exclusively with acellular pertussis vaccines.[1-5] Until recently, diphtheria-tetanus-

See also pp 746 and 750.

pertussis immunization with adsorbed vaccines containing acellular pertussis components (APDT) routinely commenced at about 2 years of age in Japan, and over 40 million doses of vaccine have been administered. Currently, epidemic pertussis is controlled in Japan, but the incidence of the disease is higher in infants than it was in the early 1970s, when diphtheria-tetanus-pertussis vaccines containing whole-cell pertussis antigens were used and immunization commenced at 3 months of age. Today, the majority of cases of pertussis in Japan occur in nonimmunized children who are younger than 2 years.[6]

This communication reports the results of a field trial with a single lot of commercially available APDT from Takeda Chemical Industries Ltd (Osaka, Japan). The study was done as a cooperative Japan–United States effort by Takeda and Lederle Biologicals, Pearl River, NY. It was designed to supply information for both the Japanese and US acellular pertussis vaccination programs.

Although the Japanese acellular pertussis vaccination program has been highly successful, it has become evident that a lowering of the age of immunization is necessary to reduce the occurrence of pertussis in infants. This report compares the reactogenicity and immunogenicity of APDT in 3- to 8-month-old infants, 9- to 23-month-old infants and children, and 2-year-old children. The results of this study should provide valuable information for the United States as well as for Japan. Since pertussis is currently well controlled in the United States through the use of whole-cell vaccines, it would be exceedingly difficult to do an efficacy trial with an acellular pertussis vaccine.

Table 1.—Antibody Responses to PT, FHA, and Agglutinogens in Vaccinated Infants and Children With Negative Preimmunization Antibody Values*

Time	Age at Immunization, mo	No.	Geometric Mean Titer (95% CI): Anti-PT, EU/mL	Anti-FHA, EU/mL	Agglutinin Titer
Before first vaccination	3-8	107	1.4 (1.3-1.5)	2.7 (2.4-3.0)	<10.0 (. . .)
	9-23	57	1.1 (1.0-1.2)	2.2 (1.9-2.6)	<10.0 (. . .)
	24-30	82	1.1 (1.1-1.2)	2.2 (1.9-2.5)	<10.0 (. . .)
Before third vaccination	3-8	87	51.0 (43.8-59.4)	49.3 (43.0-56.7)	69.8 (54.2-90.0)
	9-23	52	54.4 (45.8-64.5)	61.0 (50.0-74.4) †	86.7 (66.6-112.9)
	24-30	67	45.0 (38.7-52.3)	45.6 (38.7-53.7)	101.5 (81.6-126.2)
After third vaccination	3-8	101	74.5 (66.6-83.4)	110.3 (96.9-125.5)	156.7 (125.5-195.7) †
	9-23	55	74.6 (63.9-87.1)	114.9 (96.9-136.1)	159.7 (128.4-198.6) †
	24-30	77	74.9 (66.4-88.9)	107.1 (90.3-127.0)	225.2 (185.8-272.9)
Before booster shot	3-8	79	13.1 (11.3-15.2) †	20.9 (17.6-24.9) † ‡	22.0 (17.9-27.1)
	9-23	28	18.8 (14.3-24.7)	32.2 (24.6-42.1)	34.8 (24.5-49.5)
	24-30	54	19.0 (15.3-23.6)	40.5 (30.2-54.4)	37.0 (26.1-52.5)
After booster shot	3-8	79	67.8 (58.4-78.8) † †	149.5 (126.5-176.7) ‡ ‡	125.6 (94.3-167.3) ‡ ‡
	9-23	27	105.4 (77.9-142.6)	274.2 (210.7-357.0)	318.7 (225.9-449.7)
	24-30	52	92.9 (75.0-115.1)	251.7 (204.0-309.2)	275.8 (194.6-390.9)

*PT indicates pertussis toxin; FHA, filamentous hemagglutinin; and CI, confidence interval. Negative preimmunization antibody values were less than 10 enzyme-linked immunosorbent assay units (EU) per milliliter of anti–PT antibody, less than 10 EU/mL of anti–FHA antibody, and an agglutinin titer less than 10. The agglutinin titer is expressed as the reciprocal of the serum dilution. Extremely low concentration in most samples made calculation of the value before the first geometric mean titer impractical, and accordingly significance testing was not performed.

†$P<.05$, Tukey's Studentized Range Test, comparison between age groups at specific times.

‡$P<.01$.

Table 2.—Seroconversion Rates (%) in Vaccinated Infants and Children With Negative Preimmunization Antibody Values*

Time	Age at Immunization, mo	No.	Anti-PT, EU/mL ≥10	Anti-PT ≥20	Anti-PT ≥40	Anti-FHA, EU/mL ≥10	Anti-FHA ≥20	Anti-FHA ≥40	Agglutinin Titer ≥10	Agglutinin ≥40	Agglutinin ≥160
Before third vaccination	3-8	87	98.9	94.3	65.5	100.0	93.1	60.9	92.0	74.7 ‡	33.3
	9-23	52	100.0	98.1	69.2	98.1	96.2	73.1	96.2	88.5	36.5
	24-30	67	98.5	94.0	59.7	100.0	94.0	52.2	98.5	92.5	40.3
After third vaccination	3-8	101	100.0	98.0	88.1	100.0	100.0	96.0 †	99.0	93.1	64.1 †
	9-23	55	100.0	100.0	94.6	100.0	98.1	96.4	100.0	96.4	63.6
	24-30	77	100.0	97.4	81.8	100.0	100.0	87.0	100.0	97.4	81.8
Before booster shot	3-8	79	72.2	29.1 †	6.3	86.1	51.9 †	20.3 † ‡	79.8	33.0	7.6
	9-23	28	78.6	42.9	10.7	92.9	78.6	46.4	96.4	53.6	3.6
	24-30	54	77.8	50.0	18.5	96.3	70.4	46.3	92.6	50.0	13.0
After booster shot	3-8	79	98.8	96.2	79.8	100.0	100.0	96.2	100.0	82.3 † ‡	48.1 † ‡
	9-23	27	100.0	96.3	92.6	100.0	100.0	100.0	100.0	100.0	81.5
	24-30	52	98.1	96.2	88.5	100.0	100.0	100.0	98.1	98.1	73.1

*PT indicates pertussis toxin; EU, enzyme-linked immunosorbent assay unit; and FHA, filamentous hemagglutinin. For negative preimmunization antibody values, see Table 1.

†$P.<05$, Tukey's Studentized Range Test, comparison between age groups at specific times.

‡$P<.01$.

However, since the efficacy of Takeda's APDT vaccine in children 2 years of age or older has been demonstrated in a large household contact study in Japan,[7] the present study in Japan might provide important data that could serve as a surrogate for predicting efficacy in young infants.

SUBJECTS AND METHODS

Subjects

The study participants were healthy 3- to 30-month-old infants and children at the time of the first dose of APDT. They had neither been immunized previously with pertussis-containing vaccines nor had a history of pertussislike illness. At enrollment, the details of the study were explained to the parents or guardians, and verbal informed consent was obtained.

The vaccine was administered by the deep subcutaneous route in a volume of 0.5 mL per dose. Following the initial immunization, the children received two subsequent doses of vaccine at 6- to 10-week intervals, and a fourth dose was given 12 to 18 months after the third dose. Serum samples for antibody determination were obtained before the first inoculation and immediately before and 1 month after both the third dose and the booster (fourth) dose.

Table 3.—Antibody Responses to PT, FHA, and Agglutinogens in Vaccinated Infants and Children With Positive Preimmunization Antibody Values*

Time	Age at Immunization, mo	No.	Geometric Mean Titer (95% CI) Anti-PT, EU/mL	Anti-FHA, EU/mL	Agglutinin Titer
Before first vaccination	3-8	32	5.3 (3.8-7.5)	10.2 (7.9-13.1)	10.7 (10.0-11.4)
	24-30	17	2.3 (1.0-5.2)	12.5 (8.7-18.1)	10.2 (9.8-10.7)
Before third vaccination	3-8	32	56.6 (47.3-67.9)	63.0† (54.5-72.8)	65.1 (45.0-94.1)
	24-30	16	48.7 (27.5-86.2)	150.5‡ (90.9-249.2)	97.3 (51.3-184.6)
After third vaccination	3-8	28	77.5 (65.2-91.9)	108.7 (88.9-132.8)	157.2 (102.1-242.3)
	24-30	16	107.5 (64.3-179.6)	223.6§ (150.6-332.0)	255.9 (149.4-438.3)
Before booster shot	3-8	26	18.7 (13.8-25.3)	24.6 (18.1-33.3)	18.9 (14.1-25.4)
	24-30	10	16.6 (9.3-29.5)	34.5 (20.7-57.5)	41.4 (27.4-62.6)
After booster shot	3-8	25	62.7 (50.3-78.3)	162.1 (127.5-206.0)	102.7 (71.7-147.0)
	24-30	11	149.4 (65.3-341.9)	242.6 (174.1-337.3)	159.8 (69.9-365.6)

*For abbreviations, see footnotes to Table 1. The agglutinin titer is expressed as the reciprocal of the serum dilution. Positive preimmunization antibody values were 10 EU/mL or greater of anti-PT or anti-FHA antibody or an agglutinin titer of 10 or greater.
†$P=.02$ when compared with a similar value in infants with negative preimmunization antibody values (Table 1).
‡$P=.0001$.
§$P=.002$.

Table 4.—Antibody Responses to PT, FHA, and Agglutinogens in 3- to 8-Month-Old Infants With Negative Preimmunization Antibody Values*

Time	Age at Immunization, mo	No.	Geometric Mean Titer (95% CI) Anti-PT, EU/mL	Anti-FHA, EU/mL	Agglutinin Titer
Before first vaccination	3	35	1.6 (1.4-1.9) †	2.8 (2.2-3.4)	<10 (. . .)
	4-5	28	1.4 (1.1-1.7) †	2.7 (2.1-3.4)	<10 (. . .)
	6-8	44	1.2 (1.1-1.4) †	2.7 (2.3-3.2)	<10 (. . .)
Before third vaccination	3	32	48.8 (35.7-66.9)	50.1 (37.9-66.2)	56.5 (37.3-85.6)
	4-5	22	53.1 (42.5-66.4)	46.5 (35.4-61.0)	75.1 (41.8-134.9)
	6-8	33	51.7 (40.6-65.9)	50.61 (41.6-61.6)	87.7 (54.6-122.2)
After third vaccination	3	35	69.6 (56.8-85.3)	97.7 (77.2-123.6)	118.8 (79.5-177.7)
	4-5	25	77.4 (62.6-95.7)	115.4 (89.1-149.4)	173.9 (110.2-274.5)
	6-8	41	77.3 (64.0-93.2)	118.9 (97.0-145.8)	186.3 (132.5-261.9)
Before booster shot	3	31	11.5 (9.1-14.4)	20.5 (15.3-27.5)	14.1 (11.8-16.9) ‡
	4-5	23	13.1 (10.0-17.2)	21.3 (15.7-29.1)	20.6 (14.7-28.8) ‡
	6-8	25	15.5 (11.4-21.0)	21.1 (15.1-29.5)	40.6 (25.4-64.8) ‡
After booster shot	3	30	51.6 (40.8-64.2) †	116.4 (88.5-152.9)	70.4 (47.8-103.7) ‡
	4-5	23	70.4 (54.3-91.3) †	165.7 (116.8-235.0)	139.6 (84.4-230.9) ‡
	6-8	26	90.1 (68.8-118.0) †	182.5 (140.7-236.6)	223.3 (127.6-390.5) ‡

*For abbreviations and explanation of values, see footnotes to Table 1.
†$P<.05$, Tukey's Studentized Range Test, comparison between age groups at specific times.
‡$P<.01$.

After each immunization, the child was observed in the clinic for local and systemic symptoms for 30 minutes. Thereafter, clinical follow-up was performed by the parents or guardians. Specific observations were made 3 and 6 hours after immunization and then daily for 7 days. The following were monitored: axillary temperature; the presence or absence of fretfulness, drowsiness, anorexia, and vomiting; and local reactions. Pain and warmth at the immunization site were graded as marked (2+), present (+), or none (−). Redness and swelling were quantified as 5 cm or greater (2+), 1 to 4 cm (+), and 0 to less than 1 cm (−); induration was evaluated as clearly palpable (2+), slightly palpable (+), and none (−).

Vaccine

The adsorbed APDT vaccine used in this trial was a single lot (HJ027) of a commercially available Japanese vaccine manufactured by Takeda Chemical Industries Ltd. It contained 25 Lf/mL of diphtheria toxoid and 3.5 Lf/mL of tetanus toxoid. The pertussis component was made up of three main antigens: filamentous hemagglutinin (FHA), lymphocytosis-promoting factor hemagglutinin (LPF), which is also called pertussis toxin (PT), and agglutinogens, in an approximate ratio of 90:9:1. In addition, it has been found that the pertussis component contains a 69-kd outer-membrane protein that has protective efficacy in animal studies.[8]

Laboratory Studies

All serologic tests except for anti–69-kd studies were performed by Takeda Chemical Industries Ltd with supervision by the Japanese National Institute of Health. Agglutinating antibodies were determined by the method of Sato et al,[9] and antibodies to PT and FHA were determined by an indirect enzyme-linked immunosorbent assay.[9,10] Antibodies to 69-kd outer membrane protein were determined in a subset of serum samples by

Table 5.—Antibody Responses to Diphtheria and Tetanus Toxoids in Vaccinated Infants and Children*

Time	Age at Immunization, mo	Diphtheria Antitoxin, IU/mL No.	Diphtheria Antitoxin, IU/mL GMT (95% CI)	Tetanus Antitoxin, IU/mL No.	Tetanus Antitoxin, IU/mL GMT (95% CI)
Before first vaccination	3-8	16	<0.01 (. . .)	16	<0.01 (. . .)
	9-23	22	<0.01 (. . .)	31	<0.01 (. . .)
	24-30	19	<0.01 (. . .)	18	<0.01 (. . .)
Before third vaccination	3-8	16	0.8 (0.6-1.0)	16	1.2 (0.8-1.7)
	9-23	22	0.5 (0.3-0.7)	29	1.1 (0.8-1.5)
	24-30	19	0.7 (0.5-0.9)	18	1.5 (1.0-2.1)
After third vaccination	3-8	16	1.6 (1.2-2.1)	16	2.0 (1.5-2.8)
	9-23	22	1.5 (1.1-2.0)	31	2.1 (1.6-2.8)
	24-30	19	1.7 (1.4-2.1)	17	2.6 (1.9-3.4)
Before booster shot	3-8	45	0.3 (0.2-0.4)	45	0.2 (0.1-0.2)†
	9-23	21	0.3 (0.3-0.4)	21	0.4 (0.3-0.7)†
	24-30	34	0.3 (0.2-0.4)	34	0.2 (0.1-0.3)
After booster shot	3-8	45	6.7 (4.9-9.2)	45	3.1 (2.4-4.1)
	9-23	21	10.2 (7.2-14.5)	21	4.9 (3.6-6.7)
	24-30	34	8.3 (6.2-11.1)	34	4.3 (3.4-5.4)

*GMT indicates geometric mean titer; CI, confidence interval.
†$P<.01$, Tukey's Studentized Range Test, comparison between age groups at specific times.

Table 6.—Incidence (%) of Adverse Reactions in Vaccinated Infants and Children*

	Age at Immunization, mo	Within 24 Hours of First Vaccination	Within 24 Hours of Second Vaccination	Within 24 Hours of Third Vaccination	Within 24 Hours of Booster Vaccination	1-7 Days After First Vaccination	1-7 Days After Second Vaccination	1-7 Days After Third Vaccination	1-7 Days After Booster Vaccination
Any	3-8	36.3	42.9	52.2	64.7	6.6	11.0	6.6	7.8
adverse	9-23	28.3	40.2	44.2	66.7	9.8	5.4	3.5	10.3
reactions	24-30	38.1	54.8	50.8	64.0	13.8	4.8	4.0	10.7
Systemic	3-8	20.9	16.2	15.6	21.6	3.9	6.7	3.9	7.8
reaction	9-23	13.0	10.9	10.5	18.0	4.4	4.4	4.7	5.1
	24-30	14.4	12.1	10.7	22.7	8.8	6.4	3.3	12.0
Local	3-8	20.3	35.0†	47.5	57.8	4.0	7.8	3.4	5.2
reactions	9-23	20.2	34.8†	43.5	64.1	7.9	3.3	1.2	7.7
(+/2+)	24-30	28.6	50.8	48.0	60.0	10.3	3.2	2.4	9.3
Local	3-8	2.3	7.2	7.3	19.0	1.7	1.1	3.4	11.2
reaction	9-23	1.1	6.5	5.9	28.2	6.7	1.1	1.2	10.3
(2+)	24-30	0.8	7.9	13.0	30.7	5.6	1.6	6.5	8.0

*Local reactions were graded as marked (2+), present (+), or none (−).
†$P<.05$, Tukey's Studentized Range Test.

enzyme-linked immunosorbent assay at Lederle Biologicals by a previously described method.[11] All agglutinin titers are expressed as reciprocals of the serum dilution. Antitoxins to diphtheria and tetanus toxins were measured by the microcell culture method using VERO cells[12] and by passive hemagglutinations using tetanus toxoid–coated sheep erythrocytes,[13] respectively.

Statistical Evaluation

The geometric mean titers and their 95% confidence intervals were computed based on the log assay values at baseline and those before and after the third immunization. These values were first logarithmically transformed, then the (simple) means and 95% confidence intervals were computed, and finally the means and confidence intervals were expressed as the antilogarithms. Comparisons across age groups are based on a nonparametric version of Tukey's Studentized Range Test. Differences among the groups were reported as statistically significant if a two-sided *P* value of .05 or less was obtained.

The clinical reactions were classified into those observed within the first 24 hours and those observed between 24 hours and 7 days after injection. Clinical reactions observed among different age groups of children were analyzed using Tukey's Studentized Range Test.

Participants

A total of 454 infants and children originally entered the study. Of this group, there were four subjects under 3 months of age, 182 who were 3 to 8 months old, 92 who were 9 to 23 months old, 126 who were 24 to 30 months old, and 50 who were older than 30 months of age. Clinical reactions in subjects 3 to 30 months of age were analyzed. One hundred two children did not receive their subsequent immunizations in the allotted periods and therefore were excluded from analysis.

There were a total of 298 infants and children 3 to 30 months old immunized according to the protocol. Of this group, 246 had prevaccination antibody values that were considered negative (ie, less than 10 enzyme-linked immunosorbent assay units [EU] per milliliter of anti–PT antibody, less than 10 EU/mL of anti–FHA

Table 7.—Incidence (%) of Specific Systemic Reactions in Vaccinated Infants and Children									
		Within 24 Hours of				1-7 Days After			
	Age at Immunization, mo	First Vaccination	Second Vaccination	Third Vaccination	Booster Vaccination	First Vaccination	Second Vaccination	Third Vaccination	Booster Vaccination
Temperature									
⩾37.5°C	3-8	5.5	4.2	4.5	2.7	3.6	8.4	7.0	11.5
	9-23	4.6	3.3	9.9	8.1	6.8	10.0	4.9	10.8
	24-30	2.6	0.9	4.5	9.9	7.0	8.0	5.4	9.9
⩾38.5°C	3-8	0.0	0.0	1.3	0.9	1.8	0.6	1.3	6.2
	9-23	1.1	1.1	0.0	2.7	2.3	2.2	4.9	2.7
	24-30	0.9	0.0	0.0	0.0	4.4	3.5	2.7	4.2
Fretfulness	3-8	9.3	10.1	8.4	8.8	3.3	2.2	2.8	3.5
	9-23	5.4	5.5	4.7	10.3	3.3	3.3	3.5	2.6
	24-30	7.2	4.8	5.7	8.0	6.4	6.4	2.5	5.3
Drowsiness	3-8	17.1	7.8	8.9	8.8	3.3	3.4	0.0	3.5
	9-23	8.7*	4.4	5.9	7.7	1.1	3.3	2.4	5.1
	24-30	8.0	8.1	8.2	6.7	2.4	2.4	0.8	1.3
Anorexia	3-8	3.3	2.2	3.9	7.0	3.3	4.5	3.3	7.0
	9-23	2.2	1.1	2.4	5.1	2.2	2.2	3.5	5.1
	24-30	4.0	2.4	4.9	6.7	8.8	4.8	2.5	8.0
Vomiting	3-8	0.6	2.2	1.1	0.0	1.1	3.4	1.1	3.5
	9-23	2.2	1.1	1.2	0.0	1.1	0.0	1.2	0.0
	24-30	0.0	0.0	0.0	0.0	3.2	2.4	0.0	4.0

*$P<.05$, Tukey's Studentized Range Test, comparison between age groups at specific times.

antibody, and an agglutinin titer less than 10), and 52 had one or more positive prevaccination antibody values (ie, ⩾10 EU/mL of anti–PT or anti–FHA antibody, and an agglutinin titer of ⩾10). Data from these participants were used for the analysis. There were 107 infants 3 to 8 months old, 57 infants and children 9 to 23 months old, and 82 children 24 to 30 months old with negative preimmunization values, and 32 infants 3 to 8 months old, three infants and children 9 to 23 months old, and 17 children 24 to 30 months old with positive preimmunization values. To evaluate the immunogenicity and reactogenicity of the vaccine in a homogeneous population, it was decided that the most appropriate major analysis would involve only those subjects with negative preimmunization values. Antitoxins to diphtheria and tetanus toxins were measured in serum samples from 57 and 65 vaccinees, respectively. Some of the children in each age group returned for their booster (fourth dose) immunization, and their prebooster and postbooster antibody values were determined.

RESULTS

Serologic Responses

The serum antibody responses to PT, FHA, and agglutinogens in the immunized infants and children with negative preimmunization values are presented in Table 1. Following two doses of vaccine, the mean values of the antibodies to all three antigens were significantly higher than those before vaccination in all three age groups. There were no significant differences in responses to PT or FHA among the three age groups after two doses except that the anti–FHA antibody values in the infants and children immunized at 9 to 23 months of age were higher than those in the children immunized at 24 to 30 months of age. Following the third immunization, the values of the antibodies to the respective antigens significantly increased further in all three vaccination age groups. The increases were approximately 1.5-fold for anti–PT values and twofold for anti–FHA values and for agglutinin titers. The only significant difference between the immunized infants and younger children (3 to 23 months old) and the older children was related to agglutinin titers. The agglutinin geometric mean titer after the third dose was 156.7 in 3- to 8-month-old infants, 159.7 in 9- to 23-month-old infants and children, and 225.2 in 24- to 30-month-old children.

Marked decreases in anti–PT and anti–FHA values and agglutinin titers were observed in the samples taken before the booster dose. Greater decreases were observed in children who had received the first dose when they were 3 to 8 months of age. High antibody values and titers were observed in serum samples taken 4 weeks after the booster dose. The responses after the booster in the infants immunized at 3 to 8 months of age were relatively low compared with those immunized at the other ages.

In Table 2, the percentage of children with negative preimmunization antibody values who obtained selected antibody titers following immunization is presented. After the third immunization, the respective values of those immunized at 3 to 8 months of age with an antibody level of 40 EU/mL or greater against PT and against FHA and an agglutinin titer of 40 or greater were 88%, 96%, and 93%; the respective values in those immunized at 9 to 23 months of age were 95%, 96%, and 96%, and the respective values in those immunized at 24 to 30 months of age were 82%, 87%, and 97%.

Presented in Table 3 are the antibody responses in vaccinated infants (3 to 8 months old) and children (24 to 30 months old) with a positive preimmunization antibody value to one of the three vaccine antigens (PT, FHA, or agglutinogens). When compared with the antibody values in infants and children with negative preimmunization values (Table 1), it is noted that those with positive preimmunization antibody values had higher antibody values

Table 8.—Incidence (%) of Specific Local Reactions in Vaccinated Infants and Children*

	Age at Immunization, mo	Within 24 Hours of: First Vaccination	Second Vaccination	Third Vaccination	Booster Vaccination	1-7 Days After: First Vaccination	Second Vaccination	Third Vaccination	Booster Vaccination
Pain									
+/2+	3-8	3.4	3.3	4.6	14.4 ‡	0.0	0.6	1.1	2.7
	9-23	6.8	11.1 †	11.9 †	37.5	0.0	0.0	1.2	3.0
	24-30	9.5	18.7	18.2	24.7	1.6	1.6	0.8	4.1
2+	3-8	0.6	0.0	0.0	0.0	0.0	0.0	0.0	0.0
	9-23	0.0	0.0	0.0	0.0	0.0	0.0	0.0	0.0
	24-30	0.0	0.0	0.0	2.7	0.0	0.0	0.0	0.0
Warmth									
+/2+	3-8	5.1	10.7	12.1	30.4	1.7	2.8	1.7	1.8
	9-23	3.4	13.2 ‡	19.1 †	53.1 ‡	3.4	1.1	2.4	6.1
	24-30	3.2	21.0	29.4	37.0	4.8	4.0	1.7	8.2
2+	3-8	0.6	0.0	0.6	5.4	0.6	0.0	0.0	0.9
	9-23	0.0	2.2	0.0	12.5	0.0	0.0	1.2	3.0
	24-30	0.8	0.8	0.0	4.1	0.0	0.0	0.0	2.7
Redness									
+/2+	3-8	18.3	26.4	42.4	53.5	3.4	5.0	3.9	3.5
	9-23	14.6	28.6 ‡	35.7	61.5	5.6	4.4	1.2	7.7
	24-30	17.5	41.3	43.1	53.3	8.7	4.0	2.4	6.7
2+	3-8	1.1	4.5	3.4	11.2	0.0	0.0	1.7	10.3
	9-23	0.0	2.2	3.6	18.0	2.3	2.2	1.2	7.7
	24-30	0.0	5.6	8.1	22.7	1.6	1.6	5.7	10.7
Swelling									
+/2+	3-8	8.0	18.0	33.9	47.4	2.3	2.8	2.3	4.3
	9-23	9.0	23.1	27.4	56.4	5.6	3.3	1.2	10.3
	24-30	7.1	28.6	38.2	50.7	7.1	3.2	3.3	6.7
2+	3-8	0.6	2.8	5.1	12.1	0.0	0.0	2.3	8.6
	9-23	0.0	2.2	3.6	20.5	2.3	0.0	1.2	10.3
	24-30	0.0	4.0	8.1	20.0	0.8	0.0	4.1	9.3
Induration									
+/2+	3-8	5.8	19.7	25.4	40.5	5.1	6.7	5.1	7.8
	9-23	9.0	22.0	28.6	47.4	12.4 ‡	5.5	7.1	10.3
	24-30	7.9	27.8	33.3	41.3	13.5	4.0	4.1	9.3
2+	3-8	0.6	3.9	4.5	13.8	1.1	1.1	1.7	6.9
	9-23	1.1	5.5	1.2 ‡	18.4	5.6	1.1	1.2	7.7
	24-30	0.0	6.4	8.9	22.7	5.6	0.0	3.3	1.3

*Reactions were graded as marked (2+), present (+), or none (−).
†$P<.01$, Tukey's Studentized Range Test, comparison of age groups at specific times.
‡$P<.05$.

against PT and FHA in the following specimens: before the third immunization, anti-FHA in both the 3- to 8-month-old and the 24- to 30-month-old groups; after the third immunization, anti-FHA in the 24- to 30-month-old group; and before the booster, anti-PT in the 3- to 8-month-old group.

The mean serum antibody responses to PT, FHA, and agglutinogens in infants with negative preimmunization antibody values immunized at 3 months, 4 to 5 months, and 6 to 8 months are presented in Table 4. The following antibody responses in 3-month-old infants were less than those in 6- to 8-month-old infants: agglutinin titers before and after the booster dose and anti–PT values after the booster.

Following the third dose of vaccine, the serum samples from 23 infants 3 to 8 months of age at the time of immunization had a 69-kd antibody value of 150 EU/mL. Twenty-three children initially vaccinated at 24 to 30 months of age had a value of 138 EU/mL.

Table 5 gives the antibody responses to diphtheria and tetanus toxoids. Following two doses of vaccine, mean antitoxin levels against diphtheria and tetanus toxins in all age groups were much greater than established protective levels (0.01 IU/mL) for each antitoxin.

Clinical Reactions

During the first 24 hours after the first immunization, between 28% and 38% of the vaccinated individuals had one or more reaction complaints (Table 6). The specific complaints during the first 24 hours and between 24 hours and 7 days after immunization by age group and vaccine dose are presented in Tables 7 and 8, respectively. Fever within the first 24 hours after immunization occurred in less than 10% and fever during the next 7 days occurred in less than 12% of the vaccinated subjects. Drowsiness was notably more common after the first dose in 3- to 8-month-old infants than with any other dose in infants or children. Local reactions tended to increase in incidence and severity with each dose regardless of age. Pain and local warmth within the first 24 hours became increasingly more common after the second, third, and booster doses. Frequencies of local redness and swelling, both mild and severe, within the first 48 hours were significantly greater after the booster dose than after any of the primary injections in all three age groups. No serious side effects such as encephalopathy or convulsions were observed.

COMMENT

In Japan, there are six manufacturers of acellular pertussis vaccines, including Takeda Chemical Industries Ltd. The acellular pertussis vaccines are divided into two types, the T type and the B type. T-Type vaccines contain predominately FHA, varying amounts of PT and 69-kd protein, and small amounts of agglutinogens. B-Type vaccines, on the other hand, contain only PT and FHA.

This study and a specific efficacy trial were planned in 1986. At that time, there were no formal efficacy data for any of the six individual APDT vaccines in use in Japan, but it was clear that collectively they were effective in controlling pertussis in children 2 years of age and older. It was reasoned that the demonstration of similar antibody patterns in infants and older children would support the use of the Takeda APDT vaccine in infants.

In 1986, an efficacy trial with two acellular vaccines was under way in Sweden, and that study has subsequently been completed.[14] In the Swedish trial, two different vaccines were used. One vaccine, a two-component product, contained equal amounts of PT and FHA (B-type vaccine) and the other vaccine contained only PT. Two doses of both vaccines produced good antibody responses to the vaccine antigens. It was anticipated that the results from the Swedish trial would provide efficacy data for older infants (>6 months of age) and, more importantly, might reveal FHA and/or PT antibody levels that correlated with protection in vaccinees.

The results of the Swedish trial revealed that both vaccines were efficacious in preventing the manifestations of severe pertussis, but when mild cases of pertussis were included, the calculated efficacy was less than expected. Furthermore, it was found that the vaccinees in whom pertussis developed had postimmunization antibody levels to PT that were similar to those in vaccinees who did not get pertussis.

The Takeda vaccine used in this trial is a T-type vaccine and is different from the two vaccines used in Sweden. Specifically, the Takeda vaccine contains agglutinogens as well as PT and FHA. In addition, this vaccine also contains the recently identified 69-kd outer-membrane protein.[8,15,16] Antibodies to this protein occur following natural pertussis and after immunization with whole-cell pertussis vaccines and have had protective efficacy in animal studies.[11,15,16]

In the present trial, reactions following immunization were minimal. Except for the occurrence of drowsiness, which was most common after the first dose in infants, there were no clinically significant differences in reactions between the infants and the older children.

In the present trial, the infants and children with negative preimmunization antibody values had good antibody responses to the four antigens studied (Table 1). In general, the 24- to 30-month-old children had more vigorous responses than the 3- to 8-month-old infants. Specifically, after the third dose, the agglutinin titer was 156.7 in 3- to 8-month-old infants and 225.2 in the 24- to 30-month-old children ($P<.05$). After the booster dose, the antibody values for all three antigens were significantly greater in the older children. However, the values in the infants vaccinated at 3 to 8 months of age were comparable with those observed after natural pertussis in Japanese infants.[17]

When we analyzed infants and children who had preimmunization values for PT or FHA above 10 EU/mL or an agglutinin titer greater than or equal to 10 (positive preimmunization antibody values), the results were not considerably different from those in vaccinees with negative preimmunization values (Tables 1 and 3). Those with positive preimmunization antibody values in a few instances had better responses than those vaccinees with negative preimmunization values. With whole-cell pertussis vaccines, it has been noted in the past that in 2-month-old infants the antibody response is blunted by the presence of high antibody values in the preimmunization serum samples.[18] In a recent study, Savage et al[19] reconfirmed this finding with a whole-cell pertussis vaccine but found that vaccinees responded equally well with regard to anti–PT antibody when immunized with an acellular vaccine regardless of the preimmunization antibody value.

In the present study, the positive preimmunization antibody values were in most instances probably due to previous unrecognized infections rather than to the presence of transplacentally acquired maternal antibody. Savage and associates[19] found that most infants had no detectable antibody to PT and FHA by the age of 4 months. In our study, only a small number of infants were less than 4 months old.

When the 3- to 8-month-old immunization group is analyzed further by age (Table 4), it is noted that, in general, those vaccinated at 3 months of age had lower antibody values at all follow-up points than the infants vaccinated at the older ages. Since by study design the infants in each age group had low preimmunization antibody values, it would seem that this age-related difference in immune response may not be due to transplacentally acquired maternal antibody but instead may be associated with age-related immunologic development. In a trial in the United States with an APDT vaccine with the Takeda acellular pertussis component, immunization was initiated at 2 months of age.[20] Although it is difficult to compare immune responses in two studies in two countries in which the laboratory tests were performed in the respective countries, it appears that the US children vaccinated at 2 months of age had lower antibody values to PT, FHA, and agglutinins than the Japanese children in whom immunization commenced at 3 months of age. Except for the response to agglutinins, these differences were not great. However, even after adjustment for laboratory differences, the agglutinin response in the US children was significantly less than that in the Japanese children.

The cause of this difference is unknown, but three possibilities need to be considered. First, it may be due to the maturity of the immune system (ie, 2 vs 3 months of age). Second, it could be due to a genetic difference between the two populations. Third, it could be due to the route of vaccine administration (ie, deep subcutaneous vs intramuscular). In Japan, vaccine is administered with a longer needle than used in the United States and it is injected at a narrow angle so that the vaccine enters subcutaneous tissue. In the United States, vaccine is injected directly into a muscle mass.

It is reassuring to note that antibody to the 69-kd protein was similar after the third dose in both those vaccinated as infants and those over 2 years of age at the time of immunization. Also, in the large study in the United States, infants vaccinated with the Takeda pertussis vaccine had 69-kd antibody values similar to those of whole-cell vaccine recipients after the third and fourth vaccine doses.[20]

The efficacy of the Takeda APDT vaccine has recently been demonstrated in 2-year-old children in Japan.[7] In a household contact study with 62 Takeda APDT–vaccinated children and 62 unvaccinated children, the efficacy was found to be 98% for the prevention of typical pertussis and 81% for the prevention of mild possible pertussis and typical pertussis combined.

At present, the specific serum antibody values, types, or combinations that confer protection against pertussis after immunization are not known. However, the antibody findings in the present study in association with the efficacy data in 2-year-old children are encouraging and lead us to suggest that the Takeda APDT vaccine may be effective in infants.

Recently, a three-community epidemiologic study in Japan was presented.[21] In this study, the incidence of pertussis in two communities where immunization commenced at 2 years of age was compared with that in an area in which immunization was begun at 3 to 6 months of age. The observation period was 2 years. The incidence of pertussis in the community in which 3- to 6-month-old infants were immunized was less than one third of that in the other two communities, where vaccination was started at 2 years of age. In these communities, vaccines of several different manufacturers were used, suggesting efficacy in infants with T-type vaccines.

In December 1988, the Ministry of Health and Welfare in Japan recommended that the initiation of vaccination with APDT be lowered from 2 years to 3 months of age. The results of the present study lend support to this recommendation.

This study was supported by Lederle Laboratories.

This study was abstracted in part in *Tokai J Exp Clin Med.* 1988;13(suppl):15-19.

We are indebted to Takeda Chemical Industries Ltd for assistance in making arrangements for the study.

We also acknowledge Denise Tritt for her technical assistance.

References

1. Kimura M, Kuno-Sakai H. Developments in pertussis immunization in Japan. *Lancet.* 1990;336:30-32.
2. Kimura M, Kuno-Sakai H. Pertussis vaccines in Japan. *Acta Paediatr Jpn.* 1988;30:143-153.
3. Kimura M, Kuno-Sakai H. Experiences with acellular pertussis vaccine in Japan and epidemiology of pertussis. *Tokai J Exp Clin Med.* 1987;12:263-273.
4. Noble GR, Bernier RH, Esber EC, et al. Acellular and whole cell pertussis vaccines in Japan: report of a visit by U.S. scientists. *JAMA.* 1987;257:1351-1356.
5. Kimura M, Kuno-Sakai H. Epidemiology of pertussis in Japan. *Tokai J Exp Clin Med.* 1988;13(suppl):1-7.
6. Kimura M, Kuno-Sakai H. Immunization system in Japan: its history and present situation. *Acta Paediatr Jpn.* 1988;30:109-126.
7. Mortimer EA, Kimura M, Cherry JD, et al. Protective efficacy of the Takeda acellular pertussis vaccine combined with diphtheria and tetanus toxoids following household exposure of Japanese children. *AJDC.* 1990;144:899-904.
8. Shahin RD, Brennan MJ, Li ZM, Meade BD, Manclark CR. Characterization of the protective capacity and immunogenicity of the 69-kD outer membrane protein of *Bordetella pertussis. J Exp Med.* 1990;171:63-73.
9. Sato Y, Kimura M, Fukumi H. Development of a pertussis component vaccine in Japan. *Lancet.* 1984;1:122-126.
10. Sato Y, Sato H, Izumiya K, Cowell JL, Manclark CR. Role of antibody to filamentous hemagglutinin and to leukocytosis promoting factor-hemagglutinin in immunity to pertussis. In: Robbins JB, Hill JC, Sadoff JC, eds. *Seminars in Infectious Diseases.* New York, NY: Thieme-Stratton Inc; 1982;4:380-385.
11. Blumberg DA, Mink CM, Cherry JD, et al. Comparison of an acellular pertussis-component diphtheria-tetanus-pertussis (DTP) vaccine with a whole-cell pertussis-component DTP vaccine in 17- to 24-month-old children, with measurement of a 69-kilodalton outer membrane protein antibody. *J Pediatr.* 1990;117:46-51.
12. Miyamura K, Nishio S, Ito A, Murata R, Kono R. Micro cell culture method for determination of diphtheria toxin and antitoxin titers using VERO cells, I: studies on factors affecting the toxin and antitoxin titration. *J Biol Scand.* 1974;2:189-201.
13. Kameyama S, Kondo S. Titration of tetanus antitoxin by passive hemagglutinin, I: titration of guinea-pig antitoxins at various periods of immunization. *Jpn J Med Sci Biol.* 1975;28:127-138.
14. Ad Hoc Group for the Study of Pertussis Vaccines. Placebo controlled trial of two acellular pertussis vaccines in Sweden: protective efficacy and adverse events. *Lancet.* 1988;1:955-960.
15. Brennan MJ, Li ZM, Cowell JL, et al. Identification of a 69-kilodalton nonfimbrial protein as an agglutinogen of *Bordetella pertussis. Infect Immun.* 1988;56:3189-3195.
16. Thomas MG, Redhead K, Lambert HP. Human serum antibody response to *Bordetella pertussis* infection and pertussis vaccination. *J Infect Dis.* 1989;159:211-218.
17. Kuno-Sakai H, Kimura M, Sato Y, et al. Serum anti-PT and anti-FHA antibody levels, and agglutinin titers after administration of acellular pertussis vaccines. *Acta Paediatr Jpn.* 1989;31:120-126.
18. Baraff LJ, Leake RD, Burstyn DG, et al. Immunologic response to early and routine DTP immunization in infants. *Pediatrics.* 1984;73:37-42.
19. Savage JV, Decker MD, Edwards KM, Sell SH, Karzon DT. Natural history of pertussis antibody in the infant and effect on vaccine response. *J Infect Dis.* 1990;161:487-492.
20. Blumberg DA, Mink CM, Cherry JD, et al. Comparison of acellular and whole-cell pertussis-component diptheria-tetanus-pertussis (DTP) vaccines: a multicenter double-blind randomized longitudinal study in 2-, 4-, and 6-month-old children, with administration of acellular DTP vaccine at 18 months of age. *J Pediatr.* In press.
21. Ohkuni H, Kitaura T, Tamai T, Takasugi Y, Sugimoto T, Fukai K. Efficacy of acellular pertussis vaccines in Japan: comparison of two areas, one area where immunization started at 6 months and the other area at over 2 years of age. *Tokai J Exp Clin Med.* 1988;13(suppl):51-54.

Dose-Related Immunogenicity of *Haemophilus influenzae* Type b Capsular Polysaccharide–*Neisseria meningitidis* Outer Membrane Protein Conjugate Vaccine

Victor K. Wong, MD; Rory Quagliata, MPH, RN; Robert Adler, MD; Kwang Sik Kim, MD

• We studied the immunologic responsiveness to *Haemophilus influenzae* type b capsular polysaccharide–*Neisseria meningitidis* group b outer membrane protein conjugate vaccine (PRP-NOMP) in children 2 to 42 months of age with vaccine dosages containing 7.5, 15, or 30 μg of PRP. Overall, PRP-NOMP was highly immunogenic. Geometric mean titers of anti-PRP antibody increased from 0.09 to 3.3 mg/L and 6.6 mg/L following each dose of vaccine, respectively, in the 2- to 18-month age group. Similarly, anti-PRP antibody geometric mean titers increased from 0.12 to 5.9 mg/L in the older than 18-month age group. However, we noted an apparent inverse relationship between vaccine dosages and immune responses following two doses of PRP-NOMP in 2- to 18-month-old children. Anti-PRP antibody geometric mean titers were 12.0, 6.9, and 3.5 mg/L, respectively, after the second dose of vaccine containing 7.5, 15, or 30 μg of PRP. Additional studies are needed to understand the mechanisms responsible for this inverse relationship and also to determine the optimal dosage of PRP-NOMP for young children.

***(AJDC.* 1991;145:742-745)**

The variable immunogenicity[1,2] and efficacy[3-6] of the *Haemophilus influenzae* type b capsular polysaccharide vaccines (polyributylribitol phosphate [PRP]) has prompted the continued development of PRP–protein conjugated vaccines. One such vaccine utilizes the outer membrane protein complex of *Neisseria meningitidis* group b covalently linked to PRP (Ped-vax-HIB; Merck Sharp & Dohme Research Laboratories, West Point, Pa). Previous studies of *H influenzae* type b capsular polysaccharide—*N meningitidis* group b outer membrane protein conjugate vaccine (PRP-NOMP) utilizing dosages ranging from 7 to 15 μg of PRP have shown improved immunogenicity in children as young as 2 months of age when compared with PRP vaccines.[7-11] We undertook a study to determine the effect of varying vaccine dosages on the immunogenicity of PRP-NOMP.

Accepted for publication January 10, 1991.

From the Department of Pediatrics, Childrens Hospital of Los Angeles and the University of Southern California School of Medicine. Dr Wong is now with the Department of Pediatrics, Southern California Permanente Medical Group, Downey.

Presented in part at the 29th International Conference of Antimicrobial Agents and Chemotherapy, Houston, Tex, September 18, 1989.

Reprint requests to the Division of Infectious Diseases, Childrens Hospital of Los Angeles, 4650 Sunset Blvd, Box 51, Los Angeles, CA 90027 (Dr Kim).

PATIENTS AND METHODS

Vaccine

Each vial of a lyophilized PRP-NOMP vaccine consisted of 30.7 μg of PRP, 334 μg of partially purified outer membrane protein of *N meningitidis* (NOMP), and 4.1 mg of lactose. A single lot of vaccine (lot 1072/C-P298/37359) was utilized and reconstituted with the appropriate amount of aluminum hydroxide containing diluent (0.45 mg/mL) to provide 7.5 μg of PRP and 82 μg of NOMP, 15 μg of PRP and 163 μg of NOMP, or 30 μg of PRP and 326 μg of NOMP and 0.5-mL dose.

Study Design

Informed consent was obtained from the parents of 2- to 42-month-old children presenting to the General Pediatric Clinic at the Childrens Hospital of Los Angeles (Calif) following guidelines established by the Committee on Clinical Investigations at Childrens Hospital of Los Angeles. Children 2 to 18 months of age received two doses of 7.5 μg of PRP and 82 μg of NOMP, 15 μg of PRP and 163 μg of NOMP, or 30 μg of PRP and 326 μg of NOMP intramuscularly during a 2-month andiod, while children older than 18 months of age received a single dose of 7.5 μg of PRP and 82 μg of NOMP, 15 μg of PRP and 163 μg of NOMP, or 30 μg of PRP and 326 μg of NOMP according to a predetermined randomization.

Safety and tolerability were assessed by parental observation for temperature and local or systemic complaints (swelling, erythema, or tenderness at injection site; excessive crying; appearing tired or irritable; and diarrhea or vomiting) 5 days following immunization. Parents were also asked to record any clinical complaints on a standard report form. All forms were returned to the investigators, and a telephone follow-up interview was obtained when appropriate.

Serology

Serum was collected from children aged 2 to 18 months before each dose of vaccine and 1 month following the second dose of vaccine. Children aged 19 months or older underwent phlebotomy before and 1 month following immunization. Serum was stored at −70°C, and anti-PRP antibody levels were determined by radioimmunoassay[12] in a "blinded" fashion.

Statistical Analysis

All antibody values were converted to logarithms for statistical comparisons. Anti-PRP levels below the lower limit of our assay

Table 1.—Comparison of Geometric Mean Anti-PRP Antibody Concentrations Before and After Immunization With *Haemophilus influenzae* Type b–*Neisseria meningitidis* Outer Membrane Protein Conjugate Vaccine Among 2- to 18-Month-Old Children Who Received 7.5, 15, or 30 μg of PRP*

			After First Injection		After Second Injection	
Vaccine Dose, μg (No.)	Mean ± SD Age, mo†	Prevaccination, mg/L†	Mean ± SD Interval, wk†	Antibody Levels, mg/L†	Mean ± SD Interval, wk†	Antibody Levels, mg/L‡
7.5 (22)	8.8±5.1	0.09 (0.07-0.14)	8.5±1.3	4.1 (2.4-7.1)	5.0±1.6	12.0 (6.1-24)
15 (22)	7.3±3.8	0.08 (0.06-0.10)	8.2±0.9	2.8 (1.3-6.0)	5.1±1.5	6.9 (3.6-13)
30 (22)	7.8±4.6	0.09 (0.06-0.13)	8.3±1.0	3.1 (1.8-5.4)	4.7±1.2	3.5 (2.3-5.4)

*PRP indicates polyributylribitol phosphate. Values in parentheses are 95% confidence intervals.
†No significant difference by analysis of variance.
‡Significantly different ($P=.021$) by analysis of variance.

Table 2.—Comparison of Geometric Mean Anti-PRP Antibody Concentrations Before and After Immunization With *Haemophilus influenzae* Type b—*Neisseria meningitides* Outer Membrane Protein Conjugate Vaccine Among 19- to 42-Month-Old Children Who Received 7.5, 15, or 30 μg of PRP*

Vaccine Dose, μg (No.)	Mean ± SD Age, mo†	Prevaccination, mg/L†	Mean ± SD Interval, wk†	Antibody Levels, mg/L†
7.5 (15)	23.5±6.3	0.14 (0.10-0.22)	4.4±1.1	6.2 (2.9-13.4)
15 (21)	28.4±3.7	0.10 (0.07-0.14)	5.1±2.0	4.9 (3.0-8.1)
30 (13)	28.2±5.7	0.12 (0.06-0.25)	5.0±1.7	7.3 (4.1-13.0)

*PRP indicates polyributylribitol phosphate. Values in parentheses are 95% confidence intervals.
†No significant difference by analysis of variance.

(<0.12 mg/L) were assigned a value of 0.06 mg/L when calculating geometric mean titers (GMTs). Comparisons of anti-PRP antibody GMTs were performed with analysis of variance or Student's *t* test[13] where appropriate.

RESULTS

Patient Characteristics

Of the 115 children enrolled in the study, 66 (57%) were 2 to 18 months of age (mean±SD, 8.0±4.5 months), while 49 (43%) were 19 to 42 months of age (26.9 ±5.5 months). In the 2- to 18-month age group, 22 each received 7.5 μg of PRP and 82 μg of NOMP (seven aged 2 to 4 months, three aged 5 to 7 months, five aged 8 to 11 months, and six aged 12 to 17 months), 15 μg of PRP and 163 μg of NOMP (six aged 2 to 4 months, seven aged 5 to 7 months, four aged 8 to 11 months, and five aged 12 to 17 months), or 30 μg of PRP and 326 μg of NOMP (six aged 2 to 4 months, four aged 5 to 7 months, six aged 8 to 11 months, and six aged 12 to 17 months). This age distribution among the recipients of three different dosages was similar. The ethnic distribution was representative of our outpatient population: white, 37 (32%); Hispanic, 48 (42%); black, 24 (21%); and other, six (5%).

Clinical Observations

No serious reactions were noted, with the majority being limited to local complaints of pain, swelling, or redness at the injection site (24/115 [21%]) or appearing tired or irritable (24/115 [21%]). Fever (temperature >38.0°C) was noted in eight (7%) of the recipients. There was no apparent increase in reactions following the second vaccine dose.

Serologic Response

Anti-PRP antibody GMTs increased from 0.09 to 3.28 mg/L and 6.61 mg/L following each dose of PRP-NOMP, respectively, in the 2- to 18-month age group. In the older age group, the anti-PRP antibody GMTs increased from 0.12 to 5.88 mg/L following a single injection. Sixty-one (92%) and 58 (95%; two children failed to return for the second vaccine dose) of the 2- to 18-month-old children had postimmunization anti-PRP antibody levels greater than 1.0 mg/L following the first and second doses of the PRP-NOMP, respectively. Forty-eight (98%) in the 19- to 42-month age group had anti-PRP antibody levels greater than 1.0 mg/L 1 month following vaccination. These antibody responses between children 2 to 18 months old and 19 to 42 months old did not differ significantly.

The preimmunization and postimmunization anti-PRP antibody levels did not differ significantly when evaluated by ethnicity, preexisting anti-PRP antibody levels, or gender. A statistically significant difference was noted when anti-PRP antibody levels were compared regarding dosage of the vaccine administered in the 2- to 18-month age group. After the second dose of vaccine, anti-PRP antibody GMTs ranged from 3.5 to 12.0 mg/L, which were statistically significantly different ($P=.021$, Table 1). In addition, when we compared antibody responses of the different vaccine dosages by subtracting the prevaccination anti-PRP antibody levels from antibody levels following the second dose of vaccine, the difference was again significant ($P=.046$).

Furthermore, we noted that although the differences in anti-PRP antibody levels between those receiving 7.5 μg of PRP and 82 μg of NOMP and 15 μg of PRP and 163 μg of NOMP or 15 μg of PRP and 163 μg of NOMP and 30 μg of PRP and 326 μg of NOMP were not significant, the difference between the 7.5 μg of PRP and 82 μg of NOMP group vs the 30 μg of PRP and 326 μg of NOMP group *was* significant ($P=.05$). These differences could not be explained by the differences in the ages of each group or the differences in time interval between administration of vaccine and phlebotomy. However, anti-PRP antibody levels in the 19- to 42-month age group did not differ significantly when analyzed by the dosage of vaccine administered (Table 2).

COMMENT

The PRP-NOMP vaccine was well tolerated and found to be highly immunogenic in children 2 to 42 months of age, with 92% of children 2 to 18 months of age and 98% of the 19- to 42-month age group achieving what may be a so-called protective postimmunization antibody level (ie, ≥1.0 mg/L[14]) following a single dose of PRP-NOMP.

The intriguing finding was that the immunogenicity of PRP-NOMP in 2- to 18-month-old children appeared to be inversely related to the amount of PRP administered. This was shown by our demonstration that significantly greater anti-PRP antibody levels were achieved following the second dose in the recipients of PRP-NOMP containing 7.5 μg of PRP compared with those receiving 30 μg of PRP. The reasons for this inverse relationship between immunogenicity and vaccine dosage are unclear. Tudor-Williams et al,[15] utilizing *H influenzae* type b oligosaccharide-protein conjugate vaccine (at 3, 5, and 9 months of age), have reported rises in anti-PRP antibody GMTs from 0.11 mg/L at 3 months to 14.6 mg/L at 10 months in recipients of a 2-μg vaccine dosage vs 0.11 to 26.4 mg/L in recipients of a 10-μg vaccine dosage. These findings suggest that immunologic responsiveness to *H influenzae* type b protein conjugate vaccines may differ. It should, however, be noted that the ethnic distribution of patients recruited by Tudor-Williams et al in Oxford, England, is different from our population base and that 0.9% sodium chloride was used as a diluent instead of our aluminum hydroxide–containing diluent.

Potential explanations for our findings might relate to components of PRP-NOMP, ie, PRP, carrier protein (group b meningococcal outer membrane protein) or aluminum hydroxide–containing diluent, but no data are available at present to support or refute any of these hypotheses. Taylor and Baker[16] have demonstrated suppression of antibody response to type III pneumococcal antigen in mice when prior priming with antigen had been performed. These investigators have suggested that a soluble suppressor factor might be released from suppressor T cells after antigenic stimulation, which may later inhibit antigen-stimulating B cells or inhibit amplifier T cells when reexposed to the polysaccharide antigen. We were not able to demonstrate a soluble factor responsible for our dose-dependent phenomenon, and this hypothesis remains speculative.

Another potential explanation might be a so-called carrier-induced epitope suppression. Di John et al[17] have shown, in studies of malaria vaccines coupled with a tetanus carrier, that prior immunity against a carrier protein modulates the serologic response to injected malaria peptides attached to the same carrier in humans. A statistically significant negative correlation was observed between preimmunization tetanus antitoxin titers and postimmunization response to a malaria sporozoite antigen. In our study, 2- to 18-month-old children responded to the first injection of 30 μg of PRP, with postimmunization anti-PRP antibody levels being similar to those achieved with 7.5 or 15 μg of PRP, but did not show greater booster responses with subsequent injection. It remains to be determined whether this lack of booster response stems from epitope suppression due to prior exposure to the carrier protein or whether there may have been antigenic competition. A complicating factor to exploring this concept was that standardized assays were not available to measure antibody to the outer membrane protein carrier.

Mannhalter et al[18] have demonstrated in vitro that aluminum hydroxide, when utilized as an adjuvant with tetanus toxoid, may increase the interleukin 1 release from monocytes, resulting in increased antibody production by B cells. However, these investigators also demonstrated a decrease in cellular proliferation when booster antigen rechallenge contains aluminum hydroxide adjuvant. Similarly, Stewart-Tull,[19] in a rabbit model utilizing influenza vaccine, has noted that repetitive injections of an adjuvant substance reduce the titer of anti-influenza antibody. However, this possibility appears to be very unlikely, because aluminum hydroxide contained in each 0.5-mL vaccine would be identical (0.225 mg), regardless of dosages.

The differences in immunogenicity observed in our study after two doses of PRP-NOMP containing 7.5, 15, or 30 μg of PRP may not be clinically important, as almost all the children achieved anti-PRP antibody levels greater than 1.0 mg/L. However, further investigations of factors that may affect immune responsiveness to polysaccharide-protein conjugate vaccines are warranted to establish optimal vaccine dosage in young children.

This work was supported in part by a research grant from Merck Sharp & Dohme Research Laboratories, West Point, Pa.

We thank Dr Philip Vella of Merck Sharp & Dohme Research Laboratories for quantitation of anti-PRP antibody and Caroline Rivera and Lillian Vivona for typing the manuscript.

References

1. Ward JI, Broome CV, Harrison LH, Shinefield H, Black S. *Haemophilus influenzae* type b vaccines: lessons for the future. *Pediatrics.* 1988;81:886-893.

2. Smith DH, Peter G, Ingram DL, Harding AL, Anderson P. Responses of children immunized with the capsular polysaccharide of *Haemophilus influenzae* type b. *Pediatrics.* 1973;52:637-644.

3. Harrison LH, Broome CV, Hightower AW, et al. A day care-based study of the efficacy of *Haemophilus* b polysaccharide vaccine. *JAMA.* 1988;260:1413-1418.

4. Osterholm MT, Rambeck JH, White KE, et al. Lack of efficacy of *Haemophilus* b polysaccharide vaccine in Minnesota. *JAMA.* 1988;260:1423-1428.

5. Black SB, Shinefeld HR, Hiatt RA, Fireman BH. Efficacy of *Haemophilus influenzae* type b capsular polysaccharide vaccine. *Pediatr Infect Dis J.* 1988;7:149-156.

6. Shapiro ED, Murphy TV, Wald ER, Brady CA. The protective efficacy of *Haemophilus* b polysaccharide vaccine. *JAMA.* 1988;260:1419-1422.

7. Einhorn MS, Weinberg GA, Anderson EL, Granoff PD, Granoff DM. Immunogenicity in infants of *Haemophilus influenzae* type b polysaccharide in a conjugate vaccine with *Neisseria meningitides* outer-membrane protein. *Lancet.* 1986;2:299-302.

8. Lenoir AA, Granoff PD, Granoff DM. Immunogenicity of *Haemophilus influenzae* type b polysaccharide-*Neisseria meningitidis* outer membrane protein conjugate vaccine in 2- to 6-month-old infants. *Pediatrics.* 1987;80:283-287.

9. Weinberg GA, Einhorn MS, Lenoir AA, Granoff PD, Granoff DM. Immunologic priming to capsular polysaccharide in infants immunized with *Haemophilus influenzae* type b polysaccharide–*Neisseria meningitides* outer membrane protein conjugate vaccine. *J Pediatr.* 1987;111:22-27.

10. Shapiro ED, Capobianco LA, Berg AT, Zitt MQ. The immunogenicity of *Hemophilus influenzae* type b polysaccharide–*Neisseria meningitides* group B outer membrane protein complex vaccine in infants and young children. *J Infect Dis.* 1889;160:1064-1067.

11. Kim KS, Wong VK, Adler R, Steinberg EA. Comparative

immune responses to *Haemophilus influenzae* type b polysaccharide and a polysaccharide-protein conjugate vaccines. *Pediatrics.* 1990;85(suppl):648-650.

12. Vella PP, Staub JM, Armstrong J, et al. Immunogenicity of a new *Haemophilus influenzae* type B conjugate vaccine. *Pediatrics.* 1990;85(suppl):668-675.

13. Snedecor GW, Cochran WG, eds. *Statistical Methods.* 6th ed. Ames, Ia: Iowa State University Press; 1967.

14. Kayhty H, Peltola H, Karanko V, Makela PH. The protective level of serum antibodies to the capsular polysaccharide of *Haemophilus influenzae* type b. *J Infect Dis.* 1983;147:1100.

15. Tudor-Williams G, Frankland J, Isaacs D, et al. *Haemophilus influenzae* type b conjugate vaccine trial in Oxford: implications for the United Kingdom. *Arch Dis Child.* 1989;64:520-524.

16. Taylor CE, Baker PJ. Production of soluble suppressor factor by spleen cells from mice immunized with type III pneumococcal polysaccharide. *J Immunol.* 1985;135:2551-2556.

17. Di John D, Torres JR, Murillo, J, et al. Effect of priming with carrier on response to conjugate vaccine. *Lancet.* 1989;2:1415-1418.

18. Mannhalter JW, Neychev HO, Zlabinger GJ, Ahmad R, Eibl MM. Modulation of the human immune response by the non-toxic and non-pyogenic adjuvant aluminum hydroxide: effect on antigen uptake and antigen presentation. *Clin Exp Immunol.* 1985;61:143-151.

19. Stewart-Tull DES. The immunological activities of bacterial peptidoglycans. *Ann Rev Microbiol.* 1980;34:311-340.

In Other AMA Journals

ARCHIVES OF OTOLARYNGOLOGY—HEAD & NECK SURGERY

The Effect of Steroid Therapy on Recovery From Tonsillectomy in Children

Francis I. Catlin, MD, ScD; William J. Grimes, MD
(*Arch Otolaryngol Head Neck Surg.* 1991;117:649-652)

Fine-Needle Aspiration in Recurrent Tonsillitis

Conrad I. Timon, FRCSI, FRCSI(Oto); Mary T. Cafferkey, MD; Michael Walsh, FRCSI, FRCS(Ed)
(*Arch Otolaryngol Head Neck Surg.* 1991;117:653-656)

ARCHIVES OF NEUROLOGY

A Comparison of Daily and Alternate-Day Prednisone Therapy in the Treatment of Duchenne Muscular Dystrophy

Gerald M. Fenichel, MD; Jerry R. Mendell, MD; Richard T. Moxley III, MD; Robert C. Griggs, MD; Michael H. Brooke, MD; J. Philip Miller; Alan Pestronk, MD; Jenny Robison, MS; Wendy King, LPT; Linda Signore, RN, MS; Shree Pandya, MS; Julaine Floremance, MS; Janine Schierbecker, PT; Bradley Wilson
(*Arch Neurol.* 1991;48:575-579)

The Influence of Gender on the Susceptibility to Multiple Sclerosis in Sibships

Adele D. Sadovnick, PhD; Dennis E. Bulman; Lara Hashimoto, MS; Marie B. D'Hooghe, MD; George C. Ebers, MD
(*Arch Neurol.* 1991;48:586-588)

Literary Neurologic Syndromes: Alice in Wonderland

Loren A. Rolak, MD
(*Arch Neurol.* 1991;48:649-651)

Apparent Decreased Risk of Invasive Bacterial Disease After Heterologous Childhood Immunization

Steven B. Black, MD; James D. Cherry, MD; Henry R. Shinefield, MD;
Bruce Fireman, MS; Peter Christenson, PhD; Dominique Lampert, MS

• To investigate the possibility that there might be an increased risk of heterologous invasive bacterial disease after routine childhood immunization with measles, mumps, and rubella vaccine live; diphtheria and tetanus toxoids and pertussis vaccine; and oral poliovirus vaccine live, a case-control study was conducted within the Kaiser Permanente Northern California pediatric population. Contrary to the premise, an apparent protective effect against invasive bacterial disease was detected after all childhood vaccinations. However, when adjustment was made for frequency of well-care visits and day-care attendance, no significant relationship was seen between receipt of routine childhood immunizations and risk of invasive heterologous bacterial disease for any individual vaccine, although a statistically significant protective effect was detected within 1 or 3 months after the receipt of any vaccine. Since a decreased risk of invasive bacterial disease was also noted to be related to the receipt of routine well-child pediatric care, other preventive health care measures may be responsible for the apparent immunization protective effect.

(*AJDC.* 1991;145:746-749)

Shortly after release of the polyribosyl phosphate *Haemophilus influenzae* type b vaccine, a possible increased risk of acquiring invasive disease due to *H influenzae* during the 3-week period after receipt of the polyribosyl phosphate vaccine was reported.[1] More recently, in a field trial of two acellular pertussis vaccines in Sweden, it was observed that four vaccinees, but no controls, died of invasive bacterial disease during the follow-up period.[2,3] Because of these reports regarding the possibility of an increased risk of bacterial disease following childhood immunizations, a study was undertaken to investigate the relationship, if any, between risk of heterologous bacterial disease and receipt of diphtheria and tetanus toxoids and pertussis (DTP) vaccine; measles, mumps, and rubella (MMR) virus vaccine, and oral poliovirus (OPV) vaccine live immunizations during the first 2 years of life.

See also pp 734 and 750.

Accepted for publication December 21, 1990.

From the Northern California Kaiser Permanente Vaccine Study Center and the Permanente Medical Group Division of Research, Oakland, Calif (Drs Black and Shinefield, Mr Fireman, and Ms Lampert); Department of Pediatrics, UCLA Medical Center (Dr Cherry); and the Department of Biomathematics, UCLA School of Medicine (Dr Christenson).

Reprint requests to Kaiser Permanente Pediatric Vaccine Study Center, 280 W MacArthur Blvd, Oakland, CA 94611 (Dr Black).

PATIENTS AND METHODS

Invasive bacterial disease occurring in children between ages 1 month and 2 years in the Kaiser Permanente Medical Care Program of Northern California during the years 1986 through 1988 were identified from a computerized microbiology laboratory database. The medical records of all cases were reviewed to verify that each child had invasive bacterial disease as defined by a positive bacterial culture from a normally sterile site. Two controls were selected from the Kaiser Permanente Medical Care Program membership and matched to individual cases with respect to age (±1 month), sex, zip code of residence, and duration of health plan membership. A chart review was conducted of all cases and controls to record all immunizations within 3 months of the index date, defined as the date of onset of invasive bacterial disease for the cases and the corresponding reference date for the matched controls. The reference date for controls was the date of diagnosis for the corresponding patient. In addition, telephone interviews were conducted with the parents of cases and controls to obtain information on possible covariates, including day-care, breast-feeding, parental ethnicity, parental education, and crowding. Subsequent to the initial analysis, an additional chart review was conducted to investigate frequency of well-care visits as a possible covariate. In this review, the total number of well-care visits that had occurred for each child within 6 months before the onset of illness for cases and the corresponding reference date for controls was obtained. Possible predictors of disease include immunization within specific intervals prior to the index date and the potential covariates. Individual conditional logistic regression models that recognize case-control matching were used to assess the effect of possible predictors individually on disease. Multiple conditional logistic regression was then used to determine the adjusted effect of recent immunization on disease by controlling for significant confounding covariates. Odds ratios relating immunization and disease were calculated from the regressions.[4]

RESULTS

Between January 1986 and December 1988, 223 cases of invasive bacterial disease were identified by the Kaiser Permanente Medical Care Program Regional Microbiology Laboratory. Of these, 144 were due to *Pneumococcus*, 58 due to *H influenzae*, seven due to *Escherichia coli*, five due

Table 1.—Cases and Controls Immunized at Specified Intervals Prior to Onset of Disease*

Interval, d	Vaccine	% Immunized: Cases (n=223)	% Immunized: Controls (n=438)	Odds Ratio†: Estimate	Odds Ratio†: 95% CI	P
0-7	DTP	1.4	3.0	0.44	(0.12-1.60)	.21
	OPV	0.9	2.6	0.34	(0.07-1.59)	.17
	MMR	0	0.9	. . .	. . .	
	Any‡	1.4	4.0	0.34	(0.10-1.18)	.09
8-30	DTP	1.9	10.0	0.17	(0.06-0.47)	.001
	OPV	0.9	8.6	0.10	(0.02-0.41)	.001
	MMR	0.5	0.9	0.50	(0.06-4.47)	.53
	Any‡	2.3	11.2	0.19	(0.07-0.49)	.001
31-60	DTP	4.2	10.0	0.36	(0.16-0.78)	.01
	OPV	3.7	7.7	0.44	(0.19-1.00)	.05
	MMR	0.5	1.6	0.25	(0.03-2.19)	.21
	Any‡	4.7	11.9	0.34	(0.16-0.70)	.003
61-90	DTP	0.5	6.1	0.07	(0.01-0.51)	.01
	OPV	0	6.8	. . .	. . .	. . .
	MMR	0	2.3	. . .	. . .	. . .
	Any‡	0.5	7.9	0.05	(0.01-0.40)	.004

*DTP indicates diphtheria and tetanus toxoids and pertussis vaccine; OPV, oral polio virus vaccine live; MMR, measles, mumps, and rubella vaccine live; and CI, confidence interval.

†Ratio of the odds of disease among children vaccinated in the interval to the odds of disease among children not vaccinated in the interval, obtained from conditional logistic regression.

‡DTP, OPV, or MMR.

to *Meningococcus,* and nine due to other organisms. The age range of cases was between 1 and 20 months with most disease occurring between 5 and 15 months of age. Chart review was accomplished for 221 of 223 cases and 438 of 446 controls. Telephone interviews were completed for 202 of 223 cases and 414 of 446 controls.

The percentage of cases and controls immunized at specific intervals up to 3 months prior to onset of illness in the cases is shown in Table 1. Generally, controls were about four times more likely to have been immunized within either 1 or 3 months than were cases. Odds ratios utilizing case-control matching translate immunization rates into ratios of likelihood of disease. (An odds ratio of 1 would indicate no difference between cases and controls.) Ignoring other factors related to disease, recent DTP or OPV immunization reduces the risk of disease by a factor of 0.07 to 0.44. Table 2 shows the potential for confounding the observed results. Thirty-one percent of cases attended day-care compared with only 16% of controls ($P<.0001$). Children in day-care were at significantly greater risk of disease than those who were not (odds ratio, 2.40). In contrast, cases had significantly fewer well-care visits than controls ($P<.0001$). They had an average of 1.1 well-care visits within 6 months prior to onset of illness, whereas controls had an average of 2.6 visits during the same period. Children with fewer well-care visits were at significantly greater risk of invasive bacterial disease (odds ratio, 4.0 for none to one visit vs two visits).

Table 3 shows adjusted odds ratios for day-care and frequency of well-care visits for 484 subjects for whom this information was available. (The other 177 subjects did not

Table 2.—Comparability of Cases and Controls in Potential Confounders of the Apparent Effect of Immunization on Disease

Potential Factor	Cases, %	Controls, %	P*
Maternal ethnicity†			
White	59	57	NS
Black	21	13	
Hispanic	12	14	
Asian	8	16	
Maternal education†			
High school	62	56	NS
College	25	28	
Professional	13	16	
No. of siblings			
None	34	36	NS
1	41	39	
2	16	17	
3 or more	8	8	
Breast-feeding	65	71	NS
Day-care attendance	31	16	<.0001
Well-child visits within 6 mo			
0 or 1	73	15	<.0001
2	23	22	

*Potential confounding factors were compared between patients and their matched controls in individual conditional logistic regressions that modeled the likelihood of disease depending on the status of the factor. NS indicates not significant.

†Ethnicity and education distributions for fathers are nearly identical to those for mothers.

Table 3.—Odds of Disease Based on Recent Immunization History, Adjusted for Day-Care Status and No. of Well-Care Visits Within 6 Months*

		Receipt of Vaccine in Interval					OR†	
Interval, d	Vaccine	Cases, %	Controls, %	OR†	95% CI	*P*	Day-Care	Well Care
0-7	DTP	0.6	3.8	0.38	(0.04, 3.53)	.40	1.94	0.10
	OPV	0.6	3.2	0.44	(0.05, 4.25)	.48	1.92	0.10
	MMR	0	1.0	. . .	. . .	. . .	1.92	0.10
	Any	0.6	4.7	0.27	(0.03, 2.33)	.23	1.95	0.10
8-30	DTP	1.8	7.6	0.37	(0.10, 1.41)	.15	1.95	0.10
	OPV	0.6	3.2	0.13	(0.02, 1.11)	.06	1.84	0.10
	MMR	0.6	1.0	0.16	(0.01, 2.33)	.18	1.90	0.09
	Any	2.4	10.1	0.29	(0.09, 0.95)	.04	1.94	0.10
31-60	DTP	4.8	10.4	1.02	(0.38, 2.76)	.96	1.92	0.10
	OPV	4.2	7.3	1.41	(0.50, 3.96)	.52	1.92	0.09
	MMR	0.6	1.9	0.70	(0.06, 8.76)	.78	1.92	0.10
	Any	5.4	12.3	0.97	(0.38, 2.45)	.95	1.92	0.10
61-90	DTP	0.6	5.1	0.31	(0.04, 2.50)	.27	1.85	0.10
	OPV	0	5.7	. . .	. . .	. . .	1.83	0.11
	MMR	0	2.5	. . .	. . .	. . .	1.88	0.10
	Any	0.6	6.9	0.21	(0.03, 1.63)	0.14	1.81	0.10

*OR indicates odds ratio; CI, confidence interval; DTP, diphtheria and tetanus toxoids and pertussis vaccine; OPV, oral polio virus vaccine live; and MMR, measles, mumps, and rubella vaccine live. Day-care status, well-child care visits, and vaccine history were available for 167 patients and 317 controls.

†Ratio of the odds of disease among children vaccinated in the interval to the odds of disease among children not vaccinated in the interval, obtained from conditional logistic regression models, which adjust for day-care status and number of well-child care visits within 6 months. Odds ratios for day care (yes vs no) and well-child care (at least two visits vs at most one) are similarly adjusted for each other and for vaccination in the interval.

differ in vaccination rates from these 484 subjects.) There was still a tendency for recently immunized children to have less risk of disease, but for most vaccines and intervals the odds ratios shifted toward the no-effect value of 1.0. The apparent contradictory odds ratio of 1.41 for OPV 31 to 60 days prior to the reference date was due to proportionally more cases than controls with none or one well-care visit, and no OPV immunizations in this interval among these subjects. Among subjects with at least two well-care visits, 14% of cases and 9% of controls received OPV in this interval. A similar phenomenon occurred for DTP in this interval.

During the 0- to 30-day interval for any vaccine, 3% of cases and 15% of controls were immunized. The odds ratio was 0.26 (95% confidence interval [CI], 0.09 to 0.76; $P=.01$). Similarly, for the whole 90-day period for any vaccine, 9% of cases and 34% of controls were immunized (odds ratio, 0.31; 95% CI, 0.13 to 0.73; $P=.01$).

Day-care attendees are almost twice as likely to develop disease, and children with at least two well-care visits in 6 months are at one tenth the risk of disease as are children with at most one well-care visit.

COMMENT

We have investigated a possible increased risk of heterologous invasive bacterial disease following routine immunizations in early childhood. In this case-control study we observed an apparent protective effect of MMR, DTP, or OPV against the development of invasive bacterial disease for a 1- or 3-month period. When the data were analyzed for available information on covariates including socioeconomic indicators, race, and day-care attendance, only day-care was found to be a potential confounder. However, this possible confounding was in the direction of increasing the apparent protective effect of vaccination; children in day-care are both at increased risk of bacterial disease and more likely to be vaccinated. Subsequently, a second chart review was undertaken to determine the frequency of well-care visits among cases and controls. In this second review, it was found that children who received well care were significantly less likely to develop invasive bacterial disease than those who had few or no well-care visits. With adjustment for this confounder, the apparent protective effect of routine childhood immunization against subsequent heterologous invasive bacterial disease was greatly diminished in magnitude and precision, and became a statistically nonsignificant trend for each vaccine considered individually.

It is possible that the apparent difference in disease risk between cases and controls is the result of selection bias. That is, children who were ill at the time of their well-care visits were less likely to be immunized than children who were well. However, if this were the explanation for the observed difference, one would have expected that cases would have been less likely to be immunized, but not less likely to receive well care. If deferral of immunization in sick children accounted for the observed results, one would have expected the number of well-care visits to be the same.

The biologic plausibility of a protective effect of routine childhood immunization with DTP, OPV, and MMR must be considered. Endotoxin, a component of the pertussis portion of the DTP vaccine, is a known protective factor against experimental bacterial infections.[5] In one experiment, protection induced by *Bordetella pertussis* was still present 49 days after vaccine administration. Infection with the measles virus elicits the production of interferon, and this may offer protection against other viral infections.[6] Since invasive bacterial disease may have a relationship to respiratory viral infections it is possible that MMR immunization could also be a factor in decreasing the occurrence of invasive bacterial disease.[7] However, since the protective findings in this study were uniform over a 3-month period, it is difficult to attribute them solely to the vaccine properties discussed above.

Based on our data, we conclude that there is no evidence of an increased risk of invasive bacterial disease following any of the routine childhood immunizations investigated; on the contrary, there is a trend toward lower rates of disease among children after receiving these immunizations. Furthermore, the receipt of routine well-child pediatric care is associated with a decreased risk of invasive bacterial disease that appears to be unrelated to the receipt of childhood vaccinations and may relate to other factors such as nutrition counseling, other preventive health care measures, or an increased level of health consciousness and hygiene among parents bringing their children in for well-care visits.

Although a protective effect of the vaccines is biologically plausible, it is possible that the apparent protective effect is related to good health practices that are only partially reflected in well-child care visits.

This study was funded by an unrestricted grant from Lederle Laboratories, Pearl River, NJ, and by the Community Services Program of the Northern California Permanente Medical Group.

References

1. Black S, Shinefield H, Hiatt RA, et al. b-CAPSA 1 *Haemophilus influenzae* type b capsular polysaccharide vaccine safety. *Pediatrics.* 1987;79:321-325.
2. Ad Hoc Group for the Study of the Pertussis Vaccines. Placebo-controlled trial of two acellular pertussis vaccines in Sweden: protective efficacy and adverse events. *Lancet.* 1988;1:954-960.
3. Storsaeter J, Olin P, Berit R, et al. Mortality and morbidity from invasive bacterial infections during a clinical trial of acellular pertussis vaccines in Sweden. *Pediatr Infect Dis.* 1988;7:637-645.
4. Breslow NE, Day NE. *Statistical Methods in Cancer Research.* Lyon, France: International Agency for Research on Cancer Scientific Publications; 1980:248-279.
5. Dubos R, Schaedler R. Reversible changes in the susceptibility of mice to bacterial infections. *J Exp Med.* 1956;104:53-65.
6. Petralli JK, Merigan TC, Wilbur JR. Circulating interferon after measles vaccination. *N Engl J Med.* 1965;273:198-201.
7. Young LS, LaForce M, Head JJ, Feeley JC, Bennett JV. A simultaneous outbreak of meningococcal and influenza infections. *N Engl J Med.* 1972;287:5-9.

DTP Immunization and Susceptibility to Infectious Diseases

Is There a Relationship?

Michael Davidson, MD, MPH; G. William Letson, MD; Joel I. Ward, MD; Angela Ball, MD; Lisa Bulkow, MS; Peter Christenson, PhD; James D. Cherry, MD, MSc

• A two-part study was carried out in Alaskan Native children to evaluate the potential risk of invasive bacterial disease and the occurrence of minor illnesses after immunization with diphtheria and tetanus toxoids and whole-cell pertussis vaccine (DTP). First, a case-control comparison was performed with 186 children who had invasive *Haemophilus influenzae* type b or *Streptococcus pneumoniae* disease (cases) and 186 healthy controls matched for sex, region of residence, birth date, and number of DTP immunizations. The proportion of cases and controls immunized in the 30-day period before onset of disease for cases or reference date for controls was identical, suggesting no association with DTP immunization. In a second analysis, the occurrence of any illness, particularly infectious diseases, in 104 study subjects was compared for the period 30 days before and after 377 DTP immunizations. The rate of illness before immunization was 53%, and after immunization, 43%, again suggesting no causative effects from DTP immunization. Despite the high rates of invasive bacterial disease and nearly compete DTP immunization status in this population, no consistent relationship could be demonstrated between DTP immunization and susceptibility to infectious diseases.

***(AJDC.* 1991;145:750-754)**

Until recently, little attention has been given to the possibility that pertussis vaccination might affect the

See also pp 734 and 746.

susceptibility of children to other infectious diseases. However, in a large acellular pertussis vaccine efficacy trial conducted in Sweden in 1986 and 1987, it was observed that three pertussis vaccinees died of invasive bacterial infections.[1,2] In another recent study, infants who were immunized with diphtheria and tetanus toxoids and whole-cell pertussis vaccine (DTP) subsequently had an increased rate of fever, cough, and diarrheal illness.[3]

To examine these issues further, we evaluated in Alaska Native infants the potential risk of, or protection from, invasive bacterial disease and other minor illnesses after DTP immunization. We selected the Alaskan Native American population (Eskimo, Indian, and Aleut) for this study because they suffer the highest known incidence of invasive *Haemophilus influenzae* type b and *Streptococcus pneumoniae* disease, and detailed surveillance data for these diseases are available for the past 10 years.[4,5] Also, there is a concerted statewide effort to immunize all Alaskan children with DTP, and the state maintains computerized immunization records. In this study we performed two analyses: (1) to evaluate the temporal relationship of DTP immunization in children with and without invasive *H influenzae* type b and *S pneumoniae* disease and (2) to evaluate in those children with complete medical record reviews the occurrence of any illness, particularly infectious diseases, in the 30-day period before and after DTP immunization.

SUBJECTS AND METHODS

Study subjects were Alaskan Native American Eskimos, Indians, or Aleuts residing in two health service areas of the Alaska Area Indian Health Service: the Yukon-Kuskokwim Delta and the Anchorage service units.

Case-Control Analysis

Cases had invasive *H influenzae* type b or *S pneumoniae* disease proved by culture of specimens obtained from normally sterile body sites (blood, cerebrospinal fluid, empyema, or joint space) during the period from January 1, 1980, through April 1988 and were 2 to 24 months old with at least one previous DTP immunization. Cases were detected by both active and passive surveillance for invasive *H influenzae* type b and *S pneumoniae* diseases, as previously described.[4,5] Children who had received previous *H influenzae* type b vaccines were excluded.

For each case, one control was selected from computerized birth logs starting from the birth date of the case and matching for birth date, sex, residence within the same service unit, and the number of DTP immunizations given at the time of disease

Accepted for publication December 26, 1990.

From the Arctic Investigations Program, Center for Infectious Diseases, Centers for Disease Control, Anchorage, Alaska (Drs Davidson, Letson, and Ball and Ms Bulkow); UCLA Center for Vaccine Research, Harbor-UCLA Medical Center, Torrance, Calif (Drs Letson and Ward); Department of Biomathematics (Dr Christenson), and Department of Pediatrics (Drs Ward and Cherry) School of Medicine, UCLA.

Reprint requests to Arctic Investigations Program, 225 Eagle St, Anchorage, AK 99501 (Dr Davidson).

Table 1.—Characteristics and Comparability of Cases and Controls*

	No. (%)	
	Cases	Controls
Matched Characteristics		
Gender		
M	103 (55)	103 (55)
F	83 (45)	83 (45)
Region		
Anchorage Service Unit	42 (23)	42 (23)
Yukon-Kuskokwim	144 (77)	144 (77)
No. of DTP immunizations before disease diagnosis or reference date		
1	48 (26)	48 (26)
2	39 (21)	39 (21)
3	89 (48)	89 (48)
4	10 (5)	10 (5)
Age at disease diagnoses or reference date		
Mean±SD, mo	10.5±5.0	10.5±5.0
Under 1 y	118 (63)	118 (63)
Unmatched Characteristics		
Ethnicity (Native American)		
Eskimo	159 (85)	162 (87)
Indian	12 (6)	10 (5)
Aleut	13 (7)	13 (7)
Mixed Eskimo/Indian	2 (1)	1 (1)
Proportion Alaskan native		
<4/8	14 (10)	21 (13)
4/8	24 (17)	28 (17)
5/8-7/8	10 (7)	5 (3)
8/8	96 (67)	106 (66)
Unknown	42	26
Maternal parity at birth of study subject		
1 (1st child)	55 (30)	50 (28)
2	43 (24)	49 (27)
3	33 (18)	25 (14)
4	24 (13)	25 (14)
5	17 (9)	17 (9)
>5	9 (5)	13 (7)
Unknown	5	7
Birth weight		
<2500 g	11 (6)	8 (4)
Mean±SD, g	3423±563	3525±546
Maternal age at birth of study subjects, y (mean±SD)	26.3±5.7†	27.5±5.5

*DTP indicates diphtheria and tetanus toxoids and whole-cell pertussis vaccine.
†P=.04 when compared with age of mothers of controls. All other comparisons not significantly different.

diagnosis. When cases were from small communities (under 1000 population), controls were selected from a distant village within the same service unit. This was done to avoid overmatching, resulting from coincident immunizations in a village administered by a visiting public health nurse. Controls were excluded if they had a history of pneumonia, meningitis, cellulitis, sepsis, or arthritis diagnosed during the first 24 months of life or if they had received any *H influenzae* type b vaccines. To compare intervals from immunization, a reference date for the controls was established. This reference date was the day that the control was the same age as his or her matched case at the time of diagnosis of *H influenzae* type b or *S pneumoniae* disease.

All available medical records for both cases and controls, including the public health nurse immunization records, were reviewed to verify and identify all vaccinations, illnesses, birth weight, maternal age, and birth order. Computerized Indian Health Service medical record summaries were also searched for illness and immunization data. Cases and controls were compared with respect to the interval from the last DTP immunization to the diagnosis date of illness for cases or to the reference date for controls.

Statistical analyses included McNemar's test to compare the proportion of cases and controls having recent immunizations and the paired t test to compare mean interval differences. A conditional logistic regression analysis of case-control differences for maternal age, parity, birth weight, ethnicity, and interval since last immunization was also used to detect effects of potential confounders.[6] Odds ratios and their confidence limits were calculated for varying intervals between immunization and the date of diagnosis of invasive bacterial disease for cases or reference date for controls.[7]

Analysis of All Illnesses

The complete medical records for both outpatient and inpatient encounters were available for 104 cases and controls who resided in the communities of Bethel and Anchorage. These records were reviewed for the occurrence of all illnesses, including minor infectious diseases, during the periods 30 days before and after each DTP immunization. For all illness and selected infectious illness, McNemar's test was used to compare the occurrence of illness in the prevaccine vs postvaccine periods for cases and controls and for the two combined.

RESULTS

Cases

During the study period, there were 179 *H influenzae* type b and 94 *S pneumoniae* cases of invasive disease in Alaskan Native children between 2 and 24 months of age at the time of diagnosis. Of this group, 55 cases of invasive *H influenzae* type b and 32 cases of *S pneumoniae* disease were excluded from the study for one of three reasons: (1) they had participated in an *H influenzae* type b conjugate vaccine trial (N=37); (2) they lacked previous DTP immunization or could not be adequately matched to a control child (N=30); or (3) they had not yet been reported on by surveillance at the time of study (N=20). There were five cases with more than one episode of invasive bacterial disease; only the first illness was considered. In the final analysis, there were 124 *H influenzae* type b and 62 *S pneumoniae* cases with matched controls. Of these cases, 31.2% had meningitis, 27.4% had pneumonia, 0.6% had epiglottitis, 12.4% had arthritis, 10.1% had cellulitis, and 18.4% had septicemia/bacteremia.

Case-Control Analysis

The characteristics and comparability of cases and controls are shown in Table 1. The mean age of the mothers of cases was 26.3 years, whereas it was 27.5 years for mothers of controls (P=.04). There were no other significant differences between the groups. The birth dates of 69% of the case-control pairs were 14 days or less apart; only 3% were more than 60 days apart.

Shown in the Figure are the weekly intervals from last DTP immunization to date of disease diagnosis for cases or from last immunization to the reference date for controls. Considerable weekly variations occurred for both cases and controls. However, in the 1st month after immunization, the distribution of individuals in weekly intervals after DTP immunization was equal for cases and controls. Cases predominated intermittently over controls for the 5th through the 10th weeks after immunization. Controls predominated over cases or were equal to cases for 19 of the 30 subsequent intervals analyzed.

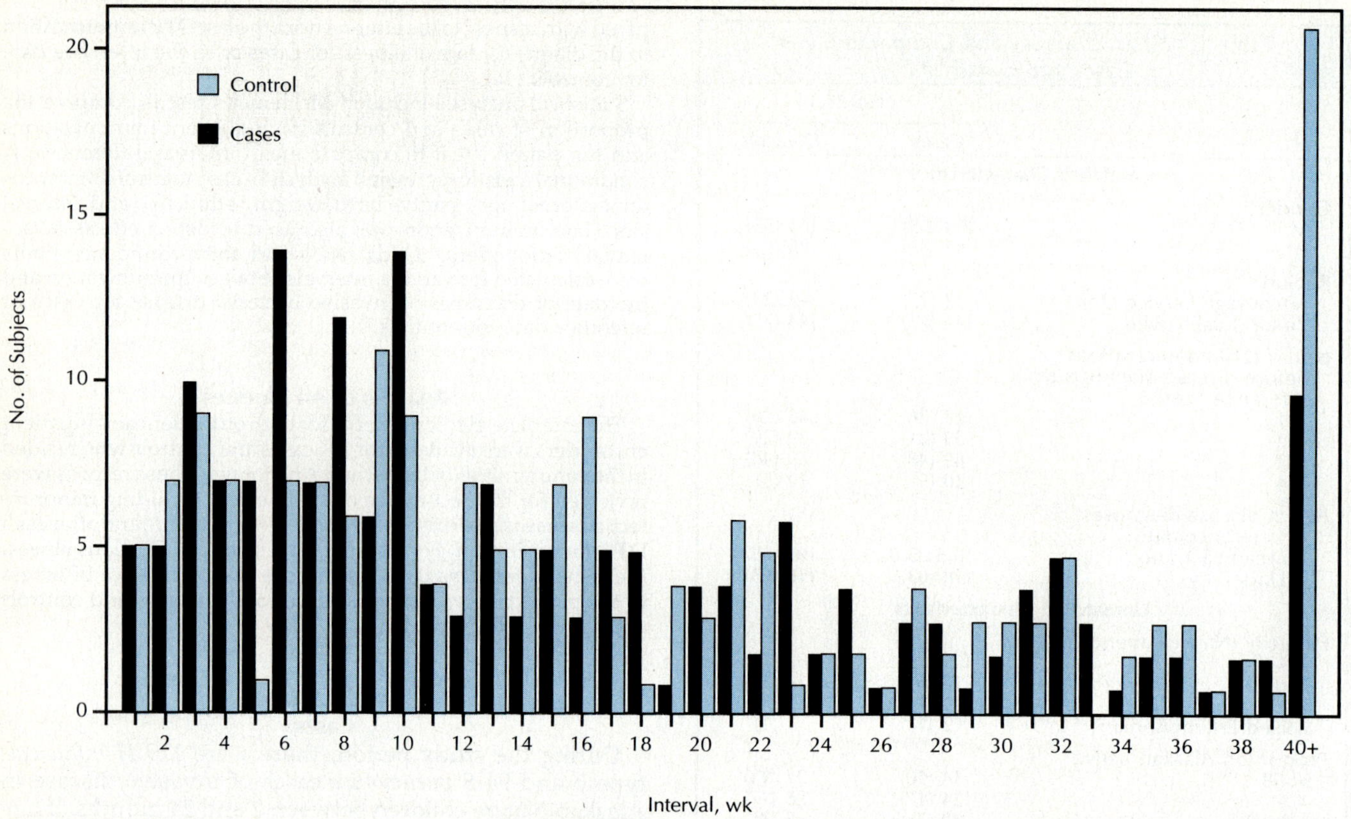

Time from the most recent immunization to the diagnosis of invasive Haemophilus influenzae *type b or* Streptococcus pneumoniae *disease for cases or the matched reference date for healthy controls.*

Analyses stratified for first, second, third, or fourth recommended DTP immunizations at approximately 2, 4, 6, and 18 months of age were also performed, and no associations were found. Therefore, only the combined data are presented.

In the categoric analysis in Table 2, the numbers of cases and controls are presented by specified intervals from the last DTP immunization to the date of disease diagnosis or reference date. The numbers of cases and controls who were immunized within 30 days of disease onset or reference date respectively were identical. Of the seven periods examined, the combined odds ratio was 1 for the first three, slightly greater than 1 for the next two, and below 1 for the final two. The only variation of note was in the 31- to 60-day period for invasive *S pneumoniae* disease. Immunization occurred in 19 cases and only 10 controls ($P = .05$; odds ratio, 3.3, with a confidence interval of 1.1 to 10). A similar trend for *S pneumoniae* disease was noted in the 61- to 90-day period.

The mean interval from the last DTP to diagnosis was 110 days for cases compared with 128 days to the reference date for controls; the corresponding medians were 80 and 101 days, respectively ($P<.05$). A similar analysis was repeated separately for meningitis, and no significant case-control differences were found, nor was there an imbalance in the 31- to 90-day interval. A multivariate logistic regression analysis of the variables shown in Table 1 and the intervals in Table 2 also revealed no additional associations between DTP vaccination and disease.

Analysis of All Illnesses

To evaluate further any possible temporal association between illness and DTP immunization, the occurrence of any illness during the 30-day period before and after DTP administration was compared for the subset of infants for whom all medical records were available (Table 3). For this analysis, there were only minor differences between cases and controls, and therefore the two were combined for the analysis in Table 3. For all categories examined, a higher proportion of the 30-day patient intervals before (rather than after) immunization had any illness. This was also true for all of the infectious disease illnesses. These differences achieved statistical significance only for all illnesses combined (53% vs 43%; $P<.004$) and likely reflects the fact that immunizations are usually withheld from ill children (well-child effect; see the "Comment" section). During the first 18 months of life, total minor infectious illnesses were more common in infants who developed invasive bacterial disease (0.98 episodes per month) than in infants without invasive bacterial disease (0.67 episodes per month).

COMMENT

In animal-model systems, pertussis vaccine and isolated pertussis antigens have been found to have an effect on the susceptibility of the animals to other bacteria and to viruses; in some systems protection is observed, and in others increased susceptibility occurs.[8-17] In most of these systems, the effects are short-lived; the bacterial or viral challenge must occur within a few days of immunization. The most persistent effect was noted in a mouse adenoviral system in which pertussis vaccine rendered the mice resistant to the virus for a period of 5 to 35 days after immunization.[15]

In a traditional case-control study, patients with a particular disease (ie, cases) are compared with randomly selected or matched controls without disease to assess the relative prevalence of some associated risk factor. One

Table 2.—Number of Hib and Sp Cases and Controls With DTP Immunization During Specified Time Intervals Before Onset of Disease in Cases and Reference Date in Controls*

Interval, d	Category	No. Cases	No. Controls	P†	Odds Ratio‡ (95% Confidence Interval)
≤3	Hib	2	2	1.0	1.0 (0.05-20.9)
	Sp	0	0	...	...
	Total	**2**	**2**	1.0	1.0 (0.05-20.9)
4-7	Hib	2	1	.6	2.0 (0.2-22.1)
	Sp	1	2	.6	0.5 (0.0-15.3)
	Total	**3**	**3**	1.0	1.0 (0.2-5.0)
8-30	Hib	19	17	.8	1.2 (0.5-2.8)
	Sp	4	6	.8	0.7 (0.2-2.4)
	Total	**23**	**23**	1.0	1.0 (0.5-2.0)
31-60	Hib	21	21	1.0	1.0 (0.5-2.0)
	Sp	19	10	.5	3.3 (1.1-10.0)
	Total	**40**	**31**	.3	1.4 (0.8-2.5)
61-90	Hib	23	21	.9	1.2 (0.6-2.4)
	Sp	9	3	.08	7.0 (0.9-57.0)
	Total	**32**	**24**	.3	1.6 (0.8-3.1)
91-120	Hib	13	18	.5	0.7 (0.3-1.5)
	Sp	4	8	.3	0.3 (0.07-1.7)
	Total	**17**	**26**	.2	0.6 (0.3-1.2)
>120	Hib	44	44	1.0	1.0 (0.5-2.2)
	Sp	25	33	.06	0.3 (0.08-1.0)
	Total	**69**	**77**	.3	0.7 (0.3-1.3)

*Hib indicates *Haemophilus influenzae* type b; Sp, *Streptococcus pneumoniae*; and DTP, diphtheria and tetanus toxoids and whole-cell pertussis vaccine.
†McNemar's test, using case-control matching.
‡Ratio of the odds of a case being immunized in the specified interval relative to the odds of its controls being immunized in the same interval.

Table 3.—Occurrence of Illnesses in 104 Study Subjects Within a 30-Day Interval Before and After 377 DTP Immunizations*

Illness Category	No. of Subject-Intervals (%) With Illness Before Immunization	No. of Subject-Intervals (%) With Illness After Immunization	P (McNemar's Test)
Any illness	198 (53)	162 (43)	.004
Any infectious disease	163 (43)	141 (37)	.084
Otitis media	78 (21)	70 (19)	.501
Other respiratory infections	77 (20)	65 (17)	.285
Temperature >38°C	50 (13)	46 (12)	.724
Hospitalization	11 (3)	7 (2)	.424

*DTP indicates diphtheria and tetanus toxoids and whole-cell pertussis vaccine.

purpose of matching is to eliminate potential confounding effects. The present study is different from a classic case-control study, because the prevalence of DTP immunization is, by design, equivalent for cases and controls. What we evaluated was the temporal proximity of DTP immunization to the occurrence of invasive bacterial disease, concentrating on the earliest time intervals. Our hypothesis is that a cause-and-effect relationship would lead to shorter intervals for the cases relative to controls.

The possibility of overmatching should be considered as a possible explanation for the lack of differences in this study. By matching too closely, one might select a control group that is too much like the cases for all factors, including timing of DTP immunizations. In our study, considerable effort was made to eliminate confounding effects by carefully defining and restricting both the study cases and controls for potential confounding factors and matching the controls only for potential confounders (factors that might influence the timing of immunization or the risk of bacterial disease). Previous DTP immunization was such a matching/confounding factor. Nearly all Alaskan Natives are immunized, and minor infectious illnesses are more common for *H influenzae* type b and *S pneumoniae* cases than controls during the first 18 months of life, frequently resulting in postponement of immunization. Without matching on the number of immunizations, cases would have received fewer DTP doses, suggesting a protective effect. Also, matching on the number of DTP doses seemed reasonable to reduce potential confounding effects related to overall health status. Importantly, we did not match for village of residence, which would have overmatched the cases and controls. The lack of rigid immunization schedules in this remote population of Alaskan Natives likely provides sufficient variability in the timing of DTP immunization to permit evaluation of time intervals as an outcome measure.

In this investigation, we found no clear temporal relationship between DTP immunization and risk of invasive bacterial infection or the risk of common pediatric illnesses. This was particularly true for the 1-month interval after immunization. The finding that immunization occurred in 19 *S pneumoniae* cases and in only 10 controls during the 31- to 60-day period deserves comment. This may be a chance occurrence, since only one significant result was observed in Table 2. It seems unlikely that a biologic effect resulting from DTP vaccine would be seen only during the 2nd month and not the 1st month. Also, there is no reason for a relationship to occur for *S pneumoniae* but not *H influenzae* type b disease, especially when there were more than twice as many *H influenzae* type b cases to evaluate. Finally, there was no evidence or trend of an increase in common illnesses, particularly infectious disease illnesses, after DTP immunization in either healthy infants or those with invasive bacterial disease.

Our results do not support the concerns raised by the Swedish acellular pertussis study of increased risk of bacterial disease and case fatality.[2] However, our study only looked at disease occurrence and not mortality, as fatal cases of *H influenzae* type b and *S pneumoniae* disease in Alaska are too rare for analysis (3% to 4% case fatality in Alaskan Native infants).[4,5]

In contrast to the findings in a small Israeli study by Jaber and associates,[3] we found no increase in common illnesses, including infectious diseases, in the month after immunization.[5] In fact, we noted more illnesses in the month before vaccination than in the subsequent month. This finding is likely influenced by the fact that immunizations are frequently deferred in children with infectious illnesses until they are well, thereby artificially increasing the rate of illnesses before immunizations are given. This "well-child effect" is the likely explanation for our observations. Recently, Joffe and colleagues[18] reported that children hospitalized with infectious illnesses in the Colorado Kaiser Foundation Health Plan had a rate of immunization in the preceding month that was equivalent to the rate in matched controls.

In conclusion, we found no consistent evidence that DTP immunization has a temporal association with the occurrence of invasive bacterial disease in children, and we found no evidence that the risk is increased for any illnesses, particularly infectious diseases, after immunization.

These studies were funded by an unrestricted grant from Lederle Laboratories, Pearl River, NY, and by contract N01-AI-32512 from the National Institute for Allergy and Infectious Disease, National Institutes of Health, Bethesda, Md.

The authors gratefully acknowledge the comments of Robert Chun, MD, and Robert Wainwright, MD, and the assistance of Alice Christian, RN, Annette Harpster, RN, Patty Schnitzer, RN, MSN, Debbie Parks, Alice Mueller, Joseph Mannion, Denise Tritt, Rose Eward, and Emily Klees.

References

1. Ad Hoc Group for the Study of the Pertussis Vaccines. Placebo-controlled trial of two acellular pertussis vaccines in Sweden: protective efficacy and adverse events. *Lancet.* 1988;1:954-960.

2. Storsaeter J, Olin P, Berit R, et al. Mortality and morbidity from invasive bacterial infections during a clinical trial of acellular pertussis vaccines in Sweden. *Pediatr Infect Dis.* 1988;7:637-645.

3. Jaber L, Shohat M, Mimouni M. Infectious episodes following diphtheria-pertussis-tetanus vaccination: a preliminary observation in infants. *Clin Pediatr.* 1988;27:491-494.

4. Ward J, Lum MK, Hall DB, et al. Invasive *Haemophilus influenzae* type b disease in Alaska: background epidemiology for a vaccine efficacy trial. *J Infect Dis.* 1986;153:17-26.

5. Davidson M, Schraer CD, Parkinson AJ, et al. Invasive pneumococcal disease in an Alaska Native population 1980-1986. *JAMA.* 1989;261:715-718.

6. Breslow NE, Day NE. *Statistical Methods in Cancer Research.* Lyon, France: International Agency for Research on Cancer;1980;1:scientific publication No. 32.1.

7. Rothman KJ. *Modern Epidemiology.* Boston, Mass: Little Brown & Co; 1986.

8. Cherry JD, Brunell PA, Golden GS, et al. Report on the task force on pertussis and pertussis immunization—1988. *Pediatrics.* 1988;81:939-984.

9. Munoz JJ, Bergman RK. *Bordetella pertussis:* immunological and other biological activities. New York, NY: Marcel Decker Inc; 1977;4:115-168. Immunology Series; 4.

10. Arch RN, Parfentjev IA. The effect of *Haemophilus pertussis* sensitization on the increase of susceptibility of mice to infection by a saprophyte. *J Infect Dis.* 1957;101:31-34.

11. Kind LS. Sensitivity of pertussis inoculated mice to endotoxin. *J Immunol.* 1959;82:32-37.

12. Dubos RJ, Schaedler RWJ. Reversible changes in the susceptibility of mice to bacterial infections, I: changes brought about by injection of pertussis vaccine or of bacterial endotoxins. *J Exp Med.* 1956;104:53-65.

13. Landy M. Increase in resistance following administration of bacterial lipopolysaccharides. *N Y Acad Sci.* 1956;66:292-303.

14. Bell JF, Munoz JJ. Enhancement of immune response to rabies virus by *Bordetella pertussis* extract: International Symposium on Rabies. *Symp Series Immunobiol Standard.* 1974;21:199-206.

15. Winters AL, Baggett DW, Benjamin WR, et al. Resistance to adenovirus infection after administration of *Bordetella pertussis* vaccine in mice. *Infect Immun.* 1985;47:487-491.

16. Parfentjev IA. Bacterial allergy increases susceptibility to influenzae virus in mice. *Proc Soc Exp Biol Med.* 1955;90:373-375.

17. Samore MH, Siber GR. Pertussis toxin increases susceptibility of infant rats to *Haemophilus influenzae* type b. Program and abstracts of the 29th Interscience Conference on Antimicrobial Agents and Chemotherapy; September 17-20, 1989. Page 158.

18. Joffe LS, Luckey DW, Glode MP, et al. Does DTP increase the risk of hospitalization with an infectious illness? *Pediatr Res.* 1990;27:174A. Abstract.

In Other AMA Journals

ARCHIVES OF INTERNAL MEDICINE

Protecting Tomorrow's Health Care Professionals Against Hepatitis B Virus Today

Dennis L. Murray, MD; Angella Goetz, RN; Victor L. Yu, MD
(*Arch Intern Med.* 1991;151:1069-1070)

National Cholesterol Education Program: Report of the Expert Panel on Population Strategies for Blood Cholesterol Reduction: Executive Summary

US Department of Health and Human Services, Public Health Service, National Institutes of Health, the National Heart, Lung, and Blood Institute, National Cholesterol Education Program
(*Arch Intern Med.* 1991;151:1071-1084)

Cost-Benefit Issues in the Practice of Internal Medicine

Richard B. Friedman, MD, Jeffery A. Katt, MD
(*Arch Intern Med.* 1991;151:1165-1168)

Objective Structured Clinical Examination in a Pediatric Residency Program

Bahman Joorabchi, MD, MEd

• **This report describes and evaluates a 42-station objective structured clinical examination (OSCE) administered to 29 pediatric residents and six medical students. In half of the stations, residents spent 5 minutes performing a clearly defined clinical task while being rated by an observer. In the other half of the stations, they answered questions based on the data just gathered. There were six interviews with real or simulated patients, four physical examinations, six laboratory tests or procedures, and one chart review. Eight rest stops were provided. The results of the OSCE were compared with those of resident performance ratings and the Pediatric Board's in-training examination. The OSCE scores could clearly separate the students from the residents and each class of residents from all others (construct validity). The in-training examination could not separate first-year postgraduate level and second-year postgraduate level residents. Resident performance ratings could distinguish only first-year postgraduate level from third-year postgraduate level residents. Residents uniformly agreed that the OSCE measured important clinical objectives attesting to its content validity. Reliability for the OSCE was calculated at the 0.8 to 0.83 range. It is concluded that valid and reliable clinical examinations in pediatrics are feasible, practical, and highly desirable.**

(*AJDC.* 1991;145:757-762)

Evaluation of clinical competence is a desired, but elusive, goal in medical education. Valid and reliable examinations are generally difficult, labor intensive, and costly. Furthermore, there is no deep-rooted tradition for clinical examination in this country. Despite pleas for reform,[1,2] the prevalent certifying examinations (from National Boards to specialty boards) and the in-training examinations (ITE) rely on paper and pencil tests that measure only cognitive objectives of generally lower taxonomic levels. This is understandable given the difficulties of conducting any form of evaluation involving patients, simulated or real. Aside from the issue of costs, organization, and manpower, one has to grapple with inadequate samplings, subjective scoring, interrater variability, and low reliabilities.

To overcome some of these problems, Harden and his associates[3] introduced the objective structured clinical examination (OSCE), a multistation format that evaluates clinical skills and attitudes as well as cognitive objectives. In half the stations of this examination, the student carries out a clearly defined task such as a patient interview or physical examination or interpretation of test results, while an observer rates the performance. In the other half of the stations, the student answers open-ended or multiple-choice questions based on the clinical task just completed.

The method has been gaining in popularity and is widely used in Europe and in the Commonwealth countries.[4-6] In the United States, only a few medical schools[7-11] and residency programs[12,13] have used it. Mounting an OSCE in pediatrics is an especially difficult task. Only one small example involving two history stations, three physical examination stations, and seven laboratory stations given to medical students in three British medical schools has been reported.[14-17] To my knowledge to date, there has been no report of an OSCE for pediatric residents.

This report details an experience in the use of OSCE to evaluate clinical competence in 29 pediatric residents and six medical students in a community-based residency

Accepted for publication November 27, 1990.

From the Wayne/Oakland Child and Adolescent Medicine Program, Pontiac (Mich) General Hospital.

Reprint requests to Wayne/Oakland Child and Adolescent Medicine Program, Pontiac General Hospital, Pontiac, MI 48341 (Dr Joorabchi).

Purpose.—*This department is intended to share information concerning educational efforts in the broad field of pediatrics. We welcome studies on the following topics: undergraduate and graduate education in medicine and allied health occupations; continuing education of health professionals; education of patients and families; and health education for the general public, the community, and organizations that contribute to the promotion and improvement of the health of children.*

Editorial Comment.—*We teach, but how do we evaluate? This is one of our system's greatest problems. Joorabchi used a testing scenario, including simulated patients, real patients, and short case situations to assess resident and student learning. The tests were tested. See if this may be a useful approach for your program.*–H.D.A.

Table 1.—Contents of the OSCE*

The following is a list of professional skills, cognitive objectives, and affective objectives measured in each of the stations. The heading for each station includes the numbers and the name of the station, whether it was a laboratory, history, or physical examination station, and whether an observer was present.

Stations 1 and 2, Urinalysis.—Laboratory, no observer
- Interprets a slide of an abnormal urinary sediment and the report of a urine culture
- Recognizes a normal IVP
- Decides on the need for further tests
- Orders appropriate antibiotics

Stations 3 and 4, Bowlegs.—Laboratory, no observer
- Detects the abnormalities in bone roentgenograms of a patient with rickets
- Correctly interprets results of urine and blood tests
- Arrives at a differential diagnosis

Stations 5 and 6, Cesarean Section.—History, observer present
- Obtains an adequate history from the lying-in nurse (per observer checklist) while an emergency cesarean section is in progress
- Arrives at a differential diagnosis on viewing four pictures of the newborn
- Answers questions on characteristics of and differences between tremors, drug withdrawal, and neonatal seizures
- Interprets the nurse's "activity chart" and growth grid recorded on the newborn
- Writes appropriate hospital admission orders for the infant

Stations 7 and 8, Hearing.—Physical examination, observer present
- Performs otoscopy and pneumotoscopy appropriately
- Detects presence or absence of abnormalities of tympanic membrane appearance and motion
- Detects conduction hearing loss in one ear grossly and by using a tuning fork
- Lists at least six risk factors predisposing to hearing loss in a child

Stations 9 and 10, Rest Stations

Stations 11 and 12, Cholesterol.—History, observer present
- Takes an appropriate history from a mother with a xanthoma diagnosed as hypercholesterolemia
- Given the results of the lipid screening tests on the children arrives at the diagnosis of familial hypercholesterolemia
- Uses appropriate interviewing skills (per observer checklist)
- Discusses prognosis and gives nutritional advice to the family
- Answers questions on the mode of inheritance (based on the family history) and on the mechanism of hypercholesterolemia

Stations 13 and 14, Swollen Ankles.—History, observer present
- Takes an appropriate history (per observer checklist) from an adolescent with swollen ankles
- Demonstrates appropriate interviewing skills (per observer checklist)
- Arrives at acute glomerulonephritis as the most likely diagnosis
- Recommends appropriate investigation
- Lists at least three possible complications

Stations 15 and 16, Wheezer.—History, observer present
- Takes an appropriate history (per observer checklist) from the mother of a child with "frequent" infections
- Uses appropriate interviewing skills (per observer checklist)
- Arrives at the most likely diagnosis and gives a differential
- Offers reassuring explanations

Stations 17 and 18, Rest Stations

Stations 19 and 20, Facies.—Physical examination, no observer
- Detects and describes at least nine of the 15 distinct abnormalities in general physical examination in this child with fetal alcohol syndrome
- Arrives at a differential diagnosis

Table 1.—Contents of the OSCE* (cont)

Stations 21 and 22, Smear.—Laboratory, no observer
- Uses a microscope appropriately
- Detects four of the six abnormalities in the morphologic features of the blood smear
- Proposes four of the six possible differential diagnoses
- Orders at least three other necessary hematologic tests and avoids invasive ones (eg, bone marrow)

Stations 23 and 24, Tachycardia.—Laboratory, no observer
- Given before-and-after ECGs, makes a diagnosis of supraventricular tachycardia in a newborn
- Points out at least four ECG characteristics that differentiate this from a ventricular tachycardia
- Proposes at least three means of emergency treatment (avoids use of verapamil)

Stations 25 and 26, Heart Murmur.—Physical examination, observer present
- Performs an appropriate cardiovascular examination (per observer checklist)
- Detects and records at least five normal or abnormal pertinent physical signs in this patient with a VSD
- Makes a correct diagnosis of VSD, including assessment of the size of shunt
- Answers questions on hemodynamics and prognosis for this child

Stations 27 and 28, Rest Stations

Stations 29 and 30, Anemia.—Physical examination, observer present
- Performs an appropriate general physical examination on a child with anemia and hepatosplenomegaly (per observer checklist)
- Detects and records at least five of the eight major abnormalities on physical examination
- Arrives at a differential diagnosis
- Answers questions on possible complications and on recommended treatment for this patient

Stations 31 and 32, Alte.—History, observer present
- Takes an appropriate history (per observer checklists, process and content) from the mother of an infant who "stopped breathing"
- Lists at least two items from the history that suggest a significant occurrence
- Answers questions on epidemiology, pathogenesis, management, and follow-up of this infant

Stations 33 and 34: FTT.—History, observer present
- Given a 9-month-old infant with FTT, takes a focused history from the mother (per observer checklists for process and content)
- Makes a differential diagnosis
- Writes hospital admission orders

Stations 35 and 36, Rest Stations

Stations 37 and 38, Chart Review.—No observer; given a copy of the history and physical examination on a 12-year-old boy with abdominal pain
- Lists information missing in the history
- Lists information missing in the physical examination
- Assesses the overall quality of the document

Stations 39 and 40, Stridor.—Laboratory station, no observer; given roentgenograms of the upper airway in a child with stridor
- Describes the radiologic findings
- Offers the most likely diagnosis
- Outlines a plan of management

Stations 41 and 42, Cough.—Laboratory station, no observer; given chest roentgenograms of a 2-year-old child with lobar consolidation and atelectasis of the left lung
- Describes the radiologic findings
- Gives the reason(s) for mediastinal shift
- Predicts the physical findings in the chest

*OSCE indicates Objective Structured Clinical Examination; IVP, intravenous pyelogram; ECG, electrocardiogram; VSD, ventricular septal defect; and FTT, failure to thrive.

program. The following hypotheses were formulated: (1) residents at an advanced level of training would score higher than the more junior residents and students (*construct validity*); (2) there would be a low but acceptable correlation between the OSCE scores and the results of the monthly resident evaluation (*concurrent validity*); and (3) residents would agree that the OSCE is a better measure of clinical competence than the other methods used (*content validity*).

METHODS

The Planning Process

A task force composed of five full-time faculty and the two chief residents created a blueprint for the examination. Selection of problems was guided by the written program objectives and according to such considerations as prevalence, priority, availability, practicality, and adequate sampling.

The Stations

Forty-two stations were created as follows: there were 17 stations for performance of a variety of well-defined clinical tasks, 17 were for answering questions, and eight were rest stops. The clinical tasks were six interviews, four physical examinations, one chart review, and six laboratory tests. In the interview sections, there were two real patients with their mothers (recurrent respiratory infections and familial hypercholesterolemia, respectively) and four simulated ones (the "mother" of an infant with failure to thrive and another of an infant with apnea, a teenager with a history of swollen ankles, and a lying-in nurse attending a mother in the process of having a cesarean section). For physical examination there were real patients with hearing loss in one ear, fetal alcohol syndrome, ventricular septal defect, and hepatosplenomegaly with anemia. In three of the laboratory stations, there were roentgenograms of patients with pneumonia, upper airway obstruction, and rickets. In one, there were before and after conversion electrocardiograms of supraventricular tachycardia and in another, there was a microscopic slide of a blood smear of a patient with hypochromic microcytic anemia. In the sixth and last laboratory station, there were results of a urinalysis, slides of urinary sediment, and roentgenograms of an intravenous pyelogram in a patient with pyelonephritis. In the chart review station, an actual history and physical examination on a patient with abdominal pain was reproduced and the resident was directed to point out its deficiencies. Table 1 shows more details on the contents of the evaluation.

Patient Selection and Preparation

Pediatric clinic patients with stable physical findings and cooperative dispositions were invited to participate. An attempt was made to find duplicate patients to provide relief. For two of the four physical examinations, duplicate patients with identical findings were found. For the third, a sister of the patient with hearing loss was taught to simulate a conduction hearing loss in one ear. She was coached and tested repeatedly and learned to be consistent in her responses. The examination of the patient with fetal alcohol syndrome required mainly inspection only and an alternative was not thought necessary. For this initial trial, there were no plans to formally assess the reliability of patients or interviewees, but every attempt was made to ensure a level of consistency. Of the total of 13 individuals used (four as duplicates), five had stable physical findings and two were mothers of patients with chronic disorders (hypercholesterolemia, frequent infections). Only six had to learn a scenario. Three of these were trained nurses simulating a lying-in nurse, the mother of a child with failure to thrive, and the mother of an infant with "apnea." The fourth was the sister of a girl with conduction hearing loss who simulated the condition and the last two were sisters simulating a history of swollen ankles and dark urine. All the patients, real or simulated, were given salient features of their case histories in writing and were asked to memorize them. They were instructed not to volunteer the information unless specifically asked. For unanticipated questions, they were to supply their own real-life experiences. Designers of each of the stations held frequent practice sessions in person or by phone until they were assured of a reasonable degree of consistency. Thus, given the stability, experience, and the background of the patients, it was believed that the interresident variability of the encounters would be minimized. Each patient or family was paid $50 as an honorarium.

Checklists and Rating Scales

For each of the history-taking and three of the examination stations, an observer checklist was developed that listed all the expected questions to be asked and maneuvers to be performed. The planning group agreed on a score for each item. An observer rating scale was similarly constructed to evaluate the process of the encounter. Finally, a rating scale was produced for the patient to assess the resident interaction and general approach.

Test Questions

For each of the 17 halfway stations, a set of written questions was prepared. These were composed of open-ended, short-answer, and multiple-choice questions. The latter had one or more correct answers with negative marks for incorrect ones. A serious attempt was made to avoid trivial questions and to concentrate on meaningful outcomes related to the case at hand. For each question, all expected answers were written out and a score was assigned for each. Finally, a minimum pass level was derived for each station. All of this work was done by committee consensus.

Resident and Observer Orientation

Two weeks before and again on the morning of the examination, a three-page orientation handout was discussed with the residents and their questions were answered. In addition to an explanation of the test procedures, they were cautioned to do exactly what was asked of them and no more. They were told to describe to the observer what they were doing and what they were finding in the physical examination stations. Otherwise they were to have no interaction with the observers. Each resident was given a sufficient number of name tags to affix to all the various rating scales and answer sheets. Another orientation handout was produced and mailed to the observers and was discussed as a group on the morning of the test. Each observer was expected to learn two stations.

The Test Administration

The examination, given over a 4½-hour period, took place in a single large hall on Saturday morning, April 7, 1990. There were enough examining rooms for each patient encounter and laboratory station. Desks and chairs were set up outside each room for answer stations. Five minutes were allowed for each station and 1 minute was allowed for changeovers. The timekeeper announced each round by a shrill whistle. At the start, one half of the residents entered the odd-numbered stations, including rest stops, while the other half waited their turn. As the first group emerged to answer their questions, the second group took their places. Runners continually collected answer sheets, rating scales, and checklists as soon as they were completed. These were then checked against a master list and filed. To avoid fatigue, three observers worked on two stations. Each rotated after four rounds in one station and took a four-round rest after eight rounds of work. Similarly, physical examination patients rotated every four rounds. Schedules were made for each patient and observer to indicate where he or she was expected to be at each round. A running count of the rounds was kept on a flip chart.

Resident Feedback

At the end of the session, each resident anonymously filled out a form evaluating the process and content of the examination. There were seven Likert-type questions with five scales ranging from "strongly agree" (5) to "strongly disagree" (1). In addition, there were three open-ended questions asking about problems

Table 2.—Analysis of Variance of the Scores Grouped According to the Level of Training*

	Students	PL-1	PL-2	PL-3	F	P
OSCE†	102	136	151	166	13.5	.000
ITE‡	...	50	57	68	11.06	.000
RPR§	...	3.71	3.79	4.29	3.85	.035

*PL-1 indicates first-year postgraduate level; PL-2, second-year postgraduate level; and PL-3, third-year postgraduate level.

†Group means of the sum of all station scores; OSCE indicates objective structured clinical examination.

‡Group means of percent correct; ITE indicates in-training examination.

§Group means of 1 year of ratings, scales 1 to 5; RPR indicates resident performance rating.

during the test, organization of the test as a whole, and overall impression.

Other Test Scores Used for Comparison

There were two other scores for comparison: resident performance ratings (RPRs) are five-point Likert-type rating scales that are completed monthly by attending physicians and by chief residents. They consist of sections assessing attitude, interpersonal relationship, clinical judgment, knowledge base, and technical skills. During the last year, each of the three hospitals' Evaluation Subcommittees met at the end of each month's rotation and compiled an overall rating that was then forwarded to the program Evaluation Committee. Participation of nursing staff was considered a significant improvement in the process. For the purpose of this study, the overall scores for the ratings of the previous year were averaged and used in the comparisons. The other test scores were those of the American Academy of Pediatrics ITE which all but three of the residents had taken the previous July.

Data Management

All answer sheets, rating scales, and checklists, including resident evaluation of the examination, were corrected by hand. All scores for each station were converted to a proportion of the maximum score that ranged from 8 to 12 based on a differential weighting system. The data were tabulated and summed in various ways using a spread sheet program. A statistical program was used to calculate one-way analysis of variance, Pearson Product-Moment and Spearman Rank-Order correlations, and α-reliability coefficient. The OSCE scores of various groups of examinees were compared with each other and with their scores in the other tests available. The level of statistical significance was taken to be P less than .05.

RESULTS

Table 2 shows the results of one-way analysis of variance of the total OSCE scores of the four groups of trainees. The residents' scores in their ITE and results of their monthly RPR are also shown. The Student-Newman-Keul method for comparison testing showed significant ($P<.05$) differences among all four groups in the OSCE scores, with scores being higher in groups with greater clinical experience. This attests to the construct validity of the OSCE. The ITE scores differed significantly between first-year postgraduate level (PGY-1) and third-year postgraduate level (PGY-3) residents, and between second-year postgraduate level (PGY-2) and PGY-3 residents, but not between PGY-1 and PGY-2 residents. The RPRs could distinguish only PGY-1 and PGY-3 residents.

Table 3 shows the results of Pearson Product-Moment correlations among OSCE scores, ITE scores, and RPRs of all the residents taken together. The correlation is strong between OSCE and ITE and between ITE and RPR, but is weaker between OSCE and RPR. This indicates that OSCE measures some of the same objectives measured by ITE and RPR. These tests were not given simultaneously but were close enough in time to still be considered a measure of concurrent validity of the OSCE.

Table 3.—Correlations Between OSCE, ITE, and RPR*

	OSCE	ITE	RPR
OSCE	1	...	...
ITE	0.71 ($P<.001$)	1	...
RPR	0.41 ($P<.05$)	0.61 ($P<.001$)	1

*OSCE indicates objective structured clinical examination; ITE, in-training examination; and RPR, resident performance rating.

Table 4.—Results of Resident Evaluation of the Examination*

Questions	Mean Score
1. The OSCE measured important outcomes not measured by other tests	4.1
2. It should be a regular part of resident evaluation	3.8
3. The distractions prevented achievement of OSCEs goals	3.2
4. I felt intensely involved in most of the stations	4.0
5. The patients and the historians were realistic	4.2
6. The laboratory stations were useful and should be continued	3.8
7. It was an enjoyable experience	4.1

*The scales are from 1 (strongly disagree) to 5 (strongly agree). OSCE indicates objective structured clinical examination.

Table 5.—Correlations Between Subsections of OSCE*

	Total Score	History	Physical	Laboratory
Total score	1	...	...	...
History stations	.88	1	...	...
Physical examination stations	.85	.81	1	...
Laboratory stations	.85	.81	.76	1

*Pearson product-moment correlations, $P<.0001$ in all instances; OSCE indicates objective structured clinical examination.

Thirty-two (94%) of 34 participants completed the anonymous resident evaluation forms. Results are shown in Table 4. As can be seen, the reactions were strongly positive. In retrospect, more than one item should have been negatively worded (item 3), but the distractions of this complex examination were of special concern to the planners who wished to highlight it. In any event, the open-ended questions invited negative comments by asking for problems with any of the stations. In the section asking for "overall comments," eight residents volunteered statements about the relevance of the examination to clinical evaluation. When asked about the organization of the event, 23 (92%) of the 25 who answered the question had laudatory comments about the smooth running of the examination despite this being a first-time experience for all. There were remarkably few complaints about the individual stations. Three residents needed more time in stations requiring psychosocial histories, while one resident felt 5 minutes was too long for each station. Two residents felt time pressures in answering questions and one would have preferred videotapes to slides of the newborn. On the whole, the resident's reaction can be taken as evidence for content validity of the OSCE.

Reliability of the examination was tested in different ways. Using each station as a test item, coefficient α was calculated to be .80. Using this figure, SE of measurement for the total OSCE score was calculated as ±12.2 points (mean [±SD] for the total group, 139.3±27.2; range, 88 to 191). Next, dividing the stations into two equivalent halves based on what was being measured, a split half reliability index of 0.83 was obtained. Finally, Table 5 shows correlations between scores derived for subsections of the OSCE (history, physical, and laboratory stations). All of this can be taken to indicate good reliability for the test as a whole.

COMMENT

Evaluation is a powerful determinant of student learning. Alterations in examination methods have been shown to change both learning and teaching behaviors.[18,19] Unfortunately, as most often practiced, examinations are also the weakest link in the educational process. In the United States, most formal examinations in medicine mainly test cognitive objectives of lower taxonomic orders. Yet Altmaier et al,[20,21] in studies involving pediatric and obstetric residents, found that only 20% to 30% of critical incidents selected as defining successful performance among residents were cognitive in nature; the remainder dealt with attitudes, communication skills, and interpersonal relations. These latter attributes are presumably measured by performance ratings, the most prevalent mode of evaluation in postgraduate training.[22] Yet these ratings generally have low reliability (subjective assessment, poor interrater relationships, central tendency) and poor validity (the halo effect, influence of irrelevant attributes, and rating of skills never directly observed).[23] Studies correlating these subjective ratings with measures of clinical competence have yielded poor results.[13,24-26]

Thus, the emerging trend toward measuring more meaningful educational objectives is a welcome development. The task is difficult but the rewards are plentiful once the inertia is overcome. This initial attempt at clinical evaluation in our program was the high point of the academic year. The willingness of the parents and the older children to get involved (there were more volunteers than needed and no cancellations) was gratifying. The smooth running of the test was remarkable and the few glitches were taken in stride and in good humor. The much-feared problems of using children in an OSCE did not materialize. The total out-of-pocket cost was less than $2000 ($57 per examinee), not counting faculty and staff time. This compares with $140 per student in a performance-based assessment of clinical skills in 72 senior students[8] and with an estimated $200 per medical resident in a full-day OSCE that used standardized patients.[12] The latter figure included administrative, developmental, and other costs. No cost figures are available for our RPR. The standard charge for the pediatric ITE has been $30 per resident.

The main purpose of this study was to check validity and reliability of the test. The rise in OSCE scores with increasing levels of training supports construct validity for the examination. The fact that the ITE did almost as well in separating the years of training (could not distinguish between PGY-1s and PGY-2s) and showed good overall correlation with the OSCE scores indicates that these two tests measured some of the same objectives. The RPR did less well: it could only distinguish PGY-1s from PGY-3s. This is understandable. Aside from the inherent weaknesses of the rating process alluded to above,[22] residents tend to be compared with those in the same year of training rather than with those above or below. In any case, the good overall correlations among OSCE, ITE, and RPR (Table 3) can be taken as evidence for concurrent validity of the OSCE. The reactions of the residents and students were encouraging and supported the content validity of the examination.

Tests measuring clinical competence suffer from low reliability. The more objective nature of the OSCE and a wider content sampling are expected to improve reliability. The reliabilities obtained on this examination were quite respectable and on a par with multiple-choice questions in other "objective" examinations. The relatively good correlations found in the present study between OSCE and the other more established examination methods (ITE and RPR) should not lead to the conclusion that these tests are equivalent and the introduction of infinitely more complex and difficult OSCE is not necessary for resident evaluation. The great advantage of OSCE and other tests directly measuring clinical competence is in the strong message conveyed to the learners of what the program values as important and desirable outcome of their education. It is not the ability to memorize details that is valued but the ability to gather data, analyze it, and make justifiable conclusions, all attributes of the skillful physician.

I gratefully acknowledge the immense amount of time, energy, and talent that were unstintingly given by the members of the OSCE Task Force (Ratnakar Kini, MD, Gregory Preston, MD, James Noble, MD, Homer Ryan, MD, Mirta Soler, MD, and Ramesh Sachdeva, MD) to the preparation and administration of this examination. Special thanks go to Michael Campbell for assistance in data processing and to Toni Kincannon for preparation of the manuscript.

References

1. Eichna LW. Medical school education 1975-1979: a student's perspective. *N Engl J Med.* 1980;303:707-734.

2. Muller S. Physicians for 21st century: report of the panel on the general professional education of physicians and college preparation for medicine. *J Med Educ.* 1984;59(pt 2):11-13.

3. Harden RM, Stevenson M, Downie WW, Wilson GM. Assessment of clinical competence using objective structured examination. *BMJ.* 1975;1:447-451.

4. Bouhuijs P, VanderVleuten C, VanLuyk S. The OSCE as part of a systematic skills training approach. *Med Teach.* 1987;9:183-191.

5. Robb K, Rothman A. The assessment of clinical skills in general internal medicine residents: comparison of objective structured clinical examination to a conventional oral examination. *Ann R Coll Phys Surg.* 1985;18:235-238.

6. Newble D. Eight years' experience with a structured clinical examination. *Med Educ.* 1988;22:200-204.

7. Stillman P, Swanson D. Ensuring the clinical competence of medical school graduates through standardized patients. *Arch Intern Med.* 1987;147:1049-1052.

8. Barrows HS, Williams RG, Moy RH. A comprehensive performance-based assessment of fourth year students' clinical

skills. *J Med Educ.* 1987;62:805-809.
9. Hoole AJ, Kowlowitz V, McGaghie WC, Sloane PD, Colindres RE. Using the objective structured clinical examination at the University of North Carolina Medical School. *N C Med J.* 1987;48:463-467.
10. Petrusa ER, Blackwell TA, Rogers LP, Saydjari C, Parcel S, Guckian JC. An objective measure of clinical performance. *Am J Med.* 1987;83:34-42.
11. Harris IB, Miller WJ. Feedback in an objective structured clinical examination by students serving as patients, teachers and examiners. *Acad Med.* 1990;65:433-434.
12. Stillman PL, Swanson BB, Smee S, et al. Assessing clinical skills of residents with standardized patients. *Ann Intern Med.* 1986;105:762-771.
13. Petrusa ER, Blackwell TA, Ainsworth MA. Reliability and validity of an objective structured clinical examination for assessing the clinical performance of residents. *Arch Intern Med.* 1990;150:573-577.
14. Waterston T, Cater JI, Mitchell RG. An objective undergraduate clinical examination in child health. *Arch Dis Child.* 1980;55:917-922.
15. Watson AR, Houston IV, Close GC. Evaluation of an objective structured clinical examination. *Arch Dis Child.* 1982;57:390-398.
16. Smith LJ, Price DA, Houston IV. Objective structured clinical examination compared with other forms of student assessment. *Arch Dis Child.* 1984;59:1173-1176.
17. Frost GJ, Cater JI, Forsyth JS. The use of objective structured clinical examination (OSCE) in paediatrics. *Med Teach.* 1986;8:261-269.
18. Frederiksen N. The real test bias: influences of testing on teaching and learning. *Am Psychol.* 1984;39:193-202.
19. Newble DI, Jaeger K. The effect of assessments and examinations on the learning of medical students. *Med Educ.* 1983;17:165-171.
20. Altmaier EM, McGuinness G, Wood P, Ross RR, Bartley J, Smith W. Defining successful performance among pediatric residents. *Pediatrics.* 1990;85:139-143.
21. Altmaier EM, Johnson SR, Tarico P, Laube D. An empirical specification of residency performance dimensions. *Obstet Gynecol.* 1988;72:126-130.
22. Heins N, Ruggill J, Baker H. Education of residents: results of a survey of pediatric training programs. *AJDC.* 1983;137:691-695.
23. Levine HG, McGuire CH. Rating habitual performance in graduate medical education. *J Med Educ.* 1971;46:306-311.
24. Kroboth FJ, Kapoor W, Brown FH, Karpf M, Levey GS. A comparative trial of the clinical evaluation exercise. *Arch Intern Med.* 1985;145:1121-1123.
25. Ginsburg AD. Comparison of intraining evaluation with tests of clinical ability in medical students. *J Med Educ.* 1985;60:29-36.
26. Lazer HL, DeLand EC, Tompkins RK. Clinical performance vs in-training examinations as measure of surgical competence. *Surgery.* 1980;87:357-362.

Effects of Obesity on Aerobic Fitness in Adolescent Females

Thomas W. Rowland, MD

• Obesity impairs performance in most athletic events, but the influence of increased body fat on cardiopulmonary function has not been clearly delineated. An understanding of the fatness-fitness relationship is important in the optimal design of exercise programs for obese subjects. In this study, 27 adolescent females with body fat levels ranging from normal to gross obesity were evaluated to determine the impact of adiposity on physiologic factors during maximal and submaximal treadmill walking. Increased skinfold measures correlated significantly with absolute maximal oxygen uptake throughout the range of body fat levels ($r=.72$), and oxygen consumption per kilogram of body weight and treadmill endurance time both declined as fatness increased ($r=-.49$ and $-.42$, respectively). Obesity did not affect submaximal walking economy. These findings indicate that increased fat levels are associated with increased cardiopulmonary exercise capacity, but that functional fitness declines because of the inert load created by excess body fat. Therefore, therapeutic exercise programs for obese adolescents are best designed to increase caloric expenditure and decrease body fat rather than to improve aerobic fitness.
(*AJDC.* 1991;145:764-768)

Excess body fat may be significantly detrimental to exercise performance, particularly in activities requiring propulsion or lifting of body weight.[1-5] Increased body fat content has been consistently reported to relate inversely to performance in events such as distance runs, sprints, pull-ups, and broad jumping regardless of age, sex, or athleticism. Watson's study of adolescent boys[2] indicated that a 46-yard decrement in distance covered in a 12-minute walk-run might be expected for each 1% increase in body fat. Boileau and Lohman[3] showed that if age, height, and weight of children were statistically constant, a decline from the 10th to 35th percentile in mile-run performance occurred when the percentage of body fat increased from 15% to 30%.

Several explanations have been offered for this negative relationship between fitness and fatness: (1) Body fat may be simply an inert load during weight-bearing activities.[6,7] According to this concept, cardiopulmonary responses to exercise are normal in obese individuals, and exercise performance is compromised by the extra "baggage" that needs to be transported. (2) Excessive body fat may interfere with normal cardiac and pulmonary function and limit maximal aerobic responses to high-exercise loads.[8,9] If so, physical capabilities in obese subjects are reduced at least partially by direct reduction of cardiopulmonary reserves during exercise. (3) Ventilatory function may be compromised by excessive body fat and thereby limit aerobic capacity. Obesity has been reported to diminish pulmonary compliance, decrease the efficiency of the ventilatory muscles, and decrease lung vital capacity.[10,11] (4) Cardiovascular fitness may be depressed by the sedentary life-style adopted by the obese individual.[12] Reduced exercise capability in this case is secondary to a decline in maximal aerobic power no different than that of any individual not engaging in normal amounts of physical activity.

An understanding of alterations in cardiopulmonary responses to exercise in obese subjects bears practical importance. If adiposity causes depression of cardiovascular fitness, measured as the maximal oxygen uptake ($\dot{V}O_2max$) therapeutic exercise programs for obese individuals should be designed to conform to guidelines of frequency,

Accepted for publication January 28, 1991.
From the Department of Pediatrics, Baystate Medical Center, Springfield, Mass.
Reprint requests to the Department of Pediatrics, Baystate Medical Center, 756 Chestnut St, Springfield, MA 01199 (Dr Rowland).

Department Editors.—*William B. Strong, MD, Augusta, Ga; Carl L. Stanitski, MD, Pittsburgh, Pa; Ronald E. Smith, PhD, Seattle, Wash; Jack H. Wilmore, PhD, Austin, Tex*
Purpose.—*This section provides current information related to the medical needs of young athletes, as pertinent to counseling young athletes and their parents regarding sports participation and practices contributing to the health maintenance of the athlete, as well as current concepts in the prevention, diagnosis, and treatment of sports-related illnesses and injuries.*
Editorial Comment.—*The National Health Promotion and Disease Prevention Objectives that have been enunciated in the 1991 edition of* Healthy People 2000 *include physical activity and fitness as well as nutrition. One of the major goals of these two objectives, especially among the young, is to reduce the prevalence of obesity. Both physical activity and nutrition interventions are necessary. This article documents the importance of physical activity as the major source for caloric expenditures and weight reduction.*
—W.B.S.

Anthropometric and Physiologic Comparisons of Obese and Nonobese Subjects*		
	Obese Subjects (n=14)	Nonobese Subjects (n=13)
Age, y	16.2±1.8	16.4±1.0
Weight, kg	76.5±16.6	51.8±6.8†
Height, cm	159±6	157±5
Skinfold sum, mm	63.9±14.9	29.7±6.0†
Submaximal exercise‡		
$\dot{V}O_2$		
L/min	1.98±0.35	1.40±0.17†
mL/kg per minute	26.1±1.8	27.0±1.3
$\dot{V}E$		
L/min	63.5±14.2	46.1±6.5†
mL/kg per minute	0.84±0.11	0.89±0.08
HR, beats/min	182±14	178±14
Oxygen pulse, $\dot{V}O_2$/HR x10[3]	10.8±1.7	7.9±1.2†
Breathing rate, breaths/min	46±9	41±8
Breathing rate: tidal volume	33.3±9.3	38.0±14.8
$\dot{V}E/\dot{V}O_2$	32.09±4.02	32.98±3.39
Maximal exercise‡		
Endurance, min	8.1±2.4	10.9†±3.6†
$\dot{V}O_2$	2.16±0.36	
L/min	2.16±0.36	1.71±0.30†
mL/kg per minute	29.2±3.8	33.1±4.7†
RER	1.05±0.05	1.02±0.05†
$\dot{V}E$		
L/min	77.4±13.6	64.8±15.0†
mL/kg per minute	1.03±0.19	1.25±0.25†
HR, beats/min	190±11	197±11
Oxygen pulse, $\dot{V}O_2$/HR x10[3]	11.3±1.8	8.7±1.5†
Breathing rate, breaths/min	52±8	51±9
Breathing rate: tidal volume	33.1±13.0	38.3±16.9
$\dot{V}E/\dot{V}O_2$	36.17±4.53	37.84±5.65
Ventilatory threshold		
mL/kg per minute	18.6±2.0	20.8±2.1†
% of $\dot{V}O_2$max	63.6±6.1	66.4±7.0

*Subjects were considered obese if the sums of their tricep and scapular skinfold measurements were above the 90th percentile. Values are means±SDs. $\dot{V}O_2$ indicates oxygen consumption per unit of time; $\dot{V}E$, expired volume per unit of time; HR, heart rate; RER, respiratory exchange ratio; and $\dot{V}O_2$max, maximum oxygen consumption.

†$P<.05$ for obese vs nonobese subjects.

‡Submaximal exercise was performed on a treadmill with an 8% grade at 5.2 km/h. Maximal exercise was performed at the same rate with 2% increases in grade every 3 minutes until exhaustion.

duration, and intensity necessary to improve aerobic fitness.[13] If a decrease in cardiopulmonary function is not characteristic of obesity, exercise programs may be of lower intensity sufficient to increase caloric output. The distinction is important, because limiting exercise intensity in managing obese patients is considered a valuable means of improving subject compliance.[14]

This study investigates the effects of obesity on cardiopulmonary function during exercise in a group of low-fit adolescent females. Specifically, information was sought concerning the relationship of adiposity and markers of maximal aerobic function, submaximal indicators of aerobic fitness (heart rate, walking economy, and anaerobic threshold), and patterns of ventilation, particularly as they relate to breathing efficiency. These factors were examined in subjects representing a continuum of body fat levels from normal to grossly obese to determine if the degree of fatness affects the qualitative features of the cardiopulmonary response to exercise.

SUBJECTS AND METHODS

Twenty-seven female high school students were recruited for treadmill testing from a physical education class designed for individuals with self-perceived low levels of physical fitness. The mean age of the subjects was 16.5 years (SD, 1.0 year; range, 15.3 to 18.8 years). None suffered chronic disease or were acutely ill at testing. All denied smoking cigarettes, and there was no history of use of medications that would affect exercise performance. Fourteen of the students were included in a previous report[15] describing the effects of walking training on aerobic fitness.

Informed consent was obtained from the parents of all subjects. This study was reviewed and approved by the research review committees of the Baystate Medical Center, Springfield, Mass.

Measures of cardiopulmonary fitness were recorded during a maximal treadmill walking test. Height and weight were determined before testing, followed by calculation of body mass index (BMI, weight divided by square of height). The BMI correlates well with other indexes of obesity; a value of 24 is believed to be the upper limit of "desirable" body fat, and a BMI of 29 indicates approximately 20% overweight.[16] Triceps and subscapular skinfolds were measured using a skinfold caliper (Holtain, Crosswell, England) that provides a constant pressure of 10 g/mm^2. Three values were obtained from the right side of the body using standard techniques.[17] The mean values were summed to create a skinfold score. This score has been shown to correlate with body density (and, thus, with body fat content) in obese and nonobese adolescents, with correlation coefficients of .77 to .95.[18,19]

Progressive, continuous treadmill walking was performed to exhaustion in an air-conditioned laboratory (20°C to 22°C). The subjects were acclimated to the treadmill with a 2-minute warm-up walk at 4.8 km/h with no grade. The initial treadmill slope was 6%, which was increased 2% every 3 minutes. A speed of 5.25 km/h was maintained, and subjects exercised until voluntary exhaustion. Grasping of handrails was not permitted except transiently during gradient changes. At peak effort, all subjects demonstrated hyperpnea, facial flushing, sweating, and unsteady gait as well as either respiratory exchange ratio of more than .98 or heart rate exceeding 190 beats per minute.

Heart rates were determined electrocardiographically during the final 30 seconds of each stage and at maximal exercise. Gas exchange values were measured using standard open-circuit techniques using a computerized metabolic cart (Q-Plex Cardio-Pulmonary Exercise System; Quinton Instrument Co, Seattle Wash). Subjects breathed through a 94-mL dead-space Rudolph valve, and minute ventilation was determined using a pneumotachometer in the expiratory line. Expired gas samples from a mixing chamber were analyzed for oxygen and carbon dioxide concentration using zirconia oxide and infrared analyzers, respectively. Data were averaged every 15 seconds, and used to calculate oxygen uptake, carbon dioxide output, expired ventilation ($\dot{V}E$), ventilatory equivalent for oxygen ($\dot{V}E/\dot{V}O_2$), respiratory rate, tidal volume, and respiratory exchange ratio. The system was calibrated before each session with standard gases of known oxygen and carbon dioxide concentrations.

Maximal values of gas exchange parameters were defined as the mean of the two highest recordings during the final minute of exercise. Submaximal values were defined as the mean during the final minute of the second stage (5.2 km/h and 8% grade).

Confusion exists concerning the proper expression of physical

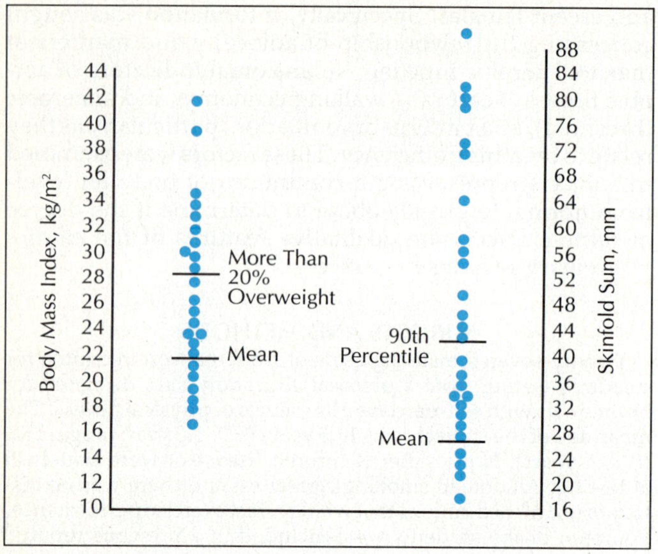

Fig 1.—*Body mass index and skinfold scores (triceps and scapular sum) of the 27 subjects.*

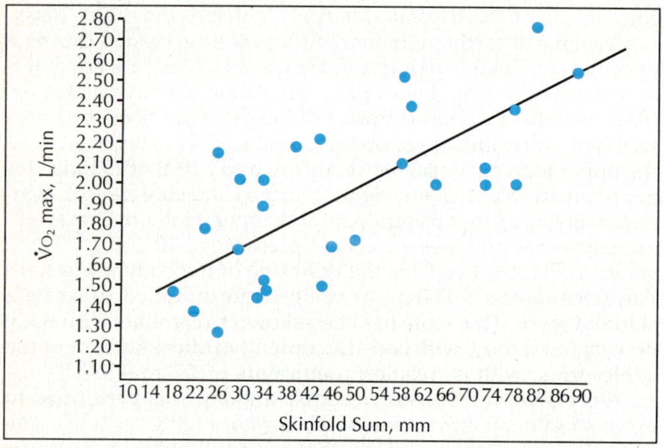

Fig 2.—*Relationship of body fat, as indicated by sum of triceps and scapular skinfold thickness, and absolute maximal oxygen uptake* ($r = .72$, $P < .01$, *and* $y = 1.33 + .014x$).

fitness of obese subjects, and definition of terms is important. In this study, absolute aerobic fitness denotes physiologic characteristics independent of body weight or composition and is indicated by measurement of oxygen uptake. Oxygen consumption is an expression of the product of cardiac output and arteriovenous oxygen difference, but several factors, including pulmonary and hematologic factors and muscle disease, can limit maximal oxygen uptake.[12] Functional aerobic fitness is the maximal oxygen uptake relative to body mass ($\dot{V}O_2$max/kg of body weight), a critical determinant of exercise capacity or performance, which refer to capabilities in physical activities (such as 1-mile run time).

Walking economy was defined as the gross oxygen cost of moving 1 kg of body mass at a given submaximal treadmill setting. The maximal and submaximal oxygen pulse ($\dot{V}O_2$/heart rate) was examined as an indicator of absolute cardiovascular fitness. Unfit individuals are characterized by a greater reliance on heart rate to increase $\dot{V}O_2$ (and lower oxygen pulse) than those who are fit.[20]

Respiratory function during exercise was assessed using maximal and submaximal $\dot{V}E$, breathing rate, ratio of breathing rate to tidal volume, and ventilatory equivalent for oxygen ($\dot{V}E/\dot{V}O_2$, an index of breathing efficiency). The ventilatory threshold was investigated as an indirect measure of anaerobic threshold. Ventilatory threshold was defined as the $\dot{V}O_2$ at the point of upward deflection of the ventilatory equivalent for oxygen without a concomitant rise in ventilatory equivalent for carbon dioxide. Ventilatory threshold was expressed as both $\dot{V}O_2$/kg and percentage of $\dot{V}O_2$max (which may reflect anaerobic capacity).[21]

Subjects were divided into obese (n = 13) and nonobese (n = 14) groups based a skinfold score above and below the 90th percentile (42 mm) for age, respectively.[22] Anthropometric and physiologic values were compared between groups using an unpaired Student's *t* test. A simple Pearson's Product-Moment Correlation Coefficient analysis was conducted between skinfold scores of the two groups as a marker of obesity and maximal absolute and weight-relative oxygen uptake and treadmill endurance time. Statistical significance was defined as $P \leq .05$.

RESULTS

The perceived low level of physical fitness of the subjects was verified by depressed levels of $\dot{V}O_2$max/kg (group mean, 30.9 mL/kg per minute; SD, 4.6; expected $\dot{V}O_2$max/kg, 40 to 45 mL/kg per minute).[23] Body mass index and skinfold scores compared with population norms are illustrated in Fig 1. A continuum of increased body fat was observed, with one half of subjects having BMI values exceeding the "desirable" range and more than one quarter having values above that estimated for 20% overweight.[16] Eighty-one percent had skinfold scores exceeding the average expected for age and sex, and measurements in 13 (48%) were greater than the 90th percentile (42 mm).[22] No association was evident between height and skinfold score ($r = .05$, $P = .8$). A correlation coefficient of .89 was observed between BMI and skinfold score.

Anthropometric and physiologic comparisons between the obese and nonobese groups during maximal and submaximal exercise are indicated in the Table. Maximal absolute oxygen uptake and ventilation were greater in the obese individuals, but were significantly less than those of the nonobese subjects when related to body weight. Corresponding to their lower $\dot{V}O_2$/kg, the obese subjects demonstrated 26% shorter treadmill endurance times than did the nonobese.

Increased body fat did not affect walking economy. Absolute values of submaximal $\dot{V}O_2$ were greater among obese subjects, but the oxygen uptake cost of moving body mass ($\dot{V}O_2$/kg) was not affected by increased body fat. Submaximal ventilation values paralleled those of oxygen uptake.

Submaximal heart rate was not affected by skinfold score. Increases in absolute $\dot{V}O_2$ to accommodate propelling larger fat mass at submaximal exercise levels were attributed to greater cardiac stroke volume and/or peripheral oxygen uptake. This is indicated by the significantly greater mean submaximal oxygen pulse value of the obese group.

Skinfold score was directly related to absolute $\dot{V}O_2$max ($r = .72$, $P < .0001$), with a linear association through the extremes of adiposity in this group of subjects (Fig 2). However, increased obesity resulted in progressive deterioration of both $\dot{V}O_2$max related to body mass ($r = -.49$, $P = .02$) and treadmill endurance time ($r = -.42$, $P = .03$). Therefore, subjects who were more obese had greater levels of absolute aerobic fitness but lower functional aerobic fitness and exercise capacity.

The obese subjects exhibited significantly higher oxygen pulses at maximum exercise, but obesity had no influence on maximal heart rate. As with submaximal exercise, the higher $\dot{V}O_2$max values associated with greater obesity reflected larger maximal cardiac stroke volumes and/or peripheral oxygen extractions.

The influence of body fat on maximal absolute and weight-relative minute ventilation during treadmill walking paralleled those of oxygen uptake. Obesity did not affect breathing rate, breathing rate–tidal volume ratio, or breathing efficiency ($\dot{V}E/\dot{V}O_2$) at either submaximal or maximal levels of walking. Ventilatory threshold could be determined in 24 (89%) of the 27 subjects. Oxygen consumption at ventilatory threshold was significantly lower in the obese subjects, but excess body fat had no effect on ventilatory threshold expressed as percentage of $\dot{V}O_2max$.

COMMENT

Cross-sectional studies of obese adults have provided a consistent picture of the influence of adiposity on cardiopulmonary function during rest.[24-28] The greater perfusion demands created by excess body fat are reflected in increased resting cardiac output. This response to adiposity is met entirely through increases in stroke volume; heart rate remains unchanged. This chronic elevation in stroke volume in the obese subject is reflected in ventricular enlargement and eccentric hypertrophy but normal myocardial function.

Until body weight becomes extreme (generally more than 135 kg), these hemodynamic changes are well tolerated.[25] With marked long-standing obesity, however, left ventricular function becomes impaired, resulting in increased end-diastolic pressure and clinical signs of hepatomegaly, peripheral edema, ascites, and dyspnea.[25,29,30] Early investigators considered these changes secondary to the direct effects of fatty infiltration in and around the heart, but most now view such congestive signs as a reflection of chronically accelerated cardiac output.[25,31] Complications of systemic and pulmonary hypertension (pickwickian syndrome) resulting from obesity may add to this cardiac compromise.

Interpretation of cardiovascular responses to excessive body fat during exercise is less certain. Buskirk and Taylor[6] contended that "the presence of excess fat per se does not have any important influence on the capacity of the cardiovascular system to deliver oxygen to muscles under maximal performance conditions." Their study of adult men exercising on treadmills indicated that absolute $\dot{V}O_2max$ related directly to percentage of body fat, while $\dot{V}O_2max/kg$ decreased with increasing obesity.

Our results confirm this conclusion. Increased adiposity in our subjects was linked to several indicators of superior absolute aerobic fitness during exercise. Maximum oxygen uptake was directly related to body fat (independent of body height) in a continuum from lean to grossly obese subjects. Maximum minute ventilation increased parallel with $\dot{V}O_2max$ as obesity increased. While the obese subjects demonstrated more cardiopulmonary functional reserve, their functional aerobic fitness and exercise capacity were impaired. That is, the augmented $\dot{V}O_2max$ in these individuals was insufficient to compensate for the load created by excessive body fat, as indicated by lower values of $\dot{V}O_2max/kg$ and shortened treadmill endurance times.

Arteriovenous oxygen difference is typically similar among obese and nonobese individuals.[28] The greater peak oxygen pulse values in the obese subjects in this study implies that the subjects' augmented oxygen delivery reflects increased maximal stroke volume. Maximal heart rates were not affected by body fat in this study or in others,[32,33] and resting left ventricular size as determined using echocardiography and roentgenographic estimation of heart volume have been reported to be greater in obese subjects even before puberty.[19,34]

The higher submaximal oxygen pulse values of our obese subjects are typical of athletes and subjects following athletic training and presumably reflect improved myocardial efficiency.[20] The relationship between heart rate and $\dot{V}O_2$ during exercise differs between obese and nonobese subjects in the same manner as between athletes and nonathletes. Farebrother[35] commented that "it could be considered that obese are fitter, due to the training effect of carrying about the excess body weight, but this implies the change is beneficial. It seems better to regard it as just appropriate to a condition of increased demand on the myocardium."

The greater muscle mass typical of young obese subjects may also contribute to increased absolute $\dot{V}O_2max$.[6,8,19,33] Sprynarova and Parizkova[36] observed changes in body composition and oxygen uptake during an obesity therapy program in a group of 11-year-old boys. Body weight, fat, and lean body mass all declined with treatment, but changes in $\dot{V}O_2max$ correlated only with those of lean body mass. Buskirk and Taylor[6] showed no significant differences in $\dot{V}O_2max$ related to fat-free mass (reflecting muscle volume) among their subjects, who demonstrated a wide range of obesity.

At submaximal levels of exercise, adiposity did not affect the walking economy of subjects in our study. Oxygen consumption increased because of the need to move excessive fat, but $\dot{V}O_2/kg$ was not affected. This implies that at this intensity of exercise the many factors that contribute to the energy cost of treadmill walking (eg, gait kinematics, elastic recoil forces, and mechanical efficiency) were not influenced by the degree of obesity in these subjects.[37]

Previous exercise studies of young obese subjects have provided conflicting data. Cooper et al[38] evaluated aerobic responses to exercise in obese children and adolescents by examining the ratio of maximal to resting oxygen uptake. The average among obese subjects was in the normal range, but six of 18 had values more than two SDs below the mean of nonobese subjects.

Zanconato et al[32] performed maximal exercise testing on 23 obese children aged 9 to 14 years.[32] Compared with lean control subjects, obese subjects demonstrated lower endurance times and $\dot{V}O_2max/kg$, but absolute $\dot{V}O_2max$ was not significantly different between the two groups. Huttunen et al[33] described similar findings among obese children and adolescents during exercise testing using cycle ergometers.

Other authors have reported a detrimental effect of obesity on cardiovascular function during exercise. Davies et al[8] found that absolute $\dot{V}O_2max$ during treadmill testing of obese females aged 6 to 25 years was no greater than that of nonobese subjects. When $\dot{V}O_2max$ was related to lean body mass or leg volume, values were lower among obese subjects. These findings implied that fat is not simply an inert load but plays "some indirect role in the etiology of relative effort intolerance of the obese."

Dempsey et al[9] reached the same conclusion in their study of obese young adult males exercising on cycle ergometers.[9] At maximum exercise, no relationship between absolute $\dot{V}O_2max$ and percentage of body fat was observed, but a negative correlation existed between $\dot{V}O_2max$ and fat-free mass. The authors concluded that "gross obesity—at least that in excess of 30% body fat—imposes a severe limitation on physical work capacity by its apparent interference with overall maximal cardiorespiratory function in addition to its burden as an inert, noncontributing load."

This study failed to identify any evidence of physiologic impairment due to obesity during maximal or submaximal treadmill walking in a group of adolescent girls with a wide range of body fat. On the contrary, obesity was associated with augmented cardiovascular and pulmonary function at maximal exercise. Reductions in relative aerobic fitness and exercise capacity appeared to result entirely from the effect of excess body fat acting as an inert load during weight-bearing activities. These results indicate that the problem for obese adolescents is not depressed aerobic fitness but rather insufficient increases in cardiovascular function to match the augmented load imposed by excessive body fat. Therefore, therapeutic exercise programs for obese teenagers would be best designed to increase caloric expenditure rather than improve aerobic fitness. Incorporation of activities to improve caloric energy output, which need not be at the high sustained intensity necessary to increase aerobic fitness, should help facilitate adherence to exercise programs for obese patients.

The author thanks Coleen Walsh, MS, and Meredith Varzeas, MEd, for their assistance with this study and Lee Cunningham, DPE, Paul Martha, MD, and Edward Reiter, MD, for their thoughtful reviews of the manuscript.

References

1. Wilmore JH. Body composition in sport and exercise: direction for future research. *Med Sci Sports Exerc.* 1983;15:21-31.
2. Watson AWS. Quantification of the influence of body fat content on selected physical performance variables in adolescent boys. *Ir J Med Sci.* 1988;157:383-384.
3. Boileau RA, Lohman TG. The measurement of human physique and its effect on physical performance. *Orthop Clin North Am.* 1977;8:563-572.
4. Slaughter MH, Lohman TG, Misner JE. Association of somatotype and body composition to physical performance in 7-12 year old girls. *J Sports Med.* 1980;20:189-198.
5. Cureton KJ, Boileau RA, Lohman TG. Relationship between body composition measures and AAHPER test performances in young boys. *Res Q.* 1975;46:218-223.
6. Buskirk E, Taylor HL. Maximum oxygen uptake and its relation to body composition, with special reference to chronic physical activity and obesity. *J Appl Physiol.* 1951;11:72-78.
7. Welch BE, Riendeau RP, Crisp CE, Isenstein RS. Relationship of maximal oxygen consumption to various components of body composition. *J Appl Physiol.* 1958;12:395-398.
8. Davies CTM, Godfrey S, Light M, Sargeant AJ, Zeidifard E. Cardiopulmonary responses to exercise in obese girls and young women. *J Appl Physiol.* 1975;38:373-376.
9. Dempsey JA, Redden W, Balke B, Rankin J. Work capacity determinants and physiologic cost of weight supported work in obesity. *J Appl Physiol.* 1966;21:1815-1820.
10. Whipp BJ, Davis JA. The ventilatory stress of exercise in obesity. *Am Rev Respir Dis.* 1984;129(suppl):S90-S92.
11. Farebrother MJB. Respiratory function and cardiorespiratory response to exercise in obesity. *Br J Dis Chest.* 1979;73:211-225.
12. Bar-Or O. *Pediatric Sports Medicine for the Practitioner: From Physiologic Principles to Clinical Applications.* New York, NY: Springer-Verlag NY Inc; 1983:66-75.
13. American College of Sports Medicine. The recommended quantity and quality of exercise for developing and maintaining cardiorespiratory and muscular fitness in healthy adults. *Med Sci Sports Exerc.* 1990;22:265-274.
14. Rowland TW. *Exercise and Children's Health.* Champaign, Ill: Human Kinetics Publishers; 1990:131-159.
15. Rowland TW, Varzeas M, Walsh CA. Aerobic responses to walking training in sedentary adolescents. *J Adolesc Health Care.* 1991;12:30-34.
16. Thomas AE, McKay DA, Cutlip MB. A nomograph method for assessing body weight. *Am J Clin Nutr.* 1976;29:302-304.
17. Tanner JM, Whitehouse RH. Revised standards for triceps and subscapular skinfolds in British children. *Arch Dis Child.* 1975;50:142-145.
18. Hoerr SL, Nelson RA, Lohman TG, Steiger D. Relation of skinfolds to body fatness in a population of obese adolescent girls. *Med Sci Sports Exerc.* 1984;16:135.
19. Parizkova J. *Body Fat and Physical Fitness.* The Hague, the Netherlands: Martinus Nijhoff Publishers; 1977:37.
20. Ekblom B, Astrand P-O, Saltin B, Stenberg J, Wallstrom B. Effect of training on circulatory response to exercise. *J Appl Physiol.* 1968;24:518-528.
21. Weymans ML, Reybrouck T, Stijns HJ, Knops J. Influence of age and sex on the ventilatory threshold in children. In: Binkhorst RA, Kemper HCG, Saris WHM, eds. *Children and Exercise XI.* Champaign, Ill: Human Kinetics Publishers; 1985;114-118.
22. Ross JD, Dotson CO, Gilbert GC, Katz SJ. New standards for fitness measurement. *JOPERD.* 1985;56:62-66.
23. Krahenbuhl GS, Skinner JS, Kohrt WM. Developmental aspects of maximal aerobic power in children. *Exerc Sport Sci Rev.* 1985;13:503-538.
24. Bray GA. Obesity and the heart. *Mod Concepts Cardiovasc Dis.* 1987;56:67-71.
25. Alexander JK. The cardiomyopathy of obesity. *Prog Cardiovasc Dis.* 1985;27:325-334.
26. Messerli FH. Cardiomyopathy of obesity: a not-so-Victorian disease. *N Engl J Med.* 1986;314:378-379.
27. Vaughn RW, Conahan TJ. Cardiopulmonary consequences of morbid obesity. *Life Sci.* 1980;26:2119-2127.
28. DeDivitiis O, Fazio S, Petitto M, Maddalena G, Contaldo F, Mancini M. Obesity and cardiac function. *Circulation.* 1981;64:477-482.
29. Romano M, Carella G, Cotecchia MR, et al. Abnormal systolic time intervals in obesity and their relationship with the amount of overweight. *Am Heart J.* 1986;112:356-360.
30. Carabello BA, Gittens L. Cardiac mechanics and function in obese normotensive persons with normal coronary arteries. *Am J Cardiol.* 1987;59:469-473.
31. Kaltman AJ, Goldring RM. Role of circulatory congestion in the cardiorespiratory failure of obesity. *Am J Med.* 1976;60:645-653.
32. Zanconato S, Baraldi E, Santuz P, et al. Gas exchange during exercise in obese children. *Eur J Pediatr.* 1989;148:614-617.
33. Huttunen NP, Knip M, Paavilainen T. Physical activity and fitness in obese children. *Int J Obesity.* 1986;10:519-525.
34. Hayashi T, Fujino M, Shindo M, Hiroki T, Arakawa K. Echocardiographic and electrocardiographic measures in obese children after an exercise program. *Int J Obesity.* 1987;11:465-472.
35. Farebrother MJB. Respiratory function and cardiorespiratory response to exercise in obesity. *Br J Dis Chest.* 1979;73:211-225.
36. Sprynarova S, Parizkova J. Changes in the aerobic capacity and body composition in obese boys after reduction. *J Appl Physiol.* 1965;20:934-937.
37. Katch V, Becque MD, Marks C, Moorehead C, Rocchini A. Oxygen uptake and energy output during walking of obese male and female adolescents. *Am J Clin Nutr.* 1988;47:26-32.
38. Cooper DM, Poage J, Barstow TJ, Springer C. Are obese children truly unfit?: minimizing the confounding effect of body size on the exercise response. *J Pediatr.* 1990;116:223-230.

Seasonal Variation in Growth During Growth Hormone Therapy

Mary C. J. Rudolf, MD; Zvi Zadik, MD; Shai Linn, MD, PhD; Zeev Hochberg, MD, DSc

• Seasonal variation in growth of normal children has been well described, although the mechanism by which it occurs has not been elucidated. The growth of 52 growth hormone–deficient children treated with synthetic human growth hormone was analyzed. A similar seasonal variation was observed, with mean (±SEM) peak growth occurring in the summer (8.2±0.3 cm/y) and winter (7.7±0.2 cm/y), and trough growth occurring in the autumn (6.9±0.3 cm/y). Forty-seven percent of subjects grew minimally during the autumn, and only two children showed peak growth in that season. Individual variations between maximal and minimal growth seasons amounted to 3.5±0.3 cm/y. The seasonal pattern was statistically significant for the group as a whole, for the prepubertal subgroup, and for the boys. The variation persisted when the first year of treatment was excluded to avoid bias of the initial growth spurt. The season of onset of therapy did not affect total growth during the first year. The demonstration of a seasonal pattern in growth of these children suggests that the seasonal variation may be mediated by peripheral rather than central factors. Paired clonidine-provoked growth hormone levels and an integrated concentration of 24-hour growth hormone levels and serum levels of insulinlike growth hormone I measured in a control group of normally growing children were also analyzed and showed no seasonal variation. This further suggests that peripheral rather than central factors are responsible for the seasonal variation in children's growth.

(*AJDC.* 1991;145:769-772)

Seasonal variation has been repeatedly, if not consistently, observed in the growth of normal children,[1-3] with variations in growth velocity between seasons amounting to as much as 5 cm/y.[2] The mechanism by which this seasonal variation occurs remains unclear.[1] No variation in growth hormone (GH) secretion through the year has been demonstrated,[4,5] thus suggesting that peripheral rather than central factors are responsible for seasonal variation. We attempted to clarify retrospectively the seasonal effect by analyzing the growth of GH-deficient children receiving constant-dose GH therapy. In addition, peak responses to clonidine-provoked testing and integrated concentration of daily GH profiles were also reviewed.

Accepted for publication May 23, 1990.

From the Departments of Pediatrics (Drs Rudolf and Hochberg) and Epidemiology (Dr Linn), Rambam Medical Center, Haifa, Israel, and the Pediatric Endocrine Unit (Dr Zadik), Kaplan Hospital, Rehovot, Israel.

Reprint requests to Rappaport Family Institute of Research in the Medical Sciences, Technion-Israel Institute of Technology, PO Box 9697, 31096 Haifa, Israel (Dr Hochberg).

PATIENTS AND METHODS

Clinical Data

The medical records of 52 patients treated for GH deficiency at Rambam Medical Center, Haifa, Israel, and Kaplan Hospital, Rehovot, Israel, were reviewed. Patients had received a constant dose of 0.3 mg/kg of human GH recombinant (BioTechnology General Ltd, Rehovot, Israel) weekly in three divided doses from the onset of treatment for 24 to 33 months and were measured at 2- to 3-month intervals using Harpenden stadiometers. Based on the respective ratios of days in each season, growth velocities were calculated for each child for four 3-month periods corresponding to Israel's seasons, namely, March through May (spring), June through August (summer), September through November (autumn), and December through February (winter). Growth velocities for each season were compared by Student's *t* test. The data were then further analyzed as follows: (1) for each sex alone; (2) for those children who were pubertal or entered puberty during the study compared with those who remained prepubertal; (3) excluding the first year of treatment, to minimize bias of the initial growth spurt at the onset of therapy; (4) for a relationship between the season of start of treatment and growth in the first year; and (5) for the seasons in which each child demonstrated peak and minimal growth.

Laboratory Data

The integrated concentration of GH was studied in 82 normally growing children (54 boys and 28 girls; mean [±SD] age, 12.5±3.0 years) as previously reported.[6] Plasma insulinlike growth factor I (IGF-I) was measured before initiation of therapy, and at the end of 2 years of therapy in all 52 patients. These results were reviewed for evidence of a seasonal variation. Data were analyzed using the Kruskal-Wallis Test. In addition, GH response to clonidine (0.15 mg/m^2) was analyzed in 82 children studied on two occasions in consecutive seasons. Results were analyzed using Student's paired *t* test.

RESULTS

Clinical Data

The medical records of 52 patients (39 boys and 13 girls) aged 5 to 17 years were reviewed. Thirty-five patients remained prepubertal throughout the study period of 24 to 33 months. The start of therapy was distributed throughout the year, as shown in Table 1. The total number of seasons of growth equaled 455.

Table 1.—Effect of Season in Which Human Growth Hormone Therapy Was Initiated on the Growth of 52 Children During the First Year of Treatment

	Spring	Summer	Autumn	Winter
No. of children starting treatment	16	28	7	1
Height gain in first year, cm*	8.2±0.5	8.2±0.4	9.1±0.6	9.2

*Values of height gain are mean±SEM. Differences were not significant.

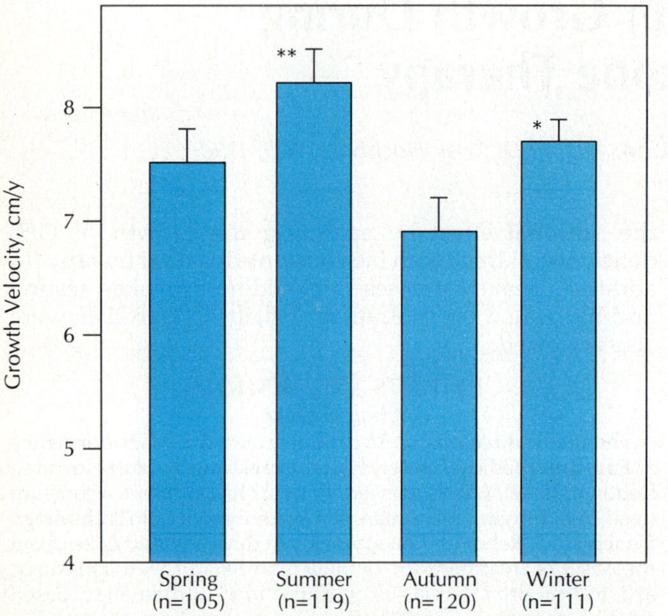

Fig 1.—*Variation in growth velocity with season for 52 growth hormone (GH)–deficient children receiving human GH therapy for at least 2 years. The numbers in parentheses indicate the number of seasons of human GH therapy. Values are mean±SEM. The asterisk indicates P<.05; double asterisk, P<.005 vs autumn.*

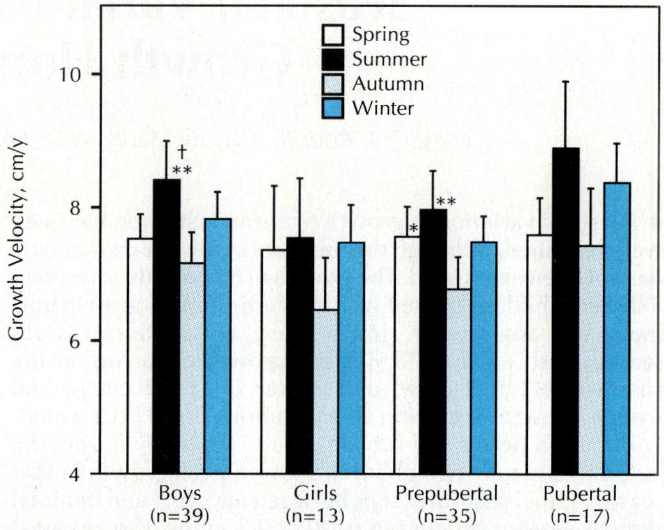

Fig 2.—*Variation in growth velocity with season, according to sex and pubertal development, for 52 children treated with growth hormone who were studied for at least 2 years. Values are mean±SEM. The asterisk indicates P<.05; double asterisk, P<.01 vs autumn; and dagger, P<.01 vs spring.*

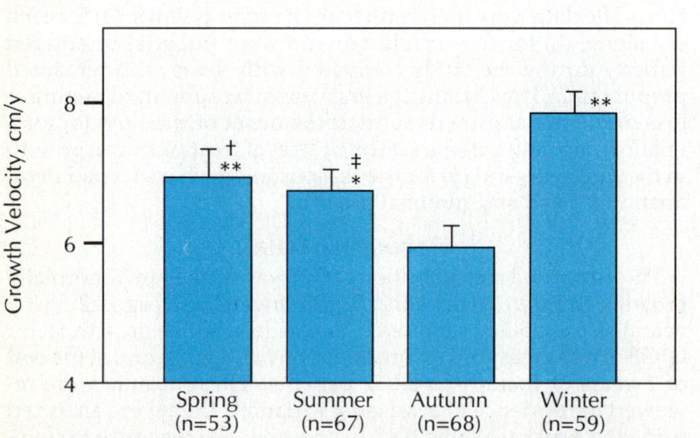

Fig 3.—*Variation in growth velocity with season, excluding the first year of therapy, for 52 children treated with growth hormone. The numbers in parentheses indicate the number of seasons of growth. Values are mean±SEM. The asterisk indicates P<.05; double asterisk, P<.01 vs autumn; dagger, P<.05; and double dagger, P<.01 vs winter.*

Growth velocities for each season are shown in Fig 1. A seasonal variation was observed, with mean (±SEM) peak growth occurring in the summer (8.2±0.3 cm/y) and, to a lesser degree, in winter (7.7±0.3 cm/y). The lowest growth velocity occurred in autumn (6.9±0.3 cm/y).

Figure 2 shows seasonal differences for the four subgroups: male, female, prepubertal, and pubertal children. The pattern remained consistent for each subgroup, although it failed to reach statistical significance for the small number of girls and pubertal children in the study.

When the first year of therapy was excluded from the study, thereby reducing the influence of growth spurts occurring at the initiation of treatment, a seasonal variation was again observed, although the summer peak was blunted (Fig 3). The trough in autumn remained constant, however.

Table 2 shows the percentage of children demonstrating their peak and trough growth for each season, again excluding the first year of treatment. Only 8% of children had their peak growth in autumn, but 47% had their trough growth in this season. Seventy percent of children demonstrated their peak growth between December and May. These were significantly different from the expected 25% of children in each season (χ^2 analysis). The differences in growth velocity between maximal and minimal growth seasons amounted to 3.5±0.2 cm/y for the group as a whole. No significant differences were seen in girls compared with boys or in pubertal compared with prepubertal children.

Finally, Table 1 shows the growth achieved during the first year of treatment as it related to the season of initiation of GH therapy. Small differences were observed between the groups, with those children starting treatment in autumn showing a slightly greater increment in growth. This, however, was not statistically significant.

Table 2.—Peak and Minimum Growth in Each Season of Children Receiving Human Growth Hormone Therapy (First Year of Treatment Excluded)	Spring	Summer	Autumn	Winter
Children showing peak growth, %	34	22	8*	36†
Children showing minimum growth, %	22	27	47*	4*

*$P<.005$ of the expected 25%.
†$P<.05$ of the expected 25%.

Table 3.—Mean (±SEM) Growth Hormone (GH) Secretion as Related to Season at Time of Testing

	No.	Spring	Summer	Autumn	Winter	Spring
Clonidine-provoked GH levels, μg/L*	24	14.9±1.4	15.5±1.4	...	...	...
	16	...	15.8±1.4	16.4±1.7	...	...
	27	...	...	14.1±1.3	16.2±1.4	...
	15	...	...	...	15.3±0.9	15.4±3.1
Integrated concentration of GH levels, μg/L†	82	5.1±0.5 (21)	4.9±0.4 (22)	5.0±0.3 (20)	4.9±0.3 (21)	... ...

*Clonidine-provoked GH response in subjects tested in two consecutive seasons. Differences were not significant.
†Integrated concentration of GH in 84 subjects tested in different seasons. No significant seasonal differences were found. Numbers in parentheses indicate numbers of tests.

Table 4.—Insulinlike Growth Hormone (GH) I Measurements in Pubertal Controls and GH-Deficient Children Receiving Human GH Therapy, as Related to Seasons*	Spring	Summer	Autumn	Winter
Controls, U/mL	1.7±1.2	1.6±1.3	1.7±1.3	1.7±1.5
GH-deficient children, U/mL	1.9±2.3	2.0±1.6	1.7±1.5	1.9±1.5

*Values are mean±SEM. Differences were not significant.

Laboratory Data

In a control group of 84 normally growing children, no significant differences were found in results of repeated clonidine tests performed in consecutive seasons in the same patient (Table 3). Furthermore, no significant change in the integrated concentration of GH was found between seasons. No significant change was found between seasons in the IGF-I level of normal control children or of GH-deficient patients receiving GH therapy (Table 4).

COMMENT

Various studies carried out in California, England, and Ohio have demonstrated a seasonal variation in growth, with peak growth observed in spring to early summer and minimal growth in fall to early winter.[1-3] Previous studies failed to demonstrate variations in GH secretion, either in spontaneous profiles or on provocative testing,[4,5] suggesting that the seasonal effect is not mediated by changes in GH secretion.

Results of the present study provide evidence that growth can substantially vary throughout the year, despite unchanging circulating levels of GH and IGF-I in children with GH deficiency treated with constant-dose GH. This is at variance with a previous study in which GH was administered intermittently during the seasons.[7] The pattern of growth in our study was remarkably similar to that described in normal children,[1-3] with peak growth occurring in summer, although we found that good growth also occurred in the mild Israeli winter months. Particularly consistent was the trough in growth occurring in autumn, which was observed in both the first and subsequent years of treatment, and in the usually more uniform growth in the prepubertal years, especially in boys.

This autumnal dip is of particular interest, given that 28 of the children started therapy in the summer. Accelerated growth is usually seen in the several months following initiation of treatment, and thus one would expect an artificially increased growth velocity in this season. This seasonal variation is further emphasized when the periods of peak and trough growth for each child are considered. The first year of growth was excluded to avoid bias of growth spurts at the start of treatment. In subsequent years, although children's peak growth was distributed through December to August, it is noteworthy that only two of our 52 children grew maximally between September and November. It is also striking that 47% of the children showed minimal growth in autumn.

The degree of variation in growth between seasons was not insignificant. Although a mean difference of 1.3 cm/y was seen between autumn and summer for the group, individuals showed greater fluctuations in their growth, with a mean of 3.5 cm/y, and differences as high as 7.4 cm/y measured between minimal and maximal growth seasons.

The question whether the season in which GH treatment is initiated affects total growth in the important first year of treatment was also addressed. The group starting treatment in the autumn showed a marginally higher growth increment than the rest of the children. Thus, although children in this group did not have an autumnal dip, this did not significantly add to their total first-year growth.

It is difficult to hypothesize the mechanism by which the seasonal variation occurs. It has been shown that duration of sunlight does not cause fluctuations in GH secretion[5]; however, this does not exclude a role in seasonal growth through other means, since totally blind children grow with minimal growth periods distributed throughout the year.[1] Temperature, on the other hand, does not seem to be a factor since children showed a seasonal pattern of growth in California, where minimal changes in temperature occur throughout the year.[1] The mild climate of Israel is likewise unlikely to mediate seasonal variations.

The autumnal dip seems to have been consistent throughout these studies.[1-3] Autumn is a season in which differences in temperature and light are not extreme and therefore are unlikely to be responsible for the seasonal variation. It has been shown that seasonal variations in weight show the converse pattern to that of height.[3] It is tempting to speculate that in late summer, when children tend to be more active and heat reduces appetites, weight gain is inadequate to promote good growth in the following season.

In concordance with previous studies, we did not demonstrate a seasonal variation in GH levels, either on provocation with clonidine or in integrated concentrations of GH; neither did we find that serum levels of IGF-I were affected by seasonal variations.

The observations in this study strongly suggest that variations in growth can occur independently of GH and IGF-I levels. Explanations for this phenomenon must invoke peripheral rather than central mechanisms; possibly an alteration in sensitivity of the end-organ or, alternatively, involvement of other hormones, such as androgens, which do vary throughout the year[8] and which might augment GH activity.

Relative resistance to treatment with human GH has been described in emotionally deprived children: when endogenous GH secretion resumes, these children respond normally.[9] Another point of special interest is the greater vulnerability of boys to the seasonal variations of growth. We recently reported that boys are also more susceptible to psychological deprivation in terms of their physical growth.[10] Whether the autumnal dip in growth rate and emotional deprivation share a similar mechanism is unkown.

Despite the fact that these fascinating aspects of growth are yet to be elucidated, important conclusions can be drawn from this study. First, evaluations of response to GH therapy cannot be made on short-term measurements, any more than they can be used in the evaluation of any child's growth.[2,11] This is certainly true until the extent of seasonal variation is defined for any climatic area, and even then individuals seem to demonstrate considerable variation. This study also indicates that the season in which GH therapy is started does not seem to have a significant effect on the growth attained in the vital first year, although this should perhaps be reassessed with a larger group of children.

We thank Ruth Singer for her expert secretarial assistance.

References

1. Lee PA. Independence of seasonal variation of growth from temperature change. *Growth*. 1980;44:54-57.

2. Marshall WA. Evaluation of growth rate in height over periods of less than one year. *Arch Dis Child*. 1971;46:414-420.

3. Reynolds EL, Sontag LW. Seasonal variations in weight, height, and appearance of ossification centers. *J Pediatr*. 1944;24:524-535.

4. Campbell IT, Jarrett RJ, Rutland P, Stimmler L. The plasma insulin and growth hormone response to oral glucose: diurnal and seasonal observations in the Antarctic. *Diabetologia*. 1975; 11:147-150.

5. Weitzman ED, deGraaf AS, Sassin JF, et al. Seasonal patterns of sleep stages and secretion of cortisol and growth hormone during 24-hour periods in northern Norway. *Acta Endocrinol (Copenh)*. 1975;78:65-76.

6. Zadik Z, Chalew SA. McCarter RJ Jr, Meistas M, Kowarski AA. The influence of age on the 24-hour integrated concentration of growth hormone. *J Clin Endocrinol Metab*. 1986;60:513-516.

7. Kollipara S, Connors MH. Lack of seasonal influence on growth hormone therapy. *Growth*. 1985;49:341-345.

8. Deslypere JP, DeBishop G, Vermeulen A. Seasonal variation of plasma dehydroepiandrosterone sulphate and urinary androgen excretion in postmenopausal women. *Clin Endocrinol*. 1983;18:25-30.

9. Frasier SD, Rallison ML. Growth retardation and emotional deprivation: relative resistance to treatment with human growth hormone. *J Pediatr*. 1972;80:603-604.

10. Rudolf MCJ, Hochberg Z. Are boys more vulnerable to psychosocial growth retardation? *Dev Med Child Neurol*. 1990; 32:1022-1025.

11. Hermanussen M, Burmeister J. Standards for the predictive accuracy of short-term body height and lower-leg length measurements on half-annual growth rates. *Arch Dis Child*. 1989;64:259-263.

A Survey of Antiemetic Use in Children With Cancer

Jack van Hoff, MD; Marilyn J. Hockenberry-Eaton, MSN, PNP;
Katherine Patterson, MN; John J. Hutter, MD

• Pediatric oncologists within Pediatric Oncology Group institutions were surveyed to determine current antiemetic practices for children receiving chemotherapy and the basis for those practices. A mean severity rating for associated nausea and vomiting was calculated and used to rank 31 chemotherapeutic agents commonly used in the treatment of childhood cancer. Antiemetics were used 17%, 79%, and 98% of the time for chemotherapeutic agents with mild, moderate, or severe associated nausea and vomiting, respectively. A median of one, two, and three antiemetics were used for mild, moderate, and severe agents, respectively. Antihistamines and phenothiazines were the drugs most commonly used for agents causing mild or moderate nausea and vomiting, and metoclopramide hydrochloride/antihistamines with lorazepam and/or corticosteroids were used most often for chemotherapeutic agents causing severe nausea and vomiting. Most oncologists based their choice of antiemetics on personal experience. Current literature addressing the treatment of nausea and vomiting in children receiving chemotherapy, as reviewed here, does not always support the present clinical practices.
(*AJDC.* 1991;145:773-778)

Chemotherapy-related nausea and vomiting remains a major adverse side effect of cancer therapy despite an increasing number of available antiemetic agents. This is due in part to the increasing use of certain highly emetogenic agents such as cisplatin or high doses of cytarabine or cyclophosphamide. Pediatric antiemetic regimens have generally been adapted from those used in adults; however, the benefit-toxicity ratio may differ substantially in children compared with adults.[1] Although some of the antiemetic regimens have been tested specifically in children, many have not, and there is no general consensus regarding optimum antiemetic regimens for children receiving chemotherapy. In fact, the perceived need and usage of any antiemetics appears to vary substantially among pediatric oncologists. Differences in the potency of chemotherapeutic agents and combinations of agents to induce nausea and vomiting are recognized but not quantified, contributing to the problem. A survey of pediatric oncologists and pediatric oncology nurses within the Pediatric Oncology Group (POG) was conducted to assess current uses of antiemetics for children receiving chemotherapy and the basis for decisions regarding choice of antiemetics. The results of that survey are presented in this article and compared with an earlier unpublished POG survey implemented in 1984, as well as with published reports of pediatric antiemetic trials. Behavioral and other nondrug therapies were not surveyed and are not discussed in this report.

Accepted for publication August 13, 1990.
From the Yale University School of Medicine, New Haven, Conn (Dr van Hoff); Emory University School of Nursing, Atlanta, Ga (Ms Hockenberry-Eaton); University of Kansas Medical Center, Kansas City (Ms Patterson); and the University of Arizona Health Sciences Center, Tucson (Dr Hutter).
Reprints not available.

MATERIALS AND METHODS

A brief questionnaire was distributed to all POG institutions via the newsletter and at the fall meeting in 1988 (Fig 1). The questionnaire focused on scoring the severity of nausea and vomiting associated with specific chemotherapeutic agents and current antiemetic practices at that institution.

The symptoms associated with specific chemotherapeutic agents were scored on a scale of 1 to 3, with 1 being least severe and 3 being most severe. The results were recorded in intervals of 0.5. A mean severity score was calculated for each agent for comparison purposes. Although these agents were often used in combination, an attempt was made to rate each agent individually. The frequency of antiemetic use and the drug or combination of drugs used to control nausea and vomiting was ascertained for mild, moderate, and severe chemotherapeutic agents. The responders were asked to specify modifications used, if any, for children younger than 5 years. In addition, the reasons for current antiemetic practices was evaluated. Responders were asked to rank two of a list of six possible reasons, including an "other" category. Differences between responses of physicians and nurses were tested with *t* tests or Wilcoxon rank sum tests where appropriate.

RESULTS

Current Usage

Responses were received from 76 individuals representing 46 POG institutions and affiliates. Seventy-one (93%) completed the entire questionnaire. Eighty-five percent (35 of 41) of member institutions and consortiums responded. Thirty-one institutions submitted a single response, 12 submitted responses from two individuals, and five submitted three or more responses. Differences in the responses were as common within as between institutions, although no formal statistical analysis was done.

Please score each of the following agents, assigning a level of associated nausea and vomiting as follows:

1 = mild or no nausea and vomiting associated with the use of this agent.
2 = moderate nausea and vomiting associated.
3 = severe nausea and vomiting associated.
X = no experience with this agent.

We realize many of these agents are used in combination, however, please attempt to rank each agent individually.

___ Dactinomycin	___ Doxorubicin
___ L-Asparaginase	___ Fluorouracil
___ 5-Azaacytidine	___ Hydroxyurea
___ Carmustine	___ Mercaptopurine orally
___ Bleomycin	___ Mercaptopurine intravenously
___ Carboplatin	___ Methotrexate 1gm/m^2
___ Lomustine	___ Methotrexate 1gm/m^2
___ Iproplatin	___ Nitrogen Mustard
___ Cis-Platinum	___ L-Phenylalanine Mustard
___ Cyclophosphamide 10mg/kg	___ Procarbazine
___ Cyclophosphamide 10mg/kg	___ Thioguanine
___ Cytosine Arabinoside Std Dose	___ Triple Intrathecal Therapy
___ Cytosine Arabinoside High Dose	___ Vinblastine
___ Dacarbazine	___ Vincristine
___ Daunomycin	___ Teniposide
	___ Etoposide

Please answer these questions for agents with each of the following scores for severity of associated nausea and vomiting.

1 = mild 2 = moderate 3 = severe

1. In what percentage of patients do you use antiemetics when giving these agents? ______ ______ ______

2. What drug or drug combination do you use in these settings? Please indicate the dose you would use for a 1 m^2 (30 kg) child. ______ ______ ______

   Do you modify these choices for children less than five years of age? If so, what agents are used? Please indicate the dose used for a 0.5 m^2 (10 kg) child. ______ ______ ______

3. How effective are these antiemetics in these settings? ______ ______ ______
   1 = Highly effective
   2 = Moderately effective
   3 = Minimally effective

4. Why have you chosen these antiemetics? Pick the two most important reasons from the following list and rank as:
   1 = Most important
   2 = Less important

   ___ Institutional policy
   ___ Past experience
   ___ Review of the literature
   ___ Parent or patient request
   ___ Advice from other oncologists or nurses
   ___ Other; please state.

Name (Optional) MD, RN, or other ____________ Institution ____________

Fig 1.—*Questionnaire scoring severity of nausea and vomiting associated with specific chemotherapeutic agents and antiemetics.*

The majority of responses (82%) were from physicians, with the remaining 18% coming from nurses or physician's assistants. There were no statistically significant differences between those two groups.

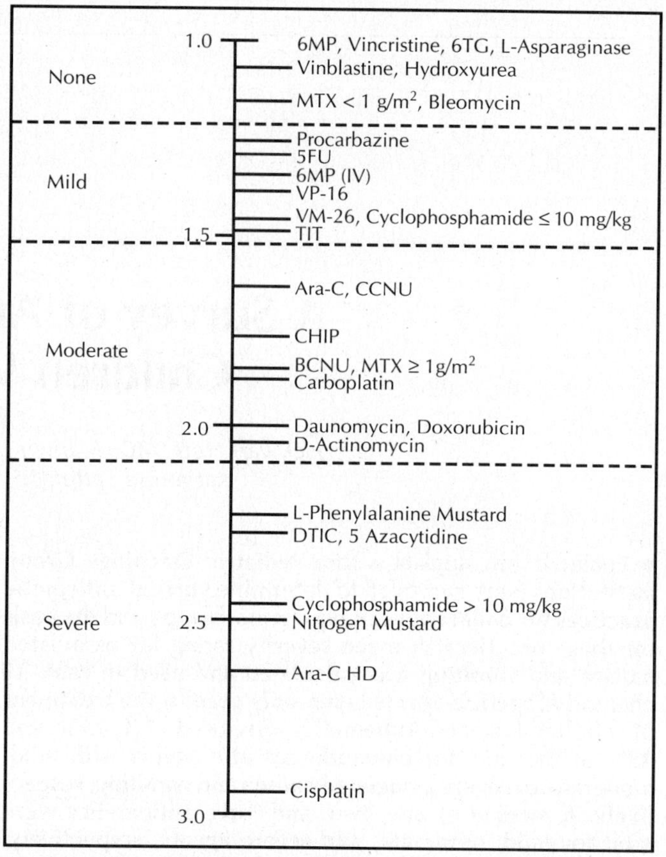

Fig 2.—*Mean severity scores of nausea and vomiting associated with chemotherapeutic agents, according to the survey, indicated in rank order using a rating scale of 1 to 3, with 1 being least severe and 3 being most severe. 6MP indicates 6-mercaptopurine; 6TG, 6-thioguanine; MTX, methotrexate; IV, intravenous; 5FU, fluorouracil; VP-16, etoposide; VM-26, teniposide; Ara-C, cytarabine; CCNU, lomustine; CHIP, iproplatin; BCNU, carmustine; DTIC, dacarbazine; and TIT, triple intrathecal therapy of methotrexate, hydrocortisone, and cytarabine.*

The mean severity rating for associated nausea and vomiting was calculated for each of 31 chemotherapeutic agents. The results are displayed in Fig 2 and are divided into four severity groups of approximately equal size.

The percentage of patients given antiemetics for chemotherapeutic agents with mild, moderate, or severe associated nausea and vomiting was determined. Antiemetics were used an average of 17% of the time with mild agents, 79% of the time with moderate agents, and 98% of the time with severe agents. The number of antiemetic drugs used also increased with the severity of expected nausea and vomiting. A median (mean) of 1 (1.4), 2 (2.0), and 3 (3.1) antiemetics were used per course for agents with mild, moderate, and severe nausea and vomiting, respectively. Several responders reported using as many as five antiemetics in combination to control symptoms associated with agents causing moderate or severe nausea and vomiting. Antihistamines and phenothiazines were the most commonly used antiemetics in children, followed closely by metoclopramide hydrochloride, steroids, and lorazepam (Fig 3). While antihistamines are often given to prevent extrapyramidal side effects of other agents, 14 responders (18%) used them alone as antiemetic agents, primarily for agents with mild associated symptoms. Diphenhydramine hydrochloride was the antihistamine used

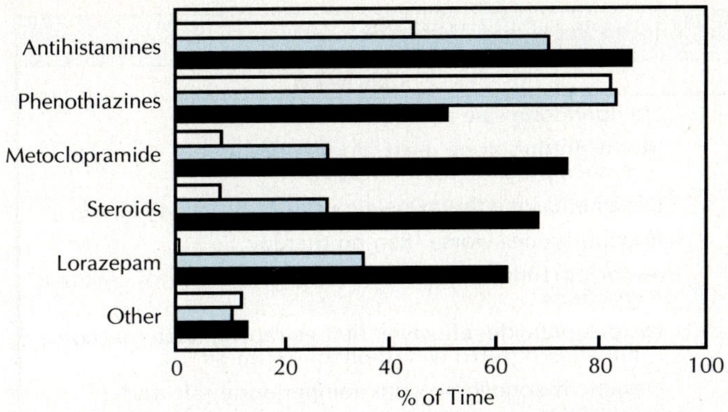

Fig 3.—*Percentage of time each drug or drug class is used as an antiemetic for chemotherapeutic agents with mild (open bars), moderate (tinted bars), or severe (closed bars) associated nausea and vomiting. The amount shown is the percentage of time that the drug is given when antiemetics are used. The total percentage for each severity level is greater than 100% as multiple antiemetics are used per course of chemotherapy. Other drugs include tetrahydrocannabinol, phenobarbitol, domperidone, trimethobenzamide, and scopolamine.*

most often, accounting for 85% of all antihistamine usage. Hydroxyzine hydrochloride accounted for 13% and dimenhydrinate for 2% of antihistamines used. Chlorpromazine was the most commonly used phenothiazine, accounting for 51% of all usage. It was followed by promethazine hydrochloride, which accounted for 28% of phenothiazine usage. The tabulation below lists the generic and product names of phenothiazines used as antiemetics.

Generic Name	Product Name
Chlorpromazine	Thorazine, Largactil
Perphenazine	Trilafon
Prochlorperazine	Compazine
Promazine	Sparine
Promethazine	Phenergin, Mepergan
Thiethylperazine	Torecan

Other phenothiazines reported in the survey included thiethyperazine (8%), prochlorperazine (6%), perphenazine (5%), and promazine (2%). Dexamethasone was used 88% of the time that corticosteroids were given as antiemetics, and methylprednisolone accounted for the remaining 12%. The most common drug combinations were phenothiazine/antihistamine and metoclopramide/antihistamine, to which lorazepam and/or corticosteroids were added. Phenothiazines with or without antihistamines were preferred for chemotherapy with mild or moderate nausea and vomiting. Metoclopramide-based combinations were preferentially used for chemotherapy with severe associated nausea and vomiting. Metoclopramide/phenothiazine, or two different phenothiazine combinations, were occasionally used. All drugs were used primarily at recommended dosages, but there was a wide dosage range for many of the agents. For example, metoclopramide hydrochloride was used in doses ranging from 3 to 90 mg/m^2 (median, 30 mg/m^2), lorazepam from 0.5 to 3 mg/m^2 (median, 1 mg/m^2), and dexamethasone from 2 to 30 mg/m^2 (median, 10 mg/m^2). Dosages used varied between responders; however, they did not vary with the severity of expected nausea and vomiting. Forty-two percent of responders made no change in choice or dose of antiemetics for children less than 5 years of age. Twenty-six percent decreased the dose per body surface area or weight to approximately 70% of the dose used for children older than 5 years. Sixteen percent of the responders reported withholding metoclopramide and lorazepam from children younger than 5 years.

Table 1.—Reasons for Choice of Antiemetic Regimen

	Ranked		
Reasons	**Most Important**	**Second Most Important**	**Not Ranked**
Experience	36	4	24
Literature review	4	13	11
Professional advice	2	9	10
Patient request	1	13	11
Other	1	1	2
Total	**44**	**40**	**25***

*Multiple reasons listed account for total less than the sum of the individual reasons.

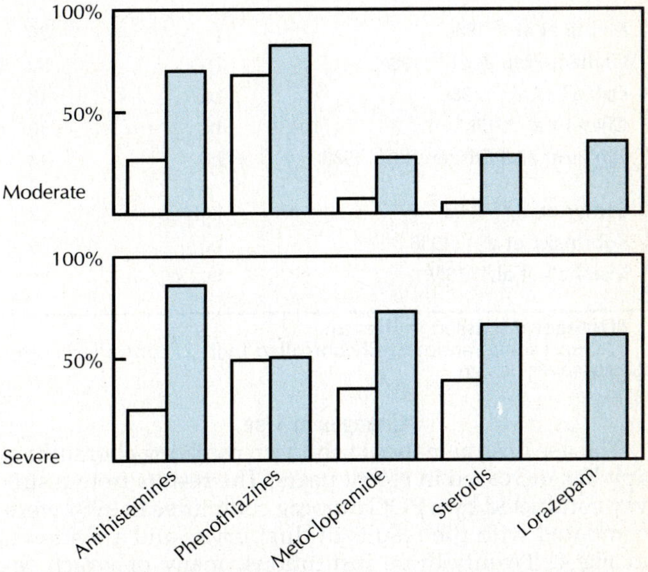

Fig 4.—*Percentage of time each drug or drug class is used as an antiemetic for chemotherapeutic agents with moderate or severe associated nausea and vomiting, comparing 1984 (tinted bars) practice with 1988 (solid bars) practice. The total percentage for each severity level is greater than 100% as multiple antiemetics are used per course of chemotherapy.*

Reasons for Use

The responders' clinical experience was the most important factor in the decision of which antiemetics to use. Thirty-six (82%) of the 44 responders who ranked their reasons for choosing a specific antiemetic regimen listed clinical experience as the most important reason (Table 1). Literature review, professional advice, and patient request were the next most frequently reported reasons for choosing particular antiemetics. Responders who reported several reasons without ranking them included experience as one of the reasons 96% of the time (Table 1), and literature review, professional advice, or patient request 40% of the time each.

Source, y	Design†	No. of Patients	Conclusion
O'Meara and Mott,[24] 1981	3	27	Domperidone safe and effective
Ise et al,[15] 1982	2	62	Methylprednisolone most, domperidone less, metoclopramide least effective
Khan et al,[21] 1983	2x	22	Dexamethasone/thorazine superior to thorazine alone
Zeltzer et al,[1] 1984	2x	23	Phenothiazines worse than no therapy
Terrin et al,[16] 1984	3	8	Metoclopramide effective but high incidence of dystonic reactions
Allen et al,[17] 1985	3	45	Metoclopramide effective but extrapyramidal reactions, not all controlled with diphenhydramine
Ekert et al,[19] 1986	3	23	Dexamethasone/lorazepam/domperidone safe and effective
Howrie et al,[18] 1986	2x	11	Metoclopramide effective, high incidence of extrapyramidal reactions
Mehta et al,[13] 1986	1	20	Methylprednisolone as effective as chlorpromazine
Graham-Pole et al,[12] 1986	1	50	Chlorpromazine superior to metoclopramide
Dalzell et al,[23] 1986	1x	18	Nabilone superior to domperidone
Chan et al,[22] 1987	1x	30	Nabilone superior to prochlorperazine
van Hoff and Olszewski,[20] 1988	2x	14	Lorazepam as effective as phenothiazine and/or methylprednisolone
Sumer et al,[10] 1988	1x	9	Dexamethasone superior to no therapy
Kobrinsky et al,[11] 1988	1x	6	Naloxone worse than placebo
Marshall et al,[14] 1989	1x	26	Metoclopramide/benztropine/dexamethasone/lorazepam superior to chlorpromazine

Table 2.—Summary of Antiemetic Trials in Children Receiving Chemotherapy*

*Dosages discussed in the text.
† 1 represents randomized controlled trial; 2, controlled comparison trial, nonrandomized; 3, single course efficacy/safety trial; and x, crossover design.

Changes in Use

The use of antiemetics in children receiving chemotherapy has increased in recent years. The results from a survey conducted by a POG nursing committee in 1984 were compared with the results of this survey and are shown in Fig 4. Twenty-three institutions, many of which responded to this survey, participated in the 1984 descriptive survey. The 1984 survey solicited the antiemetics used for individual chemotherapeutic agents. The responses were similar for all agents except cisplatin. Therefore, the cisplatin responses from 1984 were compared with the severe agent responses in 1988, and the rest of the 1984 agents were compared with the 1988 moderate agents. Comparison of the two surveys revealed a general increase in the use of all agents, implying an increase in the number of antiemetic agents used per treatment course. Increased antihistamine use reflects its incorporation into antiemetic combinations. Metoclopramide, corticosteroids, and lorazepam use increased particularly between 1984 and 1988.

COMMENT

Nausea and vomiting related to chemotherapeutic agents are major problems in the treatment of cancer at all ages. In a prospective evaluation of chemotherapy-related nausea and vomiting, 92% of children who did not receive antiemetics had symptoms.[2] A more recent survey showed that 83% of children had nausea and 78% had vomiting after receiving chemotherapy without antiemetics.[3] In both studies, the severity of symptoms varied substantially between patients and between successive courses of chemotherapy in the same patient. With repeated courses of chemotherapy, some children develop anticipatory nausea and vomiting that appears to have a different pathophysiologic mechanism than that induced directly by chemotherapeutic agents.[4] Anticipatory nausea has been noted in 28% to 36% of children; approximately 20% report anticipatory vomiting.[3,4]

A rating scale of the emetogenic potency of various chemotherapeutic agents was developed for adults from a survey of medical oncology nurses,[5] but similar data have not been previously reported for children. We present the results of an emetic potency survey in Fig 2, dividing the agents surveyed into groups with severe, moderate, mild, or no expected nausea and vomiting. Although this scoring system cannot be expected to predict each patient's response to particular chemotherapy, it can be used to help decide when to use antiemetics for children beginning chemotherapy. The emetogenicity of chemotherapeutic agents has been shown to strongly influence the severity of nausea and vomiting,[4,6] although other nondrug factors such as age, sex, behavioral traits, and even child-rearing practices also play a role.[3,4,6]

We also evaluated current antiemetic practices at 46 pediatric oncology centers. This survey was limited to pharmacologic antiemetic practices, although behavioral interventions may also be effective in children receiving chemotherapy.[7-9] The results of this survey conflict somewhat with the limited available literature on antiemetic use in children. In August 1989, a total of 16 clinical trials evaluating antiemetic agents in children could be located by a computer search (Table 2). Seven of these studies were randomized controlled trials, and the others were sequential (n=3) or single-course (n=6) trials of agents or combinations of agents. Only three studies included a "no therapy"[1,10] or placebo[11] arm and two of these concluded that the antiemetic studied exacerbated the nausea and vomiting.[1,11]

Phenothiazines ranked among the most frequently used

antiemetics for children in this survey (Fig 3), yet the literature on their efficacy is inconclusive. Chlorpromazine (0.5 mg/kg every 3 hours) appeared more effective than a relatively low dosage of metoclopromide (0.5 mg/kg every 3 hours)[12] and equal to methylprednisolone[13] in two reported randomized trials. The same drug was less effective than metoclopramide used at a higher dose (four 2-mg/kg doses) with dexamethasone, lorazepam, and benztropine in a randomized crossover trial.[14] Prochlorperazine and chlorpromazine both appeared to increase the severity and duration of nausea and vomiting compared with no antiemetics in a sequential nonrandomized study.[1] However, the majority of those patients were given relatively low doses of prochlorperazine (12.5 or 25 mg) rectally. Antihistamines are commonly used as antiemetic agents, particularly in combination with phenothiazines or metoclopramide. There are no reported studies of their efficacy as antiemetics for children receiving chemotherapy, although physicians, as reported in this survey, use them as such, even as single agents.

Metoclopramide is commonly used as an antiemetic, and in this survey was the preferred antiemetic, in combination with other drugs, for chemotherapeutic agents with severe emetogenic potential (Fig 3). Metoclopramide's use in pediatric oncology centers increased substantially from 1984 to 1988 (Fig 4), in spite of the relative lack of support from published studies. Metoclopramide hydrochloride at low doses (0.5 mg/kg every 3 hours) was shown to be less effective than chlorpromazine[12] and less effective than either methylprednisolone or domperidone[15] in comparative studies of children receiving chemotherapy. In addition, there were several reports that heavily emphasized metoclopramide's adverse side effects in children, particularly the extrapyramidal reactions.[16-18] Subsequent experience has shown that these can usually be prevented by concomitant use of diphenhydramine. The single study demonstrating superiority of metoclopramide to chlorpromazine in children (when used with dexamethasone, lorazepam, and benztropine)[14] was published after this survey was conducted. The use of lorazepam as an antiemetic also increased in spite of a paucity of literature supporting its use in children at the time of the survey. A single report mentioned its use with domperidone and dexamethasone in 1986.[19] Since this survey, however, lorazepam's efficacy in combination[14] and as a single agent at 0.05 mg/kg[20] has been reported.

Corticosteroids have been used increasingly and have received positive reports in the pediatric literature. Dexamethasone given at a dose of 1 mg/m^2 every 4 hours for 10 doses is the only agent that has been shown to be more effective than no antiemetics in a controlled trial.[10] Dexamethasone (5 to 10 mg intravenously) also decreased nausea and vomiting when added to chlorpromazine.[21] Methylprednisolone was more effective than metoclopramide or domperidone in one study,[15] and at 4 mg/kg was equal in efficacy to chlorpromazine (0.5 mg/kg) in another.[13]

Two other agents deserve mention in a discussion of antiemetics for children receiving chemotherapy, although neither was licensed for use in the United States at the time of this survey. Nabilone (0.5 to 1.0 mg orally twice a day) has been shown to be more effective than prochlorperazine (5 to 10 mg orally twice a day)[22] or domperidone (5 to 10 mg orally twice a day)[23] in randomized crossover trials. Domperidone was effective both as a single agent[24] and in combination with dexamethasone and lorazepam,[19] although it was not as effective as methylprednisolone[15] or nabilone[23] in comparative trials.

Pediatric oncologists are using an increasing number of antiemetics, often in combinations that have not been studied in children. This may incur risks, as children, particularly young children, may experience unique or more severe side effects compared with adults.[16-18,20,25] This study suggests that the choice of agents is based on experience, not on prospective controlled trials, resulting in a lack of consensus regarding appropriate antiemetic therapy for children. There are many obstacles to an organized study of antiemetics for children, the principal one being the number of available subjects. The infrequency of childhood cancer and the wide variety of types of cancer and treatment regimens make the assembly of a sizable homogeneous group difficult. Individual variation in the susceptibility to nausea and vomiting, as well as the frequent lack of complete response to pharmacologic agents in current use, are additional factors that make antiemetic studies difficult. Nonetheless, pediatric oncologists should put a priority on participating in randomized controlled trials of antiemetics to improve our present understanding of and therapy for chemotherapy-related nausea and vomiting in children. Additional studies of the four-drug regimen now in routine use (metoclopramide, diphenhydramine, dexamethasone, and lorazepam) to determine which components are the most effective would be particularly helpful. The optimal combination could then be compared with the new serotonin antagonists that are now being used in clinical trials.[26] In addition, behavioral techniques should be compared with the available pharmacologic agents. Finally, pediatric oncologists should depend more heavily on clinical trials when choosing antiemetics to quickly implement the most effective and least toxic regimens.

This study was supported in part by grant RR-125 (General Clinical Research Center) from the National Institutes of Health; and by a Clinical Oncology Career Development Award from the American Cancer Society (Dr van Hoff) (CA-205549, CA-41188, CA-33603, CA-30969). We acknowledge the members and administrative office of the Pediatric Oncology Group, St Louis, Mo, for their assistance. The following is a list of POGs participating in this study, with the principal investigators and grant number in parentheses: Alberta Pediatric Oncology Consortium, Edmonton (John Akabutu, MD); Baylor College of Medicine, Houston, Tex (Donald Fernbach, MD; CA-03161); Bowman Gray School of Medicine, Winston-Salem, NC (Richard Patterson, MD; CA-15525); Boston (Mass) Floating Hospital (Molly Schwenn, MD); Children's Hospital of Michigan, Detroit (Y. Ravindranath, MD; CA-29691); City of Hope, Duarte, Calif (Patricia Konrad, MD; CA-32278); Dana-Farber Cancer Institute, Boston, Mass (Howard Weinstein, MD; CA-41573); Duke University, Durham, NC (John Falletta, MD; CA-15525); Emory University School of Medicine, Atlanta, Ga (Abdel Ragab, MD; CA-20549); Johns Hopkins University, Baltimore, Md (Brigid Leventhal, MD; CA-28476); McGill University, Montreal, Quebec, Children's Hospital (Michael Whitehead, MD; CA-33587); Medical College of Virginia, Richmond (Harold Maurer, MD; CA-28530); Medical University of South Carolina, Charleston (Biemann Othersen, MD); Midwest Children's Cancer Center, Milwaukee, Wis (Bruce Camitta, MD; CA-32053); New England Pediatric Oncology Consortium, Providence, RI (Edwin Forman, MD; CA-29293); Mount Sinai School of Medicine, New York, NY (Jeffery Lipton, MD, PhD); Oklahoma University, Oklahoma City (R. Nitschke, MD; CA-11233); Roswell Park Memorial Institute, Buffalo, NY (Martin Brecher, MD; CA-28383); St Christopher's Hospital for Children, Philadelphia, Pa (Robert Wimmer, MD); St Jude Children's

Research Hospital, Memphis, Tenn (H-C Pui, MD; CA-31566); Stanford University, Palo Alto, Calif (Michael Link, MD; CA-33603); SUNY Health Science Center, Syracuse, NY (Ronald Dubowy, MD; CA-41721); Swiss Pediatric Oncology Group, Bern, Switzerland (Hans Wagner, MD); University of Alabama, Birmingham (R. Castleberry, MD; CA-25408); University of California, San Diego (Faith Kung, MD; CA-28439); University of Florida, Gainesville (Samuel Gross, MD; CA-29281); University of Kansas, Kansas City (Tribhawan Vats, MD; CA-28841); University of Miami (Fla) (Stuart Toledano, MD; CA-41082); University of Mississippi, Jackson (Jeanette Pullen, MD; CA-15989); University of Texas M. D. Anderson Center, Houston (Donald Pinkel, MD; CA-03713); University of Virginia, Richmond (Beverly Raney, MD); Washington University, St Louis, Mo (Vita Land, MD; CA-05587); Yale University School of Medicine, New Haven, Conn (Peter Beardsley, MD, PhD); Florida Community Clinical Oncology Program (James Talbert, MD; CA-35157).

References

1. Zeltzer LK, LeBaron S, Zeltzer PM. Paradoxical effects of prophylactic phenothiazine antiemetics in children receiving chemotherapy. *J Clin Oncol.* 1984;2:930-936.
2. Zeltzer LK, LeBaron S, Zeltzer PM. A prospective assessment of chemotherapy-related nausea and vomiting in children with cancer. *Am J Pediatr Hematol Oncol.* 1984;6:5-16.
3. Frick SB, Guzzi DelPo E, Keith JA, Davis MS. Chemotherapy-associated nausea and vomiting in pediatric oncology patients. *Cancer Nurs.* 1988;11:118-124.
4. Dolgin MJ, Katz ER, McGinty K, Siegel SE. Anticipatory nausea and vomiting in pediatric cancer patients. *Pediatrics.* 1985;75:547-552.
5. Cohen RE, Blanchard EB, Ruckdeschel JC, Smolen RC. Prevalence and correlates of posttreatment and anticipatory nausea and vomiting in cancer chemotherapy. *J Psychosom Res.* 1986;30:643-654.
6. LeBaron S, Zeltzer LK, LeBaron C, Scott SE, Zeltzer PM. Chemotherapy side effects in pediatric oncology patients: drugs, age and sex as risk factors. *Med Pediatr Oncol.* 1988;16:263-268.
7. Zeltzer L, LeBaron S, Zeltzer PM. The effectiveness of behavioral intervention for reduction of nausea and vomiting in children and adolescents receiving chemotherapy. *J Clin Oncol.* 1984;2:683-690.
8. Redd WH, Jacobsen PB, Die-Trill M, Dermatis H, McEvoy M, Holland JC. Cognitive/attentional distraction in the control of conditioned nausea in pediatric cancer patients receiving chemotherapy. *J Consult Clin Psychol.* 1987;55:391-395.
9. Hockenberry MJ, Cotanch PH. Hyphosis as adjuvant antiemetic therapy in childhood cancer. *Nurs Clin North Am.* 1985;20:105-107.
10. Sumer T, Abu-Melha A, Maqbool G, Al-Mulhim I. Dexamethasone as an antiemetic in children receiving cis-platinum. *Am J Pediatr Hematol Oncol.* 1988;10:126-128.
11. Kobrinsky NL, Pruden PB, Cheang MS, Levitt M, Bishop AJ, Tenenbein M. Increased nausea and vomiting induced by naloxone in patients receiving chemotherapy. *Am J Pediatr Hematol Oncol.* 1988;10:206-208.
12. Graham-Pole J, Weare J, Engel S, Gardner R, Mehta P, Gross S. Antiemetics in children receiving cancer chemotherapy: a double-blind prospective randomized study comparing metoclopramide with chlorpromazine. *J Clin Oncol.* 1986;4:1110-1113.
13. Mehta P, Gross S, Graham-Pole J, Gardner R. Methylprenisolone for chemotherapy-induced emesis: a double-blind randomized trial in children. *J Pediatr.* 1986;108:774-776.
14. Marshall G, Kerr S, Vowels M, O'Gorman-Hughes D, White L. Antiemetic therapy for chemotherapy-induced vomiting: metoclopramide, benztropine, dexamethasone and lorazepam regimen compared with chlorpromazine alone. *J Pediatr.* 1989;115:156-160.
15. Ise T, Ohira M, Omiya A, Hirose M, Shibata T. Clinical evaluation of antiemetics for vomiting due to cancer chemotherapy in children. *Gan To Kagaku Ryoho.* 1982;9:1108-1118.
16. Terrin BN, McWilliams NB, Maurer HM. Side effects of metoclopramide as an antiemetic in childhood cancer chemotherapy. *J Pediatr.* 1984;104:138-140.
17. Allen JC, Gralla R, Reilly L, Kellich M, Young C. Metoclopramide: dose related toxicity and preliminary antiemetic studies in children receiving cancer chemotherapy. *J Clin Oncol.* 1985;3:1136-1141.
18. Howrie DL, Felix C, Wollman M, Juhl RP, Blatt J. Metoclopramide as an antiemetic agent in pediatric oncology patients. *Drug Intelligence Clin Pharm.* 1986;20:122-124.
19. Ekert H, Carden PA, Mitchell SL. Multiple drug antiemetic therapy. *J Clin Oncol.* 1986;4:1016.
20. van Hoff J, Olszewski D. Lorazepam for the control of chemotherapy-related nausea and vomiting in children. *J Pediatr.* 1988;113:146-149.
21. Khan AB, Bucklew CA, Levanthal BG. Effectiveness of decadron and thorazine in prevention of nausea and vomiting induced by chemotherapy in pediatric patients. *Proc Am Soc Clin Oncol.* 1983;2:78. Abstract.
22. Chan HSL, Correia JA, MacLeod SM. Nabilone versus prochloperazine for control of cancer chemotherapy-induced emesis in children: a double-blind, crossover trial. *Pediatrics.* 1987;79:946-952.
23. Dalzell AM, Bartlett H, Lilleyman JS. Nabilone: an alternative antiemetic for cancer chemotherapy. *Arch Dis Child.* 1986;61:502-505.
24. O'Meara A, Mott MG. Domperidone as an antiemetic in pediatric oncology. *Cancer Chemother Pharmacol.* 1981;6:147-149.
25. Kofoed PE, Kamper J. Extrapyramidal reactions caused by antiemetics during cancer chemotherapy. *J Pediatr.* 1984;105:852.
26. Einhorn LH, Nagy C, Werner K, Finn AL. Ondansetron: a new antiemetic for patients receiving cisplatin chemotherapy. *J Clin Oncol.* 1990;8:731-735.

Injuries and Poisonings in Out-of-Home Child Care and Home Care

Walter J. Gunn, PhD; Paul F. Pinsky, MPH; Jeffrey J. Sacks, MD, MPH; Lawrence B. Schonberger, MD, MPH

• As part of a national telephone survey regarding health events associated with out-of-home child care, data regarding poisonings and injuries were collected. Of 171 reported poisonings, none occurred during out-of-home child care. The rate of injury during out-of-home child care was 1.69 per 100 000 child-hours compared with 2.66 for home care. Overall injury rates were slightly higher for children who attended out-of-home child care than for those who do not. This occurred because children who attended out-of-home child care had a higher injury rate during home care than did the children who did not attend out-of-home child care at all. Although out-of-home child care may carry an increased risk of infectious disease relative to home care, it does not appear to carry an increased risk of injury and, in fact, may confer a lower risk.
(*AJDC*. 1991;145:779-781)

Recent studies have raised concern that out-of-home child care (OHC) may expose children to an excessive risk of injury.[1-8] In the first study to document that OHC was as safe, if not safer, than home care (HC), Rivara and coworkers[9] calculated a medically attended injury rate of 2.50 per 100 000 child-hours for OHC compared with 4.88 for HC. As part of a national telephone survey conducted in 1987 about health events associated with OHC, we report herein on data we obtained about injuries and poisonings.

METHODS

The nationwide random-digit dialing clustered-sample telephone survey has been described in detail elsewhere.[10] Briefly, to compare rates of health events between OHC and HC, the study was designed to enroll at least 262 children in OHC and 262 children with no OHC in each of three age groups: 6 weeks to 17 months, 18 to 35 months, and 36 to 59 months. These age groups were chosen, in part, to facilitate separate data analysis for diapered and nondiapered children for the study of infectious disease–related issues.

Accepted for publication September 11, 1990.

From the Division of Viral and Rickettsial Diseases, Center for Infectious Diseases (Drs Gunn and Schonberger and Mr Pinsky), and the Division of Injury Control, Center for Environmental Health and Injury Control (Dr Sacks), Centers for Disease Control, Public Health Service, US Department of Health and Human Services, Atlanta, Ga.

Reprint requests to the Center for Infectious Diseases, Centers for Disease Control, MS A-32, Atlanta, GA 30333 (Dr Gunn).

For the present study, OHC was defined as spending 10 hours or more per week in any care setting outside the child's home for at least a 4-week period during the year preceding the interview. Part-year OHC was defined as attending OHC for less than 12 months during the preceding year. Home care was defined as the time not spent in OHC. A child with no exposure to OHC was classified as "HC only."

Of a total of 35 000 households called, 28 500 (81%) participated, and 2853 households had children under 5 years of age. Based on enrollment needs in each age and OHC-exposure group, detailed information regarding child care and health events was collected from 1775 households that included 2250 children under 5 years of age.

An adult respondent was asked the following questions: "During the past year, have any of your children had an accident or injury that required a visit to a doctor or hospital?" "During the past year, has there been any incident where you had to contact a doctor or poison control center about a possible poisoning of one of your children?" Information was collected regarding the nature and place of occurrence of each injury or poisoning event, but not the date or time.

Dates of enrollment and average hours per week in each OHC setting were used to calculate site-specific OHC hours at risk. Because 98% of all childhood injuries occur between 7 AM and 10 PM,[11] we assumed that a child was at risk of injury 15 hours per day (105 hours per week). Home care hours at risk were then calculated as 105 hours minus the weekly hours spent in OHC.

Overall rates per 100 child-years and site-specific rates per

Injury rate per 100 000 child-hours by age group and location. Black bars indicate home care; shaded bars, out-of-home care.

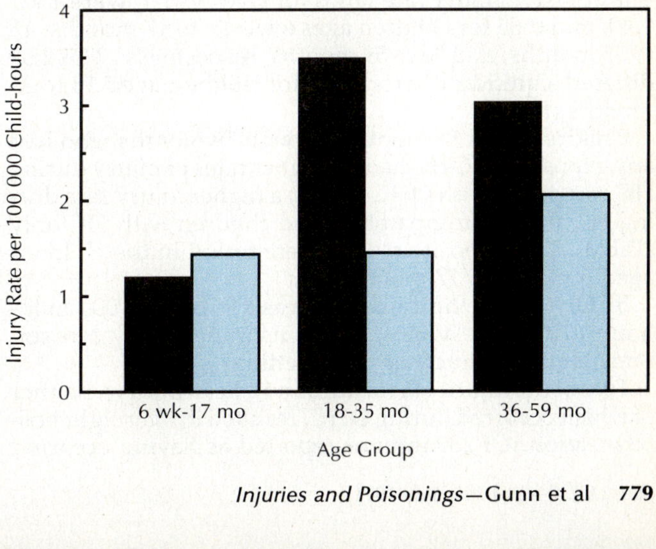

Rate of Injury per 100 000 Child-hours by Age Group and OHC Exposure*								
	Injury Rate per 100 000 Child-hours							
	6 wk-17mo		18-35 mo		36-59 mo		Total	
OHC Exposure	HC	OHC	HC	OHC	HC	OHC	HC	OHC
Any OHC	0.89	1.43	4.63	1.42	3.59	2.04	3.40†	1.69‡
HC only	1.28	. . .	3.00	. . .	2.63	. . .	2.31	. . .
Total§	1.20	1.43	3.50	1.42	3.02	2.04	2.66	1.69

*OHC indicates out-of-home care; HC, home care.
†The rate for full-year OHC=4.35; part-year OHC=2.61.
‡The OHC rate for full-year OHC=1.47; part-year OHC=2.16.
§Any OHC plus HC only.

100 000 child-hours for both injuries and poisonings were calculated for the three age groups (6 weeks to 17 months, 18 to 35 months, and 36 to 59 months) and for three OHC-exposure groups (HC only, part-year OHC, and full-year OHC). To ensure the independence of all observations within an age group, only one child, the youngest, was selected from any one household. Rates were adjusted for the probability of selection imposed by the sampling plan. Rate ratios were adjusted for age, family income, and region; 95% confidence intervals were calculated with the method of Breslow and Day.[12] Statistical comparisons were performed only within age groups.

For descriptive purposes, all eligible children in the household were used in the following analyses: injury rate by type of OHC, type of injuries during OHC and HC, and aggregate injury rates for all age groups combined. Because of the nonindependence of these observations, no statistical comparisons were made.

RESULTS

Injuries

The overall injury rate was 15.2 per 100 child-years. For those aged 6 weeks to 17 months, the overall rate was 7.3 per 100 child-years compared with 18.7 for those aged 18 to 35 months and 17.3 for those aged 36 to 59 months. For children with HC only, the injury rate was 13.6 per 100 child-years compared with 17.8 for children with any exposure to OHC (children in full-year OHC, 20.2; children in part-year OHC, 15.4). The adjusted injury rate ratios for any OHC vs HC only were 0.77, 1.32, and 1.23 for children aged 6 weeks to 17 months, 18 to 35 months, and 36 to 59 months, respectively. The 95% confidence interval for all of these ratios included one.

The injury rate for OHC was 1.69 per 100 000 child-hours compared with 2.66 for HC. The effect of OHC on injury rate differed with age (Figure); only the two older age groups showed a decreased injury rate during OHC. The adjusted injury rate ratios for OHC vs HC were 1.22, 0.40, and 0.65 for children ages 6 weeks to 17 months, 18 to 35 months, and 36 to 59 months, respectively. This risk differed significantly from one for children aged 18 to 35 months ($P=.02$).

Children aged 18 months through 59 months who had any exposure to OHC had (1) higher rates of injury during HC compared with OHC and (2) a higher injury rate during HC than in comparably aged children with HC only (Table). The opposite results were found in the children aged 6 weeks to 17 months.

By OHC type, the injury rate was 3.95 per 100 000 child-hours in day-care homes, 2.18 in institutional day-care settings, and 0.74 in other OHC settings.

Two of the injuries (a fracture and a head injury), neither of which occurred during OHC, resulted in overnight hospitalization. Of 280 injuries reported as having occurred during HC, 76.1% occurred in the child's own home or yard. Cuts and bruises were the most common injuries (40.4%) during HC, followed by head injuries (16.8%), eye injuries (7.9%), and fractures (5.7%). Of 24 injuries occurring during OHC, head injuries were the most common (37.5%), followed by cuts and bruises (25.0%) and fractures (4.2%). Six burns occurred during HC compared with none during OHC.

Poisonings

Of 171 poisonings, none occurred during OHC. The poisoning agents were medicines (50 [29.2%]), chemicals (32 [18.7%]), plants (30 [17.5%]), cleaning agents (25 [14.6%]), and other agents (34 [19.9%]). The agent differed with the age of the child; for those aged 6 weeks to 17 months, plants were the leading cause (40.0%); for those aged 18 to 35 months, chemicals (25.6%); and for those aged 36 to 59 months, medicines (45.9%). The pattern of poisoning rates was similar to that for injuries. For each age group, the HC poisoning rate for those who attended OHC was higher than that for children with HC only.

COMMENT

Our results suggest that the rate of injury and poisoning is lower during OHC than HC. However, the child who attends OHC has a higher rate of injury during HC than does the child who does not attend OHC at all. Indeed, the overall injury rate was slightly higher for children who attended OHC than for those who did not.

Injury rates during OHC and HC are not directly comparable, because the times of day and days of the week were distributed differently between the two. For children who attend OHC, HC hours are mainly during evenings and weekends; OHC hours are mainly daytime weekday hours. For the HC only group, HC hours reflect a mixture of weekday, weekend, and evening hours. Because childhood injuries are more likely to occur during daytime than evening hours and are more likely to occur on weekdays than weekends,[11] adjusting for the differing time periods would presumably further decrease the OHC rate relative to the HC rate.

Ascertainment and recall problems may have affected our results. Parents may not have been as aware of injuries and poisonings occurring during OHC as during HC. If an OHC provider's call to a poison control center determined that an exposure did not warrant treatment, the parents may not have been told about the event, and we may therefore have underestimated OHC poisonings. However, because reported injuries were medically attended ones, either the OHC provider took the child for medical care without telling the parents or parents did not recall injuries that occur during OHC as well as those that occur during HC. We think both possibilities are unlikely. For those in the full-year OHC group, the HC injury rate was markedly higher (4.35) than the OHC rate (1.47); for those in the part-year OHC group, the HC rate (2.61) was more similar to the OHC rate (2.16). Because the midpoint of OHC exposure in the year preceding the study was further from the interview date in the full-year OHC group than in the part-year OHC group, injuries that occurred during OHC presumably occurred further from the interview date for the full-year OHC group. Thus, recall problems about location may have been greater for the full-year OHC group.

Beyond recall problems, differences in supervision, behavior, and environment may explain why children with any OHC have higher injury rates during HC. After work, parents of children exposed to OHC may have to spend time preparing meals or otherwise managing the home instead of supervising the child. Parents of children in full-time HC may be able to accomplish such tasks while the child naps. On release from the structured, controlled OHC environment, children may exhibit more reckless behavior; the child in full-time HC may exhibit more constant behavior. Some parents may place hard-to-manage children in OHC. The HC environments of children in OHC may not be as completely "child-proofed" as those of children in full-time HC. Further research should verify whether the rate differences remain, explore potential explanations, and define the time and circumstances of injuries in HC.

Based on reports from child-care center directors, Sacks and coworkers[5] calculated a medically attended injury rate of 1.56 per 100 000 child-hours for children under 5 years of age in child-care centers. This figure is 28% lower than our estimate (2.18) for injuries in child-care centers. The rate estimates of Rivara et al,[9] on the other hand, are 83% higher than ours for HC (4.88 vs 2.66) and 48% higher than ours for OHC (2.50 vs 1.69). That our results are intermediate and that our findings confirm those of Rivara et al suggest that our estimates are reasonable and not grossly distorted from biases.

Despite the limitations of our study, we believe that our analysis sheds light on the relative safety of OHC and HC. The data on poisonings overwhelmingly favor OHC as being safer. Although OHC, compared with HC, may carry an increased risk of infectious disease,[13] it does not appear to carry an increased risk of injury and, in fact, may confer a lower risk of injury.

References

1. Aronson SS. Injuries in child care. *Young Children.* 1983;38:19-20.
2. Landman PF, Landman GB. Accidental injuries in children in day-care centers. *AJDC.* 1987;141:292-293.
3. Elardo R, Solomons HC, Snider BC. An analysis of accidents at a day care center. *Am J Orthopsychiatry.* 1987;57:60-65.
4. Chang A, Lugg MM, Nebedum A. Injuries among preschool children enrolled in day-care centers. *Pediatrics.* 1989;83:272-277.
5. Sacks JJ, Smith JD, Kaplan KM, Lambert DA, Sattin RW, Sikes RK. The epidemiology of injuries in Atlanta day-care centers. *JAMA.* 1989;262:1641-1645.
6. O'Connor MA, Boyle WE, O'Connor GT, Letellier R. Injury prevention practices in daycare centers. Presented at the 115th Annual Meeting of the American Public Health Association; October 20, 1987; New Orleans, La.
7. Davis WS, McCarthy PL. Safety in day-care centers. *AJDC.* 1988;142:386. Abstract.
8. Wasserman RC, Dameron DO, Brozicevic MM, Aronson RA. Injury hazards in home day care. *J Pediatr.* 1989;114:591-593.
9. Rivara FP, DiGuiseppi C, Thompson RS, Calonge N. Risk of injury to children less than 5 years of age in day care versus home care settings. *Pediatrics.* 1989;84:1011-1016.
10. Hurwitz ES, Gunn WJ, Pinsky PF, Schoenberger LB. A nationwide study of the risk of respiratory illness associated with day-care attendance. *Pediatrics.* 1991;87:62-69.
11. Westfeldt J. Environmental factors in childhood accidents: a prospective study in Goteborg, Sweden. *Acta Paediatr Scand.* 1982;291(suppl):1-75.
12. Breslow NE, Day NE. *Statistical Methods in Cancer Research.* Lyon, France: International Agency for Research on Cancer; 1982;2:scientific publications.
13. Johansen AS, Leibowitz A, Waite LJ. Child care and children's illness. *Am J Public Health.* 1988;78:1175-1177.

A Longitudinal Study of Birth Weight and Being Overweight in Late Adolescence

Daniel S. Seidman, MD; Arie Laor, MD; Rena Gale, MD; David K. Stevenson, MD; Yehuda L. Danon, MD

• A total of 33 413 infants born in Jerusalem between 1964 and 1971 were followed up at 17 years of age by matching computerized database files. A logistic regression model was used to estimate the odds ratios for being overweight at 17 years of age for 500-g birth weight categories from less than 2500 g to 4500 g or greater. Information on the ethnic origin, paternal education, birth order, maternal age, and area of residence at birth was available, and these factors were used as possible confounders. The adjusted odds ratios for being overweight (≥90th percentile; body mass index >24.6 kg/m²) and severely overweight (≥97th percentile; body mass index >27.8 kg/m²) at 17 years of age was elevated for the three birth weight categories above the normal reference category of 3000 to 3499 g, with an estimate of 2.16 and 2.30 for male subjects with a birth weight greater than 4500 g and 2.95 and 4.39 for female subjects. The data suggest that higher birth weights correlate strongly with being overweight in late adolescence independently of other factors considered. However, the predictive power of this association is poor.

***(AJDC.* 1991;145:782-785)**

Obesity is a well-established health hazard.[1] As the long-term results of treatment are discouraging, more attention is being directed toward prevention and the study of groups at particular risk. The possible association of being overweight during infancy and adult obesity is important, because it may contribute to our understanding of genetic, metabolic, and environmental predisposing factors.[2] The relationship of adult obesity with weight at 1 year of age or older has been recognized.[3,4] However, a predictive pattern for adult obesity is still not proved regarding birth weight.[2,5]

The discrepancies found between results of previous studies that examined the link between birth weight and being overweight as an adult may be due to short follow-up periods,[6,7] recall bias,[8] and limited sample size.[9,10] We examined the risk for being overweight at 17 years of age by birth weight in a sample of 33 413 subjects born in Jerusalem, Israel.

SUBJECTS AND METHODS

The study population consisted of 33 413 subjects born in Jerusalem between 1964 and 1971. Birth weights, recorded at the time of delivery, were obtained from the computerized files of the Jerusalem Perinatal Study.[11,12] The Jerusalem Perinatal Study was a population-based study that included all of the deliveries at the three major obstetric wards in Jerusalem during the years 1964 through 1976. Body weight and height measurements at 17 years of age, as well as detailed demographic data, were available from the Israel Defence Forces draft medical examination computerized records.[13] Standing body height was measured without shoes to the nearest 1 cm, and nude body weight was determined to the nearest 100 g. The data for each individual were matched with use of a seven-digit identification number. The completeness of the match was confirmed by comparing sex and maternal identity number. Females consisted of only 38.3% of our study population, because girls who declare themselves to be orthodox religious are exempt from compulsory service.[13] The results are thus presented separately for male and female subjects. Only a negligible minority of patients hospitalized for severe chronic and psychiatric diseases and long-term prisoners were not examined and consequently were not included in our data.[13]

A multiple logistic regression analysis with the Logist procedure of SAS software[14] was performed by a stepwise method to adjust for the effect of the studied independent variables. Separate models were estimated for male and female subjects. Being overweight, and being severely overweight, were used as dependent variables. Overweight was defined as a body mass index (body weight in kilograms/[height in meters]²) equal to or greater than the 90th percentile of 17-year-old male and female adolescents examined at the Israel Defence Forces draft board (>24.6 kg/m² for both male and female subjects). Severely overweight was defined as a body mass index equal to or greater than that at the 97th percentile of the same population (>27.8 kg/m² for male subjects and >27.7 kg/m² for female subjects). The independent variables used in the analysis were birth weight (500-g categories from <2500 g to ≥4500 g to provide a clinically relevant estimate of the associated risk), ethnic origin (defined according to paternal country of birth), area of residence (classified by municipal tax level areas[12]), maternal age (as a continuous variable), paternal educational attainment level, and birth order (categorized to avoid dubious assumptions about linearity). All variables that were significant at the .05 level were added to a model that contained the birth weight variable.

The results of the logistic regressions are presented as adjusted odds ratios and their 95% confidence intervals (ie, $e^{b \pm 1.96s}$, where b is the logistic regression coefficient and s is its estimated standard error). The estimates presented are based on the exclusion of cases with missing values (1.9%).

Accepted for publication January 29, 1991.

From the Department of Obstetrics and Gynecology, Sheba Medical Center, Tel-Hashomer, Israel (Dr Seidman); the Medical Statistics Branch, Israel Defence Forces Medical Corps (Dr Laor and Danon); the Department of Neonatology, Bikur Cholim Hospital, Jerusalem, Israel (Dr Gale); the Department of Pediatrics, Stanford (Calif) University School of Medicine (Dr Stevenson); and the Division of Pediatric Immunology, Belinson Medical Center, Sackler School of Medicine, Tel-Aviv (Israel) University (Dr Danon).

Reprint requests to the Department of Obstetrics and Gynecology, Sheba Medical Center, Tel-Hashomer 52621, Israel (Dr Seidman).

Table 1.—Distribution of Population Characteristics and Prevalence of Overweight and Severely Overweight at 17 Years of Age Among 33 547 Subjects Born in Jerusalem, Israel, Between 1964 and 1971*

Population Characteristics	Male (n=20 747) % of Population	Male % Overweight	Male % Severely Overweight	Female (n=12 666) % of Population	Female % Overweight	Female % Severely Overweight
All	100.0	10.2	3.0	100.0	10.1	3.1
Ethnic origin†						
Israel	14.9	12.4‡	4.2‡	13.1	9.4	3.5§
Asia	33.3	10.2	2.6	34.7	10.5	3.0
Africa	23.5	7.9	2.2	23.3	11.1	3.9
West	28.3	12.4	3.6	28.9	9.3	2.3
Paternal educational attainment, y of schooling						
<8	37.2	10.4	2.8§	36.8	11.6‡	4.0§
8-12	38.7	10.8	3.5	37.9	9.8	2.7
>12	24.1	9.5	2.8	25.3	8.1	2.1
Birth order						
1	28.2	10.6	3.3	32.7	10.0	3.3
2	23.3	9.5	2.7	26.6	9.6	2.9
3-4	26.8	10.4	3.1	26.7	10.0	2.7
≥5	21.7	10.4	3.0	14.0	11.5	3.3
Area of residence, municipal tax level						
High	26.3	10.6	3.3	26.0	8.7§	3.0
Medium	33.8	10.5	3.2	34.3	10.5	3.0
Low	39.9	9.7	2.8	39.7	10.8	3.1
Birth weight, g						
<2500	4.7	9.2‡	2.9‡	5.3	8.2§	2.6‡
2500-2999	16.3	7.9	2.0	22.8	8.4	2.6
3000-3499	41.2	9.4	2.8	45.2	9.6	2.8
3500-3999	28.8	11.3	3.4	21.7	12.5	3.8
4000-4499	7.8	15.1	4.9	4.5	13.2	4.9
≥4500	1.2	18.2	6.0	0.5	23.3	10.0

*Overweight was defined as body mass index greater than 24.6 kg/m², and severely overweight was defined as body mass index greater than 27.8 kg/m².
†Ethnic origin was defined by paternal country of birth.
‡χ^2 test comparing overweight and severely overweight groups with the total population, $P<.001$.
§χ^2 test comparing overweight and severely overweight groups with the total population, $P<.01$.

RESULTS

Table 1 gives the percentage of overweight and severely overweight 17-year-old subjects according to the independent variables included in the analyses. The table also indicates that ethnic origin, paternal educational attainment level, and area of residence are associated with significantly different rates of overweight and severely overweight subjects. A strong and apparently linear link is observed between birth weights of more than 3000 g and the prevalence of being both overweight and severely overweight, regardless of sex.

The association of the birth weight groups with being overweight was analyzed with the use of multiple logistic regression to control for the effects of confounding variables. All of the variables in Table 1 were analyzed. The final model for overweight reached by the stepwise procedure included the birth weight variable and four confounders (paternal education, area of residence, ethnic origin, and birth order) for male subjects and only one confounder (paternal education) for female subjects (Table 2). The final regression model for severely overweight eliminated all independent variables, except birth weight and two confounders (paternal education and ethnic origin for male subjects and paternal education and maternal age for female subjects) (Table 3). Logistic analysis of these data confirmed the significant ($P<.001$) positive association between birth weights of 3000 g or more and being overweight and severely overweight at 17 years of age (Tables 2 and 3).

COMMENT

Higher birth weight was found to be a risk factor for obesity in late adolescence. To our knowledge, ours is the first study of its kind based on a large data base of recorded birth weights and a long follow-up period of 17 years. The results may thus shed light on the conflicting data reported in previously published studies. Some investigators have found a clear-cut relationship between birth weight and obesity in later childhood[6,15,16]; others have found no cor-

Table 2.—Adjusted Odds Ratios for Being Overweight at 17 Years of Age Among 33 547 Subjects Born in Jerusalem, Israel, Between 1964 and 1971*

	Adjusted Odds Ratios (95% Confidence Interval)	
Birth weight, g	Males (n=20 324)	Females (n=12 672)
<2500	1.04 (0.79-1.28)	0.83 (0.62-1.10)
2500-2999	0.81 (0.69-0.94)	0.87 (0.74-1.02)
3000-3499†	1.00	1.00
3500-3999	1.25 (1.12-1.39)	1.34 (1.16-1.54)
4000-4499	1.72 (1.74-2.02)	1.35 (1.03-1.77)
≥4500	2.16 (1.54-3.04)	2.95 (1.59-5.49)

*Overweight was defined as body mass index greater than 24.6 kg/m^2.
†Reference group.

Table 3.—Adjusted Odds Ratios for Being Severely Overweight at 17 Years of Age Among 33 547 Subjects Born in Jerusalem, Israel, Between 1964 and 1971*

	Adjusted Odds Ratios(95% Confidence Interval)	
Birth Weight, g	Males (n=20 324)	Females (n=12 672)
<2500	1.09 (0.72-1.64)	0.93 (0.56-1.54)
2500-2999	0.74 (0.56-0.98)	0.94 (0.71-1.25)
3000-3499†	1.00	1.00
3500-3999	1.26 (1.04-1.54)	1.41 (1.09-1.82)
4000-4499	1.83 (1.40-2.40)	1.79 (1.36-2.76)
≥4500	2.30 (1.33-3.95)	4.39 (1.82-10.58)

*Severely overweight was defined as body mass index greater than 27.8 kg/m^2.
†Reference group.

relation between high birth weight and subsequent obesity.[5,9,10] A high correlation between birth weight and adult body mass is usually attributed to a genetic effect. The variance in birth weight has been shown to be largely determined by fetal genes.[17] Obesity has similarly been found to be strongly dependent on genetic factors.[18] Common mechanisms affecting both birth weight and adult obesity have therefore been suggested, including an inborn error in adipose tissue regulation and inherited abnormal mechanisms controlling food intake and systemic energy expenditure.[19] None of these hypotheses has been substantiated thus far, and the influence of genetic factors on the development and structure of adipose tissue in humans is poorly understood.[20]

Ethnic and environmental factors may also have an important influence on adult body weight. Medical insurance is widely available in Israel, and almost the entire population (95%) is insured in one of the nation's sick funds.[21] Virtually all of the mothers thus receive prenatal care as well as perinatal and child care at one of the Mother and Child Health Centers.[12,21] The effect of birth weight was adjusted in our study for the possible confounding effects of ethnic origin[22,23] and socioeconomic status (determined according to paternal education attainment level and area of residence).[24] However, it was not possible to control for the influence of parental body mass. We have recently shown that birth weight is significantly ($P<.001$) related in the Jerusalem population to maternal prepregnant body mass.[25]

Overweight mothers may be more likely to overfeed their infants.[26] Such a trend toward infantile overnutrition may predispose to obesity in later childhood and adulthood.[27] This suggestion is consistent with the possible causative role of adipose cell hyperplasia largely determined in early life.[20,28] Mossberg[15] has recently shown that the degree of obesity in parents is among the most important factors for weight level in adulthood.

Eid[7] suggested that infants with a lower birth weight may gain weight more rapidly than those with a higher birth weight and may therefore be at a greater risk of subsequent obesity. Binkin et al[6] have recently shown that although infants with low birth weight exhibit proportionately greater weight gain in the first year of life, they tend to remain shorter and lighter in early childhood compared with children with higher birth weights. We found the body mass at 17 years of age of low-birth-weight (<2500 g) infants not to differ from that of the reference group (birth weight 3000 to 3499 g). However, the possibility that below-average birth weight (2500 to 2999 g) may offer some long-term benefit in terms of reduced obesity in adulthood could be suggested. It should be remembered that we could not fully assess the effect of intrauterine growth retardation on future growth, as gestational age was unavailable.

Our results may increase our ability to identify those children who are more prone to becoming overweight adults and to more clearly define risk groups. However, despite the observation that in contrast to the normal-birth-weight group a greater proportion of the overweight subjects had higher birth weights, the predictive power of this association is poor. In fact, most of the overweight adults in our study had normal birth weights. The search for predictive markers for adult obesity continues as data linking high body mass index in early adulthood with mortality are accumulating.[29,30] Van Itallie[30] has suggested that being overweight during early adulthood is even more dangerous than a similar degree of being overweight in later adult life. Nevertheless, despite the increased risk for obese children of being obese as adults,[31] a weight-reducing diet very early in life could be harmful to the child's growth and development.[32] Our results imply that although being overweight at birth increases the risk of being overweight in late adolescence, it has little predictive power and may reflect body build more than adiposity.

This work was supported in part by the Doron Foundation, Tel-Aviv, Israel.

References

1. National Institutes of Health consensus development conference statement: health implications of obesity. *Ann Intern Med.* 1985;103:1073-1077.
2. Johnson FE. Health implications of childhood obesity. *Ann Intern Med.* 1985;103:1068-1072.
3. Stark O, Atkins E, Wolff OH, Douglas JWB. Longitudinal study of obesity in the National Survey of Health and Development. *BMJ.* 1981;283:13-17.
4. Charney E, Chamblee Goodman H, McBride M, Lyon B, Pratt R. Childhood antecendents of adult obesity: do chubby infants become obese adults? *N Engl J Med.* 1976;295:6-9.
5. Heald FP, Hollander RJ. The relationship between obesity in adolescence and early growth. *J Pediatr.* 1965;67:35-38.
6. Binkin NJ, Yip R, Fleshood L, Trowbridge FL. Birth weight and childhood growth. *Pediatrics.* 1988;82:828-834.
7. Eid EE. Follow-up study of physical growth of children who had excessive weight gain in first six months of life. *BMJ.* 1970;2:74-76.
8. Rimm IJ, Rimm AA. Association between juvenile onset obesity and severe adult obesity in 73,532 women. *Am J Public Health.* 1976;66:479-481.
9. Wolf OH. Obesity in childhood. *Q J Med.* 1955;24:109-123.
10. Bruch H. Obesity in childhood. *AJDC.* 1939;58:457-484.

11. Davies AM, Prywes R, Tzur B, et al. The Jerusalem Perinatal Study, I: design and organization of a continuing, community-based, record-linked survey. *Isr J Med Sci.* 1969;5:1095-1101.
12. Harlap S, Davies AM, Grover NB, Prywes R. The Jerusalem Perinatal Study: the first decade 1964-1973. *Isr J Med Sci.* 1977;13:1073-1082.
13. Kark JD, Kedem R, Revach M. Medical examination of Israeli 17-year-olds before military service as a national resource for health information. *Isr J Med Sci.* 1986;22:318-325.
14. SAS Institute Inc. *SAS User's Group International Supplemental Library Users' Guide, Version 5 Edition.* Cary, NC: SAS Institute Inc; 1986:269-293.
15. Mossberg HO. 40-year follow up of overweight children. *Lancet.* 1989;2:491-493.
16. Fisch RO, Bilek MK, Vlstrom R. Obesity and leanness at birth and their relationship to body habitus in later childhood. *Pediatrics.* 1975;56:521-528.
17. Magnus P, Berg K, Bjerkedal T, Nance WE. Parental determinants of birth weight. *Clin Genet.* 1984;26:397-405.
18. Sorensen TIA, Price RA, Stankard AJ, Schulsinger F. Genetics of obesity in adult adoptees and their biological siblings. *BMJ.* 1989;298:87-90.
19. Leible RL, Hirsch J. Metabolic characterization of obesity. *Ann Intern Med.* 1985;103:1000-1002.
20. Greenwood MRC. Adipose tissue: cellular morphology and development. *Ann Intern Med.* 1985;103:996-999.
21. Samueloff A, Mor-Yosef S, Seidman DS, et al. The 1984 National Perinatal Census: design, organization and uses for assessing obstetric services in Israel. *Isr J Med Sci.* 1989;25:629-634.
22. Shiono PH, Klebanoff MA, Graubord BI, Berendes HW, Rhoads GG. Birth weight among women of different ethnic groups. *JAMA.* 1986;255:38-52.
23. Rona RJ, Chinn S. National study of health and growth: social and biological factors associated with weight-for-height and triceps skinfold of children from ethnic groups in England. *Ann Hum Biol.* 1987;14:231-248.
24. Power C, Moynihan C. Social class and changes in weight-for-height between childhood and early adulthood. *Int J Obes.* 1988;12:445-453.
25. Seidman DS, Ever-Hadani P, Gale R. The effect of maternal weight gain in pregnancy on birth weight. *Obstet Gynecol.* 1989;74:240-246.
26. Mogan J. Parental weight and its relation to infant feeding patterns and infant obesity. *Int J Nurs Stud.* 1986;23:255-264.
27. Taitz LS. Infantile overnutrition among artificially fed infants in the Sheffield region. *BMJ.* 1971;1:315-316.
28. Brook CDG, Lloyd JK, Wolf OH. Relation between age of onset of obesity and size and number of adipose cells. *BMJ.* 1972;2:25-27.
29. Hoffmans MDAF, Kromhout D, de Lezenne Coulander C. Body mass index at the age of 18 and its effects on 32-year mortality from coronary heart disease and cancer. *J Clin Epidemiol.* 1989;42:513-520.
30. Van Itallie TB. Health implications of overweight and obesity in the United States. *Ann Intern Med.* 1985;103:983-988.
31. Rolland-Cachera MF, Deheeger M, Avons P, Guilloud-Bataille M, Patois E, Sempe M. Tracking adiposity patterns from 1 month to adulthood. *Ann Hum Biol.* 1987;14:219-222.
32. Rolland-Cachera MHF, Bellisle F. Timing weight-control measures in obese children. *Lancet.* 1990;1:918.

Guidelines for Auditing Pediatric Blood Transfusion Practices

Victor S. Blanchette, FRCP(UK), FRCP(C); Heather A. Hume, FRCP(C); Gary J. Levy, MD; Naomi L. C. Luban, MD; Ronald G. Strauss, MD

• Although transfusion of blood products is an essential and potentially life-saving measure, not all blood transfusions are beneficial to patients. The associated risks, particularly transfusion-transmitted viral illnesses, such as hepatitis and acquired immunodeficiency syndrome, require that careful consideration be given before a decision is made to transfuse any blood product. Many institutions have established a local committee to monitor transfusion practices and audit such practices regularly. To assist in this task, the Pediatric Hemotherapy Committee of the American Association of Blood Banks has developed guidelines for the conduct of pediatric blood transfusion audits. These guidelines, summarized herein, cover transfusion of red blood cells, platelets, white blood cells, fresh-frozen plasma, albumin, and clotting concentrates. The use of cytomegalovirus low-risk and irradiated blood products is also discussed. Throughout the report, special attention is given to the transfusion needs of newborn infants.

***(AJDC.* 1991;145:787-796)**

Transfusions are essential in many clinical situations. Although current blood-banking practices have reduced the risks of transfusion, transmission of infections, particularly hepatitis C, continues to be of concern.[1] Fortunately, transmission of the human immunodeficiency virus type 1, the cause of the acquired immunodeficiency syndrome, is now very rare.[2] Noninfectious risks include immune-mediated hemolytic and allergic reactions, graft-vs-host disease, and iron overload. Because of these risks, it is recommended that informed consent be obtained and documented for all nonemergency blood transfusions,[3] and decisions to transfuse blood products should reflect consideration of the risk/benefit ratio. Auditing of transfusion practices is one method of addressing this issue.

Transfusion practice guidelines, developed to assist in conducting audits, simply provide a list of acceptable clinical circumstances in which transfusions may be given without need for additional justification. However, they should not serve as absolute indications for transfusion therapy. On the one hand, not all patients eligible to receive a transfusion according to the guidelines would actually benefit from one; on the other hand, some transfusions judged inappropriate by guidelines may be justified because of special clinical circumstances. Such transfusions require explanation, a task that usually involves review of the patient's medical records or a request for additional information from the patient's physician by the local transfusion committee.

Given this background, the Pediatric Hemotherapy Committee of the American Association of Blood Banks has developed guidelines for auditing pediatric transfusions (Tables 1 through 7). These criteria apply to infants and children younger than 18 years, except when otherwise stated; statements in the tables that are underlined require additional definition by each local transfusion committee. This format was selected to permit flexibility and to ensure consistency with local standards of practice.

TRANSFUSION OF WHOLE BLOOD OR RECONSTITUTED WHOLE BLOOD

Reconstituted whole blood (red blood cells [RBCs] reconstituted with fresh-frozen plasma [FFP]) or whole blood (≤5 days old) may be given without the need for further justification in the setting of massive transfusions (Table 1). Acute blood loss (in the absence of documented coagulation abnormalities) should be treated with whole blood or reconstituted whole blood only when replacement of losses with

Table 1.—Criteria for Transfusion of Whole Blood or Reconstituted Whole Blood

1. Massive transfusion or acute blood loss (>1 blood volume* in < 24 h)
2. Exchange transfusion
3. Cardiovascular bypass surgery
4. Extracorporeal membrane oxygenation

*Estimated as 70 mL/kg of body weight.

Accepted for publication January 10, 1991.

From the Department of Paediatrics, Hospital for Sick Children, Toronto, Canada (Dr Blanchette); the Department of Pediatrics, Hôpital St Justine, Montreal, Canada (Dr Hume); Louisiana Blood Center, Shreveport (Dr Levy); the Division of Laboratory Medicine, Children's Hospital National Medical Center, Department of Pediatrics and Pathology, George Washington University School of Medicine, Washington, DC (Dr Luban); and the Department of Pathology and Pediatrics, DeGowin Memorial Blood Center, University of Iowa Hospitals and Clinics, Iowa City, Iowa (Dr Strauss).

This report expresses the opinions of the authors and does not represent official policy of the American Association of Blood Banks.

Reprint requests to the American Association of Blood Banks, 1717 N 19th St, Arlington, VA 22209.

Table 2.—Criteria for Transfusion of Red Blood Cells*
Neonates younger than 4 months
1. Venous hemoglobin level <130 g/L in neonates <24 h old
2. Hemoglobin level <130 g/L and severe pulmonary disease, cyanotic heart disease, or heart failure
3. Acute blood loss ≥10% of total blood volume
4. Phlebotomy losses ≥5%-10% of the total blood volume
5. Hemoglobin level <80 g/L in stable newborn infants with clinical manifestations of anemia
Patients 4 months of age
1. Significant preoperative anemia; intraoperative blood loss ≥15% of total blood volume; postoperative hemoglobin level <80 g/L and symptoms or signs of anemia
2. Acute blood loss with hypovolemia unresponsive to crystalloid or colloid
3. Hemoglobin level <130 g/L in patients with severe pulmonary disease requiring assisted ventilation
4. Chronic congenital or acquired anemia without an expected satisfactory response to medical therapy and a hemoglobin level <80 g/L, or a hemoglobin level <100 g/L with symptoms and/or signs of anemia
5. Chronic transfusions to suppress endogenous hemoglobin production in selected patients with sickle-cell or thalassemia syndromes
6. Induction of immune tolerance before renal transplantation

*Statements that are underlined require additional definition by each local transfusion committee.

RBCs and crystalloid or colloid would dilute coagulation factors to levels insufficient to ensure hemostasis. In adults, such dilution is thought to occur once acute blood loss exceeds one blood volume[4,5]; in the neonate and young infant, the comparable value, although unknown, is presumed to be similar. However, levels of several coagulation factors are lower in neonates,[6,7] and it is possible that very young infants may require coagulation factor replacement after smaller losses.

TRANSFUSION OF RBCs

Although RBCs are the most commonly transfused blood component, the pediatric literature (particularly outside the neonatal period) is remarkable for the paucity of carefully designed studies investigating the benefits and/or risks associated with this therapy. The guidelines that follow are therefore based, in many instances, on expert opinion and common practice rather than on the results of scientific studies.

Neonates and Infants Younger Than 4 Months

Guidelines for RBC transfusions in neonates are presented in Table 2 (hereafter, the term *neonates* refers to both neonates and infants younger than 4 months). Mean hemoglobin values (±2 SDs) in normal term and preterm (32 weeks' gestation) newborns at 24 hours of life are 193±22 g/L and 185±20 g/L, respectively.[8] A venous hemoglobin level less than 130 g/L in the first 24 hours of life indicates severe anemia, for which an RBC transfusion is generally recommended. It is also current practice to maintain the hemoglobin level greater than 130 g/L in neonates with severe respiratory or cardiac disease. While these practices seem logical, their efficacy remains to be established.[9]

Most RBC transfusions are given to replace phlebotomy losses for laboratory monitoring of ill premature infants or to treat clinically important problems attributed to the physiologic decline in hemoglobin level that occurs after birth (anemia of prematurity). Precise indications for the use of RBCs in these two clinical settings have not been determined; however, the issues involved have been extensively reviewed.[9-14]

Phlebotomy losses are generally replaced after 5% to 10% of the infant's total blood volume has been removed. Although extensive blood loss in a sick infant may justify an RBC transfusion, the decision to transfuse should not be based exclusively on the quantity of blood removed. Other considerations include the age and clinical status of the neonate, the hemoglobin level at birth, and the length of time over which the losses have occurred.

Healthy preterm infants with a physiologic decline of hemoglobin level to 70 to 80 g/L do not require RBC transfusion in the absence of signs of anemia.[13,14] However, it is difficult to define "signs of anemia" in the premature infant. Although most would include tachycardia, tachypnea, recurrent apnea, decreased vigor, and poor weight gain unexplained by other causes, controversy remains over the correlation of these signs and the response to RBC transfusions.[9-19]

Infants and Children 4 Months and Older

Guidelines for RBC transfusions in older infants and children are similar to those for adults (Table 2). In general, RBCs are indicated to (1) prevent or reverse tissue hypoxia due to a diminished RBC mass and/or (2) decrease endogenous (abnormal) hemoglobin production. In the assessment of the importance of any hemoglobin level in a child, it is important to remember that normal hemoglobin and hematocrit levels are lower in children than in adults.[8] Indications for perioperative RBC transfusions are currently being reevaluated. The National Institutes of Health Consensus Development Conference convened to address this issue advocated an individualized approach.[20] Selected adult patients can be safely managed with an intraoperative hemoglobin level of 80 g/L.[21] An individualized approach is especially important in pediatric practice, where most patients do not have associated cardiorespiratory diseases and likely do not require hemoglobin levels of greater than 100 g/L before, during, or after surgery. In particular, there should be a compelling reason to administer a postoperative RBC transfusion to a pediatric patient, as most children (without bleeding) can quickly restore their hemoglobin mass if given appropriate oral iron therapy.[8]

The development of guidelines for the replacement of acute blood loss due to nonsurgical bleeding is more difficult, because estimates of losses are frequently unreliable, and the diagnosis of impending shock in a child may be easily overlooked. The situation is further complicated by the wide range of values for heart rate and blood pressure in normal children. With adults, the most important measures in the treatment of acute hemorrhage are to control the hemorrhage and then to restore perfusion, usually with crystalloid and/or colloid. If the patient's condition remains unstable, then RBC transfusions are indicated.

In acutely ill patients with severe pulmonary disease requiring assisted ventilation, it is recommended that the hemoglobin level be maintained in the normal range.[22,23] Although this recommendation may be valid, it has not been documented by scientific studies.

With anemias that develop slowly, the decision to administer RBCs to increase tissue oxygen delivery should not be based solely on the hemoglobin concentration. Children with anemias that develop slowly may be asymptomatic despite hemoglobin levels well below 80 g/L. Patients with iron deficiency anemia, for example, often are treated with oral iron alone, even at hemoglobin levels below 50 g/L. Factors other than hemoglobin concentration to be considered in the decision to transfuse RBCs include (1) the patient's symptoms, signs, and functional capacities; (2) the presence or absence of cardiovascular, respiratory, or central nervous system disease; (3) the causes and anticipated evolution of the anemia; and (4) alternate therapies (and the ability to comply with them). In anemias that are likely to be permanent, one must also consider the effect of the anemia on growth and development as well as the effects of repeated transfusions.

Patients with sickle-cell diseases (SS, SC, or Sβ-thalassemia) without complications do not require RBC transfusions. However, there are several clinical settings in which these patients may require simple or partial exchange RBC transfusions to prevent tissue hypoxia and/or to suppress endogenous hemoglobin production.[24] A chronic RBC transfusion program is appropriate for patients with sickle-cell disease following a splenic sequestration crisis until splenectomy is performed (usually after 2 years of age)[25-27] or following a cerebrovascular accident.[27-33] There are no clear criteria to determine when it is safe to discontinue RBC transfusion following a cerebrovascular accident. Red blood cell transfusions may also be beneficial in the management of the following complications in patients with sickle cell diseases: acute chest syndrome, acute aplasia, priapism, and chronic leg ulcers.[27,33,34-37] Although prophylactic RBC transfusions have frequently been used during pregnancy, a recent study has demonstrated that omitting them is not harmful to pregnant patients with sickle-cell disease or their offspring.[38] The optimal preoperative use of RBC transfusions has been extensively discussed in the literature.[24,33,39-43] While most authors agree that the preoperative hemoglobin level should be 100 g/L, the issue of whether the hemoglobin S concentration should be lower than a predetermined level, eg, 30%, remains unresolved. Finally, RBCs are not indicated for patients with sickle-cell disease with uncomplicated episodes of pain.[27,33]

Patients with severe thalassemia syndromes are placed on long-term RBC transfusion programs to prevent the consequences of severe anemia and ineffective erythropoiesis.[8] The extent to which endogenous (ineffective) erythropoiesis is suppressed varies inversely with the minimum hemoglobin level achieved with the RBC transfusion program.[44] While most experts agree that the minimum pretransfusion hemoglobin level should be at least 90 g/L, there is controversy about the value of maintaining a higher minimum hemoglobin level.[8]

Red blood cell transfusions may also be given before renal transplantation to induce immune tolerance in patients with chronic renal failure.[45] However, in light of cyclosporine therapy, this indication for transfusion both in cadaveric and living related donor transplants is being reexamined.[46,47]

TRANSFUSION OF PLATELET CONCENTRATES

Platelet transfusions are indicated for support of children with clinically important quantitative and/or qualitative platelet disorders (Table 3). Guidelines for children are similar to those published for adults by a recent National Institutes of Health Consensus Conference on platelet transfusion therapy.[48]

Table 3.—Criteria for Transfusion of Platelet Concentrates*
Premature infants (gestational age <37 weeks)
1. Blood platelets <50x10^9/L in a stable infant
2. Blood platelets <100x10^9/L in a sick infant
All other infants and children
1. Blood platelet count <20x10^9/L and marrow failure
2. Blood platelet count <50x10^9/L with active bleeding or the need for an invasive procedure in a child with bone marrow failure
3. Blood platelet count <100x10^9/L with active bleeding plus disseminated intravascular coagulation or other coagulation abnormalities
4. Bleeding with qualitative platelet defect and marked prolongation of the bleeding time regardless of the platelet count
5. Cardiovascular bypass surgery with unexplained excessive bleeding, regardless of the platelet count

*Statements that are underlined require additional definition by each local transfusion committee.

The risk of life-threatening hemorrhage, particularly intracranial hemorrhage, relates to the severity of thrombocytopenia. Studies in thrombocytopenic leukemic patients,[49] and in a thrombocytopenic dog model,[50] indicate that mucosal bleeding increases markedly when platelet levels fall below 20 × 10^9/L. For this reason, many physicians recommend prophylactic platelet transfusions to maintain a platelet count greater than 20 × 10^9/L in children with thrombocytopenia due to bone marrow failure. This recommendation is supported by the findings of at least one randomized study.[51] When thrombocytopenia occurs in association with fever, active bleeding, the need for an invasive procedure, disseminated intravascular coagulation, or other severe clotting abnormalities, the "threshold" for platelet transfusions needs to be raised. Platelet transfusions should be used with caution and are generally contraindicated in the hemolytic-uremic syndrome and thrombotic thrombocytopenic purpura, disorders caused by the formation of platelet thrombi in small vessels.

Platelet transfusions for the newborn infant merit separate consideration. Premature infants, particularly those who are ill, are at risk for intracranial hemorrhage. The incidence of this complication is higher in thrombocytopenic than in nonthrombocytopenic infants.[52] Moreover, multiple abnormalities of hemostasis may be present in such infants. Thus, it is reasonable clinical practice to maintain a minimum platelet count of 50 × 10^9/L in premature infants, although this recommendation has not been proved scientifically. Until more data are available, the report from Andrew and colleagues[52] suggests that the threshold for platelet transfusions in sick premature infants should be even higher, of the order of 100 × 10^9/L.

Neonatal alloimmune thrombocytopenia, a condition that reflects fetomaternal incompatibility for a platelet antigen, also deserves special consideration.[53] In more than 75% of cases, the pathologic platelet antibody demonstrates specificity for the platelet-specific antigen, Pl^{A1}.[54] The therapy of choice for affected infants with severe thrombocytopenia is the infusion of compatible platelets, obtained from the mother or a known antigen-negative

Table 4.—Criteria for Transfusion of Granulocyte Concentrates*
1. Bacterial sepsis in neonates <2 weeks of age with neutrophil plus band cell counts $<3x10^9/L$
2. Bacterial sepsis unresponsive to antibiotics in patients >2 weeks of age with neutrophil plus band cell counts $<0.5x10^9/L$
3. Documented infection(s) unresponsive to antibiotics plus a qualitative neutrophil defect, regardless of the neutrophil plus band cell count

*Statements that are underlined require additional definition by each local transfusion committee.

blood donor. If maternal platelets are used, it is important that they be irradiated and that maternal plasma containing pathologic platelet alloantibodies be removed from the platelet concentrate before transfusion.[55]

Of the immune thrombocytopenic disorders encountered in pediatric practice, autoimmune thrombocytopenic purpura is the most common. In this disorder, platelets are rapidly destroyed by broadly reacting circulating platelet autoantibodies or immune complexes. The survival of donor platelets is markedly reduced, and there is general agreement that, except in the circumstance of life-threatening bleeding, platelet transfusions are not indicated. Alternate therapies (eg, steroids and high-dose intravenous IgG) are preferred.[56,57] An analogous condition, neonatal autoimmune thrombocytopenia, occurs in infants delivered to affected mothers.[58] Thrombocytopenia in this disorder is self-limiting, and therapy is administered to minimize the risk of intracranial hemorrhage in severely thrombocytopenic infants. Similar to older children with autoimmune thrombocytopenic purpura, there is little rationale for use of platelet transfusions, and infants with severe autoimmune thrombocytopenia should receive intravenous IgG and/or steroid therapy.[54,59]

Qualitative platelet disorders may be inherited or acquired, for example, in children with advanced hepatic or renal insufficiency or following cardiopulmonary bypass. In such patients, platelet transfusion therapy is justified if severe bleeding occurs. Prophylactic administration of platelets is not justified unless there are other conditions that interfere with hemostasis or if an invasive procedure is planned. In these cases, a bleeding time of greater than twice the upper limit of laboratory normal may be taken as justification for therapy,[48] and alternatives to platelet transfusions, particularly desmopressin acetate, should be considered.[60,61]

It is easier to prevent than to stop bleeding in the thrombocytopenic patient. In children with uncomplicated thrombocytopenia due to bone marrow failure, 1 U per 10 to 15 kg is sufficient to prevent bleeding.[62] Larger doses (1 U per 5 kg) may be required to achieve hemostasis in bleeding patients. It is common practice to limit the dose to 6 to 8 U of random donor platelets or one platelet pheresis concentrate (platelets obtained by apheresis of a single donor). The dose of platelets required to increase the platelet count to greater than $100 \times 10^9/L$ in newborn infants is 10 mL/kg of standard platelet concentrates prepared from single units of whole blood or by automated platelet pheresis (R. G. Strauss, MD, oral communication, 1990).

TRANSFUSION OF GRANULOCYTES

Granulocyte transfusions should be considered for infected pediatric patients in three clinical settings (Table 4). Because some patients recover with antibiotics alone, institutions should survey the outcome of infections in neonates and neutropenic children treated locally. If the response to antimicrobial drugs alone is prompt and survival approaches 100%, granulocyte transfusions are unnecessary. However, if large numbers of patients fail to respond to antibiotic therapy, the addition of granulocyte transfusions should be considered.

During the first week of life, healthy neonates exhibit both neutrophilia and neutrophil functional abnormalities.[63] In infected neonates, neutrophil counts may fall to relatively "neutropenic" values of less than $3 \times 10^9/L$, with function thus deteriorating further.[64] At least 11 reports of granulocyte transfusions in neonates exist,[65] of which six are controlled studies.[66-71] Four of the six reported a markedly better outcome for neonates receiving antibiotics plus granulocyte transfusions prepared by automated leukapheresis than for neonates receiving antibiotics alone.[66-69] In the two negative studies,[70,71] low doses of neutrophils were transfused because they were isolated from buffy coats of whole blood, rather than by apheresis. Although data are inconclusive, sepsis is likely to be fatal in neonates with a fulminant clinical picture, blood neutrophil counts of less than $3 \times 10^9/L$, and evidence of a depleted bone marrow neutrophil storage pool.[64-66] Granulocyte transfusions should be considered for these infants.

The role of granulocyte transfusions added to antibiotics for patients with severe neutropenia due to bone marrow failure is similar for both adults and children.[72] Patients in most reports have been adults with leukemia or aplastic anemia, but five studies relate exclusively to children.[73-77] Infected neutropenic patients usually respond to antibiotics alone, provided that bone marrow function recovers early in infection. Because children with newly diagnosed leukemia respond rapidly to induction chemotherapy, only rarely are they candidates for granuloctye transfusions. In contrast, infected children with sustained bone marrow failure (ie, malignant neoplasms resistant to treatment, aplastic anemia, and bone marrow transplant recipients) may benefit when granulocyte transfusions are added to antibiotics. The use of granulocyte transfusions for bacterial sepsis that is unresponsive to antibiotics in patients with severe neutropenia ($<0.5 \times 10^9/L$) is supported by most of the seven controlled studies reported to date.[78-84]

Patients with qualitative neutrophil defects (neutrophil dysfunction) usually have adequate numbers of blood neutrophils but are susceptible to serious infections because their cells kill pathogenic microorganisms inefficiently. Neutrophil dysfunction syndromes are rare, and no definitive studies have been reported to establish the efficacy of granulocyte transfusions. However, a few patients with progressive, life-threatening infections have improved strikingly with the addition of granulocyte transfusions.[65] These disorders are chronic, and granulocyte transfusions are recommended only when infections are clearly unresponsive to antimicrobial drugs.

Once the decision to provide granulocyte transfusions has been made, an adequate dose must be transfused. Neonates and infants weighing less than 10 kg should receive 1 to 2×10^9 neutrophils per kilogram per infusion. Larger infants and children should receive at least 1×10^{10} neutrophils per infusion; the preferred dose for adolescents is 2 to 3×10^{10}. Granulocyte transfusions should be continued daily until either the infection resolves or the blood neutrophil count rises to greater than $0.5 \times 10^9/L$.

TRANSFUSION OF FFP

The indications for FFP transfusion in children (Table 5) are similar to those reported for adults by the National Institutes of Health Consensus Development Conference addressing FFP transfusions.[4] Transfusion of FFP is efficacious for the treatment of deficiencies of factors II, V, VII, X, XI, and XIII.

Requirements for FFP vary with the specific factor being replaced.[85] Transfusion of FFP is no longer recommended for the treatment of patients with hemophilia A or B, because safer factor VIII and IX concentrates are available for the treatment of these disorders. An important, albeit rare, use of FFP is for the rapid reversal of anticoagulant effect of warfarin sodium in patients who are actively bleeding or who require emergency surgery and in whom functional deficiencies of factors II, VII, IX, and X cannot be rapidly reversed by the administration of vitamin K.

In clinical practice, results of screening coagulation tests (prothrombin, activated partial thromboplastin, and thrombin times) are assumed to reflect the integrity of the coagulation system, and abnormalities are often used to justify FFP transfusion. However, test results must be related to the clinical condition of the patient. Transfusion of FFP in patients with chronic liver disease and prolonged screening coagulation test times are generally not recommended unless severe bleeding is present or an invasive procedure is planned. Fresh-frozen plasma transfusions in newborn infants merit special consideration; coagulation test times are prolonged in these infants,[6,7] and FFP should only be transfused after reference to values expected for the particular patient. The indications for FFP in neonates have been reviewed[86] and include (1) reconstitution of RBC concentrates to whole blood in the setting of massive transfusions (for example, exchange transfusion or cardiovascular surgery), (2) hemorrhage secondary to vitamin K deficiency, (3) disseminated intravascular coagulation (although exchange transfusion is more often used than simple transfusion), and (4) bleeding in a patient with a congenital coagulation factor deficiency when more specific treatment is either unavailable or inappropriate. The use of prophylactic FFP transfusions to prevent intraventricular hemorrhage in premature infants is controversial,[87-89] so a firm recommendation about this practice cannot be made. Although still being used to adjust the hematocrit values for small-volume RBC transfusions to neonates, FFP offers no apparent medical benefit[90] and exposes the infant to an additional donor. This practice should be discouraged. In addition, its use in partial exchange transfusion for the treatment of neonatal hyperviscosity syndrome is unnecessary, as safer colloid solutions are available.[91]

While its major benefit has been in the treatment of bleeding associated with coagulation factor deficiencies, FFP also contains several anticoagulant proteins (antithrombin III, protein C, and protein S) whose deficiencies have been associated with thrombosis.[92] In selected situations, FFP may be appropriate as replacement therapy in patients with these disorders.[93] An alternative is a commercially produced concentrate.[94,95]

Other indications for FFP include replacement fluid during plasma exchange in patients with thrombotic thrombocytopenic purpura or other disorders in which FFP is beneficial.[96,97] Fresh-frozen plasma transfusions are not indicated for correction of hypovolemia or as immunoglobulin replacement therapy, because safer alternatives exist.[98]

Table 5.—Criteria for Transfusion of Plasma Products*

Fresh-frozen plasma
1. Bleeding, or an invasive procedure, in a patient with a coagulation factor deficiency or a markedly prolonged prothrombin, and/or partial thromboplastin times
2. Replacement therapy in antithrombin III or protein C or S deficiencies
3. Replacement therapy during therapeutic plasma exchange for disorders in which fresh-frozen plasma is beneficial
Cryoprecipitate
1. Bleeding, or an invasive procedure, in hemophilia A or von Willebrand's disease
2. Bleeding, or an invasive procedure, in hypofibrogenemia or dysfibrinogenemia
3. Replacement therapy in factor XIII deficiency
Clotting factor concentrates
1. Bleeding, active or anticipated, in patients with documented coagulation factor deficiencies, such as hemophilia A or B
2. Severe or variant forms of von Willebrand's disease
Albumin
1. Acute correction of hypoalbuminemia when clinically indicated
2. Correction of hypovolemia when colloid infusion is indicated
3. Replacement therapy in therapeutic plasma exchange procedures

*Statements that are underlined require additional definition by each local transfusion committee.

TRANSFUSION OF CRYOPRECIPITATE

Cryoprecipitate, prepared by thawing FFP at 4°C, is still used by some hemophilia programs for factor replacement of patients with hemophilia A or von Willebrand's disease. A refinement that is sometimes used is the preparation of cryoprecipitate following repetitive plasmapheresis of selected donors.[99] Alternatives to cryoprecipitate include desmopressin acetate (for patients with mild to moderate hemophilia A or von Willebrand's disease) or specific clotting factor concentrates.[100-102]

Other uses for cryoprecipitate include correction of hypofibrinogenemia or dysfibrinogenemia and replacement therapy in patients with factor XIII deficiency.[103] Its use to provide fibronectin, a substance with opsonic activity, in patients with, or at risk for, bacterial sepsis (eg, premature infants) remains uncertain.[104]

TRANSFUSION OF CLOTTING FACTOR CONCENTRATES

Factor VIII and IX concentrates are used as replacement therapy in patients with hemophilia A and B. The introduction of commercial concentrates into North America in the late 1960s markedly improved the treatment of patients with these inherited coagulation disorders. They made possible the development of cost-effective home therapy programs[105] and allowed severe hemophiliacs a degree of freedom previously not possible. For this advance, hemophiliacs have paid a high price. The majority who received repeated infusions of factor VIII or IX concentrates of

Table 6.—Criteria for Transfusion of Cytomegalovirus Low-Risk Blood Products in Seronegative Patients
1. Recipients of seronigative kidney, heart, heart-lung, or liver organ grafts
2. Recipients of seronegative bone marrow
3. Patients who are likely candidates for bone marrow transplantation
4. Pregnant women and their fetuses, if intrauterine transfusions are required
5. Neonates weighing ≤1250 g at birth
6. Patients infected with the human immunodeficiency virus

North American origin now manifest clinical and/or serologic evidence of infection with the hepatitis and acquired immunodeficiency syndrome viruses, reflecting the fact that these concentrates are prepared from pools of thousands of plasma units. Fortunately, a number of effective virus inactivation processes (super dry heat, vapor heat, pasteurization, and solvent-detergent treatment) can now be applied to factor concentrates during the manufacturing process, and the newer concentrates carry an extremely low risk of transmitting known infections, such as acquired immunodeficiency syndrome or hepatitis.[106-109] Until factors VIII and IX produced by recombinant DNA technology become available, these new plasma-derived factor concentrates are the treatment of choice for patients with severe hemophilia A or B (Table 5).

Other clotting-factor concentrates in current use include both activated and nonactivated prothrombin complex concentrates for the management of bleeding in patients with hemophilia A and a circulating inhibitor[110,111] and concentrates that are known to contain the multimeric forms of von Willebrand factor in patients with von Willebrand's disease.[112,113]

TRANSFUSION OF ALBUMIN

The major uses of albumin are listed in Table 5.[114] The most common is for the correction of hypovolemia when colloid infusion is indicated.[115] Administered with a diuretic, albumin is also used for the acute correction of hypoalbuminemia in the treatment of fluid overload[115] and in postburn fluid resuscitation.[116] It is routinely used as replacement fluid with normal saline for most therapeutic plasma exchange procedures.[96]

Albumin is available as both a 5% and 25% solution. Plasma protein fraction is equivalent to 5% albumin but is subject to fewer purification steps and in the past has been associated with more adverse reactions.[117]

TRANSFUSION OF CYTOMEGALOVIRUS (CMV) LOW-RISK BLOOD PRODUCTS

Cytomegalovirus is an ubiquitous herpes virus harbored in the white blood cells of donor blood. In the immunocompromised host, posttransfusion CMV may cause further immunosuppression, placing the patient at substantial risk for morbidity or mortality. Immunocompromised groups of patients at risk for posttransfusion CMV[118-122] are listed in Table 6. These groups are candidates for CMV low-risk (eg, seronegative) blood products. In addition, it may be prudent to transfuse CMV low-risk products until the serologic status of the following patients is known: (1) premature infants weighing less than 1250 grams at birth, (2) patients with malignant neoplasms who are likely candidates for bone marrow transplantation, and (3) patients infected with the human immunodeficiency virus type 1.

Table 7.—Criteria for Transfusion of Irradiated Blood Products*
1. Bone marrow transplant recipients
2. Neonates and children with severe known or suspected congenital or acquired immunodeficiency states
3. Fetuses who require intrauterine transfusions
4. Neonates who received intrauterine transfusions and who require transfusions postnatally
5. Recipients of cellular blood products from first-degree relatives

*Statements that are underlined require additional definition by each local transfusion committee.

There is no evidence to support the use of CMV low-risk blood products either in seropositive oncology or in solid organ transplant patients who are receiving immunosuppressive drug regimens or in other seropositive subjects.

Current practice is to utilize IgG CMV seronegative blood and blood products, with the knowledge that only a fraction of IgG seropositive units are infectious. Tests to detect IgM antibodies or CMV viral antigens are not yet sufficiently developed to replace IgG testing. Other methods to decrease CMV transmission include extreme leukodepletion of blood products by filtration or following freeze-thawing and washing.[123] Use of frozen deglycerolized washed RBCs, regardless of donor serology, has been demonstrated to reduce posttransfusion CMV in renal allograft recipients, post–cardiac surgery patients, and premature infants. Whether leukodepleted RBCs are a viable alternative to the use of CMV IgG–negative RBC merits further study.[124] Measures to reduce the risk of CMV transmission need only be applied to cellular blood products (RBCs, platelets, and granulocytes); FFP and cryoprecipitate are sufficiently acellular that CMV transmission does not present a substantial clinical problem.

TRANSFUSION OF IRRADIATED BLOOD PRODUCTS

Graft-vs-host disease occurs when donor-derived T cells engraft in an immunoincompetent recipient. Clinically important graft-vs-host disease is a rare complication[125,126] that occurs from 3 to 30 days (median, 8 days) following transfusion. It has been observed following transfusion of whole blood, RBCs, buffy coats, fresh plasma, and granulocyte or platelet concentrates but not following transfusion of cryoprecipitate or frozen plasma, probably because component preparation reduces the concentration of functional lymphocytes to less than the number critical to induce graft-vs-host disease.[127]

Posttransfusion graft-vs-host disease follows an acute course and is frequently fatal, especially in infants and children, in whom 80% to 90% mortality rates have been reported.[125] Because there is no effective treatment, the goal is to (1) recognize clinical conditions in which posttransfusion graft-vs-host disease is likely to occur, (2) employ techniques to eliminate its cause, and (3) ensure that the techniques used do not adversely affect the product to be transfused. Patients at risk should receive blood products processed to remove functional T cells or to render such cells ineffective. Filtration, sedimentation, freeze-thawing, or washing with current methods has the undesired potential to leave enough T cells to induce graft-vs-host disease or to render the product inadequate for transfusion. Current practice utilizes ionizing radiation from a cesium, cobalt, or linear acceleration source at doses ranging from 1500 to 5000 cGy to protect against graft-vs-host disease. A dose of 1500 cGy is most frequently used.[128,129] Patients at risk for graft-vs-host disease (Table 7) should receive irradiated blood products.

Premature infants are known to have immune dysfunction, but their risk of acquisition of posttransfusion graft-vs-host disease is not well established. The postnatal age of the infant, number of immunocompetent lymphocytes in the transfusion product, degree of HLA compatibility between donor and recipient, and other as yet poorly described phenomena may determine which infants should receive such products.[130] Directed donations with blood from first-degree relatives should be irradiated because of the risk of engraftment with HLA haploidentical lymphocytes in these products.[131,132] Other groups potentially at risk, but for whom no data are available, are those receiving T-cell depletion therapy (antithymocyte globulin or OKT3) and recipients of organ transplantation who are receiving chronic T-cell suppressive drug regimens.

The following persons served on the Pediatric Hemotherapy Committee during conduct of this project: Asa Barnes, Jr, MD; Christine Barrasso, MT(ASCP) SBB; Janice F. Blazina, MD; Lynn Black, MS, MT(ASCP) SBB; Susanne Butch, MT(ASCP) SBB; Ann McMican, MT(ASCP) SBB; Cirilo Sotelo-Avila, MD; Kenneth Starling, MD; Alice Werner, MD; and Alvin M. Mauer, MD (liaison from the American Academy of Pediatrics).

We thank Maureen Andrew, MD, Nancy Olivieri, MD, and Jutta Preiksaitis, MD, for their helpful comments during preparation of the manuscript, and Nancy Fair for excellent secretarial assistance. The manuscript was prepared with the assistance of Medical Publications, The Hospital for Sick Children, Toronto, Ontario.

References

1. Bove JR. Transfusion-associated hepatitis and AIDS: what is the risk? *N Engl J Med.* 1987;317:242-244.

2. Menitove JE. The decreasing risk of transfusion-associated AIDS. *N Engl J Med.* 1989;321:966-968. Editorial.

3. Rigney PR. *Informed Consent for Blood Transfusions.* Arlington, Va: American Association of Blood Banks; September 11, 1989.

4. Consensus Development Panel, National Institutes of Health. Fresh-frozen plasma: indications and risks. *JAMA.* 1985;253:551-553.

5. Murray DJ, Olson J, Strauss R, Tinker JH. Coagulation changes during packed red cell replacement of major blood loss. *Anesthesiology.* 1988;69:839-845.

6. Andrew M, Paes B, Milner R, et al. Development of the human coagulation system in the full-term newborn. *Blood.* 1987;70:165-172.

7. Andrew M, Paes B, Milner R, et al. Development of the human coagulation system in the healthy premature infant. *Blood.* 1988;72:1651-1657.

8. Nathan DG, Oski FA, eds. *Hematology of Infancy and Childhood.* 3rd ed. Philadelphia, Pa: WB Saunders Co; 1987.

9. Strauss RG. Current issues in neonatal transfusions. *Vox Sang.* 1986;51:1-9.

10. Blank JP, Sheagren TG, Vajaria J, Mangurten HH, Benawra RS, Puppala BL. The role of RBC transfusion in the premature infant. *AJDC.* 1984;138:831-833.

11. Blanchette VS, Zipursky A. Assessment of anemia in newborn infants. *Clin Perinatol.* 1984;11:489-510.

12. Philips HM, Holland BM, Abdel-Moiz A, et al. Determination of red cell mass in assessment and management of anemia in babies needing blood transfusion. *Lancet.* 1986;1:882-884.

13. Stockman JA III. Anemia of prematurity: current concepts in the issue of when to transfuse. *Pediatr Clin North Am.* 1986;33:111-128.

14. Sacher RA, Luban NLC, Strauss RG. Current practices and guidelines for the transfusion of cellular blood components in the newborn. *Transfusion Med Rev.* 1989;3:39-54.

15. Stockman JA III, Clark DA. Weight gain: a response to transfusion in selected preterm infants. *AJDC.* 1984;138:828-830.

16. Alverson DC, Isken VH, Cohen RS. Effect of booster blood transfusions on oxygen utilization in infants with bronchopulmonary dysplasia. *J Pediatr.* 1988;113:722-726.

17. DeMaio JG, Harris MC, Deuber C, Spitzer AR. Effect of blood transfusion on apnea frequency in growing premature infants. *J Pediatr.* 1989;114:1039-1041.

18. Keyes WG, Donohue PK, Spivak JL, Jones MD Jr, Oski FA. Assessing the need for transfusion of premature infants and the role of hematocrit, clinical signs, and erythropoietin level. *Pediatrics.* 1989;84:412-417.

19. Ross MP, Christensen RD, Rothstein G, et al. A randomized trial to develop criteria for administering erythrocyte transfusions to anemic preterm infants 1 to 3 months of age. *J Perinatol.* 1989;9:246-253.

20. Consensus Development Panel, National Institutes of Health. Perioperative red blood cell transfusions. *JAMA.* 1988;260:2700-2703.

21. Carson JL, Poses RM, Spence RK, Bonavita G. Severity of anemia and operative mortality and morbidity. *Lancet.* 1988;1:727-729.

22. Royall J, Leven DL. Adult respiratory distress syndrome in pediatric patients, II: management. *J Pediatr.* 1988;112:335-347.

23. Charache S, Lubin, B, Reid, CD, eds. *Management and Therapy of Sickle Cell Disease.* Washington, DC: US Dept of Health and Human Services; 1989. National Institutes of Health publication 89-2117.

24. Rogers MC, ed. *Textbook of Pediatric Intensive Care.* Baltimore, Md: Williams & Wilkins; 1987:254-255.

25. Emond AM, Collis R, Darvill D, Higgs DR, Maude GH, Serjeant GR. Acute splenic sequestration in homozygous sickle cell disease: natural history and management. *J Pediatr.* 1985;107:201-206.

26. Rao S, Gooden S. Splenic sequestration in sickle cell disease: role of transfusion therapy. *Am J Pediatr Hematol Oncol.* 1985;7:298-301.

27. Vichinsky E, Lubin BH. Suggested guidelines for the treatment of children with sickle cell anemia. *Hematol Oncol Clin North Am.* 1987;1:483-502.

28. Lusher JM, Haghighat H, Khalifa AS. A prophylactic transfusion program for children with sickle cell anemia complicated by CNS infarction. *Am J Hematol.* 1976;1:265-273.

29. Russell MO, Goldberg HI, Reis L, et al. Transfusion therapy for cerebrovascular abnormalities in sickle cell disease. *J Pediatr.* 1976;88:382-387.

30. Wilimas J, Goff JR, Anderson HR Jr, Langston JW, Thompson E. Efficacy of transfusion therapy for one to two years in patients with sickle cell disease and cerebrovascular accidents. *J Pediatr.* 1980;96:205-208.

31. Sarnaik SA, Lusher JM. Neurological complications of sickle cell anemia. *Am J Pediatr Hematol Oncol.* 1982;4:386-394.

32. Russell MO, Goldberg HI, Hodson A, et al. Effect of transfusion therapy on arteriographic abnormalities and on recurrence of stroke in sickle cell disease. *Blood.* 1984;63:162-169.

33. Serjeant GR, ed. *Sickle Cell Disease.* New York, NY: Oxford University Press; 1985.

34. Davies SC, Luce PJ, Win AA, Riordan JF. Acute chest syndrome in sickle-cell disease. *Lancet.* 1984;1:36-38.

35. Mallouh AA, Asha M. Beneficial effect of blood transfusion in children with sickle cell chest syndrome. *AJDC.* 1988;142:178-182.

36. Seeler RA. Intensive transfusion therapy for priapism in boys with sickle cell anemia. *J Urol.* 1973;110:360-361.

37. Tarry WF, Duckett JW Jr, Snyder HM III. Urological complications of sickle cell disease in a pediatric population. *J Urol.* 1987;138:592-594.

38. Koshy M, Burd L, Wallace D, Moawad A, Baron J. Prophylactic red-cell transfusions in pregnant patients with sickle cell

disease: a randomized cooperative study. *N Engl J Med.* 1988;319:147-152.

39. Holtzmann L, Finn H, Lichtman HC, et al. Anesthesia in patients with sickle cell disease: a review of 112 cases. *Anesth Analg.* 1969;48:566-572.

40. Janik J, Seeler RA. Perioperative management of children with sickle hemoglobinopathy. *J Pediatr Surg.* 1980;15:117-120.

41. Charache S. The treatment of sickle cell anemia. In: Creger WP, Coggins CH, Hanock EW, eds. *Annual Review of Medicine.* Palo Alto, Calif: Annual Reviews; 1981:195-206.

42. Coker NJ, Milner PF. Elective surgery in patients with sickle cell anemia. *Arch Otolaryngol.* 1982;108:574-576.

43. Esseltine DW, Baxter MRN, Bevan JC. Sickle cell states and the anaesthetist. *Can J Anaesth.* 1988;35:385-403.

44. Propper RD, Button LN, Nathan DG. New approaches to the transfusion management of thalassemia. *Blood.* 1980;55:55-60.

45. Perkins HA. Transfusion-induced immunologic unresponsiveness. *Transfusion Med Rev.* 1988;2:196-203.

46. Flechner SM, Kerman RH, Van Buren C, Kahan BD. Successful transplantation of cyclosporine-treated hapolidentical living-related renal recipients without blood transfusions. *Transplantation.* 1984;37:73-76.

47. Opelz G. Improved kidney graft survival in nontransfused recipients. *Transplant Proc.* 1987;19:149-152.

48. Consensus Development Panel, National Institutes of Health. Platelet transfusion therapy. *JAMA.* 1987;257:1777-1780.

49. Gaydos LA, Freireich EJ, Mantel N. The quantitative relation between platelet count and hemorrhage in patients with acute leukemia. *N Engl J Med.* 1962;266:905-909.

50. Slichter SJ. Controversies in platelet transfusion therapy. *Annu Rev Med.* 1980;31:509-540.

51. Higby DJ, Cohen E, Holland JF, Sinks L. The prophylactic treatment of thrombocytopenic leukemic patients with platelets: a double blind study. *Transfusion.* 1974;14:440-446.

52. Andrew M, Castle V, Saigal S, Carter C, Kelton JG. Clinical impact of neonatal thrombocytopenia. *J Pediatr.* 1987;110:457-464.

53. Blanchette V. Neonatal alloimmune thrombocytopenia. In: Stockman JA III, Pochedly C, eds. *Developmental and Neonatal Hematology.* New York, NY: Raven Press; 1988:145-168.

54. Mueller-Eckhardt C, Kiefel V, Grubert A, et al. 348 cases of suspected neonatal alloimmune thrombocytopenia. *Lancet.* 1989;1:363-366.

55. Adner MM, Fisch GR, Starobin SG, Aster RH. Use of 'compatible' platelet transfusions in treatment of congenital isoimmune thrombocytopenic purpura. *N Engl J Med.* 1969;280:244-247.

56. Imbach P, Wagner HP, Berchtold W, et al. Intravenous immunoglobulin versus oral corticosteroids in acute immune thrombocytopenic purpura in childhood. *Lancet.* 1985;2:464-468.

57. van Hoff J, Ritchey AK. Pulse methylprednisolone therapy for acute childhood idiopathic thrombocytopenic purpura. *J Pediatr.* 1988;113:563-566.

58. Kelton JG. Management of the pregnant patient with idiopathic thrombocytopenic purpura. *Ann Intern Med.* 1983;99:796-800.

59. Blanchette V, Andrew M, Perlman M, Ling E, Ballin A. Neonatal autoimmune thrombocytopenia: role of high-dose intravenous immunoglobulin G therapy. *Blut.* 1989;59:139-144.

60. Kobrinsky NL, Israels ED, Gerrard JM, et al. Shortening of bleeding time by 1-deamino-8-D-arginine vasopressin in various bleeding disorders. *Lancet.* 1984;1:1145-1148.

61. Janson PA, Jubelirer SJ, Weinstein MJ, Deykin D. Treatment of the bleeding tendency in uremia with cryoprecipitate. *N Engl J Med.* 1980;303:1318-1322.

62. Roy AJ, Jaffe N, Djerassi I. Prophylactic platelet transfusions in children with acute leukemia: a dose response study. *Transfusion.* 1973;13:283-290.

63. Strauss RG. Granulopoiesis and neutrophil function in the neonate. In: Stockman JA III, Pochedly C, eds. *Development and Neonatal Hematology.* New York, NY: Raven Press; 1988:87-101.

64. Christensen RD, Anstall HB, Rothstein G. Review: deficiencies in the neutrophil system of newborn infants, and the use of leukocyte transfusions in the treatment of neonatal sepsis. *J Clin Apheresis.* 1982;1:33-41.

65. Strauss RG. Granulocyte transfusions. In: Rossi EC, Simon TL, Moss GS, eds. *Principles of Transfusion Medicine.* Baltimore, Md: Williams & Wilkins; 1991:287-294.

66. Christensen RD, Rothstein G, Anstall HB, Bybee B. Granulocyte transfusions in neonates with bacterial infection, neutropenia, and depletion of mature marrow neutrophils. *Pediatrics.* 1982;70:1-6.

67. Laurenti F, Ferro R, Isacchi G, et al. Polymorphonuclear leukocyte transfusion for the treatment of sepsis in the newborn infant. *J Pediatr.* 1981;98:118-123.

68. Cairo MS, Rucker R, Bennets GA, et al. Improved survival of newborns receiving leukocyte transfusions for sepsis. *Pediatrics.* 1984;74:887-892.

69. Cairo MS, Worcester C, Rucker R, et al. Role of circulating complement and polymorphonuclear leukocyte transfusion in treatment and outcome in critically ill neonates with sepsis. *J Pediatr.* 1987;110:935-941.

70. Baley JE, Stork EK, Warkentin PI, Shurin SB. Buffy coat transfusions in neutropenic neonates with presumed sepsis: a prospective, randomized trial. *Pediatrics.* 1987;80:712-720.

71. Wheeler JC, Chauvenet AR, Johnson CA, Block SM, Dillard R, Abramson JS. Buffy coat transfusions in neonates with sepsis and neutrophil storage pool depletion. *Pediatrics.* 1987;97:422-425.

72. Strauss RG. Granulocyte transfusions: uses, abuses and indications. In: Kolins J, McCarthy LJ, eds. *Contemporary Transfusion Practice.* Arlington, Va: American Association of Blood Banks; 1987:65-83.

73. Higby DJ, Freeman A, Henderson ES, Sinks L, Cohen E. Granulocyte transfusions in children using filter-collected cells. *Cancer.* 1976;38:1407-1413.

74. Maybee DA, Milan AP, Ruymann FB. Granulocyte transfusion therapy in children. *South Med J.* 1977;70:320-324.

75. Pole JG, Davie M, Kershaw I, Barter DAC, Willoughby MLN. Granulocyte transfusions in treatment of infected neutropenic children. *Arch Dis Child.* 1976;51:521-527.

76. Steinherz PG, Reich LM. Granulocyte transfusions in infected neutropenic children with malignancies. *Med Pediatr Oncol.* 1979;6:67-76.

77. Meyerovitz MF, Fellows KE. Typhlitis: a cause of gastrointestinal hemorrhage in children. *AJR Am J Roentgenol.* 1984;143:833-835.

78. Fortuny IE, Bloomfield CD, Hadlock DC, Goldman A, Kennedy BJ, McCullough JJ. Granulocyte transfusion: a controlled study in patients with acute nonlymphocytic leukemia. *Transfusion.* 1975;15:548-558.

79. Graw RG Jr, Herzig G, Perry S, Henderson ES. Normal granulocyte transfusion therapy: treatment of septicemia due to gram-negative bacteria. *N Engl J Med.* 1972;287:367-371.

80. Herzig RH, Herzig GP, Graw RG Jr, Bull MI, Ray KK. Successful granulocyte transfusion therapy for gram-negative septicemia: a prospectively randomized controlled study. *N Engl J Med.* 1977;296:701-705.

81. Alavi JB, Root RK, Djerassi I, et al. A randomized clinical trial of granulocyte transfusions for infection in acute leukemia. *N Engl J Med.* 1977;296:706-711.

82. Vogler WR, Winton EF. A controlled study of the efficacy of granulocyte transfusions in patients with neutropenia. *Am J Med.* 1977;63:548-555.

83. Winston DJ, Ho WG, Gale RP. Therapeutic granulocyte transfusions for documented infections: a controlled trial in ninety-five infectious granulocytopenic episodes. *Ann Intern Med.* 1982;97:509-515.

84. Higby DJ, Yates JW, Henderson ES, Holland JF. Filtration leukapheresis for granulocytic transfusion therapy: clinical and

laboratory studies. *N Engl J Med.* 1975;292:761-766.
85. Smith JK, Snape TJ. Therapeutic materials in the management of hemorrhagic disorders. In: Biggs R, Rizza C, eds. *Human Blood Coagulation, Haemostasis and Thrombosis.* Boston, Mass: Blackwell Scientific Publications Inc; 1984.
86. Hume H. Pediatric Transfusions: quality assessment and assurance. In: Sacher RA, Strauss R, eds. *Contemporary Issues in Pediatric Transfusion Medicine.* Arlington, Va: American Association of Blood Banks; 1989:55-80.
87. Goldberg RN, Chung D, Goldman SL, Bancaleri E. The association of rapid volume expansion and intraventricular hemorrhage in the preterm infant. *J Pediatr.* 1980;96:1060-1063.
88. Beverley DW, Pitts-Tucker TJ, Congdon PJ, Arthur RJ, Tate G. Prevention of intraventricular hemorrhage by fresh frozen plasma. *Arch Dis Child.* 1985;60:710-713.
89. Van De Bor M, Briet E, Van Bel F, Ruys JH. Hemostasis and periventricular-intraventricular hemorrhage of the newborn. *AJDC.* 1986;140:1131-1134.
90. Sacher RA, Strauss RG, Luban NLC, et al. Blood component therapy during the neonatal period: a national survey of red cell transfusion practice, 1985. *Transfusion.* 1990;30:271-276.
91. Wu PY. Neonatal hyperviscosity syndrome. *West J Med.* 1985;142:119-120.
92. High KA. Antithrombin III, protein C, and protein S: naturally occurring anticoagulant proteins. *Arch Pathol Lab Med.* 1988;112:28-36.
93. Marlar RA, Montgomery RR, Broekmans AW, and the Working Party. Diagnosis and treatment of homozygous protein C deficiency: report of the Working Party on homozygous protein C deficiency of the Subcommittee on Protein C and Protein S, International Committee on Thrombosis and Hemostasis. *J Pediatr.* 1989;114:528-534.
94. Vukovich T, Auberger K, Weil J, Engelmann H, Knöbl P, Hadorn HB. Replacement therapy for a homozygous protein C deficiency-state using a concentrate of human protein C and S. *Br J Haematol.* 1988;70:435-440.
95. Gallus AS. Replacement therapy in antithrombin III deficiency. *Transfusion Med Rev.* 1989;3:253-263.
96. Kasprisin D. Therapeutic apheresis in children. In: Kasprisin DO, Luban NLC, eds. *Pediatric Transfusion Medicine.* Boca Raton, Fla: CRC Press; 1987:169-186.
97. Shumak KH, Rock GA. Therapeutic plasma exchange. *N Engl J Med.* 1984;310:762-771.
98. Sacher R. Intravenous gammaglobulin products: development, pharmacology and precautions. In: Garner RJ, Sacher RA, eds. *Intravenous Gammaglobulin Therapy.* Arlington, Va: American Association of Blood Banks; 1988:1-30.
99. McLeod BC, Sassetti RJ, Cole ER, Scott JP. A high-potency, single-donor cryoprecipitate of known factor VIII content dispensed in vials. *Ann Intern Med.* 1987;106:35-40.
100. del la Fuente B, Kasper CK, Rickles FR, Hoyer LW. Response of patients with mild and moderate hemophilia A and von Willebrand's disease to treatment with desmopressin. *Ann Intern Med.* 1985;103:6-14.
101. Mannucci PM. Desmopressin: a nontransfusional form of treatment for congenital and acquired bleeding disorders. *Blood.* 1988;72:1449-1455.
102. Brettler DB, Levine PH. Factor concentrates for treatment of hemophilia: which one to choose? *Blood.* 1989;73:2067-2073.
103. Forbes C. Clinical aspects of the hemophilias and their treatment. In: Ratnoff OD, Forbes CD, eds. *Disorders of Hemostasis.* New York, NY: Grune & Stratton; 1984:210-211.
104. Snyder EL, Luban NL. Fibronectin: applications to clinical medicine. *CRC Crit Rev Clin Lab Sci.* 1986;23:15-34.
105. Levine PH, Britten AFH. Supervised patient-management of hemophilia: a study of 45 patients with hemophilia A and B. *Ann Intern Med.* 1973;78:195-201.
106. Schimpf K, Mannucci PM, Kreutz W, et al. Absence of hepatitis after treatment with a pasteurized factor VIII concentrate in patients with hemophilia and no previous transfusions. *N Engl J Med.* 1987;316:918-922.
107. Mannucci PM, Zanetti AR, Colombo M, et al. Prospective study of hepatitis after factor VIII concentrate exposed to hot vapour. *Br J Haematol.* 1988;68:427-430.
108. Study Group of the UK Haemophilia Centre Directors on Surveillance of Virus Transmission by Concentrates. Effect of dry-heating of coagulation factor concentrates at 80°C for 72 hours on transmission of non-A, non-B hepatitis. *Lancet.* 1988;2:814-816.
109. Horowitz MS, Rooks C, Horowitz B, Hilgartner MV. Virus safety of solvent/detergent-treated antihemophilic factor concentrate. *Lancet.* 1988;2:186-188.
110. Lusher J. Controlled clinical trials with prothrombin complex concentrates. In: Hoyer L, ed. *Factor VIII Inhibitors: Proceedings of an International Symposium Held in Farmington, Conn., Nov 3-5, 1983.* New York, NY: Alan R Liss Inc; 1984:277-290.
111. Penner JA. Treatment of inhibitor patients with activated prothrombin complex concentrates. In: Hoyer L, ed. *Factor VIII Inhibitors: Proceedings of an International Symposium Held in Farmington, Conn., Nov 3-5, 1983.* New York, NY: Alan R Liss Inc; 1984:291-308.
112. Fukui H, Nishino M, Terada S, et al. Hemostatic effect of a heat-treated factor VIII concentrate (Haemate P) in von Willebrand's disease. *Blut.* 1988;56:171-178.
113. Berntorp E, Nilsson IM. Use of a high-purity factor VIII concentrate (Hemate P) in von Willebrand's disease. *Vox Sang.* 1989;56:212-217.
114. Pisciotto PT, ed. *Blood Transfusion Therapy: A Physician's Handbook.* 3rd ed. Arlington, Va: American Association of Blood Banks; 1989:34-35.
115. Kaufman BS, Rackow EC, Falk JL. Fluid resuscitation in circulatory shock: colloids versus crystalloids. *Curr Stud Hematol Blood Transfus.* 1986;53:186-198.
116. Hilton J. Experimental studies of the use of albumin in postburn fluid resuscitation. *Curr Stud Hematol Blood Transfus.* 1986;53:114-124.
117. Olinger GN, Werner PH, Bonchek LI, Boerboom LE. Vasodilator effects of the sodium acetate in pooled protein fraction. *Ann Surg.* 1979;190:305-311.
118. Meyers JD, Flournoy N, Thomas ED. Risk factors for cytomegalovirus infection after human marrow transplant. *J Infect Dis.* 1986;153:478-488.
119. Wreghitt TG, Hakim M, Gray JJ, Kricia S, Wallwork J, English TAH. Cytomegalovirus infection in heart and heart and lung transplant recipients. *J Clin Pathol.* 1988;41:660-667.
120. Peterson PK, Balfour HH, Marker SC, et al. Cytomegalovirus disease in renal allograft recipients: a prospective study of the clinical features, risk factors and impact on renal transplantation. *Medicine.* 1980;59:283-300.
121. Adler SP. Neonatal cytomegalovirus infections due to blood. *CRC Crit Rev Clin Lab Sci.* 1985;23:1-14.
122. Tegtmeier G. The use of cytomegalovirus-screened blood in neonates. *Transfusion.* 1988;28:201-203. Editorial.
123. Gilbert GL, Hayes K, Hudson IL, James J. Prevention of transfusion-acquired cytomegalovirus infection in infants by blood filtration to remove leucocytes. *Lancet.* 1989;1:1228-1231.
124. Lamberson HV Jr, McMillian JA, Weiner LB, et al. Prevention of transfusion-associated cytomegalovirus (CMV) infection in neonates by screening blood donors for IgM to CMV. *J Infect Dis.* 1988;157:820-823.
125. Von Fliedner V, Higby DJ, Kim U. Graft-versus-host reaction following blood product transfusion. *Am J Med.* 1982;72:951-961.
126. Woods WG. Supportive care for children with cancer: guidelines of the Childrens Cancer Study Group: prevention of graft-vs.-host disease. *Am J Pediatr Hematol Oncol.* 1984;6:283-286.
127. Brubaker DB. Human posttransfusion graft-versus-host disease. *Vox Sang.* 1983;45:401-420.
128. Leitman SF, Holland PV. Irradiation of blood products: indications and guidelines. *Transfusion.* 1985;25:293-300.

129. Pisciotto P. Irradiated blood. In: Kasprisin DO, Luban NLC, eds. *Pediatric Transfusion Medicine.* Boca Raton, Fla: CRC Press; 1987.
130. Luban NLC, Ness PM. Irradiation of blood products: indications and guidelines. *Transfusion.* 1985;25:301-303. Comment.
131. Strauss RG. Directed and limited-exposure donor programs for children. In: Sacher RA, Strauss RG, eds. *Contemporary Issues in Pediatric Transfusion Medicine.* Arlington, Va: American Association of Blood Banks; 1989:1-11.
132. Simon TL. Patient directed donations from first degree family members and graft versus host disease (GVHD). Arlington, Va: American Association of Blood Banks; November 6, 1989.

In Other AMA Journals

JAMA

Access to Health Care for the Uninsured: The Perspective of the American Academy of Family Physicians
G. F. Aukerman
(*JAMA.* 1991;265:2856)

Promoting Professionalism Through Self-Appraisal in This Critical Decade
G. D. Lundberg
(*JAMA.* 1991;265:2859)

Health Consequences of Contraceptive Use and Reproductive Patterns
J. DaVanzo; A. M. Parnell; W. H. Foege
(*JAMA.* 1991;265:2692)

Statements From the International Committee of Medical Journal Editors
The International Committee of Medical Journal Editors
(*JAMA.* 1991;265:2697)

Diagnosis and Management of Kawasaki Disease
W. M. Gersony
(*JAMA.* 1991;265:2699)

Global Trends in Adolescent Health
R. W. Blum
(*JAMA.* 1991;265:2711)

Patients Have a Right to Privacy and Anonymity in Medical Publication
R. Riis, M. Nylenna
(*JAMA.* 1991;265:2720)

***JAMA* as an International Public Health Journal: Transcending Geographic and Political Boundaries**
A. Flanagin; I. G. Thomas; G. D. Lundberg
(*JAMA.* 1991;265:2721)

The Effect of Low-Dose Dopamine Infusion on Cardiopulmonary and Renal Status in Premature Newborns With Respiratory Distress Syndrome

Lily Cuevas, MD; Tsu F. Yeh, MD; Eunice G. John, MD; Danilo Cuevas, MD; Rosita S. Plides, MD

• To study the effects of infusion of low doses of dopamine hydrochloride on cardiopulmonary and renal status in premature newborns with respiratory distress syndrome, 49 newborns were randomly assigned to three groups: group 1 (18 patients) received no dopamine and was the control group; group 2 (16 patients) was infused with a dose of dopamine measuring 1.0 μg/kg of body weight per minute for 72 hours; and group 3 (15 patients) was infused with a dose of dopamine measuring 2.5 μg/kg of body weight per minute for 72 hours. Birth weights, gestational ages, postnatal ages, and cardiopulmonary status of all groups at the start of the study were comparable. Continuous infusion of these low doses of dopamine for 3 days after birth did not significantly improve levels of blood gases, acid-base balance, or clinical outcome. In newborns with systemic hypotension, dopamine improved cardiovascular status and caused early return of blood pressure to the normal range. Infusion of low doses of dopamine produced mild to moderate natriuresis and insignificant increases in glomerular filtration rate and urine volume.

***(AJDC.* 1991;145:799-803)**

Pulmonary edema sometimes occurs in the early stages of respiratory distress syndrome (RDS) in premature newborns. Although the causes are many, vasoregulatory disturbances and poor renal function are important causes of the fluid accumulation associated with pulmonary edema.[1,2] Dopamine hydrochloride, infused in low doses, has recently been shown effective in improving circulation and promoting diuresis in premature newborns.[3-5] This prospective study investigates whether early and continuous infusion of low doses of dopamine during the first 3 days after birth improves outcome in premature newborns with RDS.

Accepted for publication August 20, 1990.
From the Division of Neonatology, Cook County (Illinois) Children's Hospital, Chicago, Ill, and the Department of Pediatrics, College of Medicine, University of Illinois, Chicago.
Presented in part before the Society for Pediatric Research, Washington, DC, May 7, 1987.
Reprint requests to Division of Neonatology, Cook County Children's Hospital, 700 S Wood St, Chicago, IL 60612 (Dr Yeh).

PATIENTS AND METHODS

This study was approved by the scientific and lay committees of the Cook County (Illinois) Hospital, Chicago, and informed consent was obtained from the parents of each participant.

Between October 1986 and September 1987, 60 newborns whose birth weights ranged from 700 to 2000 g were included in

Table 1.—Perinatal Characteristics and Biochemical Data of Patients*

	Group 1	Group 2	Group 3
Birth weight, g	1289±320	1178±187	1190±272
Gestational age, wk	31±2.0	30±1.9	31±1.4
Type of delivery			
Natural spontaneous vaginal delivery	12	12	10
Cesarean section	6	4	5
Apgar score, No. of patients			
≤3	3	4	4
4-6	12	11	10
>6	3	1	1
Age at time of study, h	5.8±1.4	6.0±1.5	5.6±1.4
Biochemical level at time of study			
Mean airway pressure, cm H_2O	10.1±1.9	10.6±3.2	10.1±2.4
Fractional inspired oxygen	0.54±.23	0.60±.26	0.66±.25
PO_2, mm Hg	74.0±48.8	99.4±87.3	110±77.7
PCO_2, mm Hg	36.5±7.4	33.7±8.3	32.0±8.5
pH	7.36±0.07	7.39±0.06	7.39±0.08
Blood pressure, mm Hg			
Systolic	46.9±10.5	42.3±6.9	43.4±7.0
Diastolic	30.0±10.4	30.4±7.3	24.7±8.4
Mean	37.0±8.2	36.0±7.0	33.0±6.4
Heart rate, beats/min	142.6±9.4	141.6±8.4	144.6±10.8

*Values are means±SDs.

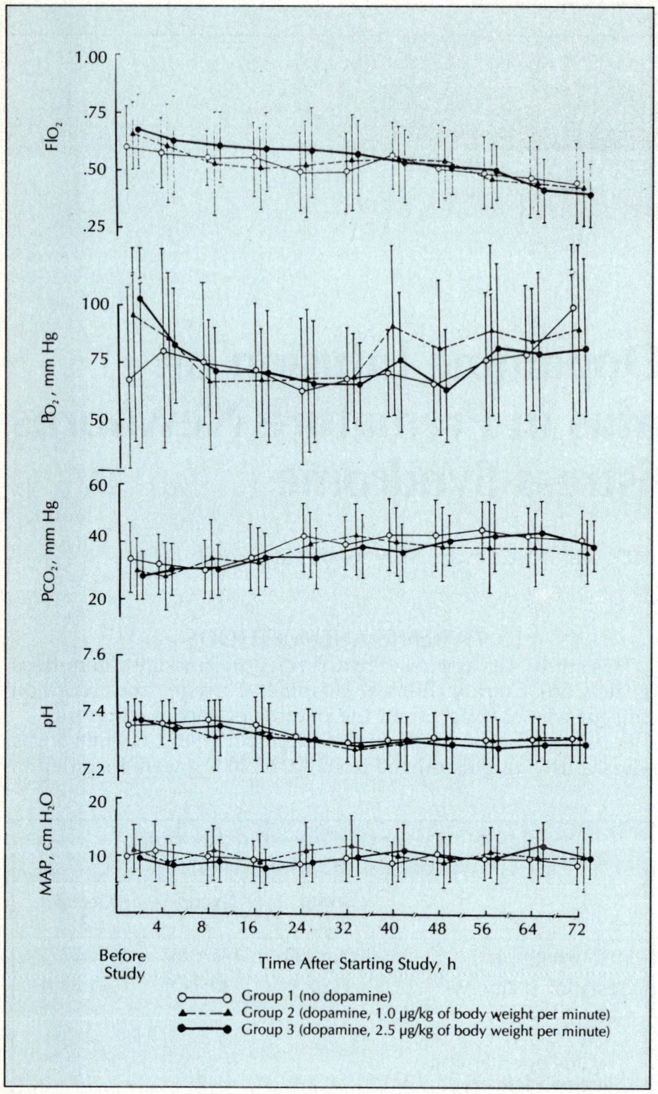

Fig 1.—*Blood gases, pH, and mean airway pressure (MAP) of mechanical ventilation during the study.*

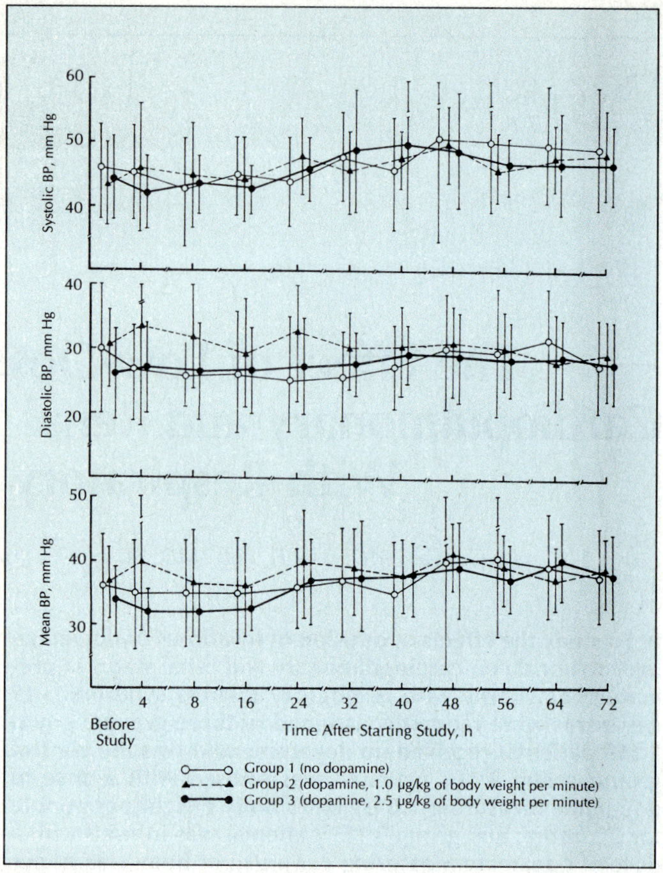

Fig 2.—*Systolic, diastolic, and mean blood pressure (BP) during the study.*

the study. Inclusion required that newborns have clinical and radiologic evidence of RDS and that they received mechanical ventilation within 4 hours of birth. On inclusion, the newborn was randomly assigned to one of the following three groups: group 1, in which patients were not administered dopamine; group 2, in which patients were administered dopamine in doses of 1.0 μg/kg of body weight per minute for 72 hours; and group 3, in which patients were administered dopamine in doses of 2.5 μg/kg of body weight per minute for 72 hours. Each group comprised 20 newborns. During the study, dopamine was infused through a peripheral vein by an intravenous pump (Micro Flogard 8500, Travenol, Deerfield, Ill). Dopamine was administered through an umbilical arterial catheter when no peripheral vein was accessible.

All newborns were treated using a standard protocol previously reported from our nursery.[6] The protocol emphasized the criteria for initiation of and weaning from mechanical ventilation and intake of fluids and electrolytes. Blood gas samples were obtained before the study began and every 4 hours after from an umbilical arterial catheter or a radial artery. Occasionally, blood gas samples were obtained by the arterialized capillary method; in these cases, only pH and P_{CO_2} levels were included for data analysis. The P_{O_2} values were then obtained by the transcutaneous method (TcP_{O_2}) (Radiometer Copenhagen TCM2 Transcutaneous Monitor, Radiometer, Copenhagen, Denmark). Blood pressure was continuously monitored through an umbilical arterial catheter on a multiple-channel neonatal monitor (HP 78834 A; Hewlett Packard, Palo Alto, Calif). Arterial hypotension was diagnosed as systolic blood pressure at least 10 mm Hg below the predicted normal value for gestational and postnatal age.[7,8]

During the study period, fluid intake was adjusted to 80, 95, and 110 mL/kg of body weight per day on days 1, 2, and 3, respectively. An additional 20 mL/kg of body weight per day was given if the infant was receiving phototherapy. The intravenous fluids consisted of 10% dextrose in water during the first day and 5% dextrose with electrolytes (25 mmol of sodium per liter of water and 20 mmol of potassium per liter of water) thereafter. No oral or nasogastric feeding was administered during the study period, and none of the newborns received diuretics or aminophylline.

All newborns were kept in incubators, and their skin temperatures were maintained by servocontrol at 36.5°C. Urine was collected in three aliquots 0 to 24, 24 to 48, and 48 to 72 hours after starting the study by attaching a U-bag (Hollister, Chicago, Ill) to the perineum. Suprapubic compression was performed at the beginning and end of each collection to ensure that the bladder was empty. The urine samples and the corresponding timed serum specimens were measured for electrolytes, creatinine, and osmolarity. The glomerular filtration rate (GFR) or creatinine clearance; fractional excretion of sodium (FE^{Na}), chloride (FE_{Cl}), and potassium (FE_K); and osmolality (Cosm) and free water clearance (C_{H_2O}) were all calculated using the conventional formulas.[6]

After completion of the study, all newborns were treated using a standard protocol currently used in our neonatal intensive care unit. Presumptive diagnosis of chronic lung disease was made if the infant had respiratory distress that required oxygen therapy and had an abnormal chest roentgenogram by the criteria of Northway et al.[9] Mortality rate and duration of oxygen therapy were also assessed.

Table 2.—Characteristics of Renal Function*

	Group No.	Time After Starting Study, h		
		0-24	24-48	48-72
Urine output, mL/kg of body weight per hour	1	2.9±1.9	4.8±2.4	4.2±2.4
	2	2.6±1.3	3.8±2.1	3.1±1.1
	3	2.3±1.2	3.2±1.6	2.9±1.5
Glomerular filtration rate, mL/min per 1.73 m^2	1	5.5±3.2	6.5±3.7	8.6±5.4
	2	5.1±1.9	8.4±5.2	7.6±3.2
	3	4.3±3.7	6.1±4.7	6.1±3.8
Fractional excretion of sodium, %	1	2.1±1.3	5.1±4.2	3.9±2.8
	2	6.6±4.4 †	6.7±4.1 ‡	6.7±5.0 ‡
	3	3.7±2.7	4.5±3.2	4.8±2.8
Fractional excretion of chloride, %	1	2.1±1.3	5.4±4.7	4.2±3.1
	2	5.0±3.2	6.0±4.7	6.5±4.8
	3	2.7±2.4	4.2±3.2	5.1±3.1
Fractional excretion of potassium, %	1	28.8±15.9	34.6±20.7	36.9±34.8
	2	39.6±19.4	45.3±35.2	36.4±22.9
	3	34.7±21.2	33.3±15.0	36.6±14.6
Osmolar clearance, mL/min per 1.73 m^2	1	.25±.13	.49±.23	.51±.30
	2	.60±.32†	.72±.34‡	.70±.26‡
	3	.24±.24	.33±.22	.39±.32
Free water clearance, mL/min per 1.73 m^2	1	.21±.13	.41±.22	.41±.35
	2	.56±.30‡	.66±.32	.64±.26
	3	.21±.24	.25±.25	.34±.31

*Values are means±SDs.
†$P<.05$, group 2 vs group 1.
‡$P<.01$, group 2 vs group 1.

The Student's *t* test was used to compare the continuous variable between the groups, and the χ^2 test to compare categorical variables between groups. The values were expressed as means±SDs. Except where otherwise indicated, the time discussed in the text was the time after entry into the study.

RESULTS

Sixty newborns were enrolled in the study, 20 in each group. Three newborns in group 2 and four newborns in group 3 were excluded from the study because of skin blanching around the infusion site. Two newborns in group 1 and one newborn each in group 2 and group 3 died of severe RDS shortly after the study began. The final numbers of newborns included for data analysis were 18 in group 1, 16 in group 2, and 15 in group 3. The perinatal characteristics and the biochemical data of all patients at entry into the study are shown in Table 1. No significant difference in any of these variables was shown.

Ventilator Set-up, Blood Gases, and Acid-Base Balance

While no significant difference was evident between the groups in mean airway pressure (Fig 1) and peak inspiratory pressure at any time during the study, newborns in group 2, compared with those in group 1, required significantly lower ventilatory rates 4 and 8 hours after entering into the study (36±12/breaths per minute vs 50±11/breaths per minute and 36±13/breaths per minute vs 49±14/breaths per minute, respectively). Ventilatory rates of groups 1 and 3 were comparable. No significant difference was evident between the groups in incidence of extubation after 72 hours (two in group 1, four in group 2, and three in group 3). Except for a temporary higher Po_2 in group 2 than in group 1 after 40 hours, FIo_2, Pco_2, and pH did not significantly differ between the groups during the study.

Blood Pressure and Heart Rate

The systolic, diastolic, and mean blood pressure changes in the groups are shown in Fig 2. The groups did not significantly differ in any of these variables during the study.

Renal Function

Glomerular filtration rate (creatinine clearance) and levels of urine output, fractional excretion of electrolytes, and Cosm and C_{H_2O} clearance are shown in Table 2. Urine volume increased as a function of age in all three groups. The increase in urine volume was onefold to twofold higher in groups 2 (120%) and 3 (90%) than in group 1 (65%) after 24 to 48 hours. The same trend, but of a lesser magnitude, was noted in groups 2 (50%) and 3 (60%) compared with group 1 (44%) after 48 to 72 hours. None of these changes were significant owing to a wide variation in individual values.

Glomerular filtration rates also increased in all three groups of newborns as a function of age. After 24 to 48 hours, the incremental change in GFR from baseline values after 0 to 24 hours was 3.6 and 2.3 times greater in groups 2 (65%) and 3 (42%), respectively, than in group 1 (18%). A similar trend of increased GFR, but to a lesser extent, was noted in groups 2 and 3 after 48 to 72 hours. However, these changes were not statistically significant.

In groups 1 and 3, increases in levels of FE_{Na} were noted after 24 to 48 and 48 to 72 hours compared with baseline values after 0 to 24 hours. These changes were not significant, but consistent. Group 2 newborns had significantly higher levels of FE_{NA} after 0 to 24, 24 to 48, and 48

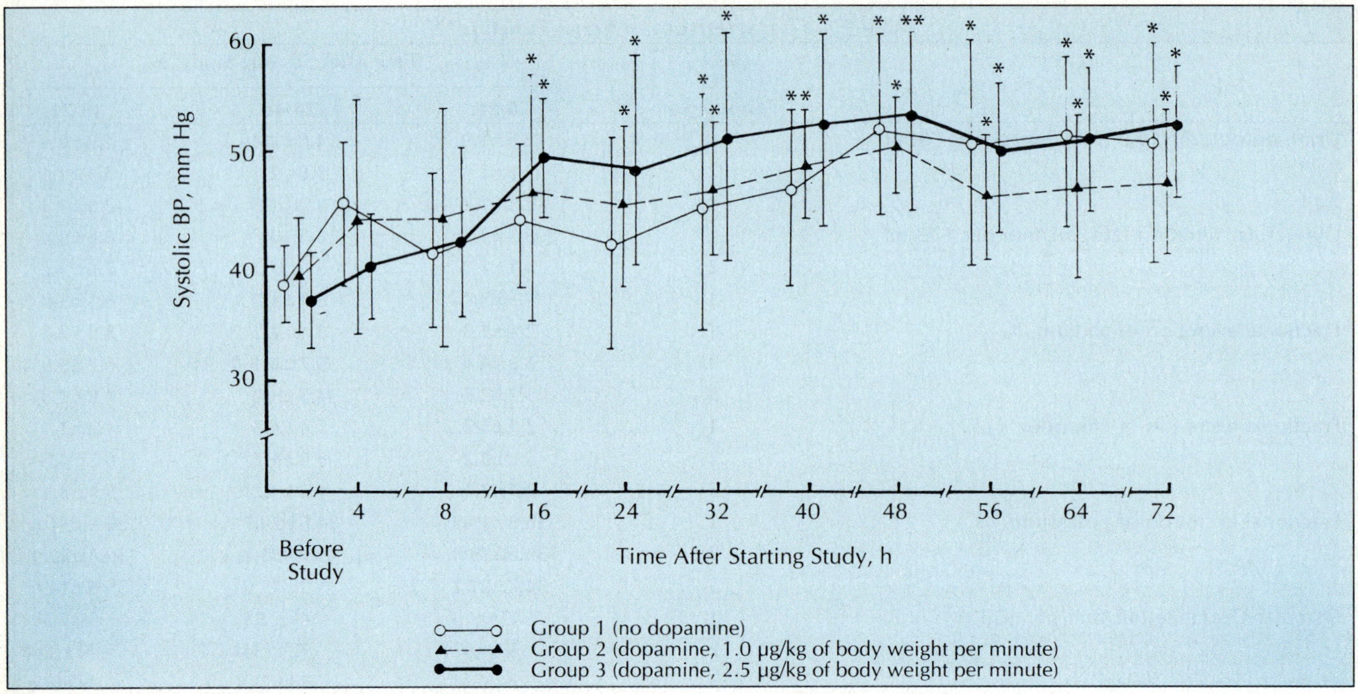

Fig 3.—*Changes in systolic blood pressure (BP) after starting the study in infants who showed initial systemic hypotension. Asterisk indicates* $P<.05$*, compared with baseline. Double asterisks indicate* $P<.01$*, compared with baseline.*

to 72 hours compared with group 1 newborns. Similar changes were noted in levels of FE_{Cl} and Cosm in group 2 newborns (Table 2).

Free water clearance also increased as a function of age, but these changes were less obvious in group 3 than in groups 1 and 2. Because these newborns were not loaded with water, interpretation of C_{H_2O} values should be made with caution. Significantly higher levels of C_{H_2O} were noted in group 2 than in group 1 throughout the study.

Levels of FE_K were not significantly different among groups or in each group compared with baseline values.

Newborns With Systemic Hypotension

Seven newborns in group 1, eight in group 2, and six in group 3 had systemic hypotension when the study began. A significant rise in systolic BP from baseline values to predicted normal values was seen after about 16 hours in groups 2 and 3 and after 32 hours in group 1 (Fig 3). However, no significant difference was evident between the groups during the study in FIO_2, PCO_2, pH, and in all parameters of ventilator set-up. Except for transient higher levels of Cosm and C_{H_2O} after 4 hours in group 2 than in groups 1 and 3, GFR and levels of urine output and fractional excretion of electrolytes did not significantly differ among groups.

Clinical Outcome

No significant difference was evident between groups 1, 2, and 3 in mortality (five of 18, four of 16, and four of 15, respectively), chronic lung disease among surviving newborns (five of 13, four of 12, and five of 11, respectively), and duration of oxygen therapy (30±18, 26±25, and 32±29 days, respectively).

COMMENT

This study demonstrates that continuous infusion of low doses of dopamine (1 µg/kg of body weight per minute and 2.5 µg/kg of body weight per minute) during the first 3 days after birth in premature newborns with RDS did not significantly improve levels of blood gases, acid-base balance, or clinical outcome. In newborns with RDS and systemic hypotension, administration of dopamine improved cardiovascular status by producing early return of blood pressure to the normal range. Infusion of low doses of dopamine produced mild to moderate natriuresis and subtle but nonsignificant increases in levels of GFR and urine volume. Considering these findings, we do not recommend general use of dopamine in newborns with RDS.

The systemic and renal effects of dopamine are complex and related to dose and age. Because sympathetic innervation may be incomplete in developing animals and newborn humans,[10] responses to dopamine may be different from those in adults. In preterm neonates, low doses of dopamine have pronounced effects on α and dopamine receptors, while it only minimally stimulates β receptors.[11] In addition to the difference in vascular receptor maturation, decreased metabolic clearance of dopamine[5] also should be considered when explaining cardiovascular and renal effects of the drug. Dopamine has been found useful in improving impaired peripheral circulation and producing diuresis in hypotensive preterm newborns with severe hyaline membrane disease and oliguria.[3,4] In these newborns, the effects of low doses of dopamine (2 µg/kg of body weight per minute) were assessed after the intravenous infusion of plasma protein (1 g/kg of body weight to 2 g/kg of body weight). Dopamine produced only transient increases in systolic BP.[3,4] In our study, administration of dopamine in doses of 1 µg/kg of body weight per minute and 2.5 µg/kg of body weight per minute did not significantly increase BP when data for all patients in each group were considered. However, the return of blood pressure to normal range in hypotensive newborns was similar to that noted by Seri et al.[3] They noted sustained and significant increases in blood pressure only after increasing the dopamine dosage to 2 μg/kg of body weight per minute. Because most of our patients were normotensive, had only mild to moderate RDS, and received only maintenance fluid, low doses of dopamine did not have an obvious effect on their blood pressures. Thus, low doses of dopamine may play a modulating role depending on the basal condition in a given newborn and may be most effective only in hypotensive patients. Seri et al also noted tachycardia during dopamine infusion only with doses of 8 μg/kg of body weight per minute.[3] In our patients, administration of low doses of dopamine (1 μg/kg of body weight per minute and 2.5 μg/kg of body weight per minute) had no effect on heart rate, a result that was also noted by Seri et al.[3]

The natriuretic effect of dopamine depends on its direct enhancement of renal blood flow and GFR, and inhibition of sodium absorption by the tubules and on its indirect inhibition of salt-retaining hormones such as aldosterone[12] and prolactin.[13] Studies by Jose et al[14] on the effects of catecholamines, including dopamine, on renal function during neonatal development indicate that the low renal blood flow of newborns is due to increased effects of α-adrenergics and decreased effects of dopaminergics.[14,15] Similar observations were made by Buckley et al[16] in newborn pigs. Felder et al[17] observed that the natriuretic and renal vasodilatory effects of dopamine also increase with age.

Alpha-adrenergic blockade increased sodium excretion in puppies and adult dogs. A greater effect was observed in older puppies. The addition of β-adrenergic blockade did not change levels of sodium excretion in younger puppies. These physiologic properties were related to low densities of β-adrenoreceptors and high densities of α-adrenoreceptor in renal tubular membranes.[17] In adults, low doses of dopamine (1 to 8 μg/kg of body weight per minute) may increase renal blood flow. In puppies, dopamine administered in doses of 5 to 10 μg/kg of body weight per minute decreased the rate of renal blood flow and GFR and increased levels of FE_{Na}.

In our studies, GFR and urine volume increased as a function of age in all three groups. However, increases in GFR were of greater magnitude in newborns who received dopamine. The nonsignificant increase in GFR and urine volume shown in this study compared with other studies[4,14] that have shown significant increases in GFR and natriuresis was most probably due to variation in values caused by age-related changes and differences in basal conditions. It is also possible that low doses of dopamine exert beneficial effects on GFR and urine volume only in patients with oliguria and impending renal failure and/or hypotension. Our patients had no evidence of impending renal failure or oliguria, and only a few patients had hypotension without administration of intravenous fluid boluses. Our studies were conducted for 72 hours, while other studies were conducted for only a few hours.[4]

In group 2 newborns, levels of FE_{Na}, FE_{Cl}, and Cosm increased significantly compared with levels in group 1 newborns despite nonsignificant increases in GFR and urine volume. This increase in sodium excretion could have been due mainly to dopamine's direct and indirect effects on tubules and partly to minor increases in GFR. In our patients, the natriuretic effect of higher doses of dopamine (2.5 μg/kg of body weight per minute) was less prominent than that of lower doses (1 μg/kg of body weight per minute). These results are different from other studies in which diuresis and natriuresis were noted with administration of both high and low doses.[3,4] It is possible that group 3 newborns were volume-depleted compared with newborns in groups 1 and 2, as proved by low levels of C_{H_2O} in group 3 newborns after 24, 48, and 72 hours. On the other hand, delayed clearance of dopamine and high plasma concentration may have decreased the effects of renal dopaminergics and increased the effects of α-adrenergics. The blunted natriuretic effect of dopamine in group 3 newborns also could have been due to different basal conditions such as intravascular volume[18]; levels of plasma aldosterone,[12] prolactin,[13,18] and vasopressin[19]; and sensitivity of renal α receptors vs dopaminergic receptors. Because we did not measure levels of plasma aldosterone, prolactin, or vasopressin, these possibilities remain speculations.

References

1. Guignard JP, Torrado A, Mazouni SM, Gautier E. Renal function in respiratory distress syndrome. *J Pediatr.* 1976;88:845-850.
2. McLaurin JC. Changes in body water distribution during the first two weeks of life. *Arch Dis Child.* 1966;41:286-291.
3. Seri I, Tulassay T, Kiszel J, Machay T, Csomor S. Cardiovascular response to dopamine in hypotensive preterm neonates with severe hyaline membrane disease. *Eur J Pediatr.* 1984;142:3-9.
4. Tulassay T, Seri I, Machay T, Kiszel J, Varga J, Csomor S. Effects of dopamine on renal function in premature neonates with respiratory distress syndrome. *Int J Pediatr Nephrol.* 1983;4:19-23.
5. Padbury JF, Agata Y, Baylen BG, et al. Dopamine pharmacokinetics in critically ill newborn infants. 1987;110:293-298.
6. Yeh TF, Shibli A, Leu ST, Raval D, Pildes RS. Early furosemide therapy in premature infants with RDS: a randomized study. *J Pediatr.* 1984;105:603-609.
7. Bucci G, Scalamadre A, Sonignoni PG. The systemic systolic blood pressure of newborns with low birth weight. *Acta Paediatr Scand Suppl.* 1972;3:229-233.
8. Kitterman JA, Phibbs RH, Tooley WH. Aortic blood pressure in normal newborn infants during the first 12 hours of life. *Pediatrics.* 1969;44:959-966.
9. Northway WH, Rosan RC, Porter DY. Pulmonary disease following respirator therapy for hyaline membrane disease. *N Engl J Med.* 1967;276:357-368.
10. Driscoll DJ, Gillette PC, Ezrailson EG, Schwartz A. Inotropic response of the neonatal canine myocardium to dopamine. *Pediatr Res.* 1978;12:42-46.
11. Jose PA, Slotkoff LM, Lilienfield L. Sensitivity of the neonatal renal vasculature to epinephrine. *Am J Physiol.* 1974;226:796-800.
12. Zariksky A, Charnow B. Use of catecholamine in pediatrics. *J Pediatr.* 1984;105:341-350.
13. Seri I, Tulassay TT, Kiszel J, et al. Effect of low-dose dopamine infusion on prolactin and thyrotropin secretion in premature infants with hyaline membrane disease. *Biol Neonate.* 1985;47:317-322.
14. Jose PA, Slotkoff LM, Montgomery S. Autoregulation of renal blood flow in the puppy. *Am J Physiol.* 1975;229:983-986.
15. Pelyayo JR, Jose PA. The influence of age on renal dopamine effects. *Pediatr Res.* 1982;16:301A.
16. Buckley NM, Brazeau P, Frasier ID. Cardiovascular effects of dopamine in developing swine. *Biol Neonate.* 1983;43:50-54.
17. Felder RA, Blechan M, Schoelkapf L. Renal dopamine receptors during maturation. *Pediatr Res.* 1983;170:148A.
18. Krishna GG, Danovitch GM, Beek FW, Sowers JR. Dopaminergic mediation of the natriuretic response to volume expansion. *J Lab Clin Med.* 1985;105:214-218.
19. Koyama S, Sasakr M, Setoyama T, Takahase K. Dopaminergic modulation of the renal effects of arginine: vasopressin in water-loaded rats. *Jpn J Pharmacol.* 1985;38:30-34.

Effect of Necrotizing Enterocolitis on Urinary Epidermal Growth Factor Levels

Susan M. Scott, MD; Cathy Rogers; Pam Angelus, RN; Conra Backstrom, RN

• The pattern of urinary epidermal growth factor/creatinine levels in necrotizing enterocolitis was examined in 75 infants (in 28 infants the diagnosis of necrotizing enterocolitis was considered; 47 infants were studied for effect of surgery or nutrition on epidermal growth factor levels). There was a consistent and significant increase in epidermal growth factor/creatinine values at the time of diagnosis of necrotizing enterocolitis compared with baseline values. Epidermal growth factor levels in infants without necrotizing enterocolitis and in early nutrition remained unchanged. These results suggested that urinary epidermal growth factor/creatinine levels may differentiate stage II and III necrotizing enterocolitis from stage I disease. The increased epidermal growth factor/creatinine levels may be related to the absorption into the circulation of preexisting gastrointestinal tract epidermal growth factor through damaged tissue or to increased synthesis by the gastrointestinal tract in response to the injury caused by necrotizing enterocolitis.

(*AJDC.* 1991;145:804-807)

Epidermal growth factor (EGF) is a polypeptide that may be involved in the growth and differentiation of the gastrointestinal tract.[1] Exogenous EGF enhances gut enzyme activity[2] while maintaining proliferation of the intestinal mucosa during total parenteral nutrition.[3] Epidermal growth factor may be available to the gut via the saliva,[4] breast milk,[5] and probable endogenous gastrointestinal tract synthesis.[6] In the mature animal, EGF appears to function primarily during periods of injury,[7] while the intact gastrointestinal tract has been inconsistently demonstrated to be responsive to the oral administration of EGF.[8,9]

Although the role of EGF in healing has been studied primarily using skin[10] and cornea,[11] recently Wright et al[12] described new EGF synthesis sites near ulcer formations in patients with Crohn's disease, and Grotendorst et al[13] demonstrated EGF-like activity in wound fluid. In the neonatal period, the most prevalent gut injury is related necrotizing enterocolitis (NEC).[14] Necrotizing enterocolitis is distinguished from immature gut motility and absorption abnormalities by its association with the loss of mucosal integrity and tissue destruction.[15,16] As such, NEC serves as a human model of gastrointestinal injury in which early healing is needed for recovery.[17]

Because of EGF's role in healing and the evidence of early healing in the process of NEC, we hypothesized that at the time of diagnosis, EGF levels would be elevated in infants with NEC in contrast to levels in infants with abnormalities of gut motility.

SUBJECTS AND METHODS

Subjects and Samples

All infants admitted to the Newborn Intensive Care Unit at the Children's Hospital of New Mexico, Albuquerque, were eligible for the study. The research protocol was approved by the Human Research Review Committee of the University of New Mexico School of Medicine and parental informed consent was obtained prior to the collection of urine samples. As part of a developmental urinary EGF study, a urine sample was collected within 24 hours of birth and then at least weekly unless the diagnosis of NEC was considered by the attending neonatologist. Daily urine samples were then collected until the diagnosis was ruled out or the therapy for NEC was completed. Some of the infants who required surgical therapy had urine samples collected until closure of their enterostomy.

Infants with NEC were staged according to the criteria of Bell et al.[18] Criteria for a diagnosis of stage I (suspect) disease included mild ileus on roentgenography with clinical evidence of feeding intolerance, temperature instability, lethargy, apnea, and/or bradycardia. Criteria for stage II (definite) disease also included gastrointestinal bleeding and abdominal roentgenograms that show bowel wall separation suggesting edema, pneumatosis intestinalis, or portal vein gas. A diagnosis of state III (advanced) disease included the above criteria as well as deterioration of vital signs and/or evidence of septic shock. Abdominal roentgenograms may demonstrate pneumoperitoneum.

A separate group of infants had urine samples collected daily for 14 days to explore the acute effect of initiation of nutrition on EGF excretion. Day-1 EGF values were compared 2 days after initiation of oral alimentation and at age 10 days, correlating to the period during which NEC was noted in the study group. The effect of surgery was also explored in infants who had a surgical ligation of a patent ductus arteriosus. All samples were separated into two aliquots and frozen at −20°C for measurement of human EGF and creatinine.

Accepted for publication January 28, 1991.

From the Pediatric Research Laboratory, Department of Pediatrics, Children's Hospital of New Mexico, University of New Mexico School of Medicine, Albuquerque.

Presented in part at the Western Society of Pediatric Research meeting, Carmel, Calif, February 9, 1989, and the Society for Pediatric Research meeting, Washington, DC, May 2, 1989.

Reprint requests to Department of Pediatrics, University of New Mexico School of Medicine, 2211 Lomas NE, Albuquerque, NM 87131 (Dr Scott).

Table 1.—Patient Clinical Description*

	Stage of NEC		
	I	II	III
Sample size	15	5	8
No. F/M	6/9	2/3	4/4
Gestational age, wk	24-42	28-32	24-40
No. SGA/AGA	1/8	0/5	4/4

*NEC indicates necrotizing enterocolitis; SGA, small for gestational age; and AGA, appropriate for gestational age.

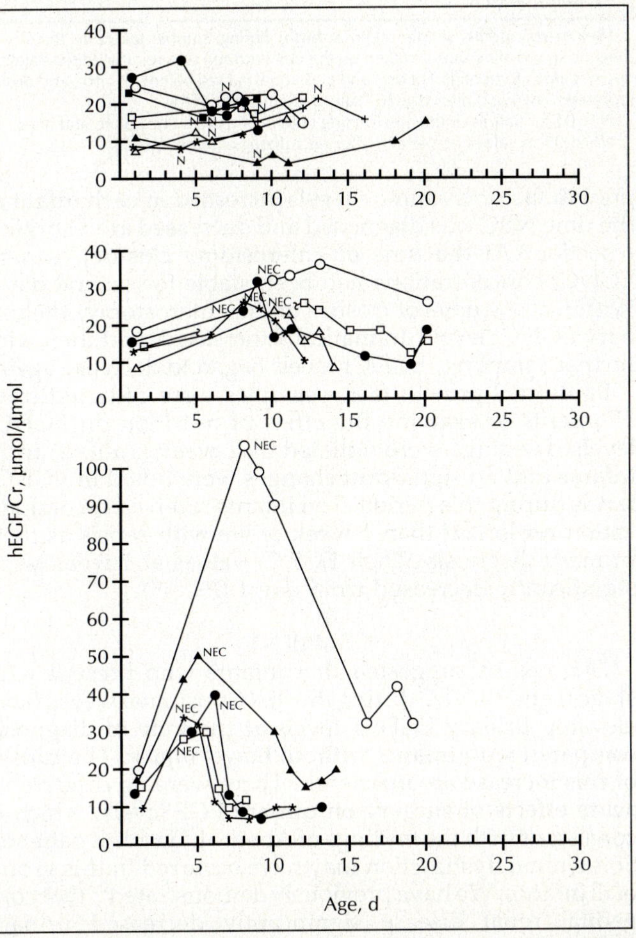

Fig 1.—*Top, Human epidermal growth factor/creatinine (hEGF/Cr) values in eight of 15 infants with stage I necrotizing enterocolitis (NEC) (from Table 2). N indicates days feedings were withheld. The last sample was collected on the day that feedings were reinitiated. Middle, EGF values in the five infants with stage II NEC (from Table 2). NEC indicates day that the diagnosis was made. Bottom, EGF values in the five infants with stage III NEC (from Table 2). NEC indicates day that the diagnosis was made.*

EGF Assay and Creatinine Measurements

Antibodies to human EGF were raised in white New Zealand rabbits using recombinant human EGF. The recombinant form of human EGF had biological activity similar to that of the native hormone.[19] Our radioimmunoassay, as previously reported,[20] used human recombinant EGF for antigen and for use in antibody production. Human EGF was stored at −20°C for use in a standard curve ranging from 10 ng through 0.01 ng. Urine control samples were added to every 50th tube. Human EGF was iodinated with fresh iodine 125 (ICN Biomedical, Inc, Irvine, Calif) using chloramine-T.[21] Repurification was done on a size separation column (Sephadex G=25, Sigma Chemical Co, St Louis, MO) before use in each assay. The homologous EGF radioimmunoassay was run as a discontinuous assay beginning on day 1 with first antibody, normal rabbit serum, bovine serum albumin, and phosphate-buffered saline added to the tubes for the standard curve and the samples to be tested. On day 3, EGF with iodine 125 was added to each tube at 10 000 counts per minute. On day 4, a second antibody (goat, antirabbit immunoglobulin antibody) was added, followed by polyethylene glycol. The samples were centrifuged (TJ-6, Beckman Centrifuge, Palo Alto, Calif) at 1500*g* for 30 minutes, and the supernatant was decanted. The pellet was counted (Searle gamma counter, Des Plaines, Ill) for 1 minute. Nerve growth factor (Sigma Chemical Co), insulin (Sigma) and transforming growth factor α (Calbiochem, La Jolla, Calif) did not cross-react in the assay at a hundredfold molar excess. Human EGF values were expressed in micrograms per liter. Creatinine levels were measured using the picric acid method.[22] Creatinine values were expressed in millimoles per liter and EGF/creatinine (EGF/Cr) values in micrograms per millimole.

Statistical Analysis

Epidermal growth factor/creatinine values in individual patients were examined with paired *t* tests for values before and after an episode of NEC and compared with the values at the time of diagnosis of NEC. One-way analysis of variance and paired *t* tests were used to examine the effect of nutrition and the effect of patent ductus arteriosus ligation surgery on EGF excretion, respectively. Comparisons between groups in which the diagnosis of NEC was considered were performed using the two-way analysis of variance followed by the Neuman-Kuel test, which demonstrates significance for unpaired results. The values at diagnosis were also compared with baseline values by percent of change from baseline, and groups were compared using unpaired *t* tests.

RESULTS

Patients

During the period from January 1986 to December 1988, the diagnosis of NEC was considered in 53 infants. We have chosen to discuss in depth only those 28 infants who presented at less than 2 weeks of age. This decision was made because of the postnatal developmental urinary EGF/Cr pattern. Epidermal growth factor/creatinine levels are relatively stable prior to age 2 weeks[23]; there is a dramatic change beginning at age 4 weeks. The absolute EGF/Cr values of the infants with NEC who were older than 2 weeks were thus different from the EGF/Cr values of the younger infants, but the change from baseline remained comparable. The values in the older infants are not included in the results.

Clinical information on the 28 infants is presented in Table 1. All of the 15 infants with stage I disease survived and were refed 1 to 5 days after the diagnosis of NEC was entertained. None progressed to stage II or III disease. All of the five infants with stage II disease continued receiving total parenteral nutrition for 7 to 10 days and were treated with intravenous antibiotics and gastric suctioning. Each of the eight infants with stage III disease manifested clinical deterioration and required operation for damaged gut. All eight infants survived.

In the older group not described in detail, three infants with stage III disease died. The changes in EGF/Cr values from baseline in those three infants were the lowest of all 13 infants with stage III disease, although they were not significantly different (eight at less than 2 weeks and five at more than 2 weeks).

EGF Values

The first three rows of Table 2 display the mean (±SEM) EGF/Cr values for the stages of NEC. Epidermal growth

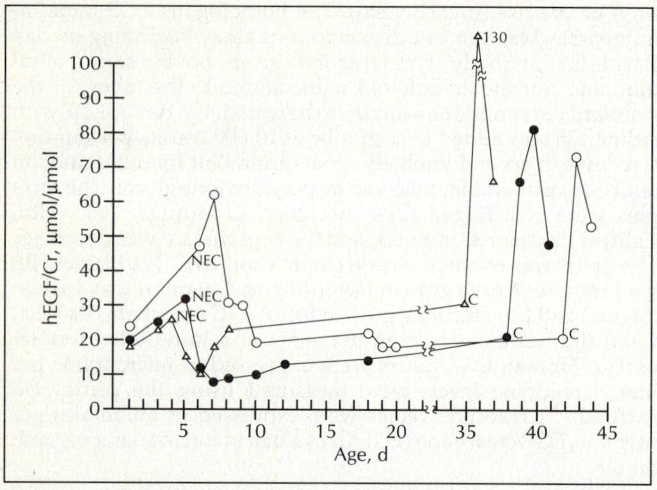

Fig 2.—*Human epidermal growth factor (hEGF) levels in three infants followed up from birth until closure of an enterostomy. NEC indicates day that the necrotizing enterocolitis was diagnosed, and C, the day that the enterostomy was closed.*

factor/creatinine values for infants with stage I disease did not demonstrate a significant change from baseline. There was a significant increase in EGF/Cr values for each patient with stage II ($P<.01$) or stage III ($P<.005$) NEC compared with values before and after the course of NEC, with an increase in EGF/Cr values for each infant ranging from 1.1 to 1.5 and 1.5 to 5.0 times above baseline values for stage II and stage III disease, respectively. There were no significant differences in the EGF/Cr values at diagnosis between patients with stages II and III NEC. The data were converted to percent change from baseline to remove the effect of the wide range of baseline values on statistical evaluation. The groups were still not statistically different ($P=.06$).

Figure 1 displays the EGF/Cr patterns for each stage of NEC. Baseline EGF values were related to gestational age and gender. Our studies have demonstrated higher EGF/Cr levels in female infants and increasing cross-sectional levels with advancing gestation.[23] There was no consistent change in EGF/Cr values in the group with stage I NEC related to the withdrawal of oral nutrition, which is the time of initiation of daily sampling and/or reinitiation of enteral feeding (upper panel). Epidermal growth factor/creatinine values for only eight of 15 infants are displayed for visual clarity. The EGF/Cr values for the other seven were not different from those displayed. For infants with stage II and stage III NEC, increased EGF/Cr values were noted on two sequential days. There was a consistent increase in EGF/Cr values in infants with stage II (middle panel) disease at diagnosis, and levels appeared to stay elevated longer than in patients with stage III disease. For stage III disease, data on all infants who did not require an enterostomy are displayed (lower panel). The increase in EGF/Cr levels usually occurred on the same day as surgery. Values dropped consistently after resection of damaged bowel.

Thirteen infants had urine samples collected for EGF/Cr levels concomitant with a surgical procedure. Values did not significantly change for the 10 infants who underwent a surgical ligation of a patent ductus arteriosus (18.4±9.1 µmol/mmol before surgery and 17.3±7.4 µmol/mmol 1 day after ligation). Figure 2 shows the EGF/Cr values in the three infants with NEC for whom samples were available when their enterostomy was closed. Epidermal growth factor/creatinine levels increased in each infant at the time NEC was diagnosed and decreased after surgical resection. At the time of enterostomy closure, urinary EGF/Cr concentrations had been stable for several days. Within a few days of closure of the enterostomy, the urinary EGF/Cr levels dramatically increased, and then with further sampling, EGF/Cr levels began to decrease again.

Table 2.—Urinary Epidermal Growth Factor Values During Necrotizing Enterocolitis*

	Epidermal Growth Factor Values, µmol/µmol		
	Before	During	After
Stage I (n=15)	17.5±4.0	20.3±2.8	21.0±2.4
Stage II (n=5)	15.0±1.6	33.1±5.2†	18.0±4.1
Stage III (n=5)	13.9±7.8	45.8±25.4‡	16.3±5.8
Oral (n=27)	14.9±8.9	15.9±10.3	13.5±12.3
Parenteral (n=10)	16.4±9.3	12.3±5.5	8.9±3.2

*Before represents sample taken at birth; during, sample taken on the day of diagnosis; and after, sample taken on the day nutrition was reinitiated for stages of necrotizing enterocolitis. For oral and parenteral values, before, at birth, and during represent day 6 and after day 10. Values are means±SEMs.
†$P<.01$ for values during necrotizing enterocolitis vs those before and after.
‡$P<.005$ vs values before and after necrotizing enterocolitis.

Epidermal growth factor samples were collected from 37 infants to examine the effect of nutrition on EGF/Cr levels. Feedings were initiated by 1 week (Table 2) in 27 infants and no significant changes were noted in EGF/Cr levels during this period. Ten infants received no oral nutrition for longer than 1 week of life with sepsis as their primary diagnosis. Their EGF/Cr values at 1 week were significantly decreased from day 1 ($P<.05$).

COMMENT

Our results suggested that infants who present with stage II and III NEC during the first 2 postnatal weeks have elevated urinary EGF/Cr levels at the time of diagnosis compared with infants without bowel injury. The causes of this increase are unknown. There were no discernible acute effects of surgery on urinary EGF levels, which is consistent with the findings of Abe et al[24] in adult patients. Some renal dysfunction may have occurred in this group of ill infants. We have previously demonstrated[20] that congenital renal disease significantly decreased urinary EGF/Cr levels, and others have also described decreased EGF excretion in acquired renal disease,[25] suggesting that our results are not related to renal dysfunction.

A consistent change in EGF/Cr levels could be related to a change in nutrition. Gale et al[26] demonstrated increased urinary EGF/Cr levels in preterm infants receiving oral nutrition compared with those receiving total parenteral nutrition. Our results demonstrated that there was a significant decrease in EGF/Cr values when oral nutrition was not initiated by 1 week. Thus, the initial acute increase in EGF/Cr levels with stages II and III NEC was not consistent with interruption of oral alimentation.

The urinary EGF/Cr pattern in stage II disease may be related to the greater production of factors involved in healing. These infants may have less severely damaged tissue that has not been removed but would then require or stimulate a constant release of factors for healing. The study of Crohn's disease demonstrated the development of a novel cell lineage that secreted EGF in response to chronic ulcer formation.[11]

The urinary EGF pattern in infants with stage III disease may initially reflect the absorption of EGF through a damaged bowel into the circulation, reflecting the loss of gastrointestinal barrier to absorption of proteins.[27] With removal of the bulk of diseased tissue followed by a prolonged cessation of oral nutrition, EGF values would drop quickly. The prolonged increase in EGF excretion from baseline in infants with stage II disease would then suggest continued absorption through the diseased bowel.

The acute increase in EGF levels after closure of the enterostomies was unanticipated. If EGF is lost through an enterostomy and is also needed for healing, gastrointestinal tract EGF production may be enhanced. With closure of the enterostomy, an increased load of EGF may be present and may lead to an acute, short-term absorption through newly anastomosed tissue.

Finally, evidence of absorption of EGF through an intact bowel into the blood stream was demonstrated by Thornburg et al,[28] and urinary excretion of blood-borne EGF was described by Jorgensen et al.[29] These results, combined with the loss of the gastrointestinal barrier to absorption of proteins and the demonstration of EGF production both in wound fluid and specifically in the ulcerated gut, suggest that the changes in EGF levels we describe with definite NEC are not unexpected.

Extremely low-birth-weight infants are at high risk of feeding intolerance and comprise the group in whom the most consistent nutrition is desirable. Also, concerns for NEC are greatest in this group. A marker that could distinguish definite NEC from bowel dysfunction may result in fewer significant interruptions in oral alimentation. Further studies are needed to define the role of EGF in the process of NEC and to clarify the usefulness of EGF as a biochemical marker of true bowel disease. Thus, although measurement of EGF remains a research tool, it may become clinically important in the treatment of the extremely low-birth-weight infant.

This work was funded in part by Basic Science grant 1-1034 from the March of Dimes, chronic disease grant 042-022-87 from the Flinn Foundation, and grant NIH 5 MOI RR00997-13 from the General Clinical Research Program, DDR, National Institutes of Health, Bethesda, Md. Dr Scott is a recipient of a Clinical Investigator Award from the National Institutes of Health.

Recombinant human EGF was donated by Carlos George-Nascimento, PhD, and Pablo Valenzuela, PhD, at the Chiron Corporation, Emeryville, Calif.

References

1. Calvert R, Beaulieu J-F, Menard D. Epidermal growth factor (EGF) accelerates the maturation of fetal mouse intestinal mucosa in utero. *Experientia.* 1982;38:1096-1097.

2. Oka Y, Ghishan FK, Greene HL, Orth DN. Effect of mouse epidermal growth factor/urogastrone on the functional maturation of rat intestine. *Endocrinology.* 1983;112:940-944.

3. Goodlad R, Wilson T, Lenton W, et al. Urogastrone-epidermal growth factor is trophic to the intestinal epithelium of parenterally fed rats. *Experientia.* 1985;41:1161-1163.

4. Mattila A, Perheentupa J, Salmi J, Viinikka L. Human epidermal growth factor concentrations in urine, but not in saliva and serum, depend on thyroid state. *Life Sci.* 1987;41:2739-2747.

5. Yagi H, Suzuki S, Noji T, et al. Epidermal growth factor in cow's milk and milk formulas. *Acta Paediatr Scand.* 1986;75:233-235.

6. Kirkegaard P, Skow Olsen P, Poulsen SS, Nexo E. Exocrine secretion of epidermal growth factor from Brunner's glands: stimulation by VIP and acetylcholine. *Regul Pept.* 1983;7:267-372.

7. Poulsen SS. On the role of epidermal growth factor in the defense of the gastroduodenal mucosa. *Scand J Gastroenterol.* 1987;22(suppl):20-21.

8. Ulshen M, Lyn-Cook L, Raasch R. Effects of intraluminal epidermal growth factor on mucosal proliferation in the small intestine of adult rats. *Gastroenterology.* 1986;91:1134-1140.

9. Goodlad R, Wilson TJG, Lenton W, Gregory H, McCullagh G, Wright N. Intravenous but not intragastric urogastrone-EGF is trophic to the intestine of parenterally fed rats. *Gut.* 1987;28:573-582.

10. Brown G, Nanney L, Griffen J, et al. Enhancement of wound healing by topical treatment with epidermal growth factor. *N Engl J Med.* 1988;18:641-646.

11. Singh G, Foster C. Epidermal growth factor in alkali-burned corneal epithelial wound healing. *Am J Ophthalmol.* 1987;103:802-807.

12. Wright N, Pike C, Elia G. Induction of a novel epidermal growth factor–secreting cell lineage by mucosal ulceration in human gastrointestinal stem cells. *Nature.* 1990;343:82-85.

13. Grotendorst G, Soma Y, Takehara K, Charette M. EGF and TGF-alpha are potent chemoattractants for endothelial cells and EGF-like peptides are present at sites of tissue regeneration. *J Cell Physiol.* 1989;139:617-623.

14. Kosloske A. Pathogenesis and prevention of necrotizing enterocolitis: a hypothesis based on personal observation and a review of the literature. *Pediatrics.* 1984;74:1086-1092.

15. Kliegman R, Fanaroff A. Necrotizing enterocolitis. *N Engl J Med.* 1984;310:1093-1103.

16. Walsh M, Kliegman R, Fanaroff A. Necrotizing enterocolitis: a practitioner's perspective. *Pediatr Rev.* 1988;9:219-226.

17. Joshi V, Winston Y, Kay S. Neonatal necrotizing enterocolitis: histologic evidence of healing. *AJDC.* 1973;126:113-116.

18. Bell M, Ternberg L, Feigin R, et al. Neonatal necrotizing enterocolitis: therapeutic decisions based upon clinical staging. *Ann Surg.* 1978;187:1-6.

19. Read L, Summer L, Gale S, George-Nascimento C, Ballard F, Wallace J. Urinary excretion of epidermal growth factor in the newborn. *Early Hum Dev.* 1986;14:277-282.

20. Scott S, Guardian C, Rogers C, Angelus P, Werner S. Effect of congenital renal disease and neonatal thyroid status on urinary human epidermal growth factor concentrations. *Acta Endocrinol.* 1989;121:505-512.

21. Greenwood F, Hunter W, Glover J. The preparation of ^{131}I-labeled human growth hormone of high specific radioactivity. *Biochem J.* 1963;89:114-123.

22. Chasson A, Grady H, Stanely MA. Determination of creatinine by means of automatic chemical analysis. *Am J Clin Pathol.* 1961;35:83-88.

23. Scott S, Guardian C, Angelus P, Backstrom C. Developmental pattern of urinary epidermal growth factor in the premature infant and the influence of gender. *J Clin Endocrinol Metab.* 1991;72:588-593.

24. Abe Y, Miyake M, Sagawa T, Kimura S. Urine human epidermal growth factor (hEGF) levels following surgery. *Jpn J Surg.* 1988;18:641-646.

25. Mattila A, Pasternack A, Vinikka I, Perheentupa J. Subnormal concentrations of urinary epidermal growth factor in patients with kidney disease. *J Clin Endocrinol Metab.* 1986;62:1180-1183.

26. Gale S, Read L, George-Nascimento C, Wallace J, Ballard F. Is dietary epidermal growth factor absorbed by premature human infants? *Biol Neonate.* 1989;55:104-110.

27. Walker W. Gastrointestinal host defence: importance of gut closure in control of macromolecular transport. *Ciba Found Symp.* 1979;70:201-219.

28. Thornburg W, Matrisian L, Magun B, Koldovsky O. Gastrointestinal absorption of epidermal growth factor in suckling rats. *Am J Physiol.* 1984;246:G80-G85.

29. Jorgensen PE, Rasmussen T, Olsen P, Raabert L, Poulsen S, Nexo E. Renal uptake and excretion of epidermal growth factor from plasma in the rat. *Regul Pept.* 1990;28:273-280.

Neutropenia in an Extremely Premature Infant Treated With Recombinant Human Granulocyte Colony-Stimulating Factor

Robert L. Roberts, MD, PhD; Cynthia M. Szelc, MD; Steven M. Scates, MD; Maria T. Boyd, RN, MN; Ken M. Soderstrom; Mark W. Davis, MS; John A. Glaspy, MD

• Neutropenia in the newborn is often associated with sepsis, maternal hypertension, or prematurity. We describe a 654-g infant born at 30 weeks' gestation by cesarean section due to severe maternal hypertension. His course was complicated by five episodes of sepsis, including three with group B streptococcus. The results of hematologic and immunologic studies were normal except that absolute neutrophil counts were low ($<1 \times 10^9/L$) with intermittent increases during sepsis. Human recombinant granulocyte colony-stimulating factor administered subcutaneously (10 μg/kg per day initially) resulted in an absolute neutrophil count of greater than $30 \times 10^9/L$ within 2 weeks. The dosage was lowered and the absolute neutrophil counts were maintained at 8 to $12 \times 10^9/L$ with no further septic episodes. The human recombinant granulocyte colony-stimulating factor therapy was discontinued after 7 months, and the patient remained healthy with an absolute neutrophil count of greater than $2 \times 10^9/L$. Thus, treatment with human recombinant granulocyte colony-stimulating factor may be useful as a temporary measure for neonatal neutropenia associated with sepsis. A controlled, clinical trial is warranted.

(*AJDC*. 1991;145:808-812)

Neutropenia in the newborn may be associated with bacterial sepsis, transplacental transfer of maternal antineutrophil antibodies, toxemia of pregnancy, and rare congenital defects in myelopoiesis.[1-7] In many cases, there is no clear cause of the neutropenia, although the decreased number of myeloid precursor cells in the normal newborn's marrow compared with adults puts the infant at much greater jeopardy of becoming neutropenic. The most common organism associated with overwhelming sepsis in the newborn is group B streptococcus (GBS), which continues to produce significant mortality despite modern antibiotic therapies.

Thus, the decrease in circulating neutrophils, the diminished myeloid reserve in the marrow, and the immaturity of the immune system of the newborn make these infants susceptible to life-threatening bacterial infections when neutropenic. These problems are accentuated by prematurity, although the neutropenia will usually resolve in both term and premature infants if they survive the early complications.

Treatment has been limited in most cases to supportive therapy with antibiotics to treat the infection when the infant is septic. Granulocyte transfusions have been used with some success, but frequent infusions are required due to the short half-life of neutrophils, and the patient is exposed to blood products from several donors with the associated risks.[8,9] Intravenous γ-globulin may be beneficial for immune-mediated neutropenia but it is ineffective for other forms.[10,11] Bone marrow transplantation has been used to treat specific forms of congenital neutropenia, such as Kostmann's syndrome, but it requires the identification of a suitable donor and further immunosuppression in an already immunocompromised infant.[12]

Several human hematopoietic growth factors that mediate proliferation and maturation of myeloid cells have been cloned with recombinant DNA technology and are now used in clinical trials.[13,14] One of these cytokines, recombinant human granulocyte colony-stimulating factor (r-metHuG-CSF), specifically stimulates the maturation of myeloid bone marrow cells into neutrophils.[15] This cytokine has been used in patients with Kostmann's syndrome and idiopathic and cyclic neutropenia.[16-18] Patients with these forms of neutropenia have responded to r-metHuG-CSF with increased neutrophil counts and decreased infections. However, daily injections are required indefinitely to maintain the neutrophil count, and the neutropenia recurs when drug therapy is discontinued. To our knowledge, r-metHuG-CSF has not been used to treat transient neutropenia in neonates.

We describe the use of r-metHuG-CSF in an extremely premature, neutropenic infant who had experienced multiple episodes of bacterial sepsis, including three episodes

Accepted for publication January 28, 1991.

From the Departments of Pediatrics (Drs Roberts and Szelc) and Medicine (Drs Scates and Glaspy and Ms Boyd), UCLA School of Medicine, Los Angeles, Calif, and Amgen Inc, Thousand Oaks, Calif (Messrs Soderstrom and Davis).

Presented in part at the annual Society of Pediatric Research meeting, Anaheim, Calif, May 10, 1990.

Reprint requests to the Department of Pediatrics, 22-387 MDCC, UCLA Medical Center, Los Angeles, CA 90024 (Dr Roberts).

Infectious Episodes Before r-metHuG-CSF Therapy*				
			Absolute Neutrophil Count (No. x 10^9/L)	
Date	Source	Organism	Before Therapy†	After Therapy‡
6/03/89	Blood, cerebrospinal fluid, urine, tracheal aspirate	*Staphylococcus aureus*	0.72	3.588
6/12/89	Blood	Coagulase-negative staphylococcus	2.835	7.938
7/01/89	Tracheal aspirate	Group B streptococcus	0.752	1.581
7/24/89	Blood	Group B streptococcus	1.484	4.554
8/12/89	Nasal swab	Group B streptococcus	0.555	6.278
8/23/89	Blood	Group B streptococcus	1.504	7.150

*r-metHuG-CSF indicates recombinant human granulocyte colony-stimulating factor.
†Twenty-four to 48 h before antibiotic therapy started.
‡Twenty-four to 72 h after antibiotic therapy started.

of GBS. This patient's neutropenia was not characteristic of Kostmann's syndrome or immune-mediated forms, but the pregnancy was complicated by severe maternal hypertension. The patient's neutrophil count rose dramatically and he experienced no further septicemia after the initiation of r-metHuG-CSF therapy. This patient, in addition to being the youngest patient, to our knowledge, to be treated with this cytokine, also differed from previously reported cases of congenitally neutropenic patients in that his neutrophil count was maintained when the r-metHuG-CSF was discontinued.

MATERIALS AND METHODS

The r-metHuG-CSF (Amgen, Thousand Oaks, Calif) used had been molecularly cloned from human cells and successfully expressed in *Escherichia coli* by Souza et al.[15] Highly purified HuG-CSF and the recombinant product have been shown to have identical in vitro biological activity.[19]

The nitroblue tetrazolium test to assess oxidative potential of neutrophils was performed on neutrophils separated from blood on gradients (Percoll, Pharmacia Fine Chemicals, Uppsala, Sweden). The cells were activated in suspension with phorbol myristate acetate (20 mg/L) and adhered to a glass slide by centrifugation. The slides were counterstained with safarine dye and the percentage of nitroblue tetrazolium–positive cells (those staining blue due to dye reduction) was determined with light microscopy.

Immunofluorescence and flow cytometry were used to detect the presence of antineutrophil antibodies in the patient's serum (Specialty Labs, Santa Monica, Calif). Neutrophils from a normal donor were incubated in a patient's serum, and fluorescently tagged rabbit antihuman IgG antisera was then employed to detect IgG on the neutrophil surface.

Flow cytometry performed by the Clinical Immunology Research Laboratory at UCLA was used to determine lymphocyte subsets (based on surface antigens CD3, CD4, CD8, and CD19). Flow cytometry using a flow cytometer (FACScan, Becton-

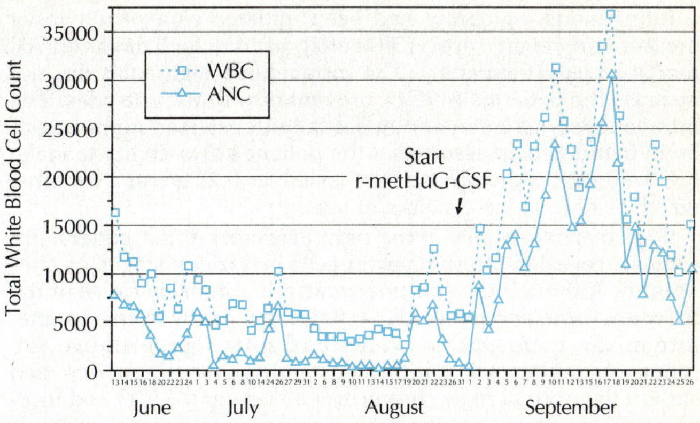

Total white blood cell (WBC) count and absolute neutrophil count (ANC) before and after recombinant human granulocyte colony-stimulating factor (r-metHuG-CSF) therapy. The increases in WBC count and ANC on June 24, July 24, and August 21 before r-metHuG-CSF therapy were associated with septic episodes. The initial dose of 10 µg/kg per day was gradually decreased; by day 20 the dose was 1 µg/kg per day due to the high ANC.

Dickinson, Mountain View, Calif) determined the presence and density of the CD11b (C3bi receptor) antigen on the surface of the neutrophils. The patient's neutrophils were assessed for the presence of the CD11b antigen both at a baseline state (blood kept at 4°C) and following stimulation with the peptide formyl-methionyl-leucyl-phenylalanine at 37°C.

REPORT OF A CASE

A 654-g boy was born at 30 weeks' gestation by cesarean section to a 38-year-old primigravida white woman. The pregnancy had been induced by in vitro fertilization, and the mother had suffered severe pregnancy-induced hypertension. The patient had an Apgar score of 8/9 at 1 and 5 minutes. He required intubation for apnea on the first day of life, and routine supportive care was initiated. Blood, cerebrospinal fluid, and urine cultures taken 3 days later were positive for *Staphylococcus aureus*. During the next 3 months, the patient suffered four additional episodes of sepsis despite treatment with appropriate courses of antibiotics and multiple infusions of intravenous γ-globulin. The causal agents included *Staphylococcus epidermidis* and three episodes of GBS sepsis, all of the same phage type.

The patient was noted to be neutropenic, with an absolute neutrophil count (ANC) of less than 1×10^9/L at age 3 days. The ANC rose to between 7 and 8×10^9/L by age 2 weeks, but then dropped to less than 1×10^9/L by age 4 weeks. The patient continued to have periods of neutropenia, with intermittent increases in his ANC to 3 to 8×10^9/L when septic (Figure).

These recurrent septic episodes and neutropenia prompted an immunologic evaluation. The patient's neutrophil oxidative respiratory burst activity was evaluated with the nitroblue tetrazolium test and the results were normal, with greater than 95% of cells staining blue, indicating dye reduction. Complement activity, as assessed with erythrocyte hemolysis (CH100), was within normal limits, as were quantitative levels of the complement components C3 and C4 (0.74 g/L and 0.24 g/L, respectively). Analysis of lymphocyte subsets showed them to be normal for gestational age, with 61% total T cells (CD3), 39% T helper cells (CD4), 11% T suppressor cells (CD8), and 24% B cells (CD20). Antineutrophil antibodies were not detected in the patient's serum by immunofluorescence assays performed using flow cytometry.

In flow cytometric assays, the baseline CD11b expression of the patient's neutrophils were within the range obtained using normal adult donors. Following stimulation with formyl-methionyl-leucyl-phenylalanine, neutrophils from both patients and controls showed an approximately 20-fold increase in antigen density of CD11b.

Intravenous γ-globulin had been initiated as a prophylactic measure to prevent sepsis (500 mg/kg per day for 5 days and 500 mg/kg weekly thereafter). The intravenous γ-globulin did not increase the patient's ANC or prevent new septic episodes. The intravenous γ-globulin and maternally transferred immunoglobulin hampered assessment of the patient's own ability to make IgG antibody, although his IgM level was 0.22 g/L at 3 months, which is normal for gestational age.

Bone marrow biopsy of the right iliac crest under general anesthesia revealed a few myeloid cells in various stages of maturation. Although the specimen was not optimal because of the technical difficulty involved in obtaining marrow from a premature infant, there was no evidence of a myeloproliferative disorder. Amniocentesis performed during the pregnancy had shown the normal male chromosome number (46,XY) and morphologic structure, but the bone marrow specimen was not adequate for chromosomal analysis.

Repeated cranial ultrasonography showed no evidence of periventricular or intraventricular hemorrhage. The patient appeared neurologically intact and in clinically stable condition between his septic episodes.

Because the patient's neutropenia appeared to precede his septicemia (Table), we believed that he might benefit from treatment with r-metHuG-CSF. His parents concurred with this therapeutic plan, and informed consent was obtained under a protocol approved by the UCLA Human Subjects' Protection Committee.

RESULTS

Within 24 hours of receiving an initial subcutaneous injection of 10 μg/kg of r-metHuG-CSF at age 3 months, the patient's white blood cell count rose dramatically from 5.8×10^9/L, with a differential cell count of 0.12 segmented neutrophils, no bands, and an ANC of 0.70×10^9/L, to a white blood cell count of 14.9×10^9/L with 0.32 segmented neutrophils, 0.29 band cells, and an ANC of 9.09×10^9/L (Figure). As the white blood cell count climbed to a peak of 37×10^9/L, with a corresponding ANC of 26×10^9/L, the daily dose of r-metHuG-CSF was gradually decreased. A maintenance dose of 1 μg/kg per day was reached on day 20 of therapy, and the white blood cell count was stabilized at between 10 and 20×10^9/L, with an ANC of 8 to 15×10^9/L.

A slight increase in irritability that was noted at the highest dose of r-met HuG-CSF (10 μg/kg) resolved at the lower dose. This irritability may have been due to bone pain reported by older patients in clinical trials of r-metHuG-CSF.[16,18] The patient had no evidence of infection for the remainder of his hospitalization. He was discharged 24 days after starting r-metHuG-CSF therapy of diuretics, theophylline, and oxygen by nasal cannula for his bronchopulmonary dysplasia.

Approximately 1 week after discharge, the patient was readmitted to UCLA for respiratory distress secondary to fluid overload. He remained afebrile; cultures of blood, cerebrospinal fluid, and urine were negative and a chest roentgenogram was consistent with chronic bronchopulmonary dysplasia. The patient was discharged after 5 days when his pulmonary status had improved.

The remainder of the patient's course was unremarkable except for three episodes of otitis media that were treated with oral antibiotics. He did not show any evidence of allergic or other adverse reactions to the r-metHuG-CSF. His quantitative immunoglobulin levels were normal for a person aged 10 months, and the functional status of his B cells was verified by a protective antitetanus toxoid titer following immunization. Abdominal ultrasonography did not show any abnormal enlargement of the spleen.

Six months after starting treatment, the patient continued to maintain an ANC of between 8 and 12×10^9/L while receiving 1 μg/kg per day of r-metHuG-CSF. The dosage was reduced to 0.5 μg/kg per day for 2 weeks, and the patient remained in clinically stable condition, with no significant drop in ANC. The r-metHuG-CSF was completely discontinued after 7 months of treatment, and the patient remained in clinically stable condition, with an ANC of greater than 2×10^9/L and with no infections 6 months after the drug therapy was discontinued.

COMMENT

Neonatal sepsis is thought to be a major cause of neonatal neutropenia, as determined by the absolute number of circulating neutrophils and their bone marrow precursors in the newborn. However, in a review by Baley et al,[1] fewer than half of 119 prospectively identified episodes of neutropenia in 87 infants could be attributed to sepsis. Other forms of neutropenia seen in the newborn include autoimmune and isoimmune neutropenia (analogous to Rh isoimmunization), congenital neutropenia (autosomal recessive or dominant), and neutropenia secondary to exchange transfusion or drug ingestion. Maternal hypertension,[3] prematurity,[2] periventricular hemorrhage,[20] severe asphyxia,[4] and extracorporeal membrane oxygenation[21] have also been associated with neonatal neutropenia. In one third of the cases of neonatal neutropenia, no cause of the neutropenia was identified.[1] Thus, the clinical cause of a low neutrophil count in the neonatal period is not clear in many cases.

Newborns have a much greater tendency to develop neutropenia when septic owing to their low bone marrow reserve of myeloid cells.[5,22] Christensen et al[23] examined the marrow of a series of neutropenic neonates and reported that only one of nine survived when the marrow was depleted of mature neutrophils. Neutropenia associated with recurrent episodes of sepsis that persists despite antibiotic therapy merits further investigative studies.

Kostmann's syndrome, or severe congenital neutropenia, is an autosomal recessive disorder in which the ANC is chronically less than 0.2×10^9/L, and bone marrow examination reveals arrested development at the promyelocyte or myelocyte stage. Most patients develop fatal infections in childhood, although a few have been treated with bone marrow transplantation.[12]

Maternal hypertension is often associated with newborn neutropenia, particularly in premature infants. In a recent study of 72 infants whose mothers experienced hypertension during pregnancy, 35 (49%) had neutropenia, which was more profound in those born prematurely or growth retarded in utero. Kinetic evaluation of neutrophil storage, margination, and proliferation suggests that diminished production is responsible for neutropenia in these newborns,[7] and evidence exists of an inhibitory factor produced by the placenta.[24] The neutropenia resolved in 83% of these infants within 60 hours after birth, and no infant was neutropenic for more than 30 days.

Two recombinant hematopoietic growth factors, r-metHuG-CSF and granulocyte macrophage (GM) CSF, have been used in clinical trials for the treatment of primary neutropenia. Although both of these cytokines stimulate neutrophils, GM-CSF also enhances proliferation of monocytes and eosinophils.[25] Granulocyte macrophage colony-stimulating factor has been used effectively in patients with aplastic anemia, chemotherapy-induced myelosuppression, autologous bone marrow transplants, and myelodysplastic syndrome.[26-29] When GM-CSF was used to treat one patient with congenital neutropenia associated with a myeloid maturation defect, the result was a profound increase in circulating eosinophils and monocytes but little change in neutrophils.[30] Other investigators[31,32] have also found that in patients with congenital neutropenia, GM-CSF has a much more pronounced effect on eosinophils than neutrophils.

Prior investigations using r-metHuG-CSF in the pediatric population have focused on treatment of severe congenital and cyclic neutropenia. In a study by Bonilla et al,[16] patients with congenital agranulocytosis (Kostmann's syndrome) responded to r-metHuG-CSF by an increase in their ANCs from less than 0.1×10^9/L to between 1.3 and 9.5×10^9/L 8 to 9 days after the appropriate dose was administered. Marrow aspirates from treated patients showed maturation to the mature neutrophil stage. Side effects of treatment included medullary pain, splenomegaly, and elevated levels of leukocyte alkaline phosphatase. Clinically, chronic infections resolved and the number of new infectious episodes as well as the requirement for intravenous antibiotics decreased.

Hammond et al[17] and others[33] found that mean neutrophil counts in patients with cyclic neutropenia increased following r-metHuG-CSF therapy. Although cycling of blood cell counts continued, the length of the cycling period decreased from 21 to 14 days and the frequencies of fever, infection, and mouth ulcers were also reduced. This cytokine has also been used successfully to treat idiopathic neutropenia[18] and myelodysplastic syndromes.[34,35] Treatment of these forms of neutropenia as well as Kostmann's syndrome and cyclic neutropenia may require indefinite administration of r-metHuG-CSF since the ANC decreases abruptly when the drug therapy is discontinued.

The cause of the neutropenia in the infant described herein is unclear, although this case demonstrated multiple factors that could be implicated, such as bacterial sepsis, maternal hypertension, and prematurity. The absence of antineutrophil antibodies and the lack of response to intravenous immunoglobulin make it unlikely that there was an immune-mediated destruction of his neutrophils. Maternal hypertension is often associated with neonatal neutropenia, but in a recent report by Koenig and Christensen,[7] the neutropenia resolved by age 30 days. Our patient continued to be neutropenic 3 months after birth.

Our patient also experienced multiple episodes of bacterial sepsis, the most commonly reported association with neutropenia. However, his neutropenia often preceded the sepsis, and the ANC actually rose during the septic episode, although not to markedly high levels. This infant's extreme prematurity (654 g at birth) also put him at greater risk of neutropenia. Although full-term infants have been reported to have high levels of G-CSF and GM-CSF at birth, the levels in premature infants are unknown.[36] It has been suggested that in some patients with congenital neutropenia the defect is in the G-CSF receptor on the myeloid cells rather than in decreased G-CSF production.[16,37] However, our patient's very rapid and profound increase in ANC after receiving just one dose of r-metHuG-CSF suggests that his cells were responding appropriately to the drug. Thus, there is no single factor to which we can attribute neutropenia in this patient.

The increased susceptibility of GBS sepsis in newborns is believed to be due to both a decreased neutrophil reserve as well as qualitative defects in the function of neonatal neutrophils.[38] Cairo et al[39] showed that simultaneous administration of r-metHuG-CSF and antibiotics to neonatal rats inoculated with GBS increased survival to 91%, compared with a 28% survival rate with antibiotics alone and a 4% survival rate with no treatment. These findings and a later study[40] in which r-metHuG-CSF was administered for a longer period suggest that G-CSF may act synergistically with antibiotics in preventing GBS sepsis. The myeloid marrow reserve is decreased in newborn rats compared with adults, as is also true in humans. Our patient had an unusual susceptibility to GBS, developing three episodes of sepsis with the same serotype prior to G-CSF therapy. Although ours is the only reported case, to our knowledge, of a premature infant treated with G-CSF, this cytokine may be useful in treating or preventing GBS sepsis in other infants who are not so severely neutropenic.

This case suggests that G-CSF may be used safely and effectively to treat premature infants with neonatal neutropenia, and a clinical trial using r-met HuG-CSF for neonatal neutropenia associated with sepsis is warranted. Although neonatal neutropenia is usually self-limited, it may contribute to a large number of infant deaths and morbidity when other risk factors, such as extreme prematurity or the need for assisted ventilation, are present.[1,4,5] Our patient, unlike those previously described with Kostmann's syndrome and cyclic neutropenia, was able to discontinue r-met HuG-CSF treatment after 7 months and maintain a stable ANC. His lungs and immune system had also matured by the time the drug therapy was discontinued, thus making him much more resistant to the usual childhood illnesses.

To our knowledge, this is the first reported case of using r-metHuG-CSF as a temporary measure to treat the self-limited but often lethal neutropenia occurring in infants. The r-metHuG-CSF caused the neutropenia to resolve within 24 hours, produced no significant side effects, and could be discontinued after 7 months. Further studies on the use of this cytokine to treat neutropenia and septicemia in these highly vulnerable infants is warranted.

The authors thank Jeffrey Smith, MD, who performed the flow cytometry assays for the C3bi receptor on neutrophils; C. T. Barrett, MD, who brought this infant to our attention; Roger Kobayashi, MD, who assisted in the immunologic evaluation; and the other physicians and nurses who helped us collect data.

We also express our appreciation to Michelle Edenfeld for her secretarial expertise and to E. R. Stiehm, MD, for his editorial assistance.

References

1. Baley JE, Stork EK, Warkentin PI, Shurin SB. Neonatal neutropenia: clinical manifestations, cause, and outcome. *AJDC.* 1988;142:1161-1166.

2. Manroe BL, Weinberg AG, Rosenfeld CR, Browne R. The neonatal blood count in health and disease, I: reference values for neutrophilic cells. *J Pediatr.* 1979;95:89-98.

3. Brazy JE, Grimm JK, Little VA. Neonatal manifestations of severe maternal hypertension occurring before the thirty-sixth week of pregnancy. *J Pediatr.* 1982;100:265-271.

4. Engle WD, Rosenfeld CR. Neutropenia in high risk neonates. *J Pediatr.* 1984;105:982-986.

5. Engle WA, McGuire WA, Schreiner RL, Yu PL. Neutrophil storage pool depletion in neonates with sepsis and neutropenia. *J Pediatr.* 1988;113:747-749.

6. Kobayashi M, Yumiba C, Satoh T, et al. Autoimmune neutropenia in infancy due to anti-NAI antibody: detection of antibody with immunofluorescence and agglutination test. *Pediatr Res.* 1989;26:246-249.

7. Koenig JM, Christensen RD. Incidence, neutrophil kinetics, and natural history of neonatal neutropenia associated with maternal hypertension. *N Engl J Med.* 1989;321:557-562.

8. Laurenti F, Ferro R, Isacchi G, et al. Polymorphonuclear leukocyte transfusion for the treatment of sepsis in the newborn infant. *J Pediatr.* 1981;98:118-123.

9. Cairo MS, Worcester C, Rucker R, et al. Role of circulating complement and polymorphonuclear leukocyte transfusion in treatment and outcome in critically ill neonates with sepsis. *J Pediatr.* 1987;110:935-941.

10. Lalezari P, Khorshidi M, Petrosova M. Autoimmune neutropenia of infancy. *J Pediatr.* 1986;109:764-769.

11. Bussel J, Lalezari P, Fikrig S. Intravenous treatment with gammaglobulin of autoimmune neutropenia of infancy. *J Pediatr.* 1988;112:298-301.

12. Rapperport JM, Parkman R, Newburger P, Camitta BM, Chusid MJ. Correction of infantile agranulocytosis (Kostmann's syndrome) by allogeneic bone marrow transplantation. *Am J Med.* 1980;68:605-609.

13. Bronchud MH, Dexter TM. Clinical use of haematopoietic growth factors. *Blood Rev.* 1989;3:66-70.

14. Glaspy JA, Golde DW. Clinical applications of the myeloid growth factors. *Semin Hematol.* 1989;26:14-17.

15. Souza LM, Boone TC, Gabrilove J, et al. Recombinant human granulocyte colony-stimulating factor: the effect on normal and leukemic myeloid cells. *Science.* 1986;232:61-65.

16. Bonilla MA, Gillio AP, Ruggeiro M, et al. Effects of recombinant human granulocyte colony-stimulating factor on neutropenia in patients with congenital agranulocytosis. *N Engl J Med.* 1989;320:1574-1580.

17. Hammond WP, Price TH, Souza LM, Dale DC. Treatment of cyclic neutropenia with granulocyte colony-stimulating factor. *N Engl J Med.* 1989;320:1306-1311.

18. Jakubowski AA, Souza L, Kelly F, et al. Effects of human granulocyte colony-stimulating factor in a patient with idiopathic neutropenia. *N Engl J Med.* 1989;320:38-42.

19. Zsebo KM, Cohen AM, Murdock DC, et al. Recombinant human granulocyte colony stimulating factor: molecular and biological characterization. *Immunobiology.* 1986;172:175-184.

20. Faix RG, Hric JJ, Naglie RA. Neutropenia and intraventricular hemorrhage among very low birth weight (less than 1500 grams) premature infants. *J Pediatr.* 1989;114:1035-1038.

21. Zach TL, Steinhorn RH, Georgieff MK, Mills MM, Green TP. Clinical and laboratory observations: leukopenia associated with extracorporeal membrane oxygenation in newborn infants. *J Pediatr.* 1990;116:440-444.

22. Wheeler JG, Chauvenet AR, Johnson CA, et al. Neutrophil storage pool depletion in septic, neutropenic neonates. *Pediatr Infect Dis J.* 1984;3:407-409.

23. Christensen RD, Rothstein G, Anstall HB, Bybee B. Granulocyte transfusions in neonates with bacterial infection, neutropenia, and depletion of mature marrow neutrophils. *Pediatrics.* 1982;70:1-6.

24. Koenig JM, Christensen RD. The mechanism responsible for decreased neutrophil production in neonates delivered after pregnancy-induced hypertension. *Pediatrics.* 1990;27:266.

25. DiPersio J, Billing P, Kaufman S, Eghtesady P, Williams RE, Gasson JC. Characterization of the human granulocyte-macrophage colony-stimulating factor receptor. *J Biol Chem.* 1988;263:1834-1841.

26. Vadhan-Raj S, Keating M, LeMaistre A, et al. Effects of recombinant human granulocyte-macrophage colony-stimulating factor in patients with myelocysplastic syndromes. *N Engl J Med.* 1987;317:1545-1552.

27. Brandt SJ, Peters WP, Atwater SK, et al. Effect of recombinant human granulocyte-macrophage colony-stimulating factor on hematopoietic reconstitution after high-dose chemotherapy and autologous bone marrow transplantation. *N Engl J Med.* 1988;318:869-876.

28. Antman KS, Griffin JD, Elias A, et al. Effect of recombinant human granulocyte-macrophage colony-stimulating factor on chemotherapy-induced myelosuppression. *N Engl J Med.* 1988;319:593-598.

29. Vadhan-Raj S, Buescher S, Broxmeyer HE, et al. Stimulation of myelopoiesis in patients with aplastic anemia by recombinant human granulocyte-macrophage colony-stimulating factor. *N Engl J Med.* 1988;319:1628-1634.

30. Vadhan-Raj S, Buescher S, LeMaistre A, et al. Stimulation of hematopoiesis in patients with bone marrow failure and in patients with malignancy by recombinant human granulocyte-macrophage colony-stimulating factor. *Blood.* 1988;72:134-141.

31. Ganser A, Ottmann OG, Erdmann H, Schulz G, Hoelzer D. The effect of recombinant human granulocyte-macrophage colony-stimulating factor on neutropenia and related morbidity in chronic severe neutropenia. *Ann Intern Med.* 1989;111:887-892.

32. Welte K, Zeidler C, Reiter A, et al. Differential effects of granulocyte-macrophage colony-stimulating factor and granulocyte colony-stimulating factor in children with severe congenital neutropenia. *Blood.* 1990;75:1056-1063.

33. Migliaccio AR, Migliaccio G, Dale DC, Hammond WP. Hematopoietic progenitors in cyclic neutropenia: effect of granulocyte colony-stimulating factor in vivo. *Blood.* 1990;75:1951-1959.

34. Negrin RS, Haeuber DH, Nagler A, et al. Treatment of myelodysplastic syndromes with recombinant human granulocyte colony-stimulating factor. *Ann Intern Med.* 1989;110:976-984.

35. Negrin RS, Haeuber DH, Nagler A, et al. Maintenance treatment of patients with myelodysplastic syndrome using recombinant human granulocyte colony-stimulating factor. *Blood.* 1990;76:36-43.

36. Laver J, Duncan E, Abboud M, et al. High levels of granulocyte and granulocyte-macrophage colony-stimulating factors in cord blood of normal full term meonates. *J Pediatr.* 1990;116:627-632.

37. Watari K, Axano S, Shirafuji N, et al. Serum granulocyte colony-stimulating factor levels in healthy volunteers and patients with various disorders as estimated by enzyme immunoassay. *Blood.* 1989;73:117-122.

38. Cairo MS. Neonatal neutrophil host defense. *AJDC.* 1989;143:40-46.

39. Cairo MS, Mauss D, Kommareddy S, Norris K, Van de Ven C, Modanlou H. Prophylactic or simultaneous administration of recombinant human granulocyte colony stimulating factor in the treatment of group B streptococcal sepsis in neonatal rats. *Pediatr Res.* 1990;27:612-616.

40. Cairo MS, Plunkett JM, Mauss D, Van de ven C. Seven-day administration of recombinant human granulocyte colony-stimulating factor to newborn rats: modulation of neonatal neutrophilia, myelopoiesis, and group B streptococcus sepsis. *Blood.* 1990;76:1788-1794.

Predictors of Neurodevelopmental Outcome Following Bronchopulmonary Dysplasia

Jean M. Luchi, MD; Forrest C. Bennett, MD; J. Craig Jackson, MD

• In infants with bronchopulmonary dysplasia, the influence of the severity of their pulmonary disease on neurodevelopmental outcome is unknown. Neurodevelopmental outcomes at a mean age of 36 months were assessed in 27 premature subjects who had bronchopulmonary dysplasia. Subjects had a mean birth weight of 940 g (range, 540 to 1690 g) and a mean gestational age of 27 weeks (range, 25 to 31 weeks). The duration of mechanical ventilation ranged from 22 to 128 days, and the duration of requirement of supplemental oxygen ranged from 34 to 1033 days. No significant correlations were found between duration of mechanical ventilation or oxygen therapy and overall neurodevelopmental outcome. In contrast, cranial ultrasound findings of intracranial hemorrhage and/or periventricular echodensity related specifically to poorer cognitive outcome. By age 3 years, severity of bronchopulmonary dysplasia is not a sufficient predictor of neurodevelopmental outcome. Intracranial hemorrhage and periventricular echodensity continue to be important predictors.

***(AJDC.* 1991;145:813-817)**

Bronchopulmonary dysplasia (BPD) is a chronic pulmonary disease that often affects very premature infants during recovery from respiratory distress syndrome (RDS). The reported incidence of BPD varies between 5% and 70% depending on investigators' varying diagnostic criteria.[1-7] Very premature infants are known to be at increased risk of poor neurodevelopmental outcome, but it is not known whether the severity of pulmonary disease in infancy further increases this risk. Outcome investigations of survivors of RDS and BPD provide differing conclusions as to the neurodevelopmental performance of these populations.[8-10] Some studies have shown that RDS and BPD are less important than birth weight, perinatal asphyxia, and other perinatal and neonatal events in predicting developmental outcome.[11-15] However, other studies have reported that severity of BPD is a more important predictor of developmental performance than birth weight, gestational age,[16,17] or intracranial hemorrhage (ICH).[18]

This report describes the neurodevelopmental outcomes at age 2 to 4 years of low-birth-weight, premature infants who experienced varying degrees of BPD. We investigated the hypothesis that there is a direct correlation between the severity of BPD as measured by the duration of mechanical ventilation and oxygen therapy and the risk of suboptimal neurodevelopmental outcome. The developmental sequelae of ICH and periventricular echodensity (PVE)/periventricular leukomalacia as identified on cranial ultrasound studies were also compared.

SUBJECTS AND METHODS

For purposes of this investigation, BPD was defined as the chronic pulmonary disease that develops in premature infants with RDS who require 30 or more days of supplemental oxygen therapy and who have abnormal chest roentgenographic findings after age 30 days. All study subjects were diagnosed using this definition of BPD by the attending neonatologist and radiologist who cared for them in the University of Washington (Seattle) Neonatal Intensive Care Unit. The clinical care of patients with BPD has been previously summarized.[19,20] Ventilator pressure, rate, and fraction of inspired oxygen (F_{IO_2}) were altered in attempts to keep Pa_{O_2} between 55 and 70 mm Hg, and arterial pH between 7.30 and 7.40. Pulse oximetry was used frequently to monitor arterial hemoglobin oxygen saturation to keep saturation between 90% and 94%. Alterations in ventilator settings were individualized for each patient. Diuretics, bronchodilators, sedatives, and steroids were used as clinically indicated.

The study population consisted of 27 infants born between January 1, 1984, and December 31, 1985, who met the described BPD criteria and were followed up longitudinally for 2 years or longer. Infants with congenital anomalies were excluded from study recruitment.

The 27 study subjects included 16 female and 11 male infants; 25 were white and two were Hispanic. The mean birth weight for the study population was 940 g (range, 540 to 1690 g), and the mean gestational age was 27 weeks (range, 25 to 31 weeks). The mean length of hospitalization was 97 days (range, 48 to 198 days). Study subjects were mechanically ventilated for a mean of 46 days (range, 22 to 128 days), and the mean total duration of oxygen therapy was 140 days (range, 34 to 1033 days).

All 27 study subjects were followed up longitudinally in the University of Washington High-Risk Infant Follow-up Program to a mean age at final evaluation of 36 months (range, 24 to 48 months). A developmental pediatrician performed a complete physical and neurodevelopmental examination of each child.

Accepted for publication February 13, 1991.

From the University of Washington School of Medicine, Seattle.

Presented in part at the annual meeting of the Western Society for Pediatric Research, Carmel, Calif, February 7, 1989.

Reprint requests to Child Development and Mental Retardation Center (WJ-10), University of Washington, Seattle, WA 98195 (Dr Bennett).

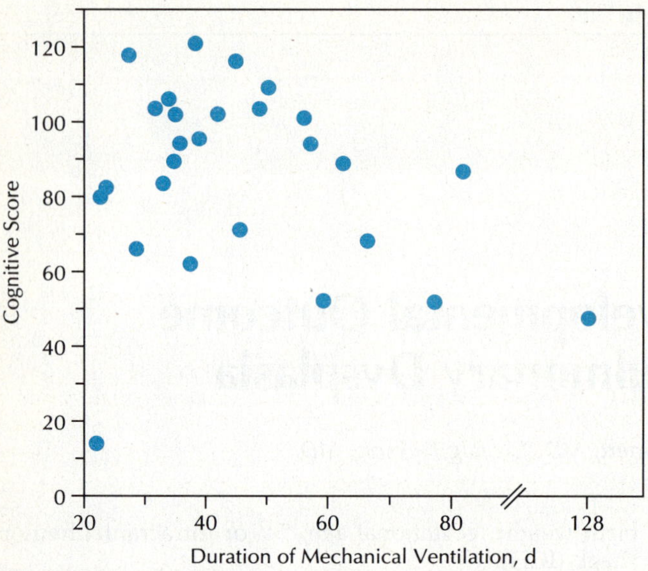

Fig 1.—*Relationship between cognitive score and the duration of mechanical ventilation.*

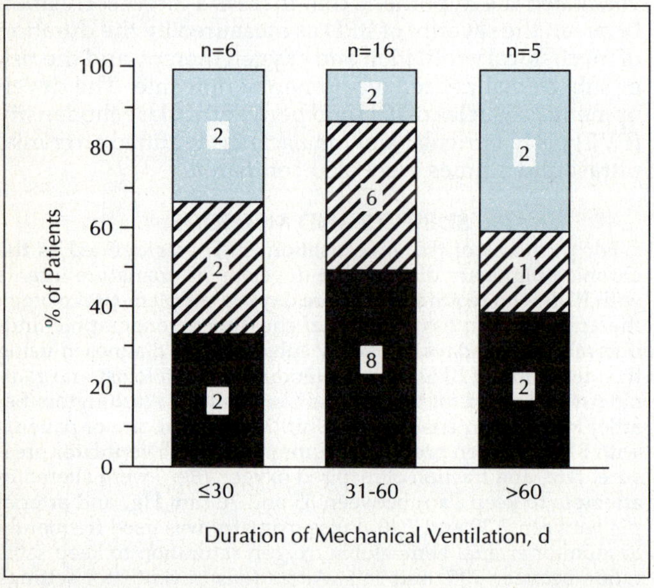

Fig 2.—*Relationship between overall neurodevelopmental outcome and the duration of mechanical ventilation. Solid area represents patients with normal neurodevelopmental outcome; hatched area, those with minor abnormalities; and shaded area, those with major abnormalities.*

Each child was evaluated by a clinical psychologist using the Bayley Scales of Infant Development, the Stanford-Binet Intelligence Scale, or the Wechsler Preschool and Primary Scale of Intelligence (WPPSI). The test administered depended on the age and developmental abilities of the subject. Both neurodevelopmental and psychological evaluations were performed using the child's conceptional age (chronologic age corrected for prematurity).

For data analysis purposes, the Bayley Mental Developmental Index, Stanford-Binet IQ, and WPPSI Full Scale IQ scores were combined to generate a "cognitive score" that describes the cognitive outcome of the group as a whole. Because these tests have similar psychometric properties with a standard mean of 100 and an SD of 15 or 16, it is acceptable to combine the scores for reporting purposes. We further combined the standardized test outcomes with findings from the neurodevelopmental examination to produce an overall summary of neurodevelopmental outcome. Overall neurodevelopmental outcome was categorized as being normal (normal neuromotor and developmental performance), demonstrating minor abnormalities (mild disturbances of muscle tone, coordination, or motor milestones, and/or borderline cognitive function as reflected by a standardized psychometric assessment between 1 and 2 SDs below the mean), or demonstrating major abnormalities (diagnosed cerebral palsy or mental retardation as reflected by a standardized psychometric

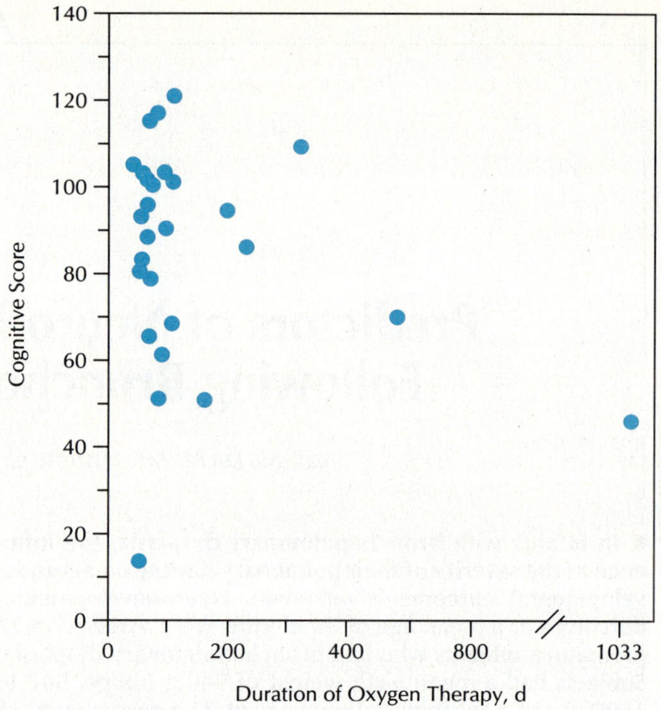

Fig 3.—*Relationship between cognitive score and the duration of oxygen therapy.*

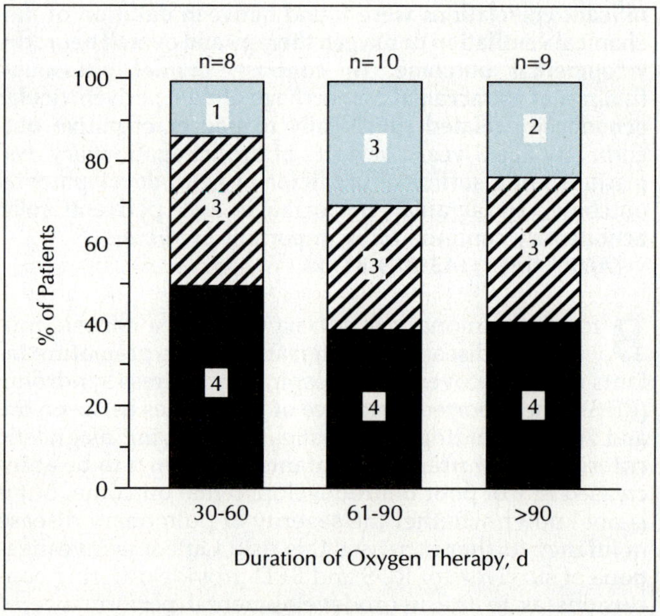

Fig 4.—*Relationship of overall neurodevelopmental outcome and the duration of oxygen therapy. Solid area represents patients with normal neurodevelopmental outcome; hatched area, those with minor abnormalities; and shaded area, those with major abnormalities.*

Relationship of Overall Neurodevelopmental Outcome and Severity of Intracranial Hemorrhage (ICH) and Periventricular Echodensity (PVE)

Grades of ICH/PVE	No. of Patients	Mean Cognitive Score	Overall Neurodevelopmental Outcome, No. (%)		
			Normal	Minor Abnormalities	Major Abnormalities
0/0	8	95	5 (63)	3 (37)	0
I-II/1,2	10	91	7 (70)	1 (10)	2 (20)
III-IV/3	9	70	0	5 (56)	4 (44)

assessment at 2 or more SDs below the mean).

All 27 study subjects underwent at least one cranial ultrasound examination during the neonatal period. Examinations were performed at the bedside with a commercially available, mechanical real-time sector scanner with a 7.5-MHz, medium internal-focused transducer. Scans were typically performed during the first week of life (most between age 2 and 5 days), second week of life (most between age 8 and 12 days), and at least once more beyond age 2 weeks (most between age 2 and 6 weeks). Thus, most subjects underwent three periodic cranial ultrasonographic examinations, with some subjects additionally examined with ultrasound and/or computed tomography at the discretion of the attending neonatologist. These ultrasound scans were reviewed for evidence of ICH and PVE. Intracranial hemorrhage was graded using a modification of the system of Papile et al[21] as follows: grade 0, no evidence of ICH; grade I, subependymal hemorrhage only; grade II, intraventricular hemorrhage; grade III, intraventricular hemorrhage with ventriculomegaly; and grade IV, intraparenchymal hemorrhage. Periventricular echodensity was graded on a numerical scale of 0 to 3, with 0 indicating absolutely no echodensities, 1 and 2 indicating increasing degrees of observed echodensities without cysts, and 3 indicating cystic formation. For purposes of this study, the highest grades of both ICH and PVE coded on any scan were used in the data analysis.

Data analyses were performed with the assistance of the Data Management Core of the University of Washington's Child Development and Mental Retardation Center. Statistical methods included analysis of variance, linear regression, and χ^2 tests. $P \leq .05$ was considered significant.

RESULTS

Six of the 27 study subjects had their cognitive development assessed by means of the Bayley Mental Developmental Index. The mean mental developmental index for this subgroup was 78 (range, 14 to 121). Nineteen subjects were able to be assessed with the Stanford-Binet Intelligence Scale; the mean IQ of this subgroup was 86 (range, 52 to 117). Two subjects completed the Wechsler Preschool and Primary Scale of Intelligence and were found to have IQ scores of 101 and 103. The mean cognitive score for the entire cohort was 85 (range, 14 to 121). Twelve (44.4%) of the 27 study subjects were determined to have normal overall neurodevelopmental outcome, nine (33.3%) demonstrated minor abnormalities, and six (22.2%) were found to have major abnormalities.

Duration of mechanical ventilation was not significantly related to cognitive score in this group of BPD survivors ($P = .09$). Figure 1 demonstrates the distribution for all 27 subjects comparing cognitive score by duration of mechanical ventilation. Likewise, duration of mechanical ventilation was not significantly correlated with overall neurodevelopmental outcome ($P = .08$, Fig 2). Two subjects in each of the three categories of duration of mechanical ventilation demonstrated major abnormalities.

Similarly, duration of oxygen therapy failed to reliably predict cognitive score ($P = .07$), as demonstrated by the data point distribution in Fig 3 ($P = .09$) in overall neurodevelopmental outcome between subjects in three categories of duration of oxygen therapy. There were the same number of subjects with normal outcome and with minor abnormalities in each of the three duration categories.

The Table summarizes the mean cognitive score and overall neurodevelopmental outcome for three subject subgroups divided by severity of ICH and PVE. In the subgroup of eight subjects with entirely normal cranial ultrasound readings, there were no subjects with major neurodevelopmental abnormalities. Of the 10 subjects with grade I or II ICH or grade 1 or 2 PVE or both, seven (70%) had normal neurodevelopmental outcome. In contrast, the subgroup of nine subjects with grade III or IV ICH, cystic grade 3 PVE, or both had no subjects with normal neurodevelopment. By analysis of variance, we found that increased severity of ICH and PVE is associated with worse neurodevelopmental outcome ($P = .002$). Mean cognitive scores were within the average range for the two study subgroups with normal or less severe cranial ultrasound findings in contrast to the mean cognitive score of 70 for the nine subjects with the most abnormal neuroimaging results ($P = .022$).

COMMENT

The present study assessed the cognitive and neuromotor outcomes at 2 to 4 years' corrected age in a cohort of children born prematurely who required extended mechanical ventilation for neonatal RDS and 30 or more days of supplemental oxygen therapy. We were unable to demonstrate a clear and consistent correlation between the severity of BPD and suboptimal neurodevelopmental outcome. No significant relationships were found in this cohort between the duration of mechanical ventilation or oxygen therapy and cognitive performance or overall neurodevelopmental outcome. While nonsignificant outcome trends were apparent for duration of both mechanical ventilation and also oxygen administration, one outlier subject (ie, 128 days of mechanical ventilation and 1033 days of oxygen therapy) exerted an unusually large influence on the two linear regressions. Exclusion of this one subject from the data analyses would have substantially diminished these suggestive trends.

These data support our previous observations that other factors related to low birth weight and prematurity may be more important contributors to eventual outcome than pulmonary disease.[13] This has also been the experience of many other investigators. Fisch et al[11] reported convergence to similar neurodevelopmental performance after the first year of life in low-birth-weight RDS survivors and control subjects without RDS matched for birth weight. More recently, Piekkala et al[14] and Ludman et al[15] have described the relative lack of impact of uncomplicated RDS on neurodevelopmental outcome at 2 and 4 years of age, respectively. In the study by Piekkala et al,[14] the factors most predictive of abnormal long-term development were ICH, hypoxic-ischemic encephalopathy, and very low birth weight. However, the majority of infants in these studies did not meet BPD criteria and the findings may not be applicable to those infants with more severe and prolonged pulmonary disease.

Markestad and Fitzhardinge[12] found perinatal/neonatal factors (eg, birth asphyxia, metabolic acidosis, intraventricular hemorrhage) to be better predictors of developmental outcome than the presence or absence of BPD in 20 premature subjects followed up to 2 years of age. In contrast, Meisels et al[16] reported that 17 survivors of BPD performed significantly worse on developmental measures in the second year of life than their 20 counterparts with less severe RDS. They also found severity of BPD to be a better predictor of developmental performance than birth weight or gestational age. In a study of 159 low-birth-weight infants, Bozynski et al[18] contrasted the effects on development of prolonged mechanical ventilation for BPD with the presence of ICH. The infants who required prolonged mechanical ventilation had uniformly poor performance on developmental scales at 4, 8, 12, and 18 months' corrected age, whereas ICH did not have consistent detrimental effects on developmental scores. These authors concluded that mechanical ventilation for more than 21 days is a powerful predictor of developmental delay up to 18 months of age, while ICH is not.

The major difference between this study and previous BPD outcome investigations is the length of follow-up. While the major recent reports in this area have described 18 to 24 months' performance, we are reporting neurodevelopmental status beyond the age at which these studies conclude, ie, from 24 through 48 months. This older follow-up age (mean, 36 months) provides two distinct study advantages. On the one hand, it allows for more comprehensive reliable developmental assessment with instruments of greater long-term predictive validity. Even more important, for recovering, medically fragile, very premature infants, it allows for an adequate period of developmental "catch-up" to have occurred before making outcome conclusions and prognostications. Borderline, mild, and even moderate developmental delays in the first 2 years of life may substantially improve and even disappear over time coincident with steady, gradual improvement in the child's health status. Of course, the more severe developmental retardation that has been reported to occur in those few infants with extremely prolonged hospitalization and assisted ventilatory requirements (ie, 6 months or longer) would be anticipated to be of a more permanent nature.[20]

While the influence of neonatal pulmonary disease on neurodevelopmental outcome appears to diminish over time, we found a persistent, deleterious impact of common intracranial complications (ie, ICH and PVE) on ultimate long-term performance. Again, one major explanation for the contrasting interpretations of Bozynski et al[18] concerning the relative developmental importance of respiratory vs certain intracranial events is their shorter follow-up. As infants slowly recover from chronic pulmonary disease, the residual and permanent neurodevelopmental effects of perinatal/neonatal intracranial complications may become more apparent.

It is encouraging that the majority of our study subjects were free of major abnormalities. Nevertheless, the observation that less than one half of this cohort could be categorized as having normal overall neurodevelopmental outcome as well as the relatively high prevalence of minor abnormalities mandates caution in terms of predicting school-age function. In time, these less severe but functionally disabling conditions are likely to be encountered with increased frequency in this vulnerable population.

This study suffers from a somewhat small BPD cohort and the lack of a matched premature contrast group without neonatal pulmonary disease. However, BPD was consistently defined, and the investigation's primary purpose was to identify the neurodevelopmental predictive utility of neonatal respiratory and intracranial complications, rather than to describe long-term outcome in BPD in general. Sociodemographic environmental variables not measured by this study also influence outcome. With these cautions in mind, our follow-up of premature BPD survivors into the preschool years confirms the complex, multifactorial nature of determining future neurodevelopmental performance. While severe BPD clearly constitutes an important risk factor for permanent central nervous system dysfunction, follow-up indicates that this risk is not a simple direct relationship and that other interactive variables may eventually prove to be more important.

This study was supported in part by a grant from the Washington Association for Retarded Citizens Research Trust Fund.

References

1. Northway WH. Observations on bronchopulmonary dysplasia. *J Pediatr.* 1979;95:815-818.

2. Bancalari E, Abdenour GE, Feller R, Gannon J. Bronchopulmonary dysplasia: clinical presentation. *J Pediatr.* 1979; 95:819-823.

3. Wung JT, Koons AH, Driscoll JM, James LS. Changing incidence of bronchopulmonary dysplasia. *J Pediatr.* 1979;95:845-847.

4. Ruiz MPD, LeFever JA, Hakanson DO, Clark DA, Williams ML. Early development of infants of birthweight less than 1000 grams with reference to mechanical ventilation in the newborn period. *Pediatrics.* 1981;68:330-335.

5. Toce SS, Farrell PM, Leavitt LA, Samuels DP, Edwards DK. Clinical and roentgenographic scoring systems for assessing bronchopulmonary dysplasia. *AJDC.* 1984;138:581-585.

6. Koops BL, Abman SH, Accurso FJ. Outpatient management and follow-up of bronchopulmonary dysplasia. *Clin Perinatol.* 1984;11:37-58.

7. Kraybill EN, Bose CL, D'Ercole AJ. Chronic lung disease in infants with very low birthweight: a population-based study. *AJDC.* 1987;141:784-788.

8. Harrod JR, L'Heureux P, Wangensteen OD, Hunt CE. Long-term follow-up of severe respiratory distress syndrome treated with IPPB. *J Pediatr.* 1974;84:277-286.

9. Fitzhardinge PM, Pape K, Arstikaitis M, et al. Mechanical ventilation of infants of less than 1505 gm birthweight: health, growth, and neurologic sequelae. *J Pediatr.* 1976;88:531-541.

10. Mayes L, Perkett E, Stahlman MT. Severe bronchopulmonary dysplasia: a retrospective review. *Acta Paediatr Scand.* 1985;72:225-229.

11. Fisch RO, Bilek MK, Miller LD, Engel RR. Physical and mental status at 4 years of age of survivors of the respiratory distress syndrome. *J Pediatr.* 1975;86:497-503.

12. Markestad T, Fitzhardinge PM. Growth and development in children recovering from bronchopulmonary dysplasia. *J Pediatr.* 1981;98:597-602.

13. Bennett FC, Robinson NM, Sells CJ. Hyaline membrane disease, birth weight, and gestational age. *AJDC.* 1982;146:888-890.

14. Piekkala P, Kero P, Sillanpaa M, Erkkola R. Growth and development of infants surviving respiratory distress syndrome: a 2-year follow-up. *Pediatrics.* 1987;79:529-537.

15. Ludman WL, Halperin JM, Driscoll JM, Driscoll YT, Belmont I. Birth weight, respiratory distress syndrome, and cognitive development. *AJDC.* 1987;141:79-83.
16. Meisels SJ, Plunkett JW, Roloff DW, Pasick PL, Stiefel G. Growth and development of preterm infants with respiratory distress syndrome and bronchopulmonary dysplasia. *Pediatrics.* 1986;77:345-352.
17. Meisels SJ, Plunkett JW, Pasick PL, Stiefel G, Roloff DW. Effects of severity and chronicity of respiratory illness on the cognitive development of preterm infants. *J Pediatr Psychol.* 1987;12:117-132.
18. Bozynski ME, Nelson MN, Matalon TAS, et al. Prolonged mechanical ventilation and intracranial hemorrhage: impact on developmental progress through 18 months in infants weighing 1200 grams or less at birth. *Pediatrics.* 1987;79:670-676.
19. Truog WE, Jackson JC, Badura RJ, Sorensen GK, Murphy JH, Woodrum DE. Bronchopulmonary dysplasia and pulmonary insufficiency or prematurity. *AJDC.* 1985;139:351-354.
20. Gibson RL, Jackson JC, Twiggs GA, Redding GJ, Truog WE. Bronchopulmonary dysplasia: survival after prolonged mechanical ventilation. *AJDC.* 1988;142:721-725.
21. Papile LA, Burstein J, Burstein R, Koffler H. Incidence and evolution of subependymal and intraventricular hemorrhage: a study of infants with birthweights less than 1500 gm. *J Pediatr.* 1978;92:529-534.

BOOK REVIEW

The H. L. Mencken Baby Book

By Howard Markel and Frank A. Oski, 194 pp, $20, Philadelphia, Pa, Hanley and Belfus Inc, 1990.

How's that again? A *baby book* by H. L. Mencken, the great Baltimore, Md, curmudgeon? An oxymoron for sure!

Amazing? Apparently not. In the summer of 1907, a physician, a magazine editor, and a reporter in Baltimore (Mencken) joined forces to prepare a series of magazine articles that culminated in a book entitled, *What You Ought to Know about Your Baby* (Butterick, 1910). The current volume, revised and updated, was prepared by Howard Markel, a pediatric intern in 1986 at The Johns Hopkins Hospital, Baltimore, and a Mencken aficionado, and Frank Oski, the chairman of Pediatrics at The Johns Hopkins University Medical School. The authors review the collaboration of Mencken, Leonard Hershberg (the physician), and Theodore Dreiser (the magazine editor), and include a complete reproduction of the original text.

Both parts of the book are fascinating. Chapters discuss the newborn, nursing, bottle feeding, milk, food for growing children, schooling, and "catching diseases." Questions for mothers are included at the end of each chapter, along with the 1910 answers and current answers with up-to-date and appropriate information for parents.

Here are some sample quotations from Mencken:

> Two considerations must be kept ever in mind in discussing the care of infants. One is the fact that silly superstitions, far from being confined to the slum mothers who give their babies beer and dress them in wadded flannels, are rampant to an astonishing degree among women otherwise intelligent and presumably sane (p 29).
>
> Next to unwise feeding, as a source of infantile ills, comes over-coddling. Kissing the baby after it has been fed, for instance, is very likely to cause it to vomit, and vomiting is even more exhausting to a child than to an adult. The desire of all aunts, cousins, sisters, grandmothers, neighbors, parlor maids, cooks, seamstresses, and other members of the affectionate sex to hold the baby and kiss it, and of all uncles, grandfathers and bachelor friends of its father to hoist it to the ceiling should be rigorously denied (p 33).
>
> I sometimes think, indeed, that the degree of civilization of a community may be judged by the contents of its average family medicine chest. In the old days this chest bulged with herbs, barks, roots, soothing syrups, headache powders, lint salves, and ointments. Paregoric was in a place of honor, and behind it stood carboise of arnica and sweet spirits of nitre. In the future, I fancy, the medicine chest will be smaller and less horrifying. It will contain a box of aseptic cotton, a bottle of carbolic Vaseline, a bottle of castor oil, a hot water bag, and very little else (p 160).

Despite my initial incredulousness at the very existence of this book, Drs Markel and Oski have provided a delightful experience for all of us interested in children and good writing. Modern pediatricians and parents will clearly enjoy this unusual compilation of the progress of infant and child care in the 20th Century.

Peggy C. Ferry, MD
Department of Pediatrics
University of Arizona
College of Medicine
1501 N Campbell
Tucson, AZ 85724

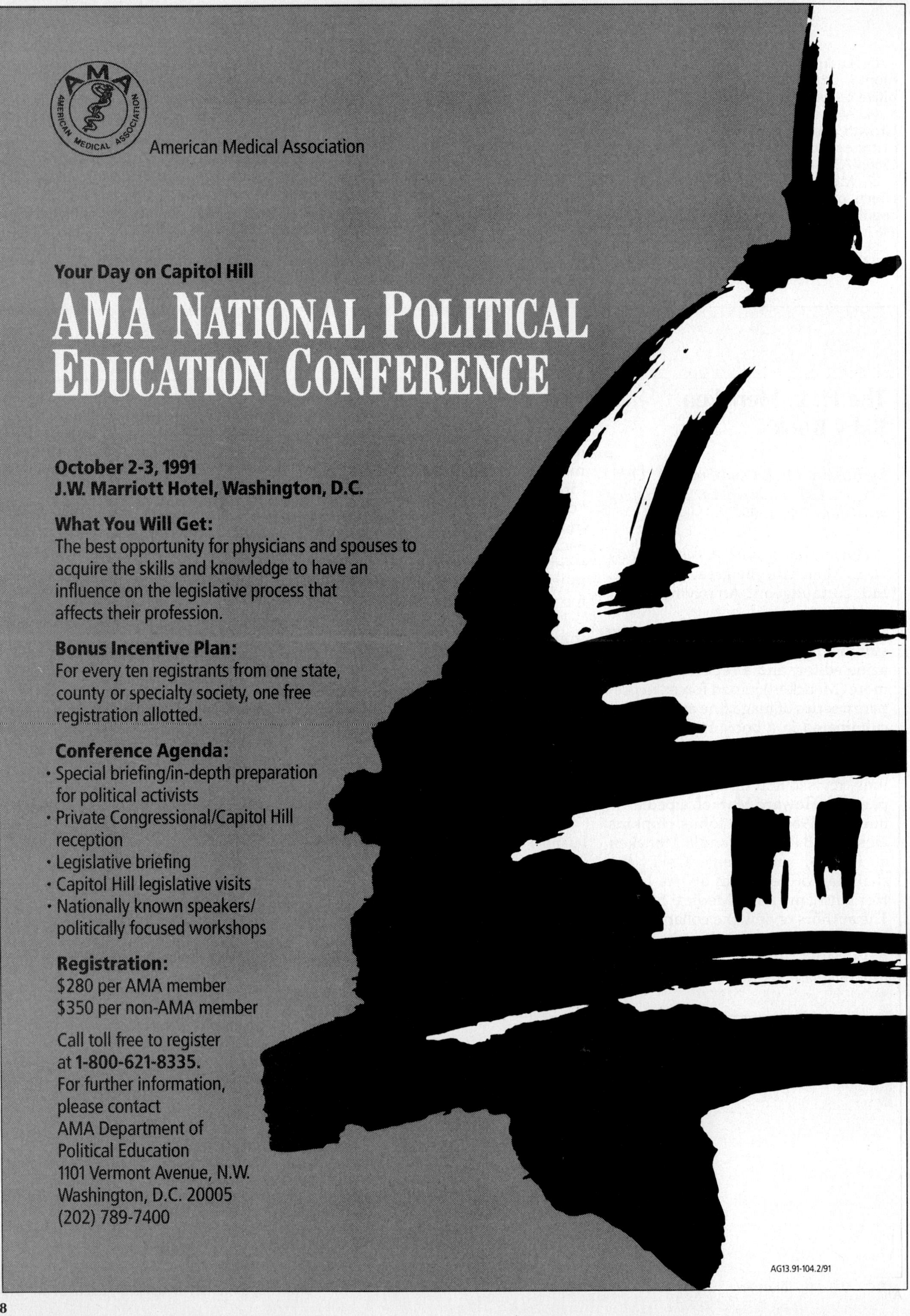
American Medical Association
AMA AMERICAN MEDICAL ASSOCIATION
Your Day on Capitol Hill
AMA NATIONAL POLITICAL EDUCATION CONFERENCE
October 2-3, 1991
J.W. Marriott Hotel, Washington, D.C.
What You Will Get:
The best opportunity for physicians and spouses to acquire the skills and knowledge to have an influence on the legislative process that affects their profession.
Bonus Incentive Plan:
For every ten registrants from one state, county or specialty society, one free registration allotted.
Conference Agenda:
· Special briefing/in-depth preparation for political activists
· Private Congressional/Capitol Hill reception
· Legislative briefing
· Capitol Hill legislative visits
· Nationally known speakers/ politically focused workshops
Registration:
$280 per AMA member
$350 per non-AMA member
Call toll free to register at 1-800-621-8335.
For further information, please contact
AMA Department of Political Education
1101 Vermont Avenue, N.W.
Washington, D.C. 20005
(202) 789-7400
AG13.91-104.2/91

SPECIAL FEATURE

Radiological Case of the Month

Ahmed H. Al-Salem, FRCSI, FICS, Chris Grant, FRCS (Contributors);
Beverly P. Wood, MD (Section Editor)

A 4-month-old male infant was admitted to the hospital because of recurrent respiratory infections that started early in the neonatal period. He had been admitted to hospitals at ages 6 days, 50 days, and 3 months for treatment of respiratory infections. His physical examination revealed respiratory distress with decreased breath sounds in the left hemithorax. The cardiac examination results were normal. A chest radiograph was obtained (Fig 1). Culture of tracheal aspirate yielded *Streptococcus pneumoniae.* The patient was treated with antibiotics and chest physiotherapy. Despite clinical improvement, there was no alteration in the chest radiographic findings. A computed tomographic scan of the chest (Fig 2), bronchoscopy, and bronchography (Fig 3) were performed. Bronchoscopy showed no inhaled foreign body.

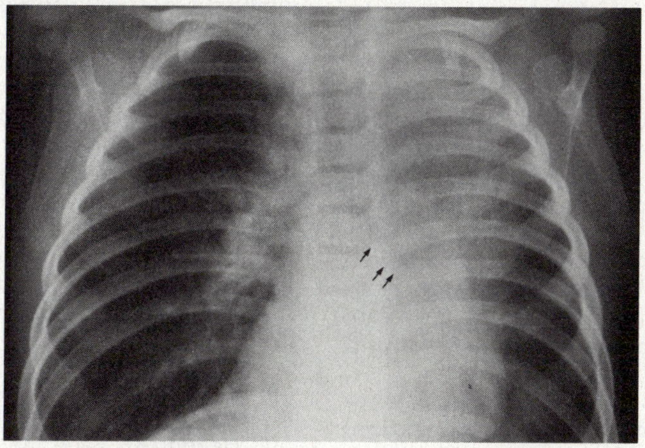

Figure 1.

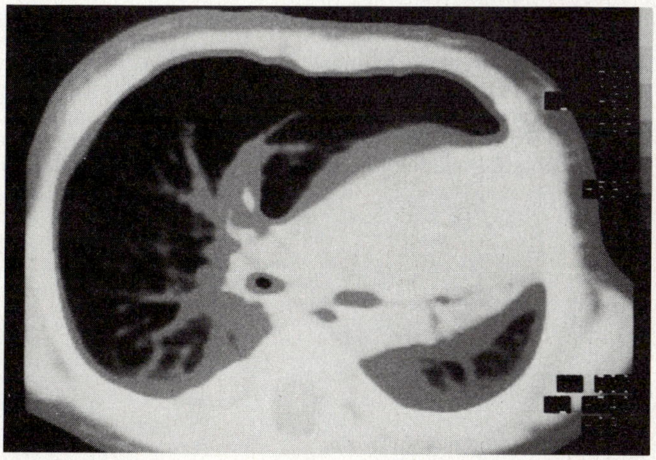

Figure 2.

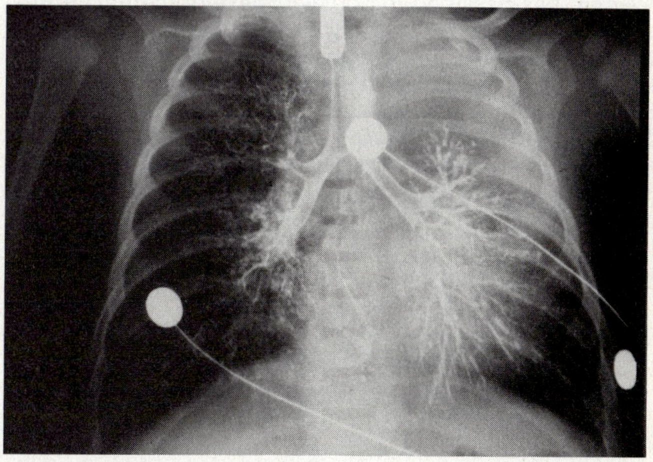

Figure 3.

Accepted for publication March 12, 1990.

Contributed from the Pediatric Surgery Division, Department of Surgery, King Fahd Hospital of the University, PO Box 2208, Al-Khobar 31952, Saudi Arabia.

Reprint requests to the Department of Radiology, Childrens Hospital of Los Angeles, 4650 Sunset Blvd, Los Angeles, CA 90027 (Dr Wood).

Denouement and Discussion

Hypoplastic Left Upper Lobe

Fig 1.—*Anteroposterior radiograph of the chest shows opacity in the left upper hemithorax, a shift of the mediastinum to the left, reflecting decreased lung volume on that side, and increased volume of the right lung. The left main-stem bronchus is low (arrows), and the pattern of density does not demonstrate the usual configuration of lobar atelectasis.*

Fig 2.—*Computed tomographic scan of the chest shows compensatory hyperinflation of the right upper lobe with midline herniation. The left hemithorax is small.*

Fig 3.—*Bronchogram shows visualization of the bronchial tree bilaterally. The upper lobe bronchi on the left are hypoplastic, and all bronchi are displaced downward. No bronchi communicate with the opacity in the left upper thorax.*

At thoracotomy, the patient was found to have a markedly hypoplastic left upper lobe that was firm, consolidated, and had fibrinous pleural adhesions. The right lung was hyperexpanded. While dissection was carried out for a left upper lobectomy, the patient developed severe bradycardia and hypotension from reflex vagal stimulation. He was resuscitated and recovered, but soon developed another such episode. The procedure was postponed and the infant was admitted to the intensive care unit. Seven days later, he experienced a cardiac arrest and died.

In the development of the respiratory tract, interference with bronchial branching, pulmonary artery arborization, and subsequent development of the lung mesenchyme result in a wide spectrum of pulmonary malformations.[1,2] Boyden[3] has classified hypoplastic developmental anomalies of the lung into the following categories: (1) agenesis, in which there is complete absence of one or both lungs, without bronchial or pulmonary arterial supply or differentiated parenchymal tissue; (2) aplasia, in which a rudimentary bronchus ends in a blind pouch with no arterial supply or parenchymal development; and (3) hypoplasia, in which the bronchus is formed but is very small and ends in a fleshy mass of undifferentiated lung mesenchyme.

Hypoplasia may involve the entire lung or a lobe. The most common association of pulmonary hypoplasia is with a congenital diaphragmatic hernia.[4] Congenital hypoplasia also results from interference with the progressive development and arborization of the bronchiolar-acinar groups during the period of rapid growth in the third trimester of gestation.[5] Acquired hypoplasia may result from severe infection, with extensive parenchymal involvement in infancy and inhibition of further development. When one lobe is hypoplastic, the patient may be asymptomatic, but common symptoms are those of recurrent respiratory infection. Although developmental defects of the lung are uncommon, awareness of the possibility is essential in prospective management.

Diagnosis by chest radiography is difficult because the appearance mimics some features of atelectasis. A computed tomographic scan of the chest is helpful in identifying hypoplasia of the thorax and hypoplastic or absent bronchi, also shown by bronchography (Fig 3). Bronchoscopy and computed tomography exclude possible extraluminal or intraluminal bronchial obstruction.

Treatment consists of antibiotics and chest physiotherapy for superimposed infection. An infected hypoplastic lobe may require resection since it lacks the usual intrinsic mechanisms for combating infection and stasis of secretions.

1. Moore KL. *The Developing Human: Clinically Oriented Embryology.* Philadelphia, Pa: WB Saunders Co; 1974:168-172.

2. Heithoff KB, Sane SM, Williams HJ, et al. Bronchopulmonary foregut malformations: a unifying etiological concept. *AJR Am J Roentgenol.* 1976;126:46-55.

3. Boyden EA. Developmental anomalies of lungs. *Am J Surg.* 1955;89:79-89.

4. Raffensperger JG. Agenesis and hypoplasia of the lung. In: *Swenson's Pediatric Surgery.* 4th ed. East Norwalk, Conn: Appleton & Lange; 1980:704-706.

5. Sabiston DC Jr, Spencer FC, eds. *Gibbon's Surgery of the Chest.* 4th ed. Philadelphia, Pa: WB Saunders Co; 1983;1:676-678.

SPECIAL FEATURE

Picture of the Month

Walter W. Tunnessenn, Jr, MD (Contributor and Section Editor)

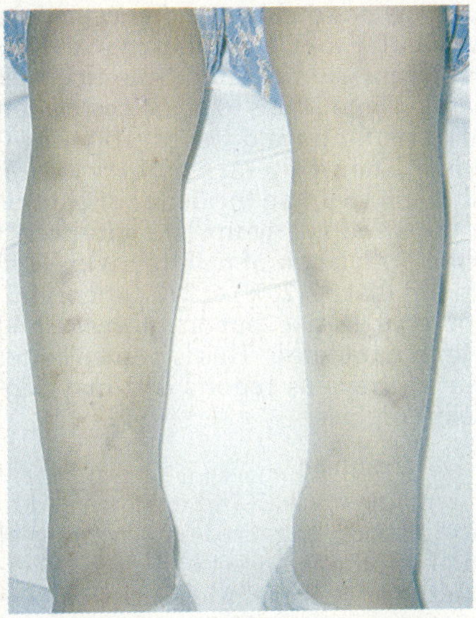

Figure 1.

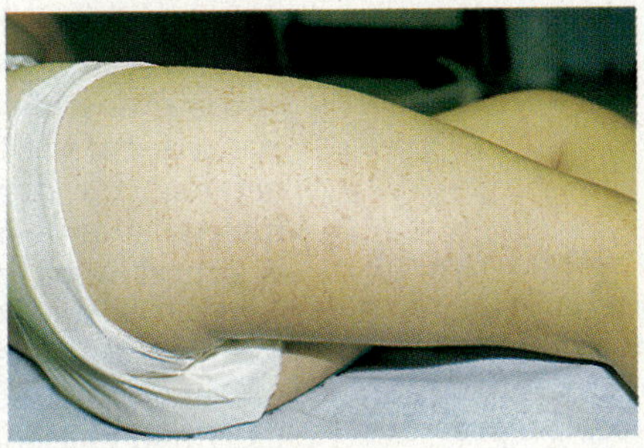

Figure 2.

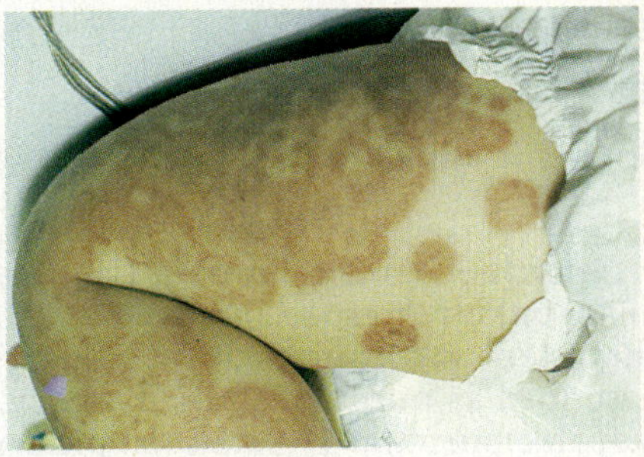

Figure 3.

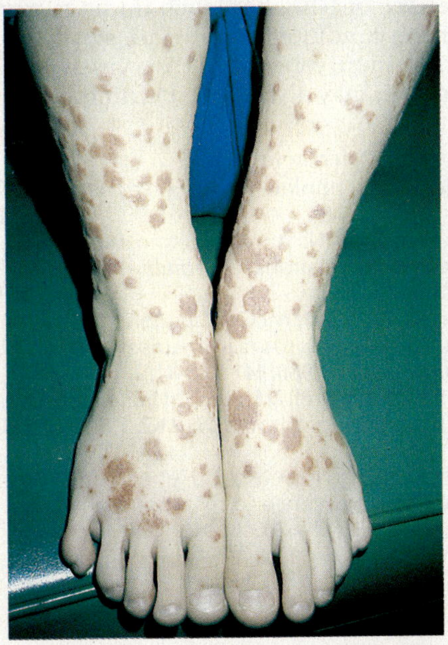

Figure 4.

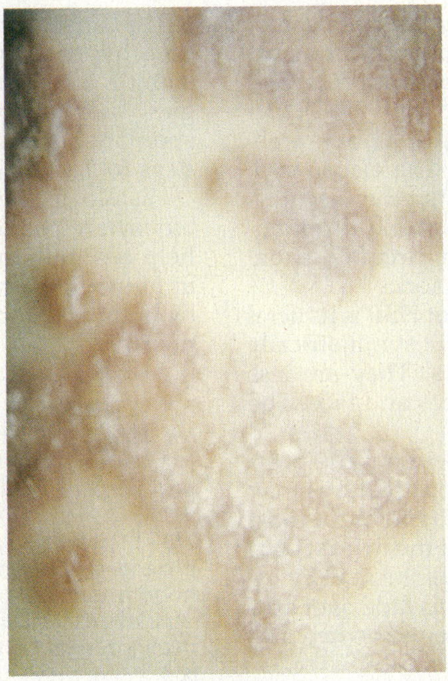

Figure 5.

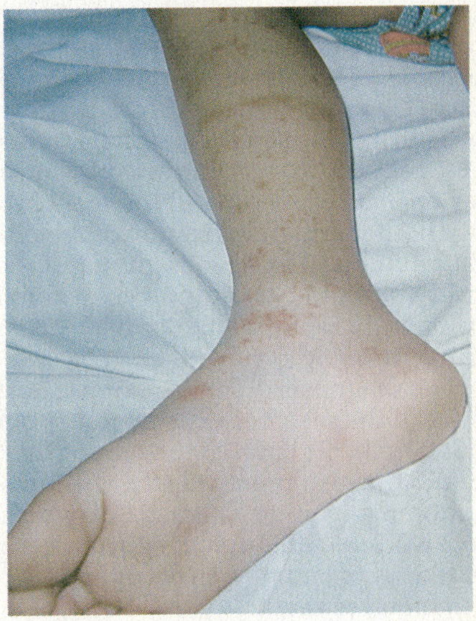

Figure 6.

The Editors welcome contributions to Picture of the Month and Radiological Case of the Month. Those who wish to contribute should send their manuscripts to Dr Tunnessen (Picture of the Month), The Children's Hospital of Philadelphia, 34th Street and Civic Center Blvd, Philadelphia, PA 19104, or Dr Wood (Radiological Case of the Month), Department of Radiology, Childrens Hospital of Los Angeles, 4650 Sunset Blvd, Los Angeles, CA 90027. Articles and photographs accepted for publication will bear the contributor's name. There is no charge for reproduction and printing of color illustrations.

Accepted for publication January 3, 1991.
Contributed from the Children's Hospital of Philadelphia (Pa).
Reprint requests to Children's Hospital of Philadelphia, 34th St and Civic Center Blvd, Philadelphia, PA 19104 (Dr Tunnessen).

Denouement and Discussion

Henoch-Schönlein Purpura

Fig 1.—*Ecchymotic lesions.*

Fig 2.—*Petechial lesions.*

Fig 3.—*Targetoid lesions.*

Figs 4 and 5.—*Vesicular lesions.*

Fig 6.—*The elastic sock sign.*

Manifestations

Henoch-Schönlein Purpura (HSP) is a systemic vasculitis of unknown cause. Involvement of the skin is the most characteristic feature of this disorder. The rash of HSP is described as purpuric and, classically, as demonstrating palpable purpura. The children pictured on the previous page all have HSP, but their skin involvements differ considerably in appearance. The variability in appearance of the rash associated with HSP may lead to confusion regarding the correct diagnosis unless associated features make other possibilities less likely.

Before the appearance of the purpura, the rash sometimes appears as erythematous maculopapules or as urticarial lesions. These lesions usually become purpuric and can be ecchymotic (Fig 1) or petechial (<3 mm, Fig 2). Occasionally, the lesions appear targetoid (Fig 3), but rarely become vesiculobullous (Figs 4 and 5). The elastic sock sign (Fig 6) is helpful in clinically separating the vasculitis of HSP from purpuric lesions associated with thrombocytopenia. The sign is created by linearly circumferential lesions corresponding to the top of the sock.

Another important feature of the rash of HSP is its acral distribution. The lesions primarily occur symmetrically over the buttocks and lower extremities. They are less commonly found on the upper extremities and face. The trunk is rarely involved.

The diagnosis of HSP is rarely made without the presence of the rash because the noncutaneous features may not be specific enough to warrant this diagnosis. In most cases, the rash precedes other features of the disease, but abdominal pain or arthralgia may precede the rash by up to 2 weeks.[1] Although the purpuric lesions fade over several days of bed rest, they commonly reappear when ambulation resumes.

Another curious cutaneous finding in HSP is the appearance of localized areas of subcutaneous swelling. The hands, feet, and scalp are the areas most often affected by edema, but facial, periorbital, scrotal, and lumbar areas may also be affected. The edema is often painful.

Noncutaneous features of HSP may also include periarticular swelling, colicky abdominal pain with melena, guaiac-positive stools, hematemesis, and intussusception, nephritis, hypertension, orchitis, and encephalopathy. Nephritis occurs in 40% to 60% of children with HSP and is almost always present within the first 3 months after the onset of the illness.[1] There seems to be no correlation between the degree of nephritis and the severity of extrarenal manifestations.[2] The long-term morbidity of HSP is generally of renal origin, with an incidence of chronic renal disease of 6% to 38% at follow-up.[3] A more recent study in an unselected population of children with HSP in Belfast, Ireland, found that 54 (20%) of 270 patients initially had evidence of renal disease, but only three (1.1%) demonstrated long-term morbidity.[3] This is a much better prognosis than those of previous reports and may represent the lack of selection bias.

Treatment

The cause of HSP remains unclear, but it is believed to be a hypersensitivity reaction triggered by a variety of stimuli, including viral infections, insect bites, food allergies, vaccinations, and drug therapy. Most cases resolve spontaneously and last an average of 3.9 weeks (range, 3 days to 2 years).[4]

Histologic findings of leukocytoclastic vasculitis on skin biopsy are characteristic of HSP, and such findings may help recognition of the condition. The demonstration of immunoglobulin deposition, especially IgA in vessel walls by immunofluorescence, may also help confirm the diagnosis.[5]

References

1. Saulsbury FT. Henoch-Schönlein purpura. *Pediatr Dermatol.* 1984;1:195-201.
2. Hurley RM, Drummond KN. Anaphylactoid purpura nephritis: clinicopathologic correlations. *J Pediatr.* 1972;81:904-911.
3. Stewart M, Savage JM, Bell B, McCord B. Long term renal prognosis of Henoch-Schönlein purpura in an unselected childhood population. *Eur J Pediatr.* 1988;147:113-115.
4. Allen DM, Diamond LK, Howell DA. Anaphylactoid purpura in children (Schönlein-Henoch syndrome). *AJDC.* 1960;99:833-854.
5. Van Hale HM, Gibson LE, Schroeter AL. Henoch-Schönlein vasculitis: direct immunofluorescence study of uninvolved skin. *J Am Acad Dermatol.* 1986;15:665-670.

Child Welfare: The Phantom of the Health Care System

Sir.—The problem of infants requiring prolonged hospitalization for lack of appropriate discharge placements has resulted in a new population of children receiving medical care. These children have been called "boarder babies," and their numbers are steadily increasing. On a given day in Philadelphia, Pa, 70 boarder babies are in hospitals awaiting discharge. They limit access to medical care for other children by occupying beds and increasing the hospitals' operating costs.

This is one of the most insidious side effects of the current crack cocaine epidemic, resulting in the abandonment of numerous infants in hospitals. It has resulted in what one author describes as "the youngest of the homeless."[1]

A June 1989 survey[1] by the Child Welfare League of America of hospitals in five American cities identified 304 boarder babies in the 54 hospitals reporting cases. At least 69% of the identified babies showed signs of impairment due to the mother's drug habits.

The reason for the continuation of hospitalization following completion of medical goals generally falls into two categories. The first is the abandonment by families unwilling to provide care. This group contains many of the cocaine-addicted mothers. In Philadelphia alone, it is estimated that 16.4% of the more than 28 000 babies born annually will have been exposed to cocaine in utero. In just 1 year, that city will have another 4500 potentially drug-damaged children for whom to plan. Approximately 10% of these children will require some form of substitute care after birth.

The second group includes the technology-dependent, medically fragile child whose family is unable to provide appropriate care at home. This group includes many single-parent, low-income families for whom medical assistance does not reimburse for sufficient support services in the home. A committed secondary care provider is unavailable in many cases, and the child welfare system is faced with the challenge of finding a medically sophisticated foster home for these children.

The number of special-needs children in Philadelphia increased from 79 in fiscal year 1986 to 467 in fiscal year 1990. The cost of providing services to these children grew from $2.9 million to approximately $16.1 million in that time.[2] The response by the state and federal legislatures for increased support for these children has been sluggish, and consequently many of these infants remain in tertiary care or intermediate care hospitals due to lack of funds.

This problem adversely affects both the health of individual children and the health of medical practice by causing inappropriate utilization of hospital beds. The pediatric community has an obligation to understand the child welfare system and advocate for its mission. Through programs such as the American Academy of Pediatrics' "Healthy Partnership for Children," pediatricians can participate in innovative programs that directly impact community issues. Pediatricians can become involved with their local child welfare system by serving on advisory boards and providing medical input to a system that is struggling with comprehending medical issues.

For too long, the child welfare system has been regarded as the "phantom of the health care system," an unseen and sinister actor in the tragedy that affects many of our sickest and most vulnerable children. It is time for pediatricians, social workers, educators, and bureaucrats to form alliances that will result not only in preventive programs to improve health, but also in "care providing" programs that offer services to children and families who desperately require aid.

Frank S. Pidcock, MD
Department of Pediatrics
Jefferson Medical College
Philadelphia, PA 19131

1. Munns JM. The youngest of the homeless: characteristics of hospital boarder babies in five cities. Presented at the Child Welfare League of America; August 2, 1989.
2. Philadelphia, Pa, City Council Operating Budget Hearings, April 23, 1990 (testimony of Joan M. Reeves, commissioner of the Department of Human Services, Philadelphia).

Resident and Nurse Practitioners: Responding to Education and Patient Care Needs

Sir.—In recent issues of *AJDC*, Bedrick[1,2] and Winter[3] address the issue of residency work demands and the overburden in terms of hours and responsibility that hinder the effectiveness and humanity of the physician education process. They suggest that to hire more house staff to limit the number of resident working hours is not the answer to the problem. Likewise, expanding the number of residents in a given program to meet the ever-increasing service demands of the current tertiary and quaternary care centers will not meet service needs or optimize a resident's educational experience. Other practical ways are needed to address the problems associated with resident overwork and hospital care needs.

The use of nonphysician primary care providers in the inpatient hospital setting bears further comment. Before a solution is implemented, physicians should analyze the available data to ensure that quality of patient care is maintained. It is also imperative to ensure that the implementation of a new care modality maintains or increases a resident's learning time and educational experience. We would like to explore the reality of using nurse practitioners and physician assistants as primary health care providers in the inpatient setting.

A number of published reports have discussed the use of nonphysicians in providing primary care. Studies show that skilled primary care providers, such as nurse practitioners, can perform specific patient care responsibilities usually assigned to house staff. Responsibilities include such functions as admitting patients, assessing the initial and subsequent status of patients, obtaining histories and performing physical examinations, and performing laboratory evaluations and therapeutic procedures. As we transfer these duties to nonphysicians and then evaluate the outcome, it may mean that fewer residents are needed to meet the increasing service demands, and the resident educational experience might be enhanced.

A necessary phase in using nonphysician health care providers is to test their effectiveness in the clinical area. We need to write job descriptions for the nurse who functions in the role of health associate or associate resident. We must document the effectiveness of this new role and its effect on patient care and resident education. Will resident time, in fact, be redirected to educational pursuits? Will quality of patient care be maintained? Will the nurse practitioners be integrated into the patient care role or will they be relegated to work not desired by the residents? The bulk of the material published to date has dealt with the issue of quality of care, and very little data exist to provide an answer to our other questions.[4,5] This is a concern in view of the impact and magnitude of the changes proposed.

The University of Colorado, Denver has been a leader in the pediatric nurse practitioner movement and in the integration of nonphysician health care providers. Silver and McAtee[6,7] have published reports in medical and nursing journals discussing the evolving role of the pediatric nurse practitioner in both the inpatient and outpatient environment. In addition, Silver et al[8] championed the development of a specially trained physician assistant, the child health associate, to provide primary care in the ambulatory setting. The reports by Silver and McAtee center on efforts to confirm the notion that nonphysicians can provide care to pediatric patients comparable with that provided by a first-year resident.

Research supports this practice in a setting in which a trained professional works with an experienced senior colleague. Nurse practitioners are effective, competent, and capable of providing high-quality care in the hospital setting as well.[9] The nurse practitioner in the University of Colorado's program for hospital-based pediatric nurse practitioners was capable of the following: (1) admitting patients; (2) assessing both initial clinical states and subsequent changes in a patient's condition; (3) writing relevant orders; (4) performing a variety of complex diagnostic and therapeutic procedures, including lumbar punctures and thoracenteses; (5) ordering and integrating laboratory studies; (6) counseling patients and family members; (7) discharging patients; and (8) performing other traditional nurse practitioner duties.

They were further trained to share primary responsibility for inpatient care and to make independent value judgments regarding the health status of the patient. Silver and McAtee[6,7] stated that the expanded hospital nurse practitioner's role can be practiced most effectively in urban nonteaching hospitals or in rural hospitals where no direct competition would occur with residents, interns, or medical students. They suggest the use of nurse associate residents. These individuals are nurse practitioners, clinical nurse specialists, or other nurse specialists who receive several months of formal preparation that equips them to substitute for house officers in teaching hospitals. Nurse associate residents would participate in all house staff activities, including regularly assigned rotations and night call. They maintain their identity as nurses and function as members of the health care team. The proposed nurse associate residents could substitute for up to 5% to 10% of the house staff in the oversupplied subspecialties.

Few data are available to suggest that using nonphysicians improves the educational experience for the resident. Major issues, such as daytime and nighttime supervision of the nonphysician, remain unanswered. Would the senior resident serve as a supervisor for these traditionally attending supervised professionals?

Sox,[4] in his review of 10 years of literature on nonphysician primary health care providers in outpatient care, found 21 articles that offered comparisons of care between the nonphysician practitioner and physicians. His finding was that nurse practitioners and physician assistants provide care that is indistinguishable from the care provided by physicians in the outpatient setting. Because of the variable research methods, there was no experimental basis on which this finding could be generalized to settings outside the office, to unsupervised care, or to care of the seriously ill patient. Once again, no data were provided to determine the impact of using such health care providers on the educational experience of the resident.

The problem of resident education needs and hospital service demands remains. This discussion demonstrates that the use of nonphysicians has potential, but not all pertinent questions have been addressed. Staffing needs may be met but resident educational needs may or may not be served. The easy solution is to use the residents for whatever is dictated by the hospital. The more difficult solution will involve a reconfiguration of the health care setting and an insistence on excellent patient care in the context of rational educational planning for residents. Rather than embracing more and more in the service area with a consequent increase in the number of residents, we need to attend to the educational needs of the residents. Decisions on hospital staffing should be based on patient care and resident education needs, not merely on economic constraints or the availability of other health care professionals.

ANGELO GIARDINO, MD, MSEd
Robert Wood Johnson Clinical Scholars Program
University of Pennsylvania School of Medicine
3615 Chestnut St
Philadelphia, PA 19104

EILEEN GIARDINO, PhD, RN
Department of Nursing
La Salle University
Philadelphia, PA 19141

1. Bedrick AD. The eighty-hour workweek: residency friend or foe? *AJDC.* 1990;144:857.
2. Bedrick AD. In reply to: Winter RJ. Neonatology and residency training. *AJDC.* 1990;144:953-954.
3. Winter RJ. Neonatology and residency training. *AJDC.* 1990;144:953.
4. Sox HC. Quality of patient care by nurse practitioners and physician's assistants. *Ann Intern Med.* 1979;91:459-468.
5. Honigfeld L, Perloff J, Barzansky B. Replacing the work of pediatric residents. *Pediatrics.* 1990;85:969-976.
6. Silver HK, McAtee P. On the use of nonphysician 'associate residents' in overcrowded specialty-training programs. *N Engl J Med.* 1984;311:326-328.
7. Silver HK, McAtee P. Should nurses substitute for house staff? *Am J Nurs.* 1988;88:1671-1673.
8. Silver HK, Ott JE, Dungy CI, Fine LL, Moore VM, Krugman RD. Assessment and evaluation of child health associates. *Pediatrics.* 1981;67:47-52.
9. Silver HK, Murphy MA, Gitterman BA. The hospital nurse practitioner in pediatrics: a new expanded role for staff nurses. *AJDC.* 1984;138:237-239.

Priorities in Academic Pediatrics

Sir.—I found it interesting to read Goetzman's comments[1] in the December 1990 issue of *AJDC* concerning the effects of selecting a new department head. As a practicing physician, I had no insight into some of what he mentioned. I was struck, however, by the comment that junior faculty members are said to "sacrifice" their careers if they are to "keep clinical programs afloat." In other words, caring for the sick will interfere with the need to publish. In the editorial by Bier et al[2] in the same issue, several editors discuss their methods for dealing with "self-plagiarism." The motivation for this activity is to enlarge the physician's list of publications.

In reality, the cause of "self-plagiarism" is the mind-set evidenced by Goetzman's comments. I have no quarrel with research. All of what I do is based on what researchers have done before me. However, I have a somewhat different perception of the reality of health care in the United States. We live in a place and time in which many children do not have access to basic health care services and immunizations. In spite of reports of various committees, it is clear that there is a profound shortage of practicing general pediatricians. The problem with pediatric practice is not money; the pay is fine and I doubt that researchers make any more. The problem is the attitude of the medical center. In my group of 25 residents at a major children's hospital, only one went into practice. The others followed their favored role models and went into academic medicine. Thus, *AJDC* can publish articles on liver transplantation, extracorporeal membrane oxygenation, and prolonged intubation in a society that cannot even properly control measles.

I harbor no ill will toward Goetzman, but I do have a suggestion for him and other department chairmen who read *AJDC.* They should start hiring and promoting physicians who want to perform clinical work. Every medical center has them, the lifelong assistant professors who are in the hospital day and night treating patients but never seem to get anything published. The residents would then see the value of clinical pediatrics and would be more likely to enter that arena. In addition, a medical center that emphasizes clinical work over research is going to get far more referrals from the "local medical doctors." Research is important, but so is caring for children who do not have rare, interesting conditions.

STEPHEN E. JACOBS, MD
Valley Oak Pediatric Associates
1325 Melrose Ave
Modesto, CA 95350

1. Goetzman B. The editorial board speaks: appointment vs anointment. *AJDC.* 1990;144:1291.
2. Bier DM, Fulginiti VA, Garfunkel JM, et al. Duplicate publication and related problems. *AJDC.* 1990;144:1293-1294.

In Reply.—The development of special academic series for faculty members heavily involved in patient care is becoming widespread in academic medical centers in this country. Faculty in such series must make creative contributions in the clinical arena, but the pressure on them is significantly reduced in recognition of their major time commitment to patient care. It is hoped that this will help alleviate the problem that Jacobs addresses. In this age of medical specialization and subspecialization, it has taken quite a while to recognize that faculty members also become more expert at one of the traditional academic modes of university service, ie, teaching, research, and public service, when clinical activities are a central part of these duties. Thus, it is becoming more and more rare in academic medicine for an individual to be excellent in all three roles. As the pendulum swings, let us hope that it swings far enough to put the emphasis on teaching that it deserves.

BOYD W. GOETZMAN, MD, PHD
Department of Pediatrics
Division of Neonatology
Research Laboratory TB 193
University of California, Davis
Davis, CA 95616

Thumb-Sucking

Sir.—Because my oldest son was a thumb-sucker who also carried a blanket and now needs orthodontic correction of malaligned teeth, I was particularly interested in the recent article by Friman.[1]

Thumb-sucking seems to be fairly common, yet Friman studied only eight patients. This seems like a very small sample size considering the prevalence of this problem. The eight patients who were followed up seem to have been preselected in a sense, not only because of the general inclusion criteria, but also because of the apparent motivation to stop thumb-sucking exhibited by both the children and their parents. Thumb-sucking, with or without other object attachment, is a very common problem. Therefore, it seems to me that Friman could have studied a much larger patient group and reached much more valid conclusions. Similar problems occur in studies in orthopedic surgery, especially those in which the natural history of a disease or a specific treatment modality is followed up. Although a number of reports purport to be long-term follow-up studies of various conditions, data from 25% to 50% of the initial group of study patients are often unavailable at the study's conclusion. One always wonders what happened to those others who are no longer represented and what effect their inclusion would have had on the final results. The size of a study group should be proportional to the prevalence of the problem and/or the importance of the problem if the conclusions are to be valid.

John P. Lubicky, MD
Shriners Hospital
2211 N Oak Park Ave
Chicago, IL 60635

1. Friman PC. Concurrent habits: what would Linus do with his blanket if his thumb-sucking were treated? *AJDC.* 1990;144:1316-1318.

In Reply.—I appreciate Dr Lubicky's interest in my study of concurrent habits, but he has misunderstood it in two ways. First, it was not a study of thumb-sucking per se, but rather of covariation between chronic thumb-sucking and object attachment (ie, the "Linus" syndrome). To study this covariation, I treated thumb-sucking and measured, but did not treat, attachment. I followed guidelines derived from a thorough literature review for treatment of thumb-sucking.[1,2] These guidelines recommend that only children aged 5 years or older be treated to reduce thumb-sucking, and then only if the habit is chronic (ie, occurs in more than one environment, such as at home and at school). Thumb-sucking is common in young children, but chronic thumb-sucking in children aged 5 years and older is not. No incidence figures are available, but my estimate, based on 9 years of research on thumb-sucking, is that about 5% to 10% of thumb-sucking children older than age 5 years have a chronic habit. I also estimate that only about one third of these children are strongly attached to an object. Thus, as a representative sample of simple thumb-sucking, eight children is quite small, as Dr Lubicky points out. But as a representative sample of children with the true "Linus" syndrome, eight is substantial. Still, additional study with larger samples is desirable.

Second, my study focused on a behavioral process, not on an actuarial outcome.[3] If I had wanted an actuarial outcome (eg, the number of children in a given population who would respond to treatment), I would have recruited a much larger sample and used a group design. Instead, I recruited a smaller sample for intensive study of the behavioral process resulting from treating thumb-sucking and ignoring concurrent object attachment. Research on covariation between childhood habits is new, and, at this stage, process questions are much more informative and important than actuarial questions. Single subject (N=1) research designs such as the multiple baseline used in my article are ideally suited to such study because they reveal the relationship between dependent and independent variables over time. These designs also have a very high degree of internal validity, the reasons for which include multiple direct observations and multiple direct replications in the study. Furthermore, in the domain of N=1 research, eight baselines (eight direct replications) is quite high.[4] Thus, contrary to Dr Lubicky's suggestion about small sample size, my sample of eight is large given the research question and design of my study. I do share Dr Lubicky's belief in the value of an actuarial outcome from treatment-based research on concurrent habits, but pursuing such an outcome without first more fully understanding the relationship between the habits would be premature. I request that he have what I must have in pursuit of my research on concurrent habits: patience.

Patrick C. Friman, PhD
Children's Hospital
of Philadelphia
Children's Seashore House
34th Street and
Civic Center Boulevard
Philadelphia, PA 19104

1. Friman PC, Schmitt BD. Thumb sucking in childhood: pediatrician's guidelines. *Clin Pediatr.* 1989;28:438-440.
2. Friman PC, Leibowitz JM. An acceptable and effective treatment alternative for chronic thumb and finger sucking. *J Pediatr Psychol.* 1990;15:57-65.
3. Johnston JM, Pennypacker HS. *Strategies and Tactics of Human Behavioral Research.* Hillsdale, NJ: Lawrence Erlbaum; 1980.
4. Kratochwill TR. *Single Subject Research: Strategies for Evaluating Change.* Orlando, Fla: Academic Press Inc; 1978.

The 80-Hour Workweek and Residency Programs: Closing Arguments

Sir.—*AJDC* recently published two commentaries by me concerning the educational goals (vs service needs) of resident rotations in the neonatal intensive care unit[1] and the implications of an 80-hour workweek for pediatric residents.[2] In these pieces, I reflected on the potential impact of these issues on the educational curricula of pediatric postgraduate programs. Now, after several months of "lively discussion," not only in *AJDC*, but with residents and faculty at my own institution, it is appropriate now for me to present some additional thoughts and "closing arguments."

Concerns that excess workloads result in overstressed physicians and ensuring that residents go home to sleep after a rigorous night on call are important as we design optimal residency educational curricula. However, dwelling on these topics at the expense of the learning process may sidestep some of the more pressing issues about postgraduate residency training.

The long working hours of practicing pediatricians (and residents) are legion. Why do these clinicians persist in their daily duties and responsibilities despite working long hours with sick patients? It is certainly not the lure of vast wealth and bankers' hours! Few of us went into pediatrics expecting to work a 40-hour week. We did so because of the profound satisfaction in and enjoyment of our chosen specialty and that special feeling that occurs when a critically ill patient or family takes that extra moment to express their gratitude.

Residency training and its inherent educational goals should not be an endurance test. Even though house officers may work long hours and stay up all night, they experience and savor the same nonremunerative rewards as do attending physicians. Residents should enjoy their work (and I believe that most do!). I believe that many residents experience some of their most valued educational moments while on call. Conversely, some house officers recall that the worst moments of their residencies occurred while on call. The reality of the situation is that being on call is not always a great experience, but we need to make the best of it. It is important to temper idealism with reality.

Residents in postgraduate education must have an appreciation and understanding of the natural history of pediatric medical disorders. A "postcall" (the period or state of mind immediately following an overnight shift of inhospital call, usually commencing at 8 AM)resident will not do himself or herself any favors by admitting a patient in diabetic ketoacidosis at 7 AM, writing admitting orders for a continuous insulin infusion, and signing out the patient at 8 AM without participating in that patient's ongoing care, let alone learning about the pathophysiology and treatment of diabetes mellitus. The timing of educational opportunities cannot be managed by punching a time clock; neither can resident work hours.

We can all recall numerous instances when residents were up all night with sick patients, but insisted on being involved in their patients' care most of the following day because of a genuine concern for their patients and an interest in their own education. These residents were indeed tired the next day, but they felt that a more significant process was occurring and that an important goal was being met. They were excited about what they were doing and learned despite a nagging fatigue. These individuals were now one rung higher on their educational ladder. Yes, they went home tired, but they had the personal satisfaction of knowing that they had done a good job. I know that not all (perhaps few) residents have felt this way; some nights on call (or postcall days) may not permit ideal educational experiences.

Residents need time to attend to personal and family needs; their call schedules need to accommodate these priorities. The "good old days" were far from perfect. Our present system is considerably better. However, we should continue making improvements in the residency educational process to prepare house officers not only for satisfying careers in pediatrics, but for a fulfilling life outside the office. The era of 36-hour shifts must end. Weary residents can make mistakes, but as educational programs improve, we can minimize such mistakes. Above all, we must not teach our residents that pediatrics can be learned and eventually practiced while punching a time clock. As educators, we will do our students and patients an injustice by conveying this type of mind-set.

Alan D. Bedrick, MD
Section of Neonatology
and Nutritional Sciences
Department of Pediatrics
University of Arizona
College of Medicine
1501 N Campbell Ave
Tucson, AZ 85724

1. Bedrick AD. Neonatology in residency curricula: how much is too much? *AJDC*. 1990;144:159.

2. Bedrick AD. The eighty-hour workweek: residency friend or foe? *AJDC*. 1990;144:857.

Child Sexual Abuse and Human Immunodeficiency Virus Transmission

Sir.—The article by Gutman et al[1] on human immunodeficiency virus (HIV) transmission by child sexual abuse in the February 1991 issue of *AJDC* can be misleading. The authors found that the incidence of sexual abuse among the 96 children who tested positive for HIV was 14.6%. The accepted incidence of sexual abuse in the general population is one in six, or 17%.[2] If one were to examine any group of children for signs of sexual abuse, leukemia, or the common cold, one would expect to come up with a similar figure. It appears that HIV-positive children are at no increased risk of abuse.

I agree with the authors that it is important to identify those children who are HIV positive and have been sexually abused, because some immediate and delayed behavioral sequelae of child sexual abuse may put the child and adult survivor at increased risk of exposure to HIV infection or transmission of HIV to others.

I have found that positive HIV test results in children abused by perpetrators at high risk for acquired immunodeficiency syndrome has been low. To date, I have found none. I have followed up four children who were abused by HIV-positive perpetrators and they have proven to be negative for HIV 2 years after the abuse. Other centers have had similar experience.

The estimated incidence of HIV positivity in the general population is about 1 in 250.[3] We have seen over 6000 sexually abused children. To date, I have not found one with evidence of HIV infection, which suggests that these children are not at increased risk of HIV infection.

James A. Monteleone, MD
St. Louis University
School of Medicine
1465 S Grand Blvd
St Louis, MO 63104-1095

1. Gutman LT, St Claire KK, Weedy C, et al. Human immunodeficiency virus transmission by child sexual abuse. *AJDC*. 1991;145:137-141.

2. Greenwood CL, Tangalos EG, Maruta T. Prevalence of sexual abuse, physical abuse, and concurrent traumatic life events in a general medical population. *Mayo Clinic Proc*. 1990;65:1067-1071.

3. Centers for Disease Control. HIV prevalence estimates and AIDS case projections for the United States. *MMWR*. 1990;39:1-31.

In Reply.—Dr Monteleone has made several points worthy of reply. First, he notes that the incidence rate of sexual abuse in the general population is 17%. Studies that lead to prevalence rates of that level define sexual abuse broadly (a definition we endorse). However, many of the abusive activities are only minimally physically invasive, such as viewing, fondling, kissing, rubbing, photographing, and so forth. These activities would not cause the traumatic injuries that resulted in the genital physical findings that were described in 13 of the 14 children in the present study. This is in contrast to the situation for the majority of sexually abused children in whom significant physical findings resulting from the abuse are not found. Therefore, compared with other groups of abused children, and as was noted in the original article, the abuse of the children in our study was unusually severe. We were not prospectively evaluating every child for all forms of sexual abuse; were we to have done so, our percentage would undoubtedly have risen to well above 14.6%.

The fact that Dr Monteleone has not yet identified an infected child in his clinic may reflect several factors. First is the maturity of the HIV epidemic in the communities from which his patients come. The median HIV seroprevalence in four St Louis women's clinics was 0.2% through 1989.[1] In a conversation with Rebecca Meriwether, MD, (winter 1990), the seroprevalence in women delivering in Durham County (North Carolina) in 1989 was higher. The increase in HIV seroprevalence in the midwest is a recent phenomenon, and the total number of infected children may consequently still be low. Furthermore, they would be less likely to have progressed to clinically apparent disease.

Another reason Dr Monteleone may have different results than ours is that patients were referred to Duke University Medical Center (Durham, NC) because they were HIV seropositive, not because they had been abused. The HIV-infected children in St Louis may be referred to a clinic other than his. Dr Monteleone does not say what proportion of his patients were tested initially for HIV or retested at the recommended interval. If he is relying on a history of an HIV-infected perpetrator or on symptoms of HIV infection to appear, he is not going to identify many of his patients who are HIV infected, since many HIV-infected patients may be asymptomatic for years.

Dr Monteleone commented that he has followed up four HIV-negative children who were abused by HIV-positive perpetrators. The type of abuse (for example, penile-anal, fondling, etc) should certainly be specified. In addition, one of the many unresolved problems regarding sexual abuse of children is that the child's right to safety may conflict with perceived rights of the suspected perpetrator. In that regard, we also wonder whether Dr Monteleone has found a means of protecting other vulnerable children from abuse by the same perpetrators, and if so, how this was accomplished. A description of the experiences would be valuable.

Our data unequivocally demonstrate that there are children who are infected with HIV by sexual abuse, and that the number is substantial. There are significant limitations in the application of our data to a general population of abused children since the denominator in our study is children who are referred because they are HIV seropositive. To clarify this issue, Dr Gellert et al[2] have begun to gather badly needed data regarding acquisition of HIV through sexual abuse from child protection teams throughout the United States. At least 26 cases have been identified, including the four we reported. Any clinician who is evaluating children for sexual abuse should evaluate the child for HIV and other sexually transmitted diseases. Transmission does occur, so the problem is only going to get worse, and to deny that HIV transmission to children is a problem does a terrible disservice to those children who are HIV infected and in need of treatment for the infection and protection from further abuse.

Laura T. Gutman, MD
Karen St Claire, MD
Marcia Herman-Giddens, MPH
Ross E. McKinney, Jr, MD
Duke University
Medical Center
Department of Pediatrics
Box 3971
Durham, NC 27710

1. *National HIV Seroprevalence Surveys: Summary of Results.* DHHS publication HIV/CID 9-90/006. Atlanta, Ga: Centers for Disease Control; 1990.

2. Gellert G, Berkowitz C, Durfee M. Situational and sociodemographic characteristics of children infected with HIV from pediatric sexual abuse. Presented at the Seventh International Congress on AIDS; Florence, Italy. June 15-21, 1991.

Anal Fissure Produced by Examination for Sexual Abuse

Sir.—The article by Bays and Jenny[1] in the December 1990 issue of *AJDC* is a valuable review of the many physical findings that can be confused with sexual abuse. The authors stated that forceful abduction of the legs may cause splitting injuries of midline structures. I would like to report a case in which forceful abduction of the buttocks coupled with misrecognition of a normal structure led to a false assumption of sexual abuse.

Report of a Case.—A 12-month-old white girl was brought to the office by her mother. The mother gave a specific history that the father, who had only weekend custody, had had rectal intercourse with her daughter. The mother stated that the child had difficulty with bowel movements after a weekend visitation. The child had already been examined by an emergency department physician and another local pediatrician. Without prompting, the mother then suddenly demonstrated how the physicians examined her daughter by violently opposing the child's buttocks, thereby opening a large anal fissure. She also pointed out a bluish circumanal discoloration that she was told was a bruise. It was a venous plexus. Reexamination 5 days later showed healing of the anal fissure. The venous plexus was unchanged. Unfortunately, the mother remained convinced that abuse had occurred and the case remained open for several years.

Comment.—This case further illustrates that examinations performed by inadequately trained personnel may be more harmful than helpful. Current controversies over the effect of false allegations[2,3] behoove us all to exercise great care and good judgment.

Robert B. Baker, MD
Kaiser Permanente
Medical Group
3955 Bonita Rd
Bonita, CA 92002

1. Bays J, Jenny C. Genital and anal conditions confused with child sexual abuse trauma. *AJDC.* 1990;144:1319-1322.

2. Paradise JE, Rosatain AL, Nathanson M. Substitution of sexual abuse charges when parents dispute custody or visitation. *Pediatrics.* 1988;81:835-839.

3. Fay RE. Allegations of sexual abuse. *Pediatrics.* 1990;86:488-489.

In Reply.—The case described by Baker is unfortunate. It is intrusive and even abusive for a child to be taken to multiple examiners for repetitive genital examinations. Herman-Giddens and Berson[1] have described parents who focus excessively on their child's genitalia, including parents who performed genital inspections or took the child for multiple examinations or procedures by professionals. Many physicians have not been trained to perform detailed genital examinations,[2] and further confusion arises if the examiner is unsure or mistaken in interpreting physical findings. It is unfortunate that the mother in the case described by Baker, and apparently the child protective authorities, "remained convinced that abuse had occurred" even after being informed that the "bruise" was a venous plexus.

Regardless of whether a child is being molested, unresolved allegations of sexual abuse in the context of a divorce or custody dispute create additional stress for the child. These disputes can create an emotionally abusive atmosphere for the child. Ideally, the parents in such cases will agree to be counseled and focus on the welfare of their child.

Jan Bays, MD
Emanuel Hospital
& Health Center
2801 N Gantenbein Ave
Portland, OR 97227
Carole Jenny, MD
Kempe National Center
1205 Oneida St
Denver, CO 80220

1. Herman-Giddens ME, Berson NL. Harmful genital care practices in children: a type of child abuse. *JAMA.* 1989;261:577-579.
2. Ladson S, Johnson CJ, Doty RE. Do physicians recognize sexual abuse? *AJDC.* 1987;141:411-415.

Gilding the Lily

Sir.—I am writing in regard to the Radiological Case of the Month on retropharyngeal abscess published in the December 1990 issue of *AJDC.*[1]

Although Fig 2 of this article is a very nice exhibit of an abscess, I fail to see the necessity of computed tomography as part of the evaluation and treatment of a peritonsillar or retropharyngeal abscess. In the discussion, the computed tomographic scan adds little to the diagnosis or treatment. I can assure you, it adds much to the high cost of medical care.

The publication of such photos can be easily misinterpreted as a demonstration of the proper procedure in handling such cases. It is not. It is, in fact, an abuse of the available technology. It is abuses such as this that bring such strong reactions to control medical practice as a means of controlling medical costs.

Harris C. Faigel, MD
Director of University Health
Services
Brandeis University
PO Box 9110
Waltham, MA 02254-9110

1. Grosso J, Myer CM, Wood BP. Retropharyngeal abscess. *AJDC.* 1990;144:1349-1350.

In Reply.—We certainly agree with Dr Faigel that in many situations there is abuse of advanced technology in the form of "overtesting."

This particular infant, however, was suspected of having retropharyngeal abscess (RPA) several days before otolaryngologic consultation was obtained. A delay in treatment of an RPA leads to an increased risk that the infectious process may spread not only within the retropharyngeal space, but also to the parapharyngeal space, carotid sheath, and mediastinum. The surgical procedure for a complicated RPA is much different from that for an uncomplicated one. Most RPAs are incised and drained with a transoral approach. If there is spread of the abscess to the parapharyngeal space or within the retropharyngeal space below the hyoid bone, for example, an external neck approach is best.

As discussed in our article, a complete medical history, physical examination, and lateral neck roentgenography are the best tools for diag-nosing an RPA. The computed tomographic scan, however, can delineate the extent of suspected spread of RPA, allowing the surgeon to plan the most appropriate surgical approach. Indeed, "overtesting" is not justified, but to reduce the morbidity and mortality associated with a disease process, such advanced technology should be used without hesitation.

Charles M. Myer III, MD
Children's Hospital
Medical Center
Pediatric Otolaryngology
Elland and Bethesda Avenues
Cincinnati, OH 45229-2899
John Grosso, MD
University of Cincinnati
College of Medicine
231 Bethesda Ave
Cincinnati, OH 45267-0528

Enfamil...

Because breast-fed infants deserve a natural transition

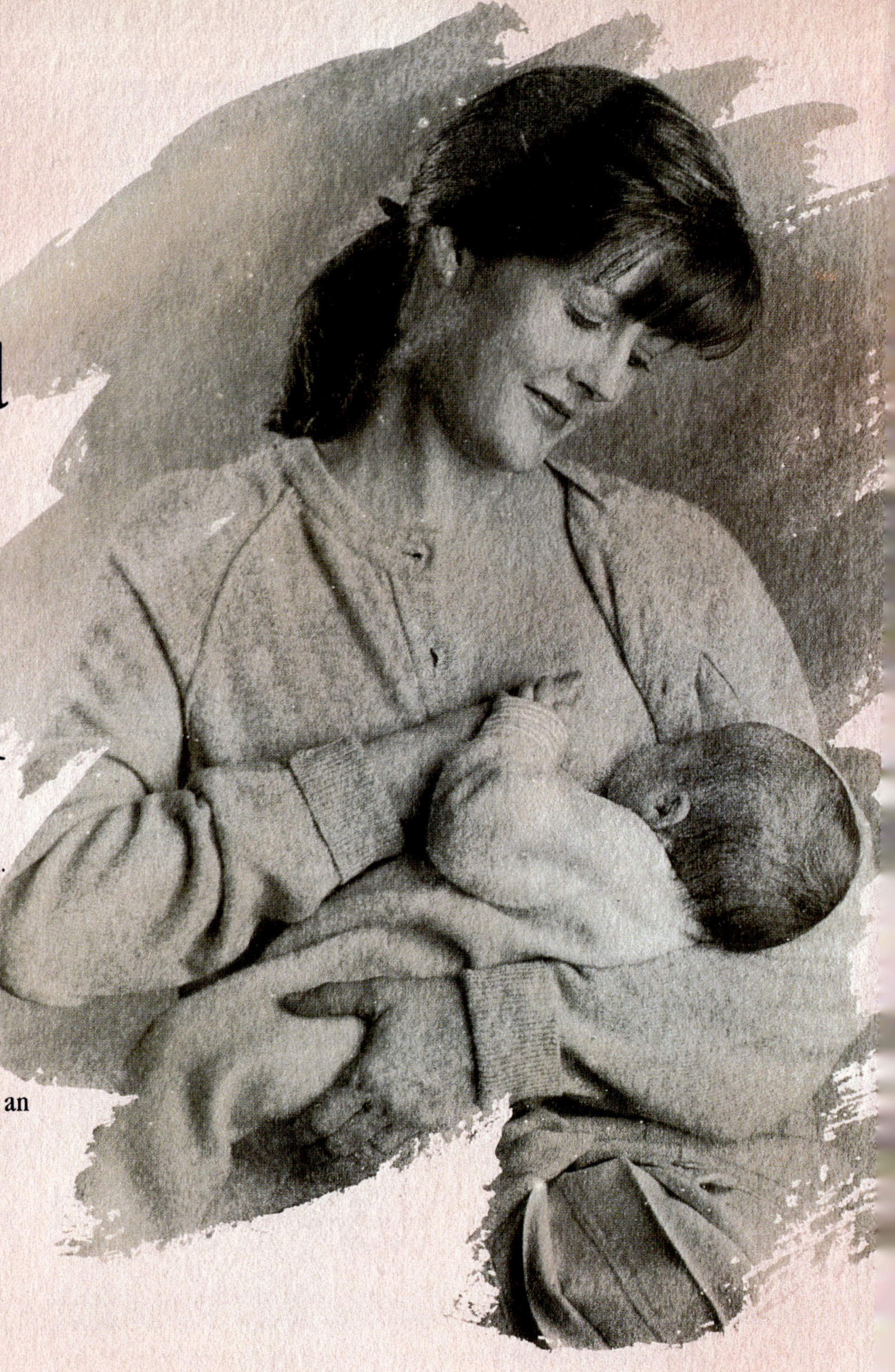

Enfamil has a 60:40 whey-to-casein ratio — similar to that of breast milk. Similac* has an 18:82 whey-to-casein ratio, similar to that of cow's milk. So when mothers need a supplementing or weaning formula, or when bottle-feeding is chosen, recommend a formula that provides an easily digestible, natural transition from breast milk. Stay with whey... stay with Enfamil.

*Similac is a registered trademark of Ross Laboratories, Columbus, Ohio.

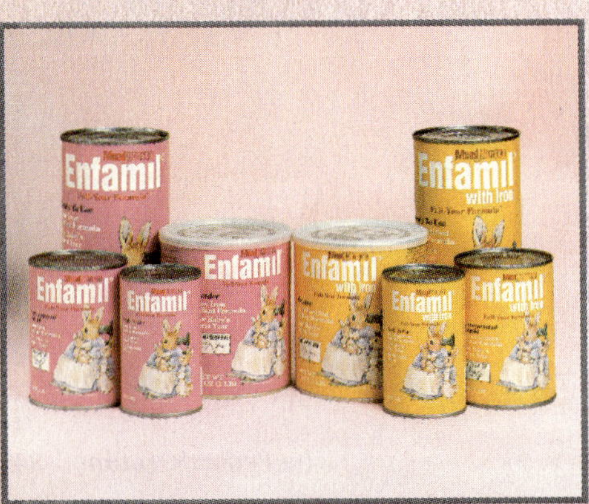

Enfamil®

Infant Formula for 0-12 Months

©1990, Mead Johnson & Company, Evansville, Indiana 47721, U.S.A.

L-K324-2-91

STAY WITH ENFAMIL® ■ STAY WITH WHEY ■ INFANT FORMULA FOR 0-12 MONTHS

EDITORIAL

Jack Metcoff Festschrift

In every field of endeavor, only a limited number of people make a major impact. Jack Metcoff has had such an influence in the fields of pediatric nephrology and body fluid physiology.

On June 11, 1990, a symposium and dinner was held in his honor. Several of the articles in this issue of the JOURNAL were presented at the symposium. Approximately 100 of his colleagues and students attended the event. Seventeen presented synopses of their experiences working with Dr Metcoff or their current research in pediatrics. Some of the presentations were submitted to and reviewed by *AJDC*, and those that were accepted appear in this issue.

Jack Metcoff was honored as an outstanding and visionary scientist, teacher, and leader. His scientific contributions include an early description of an experimental model of the nephrotic syndrome produced in the rat by injection of an aminonucleoside of puromycin and an elegant exposition of the mechanisms leading to development of the nephrotic syndrome and its renal dysfunction in that model. He also reported the early use of prednisone and diuretics for the treatment of the nephrotic syndrome in childhood. He was one of the first to use hemodialysis to treat renal failure in children, and his studies altered our understanding of renal function and fluid therapy after thermal injury. He was one of the first to integrate renal physiology and biochemistry and conducted multiple studies of renal metabolism. His international studies of protein-calorie malnutrition in pregnancy and renal failure have led to an improved understanding of the mechanisms that result in fetal malnutrition and to new approaches to therapy. In addition to his personal contributions to the scientific literature, he facilitated the growth of knowledge in pediatric nephrology by editing *The Annual Conference on the Kidney*. He was a catalyst and leader in the development and sustenance of the Nephrosis Foundation, which evolved into the National Kidney Foundation. The annual conferences on the kidney began in 1948 and concluded with a conference addressing acute glomerulonephritis in 1965. The proceedings of these conferences brought the cutting edge of the developing field of nephrology to the scientific and clinical community.

Many practicing pediatricians and pediatric academicians owe their initial stimulus and training to Jack Metcoff. The most important quality, and the one for which I believe he would most want to be remembered, is his ability and ever-present desire to be a catalyst and supporter of young academicians. He has always regarded his most important role to be that of a facilitator and stimulator of ideas and people, and he gained great satisfaction from his students' successes. The articles in this issue reflect his influence on the fields of nutrition, metabolism, and nephrology. The fields of pediatric nephrology, fluid and electrolyte physiology, and clinical nutrition owe him great gratitude. He was usually ahead of his time, elevated socratic dialogue to a new level of excellence, and stimulated many students to enter a variety of disciplines in academic pediatrics or to practice primary pediatrics in the community with an ever-present quest for knowledge and the application of scientific principles to clinical problem solving.

JOHN E. LEWY, MD
Department of Pediatrics
Tulane University
School of Medicine
1430 Tulane Ave
New Orleans, LA 70112

Part-time Peg: Who, Me?

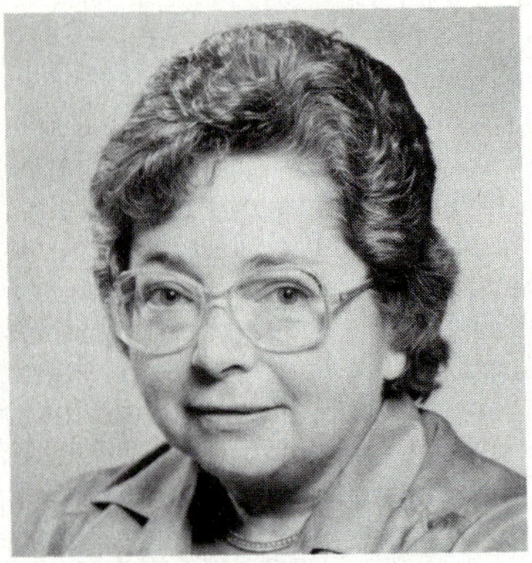

Peggy C. Ferry, MD

Peggy has been a workhorse for **AJDC**. *She has reviewed hundreds of manuscripts for us, suggested new features and procedures for* **AJDC**, *and recently implemented one of these, "Pediatric Legal Medicine." In addition, she has faithfully handled our "Book Review" section for the past 8 years. In her contribution this month, she details a change in professional life-style she has recently undergone. Having worked with Peggy during her full-time activities, I can attest to her dedication to hard work, to completion of all of her duties, no matter what she was asked to do, and to her professionally competent performance. I have no doubt that her "reduced" activity will not alter the way in which she performs, for academe and for* **AJDC**. *Even a brief glance at her curriculum vitae reveals continued high-level activity locally, regionally, and nationally.* **AJDC**, *pediatrics, and pediatric neurology have benefited from her energy, intelligence, and dedicated performance and will continue to do so, even if she is so-called part-time.*

On a recent delightful sunny Arizona Saturday afternoon, I found myself seated next to a young visiting academic pediatrician who was being actively recruited to join our department. Sitting outside amidst the splendor of blue skies and a Tucson mountain view, we discussed the rigors of academic pediatrics and the limited free time to spend with one's family. When I mentioned to the young man that I was thinking about writing an editorial on part-time work, he said, "Boy, I'd love to work part-time, but there's no way I could."

He is right. The vast majority of academic pediatric departments, as well as private practice groups, frown on hiring part-time physicians. It is almost as if they have a sign in the window: *Now Hiring–Full-Time Employees Only.*

In July 1989, after 30 years of virtually full-time practice (most of it in academic pediatric neurology), I stepped down from a full-time academic post (including associate headship of our department) and, for health reasons, began working part-time. I wrestled for a long time with the decision to make this change because I had always planned to work full-time until at least age 90 years or so. I had worked hard to achieve the professional successes for which I felt a reasonable degree of pride. Reducing my work schedule was not part of the vocabulary in my career trajectory.

I was unprepared for the reactions of my colleagues, most of whom developed a somewhat glazed look in their eyes when I told them I was going to work the "P" word (part-time). With one or two valued exceptions, they conveyed the opinion that I had dropped out of the mainstream of academic life and that my contributions were no longer valued. In retrospect, I think they were a bit jealous.

Their reactions stimulated me to think, however, about the role of part-time work in the future of pediatrics. Recently, a lot of publicity has been generated about "mommy-track" decisions that has brought needed public attention to different career tracks that competent women (and a few good men) will pursue in the years ahead. Prominent women in the public eye have spoken out forcefully on the issue, at the price of losing their jobs in some instances.

Barbara Bush also put it well in her address to the 1990 Wellesley graduating class: "At the end of your life, you will never regret not having passed one more test, winning one more verdict, or not closing one more deal. You *will* regret time not spent with a husband, a child, a friend, or a parent" (*Washington Post.* June 2, 1990:C4). In my own situation, my former husband is happily remarried to a tall, thin (sic!), younger woman; we decided years ago not to have children because it would interfere with our professional careers.

An astounding 62% of last year's PL-1s were women.[1] As noted in the title of a recent pithy *New England Journal of Medicine* editorial, "Medicine is no longer a man's profession: or, when the men's club goes coed, it's time to change the regs."[2] Change in the pediatric club is long overdue. The challenge to pediatric department chairpeople is clear: to attract and *keep* bright, competent women, academic units will need to modify their personnel policies accordingly. Otherwise, increasing numbers of these capable and caring individuals who wish to experience the joys of a good marriage, family life, and successful pediatric career will no longer enter the fast track because the price they would have to pay is too high. Successful major corporations, way ahead of the medical profession, have already learned this lesson by introducing flexible hours, extended leaves of absences, job sharing, and on-site child care. Pediatrics, of all fields, should exert leadership in academe to support issues regarding children and families, whether these children be ours, those we serve, or our colleagues'.

References

1. *AAMC Data Book.* Washington, DC: Association of American Medical Colleges; 1991. Table F1.

2. Eisenberg C. Medicine is no longer a man's profession: or, when the men's club goes coed, it's time to change the regs. *N Engl J Med.* 1989;321:1542-1544.

Zinc Deficiency

A Public Health Problem?

Harold H. Sandstead, MD

• Zinc deficiency occurs in individuals and populations whose diets are low in sources of readily bioavailable zinc such as red meat, and high in unrefined cereals that are rich in phytate and dietary fibers. Dietary zinc deficiency was described nearly three decades ago among the poor of the Middle East. It is now known to occur in children and adolescents from widely diverse areas including Egypt, Iran, Turkey, China, Yugoslavia, Canada, and the United States; and among pregnant women from Iran, Turkey, the United Kingdom, Australia, and the United States. Major manifestations include retarded growth and development and an increased incidence of pregnancy complications. Other manifestations may include suppressed immunity, poor healing, dermatitis, and impairments in neuropsychological functions. Precise information as to the numbers of people affected by dietary zinc deficiency is not available. Even so the nature of diets associated with zinc deficiency suggests that mild deficiency is common in some populations.

(*AJDC.* 1991;145:853-859)

The first unequivocal evidence of primary human zinc deficiency was reported by Prasad et al,[1,2] who studied adolescent Egyptian village boys. Subsequently, in 1967, the improved growth and sexual maturation of the boys following zinc treatment were described.[3] Coincident with the studies in Egypt, Halsted et al[4] investigated the syndrome in growth-stunted adolescents from Iranian farm villages. They found that both boys and girls were affected. They also conducted controlled therapeutic trials of zinc in village schoolboys and showed that their growth improved subsequent to zinc repletion.

See also pp 860, 865, 871 and 877.

Adolescents with the Prasad-Halsted syndrome display severe growth retardation, delayed sexual maturation, and in most instances, iron deficiency (Figure). Plasma zinc levels are generally reduced. Measurements of zinc kinetics are consistent with zinc deficiency in that isotopic tracers of zinc given intravenously rapidly disappear from the plasma, and their retention in the body is prolonged.[2] Treatment with zinc and an adequate intake of other nutrients stimulated linear growth, maturation of the skeleton, and development of the genitalia and secondary sex organs to a greater extent than treatment with diet alone or diet and iron.[3,4]

From an examination of the settings in which the Prasad-Halsted syndrome occurs, it appears that the affected individuals represent index cases of a common problem among the poor. The syndrome is associated with poverty and the consumption of diets that include large amounts of unleavened whole-meal wheat bread, a rich source of phytate. Red meat and other sources of highly bioavailable zinc are infrequently consumed. In Egypt, blood loss from hookworm and schistosomiasis infections causes further impairment of zinc nutriture. In Iran, geophagia is a common practice among village children. Clay forms insoluble complexes with iron.[5] Presumably, it also binds zinc and inhibits its absorption.

The discovery of dietary zinc deficiency in humans provided substantial stimulation to study the role of zinc in metabolism, human physiology, and disease. Before that time, the essentiality of zinc for plants[6] and experimental[7,8] and farm animals[9,10] had been established, and the impairment of zinc utilization by dietary phytate had been described in chicks.[11]

The following and many other studies established the essentiality of zinc for cell growth and differentiation. Lieberman et al[12] were among the first to show that zinc is essential for synthesis of DNA by mammalian cells. They found that the activity of DNA polymerase was reduced in zinc-deprived kidney cells in vitro. Subsequent in vivo research disclosed that the synthesis of DNA, RNA, and proteins was suppressed in zinc-deficient rats to a greater extent than in pair-fed control rats.[13-17] Similarly, zinc deficiency was found to cause reductions in activities of some enzymes that mediate these processes. Examples include thymidine kinase,[18] DNA-dependent RNA polymerase,[16] and aminoacyl-tRNA synthetase.[19] Other studies found fewer polysomes on sucrose-density gradients of brain and liver from zinc-deficient rats than control rats.[20,21] More recently the binding of zinc to strategically located cysteines and histidines in the peptide chain of auxiliary transcription factors was reported. Factor IIIA of *Xenopus laevis* was the first of those "finger proteins" to be recog-

Accepted for publication February 11, 1991.
From the Department of Preventive Medicine and Community Health, University of Texas Medical Branch, Galveston.
Presented at the Jack Metcoff Festschrift, Chicago, Ill, June 11, 1990.
Reprint requests to Department of Preventive Medicine, University of Texas Medical Branch, Ewing Hall J-09, Galveston, TX 77550-2774 (Dr Sandstead).

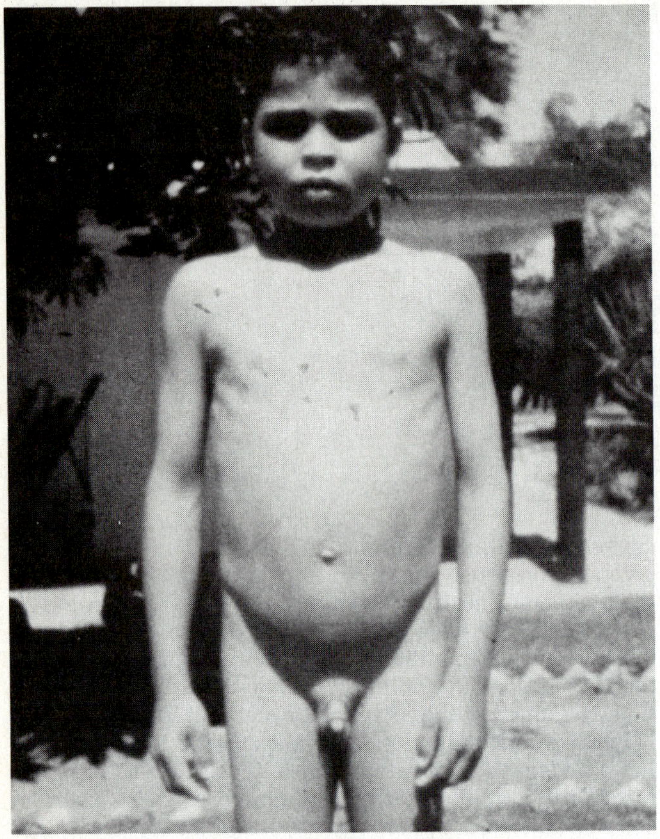

Sixteen-year-old zinc-deficient Egyptian boy with a prepubertal physical appearance and growth stunting. This subject was studied at US Naval Medical Research Unit 3 in Cairo, Egypt, in 1963.[3]

nized.[22] Other findings suggest that zinc mediates enzymes that degrade nucleic acids. The activity of ribonuclease is increased in tissues from zinc-deficient animals,[23] while the activity of nucleoside phosphorylase is depressed by zinc deficiency.[24] Further information on zinc deficiency can be found in reviews.[25-27]

Factors in the pathogenesis of primary zinc deficiency include the zinc content of the diet, the consumption of dietary and other substances that affect zinc bioavailability, and the homeostatic capacity of the individual to retain zinc. The zinc content of foods varies widely, as does its bioavailability. The zinc content of commonly consumed food in the United States is indicated in Table 1.[28] Current data[29] suggest that about 50% of zinc in US diets is provided by meat, and that beef is the principle source.[30] Dairy products provide about 20%, while cereals and legumes provide most of the remainder. In contrast to omnivorous diets, most of the zinc in lacto-ovo-vegetarian diets is provided by cereal products (26%), beans and nuts (26%), and milk and eggs (18%).[31]

A variety of substances in the diet can affect the bioavailability of zinc. Inhibitors include phytate (hexaphosphate inositol), oxalate, certain components of dietary fiber, products of Maillard browning, phosphopeptide products of the digestion of casein, ferrous iron, calcium, copper, and cadmium.[32-37] Facilitators include digestible dietary proteins, histidine, cysteine, citrate, picolinate, and ethylenediaminetetraacetic acid.[38-41]

Phytate is believed by many investigators to be the most important dietary inhibitor of zinc bioavailability. It is present in many food products that are derived from plants. Whole grain cereals and legumes are the major sources of phytate for humans. The inhibitory effects of phytate and calcium on zinc nutriture were first described in chicks and rats.[11,42] It is now known that phytate complexes with zinc and calcium together at alkaline pH to form highly insoluble compounds.[35] The inhibition of human zinc absorption by phytate was suggested by the findings of Reinhold et al,[43] in which diets rich in phytate lowered zinc retention. Subsequent zinc tolerance tests in humans confirmed that foods rich in phytate reduce zinc absorption.[44] More recently, Turnland et al[45] showed that sodium-phytate suppresses the retention of stable isotopic tracers of zinc by humans.

Semiquantitative studies by Sandström et al[46] indicate that retention of zinc is inversely related to the level of dietary phytate. They fed subjects 80-g meals of rye, barley, oatmeal, triticale, or whole wheat that were labeled with zinc 65 and measured retention of the isotope 14 days later using whole-body counting technology. The retention of zinc was inversely proportional to the amount of phytate present in the meal. For example, an intake of 600 μmol of phytate was associated with a retention of 8%, while a phytate intake of 100 μmol was associated with a retention of 25%. These investigators had previously shown that 16 hours of leavening caused a substantial reduction in phytate in whole-wheat bread and a doubling of zinc 65 retention from a standard meal.[47] Sandström et al[48] also found that the impact of phytate from beans on zinc retention was less than that of

Table 1.—Zinc Content of Common Household Portions of Selected Foods

Food	Portion	Zinc, mg	Protein, g
Fish (flounder, tuna, salmon)	3 oz	0.58	22.89
Oysters	3 oz	77.51	6.00
Crab	3 oz	6.48	16.46
Poultry			
Dark meat	3 oz	2.20	22.08
Light meat	3 oz	0.87	25.34
Beef	3 oz	4.60	26.82
Pork	3 oz	4.40	26.72
Bologna	3 oz	1.70	13.02
Liver (chicken, beef, pork)	3 oz	4.90	23.48
Whole egg	1 large	0.70	6.07
Dried beans and lentils	½ cup	0.95	7.70
Milk	1 cup	0.93	8.03
Cheese (cheddar)	1 oz	0.88	7.05
Bread			
White	1 slice	0.15	2.07
Wheat	1 slice	0.47	2.69
Rice			
White	½ cup	0.35	2.00
Brown	½ cup	0.60	1.80
Cornmeal (cooked)	½ cup	0.15	1.50
Oatmeal (cooked)	½ cup	0.58	3.00
Bran flakes (40%)	1 oz	1.16	3.20
Corn flakes	1 oz	0.03	0.95

*Source: United States Department of Agriculture; Agricultural Handbooks, 1976-1988.

Table 2.—Factorial Basis of Provisional Requirements of Dietary Zinc in Assumed Losses and Availability*

Age	Peak Daily Retention, mg	Urinary Excretion, mg	Sweat Excretion, mg	Total Required, mg	Daily Dietary Requirement as a Function of Available Zinc, mg 10%	20%	40%
Infants, mo							
0-4	0.35	0.4	0.5	1.25	12.5	6.3	3.1
5-12	0.2	0.4	0.5	1.1	11.0	5.5	2.8
Boys, y							
1-10	0.2	0.4	1.0	1.6	16.0	8.0	4.0
11-17	0.8	0.5	1.5	2.8	28.0	14.0	7.0
≥18	0.2	0.5	1.5	2.2	22.0	11.0	5.5
Girls, y							
1-9	0.15	0.4	1.0	1.55	15.5	7.8	3.9
10-13	0.65	0.5	1.5	2.65	26.5	13.3	6.6
14-16	0.2	0.5	1.5	2.2	22.0	11.0	5.5
≥17	0.2	0.5	1.5	2.2	22.0	11.0	5.5
Pregnant women, wk of gestation							
0-20	0.55	0.5	1.5	2.55	25.5	12.8	6.4
20-30	0.9	0.5	1.5	2.9	29.0	14.5	7.3
30-40	1.0	0.5	1.5	3.0	30.0	15.0	7.5
Lactating women	3.45	0.5	1.5	5.45	54.5	27.3	13.7

*The above estimates are based on the assumption that the fat-free tissue concentration of zinc in man is approximately 30 μg/g. This figure is equivalent to 2.0 g of zinc in the soft tissues of an adult male and 1.2 g in the soft tissues of an adult female, as determined from lean body mass. The zinc requirement at various ages was determined from the change in lean body mass with age. Bone zinc was not included in these calculations, because it is relatively sequestered from the metabolically active pool of body zinc. The excretion of zinc in sweat is based on an assumed zinc content in sweat of 1 mg/L. The estimated requirement for lactation is based on a zinc content in milk of 5 mg/L and a daily milk secretion of 650 mL. The urinary excretions or zinc are based on levels reported.[43]

phytate from cereal products.

The effects of relatively small intakes of wheat bran on zinc retention were shown by balance studies in which 20 normal men were fed 26 g of wheat bran daily as part of a mixed diet of conventional North American foods.[49] Zinc retention was measured in intervals of 26 to 30 days. The phytate content of the control diet was 0.29 mmol daily compared with 1.42 mmol daily in the experimental diets. Analysis of covariance, with dietary zinc as the covariate, revealed that zinc retention was reduced substantially ($P<.01$) when wheat bran was included in the diet. Regression analysis of data from 195 similar balance studies found that dietary phytate, calcium, nitrogen, and zinc were significant ($P<.05$) predictors of zinc retention. Together they accounted for 20% ($P<.0001$) of the variance in zinc retention.

Findings from a study by Solomons et al[50] support the thesis that the inhibition of zinc retention by phytate and other zinc-binding substances in foods that are commonly consumed by the poor can be severe. Solomons et al measured the increase in plasma zinc in humans after meals of oyster, oyster with beans, and oyster with tortilla. Plasma zinc rose substantially after a meal of 120 g of oyster. When 120 g of beans were fed with the oyster, the increase in plasma zinc was reduced by more than 50%. When 120 g of tortilla were fed with the oyster the increase in plasma zinc was almost completely suppressed. Thus, absorption of highly bioavailable zinc was impaired by two foods that are important constituents of diet of the poor throughout Central and South America.

Findings by Brune et al[51] indicate that humans do not adapt to habitually high intakes of phytate. Using the absorption of iron 59 from a standard meal as an index, they found that vegetarians experienced as much inhibition of iron absorption by wheat bran as did nonvegetarians. These findings indicate that it is unlikely that the poor of less developed countries adapt to the high phytate contents of their habitual diets.

Reinhold et al[32] pointed out that components of dietary fiber can also inhibit the intestinal absorption of zinc by humans. A zinc 65 tracer study by Lykken et al[52] in normal volunteers showed that increased consumption of Maillard browning products in corn flakes can reduce retention of zinc, as measured by whole-body counting of the retained isotope.

Thus, it seems clear that a number of binding substances present in foods can reduce zinc retention. Their negative impact on human zinc nutriture becomes apparent when they are eaten in large amounts, as occurs when humans depend primarily on whole-grain cereal products for their subsistence.

Factorial estimates of human zinc requirements and their relation to bioavailability are shown in Table 2.[53] For example, a 10-year-old child requiring 1.6 mg of zinc daily for growth and tissue maintenance needs to consume 4.0 mg of zinc daily if the dietary zinc is 40% bioavailable. On the other hand, if the zinc is only 10% bioavailable, an intake of 16 mg daily would be needed. From this it is apparent that food choice and food availability must have a major impact on zinc nutriture. Restricted food choices appeared to be a key factor in the pathogenesis of the Prasad-Halsted syndrome. Because of this, Waslien[54] evaluated diets of poor Egyptian village families for zinc content and the sources of zinc. She found that the average intake was 8 mg daily and that 71% was provided by bread and other cereal products while meat, poultry, and fish provided about 6%. Sandström et al,[55] as part of a recent World Health Organization committee, calculated zinc requirements similar to those in Table 2. They estimated that less than 10% to 15% of the zinc is bioavailable from diets such as those described by Waslien. In contrast, the sources, content, and bioavailability of zinc from North

Table 3.—Zinc Intakes in Diets of Children, Adults, and Vegetarians

Age	Sex	No. of Subjects	Mean ± SD Zinc Intake, mg/d*	Population†	Source, y
1 mo	M/F	35	1.90±0.20	Breast-fed, Canada	McDonald et al,[90] 1982
1 mo	M/F	25	3.60±0.60	Bottle-fed, Canada	McDonald et al,[90] 1982
6 mo	M/F	16	2.70±0.50	Breast-fed, Canada	McDonald et al,[90] 1982
6 mo	M/F	23	4.60±0.70	Bottle-fed, Canada	McDonald et al,[90] 1982
2-7 y	M/F	96	6.30±0.44	Middle income, US	Hambridge et al,[72] 1979
2-6 y	M/F	85	5.00*	Low income, US	Walravens et al,[64] 1983
3-5 y	M/F	5	6.36±0.83	Norwegian children	Schlage and Wortberg,[91] 1972
10-13 y	M/F	6	10.16±1.42	Norwegian preteens	Schlage and Wortberg,[91] 1972
14-16 y	F	15	12.00±5.00	High school, US	White,[56] 1969
18-30 y	F	21	13.80±7.27	College women, US	White,[56] 1969
14-64 y	M/F	22	8.60±0.52	Middle income, US	Holden et al,[57] 1979
30 y	F	100	10.10±3.30	Canadians, omnivorous	Gibson and Seythes,[58] 1982
Adult	F	5	6.40±1.69	Vegetarians, US	King et al,[92] 1981
Adult	M	5	20.30±8.80	Military, US	Milne et al,[93] 1980
81.7 y	M/F	21	5.53	Geriatric hospital	Thomas et al,[94] 1988
85.5 y	M/F	24	8.90±2.53	Healthy elderly	Bunker et al,[95] 1984
25-48 y	M/F	112	8.50±4.50	Vegetarians, Punjabi, Canada	Bindra et al,[96] 1986

*No readings were reported for entries with no SD values.
†Diet assessment was as follows: via 3-day records taken at home visits in breast- and bottle-fed Canadians; 24-hour recall and food checklists in middle- and low-income US subjects; 2-week food records in Norwegian children and preteens; weighed 24-hour diets with duplicate food composite in US female and high school subjects; 14-day food record and 132 diet composites in middle-income US subjects aged 14 to 64 years; 3-day food reccords and 24-hour food composite in omnivorous Canadians; 3-day food records in US vegetarians; 6 days of duplicate chemical diet composites in US military subjects; duplicate chemical diet composites in geriatric hospital subjects and the healthy elderly; and 3-day weighed records and 30 1-day duplicate composites in vegetarian Punjabi Canadians.

American mixed omnivorous diets is substantially higher. For example, a study of 21 US college women (Table 3) who ate self-selected cafeteria diets found a mean (±SD) of 13.8±7.3 mg of zinc consumed daily.[56] Another study of 22 middle-income men and women found that their home diets provided 8.6±0.1 mg zinc daily.[57] A study of 100 Canadian women found a zinc intake of 10.1±3.5 mg daily.[58] As noted previously, about 50% of the zinc in omnivorous mixed North American diets is provided by meat.[30] The availability of zinc from such diets is probably 20% to 30%.[55] This level of bioavailability will allow a dietary intake of about 12 mg to be fully adequate for adult men who consume an omnivorous mixed western diet.[53,55]

Since its discovery three decades ago, dietary zinc deficiency has been described among children of many countries. Turkish workers[59] found zinc and iron deficiencies in growth-stunted children who indulged in geophagia. Subsequently, Chinese investigators reported evidence that led them to speculate that 30% of Chinese children are stunted from zinc deficiency.[60] In a study of 187 children they found that hair zinc and relative height for age were related ($P<.002$). They treated 50 growth-retarded children with 1.2 to 2.0 mg of zinc per kilogram per day and found that their growth rate was 40% greater than that of 235 normal children who were not given zinc ($P<.001$). A study from Yugoslavia[61] of 110 children aged 9 to 12 years found strong associations of relative body height and hair with plasma zinc ($r=.95$ and .93, respectively). More recently 70% of schoolchildren from northeastern Thai villages were reported to have low plasma zinc.[62]

The first description of dietary zinc deficiency in the United States was reported from Denver, Colo, in 1972.[63] Hambidge et al[63] found short stature, low weight, and poor appetite in preschool infants and children that were associated with low levels of zinc in hair. Treatment of the children with zinc improved their appetites and growth. More recently, growth retardation associated with low zinc nutriture was found by Walravens et al[64] among poor Hispanic preschool children from Denver. Treatment with zinc improved growth. A recent survey of the US population found a 3.3%±0.91% (SE) incidence of low serum zinc (<10.7 μmol/L) in children aged 3 to 8 years, irrespective of income.[65] Stature and serum zinc were not associated, perhaps because serum zinc can be perfectly normal in mild zinc deficiency.[63,64,66] In Canada, Gibson et al[66] found an association between short stature in young boys and low levels of hair zinc. Treatment with zinc improved their growth. These investigators[67] had previously reported associations between hair zinc levels and short stature in 13 boys. All had hair zinc levels of less than the 70 ng/g found in 48 boys of more normal stature ($P<.05$). They ascribed the lower hair zinc levels in the growth-stunted boys to poor food choices. Dietary histories indicated that they consumed 15% less meat, poultry, and fish ($P<.01$), and more fluid milk ($P<.05$), than the control group.

Information on diets and requirements suggests that children with zinc intakes in the lowest quartile are at risk of zinc deficiency. Balance studies found that intakes of 7 to 8 mg of dietary zinc in a mixed omnivorous diet allowed young children to absorb 2.1 to 3.4 mg daily.[68,69] In contrast, the data of Price et al[70] indicate that 7- to 10-year-old girls fed diets similar to those consumed by low-income children in the Southeastern United States were in negative zinc balance when the diet provided about 4.6 mg of zinc and 25 g of protein daily and the estimated losses of zinc in sweat were included in the balance calculation.[71] When the zinc intake was increased to 6.8 mg and the protein intake to 46 g daily, the retention of zinc was positive.

According to surveys conducted by the United States Department of Agriculture,[29] the average zinc intake of US children is about 7.5 mg. Studies cited in Table 3 by Hambidge et al[72] and Walravens et al[64] found that mean (±SD) zinc intakes of 96 middle-income and 85 low-income children aged 2 to 7 years and 2 to 6 years, respectively, from the Denver area were 6.30±0.44mg and 5.00±0.35mg (assuming a similar coefficient of variation as the middle income group). Calculations of the zinc intakes of children who were 1 SD below the mean indicates zinc levels of 5.86 and 4.65 mg, respectively. At 20% absorption, this provides about 1.17 and 0.93 mg of zinc, respectively, amounts below the factorially estimated World Health Organization[53,55] requirement of 1.5 to 1.6 mg daily.

Pregnant women are another group at risk of zinc deficiency.[71] Factorial estimates of zinc requirements of pregnant women[71] suggest that pregnant women should retain about 400 μg of zinc daily in the second trimester and 750 μg of zinc during the third trimester. An evaluation of the reported zinc contents of self-selected diets of young women suggested that 20% to 30% of the subjects would have been at risk of zinc deficiency if they had been pregnant and the bioavailability of the zinc from their diets was 20%.[71] In a 1976 study from Sweden[73] of about 300 pregnant women, abnormal pregnancy outcomes were associated with low plasma levels of zinc in the first trimester.

Experimental studies in animals have revealed that zinc nutriture is particularly critical during pregnancy.[14,74-79] In chickens and rats, zinc deficiency retards growth and maturation of the blastula, embryo, and fetus. Death of concepti and a variety of malformations occur. Parturition is impaired and perinatal survival reduced. Surviving offspring display residual behavioral abnormalities.

The hypothesis that zinc deficiency during human pregnancy is an important problem in the Middle East was put forward by Sever and Emanuel.[80] They based their hypothesis on knowledge of the effects of zinc deficiency on pregnant animals and the clinical evidence of zinc deficiency among adolescents from Egypt and Iran. They proposed that endemic zinc deficiency among the poor is the cause of the high rates of neural tube defects among Middle Eastern babies. A report from Turkey of low levels of zinc in plasma of women who delivered anencephalic infants[81] supports Sever and Emanuel's suggestion.

Evidence consistent with the occurrence of zinc deficiency among pregnant women in the United States was provided by a 1984 report that described associations between low maternal plasma zinc levels in the second and third trimester and subsequent pregnancy complications in 394 women from Ohio.[82] Data analysis by *z* scores indicated that more complications occurred in women with plasma zinc levels in the lowest quartile than in women with plasma zinc in the highest quartile ($n=89$, $P<.02$). Fetal distress was more frequent among women with plasma zinc levels in the lowest than the highest quartile ($n=33$, $P<.002$). Step-wise discriminate analysis revealed that zinc, albumin, and transferrin were important discriminators for complications in the lowest quartile plasma zinc sub-population, and that zinc was not a discriminator in any other quartile. Associations between complications of pregnancy and plasma zinc were unique to the lowest quartile.

Evidence that maternal zinc nutriture has a profound effect on human fetal growth was provided by Meadows et al.[83] Using the concentration of zinc in a preparation that contained peripheral blood maternal leukocytes as an index of zinc status, they found that severe fetal growth failure was more common in women who, at term, had low levels of zinc in the cellular isolate. They also found that the level of zinc in the cellular isolate was highly correlated with the level of zinc in maternal muscle. Consistent with this association between low maternal tissue zinc and fetal growth failure were the findings by Favier et al[84] of an association between baby size and the zinc concentration in amniotic fluid.

The frequency with which zinc deficiency occurs in human pregnancy is uncertain. Jameson et al[85] found a 17.5% incidence of plasma zinc level of less than 10 mmol/L in 1231 Swedish women who attended a maternity clinic before the eleventh week of pregnancy. A recent study of 460 low-income women in Alabama reported that lowest quartile plasma zinc levels in the first trimester were associated with a likelihood of subsequent delivery of an infant weighing less than 2500 g that was eight times that associated with highest quartile plasma zinc levels.[86] Maternal plasma zinc at 16 weeks' gestation, adjusted for dilution, was directly related to infant birth weight ($r=0.32$, $P<.001$).

The cause-and-effect relationship between maternal zinc nutriture and pregnancy outcome has been studied in a randomized controlled trial.[87] In 295 normal-weight, primiparous, low-income, pregnant teenagers from New Orleans, La, zinc treatment (30 mg daily) reduced the rate of premature delivery by 32% ($P<.05$) and nearly eliminated the need for respiratory assistance of newborns ($P<.002$). Jameson[88] previously described 133 women with plasma zinc levels of less than 10 mmol/L at 14 weeks' gestation, of whom 64 were given zinc and 69 were given placebo. Sixty-three percent of the women given zinc delivered normally and had normal infants. In contrast, 50% of the women given placebo had complications. Further study of 1231 women given zinc or placebo showed a significant ($P<.01$) reduction in the incidence of perinatal death in the zinc-treated group compared with the placebo-treated group.[85] It should be noted that the beneficial effects of zinc treatment on pregnancy outcome were less evident in a study of Mexican-American women.[89] This study did not evaluate the response to treatment in terms of the underlying nutritional status of the subjects, as was done in the study from New Orleans. This might account for the limited evidence of treatment benefit.

In summary, the available evidence supports the hypothesis that zinc deficiency is an important public health problem both internationally and domestically. Estimates of human zinc requirements at different times in the life cycle,[53,55,71] the zinc content of human diets,[28,54] and evidence that phytate and other factors can impair the utilization of dietary zinc[28,33,36,46,49] suggest that the risk of zinc deficiency increases as economic resources and the availability of a varied diet decrease. Clinical zinc deficiency among infants, children, adolescents, and pregnant women has been described both in developing countries and industrialized countries, including the United States. These clinical examples are believed to represent index cases of a more widespread problem whose true extent is presently unknown. Experiments in humans and animal models have established the essential role of zinc in many physiologic functions, including immunity, taste acuity, dark adaptation, wound healing, lipid metabolism, sexual function, and cognition.[25,26] It is unclear how frequently these manifestations of zinc deficiency occur in humans. This issue needs clarification.

There is a need to define the prevalence of and the factors that cause human zinc deficiency more precisely. Randomized controlled trials of zinc treatment in growth-retarded infants and children and in pregnant women in populations where stunting and abnormal pregnancy outcomes are prevalent would be useful. Data from such research would provide a basis for health authorities to institute preventive measures.

References

1. Prasad AS, Miale A Jr, Farid Z, Sandstead HH, Schulert AR, Darby WJ. Biochemical studies on dwarfism, hypogonadism and anemia. *Arch Intern Med.* 1963;111:407-428.

2. Prasad AS, Miale A Jr, Farid Z, Sandstead HH, Schulert AR. Zinc metabolism in patients with syndrome of iron deficiency anemia, hepatosplemomegaly, dwarfism and hypogonadism. *Lab Clin Med.* 1963;61:537-549.

3. Sandstead HH, Prasad AS, Farid Z, et al. Human zinc deficiency, endocrine manifestations, and response to treatment. *Am J Clin Nutr.* 1967;20:422-442.

4. Halsted JA, Ronaghy HA, Abadi P, et al. Zinc deficiency in man: the Shiraz experiment. *Am J Med.* 1972;53:277-284.

5. Minnich V, Okçuoğlu A, Tarcon Y, et al. Pica in Turkey, II: effect of clay on iron absorption. *Am J Clin Nutr.* 1968;21:78-86.

6. Sommer AL, Lipman CB. Evidence on the indispensable nature of zinc and boron for higher green plants. *Plant Phys.* 1926;1:231-249.

7. Todd WR, Elvehjem CA, Hart EB. Zinc in the nutrition of the rat. *Am J Physiol.* 1934;107:146-156.

8. Hove E, Elvehjem CA, Hart EB. Further studies on zinc deficiency in rats. *Am J Physiol.* 1938;124:750-758.

9. O'Dell BL, Newberne PM, Savage JE. Significance of dietary zinc for the growing chicken. *J Nutr.* 1958;65:503-523.

10. Tucker HF, Salmon WD. Parakeratosis or zinc deficiency in the pig. *Proc Soc Exp Biol Med.* 1955;88:613-616.

11. O'Dell BL, Savage JE. Effect of phytic acid on zinc availability. *Proc Soc Exp Biol Med.* 1960;103:304-306.

12. Lieberman L, Abrams R, Hunt N, Ove P. Levels of enzyme activity and deoxyribonucleic acid synthesis in mammalian cells cultured from the animal. *J Biol Chem.* 1963;238:3955-3962.

13. Sandstead HH, Rinaldi RA. Impairment of deoxyribonucleic acid synthesis by dietary zinc deficiency in the rat. *J Cell Physiol.* 1969;73:81-83.

14. Dreosti IE, Gray PC, Wilkins PJ. Deoxyribonucleaic synthesis, protein synthesis, and teratogenisis in zinc deficient rats. *So Afr Med J.* 1972;46:1585-1588.

15. Hsu JM, Woosley RL. Metabolism of L-methionine ^{35}S in zinc deficient rats. *J Nutr.* 1972;102:1181-1186.

16. Terhune MW, Sandstead HH. Decreased RNA polymerase activity in mammalian zinc deficiency. *Science.* 1972;177:68-69.

17. Duerre JA, Ford KM, Sandstead HH. Effects of zinc deficiency on protein synthesis in brain and liver of suckling rats. *J Nutr.* 1977;107:1082-1093.

18. Prasad AS, Oberleas D. Thymidine kinase activity and incorporation of thymidine into DNA in zinc-deficient tissue. *J Lab Clin Med.* 1974;83:634-639.

19. Hicks SE, Wallwork JC. Effect of dietary zinc deficiency on protein synthesis in cell-free systems isolated from rat liver. *J Nutr.* 1987;117:1234-1240.

20. Fosmire GJ, Al-Ubaidi YY, Halas ES, Sandstead HH. Some effects of postnatal zinc deficiency on developing rat brain. *Pediatr Res.* 1975;9:89-93.

21. Fosmire GJ, Fosmire MA, Sandstead HH. Zinc deficiency in the weanling rat: effects on liver composition and polysomal profile. *J Nutr.* 1976;106:1152-1158.

22. Hanas JS, Hazuda DJ, Wu CW. Xenopus transcription factor A promotes DNA reassociation. *J Biol Chem.* 1985;260:13 316-13 220.

23. Somers M, Underwood EJ. Ribonuclease activity and nucleic acid and protein metabolism in the testes of zinc deficient rats. *Aust J Biochem Sci.* 1969;22:1277-1282.

24. Prasad AS, Rabbani P. Nucleoside phosphorylase in zinc deficiency. *Trans Assoc Am Physicians.* 1981;94:314-321.

25. Sandstead HH. Zinc in human nutrition. In: Bronner F, Coburn J, eds. *Disorders of Mineral Metabolism-2.* Orlando, Fla: Academic Press Inc; 1981:93-157.

26. Hambidge KM, Casey CE, Krebs NF. Zinc. In: Mertz W, ed. *Trace Elements in Human and Animal Nutrition.* Orlando, Fla: Academic Press Inc; 1986:1.

27. Cousins RJ, Hempe JM. Zinc. In: Brown ML, ed. *Present Knowledge in Nutrition.* Washington, DC: International Life Science Institute (ILSI), Nutrition Foundation;) 1990:251-260.

28. Sandstead HH, Darnell LS, Wallwork JC. Role of zinc and the contribution of meat to human nutrition. In: Pearson AM, Dutsoin TR, eds. *Meat and Health, Advances in Meat Research.* Amsterdam, the Netherlands: Elsevier Science Publishers; 1990:237-274.

29. United States Department of Agriculture, Food and Consumer Services. *Nutrition Monitoring in the United States: A Progress Report from the Joint Nutrition Monitoring Evaluation Committee.* Hyattsville, Md: US Dept of Health and Human Services Public Health Service; 1986.National Center for Health Statistics, Human Nutrition Information Service publication PHS 1255.

30. Welsh SO, Marston RM. Zinc levels of the US food supply 1909-1980. *Food Technol.* 1982;36:70-76.

31. Anderson BM, Gibson RS, Sabry JH. The iron and zinc status of long-term vegetarian women. *Am J Clin Nutr.* 1981;34:1042-1048.

32. Reinhold JG, Faradji B, Abadi P, Ismail-Beigi F. Binding of zinc to fiber and other solids of wholemeal bread. In: Prasad AS, ed. *Trace Elements in Human Health and Disease.* Orlando, Fla: Academic Press Inc; 1976;1:163-180.

33. Solomons NW, Pineda O, Viteri F, Sandstead HH. Studies on the bioavailability of zinc in humans: mechanism of the intestinal interaction of non-heme iron and zinc. *J Nutr.* 1983;113:337-349.

34. Harzer G, Kauer H. Binding of zinc to casein. *Am J Clin Nutr.* 1982;35:981-990.

35. Mills CF. Dietary interactions involving the trace elements. *Annu Rev Nutr.* 1985;5:173-193.

36. Sandstead HH. Requirements and availability of dietary zinc for humans. In: Prasad AS, ed. *Clinical and Public Health Significance of Trace Elements in the World Population.* New York, NY: Alan R Liss Inc; 1982:83-102.

37. Sandstead HH. Requirement of zinc in human subjects. *J Am Coll Nutr.* 1985;4:73-82.

38. Evans GW, Johnson PE. Characterization and quantitation of a zinc binding ligand in human milk. *Pediatr Res.* 1980;14:847-880.

39. Oestreicher P, Cousins RJ. Influence of intraluminal constituents on zinc absorption by isolated, vascularly perfused rat intestine. *J Nutr.* 1982;112:1978-1982.

40. Seal CJ, Heaton FW. Chemical factors affecting the intestinal absorption of zinc in vitro and in vivo. *Br J Nutr.* 1983;50:317-324.

41. Wapnir RA, Khani DE, Bayne MA, Lifshitz F. Absorption of zinc by the rat ileum: effects of histidine and other low molecular-weight ligands. *J Nutr.* 1983;113:1346-1354.

42. Oberleas D, Muhrer ME, O'Dell BL. Dietary metal-complexing agents and zinc availability in the rat. *J Nutr.* 1966;90:56-62.

43. Reinhold JG, Hedayati H, Lahimgarzadeh A, Nasr K. Zinc, calcium, phosphorus, and nitrogen balances of Iranian villages following a change from phytate rich to phytate poor diets. *Ecol Food Nutr.* 1973;2:157-161.

44. Pecoud A, Donzel P, Schelling JL. Effect of foodstuffs on the absorption of zinc sulfate. *Clin Pharmacol Ther.* 1975;17:469-473.

45. Turnland JR, King JC, Keyes WR, Gong B, Michel MC. A stable isotope study of zinc absorption in young men: effects of phytate and alpha-cellulose. *Am J Clin Nutr.* 1984;40:1071-1077.

46. Sandstrom B, Almgren A, Kivisto B, Cederblad Å. Zinc absorption in humans from meals based on rye, barley, oatmeal, triticale and whole wheat. *J Nutr.* 1987;117:1898-1902.

47. Navert B, Sandström B, Cederblad Å. Reduction of the phytate content of bran by leavening in bread and its effect on zinc absorption in man. *Br J Nutr.* 1985;53:47-53.

48. Sandström B, Almgren A, Kivistö B, Cederblad Å. Effect

of protein level and protein source on zinc absorption in humans. *J Nutr.* 1989;119:48-53.
49. Sandstead HH, Dintzis FR, Bogyo TP, Milne DA, Jacob RA, Klevay LM. Dietary factors that can impair calcium and zinc nutriture of the elderly. In: Prinsley DM, Sandstead HH, eds. *Nutrition and Aging*. New York, NY: Alan R Liss Inc; 1990:241-262.
50. Solomons NW, Jacob RA, Pineda O, Viteri F. Studies on the bioavailability of zinc in man, II: absorption of zinc from organic and inorganic sources. *J Lab Clin Med.* 1979;94:335-343.
51. Brune M, Rossander L, Hallberg L. Iron absorption: no intestinal adaptation to a high-phytate diet. *Am J Clin Nutr.* 1989;49:542-545.
52. Lykken GI, Johnson PE, Mahalko J, et al. Effect of browned and unbrowned corn products intrinsically labeled with zinc on absorption of zinc in humans. *J Nutr.* 1986;116:795-801.
53. World Health Organization (WHO). Zinc. *WHO Tech Rep Ser.* 1973;532:9-16.
54. Waslien CA. Human intake of trace elements. In: Prasad AS, ed. *Trace Elements in Human, Health and Disease*. Orlando, Fla: Academic Press Inc; 1976:347-370.
55. Sandström BM, King J, Chandra R, et al. Human zinc requirements. *WHO Tech Rep Ser.* 1991. In press.
56. White HS. Inorganic elements in weighted diets of girls and young women. *J Am Diet Assoc.* 1969;55:38-43.
57. Holden JM, Wold WR, Mertz W. Zinc and copper in self-selected diets. *J Am Diet Assoc.* 1979;75:23-28.
58. Gibson RS, Scythes CA. Trace element intakes of women. *Br J Nutr.* 1982;48:241-248.
59. Arcasoy A, Cavdar AO, Babacan E. Decreased iron and zinc absorption in Turkish children with iron deficiency and geophagia. *Acta Hematol.* 1978;60:76-84.
60. Xue-Cun C, Tai-An Y, Jin-Sheng H, Giu-Yan M, Zhi-Min H, Li-Xiang L. Low levels of zinc in hair and blood, pica, anorexia, and poor growth in Chinese preschool children. *Am J Clin Nutr.* 1985;42:694-700.
61. Buzina R, Jusic M, Sapunar J, Milanovic N. Zinc nutrition and taste acuity in school children with impaired growth. *Am J Clin Nutr.* 1980;33:2262-2267.
62. Udomkesmalee E, Dhanamitta S, Yhoung-Aree J, Rojroongwasinkul N, Smith JC Jr. Biochemical evidence suggestive of suboptimal zinc and vitamin A status in schoolchildren in Northeast Thailand. *Am J Clin Nutr.* 1990;52:564-567.
63. Hambidge KM, Hambidge C, Jacobs M, Baum JD. Low levels of zinc in hair, anorexia, poor growth and hypogeusia in children. *Pediatr Res.* 1972;6:868-874.
64. Walravens PA, Krebs NF, Hambidge KM. Linear growth of low income preschool children receiving a zinc supplement. *Am J Clin Nutr.* 1983;38:195-201.
65. Pilch SM, Senti FR. Analysis of zinc data from the Second National Health and Nutrition Examination Survey (NHANES II). *J Nutr.* 1985;115:1393-1397.
66. Gibson RS, Vanderkooy PDS, MacDonald AC, Goldman A, Ryan BA, Berry M. A growth-limiting mild zinc deficiency syndrome in some Southern Ontario boys with low height percentiles. *Am J Clin Nutr.* 1989;49:1266-1277.
67. Vanderkooy PDS, Gibson RS. Food consumption patterns of Canadian preschool children in relation to zinc and growth status. *Am J Clin Nutr.* 1987;45:609-616.
68. Scoular FL. A quantitative study by means of spectrographic analysis of zinc in nutrition. *J Nutr.* 1939;17:103-113.
69. Engle RW, Miller RF, Price NO. Metabolic patterns in preadolescent children, XIII: zinc balance. In: Prasad AS, ed. *Zinc Metabolism.* Springfield, Ill: Charles C Thomas Publisher; 1966:326-337.
70. Price NO, Bunce GE, Engel RW. Copper, manganese and zinc balance in preadolescent girls. *Am J Clin Nutr.* 1970;23:258-260.
71. Sandstead HH. Zinc nutrition in the United States. *Am J Clin Nutr.* 1973;26:1251-1260.
72. Hambidge KM, Chavez MN, Brown RM, Walravens PA. Zinc nutritional status of young middle-income children and effects of consuming zinc-fortified breakfast cereal. *Am J Clin Nutr.* 1979;37:2532-2539.
73. Jameson S. Effects of zinc deficiency in human reproduction. *Acta Med Scand Suppl.* 1976;593:4-89.
74. Blamberg DL, Blackwood WB, Supplee WC, Combs CF. Effect of zinc deficiency in hens on hatchability and embryonic development. *Proc Soc Exp Biol Med.* 1960;104:217-220.
75. Hurley LS, Swenerton H. Congenital malformation resulting from zinc deficiency in rats. *Proc Soc Exp Biol Med.* 1966;123:692-696.
76. Apgar J. Effect of zinc deprivation from day 12, 15, 18 of gestation on parturition in the rat. *J Nutr.* 1972;102:343-348.
77. Hurley LS, Shrader RE. Abnormal development of preimplantation rat eggs after three days of maternal dietary zinc deficiency. *Nature.* 1974;254:427-429.
78. McKenzie JM, Fosmire GJ, Sandstead HH. Zinc deficiency during the later third of pregnancy: effects on fetal rat brain, liver, and placenta. *J Nutr.* 1975;105:1466-1475.
79. Sandstead HH. Zinc: essentiality for brain development and function. *Nutr Rev.* 1985;43:129-137.
80. Sever LE, Emanuel I. Is there a connection between maternal zinc deficiency and congenital malformations of the central nervous system in man? *Teratology.* 1973;7:117-118.
81. Cavdar AO, Babacan E, Asik S, et al. Neural tube defects and zinc. *Nutr Res Suppl.* 1985:331-334.
82. Mukherjee MD, Sandstead HH, Ratnaparkhi MV, Johnson LK, Milne DB, Stelling HF. Maternal zinc, iron, folic acid, and protein nutriture and outcome of human pregnancy. *Am J Clin Nutr.* 1984;40:496-507.
83. Meadows NJ, Ruse W, Smith MF, et al. Zinc and small babies. *Lancet.* 1981;2:1135-1136.
84. Favier M, Yacoub M, Racinet C, Marka C, Chambert P, Benbassa A. Les ions metalliques dans le liquide amniotique au cours du troisiem trimetre de la gestation. *Rev Frn Gynecol Obstet. 1972;67:707-714.*
85. Jameson S, Bertröm M, Hellsing K. Zinc status in pregnancy, the effect of zinc therapy on perinatal mortality. Presented at the 7th International Symposium on Trace Elements in Man and Animals; May 20, 1990; Dubrovnik, Yugoslavia. Abstract.
86. Neggers YH, Cutter GR, Acton RT, et al. A positive association between maternal serum zinc concentration and birth weight. *Am J Clin Nutr.* 1990;51:678-684.
87. Cherry FF, Sandstead HH, Rojas P, Johnson LK, Batson HK, Wang XB. Adolescent pregnancy: associations among body weight, zinc nutriture, and pregnancy outcome. *Am J Clin Nutr.* 1989;50:945-954.
88. Jameson S. Zinc status and pregnancy outcome in humans. In: Prasad AS, Dreosti IE, Hetzel BS, eds. *Clinical Application of Recent Advances in Zinc Metabolism.* New York, NY: Alan R Liss Inc; 1982:39-52.
89. Hunt IF, Murphy NJ, Cleaver AE, et al. Zinc supplementation during pregnancy. *Am J Clin Nutr.* 1984;40:508-521.
90. MacDonald LD, Gibson RS, Miles JE. Changes in hair zinc and copper concentration of breast fed and bottle fed infants during the first six months. *Acta Paediatr.* 1982;71:785.
91. Schlage C, Wortberg B. Zinc in the diet of healthy preschool and school children. *Acta Paediatr Scand.* 1972;61:421-425.
92. King JC, Stein T, Doyle M. Effect of vegetarianism on the zinc status of pregnant women. *Am J Clin Nutr.* 1981;34:1049-1055.
93. Milne DB, Schnakenberg DD, Johnson HL, et al. Trace element mineral intake of enlisted military personnel. *J Am Diet Assoc.* 1980;76:41-45.
94. Thomas AJ, Bunker VW, Hinks LJ, Sodha N, Mullee MA, Clayton BE. Energy, protein zinc and copper status of twenty-one elderly inpatients: analyzed dietary intake and biochemical indices. *Br J Nutr.* 1988;59:181-194.
95. Bunker VW, Hinks LJ, Lawson MS, Clayton BE. Assessment of zinc and copper status of healthy elderly people using metabolic balance studies and measurement of leukocyte concentrations. *Am J Clin Nutr.* 1984;40:1096-1102.
96. Bindra GS, Gibson RS, Thompson LU. [Phytate] [calcium]/[zinc] ratios in Asian immigrant lacto-ovo vegetarian diets and their relationship to zinc nutriture. *Nutr Res.* 1986;6:475-483.

Paleonephrology and Reflux Nephropathy

From the 'Big Bang' to End-Stage Renal Disease

Ronald J. Kallen, MD

• Urinary tract infections, in association with ureteral reflux or dysperistalsis, may lead to invasive renal parenchymal infection and residual scarring (reflux nephropathy). Such infections in infants are often not diagnosed during the acute phase. Late sequelae of reflux nephropathy include hypertension, proteinuria, or chronic renal failure. The latter may eventuate in the subset of patients with urinary tract infection and unilateral reflux extending to a solitary kidney or bilateral reflux. Proteinuria may herald the inexorable progression of glomerular sclerosis in patients destined to progress to end-stage renal disease, despite the absence of further recurrences of urinary tract infections. The mechanism of progression is probably similar to that occurring in other forms of chronic, diffuse parenchymal renal disease, which all have similar alterations in glomerular hemodynamics (an increase in glomerular capillary flow, pressure, and filtration). The consequent hyperfiltration per nephron may be related to the level of dietary protein intake or to some derivative of the protein load. Hyperfiltration appears to recapitulate the presumed renal hemodynamic response to the relatively high level of episodic meat consumption by paleolithic hunter-gatherers. A prudent therapeutic intervention in children with progressive reflux nephropathy may be a proportional reduction in protein intake.

(*AJDC.* 1991;145:860-864)

The most common cause of end-stage renal disease (ESRD) in children and young adults is reflux nephropathy.[1] Although other morbidities, such as hypertension[2] or the Ask-Upmark kidney,[3] are associated with reflux nephropathy, the main focus of this review is the mechanism that causes a disease occurring for the first time during infancy to progress inexorably, in some individuals, to ESRD many years later.

See also pp 853, 865, 871, and 877.

URINARY TRACT INFECTIONS (UTIs), THE 'BIG BANG,' AND REFLUX NEPHROPATHY

Urinary tract infections in infants and children are commonly encountered in clinical practice. Although UTI can occur at any age, infections in young infants are especially of concern. The consensus among pediatric nephrologists is that the very first UTI in a vulnerable infant may be sufficient to cause permanent renal scarring. This vulnerability results from mechanisms for extension of infection from the lower urinary tract to the renal parenchyma. Although the resulting invasive renal infection is often referred to as "acute pyelonephritis," a more accurate term is "acute infective interstitial nephritis."

Two principal mechanisms lead to invasive renal infection: vesicoureteric reflux extending to the renal pelvis, and, in children without demonstrable reflux, ureteral dysperistalsis.[4] The latter is facilitated by a unique host-microbial interaction, which involves the attachment of certain organisms, with specific molecular groupings on their surfaces, to complementary receptors on uroepithelial cells. In particular, certain P-fimbriated strains of *Escherichia coli* have been implicated.[5] Local inflammation of the ureter may impair peristalsis, further contributing to urinary stasis. Imaging studies have shown a relationship between infection with such "pyelonephritogenic" strains of *E coli* and increased ureteral width.[6] Moreover, microbial adherence presumably allows pathogens to resist the "washout" effect of urinary flow and facilitates retrograde migration toward the kidneys.

Other host factors predisposing to focal renal scarring as a consequence of parenchymal infection include the occurrence of compound papillae and their association with intrarenal reflux.[7] Herein, renal scarring is referred to as reflux nephropathy, although it is recognized that some scars may follow UTI in the absence of reflux. Jacobson et al[8] have proposed the term "postinfectious focal renal scarring" as an alternative to reflux nephropathy.

The notion that the very first UTI can inflict permanent renal scarring has been referred to as the "big bang" theory.[7,9] According to this theory, only one infection in an infant or young child with ureteral reflux or dysperistalsis

Accepted for publication February 4, 1991.

From the Division of Pediatric Nephrology and Hypertension, Lutheran General Children's Medical Center, Park Ridge, Ill, and the Department of Pediatrics, University of Chicago–Pritzker School of Medicine, Chicago, Ill.

Presented at the Festschrift for Jack Metcoff, MD, Chicago, Ill, June 11, 1990.

Reprint requests to the Lutheran General Children's Medical Center, 1775 Dempster St, Park Ridge, IL 60068-1174 (Dr Kallen).

is sufficient to lead to scarring. Often, the first UTI is not recognized as such but has been misdiagnosed as "fever of unknown origin."

Recognition that substantial renal damage can occur in the absence of further recurrences of infection suggests that UTIs, in certain vulnerable infants, are not benign. In particular, infants with reflux extending to a solitary kidney, or bilateral high-grade reflux, are especially vulnerable to serious long-term sequelae, including ESRD.

A recent report suggested that chronic renal disease may be a more likely outcome than is generally appreciated. An extended follow-up (average, 27 years) of young adults with a history of a febrile UTI as infants and children, demonstrable renal scars on intravenous urograms, and a high prevalence of reflux in the subset studied with voiding cystograms showed that all patients had evidence of chronic renal disease.[8] Ten percent of the group already had progressed to ESRD.

THE MECHANISM OF PROGRESSION TO CHRONIC RENAL FAILURE

It is known that progression to ESRD can occur in the absence of further occurrences of UTI and despite surgical correction of reflux.[10] It is now believed that the mechanism of progression of reflux nephropathy to ESRD involves the same "final common pathway" as in other forms of diffuse renal parenchymal disease.

The "nephron hyperfiltration" hypothesis of Brenner et al[11] has been invoked as an explanation for an irreversible, progressive course. Considerable data suggest that the loss of a "critical mass" of functioning nephron units, or glomerular capillary surface area,[12] in the face of an unchanged excretory load initiates an increase in glomerular capillary flow and pressure, resulting in hyperfiltration by remnant glomeruli. The nature of endogenous vasoactive substances responsible for an increase in glomerular capillary blood flow and pressure is unknown, although it is believed that the effector substance causes a preferential increase in constrictive tone of the efferent arteriole, facilitating an increase in single-nephron glomerular filtration rate. The role of locally released vasoactive hormones is currently under study.[13] The precise stimulus to hyperfiltration is also unknown. Certain amino acids or humoral factors, such as glucagon, have been implicated.[10]

Hyperfiltration, if sustained, is injurious and leads, in some unknown way, to expansion of mesangial matrix and progressive glomerular sclerosis. As individual nephron units are rendered nonfunctional, the cycle becomes self-perpetuating. The mesangial injury, coupled with hyperfiltration, causes alterations in glomerular permselectivity, culminating in pathologic proteinuria. Microalbuminuria has been observed to correlate with increasingly severe renal scarring in children with reflux nephropathy.[14] The point in time at which this cycle of progressive disease becomes irreversible appears to correspond to a decline of renal excretory function to less than 50% of normal.[15] The emergence of nephrotic-range proteinuria is ominous and marks the development of glomerular sclerosis,[16] which progresses in parallel with the underlying initial interstitial renal disease. The pathologic term often used for the end-stage kidney of reflux nephropathy is "chronic atrophic pyelonephritis," which, however, fails to reflect the superimposed lesion of glomerular sclerosis.

Although renal hyperechogenicity on ultrasound examination is a nonspecific finding,[17] recent reports of a diffuse or nodular ("pseudotumoral") hyperechoic pattern have suggested a marker for the detection of hyperfiltration.[18,19]

Nephron hyperfiltration, if viewed teleologically as a compensatory response to an altered excretory load per nephron, makes physiologic sense. Nevertheless, sustained hyperfiltration, by producing disease, is counterproductive and is considered a "disorder of adaptation."[20] The precise relationship of hyperfiltration to the development of focal sclerosis is not fully understood. As mentioned above, Brenner et al[11] have proposed that hyperfiltration results in mesangial injury, perhaps related to an increase in transcapillary flux of macromolecules, which, in some unknown way, leads to sclerosis. Other data suggest that the key development is glomerular hypertrophy and altered growth dynamics of infiltrating or resident glomerular cells.[21,22] However, the latter mechanism may not be independent from glomerular hypertension as a risk factor for the development of progressive disease.[23]

Nevertheless, in view of the pathogenic potential of hyperfiltration, further questions arise: Why does a mechanism for hyperfiltration even exist? Was there once a survival advantage for such a mechanism? There is evidence that the evolutionary basis of hyperfiltration may lie in the food-procurement behavior of our ancestors.

PALEONEPHROLOGY

The paleolithic period of human evolution encompasses 2 million years, beginning with fabrication of rudimentary stone tools by our hominid ancestor, *Homo habilis*, and ending with the emergence of agriculture, between 5000 and 10 000 years ago. Approximately 40 000 years ago, biologically modern humans emerged (*Homo sapiens sapiens*), and during the ensuing period, brain size and the human genetic pool are believed to have changed little. Until about 10 000 years ago, it is estimated that the diet of our hunter-gatherer forebears consisted of a large proportion of meat obtained by hunting or carcass scavenging.[24] According to Brenner et al,[11] the capacity to hyperfilter was salutary for our primitive ancestors, who lived during epochs when the food supply was marginal. Until the relatively recent advent of settled human societies with knowledge of farming (some 8000 to 10 000 years ago), there were some 30 000 years of a marginal existence for hunter-gatherers. During much of this period, the planet was in the grip of the last glaciation, and the climate was colder. The expanding human population probably did not migrate beyond subtropical latitudes, increasing competition for the food supply. Survival depended on hunting ability, both for nutritional sustenance and animal skins for warmth. Reproductive success may also have depended on hunting ability; the successful hunter was more likely to mate with a receptive female.[25]

Success as a hunter depended on physical strength, at least for predation of large animals. The requisite physical strength, in turn, mandated sufficient protein intake to maintain muscle mass. A successful hunt of large game depended on a close approach to an animal. The hunter, using a spear, then had to lunge with considerable thrust to mortally injure the animal. The imperative to maintain muscle mass is consistent with evidence that the paleolithic diet consisted of a high proportion of animal protein, probably derived from large grazing animals.[24] Despite the abundance of vegetation in the tropical savannas that supported herds of grazing animals, the supply of edible

Renal Solute Load of Late Paleolithic Humans*	
Solute	**Load, mmol (or mOsm)/d**
Urea†	1487
Sodium	30
Potassium	285
Ammonium‡	70
Anions§	385
Total	**2257**

*Based on estimates of dietary intake of late paleolithic humans (10 000 to 40 000 years ago) by Eaton and Konner.[24] The renal solute load for a 70-kg human is 32 mOsm/kg per day.

†Urea derived from the daily dietary protein intake of 251.1 g,[24] assuming zero net nitrogen balance.

‡Assuming net hydrogen ion excretion as ammonium to be 1.0 mmol/kg per day and ignoring net acid excretion as titratable acid.

§Assuming 1:1 cation-anion equivalence (a slight overestimate, as this assumption ignores the minor effect of divalent anions).

plants was probably meager, and hunting of large mammals persisted as the major means of food procurement.[26]

A successful hunt yielding sufficient meat for the clan was probably not accomplished on a daily basis. It is likely that the animal protein intake of the clan oscillated between "feast" and "famine." During several successive days of limited food intake, demands on renal excretory function would have been minimal, and glomerular filtration would have declined to a "resting" level,[11] perhaps analogous to the low filtration rate now observed in chronic malnutrition.[27] On the day of a successful hunt, the clan gorged themselves. Consequently, there was a sudden need to modulate renal glomerular hemodynamics in support of a glomerular filtration rate commensurate with the excretory load of urea and electrolytes.

Based on the assumption that the diet of hunter-gatherers contained 35% meat, the nutrient composition[24] and the renal solute load can be estimated (Table). The paleolithic meat eater had a relatively high potassium intake relative to sodium. Moreover, the overall renal solute load was relatively high (32 mOsm/kg per day).

The estimates of the paleolithic diet[24] are based on the assumption of a readily available food supply in terms of predation on a day-to-day basis. Given an alternative assumption that the availability of big game on a day-to-day basis was marginal and that consumption of meat occurred on an intermittent basis with binge-type meals, the consequent solute and potassium load presented an enormous excretory challenge to the kidneys. Thus, the intermittent nature of food intake of our ancestors resulted in the gradual evolutionary development of a mechanism for up- and down-regulation of intraglomerular hemodynamics, especially the filtration rate. In essence, nephron hyperfiltration, evolving over tens of thousands of years of intermittent intake and binge-eating, was an appropriate adaptation to conditions of precarious nutrition at the time. This vestigial primitive reflex became encoded in the genetic memory of our species. Thus, reflex glomerular hyperfiltration to a protein meal persists to this day.[28,29]

After the last glacial retreat, beginning 14 000 years ago,[30] and as the climate became more hospitable and grazing animals migrated to latitudes formerly covered by ice, primitive human societies were less preoccupied with mere survival. Between 8000 and 10 000 years ago, humans learned to plant seed, cultivate wheat, and raise livestock for milk, meat, blood, and, in the instance of sheep, wool for clothing. Thus, the transition from hunter-gatherer to farmer-herder marked the beginning of some degree of control over the food supply, favoring more frequent meals. According to Bronowski,[31] the signal event in the meteoric ascent of human civilization was a genetic mutation (a tripling of the chromosome complement) of a species of wild grass, leading to the evolution of wheat. The seeds of this mutant, instead of being scattered by the wind, had to be manually collected and sowed. Thus, the emergence of farming lessened dependence on big-game hunting, and, for the first time, grain became an important component of the diet. Humans were now able to provide meals for themselves more frequently, although the effects of climatic events on the availability of food probably continued to impose a considerable degree of episodicity on meals.

After the emergence of the Bronze Age, tools and weapons were more efficient, and hunting strategies, including trapping and stampeding, became more refined. Because there was now less of a need for brute strength for the purpose of hunting, coupled with the development of agriculture, humans began to consume less animal protein. In fact, this transition was apparently accompanied by a decline in stature (of about 15 cm) compared with the height of the hunter-gatherer.[24] Because humans were now able to provide meals for themselves on a regular, frequent basis, it is likely that the average level of glomerular perfusion reached a higher "set point" to cope with frequent, repeated excretory loads.

The most important electrolyte accompanying a high-protein meat meal, consumed in raw form along with animal blood erythrocytes, is potassium. If the glomerular filtration rate were not appropriately up-regulated from the resting state, dangerous hyperkalemia after a binge meal might have ensued. Because urea, the major excretory product of protein metabolism in humans, is not directly toxic, it is tempting to speculate that hyperfiltration evolved as an adaptation to the most compelling excretory challenge of protein intake: the rapid elimination of potassium. Because hyperfiltration probably results in increased distal delivery of sodium, which provides the sodium necessary for exchange with secreted potassium, it may serve as the first line of defense against an acute potassium load. In the face of a sustained potassium load, the regulatory loop is completed by stimulating renin release, ultimately leading to increased aldosterone secretion. Given the relatively low sodium content of the paleolithic diet (Table), the dual imperatives of sodium conservation and potassium elimination are perfectly conjoined by means of aldosterone-regulated distal sodium-potassium exchange. In fact, according to one view, the renin-angiotensin-aldosterone mechanism primarily functions as a defense against potassium excess.[32] Remarkably, a recent review does not cite data as to the pure effect of an acute potassium load on whole-kidney or single-nephron glomerular filtration rate.[33] The hypothesis that the artifice of hyperfiltration evolved as an adaptation to cope with intermittent binge eating and, in particular, the imperative to eliminate potassium remains speculative.

The critical balance of excretory load and renal mass is changed in renal disease. Although the absolute excretory load is in the usual range, the nephron complement, reduced by disease, is now burdened with an increased load per nephron. The primitive reflex of renal glomerular hyperfiltration is activated. Thus, for some infants and young children with UTI and renal scarring, the progression to

ESRD many years later is a recapitulation of an evolutionary adaptation to the binge-meal, meat-eating dietary habits of our paleolithic ancestors.

IMPLICATIONS OF PALEONEPHROLOGY FOR PEDIATRIC PRACTICE

The central biologic process of infant and child health is growth. The level of protein intake is a critical determinant of optimal growth. Current recommendations of infant nutrition have resulted in levels of protein intake commensurate with that ingested naturally by means of breast-feeding. One can only speculate whether higher levels of protein intake by infants during the era that nonhumanized milk formula was widely used had adverse renal effects, perhaps subtly in the form of glomerular sclerosis. It is known that a gradual process of glomerular senescence attends the aging process. It is possible that this process is not normal or physiologic but reflects the sustained high level of excretory demands on the kidney throughout one's life.[34]

Focal glomerular sclerosis culminating in chronic renal failure has been reported in children with a single kidney.[35] A recent case report documented focal glomerular sclerosis in a child with a solitary kidney affected by oligomeganephronia and a supernormal creatinine clearance.[36] Studies in adults with a single kidney since childhood have shown a gradual decline in renal excretory function from a baseline of higher-than-expected values and the emergence of microalbuminuria.[37] The question arises: Should children with a solitary kidney due to congenital absence, disease, or trauma of the contralateral kidney or surgical removal have a reduction in dietary protein intake? A definitive answer is not currently available, but a proportional reduction of protein intake may be prudent if a collaborative study currently in progress yields data supporting such intervention.[38]

A common recommendation in the management of the nephrotic syndrome in children is to increase the dietary intake of protein as compensation for urinary losses of albumin. Is it possible that "supernormal" glomerular filtration rates observed in some nephrotic children[39] and the common pathologic lesion of focal glomerular sclerosis are consequences of high exogenous protein intake or augmented endogenous protein synthesis by the liver? Is the development of focal sclerosis related to renal vasodilatory effects of glucocorticoids?[40]

Should children known to have chronic renal disease, including those with reflux nephropathy, have dietary limitations imposed early in life? If protein restriction is employed, is there a concomitant risk of impaired somatic growth?[41] If data emerge supporting the salutary effect of dietary protein restriction, the possible impairment of growth may be a reasonable tradeoff for a delay in the progression to ESRD. Preliminary data suggest that dietary protein restriction lessens urinary protein excretion in children with reflux nephropathy.[14]

The implications of diet modification for patients with chronic renal disease are so far reaching in terms of the enormous demand currently for ESRD treatment that a multicenter, collaborative study of protein and phosphorus limitation is currently in progress.[38] Although the efficacy of therapeutic strategies aimed at interdicting the development of sustained hyperfiltration and progressive glomerular sclerosis is controversial,[42,43] recent studies suggest that protein restriction may be beneficial.[44-46] A feasibility study of dietary protein restriction in infants with chronic renal insufficiency has yielded preliminary data.[47]

Because angiotensin-converting enzyme inhibitors have a predominant effect on the glomerular efferent arteriole, the possible benefit of such agents in the amelioration of progressive renal disease has been considered.[48] A short-term study involving children, most of whom had primary glomerular diseases, showed that therapy with angiotensin-converting enzyme inhibitors was efficacious in reducing proteinuria.[49] The long-term benefit of such pharmacotherapy remains to be established.

The question of the possible risk of focal glomerular sclerosis in the remaining kidney of individuals donating a kidney has been raised.[10] Although follow-up studies generally show stable renal function, available preliminary data suggest that some donors may develop proteinuria, microalbuminuria, or hypertension.[50-55] If long-term follow-up indicates a substantial risk to kidney donors, transplant programs will have the ethical obligation to inform prospective donors of such risks.

References

1. Goldraich NP, Barratt TM. Vesicoureteric reflux and renal scarring. In: Holliday MA, Barratt TM, Vernier RL, eds. *Pediatric Nephrology*. 2nd ed. Baltimore, Md: Williams & Wilkins; 1986:647-666.
2. Savage JM, Koh CT, Shah V, Barratt TM, Dillon MJ. Five year prospective study of plasma renin activity and blood pressure in patients with longstanding reflux nephropathy. *Arch Dis Child.* 1987;62:678-682.
3. Arant BS, Sotelo-Avila C, Bernstein J. Segmental 'hypoplasia' of the kidney (Ask-Upmark). *J Pediatr.* 1979;95:931-939.
4. Roberts JA. Pathogenesis of nonobstructive urinary tract infections in children. *J Urol.* 1990;144(pt 2):475-479.
5. Winberg J, Bollgren I, Kallenius G, Mollby R, Svenson SB. Clinical pyelonephritis and focal renal scarring: a selected review of pathogenesis, prevention, and prognosis. *Pediatr Clin North Am.* 1982;29:801-814.
6. Marild S, Heilstrom M, Jacobsson B, Jodal U, Eden CS. Influence of bacterial adhesion on ureteral width in children with acute pyelonephritis. *J Pediatr.* 1989;115:265-268.
7. Ransley PG, Risdon RA. The renal papilla, intrarenal reflux, and chronic pyelonephritis. In: Hodson CJ, Kincaid-Smith P, eds. *Reflux Nephropathy.* New York, NY: Masson Publishing USA Inc; 1979.
8. Jacobson SH, Eklof O, Eriksson CG, Lins L-E, Tidgren B, Winberg J. Development of hypertension and uraemia after pyelonephritis in childhood: 27 year followup. *BMJ.* 1989;299:703-706.
9. Lerner GR, Fleischmann LE, Perlmutter AD. Reflux nephropathy. *Pediatr Clin North Am.* 1987;34:747-770.
10. Dunn BR, Anderson S, Brenner BM. The hemodynamic basis of progressive renal disease. *Semin Nephrol.* 1986;6:122-138.
11. Brenner BM, Meyer TW, Hostetter TH. Dietary protein intake and the progressive nature of kidney disease: the role of hemodynamically mediated glomerular injury in the pathogenesis of progressive glomerular sclerosis in aging, renal ablation, and intrinsic renal disease. *N Engl J Med.* 1982;307:652-659.
12. Brenner BM, Garcia DL, Anderson S. Glomeruli and blood pressure: less of one, more of the other? *Am J Hypertens.* 1988;1(pt 1):335-347.
13. Pelayo JC, Quan AG. Pathophysiology of glomerular hemodynamic adaptations to nephron loss. *Semin Nephrol.* 1989;9:10-13.
14. White RHR. Vesicoureteric reflux and renal scarring. *Arch Dis Child.* 1989;64:407-412.

15. Brenner BM. Hemodynamically mediated glomerular injury and the progressive nature of kidney disease. *Kidney Int.* 1983;23:547-655. Nephrology Forum.

16. El-Khatib M, Becker GJ, Kincaid-Smith PS. Reflux nephropathy and primary vesicoureteric reflux in adults. *Q J Med.* 1990:77(New Series):1241-1253.

17. Krensky AM, Reddish JM, Teele RL. Causes of increased renal echogenicity in pediatric patients. *Pediatrics.* 1983;72:840-846.

18. Enriquez G, Lucaya J, Nieto J, Aso C. Hyperechogenic renal hypertrophy in glomerulosclerosis. *Pediatr Radiol.* 1989;19:441.

19. Avni EF, Van Sinoy ML, Hall H, Stallenberg B, Matos CL. Hypothesis: reduced renal mass with glomerular hyperfiltration, a cause of renal hyperechogenicity in children. *Pediatr Radiol.* 1989;19:108-110.

20. Anderson S, Brenner BM. Progressive renal disease: a disorder of adaptation. *Q J Med.* 1989;70(New Series):185-189.

21. Klahr S, Schreiner G, Ichikawa I. The progression of renal disease. *N Engl J Med.* 1988;318:1657-1666.

22. Fogo A, Ichikawa I. Evidence for the central role of glomerular growth promoters in the development of sclerosis. *Semin Nephrol.* 1989;9:329-342.

23. Lafferty HM, Brenner BM. Are glomerular hypertension and 'hypertrophy' independent risk factors for progression of renal disease? *Semin Nephrol.* 1990;10:294-304.

24. Eaton SB, Konner M. Paleolithic nutrition: a consideration of its nature and current implications. *N Engl J Med.* 1985;312:283-289.

25. Hill K. Hunting and human evolution. *J Hum Evolut.* 1982;11:521-544.

26. Foley R. A reconsideration of the role of predation on large mammals in tropical hunter-gatherer adaptation. *Man.* 1982;17:393-402.

27. Klahr S, Tripathy K. Evaluation of renal function in malnutrition. *Arch Intern Med.* 1966;118:322-325.

28. Hostetter TH. Human renal response to meat meal. *Am J Physiol.* 1986;250:F613-F618.

29. Herrera J, Rodriguez-Iturbe B, Parra G, et al. Urinary prostaglandin E and kallikrein activity in glomerular hyperfiltration induced by a meat meal in man. *Clin Nephrol.* 1988;30:151-157.

30. Broecker WS, Denton GH. What drives glacial cycles? *Sci Am.* 1990;262:48-56.

31. Bronowski J. *The Ascent of Man.* Boston, Mass: Little Brown & Co Inc; 1973:65-68.

32. Itskovitz HD. The renin-angiotensin system. In: Kurtzman NA, Martinez-Maldonado M, eds. *Pathophysiology of the Kidney.* Springfield, Ill: Charles C Thomas Publisher; 1977:391-445.

33. Giebisch G, Malnic G, Berliner RW. Renal transport and control of potassium excretion. In: Brenner BM, Rector FC Jr, eds. *The Kidney.* 3rd ed. Philadelphia, Pa: WB Saunders Co; 1986:177-205.

34. Meyer TW, Anderson S, Brenner BM. Dietary protein intake and progressive glomerular sclerosis: the role of capillary hypertension and hyperperfusion in the progression of renal disease. *Ann Intern Med.* 1983;98(pt 2):832-838.

35. Thorner PS, Arbus GS, Celermajer DS, Baumal R. Focal segmental glomerulosclerosis and progressive renal failure associated with a unilateral kidney. *Pediatrics.* 1984;73:806-810.

36. Nomura S, Osawa G. Focal glomerular sclerotic lesions in a patient with unilateral oligomeganephronia and agenesis of the contralateral kidney: a case report. *Clin Nephrol.* 1990;33:7-11.

37. Wikstad I, Celsi G, Larsson L, Herin P, Aperia A. Kidney function in adults born with unilateral renal agenesis or nephrectomized in childhood. *Pediatr Nephrol.* 1988;2:177-182.

38. Klahr S. The modification of diet in renal disease study. *N Engl J Med.* 1989;320:864-866. Sounding Board.

39. Metcoff J, Kelsey WM, Janeway CA. The nephrotic syndrome in children: an interpretation of its clinical, biochemical, and renal hemodynamic features as a variation of a single type of nephron disease. *J Clin Invest.* 1951;30:471-491.

40. Garcia DL, Rennke HG, Brenner BM, Anderson S. Glucocorticoids amplify glomerular injury in rats with renal ablation. *Am J Hypertens.* 1988;1:54-57.

41. Friedman AL. Dietary manipulation and progression of renal disease: strategies for the growing animal. *Semin Nephrol.* 1989;9:14-18.

42. Fine LG. Preventing the progression of human renal disease: have rational therapeutic principles emerged? *Kidney Int.* 1988;33:116-128.

43. Hunsicker LG. Studies of therapy of progressive renal failure in humans. *Semin Nephrol.* 1989;9:380-394.

44. Acchiardo SR, Moore LW, Cockrell S. Does low protein diet halt the progression of renal insufficiency? *Clin Nephrol.* 1986;25:289-294.

45. Ihle BU, Becker GJ, Whitworth JA, Charlwood RA, Kincaid-Smith PS. The effect of protein restriction on the progression of renal insufficiency. *N Engl J Med.* 1989;321:1773-1777.

46. Zeller K, Whittaker E, Sullivan L, Raskin P, Jacobson HR. Effect of restricting dietary protein on the progression of renal failure in patients with insulin-dependent diabetes mellitus. *N Engl J Med.* 1991;324:78-84.

47. Uauy R, Hogg RJ, Holliday M. Protein-energy requirements of children with chronic renal insufficiency: report from the Southwest Pediatric Nephrology Study Group and the Infant Diet Protein Study Group. *Semin Nephrol.* 1989;9:24-30.

48. Keane WF, Anderson S, Aurell M, de Zeeuw D, Narins RG, Povar G. Angiotensin converting enzyme inhibitors and progressive renal insufficiency. 1989;111:503-516.

49. Trachtman H, Gauthier B. Effect of angiotensin-converting enzyme inhibitor therapy on proteinuria in children with renal disease. *J Pediatr.* 1988;112:295-298.

50. Miller IJ, Suthanthiran M, Rigio RR, et al. Impact of renal donation: long-term clinical and biochemical follow-up of living donors in a single center. *Am J Med.* 1985;79:201-208.

51. Anderson CF, Velosa JA, Frohnert PP, et al. The risks of unilateral nephrectomy: status of kidney donors 10 to 20 years postoperatively. *Mayo Clin Proc.* 1985;60:367-374.

52. Chavers BM, Michael AF, Weiland D, Najarian JS, Mauer SM. Urinary albumin excretion in renal transplant donors. *Am J Surg.* 1985;149:343-346.

53. Williams SL, Oler J, Jorkasky DK. Long-term renal function in kidney donors: a comparison of donors and their siblings. *Ann Intern Med.* 1986;105:1-8.

54. Talseth T, Fauchald P, Skrede S, et al. Long-term blood pressure and renal function in kidney donors. *Kidney Int.* 1986;29:1072-1076.

55. Bay WH, Hebert LA. The living donor in kidney transplantation. *Ann Intern Med.* 1987;106:719-727.

X-linked Hypophosphatemia

Genetic and Clinical Correlates

James D. Hanna, MD; Kazuhiko Niimi, MD; James C. M. Chan, MD

• X-linked hypophosphatemia is a hereditary form of rickets that results from an isolated renal tubular wasting of phosphate. The clinical features unique to this disorder, and the recent advances in our understanding of vitamin D metabolism and molecular genetics in X-linked hypophosphatemia are reviewed. Finally, a succinct critique of the controversial treatment modalities round up this review.

(*AJDC.* 1991;145:865-870)

X-linked hypophosphatemia, previously regarded as a rare disease, is the most frequent cause of familial rickets, with an incidence of one in 20 000 births.[1] This disorder is an isolated phosphate transport defect at the renal tubule that is inherited by X-linked dominant trans

See also pp 853, 860, 871, and 877.

mission and characterized clinically by hypophosphatemia, growth retardation, and rickets, most pronounced in male patients.[2] It has been repeatedly demonstrated that the degree of hypophosphatemia is not correlated to the severity of skeletal lesions,[3-5] which supports the suggestion of an associated primary defect in the osteoblasts[6] in patients with X-linked hypophosphatemia as well as in the Hyp mouse, the murine homologue of the human disease. As the affected patient ages, osteomalacic bone pain, pseudofractures, skeletal deformities, progressive ankylosis, and dental caries occur.[7] Herein, we review the progress made in the last decade concerning both biochemical and genetic aspects of this disease and examine the strengths and weaknesses of new treatment modalities with vitamin D metabolites, phosphate, and diuretics. The use of magnetic resonance spectroscopy in a clinical setting to study intracellular phosphate metabolism, the evidence of an as yet unidentified phosphaturic factor as suggested by parabiosis experimentation, and a review of the powerful tools of molecular genetics with the potential to identify the gene defect in this disorder will form the final focus of our report.

Accepted for publication January 24, 1991.

From the Department of Pediatrics and Children's Medical Center, Virginia Commonwealth University's Medical College of Virginia, Richmond.

Reprint requests to Box 498, MCV Station, Richmond, VA 23298-0498 (Dr Chan).

TREATMENT REGIMENS

As recently as 1980, the standard therapy for X-linked hypophosphatemia consisted of high doses of vitamin D_2 (10 000 to 50 000 U/d) and phosphate supplementation (1.5 to 2.0 g/d in five divided doses) to maintain the serum phosphate concentration above 1 mmol/L. Hypercalcemia, a frequent complication associated with high doses of vitamin D_2, was often prolonged because of the ongoing storage of vitamin D_2 in adipocytes. Consequently, constant concerns among physicians who treat these patients[8] are the complications of hypercalcemia, hypercalciuria, nephrocalcinosis, and nephrolithiasis, some or all of which are associated with progressive deterioration of renal function.

Despite earlier reports[9,10] of a lack of response to 1,25-dihydroxyvitamin D_3, Hirschman et al[11] reasoned that there must be a defect in the regulation of 1α-hydroxylase in X-linked hypophosphatemia and proved their hypothesis in 1978 by treating an affected child with pharmacological doses of 1,25-dihydroxyvitamin D_3, thereby reversing rickets and growth retardation. Concurrent and subsequent studies[12-15] in the early 1980s continued to confirm these initial observations. In addition, intensive efforts by a number of investigators in the mid-1980s substantiated this 1α-hydroxylase defect in humans[16-19] as well as in the Hyp mouse, the murine homologue of the human disease.[20,21]

The principal therapy for X-linked hypophosphatemia is phosphate supplementation in five or more daily doses to compensate for the renal phosphate wasting. However, phosphate supplementation alone is often associated with secondary hyperparathyroidism,[22,23] especially in patients with low concentrations of circulating 1,25-dihydroxyvitamin D_3. These advances in our understanding of disordered vitamin D metabolism in X-linked hypophosphatemia provide the rationale for the use of pharmacologic doses of 1,25-dihydroxyvitamin D_3 in the treatment of this disease. The initial clinical impression[22] in 1980 that 1,25-dihydroxyvitamin D_3 was superior to vitamin D_2 or 25-hydroxyvitamin D_3 (Fig 1) received unequivocal support in 1990 when a clinical trial[23] of almost a decade's duration involving 40 patients demonstrated that 1α-hydroxyvitamin D_3 (1 to 3 μg/d) promoted substantial improvement in linear growth when compared with treatment with 25-hydroxyvitamin D_3 (50 to 200 μg/d) or vitamin D_2 (0.5 to 2 mg/d). Each of these treatment

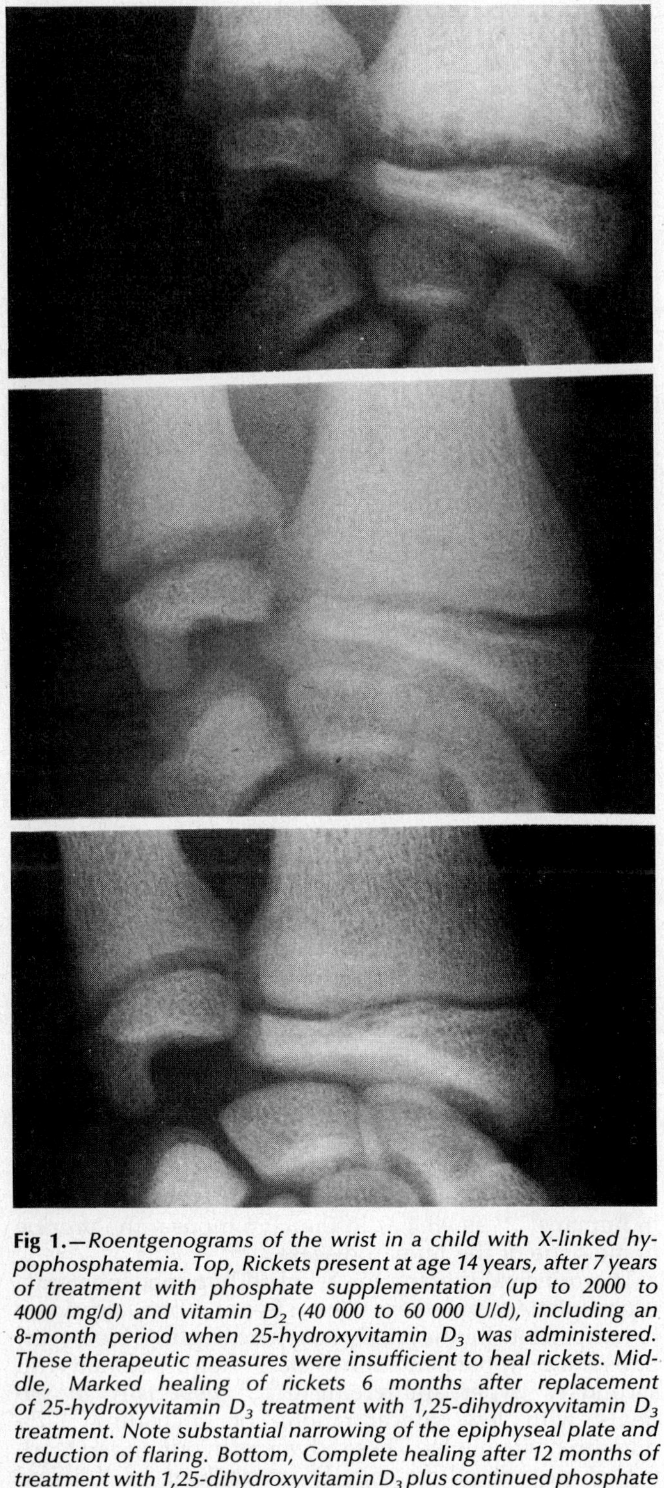

Fig 1.—*Roentgenograms of the wrist in a child with X-linked hypophosphatemia. Top, Rickets present at age 14 years, after 7 years of treatment with phosphate supplementation (up to 2000 to 4000 mg/d) and vitamin D_2 (40 000 to 60 000 U/d), including an 8-month period when 25-hydroxyvitamin D_3 was administered. These therapeutic measures were insufficient to heal rickets. Middle, Marked healing of rickets 6 months after replacement of 25-hydroxyvitamin D_3 treatment with 1,25-dihydroxyvitamin D_3 treatment. Note substantial narrowing of the epiphyseal plate and reduction of flaring. Bottom, Complete healing after 12 months of treatment with 1,25-dihydroxyvitamin D_3 plus continued phosphate supplementation (from Chan et al[22]).*

regimens was coupled with oral phosphate supplementation (0.7 to 2.1 g/d in four or five divided doses). According to this clinical trial by Balsan and Tieder,[23] 75% of the 1α-hydroxyvitamin D_3– and phosphate-treated group achieved normal stature, with accelerated and catch-up growth occurring primarily between the age of 2 years and puberty; this is in distinct contrast to the lack of response in the majority of those treated with vitamin D_2 or in the group treated with 25-hydroxyvitamin D_3 plus phosphate. These provocative observations can be interpreted in several ways. The effectiveness of 1α-hydroxyvitamin D_3 is unlikely due to more effective bone healing because radiologic findings were found to be similar among the three treatment groups. It is possible that pharmacologic dosages of vitamin D_2 and 25-hydroxyvitamin D_3 have a more toxic effect than does 1α-hydroxyvitamin D_3 on the growth of chondrocytes. Alternatively, 1α-hydroxyvitamin D_3 and 1,25-dihydroxyvitamin D_3 may directly and specifically enhance growth plate and chondrocyte multiplication.

In addition, whereas rickets are controlled with phosphate supplementations and vitamin D_2, endosteal bone lesions are controlled only with phosphate supplementation and 1,25-dihydroxyvitamin D_3. It is hypothesized that pharmacologic doses of 1,25-dihydroxyvitamin D_3 are needed to overcome the bone resistance. The fact that vitamin D_2 in pharmacologic doses fails to increase 1,25-dihydroxyvitamin D_3 concentrations has been taken as further support of this hypothesis.[8]

Hypercalcemia and hypercalciuria were encountered by a number of patients[24] following the administration of 1,25-dihydroxyvitamin D_3 at dosages of 30 to 40 ng/kg per day plus phosphate supplementation, the dosage required to maintain normal serum phosphate concentrations. However, on reducing the dosage of 1,25-dihydroxyvitamin D_3, radiologic evidence of bone lesions was again observed. In this subset of patients, the addition of a diuretic regimen to contract the extracellular volume, to enhance tubular reabsorption of phosphate, and to reduce urinary calcium excretion[24] has permitted an adequate dosage of 1,25-dihydroxyvitamin D_3 to promote bone healing without hypokalemia, metabolic alkalosis, and other observable side effects. The recommended diuretic regimen consists of hydrochlorothiazide and amiloride hydrochloride.[25] The latter medication is a potassium-sparing diuretic that prevents the hypokalemic metabolic alkalosis sometimes encountered with the use of hydrochlorothiazide alone.

The current recommendations for the treatment of X-linked hypophosphatemia can be summarized as follows: (1) 1,25-dihydroxyvitamin D_3, calcitriol (Rocaltrol, 0.25 μg or 0.5 μg per capsule), in an initial dose of 15 to 20 ng/kg per day with subsequent increases to 30 to 60 ng/kg per day during several months to achieve a maintenance serum phosphate concentration of at least 1 mmol/L. It should be noted that the dosage of 1,25-dihydroxyvitamin D_3 should be modified upward according to the severity of the rickets and the growth velocity. Hypercalciuria prevents the use of higher doses of 1,25-dihydroxyvitamin D_3. During the first 5 years of life and during puberty, the dosage is usually higher on a per-kilogram—body weight basis. The dosage is usually lower in patients 5 to 12 years of age. (2) Phosphate salts (Neutro-Phos, 1000 mg per 300 mL, or four capsules) to supply a total dose of 2000 to 4000 mg of phosphate per day in five to six divided doses until bedtime. The phosphate supplements are begun in small doses (30 to 40 mg/kg per day in five to six divided doses) to alleviate the gastrointestinal side effects of nausea and diarrhea. The dose is increased over several months to maintain the serum phosphate concentration at or above 1 mmol/L. (3) Patients are monitored with monthly serum calcium and phosphorus determinations as well as urine calcium/creatinine ratios. A urinary calcium/creatinine (both in milligrams per deciliter) ratio above 0.25 is indicative of hypercalciuria. When this is encountered, the dosages of calcitriol must be decreased or phosphate supplementation increased, or hydrochlorothiazide and amiloride must be added. The two diuretics are in a 5:1 proportion, with the initial dose of hydrochlorothiazide at 1.5 to 2.5 mg/d and amiloride at 0.3 to 0.5 mg/kg per day.

To evaluate the bone status, roentgenograms of the hands, wrists, ankles, and knees should be obtained every 1 to 3 years. To evaluate the risk of nephrocalcinosis, a renal ultrasound[26] scan is obtained every 12 months. To avoid the risk of hyperparathyroidism that is occasionally encountered due to phosphate supplementation without the suppressive effects of concomitant 1,25-dihydroxyvitamin D_3 administration, intact (I-84) parathyroid hormone concentrations should be determined semiannually or yearly. To assess the effect of treatment on linear growth, the patients' heights should be measured annually. For the sporadic cases, the heights of the parents should be obtained for the midparental height calculations,[27] to provide an estimation of the target height for the treated patients. It is difficult to use the midparental heights in the familial cases, because the final height of the affected parent is determined by the success of treatment.

In the 1990s and beyond, the powerful tools of molecular biology will surely reveal the gene defect and eventually lead the way to gene therapy, which will be the definitive treatment. In the meantime, the wider availability of recombinant human growth hormone may lead to a new therapeutic approach.[28] The rationale for this belief is that exogenous growth hormone can promote tubular reabsorption of phosphate alone or in conjunction with 1,25-dihydroxyvitamin D_3 plus phosphate treatments and can promote normalization of serum phosphate, healing of the rachitic process, and acceleration of linear growth, while avoiding some of the treatment-related complications currently being encountered.

TREATMENT COMPLICATIONS

The treatment of X-linked hypophosphatemia, in the past with pharmacologic doses of vitamin D_2, 25-hydroxyvitamin D_3 plus phosphate supplementation and more recently with 1,25-dihydroxyvitamin D_3 plus phosphate supplementation has been fraught with controversy. While low-dose vitamin D treatment regimens have little chance of reversing the rachitic and osteomalacic processes or preventing dental caries and osteoarthritis, high-dose treatment regimens increase the risk of hypercalcemia, hypercalciuria, and renal damage.[29-32]

The initial ultrasonographic demonstration of nephrocalcinosis in treated children with this disorder by Alon et al[26] in 1983 led to later documentation in 1987 by Goodyer et al[30] that 47% of a large series of children with this disorder treated with 1,25-dihydroxyvitamin D_3 had evidence of nephrocalcinosis. Such a high risk of potential kidney damage has given rise to the contention that children with X-linked hypophosphatemia should never be treated at all[33]; in a retrospective study that lasted almost 50 years, the final adult heights of untreated patients were not significantly different from those of the treated patients.[33] Furthermore, in an earlier report, Stickler et al[34] demonstrated that the treated affected twin suffered pseudofractures, whereas the untreated affected twin escaped this complication of X-linked hypophosphatemia. However, the intense efforts by a number of investigative teams in the past decade have clearly demonstrated a 1α-hydroxylase defect in both X-linked hypophosphatemic humans and mice.[17-21] Finally, the extensive studies by Hardy et al[7] and Reid et al[35] in 1989 of a large series of affected adults further demonstrate the high prevalence of the progressive ankylosis of the spine and major joints, dental caries, pseudofractures, and other complications in the essentially untreated patients. Based on the strength of such data, most physicians are unwilling to subscribe to the provocative suggestion to withhold treatment from affected patients.

Several lines of evidence[36-41] suggest that 1,25-dihydroxyvitamin D_3 directly suppresses parathyroid hormone secretion and that the use of phosphate alone leads to continuous stimulation of the parathyroid glands, resulting in hyperparathyroidism. To avoid this complication, Alon et al[29] recommended that when hypercalcemia or hypercalciuria is encountered, vitamin D and phosphate supplements should be simultaneously withheld until normal calcium values are reestablished. The continued administration of phosphate supplements as before, while withholding 1,25-dihydroxyvitamin D_3 because of hypercalcemia, is no longer tenable in light of the current understanding of the parathyroid suppressive effects of 1,25-dihydroxyvitamin D_3.[32-37]

MAGNETIC RESONANCE SPECTROSCOPY AND MUSCLE PHOSPHORUS

X-linked hypophosphatemia has reportedly been distinguished from all other forms of hypophosphatemia by the absence of muscle weakness.[42] Inorganic phosphate, a substrate in the formation of high-energy phosphate compounds, is used by muscle in anaerobic and aerobic metabolism. It also acts to modulate the kinetic rates of several key enzymes in metabolism. In view of the universal finding of a reduced serum phosphate concentration associated with this disorder, a disturbance of intracellular inorganic phosphate concentration and metabolism is also likely in X-linked hypophosphatemia. With the use of magnetic resonance spectroscopy (Fig 2), Clarke et al[43] demonstrated a subnormal concentration of intramyocellular inorganic phosphate in five patients with X-linked hypophosphatemia compared with those of five age- and sex-matched control subjects. Furthermore, intramyocellular phosphate concentrations increased within 24 hours in patients after initiation of standard 1,25-dihydroxyvitamin D_3 therapy without phosphate supplementation (Fig 2). These results contrast with those of Smith et al[44] in four adult female patients in whom intracellular phosphate concentrations were normal, which could account for the preservation of muscle strength despite severe systemic hypophosphatemia. However, there is no evidence to indicate an active transport mechanism, specific to the myocytes of X-linked hypophosphatemia, to maintain intracellular phosphate values greater than serum values. Therefore, previously reported data[43] are more in agreement with those reported in magnetic resonance spectroscopy studies of other forms of chronic hypophosphatemia and are consistent with the current understanding of disordered vitamin D metabolism in this disease.

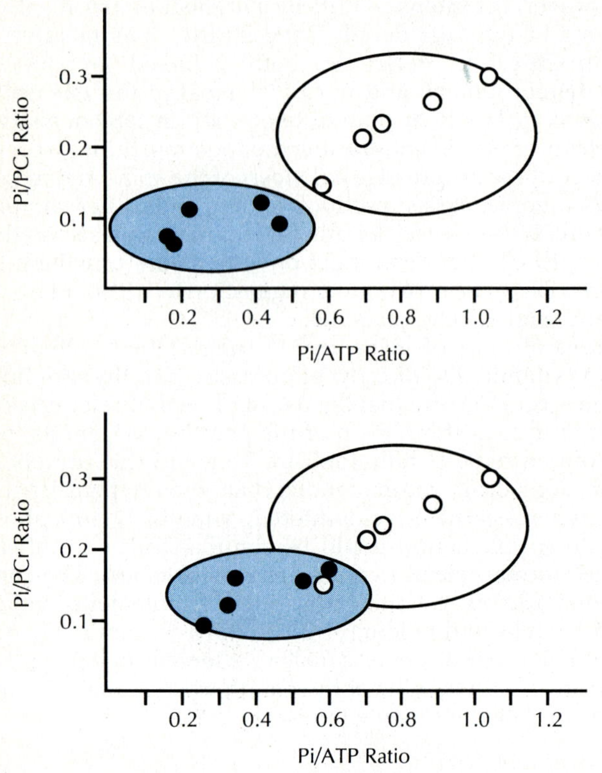

Fig 2.—*Ratio of intracellular phosphate (Pi) to phosphocreatine (PCr) concentrations before and after treatment with 1,25-dihydroxyvitamin D_3 in X-linked hypophosphatemia compared with that of age- and sex-matched control subjects. Scatterplots depict the Pi/PCr ratio vs the Pi to adenosine triphosphate (Pi/ATP) ratio measured for each patient (solid symbols) and control subjects (open circles). The ellipses are centered at the mean value for each group and their semiaxes are ±2 SDs from the mean. Top, Control group compared with patients not receiving medication. Bottom, Control group compared with patients receiving medication. Data are from Clarke et al.*[43]

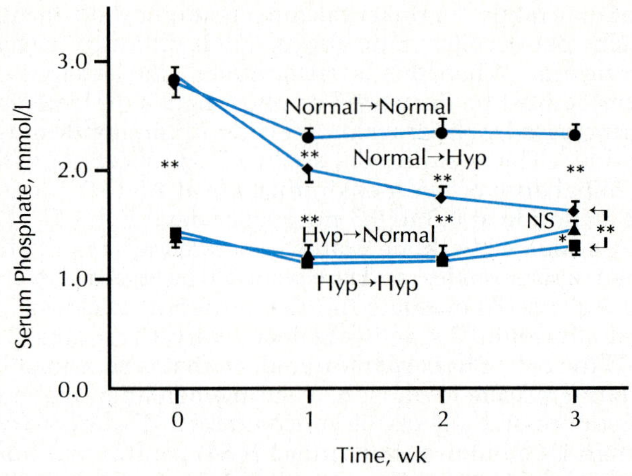

Fig 3.—*Parabiosis experiment in Hyp mice and normal mice. Note the substantial hypophosphatemia in the normal mice after 3 weeks of parabiosis with the Hyp mice. Double asterisks indicate* P<.01*; single asterisk,* P<.05*. These are significant differences compared with the values above and below the symbols. NS indicates not significant. Data are from Meyer et al.*[45]

PARABIOSIS IN THE HYP MOUSE

Meyer et al[45,46] recently demonstrated a humoral factor, unrelated to parathyroid hormone, in the development of phosphate wasting in the Hyp mouse. Within 3 weeks of parabiotic union through the peritoneal space between a Hyp mouse and a normal mouse, renal phosphate wasting and hypophosphatemia were documented in the normal mouse (Fig 3). After separation of the parabiotic union, the renal phosphate wasting ceased and normophosphatemia was restored in the normal mice.

In studies of the brushborder membrane vesicles of the normal mouse joined by parabiosis with the Hyp mouse,[45] a defective phosphate transport was demonstrated, again attesting to the transfer of a humoral substance to cause hyperphosphaturia in the normal animals. It is unlikely that parathyroid hormone is unlikely the cause of the phosphaturia, because parathyroidectomy did not affect the phosphate transport defect. Glucose uptake in brushborder membrane vesicles was unaffected by genotype or parabiosis. These studies point to the possibility of a humoral factor other than parathyroid hormone to account for the hypophosphatemia in the Hyp mouse.

ADVANCES IN MOLECULAR GENETICS

In the last decade, illuminating molecular genetic research in the Hyp mouse,[47] the murine homologue of the human disease, stimulated Reade et al[48] and Machler et al[49] in 1986 to localize the human hypophosphatemic gene to the distal end of the X-chromosome at the Xp22 region or band.

The building blocks of DNA are called nucleotides. Each DNA nucleotide includes one sugar-phosphate backbone and one base. The 100 restriction enzymes currently available can cut the double-stranded DNA molecule into fragments at specific recognition sites consisting of specific base pair sequences. Each restriction enzyme cuts the DNA molecule at each site where the specific base pair sequence appears. The resulting DNA fragments, after exposure to a specific restriction enzyme, can vary in length. These variations in the length ("polymorphism") between recognition sites are inherited in a mendelian fashion.[50] Molecular genetics has taken advantage of this restriction fragment length polymorphism to test whether a particular gene defect may also be inherited together with the same fragment. Linking these DNA fragments to a gene defect within a large family narrows the search to a fragment of the 6 million base pairs in human DNA. The probes most often linked to an affected family provide a better idea of the location of the gene defect.[51] Such statistical analysis of linkage is vastly enhanced by special computer programs and the availability of large affected families for study. With the use of X-chromosomal probes, restriction fragment length polymorphism, and linkage statistical analysis, the hypophosphatemic gene has now been localized to the Xp22 chromosomal band,[43-45] in close proximity to the recently identified Duchenne/Becker muscular dystrophy gene.

Recently, a second murine hypophosphatemic gene closely linked to the Hyp gene, the Gy gene (named for the Gyro mouse), has been reported[52] with cochlear and vestibular defects. The discovery of the Gy gene will help in the further identification of the gene defect in the human disorder.[52] The presence of two related defects in the mouse—the hypophosphatemia and the cochlear-vestibular abnormalities associated with hypophosphatemia—raises the possibility of two linked disease loci in humans. It is hoped that work in progress with newer markers, subtraction hybridization, automated DNA sequencing, and the polymerase chain reaction technique will "close in" on the hypophosphatemic gene in humans in the near future.

QUESTIONS FOR THE FUTURE

Many questions remain unanswered. The use of magnetic resonance spectroscopy[43] will examine intracellular phosphate and energy metabolism in various test conditions; isolation and characterization of the humoral factor[46] will substantially advance our understanding of phosphate metabolism. Linkage studies[47-51,53] to characterize the two phenotypes[52] will assist in the isolation of the gene and eventually lead to the delineation of its protein expression product for early diagnosis. With the rapid advances in molecular biology, it is conceivable that gene therapy will be available in the next generation for affected individuals. This is one example of how basic research can lead to definitive treatment.

We thank Marilyn Reilly for secretarial assistance and Martha D. Massie, RD, and Martha D. Wellons for editorial assistance.

References

1. Davis M, Stanbury SW. The rheumatic manifestation of metabolic bone disease. *Clin Rheum Dis.* 1981;7:595-646.

2. Rasmussen H, Tenenhouse HS. Hypophosphatemias. In: Scriver CR, Beaudet AC, Sly W, Valle D, eds. *Metabolic Basis of Inherited Disease.* 6th ed. New York, NY: McGraw-Hill International Book Co; 1989:2581-2604.

3. Engfeldt B, Zetterstrom R, Winberg J. Primary vitamin D–resistant rickets, III: biophysical studies of skeletal tissues. *J Bone Joint Surg Am.* 1956;38:1323-1334.

4. Frost HM. A unique histological feature of vitamin D–resistant rickets observed in four cases. *Acta Orthop Scand.* 1963;33:220-226.

5. Steendijk R, van den Hooff A, Nielsen HKL, Jowsey J. Lesion of bone matrix in vitamin D–resistant rickets. *Nature.* 1965;207:426-427.

6. Ecarot-Charrier B, Glorieux FH, Travers R, Desbarats M, Bouchard F, Huick A. Defective bone formation by transplanted Hyp mouse bone cells into normal mice. *Endocrinology.* 1988;123:768-773.

7. Hardy DC, Murphy WA, Siegel BA, Reid IR, Whyte MP. X-linked hypophosphatemia in adults: prevalence of skeletal radiographic and scintigraphic features. *Radiology.* 1989;171:403-414.

8. Chan JCM, Alon U, Hirschman GM. Renal hypophosphatemic rickets. *J Pediatr.* 1985;106:533-544.

9. Brickman AS, Coburn JW, Kurokawa K, Bethune JE, Harrison HE, Norman AW. Actions of 1,25-dihydroxycholecalciferol in patients with hypophosphatemic, vitamin D–resistant rickets. *N Engl J Med.* 1973;289:495-498.

10. Glorieux FH, Scriver CR, Reade TM, Goldman H, Roseborough A. Use of phosphate and vitamin D to prevent dwarfism and rickets in X-linked hypophosphatemia. *N Engl J Med.* 1972;287:481-487.

11. Hirschman GH, DeLuca HF, Chan JCM. Hypophosphatemic vitamin D–resistant rickets: metabolic balance studies in a child receiving 1,25-dihydroxyvitamin-D_3, phosphate and ascorbic acid. *Pediatrics.* 1978;61:451-457.

12. Glorieux FH, Marie PJ, Pettifor JM, Delvin EE. Bone response to phosphate salts, ergocalciferol, and calcitriol in hypophosphatemic vitamin D–resistant rickets. *N Engl J Med.* 1980;303:1023-1031.

13. Kristiansen JH, Pedersen VF. Hypophosphatemic vitamin D–resistant rickets treated with 1 alpha-hydroxyvitamin D_3. *Int J Pediatr Nephrol.* 1981;2:245-247.

14. Chesney RW, Mazess RB, Rose P, Hamstra AJ, DeLuca HF, Breed AL. Long-term influence of calcitriol (1,25-dihydroxyvitamin D) and supplemental phosphate in X-linked hypophosphatemic rickets. *Pediatrics.* 1983;71:559-567.

15. Rasmussen H, Pechet M, Anast C, Mazur A, Gertner J, Broadus AE. Long-term treatment of familial hypophosphatemic rickets with oral phosphate and 1 alpha-hydroxyvitamin D_3. *J Pediatr.* 1981;99:16-25.

16. Chesney RW, Mazess RB, Rose P, Hamstra AJ, DeLuca HF. Supranormal 25-hydroxyvitamin D and subnormal 1,25-dihydroxyvitamin D: their role in x-linked hydrophosphatemic rickets. *AJDC.* 1980;134:140-143.

17. Lyles KW, Clark AG, Drezner MK. Serum 1,25-dihydroxyvitamin D levels in subjects with X-linked hypophosphatemic rickets and osteomalacia. *Calcif Tissue Int.* 1982;34:125-130.

18. Lyles KW, Clark AG, Drezner MK. Parathyroid hormone effects on serum 1,25-dihydroxyvitamin D levels in patients with X-linked dominant hypophosphatemic rickets: evidence for abnormal 25-hydroxyvitamin D-1-hydroxylase activity. *J Clin Endocrinol Metab.* 1982;54:638-644.

19. Mason RS, Rohl PG, Lissner D, Posen S. Vitamin D metabolism in hypophosphatemic rickets. *AJDC.* 1982;136:909-913.

20. Meyer RA Jr, Gray RW, Meyer MH. Abnormal vitamin D metabolism in the X-linked hypophosphatemic mouse. *Endocrinology.* 1980;107:1577-1581.

21. Tenenhouse HS. Abnormal mitochondrial 25-hydroxyvitamin D_3-1-hydroxylase activity in the vitamin D and calcium deficient X-linked Hyp mouse. *Endocrinology.* 1983;113:816-818.

22. Chan JCM, Lovinger RD, Mamunes P. Renal hypophosphatemic rickets: growth acceleration after long-term treatment with 1,25-dihydroxyvitamin D_3. *Pediatrics.* 1980;66:445-454.

23. Balsan S, Tieder M. Linear growth in patients with hypophosphatemic vitamin D–resistant rickets: influence of treatment regimen and parental height. *J Pediatr.* 1990;116:365-370.

24. Alon U, Chan JCM. Effects of hydrochlorothiazide and amiloride in renal hypophosphatemic rickets. *Pediatrics.* 1985;75:754-763.

25. Alon U, Costanzo LS, Chan JCM. Additive hypocalciuric effects of amiloride and hydrochlorothiazide in patients treated with calcitriol. *Miner Electrolyte Metab.* 1984;10:379-386.

26. Alon U, Brewer WH, Chan JCM. Nephrocalcinosis: detection by ultrasonography. *Pediatrics.* 1983;71:970-973.

27. Tanner JM, Whitehouse RH, Marshall WA, Carter BS. Prediction of adult height, bone age, and occurrence of menarche at ages 4 to 6 with allowance for midparent height. *Arch Dis Child.* 1975;50:14-26.

28. Wilson DM, Lee PDK, Marcus R, et al. Growth hormone therapy in familial hypophosphatemia. *Pediatr Res.* 1990;27:195. Abstract.

29. Alon U, Newsome H, Chan JCM. Hyperparathyroidism in patients with X-linked dominant hypophosphatemic rickets: application of the calcium infusion test as an indication for parathyroidectomy. *Int J Pediatr Nephrol.* 1984;5:39-43.

30. Goodyer PR, Kronick JB, Jequier S, Reade TM, Scriver CR. Nephrocalcinosis and its relationship to treatment of hereditary rickets. *J Pediatr.* 1987;111:700-704.

31. Moncrieff MW, Change GW. Nephrotoxic effect of vitamin D therapy in vitamin D refractory rickets. *Arch Dis Child.* 1969;44:571-579.

32. Weber G, Cazziffo MA, Frisone F, et al. Nephrocalcinosis in children and adolescents: sonographic evaluation during long-term treatment with 1,25-dihydroxycholecalciferol. *Child Nephrol Urol.* 1988-1989;9:273-276.

33. Stickler GB, Morgenstern BZ. Hypophosphataemic rickets: final height and clinical symptoms in adults. *Lancet.* 1989;2:902-905.

34. Stickler GB, Jowsey J, Bianco AJ Jr. Possible detrimental effect of large doses of vitamin D in familial hypophosphatemic vitamin D–resistant rickets. *J Pediatr.* 1971;79:68-71.

35. Reid IR, Hardy DC, Murphy WA, Teitelbaum SL, Bergfield MA, Whyte MP. X-linked hypophosphatemia: a clinical, biochemical, and histopathologic assessment of morbidity in adults. *Medicine.* 1989;68:336-352.

36. Slatopolsky E, Weerts C, Thielan R, Horst R, Harter H, Martin K. Marked suppression of secondary hyperparathyroidism by intravenous administration of 1,25-dihydroxycholecalciferol in uremic patients. *J Clin Invest.* 1984;74:2136-2143.

37. Silver J, Naveh-Many T, Mayer H, Schmelzer H, Popovtzer M. Regulation by vitamin D metabolites of parathyroid hormone gene transcription in vivo in the rat. *J Clin Invest.* 1986;78:1296-1301.

38. Burmester JK, Weise RJ, Maeda N, DeLuca HF. Structure and regulation of the rat 1,25-dihydroxyvitamin D_3 receptor. *Proc Natl Acad Sci U S A.* 1988;85:9499-9502.

39. Minghetti PP, Norman AW. 1,25$(OH)_2$-vitamin D_3 receptors: gene regulation and genetic circuitry. *FASEB J.* 1988;2:3043-3053.

40. DeLuca HF. The vitamin D story: a collaborative effort of basic science and clinical medicine. *FASEB J.* 1988;2:224-236.

41. Kainer G, Bell NH, Chan JCM. Disorders of calcium metabolism. In: Chan JCM, Gill JR Jr, eds. *Kidney Electrolyte Disorders.* New York, NY: Churchill Livingstone Inc; 1990:171-222.

42. Rasmussen H, Anast C. Familial hypophosphatemic and vitamin D dependent rickets. In: Stanbury JB, Wyngaarden JB, Frederickson DS, Goldstein JL, Brown MS, eds. *Metabolic Basis of Inherited Disease.* 5th ed. New York, NY: McGraw-Hill International Book Co; 1983:1743-1773.

43. Clarke GD, Kainer G, Conway WF, Chan JCM. Intramyocellular phosphate metabolism in X-linked hypophosphatemic rickets. *J Pediatr.* 1990;116:288-292.

44. Smith R, Newman RJ, Radda GK, Stokes M, Young A. Hypophosphatemic osteomalacia and myopathy: studies with nuclear magnetic resonance spectroscopy. *Clin Sci.* 1984;67:505-509.

45. Meyer RA Jr, Meyer MH, Gray RW. Parabiosis suggests a humoral factor is involved in X-linked hypophosphatemia in mice. *J Bone Miner Res.* 1989;4:493-500.

46. Meyer RA Jr, Conway GD, Chan JCM. X-linked hypophosphatemia. *Semin Nephrol.* 1989;9:56-61.

47. Lyon MF, Scriver CR, Baker LRT, Tenenhouse HS, Kronick J, Mandla S. The Gy mutation: another cause of hypophosphatemia in mouse. *Proc Natl Acad Sci U S A.* 1986;83:4899-4903.

48. Reade AP, Thakker RV, Davis KE, et al. Mapping of human X-linked hypophosphatemic rickets by multilocus linkage analysis. *Hum Genet.* 1986;73:267-270.

49. Machler M, Frey D, Gal A, et al. X-linked dominant hypophosphatemia is closely linked to DNA markers DX 41 and DX 43 at Xp22. *Hum Genet.* 1986;73:271-275.

50. Kainer G, Clarke GD, Spence JE, Chan JCM. X-linked hypophosphatemia: an 'experiment of nature' on phosphate transport. In: Strauss J, ed. *Growth Immunosuppression and Renal Disorders in Neonates and Children.* Coral Gables, Fla: University of Miami Press; 1989:59-66.

51. Spence JE, Kainer G, Chan JCM. Genetics of vitamin D resistant rickets. In: Spitzer A, Avner E, eds. *Inheritance of Kidney and Urinary Tract Disease.* Boston, Mass: Kluwer Academic Publishers; 1989:167-176.

52. Boneh A, Reade TM, Scriver CR, Rishikof E. Audiometric evidence for two forms of X-linked hypophosphatemia in humans, apparent counterpoints of Hyp and Gy mutations in mouse. *Am J Med Genet.* 1987;27:997-1003.

53. Kainer G, Spence JE, Chan JCM. X-linked hypophosphatemia: progress in characterization of genetic and metabolic defects. *Nephron.* 1989;51:449-453.

Studies in Fetal Malnutrition

Warren M. Crosby, MD

• Fetal malnutrition, a worldwide problem, is accompanied by varying degrees of lifelong morbidity for the child. Only 25% of fetal malnutrition is accomplished by maternal risk factors known to cause intrauterine growth retardation (ie, chronic hypertension, advanced diabetes mellitus, or severe preeclampsia). If the malnourished fetus could be detected early in pregnancy, nutritional intervention might be successful in improving fetal growth rate and in avoiding the morbidity due to malnutrition. This communication reviews the almost 40 years of studies by Jack Metcoff, MD, and coworkers to unravel the causes of fetal malnutrition and their efforts to prevent it.

(*AJDC.* 1991;145:871-876)

Fetal malnutrition, a term coined by Usher, can be found in every country and culture and at every socioeconomic level.[1] The effect of nutritional deprivation in utero is to decrease the child's potential for a normal productive life after birth. Specifically, increased perinatal morbidity,[2] poor postnatal growth,[3] reduced numbers of brain cells,[4] altered myelin,[5] neurologic difficulties,[6] and impaired learning ability[7,8] have each been shown to be associated with fetal malnutrition. Fetal malnutrition can be identified in 2% to 3% of newborns in the United States and has been estimated to be as frequent as 8% to 10% in developing countries.[9] Fetal malnutrition is not simply dependent on maternal malnutrition, although the latter plays a role. Other maternal diseases besides malnutrition are known to be associated with undergrown newborns. That maternal hypertension, chronic and the acute form of preeclampsia-eclampsia, and advanced diabetes mellitus regularly produce small-for-date babies, implies that the vascular component of these diseases can reduce uteroplacental blood flow sufficiently to restrict the normal flow of nutrients to the fetus. However, only about 25% to 30% of undergrown newborns occur in mothers with such diseases.[10] It is clear that fetal malnutrition is a complex disease, and one with many causes. Fetal malnutrition that occurs in an apparently uncomplicated pregnancy in an apparently healthy mother with a diet consistent with her peers whose babies are not malnourished cries out for an explanation and prevention.

See also pp 853, 860, 865, and 877.

During World War II, Jack Metcoff, MD, was trained in nutrition at the Harvard School of Public Health, Boston, Mass. Following completion of this training he was assigned to the United Nations Relief and Rehabilitation Administration as a public health service officer. He spent a year in Italy surveying the nutritional status of high-risk groups in anticipation of the initiation of the Marshall Plan. After this assignment he returned to Boston. Both in Italy and in Mexico City's Hospital Infantile, Metcoff studied children with severe malnutrition and found that simply refeeding and rehydrating severely malnourished children did not always prevent their death. Indeed, one of the early publications[11] reported that eight of 13 children hospitalized with severe protein energy malnutrition in the study died of their disease. One of the first to study intracellular changes in this condition, Metcoff found in the muscle cells of these starved children differences from those obtained from normal children. It had been shown previously by Metcoff and others[11] that muscle cells obtained by small percutaneous needle biopsies from children with kwashiorkor contained more water and sodium content with depleted concentrations of sodium, potassium, and magnesium. Because these differences widen just prior to death, it was believed that rapid decline in intracellular energy production would account for the findings. Investigation of intracellular energy production offered promise of finding a way to prevent death if the intracellular processes could be reversed. The first report using newer microanalytic methods that allowed simultaneous analysis of more components of cellular energy metabolism was published in *Medicine* in 1966,[11] and reported successful measurement of pyruvate kinase, lactate, malic, and isocitric dehydrogenase enzymes and concentrations of sodium, potassium, chloride, phosphoenol pyruvate, pyruvate, alphaketoglutarate, and oxaloacetate. As expected, muscle cells from these 13 starving children contained increased water and sodium, with significant reduction in the concentration of potassium, phosphoenol pyruvate, and oxaloacetate. The activities of each of these intracellular enzymes, except lactate dehydrogenase, were substantially lower in the starving children as compared with normal controls. Kinetic studies of pyruvate kinase were carried out in three children, all of whom showed that the enzyme was both quantitatively and qualitatively deficient in starving children.

Accepted for publication December 26, 1990.
From the Department of Obstetrics and Gynecology, The University of Oklahoma College of Medicine, Oklahoma City.
Reprints not available.

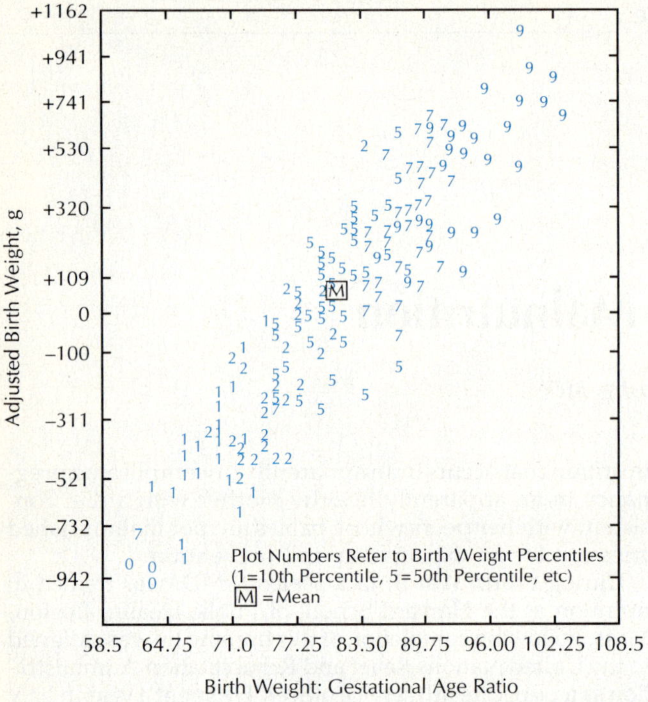

Fig 1.—*The relationship between the adjusted birth weight, birth weight–gestational age ratio, and actual birth weight percentiles (Lubchenko[2]). The clear linearity shows an excellent correlation between all three criteria for appropriate size at birth and confirms the concept that fetal growth is a continuum with malnourished babies on one end and overgrown babies at the other.*

Table 1.—Differences Between Smokers and Nonsmokers

Variable	No.	Mean smokers	No.	Mean nonsmoker	P
Adjusted birth weight	59	−94	99	+56	<.05
Adjusted baby length	59	−0.57	99	+0.34	<.05
Maternal height	77	163	129	160	<.01
Pyruvate kinase	47	11,197	70	12,414	<.05
RNA synthesis	43	18	67	23	<.01
Total carotene	42	96	67	115	<.01
Amino acids					
Aspartic acid*†	13	42	39	57	<.01
Threonine*‡	13	166	39	211	<.001
Serine*	13	139	39	173	<.01
Proline	12	176	39	247	<.01
Alanine	12	310	39	388	<.01
Valine‡	12	149	39	190	<.001
Isoleucine‡	13	60	38	77	<.001
Leucine*‡	13	105	38	138	<.001
Tyrosine*‡	13	58	38	69	<.01
Phenylalanine*†‡	13	64	38	80	<.001
Lysine*†‡	13	143	38	191	<.001
Histidine*†‡	13	90	39	102	<.05
Arginine*†	13	132	39	164	<.01
Ornithine*	12	34	39	43	<.001

*Correlated with adjusted birth weight (entire group).
†Correlated with adjusted birth weight of nonsmokers.
‡Essential amino acid.

Performing muscle biopsies or liver biopsies on dying children is an onerous task and also may have been harmful. The next year, Metcoff et al[12] reported that leukocytes obtained by simple venipuncture in starving children had alterations in energy metabolism similar to muscle cells obtained by biopsy. While muscle cells account for the largest part of the body's production and consumption of energy, it appeared that leukocytes could serve as biochemical surrogates for muscle cells in studies of protein energy malnutrition.[13] Leukocytes from 16 severely and four moderately malnourished children were studied and compared with leukocytes from normal controls. Substantial decreases in the cellular content of oxaloacetate, pyruvate, and lactate were found. However, in the moderately malnourished children, only minor changes were seen, suggesting that alterations in cellular energy metabolism can be detected only in leukocytes from severely malnourished children. Adenosine diphosphate levels in the leukocytes from the most severely malnourished children were markedly decreased, while the decrease in adenosine triphosphate and adenosine monophosphate concentrations was not significant. It was believed that the data indicated that severe protein energy malnutrition produces significant alteration in cellular energy production characterized by inhibition of the terminal step in glycolysis: the production of adenosine triphosphate by the enzyme pyruvate kinase.[13]

Krebs and Eggleston[14] had shown that starvation decreases the activity of pyruvate kinase in the liver and refeeding with carbohydrates induces biosynthesis of the enzyme. Severely malnourished children composed a substantial part of infant mortality in Mexico City. It became apparent that small-for-date babies born in that city frequently displayed many of the clinical and biochemical characteristics of malnutrition previously identified in starving children. In addition, analysis of leukocytes from these newborns showed intracellular changes in energy metabolism that were comparable to those changes seen in older children with malnutrition. Studies of leukocytes from the fetus obtained from cord blood samples at birth and compared with studies of the mother's leukocytes drawn at the same time showed changes in energy metabolism of the leukocytes in the mother that were similar to those found in the malnourished fetus. Comparing mothers' leukocyte energy metabolism with the leukocyte energy metabolism of their neighbors who had recently given birth to normal-sized children showed that the mothers of malnourished newborns were different from the mothers of normal children despite the fact that the mothers generally lived in the same area and ate similar diets. Thus, in an overview of malnutrition published in the *Annual Review of Medicine*, Metcoff[9] stated "in all probability the maternal environment is more important to fetal growth than genetic factors." These findings—altered cellular energy metabolism in children with severe protein energy malnutrition; that these alterations were found in leukocytes and muscle and liver cells obtained from these children; and similar alteration of energy metabolism in leukocytes from small-for-date newborns and their mothers—raised the possibility that analysis of maternal leukocyte energy metabolism might permit antepartum diagnosis of fetal malnutrition.

This concept was pursued in Mexico City, where a study was carried out to see if it were possible to identify those

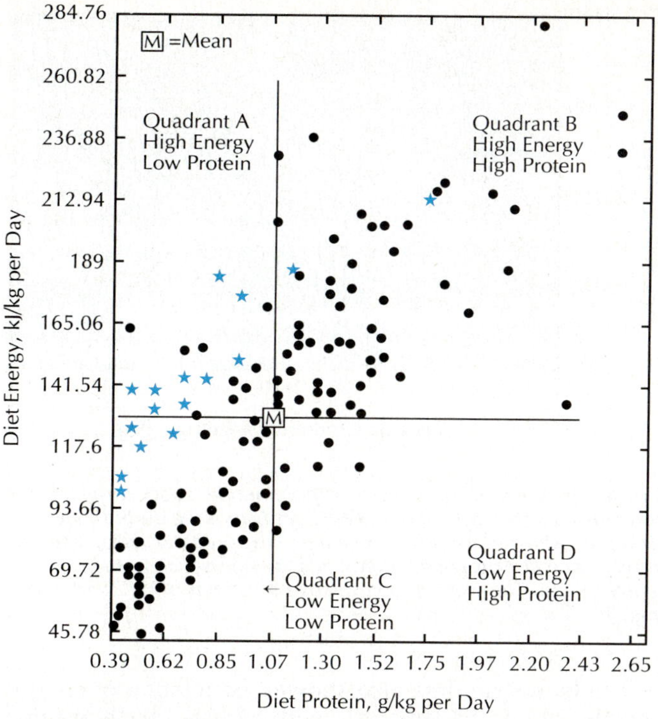

Fig 2.—*The relationship between maternal intake of protein and energy at midpregnancy and the adjusted birth weight. The general linear relationship shows a strong correlation between maternal intake and adjusted birth weight. Dot indicates mothers of babies whose adjusted birth weights were normal; star, those mothers whose babies had adjusted birth weights that were below 1 SD. Nine of the 15 undergrown babies were in the low energy–low protein quadrant.*[15]

mothers who were to have malnourished fetuses and identify them early in pregnancy so that a nutritional intervention might prevent the fetal malnutrition.[12] This study suggested that the normal metabolic activity of leukocytes is altered somewhat in late pregnancy, prior to labor, in mothers carrying malnourished fetuses.[12] Similar alteration was reported for leukocyte RNA synthesis. It was suggested that whatever factor[s] was responsible for this alteration of maternal leukocytes also altered the energy metabolism of fetal cells. Thus, this pilot study confirmed that study of the mother's leukocytes in midpregnancy identified fetuses with a high likelihood of protein energy malnutrition; with in utero diagnosis, it should be possible to provide nutritional intervention for the mother in an attempt to decrease malnutrition in her fetus.

This concept was pursued by a controlled prospective study of the relationship between a large number of maternal factors and fetal malnutrition. This study also introduced the concept of "adjusted birth weight" to allow for more definitive identification of the malnourished fetus. This concept depends on adjusting the actual birth weight of the fetus to those demographic factors of the parents that are known to affect birth weight.

Reported were the cases of 182 patients from the University of Oklahoma (Oklahoma City) prenatal clinics whose length of gestation clinically matched their ultrasound measurements, and who had otherwise normal pregnancies that resulted in deliveries between 35 and 43 weeks of gestation.[15] The length of pregnancy was corroborated by a Dubowitz score following birth. To account for the genetic variability in birth weight adjustments for

Table 2.—Multiple Regression (Dependent Variable: Adjusted Birth Weight)*

Independent Variable
Total carotenes
Family income
Maternal weight at 24 wk
Leukocyte adenosine diphosphate
α_1 globulin
Leukocyte phosphofructokinase
Cigarette smoking (−)
Leukocyte protein: DNA ratio (cell size)
Leukocyte RNA synthesis

*$R=.4982$: $P<.05$. Thirty independent variables were analyzed (amino acid concentration not included). All Correlations were positive except maternal smoking.

maternal age, race, parity, height, prepregnancy weight, and weight gain during pregnancy as well as the week of gestation of birth and the sex of the babies were combined to produce an adjusted birth weight that was calculated for each newborn. Each adjustment was made according to previously reported influences of these factors on birth size adjusted by multiple regression analysis of those factors in the study mothers. The adjusted birth weight, thus, was what a given sex baby in a given mother at a particular week of gestation *should* weigh. This was compared with what the newborn actually did weigh and its actual sex and birth week.

The formula used for calculation of adjusted birth weight is as follows:

$$\begin{aligned}&\text{Adjusted Birth Weight} = 1491.9 + 126.1 \times \\ &\text{Gestational Age in Weeks} - 101.5 \times \\ &\text{Sex (Males} = 1\text{, Females} = 0) - 150.3 \times \\ &\text{Week of Gestation at Entry} - 130.3 \times \\ &\text{Race (White} = 0\text{, Nonwhite} = 1) + \\ &72.0 \times \text{Height (cm)} + 98.0 \times \\ &\text{Weight at Entry (kg)} + 87.1 \times \\ &\text{Nonpregnant Weight (kg)} - 108.3 \times \\ &\text{Smoking (No Smoking} = \\ &0\text{, Up to 10 Cigarettes/d} = \\ &1\text{, 11 to 20 Cigarettes/d} = \\ &2\text{, 21 to 30 Cigarettes/d} = 3, \\ &\text{and} \geq 31 \text{ Cigarettes/d} = 4) + 119.5 \times \\ &\text{Fundal Height at Entry (cm)} + 43.5 \times \\ &\text{Parity Including This Pregnancy (No.)}\end{aligned}$$

The differences between the adjusted birth weight and the actual one thus reflected the degree of overgrowth or undergrowth of the baby. It became clear that there is a continuum of appropriate fetal growth from very small to very large. For statistical purposes, the study defined a fetus whose adjusted birth weight was 1 SD below the mean as having fetal malnutrition, while those that weighed more than 1 SD above the mean were termed "macrosomic." A small-for-gestational-age baby, one that was termed as having fetal malnutrition, could thus be defined with more precision than previously. Figure 1 shows there is a linear relationship between three different criteria of appropriate fetal size at birth.

This study[15] introduced the important concept of the adjusted birth weight and showed that it correlated with biochemical factors measured in maternal leukocytes.

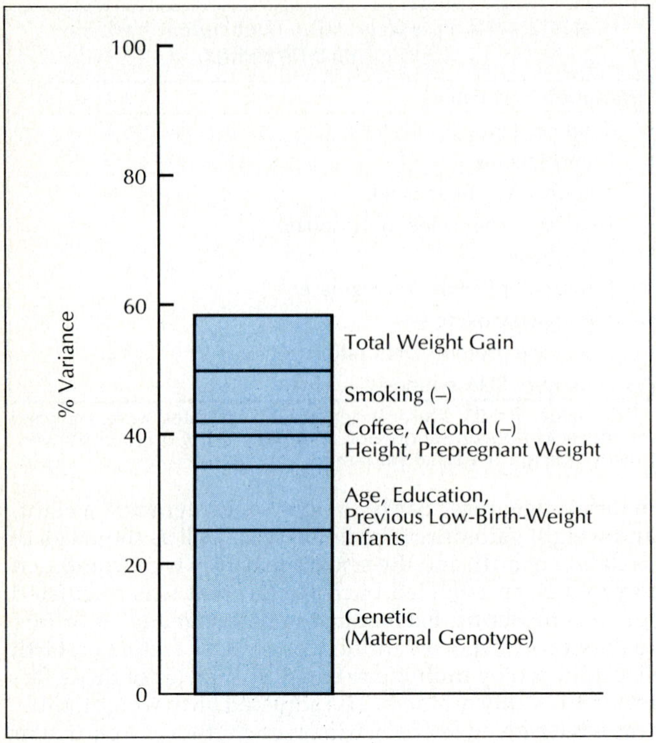

Fig 3.—*Percent variance in birth weight due to various characteristics by multiple regression analysis*

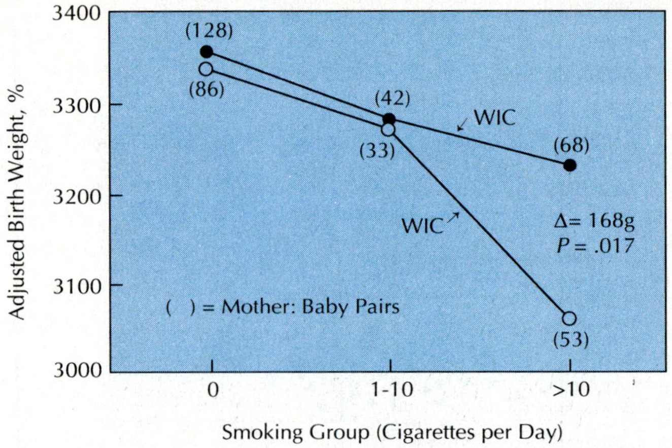

Fig 4.—*Interaction of special supplemental food program for women, infants, and children (WIC) and smoking on birth weight. This was adjusted for gestational age, sex, prenatal visits, race, interval since last pregnancy, previous low-birth-weight babies, and entry weight. The graph shows the overall effects of WIC and smoking.*

From this study, the largest contributor to fetal size at birth was length of gestation. Smoking had a clear negative effect on adjusted birth weight. So much so in fact, that to study the relationship of the many factors measured in the plasma and leukocytes and comparing them with adjusted birth weight, the initial study group was divided into smokers and nonsmokers. The relationship between the two is shown in Table 1.

The plasma constituent measured at midpregnancy that most highly correlated with fetal malnutrition was carotene. This finding was entirely unexpected. The maternal serum carotene level was negatively correlated with maternal smoking, but the correlation with fetal malnutrition was even greater in nonsmoking mothers. Similarly, plasma zinc level was also correlated directly with adjusted birth weight. Maternal serum concentration of amino acids, like carotene and zinc, was found to correlate with fetal growth. Ten amino acid levels in maternal serum had a statistically significant correlation with adjusted birth weight.[15]

The data in this study were analyzed by linear and by multiple regression techniques. Linear regression identified the rank order of factors that make up the contributions to adjusted birth weight. Figure 2 shows the relationship between maternal protein and energy intake and the adjusted birth weight of the baby.

Multiple regression analysis identified the effect of several variables on a single variable. In this analysis, nine variables contributed at the .05 level to adjusted birth weight. Table 2 shows this relationship. Beta-carotene and smoking headed the list, followed by family income. While some of these correlations had been observed by others, the mechanism by which an individual factor influences fetal growth is entirely unknown.

The leukocyte data also showed correlation of energy metabolism of the leukocyte with adjusted birth weight. The adenosine diphosphate generation, phosphofructokinase activity, RNA synthesis, and cell size each correlated with adjusted birth weight at a .05 level of significance.[15]

It is clear from this study that many things that control leukocyte metabolism also relate to the growth of the fetus. This study identified those factors that can be measured in maternal blood in midpregnancy that correlate significantly with the presence of a malnourished fetus at birth.

Further studies by McClain et al[16] continued to demonstrate positive correlations between serum amino acid levels in midpregnancy and the baby's size at birth. They showed that the concentration of total free amino acids in plasma from mothers carrying malnourished fetuses was significantly lower than from mothers having normal-sized fetuses at birth. Abnormally low levels of aspartic acid, serine, alanine, tyrosine, ornithine, and arginine correlated with fetal malnutrition. The branched chain amino acids, isoleucine and valine, were at normal levels in mothers with malnourished fetuses.[16]

From the enormous complexity indicated by the relationship of this multitude of serum and intracellular metabolic components with fetal growth, the concept of nutritional interrelationships interfering with normal fetal growth began to emerge. In a lecture to the symposium on The Year of the Child in Ontario, Canada, in 1979, Metcoff[17] reported that the various maternal supplemental feeding experiments that had been performed in developing countries had a small influence on average birth weight. An increase of 60 to 80 g was seen to be hardly worth the effort. But Metcoff pointed out in these studies that every mother in the experimental group was given supplemental nourishment. Because most of the fetuses in that group of women were not malnourished in the first place, the supplement would be expected to have little effect on them. The weight gain for malnourished fetuses produced by maternal feeding is thus diluted by the weight of the normal fetuses for which maternal feeding was not necessary. Mothers of most malnourished fetuses are not malnourished themselves; supplementation of diet in an across-the-board study might be predicted to have little detectable effect on the mean birth weight for the entire group. Nutritional imbalances are probably as important as a simple deficiency, and simple deficiencies in maternal diets, except in rare instances, are not found in developed countries.

The concept that complex interrelationships between various nutrients that affect fetal growth was tested in a study using inbred rats in 1981.[18] In this study, three groups of pregnant rats were fed similar diets containing narrowly similar amounts of protein and energy. The two experimental groups were provided diets containing excess disposable amino acids with adequate net protein and energy intakes. One of the two experimental groups differed by having threonine limited from the otherwise normal protein and energy diet. Fetal growth retardation occurred in both of the experimental groups and was greatest in the threonine-restricted group. The conclusion of the study was that a relative excess of small neutral amino acids which, along with the larger neutral amino acids, competes with threonine for transport into cells. When there is adequate threonine concentration in the serum, the excess of small neutral amino acids limits entry of threonine into cells. By further limiting intake of threonine, an essential amino acid, the effect is augmented and fetal growth retardation becomes worse. Furthermore, this study was designed to test the concept that maternal catabolism would be able to correct the imbalance by the provision of the diminished amino acid supplies from the mother's protein stores. This did not occur and, at least in this instance, it appears that maternal protein catabolism cannot make up the difference when imbalance rather than a deficiency occurs in her diet.

In a later article, Metcoff et al[19] state "maternal genetic factors account for about 25% of variance in birth weight" and "the fathers genetic contribution to the variance is only about 1 to 2%." As shown in Fig 3, the proportions of variance in birth weight accounted for by some maternal characteristics and environmental factors are as follows: maternal age, education, and previous delivery of low-birth-weight infant account for 8% of the variance; maternal height and prepregnant weight explain another 8%. Coffee and alcohol consumption have a negative influence on fetal growth and contribute about 2% of the variance. Cigarette smoking has a major deleterious influence and accounts for 3% to 6% of the variation and the effect is related to the number of cigarettes smoked per day.

Maternal weight gain from midpregnancy to term contributes about 3% of the variance, and total weight gain during pregnancy contributes another 3% to 6%. Metcoff goes on to say that this report shows that birth weight is related to maternal nutrition and can be predicted from a set of maternal characteristics and nutrition-related measurements obtained in midpregnancy.

During the 1970s and early 1980s, the registration of patients from the prenatal clinics at the University of Oklahoma Hospitals continued. The next study of these women was supported by the US Department of Agriculture and was based on the food supplementation program of that department (Special Supplemental Food Program for Women, Infants and Children [WIC]) and was designed to test the hypotheses that women destined to have malnourished newborns could be identified at midpregnancy with the prediction equation based on previous subjects drawn from the same population using both demographic and biochemical data.[20] This study enrolled patients based on predicted fetal malnutrition. (The prediction was based on those maternal demographic factors that had been correlated with fetal malnutrition in previous studies.) The demographic equation identified 226 women who were predicted to have either large or small babies of the 410 enrolled in the study. One third of all of the mothers' diets were unsupplemented and two thirds of the mothers were given standard WIC supplementations. The results of this study indicated that, aside from the week of gestation during which birth occurred, the strongest maternal effect on adjusted birth weight was smoking. Of interest, however, is that WIC supplementation ameliorated the negative effect of smoking on birth weight (Fig 4). The effect was dose dependent, ie, the greatest effect of smoking on unsupplemented mothers increased with the number of cigarettes smoked per day, but the difference could be seen only at a daily smoking level of more than 10 cigarettes per day.

Because of previous findings that carotene and, to a lesser extent, cholesterol, correlated with fetal malnutrition, the next study, again supported by the US Department of Agriculture, reported the relationships between midpregnancy maternal plasma levels of carotene and cholesterol in relationship to birth weight in smoking and nonsmoking mothers.[21] The outcome of these studies is curious, but it reflects the complex interaction of levels of plasma nutrients and fetal malnutrition. The heavy hand of cigarette smoking can also be seen. This study indicated that smoking not only reduced the birth weight of malnourished fetuses, but it also altered the relationship between carotene, cholesterol, and birth weight. Smoking continued to show a negative effect on fetal growth, and in nonsmokers there was a clear relationship between plasma cholesterol level and adjusted birth weight. The interactive effect of smoking, cholesterol, and carotene on birth weight was significant ($P = .017$) after adjusting for the demographic factors and gestational age.

From these studies and from the observations of others, our understanding of the relationship between maternal nutrition and fetal growth and development leaves a lot to be desired. The growth and reproductive functions of the billions of cells in the body and the biochemical interactions across cellular membranes are poorly understood because of the enormous complexity between the various molecules that are transported across cell membranes and what happens to them in the process of metabolism. This complexity is made considerably more difficult when one tries to study the process in the developing fetus because of the interposition of both maternal nutrition, the placenta, and changes in cellular metabolism of the fetus as it matures.

The contributions of Jack Metcoff to the understanding of the relationship between maternal nutrition and fetal growth and development during a 40-year period has enabled us to recognize the complexity and to identify those relationships that can be measured so that the likelihood for fetal malnutrition can be quantified by studying the mother in midpregnancy. Since we still do not understand the relationship between maternal nutrition and fetal development directly, nutritional intervention is still confined to "shotgun" approaches.

From this professional lifetime of study, several salient points are evident: (1) Fetal malnutrition resembles postnatal malnutrition and appears to have many of the same cellular changes. (2) Fetal malnutrition is a complex disorder and has many causes, including genetic, placental insufficiency caused by maternal vascular and other diseases, and, as Metcoff's studies have shown, by derangements and imbalances of various nutrients in the maternal biochemical milieu that are apparently entirely apart from known maternal diseases. (3) The concept of adjusted birth weight is an important tool to increase the precision by which we can identify malnutrition in the newborn.

The clinical observation of subjective factors such as wrinkled skin and apparent deficiency of subcutaneous fat is entirely too crude a variable on which to compare the outcome of nutritional interference. Similarly, actual birth weight is so much dependent on racial and demographic factors that raw birth weight itself is also too crude a measurement for appropriate use. Metcoff has shown that fetal nutrition, like normal growth and development, is a continuum from inadequate to excessive and that the inadequacies and excesses are not just simply related to the dietary intake of the mother. By using the adjusted birth weight, a calculation based on demographic factors that indicates what a given fetus in a given mother should weigh at a given week of gestation, the researcher acquires the opportunity to be more precise in studying the relationship of maternal nutrition to fetal growth.

The use of the leukocyte as a surrogate for the rapidly growing and developing cells of the fetus was also a major contribution to our ability to study fetal malnutrition. Metcoff's illustration of the relationships between maternal leukocyte biochemistry and fetal growth is important. However, there are differences between leukocytes and developing cells and perhaps these differences limited our capability for drawing direct inferences from the findings of leukocyte metabolism and that of the cells of the growing fetus.

Of most importance, perhaps, is Metcoff's demonstration of the enormous complexity of the system. His rat study pointed out that even with excess availability of amino acids in the maternal serum, fetal malnutrition still could occur when combinations of these amino acids interfered with the transfer mechanisms of other amino acids across cell membranes. Our understanding of individual mechanisms that only alter cellular metabolism, but do not kill the cell, is sparse. In most cases we do not know precisely what the effect of halving or doubling of the concentration of a molecule such as carotene will do to cellular growth and development, whether we are measuring that concentration in the maternal serum, the fetal serum, the fetal interstitial space, or within the fetal cells themselves. If we are ever to develop the capability of reversing fetal malnutrition prior to birth, we will need to better understand these complex interrelationships. Jack Metcoff has laid some of the groundwork for this process. By the use of Metcoff's concepts, we should be able to identify those fetuses at greatest risk for malnutrition and apply an appropriate nutritional intervention. Sooner or later this will become possible with precision. Those malnourished fetuses should, with prenatal treatment, be able to start independent life with a healthier set of organs and a better capability to become contributing rather than dependent citizens.

The following persons have played major roles in the series of studies of fetal malnutrition performed in Dr Metcoff's laboratories: Paul Costiloe, PhD; Harold Sandstead, MD; C. E. Bodwell, PhD; Joan Wikman-Coffelt, PhD; Alfonso Bernal, MD; Pablo Yoshida, MD; Silvestre Frank, MD; Luis Velasco, MD; A. Sosa; Gail Jacobson; Carolyn Johnson; Larry Bentle, PhD; Timothy Cole; Carmen de la Pena; Elizabeth Kaiser, PhD; Dutta Seshachalam, PhD; David Milne, PhD; Stephen Majors; Takashi Yoshida, MD; Adolfo Rosado, MD, PhD; Juan Urrusti, MD; Ricardo Madrazo, MD; Myriam Morales, MS; M. Mameesh; Philip McClain, PhD; James Gable; Frances Weaver, RD; Richard Luff; Ramon Torres Pinedo, MD; John Hansen, MD.

References

1. Metcoff J. Intrauterine detection of fetal malnutrition. In: Hake ESE, ed. *The Mammalian Fetus: Comparative Biology and Methodology*. Springfield, Ill: Charles C Thomas Publisher; 1975:213-235.

2. Lubchenko LO. *The High Risk Infant*. Philadelphia, Pa: WB Saunders Co; 1976.

3. Cruise MD. A longitudinal study of the growth of low birth weight infants. *Pediatrics*. 1973;51:260-268.

4. Rosso P, Winick M. The effect of severe malnutrition on weight, cholesterol, phospholipid and DNA content of the developing human brain. *Fed Proc*. 1970;29:495. Abstract 1414.

5. Chase HP. Alterations in human brain biochemistry following intrauterine growth retardation. *Pediatrics*. 1972;50:403.

6. Drillien CM. The small for date infant: etiology and prognosis. *Pediatr Clin North Am*. 1970;17:9-24.

7. Fitzhardinge PM, Steven EN. The small for date infant, II: neurological and intellectual sequelae. *Pediatrics*. 1972;50:50-57.

8. Fancourt R, Campbell S, Harvey D, Norman AP. Follow up study of small for dates babies. *BMJ*. 1976;1:1435-1437.

9. Metcoff J. Biochemical effects of protein-calorie malnutrition in man. *Annu Rev Med*. 1967;18:377-422.

10. Altshuler G, Russell P, Ermocilla R. The placental pathology of small-for-gestational age infants. *Am J Obstet Gynecol*. 1975;121:351-359.

11. Metcoff J, Frank S, Yoshida T, Torres-Pineda R, Kaiser E, Hansen JDL. Cell composition and metabolism in kwashiorkor (severe protein-calorie malnutrition in children). *Medicine*. 1966;45:365-390.

12. Metcoff J, Wikman-Coffelt, Yoshida T, et al. Energy metabolism and protein synthesis in human leukocytes during pregnancy and in placenta related to fetal growth. *Pediatrics*. 1973;51:866-877.

13. Yoshida T, Metcoff J, Frank S, de la Pena C. Intermediary metabolites and adenine nucleotides in leukocytes of children with protein calorie malnutrition. *Nature*. 1967;214:525-526.

14. Krebs HA, Eggleston LV. The role of pyruvate kinase in the regulation of gluconeogenesis. *Biochem J*. 1965;94:3C-4C.

15. Crosby WM, Metcoff J, Costiloe JP, et al. Fetal malnutrition: an appraisal of correlated factors. *Am J Obstet Gynecol*. 1977;128:22-31.

16. McClain PE, Metcoff J, Crosby WM, Costiloe JP. Relationship of maternal amino acid profiles at 25 weeks gestation to fetal growth. *Am J Clin Nutr*. 1978;31:401-407.

17. Metcoff J. Maternal nutrition and fetal development. *J Early Hum Dev*. 1980;4:99-120.

18. Metcoff J, Cole TJ, Luff R. Fetal growth retardation induced by dietary imbalance of threonine and dispensable amino acids with adequate energy and protein-equivalent intakes in pregnant rats. *J Nutr*. 1981;111:1411-1424.

19. Metcoff J, Costiloe JP, Crosby WM, et al. Maternal nutrition and fetal outcome. *Am J Clin Nutr*. 1981;34:708-721.

20. Metcoff J, Costiloe JP, Crosby WM, et al. Effect of food supplementation (WIC) during pregnancy on birth weight. *Am J Clin Nutr*. 1985;41:933-947.

21. Metcoff J, Costiloe JP, Crosby WM, Sandstead H, Milne D. Smoking in pregnancy: relation of birth weight to maternal plasma, carotene and cholesterol levels. *Obstet Gynecol*. 1989;74:302-309.

Partial Hypoparathyroidism

A Variant of Transient Congenital Hypoparathyroidism

Sang Whay Kooh, MD, FRCPC, Ann Binet, BSc, RN

• We encountered three children who had neonatal hypocalcemia followed by a period of normocalcemia and recurrence of hypocalcemia later in childhood. They were full-term infants with normal birth weights who developed hypocalcemia within the first 48 hours after birth. The hypocalcemia resolved in 1 week, 3 months, and 14 months in the three patients. The recurrences of hypocalcemia occurred at 4, 7, and 12 years of age. Their plasma parathyroid hormone concentrations were consistently low but detectable. We suggest that partial hypoparathyroidism is the underlying abnormality in these patients and that neonatal hypocalcemia in otherwise healthy infants indicates the need for calcium measurements during childhood and adolescence.

(*AJDC.* 1991;145:877-880)

Most cases of hypocalcemia during the neonatal period are transient.[1] It seldom signals the onset of a permanent disorder of calcium homeostasis, such as primary hypoparathyroidism. However, some children who develop symptomatic hypocalcemia during the neonatal period that requires treatment for weeks to months ultimately recover from hypocalcemia. The diagnosis of transient congenital hypoparathyroidism has been applied to this condition.[2,3] Bainbridge et al[4] questioned whether these patients truly recover from hypoparathyroidism and speculated that the patients who recover from the neonatal hypocalcemia have a compensated form of hypoparathyroidism. Herein, we describe three patients who had neonatal hypocalcemia followed by a period of normocalcemia and then a recurrence of hypocalcemia later during childhood.

See also pp 853, 860, 865, and 871.

METHODS

Plasma calcium, magnesium, and phosphate levels were measured with a Kodak Ektachem 400 analyzer (Eastman Kodak Co, Rochester, NY) from 1984 to 1988 and a Kodak Ektachem 700 analyzer since 1989. The ionized calcium level was analyzed with a Nova Stat Profile 4 (Nova Biochemical, Waltham, Mass). The reference ranges and conversion factors from millimoles per liter to milligrams per deciliter are shown in the Table. Plasma parathyroid hormone (PTH) was assayed until 1986 by radioimmunoassay with antisera directed toward the N- and C-terminals of the PTH molecule and from 1987 to the present by an immunoradiometric method with the intact PTH kit (ALLEGRO, Nichols Institute, Los Angeles, Calif). The normal reference range for the intact PTH assay was 10 to 65 ng/L, and the sensitivity of the assay was 1 ng/L. The reference range for the assays performed before 1987 was adjusted so that these values also ranged from 10 to 65 ng/L.

PATIENTS

PATIENT 1.—Patient 1 was born June 29, 1974. The biochemical findings and treatment of this female patient are presented in Fig 1. The patient was born at a local hospital at 38 weeks' gestation with a birth weight of 2930 g. She became irritable and developed tonic-clonic convulsions on the first day of life. Plasma chemistry levels were as follows: calcium, 1.43 mmol/L; magnesium, 0.86 mmol/L; and phosphate 1.95 mmol/L. Intravenous and oral calcium treatment improved the hypocalcemia, and the patient was sent home without medication at 1 week of age. The plasma calcium level at the time of discharge was 2.15 mmol/L. The plasma calcium and phosphate levels were normal in both parents. She was hospitalized again at 4 weeks of age for investigation of asymptomatic hypocalcemia and was subsequently transferred

Reference Ranges and Conversion Factors for Calcium, Magnesium, and Phosphate Level

Variable	Reference Value mmol/L	Conversion Factor	Value, mg/dL
Calcium	2.25-2.59	4.0	9.00-10.36
Magnesium			
Newborn	0.75-1.15	2.4	1.80-2.67
Children	0.70-0.94		1.68-2.28
Adults	0.65-1.00		1.56-2.40
Phosphate			
Birth-1 mo	1.62-3.10	3.1	5.02-9.61
1-4 mo	1.55-2.62		4.81-8.12
			4.03-6.82
4 mo-1 y	1.30-2.20		
1-4 y	1.16-2.10		3.60-6.51
4-8 y	1.16-1.81		3.60-5.61
9-14 y	1.07-1.71		3.32-5.30
15 y+	0.87-1.52		2.70-4.71

Accepted for publication April 21, 1991.
From the Department of Paediatrics, The Hospital for Sick Children, Toronto, Ontario.
Reprint requests to the Division of Endocrinology, The Hospital for Sick Children, 555 University Ave, Toronto, Ontario M5G 1X8 Canada (Dr Kooh).

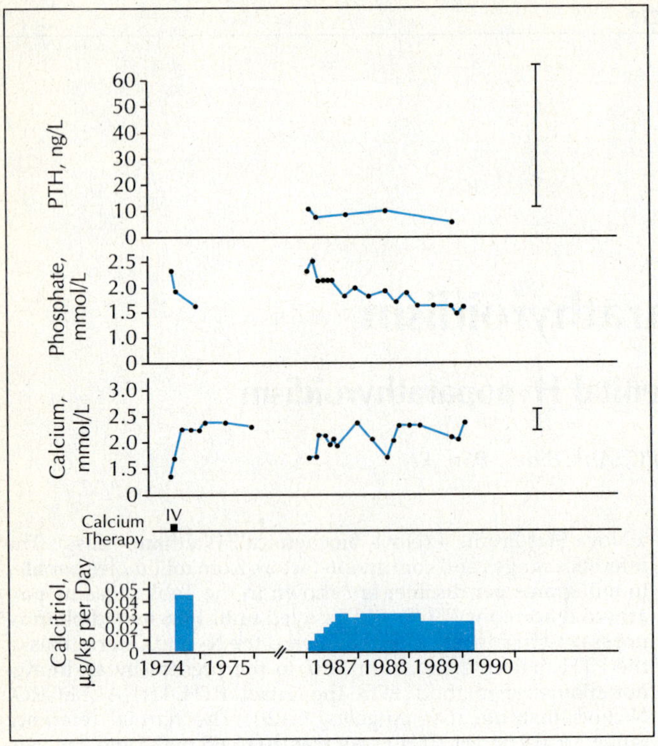

Fig 1.—*Case 1. Plasma parathyroid hormone (PTH), phosphate, and calcium concentrations and treatment. Vertical bars indicate normal reference range; IV, intravenous.*

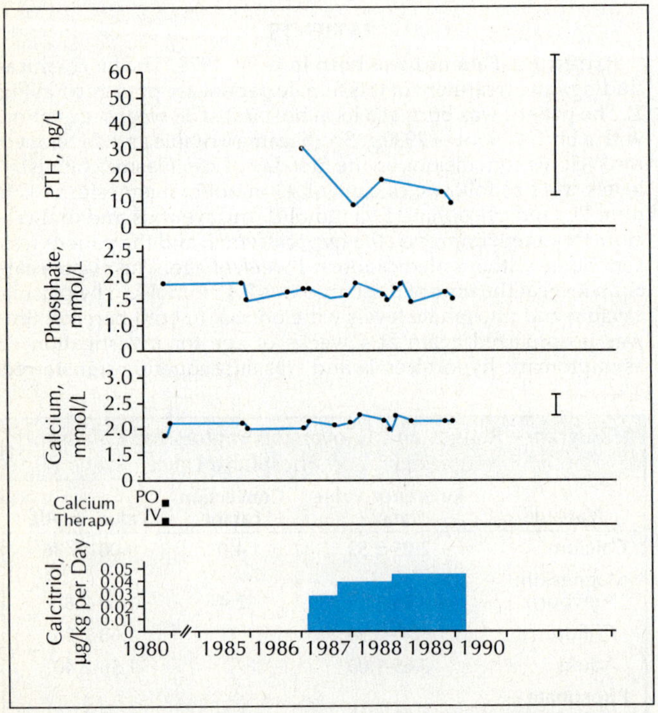

Fig 2.—*Case 2. Plasma parathyroid hormone (PTH), phosphate, and calcium concentrations and treatment. Vertical bars indicate normal reference range; PO, by mouth; and IV, intravenous.*

to our hospital on July 31, 1974. The plasma calcium level was 1.70 mmol/L, and the phosphate level was 2.80 mmol/L. She was treated with intravenous calcium and oral calcitriol (1,25-dihydroxyvitamin D_3), which was later changed to 1α-hydroxyvitamin D_3. Results of immunologic studies were normal. She was discharged from the hospital at 3 months of age

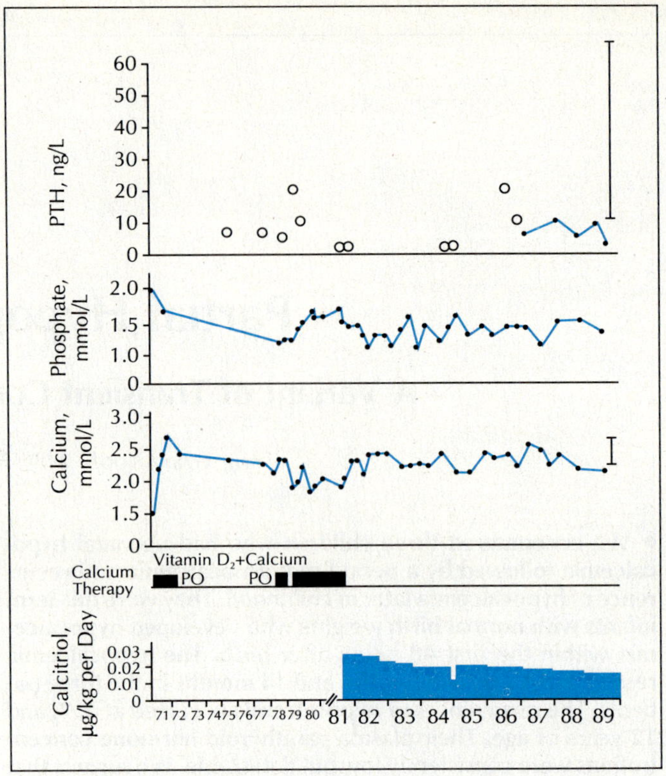

Fig 3.—*Case 3. Plasma parathyroid hormone (PTH), phosphate, and calcium concentrations and treatment. Open circles indicate PTH values before 1987, adjusted to represent their relative value equivalent to those determined by the present immunoradiometric assay (see "Methods" section); closed circles, PTH values determined with presently used radiometric method (see "Methods" section); and vertical bars, normal reference range; PO, by mouth; and IV, intravenous.*

when the plasma calcium levels could be maintained above 2.00 mmol/L. Shortly thereafter, 1α-hydroxyvitamin D_3 therapy was discontinued, with frequent monitoring of plasma calcium levels; plasma calcium levels were maintained above 2.25 mmol/L. At 18 months of age, the calcium level was 2.45 mmol/L and the phosphate level was 1.77 mmol/L.

Except for a generalized developmental delay, first noted at 7 months of age, the patient had no clinically important illnesses until she was 12 ½ years of age in 1986, at which time she began to experience difficulty bending her fingers and numbness of her hands and feet. Several months later, following a minor viral illness, she lost consciousness while watching television. On admission to a local hospital, she had a plasma calcium concentration of 1.35 mmol/L, an ionized calcium level of 0.69 mmol/L (reference range, 1.10 to 1.30 mmol/L), a phosphate level of 2.45 mmol/L, and a PTH level of 28 pmol/L (reference range, 29 to 85 pmol/L). The electroencephalogram was interpreted as showing "abnormalities consistent with a metabolic disorder."

During the last 3 years, she has received therapy with calcitriol, ranging from 0.02 to 0.03 µg/kg per day, and has maintained a plasma calcium concentration between 2.05 and 2.35 mmol/L, a phosphate level between 1.40 and 1.65 mmol/L, and a PTH level of 5 to 9 ng/L. She has had frequent minor viral illnesses but no bacterial infections. She attends a special class for the learning impaired. The renal responses to exogenous PTH were tested in 1990. Injection of human PTH (1-38, Bissendorf Peptide GmbH, Wedemark, Germany) raised the cyclic adenosine monophosphate excretion rates 55-fold and decreased the tubular reabsorption of phosphate from 93% to 67%.

Patient 2.—Patient 2 was born November 20, 1980. The biochemical findings and treatment of this female patient are shown in Fig 2. She was born after a normal pregnancy at a birth weight

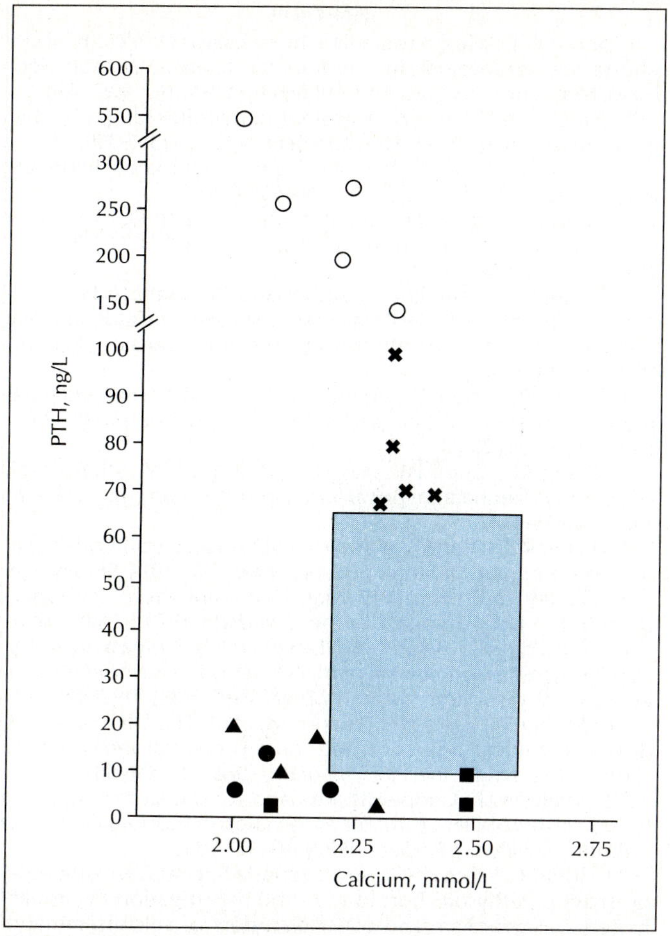

Fig 4.—*Plasma calcium and parathyroid hormone (PTH) concentrations of various parathyroid disorders. Solid circles indicate partial hypoparathyroidism; open circles, pseudohypoparathyroidism type I (A and B); X's, secondary hyperparathyroidism (X-linked hypophosphatemia treated with phosphate); solid squares, MEDAC (multiple endocrine deficiency, Addison's disease, and candidiasis); triangles, DiGeorge syndrome; and large shaded square area, normal calcium and PTH values.*

of 2860 g. On the second day of life, she was noted to be "dusky" around the mouth. A chest roentgenogram and an electrocardiogram were normal. The plasma calcium concentration was found to be 1.55 mmol/L, the magnesium level was 0.75 mmol/L, and the phosphate level was 2.42 mmol/L. The maternal plasma calcium, phosphate, and PTH concentrations were normal.

The hypocalcemia resolved after intravenous and oral calcium administration, skin color improved, and she was discharged from hospital at 7 days of age without medication. The plasma calcium and phosphate levels at the time of discharge were 2.25 and 2.42 mmol/L, respectively. Plasma calcium and phosphate concentrations at 4 months and 18 months of age were normal. She remained in good health, except for episodes of otitis media and skin allergy.

At 4 years of age, in 1985, she began to complain of cramps in her hands and feet. The plasma calcium level was 2.01 mmol/L, the ionized calcium level was 1.04 mmol/L, the phosphate level was 1.41 mmol/L, the magnesium level was 0.64 mmol/L, and the PTH level was 31 ng/L (reference range, 10 to 65 ng/L). Immunologic studies yielded normal results.

The patient has been treated with calcitriol since 1987. The plasma calcium levels have been borderline normal to mildly hypocalcemic. Plasma magnesium levels were also mildly low, at 0.53 to 0.64 mmol/L (reference range, 0.70 to 0.95 mmol/L), and the plasma PTH level was 7 to 17 ng/L.

Patient 3.—Patient 3 was born December 22, 1970. The biochemical findings and treatment of this female patient are shown in Fig 3. The patient, now 20 years of age, was born at 39 weeks' gestation by cesarean section due to irregular labor. Her birth weight was 3750 g. She had an Apgar score of 2 and required resuscitation and oxygen therapy. Her condition improved promptly. However, she suffered generalized convulsions on the second day of life. The plasma calcium level was 1.55 mmol/L, the magnesium level was 0.95 mmol/L, and the phosphate level was 2.01 mmol/L. No other cause of the seizure disorder was found, and no evidence of cardiac or immunologic abnormalities was found. She had a high-pitched, shrill cry that was later diagnosed as laryngomalacia. Repeated injections of parathyroid extracts increased the plasma calcium concentrations. Maternal plasma calcium and phosphate concentrations were normal. She was treated with 8400 U of vitamin D_2 and oral calcium supplementation.

At 12 months of age, the vitamin D_2 treatment was reduced, and it was stopped completely at age 14 months in 1972. The subsequent course, as shown in Fig 3, indicates that she remained normocalcemic until she was 7 years of age in 1977, when the plasma calcium started to fall below the normal value. Plasma PTH values were either at the lower end of normal or below the normal range. During a trial period of oral calcium supplementation, the plasma calcium level decreased further. Calcitriol therapy, which was started at 10 years of age, has been maintaining the plasma calcium level within the normal range. Plasma PTH concentrations continue to be below normal. In addition to hypoparathyroidism, she has adolescent exogenous obesity and residual hoarseness of the voice.

COMMENT

Substantial hypocalcemia during the early neonatal period is uncommon in full-term normal infants. Most patients with early neonatal hypocalcemia are premature, have birth asphyxia, or are born to diabetic mothers.[5-8] All of our patients were born at term with normal birth weights to nondiabetic mothers. Patient 3 had a history of neonatal distress, but her only outstanding problem was related to hypocalcemia.

The hypocalcemia resolved within a week in patient 2, and before 3 and 14 months of age in patients 1 and 3, respectively. These patients would have been diagnosed as having either neonatal hypocalcemia or transient congenital hypoparathyroidism had they not returned with a recurrence of hypocalcemia later in childhood.

It is not difficult to understand the cause of hypocalcemia during the neonatal period. The limited capacity of the parathyroid glands in these infants rendered them unable to respond adequately to decreases in plasma calcium concentration caused by the abrupt cessation of maternal supply of calcium and the accumulation of phosphate load from the endogenous source. It is more difficult, however, to understand what brought about the recurrence of hypocalcemia. Patient 1 had hypocalcemic convulsions following a minor respiratory illness. However, this patient had had symptoms suggestive of hypocalcemia for at least several months before the convulsions. The childhood hypocalcemia developed gradually over several years in patients 2 and 3. It appears that the parathyroid reserve was inadequate to meet the normal demands of childhood.

In all three patients, the PTH levels were either at the low end of or below the normal range, but they were consistently detectable by a sensitive assay. In patient 3 only, PTH levels were measured during the normocalcemic period; the levels were consistently low but were detectable. This patient, and most likely the other two patients, had permanent partial hypoparathyroidism regardless of their plasma calcium concentrations.

Among disorders of calcium homeostasis encountered

during the neonatal period, the DiGeorge syndrome most closely resembles congenital partial hypoparathyroidism as far as the parathyroid function is concerned. A number of reports indicate that the DiGeorge syndrome is heterogeneous and may be partial in immunologic, cardiac, and parathyroid abnormalities.[9-11] The PTH concentrations of the three patients with partial DiGeorge syndrome followed up in our clinic are within the range found in congenital partial hypoparathyroidism reported herein (Fig 4). Mallette et al[12] described four neonates who had transient congenital hypoparathyroidism with anomalies of the pulmonary valve. Our patients had no cardiac or immunologic abnormalities.

Some acquired forms of hypoparathyroidism may also be partial. For example, during the progression of MEDAC syndrome (multiple endocrine deficiency, Addison's disease, and candidiasis), the patient may have partial PTH deficiency (Fig 4). Similarly, in the course of iron storage disease in thalassemia, the patient may go through a phase of partial hypoparathyroidism before developing complete hypoparathyroidism. In these acquired conditions, however, the underlying disease is usually obvious, and the disease involves other organs in addition to the parathyroid gland. In all of these conditions, the degree of PTH deficiency will be better defined in the future, as sensitive assays for plasma PTH measurements become more readily available.[13,14] It is possible that the patients described herein are unusual examples of patients with transient congenital hypoparathyroidism. We rather believe, however, that partial hypoparathyroidism is a problem shared by all patients with transient congenital hypoparathyroidism, to a greater or lesser degree. There are lessons to be learned from our patients for physicians caring for newborns and children: (1) transient congenital hypoparathyroidism is not always transient, (2) neonatal hypocalcemia may signal permanent partial hypoparathyroidism, and (3) hypocalcemia in an otherwise normal neonate should be followed up with blood calcium measurements during childhood and adolescence.

References

1. Senterre J, Salle B. Problems in homeostasis of calcium, phosphorus and magnesium. In: Stern L, Vert P, eds. *Neonatal Medicine*. New York, NY: Masson Publishing USA Inc; 1987:836.
2. Fanconi A, Prader A. Transient congenital idiopathic hypoparathyroidism. *Helv Paediatr Acta*. 1967;22:342-359.
3. Rosenbloom AL. Transient congenital idiopathic hypoparathyroidism. *South Med J*. 1973;66:666-670.
4. Bainbridge R, Maghai Z, Mimouni F, Tsang RC. Transient congenital hypoparathyroidism: how transient is it? *J Pediatr*. 1987;111:866-868.
5. Tsang RC, Kleinman LI, Sutherland JM, Light IJ. Hypocalcemia in infants of diabetic mothers: studies in Ca, P, and Mg metabolism and in parathormone responsiveness. *J Pediatr*. 1972;80:384-395.
6. Tsang RC, Chen IW, Friedman MA, Chen I. Neonatal parathyroid function: role of gestational and post-natal age. *J Pediatr*. 1973;83:728-738.
7. Tsang RC, Chen IW, Hayes W, Atkinson W, Atherton H, Edwards N. Neonatal hypocalcemia in birth asphyxia. *J Pediatr*. 1974;84:428-433.
8. Tsang RC, Chen IW, Friedman MA, et al. Parathyroid function in infants of diabetic mothers. *J Pediatr*. 1974;86:399-404.
9. Conley ME, Beckwith JB, Mancer JF, Tenckhoff L. The spectrum of the DiGeorge syndrome. *J Pediatr*. 1979;94:883-890.
10. Gidding SS, Minciotti AL, Langman CB. Unmasking of hypoparathyroidism in familial partial DiGeorge syndrome by challenging with disodium edetate. *N Engl J Med*. 1988; 319:1589-1591.
11. Müller W, Peter HH, Wilken M, et al. The DiGeorge syndrome, I: clinical evaluation and course of partial and complete form of the syndrome. *Eur J Pediatr*. 1988;147:496-502.
12. Mallette LE, Cooper JB, Kirkland JL. Transient congenital hypoparathyroidism: possible association with anomalies of the pulmonary valve. *J Pediatr*. 1982;101:928-931.
13. Blind E, Schmidt-Gayle H, Scharla S, et al. Two-site assay of intact parathyroid hormone in the investigation of primary hyperparathyroidism and other disorders of calcium metabolism compared with a mid region assay. *J Clin Endocrinol Metab*. 1988;67:353-360.
14. Nussbaum SR, Zahradnik RJ, Lavigne JR, et al. Highly sensitive two-site immunoradiometric assay of parathyrin, and its clinical utility in evaluating patients with hypercalcemia. *Clin Chem*. 1987;33:1364-1367.

In Other AMA Journals

JAMA

Adolescent Medicine

I. F. Litt (*JAMA*. 1991;266:3100)

Allergy and Immunology

S. C. Bukantz, F. R. Lockey (*JAMA*. 1991;266:3102)

Ethics

E. D. Pellegrino (*JAMA*. 1991;266:3118)

Clinic-Based Intervention to Promote Literacy

A Pilot Study

Robert Needlman, MD; Lise E. Fried, MSPH; Debra S. Morley, MA; Sunday Taylor; Barry Zuckerman, MD

• **Educational research has shown that children become literate more easily if their parents read to them. A clinic-based program was designed to encourage early book use among parents of children at risk. It included (1) waiting room readers, (2) guidance about literacy development, and (3) provision of children's books at each visit. Seventy-nine parents of children aged 6 to 60 months were interviewed. Parents who had previously received a book were more likely to report looking at books with their children or that looking at books was a favorite activity (adjusted odds ratio, 4.05). This association was strongest among parents receiving Aid to Families With Dependent Children (odds ratio, 7.8). This preliminary study suggests that pediatricians can play a role in enriching children's early literacy environments, especially for children at high risk of school failure.**

(*AJDC.* 1991;145:881-884)

Reading failure disproportionately affects children from socially disadvantaged homes and contributes to the propagation of the cycle of poverty.[1] Pediatricians have a special opportunity to encourage behaviors that improve the child's chances to become literate. Parents come to the clinic regularly throughout their children's early years, and they expect to receive guidance that is important to the well-being of their children. Guidance from the pediatrician occurs within the context of a personal relationship and can be tailored to the individual child and family.

Current research on literacy acquisition assigns a critical role to the child's early literacy environment. Young children learn about the form and function of written language through daily exposure to print mediated by their parents or other adults. The quality of these early experiences affects the child's ability to profit from formal reading instruction once in school.[2] Thus, interventions that enhance the child's early exposure to literacy may increase the chances of reading success, even in the face of other risk factors associated with poverty.

While a variety of experiences contribute to the preschool child's emerging literacy, there is consensus among researchers that exposure to children's books is particularly important.[3-7] Children who are read to learn that printed words convey information they want to know. This realization motivates them to master reading, a task that, by nature, is repetitious and often frustrating.[8] Book sharing routines also familiarize children with the question-and-answer format prevalent in elementary schools, smoothing the transition from home-based to school-based learning.[9]

For infants and toddlers as well as preschool children, books provide a context for language and cognitive developments related to literacy acquisition and school success. Rhythmic speaking and holding enhance infant attention.[10] Parents are more responsive to their children's utterances while looking at books together than during free play or play with a toy.[11] With repeated "reading," increasingly complex language routines develop, from the simple labeling of objects to descriptions of events to the child's creation of fictions about his or her own experiences relating to the book.[12-14] As a group, children from underprivileged homes experience fewer of these important book-sharing interactions than do their more advantaged peers.[2,7] Because of the benefits of early book sharing and the special potential for parent education in the pediatric clinic, we implemented a program in the Pediatric Primary Care Clinic at Boston (Mass) City

Department Editors.—*Hugh D. Allen, MD, Columbus, Ohio; Fredric Burg, MD, Philadelphia, Pa; Harold Levine, MPA, Galveston, Tex; Barbara Starfield, MD, Baltimore, Md; Larrie W. Greenberg, MD, Washington, DC*
Purpose.—*This department is intended to share information concerning educational efforts in the broad field of pediatrics. We welcome studies on the following topics: undergraduate and graduate education in medicine and allied health occupations; continuing education of health professionals; education of patients and families; and health education for the general public, the community, and organizations that contribute to the promotion and improvement of the health of children.*
Editorial Comment.—*Promotion of literacy is an important national issue, but how can pediatricians be effective in this effort? Needlman et al present a clinic-based program that offers us suggestions that worked. See if you can apply this to your practice.*—H.D.A.

Accepted for publication January 14, 1991.

From the Division of Developmental and Behavioral Pediatrics, Department of Pediatrics, Boston (Mass) City Hospital and Boston University School of Medicine.

Read in part before the 31st Annual Meeting of the Ambulatory Pediatric Association, New Orleans, La, May 1, 1991.

Reprint requests to the Division of Developmental and Behavioral Pediatrics, Boston City Hospital, 818 Harrison Ave, Boston, MA 02118 (Dr Needlman).

Characteristic	% of Patients
Gender of child	
M	48
Childs age, mo	
6-12	41
>12-24	32
>24-60	28
Parents' country of origin	
United States	49
Haiti	17
Puerto Rico	10
Other	24
Parents' educational level (n=76)*	
0-8th grade	5
9-11th grade	20
High school graduate	40
Post-high school	36
Government support (n=77)*	
AFDC	39
No AFDC	61
Marital status (n=62)*	
Single	40

Table 1.—Sample Characteristics (n=79)

*Patient numbers are less than 79 due to missing data. AFDC indicates Aid to Families With Dependent Children.

Hospital to promote literacy development by encouraging parent-child book sharing.

The purpose of this pilot study was to assess parental response to the clinic-based literacy program. We hypothesized that exposure to the literacy program would be associated with increased book use by the parents and children.

SUBJECTS AND METHODS

Intervention

The clinic-based literacy program began in March 1989. The program included three components: (1) volunteers who read aloud to children in the waiting room, (2) counseling by the pediatrician about literacy development, and (3) book distribution. The program was designed so that a child would spend time with the reader in the waiting room and then move to the examination room where parent education about literacy development and a free book would be delivered together as part of anticipatory guidance.

Volunteers from the hospital and surrounding community underwent a 1-hour training session that focused on flexibility in approaching children of different ages and interests (eg, not always sticking to the printed text as well as encouraging participation) and supporting positive parental responses (eg, commenting on the child's level of interest). In practice, the content of the reading sessions varied depending on the particular reader, child, and level of activity in the waiting room.

Pediatricians, residents, and nurse-practitioners were trained via a combination of lectures on literacy development and workshops. The workshops focused on ways to support parents' appropriate desire to perceive their children as "smart" without encouraging undue pressure to "learn to read" too early. No set content for the anticipatory guidance was established, and in practice the counseling varied depending on the particular practitioner and family.

A selection of developmentally and ethnically appropriate books was obtained in sufficient quantity that every child from 6 months through 6 years of age could take home a free book after each visit. A stock of books was kept in the clinic for pediatricians to distribute to their patients.

Subjects

Between January and April 1990, parents bringing their children to the Boston City Hospital Pediatric Primary Care Center for routine care were recruited for the study. Parents present in the waiting room during the hours that the interviewer worked were asked to participate. Parents who were conversant in either English or Spanish and whose children were between the ages of 6 and 60 months were included in the study. Parents were excluded if the children were acutely ill or had not received routine care in the clinic within the past 6 months. Few parents who met the study criteria refused to participate; however, no record of refusals was kept.

Survey Design

The study employed a 15-minute structured interview administered by a research assistant who was not otherwise associated with the literacy program. Respondents consented to answer a series of questions about how their child "spends his/her time." They were not told at the outset that the focus of the questions was literacy, although this was made clear after information regarding the principal outcome had been elicited. The study was approved by the Boston City Hospital Human Investigations Committee.

After demographic data were obtained, parents were asked to provide a 24-hour "activity recall," modeled after a 24-hour diet recall, including everything they did with their child during that period. To increase the recall of details, the day was broken down into three periods: waking to lunch, lunch to dinner, and dinner to bedtime. If parents responded "We played," they were asked to describe what they actually did. Parents were then asked what their child's three favorite activities were, excluding eating and sleeping. These questions were presented in an open-ended format and at a point in the interview when no mention had yet been made of books or reading. Thus, the parents' responses were not likely to have been biased by any tendency to give answers they thought were desirable or expected. "Literacy orientation" was scored as positive if the parent mentioned looking at books or magazines with the child during the past 24 hours or included looking at books among the child's three favorite activities. This measure was designed to reflect parent-and-child behaviors believed to be particularly literacy-promoting and to be least subject to reporting bias.

After these open-ended questions, parents were asked specific questions regarding their use of books with their child and the number of books in the home. Parental reading habits and a history of having been read to during childhood were then assessed. As a way of gauging parental literacy, parents were asked to choose which one of three statements best described their reading ability: (1) "I can read anything easily." (2) "I can read enough to get by." (3) "Reading is difficult for me."

Finally, parents were asked to recall whether during previous visits they had seen the volunteer readers, had spoken with their pediatrician or nurse-practitioner about books or reading, or had been given a free book by their pediatrician or nurse practitioner. Parental report of exposure to each of these components of the literacy program constituted the independent variables for the study. As noted, the actual content of the waiting room reading experience and anticipatory guidance varied depending on the reader, pediatric provider, and family.

Analysis

Because the study was designed to evaluate an ongoing program, we were unable to assign subjects randomly to an intervention or nonintervention group. Instead, we compared parents who reported prior exposure to each of the components of the literacy program with those who denied such exposure. Characteristics of exposed and nonexposed parents were compared to determine whether they were similar. In form, this was a nested case-control design.

Literacy orientation, defined above, was the dependent variable used in both bivariate (unadjusted) and multivariate (adjusted) analyses. χ^2 Tests were used in the bivariate analyses. $P<.05$ was considered statistically significant. A logistic regression analysis (SAS computer program) was used to assess adjusted relationships for the dichotomous outcome. Odds ratios and 95% confidence intervals were calculated from these analyses.[15]

RESULTS

Seventy-nine parents participated in the study. Demographic characteristics of the sample appear in Table 1. Thirty-eight percent (30/79) reported having seen a volunteer reader in the waiting room during a previous visit;

Table 2.—Associations Between Exposure to Program Components and Reported Literacy Orientation

Program Component	% Reporting Literacy Orientation	
Saw waiting-room reader (n=78)*		
Yes	40	P=.9
No	42	
Guidance on literacy development (n=76)*		
Yes	43	P=.9
No	42	
Received book (n=77)*		
Yes	53	P=.06†
No	32	

*Patient numbers are less than 79 due to missing data.
†Odds ratio, 2.4; 95% confidence interval, 0.95 to 6.1.

Table 3.—Association Between Having Received a Book and Literacy Orientation: Stratification by Income (AFDC Status) (n=77)*

Variable	% Reporting Literacy Orientation	
Parents receiving AFDC (n=30)		
Received book		
Yes (n=14)	64	P=.011
No (n=16)	19	(odds ratio, 7.8)†
Parents not receiving AFDC (n=47)		
Received book		
Yes (n=22)	46	P=.7
No (n=25)	40	(odds ratio, 1.25)

*AFDC indicates AID to Families With Dependent Children.
†Confidence interval, 1.48 to 41.2.

27% (21/79) reported having talked with their pediatrician about literacy development; and 46% (36/79) had been given one or more books by their pediatrician. Although the program was designed to incorporate readers, anticipatory guidance, and books, only 6% (5/79) reported having been exposed to all three components of the program. Therefore, each component was considered separately. Parents exposed to the readers, anticipatory guidance, or books did not differ from unexposed parents in any of the following characteristics: child's gender, child's age, parent's country of origin, parent's educational level, government support, or marital status.

Bivariate analyses showed no statistically significant relationships between literacy orientation and exposure to any of the three components of the program, taken singly or in combination. Trends linking exposure to the readers or anticipatory guidance were not evident; therefore, these program components were omitted from subsequent analyses. There was, however, an association between literacy orientation and having been given a book at a previous visit that approached statistical significance (Table 2). Further exploration of this one component (books) was performed.

To assess the independent effect of having been given a book and to control for possible confounding variables, a logistic regression procedure was performed, which included the following: age of the child, parental ethnicity, parental educational level, parental reading habits, government support (whether receiving Aid to Families With Dependent Children [AFDC]), and whether the child had been given a book by their pediatrician. In this model, having been given a book was associated with literacy orientation ($\beta = 1.40$; odds ratio, 4.05; $P = .028$; 95% confidence interval, 1.12 to 14.6). This finding shows that parents who were given books were approximately four times more likely to report literacy orientation than parents who did not receive books, when other factors were controlled for. The fact that the odds ratio increased from 2.4 in the unadjusted analysis (Table 2) to 4.05 in the adjusted analysis indicates the effect of uncontrolled confounders in the unadjusted analysis.

Given the diversity of the sample, further analyses were performed to investigate whether receiving books had a positive effect for a specific subgroup of parents. Three factors were chosen as likely to influence parental response to the intervention: whether the family received AFDC (used as a proxy for income), parental education, and the child's age. Stratified analyses were performed for each of these variables.

Stratification by income revealed a strong effect (Table 3). Among parents receiving AFDC, 64% of those who had been given books reported literacy orientation compared with 19% of those who had not been given books ($P = .011$). Among parents not receiving AFDC, literacy orientation was not significantly different between parents who had or had not been given books (46% vs 40%, $P = .7$). Stratification by parent's education or child's age did not result in significant associations between literacy orientation and having been given a book.

COMMENT

The main finding of our study is that parents who had been given a children's book during a previous visit were approximately four times more likely to report positive literacy orientation, after controlling for confounding factors. This result supports the contention that a simple, inexpensive, clinic-based intervention can lead to positive changes in the home literacy environment, as reported by parents. Such changes may result in increased success in acquiring reading skills in early elementary school. It is encouraging that the benefits of the intervention were especially apparent among families at highest risk for reading failure, ie, those receiving AFDC.

Our findings are consistent with the single other published evaluation of a clinic-based literacy program. In Pittsburgh, the percentage of parents who reported daily reading with their child rose from 47% to 69% 6 months after having been given a packet of books and information by a volunteer in the clinic. However, details of sample selection and data collection were not reported.[16]

Several potential sources of error need to be considered in interpreting our findings. First, although the interviewer attempted to enroll all eligible parents, it is possible that parents less responsive to the intervention were missed with greater frequency. This bias would have led to overestimation of intervention effects.

Second, the study relied on parental self-reporting, raising the possibility that observed differences may have reflected parental perceptions or priorities rather than their actual behavior. The possibility of biases introduced because of systematic differences in reporting between groups of parents cannot be excluded. However, information for the principal dependent variable was obtained by spontaneous recall, without the parent knowing the specific purpose of the question.

Third, the fact that patients were not randomized increases the chance that observed associations resulted from confounding. Although several factors likely to be confounders were included in the logistic regression model, we cannot exclude confounding by unmeasured factors. For example, parents who were more highly motivated to provide literacy stimulation for their children might also have been more vocal in requesting books, which could explain the apparent association between taking home a book and literacy orientation; however, it cannot easily account for the large increase in literacy orientation associated with taking home a book among parents receiving AFDC compared with the negligible increase among parents not receiving AFDC.

Finally, small sample size may have resulted in type II errors in the stratified analyses. It is possible that with larger sample sizes, additional subgroups of parents who responded positively to the program would be identified.

While the present study suggests a positive effect of book distribution on the reported frequency of literacy orientation, similar effects were not found for the volunteer readers or the anticipatory guidance. Parents' ability to remember having seen a volunteer or having spoken about reading with their pediatrician may be more subject to recall bias than whether they were given a book to take home. Some parents may have been affected by the modeling or counseling but may have failed to report the exposures. Another explanation may be that modeling and anticipatory guidance influence the quality of the parent-child book interaction more than they do its quantity. Qualitative aspects of early literacy interactions have been shown to differ between social classes,[17] and such differences may be more important than the mere quantity of book use.

It may be that for the poorest children, the lack of books poses the greatest barrier to literacy-promoting experiences. By supplying books in those homes, we may have been not only communicating the importance of book sharing to parents but also providing them with the means to act on the information. Informal discussions with parents indicate that the books often provided a vehicle for the child to secure parental attention: "He's always bringing me a book to read for him." The fact that the books were given by the pediatrician or nurse practitioner was meaningful to some parents: "Every time I brought her to the clinic, the doctor gave us a book, so I figured he must want me to *do* something with them."

Future Research

Further work needs to be done to confirm these findings. Future evaluations of clinic-based literacy programs should include randomized, controlled trials employing standardized modeling and pediatric guidance, observation of the parent-child book interaction before and after the intervention, and testing of the child's verbal and written language skills. It will be necessary to follow a group of intervention and control children longitudinally to discover whether early pediatric intervention can indeed affect elementary school performance for children at risk. One published study suggested that preschoolers who are given books do indeed perform better in first grade.[7]

Implications

This preliminary study suggests that the pediatric primary care clinic can serve as an effective site for interventions to enrich children's early literacy development, particularly for those children at greatest risk for school failure. Pediatricians can develop such programs themselves or invite community literacy groups to provide the services and books in the clinic. Medical-educational collaborative programs are more likely to meet the needs of children than is either type of intervention alone. Specific support for literacy development may complement other efforts by pediatricians to combat the biologic and social risk factors for school failure.[18]

This work was supported in part by grant MCJ 009094 from the Bureau of Health Care Delivery and Assistance, Maternal and Child Health Branch. The Reach Out And Read program was supported by grants from The Old South Church Fund, Boston, Mass, The Polaroid Foundation, Cambridge, Mass, The Francis R. Dewing Foundation, Wellesley, Mass, and Ronald McDonald Children's Charities, Boston-Providence Chapter, Boston, Mass, The Boston Globe Foundation, Boston Mass, and Wordsworth Books, Cambridge, Mass.

We thank Howard Bauchner, MD, for his helpful comments and Kathleen Fitzgerald, MA, for codirecting the literacy program.

References

1. Anastasiou N, Hanes ML, Hanes M. *Language and Reading Strategies for Poverty Children*. Baltimore, Md: University Park Press; 1982.

2. Teale W, Sulzby E. Emergent literacy as a perspective for examining how young children become writers and readers. In: Teale W, Sulzby E, eds. *Emergent Literacy: Writing and Reading*. Norwood, NJ: Ablex Publishing Corp; 1986.

3. Anderson AB, Stokes SJ. Social and institutional influences and the development and practice of literacy. In: Goelman H, Oberg A, Smith F, eds. *Awakening to Literacy*. Exeter, NH: Heinemann; 1984:23.

4. Goldfield BA, Snow C. Reading books with children: the mechanics of parental influence on children's reading achievement. In: Flood J, ed. *Promoting Reading Comprehension*. Newark, Del: International Reading Association; 1984.

5. Hiebert EH. Issues related to home influences on young children's print-related development. In: Yaden DB, Templeton S, eds. *Metalinguistic Awareness and Beginning Literacy*. Portsmouth, NH: Heinemann Educational Books; 1986.

6. Durkin D. *Children Who Read Early: Two Longitudinal Studies*. New York, NY: Teachers College Press; 1966.

7. McCormick C, Mason J. Intervention procedures for increasing preschool children's interest in and knowledge about reading. In: Teale W, Sulzby E, eds. *Emergent Literacy: Writing and Reading*. Norwood, NJ: Ablex Publishing Corp; 1986:90-116.

8. Bettelheim B, Zelan K. *On Learning to Read*. New York, NY: Random House; 1982.

9. Heath SB. *Ways With Words: Language Life and Work in Communities and Classrooms*. Cambridge, Mass: Cambridge University Press; 1983.

10. Brown DR, Ottinger DR. *The Perceptual Basis of Developing Reading Skill: Final Report*. Washington, DC: Office of Education, Bureau of Research; 1970. US Department of Health, Education, and Welfare publication RMQ66004.

11. Lewis C, Gregory S. Parents' talk to their infants: the importance of context. *First Language*. 1987;7:201-216.

12. Ninio A, Bruner JS. The achievement and antecedents of labelling. *J Child Lang*. 1978;5:1-15.

13. Snow C, Ninio A. The contracts of literacy: what children learn from learning to read books. In: Teale W, Sulzby E, eds. *Emergent Literacy: Writing and Reading*. Norwood, NJ: Ablex Publishing Corp.; 1986:116-138.

14. Heath SB, Branscombe A. The book as narrative prop in language acquisition. In: Schieffelin B, Gilmore P, eds. *The Acquisition of Literacy: Ethnographic Perspectives*. Norwood, NJ: Ablex Publishing Corp.; 1986:16-34.

15. Kleinbaum DG, Kupper LL, Morgenstern H. *Epidemiologic Research*. New York, NY: Van Nostrand Reinhold; 1982.

16. Locke J. Pittsburgh's Beginning With Books Project. *School Library J*. February 1988:22-24.

17. Ninio A. Picture-book reading in mother-infant dyads belonging to two subgroups in Israel. *Child Dev*. 1980;51:587-590.

18. Parker S, Greer S, Zuckerman B. Double jeopardy: the impact of poverty on early child development. *Pediatr Clin North Am*. 1988;45:1227-1240

Immunization Response Varies With Intensity of Acute Lymphoblastic Leukemia Therapy

Derry Ridgway, MD; Lawrence J. Wolff, MD; Adamadia Deforest, PhD

• Twenty-four children receiving maintenance chemotherapy for acute lymphoblastic leukemia were given booster doses of tetanus-diphtheria combined toxoids. One month later, 19 of the 24 children were given *Haemophilus influenzae* B oligosaccharide–cross-reacting material conjugate vaccine. Following immunization, all patients had protective antibody titers against tetanus, 92% had protective antidiphtheria titers, and 84% had protective titers against *H influenzae*. Preimmunization titers, postimmunization titers, and response to immunization varied according to the intensity of therapy. There was no correlation with duration of therapy or quantitative hematologic values in the peripheral blood. These observations support the recommendation that children treated for acute lymphoblastic leukemia should be immunized against *H influenzae* B.

***(AJDC.* 1991;145:887-891)**

The role of immunization in the treatment of children receiving chemotherapy for malignant disease remains controversial. Concerns about the persistence of protection provided by previous immunizations and about the efficacy of immunization or reimmunization during chemotherapy make clinical decisions difficult. Few studies have examined antibody titer levels or the response to immunization in this population.[1-7] Most previously immunized children receiving anticancer chemotherapy have protective antibody titers against both tetanus and diphtheria, and most children respond with fourfold or greater increases after booster immunization. All studies report a few exceptions to these generalizations. Kung and coworkers[1] noted that for both diphtheria and tetanus, antibody levels and response to immunization were lower among children with leukemia than among children receiving chemotherapy for other forms of cancer.

Current approaches to therapy in children with acute lymphoblastic leukemia (ALL), the most common form of childhood cancer, use different intensities of therapy depending on prognostic characteristics.[8] While some children with favorable initial characteristics may be treated with low-intensity chemotherapy, others receive much more aggressive initial therapy, and then receive either continuous or periodic cyclic aggressive therapy. We sought to determine if the intensity and/or duration of therapy was related to the baseline antibody titer or to the response to immunization among children receiving therapy for leukemia. We compared the preimmunization and postimmunization titers against tetanus, diphtheria, and *Haemophilus influenzae* in a group of children receiving chemotherapy for ALL of the "standard" protocol, an "aggressive induction-consolidation with intensification and standard maintenance" protocol, and an "aggressive induction-consolidation with aggressive maintenance" protocol.

MATERIALS AND METHODS

Subjects

Twenty-four children (17 boys and seven girls) receiving maintenance chemotherapy for ALL were entered in the study after permission was obtained in accordance with the requirements of the Human Subjects Research Committee of the Oregon Health Sciences University, Portland. The patients ranged in age from 3 to 13 years (mean age, 7.3 years). Each patient had been immunized in infancy with four injections of diphtheria and tetanus toxoids. Eight patients had received an additional booster dose of both toxoids before school entry and two other patients had received an additional booster dose after the completion of an initial 2- or 3-year course of antileukemic chemotherapy. No patient had been immunized against *H influenzae* B or been treated for known or suspected invasive *Haemophilus* infection.

All subjects were in complete remission at the time of entry, with remission durations ranging from 6 to 35 months (mean remission, 16.2 months). Prognosis (ie, favorable, intermediate, or unfavorable) was determined using the standard criteria of age, white blood cell (WBC) count, morphologic cell features, and mass disease.[8] Seventeen patients were in first remission of their disease, three patients were in second remission after sustaining marrow relapses while not receiving therapy, one patient was in third remission after sustaining two marrow relapses while not receiving therapy, and two patients were in first continuous marrow remission after sustaining extramedullary relapses treated with local therapy and systemic reinduction.

Six patients were treated with standard therapy protocol (STD); 12 patients were treated with the Children's Cancer Study Group modification of the Berlin-Frankfurt-Munster protocol (BFM)[8]; and six patients were treated with the Children's Cancer Study Group modifications of the New York protocol or the very similar

Accepted for publication April 9, 1991.

From the Department of Pediatrics and the Doernbecher Memorial Hospital for Children of the Oregon Health Sciences University, Portland (Drs Ridgway and Wolff) and St Christopher's Hospital for Children, Philadelphia, Pa (Dr Deforest).

Reprints not available.

Table 1.—Treatment Protocols for Acute Lymphoblastic Leukemia

Stage	Protocol* STD	BFM	NY/L
Induction (weeks 1-4)	Vincristine, L-asparaginase, Intrathecal (IT) methotrexate, prednisone	Vincristine, daunorubicin, L-asparaginase, IT methotrexate, prednisone	Cyclophosphamide, daunorubicin, vincristine, IT methotrexate, prednisone
Consolidation (weeks 5-9)	Prednisone, 6-mercaptopurine, IT methotrexate	Prednisone, 6-mercaptopurine, IT methotrexate, cyclophosphamide, cytosine arabinoside (+/−cranial irradiation)	Prednisone, L-asparaginase, IT methotrexate, carmustine, cytosine arabinoside, cranial irradiation, 6-thioguanine
Maintenance (week 9 through year 2 or 3)	Vincristine, 6-mercaptopurine, IT methotrexate, prednisone methotrexate	Vincristine, 6-mercaptopurine, IT methotrexate, prednisone methotrexate	Vincristine, daunorubicin, IT methotrexate, cytosine arabinoside, 6-thioguanine, prednisone or hydroxyurea, cyclophosphamide, carmustine (+/−)
Reintensification (interrupts maintenance weeks 20-28, BFM only)	. . .	Vincristine, dexamethasone, 6-thioguanine, doxorubicin, cyclophosphamide, cytosine arabinoside, L-asparaginase	Methotrexate

*STD indicates standard therapy; BFM, Berlin-Frankfurt-Munster; NY/L, New York protocol or LSA2L2; plus sign, with; and minus sign, without.

LSA2L2 (NY/L) protocol[8] (Table 1). Nine of the patients in the BFM protocol also received cranial irradiation (18 to 24 Gy) during the second month of therapy or during a previous period of therapy, and two patients received spinal irradiation (12 Gy) as well.

Study Design

Immunization histories were recorded and the patients were immunized with diphtheria-tetanus vaccine (diphtheria and tetanus toxoids for pediatric use [DT] for children aged 5 years and younger or tetanus and diphtheria toxoids for adult use [Td] for older children [Connaught Laboratories, Swiftwater, Pa]) on the first day of the study. Twenty-eight days later, 19 subjects were immunized against *H influenzae* B by administration of *H influenzae* B oligosaccharide–cross-reacting material conjugate vaccine (HbOC). Four subjects did not receive the HbOC immunization for reasons unrelated to this study. Serum was obtained immediately before each immunization and 28 days after the HbOC injection, frozen, and stored at −70°C. A complete blood cell count was performed in the clinical laboratories of the Oregon Health Sciences University every time serum was drawn.

Antibody Measurement

Serum antibody titers to tetanus toxin were determined with passive hemagglutination as described by Deforest et al[9] and Hardegree et al.[10] Antibody titers against diphtheria toxin were determined by toxin neutralization in VERO cells as described by Deforest et al [9] and Miyamura et al.[11] Serum antibodies against capsular polysaccharide polyribosylribitol phosphate were determined with a Farr precipitation assay using radiolabeled antigen.[12,13]

Statistical Analysis

Comparisons of antibody titers among groups or between the prognostic group and titer level were made using the Kruskal-Wallis H test. Correlations among other values were examined with the Pearson *r* test.

RESULTS

Hematologic Values

The mean total WBC counts and absolute lymphocyte counts (ALCs) for patients receiving standard therapy were 4.4×10^9/L (range, 2.0 to 7.1×10^9/L) and 1.3×10^9/L (range, 0.1 to 2.5 $\times 10^9$/L), respectively. The corresponding values for patients receiving the BFM or NY/L protocols were lower, but the differences did not achieve statistical significance. The mean WBC count for patients receiving the BFM protocol was 3.3×10^9/L (range, 1.5 to 7.5×10^9/L), and the mean ALC was 0.5×10^9/L (range, 0.1 to 2.5×10^9/L). The mean WBC count for patients receiving the NY/L protocol was 4.4×10^9/L (range, 0.2 to 23.7×10^9/L), and the mean ALC was 0.7 (range, 0 to 2.6×10^9/L). The WBC and ALC levels were similar during the 3-month study period.

Tetanus Antibody Levels

The preimmunization and 28-day postimmunization tetanus antibody titers for the three patient groups are shown in Table 2. All patients had protective tetanus antibody titers (≥0.01 U/mL)[9,14] before immunization with DT or Td. Initial titers for children receiving the BFM protocol were lower than for children receiving STD therapy or the NY/L protocol ($P \leq .005$). Similarly, postimmunization titers were lower for patients in the BFM group ($P \leq .005$). Only seven of 12 patients in the BFM group had a fourfold or greater increase in antibody titers after immunization, in contrast to eight of nine assessable patients in the STD or NY/L groups.

No correlation existed between either the WBC count or ALC and initial titers, postimmunization titers, or antibody changes. Five children had ALC levels below

Table 2.—Response of Patients to Immunization*							
		Tetanus Antibody Titers (Protective Titers ≥0.01 U/mL)		Diphtheria Antibody Titers (Protective Titers ≥0.1 U/mL)		*Haemophilus influenzae* Antibody Titers (Protective Titers ≥1.0 mg/L)	
Patient No./ Age, y/ Prognosis/ Relapses†	Months Receiving Therapy	Pre-immunization	Post-immunization	Pre-immunization	Post-immunization	Pre-immunization	Post-immunization
STD							
1/ 4/ intermediate	10	5	20	2.8	11.2	0.31	8.04
2/ 3/ intermediate	12	5	20	0.7	1.4	0.23	2.25
3/ 6/ intermediate	22	1.25	20	0.7	11.2	. . .	. . .
4/ 5/ intermediate	12	5	10	1	2	0.13	24.32
5/ 4/ favorable	23	0.31	20	0.02	5.6	0.25	12.23
6/ 3/ favorable	12	0.31	10	0.09	1.4	0.1	4.77
Mean (age, 4.2 y)	15.2	2.8	16.6	0.88	5.46	0.194	10.3
BFM							
7/ 4/ intermediate	20	0.625	10	0.18	2.8	0.1	3.66
8/ 6/ intermediate	26	2.5	20	0.7	2.8	0.1	0.62
9/ 8/ favorable/ testicular relapse	11	0.31	0.16	0.09	0.06	. . .	. . .
11/ 6/ intermediate	13	2.5	5	2	2.8	0.1	0.1
12/ 4/ intermediate	13	0.31	0.625	0.125	0.125	0.1	0.1
13/ 10/ unfavorable	14	0.31	20	0.25	2.8	0.15	1.15
14/ 12/ intermediate/ two relapses	25	0.16	5	0.045	0.7	0.064	15.44
15/ 4/ unfavorable	25	0.16	2.5	0.015	0.25	0.1	20.02
16/ 13/ intermediate/ one relapse	19	1.25	20	0.35	22.4	0.1	60.66
23/ 6/ intermediate	14	0.16	5	0.0075	0.18	0.21	12.14
25/ 13/ intermediate/ central nervous system	31	5	5	1.4	1.4	. . .	. . .
26/ 12/ intermediate/ one relapse	35	0.31	0.625	0.01	0.01	10.63	10.16
Mean (age, 8.2 y)	20.5	1.18	7.82	0.43	3	1.14	12.4
NY/L							
17/ 7/ unfavorable	23	10	20	2.8	2.8	0.1	669.28
18/ 8/ unfavorable	19	20	20	1.4	22.4	1.28	64.93
19/ 10/ unfavorable	10	5	20	0.5	0.7	0.1	7.29
20/ 10/ intermediate/ one relapse	15	1.25	20	0.7	11.2	1.63	586
21/ 9/ unfavorable	21	20	20	0.7	0.7	. . .	. . .
22/ 8/ unfavorable	11	5	20	2.8	5.6	. . .	. . .
Mean (age, 8.7 y)	16.5	10.2	20	1.48	7.23	0.75	331.8

*The upper limits of laboratory determination for antibody titers were 20 U/mL for tetanus and 22.4 U/mL for diphtheria. Values at or exceeding these limits were averaged as the limit value. The lower limit of detection for diptheria was 0.0075 U/mL; for *Haemophilus influenzae* it was 0.1 mg/L. Values below these limits were averaged as one half the limit value.

†STD indicates standard therapy; BFM, Berlin-Frankfurt-Munster; and NY/L, New York protocol or LSA2L2.

0.2×10^9/L; four were receiving BFM therapy, two of whom had fourfold or greater titer rises, and two of whom did not respond. There was no correlation between the initial titers, postimmunization titers, or titer changes and age, prognosis, or the number of months receiving chemotherapy.

Diphtheria Antibody Titers

The preimmunization and 28-day postimmunization diphtheria antibody titers are shown in Table 2. Prior to immunization, 17 patients (seven of 12 patients in the BFM group, four of six patients in the STD group, and all six patients in the NY/L group) had protective diphtheria antibody titers (≥0.10 U/mL).[9,14] Three patients in the BFM group and the remaining two patients in the STD group had marginally protective titer levels (between 0.01 U/mL and 0.10 U/mL). Two patients in the BFM group had titers less than or equal to 0.01 U/mL. Patients receiving BFM therapy had lower initial titers than the other patients ($P \leq .02$). There were no significant differences in postimmunization antibody titers or in response to immunization among groups. There was no correlation between WBC count or ALC and initial or postimmunization antibody titers or response to diphtheria toxoid administration.

As with tetanus, two patients in the BFM group with an ALC of less than 0.2×10^9/L responded with fourfold or greater increases in antibody titers, and two had no response. The two diphtheria toxoid nonresponders were the same patients as the two tetanus toxoid nonresponders. There was no correlation between age, prognosis, or duration of chemotherapy and initial or postimmunization antibody titers or response to immunization. There was a positive correlation between changes in tetanus antibody titers and changes in diphtheria antibody titers following immunization, whether measured as absolute change in titers ($r = .588$; $P \leq .01$) or as a multiple of the initial titer level ($r = .426$; $P \leq .05$).

H influenzae B Antibody Titers

Preimmunization and 28-day postimmunization *H influenzae* antibody levels for the three groups are shown in Table 2. There were no statistically significant differences among groups for preimmunization or postimmunization antibody titers. As shown, six of the 10 patients in the BFM group and all patients in the STD and NY/L groups had protective titers after immunization.

There was no correlation between age, prognosis, WBC count, ALC, or duration of therapy and initial or postimmunization antibody titers or response to immunization. The response to HbOC immunization did not correlate with the response to DT or Td.

COMMENT

The 24 leukemic children examined in this study all had protective antibody levels against tetanus. The protective levels were presumably established during the initial series of infant immunizations and were preserved in many cases without the booster effect of a fifth immunization for as long as 10 years. This observation agrees with the reports by Nyerges et al,[3] who found protective titers in all 10 leukemic children receiving chemotherapy and in seven leukemic children after elective discontinuation of chemotherapy, and van der Does-van den Berg et al,[4] who observed protective titers in 48 of 49 leukemic children at the end of 2 to 3 years of chemotherapy. Twenty-two of the 24 children described in the present study had at least marginally protective titers against diphtheria, an observation similar to that of van der Does et al,[4] who observed protective titers in 48 of 49 leukemic children at the end of chemotherapy, and Kung et al,[1] who examined 12 leukemic children receiving chemotherapy and found seven with protective titers, four with marginal titers, and one with no detectable antibody. Only three of 20 children in this study developed anti–*H influenzae* antibody titers before immunization. Weisman et al[6] found that five of 21 leukemic patients receiving chemotherapy had anti–*H influenzae* antibody titers greater than or equal to 1.0 mg/L before immunization. With a lower standard for protection (150 mg/L), Feldman et al[2] reported that 12 of 34 leukemic children receiving chemotherapy had a protective level before immunization against *H influenzae*.

Following immunization, 100% of subjects had protective titers against tetanus, 92% had protective titers against diphtheria, and 84% had protective titers against *H influenzae*. Nineteen of 21 assessable patients responded to tetanus toxoid by at least a doubling of antibody titers, and 17 of 19 patients responded to HbOC with at least a doubling of measurable titers, but only 16 of 24 patients responded to diphtheria toxoid. In comparison, 25 (86%) of 29 previously described leukemic children (data combined from the reports of Nyerges et al[3] and Kung et al[1]) responded to tetanus toxoid booster, 60% of previously described leukemic children responded to immunization against *H influenzae*,[2,6,7] and 83% of previously described leukemic children responded to diphtheria booster immunization.[1] While increases in antibody titers in children with protective levels are of immunologic relevance, they have no known clinical significance. We were unable to observe a statistically significant correlation between total WBC count or ALC on the day of immunization and the response to immunization, although the two children who did not respond to either tetanus or diphtheria toxoid had an ALC of less than 0.2×10^9/L. In contrast to the report by Feldman et al,[2] we found no relationship between duration of therapy and antibody levels or response to immunization.

We hypothesized that differences in chemotherapy regimens might be reflected in differences in baseline antibody levels and in response to booster doses of DT vaccine or HbOC. We observed that patients treated with more aggressive induction and consolidation therapy, late intensification therapy, and then continuous standard-dose maintenance therapy (BFM) had lower baseline antibody titers for both diphtheria and tetanus and were less likely to respond to immunization with each of the three agents than patients receiving STD therapy. Patients treated with aggressive induction and consolidation followed by cyclic high-dose maintenance therapy (NY/L) had intermediate values.

Although the precise explanation for these differences remains unclear, it may be that aggressive induction therapies cause a more profound defect in the antibody-forming mechanisms of the immune system. Cyclic maintenance regimens may permit sufficient time for recovery, while the less intense but continuous maintenance regimens do not.

Thirteen of 16 unprotected leukemic children achieved titer levels greater than 1.0 mg/L 1 month after immunization with HbOC. This success rate is slightly higher than that previously reported.[2,6,7] The difference may be due to increased immunogenicity of HbOC in comparison with previous immunizing agents or to differences in chemotherapy protocols. Our patients were all older than 3 years, older than the patients in the study by Lange et al[7] but similar to the populations described by Feldman et al[2] and Weisman et al.[6] We failed, as did Lange et al,[7] to confirm the observation by Feldman et al[2] that longer durations of chemotherapy correlated with lower baseline titers or with poorer response to immunization. Although the number of subjects in this study was small, the results suggest that patients receiving the BFM protocol respond less well than other leukemic children to HbOC immunization.

Several clinically relevant conclusions can be drawn from these results. The presumption that previously immunized leukemic children receiving chemotherapy have antibody protection against both tetanus and diphtheria is supported. This appears to be true even for children who completed only part of their initial immunization schedule before the discovery and initiation of therapy for leukemia. The majority, but not all, of such children will respond to booster immunization with tetanus or diphtheria toxoids. Thus, the "routine" use of DT or Td immunization, as suggested by Nyerges et al,[3] cannot be depended on to boost immune status. This caution is particularly applicable to children treated with protocols modeled after the BFM regimen.

The risk of invasive *H influenzae* disease among children treated for acute leukemia (up to 5% of bacteremic episodes[6,15,16]), the low rate of naturally acquired immunity, and the 84% efficacy of immunization with HbOC support the recommendation that all leukemic children should be immunized against *H influenzae* during therapy.[17] Clinicians should be aware that immunization is not uniformly effective in this population and that invasive *H influenzae* remains a risk, particularly for leukemic patients receiving BFM-like protocols.

The authors gratefully acknowledge the generous support of Praxis Biologics Corp, Rochester, NY, which provided the HbOC vaccine and performed the *Haemophilus influenzae* antibody studies; the assistance of Anita R. Gessner, MS, who performed the diphtheria and tetanus antibody titer tests; and Rosemary Allen, who prepared the manuscript.

References

1. Kung FH, Orgel HA, Wallace WW, Hamburger RN. Antibody production following immunization with diphtheria and tetanus toxoids in children receiving chemotherapy during remission of malignant disease. *Pediatrics.* 1984;74:86-89.
2. Feldman S, Gigliotti F, Shenep JL, Roberson PK, Lott L. Risk of *Haemophilus influenza* type b disease in children with cancer and response of immunocompromised leukemic children to a conjugate vaccine. *J Infect Dis.* 1990;161:926-931.
3. Nyerges G, Zimonyi I, Nyerges G, Meszner Z, Marosi A. Efficiency of tetanus toxoid booster in leukemic children. *Acta Paediatr Acad Scientiarum Hung.* 1981;22:237-241.
4. van der Does-van den Berg A, Hermans J, Nagel J, van Steenis G. Immunity to diphteria, pertussis, tetanus, and poliomyelitis in children with acute lymphocytic leukemia after cessation of chemotherapy. *Pediatrics.* 1981;67:222-229.
5. Feldman S, Gigliotti F, Bockhold C, Naegele R. Measles and rubella antibody status in previously vaccinated children with cancer. *Med Pediatr Oncol.* 1988;16:308-311.
6. Weisman SJ, Cates KL, Allegretta GJ, Quinn JJ, Altman AJ. Antibody response to immunization with *Haemophilus influenza* type B polysaccharide vaccine in children with cancer. *J Pediatr.* 1987;111:727-729.
7. Lange B, Jakacki R, Nasab AH, Luevy N. Immunization of leukemic children with *Haemophilus* conjugate vaccine. *J Pediatr Infect Dis.* 1989;8:883-884.
8. Gaynon PS, Steinherz PG, Reaman GH, Bleyer WA, Sather H, Hammond GD. Strategies for the treatment of children with acute lymphoblastic leukemia and unfavorable presenting features. *Haematol Blood Transfus.* 1987;30:167-172.
9. Deforest A, Long SS, Lischner HW, et al. Simultaneous administration of measles-mumps-rubella vaccine with booster doses of diphtheria-tetanus-pertussis and poliovirus vaccines. *Pediatrics.* 1988;81:237-246.
10. Hardegree MC, Barile MF, Pittman M, Maloney CJ, Schofield F, Maclennan R. Immunization against neonatal tetanus in New Guinea, IV: comparison of tetanus antitoxin titres obtained by haemagglutination and toxin neutralization in mice. *Bull WHO.* 1970;43:461-468.
11. Miyamura K, Nishio S, Ito A, Murata R, Kono R. Micro cell culture method for determination of diphtheria toxin and antitoxin titres using VERO cells, I: studies on factors affecting the toxin and antitoxin titration. *J Biol Stand.* 1974;2:189-201.
12. Farr RS. A quantitative immunochemical measure of the primary interaction between I*BSA and antibody. *J Infect Dis.* 1958;103:239-262.
13. Anderson P. Intrinsic tritium labeling of the capsular polysaccharide antigen of *Haemophilus influenza* type B. *J Immunol.* 1978;120:866-870.
14. Orenstein WA, Weisfeld JS, Halsey NA. *Diphtheria and Tetanus Toxoids and Pertussis Vaccine, Combined.* Washington, DC: Pan American Health Organization, World Health Organization; 1983. Publication 451:30-51.
15. Saarinen UM. Severe infections in childhood leukemia: a follow-up study of 100 consecutive ALL patients. *Acta Paediatr Scand.* 1984;73:515-522.
16. Siber GR. Bacteremias due to *Haemophilus influenza* and *Streptococcus pneumonia*: their occurrence and course in children with cancer. *AJDC.* 1980;134:668-672.
17. Immunization Practices Advisory Committee. Update: prevention of *Haemophilus influenza* type B disease. *AJDC.* 1988;142:419-420.

In Other AMA Journals

ARCHIVES OF DERMATOLOGY

Bullous Eruption in an Infant

A. J. G. McDonagh, MB, ChB, MRCP; A. G. Messenger, MD, MRCP; B. L. Priestly, MD, BS, FRCP
(*Arch Dermatol.* 1991;127:1049)

Vesiculopapular Eruption in an Infant

Jay M. Weitzner, MD; Marti J. Rothe, MD; Lawrence Schachner, MD; Edwin Gould, MD
(*Arch Dermatol.* 1991;127:1049)

Diffuse Papular Eruption With Swelling of Joints in a Preschooler

Francine Bruyneel-Rapp, MD, Susan B. Mallory, MD
(*Arch Dermatol.* 1991;127:1049)

Immunogenicity of Tetravalent Rhesus Rotavirus Vaccine Administered With Buffer and Oral Polio Vaccine

Donna J. Ing, MPH; Roger I. Glass, MD; Patricia A. Woods; Murri Simonetti; Mark A. Pallansch, PhD; Wallace D. Wilcox, MD; Bruce L. Davidson, MD; Alan J. Sievert, MD

• Between January and November 1989, we studied 174 infants aged 6 to 16 weeks in a randomized clinical trial to (1) determine the immunogenicity of a single dose of tetravalent rhesus rotavirus vaccine (RRV-TV) when administered with three different buffer regimens: no antacid buffer and small-volume (2.5-mL) and large-volume (30-mL) antacid buffer; and (2) examine the potential interference of RRV-TV on the immune response to oral polio vaccine. Immunogenicity of RRV-TV, measured as a fourfold rise in antibody titers to rotavirus, was similar in the groups receiving small- and large-dose buffer (45% and 49%, respectively) and significantly less in the group that received RRV-TV alone (23%). Administration of RRV-TV with oral polio vaccine did not significantly interfere with the neutralization response of oral polio vaccine poliovirus serotypes 1, 2, or 3, and overall, 29%, 87%, and 24% of the infants had a fourfold rise in titer to each serotype, respectively.

(*AJDC.* 1991;145:892-897)

Worldwide, rotavirus (RV) is one of the most important causes of severe dehydrating diarrhea and vomiting in infants and children.[1,2] Many researchers have emphasized the need for a vaccine that can be incorporated into routine childhood immunization programs.[2,3] Several vaccines have been developed and tested that have shown promising results in small field trials.[4-7] One, the oral tetravalent rhesus rotavirus vaccine (RRV-TV), has advanced to a large-scale trial at 22 centers in the United States involving nearly 1000 infants who are receiving three oral doses. If this trial demonstrates significant efficacy, this vaccine might be considered for incorporation into routine childhood immunization programs in the United States.

In vaccine studies conducted to date, RV vaccines have been administered with large volumes of buffer and separated by periods of 2 weeks from oral poliovirus vaccine (OPV) immunization. Each of these conditions would make the incorporation of RV vaccine into the routine schedule of childhood immunizations logistically difficult: administration separate from that of the OPV would require extra visits, and the large-dose buffer is more difficult to administer than the vaccine itself. In previous studies, buffer was shown to be important to ensure a good immunogenic response, but the dose of buffer has never been titered against the immunogenicity of the RRV-TV vaccine to determine if a smaller dose would have a comparable effect.[8] Furthermore, since rotavirus vaccine should optimally be administered before 2 to 3 months of age, it could ideally be given together with OPV if there were no interference in the immunogenicity of either vaccine. This issue has been addressed in previous studies[9-12] but has not been adequately resolved.

This study was conducted (1) to determine the immunogenicity of RRV-TV vaccine when administered with one of three different buffer regimens (large-volume [30-mL], small-volume [2.5-mL], and no buffer) and (2) to examine the interference of RRV-TV in the immune response to OPV.

Accepted for publication January 3, 1991.

From the Department of Pediatrics, Emory University School of Medicine, Atlanta, Ga (Ms Ing, Drs Glass and Wilcox, and Ms Simonetti); Viral Gastroenteritis Unit, Respiratory and Enteric Virus Branch, Division of Viral and Rickettsial Diseases, Center for Infectious Diseases, Centers for Disease Control, US Department of Health and Human Services, Public Health Service, Atlanta (Drs Glass and Pallansch and Ms Woods); Wyeth-Ayerst Research, Clinical Research and Development, Philadelphia, Pa (Dr Davidson); and Division of Physical Health, DeKalb County Board of Health, Decatur, Ga (Dr Sievert).

Use of trade names is for identification only and does not constitute endorsement by the Public Health Service or the US Department of Health and Human Services.

Reprint requests to Division of Viral and Rickettsial Diseases, Centers for Disease Control, 1600 Clifton Rd, Atlanta, GA 30333 (Dr Glass).

SUBJECTS AND METHODS

Subjects

The study was conducted at five well-baby and immunization clinics of the DeKalb County Board of Health, Decatur, Ga, during the period between January and November 1989. Healthy infants 6 to 16 weeks of age who came to the clinic for their first well-baby visit and immunization (diphtheria-pertussis-tetanus and OPV) were recruited into the study. A pediatrician or study nurse reviewed each infant's medical history and examined the child. Infants were excluded if they (1) had had diarrhea, vomiting, or fever within the past week, (2) had been exposed to chickenpox within the past 3 weeks, (3) had had any serious illness since birth, (4) lived in a home with no telephone, or (5) had anyone in the household who was pregnant or immunocompromised. The study was explained to parents, and written informed consent was obtained. The study was approved by the Human Investigations Committee of Emory University, School of Medicine, Atlanta, Ga, by the Human

Table 1.—Characteristics of Participants in Four Study Groups*

Characteristic	RRV-TV/OPV, No Buffer (N=44)	RRV-TV/OPV, Small Buffer (N=44)	RRV-TV/OPV, Large Buffer (N=47)	OPV Alone (N=39)	Total (N=174)
	No. (%)				
Age, wk					
7-8	7 (16)	15 (34)	10 (21)	11 (28)	**43** (25)
9-10	26 (59)	16 (36)	25 (53)	18 (46)	**85** (49)
≥11	11 (25)	13 (30)	12 (26)	10 (26)	**46** (26)
Sex					
M	23 (52)	27 (61)	28 (60)	22 (56)	**100** (57)
F	21 (48)	17 (39)	19 (40)	17 (44)	**74** (43)
Race					
W	4 (9)	7 (16)	5 (11)	3 (8)	**19** (11)
B	37 (84)	33 (75)	42 (89)	35 (90)	**147** (84)
Other	3 (7)	4 (9)	0 (0)	1 (3)	**8** (5)
Birth weight, g					
<2500	4 (9)	3 (7)	3 (6)	2 (5)	**12** (7)
≥2500	40 (91)	41 (93)	44 (94)	37 (95)	**162** (93)
Breastfed					
Yes	5 (11)	6 (14)	5 (11)	4 (10)	**20** (11)
No	39 (89)	38 (86)	42 (89)	35 (90)	**154** (89)

*Infants who had preimmunization and postimmunization serum samples tested for rotavirus antibodies. There was no significant difference among study groups for the characteristics tested (by χ^2 or Fisher's Exact Test). RRV-TV indicates tetravalent rhesus rotavirus vaccine; OPV, oral polio vaccine.

Research Review Board of Georgia Department of Human Resources, and by the Institutional Review Board for Human Subjects of the Centers for Disease Control, Atlanta.

Study Design and Vaccine Administration

Participants were assigned to one of four groups according to a prepared randomization schedule and enrolled by the study nurse immediately after receiving their first OPV and diphtheria-pertussis-tetanus immunizations. The clinical trial was not blinded because of the difference in volumes of the buffer used and because the group receiving OPV alone did not receive a placebo. At the same time, and to avoid any possible biases, the study nurses who monitored adverse reactions did not know the vaccine group to which each child had been assigned. The laboratory staff who measured immune response to the vaccines received numbered specimens only.

In three of the four groups, infants received RRV-TV with no buffer (group 1), with a small volume of buffer (64 mg of sodium bicarbonate plus 24 mg of sodium citrate in 2.5 mL of water) (group 2), or with a large volume of buffer (400 mg of sodium bicarbonate in 25 mL of soybean formula [Prosobee; Mead Johnson Nutritionals, Evansville, Ind]) (group 3). The buffer doses were chosen empirically. The large dose had been administered in most previous trials with the rhesus RV vaccine. The smaller buffer (with citrate) had been successfully used in the oral cholera vaccine trials in Bangladesh[8] and was theoretically preferred because it produced more prolonged buffering without the reflex stimulation of stomach acid (David Sack, MD, oral communication, January 23, 1991). A control group received no RRV-TV (group 4). In groups 2 and 3, the antacid was administered 5 minutes before RRV-TV. All parents were instructed not to feed their infants for 1 hour before and 30 minutes after immunization. The infants remained in the clinic for approximately 30 minutes after vaccination for evaluation of any immediate reactions.

To monitor the immune responses to RRV-TV and OPV, the nurse collected blood samples on the day of and 56 days after vaccine administration. Serum samples were inactivated at 56°C for 30 minutes and stored at −20°C until analyzed.

Vaccine

The RRV-TV was prepared by Wyeth-Ayerst Research, Philadelphia, Pa, and contained the rhesus RV serotype 3 strain and genetic reassortants for human serotypes 1, 2, and 4.[4] The vaccine was stored at 2°C to 8°C as a lyophilized product and was reconstituted immediately before use. Each 1.0-mL dose of oral RRV-TV consisted of 10 000 plaque-forming units (PFU) of the parent rhesus RV and each of the three reassortant strains (total, 40 000 PFU).

Surveillance for Adverse Reactions

After the administration of RRV-TV, parents received a digital thermometer, a bottle of oral rehydration solution, and acetaminophen drops to treat fever resulting from the diphtheria-pertussis-tetanus vaccine, a Board of Health recommendation at that time. The parents were instructed on how to take the infant's rectal temperature.

For the 5 days after vaccination, parents were instructed to record in a structured diary the infant's afternoon temperature and the occurrence of loose stools or vomiting. For the 2-month period after vaccination, they were instructed to call the study nurse if the infant became ill, had loose stools, or developed diarrhea, defined as three or more stools judged to be looser than normal in a 24-hour period.

The nurse contacted the parent by telephone every other day and reviewed the signs or symptoms reported. For any problems, including diarrhea, the nurse made a home visit to evaluate the infant's condition, collected a stool specimen, and, when necessary, referred the parent to a physician.

RV Antibody Assay

IgA and IgG serum antibodies to RV were measured by enzyme-linked immunosorbent assay, by means of a procedure modified from that described previously.[9] Serum samples were tested in an initial dilution of 1:25, and alkaline phosphatase conjugate (Kierkegaard and Perry Laboratory, Gaithersburg, Md) replaced the peroxidase conjugate used before. Seroconversion was measured as a fourfold or greater rise in titer between preimmunization and postimmunization serum samples.

Polio Antibody Testing

Serum antibodies to poliovirus serotypes 1, 2, and 3 were measured by a microneutralization test[13,14] in which (1) twofold serial dilutions starting at 1:8 were performed, (2) 25 μL of HeLa cells at 300 000 cells per milliliter was added to the wells, and (3) 25 μL (100 times median tissue culture infective dose) of Sabin 1, 2, and 3 poliovirus was dispensed into plates. Seroconversion was defined as a fourfold or greater increase in titers between preimmunization and postimmunization serum samples.

Data Analysis

To evaluate the immunogenicity of RRV-TV with different doses of buffer and to examine the immune response to OPV, we compared the rates of seroconversions and plotted the cumulative distributions of rises in titer to polio (serotypes 1 through 3) and RV IgA and IgG titer rises for each of the study groups. We estimated that rates of seroconversion to RV in the range of 30% to 70% would be needed to demonstrate a statistically significant effect of the buffer. We anticipated rates of seroconversion to poliovirus serotypes 1, 2, and 3 to range from 10% (serotype 3) to 90% (serotype 2), allowing assessment of interference most sensitively with serotype 2. Fisher's Exact Test and χ^2 test were used to test the statistical significance of differences in seroconversions, and the Kolmogorov-Smirnov test was used to examine differences in the cumulative frequency distribution of titer rises between groups.

RESULTS

Characteristics of Participants

Between January 12 and August 31, 1989, a total of 174 infants recruited into the study were monitored for the full 2 months of follow-up and provided serum samples of sufficient quantity for analysis. Of these, 49% were between 9 and 10 weeks of age, 57% were male, 84% were black, 11% were breastfed, and only 7% were of low birth weight (<2500 g) (Table 1). The four groups did not differ significantly by age, sex, race, birth weight, or feeding status.

Table 2.—Clinical Reactions Within 5 Days of RRV-TV Vaccination in Four Study Groups*

	No. (%)			
Clinical Reaction	RRV-TV/OPV, No Buffer (N=44)	RRV-TV/OPV, Small Buffer (N=44)	RRV-TV/OPV, Large Buffer (N=47)	OPV Alone (N=39)
Temperature, °C†				
≤38.0	34 (80)	39 (89)	42 (93)	33 (92)
38.1-39.0	7 (16)‡	5 (11)	2 (4)	1 (3)
≥39.1	2 (5)	0 (0)	1 (2)	2 (6)
Vomiting				
None	43 (98)	39 (89)	40 (85)	38 (97)
Once or more	1 (2)	5 (11)	7 (16)§	2 (5)
Loose stools, No./d				
≤2	41 (93)	38 (86)	40 (85)	36 (92)
≥3	3 (7)	6 (14)	7 (15)	3 (8)
Watery stools				
None	42 (95)	42 (95)	45 (96)	37 (95)
Once or more	2 (5)	2 (5)	2 (4)	2 (5)

*RRV-TV indicates tetravalent rhesus rotavirus vaccine; OPV, oral polio vaccine.
†There were 1, 0, 2, and 3 infants with unknown temperatures in the four groups, respectively.
‡$P=.06$ vs group receiving OPV alone, by Fisher's Exact Test.
§$P=.06$ vs group receiving RRV-TV/OPV with no buffer, by Fisher's Exact Test.

Table 3.—Infants in Each Study Group With Fourfold Rise in Serum IgA and IgG Titers*

	No. (%)			
Serum IgA/IgG	RRV-TV/OPV, No Buffer (N=44)	RRV-TV/OPV, Small Buffer (N=44)	RRV-TV/OPV, Large Buffer (N=47)	OPV Alone (N=39)
IgA	10 (23)†	20 (45)‡	23 (49)‡	5 (13)
IgG	5 (11)	7 (16)§	7 (15)	1 (3)‖
Both IgA and IgG	2 (5)	6 (14)	6 (13)	1 (3)‖
Either IgA or IgG	13 (30)†	21 (48)‡	24 (51)‡	5 (13)‖

*RRV-TV indicates trivalent rhesus rotavirus vaccine; OPV, oral polio vaccine.
†$P<.05$ vs groups receiving RRV-TV/OPV with buffer (small or large), by χ^2 test.
‡$P<.005$ vs group receiving OPV alone, by χ^2 test.
§$P=.06$ vs group receiving OPV alone, by χ^2 test.
‖No IgG titer available for one specimen.

Side Effects of RRV-TV

Clinical reactions were recorded for 5 days after administration of RRV-TV and/or OPV (Table 2). No serious adverse reactions were reported by parents or physicians after vaccination in any of the study participants, and none of the children was hospitalized. The rate of minor adverse reactions in the total study group was low, and, except for a minor increase in vomiting among the infants receiving RRV-TV with large buffer, no significant differences were observed between groups. Nonetheless, children receiving RRV-TV with buffer tended to have more vomiting and loose stools, although reaction rates were so low that a much larger sample would have been required to look for significance.

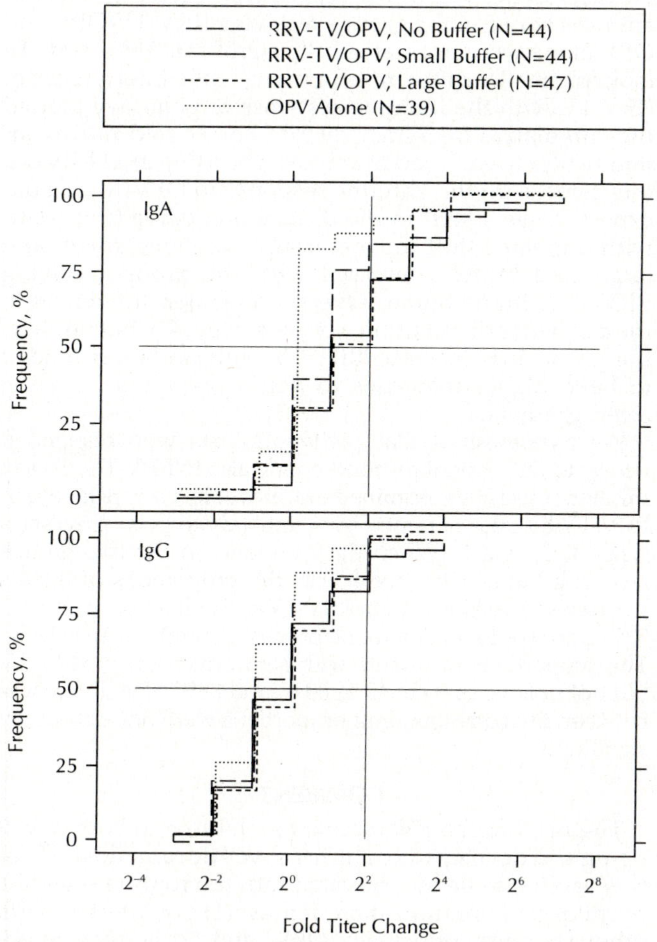

Fig 1.—*Cumulative distributions of IgA and IgG titer fold changes in each study group. Vertical line denotes fourfold rise in titer. Horizontal line represents median for the groups. Increased immunogenicity of tetravalent rhesus rotavirus vaccine (RRV-TV) is reflected as a shift in the curve to the right compared with the curve for oral polio vaccine (OPV) alone. Groups that received RRV-TV with small or large buffer had significantly greater titers than the control group (P<.01) and the group that received no buffer (P<.05) (Kolmogorov-Smirnov test).*

Seroresponse to RRV-TV Vaccine

The IgA seroconversion rate for infants receiving small-volume buffer with RRV-TV was comparable with that for infants receiving large-volume buffer (45% and 49%, respectively) (Table 3). These seroconversion rates were significantly higher than those for infants receiving RRV-TV with no buffer (23%) or OPV alone (13%). The difference in seroconversion rates between the group receiving RRV-TV with no buffer and that receiving OPV alone was not statistically significant.

The cumulative frequency distributions of fold rises in IgA and IgG titer were plotted for each of the study groups (Fig 1). Seroconversions of IgA were significantly more common among the groups receiving some buffer. The addition of IgG added little to the overall rates of seroconversion.

Five (13%) of the infants in the control group showed IgA seroconversion, indicating possible exposure to natural RV infection during the study period (Table 3). One of them had an IgA titer rise from 50 to 800, an IgG titer rise from 400 to 1600, and a stool specimen collected for diarrhea 7 days after OPV vaccination that was positive for RV by enzyme-linked immunosorbent assay. Assuming a 16-fold rise in IgA and a postvaccination IgA titer of 800 or higher to represent possible infection with wild-type RV, one infant each in the groups receiving no buffer, small buffer, and OPV alone met these criteria. These cases were not excluded from subsequent data analyses.

Effect of Breastfeeding and Maternal Antibody

Since breastfeeding may interfere with the response to RV vaccines, we compared rates of seroconversion by breastfeeding status combining all RV vaccine groups. Seroconversion by IgA was observed in 38% (6/16) of infants who were breastfed and 39% (47/119) of those who were not breastfed (χ^2, not significant).

Table 4.—Infants in Each Study Group Demonstrating Fourfold Rise in Serum Neutralizing Antibody to Three Serotypes of Poliovirus*

	No. (%)				
Serotype	**RRV-TV/OPV, No Buffer (N=39)**	**RRV-TV/OPV, Small Buffer (N=34)**	**RRV-TV/OPV, Large Buffer (N=38)**	**OPV Alone (N=31)**	**Total (N=142)**
Poliovirus 1	17 (44)†	8 (24)	8 (21)	8 (26)	**41** (29)
Poliovirus 2	35 (90)	27 (79)	35 (92)	27 (87)	**124** (87)
Poliovirus 3	9 (23)	9 (26)	7 (18)	9 (29)	**34** (24)

*RRV-TV indicates tetravalent rhesus rotavirus vaccine; OPV, oral polio vaccine.
†*P*<.05 vs group receiving RRV-TV/OPV with large buffer, by χ^2 test.

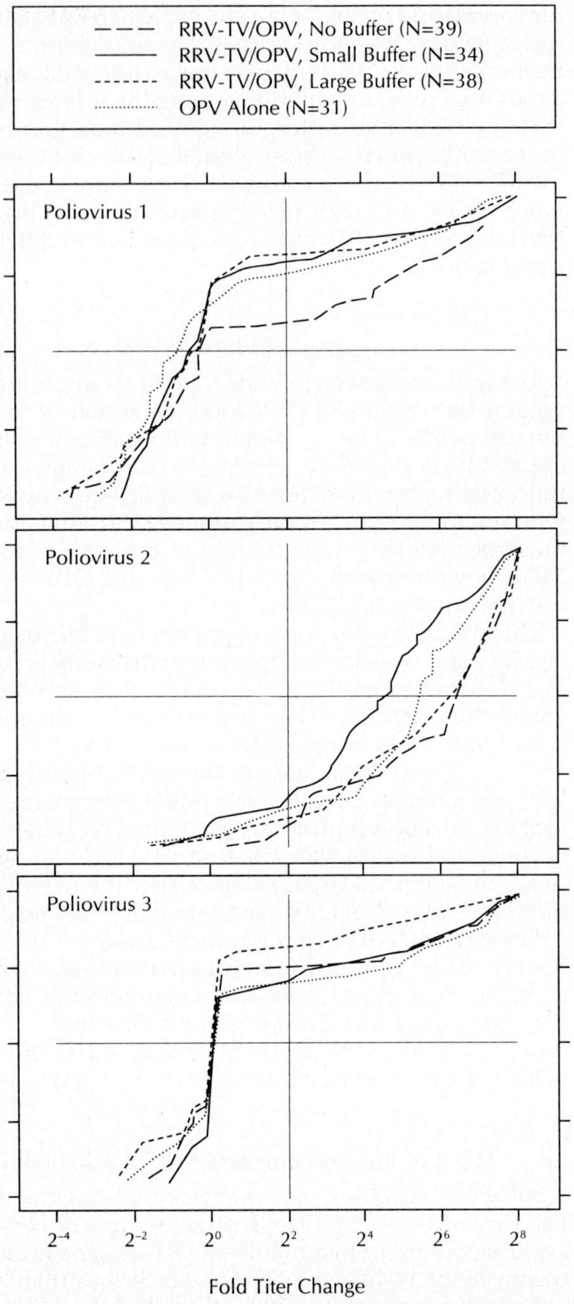

Fig 2.—*Cumulative distributions of titer fold changes in serum neutralizing antibody to three serotypes of poliovirus in each study group. Interference by tetravalent rhesus rotavirus vaccine (RRV-TV) in the immune response to poliovirus would be represented by a shift in the group's curve to the left compared with the curve for oral polio vaccine (OPV) alone. We hypothesized that if interference occurred, it would be greatest in the groups that received rotavirus vaccines with the small or large buffer (in which the immune response to rotavirus vaccine was greatest) and would be present for each of the serotypes of OPV used in the neutralizing assays. No consistent or significant trends in the immune response to poliovirus was observed according to the dose of buffer administered with the RRV-TV or for individual poliovirus serotypes used for neutralization.*

We also examined whether maternal antibody measured as the infant's initial IgG titer was associated with seroconversion by IgA. Seroconversion was observed in 38% (27/72) of infants with a low initial IgG titer (≤800) vs 36% (26/73) of infants with a high initial titer (≥1600) (χ^2, not significant).

Lack of Interference of RRV-TV With the Immune Response to OPV

Polio titers were available for 142 infants whose serum was collected at the time of OPV immunization and 8 to 10 weeks later. Overall, 29%, 87%, and 24% of infants had a fourfold rise in serum neutralizing antibodies to poliovirus serotypes 1, 2, and 3, respectively (Table 4). The differences between the groups receiving RRV-TV/OPV and OPV alone were not statistically significant by χ^2 test. To look for smaller differences or more subtle interference of RRV-TV with the immune response to polio, we plotted the cumulative frequency distribution of fold rise in antibody titer to each vaccine study group (Fig 2). If RRV-TV interfered with the immune response to OPV, we would expect to see a shift in the distribution curve to the left, with a greater shift for the groups receiving small- and large-dose buffer compared with the group receiving RRV-TV with no buffer. Overall, no major differences in the frequency distribution were observed. To the contrary, the group that received RRV-TV with no buffer tended to have higher fold rises to poliovirus 1 than did the other groups.

We hypothesized that perhaps infants who responded poorly to OPV might respond poorly also to RRV-TV. To test this hypothesis, we examined the rates of IgA seroresponse to RRV-TV by rates of neutralizing antibody to polio virus serotypes 1, 2, and 3. When the 72 infants in the two groups receiving buffer were combined, the proportions of infants with seroconversion to both RRV-TV and poliovirus were 31%, 37%, and 50% for poliovirus serotypes 1, 2, and 3, respectively. The proportions of infants with seroconversion to RRV-TV but not poliovirus were 43%, 60%, and 38%. The differences between the corresponding proportions were not statistically significant.

COMMENT

The need for an RV vaccine for children in both developing and developed countries is well documented.[3,9] For this vaccine to be incorporated into the routine schedule of childhood immunization, it must (1) not interfere with other vaccines, principally OPV, and (2) be easy to administer and not require a large volume of antacid (30 mL). This study demonstrates that antacid is important for achieving a good immune response to the RRV-TV vaccine and that the small (2.5-mL) dose of antacid, which is easy to administer, is as effective as the large volume of antacid, which would be difficult and logistically impractical for use in immunization programs. The addition of a small amount of buffer made a striking difference in immunogenicity of RRV-TV, but the vaccine was essentially nonimmunogenic in the group that received no buffer, suggesting that the original estimates of the amount of acid produced in the infant stomach were excessive.[8,15] Only half of the children who received RRV-TV with buffer had an immune response as measured by IgA and IgG. The extreme sensitivity of the vaccine to acid might be overcome by giving a larger inoculum of the vaccine, multiple doses of the same vaccine, or both. In fact, when this study was initiated, many investigators believed that one dose of the vaccine should be sufficient and that a 40 000-PFU inoculum would be adequate. In more recent trials, a three-dose regimen has been adopted to increase immunogenicity and to improve the potential efficacy of the vaccine. In two of these efficacy trials, the inoculum dose was increased to 400 000 PFU.

Second, this study demonstrates that RRV-TV in its current formulation (40 000 PFU) administered within 1 hour of OPV does not interfere with the immune response to OPV. In most field trials to date, the administration of RV vaccines has been separated from OPV by an interval of at least 2 weeks, in part because of theoretical concerns about the possible interference of these two live oral vaccines. This concern may be unwarranted, since OPV will remain in a child's gut for weeks and be shed by a majority of children for 1 month after first immunization. Also, polio and RV attack different cells in the gut, so interference at the level of cellular attachment or receptors is unlikely. This lack of interference would have to be reassessed if a higher inoculum of RRV-TV were used in future formulations.

The results of this study confirm and extend those of two earlier studies that examined the possible interference of the monovalent RV vaccines and OPV. In a previous study in Atlanta,[9] blood drawn at 3 to 4 weeks to monitor response to RV vaccines demonstrated an incomplete immune response to OPV. Since immune response to OPV peaks at 6 to 8 weeks, we tested convalescent-phase serum at 8 weeks to maximize our ability to detect a complete response to OPV. As expected, we observed a higher rate (87%) of seroconversion to poliovirus 2 (measured in the same laboratory) compared with 60% reported in the previous study.

In this study we also compared the cumulative distribution of titer rises between groups, a more statistically robust method to look for small differences; none was observed. Moreover, small differences in the immune response to polio that might be missed here would potentially be eliminated with the second or third doses of OPV. Consequently, in future trials, RRV-TV in its current formulation can be given safely with OPV without fear of interference in the immune response to OPV.

We did not examine whether OPV might interfere with the immune response to RRV-TV. This was observed with the RIT 4237 vaccine[10,12] but could not be demonstrated in our previous trial with monovalent RV vaccines.[9,16] Considering that most children who receive OPV have poliovirus in their intestines for long periods, the ability to test this interference would require trials substituting inactivated poliovirus vaccine for OPV or delaying the administration of the first OPV immunization, neither of which could be conveniently or ethically examined in our setting.

Although this trial could not be completely blinded, special attention was paid to ensure proper randomization in assignment to groups, to biases in assessing side effects, and to blinding in performing the laboratory studies. Randomization did ensure that the characteristics of the participants in the four study groups were not different, and rates of clinical reactions among vaccinees were so low that a very large sample would have been required to observe significant differences from the control group if they were present. Laboratory specimens were run in bulk without regard to the individual infants' vaccine group.

Some of the recruitment for this trial occurred during the RV season, and 13% of the infants who received no RRV-TV had an immune response to RV. In one such infant, a wild-type infection was documented during the week after enrollment. The infant's immune response to this infection was unlike that of the routine vaccinees, since he had a very large 16-fold rise in IgA, his convalescent-phase IgA titer was unusually elevated (800), and he had a fourfold rise in IgG (400 to 1600). Using the first two criteria (ie, 16-fold rise in IgA and convalescent IgA titer ≥800), we estimated that three infants in the study may have had wild-type infections. The marked difference in the immune response to wild-type infection vs the vaccine suggests that the vaccine may still require a more immunogenic combination of antigens. Wild-type infection is a far better immunogen than oral RRV-TV, and whether the reduced immunogenicity of oral RRV-TV results in reduced protection against symptomatic infection remains to be determined.

This study was funded in part by Wyeth-Ayerst Research.

We acknowledge the support and assistance provided by Paul J. Wiesner, Lynne McIntyre, Bob Davies, Jenine Clifford, Rebecca Gerrard, Rachel Cowley, Barbara Hester, Georgina Howard, Betty Jones, Beverly Waters, Claudette Williams, and the nursing staff at the clinics of the DeKalb County Board of Health.

References

1. Kapikian AZ. Approaches to immunization of infants and young children against gastroenteritis due to rotaviruses. *Rev Infect Dis.* 1980;2:459-469.

2. De Zoysa I, Feachem RG. Interventions for the control of diarrhoeal diseases among young children: rotavirus and cholera immunization. *Bull WHO.* 1985;63:569-583.

3. Institute of Medicine. Prospects for immunizing against rotavirus. In: *New Vaccine Development: Establishing Priorities.* Washington, DC: National Academy Press; 1985;1:410-423.

4. Kapikian AZ, Flores J, Hoshino Y, et al. Rotavirus: the major etiologic agent of severe infantile diarrhea may be controllable by a 'Jennerian' approach to vaccination. *J Infect Dis.* 1986;153:815-822.

5. Gothefors L, Wadell G, Juto P, et al. Prolonged efficacy of rhesus rotavirus vaccine in Swedish children. *J Infect Dis.* 1989;159:753-757.

6. Flores J, Perez-Schael I, Gonzalez M, et al. Protection against severe rotavirus diarrhoea by rhesus rotavirus vaccine in Venezuelan infants. *Lancet.* 1987;1:1882-1884.

7. Clark HF, Borian FE, Plotkin SA. Immune protection of infants against rotavirus gastroenteritis by a serotype 1 reassortant of bovine rotavirus WC-3. *J Infect Dis.* 1990;161:1099-1104.

8. Clemens J, Jertborn M, Sack D, et al. Effect of neutralization of gastric acid on immune responses to oral B-subunit killed whole-cell cholera vaccine. *J Infect Dis.* 1986;154:175-178.

9. Ho MS, Floyd RL, Glass RI, et al. Simultaneous administration of rhesus rotavirus vaccine and oral poliovirus vaccine: immunogenicity and reactogenicity. *Pediatr Infect Dis J.* 1989;8:692-696.

10. Giammanco G, DeGrandi V, Lupo L, et al. Interference of oral poliovirus vaccine on RIT 4237 oral rotavirus vaccine. *Eur J Epidemiol.* 1988;4:121-123.

11. Hanlon P, Marsh V, Shenton F, et al. Trial of an attenuated bovine rotavirus vaccine (RIT 4237) in Gambian infants. *Lancet.* 1987;1:342-345.

12. Vodopija I, Baklaic Z, Vlatkovic R. Combined vaccination with live oral poliovirus vaccine and the bovine rotavirus RIT 4237 strain. *Vaccine.* 1988;4:233-236.

13. Wulff H, Anderson LJ, Pallansch MA, et al. Diagnosis of enterovirus 70 infection by demonstration of IgM antibodies. *J Med Virol.* 1987;21:321-327.

14. Schmidt NJ. Diagnostic procedures for viral, rickettsial and chlamydial infections. In: Lennette EH, Schmidt NJ, eds. *Cell Culture Techniques for Diagnostic Virology.* 5th ed. Washington, DC: American Public Health Association; 1979:65-139.

15. Weiss C, Clark HF. Rapid inactivation of rotaviruses by exposure to acid buffer or acidic gastric juice. *J Gen Virol.* 1985;66:2725-2730.

16. Jalil F. Immunogenicity and reactogenicity rhesus rotavirus vaccine given in combination with oral or inactivated poliovirus vaccine and diptheria tetanus and pertussis vaccine. *Trans R Soc Trop Med Hyg.* In press.

Response of 7- to 15-Month-Old Infants to Sequential Immunization With *Haemophilus influenzae* Type b-CRM_{197} Conjugate and Polysaccharide Vaccines

Edward P. Rothstein, MD; Ruth P. Schiller, MD; Joseph A. C. Girone, MD; Thomas J. Hipp, MD; Ronald L. Souder, MD; Henry H. Bernstein, DO; Dace V. Madore, PhD; Cynthia L. Johnson; David H. Smith, MD

• *Objective.*—To evaluate the immunologic potential of infants 7 to 15 months of age to respond to *Haemophilus influenzae* type b polysaccharide vaccine following immunization with *H influenzae* b oligosaccharide-CRM_{197} conjugate vaccine.

***Study Design.*—One hundred seventy-one infants, aged 7 to 15 months, were consecutively and alternatively assigned to one of three immunization protocols. Group 1 (n=71) received three doses of *H influenzae* b oligosaccharide-CRM_{197} conjugate vaccine, group 2 (n=47) received two doses of *H influenzae* b oligosaccharide-CRM_{197} conjugate vaccine followed by one dose of *H influenzae* type b polysaccharide vaccine, and group 3 received one dose of *H influenzae* b oligosaccharide-CRM_{197} conjugate vaccine followed by two doses of *H influenzae* type b polysaccharide vaccine. Immunizations were given on day 0 and at 2 months and 6 months. Anti–*H influenzae* type b polysaccharide antibody levels were measured on day 0 and 2, 3, 6, 7, and 12 months after the study began.**

***Results.*—*Haemophilus influenzae* type b polysaccharide vaccine given as a second dose stimulated an antibody rise but did so less effectively than *H influenzae* b oligosaccharide-CRM_{197} conjugate vaccine. Two doses of *H influenzae* b oligosaccharide-CRM_{197} conjugate vaccine were highly immunogenic; geometric means were 31 and 35 μg/mL in the 7- to 11-month and 12- to 15-month age groups, respectively. Following two doses of *H influenzae* b oligosaccharide-CRM_{197} conjugate vaccine, both immunization protocols resulted in (1) equally high geometric mean antibody levels 1 month after immunization and (2) similar geometric mean antibody levels 6 months after immunization.**

***Conclusions.*—*Haemophilus influenzae* b oligosaccharide-CRM_{197} conjugate vaccine induces antibody levels that would be expected to protect infants from initial invasion and primes the immune system for an anamnestic response. Our data indicate that if a booster immunization is needed, *H* influenzae type b polysaccharide vaccine could be an alternative to *H influenzae* b oligosaccharide-CRM_{197} conjugate vaccine.**

(*AJDC*. 1991;145:898-900)

The originally licensed *Haemophilus influenzae* type b (Hib) vaccine, *H influenzae* type b polysaccharide (HbPs) vaccine, is poorly immunogenic in children younger than 18 to 24 months and does not induce immunologic memory.[1-4] Vaccines that link the capsular saccharide of Hib to a protein (conjugate vaccines) have two goals. The primary goal is to stimulate an infant's immature immune system to produce anti-HbPs antibody levels that are high enough and last long enough to prevent invasive disease. The second is to prime the immune system so that exposure to Hib can rapidly stimulate clonal expansion of already-primed B cells. Two conjugate vaccines, *H influenzae* b oligosaccharide-CRM_{197} conjugate vaccine (HbOC) (HibTITER; Praxis Biologics Inc, Rochester, NY) and *Haemophilus* b Conjugate Vaccine (Meningococcal Protein Conjugate) (PedvaxHIB; Merck Sharp & Dohme Laboratories, West Point, Pa), are licensed for use beginning at 2 months of age.[5,6] Our study documents the immunogenicity of various sequential combinations of HbOC and HbPs vaccines in infants aged 7 to 15 months of age and the ability of HbOC to prime these infants for a response to HbPs vaccine.

SUBJECTS AND METHODS

Subject Selection

Children aged between 7 and 15 months were eligible to participate if they had no serious chronic illness, no history of Hib disease, no previous immunization with either HbPs vaccine or a conjugate Hib vaccine, and no history or physical findings suggestive of an acute febrile illness. Children were enrolled in the study, approved by the Institutional Review Board of Grand View Hospital, Sellersville, Pa, after parental written informed consent was obtained.

Vaccines and Vaccine Administration

The HbPs vaccine (b-Capsa I, lot 038AL; Praxis Biologics Inc), containing 25 μg/mL of capsular polysaccharide per 0.5 μg/mL, or the HbOC vaccine (HibTITER, lots BRH512 and A2K61), containing

Accepted for publication March 3, 1991.

From Pennridge Pediatrics Associates, Sellersville, Pa (Drs Rothstein, Schiller, Girone, Hipp, Souder, and Bernstein); St Christopher's Hospital for Children and Temple University School of Medicine, Philadelphia, Pa (Drs Rothstein, Schiller, Girone, Hipp, Souder, and Bernstein); and Praxis Biologics Inc, Rochester, NY (Drs Madore and Smith and Ms Johnson).

Reprint requests to 711 Lawn Ave, Sellersville, PA 18960 (Dr Rothstein).

Table 1.—Comparison of Anti–*Haemophilus influenzae* Type b Polysaccharide (HbPs) Antibody Responses of 7- to 11-Month-Old Infants According to Different Vaccination Protocols

Vaccination Schedule†	Months After First Vaccination	GM Anti-HbPs Antibody, μg/mL*					
		No.	HbOC/HbOC/HbOC	No.	HbOC/HbOC/HbPs	No.	HbOC/HbPs/HbPs
P/V	0	48	0.11 (0.08-0.15)	33	0.11 (0.08-0.17)	39	0.12 (0.08-0.17)
P/V	2	48	2.91 (0.64-13.30)	33	4.86 (1.74-13.58)	39	3.84 (0.91-16.25)
P	3	48	29.05 (12.35-68.35)	33	34.57 (25.49-46.88)	38	9.83‡ (2.58-37.51)
P/V	6	47	15.97 (5.50-46.41)	33	19.04 (8.47-42.83)	39	3.72‡ (0.98-14.17)
P	7	48	37.93 (32.32-44.52)	33	37.52 (32.06-43.91)	38	11.89‡ (2.91-48.59)
P	12	48	16.38 (7.82-34.33)	33	16.76 (7.80-36.02)	33	6.76‡ (2.22-20.62)

*GM indicates geometric mean; HbOC, *H influenzae* b oligosaccharide-CRM_{197} conjugate. Numbers in parentheses are SDs.
†P indicates phlebotomy; V, vaccination.
‡Significantly different from response in HbOC/HbOC/HbOC and HbOC/HbOC/HbPs groups ($P < .05$).

Table 2.—Comparison of Anti–*Haemophilus influenzae* Type b Polysaccharide (HbPs) Antibody Responses of 12- to 15-Month-Old Infants According to Different Vaccination Protocols

Vaccination Schedule	Months After First Vaccination	GM Anti-HbPs Antibody, μg/mL*					
		No.	HbOC/HbOC/HbOc	No.	HbOC/HbOC/HbPs	No.	HbOC/HbPs/HbPs
P/V	0	23	0.15 (0.09-0.26)	14	0.16 (0.09-0.29)	14	0.13 (0.10-0.16)
P/V	2	23	10.91 (3.24-36.71)	14	12.10 (4.70-31.81)	13	8.31 (2.65-26.04)
P	3	23	33.37 (21.78-51.14)	14	37.27 (28.62-48.54)	14	9.34‡ (1.62-53.86)
P/V	6	23	22.86 (12.50-41.81)	14	26.79 (16.24-44.20)	14	5.10‡ (1.38-18.82)
P	7	23	39.55 (38.07-41.10)	14	37.97 (31.23-46.15)	14	17.48‡ (5.00-61.05)
P	12	22	25.39 (13.96-46.18)	14	27.28 (16.99-43.18)	14	10.83‡ (2.57.45.65)

*GM indicates geometric mean; HbOC, *H influenzae* b oligosaccharide-CRM_{197} conjugate. Numbers in parentheses are SDs.
†P indicates phlebotomy; V, vaccination.
‡Significantly different from response in HbOC/HbOC/HbOC and HbOC/HbOC/HbPs groups ($P < .05$).

10 μg/mL of capsular derived oligosaccharide and 25 μg/mL of CRM_{197} per 0.5 μg/mL, was administered as a 0.5-mL intramuscular dose, as recommended by the manufacturer. A three-dose sequential schedule was used to immunize infants on study day 0 and at 2 and 6 months after initial immunization.

Study Design

Subjects were consecutively and alternately assigned to one of three immunization protocols. As shown in Tables 1 and 2, subjects were immunized with three doses of HbOC, two doses of HbOC followed by one dose of HbPs, or one dose of HbOC followed by two doses of HbPs. Further enrollment in the HbPS groups was terminated after it became apparent that the antibody response to HbPs in one of the groups was statistically significantly less than that to HbOC (Tables 1 and 2). Therefore, more infants were enrolled in the group that received three doses of HbOC than in the other two groups.

Specimen Collection

Venous blood was obtained before each immunization, 1 month after the second and third immunizations, and 6 months after the third immunization. Blood was separated within 4 hours of collection, and serum samples were frozen until they were analyzed for anti-HbPs antibodies.

Serologic Assays

All serum samples were coded so that Praxis Biologics Inc laboratory personnel were unaware of the subjects' protocol assignment. Total serum antibody to HbPs was quantitated by a Farr-type radioantigen binding assay, as previously described.[7] The anti-HbPs antibody levels in each group were evaluated by determining the geometric mean (GM). Values at or below 0.10 μg/mL were recorded as 0.10 μg/mL and those equal to or greater than 40.00 μg/mL were recorded as 40.00 μg/mL. The significance of differences in the GM between groups was determined by least square means analysis.

RESULTS

One hundred eighty-one white infants 7 to 15 months of age were enrolled. One hundred seventy-five infants (96.4%) completed the study. Four infants with initial anti-HbPs antibody levels of greater than 1 μg/mL were eliminated from further analysis. Of the remaining 171 infants, 82 were female and 89 were male. The sex distribution and mean ages of the immunization groups were similar within each age group. The mean age at the time of first immunization for each group was between 8.3 and 9.2 months and 13.1 and 13.3 months for the younger and older groups, respectively.

Analysis of Anti-HbPs Antibody Response

The immunologic response to each immunization protocol was evaluated in infants aged 7 to 11 months (Table 1) and 12 to 15 months (Table 2). Within each age group, the GM anti-HbPs antibody levels before and after one dose of HbOC vaccine were not statistically different. Older infants (12 to 15 months old) responded to one dose of HbOC with greater GM antibody levels than younger infants (7 to 11 months old). Eighty-five percent of 7- to 11-month-old and 98% of 12- to 15-month-old infants had anti-HbPs antibody values greater than 1 μg/mL after a single dose of HbOC.

Following a second dose of HbOC, the GM anti-HbPs antibody of the 7- to 11-month-old infants rose sevenfold to 10-fold further (Table 1). In the older group, the second dose of HbOC increased the GM threefold further (Table 2). Irrespective of the age of the infant at the time of the initial immunization, the GM anti-HbPS antibody level was high (29 to 37 μg/mL) following two doses of HbOC. Two doses of HbOC resulted in a greater than 200-fold increase in GM anti-HbPs antibodies over the preimmunization levels. Ninety-nine percent of the infants had anti-HbPs levels greater than 1 μg/L. Ninety-six percent had levels greater than 10 μg/mL.

In contrast, infants who were immunized with one dose of HbOC followed by HbPs 2 months later showed a 72- to 82-fold increase over the preimmunization antibody level. This increase was seen irrespective of age at initial immunization. The GM anti-HbPs antibody levels were 9.83 μg/mL (92% ≥1 μg/mL) and 9.34 μg/mL (86% ≥1 μg/mL) in the younger and older groups, respectively.

Further evaluation of the individual responses in the younger age group indicates that 21 of the 39 individuals given HbPs 2 months after an initial dose of HbOC showed a greater than twofold increase in GM anti-HbPs antibody. The GM of these 21 responders rose from 2.41 to 17.01 μg/mL (SD, 7.2 to 40.2 μg/mL) after the HbPs immunization. The mean age of this 7- to 11-month-old responder subgroup was 10.6 months (range, 9 to 13 months) at the time of their HbPs immunization. In contrast, the pre- and post-HbPs immunization GM antibody level in the nonresponders (those having less than twofold antibody rise) was 5.94 and 4.75 μg/mL, respectively. These two groups (responders and nonresponders) were not distinguishable by preimmunization anti-HbPs levels (nonresponder GM, 0.11) or by age (nonresponder mean age, 10.8 months; range, 9 to 13 months). When these nonresponders to HbPs received a second dose of HbPs 4 months later, 13 of the 17 showed a greater than twofold increase (one child's specimen was unavailable). At the time of their third immunization (one dose of HbOC followed by two doses of HbPs), the ages of the four remaining nonresponders were 13.2, 13.6, 14.8, and 15.5 months.

Two primary doses of HbOC resulted in high-GM anti-HbPs antibody levels, approaching the upper limit of data analysis (40.0 μg/mL) in both age groups. In those in whom antibody levels declined after the second dose of HbOC, a third dose of either HbOC or HbPs boosted the anti-HbPs antibodies back to levels that approached the upper limit of the assay.

Irrespective of the immunization schedule or the age at the time of initial examination, high anti-HbPs antibody levels were sustained over time. Six months following the third immunization, when children were 19 to 27 months of age, all who were in the groups that received three doses of HbOC or two doses of HbOC followed by one dose of HbPs had antibody levels greater than 1 μg/mL. Of those who received one dose of HbOC followed by two doses of HbPs, 93% had levels greater than 1 μg/mL, irrespective of age group.

COMMENT

To our knowledge, ours is the first study to use HbPs in a primary immunization series following an initial dose with an Hib conjugate vaccine in infants younger than 15 months. Our observations show that, following a single dose of HbOC, (1) HbPs can boost anti-HbPs antibody levels in infants who, because of age, would not be expected to respond with this frequency or to this level; (2) HbPs boosts anti-HbPs antibody to the same GM antibody level in infants who received their primary dose of HbOC whether they were 7 to 11 or 12 to 15 months of age; (3) a second vaccination with HbOC results in a greater GM anti-HbPs antibody level than when the second vaccination is HbPs; and (4) when given after two doses of HbOC, both HbPs and HbOC boost GM antibody levels to the same high value, the values decline to the same levels 6 months after immunization, and in all the children levels were maintained that have been correlated with long-term immunity after immunization with an HbPs vaccine (≥1 μg/mL).[8]

The greater response when the second dose is HbOC rather than HbPs may reflect recruitment of new clones of B cells (T-cell dependent) along with better stimulation of already-primed B cells. The HbPs, as a second dose in these young infants, probably only stimulates already-primed B cells. It appears that some children may not be primed within 2 months after a single dose of HbOC, as evidenced by their lack of response to HbPs. However, almost all of these children responded to a second dose of HbPs administered 4 months later, and all had anti-HbPs antibody concentrations of greater than 1 μg/mL when evaluated 6 months after their last immunization. The response to the second dose of HbPs may be related to both age and prior immunization.

While current recommendations for immunization of infants 7 to 11 months of age include a booster, the data from this study indicate that two doses of HbOC stimulate high antibody levels. There may not be an advantage to vaccinating this age group with three doses of HbOC. If three doses are desirable, HbPs could be a reasonable alternative following two doses of HbOC.

The more important implication of these data is that in the months after successful primary immunization, as the expected decline in antibody levels occurs, exposure to the polysaccharide (probably representative of the organism) should elicit an accelerated memory response that will aid in protection against invasive *Haemophilus* disease and help to maintain immunity. The HbOC not only generates high levels of anti-HbPs antibodies following one or two doses, but it appears to prime, as evidenced by a further antibody rise when HbPs vaccine is administered 2 to 4 months later.

The helpful review by Sarah S. Long, MD, is thoroughly appreciated. We acknowledge the superb support of Dorothy Kratz, RN, and Jean Bitner, RN, as well as the rest of the staff of Pennridge Pediatrics Associates, Sellersville, Pa. The dedication of the staff of the Immunobiologic Service Department and the Clinical Studies Department at Praxis Biologics Inc, especially Donna Phipps, MS, Carolyn Cimino, and Kim Kukfa, MS, are also deeply appreciated.

References

1. Granoff DM, Cates KL. *Haemophilus influenzae* type b polysaccharide vaccines. *J Pediatr.* 1985;107:330-335.
2. Käyhty H, Karanko V, Peltola H, Mäkelä PH. Serum antibodies after vaccination with *Haemophilus influenzae* type b capsular polysaccharide and responses to reimmunization. *Pediatrics.* 1984;74:857-865.
3. Anderson P, Pichichero M, Edwards K, Porch CR, Insel RA. Priming and induction of *Haemophilus influenzae* type b capsular antibodies in early infancy by Dpo20, an oligosaccharide-protein conjugate vaccine. *J Pediatr.* 1987;111:644-650.
4. Ward J. Newer *Haemophilus influenzae* type b vaccines and passive prophylaxis. *Pediatr Infect Dis J.* 1987;6:799-803.
5. Centers for Disease Control. Food and Drug Administration approval of use of a *Haemophilus* b conjugate vaccine for infants. *MMWR.* 1990;39:925-926.
6. Centers for Disease Control. Food and Drug Administration approval of use of a *Haemophilus* b conjugate vaccine in infants. *MMWR.* 1990;39:698-699.
7. Madore DV, Johnson CL, Phipps DC, et al. Safety and immunologic response to *Haemophilus influenzae* type b oligosaccharide-CRM_{197} conjugate vaccine in 1- to 6-month-old infants. *Pediatrics.* 1990;85:331-337.
8. Käyhty H, Peltola H, Karenko V, Mäkelä PH. The protective level of serum antibodies to the capsular polysaccharide of *Haemophilus influenzae* type b. *J Infect Dis.* 1983;147:1100.

Transfusion Therapy in Neonates

Ronald G. Strauss, MD

• Infants, particularly those who were very small premature neonates, are among the most common of all patient groups to undergo extensive transfusion. It is estimated that approximately 300 000 neonates undergo transfusions annually. Most infants who undergo transfusion are exposed to multiple blood donors, and although each exposure poses only a small risk, the potential for adverse effects of multiple transfusions is not trivial. Transfusion practices for neonates are controversial, variable, and based on scanty scientific information. For the most part, controlled scientific studies have not been performed to clearly establish the indications for the transfusion of blood components to neonates. Considering these limitations, guidelines are offered for the transfusion of red blood cells, platelets, and neutrophils into neonates.

(*AJDC.* 1991;145:904-911)

Some neonates require multiple blood transfusions, and the risks of transfusion, although infrequent, are not trivial. Thus, knowledge of neonatal transfusion medicine is crucial for optimal pediatric practice.

THE NEED FOR MULTIPLE TRANSFUSIONS

Infants, particularly those who were very small premature neonates, are among the most common of all patient groups to undergo extensive transfusions. Of the 38 000 premature neonates with birth weights (BWs) of less than 1500 g estimated to be born annually in the United States,[1,2] 80% will require multiple red blood cell (RBC) transfusions—many infants will receive cumulative transfusion volumes exceeding their total blood volumes.[3,4] Based on a review of eight studies, Sacher et al[4] concluded that infants undergoing multiple transfusions typically are exposed to eight to 10 different donors (range, two to 18 donors). Likewise, results of a study conducted at our institution between 1983 and 1984[5] showed a substantial use of RBC transfusions from multiple donors: 53 infants received 683 RBC transfusions from 503 different donors (mean number of donors per neonate, 9.5). In an unpublished study (R.G.S., unpublished data, 1989) performed between 1988 and 1989 to assess current practices, a similar rate was documented: 38 (78%) of 49 infants with BWs of less than 1500 g received an average of 10 RBC transfusions per infant, with a mean exposure to slightly more than six donors per neonate (Table 1). In addition, about 16% of infants underwent transfusions of other blood components. Thus, concerns about transfusion-associated diseases have not caused a major reduction in blood transfusions by neonatologists—presumably because RBC transfusions are perceived to be mandatory for the optimal care of sick premature infants.

Assuming my data (Table 1) and that of others[3,4,6] are representative of current national practices, approximately 29 640 low-BW infants will receive 296 400 RBC transfusions annually. Importantly, the long-term survival of infants with BWs of less than 1500 g continues to improve, which results in an increasing number of infants requiring multiple RBC transfusions. In addition, occasional transfusions are given to infants with BWs of greater than 1500 g. It is very alarming that, by current practices, many infants will be exposed to different donors for most transfusions. Thus, the importance of sound knowledge about neonatal transfusion practices is emphasized by the mandatory and crucial role of blood component transfusions in the treatment of extremely small, premature neonates.

THE RISK OF TRANSFUSIONS

It is logical to conclude that exposure to multiple blood donors will increase the potential for adverse effects, particularly transfusion-associated infections. The rate of transfusion-associated infections, although not always directly proportional to the frequency of donor exposure, increases when multiple transfusions are given.[7,8] To eliminate the transmission of infections from donors, blood banks continuously improve medical screening of blood donors and laboratory testing of donated blood. For every donation, donors are advised that they are not to donate if they are in high-risk groups (eg, intravenous drug abusers). Donors are directly questioned about high-risk behavior, and they must give written confirmation that they are not involved in such behavior. A complete medical history is recorded and, if needed, a physical examination is conducted. Laboratory testing is performed to detect hepatitis, syphilis, and retrovirus (human immunodeficiency virus [HIV] type 1 and human T-cell leukemia/lymphoma virus type I or II) infections. However, to ensure maximum safety, these measures employed to

Accepted for publication April 1, 1991.

From the Departments of Pathology and Pediatrics, University of Iowa College of Medicine, and the DeGowin Blood Center, University of Iowa Hospitals and Clinics, Iowa City.

Reprint requests to the Department of Pathology, University of Iowa Hospitals and Clinics, Newton Road, Iowa City, IA 52242 (Dr Strauss).

Table 1.—RBC Transfusions in Preterm Infants at the University of Iowa—1988-1989*	
Clinical Characteristics of Infants	**Data**
All Infants Reviewed (n = 49)	
No. (%) who underwent RBC transfusions	38 (78)
No. (%) who underwent transfusions of other components	8 (16)
Infants Who Underwent Transfusion (n = 38)	
No. of RBC transfusions (mean ± SD)	10.0 ± 8.3
No. of RBC donors (mean ± SD)	6.2 ± 5.3
No. (%) who underwent >4 RBC transfusions	31 (82)
No. (%) who underwent >15 RBC transfusions	10 (26)
Maximum No. of RBC transfusions undergone	40

*RBC indicates red blood cell. All infants weighed less than 1500 g at birth.

improve transfusion safety must be coupled with efforts to diminish the need for homologous transfusions.

The percentage of infants and children who acquire HIV via transfusion is disproportionately high compared with the number of adults thus infected. In one survey[9] excluding hemophiliacs, 15% of childhood cases of HIV infection were due to blood transfusions compared with 2% of adulthood cases of HIV infection.[9] These rates were determined before current methods of donor screening and testing were used, and, thus, are overestimates of the current rate of transfusion-associated HIV infection. However, the data illustrate the importance of transfusions as a route for transmitting blood-borne organisms to neonates. The current risk of an infected donor not being detected with testing is estimated to be about one in 1 million.[10] Because the exact figure is unknown, some controversy exists, and most experts accept a rate of between one and 20 per million.

The current rate of transfusion-associated hepatitis has not been determined accurately in infants. Although the incidence of non-A, non-B hepatitis (which, in most cases, is presumed to be due to the hepatitis C virus) is believed to be low,[11] the rate is difficult to establish because, until very recently, the diagnosis was made by documenting an unexplained elevation in serum alanine aminotransferase occurring within 6 months of transfusion. Long-term serial measurements of alanine aminotransferase during the perinatal period have been rarely reported, and alanine aminotransferase values are higher and more variable in infants who apparently are healthy than are values in subjects of other ages.[12] Nonetheless, non-A, non-B hepatitis is of concern because it is the most common transfusion-related viral infection and has the potential for long-term toxic effects.[13] Disorders leading to long-term morbidity (eg, posthepatic cirrhosis and hepatic cancer) are particularly alarming when they occur during infancy because of the potential for an extended disability requiring costly care.

The importance of transfusion-associated cytomegalovirus (CMV) infection in neonates is controversial. Studies conducted during the 1970s and early 1980s reported a disturbingly high incidence (25% to 50%) of CMV infection in neonates who had undergone transfusion.[14] This was particularly true in those who underwent the most extensive transfusions, some of whom died. Several recent studies indicate a diminishing, almost negligible risk.[14] However, these studies have been criticized,[15] and the importance of transfusion-associated CMV infection and the need for special precautions (use of CMV-seronegative donors or components markedly depleted of leukocytes) when conducting transfusions in neonates remains controversial. The American Association of Blood Banks, in its *Standards for Blood Banks and Transfusion Services*,[16] has recommended that cellular blood products with low risks of transmitting CMV infection be given to infants with BWs of less than 1200 g who are seronegative for antibody to CMV or of unknown serostatus if they are being managed in hospitals in which CMV is known to be a problem. The transmission of CMV to infants has implications beyond immediate infant morbidity and mortality. Infected infants can transmit CMV to their mothers and to other susceptible contacts.

Other transfusion-associated conditions of noninfectious natures that may occur in infants include fluid overload, graft-vs-host disease,[17,18] electrolyte and acid-base imbalances, iron overload,[19] increased susceptibility to oxidant damage,[20] exposure to plasticizers,[21] hemolysis when T-antigen activation of RBCs has occurred,[22] immunosuppression,[23] and alloimmunization,[11] although, in limited studies,[5] alloimmunization to RBC and leukocyte antigens has been shown to be uncommon in infants. Regarding graft-vs-host disease and techniques for irradiation, the American Association of Blood Banks[16] recommends that cellular blood products be irradiated with a minimum of 15 Gy to prevent graft-vs-host disease in fetuses (intrauterine transfusion), in selected immunocompromised recipients, and in patients receiving transfusion products from first-degree relatives. In practice, "selected immunocompromised recipients" are usually defined as bone marrow transplant recipients, patients with congenital defects of cell-mediated immunity, and patients with disseminated reticuloendothelial cancer undergoing therapy. Although enthusiasm for the transfusion of irradiated blood components is variable, it is difficult to justify scientifically the exclusive use of these products in neonates in general, even if they are premature or infected with HIV. Some adverse effects occur only with massive transfusions, such as exchange transfusions, and are rare in the usual, small-volume RBC transfusion. The relationship of some alleged adverse effects to transfusions is controversial.[24] Nonetheless, the risks of transfusion are significant, and blood components should be transfused only when necessary.

INDICATIONS FOR NEONATAL TRANSFUSION

The lack of a rational approach to transfusion practices[4,25,26] stems from limited knowledge of the cellular and molecular biology of hematopoiesis during the perinatal period as well as from a lack of understanding of the infant's response to severe cytopenia. Data from clinical studies of infants are sparse and difficult to interpret because of the precarious and heterogeneous medical condition of these patients. Even the deceptively simple task of obtaining sufficient blood to conduct definitive studies is a major impediment because of small total blood volumes and difficult vascular access. Although, in some instances, the value of transfusions is clear (eg, transfusing RBCs to treat anemia that has caused congestive heart failure and transfusing platelets to treat severe thrombocytopenia with bleeding), in others, it is not. Following are reasonable guidelines for the transfusion of the three most frequently used cellular components—RBCs, platelets, and neutrophils (granulocytes).

RBC Transfusions

Generally, RBC transfusion is performed to maintain a level of hematocrit believed to be most desirable for each neonate's clinical status.[27] It is widely recognized that this clinical approach is imprecise, and consideration of more physiologic indications such as RBC mass, available oxygen, and measurements of oxygen delivery and tissue extraction has been suggested. However, the means by which these techniques can best be applied to everyday practice are undefined. Clearly established indications for neonatal RBC transfusions, based on controlled scientific studies, do not exist. In many clinical situations, the need for RBC transfusion seems logical, but often efficacy has not been established, and a complete understanding of the risks is lacking. Because of the limited data available, it is important that pediatricians critically evaluate the following recommendations in light of neonatal practice at their institutions. Most RBC transfusions performed in neonates are of small volume (5 to 15 mL of RBCs per kilogram of body weight) and are repeated frequently.[27] The usual indications for small-volume transfusions are discussed separately.

Replacement of Blood Drawn for Laboratory Studies.—This indication accounts for about 90% of all RBC transfusions in neonates.[28] Although laboratory micromethods can be used, cumulative blood losses due to laboratory sampling are proportionately very large.[4] Attempts are being made to limit blood sampling via the use of indwelling catheters with specific transducers, transcutaneous electrodes, and monitors. Until these are available for routine use, the practice of replacing drawn blood with transfused RBCs will continue.[29] Often, RBCs are replaced when 5% of the estimated total blood volume has been removed from neonates requiring frequent monitoring. Replacement is frequently performed if the hematocrit has decreased rapidly and/or if mechanical ventilation is required. Some physicians do not replace RBCs until about 10% of the blood volume has been drawn if the neonate is relatively stable and the hematocrit level reasonable.

Maintenance of Hematocrit Levels of Greater Than 0.40 During Severe Respiratory Disease.—In neonates with severe respiratory disease, particularly those requiring oxygen and/or ventilator support, it is customary to maintain the hematocrit level at greater than 0.40 (blood hemoglobin, >130 g/L). Proponents believe that transfused RBCs containing adult hemoglobin are most likely to provide satisfactory oxygen delivery throughout the period of diminished pulmonary function. Although this practice is widely recommended, little evidence is available to establish its efficacy, define its optimal use (ie, the best hematocrit level during each clinical situation), or document its risks.[25] A recent study[30] of 10 infants with severe (oxygen-dependent) bronchopulmonary dysplasia demonstrated improvement of physiologic end points (increased systemic oxygen transport and decreased oxygen use) after small-volume RBC transfusions. It is notable that the blood hemoglobin levels alone did not predict which infants would benefit from transfusion.[30] More information is needed to define the precise indications for and benefits of RBC transfusions as based on measurements of tissue oxygenation rather than on hematocrit levels alone.

Maintenance of Hematocrit Levels of Greater Than 0.40 in Neonates With Symptomatic Heart Disease.—Consistent with the rationale for optimal oxygen delivery discussed above, it seems logical to maintain hematocrit levels of greater than 0.40 in neonates with severe congenital heart disease leading to either cyanosis or congestive heart failure. Regarding the latter, isovolumic exchange transfusions were used to treat nine infants with ventricular septal defects and large left-to-right shunts.[31] The postpartum decreases in hematocrit levels had produced decreases in blood viscosity that resulted in decreased pulmonary vascular resistance and increased left-to-right shunting. Exchange transfusion increased the mean blood hemoglobin level from 99 to 146 g/L—a change that increased pulmonary vascular resistance and decreased both left-to-right shunting and pulmonary blood flow. These changes lowered heart rate and left ventricular stroke volume without compromising oxygen transport to the tissues. Extending these observations to neonatal patients with patent ductus arteriosus, Rosenthal[32] suggested that RBC transfusions might increase pulmonary vascular resistance, enhance ductal closure, and alleviate high-output cardiac failure. This indication seems tenuous. Because transfusions may transiently increase blood volume and exacerbate cardiac failure, the precise role of RBC transfusions in the treatment of severe patent ductus arteriosus requires more study.

Maintenance of Hematocrit Levels of Greater Than 0.30 in Neonates With Cardiopulmonary Problems.—Neonates who are relatively stable do not require RBC transfusions unless they exhibit clinical problems that are presumed to be related to the degree of anemia present. Proponents of transfusion therapy believe that anemia contributes to tachypnea, dyspnea, apnea, tachycardia, bradycardia, feeding difficulties, and lethargy and that these problems can be alleviated with RBC transfusions. Tachypnea, dyspnea, and apnea could be exacerbated by anemia as a consequence of decreased oxygen delivery to the respiratory center of the brain.[33] Generally, by the time healthy, premature infants reach the physiologic nadir of hemoglobin concentration, the respiratory center has become more mature and less sensitive to hypoxemia so that apnea is no longer a major problem. However, sick, premature infants become anemic earlier, and when anemia and severe apnea occur together it is tempting to believe that transfusion of RBCs might decrease the frequency of apneic episodes via an improvement in oxygen delivery to the central nervous system. Confirming the validity of this practice, RBC transfusions were shown to diminish irregular breathing patterns and episodes of bradycardia in anemic preterm infants when their mean hematocrit levels were increased from 27% to 36%.[34] However, beneficial effects of RBC transfusions on breathing patterns have not been found by all investigators.[35]

Maintenance of Hematocrit Levels of Greater Than 0.30 in Neonates With Growth Failure.—Some neonatologists consider poor weight gain to be an indication for RBC transfusion, particularly if the hemoglobin concentration is below 100 g/L (hematocrit level, less than 0.30) and other signs of distress (eg, tachycardia, respiratory difficulty, weak suck, less vigorous cry, and less activity) are evident. The validity of this practice was confirmed by studies of infants with bronchopulmonary dysplasia in whom growth failure was ascribed to increased metabolic expenditure.[36] Stockman and Clark[37] investigated the effects of

RBC transfusion on weight gain in relatively stable, low-BW infants. Thirteen infants with BWs of less than 1500 g were studied for 1 week before and after transfusion. The mean (±SD) hemoglobin concentration increased from 85±16 to 114±21 g/L by transfusion, and mean daily weight gain increased from 20.8±4.6 to 28.0±6.3 g. Infants with the lowest hemoglobin values before transfusion exhibited the greatest increase in weight. Increased weight gain was associated with decreased metabolic rates (measured by oxygen consumption). The authors considered anemia as only one of several possible causes of growth failure, and they recommended RBC transfusions for treatment of growth failure in infants with low-normal or subnormal hemoglobin levels, providing nothing else could explain the poor weight gain.[37]

Blank et al[38] found no advantage for the prophylactic use of small-volume RBC transfusions in otherwise well, growing, premature infants. Fifty-six premature infants were randomly assigned to either a mandatory (prophylactic) transfusion group (hemoglobin maintained at greater than 100 g/L) or an elective (nontransfusion) group in which RBC transfusions were permitted only for treatment of marked clinical manifestations of anemia. Only four (13%) of 30 infants in the latter group underwent transfusion electively (once each for treatment of apnea). Characteristics of all patients at birth were similar to those of fetuses at about 30 weeks' gestation, and mean BWs were 1196±279 g and 1145±251 g for mandatory and elective transfusion groups, respectively. At discharge, the infants in the elective transfusion group exhibited significantly greater anemia and reticulocyte counts than did those receiving mandatory transfusions ($P<.01$; mean hemoglobin level, 91.0±16.7 vs 117.5±17.2 g/L; and mean reticulocyte count, 6%±3% vs 3%±2%). Despite these differences, both groups were comparable in the number of days required to regain BW, discharge weight, length and cost of hospitalization, and frequency and severity of clinical problems. Thus, this study did not indicate benefits of mandatory, small-volume RBC transfusions to maintain hematocrit levels of greater than 0.30 in stable, growing, premature infants who were otherwise healthy.[38]

In a similar study, Ross et al[39] randomly assigned 16 preterm, clinically stable infants aged older than 1 month to either an RBC transfusion or a nontransfusion group. Infants with hematocrit levels of less than 0.29 were studied for 3 days before and after receiving either 10 mL of packed RBCs per kilogram of body weight or no transfusions for signs of improvement, as indicated by measures of cardiopulmonary function. Factors that identified infants most likely to benefit from RBC transfusions included pretransfusion heart rates of more than 152 beats per minute, presence of apnea/bradycardia requiring intervention, and elevated blood lactate levels.[39] Additional studies of this nature may help identify infants for whom RBC transfusions are indicated.

RBC Product for Transfusion.—The RBC product of choice for small-volume neonatal transfusions is sedimented RBC concentrate. Fresh units of whole blood are centrifuged, plasma is removed, storage additives are added as needed, and the RBC units are stored in an inverted position so that RBC concentrates with hematocrit levels approximately equal to 0.80 can be issued for transfusion. Most RBCs are infused at a dose of 5 to 15 mL/kg of body weight over 3 to 6 hours. Because of the small quantity of extracellular fluid infused (hematocrit level, ≈0.80) and the slow rate of transfusion, the type of storage medium selected is not believed to pose risks to most premature infants.[40] Based on data calculated using RBCs stored in a chemical solution (Adsol; Fenwal Laboratories, Roundlake, Ill),[40] Table 2 shows the doses of additives infused with small-volume transfusions.

Table 2.—Quantity of Additives in 10 mL of RBC Storage Solution*

Additive	Standard RBCs	Sedimented RBC Concentrate	Total Dose, mg/kg/h†	Estimated Toxic Dose
Glucose	86.0	86.0	17.20	240 mg/kg/h
Phosphate	1.3	1.3	0.26	60 mg/kg/d
Adenine	0.7	0.7	0.14	15 mg/kg/dose
Sodium	28.0	14.0	2.80	137 mg/kg/d
Citrate	6.5	3.3	0.66	180 mg/kg/h
Mannitol	22.0	11.0	2.20	360 mg/kg/d

*Data are from Luban et al.[40] RBC indicates red blood cell. Standard RBCs had hematocrit levels of 0.60, and sedimented RBC concentrate had a hematocrit level of 0.80. Values of additives in columns 2 and 3 are in milligrams. Sodium, citrate, and mannitol are confined to the extracellular fluid. Thus, the quantity infused decreases as the hematocrit level increases at the expense of a decreased extracellular fluid volume. In contrast, glucose, phosphate, and adenine are distributed throughout RBCs and the extracellular fluid and remain constant as long as the total volume infused is constant.

†Values are for 10 mL of sedimented RBC concentrate per kilogram of body weight infused over 5 hours.

As an additional consideration, the traditional use of relatively fresh RBCs (less than 7 days of storage) is being challenged in hopes that donor exposure can be diminished by using a single unit of RBCs for each infant, regardless of the duration of RBC storage.[27] Neonatologists who object to this insist on transfusing fresh RBCs generally raise two objections: the increase in plasma potassium (K^+) levels and the decrease in RBC 2,3-diphosphoglycerate levels during extended storage. After 42 days of storage, plasma K^+ levels are approximately 50 mmol/L, a value that, at first glance, seems alarmingly high. With simple calculations, however, the dose of bioavailable plasma K^+ transfused is shown to be quite small. An infant weighing 1 kg undergoing a 10–mL/kg of body weight transfusion of packed RBCs (hematocrit level, ≈0.80) will receive 2 mL of plasma, or only 0.1 mmol/L of K^+, via slow infusion. This dose is quite small compared with the usual daily K^+ requirement of 2 to 3 mmol/L per kilogram of body weight. As for the second objection, 2,3-diphosphoglycerate is totally depleted from RBCs by the 21st day of storage, and this is reflected in a p50 value that decreases from about 27 mm of Hg in fresh blood to 18 mm of Hg at outdate. The last value corresponds to the p50 in RBCs obtained from the blood of many normal premature infants at birth. Thus, the p50 of older transfused RBCs is comparable with that of RBCs produced by the infant's own bone marrow. Moreover, these older RBCs provide an advantage because the p50 of transfused RBCs (but not endogenous cells) increases rapidly after transfusion as 2,3-diphosphoglycerate regenerates within hours. Thus, small-volume transfusions with older RBCs appear to pose no substantive risks to relatively stable, premature infants, and their acceptance as a suitable blood component likely will diminish donor exposure.

Platelet Transfusions

To my knowledge, no controlled clinical trials have been reported in the literature to establish the efficacy of platelet transfusions in high-risk, thrombocytopenic infants. Based on general knowledge of the risks of thrombocytopenia and the success of platelet transfusions,[41] it seems logical for thrombocytopenic infants to undergo platelet transfusions.[42] A major indication for platelet transfusion during the perinatal period is hemorrhage in infants with blood platelet counts of less than 50×10^9/L. Platelet transfusions are also sometimes recommended for infants to treat bleeding that occurs with higher platelet counts (between 50×10^9/L and 100×10^9/L), to diminish risk of intracranial hemorrhage in high-risk premature infants with platelet counts of less than 100×10^9/L, or to prevent bleeding when platelet levels are below a predetermined value—usually between 20×10^9/L and 100×10^9/L, depending on the status of the infant being treated (prophylactic platelet transfusion).

Although the underlying cause of thrombocytopenia must be identified and treated, it seems logical, for several reasons, for neonates to undergo platelet transfusion when the blood platelet count is less than 20×10^9/L, regardless of whether overt bleeding is present. One reason is that this severity of thrombocytopenia is the level at which other patients are known to be at greatest risk of experiencing spontaneous hemorrhage.[41] Another reason is that even healthy neonates exhibit hemostatic abnormalities of both platelets and clotting proteins. Almost any type of stress can accentuate these abnormalities and/or precipitate thrombocytopenia. Neonatal platelet dysfunction and the other abnormalities of hemostasis at this age might increase the potential for actual hemorrhage beyond that expected for the severity of thrombocytopenia.[43] A third reason is that severe thrombocytopenia occurs most often in sick infants who are receiving medications that may compromise platelet function; platelet transfusion may reverse some of these adverse effects. Because all of these factors are accentuated in low-BW infants, some neonatologists prefer platelet transfusion when the platelet count is less than 50×10^9/L in stable premature neonates or less than 100×10^9/L in sick, premature neonates.[44] Intracranial hemorrhage occurs frequently during the neonatal period in sick, low-BW neonates, and although the etiologic role of thrombocytopenia and the therapeutic benefit of platelet transfusion have not been conclusively established in this disorder, it seems logical to treat severe thrombocytopenia when it occurs in high-risk infants.[44,45]

The goal of most platelet transfusions is to increase the platelet count to greater than 100×10^9/L. This can be achieved, consistently, with the infusion of 10 mL of standard platelet concentrates per kilogram of BW. These concentrates are obtained either via centrifugation of fresh units of whole blood or via automated plateletpheresis.[42] These procedures are based on the following assumptions and calculations.

1. A 50-mL platelet concentrate from whole blood contains approximately 5×10^{10} platelets. If a 300-mL apheresis platelet unit contains approximately 3×10^{11} platelets, 50 mL will contain 5×10^{10} platelets. Thus, 10 mL of most platelet concentrates will contain approximately 1×10^{10} platelets.
2. The total blood volume of a 1-kg neonate is between 80 and 100 mL. For ease of calculations, 100 mL is assumed as the blood volume into which the platelet concentrate will be infused. With a hematocrit level of 0.50, the plasma volume will be 0.05 L.
3. An infusion of 10 mL of platelet concentrate (10×10^9 platelets) into a 1-kg neonate with a 0.1-L blood volume will increase the blood platelet count by 100×10^9/L. Using the plasma volume as the volume of distribution, the platelet count would increase about 200×10^9/L. Because recovery in the bloodstream is always less than 100% of the dose infused, the yield of platelets in the concentrate is variable, and turnover is often accelerated, a postinfusion platelet count should always be obtained to determine whether additional platelet transfusions are needed.

Platelet concentrates should be transfused as rapidly as the neonate's overall condition permits, certainly within 2 hours. Generally, 10 mL/kg of BW is not an excessive volume—providing intakes of other intravenous fluids, medications, and nutrients are monitored and adjusted as needed. Although proven methods exist to reduce the volume of platelet concentrates,[46,47] additional processing should be performed with great care because of possible platelet loss, clumping, and dysfunction caused by the additional handling. Platelet concentrates contain viable lymphocytes, and, like all cellular blood products, they should be considered for irradiation to prevent graft-vs-host disease, especially when the donor and neonate recipient are first-degree relatives.

Granulocyte (Neutrophil) Transfusions

Neonates are susceptible to severe bacterial infections, and several defects of neonatal body defenses have been reported as possible contributing factors. Abnormalities of neonatal neutrophils (polymorphonuclear neutrophil leukocytes [PMNs]) include absolute and relative neutropenia, diminished chemotaxis, abnormal adhesion and aggregation, defective cellular orientation and receptor capping, decreased deformability, inability to alter membrane potential during stimulation, imbalances of oxidative metabolism, and diminished ability to withstand oxidant stress.[48] The age at which neonatal PMN defects disappear, and whether the change is abrupt or gradual, are unknown.

Neutropenia can occur during neonatal bacterial infections, particularly with fulminant sepsis. When contrasted with the neutrophilia of normal neonates, it is considered abnormal for the absolute blood PMN count to be less than 3×10^9/L during the first week of life. Although an abnormally low PMN count can occur in neonates with disorders as diverse as sepsis, asphyxia, and maternal hypertension, suspicion of severe bacterial infection must always be high when relative neutropenia (neutrophil count, less than 3×10^9/L) occurs. The mechanisms responsible are only partially known, but abnormalities of neonatal granulopoiesis frequently are involved. Committed precursors to PMN development are fewer in neonatal marrow than in the marrow of older subjects, and they proliferate at a rate close to capacity even when studied during an apparently basal state. Thus, neonatal marrow is unable to rapidly increase and sustain PMN output in response to an infection.

Granulocyte transfusions have been used to treat infections in patients of all ages exhibiting either neutropenia or PMN dysfunction. Thus, a rationale exists for combining granulocyte transfusions with antibiotics to treat septic neonates—subjects in whom both neutropenia and PMN dysfunction have been demonstrated. This topic was recently reviewed,[49] and only information particularly germane to the transfusion medicine aspects of this topic are discussed herein.

Granulocyte transfusions have been used to treat neonatal sepsis regardless of whether neutropenia is present. Neonates exhibiting fulminant sepsis, relative neutropenia (less than 3×19^9 PMNs per liter of blood during the first week of life), and severely diminished PMN marrow storage pools (less than 10% of nucleated marrow cells being postmitotic PMNs) are at particularly high risk of dying if treated only with antibiotics. Eleven publications[50-60] report the use of granulocyte transfusion to treat infected neonates. Six were designed as controlled studies.[50-53,58,59] That four of these six studies found granulocyte transfusion to be significantly beneficial is encouraging.[30-53] Although five of the six controlled studies incorporated randomized trials, two included subjects who did not undergo transfusion and who were deemed ineligible for randomization.[50,59] One study is described in two reports. It was reported first as a somewhat preliminary trial[52] and again after expansion and slight modification.[53] Although the controlled studies contained obvious flaws, they had important features.

Laurenti et al[51] studied mostly premature neonates, many of whom were infected with an antibiotic-resistant *Klebsiella* bacteria. Neutropenia was not a criterion for entry. Neonates received two to 15 daily transfusions of granulocytes prepared via filtration leukapheresis at a dose of 0.5×10^9 to 1.0×10^9 per kilogram of body weight and fared strikingly better (90% survival rate) than did those receiving only antibiotics (28% survival rate). One lesson of this study is that supplementing antibiotic therapy with granulocyte transfusion may help eradicate a resistant organism anticipated to be poorly responsive to antibiotics alone.

Christensen et al[50] studied 26 infants, all of whom had proven sepsis with some degree of neutropenia (less than 2900 PMNs per microliter).[50] All underwent bone marrow examinations, and 10 neonates were determined to have had adequate marrow PMN storage pools. These 10 were not considered to be candidates for granulocyte transfusion because of adequate marrow reserves. They were not randomized, and all survived with standard therapy that included antibiotics. The remaining 16 infants were documented to have had markedly diminished marrow PMN storage pools (less than 7% of nucleated marrow cells were postmitotic PMNs) on entering the controlled study. Neonates who underwent transfusion received one granulocyte transfusion containing 0.2×10^9 to 1.0×10^9 PMNs per kilogram of body weight (mean, 0.7×10^9) collected via intermittent-flow centrifugation leukapheresis. All seven neonates in the transfusion group survived, compared with only one of the nine control neonates, indicating that granulocyte transfusion benefits septic neonates who exhibit both relative neutropenia and severely diminished marrow PMN storage pools.

Infants received extensive granulocyte transfusion therapy in the studies by Cairo et al.[52,53] Those in the granulocyte transfusion group received a course of five transfusions (one every 12 hours); each contained 0.5×10^9 to 1.0×10^9 PMNs per kilogram of body weight collected via continuous-flow centrifugation leukapheresis. In the expanded study,[53] survival of infants in the transfusion group (95%) was significantly greater than that of controls. The results were similar whether considering all infants or only those with culture-proven sepsis. To identify prognostic features, infants who died were found to exhibit lower levels of total hemolytic complement in serum than did survivors ($P<.03$).

Results of two of the controlled trials, reported by Baley et al[58] and Wheeler et al,[59] indicated no advantage of antibiotic therapy supplemented with granulocyte transfusion compared with antibiotic therapy alone. Unlike the trials reporting the benefits of granulocyte transfusion, all of which used granulocyte concentrates prepared via automated leukapheresis, both of these studies involved the infusion of granulocytes harvested from units of whole blood. Baley et al[58] isolated PMNs via centrifugation of fresh, whole blood units, and infused 0.1×10^9 to 0.9×10^9 PMNs per kilogram of body weight (mean, 0.35×10^9) per granulocyte transfusion. Transfusion did not improve survival when results were analyzed for the entire group or for only infants with positive cultures. The study by Wheeler et al[59] can be easily criticized (few patients were randomized, doses of PMNs were small, and the quality of the PMNs were unsatisfactory). However, two lessons can be learned from this study. First, refrigerated whole blood units are likely to provide unsatisfactory products for transfusion; the mean dose of PMNs per transfusion was only 0.4×10^9 per kilogram of body weight, and the PMNs collected were of poor quality. Second, it is nearly impossible for one institution, despite the best intentions of the investigators, to provide definitive, clinical information. A carefully designed and conducted multicenter trial seems mandatory to provide clear guidance.

Granulocyte transfusions cannot now be firmly recommended to treat neonatal sepsis. However, until more information is available, it seems reasonable to consider supplementing antibiotic therapy with granulocyte transfusion for certain neonates exhibiting strong evidence (either clinically or microbiologically) of bacterial septicemia. To consider granulocyte transfusion, relative neutropenia (less than 3000 PMNs per microliter) must be present, and, in most cases, the marrow PMN storage pool should be diminished (less than 10% of marrow nucleated cells being postmitotic PMNs). The last condition can best be demonstrated with direct examination of the bone marrow. Because it is impractical to always perform a bone marrow examination, some suggest that a tentative estimate can be made indirectly using the differential white blood cell count; thus, diminished storage pools would be indicated when greater than 70% of circulating blood PMNs are immature forms, such as band cells, stabs, or metamyelocytes.[48,55,61] However, not all agree on the accuracy of this indirect method, and the precise role of the differential white blood cell count in predicting marrow storage pool size requires further study.

The ideal granulocyte product for neonatal transfusions is considered to have these characteristics: volume for infusion of 10 to 15 mL/kg of body weight; dose of PMNs per infusion, 1×10^9 to 2×10^9 per kilogram of body weight; donor seronegativity for hepatitis, cytomegalovirus, human immunodeficiency virus, human T-cell leukemia/lymphoma virus types I and II, and syphilis; and erythrocyte compatibility between donor and neonate. Until more information is available, the granulocyte product of choice is a PMN concentrate prepared via automated leukapheresis.[60,61] Local practices should be followed regarding the need to irradiate cellular blood products for use in neonates. Granulocyte concentrates must be infused promptly, certainly within a few hours of donation.

COMMENT

Transfusions of blood components are indispensable to the modern care of critically ill, premature infants. In the future, treatment with recombinant growth factors may decrease the need for homologous blood products. In particular, the treatment of neonatal anemia with erythropoietin seems promising. However, several small studies of such treatment have demonstrated little success.[62,63] Once problems are resolved to establish the optimal dose, schedule, and route of administration of erythropoietin and to ensure the availability of iron, it seems likely that the need for RBC transfusions will diminish with this treatment.

The best approach now is to transfuse blood components only when they are highly likely to benefit the neonate. Attempts must also be made to select the most effective products from the fewest donors possible. All homologous blood products pose risks, although very small, to the recipient. Remarkable strides have been made recently to diminish these risks in the standard blood supply. These improvements, coupled with the possibility that blood from directed (designated) donors may be less safe than that from volunteer donors, make it mandatory that directed donors be selected with extreme caution.[17,64] The selection of biological parental donors for neonates may be particularly dangerous because of the alloimmunization of the mother to blood cell antigens inherited by the neonate from the father.[64,65] Although some would disagree, it is my opinion that directed donors should be avoided whenever possible.[64] Obviously, this option must be made available when mandated by law and, occasionally, is the most reasonable medical approach (eg, limited-exposure donor programs and difficult compatibility problems). Finally, continued research into the pathophysiology of fetal and neonatal hematopoiesis, the effects of cytopenia (eg, anemia and thrombocytopenia) and the risk-benefit ratio of transfusion therapy is needed to ensure optimal neonatal transfusion practice.

Dr Strauss' research is supported in part by Research Career Development Award K04 HD00255 and Transfusion Medicine Academic Award K07 HL01426 from the National Institutes of Health, Bethesda, Md.

References

1. Wegman WE. Annual summary of vital statistics—1988. *Pediatrics.* 1989;84:943-955.

2. Guyer B, Wallach LA, Rosen SL. Birth-weight-standardized neonatal mortality rates and prevention of low birth weight: how does Massachusetts compare with Sweden? *N Engl J Med.* 1982;306:1230-1233.

3. Kim HC. Red blood cell transfusion in the neonate. *Semin Perinatal.* 1983;7:159-174.

4. Sacher RA, Luban NLC, Strauss RG. Current practice and guidelines for the transfusion of cellular blood components in the newborn. *Transfusion Med Rev.* 1989;3:39-54.

5. Floss AM, Strauss RG, Goeken N, Knox L. Multiple transfusions fail to provoke antibodies against blood cell antigens in human infants. *Transfusion.* 1986;26:419-422.

6. Brown MS, Berman ER, Luckey D. Prediction of the need for transfusion during anemia of prematurity. *J Pediatr.* 1990;116:773-778.

7. Council on Scientific Affairs. Autologous blood transfusions. *JAMA.* 1983;256:2378-2380.

8. Czaja AJ, Davis GL. Hepatitis non-A, non-B: manifestations and implications of acute and chronic disease. *Mayo Clin Proc.* 1982;57:639-652.

9. Rogers MF, Thomas PA, Starcher ET, Noa MC, Bush TJ, Jaffe HW. Acquired immunodeficiency syndrome in children: report of the Centers for Disease Control national surveillance, 1982 to 1985. *Pediatrics.* 1987;79:1008-1014.

10. Strauss RG. Safety of Iowa's blood supply. *Iowa Med.* 1990;80:195-198.

11. Blajchman MA, Sheridan D, Rawls WE. Risks associated with blood transfusion in newborn infants. *Clin Perinatol.* 1984;2:403-415.

12. Howell RR. The diagnostic value of serum enzyme measurements. *J Pediatr.* 1966;68:121-134.

13. Alter HJ, Purcell RH, Shih JW, et al. Detection of antibody to hepatitis C virus in prospectively following transfusion recipients with acute and chronic non-A, non-B hepatitis. *N Engl J Med.* 1989;321:1494-1500.

14. Tegtmeier GE. The use of cytomegalovirus-screened blood in neonates. *Transfusion.* 1988;28:201-203.

15. Adler SP. Transfusion-acquired CMV infection in premature infants. *Transfusion.* 1989;29:278-279.

16. American Association of Blood Banks. 13th ed. *Standards for Blood Banks and Transfusion Services.* Arlington, Va: American Association of Blood Banks; 1989:31-35.

17. Strauss RG, Barnes A, Blanchette VS, et al. Directed and limited-exposure blood donations for infants and children. *Transfusion.* 1990;30:68-72.

18. Sanders MR, Graeber JE. Posttransfusion graft-versus-host disease in infancy. *J Pediatr.* 1990;117:159-163.

19. Shaw JCL. Iron absorption by the premature infant: the effect of transfusion and iron supplements on the serum ferritin levels. *Acta Paediatr Scand.* 1982;299(suppl):83-89.

20. Adamkin DH, Shott RJ, Cook LN, Andrews BF. Nonhyperoxic retrolental fibroplasia. *Pediatrics.* 1977;60:828-830.

21. Sjoberg POJ, Bondesson UG, Sedin EG, Gustafsson JP. Exposure of newborn infants to plasticizers. *Transfusion.* 1985;25:424-428.

22. Williams RA, Brown EF, Hurst D, Franklin LC. Transfusion of infants with activation of erythrocyte T antigen. *J Pediatr.* 1989;115:949-953.

23. Pahwa S, Sia C, Harper R, Pahwa R. T lymphocyte subpopulations in high-risk infants: influence of age and blood transfusions. *Pediatrics.* 1985;76:914-917.

24. Sullivan JL. Iron, plasma antioxidants, and the 'oxygen radical disease of prematurity.' *AJDC.* 1988;142:1341-1344.

25. Strauss RG. Current issues in neonatal transfusions. *Vox Sang.* 1986;51:1-9.

26. Blanchette VS, Zipursky A. Assessment of anemia in newborn infants. *Clin Perinatol.* 1984;11:489-510.

27. Strauss RG, Sacher RA, Blazina JF, et al. Commentary on small-volume red cell transfusions for neonatal patients. *Transfusion.* 1990;30:565-570.

28. Lenes BA, Sacher RA. Blood component therapy in neonatal medicine. *Clin Lab Med.* 1981;1:285-309.

29. Stockman JA. Anemia of prematurity. Current concepts in the issue of when to transfuse. *Pediatr Clin North Am.* 1986;33:111-128.

30. Alverson DC, Isken VH, Cohen RS. Effect of booster blood transfusions on oxygen utilization in infants with bronchopulmonary dysplasia. *J Pediatr.* 1988;113:722-726.

31. Lister G, Hellenbrand WE, Kleinman CS, Talner NS. Physiologic effects of increasing hemoglobin concentration in left-to-right shunting in infants with ventricular septal defects. *N Engl J Med.* 1982;306:502-506.

32. Rosenthal A. Hemodynamics in physiologic anemia of infancy. *N Engl J Med.* 1982;306:538-540.

33. Kattwinkel J. Neonatal apnea: pathogenesis and therapy. *J Pediatr.* 1977;90:342-347.

34. Joshi A, Gerhardt T, Shandloff P, Bankalari E. Blood transfusion effect on the respiratory pattern of preterm infants. *Pediatrics.* 1987;80:79-84.

35. Keyes WG, Donohue PK, Spivak JL, Jones MD Jr, Oski FA. Assessing the need for transfusion of premature infants and role of hematocrit, clinical signs, and erythropoietin level. *Pediatrics.* 1989;84:412-417.
36. Kurzner SI, Garg M, Gautista DB, et al. Growth failure in infants with bronchopulmonary dysplasia: nutrition and elevated resting metabolic expenditure. *Pediatrics.* 1988;81:379-384.
37. Stockman JA, Clark DA. Weight gain: a response to transfusion in selected preterm infants. *AJDC.* 1984;138:828-830.
38. Blank JP, Sheagren TG, Vajaria J, Mangurten HH, Benawra RS, Puppala BL. The role of RBC transfusion in the premature infant. *AJDC.* 1984;138:831-833.
39. Ross MP, Christensen RD, Rothstein G, et al. A randomized trial to develop criteria for administering erythrocyte transfusions to anemic preterm infants 1 to 3 months of age. *J Perinatol.* 1989;9:246-253.
40. Luban NLC, Strauss RG, Hume HA. Commentary on the safety of red blood cells preserved in extended storage media for neonatal transfusions. *Transfusion.* 1990;31:229-235.
41. Strauss RG. The risks of thrombocytopenia and the standard uses of platelet transfusions. *Plasma Ther Transfusion Technol.* 1986;7:279-285.
42. Strauss RG. Perinatal platelet and granulocyte transfusions. In: Kennedy MS, Wilson S, Kelton J, eds. *Perinatal Transfusion Medicine.* Arlington, Va: American Association of Blood Banks; 1990:123-144.
43. Gibson B. Neonatal haemostasis. *Arch Dis Child.* 1989;64:503-506.
44. Andrew M, Castle V, Saigal S, Carter C, Kelton JG. Clinical impart of neonatal thrombocytopenia. *J Pediatr.* 1987;110:457-464.
45. Lupton BA, Hill A, Whitfield MR, Carter CJ, Wadsworth LD, Roland EH. Reduced platelet count as a risk factor for intraventricular hemorrhage. *AJDC.* 1988;142:1222-1224.
46. Moroff G, Friedman A, Robkin-Kline L, Gautier G, Luban NLC. Reduction of the volume of stored platelet concentrates for use in neonatal patients. *Transfusion.* 1984;24:144-146.
47. Simon TL, Sierra ER. Concentration of platelet units into small volumes. *Transfusion.* 1984;24:173-175.
48. Strauss RG. Granulopoiesis and neutrophil function in the neonate. In: Stockman JA, Pochedly C, eds. *Developmental and Neonatal Hematology.* New York, NY: Raven Press; 1988:88-101.
49. Cairo MS. Neonatal neutrophil host defense. *AJDC.* 1989;143:40-46.
50. Christensen RD, Rothstein G, Anstall HB, Bybee B. Granulocyte transfusions in neonates with bacterial infection, neutropenia and depletion of mature marrow neutrophils. *Pediatrics.* 1982;70:1-6.
51. Laurenti F, Ferro R, Isacchi G, et al. Polymorphonuclear leukocyte transfusion for the treatment for sepsis in the newborn infant. *J Pediatr.* 1981;98:118-123.
52. Cairo MS, Rucker R, Bennetts GA, et al. Improved survival of newborns receiving leukocyte transfusions for sepsis. *Pediatrics.* 1984;74:887-892.
53. Cairo MS, Worcester C, Rucker R, et al. Role of circulating complement and polymorphonuclear leukocyte transfusion in treatment and outcome in critically ill neonates with sepsis. *J Pediatr.* 1987;110:935-941.
54. DeCurtin M, Romano G, Scarpato N, D'Antonia F, Paludetto R, Ciccimara F. Transfusions of polymorphonuclear leukocytes (PMN) in an infant with necrotizing enterocolitis (NEC) and a defect of phagocytosis. *J Pediatr.* 1981;99:665-668.
55. Christensen RD, Anstall H, Rothstein G. Neutrophil transfusion in septic neutropenic neonates. *Transfusion.* 1982;22:151-154.
56. Laing IA, Boulton FE, Hume R. Polymorphonuclear leukocyte transfusion in neonatal septicemia. *Arch Dis Child.* 1983;58:1003-1005.
57. Laurenti F, LaGreca G, Ferro R, Bucci G. Transfusion of polymorphonuclear neutrophils in premature infant with *Klebsiella* sepsis. *Lancet.* 1978;2:111-112.
58. Baley JE, Stork EK, Warkentin PI, Shurin SB. Buffy coat transfusions in neutropenic neonates with presumed sepsis: a prospective, randomized trial. *Pediatrics.* 1987;80:712-720.
59. Wheeler JC, Chauvenet AR, Johnson CA, et al. Buffy coat transfusions in neonates with sepsis and neutrophil storage pool depletion. *Pediatrics.* 1987;97:422-425.
60. Newman RS, Waffarn F, Simmons GE, Goldsticker RD, Pcariz JA. Questionable value of saline prepared granulocytes in the treatment of neonatal septicemia. *Transfusion.* 1988;28:196-197.
61. Strauss RG. Current status of granulocyte transfusions to treat neonatal sepsis. *J Clin Apheresis.* 1989;5:25-29.
62. Halpern DS, Wacher P, Lacourt G, et al. Effects of recombinant human erythropoietin in infants with the anemia of prematurity: a pilot study. *J Pediatr.* 1990;116:779-786.
63. Shannon KE, Mentzer WC, Abels RI, et al. Recombinant human erythropoietin (r-Hu-EPO) in anemia of prematurity (ACP): preliminary results of a double-blind placebo controlled pilot study. *Pediatr Res.* 1990;27:269A. Abstract.
64. Strauss RG. Directed and limited-exposure donor programs for children. In: Sacher RA, Strauss RG, eds. *Contemporary Issues in Pediatric Transfusion Medicine.* Arlington, Va: American Association of Blood Banks; 1989:1-11.
65. Elbert C, Strauss RG, Barrett F, Goeken NE, Pittner B, Cordle D. Biological mothers may be dangerous donors for their neonates. *Acta Haematol.* 1991. In press.

An Optimal Balance

Innovation through acellular pertussis technology

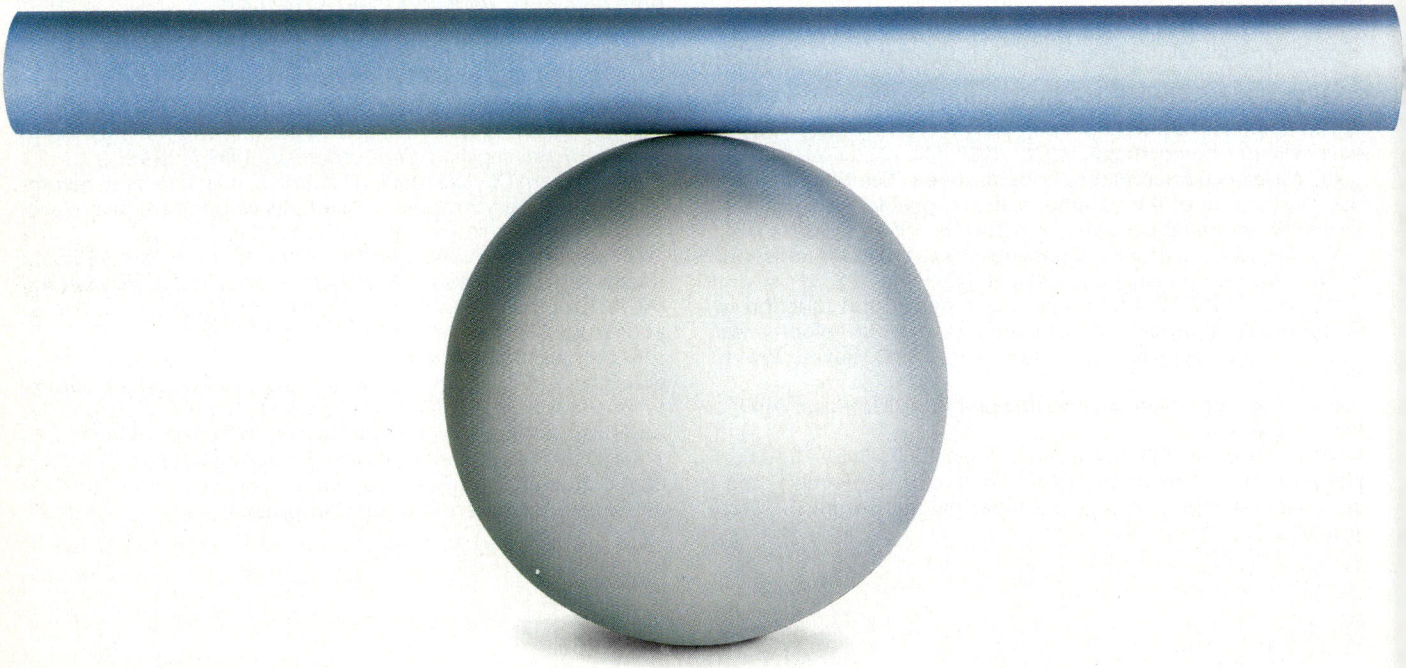

CONNAUGHT LABORATORIES, INC.
A PASTEUR MÉRIEUX COMPANY

Testing the Psychogenic Vomiting Diagnosis

Four Pediatric Patients

Joseph Gonzalez-Heydrich, MD; John Alan Kerner, Jr, MD; Hans Steiner, MD

• We treated four patients with chronic vomiting during childhood in whom a tentative diagnosis of psychogenic vomiting was made after an extensive evaluation. In each case, the diagnosis was reconsidered during the course of treatment, as observations about the patients and their response to interventions accumulated. In three instances, these observations did not fit those expected if the diagnosis of psychogenic vomiting was correct. This led to a reexamination of the organic evaluation and the discovery of an undiagnosed organic contribution to the vomiting. In the fourth patient, gastric emptying studies confirmed that there was a strong psychological contribution to the vomiting, and helped to more carefully define this contribution. Family and individual psychotherapy and treatment were aided by the greater clarity in diagnosis.

(*AJDC.* 1991;145:913-916)

Chronic unexplained vomiting presents a difficult diagnostic challenge. The differential diagnosis includes organic causes, yet psychogenic disorders are among the most commonly diagnosed. Diagnostic tests, hospitalization, and psychiatric evaluation are associated with certain risks and morbidity, especially in pediatric patients. Thus, the decision as to what tests to perform and when to stop the search for an organic cause is a difficult one. In the presence of obvious psychiatric disease, consideration of organic causes and further diagnostic evaluation may come to a halt. A recent article on the diagnosis and treatment of unexplained vomiting illustrates both the conventional wisdom and some of its difficulties.[1] After a very thorough history, physical examination, blood tests, and radiologic or endoscopic examinations of the upper gastrointestinal (GI) tract, Malagelada and Camilleri[1] recommended, "in the absence of obvious central, labyrinthine, or psychiatric disease, one may proceed with therapeutic trials as outlined above or move on to more specialized investigations, such as gastric emptying studies and gastrointestinal manometry." Despite a warning in their article that "the presence of neurosis in a patient may be a consequence of the chronic vomiting rather than the cause," in our experience the diagnostic evaluation often does come to a halt when substantial psychopathology is identified. In many instances, this termination of the physical evaluation is appropriate, yet in three of the four patients described herein, all cared for within a 4-month period in the psychosomatic unit at Children's Hospital at Stanford (Calif) University Medical Center, it would not have been. For the fourth patient, continued diagnostic evaluation provided strong evidence of a psychogenic influence on the vomiting and helped direct treatment toward that influence.

Accepted for publication October 8, 1990.

From the Departments of Psychiatry and Neurology (Dr Gonzalez-Heydrich), Pediatrics (Dr Kerner), and Psychiatry, Division of Child Psychiatry (Dr Steiner), Stanford (Calif) University Medical Center. Dr Gonzalez-Heydrich is now in private practices in Los Angeles.

Reprint requests to Packard Children's Hospital at Stanford, 725 Welch Rd, Palo Alto, CA 94304 (Dr Steiner).

PATIENT REPORTS

Patient 1.—The first patient was a previously healthy 8-year-old girl whose illness began with substernal pain. She was diagnosed as having bronchitis and was treated with anhydrous ampicillin. One day later, she began to have protracted emesis, syncope, and headache. She was admitted to a community hospital for 2 weeks and was then readmitted for 1 month because of the same symptoms. An initial upper GI series showed a partial small-bowel obstruction, but subsequent upper endoscopy yielded normal findings, except for "increased mucus in the esophagus." Two weeks after her initial radiologic examination, she underwent a complete upper GI series with small-bowel follow-through, the findings of which were interpreted as normal. She underwent extensive evaluation at her community hospital and subsequently at a tertiary care pediatric hospital before she was transferred to the psychosomatic unit at Stanford University Medical Center. These evaluations included abdominal and pelvic computed tomography, abdominal ultrasound examination, electroencephalography, and magnetic resonance imaging of the head, as well as numerous blood chemistry evaluations; all yielded normal findings. At the tertiary care pediatric hospital, the impression of the pediatric GI and neurology services was that the cause of the vomiting was psychogenic. The neurologist suggested to the family that their child might have been sexually abused.

She was transferred to the psychosomatic unit at Children's Hospital at Stanford University Medical Center, a combined psychiatric and pediatric ward. She was receiving nasogastric (NG) tube feeding; previous total parenteral nutrition through a central line had been discontinued because of septicemia. Repeated electroencephalography and a gastric emptying study were performed; both yielded normal findings. A careful physical examination to identify signs of sexual abuse was unrevealing. The patient and her family were evaluated by the family therapy team. The mother was judged to have a borderline personality disorder, and the child was noted to be very depressed. A behavioral "loop" was identified that was thought to explain the child's vomiting. It was observed that when the patient made reasonable demands for her mother's support during conflicts with a sibling, she was reprimanded; however, when she vomited or had abdominal pain, her mother would comfort her. A behavioral program seeking to discourage regressed behavior and reward age-appropriate behavior was instituted, which resulted in some improvement in the child's functioning on the unit; however, the vomiting and complaints of severe substernal pain continued. Meanwhile NG tubes became increasingly difficult to place. The psychiatric resident observed that while treatment directed toward correction of the behavioral loop had resulted in the child exhibiting less regressed behavior, it had not affected the severity of the vomiting. He noted the tremendous difficulty the pediatric team was having placing the NG tubes and did not believe that this could be explained by the child's lack of cooperation. He ordered a barium swallow examination and enlisted the mother's cooperation in getting the child to drink the contrast agent. The barium swallow showed a dilated, residue-filled esophagus with apparent tapering at the gastroesophageal junction. Upper esophagoscopy and esophageal manometry confirmed the diagnosis of achalasia. A review of the radiologic studies from the referring hospitals showed that the two upper GI contrast studies had been performed through an NG tube because the child would not cooperate; thus, the esophagus had not been visualized. On our own unit, the presence of a clear psychiatric disorder in the mother and disturbed family relations delayed the discovery of the diagnosis by 2 months.

Patient 2.—The second patient was a 6-year-old girl who was transferred from another tertiary care hospital for investigation of intractable vomiting and abdominal pain that were thought to be psychogenic. During the 15 months before her arrival at Stanford University Medical Center, she was hospitalized four times for abdominal pain, vomiting, and dehydration. Abdominal and head computed tomography, electroencephalography, upper and lower GI series, and blood studies had been performed, but the findings were normal.

During the child's first episode of vomiting, she had been noted to be depressed and was referred to a child psychiatrist. It was noted that her symptoms began soon after the birth of her sister. Also, her mother was depressed for approximately 1 year after the birth and was treated with antidepressant medication. One of the episodes of vomiting that led to hospitalization began the night of her parents' marriage; they had lived together, unmarried, for 10 years. She underwent psychotherapy and was treated with 25 mg/d of imipramine hydrochloride without improvement.

On admission to our psychosomatic unit, she was noted to be very anxious and to have a major depression. She required NG tube feedings and intravenous fluids. A gastric emptying study showed a half-life of 3 hours (markedly delayed), so treatment with metoclopramide hydrochloride was initiated, eventually reaching 0.2 mg/kg per day. Her emesis initially decreased but then worsened. She confided to the nursing staff that her parents beat her and that her father petted her in the genital area. A physical examination revealed bruises on her back, but the genital examination revealed no abnormal findings. The Child Protective Services was called, and the child placed in protective custody.

At this point, the parents became very uncooperative and menacing, and the child's vomiting increased in frequency. Given the allegations of child abuse, the parents' behavior, and the previous organic evaluation that yielded normal findings, a diagnosis of psychogenic vomiting was considered to be likely. It was believed that the vomiting was a symbolic communication and anxiety-binding compromise to deal with the trauma of sexual and physical abuse and/or a somatic manifestation of intense anxiety brought about by the disordered family system and the abuse. The characteristics of the child's vomiting were then reexamined to see if they fit the above psychogenic diagnosis. The child psychiatry fellow noted the child's complaints of abdominal pain just before vomiting and believed they were not typical of psychogenic vomiting. Thus, she ordered further GI evaluation. A repeated gastric emptying study while the patient was receiving metoclopramide showed delayed emptying, and an upper GI series showed markedly reduced gastric motility. Endoscopy showed esophagitis and reverse peristalsis of the duodenum. As the parents became more calm, the frequency of the child's vomiting decreased so that despite the finding of a physical abnormality, her psychological state also seemed to influence her symptoms. Child Protective Services' protective custody of the child was lifted by court order, and the parents decided to transfer her to another hospital for further evaluation of her vomiting.

Follow-up information from the other hospital revealed a continued pattern of vomiting during the next 2 years, difficulties within the family, and anxiety and depression in the child. The vomiting had resulted in an additional nine hospitalizations during those 2 years, despite continued psychiatric and pediatric interventions. Subsequent to leaving our unit, the patient's esophageal manometry revealed normal findings, but radiologic examinations of the upper GI tract showed a very atonic stomach and a very slow transit time through the small bowel.

Patient 3.—The third patient was an 8-year-old girl who suffered from glycogen storage disease type IB, the diagnosis of which had been made at birth. She presented to our child psychosomatic unit after a 2-year history of behavioral problems, culminating in a suicide attempt by disconnecting her NG tube feeding machine. Because of her glycogen storage disease, she was unable to maintain an adequate serum glucose concentration without constant NG tube feedings during the night. Thus, when she disconnected her tube, it resulted in severe hypoglycemia, seizures, and respiratory arrest.

After physical stabilization, she was transferred to our psychosomatic unit. There the myriad of family, social, and individual problems that she was experiencing became apparent; the child psychiatry staff engaged her and her family around these issues. Both the pediatric and pediatric GI services monitored the patient daily and managed her multiple medical problems, which included her glycogen storage disease and its resulting cyclic neutropenia, hyperuricemia, anemia, and multiple infections. Before transfer to the psychosomatic unit, she was noted to have vomiting and abdominal pain. Multiple gastric emptying studies showed either slow but steady emptying or normal emptying. Abdominal ultrasound examinations revealed no abnormalities. Despite treatment with metoclopramide, she continued to vomit two to three times per day, to complain of abdominal pain, and to have diarrhea. Her stools were guaiac positive. Stool examinations for viral and bacterial pathogens yielded normal findings. However, as repeated examinations by both pediatric and pediatric GI teams showed no cause for the emesis and as it remained unresponsive to any treatment, it was ascribed to psychological factors. The milieu staff noted that she vomited when upset about limit setting or about her mother's visits. The vomiting was seen as an expression of her desire to strike out at milieu staff and at her mother. She was encouraged to express her feelings verbally instead of by vomiting.

This situation continued until 2 months after admission. The psychiatry resident made a flow chart of the number of emesis episodes and stools per day vs maternal visits. When no correlation was found, the resident asked the pediatricians to reexamine the child for organic causes of vomiting. When a physical examination revealed no organic cause, the psychiatry resident again reviewed the results of the studies performed to date and, noting that it had not been done yet, he ordered a stool ova and parasite examination. The stool was shown to be harboring *Giardia lamblia,* and the patient was treated with oral furazolidone for 7 days. Her emesis and diarrhea improved, but her psychiatric difficulties persisted. She was not discharged from the unit for another 2 months.

Patient 4.—The fourth patient was a previously healthy 7-year-old girl who was admitted to our psychosomatic unit after four hospitalizations and an extensive pediatric evaluation in her community failed to identify a cause of her vomiting. Her weight had decreased from 21.6 to 15.3 kg since the onset of her illness. The only abnormal finding from her diagnostic evaluation was some mild inflammation of the gastroesophageal junction found at biopsy with otherwise normal endoscopic findings. A stool examination revealed no parasites but was positive for rotavirus 1 month after the illness onset. Head computed tomography demonstrated an Arnold-Chiari malformation type I, and magnetic resonance imaging of the head showed slightly enlarged cerebellar tonsils. On admission to our pediatric psychosomatic unit, it was noted that since the onset of this child's illness, there had been increased stress at home. A mental status examination revealed a tearful, very withdrawn, and anxious child. She continued to vomit to the point that she needed parenteral nutrition. A gastric emptying study showed mild delay, and metoclopramide was prescribed. Because her father was perceived to be intrusive, sexual abuse was suspected. An investigation revealed no evidence of sexual abuse. However, during the investigation, which lasted 1 week, her parents were not allowed to visit her. During this time, she stopped vomiting, began to eat, and became outgoing, active, and assertive. After the parents were allowed to visit again, vomiting resumed, and she became withdrawn. A repeated gastric emptying study showed marked delay. Because the father was present during the test and was noted to be extremely intrusive and anxious, the gastroenterologist requested that it be repeated with the father absent. This was done, and the test revealed normal findings just a few hours after the previous test. The father's level of intrusiveness and the family's general level of stress were addressed in family therapy, with improvement in the child's vomiting. A couple of days before discharge, the child expressed apprehension and began vomiting again. She was transferred back to her community hospital, where she and her family continued individual and family therapy.

COMMENT

Although psychogenic vomiting is frequently diagnosed, it has received relatively little attention in the literature. Those reports that have been published seem to fall into one of two categories: (1) case reports and commentaries emphasizing psychodynamic, family systems and cultural causes, with the treatments targeted accordingly,[2-7] and (2) case series demonstrating organic disease in individuals diagnosed as having psychogenic vomiting.[8] The researchers in the first category have emphasized the role of stress in causing psychogenic vomiting and have described many sources of that stress. These investigators have called attention to the presence in some of their patients of a perception of being trapped in a hostile relationship,[2] cultural or family dynamic conflicts,[3] and emotional upset or profound psychic disturbance within the vomiting individual.[4] They have also proposed some predisposing factors, including parental loss, a family history of vomiting,[2] and prolonged symbiotic relationships with a failure of separation individuation in the child.[5] In addition Rosenthal et al[6] and Wruble et al[7] have described the natural history of psychogenic vomiting and noted that, at the time of follow-up, almost all patients are improved but still vomiting, regardless of whether or not they received psychotherapy. There are several problems with this literature, however. There is no way offered to distinguish whether the conflicts described above in the individual and the family are causing the vomiting, are themselves the result of the chronic vomiting, or simply coincident with it. Another problem is in the definition of psychogenic vomiting as vomiting for which no physical cause can be found.[4] This presumes that, with our present technology, we are able to detect all organic abnormalities that can cause vomiting.

Among authors who are skeptical of the diagnosis of psychogenic vomiting, Stacher[8] describes 58 patients referred for either dysphagia or chronic vomiting and in whom the condition was thought to be psychogenic by the referring physicians. He reported that all were found to be suffering from organic disorders: achalasia, esophageal motility disorders, gastric ulcer, or gastroesophageal reflux. A problem with this analysis is that it is unclear whether the motility disorders are the only factor influencing the vomiting or whether psychological factors could be influencing the vomiting despite the presence of organic disease.

Recently, Abell and coworkers[9] examined eight adults with recurrent cyclic vomiting in whom no demonstrable lesions were found either in the gastrointestinal tract by endoscopy and barium studies or in the central nervous system by computed tomography or electroencephalography. All eight had abnormalities of gastrointestinal motility during an asymptomatic period—gastric hypomotility in five, small-bowel dysmotility in six, delayed gastric emptying in two, and gastric dysrhythmia in two. Abell and coworkers concluded that idiopathic cyclic nausea and vomiting may be related to altered gastrointestinal motility. However, of five patients who underwent psychological evaluation, one was diagnosed as having depression and two others were thought to have psychosomatic preoccupation on the basis of the Minnesota Multiphasic Personality Inventory. An editorial[10] in the same journal issue described the confusion that exists in the basic concept of "functional" gastrointestinal disease, especially in light of recent data that an organic basis, such as vagal neuropathy[11] or autonomic denervation,[12] may exist for the development of the irritable bowel syndrome. As stated previously, even in patients with documented motility abnormalities, it may be that these are not the only cause of the recurrent vomiting symptoms.

As the above-mentioned reports illustrate, the literature on psychogenic vomiting parallels the archaic organic/functional dichotomy that until recently dominated medicine and psychiatry. Interactions between stress and a gastrointestinal system with a low threshold for vomiting are not emphasized. The implication is that cases can be neatly separated into organic or functional vomiting and that the diagnosis of psychogenic vomiting is strictly one of exclusion. No way of making the diagnosis of psychogenic vomiting on the basis of an abnormal finding is offered nor are criteria offered for the rejection of the psychogenic diagnosis when the organic evaluation yields normal findings.

An underlying assumption of the articles that discuss psychogenic vomiting from a psychological perspective seems to be that we are able, with our present technology, to detect all organic contributions to the vomiting. The assumption of the article discussing psychogenic vomiting as misdiagnosed organic vomiting seems to be that if an abnormality is found on a physical test, then there is no psychogenic contribution to the vomiting. In our opinion, neither of these assumptions is warranted. The four patients described above demonstrate some of the pitfalls of these assumptions and the dualistic paradigm underlying them. They also illustrate some different ways to proceed diagnostically.

All four patients underwent extensive inpatient pediatric scrutiny for several months before objective evidence for an organic contribution to their vomiting surfaced. For the first patient, the substantial psychiatric dysfunction in the family and child contributed to the omission of an important early step in the evaluation of chronic unexplained vomiting: visualization of the esophagus during the upper GI study. Our patient would not swallow the contrast material, and the child psychiatry team needed to enlist the mother's help in getting the child to cooperate. Moreover, the psychiatry resident had to draw on his experience in psychiatrically and medically treating children to realize that the psychogenic hypothesis could not explain how a child (no matter how oppositional and stubborn) could impede the downward progress of an NG tube once it was in the esophagus. In this case, psychiatric and organic disease coexisted. It should be noted that the endoscopy at our hospital during which achalasia was noted took place 3 months after the study performed at the outside hospital, during which only increased mucus was noted. Either the outside hospital study was in error or the achalasia was very early in its evolution at the time of the initial study.

For the second child, objective evidence of a physical abnormality was also found. Again, the preponderance of psychiatric disease in the child and family as well as the timing of the onset of symptoms would have led many reasonable clinicians to abandon the consideration of an organic cause after the extensive initial evaluation revealed no abnormality. Yet the physician treating the child, because she had pediatric and psychiatric experience treating children, was able to press for further work-up when the psychogenic hypothesis could not fully explain the observed characteristics of the child's vomiting. The third child's history, in addition to illustrating the above points again, also shows the dangers of relying too heavily on correlations between variables such as maternal visits and vomiting that are casually observed rather than formally tested against the documentation in the chart.

The findings of the fourth child's evaluation illustrate how vomiting can be a somatic manifestation of stress. The gastroenterologist subjected this hypothesis to a rigorous test. The reasoning behind this test is as follows: if the stress the child is feeling is contributing to her vomiting because it is slowing the transit through her stomach and if a major part of her stress is being caused by the immediate intrusiveness of her father, then one may predict that if the father leaves the room, then the child's gastric emptying might improve. The findings confirmed the hypothesis and aided in guiding treatment and strengthening the treatment alliance with the family. For all four children, the child's psychologic state and the contingencies impinging on their behavior were observed to influence the severity of the vomiting. Thus, one should avoid the trap of reductionism.

If the history of these four children and our review of the literature contain any lessons for those faced with similar diagnostic conundrums, they might be as follows: First, constantly rethink the diagnosis. If the primary diagnosis is organic, can dynamic, interpersonal, or environmental factors be contributing as well? If the primary diagnosis is psychogenic, could psychopathology in the patient or family have sabotaged the organic evaluation? Could the limitations of the available technology allow one to miss an organic disease? Could a previously undiagnosable disease, organic or psychologic, become more apparent with time? Thus, it is imperative that the clinician supervising the care of these patients have a firm grasp of physical medicine and psychology. Also, it is important that psychiatry and pediatrics work together as a team and pool their experience to think through these patients' evaluations.

Second, make predictions based on the diagnosis of what you would expect to see in the history, presentation, laboratory examinations, and response to treatment; then, test these predictions. If the diagnosis is psychogenic, three constellations need to be distinguished and looked for, alone and in combination: (1) vomiting as a symbolic communication and anxiety-binding compromise (for this constellation, one needs to be able to demonstrate a conflict, a traumatic event and primary and secondary gain); (2) vomiting as a willful, manipulative act (malingering, Munchausen syndrome, and Munchausen syndrome by proxy); and (3) vomiting as a somatic equivalent of anxiety, ie, a nonspecific, nonsymbolic expression of current conflict.

The possibility must always be entertained that psychiatric and pediatric diseases coexist and interact without any causal connection. Positive evidence for each of these should be looked for, and the clinician should also think about what would suffice to convince him or her to abandon the diagnosis. Last, we would emphasize again that as true psychiatric disease makes the orderly pursuit of an evaluation much more difficult, the presence of definable psychiatric disease should lead the clinician to intensify rather than relax his or her scrutiny of the differential diagnosis and adequacy of the organic evaluation.

The authors thank Mark Perl, MD, for his advice and comments on the manuscript and Darcia Elliott for editorial assistance.

References

1. Malagelada JR, Camilleri M. Unexplained vomiting: a diagnostic challenge. *Ann Intern Med.* 1984;101:211-218.

2. Hill WH. Psychogenic vomiting. *Gut.* 1968;9:348-352.

3. Clarke DJ, Salmons PH, Harrison T. Psychogenic vomiting among female Asian migrants to the United Kingdom. *Int J Soc Psychiatry.* 1988;34:221-229.

4. Leibovich MA. Psychogenic vomiting. *Psychother Psychosom.* 1973;22:263-268.

5. Reinhart JB. Disorders of the gastrointestinal tract in children: consultation-liaison experience. *Psychiatr Clin North Am.* 1982;5:387-397.

6. Rosenthal RH, Webb WL, Wruble LD. Diagnosis and management of persistent psychogenic vomiting. *Psychosomatics.* 1980;21:722-730.

7. Wruble LD, Rosenthal RH, Webb WL. Psychogenic vomiting: a review. *Am J Gastroenterol.* 1982;77:318-321.

8. Stacher G. Differentialdiagnose psychosomatischer Schluckstorungen. *Wien Klin Wochenschr.* 1986;98:658-663.

9. Abell TL, Kim CH, Malagelada JR. Idiopathic cyclic nausea and vomiting: a disorder of gastrointestinal motility? *Mayo Clin Proc.* 1988;63:1169-1175.

10. Camilleri M. Organic basis for symptoms in functional gastrointestinal disease? *Mayo Clin Proc.* 1988;63:1256-1257.

11. Smart HL, Atkinson M. Abnormal vagal function in irritable bowel syndrome. *Lancet.* 1987;2:475-478.

12. Camilleri M, Fealey RD. Idiopathic autonomic denervation (AD): an unrecognized cause of dysmotility in patients with apparently functional bowel disorders. *Gastroenterology.* 1988;95:858. Abstract.

A Practical Guide to Successful Breast-feeding Management

Gary L. Freed, MD; Susan Landers, MD; Richard J. Schanler, MD

• It is often difficult for new mothers to know whom to approach for the necessary guidance and practical problem solving required for successful long-term lactation. Although obstetricians are familiar with the care of the breast, they may not maintain the degree of postpartum follow-up necessary to ensure its proper function nor is it their responsibility to ensure that the infant receives proper nourishment. Pediatricians are expected to offer advice and information regarding not only the advantages and disadvantages of breastfeeding but also practical management of this art. We provide a guide for practitioners who wish to assist breast-feeding mothers and their infants.
(*AJDC.* 1991;145:917-921)

Demonstrable knowledge regarding breast-feeding and experience in counseling nursing mothers are important to parents and contribute to their selection of a primary care pediatrician. Unfortunately, few house staff training programs provide sufficient education about this physiologic function. As a result, most pediatricians today enter practice unaware of how to manage the common problems of breast-feeding, such as cracked nipples, poor latch-on, mastitis, and supplemental feeding. When confronted with lactation difficulty in a new mother, many find it easiest to recommend formula to prevent further problems.

Historically, it has not always been incumbent on the pediatrician to be well versed in the practical management of lactation. In past generations, breast-feeding was handled within the extended family, and the art was passed from mother to daughter. However, in the early 1950s, the incidence of breast-feeding in the United States began to decrease, and formula feeding became the predominant mode of infant feeding. This was a result of the development of safe and affordable infant formulas, complex social and cultural pressures influencing women, and the failure of the medical profession to promote the benefits of breast-feeding.[1] The incidence of breast-feeding increased during the 1970s and peaked in the mid-1980s. Nationwide figures for 1983 indicated that 62% of women chose to breast-feed their newborns.[2] These figures may be somewhat misleading, as studies tend to define breast-feeding as nursing at least once per day. Therefore, the incidence of exclusive breast-feeding in the first few months after birth may be lower. To increase the incidence of breast-feeding, pediatricians must possess greater knowledge of the practice of this art, the difficulties that may be encountered, and the solutions to those difficulties.

Our objective is to provide resident physicians-in-training with a practical guide for counseling about breast-feeding in the prenatal and postnatal periods.

Accepted for publication January 3, 1991.
From the Department of Pediatrics, Baylor College of Medicine, Houston, Tex.
Reprint requests to the Department of Pediatrics, Baylor College of Medicine, CNRC, 1100 Bates St, Houston, TX 77030 (Dr Schanler).

PREPARATION FOR BREAST-FEEDING

The initial contact pediatricians have with a new mother is usually during the third trimester of pregnancy at the prenatal interview. This is an ideal time to inquire about choice of infant feeding and to reinforce breast-feeding when appropriate. Although some studies have shown that infant feeding decisions are made before the third trimester,[3] choices may have been influenced by certain misconceptions or fears held by the expectant mother or father. Some of these commonly held misconceptions and fears regarding breast-feeding are summarized in Table 1. Pediatricians should discuss these fears and any differences of opinion between parents over preferred feeding methods. The parents' attitudes and opinions should be explored so that myths can be openly dispelled.

The American Academy of Pediatrics recommends exclusive breast-feeding during the first 6 months of life. Benefits to the child from breast-feeding, such as improved mother-infant bonding; reduced incidence of gastroenteritis and otitis media; reduced frequency of hospital admissions; protective immunity against fungal, viral, and bacterial infections; and reduced incidence of allergic diseases, should be presented.[4-8] However, when informed parents decide against breast-feeding, it is important for the pediatrician to support them. Pediatricians should encourage prospective mothers to attend classes on breast-feeding, because the likelihood of breast-feeding success is increased by providing mothers with specific knowledge about breast-feeding and the support of other nursing mothers.[9] Pediatricians should become familiar with

Table 1.—Some Commonly Held Misconceptions and Fears Regarding Breast-feeding
1. Inadequate milk supply secondary to small breast size.
2. Loss of sexual breast activity during lactation.
3. Cosmetic breast changes as a result of lactation.
4. Previous generation failure of breast-feeding.
5. Poor nutritional content of breast milk ("not rich enough").
6. Difficulty in learning how to breast-feed.
7. Disapproval of spouse.
8. Poor public acceptance.
9. Loss of freedom or spontaneity.

local community breast-feeding support groups and encourage parental participation. Pediatricians should advocate the assistance of lactation support teams that are currently employed in many hospitals to assist new mothers before discharge. Frequently, the pediatrician's office personnel are the initial contact for mothers who call with lactation problems. Therefore, the office staff should be appropriately trained regarding lactation management.

A thorough understanding of specific problems commonly encountered by breast-feeding mothers, together with proper intervention and treatment, is required to provide adequate support and counseling to breast-feeding mothers.[10] Prenatal interviews and discussions with expectant mothers will serve to define their knowledge base and to uncover potential problems.

PRENATAL CONCERNS

Inverted Nipples

Although a substantial number of problems encountered in breast-feeding are due to variant nipple morphologic features, such as flat or inverted nipples, pediatricians do not examine the breasts of an expectant mother during a prenatal interview. The normal nipple may be flush or confluent with the areola but will become erect with the stimulation provided by the newborn's sucking. The inverted nipple will retract into the areola when pinched between the thumb and index finger. Ideally, this condition should be identified prenatally so that proper measures can be instituted to prepare the nipple.[11]

Pediatricians may elicit a history of inverted nipples by asking if there have been difficulties with nursing previous infants, or they may wish to show mothers pictures or drawings of different types of nipples and ask which type appears most similar to their own. If a history of any nipple and/or breast abnormality is elicited, communication with the mother's obstetrician should be considered.

Breast shields and breast shells are corrective devices that fit over the nipple and are worn underneath the bra. They are readily available at pharmacies or maternity stores and should be worn daily during the third trimester by women with inverted nipples. Hoffman's[12] exercise is a useful additional therapy, in which the forefingers are placed at opposite locations on the areola margins and then pulled outward. This procedure should be performed several times daily. Both of these interventions may be continued after birth should flat or inverted nipples not be fully corrected by the time of delivery. Occasionally, changes in nipple contour will not occur until after suckling has begun.

Nipple Preparation

Preparation of the nipple has been recommended by various sources, although the efficacy of such practices has not been shown.[11,13] Some popular techniques, including harsh rubbing or the use of soaps containing irritants, can dry or crack nipples. Creams and lotions for the breast may also be detrimental. In reality, specific intervention for the normal nipple is unnecessary.

Previous Breast-feeding Experience

For various reasons, some mothers may have experienced difficulty breast-feeding an infant in the past. This can produce anxiety or reluctance regarding their future attempts. A careful history to elucidate the nature of the previous problem and evaluation of its relevance to future attempts is essential. These mothers may be insecure and may question the physician frequently regarding whether the infant is receiving sufficient milk. These mothers will benefit from additional support and positive reinforcement.

POSTPARTUM PERIOD

Duration and Frequency

Suggested durations for nursing at each breast range from 3 minutes to 20 minutes.[1,12] The American Academy of Pediatrics recommends a nursing duration of up to 10 minutes on the first breast and up to 20 minutes on the second breast. However, exact times should not be recommended, as time may vary with each individual infant and many newborns are too sleepy in the first few days after birth to achieve long nursing durations. Proper latch-on techniques are important to facilitate breast stimulation and to hasten the let-down reflex.[14] Although glucose water following nursing continues to be routine on (too) many neonatal services, it is unnecessary, because breast milk contains sufficient water for the normal newborn infant. In fact, supplemental feedings of sterile or glucose water should be discouraged during the first few days of nursing, as they may reduce milk production and increase neonatal jaundice. Instead, mothers should be instructed to nurse more frequently to enhance milk supply, even as often as every 2 to 3 hours (eight to 12 times per day). In addition, the early introduction of a bottle may result in nipple confusion.

In most cases, supplemental feeding should be avoided to prevent nipple confusion and suppression of milk production. However, a mother who experiences extreme exhaustion or who has received medication before or during delivery may be physically unable to nurse her child eight to 12 times per day. Also, certain infants (such as those with low birth weight) may be at increased risk for hypoglycemia if feedings are diminished. In those situations, supplemental feeding with formula may be necessary. If supplemental feedings are begun, they should be rapidly weaned once the specific indication for their initiation has resolved.

Initially, infants should be nursed on demand. Both breasts should be nursed at each feeding to ensure bilateral breast stimulation and sufficient infant intake. To prevent engorgement, the first breast for each feeding should be the last breast offered during the prior feeding. Many mothers find that placing a small safety pin on the side of the bra on which the next feed will begin is a helpful reminder. Newborns demand feedings every 1.5 to 3 hours throughout the day and night. Long intervals between feedings should be discouraged initially. Most mothers need reassurance during the early postpartum period that a better schedule will occur later.

Positioning

Fortunately, several available brochures and manuals contain photographs and illustrations of proper nursing

Table 2.—Management of Breast-feeding Jaundice[15]*
A. Early onset (starts 3 to 4 days post partum): "jaundice in a breast-fed infant"
1. Encourage mothers to nurse frequently (minimum 8 times per day).
2. Avoid formula supplementation, unless milk production is inadequate.
3. Do not use glucose water or sterile water supplementation.
4. Monitor serum bilirubin concentrations daily on an outpatient basis.
5. Mothers may use mechanical or manual methods to express their milk after feedings to increase milk volume.
B. Late onset (starts 7 to 10 days post partum): "breast milk jaundice"
1. If the bilirubin concentration reaches 290 to 342 μmol/L, breast-feeding should be interrupted for 48-96 hours with formula given as a diagnostic test.
2. Instruct mothers to maintain lactation with manual or mechanical methods of milk expression during the interruption.
3. Monitor serum bilirubin concentrations every 12 to 24 hours.
4. Resume breast-feeding after a decrease in serum bilirubin concentration confirms the diagnosis.

*For conversion of serum bilirubin, 1 μmol/L = 0.06 mg/dL.

positioning.[1,12,14] The most commonly used position involves cradling the infant in the crook of the mother's arm, with the infant's head aligned with the breast. The infant should be lying on his or her side with the mouth directly in front of the nipple. The infant's lower arm can be tucked under the torso or around the mother's side to keep the area clear of distraction or obstacle. The breast should be cupped with the mother's free hand with use of the first and second fingers to grasp behind (posterior to) the areola. The nipple alone should not be offered to the infant; instead, both the nipple and areola should be offered. Alternate positions for nursing include the "football hold" (head in the palm of the hand with the infant's body supported by the mother's forearm and the side of the torso) and the recumbent position.

Latch-on

As much of the nipple and areola as possible should be inserted into the infant's mouth. Allowing the infant to suck only on the nipple leads to cracked, sore, and bleeding nipples (problems discussed in the following section). After latch-on, the mother may use her free hand to gently press down on the part of her breast near the infant's nose to ensure adequate clearance for unlabored respiration. Removal of the infant from the breast is accomplished best by inserting a finger into the infant's mouth between the gums to break suction. This technique effectively prevents nipple traction or trauma.

EARLY PROBLEMS

Jaundice

Breast-feeding jaundice can be categorized as early-onset jaundice in a breast-fed infant (occurring 3 to 4 days post partum) and late-onset breast milk jaundice (occurring 7 to 10 days post partum). The cause of early-onset breast-feeding jaundice, "jaundice in a breast-fed infant," is related to infrequent feedings, lack of demand feedings, and inadequate energy intake.[15] Frequent feedings will stimulate gut motility and decrease the intestinal absorption of bilirubin by decreasing enterohepatic circulation. Contrary to common belief, sterile water or glucose water supplementation of breast-fed infants does not reduce bilirubin concentrations.[16]

This condition should be anticipated when mother and infant are discharged from the hospital within 48 hours of delivery. Often, it can be prevented with appropriate lactation counseling. It is very important for diagnosis to obtain a detailed history, which should include the number of feedings in the last 24 hours, the number of wet diapers, the number of stools, feeding vigor, and the amount of supplementation, if any.

The management strategies for early and late breast-feeding jaundice are summarized in Table 2. Mothers of infants with early-onset jaundice should be encouraged to nurse as frequently as possible, especially if the bilirubin level is rising.[17] In an otherwise healthy infant, outpatient bilirubin determinations may be obtained if other causes of pathologic jaundice are excluded. It is important not only to determine the bilirubin concentration but also to ensure adequate milk intake by the infant. If there is a concern that the mother's milk supply is inadequate, she should be encouraged to express her milk manually or mechanically after each nursing episode to increase stimulation and thus milk production. During that time, the infant should receive a milk-based formula after each suckling. This should be continued until it is determined that the mother has an adequate milk supply.

The cause of late-onset breast-feeding jaundice, "breast milk jaundice," originally was attributed to a hormone in breast milk that inhibited glucuronyl transferase. Studies have been contradictory, with some supporting this association and others failing to do so. Recently, other studies have demonstrated an enhancement of enteric bilirubin absorption in breast-fed infants with jaundice as a result of increased concentrations of long-chain nonesterified fatty acids and human milk lipoprotein lipase. The timing of onset is probably related to the fact that lipoprotein lipase level is not elevated in human milk until after the fourth postpartum day.[17] It has also been demonstrated that the milk from mothers of infants with breast milk jaundice will enhance intestinal bilirubin absorption.[17] The process can be blocked with milk-based formula feeding.[17] It appears that the causes may include an abnormality in the milk and in the recipient host, so that bilirubin absorption continues unimpeded.[17] A definite cause, however, has not been firmly established.

Late-onset breast-feeding jaundice usually peaks by days 10 to 15 and is noted clinically during the second and third week of life. Jaundice may persist for 27 to 80 days,[18] but usually the serum bilirubin is below 86 μmol/L by the end of the third week. When the serum bilirubin level exceeds 290 μmol/L, breast-feeding should be interrupted for 1 to 4 days (usually 48 hours) and a milk-based formula substituted as a diagnostic test. Serum bilirubin will decline by 50% during this period if the elevation was a result of breast milk jaundice. Realizing that kernicterus has never been reported in an infant with breast-feeding jaundice, some physicians prefer waiting until the serum bilirubin concentration approaches 342 μmol/L before interrupting nursing.[17,19] If the serum bilirubin level does not decline as a result of interruption of nursing, breast-feeding should be resumed during the search for a cause of the jaundice. Nursing should not be interrupted if a separate cause for hyperbilirubinemia is identified. Again, during any period of nursing interruption, mechanical methods of milk expression should be utilized. In all situations, documentation of the rationale for continuing breast-feeding in the presence of jaundice should be made in the patient's chart.

Engorgement

Breast engorgement is an uncomfortable and sometimes painful swelling of the breasts that occurs commonly on the second to seventh postpartum days. It is due to increased blood and lymph flow to the breast at the onset of lactogenesis. Poor or infrequent emptying of the breast can compound this problem. Fortunately, this condition is easily managed by frequent emptying of the breast by feeding or by mechanical or manual methods of milk expression during times of mother-infant separation. Additional comfort may be provided by warm, moist compresses and warm showers, which aid in milk flow, and by hand expression of milk before nursing, which softens the areola and allows for easier infant latch-on.

Sore Nipples

Commonly, the initial grasp and suck of the nipples will cause pain during the first few days of lactation. This sensation is the result of negative pressure on the still-empty ductules. Sore nipples can be exacerbated by incorrect latch-on or impairment of milk let-down. Usually, this condition begins during the first few days of lactation and is greatest at the beginning of feeds. Once lactation is well established, the tenderness diminishes; therefore, treatment is simply supportive.

Cracked or fissured nipples are usually the result of improper latch-on, improper disengagement, or the use of abrasive soaps or alcohol. Treatment of this condition involves rinsing the nipples with water and allowing thorough air drying after nursing. Once the nipples are dry, a small amount of milk should be expressed, gently rubbed onto the nipples, and allowed to air dry. Prolonged nipple exposure to air will augment healing. When severe discomfort from fissuring occurs, nipple shells with a large back may be worn between feedings to prevent the nipple from rubbing on the bra. If infection of the nipple is a possibility, topical antibiotics may be applied but should be washed off before nursing.

Late onset (>1 month postpartum) or chronically sore nipples causing burning pain throughout the breast is often the result of *Monilia* infection. There is often concomitant thrush or fungal diaper rash in the infant. Treatment of both maternal and infant sources of infection with topical antifungal agents, coupled with meticulous air drying of the nipples, is required.[1]

Appetite Spurts

Appetite spurts are periods of crying and apparent insatiability on the part of the infant. The infant nurses more frequently and for longer periods but still seems hungry.[20] The episodes usually occur at 8 to 12 days, 3 to 4 weeks, and 3 months of age, and at variable times thereafter. Appetite spurts can be very frustrating for the mother, who may feel inadequate because she perceives herself as failing to satisfy her child. They are usually able to be differentiated from colic based on their occurrence at the previously stated ages. Many physicians are tempted to recommend supplemental formula feeding at this time, but this will only intensify the problem. The mother's milk production should meet the increased demand within 3 to 5 days of increased stimulation from the hungry infant. Supplemental formula feedings will satiate the infant but decrease the suckling time, resulting in insufficient stimulation of the breast and inadequate milk production. Physicians should recommend frequent feedings of eight to 10 times per day during these periods.

Table 3.—Danger Signs of Possible Inadequate Milk Supply in First 2 Weeks

1. Less than 6 wet diapers per day (normal, 6 to 8/d).
2. Stool frequency of less than 4 per day (normal, 6 to 10/d).
3. Continual crying and apparent hunger.
4. Infant refusal to latch on.
5. Continually sleepy infant.
6. Nursing frequency of less than 7 feedings per day.
7. Frequent formula supplementation.
8. Jaundice.
9. Body weight loss of ≥10%.
10. Long nighttime intervals without feeding.
11. Maternal fatigue/anxiety.

Plugged Ducts

Plugged ducts are focal areas of breast engorgement usually caused by stasis of milk. The condition results from irregular nursing, skipped feedings, or inadequate emptying of the entire breast and may occur at any time during lactation, although it is most common during the first 3 months. Treatment involves starting consecutive feeds on the affected side and changing nursing position often to help facilitate emptying of different lobes of the breast. Additional relief is provided by gently massaging the affected area during nursing or pumping while applying moist heat. Frequent nursing should also be recommended.

Mastitis

Mastitis is a cellulitis of the interlobar connective tissue of the breast. Affected women will experience breast pain, swelling, erythema, and fever. The infection is usually due to *Staphylococcus aureus* and occasionally to *Streptococcus* species. Mastitis may occur anytime during lactation but rarely occurs before 2 weeks post partum. A plugged duct is a frequent precursor of infection.

Antibiotic therapy with oral antistaphylococcal medication should be instituted promptly. Bed rest and moist heat application provide symptomatic relief. Most important, nursing should not be stopped during treatment. Feedings should be initiated on the unaffected breast and the infant switched to the affected side only after let-down occurs.

DANGER SIGNS

The danger signs manifested by an infant who is not receiving an adequate milk supply are summarized in Table 3. These signs often become apparent during the interval between hospital discharge and the first physician's office visit, 1 to 2 weeks after birth. Therefore, telephone or office contact with a knowledgeable source at approximately 3 to 5 days after birth is essential to determine the adequacy of the mother's milk supply, to provide support and encouragement to the lactating mother, and to identify any problems. It is essential that a nursing mother's initial contact be with personnel trained in breast-feeding management. Therefore, pediatric office staff should be encouraged to attend lactation seminars to develop and maintain their skills at recognizing danger signs.

CONCLUSION

Health professionals in general, and pediatricians in particular, are expected to provide guidance before and during lactation to increasing numbers of breast-feeding mothers. This need for professional guidance will continue as long as traditional and historical support systems for new mothers remain generally unavailable. We, as pediatricians, need to become familiar and comfortable with the role of counselor and adviser for nursing mothers. This role will allow us to place an increased emphasis on well-child and preventive care. It will give us another avenue to help prevent disease, rather than only treat it once it occurs. Moreover, the role will offer us participation in one of the most rewarding experiences in the lives of parents and their infants.

References

1. Neifert M, Secat J. Medical management of successful breastfeeding. *Pediatr Clin North Am.* 1986;30:743-762.
2. Koop CE, Brannin ME. Breastfeeding—the community norm: report of a workshop. *Public Health Rep.* 1984;99:550-558.
3. Sarett P, Bain KR, O'Leary JC. Decisions on breastfeeding or formula feeding and trends in infant feeding practices. *AJDC.* 1983;137:719-725.
4. Palti H, Mansbuck I, Pridan H, et al. Episodes of illness in breastfed and bottle-fed infants in Jerusalem. *Isr J Med Sci.* 1984;20:395-399.
5. Cunningham AS. Morbidity in breastfed and artificially-fed infants. *J Pediatr.* 1977;90:726-729.
6. Cunningham AS. Morbidity in breastfed and artificially-fed infants, II. *J Pediatr.* 1979;95:5:685-689.
7. Fergusson DM, Horwood LJ, Shannon FT, Taylor B. Breastfeeding, gastrointestinal and lower respiratory illness in the first two years. *Aust Peditar J.* 1981;17:191-195.
8. Habicht JP, DaVanzo J, Butz WP. Does breastfeeding really save lives, or are apparent benefits due to biases. *Am J Epidemiol.* 1986;123:279-290.
9. Beske E, Garvis M. Important factors in breastfeeding success. *Matern Child Nurs J.* 1982;7:174-149.
10. Hill R. *A Passage Into Life: Breastfeeding.* Houston, Tex: Texas Children's Hospital Press; 1981:2.
11. Hoffman JB. A suggested treatment for inverted nipples. *Am J Obstet Gynecol.* 1953;66:346-348.
12. Brown MS, Hurlock JT. Preparation of the breast for breastfeeding. *Nurs Res.* 1975;24:448-451.
13. American Academy of Pediatrics. *Breastfeeding.* Evanston, Ill: American Academy of Pediatrics Publications Department; 1984.
14. Lawrence RA. Breastfeeding: a guide for the medical profession. St Louis, Mo: CV Mosby Co; 1980:123.
15. Lascari A. 'Early' breastfeeding jaundice: clinical significance. *J Pediatr.* 1986;108:156-158.
16. DeCarvalho MD, Hall M, Harvey D. Effects of water supplementation on physiological jaundice in breastfed babies. *Arch Dis Child.* 1989;56:568-569.
17. Gartner LM, Auerbach KG. Breastfeeding and human milk: their association with jaundice in the neonate. *Clin Perinatol.* 1987;14:89-107.
18. Winfield CR, MacFaul R. Clinical study of prolonged jaundice in breast and bottle-fed babies. *Arch Dis Child.* 1978;53:506-507.
19. Maisels MJ. Hyperbilirubinemia. In: Nelson NM, ed. *Current Therapy in Neonatal-Perinatal Medicine, 1985-86.* St Louis, Mo: CV Mosby Co; 1985.
20. Neifert MR, Seacat JM. Contemporary breast-feeding management. *Clin Perinatol.* 1985;12:319-342.

In Other AMA Journals

ARCHIVES OF GENERAL PSYCHIATRY

Criminality and Childhood Hyperactivity

M. Menuck, MD, FRCPC
(*Arch Gen Psychiatry.* 1991;48:667-675)

ARCHIVES OF OTOLARYNGOLOGY—HEAD & NECK SURGERY

Otitis Media With Effusion in Children: Binaural Hearing Before and After Corrective Surgery

Harold C. Pillsbury, MD; John H. Grose, PhD; Joseph W. Hall III, PhD
(*Arch Otolaryngol Head Neck Surg.* 1991;117:718-723)

Predicting Risk of *Pneumocystis carinii* Pneumonia in Human Immunodeficiency Virus–Infected Children

Richard M. Rutstein, MD

• Effective prophylaxis exists against *Pneumocystis carinii* pneumonia, a major cause of illness and death among human immunodeficiency virus–infected children and adults. While adults with CD4 counts less than $0.2 \times 10^9/L$ are at highest risk for *Pneumocystis carinii*, clinical or laboratory markers of high risk in children infected with the human immunodeficiency virus have not yet been established. A chart review of 13 infants with perinatally acquired human immunodeficiency virus infection and children with *Pneumocystis carinii* pneumonia revealed that infants younger than 12 months developed *Pneumocystis carinii* pneumonia despite CD4 counts that were normal by adult standards. In contrast to the markedly increased serum IgG levels seen in most children infected with the human immunodeficiency virus, five children with *Pneumocystis carinii* pneumonia had IgG levels less than 3.0 g/L. Twelve patients had preexisting symptoms consistent with human immunodeficiency virus infection before the episode of *Pneumocystis carinii* pneumonia. In addition to clinical symptoms, low IgG levels and CD4 counts adjusted for age may serve to identify those children who are most at risk for *Pneumocystis carinii* pneumonia and therefore candidates for prophylaxis. Prophylaxis should be offered to all infants under age 12 months with proven, or clinical symptoms compatible with, human immunodeficiency virus infection. For children older than 12 months, CD4 counts less than $0.3 \times 10^9/L$ appear to be predictive of risk for *Pneumocystis carinii* pneumonia, and these children should also receive prophylaxis.

(*AJDC*. 1991;145:922-924)

Pneumocystis carinii pneumonia (PCP) represents a leading cause of morbidity and mortality in individuals infected with human immunodeficiency virus (HIV). More than 75% of adults with HIV will ultimately develop PCP[1]; as many as 20% will succumb during the first episode. In children with HIV infection, PCP is the most common opportunistic infection and associated with a median survival of only 1 month from the time of diagnosis.[2]

Effective prophylaxis against PCP has been demonstrated in studies of adults with HIV infection and children with cancer undergoing chemotherapy.[3-7] The agents most commonly employed are aerosolized pentamidine and oral trimethoprim/sulfamethoxazole.

Optimal treatment of HIV-infected individuals includes the determination of relative risk for a first episode of PCP and the initiation of chemoprophylaxis if indicated. The adults at greatest risk, with a 20% yearly incidence of PCP, have absolute CD4 counts lower than $0.2 \times 10^9/L$.[8] For these patients, the Centers for Disease Control advises prophylaxis with aerosolized pentamidine or trimethoprim/sulfamethoxazole.[9] In children with HIV, there are no published data on primary prophylaxis against PCP or on markers for those most at risk of developing the disease. One recent article and several abstracts indicate that the CD4 count is not as useful in children as in adults.[10-13]

To further investigate clinical and laboratory markers useful as indicators of risk of PCP in HIV-infected children, a retrospective chart review was conducted.

SUBJECTS AND METHODS

I reviewed the charts of patients congenitally infected with HIV who were treated at the Children's Hospital of Philadelphia (Pa) from January 1985 to March 1990. Thirteen patients had histologically proven PCP (by bronchopulmonary lavage or biopsy). T-cell ratios, absolute CD4 counts, IgG levels, and presence of HIV-related preexisting symptoms were noted. T-cell subsets were determined using whole blood specimens stained with monoconal antibody directed against the desired subset. The specimen was then run through a flow cytometer and the number of stained cells counted. Patients were classified according to the Centers for Disease Control pediatric HIV guidelines.[14] In 11 of the 13 patients, the CD4 counts and IgG levels were obtained 1 week to 3 months before the diagnosis of PCP. In two patients who first presented with acute PCP, the studies were performed at the time of hospitalization and diagnosis of PCP.

RESULTS

Age at diagnosis of PCP ranged from 3 months to 9 years. These 13 patients represented 26% of the HIV-infected symptomatic children (P2A symptomatic, nonspecific findings or acquired immunodeficiency syndrome–defining illness)[14] followed up at our institution during the study period. Five patients died of PCP. All three children older than 12 months had absolute CD4 counts of less than $0.3 \times 10^9/L$ at the time of PCP diagnosis (at ages 14, 31, and 102 months).

All 10 patients younger than 12 months had CD4 counts higher than $0.25 \times 10^9/L$; eight had absolute CD4 counts

Accepted for publication January 28, 1991.
From the Division of General Pediatrics, Children's Hospital of Philadelphia, Pa, and the University of Pennsylvania School of Medicine, Philadelphia.
Reprints not available.

Table 1.—Signs or Symptoms of Human Immunodeficiency Virus in 13 Patients Before Presentation With *Pneumocystis carinii**

Patient No./ Age, mo†	Symptoms‡	CDC Classification§	CD4-CD8 Ratio	Absolute CD4, x10⁹/L	IgG, g/L	Outcome
1/3	FTT, UTI	P2A	0.3	0.712	2.94	Died
2/3	None	P-O	0.5	0.350	19.00	Died
3/5	Recurrent *Salmonella* bacteremia	P2D1	2.4	1.600	2.69	Survived
4/6	Recurrent bacterial disease	P2D2	0.8	1.030	2.36	Survived
5/6	Recurrent thrush	P-O	0.2	0.284	13.80	Survived
6/7	FTT, thrush, *Candida* esophagitis	P2D1	1.8	1.000	1.90	Died
7/7	FTT, adenopathy, hepatomegaly	P2A	2.2	0.700	6.78	Survived
8/8	FTT, UTI, thrush	P2A	0.7	2.000	23.00	Survived
9/9	CMV retinitis	P2D1	0.3	0.770	4.38	Died
10/9	Adenopathy, heptomegaly	P2A	0.5	1.875	20.80	Survived
11/14	Hepatitis, *Candida* esophagitis	P2D1	0.1	0.130	1.95	Died
12/31	FTT, CNS, LIP	P2BC	0.3	0.269	32.00	Survived
13/102	MAI, LIP	P2CD1	0.1	0.108	10.20	Survived

*FTT indicates failure to thrive; UTI, urinary tract infection; CMV, cytomegalovirus; CNS, progressive encephalopathy; MAI, disseminated *Mycobacterium avium/intracellulare;* and LIP, lymphocytic interstitial pneumonitis.
†At time of diagnosis of *Pneumocystis carinii* pneumonia.
‡Noted before diagnosis of *Pneumocystis carinii* pneumonia.
§Center for Disease Control classification at time of presentation of respiratory distress.[14]

Table 2.—Age at Diagnosis of *Pneumocystis carinii* Pneumonia and Absolute CD4 Count

	Age <12 mo CD4 Count, x10⁹/L				Age >12 mo CD4 Count, x10⁹/L			
Source, y	**No.**	**<.20**	**200-1.00**	**>1.00**	**No.**	**<.200**	**.200-.300**	**>.300**
Present study	10	0	5	5	3	2	1	0
Leibovitz et al,[13] 1990	15	7	2	6	6	6	0	0
Total	**25**	**7** (28%)	**7** (28%)	**11** (44%)	**9**	**8**	**1**	**0**

higher than 0.7×10^9/L, three had a CD4-CD8 ratio higher than 1.0, and seven had a CD4-CD8 ratio lower than 1.0. Five children had IgG values of less than 3.0 g/L. Twelve children, including nine of 10 younger than 12 months, had signs or symptoms of HIV infection prior to presentation with PCP (Table 1).

COMMENT

Reliance on adult values of CD4 counts to predict risk of PCP would have caused us to miss all of the 10 infants with PCP younger than 1 year; these infants had CD4 counts in excess of 0.25×10^9/L. Seventeen of the 18 patients described by Bernstein et al[10] had previous CD4 counts measured. Nine (50%) of these patients had CD4 counts greater than 0.6×10^9/L. Unfortunately, the CD4 counts were not stratified by age.

Leibovitz et al[13] recently described 22 HIV-infected children who developed PCP. Fifteen were younger than 12 months at the time of PCP diagnosis. Combining the patients in their study and ours, all nine patients older than age 12 months with available CD4 counts had absolute CD4 counts lower than 0.27×10^9/L (Table 2). Of the 25 patients younger than 1 year, seven (28%) had absolute CD4 counts less than 0.2×10^9/L, seven (28%) had CD4 counts between 0.2×10^9/L and 1.0×10^9/L, and 11 (44%) had CD4 counts greater than 1.0×10^9/L. Almost half of the 35 patients died during the first episode of acute PCP.

Two additional studies[11,12] also report that high CD4 counts do not prevent the occurrence of PCP in HIV-infected children.

All these findings illustrate the lack of utility of using adult standards of CD4 counts in predicting risk of PCP in infants with HIV infection. Part of the difficulty may be the absence of normative data on T-cell counts among noninfected children. Since infants typically have relative lymphocytosis (compared with older children and adults), the criteria for a low absolute CD4 count are not yet established.

A recent abstract[15] noted average CD4-CD8 ratios of 2.72 in 11 normal children younger than 18 months, with a mean absolute CD4 count of 1.8×10^9/L. A second abstract[16] described a larger group of normal infants. In the 100 infants younger than age 6 months, the mean CD4-CD8 ratio was 2.3 with a mean absolute CD4 count of 3.17×10^9/L. In 70 6- to 12-month-old children, the mean ratio was 2.0 and the mean absolute CD4 count was 2.83×10^9/L. Three of our 10 infants with PCP had CD4-CD8 ratios in this range, although all had absolute CD4 counts less than 2.00×10^9/L. Larger studies are needed to stratify normal CD4 counts and CD4-CD8 ratios according to age, especially in the patients younger than 12 months.

That five of 13 children with PCP had IgG levels less than 3.0 g/L was unexpected. The vast majority of children with documented HIV infection have elevated IgG levels at the time of diagnosis.[17,18] In normal children, IgG levels increase with age during the first year of life. The rate of increase of IgG in HIV-infected children in the first year of life has not been documented, although in one study, four of eight children had increased IgG levels by age 4 months, and six of eight by age 9 months.[19] Because host defense mechanisms for PCP are still not elucidated, the CD4 count may be only one of several relevant immunologic markers of susceptibility to PCP in infancy, and other surrogate markers should be examined. For instance, congenitally hypogammaglobulinemic infants are at risk for PCP despite normal T-cell counts.[20] Human immunodeficiency virus–positive infants with low IgG levels may represent a subgroup at high risk for PCP.

Half of all HIV-infected infants will have associated symptoms or diseases by age 12 months, and over 75% will be symptomatic by age 2 years.[2] All 18 HIV-infected patients with PCP previously reported[14] experienced failure to thrive at the time of PCP diagnosis. Twelve of our 13 patients had preexisting symptoms or illnesses consistent with HIV infection before the diagnosis of PCP. In five of the 13 patients and four of the 10 infants, failure to thrive was noted before the diagnosis of PCP. Early development of HIV-related symptoms, especially the failure to thrive, may serve as a marker for infants at high risk for PCP.

Prompt identification and assessment of infants at risk for HIV infection is important because PCP may occur as early as the second month of life. Since only 30% to 40% of HIV antibody–positive newborns are actually infected, optimal care would include determining each child's immune and infectious status. Infants at risk, or those already known to be HIV antibody–positive, should be referred to a pediatric HIV center with the capability to perform HIV DNA polymerase chain reaction (PCR) and blood culture testing for HIV. Infants younger than 15 months with proven HIV infection (positive PCR or HIV blood culture) should receive prophylaxis. Because the rate of false-negative HIV cultures and PCR in childhood is not well established, infants younger than 12 months with negative results but evidence of immune dysfunction (abnormal IgG levels or CD4 counts), or compatible symptoms (failure to thrive, adenopathy, and hepatosplenomegaly), should be considered for prophylaxis. When direct HIV testing is unavailable, or the results are pending, it would be prudent to begin prophylaxis for HIV antibody–positive infants through age 12 to 15 months.

Data from this study and others suggest that an absolute CD4 count less than 0.3×10^9/L is helpful in predicting risk of PCP in children older than 12 months, and these children should receive prophylaxis. Low IgG levels may serve as an additional marker for increased risk of PCP.

Trimethoprim/sulfamethoxazole provides relatively inexpensive and effective prophylaxis. Unfortunately, 20% to 40% of HIV-infected adults treated with trimethoprim/sulfamethoxazole develop allergic reactions.[21,22] Of the last 15 HIV-positive children at our center who started receiving trimethoprim/sulfamethoxazole, seven developed allergic reactions requiring discontinuation of the medication (one case of erythema multiforme, two cases of acute anaphylactic reaction, and four cases of recurrent severe urticarial rashes). The use of aerosolized pentamidine for HIV-infected children allergic to trimethoprim/sulfamethoxazole is currently under investigation.

Further research needs to be devoted toward establishing normative T-cell subset data in infants. In addition, the effectiveness of alternative therapies for PCP prophylaxis in HIV-infected children remains to be determined.

I am grateful to S. Plotkin, S. Douglas, and W. Schwartz for their editorial assistance.

References

1. Centers for Disease Control. *AIDS Weekly Surveillance Report.* January 30, 1989;1-5.

2. Scott GB, Hutto C, Makuch RW, et al. Survival in children with perinatally acquired human immunodeficiency virus type 1 infection. *N Engl J Med.* 1989;321:1791-1796.

3. Hughes WT, Kuhn S, Chaudhary S, et al. Successful chemoprophylaxis for *Pneumocystis carinii* pneumonia. *N Engl J Med.* 1977;297:1419-1426.

4. Hughes WT, Rivera GK, Schell MJ, Thornton D, Lott L. Successful intermittent chemoprophylaxis for *Pneumocystis carinii* pneumonitis. *N Engl J Med.* 1987;316:1627-1632.

5. Leoung GS, Montgomery AB, McGinty E, Feigal DW, LymphoMed Consortium Investigators. Double-blinded randomized trial of aerosol pentamidine for secondary prophylaxis of *Pneumocystis carinii* pneumonia. Proceedings of the Fifth International Conference on AIDS; June 4-9, 1989; Montreal, Canada. Abstract.

6. Fischl MA, Dickinson GM, La Voie L. Safety and efficacy of sulfamethoxazole and trimethoprin chemoprophylaxis for *Pneumocystis carinii* pneumonia in AIDS. *JAMA.* 1988;259:1185-1189.

7. Kovacs JA, Masur H. Prophylaxis of *Pneumocystis carinii* pneumonia: an update. *J Infect Dis.* 1989;160:882-886.

8. Phair JP, Munoz A, Detels R, et al. The risk of *Pneumocystis carinii* pneumonia among men infected with human immunodeficiency virus type 1. *N Engl J Med.* 1990;322:161-165.

9. Centers for Disease Control. Guidelines for prophylaxis against *Pneumocystis carinii* pneumonia for persons infected with human immunodeficiency virus. *MMWR.* 1989;38:1-9.

10. Bernstein LA, Bye MR, Rubinstein A. Prognostic factors and life expectancy in children with acquired immunodeficiency syndrome and *Pneumocystis carinii* pneumonia. *AJDC.* 1989;143:775-778.

11. Sanders-Laufer D, Burroughs M, Marshall F, et al. *Pneumocystis carinii* pneumonia in "low risk" HIV-infected children. *Pediatr Res.* 1990;27:183. Abstract.

12. Bagarazzi ML, Connor E, McSherry GD, Oleske JM. PCP among HIV infected children: ten years experience. *Pediatr Res.* 1990;27:166. Abstract.

13. Leibovitz E, Riguard M, Pollack H, et al. *Pneumocystis carinii* pneumonia in infants with the human immunodeficiency virus with more than 450 CD4 lymphocytes per cubic millimeter. *N Engl J Med.* 1990;323:531-533.

14. Centers for Disease Control. Classification system for human immunodeficiency virus (HIV) in children under 13 years of age. *MMWR.* 1987;36:225-230.

15. O'Rouke S, Plaeger-Marshall S, Gillespie S, et al. T cell parameters by age in normal and HIV-infected children. Presented at the Sixth International Conference on AIDS; June 1990; San Francisco, Calif.

16. Denn TN, Niven P, Skuia C, et al. Age related changes of lymphocyte phenotypes in healthy children. *Pediatr Res.* 1990;27:155. Abstract.

17. Rubinstein A. Pediatric AIDS. *Curr Probl Pediatr.* 1986; 26:387-392.

18. Blanche S, Le Deist F, Fischer A, et al. Longitudinal study of 18 children with perinatal LAV/HTLV III infection. *J Pediatr.* 1986;109:965-970.

19. Johnson JP, Nair P, Hines SF, et al. Natural history and serologic diagnosis of infants born to human immunodeficiency virus infected women. *AJDC.* 1989;143:1147-1153.

20. Rao CP, Gelfand EW. *Pneumocystis carinii* pneumonitis in patients with hypogammaglobunemia and intact T cell immunity. *J Pediatr.* 1983;103:410-412.

21. Gordin FM, Simon GL, Wofsky CB, Mills J. Adverse reactions to trimethoprin-sulfamethoxazole in patients with acquired immunodeficiency syndrome. *Ann Intern Med.* 1984;100:495-499.

22. Sattler FR, Cowan R, Nielsen DM, Ruskin J. Trimethoprin-sulfamethoxazole compared with pentamidine for treatment of *Pneumocystis carinii* pneumonia in the acquired immunodeficiency syndrome. *Ann Intern Med.* 1988;109:280-287.

Measurement of Serum Granulocyte Colony-Stimulating Factor in a Patient With Congenital Agranulocytosis (Kostmann's Syndrome)

Lewis Glasser, MD; Burris R. Duncan, MD; James J. Corrigan, Jr, MD

• A 12-month-old boy with Kostmann's syndrome was admitted with cavitary pulmonary disease. He had also had bacterial conjunctivitis, periorbital cellulitis, pneumonitis, and otitis media since the age of 10 days. His umbilical cord had not fallen off until he was 3 weeks old. Neutropenia was diagnosed at 4 weeks of age. Antineutrophil antibody studies were negative. A bone marrow aspirate showed granulocytic hypoplasia and a maturation arrest at the promyelocyte stage. Hematopoietic cell culture showed normal numbers of colony-forming units–granulocyte macrophage. Serum granulocyte-macrophage colony-stimulating factor level, was 0.24 ng/mL (normal, >0.05 ng/mL). Serum granulocyte colony-stimulating factor levels, measured by enzyme immunoassay, were undetectable. The patient was successfully treated with filgrastim (granulocyte colony-stimulating factor), with an increase in the absolute neutrophil count to 10.0 × 10⁹/L. Thus, our case of Kostmann's syndrome appears to represent a defect in regulation or production of granulocyte colony-stimulating factor.

(*AJDC.* 1991;145:925-928)

Granulocyte colony-stimulating factor (G-CSF) is a recently discovered hematopoietic growth factor, and our understanding of its role in normal physiology and disease is beginning to emerge. It is primarily a neutrophilopoietin,[1] important in the regulation of granulopoiesis. It now appears evident that a defect in its production or regulation causes Kostmann's syndrome,[2] a congenital neutropenia that not only has benefited from G-CSF therapy[3] but is an experiment of nature that provides a rare opportunity to study the homeostatic mechanisms involved in granulopoiesis. In this report, we describe the application of measuring the serum G-CSF level to the pathogenesis, diagnosis, and subsequent successful treatment of a patient with congenital agranulocytosis (Kostmann's syndrome).

Accepted for publication February 11, 1991.

From the Departments of Pathology (Dr Glasser) and Pediatrics (Dr Duncan and Dr Corrigan), University of Arizona Health Sciences Center, College of Medicine, Tucson.

Presented in part at the annual meeting of the American Society of Hematology, Boston, Mass, December 3, 1990.

Reprint requests to Clinical Pathology, Arizona Health Sciences Center, Tucson, AZ 85724 (Dr Glasser).

PATIENT REPORT

A 3830-g boy was the product of a full-term pregnancy. He was born to a 30-year-old, gravida 5, para 3, abortus 1 mother. His mother stated that his umbilical cord did not fall off until he was 3 weeks old. At 10 days of life, he had *Chlamydia* conjunctivitis that was treated with erythromycin. At 4 weeks he had periorbital cellulitis and was found to have severe neutropenia. *Pseudomonas* grew from a culture from his conjunctivas, and he was treated for 10 days with intravenous antibiotics. He subsequently developed persistent otitis media requiring multiple courses of antibiotics, without benefit.

At 12 months of age, he developed cough and fever. A chest roentgenogram showed right-upper-lobe consolidation with cavitary lesions, and he was placed on a regimen of intravenous antibiotics. His weight and length had decreased from the 50th percentile at 4 weeks of age to below the fifth percentile at 12 months. Laboratory studies at 4 weeks of age had showed a normal hemoglobin level (113 g/L) that progressively decreased throughout his illness to a low value of 76 g/L before filgrastim (G-CSF) therapy. Platelet counts were consistently elevated at 362 to 936 × 10^9/L. Leukocyte counts before filgrastim therapy were as follows: white blood cells, 4.6 to 12.3 × 10^9/L; neutrophils, 0 to 0.32 × 10^9/L; eosinophils, 0 to 0.592 × 10^9/L; basophils, 0 to 0.327 × 10^9/L; monocytes, 1.0 to 5.5 × 10^9/L; and lymphocytes, 3.5 to 9.1 × 10^9/L.

After informed consent was obtained, treatment with filgrastim (Neupogen, Amgen Inc, Thousand Oaks, Calif) therapy (6 μg/kg twice daily subcutaneously) was started at the age of 12 months for treatment of pneumonitis. Absolute neutrophil counts exceeded 5.0 × 10^9/L. The right-upper-lobe cavitation gradually cleared. The patient was placed on a regimen of maintenance filgrastim therapy; however, absolute neutrophil counts were consistently less than 1.0 × 10^9/L. During the next 7 months, he continued to have patchy parenchymal densities. At 18 months of age, he was readmitted for evaluation of chronic pulmonary changes and failure to thrive. Episodes of obstructive apnea prompted a tonsillectomy and adenoidectomy. Cultures of bronchoalveolar washings yielded cytomegalovirus. Increasing the dose of filgrastim to 12 μg/kg twice daily increased the absolute neutrophil count to 3.0 × 10^9/L. In the hospital he was also given nasogastric feedings of a high-energy formula. The patient's condition responded, and he showed significant clinical improvement.

MATERIALS AND METHODS

Neutrophil Antibody Assays

The indirect immunofluorescence and neutrophil agglutination tests were done as described by Lalezari and Pryce.[4]

Clonogenic Assays for Bone Marrow Progenitor Cells

These assays were done as previously described.[5-7] Bone marrow light density cells were separated by density gradient centrifugation using Ficoll-Hypaque (specific gravity 1.077 g/mL). Erythrocytes were removed by hypotonic lysis. For the colony-forming unit–granulocyte macrophage assay, 1×10^5 cells were plated in 0.3% semisolid agar containing recombinant human GM-CSF. Burst-forming units–erythroid were cultured in 1.5% methylcellulose containing Iscove's modified Dulbecco's medium, 5% phytohemagglutinin–leukocyte-conditioned medium, 30% fetal bovine serum, 10^{-4}-mol/L 2-mercaptoethanol, and 2 units of erythropoietin. Each plate was seeded with 5×10^4 cells. Cultures were done in quadruplicate. Plates were cultured at 37°C, in 5% carbon dioxide with humidity. Colonies (>40 cells) were counted at 14 days by means of an inverted microscope.

Serum G-CSF and Granulocyte-Macrophage Colony-Stimulating Factor (GM-CSF) Assays

Serum G-CSF was measured by enzyme immunoassay (Amgen Inc, Boulder, Colo).[8,9] The method uses microtiter wells coated with a rabbit polyclonal anti G-CSF antibody. After overnight incubation, monoclonal anti–G-CSF conjugated with horseradish peroxidase was added to the wells and incubated at 37°C for 2 hours. Substrate (tetramethylbenzidine) was added, and the chromogen was read at an absorbance of 450 nm. The level of sensitivity of this assay is 50 pg/mL.

Serum samples were tested for GM-CSF (Immunex, Seattle, Wash) by means of the GM-CSF human bone marrow assay.[10] Test serum samples were titered through a duplicate series of threefold dilutions. Human bone marrow cells were added to wells containing the test serum. Plates were incubated at 37°C in 10% carbon dioxide for 4 days. Tritiated thymidine was added, and plates were incubated for 4 hours. The well contents were harvested, and radioactivity was measured on a beta counter.

RESULTS

Blood Counts

Before treatment, absolute neutrophil counts ranged from 0 to 0.32×10^9/L. Most counts were 0×10^9/L, and the highest count occurred when the patient had a severe cavitary pulmonary infection. After filgrastim treatment, a consistent increase in the absolute neutrophil count occurred on the 8th day (Fig 1). There was an absolute increase in numbers of band and segmented neutrophils; the neutrophils had toxic granules and Dohle bodies. Monocytosis was present, with counts ranging from 1.0 to 5.5×10^9/L, and persisted after filgrastim treatment, with counts ranging from 1.6 to 8.6×10^9/L. Before filgrastim therapy, eosinophils were seen in the blood despite severe neutropenia. After therapy, the eosinophil count did not increase significantly, ranging from 0% to 6% (0 to 0.5×10^9/L) during the first 30 days.

Bone Marrow Morphologic Characteristics

Bone marrow studies were done at the ages of 7 months (before filgrastim therapy) and approximately 13 months (23 days after filgrastim therapy). Informed consent was obtained. Before G-CSF therapy, the granulocytic series showed myeloblasts and promyelocytes but an absence of neutrophils. Eosinophils and basophils were normally present. A reactive plasmacytosis was present, presumably a reflection of chronic infections. The myeloid-erythroid ratio was markedly decreased to 0.5. Cellularity was normal. After filgrastim therapy, neutrophilic differentiation was seen, and the myeloid-erythroid ratio significantly increased to 1.1. A comparison between pretreatment and posttreatment marrow findings is shown in the Table.

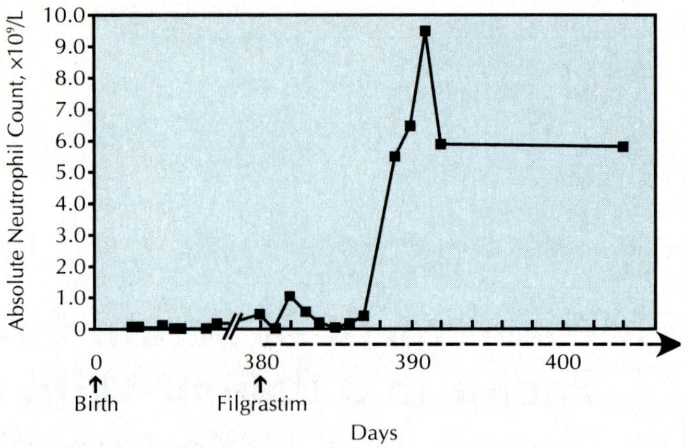

Fig 1.—*Absolute neutrophil counts before and after treatment with filgrastim (granulocyte colony-stimulating factor). The dose given was 6 μg/kg subcutaneously twice daily.*

Bone Marrow Differential Counts Before and After Filgrastim (Granulocyte Colony-Stimulating Factor) Therapy

	Count, %	
	Before Therapy	After Therapy
Myeloblasts	4	2
Promyelocytes	5	7
Neutrophils		
Myelocytes	0	3
Metamyelocytes	0	3
Bands	0	9
Segmented	0	3
Eosinophils		
Myelocytes	2	1
Metamyelocytes	1	2
Bands	1	2
Segmented	2	2
Basophils	0.5	0.6
Monocytes	20	5
Pronormoblasts	1	3
Normoblasts		
Basophilic	2	2
Polychromatic	21	19
Orthochromatic	8	8
Lymphocytes	24	23
Plasma cells	6	3

Neutrophil Antibodies

Serum samples from the infant and mother were analyzed. The sample from the infant was obtained at 6 weeks of age. Results of the indirect immunofluorescence (against neutrophils from three normal donors) and neutrophil agglutination (against neutrophils from 10 donors) tests were negative.

Serum G-CSF and GM-CSF Levels

Serum samples were obtained at 8 months of age. No G-CSF was detected in the serum of the patient or four pediatric controls (7 to 35 months old). The GM-CSF level was 0.24 ng/mL (six replicates) by the bioassay (normal, >0.05 ng/mL).

Colony-Forming Unit–Granulocyte Macrophage and Burst-Forming Unit–Erythroid Assays

The bone marrow (before treatment) at 7 months of age showed normal progenitors, with 50 colony-forming units–granulocyte macrophage per 10^5 cells and 46 burst-forming units–erythroid per 10^5 cells.

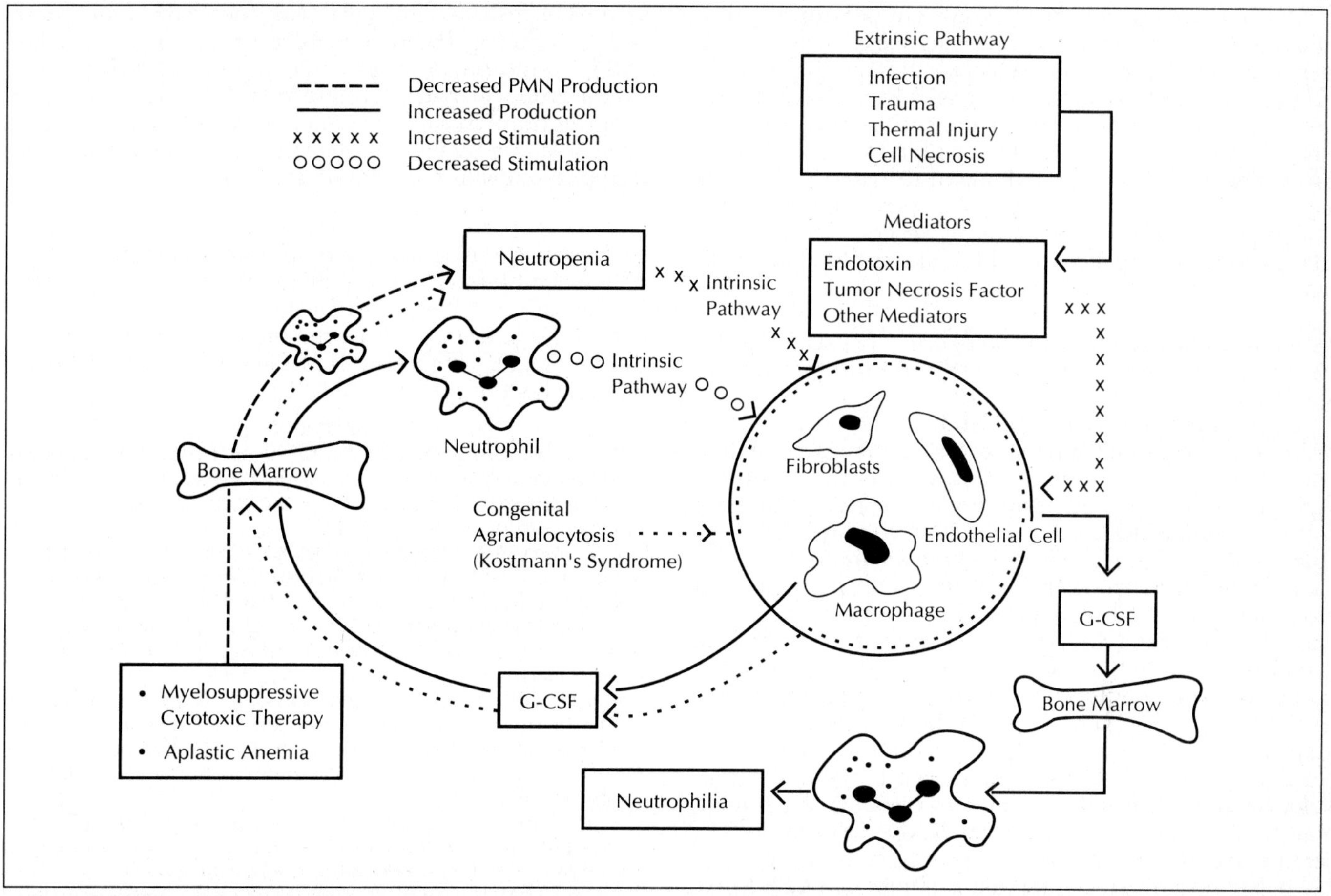

Fig 2.—*Hypothetical model of the regulatory mechanisms controlling neutrophil (PMN) granulopoiesis. An intrinsic circuit is postulated that is responsible for normal neutrophil homeostasis. Low numbers of neutrophils increase the stimulation for granulocyte colony-stimulating factor (G-CSF) production; as neutrophils are produced, the stimulus for G-CSF production decreases. In disease, myelosuppressive chemotherapy and aplastic anemia are associated with low absolute neutrophil counts, stimulating the production of G-CSF from macrophages, fibroblasts, and endothelial cells. In congenital agranulocytosis (Kostmann's syndrome) there is a primary defect in the production or regulation of G-CSF, causing a low absolute neutrophil count. An extrinsic pathway also exists that bypasses the intrinsic feedback loop. In this pathway, infection, injury, or cell necrosis results in the increased production of mediators that stimulate producer cells to increase G-CSF production, promoting granulopoiesis and neutrophilia.*

COMMENT

Neutropenias are caused by underproduction, excessive destruction, or increased utilization. Underproduction can be caused by cytotoxic drugs, irradiation, neoplastic infiltration of the bone marrow, nutritional deficits, or stem cell failure. Recently, hematopoietic growth factors have been identified and characterized,[11] and it is becoming clear that abnormal regulation or production of growth factors also causes underproduction of neutrophils. The regulation of neutrophil production is not fully understood; however, it is established that G-CSF is primarily a neutrophilopoietin without much effect on other granulocytes.[1,3,12] In our patient, the presence of eosinophils in the bone marrow and blood with an absolute neutrophil count of 0×10^9/L and the absence of eosinophilia during filgrastim therapy is similar to the observations of others, providing strong evidence that separate regulatory mechanisms control each of these cell types even though both are granulocytes. Thus, the term *G-CSF* is a misnomer, and *neutrophil–colony-stimulating factor* would be more appropriate. In contrast, GM-CSF is known to stimulate the production of eosinophils as well as neutrophils and monocytes. In addition to GM-CSF, the humoral regulation of eosinophils is influenced by interleukin 3 and interleukin 5.[13]

A proposed hypothetical model for the control and regulation of neutrophil granulopoiesis is shown in Fig 2. Granulocyte colony-stimulating factor is produced by monocytes, fibroblasts, and endothelial cells.[11] There is evidence suggesting that both intrinsic and extrinsic pathways may control secretion of G-CSF from producer cells. Although evidence of a feedback mechanism controlling G-CSF production was previously lacking, a recent study supports the hypothesis that an intrinsic feedback system regulates neutrophil homeostasis.[1] In aplastic anemia, there was an inverse relationship between the absolute neutrophil count and G-CSF levels; in cyclic neutropenia, G-CSF levels increased during the neutropenic phase and decreased during the neutrophilic phase; during myelosuppressive therapy, G-CSF levels rose as the absolute neutrophil count decreased.[1] On the other hand, an extrinsic pathway appears to be primarily involved in the host's response to infection and inflammation. In these conditions, mediators (eg, endotoxin, tumor necrosis factor) directly stimulate producer cells to secrete G-CSF.[11] This extrinsic circuit bypasses the intrinsic homeostatic feedback mechanism, stimulating producer cells to secrete G-CSF. Thus, the absolute neutrophil count varies directly with serum G-CSF levels in bacterial infections and lung cancer.[1]

Deciphering the variables involved in neutrophil granulopoiesis is dependent on a sensitive and reliable assay for serum G-CSF. Biologic assays are nonspecific, and immunoassays still lack sufficient sensitivity to detect serum levels in normal individuals. A previous report indicated that G-CSF was not detectable or within the normal range in patients with congenital agranulocytosis. Unfortunately, the level of sensitivity of the assay was 0.8 ng/mL, too high for critical evaluation.[12] Recent modifications have improved the assay, and the present limit of sensitivity is 30 or 50 pg/mL.[9] The assay is capable of detecting G-CSF in only 12% of healthy adults; the highest reported level in healthy adults was 163 pg/mL.[1] Levels of G-CSF were undetectable (<50 pg/mL) in four normal infants, 7 to 35 months of age, in our study.

The inappropriately low serum G-CSF level in our patient with congenital agranulocytosis is consistent with a defect in regulation or production, since G-CSF levels are typically elevated in other neutropenic states.[1] There are several possible explanations for the failure of G-CSF regulation or production. These include an abnormal or deleted gene on chromosome 17 with an inability of the cell to synthesize G-CSF, inability to synthesize a normal functional molecule of G-CSF, failure to synthesize normal amounts of G-CSF analogous to thalassemia, abnormal producer cell receptors that do not recognize cytokines functioning as mediators in either the intrinsic or extrinsic pathways, or target cells with decreased responsiveness to G-CSF. The last is less likely, since congenital agranulocytosis responds to exogenous recombinant human G-CSF. More than one cause may be operative in cases of congenital agranulocytosis.

In our case of congenital neutropenia, GM-CSF levels were difficult to interpret. Monocytosis was present throughout the patient's course, suggesting normal GM-CSF production. Serum GM-CSF was normal by the bioassay; however, the assay is nonspecific and also detects G-CSF, interleukin 3, interleukin 4, and interleukin 7. Immunologic methods for measuring serum GM-CSF lack sensitivity in the normal range. It is probable that when the sensitivity of the more specific immunoassay method is improved, GM-CSF levels of body fluids will be found to be either normal or increased in Kostmann's syndrome.

The causes of isolated congenital neutropenia include immune neonatal neutropenia, congenital agranulocytosis (Kostmann's syndrome), cyclic neutropenia, and chronic idiopathic neutropenia. In immune neonatal neutropenia, the neutropenia is secondary to transplacental transfer of antibodies from mother to fetus. Serum G-CSF levels have not been reported. In Kostmann's syndrome, progenitor cells are present, as shown by normal growth of colony-forming units–granulocyte macrophage in our patient and as reported by others[14]; in our patient, the serum G-CSF level was inappropriately low. Pietsch et al[15] showed that monocytes from patients with Kostmann's syndrome produce G-CSF. This suggests a defect in regulation but does not exclude a primary defect in production. In our patient, absolute neutrophil counts were low in both the infected and noninfected state. The highest neutrophil count was obtained when the patient had a severe cavitary pulmonary infection, perhaps indirectly suggesting an abortive response to inflammatory stimuli. Serum G-CSF levels were not measured at this time. In contrast to Kostmann's syndrome, in cyclic neutropenia there is a defect in the regulation of granulopoiesis, and serum G-CSF levels are high during the neutropenic phase and low during the neutrophilic phase.[1] Chronic idiopathic neutropenia most likely represents a heterogeneous group of patients. Serum G-CSF levels have not been reported in these patients but would be of interest and could potentially elucidate the various causes and aid in the classification of this diverse group.

CONCLUSION

The cause of Kostmann's syndrome is not known. Our patient had severe neutropenia with an inappropriately low serum G-CSF level, suggesting that the cause of this disorder is a defect in either the regulation or the production of G-CSF. The defect is isolated to G-CSF and does not involve the cytokine GM-CSF.

References

1. Watari K, Shigetaka A, Shirafuji N, et al. Serum granulocyte colony-stimulating factor levels in healthy volunteers and patients with various disorders as estimated by enzyme immunoassay. *Blood.* 1989;73:117-122.
2. Kostmann R. Infantile agranulocytosis: a review with presentation of ten new cases. *Acta Paediatr Scand.* 1975;64:362-368.
3. Welte K, Zeidler C, Reiter A, et al. Differential effects of granulocyte-macrophage colony-stimulating factor and granulocyte colony-stimulating factor in children with severe congenital neutropenia. *Blood.* 1990;75:1056-1063.
4. Lalezari P, Pryce SC. Detection of neutrophil and platelet antibodies in immunologically induced neutropenia and thrombocytopenia. In: Rose NR, Friedman H, eds. *Manual of Clinical Immunology.* Washington, DC: American Society for Microbiology; 1980:744-749.
5. Kurland JI. Granulocyte-monocyte progenitor cells. In: Golde DW, ed. *Methods in Hematology, 11: Hematopoiesis.* New York, NY: Churchill Livingstone; 1984:87-122.
6. Iscove NN, Sieber F, Winterhalter KH. Erythroid colony formation in cultures of mouse and human bone marrow: analysis of the requirement for erythropoietin by gel filtration and affinity chromatography on agarose-concavalin A. *J Cell Physiol.* 1974;83:309-320.
7. Ogawa M, Leary AG. Erythroid progenitors. In: Golde DW, ed. *Methods in Hematology, 11: Hematopoiesis.* New York, NY: Churchill Livingstone; 1984:123-132.
8. Tsu TT, Hertzenberg LA. Solid-phase radioimmune assays. In: Mishell BB, Shiigi SM, eds. *Selected Methods in Cellular Immunology.* San Francisco, Calif: WH Freeman; 1980:373-397.
9. Motojima H, Kobayashi T, Shimane M, Kamachi S, Fukushima M. Quantitative enzyme immunoassay for human granulocyte colony stimulating factor (G-CSF). *J Immunol Methods.* 1989;118:187-192.
10. Cantrell MA, Anderson D, Cerretti DP, et al. Cloning, sequence, and expression of a human granulocyte/macrophage colony stimulating factor. *Proc Natl Acad Sci U S A.* 1985;82:6250-6254.
11. Groopman JE, Molina JM, Scadden DT. Hematopoietic growth factors. *N Engl J Med.* 1989;321:1449-1459.
12. Bonilla MA, Gillio AP, Ruggeiro M, et al. Effects of recombinant human granulocyte-stimulating factor on neutropenia in patients with congenital agranulocytosis. *N Engl J Med.* 1989;320:1574-1580.
13. Sonoda Y, Arai N, Ogawa M. Humoral regulation of eosinophilopoiesis in vitro: analysis of the targets of interleukin-3, granulocyte/macrophage colony-stimulating factor (GM-CSF), and interleukin-5. *Leukemia.* 1989;3:14-18.
14. Kawaguchi Y, Kobayashi M, Tanabe A, et al. Granulopoiesis in patients with congenital neutropenia. *Am J Hematol.* 1985;20:223-234.
15. Pietsch T, Buhrer C, Mempel K, et al. Blood mononuclear cells from patients with severe congenital neutropenia are capable of producing granulocyte colony-stimulating factor. *Blood.* 1991;77:1234-1237.

Use of Infant Walkers

Board of Trustees

• Infant walkers are used by many parents because of the convenience they provide in keeping children occupied. Unfortunately, parents may develop a false sense of security that leads to diminished vigilance over the safety of their infant. Although most injuries that result from walkers are minor, serious trauma from head injuries, lacerations, and burns does occur occasionally. The American Medical Association recommends that physicians counsel parents on the risk of injury that can occur from the use of infant walkers and inform parents that these devices do not either promote bipedal ambulation or offer a substitute for careful parental supervision.

(*AJDC.* 1991;145:933-934)

Concern for the safety of infants who use walkers first surfaced in the early 1970s when the federal government developed standards under the Federal Hazardous Substance Act (1971) that regulated the construction of walkers and jumpers to prevent the crushing of fingers or toes. The Consumer Product Safety Commission, in a 1974 study involving review of visits to 176 emergency departments and personal interviews, found that 3700 children had received treatment for trauma resulting from use of infant walkers.[1,2] Most of these were infants under age 2 years. From a follow-up survey in 1980, the Consumer Product Safety Commission reported that 24 000 infants had sustained an injury related to use of walkers resulting in 8600 emergency department visits; 54% of these involved trauma from falling down stairs.[3] Although the results of other studies have confirmed the initial concerns, the samples investigated have been relatively small and there have been no efforts to compare the rates and types of injuries between infants who use walkers and those who do not.[4-8] With these limitations in mind, the epidemiology of walker injuries may be summarized as follows:

1. Between 70% and 80% of infants will use a walker, mostly between ages 5 and 12 months; twice as many boys use walkers as girls.
2. Of infants who use walkers, 30% to 40% will have an accident.
3. Most walker accidents are minor and relatively few result in contact with a physician.
4. The most common types of accident involve falling down stairs, tipping over, and finger entrapment. Other injuries result from infants pulling objects down onto themselves.
5. Of infants seen in emergency departments for a walker injury, almost all *serious* trauma results from falling down stairs. Over 90% of all stairwell injuries among infants less than 12 months of age are related to use of walkers. Closed head injury is the most common serious walker injury, followed by fractures (skull, arm, clavicle) and other trauma, such as burns, dental injuries, and lacerations.
6. Of infants with serious injury, about one third stop walker use immediately, one third stop use within 2 months (usually because infants begin walking on their own), and one third are still using a walker 2 months after the injury.
7. Most walker injuries occur in the home with one or both parents present. Of injuries involving stairs, about half occur in houses *with* stairwell gates.
8. Although the occurrence of trauma is unrelated to the age at first use, number of siblings, and parents' occupations, it is related to the amount of time spent in the walker. Fewer than 30% who spend less than 2 hours a day in a walker suffer a nonserious fall, compared with approximately 55% of infants who spend more than 2 hours per day in a walker.
9. The types of walkers involved in serious injury are fairly evenly divided between the X-frame, in which the steel support bars form an X, and the circular frame, in which the support bars go up in a straight vertical pattern to reach the upper tray.

An estimated one million infant walkers are sold each year.[3] The most common reason given by parents is to keep the infant quiet, occupied, and happy. Although many parents use these devices to stimulate ambulation, there is no supportive evidence that walkers help babies learn to walk sooner.[9] Because the type of leg movement stimulated by walkers is different from that found with nonassisted locomotion, there is some concern that they may actually impede ambulation among infants with spastic cerebral palsy.[10] No studies, however, have confirmed the concern that use of walkers adversely affects development of either apparently normal infants or those who have or who are at high risk for neurologic delay in ambulation.

Walkers are popular among some parents because of the convenience they provide in keeping children occupied.

Accepted for publication January 3, 1991.

From the Board of Trustees, American Medical Association, Chicago, Ill.

Reprint requests to 515 N State St, Chicago, IL 60610 (Jerrod Loeb, PhD).

Unfortunately, this convenience creates, among some parents, a false sense of security resulting in diminished vigilance over the safety of the infant. Injuries among infants who use walkers are common, but usually minor. Although relatively rare, such serious trauma as head injuries, lacerations, and burns do occur occasionally. Parents also have a mistaken belief that walkers promote bipedal ambulation.

However, because the use of infant walkers provides some degree of danger to unsupervised infants, the American Medical Association recommends that "physicians counsel parents on the risk of injury that can occur from the use of infant walkers and inform parents that these devices do not either promote bipedal ambulation or offer a substitute for careful parental supervision."

This report was passed by the AMA House of Delegates in June 1990.

References

1. US Consumer Product Safety Commission. *Baby Walker Injuries: Hazard Analysis.* Washington DC: US Bureau of Epidemiology; 1974.
2. US Consumer Product Safety Commission. *Baby Walkers.* Washington DC: US Bureau of Epidemiology; 1975. US Consumer Product Safety Commission Fact Sheet 66.
3. US Consumer Product Safety Commission. *Baby Walkers.* Washington DC: US Bureau of Epidemiology; 1980. US Consumer Product Safety Commission Fact Sheet 66 Revised.
4. Fazen LF, Felizberto PI. Baby walker injuries. *Pediatrics.* 1982;70:106-109.
5. Kavanagh CA, Banco L. The infant walker: a previously unrecognized health hazard. *AJDC.* 1982;136:205-206.
6. Stoffman JM, Bass MJ, Fox AM. Head injuries related to the use of baby walkers. *Can Med Assoc J.* 1984;131:573-575.
7. Greensher J, Mofenson HC. Injuries at play. *Pediatr Clin North Am.* 1985;32:136-139.
8. Rieder MJ, Schwartz C, Newman J. Patterns of walker use and walker injury. *Pediatrics.* 1986;78:488-493.
9. Kauffman IB, Ridenour M. Influences of infant walker on onset and quality of walking pattern of locomotion: an electromyographic investigation. *Percept Mot Skills.* 1977;45:1323-1329.
10. Holm VA, Harthun-Smith L, Tada WL. Infant walkers and cerebral palsy. *AJDC.* 1983;137:1189-1190.

In Other AMA Journals

ARCHIVES OF PATHOLOGY & LABORATORY MEDICINE

Influence of Laboratory Test Volume and Geographic Location on Maternal α-Fetoprotein Results: Information From the College of American Pathologists Maternal α-Fetoprotein Survey

John H. Eckfeldt, MD, PhD, Thomas A. Long, MPH
(*Arch Pathol Lab Med.* 1991;115:647-653)

A Brief Review of the Anatomy, Histology, and Ultrastructure of the Full-Term Placenta

Richard F. Novak, MD
(*Arch Pathol Lab Med.* 1991;115:654-659)

College of American Pathologists Conference XIX on the Examination of the Placenta: Introduction

Henry Travers, MD, Waldemar A. Schmidt, PhD, MD
(*Arch Pathol Lab Med.* 1991;115:660-662)

Rice Solution and World Health Organization Solution by Gastric Infusion for High Stool Output Diarrhea

Felipe Mota-Hernández, MD, PhD; Daniel Bross-Soriano, MD; Maria L. Pérez-Ricardez, MD, PhD; Luis Velásquez-Jones, MD, PhD

• We sought to determine the efficacy of three different types of treatment in children with acute diarrhea who, during the oral rehydration period, had high stool output (>10 mL/kg per hour). Sixty-six children, aged 1 to 18 months, with an average stool output of 22.6 mL/kg per hour were randomly distributed into three groups: group 1 received a rice flour solution, group 2 received the World Health Organization rehydration solution by gastric infusion, and group 3 continued to receive this solution orally. In all three groups, a decrease in stool output was observed, with the higher decrease observed in group 1 patients. Such a decrease facilitated rehydration of all 22 patients in group 1 (100%) in 3.3±1.5 hours, 16 (73%) in group 2 in 4.3±2.1 hours, and 15 (69%) in group 3 in 4.9±2.0 hours. No complications were observed. These data indicate that the rice flour solution is effective in children with high stool output diarrhea.

(*AJDC.* 1991;145:937-940)

The use of the oral rehydration therapy (ORT) with the formula recommended by the World Health Organization (WHO)[1] has constituted a great advance for the treatment of dehydration secondary to diarrhea. A successful outcome in more than 90% of patients treated for 4 to 6 hours has been reported.[2,3] Unfortunately, this treatment usually fails in the high stool output state and hydration by the intravenous route is usually required.[3] Some authors[4] have proposed the use of a nasogastric tube (gastric infusion) as an alternate mode of therapy. This method of delivering lower volume at a constant rate may increase intestinal absorption of water, thus circumventing the intravenous route.

It has been proposed that products of rice starch hydrolysis, such as amylose and amylopectin (which ultimately break down into glucose), amino acids (glycine), dipeptides (glycil-glycine), and short-chain oligosaccharides (<10 molecules of glucose), enhance the absorption of sodium and water through an active membrane transport mechanism at the intestinal level without presenting an unwanted osmotic charge.[5-8] This might then account for the beneficial effect of oral rice solution on stool output during the correction of dehydration in children with liquid diarrhea.[9-12]

Our purpose was to compare the usefulness of rice flour solution with no electrolytes added (RFS) with the WHO formula administered either by the oral route (WHO) or through gastric infusion. The aim was to reduce the stool output in children in whom a high stool output was documented during the initial period of ORT.

PATIENTS AND METHODS

Sixty-six children whose ages ranged from 1 to 18 months, who presented with dehydration due to acute diarrhea of less than 17 days' duration and a persistent high stool output (>10 mL/kg per hour for 2 consecutive hours) during the oral rehydration period, were included in the trial. Stool output was calculated as the volume of feces in 1 hour divided by the patient's weight. The patients were seen between March 1988 and April 1989 at the Oral Hydration Ward of the Hospital Infantil de México "Federico Gómez, Mexico City."

Patients were excluded from the study if they had the following associated problems: acute renal failure, septicemia, meningitis, bronchopneumonia, third-degree malnutrition, persistent or progressive abdominal distention with suspicion of ileus or intestinal perforation, and those who had received gastric infusion in the preceding 12 hours or with an altered state of consciousness or in shock.

Before the children were admitted into our study and according to the routine management for dehydrated children at our hospital, all patients received ORT with the citrate WHO formula containing 90 mmol/L of sodium, 80 mmol/L of chloride, 20 mmol/L of potassium, 10 mmol/L of citrate, and 111 mmol/L of glucose.[13] The initial dose (100 mL/kg) was calculated for a 4-hour period. If, at any point during the observation period (at 1-hour intervals), the stool output was greater than the oral ingestion, the amount of oral solution offered in the next hour was increased to the equivalent of the stool loss during the previous hour plus 10%. All patients received 50 to 100 mL/kg of oral rehydration solution with the WHO formulation, given at a rate of 25 mL/kg per hour before entering the study. Not all the patients continued to receive the WHO formula during all 4 hours of this period because the criteria for their inclusion was that they had high stool outputs during 2 consecutive hours, and this requirement was reached after 2, 3, or 4 hours.

Accepted for publication December 12, 1990.

From the Servicio de Hidratación Oral, Hospital Infantil de México, "Frederico Gómez," México.

Read before the 19th International Congress of Pediatrics, Paris, France, July 28, 1989.

Reprint requests to the Servicio de Hidratación Oral, Hospital Infantil de México, "Frederico Gómez," Dr Marquez No. 162, Col. Doctores, 06720 Mexico D. F., Mexico (Dr Mota-Hernández).

Table 1.—Clinical Characteristics of 66 Children With High Stool Output Diarrhea Treated With Rice Flour Solution (Group 1), World Health Organization Solution by Gastric Infusion (Group 2), or by Oral Route (Group 3)*			
Characteristics	Group 1 (n=22)	Group 2 (n=22)	Group 3 (n=22)
Sex Ratio, M/F	13/9	12/10	14/8
Age, mo	8.54±3.6	8.18±3.9	10.36±5.1
Malnourished, No.	1	0	3
Evolution, h	89.7±75.6	124.9±103.2	96.9±115.9
Dehydration, %	5.9±2.5	7.2±2.6†	5.5±2.2†
Stool output, mL/kg per h	22.2±8.7	25.5±10.6	20.5±9.0

*Values are mean±SD, unless otherwise stated.
†$P<.05$ between groups B and C.

Table 2.—Previous Stool Output and During Treatment With Rice Flour Solution (Group 1), World Health Organization Solution by Gastric Infusion (Group 2), or by Oral Route (Group 3) in 66 Children With High Stool Output Diarrhea*

Group	Outcome	No.	Stool Output: Previous	Stool Output: During Treatment
1	Success	22	22.2±8.7	4.2±1.9†
2	Success	16	† 23.1±7.3	† 5.3±2.7†
	Failure	6	31.2±7.3	12.2±3.5†
3	Success	15	18.7±4.8	† 5.6±1.9†
	Failure	7	24.4±11.7	19.3±8.7

*Values are mean±SD.
†$P<.05$.

Table 3.—Rehydration Time in 53 Children With High Stool Output Diarrhea and Favorable Outcome With Rice Flour Solution (Group 1), World Health Organization Solution by Gastric Infusion (Group 2), or by Oral Route (Group 3)

Group	Rehydration	Time, h*	No.
1	3.3±1.5†	(1-6)	22
2	4.3±2.0	(1-8)	16
3	4.9±2.0†	(2-8)	15
Total	4.0±1.9	(1-8)	53

*Values are mean±SD (range).
†$P<.05$ between groups 1 and 3.

All eligible patients with persistent high stool output during the oral rehydration period, independently of the degree of dehydration, were divided into three groups by a list of random treatment assignments[14]: patients in group 1 received RFS, patients in group 2 received the WHO solution via gastric infusion, and patients in group 3 (the control group) continued to receive the WHO formula orally. The RFS was prepared with 50 g of rice flour and cooked for 10 minutes in water. If necessary, water was added to complete 1 L. The RFS analysis (22 samples) showed a sodium concentration of 1.4±1.0 mmol/L (mean±SD), a potassium concentration of 2.0±0.9 (mean ±SD), and an osmolarity of 47.1±10.3 mmol/L (mean ±SD).

In the three groups, a constant balance of fluid was measured, body weight was determined, and the evolution of the clinical signs of dehydration were recorded every hour. The patients received the same volume calculated previously. If, during any of the observation periods, the feces excretion was greater than the amount of ingestion, the volume of solution offered the following hour was increased in the same way as before entering the study.

If, during the first 2 hours of the study, the rate of stool loss decreased by 30% or more in relation to the previous average rate output during the 2 hours before entering the study, the administration of the same solution was continued through the same route in the required volumes until a normal state of hydration, assessed separately by two physicians, was obtained. Patients were closely monitored for clinical changes. The treatment was judged to be successful if there was both clinical response with decreased stool volume and correction of dehydration within 8 hours of initiation of ORT when admitted to our service.

In patients in whom fecal output did not decrease more than 30% during the first 2 hours of the study, treatment was considered to be a failure. In those in whom hydration was not attained in less than 8 hours, treatment was also considered to be a failure independently of the decrease in fecal output. All patients in whom treatment failed were hydrated by the intravenous route.

In admitting the patients to the study, the following laboratory values were determined: sodium, potassium, and osmolarity in serum and stool; serum glucose; and hemoglobin. Stool culture, investigation for rotavirus (by rotaphoresis), and assessment for ova and parasites were also performed.[15] When the state of dehydration was corrected or the patients were withdrawn from the study because of treatment failure, serum sodium, potassium, and hemoglobin levels were determined.

The sample size was determined by seeking a decrease of 30% in the rate of diarrhea output to be obtained with the use of RFS or gastric infusion. The mean value previously observed in our hospital for a group of 24 infants with high stool output requiring intravenous fluids was 17.89±7.04 mL/kg per hour (mean ±SD). Therefore, the expected decrease would be 6 mL (30%). The calculated sample sizes included 22 cases in each group with use of a two-tailed test,[14,16] as follows: $[2(SD)^2/(\text{expected difference})^2] \times 80\%$ of weight of the expected probability ($P<.05$), or $[2(7.04)^2/(6)^2] \times 7.9 = 22$ cases in each group.

The Mann-Whitney *U* Test, Wilcoxon Matched-Pairs Signed-Rank test, and Student's paired *t* test were used for statistical analysis.[17] The study was approved by the Hospital Infantil de México "Federico Gómez" Ethics Committee. Signed informed consent was obtained from the parents.

RESULTS

A summary of the characteristics of patients included in the three groups is shown in Table 1. The groups were comparable with respect to age, sex, duration of diarrheal state, and stool output volume. Except for four children with second-degree malnutrition, the patients were well nourished. The mean percentage (±SD) of dehydration, defined by the recuperation of weight observed when obtaining the state of normohydration, was 6.4%±2.7%, with a range from 2% to 13%; three patients in each group were severely dehydrated (>10%). There was a greater degree of dehydration in those patients in group 2, but these differences only became significant ($P<.05$) when compared with group 3, but not with group 1. In one third of the cases, the stool output was higher than 25 mL/kg per hour, distributed as follows: eight in group 1, 10 in group 2, and four in group 3.

A reduction in stool output of more than 30% was observed in all three groups since the first hour of the study. This reduction, as shown in Table 2, facilitated the rehydration of all 22 patients in group 1, 16 of 22 patients in group 2, and 15 of 22 patients in group 3. The failure rate in the patients rehydrated by gastric infusion was 27% (group 2) and 31% in the group hydrated by the oral route (group 3). Moreover, the stool output reduction was

Table 4.—Initial Laboratory Data From 66 Dehydrated Children With Diarrhea Treated With Rice Flour Solution (Group 1), World Health Organization Solution by Gastric Infusion (Group 2), or by Oral Route (Group 3)*

Examination	Total Patients (N=66)	Group 1 (n=22)	Group 2 (n=22)	Group 3 (n=22)
Stool				
Sodium, mmol/L	50.7±33.9 (8-182)	41.4±26.5 (8.1-75)	50.5±34.4 (13.5-94)	60.4±37.7 (20-182)
Potassium, mmol/L	18.8±9.4 (3.5-54)	19.8±10.7 (3.5-46)	19.1±13.1 (7.2-54)	18.3±7.1 (8-33)
Osmolarity, mosm/kg	200.6±65.1 (63-387)	212.9±76.2 ((114-320)	214.0±75.3 (63-322)	183.5±51.3 (131-387)
Serum				
Glucose, mmol/L	5.6±1.5 (2.8-11.1)	5.3±1.3 (3.8-7.8)	5.5±5.2 (2.8-8.3)	6.0±1.7 (3.5-11.1)
Hemoglobin, g/L	120±16 (90-164)	126±18 (90-146)	116±12 (98-142)	120±14 (92-164)
Hemoglobin, (post† rehydration), g/L	112±13 (84-135) [53]	117±13 (93-135) [22]	112±10 (91-131) [16]†	107±14 (84-130) [15]†

*Values are mean±SD (range) [number].
†Successful cases.

greater in those patients who were successfully rehydrated with RFS (group 1) than in patients in groups 2 and 3. During analysis of the average stool output of those patients in groups 2 and 3 in whom treatment failed, it was observed that the previous stool output was higher in group 2, showing a statistically significant difference (Table 2).

The time required to achieve hydration was shorter in the 22 patients hydrated successfully in group 1 than in the 16 patients in group 2 and in the 15 patients of group 3, with $P<.05$ between groups 1 and 3 (Table 3). In contrast, the quantity of solution required to obtain normohydration (mean±SD) was lower in group 1 than in groups 2 and 3 (65.8±36.2, 85.0±38.4, and 93.1±45.7 mL/kg, respectively), but the differences were not statistically significant. None of the patients in the study suffered a relapse, and none of those in whom treatment was considered to be successful required intravenous therapy.

No statistically significant differences were observed in the laboratory results of the three groups (Table 4). In the three groups, a nonsignificant decrease in the final concentration of serum sodium and potassium occurred when the state of normohydration was achieved (Table 5). No cases of symptomatic hyponatremia or hypokalemia were observed.

As to the causative agents, enteropathogens were identified or isolated in 25 (38%) of 66 children (Table 6). No causative agent was observed in the remaining 62% of the patients studied. No correlation was found between cause and the clinical evolution.

Table 5.—Serum Sodium and Potassium Concentrations Before and After Rehydration in 53 Dehydrated Children With Diarrhea Treated With Rice Flour Solution (Group 1), World Health Organization Solution by Gastric Infusion (Group 2), or by Oral Route (Group 3)*

	Serum Levels, mmol/L			
	Initial (N=66)		Final (n=53)	
Group	Sodium	Potassium	Sodium	Potassium
1	146.3±6.2 (138-161)	4.2±0.7 (3.5-5.9)	141.7±4.5 (135-148)	3.9±0.7 (2.8-5.6)
2	148.9±8.2 (134-160)	4.2±0.8 (3.0-6.5)	145.4±7.2 (141-158)	4.1±0.4 (3.4-4.5)
3	145.8±6.9 (132-170)	4.0±0.9 (2.4-6.3)	141.2±6.0 (127-143)	3.6±0.9 (2.1-4.6)

*Values are mean±SD (range).

Table 6.—Causes of Diarrhea in 25 Dehydrated Children Treated With Rice Flour Solution (Group 1), World Health Organization Solution by Gastric Infusion (Group 2), or by Oral Route (Group 3)*

Cause	Group 1	Group 2	Group 3	Total
Rotavirus	6	2	3	11
Escherichia coli	1	2	...	3
Shiqella flexneri	1	1	1	3
Campylobacter	1	...	...	1
Candida albicans	1	...	...	1
Klebsiella species	...	1	...	1
Pseudomonas	...	1	...	1
Cryptosporidium	...	...	1	1
Giardia lamblia	1	1	1	3
Total	**11**	**8**	**6**	**25 (38%)**

COMMENT

The most important finding in our study was that correction of high stool output permitted rehydration in all 22 patients treated with RFS. In contrast, in almost one third of the cases managed with WHO solution (by oral route or by gastric infusion), the high stool output persisted, thereby hindering the correction of dehydration. Previous studies of ORT[18,19] have shown that the most frequent cause of failure was precisely the presence of a high stool output.

It has been suggested that the osmolarity of a solution is inversely related to its intestinal absorption and that it enhances active intestinal secretion that in turn increases stool output.[20] Based on this knowledge, no electrolytes were added to the RFS in our study. The widespread use of RFS without electrolytes for the management of all cases of dehydration secondary to diarrhea has some inconveniences, such as fast fermentation and the hardware needed to cook the rice before its administration,[18,21,22] but the most important drawback is the risk of hyponatremia. To explain why hyponatremia was not induced in our patients, we assume that the initial treatment with the WHO solution for 2 to 4 hours may have provided sufficient electrolytes to maintain their normal serum levels during and after the RFS treatment period. Furthermore, at the beginning of the study, most of the patients included had an improved state of hydration.

An advantage of RFS over the WHO formula is that lower amounts of starch are required to correct dehydration and diminish the rate of diarrhea.[9,11] This advantage was also demonstrated in our study, even in patients with severe dehydration. Our study is the first we know of in which RFS without electrolytes has been used specifically for the treatment of children with persistent high stool output diarrhea and provides evidence that this condition may be an indication for RFS.

Whether the use of RFS powder solution plus electrolytes is equally effective in diminishing the stool output in children with persistent high output diarrhea remains to be clarified. Also left to be elucidated is the usefulness of RFS in children who, in addition to dehydration and high stool output rate, have third-degree malnutrition. In these patients, a subnormal intestinal hydrolytic process may interfere with rice starch digestion, as has been shown in children younger than 4 months.[9] In our study, however, a 3-month-old infant was adequately hydrated with RFS during a 2-hour period. Finally, we cannot determine the value of RFS in patients with chronic diarrhea, because they were not included in our study.

In the gastric infusion group, the six treatment failures occurred in those patients who had the highest stool output, and the decreased stool output in the 16 patients in whom treatment was successful was similar to that observed in the RFS group. One could speculate, then, that the efficiency of the RFS could be similar to that of the WHO formula administered by gastric infusion, except in those cases with the highest stool output. The success achieved in some patients who continued to receive the WHO formula by the oral route suggests that in some patients with high stool output, the administration of oral rehydration salts can diminish the stool output and correct the dehydration if one waits the required time to achieve it.

Although no cases of hyponatremia or hypokalemia were observed, and despite the good results obtained with the use of RFS in our study, we cannot dismiss the possibility that in patients with severe depletion of these cations, the prolonged administration of electrolyte-free RFS could worsen these complications. Its indiscriminate or prolonged use—mainly in malnourished children—should be avoided.

We conclude that RFS administered orally for short periods and after ORT may be useful in the treatment of well-nourished children with acute high stool output diarrhea and dehydration.

We thank Drs E. Aguilar-Parada, PhD, J. I. Santos, PhD, J. J. Urrutia, PhD, and M. Merson, PhD, for reading and revising the manuscript and Laura Leon for manuscript transcription. We also thank the Hospital Infantil de México "Federico Gómez" pharmacy, laboratory, resident physicians and interns, and Oral Hydration Department nursing staff for their invaluable support and cooperation in conducting our study.

References

1. World Health Organization. *A Manual for the Treatment of Acute Diarrhea: For Use by Physicians and Other Senior Health Workers.* Geneva, Switzerland: Program for Control of Diarrhoeal Diseases, World Health Organization; 1984. WHO/CDD/SER/80.2, Rev 1.

2. Santosham M, Daum RS, Dillman L, et al. Oral rehydration therapy of infantile diarrhea. *N Engl J Med.* 1982;306:1070-1076.

3. Velásquez JL, Llausás ME, Mota HF, Quiroz RB. Tratamiento ambulatorio del ninõ deshidratado por diarrea aguda. *Bol Med Hosp Infant Mex.* 1985;42:220-225.

4. Pizarro D, Posada G, Mahalanabis D, Sandi L. Comparison of efficacy of a glucose/glycine/glycil-glycine electrolyte solution versus the standard WHO/ORS in diarrheic dehydrated children. *J Pediatr Gastroenterol Nutr.* 1988;7:882-888.

5. Mahalanabis D. *Development of an Improved Formulation of Oral Rehydration Salts (ORS) With Antidiarrhoeal and Nutritional Properties: A 'Super ORS.'* Geneva, Switzerland: World Health Organization; 1985. WHO/CDD/DDM/85.3.

6. Murtaza A, Zulbigan I, Khan S, Lindblod BS, Sahlgren BA, Aperia A. The benefits of the very early introduction of powdered rice and dried edible seeds (Dal moong) in the oral rehydration solution during the treatment of acute infectious diarrhoea of infancy. *Acta Paediatr Scand.* 1987;76:861-864.

7. Carpenter CH, Greenough WB, Pierce N. Oral-rehydration therapy: the role of polymeric substrates. *N Engl J Med.* 1988;319:1346-1348.

8. Velásquez JL. Nuevas soluciones de hidratación oral en diarrea aguda. *Bol Med Hosp Infant Mex.* 1988;45:781-786.

9. Wong HB. Rice water in the treatment of infantile infectious gastroenteritis. *Lancet.* 1981;2:102-103.

10. Molla AM, Sarker SA, Holssain M, Greenough WB. Rice powder electrolyte solution as oral therapy in diarrhea due to *Vibrio cholerae* and *Escherichia coli. Lancet.* 1982;1:1317-1319.

11. Mehta MN, Subramanian S. Comparison of rice water, rice eletrolyte solution, and glucose electrolyte solution in the management of infantile diarrhoea. *Lancet.* 1986;1:843-845.

12. Bhan MK, Ghut OP, Knoshoo V, et al. Efficacy of mung bean (lentil) and pop rice based rehydration solutions in comparison with the standard glucose electrolyte solution. *J Pediatr Gastroenterol Nutr.* 1987;6:392-399.

13. World Health Organization. *Oral Rehydration Salts (ORS) Formulation Containing Trisodium Citrate.* Geneva, Switzerland: Program for Control of Diarrhoeal Diseases, World Health Organization; 1984. World Health Organization/Control Diarrhoeal Diseases/SER/84.7.

14. Pocock SJ. Clinical trials: a practical approach. New York, NY: John Wiley & Sons Inc; 1983:123.

15. Mota HF. *Diagnóstico en Pediatría: Interpretación Clínica de Exámenes de Laboratorio y Gabinete.* México, D.F.: Ed. Méndez Cervantes; 1985.

16. Brown G. Sample size. *AJDC.* 1988;142:1213-1215.

17. Bradford H. *Principios de Estadística Médica.* 3rd ed. Buenos Aires, Argentina: Ed. El Ateneo; 1965.

18. Velásquez JL, Mota HF. Procedimientos médicos para la hidratación oral en ninõs con diarrea. *Bol Med Hosp Infant Mex.* 1984;41:505-511.

19. Velásquez JL, Mota HF, Kane QJ, Puente TME, Llausás ME. Frecuencia de vómitos en ninõs con diarrea hidratados por vía oral. *Bol Med Hosp Infant Mex.* 1986;43:353-358.

20. Lifshitz F, Wapnir RA. Oral hydration solutions: experimental optimization of water and sodium absorption. *J Pediatr.* 1985;106:383-386.

21. Rahman ASMM, Bari A, Molla AM, Greenough WB. Mothers can prepare rice and use rice-salt oral rehydration solution in rural Bangladesh. *Lancet.* 1985;2:539-541.

22. De Vizia B, Ciccimarra F, DeCicco N, Auricchio S. Digestibility of starches in infants and children. *J Pediatr.* 1975;86:50-55.

Low Serum Calcium and High Parathyroid Hormone Levels in Neonates Fed 'Humanized' Cow's Milk–Based Formula

Bonny L. Specker, PhD; Reginald C. Tsang, MBBS; Mona L. Ho, MS; Theresa M. Landi, MSN; Teresa L. Gratton, MS

• We previously suggested that "late" neonatal hypocalcemia is related to a low calcium-phosphorus ratio of current cow's milk–based formula compared with human milk. However, there are no longitudinal studies of ionized calcium and parathyroid hormone concentrations in neonates receiving formulas with varying Ca/P ratios. Sixty-nine term neonates were studied through 2 weeks of age, and formula-fed neonates were randomized at birth to receive formula with molar ratios of 0.9, 1.2, or 1.4. Serum phosphate concentrations on days 2 and 6 of age were higher, and ionized calcium levels lower on days 6 and 14, in formula-fed vs human milk–fed neonates. Serum intact parathyroid hormone level increased between days 2 and 6 in formula-fed neonates compared with a decrease in human milk–fed neonates. Serum parathyroid hormone level on day 6 correlated with phosphorus intake among formula-fed neonates. No differences were noted in serum mineral or hormone levels among formula-fed groups. We speculate that the lowering of serum ionized calcium concentrations in neonates fed a modern "humanized" cow's milk formula may be a factor in late neonatal hypocalcemia.

(*AJDC.* 1991;145:941-945)

Standard cow's milk–based infant formulas have a calcium-phosphorus molar ratio of approximately 1.0. Although it is generally assumed that these formulas are sufficiently "humanized" with respect to calcium and phosphorus content, we have observed that neonates fed these formulas occasionally suffer hypocalcemic convulsions and apparent secondary hyperparathyroidism within the first weeks of age.[1] Hypocalcemia in neonates presumably is related to the higher phosphate load of these formulas when compared with human milk (Ca/P molar ratio, approximately 1.6), and a more optimal Ca/P ratio theoretically might be between 1.2 and 1.6, closer to that of human milk.

There are no longitudinal studies of serum calcium, phosphorus, and parathyroid hormone (PTH) changes in normal neonates fed formulas with varying Ca/P ratios compared with neonates fed human milk. We undertook such a study to determine the effect of cow's milk–based formulas containing varying Ca/P ratios (0.9, 1.2, and 1.4) on indicators of calcium and parathyroid status during the first 2 weeks of age. These results were compared with those obtained from neonates receiving human milk.

The major hypotheses tested were that during the neonatal period, (1) serum calcium concentrations would be lower, and serum phosphorus and PTH concentrations higher, in neonates fed cow's milk–based formula compared with neonates fed human milk; and (2) neonates fed formula with a higher Ca/P ratio than that in standard infant formula would have calcium indices more similar to those in neonates fed human milk.

SUBJECTS AND METHODS

A total of 69 term, white neonates were studied from birth and completed the 14-day study period. Four parallel groups were studied longitudinally: a group of 20 neonates fed human milk (approximate concentrations of calcium and phosphate, 8.2 and 4.8 mmol/L; Ca/P molar ratio, 1.6; Ca/P weight ratio, 2.0) and three groups of neonates fed cow's milk–based formula identical in composition except for the amount and ratio of calcium and phosphorus. Commercially available formula (Similac, Ross Laboratories, Columbus, Ohio) was used as the low Ca/P ratio formula; the two additional formulas were developed by Ross Laboratories, Columbus, Ohio, and contained different amounts of calcium and phosphorus. The measured concentrations of the lots used for the three formula-fed groups were as follows: Ca/P molar ratio, 0.9 (calcium, 14.2 mmol/L; phosphate, 15.3 mmol/L; Ca/P weight ratio, 1.2; n = 16); Ca/P molar ratio, 1.2 (calcium, 17.5 mmol/L; phosphate, 14.6 mmol/L; Ca/P weight ratio, 1.5; n = 17); and Ca/P molar ratio, 1.4 (calcium, 20.3 mmol/L; phosphate, 14.9 mmol/L; Ca/P weight ratio, 1.7; n = 15).

Investigators and mothers of the formula-fed neonates were "blinded" to the formula that was being used. All neonates were above the 10th percentile in birth weight and birth length and had 1- and 5-minute Apgar scores of 7 or greater and 8 or greater.

Accepted for publication April 18, 1991.

From the Division of Neonatology, Department of Pediatrics, University of Cincinnati (Ohio) Medical Center, Cincinnati Children's Hospital Medical Center, and Perinatal Research Institute, Cincinnati.

Presented in part at the Society for Pediatric Research Annual Meeting, Washington, DC, May 5, 1988.

Reprint requests to Department of Pediatrics, ML 541, University of Cincinnati Medical Center, Cincinnati, OH 45267-0541 (Dr Specker).

Serum Mineral and PTH Concentrations Over First 2 weeks of Age by Type of Feeding*

	Human Milk	Formula 0.9 Ca/P	Formula 1.2 Ca/P	Formula 1.4 Ca/P
Calcium, mmol/L				
Day 2	2.30±0.18 (25)	2.32±0.14 (12)	2.62±0.14 (17)	2.42±0.12 (15)
Day 6	2.59±0.16 (20)	2.52±0.23 (16)	2.42±0.25 (12)	2.54±0.15 (11)
Day 14	2.67±0.15 (15)	2.62±0.10 (13)	2.64±0.16 (16)	2.62±0.15 (14)
Ionized calcium, mmol/L				
Day 2	1.25±0.08 (26)	1.23±0.08 (15)	1.25±0.09 (18)	1.28±0.06 (16)
Day 6	1.44±0.10 (18)	1.34±0.04 (11)	1.28±0.08 (12)	1.34±0.05 (15)
Day 14	1.46±0.06 (17)	1.40±0.06 (14)	1.39±0.04 (14)	1.43±0.03 (13)
Phosphate, mmol/L				
Day 2	1.71±0.40 (25)	2.09±0.11 (11)	2.13±0.24 (17)	1.94±0.42 (16)
Day 6	1.61±0.29 (19)	2.32±0.36 (14)	2.45±0.21 (12)	2.32±0.36 (12)
Day 14	1.94±0.29 (15)	2.13±0.27 (14)	2.29±0.55 (16)	2.00±0.38 (13)
Intact PTH, μL Eq/mL				
Day 2	84±34 (18)	70±52 (6)	53±20 (9)	86±55 (12)
Day 6	50±19 (14)	96±72 (8)	70±37 (7)	87±69 (9)
Day 14	54±21 (12)	63±35 (10)	73±17 (8)	65±22 (6)

*PTH indicates parathyroid hormone. Molar ratios of calcium to phosphorus are given for three formulas given formula-fed groups. Values are mean±SD (number of subjects).

None of the neonates had evidence of cardiac, respiratory, gastrointestinal, or other systemic disease. There were no significant maternal medical histories that could affect fetal growth, such as diabetes or perinatal infections.

Mothers were recruited prenatally, and if the mother intended to feed the neonate formula, provided the neonate met the eligibility requirements at birth, the neonate was randomized after stratification by sex. For ethical and pragmatic reasons, neonates were not randomized to human milk or formula feeding. All formula-fed neonates received only the study formula immediately from birth through 2 weeks of age. Human milk–fed neonates did not receive supplemental formula at any time through 2 weeks of age. All neonate groups were concurrently studied to minimize any possible seasonal effects on calcium metabolism.[2,3]

Each neonate had blood samples collected at 36 to 48 hours of age and on days 6 and 14 (±1 day) of age. When possible, blood samples were drawn by venipuncture in the late morning 2 hours postprandially. Samples were collected in 5% carbon dioxide tubes to stabilize pH, and serum was separated for immediate ionized calcium measurement. The rest of the serum was frozen and analyzed in one batch for total calcium, phosphorus, and PTH concentrations. Serum ionized calcium concentrations were measured using an ion-selective electrode (Radiometer, Copenhagen, Denmark). The intra-assay and interassay coefficients of variation (CVs) on normal control serum are 0.8% and 2.5%, respectively. Serum total calcium concentrations were measured by atomic absorption spectrophotometry; the interassay CV is 2.1% to 2.5%. Serum phosphate concentrations were measured on an autoanalyzer (ABA-100, Abbott Diagnostics, Abbott Park, Ill). Our intra-assay and interassay CVs are 1.5% and 2.5%, respectively.

Intact PTH concentrations were measured using a modification of the method of Arnaud[4] using guinea pig antiserum produced in our laboratory that recognizes the entire PTH molecule with no cross-reactivity with the 65-85 fragment or the 1-34 fragment. The intra-assay and interassay CVs are 8.4% and 16.3%, respectively.

Anthropometric measurements were obtained on days 2 and 14 of age. Dietary intakes were recorded daily for the first 14 days of life. The average daily phosphorus intake for days 1 to 6 and days 7 to 14 were calculated as the product of volume consumed and the phosphorus content of the formula divided by the number of days. The relationships between serum measurements at 6 and 14 days of age, and average phosphorus intakes during the week preceding the collection of blood samples, were determined. A specialized form of analysis of variance (ANOVA) techniques (nested) was performed that takes into account the repeated measurements obtained from a neonate.[5] The factors included in the statistical model were diet, time, and the diet-by-time interaction. If this interaction is significant, it implies that the relationship, or changes over time, in the measurement differs depending on the diet of the neonate. In addition, Student's t test was performed to compare formula-fed and human milk–fed neonates at each time point. Analysis of variance was performed to determine whether there were differences between the three formula-fed groups at each time point. Biochemical measurements were normally distributed among human milk–fed neonates. However, serum PTH concentrations had a log normal distribution among formula-fed neonates. Statistical analyses using the log PTH concentration did not alter the findings. Data are presented as mean±SD.

RESULTS

The four groups were similar in weight and length at birth and 14 days of age, as well as in the percent of male neonates.

Formula-fed neonates had significantly lower serum ionized calcium concentrations than human milk–fed neonates (nested ANOVA, $P<.001$), and ionized calcium concentrations significantly increased over time (nested ANOVA, $P<.001$). The changes over time differed depending on the diet of the neonate (nested ANOVA interaction term, $P<.001$). Ionized calcium concentrations were lower in formula-fed neonates compared with human milk–fed neonates at both 6 and 14 days of age compared with human milk–fed neonates (Student's t test, $P<.001$ and $P=.001$, respectively; Fig 1). No differences were noted among the formula-fed groups (nested ANOVA, $P=.10$) in serum ionized calcium concentrations, and changes over time were similar among the groups (nested ANOVA interaction term, $P=.26$).

Serum total calcium level did not differ between formula- and human milk–fed neonates (nested ANOVA, $P=.10$) but did increase significantly with time (nested

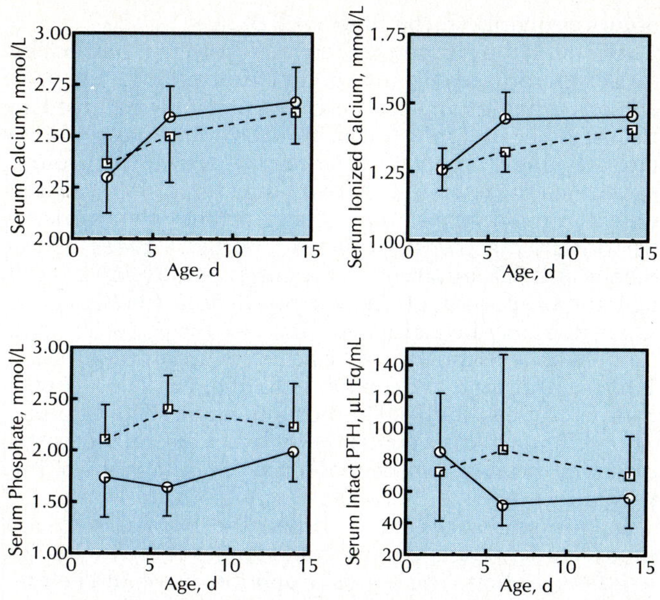

Fig 1.—*Serum phosphate, calcium (total and ionized), and intact parathyroid hormone (PTH) concentrations in formula-fed neonates (squares) and human milk–fed neonates (circles). Data are presented as mean±SD. Overall, there was a significant effect of diet on serum ionized calcium (P<.001) and phosphate (P<.001) concentrations. Significant age effects were observed for serum ionized calcium (P<.001), total calcium (P<.001), and phosphate (P<.001) concentrations. The changes with age differed significantly by diet for serum ionized calcium (P<.001), total calcium (P=.005), phosphate (P<.001), and intact PTH (P=.002) concentrations.*

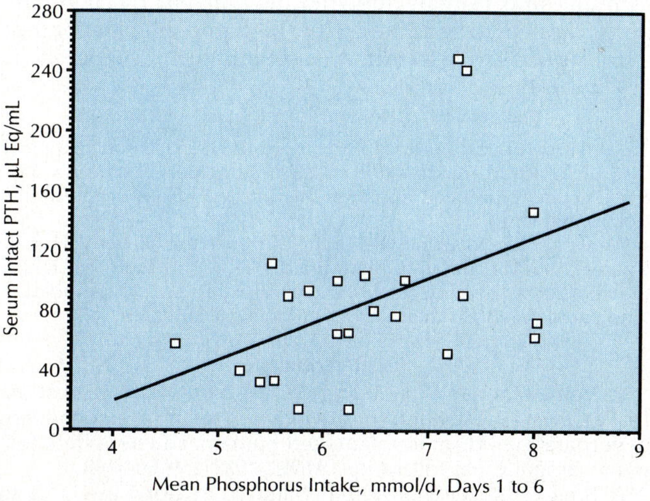

Fig 2.—*Serum intact parathyroid hormone (PTH) level at 6 days of age was associated with average daily phosphorus intake from days 1 to 6 of age (r=.436, P=.03).*

ANOVA, *P*<.001). This change over time differed between the formula- and human milk–fed groups (Fig 1; nested ANOVA interaction term, *P*=.005). There were no significant differences among the three formula-fed groups (nested ANOVA, *P*=.92) in serum total calcium concentrations (Table), and changes over time were similar among the groups (nested ANOVA interaction term, *P*=.17).

Neither serum ionized nor total calcium concentrations on days 6 or 14 of age were related to the amount of phosphorus consumed (average in milligrams per day) during the first 6 or 14 days of age.

Formula-fed neonates had higher serum phosphate concentrations than human milk–fed neonates (nested ANOVA, *P*<.001), and serum phosphate concentrations changed significantly over time (nested ANOVA, *P*<.001). This change over time differed depending on the diet of the neonate (nested ANOVA interaction term, *P*<.001). Formula-fed neonates had higher serum phosphate levels on days 2 (*P*<.001) and 6 (*P*<.001) of age (Fig 1). No significant differences were noted among the three formula-fed groups (nested ANOVA, *P*=.19) in serum phosphate concentrations (Table), and changes over time were similar among the groups (nested ANOVA, *P*=.88). Serum phosphate concentrations on days 6 or 14 of age were not related to the phosphorus consumed during the first 6 or 14 days of age.

Overall, there was no difference in intact PTH concentrations between formula- and human milk–fed neonates (nested ANOVA, *P*=.20), and for all neonates combined there was no difference with time (nested ANOVA, *P*=.13). However, changes in serum PTH concentrations over time were different in formula-fed compared with human milk–fed neonates (nested ANOVA interaction term, *P*=.002): concentrations decreased between days 2 and 6 in neonates fed human milk, while they increased in neonates fed formula. There were no significant differences among the three formula-fed groups (nested ANOVA, *P*=.87) in serum intact PTH concentrations (Table), and changes over time were similar among the groups (nested ANOVA, *P*=.34). Serum C-terminal PTH concentrations were also measured. No significant results were found, and since C-terminal PTH represents inactive PTH fragments, the results are not presented.

Serum PTH concentration on day 6 of age was related to the phosphorus intake during the first 6 days of age (*r*=.436, *P*=.03; Fig 2). Serum PTH concentrations on day 14 of age were not related to the average phosphorus intake during the preceding 7 or 14 days (*r*=.155, *P*=.47 and *r*=.121, *P*=.57, respectively).

COMMENT

In a previous study, our laboratory reported the anecdotal occurrence of hypocalcemic convulsions, hyperphosphatemia, and elevated serum PTH concentrations in neonates fed modern humanized cow's milk–based formula.[1] Although secondary hyperparathyroidism is thought to occur in such neonates as a result of the lowering of serum calcium concentrations resulting from the high phosphate load, there have been no prospective studies evaluating sequential serum mineral and PTH concentrations in this situation.

Early reports from the United Kingdom linked the occurrence of "late" neonatal hypocalcemia and tetany to neonates receiving cow's milk–based formulas with high phosphorus content.[6,7] Lealman and coworkers in Glasgow, Scotland,[8] reported lower serum calcium and higher serum phosphate concentrations at 6 days of age in term neonates fed a humanized cow's milk–based formula (Cow and Gate V formula; phosphorus, 16 mmol/L; Ca/P molar ratio, 1.1) compared with neonates fed human milk (phosphorus, 4.8 mmol/L; Ca/P molar ratio, 1.6). Serum phosphate concentrations were not as high, and serum calcium concentrations not as low, as those respective measurements in neonates receiving an even higher phosphorus–containing cow's milk–based formula (Ostermilk; phosphorus, 20.6 mmol/L; Ca/P molar ratio, 1.0). Bagnoli and coworkers[9] in Italy found that neonates fed cow's milk–based formula (phosphorus, 11.6 mmol/L; Ca/P molar ratio, 1.0) had lower total calcium and higher serum phosphate concentrations by 48 hours of age than human milk–fed neonates. In none of the above studies were serum PTH concentrations determined.

In the United States, late infantile tetany apparently has become less common since the introduction of humanized cow's milk–based proprietary formulas with lower phosphorus content. However, these humanized formulas still contain a higher phosphorus load and lower Ca/P molar ratio than that provided by human milk. It has been impossible to lower the phosphorus content further because of the phosphorus present in the protein, and owing to the low solubility of calcium, it has been difficult to incorporate higher amounts of calcium into formula to increase the Ca/P ratio. Thus, theoretically, since humanized cow's milk–based formulas still contain a phosphorus content relatively higher than that in human milk, the potential for high serum phosphate and low serum calcium concentrations in neonates fed these formulas still exists.

The phosphorus content in formula theoretically may affect calcium homeostasis either by forming insoluble calcium salts in the intestine, thereby reducing the availability of calcium, or by increasing serum phosphate concentrations once absorption has occurred.[10] This increase in serum phosphate concentration would increase the calcium × phosphate product in blood, promoting efflux of calcium and phosphate into bone, theoretically resulting in a lowering of blood ionized calcium concentrations. An increase in serum PTH concentrations theoretically will reduce (normalize) the high serum phosphate concentrations through its phosphaturic action and elevate (normalize) the low serum calcium concentrations through its bone and renal actions.

In this study, we observed a significant difference between formula- and human milk–fed neonates with respect to serum phosphate (higher in formula-fed neonates) and ionized calcium (lower in formula-fed neonates) concentrations. However, a dose-response relationship of increasing calcium concentrations or decreasing phosphorus concentrations with formulas of increasing Ca/P ratios was not observed. In addition, we observed a positive relationship between intact PTH concentrations on day 6 of age and the average amount of phosphorus consumed during the first 6 days of age. We suggest from our results that the amount of phosphorus consumed, rather than the Ca/P ratio of the formula, may be more important in altering calcium homeostasis in infancy. Larger amounts of phosphorus ingested thus indirectly trigger a PTH response, which normalizes serum calcium and phosphate concentrations.

Enhanced phosphate reabsorption by the immature kidney has been reported. It has been suggested that the mechanism for this enhanced renal phosphate reabsorption is the high concentration of growth hormone in the neonatal period[11] or possibly intracellular phosphate depletion in immature renal cells, thereby increasing apical membrane phosphate transport.[12] Thus, this maximal reabsorption of phosphate in the immediate neonatal period may in part explain the significant increase in serum phosphate concentrations related to a high phosphorus intake. This also might explain why late neonatal hypocalcemia occurs primarily in the first week of age.

Although the differences between the means, especially for serum ionized calcium, do not appear large, the variation is small owing to the inherent biological need to maintain serum ionized calcium concentrations within a narrow range. These differences are significant from a public health viewpoint. A lower limit for ionized calcium of 1.10 mmol/L at 24 hours of age, a time when concentrations are the lowest, has been reported.[13] Based on the means and SDs observed in the current study at 6 days of age, the proportion of the two populations that lie below this value may be estimated. The risk for hypocalcemia, defined as a serum ionized calcium concentration below 1.10 mmol/L, among neonates fed human milk is 1/10 000, compared with 30/10 000 among neonates fed formula. This difference may explain why hypocalcemic tetany is observed primarily in neonates fed formula and not human milk.

In this study, we have chosen the human milk–fed group as the reference, or "gold standard," with respect to infant feeding. The opposite opinion also could be presented: the volume of intake of formula-fed neonates could be considered the norm, and human milk–fed neonates could be receiving lower, inadequate intakes of phosphorus during the first week of age.

In summary, cow's milk–based formula feeding results in increased serum phosphate, decreased serum ionized calcium, and increased PTH levels compared with human milk feeding in the neonatal period. We speculate that late neonatal hypocalcemia, which can develop in some term neonates, may be related to use of cow's milk–based formula. Differences in calcium homeostasis between formula- and human milk–fed neonates in the neonatal period appear to be related to the high phosphorus content of formula relative to human milk rather than differences in Ca/P ratio.

This study was supported in part by grant 11725 from the National Institute of Child Health and Human Development, Bethesda, Md; the Cincinnati Perinatal Research Institute; and Ross Laboratories, Columbus, Ohio.

We would like to acknowledge the nurses in the Obstetric Unit of University of Cincinnati (Ohio) Medical Center for their assistance; the laboratory personnel for their technical expertise; and the mothers who participated for their support of medical research.

References

1. Venkataraman PS, Tsang RC, Greer FR, Noguchi A, Laskarzewski P, Steichen JJ. Late infantile tetany and secondary hyperparathyroidism in infants fed humanized cow's milk formula: longitudinal follow-up. *AJDC*. 1985;139:664-668.

2. Specker BL, Lichtenstein P, Mimouni F, Gormley C, Tsang RC. Calcium-regulating hormones and minerals from birth to 18 months of age: a cross-sectional study, II: effects of sex, race, age, season, and diet on serum minerals, parathyroid hormone, and calcitonin. *Pediatrics*. 1986;77:891-896.

3. Lichtenstein P, Specker BL, Tsang RC, Mimouni F, Gormley C. Calcium-regulating hormones and minerals from birth to 18 months of age: a cross-sectional study, I: effects of sex, race, age, season, and diet on vitamin D status. *Pediatrics*. 1986;77:883-890.

4. Arnaud C, Tsao J, Littledike T. Radioimmunoassay of human parathyroid hormone in serum. *J Clin Invest*. 1971;50:21.

5. Hicks CR. *Fundamental Concepts in the Design of Experiments*. 2nd ed. New York, NY: Holt Rinehart & Winston; 1973.

6. Bakwin H. Tetany in newborn infants. *AJDC*. 1937;54:1211-1226.

7. Baum D, Cooper L, Davies PA. Hypocalcemic fits in neo-

nates. *Lancet.* 1968;1:598-599.
8. Lealman GT, Logan RW, Hutchinson JH, Kerr MM, Fulton AM, Brown CW. Calcium, phosphorus and magnesium concentrations in plasma during first week of life and their relation to type of milk feed. *Arch Dis Child.* 1976;51:377-384.
9. Bagnoli F, Bruchi S, Sardelli S, et al. Calcium homeostasis in the first days of life in relation to feeding. *Eur J Pediatr.* 1985;144:41-44.
10. Allen LH. Calcium bioavailability and absorption: a review. *Am J Clin Nutr.* 1982;35:783-808.
11. Mulroney SE, Lumpkin MD, Haramati A. Antagonist to GH-releasing factor inhibits growth and renal P_i reabsorption in immature rats. *Am J Physiol.* 1989;257:F29-F34.
12. Johnson A, Spitzer A. Renal reabsorption of phosphate during development: whole-kidney events. *Am J Physiol.* 1986;251:F251-F256.
13. Loughead JL, Mimouni F, Tsang RC. Serum ionized calcium concentrations in normal neonates. *AJDC.* 1988;142:516-518.

BOOK REVIEW

An Introduction to Clinical Research

By Catherine DeAngelis, 183 pp, with illus, $24.95, Stoneham, Mass, Butterworth Publishers Inc, 1991.

This is a clear, well-written book that walks the reader through a clinical research project. It begins with defining the research question and ends with critiquing the published project description. The author has consulted respected clinical researchers in writing this text, and her introduction is an excellent précis of the journey from the beginning to the end of a research project. Chapter 1, which discusses the scientific method, is the most difficult chapter to understand and could be simplified in the next edition. Chapters 2 and 3 review the definition of the research question and selection of subjects. Chapter 4 ("Types of Research Models and Methods") is particularly good. It clarifies such difficult concepts as varied study designs by using excellent tables and figures. Chapter 5 discusses data collection, management, and analysis; like chapter 4, its clarification of topics such as statistical tests of significance and data collection methods is excellent. Chapter 6 discusses frequently asked questions about finding sources and about ethical standards for research involving human subjects, including federal regulations and criteria of institutional internal review boards.

A particular strength of this book is its success at remaining an *introduction* to clinical research. Each chapter contains references to books and articles that address particular issues more comprehensively. In addition, chapter 8 is an annotated bibliography providing a synopsis of books with particular relevance to research methods and development, statistics, clinical research funding, and critical appraisal of the medical literature.

This book should be a valued addition to the library of junior faculty, physicians on fellowship, residents, and any student in the health profession who is interested in understanding and performing clinical research.

Jessie R. Groothuis, MD
Department of Pediatrics
Children's Hospital
1056 E. 19th Ave
Denver, CO 80218-1088

Evaluation of Intraosseous vs Intravenous Antibiotic Levels in a Porcine Model

David G. Jaimovich, MD; Ashir Kumar, MD; Steve Francom, PhD

• *Objectives.*—To compare intraosseous vs intravenous routes of administration and their effects on serum levels of four antibiotics in an animal model.
Design.—Prospective controlled study comparing two routes of drug administration.
Setting.—Research laboratories of a large pharmaceutical company.
Participants.—Twenty male and female domestic swine weighing 10 to 20 kg.
Interventions.—The animals were anesthetized and treated with controlled ventilation. The animals were divided into one of four groups: (1) intravenous and intraosseous cefotaxime sodium (50 mg/kg), (2) intravenous and intraosseous chloramphenicol sodium succinate (25 mg/kg), (3) intravenous and intraosseous vancomycin hydrochloride (15 mg/kg), or (4) intravenous and intraosseous tobramycin sulfate (2.5 mg/kg). There was a 24-hour clearance period for groups 1 and 2 and a 48-hour clearance period for groups 3 and 4. Serum drug levels were measured at 1, 15, 30, 45, 60, 90, and 120 minutes after intravenous and intraosseous administration of the respective antibiotics. Control and treated tibias were sampled for drug levels at the end of the experiment.
Measurements and Main Results.—Peak serum concentrations for intravenously administered antibiotics were within the therapeutic range. Peak serum levels after intravenous and intraosseous administration were 102 and 82 mg/L, respectively for cefotaxime; 13.9 and 6.3 mg/L, respectively, for chloramphenicol; 24.5 and 3.8 mg/L, respectively, for vancomycin; and 7.1 and 1.3 mg/L, respectively, for tobramycin.
Conclusions.—Cefotaxime may be administered intraosseously when intravenous access is not possible. We cannot recommend chloramphenicol or vancomycin for intraosseous administration, because serum levels were not comparable with those following intravenous administration. Findings with tobramycin suggested a lack of achievement of serum levels comparable with those following intravenous administration.

(*AJDC*. 1991;145:946-949)

Infants and children with fulminant bacterial infection often present in septic shock.[1] If intravenous (IV) access is not readily available for administration of volume expanders and antimicrobial agents, morbidity and mortality are adversely affected.[2] In recent years, there has been a resurgence of the intraosseous (IO) route for the administration of a variety of drugs that may need to be administered urgently.[3-5] The IO route was first utilized for administration of fluids and blood almost half a century ago but was virtually abandoned because of the availability of "fine butterfly" needles and IV catheters.[6,7] Some drugs, when administered IO, achieve therapeutic serum levels; others, however, fail to do so.[8] Recently, Jaimovich et al[8] reported that serum levels of phenobarbital sodium and phenytoin sodium, when administered IO, were markedly lower than when these anticonvulsant drugs were administered IV. Furthermore, phenytoin, when administered IO, failed to achieve therapeutic serum levels and therefore could not be recommended for IO administration. Despite a large number of antimicrobial drugs available today, no data regarding serum levels achieved after the IO administration of an antibiotic are readily available. We compared IO vs IV routes and their effects on serum levels of four antibiotics in an animal model.

Accepted for publication February 4, 1991.

From the Department of Pediatrics, Division of Pediatric Critical Care Medicine, University of Illinois at Chicago (Dr Jaimovich); Department of Pediatrics, Division of Infectious Disease, Michigan State University School of Human Medicine, Lansing, Mich (Dr Kumar); and the Division of Biostatistics, The Upjohn Company, Kalamazoo, Mich (Dr Francom).

Reprint requests to the Department of Pediatrics (M/C 856), Division of Critical Care, University of Illinois, 840 S Wood St, Chicago, IL 60612 (Dr Jaimovich).

MATERIALS AND METHODS

The animals were housed in the animal care facility of the Upjohn Research Facility, Kalamazoo, Mich, in accordance with their institutional animal care guidelines. Twenty domestic swine weighing 10 to 20 kg were anesthetized with ketamine hydrochloride (20 mg/kg given intramuscularly). The animals were then given inhalation anesthesia with halothane. Subsequently, the trachea was intubated with a No. 5 or 6 endotracheal tube, ventilation was controlled, and halothane anesthesia was continued. Lead II electrocardiography monitored heart rate and rhythm throughout the experiment. Two peripheral hind limb veins were cannulated with 20-gauge catheters for administration of IV fluids as necessary and for administration of the antibiotics, respectively. The jugular vein was catheterized to obtain serum samples for antibiotic levels. Intravenous fluids were administered as 5% dextrose in water at a rate of 4 mL/kg per hour; temperature was maintained between 37°C and 38°C. The animals were randomly assigned to one of the four study groups: (1) IV and IO cefotaxime sodium, (2) IV and IO chloramphenicol sodium succinate, (3) IV and IO vancomycin hydrochloride, and (4) IV and IO tobramycin sulfate.

After skin preparation, a 16-gauge adjustable-length bone marrow aspiration needle (Monoject Illinois Sternal-Iliac, Sherwood Medical, St Louis, Mo) was inserted into the broad, flat, anteromedial surface of the tibia 1 cm below the tibial tuberosity. Once the needle was advanced into the bone marrow, the obturator was removed, and the IO position of the needle was confirmed by free aspiration of blood and bone marrow contents, such as fat and bone spicules. All animals received a 10-mL saline solution flush to clear the cannula of the antibiotic after IO administration.

The first study group (n=5) was given cefotaxime sodium (50 mg/kg) through a peripheral IV line, and a similar dose was administered via the IO route. The second group (n=5) was given chloramphenicol sodium succinate (25 mg/kg) IV and IO. There was a 24-hour serum clearance period between the IV and IO administrations of cefotaxime and chloramphenicol. The third group (n=5) was administered vancomycin hydrochloride (15 mg/kg) IV and IO. The fourth group (n=5) received tobramycin sulfate (2.5 mg/kg) IV and IO. There was a 48-hour serum clearance period between the IV and IO administrations of vancomycin and tobramycin. The animals were allowed to recover in their pens and were reanesthetized in similar fashion for the IO phase of the study. Cefotaxime, chloramphenicol, and tobramycin were administered during a 30-minute period, and vancomycin was administered during a 60-minute period. Blood, to measure serum antibiotic levels for each drug, was drawn from the jugular venous line at 1, 15, 30, 45, 60, 90, and 120 minutes after the administration of the respective antibiotics by both the IV and the IO routes. An additional pretreatment serum level, before IO administration, was measured to verify drug clearance from the serum. All animals were killed at the end of the experiment per Upjohn Research facility protocol.

Cefotaxime serum levels were assayed by high-pressure liquid chromatography by solvent delivery system (Water's 501 Pump), with a sample injector (Water's U6K Injector), cefotaxime levels were detected by a UV spectrophotometer (Water's 481 Spectrophotometer Water's Associates, Milford, Mass), and recorded on a strip chart recorder (Omniscribe Inc, Houston, Tex). Serum samples and standards were processed by phase extraction and injected into the system with a mobile phase of 8% acetonitrile and 92% 0.1-mol/L potassium phosphate buffer. Peak heights were measured and specimen valleys were calculated according to the standard curve. Validation of the procedure yielded within-batch and between-batch reproducibility of greater than 95%. Serum for chloramphenicol was analyzed by submitting samples into a delivery system (SYVA Auto Carousel, SYVA Company, Palo Alto, Calif). Chloramphenicol levels were detected by a UV spectrophotometer (S-III Spectrometer, SYVA Company), and drug level calcaluations were computer analyzed (Lab Processor 6500, SYVA Company). Samples were analyzed along with standards and quality control materials with emit reagents (SYVA Emit Assay, SYVA, Company). This assay is a homogeneous enzyme immunoassay technique based on competition between drug in the sample and enzyme-labeled drug. This assay has a within-run coefficient of variance of 4% and a between-run coefficient of variance of 5%. Tobramycin and vancomycin were tested by fluorescent polarization (TDX Analyzer, Abbott Diagnostics, North Park, Ill). Samples were analyzed along with quality control materials with the use of reagent packs (Abbott Diagnostics) according to the manufacturer's specifications. The analyzer utilizes fluorescent polarization immunoassay technology. Both assays have between- and within-run coefficients of variance of less than 5%.

Control contralateral tibias and the tibias into which antibiotics were administered were frozen in liquid nitrogen, crushed, and then homogenized. The tibia into which chloramphenicol was administered was placed in a 100-mL solution of methanol and extracted with a high-speed tissue homogenizer. The extract was centrifuged at 2000g for 10 minutes. The resulting supernatant was then submitted for enzyme immunoassay, and the concentration was determined by UV spectrophotometry and computer analysis. Samples from the tibias that received intraosseous tobramycin and vancomycin infusions were prepared with a similar procedure, with the exception of the solvent. The frozen, crushed tibias were homogenized with 200 mL of a 0.01-mol/L sodium phosphate (pH 8.0) and placed in a refrigerated continuous rotor device that stirred the solution for 24 hours. The resulting supernatants were submitted and the concentrations were determined by fluorescent polarization immunoassay.

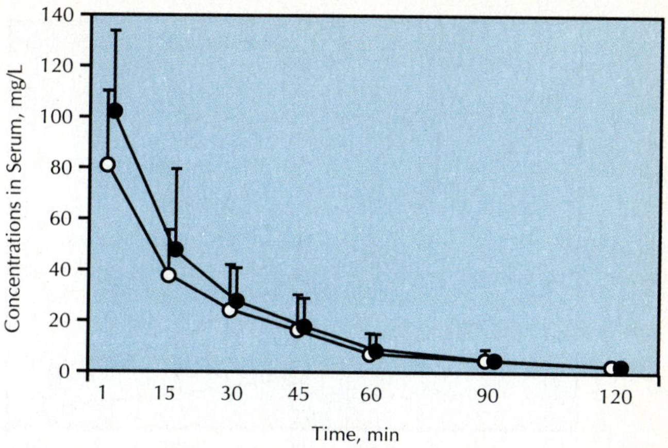

Fig 1.—*Serum concentrations of cefotaxime over time following intravenous (solid circles) and intraosseous (open circles) routes of administration.*

Pharmacokinetic Data Following Intravenous and Intraosseous Routes of Administration*

Drug	Intravenous	Intraosseous	*P*
Cefotaxime			
AUC	2673 ± 923	2347 ± 931	NS
C^{max}	102 ± 32	82 ± 27	NS
T^{max}	1.0 ± 0.0	1.0 ± 0.0	NS
Tobramycin (n=4)			
AUC	268 ± 182	62 ± 38	NS
C^{max}	7.1 ± 5.4	1.3 ± 0.7	NS
T^{max}	1.0 ± 0.0	12 ± 22	NS
Chloramphenicol			
AUC	753 ± 182	299 ± 138	.006
C^{max}	14.0 ± 1.8	6.4 ± 3.3	.005
T^{max}	1.0 ± 0.0	1.0 ± 0.0	NS
Vancomycin			
AUC	1598 ± 876	234 ± 281	.025 (n=4)
C^{max}	25 ± 13	3.8 ± 3.2	.023
T^{max}	1.0 ± 0.0	28 ± 52	NS

*Values are mean ± SD. AUC indicates area under the plasma concentration time curve; C^{max}, T^{max}, ; and NS, not significant.

Statistical analysis was used to compare the means of the serum levels at each time point between the two routes of administration for each antibiotic. This was performed by using an analysis of variance model that incorporated factors for animals and route of administration. The pharmacokinetic data associated with antibiotic serum levels, maximum concentration (C_{max}), and the time to peak plasma concentration (T_{max}) were determined by inspection. The area under the plasma concentration time curve (AUC) was estimated with the trapezoid rule.

RESULTS

All animals survived the experiment with no adverse effects noted clinically from the IV and IO administration of antibiotics. At no time during the experiment did any

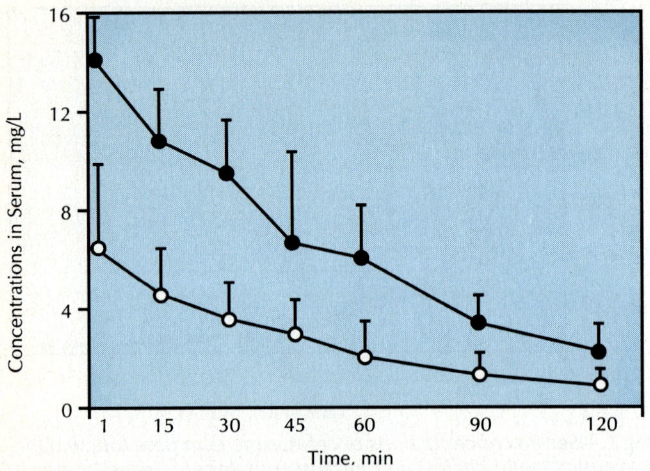

Fig 2.—*Serum concentrations of chloramphenicol over time following intravenous (solid circles) and intraosseous (open circles) routes of administration.*

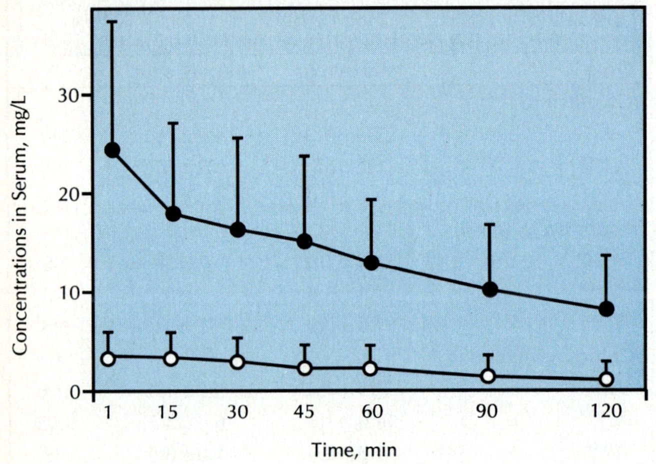

Fig 3.—*Serum concentrations of vancomycin over time following intravenous (solid circles) and intraosseous (open circles) routes of administration.*

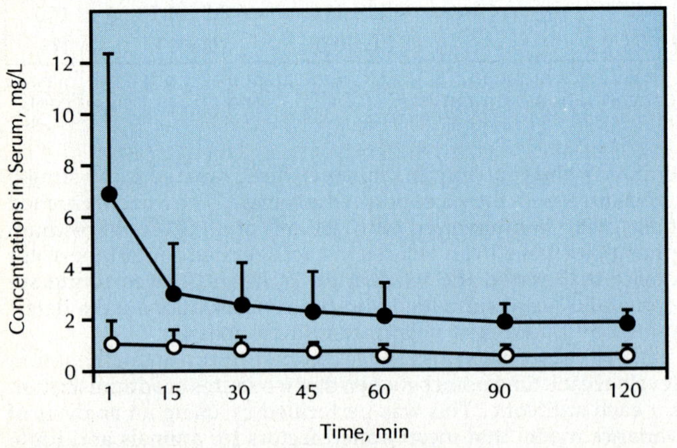

Fig 4.—*Serum concentrations of tobramycin over time following intravenous (solid circles) and intraosseous (open circles) routes of administration.*

of the animals exhibit signs of deterioration in cardiovascular, hemodynamic, or pulmonary status.

The means, SDs, and *P* values associated with the various drugs, routes of administration, and pharmacokinetic data are seen in the Table. Serum cefotaxime levels following the IV and IO routes of administration showed the curve to be nearly identical, and there were no significant differences (Fig 1, Table, $P<.01$) and vancomycin ($P<.05$) showed significant differences between the IV and the IO routes of administration for C_{max} and AUC (Table, Figs 2 and 3). Although the differences for C_{max} and AUC were not statistically significant ($P>.15$) between the two routes, for tobramycin, the peak achieved after the IO route of administration was only 1.3 mg/L (Fig 4). Tobramycin had a lower power due to one less subject in the study group.

The level of chloramphenicol in the tibia receiving the IO administration after 120 minutes of infusion was 253.8 mg/L, and the contralateral (control) tibia showed a level of 42.4 mg/L. The vancomycin level in the tibia at 120 minutes after the IO infusion was 28.6 mg/L, and the control tibia showed a level of 3.08 mg/L. Similarly, the tobramycin level in the tibia at 120 minutes after the IO infusion was 0.81 mg/L, and the control tibia showed a level of 0.20 mg/L. Bones for cefotaxime levels were not assayed due to the near-identical serum levels achieved following the IO and IV routes of administration of cefotaxime.

COMMENT

The peak serum concentration achieved following the administration of recommended IV dosages was within the therapeutic range and was also similar to the levels achieved in infants and children after the administration of a single dose for all four antibiotics.[9] Serum levels achieved after IO administration were subtherapeutic for vancomycin, chloramphenicol, and tobramycin; however, the serum concentration of cefotaxime was comparable with the levels measured following IV administration. This subtherapeutic phenomenon has also been demonstrated when phenytoin was administered IO.[8] Severalfold higher concentrations of chloramphenicol (sixfold), tobramycin (fourfold), and vancomycin (ninefold) were detected, even after 120 minutes in the respective tibias where these antibiotics were administered IO. These observations indicate that these three antibiotics were not fully distributed into the systemic circulation from the site of the administration. Chemical characteristics of antibiotics (ie, fat solubility, protein binding, and calcium binding) may influence the distribution of antibiotic from the IO space to the systemic circulation. These factors remain poorly understood. In critically ill children, the IO administration provides an alternate route to obtain vascular access when IV access is not readily available. The IO route is used to administer a variety of drugs; however, very limited data are available regarding serum concentrations of drugs achieved after I0 administration.[4,8,10] Domestic swine were chosen as the experimental model because of similarities between their tibias and those of infants. The weight and development of the bone marrow of 10- to 14-week-old swine are similar to those of infants or small children.[3] In our study, only one of the four antibiotics evaluated achieved a comparable serum concentration when administered IO; therefore, we recommend that pharmacokinetic data be obtained for the drugs that may need to be administered through the IO route in an emergency. Our study demonstrated that cefotaxime, a third-generation cephalosporin with a broad spectrum of activity and that is capable of good central nervous system penetration in the presence of meningeal inflammation, achieved comparable levels in serum after IO administration. A large number of third-generation cephalosporins and other antimicrobial drugs are available to pediatricians to treat critically ill infants and children. The physician should be aware that cefotaxime achieved comparable levels in the serum after IO and IV routes of administration.

This investigation was funded by the Bronson Clinical Investigation Unit Community Research Fund.

References

1. Gotoff SP, Behrman RE. Neonatal septicemia. *J Pediatr.* 1970;76:142-153.
2. Hodes HL. Care of the critically ill child: endotoxic shock. *Pediatrics.* 1969;44:248-260.
3. Spivey WH, Unger HD, Lathers CM, McNamara RM. Intraosseous diazepam suppression of pentylenetetrazol-induced epileptogenic activity in pigs. *Ann Emerg Med.* 1987;16:156-158.
4. Spivey WH, Lathers CM, Malone DR, et al. Comparison of intraosseous, central, and peripheral routes of sodium bicarbonate administration during CPR in pigs. *Ann Emerg Med.* 1985;14:1135-1140.
5. Berg RA. Emergency infusion of catecholamines into bone marrow. *AJDC.* 1984;138:810-811.
6. Rosetti VA, Thompson BM, Miller J, Mateer JR, Aprahamian C. Intraosseous infusion: an alternative route of pediatric intravascular access. *Ann Emerg Med.* 1985;14:885-888.
7. Spivey WH. Intraosseous infusions. *J Pediatr.* 1987;111: 639-643.
8. Jaimovich DG, Shabino CL, Ringer TV, Peters GR. Comparison of intraosseous and intravenous routes of anticonvulsant administration in a porcine model. *Ann Emerg Med.* 1989;18:842-846.
9. McCracken GH, Nelson JD. Clinical pharmacology and dosage. In: McCracken GH, Nelson JD, eds. *Antimicrobial Therapy for Newborns: Practical Application of Pharmacology to Clinical Usage.* New York, NY: Grune & Stratton; 1977:5-68.
10. Orlowski JP, Porembka DT, Gallagher JM, van Lente F. Comparison study of intraosseous, central intravenous, and peripheral intravenous infusions of emergency drugs. *AJDC.* 1990;144:112-117.

In Other AMA Journals

JAMA

Treatment Choice for Infants in the Neonatal Intensive Care Unit at Risks for AIDS

B.W. Levin; J.M. Driscoll, Jr; A.R. Fleischman (*JAMA.* 1991;265:2976)

Health, Health Insurance, and the Uninsured

R.H. Brook (*JAMA.* 1991;265:2998)

The Case Against 'the Case Against Childhood Cholesterol Screening'

K. Resnicow; G. Berenson; S. Shea; S. Srinivasan; W. Strong; E.L. Wynder (*JAMA.* 1991;265:3003)

Family Practice

R.E. Rakel (*JAMA.* 1991;265:3120)

Neurology

R.J. Joynt (*JAMA.* 1991;265:3134)

Classified Advertising

All classified advertising orders, correspondence and payments should be directed to: American Journal of Diseases of Children, P.O. Box 1510, Clearwater, Florida 34617. Our telephone numbers are: 800-237-9851; 813-443-7666. Please do not send classified ads, payments or related correspondence to the AMA headquarters in Chicago. This causes needless delay.

Inquiries about "BOX NUMBER" advertisements: All replies must be in writing and must cite the box number in the ad. Example: Box ____, c/o AJDC, P.O. Box 1510, Clearwater, Florida 34617. We are not permitted to divulge the identity of advertisers who wish their mail sent in care of American Journal of Diseases of Children .

CLASSIFIED INFORMATION

Regular Classified	1 Time	3 times or more*
Cost per word	$1.85	$1.70
Minimum ad: 20 words		per issue

**In order to earn the three-time rate, your ad must be placed and prepaid at the same time for three or more issues.*

Counting Words: Two initials are considered one word, each abbreviation is considered one word, and figures consisting of a dollar sign and five numerals or less are considered one word. Cities and states consisting of two words or more are counted as one word: i.e., "New York" and "Salt Lake City". Zip code is considered one word and must appear in all ads. Telephone number with area code is considered one word. When box numbers are used for replies, the words "Box ____, c/o AJDC" are to be counted as three words.

Classified Display	1 Time	3 times or more*
Full page	$1,155	$1,005
Two-thirds page	985	856
One-half page	809	704
One-third page	638	554
One-sixth page	295	257
Column inch	80	65

Minimum display ad: one column inch
12-time and 24-time rates available on request.

Display Production Charge: The publication will pub-set advertisements upon request. The typesetting fee is 10% of the one-time ad cost shown above. Special requests will be billed to the advertiser and/or agency at the then prevailing rates.

Box Service

Available for all ads. The cost is $15.00 for the first issue only. Responses to your ad will be consolidated in our office and promptly mailed directly to you.

Closing Date

The 25th of the second month prior to the issue date. Example: The November issue closes September 25th. No ads can be cancelled after the closing date.

Send all copy, correspondence, production materials and payments to:

AMERICAN JOURNAL OF DISEASES OF CHILDREN

AJDC

Classified Department
P.O. Box 1510, Clearwater, Florida 34617

For assistance with your ad schedule call toll free:
800-237-9851 ◆ 813-443-7666

Professional Opportunities

NEONATOLOGIST to join five-member BC/BE group in a Level III perinatal center with academic affiliation. For further information, contact: B.T. Bloom, MD, 550 North Hillside, Wichita, KS 67214. (316) 688-2360.

IMMEDIATE OPENING for BC/BE pediatrician to associate with well-established, rapidly growing, 32-MD multi-specialty group. Located in the San Francisco Bay area in a growing community serving 170,000. Patients include both fee-for-service and prepaid health plan. Attractive compensation and benefits. Malpractice provided. California license required. Send CV to: Bart Bona, Administrator, Fairfield Medical Group, Caller Box 4020, Fairfield, CA 94533-0410. (707) 426-3911.

MAINE: Immediate opportunity for a fourth BC/BE pediatrician with general and/or subspecialty interests to join a multi-specialty group affiliated with a 250-bed regional referral hospital. Enjoy the professional challenge offered in a sophisticated medical community along with the wonderful recreational opportunities and quality of life in Maine. Please send CV to: Richard Marsh, MD, 76 High Street, Suite 203, Lewiston, ME 04240. Or call: (207) 795-2389; (800) 445-7431, ask for Shannon Tamminen.

TWO PEDIATRICIANS seeking third BC/BE pediatrician to join two site, growing practice. Ideal all season recreational area. Ideal site for young family. Please contact: Tahoe City Pediatrics, P.O. Box 6959, Tahoe City, CA 95730.

ROCHESTER, NEW YORK – Opportunity for a general pediatrician to develop their practice as part of the Rochester Medical Group pediatric department. Rochester Medical Group is a multi-specialty group practice which cares for fee-for-service as well as prepaid patients. In addition to full-time position, willing to consider part-time or job-share opportunities. Subspecialty interests possible. University affiliation encouraged. Competitive salary and benefits. Located in attractive metropolitan area with many cultural and recreational advantages. Send resume or call: Rochester Medical Group, P.C. Attention: James Tobin, MD, 800 Carter Street, Rochester, NY 14621. (716) 338-1400. EOE, M/F.

NEONATOLOGIST: Marshfield Clinic, a 350 physician multi-specialty private group practice in central Wisconsin, is seeking a fourth BC/BE neonatologist to join its 20-member pediatric department. Adjacent 524-bed acute care teaching hospital includes a 24-bed, Level III Neonatal Unit. Full pediatric support subspecialties are available on-site. Pediatric Residency Program, University of Wisconsin Medical School affiliation, Medical Research Foundation and large regional referral base contribute to a very stimulating environment. Marshfield, a community of 20,000, was recently designated as "one of the best small cities in the Midwest." Send curriculum vitae plus the names of several references to: James C. Opitz, MD, Marshfield Clinic, 1000 North Oak Avenue, Marshfield, WI 54449. Or call collect: (715) 387-5016.

WASHINGTON – Established, five full-time, one part-time pediatric group seeking full-time BC/BE pediatrician. Beautiful, rapidly growing community in midst of mountains and water, one hour from Seattle. Local hospital and nearby childrens' hospitals. Opportunity to practice a wide range of pediatric skills. Competitive salary; early partnership. Reply with cover letter and CV to: Medical Director, Kitsap Children's Clinic, 2625 Wheaton Way, Suite A, Bremerton, WA 98310. (206) 479-1651.

Professional Opportunities

LARGE MULTI-SPECIALTY GROUP in northern Virginia area needs bilingual (Spanish) pediatrician to replace retiring physician of forty years. Send CV to: Medical Director, Falls Church Medical Center, 6060 Arlington Boulevard, Falls Church, VA 22044.

PEDIATRICIAN – SEATTLE: Outstanding pediatric practice seeking an associate. Busy practice, affiliated with excellent 300-bed general hospital. Must be board-certified or board-eligible. Contact: Richard G. Wedig, Highline Hospital, 12844 Military Road South, Seattle, WA 98168. (206) 248-4561.

SAVANNAH, GEORGIA – General pediatrician wanted to join four-member group. Growing practices include a satellite office. Guaranteed salary, productivity incentive and early buy-in offered. Personal and professional life in Savannah can be very rewarding. Contact: William Hutcheson, MD, (912) 354-5814.

PEDIATRICIAN
which do you prefer?

Generous Salary and Benefits
Modern Facility
Group Practice
Flexible Working Schedule
Community Oriented Primary Care
Computerized Office
Experienced Management Team
Friendly Patients and Staff
Shared Call Schedule
Social Worker
WIC Program
Federally Funded Migrant Program
Sliding Fee
Excellent Local Hospital
Diversified Practice
Eligible for Loan Forgiveness
Medical School Affiliation and Faculty Appointment Possible

We've got it all!

Send CV to: James Goetz, MD, Medical Director,
Oak Orchard Community Health Center
80 West Avenue, Brockport, New York, 14420

PHILADELPHIA – Two pediatricians seeking BE/BC third for growing practice in southwest Philadelphia. Full partnership opportunity after two years. Send CV to: Fredric Nelson, MD, 2801 Island Avenue, Philadelphia, PA 19153.

BC/BE PEDIATRICIAN NEEDED. Busy office practice. Guaranteed salary, benefits. Mountain local. CV to: Mike McCraley, Ogden Clinic, 4650 Harrison Boulevard, Ogden, UT 84403. (801) 479-4621.

PARTNER NEEDED IN 1992 for three physician practice. Join two BC pediatricians: a 1980 MD of University of Pittsburgh and residency at Children's Hospital, Pittsburgh and a 1984 MD of Pennsylvania State School of Medicine, Hershey and residency at the University of Chicago. Opportunity is close to New York and Ohio in the greater lakeland area of Meadville, Pennsylvania. This college community is family oriented with excellent schools. First year guarantee and benefits. For further information call: (800) 283-8321, Extension 5705. Or send curriculum vitae to: Brenda Lewis, Meadville Medical Center, 1034 Grove Street, Meadville, PA 16335.

PLEASE NOTE – Address replies to box number ads as follows: Box number ________ , c/o AJDC, P.O. Box 1510, Clearwater, FL 34617.

Family Physicians and Neonatology

Sir.—It is regrettable that the editor who edits this section of THE JOURNAL is so ignorant of interspecialty relations that he or she would not have purged the slur to family practitioners in the letter by DiTraglia[1] that appeared in the November 1990 issue.

All specialties contribute in unique ways to the care of the patient. I am convinced that there are medical and family issues that family practitioners handle better than pediatricians, because of the family physician's involvement with other family members and in other acute care settings. One example is of a 4-year-old girl who presented with chest pains and was recognized by her family physician to have an acute myocardial infarction, despite the pediatricians' diagnoses. I guess I have participated in the resuscitation of more newborns in the last 10 years than many pediatric oncologists, yet I would not disparage another specialty because of disparate practice patterns.

The general pediatricians and pediatric subspecialists who trained me were intent on spreading good pediatric care to the most children who could be reached. This should remain our common goal rather than slandering each other, especially in eminent journals.

FLOYD L. MCINTYRE, MD
Family Medicine
76 Airline Rd
South Dennis, MA 02660

1. DiTraglia J. Neonatology blues. *AJDC.* 1990;144:1180.

In Reply.—I am sorry that McIntyre considers my statement a slur. It was not intended to be derogatory.

He states that we all offer unique care to children; this is what I meant. Even within specialties, different individuals have different strengths and training backgrounds.

I am comfortable with my role as a pediatrician and with the unique contribution I make to the care of patients. I hope McIntyre is not insecure with his role as a family practitioner in his community.

JOHN DITRAGLIA, MD
1835 Oakland Ave Bldg A
Portsmouth, OH 45662

Your Child's Best Friend: TV or Not TV?

Sir.—In the March 1991 issue of *AJDC*,[1] Dr Stiehm described his experience with strict curtailment of his three daughters' TV viewing so that they would devote more time to schoolwork, reading, music, and exercise. This worked out well for his family, but it might not for others who have different interests and/or lack entertainment and learning alternatives.

Television has been stigmatized as the "boob tube," yet it also provides fine educational, news, public affairs, sports, music, and general entertainment programs. One must be selective to find good books in a library and good music on the radio; this also applies to TV programs. Thus, rather than proscribe TV, parents might be better advised to review the coming weeks' TV fare, go over it with their children, and help them decide which programs of value to watch. Clearly, there is nothing wrong with children viewing "Sesame Street"; "Mister Rogers"; "NoVA"; "The National Geographic Explorer"; telecourses; plays, such as *The Grapes of Wrath* and *Hamlet*; selected well-regarded movies and docudramas; operas, concerts, "Live From Lincoln Center"; "Evening at Pops"; "20/20"; "60 Minutes"; "The Civil War" series; "The Cosby Show"; a sports event or two; and the news, including Cable News Network's coverage of events such as the Persian Gulf war.

Television is a major educational tool for many people and may be their only real contact with the outside world. (About 30% of US families do not subscribe to a newspaper.) It is the only entertainment many families can afford. A large number of TV viewers are latchkey kids whose neighborhoods are unsafe and drug infested (*Wall Street Journal.* March 25, 1991: A-1). Their parents are often poor and single. It would be nice if those children had more recreational and educational options, but the reality is that they frequently do not.

As they grow up, our children must adjust to the electronic age and put TV into reasonable perspective. We must teach them this without simply turning off the TV. My experience with my three teenaged daughters has been that they tend to watch TV when there seems to be nothing better to do; they much prefer socializing with their friends, shopping, and engaging in more active pursuits. Also, their taste in music is not Brahms, which would put them to sleep when they do their homework. They prefer the Hot 30 Countdown, featuring Timmy T; Tara Kemp; Escape Club; Styx; and Jellyfish (DP).

MAX BADER, MD
2 SW Del Prado
Lake Oswego, OR 97035

1. Stiehm ER. Your child's best friend: TV or not TV? *AJDC.* 1991;145:257.

In Reply.—I agree with Dr Bader that there are worthwhile things on TV and that monitored, selective viewing is harmless, amusing, and sometimes educational. Such monitored viewing did not work at our house; nor, I daresay, does it work in most houses, so the choice is no monitoring or no TV.

For the alcoholic, abstinence is necessary; for the nonalcoholic, abstinence is harmless. I have yet to see any adverse emotional, social, or physical consequences of "hypotelevisionemia." Has anyone?

E. Richard Stiehm, MD
Division of Allergy/Immunology
Department of Pediatrics
UCLA School of Medicine
10833 Le Conte Ave
Los Angeles, CA 90024-1752

Misdiagnosis of Reye's-like Illness

Sir.—There are a number of case reports in the literature describing children with inborn errors of metabolism who have previously been misdiagnosed as having Reye's syndrome.[1-4] It is not known, however, whether these cases represent rare events or whether the misdiagnosis of Reye's syndrome is common in clinical practice.

We previously reported[5] the results of an epidemiologic study in which we demonstrated that the association between Reye's syndrome and prior exposure to aspirin was not accounted for by bias. In that study, potential cases of Reye's syndrome were reported to the investigators from a network of 108 pediatric tertiary care centers throughout the United States and Canada. The purpose of the present report is to describe the potential for misdiagnosis of Reye's syndrome in clinical practice by comparing the final diagnoses made by physicians who cared for the patients with the diagnoses made by a panel of three physicians with extensive knowledge and expertise in Reye's syndrome. We also investigated whether the age of the patient, the severity of the illness, and a history of aspirin exposure might contribute to the misdiagnosis of Reye's syndrome.

The results of liver biopsies are often accepted as conclusive evidence in either confirming or excluding the diagnosis of Reye's syndrome.[6] However, abnormalities demonstrated by light microscopy are not specific to Reye's syndrome and cannot be relied on to confirm the diagnosis.[7,8] Electron microscopy is now widely recommended to confirm the diagnosis, although, to our knowledge, no one has reported on the validity or reliability of this technique as it is used in clinical practice.

Table 1.—Agreement Between Diagnoses of Reye's Syndrome by Hospital Physicians and Expert Panel*

Hospital Physicians	Expert Panel: Definite	Uncertain	Definitely Not	Total
Definite	22	7	5	**34**
Uncertain	2	7	4	**13**
Definitely not	1	5	10	**16**
Total	**25**	**19**	**19**	**63**

*Overall agreement equals 62% (39 of 63 patients). $\kappa_w = .48$.

Research Methods.—Identification and Enrollment of Subjects.—Between January 1986 and July 1987, surveillance clinicians at each of 108 hospitals were asked to notify the researchers as soon as a patient was admitted for whom the diagnosis of Reye's syndrome could be considered, even if the diagnosis had already been ruled out. Subjects were ineligible if they had a history of Reye's syndrome, chronic liver disease, chronic encephalopathy, or a chronic disorder for which salicylates or acetaminophen were strongly indicated or contraindicated (eg, juvenile rheumatoid arthritis). After receiving reports of potential subjects, physician-researchers (B.W.F., R.I.H., and E.D.S.), blind to the medication history of the subject, decided on eligibility using predetermined guidelines. The guidelines had two purposes. The first was to allow for the early exclusion of children for whom there were already sufficient data to rule out conclusively the diagnosis of Reye's syndrome (eg, normal aminotransferase and ammonia levels). Second, the guidelines were intended to ensure that children were enrolled whenever there was any possibility that they might have Reye's syndrome.

Diagnostic Classification.—The "hospital diagnosis" was recorded as the discharge diagnosis on the hospital discharge summary sheet. This diagnosis was categorized as either definite Reye's syndrome, uncertain Reye's syndrome, or definitely not Reye's syndrome. The uncertain category included those cases in which terms were used that suggested uncertainty, such as "possible Reye's syndrome," and indeterminate expressions, such as "rule out Reye's syndrome." The category "definitely not" Reye's syndrome included those patients for whom an alternative diagnosis was recognized.

Three physicians who have extensive research experience and clinical expertise in Reye's syndrome were chosen to form an expert panel. The panel reviewed all data from each subject. These included a copy of the complete hospital record and a detailed account of the illness prior to hospitalization obtained through interviews of all persons who had cared for the child. The panel then assigned each subject to one of the three categories described above. Individual judgments were made by panel members before a consensus was reached. All references in the records to medications administered before hospitalization were removed before review.

The stage of severity of Reye's syndrome was classified according to the criteria developed by the National Institutes of Health Consensus Conference on Reye's syndrome: stage 1 includes children with lethargy, and stage 2 requires evidence of combative behavior or delirium. Stages 3 through 5 include coma with increasingly severe neurologic deficits.[9]

Review of Electron Micrographs of Liver Biopsy Specimens.—Whenever electron micrographs of liver biopsy specimens were available, copies were reviewed by John Partin, MD, a member of the panel and an authority on abnormalities of liver ultrastructure in Reye's syndrome.[6,10] The results of these reviews were made available to the panel before they reached their consensus.

Methods of Analysis.—The extent of agreement between the expert panel and the hospital physicians was assessed using the percentage of observed agreement. We also calculated a weighted κ statistic (κ_w) to correct for chance agreement. Individual weights were assigned as follows: 1 for complete agreement between the hospital discharge diagnosis and the consensus of the expert panel; ½ for a disagreement that is one category apart; and 0 for a disagreement that is two categories apart. The value of κ_w can vary from +1, indicating perfect agreement, to 0, indicating no better than chance agreement. The κ_w value was interpreted as follows: when the value of the index was less than .4, the rating of agreement was poor; when the index was between .4 and .59, the rating was fair; when the index was between .60 and 0.75, the rating was good; and when the index was greater

Table 2.—Agreement Between Diagnoses of Reye's Syndrome by Hospital Physicians and Expert Panel for Different Age Groups

	Expert Panel					
	Patient Age ≤ 3 y*			Patient Age > 3 y†		
Hospital Physicians	Definite	Uncertain	Definitely Not	Definite	Uncertain	Definitely Not
Definite	2	6	3	20	1	2
Uncertain	0	3	2	2	4	2
Definitely not	0	3	7	1	2	3

*Overall agreement equals 46% (12 of 26 patients). $\kappa_w = .29$.
†Overall agreement equals 73% (27 of 37 patients). $\kappa_w = .54$.

than .75, the rating of agreement was excellent.[11]

Results.—One hundred twenty-nine patients who met the eligibility criteria were reported to the investigators. Of these, 63 patients fulfilled the screening criteria as candidate case subjects, and complete data about them were obtained. These 63 patients were from 46 medical centers: 34 centers reported one case only, nine centers reported two cases, and three centers reported three or more cases. Nineteen subjects (30%) were classified as having stage 1 severity; 17 (27%) had stage 2; and 27 (43%) had stage 3 or greater.

Comparison of Hospital Diagnoses With Diagnoses of Expert Panel.—The comparison between the final diagnoses made by hospital physicians and the diagnoses made by the expert panel are shown in Table 1. The panel confirmed the diagnosis of definite Reye's syndrome in only 22 (65%) of the 34 hospital-diagnosed cases, and made the diagnosis of definite Reye's syndrome in three other cases not considered to be definite Reye's syndrome by the hospital physicians. Only 10 (53%) of the 19 subjects considered by the expert panel to definitely not have Reye's syndrome had been similarly classified by the hospital physicians. Overall agreement was 62% and κ_w was .48, indicating only fair agreement.

Substantial differences in levels of agreement existed between the expert panel and hospital physicians depending on whether the child was aged 3 years or younger (26 subjects) or older than age 3 years (37 subjects) (Table 2). For the younger children, the overall agreement rate was only 47% ($\kappa_w = .29$); for the older children, the overall agreement rate was 73% ($\kappa_w = .54$). The expert panel confirmed the diagnosis for only two (18%) of the 11 younger children compared with 20 (87%) of the 23 older children diagnosed by the hospital as having definite Reye's syndrome ($\chi^2 = 15.41$; $P < .0001$).

As might be expected, there was less agreement between the hospital physicians and the expert panel for those children classified as having stage 1 disease severity (overall agreement, 53% [10 of 19 patients]; $\kappa_w = .23$) than for those children in stage 2 (overall agreement, 76% [13 of 17 patients]; $\kappa_w = .66$), or stage 3 and greater (overall agreement, 59% [16 of 27 patients]; $\kappa_w = .43$).

Hospital physicians often made the diagnosis of definite Reye's syndrome even when a child had not received aspirin: 11 (33%) of the 33 subjects who did not receive aspirin were considered to have definite Reye's syndrome by the physicians who cared for them at the hospital. However, in only two (18%) of these 11 cases was the diagnosis confirmed by the expert panel who were blind to information about exposure to aspirin.

Use of Liver Biopsy Specimens and Comparison of Results With Experts' Review.—Liver biopsies were performed on 13 subjects and postmortem liver specimens were available for five other patients. Biopsies were performed no more frequently for those children aged 3 years or younger than for those children older than 3 years (31% vs 27%). Electron microscopy was performed on 14 specimens and photomicrographs of 13 of these specimens were available for review by the expert physician. Of the seven cases considered by hospital pathologists to be diagnostic of Reye's syndrome, only two were considered diagnostic by the experts; two others were questionable, and three were considered inconsistent with Reye's syndrome. Overall agreement was only 46%, and κ_w was .27, indicating poor agreement.

Comment.—The results of this study demonstrate that a diagnosis of Reye's syndrome in pediatric tertiary care hospitals was often not confirmed when the data were reviewed by a panel of experts. One third of cases were considered by an expert panel to be misdiagnosed. The study was performed between 1986 and 1987 when the incidence of Reye's syndrome was declining. As the incidence of true cases of Reye's syndrome declines further, a greater proportion of those patients given the diagnosis will likely be misdiagnosed.

Of the 12 patients considered to have false-positive diagnoses, nine were younger than age 3 years. The reluctance of the expert panel to make the diagnosis of Reye's syndrome in a young child is almost certainly due to their concern that inborn errors of metabolism had not been excluded as an alternative diagnosis. At the same time, in only one (2%) of the 63 subjects was a definitive diagnosis of an inborn error of metabolism made, and in only five (19%) of the 26 children aged 3 years or younger were investigations requested that were specific for these disorders. It appears from these data that the warnings to clinicians to consider the possibility of inborn errors of metabolism when faced with a young child with a Reye's-like illness are going largely unheeded.

Even as the incidence of Reye's syndrome declines, physicians need to be careful that children who present with a Reye's-like illness are not misdiagnosed. Young children, in particular, may require biochemical investigations for inborn errors of metabolism, and a liver biopsy may be indicated. In addition, review of the biopsy specimen by someone who is experienced in interpreting electron micrographs in patients with Reye's syndrome may help to avoid misdiagnoses.

Brian W. Forsyth, MB, ChB
Eugene D. Shapiro, MD
Department of Pediatrics
Ralph I. Horwitz, MD
Department of Medicine and Epidemiology
Catherine M. Viscoli, PhD
Denise Acampora, MPH
Department of Medicine
Yale University School of Medicine
Room IE-61 SHM
PO Box 3333
New Haven, CT 06510

This research was supported in part by the American Home Products Corp, Bristol-Myers Co, and Sterling Drug Co, New York, NY; Miles Laboratories Inc, West Haven, Conn; and Procter and Gamble Co, Cincinnati, Ohio.

The authors have no ongoing affiliation or financial involvement with any of these companies or with any other organization or entity with a direct financial interest in the subject matter or material of the research discussed in this letter.

Reprint requests to Yale University School of Medicine, Room IE-61 SHM, PO Box 3333, New Haven, CT 06510 (Dr Horwitz).

Members of Expert Panel

Darryl C. De Vivo, MD, director, Pediatric Neurology, Columbia-Presbyterian Medical Center, New York, NY; Morey W. Haymond, MD, chief, Endocrine Research Unit, Department of Pediatrics and Medicine, Mayo Clinic, Rochester, Minn; and John C. Partin, MD, Department of Pediatrics, State University of New York at Stony Brook.

1. Traumer DA. Reye's syndrome. *Curr Probl Pediatr.* 1982;12:23-24.
2. Glasgow AM, Eng G, Engel AG. Systemic carnitine deficiency simulating recurrent Reye syndrome. *J Pediatr.* 1980;96:889-891.
3. Bougneres PF, Rocchicciol F, Kolvraa S, et al. Median chain acyl CoA dehydrogenase deficiency in two siblings with a Reye-like syndrome. *J Pediatr.* 1984;106:918-921.
4. Roe CR, Millington DS, Maltby DA, Kinneclerew P. Recognition of medium chain acyl-CoA dehydrogenase deficiency in asymptomatic siblings of children dying of sudden infant death or Reye-like syndromes. *J Pediatr.* 1986;108:13-18.
5. Forsyth BW, Horwitz RI, Acampora D, et al. New epidemiologic evidence confirming that bias does not explain the aspirin/Reye's syndrome association. *JAMA.* 1989;261:2517-2524.
6. Partin JC, Schubert WK, Partin JS. Mitochondrial ultrastructure in Reye's syndrome. *N Engl J Med.* 1971;285:1339-1343.
7. Taubman B, Hale DE, Kelley RI. Familial Reye-like syndrome: a presentation of medium-chain acyl-coenzyme A dehydrogenase deficiency. *Pediatrics.* 1987;79:382-385.
8. Bonnell HJ, Beckwith JB. Fatty liver in sudden childhood death: implications for Reye's syndrome. *AJDC.* 1986;140:30-33.
9. Dodge PR, Brown SB, Ector WL, et al. Consensus conference: diagnosis and treatment of Reye's syndrome. *JAMA.* 1981;246:2441-2446.
10. Partin JS, Daugherty CC, McAdams AJ, Partin JC, Schubert WK. A comparison of index ultrastructure in salicylate intoxication and Reye's syndrome. *Hepatology.* 1984;4:687-690.
11. Fleiss JL. The measure of inter-rate agreement. In: *Statistical Methods for Rates and Proportions.* 2nd ed. New York, NY: John Wiley & Sons Inc; 1981: chap 13.

Syringomas in Down Syndrome

Sir.—Syringomas are small, skin-colored or slightly yellow, firm papules that frequently appear in crops and are usually located in the periorbital area (Figure). They may also appear on the side of the neck, cheeks, thorax, abdomen, axilla, and pubic area. An association between Down syndrome (DS) and syringomas was first reported by Butterworth et al[1] in 1964. They studied a residential population whose ages ranged from 10 to 52 years; the majority of the patients were adults. The incidence of syringomas in the population with DS was 18.5%, with 26% of the women and 13% of the men having syringomas. The comparison group, 1001 mentally retarded individuals without DS, had a 0.6% incidence of syringomas. Another study in 1976,[2] also of institutionalized residents with DS, reported an incidence of syringomas in 26.6% of the male and 58.1% of the female subjects. There are no reports concerning the association of DS and syringomas in a younger population.

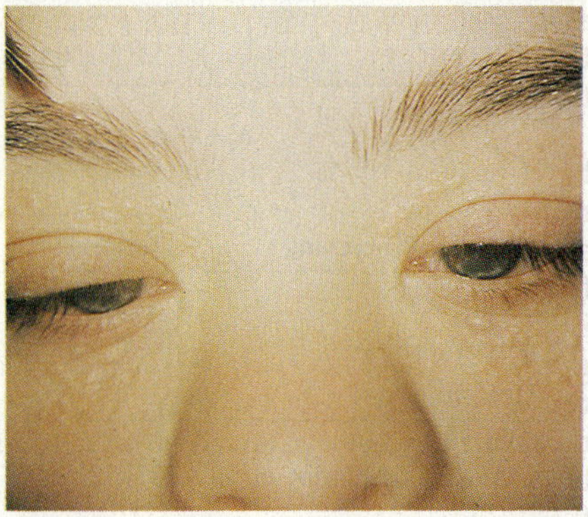

Syringomas seen in child with Down syndrome.

Patients and Methods.—In an attempt to confirm the results of previous studies, but in a younger population, 32 patients with DS between ages 14 and 25 years who were being seen for routine follow-up in our DS clinic were evaluated for facial syringomas. Because syringomas usually do not appear before puberty, only patients with DS aged 14 years or older were included in the study. These patients were followed up for an average of 13 years. A comparison group of 50 children without DS with and without mental retardation and matched for age was examined for the presence of syringomas. The syringomas in both groups were restricted to the face.

Results.—Fifteen (46.9%) of the 32 patients with DS examined had syringomas. The majority of patients studied (62.5%) were in the 14- to 20-year age group and 21 (65.6%) of the 32 patients were men. Eight (38%) of the men and seven (63.6%) of the women had syringomas. Patients with syringomas did not have a greater incidence of congenital heart disease, hypothyroidism, or other abnormalities associated with DS than the group with DS without syringomas, although one did have diabetes mellitus. One of the 50 patients of the control group matched for age (a patient with Williams syndrome) had facial syringomas.

Comment.—The results of this study substantiate the findings of two prior reports concerning an association of syringomas with DS. The rate of occurrence in our patients was higher than anticipated because of the preponderance of men and younger individuals in our study group (syringomas appear more commonly in women and older individuals). However, this may be spuriously high due to the relatively small number of patients in the study group.

Syringomas were first described by Kaposi in 1876. They are uncommon, appear usually during puberty, and have been reported to occur in families. They are usually 1 to 3 mm in diameter but can be larger. Syringomas are benign, and there are no reports of them undergoing malignant degeneration. Histologic, histochemical, and electron microscopic findings show a close relationship between syringomas and intraepithelial eccrine sweat gland ducts. Brownstein[3] described syringomas as adenomas of the intraepidermal portions of the eccrine duct. Small cystic ducts as well as solid epithelial strands embedded in fibrous stromas are seen on histologic examination of the upper and middle area of the dermis.

Syringomas may be mistaken for xanthomas because of their location around the eyes. However, xanthomas are somewhat larger and yellowish in color, while syringomas have a flesh-like or light yellow color.

Treatment is usually not necessary except for cosmetic reasons. Isotretinoin has recently been used to treat syringomas, but it is not recommended for routine treatment because of the benign nature of these skin lesions and the possible risks of the medication.[4]

The association of syringomas and DS has not previously been reported in the pediatric literature. It is important for pediatricians to be aware of the significance of syringomas in patients with DS so that they can inform the patient and family of the benign nature of these lesions and not subject the patient to an unnecessary evaluation.

Murray Feingold, MD
National Birth Defect Center
Franciscan Children's Hospital
30 Warren St
Boston, MA 02135

This study was supported by a grant from the Genesis Fund.

1. Butterworth T, Strean LP, Berman H, Wood MG. Syringoma and mongolism. *Arch Dermatol.* 1964;90:483-487.
2. Carter DM, Jegasothy BV. Alopecia areata and Down syndrome. *Arch Dermatol.* 1976;112:1397-1399.
3. Brownstein MN. The sweat gland adenomas. *Int J Dermatol.* 1975;14:397.
4. Maintitz M, Schmidt JB, Gebhardt W. Response of multiple syringomas to isotretinoin. *Arch Dermatol Venereol.* 1986;16:51-55.

Congenital Syphilis Associated With Negative Results of Maternal Serologic Tests at Delivery

Sir.—The incidence of congenital syphilis has steadily increased in the last decade. In 1988, 691 cases of early congenital syphilis were reported to the Centers for Disease Control.[1] This is the largest number of cases reported to the centers since the early 1950s, when penicillin became widely used to treat syphilis in pregnant women.[1] Because congenital syphilis generally can be prevented by detection and treatment of syphilis early in pregnancy, failure to obtain adequate prenatal care is believed to be the most important factor associated with congenital syphilis.[1,2]

Current recommendations from the Centers for Disease Control require that all states perform serologic screening tests for detecting syphilis at the beginning of prenatal care. Additional screenings at the beginning of the third trimester (28 weeks) and at delivery also are recommended for mothers who live in areas with high incidences of syphilis.[2-4] This approach will reveal almost all cases of antepartum infection. However, it may not detect infection acquired immediately before delivery when results of serologic tests may be negative.[3-10] We describe three infants born to mothers with peripartum syphilis that was not diagnosed by routine serologic screening at delivery. Two mothers were seronegative at delivery, but their infants later developed evidence of congenital syphilis. The third infant was born to a seronegative mother with primary syphilis diagnosed post partum; this infant was asymptomatic and received prophylactic antimicrobial therapy after delivery. These cases underscore the limitations of current prenatal screening methods.

Patient Reports.—Patient 1.—A 2385-g male was delivered vaginally at 36 weeks' gestation to a 20-year-old black woman. The pregnancy was uncomplicated and the result of a maternal rapid plasma reagin (RPR) test did not show reactivity at delivery. No maternal genital lesions were noted. Results of physical examination of the infant were normal, and he and his mother were discharged from the hospital. Two months after delivery, the mother was diagnosed with salpingitis due to *Neisseria gonorrhoeae* and received ceftriaxone sodium and doxycyclinehyclate. No genital lesions were noted; a serologic test to detect syphilis was not performed at that time.

The infant was in good health until age 2½ months, when he developed clear rhinorrhea and a generalized maculopapular rash with oval red lesions and superficial desquamation. On presentation at the emergency department, hepatosplenomegaly and axillary adenopathy were noted. Roentgenograms of the long bones revealed symmetric osteochondritis and periostitis. Laboratory evaluation revealed a hemoglobin level of 90 g/L, hematocrit of 0.27, and a platelet count of 422×10^9/L. The alanine aminotransferase, aspartate aminotransferase, and γ-glutamyltransferase (GGT) levels were 65, 140, and 128 U/L, respectively. The total bilirubin level was 6 μmol/L. The serum VDRL titer was 1:128, and the result of the microhemagglutination assay to detect *Treponema pallidum* (MHA-TP) antibody showed reactivity. Laboratory test results of the infant's cerebrospinal fluid showed no white blood cells and normal glucose and protein concentrations. The cerebrospinal fluid was nonreactive during VDRL testing. The IgM reactivity of whole serum with *T pallidum* antigens was examined using Western blotting[11]; an IgM resonse to *T pallidum* antigens with apparent molecular masses of 47, 45, and 17 kd was observed. The infant was diagnosed as having congenital syphilis and received 200 000 U/kg of intravenous penicillin G daily for 10 days. There was no history or physical signs of sexual abuse.

The mother's VDRL titer was 1:8, and the result of an MHA-TP assay showed reactivity. Antibody to the human immunodeficiency virus (HIV) was not detected. She was diagnosed as having early latent syphilis and was treated with 2.4 million U of benzathine penicillin G intramuscularly.

Patient 2.—A 3550-g female was delivered vaginally at 40 weeks' gestation to a 20-year-old black woman following an uncomplicated pregnancy. The result of a maternal RPR test at delivery did not show reactivity, and there were no signs of 1° or 2° syphilis. Results of physical examination of the newborn were normal.

At age 2 months, the infant appeared to experience pain when lifted at the shoulders, and subsequently the parents noted decreased movement of the left arm. The infant was taken to the emergency department for evaluation. Roentgenograms of the long bones revealed symmetric osteochondritis and periostitis of the upper and lower extremities and osseous destruction of the proximal medial tibial metaphysis (Wimberger's sign). There was no associated rash or hepatosplenomegaly; bilateral axillary lymphadenopathy was present. Laboratory evaluation revealed a hemoglobin level of 80 g/L, hematocrit of 0.25, reticulocyte count of 34×10^{-3}, and a platelet count of 724×10^9/L Results of liver function tests were normal. The serum VDRL titer was 1:128, and the result of the MHA-TP assay showed reactivity. Examination of the cerebrospinal fluid revealed the following values: red blood cell count, 16×10^6/L; white blood cell count, 25×10^6/L (0.24 mononuclear, 0.69 lymphocytes, and 0.07 segmented cells); and a protein level of 0.51 g/L. The result of a VDRL test did not show reactivity. The infant was hospitalized and diagnosed as having congenital syphilis. She was treated with 150 000 U/kg of intravenous penicillin G daily. A dose of 37 500 U/kg was administered every 6 hours for 10 days. Western blot analysis[11] revealed serum IgM reactivity with the 47- and 45-kd antigens of *T pallidum*. There was no evidence of physical or sexual abuse.

The mother's VDRL titer was 1:512; the result of an MHA-TP assay did not show reactivity. She had palmar and plantar rashes consistent with secondary syphilis and received 2.4 million U of benzathine penicillin G. She lacked antibody to HIV.

PATIENT 3.—A 2550-g female was delivered vaginally at 36 weeks' gestation to a 28-year-old black woman who had received no prenatal care. The result of an RPR test of the mother at delivery did not show reactivity. However, on the second day after delivery, an ulcerated perineal lesion was noted that contained motile spirochetes detected with darkfield microscopy. The result of an MHA-TP assay did not show reactivity. The mother's serum did not exhibit a prozone reaction; diluted serum was nonreactive during VDRL testing. She was diagnosed as having primary syphilis and was treated with 2.4 million U of benzathine penicillin G intramuscularly. The result of a test to detect antibody to HIV was negative. Results of physical examination of the infant were normal. Roentgenograms of the long bones and results of complete blood cell count and liver function tests were also normal. The result of a VDRL test performed on umbilical-cord blood did not show reactivity. No specific fetal IgM antibody to *T pallidum* antigens in whole serum was detected using Western blot analysis.[11] The infant received an intramuscular injection of benzathine penicillin G (50 000 U/kg).

Comment.—Routine serologic testing of mothers during pregnancy and at delivery is essential to prevent congenital syphilis.[2] However, limitations on the usefulness and reliability of such screening tests exist. Serologic tests are poor diagnostic tools during the incubation or early primary stage of syphilis. During those times, results of the nontreponemal (RPR or VDRL) tests may not show reactivity because reactivity occurs approximately 4 to 8 weeks after the infection is acquired and several days to 1 week after the development of a chancre.[10,12] In primary syphilis, nonreactivity to nontreponemal tests is reported to occur in approximately one fourth to one third of cases.[5,8] Nonreactivity during the MHA-TP assay and the fluorescent treponemal antibody absorption test occurs in as many as 36% and 18% of cases of primary syphilis, respectively.[9] It is clear that no single test or combination of tests will detect all cases of maternal syphilis and prevent neonatal infection. Our cases highlight these limitations, which are due to the natural history of the development of clinical signs of syphilis and production of antibody to that infection. As shown in the mothers of patients 1 and 2, the mother may transmit infection to the fetus during the period of seronegativity in early primary or incubating syphilis. The importance of diligent physical examination to detect suspicious lesions supplemented by darkfield or immunofluorescence microscopic[13] examination in the diagnosis of primary syphilis is demonstrated in the mother of patient 3.

Another possible explanation for the nonreactivity during nontreponemal tests is the prozone phenomenon.[5,8,12] Less than 2% of serum samples from patients with secondary syphilis will exhibit a prozone effect.[5,8,12] This phenomenon is due to excess reagin antibody, which prevents flocculation in the undiluted serum sample. When diluted, the serum will usually exhibit titers of 1:16 or greater. The prozone reaction was not specifically sought in serum samples from the mothers of patients 1 and 2. It is unlikely, however, that it contributed to the nonreactivity during nontreponemal testing in our patients. Serum exhibiting a prozone phenomenon will show a nonreactive, rough appearance or be weakly reactive during nontreponemal testing.[8] Serum samples with such equivocal reactions are diluted routinely in our laboratory and, if the prozone effect were present, it would have been detected in our patients.

There was no history or physical evidence of sexual abuse in patients 1 and 2. Moreover, syphilitic osteochondritis and periostitis require approximately 5 and 16 weeks, respectively, to become demonstrable on long bone roentgenograms.[14] This period is consistent with perinatal acquisition of *T pallidum* in both infants.

With the dramatic increase in the incidence of congenital syphilis, areas with a high prevalence of infectious syphilis in women of childbearing age may need to screen women post partum to detect prior incubating or seronegative primary infection at delivery. Moreover, if a woman with a child younger than 1 year is diagnosed to have primary, secondary, or early latent syphilis, that child should be fully evaluated for signs of congenital syphilis, tested serologically, and treated accordingly. When a woman is treated for late syphilis, all of her young children should also be evaluated. Only with adequate prenatal care and postpartum evaluation will congenital syphilis be prevented.

PABLO J. SÁNCHEZ, MD
Department of Pediatrics
GEORGE D. WENDEL, MD
Department of Obstetrics and Gynecology
MICHAEL V. NORGARD, PhD
Department of Microbiology
University of Texas
Southwestern Medical Center
Dallas, TX 75235

We thank the staff of the Immunology Laboratory of Parkland Memorial Hospital, Dallas, Tex, for assisting in handling specimens and performing serologic testing and the Transfusion Service staff of PMH for assistance in collection of umbilical-cord blood specimens.

1. Congenital syphilis—New York City, 1986-1988. *MMWR.* 1989;38:825-829.

2. Guidelines for the prevention and control of congenital syphilis. *MMWR.*

1988;37(suppl):1-13.
3. Hallock J, Tunnessen WW. Congenital syphilis in an infant of a seronegative mother. *Obstet Gynecol.* 1968;32:336-338.
4. Ewing CI, Roberts C, Davidson DC, Arya OP. Early congenital syphilis still occurs. *Arch Dis Child.* 1985;60:1128-1133.
5. Sparling PF. Diagnosis and treatment of syphilis. *N Engl J Med.* 1971;284:642-653.
6. Monif GRG, Williams BR, Shulman ST, Baer H. The problem of maternal syphilis after serologic surveillance during pregnancy. *Am J Obstet Gynecol.* 1973;117:268-270.
7. Taber LH, Huber TW. Congenital syphilis. In: Krugman S, Gershon AA, eds. *Infections of the Fetus and the Newborn Infant.* New York, NY: Alan R Liss Inc; 1975:183-190.
8. Felman YM, Nikitas JA. Syphilis serology today. *Arch Dermatol.* 1980; 116:84-89.
9. Larsen SA, Hambie EA, Pettit DE, Perryman MW, Kraus SJ. Specificity, sensitivity, and reproducibility among the fluorescent treponemal antibody-absorption test, the microhemagglutination assay for *Treponema pallidum* antibodies, and the hemagglutination treponemal test for syphilis. *J Clin Microbiol.* 1981;14:441-445.
10. Felman Y. How useful are the serologic tests for syphilis? *Int J Dermatol.* 1982;21:79-81.
11. Sanchez PJ, McCracken GH, Wendel GD, Olsen K, Threlkeld N, Norgard MV. Molecular analysis of the fetal IgM response to *Treponema pallidum* antigens: implication for improved serodiagnosis of congenital syphilis. *J Infect Dis.* 1989;159:508-517.
12. Spangler AS, Jackson JH, Fiumara NJ, Warthin TA. Syphilis with a negative blood test reaction. *JAMA.* 1964;189:113-116.
13. Wendel GD, Maberry MC, Christmas JT, Goldberg M, Norgard MV. Examination of amniotic fluid in diagnosing congenital syphilis with fetal death. *Obstet Gynecol.* 1989;74:967-970.
14. Schulz KF, Murphy FK, Patamasucon P, Meheus AZ. Congenital syphilis. In: Holmes KK, Mardh P-A, Sparling PF, et al, eds. *Sexually Transmitted Diseases.* New York, NY: McGraw-Hill International Book Co; 1990:821-842.

Response of Seronegative Adults to Measles Immunization

Sir.—In March 1990 we published a study in *AJDC*[1] indicating that adult hospital employees, with significant frequency, tested seronegative to measles. We identified 16 such workers whom we subsequently immunized with monovalent measles vaccine. We further recommended and initiated a screening program to test new employees for immunity to measles and to immunize those who tested seronegative.

Correspondents have suggested to us that these seronegative individuals might represent primary immunization failures, and, therefore, a significant number might not seroconvert following the administration of vaccine. Some expressed interest in follow-up data on this population.

Accordingly, we solicited and were able to obtain serum samples from 15 seronegative individuals and study them by the methods described in our article.[1] Of these 15 employees who were subsequently vaccinated, 13 were members of the original group of 16 and two were employees identified in our ongoing screening program.

All 15 employees tested developed immunity to measles following vaccination. These data suggest that seronegative adults do not represent individuals who fail to respond to measles vaccination. Although the group we studied was small, their response to vaccination does not appear to differ significantly from that of the population at large.[2]

Herbert Braunstein, MD
Susan Thomas, MT(ASCP)
Ray Ito, MT(ASCP)
Carole Jarman, MA, RN
San Bernardino County
Medical Center
780 E Gilbert St
San Bernardino, CA 92404

1. Braunstein H, Thomas S, Ito R. Immunity to measles in a large population of varying age: significance with respect to vaccination. *AJDC.* 1990;144:296-298.
2. Cherry JD. Measles. In: Felgin RD, Cherry JD, eds. *Textbook of Pediatric Infectious Diseases.* 2nd ed. Philadelphia, Pa: WB Saunders Co; 1987:1607-1628.

Improvement of Leukemic Hyperleukocytosis With Only Fluid and Allopurinol Therapy

Sir.—Children with leukemic hyperleukocytosis ($>100 \times 10^9$/L) may have manifestations of hyperviscosity with disseminated intravascular coagulation, intracranial hemorrhage, and pulmonary insufficiency as well as the tumor lysis syndrome.[1] Initial treatment before chemotherapy includes vigorous intravenous fluid therapy, allopurinol, and intravenous sodium bicarbonate to decrease the risk of uric acid nephropathy. Some patients have received leukapheresis, exchange transfusion, or cranial irradiation to treat or prevent the manifestations of hyperviscosity.[1-5] A current protocol recommends leukapheresis or exchange transfusion if the cytocrit (volume of packed red blood cells and volume of packed white blood cells) is greater than 0.30.[6]

Three patients had a marked drop (52% to 89%) in leukocyte count during 1 to 2 days while receiving intravenous hydration, sodium bicarbonate, and allopurinol therapy and before receiving any chemotherapy. Thus, the more aggressive measures may be avoided in some patients who have no symptoms of hyperviscosity and whose leukocyte counts decrease to levels at which there is no longer a concern about hyperviscosity.

Patient Reports.—Data from the three patients are outlined in the Table. No patient had any manifestations of the hyperviscosity syndrome and no child was clinically dehydrated or had laboratory evidence of dehydration as assessed by tests of urine specific gravity and blood urea nitrogen. The liver and spleen in patient 1 were palpable 7 cm below the costal margins; the spleen in patient 2 was palpated down to the umbilicus, and the liver was not enlarged; and the liver and spleen in patient 3 were palpated down 6 and 4 cm, respectively.

The uric acid and creatinine levels were normal and remained normal during the hydration period. Only patient 1 had a cytocrit determination (0.20). Manual counts were done when the leukocyte count was greater than 100×10^9/L, and immunologic typing and cytochemistry confirmed the type of leukemia. All patients were treated with Children's Cancer Study Group protocols. Patient 1 received an autologous transplant and 8 months later was free of disease; patient 2 received treatment for 3 years and has not been receiving treatment for 1 year; and patient 3 remained in remission 5 months after she completed 2 years of chemotherapy.

Comment.—The observation of a significant decrease in the leukocyte count in children with leukemia shortly after admission and before receiving chemotherapy has been observed by others but not documented in the literature, to my knowledge.[7,8] The changes were attributed to the stress of hospitalization and the resulting secretion of corticosteroids.

Patient Data

Patient No./ Age	Type of Leukemia	Initial: WBC Count, × 10⁹/L	Initial: Blasts	Interval Between Fluid Administration, h	After Hydration: WBC Count, × 10⁹/L	After Hydration: Blasts	Decrease in WBC Count, %	Hemoglobin, g/L	Platelets, × 10⁹/L
1/5 mo	AML	129	0.74	18	62.4	0.68	52	40	61
2/5 mo	ALL	572	0.80	32	179	0.74	69	90	78
3/3.5 y	ALL	121	0.86	50	16.3	0.45	89	60	18

*AML indicates acute myelocytic leukemia; ALL, acute lymphocytic leukemia; and WBC, white blood cell.

Some children with acute lymphocytic leukemia are exquisitely sensitive to small doses of corticosteroids, and this theory is perhaps plausible. It would not, however, explain the 52% decrease in leukocyte count of patient 1 who had acute myelocytic leukemia. Such marked sensitivity to corticosteroids would be most unusual in that form of leukemia.

The infrequent temporary remissions following blood transfusions have also been attributed to a stress reaction.[7] Two of the three patients (patients 1 and 3) received packed red blood cells during the hydration period, but I believe that this is an unlikely explanation. Only patient 3 had evidence of infection (sepsis) that could also be associated with temporary remissions.[9] No antileukemic effect has ever been attributed to allopurinol, sodium bicarbonate, or intravenous fluids, to my knowledge.

It is not known whether the decreases in leukocyte count reflect an actual decrease in leukemic cell mass or are only the result of redistribution, ie, into the marginal leukocyte pool, spleen, or liver. The three patients had very large spleens and, conceivably, expansion of the blood volume with intravenous fluids may have increased the circulation in the enlarged spleens, resulting in increased sequestration of the leukemic cells. Marginal pools have not been studied in leukemic patients, to my knowledge, but it seems unlikely that this explains the shifts of the magnitude observed in these patients.

Allopurinol is a xanthine oxidase inhibitor that reduces the production of uric acid by inhibiting the biochemical reactions immediately preceding its formation. It acts on purine catabolism without disrupting the biosynthesis of purines and has no known antileukemic effect. The absence of an elevated uric acid level during the hydration period does not rule out leukemic cell destruction since the patients were receiving allopurinol and sodium bicarbonate to decrease the risk of uric acid nephropathy.

Thus, there appears to be no obvious explanation for this phenomenon, but it does occur in some patients and has clinical relevance. I suggest that a 24- to 48-hour regimen of intravenous fluid, allopurinol, and sodium bicarbonate be administered to a child with leukemic hyperleukocytosis who has no signs or symptoms of hyperviscosity. Following this trial, a decision could be made about whether more aggressive measures, ie, exchange transfusion or leukapheresis, are necessary depending on the change in leukocyte count or the development of manifestations of hyperviscosity. The decreased viscosity associated with anemia often helps to compensate for the increased viscosity due to the hyperleukocytosis; therefore, blood transfusions should be avoided, if possible.[10]

It should be noted that in a series of 124 children with acute lymphoblastic leukemia and leukocyte counts greater than $200 \times 10^9/L$, the incidence of intracranial hemorrhage was only 3% and hemorrhages in three of the four patients occurred before presentation.[1] Patients who present with symptoms of hyperviscosity should be treated with exchange transfusion or leukapheresis to immediately correct the hyperviscosity. Further studies would help to verify these changes in leukocyte counts before chemotherapy and to explain the mechanism.

André D. Lascari, MD
Children's Hospital
Albany Medical College
New Scotland Ave
Albany, NY 12208

1. Maurer H, Steinherz P, Gaynon P, et al. The effect of initial management of hyperleukocytosis on early complications and outcome of children with acute lymphoblastic leukemia. *J Clin Oncol.* 1988;6:1425-1432.

2. Carpentiere U, Patten E, Chamberlin P, Young A, Hitter M. Leukophoresis in a 3-year-old-child with lymphoma in leukemic transformation. *J Pediatr.* 1979; 94:919-921.

3. Kamen B, Sommers C, Pearson H. Exchange transfusion as a treatment for hyperleukocytosis, anemia, and metabolic abnormalities in a patient with leukemia. *J Pediatr.* 1980;96:1045-1046.

4. Dickerman J. Extreme leukocytosis successfully managed by double-volume exchange transfusion in an infant with T-cell leukemia. *AJDC.* 1982;36:643-644.

5. Gilchrist G, Fountain K, Dearth J, Smithson W, Burgert E. Cranial irradiation in the management of extreme leukemic leukocytosis complicating childhood acute lymphocytic leukemia. *J Pediatr.* 1981;98:257-259.

6. Treatment of newly diagnosed acute lymphoblastic leukemia in infants less than 12 months of age. Children's Cancer Study Group CCG-1883; 1988.

7. Darte J, Snelling C, Donohue W. The effect of plasma infusions in acute leukemia in children. *Can Med Assoc J.* 1952;66:576-578.

8. Wetherley-Mein G, Cottom D. Fresh blood transfusion in leukemia. *Br J Haematol.* 1956;2:25-31.

9. Bierman H, Crile M, Dod K, et al. Remissions in leukemia of childhood following acute infectious disease. *Cancer.* 1953;6:591-605.

10. Lichtman M, Heal J, Rowe J. Hyperleukocytic leukemia: rheological and clinical features and management. *Baillieres Clin Haematol.* 1987;1:725-746.

Myopathy Associated With Ketoconazole Treatment

Sir.—Ketoconazole is an imidazole-derivative, broad-spectrum antimycotic agent, with relatively limited toxicity compared with other antifungal medications. However, gastrointestinal disturbances, hepatotoxicity, impaired adrenal steroidogenesis, gynecomastia, and immune hemolytic anemia have been reported in association with ketoconazole treatment.[1,2] We noticed myopathy with a significant increase of serum creatine phosphokinase during ketoconazole treatment, indicating a possible drug-induced myositis. To our knowledge, there has been no fully documented report of myopathy associated with the use of this drug, although myalgia has been reported in two patients[3] and muscular weakness in one patient.[4]

Patient Report.—A 17-year-old boy afflicted with autoimmune polyglandular syndrome type I presented with hypoparathyroidism, Addison's disease, alopecia universalis, and mucocutaneous candidiasis was treated with ketoconazole (200 mg/d) because of worsening oral candidiasis. Within a week, doctors noticed clinical improvement of the oral lesions, but concomitantly, the patient developed significant weakness and diffuse myalgia, particularly of the shoulder girdle muscles. The serum creatine phosphokinase level, which had been normal 2 months earlier, rose to 5200 U/L (normal range, 24 to 200 U/L), and of this, 96% was isoenzyme of skeletal muscle origin. Liver enzyme levels remained unchanged, serum electrolyte levels were normal, and no antiskeletal muscle antibodies were found. The electrocardiogram was normal, but the electromyogram revealed a distinct myopathic pattern. Ketoconazole therapy was discontinued 8 days after its start, and rapid clinical improvement followed with eventual disappearance of myalgia and weakness. One week after withdrawal of the drug therapy, the serum creatine phosphokinase level had decreased to 480 U/L, and after 3 weeks to 96 U/L. Repeated electromyogram obtained 5 weeks after withdrawal of ketoconazole therapy was normal; viral cultures were negative. Results of serologic tests for influenza A, influenza B, adenovirus, enterovirus, cytomegalovirus, herpesvirus, hepatitis A virus, hepatitis B virus, Epstein-Barr virus, mycoplasma, streptococci, and *Toxoplasma* remained unchanged.

Results of a macrophage inhibiting factor test[5] for ketoconazole were negative, and results of a mast cell degranulation test[6] for ketoconazole were positive, indicating the possible presence of IgE antibodies to the drug. However, the relationship of this finding to the myositis is questionable.

Comment.—There have been reports of myositis or myasthenia in patients with mucocutaneous candidiasis, but these cases were usually associated with long-standing muscle disease or thymoma.[7] Chest roentgenography failed to show an enlarged thymus in our patient. Moreover, the temporary relationship between clinical symptoms and laboratory evidence of myositis shortly after the start of ketoconazole treatment, and their rapid resolution after discontinuation of this medication, suggest a drug-related myopathy.

Ben-Zion Garty, MD
Rivka Kauli, MD
Ella Livni, PhD
Zvi Laron, MD
Menachem Nitzan, MD
Department of Pediatrics
Beilinson Medical Center
Petah Tiqva 49100, Israel

1. Smith EB, Henry FC. Ketoconazole: an orally effective antifungal agent: mechanism of action, pharmacology, clinical efficacy and adverse effects. *Pharmacotherapy.* 1984;4:199-204.

2. Umstead GS, Babiak LM, Tejwani S. Immune hemolytic anemia associated with ketoconazole therapy. *Clin Pharm.* 1987;6:499-500.

3. National Institute of Allergy and Infectious Disease Mycoses Study Group. Treatment of blastomycosis and histoplasmosis with ketoconazole. *Ann Intern Med.* 1985;103:861-872.

4. Hersle K, Mobacken H, Moberg S. Long-term ketoconazole treatment of chronic acral dermatophyte infections. *Int J Dermatol.* 1985;24:245-248.

5. Aderka D, Livni E, Sharon S, Pinkhas J. The migration inhibition factor test for identification of hypersensitivity reactions to drugs. *Ann Allergy.* 1986;56:341-344.

6. Schwartz J, Klopstock A, Zibert Duvdevani P, Honig S. Detection of hypersensitivity by indirect rat mast cell degranulation. *Int Arch Allergy.* 1965;26:333-339.

7. Kirkpatrick CH, Windhort DB. Mucocutaneous candidiasis and thymoma. *Am J Med.* 1979;66:939-945.

Gallstones in Children

Sir.—Recently, Reif et al[1] described 50 children and adolescents with gallstones and discussed the conditions associated with the development of gallstones in children, with the exception of erythropoietic protoporphyria (EPP). Of the two most common porphyrias, EPP rivals porphyria cutanea tarda in prevalence, and is characterized clinically by photosensitivity commencing in childhood and biochemically by excessive amounts of red blood cell protoporphyrins.[2] Protoporphyrin is excreted in the bile and gallstones, which are partially composed of protoporphyrin and have been reported in about 12% of patients with EPP who are liable to produce symptoms at an unusually early age.[3] Determination of the protoporphyrin solubility in the bile and the mechanism by which gallstones form in patients with EPP is poorly understood. Results of scientific research on rat models have shown that biliary protoporphyrin excretion depends on bile acids and, if bile acid excretion rates decrease, biliary concentration of protoporphyrin increases, which may predispose to gallstones.[4]

Ten of the 50 patients described by Reif et al had no associated conditions, and their disease was categorized as idiopathic. Patients with EPP may experience photosensitivity without any objective physical signs; if their complaint is initially dismissed by their family physician, they may fail to mention it to future physicians.[5] It is important not to miss the diagnosis of EPP because a number of patients may develop fatal liver disease and there is evidence that early detection can improve the outcome.[6] Therefore, I suggest that a medical history should be taken for photosensitivity for those children with idiopathic gallstones; if present, red blood cell protoporphyrin levels should be determined. If cholecystectomy is performed, sections of the gallstones can also be examined with fluorescence microscopy to detect protoporphyrins.[7]

David J. Todd, MRCP(UK)
Department of Dermatology
Royal Victoria Hospital
Grosvenor Road
Belfast BT12 6BA,
Northern Ireland

1. Reif S, Sloven DG, Lebenthal E. Gallstones in children: characterization by age, etiology, and outcome. *AJDC.* 1991;145:105-108.

2. Poh-Fitzpatrick M. The erythropoietic porphyrias. *Dermatol Clin.* 1986;4:291-296.

3. DeLeo VA, Poh-Fitzpatrick M, Matthews-Roth M, Harber LC. Erythropoietic protoporphyria: 10 years experience. *J Am Acad Dermatol.* 1976;60:8-22.

4. Avner DL, Lee RG, Berenson MM. Protoporphyrin-induced cholstasis in the isolated in situ perfused rat liver. *J Clin Invest.* 1981;67:385-394.

5. Todd DJ, Nesbitt GS, Lavery TD, Trimble ER, Burrows D. Erythropoietic protoporphyria: the problem of a suitable screening test. *Acta Derm Venereol (Stockh).* 1990;70:347-350.

6. Matthews-Roth MM. The consequences of not diagnosing erythropoietic protoporphyria. *Arch Dermatol.* 1980;116:407.

7. Cripps DJ, Scheuer PJ. Hepatobiliary changes in erythropoietic protoporphyria. *Arch Pathol Lab Med.* 1965; 80: 500-508.

Obesity and Body-Mass Index

Sir.—The discussion on the percentile curves of body-mass index (BMI) by Hammer et al[1] alerts the pediatrician to another method of getting more involved in clinical nutrition. Pediatricians see a significant amount of nutritional problems, especially obesity, and can apply these curves to help improve the patient's weight per height. However, the authors hedge on the diagnosis of obesity by saying " . . . we have found the 95th percentile BMI to be a conservative cutoff point for defining obesity in childhood." There are better criteria for defining obesity, especially for adolescents. These can be extracted from the National Center for Health Statistics[2] and were recently reprinted.[3] Using these tables for ages 12 to 17 years, the ideal body weight can be estimated, and obesity can be defined as greater than 20% above the ideal body weight. We recommend that clinicians post these tables in their offices and refer to them when estimating the ideal body weight and percentile of ideal body weight.

With respect to estimation of body fat, skinfold measurements can be imprecise and inaccurate, but in trained hands, skinfold measurements can add an important step in assessing body fat. In 1988, Slaughter et al[4] published equations for estimating the percentile of body fat in preteens and teenagers using two simple skinfold measurements with a standard error of about 3.8%. The value of these equations is that they were established using a four-component model and represent the best method of computation available.

The BMI graphs and table provided by Hammer et al are an important step in getting the pediatrician to make a more accurate assessment of the patient's weight per height, and the authors should be congratulated in providing the pediatrician with a tool to get more involved in clinical nutrition. In addition, the tables for estimating the percentile of ideal body weight for the National Center for Health Statistics in using skinfold measurements and the equations developed by Slaughter et al might increase the pediatrician's skill in diagnosing obesity even further.

Albert C. Hergenroeder, MD
Baylor College of Medicine
Adolescent Medicine
6621 Fannin
Houston, TX 77030

1. Hammer LD, Kraemer HC, Wilson DM, Ritter PL, Dornbusch SM. Standardized percentile curves of body-mass index for children and adolescents. *AJDC.* 1991;145:259-263.

2. National Center for Health Statistics. Plan and Operation of a Health Examination Survey of US Youths 12-17 Years of Age. Rockville, Md: Health Resources Administration; 1974. National Center for Health Statistics series 1, No. 8, publication HRA 75-1018.

3. Hergenroeder AC, Klish WJ. Body composition in adolescent athletes. *Pediatr Clin North Am.* 1990;37:1057-1083.

4. Slaughter MH, Lohman TG, Boileau RA, et al. Skinfold equations for estimation of body fatness in children and youth. *Hum Biol.* 1988; 60:709-723.

In Reply.—We agree with Dr Hergenroeder's contention that pediatricians should become more involved in problems of clinical nutrition. In our article, we chose not to recommend a specific BMI or percentile of BMI as a criterion for the diagnosis of obesity. Until a level of BMI is identified that is either associated with an increase in morbidity, or predictive of later morbidity or mortality, the specification of a diagnostic cutoff point for obesity during childhood remains somewhat arbitrary.[1] Rather than emphasizing the diagnosis of obesity, we recommend that clinicians use longitudinal assessments of BMI to monitor changes in weight relative to height and age, and that investigators continue to study the pattern of development of BMI and its relevance as a predictor of obesity. For example, Rolland-Cachera et al[2] have identified the timing of the adiposity rebound as a predictor of later obesity.

Further research is needed to demonstrate increased morbidity in association with either elevation of BMI, as identified for adults by the National Institute of Health Consensus Development Conference on Obesity (26.9 kg/m^2 for women and 27.2 kg/m^2 for men),[3] or percentiles of BMI during childhood or adolescence.

Since BMI is influenced by lean and fat tissue, it should not be construed as a measure of fatness. Measurement of skinfold thickness provides an estimate of subcutaneous fat deposition, which is correlated with BMI.[4] In those circumstances that require an estimate of body fatness, skinfold thickness or other indirect measures of fatness should be employed.

Lawrence D. Hammer, MD
Darrell M. Wilson, MD
Department of Pediatrics
Helena C. Kraemer, PhD
Philip L. Ritter, PhD
Sanford M. Dornbusch, PhD
Department of Sociology
Stanford University
School of Medicine
750 Welsh Rd
Palo Alto, CA 94304

1. Kraemer HC, Berkowitz RI, Hammer LD. Methodological difficulties in studies of obesity, I: measurement issues. *Ann Behav Med.* 1990;12:112-118.

2. Rolland-Cachera MF, Deheeger M, Bellisle F, Sempe M, Guilloud-Bataille M, Patois E. Adiposity rebound in children: a simple indicator for predicting obesity. *Am J Clin Nutr.* 1984; 39:129-135.

3. Burton BT, Foster WR, Hirsch J, Van Italie TB. Health implications of obesity: an NIH consensus development conference. *Int J Obes.* 1985; 9:155-169.

4. Roche AF, Siervogel RM, Chumlea WC, Webb P. Grading body fatness from limited anthropometric data. *Am J Clin Nutr.* 1981;34:2831-2838.

The Clinic Attending: Teaching Strategies for Patient Encounters

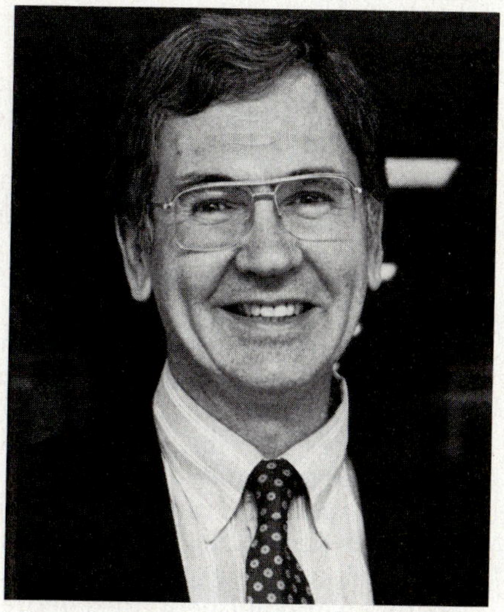

Barton Schmitt, MD

Bart recently left the board after 10 years of dedicated effort. This contribution reflects his observations on an important academic function, appropriate teaching objectives for the instructor and learner.

Bart comes to this discipline with superb credentials. He has directed the General Consultative Services at the University of Colorado and Children's Hospital in Denver since 1986. He has also directed the telephone triage program since 1988, which enables the nursing staff in the emergency department to respond to parental inquiries. He also established a weekly conference series for practicing pediatricians that covers topics of direct applicability to office practice; the success of this venture is attested by the constant active attendance of between 40 and 50 community pediatricians.

The second edition of his well-regarded book, **Your Child's Health,** *will be distributed in September 1991, and in 1992, the second edition of his text for providers,* **Pediatric Telephone Advice,** *will appear.*

Bart served **AJDC** *extremely well in his decade of board membership. We shall miss his wisdom and participation.*

—V.A.F.

Most of us in academic general pediatrics use continuity clinics, walk-in clinics, or emergency departments as our teaching turf. When I am working in these settings, my overriding goal is ensuring quality of care for all patients. My main educational goal is teaching residents how to think better about patient care. Knowing that we cannot teach everything in 3 years, I try to help residents approach problems in an organized and logical way that will provide a foundation for independent decision making. Here are some guidelines that help me fulfill my teaching responsibilities:

1. *Treat residents as adult learners:* Keep the learning environment respectful and nonthreatening. Challenge residents' thinking without challenging their status or self-esteem. Question learners to help themselves, not to reveal their uncertainties. Do not compete with residents, for they are the learners. Be open to disagreement. Never retaliate with verbal abuse of residents (eg, blaming, belittling, insulting, or demeaning comments).

2. *Use questions as the main vehicle for teaching:* The question-answer format is in contrast to the straight information giving, mini-lectures, or "this is what I would do" approaches. Questions stretch people. Questions help people crystallize and declare their position. Questions help people appreciate what they do know and do not know. Unless they are encouraged to speak first, junior people may be intimidated by their senior colleagues. Some useful questions to stimulate discussion include the following: What do you think? How do you add it up? What is your differential diagnosis? Given this chief complaint, what is the one thing you must rule out (eg, epiglottitis in children with stridor)? What is your leading diagnosis? Is it confirmed or tentative? Which laboratory studies, if any, are indicated? Will the diagnosis or treatment be changed by the results? What is your treatment plan? What is your follow-up plan? How can we prevent recurrences?

3. *Encourage the resident to ask you questions:* If the diagnosis is straightforward (eg, conjunctivitis) and the resident has previous experience with the condition, bypass the usual case presentation and go directly to the resident's agenda or needs. If necessary, trigger this discussion with "How can I help you?" or "What are your questions?" Encourage the resident to clarify the information he or she needs to help the patient and to tap into the consultant's experience. The attending physician functions as a computerized encyclopedia of pediatrics. When residents ask questions, we should assume they do not know the answers, and we should answer them directly rather than countering with other questions. This approach is called resident-driven learning. As the clinic becomes busier, we can become more efficient by using this approach. Although teaching time decreases, teaching is never completely set aside.

4. *Recommend additional questions for the resident to ask the parent:* In patients with complicated symptoms (eg, chronic cough or syncope), the

database is often incomplete. Any unanswered questions that come up during the case discussion should be saved until later. The resident can then return to the parent and pursue these pertinent questions. Occasionally, the resident will be requested to perform an additional examination, such as a rectal or neurologic examination.

5. *See the resident's patients:* For medical liability and billing purposes, we need to see all patients. When the clinic is busy, however, we need to be selective about which patients we evaluate in depth. Anyone who has an unknown diagnosis or might be seriously ill needs our full attention. In addition, I perform a careful physical examination of any patient who might have a physical finding that could easily be missed by an inexperienced physician, eg, asymmetrical breath sounds with a foreign body, an enlarged spleen in a child with exudative tonsillitis, or an inflamed uvula in a child who is drooling.

6. *Bring the resident with you into the examining room:* Why this does not happen automatically, I am not certain. Some residents may believe they are already on top of everything and that we cannot add anything. However, if we are to teach by example, residents must be with us. In a way, they are right—we usually do not turn up a new physical finding—but we may trigger a line of questioning that leads to considering a new diagnosis (such as diarrhea from excessive consumption of pear juice, weight loss from an overly diluted formula, or passive smoking as a cause of out-of-control asthma). We can ask, "What are you most concerned about?" and more than 30% of the time we will turn up a "hidden agenda" that needs some education and reassurance. The nuances of obtaining medical histories could easily take an additional 3 years of training.

Other aspects of pediatrics that we can demonstrate are interactions with children: how to include them, interview them, put them at ease, or motivate them. We can show how to make the return visit easier by telling the fearful child how good he or she was following a painful procedure. There is always something to teach.

7. *Protect the resident's role as primary physician for this encounter:* One of our goals is to help the resident treat patients independently. This is the role they have been studying for. We are the consultants for residents' cases. We do not replace residents unless we have their permission. If we agree with the residents' findings, we should commend them (eg, "good pick up") or concur with them ("I agree with your plan") in front of the parents. If we disagree, we should discuss our differences in the hallway. If they have never "defused" an angry parent, it may be more educational to "see one" before they "do one." The same holds true for removing a stubborn foreign body from the nose. However, if we rehearse appropriate advice with residents, they can provide the counseling (eg, for a colicky baby). Whenever we can talk a resident through the procedure, we should do so (eg, the reduction of a subluxed radius).

8. *Encourage the resident to convey all joint decisions to the parents:* Providing the the parent with the diagnosis, treatment recommendations, and follow-up plan (ie, debriefing) is more complicated than obtaining the standard medical history and performing the physical examination. It requires a sensitivity to what the parent is able to understand and absorb. The parent needs an opportunity to respond to the advice. When time permits, try to observe this challenging part of the encounter. Also, encourage residents to give written information or instructions to parents. It can be handwritten, preprinted, or computer generated. Feedback about the resident's technique is helpful after the parent has departed (including interviewing skills).

9. *Encourage 5-minute reading breaks regarding disorders that are new to them:* The best learning combination is a patient with a disease the resident has not seen before, a knowledgeable attending physician, and a short article on the topic. Our learning curve peaks with a patient who needs our help. The new information is more likely to get into the permanent memory if the learner also reads a short description of the disease (eg, torticollis is just a few paragraphs in most texts). This is especially true for visual learners or people who mainly believe what they read. After the patient leaves and before the resident becomes involved with another patient, we can direct him or her to a selected textbook or key article file. Reading about cases at the end of a long day is difficult.

10. *Bring all the residents in to see interesting physical findings:* This is one of the attending's responsibilities. We all like to say that we have seen "one of those" (eg, spider bite, labial adhesions, herpes whitlow, or urticaria pigmentosa). First, we need the parents' and patient's permission. Second, we need to round up the residents for a few minutes.

11. *Encourage 15-minute meal breaks, even if patients are waiting:* The statement, "We can't eat until everyone is seen" came from clinics that closed for lunch. If we are running an emergency department or walk-in clinic, we need to be sure our staff eats before the cafeteria closes. Some dedicated individuals (future victims of burnout?) actually need to be ordered to take a break. As long as all emergencies are handled, people should be sent for a quick bite to eat. Without food and fluids, residents lose efficiency, focus, judgment, and compassion. If the parents did not call for an appointment, the children are not seriously ill, and there is no end in sight, it is time to address the basic needs of the health care providers.

12. *Affirm the resident's strengths:* Sometimes our only responses to residents relate to areas in which they need to improve. We tend to forget that they are already self-critical people and usually well aware of their weaknesses. Do not forget to remind them of their many strengths, eg, curiosity, questioning, healthy skepticism, intellectual honesty about their limitations, initiative, willingness to see difficult families, decisiveness, openness to change, good documentation of information on medical records, good follow-through, and people skills (rapport). Knowing in which areas they are strong gives residents the courage to persevere in the crosscurrents of medicine.

My heartfelt thanks to house staff of 23 years who have taught me and continue to teach me to be an effective teacher. My special thanks go to the dedicated members of our section of general pediatrics for reviewing these comments.

EDITORIAL

Water Intoxication

A Prevalent Problem in the Inner City

The article in this issue of *AJDC* by Keating et al[1] from St Louis, Mo, adds to our warning in 1986 that the incidence of water intoxication in infants has risen during the last 15 years.[2] Four additional issues not extensively addressed by Keating et al are worth comment.

See also p 985.

First, why has there been a sharp increase in the number of patients with water intoxication? Families living in poverty have diluted formulas and fed water to hungry infants as long as any of us can remember, yet before about 1970 we clinicians working in inner-city hospitals rarely encountered water intoxication as a result. On the contrary, we encountered a high incidence of hypernatremic dehydration between 1945 and 1970.[3] I believe the most important factor in bringing about this reversal was the deliberate reduction in the salt (and other "renal solute") content of infant formulas and foods because of concerns about hypertension in later life. Older pediatricians will remember evaporated milk formulas with high solute content. Whether we have achieved a clinically important goal in preventing hypertension remains unknown, but clearly the hypernatremic variety of dehydration is much less common; the percentage of infants hospitalized owing to dehydration decreased from 25% before changes in salt content of formulas to about 2% after these changes were made. This is a welcome outcome because permanent brain damage occurred in 8% to 10% of infants after severe hypernatremic episodes.[4] On the other hand, water intoxication with convulsion has partially replaced hypernatremia. Patients with cystic fibrosis are especially vulnerable to a low salt intake. Fortunately, permanent neurologic damage is uncommon after water intoxication, so the change in salt content of formulas is ultimately a gain.

A second issue is an understanding of the pathophysiologic aspects of water intoxication, which involves the same physiochemical process, but in reverse, of serious hypernatremic dehydration. For water intoxication to occur, there must be a rapid decline in extracellular solute concentration (osmolality), creating a concentration gradient between extracellular fluid and cell water generally and a gradient between the vascular fluid of the brain and the rest of the brain fluids in particular. The brain is affected differently because, unlike other tissues, the endothelial cells of the cerebral blood vessels are joined by tight junctions (the so-called blood-brain barrier). This means that when an osmolal gradient is produced, relief of the gradient in the brain cannot be quickly achieved by rapid diffusion of sodium and chloride ions from the extracellular fluid of the brain, but must be equilibrated by movement of water molecules into both the extracellular fluid and cells of the brain. Consequently, the brain picks up disproportionately more water than other organs; such swelling causes the convulsion, but *only* if the dilution occurs over a few hours. If the change is gradual (a few milliosmoles every 12 hours or so), enough sodium chloride diffusion occurs, keeping the respective volumes constant, preventing a convulsion. This rate of change is a key element in the clinical picture of convulsion in hyponatremic states, and it is more important than the degree of hyponatremia. There are other aspects to the adaptation to an osmolal gradient, but none so relevant to the clinical picture.

A third point concerns which patients present with water intoxication. The St Louis group has identified families in which formula dilution or water substitution for formula was most important. In Brooklyn, we have also encountered patients from such families, but formula dilution and water substitution most commonly occurs in patients with mild diarrhea. Often, a physician (sometimes the mother herself, remembering a previous episode of diarrhea) prescribes dilute beverages to replace formula already low in solute. Thus, there is an iatrogenic component to the increased incidence of water intoxication. The lesson is that use of fluids to prevent or correct dehydration should be based on physiologic principles and prescribed with considerable care. The common suggestion of "drink juices, soda, water, and/or an athletic replacement solution" does not suffice.

Finally, how should the patient with water intoxication be treated? The convulsions are usually fairly brief and should be cared for as any others. The hyponatremia can be corrected in many ways. The St Louis group recommends hypertonic saline (0.5 mol/L or 3%) corrected to about 125 mmol/L. While this is a safe procedure if done correctly, it can be very dangerous if an error is made. Having hypertonic solution in the same cabinet with others may also lead to erroneous administration of the solution to a different patient. Patients with water intoxication who do not have renal damage (those discussed in the article by Keating et al do not) will also recover by simple expenditure of insensible water while being given higher than usual amounts of sodium (100 to 150 mmol/L) in fluids. Some may be dehydrated despite water intoxication and need deficit replacement as well as intake of maintenance fluid. I recommend not using hypertonic solutions for this purpose except when an expert is available to direct the therapy. Our patients with water intoxication (about 10 to 12 per year) thus treated have all recovered well.

LAURENCE FINBERG, MD
Children's Medical Center
of Brooklyn
450 Clarkson Ave, Box 49
Brooklyn, NY 11203-2098

References

1. Keating JP, Schears GJ, Dodge PR. Oral water intoxication in infants: an American epidemic. *AJDC.* 1991;145: 985-990.
2. Finberg L. Too little water has become too much. *AJDC.* 1986;140:524.
3. Finberg L, Kravath R, Fleischman, A. *Water and Electrolytes in Pediatrics.* Phildelphia, Pa; WB Saunders Co; 1982:79.
4. Macauley D, Watson M. Hypernatremia in infants as a cause of brain damage. *Arch Dis Child.* 1967;42: 485-488.

CORRECTION

Incorrect Unit of Measure

In the article entitled "Effect of Necrotizing Enterocolitis on Urinary Epidermal Growth Factor Levels" in the July 1991 issue of *AJDC* (1991;145:804-807), there were some errors in the units of measure used to report EGF and creatinine values. The unit of measure for human EGF values cited five lines from the end of the text under the subhead "EGF Assay and Creatinine Measurements" on page 805 should have read micromoles per liter, and three lines below, the unit of measure for EGF/creatinine values should have read micromoles per micromole. Also, in the last paragraph in the left column of the next page, four lines from the bottom, the values in parentheses should have read µmol/µmol, not µmol/mmol.

Oral Water Intoxication in Infants

An American Epidemic

James P. Keating, MD, MSci(Epidem); Gregory J. Schears, MD; Philip R. Dodge, MD

• Between 1975 and 1990, a total of 34 patients with water intoxication were treated at St Louis (Mo) Children's Hospital, 24 of these in the last 3 years, indicating a marked increase in incidence of this previously rare condition. Thirty-one were infants living in poverty who ingested excessive amounts of water offered at home by their caretakers. Exhaustion of the supply of infant formula was the most common reason given for this substitution. Infants were treated by a single infusion of hypertonic saline or a slow infusion of isotonic saline. Central pontine myelinolysis was not observed as a complication of hypertonic saline therapy. Modification of the Special Supplemental Food Program for Women, Infants, and Children to provide sufficient formula for the growing infant and better education of mothers as to the hazards of excessive water ingestion might reduce the incidence of this preventable and life-threatening condition.

(*AJDC.* 1991;145:985-990)

In 1922, Larson et al[1] described the acute neurologic disturbance that results from rapid, excessive water intake. Water intoxication has been considered a rare clinical event that follows excessive parenteral or enteral water administration by medical personnel,[2] malicious forcing of water on a child,[3] repeated immersion (infant swimming lessons),[4] or voluntary ingestion of iced water to control toothache[5] or occurs during marathon runs,[6] after drug testing,[7] or as a manifestation of psychosis.[8] In 1967, Dugan and Holliday[9] provided the first description of infants who developed water intoxication after the voluntary ingestion of dilute formula. During the following decade and a half, 21 additional examples of healthy infants suffering from water intoxication by the oral route in institutions in five US cities appeared in the medical literature.[10-14] In 1987, Medani[15] described 19 such infants at a single Baltimore (Md) hospital. The possibility that an epidemic is occurring is suggested by these reports and our own experience in the years 1975 through 1990. The details of the clinical syndrome are provided to guide clinicians in the recognition and treatment of the illness. Preventive interventions applicable to the population at risk are discussed.

See also p 981.

Accepted for publication April 18, 1991.

From the Divisions of Gastroenterology and Nutrition (Dr Keating) and Neurology (Dr Dodge), Edward Mallinckrodt Department of Pediatrics (Drs Schears, Dodge, and Keating), Washington University School of Medicine and St Louis Children's Hospital, St Louis, Mo.

Reprint requests to 400 S Kingshighway Blvd, St Louis, MO 63110 (Dr Keating).

PATIENTS AND METHODS

St Louis (Mo) Children's Hospital is a 235-bed facility with 50 000 emergency room visits per annum that serves the health needs of a large geographic region. Approximately 60% of patients have private insurance, and 40% are enrolled in Medicaid. There was a modest increase in the number of urban poor cared for when two small pediatric services in municipal hospitals closed 5 to 10 years ago. A second children's hospital (Cardinal Glennon Memorial Children's Hospital) also serves the region's pediatric needs, but no fluctuation in the acute care activities of either children's hospital occurred during the study period of a magnitude that would explain the first appearance and recent increase in the number of infants with oral water intoxication described in this report.

The records of all patients diagnosed as having water intoxication (*International Classification of Diseases, Ninth Edition,* 276.6) were obtained from the Medical Records Department and the Pediatric Gastroenterology Registry at St Louis Children's Hospital for the period from January 1975 through July 1990. All records that contained a description of an acute neurologic syndrome occurring in association with hyponatremia were selected for detailed review and analysis. Information was abstracted from notes of physicians, social workers, emergency medical technologists, and nurses. Follow-up information was sought by telephone interview with each child's current physician or parent if adequate information was not present in the child's chart.

The 34 patients identified by this process were divided into group 1 (infants) (n = 31) and group 2 (children) (n = 3) for further analysis and to facilitate discussion. The infants were further subdivided by the treatment given (hypertonic saline [group 1a] or a slow infusion [1.0 L/m^2 per day] of isotonic fluid [group 1b]). A patient's treatment was chosen by the clinicians at the time rather than by randomized assignment as would be done in a prospective study of the efficacy of the therapies. Infants in group 1b were more likely to have been recognized to have water intoxication late in their course; a brisk water diuresis had already occurred. Infants in group 1a received a single infusion of 3% saline given during 30 to 90 minutes. The dose was calculated

Table 1.—Infants and Children With Water Intoxication (n=34)*						
		Serum Sodium				
Patient/Age, mo	Treatment	Admission, mmol/L	Rate of Increase, mmol·L⁻¹·h⁻¹	Time Until Normal, h	Temperature, °C†	Respiratory Failure
Group 1a (n=17)						
1/3	3%	116	10.0	2	36.0	−
2/9	3%	114	2.5	8	35.4	−
3/6	3%	114	2.0	8	36.7	+
4/1	3%	116	1.7	14	35.0	−
5/3	3%	114	3.0	6	35.0	+
6/4	3%	116	2.5	12	36.5	−
7/6	3%	115	1.7	14	35.0	+
8/4	3%	119	1.8	10	35.0	+
9/4	3%	112	1.7	13	34.0	+
10/3	3%	112	1.7	15	35.2	+
11/4	3%	115	2.8	15	35.2	−
12/3	3%	112	2.2	8	35.0	−
13/4	3%	118	3.6	5	36.4	−
14/4	3%	116	4.4	5	35.4	+
15/4	3%	117	4.4	5	34.2	+
16/4	3%	114	2.7	8	36.7	+
17/10	3%	115	3.3	6	34.0	−
Mean±SD 4.5±2.2 (range) (1-10)	. . .	115.0±2.0 (112-119)	3.05±2.0 (1.7-10.0)	9.06±4.1 (2-15)	35.3±0.9	9 (53%)
Group 1b (n=14)						
18/4	NS	118	3.0	5	34.0	+
19/4	0.25 NS	117	2.0	10	35.4	+
20/10	RL	119	1.8	10	36.0	−
21/3	RL	112	1.2	16	34.0	+
22/2	RL	122	2.0	2	36.7	−
23/4	NS	116	3.0	15	36.0	−
24/4	NS	125	1.5	10	36.4	−
25/3	NS	119	1.4	11	35.5	−
26/2	RL	117	2.0	12	36.5	−
27/5	NS	119	1.2	10	35.4	+
28/4	PO	123	3.0	4	36.4	+
29/5	RL	116	1.5	12	37.0	+
30/2	PO	127	1.0	8	36.0	−
31/2	NS	111	1.8	12	35.5	+
Mean±SD 3.86±2.07 (range) (2-10)	. . .	118.6±4.5 (111-127)	1.89±0.68 (1.0-3.0)	9.79±3.95 (2-16)	35.8±0.9	6 (43%)
Group 2 (n=3)						
32/8 y	0.5 NS	120	3.0	5	36.2	−
33/3 y	5%	114	2.6	8	34.7	+
34/2 y	3%	112	7.0	30	<34.0	+

*Group 1a consisted of infants intoxicated by the oral route, treated by infusion of 3% saline. Group 1b consisted of infants intoxicated by the oral route, treated with normal saline (NS), Ringer's lactate (RL), or infant formula (PO). Group 2 consisted of children intoxicated by the parenteral or oral route. The difference (1a vs 1b) in initial serum sodium level (115.0 vs 118.6 mmol/L) was statistically significant ($P<.05$). The differences (1a vs 1b) in age, sex, race, rate of serum sodium level increase, time until sodium level was normal, temperature, and proportion of patients with respiratory failure failed to reach statistical significance.

†Temperatures are given as rectal. In seven infants, rectal temperatures were not measured; the number given is their axillary temperature transformed to rectal. In the three infants with temperatures of 34°C, that was the lowest reading possible on the thermometer; they may have been colder.

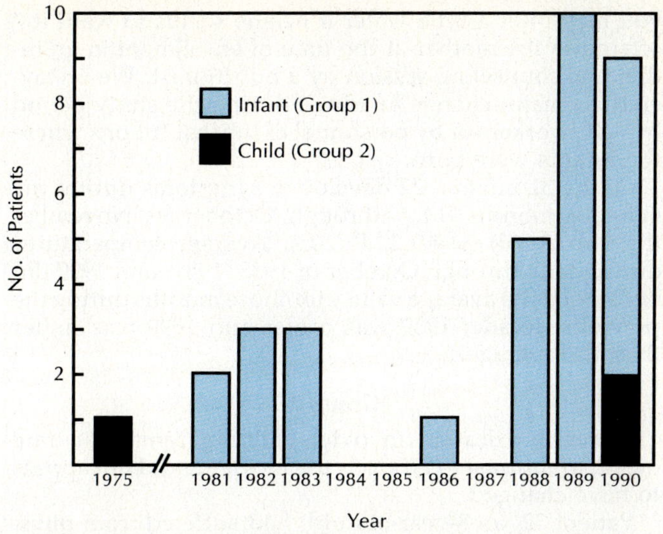

Fig 1.—*Frequency distribution by calendar year of all patients diagnosed as having water intoxication between January 1975 and December 1990.*

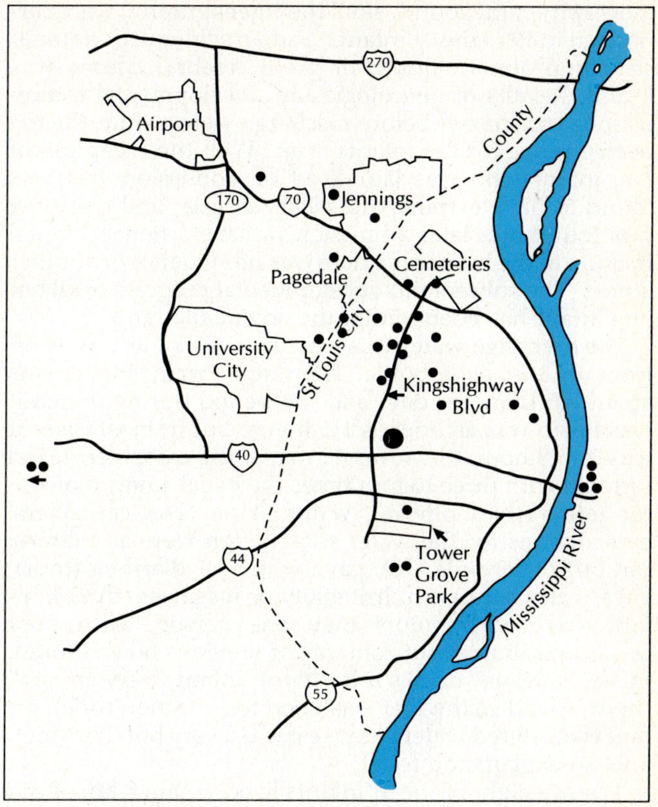

Fig 2.—*Map of the St Louis (Mo) metropolitan area. St Louis Children's Hospital (star) is within the city limits. The dots to the extreme right represent infants from East St Louis, Ill. The two dots to the extreme left are two white infants, one from a small city 112 km from St Louis, the other from a suburb 24 km from the hospital. Kingshighway Boulevard is the main north-south traffic artery through a densely populated, poor, residential area.*

as follows: (body weight in kilograms)(125 mEq/L − initial serum sodium level)(0.6), or about 10 mL of 3% saline per kilogram of body weight.

We obtained records of ambient temperature in St Louis during the years 1988, 1989, and 1990 from the National Oceanic and Atmospheric Administration, US Department of Commerce (Asheville, NC) and compared these with the average temperatures in this area during the last three decades.

The local offices of the Supplemental Food Program for Women, Infants, and Children (WIC) of the State of Missouri/US Department of Agriculture were visited to gather data concerning the availability of food supplements and nutritional advice provided to families in our area during the period of the study. The instructions provided to new mothers by physicians and nurses at St Louis Regional, St Louis Jewish, and Barnes Hospitals (hospitals where most of the infants had been born) were reviewed. Particular attention was paid to changes in allotments of formula and to any advice that might have fostered the substitution of water for formula.

Availability of a clinical microchemistry laboratory and the practice of measuring serum electrolytes in the first sample taken from a convulsing child had not changed during the period of the study.

Descriptive and comparative statistics were calculated by conventional methods, and comparison of means was carried out by *t* test. Comparison of ratios of discrete variables was carried out with the χ^2 test. All tests were two tailed. $P<.05$ was considered statistically significant.

RESULTS

Thirty-four patients were treated for water intoxication, the first infant in 1982 and 24 during the last 3 years (1988 through 1990) (Fig 1). Selected data from each patient are seen in Table 1.

Group 1

The mean±SD age of the 31 infants was 4.2±2.1 months; 17 were male. The illness started suddenly with convulsions or apnea. Seizures occurred in all infants and usually (28 of 31 cases) consisted of generalized tonic-clonic activity. Opisthotonic posturing was common (10 of 31 cases). Seizures persisted from 15 minutes to 6 hours, often intermixed with periods of reduced responsiveness. The possibility of continuing, clinically inapparent seizures, the postictal state, and the depressant effect of anticonvulsant medications made determination of causality of the depressed level of consciousness difficult. In several infants, physicians noted rapid improvement in neurologic signs as hypertonic saline was administered. Bulging of the fontanelle and radiologic evidence of increased intracranial pressure were notably absent.

Respiratory failure, neither preceded nor obviously caused by seizure, occurred in six patients, either at home (five patients) or in the radiology suite (one patient). Others stopped breathing in the emergency room (nine patients). The overall rate of respiratory failure was 15 of 31 (48%). Except in one infant who developed noncardiologic pulmonary edema, mechanical ventilation was withdrawn within 24 hours of admission.

Mean±SD laboratory values (Table 1) included the following: urine specific gravity (31 of 31 patients), 1.004±0.001; serum urea nitrogen (31 of 31 patients), 1.4±0.4 mmol/L; serum calcium (31 of 31 patients), 2.40±0.07 mmol/L; serum magnesium (29 of 31 patients), 0.88±0.03 mmol/L; and serum glucose (31 of 31 patients), 5.5±0.67 mmol/L. Cerebrospinal fluid (29 of 31 patients) was sterile and contained a nucleated cell count of less than 8×10^6/L. The serum cortisol level (24 patients) was within the normal reference range, as was the blood ammonia level (25 patients). A urine toxic screen (26 patients) failed to reveal substances capable of causing seizures, respiratory failure, or hyponatremia. The mean platelet count (31 of 31 patients) was 615×10^9/L (range, 250 to 1300×10^9/L). Imaging studies of the brain (computed tomography, ultrasound, skull roentgenography) were carried out in 19 of the 31 infants, and no evidence of trauma, structural abnormalities, or gross cerebral edema was found. Results of neurologic and developmental examinations carried out before discharge were within the expected range for the infants' ages. With the exception of one infant who was jaundiced on admission and was found to have extrahepatic biliary atresia, and one who was found at a later admission to have a nonaccidental fracture of the humerus, there was no evidence of another illness. The subsequent developmental progress of all but one infant has been within the acceptable range.

The excessive water was usually ingested as tap water from an 8-oz baby bottle. The rate of water intake was about 7.5 L/m^2 per day, and the period during which it was taken was as brief as 1½ hours, but in most cases it was 2 to 8 hours. In several infants, the caregiver mixed formula with three to four times the usual amount of water rather than offering water alone. The caregivers' explanations for the water substitution were as follows: ran out of formula (16), gave water for diarrhea (four), gave water because of irritability or fussiness (three), infant was fed by more than one person, with poor communication about contents of previous bottles (one), infant "always" drinks a lot (two), infant "very thirsty" (two), friend said water was good for infection (one), infant was offered water because it was a very hot day (one), and no explanation (one).

Twenty-eight of the 31 infants lived within 8 km of our hospital (Fig 2), most in residential areas known to have high lead exposure risk, high crime rates, and poverty. Twenty-seven infants were black. Twenty-seven were enrolled in WIC, Aid to Families With Dependent Children, and the food stamp program. Only one mother was married; three were addicted to crack cocaine and alcohol. Most of the mothers were in their 20s and 30s and had older children (one had seven).

Since the WIC program began in 1976, the maximum provision of infant formula has been one can of formula per day per infant (403 fl oz of concentrated liquid formula per month) through the first 12 months of life. In some areas this is provided as an equivalent amount of powdered or ready-to-feed formula. This allotment provides 2293 kJ, or a little more than three 8-oz bottles per infant per day. Based on the average body weight of 4-month-old infants, this provides 378 kcal/kg per day, which is approximately the 50th percentile of observed intake of healthy 4-month-old infants. A small amount of juice and cereal is provided after age 4 months. The mothers of many of our patients found themselves using more than one can per day and exhausted the WIC-supplied formula before the end of the month. The WIC nutritionists, and our hospital social workers, reported a disappearance of alternate (non-WIC) sources of free infant formula and a sharp increase in the cost of formula in retail outlets during the last decade. Sources of additional formula, which in the past were manufacturers' representatives, food pantries, and local churches, appear to have been eliminated. The WIC workers emphasize the word *supplemental* in the program title, but they recognize that many mothers presume that WIC provides everything the infant needs and are reluctant or unable to use their food stamps or cash to buy infant formula. Advice concerning water feeding has been the same since the program began in 1976: "After the infant has taken the breast or formula, you may offer a little water if he/she seems to want it," offered to the mother at the time of enrollment in an individual counseling session by a nutritionist. We uncovered no major change in advice during the study period by WIC workers or by personnel of the institutions where the infants were born.

Of the 31 infants, 22 developed symptoms during the summer months (May through October vs November through April) ($\chi^2=9.2$, $P<.05$). Average temperatures during May through October of 1988, 1989, and 1990 did not exceed the average values for those months during the previous decade; 1989 was cooler and 1990 was hotter than the average.

Group 2

Water intoxication in older children remains a rare event; in contrast to group 1, the incidence did not appear to have changed.

Patient 32, an 8-year-old girl, had suffered from physical abuse as an infant and had openly stated her intention to stab to death a foster parent. Her foster parents, after much counseling, chose water drinking as a method of punishment. When forced to stand in the kitchen and drink 12 glasses of water, the patient lost consciousness. Her recovery was complete.

Patient 33, a 3-year-old girl, was admitted to an outlying hospital with severe dehydration (serum urea nitrogen level, 23.6 mmol/L) due to gastroenteritis. Fluid resuscitation (40 mL/kg) was carried out with the use of 5% glucose in water instead of the intended 5% glucose in saline. As the 4-hour infusion ended, the patient lost consciousness, serum sodium level decreased from 133 to 114 mmol/L, and apnea and coma ensued; hypertonic saline and nonspecific measures were of no avail, and the patient died. Autopsy showed only brain swelling.

Patient 34, who was 2 years old, became comatose 4 hours after elective hip surgery. Serum sodium level had decreased to 112 mmol/L while dilute intravenous fluids were infused. Again, therapy had no apparent effect, and autopsy showed brain swelling. The vulnerability of postoperative patients to water intoxication has been emphasized,[2,16] and the devastating course in such patients has recently been described.[17]

COMMENT

Oral water intoxication is a recognizable clinical syndrome. The victim is usually 3 to 6 months old, comes from a poor family, and presents to the ambulance service or emergency room with apnea or seizures. Body temperature is low, even in hot weather, and the majority of episodes occur in the summer months. Respiratory failure, if not the presenting complaint, may occur as the seizures are treated. After documentation of hyponatremia and the infusion of hypertonic saline, the neurologic disturbance abates. In some infants, spontaneous water diuresis occurs so rapidly that treatment with hypertonic saline may be unnecessary. Ventilatory support is seldom needed for more than 12 hours, and recovery appears complete within a few days. The infants' salt and water homeostatic mechanisms are intact, and, with appropriate feeding instructions, recurrence can be avoided. There is clearly some risk of death or hypoxic organ damage, although this did not occur in our patients (group 1).

The controversy[18,19] that surrounds the treatment of chronically hyponatremic adults and the belief that ex-

Table 2.—Oral Water Intoxication in 85 Healthy Infants

Source, y	City	No. of Patients	Age, mo	Comments
Dugan and Holliday,[9] 1967	Pittsburgh, Pa	1	3	Errors in mixing; ⅙ strength formula
Dugan and Holliday,[9] 1967	Oakland, Calif	1	5	Ten 8-oz bottles of water over 20 h
Nickman et al,[10] 1968	Philadelphia, Pa	2	4, 14	Fed water
Crumpacker and Kriel,[11] 1973	Minneapolis, Minn	5	5.8±4.1	Short of money; gave 12 8-oz bottles of tap water in 1 d; "Hunger is probably the main force that would compel a baby to accept a solute-poor diet . . ."
Schulman,[12] 1980	Albany, NY	2	5, 6	Ran out of milk; gave 64 oz of tap water
David et al,[13] 1981	Pittsburgh	8	3.4±1.0	Authors focused on antidiuretic hormone secretion
Partridge et al,[14] 1981	Cincinnati, Ohio	4	4.1±1.5	Two sibling pairs; water given after each feeding for irritability; physical abuse in one family
Lipsitz,[26] 1984	Pueblo	1	2.5	Water and tea substituted due to coryza
O'Connor,[27] 1985	Wilmington, Del	1	2	Water fed because of diarrhea
Corneli et al,[28] 1985	Cincinnati	7	6.7±1.8	All occurred in 6-wk period, summer 1983
Gold and Koenigsberg,[29] 1986	Chicago, Ill	1	4	Tap water given because of summer heat
Borowitz and Rocco,[30] 1986	Nashville, Tenn	2	5, 3	Considered previous salt restriction important
Medani,[15] 1987	Baltimore, Md	19	5.1±4.3	Water supplements
Schaeffer and Ditchek,[31] 1991	Brooklyn, NY	3	4, 6, 10	. . .
Present report	St Louis, Mo	31	4.2±2.1	. . .

cessively rapid administration of hypertonic saline may cause central pontine myelinolysis should not unduly influence physicians caring for acutely hyponatremic children. The rate of increase in serum osmolality/sodium recommended in the former group of patients (less than 0.5 mmol/h)[18] is inappropriate in acutely hyponatremic patients, such as those described in this report. For symptomatic patients with acute hyponatremia, the rate of increase should be at least 1 mmol/L per hour[19]; the rate of 2 to 3 mmol/L per hour that occurred in our patients (Table 1) was associated with an excellent overall outcome. The rate of increase in serum osmolality in the infants who had spontaneous diuresis (group 1b) was threefold faster than the maximal recommended rate of correction in the chronically hyponatremic adult. The safety and efficacy of prompt infusion of hypertonic saline in the amounts recommended by current pediatric authorities[20-22] is supported by our experience. We recognize the limits of our retrospective study and cannot reject the possibility that isotonic fluids at a restricted infusion rate may be effective therapy for many infants, although we think that a more rapid reversal of the movement of water into the brain may be lifesaving in some.

Incidence figures for water intoxication are not available. Since 1935, when the first report[23] of fatal water intoxication appeared, until 1958, only seven patients, of all ages, were noted in the literature.[23-25] In 1959, Crawford and Dodge[2] described five children, three intoxicated by parenteral fluids, one by gastrostomy, and one by enemas. After the first report of infants who took excessive water by mouth appeared in 1967,[9] only seven similar infants were observed in the next decade,[10,11] but, during the last 5 years, 33 examples[15,26-30] have appeared. Table 2 summarizes 85 reported cases of water intoxication.[9-15,26-31] An article in the lay press in 1981 mentioned 17 Milwaukee (Wis) infants who were not described in the medical literature.[32] We found only three reports[33-35] of infants with oral water intoxication from other countries. The ages of those infants were more evenly distributed through the 1st year of life than in the American patients; withdrawal of formula or breast before excessive water ingestion was a consistent theme in these reports.

The reason for the striking increase in the occurrence of oral water intoxication is not clear. Although other investigators have suggested that abusive caretakers,[14] excessive secretion of antidiuretic hormone,[13] or previous salt restriction may have played a role in their patients, we share Crumpacker and Kriel's view[11] that hunger overwhelms the infants' innate protective mechanisms and is the most important cause of infantile water intoxication. Three facts strongly suggest that unavailability of formula plays a major causative role: (1) the current volume of formula provided by WIC meets the needs of most 3-month-olds and fails to satisfy many 4- and 5-month-old healthy infants; (2) in our study, and in most US reports (Table 2), the ages of the infants are 4 to 6 months; and (3) the majority of mothers said that exhaustion of their supply of formula was the reason they were feeding water. Even when another explanation for water feeding was recorded in the patient's chart, specific history concerning the family's formula supply may not have been sought or offered. We also speculate that the summer clustering may be due to the added burden placed on the families' limited resources by the interruption of the school lunch program for the older siblings and other children in the home.

We are convinced that oral water intoxication is a new, probably underreported, entity. A prospective, national, epidemiologic study is needed to ascertain the incidence of and causative factors responsible for this illness. Immediate consideration should be given to increasing the availability of formula to infants living in poverty. Increased education concerning the dangers of excessive water intake in infants who are denied formula or breast-feeding is also needed,[36] both for medical personnel and for infant caregivers.

Our gratitude to the pediatric interns, residents, nurses, and staff physicians in the emergency room, pediatric intensive care unit, and floors of St Louis Children's Hospital, and to the medical record room staff, the social workers, WIC nutritionists, and the child neurology staff, all of whom saw the infants' needs and met them, documenting what they saw and did. The suggestion concerning the cause of summer clustering came from Rebecca Graves, the able director of the St Louis Children's Hospital social work department. Thanks to Aileen Derhake, whose transformation of handwritten gibberish into clean prose raises the skill of typing to a profession.

References

1. Larson EE, Rowntree LG, Weir JF. Studies in diabetes insipidus, water balance, and water intoxication. *Arch Intern Med.* 1922;29:306-330.
2. Crawford JD, Dodge PR. Complications of fluid therapy in patients with neurologic disease with special emphasis on water intoxication and hypertonic dehydration. *Pediatr Clin North Am.* 1959;6:257-279.
3. Mortimer JG. Acute water intoxication as another unusual manifestation of child abuse. *Arch Dis Child.* 1980;55:401-403.
4. Kropp RM, Schwartz JF. Water intoxication from swimming. *J Pediatr.* 1982;101:947-948.
5. Pickering LK, Hogan GR. Voluntary water intoxication in a normal child. *J Pediatr.* 1971;78:316-318.
6. Frizzell RT, Lang GH, Lowance DC, Latham SR. Hyponatremia and ultramarathon running. *JAMA.* 1986;255:772-774.
7. Klonoff DC, Jurow AH. Acute water intoxication as a complication of urine drug testing in the workplace. *JAMA.* 1991;265:84-85.
8. Cheng JC, Zikos D, Skopicki HA, Peterson DR, Fisher KA. Long-term neurologic outcome in psychogenic water drinkers with severe symptomatic hyponatremia: the effect of rapid correction. *Am J Med.* 1990;88:561-566.
9. Dugan S, Holliday MA. Water intoxication following the voluntary ingestion of excessive fluids. *Pediatrics.* 1967;39:418-420.
10. Nickman SL, Buckler JM, Weiner LB. Further experience with water intoxication. *Pediatrics.* 1968;41:149-151.
11. Crumpacker RW, Kriel RL. Voluntary water intoxication in normal infants. *Neurology.* 1973;23:1251-1255.
12. Schulman J. Infantile water intoxication at home. *Pediatrics.* 1980;66:119-120.
13. David R, Ellis D, Gartner JC. Water intoxication in normal infants: role of antidiuretic hormone in pathogenesis. *Pediatrics.* 1981;68:349-353.
14. Partridge JC, Payne ML, Leisgang JJ, Randolph JF, Rubinstein JH. Water intoxication secondary to feeding mismanagement, a preventable form of familial seizure disorder in infants. *AJDC.* 1981;135:38-40.
15. Medani CR. Seizures and hypothermia due to dietary water intoxication in infants. *South Med J.* 1987;80:421-425.
16. Arieff AI. Hyponatremia, convulsions, respiratory arrest, and permanent brain damage after elective surgery in healthy women. *N Engl J Med.* 1986;314:1529-1535.
17. Arieff AI, Fraser CL. Detrimental consequences of untreated hyponatremia in children. *Kidney Int.* 1987;31:290. Abstract.
18. Sterns RH. The treatment of hyponatremia: unsafe at any speed? *Am Kidney Found Nephrol Lett.* 1989;6:1-10.
19. Cluitmans FHM, Meinders AE. Management of severe hyponatremia: rapid or slow correction? *Am J Med.* 1990;88:161-166.
20. Fleisher GR, Ludwig S. *The Textbook of Pediatric Emergency Medicine.* Baltimore, Md: Williams & Wilkins;1983:419.
21. Black JA. *Paediatric Emergencies.* 2nd ed. London, England: Butterworths;1987:125.
22. Feld LG, Kaskel FJ, Schoeneman MJ. The approach to fluid and electrolyte therapy in pediatrics. In: Barness LA, DeVivo DC, Morrow G, Oski F, Rudolph AM, eds. *Advances in Pediatrics.* Chicago, Ill: Mosby Year Book Medical Publishers Inc; 1988:526.
23. Helwig FC, Schutz CB, Curry DE. Water intoxication, report of a fatal human case. *JAMA.* 1935;104:1569-1575.
24. Swanson AG, Iseri OA. Acute encephalopathy due to water intoxication. *N Engl J Med.* 1958;258:831-834.
25. Baskin JL, Keith HM, Scribner BH. Water metabolism in water intoxication. *AJDC.* 1958;83:618-627.
26. Lipsitz DJ. Herbal teas and water intoxication in a young child. *J Fam Pract.* 1984;18:933-937.
27. O'Connor RE. Water intoxication with seizures. *Ann Emerg Med.* 1985;14:71-73.
28. Corneli HM, Gormley CJ, Baker RC. Hyponatremia and seizures in the first two years of life. *Pediatr Emerg Care.* 1985;1:190-193.
29. Gold I, Koenigsberg M. Infantile seizures caused by voluntary water intoxication. *Am J Emerg Med.* 1986;4:21-27.
30. Borowitz SM, Rocco M. Acute water intoxication in healthy infants. *South Med J.* 1986;79:1156-1158.
31. Schaeffer AV, Ditchek S. Current social practices leading to water intoxication in infants. *AJDC.* 1991;145:27-28.
32. Heyrman K. Baby doctors warn of diluted formula. *Milwaukee J.* August 11, 1981:1.
33. Etzioni A, Benderly A, Levi Y. Water intoxication by the oral route in an infant. *Arch Dis Child.* 1979;54:551-553.
34. Lingh HF, Hsu CH, Chyou SC, Lee YJ, Chang KL. Neonatal water intoxication secondary to feeding mismanagement. *Chung Hua I Hsueh Tsa Chih.* 1987;39:131-134.
35. Vanapruks V, Prapaitvakul K. Water intoxication and hyponatremic convulsions in neonates. *Arch Dis Child.* 1989;64:734-735.
36. Finberg L. Too little water has become too much. *AJDC.* 1986;140:524.

Vasopressin Levels in Infants During the Course of Aseptic and Bacterial Meningitis

Guadalupe Padilla, MD; M. Gore Ervin, PhD; Michael G. Ross, MD; Rosemary D. Leake, MD

• We measured urine vasopressin (VP) once daily on days 1 through 3 in 18 patients hospitalized with meningitis. Urine VP values were 215±100, 116±44, and 69±23 pg/mL on days 1 through 3, respectively, for children with bacterial meningitis and 34±14, 20±4, and 15±4 pg/mL for those with aseptic meningitis. Urinary VP levels of infants with bacterial meningitis were significantly greater than those of healthy ambulatory subjects (n=18) on all three study days; VP values of infants with bacterial meningitis were also greater than those of infants with aseptic meningitis on study days 2 and 3. The VP levels for the subjects with aseptic meningitis were significantly greater than those of the controls on day 1 only. None of the infants exhibited the clinical syndrome of inappropriate antidiuretic hormone secretion.

(*AJDC*. 1991;145:991-993)

The occurrence of the clinical syndrome of inappropriate secretion of antidiuretic hormone (SIADH) in meningitis implies that circulating vasopressin (VP), or antidiuretic hormone, levels are elevated in this condition. Limited data are available, however, reporting only single values of serum, urine, or spinal fluid VP levels in pediatric patients with meningitis.[1-7] These reports suggest that SIADH is a risk for children with meningitis but do not document the time course of increased VP secretion during the illness. In this study, we measured urinary VP levels by radioimmunoassay,[8] as well as serum and urinary sodium levels and osmolality, in infants with bacterial meningitis (BM) and aseptic meningitis (AM). These data quantify VP during the initial 3 days of illness, relate values to responses in serum and urinary sodium levels and osmolality, and allow a comparison of VP levels in BM and AM over time.

PATIENTS AND METHODS

Consent for the study before its initiation was obtained from the Human Subjects' Protection Committee. During the period from March 1985 to April 1988, we studied 18 infants during the first 3 days of their hospitalizations for meningitis at the Harbor-UCLA Medical Center, Torrance, Calif. Ten patients were diagnosed as having BM, and eight had AM. Patients with hypovolemia, dehydration, or renal, cardiac, pulmonary, or central nervous system diseases other than meningitis were excluded from the study.

The cerebrospinal fluid evaluation consisted of cell count, glucose, protein, and latex agglutination determinations and bacterial/viral cultures. The patients with BM had positive culture and/or latex agglutination results. *Haemophilus influenzae* was cultured in eight infants and meningococcus in two patients. Those diagnosed as having AM had negative culture and latex agglutination results but demonstrated cerebrospinal fluid cell numbers and types consistent with AM. Viral cultures yielded echovirus 17, coxsackievirus B_2, or no growth (n=6). No infant received antibiotic therapy before lumbar puncture; all received ampicillin, gentamicin, chloramphenicol, and/or cefotaxime throughout the 3 study days.

A single urine sample was collected from a bladder catheter or spontaneous void within the first 24 hours of hospitalization and for 2 days thereafter for urinary osmolality, sodium, and VP determinations. Urinary VP levels were also measured in single, freely voided urine samples from 18 healthy nonhospitalized children of similar age receiving fluid ad libitum. Serum sodium and urea nitrogen levels were measured daily within 8 hours of the urine sample collection in the patients with meningitis. Serum osmolality was measured directly or calculated by means of the following formula: osmolality=2(sodium)+serum urea nitrogen/2.8+glucose/18.

The infants' charts were reviewed daily for fluid and sodium intake, for evidence of the clinical syndrome of SIADH, and specifically for a history of hypoxia, pneumothorax, seizures, ventilator therapy, use of volume expanders, and drug administration.

Initial fluid management consisted of 0.9% sodium in 5% glucose infused at rates calculated to provide maintenance needs for all infants. As tolerance allowed, enteral feedings were begun at rates calculated to provide fluid maintenance.

Urine VP levels were measured by radioimmunoassay by means of a method previously described in our laboratory.[8] Urine samples were collected in plain glass tubes containing 1N hydrochloric acid and stored frozen at −20°C until extraction with disposable columns (C18 SepPak, Milford, Mass). Each sample was assayed in duplicate. Standardized samples were assayed to determine the amount of VP recovered per assay; all values were corrected for recovery rate. Intercoefficients and intracoefficients of variation of the VP assay were 3% and 9%, respectively. Urinary sodium was measured by flame photometry (Instrumentation Laboratories, Watertown, Mass). Urine osmolality was determined by freezing-point depression by means of

Accepted for publication April 10, 1991.

From the Departments of Pediatrics (Drs Padilla and Leake) and Obstetrics (Drs Ervin and Ross), UCLA School of Medicine, Harbor-UCLA Medical Center, Torrance, Calif.

Reprint requests to Department of Pediatrics, Harbor-UCLA Medical Center, 1000 W Carson St, RB-1, Torrance, CA 90509 (Dr Leake).

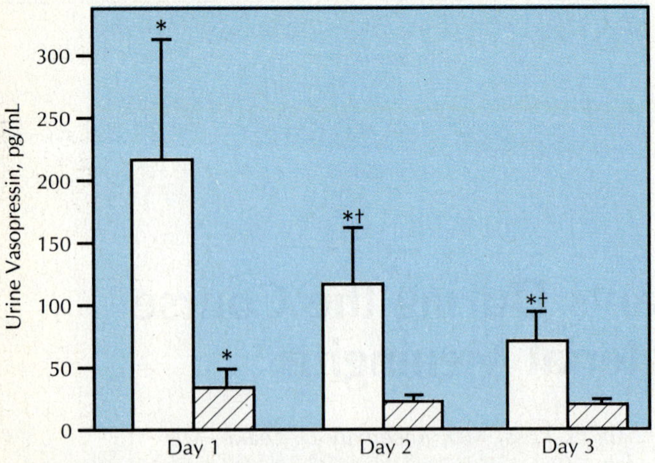

Fig 1.—*Mean (±SEM) urine vasopressin levels over the 3 study days for infants with bacterial (open bars) and aseptic (crosshatched bars) meningitis (n=18). Mean value for a single vasopressin measurement in 18 healthy, age-matched controls was 16.3±2 pg/mL. Asterisk indicates* P<.05, *greater than controls; dagger,* P<.05, *bacterial meningitis greater than (time-matched) aseptic meningitis values.*

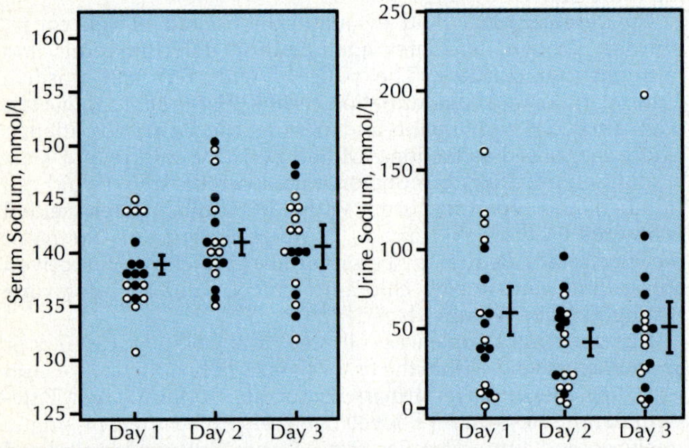

Fig 2.—*Serum and urine sodium levels during the 3 study days for patients with bacterial (open circles) and aseptic (closed circles) meningitis. Bars show mean (±SEM) for each day.*

an osmometer (Digimatic, Advanced Instruments, Needham Heights, Mass). Serum sodium and urea nitrogen concentrations were measured in the hospital laboratory by standard methods.

The VP values for the three study groups were compared by analysis of variance with pairwise comparisons between groups. To achieve a normal distribution with equal variances in each group, log values of the vasopressin levels were used for statistical comparisons. Log VP values were also compared by linked correlation with urinary osmolality (linear regression analysis).

RESULTS

Mean (±SEM) ages of the patients with BM and AM were 10.3±2 months and 2.8±1 months, respectively. The mean age of the healthy controls was 7.2±1 months. One patient with BM required placement of a subdural catheter on study day 3. Two patients had single generalized seizures; one required intubation for several hours after the seizure but was not hypoxemic. Two patients with BM received phenytoin for seizure activity, and two patients with BM received furosemide; however, all doses were given 8 to 12 hours after urine samples were obtained. One patient received dexamethasone and one received prednisolone sodium succinate throughout the hospital course.

Urine VP levels in patients with BM and AM are shown in Fig 1. In subjects with BM, mean (±SEM) VP values were 215±100 pg/mL on study day 1, 116±44 pg/mL on day 2, and 69±23 pg/mL on day 3. The VP values for the subjects with AM were 34±14, 20±4, and 15±4 pg/mL on days 1, 2, and 3, respectively. The urine VP level for the control subjects was 16.3±2 pg/mL. The VP levels of patients with BM were significantly greater (*P*<.01) than those of the control subjects on all 3 study days; the VP values in BM were also greater than those in AM (*P*<.05) on study days 2 and 3. The VP levels of the infants with AM were significantly greater (*P*<.05) than those of the controls on day 1 only.

Maintenance daily fluid requirements were provided for all subjects, and all infants were clinically euvolemic. Mean (±SEM) fluid intake in the patients with BM was 88±9 mL/kg per day on day 1, 100±11 mL/kg per day on day 2, and 110±11 mL/kg per day on day 3; thus, there was a gradual increase in intake amounting to 25% by the 3rd day of the study. Fluid intake in the patients with AM was 97±13, 113±15, and 109±10 mL/kg per day on days 1, 2, and 3, respectively.

Mean sodium intake was 5.6±1, 6.6±2, and 4.6±1.3 mEq/kg per day for patients with BM. Infants with AM received 3.3±1 mEq/kg per day on day 1; oral feedings were resumed on day 2 or 3. Serum and urine sodium levels of patients with BM and AM are shown in Fig 2. Mean serum sodium level was 139±1.5, 141±1.4, and 140±1.5 mmol/L for patients with BM on days 1 through 3, respectively, and 138±0.6, 141±1.9, and 140±2.4 mmol/L for patients with AM. Only one subject (with BM) exhibited a serum sodium level below 135 mmol/L, and then only on day 1. Mean urine sodium values were 64±18, 30±7.8, and 50±7 mmol/L on days 1 through 3, respectively, for patients with BM and 52±11, 52±10, and 51±13 mmol/L for patients with AM. Mean serum osmolality was 282±3, 285±2, and 284±2 mmol/kg for the patients with BM and 282±2.5, 288±5.7, and 287±1 mmol/kg for the patients with AM on days 1 through 3, respectively. Urine osmolality was 578±87, 664±100, and 469±46 mmol/kg for the patients with BM and 461±66, 369±33, and 491±79 mmol/kg for the patients with AM. There was a significant correlation coefficient ($r=.6$) of log VP and urine osmolality but no correlation with serum or urinary sodium level.

COMMENT

The VP levels in this study represent, to our knowledge, the first reported serial values during the course of meningitis and the first comparisons of VP values and fluid intake, serum and urinary sodium levels, and osmolality in this study population.

Urinary VP levels provide a noninvasive, integrated index of VP secretion. Plasma and (extracted) urine VP correlate linearly, whether compared as urinary VP concentration or rate of VP excretion.[9] The source of urinary VP is glomerular filtration[10]; urinary VP levels correlate significantly with creatinine clearance.[11,12] Urinary VP levels increase with hypoxia, mask ventilation, the occurrence of pneumothorax, intraventricular hemorrhage in the newborn period, and head trauma in pediatric patients.[13,14]

With the use of urinary VP determination, we confirmed that during the 1st day of illness, patients with both BM and AM exhibit markedly elevated VP levels. On subsequent days, VP levels return toward normal, more rapidly for patients with AM than BM.

The stimulus for increased VP secretion in meningitis is unclear. The VP values cannot be explained on the basis of the therapies administered for meningitis, since phenytoin inhibits VP secretion,[15] and dexamethasone has been reported to increase sodium excretion and produce diuresis or to have no effect.[16]

Urine osmolality correlated well with log VP levels in our study; with urine VP measured in unextracted urine,[4] urine osmolalities were not increased despite high VP levels. We previously reported that a urine osmolality greater than 800 mmol/kg was associated with markedly increased urine VP levels (200 to 1650 pg/mL) in pediatric head trauma[14] (mean age, 7.5±1.6 years). In the younger subjects included in this study, a urine osmolality of greater than 600 mmol/kg was associated with urinary VP levels ranging from 98 to 1038 pg/mL, perhaps reflecting the limitation in any additional urinary concentrating ability of our younger subjects.

Despite the elevated VP and urine osmolality levels and the lack of fluid restriction, none of the patients demonstrated the complete clinical SIADH (hyponatremia, increased urinary sodium concentration, diminished serum osmolality, and urine osmolality greater than serum osmolality). The reported incidence of SIADH varies from 4% to 88% and from 9% to 64% for bacterial and viral meningitis, respectively.[1-7] In most studies, however, VP blood and urine levels were not measured. There are a number of possible explanations for our low incidence of SIADH. Our series may have been too limited, the VP increase insufficient or too short-lived, and/or the fluid administration inadequate to produce SIADH in this group of moderately ill patients with meningitis. It remains unclear whether patients who are older or experience meningitis associated with asphyxia,[17] cerebral edema,[14] or effusion[18] might secrete more VP and/or respond differently. Moreover, the age at study differed significantly for our patients with BM vs AM (10.3±2 vs 2.8±1 months, respectively). This may have affected VP secretion, although previous studies suggest an intact, appropriate response from birth onward.[11-13,17,19] Developmental changes in renal response to elevated VP levels, however, have not been well studied in infancy. Thus, our series represents a limited examination of the entire question of VP secretion in childhood meningitis, since our study subjects were too few to analyze by organism, adjunctive therapies, or severity of disease, for example. It is clear from our serial measurements that VP secretion continues despite treatment of meningitis, and although several of our subjects appeared well enough to be discharged on day 4 of hospitalization, their VP levels remained elevated and continued to be a potential risk for development of SIADH.

This work was supported in part by grant HD-06355 from the National Institute of Child Health and Human Development, Bethesda, Md, and by grant RR-00425 (General Clinical Research Center) from the National Institutes of Health, Bethesda.

References

1. Feigin RD, Kaplan S. Inappropriate secretion of antidiuretic hormone in children with bacterial meningitis. *Am J Clin Nutr.* 1977;30:1482-1484.

2. Kaplan SL, Feigin RD. The syndrome of inappropriate secretion of antidiuretic hormone in children with bacterial meningitis. *J Pediatr.* 1978;92:758-761.

3. Garcia H, Kaplan SL, Feigin RD. Cerebrospinal fluid concentration of arginine vasopressin in children with bacterial meningitis. *J Pediatr.* 1981;98:67-70.

4. Fajardo JE, Staford EM, Bass JW, Poscelli JD, Sato AK, Claybough JR. Inappropriate antidiuretic hormone in children with viral meningitis. *Pediatr Neurol.* 1989;5:37-40.

5. Chemtob S, Reece ER, Mills EL. Syndrome of inappropriate secretion of antidiuretic hormone in enteroviral meningitis. *AJDC.* 1985;139:292-294.

6. Prince AS, Neu HC. Fluid management in *Haemophilus influenzae* meningitis. *Infection.* 1980;8:5-7.

7. Feigin RD, Stechenberg BW, Chang MJ, et al. Prospective evaluation of treatment of *Haemophilus influenzae* meningitis. *J Pediatr.* 1976;88:542-548.

8. Tausch A, Stegner H, Leake RD, Artman HG, Fisher DA. Radioimmunoassay of arginine vasopressin in urine: development and application. *J Clin Endocrinol Metab.* 1983;57:777-781.

9. Moses AM. Osmotic thresholds for AVP release with the use of plasma and urine AVP and free water clearance. *Am J Physiol.* 1989;256:R892-R897.

10. Baumann G, Dingham JF. Distribution, blood transport and degradation of antidiuretic hormone in man. *J Clin Invest.* 1976;57:1109-1115.

11. Godard C, Gearing J-M, Geering K, Vallotton MB. Plasma renin activity related to sodium balance, renal function, and urinary vasopressin in the newborn infant. *Pediatr Res.* 1979;13:742-745.

12. Godard C, Vallotton MB, Favre L. Urinary prostaglandins, vasopressin and kallikrein excretion in healthy children from birth to adolescence. *J Pediatr.* 1982;100:898-901.

13. Rees L, Brook CGD, Shaw JCL, Forsling ML. Hyponatremia in the first week of life in preterm infants. *Arch Dis Child.* 1984;59:416-422.

14. Padilla G, Leake JA, Castro R, Ervin MG, Ross MG, Leake RD. Vasopressin levels in pediatric head trauma. *Pediatrics.* 1989;83:700-750.

15. Fishman MP, Kleeman CR, Bethune JE. Inhibition of antidiuretic hormone secretion with diphenylhydantoin. *Arch Neurol.* 1970;22:45-53.

16. Shenkin HA, Gutterman P. The analysis of body water compartments in postoperative craniotomy patients, part 3: the effects of dexamethasone. *J Neurosurg.* 1969;31:400-407.

17. Moylan MB, Herrin JT, Krishnamorrthy K, Todres ID, Shannon DC. Inappropriate antidiuretic hormone secretion in premature infants with cerebral injury. *AJDC.* 1978;123:399-402.

18. Gaufin L, Skowsky WR, Goodman SJ. Release of antidiuretic hormone during mass-induced elevation of intracranial pressure. *J Neurosurg.* 1977;46:627-637.

19. Leake RD, Weitzman RE, Weinberg JA, Fisher DA. Control of vasopressin in the newborn lamb. *Pediatr Res.* 1979;13:257-260.

Demographic and Risk Factors Associated With Chronic Dieting in Adolescents

Mary Story, PhD; Kim Rosenwinkel, MPH; John H. Himes, PhD; Michael Resnick, PhD; Linda J. Harris; Robert Wm. Blum, MD, PhD

• A comprehensive, school-based survey was administered to 36 320 Minnesota public school students in grades 7 through 12 during the 1987-1988 school year. Self-reported chronic dieting was much higher in girls than in boys (12.1% of all girls vs 2.1% of boys). For girls, the percentage of chronic dieters was significantly less in grades 7 and 8 (7.8%) than in grades 9 and 10 (13.5%) or grades 11 and 12 (14.3%). There were no differences among urban, suburban, or rural youth. Black girls were less likely to diet compared with white girls. Chronic dieters were more likely than other students to report maladaptive weight-loss techniques, such as self-induced vomiting (relative risk, 9.92 for girls and 9.40 for boys), laxative use (relative risk, 7.18 for girls and 11.00 for boys), ipecac use (relative risk, 8.33 for girls and 11.00 for boys), and diuretic use (relative risk, 7.30 for girls and 13.5 for boys). It is suggested that chronic dieting may serve as a screening marker for more severe eating and weight-loss behaviors.

(*AJDC.* 1991;145:994-998)

During adolescence, both boys and girls become preoccupied with and sensitive about their size and physical appearance. Studies have consistently shown a high prevalence of dissatisfaction with body weight or shape among male and female adolescents.[1-5] The cultural pressure to be thin, especially for female adolescents, coupled with the societal stigma of obesity, may predispose weight-conscious youth to abnormal eating patterns and eating disorders.[6,7] Disordered eating behaviors—unhealthy preoccupation with weight and food, crash diets, fasting, binge eating, and purging—appear to be quite common, especially among female adolescents and young adults.[1-5] The National Adolescent Health Survey (1988) found that 61% of adolescent girls and 28% of adolescent boys had dieted during the previous year. Unhealthy weight control methods were common among the dieters: 51% reported fasting, 16% used diet pills, and 12% reported vomiting to control their weight.[8] Johnson et al[9] surveyed 1268 high school girls and found that 36% were currently dieting and 14% were chronically dieting. Killen et al[10] found that 10.6% of female teenagers reported self-induced vomiting for weight control, while 13% reported some form of purging behavior (vomiting and use of laxatives or diuretics). Recent studies indicate that weight concerns and dieting practices are now occurring with greater frequency than was previously reported among older children and very young teenagers.[11,12] Maloney et al[11] found that 45% of 8- to 13-year-old boys and girls wanted to be thinner and that 37% had already tried to lose weight.

Several authors have proposed that dieting is a predisposing factor in the development of bulimic symptoms as well as the more serious eating disorders anorexia nervosa and bulimia nervosa.[6,7,9,13,14] Little is known, however, about the prevalence of excessive dieting or if it is associated with other unhealthy eating or weight-loss behaviors. Research on prevalence rates of abnormal eating and of attending demographic risk factors is necessary for the nature and extent of these problems to be understood. Although there are a number of descriptive studies of prevalence of dieting and disordered eating patterns among adolescents and young adults, these tend to be based on relatively small and very select samples, often in private schools or on university campuses, and focus primarily on girls. Therefore, little is known about dieting in relation to sociodemographic characteristics.

We present a descriptive study of unhealthy eating and dieting behaviors based on 34 196 Minnesota youth 12 to 18 years of age. Because repeated dieting constitutes a risk factor for eating disorders as well as inappropriate eating behavior among adolescents, we selected chronic dieting as our chief dependent variable. The distinctive feature of our study is that the sample size of youth from throughout the state of Minnesota is large enough to determine, with some confidence, the relationships of chronic dieting to important sociodemographic characteristics, such as school grade, sex, race, socioeconomic status (SES), and geographic location (urban, suburban, and rural). Furthermore, we examined the relationships of chronic dieting to other disordered eating behaviors.

Accepted for publication January 28, 1991.

From the Adolescent Health Program, Department of Pediatrics, and School of Public Health, University of Minnesota, Minneapolis (Drs Story, Himes, Resnick, and Blum and Ms Harris), and the Division of Maternal and Child Health, Minnesota Department of Health (Ms Rosenwinkel).

Reprint requests to the University of Minnesota, Box 197, Mayo Building, 420 Delaware St SE, Minneapolis, MN 55455 (Dr Story).

Table 1.—Dieting and Weight-Related Questions From the Minnesota Adolescent Health Survey

How often have you gone on a diet during the last year? By "diet," we mean changing the way you eat so you can lose weight.
- Never
- 1-4 times
- 5-10 times
- More than 10 times
- Am always dieting

At the present time, do you feel like you are:
- Underweight
- About the right weight
- Overweight

At this time, how satisfied are you with your weight?

Very satisfied						Not at all satisfied
1	2	3	4	5	6	7

At this time, how proud are you of your body?

Very proud						Not at all proud
1	2	3	4	5	6	7

How often do you vomit (throw up) on purpose after eating?
- Never
- Once a month or less
- 2-3 times a week
- Once a week
- 2 or more times a week

Do you use any of the following to lose weight?
- Laxatives
- Ipecac
- Diuretics (water pills) not just for your period
- None of the above

Have you ever eaten so much food in a short period of time that you felt out-of-control and would be embarrassed if others saw you (binge-eating, gorging, or bulimia)?
- Yes No

Are you ever afraid to start eating because you think you won't be able to stop?
- Yes No

SUBJECTS AND METHODS

The Minnesota Adolescent Health Survey was administered from September 1987 to May 1988 and involved 36 320 Minnesota public school students in grades 7 through 12 in 86 school districts. Schools were selected to elicit participation from different ethnic and geographic groups after stratifying for size of school districts. This sample, however, cannot be considered statistically representative of all of Minnesota in a technical sense. Nevertheless, to our knowledge, it is the largest study ever undertaken on youth in America. After the exclusion of obvious errors and inconsistent and incomplete data, usable data were obtained for 34 196 subjects.

The Minnesota Adolescent Health Survey questionnaire covered a broad range of subject areas related to adolescent health. Questions included health care utilization, major worries and concerns, sexuality, emotional stress, suicide attempts, and substance use. A series of questions dealt with body image, weight satisfaction, and eating and weight-loss behaviors (Table 1).

Adolescents were considered "chronic dieters" if they reported that they had been on a diet more than 10 times during the past year or were always dieting during the past year. Because the percentage of chronic dieters among boys was so different from that among girls, analyses were performed for boys and girls separately. Other variables of interest included race/ethnicity, geographic location (urban, suburban, rural), and a measure of parental SES, based on educational attainment and work status. A variable concerning body image was derived from satisfaction with current weight and the response to the question "How proud are you of your body?" Those with high levels of dissatisfaction and low body pride were considered to have a poor body image. Self-reported height and weight were used to calculate the body mass index (in kilograms per square meter) as an indicator of actual body size and weight status. The distribution categories of body mass index were obtained from the National Health and Nutrition Examination Survey.[15]

Table 2.—Selected Characteristics of Minnesota Youth in the Adolescent Health Survey

Variable	No. (%)
Sex	
M	16 725 (48.9)
F	17 471 (51.1)
Grade	
7 and 8	10 445 (30.6)
9 and 10	11 613 (34.0)
11 and 12	12 138 (35.4)
Location	
Urban	16 772 (49.0)
Suburban	5660 (16.6)
Rural	11 764 (34.4)
Parental socioeconomic status	
Low	3937 (12.8)
Moderate	16 681 (54.2)
High	10 165 (33.0)
Ethnicity	
W	28 901 (86.4)
B	2603 (7.8)
Hispanic	343 (1.1)
American Indian	551 (1.6)
Asian	1053 (3.1)
Dieted during the last year	
F	10 832 (61.9)*
M	3512 (20.1)*
Chronic dieters	
F	2104 (12.0)*
M	364 (2.1)*

*Percent of sex class who dieted or were chronic dieters.

Table 3.—Percent of Chronic Dieting by Selected Characteristics Among Adolescent Male and Female Subjects*

	Female Subjects		Male Subjects	
	%	95% CI	%	95% CI
Grade				
7 and 8	7.8	(7.1, 8.5)	1.6	(1.3, 2.0)
9 and 10	13.5	(12.6, 14.4)	2.5	(2.1, 2.9)
11 and 12	14.3	(13.4, 15.2)	2.4	(2.0, 2.8)
Location				
Urban	11.1	(10.5, 11.8)	2.2	(1.9, 2.5)
Suburban	13.8	(12.5, 15.1)	1.8	(1.3, 2.3)
Rural	12.5	(11.7, 13.4)	2.3	(1.9, 2.7)
Parental socioeconomic status				
Low	10.2	(9.0, 11.5)	2.0	(1.4, 2.7)
Moderate	12.6	(11.9, 13.3)	2.2	(1.9, 2.5)
High	12.1	(11.2, 13.0)	2.0	(1.6, 2.4)
Race/Ethnicity				
W	12.5	(11.9, 13.0)	2.1	(1.8, 2.3)
B	8.1	(6.7, 9.6)	2.1	(1.3, 3.0)
Hispanic	14.9	(10.0, 26.9)	3.0	(0.9, 6.0)
Native American	10.8	(7.5, 14.6)	2.3	(0.8, 4.4)
Asian	10.5	(7.9, 13.3)	3.3	(0.9, 6.1)

*CI indicates confidence interval.

Table 4.—Relative Risks of Inappropriate Eating and Weight Loss Behaviors and Body Image Concerns Among Adolescent Chronic Dieters Compared With Other Adolescents*

	Female Subjects				Male Subjects			
	Chronic Dieters, %	Others, %	RR	95% CI	Chronic Dieters, %	Others, %	RR	95% CI
Feel overweight	75.7	38.4	1.97	(1.91, 2.03)	42.7	16.3	2.62	(2.18, 2.97)
Poor body image	44.2	14.7	3.01	(2.83, 3.20)	18.1	4.7	3.86	(3.06, 4.84)
Self-induced vomiting weekly or more	11.9	1.2	9.92	(8.45, 11.64)	4.7	0.5	9.40	(5.61, 15.74)
Use of laxatives to lose weight	7.9	1.1	7.18	(5.83, 8.85)	4.4	0.4	11.00	(6.44, 18.80)
Use of ipecac to lose weight	2.5	0.3	8.33	(3.13, 22.18)	1.1	0.1	11.00	(3.71, 32.65)
Use of diuretics to lose weight	7.3	1.0	7.30	(5.86, 9.09)	2.7	0.2	13.50	(6.67, 27.32)
Ever been on food binge	54.8	26.4	2.08	(1.98, 2.18)	27.7	12.3	2.25	(1.90, 2.67)
Fear of uncontrolled eating	42.7	13.7	3.12	(2.92, 3.33)	18.2	4.1	4.44	(3.52, 5.59)
Binge eating and fear of uncontrolled eating	32.2	8.7	3.70	(3.47, 3.95)	11.0	1.9	5.79	(2.26, 14.84)
Self-reported weight for height								
<25th percentile BMI	13.1	22.6	0.58	(0.51, 0.66)	11.9	16.2	0.74	(0.54, 1.00)
25th-75th percentile BMI	63.9	60.7	1.05	(1.02, 1.09)	49.0	56.4	0.87	(0.77, 0.98)
>75th percentile BMI	23.0	16.7	1.38	(1.26, 1.51)	39.0	27.3	1.43	(1.24, 1.65)

*RR indicates relative risk; CI, confidence interval; and BMI, body mass index.

Two types of analyses were performed. First, demographic characteristics of chronic dieters were described. Proportions of chronic dieters and 95% confidence intervals were calculated within categories of grade, geographic location, and parental SES. Because many of the proportions were extremely small, the arc sine transformation for proportions was used to calculate confidence intervals.[16]

Second, chronic dieters were compared with other adolescents in terms of feeling overweight, poor body image, weekly self-induced vomiting, food bingeing, and use of laxatives, ipecac, or diuretics to lose weight. For boys and girls separately, the risks of having a particular characteristic among chronic dieters were compared with the risks of having that characteristic among adolescents not considered chronic dieters. Relative risks were calculated, and 95% confidence intervals were calculated with Taylor's Series Approximation.[17]

For each analysis, the actual sample size varied slightly depending on the number of missing values for each variable. Table 2 presents the numbers and proportions of youth included, according to key characteristics.

RESULTS

The percentages of chronic dieters according to grade in school, location, parental SES, and ethnicity are presented in Table 3. The percentages of chronic dieters among the female adolescent group are five to more than seven times greater than corresponding rates among male adolescents. Among both female and male adolescents, chronic dieting is more frequent in grades 9 through 12 than in the lower grades, but its reported occurrence does not increase appreciably after grade 9. There are small but detectable differences among geographic locations in occurrence of chronic dieting among girls but not among boys. Girls in suburban schools have the highest percent of chronic dieters (13.8%), followed by those in rural (12.5%) and urban (11.1%) settings. Female youth from low SES have greatly elevated frequency of chronic dieting compared with their male counterparts but have slightly, though significantly, lower rates than other female youth of moderate or high SES. No differences among boys according to SES are apparent. Black girls had the lowest prevalence of chronic dieting compared with other ethnic groups. No differences existed among boys in the different racial groups.

The relative risks for inappropriate eating and weight-loss behaviors, concerns about body image, and body mass index status among chronic dieters compared with other adolescents are presented in Table 4. Chronic dieters are more likely to report other maladaptive eating behaviors compared with those teenagers who are not chronic dieters. Although the percent of chronic dieters was much higher for female adolescents, both male and female chronic dieters exhibit similar risk behaviors. Both male and female chronic dieters were about twice as likely as other adolescents to report binge eating. Three times as many female and five times as many male chronic dieters reported binge eating combined with the fear of not being able to stop eating. Female chronic dieters were seven to nine times more likely to report purging behaviors (ie, vomiting, laxative, diuretic, or ipecac use) for weight control relative to other adolescent girls. Chronic dieters were also more likely to feel overweight and have a poor body image. While there was a much smaller proportion of adolescent male chronic dieters compared with female chronic dieters, male dieters were 11 to 13 times more likely than male nondieters to purge to control their weight and nine times more likely to report vomiting on at least a weekly basis.

COMMENT

We found that dieting is a common occurrence among adolescent girls, with almost two thirds reporting having been on a diet during the previous year. This finding agrees closely with findings of other recent studies.[1,8,13,18,19] In the survey by Johnson et al,[9] 14% of teenage girls were chronically dieting, which was consistent with our finding that 12% of Minnesota girls were chronic dieters.

Our results are also similar to those of previous studies[4,8,10,18] in that large and significant gender differences were found. We found that for all the aspects of chronic dieting, eg, inappropriate eating, weight-loss behaviors, and body image concerns (Table 4), the rates of occurrence were greater in girls than boys. This gender disparity has frequently been explained by sociocultural variables that equate thinness with greater attractiveness and social approval. Numerous reports suggest that these social norms are applied more strongly to women than men.[6,7] The cultural overemphasis on thinness and weight may predispose young women to excessive dieting and abnormal eating patterns.[7]

Although more young women are affected by dieting behaviors, it is important that boys not be overlooked. While the number of male chronic dieters is small (n=364), they were nine to 13 times more likely to use unhealthy weight-reduction techniques compared with other male adolescents, and their likelihood of bingeing and experiencing uncontrolled eating was four to five times greater. Therefore, a small but significant portion of adolescent male chronic dieters show evidence of disturbed eating and weight-loss patterns.

We found that the percentage of chronic dieters was significantly lower in school grades 7 and 8 than in grades 9 through 12. From a developmental perspective, teenagers in their middle adolescent years may be more conscious of appearance, weight, and peer opinions than in the early adolescent years. The major increase in subcutaneous and total body fat during puberty in girls may lead to perceptions of being overweight and weight-loss attempts. For both the male and female adolescents in our study, the occurrence of chronic dieting did not increase appreciably after grade 9, suggesting that prevention efforts may need to be established well before this time.

We found few appreciable SES or location (urban, suburban, or rural) differences in the prevalence of chronic dieting for either boys or girls, suggesting that these behaviors have permeated all levels of social status and locations of residence. While the vast majority of studies on the prevalence of dieting and weight-control practices have been conducted in urban areas, one recent study[20] of 547 teenage girls from a rural community found that extreme dieting behaviors and symptoms associated with bulimia nervosa were fairly common, with a prevalence of bulimia of 1.7%. Similar to nonurban areas, low social class has been underrepresented in the majority of studies on weight-reducing behaviors and bulimia. Still, the majority of studies[18,21] have not found social class to be a correlate of bulimia in adolescents.

Few studies have examined ethnic differences in dieting practices. We found that black girls were less likely to diet compared with white girls. Other investigators[22-24] have also reported that black teenage girls were less likely to think about their weight or diet compared with white adolescent girls and that bulimia is less common in black teenage girls. Some authors have speculated that there may be differing cultural attitudes toward weight and standards of beauty and that the black culture may be more tolerant of higher weight levels and less likely than whites to equate attractiveness with thinness.[22,23] We found no significant differences in the prevalence of chronic dieting among white, Hispanic, Native American, or Asian female adolescents. However, there is a conspicuous gap in the literature on dieting and eating behaviors among these different ethnic groups.

Our data indicate that chronic dieters were more likely to be heavier or of normal weight than were those who were not chronic dieters. Although both male and female chronic dieters were significantly heavier than other students, the relative risks were not large. Several other studies[1-3] have found that adolescent boys and girls who diet tend to be heavier than other adolescents. Killen et al[10] found that young male adolescent purgers were heavier and had greater triceps skinfold thickness than nonpurgers, but there was no corresponding difference among girls. There is a major limitation to the use of self-reported heights and weights for adolescents, as few validity studies have been performed. It may be that overweight teenagers underestimate their weight or that young teenagers or those in a rapid phase of growth might not know their actual weights or heights.

Our findings suggest that dissatisfaction with weight and a poor body image are much more pronounced among adolescent chronic dieters than in other teenagers. In addition, chronic dieters are more likely to experience abnormal eating patterns and to engage in unhealthy weight-loss methods compared with other teenagers. While the overall percentage of chronic dieters using purging techniques tended to be small (<12%), the relative risks associated with these behaviors were very high, with chronic dieters being seven to 13 times more likely to use these methods compared with other teenagers (relative risks >2 are considered strong relationships).

Our data indicate a strong relationship between excessive dieting and symptoms associated with bulimia (binge eating and purging techniques). This relationship has been noted in other studies. Wardle[19] found that the incidence of binge eating was much higher among dieting than nondieting medical students. Johnson et al[9] found that 47% of bulimic students were chronic dieters in contrast to 9% of the nonbulimic group. In his study of 895 male adolescents, Moore[2] found that there was a higher prevalence of binge eating among boys who wanted to lose weight or were dissatisfied with their weight compared with other boys.

Our results indicate that chronic dieting is not a benign or innocuous process and that associated with it are considerable risks for unhealthy eating and weight-control behaviors. Weight-reducing attempts are important in that these behaviors can become self-perpetuating and appear to be a risk factor for the development of eating disorders. While only a minority of chronic dieters will likely develop the clinical syndromes of anorexia nervosa or bulimia nervosa, the larger group may have health effects from chronic dieting. Health hazards associated with weight-reduction attempts for teenagers include retardation of physical growth, menstrual irregularities, weakness, persistent irritability, constipation, poor concentration, sleep difficulties and impulses to binge eat.[25,26]

One of the most important findings from our study is that chronic dieting may serve as a screening marker for more severe eating and weight-reduction behaviors. In a clinical setting, asking how often the adolescent diets may help to identify those who are engaging in unhealthy methods of weight regulation or those who may have an eating disorder. Therefore, clinicians involved in health assessments of adolescents should inquire about dieting practices. If the patient is dieting or has a history of repeated dieting, further history should be obtained on methods of weight control and eating practices.

Finally, efforts are needed in school, health care settings, and the community to provide appropriate education and guidance, especially for preadolescent and adolescent girls. Information should be provided about the normal changes during puberty and the increased deposition of fat tissue. Efforts should be directed toward helping adolescents adopt healthy eating and exercise habits, understanding the physiologic and psychological effects of food restriction and chronic dieting as well as discouraging drastic weight-loss techniques.[27] Such education should begin before grade 9.

References

1. Moore DC. Body image and eating behavior in adolescent girls. *AJDC.* 1988;142:1114-1118.
2. Moore DC. Body image and eating behavior in adolescent boys. *AJDC.* 1990;144:475-479.
3. Desmond SM, Price JH, Gray N, O'Connel JK. The etiology of adolescents' perceptions of their weight. *J Youth Adolesc.* 1986;15:461-473.
4. Greenfield D, Quinlan DM, Harding P, Glass E, Bliss A. Eating behavior in an adolescent population. *Int J Eating Disord.* 1987;6:99-111.
5. Fabian LJ, Thompson JK. Body image and eating disturbance in young females. *Int J Eating Disord.* 1989;8:63-74.
6. Yates A. Current perspectives on the eating disorders, I: history, psychological and biological aspects. *J Am Acad Child Adolesc Psychiatry.* 1989;28:813-828.
7. Striegel-Moore RH, Silberstein LR, Rodin J. Toward an understanding of risk factors for bulimia. *Am Psychologist.* 1986;41:246-263.
8. American School Health Association, Association for the Advancement of Health Education, Society for Public Health Education, Inc. *The National Adolescent Student Health Survey: A Report on the Health of America's Youth.* Oakland, Calif: Third Party Publishing Co; 1989.
9. Johnson CL, Lewis C, Love S, Lewis L, Stuckey M. Incidence and correlates of bulimic behavior in a female high school population. *J Youth Adolesc.* 1984;13:15-26.
10. Killen JD, Taylor CB, Telch MH, Saylor KE, Maron DJ, Robinson TN. Self-induced vomiting and laxative and diuretic use among teenagers: precursors of the binge-purge syndrome? *JAMA.* 1986;255:1447-1449.
11. Maloney MJ, McGuire J, Daniels SR, Specker B. Dieting behavior and eating attitudes in children. *Pediatrics.* 1989; 84:482-489.
12. Feldman W, Feldman E, Goodman JT. Culture versus biology: children's attitudes toward thinness and fatness. *Pediatrics.* 1988;81:190-194.
13. Rosen J, Tacy B, Howell D. Life stress, psychological symptoms and weight reducing behavior in adolescent girls: a prospective analysis. *Int J Eating Disord.* 1990;9:17-26.
14. Shisslak CM, Crago M, Neal ME, Swain B. Primary prevention of eating disorders. *J Consult Clin Psychol.* 1987;55:660-667.
15. Cronk CE, Roche AF. Race- and sex-specific reference data for triceps and subscapular skinfolds and weight/stature. *Am J Clin Nutr.* 1982;35:347-354.
16. Snedecor GN, Cochran WG. *Statistical Methods.* 7th ed. Ames, Ia: Iowa State University Press; 1980:290.
17. Kleinbaum DG, Kupper LL, Morgenstern H. *Epidemiologic Research: Principles and Quantitative Methods.* Belmont, Calif: Wadsworth Inc; 1982:296-300.
18. Gross J, Rosen JC. Bulimia in adolescents: prevalence and psychosocial correlates. *Int J Eating Disord.* 1988;7:51-61.
19. Wardle J. Dietary restraint and binge eating. *Behav Analysis Modification.* 1980;4:201-209.
20. Stein DM, Brinza SR. Bulimia: prevalence estimates in female junior high and high school students. *J Clin Child Psychol.* 1989;18:206-213.
21. Pope HG, Champoux RF, Hudson JI. Eating disorder and socioeconomic class: anorexia nervosa and bulimia in nine communities. *J Nerv Ment Dis.* 1987;175:620-623.
22. Gray JJ, Ford K, Kelly LM. The prevalence of bulimia in a black college population. *Int J Eating Disord.* 1987;6:733-740.
23. Desmond SM, Price JH, Hallinan C, Smith D. Black and white adolescents' perceptions of their weight. *J Sch Health.* 1989;59:353-358.
24. Hsu LKG. Are the eating disorders becoming more common in blacks? *Int J Eating Disord.* 1987;6:113-124.
25. Mallick MH. Health hazards of obesity and weight control in children: a review of the literature. *Am J Public Health.* 1983;73:78-82.
26. Lifshitz F, Moses N. Nutritional dwarfing: growth, dieting and fear of obesity. *J Am Coll Nutr.* 1988;7:367-376.
27. Adams LB, Shafer MAB. Early manifestations of eating disorders in adolescents: defining those at risk. *J Nutr Educ.* 1988;20:307-313.

The Effect of Valproic Acid on Plasma Carnitine Levels

Grzegorz Opala, MD, PhD; Susan Winter, MD; Carol Vance, MD; Hugh Vance, PhD;
H. Terry Hutchison, MD, PhD; Lawrence S. Linn

• Plasma total, free, and acyl carnitine levels were determined in four groups of children: (1) those treated with valproic acid as monotherapy (n=43), (2) those treated with valproic acid plus other antiepileptics as polytherapy (n=91), (3) those treated with other antiepileptic drugs alone (n=43), and (4) normal patients (n=89). The mean free carnitine level was significantly lower in both the valproic acid monotherapy (29.9 μmol/L) and polytherapy (21.4 μmol/L) groups compared with normal subjects (36.8 μmol/L); it was also significantly lower than that in patients treated with other antiepileptic drugs (36.7 μmol/L). Comparison of valproic acid polytherapy and monotherapy yielded significantly lower free carnitine levels in the polytherapy group. The ratios of acyl to free carnitine for monotherapy (0.41) and polytherapy (0.45) were significantly higher than that in the normal group (0.25). This study indicates that a general decrease in the carnitine pool should be anticipated in patients taking valproic acid polytherapy and, to a lesser degree, monotherapy. Carnitine levels in the group taking other drugs did not differ from normal.

(*AJDC.* 1991;145:999-1001)

Valproic acid (VPA) is a branched-chain aliphatic acid, 2-*n*-propylpentanoic acid, commonly used as an antiepileptic drug in the United States since 1978.[1] An effective anticonvulsant for a broad spectrum of epileptic disturbances, valproic acid continues to increase in use, especially in lower-risk patient groups.[2]

Valproic acid is safe relative to the problems it is used to treat, but clinical experience indicates that patients receiving valproic acid exhibit a variety of side effects. Three important observations relate valproic acid and carnitine. First, complications of valproic acid therapy and carnitine deficiency both mimic Reye's syndrome.[3,4] Second, valproic acid is toxic to isolated liver mitochondria, with effects similar to accumulating acyl–coenzyme A compounds. Demonstration of carnitine's ability to prevent in vitro mitochondrial toxic effects led to the hypothesis that carnitine converts acyl–coenzyme A compounds to less toxic acylcarnitine derivatives.[5] Finally, valproylcarnitine is excreted in urine of patients receiving valproic acid.[6] Millington et al[6] hypothesized that the synthesis and subsequent excretion of valproylcarnitine could contribute to the development of carnitine deficiency in valproic acid–treated patients. However, analysis of urine concentrations does not yield valproylcarnitine as the predominant acylcarnitine excreted by valproic acid–treated patients.

The impact of anticonvulsants on carnitine levels has been explored since first addressed by Ohtani et al in 1982.[4] Carnitine level is lower in patients treated with valproic acid as a monotherapy than in controls.[7] Patients treated with valproic acid and other anticonvulsants as polytherapy reportedly have lower carnitine levels than patients receiving valproic acid monotherapy[8] and/or control patients.[8-11] Decreased carnitine levels may also fol- low treatment with other antiepileptic drugs (OADs) alone.[12,13]

Some investigators have not found differences in free carnitine levels between patients treated with OADs and controls[4,10] or between patients given valproic acid monotherapy, those treated with OADs, and controls.[8,11] Other studies finding decreased free carnitine levels did not divide patients receiving valproic acid into monotherapy and polytherapy subgroups.[4,12-16] Generally, most studies involved small samples of valproic acid–treated patients and/or patients older than 3 years.[4,7-10,12,13,15,16] We assessed the effect of therapy with valproic acid monotherapy, valproic acid polytherapy, and OADs on the plasma carnitine pool between all four groups (including a normal group for comparison) in a relatively large population of pediatric-age patients.

PATIENTS AND METHODS

A total of 266 patients had plasma total, free, and acyl carnitine levels determined. The four groups were as follows: (1) patients treated with valproic acid monotherapy (n=43), (2) patients treated with valproic acid polytherapy (n=91), (3) patients treated with OADs (n=43), and (4) normal, healthy patients who served as controls (n=89). The groups of patients treated with anticonvulsants (valproic acid monotherapy, valproic acid polytherapy, and OADs) included 26, 48, and 19 female patients and 17, 43, and 24 male patients, respectively. The normal group had 47 female patients and 42 male patients. The mean age of the patients treated with valproic acid monotherapy was 8.1 years (range, 1.3 months to 20.3 years); of those treated with valproic acid polytherapy, 8.2 years (1 month to 21.6 years); of the OAD

Accepted for publication April 22, 1991.
From Metabolic Research and Analysis Inc, Fresno, Calif (Drs Opala and H. Vance and Mr Linn), and Valley Children's Hospital and University of California, San Francisco, Fresno (Drs Winter, C. Vance, and Hutchison).
Reprint requests to Metabolic Research and Analysis Inc, 3150 E Shields Ave 104, Fresno, CA 93726 (Dr Opala).

Plasma Carnitine Total, Free, Ester, and Ratio Levels in Patients Treated With Monotherapy, Polytherapy, and Other Antiepileptic Drugs and in Normal Subjects

Group	n	Carnitine, μmol/L			
		Total	Free	Ester	Ester-Free Ratio
Valproic acid monotherapy	43	40.8* ± 14	29.9† ± 10	10.9‡ ± 9	0.41§ ± 0.5
Valproic acid polytherapy	91	29.3‖ ± 14	21.4‖ ± 12	8.0 ± 4	0.45¶ ± 0.3
Other antiepileptic drugs	43	48.1 ± 11	36.7 ± 10	11.5 ± 7	0.34 ± 0.3
Normal subjects	89	44.2 ± 10	36.8 ± 7	8.9 ± 5	0.25 ± 0.1

*$P<.05$ vs other antiepileptic drug, $P<.01$ vs valproic acid polytherapy. All values expressed as mean ± SD.
†$P<.01$ vs normal subjects, $P<.01$ vs other antiepiliptic drugs, $P<.01$ vs valproic acid polytherapy.
‡$P<.05$ vs valproic acid polytherapy.
§$P<.05$ vs normal subjects.
‖$P<.01$ vs normal subjects, $P<.01$ vs other antiepileptic drugs.
¶$P<.01$ vs normal subjects.

group, 8.3 years (1.4 months to 17.1 years); and of the normal subjects, 6.7 years (1.3 months to 17.2 years). Mean age differences between the four groups were not significantly different by analysis of variance procedure.

Patients receiving anticonvulsants (valproic acid monotherapy, valproic acid polytherapy, and OADs) were treated for different types of epilepsy. The OADs included carbamazepine (n = 18), phenobarbital (n = 10), phenytoin (n = 9), and ethosuximide (n = 1) as monotherapy or in combinations (n = 5). Patients were selected for determination of plasma carnitine level from the practices of two pediatric neurologists on the basis of one of the specific drug regimens. Blood samples were randomly drawn after initiation of valproic acid and OAD therapy, with a minimum elapsed time of 5 days. Plasma samples from the valproic acid monotherapy and polytherapy groups were obtained from 1984 to 1990, and from the OAD group, between 1986 and 1990.

All samples were collected at Valley Children's Hospital, Fresno, Calif, and frozen plasma was sent to the Metabolic Analysis Laboratories Inc in Madison, Wis. Plasma carnitine levels were assayed by the method of Parvin and Pande.[17] In most cases, only one level was available after the introduction of valproic acid therapy but before carnitine supplementation. Occasionally, however, more than one level was available as a result of clinical laboratory orders. The lowest free level was selected, and this almost always corresponded to the last available level before carnitine supplementation. Of note, this supports other findings of a dose-response (ie, time-dependent) relationship. Patients with a known metabolic disorder were excluded. The nonretrospective portion of this study, plasma level determination in normal subjects, was approved by both the Valley Medical Center Human Investigation Review Committee and the Valley Children's Hospital Human Subjects Committee. Informed consents were obtained from either the patient or the parent/guardian if the patient was a minor.

RESULTS

Mean total, free, and esterified plasma carnitine levels and the esterified-to-free carnitine ratio are presented for the four groups in the Table. Data for the four different groups and four variables were analyzed by means of a one-between multivariate analysis of variance procedure. Post hoc tests were performed on resultant univariate analyses by Scheffe's procedure.

The mean total carnitine level was significantly lower only in patients given valproic acid polytherapy compared with normal subjects. However, the levels in both the valproic acid monotherapy and polytherapy groups were significantly lower than those in the OAD group ($P<.05$ and $P<.01$, respectively). In addition, the mean total carnitine level in the valproic acid polytherapy group was significantly lower than that in the valproic acid monotherapy group ($P<.01$).

The mean free carnitine level was significantly lower in both the valproic acid monotherapy and polytherapy groups than in the normal subjects ($P<.01$ for both) and also significantly lower than in the OAD group ($P<.01$ for both). Comparison of valproic acid polytherapy and valproic acid monotherapy also yielded a significantly lower plasma free carnitine level ($P<.01$).

The mean acylcarnitine level was significantly lower in patients receiving valproic acid polytherapy than in those receiving OADs ($P<0.01$) and also was significantly lower than that in the group receiving valproic acid monotherapy ($P<.05$).

The ratio of acylcarnitine to free carnitine levels was significantly higher in both the valproic acid monotherapy and valproic acid polytherapy groups than in the normal subjects ($P<.05$ and $P<.01$, respectively).

COMMENT

Our study supports previous findings that administration of valproic acid results in a lowering of carnitine levels.[3,4,7-15] Both groups of our patients receiving valproic acid had plasma free carnitine levels significantly lower than those of patients receiving OADs and controls; moreover, plasma free carnitine levels in the valproic acid polytherapy group were significantly lower than those in the valproic acid monotherapy group.

In contrast to our data, Laub et al,[10] Komatsu et al,[8] and Beghi et al[11] did not find the free carnitine levels in the valproic acid monotherapy group significantly lower than those in the controls. Only Komatsu et al[8] found, as we did, a significant difference between free carnitine levels in the valproic acid polytherapy and valproic acid monotherapy groups. Consistent with the findings of Ohtani et al,[4] Laub et al,[10] Komatsu et al,[8] and Beghi et al,[11] we did not find significant differences in free carnitine levels between the OAD and normal groups, suggesting that reduction of plasma carnitine level is associated with valproic acid therapy but is not associated with antiepileptic therapy in general. Moreover, the lowest mean free carnitine level during valproic acid polytherapy in comparison with the valproic acid monotherapy, OAD, and normal groups suggests that treatment with valproic acid in combination with antiepileptic drugs other than valproic acid increases the reduction of carnitine level.

In general, carnitine deficiency should be anticipated in patients taking anticonvulsant medications that include valproic acid (particularly if these medications induce microsomal enzyme systems); why the lowest plasma free and total carnitine levels were found in the group treated with valproic acid polytherapy remains speculative. It is likely that drug interactions can lead to enhanced valproic acid metabolism and further impairment of carnitine values. This is particularly true of phenobarbital, which may result in increased conversion of valproic acid to toxic metabolites.[11] Another possibility is that patients receiving polytherapy are more severely neurologically affected and may have an underlying metabolic disorder predisposing them to carnitine deficiency.

It is also important to consider alternative mechanisms of decreasing plasma free carnitine level during valproic acid therapy. Suggestions from other investigators include increased renal loss of free carnitine,[18,19] insufficient endogenous carnitine synthesis, or a decreased dietary carnitine intake.[7]

Thoughtful analysis of the relationships among the variables and cited hypotheses may yield some insight into an overall mechanism of valproic acid–induced decreased carnitine levels. Significantly lower acyl, free, and total plasma carnitine levels in valproic acid polytherapy in comparison with valproic acid monotherapy indicate that the total carnitine pool in the valproic acid polytherapy group of patients is significantly decreased. Also, ratios of acyl to free carnitine in both valproic acid monotherapy and valproic acid polytherapy groups were the same and significantly higher than in normal subjects. These observations are in agreement with the hypothesis that (1) elevated production of acylcarnitine increases the excretion of acylcarnitine; (2) this reduces the free carnitine level[6,9]; and (3) the decreased free carnitine level results in a relative increase in acylcarnitine level, compared with the free carnitine level, which constitutes an increase in the acyl-free carnitine ratio.

It is also important to evaluate overall findings in the context of methodologic considerations. Differences in levels of esterified carnitine in our data may be due to varying durations of therapy before carnitine assay. In addition, elevated urinary excretion of acylcarnitines during an initial period of valproic acid administration leads to insufficient quantities of ingested and endogenously produced carnitine necessary to maintain tissue and plasma stores at normal levels[16]; later, as free carnitine levels become low, esterified carnitine levels may also decrease because of inadequate free carnitine available to combine with acyl groups.

The absence of carnitine determinations before valproic acid therapy leads to the possibility that low carnitine levels may have preexisted in the population. Indeed, the low free carnitine levels in the group treated with valproic acid polytherapy, instead of the preferred monotherapy, coincide with the group we expect to present the most difficult seizure control problems and therefore be the most involved neurologically. However, the absence of a significant difference between the OAD and normal groups indicates that the patient sample did not have low carnitine levels before therapy.

CONCLUSION

The sample size of the four groups of patients in our study, valproic acid monotherapy, valproic acid polytherapy, OADs, and normal, allows for establishment of reliable statistics indicating that a general decrease in the carnitine pool should be anticipated in patients taking valproic acid polytherapy and, to a lesser degree, valproic acid monotherapy. Carnitine levels in the OAD group did not differ from normal.

This research was supported in part by a grant from Sigma Tau Pharmaceuticals Inc, Gaithersburg, Md.

We to thank the University of California, San Francisco, library staff for their support; the Valley Children's Hospital laboratory staff, Tim O'Hara, and Steven Szabo-Aczel, MD, for project consultation; and Any Szabo for data compiling.

References

1. Penry JK, Dean JC. The scope and use of valproate in epilepsy. *J Clin Psychiatry.* 1989;50:17-22.

2. Dreifuss FE, Langer DH, Moline KA, Maxwell JE. Valproic acid hepatic fatalities, II: US experience since 1984. *Neurology.* 1989;39:201-207.

3. Bohles H, Richter K, Wagner-Thiessen E, Schafer H. Decreased serum carnitine levels in valproate induced Reye's syndrome. *Eur J Pediatr.* 1982;139:185-186.

4. Ohtani Y, Fumio E, Matsuda I. Carnitine deficiency and hyperammonemia associated with valproic acid therapy. *J Pediatr.* 1982;101:782-785.

5. Stumpf DA, Parker DW, Hass R. Carnitine deficiency with valproate therapy. *J Pediatr.* 1983;103:175-176.

6. Millington D, Bohan T, Roe C, Yergey AL, Liberato DJ. Valproylcarnitine: a novel drug metabolite identified by fast atom bombardment and thermospray liquid chromatography mass spectrometry. *Clin Chim Acta.* 1985;145:69-76.

7. Melegh B, Kerner J, Kispal G, Acsadi A, Dani M. Effect of chronic valproic acid treatment on plasma and urine carnitine levels in children: decreased urinary excretion. *Acta Paediatr Hung.* 1987;28:137-142.

8. Komatsu M, Kodoma S, Yokoyama S, et al. Valproate-associated hyperammonemia and DL-carnitine supplement. *Kobe J Med Sci.* 1987;33:81-87.

9. Matsuda I, Ohtani Y, Ninomiya N. Renal handling of carnitine in children with carnitine deficiency and hyperammonemia associated with valproate therapy. *J Pediatr.* 1986;109:131-134.

10. Laub MC, Paetzke-Brunner I, Jaeger G. Serum carnitine during valproic therapy. *Epilepsia.* 1986;27:559-562.

11. Beghi E, Bizzi A, Codegoni AM, Trevisan D, Torri W, Collaborative Group for the Study of Epilepsy. Valproate, carnitine metabolism, and biochemical indicators of liver functions. *Epilepsia.* 1990;31:346-352.

12. Morita J, Yuge K, Yoshino M. Hypocarnitinemia in the handicapped individuals who receive a polypharmacy of antiepileptic drugs. *Neuropediatrics.* 1986;17:203-205.

13. Rodriguez-Segade S, Alonso de la Pena C, Tutor JC, et al. Carnitine deficiency associated with anticonvulsant therapy. *Clin Chim Acta.* 1989;181:175-182.

14. Winter SC, Szabo-Aczel S, Curry CJS, et al. Plasma carnitine deficiency: clinical observations in 51 pediatric patients. *AJDC.* 1987;141:660-665.

15. Murphy JV, Marquardt KM, Shug AL. Valproic acid associated abnormalities of carnitine metabolism. *Lancet.* 1985;1:820-821.

16. Melegh B, Kerner J, Acsadi G, Lakatos J, Sandor A. L-carnitine replacement therapy in chronic valproate treatment. *Neuropediatrics.* 1990;21:40-43.

17. Parvin R, Pande SV. Microdetermination of (−) carnitine and carnitine acetyltransferase activity. *Anal Biochem.* 1977;79:190-201.

18. Thurston JH, Caroll JE, Dodson WE, Hauhart RE, Tasch V. Chronic valproate administration reduces fasting ketonemia in children. *Neurology.* 1983;33:1348-1355.

19. Ohtani Y, Matsuda I. Valproate treatment and carnitine deficiency. *Neurology.* 1984;34:1128-1129.

Support Services for Pediatric Trainees

A Survey of Training Program Directors

Anne Sturmthal Bergman, LCSW, DrPH, Robert Adler, MD, MSEd

• **We conducted a survey of pediatric training program directors (75% response rate) regarding program support services for house staff, directors' attitudes about stress in training, and program plans to ameliorate such stress. Support services included explicit measures to alleviate stress, policies that may minimize stress, evaluation of house staff performance, feedback regarding career concerns, and benefits (eg, medical insurance and child care). Most programs offered services to reduce stress from training, but few offered preventive services. Support policies were reported to be inadequate, especially in the areas of coverage for leaves of absence. Maternity leave represented most leaves of absences, as 10% of the female house staff and 11% of the male house staff members became parents. Program directors' terms were short, and only 30% perceived these roles to be their primary roles. Male directors believed that female house officers had a harder time adjusting to their programs. We suggest changes and present a simple way for program directors to evaluate their support services.**

(*AJDC.* 1991;145:1002-1005)

Stress in postgraduate medical training concerns training directors, trainees, and the general public. Many support services to reduce stress in training have been proposed, but information about these services in pediatric training programs is lacking.[1-8] A committee of program directors of internal medicine has outlined what services should be included in a supportive program.[9] Berg and Garrard[10] have categorized support services available in family practice programs. Our study was designed to document support services offered in pediatric training programs.

MATERIALS AND METHODS

A questionnaire was developed that addressed several topics and included both closed- and open-ended questions. A test questionnaire was sent to six pediatricians who were either training directors or involved in pediatric education. Information was solicited about the services available to reduce stress (Table 1). The study population included every training director (n = 232) in an accredited pediatric training program on July 1, 1987, from a list provided by the Association of Pediatric Program Directors.

There were two mailings separated by 4 weeks. Eight programs were excluded from the original 232 because they had merged with other programs or were no longer training pediatricians. Sixty-one percent of the responses came from the first mailing and another 14% from the second, for a total response rate of 75%. Data from both mailings were combined. The only difference between data from the two mailings was that respondents to the second mailing spent more time (30%) functioning as training directors ($P<.05$) and had been in the position less time (4 years or less) ($P=.01$) than directors responding to the first mailing.

Demographic data included program affiliation, the presence of a designated training director, gender of director, number of years as training director, and percentage of time spent fulfilling duties as training director. Inquiries were made about number and gender of the trainees, number of leaves of absence, number of pregnancies, and number of referrals for counseling during the training year. Training directors were asked about their attitudes toward support services, and responses were coded using a 5-point Likert Scale.

Department Editors.—*Hugh D. Allen, MD, Columbus, Ohio; Fredric Burg, MD, Philadelphia, Pa; Harold Levine, MPA, Galveston, Tex; Barbara Starfield, MD, Baltimore, Md; Larrie W. Greenberg, MD, Washington, DC*

Purpose.—*This department is intended to share information concerning educational efforts in the broad field of pediatrics. We welcome studies on the following topics: undergraduate and graduate education in medicine and allied health occupations; continuing education of health professionals; education of patients and families; and health education for the general public, the community, and organizations that contribute to the promotion and improvement of the health of children.*

Editorial Comment.—*Bergman and Adler present a survey of program directors that addresses management of house officer stress. Most directors deal with crises, but few deal with problems through prevention. The authors discuss various problems and offer a way for programs to evaluate their support services. This is a good start.*—H.D.A.

Accepted for publication December 14, 1990.
From the Department of Psychiatry, Stanford (Calif) Medical School (Dr Bergman), and Childrens Hospital of Los Angeles (Calif) and the UCLA School of Medicine (Dr Adler).
Reprints not available.

Support Services for Pediatric Trainees	
Pediatric Support Service	**% of Pediatric Training Programs Reporting Services**
Explicit measures to alleviate stress	
Orientation	98
Social events	98
Psychiatric services	92
Specific counseling for stress	61
Retreats	44
Counseling for house staff member's families	53
Support groups	35
Ombudsman	30
Drug/alcohol education	33
Supportive policies to minimize stress	
Maternity leave policy	95
Ward on-call—every 4th night or less frequently	49
NICU on-call—every 4th night or less frequently	40
House staff goes home after call before 5 pm	31
Limit on maximum consecutive hours worked	30
More than 4 weeks of vacation for all years	28
Coverage by faculty and house staff	12
Evaluation and feedback	
Evaluation of house staff	100
Feedback from house staff to faculty	92
Disciplinary policy and grievance procedure	88
Review of program	84
Career counseling	80
Faculty advisor	77
Benefits	
Medical insurance	100
Mental health insurance	89
Disability coverage	81
Payment for counseling	52
Child care	19

RESULTS

Our data on characteristics of the respondents were compared with data available about pediatric training programs from the American Medical Association's 1988-1989 *Directory of Graduate Medical Education Programs.*[11] There was no difference between the two groups of data in geographic distribution or percentage of women house staff members.

Characteristics of Program Respondents and Trainees

Most programs were university based (101 [45%]) or affiliated (90 [40%]). The remaining 33 programs included those that were not university affiliated and those that were affiliated with military bases or religious institutions. Size was associated with affiliation; the largest programs were university based. Seventy-eight programs (35%) had 17 or fewer house staff members, 70 (31%) had 18 to 35 house staff members, and 76 (34%) had 36 or more house staff members. Sixty-seven program directors (30%) reported that house staff members trained in only one hospital; 76 (34%), two hospitals; 63 (28%), three hospitals; and 18 (8%), four or more hospitals.

Most programs (217 [97%]) had a designated program director, 65 (30%) of whom were department chairs and 22 (10%) of whom had another title related to training (eg, residency manager). Only 65 (30%) considered themselves primarily program directors. Forty-seven respondents (21%) were women. Half of the respondents graduated from medical school before 1968, and half spent 30% or less time in their roles as program directors. Half were program directors for 4 years or less.

The survey comprised 4424 house staff members, 2300 (52%) of whom were women. This is consistent with the ratio reported in the American Medical Association's *1988-1989 Directory of Graduate Medical Education Programs.*[11]

How Supportive Are Pediatric Training Programs?

We inquired about explicit measures to alleviate stress in residency training programs. Social events and orientation programs were nearly universal (220 [98%]). Almost half (99 [44%]) of all programs had retreats for house staff. The majority of the retreats were for postgraduate-year-1 interns alone. In most programs, a variety of individuals ran the retreat, including chief residents, faculty, and consultants. A smaller number (78 [35%]) of responding programs offered support groups, of which 17 (22%) were run by faculty and nine (12%) by consultants. Only 23 program directors (29%) who offered support groups perceived them as helpful. Individual counseling was available in 206 programs (92%), and specific psychiatric services directed to issues of stress in residency training were offered by 137 programs (61%). Family counseling was offered by 119 programs (53%), and an ombudsman was available in 74 programs (30%). Only 74 programs (33%) provided drug and alcohol abuse education.

Two hundred six programs (92%) offered counseling for house officers. In 90 programs (44%), it was provided by the psychiatric staff of the training program. Counseling in the remaining 116 programs was provided by the program director (24 programs [21%]), behavioral science staff (14 programs [12%]), employee assistance programs (12 programs [10%]), private psychiatric and pastoral counselors (six programs [5%]), and social workers and behavioral pediatricians (11 programs [5%]). Directors of the remaining programs did not note who provided counseling. Between 1987 and 1988, 106 house staff members (2.4%) were referred to counseling owing to poor performance.

We also explored on-call schedules. On-call duties every fourth night or less often for ward rotations were reported by 110 respondents (49%). On-call duties of similar frequency, but for rotation into the neonatal intensive care unit, were reported by 90 respondents (40%). Sixty-nine programs (31%) sent house staff members home around or before 5 PM the night after being on call, and 67 programs (30%) limit the maximum number of consecutive hours worked to 32. Half the programs reported that their house staffs worked 33 to 39 consecutive hours, and 45 respondents (20%) said there was no limit on work hours.

Coverage for absent house staff members was most often provided by other house staff members (179 programs [80%]) or occasionally by a mixture of faculty and other house staff members (27 programs [12%]). In one program, the faculty alone covered for absent house staff members. A maternity leave policy was in place in 213 programs (95%), and time off ranged from less than 6 weeks (98 programs [46%]) to 8 weeks, to 3 months (38 programs [18%]). From 1987 to 1988, 230 female house staff members (10%) and 233 male house staff members (11%) became parents. Most programs (134 [60%]) had leave of absence policies, and 110 programs (49%) granted at least one leave of absence during the year. Of these leaves of absence, 30 (27%) were maternity leaves, 12 (11%) were because of personal stress, six (5%) were because of family illness, and 8 (7%) were because of personal illness. No significant correlations were noted between leaves of absence and characteristics of the program, the director, or trainees. All programs had specific vacation policies, and 63 (28%) offered 4 or more weeks of vacation for all years of training. A shared-residency program was offered by 65 programs (29%), but of those only four (6%) had individuals actually in a shared residency.

Written disciplinary policies were provided by 199 programs (89%), feedback to faculty by 206 (92%), faculty advisers by 172 (77%), specific career counseling by 179 (80%), and a committee to review the program by 188 (84%).

Medical insurance was offered to house staff by all programs, mental health insurance by 199 (89%), and disability insurance by 181 (81%). Specific payment for counseling was reported by most programs (107 of 206 [52%]), and a few programs (43 of 206 [19%]) offered child care.

We explored one tangential measure of stress by asking why house staff members left their training programs. Sixty-six house officers (29%) had left their programs unexpectedly. Of the house staff members who left, 45 (69%) changed their specialties, seven (10%) left because of family reasons, five (7%) left because of illness, and the rest (nine [14%]) reportedly left because of religious reasons, feelings of inadequacy, and other reasons.

Program Directors' Attitudes Toward Training

A series of questions was asked of the program directors exploring their attitudes toward support services. Most training directors (201 [90%]) believed that house staff support was a priority in the program, that their house staff members were happy with the program, and that the patients benefited from house staff support services. Training directors who believed that house staff support was a priority in their programs also believed that support programs helped recruitment ($r = .35$ and $P = .0001$). To a lesser degree, they believed that access to support services made trainees better pediatricians (181 respondents [81%]) and that the faculty generally cared about the house staff. One hundred fifty-nine respondents (71%) believed their programs provided more support than other programs. Only 83 program directors (37%) believed that house staff training was easier now than when they were in training, and half believed that the house staff worked too many hours per week. Most directors (130 [58%]) believed that female house staff members should be able to plan a pregnancy during training, and 58 (26%) believed that, in general, female house staff members had a harder time adjusting to training than did male house staff members.

The training directors noted the following greatest sources of stress among house staff members (some respondents listed more than one item): workload (72 [32%]), caring for very sick or difficult patients (60 [27%]), conflicts between work and home life (54 [24%]), high expectations of themselves (25 [11%]), concern about lack of knowledge (18 [8%]), work relationships (nine [4%]), money (seven [3%]), and quality of teaching (two [1%]). In response to an open-ended question, 40 program directors (18%) anticipated making the program more supportive, reducing the number of working hours, or planning a retreat. A small percentage (20 respondents [9%]) were planning to encourage more faculty involvement, while 13 respondents (6%) were planning to add an advisory system.

Program directors were also asked about recruitment. Slightly over half the programs (114 [51%]) had increasing numbers of applicants, 25 (11%) had decreasing numbers of applicants, and 85 (38%) had stable levels of applicants. One hundred fifty programs (67%) recruited enough residents to fill all their positions, 27 (12%) had one vacant position, and 47 (21%) had two vacant positions.

COMMENT

This study describes a way to measure the level of house staff services that may reduce stress in pediatric training programs. Program directors may not wish to include the specific services listed, but this data makes comparisons of the programs with a 1988 national data base possible. These comparisons may be helpful in discussions with hospital administrations regarding the institution of new services.

Although this study mostly catalogs existing programs and services, some interesting observations can be made. Those services required by the Accreditation Council for Graduate Medical Education were almost universally provided. Others, such as social events and orientation, were also offered by all training programs. Availability of services to reduce or help cope with the stress of the program showed an interesting pattern. While 92% of the programs offered various counseling options for treatment of stressed house staff members, preventive measures such as support groups and retreats were offered by only 78 programs (35%) and 99 programs (44%), respectively. Fewer than one third of the directors whose programs offered support groups thought that they were helpful. Although there is considerable concern regarding physician impairment due to chemical dependency, only 74 programs (33%) offered alcohol and drug abuse education.

Program directors and the hospital administration set policies for house staff and have considerable control in this area. Despite this, specific policies that might alleviate house staff stress were absent from most programs. Although trainees in 49% of the programs were on call every fourth night or less often, fewer than one third of the programs limited consecutive working hours to less than 32. Four weeks of vacation each year were offered by

28% of programs. Vacation time was distributed unequally through the 3 years of training in most programs, and the largest amount of vacation time was in the later years, although the internship year is clearly the most stressful. Support policies may change in response to legislation, but in most hospitals these policies are under institutional and program control and do not need legislative approval to be reevaluated.

Coverage for absent house staff members was almost exclusively provided by other house staff members. Coverage by faculty and innovative methods of coverage were rare. House staff members' absences are disruptive to all programs and, in light of the data, it becomes increasingly clear that program directors need to plan prospectively for absences, the most common of which is maternity leave. Change in assigned rotations and electives is stressful to the remaining house staff members and can significantly affect the educational program. The program director and administration must explore methods of coverage that do not increase burdens on house staff members.

Most programs had maternity leave policies, but they varied considerably. Ten percent of the female house staff members and 11% of the male house staff members became parents during the year studied. This is consistent with a recent study by Sinal et al[12] in which 11% of 904 female physicians became pregnant during their internships, and 32% became pregnant during their residency programs. Regardless of when their babies were born, 60% had maternity leaves of 6 weeks or less. Parental leave should be planned prospectively and anticipated by program staff. Costs of providing a method to deal with such absences should be included in the budgets of training programs. There will always be exceptional situations for which prospective planning will be inadequate, but house staff members and program directors should plan for what seems to be a consistent use of the leave of absence policy.

The issue of maternity leave also brings up the issue of gender in residency training. More than 50% of trainees in pediatric training programs are women. Only 21% of the program directors were women, and 52% of the pediatric house staff members in our study were women. The attitudes of program directors toward house staff support programs did not differ on the basis of gender, except that male directors believed that female house officers had a harder time adjusting to stress in training ($P = .0004$). The view that female house officers should be able to plan pregnancies during training was equally held by both male and female program directors.

Most training directors perceived that their house staffs were happy with their programs. They considered their training programs to be more supportive than other programs and believed that patients benefited from house staff support services. Another reflection of the program directors' general comfort level with support services was that only 18% of the program directors anticipated adding support services to their programs. Program directors identified the greatest sources of stress among house staff members as workload, caring for sick or difficult patients, and conflict between work and home life. This differed somewhat from a previous report[8] in which interns stated that fatigue, lack of time for family and personal activities, and making a mistake were the greatest sources of stress.

The role of the program director will need to be reexamined as programs struggle with the difficult issues of meeting the dual responsibilities of the programs' educational requirements and of the service requirements of their institutions. A consistent and long-term commitment from program directors will allow the examination and achievement of these often conflicting goals and investigation of preventive strategies to reduce stress. Such strategies should include the planning and evaluation of administration policies to reduce stress. A policy that anticipates leaves of absences (including parental leave for male and female house staff members) should be considered by each program, and policies that deal with frequency of on-call duties, number of consecutive working hours, benefits (eg, disability and life insurance), and other issues affecting trainee stress should be evaluated. These issues are under the control of individual program directors and their administrations. Changing policy in an institution often takes a long time, and a consistent spokesperson with a strong support base who advocates for change is necessary. In return, chairmen in pediatrics need to support program directors financially and academically.

This simplified way for programs to evaluate the support services available to their trainees should be a good starting point for directors who are contemplating changes in their programs. It might also stimulate program directors to evaluate the effectiveness of existing services and to explore innovative ways to reduce stress in training programs. Clearly, the ability to provide support services to pediatric residents will provide programs with a competitive edge in an increasingly tight market for potential applicants.

This study was supported in part by a grant from the Childrens Hospital of Los Angeles General Pediatric Research Fund.

We thank Evan Charney, MD, and the Association of Pediatric Training Program Directors for their participation in and support of this survey.

References

1. Asken MJ, Raham D. Resident performance and sleep deprivation: a review. *J Med Educ.* 1983;58:382-388.
2. Reuben D. Psychological effects of residency. *South Med J.* 1983;76:380-383.
3. Bergman AB. Resident stress. *Pediatrics.* 1988;82:260-263.
4. Werner ER, Adler R, Robinson R, Korsch B. Attitude and interpersonal skills during pediatric internship. *Pediatrics.* 1979;63:491-499.
5. Friedman RC, Bigger JT, Kornfield DS. The intern and sleep loss. *N Engl J Med.* 1971;281:201-203.
6. Ford CV, Wents DK. The internship year: a study of sleep, mood states and physiologic parameters. *South Med J.* 1984;77:1435-1442.
7. Garrard DE, Elliot DL, Hickam DH, et al. The internship: a prospective investigation of emotions and attitudes. *West J Med.* 1986;144:93-98.
8. Adler R, Werner ER, Korsch B. Systematic study of four years of internship. *Pediatrics.* 1980;66:1000-1008.
9. Resident Services Committee. Association of program directors in internal medicine, stress and impairment during residency training: strategies for reduction, identification and management. *Ann Intern Med.* 1988;109(2):154-161.
10. Berg J, Garrard J. Psychosocial support in training programs. *J Med Educ.* 1980;55:851-857.
11. *1988-1989 Directory of Graduate Medical Education Programs.* Chicago, Ill: American Medical Association; 1988.
12. Sinal S, Weavil P, Camp MG. Survey of women physicians on issues relating to pregnancy during a medical career. *J Med Educ.* 1988;63:531-538.

Optimal Positioning of Endotracheal Tubes for Ventilation of Preterm Infants

Avi Rotschild, MD; David Chitayat, MD; Martin L. Puterman, PhD; Min S. Phang, MB; Emily Ling, MB, BS; Virginia Baldwin, MD

• Accurate knowledge of upper-airway dimensions is required to prevent malpositioning of endotracheal tubes in preterm infants. We measured vocal cord–carina, oral-carina, and nasal-carina distances in situ at autopsy of two groups of infants (<1000 and ≥1000 g). In all 24 infants, crown-heel length, crown-rump length, and occipitofrontal circumference were better than weight in predicting upper-airway dimensions. Flexion of the neck decreased and extension increased both nasal-carina and oral-carina distances. Lateral rotation produced no significant changes. The postmortem data were not different from nasal-carina distances measured radiologically in 40 living, nasally intubated and ventilated infants, confirming the clinical validity of our findings. Regression equations were derived to predict optimal endotracheal tube lengths based on the external measurements of crown-rump length and crown-heel length.

(*AJDC.* 1991;145:1007-1012)

With the advent of neonatal intensive care, endotracheal intubation and mechanical ventilation of very-low-birth-weight infants is now common. However, malpositioning of the endotracheal tube (ETT) is still a well-recognized and, unfortunately, frequent complication of mechanical ventilation.[1,2] To minimize the risk of this complication, accurate knowledge of the upper-airway dimensions is essential. Earlier studies used various methods to measure the dimensions and topographic locations of the important anatomic landmarks in the upper airway and attempted to predict optimal ETT lengths. These methods included anatomic measurements of excised tissues from autopsies,[3,4] observations at bronchoscopy in live infants,[5,6] and radiologic evaluations[1,2,7-9] that included the effect of respiratory movements[1] and alterations of head position.[1,10-12] However, few data are available from direct measurements of upper-airway dimensions in neonates, and practically no data are available for infants who weigh less than 1000 g.

Our study was carried out to formulate a reliable method of predicting the optimal ETT length from data obtained from direct measurements of upper-airway dimensions in the neonatal population, including very-low-birth-weight infants, using an in situ postmortem method. We also studied the changes in these dimensions with different head positions. The clinical relevance of the postmortem data was tested by comparing the results of the postmortem study with those obtained radiologically in living, nasally intubated and ventilated infants.

SUBJECTS AND METHODS

Study Population

Postmortem measurements of upper-airway dimensions were performed in 24 infants whose parents had given consents for autopsies and who met either of the following two criteria: (1) nonmacerated stillborn infants over 22 weeks of gestation with birth weights of 400 g or more and (2) infants who died in the neonatal period or during the first 4 months of life. Radiologic determination of nasal-carina (NC) distances was carried out in a separate group of 40 living, nasally intubated and ventilated infants. Infants with hydrops fetalis, congenital malformations, or chromosomal abnormalities or who were small for gestational age were excluded from both study groups.

Postmortem Study

Postmortem crown-heel length (CHL), crown-rump length (CRL), occipitofrontal head circumference (OFC), and body weight were measured before autopsy dissection. To study upper-airway dimensions, the body cavity was entered with the usual Y-shaped incision, and the anterior part of the rib cage was removed. The trachea was then exposed in situ by removing the thymus and dissecting the blood vessels. A short transverse incision was made in the anterior wall of the trachea at the level of the carina. To measure the distances from the carina to the naris and to the upper lip, each infant was intubated alternately nasally and orally with a pediatric suction catheter marked at centimeter intervals (Argyle, Sherwood Medical, Petit-Techain, Belgium). The catheter was advanced to the carina and secured under direct vision at the level of the carina. Nasal-carina and oral-carina (OC) distances were taken as the lengths of the suc-

Accepted for publication February 25, 1991.

From the Division of Neonatology, Departments of Pediatrics (Drs Rotschild, Phang, and Ling) and Medical Genetics (Dr Chitayat), Faculty of Commerce (Dr Puterman), and Department of Pathology (Dr Baldwin), University of British Columbia, B.C.'s Children's Hospital, Vancouver.

Read in part before the Joint Scientific Meeting of the Australian College of Paediatrics and the Singapore Paediatric Society with the Canadian Paediatric Society, Singapore, May 18, 1990; and presented as a poster exhibit at the American Academy of Pediatrics District VIII Perinatal Pediatrics Conference, Keystone, Colo, May 25 to 27, 1990.

Reprint requests to B.C.'s Children's Hospital, Room 1N1, 4480 Oak St, Vancouver, British Columbia, Canada V6H 3V4 (Dr Ling).

Table 1.—Population Description

	Mean ± SD (Range)	
	Postmortem Study (N=24)	Radiologic Study (N=40)
Gestational age, wk		
At birth	31±6.1 (23-42)	27.7±3.6 (23-34)
At study	32±7.2 (23-48)	29.4±4.5 (23-42)
Weight, g		
At birth	1937±1365 (415-4920)	1197±651 (500-3620)
At study	2203±1628 (415-5355)	1403±810 (500-3965)
No. of infants weighing <1000 g	9	19
Crown-rump length, cm	32±8.3 (20-45.5)	26.8±4.8 (20.4-38.0)
Crown-heel length, cm	45±10.6 (28.1-62.5)	39.2±6.2 (30.3-54.0)
Head circumference, cm	31±6.6 (21.5-43)	26.8±4.2 (22-37.8)
Vocal cord–carina length, cm	4.1±1.1 (2.2-6.5)	. . .
Oral-carina length, cm	9.3±2.4 (5.8-13.5)	. . .
Nasal-carina length, cm	10.8±2.5 (7-15.6)	9.4±1.5 (6.8-13.9)

tion catheter at the naris and upper lip, respectively, the catheter tip at the carina being 0 cm. These two measurements were taken for each infant in five different positions of the head relative to the body. These positions were the midline neutral, lateral rotation 90° to the right, lateral rotation 90° to the left, maximum flexion, and maximum extension.

To determine the vocal cord–carina (VC) distance, the distance from the thyroid cartilage notch to the carina was first measured in situ with the head in the neutral position. The lungs and trachea were then removed from the body en bloc. The trachea was incised posteriorly longitudinally, and the distance from the thyroid cartilage notch to the vocal cords was measured. The VC distance was obtained by subtracting the distance from the thyroid cartilage notch to the vocal cords from the distance from the thyroid cartilage notch to the carina.

In two of the autopsies, the VC measurement was repeated after the trachea was removed from the thoracic cage.

Radiologic Study

The NC distances were determined in a separate group of living, nasally intubated infants by means of clinical and radiologic data. The nasal route is the preferred route for intubation of infants in our nursery. The ETT length from its tip to the subject's nares was recorded just before or after clinically indicated anteroposterior chest roentgenograms. All chest roentgenograms were performed with the infant's head held in the neutral position and the infant lying directly on the roentgenographic film at a focal film distance of 101.6 cm. Infants with conditions causing displacement of the trachea and main-stem bronchi were excluded from the study. The distance of the ETT tip to the carina was measured on the chest roentgenogram only if the carina and main-stem bronchi were clearly visible and the chest was well centered during exposure. The NC distance was the sum of the ETT length and the ETT tip to carina distance. The magnification on roentgenogram of the ETT tip to carina distance was shown to be negligible by taking roentgenograms at the same focal film distance of a metal grid placed at different distances of up to 5 cm from the film cassette to simulate the different depths of the trachea in infants of different weights.

On the same day, OFC, CHL, CRL, and weight were measured by standard methods. Only one set of measurements was obtained for each subject.

Statistical Analysis

For data from the postmortem study, multiple linear regression was used to investigate the relationship of VC, NC, OC, nasal-midtrachea, and oral-midtrachea lengths with potential predictors, including corrected gestational age, weight at autopsy, CHL, CRL, and OFC. All subset regression with adjusted R^2 criterion was used for model selection. We investigated whether transformations[13] to logarithmic, polynomial, and piecewise linear (straight lines with different slopes on different ranges of the explanatory variable) functions of explanatory variables produced improved estimates and assessed the quality of the fits by residual analysis. We computed 95% prediction intervals as the predicted value determined by the regression equation $\pm t(n-2, 0.975)$ times the SE of prediction.[13] Simple regression was used to determine whether the changes in NC and OC lengths due to alterations in head position relative to the body were dependent on the NC and OC measurements with the head in the neutral anatomic position.

Subjects were divided into two groups on the basis of weight at autopsy (<1000 g and ≥1000 g). Standard univariate methods were used to obtain ranges for the effects of head positioning on the measurements in each group. Measurements in the two groups were compared by means of two-sample t tests adjusted for unequal variances. Effects of position changes within subjects were analyzed by paired t tests. Bonferroni adjustments were taken into account when statistical significance was assessed. For the radiologic study, multiple linear regression was used to investigate the relationship of NC distance with corrected gestational age, weight, CHL, CRL, and OFC and to compare relationships in postmortem and radiologic studies. All statistical calculations were performed with the Number Cruncher statistical software.

RESULTS

Postmortem Study

Postmortem measurements of upper-airway dimensions were performed in 24 infants, whose corrected gestational age at autopsy ranged from 23 weeks to term plus 8 weeks. Nine infants weighed less than 1000 g. The basic descriptors of the study population are provided in Table 1. There was a significant linear relationship between each of the three inner airway measurements and

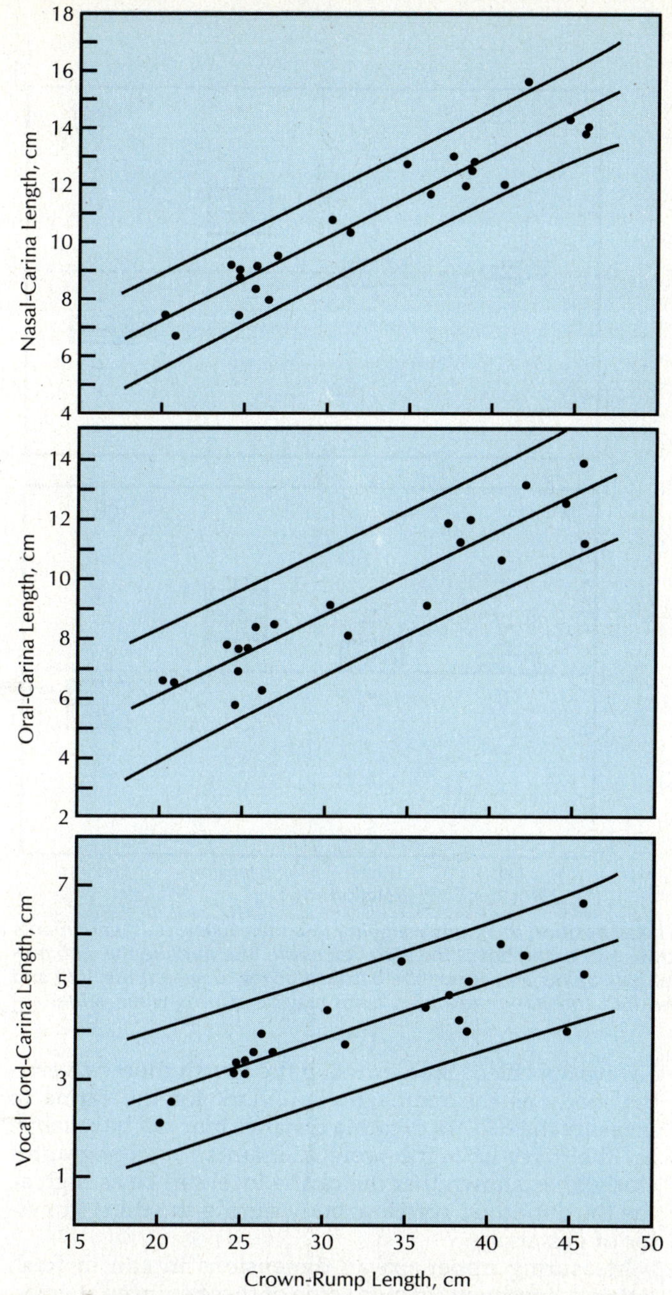

Fig 1.—*Relationships of nasal-carina, oral-carina and vocal cord–carina lengths with crown-rump length. Center lines are the regression estimates; outside curves are 95% prediction intervals, based on SEs of prediction. Some points are obscured because of nearly concurrent values.*

each of the four external anthropometric measurements, as demonstrated by the estimation equations (Table 2). We found that the use of polynomials, other transformations, or additional predictor variables did not provide any better explanatory relationship based on the adjusted R^2 criterion and residual analysis.

The CRL was the best single anthropometric measurement for predicting the inner airway dimension for all three upper-airway measurements. The relationships between each of NC, OC, and VC to CRL, together with 95% prediction intervals, are displayed in Fig 1. Corresponding graphs for the relationships of upper-airway measurements with CHL, weight, and OFC are similar and, therefore, not shown. The CHL and OFC, but not weight, were as good as CRL for predicting upper-airway distances.

The effect of head orientation on NC and OC measurements is depicted in Fig 2. In both weight groups, flexion significantly decreased ($P<.005$) and extension increased ($P<.0001$) OC and NC distances, while left and right rotation did not alter the measurements. We looked at the effect of head position on changes in NC and OC lengths based on the 90th percentile in the two weight groups. In infants weighing less than 1000 g, maximum flexion decreased NC distance by 1.0 cm and OC distance by 1.5 cm, whereas maximum extension increased NC distance by 0.8 cm and OC distance by 1.3 cm. In infants weighing 1000 g or more, maximum flexion decreased NC distance by 1.6 cm and OC distance by 1.0 cm, while maximum extension increased NC distance by 1.7 cm and OC distance by 1.5 cm. The effects of head positioning on NC distance were not statistically different from its effects on OC distance.

In the two infants (26 and 41 weeks of gestation) in whom measurements were taken both in situ and after removal of the trachea at postmortem examination, the VC lengths were longer when measured in situ than after removal of the trachea (3.5 vs 2.8 cm in one infant and 5.0 vs 4.0 cm in the other).

Radiologic Study

Radiologic measurements of NC distances were performed in 40 infants whose corrected gestational ages ranged from 23 to 42 weeks. Population descriptors are given in Table 1. Simple linear regressions of NC distance with CRL, CHL, and OFC each provided highly significant linear relationships ($P<.0001$). The estimated equations obtained from the radiologic study did not differ significantly from those obtained from the postmortem study. Neither the slope ($P=.11$) nor the intercept ($P=.20$) in the relationship between NC distance and CRL differed between these two methods (Fig 3).

COMMENT

Tracheal length is a physiologic and functional dimension that is affected by both respiratory movements[1] and changes in head posture.[1,10] The trachea lengthens and widens during inspiration and shortens and narrows during expiration.[14] The results of our study concur with those of others[10-12,15] that significant changes in tracheal length are associated with extension and flexion of the head, while lateral rotation produces minimal changes. Thus, these functional changes must be considered when attempting to define the optimal length of the ETT during intubation.

Discrepancies in tracheal dimension (VC length) reported in different studies are probably related to the limitations of the various methods used. Due to changes in tissue elasticity after death and during preservation, measurements of tissues removed from cadavers[3,4] may not reflect the true tracheal length in a live infant. Also, direct measurements on excised airways at autopsy[3,4] may be shorter than normal once tissue attachments are severed. This is suggested by our finding of shorter VC lengths in excised trachea. Conversely, measurements by direct rigid bronchoscopy[5] may produce longer than normal tracheal lengths due to relative extension of the head during this procedure. Results from radiologic studies[1,2,7-9]

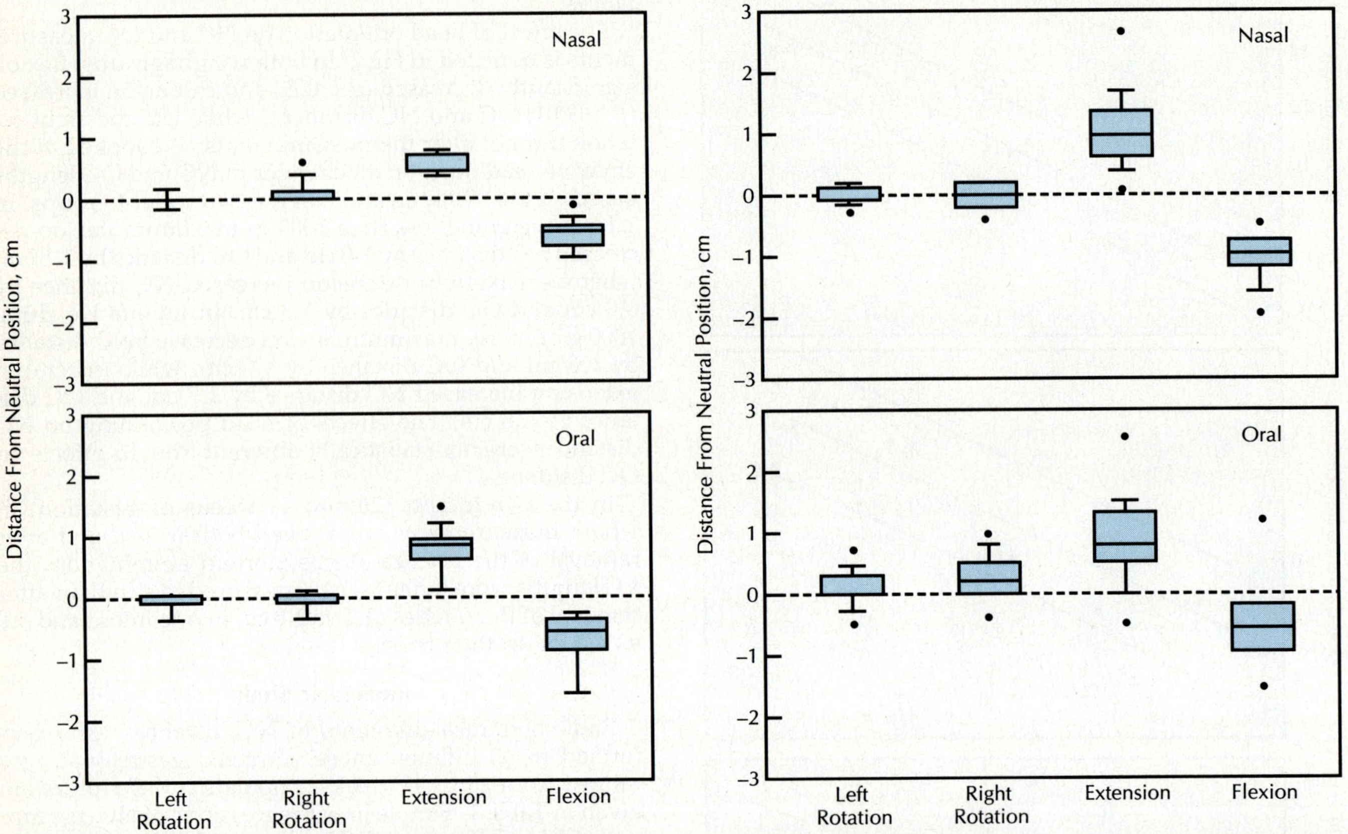

Fig 2.—*Changes in nasal-carina and oral-carina lengths with changes in head position in infants weighing less than 1000 g (left) and infants weighing 1000 g or more (right). Data are displayed by box plots. The lower line of the box is the 25th percentile, the midline the 50th percentile (median), and the upper line the 75th percentile. The horizontal bars below and above the hatched boxes represent the 10th and 90th percentiles, respectively. Dots represent measurements beyond the 10th and 90th percentiles. Lines may be missing when values are the same.*

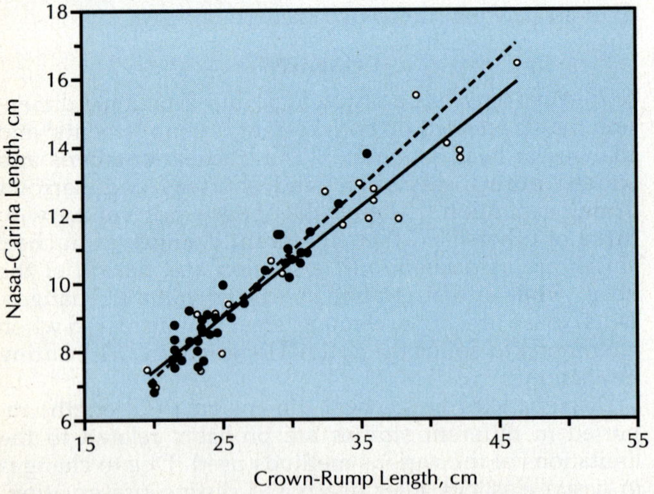

Fig 3.—*Relationship between nasal-carina (NC) distance and crown-rump length (CRL) from radiologic (broken line and closed circles) and postmortem (solid line and open circles) data. Regression equations are NC=0.52+0.33CRL (radiologic data) and NC=1.52+0.29CRL (postmortem data). Slopes and intercepts were not significantly different between these two data sources.*

may also be affected by several potential sources of error. In the retrospective studies, the position of the infant's head during exposure for the roentgenogram is not always specified. Studies using the fourth thoracic vertebral body as the radiologic landmark for the carina to measure the ETT tip to carina distance may not be reliable. In the very-low-birth-weight infants, a topographic study[16] has shown that the carina level can be as high as the third thoracic vertebral body during the third trimester of gestation.

Measuring upper-airway dimensions in situ in fresh autopsy specimens avoids some of these sources of error. Moreover, obtaining these measurements with the head in different positions may demonstrate the effect of head movement on the length of the airway.

Although other studies have found linear relationships of upper-airway dimensions to CHL[7,8] and weight,[3] we found that the best correlation of all three dimensions—VC, OC, and NC distances—was with CRL and CHL. The linear relationship of NC distance with CRL, OFC, and CHL from the radiologic study was almost identical to that from the postmortem study, thus confirming that the results from our postmortem study are applicable clinically.

Weight is a routine measurement, but it does not give the best correlation. Of interest, for infants weighing less than 1000 g, the optimum ETT length for nasal intubation varied only from 6.9 to 7.4 cm for weights between 600 and 1000 g (Table 2).

When we looked at the effect of head positioning on

Anthropometric Measurements	Regression Equations		
	NC Distance	OC Distance	VC Distance
CRL	1.659+0.285CRL (R^2-.91)†	0.933+0.261CRL (R^2-.84)	0.708+0.106CRL (R^2-.71)
CHL	0.735+0.225CHL (R^2-.91)	0.262+0.202CHL (R^2-.81)	0.423+0.082CHL (R^2-.69)
WT	7.738+0.0014WT (R^2-.82)	6.479+0.0013WT (R^2-.76)	3.005+0.0005WT (R^2-.62)
OFC	0.437+0.332OFC (R^2-.90)	0.441+0.313OFC (R^2-.82)	0.306+0.123OFC (R^2-.62)

Table 2.—Regression Equations*

*Regression equations were derived from the postmortem anthropometric measurements of each of crown-rump length (CRL), crown-heel length (CHL), weight (WT) and occipitofrontal head circumference (OFC) with each of the upper airway dimensions of nasal-carina (NC), oral-carina (OC), and vocal cord–carina (VC) distances. All lengths and distances are in centimeters, and weights are in grams.

†The quantity R^2 measures the fractions of total variation around the mean explained by the regression equation. In simple regression it provides *one* measure for comparing the quality of the estimation.

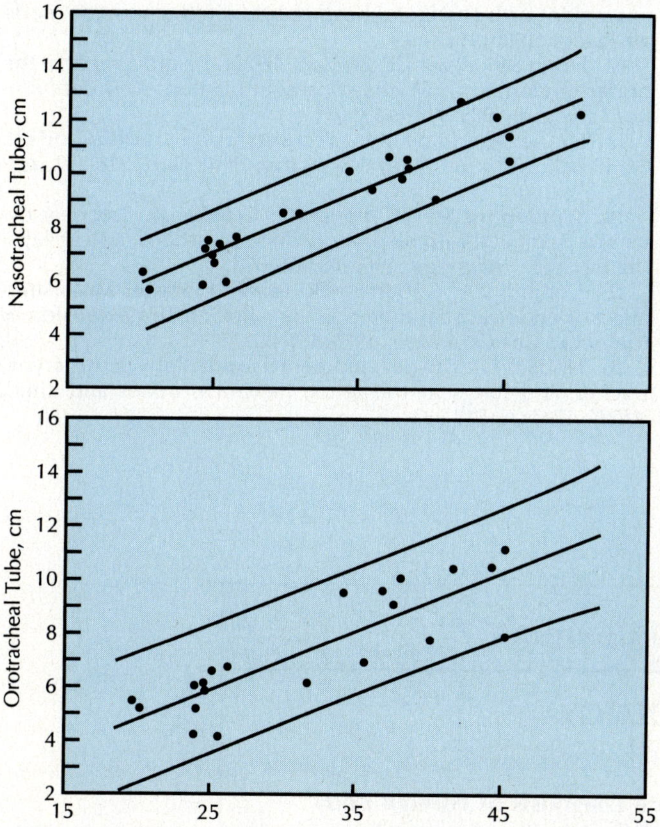

Fig 4.—*Graph for prediction of optimal endotracheal tube lengths for nasotracheal and orotracheal intubation based on the external measurement of crown-rump lengths. Center line is the regression estimate; outside curves are 95% prediction intervals, based on SEs of prediction. Some points are obscured because of nearly concurrent values.*

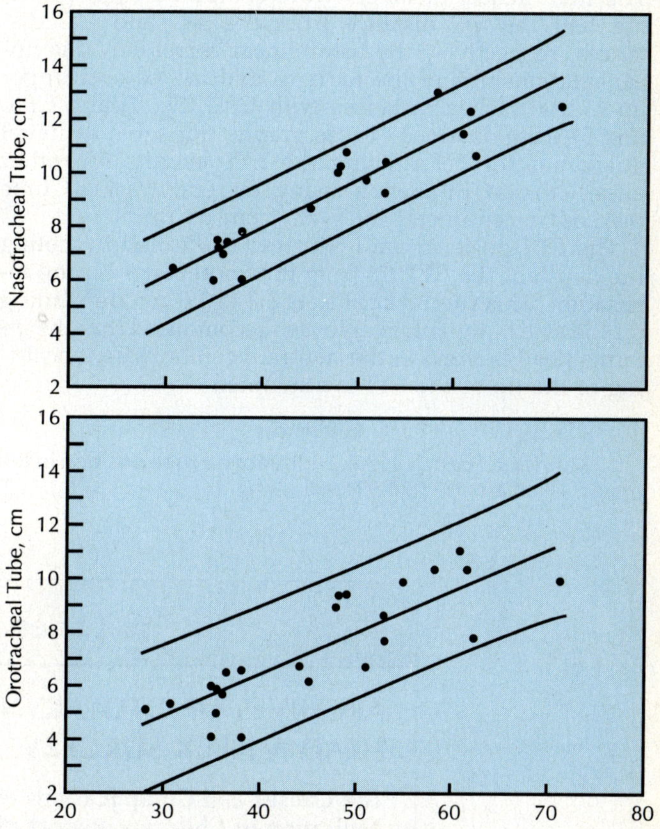

Fig 5.—*Graph for prediction of optimal endotracheal tube lengths for nasotracheal and orotracheal intubation based on the external measurement of crown-heel lengths. Center line is the regression estimate; outside curves are 95% prediction intervals, based on SEs of prediction. Some points are obscured because of nearly concurrent values.*

upper-airway measurement, flexion decreased whereas extension increased both the NC and OC lengths. We can deduce that with either nasal or oral intubation, flexion pushes the ETT tip toward the carina and extension retracts the tip away from the carina. This information will be useful for the nursing care of intubated infants. Based on the 90th percentile of changes in ETT position with maximum flexion and extension, a safe position of the ETT tip for infants weighing less than 1000 g is defined as at least 0.8 cm below the vocal cords and more than 1.0

cm above the carina during nasal intubation, and 1.3 and 1.5 cm, respectively, during oral intubation. The corresponding safe ETT tip position for infants weighing 1000 g or greater should be at least 1.7 cm below the vocal cords and at least 1.6 cm above the carina during nasal intubation, and 1.5 cm below the vocal cords and 1.0 cm above the carina during oral intubation. It can be deduced from these figures that the ideal safe position for the ETT tip with both routes of intubation is the midtracheal position for both groups of infants.

In this study, although maximum flexion and extension of the head produced a wider scatter in OC length changes than NC length changes, there was no statistically significant difference in the changes whether the infant was intubated nasally or orally. This finding contrasted with that of Donn and Blane,[12] who found greater ETT movement with nasotracheal intubation in their postmortem study of a single infant weighing 1100 g at birth.

Based on our findings, we have formulated a method of predicting the optimal ETT lengths from naris or upper lip to midtrachea during nasotracheal and orotracheal intubation based on CRL and CHL. The midtracheal distances were computed by subtracting half the VC distance from the NC and OC distances, respectively. By using linear regression, the linear relationships of the naris to midtrachea and upper lip to midtrachea distances with CRL (Fig 4) and CHL (Fig 5) were obtained. These graphs can serve as initial guidelines for determining the ETT lengths for either nasal or oral intubation using an endotracheal tube marked at centimeter intervals from its tip.

The ETT position can be further confirmed by noting the depth of the ETT tip from the vocal cords during intubation. This should be at least 1.3 to 2.0 cm, depending on the size of the infant. We also recommend that the infant's head be held in the neutral position when localizing of the tip of the ETT is attempted.

References

1. Kuhns LR, Poznanski AK. Endotracheal tube position in the infant. *J Pediatr.* 1971;78:991-996.
2. Curran JE, Doust BD, Doust VL. The length of the upper airway in infants and neonates: a study to determine the optimal length for endotracheal tubes. *Aust Radiol.* 1975;19:161-163.
3. Coldiron JS. Estimation of nasotracheal tube length in neonates. *Pediatrics.* 1968;41:823-828.
4. Butz RO. Length and cross-section growth patterns in the human trachea. *Pediatrics.* 1968;42:336-415.
5. Fearon B, Whalen JS. Tracheal dimensions in the living infant. *Anat Otol.* 1967;76:964-974.
6. Morgan GAR, Steward DJ. Linear airway dimensions in children: including those with cleft palate. *Can Anaesth Soc.* 1982;29:1-8.
7. Matilla MAK, Heikel PE, Suutarinen T, Lindfors EL. Estimation of a suitable nasotracheal tube length for infants and children. *Acta Anaesthesiol Scand.* 1971;15:239-246.
8. Loew A, Thibeault DW. A new and safe method to control the depth of endotracheal intubation in neonates. *Pediatrics.* 1974;54:506-508.
9. Tochen ML. Orotracheal intubation in the newborn infant: a method for determining depth of tube insertion. *J Pediatr.* 1979;95:1050-1051.
10. Todres ID, deBros F, Kramer SS, Moylan FMB, Shannon DC. Endotracheal tube displacement in the newborn infant. *J Pediatr.* 1976;89:126-127.
11. Donn SM, Kuhns LR. Mechanism of endotracheal tube movement with change of head position in the neonate. *Pediatr Radiol.* 1980;9:37-40.
12. Donn SM, Blane CE. Endotracheal tube movement in the preterm neonate: oral versus nasal intubation. *Ann Otol Rhinol Laryngol.* 1985;94:18-20.
13. Draper N, Smith H. *Applied Regression Analysis.* 2nd ed. New York, NY: John Wiley & Sons Inc; 1981:30-31, 218-222, 252-257.
14. Wittenborg MH, Gyepes MT, Crocker D. Tracheal dynamics in infants with respiratory distress, stridor, and collapsing trachea. *Radiology.* 1967;88:653-662.
15. Conrady PA, Goodman LR, Lainge F, Singer MM. Alteration of endotracheal tube position: flexion and extension of the neck. *Crit Care Med.* 1976;4:8-12.
16. Noback GJ. The developmental topography of the larynx, trachea and lungs in the fetus, newborn, infant and child. *AJDC.* 1923;26:515-533.

In Other AMA Journals

ARCHIVES OF OTOLARYNGOLOGY—HEAD & NECK SURGERY

The Causes and Complications of Late Diagnosis of Foreign Body Aspiration in Children: Report of 210 Cases

Liancai Mu, MD; Ping He, MD; Deqiang Sun, MD
(*Arch Otolaryngol Head Neck Surg.* 1991;117:876-879)

Oral Vaccine Therapy for Pneumococcal Otitis Media in an Animal Model

Hiroyuki Yoshimura, MD; Noritake Watanabe, MD; Junichi Bundo, MD; Mitsunori Shinoda, MD
(*Arch Otolaryngol Head Neck Surg.* 1991;117:889-894)

Evaluation of Auditory Brain-stem Response in Full-term Infants of Cocaine-Abusing Mothers

Ronald P. Carzoli, MD; Suzanne P. Murphy, PhD; Judy Hammer-Knisely, MA, CCC-A; Jean Houy, ARNP

• The purpose of this study was to examine the association between perinatal cocaine exposure and the prevalence of hearing deficit in the newborn. Auditory brain-stem response testing was performed on 50 infants of cocaine-abusing mothers and 50 control infants. All infants were born at full term. Cocaine-exposed infants had lower birth weights and a greater incidence of maternal tobacco and alcohol use. No differences were found in size, method of delivery, Apgar scores, or use of other illicit substances. Four infants of cocaine-abusing mothers and two control infants failed initial auditory brain-stem response testing. There were no differences in absolute or interpeak latencies of waveforms noted between the two groups. These data suggest that there is no increased incidence of hearing deficit as determined by auditory brain-stem response in newborns of cocaine-abusing mothers born at term and without other risk factors.

(*AJDC.* 1991;145:1013-1016)

Cocaine abuse during pregnancy has increased dramatically in recent years, paralleling the increased use in the general population. Seventeen percent of pregnant women have been estimated to use cocaine at least once during pregnancy.[1] Cocaine is a potent vasoconstrictor that has been shown in animal studies to decrease uterine blood flow, resulting in fetal hypoxemia, hypertension, and tachycardia.[2,3] In infants of cocaine-abusing mothers (ICAMs), a variety of perinatal and neonatal complications have been reported, including relative or absolute microcephaly and a high prevalence of small-for-gestational-age infants.[4-7] Neurologic problems include perinatal cerebral infarction, cranial ultrasound abnormalities such as intraventricular hemorrhage, brain necrosis, and cavitary lesions, transient electroencephalographic changes, and retinal and other ocular anomalies.[8-11] In addition, cardiorespiratory pattern abnormalities such as increased incidence of periodic breathing and apnea have been reported.[12] Finally, using the Brazelton Neonatal Behavioral Assessment Scale, depression of interactive behavior and poor organizational response to environmental stimuli have been noted.[13] However, the effect of perinatal cocaine exposure on the auditory system in the neonate has remained largely unexplored, and in view of the aforementioned effects on neurodevelopmental outcome, needs to be examined. The present study was designed to determine whether the prevalence of sensorineural hearing deficit, using the auditory brain-stem response (ABR), is greater in full-term infants exposed to cocaine prenatally than in age-matched control infants of mothers who did not use cocaine.

SUBJECTS AND METHODS

All infants enrolled in the study were born at the University of Florida Health Science Center, Jacksonville, between April 1989 and February 1990, and were admitted directly to the normal newborn nursery. Only apparently healthy, full-term infants, of at least 37 weeks' gestation, were included in the study population. The cocaine-exposed group consisted of ICAMs, as determined either by maternal history of cocaine use during pregnancy or infants in whom maternal cocaine abuse was suspected and results of urine toxicology examination for cocaine metabolites were positive. Infants were routinely screened for urine cocaine metabolites if pregnancy was complicated by a known history of maternal substance abuse, no prenatal care, abruptio placentae, precipitous delivery, home delivery, or the presence of certain congenital malformations.

Infants in the control group were born to women with uncomplicated pregnancy including no maternal history of cocaine use, and had no detectable cocaine metabolites on urine screening. Infants with known or suspected risk factors for hearing loss (family history of hearing impairment before age 6 years; congenital toxoplasmosis, other [syphilis, hepatitis, zoster], rubella, cytomegalovirus, and herpes simplex [TORCHES] infection; sepsis; bilirubin levels of 256.5 μmol/L or more; Apgar scores less than or equal to 6 at 5 minutes; intraventricular hemorrhage; seizures; birth weight less than 1500 g; aminoglycoside use longer than 10 days; craniofacial anomalies; renal malformations; or other congenital malformation) were excluded from the study.[14,15]

Other information obtained on all infants included birth weight, gestational age, size for gestational age, 1- and 5-minute Apgar scores, and method of delivery. Gestational age was based on maternal dates if within 2 weeks of the Dubowitz score, or otherwise as assessed with the Dubowitz scale.[16] Mothers

Accepted for publication March 21, 1991.

From the Department of Pediatrics and the Infant Hearing Program, University Medical Center, University of Florida Health Science Center, Jacksonville (Dr Carzoli and Mss Hammer-Knisely and Houy), and Nemours Children's Clinic, Jacksonville (Dr Murphy).

Reprint requests to Department of Pediatrics, University of Florida Health Science Center, 655 W Eighth St, Jacksonville, FL 32209 (Dr Carzoli).

Table 1.—Frequency Distributions of Background Variables of 50 Cocaine-Exposed and 50 Nonexposed Newborns*

Variable	Cocaine-Exposed Infants, No. (%)	Nonexposed Infants, No. (%)	χ^2	P<
Sex				
M	20 (40)	20 (40)	0	.99
F	30 (60)	30 (60)		
Race				
W	11 (22)	20 (40)	3.79	.10
B	39 (78)	30 (60)		
Size				
SGA	11 (22)	3 (6)		
AGA	37 (74)	43 (86)	5.69	.10
LGA	2 (4)	4 (8)		
Delivery				
Vaginal	44 (88)	41 (82)	0.71	.50
C-Section	6 (12)	9 (18)		
Maternal substance use				
Tobacco	38 (76)	14 (28)	23.08	.001
Alcohol	17 (34)	6 (12)	6.83	.01
Marijuana	6 (12)	3 (6)	1.10	.30

*SGA indicates small for gestational age; AGA, appropriate for gestational age; LGA, large for gestational age; and C-section, cesarean section.

Table 2.—Comparison of Background Characteristics Between Cocaine-Exposed and Nonexposed Infants*

Variable	Values: Mean (SD)	Median	Range
Gestational age, wk			
Cocaine-exposed	39.36 (1.22)	40	37-42
Nonexposed	39.10 (1.03)	39	37-42
Birth weight, g			
Cocaine-exposed	2844 (465.99)	2745	2015-3884
Nonexposed	3140 (428.32)	3230	2065-4040
Apgar score			
1 minute			
Cocaine-exposed	7.80 (1.27)	8	4-9
Nonexposed	7.84 (1.60)	8	1-9
5 minutes			
Cocaine-exposed	8.94 (0.47)	9	7-10
Nonexposed	8.98 (0.47)	9	7-10

*The results of independent *t* tests indicated a significant difference between cocaine-exposed and nonexposed infants for birth weight ($P\leq.001$), but not for gestational age ($P\leq.25$), 1-minute Apgar score ($P\leq.88$), or 5-minute Apgar score ($P\leq.66$).

Table 3.—Frequency of Maternal Cocaine Use by Trimesters

Trimester	No. Admitted Use	Positive Urine Screen	Adjusted Usage*
1 only	12	3	9
2 only	2	1	1
3 only	2	2	2
1 and 2	8	5	3
2 and 3	1	1	1
1, 2, and 3	22	18	34
Denied use	. . .	3	. . .

*Adjusted use indicates that any mother who denied use during the third trimester, but had an infant whose urine sample showed positive results, was presumed to have used cocaine during all three trimesters. This included a total of 12 women, three of whom denied cocaine use at any time during pregnancy.

were questioned as to their use of tobacco, alcohol, marijuana, and other illicit drugs during pregnancy. Cocaine use was divided into first, second, and/or third trimester usage.

Cocaine urine screening was performed in all infants with a cocaine metabolite assay (ADx, Abbott Laboratories, Abbott Park, Ill), and was considered positive when 0.3 µg/dL or more was detectable.

Hearing was screened in all infants within the first week of life using the ABR. Infants who failed initial ABR testing were scheduled for repeated ABR testing after postconceptual age 44 weeks, because thresholds do not change significantly after this age.[17] The sensitivity of the ABR test has been predicted to be as high as 100%, and specificity, 86%. The predictive value of a positive test is 5.3% and of a negative test is 100% in a high-risk population.[18] Although the ABR test is not considered a definitive predictor of hearing loss later in life, it is currently considered the most reliable instrument for assessing the integrity of the auditory system in infancy.[19,20]

The test was administered by a certified audiologist who was blinded to the infant's group. Testing was done using an auditory evoked potential electrodiagnostic computer and averaging system (Nicolet Compact Four, Nicolet Biomedical Instruments, Madison, Wis). Electrode placement consisted of three silver 6-mm cup electrodes. Placement of the active (noninverting) electrode was at the forehead, with the reference (inverting) electrode attached to the earlobe of the test ear and the ground electrode attached to the contralateral earlobe. Click stimuli were presented to each ear separately at a repetition rate of 21.1 clicks per second through tubal insert phones and immittance tip adaptors at an intensity level of 30 dB relative to normal hearing threshold (dBnHL). To obtain a quiet recording, filters were used to eliminate background electroencephalographic noise below 150 Hz and above 3000 Hz. Recordings were obtained by averaging 2000 stimulus presentations, with reproducible waveforms obtained in at least two separate trials. All testing was performed in a sound-treated chamber (model RS 2425, Acoustic Systems, Austin, Tex).

Hearing evaluations were scored on a pass/fail basis. Infants were considered to have passed the ABR test if waves I, III, and V were present at 30 dBnHL with good wave replicability, interaural agreement, and morphologic features. Latencies of waves were recorded at 30 dBnHL for comparison between study and control groups. In infants who failed the initial ABR, follow-up testing included latency intensity function and immittance, in an attempt to distinguish conductive from sensorineural hearing loss.

RESULTS

Consents were obtained for a total of 112 infants, but 12 were excluded due to incomplete data, other risk factors for hearing impairment, or ABR test not being performed within the first week of life. Therefore, a total of 50 ICAMs and 50 control infants were enrolled in the study and underwent ABR examinations.

Urine samples of all infants were screened for cocaine

metabolites within the first 48 hours after delivery. Results of urine toxicologic tests were positive (greater than 0.3 μg/dL) in 33 of the 50 infants in the cocaine-exposed group. No control infants had detectable cocaine metabolites on urine screening.

In the cocaine-exposed newborns, 46 passed the initial ABR test and four failed, compared with 48 passes and two failures in the control group. Using χ^2 analysis with Yates' correction for continuity, this difference was not significant ($\chi^2=0.18$ [$df=1$]). Using one-tailed independent t tests, no significant differences were noted between the two groups in absolute latencies of waves I, III, and V or III to V and I to V interpeak latencies for either the left or right ear.

Background characteristics of infants in the two groups are presented in Tables 1 and 2. Cocaine-exposed infants had a lower mean birth weight ($P<.001$) and a higher incidence of maternal use of tobacco ($P<.001$) and alcohol ($P<.01$). There were no significant differences found in size, method of delivery, 1- or 5-minute Apgar scores, or use of other illicit substances.

Table 3 depicts the estimated pattern of maternal cocaine use by trimester. Adjusted use in pregnancy was greater than admitted use, based on the number of positive infant urine screens. A total of 12 women denied third trimester cocaine use, yet cocaine metabolites were found in their infants' urine samples. These women were considered to have used cocaine during all three trimesters, as historical information obtained was considered unreliable.

In all, at least 46 women used cocaine during the first trimester, 39 were second trimester users, and 37 women used cocaine during the last trimester of pregnancy. According to adjusted usage rates, the majority of women who used cocaine did so throughout pregnancy. The second largest group comprised first trimester users only. Based on histories obtained from these women in the latter group, most indicated attempting to stop cocaine use once they discovered they were pregnant, due to concerns of effects on the developing fetus. Several of the women had voluntarily entered treatment programs in an attempt to overcome their addiction.

Of the six infants who failed initial ABR testing, all were appropriate for gestational age in size. Five of six mothers whose infants failed initial ABR testing used tobacco during their pregnancy. Results of repeated ABR tests were normal in five of the six infants. The only infant who failed follow-up testing had latency intensity curves and immittance measurements indicative of a conductive rather than sensorineural hearing loss. This infant had a history of recurrent otitis media, and was referred for further evaluation.

COMMENT

Based on previously published reports on neurodevelopmental problems in ICAMs, abnormalities on infant hearing evaluation by ABR testing were expected, but no such abnormalities were found. In this study, no significant increase in sensorineural hearing loss was observed in ICAMs compared with control infants. The relatively high false-positive rate on initial testing found in this study has also been reported by others.[18,21] The one infant who did fail repeated ABR testing was diagnosed to have a conductive rather than sensorineural hearing loss, which was presumed secondary to recurrent otitis media and not due to perinatal cocaine exposure. Although no differences between the two groups were noted, further study with larger samples will be needed to confirm these results. Confirmed hearing loss in high-risk populations, most notably infants in neonatal intensive care units with various risk factors, has been estimated at between 2% and 4% and higher.[18,21] The estimated incidence of hearing loss in the general population is approximately one in 750 infants.[15]

These findings are in contrast to a previously published report by Shih et al,[22] which indicated prolonged interpeak and absolute latencies in 18 ICAMs compared with 18 control infants. However, the increase in absolute latencies reported in the study by Shih et al occurred only at high intensities (80 dBnHL) and only for wave V. Prolonged interpeak latencies were seen at 40 and 80 dBnHL for the wave III to V interval, and for the wave I to V interval at 80 dBnHL, indicating possible slower brain-stem transmission times at higher intensities. Higher stimulus rates were used (60 per second), and the latency prolongation seen may indicate prolonged brain-stem neuronal refractory periods in cocaine-exposed infants. However, their population of cocaine-exposed infants had gestational ages ranging from 32 to 40 weeks. It has been shown that there is a progressive neuromaturational decrease in wave latencies and hearing threshold with increasing gestational age.[17,23,24] Therefore, the latencies reported by Shih et al may have been prolonged as a result of the preterm infants, thus biasing the results, although it may indicate subtle auditory brain-stem dysfunction at higher stimulation rates.

Compared with the control group, the ICAM population in the present study was found to have significantly lower birth weights, as has been reported by others,[4-7,13] although no cause-and-effect relationship can be proposed. A variety of other factors may influence the intrauterine growth of ICAMs, including maternal smoking and nutritional and socioeconomic status. Mothers who used cocaine during the pregnancy were also more likely to use tobacco and alcohol, although there was no reported difference in other illicit drug use. There was also no difference in Apgar scores at 1 and 5 minutes or method of delivery between the two groups. The lack of difference in size between infants who were exposed to cocaine and those who were not may be partly explained by the fact that only apparently healthy infants of over 37 weeks' gestation were chosen for the study.

Therefore, despite numerous other neurologic complications reported in ICAMs,[4-13] the present results suggest that there was no apparent effect on the developing auditory system in otherwise healthy, full-term infants due to maternal cocaine abuse. It remains to be seen whether infants born prematurely or with congenital abnormalities directly attributable to maternal cocaine use will be similarly unaffected.

This study was supported by a grant from the Department of Sponsored Research, University of Florida, Gainesville.

We are grateful to Kathy Beaulieu and Karen Richard for their help in preparation of this article.

References

1. Frank DA, Zuckerman BS, Amaro H, et al. Cocaine use during pregnancy: prevalence and correlates. *Pediatrics.* 1988;182:888-895.

2. Moore TR, Sorg J, Miller L, Key T, Resnik R. Hemodynamic

effects of intravenous cocaine on the pregnant ewe and fetus. Am J Obstet Gynecol. 1986;155:883-888.
3. Woods JR, Plessinger MA, Clerk KE. Effect of cocaine on uterine blood flow and fetal oxygenation. *JAMA.* 1987;257:957-961.
4. Hadeed AJ, Siegel SR. Maternal cocaine use during pregnancy: effect on the newborn infant. *Pediatrics.* 1989;84:205-210.
5. Cherukuri R, Minkoff H, Feldman J, Parekh A, Glass L. A cohort study of alkaloid cocaine ('crack') in pregnancy. *Obstet Gynecol.* 1988;72:147-151.
6. Ryan L, Erich S, Finnegan L. Cocaine abuse in pregnancy: effects on the fetus and newborn. *Neurotoxicol Teratol.* 1987;9:295-299.
7. Mitchell M, Sabbagha RE, Keith L, MacGregor S, Mota JM, Minoque J. Ultrasonic growth parameters in fetuses of mothers with primary addiction to cocaine. *Am J Obstet Gynecol.* 1988;159:1104-1109.
8. Chasnoff IJ, Bussey ME, Sauich R, Stack C. Perinatal cerebral infarction and maternal cocaine use. *J Pediatr.* 1986;108:456-459.
9. Dixon SD, Bejar R. Echoencephalographic findings in neonates associated with maternal cocaine and metamphetamine use: incidence and clinical correlates. *J Pediatr.* 1989;115:770-778.
10. Doberczak TM, Shanzer S, Senie RT, Kendall SR. Neonatal neurologic and electroencephalographic effects of intrauterine cocaine exposure. *J Pediatr.* 1988;113:354-358.
11. Teske MP, Trese MT. Retinopathy of prematurity-like fundus and persistent hyperplastic primary vitreous associated with maternal cocaine use. *Am J Ophthalmol.* 1987;103:719-720.
12. Chasnoff IJ, Hunt CE, Kletter R, Kaplan D. Prenatal cocaine exposure is associated with respiratory pattern abnormalities. *AJDC.* 1989;143:583-587.
13. Chasnoff IJ, Burns WJ, Schnoll SH, Burns KA. Cocaine use in pregnancy. *N Engl J Med.* 1985;313:666-669.
14. Joint Committee on Infant Hearing, American Academy of Pediatrics. Position statement 1982. *Pediatrics.* 1982;70:496-497.
15. Epstein S, Reilly JS. Sensorineural hearing loss. *Pediatr Clin North Am.* 1989;36:1501-1520.
16. Dubowitz LMS, Dubowitz V, Goldberg C. Clinical assessment of gestational age in the newborn infant. *J Pediatr.* 1970;77:1-10.
17. Lary S, Briassoulis G, deVries L, Dubowitz LM, Dubowitz V. Hearing threshold in preterm and term infants by auditory brainstem response. *J Pediatr.* 1985;107:593-599.
18. Shannon DA, Felix JK, Krumholz A, Goldstein PH, Harris KC. Hearing screening of high-risk newborns with brainstem auditory-evoked potentials: a follow-up study. *Pediatrics.* 1984;73:22-26.
19. Committees on Hearing, Bioacoustics, and Biomechanics, Commission on Behavioral and Social Sciences, and Education National Research Council. Brainstem audiometry of infants. *ASHA.* 1987;29:47-55.
20. Warren MP. The auditory brainstem response in pediatrics. *Otolaryngol Clin North Am.* 1989;22:473-500.
21. Stein L, Ozdamar O, Kraus N, Paton J. Follow-up of infants screened by auditory brainstem response in the neonatal intensive care unit. *J Pediatr.* 1983;103:447-453.
22. Shih L, Cone-Wesson B, Reddix B. Effects of maternal cocaine abuse on the neonatal auditory system. *Int J Pediatr Ortorhinolaryngol.* 1988;15:245-251.
23. Murray AD. Newborn auditory brainstem evoked responses (ABRs): longitudinal correlates in the first year. *Child Dev.* 1988;59:1542-1554.
24. Eggermont JJ, Salamy A. Development of ABR parameters in a preterm and a term born population. *Ear Hear.* 1988;9:283-289.

In Other AMA Journals

ARCHIVES OF OPHTHALMOLOGY

Persistent Hyperplastic Primary Vitreous With Glaucoma Presenting in Infancy

Wallace L. M. Alward, MD; Michael A. Krasnow, DO; Ronald V. Keech, MD; Jose S. Pulido, MD; Gregory L. Sutton, MD
(*Arch Ophthalmol.* 1991;109:1063-1066)

Ductal Patency in Neonates With Respiratory Distress Syndrome

A Randomized Surfactant Trial

Mark D. Reller, MD; Donald C. Buffkin, MD; Michael A. Colasurdo, MD; Mary J. Rice, MD; Robert W. McDonald, RCPT, RDMS

• The purpose of this study was to evaluate in a controlled study the effect of exogenous surfactant on various manifestations of ductal patency. Premature infants with respiratory distress syndrome were randomized to receive surfactant (Survanta) (n=22) or air (n=14). In neonates receiving surfactant, there was a greater tendency for an audible murmur to develop (13 of 22 vs four of 14). In spite of this, the clinical use of indomethacin was similar for the two groups, 10 (45%) of 22 vs six (43%) of 14. Excluding neonates given indomethacin early, a comparable number of surfactant-treated neonates (9/17 [53%]) vs control neonates (6/12 [50%]) demonstrated spontaneous closure of the ductus within a physiologic time frame (on or before day 4). For the gestational ages studied, the beneficial effects of exogenous surfactant were not associated with either an increased risk for delayed closure of the ductus arteriosus or a greater incidence of indomethacin usage. Utilization of exogenous surfactant does not appear to have an adverse impact on ductal patency.

(*AJDC.* 1991;145:1017-1020)

Premature neonates with respiratory distress syndrome are at well-recognized risk for persistent shunting through the ductus arteriosus. Currently, the treatment of premature neonates frequently includes the use of exogenous surfactant to reduce the severity and complications of respiratory distress syndrome.[1-6] However, little objective information exists regarding the effect of surfactant administration on ductal patency. Symptoms of ductal shunting have been reported to be more frequent after surfactant treatment,[1] and concerns exist that this shunting could either affect the resolution of respiratory distress[1] or be associated with a transient or poor response to surfactant.[7] Additionally, surfactant therapy has been reported to be associated with a greater need to treat symptomatic patent ductus arteriosus.[8] While several other investigational trials have not reported an increased incidence of clinically significant patent ductus arteriosus,[4,9-13] the assessment of ductal patency was not the primary focus in any of these studies. Additionally, because no uniform or objective criteria exist for determining significant ductal shunting, the "incidence" of patent ductus in most of these randomized trials has depended on a variety of clinical and/or subjective echocardiographic criteria.

In previous studies evaluating ductal patency,[14,15] we have utilized duration of ductal patency (ie, timing of functional closure) as one objective end point and have established normative data for the timing of spontaneous ductal closure in premature neonates.[14] The purpose of the current study was to systematically evaluate the impact of surfactant, administered in a randomized prospective trial, as to its impact on the timing of spontaneous ductal closure. Because indomethacin sodium trihydrate administration obviously affects the timing of ductal closure, we specifically analyzed a subgroup of neonates who did not receive indomethacin during the first 4 days of life (the normal time frame of physiologic ductal patency) as to the risk factors associated with delayed ductal closure. We separately analyzed two clinical manifestations of ductal patency: the need for indomethacin (as clinically determined by the neonatal attending staff), and the incidence of cardiac murmurs in neonates with ductal patency confirmed by echocardiography.

PATIENTS AND METHODS

Thirty-seven neonates were enrolled into this investigation over a 19-month period between March 31, 1988 and October 15, 1989. Of these, 28 neonates were delivered at the Oregon Health Sciences University Hospital, Portland, while nine were outborn referrals. Criteria for inclusion into this study were (1) birth weight below 1750 g; (2) gestational age greater than 26 weeks (confirmed by a neonatal modified Ballard examination); (3) positive-pressure ventilatory support with fraction of inspired oxygen (FIO_2) of 0.40 or greater (with PaO_2, ≤80 mm Hg); (4) absence of congenital malformation; and (5) signed parental consent.

Accepted for publication March 28, 1991.

From the Department of Pediatrics, Oregon Health Sciences University, Portland.

Presented before the Society for Pediatric Research, Anaheim, Calif, May 10, 1990.

Reprint requests to Department of Pediatrics, OHSU, 3181 SW Sam Jackson Park Rd, Portland, OR 97201-3042 (Dr Reller).

Table 1.—Factors Associated With Delayed Closure of the Ductus Arteriosus*

	Normal Closure (n=15)	Delayed Closure (n=14)
Birth weight, g	**1355±304**	**1286±258**
Gestational age, wk	29.8±1.2	28.7±1.6†
Apgar score		
1 min	5.9±1.8	3.4±2.3‡
5 min	7.4±1.3	5.6±2.3†
Positive pressure ventilation (day 4)	6 (40)	11 (79)†
Exogenous surfactant	9 (60)	8 (57)

*Data for the subgroup of infants who did not receive indomethacin in the first 4 days of life. Values are mean±SD or number (percent).
†$P<.05$.
‡$P<.01$.

All neonates entered into this study had previously been enrolled in a prospective, randomized, blinded trial to assess the effects of surfactant administration in premature neonates with respiratory distress syndrome and assisted positive-pressure ventilation (for which a separate signed consent was obtained). The surfactant preparation used in this study was an organic solvent extract of minced cow lung supplemented with dipalmitoyl phosphatidylcholine, palmitic acid, and tripalmitin (Survanta, Ross Laboratories, Division of Abbott Laboratories, Columbus, Ohio). The initial dose was administered between 1 and 8 hours of life. The dose of surfactant was 100 mg/kg (4 mL/kg). Control neonates were administered air. Subsequent doses up to a total of four could be given in the first 48 hours of life if continued ventilatory support and FiO_2 above 0.30 were required. The minimum dose interval was 6 hours.

Neonates enrolled into this investigation were treated by the neonatal attending staff. When criteria for surfactant dosing were met, the surfactant was administered by a separate group of workers not directly involved with care of the neonate. Thus, both the attending staff and our investigational group were "blinded" as to the medication given to the neonates enrolled into the study.

After initiation of the investigational protocol and administration of the first dose of surfactant (or air), a complete two-dimensional echocardiographic study was performed. The initial study was performed in the first 16 hours of life. All subsequent studies were limited to high parasternal and suprasternal notch imaging to optimize visualization of the ductus arteriosus.

For detection of left-to-right ductal shunt flow, color flow Doppler imaging was utilized. With this extremely sensitive tool, ductal flow is noted to originate near the orifice of the left pulmonary artery and generally produces a mosaic pattern. With use of current color flow Doppler imaging techniques, the detection and confirmation of even small left-to-right ductal jets are easily obtained.[14-18]

The echocardiograms were obtained using an ultrasound imaging system (Hewlett-Packard Color Flow Ultrasound imaging system, model HP77020A, Hewlett-Packard Co, Andover, Mass). The two-dimensional images and color flow signals were obtained with a 5-MHz short-focus transducer. The two-dimensional and color flow Doppler images were recorded on a videocassette recorder (Panasonic).

For all neonates, daily sequential ductal shunt flow studies were obtained at roughly 24-hour intervals until no shunt flow could be detected on two consecutive studies, signifying that functional closure of the ductus arteriosus had occurred. Functional closure was defined as occurring on the first day that no shunt flow was detected. Studies were also continued following indomethacin administration or ligation until closure of the ductus was confirmed.

A daily cardiac examination was made by a member of our investigational group. This person was blinded to both the medication given as well as the results of the daily echocardiographic evaluation. By design, it was the goal of this study not to alter standard care in the neonatal unit. Thus, to avoid introduction of bias, the results of our daily investigational echocardiograms were not made available to the neonatal staff. In addition, no set criteria were established for the utilization of indomethacin. The decision to administer indomethacin was made solely by the attending neonatal staff. Clinical concerns suggesting significant ductal shunting (ie, new onset murmur, worsening chest roentgenogram, deterioration in ventilatory requirements) usually resulted in cardiology consultation for the assessment of ductal status. As it is not standard practice in our nursery, no neonate received prophylactic indomethacin.

Intravenous fluid administration was not prospectively controlled in this study. However, all neonates were treated using a standard fluid management of 80 mL/kg for 2 days, then 100 mL/kg increasing to 120 mL/kg by day 5. Daily weights were subsequently evaluated.

Statistical differences between the two groups were analyzed using Student's t test or by the Mann-Whitney U test.

RESULTS

The mean birth weight and gestational ages for the 22 surfactant-treated neonates and 15 control neonates were 1344±291 vs 1270±313 g and 29.3±1.7 vs 29.0±1.5 weeks, respectively (not significant). One of the control neonates died at 20 hours of life and was eliminated from the study. Both groups were maintained in a negative fluid balance and demonstrated comparable weight losses. By day 4, surfactant-treated neonates weighed 8.2%±4.5% less than birth weight, compared with 9.2%±7.1% less for control neonates.

The echocardiographic evaluations for the two groups of neonates were performed at comparable times. The average age for the two groups on the first 5 days of life for surfactant-treated and control neonates were 10.4 vs 10.3 hours, 33.0 vs 32.8 hours, 57.9 vs 58.0 hours, 83.0 vs 83.0 hours, and 107.1 vs 106.6 hours, respectively.

Healthy premature neonates without respiratory distress undergo spontaneous closure of the ductus arteriosus in the first 4 days of life.[14] To examine the extent to which respiratory distress syndrome and exogenous surfactant affect the timing of ductal closure, we excluded neonates who received indomethacin during the first 4 days of life (five surfactant-treated, two control). Of the 17 surfactant-treated neonates not receiving indomethacin early in life, nine (53%) demonstrated evidence for spontaneous ductal closure by the fourth day of life. For the 12 control neonates not receiving indomethacin early in life, the ductus in six (50%) closed spontaneously by the fourth day of life. For the eight surfactant-treated neonates whose ductus did not close by the fourth day, the ductus in three subsequently closed spontaneously on days 8, 10, and 11, while the other five required either indomethacin or ligation for closure. For the remaining six control neonates, the ductus in two also closed spontaneously on days 5 and 9, while four neonates required indomethacin or ligation for closure. For both groups of neonates, ductal closure occurred within 1 to 3 days of initiation of indomethacin treatment. Thus, surfactant did not appear to alter either the response to indomethacin or the need for ligation.

Approximately 50% of the neonates not receiving indomethacin early in life had delayed closure of the ductus arteriosus (ie, persistent patency). Of the 29 neonates

Table 2.—Ventilator Settings (Day 4) for Infants With Delayed Closure of Ductus Arteriosus and Continued Need for Positive-Pressure Ventilatory Assistance.*

	Surfactant (n=5)	Control (n=6)
Peak inspiratory pressure, cm H_2O	15.2±4.7	24.0±7.4
Respiratory rate/min	17.8±11.6	37.2±16.4

*Three of the 14 infants with delayed closure from Table 1 were extubated (all received exogenous surfactant). For both variables, $P<.05$.

(from both treatment groups), 15 (nine surfactant-treated, six control) demonstrated ductal closure within the physiologic time frame, while 14 (eight surfactant-treated, six control) did not (Table 1). Delayed ductal closure was associated with lesser gestational age, lower Apgar scores, and continued need for positive-pressure ventilatory therapy.

In this study, two clinical manifestations of ductal patency were evaluated: the presence of a murmur and the need for indomethacin. Of the 22 neonates who received surfactant, 13 had a detectable cardiac murmur coinciding with confirmed ductal patency by echocardiography. Only four of 14 control neonates had a detectable murmur ($P=.07$). The decision to give indomethacin was determined independently by the neonatal attending staff. Of the 22 neonates receiving surfactant, a total of 10 (45%) required indomethacin, three of whom subsequently required ligation of the ductus arteriosus. Of the 14 control neonates, six (43%) received indomethacin with one subsequent ligation. Thus, the clinically determined need for indomethacin was comparable for the two groups.

While it was not the purpose of this study to evaluate the ventilatory effects of exogenous surfactant, the concurrent ventilator settings were noted at the time of our daily echocardiographic studies. Our initial echocardiographic evaluation always followed the first randomized administration of surfactant (or air). At the time of this study (mean, 10.4 hours), the oxygen requirements were significantly lower for the surfactant-treated neonates (FIO_2, 0.42±0.22 vs 0.70±0.21; $P<.01$). This finding persisted on the day 2 study (at about 33 hours) (FIO_2, 0.36±0.18 vs 0.77±0.23; $P<.01$). In addition, at the time of the day 2 study, neonates receiving surfactant required a lower peak inspiratory pressure (15.9±3.1 vs 22.9±6.2 cm H_2O; $P<.01$). This finding persisted even in the subgroup with delayed closure of the ductus arteriosus (Table 2). Last, neonates receiving surfactant were extubated from positive-pressure ventilatory assistance more rapidly. The median duration of ventilatory therapy was through the third day for surfactant-treated neonates (range, 1 to 32 days) vs 8 days for control neonates (range, 1 to 26 days) ($P=.023$). By the fourth day of life, 11 (50%) of 22 surfactant-treated neonates were extubated, while only two (14%) of 14 control neonates were extubated ($P<.05$).

COMMENT

The purpose of this study was to assess the effect of exogenous surfactant on several well-defined manifestations of ductal patency, and to evaluate the risk factors associated with delayed closure of the ductus arteriosus. The primary limitation of this and all studies evaluating ductal patency is the difficulty in defining clinically significant ductal shunting. Unfortunately, no reliable criteria exist with which to make this determination. Left-sided cardiac dimension measurements (left ventricular dimensions, left atrial–aortic root ratios) are known to be insensitive.[19] On the other hand, simple echocardiographic detection of ductal patency in the first days of life fails to differentiate between pathologic (significant) ductal shunting and physiologic patency before normal closure. We have previously established normative data for the timing of spontaneous ductal closure in healthy premature neonates and have utilized delayed closure as an objective end point that is readily evaluable. Using this end point in the current study, the risk factors associated with persistent ductal patency were lower gestational age, lower Apgar scores, and continued positive-pressure ventilatory assistance, while exogenous surfactant was not associated with delayed ductal closure.

In a previous study, we found a relatively low incidence of persistent patency in premature neonates with respiratory distress syndrome.[15] In that study, however, we only evaluated neonates greater than or equal to 30 weeks gestational age and excluded neonates with low Apgar scores (ie, birth asphyxia). In the current study, the higher incidence of delayed closure would appear to be due to inclusion of neonates both sicker (ie, lower Apgar scores) and gestationally less mature, all of whom required ventilatory assistance. That these were the specific risk factors associated with delayed ductal closure in this study confirms this impression. In evaluating the overall group, approximately 50% demonstrated spontaneous closure of the ductus within the physiologic time frame.

Animal models have suggested that exogenous surfactant might lower pulmonary vascular resistance.[20,21] Thus, it is possible that although ductal closure rates were comparable, the volume of ductal shunting could be greater in those neonates who received surfactant. Evidence that this was not the case is indirect. First, because the attending staff was blinded as to which patients received surfactant as well as to the results of the daily investigational echocardiograms, the decision to give indomethacin was made independently, usually in conjunction with cardiology consultation. That the utilization of indomethacin was nearly identical would argue against clinically significant differences in ductal shunting. In addition, the reductions in both initial oxygen requirements and peak inspiratory pressure, in conjunction with earlier extubation, argue against the development of greater left-to-right ductal shunts in those neonates who received surfactant. Last, this reduction in ventilatory support with surfactant was present even in the subgroup with persistent ductal patency (Table 2). If differences in ductal shunting existed in neonates receiving surfactant, the shunt volume was not sufficiently large to blunt these beneficial ventilatory effects.

Our conclusion that surfactant does not have an adverse impact on ductal patency differs from that of Charon and colleagues,[7] who found surfactant-receiving neonates to have a higher incidence of patent ductus arteriosus. In their study, patent ductus arteriosus was diagnosed using only clinical signs, including the presence of a systolic or continuous murmur. Neonates receiving surfactant in our study had a similar tendency for a murmur to develop. Our results also differ from a recent publication by Heldt and coworkers,[8] who reported an increased incidence of patent ductus. Their study differed from ours, however, in that their surfactant-treated group included both a prophylactically treated group and a later "rescue" group that experienced mechanical ventilatory assistance and clinical deterioration. This latter group introduced a selection bias not present in their control group. Their study also included a smaller (450 to 1580 g) and gestationally less mature (24 to 29 weeks) group of neonates than included in our study. However, similar to the study of Heldt and coworkers, surfactant utilization was not found to alter either the ductal response to indomethacin or the subsequent need for ligation.

We conclude that the beneficial effects of surfactant administration on oxygenation and duration of ventilatory therapy are not associated with either a greater need for indomethacin or any increased risk for delayed closure of the ductus arteriosus. For the gestational ages studied, while the standard risk factors for delayed ductal closure were confirmed, surfactant does not appear to have had an adverse impact on ductal patency.

References

1. Fujiwara T, Maeta H, Chida S, Morita T, Watabe Y, Abe T. Artificial surfactant therapy in hyaline-membrane disease. *Lancet.* 1980;1:55-59.
2. Hallman M, Merritt TA, Jarvenpaa A, et al. Exogenous human surfactant for treatment of severe respiratory distress syndrome: a randomized prospective clinical trial. *J Pediatr.* 1985;106:963-969.
3. Merritt TA, Hallman M, Bloom BT, et al. Prophylactic treatment of very premature infants with human surfactant. *N Engl J Med.* 1986;315:785-790.
4. Enhorning G, Shennan A, Possmayer F, Dunn M, Chen CP, Milligan J. Prevention of neonatal respiratory distress syndrome by tracheal instillation of surfactant: a randomized clinical trial. *Pediatrics.* 1985;76:145-153.
5. Raju NKR, Vidyasagar D, Bhat R, et al. Double-blind controlled trial of single-dose treatment with bovine surfactant in severe hyaline membrane disease. *Lancet.* 1987;1:651-656.
6. Couser RJ, Ferrara TB, Ebert J, Hoekstra RE, Fangman JJ. Effects of exogenous surfactant therapy on dynamic compliance during mechanical breathing in preterm infants with hyaline membrane disease. *J Pediatr.* 1990;116:119-124.
7. Charon A, Taeusch HW, Fitzgibbon C, Smith GB, Treves ST, Phelps DS. Factors associated with surfactant treatment response in infants with severe respiratory distress syndrome. *Pediatrics.* 1989;83:348-354.
8. Heldt GP, Pesonen E, Merritt TA, Elias W, Sahn DJ. Closure of the ductus arteriosus and mechanics of breathing in preterm infants after surfactant replacement therapy. *Pediatr Res.* 1989;25:305-310.
9. Collaborative European Multicenter Group. Surfactant replacement therapy for severe neonatal respiratory distress syndrome: an international randomized clinical trial. *Pediatrics.* 1988;82:683-690.
10. Kendig JW, Notter RH, Cox C, et al. Surfactant replacement therapy at birth: final analysis of a clinical trial and comparisons with similar trials. *Pediatrics.* 1988;82:756-762.
11. Kwong MS, Egan EA, Notter RH, Shapiro DL. Double-blind clinical trial of calf lung surfactant extract for the prevention of hyaline membrane disease in extremely premature infants. *Pediatrics.* 1985;76:585-592.
12. Gitlin JD, Soll RF, Parad RB, et al. Randomized controlled trial of exogenous surfactant for the treatment of hyaline membrane disease. *Pediatrics.* 1987;79:31-37.
13. Lang MJ, Hall RT, Reddy NS, Kurth CG, Merritt TA. A controlled trial of human surfactant replacement therapy for severe respiratory distress syndrome in very low birth weight infants. *J Pediatr.* 1990;116:295-300.
14. Reller MD, Ziegler ML, Rice MJ, Solin RC, McDonald RW. Duration of ductal shunting in healthy preterm infants: an echocardiographic color flow Doppler study. *J Pediatr.* 1988;112:441-446.
15. Reller MD, Colasurdo MA, Rice MJ, McDonald RW. The timing of spontaneous closure of the ductus arteriosus in infants with respiratory distress syndrome. *Am J Cardiol.* 1990;66:75-78.
16. Sherman FS, Sahn DJ. Pediatric Doppler echocardiography, 1987: major advances in technology. *J Pediatr.* 1987;110:333-342.
17. Swensson RE, Sahn DJ, Valdes-Cruz LM. Color flow mapping in congenital heart disease. *Echocardiography.* 1985;2:545-549.
18. Swensson RE, Valdes-Cruz LM, Sahn DJ, et al. Real-time Doppler color flow mapping for detection of patent ductus arteriosus. *J Am Coll Cardiol.* 1986;8:1105-1112.
19. Valdes-Cruz LM, Dudell GG. Specificity and accuracy of echocardiographic and clinical criteria for diagnosis of patent ductus arteriosus in fluid-restricted infants. *J Pediatr.* 1981;98:298-305.
20. Clyman RI, Jobe A, Heymann M, et al. Increased shunt flow through the patent ductus arteriosus after surfactant replacement therapy. *J Pediatr.* 1982;100:101-107.
21. Vidyasagar D, Maeta H, Raju TNK, et al. Bovine surfactant (Surfactant TA) therapy in immature baboons with hyaline membrane disease. *Pediatrics.* 1985;75:1132-1142.

Safety of a Preadolescent Basketball Program

Margaret E. Gutgesell, MD, MPH

• **A preadolescent youth basketball program was prospectively studied to determine injury rates and the kinds of injuries sustained. The overall injury rate was 7.6% (39 injuries among the 510 children aged 5 to 12 years). Girls had a higher injury rate than boys (*P*<.02). Only 12 children (2.4%) suffered significant injuries as defined by the inability to play for at least one session. Most injuries were contusions (35.9%), followed by strains or sprains (28.2%), epistaxis (12.8%), lacerations (5.1%), and one finger fracture (2.6%), the most significant injury. Games were more likely to produce injuries than practice sessions; most injuries occurred in the second half of game play. This study documents a low injury rate in an organized preadolescent basketball program.**

(*AJDC*. 1991;145:1023-1025)

Organized athletics for preadolescent children are an established fact in the United States. The American Academy of Pediatrics' committees on Sports Medicine and School Health have endorsed such programs if appropriate safeguards are followed.[1] Many communities have well-organized basketball programs for this age group. Although injury rates of athletes participating in high school basketball programs have been reported,[2-7] little is known about injury rates in preadolescent basketball programs. A local YMCA youth basketball program with multiple levels of organized play for preadolescents was prospectively studied for one season to determine acute traumatic injury rates and kinds of injuries sustained.

SUBJECTS AND METHODS

The Charlottesville-Albemarle (Va) YMCA youth basketball program has three preadolescent play levels: introductory, grades kindergarten through second (aged 5 to 8 years); grades third through fourth (aged 8 to 10 years); and grades fifth through sixth (aged 10 to 12 years). Each level was divided into teams composed of six to eight children with at least one coach, frequently a parent or a college student. The youngest group of children had eight 1-hour sessions, with each child participating for the full hour. The middle-level youths had 10 1-hour practice sessions and either seven or eight games. Each child played for at least 30 minutes per game. The oldest group had 11 1-hour practice sessions and eight or nine games, with each child playing for at least 30 minutes per game. Mean minimum participation time for the entire group of children was 1.27 h/wk. Participation time was the same for boys and girls. Because of limited YMCA facilities, all practice sessions and games were held in Albemarle County elementary and junior high schools.

Age, sex, school level, telephone number, team, and coach's name and telephone number were available for all children through registration. Coaches were asked to complete a practice/game report for each week of the season with regard to injury occurrence. For this study, an injury was defined as an acute traumatic event occurring during a practice or game that caused the youth to miss the remaining time in practice or in the game or required the youth to have first aid administered or seek an injury assessment before returning to play. If no injuries occurred, the coach stated such.

If an injury did occur, the coach listed the child's name, how the injury happened, the nature of the injury, and any first aid administered. The coach also noted if the injury had occurred in a practice or a game and, if in a game, in which quarter. For those children listed, the parent was contacted to confirm the injury and to obtain other information, such as exact nature of injury, necessity of a physician visit, and missed school and/or practice or games. If a team's weekly game report was not turned in, the coach was contacted by telephone. Confirmatory evidence of fracture was obtained through the child's physician. This project was approved by the Human Investigation Committee of the University of Virginia Health Sciences Center.

RESULTS

The overall injury rate was 7.6% (39 injuries among the 510 children participating in the 1989-1990 season). Girls

Accepted for publication May 3, 1991.
From the Department of Pediatrics, University of Virginia Health Sciences Center, Charlottesville.
Reprints not available.

Department Editors.—*William B. Strong, MD, Augusta, Ga; Carl L. Stanitski, MD, Pittsburgh, Pa; Ronald E. Smith, PhD, Seattle, Wash; Jack H. Wilmore, PhD, Austin, Tex*

Purpose.—*This section provides current information related to the medical needs of young athletes, as pertinent to counseling young athletes and their parents regarding sports participation and practices contributing to the health maintenance of the athlete, as well as current concepts in the prevention, diagnosis, and treatment of sports-related illnesses and injuries.*

Editor's Comment.—*Physical education, unfortunately, is being reduced in many schools. Community recreation programs are becoming the major source of physical activity for many children. A knowledge of the expected injury rates and their epidemiology will be useful in reducing their incidence. This is the second study to demonstrate greater injury rates in girls than in boys. This suggests that more attention to the development of the proper motor skills and to conditioning could eliminate some of the injuries.*—W.B.S.

Table 1.—Injury Rates in a Preadolescent Basketball Program

Grade	No. of Participants, M/F	Total
K-2	105/14	119
3-4	143/41	184
5-6	158/49	207
Total	406/104	510
	No. (%) of Injuries, M/F	Total No. (%) of Injuries
K-2	0	0
3-4	15 (10.5)/8 (19.5)	23 (12.5)
5-6	10 (6.3)/6 (12.2)	16 (7.7)
Total	25 (6.2)/14 (13.5)*	39 (7.6)

*$\chi^2=6.131$; $P<.02$.

Table 2.—Types of Injuries Among 510 Children in a Preadolescent Basketball Program

Injury	No. (%) of Cases
Contusion	14 (35.9)
Strain/sprain	11 (28.2)
Epistaxis	5 (12.8)
Laceration	2 (5.1)
Finger fracture	1 (2.6)
Miscellaneous	6 (15.4)
Total	39 (100)

had a higher injury rate than boys (14 of 104 [13.5%] vs 25 of 406 [6.2%]; $\chi^2=6.131$, $P<.02$) (Table 1). None of the introductory-group children sustained injuries in the eight hours of play.

Most injuries (35 of 39 [90%]) occurred in games rather than in practice, and in those injury reports indicating the quarter in which injury occurred, most (19 of 27 [70.4%]) occurred in the second half. Fourth-quarter injuries accounted for 40.7% of all injuries.

The types of injuries are shown in Table 2. The most common type was contusion (35.9%). Strains and sprains accounted for 28.2% of injuries. There were five finger injuries, four finger "jams," and one fracture of a fifth finger near the distal interphalangeal joint. A finger "jam" is a mild sprain of the proximal interphalangeal joint. The five episodes of epistaxis occurred in the third through fourth–grade group. These were all secondary to direct trauma. Miscellaneous injuries included minor eye trauma and a swollen lip. Lower extremity trauma accounted for 14 injuries, half of which were to the knee. There were two knee injuries listed as sprains or strains and five contusions. There were four ankle injuries.

First aid, most commonly application of an ice pack, was administered in 22 of the 39 cases of injury. Ten children sustained injuries that required them to sit out the remainder of the game/practice session. Additionally, two children sustained injuries, returned to the game/practice session, but missed two subsequent sessions (one practice session and one game each) because of their injuries. Only five injuries prompted physician assessment, including the finger fracture. This injury, in a 10-year-old boy, necessitated a visit to a hospital emergency department, roentgenography, splinting, a follow-up physician visit, and a second roentgenogram. The child missed 3 weeks (six sessions) of play. Only one of the other four children with physician-assessed injuries missed playing time (one session).

If missed playing time is used as the definition of a significant injury, the overall injury rate was only 2.4% (12 of 510). Boys had eight of these injuries. Although most injuries (36 of 39) occurred on a linoleum-tile playing surface, not in a standard wood-floor gymnasium, this was not out of proportion with the number of players participating in games played on linoleum (453 of 510 children [89%]).

COMMENT

The rates of injury in this preadolescent population are much lower than those reported among high school athletes participating in basketball and soccer, both limited-contact sports. McLain and Reynolds[6] reported injury rates of 37% for boys and 31% for girls, defining an injury as an incident resulting from athletic participation that kept an athlete from completing a practice or game or that caused the athlete to miss a subsequent practice or game. Powell[7] reported that approximately 22% of both boys and girls playing high school basketball sustained at least one time-loss injury per year. However, Austin and colleagues[4] noted only 3.6 injuries per 100 participants in twice-weekly high school physical education classes. In a study of soccer injuries in youths ages 6 to 17 years, Backous et al[8] compared injury rates by age group and found that older youths had higher injury rates than did younger ones in a one-week soccer camp. They believed more aggressive play and greater risk-taking contributed to the older soccer athletes' higher injury rate. The low injury rates in this study are probably related to the total amount of time spent in practice and game sessions. Although the study design did not allow the detection of overuse injuries, it is unlikely that they would have occurred because of the limited playing time.

The data in this report might underestimate the total number of injuries if a coach did not document all injuries. Using the missed time and/or first aid requirement as an injury definition should have eliminated underreporting of injuries. If anything, the coaches probably overreported injuries.

Although girls had a higher overall injury rate, their rate of significant injury was similar to that of boys. This is in contrast to data from McLain and Reynolds' study,[6] in which girls had fewer but more severe injuries. Their data were skewed by one girl who was out of play for 300 days due to an anterior cruciate ligament tear. It is not clear why girls in our study had a higher injury rate.

The fact that more injuries occurred in games rather than in practice is not surprising owing to the competitive nature of a game. Increased frequency of injuries in the second half has also been reported.[7] This may be related to the young athlete becoming tired near the end of the game.

The types of acute traumatic injuries sustained by this group of young athletes were similar to those described by McLain and Reynolds,[6] even in the absence of an athletic trainer in our study. Because of the nature of basketball, a considerable number of finger injuries would be expected. Most, however, would fall into the "lumps, bumps, and bruises" category of injuries and probably would have few sequelae.

This study documents a low injury rate in a local preadolescent basketball program. Youth basketball is not a hazardous sport even when played on linoleum floors. A simple first aid kit should be sufficient to treat most acute traumatic injuries. It is important for such programs to be safe for young athletes so that the goals of the program are achieved. These include the enjoyment of the sport and the development of a positive self-image.[1]

I thank Stephanie Roberts of the Charlottesville-Albemarle YMCA and the coaches and site supervisors in the youth basketball program for making this study possible. Jacob Lohr, MD, provided valuable encouragement and editorial suggestions.

References

1. American Academy of Pediatrics, Committee on Sports Medicine, Committee on School Health. Organized athletics for preadolescent children. *Pediatrics.* 1989;84:583-584.

2. Garrick JG, Requa RK. Girls' sports injuries in high school athletics. *JAMA.* 1978;239:2245-2248.

3. Chambers RB. Orthopaedic injuries in athletes. *Am J Sports Med.* 1979;7:195-197.

4. Austin GJ, Rogers KD, Reese G. Injuries in high school physical education classes. *AJDC.* 1980;134:456-458.

5. DeHaven KE, Lintner DM. Athletic injuries: comparison by age, sport, and gender. *Am J Sports Med.* 1986;14:218-224.

6. McLain LG, Reynolds S. Sports injuries in a high school. *Pediatrics.* 1989;84:446-450.

7. Powell JW. 22% of boys hurt in high school basketball. *Pediatr News.* 1989;23:32.

8. Backous DD, Friedl KE, Smith NJ, Parr TJ, Carpine WD. Soccer injuries and their relation to physical maturity. *AJDC.* 1988;142:839-842.

BOOK REVIEW

Parenteral Nutrition in Infants and Children: Basic Principles and Practical Guidelines

By T.M. Ramanujam, 185 pp with illus, $20, Madras, India, Password Process Pvt Ltd, 1989.

This book provides a stepwise approach to the use of safe parenteral nutrition (PN) in developing countries and presents an overview of PN topics at an elementary level.

The book is divided into two sections. Section 1, "Basic Principles," includes chapters on consequences of malnutrition, general principles of PN, evaluation of nutritional status and requirements, technical considerations in PN, venous access, administration of PN, metabolic response to PN, monitoring, complications, and the role of the nursing staff. The chapters are typically four- or five-page synopses of generally accepted information written in a simple format.

Unfortunately, however, certain information is inaccurate. For example, the statement "[Intravenous dextrose] has a caloric value of 4 kcal/gm [16.8 kJ/g]" is of concern in a book written for persons with a minimal knowledge of PN, because it could lead to undernutrition; carbohydrates have a caloric value of 16.8 kJ/g, but intravenous dextrose has only 14.3 kJ/g. Likewise, the suggestion that solubility problems of calcium and phosphate can be overcome by adding them to alternate bags of PN is disturbing, since this practice has been shown to result in poor retention of both minerals and is, thus, not currently recommended. Stating that insulin can be added to PN is appropriate, but it is an error of omission not to specify that only regular insulin should be used. Statements such as "some administer amphotericin B along with Intralipid" infers that this practice is acceptable, despite no data in current literature to support the compatibility or stability of either component during such administration.

The author provides a discussion and illustrations of the PN preparation method that he uses. This description serves its purpose of providing a guide for practitioners in developing countries, and for others, it provides insight into the conditions faced by these practitioners. More detailed information on types, rates, and management of complications, especially infections, would have complemented the brief discussion of complications. Good diagrams and photographs are included in the chapters on venous access and monitoring, although safer approaches are now used for some of the techniques demonstrated (eg, femoral access).

Section 2, "Special Problems," includes chapters on management of PN in neonates, diarrhea, inflammatory bowel disease, and gastrointestinal fistulas. Recent advances in PN and the views of the author on PN in developing countries are also presented. The chapters on intractable diarrhea and gastrointestinal fistulas present good, but brief reviews of the subjects. These chapters are greatly enhanced by the pictures of patients before and after PN therapy. The discussion of intestinal tuberculosis is also highlighted by such pictures. Better references, however, would be of benefit in these chapters.

Overall, *Parenteral Nutrition in Infants and Children* would be of limited value to most practitioners. However, the book provides insight into practice conditions and a basic guide for PN preparation in developing countries. Here again, the highlights of the book are the pictures of children before and after PN therapy.

Carol J. Rollins, MS, RD, PharmD
Arizona Health Sciences Center
Department of Pharmacy
1501 N Campbell
Tucson, AZ 85724

Decreasing Severity of Chronic Uveitis in Children With Pauciarticular Arthritis

David D. Sherry, MD; Elizabeth D. Mellins, MD; Ralph J. Wedgwood, MD

• We compared the current prevalence and severity of chronic uveitis in children with pauciarticular juvenile rheumatoid arthritis in Seattle, Wash, with that of children with the same condition in the same area in 1975. The prevalence of eye disease decreased from 45% in 1975 to 13% in 1989, and the proportion of patients with severe visual loss decreased from 21% in 1975 to none in 1989. We could not attribute these findings to differences in known risk factors for iritis, such as age, sex, or presence of antinuclear antibodies. There was no difference in the duration of follow-up between the two groups. It is possible that the decline in prevalence of uveitis reflects a referral bias for eye disease in the 1975 population. However, the decrease in disease severity remains unexplained and may represent more effective treatment, earlier surveillance for ocular disease, or a change in the frequency of ocular manifestations of this disease in the 1989 group.

(*AJDC.* 1991;145:1026-1028)

Chronic uveitis may occur in association with juvenile rheumatoid arthritis (JRA) and is most often observed in young girls with pauciarticular-onset JRA and antinuclear antibodies.[1-3] Initially, JRA-associated uveitis is asymptomatic and can only be detected using slit-lamp ophthalmologic examination. However, if untreated, chronic uveitis may lead to synechiae, cataracts, and band keratopathy, all of which can obscure vision.[4] Past studies suggest that approximately 16% of the eyes affected with JRA-associated uveitis will become blind.[4-6]

In the 1960s and 1970s, the prevalence of chronic uveitis in patients with pauciarticular JRA varied from 14% to 34% in North American centers other than that in Seattle, Wash (Table 1).[4,6-10] We were interested in determining whether the prevalence or the severity of JRA-associated uveitis was changing over time. Therefore, we compared the prevalence and severity of chronic uveitis in children with pauciarticular JRA followed up by the University of Washington Pediatric Rheumatology Clinic during 1975 with the prevalence and severity of those followed up by the clinic in 1989.

Accepted for publication January 31, 1991.

From the Department of Pediatrics, University of Washington, Seattle.

Reprint requests to the Division of Rheumatology, Children's Hospital and Medical Center, Seattle, WA 98105 (Dr Sherry).

PATIENTS AND METHODS

All study patients met the American Rheumatism Association's criteria of JRA.[11] We restricted this study to children with pauciarticular-onset disease because most patients with JRA-associated uveitis have this type of disease onset.[1-10] The patients were evaluated for evidence of uveitis through periodic ophthalmologic examinations, generally at 3- to 4-month intervals. These examinations were performed by a variety of ophthalmologists; methods of detection of uveitis have not changed during the period of this study. Uveitis was determined by the presence of inflammatory cells or by increased levels of anterior-chamber protein as detected by light refraction during any ocular examination. Data on the prevalence of uveitis in 1975 were derived from data in a previously published report[8] of children presenting to the Seattle, Wash, clinic. Data on prevalence in 1989 were compiled from records of all active patients with pauciarticular JRA. None of the 1989 patients was an active patient in 1975.

Assays to determine the presence of antinuclear antibodies were performed using standard methods; rat liver was used as substrate in 1975 assays, and Hep-2 cells were used in 1989 assays. Immunoglobulin M rheumatoid factor was assayed using the latex agglutination method.

Data were subjected to χ^2 analyses with Yates' correction using the Statistical Package for the Social Sciences (SPSS Inc, Chicago, Ill).

RESULTS

The 33 patients from 1975 were compared with 134 active patients in 1989 (Table 2). The median age of both groups was less than 4 years, and the percentages of female or antinuclear antibody–positive patients were similar. Thus, the patient groups were comparable in terms of known risk factors of uveitis.[1-3] Data on time of onset of uveitis relative to onset of arthritis were unavailable, but duration of follow-up was similar between groups. In 1989, however, the prevalence of chronic uveitis decreased significantly, and the decrease in the prevalence of impaired vision due to uveitis was even more marked. In 1975, seven patients experienced substantial visual impairment, and of these five experienced unilateral or bilateral blindness. In contrast, no child studied in 1989 experienced significant visual loss ($P<.00005$).

COMMENT

Strikingly, severe visual impairment was absent among the children with JRA-associated uveitis seen in 1989 compared with a similar group of children treated in 1975. This is surprising because the 1989 patient group did not

Table 1.—Reports of Prevalence of Chronic Uveitis in Children With Pauciarticular Juvenile Rheumatoid Arthritis in the United States

Location of Center	Years of Study	Prevalence (%)	Source, y
Seattle, Wash	1964-1968	7/24 (29)	Schaller et al,[7] 1969
Seattle, Wash	1974-1975	15/33 (45)	Schaller,[8] 1977
Ann Arbor, Mich	1961-1974	24/133 (18)	Cassidy et al,[9] 1977
Boston, Mass	1963-1974	28/83(34)	Chylack,[4] 1977
Dallas, Tex	1974-1975	12/88 (14)	Fink,[10] 1977
Jersey City, NJ	1960-1970	6/32 (19)	Calabro et al,[5] 1970

Table 2.—Comparison of Past and Present Patients With Pauciarticular JRA in Seattle, Wash*

	1974 Patients	1989 Patients	Results of χ^2 Analysis	P
N	33	134	. . .	. . .
Median age, y	2.2	3.2	. . .	. . .
Mean follow-up, y	6.0	5.9	. . .	. . .
Patient characteristics, %				
Female	88	75	1.73	NS
ANA positive	52	70	3.33	NS
RF positive	None	3	0.17	NS
Uveitis	45	13	15.16	.0001
Visual loss	21	None	24.62	<.00005

*JRA indicates juvenile rheumatoid arthritis; NS, not significant; ANA, antinuclear antibody; and RF, rheumatoid factor.

differ from the 1975 group in variables known to confer increased risk of eye disease. There are several possible explanations for this trend. The first is that uveitis may have been identified and treated earlier in the 1989 group than in the 1975 group. Uveitis diagnosed simultaneously with JRA has been associated with a higher risk of visual impairment in the patient; this is thought to be due to the fact that the uveitis has gone untreated for some time.[12,13] We had no data concerning the onset of uveitis in the 1975 group. Therefore, no precise evaluation of this risk factor could be made. Duration of follow-up is another important variable because visual impairment usually develops over a long period. There was no difference in duration of follow-up between the two groups of patients. It is possible that prompt treatment of uveitis effectively decreased the prevalence of visual impairment. Another possibility is that current techniques of treatment of JRA are modifying the associated eye disease. Although there is no relationship between flares of ocular and articular disease in JRA,[12,13] anti-inflammatory medications given to treat JRA may reduce ocular inflammation.[14] Thus, earlier referral and more aggressive treatment of arthritis among patients with JRA in 1989 might have reduced the severity of uveitis. It is postulated that autoimmune diseases are initiated by an environmental trigger interacting with a susceptible host. If this paradigm applies to JRA-associated uveitis, the change in severity of uveitis may reflect a change in the virulence of the environmental trigger. In this regard, it is interesting that in New Zealand between 1971 and 1980 there was only one case of mild, remitting iritis among 38 children with pauciarticular JRA.[15] Alternatively, patients with aggressive uveitis may represent a clinical subgroup.[16,17] Such a subgroup might be associated with a particular human leukocyte antigen type; an association between B15/w62 and severe uveitis has been reported.[16] Other immunologic characteristics, such as titer or class of antibodies to retinal antigen S, may also identify a subgroup of patients with chronic uveitis and poor prognoses.[18,19]

This study also revealed a reduction in the prevalence of chronic uveitis in children with JRA in the 1989 group. Prevalence of chronic uveitis in children with pauciarticular JRA in Seattle in 1975 was particularly high compared with that of patients in other pediatric rheumatology centers (Table 1) in other years, raising the possibility that 1975 was an unusual year in this regard. However, the prevalence of uveitis in the 1989 group was also less than half of the 29% prevalence observed in patients of an earlier study conducted in Seattle between 1964 and 1968 (Table 1). During the 14-year span between groups examined in our study, the composition of our patient population likely changed. Most children diagnosed with JRA in our community receive medical attention; this includes those with mild, uncomplicated disease. It is likely that only complicated cases of JRA were referred for medical attention at both earlier reports; chronic uveitis would have constituted such a complication, thus increasing its apparent prevalence in the population with JRA. This is corroborated by the increase in the number of children presenting at our clinic with pauciarticular JRA from 3.22 children per 100 000 children in Washington in 1975 to 11.85 per 100 000 in 1989.[20] Given present referral practices, we believe the data from 1989 accurately reflect the current prevalence of chronic uveitis associated with pauciarticular JRA in our region. This level (13%) is similar to earlier findings from several other geographic locations (Table 1). These results suggest that the prevalence of chronic uveitis among patients with pauciarticular JRA is relatively constant.

Data from other centers are necessary to determine if our findings are unique to our region. Rigorous surveillance for asymptomatic chronic uveitis and prompt treatment are still recommended because blindness remains a potential sequela of this disease. Nonetheless, the decreasing severity of JRA-associated uveitis in the Pacific Northwest is reminiscent of milder carditis associated with acute rheumatic fever in the 1960s compared with earlier years[21] and may indicate that pauciarticular JRA is a dynamic disease with changing manifestations.

References

1. Petty RE, Cassidy JT, Sullivan DB. Clinical correlates of antinuclear antibodies in juvenile rheumatoid arthritis. *J Pediatr.* 1973;83:386-389.

2. Schaller JG, Johnson GD, Hulborow EJ, Ansell BM, Smiley WK. The association of antinuclear antibodies with the chronic iridocyclitis of juvenile rheumatoid arthritis (Still's disease). *Arthritis Rheum.* 1974;17:409-416.

3. Rosenberg AM. Uveitis associated with juvenile rheuma-

toid arthritis. *Semin Arthritis Rheum.* 1987;16:158-173.
4. Chylack LT Jr. The ocular manifestations of juvenile rheumatoid arthritis. *Arthritis Rheum.* 1977;20:217-223.
5. Calabro JJ, Parrino R, Atchoo PD, Marchesano JM, Goldberg LS. Chronic iridocyclitis in juvenile rheumatoid arthritis. *Arthritis Rheum.* 1970;13:406-413.
6. Wolf MD, Lichter PR, Ragsdale CG. Prognostic factors in the uveitis of juvenile rheumatoid arthritis. *Ophthalmology.* 1987;94:1242-1248.
7. Schaller JG, Kupfer C, Wedgwood RJ. Iridocyclitis in juvenile rheumatoid arthritis. *Pediatrics.* 1969;44:92-100.
8. Schaller JG. Juvenile rheumatoid arthritis: series 1. *Arthritis Rheum.* 1977;20:165-170.
9. Cassidy JT, Sullivan DB, Petty RE. Clinical patterns of chronic iridocyclitis in children with juvenile rheumatoid arthritis. *Arthritis Rheum.* 1977;20:224-226.
10. Fink CW. Patients with juvenile rheumatoid arthritis: a clinical study. *Arthritis Rheum.* 1977;20:183-184.
11. Brewer EJ, Bass J, Baum J, et al. Current proposed revision of JRA criteria. *Arthritis Rheum.* 1977;20:195-199.
12. Rosenberg AM, Oen KG. The relationship between ocular and articular disease activity in children with juvenile rheumatoid arthritis and associated uveitis. *Arthritis Rheum.* 1986;29:797-800.
13. Leak AM, Ansell BM. The relationship between ocular and articular disease activity in juvenile rheumatoid arthritis complicated by chronic anterior uveitis. *Arthritis Rheum.* 1987;30:1196-1197.
14. Olson NY, Lindsley CB, Godfrey WA. Nonsteroidal anti-inflammatory drug therapy in chronic childhood iridocyclitis. *AJDC.* 1988;142:1289-1292.
15. McGill NW, Gow PJ. Juvenile rheumatoid arthritis in Auckland: a long term follow-up study with particular reference to uveitis. *Aust N Z J Med.* 1987;17:305-308.
16. Leak AM, Ansell BM, Burman SJ. Antinuclear antibody studies in juvenile chronic arthritis. *Arch Dis Child.* 1986;61:168-172.
17. Smiley WK. The eye in juvenile chronic polyarthritis. *Clin Rheum Dis.* 1976;2:413-428.
18. Petty RE, Hunt DWC, Rollins DF, Schroeder ML, Puterman ML. Immunity to soluble retinal antigen in patients with uveitis accompanying juvenile rheumatoid arthritis. *Arthritis Rheum.* 1987;30:287-293.
19. Uusitato RJ, Stjernschantz J, Mahlberg K, et al. Serum antibody level to S-antigen in children with chronic uveitis. *Br J Ophthalmol.* 1985;69:212-216.
20. *Population Estimate.* Office of Financial Management, State of Washington.
21. Markowitz M, Gordis A. *Rheumatic Fever.* 2nd ed. Philadelphia, Pa: WB Saunders Co; 1972:1-13.

Family History of Myocardial Infarction and Hemodynamic Responses to Exercise in Young Black Boys

Frank A. Treiber, PhD; William B. Strong, MD; Frederick W. Arensman, MD; Thomas Forrest, MD; Harry Davis, MS; Linda Musante, PhD

• The influence of family history of coronary artery disease on children's hemodynamic responses to exercise was examined with 25 black boys aged 7 to 10 years. Blood pressure, heart rate, cardiac output, stroke volume, and total peripheral resistance were evaluated during preexercise, peak exercise, and recovery stages. Children with a family history of CAD exhibited greater systolic blood pressure and total peripheral resistance during preexercise and peak exercise stages than did those without a family history of coronary artery disease. After controlling for preexercise differences, the group with a family history of coronary artery disease exhibited greater increases in systolic blood pressure and less attenuation of total peripheral resistance to peak exercise than the group without a family history of coronary artery disease. Cardiac output indexed by body surface area and stroke volumes were higher at all times in the group without a family history compared with the group with a family history of coronary artery disease. Findings are compared with those of adult studies in terms of influence of family history of coronary artery disease on cardiovascular reactivity to stress.

(*AJDC*. 1991;145:1029-1033)

Coronary artery disease (CAD) continues to be the leading cause of death among black adults in the United States, with mortality rates comparable in black and white men and greater in black women compared with white women.[1,2] Research indicates that cardiovascular reactivity to stress may play a role in the cause and/or clinical manifestations of CAD.[3,4] Prospective studies involving both humans and animals indicate that blood pressure (BP) and heart rate (HR) reactivity to laboratory stressors are predictive of atherosclerotic development and CAD-related mortality.[5,6]

Studies involving children and adults have found that blacks exhibit greater BP responses to physical (eg, dynamic exercise and cold pressor task) and psychological (eg, video game challenge task) stressors than do white cohorts.[7-12] Recent findings indicate that greater levels of total peripheral resistance (TPR) may account for the racial differences in BP reactivity, regardless of whether the stressor is primarily α-adrenergically[8,12] or β-adrenergically[9,10] mediated.

A major risk factor for CAD is a family history of the disease.[13,14] Cardiovascular hyperactivity in response to stress has been associated with family history of CAD in young white adults.[15,16] To our knowledge, no published studies have assessed this relationship among blacks. Such an evaluation is needed because CAD is a substantial problem among blacks, and blacks exhibit greater reactivity than whites to many stressors.

In this study, we evaluated the cardiovascular responses to dynamic exercise in a healthy group of black children with or without a family history of CAD. Because premature myocardial infarction among first- and second-degree relatives has been strongly associated with later development of CAD,[14] children were classified by presence or absence of myocardial infarction among one or more biological parents or grandparents before 55 years of age. Given on the above findings, we predicted that the black boys with a family history of CAD would exhibit greater increases in BP in conjunction with less attenuation of TPR.

SUBJECTS AND METHODS

Twenty-eight healthy 7- to 10-year-old black boys (14 with and 14 without a family history of CAD) were selected from family health history records obtained from a countywide public school screening of families interested in participating in a longitudinal study of cardiovascular health.[17] The family health history form completed by the parent(s) assessed cardiovascular disease history in the child's biologic parents and grandparents. This questionnaire has been used in previous research from our laboratory and validated with substantial agreements noted between physician records and parental self-reports of family health history.[12,17]

On arrival at the laboratory, a parent granted informed consent and the child granted assent to participate as approved by our institutional human assurance committee. The parent again completed the family health history questionnaire. Given the age range of the children, parents were relatively young (mean age,

Accepted for publication March 28, 1991.

From the Departments of Psychiatry and Health Behavior (Dr Treiber) and Pediatrics (Drs Strong and Treiber), the Georgia Institute for the Prevention of Human Disease and Accidents (Drs Treiber, Strong, and Forrest), and the Office of Biostatistics (Mr Davis), Medical College of Georgia, Augusta; the Department of Pediatrics, University of Louisville (Ky) (Dr Arensman); and the Department of Psychology, University of Tampa (Fla) (Dr Musante).

Reprints not available.

Table 1.—Anthropometric Variables by Coronary Artery Disease (CAD) History Group*

Anthropometric Variables	CAD− (n=13)	CAD+ (n=12)
Age, y	8.80 (0.86)	8.64 (1.05)
Height, cm	135.30 (7.60)	135.21 (4.81)
Weight, kg	33.80 (5.20)	32.78 (5.29)
Body surface area, m^2	1.11 (0.08)	1.11 (0.18)
Quetelet index, kg/m^2	18.40 (1.80)	17.90 (2.40)

*CAD− indicates no family history of CAD; CAD+, family history of CAD. Values are mean (SD).

33.2 years for those without and 35.7 years for those with a family history of CAD, $P>.15$), and all biologic grandparents were older than 55 years. None of the children's biologic parents or siblings were reported to have experienced a myocardial infarction. Parents of two subjects were unsure of the age at the time of myocardial infarction in the child's grandparent. Therefore, these children's data were excluded from the analyses. Complete information concerning history of myocardial infarction was obtained for all parents and grandparents of the remaining subjects.

Although family history of essential hypertension has been associated with greater cardiovascular reactivity to laboratory stressors among white children and adults, only a few studies have evaluated this issue among blacks.[18] A family history of hypertension has not been associated with increased reactivity in black adults in response to β-adrenergic–mediated stressors.[19] However, Musante et al[18] recently found that among black male children, those with family histories of hypertension exhibited greater cardiovascular reactivity to an α-adrenergic–mediated stressor of forehead cold stimulation.

Given the high prevalence rates of essential hypertension among blacks, especially in the Southeast,[20] it was not feasible to exclude from recruitment children from families with hypertension. Thus, 50% of the subjects with a positive family history had at least one parent with hypertension, as did 23% of subjects with a negative family history. Likewise, 93% of the subjects with a family history and 31% of subjects without a family history of CAD had at least one grandparent with hypertension. By using the classification system previously described, a more conservative approach is being used, ie, if family history of hypertension is related to reactivity to the β-mediated stressor of exercise, there is less likelihood of finding substantial differences because the negative history group included children from families with parents and/or grandparents with hypertension.

Each child received a complete cardiovascular examination by a pediatric cardiologist to help exclude cardiac disease. No child was a trained athlete. Children's height and weight were measured, and hematocrit readings were assessed. Body surface area was calculated with the formula of DuBois and DuBois.[21] Criteria for exclusion included body surface area less than the third or greater than the 97th percentile for age[22]; current illness, including sickle-cell disease and/or anemia (ie, hematocrit <0.32); and a resting BP greater than the 90th percentile for age.[23] Based on these criteria, one child was excluded from participation.

Exercise was performed on an exercise table with an electronically braked cycle ergometer (Quinton Table Ergometer Model 8464, Quinton Inc, Seattle, Wash). Children were placed in the supine position, and an appropriate-sized BP cuff for use with an automated BP monitor (Dinamap Monitor Model 1165, Critikon Inc, Tampa, Fla) was placed on the right arm. Electrocardiographic leads for monitoring and timing of the HR and echocardiographic and Doppler measurements (Hewlett-Packard Model 7020AC, Hewlett Packard Inc, Atlanta, Ga) were also attached. The supine position was chosen because it provides a better acoustic window for ultrasound evaluation, because the ascending aorta remains posterior and the subject is relatively immobile. With the use of this technique, the findings obtained were comparable with those of other child studies involving upright cycle ergometer exercise with similar peak responses for physical working capacity index.[24]

Following a 5-minute rest period, preexercise measurements of HR, BP, aortic valve systolic area, and velocity of ascending aortic blood flow were made. Children were then urged to pedal an electronically braked ergometer until exhausted with use of a graded protocol previously established in our laboratory. The protocol included increasing workloads of 3 minutes' duration that were predetermined on the basis of body weight.[7]

Systolic and diastolic BP (SBP and DBP) were assessed during the last 30 seconds of the preexercise rest period, during each exercise stage, and 3 to 5 minutes following cessation of exercise. Mean arterial pressure (MAP) was calculated as follows: $[SBP+(2\times DBP)]/3$. The BP monitor has been validated for use during dynamic exercise testing with children of this age range.[25] Heart rates were recorded at the same points in time described above from electrocardiography with the R-R interval.

The Doppler echocardiographic assessment technique has been used by other investigators[26,27] and is presented in detail in reports of other studies from our laboratory.[12,24] Briefly, during the preexercise stage, two-dimensional guidance directed an M-mode beam for measurement of aortic leaflet separation at the sinuses of Valsalva during systole. This measurement of aortic leaflet separation was used for calculation of all cardiac output (CO) values. Aortic flow area (AA) was calculated as follows: $AA=[(1/2)\ \text{diameter}]^2\times 3.14$ (reported in square centimeters). Doppler examination was performed concurrently with the BP and HR assessments with the use of a 1.9-mHz continuous-wave transducer placed in the suprasternal notch and directed toward the aortic valve with the beam positioned to achieve maximum flow velocity. Measurement of maximum flow velocity was made simultaneously with the other cardiovascular measurements. Computer analysis of the Doppler reading was employed to measure the peak velocity, flow velocity integral, and mean velocity at each assessment point along with the corresponding ejection times. From these values, CO was calculated as follows: $CO=(V/2)(ET\times HR)\times AA$ (where V indicates velocity in centimeters per second [$V/2$=average velocity]; ET, ejection time in seconds; and HR in beats per minute, with AA reported in square centimeters and CO reported in millimeters per minute). Cardiac index (CI) was calculated by dividing CO by body surface area. Rate pressure product (RPP) was calculated as follows: $RPP=HR\times SBP$ (expressed in beats per minute per millimeters of mercury). Stroke volume was calculated by dividing CO by HR. Total peripheral resistance was recorded in Wood units (ie, $TPR=MAP/CI$) and reported as millimeters of mercury per liter per minute per square meter.

RESULTS

Anthropometric Data

Means and SDs of anthropometric data for the two groups are presented in Table 1. Analyses revealed no significant differences between the groups in age, height, weight, body surface area, or body mass (ie, Quetelet Index) (all $P>.54$).

Physical Working Capacity

The maximum physical working capacity (aerobic power) was indexed by body weight in kilograms and was not significantly different between the groups (group without a family history of CAD, 17.8±2.7 kg/min per kilogram [mean±SD]; group with a family history of CAD, 17.9±2.5 kg/min per kilogram; $P>.96$). These values are consistent with the 50th to 75th percentile values obtained in previous upright cycle ergometer studies in our laboratory with boys of this age range.[7]

Table 2.—Hemodynamic Responses During Preexercise, Peak Exercise, and Recovery Stages by Coronary Artery Disease (CAD) History Group*

Hemodynamic Variable	Preexercise		Peak		Recovery		Effects†
	CAD−	CAD+	CAD−	CAD+	CAD−	CAD+	
Heart rate, BPM	74.7 (9.9)	80.8 (14.4)	178.8 (23.7)	174.3 (18.1)	107.4 (13.8)	110.0 (15.1)	B
Blood pressure, mm Hg							
Systolic	109.8 (10.1)‡	120.9 (10.7)	147.6 (16.3)§	166.0 (23.1)	123.5 (16.1)	119.9 (11.5)	B, C
Diastolic	72.8 (9.9)	75.3 (12.8)	78.3 (13.4)	77.9 (16.3)	68.3 (12.0)	65.9 (10.5)	B
MAP	85.2 (7.8)	90.5 (10.5)	101.4 (9.4)	107.9 (11.8)	86.7 (12.0)	83.9 (8.8)	B
Cardiac index, L/min per m^2	2.46 (0.43)‡	2.04 (0.48)	5.88 (1.28)	4.93 (1.26)	4.15 (0.99)	3.47 (0.91)	A, B
Total peripheral resistance, mm Hg/L per min per m^2	29.06 (5.79)‡	38.6 (12.5)	14.7 (4.45)§	19.7 (5.88)	18.02 (5.55)	21.72 (6.83)	A, B
Stroke volume, mL/BPM	37.4 (9.2)‡	29.4 (8.2)	37.1 (9.8)§	30.9 (5.8)	43.8 (12.8)	35.6 (8.7)	A, B
Rate pressure product, BPM mm Hg	8394.7 (886.3)‡	9747.2 (1829.9)	26 500.8 (4972.1)	28 969.4 (5502.9)	13 391.9 (3090.6)	12 863.2 (1703.4)	B

*CAD− indicates no family history of CAD; CAD+, family history of CAD; BPM, beats per minute; and MAP, mean arterial pressure. Values are mean (SD).

†A indicates main effect for family history of CAD (all $P<.05$); B, main effect for stage of exercise (all $P<.01$); and C, family history by stage of exercise interaction effect ($P<.01$).

‡Significant difference at preexercise stage, as determined by univariate testing (all $P<.05$).

§Significant difference at peak exercise, as determined by univariate testing (all $P<.05$).

Hemodynamic Responses to Exercise

The means and SDs for all hemodynamic responses during preexercise, peak exercise, and recovery stages for each group are presented in Table 2. A series of 2 (negative and positive family history) × 3 (preexercise, peak exercise, and recovery) repeated measures analyses of variance with Greenhouse-Geiser corrections[28] were conducted for each hemodynamic response. With these two-way analyses of variance, three terms are tested for statistical significance (ie, family history [negative or positive], stage of exercise [preexercise, peak, or recovery], and the family history × stage of exercise interaction). If the interaction is significant, it means that the two groups do not show the same pattern of response across the various stages of exercise. A significant main effect for family history would (in the absence of a significant interaction) mean that one group showed a higher level of response at all stages of exercise. A significant main effect for stage of exercise would indicate that both family history groups exhibited the same pattern of significant changes in cardiovascular responses to exercise.

As illustrated in Table 2, exercise produced the expected changes in all hemodynamic responses. This was verified by significant stage of exercise main effects for all hemodynamic responses (all $F>5.3$, all $P<.01$), indicating that exercise caused significant increases in SBP, DBP, MAP, HR, stroke volume, RPP, and CI, while TPR decreased.

HR

No significant differences were obtained between the groups at preexercise, peak exercise, or recovery stages (all $P>.20$). Likewise, the group × stage interaction was not significant ($P>.26$).

BP

A significant interaction effect was observed between family history and stage of exercise for SBP ($F[2,42]=6.2$, $P<.005$), with the positive family history group exhibiting greater SBP at preexercise ($P<.02$) and peak exercise ($P<.03$) stages, but not at recovery ($P>.53$). No family history × stage interaction or family history main effect approached significance for DBP or MAP (all $P>.18$). No significant differences between the groups were noted for DBP or MAP at preexercise, peak exercise, or recovery stages (all $P>.13$).

CI

A significant family history main effect was obtained ($F[1,23]=5.9$, $P<.02$). As shown in Table 2, the negative family history group exhibited a greater CI at all times. These differences were 0.42 L/min per square meter at preexercise, 0.95 L/min per square meter at peak exercise, and 0.68 L/min per square meter at recovery.

TPR

A significant family history main effect was noted ($F[1,21]=6.1$, $P<.02$). The positive family history group produced greater TPR with mean differences greatest during preexercise (9.5 mm Hg/L per minute per square meter) followed by peak exercise and recovery (5.0 and 3.7 mm Hg/L per minute per square meter, respectively). The group × stage interaction was not significant ($P>.25$).

Stroke Volume

A significant family history main effect was observed ($F[1,23]=6.0$, $P<.02$), with the negative family history group found to exhibit higher stroke volume across all phases, as illustrated in Table 2. Mean differences between the two groups at preexercise, peak exercise, and recovery stages were 8.0, 6.2, and 8.2 mL per beats per minute, respectively. The group × stage interaction was not significant ($P>.64$).

RPP

The positive family history group exhibited higher RPP during preexercise only ($P<.05$). Neither family history nor the family history × stage interaction approached significance (both $P>.24$).

Additional Analyses

Because there were preexercise differences between the groups in terms of SBP, TPR, and stroke volume, data from peak exercise and recovery stages were reanalyzed with analyses of covariance using the respective preexercise values as covariates. For SBP and TPR, the results were similar to those of the unadjusted analyses with the positive family history group exhibiting larger increases in SBP ($F[1,20]=9.73$, $P<.005$) and less attenuation of TPR ($F[1,20]=4.5$, $P<.05$). No significant differences were observed for stroke volume ($P>.51$).

COMMENT

Individuals with a positive family history of CAD have been found to exhibit greater hemodynamic reactivity to laboratory stressors.[15,16] These studies have typically involved young white adults.[15,16] Seven- to 10-year-old black boys were the subjects of our study. Boys who had a family history of CAD exhibited greater SBP and TPR at preexercise and peak exercise stages than did boys who had no family history of CAD. Adjustment for these preexercise differences indicated that the positive family history group exhibited greater increases in SBP and less attenuation in TPR in response to exercise.

Total peripheral resistance is a calculated value; it is inversely related to CO and is directly related to MAP. The greater TPR of the boys in the positive family history group at preexercise and peak exercise was associated with a lower CO. Although the boys in the positive family history group had a lower CI at peak exercise than those in the negative family history group, their power output was the same. This suggests the possibility of a more efficient cardiovascular system in the boys in the positive family history group. However, because their SBP and myocardial tension were higher, as expressed by the RPP, myocardial oxygen consumption should have been higher as well. Sarnoff et al[29] has demonstrated that myocardial tension is directly related to the RPP. At peak exercise, the RPP in boys with a family history of CAD was comparable with the boys without a family history of CAD. This suggests that each group achieved the same functional result through different mechanisms. The boys in the positive family history group achieved their power output with a lower HR response. Their peak HR response was slightly less than that in boys in the negative family history group, but their SBP was significantly greater. These responses are consistent with a baroreceptor hypothesis that suggests that individuals with a family history of CAD may possess an intrinsically greater vascular tone. The prolonged effect of long-term increased myocardial tension on a child's myocardium is unclear.

Because the boys with a positive family history demonstrated greater SBP at preexercise related to both lower CI and higher TPR, there is a strong suspicion that there is an inherent difference in autonomic regulation of the circulatory responses. The consistency of these findings with those of a previous study[24] strongly suggests differences in autonomic control of the circulatory system. In that study 10-year-old black boys exhibited greater TPR during preexercise, peak exercise, and recovery stages than white boys. The influence of family history on the hemodynamic response differences was not assessed.[24]

There was a trend toward greater CI in the boys with a negative family history than in those with a positive family history at peak exercise and recovery. The magnitude of change in CI from resting to peak and from peak to recovery were similar in the two groups. For the negative family history group, CI increased by 239% from resting to peak, and for the positive family history group the increase was 242%. This suggests that the two groups responded similarly in their CI response to the demands of exercise, although the positive family history group began at a lower level. From peak exercise to recovery, CI in both groups decreased by 30%. This reinforces the likelihood that their CI responses to the metabolic requirements of the task were similar. Therefore, the elevation in the TPR of the boys in the positive family history group may be secondary to an increase of vascular tone (resistance). This suggests that the primary difference in the boys with a positive family history of CAD is increased TPR secondary to increased vascular tone and is not caused by a lower CI, which appears to vary appropriately with the metabolic requirement.

Differences in cardiovascular responses between the two groups may be due in part to factors related to family history of essential hypertension. However, this is unlikely, as several subjects in the negative family history group had family histories of hypertension and not all subjects in the positive family history group had a positive family history of hypertension. On the other hand, perhaps combined effects of family history of early myocardial infarction and essential hypertension have additive, multiplicative, or symbiotic effects on children's cardiovascular responses to stress. The sample size of our study does not permit adequate evaluation of this issue. Research is warranted to address the separate and combined effects of a history of both CAD and essential hypertension in first- and second-degree relatives on children's hemodynamic responses to laboratory stressors.

Perhaps the blacks with a positive family history in our study are not only more likely to exhibit exaggerated BP reactivity to stress but are also more prone to exhibit physiologic reactivity to the laboratory conditions and situations surrounding the test itself. Other findings indicate that blacks compared with whites exhibit greater pressor responses to the mere presence of laboratory personnel and the surrounding laboratory environment.[9,19] Young adults who have a positive family history have been found to exhibit higher prestressor BP during competitive stressor tasks compared with negative history cohorts.[16] Thus, prestressor cardiovascular response differences may be due to the positive family history group experiencing greater anticipatory anxiety and relaxation difficulties.

The possibility also exists that the preexercise BP differences were due to differences in hemodynamic regulatory mechanisms between the two groups. Structural changes in the vasculature may have already occurred in the positive family history group, possibly due to genetic predisposition and/or early effects of environmental stress. Other differences between the two groups might be responsible for the preexercise BP differences, including differences in sodium, potassium, and calcium intakes and their influence on arteriolar smooth-muscle activity.[30]

Future studies should address these possibilities with attention to the establishment of adequate baseline levels before subjects are exposed to various stressors. One approach that would alleviate prestressor differences between groups related to anticipatory anxiety is that used by Obrist et al[31] in which subjects' baseline measures are established in a separate session after exposure to the stressor.

The current findings add to the accumulating evidence[8-10,12,24] that greater BP responses to physical and psychological stress among blacks may be due to greater TPR, even if the stressor is primarily β-adrenergic mediated, as in our study. Prospective studies are needed to determine whether individuals with a family history of cardiovascular diseases (ie, CAD and/or essential hypertension) who also exhibit exaggerated cardiovascular reactivity to stress are more likely to develop earlier clinical manifestations of other markers of cardiovascular disease (eg, left ventricular hypertrophy and S-T segment changes on echocardiography). Such studies will help identify mechanisms involved in the development of cardiovascular diseases and will permit the development of effective intervention programs (eg, physical activity and stress management as buffers against hemodynamic reactivity to stress) that could be incorporated into the pediatrician's armamentarium to promote a healthier population of children and to help prevent adult onset of cardiovascular diseases.

This research was supported by grants HL41781 and HL35073 from the National Institutes of Health, Bethesda, Md, and research grant awards from the Research Institute and Department of Pediatrics at the Medical College of Georgia, Augusta, and the Fraternal Order of Eagles Chapter 1197, Augusta, Ga.

The authors thank Pamela Hawkins for secretarial assistance, Thomas Rhodes for statistical support, and Bonnie Hadden, RCT, Pauline Asihene, Jennifer Kenrick, Leonteen McNeal, Jinny Smith, Paula Williams, and Ellen Wilson, MS, for assistance in data collection.

References

1. Gillum RF, Liu KC. Coronary heart disease mortality in United States' blacks, 1940-1978: trends and unanswered questions. *Am Heart J.* 1984;108:728-732.

2. Leaverton PE, Feinleib M, Thom T. Coronary heart disease mortality in United States' blacks, 1968-1978: interstate variation. *Am Heart J.* 1984;108:732-737.

3. Schneiderman N. Psychophysiologic factors in atherogenesis and coronary artery disease. *Circulation.* 1987;76(suppl 1):41-47.

4. Manuck SB, Krantz DS. Psychophysiologic reactivity in coronary heart disease and essential hypertension. In: Matthews KA, Weiss SM, Detre T, et al, eds. *Handbook of Stress, Reactivity, and Cardiovascular Disease.* New York, NY: John Wiley & Sons Inc; 1986:11-34.

5. Keys A, Taylor HL, Blackburn H, Brozek J, Anderson JT. Mortality and coronary heart disease among men studied for 23 years. *Arch Intern Med.* 1971;128:201-204.

6. Manuck SB, Kaplan JR, Clarkson TB. Behaviorally-induced heart rate reactivity and atherosclerosis in cynomolgus monkeys. *Psychosom Med.* 1983;45:95-108.

7. Alpert BS, Flood NL, Strong WB, et al. Responses to ergometer exercise in a healthy biracial population of children. *J Pediatr.* 1982;101:538-545.

8. Anderson NB, Lane JD, Muranaka M, Williams RB, Houseworth ST. Racial differences in blood pressure and forearm vascular responses to the cold face stimulus. *Psychosom Med.* 1988;50:57-63.

9. Light KC, Obrist PA, Sherwood A, James SA, Strogatz DS. Effects of race and marginally elevated blood pressure on responses to stress. *Hypertension.* 1987;10:555-563.

10. Light KC, Sherwood A. Race, borderline hypertension and hemodynamic responses to behavioral stress before and after beta-adrenergic blockade. *Health Psychol.* 1989;8:577-595.

11. Murphy JK, Alpert BS, Moes DM, Somes GW. Race and reactivity. *Hypertension.* 1986;8:1075-1083.

12. Treiber FA, Musante L, Braden D, et al. Racial differences in hemodynamic responses to the cold face stimulus in children and adults. *Psychosom Med.* 1990;52:286-296.

13. Nora JJ, Lortscher RM, Spangler RD, Nora AH, Kimberling WJ. Genetic epidemiology of early-onset ischemic heart disease. *Circulation.* 1980;61:503-508.

14. Barrett-Conner E, Knaw K. Family history of heart attack as an independent predictor of death due to cardiovascular disease. *Circulation.* 1984;69:1065-1069.

15. Stoney CM, Matthews KA. Parental history of hypertension and myocardial infarction predicts cardiovascular responses to behavioral stressors in middle-aged men and women. *Psychophysiology.* 1988;25:269-277.

16. Lawler KA, Schmied LA. Cardiovascular responsivity, type A behavior, and parental history of heart disease in young women. *Psychophysiology.* 1986;23:28-32.

17. Treiber FA, Mabe PA, Riley WT, McDuffie M, Strong WB, Levy M. Children's type A behavior: the role of parental hostility and family history of cardiovascular disease. *J Soc Behav Personality.* 1990;5:183-199.

18. Musante L, Treiber FA, Strong WB, Levy M. Family history of hypertension and cardiovascular reactivity to forehead cold stimulation in black male children. *J Psychosom Res.* 1990;34:111-116.

19. Anderson NB, Lane JD, Taguchi F, Williams RB. Patterns of cardiovascular responses to stress as a function of race and parental hypertension in men. *Health Psychol.* 1989;8:525-540.

20. Roberts J, Rowland M. Hypertension in adults 25-74 years of age, United States, 1971-1975. *Vital Health Stat 11.* 1981; 221:10-15.

21. DuBois D, DuBois EF. A formula to estimate the approximate surface area if height and weight be known. *Arch Intern Med.* 1916;17:863-871.

22. Vaughn VC, McKay RJ, eds. *Nelson Textbook of Pediatrics.* 10th ed. Philadelphia, Pa: WB Saunders Co; 1975:43.

23. Report of the second task force on blood pressure control in children. 1987 task force on blood pressure control in children from the National Heart, Lung and Blood Institute, Bethesda, Maryland. *Pediatrics.* 1987;79:1-25.

24. Arensman FW, Treiber FA, Gruber MP, Strong WB. Exercise induced differences in cardiac output, blood pressure and systemic vascular resistance in a healthy biracial population of ten-year-old boys. *AJDC.* 1989;143:212-216.

25. Alpert BS, Flood NL, Balfour IC, Strong WB. Automated blood pressure measurement during ergometer exercise in children. *Cathet Cardiovasc Diagn.* 1982;8:525-533.

26. Marx GR, Hicks RW, Allen HD, Kinzer SM. Measurement of cardiac output and exercise factor by pulsed Doppler echocardiography during supine bicycle ergometry in normal young adolescent boys. *J Am Coll Cardiol.* 1987;10: 430-434.

27. Daley PJ, Sagar KB, Wann LS. Doppler echocardiographic measurement of flow velocity in the ascending aorta during supine and upright exercise. *Br Heart J.* 1985;54:562-567.

28. Vasey MW, Thayer JF. The continuing problem of false positives in repeated measures ANOVA in psychophysiology. *Psychophysiology.* 1987; 24:479-486.

29. Sarnoff SJ, Braunwald GH, Welch GH, Case RB, Stainsby WN, Macruz R. Hemodynamic determinants of oxygen consumption of the heart with special reference to the tension-time index. *Am J Epidemiol.* 1958;192:148-156.

30. Falkner B. Is there black hypertension? *Hypertension.* 1987;10:551-553.

31. Obrist PA, Light KC, James SA, Strogatz DS. Cardiovascular responses to stress, I: measures of myocardial response and relationships to high resting systolic pressure and parental hypertension. *Psychophysiology.* 1987; 24:65-78.

Physiologic Responses to Playing a Video Game

Karen R. Segal, EdD, William H. Dietz, MD, PhD

• The displacement of sports and other physical activities by television and video may contribute to the associations among television viewing, obesity, and reduced physical fitness. Because video games are widely played by children and adolescents, we assessed the metabolic and cardiovascular responses to video game playing. Heart rate, blood pressure, and oxygen consumption were measured serially over 30 minutes in 32 males and females aged 16 to 25 years (mean±SEM, 20±1 years) while they played the "Ms Pac-Man" video game under standard laboratory conditions and compared with measurements made in a standing but inactive position. Playing the video game significantly increased heart rate, systolic and diastolic blood pressure, and oxygen consumption. Energy expenditure increased from 6.08±0.24 kJ/min while the subjects stood inactive to 10.94±0.49 kJ/min while they played. The increase in metabolic rate and cardiovascular stimulation was similar in magnitude to mild-intensity exercise.
(*AJDC*. 1991;145:1034-1036)

Reduced physical activity has been associated with obesity in childhood and adolescence, although the question of whether obesity precedes or is a consequence of inactivity remains.[1] Television viewing may indirectly contribute to obesity in American youth by several means, including sedentary behavior with the associated reduction in energy expenditure, as well as increased food consumption.[2,3] Also, in settings that lacked television, the introduction of television displaced sports.[4,5]

American children and adolescents spend more than 20 hours per week watching television.[6] In addition, they spend considerable time playing arcade and home video games. The recent increase in sales of home video games suggests that the time spent playing these games has also increased substantially, although firm estimates are lacking. In contrast to the experience with video games a decade ago,[7] the newer video games appear to retain their users' interest over time.

In view of the current popularity of video games, a quantitative assessment of the metabolic and cardiovascular stimulation associated with playing these games is warranted. To our knowledge, no evidence exists that suggests a linkage between obesity and video games. These games involve a degree of isometric muscular contraction and mental stress, both of which could elevate energy expenditure, heart rate, and blood pressure. Previous studies have documented the increases in heart rate and blood pressure induced by playing a television video game,[8,9] but the energy expended while playing one of these games has not been studied previously, to our knowledge. The objective of this study was to quantify the energy cost and cardiovascular responses to video game playing.

SUBJECTS AND METHODS

Subjects

Twenty males and 12 females between ages 16 and 25 years (mean±SEM age, 20±1 years) participated in this study. The subjects were healthy, normotensive nonsmokers. All subjects had some experience playing video games. The study protocol was approved by the Institutional Review Board.

Procedures

The arcade version of "Ms Pac-Man" (Bally Midway Corp, Franklin Park, Ill) was used in this study. Prior to the test session, time was allotted for the subjects to become familiar with playing while breathing through the mouthpiece and breathing valve used for metabolic measurements. Baseline resting measurements were obtained while the subjects stood quietly in front of the video machine for 30 minutes. Oxygen consumption ($\dot{V}O_2$) was measured with open circuit respirometry. The assessment consisted of three measures of 5 minutes' duration each at 5, 15, and 25 minutes within the 30-minute baseline period. The subjects breathed through a low-resistance, one-way valve (Hans Rudolph, Kansas City, Mo). The volume of air was measured with a spirometer (Parkinson-Cowan CD-4, Braintree, Mass), and the expired air was collected in meteorological bags and passed through an infrared carbon dioxide (Beckman LB-2, Fullerton, Calif) and polarographic oxygen (Applied Electrochemistry S-3A, Sunnyvale, Calif) analyzer. Oxygen consumption, carbon dioxide production ($\dot{V}CO_2$), minute ventilation, and the respiratory quotient ($RQ = \dot{V}O_2/\dot{V}CO_2$) were calculated following standard procedures. Energy expenditure was estimated using the nonprotein energy equivalent for oxygen derived from the Weir equation[10]: $kJ = 4.2 \times \{[(RQ \times 1.1) + 3.9] \times \dot{V}O_2\}$.

Brachial artery blood pressure was measured using an aneroid sphygmomanometer, and heart rate was measured with electrocardiography.

The subjects were familiar with the objectives of the game. After a 15-minute warm-up, the subjects played continuously for

Accepted for publication January 23, 1991.
From the Division of Pediatric Cardiology, Department of Pediatrics, Mount Sinai School of Medicine, New York, NY (Dr Segal), and Division of Gastroenterology and Nutrition, New England Medical Center, Boston Mass (Dr Dietz).

Reprint requests to Mount Sinai School of Medicine, Division of Pediatric Cardiology, Box 1201, 1 Gustave Levy Pl, New York, NY 10029 (Dr Segal).

Physiologic Responses to Playing a Video Game		
Response	Resting (Mean ± SEM)	Playing (Mean ± SEM)
Metabolic rate, kJ/min*†		
All subjects	6.08 ± 0.24	10.94 ± 0.49
Males	6.67 ± 0.23	11.71 ± 0.59
Females	5.10 ± 0.25	9.68 ± 0.73
Oxygen consumption (Vo_2), mL/kg per min		
All subjects	4.34 ± 0.09	7.82 ± 0.29
Males	4.41 ± 0.12	7.76 ± 0.36
Females	4.21 ± 0.14	7.93 ± 0.48
Heart rate, beats/min*		
All subjects	75 ± 2	103 ± 2
Males	73 ± 2	99 ± 2
Females	78 ± 3	109 ± 3
Blood pressure, mm Hg		
Systolic*		
All subjects	121 ± 2	138 ± 3
Males	122 ± 2	139 ± 2
Females	120 ± 4	137 ± 3
Diastolic*		
All subjects	83 ± 2	89 ± 2
Males	83 ± 2	89 ± 2
Females	81 ± 3	88 ± 2

*$P<.05$ for resting vs playing.
†$P<.05$ for males vs females.

a 30-minute test period, during which three 5-minute measurements of oxygen consumption were made, beginning at 5, 15, and 25 minutes. The validity and reliability of indirect calorimetry in our laboratory have been described previously.[11] Heart rate and blood pressure were measured during each of the three oxygen consumption measurement periods. In some cases, the timing of the measurements was adjusted to accommodate interruptions in the players' activity, such as lulls between stages in the game or between games. The scores achieved for complete games were recorded and averaged for each subject.

Design and Statistical Analyses

Analyses of variance performed with repeated measures on the data obtained from the three 5-minute measurements during the periods while the subjects either stood but were inactive or played the video game indicated that time had no significant effect on the physiologic responses (ie, heart rate, blood pressure, and oxygen consumption). Therefore, the mean values of the three measurements were used in subsequent data analyses. Two-way analyses of variance with repeated measures,[12] using sex (male vs female) and activity (resting or playing), were applied to the data to test whether heart rate, systolic and diastolic blood pressure, and energy expenditure were significantly different while the subjects were playing the game than when they stood in front of the machine but were inactive. Pearson's product-moment correlation coefficients[12] were computed to study the relationships among such variables as age, game score, and the increases in heart rate, blood pressure, and energy expenditure.

RESULTS

Heart rate, systolic and diastolic blood pressure, and Vco_2 were significantly higher when the subjects were playing the game than when they stood quietly in front of the machine (Table). No differences were found between males and females with respect to heart rate or blood pressure either at rest or while playing the video game. Although absolute energy expenditure at rest and while playing the video game was greater for males than females because of their greater body weight (mean ± SEM body weight, 74 ± 3 kg vs 60 ± 3 kg), the magnitudes of the differences between the resting and active values were similar for males and females. Also, when the data were expressed relative to body weight, the responses of the males and females were similar (Table). The energy expended by males and females during 30 minutes of resting and playing the video game is shown in the Figure.

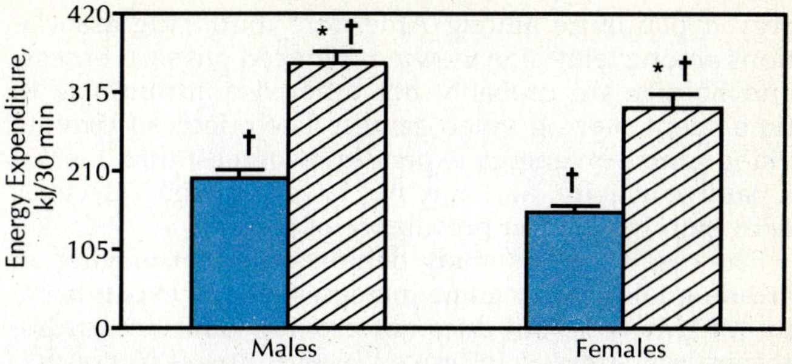

Energy expenditure of males and females during 30 minutes of standing at rest (open bars) and playing a video game (hatched bars). Energy expenditure was greater for males than females under both conditions because of their greater body weight, but the proportional increase in metabolic rate was similar. The asterisk indicates P<.01 for rest vs playing; and dagger, P<.05 for males vs females.

The increase in energy expenditure while playing was correlated with the increase in systolic blood pressure ($r=.64$, $P<.001$), perhaps because of the isometric activity and small muscle mass involved. Game score, an index of performance, and age were uncorrelated with any of the physiologic response variables.

COMMENT

The primary finding of this study was that video games are not a passive activity and the energy cost of the game approximates mild-intensity exercise. The energy cost of playing the video game was similar to that of walking at a pace of ≈2.0 mph.[13] Despite the potentially beneficial effects of video games on energy expenditure, video games are clearly not a substitute for more intensive exercise because the level of cardiorespiratory stress from playing the video game is not sufficient to improve cardiorespiratory fitness.[13] Furthermore, other aspects of video games may have adverse effects, such as "Nintendo epilepsy,"[14] a photoconvulsive response to the video game image, or "nintendinitis,"[15] tendinitis attributable to excessive playing of video games.

The increase in energy expenditure while playing was correlated with the increase in systolic blood pressure ($r=.64$, $P<.001$), perhaps a result of the relatively small muscle mass and isometric activity of hand grip involved in playing the video game. The increase in systolic blood pressure from playing the video game was greater than would be observed for the same degree of Vo_2 during an exercise that involves the whole body, such as walking.[16]

Although television video games may displace sports and other physical activities that involve a far greater energy expenditure among American youth, the associations among television viewing, reduced physical fitness, and obesity are probably not otherwise attributable to time spent playing video games. The effects of playing video games on energy expenditure suggest that it is not a passive activity, and may not have the same effects as television has on the prevalence of obesity.

The results of this study demonstrate that playing an arcade-quality video game increases energy expenditure by roughly 80%, but does not provide sufficient cardiorespiratory stress to improve physical fitness in youth.

References

1. Rosenbaum R, Leibel RL. Pathophysiology of childhood obesity. *Adv Pediatr.* 1988;35:73-138.
2. Dietz WH, Gortmaker SL. Do we fatten our children at the TV set? Television viewing and obesity in children and adolescents. *Pediatrics.* 1985;75:807-812.
3. Taras HL, Sallis JF, Patterson TL, Nader PR, Nelson JA. Television's influence on children's diet and physical activity. *J Dev Behav Pediatr.* 1989;10:176-180.
4. Williams TM, Handford AG. Television and other leisure activities. In: Williams TM, ed. *The Impact of Television: a Natural Experiment in Three Communities.* Orlando, Fla: Academic Press Inc; 1986:143-213.
5. Murray JP, Kippox S. Children's social behavior in three towns with differing television experience. *J Commun.* 1978;30:19-29.
6. AC Nielsen Company. *Nielsen Report on Television 1989.* Northbrook, Ill: Nielsen Media Research; 1989.
7. Creasey GL, Myers BJ. Video games and children: effects on leisure activities, schoolwork, and peer involvement. *Merrill-Palmer Quart.* 1986;32:251-262.
8. Murphy JK, Alpert JS, Willey ES, Somes GW. Cardiovascular reactivity to psychological stress in healthy children. *Psychophysiology.* 1988;25:144-152.
9. Dembrowski TM, MacDougall JM, Shields JL, Petitto J, Lushene R. Components of the type A coronary-prone behavior pattern and cardiovascular responses to psychomotor performance challenge. *J Behav Med.* 1978;1:159-176.
10. Weir JB. New method for calculating metabolic rate with special reference to protein metabolism. *J Physiol.* 1949;109:1-9.
11. Segal KR. Comparison of indirect calorimetric measurements of resting energy expenditure with a ventilated hood, face mask, and mouthpiece. *Am J Clin Nutr.* 1986;45:1420-1423.
12. Winer BJ. *Statistical Principles in Experimental Design.* 2nd ed. New York, NY: McGraw-Hill International Book Co; 1971.
13. McArdle WD, Katch FI, Katch VI. *Exercise Physiology: Energy, Nutrition, and Human Performance.* Philadelphia, Pa: Lea & Febiger; 1981:80-117.
14. Hart EJ. Nintendo epilepsy. *N Engl J Med.* 1990;322:1473.
15. Brasington R. Nintendinitis. *N Engl J Med.* 1990;322:1473-1474.
16. Astrand PO, Ekblom B, Messin R, Saltin B, Stenberg J. Intra-arterial blood pressure during exercise with different muscle groups. *J Appl Physiol.* 1965;20:253-256.

Arterial Catheter–Related Infections in Children

A 1-Year Cohort Analysis

Susanna Furfaro, MD; Marie Gauthier, MD; Jacques Lacroix, MD; Daniel Nadeau, MD; Lucette Lafleur, MD; Sylvain Mathews, MD

• To determine the incidence of infection secondary to arterial catheterization in children as well as the risk markers, we prospectively evaluated, during a 1-year period, all arterial catheters installed in children admitted to the pediatric intensive care unit. A total of 340 cannulas were placed in 310 children aged 80±4 months (mean±SEM) for a period of 64±4 hours. Most catheters were inserted percutaneously (99%) in the radial artery (86.5%). Ninety-two percent (313/340) of the catheters were sterile (group 1), 5% (17/340) were contaminated (<10 colony-forming units on semiquantitative culture) (group 2), and 3% (10/340) were considered either locally infected (ie, ≥10 colony-forming units) (eight of 10) or associated with a possible catheter-related sepsis (two of 10) (group 3, or infected group). The incidence of local inflammation at the insertion site was higher in group 2 than in group 1 (18% vs 2.9%) but not statistically different between groups 3 and 1 (10% vs 2.9%). The duration of arterial catheterization was longer in group 3 than in group 1 (125±31 vs 61±4 hours). The risk of infection was nonexistent in the first 48 hours of catheterization. Thereafter it was calculated as being 6.2% (10/161), but it correlated poorly with the duration of arterial catheterization. These results confirm the very low incidence of infection related to arterial catheterization in children. Thus, routine catheter reinsertion is, in our opinion, unjustified.

(*AJDC.* 1991;145:1037-1043)

Patients in intensive care units are at an elevated risk of developing nosocomial infections compared with the general hospital population; this is particularly true for young children.[1,2] These infections are mainly associated with some type of invasive monitoring or lifesupport system.[1,2] It thus becomes very important to de-termine the infectious risk associated with each of these procedures.

Arterial catheters are now considered a significant cause of catheter-related infection and septicemia in adults.[3] In the pediatric intensive care unit (PICU), arterial catheterization has become indispensable for hemodynamic monitoring purposes, and its use has increased sharply in the past 10 to 15 years. No prospective study with systematic cultures of arterial cannulas was available in the pediatric literature except for one performed during the neonatal period,[4] until we showed that the incidence of infection related to arterial catheterization was low in children.[5] However, this preliminary study was performed on a small sample of arterial catheters (70 catheters). This study was undertaken to determine more precisely the incidence of infection related to arterial catheterization in children and to characterize the risk markers.

PATIENTS AND METHODS

From September 15, 1988, through September 14, 1989, all children admitted to the St-Justine Hospital PICU and who required an arterial catheterization were included in this study.

Catheter Management

All catheter insertions were performed in the PICU or in the operating room. In most cases, an attempt was made to cannulate the radial artery percutaneously with a 2.5-cm, 22-gauge or a 3.2-cm, 20-gauge Teflon-coated catheter. If radial insertion was impossible, other sites were tried, usually the pedal, femoral, or brachial arteries. When percutaneous cannulation failed, the catheter was inserted by surgical cutdown. Techniques of insertion and site dressing have previously been described[5]; after insertion, catheters were covered with an adhesive taping without topical antibiotic or antiseptic ointments.

Catheter patency was ensured by the continuous infusion of heparinized saline solution (3 mL/h) through a continuous flow device located just distal to the transducer (Fig 1).[5] As in our previous study, two different arterial blood sampling systems were used: an extension set with T-connection (system A) or a check valve extension set with T-connection (system B).[5]

No component of the entire system, including the dressing, was changed during the study period unless it was found defective.

Accepted for publication January 28, 1991.

From the Departments of Pediatrics (Drs Furfaro, Gauthier, Lacroix, and Nadeau), Microbiology (Dr LaFleur), and Anesthesia (Dr Mathews), St-Justine Hospital, University of Montreal (Canada).

Presented in part at the 10th International Symposium on Intensive Care and Emergency Medicine, Brussels, Belgium, March 1990.

Reprint requests to Department of Pediatrics, St-Justine Hôpital, 3175 Côte St-Catherine, Montreal, Quebec, Canada H3T 1C5 (Dr Gauthier).

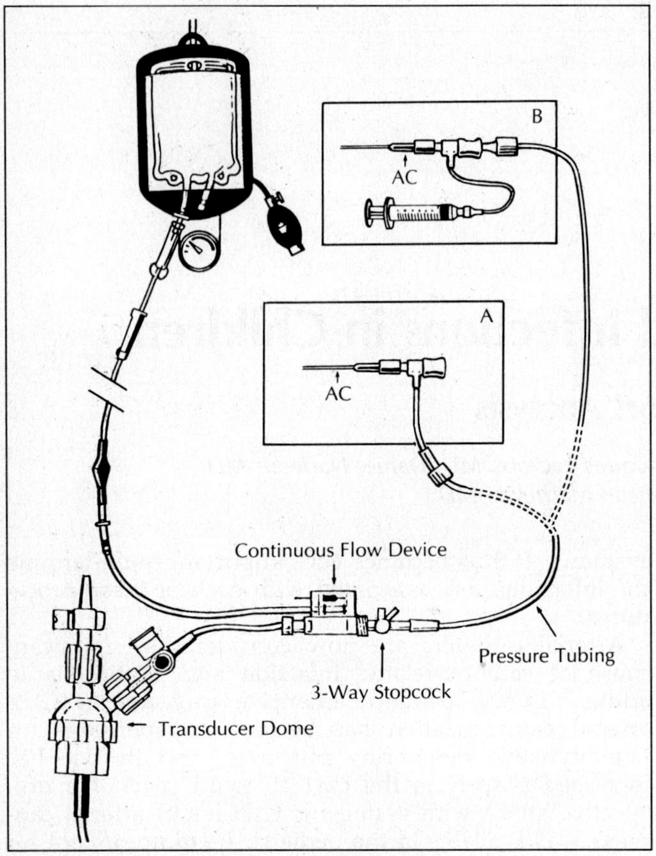

Fig 1.—*Diagram of the arterial line system (modified from Ducharme et al[5]). AC indicates arterial catheter.*

Study Protocol

The decision to remove the catheter was made by the patient's physician. When the catheter was no longer required, it was removed aseptically by an attending intensive care unit physician or nurse after local cutaneous disinfection with a 70% alcohol swab. The site was examined for the presence of local inflammation and purulence. The distal 2-cm segment of the catheter was cut with sterile scissors and placed in a sterile transport tube. If within 4 hours before catheter removal, a body temperature over 38.3°C was noted or clinical sepsis was suspected, a blood culture was obtained by venipuncture and 6 mL of infusion fluid was sampled from the nearest stopcock. Both were sent to the laboratory in broth blood culture bottles (Columbia; Chemical Products BDH Inc, Darmstadt, Germany).

In the laboratory, the 2-cm catheter segment was rolled on a blood agar plate by means of the semiquantitative (SQ) method described by Maki et al.[6] Our protocol for culturing the catheters has already been reported.[5]

For each catheter, the following data were noted: demographic information; conditions predisposing to infections, such as neutropenia (neutrophil count, $<1.0 \times 10^9$/L on any complete blood cell count during catheter insertion), documented immunodeficiency, corticosteroid therapy (more than 7 consecutive days of systemic steroid use within the month before catheter insertion), or other immunosuppressive therapy (more than 7 consecutive days of immunosuppression within the month before catheter insertion); systemic antimicrobial therapy given while the catheter was in place; all data on any suspected or proved infections of other sites; the mode (percutaneous vs cutdown), location (operating room or PICU), and site (radial, etc) of insertion; the system of arterial blood sampling (see above); the reason for removal; and the number of hours the catheter had been in place. The number of cannulation attempts required before each insertion was not recorded.

Definitions

Inflammation of the catheter site was diagnosed in the presence of lymphangitis, purulence, or at least two of the following: erythema, tenderness, increased warmth, or induration.[7] Local infection of the catheter site was defined as a positive SQ culture of the distal segment that yielded 10 or more colony-forming units (CFUs). A catheter was considered contaminated if between 1 and 9 CFUs were identified on SQ culture. A catheter tip with a positive broth culture but a negative SQ culture was considered neither infected nor contaminated and was therefore classified as negative. Catheter-related septicemia (CRS) was characterized by all the following criteria: (1) isolation of the same species of microorganism in significant number ($\geq$10 CFUs) on SQ culture of the catheter and blood cultures obtained by separate veni-puncture; (2) clinical and microbiologic data that disclosed no other apparent source of the bacteremia or fungemia; and (3) clinical features consistent with bloodstream infection.[7] Possible CRS was defined as follows: (1) isolation of a microorganism in significant number ($\geq$10 CFUs) on SQ culture of the catheter; (2) clinical and microbiologic data disclosing no other apparent source of infection; and (3) clinical features consistent with bloodstream infection. Clinical features were considered consistent with a bloodstream infection if a patient was sufficiently ill to warrant a septic workup, including at least a blood culture, and the introduction of systemic antibiotics while culture results were awaited. To diagnose a septicemia due to contaminated infusate and a catheter-related septicemia from other infected sites, we used the definitions of our previous study.[5]

Statistical Analysis

The significance of differences in characteristics among the various groups (cultured and noncultured, with and without contamination, with and without catheter-related infection) was determined by means of χ^2 with Yates' correction for discrete data (χ^2 without Yates' correction if df>1) and two-tailed Student's t test for continuous data. $P<.05$ was considered adequate to reject the null hypothesis. Mean values are presented with SEM.

Epidemiologic Analysis

Cumulative survival analysis[8] and calculations of the density of incidence of infectious complications[9] were based on epidemiologic methods described previously. For the cumulative survival analysis, the starting event was catheter placement and the terminal event was catheter infection. By definition, catheter infection was diagnosed on removal. The density of incidence of infectious complications per 10 000 hours of insertion was calculated for each day of insertion as follows: Density of incidence of infectious complications = ([cumulative number of infections] × 10 000)/cumulative number of hours of insertion. For example, up to day 4, five infections (local infection of the catheter site and possible CRS) had been diagnosed. For day 4, the density of incidence of infectious complications was thus the following: $(5 \times 10\,000)/(1255+3386+4205+2559)$, or 4.4. In this equation, the four numbers of the denominator represent the total number of hours of insertion for the catheters removed on days 1, 2, 3, and 4.

RESULTS

During the 1-year study period, 411 arterial catheters were inserted in 361 children. Of these catheters, 71 (17.5%) were not cultured because of accidental removal, contamination on withdrawal, or a failure to send the distal segment of the catheter to the laboratory. Table 1 compares the clinical characteristics of the cultured and noncultured catheters. There were no significant differences in both groups except for an increased rate of neutropenia (11.3% vs 2.4%; $P<.0015$), as well as an increased mortality (16.9% vs 5%; $P<.008$) in the noncultured group.

Table 1.—Characteristics of Cultured and Noncultured Catheters*

Characteristic	Cultured (n=340)	Noncultured (n=71)	*P*
Patient age, mo (mean±SEM)	80.9±3.6	68.8±3.7	NS
Duration of insertion, h (mean±SEM)	64.1±4.1	66.9±9.0	NS
Predisposing factors to infection, No. (%)			
Steroids	43 (12.7)	12 (16.9)	NS
OIA	35 (10.3)	12 (16.9)	NS
Neutropenia	8 (2.4)	8 (11.3)	<.0015†
Immune defect	2 (0.6)	0 (0)	NS
Percutaneous insertion, No. (%)	337 (99.1)	69 (97.2)	NS
Radial artery insertion site, No. (%)	294 (86.5)	63 (88.7)	NS
Use of antibiotics, No. (%)	281 (82.7)	61 (85.9)	NS
Local inflammation, No. (%)	13 (3.8)	1 (1.4)	NS
Reason for removal, No. (%)			
Malfunction	80 (23.5)	21 (29.6)	NS
Death	17 (5)	12 (16.9)	<.001†
Due to infection	3	2	NS
Without autopsy	5	6	NS

*OIA indicates other immunosuppressive therapy; NS, not significant.
†Significant (*P*<.05) by χ^2 test with Yates' correction.

Table 2.—Characteristics of Catheters With Negative Cultures and of Catheters Associated With Local Infection (LINF) and Possible Catheter-Related Septicemia (PCRS)*

Characteristic	Negative (n=313)	LINF+PCRS (n=10)	*P*
Patient age, mo (mean±SEM)	80.0±3.8	80.2±23.1	NS
Duration of insertion, h (mean±SEM)	61.4±4.1	125.4±31.0	<.008†
Predisposing factors to infection, No. (%)	47 (15)	2 (20)	NS
Percutaneous insertion, No. (%)	311 (99.4)	9 (90.0)	NS
Location of insertion, No. (%)			
Operating room	245 (78.2)	6 (60.0)	NS
PICU	68 (21.8)	4 (40.0)	. . .
Site of insertion, No. (%)			
Radial	269 (85.9)	9 (90.0)	NS
Dorsalis pedis	30 (9.6)	1 (10.0)	. . .
Femoral	12 (3.9)	0 (0.0)	. . .
Brachial	2 (0.6)	0 (0.0)	. . .
Arterial line system, No. (%)			
System A	113 (36.1)	8 (80.0)	<.013‡
System B	200 (63.9)	2 (20.0)	. . .
Use of antibiotics, No. (%)	259 (82.8)	8 (80.0)	NS
Local inflammation, No. (%)	9 (2.9)	1 (10.0)	NS
Reason for removal, No. (%)			
End of medical indication	206 (65.8)	5 (50.0)	NS
Malfunction	73 (23.3)	2 (20.0)	NS
Death	16 (5.1)	1 (10.0)	NS

*NS indicates not significant; PICU, pediatric intensive care unit.
†Significant (*P*<.05) by two-tailed T test.
‡Significant (*P*<.05) by χ^2 test with Yates' correction.

The 340 cultured catheters were placed in 310 children aged 80.9±3.6 months (range, 0.1 to 216 months) for a period of 64.1±4.1 hours (range, 4 to 665 hours) (Table 1). The sex distribution was 62% (210/340) boys and 38% (130/340) girls. Most catheters (99%) were inserted percutaneously in a radial artery (86.5%); 78% (266/340) were placed in the operating room and 22% (74/340) in the PICU. Seventy-six percent (257/340) of the catheters were collected from surgical patients after major operations, 9% (32 /340) from children with severe traumatic injuries, 8% (28/340) from medical patients with respiratory failure, and 7% (23/340) from children with other various medical diseases. No burned patients were studied. The end of medical indication was the reason for cannula removal in 66% of cases, followed by malfunction (24%), death (5%), and local ischemia (3%). Thirty-eight catheters (11%) were collected from patients with a culture-proved focus of infection unrelated to the catheter, such as pneumonia, epiglottitis, or pyelonephritis; 17 (46%) of these catheters were exposed to documented bacteremia. Eighty-three percent of the study population received systemic antibiotics during the time the catheter remained in place.

Cultures were negative in 92% (313/340) of the cultured cannulas (group 1). Five percent (17/340) were contaminated (group 2), and 3% (10/340) were considered either locally infected (eight) or associated with a possible catheter-related septicemia (two) (group 3, or infected group). No cases of CRS were identified.

There were no significant differences in patient characteristics between group 1 and group 2 with respect to age (80.0±3.8 months vs 97.3±15.8 months), duration of insertion (61.4±4.1 hours vs 76.5±21.5 hours), the presence of at least one predisposing factor to infection (15% vs 24%), diagnosis on admission, site of insertion, percutaneous insertion, antibiotic use (83% vs 82%), or reason for removal. The only statistically significant difference was a lower incidence of local inflammation at the insertion site for negative catheters (3% vs 18%, *P*=.012). Eighteen microorganisms were recovered from the 17 contaminated cannulas, among which *Staphylococcus epidermidis* (four catheters), viridans *Streptococcus* (three catheters), *Staphylococcus capitis* (two catheters), and *Staphylococcus simulans* (two catheters).

Table 2 depicts the characteristics of catheters with negative cultures (group 1) compared with group 3 catheters. No significant difference was noted with respect to age, predisposing factors to infection, site of insertion, percutaneous insertion, use of antibiotics, and justification for removal. The incidence of local inflammation at the insertion site was not higher in group 3 catheters. Two factors were associated with an increased rate of catheter-related infection: type A system for arterial blood sampling and duration of insertion. Catheters with system A were not left in place for a longer period than cannulas with system B (63.2±5.4 hours vs 65.9±5.5 hours, *P*=.76).

The relationship between infection and duration of catheter placement is shown in Figs 2 through 4. Figure

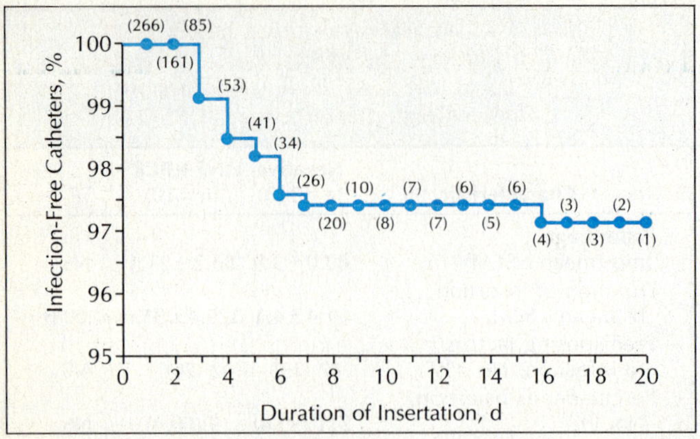

Fig 2.—*Proportion of catheters free of infectious complications among the total group of 340 catheters. Percentages are expressed by cumulative survival analysis. Numbers in parentheses represent the numbers of cannulas still in place at the end of each interval.*

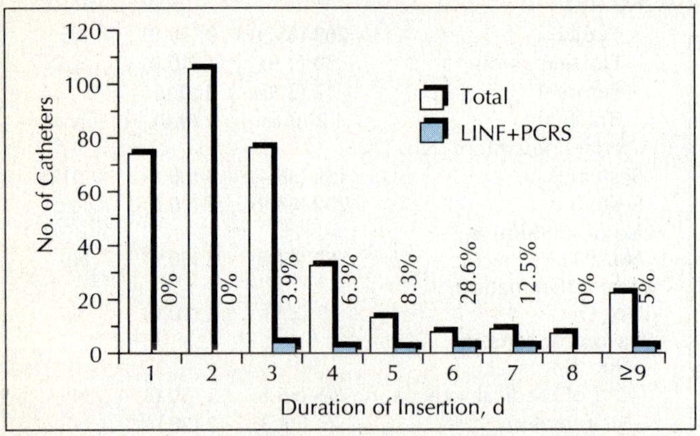

Fig 3.—*Relationship of infection caused by arterial catheters to duration of catheter insertion. LINF indicates local infection of the catheter site; PCRS, possible catheter-related septicemia. Percentages indicate the proportions of catheters with LINF or PCRS vs the numbers of catheters removed.*

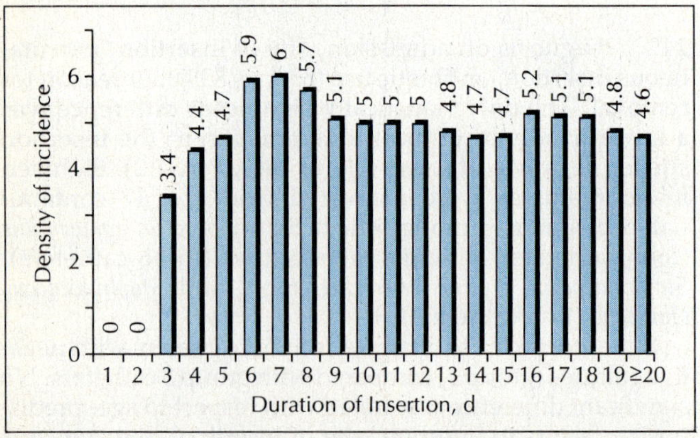

Fig 4.—*Density of incidence of arterial catheter–related infectious complications. The daily probability of infectious complications per 10 000 hours of insertion is represented for days 1 through 20.*

2 depicts the cumulative survival rate of catheters that remained free of infectious complications (ie, groups 1 and 2) from days 1 through 20. Most catheters (99.1% [337/340]) remained infection free even if left in place up to 72 hours, and 97.1% (330/340) were infection free even if in place for up to 20 days. No catheters became infected within the first 2 days of insertion (Fig 3). After the first 48 hours, the risk of infection was 6.2% (10/161), with no precise correlation existing between duration of catheterization and infection; the incidence of infection increased after day 2 and then reached a plateau, with continued catheter use not being associated with significantly more infectious complications. The density of incidence of infectious complications describes the number of infections per 10 000 hours of insertion for each of days 1 through 20 (Fig 4). It is another representation of the same phenomenon: the density of incidence of infections increased from 3.4 per 10 000 hours of insertion on day 3 to 5.9 on day 6 and decreased to 4.6 thereafter.

Nine of the 10 infected catheters yielded *S epidermidis*, and one catheter yielded both *S epidermidis* and *S simulans*.

No contamination of infusate was detected in the 13 infusions sampled. Of the 18 catheters exposed to bacteremia or fungemia from unrelated sites of infection, not one was subsequently positive on SQ culture for the bloodstream pathogen. No case of septicemia due to contaminated infusate or of CRS from other infected sites was thus identified.

Six broth cultures were positive while the SQ culture remained negative. The organisms identified were *S epidermidis* (three cases), *Corynebacterium* species (one case), streptococcus MG intermedius (one case), and *Escherichia coli* (one case).

COMMENT

We had already shown in a previous report that the incidence of infection related to arterial catheterization in children is low[5]; indeed, not one of the 70 catheters studied was identified as being infected or as being the source of a CRS. Our present study confirms these preliminary results. It shows a 2.3% incidence of catheter-related local infection and a 0.6% incidence of possible CRS. This slightly higher incidence compared with our first study may simply be due to the larger sample (340 vs 70 cannulas). Furthermore, as the previous study took place during a much shorter period, its principal investigator (F.D.[5]) personally supervised the local disinfection of the skin at the catheterization site on catheter removal. Practically, this was not feasible for the present study, and a certain number of the so-called infected catheters may have actually become positive on withdrawal.

In adults, arterial catheters are a well-established source of nosocomial infection. The incidence of catheter-related infection and septicemia varies according to the study, ranging from 4% to 35% and from 0% to 5.4%, respectively.[3,10-14] Our results show that the incidence of infection related to arterial catheterization in children is surely not higher than that in adults.

Many factors may contribute to the low incidence of infectious complications in this series, but these factors are not specific to the pediatric population. Less than 1% of the catheters were inserted by cutdown, which is associated with a higher risk of infection.[3] No burned patients were studied, and these patients are more susceptible to catheter infection.[12] Furthermore, 87% of the catheters were inserted in the radial artery, which is an area of easy access, and only 11% were exposed to a focus of infection unrelated to the catheter.

The noncultured catheters and the criteria we used to diagnose infection also warrant discussion. It is unlikely that the loss of 71 catheters significantly biased the data. The patients in whom catheters were cultured were similar to the group in whom the catheters were not cultured for all aspects but the mortality and the incidence of neutropenia, which were higher in the noncultured group. The higher mortality in the noncultured group may in itself explain why these catheters were not included; often, in these circumstances, the person who normally would have aseptically removed the catheter and sent it for culture had other priorities than culturing the catheter tip. The percentage of autopsies performed in the noncultured compared with the cultured group was similar (Table 1), as was the number of deaths due to infection (Table 1). The majority of deaths were not due to infection (Table 1), and infectious deaths were all caused by well-identified sources unrelated to the catheter. Furthermore, 77% (8/12) of deaths in the noncultured group occurred less than 48 hours after catheter insertion, rendering catheter-related infections most improbable in these patients. Among the four predisposing factors to infection recorded, neutropenia was the only one that occurred more frequently in the noncultured than the cultured group. Eight of the 71 noncultured catheters were placed in patients with neutropenia; it would be unlikely that more than one or two were infected, considering that all the catheters (eight) placed in patients with neutropenia and that were cultured were negative. We were, to our knowledge, the first group to publish the results of a prospective study on the incidence of arterial catheter-related infection and actually to compare cultured and noncultured groups.[5] Surprisingly, many studies did not even consider the catheters lost during the study period,[3,11,14,15] while some investigators only mentioned the lost catheters without taking them into consideration in their analyses.[4,12,13,16]

There is no gold standard or unquestionable diagnostic criteria for catheter-related infection.[13] This situation is attributable to two factors: the pathogenesis of intravascular catheter infection is multifactorial and the diagnostic tools are imperfect. The majority of infections are due to organism multiplication at the insertion site, with subsequent multiplication around the catheter in the subcutaneous space and then the bloodstream.[6] Other mechanisms leading to catheter sepsis are infusate contamination, hematogenous seeding of the catheter tip, and hub contamination.[12] To obviate false-negative results, each of these mechanisms should theoretically be considered, with the inherent risk of infection overdiagnosis.

We took into account the first three of these mechanisms in our study. We did not culture the internal surface of the catheter hub[17,18]; catheter hub cultures are still not routinely used to diagnose arterial catheter-related infection,[13,15] and false-positive hub cultures have been reported.[12] Our criteria for diagnosing catheter-related infection were based on SQ culture, and they were rather stringent. We used 10 CFUs on SQ culture as the cutoff point for diagnosing infection, instead of 15 CFUs as proposed by Maki et al,[6] with the risk of false-positive results that this implies. The 10-CFU cutoff point was adopted because, with pediatric catheters, only the distal 2 cm of the arterial catheter was available for culture, as opposed to the distal 5.7 cm in the study by Maki et al.[6] We did not use 5 CFUs, as suggested by Collignon et al,[19] because this only increases the number of false-positive results and probably offers no substantial advantage in terms of diagnosing bacteremia.[17,20] Because even a minute bacterial inoculum from skin flora can give a falsely positive broth culture,[18] we did not consider as significant a positive broth culture in the face of a negative SQ culture. We did not perform quantitative cultures of the tip of the catheters because this technique had not been validated in our laboratory. Cleri et al[21] recently proposed that this method, by taking into account the culture of the internal surface, is more precise and eliminates the false-negative results that can be obtained with the SQ culture. Nonetheless, the experience with this technique is still limited.

One may argue that the almost universal use of antibiotics in our patients, either prophylactically or as therapeutic agents, may have aborted CRSs, the catheters being falsely negative on removal. The same argument could be advocated for every study using positive SQ or quantitative cultures, instead of clinical criteria, to diagnose catheter-related infection.[11-13,15] In our series, only 18 catheters (5%) were exposed to documented bacteremia during their insertion. In 14, the positive blood culture was obtained less than 6 hours after catheter insertion, rendering the diagnosis of CRS very unlikely. In three cannulas among the four others, a source of infection unrelated to the catheter was identified. In only one case, no focus of infection except the catheter itself could be found to explain the bacteremia: the blood culture was sampled through a subclavian line 51 hours after insertion of the arterial catheter and yielded *S simulans*. The arterial catheter was removed 3 days after this sampling and was sterile. This isolated case could have been a false-negative CRS, but this is very unlikely considering (1) the short interval between catheter insertion and blood culture sampling (51 hours) and (2) the fact that this blood culture was done through a central venous line that was very possibly contaminated itself, but was not cultured because of accidental removal. Taking into account the limits of the criteria we used to diagnose catheter-related infections (see above), we are convinced that the very low incidence of infection reported is real.

In our study, two factors were associated with an increased rate of possible catheter-related infection: type A system for arterial blood sampling and the duration of insertion.

The major differences between systems A and B for arterial blood sampling were the following: (1) system A has 120 cm of pressure tubing through which blood is drawn back to clear the line of heparin before sampling, whereas system B has a one-way valve that does not allow blood backflow into the tubing; (2) a stopcock in system A facilitates blood sampling; and (3) the blood sampling procedure with system B necessitated more manipulations than system A. Obviously, the present study was not designed to analyze this question specifically. Nonetheless, considering that stopcocks are probably one of the sources of catheter-related infections[22] and that system A as used in our unit is by far the most widely used in North America for arterial blood sampling, a prospective study focusing on this aspect of catheter maintenance appears warranted.

The duration of cannulation, as a factor influencing the incidence of colonization (or local infection of the catheter site), has been studied by many investigators; the majority found that duration did increase the risk of colonization,[3,11,16,23] while others concluded the contrary.[13,14] In this study, the risk of infection and duration of catheter placement were related, but in a peculiar way. The risk of infection was nonexistent for the first 48 hours of catheter placement. After that period, it was 6.2% but correlated poorly with duration of insertion, ie, it did not increase in proportion with duration. The density of incidence of infectious complications is another way to represent the same observation. It shows two different phases: a first phase of zero risk lasting 48 hours followed by a second phase, characterized by a nonsignificantly fluctuating infectious risk up to day 20. This phenomenon has been described, although not discussed, by almost all investigators who have so far studied arterial catheter-related infections in adults with systematic cultures[3,11,13,23]; the "no-risk" period varies between 24[3,11] and 48[13,23] hours, and during the second phase, the risk of local and systemic infection increases severalfold but, again, not significantly from day to day.

These observations surely allow us to hypothesize that the zero-risk period corresponds to an incubation phase after which infection may happen; they are in agreement with the multifactorial pathogenesis of catheter-related infection discussed above. Indeed, the density of incidence of infections over time observed in this study is almost unexplainable by a single mechanism. As already mentioned, organism multiplication at the insertion site is possibly the major mechanism leading to infection. The fact that the density of the incidence of infectious complications did not vary significantly after the first 48 hours of insertion might indicate that spread of organisms down the transcutaneous tract may begin at any time after insertion, with the risk factors still to be determined; if this organism multiplication was mostly determined by the procedure of insertion itself, nosocomial infections should have decreased significantly after day 3 to 4, and clearly this was not the case. If contamination of the infusate or hematogenous seeding of the catheter site was the most important factor leading to infection, the density of the incidence of infectious complications should have increased proportionately with duration of insertion, and, here again, this was not the case. All these mechanisms could be causative factors, acting in sequence at different periods during insertion.

Routine replacement of the tubing and continuous flow device every 48 hours and of the infusion fluid and dressing every 24 hours is recommended by the Centers for Disease Control (Atlanta, Ga).[24] We had already questioned the merits of these recommendations.[5] The results reported here reinforce our opinion. Considering the very low rate of infection reported without these routine replacements, the significant costs involved, and the fact that minimum manipulation of the system may decrease the risk of unwanted contamination of both infusate and insertion site,[14,16] we still consider routine changes of tubing, infusion fluid, and continuous flow device debatable. Less frequent changes of the monitoring system have not been prospectively studied so far, and this should be done, particularly for financial reasons.

More than 10 years ago, Band and Maki[3] recommended systematic replacement of arterial catheters every 4 days in adults. According to our results, this replacement should be done every 48 hours, instead of every 4 days, to be fully effective in minimizing the infection risk. Indeed, this would be the ideal arterial catheter policy. Exchanging the catheters over a guidewire could be another alternative in preventing nosocomial infections.[15] However, considering (1) the low rate of infection demonstrated here (not a single case of proved CRS was identified); (2) the fact that, after the first 48 hours, the density of the incidence of infectious complications did not increase with time; (3) the much greater technical difficulties of replacing or exchanging catheters in children; and (4) the suffering incurred by such manipulations, we strongly suggest that arterial catheters should not be replaced routinely in children.

This study would not have been possible without the invaluable help of the nursing staff of St-Justine Hospital PICU. We thank Nancy Haley, MD, for reviewing the manuscript.

References

1. Riggs CD, Lister G. Adverse occurrences in the pediatric intensive care unit. *Pediatr Clin North Am.* 1987;34:93-117.
2. Milliken J, Tait GA, Ford-Jones EL, Mindorff CM, Gold R, Mullins G. Nosocomial infections in a pediatric intensive care unit. *Crit Care Med.* 1988;16:233-237.
3. Band JD, Maki DG. Infections caused by arterial catheters used for hemodynamic monitoring. *Am J Med.* 1979;67:735-741.
4. Adams JM, Speer ME, Rudolph AJ. Bacterial colonization of radial artery catheters. *Pediatrics.* 1980;65:94-97.
5. Ducharme FM, Gauthier M, Lacroix J, Lafleur L. Incidence of infection related to arterial catheterization in children: a prospective study. *Crit Care Med.* 1988;16:272-276.
6. Maki DG, Weise CE, Sarafin HW. A semiquantitative culture method for identifying intravenous-catheter–related infection. *N Engl J Med.* 1977;296:1305-1309.
7. Plit ML, Lipman J, Eidelman J, Gavaudan J. Catheter related infection. *Intensive Care Med.* 1988;14:503-509.
8. Jenicek M, Cléroux R. Epidémiologie clinique: applications à la pratique générale quotidienne et à la recherche clinique; diagnostic, thérapeutique, pronostic. In: Jenicek M, Cléroux R, eds. *Epdiemiologie: Principes, Techniques, Applications.* Paris, France: Maloine SA; 1982:339-362.
9. Jenicek M, Cléroux R. Mesure de la santé de la collectivité: indicateurs de santé. In: Jenicek M, Cléroux R, eds. *Epidemiologie: Principes, techniques, applications.* Paris, France: Maloine SA; 1982:43-78.
10. Maki DG, Hassemer CA. Endemic rate of fluid contamination and related septicemia in arterial pressure monitoring. *Am J Med.* 1981;70:733-738.
11. Pinilla JC, Ross DF, Martin T, Crump H. Study of the incidence of intravascular catheter infection and associated septicemia in critically ill patients. *Crit Care Med.* 1983;11:21-25.
12. Franceschi D, Gerding RL, Phillips G, Fratianne RB. Risk factors associated with intravascular catheter infections in burned patients: a prospective, randomized study. *J Trauma.* 1989;29:811-816.
13. Leroy O, Billiau V, Beuscart C, et al. Nosocomial infections associated with long-term radial artery cannulation. *Intensive Care Med.* 1989;15:241-246.
14. Singh S, Nelson N, Acosta I, Check FE, Puri VK. Catheter colonization and bacteremia with pulmonary and arterial catheters. *Crit Care Med.* 1982;10:736-739.
15. Norwood SH, Cormier B, McMahon NG, Moss A, Moore V. Prospective study of catheter-related infection during prolonged arterial catheterization. *Crit Care Med.* 1988;16:836-839.
16. Thomas F, Burke JP, Parker J, et al. The risk of infection related to radial vs femoral sites for arterial catheterization. *Crit Care Med.* 1983;11:807-812.
17. Sitges-Serra A, Linares J. Limitations of semiquantitative method for catheter culture. *J Clin Microbiol.* 1988;26:1074.
18. Linares J, Sitges-Serra A, Garau J, Pérez JL, Martin R. Pathogenesis of catheter sepsis: a prospective study with quantitative and semiquantitative cultures of catheter hub and segments. *J Clin Microbiol.* 1985;21:357-360.
19. Collignon PJ, Soni N, Pearson IY, Woods WP, Munro R, Sorrell TC. Is semiquantitative culture of central vein catheter tips useful in the diagnosis of catheter-related septicemia? *J Clin Microbiol.* 1986;24:532-535.
20. Brun-Buisson C. Limitations of semiquantitative method for catheter culture. *J Clin Microbiol.* 1988;26:1074.
21. Cleri DJ, Corrado ML, Seligman SJ. Quantitative culture of intravenous catheters and other intravascular inserts. *J Infect Dis.* 1980;141:781-786.
22. Parham AM. Catheter-related infections. *Crit Care Med.* 1989;17:109-110.
23. Kaye W, Wheaton M, Potter-Bynoe G. Radial and pulmonary artery catheter-related sepsis. *Crit Care Med.* 1983;11:249.
24. Centers for Disease Control. Guidelines for the prevention of intravascular infections. *Am J Infect Control.* 1983;11:183-193.

SPECIAL FEATURE

Radiological Case of the Month

George P. Giacola, MD (Contributor), Beverly P. Wood, MD (Section Editor)

A 2050-g newborn of 36 weeks' gestation was born by vaginal vertex delivery with low forceps assistance after 16 hours of labor. The newborn's Apgar scores were 4 and 8 at 1 and 5 minutes, respectively. The mother, a 14-year-old girl, had received no prenatal care. The infant forcefully vomited the first formula feeding, given at age 12 hours.

Results of physical examination showed the newborn to be active and in no distress. The newborn's length was 49 cm, and the head circumference, 35 cm. An extensive left parietal cephalohematoma was present. The white blood cell count was 14.9×10^9/L, and the differential count was as follows: neutrophils, 53%; lymphocytes, 37%; and monocytes, 10%. The hemoglobin value was 120 g/L, and the bilirubin value was 128 μmol/L.

Because of continued vomiting and regurgitation of feedings, a frontal roentgenogram of the abdomen was obtained after insertion of a nasogastric tube (Figs 1 and 2).

Accepted for publication June 19, 1991.
From the Division of Neonatology, Department of Pediatrics, The University of Oklahoma, 6161 S Yale, Tulsa, OK 74136.

Reprint requests to the Department of Radiology, Childrens Hospital of Los Angeles, 4650 Sunset Blvd, Los Angeles, CA 90027 (Dr Wood).

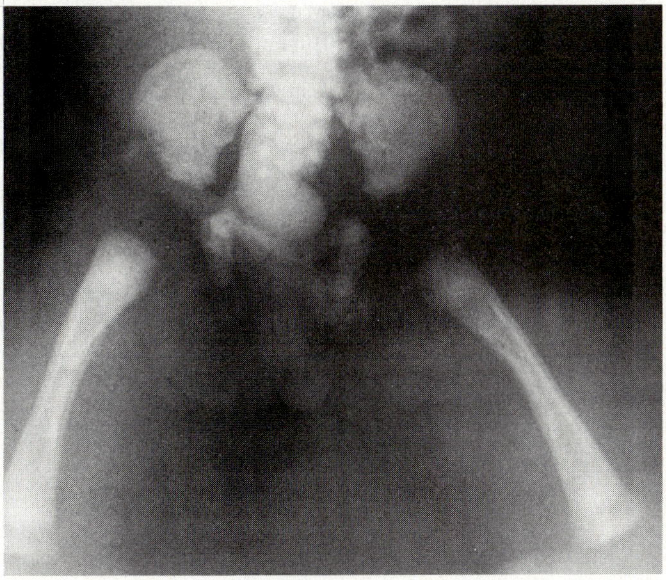

Figure 1.

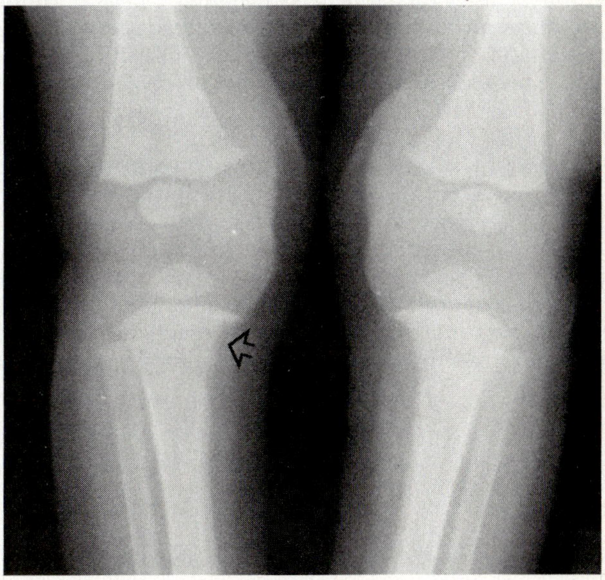

Figure 2.

Denouement and Discussion

Congenital Syphilis

Fig 1.—*Symmetric radiolucent metaphyseal bands involve the femora and ilia. Periosteal new bone is present along the shafts of the long bones (results of VDRL test, 1:32; results of a fluorescent treponemal antibody absorption test were positive).*

Fig 2.—*Roentgenogram of legs showing periosteal new bone and Wimberger's sign (arrow).*

Congenital syphilis is an important perinatal complication that has recently increased substantially in occurrence.[1] The roentgenographic characteristics of congenital syphilis usually precede clinical manifestations and may identify the condition when results of conventional serologic tests are inconclusive.[2] In a small number of affected neonates, florid clinical signs and abnormal results of serologic tests occur without demonstrable skeletal abnormality. Characteristically, diffuse bony involvement affecting the metaphyses and diaphyses is present.[3] The metaphyseal lesions appear as irregular bands of diminished mineralization or focal circumscribed areas of metaphyseal and cortical bone destruction. Disruption in the orderly progression of calcification of cartilaginous osteoid to normal bone is evidenced as transverse lucent bands at the metaphyseal ends with or without an adjacent band of sclerosis. Destructive metaphysitis takes several forms. Focal erosion of the semilunar notch of the ulna denotes congenital luetic infection. Destruction of the medial aspect of the proximal tibial metaphysis (Wimberger's sign) is characteristic but not pathognomonic of congenital syphilis. Wimberger's sign also occurs in osteomyelitis, hyperparathyroidism, and infantile generalized fibromatosis.[4] Longitudinal metaphyseal bands of decreased density, "celery stalks," occur in syphilis, congenital rubella syndrome, cytomegalovirus infection, and other viral transplacental infections.[5] Subperiosteal inflammation in the diaphysis produces cortical destruction and periosteal elevation in single or multiple layers, with new bone formation along the length of the diaphysis. Polyostotic, symmetric bone involvement is characteristic of congenital syphilis.[6] The long bones, pelvis, vertebrae, and small tubular bones are all susceptible to involvement. Lytic lesions of the crania mimic those of Langerhans' cell histiocytosis. A delay of approximately 5 weeks between initial infection of the fetus and radiologic evidence of osteitis is typical, with periostitis occurring later.[7] The pathogenesis of bone changes is focal inflammation produced directly by spirochetal infection or dystrophic alteration in endochondral bone formation secondary to generalized sepsis.

References

1. Centers for Disease Control. Guidelines for the prevention and control of congenital syphilis. *MMWR.* 1988;37:1-13.
2. Olansky S, Norins LC. Current serodiagnosis and treatment of syphilis. *JAMA.* 1966;198:185-188.
3. Caffey J. *Pediatric X-ray Diagnosis.* St Louis, Mo: Mosby–Year Book; 1985:835-836.
4. Swischuk LE. *Radiology of the Newborn and Young Infant.* Baltimore, Md: William & Wilkins; 1973.
5. Cremin BJ, Fisher RM. The lesions of congenital syphilis. *Br J Radiol.* 1970;43:333-341.
6. McLean S. Congenital osseous syphilis. *AJDC.* 1931;41:130-152.
7. Ingraham NR Jr. Lag phase in early congenital osseous syphilis: roentgenographic study. *Am J Med Sci.* 1936;191:819-827.

Picture of the Month

Luis A. Vera, MD; Nayere Zaeri, MD; Hallam Hurt, MD (Contributors);
Murray Feingold, MD (Editor for This Case); *Walter W. Tunnessen, Jr, MD* (Section Editor)

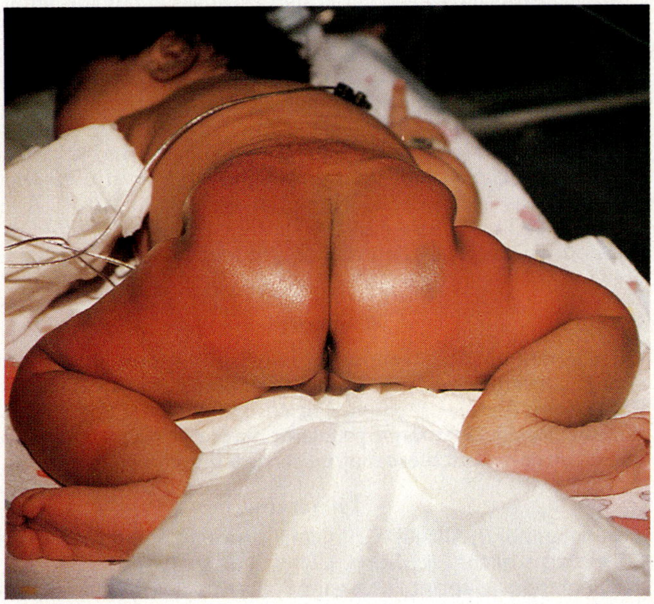

Figure 1.

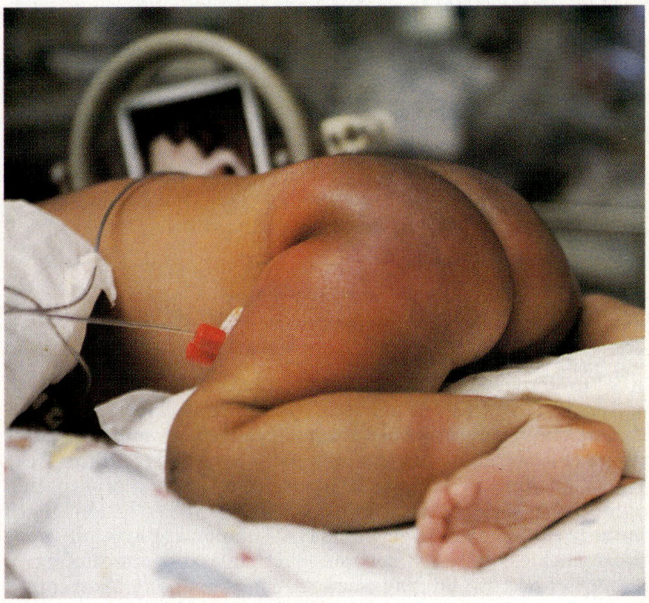

Figure 2.

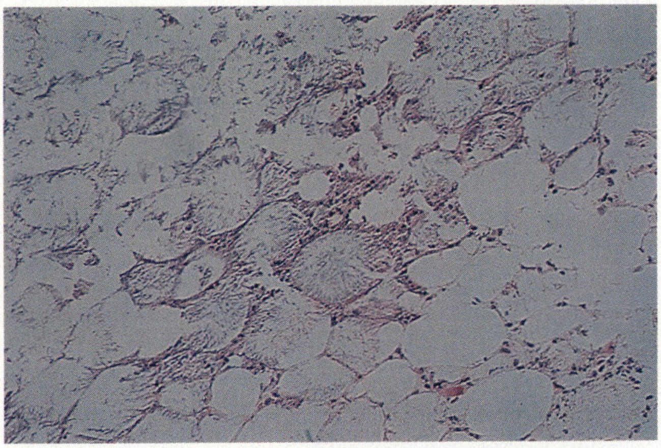

Figure 3.

The Editors welcome contributions to Picture of the Month and Radiological Case of the Month. Those who wish to contribute should send their manuscripts to Dr Tunnessen (Picture of the Month), *The Children's Hospital of Philadelphia, 34th Street and Civic Center Boulevard, Philadelphia, PA 19104, or Dr Wood* (Radiological Case of the Month), *Department of Radiology, Childrens Hospital of Los Angeles, 4650 Sunset Blvd, Los Angeles, CA 90027. Articles and photographs accepted for publication will bear the contributor's name. There is no charge for reproduction and printing of color illustrations.*

Accepted for publication January 10, 1991.

Contributed from the Division of Neonatology, Albert Einstein Medical Center, Philadelphia, Pa.

Reprint requests to National Birth Defects Center, Franciscan Children's Hospital, 30 Warren St, Brighton, MA 02135 (Dr Feingold).

Denouement and Discussion

Subcutaneous Fat Necrosis of the Newborn

Fig 1.—*At initial presentation, skin is taut, erythematous, and indurated.*

Fig 2.—*In 24 to 28 hours, the skin acquires a purple hue.*

Fig 3.—*Results of biopsy of the involved skin show the characteristic fat cell necrosis with central needle-shaped crystal formation in the fat cells.*

Manifestations

Subcutaneous fat necrosis of the newborn is a benign condition of unknown origin affecting the subcutaneous fat tissue in the first weeks of life. It is characterized clinically by multiple subcutaneous, indurated, erythematous plaques and nodules that are neither tender nor warm to palpation. The condition begins as an area of edema at the affected sites and rapidly progresses to variably circumscribed, confluent, red lesions that change to a purple hue in several days. The skin appears taut and shiny. The lesions may become fluctuant, and spontaneous drainage of necrotic fat may occur. Areas of the body most commonly involved are the buttocks, back, arms, thighs, legs, and shoulders.

Results of histologic examination of the condition typically include necrosis of subcutaneous fat with needle-shaped crystal formation in the fat cells. Calcium deposits are sometimes seen in the central part of the degenerating fat cells. The epidermis and dermis appear normal on microscopic examination.

Many factors have been implicated as causes of this condition, with the most likely being hypothermia, obstetric trauma, and perinatal asphyxia. Hypercalcemia and thrombocytopenia have been observed in several cases; however, in general, laboratory findings are nonspecific and, in most cases, within normal limits.

Differential diagnosis should include cellulitis and sclerema neonatorum. Sclerema neonatorum is very often confused with subcutaneous fat necrosis of the newborn; however, it is characterized by diffuse hardening of the skin, and is often associated with sepsis. The prognosis of sclerema neonatorum is grave.

Treatment

Treatment of subcutaneous fat necrosis is symptomatic, and should concentrate on other concurrent illnesses such as sepsis. Prognosis is good, with gradual resolution of the lesions in a few months. Residual cosmetic problems may arise from subcutaneous fat atrophy, but these may be corrected with plastic surgery.

References

1. Mogilner B, Alkalay A, Nissim F, Frumkin A. Subcutaneous fat necrosis of the newborn. *Clinic Pediatr.* 1981;20:748-750.
2. Katz OA, Huerter C, Bogard P, Braddock SW. Subcutaneous fat necrosis of the newborn. *Arch Dermatol.* 1984;120:1517-1518.
3. Fretzin DF, Arias AM. Sclerema neonatorum and subcutaneous fat necrosis of the newborn. *Pediatr Dermatol.* 1987;4:112-122.

A Variant Form of Thrombasthenia

Michael D. Tarantino, MD; James J. Corrigan, Jr, MD; Lewis Glasser, MD;
Claire M. Payne, PhD; Monette A. Jeter, PhD

• We encountered two siblings with abnormal bruising since infancy. Studies revealed functional platelet defects characterized by a lack of platelet aggregation and adenosine triphosphate release on exposure to adenosine diphosphate and collagen as well as variable responses with ristocetin (at concentrations of ≤1.25 g/L) and arachidonic acid. In addition, little or no platelet aggregation was observed after exposure to hexadimethrine bromide (Polybrene), the calcium ionophore A23187, and the thromboxane/endoperoxide analogue U46619. The membrane proteins IIIa and Ib were present, as determined with monoclonal antibody testing, and no platelet-associated IgG was found. Platelet analysis with routine electron microscopy and ultrastructural cytochemistry revealed normal morphologic features and no deficiencies in the number of alpha granules dense bodies and other organelles. The platelet abnormality may represent a new variant of thrombasthenia.

(*AJDC.* 1991;145:1053-1057)

Congenital or inherited abnormalities in the function of blood platelets produce a clinical bleeding picture similar to quantitative defects (thrombocytopenia), ie, mucus membrane and skin petechiae, ecchymoses, and the immediate onset of bleeding with trauma. The congenital defects have been classified into disorders of platelet adhesion (eg, von Willebrand disease and Bernard-Soulier syndrome), primary aggregation (eg, thrombasthenia), secretion (eg, storage pool disease and release defects), and procoagulant activities (eg, platelet factor 3 deficiency).[1]

Glanzmann thrombasthenia is an autosomal recessive disorder characterized by a deficiency or an abnormality of the platelet membrane glycoprotein IIb-IIIa complex. Patients with this disorder have a normal platelet count, normal platelet morphologic features, prolonged bleeding time, absent or substantially reduced platelet aggregation by adenosine diphosphate (ADP) and other agonists, normal platelet aggregation (agglutination) in response to ristocetin, and normal results of plasma coagulation studies. Clot retraction may or may not be impaired.[2-5]

The patient described herein had the usual laboratory findings of thrombasthenia, but his platelets also reacted poorly to ristocetin, and GP IIIa and GP Ib were detected in his platelets. His sister had similar findings. We report this unusual variant of thrombasthenia.

PATIENT REPORTS

A 7-year-old Mexican boy had excessive skin bruising, prolonged bleeding with skin lacerations, and frequent epistaxis since the age of 1 year. There was no history of joint pain or swelling. The patient took no medications, and his growth and development were normal.

The physical examination revealed normal findings, except for the skin findings. Examination of the skin revealed scattered ecchymoses, the largest of which was 3 cm in diameter. Petechiae were noted over the patella, elbows, and sternum.

Laboratory studies revealed normal red blood cell, white blood cell, and platelet counts. Prothrombin and partial thromboplastin times were within the normal range. The bleeding time was greater than 20 minutes on three separate occasions.

At the initial evaluation, the patient was treated empirically with oral prednisone (1 mg/kg of body weight per day). After 1 month, the studies were repeated, and the results revealed no change. The bleeding time remained prolonged, and the platelet count remained normal.

The boy's 3-year-old sister was also noted to have excessive skin bruising and prolonged bleeding after skin lacerations since the age of 1 year. Likewise, she had no joint symptoms and took no medications.

The family history revealed that the biologic father of the children also suffered from skin bruising since childhood and had experienced prolonged bleeding after shaving cuts. The father has three half-sisters who do not experience these symptoms but also has two brothers who have skin bruising. The paternal grandfather also has a history of excessive skin bruising. The family history revealed no consanguinity. However, the coagulation and platelet studies yielded normal findings in the father and mother (see the "Results" section).

MATERIALS AND METHODS

Initial Tests

A complete blood cell count, platelet count, prothrombin time, activated partial thromboplastin time, and template bleeding time were determined with use of standard methods in each case. Plasma von Willebrand antigen and activity and factor VIII activity were measured in the index case.[6-8] Platelet-associated immunoglobulin was determined by the method of Finley et al.[9]

Accepted for publication February 19, 1991.

From the Departments of Pediatrics (Drs Tarantino, Corrigan, and Jeter) and Pathology (Drs Glasser and Payne) and The Children's Research Center, The University of Arizona Health Sciences Center, Tucson. Dr Corrigan is now with Tulane University School of Medicine, New Orleans, La. Dr Tarantino is now with the University of Wisconsin Medical School, Madison.

Reprint requests to Tulane University School of Medicine, 1430 Tulane Ave, New Orleans, LA 70112 (Dr Corrigan).

Platelet Aggregation and Adenosine Triphosphate (ATP) Release

Blood was collected by venipuncture into plastic tubes containing 3.8% sodium citrate. The ratio of blood to anticoagulant was 9:1. Platelet-rich plasma (PRP) was obtained by centrifugation of the blood at 180*g* for 10 minutes at room temperature. Platelet-poor plasma was obtained by centrifugation of the remaining blood at 1500*g* for 10 minutes. The concentration of platelets in the PRP platelet count was adjusted to approximately 250×10^9/L for all tests. A lumiaggregometer was used to measure platelet aggregation and ATP secretion (Chrono-log Corp, Havertown, Pa).[10] Adenosine triphosphate–generated chemiluminescence was measured with firefly luciferase–luciferin (Chronolume, Chrono-log Corp).[11] The reaction mixture contained 0.4 mL of PRP and 0.1 mL of agonist. The agonists used (and their final concentration in the reaction mixture) were as follows: ADP (4.6, 23, and 46 μmol/L; Sigma Chemical Co, St Louis, Mo), collagen (Sigma Chemical Co), arachidonic acid (5.0 and 7.0 mmol/L, Chrono-log Corp), ristocetin (1.25, 1.0, 0.5 g/L; Pacific Hemostasis Laboratories, Ventura, Calif), calcium ionophore A23187 (19 μmol/L; Sigma Chemical Co), thromboxane/endoperoxide analogue U46619 (0.5 μmol/L; Caymer Chemicals, Ann Arbor, Mich), hexadimethrine bromide (Polybrene), (1 g/L; Abbott Laboratories, Chicago, Ill), snake venom (*Crotalus atrox*, 1 g/L).

Platelet Glycoprotein Antigens

Glycoprotein Ib and IIIa were analyzed by flow cytometry.[9] Mouse monoclonal antihuman platelet glycoprotein Ib and IIIa antibodies were obtained from Dako Corp, Santa Barbara, Calif. Platelets were washed, resuspended, and analyzed with the Epics V (Coulter Electronics Inc, Hialeah, Fla). Mouse antihuman platelet glycoprotein was added to the normal control and to the patient's platelet suspension and incubated for 30 minutes at 22°C. After washing, fluorescein isothiocyanate–conjugated goat antimouse IgG was added and incubated for 30 minutes in the dark at 22°C. A positive reaction was measured using the log of green fluorescence.

Ristocetin Cofactor

Ristocetin cofactor was measured in platelet-poor plasma by the method of Allain et al.[8] Briefly, 0.05 mL of a 1:2 dilution of plasma was added to a 0.40-mL suspension of lyophilized platelets (Helena Laboratories, Beaumont, Tex) and 0.05 mL of ristocetin. Platelet aggregation was measured with an aggregometer (Chrono-log Corp). The maximum slope of the aggregation curve was calculated, and the activity of the patient's ristocetin cofactor was determined.

Electron Microscopy

One milliliter of blood from the patient and each control was spun in a Wintrobe tube at 2500 rpm for 10 minutes in a swinging bucket clinical centrifuge clinical centrifuge (Beckman TJ-6, Beckman Instruments Inc, Fullerton, Calif). The plasma was removed, and the buffy coat was fixed in situ with 3% glutaraldehyde in 0.1 mol/L of phosphate buffer (pH 7.3). One-millimeter slices of the buffy coat plug were prepared, postfixed for 1 hour in 1% osmium tetroxide, dehydrated in a graded series of ethanols, and embedded in Spurr's epoxy resin. One-micron sections were prepared, stained with toluidine blue O, and examined for proper orientation of the platelet layer. Ultrathin sections were prepared with an ultramicrotome (Dupont-Sorvall MT-5000, Dupont-Sorvall, Boston, Mass) and counterstained with uranyl acetate–lead citrate before examination under an electron microscope (JEOL 100 CX, JEOL USA Inc, Peabody, Mass).

Ultrastructural Cytochemical Reactions.—Three different platelet preparations were prepared (with only plastic tubing and plastic tubes) for the following three cytochemical reactions that stain different components of the dense bodies: uranaffin reaction stains the nucleotides (ADP/ATP),[12-14] the chromaffin reaction[15] stains the amines (serotonin or 5-hydroxytryptamine), and Weiss' fixation[16] procedure (contains 2.25 mmol/L of calcium chloride) with postosmication allows the visualization of the calcium ions.

Table 1.—Preliminary Studies

Variable	Patient	Normal Control
Platelet count, x 10^9/L	351	150-350
Platelet morphologic features	Normal	Normal
Prothrombin time, s	11.5	10.7-12.3
Partial thromboplastin time, s	29.1	25.8-35.2
Fibrinogen, g/L	3.07	1.5-3.5
Bleeding time, min	>20	1-10.5
Euglobulin lysis time, h	>2.0	>2.0
Ristocetin cofactor assay, % of normal	77	44-160
Factor VIII activity, U/dL	63	50-150
von Willebrand factor antigen, % of normal	68	60-150
Clot retraction	Fair	Good to excellent

Table 2.—Platelet Aggregation and Adenosine Triphosphate Release

Reagent	Aggregation, % Patient	Aggregation, % Normal Range	ATP Release, μmol/L Patient	ATP Release, μmol/L Normal Range
ADP, μmol/L*				
4.6	0	47-74	0.07	0.18-2.7
23	0	>60	0.17	0.18-2.7
46	0	100	>3.35	>3.35
Collagen	0	42-70	0.03	0.5-2.1
Arachidonic acid, mmol/L				
2.5	0	35-80	0.30	0.07-1.3
5.0	32	>50	0.39	0.18-2.0
Thrombin, 1.0 U/mL	0	>70	1.09	>0.5
Ristocetin, g/L				
1.5	62	>80	. . .	. . .
1.25	52	>54	. . .	. . .
	0	. . .	. . .	. . .
	42	. . .	. . .	. . .
1.0	30	54-75	. . .	. . .
	0	. . .	. . .	. . .

*ADP indicates adenosine diphosphate.

Quantitation of Platelet Dense Bodies.—All platelets were evaluated for reactive sites with the use of grids that were not counterstained with uranyl acetate–lead citrate. The platelets were viewed and scored at a microscopic magnification of ×10 000; the number of reactive sites in each of 100 consecutive platelet profiles were determined. A reactive site was defined as

Table 3.—Quantitation of Platelet-Dense Bodies by Electron Microscopy*

Subject	Cytochemical Stain		
	Ca^{++}†	Nucleotides‡	Amines (Serotonin)§
Patient	1.47	0.84	0.33
10-year-old male control	1.05	0.64	0.45
8-year-old female control	0.73	0.57	0.23
Adult male			
1	0.30	0.51	0.36
2	0.82	0.81	0.53
Adult female	0.72	0.64	0.29

*Values are number of reactive sites per platelet profile (100 platelet profiles were examined).
† Weiss' fixative.
‡Uranaffin reaction.
§Chromaffin reaction.

any electron-dense precipitate that was visually more electron dense than the surrounding noncounterstained platelet organelles. These reactive sites had either a solid, punctate, or crystalline appearance. In the case of the uranaffin reaction, a platelet dense body was also scored as positive if the granule membrane alone was stained; this membrane staining was only seen with the uranaffin reaction.[13]

RESULTS

Initial Test Results

All of the results (Table 1) were noted to be in the normal range, except for the bleeding time, which was greater than 20 minutes. The bleeding time was remeasured 1 month later, and the same result was obtained. Bleeding times of the patient's mother and father were noted to be 4.5 and 6 minutes, respectively. The bleeding time was not determined for the patient's sister. The platelet-associated immunoglobulin test result was negative in the patient. The paternal uncles and paternal grandfather were not available for testing. As noted, the patient's plasma level of factor VIII activity, von Willebrand factor protein, and von Willebrand factor activity (ristocetin cofactor) were normal.

Platelet Aggregation and ATP Release

The degree of platelet aggregation to various agents is shown in Table 2. No aggregation was seen in the patient's platelets when exposed to either increasing concentrations of ADP or with collagen. Arachidonic acid at 5.0 mmol/L induced minimal aggregation (32%). The response to ristocetin showed an inconsistent pattern, being 0% and 42% with the use of 1.25 g/L of the antibiotic.

Aggregation studies with other agonists showed no response with thrombin (1 U/mL), A23187 (a calcium ionophore), and U46619 (a thromboxane/endoperoxide analogue) and only a 15% response with 1.0 g/L polybrene (normal control, 75%).[17,18] *Crotalus atrox* venom, however, caused 100% clumping.[19] The release of ATP was evident with 46 μmol/L of ADP and with thrombin (1.0 U/mL).

Aggregation and ATP release studies performed in the 3-year-old sister revealed no aggregation on exposure of PRP to ADP (4.6 μmol/L), collagen, and epinephrine. However, platelet aggregation was noted after the addition to ristocetin, ranging from 7% aggregation in a 0.5-g/L solution to 51% aggregation in a 1.25-g/L solution of ristocetin. Release of ATP was not observed when the sister's platelets were exposed to epinephrine, ADP, or collagen.

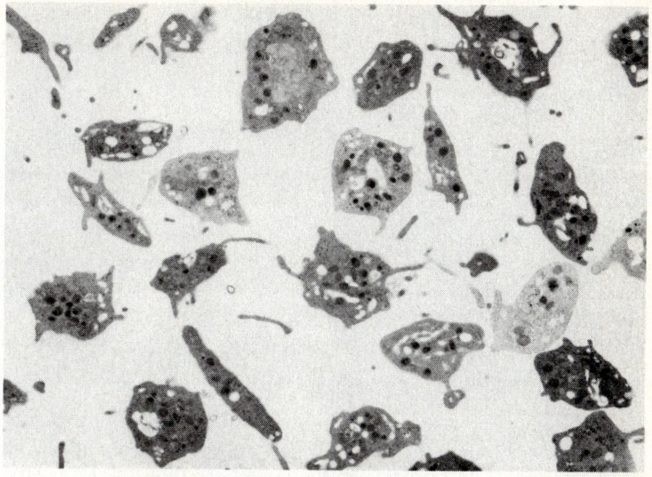

Fig 1.—*Low-power electron micrograph of platelet profiles obtained from patient with abnormal bruising and defective platelet aggregation. Platelets are of normal size and show no deficiencies of organelles. Some of the platelets have a discoid shape and others exhibit pseudopodal extensions, the latter of which is indicative of platelet activation (uranyl acetate–lead citrate, original magnification ×8700).*

Studies of platelet aggregation and ATP release in PRP from the parents revealed normal aggregation with collagen, ristocetin (1.25 g/L), arachidonic acid (5 mmol/L), and ADP (23 μmol/L).

Platelet Antigens

Platelets from the index case fluoresced after incubation with monoclonal antibodies against both platelet glycoproteins Ib and IIIa, indicating the presence of these glycoproteins in the platelet membrane. These tests were not performed on other family members.

Electron Microscopic Findings

Examination of the patient's platelets with transmission electron microscopy revealed a normal content and complement of organelles[20] (Fig 1). Compare the patient's platelets (Fig 1) with those of an age-matched control (Fig 2). Alpha granules were present and were of normal size and shape. Quantitative cytochemical studies with the use of Weiss' fixative (Fig 3) and the uranaffin and chromaffin reactions revealed no deficiency in the number or content of dense bodies (Table 3). The apparent increase in vacuolization in the patient's platelets (Fig 1) compared with the control platelets shown in Fig 2 is within the range of ultrastructural changes seen in control platelets prepared in the same manner. This dilation of the open canalicular system and the increase in microvilli (Fig 1) are commonly seen in activated platelets (ie, those exposed to glass). In contrast to the Wintrobe tube preparations, used for routine electron microscopy, the patient's platelets that were prepared for quantitative ultrastructural cytochemistry, with the use of only plastic tubing and plastic tubes, do not show this degree of vacuolization (Fig 3).

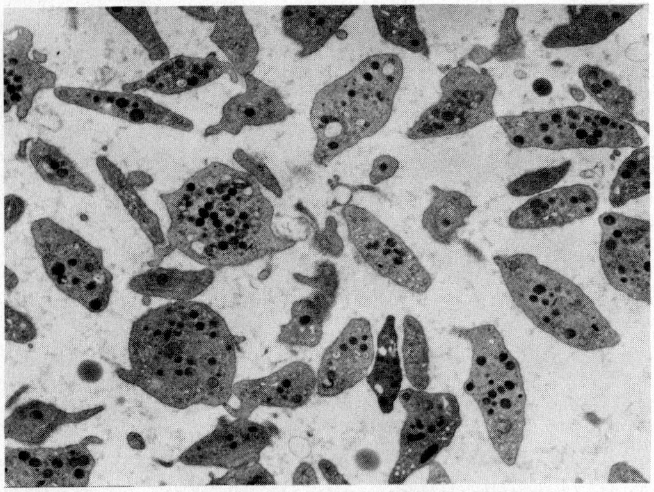

Fig 2.—*Low-power electron micrograph of platelet profiles obtained from an age-matched control subject with no evidence of a bleeding disorder. Platelets contain a normal complement of organelles. Some of the platelets have a discoid shape and others exhibit pseudopodal extensions, the latter of which is indicative of platelet activation (uranyl acetate–lead citrate, original magnification ×8700).*

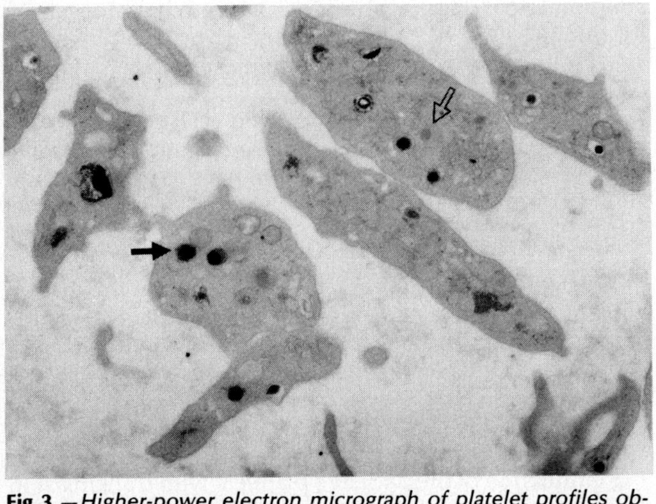

Fig 3.—*Higher-power electron micrograph of platelet profiles obtained from the patient and fixed in a calcium-containing fixative for better visualization of the abundant platelet dense bodies (solid arrow). Alpha granules with their eccentric cores (open arrow) are readily identified (Weiss' fixative, postosmicated, no counterstain; original magnification ×18 100).*

COMMENT

The initial laboratory test results in our patient of normal platelet count, prothrombin time, and partial thromboplastin time and prolonged bleeding time suggested that he had a disorder of platelet function. Further ex vivo platelet studies revealed abnormalities consistent with Glanzmann's thrombasthenia.

Glanzmann's thrombasthenia is a bleeding disorder characterized by platelets that fail to aggregate following stimulation with many agonists (eg, ADP, collagen, thrombin, and hexadimethrine bromide).[5,21] The platelets generally have a low amount of glycoprotein IIb-IIIa, although a few patients with near-normal amounts of the complex have been described.[2,22,23] The glycoprotein IIb-IIIa complex is made available on activated platelets, and this complex can bind different adhesive proteins, such as fibrinogen, von Willebrand factor, fibronectin, and vitronectin.[3,24,25] Fibrinogen binding appears to be a prerequisite for normal platelet aggregation.[24-26] Platelet membrane glycoprotein Ib is the major receptor for von Willebrand factor.[3,4] This receptor is present and functions normally in platelets from patients with thrombasthenia. Thus, activated thrombasthenic platelets will not aggregate (cell-to-cell interaction) because of either a deficiency or an abnormality of the glycoprotein IIb-IIIa complex. However, if the agonist is strong enough (eg, thrombin or a high concentration of ADP), the platelets will undergo a release/secretion reaction, but they will not aggregate.[5]

In the patient described herein, the platelets would not aggregate normally with the addition of a variety of agonists, including ADP and collagen. However, ATP release could be induced with thrombin and arachidonic acid. Electron microscopic studies of his platelets revealed normal morphologic features, dense body numbers and content of nucleotides, amines, and calcium. These findings eliminate storage pool disease as a cause of the platelet defect.

The patient's impaired response to ristocetin was unexpected. The inability of platelets to agglutinate with the addition of ristocetin is seen in von Willebrand's disease, which is due to reduced or an abnormal von Willebrand factor; the Bernard-Soulier syndrome, which is due to a deficiency of platelet glycoprotein Ib; and in storage pool/release defect diseases.[3,4,27] Our patient had normal plasma levels of von Willebrand factor protein, von Willebrand factor activity (ristocetin cofactor assay), the presence of glycoprotein Ib on his platelets, normal numbers of dense bodies in his platelets, and the ability to release ATP with thrombin. Thus, his platelet aggregation after exposure to the antibiotic ristocetin should be the same as that of normal platelets.

Although platelet aggregation is primarily mediated by fibrinogen interactions with glycoprotein IIb-IIIa, von Willebrand factor can also function as a ligand to allow platelet aggregation.[25] The suboptimal response of our patient's and his sister's platelets to ristocetin (which is mediated through von Willebrand factor) may be a manifestation of an abnormal glycoprotein IIb-IIIa complex.

The only platelet agonist that caused platelet clumping was *C atrox* snake venom. Rattlesnake venom causes a generalized membrane injury and probably does not act through a specific receptor site.[19]

The authors kindly acknowledge Douglas W. Cromey, MS, and Charles G. Bjore, Jr, MBA, for their excellent technical assistance.

The snake venom used in this study was a gift of Finley Russell, PhD, University of Arizona, Tucson.

References

1. Handin RI. Physiology of coagulation: the platelet. In: Nathan DG, Oski FA, eds. *Hematology in Infancy and Childhood.* Philadelphia, Pa: WB Saunders Co; 1987:1271-1292.

2. Holahan JR, White GC. Heterogeneity of membrane surface proteins in Glanzmann's thrombasthenia. *Blood.* 1981;57:174-181.

3. Kunicki TJ. Platelet membrane glycoproteins and their function: an overview. *Blut.* 1989;59:30-34.

4. McEver RP. The clinical significance of platelet membrane glycoproteins. *Hematol Oncol Clin North Am.* 1990;4:87-105.

5. George JN, Caen JP, Nurden AT. Glanzmann's thrombas-

thenia: the spectrum of clinical disease. *Blood.* 1990;85:383-395.

6. Simone JV, Vanderheiden J, Abilgaard CF. Semiautomatic one-stage factor VIII assay with commercially prepared standard. *J Lab Clin Med.* 1967;69:706-712.

7. Laurell CB. Electroimmunoassay. *Scand J Clin Lab Invest.* 1972;29(suppl 24):21-37.

8. Allain JP, Cooper HA, Wagner RH, Brinkhous KM. Platelets fixed with paraformaldehyde: a new reagent for assay of von Willebrand factor and platelet aggregating factor. *J Lab Clin Med.* 1975;85:318-327.

9. Finley PR, Williams JR, Fletcher C. Flow cytometry of platelet antibodies. *J Clin Lab Anal.* 1988;2:249-255.

10. Feinman RD, Lubowsky J, Caro IF, Zabinski MP. The lumi-aggregometer: a new instrument for simultaneous measurement of secretion and aggregation. *J Lab Clin Med.* 1977;90:125-129.

11. Holmsen H, Holmsen I, Bernhardsen A. Microdetermination of adenosine diphosphate and adenosine triphosphate in plasma with the firefly luciferase system. *Analyt Biochem.* 1966;17:456-473.

12. Richards JG, Da Prada M. Uranaffin reaction: a new cytochemical technique for the localization of adenine nucleotides in organelles storing biogenic amines. *J Histochem Cytochem.* 1977;25:1322-1336.

13. Payne CM. A quantitative ultrastructural evaluation of the cell organelle specificity of the uranaffin reaction in normal human platelets. *Am J Clin Pathol.* 1984;81:62-70.

14. Payne CM. Phylogenetic considerations of neurosecretory granule contents: role of nucleotide and basic hormone/transmitter packaging mechanisms. *Arch Histol Cytol.* 1989;52:277-292.

15. Tranzer J-P, Richards JG. Ultrastructural cytochemistry of biogenic amines in nervous tissue: methodologic improvements. *J Histochem Cytochem.* 1976;24:1178-1193.

16. Weiss HJ, Witte LD, Kaplan KL, et al. Heterogeneity in storage pool deficiency: studies on granule-bound substances in 18 patients including variants deficient in α-granules, platelet factor 4, β-thromboglobulin, and platelet-derived growth factor. *Blood.* 1979;54:1296-1319.

17. White JG. Effects of cationic polypeptides on thrombasthenic and afibrinogenemic blood platelets. *Am J Pathol.* 1972;68:447-460.

18. Lages B, Holmsen H, Weiss H, Dangelmaier C. Thrombin and ionophore A23187–induced dense granule secretion in storage pool deficient platelets: evidence for impaired nucleotide storage as the primary dense granule defect. *Blood.* 1983;61:154-162.

19. Corrigan JJ Jr, Jeter M, Ferlan I. In vitro effect of *Crotalus molossus molossus* (blacktail rattlesnake) venom on human platelets, fibrinolysis and fibrinogen: comparison with *C. atrox* and *C. adamanteus*. *Toxicon.* 1983;suppl 3:77-80.

20. White JG. Current concepts of platelet structure. *Am J Clin Pathol.* 1979;71:363-378.

21. Nurden AT. Congenital abnormalities of platelet membrane glycoproteins. In: Kunicki TJ, George JN, eds. *Platelet Immunobiology.* Philadelphia, Pa: JB Lippincott; 1989:63-96.

22. Phillips DR, Charo IF, Parise LV, Fitzgerald LA. The platelet membrane glycoprotein IIb-IIIa complex. *Blood.* 1988;71:831-843.

23. Jung SM, Yoshida N, Aoki N, Tanoue K, Yamazaki H, Moroi M. Thrombasthenia with abnormal membrane glycoprotein IIb of different molecular weight. *Blood.* 1988;71:915-922.

24. George JN. The role of membrane glycoproteins in platelet function. *Transfusion Med Rev.* 1987;1:34-46.

25. DeMarco L, Girolami A, Zimmerman TS, Ruggeri ZM. Von Willebrand factor interaction with glycoprotein IIb-IIIa complex: its role in platelet function as demonstrated in patients with congenital afibrinogenemia. *J Clin Invest.* 1986;77:1272-1277.

26. Coller BS. Interaction of normal, thrombasthenic and Bernard-Soulier platelets with immobilized fibrinogen: defective platelet-fibrinogen interaction in thrombasthenia. *Blood.* 1980;55:169-178.

27. Weiss HJ. Abnormalities of factor VIII and platelet aggregation: use of ristocetin in diagnosing the von Willebrand syndrome. *Blood.* 1975;45:403-412.

Lichen Sclerosus et Atrophicus in Children

Vera Loening-Baucke, MD

• The symptoms, findings, associated conditions, and treatment of lichen sclerosus et atrophicus were studied in 10 girls and one boy. Lichen sclerosus et atrophicus is a benign but chronic condition of the anogenital area of girls and, less frequently, of boys. The characteristic lesions are hypopigmented plaques in a figure-of-8 pattern surrounding the vulva and anus and often involving the natal cleft. The affected hypopigmented skin is sharply demarcated from the normal skin. Hemorrhagic, bullous lesions are uncommon. Fissures and ulcers are seen on the labia, between the labia, and on the perineum, anus, and natal cleft in many children and on the glans penis in boys. Lichen sclerosus et atrophicus causes painful defecation and anal and vulval bleeding. In two patients, one girl and one boy, anal stenosis due to lichen sclerosus et atrophicus and laxative treatment developed. Lichen sclerosus et atrophicus mimics sexual abuse and has led to false accusation and investigations. The anogenital lesions cleared in three patients at the ages of 9, 11, and 12 years, but lesions can persist into adulthood.

(*AJDC.* 1991;145:1058-1061)

Lichen sclerosus et atrophicus (LSA) is a benign but chronic condition of the epithelium and dermis and is characterized by ivory or white, shiny macules and papules that coalesce to form homogeneous hypopigmented plaques. The condition affects the vulvar and perianal areas of prepubertal girls and premenopausal women. It is most frequently seen in postmenopausal women. Boys as well as men can be affected. The major symptom in males is phimosis. The condition in females outnumbers that in males 10:1.[1]

Lichen sclerosus et atrophicus is more common than is currently recognized, with 10% to 15% of all cases occurring in children. Anogenital LSA can mimic sexual abuse and has led to false accusations and investigations for sexual abuse.[2-6] The mode of onset, clinical features, associated conditions, and treatment of this disease have received little attention in the pediatric literature. I report the symptoms, findings, associated conditions, and treatment in 10 girls and one boy to familiarize physicians with the range of appearances and the treatment of childhood LSA.

Accepted for publication February 4, 1991.
From the Department of Pediatrics, University of Iowa, Iowa City.
Reprints not available.

PATIENTS AND METHODS

Ten girls and one boy, 3 to 11 years of age, with skin changes of the anogenital region consistent with LSA were examined during a period of 3 years. These children had come to the General Pediatric Clinic or to the Encopresis Clinic at the University of Iowa, Iowa City, for evaluation of fecal soiling, constipation, severe pain with defecation, vulvar itching, vulvar bleeding, and dysuria. All patients had been studied previously, some on multiple occasions, but none had been diagnosed as having LSA before I examined them. All patients were reexamined at least once to make sure the skin lesions had responded to therapy, and their parents were interviewed by telephone at the time of this report, 3 months to 3.3 years later (mean, 1.8 years), to elicit information concerning the course of LSA, results of treatment, and the general health of the patients.

RESULTS

Clinical Features

The demographics and physical findings of these children, all of whom were white, are listed in the Table. Nine of the 11 patients had been symptomatic for more than 1 year. In two patients (patients 1 and 8), the symptoms had been present for only 3 and 4 months. The onset of LSA could not be assessed with certainty because many parents were not aware of the presence of skin lesions. One case (patient 1) had been reported for sexual abuse. In addition, the families of three girls (patients 2, 4, and 7) were intensively questioned about sexual abuse by multiple examiners. Problems with defecation, including painful bowel movements, constipation, fecal soiling, anal fissures, and anal stenosis, were the chief complaints in nine of 11 patients. Another patient had had severe difficulties with anal fissures 2 years before but not at the time of the diagnosis of LSA. One girl (patient 5) and one boy (patient 11) had been taking daily laxatives for years; they reported pencil-like stools and had developed anal stenosis. Both gave a history of large-caliber stools and painful bowel movements before the start of laxative treatment. The boy had fecal soiling frequently during the day and was also incontinent of stool at night.

Two patients complained of vulvar bleeding, three of perineal itching, and two of painful urination. The two youngest patients had severe itching of the perineum. Patient 7 complained of dysuria and spots of blood on her underwear for the last 8 months. She had two erythematous, excoriated, and desquamated fissures, 1.5 and 2 cm in length, between her labia minora and majora. These lesions had partially healed on several

Presentation of Lichen Sclerosus et Atrophicus in 11 Children

	Symptoms							Involvement on Physical Examination					
Patient/ Sex/ Age, y	Vulvar Bleeding	Perineal Itching	Dysuria	Painful Defecation	Bloody Stools	Constipation	Encopresis	Figure-of-8*	Labial Sores	Perineum	Anal Canal	Natal Cleft	Anal Fissure
1/F/3.3	+†‡	+	−	++	+†	+/−	−	+	+	+	+	−	+
2/F/4.1	−	+†‡	−	−	−	−	−	+/−	+	−	−	−	−
3/F/4.4	−	−	+‡	++‡	−	+†	+‡	+	−	+	+	+	−
4/F/4.7	−	−	−	++‡	+	−	−	+	−	+	+	−	+
5/F/5.8	−	−	−	++‡	+	−§	−	+	−	+	+/Tight	−	−
6/F/7.7	−	−	−	++†‡	+	++†‡	++†‡	+	−	+	+	+	+
7/F/8.2	+‡	+	+‡	+†	+†	+†	−	+	+	+	+	−	+†
8/F/8.4	−	−	−	++	−	++	+‡	+	−	+	+	+	+
9/F/10.2	−	−	−	++‡	−	+‡	++	+	−	+	+	−	−
10/F/11.8	−	−	−	+	+	++	++†‡	+	−	+	+	−	−
11/M/6.7	−	−	−	+†§	−	−§	++‡	+/−	Penile sores	. . .	+/Tight	+	−

*Figure-of-8 appearance of a hypopigmented and sclerotic area seen anterior to the clitoris, involving the clitoris, the labia, and the perineum and encircling the anal canal.
†Initial symptom.
‡Reason for visit.
§Receiving laxative treatment.

occasions but recurred. She had been examined by several specialists and treated with a multitude of creams containing estrogen, antibiotics, and polymyxin B sulfate–bacitracin zinc–neomycin sulfate–hydrocortisone; antibacterial detergents; and a course of oral cephalosporin before being diagnosed as having LSA. No patient gave a family history of LSA.

Physical Examination

In 10 of the 11 patients, the results of physical examination were entirely normal except for the skin changes in the anogenital area. Details on symptoms and anogenital skin changes are presented in the Table. All female patients showed the classic feature of hypopigmented plaques producing an hourglass or figure-of-8 pattern encircling the vulva and anus (Figure). Hemorrhagic, bullous lesions were seen in patient 1. Fissures and ulcers were seen on the labia, between the labia, on the perineum, and in the anal canal and natal cleft in many children and on the glans penis in the boy. In 10 children, the anus showed the same sclerotic plaques along the anal rugae, often reaching into the anal canal. Four children had anal fissures. In two patients (patients 5 and 11), the anal sphincter was very tight, and anal examination was possible only after dilation. One patient (patient 11) had extragenital LSA involving his fingers. His initial anogenital examination revealed a penis that was circumcised and free of lesions. The anus appeared hypopigmented, was surrounded by excorations, and had prominent rugae. He had anal stenosis. The hypopigmented sclerotic lesions around the anus and in the natal cleft persisted, fissuring at times, and at times extended along the raphe toward the scrotum. He later developed sores on the glans penis. All lesions responded to 1% hydrocortisone ointment.

Treatment

All of the patients were treated with 1% hydrocortisone ointment twice daily until fissures and erosions had healed. Subsequently, patients applied the ointment to their anogenital area only when symptoms recurred. The treatment was not curative, but it improved the skin condition. In the two patients with anal stenosis (patients 5 and 11), treatment with milk of magnesia was continued for 1 month and then stopped after the anogenital skin lesions had improved. The stools were normal in diameter, consistency, and frequency at follow-up 1.5 and 2.5 years later, respectively.

Course

These 11 children were followed up for 3 months to 3.3 years (mean, 1.8 years). In three, the anogenital lesions cleared completely (in patient 9 at age 12.2 years, in patient 10 at age 11.3 years, and in patient 11 at 8.8 years, respectively). The fissures healed in all patients, but the hypopigmented areas in the figure-of-8 configuration were still visible in seven, and 1% hydrocortisone ointment was used intermittently for anogenital irritation. In patient 2, the symptoms persisted 3 months later. None of the girls had had menarche on follow-up. Lichen sclerosus et atrophicus involving the fingers only persisted in patient 11.

COMMENT

Lichen sclerosus et atrophicus in childhood is more common than is currently recognized. It can occur at any age and in any race.[2,7] It is most common in the anogenital region, but extragenital involvement has been reported, with involvement of the upper part of the trunk, forearm, neck, and face.[8] The initial lesions of anogenital LSA are irregular ivory macules or papules that coalesce to form homogeneous, hypopigmented plaques producing a figure-of-8 pattern encircling the vulva and anus. The affected skin is sharply demarcated from the normal skin. The hymen is not involved. The skin becomes thin and fissured, is frag-

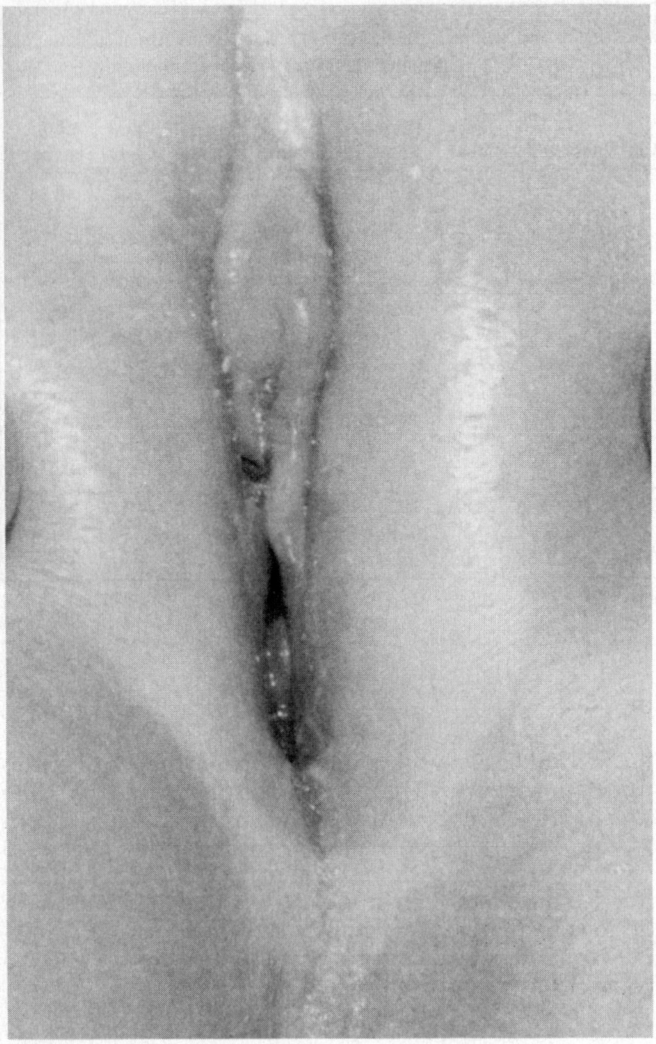

Anogenital area of patient 4. The typical hypopigmented, sclerotic figure-of-8 appearance encircling the genital and anal area is shown. The affected skin is sharply demarcated from the normal skin. A superficial perineal fissure from the posterior commissure to the anus occurred during the physical examination.

ile, and is easily traumatized by minimal pressure, resulting in bruising or bleeding. Trauma is often caused by the inexperienced examiner trying to pull the labia and buttocks apart for inspection. In particular, fissures in the midline of the perineum are easily produced. Purpura, telangiectasia, erosions, excoriations, blistering (usually hemorrhagic), and bleeding can be seen. The appearance of thinned skin with erosions and purpura may be mistaken for trauma, in particular for sexual abuse. Lichen sclerosus et atrophicus mimicking sexual abuse and leading to false accusations has been reported previously.[2-6] The presence of LSA does not exclude sexual abuse, because LSA does occur at sites of trauma, and the trauma may be caused by sexual abuse.[9,10]

The typical symptoms of anogenital LSA are itching, bleeding, and hemorrhagic blisters. Defecation problems have not been observed with the same frequency by other investigators. This could be due to several reasons: (1) my particular interest in childhood constipation and encopresis (six of the 11 patients had been referred to the Encopresis Clinic at the University of Iowa), (2) the possibility that the skin lesions in children with fecal soiling were overlooked because of feces covering the macerated area, and (3) attribution of the skin changes to chronic irritation by feces. Anal fissures, even with enormous large-diameter stools, are rarely seen in children older than 4 years and should raise suspicion of an underlying skin condition. A history of severe anal pain with defecation or anal bleeding should lead to a thorough anorectal examination.

Anogenital LSA is most often diagnosed clinically, but histologic examination of the involved skin can confirm the diagnosis in uncertain cases. Light microscopy shows hyperkeratosis with follicular plugging, atrophy of the malpighian layer, hydropic degeneration of the basal layer, edema and homogenization of collagen in the upper dermis, and an inflammatory infiltrate in the middermis.[11] The differential diagnosis of LSA includes vitiligo, morphea, perianal dermatitis, and postinflammatory hypopigmentation, eg, due to atrophic vulvitis or diaper dermatitis.

The cause of LSA is unknown and is most likely multifactorial. Enzyme deficiencies (elastase-type protease, 5-α-reductase), infection, and an immunologically mediated response to a variety of infectious processes, trauma, or friction have been discussed.[11]

Lichen sclerosus et atrophicus in prepubertal boys is very uncommon.[3] It has been suggested that LSA is the most common cause of phimosis in boys.[12,13] In the uncircumcised patient, a thickened, constricting band forms 1 to 2 cm from the distal edge of the prepuce, commonly resulting in phimosis and adhesions. Lichen sclerosus et atrophicus of the glans penis has been less frequently observed in circumcised males.[3] The involvement of the glans can lead to stenosis of the urethral meatus and urinary obstruction.[14] Carcinoma can arise in preexisting LSA.[3,15]

There is no established specific treatment for LSA. Topical corticosteroids are often of benefit, particularly for pruritus, soreness, and pain. They generally relieve symptoms and may retard the course of the disease. We used 1% hydrocortisone ointment twice daily, with improvement in all children. Fluorinated steroids have been suggested for those whose itching cannot be controlled with unfluorinated steroids.[11] The use of topical estrogen, progesterone, and androgens is not indicated in young children because of possible systemic effects.[5] Others have suggested that especially progesterone in oil or estrogen can be used safely and sometimes effectively in prepubertal girls.[16]

It is anticipated that approximately two thirds of premenarchal girls will have improvement or clearing of their lesions before or about the time of menarche.[17] Long-term prospective studies are still lacking in childhood LSA. Children with persistence of the anogenital LSA will have to be followed up because complications due to atrophy of the labia minora and clitoris and constriction of the vaginal introitus or urethral meatus can occur. The cancer risk in LSA lesions in childhood is probably insignificant, but it is suggested to be 5% in adult women.

I have not seen previous reports of anal stenosis due to LSA. Two of my patients had developed anal stenosis. I think that the laxative treatment allowed the anal stenosis to develop and that daily anal dilation by a normal-sized stool would have prevented the development of stenosis in anal LSA. In addition, the observation of anal involvement in male patients has not been previously reported.

References

1. Rook A, Wilkinson DS, Ebling FJG, Champion RH, Burton JL. *Textbook of Dermatology.* 4th ed. Boston, Mass: Blackwell Scientific Publications Inc; 1986;2:1368-1374.
2. Davidson DC, Clarke MDB, Kean HB. Lichen sclerosus et atrophicus in children misdiagnosed as sexual abuse. *BMJ.* 1987;295:211.
3. Wallace HJ. Lichen sclerosus et atrophicus. *Trans St John's Hosp Dermatol Soc.* 1971;57:9-30.
4. Handfield-Jones SE, Hinde FRJ, Kennedy CTC. Lichen sclerosus et atrophicus in children misdiagnosed as sexual abuse. *BMJ.* 1987;294:1404-1405.
5. Jenny C, Kirby P, Fuquay D. Genital lichen sclerosus mistaken for child sexual abuse. *Pediatrics.* 1989;83:597-599.
6. Berth-Jones J, Graham-Brown RAC, Burns DA. Lichen sclerosus. *Arch Dis Child.* 1989;64:1204-1206.
7. Barclay DL, Macey HB, Reed RJ. Lichen sclerosus et atrophicus of the vulva in children. *Obstet Gynecol.* 1966;27:637-642.
8. Clark JA, Muller SA. Lichen sclerosus et atrophicus in children: a report of 24 cases. *Arch Dermatol.* 1967;95:476-482.
9. Harrington CI. Lichen sclerosus. *Arch Dis Child.* 1990;65:335.
10. Priestley BL, Bleehen SS. Lichen sclerosus and sexual abuse. *Arch Dis Child.* 1990;65:335.
11. Tremaine RDL, Miller RAW. Lichen sclerosus et atrophicus. *Int J Dermatol.* 1989;28:10-16.
12. Rickwood AMK, Hemalatha V, Batcup G, Spitz L. Phimosis in boys. *Br J Urol.* 1980;52:147-150.
13. Chalmers RJG, Burton PA, Bennett R, Goring CC. Lichen sclerosus et atrophicus: a distinctive and common cause of phimosis in boys. *Br J Dermatol.* 1982;107(suppl 22):29-30.
14. Laymon CW, Freeman C. Relationship of balanitis xerotica obliterans to lichen sclerosus et atrophicus. *Arch Dermatol.* 1944;49:57-59.
15. Weber P, Rabinovitz H, Garland L. Verrucous carcinoma in penile lichen sclerosus et atrophicus. *J Dermatol Surg Oncol.* 1987;13:529-532.
16. Hebert AA, Esterly NB. Mucous membrane disorders. In: Schachner LA, Hansen RC, eds. *Pediatric Dermatology.* New York, NY: Churchill-Livingstone Inc; 1988;453-454.
17. Török E, Orley J, Gorácz G, Daróczy J. Lichen sclerosus et atrophicus in children: clinical and pathological analysis of 33 cases. *Mod Probl Paediatr.* 1975;17:262-271.

In Other AMA Journals

ARCHIVES OF NEUROLOGY

Spinal Tumors in Children and Adolescents: The International Review of Child Neurology

Ignacio Pascual-Castroviejo, Reviewed by Henry S. Schutta, MD
(*Arch Neurol.* 1991;48:786)

Diagnostic Criteria for Multiple Sclerosis Research Involving Multiply Affected Families

Donald E. Goodkin, MD; Teresa H. Doolittle, PA-C, MHP; Stephen S. Hauser, MD; Richard M. Ransohoff, MD; Allen D. Roses, MD; Richard A. Rudick, MD
(*Arch Neurol.* 1991;48:805-807)

Treatment of Ulcerated Hemangiomas With the Pulsed Tunable Dye Laser

Joseph G. Morelli, MD; O. T. Tan, MD; William L. Weston, MD

• **Hemangiomas are the most common tumor of infancy and are characterized by rapid growth during the first 6 months of life. During the rapid growth phase, approximately 5% to 10% of the hemangiomas ulcerate. Ulcerated lesions are painful, may bleed, and are at risk for bacterial infection. Previous therapy has included daily local wound care, topical antibiotics, and local and systemic steroids. We treated nine infants (eight female and one male) with ulcerated hemangiomas by means of a vascular-specific (585-nm) pulsed (450-microsecond) tunable dye laser. Eight of the nine patients had a single ulceration, whereas one patient had two ulcerations within a large hemangioma. Six of the ulcerations healed with a single laser treatment. One ulceration required two treatments to heal, and the remaining two required three treatments. Pain was subjectively decreased within 2 to 3 days in all patients after a single treatment. The pulsed tunable dye laser should be considered in the treatment of all ulcerated hemangiomas.**

(*AJDC.* 1991;145:1062-1064)

Hemangiomas are common tumors of infancy. They have a well-defined course consisting of an early rapid growth phase, followed by slow involution in most cases.[1-3] Since most hemangiomas regress, many authorities recommend treatment only for those hemangiomas that cause medical complications, such as obstruction (vision, breathing, defecation, or urination), high-output cardiac failure, and consumption coagulopathy. The treatment of choice in these situations is high-dose systemic glucocorticosteroids.[4]

Most hemangiomas do not fit into any of the above categories, do not require treatment with systemic steroids, and do not produce systemic complications. However, they are not without local complications. These include ulceration and infection during the rapid growth phase, and redundant skin folds, pigmentary changes, and fibrofatty deposits remaining after involution.[5] Ulceration of the hemangiomas occurs in 5% to 10% of cases.[5] This may cause severe discomfort for the child, scarring of the affected area, and an increased likelihood of infection and hemorrhage. Treatment of ulcerated hemangiomas is often difficult and has consisted of topical antibiotics, occlusive or semiocclusive barriers, and locally injected glucocorticosteroids, as well as systemic steroids.[5]

Pulsed tunable dye lasers were developed for the treatment of port-wine stains.[6,7] They are also approved by the Food and Drug Administration for the treatment of hemangiomas and have been reported to be effective in selected cases.[8,9] Because of the pain with ulcerated hemangiomas and the lack of fully effective therapy, we treated ulcerated hemangiomas with the pulsed tunable dye laser.

PATIENTS AND METHODS

Nine patients with ulcerated hemangiomas presented to either the Birthmark Treatment Center at the University of Colorado School of Medicine, Denver, or the Laser Center at Boston (Mass) City Hospital. The results are summarized in the Table. All of the hemangiomas ulcerated and became painful during the rapid growth phase, and the patients were brought in for treatment between 2 and 6½ months of age. Eight of the nine lesions were in the diaper area. Most of the patients had a single ulceration, while one female infant had two distinct ulcerations within a large hemangioma. The ulcerations were 3 to 35 mm in diameter and had been present for between 3 and 12 weeks before treatment.

All patients were treated with a vascular-specific (585-nm) pulsed (450-microsecond) dye laser (Candela SPTL-1, Candela Corp, Wayland, Mass). The entire hemangioma, not just the ulcerated portion, was treated during each visit. All of the ulcer bases were clean at the time of treatment.

All treatments were performed with a laser energy of 6.0 to 6.5 J/cm^2. Patients were treated every 2 to 4 weeks without anesthesia. Posttreatment care consisted of frequent application of bacitracin ointment. None of the patients received any previous or concomitant treatment.

RESULTS

Six of the 10 ulcers healed within 2 weeks with a single treatment, two healed after two treatments, and the other two required three treatments. In each of our patients, before the initial laser treatment, the parents reported the child to be in pain. Pain was subjectively eliminated in all patients after a single treatment. Parents reported that as early as the day after treatment the child's pain had subsided. Pain relief lasted as long as the patients were followed up. No injections after the treatments were re-

Accepted for publication April 4, 1991.

From the Department of Dermatology, Birthmark Treatment Center, University of Colorado School of Medicine, Denver (Drs Morelli and Weston); and Laser Center, Boston (Mass) City Hospital (Dr Tan).

Reprint requests to Department of Dermatology B-153, University of Colorado School of Medicine, 4200 E Ninth Ave, Denver, CO 80262 (Dr Morelli).

Patients With Ulcerated Hemangiomas					
Patient/Sex	Location	Age at 1st Treatment, mo	No. and Size (mm) of Ulcerations	Time Ulcerated Before Treatment, wk	No. of Treatments to Healing
1/F	L buttock	5	2, 35, and 15	6 and 4	2 and 1
2/F	Vulva	3.5	1, 9	8	1
3/M	Neck	6.5	1, 25	3	3
4/F	Perianal	5	1, 21	12	1
5/F	Perineal	4.5	1, 3	3	1
6/F	Vulva	6.5	1, 20	4	2
7/F	R buttock	3	1, 5	3	1
8/F	Vulva	4	1, 25	4	3
9/F	Perineal	2	1, 5	6	1

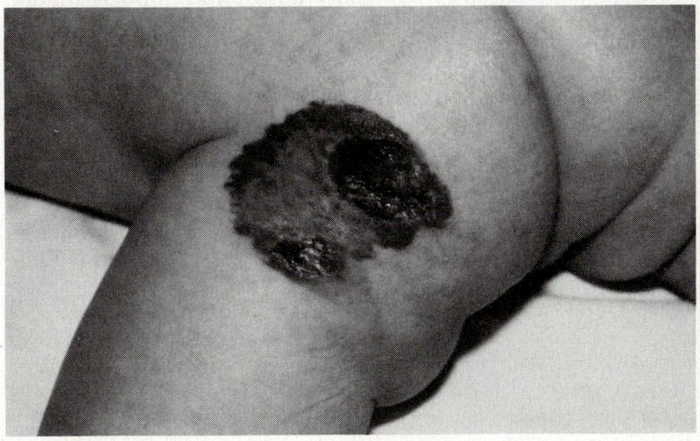

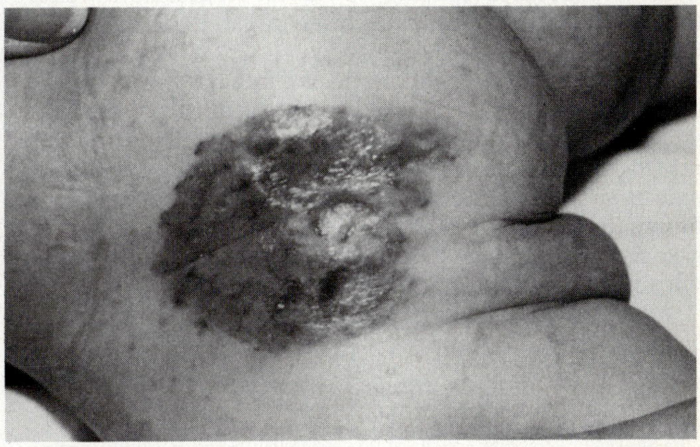

Fig 1.—*Left, Ulcerated hemangioma of the buttock in a 5-month-old white girl. Right, Same hemangioma 1 month later after two laser treatments.*

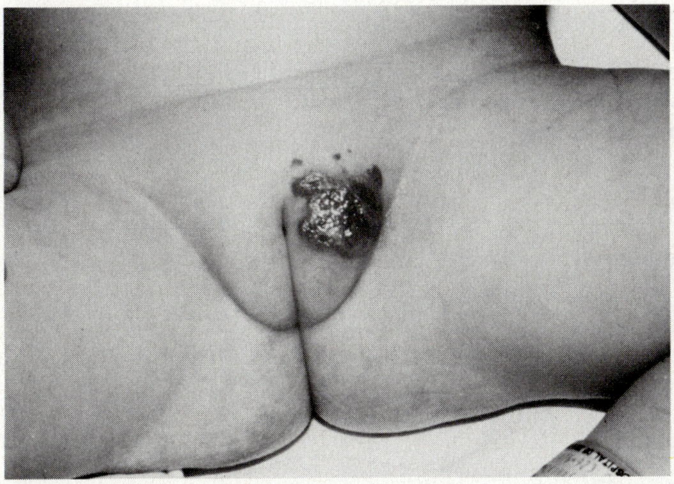

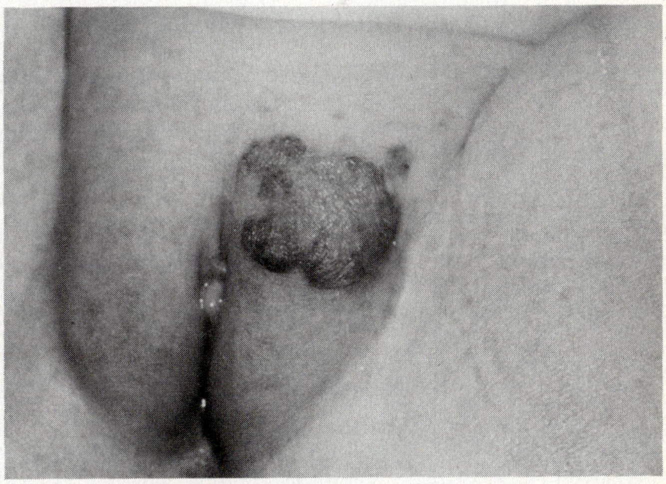

Fig 2.—*Left, Ulcerated hemangioma of the vulva in a 6½-month-old white girl. Right, Same hemangioma 1 month later after two laser treatments.*

ported. Figures 1 and 2 show patients 1 and 6, respectively, before and after treatment.

COMMENT

Ulceration of these lesions is a relatively common problem for which only supportive therapy has been available. Treatment of ulcerated hemangiomas with a vascular-specific pulsed dye laser leads to rapid healing of the ulcerated area. This therapy also decreases the associated pain, minimizes the risk of infection, and decreases the eventual scarring by preventing enlargement of the ulceration.

The mechanism of hemangioma ulceration is poorly understood. These lesions almost always ulcerate during their rapid growth phase. Ulceration also tends to occur in mixed superficial and deep hemangiomas located in areas of trauma and frequent movement. Eight of the nine ulcerated hemangiomas that we treated were located in the diaper area.

The mechanism of wound healing in ulcerated hemangiomas is also poorly understood. Vascular-specific pulsed dye lasers function by selective photothermolysis of capillary-sized blood vessels. It is possible that thermal damage to the vessels at the surface of the ulcerated hemangioma leads to the release of factors that stimulate wound healing, although this is speculative.

All of the ulcerations that were less than 20 mm healed completely within 2 weeks after a single treatment. The very large (>20 mm) ulcerations required two to three treatments, but all had begun healing after one treatment. It is possible that, given more time, they would have resolved with a single treatment. No side effects were noted.

This form of tumor destruction appears to accelerate the natural processes leading to tumor regression. After treatment, the hemangiomas often began to develop central pallor.

We suggest that vascular-specific pulsed dye lasers are safe and effective for the treatment of mixed superficial and deep hemangiomas that have ulcerated during the rapid growth phase. It is optimal to treat the hemangiomas as soon as an ulceration is noted, because ulcerations of less than 20 mm may heal within 2 weeks, and the pain associated with the ulcerated hemangioma diminishes within 24 hours after a single treatment. We believe that pulsed dye laser therapy should be considered as a treatment option for ulcerated hemangiomas.

References

1. Lister WA. The natural history of strawberry naevi. *Lancet.* 1938;1:1429-1434.
2. Simpson JR. The natural history of cavernous haemangiomata. *Lancet.* 1959;2:1057-1059.
3. Mulliken JB. Diagnosis and natural history of hemangiomas. In: Mulliken JB, Young AE, eds. *Vascular Birthmarks: Hemangiomas and Malformations.* Philadelphia, Pa: WB Saunders Co; 1988:41-62.
4. Fost NC, Esterly NB. Successful treatment of juvenile hemangiomas with prednisone. *J Pediatr.* 1968;72:351-357.
5. Mulliken JB. Diagnosis and natural history of hemangiomas. In: Mulliken JB, Young AE, eds. *Vascular Birthmarks: Hemangiomas and Malformations.* Philadelphia, Pa: WB Saunders Co; 1988:77-103.
6. Anderson RR, Parrish JA. Selective photothermolysis: precise microsurgery by selective absorption of pulsed radiation. *Science.* 1983;220:524-527.
7. Tan OT, Sherwood K, Gilchrest BA. Treatment of children with port wine stains using the flashlamp-pulsed tunable dye laser. *N Engl J Med.* 1989;320:416-421.
8. Glassberg E, Lask G, Rabinowitz LG, et al. Capillary hemangiomas: case study of a novel laser treatment and a review of therapeutic options. *J Dermatol Surg Oncol.* 1989;15:1214-1223.
9. Sherwood K, Tan OT. Treatment of a capillary hemangioma with the flashlamp pumped-dye laser. *J Am Acad Dermatol.* 1990;22:136-137.

In Other AMA Journals

ARCHIVES OF INTERNAL MEDICINE

Drug Abuse Treatment as a Strategy to Prevent Human Immunodeficiency Virus Infection Among Intravenous Drug Users: How Can We Maximize Prevention of Infection?

A. Preston West
(*Arch Intern Med.* 1991;151:1493-1496)

Legal Myths About Terminating Life Support

Alan Meisel, JD
(*Arch Intern Med.* 1991;151:1497-1502)

New Mexicare

Arthur Vall-Spinosa, MD
(*Arch Intern Med.* 1991;151:1503-1509)

The Adverse Effects of Hospitalizaton on Drug Regimens

Deborah M. Omori, MD; Roger P. Potyk, PharmD; Kurt Roenke, MD
(*Arch Intern Med.* 1991;151:1562-1564)

Call for Abstracts

The American Pediatric Society and The Society for Pediatric Research announce that the abstract deadline for the 1992 Annual Meeting (May 4-7, 1992, Convention Center, Baltimore, Md) has been set as *January 3, 1992*. For further information, contact the APS/SPR Association Headquarters, 141 Northwest Point Blvd, PO Box 675, Elk Grove Village, IL 60009-0675; (708) 427-0205; FAX (708) 427-1305.

Health Care for Uninsured and Underinsured Children

Sir.—The May issue of *AJDC* was depressing to say the least. The problems were well elucidated by all of the authors, but when it came to offering solutions, it was a different story. Some offered no concrete plans for improvement. Those with proposals did not come to a consensus. Surprisingly, I found the recommendations offered by Steve Kohl, MD, an infectious disease researcher, to be the broadest and most sensible of them all.

It seems to me that it is time for another White House Conference on Children and Youth that would, I hope, make recommendations for a major overhaul in the way our country is dealing with this problem. Certainly, the "defense" of our children is every bit as important as, if not more important than, the defense of our country with our tremendous expenditures for the military.

Joseph H. Davis, MD
Palo Alto Medical Clinic
40 Anderson Way
Menlo Park, CA 94025

Sir.—I commend you for the in-depth discussion in the May 1991 issue of *AJDC* concerning the increasing difficulty in providing adequate, not to mention equitable, care to children and adolescents in this country.

As a pediatric gastroenterologist who treats many children with chronic disease, I am only too aware of the numerous obstacles faced by their families, many of which are alluded to in the articles by Miller and White[1] and Allen et al.[2] Families cannot afford appropriate medications or continuity of care and cannot obtain medical insurance coverage. Problems mount as industrious older adolescents and young adults are refused employment because the employer would face higher medical insurance costs if they were hired.

Pediatric teaching hospitals that, in the past, championed the needs of the disadvantaged are under increasing pressures to subvert ethical concerns in the interest of fiscal success. The message we are giving to medical students and house staffs, our physicians of the future, is very disturbing.

Clearly, these issues are well recognized by pediatricians and need to be shared with the broader community. A copy of this edition of the *AJDC* should be sent to the office of each member of the US Senate and House of Representatives.

Escalating health costs are affecting not only the poor, but also large segments of the middle class. National legislation to address these problems is urgently needed.

Barbara S. Kirschner, MD
Department of Pediatrics
Section of Gastroenterology,
Hepatology, and Nutrition
The University of Chicago
Hospital Box 107
5841 S Maryland Ave
Chicago, IL 60637-1470

1. Miller ML, White PH. The challenge of caring for indigent children with rheumatologic diseases. *AJDC*. 1991; 145: 554-558.
2. Allen HD, Taubert KA, Deckelbaum RJ, et al. Poverty and cardiac disease in children. *AJDC*. 1991;145:550-553.

Sir.—I read with interest the May 1991 issue of *AJDC* devoted to the desperate plight of health care for poor children in the United States. As a pediatrician serving a low-income rural population, with 75% of my patients receiving Medicaid, 20% being uninsured, and 5% being insured (figures reflecting the area's pediatric population as a whole), I concur with Fulginiti's editorial statement, "The reasons for the lack of medical care are legion; the most often cited . . . are financial."[1] However, one aspect of the pediatric care crisis not addressed is the impact on providers of care outside of metropolitan areas.

In his article, Nelson[2] overlooks the problem in rural areas, stating that "the most serious deficits are, . . . to a great extent, concentrated in our large metropolitan areas." It is an oversight to ignore poor children in rural areas who face enormous obstacles in obtaining access to medical care.

In her article, Berkowitz states " . . . the underserved represent a diverse group, including a large portion of financially disadvantaged and/or geographically isolated children (rural and migrant farm workers). Care of these children . . . often falls into the bailiwick of pediatricians in training."[3] While this might be true in some areas near training programs, the care of rural and migrant children is usually provided by federally subsidized clinics, private pediatricians, family practitioners, and midlevel practitioners. The shortage of providers where I work is so severe that essentially all practices are closed to new patients. There are no training programs within 180 miles, and recruitment of practitioners to the area is extremely difficult. An indication of the shortage is that most of the 2500 babies born annually at our regional medical center are discharged within 24 hours of life without an identified source of pediatric care.

The immediate physician shortage crisis in medically underserved rural areas will not be alleviated without compensation to providers that is truly competitive with more "attractive" areas. Without the luxury of local training programs and well-staffed hospitals, rural pediatricians are frequently the intravenous therapy team, phlebotomists, resuscitators of neonates, emergency room code team, and trauma team. Medicaid compensates physicians for these activities at rates that are approximately 30% to 40% of usual and customary fees. Salaried physicians in rural areas generally fare poorly in terms of compensation compared with physicians in metropolitan areas. The starting salary for an experienced pediatrician at my place of employment in 1991 is $10 000 less than the average starting salary of a pediatrician just out of residency in 1988. There should be no surprise that recruitment in this setting is difficult when physicians would find themselves working long hours in a comparatively primitive medical setting, in which they are often socially and professionally isolated, for a fraction of the income possible in larger cities. Until the economic needs of rural practitioners are recognized and addressed, the physician shortage will continue, and the care of children will suffer.

STEPHEN JAMES PEARSON, MD
110 S Date St
Toppenish, WA 98948

1. Fulginiti VA. Far from the ideal: the plight of poor children in the United States. *AJDC.* 1991;145:489-490.
2. Nelson WE. A regional pediatric approach to the epidemic of social ills within our cities. *AJDC.* 1991;145:505-506.
3. Berkowitz CD. Serving the underserved: impact on resident education. *AJDC.* 1991;145:544-545.

Sir.—The May 1991 issue of *AJDC*, with the impressive articles by outstanding leaders in the field, was most interesting. Unfortunately, most wanted to put more money and effort into the plight of children without asking anything in return! Twenty-five years after a marked increase in social expenditures, we are worse off because we did not ask anything in return!

Hinman[1] was the only author who suggested it may not be just money, but "incentives, either positive or negative." Cleveland,[2] Stahlman,[3] Haggerty,[4] and Blum and Blank[5] touched on rationing, jobs, and lack of accountability. Conspicuously absent was Louis Sullivan, Secretary of Health and Human Services of the United States, who is outspoken on changing life-styles for better health and on individuals taking some responsibility. Many nationally prominant persons have pointed out our finite resources as a reminder that spending here means taking away there.

While I agree that more needs to be done for children's health care, their education and life values need attention too. Society cannot do all things for everyone. We have put individual rights and freedoms on such a pedestal that we are quickly destroying the society that made it possible. To loosely paraphrase John F. Kennedy, we need to ask what people can do for themselves (to show responsibility to society) and not what society can give to them (with no strings attached). Delayed gratification has given way to the current "me first" attitude of "Do it! Do it now!" (without thought of the consequences to society today and in the future). More money and effort alone are not going to solve the problems. We also need accountability and responsibility.

JAMES A. HECKER, MD
Cheyenne Children's Clinic, PC
433 E 19th St
Cheyenne, WY 82001

1. Hinman AR. What will it take to fully protect all American children with vaccines? *AJDC.* 1991;145:559-562.
2. Cleveland WW. Redoing the health care quilt: patches or whole cloth? *AJDC.* 1991;145:499-504.
3. Stahlman MT. Improving health care provision to neonates in the United States. *AJDC.* 1991;145:510-512.
4. Haggerty RJ. Care of the poor and underserved in America: older adolescents: a group at special risk. 1991; 145:569-571.
5. Blum BB, Blank S. Children's services in an era of budget deficits. *AJDC.* 1991;145:575-578.

Sir.—The May 1991 issue of *AJDC* clearly documents the deficiency of health care of poor children in the United States. Many address the issues of access to medical attention and the importance of insurance. A few[1-4] suggest successful innovative processes that might be more widely adopted.

Johnston[5] mentions a factor that is frequently overlooked, which is that "health is not a survival issue for poor people." Some have found that food, shelter, and jobs have much higher priority than health care and schooling. Certainly, " . . . we need a fundamental change in our national commitment. We need to behave as if children are really our most valuable resource and our future."[6]

One way to change is to encourage people to seek health care. Services that clearly benefit health should be rewarded. For example, parents should receive nominal amounts of cash each time they bring a child for timely immunizations or prenatal visits. Several precedents are known. A pediatrician is said to have started a lottery for women who attend prenatal clinics and has improved pregnancy outcome. Mothers in South Africa attend public clinics to obtain birth control pills because this is something they perceive as immediate benefit, but do not bring their children to these same clinics for free immunizations because they do not recognize an immediate benefit in doing so.

Such programs should not be expensive. Several approaches to lower the cost of health care that might be applicable have been suggested (*The New York Times.* May 14, 1991.). These include revamping the malpractice system, developing better competition for managed care plans, closing hospitals with low occupancy, and requesting doctors only for those procedures for which they are uniquely trained. Norman Fost, MD, has indicated (oral communication, April 1991) that many routine procedures and practices could be performed equally well by less qualified medical personnel and at lower cost than that of health care provided by physicians. Other funds could be obtained by taxing administrators and those duplicative procedures that raise medical costs. The shift of health care costs from physicians to administrators apparently confirms that not only governments, but also other bureaucracies, can be inefficient, wasteful, and slow.

Something has to be done while we await an improved health system with universal access.[7] Carefully selecting factors that improve health and rewarding those who participate might improve the health status of our children.

LEWIS A. BARNESS, MD
Waisman Center
University of Wisconsin-Madison
1500 Highland Ave
Madison, WI 53705-2280

1. Miller ML, White PH. The challenge of caring for indigent children with rheumatologic diseases. *AJDC*. 1991;145:554-558.
2. Udow M, Smith VK, Mason MH. The Caring Program for Children: the Michigan experience. *AJDC*. 1991;145:579-580.
3. Blum BB, Blank S. Children's services in an era of budget deficits. *AJDC*. 1991;145:575-578.
4. Porter PJ, Butler JC. Healthy children: an assessment of community-based primary health care programs for children and their impact on access, cost, and quality. *Adv Pediatr*. 1987;34:379-410.
5. Johnston RB Jr. Poverty and the health of American children: implications for academic pediatrics. *AJDC*. 1991;145:507-509.
6. Fulginiti VA. Far from the ideal: the plight of poor children in the United States. *AJDC*. 1991;145:489-490.
7. Strain JE. The American Academy of Pediatrics response to the growing health needs of children. *AJDC*. 1991;145:536-539.

Parental Drinking Habits

Sir.—More than 20 000 people die in the United States each year as a result of alcohol-related motor vehicle accidents. Since children form their own habits and life-styles based on their parents' examples, it is prudent that parents set high standards regarding alcohol and limits on its consumption. One instance of setting poor examples occurs during the holiday season, when some parents, for their children to more actively participate in the festivities, give them nonalcoholic wine and beer while the parents imbibe the real thing. This behavior can give a child the impression from an early age that since Mom or Dad gave me a beverage like their own it must be acceptable. This can only increase a child's perception that alcohol consumption in our society is part of the norm. Pediatricians should be aware of this problem and dissuade parents from this behavior, since it promotes in the child an association of the holiday season with alcohol consumption.

JOSEPH J. WELLS, MD
Maryvale Pediatric Clinic
4700 N 51 Ave
Phoenix, AZ 85031

MICHAEL A. VILLANI, MD
Temple University Hospital
Broad and Tioga Streets
Philadelphia, PA 19140

Cholesterol Testing in the Physician's Office: Accuracy Assessment

Sir.—To assess the quality of cholesterol testing performed outside hospital laboratories and reference clinical laboratories, we evaluated the accuracy of cholesterol measurement in 33 pediatricians' offices in the Washington, DC, metropolitan area. The participating pediatricians responded to a survey we conducted locally to determine the number of pediatricians performing cholesterol testing. Seventy-one of the 116 responding pediatricians performed cholesterol testing routinely in their practices. Sixty-five percent of those pediatricians participated in this study.

Materials and Methods.—Four frozen specimens, duplicate sets of two samples with cholesterol concentrations of 4.46 and 6.55 mmol/L, were sent to every participating pediatrician. The cholesterol concentrations of the samples were unknown to the pediatricians. The cholesterol concentrations of these sets were determined using an analyzer (Kodak Ektachem 700, Eastman Kodak Co, Rochester, NY) certified by the Centers for Disease Control–Reference Method Laboratory Network for cholesterol testing. Physicians were asked to thaw and twice analyze one set (one low and one high concentration) on the day the samples were received and repeat the same procedure the next day with the second set. Cholesterol was previously shown to be stable in frozen pooled serum for up to 5 years.[1]

Results.—Twenty-five of the 33 participating laboratories used either the DT-60 (Eastman Kodak; 16 laboratories) or the REFLOTRON (Boehringer-Mannheim Diagnostics, Indianapolis, Ind; nine laboratories) analyzer. Sixteen laboratories used medical technologists (nine) or laboratory technicians (seven) to perform the testing. At least one quality control specimen was used by 31 laboratories, and the remaining two laboratories did not use any control materials. Two or three samples with different cholesterol values are normally used for quality control. For the target value 4.46 mmol/L, the range of reported results was 3.57 to 7.74 mmol/L, and for the target value 6.55 mmol/L, the range was 5.49 to 8.13 mmol/L. According to the National Cholesterol Education Program's ideal criterion of ±8.9% total allowable error for one cholesterol measurement,[1] 83% of reported measurements of both samples were acceptable. When the total allowable error was increased to the currently adopted criterion of ±14.2%,[2] more than 95% of reported measurements were acceptable. All results from three laboratories were outside the ±8.9% limit. However, when a ±14.2% limit was employed, only one laboratory reported all unacceptable values. Although only one laboratory used QuickRead (Photest Diagnostics, Mahwah, NJ) and one used CHEMCARD (Chematics Inc, North Webster, Ind), we are concerned about the inaccurate measurements associated with the use of these two devices. QuickRead and CHEMCARD results were 74% to 31% higher than the target value of 4.46 mmol/L, respectively. Variations in cholesterol values from target concentrations, determined with the various methods, are listed in the Table.

Comment.—Although most pediatricians fulfilled the current National Cholesterol Education Program's requirements for cholesterol testing, the range of reported results, especially at the critical concentration of 4.46 mmol/L, remained wide. The diagnosis of hypercholesterolemia in children, according to the American Academy of Pediatrics, is based on cholesterol concentrations higher than 4.56 mmol/L (the average concentration in males and females up to age 19 years).[3] Twenty-seven percent of the reported measurements of the 4.46-mmol/L concentration sample were higher than 4.56 mmol/L. Misdiagnosis of hypercholesterolemia

Variations of Cholesterol Values From Target Concentrations*

Instrument	No. of Laboratories	4.46-mmol/L Sample: Mean ± SD (Range), mmol/L, on Day 1	4.46-mmol/L Sample: Mean ± SD (Range), mmol/L, on Day 2	6.55-mmol/L Sample: Mean ± SD (Range), mmol/L, on Day 1	6.55-mmol/L Sample: Mean ± SD (Range), mmol/L, on Day 2
DT-60 (Eastman Kodak Co, Rochester, NY)	16	0.17 ± 0.16 (0-0.62)	0.18 ± 0.12 (0-0.49)	0.39 ± 0.53 (0-2.72)	0.36 ± 0.30 (0-1.11)
Reflotron (Boehringer-Mannheim Diagnostics, Indianapolis, Ind)	9	0.25 ± 0.24 (0.03-0.80)	0.28 ± 0.21 (0.08-0.88)	0.41 ± 0.40 (0.08-1.58)	0.26 ± 0.22 (0.08-0.91)
Unimeter 300 (BioDynamics Inc, Indianapolis, Ind)	3	0.25 ± 0.20 (0.05-0.60)	0.19 ± 0.15 (0.05-0.41)	0.21 ± 0.09 (0.08-0.31)	0.28 ± 0.22 (0.05-0.57)
Seralyzer (Miles Laboratories, Ames Division, Elkhart, Ind)	3	0.25 ± 0.15 (0-0.47)	0.32 ± 0.10 (0.21-0.41)	0.39 ± 0.39 (0.03-0.98)	0.61 ± 0.36 (0.03-0.91)
QuickRead (Photest Diagnostics, Mahwah, NJ)	1	3.29	2.93	NA	NA
CHEMCARD (Chematics Inc, North Webster, Ind)	1	1.70 ± 0.37 (1.37-2.02)	1.70 ± 0.37 (1.37-2.02)	1.22	1.22
Mean	...	0.31 ± 0.51 (0-3.29)	0.33 ± 0.47 (0-2.93)	0.47 ± 0.69 (0-2.72)	0.44 ± 0.06 (0-1.22)

*Variation was defined as the difference of reported cholesterol values from the target values. NA indicates values higher than the detectable limit of the assay.

because of erroneous cholesterol measurements could precipitate unnecessary, stringent dietary modifications and parental anxiety or could prevent a true hypercholesterolemic child from receiving the appropriate therapy. Furthermore, a complete lipoprotein profile (including measurement of triglyceride, total cholesterol, high-density lipoprotein cholesterol, and low-density lipoprotein cholesterol levels) is required to adequately assess the hypercholesterolemic status of a child.

Cholesterol testing in physicians' offices is not as well regulated as that performed in clinical laboratories. State and federal regulatory agencies are beginning to address regulatory issues concerning in-office testing by physicians. The National Cholesterol Education Program's Laboratory Standardization Panel has recently issued recommendations regarding cholesterol testing outside clinical laboratories.[4] These recommendations include the use of accurate and precise analyzers that can determine cholesterol concentration within 3% bias of reference values and with ±3% precision, the use of a properly trained operator (ideally, a trained medical technician or technologist), the institution of a quality control system, participation in proficiency surveys, and the use of a system of split-sample analyses to routinely compare cholesterol testing performed in the physician's office with that performed in a qualified laboratory. Such actions will ensure that the quality of testing performed in physicians' offices is comparable with that performed in hospitals or reference laboratories.

Nader Rifai, PhD
Mariet Iosefsohn, MS
Jocelyn M. Hicks, PhD
Department of Laboratory Medicine
Children's National Medical Center
The George Washington University Medical Center
111 Michigan Ave, NW
Washington, DC 20010

1. Kuchmak M, Taylor L, Olansky AS. Suitability of frozen and lyophilized reference sera for cholesterol and triglyceride determinations. *Clin Chim Acta.* 1982;120:261-271.

2. Laboratory Standardization Panel. Current status of blood cholesterol measurement in clinical laboratories in the United States: a report from the Laboratory Standardization Panel of the National Cholesterol Education Program. *Clin Chem.* 1988;34:193-201.

3. American Academy of Pediatrics Committee on Nutrition. Indications for cholesterol testing in children. *Pediatrics.* 1989;83:141-142.

4. Laboratory Standardization Panel. *Recommendations for Improving Cholesterol Measurement: A Report From the Laboratory Standardization Panel of the National Cholesterol Education Program.* Bethesda, Md: National Institutes of Health; 1990. NIH publication 90-2964.

Formula Companies and the Medical Profession

Sir.—I enjoyed reading the article by Greer and Apple[1] detailing the historical development of formulas and the previous adverse effect of advertising on the laity. However, I must take issue with the statement "direct public advertising . . . will once again remove the realm of infant feeding from the supervision of the physician and will likely have a negative impact on the incidence and duration of breastfeeding." This opinion (and it is strictly an opinion with no factual basis) has been expressed elsewhere. It implies that the pediatrician cannot effectively influence mothers and advise and guide them as to the advantages of breastfeeding.

In my experience, mothers either do not breastfeed initially or discontinue nursing early not because of free formula coupons but because they plan to return to full-time work. Continuation of adequate nursing then poses a real problem. Formula advertising may make it easier for mothers to select a preferred formula rather than be influenced by the hospital's use of a certain formula or the contents of the give-away pack.

If a mother is really interested in breastfeeding and is encouraged to do so by her pediatrician, she will not be dissuaded by formula advertising.

H. WILLIAM FINK, MD
Department of Pediatric Education
DePaul Medical Center
150 Kingsley Ln
Norfolk, VA 23505

1. Greer FR, Apple RD. Physicians, formula companies, and advertising: a historical perspective. *AJDC*. 1991;145:282-286.

Sir.—Greer and Apple's interesting article[1] pointing out the relationship between formula companies and the medical profession tells only part of the story. In alluding to the formula companies working out of self interest, as expressed by Mead Johnson, they did not point out that the medical profession was also acting in its own economic interest when it helped establish that "comfortable, symbiotic relationship" with the formula companies. The financial benefit accrued by physicians when parents require medical assistance to feed their infants is hardly mentioned. (It is unlikely that many mothers 80 or 100 years ago would have consulted the doctor on how to breastfeed, since they knew that most doctors—almost all men—would not have been able to help them. Mothers now do consult doctors about breastfeeding, but, unfortunately, the medical curriculum is such that doctors still do not know how to help them. Indeed, doctors usually hinder mothers seeking advice). Greer and Apple's article gives the impression that the physicians were only interested in the welfare of the infants. If this were so, however, the medical profession would have promoted breastfeeding as the only proven adequate method of feeding infants, with alternatives to be used only when absolutely necessary as therapeutic modalities, not as "normal" feeding methods.

It is that direct television or magazine advertising encourages mothers to feed their babies a particular formula, which most mothers then realize can be made without physician supervision. This is the real sticking point. Greer and Apple state as a given the debatable point that infant feeding must be supervised by a physician. Thus, physicians who are enraged by television advertising of formula willingly give out starter packages of formula, which Gerber quite rightly argues is advertising, just as is a 30-second spot on television or the equally abominable practice of mailing out coupons. Starter packages have the implied backing of the physician or hospital, which is very powerful persuasion indeed. The information booklets usually contained in these starter packages subtly, and not so subtly, inform mothers that "breast is best," but that breastfeeding can be tiring, difficult, painful, complex, and possibly even dangerous, and that the mother is likely to fail at breastfeeding. In fact, the scanty information on breastfeeding is often dated, inaccurate, and likely to cause problems rather than solve them. Rarely do the information booklets warn the mother that giving bottles to young breastfeeding babies may result in serious breastfeeding problems, including breast rejection and failure to thrive. Indeed, the booklets usually encourage the "occasional" bottle feed. And they strongly reinforce the unproved notion that formula and breast milk are virtually the same. Just as the formulas of 1924 were the same as breast milk, I suppose.

Studies[2,3] have shown that the simple act of giving starter packages in hospitals results in decreased duration of breastfeeding. How anyone can turn logic on its head and suppose that starter packages do not constitute direct advertising to the lay public is beyond comprehension. There is no doubt that the starter packages are designed to "hook" the mother and baby onto formula feeding and then . . . Well, the cost of starter packages is cheap for the formula company compared with the payoff of several hundred dollars per baby of virtually guaranteed sales. Physicians willingly, happily, give free formula, even to women who prenatally expressed no interest in formula feeding—just in case they change their minds. Physicians do this instead of informing them of the benefits of breastfeeding and how to avoid problems with breastfeeding. Doctors may even believe they are doing a good deed, particularly if the pregnant woman is poor, because giving the starter packages means the mother saves money by initially buying less formula. If physicians really wanted to save the mother money, they would encourage her to breastfeed. Breastfeeding might save her some doctor's bills, too.

Greer and Apple are also too kind to the formula companies when they say that the companies have largely complied with the World Health Organization code in distributing their products in developing countries. The companies have complied only when governments have forced them to comply. In most countries, governments have not taken strong stands on distribution of formula. I do not know if Greer and Apple have firsthand knowledge in this area, but I have.

Breastfeeding should almost always work, and work well, but interference with normal breastfeeding results in many mothers failing at breastfeeding. Physicians have responded to suggestions of interference with an indifference that has been cultivated by years of formula company advertising that strives to convince us that their products are almost as good as breast milk. It is time that the health professions cut the too comfortable cord with the formula companies and refuse to be marketing agents for an inferior, expensive product that should only occasionally be necessary. The plentiful money given by the companies to doctors and their associations makes the skeptical scrutinizing of formula claims inconvenient. Physicians at the beginning of the 20th century did not think themselves less wise, or less informed, than we think ourselves to be now, yet many accepted that the concoctions marketed as infant formula were very similar to breastmilk. Are we that different, when, as a group, we accept the same line, despite the fact that we hardly know the importance of the very great differences between formulas and breastmilk?

JACK NEWMAN, MD, FRCPC
The Hospital for Sick Children
Breastfeeding Support Programme
555 University Ave
Toronto, M5G 1X8
Ontario, Canada

1. Greer FR, Apple RD. Physicians, formula companies, and advertising: a historical perspective. *AJDC*. 1991;145:282-286.

2. Bergevin Y, Dougherty C, Kramer MS. Do infant formula samples shorten the duration of breastfeeding? *Lancet*. 1983;1:1148-1151.

3. Frank DA, Wirtz SJ, Sorenson JR, Heeren T. Commercial discharge packs and breastfeeding counselling: effects on infant feeding practices in a randomized trial. *Pediatrics*. 1987;80:845-854.

In Reply.—We thank Dr Newman for his comments, with which we have no major disagreement. It is true that physicians have benefited economically from the historic relationship between formula companies and physicians, and we implied that in our article. However, we cannot jump to the conclusion that this potential economic benefit was a primary motivating factor for our predecessors. As is usually the case, there are those who benefit economically from every humanitarian cause.

We also agree with Dr Newman that take-home starter packages supplied by formula companies and distributed by hospital employees are a form of advertising, especially with accompanying toys and nursing bottles. Ironically, the vast majority of the information contained in these starter packets are guides to breastfeeding. The starter packet information also emphasizes that mothers should consult their physicians for advice on infant nutrition. A discussion of this form of advertising was inadvertently left out of our manuscript and is important when one considers that its existence has been used by Gerber and Carnation to justify their advertising campaigns.

We do not have any firsthand information regarding the formula companies' present operations in developing countries. The companies have all agreed in principal to comply with the World Health Organization code. It is noteworthy that a new organization (Action for Corporate Responsibilities) has instituted a boycott against both Nestle and American Home Products for distributing gifts of infant formula. The organization maintains that such gifts are primarily marketing tools rather than charity items and that the World Health Organization code should not allow such gifts.[1]

Finally, we agree with Dr Newman that breastfeeding is superior to bottle feeding. However, there will always be a need for safe, reliable substitutes for human milk, and we are grateful for them. They should not, however, be marketed in a way that will discourage breastfeeding.

FRANK R. GREER, MD
Department of Pediatrics
RIMA D. APPLE, PHD
Department of History of Medicine
University of Wisconsin
Madison, WI 53706

1. Infant formula: action at last. *Inside PR*. 1991:5.

Scoring Systems for Accurate Prognosis of Patients With Meningococcal Infections

Sir.—We agree with Tesoro and Selbst[1] that prognostic factors developed 30 years ago by Stiehm and Damrosch[2] are no longer helpful in treating meningococcal infections. Like Tesoro and Selbst, we observed[3] that, of 27 children with severe purpura, 17 (63%) had Stiehm-Damrosch scores of 3 or greater (sedimentation rate was not analyzed), and seven (41%) of these 17 survived. (Five [55%] of nine patients who had Stiehm-Damrosch scores of 3 or greater in the study by Tesoro and Selbst survived.) The main problem with most scores proposed in the literature is that they were defined in patients of different ages (adults and children) and with different diseases (septicemia, with or without shock; purpura with meningitis; and meningitis without septicemia).[4] Scores for all forms of meningococcal infections are helpful, especially in the emergency department, for indicating early transfer in an intensive care unit. However, for all physicians, shock is the main prognostic factor in meningococcal diseases, and mortality is low when shock is absent (eg, 1.8%[1] and 5.7%[4]). So, we have to better define shock (in literature it is defined as hypotension, decreased peripheral perfusion, low urine output, lactic acidosis, need for fluid resuscitation or pressor therapy, or association of several of these features) and propose pronostic scores for children in shock who are admitted to intensive-care units.

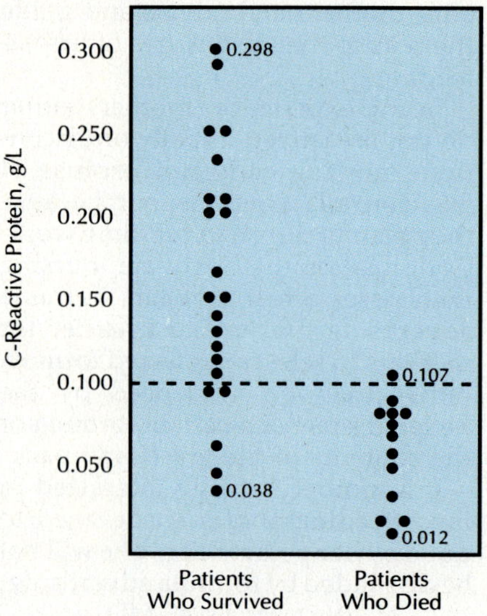

Survival related to C-reactive protein levels on admission. The dashed line indicates the cutoff point that best indicates whether a patient survives.

We studied the prognostic value of the C-reactive protein (CRP) level (determined using laser nephelometry) on admission in patients with infectious purpura of proved or suspected bacterial origin. In children who were not in shock, CRP level had no prognostic value; in children who were in shock, CRP level predicted outcome accurately, and the cutoff point of 0.100 g/L appeared highly discriminant.[5] (Shock was defined by the presence of two of the following features: blood pressure, <2 SDs of the age-related normal value; capillary refill time, >3 seconds; and urine output, <1 mL/kg per hour.) This was confirmed in a larger study of 35 children who were in shock (Figure). The positive predictive value was 94% (17 of 18 children with a CRP value >0.100 g/L survived); the negative predictive value, 71% (12 of 17 children with a CRP value <0.100 g/L died); sensitivity, 92% (12 of 13 children); and specificity, 77% (17 of 22 children).[6] In this last study, the prognostic values of eight previously reported scores were compared. C-reactive protein level on admission predicted outcome more accurately than did two other scoring systems proposed for children in shock in which multivariate analysis was used to determine scores.[4,7] Therefore, we believe that determining CRP level on admission, which can be done easily and quickly, may facilitate accurate prognosis in children with shock. Like other scoring systems, it may be helpful in the evaluation of new forms of treatment.

FRANCIS LECLERC, MD
VALÉRIE HUE, MD
ALAIN MARTINOT, MD
FLORENCE DELEPOULLE, MD
Service de Réanimation
Hôpital Calmette
Bd du Pr J Leclercq
59037 Lille, France

1. Tesoro LJ, Selbst SM. Factors affecting outcome in meningococcal infections. *AJDC*. 1991;145:218-220.
2. Stiehm ER, Damrosch DS. Factors in the prognosis of meningococcal infection. *J Pediatr*. 1966;68:457-467.
3. Leclerc F, Delepoulle F, Duhamel A, Chenaud M, Hue V, Martinot A. A comparison of 11 prognostic scores in children with infectious purpura shock. *Intensive Care Med*. 1990;16(suppl 1):S73. Abstract.
4. Leclerc F, Beuscart R, Guillois B, et al. Prognostic factors of severe infectious purpura in children. *Intensive Care Med*. 1985;11:140-143.
5. Chenaud M, Leclerc F, Meuriot S, Martinot A, Leblond B. Intérêt du dosage de la C-réactive protéine dans le purpura infeciteux sévère de l'enfant. *Presse Med*. 1987;16:1846-1849.
6. Leclerc F, Chenaud M, Delepoulle F, et al. Prognostic value of C-reactive protein level in severe infectious purpura: a comparison with 8 other scores. *Crit Care Med*. 1991;19:430-432
7. Emparanza JI, Aldamiz-Echevarria L, Perez-Yarza EG, et al. Prognostic score in acute meningococcemia. *Crit Care Med*. 1988;16:168-169.

Association of Alkaline Urine With Eating Disorders

Sir.—We read with interest the letter by Arden et al[1] on the association of alkaline urine with eating disorders. Seventeen (37%) of 46 patients with eating disorders had an alkaline urine pH compared with only one (4%) of 28 control subjects. Arden et al suggest a number of possible causes of the alkaline urine pH, including self-induced vomiting, "alkaline tide," diet, osteoporosis from estrogen deficiency, and hypochloremic alkalosis due to diuretic or laxative abuse. Several of these causes would not explain an alkaline urine pH. Chronic, self-induced vomiting and diuretic or laxative abuse are usually associated with mild extracellular fluid volume contraction and an acid urine pH. This aciduria, referred to as "paradoxical aciduria" when a metabolic alkalosis is present, develops consequent to secretion of a hydrogen ion in the distal nephron when a sodium ion is reabsorbed to replenish the volume of extracellular fluid.

The evaluation of the urine pH and sodium and chloride levels, and a clinical assessment of the hydration status of a patient, will allow differentiation of the problems in patients with eating disorders (Table).[2]

WILLIAM LANE M. ROBSON, MD, FRCPC
ALEXANDER K. C. LEUNG, MBBS, FRCPC, FRCP(EDIN)
Department of Pediatrics
University of Calgary
Alberta Children's Hospital
Calgary, Alberta, Canada
T2T 5C7

1. Arden MR, Budow L, Bunnell DW, Nussbaum MP, Shenker IR, Jacobson MS. Alkaline urine is associated with eating disorders. *AJDC*. 1991;145:28-30.
2. Kamel KS, Ethier JH, Richardson RMA, Bear RA, Halperin ML. Urine electrolytes and osmolality: when and how to use them. *Am J Nephrol*. 1990;10:89-102.

In Reply.—Drs Robson and Leung's analysis of our findings is most welcome. As they correctly point out, chronic states associated with increased aldosterone levels will not result in alkaline urine. This decreases the number of possible causes of alkaline urine in our patients, allowing us to concentrate on fewer possible causes, including recent acute vomiting, "alkaline tide," alkaline-ash diet, and osteoporosis. We appreciate their contribution and

Urine Tests and Hydration Status in the Evaluation of Eating Disorders

		Vomiting			
	Alkaline Ash Diet	Acute	Chronic	Diuretic Abuse	Laxative Abuse
Urine pH	Alkaline*	Alkaline	Acid†	Acid	Acid
Urine sodium	High‡	High	Low§	High	Low
Urine chloride	High	Low	Low	High	High
ECF‖ volume	Normal	Normal	Decreased	Decreased	Decreased

*Urine pH greater than or equal to 7.
†Urine pH less than 7.
‡Urine sodium greater than 15 mmol/L.
§Urine sodium less than 15 mmol/L.
‖ECF indicates extracellular fluid.

hope to use this information in further studies of this phenomenon.

MARTHA R. ARDEN, MD
MICHAEL P. NUSSBAUM, MD
MARC S. JACOBSON, MD
Schneider Children's Hospital
Division of Adolescent
Medicine
New Hyde Park, NY 11042

Reexpansion Pulmonary Edema

Sir.—Reexpansion pulmonary edema (REPE) is an uncommon problem that afflicts the reexpanded lung after evacuation of a large pneumothorax or pleural effusion. There are many accounts of REPE occurring in adults, but to my knowledge, this problem has not been reported in the pediatric population. A boy is described in whom severe unilateral pulmonary edema occurred after evacuation of a large pleural effusion.

Patient Report.—An 8-year-old boy weighing 40 kg was admitted for treatment of steroid-resistant nephrotic syndrome. He had no previous neurologic abnormality. The patient's medical history was remarkable for multiple bouts of infection, including a right-sided pneumococcal pneumonia 3 months before admission. One month after the pneumonia, he underwent a right pleural decortication because of recurrent pleural effusion. Two weeks before admission, a chest roentgenogram showed moderate right- and left-sided pleural effusions. During these 2 weeks, he experienced worsening shortness of breath.

On admission, the patient was suffering from marked peripheral edema and moderate respiratory distress. His total serum protein value was 40 g/L (normal range, 60 to 80 g/L), and his albumin value was 19 g/L (normal range, 38 to 54 g/L). A chest roentgenogram obtained shortly after admission showed a 100% left-sided pleural effusion and a small right-sided pleural effusion (Fig 1).

To treat the patient's peripheral edema and pleural effusion, repeated doses of 25% albumin followed by furosemide were administered. Serum electrolytes were carefully monitored during therapy. Following a brief grand mal seizure on the second day of hospitalization, the patient was admitted to the intensive care unit. His mental status quickly returned to normal. Hypoxia and electrolyte abnormalities were eliminated as possible causes of the seizure. (Arterial oxygen saturation measured with a pulse oximeter was 95% using 2 L of oxygen delivered via nasal cannula; serum sodium was 139 mmol/L.) Vital signs on admission included the following: pulse, 110 beats per minute; blood pressure, 125/82 mm Hg; temperature, 37°C (measured orally); respiratory rate, 32 breaths per minute. He had no additional seizures after receiving phenytoin (20 mg/kg of body weight). The patient's only electrolyte abnormality, a mild hypocalcemia (ionized Ca^{++}, 1.9 mmol/L [normal range, 2.35 to 2.6 mmol/L]), was treated.

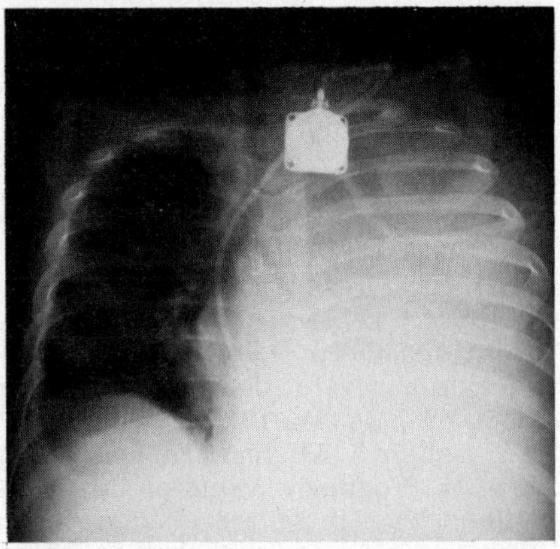

Fig 1.—*Chest roentgenogram before thoracentesis demonstrating left-sided pleural effusion occupying the entire left hemithorax.*

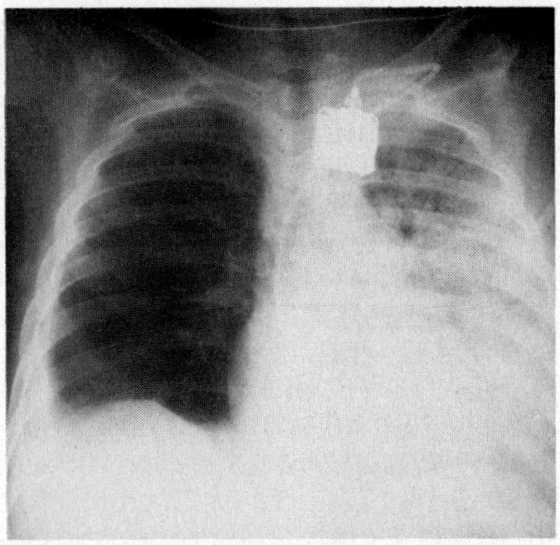

Fig 2.—*Chest roentgenogram after thoracentesis. Left-sided pleural effusion is almost entirely resolved. Widespread alveolar infiltrates on the left are consistent with unilateral pulmonary edema.*

The large left-sided pleural effusion was evacuated because the patient was in moderate respiratory distress and needed 2.5 liters per minute of oxygen via nasal cannula to maintain arterial oxygen saturation (SaO_2) of ≥0.95 (measured using a pulse oximeter). Over 30 minutes, the effusion was evacuated through a 16-gauge flexible plastic catheter placed in the midaxillary line at the seventh intercostal space. A total of 1900 mL of opalescent fluid was removed. The fluid laboratory values were as follows: glucose, 5.8 mmol/L; protein, <10 g/L; lactate dehydrogenase, 352 U/L; red blood cell count, 3.8×10^9/L; and white blood cell count, 1.2×10^9/L. Results of fluid cultures were negative for bacteria. Midway through the procedure, the patient began to cough repeatedly. Near the end of the procedure, he began to expectorate pink-tinged sputum. A chest roentgenogram was obtained because pulmonary edema was suspected. The roentgenogram showed 95% evacuation of the pleural fluid, with widespread alveolar infiltrate on the left side consistent with pulmonary edema (Fig 2). The right lung was clear.

The patient experienced progressive hypoxemia and ultimately needed 75% FIO_2 delivered via a nonrebreathing face mask to maintain $SaO_2 \geq 0.95$. After being placed in a 45-degree upright position with his left side dependent, he appeared more comfortable. The patient's distress resolved over the next 6 hours. Twelve hours after thoracentesis, the FIO_2 had decreased to 0.5 L/min via nasal cannula. A follow-up chest roentgenogram obtained 24 hours after thoracentesis showed partial resolution of the pulmonary edema and a 50% reaccumulation of the left-sided pleural effusion. The procedure was not repeated. During the 48 hours after the thoracentesis, the patient's maximum temperature was 38°C (measured orally).

Comment.—More than 60 cases of REPE have been described in adults.[1] Most cases of REPE have occurred after evacuation of pneumothorax or pleural effusion, although REPE has been reported after the rapid reexpansion of atelectasis. There does not appear to be a technique for reexpansion of a collapsed lung that is free of risk of developing REPE. Reexpansion pulmonary edema has occurred after low- or high-negative pressure use, needle aspiration, placement of a chest tube and Heimlich valve (without negative pressure), and application of positive pressure to an atelectatic lung via an endotracheal tube.[2] Although REPE is well described in the literature, it is rarely seen in clinical practice. No REPE was reported in two large series examining the evacuation of pneumothoraces in a total of 775 patients.[3,4] Despite the infrequent occurrence of this complication, it may be life threatening, with a mortality rate approaching 20%.[2] Death usually is attributable to intractable hypoxemia or heart failure.[5-8]

The pathologic derangement leading to REPE has not been characterized, but evidence suggests that increased pulmonary capillary permeability may be the primary aberration. Data from adult patients show that, after reexpansion of a collapsed lung, pulmonary edema may develop in the presence of normal pulmonary artery and pulmonary capillary wedge pressures.[1,7,9] This suggests that fluid crosses capillary membranes because of loss of vascular integrity. In REPE, the protein content of alveolar fluid is high, indicating capillary leakage.[1,9,10] A rabbit model of REPE in which radiolabeled albumin was used showed increased pulmonary vascular permeability after reinflation of the lung.[11] In addition to these abnormalities, tissue surfactant diminished after 24 hours of atelectasis induced by pneumothorax in animals.[12]

Studies of REPE in animals suggest that greater duration of collapse and the use of negative pressure to reexpand the lung may favor the development of REPE.[12-14] Nevertheless, authors have occasionally described REPE in humans experiencing collapses of short duration[2] and in whom limited negative pressure ($\geqslant$20 cm H_2O) was used.[2,15] Although it has been suggested that slower reexpansion of the lung may prevent the development of REPE,[2,5,6,8,9,12,13,16] no firm evidence exists to validate this contention.

Several mechanisms previously suspected to contribute to the formation of REPE have been shown to be unimportant. It has been postulated that capillary leakage may be caused by increased blood flow after reexpansion of the lung.[17] Subsequent investigation has refuted this hypothesis. Atelectasis elevates pulmonary vascular resistance and decreases blood flow shortly after the onset of collapse.[18] After evacuation of a pneumothorax in adults, blood flow has been shown to remain diminished for several days in the reexpanded lung.[19]

Activation of neutrophils in some diseases (eg, adult respiratory distress syndrome) results in pulmonary capillary injury and extravasation of plasma into the alveoli.[20] Although large numbers of neutrophils accumulate in reexpanded lung tissue, the role of neutrophils in REPE appears to be limited. Reexpansion pulmonary edema can be induced in neutropenic animals,[21] implying that neutrophils are not essential in the pathogenesis of REPE.

With few exceptions, REPE is a unilateral problem, occurring only in the reinflated lung. Despite the normal appearance of the contralateral lung, most patients experience hypoxemia and need treatment with supplemental oxygen or endotracheal intubation. If endotracheal intubation is necessary, the administration of positive end expiratory pressure may hasten the resolution of REPE by reversing alveolar collapse, restoring functional residual capacity, decreasing ventilation/perfusion mismatching, and lessening intrapulmonary shunting. For unknown reasons, REPE is occasionally accompanied by hypotension and low cardiac output necessitating therapy with volume replacement and inotropic agents.[22]

Our patient suffered from hypoalbuminemia. He undoubtedly had a low plasma oncotic pressure, which increased his risk of developing REPE by favoring the loss of plasma across altered capillary membranes in the reexpanded lung. He was fortunate because he did not need endotracheal intubation or vasopressors, although delivery of high levels of FIO_2 was necessary to avoid hypoxemia. This patient demonstrated several of the key features of REPE: rapid onset of respiratory distress, productive cough, unilateral pulmonary edema, and increased alveolar-arterial oxygen gradient. Previous reports document elevated blood-sputum protein ratios in REPE.[1,9,10] Unfortunately, the protein content of this patient's sputum was not measured.

Other causes of respiratory distress and unilateral pulmonary edema need to be considered in this setting. Pulmonary thromboembolism and air embolus from the central venous catheter can cause rapid onset of respiratory distress and may occasionally occur with unilateral abnormalities as shown in a chest roentgenogram. However, neither of these problems is accompanied by severe pulmonary edema. In this case, it is extremely unlikely that a pulmonary thromboembolus of such severity would resolve so rapidly. The fluid administered through the patient's central venous line was closely monitored by the nurse and was delivered by an infusion pump that automatically alarms and interrupts the infusion if air is detected in the line. These precautions make it extremely unlikely that an air embolus could have caused this patient's distress. Infection is a frequent cause of respiratory distress when unilateral pulmonary infiltrates are present, but the rapid onset and resolution of such severe symptoms in an afebrile patient indicate that an infectious cause was very unlikely.

Physicians caring for children with respiratory compromise caused by pleural effusion or pneumothorax must be aware of REPE. Although it is uncommon, this problem may be life threatening. When it occurs, REPE may appear during reinflation of the lung or several hours later.[2] Aggressive respiratory and cardiovascular intervention may be necessary to avoid patient harm. To permit early identification of this problem, appropriate monitoring and observation should be employed during and after the evacuation of a large pneumothorax or pleural effusion.

David S. Jardine, MD
Department of Anesthesiology
Children's Hospital and Medical Center
University of Washington
4800 Sand Point Way NE
Seattle, WA 98105

Reprint requests to Children's Hospital and Medical Center, 4800 Sand Point Way NE, Seattle, WA 98105 (Dr Jardine).

1. Marland AM, Blauser FL. Hemodynamic and pulmonary edema protein measurements in a case of reexpansion pulmonary edema. *Chest.* 1982;81:250-251.
2. Mahfood S, Hix WR, Aaron BL, Blaes P, Watson DC. Reexpansion pulmonary edema. *Ann Thorac Surg.* 1988; 45:340-345.
3. Mills M, Baisch BF. Spontaneous pneumothorax. *Ann Thorac Surg.* 1965; 1:286-297.
4. Brooks JW. Open thoracotomy in the management of spontaneous pneumothorax. *Ann Surg.* 1973;177:798-804.
5. Fanning J, Lettieri L, Piver MS. Fatal recurrent reexpansion pulmonary edema. *Obstet Gynecol.* 1989;74:495-497.
6. Grant MJA. Acute unilateral pulmonary oedema following re-expansion of a spontaneous pneumothorax: case re-

port. *N Z Med J.* 1971;74:250-251.
7. Kernodle DS, DiRaimondo CR, Fulkerson WJ. Reexpansion pulmonary edema after pneumothorax. *South Med J.* 1984;77:318-322.
8. Peatfield RC, Edwards PR, Johnson NM. Two unexpected deaths from pneumothorax. *Lancet.* 1979;1:356-358.
9. Sprung CL, Loewenherz JW, Baier H, Hauser MJ. Evidence for increased permeability in reexpansion pulmonary edema. *Am J Med.* 1981;71:497-500.
10. Buczko GB, Grossman RF, Goldberg M. Re-expansion pulmonary edema: evidence for increased capillary permeability. *Can Med Assoc J.* 1981;125:460-461.
11. Pavlin DJ, Nessly ML, Cheney FW. Increased pulmonary vascular permeability as a cause of re-expansion edema in rabbits. *Am Rev Respir Dis.* 1981;124:422-427.
12. Sewell RW, Fewel JG, Grover FL, Arom KV. Experimental evaluation of reexpansion pulmonary edema. *Ann Thorac Surg.* 1978;26:126-132.
13. Miller WC, Toon R, Palat H, Lacroix J. Experimental pulmonary edema following reexpansion of pneumothorax. *Am Rev Respir Dis.* 1973;108:664-666.
14. Pavlin J, Frederick W, Cheney J. Unilateral pulmonary edema in rabbits after reexpansion of collapsed lung. *J Appl Physiol.* 1979;46:31-35.
15. Light RW, Jenkinson SG, Minh V-D, George RB. Observations on pleural fluid pressures as fluid is withdrawn during thoracentesis. *Am Rev Respir Dis.* 1980;121:799-804.
16. Shanahan MX, Monk I, Richards HJ. Unilateral pulmonary oedema following reexpansion of pneumothorax. *Anaesth Intensive Care.* 1975;3:19-30.
17. Ziskind MM, Weill H, George RA. Acute pulmonary edema following the treatment of spontaneous pneumothorax with excessive negative intrapleural pressure. *Am Rev Respir Dis.* 1965;92:632-636.
18. Glasser SA, Domino KB, Lindgren L, Parcella P, Marshall C, Marshall BE. Pulmonary blood pressure and flow during atelectasis in the dog. *Anesthesiology.* 1983;58:225-231.
19. Yamazaki S, Ogawa J, Shohzu A, Suzuki A. Pulmonary blood flow to rapidly reexpanded lung in spontaneous pneumothorax. *Chest.* 1982;81:118-120.
20. Nichols DG, Rogers MC. Adult respiratory distress syndrome. In: Rogers MC, ed. *Textbook of Pediatric Intensive Care.* Baltimore, Md: Williams & Wilkins; 1987;1:237-272.
21. Jackson RM, Veal CF, Alexander CB, Brannen AL, Fulmer JD. Neutrophils in reexpansion pulmonary edema. *J Appl Physiol.* 1988;65:228-234.
22. Pavlin DJ, Raghu G, Rogers TR, Cheney FW. Reexpansion hypotension, a complication of rapid evacuation of prolonged pneumothorax. *Chest.* 1986;89:70-74.

Nintendo Enuresis

Sir.—Isolated daytime enuresis is an uncommon problem for primary school children, with a prevalence of only 1.8%.[1] I have recently seen three related boys, ages 3½ years, 5 years, and 7 years, who developed enuresis after receiving the Nintendo (Nintendo of America Inc, Redmond, Wash) arcade game. These boys lacked the known risk factors for enuresis, such as delayed maturation, low birth weights, and family stress. In each case, the child was fascinated by the Mario Brothers game, and apparently ignored his urge to micturate.

Anecdotal reports suggest that some of their peers have had similar episodes of enuresis. No formal examination was performed because the problem resolved after 1 to 2 weeks when the children learned to use the pause button. Since operant conditioning approaches, such as "the dry bed method," are effective therapy for enuresis, the Nintendo company may find a market for a wet sensor that causes the game to abort if the player loses bladder control.[2]

Pants wetting is generally behavioral, and may manifest when the child is preoccupied by play.[3,4] Although these three boys are related, daytime enuresis unaccompanied by nocturnal enuresis is exceptional in that it is not genetically determined.[5]

"Nintendo enuresis" is a short-lived disorder, but it may affect many households since these games are increasingly common. Parents should be encouraged to demonstrate the game's pause button to their children or tolerate occasional Nintendo enuresis as their youngsters develop the ability to concentrate intently on the game's goal-oriented tasks.

Julian C. Schink, MD
Northwestern University
Medical School
333 E Superior St, Suite 420
Chicago, IL 60611

1. Jarvelin MR, Vikevainen-Tervonen L, Moilanen I, Huttunen NP. Enuresis in seven-year old children. *Acta Paediatr Scand.* 1988;77:148-153.
2. Kaplan SL, Breit M, Gauthier B, Busner J. A comparison of three nocturnal enuresis treatment methods. *J Am Acad Child Adolesc Psychiatry.* 1989;28:282-286.
3. MacKeith R, Meadow R, Turner RK. How children become dry. In: Kolvin I, MacKeith RC, Meadow SR, eds. *Bladder Control and Enuresis: Clinics in Developmental Medicine.* Philadelphia, Pa: JB Lippincott; 1973; 48, 49:3-13.
4. Bakwin H. The genetics of enuresis. In: Kolvin I, MacKeith RC, Meadows SR, eds. *Bladder Control and Enuresis: Clinics in Developmental Medicine.* Philadelphia, Pa: JB Lippincott; 1973; 48, 49:73-77.
5. Hurley RM. Enuresis: the difference between night and day. *Pediatr Rev.* 1990;12:167-170.

Mitral Valve Prolapse: Back to the Basics

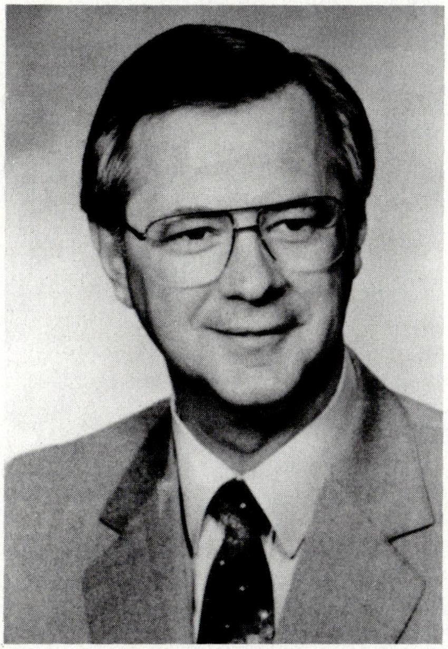

Hugh D. Allen, MD

Hugh has been with AJDC for 8 years. During that interval he has served as associate editor, editor of the Educational Interventions Department, and reviewer. In each position he has functioned competently and on time and has provided ideas for improvement of the journal and crisp comments for authors of submitted manuscripts. His work with "Educational Interventions" deserves special mention, since he developed this concept and has received a large number of manuscripts as a result of its success. It is a unique place in the pediatric literature for experiments and observations on the educational process.

Hugh has been professor of Pediatrics, vice chairman of the Department of Pediatrics, director of the Division of Cardiology, acting director of Emergency Medical Services, and associate director of Ambulatory Services at The Ohio State University, Columbus, since 1988. Prior to that, Hugh was a faculty member at the University of Arizona, Tucson, from 1973 to 1988. He has been acclaimed as a superb clinician, excellent teacher, and innovative investigator. He has won a number of teaching awards for his efforts with medical students and resident physicians.

Hugh is a prolific author with more than 120 peer-reviewed publications, many authoritative chapters in textbooks, and a number of coauthored textbooks in pediatric cardiology. His most recent contributions have dealt with fetal echocardiography, use of Doppler echocardiography in critical care, and guidelines for cardiac catheterization. Hugh is married to Elizabeth and they have three boys, Clark, Carl, and Lloyd.

—V.A.F.

Prolapse of the mitral valve is a real disorder. Primary prolapse[1] occurs when laxity of the chordal or valvular structure, often seen in patients with pectus or collagen vascular disorders and/or ischemia of the papillary muscles, causes the mitral valve to billow back into the left atrium as the left ventricular pressure rises during systole. If the valve loses its ability to coapt, a jet of blood regurgitates into the left atrium. A secondary form also exists in which the valve apparatus is normal but left ventricular volume is less than normal (frequently observed in anorexic patients). This "acquired" form of prolapse may be transient. Each of these forms can have serious complications, including death from arrhythmia, endocarditis,[2] or heart failure. Although the etiology for arrhythmias is uncertain, they can be serious if supraventricular in origin or fatal if ventricular in origin. Endocarditis can result when bacteremia is present and a jet of regurgitation creates a nidus for implantation of organisms, usually onto the valve or the left atrium. If regurgitation is severe, the left ventricle can dilate and fail, requiring valve replacement.

Mitral valve prolapse has characteristic physical findings of a midsystolic click, or multiple clicks, heard best at the cardiac apex. These may or may not be accompanied by a murmur initiated by the click. The findings are accentuated when the patient stands after squatting, a maneuver that leads to the least ventricular filling and thus exaggerates the findings. Squatting, which fills the ventricle, may diminish or erase the findings. Patients should be examined lying, sitting, standing, squatting, and standing after squatting before the examiner can be satisfied that prolapse is not present. If the examiner is uncertain as to the origin of the findings, eg , when considering a differential diagnosis of aortic valve stenosis, an echocardiography-Doppler study can be done to confirm the presence of prolapse by detecting superior-posterior mitral leaflet billowing into the left atrium, and, if regurgitation is present, the pulsed or color flow Doppler study will demonstrate a jet into the left atrium during systole.

The recent American Heart Association recommendations[2] regarding endocarditis prophylaxis suggest using amoxicillin prophylaxis if the patient has a click and murmur, but also agree that patients with clicks may also require prophylaxis. This is important in that these findings can vary and no one can say that the patient who has an isolated click in the office will not have a click and murmur (due to regurgitation) later that day.

Mitral prolapse is said to be very common. Certainly, many patients have this problem,[1] but many others who carry the diagnosis do not have it. This is a result of our misinterpreting ultrasonographic study results and paying too little attention to the basic physical examination.

I will therefore take the liberty of naming a third, most common form, ie, pseudoprolapse of the mitral valve. This is usually defined by echocardiography, often interpreted but not performed by a physician who also did not examine the patient. It can also be found in patients who had neither physical nor echocardiographic findings, but who insist that they have it anyway. This is a socially acceptable disease that makes great, or at least frequent, cocktail conversation about one's teenaged daughter. However, this diagnosis has a negative impact on life-style, insurability, endocarditis prophylaxis, pregnancy, and the young person's self-image.

The implications are important. We do not have a sudden epidemic of a disease; we have an epidemic of overdiagnosis. As pediatricians, we owe our patients accuracy in this diagnosis since prolapse is a potentially serious problem. Mitral valve prolapse is a clinical diagnosis with ultrasonographic corroboration, not the other way around. If the click and/or murmur is not heard, one should be suspect of all other methods of diagnosis and not hesitate to obtain another opinion from a cardiologist who has a stethoscope.

References

1. Boudoulas H, Wooley CF, eds. *Mitral Valve Prolapse and the Mitral Valve Prolapse Syndrome.* Mount Kisco, NY: Futura Publishing Co Inc; 1988.
2. Dajani AS, Bisno AL, Chung KJ, et al. Prevention of bacterial endocarditis: recommendations by the American Heart Association. *JAMA.* 1990;264:2919-2922.

In Other AMA Journals

ARCHIVES OF PATHOLOGY & LABORATORY MEDICINE

Use of Polymorphic DNA Probes to Test the Lymph Nodes of Infants and Fetuses for Spontaneous Chimerism

Richard C. Hard, Jr, MD; Angela M. Slosberg, MT(ASCP); Arnold M. Salzberg, MD (*Arch Pathol Lab Med.* 1991;115:891-894)

Endotoxin Concentrations in Cerebrospinal Fluid Correlate With Clinical Severity and Neurologic Outcome of *Haemophilus influenzae* Type B Meningitis

Jussi Mertsola, MD; William A. Kennedy, MD; David Waagner, MD; Xavier Sáez-Llorens, MD; Kurt Olsen; Eric J. Hansen, PhD; George H. McCracken, Jr, MD

• Endotoxin concentrations were measured in paired samples of cerebrospinal fluid from 38 patients with *Haemophilus influenzae* type b meningitis. On admission, the median concentration of endotoxin in cerebrospinal fluid was 104 ng/mL and decreased rapidly in follow-up samples. From 17 to 48 hours after admission, 50% of the patients had concentrations of less than 1 ng/mL. Endotoxin concentrations correlated significantly with concentrations of interleukin 1β, protein, and glucose in cerebrospinal fluid, duration of secondary fever, and neurologic abnormalities during hospitalization and on follow-up examinations. Twenty-eight percent of patients with endotoxin concentrations of 100 ng/mL or more on admission had long-term complications, compared with none of those with lower endotoxin concentrations (relative risk, 2.31; 95% confidence interval, 1.53 to 3.48). These results indicate that quantitation of endotoxin in cerebrospinal fluid could be a valuable aid in identifying those children at increased risk of complications during *Haemophilus influenzae* type b meningitis and provide additional evidence that the *Haemophilus influenzae* type b meningitis lipo-oligosaccharide is important in the pathogenesis of meningitis.

(*AJDC.* 1991;145:1099-1103)

Endotoxins or lipopolysaccharides (LPSs) are one of the major constituents of the outer membrane of gram-negative bacteria. These molecules are potent toxins and are considered to play a pivotal role in the initiation of the inflammatory cascade involving release of various cytokines and accumulation of leukocytes locally in the site of infection.[1,2] When injected intracisternally in rabbits, minute quantities of purified endotoxin caused disruption of the blood-brain barrier, meningeal inflammation, intracranial hypertension, and brain edema.[2-4]

Accepted for publication June 17, 1991.

From the Departments of Microbiology (Drs Mertsola and Hansen) and Pediatrics (Drs Kennedy, Waagner, Sáez-Llorens, Olsen, and McCracken), University of Texas Southwestern Medical Center, Dallas. Dr Waagner is currently with the University of Texas Health Sciences Center, Houston, and Dr Kennedy is with the University of Alberta (Edmonton) Hospitals.

Reprint requests to Department of Pediatrics, University of Texas Southwestern Medical Center, 5323 Harry Hines Blvd, Dallas, TX 75235-9063 (Dr McCracken).

The classic method of quantifying endotoxins is the *Limulus* amebocyte lysate assay. This test is based on the ability of endotoxin to activate a protease system in the amebocyte lysate, an extract prepared from the blood cells of the horseshoe crab *Limulus polyphemus*.[5] The activated enzyme can initiate gel formation and also hydrolyze certain peptides to colored substances. This property was used in the development of a new chromogenic *Limulus* assay.[6] Lipopolysaccharides of enteric gram negative bacteria have usually been used as standards in these assays. A potential problem with this practice, however, is that endotoxins from different bacterial species exhibit marked variation in their relative abilities to activate the *Limulus* assay.[7] *Haemophilus influenzae* type b (Hib) LPS differs from the classic enteric LPS molecule primarily in that the former lacks an O antigen repeat unit and consists only of lipid A and a structure equivalent to the core oligosaccharide of enteric LPS. This smaller endotoxin molecule has been referred to as lipo-oligosaccharide (LOS).

In this study, we measured endotoxin levels in patients with Hib meningitis using purified LOS of Hib as a standard in the chromogenic *Limulus* assay. The LOS concentrations from paired CSF samples were compared with the indices of meningeal inflammation, the concentrations of cytokines in the CSF, and the clinical condition and neurologic outcome of the patients. In addition, we measured the clearance of LOS from CSF in experimental meningitis.

PATIENTS AND METHODS

Patients

Children admitted consecutively from August 1988 to October 1989 to Children's Medical Center or Parkland Memorial Hospital, Dallas, Tex, with Hib meningitis were prospectively studied. The protocol for the study was approved by the Institutional Review Board of the University of Texas, and written informed consent for participation in the study was obtained from the parents of the patients. The following criteria were used for inclusion in this analysis: (1) age between 6 weeks and 13 years; (2) growth of Hib in the CSF; (3) no parenteral antibiotic therapy before the first lumbar puncture; and (4) a second lumbar puncture done between 17 and 48 hours after initiation of therapy.

The patients were treated with cefotaxime sodium (225 mg/kg per day intravenously for 10 days) and dexamethasone sodium phosphate (0.60 mg/kgper day for 4 days). Twenty-one of the 38 patients studied were male; 15 were white, 13 were black, nine were Hispanic, and one was Asian. The mean age of the patients was 11 months (range, 2 to 34 months).

Follow-up

The clinical severity of meningitis was assessed using the scoring system developed by Herson and Todd,[8] and clinical conditions of the patients were evaluated daily in the hospital. Hearing was assessed at the time of discharge from the hospital by means of brain-stem auditory evoked response testing, which was repeated 4 to 6 months later if results were abnormal.[9] Neurologic outcome was clinically evaluated 6 weeks and 4 to 6 months after discharge from the hospital. Neurologic abnormalities included abnormal state of consciousness (obtunded, semiconscious, or conscious), hemiparesis, cranial nerve palsy, seizures, or a lack of response to 50 dB or more on brain-stem auditory evoked response audiologic examination (with normal tympanogram) indicating a moderate or greater neurosensory hearing loss.[9] These neurologic complications were considered transient if they resolved within 4 to 6 months after the Hib meningitis.

Laboratory Tests

White blood cell (WBC) counts and protein and glucose concentrations in the CSF were routinely determined. Based on earlier findings that the number of bacteria per oil immersion field in a Gram-stained specimen correlated well with the concentration of bacteria in CSF,[10] a semiquantitative analysis of Gram-stained samples was used as an estimate of the number of bacteria in CSF. All fields were screened for stained organisms and the mean quantity per oil immersion field was recorded. Cerebrospinal fluid samples were centrifuged at 5000 rpm for 5 minutes, and aliquots were frozen at −70°C until tested for LOS and cytokine concentrations.

Lipo-oligosaccharide concentrations in the CSF were measured by a chromogenic *Limulus* assay with some modifications for use with microtiter plates.[11] Purified Hib DL 42 LOS was used as a standard in all microtiter plates, and all the samples and standards were heated at 75°C for 12 minutes to inactivate the possible inhibitors and nonspecific activators of the *Limulus* enzyme.[12] The lower limit of the assay was 10 pg/mL, but because the human CSF samples were diluted 1:100 in pyrogen-free phosphate-buffered saline, the assay detected LOS when concentrations were greater than or equal to 1 ng/mL. All the standards and samples were tested in duplicate wells and paired CSF specimens were always analyzed on the same microtiter plate.

Tumor necrosis factor α (TNF α) was measured by means of a bioassay with a lower limit of sensitivity of 10 pg/mL, and interleukin 1β (IL-1β) was measured with an enzyme-linked immunosorbent assay with a sensitivity within 20 pg/mL.[13]

Disappearance of LOS From CSF

An experimental meningitis model was used for evaluation of the effect of dexamethasone on the clearance of LOS from the CSF.[14] Twelve rabbits were given intracisternal injections of 200 ng of Hib DL42 LOS in pyrogen-free saline. Six rabbits received dexamethasone (1 mg/kg) intravenously immediately before the intracisternal inoculation of LOS, and six rabbits served as controls. The CSF samples (0.2 mL) obtained at various times were centrifuged at 5000 rpm for 5 minutes, and the supernatants were frozen at −70°C until tested. Before the assays were begun, the CSF samples were diluted 1:10 in pyrogen-free phosphate-buffered saline. Thus the chromogenic *Limulus* assay detected LOS when the concentrations in the original samples were greater than or equal to 100 pg/mL. To evaluate the clearance of LOS from the CSF, the LOS concentrations were fitted to a nonlinear computer program model using PCNONLIN version 3.0 (SCI Software, Lexington, Ky). The concentration time curves of the LOS obtained in the CSF were fitted to a one-compartment model with bolus input and first-order output (model 1).

Statistical Analysis

The Fisher Exact Test was used for comparisons of groups, Student's *t* test for continuous variables, and Mann-Whitney *U* test when the data were not normally distributed. The probability of a difference was calculated using two-tailed analyses. Spearman correlation coefficients were used to determine significant correlations between the variables. The results are shown as means and SDs unless otherwise stated. Differences were considered significant at $P<.05$.

Table 1.—Correlations Between Lipo-oligosaccharide (LOS), Interleukin-1_β White Blood Cell Count, Protein, and Glucose Concentrations in Correspondent Cerebrospinal Fluid Samples

	LOS Concentrations*	
Index	At Diagnosis	At 17 to 48-h Follow-up
Tumor necrosis factor α	+.14 (NS)	+.31 (.09)
Interleukin-1β	+.36 (.04)	+.39 (.03)
White blood cell count	+.30 (.10)	+.48 (.008)
Protein	+.33 (.05)	+.29 (NS)
Glucose	−.50 (.006)	−.39 (.03)

*Values are Spearman coefficients and those in parentheses are *P* values; NS indicates not significant.

RESULTS

Analysis of CSF 1

At the time of diagnosis, 35 (92%) of 38 patients had detectable concentrations (≥1 ng/mL) of LOS in the CSF. The mean concentration was 550±1352 ng/mL, with a median of 104 ng/mL. Nineteen patients had LOS concentrations of 100 ng/mL or more (high endotoxin group) and 19 had less than 100 ng/mL (low endotoxin group). Patients with high LOS concentrations in the CSF on admission significantly more often had more than 10 organisms per microscopic field in a Gram-stain analysis than those with low concentrations (16 [84%] vs 5 [26%]); $P=.0008$). Patients in the high LOS group also had lower concentrations of glucose (0.8±0.9 mmol/L) in CSF than those in the low LOS group (1.8±1.0 mmol/L) ($P=.01$). Abnormal state of consciousness was recorded in 42% of the patients in the high LOS group compared with 5% of those in the low LOS group ($P=.019$).

Interleukin 1β was found in CSF 1 in 35 (97%) of the 36 patients tested; mean concentration was 3350±7279 pg/mL (median, 564 pg/mL). Tumor necrosis factor α activity was found in 28 (76%) of the 37 samples tested; mean concentration was 2089±5412 pg/mL (median, 275 pg/mL). Tumor necrosis factor α activity was detected in 15 (83%) of 18 samples in the high LOS group (mean, 4333±8944 pg/mL) and in 13 (68%) of 19 samples in the low LOS group (1189±1295 pg/mL) ($P>.10$). The only patient who did not have detectable IL-1β also did not have detectable LOS or TNF α in the CSF at the time of diagnosis. There were statistically significant positive correlations between the LOS, IL-1β, and protein concentrations and negative correlation between LOS and glucose concentrations in CSF (Table 1).

Analysis of CSF 2

There was a rapid decrease in the concentrations of LOS in the CSF (Figure). Lipo-oligosaccharide was detectable in the second CSF samples from 19 of the 38 patients. Concentrations ranged from 1.1 to 59.6 ng/mL (mean, 10.2±14.0 ng/mL; median, 6.8 ng/mL). There was a significant correlation between the concentrations of LOS in the CSF 1 and CSF 2 samples ($r=.675$; $P<.001$). The correlations were also significant for the LOS and IL-1β and WBC concentrations (positive correlation) and for LOS and glucose concentrations (negative correlation) in the CSF 2 of these patients (Table 1). No significant correlations were found between LOS and TNF α concentrations. The lack of detection of TNF α activity in CSF 2 of 26 of 38 patients could affect this analysis. In the remaining 12 patients, TNF α concentrations in CSF 2 ranged from 300 to 1000 pg/mL (mean, 259±306 pg/mL). Patients with detectable LOS in CSF 2 were usually younger, more often had seizures, had longer duration of fever, neuro-

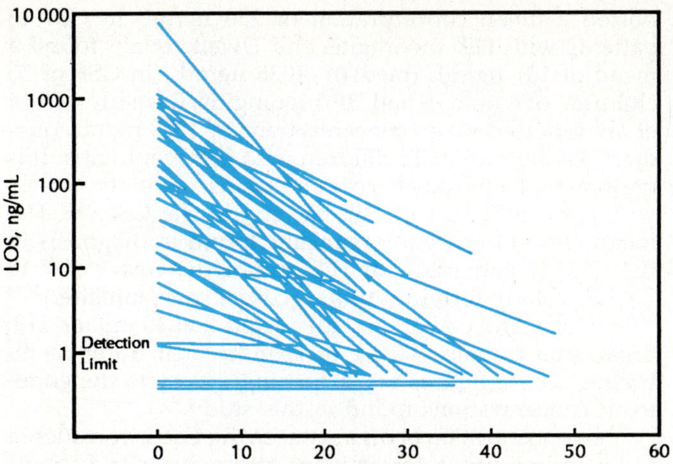

Lipo-oligosaccharide (LOS) concentrations in paired cerebrospinal fluid samples from 38 patients with Haemophilus influenzae *type b meningitis. Samples were obtained at the time of admission to the hospital and 17 to 48 hours later.*

logical abnormalities, low glucose levels, and high IL-1β concentrations in CSF 2 than those with undetectable LOS in CSF 2 (Table 2). All patients who had detectable bacteria in the CSF 2 also had detectable endotoxin.

Secondary Fever

Secondary fever, defined as a rectal temperature of 38.0°C or higher after at least 24 hours of maximal daily temperature of 37.9°C, occurred in 27 patients (71%). There was a significant correlation between the duration of secondary fever and concentration of LOS in CSF 1 ($r=.384$; $P=.017$) and CSF 2 ($r=.581$; $P=.0001$), whereas no significant correlations were found between presence of secondary fever and cytokine or WBC concentration in either CSF sample. Secondary fever was significantly longer in patients with high LOS concentrations in CSF 1 than in those with low LOS concentrations (3.4±3.3 vs 1.6±1.8 days; $P=.04$) and in those with detectable LOS compared with undetectable LOS in CSF 2 (3.8±3.0 vs 1.2±1.7; $P=.001$). In addition, secondary fever was significantly longer in the 15 patients who had transient or permanent neurologic abnormalities (3.4±2.5 days) than in those 20 patients without any neurologic complications (2.0±1.7) ($P=.004$).

Neurologic Complications

Thirty-five patients were followed up for at least 4 to 6 months after completion of treatment, and three patients were unavailable for follow-up. Two of these latter patients had no examinations after discharge from the hospital, when they both were considered neurologically normal. One of these patients had low and the other had high LOS concentrations in the CSF on admission. The third patient had low LOS in CSF on admission and was normal at 6 weeks' follow-up.

The neurologic abnormalities in the hospital and during the follow-up were significantly associated with high LOS concentrations in CSF 1 specimens (Table 3). Patients with transient or permanent neurologic abnormalities had had a longer mean duration of symptoms before admission (54±20 hours vs 30±18 hours; $P=.073$), had a higher Herson-Todd score, had more bacteria and higher concentration of LOS in CSF 1, and more often had detectable bacteria or LOS in CSF 2 (Table 4). Five (83%) of the six patients with detectable organisms in CSF 2 had had symptoms at least 48 hours before admission compared with 12 (40%) of the 30 with no detectable organism in CSF 2 ($P=.07$). At the end of antibiotic therapy, four patients in the high endotoxin group had hemiparesis, one had, in addition, bilateral severe to profound hearing loss, and two other patients had bilateral hearing loss without other neurologic complications. One patient in the low endotoxin group had hemiparesis at this time. Five patients had long-term neurologic complications and all these patients had LOS concentrations of 100 ng/mL or more in CSF 1. Two of these patients had severe bilateral hearing loss, one had unilateral moderate to severe hearing loss associated with speech and language delay, one had hemiparesis, and one had microcephaly with a developmental delay.

Table 2.—Lipo-oligosaccharide (LOS) Concentrations in Second Cerebrospinal Fluid (CSF) Samples at 17- to 48-hour Follow-up*

Clinical and Laboratory Findings	LOS Concentration ≥1 ng/mL (n=19)	LOS Concentration <1 ng/mL (n=19)	P
Ages ≤6 mo	11 (58)	3 (16)	.17†
Seizures	5 (26)	0	.046†
Duration of fever, d	5.2±3.2	1.8±1.7	.001‡
Transient neurologic abnormality	12 (63)	3 (16)	.007†
LOS concentration in CSF 1, ng/mL	924±1762	89±152	<.001§
Gram- and/or culture-positive	6 (32)	0	.020†
White blood cell count, ×10⁹/L	8.0±9.3	2.6±4.9	.011§
Glucose level <2.2 mmol/L	10 (53)	1 (5)	.003†
Interleukin 1β, pg/mL	284±528	36±47	.050§
Tumor necrosis factor α, pg/mL‖	92±104	82±123	NS

*Entries are numbers of patients except where otherwise indicated. Values in parentheses are percentages and all others are means±SDs. NS indicates not significant.
†Fisher Exact Test.
‡Student's *t* test.
§Mann-Whitney *U* test.
‖Tumor necrosis factor α activity was detected in eight patients (42%) when LOS concentration was greater than 1 ng/mL, and in four patients (21%) when LOS concentration was less than 1 ng/mL.

Table 3.—Presence of Neurologic Abnormalities as Related to Lipo-oligosaccharide (LOS) Concentrations in Cerebrospinal Fluid at Diagnosis

Time Abnormalities Were Present	LOS Concentration, No. (%) ≥100 ng/mL (n=19)	LOS Concentration, No. (%) <100 ng/mL (n=19)	P*
On admission	8 (42)	1 (5)	.019
During hospitalization	13 (68)	2 (11)	<.001
6 wk after illness	6/18 (33)	0/18	.019
4-6 mo after illness	5/18 (28)	0/17	.045

*Fisher Exact Test.

Disappearance of LOS From CSF

The rate of disappearance of LOS from CSF and the effect of dexamethasone on this clearance was tested by injecting LOS intracisternally into 12 rabbits. Lipo-oligosaccharide concentrations decreased rapidly and at the same rate in both steroid-treated and nontreated rabbits (data not shown). With the PCNONLIN estimation program, the half-life values were 57 minutes in the dexamethasone-treated animals and 60 minutes in the untreated animals. At 24 hours, two of six dexamethasone-treated and three of six nontreated rabbits had detectable levels of LOS in the CSF. Although dexamethasone treatment significantly reduced the pleocytosis compared with control animals, this had no effect on the clearance of LOS from the CSF in this experimental model.

Table 4.—Presence of Neurologic Abnormalities and Associated Statistically Significant Clinical and Cerebrospinal Fluid (CSF) Findings in Patients Followed up for 4 to 6 Months*

Index	Transient or Permanent Neurologic Abnormalities: Yes (n=15)	No (n=20)	P
Herson-Todd score	2.9±1.4	1.7±1.2	.006†
Altered level of consciousness on admission	7 (47)	0	.001‡
Duration of fever, d	4.3±2.9	1.8±1.8	.004†
Lipo-oligosaccharide concentration in CSF 1 on admission, ng/mL	1056±1957	143±294	.006§
Gram stain showing >10 organisms per field	15 (100)	6 (30)	<.001‡
Glucose concentration, mmol/L	0.6±0.7	1.7±1.1	.005§
Lipo-oligosaccharide concentration CSF 2 at 17- to 48-h follow-up ≥1 ng/mL	12 (86)	5 (9)	.002‡
Gram- and/or culture-positive	6 (40)	0	.003‡

*Entries are numbers of patients except where otherwise indicated. Values are means±SDs and values in parentheses are percentages.

†Student's *t* test.

‡Fisher Exact Test.

§Mann-Whitney *U* test.

COMMENT

Recent studies suggest that endotoxin is involved in the development of Hib meningitis in at least two ways. First, LOS appeared to be instrumental in producing bacteremia after intranasal inoculation in mice.[15,16] Preinoculation of Hib LOS intranasally can also enhance the ability of these organisms to cause bacteremia.[17] In addition, when purified Hib LOS was injected intracisternally in rabbits, a dose-dependent increase in meningeal inflammation was observed. This specific response was blocked by the use of agents that interfere with activity of the lipid A region of the LOS molecule.[2] No inflammation occurred after inoculation of purified Hib capsular polysaccharide, suggesting that LOS is responsible for the inflammatory changes observed in patients with Hib meningitis. Endotoxins can damage vascular endothelium by either direct or indirect means.[18] Intracarotid injection of *Escherichia coli* LPS into rabbits caused a diffuse breakdown of the blood-brain barrier.[19] Second, in addition to the effects of Hib LOS in the initial phase of systemic infection, LOS is a potent inflammatory agent. Intracisternal injections of purified LOS in picogram quantities in rabbits caused meningeal inflammation.[4] There is increasing evidence that endotoxins can stimulate endothelial cells and astrocytes and microglia cells in the central nervous system to release cytokines, such as IL-1β and TNF α.[2,20,21] These proinflammatory molecules can then either alone, or together in a synergistic fashion, induce meningitis.[21]

The mean (550 ng/mL) and median (104 ng/mL) concentrations of LOS found in the present study were comparable with those reported earlier. Berman et al[22] reported a mean concentration of 250 ng/mL in CSF of patients with Hib meningitis and Dwelle et al[23] found a mean of 101 ng/mL (median, 1028 ng/mL) in CSF of 33 children, of whom 29 had Hib meningitis. Recently, Arditi et al[24] reported mean concentrations of 1318 ng/mL (median, 440 ng/mL) in 22 children with Hib meningitis. It is known that endotoxin concentrations correlate closely with concentrations of Hib bacteria in the CSF.[24,25] The mean concentration of organisms found at diagnosis in the CSF of patients with Hib meningitis was 1×10^7 to 2×10^7 colony-forming units (CFUs) per milliliter.[24,26] Wispelwey and coworkers[3] calculated that 10 million Hib organisms contain 100 ng of LOS in their outer membranes. These figures are surprisingly close to the endotoxin concentrations found in this study.

The concentration of organisms in the CSF is considered to be an important determinant of prognosis in patients with Hib meningitis. Patients with greater than or equal to 10^7 CFUs/mL of Hib in CSF before treatment were more likely to have complications or clinically severe disease.[26] Five (28%) of 18 of our study patients with LOS levels greater than or equal to 100 ng/mL in CSF on admission (relative risk, 2.31; 95% confidence interval, 1.53 to 3.48) developed long-term neurologic complications, whereas none of those with LOS levels less than 100 ng/mL had sequelae. Although the follow-up period was relatively short, recently published data indicate that most patients recovering from meningitis who are normal at short-term follow-up will remain so, whereas some with neurologic abnormalities will improve.[27] Other studies have also shown that the measurement of endotoxin in the CSF has prognostic value in patients with gram-negative meningitis.[23,24,28] A recent experimental study by Tarlow and colleagues[29] showed that endotoxin-mediated lesions may be the mechanisms by which hearing loss occurs in meningitis.

Humans are exquisitely sensitive to the effects of endotoxin. The usual response to intravenously administered endotoxin is fever, arthralgias, myalgias, headache, and nausea that occur within 2 or 3 hours.[30] Endotoxin can also serve as a mediator of the cardiovascular dysfunction that develops during human septic shock.[30] When studying systemic meningococcal disease, Brandtzaeg et al[31] showed that plasma LOS concentrations of greater than 700 pg/mL correlated significantly with development of severe septic shock, adult respiratory distress syndrome, and death. The half-life of endotoxin after initiation of antibiotic therapy was 1 to 3 hours. Increasing plasma concentrations were not found during antibiotic therapy, which contrasts with recent experimental and clinical findings with bacterial meningitis.[24,32-34] Arditi et al[24] found increased concentrations of "cell free endotoxin" in the CSF of six patients from whom they obtained second CSF samples 2 to 6 hours after the initial CSF sample and start of antibiotic therapy. In this study, we obtained second CSF samples 17 to 48 hours after the first and found a rapid decrease of endotoxin concentrations. Dexamethasone therapy in experimental Hib meningitis did not affect clearance of LOS from the subarachnoid space. The half-life of LOS in CSF was approximately 1 hour in both groups.

All our patients were treated with dexamethasone, which has been shown to reduce significantly the incidence of neurologic sequelae, including bilateral hearing loss in patients with bacterial meningitis.[9,35,36] Dexamethasone-treated patients became afebrile earlier than those who were not treated with steroids (1.6 vs 5.0 days).[9,36] However, approximately two thirds of patients in the Dallas studies had a short period of secondary fever. In this study, we showed significant correlations between LOS concentrations and the presence and duration of secondary fever. The correlations were more significant when the results from the second CSF samples were analyzed, suggesting indirectly that those patients might still have low concentrations of LOS in CSF when steroid treatment was stopped.

We conclude that patients with high endotoxin concentrations in CSF at the time of diagnosis have an increased risk of permanent neurologic complications. Although endotoxin is cleared from the CSF rapidly during the first 48 hours after start of antibiotic treatment, significant amounts can still be present at this time in some patients, underscoring the need for further studies to determine the optimal duration of dexamethasone treatment.

This study was supported by Public Health Service Grant HD 27766 (Dr Hansen); and in part by the Academy of Finland and the Paulo and Hoechst-Fennica Foundations (Dr Mertsola).

The pediatric house staff at Children's Medical Center and Parkland Memorial Hospital, Dallas, Tex, provided invaluable help with this study.

References

1. Cybulsky MI, Chan MKW, Movat HZ. Acute inflammation and microthrombosis induced by endotoxin, interleukin-1, and tumor necrosis factor and their implication in gram-negative infection. *Lab Invest.* 1988;58:365-378.

2. Sáez-Llorens X, Ramilo O, Mustafa MM, Mertsola J, McCracken GH Jr. Molecular pathophysiology of bacterial meningitis: current concepts and therapeutic implications. *J Pediatr.* 1990;116:671-684.

3. Wispelwey B, Lesse AJ, Hansen EJ, Scheld MW. *Haemophilus influenzae* lipopolysaccharide-induced blood-brain barrier permeability during experimental meningitis in the rat. *J Clin Invest.* 1988;82:1339-1346.

4. Syrogiannopoulos GA, Hansen EJ, Erwin AL. *Haemophilus influenzae* type B lipooligosaccharide induces meningeal inflammation. *J Infect Dis.* 1988;157:237-244.

5. Levin J, Bang FB. The role of endotoxin in the extracellular coagulation of Limulus blood. *Bull Johns Hopkins Hosp.* 1964;115:265-274.

6. Nakamura S, Morita T, Iwanaga S, Niwa M, Takahashi K. A sensitive substrate for the clotting enzyme in the horse-shoe crab hemocytes. *J Biochem (Tokyo).* 1977;81:1567-1569.

7. Friberger P, Sörskog L, Nilsson K, Knös M. The use of a quantitative assay in endotoxin testing. In: Watson SW, Levin J, Novitsky T, eds. *Detection of Bacterial Endotoxins With the Limulus Amebocyte Lysate Test.* New York, NY: Alan R Liss Inc; 1987:149-169.

8. Herson VC, Todd JK. Prediction of morbidity in *Haemophilus influenzae* meningitis. *Pediatrics.* 1977;59:35-39.

9. Lebel MH, Freij BJ, Syrogiannopoulos GA, et al. Dexamethasone therapy for bacterial meningitis: results of two double-blind, placebo-controlled trials. *N Engl J Med.* 1988; 319:964-971.

10. Feldman WE. Concentrations of bacteria in cerebrospinal fluid of patients with bacterial meningitis. *J Pediatr.* 1976; 88:549-552.

11. Mertsola J, Munford RS, Ramilo O, et al. Specific detection of *Haemophilus influenzae* type B lipooligosaccharide by immunoassay. *J Clin Microbiol.* 1990;28;2700-2706.

12. Elin RJ, Wolff SM. Nonspecificity of the *Limulus* amebocyte lysate test: positive reactions with polynucleotides and proteins. *J Infect Dis.* 1973;128:349-352.

13. Mustafa MM, Lebel MH, Ramilo O, et al. Correlation of interleukin-1B and cachectin concentrations in cerebrospinal fluid and outcome from bacterial meningitis. *J Pediatr.* 1989;115:208-213.

14. Dacey RG, Sande MA. Effects of probenecid on cerebrospinal fluid concentrations of penicillin and cephalosporin derivatives. *Antimicrob Agents Chemother.* 1974;6:437-441.

15. Cope LD, Yogev R, Mertsola J, Argyle JR, McCracken GH Jr, Hansen EJ. Effect of mutations in lipopolysaccharide biosynthesis genes on the virulence of *Haemophilus influenzae* type b. *Infect Immun.* 1990;58:2343-2351.

16. Weiser JN, Williams A, Moxon R. Phase-variable lipopolysaccharide structures enhance the invasive capacity of *Haemophilus influenzae. Infect Immun.* 1990;58:3455-3457.

17. Kaplan SL, Hawkins EP, Inzana TJ, Patrick CC, Mason EO Jr. Contribution of *Haemophilus influenzae* type b lipopolysaccharide to pathogenesis of infection. *Microb Pathog.* 1988;5:55-62.

18. Harlan JM, Harber LA, Striker SE, Weaver LT. Effect of lipopolysaccharide on human endothelial cells in culture. *Thromb Res.* 1983;29:15-26.

19. Eckman PL, King WM, Brunson JG. Studies on the blood brain barrier, I: effects produced by a single injection of gram-negative endotoxin on the permeability of the central vessels. *Am J Pathol.* 1858;34:631-639.

20. Mustafa MM, Ramilo O, Olsen KD, et al. Tumor necrosis factor in mediating experimental *Haemophilus influenzae* type b meningitis. *J Clin Invest.* 1989;84:1253-1259.

21. Ramilo O, Sáez-Llorens X, Mertsola J, et al. Tumor necrosis factor α/cachectin and interleukin 1β initiate meningeal inflammation. *J Exp Med.* 1990;172:497-507.

22. Berman NS, Siegel SE, Nachum R, Lipsey A, Leedom J. Cerebrospinal fluid endotoxin concentrations in gram-negative bacterial meningitis. *J Pediatr.* 1976;88:553-556.

23. Dwelle TL, Dunkle LM, Blair L. Correlation of cerebrospinal fluid endotoxin-like activity with clinical and laboratory variables in gram-negative bacterial meningitis in children. *J Clin Microbiol.* 1987;25:856-858.

24. Arditi M, Ables L, Yogev R. Cerebrospinal fluid endotoxin levels in children with *H influenzae* meningitis before and after administration of intravenous ceftriaxone. *J Infect Dis.* 1989;160:1005-1011.

25. Schefele DW, Daum R, Syriopoulou, Smith AL. CSF endotoxin in primates with *Haemophilus influenzae* b meningitis. *Clin Res.* 1978;26:188. Abstract.

26. Feldman WE. Relation of concentrations of bacteria and bacterial antigen in cerebrospinal fluid to prognosis in patients with bacterial meningitis. *N Engl J Med.* 1977;296:433-435.

27. Pomeroy SL, Holmes SJ, Dodge PR, Feigin RP. Seizures and other neurologic sequelae of bacterial meningitis in children. *N Engl J Med.* 1990;323:1651-1657.

28. McCracken GH Jr, Sarff LD. Endotoxin in cerebrospinal fluid. *JAMA.* 1976;235:617-620.

29. Tarlow MJ, Comis SD, Osborne MP. Endotoxin induced damage to the cochlea in guinea pigs. *Lancet.* 1990;2:181-184.

30. Parrillo JE. Septic shock in humans: advances in the understanding of pathogenesis, cardiovascular dysfunction and therapy. *Ann Intern Med.* 1990;113:227-242.

31. Brandtzaeg P, Kierulf P, Gaustad P, et al. Plasma endotoxin as a predictor of multiple organ failure and death in systemic meningococcal disease. *J Infect Dis.* 1989;159:195-204.

32. Tauber MG, Shibl AM, Hackbarth CJ, Larrick JW, Sande MA. Antibiotic therapy, endotoxin concentration in cerebrospinal fluid, and brain edema in experimental *Escherichia coli* meningitis in rabbits. *J Infect Dis.* 1987;156:456-462.

33. Mustafa MM, Ramilo O, Mertsola J, et al. Modulation of inflammation and cachectin activity in relation to treatment of experimental *Haemophilus influenzae* type b meningitis. *J Infect Dis.* 1989;160:818-825.

34. Mertsola J, Ramilo O, Mustafa MM, Sáez-Llorens X, Risser RC, McCracken GH Jr. Release of endotoxin after antibiotic treatment of gram negative bacterial meningitis. *Pediatr Infect Dis J.* 1989;8:904-906.

35. McCracken GH Jr, Lebel MH. Dexamethasone therapy for bacterial meningitis in infants and children. *AJDC.* 1989;143:287-289.

36. Odio CM, Faingezicht I, Paris M, et al. The beneficial effects of early dexamethasone administration on CSF pressure, meningeal inflammation and clinical outcome in infants and children with bacterial meningitis. *N Engl J Med.* 1991;324:1525-1531.

House Staff Work Hours and Moonlighting: What Do Residents Want?

A Survey of Pediatric Residents in California

Tina L. Cheng, MD, MPH

• In the autumn of 1988, pediatric residents were surveyed on attitudes toward work hours, moonlighting, and priorities in regulation of working conditions. Questionnaires for all 756 California residents in accredited pediatric programs were sent to chief residents. Of these, 676 questionnaires were distributed to residents and 319 (47%) were returned. Respondents indicated strong support for limits on house staff working hours, and most approved of the reduction regulations proposed in New York State. Most believed that individual departments, hospitals, or subspecialties should regulate hours. By a ratio of 4.3:1, however, respondents favored legislative intervention if such limits were not set by the profession. Moonlighting was generally considered to be an individual's choice and responsibility, but a majority were willing to restrict moonlighting if total house staff hours were also limited.

(*AJDC.* 1991;145:1104-1108)

The association between the stress of house staff training and the quality of patient care has been hotly debated. Discussion regarding regulation of house staff hours has received much attention, especially in light of New York State's regulation on residency work hours in 1988. The Accreditation Council for Graduate Medical Education, the American Medical Association, and other organizations have addressed the issue, task forces have been formed, recommendations have been made, and legislation has been introduced in nine other states, with active bills in California, Connecticut, and Michigan (*American Medical News*. March 11, 1991:49). The editorial views of some New York pediatric chairpersons and program directors, opposing their state's regulation of hours, appeared in the February 1989 issue of *AJDC*.[1] In the same issue, Hoekelman[2] recommended several methods to reduce resident stress. These included the following: provide faculty advisor systems, set limits on work hours and moonlighting, establish policies for maternity and sick leave, conduct retreats and other support systems and social events, and provide creative scheduling.

Amid all the discussion, however, there has been little systematic evaluation of the perspectives and experience of house staff currently in training. There are numerous suggestions and proposals to decrease resident stress, but what do residents want? A questionnaire was developed and distributed to pediatric residents in California to ask: Do residents support limits on working hours? Who should regulate, and how? How should moonlighting fit into the regulation of hours? What other means are there to reduce resident stress?

SUBJECTS AND METHODS

In September 1988, a two-page questionnaire was sent to all California pediatric residents in accredited pediatric training programs listed in the "1987-1988 Directory of Graduate Medical Education Programs."[3] Packets of surveys were sent to chief residents to distribute to each house officer. Respondents were asked to return the surveys anonymously in an enclosed, postage-paid envelope. Programs were contacted subsequently by telephone to confirm the distribution of the surveys and the actual number of residents, and to encourage questionnaire completion and return. A second mailing was sent to chief residents in early 1989.

The survey included sections on house staff working hours and moonlighting. Structured questions on work hours asked whether hours should be limited, and how, and whether the New York regulations were acceptable. The survey also solicited responses on specific proposals regarding moonlighting, including proposals to restrict moonlighting and to require reporting of such activity. General comments were also encouraged, with space provided on the form.

RESULTS

Surveys were sent to 756 pediatric residents in California. Responses were received from 22 of 23 accredited and functioning programs. Forty-seven percent (319 of 676) of the surveys that were distributed were returned. Respondents were well distributed, with no particular concentration of responses from one geographic area or program. Demographic data on respondents compared with the resident population as a whole are presented in Table 1. The gender and level of training of respondents were not significantly different from those of the overall resi-

Accepted for publication June 3, 1991.

From the Department of Pediatrics, University of California, San Francisco, and San Francisco (Calif) General Hospital.

Reprint requests to the Department of Pediatrics, University of Massachusetts Medical Center, 55 Lake Avenue N, Worcester, MA 01655 (Dr Cheng).

Table 1.—Demographic Information on Resident Respondents Compared With California and Nationwide Data

Characteristic	Survey Respondents, % (No.)	California Residents, % (No.)*	US Residents, % (No.)*
Sex			
F	53.5 (121)	52.7 (403)	51.1 (3979)
M	46.5 (105)	47.3 (361)	48.9 (3808)
Level of training†			
PL-1	36.6 (104)	34.9 (267)	33.0 (2573)
PL-2	29.2 (83)	31.2 (238)	29.5 (2296)
PL-3	30.3 (86)	29.8 (228)	28.1 (2188)
PL-4 (chief resident)	3.9 (11)	4.1 (31)	9.4 (730)

*1988-1989 data from the American Academy of Pediatrics, Pediatrics Review and Education Program (PREP).
†PL indicates postgraduate level.

dent population in California and nationwide.

Most respondents (73%) believed that house staff hours should be controlled internally, by individual departments, hospitals, or subspecialties, while 24% favored some involvement by the state. Seventy-six percent thought the legislatures should intervene if individual departments, hospitals, or the medical establishment did not set limits on house staff hours; 18% responded "no"; and 6% gave no response.

Respondents were asked to evaluate the regulations to limit house staff hours, including parts of the New York guidelines (Table 2). The majority of residents thought that regulation similar to the New York guidelines was acceptable. On a subsequent question, those favoring regulation marked the number of hours per week they thought to be reasonable. Among the 20% of respondents who believed the 80-hour-per-week limit was unacceptable, more than half (37 of 61) preferred consecutive hour limits of *fewer* than 80 hours per week on the latter question. More than half (17 of 29) of those rejecting the 12-hour emergency department shifts expressed a desire for shorter shifts. Finally, almost all (43 of 47) of those rejecting the limitation of call nights to no more than every third night wanted fewer call nights.

Residents were also asked about the use of different strategies for regulating work hours, including limits on the total number of hours per week, consecutive hours per shift, and number of call nights. When those favoring limits on specific hours were asked to specify what they considered reasonable hours limits, the average number of hours per week proposed by respondents was 74.8 (SD, 10.7 hours; range, 40 to 100 hours; n = 174). Respondents proposed limiting consecutive hours of work to an average of 13 hours per emergency department shift (SD, 4.1 hours; range, 8 to 36 hours; n = 225) and 24.3 hours per shift on non–emergency department rotations (SD, 4.8 hours; range, 8 to 36 hours; n = 198). The average suggested frequency of call was once every 3.7 nights (SD, 0.57; median, every four nights; range, every three to seven nights on-call; n = 272).

With respect to moonlighting, a majority of respondents thought restrictions on moonlighting were not acceptable. Survey questions and results are presented in Table 3. When asked about mandatory reporting of moonlighting activity to program directors, however,

Table 2.—Attitudes of California Residents Regarding Regulation of Work Hours* (N = 319)

Regulation	Acceptable, % (No.)	Unacceptable, % (No.)†	No Answer, % (No.)
New York regulations			
80 h/wk, averaged over a 4-wk period	77.4 (247)	19.1 (61)	3.4 (11)
12 h per shift in emergency department	87.5 (279)	9.1 (29)	3.4 (11)
24 h per shift in nonemergency department rotations with no new work after 16 h	81.5 (260)	13.5 (43)	5.0 (16)
One 24-h period off every 7 d, averaged over 28 d	83.7 (267)	11.6 (37)	4.7 (15)
Call limitation			
No more than every third night on call	82.8 (264)	14.7 (47)	2.5 (8)

*Percentages not adding to 100% are due to rounding.
†Includes many respondents who thought that the regulations were unacceptable because regulations were not stringent enough.

Table 3.—Attitudes of California Residents Toward Moonlighting (N = 319)*

Proposed regulation	Acceptable, % (No.)	Unacceptable, % (No.)	No Answer, % (No.)
"Moonlighting should be allowed only if total hours worked do not exceed a specified total per week (eg, moonlighting plus house staff hours = 80 h/wk)"	38.9 (124)	44.5 (142)	16.6 (53)
"Moonlighting hours should be limited per week or per month"	37.3 (119)	43.3 (138)	19.4 (62)
"House staff must inform program directors of moonlighting activities"	48.0 (153)	38.6 (123)	13.5 (43)

*Percentages not adding to 100% are due to rounding.

most found this to be acceptable. When asked, "Which would you rather see: house staff work hours limited inclusive of moonlighting hours or no restriction on house staff working hours?" 59% preferred limits on total hours, including moonlighting, while 19% preferred no restrictions on total hours; 22% expressed no preference or gave no response.

Although the survey did not ask why hours should or should not be limited, many respondents offered opinions in the "Comments" section of the survey. Some residents believed that work hours were excessive and that patient care suffered as a direct result. While some expressed the belief that medical judgment suffered as a result of fatigue, others expressed concern regarding the development of cynicism toward patients and loss of compassion as a result of overwork. One resident stated that:

> As much as people worry about overwork leading to medical errors, what actually seems to suffer is the doctor-patient interaction. Admissions are "hits," [slang referring to hospital admissions] and how compassionate can anybody be when they are irritable from sleep deprivation?

The notion that continuous hours produce continuity of patient care and optimal learning was challenged. One respondent stated, "There *is no* continuity of care after 24 hours on call. There *is* very little continuity of thought" (emphasis in original). Another said, "No one sits with a patient to watch the evolution of the disease. You are generally too tired, stressed, and overworked to care."

House staff quality of life was frequently mentioned. Physical and mental health, as well as family and personal life, were thought to suffer from the combination of long hours and high stress levels. One resident said:

> Our perception of reality becomes tainted by the limited time to interact with family, friends, and the general public in a social setting. Also, family life suffers and health matters are ignored. House staff are expected to work despite fever and other acute illnesses (for) which we, as physicians, advise our patients to stay home.

Finally, resident learning was believed to be compromised by long hours. Some reported that postcall conferences and medical rounds were often seen as a chance to rest rather than a time to learn. One stated that "it makes residents worse doctors, not better, to deprive them of essential sleep, private time, and time to read."

Many respondents thought that outside employment should be an individual's choice and responsibility. Comments reiterated the point that "moonlighting is a separate and personal decision" and "as long as it does not affect clinical performance, it should be nobody's business but the resident's." Some respondents reported that their reason for moonlighting was the need for added income, as a "necessary evil to meet student loans," or as an adjunct to support their families. Others cited the value of moonlighting in exposing the resident to different hospital systems, clinical practices, and patients. Some respondents expressed the need to monitor moonlighting to ensure resident performance and quality of patient care.

COMMENT

The results indicate that many pediatric house staff in California strongly support the concept of limitation of residency hours. In addition, if the profession fails to regulate hours, respondents favor legislative intervention. A majority supports efforts to limit hours even if this would restrict the ability to moonlight. Residents' support for regulation of work hours is not surprising; the strength of the support for regulation and the ideas for change, however, are most revealing.

One clear drawback of the survey was the low response rate. It is unclear whether the surveys were incompletely distributed or were not completed and returned. With the many demands on residents' time, the low response rate was not unexpected, but may bias the results by overrepresenting respondents who believed particularly strongly about the issue. California pediatric residents represent approximately 10% of all pediatric residents in the United States (American Academy of Pediatrics, Pediatrics Residency Education Program, unpublished data, 1991), and responses were received from all but one program. Demographic data presented in Table 1 demonstrate that the gender and level of training of respondents were not significantly different from those of the overall resident population, lending some support to the generalization of the results. The sheer number and consistency of the responses show that many residents desire change and suggest a starting point for future research.

Only two other studies have addressed resident attitudes toward work hour reform, and generally support the findings of this study. In a survey of surgical residents in New England by Ruby et al,[4] 72% of respondents thought that there was a need for reform of resident work schedules and 76% thought that long hours impaired education. Most thought that reform should occur through residency review committees, as did the pediatric residents in this survey. The surgical residents, however, were not asked whether legislatures should intervene in the absence of action by the medical community.

In a recently published general survey, 23% of postgraduate level 2 and postgraduate level 3 pediatric residents addressed some issues regarding work hours.[5] They found that three fourths of all respondents believed that working for extended periods "moderately" or "greatly" hindered their performance. Only 2% indicated that prolonged periods on-duty does not affect quality of care. Forty-four percent believed that future limits should be placed on total hours worked per week and 34% were willing to exchange an extra year of residency for a 60-hour work schedule.

Regulation of Work Hours

Restricting residency hours has gained prominence since the Libby Zion[6] case in New York and subsequent regulations on work hours in New York State. Advances in medicine and increased complexity of patient care have added significantly to the burden on house staff. Many believe that the lives of residents have become too stressful, with untoward effects on health, training, and patient care necessitating regulation of hours. Others have argued that restricting hours would hinder continuity of care, which benefits both the patient and house staff learning. Also, staffing needs of clinical services may not be met if house staff hours are restricted, and the cost of replacing resident hours may be enormous.

Regulation of hours was acceptable to a majority of respondents. Most believed that the New York regulations and limitation on the number of call nights were reasonable means to limit hours. Many of those stating that the New York guidelines were unacceptable believed that these limits were not stringent enough. The 4.3:1 ratio in favor of legislative intervention in the event "that individual departments, hospitals, or the medical establishment do not set limits on house staff hours" indicates the uniformity of resident opinion in favor of controlling house staff hours. The next logical question, the point at which residents believe legislation or state regulation would be justified, is difficult to assess. Most respondents would prefer that the profession police itself; many, however, were sufficiently frustrated with the current system to call for regulation. One respondent's comments reflected these mixed feelings:

Although I would like to see working conditions monitored by the medical establishment, (it) has been pathetically unable to do this. . . . Because of this, I am not totally opposed to allowing lawmakers to decide working conditions.

Moonlighting

The issue of moonlighting has also come under scrutiny, in part, as a result of the attention on house staff hours. There has been discussion in favor of limiting or eliminating outside employment by residents to relieve house staff overwork. The New York regulations restrict moonlighting. New York house staff must notify their hospitals of any employment outside their residency and are prohibited from working beyond the maximum number of hours under the new regulations.

Results from national surveys of residents reveal that a significant proportion of house staff seek outside employment.[7-11] In a 1987 survey,[12] 23% of residents reported moonlighting, although only approximately 6% of pediatric residents did so. The average number of hours spent in moonlighting was 13.4 hours per month.[12] Other surveys[13] have found that while many residents moonlight, the actual hours worked are small and concentrated during less demanding rotations.

A survey of pediatric residency programs found that 30% did not permit moonlighting and almost half retained the right to review or approve the frequency and content of the activity.[7] Compliance with and enforcement of these rules, however, is unclear, and one survey found that of pediatric program directors who do not permit moonlighting, 30% acknowledged that it may exist.[7]

Several questionnaires have documented the number of residents who moonlight and the advantages of the opportunity; none, however, have asked residents whether they place greater priority on work hour reduction or the freedom to moonlight. In this survey, most believed that moonlighting "should be left to an individual's discretion," but respondents were willing, by a ratio of more than 2:1, to restrict moonlighting if total house staff hours were also limited. This indicates a strong desire for work hour limits and a willingness to trade the opportunity to moonlight for work hour reductions. As resident indebtedness increases, however, it is unclear whether this sentiment will remain.[8]

Suggestions for Change

The following were among suggestions given by survey respondents that appear to merit consideration.

Ancillary Services.—The lack of ancillary services was frequently mentioned by respondents as a cause of added work and stress in residency. Many hours are spent on paperwork, phlebotomy and intravenous placement, coordination of consultant activities, scheduling procedures, dictations, and other tasks with little educational value. Nursing shortages have also added to the burden on residents in many hospitals. A study of internal medicine house staff on call discovered that residents spent only 1 to 2.5 hours per night per shift in direct patient contact, with a considerable amount of time spent in administrative and communicative activities and repetitive performance of procedures.[14]

Suggested efforts to address this problem include provision of ward clerks, dictation systems, intravenous services, and phlebotomy and messenger transport teams. Computerized medical records, laboratories, and other automated data systems could also contribute significantly by improving communication and reducing or speeding clerical tasks.

Policies for Sick Coverage and Parental Leave.—The inadequacy or lack of sick leave and maternity and paternity leave policies were identified as areas of stress. Residents often feel guilty while resting when they are sick or while pregnant because of the added burden on their fellow house staff; colleagues become resentful of the increased workload. A system of coverage and a clearly delineated policy of illness or maternity and paternity leave is needed and desired by many residents. Departments must attempt to estimate their manpower needs so that rotation schedules have flexibility to accommodate unexpected situations without undue stress on the absent member or on other house staff.

Night-Float System.—Night-float systems have been instituted at some residency programs[15] and were favorably mentioned by some survey respondents. Providing a night shift of residents or attendants to help the on-call residents with night duties and admissions may aid in reducing fatigue. This system may not be feasible in all types of programs, but deserves consideration and has been endorsed by some residents and program directors in the literature.[15-19]

Beeper Moratorium.—Some residents noted that they are often interrupted on numerous occasions during the day and feel harassed by nonemergency pages. Frequent interruptions were a notable feature of the house staff work environment found in a time study of internal medicine residents on call.[14] In this study, it was found that while residents obtained a new patient history, the mean time before a house officer was interrupted was 7 to 11 minutes. Most interruptions were nonemergency pages or phone calls.

The idea of "silencing the pagers" was raised by Bergman[20] in his article on resident stress. He suggested that a small number of residents could answer the emergency pages, thereby allowing others to give their undivided attention to patient care activities or educational conferences. Providing guidelines on the appropriate use of the pagers or a triage system for paging may alleviate some of this source of stress.[21] One study of paging patterns found that decreasing the number of unnecessary pages and postponing non-urgent interruptions could reduce disruptions by up to 42%.[16]

Involvement in Planning.—Some residents expressed a desire for involvement in residency program planning at both the department or hospital level and within organized medicine as a whole. Residency training is transitory in nature, and many programs consider house staff to be students rather than employees, although some court decisions have ruled otherwise.[22] Residents are often excluded from program planning and believe they lack the leverage and opportunity to represent themselves effectively. Residents have much to contribute and may gain an important sense of control and autonomy by becoming involved in the direction of their residency programs.

An organized voice for house staff has been established through various residency associations and through the National Federation of House Staff Organizations, the American Medical Association's Resident Physician's Section, and the American Academy of Pediatrics Resident Section. These groups, together with increased resident involvement in decision-making bodies at the department and hospital level, seem to offer potential opportunities for increasing resident input.

Resident life has changed and is currently under greater scrutiny by both the medical community and the public. Understanding the attitudes of house staff and their involvement is crucial in determining strategies to address issues of resident stress. Further research is needed to understand the realities of resident work schedules, reasons for moonlighting, differences among programs, effect of stress on patient care, and the perceptions of residents regarding different approaches to stress reduction including, but not limited to, the limitation of work hours. The survey results indicate a clear desire on the part of residents for the structure of residency training to reflect the changing nature of medicine so as to improve the value of the residency experience and the quality of patient care.

The mailing of the survey was supported in part by the California Association of Interns and Residents.

The author thanks Ken Conca; Peter Lurie, MD, MPH; Thomas Newman, MD, MPH; Jonathan Klein, MD, MPH; Jay Tureen, MD; and Helen Loeser, MD, MPH, for their critical reviews of this article.

References

1. Cohen MI, Dancis J, Finberg L, Hirschhorn K, Katz M, Wasserman E. Patient care, resident stress, and government regulation. *AJDC.* 1989;143:181-182.

2. Hoekelman RA. Stress experienced during pediatric residency training: its causes, consequences, recognition, and solutions. *AJDC.* 1989;143:177-180.

3. American Medical Association. 1987-1988 Directory of Graduate Medical Education Programs. Chicago, Ill: 1987:351-352.

4. Ruby ST, Allen L, Fielding LP, Deckers PJ. Survey of residents' attitudes toward reform of work hours. *Arch Surg.* 1990; 125:764-768.

5. Forster J, ed. The pediatric residency survey: the residents talk back. *Contemp Pediatr.* 1991(May suppl):6-16.

6. Asch DA, Parker RM. The Libby Zion case. *N Engl J Med.* 1988;318:771-775.

7. Moss AJ. Moonlighting house officers: the silent majority. *N Engl J Med.* 1984;311:1375-1377.

8. McCue JD, Janiszewski M, Stickley WT. Residents' views of the value of moonlighting. *Arch Intern Med.* 1990;150:1511-1513.

9. Hough DE, Bazzoli GJ. The economic environment of resident physicians. *JAMA.* 1985;253:1758-1762.

10. Silliman RA, Dittus RS, Velez R, Wartman SA, Young MJ, Fletcher RH. Debt, moonlighting, and career decisions among internal medicine residents. *J Med Educ.* 1987;62:463-469.

11. Stange KC, Sutherland JE, Moonlighting policy and practice in family practice residencies, *J Fam Prac.* 1987;24:63-65.

12. Burkhart J, ed. American Medical Association Resident Physician Section: Survey looks at moonlighting by residents. *Resident Staff Physician.* 1987;33:118-119.

13. Cohen SN, Leeds MP. The moonlighting dilemma. *JAMA.* 1989;262:529-531.

14. Lurie N, Rank B, Parenti C, Woolley T, Snoke W. How do house officers spend their nights? a time study of internal medicine house staff on call. *N Engl J Med.* 1989;320:1673-1677.

15. Lieu TA, Blum N, Forrest C, Cornfeld D, Polin R. Late-night admissions: resident education and sleep patterns. *JAMA.* 1990;264:2124.

16. Foster HW, Seltzer VL. Accommodating to restrictions on residents' working hours. *Acad Med.* 1991;166:94-97.

17. Schwartz AJ, Black ER, Goldstein MG, Jozefowicz RF, Emmings FG. Levels and causes of stress among residents. *J Med Educ.* 1987;62:744-753.

18. Carey JC, Fishburne JI. A method to limit working hours and reduce sleep deprivation in an obstetrics and gynecology residency program. *Obstet Gynecol.* 1989;74:668-672.

19. Seltzer V, Foster HW Jr, Gordon M. Resident scheduling: night float programs, *Obstet Gynecol.* 1991;77:940-943.

20. Bergman AB. Resident stress. *Pediatrics.* 1988;82:260-263.

21. Katz MH, Schroeder SA. The sounds of the hospital: paging patterns in three teaching hospitals. *N Engl J Med.* 1988; 319:1585-1589.

22. *Regents of University of California vs Public Employment Relations Board*, 41 Cal3d 601 (Cal.Rptr. 631) (1986) also cites *House Officers, etc vs University of Nebraska Medical Center*, 198 Neb. 697 [255 NW2d 258] (1977) and *Regents of University of Michigan vs Michigan Employment Relations Commission*, 389 Mich. 96 [204 NW2d 218] (1973), and several other decisions.

Barriers to Medical Care for Homeless Families Compared With Housed Poor Families

David Wood, MD, MPH, R. Burciaga Valdez, PhD, MHSA

• To evaluate health access and health services utilization of homeless families we selected a systematic sample of 194 homeless families from 10 shelters in Los Angeles and 196 housed poor families from the same geographic regions of Los Angeles selected from welfare offices. Both samples relied primarily on Medicaid for their health insurance (61% and 96%). However, more homeless families than housed poor families were currently uninsured (26% vs 2%), had lost health insurance over the past year (50% vs 21%), and had spent a greater percentage of the past year uncovered by health insurance (22% vs 6%). Homeless families were much less likely to report a regular provider for preventive care (81% vs 94%) or for sick care (72% vs 95%). Moreover, of those reporting a regular provider, homeless families were more likely than housed poor families to use emergency departments or clinics rather than private offices for both preventive care (35% vs 15%) and sick care (37% vs 26%). Barriers to health care more frequently prevented homeless families from obtaining care (38% vs 28%). These findings suggest that homeless families have greater problems of access to health care than other poor families, related to lack of insurance, lack of a regular primary care provider, and other barriers. Programs to address these barriers for homeless families are presented.

(*AJDC.* 1991;145:1109-1115)

Health and social programs are often intended to serve as a "safety net," insuring the poor and homeless with basic needs. Numerous bureaucratic, economic, and social barriers, however, impede families most in need from receiving services.[1-4]

Homeless families, for example, are among the most needy families in our communities. They experience extreme poverty, unstable living environments, and serious family problems.[5-8] Furthermore, homeless children suffer from high rates of health problems such as acute infectious illnesses,[9-12] chronic medical problems,[6] nutritional problems,[10,11,13] developmental delay,[10,14] academic failure,[10,12,14-16] and serious emotional and behavior problems.[10,14] Despite these needs for health and social services, preliminary studies in Boston, Mass, and New York, NY, indicate that homeless families and children do not have adequate access to health or social services.[5,12,17]

Bureaucratic and other system barriers have been implicated as major impediments that prevent homeless children from receiving health and social services.[15,18] However, no studies to date have indicated whether these barriers affect homeless families and poor domiciled families differently. Understanding the similarities and differences in access barriers experienced by domiciled and nondomiciled families provides the basis for program modifications necessary to improve our "safety net."

To document the health and social needs of homeless children and the access of their families to health and social services, we surveyed 194 homeless families in shelters and 196 poor, stably housed families. In previous publications we presented our findings contrasting family composition and function, housing costs, economic and social problems,[8] and child health status[10] for homeless and housed poor families. In this report we compare their access to health care services and document barriers experienced by these families in seeking health and social services for their children.

SUBJECTS AND METHODS

Homeless families composed of at least one female parent and minor child (n = 194) and a comparison group of stably housed poor families (n = 196) were interviewed from March 1987 through early 1988 in Los Angeles, Calif.

Homeless Family Sample

We followed a three-stage sampling strategy in selecting our homeless families: (1) a purposive sample of 10 shelters, (2) a systematic sample of families in shelters, and (3) a random sample of one child in each family. In the first stage we selected the 10 largest shelters in Los Angeles County from a universe of 25 shelters that housed families. These shelters received 80% of all shelter referrals for families in Los Angeles in early 1987. We visited each shelter weekly during the interview period.

We sampled families from among those who had come to the shelter within the past week. Families had been homeless an average of 6 months (SD, 13.6 months; median, 2 months) before arriving at the shelter. Our interviews were conducted within 1 week after families arrived at the shelter; interviews were conducted independent of shelter staff and were not part of the shel-

Accepted for publication June 24, 1991.

From the RAND/UCLA Center for Health Policy Study; the Department of Pediatrics, Cedars-Sinai Medical Center; and the Department of Health Services, University of California, Los Angeles.

The opinions and conclusions expressed herein are solely those of the authors and should not be construed as representing the policies or opinions of The RAND Corp, Cedars-Sinai Medical Center, or the University of California.

Reprint requests to Department of Pediatrics, Room 4428, Cedars-Sinai Medical Center, 8700 Beverly Blvd, Los Angeles, CA 90048 (Dr Wood).

ter's intake protocol. All new residents in the five smaller shelters and every other family from the larger shelters were selected for interviews. After two failed attempts to locate a family, we approached the next family on the shelter's list of new residents.

One child in each family was randomly selected as the reference child by (1) fully listing all children in the family, (2) grouping them into two age groups of 0 through 5 years of age or 6 through 18 years of age, (3) using a random-number table to select from the two age groups, and, (4) if more than one child were in the age group, using a random-number table to select the child who was to be the focus of the interview.

No families were excluded on the basis of language or race (three interviews were conducted in Spanish). Two single-parent, male-headed families were interviewed and subsequently eliminated from our analysis. Of the nearly 200 families approached for an interview, only three families refused to participate.

Housed Poor Family Sample

The housed poor families were systematically sampled from families presenting to four welfare offices. The four welfare offices were selected based on the geographic areas of Los Angeles in which homeless families were living before becoming homeless. Over 70% of the homeless families previously lived in the combined catchment area of the selected welfare offices. We screened all presenting families and requested an interview from those who had lived in their current residence at least 6 months and had received welfare benefits continuously for at least 1 year. Of the 240 families we sought to interview, 46 refused to participate. No differences were observed in the age or ethnicity of the mothers who refused compared with the respondents.

Interview and Questionnaire

A structured interview focusing on a single child per family was conducted with the mother by a trained interviewer. The interview lasted approximately 45 minutes. Interviews were conducted in private rooms in both the shelters and the welfare offices.

Our survey asked about housing history, income, and other family characteristics. Family housing arrangements over the past 5 years were described by the number of moves and the amount of time spent in specific living arrangements, such as living in their own apartment, doubling up with strangers, living in a hotel or motel, and living in a car or on the street. Family income was a summation of the total household income contributed by all family members over the past year. The poverty level was calculated based on total family income adjusted for family size compared with the federal poverty guidelines for 1987. In 1987, the federal poverty level for a family of three was $8940.[19]

Ethnicity was determined by self-report and categorized as African-American, non-Latino white, Latino, and other. Families were defined as single-parent (female-headed) or two-parent families based on whether the mother reported that she was currently with an adult male partner. Mothers were asked about years of education completed and were categorized into 0 to 11 years and 12 or more years of education. Mothers were asked to assess their child's general health status as excellent, good, fair, or poor.

Access to Medical Care

Access to medical care was measured by (1) whether the child had a regular provider for preventive and illness care, (2) the type of regular provider (private physician's office or health maintenance organization vs emergency department, hospital outpatient clinic, or free, community, or public health clinic), and (3) barriers to care reported by the family that "made care difficult to obtain," such as cost, transportation, wait for an appointment, or lack of knowledge about available services. If interviewees named a barrier that "made health care difficult to obtain," they were asked whether the barrier actually prevented them from obtaining care. These questions were adapted from the 1982-1984 National Hispanic Health and Nutritional Examination Survey, which was designed for administration to primarily poor and less-educated populations.[20]

Questions were also developed to assess the families' current health insurance coverage (no insurance, Medicaid, private, or other) and loss of health insurance over the past 12 months. Using an open-ended format, mothers were asked the reason for loss of health insurance over the past year. The responses were abstracted into the following categories: (1) The family's health insurance was through an employer and the job was lost. (2) The head of family was employed in a job that provided no health benefits. (3) The family's health insurance was through Medicaid but was lost because of a change in the family's eligibility—usually due to a parent finding employment that provided no health benefits. (4) The family's health insurance was through Medicaid but was lost because of administrative problems. Parents were asked to estimate the time the family was uninsured over the past 12 months. No other data sources (eg, Medicaid files) were examined to confirm the study information obtained by parental report.

Analysis Methods

Differences in means and proportions for the homeless and housed samples were compared using simple two-tailed t test and χ^2 analysis. Differences in proportions are reported as the absolute differences between the two groups and the 95% confidence intervals around those differences. Confidence intervals that include zero indicate that the observed differences in proportions may be a result of chance variations. The tighter the confidence intervals around the differences in proportions, the more precise the estimates of the differences between the two groups.

We used logistic regression to test associations between access indicators and homelessness while statistically controlling for population differences in child sex, race, maternal education, child health status, health insurance status (insured vs uninsured), family size, family structure, and family income. A logistic regression model describes the associations between a dependent variable with two or more discrete values (experienced an access barrier vs did not experience an access barrier) and each independent factor (eg, homelessness, family poverty), adjusted for all other factors in the model. The 95% confidence interval around the odds ratio describes limits within which the odds ratio will fall 95% of the time. Therefore, if the 95% confidence interval includes "1," there is no significant association between the dependent and independent factor at $P = .05$.

Study Limitations

The cross-sectional design of our study does not allow determination of a causal relationship between homelessness, health insurance loss, and access to medical services. We identified other factors, such as family dysfunction and economic stress, that are common among homeless families and also affect access to medical care. Moreover, there are other factors associated with poor access to medical care that we did not assess.

The medical care access and health insurance measures used in this study depend on parental reports and are subject to reporting biases. No other information sources, such as Medicaid files, were used to confirm the families' reports. Furthermore, the acute stress of homelessness may have an important effect on the families' recall of health-related events over the past year. To minimize the potential recall bias imposed by the acute stress of homelessness, homeless families were approached for an interview only after they had 2 or 3 days to adjust to the shelter setting.

Our three-stage sampling strategy included a selection of the busiest shelters in Los Angeles, and we systematically sampled families. This approach may have overrepresented newly homeless families and underrepresented families who had been homeless in the same shelter for longer periods. Due to numerous logistical problems in the field, the sampling in some shelters often amounted to a convenience sample of families, although the selection of the child remained random. The housed poor family sample overrepresented blacks and underrepresented Latinos compared with the overall population in Los Angeles receiving

Table 1.—Demographic Characteristics of Homeless and Housed Families

Characteristic	Homeless Families (n=194)	Housed Families (n=193)	*P**
Maternal age†	29 (0.5)	29 (0.6)	.55
No. of children†	2.7 (0.1)	2.3 (0.1)	.01
Children rated in fair or poor health, %	17	13	.27
Maternal ethnicity, %			
Black	57	70	<.01
Non-Latino white	30	15	
Latino	8	11	
Maternal educational level, %			
None to 11th grade	43	28	.01
High school graduate/ some college	57	72	
Family structure, %			
Female head, one parent	53	62	.08
Two parents	47	38	
Family income, $†	9739 (401)	8150 (226)	.01
Families living below federal poverty level, %‡	82	88	.08

**P* values are from χ^2 tests of proportions or two-tailed *t* tests for means.
†Values are mean (SE).
‡Income levels were adjusted for family size.

Aid to Families With Dependent Children (AFDC). This difference results largely from our selection of welfare offices that represented the homeless families' neighborhoods of origin.

RESULTS

Homeless families were more likely to be headed by two parents and were likely to have more children than poor housed families (Table 1). Homeless mothers were more likely to be white and to have dropped out of high school. The vast majority of families from both groups had household incomes below the federal poverty level (Table 1). Homeless and housed children were equally likely to be rated in fair or poor health, but at a level three to four times higher than that observed in the general child population (approximately 4%).[21] More detailed family demographic and economic characteristics are presented elsewhere.[7,8]

Insurance Status and Loss of Insurance

Over one fourth of the homeless families reported having no health insurance (26%) compared with only 2% of the housed poor families (Table 2). The majority of families in the homeless and housed groups relied on Medicaid for health insurance coverage (67% and 96%, respectively). A small percentage of homeless families reported private health insurance (7%). Over the past year, homeless families were twice as likely to have lost their insurance coverage (50% vs 21%, $P<.001$), and they remained uninsured for a longer period than housed poor families (2.6 vs 0.66 months, $P<.001$, Table 2).

When asked why they had lost their health insurance over the past year, homeless and housed families described similar scenarios, including, in order of the frequency of response: (1) The family was dropped from AFDC and Medicaid for administrative reasons, usually due to failure to file the AFDC monthly eligibility reporting form. (2) The head of family was employed during the past year but the job did not provide health insurance or the family could not affort the added cost of dependent health insurance coverage. (3) The head of family lost employment and, with it, lost health insurance. (4) The family was dropped from AFDC/Medicaid due to a change in eligibility. Families in this category typically reported obtaining employment that did not offer health insurance as a benefit.

Table 2.—Health Insurance Coverage and Health Insurance Loss Among Homeless and Housed Families

Indicator	Homeless Families	Housed Families	*P**
Current health insurance, %†			
None	26	2	<.001
Medicaid	67	96	
Private insurance	7	2	
Lost health insurance over the previous year, %‡	50	21	<.001
Time without health insurance coverage during the previous year, mo§	2.58 (0.3)	0.66 (0.1)	<.001
Reasons reported for losing health insurance during the previous year, %‖			
Lost Medicaid due to administrative problems¶	43	59	.201
Lost eligibility for Medicaid due to employment, and job provides no health insurance	16	8	
Employed, but no health insurance benefits	15	14	
Lost health insurance with loss of job	11	16	
Other#	14	3	

**P* values are from χ^2 tests of proportions or two-tailed *t* tests for means.
†For homeless families, n=194; for housed families, n=193.
‡For homeless families, n=192; for housed families, n=194.
§For homeless families, n=192; for housed families, n=194. Values are mean (SE).
‖For homeless families, n=92: for housed families, n=37.
¶Usually due to failure to file monthly reporting forms.
#Includes change in family composition and reasons unclear to the respondent.

Access to Regular Health Providers

Homeless families were less likely than housed poor families to report a regular provider (Table 3) for either preventive care (81% vs 94%) or illness care (72% vs 95%). The most common reasons the homeless families gave for having no regular provider included frequent moves and housing instability (53%), no need for a regular physician (19%), a financial barrier (14%), and transportation problems (11%).

Table 3.—Proportion of Homeless and Housed Families Reporting a Regular Provider for Preventive and Illness Care

Access Indicator	Proportion of Homeless Families	Proportion of Housed Families	Difference of Proportions (95% Confidence Limits)
Regular provider for preventive care*	81	94	−13 (−19, −7)
Regular provider for illness care†	72	95	−23 (−30, −16)
Regular provider for both preventive and illness care‡	67	91	−24 (−32, −16)
Regular provider for well-child care is an emergency department, community clinic, or hospital outpatient clinic§	35	15	20 (11, 29)
Regular provider for illness care is an emergency department, community clinic, or hospital outpatient clinic‖	37	26	11 (1, 21)

*For homeless families, n=194; for housed families, n=1192.
†For homeless families, n=195; for housed families, n=193.
‡For homeless families, n=194; for housed families, n=192.
§Respondents were restricted to families that reported a regular provider. For homeless families, n=158; for housed families, n=181.
‖Respondents were restricted to families that reported a regular provider. For homeless families, n=139; for housed families, n=182.

Among families reporting a regular provider, the regular provider of preventive and sick care for homeless families was more likely to be an emergency department, hospital outpatient clinic, community clinic, or other public provider than a private physician's office or a health maintenance organization. Among families using public providers for preventive care, compared with housed poor families, homeless families relied more on emergency departments (6% vs 0%) and on free or community clinics (19% vs 4.5%) than on hospital outpatient departments. Among the families using public providers for illness care, homeless families relied on free or community clinics to a greater extent than housed poor families (11% vs 2.5%).

Barriers to Care

Approximately half of the families from both groups reported experiencing at least one specific barrier to health care (Table 4). Homeless families, however, more frequently reported that these barriers prevented them from obtaining care (38% vs 28%). Barriers more frequently preventing homeless families from obtaining health care included (1) not having transportation to get to care (21% vs 11%), (2) the cost of care (16% vs 8%), (3) not knowing where to go for care (11% vs 5%), and (4) waiting too long for an appointment (9% vs 3%).

Table 4.—Proportion of Homeless and Housed Families Prevented From Obtaining Medical Care by Access Barriers

Access Indicator	Proportion of Homeless Families	Proportion of Housed Families	Difference of Proportions (95% Confidence Limits)
Experienced at least one barrier in seeking care*	56	57	1 (−9, 11)
Barrier actually prevented child from obtaining care†	38	28	10 (1, 19)
Barriers that prevented care when parent felt a child needed care			
Had no transportation to the care provider‡	21	11	10 (3, 17)
Care was too expensive§	16	8	8 (2, 14)
Did not know where to go to seek care‖	11	5	6 (1, 11)
Had to wait too long for an appointment¶	9	3	6 (1, 11)

*For homeless families, n=194; for housed families, n=196.
†For homeless families, n=194; for housed families, n=196.
‡For homeless families, n=193; for housed families, n=191.
§For homeless families, n=193; for housed families, n=193.
‖For homeless families, n=193; for housed families, n=193.
¶For homeless families, n=193; for housed families, n=193.

Multivariate Analyses

After adjusting comparisons for population differences, such as race, child health status, child age, child sex, health insurance coverage, maternal education level, family income, family size, and family composition, homeless children were three times more likely than housed poor children to lack a regular provider for well-child care (Table 5) and 5.5 times more likely to lack a regular provider for illness care. Among the families reporting regular providers, homeless children were 2.5 times more likely than housed poor children to depend on public providers rather than private providers.

After adjusting comparisons for population differences, we found that barriers were 70% more likely to prevent homeless children from receiving care than housed poor children (Table 6). Specific barriers preventing homeless children from receiving medical care included lack of transportation to health care visits, having to wait too long for an appointment, and not knowing where to go for care.

COMMENT

Both the homeless and housed populations in our comparison study experienced severe problems gaining access to medical care; more than half the families in each group reported barriers to care. Nevertheless, compared with domiciled children, homeless children were more likely to have lost health insurance and less likely to have

Table 5.—Logistic Regression Analyses of Access Indicators for Homeless and Housed Families

Access Indicator	Homeless vs Housed Odds Ratio (95% Confidence Limits)*
Child lacks a regular provider for well-child care†	3.4 (1.4, 8.3)
Child lacks a regular provider for illness care‡	5.6 (2.5, 12.6)
Regular provider of well-child care is an emergency department, community clinic, or hospital outpatient clinic§	2.6 (1.4, 4.6)
Regular provider of illness care is an emergency department, community clinic, or hospital outpatient clinic‖	1.4 (0.8, 2.4)

*Odds ratios for access indicators were calculated from logistic regression analyses for children in homeless families compared with housed families, controlling for differences in race, child health status, child age, child sex, family medical insurance, maternal education, family size, family composition, and family income.

†For homeless families, n=180; for housed families, n=183.

‡For homeless families, n=180; for housed families, n=185.

§Respondents were restricted to families that reported a regular provider. For homeless families, n=147; for housed families, n=174.

‖Respondents were restricted to families that reported a regular provider. For homeless families, n=129; for housed families, n=175.

Table 6.—Logistic Regression Analyses of Access Barriers for Homeless and Housed Families

Access Indicator	Homeless vs Housed Odds Ratio (95% Confidence Limits)*
Barrier actually prevented child from obtaining care†	1.7 (1.0, 2.8)
Care was too expensive‡	1.8 (0.8, 3.9)
Had to wait too long for an appointment§	5.7 (1.9, 17.4)
Did not know where to go to seek care‖	2.1 (0.8, 5.1)
Had no transportation to the care provider¶	2.3 (1.2, 4.4)

*Odds ratios for access indicators were calculated from logistic regression analyses for children in homeless families compared with housed families, controlling for differences in race, child health status, child age, child sex, family medical insurance, maternal education, family size, family composition, and family income.

†For homeless families, n=194; for housed families, n=196.

‡For homeless families, n=193; for housed families, n=193.

§For homeless families, n=193; for housed families, n=193.

‖For homeless families, n=193; for housed families, n=193.

¶For homeless families, n= 193; for housed families, n=191.

a regular health provider for both preventive care and illness care. Moreover, homeless children were more likely to rely on emergency departments and other public providers for much of their care. Furthermore, while barriers to care were encountered with similar frequency in each group, barriers more frequently prevented homeless children from obtaining medical care.

Medicaid was the primary health insurance for both the housed and homeless families in our study. Few private health providers accept Medicaid patients, making it hard for homeless or poor families to find a provider.[22-25] Therefore, they become completely dependent on the public system of medical care.

During the last decade the number of medically indigent in Los Angeles has grown dramatically,[26] further increasing the burden on public hospitals and clinics. The overcrowding of public facilities has resulted in increased barriers and decreased quality of care for the poor and indigent (*Los Angeles Times*. June 20, 1990:B7).[27,28] This has an adverse impact on access to care for homeless families because they are less familiar with where services can be found, they are unable to travel long distances to care, and their living conditions are not stable enough for them to wait long periods of time for appointments.

Furthermore, for homeless children dependent on the overburdened system of public clinics and emergency departments for care, acute health problems may be adequately treated, but more serious health problems may go undiagnosed and untreated (*Los Angeles Times*. June 20, 1990:B7).[27-29] For example, a homeless child presenting to an emergency department with otitis media will most likely receive adequate treatment for the acute illness; however, the child may not undergo assessment for a history of otitis media or be evaluated for the presence of hearing loss or speech delay, which are common problems among homeless children.[10] Even when addressing acute health problems, the emergency department provider may fail to take into consideration the complex social setting of the homeless child and family. As a result, treatments may be inappropriate or ineffective (eg, for a child with otitis media, prescribing an antibiotic that requires refrigeration to a family living in a car without access to a refrigerator).[5,10,12]

Access to health care for homeless families is further impaired by their frequent loss of Medicaid coverage and long periods of being uninsured.[30] Both the homeless and housed families in our study described administrative problems, *not* loss of eligibility, as the primary reason they lost Medicaid coverage. Most of the disentitled homeless families in our study lost their mailing address when they became homeless. This in itself does not disqualify a family from receiving Medicaid or AFDC; in fact, the 1987 Omnibus Budget Reconciliation Act (OBRA) mandates states to develop procedures to assure continued Medicaid coverage for families without a permanent address.[31] However, families in the crisis of homelessness are unlikely to receive or return the monthly eligibility report required to maintain AFDC eligibility, and, therefore, both their AFDC and Medicaid benefits are discontinued.

The 1988 Omnibus Budget Reconciliation Act mandates that states continue to provide Medicaid coverage for families dropped from the AFDC program.[31] However, provisions such as these are rendered ineffective because of Medicaid's complex, time-consuming application and benefit maintenance procedures and problems of access to welfare facilities, such as transportation, long waiting times for appointments, long waits at the welfare offices, etc. Despite legislation broadening eligibility for Medicaid in the past several years, these barriers continue to prevent eligible poor families from obtaining Medicaid coverage or from regaining their benefits. Almost one third of all families in California lose Medicaid benefits each year without any change in their eligibility status.[32]

Nationally, the average family on Medicaid spends one fourth of the year uncovered.[33]

Half of the homeless families had been disqualified from AFDC and Medicaid over the previous year. The policy of rapid disqualification of potentially needy families is encouraged by federal law that imposes severe financial penalties on agencies if they are found to continue coverage to ineligible families. No penalties are imposed for the wrongful denial or termination of benefits to needy, eligible families, creating organizational pressure to prematurely disqualify families.[33] Once AFDC and Medicaid benefits are lost, a family must complete the complex task of reapplying for AFDC and Medicaid (the California application is 20 pages long!) and resubmit birth and financial documentation, much of which is frequently unavailable to homeless families. "Even for the . . . most capable persons, applying for Medicaid is a travail. For homeless families . . . the effort is simply overwhelming."[33]

Homeless families' access to medical care is further undermined by several issues that are associated with or caused by the condition of homelessness. First, homelessness uproots family members and separates them from their regular health care system, personal physician, and network of social supports.[6,7] The poor family's social support network often plays an important role in overcoming barriers to medical care, such as transportation, child care, and cost of care. For example, grandparents may pay for the child's health visit or care for the other children while the mother is at the physician's office.

Second, homeless families are struggling daily to provide housing, food, and protection for their children. The family energies are focused on getting through each day and meeting the most basic needs. Making an appointment for medical care for a child's health problem, even a serious health problem, may be delayed because it is not as urgent as the family's basic needs for food and shelter. This is consistent with our finding that homeless and housed families experienced barriers to care with similar frequency, but homeless families more frequently did not obtain care.

Third, homeless families are frequently dysfunctional and experience serious family problems, such as family violence, family separation, and alcohol or drug abuse.[6-8,34,35] Family dysfunction impairs the child's access to health services by decreasing the parents' ability to perceive and respond to the child's needs and by further limiting the family's ability to overcome common barriers to care. Ironically, these same factors increase the child's need for medical care by increasing the risk of serious medical, developmental, educational, and behavioral problems.[36]

POLICY IMPLICATIONS

The growing numbers of homeless families and their glaring unmet needs are a powerful indictment of our nation's "safety net."[37,38] The first step in meeting the health care needs of homeless families and children is to provide decent affordable housing. Unfortunately, even with substantial political will, it may take many years to create sufficient low-income, affordable housing to eliminate family homelessness. In the interim, the health care needs of homeless families should be addressed by increasing access to comprehensive medical care services through the elimination of barriers caused by financial and transportation problems and by a lack of knowledge. The health care system must remove these barriers rather than expect homeless families to overcome them.

These barriers can be removed through targeted programs for homeless families, such as special health care outreach projects. Special outreach projects around the country have been funded under the federal McKinney Act to provide health and social service to the homeless.[39] Transportation barriers have been overcome in some communities through outreach clinics that go to homeless shelters, welfare hotels, soup kitchens, and parks. Medical services and prescriptions are provided without charge, removing financial barriers. Furthermore, the McKinney Health Projects actively reach out to families and educate them about the availability of health and social services, removing knowledge barriers. The projects seek to stabilize families and increase medical compliance through family-centered case management that offers social support; referrals for food, clothing, and housing; and crisis intervention and other mental health services.

These special projects, however, cannot begin to meet the demand for services, as the number of homeless families continues to increase rapidly.[37,38] Moreover, outreach programs to special at-risk populations such as homeless children are most successfully implemented only in the context of a health system that is functional and accessible for all poor families. Recently, Congress has addressed disparities in access to care for poor children by expanding eligibility for Medicaid and decreasing the categorical linkage with AFDC.[40] However, despite expansion of Medicaid eligibility, there are almost 4 million uninsured children living in poverty who are not eligible and many who are eligible but not enrolled in Medicaid.[41]

At the federal level, Medicaid eligibility should be expanded further by completely eliminating the categorical linkage with AFDC and by raising family income eligibility levels and requiring states to adopt federal eligibility levels for local programs. For the unwieldy Medicaid program to be effective for poor and homeless families and children, reforms must go further.

1. The complex application and documentation requirements should be simplified substantially.
2. Presumptive eligibility, as in the present law for eligible pregnant women, should be instituted for families. This would eliminate long periods of uninsurance when Medicaid coverage is temporarily lost.
3. Outreach personnel and Medicaid eligibility workers should be placed outside welfare institutions at Women, Infants, and Children (WIC) sites; Head Start sites; public health clinics; and private hospitals and clinics. These outreach personnel could educate families eligible for the Medicaid program and assist them with enrollment and benefit maintenance.
4. Federal law and federal-state financial incentives should be changed to promote enrollment of eligible families and prevent unwarranted terminations, rather than the contrary.

Even if all poor and homeless families are enrolled in Medicaid through expanded eligibility and outreach efforts, they will not be assured of access to high-quality health care unless the number of providers participating in the Medicaid program is dramatically increased.[42] To induce providers such as pediatricians to participate in Medicaid, the following reforms should occur: (1) Raise reimbursement rates to adequate levels (the American Academy of Pediatrics[42] recommends 90% of the usual, customary, and reasonable fees for a given geographic area). (2) Eliminate bureaucratic complexities experienced by providers (eg, simplify billing procedures, make payments within shorter time periods). (3) Eligibility for families should be granted for longer time periods to prevent frequent loss of coverage and discontinuity of insurance.[41-45]

References

1. Burt MR, Cohen BE. Who is helping the homeless? local, state, federal responses. *J Federalism*. 1989;19:111-128.
2. Steinhardt B, Uslan B, Wellhouse D, Williams P. *The Tattered Safety Net: A Look at the General Assistance Programs in California's Counties*. Sacramento, Calif: Assembly Office of Research; 1985.
3. *Barriers to Participation in Benefit Programs: A 38-City Survey*. Washington, DC: US Conference of Mayors; 1988.
4. Wright JD, Weber E. Determinants of benefit-program participation among the urban homeless. *Eval Rev*. 1988; 12:376-393.
5. Alperstein G, Arnstein E. Homeless children: a challenge for pediatricians. *Pediatr Clin North Am*. 1988;35:1413-1426.
6. Bassuk EL, Rubin AL. Characteristics of sheltered homeless families. *Am J Public Health*. 1986;76:1097-1101.
7. Wood D, Hayashi T, Schlossman S, Valdez RB. *Over the Brink: Homeless Families in Los Angeles*. Sacramento, Calif: Assembly Office of Research; 1989.
8. Wood D, Valdez RB, Hayashi T, Shen A. A comparison study of homeless and housed families and their demographic, economic and family function characteristics. *Am J Public Health*. 1990;80:1049-1052.
9. Miller DS, Lin EHB. Children in sheltered homeless families: reported health status and use of health services. *Pediatrics*. 1988;81:668-673.
10. Wood D, Valdez R, Hayashi T, Shen A. A study comparing the health of homeless children and other poor children. *Pediatrics*. 1990;86:858-866.
11. Alperstein G, Rappaport C, Flanigan J. Health problems of homeless children in New York City. *Am J Public Health*. 1988;78:1232.
12. Bass JL, Brennan P, Mehta KA, Kodzis S. Pediatric problems in a suburban shelter for homeless families. *Pediatrics*. 1990;85:33-38.
13. Acker P, Fierman A, Dreyer B. Health: an assessment of parameters of health-care and nutrition in homeless children. *AJDC*. 1987;141:388. Abstract.
14. Bassuk E, Rosenberg L. Psychosocial characteristics of homeless children and children with homes. *Pediatrics*. 1990; 85:257-261.
15. Rafferty Y, Rollins N. *Learning in Limbo: The Education Deprivation of Homeless Children*. New York, NY: Advocates for Children of New York; 1989.
16. Gewirtzman R, Fodor I. The homeless child at school: from welfare hotel to classroom. *Child Welfare*. 1987;66:237-245.
17. Fine J, Foltin G, Tunik M, Fierman A, Dreyer B. Ambulance utilization by homeless children. *AJDC*. 1990;144:433.
18. *Over the Edge: Homeless Families and the Welfare System*. New York, NY:National Coalition for the Homeless; 1988.
19. *A Children's Defense Budget: FY 1990*. Washington, DC: Children's Defense Fund; 1990.
20. *The Plan and Operation of the Hispanic Health and Nutrition Examination Survey, 1982-1984: Programs and Collections Procedures*. Washington, DC: National Center for Health Statistics; 1985. Vital and Health Statistics, ser 1, No. 19.
21. Newacheck P, Halfon N. Access to ambulatory care services for economically disadvantaged children. *Pediatrics*. 1986;78:813-819.
22. Rosenbach M. The impact of Medicaid on physician use by low-income children. *Am J Public Health*. 1989;79:1220-1224.
23. Perloff J, Kletke P, Neckerman K. Recent trends in pediatrician participation in Medicaid. *Med Care*. 1986;24:749-760.
24. Davidson S, Perloff J, Kletke P, Schiff D, Connelly J. Full and limited Medicaid participation among pediatricians. *Pediatrics*. 1983;72:552-559.
25. Yudkowsky B, Cartland J, Flint S. Pediatrician participation in Medicaid: 1978-1989. *Pediatrics*. 1990;85:567-577.
26. Brown ER, Valdez RB, Morgenstern H, Nourjah P, Hafner C. *Changes in Health Insurance Coverage of Californians, 1979-1986*. Sacramento, Calif: California Policy Seminar; 1988.
27. Dallek G, Brown ER. *The Quality of Medical Care for the Poor in Los Angeles County's Health and Hospital System*. Los Angeles, Calif: Legal Aid Foundation of Los Angeles; 1987.
28. Valdez RB, Dallek G. *Variations in Preventable Hospitalizations in Los Angeles County*. Claremont, Calif: Tomás Rivera Center. In press.
29. Lion M, Altman S. Case-mix differences between hospital OPDs and private practice. *Health Care Financ Rev*. 1982; 4:89.
30. Wood D, Hayward R, Freeman H, Covey C, Shapiro M. Access to medical care for children in the United States. *Pediatrics*. 1990;86:666-673.
31. Family Support Act, 1988. Pub L No. 100-485, 102 Stat 2343 *et seq*.
32. *Quarterly Public Assistance Statistics: FY 1986*. Washington, DC: Family Support Administration, Office of Family Assistance; 1986.
33. Rosenbaum S. *Opening Doors to Benefit Programs: A Medicaid Resource Guide for Health Programs Serving the Homeless*. Washington, DC: National Association of Community Health Centers; 1990.
34. *Homeless Families: A Neglected Crisis*. Washington DC: US Government Printing Office; 1986. Report of the Committee on Government Relations to Congress.
35. Kozol J. *Rachel and Her Children: Homeless Families in America*. New York, NY: Crown Books; 1988.
36. Parker S, Greer S, Zuckerman B. Double jeopardy: the impact of poverty on early child development. *Pediatr Clin North Am*. 1988;35:1227-1240.
37. *The Status Report on Hunger and Homelessness in America's Cities: 1988, a 27-City Survey*. Washington, DC: US Conference of Mayors; 1989.
38. *Homelessness, Health and Human Needs*. Washington, DC: Institute of Medicine, National Academy Press; 1988.
39. Brickner PW, Scharer LK, Conanan BA, Savarese M, Scanlan BC, eds. *Under the Safety Net: The Health and Social Welfare of the Homeless in the United States*. New York, NY: WW Norton & Co Inc; 1990.
40. Waxman H. Kids and Medicaid: progress but continuing problems. *Am J Public Health*. 1989;79:1217-1218.
41. Rimkunas R. Medicaid and the poor. In: *Medicaid Source Book: Background Data and Analysis*. Washington, DC: Congressional Research Service. 1988:281-290. Energy and Commerce Committee print 100-AA.
42. Kutnik LA. *Testimony Before Physician Payment Review Commission on Physician Payment Reform, December 5, 1990*. Washington, DC: Department of Government Liaison, American Academy of Pediatrics; 1990.
43. *Health Policy Agenda for the American People: The Final Report of the Ad Hoc Committee on Medicaid*. Chicago, Ill: American Medical Association; 1989.
44. Rosenbaum S. Providing health for low-income children: reconciling child health goals with child health financing realities. *Milbank Mem Fund Q*. 1986;64:442-478.
45. Moscovice I, Davidson G. Health care and insurance loss of working AFDC recipients. *Med Care*. 1987;25:413-425.

Adolescents' Attrition From School-Sponsored Sports

Robert H. DuRant, PhD; Robert A. Pendergrast, MD, MPH; Josh Donner, MD, MPH; Carolyn Seymore, MD; Gregory Gaillard

• This study investigated reasons for adolescents' attrition from school-sponsored sports teams and the relationship between attrition and intention to participate in organized and nonorganized sports in the future. Of 674 high school student athletes, 26% dropped off at least one team in 1989-1990, and overall attrition increased to 29.8% when attrition from more than one sport was considered. Attrition was higher among black students, students reporting an athletic injury, those injured playing football, and those sustaining a knee injury. Injury was cited as the most frequent reason for attrition, followed by being cut from the team, "other reasons," needing to get a job, inconvenient game or practice schedule, and needing more time to study, although the main reason for attrition also varied by sport. When athletes were classified according to externally precipitated attrition, athlete-initiated attrition, or completion of the sports season, no differences were noted in the three groups' intent to engage in organized sports in the future. However, the group with externally precipitated attrition expressed a stronger intent to engage in nonorganized sports in the future than the other two groups.

(*AJDC.* 1991;145:1119-1123)

A substantial number of adolescents living in western industrialized nations participate in organized athletic programs. In the United States alone, 17 million children and adolescents between the ages of 6 and 16 years participate in a multitude of non–school-sponsored sports programs,[1] while 6 to 7 million high school students are estimated to be involved in interscholastic athletics.[2] Participation in athletics provides structure for engaging in regular physical activity, helping adolescents to develop life-style patterns that often continue into adulthood.[3-6]

Although a large number of children and adolescents participate in organized sports and other forms of physical activity, the high rate of attrition from youth sports programs has become an area of concern. Descriptive studies report that between one fourth and half of the youths involved in organized sports discontinue participation each year.[7] The State of Michigan's Youth Sports Institute found an attrition rate of 35% among 11- to 18-year-old adolescents.[8] Studies of Canadian children and adolescents have reported levels of attrition of 22% among soccer players,[9] 35% among swimmers,[10] and 29% to 37% among hockey players.[11]

Little is known about the reasons for adolescents' attrition from sports.[7] The most consistently cited motives for withdrawal from sports are interests in other sports and activities, a lack of playing time, overemphasis on competition, boredom, competitive stress, dislike of the coach, or lack of fun.[8,9,12-14] Although these studies indicate that youth sports attrition is a complex phenomenon influenced by a variety of personal and situational variables,[15] several important questions remain.[7] For example, do adolescents who drop out of sports become reinvolved in other scholastic sports, do they participate in nonscholastic organized sports, do they initiate participation in nonorganized sports, or do they discontinue all physical activity?

Most of the research on sports attrition has focused on athlete-initiated attrition from sports and has not addressed withdrawal due to external factors or its effect on future sports involvement and/or participation in regular physical activity.[7] For example, the experience of being cut from a team, no longer being able to afford the financial costs of participating in a sport, or suffering a temporarily disabling injury may be so devastating for some adolescents that they may permanently discontinue athletic participation.[16]

This study investigated factors associated with attrition

Accepted for publication March 18, 1991.

From the Section of General Pediatrics and Adolescent Medicine, Department of Pediatrics, Medical College of Georgia, Augusta.

Presented at the Southern Society for Pediatric Research Meeting, New Orleans, La, January 30, 1991; and before the Society for Pediatric Research, New Orleans, April 30, 1991.

Reprint requests to Section of General Pediatrics and Adolescent Medicine, Department of Pediatrics, CE-112, Medical College of Georgia, Augusta, GA 30912-3770 (Dr DuRant).

Table 1.—Percent of Students Who Discontinued Participation in School-Sponsored Sports

Sport	No. Who Started Season	No. (%) Who Discontinued Participation
Basketball	228	59 (25.9)
Baseball	108	22 (20.4)
Football	300	61 (20.3)
Track and field	160	31 (19.4)
Softball	99	13 (13.1)
Soccer	58	7 (12.1)
Tennis	46	5 (10.9)
Golf	30	3 (10.0)
Cheerleading	15	0 (0.0)
Rifle	1	0 (0.0)
Total	**1045***	**201** (19.2)

*Total sample size is 674. Many students participated in more than one sport; 26% quit at least one sport.

in high school–sponsored sports teams and the relationships between the reasons for attrition and intention to participate in both organized and nonorganized sports in the future.

SUBJECTS AND METHODS

Survey Design

All public high school students in grades 9 to 12 in Richmond County, Georgia, who plan to participate in interscholastic sports are required to receive a preparticipation athletic examination (PAE) at the beginning of the sports season. A standardized PAE form, which includes parental consent, biographical data, home address and telephone number, medical and health history, and physical examination sections, was used for all athletes.[2,17,18] This PAE form has been recommended by the American Academy of Pediatrics' Committee on Practice and Ambulatory Medicine.[19] The target sample consisted of all (N = 1204) adolescents who received a PAE during the 1989-1990 academic year.

Letters were sent to the parents of all athletes explaining the purpose of the study. Using the telephone numbers provided by the students on the PAE forms, we attempted to contact all students who participated in interscholastic athletics during the academic year. If a parent or guardian answered the telephone, we asked permission to conduct a short interview with his or her child concerning participation in sports. If the parent agreed, then the adolescent was asked the same question. If the adolescent answered the telephone, permission was first obtained from the adolescent and then from the parent. All telephone contacts were made between 5 and 9 PM, when we thought that both the adolescent and his or her parent would most likely to be at home, and were conducted during April and May 1990. Only 242 adolescents were at home during the period that the telephone interviews were conducted. No parents or adolescents refused to be interviewed. In May 1990, all adolescents (n = 962) not interviewed by telephone were mailed an identical questionnaire with a stamped, self-addressed return envelope. Four hundred thirty-two adolescents returned the questionnaire, resulting in 674 (56.0%) completing either the mailed questionnaire or the telephone interview.

Subjects

The subjects ranged in age from 13 to 20 years (mean ± SD, 16.1 ± 1.2 years). The sample consisted of 470 (69.7%) males, 408 (60.5%) blacks, 243 (36.1%) whites, and 23 (3.4%) other race, and was slightly skewed toward the 9th grade (36.6%), with fewer

Table 2.—All Reasons and Main Reason for Discontinuing Participation in School-Sponsored Sport Before End of Season

Reasons for Not Completing Sports Season	All Reasons, No. (%)*	Main Reason, No. (%)*
Injury that required student to stop playing	44 (25.1)	37 (21.1)
Quit to get job	22 (12.6)	14 (8.0)
Cut from team for other reasons	20 (11.4)	15 (8.6)
Inconvenient game or practice schedule	20 (11.4)	10 (5.7)
Needed more time to study	17 (9.7)	15 (8.6)
Cut from team because of bad grades	14 (8.0)	13 (7.4)
Not enough playing time	14 (8.0)	6 (3.4)
Student felt that he/she did not have adequate skill to play sport	13 (7.4)	6 (3.4)
Did not like teammates	9 (5.1)	6 (3.4)
Not enough free time	9 (5.1)	4 (2.3)
Disliked coach	9 (5.1)	2 (1.1)
Quit to play in another school-sponsored sport	7 (4.0)	6 (3.4)
Felt that it was boring or no fun	6 (3.4)	2 (1.1)
Felt too much emphasis was placed on competition and winning	4 (2.3)	1 (0.6)
Sport was too expensive to play	0 (0.0)	0 (0.0)
Quit to participate in other non–school-sponsored athletic program	3 (1.7)	0 (0.0)
Reasons other than specified above	26 (14.9)	24 (13.7)
Did not specify 1 main reason	...	14 (8.0)

*Based on 175 athletes who responded to both questions; percent represents the proportion of sports dropouts who cited this particular reason.

12th graders (14.5%). The demographic data of the sample of 674 did not differ from that of the 530 adolescents receiving PAEs who were not interviewed.

Questionnaire

The questionnaire consisted of items that had been found to be associated with sports attrition in previous studies. The questionnaire was first pretested on a small group of male and female adolescents, and revisions were made in the wording of ambiguous items. The questionnaire obtained information about demographic variables, the sport for which the initial PAE was conducted (Table 1), attrition from any sport and the reasons for attrition (see Table 2 for specific choices), attrition from a sport to participate in another school-sponsored sport, level of participation (3 d/wk, 20 min/d) in any of 17 different nonscholastic sports or nonorganized physical activities during the previous 4 weeks, sustaining an injury that required a physician visit and/or caused the adolescent to miss one or more games, sport in which injury was sustained, area of body injured, and level of intent to participate in organized and nonorganized athletic activity in the future. These last two questions were measured on five-point scales ranging from "not at all likely" to "absolutely likely."

Table 3.—Factors Associated With Attrition From School-Sponsored Sports

	Started Sports Season, No.	Completed Sports Season, No. (%)	Discontinued Participation, No. (%)	P
Injured playing sport	300	210 (70.0)	90 (30.0)	.032
No injury	374	289 (77.3)	85 (22.7)	
Injured playing football	109	67 (61.5)	42 (38.5)	.0011
No football injury	565	432 (76.5)	133 (23.5)	
Received knee injury	61	36 (59.0)	25 (41.0)	.005
No knee injury	613	463 (75.5)	150 (24.5)	
Race				
W	243	200 (82.3)	43 (17.7)	.0001
B	408	277 (67.9)	131 (32.1)	
Other	23	22 (95.7)	1 (4.3)	

Statistical Analysis

Categorical data are presented as frequency and percent. Interval level data are presented as mean±SD. Because of the large sample size and the uniform or normal distributions of the items measured on ordinal scales, these items are presented as mean±SD to simplify summation and interpretation of the data. Data were analyzed with χ^2, analysis of variance (ANOVA), Kruskall-Wallis ANOVA, and Kendall's τ.

RESULTS

Because 310 of the athletes participated in between two and five sports, 674 adolescents accounted for 1045 sports participants. Overall, 19.2% of the 1045 participants discontinued participation on sports teams. Twenty-six percent of the 674 adolescents withdrew from at least one sports team. Since 22 (12.6%) of these adolescents withdrew from more than one team, the overall attrition of the 674 was 29.8% (Table 1). Attrition from school-sponsored sports varied from 0% for cheerleading and rifle team to 25.9% for basketball (Table 1). Lower levels of attrition were also found in golf (10.0%), tennis (10.9%), soccer (12.1%), and softball (13.1%).

The proportion of athletes discontinuing participation on a sports team was significantly higher among black students, students reporting an athletic injury during the season, those injured playing football, and those sustaining a knee injury (Table 3). The mean number of injuries sustained by adolescents who stopped participating in sports was significantly higher than the mean number of injuries among those who completed the sports season (Table 4). When racial differences in attrition were examined by sport, blacks had significantly higher attrition than whites and adolescents of other races in basketball (28.2%, $P\leq.001$), soccer (26.1%, $P\leq.001$), track and field (23%, $P\leq.001$), and golf (22.2%, $P\leq.001$). There were no racial differences in any other sport and no gender differences in any of the sports in which both male and female adolescents participated.

The adolescents who withdrew from a sports team were asked to list all the reasons why they stopped participating. The athletes could choose one or more reasons for attrition from 17 possible reasons. Injury was cited most frequently (25.1%), followed by being cut from the team for academic or other reasons (19.4%), "other unspecified reasons" (14.9%), the need to get a job (12.6%), inconvenient game or practice schedule (11.4%), and the need for more time to study (9.7%; Table 2). When asked to cite the primary reason for attrition, the six reasons cited above continued to be listed most frequently. Reasons for attrition did not vary by race or gender. Also, there was not a clustering of specific reasons within different schools.

Table 4.—Factors Associated With Attrition From School-Sponsored Sports

	Completed Sports Season, Mean±SD	Discontinued Participation, Mean±SD	P
No. of injuries	0.31±0.61	0.42±0.61	.021*
Likelihood to participate in future organized sports	4.56±0.96	4.36±1.19	.032†

*Kruskal-Wallis analysis of variance.
†Analysis of variance.

The adolescents' reasons for attrition varied by sport. Injuries were cited by 50.8% of football, 18.2% of baseball, and 16.2% of track and field dropouts. Being cut from the team for either academic or other reasons was a major cause of attrition in basketball (39.0%) and baseball (22.7%). Inconvenient practice or game schedule was cited by 40.0% of tennis, 30.8% of softball, and 19.8% of track and field dropouts. Other reasons for attrition included lack of free time (softball, 38.5%), more time for study (soccer, 42.9%), and employment (baseball, 18.2%).

Adolescents who discontinued participation on a sports team were less likely to indicate they would participate in organized sports in the future (Table 4). However, no differences were noted between the attrition and nonattrition groups in the percentage who indicated that they would participate in a nonorganized athletic activity during the next year. Among adolescents who dropped off a team, lower intent to engage in organized sports in the future was associated with being black ($P\leq.04$); being female ($P\leq.011$); being older ($P\leq.012$); and citing as the reason for attrition lack of playing time in the discontinued sport ($P\leq.012$), lack of skill ($P\leq.002$), or lack of free time ($P<.04$).

When subjects were classified by externally precipitated attrition (cut from the team or injury), athlete-initiated attrition, or nonattrition (completion of the sports season), there were no longer any significant differences in their level of intent to engage in school-sponsored sports in the future (tested with both ANOVA and Kruskall-Wallis ANOVA). However, subjects in the externally controlled attrition group were significantly ($P \leq .0097$) more likely to indicate that they intended to engage in nonorganized athletic activity during the next year, followed in order by subjects in the nonattrition group and the athlete-initiated attrition group.

COMMENT

Our finding that 26% of the 674 athletes dropped off at least one sports team was lower than the 35% reported in the study of Michigan adolescents by Sapp and Haubenstricker.[8] The primary reason for this difference is that Sapp and Haubenstricker measured attrition as athletes' intention not to engage in the same sport during the next sports season, while we measured attrition during the current sports season. Another reason for this difference may be sampling error resulting from the possibility that students who quit a sports team were less inclined to return the mailed questionnaire. However, the level of attrition did not differ among athletes interviewed by telephone and those returning the mailed questionnaire. Consequently, we do not suspect that adolescents who quit a sports team were less likely to return our mailed questionnaire. A more likely explanation is that attrition rates vary by geographic location owing to differences in weather, size of town or city, level of organization of the school system's athletic program, etc.

Of the athletes in the Michigan study who indicated that they would not participate in the same sport during the next season, 64% said that their major motive for dropping out was involvement in other activities, 44% that it was work, and 34% that it was disinterest.[8] Fewer than 15% of the athletes rated lack of participation, dislike of the coach, injury, expense, and dislike of teammates as important. In comparison, we found that injury (25.1%), being cut from the team (19.4%), employment (12.6%), inconvenient game or practice schedule (11.4%), and needing time for study (9.7%) were the most frequently listed reasons for attrition. Other previously cited reasons accounted for little attrition.[8]

Few studies have examined reasons for attrition within specific sports. Robinson and Carron[15] studied a small sample of high school football players who were classified as dropouts (n=26), starters (n=33), or nonstarters (n=39). They found that dropouts felt less a part of the team, enjoyed participation less, felt they had less support from their fathers for participation, often attributed their poor performance to ability, and often viewed the coach as an autocrat. Among the football players in our study who dropped off their teams, only two (3.3%) indicated they lacked the skill to play football, one (1.6%) disliked the coach, one (1.6%) disliked his teammates, and none felt football was boring or not fun. Injury, needing to get a job, and needing time to study were the major reasons for football attrition. The levels of emphasis that communities, schools, and families place on specific sports differ geographically and could account for the differences in the reasons for attrition in sports such as football. We are aware of no studies examining specific reasons for attrition in basketball, baseball, soccer, softball, track and field, tennis, and golf.

Several investigators have hypothesized that many athletes quit sports teams to participate in other athletic activity. They argue that switching from sport to sport is a normal trial-and-error sampling process to determine what activities are enjoyed the most or performed best.[7,20] While this may be true for younger children, our data do not support this hypothesis among adolescents. Only seven (4.0%) of the athletes who dropped off a team indicated that they withdrew to play another school-sponsored sport. Also, athletes who discontinued participation were less likely to indicate that they would participate in organized sports in the future. Among adolescents who dropped off a team, blacks, girls, and older athletes were less likely to indicate that they intended to participate in organized athletics in the future. This may be due either to motivational factors or to the perception by these groups of athletes that there are fewer opportunities to participate in organized athletics once they have quit the sport they initially started playing. Among older athletes this may be due to the perception that there are fewer opportunities to participate competitively in varsity athletics during the latter years of high school, and even less opportunity to participate in organized athletics once high school has been completed. Although the number of scholastic sports offered for girls is close to the number available to boys, female athletes who discontinue participation in one sport may also believe that there are fewer opportunities to participate competitively in another sport. This explanation would not apply to the black students, who have the same opportunity to participate in all the school-sponsored sports as students from other racial and ethnic groups.

Unfortunately, most of the existing research has focused on adolescent-initiated withdrawal from sports. It has been hypothesized that having to withdraw unwillingly from a team because of injury, being cut from the team for academic reasons or lack of skill, or not being able to afford the financial costs of a sport may have a negative influence on an adolescent's willingness to participate in sports in the future.[7,16] Our data did not support this hypothesis. None of the athletes dropped out of sports for financial reasons. There were no differences in intent to engage in future organized sports among adolescents who quit owing to injury or being cut from the team, those whose attrition was self-initiated, and those who did not quit a sport. In fact, adolescents experiencing externally precipitated attrition were significantly more likely to indicate that they would engage in nonorganized athletic activity in the future. In comparison, adolescents whose attrition was self-initiated expressed the lowest intent to engage in nonorganized athletic activity in the future.

We found that approximately one fourth of the high school athletes participating in sports in our school system withdrew from at least one sports team during the school year. This is less than the average of 35% that has been reported previously.[7] We also found that the reasons our athletes dropped off teams were quite different than the reasons cited in previous, smaller descriptive studies.[7-9,12-14] Since 25% of the athletes who quit a team cited injury as a precipitating factor, aggressive preventive measures are needed if we wish to stop this interruption in the regular physical activity of adolescent athletes. Since many pediatricians and family physicians are currently involved in both conducting PAEs and serving as high school team physicians, they can be involved in designing and implementing athletic injury prevention programs. Also of concern is that many of these athletes were cut from sports teams for academic reasons, and others voluntarily withdrew because they needed more time to study. These athletes in academic difficulty represent a unique group of students who may be more receptive to extra remedial work and tutorial help if it means that they could resume sports participation. If appropriate educational intervention programs were instituted, both increases in academic achievement and continued structured physical activity for these students could occur. If not dealt with adequately, these students may continue to perform poorly in school and also be excluded from school-sponsored programs that may help them develop life-styles that include regular physical activity.

We thank Wayne Wiggins with the Richmond County Board of Education for his help on this project.

References

1. Marlens R. Youth sports in the USA. In: Weiss MR, Gould D, eds. *Sport for Children and Youths.* Champaign, Ill: Human Kinetics; 1986:27-33.
2. DuRant RH. The preparticipation examination of athletes. *AJDC.* 1985;139:657-661.
3. Dennison BA, Straos JH, Mellits ED, Charney E. Childhood physical fitness tests: predictors of adult physical activity levels? *Pediatrics.* 1988;82:324-330.
4. Skinner A. Time out: criticism not withstanding school sports still are the best game in town. *Am School Board J.* July 1988:22-23.
5. Vaughn LK. Psychological impact of organized sports on children. In: Micheli LJ, ed. *Pediatrics and Adolescent Sports Medicine.* Boston, Mass: Little Brown & Co Inc; 1988:144-166.
6. Roberts GC, Klebe DA, Doda JL. An analysis of motivation in children's sport: the role of perceived competency in participation. *J Sport Psychol.* 1981;3:206-216.
7. Gould D. Understanding attrition in children's sport. In: Gould D, Weiss MR, eds. *Advances in Pediatric Sport Series.* Champaign, Ill: Human Kinetics; 1987:61-84.
8. Sapp M, Haubenstricker J. Motivation for joining and reasons for not continuing in youth sport programs in Michigan. Presented at the Meeting of the American Alliance for Health, Physical Education, Recreation, and Dance; 1978; Kansas City, Mo.
9. Pooley JC. Drop-outs from sport: a case study for boys: age group soccer. Presented at the Meeting of the American Alliance for Health, Physical Education, Recreation, and Dance; 1981; Boston, Mass.
10. Seftan JM, Fry DA. *A Report on Participation in Competitive Swimming.* Saskatoon, Saskatchewan: Canadian Amateur Swimming Association; 1981.
11. Fry DA, McClements JD, Seftan JM. *A Report on Participation in the Saskatoon Hockey Association.* Saskatoon, Saskatchewan: SASK Sport; 1981.
12. Feigley DA. Psychological burnout in high-level athletes. *Physician Sports Med.* 1984;12:108-119.
13. Orlick TD. Children's sport: a revolution is coming. *Can Assoc Health Phys Educ Recr J.* January/February 1978:12-14.
14. Orlick TD, Botteril C. *Every Kid Can Win.* Chicago, Ill: Nelson-Hall Publishers; 1975.
15. Robinson T, Carron A. Personal and situational factors associated with dropping out versus maintaining participation in competitive sport. *J Sport Psychol.* 1982;4:364-378.
16. Ogilvie BC, Howe MA. Career crisis in sport. In: Orlick T, Partington JT, Salmela JH, eds. *Mental Training for Coaches and Athletes.* Ottawa, Ontario: Coaching Association of Canada; 1982:176-183.
17. Linder CW, DuRant RH, Strong WB, Secklecki RO. Preparticipation health screening of young athletes: results of 1268 examinations. *Am J Sports Med.* 1981;9:187-191.
18. DuRant RH, Linder CW, Sanders JM, Jay S, Brantley G, Bedgood R. Adolescent females' readiness to participate in sports: sex and race differences in the preparticipation athletic examination. *J Adolesc Health Care.* 1988;9:310-314.
19. Saltzman EL, Shea DW, eds. *Management of Pediatric Practice.* Elk Grove Village, Ill: American Academy of Pediatrics; 1986:59-60.
20. Burton D, Martens R. Penned by their goals: an exploratory investigation into why kids drop out of wrestling. *J Sports Psychol.* 1986;8:183-197.

Sun Protection in Newborns

A Comparison of Educational Methods

Jean L. Bolognia, MD; Marianne Berwick, PhD; Judith A. Fine; Pamela Simpson, MPH; Marjorie Jasmin, RN

• We investigated the effect of education on the sun exposure of newborns. Mothers of healthy newborns (n = 275) were enrolled in the spring of 1989 and interviewed by telephone in the fall of 1989. The mothers were divided into a control group, a low-level intervention group, and a high-level intervention group. Both the low-level and high-level interventions succeeded in reducing the amount of time the newborns were allowed to spend in direct sunlight. Both types of intervention also resulted in reduced sun exposure time for the mothers. Although the number of mothers who used sunscreen was approximately the same in all three groups, when sunscreen use was controlled for, the intervention groups spent significantly less unprotected time in the sun than the control group. The mothers and newborns in both intervention groups simply spent less time outdoors.

(*AJDC.* 1991;145:1125-1129)

An association between the amount of exposure to UV light and the development of cutaneous malignancies, such as basal cell carcinomas and squamous cell carcinomas, is relatively clear.[1,2] In the case of cutaneous melanoma, there is likely to be an interplay of several factors, including history of sunburns during childhood, number of nevocellular nevi, and number of family members with a history of melanoma.[3-5] Stern et al[6] have estimated that up to 80% of an individual's cumulative sun exposure occurs before age 18 years, and if youngsters were to routinely use a sunscreen with a sun protection factor (SPF) of 15, approximately 78% of cases of nonmelanoma skin cancer could be prevented.[6] While this estimate has not been empirically demonstrated, it does emphasize the importance of this period for cumulative exposure to sunlight. Therefore, it is imperative that educational programs that emphasize using sunscreen and limiting sun exposure target children and their parents.

Several groups have begun to establish sun awareness programs, but more work is obviously needed given the evidence that behavior and attitudes toward sun exposure are changing slowly.[7] The American Academies of Pediatrics and Dermatology as well as the Skin Cancer Foundation have produced pamphlets, such as "For Every Child Under the Sun," that are geared toward establishing sensible sun exposure habits in children. In Queensland, Australia, where the highest incidence of melanoma in the world is found (39/100 000 females and 47/100 000 males), children are taught about skin cancer in school, and educational pamphlets are provided in medical and public settings.[8] The media, including national television, radio, and billboards, have also been employed; even the libraries hand out bookmarks with educational messages.

In Arizona, a "sun intensity index" is reported daily on television weather reports, and educational programs on sunscreen use are aimed at children and newcomers to the area.[9] More recently, the American Academy of Dermatology in cooperation with the American Cancer Society developed and distributed a sun protection curriculum for children in kindergarten through third grade. The program is simple and teaches the "ABCs for fun in the sun." The "A" is "stay Away from midday sun"; "B," "Block with a sunscreen of at least SPF 15"; "C," "Cover up with a hat and shirt"; and "S," "Speak out." For example, avoiding midday sun is taught by advising children not to play outdoors when their shadow is shorter than they are.

Accepted for publication January 15, 1991.

From the Departments of Dermatology (Drs Bolognia and Berwick) and Epidemiology and Public Health (Dr Berwick and Ms Simpson), and the Cancer Prevention Research Unit for Connecticut at Yale (Mss Fine and Jasmin), Yale University School of Medicine, New Haven, Conn.

Reprint requests to the Department of Dermatology, Yale University School of Medicine, 333 Cedar St, New Haven, CT 06510 (Dr Bolognia).

Purpose.—*This department is intended to share information concerning educational efforts in the broad field of pediatrics. We welcome studies on the following topics: undergraduate and graduate education in medicine and allied health occupations; continuing education of health professionals; education of patients and families; and health education for the general public, the community, and organizations that contribute to the promotion and improvement of the health of children.*

Editorial Comment.—*Sun exposure is one area where preventive pediatric care is important. This study shows where early educational intervention was useful. This could easily be a template for any preventive program.—H.D.A.*

Keep Your Baby's Skin Healthy

1. Prevent sunburns in your children. Begin using sunscreens at age 6 months and allow sun exposure with moderation. Before the age of 6 months, use bonnets and sun umbrellas or put your baby in the shade when outdoors for a long time.

2. Teach children sun protection early. Sun damage adds up over the years and the majority of sun exposure occurs by age 20 years.

3. Decrease sun exposure during the hours of 11 AM to 3 PM when the sun is the strongest. Try to plan outdoor activities for the early morning or the late afternoon.

4. Both children and adults should put on a sunscreen before sun exposure, and again at least every 2 hours, as long as you stay in the sun. The sunscreen should be applied again after swimming or perspiring heavily. We recommend that you use a sunscreen with an SPF (sun protection factor) 15.

5. Don't forget to use your sunscreen on cloudy days. The sun's rays can be as strong on cloudy, hazy days as they are on sunny days.

6. If you have a reaction to your sunscreen, change sunscreens. One of the many products on the market today should be right for you.

7. Beware of the things that reflect! Sand, snow, concrete, and water can reflect as much as half the sun's rays onto your skin.

8. Avoid tanning parlors.

Sponsored by the Yale-New Haven Hospital Auxiliary and the Yale Comprehensive Cancer Center

Fig 1.—*Sheet of simple guidelines distributed to experimental groups (adapted from original by A. Kopf, MD, Skin Cancer Foundation).*

To establish behavioral patterns at an early age, our goal was to target parents of newborns at a time when they are apt to be open to suggestions. Mothers were chosen because of evidence supporting their role as primary determiners of children's health practices.[10] In addition, two interventions, one low level and one high level, were compared to determine if a simple, less expensive method would be as effective as a more costly and complex method.

MATERIALS AND METHODS

The participants in this study were mothers of infants born at Yale–New Haven (Conn) Hospital between March and June 1989. They were eligible if their infants were born full term, apparently healthy, and weighed at least 2.27 kg. Permission to participate in the study was obtained verbally and information regarding race, date of birth, and gender was recorded at the time of enrollment. Blacks and Hispanics were limited to 10% of the sample population due to their significantly lower risk of sunburn and skin cancer.[11,12] Prior to the start of enrollment, attending pediatricians at the hospital were sent a letter informing them of the study and requesting that they not alter their routine advice on sun exposure.

The mothers were assigned to one of three groups to evaluate the influence of education on their behavior: a control group, a low-level intervention group, and a high-level intervention group. The control group received only an invitation to participate in the study. The low-level intervention group received at enrollment a sheet of simple guidelines on minimizing sun exposure (Fig 1), and during August 1989 they received a postcard with the message to limit sun exposure (Fig 2). Written material was adjusted to an eighth grade reading level, and a Spanish translation was provided if indicated.

The high-level intervention group received the simple guidelines at enrollment as well as the pamphlets "For Every Child Under the Sun," prepared by the Skin Cancer Foundation, and "The Sun and Your Skin," prepared by the American Academy of Dermatology, sunscreen samples for the mother and other family members, a baby sun hat, and a sun umbrella. This group also received the postcard during August, with the message to limit sun exposure. Because the high-level intervention group received "gifts," half of the participants in each intervention group were enrolled in two consecutive periods rather than in a totally random order. In this way, no misunderstanding was created among the mothers on the maternity service.

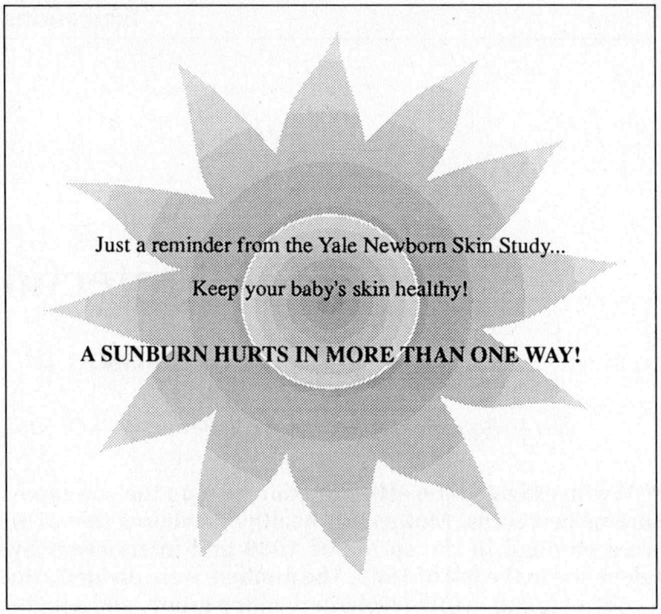

Fig 2.—*Postcard sent to experimental groups.*

To control for baseline differences in sun exposure behavior, an assessment of sun exposure habits was made for the mothers at the start of the study. Based on the reported number of days spent at the beach during the summer and vacations, the mothers were assigned to a low (no days at the beach, 33%), moderate (1 to 9 days at the beach, 32%), or high (more than 9 days, 35%) sun exposure category.

From September through December 1989, participants were interviewed by telephone by two of the authors (P.S. and M.J.). A standard questionnaire was used and the following information was obtained: amount of exposure to direct sunlight for the newborn and mother during summer weekdays and weekends, amount of time outdoors in the shade, sunscreen use by the mother, use of physical barriers to the sun for the newborn, hair and eye color of the infant, father's occupation, and advice of the pediatrician regarding sun exposure. A distinction was made between sun exposure on weekdays and weekends because of the possibility of different patterns of behavior during these periods. The values were then totaled for the entire week to form an index for the amount of time spent outdoors in direct sunlight: 0 indicates none; 1, 1 to 5 hours per week; and 2, 5 or more hours per week. The same procedure was used to estimate the amount of time spent outdoors in the shade. To estimate the amount of time mothers spent in the sun without sunscreen, we stratified the groups by sunscreen use.

Data were analyzed by χ^2 analysis[13] comparing each intervention group separately with the control group. The groups were also stratified by sunscreen use (yes/no), paternal occupation (as a proxy for socioeconomic status), and family size.

RESULTS

Of the 300 mothers invited to participate, 92% (n = 275) accepted and were followed during the entire period.

Table 1.—Ages of Parents in Yale Newborn Study

Age, y	No. of Mothers	No. of Fathers
<20	5	4
20-24	28	14
25-29	85	58
30-34	115	111
35-39	38	63
⩾40	4	25

Table 2.—Comparison of the Amount of Time Infants and Their Mothers in Three Experimental Groups Spent in Direct Sunlight

	Time, h/wk		
Experimental Group	None	⩾5	*P*
Infants			
Controls	0	99	. . .
Low intervention	75	22	<.001
High intervention	96	2	<.001
Mothers			
Controls	0	85	. . .
Low intervention	15	42	<.001
High intervention	47	17	<.001

Table 3.—Pattern of Sun Exposure in Mothers Reported at Enrollment

	Time in Direct Sunlight		
Experimental Group	Low	Moderate	High
Controls, %	29	38	33
Low intervention, %	29	34	42
High intervention, %	43	32	25

Table 4.—Change in Pattern of Sun Exposure in Mothers and Infants Reported After Intervention

	Change in Amount of Time in Direct Sunlight			
Experimental Group	Increased	Decreased	Same	*P*
Infants, %				
Controls	65	0	35	. . .
Low intervention	14	70	16	<.001
High intervention	0	53	47	<.001
Mothers, %				
Controls	67	0	33	. . .
Low intervention	32	38	33	<.001
High intervention	26	35	37	<.001

There were 149 male and 126 female infants; 94% were white. There were no differences in any of the reported behaviors by race, so the results are presented for all members of each group. Eighty-five infants were in the control group, 96 in the low-level intervention group, and 94 in the high-level intervention group. The three groups were similar in terms of hair color, eye color, paternal occupation, day-care attendance (22%), and family size (for 46% of parents, the child was their first). The mothers' ages ranged from 14 to 41 years (Table 1) and the fathers' ages ranged from 17 to 51 years; parental age was similar among the three groups.

Table 5.—Comparison of the Amount of Time Mothers Spent in Direct Sunlight Without Sunscreen

	Amount of Time, h/wk		
Experimental Group	None	⩾5	*P*
Controls	0	35	. . .
Low intervention	8	18	<.001
High intervention	24	8	<.001

Table 6.—Comparison of the Amount of Time Infants and Mothers in Three Experimental Groups Spent Outdoors (Direct Sunlight Plus Shade)

	Amount of Time Outdoors, h		
Experimental Group	⩽1	>1	*P*
Infants			
Weekdays			
Controls	1	99	. . .
Low intervention	40	60	<.001
High intervention	46	54	<.001
Weekends			
Controls	0	100	. . .
Low intervention	39	61	<.001
High intervention	49	51	<.001
Mothers			
Weekdays			
Controls	0	100	. . .
Low intervention	25	75	<.001
High intervention	58	42	<.001
Weekends			
Controls	1	99	. . .
Low intervention	5	95	.17
High intervention	23	77	<.001

Table 7.—Advice of Pediatricians As Recalled by Mothers

Advice	No. of Mothers Reporting
Stay out of the sun	46
Be cautious; limit sun exposure	23
Use protection in the sun*	19
Other†	3

*Included physical barriers (five mothers) and sunscreens (12 mothers).

†Included distributing pamphlets (two mothers) and admonishing against sunscreens.

Compared with the control group, the infants and mothers in both intervention groups spent significantly less time outdoors in direct sunlight ($P<.001$; Table 2). For ease of comparison, the values are presented as either none or 5 or more hours per week. Intermediate values of 1 to 5 hours per week were calculated, but only five infants were in this category (one in the control group and two in each intervention group). More mothers than infants were in the intermediate sun exposure category (n=46; none in the control group, 19 in the low-level intervention group, and 27 in the high-level intervention group).

Baseline sun exposure habits of the mothers were assessed to control for differences between the three groups prior to the study; the results are shown in Table 3. There were no statistically significant differences among the groups. The baseline sun exposure behavior of the mothers was then compared on an individual basis with the results reported at the end of the summer, and the percentage of mothers in each group with a change in behavior was calculated (Table 4). More of the mothers and infants in both intervention groups reduced their amount of sun exposure time than did the subjects in the control group ($P<.001$). The amount of time newborns spent in direct sunlight was also analyzed with respect to the use of physical barriers, although several of these barriers may have been inadequate (eg, stroller hoods), depending on the degree of reflectance of the UV light. There were no significant differences among the three groups in the use of hats (control, 96%; low-level intervention, 90%; and high-level intervention, 86%), stroller hoods (49%, 42%, and 48%, respectively), umbrellas (5%, 8%, and 10%, respectively), and loose-fitting clothing (2%, 3%, and 7%, respectively).

Although the number of mothers who used sunscreen was approximately the same in all groups, when the groups were controlled for sunscreen use, the intervention groups spent significantly less *unprotected* time in the sun ($P<.001$; Table 5). In calculating the *unprotected* time for a particular group, mothers who wore sunscreen were excluded (control group, 48; low-level intervention group, 48; and high-level intervention group, 52). For the mothers and infants, time in direct sunlight, time in the shade, and total time outdoors (direct sunlight plus shade) were determined (Table 6). In comparison with the control group, the intervention groups spent less time in direct sunlight (see above), less time in the shade, and significantly less time outdoors altogether (direct sunlight plus shade) ($P<.001$). The exception to this was the mothers in the low-intervention group on the weekends.

The mothers were asked to recall advice given to them by their pediatricians with regard to sun exposure for their newborns. Table 7 outlines this advice; the control group and the intervention groups received similar advice ($P=.45$).

COMMENT

Several recent studies have provided evidence that sun exposure during childhood and adolescence plays a major role in the development of skin cancer in susceptible individuals.[14] In an Australian study, 54% of melanomas were seen in individuals with five risk factors; one of these was being born in or having immigrated to Australia before age 10 years.[15] A nested case-control analysis of 130 nurses in the United States with nonfamilial cutaneous melanoma found that blistering sunburns occurring between ages 15 and 20 years were associated with an increased risk of melanoma (relative risk [RR], 2.2 for five or more burns vs none).[16] In contrast, no association was found between blistering sunburns after age 30 years and the development of melanoma. Results from a third study showed that persons aged 65 years or older who arrived in Australia between ages 1 and 20 years developed the same number of actinic keratoses as those individuals born in Australia.[17] However, individuals who immigrated after age 20 years had significantly fewer actinic keratoses than native Australians of the same age. For example, in the age group of 65 to 69 years, 25% of the adult immigrants had keratoses compared with 64% of the natives.

Changing the sun exposure behavior of adolescents may be difficult given their need for peer acceptance and their perception of what constitutes an attractive appearance.[18] A survey of 2000 students in the ninth and 10th grades showed that 70% were not using adequate protection against the sun.[19] Inadequate protection was defined as being outdoors for a 2-hour period and not wearing a hat and shirt, applying a sunscreen, or staying in the shade. Those who did not use sun protection measures were more concerned about the image that they projected to peers and were more likely to believe that "only jerks wear shirts in the sun" and covering up in the sun "makes you look like a wimp."[19] In addition, a 1989 survey of 500 young women found that 68% felt healthier and more attractive with a suntan (*Self*. 1989;5:144-149). Given the more difficult task of changing behavior during adolescence, we decided to target mothers of infants with the intent of establishing sensible sun habits at an earlier age.

In our study, both the low-level and high-level interventions succeeded in significantly reducing the amount of time the newborns were allowed to spend in direct sunlight in comparison with the control group ($P<.001$; Table 2). When the groups were controlled for total time spent outdoors (direct sunlight plus shade), both intervention groups spent less time in the shade compared with the control group and less total time outdoors (direct sunlight plus shade) ($P<.001$; Table 6). Because the current recommendation is to begin sunscreen use at age 6 months[20] and this study focused on newborns, sunscreen use in the infants was not evaluated.

Concern has been raised about the possibility of vitamin D deficiency developing in infants who are exclusively breast-fed and who have limited sun exposure. It has been estimated that spending 30 minutes per week outdoors wearing only a diaper or 2 hours a week fully clothed without a hat is sufficient to maintain serum calcifediol levels above the lower limit of normal.[21] This amount of sun exposure is required *only* while the infant is exclusively breast-fed.

To have an impact on the behavior of children and adolescents, it is also important to change the attitudes of their parents toward sun exposure and suntanning.[22] A survey for the Arizona Sun Awareness Project found that 39% of parents reported practicing no photoprotection at all for their children.[23,24] We found that both levels of intervention significantly reduced direct sun exposure time for the mothers ($P<.001$; Table 2). Although the number of mothers who applied sunscreen was similar in all three groups, when sunscreen use was controlled for, both intervention groups spent less *unprotected* time in the sun than did the control group ($P<.001$; Table 5). Mothers and their infants in both experimental groups simply spent less time outdoors ($P<.001$ except for the low-level intervention group on weekends; Table 6).

We should emphasize that the data reported in this study were collected via a survey and were based on recall that may be inaccurate. In addition, there is always the possibility of a study effect in which participants try to please the interviewer. Finally, the interviews were conducted by telephone; however, evidence indicates that telephone interviews may actually be more accurate than personal interviews.[25]

The most effective time for educating parents on sun exposure habits may be not the immediate postpartum period, but perhaps during the first or second visit to the pediatrician. This specific recommendation awaits further investigation, as does the need for continued reinforcement of the educational message. Larson et al[26] found that those individuals receiving a postcard reminder about influenza vaccination had a 59.7% vaccination rate compared with the 30.0% rate among those who did not receive a reminder. To our knowledge, no systematic study has been conducted on the duration of effect of postcard reminders. In studies in which the parents of newborns were educated on poison prevention strategies[27] or the use of car safety devices,[28] a combination of verbal and written information plus syrup of ipecac in the former study was shown to be effective, as was a longitudinal approach with multiple interactions in the latter study.

A survey of general pediatricians was conducted in Florida, and of the 349 physicians who returned the questionnaire, 71% recommended the use of sunscreens to most patients.[23] For 62% of the respondents, a discussion of photoprotection was already a part of their well-child care programs. Although 31% received written information to distribute to patients, only 7% reported using it. Therefore, if guidelines and postcard reminders on minimizing sun exposure are to be distributed by pediatricians, more of them need to receive educational materials from nonprofit organizations, such as the Skin Cancer Foundation and the American Academies of Pediatrics and Dermatology, and an emphasis should be placed on changing pediatricians' behavior. In contrast, the distribution of sun umbrellas and sunbonnets did not increase their use by mothers.

Another important point is the ability to identify youngsters who are at higher risk for the development of melanoma and nonmelanoma skin cancer.[29] Risk factors, such as fair skin that burns easily and does not tan, family history of skin cancer, and number of nevocellular nevi, can be assessed. Supplemental education and verbal and written reminders should be given to these children and their parents. However, the message of pediatricians and dermatologists should be to decrease unprotected time in the sun, not to avoid the outdoors and outdoor activities, as was demonstrated by the mothers and infants in the intervention groups in this study.

This study was supported in part by the Yale New Haven Hospital Auxiliary; BRSG SO7 RR05443 awarded by the Biomedical Research Support Grant Program, the Division of Research Resources, National Institutes of Health; and grant 2PO1-CA42101 from the National Cancer Institute.

Baby hats were donated by Paul Gotkin at Dainty Kiddie Kaps, Brooklyn, NY. Sunscreen samples were provided by Schering-Plough Corp, Memphis, Tenn.

References

1. Engel A, Johnson M-L, Haynes SG. Health effects of sunlight exposure in the United States: results from the first National Health and Nutrition Examination Survey, 1971-1974. *Arch Dermatol.* 1988;124:72-79.

2. Silverstone H, Searle JH. The epidemiology of skin cancer in Queensland: the influence of phenotype and environment. *Br J Cancer.* 1970;24:235-252.

3. Rigel DS, Rivers JK, Kopf AW, et al. Dysplastic nevi: markers for increased risk for melanoma. *Cancer.* 1989;63:386-389.

4. Holly EA, Kelly JW, Shpall SN, Chiu S-H. Number of melanocytic nevi as a major risk factor for malignant melanoma. *J Am Acad Dermatol.* 1987;17:459-468.

5. Lew RA, Sober AJ, Cook N, Marvell R, Fitzpatrick TB. Sun exposure habits in patients with cutaneous melanoma: a case control study. *J Dermatol Surg Oncol.* 1983;9:981-985.

6. Stern RS, Weinstein MC, Baker SG. Risk reduction for nonmelanoma skin cancer with childhood sunscreen use. *Arch Dermatol.* 1986;122:537-545.

7. Johnson EY, Lookingbill DP. Sunscreen use and sun exposure. *Arch Dermatol.* 1984;120:727-731.

8. Smith T. The Queensland melanoma project: an exercise in health education. *BMJ.* 1979;1:253-254.

9. Schreiber MM, Moon TE, Meyskens FL, Murdon JA. Solar ultraviolet radiation and skin cancer: a public education program. *Cutis.* 1982;30:516-526.

10. Litman TJ. The family as a basic unit in health and medicine: a social-behavioral overview. *Soc Sci Med.* 1974;8:495-519.

11. Hazen HH, Freeman CW. Skin cancer in the American negro. *Arch Dermatol.* 1950;62:622-623.

12. Oettle AG. Skin cancer in Africa. *Natl Cancer Inst Monogr.* 1963;10:197-214.

13. Feinberg SE. *The Analysis of Cross-Classified Data.* Cambridge, Mass: MIT Press;1977:9.

14. Marks R. Role of childhood in the development of skin cancer. *Aust Paediatr J.* 1988;24:337-338.

15. English DR, Armstrong BK. Identifying people at high risk of cutaneous malignant melanoma: results from a case-control study in Western Australia. *BMJ.* 1988;296:1285-1288.

16. Weinstock MA, Colditz GA, Willett WC, et al. Nonfamilial cutaneous melanoma incidence in women associated with sun exposure before 20 years of age. *Pediatrics.* 1989;84:199-204.

17. Marks R, Jolley D, Lectsas S, Foley P. The role of childhood exposure to sunlight in the development of solar keratoses and non-melanocytic skin cancer. *Med J Aust.* 1990;152:62-65.

18. Marks R, Hill D. Behavioural change in adolescence: a major challenge for skin-cancer control in Australia. *Med J Aust.* 1988;149:514-515.

19. Cockburn J, Hennrikus D, Scott R, Sanson-Fisher R. Adolescent use of sun-protection measures. *Med J Aust.* 1989;151:136-140.

20. Hurwitz S. The sun and sunscreen protection: recommendations for children. *J Dermatol Surg Oncol.* 1988;14:657-660.

21. Specker BL, Valanis B, Hertzberg V, Edwards N, Tsang RC. Sunshine exposure and serum 25-hydroxyvitamin D concentrations in exclusively breast-fed infants. *J Pediatr.* 1985;107:372-376.

22. Marks R. Skin cancer: childhood protection affords lifetime protection. *Med J Aust.* 1987;147:475-476.

23. Pupo RA, Sherertz EF, Flowers FP. Sun protection in well-child care: results of a survey of Florida pediatricians. *Pediatr Dermatol.* 1986;3:390-394.

24. Euler PG. *Marketing Research Study: Arizona Sun Awareness Project.* Tucson, Ariz: University of Arizona Cancer Center; 1982.

25. Weeks MF, Kulka RA, Lessler JT, Whitmore RW. Personal versus telephone surveys for collection of household health data at the local level. *Am J Public Health.* 1983;73:1389-1394.

26. Larson EB, Olsen E, Cole W, Shortell S. The relationship of health beliefs and a postcard reminder to influenza vaccination. *J Fam Pract.* 1979;8:1207-1211.

27. Cooper JM, Widness JA, O'Shea JS. Pilot evaluation of instructing parents of newborns about poison prevention strategies. *AJDC.* 1988;142:627-629.

28. Berger LR, Saunders S, Armitage K, Schauer L. Promoting the use of car safety devices for infants: an intensive health education approach. *Pediatrics.* 1984;74:16-19.

29. Williams ML, Sagebiel RW. Sunburns, melanoma, and the pediatrician. *Pediatrics.* 1989;84:381-382.

Gastroesophageal Reflux and Apnea in Prematurely Born Infants During Wakefulness and Sleep

Mikel de Ajuriaguerra, MD; Marie-France Radvanyi-Bouvet, MD; Catherine Huon, MD; Guy Moriette, MD

• The hypothesis that acid gastroesophageal reflux may be responsible for the persistence of apnea was tested on 20 prematurely born infants, at a median conceptional age of 38.7 weeks. Gastroesophageal reflux was identified using distal esophageal pH monitoring. Apneas of durations greater than 10 seconds were identified and classified as either central or obstructive and mixed, using recordings of respiration. Wakefulness, active sleep, and quiet sleep were identified using electroencephalography and by assessing eye movements. Of 134 episodes of acid gastroesophageal reflux in the 20 subjects, more occurred during wakefulness and during active sleep than during quiet sleep. A total of 139 apneas, predominantly of the obstructive and mixed type, occurred. No relationship could, however, be demonstrated, in this rather small number of patients, between the occurrence of gastroesophageal reflux and that of apneas.

(*AJDC*. 1991;145:1132-1136)

Apneas of prematurity, which usually cease at full term (37 weeks), may occur later, mostly following neonatal diseases.[1] Relationships have been established between a distinct type of apnea that may occur weeks after birth, apnea of infancy, and gastroesophageal reflux (GER).[2-4] We designed the present study to test the hypothesis that GER may similarly account for the persistence of apneas of prematurity after full term (37 weeks) has been reached.

PATIENTS AND METHODS

Twenty infants who had been admitted to our intensive care unit following premature (before 37 weeks' gestation) birth were studied after they reached full term (gestation of 37 weeks or more). The median values for birth weight, gestational age at birth, and postconceptional age (PCA, gestational age plus postnatal age) were 1490 g (range, 1000 to 3990 g), 31 weeks (range, 27.5 to 36.5 weeks), and 38.7 weeks (range, 37 to 43 weeks), respectively. Gestational age was determined within 3 days from birth, using the following prenatal and postnatal criteria[5]: the maternal menstrual history, data from ultrasound examinations during early pregnancy, and clinical, and in some cases electroencephalographic evaluation of the newborn. There were nine female and 11 male newborn infants whose birth weights were appropriate for gestational age (>10th percentile of Lubchenco's growth chart). Fourteen "symptomatic" infants were selected because cardiorespiratory monitoring still detected apneas (>10-second duration) and/or bradycardias (<95 beats per minute) or because regurgitations associated or not with bradycardia occurred after feeding. Six "asymptomatic" infants whose recent clinical course was uneventful, without any of the abnormalities observed in symptomatic infants, and whose discharge from the hospital within a few days was considered, were studied to assess the possible occurrence of asymptomatic GER[6-9] and/or that of undetected apneas.[10] The birth weights, gestational ages, and PCAs of both symptomatic and asymptomatic infants were similar.

In the neonatal period, respiratory distress, observed in 12 of the 14 symptomatic infants and four of the six asymptomatic infants, required mechanical ventilation for durations ranging from 28 hours to 70 days. Four symptomatic and two asymptomatic infants developed bronchopulmonary dysplasia.[11] Apneas of prematurity were treated, when necessary, with caffeine citrate,[12,13] administration of which was stopped at least 7 days before the study. Cranial ultrasonography identified stage 2 intraventricular hemorrhage in one asymptomatic infant and no significant abnormality in the rest of the population. Clinical evaluations and electroencephalograms (EEGs) were considered normal in the 20 patients at the time of study.

Measurement of Esophageal pH

Intraesophageal pH was monitored using an esophageal flexible glass microelectrode 1.6 mm in outer diameter (MI 506, Microelectrodes Inc, Londonderry, NH), with a response time between 5 and 15 seconds,[6] a reference electrode (MI 502), and a pH-meter ionometer millivoltmeter (P500 type, Solea-Tacussel, Villeurbanne, France). The data were recorded on both a recorder (Ecoscript, Solea-Tacussel) and a polygraph (see below). Before and after each session, the pH probe was calibrated using solutions of 1.1 and 7 pH. The glass electrode, introduced through the nose, was initially pushed into the stomach, where low values of pH were recorded. It was thereafter pulled carefully and positioned 3 to 4 cm above the lower esophageal sphincter, whose estimated position corresponded to the point of increase in pH. Proper positioning was checked using the data of Strobel et al.[14] Gastroesophageal reflux was defined as a pH decrease to below 4 for at least 15 seconds.[3,6] We identified GER as "pathologic" in the supine position, when the esophageal pH value was below 4 during more than 10.4% of the duration of re-

Accepted for publication April 8, 1991.

From the Service de Médecine Néonatale (Drs Ajuriaguerra, Radvanyi-Bouvet, Huon, and Moriette), and INSERM U 29 (Drs Radvanyi-Bouvet and Moriette), Maternité Port-Royal, Groupe Hospitalier Cochin, Paris, France.

Presented in part at the European Society for Pediatric Research Annual Meeting, Vienna, Austria, September 24, 1990.

Reprint requests to Service de Médecine Néonatale, Maternité Port-Royal, 123 Blvd de Port-Royal, 75674 Paris, France (Dr Moriette).

Table 1.—Individual Data of the 20 Infants*

Infant No.	No. of Apneas CA	No. of Apneas OMA	No. of IBs	GER No.	GER Duration
Symptomatic					
1	...	0.67	...	2.66	5.86
2	...	6.37	...	6.68	34.12†
3	...	0.84	0.28	3.09	22.20†
4	0.51	0.25	0.76	2.54	14.38†
5	0.25	...	...	2.54	12.01†
6	1.47	2.45	...	2.93	12.99†
7	...	2.65	0.81	0.80	10.52†
8	0.26	...	0.26	1.83	8.72
9	...	...	...	3.00	30.66†
10	0.50	5.54	0.25	1.26	15.70†
11	...	...	...	0.31	0.21
12	...	1.03	...	5.16	28.08†
13	3.50	5.54	...	0.58	4.53
14	...	0.42	16.44	3.79	29.98†
Asymptomatic					
15	...	...	...	2.27	5.53
16	...	...	...	1.93	3.20
17	...	5.66	...	1.23	1.85
18	...	...	...	2.59	25.70†
19	...	...	...	1.51	14.10†
20	...	...	...	1.92	6.80

*CA indicates central apneas; OMA, obstructive or mixed apneas; IBs, isolated bradycardias; and GER, gastroesophageal reflux. All numbers represent values per 100 minutes.

†"Pathologic" GER. See text for explanation.

cording. This cutoff value of 10.4% of recording time corresponds approximately to the mean±2 SD of one study performed in normal preterm and full-term infants[7] and is above the mean±2 SD of another study performed in normal full-term newborns.[6]

Study of Respiration

Respiration was recorded using two mercury strain gauges that assessed the thoracic and the abdominal movements, and a thermistor attached between the nostrils that assessed nasal airflow.[15] In addition, we monitored heart rate, performed surface diaphragmatic electromyography using electrodes attached in a subcostal position on the mamillary line, and monitored transcutaneous PO_2.

Apneas (only those lasting at least 10 seconds) were classified[15] as central, when there was simultaneous cessation of respiratory movements and of nasal airflow; obstructive, when nasal airflow stopped in spite of the persistence of respiratory movements; and mixed, when central and obstructive mechanisms occurred successively. Obstructive and mixed apneas were combined in one group. When analyzing the recordings, we ruled out the possibility of artefactual loss of the nasal airflow signal by assessing the simultaneous signals of heart rate, transcutaneous PO_2 and surface diaphragmatic electromyogram.

In addition to apneas, we also assessed the occurrence of bradycardias (<80/min). Bradycardias that occurred simultaneously with apneas were not studied separately, as opposed to those that occurred without apneas. "Bradycardias" will hereafter refer only to those "isolated" bradycardias.

Identification of States

Electroencephalograms were recorded on two channels, using right frontal, rolandic, and occipital electrodes. Eye movements were recorded on one channel, using a piezoelectric quartz transducer. Electroencephalography and behavioral criteria allowed for identification of the following three states: (1) wakefulness, characterized by open eyes and body movements; (2) active sleep (AS), characterized by low-voltage continuous EEG and presence of rapid eye movements; and (3) quiet sleep (QS), characterized by "tracé alternant" on EEG and absence of rapid eye movements. Identification of one state required that the corresponding criteria be present for at least 1 minute.[16] Sleep states that did not meet the criteria of AS or QS were identified as "intermediate" sleep. The signals corresponding to respiration, heart rate, transcutaneous PO_2, surface diaphragmatic electromyogram, EEG, and esophageal pH were recorded on a 10-channel polygraph (Alvar Electronique, Montreuil, France).

Experimental Design

The infants were kept under constant observation, and studied in the supine position for a period of 6 hours beginning 90 minutes after feeding. The leads, strain gauges, transcutaneous PO_2 electrode, esophageal glass, and reference (fixed on the leg) electrodes were appropriately placed toward the end of these 90 minutes, and recording was begun. The infants were fed once during the recording period.

Analysis of the Results

The results were first standardized to take into account the differences in the durations of the states of consciousness in the different infants. This was achieved by expressing them in percentages of the recording durations. For GER, whose durations may vary widely, we standardized both the number of events (number of decreases in pH to below 4 per 100 minutes of recording) and their duration (duration of acid GER per 100 minutes of recording). For apneas of more than 10-second duration, and for bradycardias, whose durations vary in a narrow range, we used only the standardized number of events.

Because most of our data were skewed, the results are expressed as medians and ranges. Differences were evaluated using the following nonparametric tests: (1) the Kruskal-Wallis test for comparing values obtained during AS, QS, and wakefulness, followed, only when significant, by Wilcoxon signed rank test for paired values; (2) Mann-Whitney *U* test for unpaired values for comparing two groups (symptomatic vs asymptomatic patients); and (3) the Spearman rank correlation coefficient for assessing relationships between the number or duration of episodes of acid GER and the number of apneas or bradycardias. Probability values of $P<.05$ were considered significant.

Informed consent was obtained from the parents of asymptomatic infants prior to each study. Since polygraphic recording and measurement of esophageal pH are routinely performed when evaluating patients with symptoms similar to those seen in our symptomatic infants, we did not ask the parents of those infants for a formal consent, but explained to them the clinical problems of their child, and the purpose of our planned investigations.

RESULTS

The median duration of recording was 371 minutes (range, 237 to 408 minutes). The median durations of recording during wakefulness and during sleep were 116.5 minutes (range, 54 to 195 minutes) and 253 minutes (range, 152 to 311 minutes), respectively. The median durations of recording during the different sleep states were as follows: (1) 152 minutes (range, 74 to 224 minutes) for AS; (2) 62 minutes (range, 17 to 95 minutes) for QS; and (3) 13 minutes (range, 3 to 86 minutes) for intermediate sleep.

Table 2.—Number of Episodes of Acid Gastroesophageal Reflux During the Different States of Consciousness

	Episodes, No. per 100 min	
	Median	Range
Active sleep	2.64*	0-8.69
Quiet sleep	1.11	0-8.33
Awake	2.17†	0-6.54
Combined	2.40	0.31-6.68

*$P<.01$ for active vs quiet sleep.
†$P<.02$ for awake vs quiet sleep.

GER

All 20 infants demonstrated episodes of acid GER. The total number of these episodes was 134. "Pathologic" GER (esophageal pH <4 during more than 10.4% of recording duration)[6,7] was observed in 10 of the 14 symptomatic infants (infants 2 through 7, 9, 10, 12, and 14; Table 1) and in two of the six asymptomatic infants (infants 18 and 19; Table 1).

The median number of acid GER episodes, in all 20 infants, in all states of consciousness combined, was 2.40 per 100 minutes (Table 2). There was no significant difference between symptomatic infants (median, 2.6 per 100 minutes; range, 0.31 to 6.68 per 100 minutes) and asymptomatic infants (median, 1.92 per 100 minutes; range, 1.23 to 2.59 per 100 minutes). These episodes were more frequent during AS (median, 2.64 per 100 minutes) and during wakefulness (median, 2.17 per 100 minutes) than during QS (median, 1.11 per 100 minutes) ($P<.01$ for AS vs QS; $P<.02$ for wakefulness vs QS; Table 2).

The median duration of GER episodes in the 20 infants, in all states of consciousness combined, was 12.50 per 100 minutes (Table 3). It was not significantly different in symptomatic (median value, 13.68 minutes) vs asymptomatic infants (6.16 per 100 minutes) (Table 3). There were no significant differences, either, in the durations of GER in the different states of consciousness between any of the two subsets of infants considered separately or in the 20 infants together (Table 3).

Apneas and Bradycardias

Twenty-six central apneas ranging in duration from 10 to 15 seconds were recorded in six symptomatic infants and in none of the asymptomatic infants (Table 1). This number was too small to enable more detailed studies to be performed. A total of 113 obstructive and mixed apneas were recorded in 10 symptomatic infants (range of duration, 10 to 28 seconds) and in one asymptomatic infant (range of duration, 10 to 20 seconds) (Table 1).

Table 3 shows the occurrence of apneas in the different groups of infants and in the different states. Obstructive and mixed apneas appeared to occur more during AS than during the other states of consciousness, when considering all 20 infants together as well as the symptomatic infants separately. The difference, however, was not significant.

Forty-six bradycardias were recorded in six symptomatic subjects (Table 1), of which 39 were recorded in the same infant who experienced only one apnea. They were not significantly more frequent during AS than during the other states. No bradycardia was recorded in asymptomatic infants.

Table 3.—Obstructive and Mixed Apneas (OMAs) and Acid Gastroesophageal Reflux (GER) in Relation to States of Consciousness*

	OMAs, No.		GER, Duration	
	Median	Range	Median	Range
Symptomatic infants (n = 14)				
AS	1.32	0-11.21	17.58	0-41.88
QS	0	0-8.33	9.51	0-50.30
Awake	0.25	0-5.50	13.65	0-34.86
Combined	0.75	0-6.37	13.68	0.21-29.98
Asymptomatic infants (n = 6)				
AS	0	0-6.32	8.37	1.40-35.90
QS	0	0-1.73	0.96	0-13.20
Awake	0	0-7.01	4.83	1.78-29.10
Combined	0	0-5.66	6.16	1.85-27.70
All infants				
AS	0.56	0-11.21	14.46	0-41.88
QS	0	0-8.33	4.02	0-50.3
Awake	0	0-7.01	9.39	0-34.86
Combined	0.33	0-6.37	12.50	0.21-34.12

*AS indicates active sleep, and QS, quiet sleep. All numbers represent values per 100 minutes.

Relationships Between Acid GER and Apneas

Two of 26 central apneas and 11 of 113 obstructive and mixed apneas occurred during acid GER. Only one apnea, of the latter type, began within 1 minute of the onset of acid GER.

Similar numbers of obstructive and mixed apneas were seen in infants with (n = 12) and without (n = 8) "pathologic" GER (median, 0.63 and 0 per 100 minutes, respectively). They were also similar between infants who had an episode of acid GER and those who did not.

Using the data listed in Table 1, we could not demonstrate any correlation between the number of obstructive and mixed apneas and that of acid GER in either the 14 symptomatic infants separately or the 20 infants together; or during all the states of consciousness combined or only during sleep. There was also no correlation between the number of obstructive and mixed apneas and the total duration of acid GER.

Relationships Between Bradycardias and Acid GER

Eight of the 46 bradycardias occurred during episodes of acid GER. One of them occurred within 1 minute of the onset of acid GER. The number of bradycardias was not different between infants with or without "pathologic" GER, or between infants with or without episodes of acid GER.

In symptomatic infants, there was no correlation between the number of bradycardias and the number or the duration of acid GERs (Table 1). The distribution of bradycardias in our population, however, was highly skewed; of the six symptomatic infants in whom they occurred (Table 1), five had fewer than one episode per 100 minutes and the last one had 16.4 per 100 minutes (infant 14). In this last patient, these very frequent bradycardias were associated with a particularly long duration of acid GER (30 per 100 minutes), which, however, was also observed in three other infants (infants 2, 9, and 12) who did not have bradycardias.

COMMENT

In prematurely born infants, apnea occasionally persists after reaching a PCA of 37 weeks. Gastroesophageal reflux has been reported to occur frequently in this population.[8,9] At 37 weeks' PCA, on assessing the possible relationships between GER and persisting apneas in 20 prematurely born infants referred to our intensive care unit, we observed frequent episodes of both acid GER, which were predominant during AS and wakefulness, and obstructive and mixed apneas; we could not distinguish any relationship between the two types of events.

The polygraphic method that enabled respiration to be studied and sleep states to be identified could not be used for more than 6 hours. Although 24 hours of recording would have been preferable,[7] we had to assess the occurrence of GER, using recording of esophageal pH, based on this rather short period of time that could have underestimated the occurrence of GER. We believe, however, that we recorded enough episodes of GER to properly evaluate their relationships with apneas.

Previous studies[6,7] in "normal" newborns evaluated for 17 to 24 hours have assessed the duration of acid GER, in percentage of recording duration. They provided criteria for "pathologic" GER, which were met by 10 of 14 symptomatic infants and by two of six of our asymptomatic infants. Thus, our data confirm that acid GER, which occurs quite frequently, may be completely asymptomatic in premature infants.[7-9] The number of acid GER episodes appears greater in the present study than in the study by Newell et al,[9] who also studied preterm infants requiring intensive care. Differences in the positions of the infants studied may account for the difference in results. Our infants were studied supine, in spite of our usual preference for nursing in prone position, because the supine position increases GER,[6,17] and is the most convenient for both observation and polygraphic recordings. Infants were in lateral or prone position in the study by Newell et al,[9] which also demonstrated a shorter total duration of acid GER than ours.

The relationship of GER with states of consciousness has rarely been evaluated in the neonatal period. In both our newborn infants and in somewhat older infants studied by others,[18-22] acid GER occurred frequently during wakefulness. During sleep, contrary to the findings of Walsh et al,[18] and in agreement with others,[19,21] we found GER to occur more frequently during AS than during QS.

We observed, as expected, more obstructive and mixed apneas in symptomatic than in asymptomatic infants. Numerous apneas, however, were recorded in one asymptomatic infant (infant 17; Table 1), confirming that apneas may not be detected with routine cardiorespiratory monitoring.[10] In addition, cardiorespiratory monitoring does not disclose obstructive apneas in the absence of bradycardia.

Most studies of "healthy" preterm and full-term newborn infants[15,23,24] have shown that apneas are rare, or of short duration (<10 seconds) and predominantly central at a postconceptional age corresponding to term. In our infants who required intensive care we found apneas of more than 10-second duration to be rather frequent, with a predominance of obstructive and mixed over central apneas. This finding confirms previous observations. Mixed apneas, indeed, have been reported to predominate in infants recovering from respiratory distress,[25] and their proportion has been shown to increase with the duration of apnea.[1] Apneas have been reported to occur more frequently during AS than during the other states of consciousness.[15,26-28] In our study, this trend was not significant, because of the Kruskal-Wallis test being used for comparison of three states of consciousness (AS, QS, and wakefulness) together (see "Patients and Methods"). If we, however, consider only two sleep states (AS and QS), as in these reports,[15,26-28] we also observe apneas occurring more often during AS than during QS ($P<.01$).

We could not find any evidence supporting the existence of a relationship between apneas of more than 10-second duration and acid GER in the distal esophagus.

The implication of GER as a possible cause of infant apnea, of apparent life-threatening events, or of sudden infant death syndrome, is still a matter of controversy.[2-4,20,22] In 14 cases of multiple and severe episodes of prolonged (of >20-second duration) apneas, selected over a 4-year period, the cessation of apnea was achieved after control of GER, and a temporal relationship between the occurrence of obstructive apnea and the onset of GER was observed in five patients.[3] Two carefully designed studies,[18,29] however, failed to demonstrate a temporal relationship between GER and short apneas, in the majority of the cases, although short obstructive apneas were found to occur more frequently during GER, in one of the two studies.[18]

In contrast with these studies, our aim was not to study apnea of infancy, but was limited to assessing the possible relationships between persisting apneas and GER in prematurely born infants. In a similar population, an increased frequency of apnea has been reported during and immediately after regurgitations,[30] which did not occur in our infants. In an earlier study on premature infants (median for gestational age, 28 weeks) (median age, 2 weeks), the reflux index (total duration of GER) in the patients with frequent severe apneas was similar to that in those without apneas.[9] Our results are in agreement with this finding. Thus, in the absence of regurgitations, no direct relationship appears to exist usually between acid GER in the distal esophagus and apnea. We, however, did not evaluate the effect of treating GER on the frequency of both apneas or bradycardias. We did not evaluate the possibility of GER being responsible for either apneas or bradycardias via stimuli other than acidic stimulation of the distal esophagus. Assessing, for example, the role of proximal GER[31] or that of dilatation of the lower esophagus[32] may help understand the recent observation of "pronounced reduction in the frequency of apneas" in infants with both xanthine-resistant apneas and elevated reflux index.[9]

The following limitations of our study, however, must be acknowledged: (1) prolonged severe apneas did not occur during our recordings; therefore, our result should not be extrapolated to that sort of event[33]; (2) we studied a small number of patients. Larger numbers of both patients and events might possibly enable relationships between apnea and GER to be demonstrated.

Although our results show that apneas of prematurely

born infants may often persist in the absence of GER, we suggest that the occurrence of GER, which is frequent in this population and may be dangerous, should be routinely assessed before discharge.

We gratefully acknowledge the contribution of A. Mlika, MD, (INSERM U 149) in the statistical aspects of the study, and the help of F. Morel-Kahn, M. Barclay, L. Rapin, and L. Salignac for polygraphic recordings. We are indebted to P. Bitoun, MD, for reviewing the manuscript.

References

1. Butcher-Puech MC, Henderson-Smart DJ, Holley D, Lacey JL, Edwards DA. Relation between apnea duration and type and neurological status of preterm infants. *Arch Dis Child.* 1985;60:953-958.
2. Leape LL, Holder TM, Franklin JD, Amoury RA, Aschcraft RW. Respiratory arrest in infants secondary to gastroesophageal reflux. *Pediatrics.* 1977;60:924-927.
3. Herbst JJ, Minton SD, Book LS. Gastro-oesophageal reflux causing respiratory distress and apnea in new born infants. *J Pediatr.* 1979;95:763-767.
4. Spitzer AR, Boyle JT, Tuchmann DN, Fox WW. Awake apnea associated with gastroesophageal reflux: a specific clinical syndrome. *J Pediatr.* 1984;104:200-205.
5. Moriette G, Chaussain M, Radvanyi-Bouvet MF, Walti H, Pajot N, Relier JP. Functional residual capacity and sleep states in the premature newborn. *Biol Neonate.* 1983;43:125-133.
6. Vandenplas Y, Sacre-Smits L. Seventeen-hour continuous esophageal pH monitoring in the newborn: evaluation of the influence of position in asymptomatic and symptomatic babies. *J Pediatr Gastroenterol Nutr.* 1985;4:356-361.
7. Gouyon JB, Boggio V, Athias P. Frequency of gastro-oesophageal reflux in neonates as assessed by 24 hours pH monitoring. *Helv Paediatr Acta.* 1986;41:301-310.
8. Saint Martin J, Choulot JJ, Leblond C. Etude de la pHmétrie oesophagienne chez le nouveau-né moins de 1700 g. *Arch Fr Pédiatr.* 1986;43:249-252.
9. Newell SJ, Booth IW, Morgan MEI, Durbin GM, McNeish AS. Gastro-oesophageal reflux in preterm infants. *Arch Dis Child.* 1989;64:780-786.
10. Southall DP, Levit GA, Richards JM, et al. Undetected episodes of prolonged apnea and severe bradycardia in preterm infants. *Pediatrics.* 1983;72:541-551.
11. Bancalari E, Abdenour GE, Feller R, Gannon J. Bronchopulmonary dysplasia: clinical presentation. *J Pediatr.* 1979;95:819-823.
12. Murat I, Moriette G, Blin MC, et al. The efficacy of caffeine in the treatment of recurrent idiopathic apneas in premature infants. *J Pediatr.* 1981;99:984-989.
13. Brouard C, Moriette G, Murat I, et al. Comparative efficacy of theophylline and caffeine in the treatment of idiopathic apnea in premature infants. *AJDC.* 1985;139:698-700.
14. Strobel CT, Byrne WJ, Ament ME, Euler AR. Correlation of esophageal lengths in children with height: application to the Tuttle test without prior esophageal manometry. *J Pediatr.* 1979;94:81-84.
15. Flores-Guevara R, Plouin P, Curzi-Dascalova L, et al. Sleep apneas in normal neonates and infants during the first three months of life. *Neuropediatrie.* 1982;13:21-28.
16. Dreyfus-Brisac C. Ontogenesis of brain bioelectrical activity and sleep organization in neonates and infants. In: Falkner F, Tanner JM, eds. *Human Growth.* New York, NY: Plenum Publishing Corp; 1979;3:157-182.
17. Blumenthal I, Lealman GT. Effect of posture on gastro-oesophageal reflux in the newborn. *Arch Dis Child.* 1982;57:555-556.
18. Walsh JK, Farrell MK, Keenan WJ, Lucas M, Kramer M. Gastroesophageal reflux in infants: relation to apnea. *J Pediatr.* 1981;99:197-201.
19. Jeffery HE, Reid I, Rahilly P, Read DJC. Gastroesophageal reflux in 'near-miss' sudden infant death infants in active but not quiet sleep. *Sleep.* 1980;3:393-399.
20. Ariagno RL, Guilleminault C, Baldwin R, Owen-Boedikker M. Movement and gastroesophageal reflux in awake term infants with 'near-miss' SIDS, unrelated to apnea. *J Pediatr.* 1982;100:894-897.
21. Paton JY, Macfadyen UM, Simpson H. Sleep phase and gastro-oesophageal reflux in infants at possible risk of SIDS. *Arch Dis Child.* 1989;64:264-269.
22. Kahn A, Rebuffat E, Sottiaux M, Blum D, Yasik EA. Sleep apneas and acid esophageal reflux in control infants with an apparent life-threatening event. *Biol Neonate.* 1990;57:144-149.
23. Curzi-Dascalova L, Christova-Gueorguieva E. Respiratory pauses in normal prematurely born infants. *Biol Neonate.* 1983;44:325-332.
24. Curzi-Dascalova L, Christova-Gueorguieva E, Lebrun F, Firtion G. Respiratory pauses in very low risk prematurely born infants reaching normal term. *Neuropediatrics.* 1984;15:13-17.
25. Thach BT, Brouillette RT, Abu-Osba YK, Wilson SL, Matew OP. Prevalence of mixed and obstructive apneic spells in preterm infants. *Pediatr Res.* 1980;14:637. Abstract.
26. Lee DR, Caces R, Kwiatkowsi K, Cates D, Rigatto H. A developmental study on types and frequency distribution of short apneas (2 to 15 seconds) in term and preterm infants. *Pediatr Res.* 1987;22:344-349.
27. Gabriel H, Albani M, Schulte FJ. Apneic spells and sleep states in preterm infants. *Pediatrics.* 1976;57:142-147.
28. Haddad GG, Lai TL, Mellins RB. Determination of the ventilatory pattern in REM sleep in normal infants. *J Appl Physiol.* 1982;53:52-56.
29. Rosen CL, Frost JD, Harrison GM. Infant apnea: polygraphic studies and follow-up monitoring. *Pediatrics.* 1983;71:731-736.
30. Menon AP, Schefft GL, Thach BT. Apnea associated with regurgitation in infants. *J Pediatr.* 1985;106:625-629.
31. Sindel BD, Maisels MJ, Ballantine TVN. Gastroesophageal reflux to the proximal esophagus in infants with bronchopulmonary dysplasia. *AJDC.* 1989;143:1103-1106.
32. Ramet J, Praud JP, d'Allest AM, Dehan M, Guilleminault C, Gaultier C. Cardiac and respiratory responses to esophageal dilatation during REM sleep in human infants. *Biol Neonate.* 1990;58:181-187.
33. Leape LL, Holder TM, Ashcraft KW. Gastro-oesophageal reflux and apnea. *J Pediatr.* 1982;101:481.

Oxygen Saturation by Pulse Oximetry in Healthy Infants at an Altitude of 1610 m (5280 ft)

What Is Normal?

Elizabeth H. Thilo, MD; Beverly Park-Moore, CRTT; Edward R. Berman, MD; Bonita S. Carson, MD

• Pulse oximetry is a valuable, noninvasive technique for assessing oxygen saturation that has gained wide clinical acceptance despite little available information concerning normal values in the newborn, especially at an altitude different than sea level. We performed serial pulse oximetry studies on 150 term, appropriate-weight-for-gestational-age, clinically healthy infants at an altitude of 1610 m (5280 ft) at 24 to 48 hours, 1 month, and 3 months of age to define a reference range for oxygen saturation as a guideline in clinical care. We found that mean oxygen saturation at 24 to 48 hours of age is 92% to 93% and varies little with infant activity. With increasing postnatal age, there is a tendency for increased oxygen saturation during the awake states to 93% to 94%, while oxygen saturation during sleep stays the same or even decreases slightly. The lower end of the reference range (2 SDs below the mean) is as low as 85% during feeding at 24 to 48 hours of age, and as low as 86% during quiet sleep at 1 and 3 months of age, with 88% to 89% the lower limit in other activities at all ages.

(*AJDC.* 1991;145:1137-1140)

Clinicians are constantly faced with the need to make decisions regarding the need for and adjustment of supplemental oxygen in the newborn patient, yet information concerning their "normal" oxygenation is inconsistent. Older data obtained from umbilical artery catheters placed into healthy newborns at sea level showed left atrial or descending aorta oxygen saturation of 94% to 95% or a Pa_{O_2} of approximately 75 mm Hg during the first hours and days of life.[1-3] Most recently, pulse oximetry performed on healthy newborns at sea level has shown a wide variation in oxygen saturation, with some infants having saturations well below 90%, especially during the first days of life.[4]

There are approximately 150 000 infants born at altitudes of 1500 m (4918 ft) or more each year in the Rocky Mountain region,[5] yet there are no data for oxygen saturation in healthy infants at these altitudes. We have observed a significant number of infants who have been supplied with small amounts of supplemental oxygen to maintain a minimum Pa_{O_2} of 55 mm Hg or oxygen saturation by pulse oximetry (Sp_{O_2}) of 90% or more at our altitude of 1610 m, despite the absence of specific clinical or radiographic signs of pulmonary disease.[6] While 1610 m is only a moderate altitude (barometric pressure, approximately 630 mm Hg; alveolar P_{O_2}, approximately 80 mm Hg), normal adult Pa_{O_2} and oxygen saturation are reduced significantly, from a range of 95 to 105 mm Hg and greater than 96% at sea level, to 65 to 75 mm Hg and 92% to 94%, respectively.[7,8] In light of this, we wondered if this arbitrarily selected minimum Sp_{O_2} of 90% might be too high.

The purpose of our study therefore was to define a reference range for Sp_{O_2} in a population of healthy, full-term infants in Denver, Colo, at an altitude of 1610 m above sea level, and to determine if Sp_{O_2} varies significantly during different infant activities. Ultimately, we hoped to define guidelines that could have a wider application both to convalescing infants and to infants with significant chronic lung disease.

SUBJECTS AND METHODS

Subjects

The study protocol was approved by the Institutional Research Review Board of Rose Medical Center, Denver. One hundred fifty full-term, appropriate-weight-for-gestational-age infants were enrolled in the study after informed parental consent was obtained. All infants had a normal cardiopulmonary examination and were judged to be clinically healthy by their physicians before being enrolled. Specifically excluded from enrollment were any infants who had Apgar scores of less than 7 at 1 or 5 minutes, infants who clinically required supplemental oxygen for more than 1.5 hours after birth (ie, had signs of a difficult transition), infants who lived outside the Denver metropolitan area (at an altitude <1560 or >1660 m), or infants with signs of respiratory distress or heart disease.

Study Techniques

Oximetry was performed using an Ohmeda Biox 3700 pulse oximeter (Ohmeda, Louisville, Colo) with a Neonatal Flex II probe (Ohmeda) applied to a foot at 24 to 48 hours after birth,

Accepted for publication January 28, 1991.

From the Department of Pediatrics, Division of Neonatology, University of Colorado School of Medicine, The Children's Hospital, and the Department of Pediatrics and Newborn Medicine, Rose Medical Center, Denver.

Presented at the 14th Annual Conference on Neonatal-Perinatal Medicine, American Academy of Pediatrics District VIII Section on Perinatal Pediatrics, Anchorage, Alaska, May 25, 1989.

Reprint requests to Division of Neonatology, The Children's Hospital, 1056 E 19th Ave, Denver, CO 80218 (Dr Thilo).

and again at 1 and 3 months of age. A simultaneous electrocardiogram was monitored to confirm the pulse oximeter waveform and Spo_2 reading. Only if the electrocardiographically determined heart rate and the oximetry-determined pulse rate were within 5 beats per minute of each other with a clear pulse waveform on the oximeter's oscilloscope screen was the Spo_2 reading considered reliable.

To assess the effects of different infant activities on Spo_2, a stable 10-minute period in each of four activities (awake, feeding, quiet sleep, and active sleep) was studied at each age whenever possible. Sleep states were assessed clinically using the criteria of Prechtl,[9] and indeterminate states were not included or analyzed. The infant was observed, but no recordings were made, until at least 3 minutes into a definable state. Quiet sleep was defined as a relaxed state, eyes closed and still, with regular respirations and heart rate, and no gross body movements except for occasional startles. Active sleep was defined as a sleep state with eyes closed but eye movements present, as well as frequent small movements of the limbs, face, and head, along with irregular respirations and a more variable heart rate. Awake was defined as the infant having eyes open and not crying. Feeding was defined as being held during active nursing or bottle feeding.

Oxygen saturation, pulse rate, and heart rate were monitored continuously by one of us (E.H.T., E.R.B., or B.P.-M.) (79% of all studies by B.P.-M.), and an average value for each minute in each activity was recorded. Once a definable state as described was achieved, there was little variation in Spo_2 noted, other than intermittent movement artifacts that were easily ignored, and it was quite easy to assign a mean Spo_2 to each minute of each activity, to a maximum of 10 minutes whenever possible. Subsequently, a mean for each infant in each activity at each age was calculated, then used to arrive at a group mean Spo_2 for each activity at each age. Each pulse oximetry study lasted for a mean (±SE) of 77±1.3 minutes.

Statistical Analysis

The initial approach to establishing normal values was to choose the 2.5 and 97.5 percentiles from the sample. These percentiles, derived directly from the data, showed excellent agreement with those calculated from the mean assuming a gaussian distribution (ie, mean±1.96 SDs). The data comparing infants who were studied at only the first period with those studied two or three times were analyzed using one-way analysis of variance. Because of the large amount of data lost and the relatively low consistency in oximetry results between periods for those infants who were repeatedly studied, a one-way analysis of variance was performed on all the data, ignoring the within-subject effects.

RESULTS

Patient Characteristics

A total of 313 pulse oximetry studies were performed on the 150 infants, of whom there were 81 male and 69 female infants. Birth weight (mean±SE) was 3285±25 g (range, 2565 to 3858 g), and gestational age was 39.6±0.1 week (range, 37 to 42 weeks). The infants were predominantly white and middle class, as is the typical population at Rose Medical Center. Of the original 150 infants studied at 24 to 48 hours of age, 100 (67%) returned for study at 1 month, and 63 (42%) returned at 3 months of age. There were no statistical differences in birth weight, gestational age, or mean Spo_2 during any infant activity at 24 to 48 hours of age between those infants who did return for serial studies and those who did not, making it likely that those who returned were representative of the group as a whole. We therefore included all subjects who were studied at each age together. One infant died of sudden infant death syndrome at 3 months of age. Her initial and 1-month studies revealed Spo_2 values similar to those of the other infants. The remaining infants continued to be clinically well at their subsequent visits.

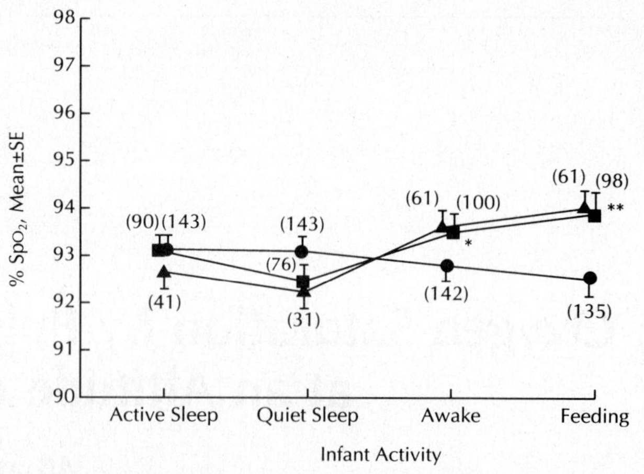

Oxygen saturation values by pulse oximetry (Spo_2) at 1610 m altitude by postnatal age and infant activity. Circles indicate 24 to 48 hours of age; squares, 1 month of age; and triangles, 3 months of age. Symbols are staggered for clarity. Values in parentheses indicate number of subjects studied in that activity; asterisk, P<.01 vs 24 to 48 hours; and double asterisk, P<.001 vs 24 to 48 hours and vs quiet sleep at 1 and 3 months.

Spo_2 and Postnatal Age

Mean Spo_2 for each age and infant activity is shown in the Figure. Mean Spo_2 was between 92% and 94% at all times. Between 24 to 48 hours and 1 month of age, saturations during the awake states (awake and feeding) increased slightly, but significantly, from 92.7%±0.2% to 93.4%±0.2% awake ($P<.01$) and from 92.4%±0.2% to 93.8%±0.2% feeding ($P<.001$). There was no further increase in Spo_2 with age after 1 month.

Spo_2 and Infant Activity

At 24 to 48 hours of age, there was no effect of infant activity on saturation (Figure). At 1 and 3 months of age, Spo_2 tended to be higher during the awake states (awake and feeding) than during sleep. This difference reached statistical significance for quiet sleep vs feeding at both 1 (92.3%±0.3% vs 93.8%±0.2%, $P<.001$) and 3 months of age (92.2%±0.4% vs 93.9%±0.3%, $P<.001$).

Reference Range of Spo_2

The 95% confidence limits for Spo_2, along with mean Spo_2 and actual ranges, are given in the Table. The lower end of the reference range (2 SDs below the mean) is as low as 85% during feeding at 24 to 48 hours of age and as low as 86% during quiet sleep at 1 and 3 months of age, with 88% to 89% being the lower limit in other activities.

COMMENT

There was a large attrition rate in our study population, with only 42% returning for study at 3 months of age despite many attempts to reschedule these visits. There were no differences in birth weight, gestational age, or Spo_2 in any activity at the time of the first study between the infants who returned and those who did not, supporting our belief that those who returned were a representative sample of the entire group.

Postnatal Age and Activity	Spo_2, % Mean ± SE	Range	95% Confidence Limits
24-48 h			
A	92.7±0.2†	83.0-98.2	88.8-97.0
F	92.4±0.2‡	83.3-98.3	85.3-96.1
AS	92.9±0.2	82.1-96.6	87.2-96.3
QS	93.0±0.2	79.1-97.6	88.0-97.0
1 mo			
A	93.4±0.2	89.7-99.2	90.2-97.2
F	93.8±0.2	87.7-98.4	89.0-98.0
AS	93.1±0.2	86.2-97.2	89.1-97.0
QS	92.3±0.2§	84.3-98.9	86.5-98.4
3 mo			
A	93.5±0.3	86.9-99.8	90.5-98.8
F	93.9±0.3	80.3-98.9	88.1-98.0
AS	92.6±0.3	87.1-95.4	89.4-94.6
QS	92.2±0.4§	85.6-97.1	85.6-97.1

Spo_2 by Age and Infant Activity*

*Spo_2 indicates oxygen saturation by pulse oximetry; A, awake; F, feeding; AS, active sleep; and QS, quiet sleep.
†$P<.01$ compared with A at 1 or 3 months.
‡$P<.001$ compared with F at 1 or 3 months.
§$P<.001$ compared with F at 1 and 3 months.

Pulse oximetry is thought to be a simple, safe, and accurate means of assessing oxygenation.[10-13] Pulse oximetry–derived saturation values have been shown to be reliable and accurate if the heart rate and pulse rate are within 5 bpm of each other, as was required in this study. The pulse oximeter used in this study has been shown to have a correlation coefficient as high as .99 with measured saturations on catheter-obtained samples.[13] For these reasons, we believe the data presented herein are a reasonable reflection of arterial saturation.

There are no published studies of oxygen saturation in healthy newborns at an altitude different from sea level with which to compare our data. Comparison of our data with those obtained at sea level, using a different brand of instrument,[4] would not be valid. Although each brand of oximeter correlates well independently with measured arterial saturations, studies comparing different instruments with each other are limited,[14,15] and only one has compared different instruments simultaneously on the same patients.[16] Certain manufacturers account for the small amounts of carboxyhemoglobin and methemoglobin present in most healthy adults in their calibration algorithms, leading to a lower Spo_2 reading than for those who do not do so.[17] Therefore, identical readings on two different brands of instrument are not necessarily interchangeable.

In looking at our own data, it is seen that there is much less variation in mean Spo_2 with infant behavior at 24 to 48 hours of life than at 1 or 3 months of age. This is unexpected in view of the desaturation that usually occurs during rapid eye movement sleep and feeding, particularly early in life.[18] Additionally, exaggerated variability in Spo_2 with infant behaviors was found at sea level in the first week of life,[4] with a significant decrease in saturation during sleep and feeding compared with the awake state, as expected (91% to 93% vs 96%). Confirmation of this lack of variability in the first days of life at altitude as well as the exploration of possible mechanisms await further study.

It is expected that oxygen saturation will decrease as altitude above sea level increases, which decreases barometric pressure (P_B) and, therefore, ambient oxygen (fraction of inspired oxygen $[Fio_2] \times P_B$). Inspired gas is then fully humidified in the upper airways, such that inspired oxygen (Pio_2) = Fio_2(PB − 47 mm Hg), 47 mm Hg being water vapor pressure at body temperature. Finally alveolar oxygen is further reduced by the presence of carbon dioxide, such that $Pao_2 = Fio_2(P_B - 47 \text{ mm Hg}) - Paco_2/0.8$, assuming a respiratory quotient of 0.8 and that alveolar Pco_2 is equal to $Paco_2$. Hyperventilation occurs to a variable degree as altitude increases, leading to a smaller drop in Pao_2 than might be expected and shifting the oxyhemoglobin dissociation curve to the left as pH increases. For these reasons, change in saturation with altitude is not linear, and accurate prediction of arterial oxygen percent saturation for a given altitude is not possible. For a complete discussion of these issues, the reader is referred to Ward et al.[19] Nomograms for P_B at different altitudes are present in standard texts.[7]

We have described a reference range for Spo_2 in healthy infants at an altitude of 1610 m. It is not clear whether infants who are clinically well at a moderate altitude of 1610 m but who have saturations below this range should be treated with supplemental oxygen. There are, to our knowledge, no studies showing that it is harmful to have oxygen saturations below this range if the infant is otherwise healthy. However, it is known that pulmonary arterial pressures fall more slowly after birth at high altitude, and that the incidence of significant pulmonary hypertension in older individuals is increased at high altitude.[20] Whether these same trends are seen at more moderate altitudes, whether one predisposes to the other, and whether treatment with supplemental oxygen in infancy might affect such a relationship, if present, will require further study.

This information should not serve as a guideline for oxygenation in infants with significant chronic lung disease at altitude. In such infants, there is evidence to support the use of supplemental oxygen to maintain saturations well above the lower end of this reference range to prevent or treat pulmonary hypertension. Both Abman et al[21] and Goodman et al[22] have shown that, at cardiac catheterization in infants with severe bronchopulmonary dysplasia, maximal pulmonary vasodilation occurs at measured arterial oxygen saturations of 93% to 95%, and that pulmonary artery pressure increases significantly at saturations as high as 89%.[21] Based on these data, it would seem appropriate to treat infants with chronic lung disease, particularly at altitude, with enough supplemental oxygen to keep Spo_2 at least at the mean (92% to 94%) rather than at the lower end of the reference range to minimize the likelihood of pulmonary hypertension.

This study describes Spo_2 in a population of clinically healthy, term infants from 24 hours to 3 months of age at an altitude of 1610 m above sea level. The mean Spo_2 at 24 to 48 hours of age is 92% to 93% and varies little with infant activity. There is a tendency for increased saturations during the awake states compared with the sleep states by 1 and 3 months of age, reaching statistical significance for quiet sleep compared with feeding. The lower end of the reference range (2 SDs below the mean) is as low as 85% during feeding at 24 to 48 hours of age and as low as 86% during quiet sleep at 1 and 3 months of age, with 88% to 89% being the lower limit in other activities.

This research was performed at Rose Medical Center and was supported by a grant from The Rose Foundation. The pulse oximeter and probe were provided by Ohmeda.

We thank Lorna G. Moore, PhD, for her review of the manuscript, Dennis Luckey, PhD, for his advice and help with the statistical analyses, and Jean Hoffman, Tammy Muehe, and Pat Winter for their secretarial assistance.

References

1. Weisbrot IM, James LS, Prince CE, Holaday DA, Apgar V. Acid-base homeostasis of the newborn infant during the first 24 hours of life. *J Pediatr.* 1958;52:394-403.
2. Oliver TK, Demis JA, Bates GD. Serial blood-gas tensions and acid-base balance during the first hour of life in human infants. *Acta Pediatr Scand.* 1961;50:346-360.
3. Koch G. Lung function and acid-base balance in the newborn infant. *Acta Pediatr Scand.* 1968;181:5-41.
4. Mok JYQ, McLaughlin K, Pintar M, et al. Transcutaneous monitoring of oxygenation: what is normal? *J Pediatr.* 1986; 108:365-371.
5. National Center for Health Statistics. *Vital Statistics of the United States, 1986,* vol 1: *Natality.* Washington, DC: Public Health Service; 1988. US Dept of Health and Human Services publication PHS 88-1123.
6. Thilo EH, Comito J, McCulliss D. Home oxygen therapy in the newborn: costs and parental acceptance. *AJDC.* 1987; 141:766-768.
7. Billings CE. Effects of physical agents. In: Sodeman WA, Sodeman TM, eds. *Pathologic Physiology: Mechanisms of Disease.* Philadelphia, Pa: WB Saunders Co; 1985:1059-1066.
8. Broughton JO. Assessment: respiratory system. In: Hudak CM, Gallo BM, Lohr T, eds. *Critical Care Nursing: A Holistic Approach.* Philadelphia, Pa: JB Lippincott; 1986:269.
9. Prechtl HFR. The behavioral states of the newborn infant (a review). *Brain Res.* 1974;76:185-212.
10. Solimano AJ, Smyth JA, Mann TK, Albersheim SG, Lockitch G. Pulse oximetry advantages in infants with bronchopulmonary dysplasia. *Pediatrics.* 1986;78:844-849.
11. Durand M, Ramanathan R. Pulse oximetry for continuous oxygen monitoring in sick newborn infants. *J Pediatr.* 1986; 109:1052-1056.
12. Dziédzick K, Vidyasagar D. Pulse oximetry in neonatal intensive care. *Clin Perinatol.* 1989;16:177-197.
13. Hay WW, Brockway JM, Eyzaguirre M. Neonatal pulse oximetry: accuracy and reliability. *Pediatrics.* 1989;83:717-722.
14. Bucher H, Fanconi S, Baeckert P, Duc G. Hyperoxemia in newborn infants: detection by pulse oximetry. *Pediatrics.* 1989; 84:226-230.
15. Severinghaus JW, Naifeh KH. Accuracy of response of six pulse oximeters to profound hypoxia. *Anesthesiology.* 1987; 67:551-558.
16. Russell RIR, Helms PJ. Comparative accuracy of pulse oximetry and transcutaneous oxygen in assessing arterial saturation in pediatric intensive care. *Crit Care Med.* 1990;18:725-727.
17. Wukitsch MW, Petterson MT, Tobler DR, Pologe JA. Pulse oximetry: analysis of theory, technology and practice. *J Clin Monit.* 1988;4:290-301.
18. Nelson NM. The onset of respiration. In: Avery GB, ed. *Neonatology: Pathophysiology and Management of the Newborn.* Philadelphia, Pa: JB Lippincott; 1987:189.
19. Ward MP, Milledge JS, West JB, eds. *High Altitude Medicine and Physiology.* Philadelphia, Pa: University of Pennsylvania Press; 1989:83-98, 179-200.
20. Reeves JT, Grover RF. High-altitude pulmonary hypertension and pulmonary edema. *Prog Cardiol.* 1975;4:99-118.
21. Abman SH, Wolfe RR, Accurso FJ, Koops BL, Bowman M, Wiggins JW. Pulmonary vascular response to oxygen in infants with severe bronchopulmonary dysplasia. *Pediatrics.* 1985; 75:80-84.
22. Goodman G, Perkin RM, Anas NG, Sperling DR, Hicks DA, Rowen A. Pulmonary hypertension in infants with bronchopulmonary dysplasia. *J Pediatr.* 1988;112:67-72.

Posthemorrhagic Hydrocephalus

Use of an Intravenous-Type Catheter for Cerebrospinal Fluid Drainage

Peter J. Marro, MD; Douglas A. Dransfield, MD; Stephen H. Mott, MD; Walter C. Allan, MD

Study Objective: **To report a 9-year experience with the treatment of posthemorrhagic hydrocephalus (PHH) with the use of an easily inserted external ventricular drain.**

Design: **A case series with a retrospective review of hospital records and cranial ultrasound results, from 1981 through 1989, in all infants with PHH.**

Intervention: **A previously defined method of identification and bedside management of PHH was applied. If infants reached 2 kg of body weight and PHH recurred, a ventriculoperitoneal shunt was inserted.**

Results: **A total of 70 procedures were performed in 24 patients, and all were associated with a decrease in head circumference and ventricular size on ultrasound scan. One infection occurred, and only 12 infants required a ventriculoperitoneal shunt.**

Conclusions: **This technique compared favorably with other methods of intervention to avoid early placement of a ventriculoperitoneal shunt in preterm infants and offered the advantage of consistently decreasing ventricular size. A multicenter-controlled trial will be needed to compare the safety and efficacy of therapies for PHH.**

(*AJDC.* 1991;145:1141-1146)

The treatment of posthemorrhagic hydrocephalus (PHH) is an unresolved clinical problem in the management of preterm infants with intraventricular hemorrhage (IVH). The placement of a ventriculoperitoneal (VP) shunt is the treatment of hydrocephalus in general, but the timing of its use in PHH is quite variable. Some authors will elect VP shunting in extremely preterm infants (weight, <1200 g),[1-4] while others will attempt to delay this procedure with various treatments.[5-13] Those investigators who temporize usually introduce a treatment based on the appearance of "progressive" ventricular dilation on cranial ultrasound (US) scan. However, there is no agreement on criteria that would quantify ventricular dilation, and some authors judge this by appearance alone, while others make various measurements and compare them with standard curves. Without a uniform definition, it is difficult to evaluate the results of the many studies of temporizing treatment of PHH.

Because we were unconvinced that early treatment methods were successful, we wished to introduce a treatment only in the setting in which we might consider a VP shunt. Ventricular dilation that caused increased intracranial pressure (ICP) was the criteria for treatment. Signs of increased ICP in premature infants, eg, obtundation or pupillary or other eye signs, are not reliably present. However, the open fontanelles and lack of cranial suture diastasis in preterm infants allow significant intracranial hypertension to be quantified by a simple measurement—the occipital-frontal circumference (OFC). This fact was demonstrated by Hill and Volpe[14] in a study of transfontanelle and lumbar puncture (LP) pressures that were correlated with OFC changes. Thus, we defined PHH as rapid head growth and marked ventricular dilation on US scan. Since it was imperative in this setting to produce ventricular decompression, we arrived at a bedside method of external ventricular drainage (EVD) that utilized an intravenous catheter and a closed drainage system.

This report presents a 9-year experience in treating PHH with percutaneous EVD. We wished, in addition, to contrast our approach to that of other published therapies for PHH, and we present reasons for a controlled trial of PHH treatment.

PATIENTS AND METHODS

Patient Selection

Since 1979, all infants aged younger than 35 weeks' gestation who were admitted to the neonatal intensive care unit of the Maine Medical Center, Portland, and who survived and remained in the neonatal intensive care unit were examined by cranial US scan on the second or third day of life and again a week later. Follow-up scans were performed weekly if IVH had occurred. The prospective collection of these examinations that were recorded on videotape has been ongoing. Throughout the period from 1981 through 1989, consistent definitions of grade of hemorrhage, ventriculomegaly, and PHH have been utilized. To prepare this report, the patients in whom PHH developed were identified with the use of the Cranial US Database of the Maine Medical Center, and their hospital medical records were reviewed. All records were analyzed for the same information about the circumstances of treatment with EVD, its complications, and hospital course to either discharge or VP shunt placement.

Definitions of Cranial US Abnormalities

The system for classification of US abnormalities has previously been reported.[15] Hemorrhage was graded as a germinal matrix hemorrhage (GMH), small IVH, large IVH, and IVH with intraparenchymal hemorrhage (IVH/IPH). A GMH was defined

Accepted for publication June 24, 1991.

From the Department of Pediatrics, Maine Medical Center, Portland.

Presented in part at the annual meeting of the Child Neurology Society, Atlanta, Ga, October 19, 1990.

Reprint requests to 180 Park Ave, Portland, ME 04102 (Dr Allan).

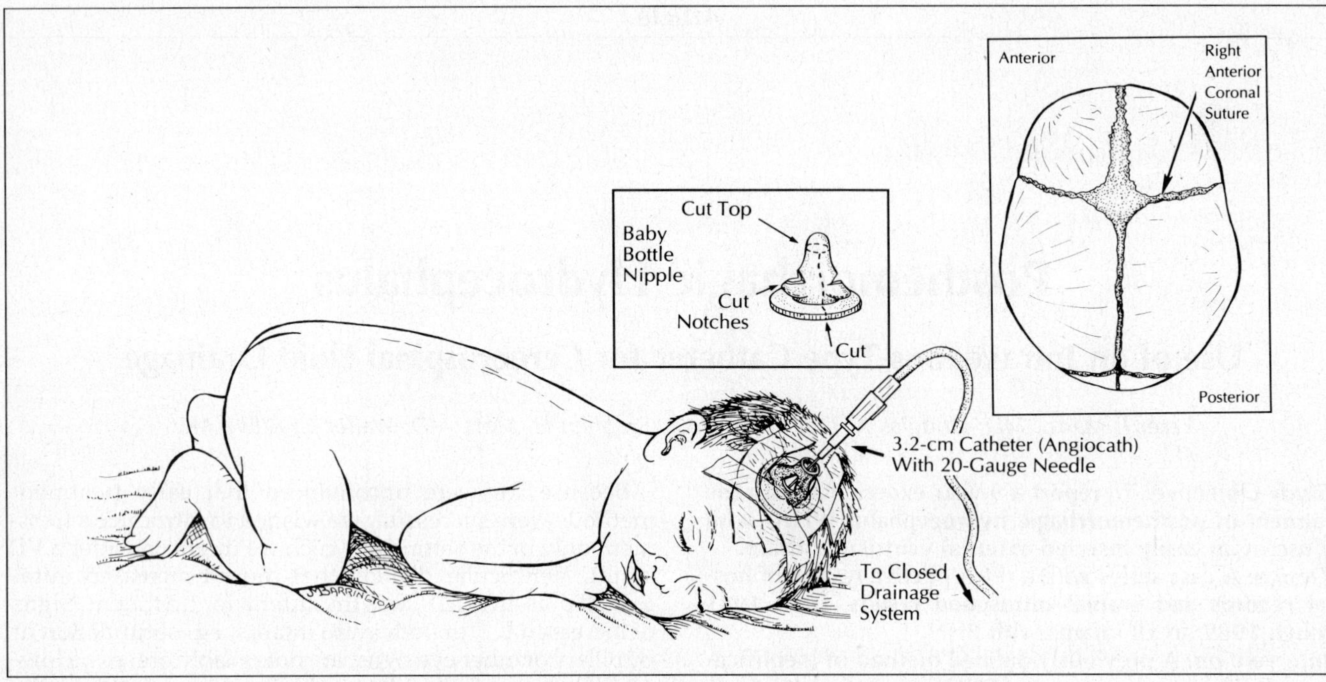

Fig 1.—*Placing and securing the catheter for external ventricular drainage. The venous catheter is shown separate from the collar for illustration. How the nipple is cut to provide the collar for securing the catheter is shown in the inset.*

as an echodensity that was limited to the germinal matrix. A small IVH was defined as an echodensity that occupied less than 50% of a normal-sized lateral ventricle, usually accompanied by a GMH. A large IVH was defined as an echodensity that occupied greater than 50% of a dilated lateral ventricle. The category IVH/IPH constituted an echodensity in the parenchyma contiguous to a GMH and usually a large IVH.

Follow-up scans were performed weekly if a small or large IVH or IVH/IPH had occurred. Ventricular dilation following IVH was quantified by measuring the ventricular diameter on the sagittal scan as previously described.[10] If the ventricular diameter increased beyond 1 cm, clinical criteria were applied to divide the dilation into the two groups: ventriculomegaly and PHH. Ventriculomegaly was defined as increased size of one or both of the lateral ventricles *without* signs of increased ICP or an increase in the OFC of less than 2 cm/wk. Posthemorrhagic hydrocephalus was defined as increased ventricular size by cranial US scan, measuring greater than 1.5 cm at the midbody on sagittal scan, *and* an increase in the OFC greater than 2 cm/wk with or without other signs of increased ICP. No treatment occurred unless the criteria for PHH were met. That is, we did not treat ventriculomegaly.

Therapy for PHH

For all infants, the same approach to clinical management of hemorrhage was applied. Assessment of the lateral ventricular size and therapy needed for PHH were also standardized. If the infant had IVH or IVH/IPH on initial study, daily measurement of the OFC was started, and weekly repeated US scans were done until 1 month of age. When dilation of either lateral ventricles was present, and the criteria for PHH were met, an initial LP was done in all infants. If LP produced greater than 10 mL of cerebrospinal fluid (CSF), a repeated OFC measurement and US scan were done. If ventricular dilation was improved, attempts at management by repeated LP was begun. In our experience, this eventually proved to be unsatisfactory in all patients because they could not tolerate prolonged handling to collect CSF by LP, or the amount of fluid decreased to an amount that did not improve ventricular size. When initial or subsequent LP was ineffective, percutaneous EVD was started. The method of insertion and criteria for removal are described below. After removal of the EVD catheter, the infant was reassessed for continued PHH. A repeated EVD was performed as soon as 3 days later if rapid reexpansion of the lateral ventricles to the size at onset of EVD occurred, accompanied by a rapid increase in the OFC. Recurrent PHH was managed with repetitive EVD unless the infant weighed more than 2 kg of body weight at which time a VP shunt was employed. Patients who had been treated with EVD were no longer candidates for drainage if ventricular enlargement resolved or if ventricular enlargement persisted but rapid head growth or signs of increased ICP were no longer present. All patients with enlarged ventricles regardless of whether they met criteria for EVD continued to have daily OFC measurements to monitor for late PHH.

Technique for EVD

The site of insertion for the catheter was the right coronal suture at the edge of the anterior fontanelle (Fig 1). With the use of a sterile technique, including shaving the scalp and skin preparation with povidone-iodine, a 3.2-cm intravenous catheter with a 20-gauge needle for insertion was introduced percutaneously in a manner similar to that used for ventricular tap. However, the catheter was not angled toward the inner canthus of the ipsilateral eye. Rather, it was passed directly toward the midbody of the lateral ventricle so that it protruded at a 90° angle to the plane of the skull. This facilitated securing it in place. With return of CSF, the catheter was advanced over the needle slightly, and the needle was removed. After collecting CSF for laboratory tests, a ventriculostomy drainage collection bag and tubing set were connected to the catheter hub. Because there was usually about 1.5 cm of catheter exposed beyond the skin, the catheter and tubing were supported by a collar that was made from a standard feeding nipple. The collar was taped in place, and the hub of the catheter and the tubing were secured to the collar. In Fig 1, to illustrate the connection of the catheter to the tubing, the final position of the supporting nipple collar is not shown. In its final position, the nipple completely encircled the end of the hub of the catheter and the tubing connector. At initial insertion and fluid drainage, some infants became pale or mottled, perhaps caused by a rapid drop in ICP. This responded to temporary interruption of fluid drainage. Part of the collection-tubing system was a one-way valve and drip chamber. The position of this valve could be adjusted to correspond to centimeters of water pressure in the lateral ventricle. A level that was 2 to 4 cm above the insertion site was usually

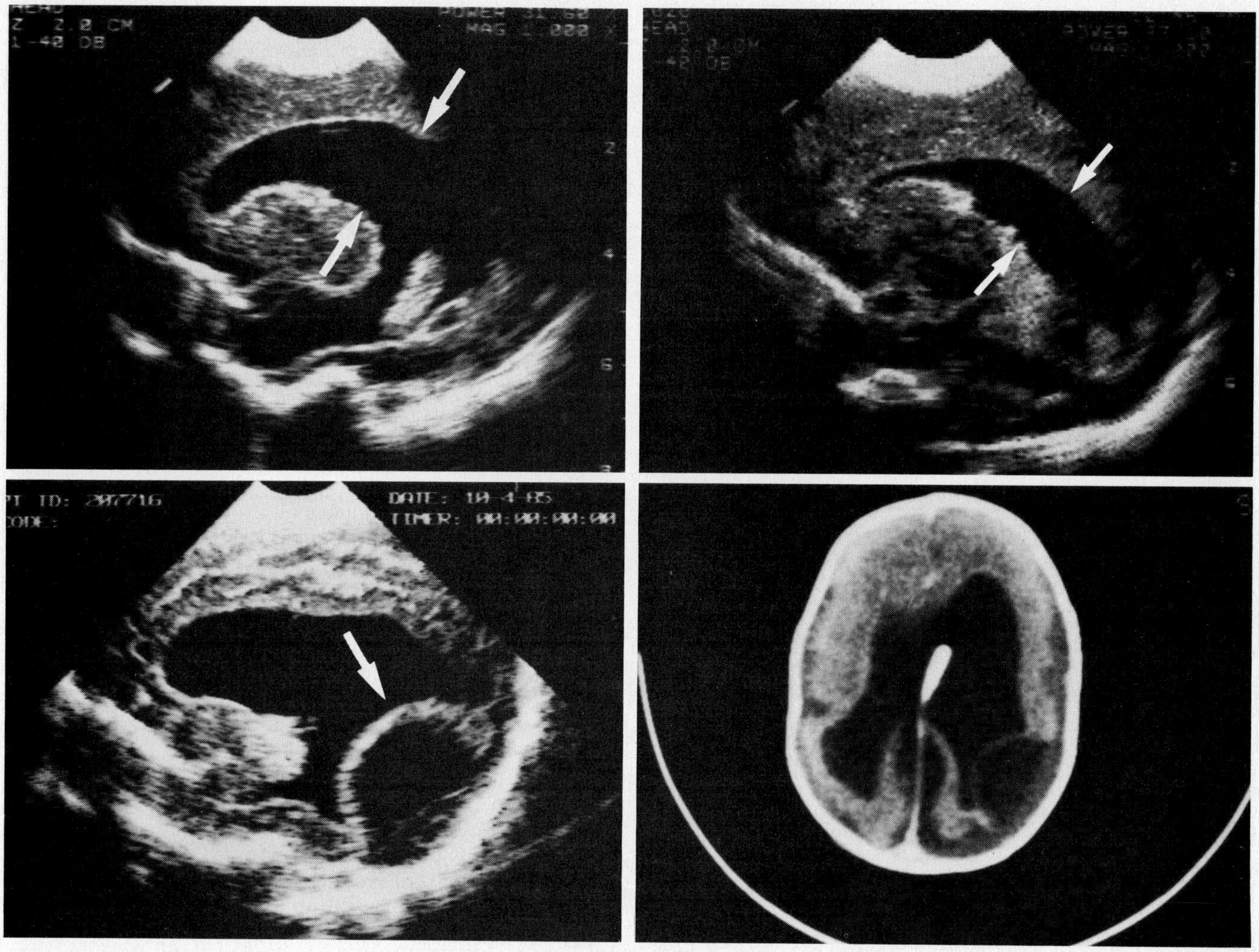

Fig 2.—*Top left, Sagittal cranial ultrasound scan of the left lateral ventricle in an infant with posthemorrhagic hydrocephalus prior to external ventricular drainage. The arrows point to the ventricular diameter that measured 1.8 cm at this point. Top right, Sagittal scan of the left lateral ventricular in the same infant following external ventricular drainage. The arrows point to the ventricular diameter that measured 1.2 cm at the midbody with much improved anterior horn dilation. Bottom left, Sagittal cranial ultrasound scan of the left lateral ventricle in an infant treated with a ventriculoperitoneal shunt that required three revisions over a period of 4 weeks. The child was transferred to the Maine Medical Center, Portland, with a ventricular reservoir in place. The scan was obtained following external ventricular drainage at the Maine Medical Center. The arrow points to the occipital cortex that failed to reexpand with drainage of ventricular fluid. Bottom right, Computed tomographic scan demonstrates the subdural fluid collection over the left hemisphere in this infant that accumulated due to lack of reexpansion of the occipital cortex.*

needed to achieve a flow of 5 to 20 mL/8 h. The amount of CSF that drained in each 8 hours was replaced milliliter for milliliter with 5% dextrose and normal saline solution during the next 8 hours. Subsequent readjustments were made as the infant's condition changed. Success of EVD is dependent on nursing care that can monitor a patient's condition without allowing the infant to disrupt the EVD. Further information about the technique of insertion and the care of infants with EVD is available from the authors.

Criteria for Removal

The catheter was removed for any of the following five reasons: (1) failure to drain CSF for 8 hours that could not be corrected by lowering the level of the valve or slight withdrawal of the catheter; (2) any leakage of blood or CSF *around* the catheter at the insertion site; (3) excessive blood draining through the catheter (almost all patients had a small amount of blood in the fluid, and this continued intermittently during the drainage—blood that filled the tubing was excessive); (4) any change in the infant's condition that could have been consistent with infection was reason for culture of the fluid in the tubing and removal of the catheter; and (5) successful completion of 7 days of CSF drainage.

RESULTS

Patient Population

There were 1498 infants born at under 35 weeks' gestation who were admitted to the neonatal intensive care unit of Maine Medical Center from January 1981 through the end of December 1989. Of these, 110 died before initial evaluation by cranial US, leaving 1388 infants. A GMH only occurred in 92 infants. A small IVH was present in 85. None of these 177 infants experienced PHH. An IPH with or without IVH was found in 34 infants. Of these, 19 survived to 1 month of age, and PHH developed in 10 (53%) of them. A large IVH was found in 60 infants; 46 survived to 1 month of age, and PHH developed in 14 (30%). Posthemorrhagic hydrocephalus was seen only in infants who had a previous IPH or large IVH and developed in 37% (24/65) of such infants who survived to 1 month of age. No infant who survived less than a month was treated for PHH during this period.

Table 1.—Problems Encountered During 70 EVDs*	
Problem	No.
Resaons for removal of EDVs	
Placement unsuccessful	5
Suspected infection	5
Leaking	17
Excessive bleeding	18
Nonfunctioning	30
Patient complications	
Confirmed infection	1
Hyponatremia	1
Apnea	2
Bradycardia	2

*EVDs indicate external ventricular drainages.

Table 2.—Summary of Outcome in PHH*

Grade IVH	No. of EVDs			VP Shunt		Died, <2 kg†	Total
	1	2-3	≥4	No	Yes		
Large IVH	4	6	4	7	6	1	14
IVH/IPH	1	5	4	2	6	2	10
Total	**5**	**11**	**8**	**9**	**12**	**3**	**24**

*PHH indicates posthemorrhagic hydrocephalus; IVH, intraventricular hemorrhage; EVDs, external ventricular drainages; VP, ventriculoperitoneal; and IPH, intraparenchymal hemorrhage. Data are given as number of infants, except for EVDs.

†Weight of infant.

The 24 infants in whom PHH developed had a mean gestational age of 29 weeks (range, 25 to 34 weeks) and a mean birth weight of 1.31 kg (range, 0.7 to 1.95 kg). The number of EVD procedures per patient ranged from 1 to 7. Most patients (14/24) had three or fewer episodes of EVD. The age at insertion of the first EVD (ie, failure to control PHH by LP) had a range of 11 to 105 days, with 22 infants having their first procedure by 27 days. Two patients were initially treated by EVD at 53 and 105 days. The mean age for all 24 patients was 23 days, but for the 22 infants with a more typical onset of PHH, the mean age was 18 days.

Efficacy of EVD

The purpose of EVD was to (1) reverse the signs of ICP (ie, the rapid rise in the OFC) and (2) drain temporarily CSF, allowing reexpansion of the brain. Therefore, three measures of the effectiveness of EVD were (1) the change in the OFC during the time of drainage, (2) the change in ventricular diameter at the midbody on sagittal scan,[10] and (3) the volume of CSF removed on the first day (not all catheters functioned more than 1 day). The measurement of ventricular diameter and its improvement following EVD are illustrated in Fig 2. The example of an infant we encountered who no longer had reexpansion of the cortex with EVD is also shown in Fig 2 for comparison.

With regard to the results of EVD, there were a total of 70 procedures performed on this group of 24 infants; the mean duration of these EVD procedures was 3.5 days (range, 1 to 7 days). The decrease in the OFC before and after insertion in these 70 episodes of EVD (n=66) had a mean±SD of 0.85±0.53 cm (range, 0.1 to 1.75 cm). The volume of CSF that was drained on the first day (n=65) had a mean±SD of 42 (exactly 41.3)±21.4 mL (range, 23 to 72 mL). For 47 of the 70 EVD procedures, it was possible to obtain a cranial US scan within 12 hours after removal of the catheter. The size of the lateral ventricle before and after EVD was compared to assess ventricular decompression. The lack of ventricular decompression during EVD only occurred if the system was nonfunctioning. That is, as long as CSF drainage was in the range of the SD given above, the ventricles decreased in size with an increase in the width of the cortical mantle. The amount of decrease in ventricular size (diameter) per EVD (n=47) was 0.93±0.56 cm (mean±SD).

The intent at insertion of an EVD was to keep it in place for 7 days. The reasons for removal of the ventricular catheter in each of these procedures are listed in Table 1. Of the 70 procedures, five times the fluid would not continue to drain after the tubing was taped in place, and the catheter was removed immediately. This was followed by a repeated procedure on the next day. These five procedures were the equivalent of a ventricular tap with the removal of 15 to 20 mL of CSF. Forty-three of the 70 EVDs lasted 4 or more days, with 13 lasting all 7 days. Of the 57 removed before 7 days, the reasons for removal are shown in Table 1.

The complications that were encountered are also listed in Table 1. There was one confirmed infection. This infant had coagulase-negative *Staphylococcus* that was grown from the CSF when EVD was removed for suspected infection. The patient was successfully treated with vancomycin. Two infants had apnea; two had episodes of bradycardia but did not have bacterial infection. One infant with apnea died after progressive respiratory failure. Hyponatremia developed in one infant during EVD, but this was corrected with increased sodium replacement.

The eventual need for a VP shunt in this group of infants is shown in Table 2. The 24 infants with PHH are listed by whether the initial hemorrhage had been an isolated large IVH (n=14) or IVH/IPH (n=10). These two groups were compared as to the number of EVDs per patient and treatment with a VP shunt. Overall, three infants died before reaching 2 kg of body weight. All deaths were a result of respiratory complications. There was a tendency for the infants who had IVH/IPH with subsequent PHH to need multiple EVDs and to require a VP shunt eventually.

Figure 3 shows the number of EVDs per patient compared with the need for eventual treatment with a VP shunt. Of the 21 survivors, nine were treated with EVD only, and 12 eventually were treated with a VP shunt. In the nine survivors who were treated with EVD only, the number of EVD procedures per patient ranged from one to five. It is interesting to note that even when five procedures were required, a VP shunt was avoided in one infant. The patient who had one EVD before a VP shunt did not have rapid head growth despite ventricular enlargement and a porencephalic cyst on a cranial US scan until the age of 105 days; at that point, he met criteria for EVD placement when the OFC increased 2 cm in 1 week. A single treatment with EVD was elected although the infant weighed 2880 g. When PHH recurred, he was treated with a VP shunt.

COMMENT

Treatment of PHH should promptly relieve intracranial hypertension with resolution of clinical signs and reexpansion of the cortical mantle. Ideally, the method used should be safe and easy to apply. A VP shunt is the standard method of hydrocephalus treatment, and although it is possible to use a VP shunt in preterm infants with PHH, there is a high failure rate in this population. Because assessment of VP shunt function is difficult in these patients, lack of function may go undetected with return of intracranial hypertension, leading to permanent injury of the cortical mantle. The cranial US scans in Fig 2 demonstrate differing cortical mantle responses to CSF drainage in PHH. The child who had multiple VP shunt revisions no longer had the response illustrated by our patient following EVD.

Shankaran et al[4] recently reviewed their experience, including neurodevelopmental outcome, in infants who had early insertion of a VP shunt following PHH. Infants were shunted if the OFC increased greater than 2 cm/wk as in our group. The mean age at shunt insertion was 26 days, and the mean weight was 1018 g in 23 infants who met the criteria. Multiple revisions were required in 18 (78%), and they found that ventricular decompression did not occur in 16 (70%) following the first procedure. Their protocol called for a repeated shunt insertion after 2 or 3 weeks if ventricular size had not decreased. This failure of ventricular decompression was found to be the most important predictor of outcome in their study. Whether the authors thought cortical injury had occurred as a result of nonfunctioning of the shunt was not stated. Other reports also have documented the high incidence of failure of early VP shunting and the high infection rate.[1-3]

Because of the difficulties encountered with early VP shunting, multiple treatments have been tried. Various drugs have been used in an attempt to control CSF production. These include isosorbide, glycerol, acetazolamide, and furosemide.[5,6,13] These treatments were started with varying degrees of ventricular dilation. In many cases, treatment was used in patients who would not be considered to have hydrocephalus by our criteria, and for whom spontaneous resolution without treatment might have occurred. Therefore, these treatments remain of uncertain value in preventing the necessity of a VP shunt for hydrocephalus.

The other major treatment, repeated LP, has been evaluated in controlled trials. The design of these studies has evaluated repeated LP as both a prophylactic treatment before development of ventricular dilation, as well as a treatment designed to reverse progression of established ventricular dilation. Both Mantovani and colleagues[9] and Anwar et al[16] introduced serial LPs in the first 1 to 2 weeks following the diagnosis of IVH by a US or computed tomographic scan. The use of repeated LP failed to decrease the incidence of ventricular dilation or the eventual need for a VP shunt compared with that for control groups.

Two recent studies evaluated repeated LP as a treatment of established ventricular dilation following IVH. Dykes et al[17] utilized simple inspection of weekly follow-up computed tomographic or US scans to categorize ventricular dilation as mild, moderate, or severe. Infants with severe ventricular dilation were randomized to treatment (daily LP) or to control groups. If infants in the control group experienced a progressive decrease in the cortical mantle, signs of increased ICP, or an OFC increase greater than 2 cm/wk, they were treated with LP. If these findings occurred despite daily LP, the infants were treated with EVD if they weighed less than 1701 g or with a VP shunt if they weighed greater than 1800 g. They found no difference between control and treatment groups with regard to eventual need for a VP shunt. In addition, follow-up data, available at 3 to 6 years, were no different between control and treatment groups. Despite this, the authors stated that they have continued to use LP to avoid or postpone ventricular shunting. Analysis of their data would suggest daily LP was not very good at avoiding VP shunting. Of 50 infants who were studied, 19 (12 in the symptomatic severe PH group and seven in the close-observation group who subsequently required LP) eventually satisfied criteria similar to those that we applied for the diagnosis of PHH. Of these, 15 (74%) were eventually shunted. By the combined use of LP and EVD, they were able to get infants to a weight of 1800 g before shunting.

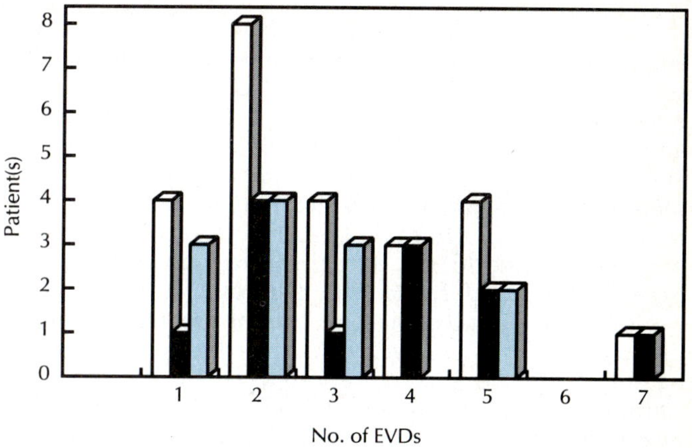

Fig 3.—*Bar graph of the number of external ventricular drainages (EVDs) compared with outcome with or without a ventriculoperitoneal shunt. Open bars indicate total; closed bars, shunted; and shaded bars, not shunted.*

A multicenter-controlled trial of repeated LP was recently published.[18] The Ventriculomegaly Trial Group consisted of 15 neonatal units in Great Britain and Ireland. They enrolled 157 infants with progressive ventricular dilation on cranial US scans. Their criteria for progression was based on measurement of ventricular size on coronal US scans to quantify ventricular dilation before enrollment. As part of their protocol, ventricular taps were instituted if LP failed to produce 2 mL of CSF. The control group went on to have LP and/or ventricular taps if there was an increase in the OFC greater than 2 cm/wk; this is the same definition that we used for PHH. Interestingly, ventricular tap was required in 65 of 134 infants who were treated initially by LP. They found no difference in the rate of VP shunting in treatment vs the control group. Their outcome results suggested that in infants with parenchymal hemorrhage, early LP (ie, institution of LP at the time that they met ventricular dilation criteria) improved some outcome parameters. Thus, they tentatively recommended LP in this group. As with Dykes et al,[17] comparison with our protocol is possible only in the control group that failed conservative management. Of the initial 78 infants who were randomized to this group, 55 experienced rapid head growth of greater than 2 cm/wk. Despite LP alone in 22 and LP and ventricular taps in 33, a VP shunt was eventually required in 42 (76%). This percentage was similar to that observed by Dykes et al.[17]

There are four methods of ventricular drainage available: two surgical and two percutaneous methods. The surgical methods are indwelling (subcutaneously tunneled) ventriculostomy that is meant to be long-standing and ventricular fluid withdrawal via a surgically placed ventricular catheter with a reservoir. The percutaneous methods are repeated direct ventricular taps and intermittent EVD. The major difference between these methods is largely technical, and thus, various authors feel more or less comfortable with each on that basis. Published rates of infection per patient treated for each method are as follows: indwelling ventriculostomy (Harbaugh et al[19]), none of 11; repeated ventricular tap (The Ventriculomegaly Trial Group[18]), eight of 65; ventricular reservoir (Anwar et al[20]), two of 19, and (Leonhardt et al[21]), none of 13; and intermittent EVD (present study), one of 24. The eventual incidence of VP shunting in these reports are as follows: Harbaugh et al,[19] 78% (7/9); The Ventriculomegaly Trial Group,[18] 76% (42/55); Anwar et al,[20] 83% (15/18); Leonhardt et al,[21] 92% (12/13); and the present study, 57% (12/21).

Thus, we believe that intermittent EVD appears to be as effective and safe as other methods. In addition, as our results have shown, EVD offers a reliable method of ventricular decompression that can be applied at the bedside. The ease of insertion of the catheter encourages removal if any problem occurs, thus minimizing the dangers of infection, rebleeding, and nonfunctioning. As was pointed out by The Ventriculomegaly Trial Group,[18] because of the low incidence of PHH, only a multicenter-controlled trial will be capable of critically evaluating whatever treatment is proposed. A more convincing demonstration of the value of our method of EVD would require such a controlled trial.

We would like to thank Donald Wilson, MD, and Thomas Mehalic, MD, for their neurosurgical expertise in perfecting this method; Ken Allan for maintenance of the Cranial Ultrasound Database; Judy Barrington for the illustration; Alistair Philip, MD, for reading the manuscript and making helpful suggestions; and Gloria Fiore for typing the manuscript.

References

1. Bada HS, Salmon JH, Pearson DH. Early surgical intervention in posthemorrhagic hydrocephalus. *Childs Brain.* 1979;5:109-115.

2. James HE, Bejar RF, Gluck L, et al. Ventriculoperitoneal shunts in high risk newborns weighing under 2000 grams: a clinical report. *Neurosurgery.* 1984;15:198-202.

3. Boynton BR, Boynton CA, Merritt TA, Vaucher YE, James HE, Bejar RF. Ventriculoperitoneal shunts in low birth weight infants with intracranial hemorrhage: neurodevelopmental outcome. *Neurosurgery.* 1986;18:141-145.

4. Shankaran S, Koepke T, Woldt E, et al. Outcome after posthemorrhagic ventriculomegaly in comparison with mild hemorrhage without ventriculomegaly. *J Pediatr.* 1989;114:109-114.

5. Lorber J. Isosorbide in treatment of infantile hydrocephalus. *Arch Dis Child.* 1975;50:431-436.

6. Volpe JJ. Neonatal intracranial hemorrhage: pathophysiology, neuropathology and clinical features. *Clin Perinatol.* 1977;4:77-81.

7. Goldstein GW, Chaplin ER, Maitland J, Norman D. Transient hydrocephalus in premature infants: treatment by lumbar punctures. *Lancet.* 1976;1:512-514.

8. Papile LA, Burstein R, Burstein J, Koffler H, Hoops BL, Johnson JD. Posthemorrhagic hydrocephalus in low birth weight infants: treatment by serial lumbar punctures. *J Pediatr.* 1980;97:273-277.

9. Mantovani JF, Pasternak JF, Mathew OP, et al. Failure of daily lumbar punctures to prevent the development of hydrocephalus following intraventricular hemorrhage. *J Pediatr.* 1980;97:278-281.

10. Allan WC, Holt PJ, Sawyer LR, Tito AM, Meade SK. Ventricular dilation after neonatal periventricular intraventricular hemorrhage. *AJDC.* 1982;136:589-593.

11. Kreusser KL, Tarby TJ, Taylor D, et al. Rapidly progressive posthemorrhagic hydrocephalus: treatment with external ventricular drainage. *AJDC.* 1984;138:633-637.

12. Kreusser KL, Tarby TJ, Kovnar E, Taylor DA, Hill A, Volpe J. Serial lumbar punctures for at least temporary amelioration of neonatal posthemorrhagic hydrocephalus. *Pediatrics.* 1985;75:719-725.

13. Shinnar S, Gammon K, Bergman EW, Epstein M, Freeman JM. Management of hydrocephalus in infancy: use of acetazolemide and furosemide to avoid cerebrospinal fluid shunts. *J Pediatr.* 1985;107:31-37.

14. Hill A, Volpe JJ. Normal pressure hydrocephalus in the newborn. *Pediatrics.* 1981;68:623-629.

15. Allan WC. Intraventricular hemorrhage. *J Child Neurol.* 1989;4:S12-S22.

16. Anwar M, Kadam S, Hiatt IM, Hegyi T. Serial lumbar punctures in prevention of post-hemorrhagic hydrocephalus in preterm infants. *J Pediatr.* 1985;107:446-450.

17. Dykes FD, Dunbar B, Lazarra A, Ahmann PA. Posthemorrhagic hydrocephalus in high-risk preterm infants: natural history, management and long-term outcome. *J Pediatr.* 1989;114:611-618.

18. The Ventriculomegaly Trial Group. Randomized trial of early tapping neonatal posthaemorrhagic ventricular dilatation. *Arch Dis Child.* 1990;65:3-10.

19. Harbaugh RE, Saunders RL, Edwards WH. External ventricular drainage for control of posthemorrhagic hydrocephalus in premature infants. *J Neurosurg.* 1981;55:766-770.

20. Anwar M, Doyle AJ, Kadam S, Hiatt IM, Hegyi T. Management of posthemorrhagic hydrocephalus in the preterm infant. *J Pediatr Surg.* 1986;21:334-337.

21. Leonhardt A, Steiner H-H, Linderkamp O. Management of posthaemorrhagic hydrocephalus with a subcutaneous ventricular catheter reservoir in premature infants. *Arch Dis Child.* 1989;64:24-28.

How Much Vitamin D for Neonates?

William B. Pittard III, MD; Kitty M. Geddes, RN, BSN; Thomas C. Hulsey, MSPH, ScD; Bruce W. Hollis, PhD

• To assess the adequacy of different dosages of neonatal vitamin D, 25–hydroxyvitamin D serum concentrations were longitudinally monitored in 27 low-birth-weight and 25 full-term well infants from birth to 16 weeks after delivery. The infants were randomly assigned to receive either 10 μg/d (400 IU/d) or 20 μg/d (800 IU/d) of vitamin D or 0.85 or 1.5 μg/d of 25–hydroxyvitamin D_3. In each infant who received 10 or 20 μg/d of vitamin D 25–hydroxyvitamin D, serum concentrations greater than 20 ng/mL were maintained, with some low-birth-weight infants reaching 60-ng/mL concentrations. Similarly, in the low-birth-weight infants receiving 1.5 and 0.85 μg/d of 25–hydroxyvitamin D_3, serum 25–hydroxyvitamin D levels greater than 12 ng/mL were maintained. In the full-term infants who received 1.5 μg/d of 25–hydroxyvitamin D_3, serum 25–hydroxyvitamin D concentrations of greater than 12 ng/mL were maintained, but in those who received 0.85 μg/d, serum 25–hydroxyvitamin D concentrations of 10 ng/mL could not be maintained. These vitamin D status data document that 10 μg (400 IU) of vitamin D represents a sufficient daily intake for both premature and full-term well infants. These data also indicate that while as little as 0.85 μg/d of 25–hydroxyvitamin D_3 may facilitate vitamin D sufficiency in low-birth-weight neonates, it does not do so in full-term infants.

(*AJDC*. 1991;145:1147-1149)

The understanding of vitamin D metabolism and its antirachitic role has dramatically expanded during the last decade.[1,2] Despite this improved metabolic understanding, there are few tangible data regarding the vitamin D status of full-term or premature infants receiving different doses. Thus, recommendations for daily neonatal vitamin D intake have been and continue to be based on estimated requirements based on indirect investigational data.[3,4] To provide tangible status data, four different daily vitamin D dosages were randomly assigned to 27 well, low-birth-weight, premature infants and 25 well full-term infants from birth to 16 weeks after delivery. During this time, the serum 25–hydroxyvitamin D (25[OH]D) concentration was monitored to assess vitamin D sufficiency.

Accepted for publication February 11, 1991.

From the Department of Pediatrics, Medical University of South Carolina, Charleston.

Reprint requests to the Department of Pediatrics, Medical University of South Carolina, 171 Ashley Ave, Charleston, SC 29425-3313 (Dr Pittard).

METHODS

This investigation was approved by the Medical University of South Carolina (Charleston) Human Investigation Committee, and written parental consent was obtained for each newborn before the study began. Low-birth-weight infants (n = 27) were chosen randomly within 12 hours of birth after the presence of minimal lung disease had been established based on clinical examination findings. Similarly, term infants (n = 25) were selected at random within 12 hours of birth from among those who had no clinically apparent problem. Gestational age was initially determined from the history of the mother's last menstrual period and was confirmed with a Ballard examination within 36 hours of birth.[5] Weight was determined at birth and biweekly with a standard balance scale (Detecto Scale Company, Webb City, Mo).

To facilitate a consistent daily intake of vitamin D, each neonate was given throughout the study an 84 J/30 mL formula that contained 12.8 mmol/L of calcium, 12.6 mmol/L of phosphorus, and no added vitamin D (Ross Laboratories, Columbus, Ohio). The randomly assigned vitamin D dosages included 10 or 20 μg/d of vitamin D (400 or 800 IU/d, respectively) or 0.85 or 1.5 μg/d of 25–hydroxycholecaliferol (25[OH]D_3 or calcidiol). The vitamin D was given to each infant in a glycerol carrier as a daily oral supplement. Serum 25(OH)D concentrations as well as parathyroid hormone, calcium, and phosphorus concentrations were measured biweekly. Maternal 25(OH)D concentration was measured in serum drawn at delivery.

Initially, ionized calcium concentration was measured in both premature and term infant serum. However, after ionized calcium was measured in seven low-birth-weight infants and 17 term infants, because of serum volume requirements for measuring ionized calcium, total calcium was measured in the remaining 20 premature and eight term infants. Total calcium and phosphorus measurements as well as vitamin D metabolite concentrations were determined according to previously published techniques.[6-8] Serum ionized calcium concentrations were measured with an ionized calcium analyzer (Radiometer ICA1, Radiometer Inc, West Lake, Ohio). Midmolecule parathyroid hormone was measured via radioimmunoassay.[9] Pearson's Product-Moment Correlation Coefficients were used to assess the associations of variables.

RESULTS

The study patients included five term and four premature white infants and 20 term and 23 premature black infants. Eleven of the term and eight of the premature infants were male. The mean(±SD) gestational ages for the term and premature study infants were 39.8±1.1 and 30.9±1.5 weeks, respectively. Similarly, the mean(±SD) birth weights for these infants were 3398±351 and 1307±212 g, respectively. All infants were of appropriate size for their gestational age and were free of con-

Week	Weight, g	
	Premature Infants	Term Infants
0	1307±212	3398±351
2	1261±188	3706±345
4	1644±419	4298±392
6	2151±637	4732±581
8	2788±659	5198±657
10	3185±648	5698±751
12	3802±772	6170±736
14	4031±586	6502±879
16	4619±626	7033±799

Table 1.—Weight From 0 to 16 Weeks in Premature (n=27) and Term (n=25) Study Infants*

*Values are mean±SD.

genital abnormalities. Their postnatal weight gain shown in Table 1 was consistent with reported normal values.[10]

The premature infants were fed via orogastric tube supplemented with intravenous glucose water during the first 2 weeks of life; otherwise, all infants were nipple fed. No infant received parenteral fluid containing amino acids, calcium or phosphate salts, lipids, or vitamin D.

None of the study infants required major medical support, such as ventilator therapy or parenteral nutrition, and none had sepsis or intraventricular hemorrhage. Similarly, none of the premature infants studied had respiratory distress syndrome or a documented blood pH level less than 7.3. Each premature neonate initially required an incubator for warmth. Three and 12 premature infants, respectively, experienced apnea (none requiring therapy) and transient oxygen therapy (<40% for <48 hours).

All infants received solely enteral feeding—420 J/kg per day or more by 2 weeks of age. The biweekly serum calcium (total or ionized), phosphorus, and parathyroid hormone concentrations for the premature and term infants throughout the study are shown in Tables 2 and 3.

Tables 4 and 5 show the neonatal 25(OH)D serum concentrations in the premature and term infants measured in each of the four vitamin D dose groups from birth to 16 weeks of age. The mean(±SD) serum 25(OH)D concentrations for mothers of the 27 premature and 25 term infants at the time of delivery were 19.2±7.7 and 18.5±9.2 ng/mL, respectively.

The cord blood 25(OH)D concentrations for both the premature and term infants significantly ($P<.001$) correlated with their mother's 25(OH)D serum concentrations ($r=.707$ and .762, respectively).

COMMENT

Based on available data from both human and animal studies, the Committee on Nutrition of the American Academy of Pediatrics reported in 1963 that 250 IU/d of vitamin D was as effective as 400 IU/d in the prevention of rickets and the promotion of linear growth in infants.[4] The committee recommended that premature infants not receive greater than 100 to 200 IU/d of vitamin D. These recommendations were not based on vitamin D status data but were strikingly close to the recommendations that might be anticipated based on the data presented herein.

Table 2.—Longitudinal Assessment of Serum Calcium in Premature and Term Infants*

Week	Premature Infants		Term Infants	
	Ionized (n=7)	Total n=20)	Ionized (n=17)	Total (n=8)
0	1.3±0.3	2.1±0.3	1.4±0.2	2.2±0.2
2	1.1±0.1	2.2±0.2	1.2±0.1	2.4±0.2
4	1.2±0.1	2.2±0.2	1.3±0.2	2.4±0.3
6	1.2±0.1	2.2±0.2	1.3±0.2	2.4±0.3
8	1.2±0.1	2.3±0.2	1.3±0.2	2.3±0.2
10	1.3±0.1	2.2±0.2	1.4±0.2	2.3±0.1
12	1.3±0.1	2.4±0.2	1.3±0.1	2.4±0.2
14	1.3±0.1	2.3±0.2	1.3±0.1	2.4±0.2
16	1.3±0.1	2.4±0.2	1.3±0.1	2.3±0.2

*Values are mean±SD ionized or total calcium concentrations in millimoles per liter.

Table 3.—Longitudinal Assessment of Serum Phosphorus and Parathyroid Hormone (PTH) in Premature and Term Infants*

Week	Phosphorus, mg/L		PTH, μg/L	
	Premature (n=27)	Term (n=25)	Premature (n=27)	Term (n=25)
0	63±29	59±16	0.7±0.3	0.5±0.3
2	75±19	75±20	1.0±1.2	0.7±0.4
4	68±13	78±19	0.8±0.3	0.7±0.3
6	66±12	82±20	0.8±0.3	0.6±0.1
8	71±34	77±20	0.7±0.2	0.6±0.2
10	65±15	74±14	0.7±0.3	0.6±0.2
12	66±17	70±12	0.7±0.3	0.6±0.3
14	75±33	71±12	0.6±0.2	0.6±0.2
16	69±16	69±18	0.7±0.4	0.5±0.2

*Values are mean±SD.

Normal 25(OH)D serum concentration in both adults and infants (during the first month of life) is approximately 10 to 30 ng/mL.[11] Furthermore, neonatal 25(OH)D serum concentrations have been reported to vary widely with different vitamin D intakes.[12]

The cord blood 25(OH)D concentrations in our study were less than 20 ng/mL in all infants, both premature and term. Although the serum 25(OH)D concentrations at birth were low-normal, they were, as previously reported, significantly ($P<.001$) correlated with the maternal serum 25(OH)D concentrations and were clearly within the normal range.[8,11] Furthermore, the 25(OH)D concentrations increased after delivery with enteral vitamin D administration in both term and premature neonates.

More than 80% of our study patients were black. Because black women and their newborns have been reported to have lower serum 25(OH)D concentrations at the time of delivery than white mother/infant pairs, this may have been related to the low 25(OH)D serum concentrations at birth.[8] No evidence, however, has been reported to suggest that black neonates absorb or metabolize vitamin D differently than do white neonates.

To summarize the data recorded in our study, in term

Table 4.—Longitudinal Assessment of Serum 25-Hydroxyvitamin D (25[OH]D) Concentrations in Premature Infants According to Vitamin D Enteral Intake Group*

	Vitamin D		Calcidiol*†	
Week	10 μg of 25(OH)D (n=8)	20 μg of 25(OH)D (n=9)	0.85 μg of 25(OH)D (n=6)	1.5 μg of 25(OH)D (n=4)
0	11±5	17±8	13±11	12±9
2	24±5	38±23	23±11	41±13
4	24±5	48±31	27±9	39±12
6	27±9	54±30	18±4	38±10
8	26±10	60±34	19±11	29±11
10	27±7	61±37	16±7	25±13
12	31±9	60±39	17±7	17±10
14	34±13	53±35	15±7	12±8
16	51±19	49±25	13±8	12±10

*Values are mean±SD serum 25(OH)D concentrations in nanograms per milliliter.
†25–Hydroxycholecalaterol.

Table 5.—Longitudinal Assessment of Serum 25-Hydroxyvitamin D (25[OH]D) Concentrations in Term Infants According to Vitamin D Enteral Intake Group*

	Vitamin D		Calcidiol†	
Week	10 μg of 25(OH)D (n=11)	20 μg of 25(OH)D (n=5)	0.85 μg of 25(OH)D (n=4)	1.5 μg of 25(OH)D (n=5)
0	11±9	9±5	8±3	12±3
2	23±8	21±5	13±3	22±7
4	21±8	26±8	12±2	34±18
6	25±10	28±6	12±2	34±18
8	28±13	28±9	10±3	23±6
10	27±9	33±13	7±2	18±3
12	27±9	34±16	10±2	19±8
14	29±13	33±16	17±10	20±11
16	26±12	35±14	15±8	24±7

*Values are mean±SD serum 25(OH)D concentrations in nanograms per milliliter.
†25–Hydroxycholecalciferol.

and premature infants receiving 10 or 20 μg/d of vitamin D postdelivery 25(OH)D serum concentrations were consistently maintained at greater than 20 ng/mL. Furthermore, in the premature infants, 25(OH)D serum concentrations were maintained at greater than 12 ng/mL with both 1.5 and 0.85 μg/d of calcidiol. In the term infants, however, while serum 25(OH)D levels were maintained at greater than 12 ng/mL with 1.5 μg/d of calcidiol, concentrations of 10 ng/mL could not be consistently maintained with 0.85 μg/d of calcidiol.

The 25(OH)D serum concentrations were lower in the latter portion of the study in both term and premature infants receiving calcidiol supplements than in those receiving either 400 or 800 IU/d of vitamin D. Although the equivalent of 1.5 or 0.85 μg of calcidiol in terms of international units of vitamin D is uncertain, it probably represents less than 400 IU. Thus, perhaps the lower serum 25(OH)D concentrations merely reflect a lower vitamin D dosage with the calcidiol intake.

Because all mothers indicated verbally that the daily vitamin D dose was routinely administered, these observations could reflect an aberration in neonatal vitamin D absorption. More likely, however, the falling serum concentrations of 25(OH)D indicate a lack of dosing compliance. Lack of compliance is suggested by the fact that the serum 25(OH)D concentrations in the low-birth-weight infants in all groups but the group receiving 400 IU/d of vitamin D decreased after hospital discharge.

Nevertheless, these data document that an enteral intake of 10 μg/d of vitamin D (400 IU/d) (even if inconsistently consumed) facilitates sufficient and nontoxic serum vitamin D concentrations for well neonates. Simultaneously, they suggest that while as little as 0.85 μg/d of calcidiol may be an adequate intake for premature infants, it may not be adequate for term neonates. Perhaps the most remarkable conclusion to be drawn from these data is that the 400 IU/d of vitamin D recommended for neonates 30 years ago without the support of vitamin D status data not only results in vitamin D sufficiency but does so with minimal or no toxic effects.

This study was partially supported by grant HD22542 from the National Institutes of Health, Bethesda, Md. The authors gratefully acknowledge the support of Ross Laboratories, Columbus, Ohio, for providing the 84 J/30 mL formula with no added vitamin D for this study.

References

1. Salle BL, Glorieux FH, Delvin EE. Perinatal vitamin D metabolism. *Biol Neonate.* 1988;54:181-187.
2. Tsang RC, Greer R, Steichen J. Perinatal metabolism of vitamin D: transition from fetal to neonatal life. *Clin Perinatol.* 1981;8:287-306.
3. Chesney RW. Requirements and upper limits of vitamin D intake in the term neonate, infant, and older child. *J Pediatr.* 1990;116:159-166.
4. American Academy of Pediatrics, Committee on Nutrition. The prophylactic requirement and the toxicity of vitamin D. *Pediatrics.* 1963;31:512-525.
5. Ballard J, Novak K, Driver M. A simplified score for assessment of fetal maturation of newly born infants. *J Pediatr.* 1979;95:769-774.
6. Sarker B, Chauhan U. A new method for determining micro quantities of calcium in biological materials. *Anal Biochem.* 1967;20:155-166.
7. Goldenburg H, Fernandez A. Simplified method for the estimation of inorganic phosphorus in body fluids. *Clin Chem.* 1966;12:871-882.
8. Hollis B, Pittard W. Evaluation of the total fetomaternal vitamin D relationship at term: evidence for racial differences. *J Clin Endocrinol Metab.* 1984;59:652-657.
9. Roos B, Lindall A, Aron D, et al. Detection and characterization of small mid-region parathyroid hormone fragment(s) in normal and hyperparathyroid glands and sera by immunoextraction and region-specific radioimmunoassays. *J Clin Endocrinol Metab.* 1981;53:709-721.
10. Shaffer SG, Auimiro CL, Anderson JV, Hall TR. Postnatal weight changes in low birthweight infants. *Pediatrics.* 1987;79:702-705.
11. Kuroda E, Okano T, Mizuno N, et al. Plasma levels of 25–hydroxyvitamin D_2 and 25–hydroxyvitamin D_3 in maternal cord blood and neonatal blood. *J Nutr Sci Vitaminol (Tokyo).* 1981;27:55-65.
12. Greer F, Tsang R. Calcium, phosphorus, magnesium and vitamin D requirements for the preterm infant. In: Tsang RC, ed. *Vitamin and Mineral Requirements in Preterm Infants.* New York, NY: Marcel Dekker Inc; 1985:99-136.

Legalization of Drugs of Abuse and the Pediatrician

Richard H. Schwartz, MD

• Growing numbers of individuals are proposing that drugs be legalized in the United States, with claims that federal, state, and local efforts to prohibit the use of illicit drugs are irrational and unenforceable. "Drug reform" advocates include persons of all political persuasions. Ironically, the call for drug reform comes at a time when trends in drug abuse, as reflected in national and state surveys, show a promising decline. It also is contradictory to at least one recent public opinion poll, in which respondents opposed the legalization of marijuana by a five-to-one margin. While their position is by no means unanimous, proponents of drug reform generally base their arguments on several key premises, such as elimination of or reductions in drug trafficking, enforcement, and interdiction expenditures; increased tax revenues from the legal sale of drugs; and reductions in health-care expenses associated with drug treatment. Reform advocates further claim that legalization would not be followed by an increase in drug use. The validity of each of these arguments is highly questionable. Legalization is a simplistic, short-sighted solution to a complex issue with public health, economic, criminal justice, and societal ramifications. Legalization would, moreover, abrogate the position taken in 1961 by the United States and 114 other nations in ratifying the United Nations Single Convention on Narcotic Drugs. The impact of drug reform merits an unbiased study by an independent agency. Until that time, pediatricians should inform themselves of the arguments for and against drug reform and be prepared to educate patients and their families about the issue.

(*AJDC.* 1991;145:1153-1158)

The alleged ineffectual result of the American "war on drugs" has engendered the resurgence of a well-financed, orchestrated movement to legalize drugs in the United States. One spokesperson for legalization of nonprescription, potent, psychoactive drugs has stated: "The call for legalization of drugs is a prayer for an end to the hatred, demagoguery, crime, violence, and harm to personal health caused by the drug war" (*Washington Post.* January 2, 1989; Health Section:12).

Nationally prominent and articulate spokespersons, such as economist Milton Friedman (*New Dimensions.* June 1990:56), have appealed to the American people to solve the problem by decriminalizing the distribution and personal use of drugs. Some of these arguments are undeniably appealing, and offer rapid salvation with few stated risks to our currently waning epidemic of drug abuse. The Drug Policy Foundation, a special-interest group based in Washington, DC, is almost exclusively dedicated to legalizing drugs ("drug policy reform") in the United States. This group has strong financial backing, amounting to at least $500 000 annually (*Chicago Sun Times.* August 31, 1989:22). The Drug Policy Foundation publishes a newsletter, *The Drug Policy Letter,* and it has sponsored four international conferences on drug policy reform held annually in Washington, DC. A 13-part series entitled "America's Drug Forum," produced by the foundation, has been televised by the Public Broadcasting System.[1] Books containing emotionally moving vignettes about people who were harmed by being denied access to marijuana or deprived of civil liberties for using illicit drugs,[2] prolegalization articles in magazines (*The Atlantic Monthly.* November 1990:126; *The Public Interest.* Summer 1988;92:3; and *International Journal on Drug Policy* (July/August 1989), and op-ed columns in newspapers (*New York Times.* May 15, 1988:1 and *USA Today.* October 30, 1989;Inquiry Section:11A) have led proponents to the conclusion that popular opinion is in favor of legalization of drugs. At least two privately funded institutes, the CATO Institute (Washington, DC), which is libertarian in philosophy, and the Hoover Institution of Stanford Uni-

Accepted for publication April 4, 1991.

From the Department of Pediatrics, Fairfax Hospital, Falls Church, Va.

Reprint requests to 410 Maple Ave, West Vienna, VA 22180 (Dr Schwartz).

Edited by Peggy C. Ferry

Editorial Comment.—*The following thought-provoking and stimulating article was written in response to situations encountered in a busy private pediatric practice outside Washington, DC. The author, a pediatrician and adolescent medicine specialist, has had firsthand experience in dealing with adolescent drug abuse, both personally and in his practice.*

Dr Schwartz is Clinical Professor of Pediatrics at Georgetown University School of Medicine and at George Washington University School of Medicine. For his work in the field of adolescent drug abuse, he was given the American Academy of Pediatrics Research Practitioner Award in 1989 and the American Medical Association Adolescent Health Award for Outstanding Services by a Practicing Physician in 1990.—P.C.F.

versity, which is conservative, have funded policy analyses of the legalization of drugs in the United States.[3-5]

No firm conclusions have emerged as yet from the latter. Adolescent patients, parents, school administrators, and reporters from the printed and broadcast media may want to interview pediatricians for their perception of the advantages and disadvantages of this vital topic. This report will review the current status of legalization efforts, and assess the possible impact of "drug reform" on the practicing pediatrician. Arguments favoring legalization are described. These arguments fall into three broad avenues of persuasion: civil libertarian, including antiprohibitionist and criminal justice arguments; economic, based on a cost-benefit analysis of drug prohibition; and medical. Facts and concerns are presented to counter many of the prolegalization arguments.

SUBSTANCE ABUSE: BIOLOGICAL, PSYCHOSOCIAL, AND SOCIETAL CONCERNS

Adolescents who drink alcohol in a social setting often overindulge. It is almost the norm for 17- to 20-year-old adolescent males to drink six or more cans of beer within the first 90 minutes of a party.[6] This is a drinking pattern vastly different from that of most adults. Personal interviews with high school and college students who use illicit drugs reveal similar patterns of overindulgence and risk-taking behavior. All drug users are not created equal. There is a proven biological susceptibility to alcohol dependence,[7-9] and many professionals in the specialty of chemical dependency believe that this also holds true for other drugs. The cost of drug abuse is enormous, encompassing much more than financial or criminal costs.[4,5] These costs are most likely to be borne by certain individuals, such as the biologically susceptible,[7-9] the economically and educationally disadvantaged, and the learning disabled. Drug use diminishes school performance[10] and job stability.[11] Moreover, frequent drug users often convince a previously non–drug-using sibling or friend to share in the pleasures of "partying."[12] Finally, there is an indescribable toll of depression and despair suffered by the non–drug-using family members,[13] adversely affecting their own performance at home, in their social network, and in the workplace. Would any of these social, psychological, scholastic, and vocational costs be reduced if drugs were legalized?

The groups likely to suffer the most if drugs were legalized, are those most affected by currently illegal drugs: youth; the underprivileged; and minority groups, especially those in our inner cities and Native American reservations and villages. Peter Bell, former director of the Institute on Black Chemical Abuse, has stated: "I cannot think of one problem that exists in the black community—teenage pregnancy, undereducation, unemployment, infant mortality, health care—that would not be negatively impacted by legalizing drugs."[14] In the Netherlands, long held to be a model of successful drug policy "reform," the poor and the immigrants from former Dutch colonies in Asia and South America constitute a disproportionately large number of the heroin addicts.[15]

PHARMACOLOGIC EFFECTS OF DRUG ABUSE

Legalizing drugs will do nothing to change the pharmacologic effects of the drugs. Stimulant drugs of high potency, such as "crack" and "ice," reach the pleasure centers of the brain in 8 seconds and are powerful reinforcers of euphoria. For many users of such drugs, there is a compelling urge to binge on these drugs repeatedly, until they are used up or the user collapses. Unlike tobacco abuse, which is equally addicting, the crack abuser often walks a pharmacologic tightrope, attempting to balance the overstimulating effect of cocaine with the depressive effects of alcohol, marijuana, or tranquilizers. This results in multiple drug abuse. Suspicion,[16] aggressiveness,[17,18] and violence[19,20] are inherently associated with use of certain drugs such as cocaine and phencyclidine,[21] and anger is difficult to suppress under their influence. There is an association between dependent or binge use of crack and the neglect and abuse of children[22,23]; many municipal and child protective service professionals are overwhelmed with caseloads related to parental crack use.

TRENDS IN DRUG ABUSE: A PROMISING DECLINE

Although the current wave of hedonistic psychoactive drug use is far from over, there has been a dramatic and sustained reduction in lifetime, annual, monthly, and daily use of almost every illicit drug by junior and senior high school students.[24,25] Latest national[24,25] and all state surveys of drug use by adolescents (except Alaska) show an impressive and statistically significant decline for all illicit drugs and early trends of decline in use of the two socially accepted legalized drugs—alcohol and tobacco. Response to the 1990 National Household Survey[24] of 12- to 17-year olds and 18- to 25-year olds, the annual survey of 16000 high school seniors,[25] and the most recent surveys from the states of Oregon,[26] Virginia,[27] Maryland,[28] New Jersey,[29] and California[30] show that more adolescents are saying "no" to drugs than at any time since the surveys began. This trend is of major importance not only because of the intermediate consequences of smoking, snorting, ingesting, or injecting drugs, but also because binge or chronic drug use is closely associated with mortality due to accidents,[31,32] homicide,[33] and suicide,[34] morbidity with injuries, sexually transmitted diseases,[35-37] injury to fetuses and newborns,[38] and overdoses. Added to all of the above is the newest risk, that of acquired immunodeficiency syndrome.[39,40]

Moreover, there are also encouraging, yet little acknowledged, trends in reduction of drug use by new arrestees. In the first 3 months of 1990, male arrestees in New York, NY; New Orleans, La; Washington, DC; and Chicago, Ill had at least a 15% reduction in positive urine test results compared with their peak frequencies during the previous 2 years.[41] In several cities, including the District of Columbia, prison inmate population in area jails has dropped sharply since March 1990 (10-month period). This is primarily due to a significant reduction in drug-related arrests. Several jurisdictions plan to eliminate or curtail projected increases in jail space because of the declining new arrests (*Washington Post.* February 11, 1991:1).

One must consider the possibility that these dramatic reductions in drug use might be reversed if drugs were legalized.

UNITED STATES INTERNATIONAL TREATY OBLIGATIONS

A final argument against drug legalization is legal rather than personal or social. In 1961, the United States and 114 other nations ratified the United Nations Single Convention on Narcotic Drugs, which maintains the illegal status of narcotics, cocaine, and cannabis derivatives, including marijuana. Because of this binding international agreement, no signatory country may legalize any of the above drugs without abrogating and violating its pledge.

THE MOVE FOR LEGALIZATION OF DRUGS

Some advocates of drug legalization maintain that prohibition laws, as exemplified by the current "war on drugs" policy, are inherently irrational, draconian, and unenforceable (*Hermes.* 1990;28:12).[42] As cited above (*Washington Post, Chicago Sun Times, The Atlantic Monthly, The Public Interest, New York Times, USA Today,* and *Hermes*), proponents say that the fundamental flaw is not one of drug use, but of enforcement of drug prohibition laws.[1-3,42] Not credited with success by the antiprohibitionists are the strict and very successful laws regulating alcohol in Norway, and amphetamines in Japan[43] and Sweden.[44] Those who espouse drug reform rarely give credit for the 70% reduction in daily marijuana use by high school students since the peak use year of 1978. Among high school seniors nationwide, there have been significant reductions in lifetime, monthly, and daily use of marijuana, cocaine, and amphetamine-type drugs, and virtual elimination of methaqualone hydrochloride as a popular drug of abuse.[25]

Proponents of drug reform have no unified position; some would have no government restraints on the production of psychoactive drugs and their sale to all except children and pregnant women.[42] How such restrictions would be enforced with teenagers, now estimated to comprise 20% of drug users, has not been spelled out. Unpublished data from my recently completed study of the frequency of use of fake identification cards by high school and college students demonstrate clearly that underage adolescents have easy access to alcohol by asking an older friend or sibling to purchase it for them or by using counterfeit or borrowed and altered identification cards. Access to cigarettes and smokeless tobacco, currently illegal for purchase by minors, is obviously no problem for underage youth.

Some proponents of drug legalization would limit the distribution of such drugs to licensed physicians who would have the authority to prescribe drugs such as cocaine and heroin (*Hermes*) for medical reasons, for example, for the palliation of cancer-related pain or control of chemotherapy-induced vomiting. More controversial criteria for use of medically prescribed amphetamines, cocaine, or marijuana might include maintenance of drug addiction as well as subjective "justifications," such as aids to weight reduction and treatment for inertia or depression. One can imagine the intense pressures exerted by streetwise, drug-using older adolescents on well-meaning, but naive, primary care physicians to prescribe the maximal amount of legal drugs; the excess might well be resold to minors for a profit. A potentially rich malpractice harvest could occur if physician-dispensed heroin or crack should lead to an overdose, an adverse reaction, a motor vehicle accident, or death.

DRUG LEGALIZATION: SEVEN ARGUMENTS FOR AND AGAINST

Advocates of drug reform generally propose seven basic arguments to support their stance. An examination of these arguments and of evidence from countries where certain drugs are legal may place the debate in perspective.

Elimination or Drastic Reduction in Drug Trafficking

Some proponents estimate that legalization would eliminate or reduce drug trafficking by $8 billion per year.[3] Legalization, some proponents claim, would take the profit out of a now-criminal enterprise and eliminate the drug pushers, gangs, and associated bloodshed and crime. This argument, seemingly logical and appealing, remains highly speculative and untested. Heavily counterbalancing it is the high probability of a marked increase in adolescent drug use. Moreover, if drugs were legalized, it is highly unlikely that South American, Caribbean, and Asian drug traffickers would simply fold up their suitcases and go back to their countries of origin.

There are already indications that dispensing legal methadone hydrochloride to addicts does not eliminate their trafficking in illicit drugs such as marijuana and cocaine. In a study of 100 patients receiving legally prescribed methadone, 70% of those who had been in treatment for 6 to 8 months continued to use illicit drugs, especially heroin and cocaine.[45] In the largest methadone program in New York City, approximately 40% of patients receiving methadone had urine specimens that tested positive for heroin, cocaine, or marijuana (personal observation from visit to the Beth Israel Hospital program and review of urine test results). If government regulation of marijuana is set at a maximum of 3% Δ-9-tetrahydrocannabinol, illicit growers and traffickers would probably offer a product with 8% Δ-9-tetrahydrocannabinol, a strength commonly found in superior grades of marijuana grown in the United States.

Reduction in the Number of Persons Arrested for Minor Drug-related Offenses

These drug-related cases obstruct our criminal justice system and overcrowd our jails.[46] Advocates believe that legalization of drugs would return these individuals to productive lives (*The Public Interest*).

Legalizing any criminal act, for example, violations of weapons laws, would obviously reduce the prison population. Nevertheless, after reviewing several studies of the criminal patterns of heroin users, the government of the Netherlands concluded that legalization of heroin would not appreciably reduce crime in that country.[47] In the Netherlands, almost half of the present 5500 inmates were imprisoned for a drug-related crime, and an estimated 60% of 1800 new jail cells under construction are expected to contain drug offenders.[48] These percentages closely parallel those in the United States.

While 50% to 80% of new arrestees in the United States have positive results on urine drug screening, urinary metabolites of cocaine, not marijuana, are found most often.[41] Many, perhaps the majority of, drug users in custody have serious antisocial problems that are independent of and antedate their drug use. Legalizing drugs would, in no way, address such antisocial traits.

Billions of Dollars Saved Annually in Law-Enforcement and Interdiction Expenditures

This estimate by *The Public Interest* assumes that no funds whatsoever would be spent on interdiction efforts at our borders or within our states, cities, and communities. The Netherlands, where use of selected drugs is decriminalized, has not abandoned drug interdiction efforts. Without surveillance, how could we prevent drug trafficking in our neighborhoods and in the vicinities of our schools? Cheap marijuana and heroin from Mexico could easily flood the country and be sold at prices lower than in government-regulated shops.

Production of a Huge Tax Revenue

Illicit and currently untaxed drugs would be taxed in the same manner as beverage alcohol and tobacco. This is a powerful argument, especially during our current economic recession. However, no country has ever been able to collect tax revenues from the sale of marijuana, cocaine, or heroin. Moreover, heavily taxed drugs might not successfully compete in the marketplace with illegal, tax-free drugs. In the Netherlands, where the possession and use of cannabis are decriminalized, the Dutch government has been unsuccessful in raising revenues from taxation of the cannabis that is sold at 300 shops in the largest Dutch cities.[49] The effort to impose a tax was blocked in the Dutch court, based on the fact that the Netherlands was a signatory to the United Nations Single Convention and was not permitted by international law to tax the sale of an illegal drug.[50]

As noted above, the United States is also a signatory to the United Nations Convention. Should a United States tax law be passed to include cannabis, cocaine, and heroin, how would interstate differences in taxation be regulated so as to prevent illegal interstate or international commerce? How could one prevent a trafficker from reselling low-taxed drugs purchased in Nevada or Mexico to adolescents in California?

Reduction in Drug-related Medical Complications

Proponents predict that the guaranteed purity of government-supervised drugs would reduce drug-related medical complications. The numbers of infections caused by adulteration and deaths due to unexpectedly high-potency cocaine or heroin would indeed decrease. However, most drug-related visits to emergency departments are not caused by adulterants, but by the pharmacologic action of the drugs themselves.[18,51] Neurologic[52,53] (strokes and seizures) and cardiovascular[54,55] (arrhythmias and myocardial infarcts) complications of cocaine would not decrease if its purity and potency were guaranteed by the government. For the majority of experienced adolescent crack smokers, the almost-irresistible compulsion to binge would not be lessened by the purchase and use of pure crack.[12] The three major causes of death and disability in adolescents—accidents, homicide, and suicide—are strongly associated with alcohol and drug use.[18-21,31-33] Drug use, moreover, has psychological and social sequelae that increase medical costs and human suffering. Government-certified pure drugs would be unlikely to reduce the cause-and-effect relationship between crack and syphilis, unwanted adolescent pregnancy, acquired immunodeficiency syndrome, and violence toward rivals, friends, lovers, spouses, and babies. Although pure drugs might, in theory, reduce some of the acute adverse effects of drug use, this advantage would almost certainly be outweighed by a large increase in long-term effects such as the health risks associated with tobacco and alcohol.

No Increase in Drug Use if Drugs Were Legalized

Recent experience in Great Britain,[56] Italy (*New York Times*. October 8, 1989:14), and Oregon[26] and Alaska,[57(Table)] clearly shows that free and unencumbered access to drugs of abuse by adolescents is associated with rapid increases in the numbers of drug users and with progressive chemical dependency. In 1975, Italy rescinded its previously liberal laws on possession and use of heroin after the number of adult heroin addicts in that country multiplied exponentially. There are approximately 100 000 heroin users in Milan, a city that the police now call the heroin capital of Europe. In 1988, there were 800 deaths from heroin overdoses in Milan, almost three times the number in 1986 (*New York Times*. October 8, 1989). In Alaska, where personal possession of up to 112 g of marijuana is legal, twice as many high school students smoke the drug frequently[57] as the national average.[58] Moreover, in 1988, the use of marijuana by Alaskan high school students stabilized since 1983 (the year of the only previous statewide survey)[59] at the same time that the use of marijuana by high school students decreased dramatically nationwide. In 1983, 70% of high school students in Alaska noted lifetime (use at least once) use of marijuana compared with 55% of seniors in the National Institute on Drug Abuse annual survey. By 1988, use by Alaskan high school seniors remained at 68% compared with the much reduced nationwide figure of 4%. Oregon, whose state laws concerning possession of marijuana were relatively liberal until their revocation in 1989, has more severe adolescent drug problems than the nearby Pacific Coast province of British Columbia, Canada,[60] and Washington state,[61] both of which have stricter laws regarding possession and use of marijuana. The move to legalization runs the risk of undermining current prevention efforts. High school drug education courses are most effective when social disapproval is strong and certain psychoactive drugs are illegal.[62] A 1990 study of the efficacy of school-based drug use prevention programs conducted by The Rand Corporation (Santa Monica, Calif) concluded that "The importance of prevailing social norms for successful prevention [programs] implies that legalizing marijuana and other illicit drugs could undermine prevention efforts. Changing the legal classification of presently illegal substances could convey the message that those substances are acceptable and thus alter the social climate that currently restricts their use."[62]

In the Netherlands, results of a drug use survey published more than 6 years ago noted that only 4% of adolescents of all ages ever tried cannabis (marijuana). A more recent survey of Amsterdam residents revealed that 32% of boys and 24% of girls between the ages of 16 and 19 years had ever tried cannabis.[63] The largest increase in use of cannabis occurred in adolescents aged 16 years, the minimum age for purchase and consumption of cannabis in the Netherlands. In the past 6 years, while lifetime use of cannabis by American high school seniors declined from 55% to 41%,[25] it appears to have increased in the Netherlands.

We Have Learned to Make Peace With the Most Dangerous of Drugs, ie, Alcohol and Tobacco

It is difficult to understand how legalization of other drugs would reduce the public health toll from alcohol and tobacco abuse. Among youth, there would likely be a marked increase, rather than the implied reduction, in nicotine and alcohol use, if drugs were legalized. One drug does not simply replace another; new drugs are superimposed on old ones; the vast majority of marijuana smokers are also cigarette smokers.

THE CONSEQUENCES OF DRUG REFORM: SOME UNANSWERED QUESTIONS

Additional consequences of drug legalization exist. How would we prohibit violent or antisocial adolescents from purchasing legal drugs? What would be the feasibility and cost of selling and safeguarding drugs at convenience stores or state- or municipality-regulated shops? How could sale be made sufficiently convenient to compete with round-the-clock street access? Would users be required to register? Would registration result in school, job, or insurance discrimination? Those who treat chemically dependent adolescents know that such persons usually want to purchase drugs at all times (including holidays such as New Year's Eve), close to their usual hangouts (at social gatherings such as parties or at beach resorts and rock concerts) easily, and certainly with no proof of identification or official documentation of the sale. How could the sale of unregulated drugs, which might come in appealing packages or exotic mixtures (crack and phencyclidine) carrying enticing names such as "Ghost Busters," be prevented? How could potency be regulated? Should we allow diazepam (Valium) to be purchased without prescription for modulation of cocaine-induced anxiety? If not, why? If drugs are legalized, what would prevent a multitude of vendors from displaying and selling instruments such as bongs (smoking chambers cooled by air or water); crack pipes; and records, tapes, and videocassettes that contain pro-drug material? How could we prevent foreign visitors, including Canadians and Mexicans, from purchasing drugs if they were legalized? Would advertising for marijuana be permitted? A legal challenge would possibly be posed if advertising of legal drugs were banned.

COMMENT

Drug abuse is a public health– and criminal justice–related, social, *and* economic problem, all interrelating with each other. The modest successes and glaring failures of the present policy on illegal drugs should stimulate serious discussion by individuals in different disciplines. Substantial reductions in drug use by the economically privileged has been demonstrated and is continuing. Much work needs to be done to effect similar reductions among the disenfranchised in inner cities, in some economically deprived rural areas, in barrios, and on Native American enclaves and reservations. We now know who is likely to initiate drug use even before it starts. We should develop programs to target these high-risk populations.

Legalization of drugs would abrogate the position we took with 114 other nations in 1961 in signing the United Nations Single Convention on Narcotic Drugs. It would also be contrary to current public opinion, as recently recorded in a poll sponsored by the Drug Policy Foundation of 1400 adults. Respondents to this telephone survey opposed the legalization of marijuana by a five-to-one margin.[64]

Legalization is a simplistic and shortsighted legislative solution to an incredibly complex issue. Many of the arguments against the legalization of drugs are succinctly summarized in a recent editorial by Frances.[65]

Perhaps the National Academy of Science or the National Academy of Medicine could examine in detail all the evidence for and against legalization of drugs. Until then, pediatricians should remain apprised of the arguments for and against drug legalization and inform their adolescent patients and their families accordingly.

References

1. The Drug Policy Foundation. *Drug Prevention Newsletter.* 1990.
2. Trebach AS. *The Great Drug War.* New York, NY: Macmillan Publishing Co; 1987.
3. Ostrowski J. Thinking about drug legalization. *CATO Institute Policy Analysis.* Washington, DC: CATO Institute; 1989;121.
4. Hay JW. The harm they do to others: a primer on the external costs of drug abuse. Presented at the Hoover Institution Conference on US Drug Policy; November 15, 1990; Stanford, Calif.
5. Rosenthal MS. The logic of legalization: a matter of perspective. Presented at the Hoover Institution Conference on US Drug Policy; November 15, 1990; Stanford, Calif.
6. Schwartz RH, Hayden GF, Getson PR, DiPaola A. Drinking patterns and social consequences: a study of middle-class adolescents in two private pediatric practices. *Pediatrics.* 1986;77:139-143.
7. Bohman M, Cloninger R, Sigvardsson S, Von Knorring A-L. The genetics of alcoholism and related disorders. *J Psychiatry Res.* 1987;21:447-452.
8. Cloninger CR, Bohman M, Sigvardsson S. Inheritance of alcohol abuse. *Arch Gen Psychiatry.* 1981;38:861-868.
9. Goodwin DW. Adoption studies of alcholism. *Prog Clin Biol Res.* 1981;69:71-76.
10. Friedman AS, Glickman N, Utada U. Does drug and alcohol use lead to failure to graduate from high school? *J Drug Educ.* 1985;15:353-364.
11. Zwerling C, Ryan J, Endel JO. The efficacy of preemployment drug screening for marijuana and cocaine in predicting employment outcome. *JAMA.* 1990;264:2639-2643.
12. Schwartz RH, Luxenberg MG, Hoffman NG. 'Crack' use by American middle-class adolescent polydrug abusers. *J Pediatr.* 1991;118:150-155.
13. Jenny L, Schwartz RH. Adolescent drug dependency and the family. *Va Med.* 1985;112:711-713.
14. Bell P. Arguments against legalizing drugs. *Drug Abuse Update.* 1988;26:18-19.
15. Van de Wijngaart GF. A social history of drug use in the Netherlands: policy outcomes and implications. *J Drug Issues.* 1988;18:481-495.
16. Sherer MA, Kumor KM, Cone EJ, Jaffe JH. Suspiciousness induced by four-hour intravenous infusions of cocaine: preliminary findings. *Arch Gen Psychiatry.* 1988;45:673-677.
17. Gawin FH, Ellinwood EH Jr. Cocaine and other stimulants: actions, abuse, and treatment. *N Engl J Med.* 1988;318:1173-1182.
18. Deriet RW, Albertson TE. Emergency department presentation of cocaine intoxication. *Ann Emerg Med.* 1989;18:182-186.
19. Tardiff K, Gross E, Wu J, Stajie M, Millman R. Analysis of cocaine-positive fatalities. *J Forensic Sci.* 1989;34:53-63.
20. Budd RD. Cocaine abuse and violent death. *Am J Drug Alcohol Abuse.* 1989;15:375-382.
21. Schwartz RH, Hoffman NG, Smith D, Hayden GF, Riddile N. Use of phencyclidine among adolescents attending a suburban drug treatment facility. *J Pediatr.* 1987;110:322-324.
22. Regan DO, Ehrlich SM, Finnegan LP. Infants of drug addicts: at risk for child abuse, neglect, and placement in foster care. *Neurotoxicol Teratol.* 1987;9:315-317.
23. Bays J. Substance abuse and child abuse. *Pediatr Clin North Am.* 1990;37:881-904.
24. Summary of trend analysis from 1990 National Household Survey on Drug Abuse. *NIDA Capsules.* December 1990.
25. Facts about teenagers and drug abuse. *NIDA Capsules.* January 1991.
26. Office of Alcohol and Drug Abuse Programs. *Oregon Public School Drug Use Survey: 1990.* Salem, Ore: Department of Human Resources, State of Oregon; 1990.
27. Wayne S. *1989 Virginia Youth Survey: Main Findings.* Richmond, Va: Governor's Council on Alcohol and Drug Abuse Problems; 1990.
28. Maryland Department of Health and Mental Hygiene. *1989-1990 Survey of Substance Abuse Among Maryland Adolescents.* Baltimore, Md: Alcohol and Drug Abuse Administration and the Juvenile Advisory Council of Maryland; 1989.
29. *Drug and Alcohol Use Among New Jersey High School Students: 1990.* Trenton, NJ: New Jersey Department of Law and Public Safety; 1990.
30. Report to the Attorney General. *Biennial Survey of Drug and Alcohol Use Among California Students in Grades 7, 9, and 11: Winter 1989-90.* Sacramento, Calif: Office of the Attorney General, Crime Prevention Center; 1991.
31. Lindenbaum GA, Carroll SF, Daskal I, Kapusnick R. Patterns of alcohol and drug abuse in an urban trauma center: the increasing role of cocaine abuse. *J Trauma.* 1989;29:1654-1658.
32. Soderstrom CA, Triffilis AL, Shankar BS, Clark WE, Cowley RA. Marijuana and alcohol abuse among 1023 trauma patients. *Arch Surg.* 1988;123:733-737.
33. Harruff RC, Francisco JT, Elkins SK, Phillips AM, Fernandez GS. Cocaine and homicide in Memphis and Shelby County: an epidemic of violence. *J Forensic Sci.* 1988;33:1231-1237.
34. Berman AL, Schwartz RH. Suicide attempts among adolescent drug users. *AJDC.* 1990;144:310-314.
35. Fullilove RE, Fullilove MT, Bowser BP, Gross SA. Risk of sexually transmitted disease among black adolescent crack users in Oakland and San Francisco, Calif. *JAMA.* 1990;263:851-855.
36. Jenny C. Adolescent risk-taking behavior and the occurrence of sexual assault. *AJDC.* 1988;142:770-772.
37. Hingson RW, Strunin L, Berlin BM, Heeren T. Beliefs about AIDS, use of alcohol and drugs, and unprotected sex among Massachusetts adolescents. *Am J Public Health.* 1990;80:295-299.
38. Chasnoff IJ. Drug use in pregnancy: parameters of risk. *Pediatr Clin North Am.* 1988;82:888-895.
39. Novick LF, Berns D, Stricof R, Stevens R, Pass K, Wethers J. HIV seroprevalence in newborns in New York State. *JAMA.* 1989;261:1745-1750.
40. Nicholas SW, Sondheimer DL, Willoughby AD, Yaffe SJ, Katz SL. Human immunodeficiency virus infection in childhood, adolescence, and pregnancy: a status report and national research agenda. *Pediatrics.* 1989;83:293-308.
41. National Institute of Justice. *Drug Use Forecasting: January to March 1990, October 1990.* Washington, DC: National Institute of Justice (Research and Action), US Department of Justice; 1990.
42. Nadelmann EA. Drug prohibition in the United States: costs, consequences, and alternatives. *Science.* 1989;245:939-947.
43. Tamura M. Japan: stimulant epidemics, past and present. *Bull Narcotics.* 1989;41:83-93.
44. Bejerot N. Drug abuse and drug policy. *Acta Psychiatr Scand.* 1975;256(suppl):27-42.
45. Dobbs WH. Methadone treatment of heroin addicts. *JAMA.* 1971;218:1536-1541.
46. Zeese KB. Marijuana: time to end the misunderstanding. *The Drug Policy Letter.* 1990;2:1-3.
47. Van Mastrigt H. Review of literature. *Newsletter of the European Movement for the Normalization of Drug Policy.* 1989;6:March 19, 1989:17-19.
48. Van Capelle MAA. Het Nederlandse Drugs befeid in hoofdlijnen (In Dutch). *Algemeen Politieblad.* 1988;13:291-296.

49. Wikesjo R. Recruiting drug addicts in the name of the law. *Parents Resource Institute on Drug Education (PRIDE).* April 1990.
50. Schwartz RH. Decriminalization of drugs of abuse: the Dutch experience. *Hosp Pract.* 1991;26:93-100.
51. Shannon M. Clinical toxicity of cocaine adulterants. *Ann Emerg Med.* 1988;17:1243-1247.
52. Levine SR, Brust JCM, Futrell N, et al. Cerebrovascular complications of the use of the 'crack' form of alkaloidal cocaine. *N Engl J Med.* 1990;323:699-704.
53. Spivey WH, Everle B. Neurologic complications of cocaine abuse. *Ann Emerg Med.* 1990;19:1422-1428.
54. Dressler FA, Malekzadeh S, Roberts WC. Quantitative analysis of amounts of coronary arterial narrowing in cocaine addicts. *Am J Cardiol.* 1990;65:303-308.
55. Virmani R, Robinowitz M, Smialek JE, Smyth DF. Cardiovascular effects of cocaine: an autopsy study of 40 patients. *Am Heart J.* 1988;115:1068-1076.
56. Stimson GV. British drug policies in the 1980s: a preliminary analysis and suggestions for research. *Br J Addict.* 1987;82:477-488.
57. Segal B. *Drug-Taking Behavior Among Alaskan Youth-1988: A Follow-Up Study.* Anchorage, Alaska: The Center for Alcohol and Addiction Studies, University of Alaska; 1988.
58. Johnston LD, O'Malley PM, Bachman JG. *Drug Use, Drinking, and Smoking: National Survey Results from High School, College, and Young Adult Populations: 1975-1989.* Rockville, Md: National Institute on Drug Abuse; 1990.
59. Segal B. Prevalence of drug-taking behavior among Alaskan youth: comparisons with national findings. *Alaska Med.* 1987;29:9-14.
60. Ministry of Health, Province of British Columbia. *British Columbia Alcohol and Drug Programs Adolescent Survey: 1987.* Victoria, British Columbia: Ministry of Health; 1988.
61. Billings JA. *A Statewide Report on Substance Use among Public School Students in Washington.* Portland, Ore: Northwest Regional Educational Laboratory; 1989.
62. Ellickson PL, Bell RB. *Prospects for Preventing Drug Use Among Young Adolescents.* Santa Monica, Calif: Rand Corp; 1990:V111.
63. Sandwijk JP, Westerterp I, Musterd S. *Het Gebruik Van Legale en Illegale Drugs in Amsterdam* (in Dutch). Amsterdam, the Netherlands: Universiteit van Amsterdam, Instituut Sociale Geografie; 1988:110-113.
64. The Drug Policy Foundation. *The American People Talk About Drugs: A Nationwide Survey.* Washington, DC: The Drug Policy Foundation; 1990.
65. Frances RJ. Should drugs be legalized?: implications of the debate for the mental health field. *Hosp Community Psychiatry.* 1991;42:119-120, 125.

Radiological Case of the Month

K. Kozlowski, MD, M. Glasson, MD (Contributors); *Beverly P. Wood, MD* (Section Editor)

This 3½-year-old girl was referred with a provisional diagnosis of osteomyelitis of the right tibia. She had painless swelling over the upper, medial aspect of the right tibia lasting several months. On physical examination, the swelling was soft, nontender, and extended over 4 cm. Six months earlier, the skin in this area had been penetrated by a palm frond, which had been removed. There was no identifiable skin lesion at the injury site.

Frontal and lateral roentgenograms of the lower leg were obtained (Fig 1) and ultrasonography (Fig 2) of the same region was later performed.

Accepted for publication June 8, 1990.

Contributed from the Departments of Radiology (Dr Kozlowski) and Surgery (Dr Glasson), Royal Alexandra Hospital for Children, Sydney, New South Wales, Australia.

Reprint requests to the Department of Radiology, Childrens Hospital of Los Angeles, 4650 Sunset Blvd, Los Angeles, CA 90027.

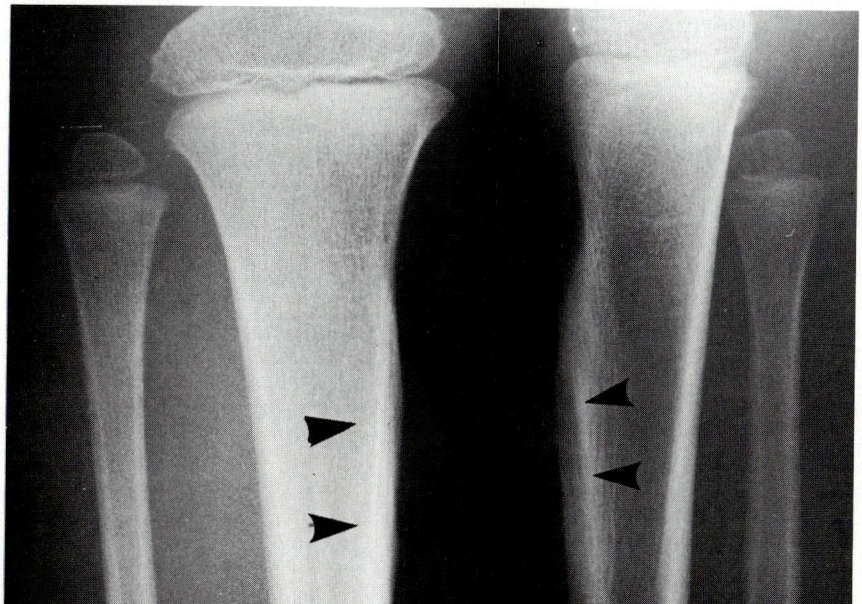

Figure 1.

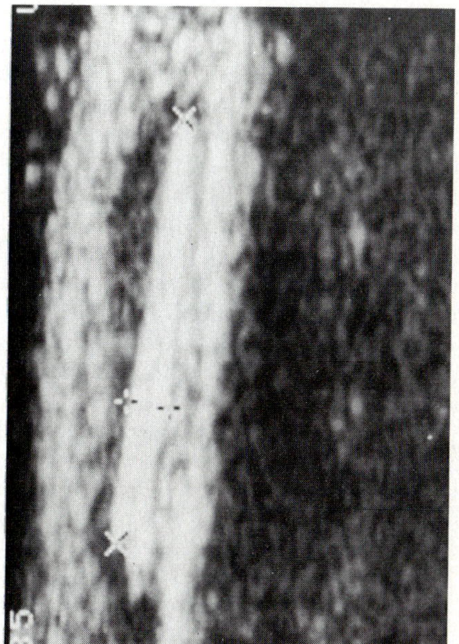

Figure 2.

Denouement and Discussion

Thorn-Induced Pseudotumor of the Tibia

Fig 1.—*Periosteal thickening at the anteromedial aspect of the right tibia (arrows) seen on frontal (left) and lateral (right) roentgenograms of the proximal tibia.*

Fig 2.—*A reflective foreign body (outlined by cursors) adjacent to the periosteum with dimensions of 22.4 mm × 2.2 mm is demonstrated on ultrasound. This is homogeneously echogenic without acoustic shadowing.*

Roentgenography showed a periosteal soft-tissue mass with secondary reactive periosteal thickening. The history of palm frond injury was strongly suggestive of soft tissue and periosteal response (pseudotumor) to an organic foreign body. This supposition was confirmed with ultrasound and operation. At surgery, a retained palm thorn was found embedded in the length of the periosteum. No pus, but a small amount of fluid, was present.

It is well known that organic foreign bodies produce changes in soft tissue and/or bone.[1] The former include cellulitis, synovitis, bursitis, soft-tissue cysts, and foreign body granuloma. The bony reaction presents as sclerosing or onionlike lamellated periostitis. This appearance is sometimes mistaken for a malignant tumour.[2,3] Osteolytic changes have also been reported.

Causes of the soft tissue and bone changes include toxic substances, mechanical irritation, and associated infection.[3]

The clinical history is most important for proper recognition of this disorder, particularly if a thorn, twig, or wooden splinter injury to soft tissue is suspected. The original puncture wound is no longer present, but local swelling, tenderness, and periosteal thickening is usually identified.

Ultrasonography is well recognized as a reliable, prompt, and low-cost method of superficial soft tissue examination. In a patient suspected to harbor a foreign body in soft tissue, roentgenography is a useful primary method of examination for detecting a radiopaque object. If a radiopaque foreign body is not identified, an ultrasound study should be performed using a high-frequency, linear-array transducer for detail.[2] This technique indicates the precise location and size of the nonopaque foreign body.

In the available literature, we found several cases of thorn-induced "tumor" of the long bones. A 6-year-old boy and 11-year-old girl both showed midfibular periosteal thickening suggestive of a malignant tumor.[4,5] Both patients had had penetrating injuries, and an organic foreign body was found at operation.

References

1. Gerle RD. Thorn-induced pseudo-tumours of bone. *Br J Radiol.* 1971;44:642-645.

2. Gooding GAW, Hardiman T, Sumers M, Stess R, Graf P, Grunfeld C. Sonography of the hand and foot in foreign body detection. *J Ultrasound Med.* 1988;6:441-447.

3. Maylahn DJ. Thorn-induced 'tumors' of bone. *J Bone Joint Surg.* 1952;48-B:386-389.

4. Schuz W, Mockwtz. Fremdkorper im Kniegelenk-eine sehr selten Verletzung bei Kindern. *Unfallchirurgie.* 1987;13:45-47.

5. Tanguy A, Penavayree JL, Raux PH, Fabre JL, Vanneuville G. Masque trompeur de corps etrangers vegetauz des mambres chez l'enfant: a propos de trois observations. *Chir Pediatr.* 1986;27:323-326.

SPECIAL FEATURE

Picture of the Month

Walter W. Tunnessen, Jr, MD (Contributor and Section Editor)

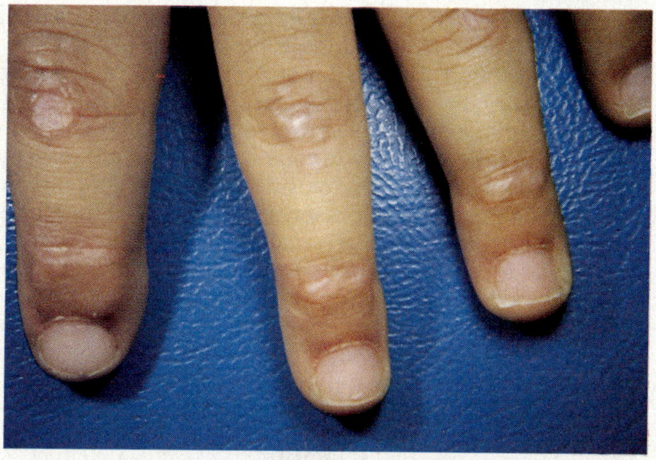

Figure 1.

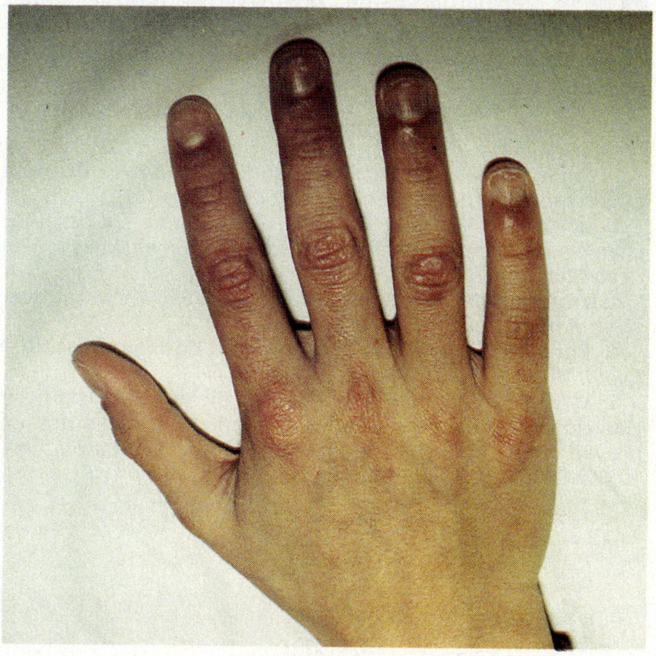

Figure 2.

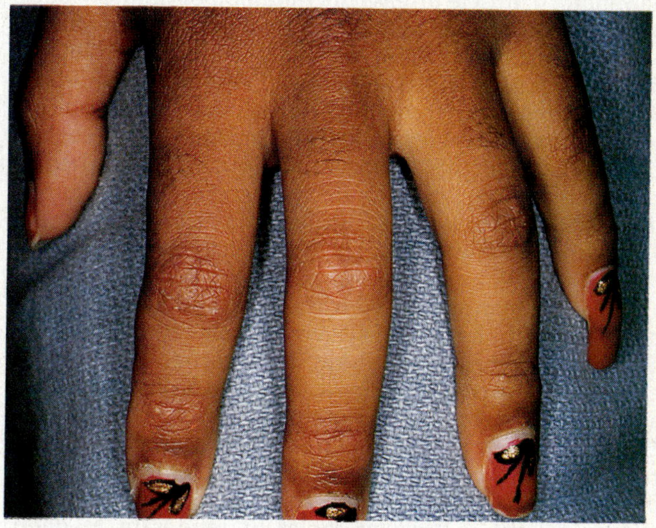

Figure 3.

Figs 1 through 3.—*The skin over the interphalangeal and metacarpalphalangeal joints is erythematous and hypertrophic. The hands of the child (Fig 1) and two teenagers (Figs 2 and 3) show the characteristic rash associated with a disorder characterized by progressive muscle weakness.*

The Editors welcome contributions to Picture of the Month *and* Radiological Case of the Month. *Those who wish to contribute should send their manuscripts to Dr Tunnessen* (Picture of the Month), *The Children's Hospital of Philadelphia, 34th Street and Civic Center Boulevard, Philadelphia, PA 19104, or Dr Wood* (Radiological Case of the Month), *Department of Radiology, Childrens Hospital of Los Angeles, 4650 Sunset Blvd, Los Angeles, CA 90027. Articles and photographs accepted for publication will bear the contributor's name. There is no charge for reproduction and printing of color illustrations.*

Accepted for publication January 3,1991.
Contributed from The Children's Hospital of Philadelphia (Pa).
Reprint requests to The Children's Hospital of Philadelphia, 34th St and Civic Center Blvd, Philadelphia, PA 19104 (Dr Tunnessen).

Denouement and Discussion

Juvenile Dermatomyositis

Manifestations

Juvenile dermatomyositis is a chronic, progressive, inflammatory muscle disease of childhood of unknown etiology. A number of cutaneous changes are associated with this disorder that are extremely helpful in arriving at the correct diagnosis. The hands of these three children (Figs 1 through 3) show the erythematous, red-to-pink, hyperkeratotic papules, known as Gottron's sign, that are characteristic of this disorder. Although the cutaneous changes over the knuckles are most commonly elevated, the involved skin may be colorless and atrophic at times. The skin over the phalanges is generally spared of this rash.

The facial rash associated with dermatomyositis may be confused with the rash of systemic lupus erythematosus. The malar areas may show a butterflylike band of erythema. The periorbital areas may also be enveloped by a similar erythema and sometimes appear edematous. The rash may be precipitated by sun exposure, but it does not fade like a sunburn does. The eyelids may turn a violaceous blue, often referred to as a heliotrope, which means a light to brilliant violet or moderate to deep reddish-purple discoloration.

The elbows, knees, and medial malleoli may show nondiscrete areas of erythematous or violaceous, scaly, and, occasionally, lichenified skin. At times, similar rashes may be seen on other parts of the extremities. The nailfold capillaries offer the best noninvasive view of the underlying microangiopathy associated with dermatomyositis. At times, enlarged, hemorrhagic capillaries can be seen without magnification of the nailbeds, but a better, more accurate assessment of the status of the capillaries can be made by using the office ophthalmoscope. A drop of microscopic immersion oil is placed on the nailfold. The lens of the ophthalmoscope is set at +40, and the capillaries are brought into focus by bringing the instrument within millimeters of the nailfold. The degree of morphologic changes of the capillaries correlates with the clinical course of the dermatomyositis.[1]

The cutaneous changes of dermatomyositis may precede the onset of muscle weakness, sometimes by more than 1 year.[2] Systemic symptoms and signs of this disorder may also include fatigability, lethargy, irritability, arthralgia, myalgia, weight loss, and dysphagia.

Five criteria are used to develop the diagnosis of dermatomyositis: (1) symmetric proximal muscle weakness; (2) elevated muscle-derived enzymes (ie, creatine kinase, aspartate aminotransferase, lactate dehydrogenase, and aldolase); (3) electromyographic changes consistent with inflammatory myopathy; (4) a muscle biopsy specimen consistent with myositis; and, (5) characteristic cutaneous changes. The presence of the typical rash plus three of the other four criteria make the diagnosis definite, the rash plus two other criteria make it probable, and the rash plus one other criterion make dermatomyositis possible.[3,4] It is important to remember that only one of the muscle enzyme levels may be elevated; therefore, it is necessary to obtain a panel of enzyme measurements at the time of the initial investigation.

Treatment

Systemic steroids are the drug of choice in the management of dermatomyositis. Hydroxychloroquine sulfate may be of help if cutaneous changes persist.[5] Methotrexate and cyclosporine have some efficacy in steroid-resistant cases.

References

1. Silver RM, Maricq HR. Childhood dermatomyositis: serial microvascular studies. *Pediatrics.* 1989;83:278-283.

2. Rockerbie NR, Woo TY, Callen JP, Giustina T. Cutaneous changes of dermatomyositis precede muscle weakness. *J Am Acad Dermatol.* 1989;20:629-632.

3. Pachman LM. Juvenile dermatomyositis: a clinical overview. *Pediatr Rev.* 1990;12:117-125.

4. Bohan A, Peter JB. Polymyositis and dermatomyositis. *N Engl J Med.* 1975;292:344-347, 403-407.

5. Woo TY, Callen JP, Voorhess JJ, Bickers DR, Hanno R, Hawkins C. Cutaneous lesions of dermatomyositis are improved by hydroxychloroquine. *J Am Acad Dermatol.* 1984;10:592-600.

Growth Hormone Therapy in Hypophosphatemic Rickets

Darrell M. Wilson, MD; Phillip D. K. Lee, MD; Alan H. Morris, MD; Edward O. Reiter, MD;
Joseph M. Gertner, MB, MRCP; Robert Marcus, MD; Valerie E. Quarmby, PhD; Ron G. Rosenfeld, MD

• The effects of growth hormone therapy on the biochemical measures of bone metabolism were studied in 11 children aged 3.5 to 17 years who had familial hypophosphatemic rickets; five were male. Subjects were maintained on a regimen of stable doses of conventional therapy (calcitriol and phosphate). Subjects were studied at baseline receiving conventional therapy and during three sequential treatment periods: no therapy (4 weeks), growth hormone only (0.05 mg/kg per day for 4 weeks), and conventional therapy plus growth hormone (2 weeks). The nine youngest subjects were continued on a regimen of triple therapy for an additional 24 weeks. Serum phosphate averaged 0.93±0.13 mmol/L (mean±SD) at entry and decreased when the subjects were not receiving any therapy. During the 4 weeks of growth hormone only treatment, phosphate rose in all 11 subjects (0.70±0.08 mmol/L to 0.83±0.08 mmol/L). With triple therapy, phosphate remained higher than with no therapy. Calcitriol, osteocalcin, and parathyroid hormone increased as the subjects received growth hormone alone. Insulinlike growth factor I *z* scores rose significantly in response to growth hormone therapy alone. All nine subjects receiving 6 months of triple therapy increased their growth rate *z* scores. Exogenous growth hormone therapy may be useful in familial hypophosphatemic rickets.

(*AJDC.* 1991;145:1165-1170)

Familial hypophosphatemic rickets (FHPR) is an uncommon disorder characterized by defective renal tubular phosphate transport, intractable hypophosphatemia, rickets, normocalcemia, defective bone mineralization, and short stature.[1,2] Affected individuals have normal intelligence, but they can suffer significant limitation due to the short stature and bone deformities. X-linked dominant inheritance is supported by linkage studies, although other patterns have been noted and a large proportion of cases are apparent spontaneous mutations. The pathogenetic mechanism for the hypophosphatemia is unknown. Calcitriol levels are inappropriately normal for the degree of hypophosphatemia,[3] and a defect in this regulatory system has been postulated.

Current conventional therapy for FHPR consists of high doses of oral phosphate and calcitriol.[4,5] Although an improvement in bone mineralization and linear growth can be achieved with this therapy, the hypophosphatemia is never fully corrected and most patients fail to achieve expected adult heights. Furthermore, the phosphate therapy is often limited by adverse gastrointestinal symptoms, and the high doses of calcitriol can lead to hypercalciuria and nephrocalcinosis.[6]

Early observations that administration of exogenous growth hormone increases renal phosphate resorption and calcitriol levels[7,8] led to speculation regarding the role of growth hormone in phosphate homeostasis and the possible beneficial effects of growth hormone therapy in FHPR. We report results from a pilot investigation of growth hormone therapy in 11 children and adolescents with FHPR. Biochemical measures were monitored with conventional therapy consisting of phosphate and calcitriol and during a 10-week period of sequential regimens of no therapy; growth hormone only; and growth hormone, phosphate, and calcitriol. Nine subjects were continued on a regimen of growth hormone plus conventional therapy for an additional 6-month period to determine possible longer-term biochemical and linear growth effects.

PATIENTS AND METHODS

Patient Population

Eleven children and adolescents with FHPR (3.5 to 17.2 years old, five male) were enrolled from four institutions (Table). At least 6 months of accurate previous linear growth data while receiving stable conventional therapy (vide infra) were required at entry. All subjects were required to meet one of these diagnostic criteria for FHPR: (1) overt rickets *and* positive family history of FHPR; (2) overt rickets *and* normocalcemia *and* normal serum 25-hydroxyvitamin D level *and* tubular maximum reabsorption rate of phosphate per liter of glomerular filtrate less than 0.84 mmol/L (vide in-fra); or (3) positive family history of FHPR *and* tubular maximum reabsorption rate of phosphate per liter of glomerular filtrate less than or equal to 0.84 mmol/L. One patient (subject 8) had cerebral palsy and central precocious puberty secondary to

Accepted for publication May 20, 1991.

From the Departments of Pediatrics, Stanford (Calif) University (Drs Wilson and Rosenfeld); University of Colorado Health Science Center, Denver (Dr Lee); The City of Hope Hospital, Duarte, Calif (Dr Morris); Baystate Medical Center, Tufts University of School of Medicine, Springfield, Mass (Dr Reiter); Cornell University Medical College, New York, NY (Dr Gertner); the Department of Medicine, Stanford University (Dr Marcus); and Peptide Section, Endocrine Sciences, Calabasas Hills, Calif (Dr Quarmby). Dr Lee is now with the Department of Pediatrics, Baylor College of Medicine, Houston, Tex.

Read in part before the Eighth Congress of the International Pediatric Nephrology Association, Toronto, Ontario, August 31, 1989, the Society of Pediatric Research, Anaheim, Calif, May 10, 1990, and the Third Eli Lilly International Symposium on Endocrine Disorders, Stanford, Calif, May 9, 1990.

Reprints not available.

Baseline Values for Subjects Not Receiving Any Therapy												
	Serum				Pretreatment z Scores				Conventional Therapy			
									Calcitriol		Phosphate	
Subject No/ Age, y/Sex	Phosphate, mmol	Calcium, mmol	Alkaline Phosphatase U/L	Osteocalcin, nmol	Height, cm	Growth Rate	Weight, kg	Growth Hormone Peak, μg/L	ng/d	ng/kg-d	mg/d	mg/kg-d
1/5/F	0.87	2.32	569	1.69	−3.78	−1.82	15	7.6	250	17	1000	69
2/5.7/F	0.61	2.47	462	3.38	−3.63	−1.07	16	12.3	500	31	500	31
3/7.4/F	0.68	2.62	371	5.38	−1.61	−1.05	27	. . .	750	27	650	24
4*/8.6/F	0.65	2.50	422	4.61	−2.45	+0.09	22	6.4	750	35	2000	92
5*/8.6/F	0.61	2.42	433	4.31	−2.31	+1.12	23	5.8	750	33	2000	88
6/10.3/F	0.71	2.37	660	3.23	−2.43	−1.66	29	9.1	500	17	1050	37
7/3.5/M	0.77	2.59	407	4.15	−2.56	−2.22	14	. . .	250	18	1000	70
8/6.1/M	0.77	2.42	334	4.92	−2.45	−4.07	21	2.3	250	12	1600	77
9/6.6/M	0.65	2.20	480	1.34	−3.08	−0.72	18	7.9	250	14	1000	54
10†/16.9/M	0.68	2.57	843	3.69	−3.04	. . .	47	8.4	1000	21	2000	42
11†/17.2/M	0.71	2.47	234	4.15	−1.54	. . .	59	. . .	500	8	2500	42
Mean 8.7	0.70	2.45	474	3.71	−2.63	−1.27	26	7.5	523	21	1391	57
SD 4.5	0.08	0.13	166	1.26	0.72	1.46	14	2.7	249	8	656	22

*Twins.
†Adults.

infantile meningitis. He was maintained on a regimen of stable doses of leuprolide acetate (Lupron) with suppression of gonadotropin and testosterone levels before and during the study. No other study subjects received any other hormone therapy before or during the investigations. Two patients were identical twins (subjects 4 and 5). No subjects received surgery during the study.

All patients were required to have been receiving stable conventional therapy, consisting of oral calcitriol and phosphate for at least 6 months prior to entry into the study. The calcitriol doses were adjusted in an attempt to maintain the urinary calcium to creatinine ratio between 0.1 and 0.2, and a serum calcium level of less than 2.72 mmol/L. Prescribed phosphate doses were generally calculated to provide 2.0 g of elemental phosphate per day divided into four to five doses. The actual baseline doses of calcitriol and phosphate and other baseline data are listed in the Table. The study protocol was approved by the respective institutional review boards at each of the four participating centers.

Study Design

Prior to entry into the study, eight patients had documentation of endogenous growth hormone response to standard provocative testing using clonidine hydrochloride.[9] Following an overnight fast, a single oral dose of clonidine hydrochloride (5 μg/kg) was administered and serum growth hormone levels were measured at 0, 60, and 90 minutes by radioimmunoassay at each center.

On day 0, baseline studies were performed and the conventional phosphate and calcitriol therapy was stopped. After 4 weeks of no therapy, subjects returned for retesting and were then started on a regimen of exogenous biosynthetic natural-sequence somatropin (human growth hormone) (Genentech Inc, South San Francisco, Calif) 0.05 mg/kg daily as a subcutaneous injection. Use of this preparation for this study was approved by the Food and Drug Administration (IND 29,518). Four weeks later, oral calcitriol and phosphate therapy was added at the previous dosages; subjects were studied 2 weeks later while receiving all three medications. The calcitriol therapy was monitored as described above. The two adults discontinued the study at this point. The nine youngest patients continued to receive all three medications for an additional 6-month period, with monitoring at 2-month intervals. Using direct reading stadiometers, experienced personnel measured standing height to the nearest millimeter at least twice at each visit.

Each subject was instructed to continue his/her regular diet during the course of the study. Nutritional intake of calcium, phosphorus, protein, carbohydrate, fat, and total energy was monitored by the Clinical Research Center dietitian at each institution.

Assays

Growth hormone levels were determined by immunoassay. Serum and urine phosphate and calcium levels, serum alkaline phosphatase levels, and other biochemical measures were determined by standard methods (at SmithKline Bio-Sciences Laboratory, Richmond, Calif). Insulinlike growth factor I (IGF-I) serum concentrations were determined by radioimmunoassay using a rabbit polyclonal antiserum (UBK487).[10] All serum samples were acidified and chromatographed (Sephadex G-50) in 1% formic acid. As previously described,[11] this procedure eliminates interfering IGF-binding proteins. Insulinlike growth factor I used for standard and iodination was purchased (from Amgen Inc, Thousand Oaks, Calif). This assay's lower limit of sensitivity (defined as 15% displacement of radioligand) is 0.4 μg/L, and half maximum displacement occurs at 3.3 μg/L. We have previously reported normal ranges for this assay.[12]

Parathyroid hormone (PTH) levels were determined by radioimmunoassay, using a goat anti-human PTH (hPTH) antiserum directed against the midregion of the PTH molecule and $[^{125}I][Tyr_0]$hPTH(44-68) as the radioligand.[13] Detection limit is 8 ng/L, with more than 96% of normal individuals having detectable levels.

Calcitriol was assayed by the method of Reinhardt et al,[14] as modified by Hollis.[15] This nonequilibrium competitive protein-binding assay (INCSTAR, Stillwater, Minn) used a fraction of calf thymus cytosol as a binding protein and 25-26 tritium-labeled calcitriol as radioligand. Bound and free radioligand were separated with dextran-coated charcoal and the bound radioactivity was counted in the tritium channel of a liquid scintillation counter. Plasma was extracted with acetonitrile and prepurified on C18 Sep-Pak columns before assay. The interassay coefficient of variation for this assay is less than 7% and the intra-assay coefficient of variation is 9.4%.

Osteocalcin concentrations were determined by radioimmu-

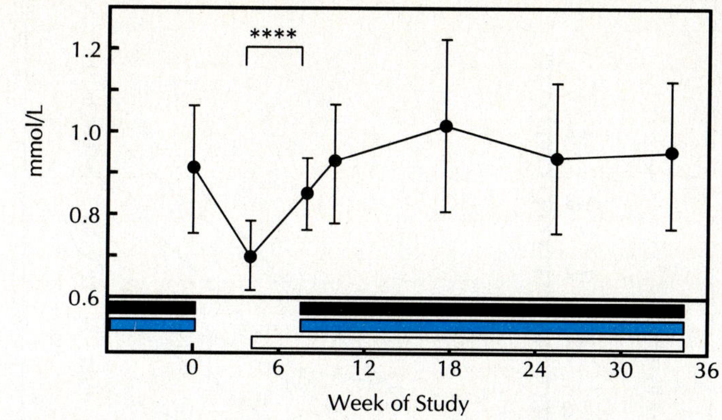

Fig 1.—*Mean (±SD) concentrations of serum phosphate at each evaluation through the study. Horizontal bars below the graph indicate the therapy at the time of each evaluation. Bold brackets over the data denote statistical significance (four asterisks indicate P<.0001, paired t test). The normal range for serum phosphate concentrations in this age group is 1.29 to 2.26 mmol/L. Closed bar indicated calcitriol; shaded bar, phosphate; and open bar, growth hormone.*

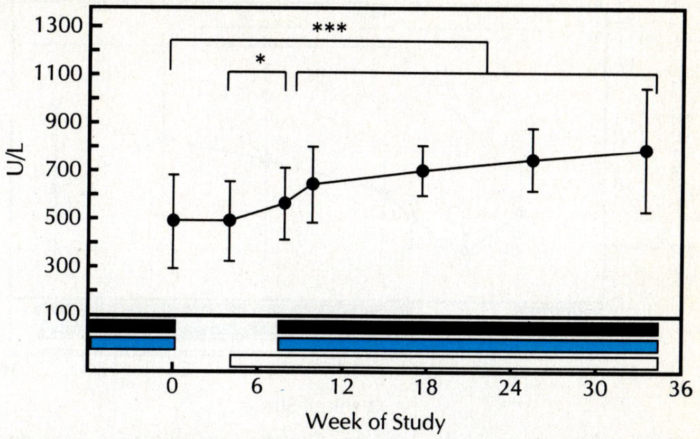

Fig 2.—*Serum alkaline phosphatase values. See the legend for Fig 1 for details. The light bracket indicates that all visits during which the subjects were receiving triple therapy were averaged together (see text). The normal range for serum alkaline phosphatase concentrations in this age group is 60 to 417 U/L. One asterisk indicates P<.05; three asterisks, P<.001. Closed bar indicates calcitriol; shaded bar, phosphate; and open bar, growth hormone.*

noassay at two dilutions using a highly specific rabbit polyclonal antibody directed against bovine osteocalcin and ^{125}I-bovine osteocalcin as radioligand.[16] The detection limit of this assay is 0.08 nmol/L.

Data Analysis

Data were analyzed using a statistical system (Statistical Analysis System) for the personal computer (SAS Institute, Cary, NC). Descriptive data are expressed as the mean±SD. For analysis, data were placed into four therapeutic categories: conventional therapy (baseline data), no therapy (week 4 data), growth hormone only (week 8 data), and combination therapy (weeks 10, 18, 26, and 34). For each biochemical variable, we statistically tested two hypotheses: (1) Did the concentration with combination therapy differ from the concentration with conventional therapy? (2) Did growth hormone therapy alone result in a change in the concentration (week 4 vs week 8 data)? Comparisons of linear growth were between the baseline data with conventional therapy and the data collected with triple therapy during the final 6-month period. Paired *t* tests were used for these comparisons. *P*<.05 was considered significant.

Insulinlike growth factor I levels were log normalized and *z* scores were calculated according to age-related normal values for the assay.[10] The *z* scores for height and growth velocity were determined using the National Health Examination Survey data.[17]

RESULTS

At entry into the study, all patients had short stature, with a mean height *z* score of −2.63 SD (range, −1.54 to −3.78 SD, Table). Growth velocities for the nine children involved in the long-term phase of the study ranged from −4.07 to +1.12 SD (mean −1.20 SD). Eight of the nine youngest patients were prepubertal. Patient 8 had a stable Tanner pubertal stage of P2G2 and low, prepubertal testosterone concentrations for the duration of the study. Three of eight subjects had a peak growth hormone response to clonidine of less than 7 μg/L.

Serum phosphorus (Fig 1) concentrations were initially low and alkaline phosphatase concentrations (Fig 2) were elevated despite conventional therapy. Calcium concentrations were normal while PTH concentrations were extremely variable at baseline. Insulinlike growth factor I *z* scores (Fig 3) ranged from −2.21 to +0.91 (mean −0.58). Calcitriol concentrations were also within the normal

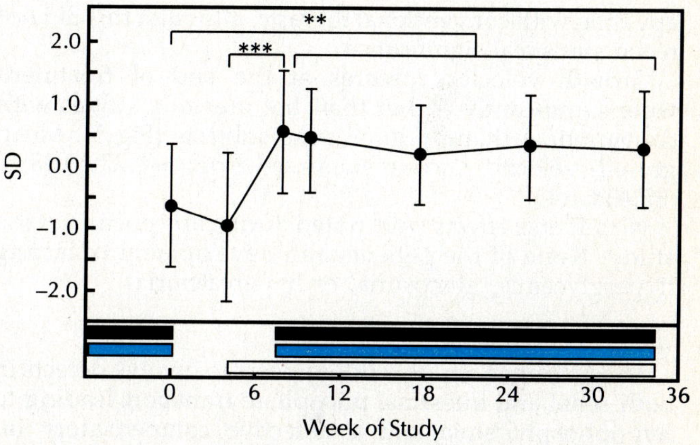

Fig 3.—*Mean (±SD) of the age-adjusted z score of the log-normalized serum insulinlike growth factor I concentrations at each evaluation through the study. See the legend for Fig 1 for details. Two asterisks indicate P<.01; three asterisks, P<.001.* Closed bar indicates calcitriol; shaded bar, phosphate; and open bar, growth hormone.

range. Osteocalcin concentrations, a sensitive indicator of bone turnover, were moderately elevated at baseline. There was no correlation between serum osteocalcin and alkaline phosphatase concentrations (*P*=.89, Spearman).

After 4 weeks of no therapy, serum PTH, calcitriol, phosphate, osteocalcin, and IGF-I *z* scores decreased. During the 4 weeks of growth hormone only treatment, all biochemical measures except calcium rose significantly (paired *t* test).

The means for the variables at each evaluation are shown in the figures. Since analysis of variance demonstrated that the means for each individual biochemical variable at all four evaluations with triple therapy (growth hormone+calcitriol+phosphate) were not different, the four values were combined for statistical analysis. Compared with conventional therapy, serum alkaline phosphatase, log normalized IGF-I, and osteocalcin concentrations were significantly higher while the subjects received all three medications (Figs 2 through 4). Calcitriol concentrations also tended to be higher with triple ther-

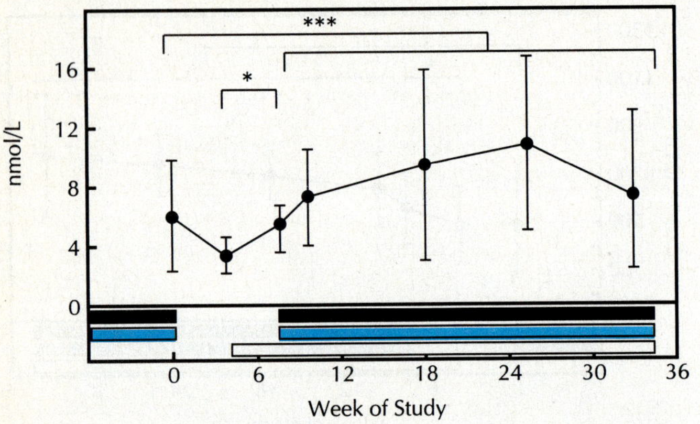

Fig 4.—*Serum osteocalcin values. See the legend for Fig 1 for details. The normal range for serum calcitriol concentrations in adults is 0.31 to 3.38 nmol/L. In normal children, osteocalcin concentrations increase markedly, reaching peak concentrations in puberty 5 to 10 times higher than seen in adults. The upper limit of normal in children is 6.61 nmol/L.*[47] *One asterisk indicates* P<.05; *three asterisks,* P<.001. *Closed bar indicates calcitriol; shaded bar, phosphate; and open bar, growth hormone.*

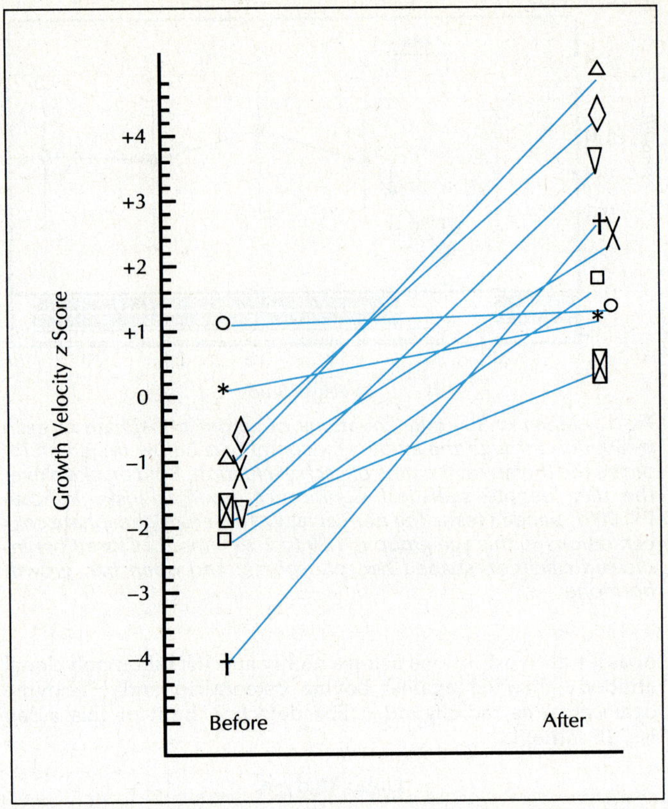

Fig 5.—*Growth response to growth hormone therapy. Growth velocity z scores before and after 6 months of growth hormone therapy. The symbols indicate individual subjects.*

apy than with conventional therapy, although this did not reach statistical significance.

Growth velocity *z* scores at the end of treatment were significantly higher than the prestudy values with conventional therapy in all nine subjects (Fig 5). Mean growth velocity *z* scores increased from −1.27±1.38 to +2.43±1.43.

No adverse effects were noted during any portion of the study. None of the patients had development of fasting hyperglycemia, glucosuria, or hypercalciuria.

COMMENT

The pathogenesis of FHPR appears to involve defects in both renal and intestinal phosphate transport leading to hypophosphatemia and a defective compensatory increase in renal 1-alpha-hydroxylation of 25-hydroxyvitamin D_3. In addition, although PTH levels are usually within the normal range in FHPR, there may be an enhanced phosphaturic response to PTH.[18] The etiology for these defects is unknown.

Clinically, severe hypophosphatemia leads to defective bone mineralization and short stature.[2,19,20] Although treatment with phosphate and calcitriol results in improved phosphate balance and alleviation of rickets, conventional therapy is limited by hypercalcemia and nephrotoxicity,[4,6,21] and normal phosphate balance is virtually never achieved. With combined calcitriol and phosphate therapy, improvements in childhood linear growth and final adult stature have not been observed consistently. Most adults with FHPR are short,[2,22] although recent reports indicate an improved height outcome using combined oral phosphate and 1-alpha-hydroxyvitamin D_3.[23,24] One group has reported that the linear growth retardation is proportionate, with a final adult height averaging 1.82 SD below the adult mean.[25,26] Although FHPR clearly plays a role, other factors, such as deformity or parental height, may also contribute to the short stature found in these patients.

Several lines of investigation indicate that growth hormone may play a role in phosphate regulation. Growth hormone administration to normal and growth hormone–deficient humans increases renal tubular phosphate reabsorption and serum phosphate levels.[7,8,27-29] Similar results have been reported in rats,[30] cattle,[31] and dogs.[32] Growth hormone therapy stimulates 1-alpha-hydroxylation of 25-hydroxyvitamin D in phosphate-deprived rats, while hypophysectomy reduces calcitriol levels,[33-35] although these effects are less consistently observed in humans.[29,36] The increase in calcitriol production may be mediated by the IGFs.[37,38] These investigations indicate that growth hormone may positively affect phosphate balance by increasing 1-alpha-hydroxylation of vitamin D, and that an endocrine feedback loop may be operative.

Although abnormalities in growth hormone secretion probably do not play a primary pathogenetic role in FHPR,[39] exogeneous growth hormone may have physiologic effects and possible therapeutic efficacy. In a short-term study conducted in 1964,[40] three children with FHPR were treated with growth hormone; two were treated for 9 days and one was treated for 4 months. Renal phosphate reabsorption improved in two of three patients, but the linear growth rate did not increase in the individual treated for 4 months. The cases of two other patients with FHPR treated with growth hormone were reported incompletely as part of a review article published in 1973.[41] Thus, previous data relating to the effects of growth hormone in FHPR are limited and inconclusive.

In the present investigation, 4 weeks of exogenous growth hormone therapy resulted in elevations of serum phosphate levels in all subjects to levels that were not significantly different from those seen with conventional exogenous calcitriol and phosphate therapy. Growth hormone therapy also increased alkaline phosphatase and osteocalcin concentrations over the untreated and conventional therapy levels. This is the second report of osteocalcin concentrations in FHPR.[42] Osteocalcin is a noncollagen bone matrix protein probably produced by osteoblasts. Osteocalcin concentrations are generally thought to reflect bone formation.[43] Previous studies indicate that calcitriol[44] and growth hormone[45] positively affect osteocalcin production. The increases in osteocalcin during growth hormone therapy occurred in the presence of an increased linear growth rate, suggesting that osteocalcin may reflect positive bone turnover.

During the 6 months of triple therapy, all nine subjects showed increased growth rate *z* scores as compared with conventional therapy. Since this was a pilot investigation, we did not investigate growth rates with growth hormone only, nor did we attempt to alter the phosphate and calcitriol dosages during the 6-month period. The observed effect, however, suggests that growth hormone stimulates skeletal growth in FHPR. The mechanism of this action is not clear but may involve growth hormone–induced improvements in phosphate balance on a direct effect of growth hormone to increase IGF-I levels in bone.

Our results support previous data that growth hormone, possibly through stimulation of IGF production, has a positive effect on serum phosphate concentrations. The apparent magnitude of this effect is of a degree that may be therapeutically beneficial in individuals with FHPR, and suggests that growth hormone therapy may supplement exogenous phosphate and calcitriol therapy. These findings gain additional clinical significance when one considers the significant morbidity associated with exogenous high-dose calcitriol and phosphate as opposed to the extremely low occurrence of adverse side effects with biosynthetic growth hormone.[46] Growth hormone therapy will also have the additional benefit of stimulating growth, but the data are too preliminary to determine if this response can be sustained or if growth hormone therapy can alter final adult height. Although our data are too limited to recommend growth hormone therapy for routine treatment of FHPR, the need for a more extensive and long-term investigation of both phosphate metabolism and growth is clearly indicated.

This investigation was supported in part by Orphan Drug grant FD-R-000120 from the US Food and Drug Administration, Washington, DC, and by Genentech Inc. Investigations at the individual study centers were supported in part by Clinical Research Center awards from the National Institutes of Health (Bethesda, Md) to Stanford University (RR00070), the Department of Pediatrics, University of Colorado Health Sciences Center (RR00069), and Cornell University (CA29502 and RR06020).

The nursing, dietary, and clerical staff of each clinical research center provided technical assistance, and the following provided clinical contributions: G. Klingensmith, MD; Ian Ocrant, MD; Albert DiNicola, MD; Lois Rountree, RN; Raymond L. Hintz, MD; and Yun Kee. James Frane, PhD, and Peter Compton, PhD, provided statistical suggestions.

Louis Underwood, MD, and Judson J. Van Wyk, MD, University of North Carolina, Chapel Hill, provided the rabbit polyclonal antiserum used in this study that was distributed by the National Hormone and Pituitary Program.

References

1. Burnett CH, Dent CE, Harper C, Warland BJ. Vitamin D-resistant rickets: analysis of 24 pedigrees with hereditary and sporadic cases. *Am J Med.* 1964;36:222-232.

2. Reid IR, Hardy DC, Murphy WA, Teitelbaum SL, Bergfeld MA, Whyte MP. X-linked hypophosphatemia: a clinical, biochemical and histopathologic assessment of morbidity in adults. *Medicine.* 1989;68:336-352.

3. Rasmussen H, Tenehouse HS. Hypophosphatemia. In: Scriver CR, Beaudet AL, Sly WS, Valle D, eds. *The Metabolic Basis of Inherited Disease.* 6th ed. New York, NY: McGraw-Hill International Book Co; 1989:2581-2604.

4. Chesney RW, Mazess RB, Rose P, Hamstra AJ, DeLuca HF, Breed AL. Long-term influence of calcitriol (1,25-dihydroxyvitamin D_3) and supplemental phosphate in X-linked hypophosphatemic rickets. *Pediatrics.* 1983;71:559-567.

5. Rasmussen H, Pechet M, Anast C, Mazur A, Gertner J, Broadus AE. Long-term treatment of familial hypophosphatemic rickets with oral phosphate and 1-alpha-hydroxyvitamin D_3. *J Pediatr.* 1981;99:16-25.

6. Goodyer PR, Kronick JB, Jequier S, Reade TM, Scriver CR. Nephrocalcinosis and its relationship to treatment of hereditary rickets. *J Pediatr.* 1987;111:700-704.

7. Gershberg H. Metabolic and renotropic effects of human growth hormone in disease. *J Clin Endocrinol.* 1960;20:1107-1119.

8. Henneman PH, Forbes AP, Moldawer M, Dempsey EF, Carroll EL. Effects of human growth hormone in man. *J Clin Invest.* 1960;39:1223-1238.

9. Alsever RN, Gotlin RW. *Handbook of Endocrine Tests in Adults and Children.* 2nd ed. Chicago, Ill: Year Book Medical Publishers Inc; 1978:5-14.

10. Wilson DM, Bennett A, Adamson GD, Nagashima RJ, Liu F, DeNatale ML, et al. Somatomedins in pregnancy: a cross-sectional study of insulin-like growth factors I and II and somatomedin peptide content in normal human pregnancies. *J Clin Endocrinol Metab.* 1982;56:858-861.

11. Horner JM, Liu F, Hintz RL. Comparison of 125-I somatomedin A and 125-I somatomedin C radioreceptor assays for somatomedin peptide content in whole and acid-chromatographed plasma. *J Clin Endocrinol Metab.* 1978;47:1287-1295.

12. Rosenfeld RG, Wilson DM, Lee PDK, Hintz RL. Insulin-like growth factors I and II in evaluation of growth retardation. *J Pediatr.* 1986;109:428-433.

13. Young G, Marcus R, Minkoff JR, Kim LY, Segre GV. Age-related increase in parathyroid hormone in man. *J Bone Miner Res.* 1987;2:367-374.

14. Reinhardt TA, Horst RL, Orf JW, Hollis BW. A microassay for 1,25-dihydroxyvitamin D not requiring high performance liquid chromatography: application to clinical studies. *J Clin Endocrinol Metab.* 1984;58:91-98.

15. Hollis BW. Assay of circulating 1,25(OH2) vitamin D involving a novel single cartridge extraction and purification procedure. *Clin Chem.* 1986;32:2060.

16. Price PA, Nishimoto SK. Radioimmunoassay for the vitamin K dependent protein of bone and its discovery in plasma. *Proc Natl Acad Sci U S A.* 1980;77:2234-2238.

17. Hamill PVV, Drizd TA, Johnson CL, Reed RR, Roche AF. NCHS growth curves for children from birth to 18 years. *Vital Health Stat.* 1977;165:1-74.

18. Short E, Morris RC, Sebastian A, Spencer M. Exaggerated phosphaturic response to circulating parathyroid hormone in patients with familial X-linked hypophosphatemic rickets. *J Clin Invest.* 1976;58:152-163.

19. Glorieux FH, Marie PJ, Pettifor J, Delvin EE. Bone response to phosphate salts, ergocalciferol, and calcitriol in hypophosphatemic vitamin D-resistant rickets. *N Engl J Med.* 1980;303:1023-1031.

20. Chan JCM, Alon U, Hirschman GM. Renal hypophosphatemic rickets. *J Pediatr.* 1985;106:533-544.

21. Chan JCM, Young RB, Alon U, Mamunes P. Hypercalcemia in children with disorders of calcium and phosphate metabolism during long-term treatment with 1,25-dihydroxyvitamin D_3. *Pediatrics.* 1983;72:225-233.

22. McNair SL, Stickler GH. Growth in familial hypophosphatemic vitamin-D-resistant rickets. *N Engl J Med.* 1969;281:511-516.

23. Balsan S, Tieder M. Linear growth in patients with

hypophosphatemic vitamin D-resistant rickets: influence of treatment regimen and parental height. *J Pediatr.* 1990;116:365-371.
24. Tsuru N, Chan JCM, Chinchilli WM. Renal hypophosphatemic rickets. *AJDC.* 1987;141:108-110.
25. Steendijk R, Herweijer TJ. Height, sitting height and leg length in patients with hypophosphatemic rickets. *Acta Paediatr Scand.* 1984;73:181-184.
26. Herweijer TJ, Steendijk R. The relation between attained adult height and metaphyseal lesions in hypophosphatemic vitamin D-resistant rickets. *Acta Paediatr Scand.* 1985;74:196-200.
27. Corvilain J, Abramow M. Some effects of human growth hormone on renal hemodynamics and on tubular phosphate transport in man. *J Clin Invest.* 1962;41:1230-1235.
28. Gertner JM, Horst RL, Broadus AE, Rasmussen H, Genel M. Parathyroid function and vitamin D metabolism during human growth hormone replacement. *J Clin Endocrinol Metab.* 1979;49:145-148.
29. Marcus R, Butterfield G, Holloway L, Gilliland L, Baylink DJ, Hintz RL, et al. Effects of short term administration of recombinant human growth hormone to elderly people. *J Clin Endocrinol Metab.* 1990;70:519-527.
30. Lee DBN, Brautbar N, Walling MW, Silis V, Carlson HE, Grindeland RE, et al. Role of growth hormone in experimental phosphorus deprivation in the rate. *Calcif Tissue Int.* 1980;32:105-112.
31. Westby GR, Goldfarb S, Goldberg M, Agus ZS. Acute effects of bovine growth hormone on renal calcium and phosphate excretion. *Metabolism.* 1977;26:525-530.
32. Corvilain J, Abramow M. Effect of growth hormone on tubular transport of phosphate in normal and parathyroidectomized dogs. *J Clin Invest.* 1964;43:1608-1612.
33. Gray RW, Garthwaite TL. Activation of renal 1,25-dihydroxyvitamin D_3 synthesis by phosphate deprivation: evidence for a role for growth hormone. *Endocrinology.* 1985;116:189-193.
34. Gray RW, Garthwaite TL, Phillips LS. Growth hormone and triiodothyronine permit an increase in plasma $1,25(OH)_2D$ concentrations in response to dietary phosphate deprivation in hypophysectomized rats. *Calcif Tissue Int.* 1983;35:100-106.
35. Wongsurawat N, Ambrecht HJ, Zenser TV, Forte LR, Davis BB. Effects of hypophysectomy and growth hormone replacement treatment on renal hydroxylation of 25-hydroxycholecalciferol in rats. *J Endocrinol.* 1984;101:333-338.
36. Spanos E, Barrett D, MacIntyre I, Pike JW, Safilian E, Haussler MR. Effect of growth hormone on vitamin D metabolism. *Nature.* 1973;273:246-247.
37. Gray RW. Evidence that somatomedins mediate the effect of hypophosphatemia to increase serum 1,25-hydroxyvitamin D_3 levels in rats. *Endocrinology.* 1987;121:504-512.
38. Halloran BP, Spencer EM. Dietary phosphorus and 1,25-dihydroxyvitamin D metabolism: influence of insulin-like growth factor. *J Endocrinol.* 1988;123:1225-1229.
39. Jasper HG, Cassinell H. Evaluation of the growth hormone-somatomedin C axis in patients with hypophospatemic rickets. Published in the 72nd Annual Program of the Endocrine Society, 1990. Abstract 300A.
40. Gershberg H, Neumann LL, Mari S. Studies on vitamin D-resistant rickets: effects of growth hormone. *Metabolism.* 1964;13:636-649.
41. Crawford JD, Bode HH, Botstein PM. Human growth hormone and nonhypopituitary disorders. In: Raiti S, ed. *Human Growth Hormone Research.* Bethesda, Md: National Institutes of Health; 1973:757-785. US Dept of Health, Education, and Welfare publication 74-612.
42. Cole ECD, Gundberg CM. Changes in serum osteocalcin associated with parathyroid hormone infusion in X-linked hypophosphatemic rickets. *Clin Chim Acta.* 1985;151:1-7.
43. Hauschka PV, Lian JB, Cole DE, Gundberg GM. Osteocalcin and matrix Gla protein: vitamin K-dependent proteins in bone. *Physiol Rev.* 1989;69:990-1047.
44. Ozono K, Liao J, Kerner SA, Scott RA, Pike JW. The vitamin D-responsive element in the human osteocalcin gene. *J Biol Chem.* 1990;265:21881-21888.
45. Johansen JS, Jensen SB, Riis BJ, Rasmussen L, Zachman M, Christiansen C. Serum bone Gla protein: a potential marker of growth hormone (GH) deficiency and the response to GH therapy. *J Clin Endocrinol Metab.* 1990;71:122-126.
46. Laron Z, Butenandt O, Raiti S. Clinical use of growth hormone: which and to whom. *Eur J Pediatr.* 1987;146:194-195.
47. Tarallo P, Henny J, Fournier B, Siet G. Plasma osteocalcin: biological variations and reference limits. *Scand J Clin Lab Invest.* 1990;50:649-655.-

In Other AMA Journals

ARCHIVES OF SURGERY

Trauma During Pregnancy: A Review of 79 Cases

Thomas J. Esposito, MD, MPH; David R. Gens, MD; Lynn Gerber Smith, RN, MS; Ronald Scorpio, MD; Timothy Buchman, MD (*Arch Surg.* 1991;126:1073-1078)

Trauma in Pregnancy: Predicting Pregnancy Outcome

David P. Kissinger, MD; Grace S. Rozycki, MD; John A Morris, Jr, MD; M. Margaret Knudson, MD; Wayne S. Copes, PhD; Sue M. Bass, ScM; H. Kendle Yates; Howard R. Champion, FRCS(Edin)FACS (*Arch Surg.* 1991;126:1079-1086)

Multilevel Model to Assess Appropriateness of Pediatric Serum Drug Concentrations

Donna M. Kraus, PharmD; Ina Lee Stile Calligaro, PharmD; Hind T. Hatoum, PhD

• A multilevel model reviewing four assessment levels for pediatric serum drug concentrations was developed. Criteria for appropriate indication, sample collection, documentation, and utilization were based on therapeutic drug monitoring principles. The model was applied to 222 pediatric serum drug concentrations. Inadequate documentation was a major problem, but it occurred at a lower rate (37%) than previously reported. The rates of inappropriateness for indication (15%), sample collection (16%), and utilization (10%) were well within reported ranges but were significantly lower with pharmacy input. Overall, 48.2% of drug concentrations were inappropriate. Digoxin, phenobarbital, and aminoglycosides had the highest error rates. The annualized cost of inappropriate serum drug concentrations was $12 325. The described method allows for targeting of educational programs with defined areas for improvement. The findings of this study also support the involvement of clinical pharmacists in the therapeutic drug monitoring process.

(*AJDC.* 1991;145:1171-1175)

The ability to measure drug concentrations in small quantities of serum has provided clinicians with a valuable tool to adjust drug doses accurately in pediatric patients. Measuring the serum drug concentration and using this information to evaluate and adjust drug therapy is a complex process commonly referred to as therapeutic drug monitoring (TDM). The appropriate use of serum drug concentrations involves four components: (1) identification of the correct indication for sample obtainment, (2) selection of an appropriate sample time, (3) documentation of the sampling time and the laboratory value in the patient's medical record, and (4) correct utilization of the measured serum drug concentration in conjunction with a proper assessment of the patient's clinical condition.

Several studies have evaluated the use of various aspects of TDM in adult[1-11] and pediatric[3,12-15] patients, but few of these studies evaluated each individual step of the process. Most studies were retrospective and assessed only one drug or a specific class of drugs. A prospective analysis of each of the four components of TDM, including all medications in which serum concentrations are routinely obtained in the pediatric population, has not previously been described, to our knowledge.

The purpose of this study was to develop and implement a serum drug concentration evaluation process specifically designed to review each step involved in optimal TDM. The study was also designed to identify drugs associated with a high incidence of inappropriateness, determine the type of common TDM errors, and assess potential benefits from clinical pharmacy input. In addition, the cost of inappropriate serum drug concentrations based on an overall evaluation was determined.

MATERIALS AND METHODS

This study was conducted at a university teaching hospital that uses pediatric attending physicians, resident physicians in training, and medical students for patient care. In addition, comprehensive clinical pharmacy services are provided to the pediatric inpatients by College of Pharmacy faculty who specialize in pediatric pharmacotherapy. Pediatric clinical pharmacists' training consists of a doctor of pharmacy degree and a specialized pediatric pharmacy residency or equivalent years of pediatric experience. Clinical pharmacists routinely make rounds with the health care team, recommend regimens to optimize patient pharmacotherapy and parenteral nutrition, provide TDM and pharmacokinetic consultations, answer drug-related questions, and help solve pharmacotherapeutic problems.[16] At the time of the study, the pediatric floor had an average daily census of 32.3 patients.

Hospitalized pediatric patients receiving any of the following medications were enrolled in the study: aminoglycoside antibiotics, carbamazepine, digoxin, ethosuximide, phenobarbital, phenytoin, primidone, theophylline, valproic acid, and vancomycin. The pediatric areas evaluated in this study included the pediatric intensive care unit, one of two general pediatric services, and the pediatric surgery service. In the pediatric intensive care unit, blood samples for TDM are drawn by the nurses acting on a physician order, while in the general pediatric area, blood samples are usually drawn by the resident physicians. General criteria for the multilevel evaluation of serum drug concentrations were developed by literature analysis[4,14,17] and consultation with two pediatric pharmacy clinicians. Acceptable standards for sample times, time to steady state, and therapeutic serum concentrations for each drug were included. The model was designed to evaluate the appropriateness of serum drug concentration determinations at each of four assessment levels: (1) indication, (2) sample collection, (3) documentation, and (4) utilization.

During the study period, the two clinical pharmacists cover-

Accepted for publication May 13, 1991.

From the Departments of Pharmacy Practice and Pediatrics, Colleges of Pharmacy and Medicine (Dr Kraus), and Departments of Pharmacy Administration and Pharmacy Practice, College of Pharmacy (Dr Hatoum), University of Illinois at Chicago; and Department of Pharmacy Practice, Temple University School of Pharmacy, Philadelphia, Pa (Dr Calligaro).

Reprint requests to Department of Pharmacy Practice, College of Pharmacy, University of Illinois at Chicago, 833 S Wood, Room 244 (m/c 886), Chicago, IL 60612 (Dr Kraus).

Table 1.—Distribution of Serum Drug Concentration Determinations (n = 222)

Drug	Absolute Frequency, No.	Relative Frequency, %
Theophylline	66	29.7
Aminoglycoside antibiotics	59	26.6
Phenytoin	36	16.2
Phenobarbital	26	11.7
Digoxin	25	11.3
Valproic acid	3	1.4
Vancomycin	6	2.7
Carbamazepine	1	0.5

Table 2.—Effect of Clinical Pharmacy Input on Serum Drug Concentration Monitoring

	No. (%)		
	Appropriate	Inappropriate	*P*
Indication			
Without pharmacy input	122 (85)	22 (15)	<.01
With pharmacy input	78 (100)	0 (0)	
Sample collection*			
Without pharmacy input	100 (84)	19 (16)	<.01
With pharmacy input	57 (100)	0 (0)	
Utilization†			
Without pharmacy input	138 (91)	14 (9)	<.05
With pharmacy input	67 (100)	0 (0)	

*Appropriateness of sample collection in 46 serum concentrations could not be evaluated due to lack of documentation. Four of these samples had pharmacy input.

†The utilization of three serum concentrations could not be evaluated.

ing the pediatric services prospectively recorded all pharmacy input relating to TDM. Satellite pharmacy staff and pharmacy residents also recorded any input they had while covering the pediatric services. Clinical pharmacy input was also categorized according to the four assessment levels. Input was further classified within each assessment area, according to the specific type of recommendation. For ease of interpretation, pharmacy input that was not followed was categorized in the "without pharmacy" input group.

Each patient's medical record, including the nurses' bedside monitoring sheet, was prospectively reviewed, and a drug monitoring form containing the information listed as follows was completed: patient variables: hospital addressograph, height, weight, sex, birth date, diagnosis, diet, and the dose, start date, and stop date of all other medications; study drug: drug, dose, dose per kilogram of body weight, route, dosing interval, start date, date and time of any missed doses, date and time of last dose before sample, sample time and date, source of sample time (chart, verbal, nurse, physician, or pharmacist), and sample result.

Each serum concentration was then evaluated for appropriateness in each of the four assessment areas. Errors made within each assessment area were further classified on the basis of the following defined criteria.[14,17]

- Incorrect indication
  - Level not indicated but drawn
    - Recent level available and patient's condition stable
    - Dose missed and steady-state level desired
    - Service plans to discontinue drug
  - Level indicated but not drawn
    - Confirm adequacy of treatment
    - Suspected toxic reaction
    - Suspected noncompliance
    - Concomitant disease that may alter drug disposition
    - Concomitant drug that may alter drug disposition
    - Establish baseline value when patient exhibits satisfactory response
    - Adjustment of dosage regimen or change in dosage formulation
    - Determination of effect of maturation on drug disposition
- Incorrect sample time
  - Administration schedule changed but level drawn
  - Drug administration problem
    - Total intravenous dose not infused
    - Incorrect rate of infusion
    - Emesis of dose
  - Incorrect sample time
    - Relation to dose
    - Relation to duration of therapy (steady-state level desired but non–steady-state level drawn)
- Insufficient documentation
  - Sample time
    - No documentation of sample time in patient chart
    - No documentation of sample time in chart but time verbally established by health professional (physician, nurse, pharmacist)
  - Drug serum concentration not reported in chart

The clinical status of the patient and physician intent (as could be determined by participation in morning report, patient rounds, and chart review) were taken into consideration in determining error classification. An individual serum sample may have contained more than one error at each assessment level, and more than one assessment level may have been in error. On the basis of the observed error type, one of the following overall evaluations was assigned to each serum drug concentration: (1) appropriate, (2) inappropriate, or (3) unassessable. A serum drug concentration with one or more errors at any assessment level was deemed *inappropriate. Unassessable* was defined as insufficient information to determine appropriateness. Physicians and nurses were not informed of the study during the time of data collection. The χ^2 statistical analysis was performed for each of three assessment areas (indication, collection, and utilization) to compare the incidence of appropriateness with clinical pharmacy input vs that without clinical pharmacy input. The number of inappropriate serum drug concentrations was tabulated according to the prescribed medication, and cost was calculated. The study was approved by the Institutional Review Board.

RESULTS

We evaluated 222 serum drug concentrations in 49 patients during the 3-month period of data collection. Approximately 43% of the average daily pediatric census received at least one drug that required TDM. Additionally, these patients received an average of 1.36 TDM medications per patient per day. Both absolute and relative frequencies of serum drug concentration determinations according to specific drug are listed in Table 1. Theophylline, gentamicin, phenytoin, phenobarbital, and digoxin accounted for 90% of the serum drug concentration determinations.

Documentation errors occurred more commonly than errors in the other three assessment areas. Written documentation of the sample time was missing from the patient's medical record for 37% (78/210) of the assessable serum samples drawn. In approximately 4% of the cases with a documentation error, neither the sample time nor the laboratory result were documented in the physician's progress notes. The sample time was verbally established by a physician, nurse, or clinical pharmacist in 49% (38/78) of the cases lacking written documentation.

The results of appropriateness of indication, sample collection, and utilization are listed in Table 2. There was a significant difference in each assessment area in the frequency of inappropriate serum concentrations when

Table 3.—Utilization Errors With Nontherapeutic Serum Concentrations

Drug	Serum Concentrations	Physician Action
Digoxin	<0.25 nmol/L	Dose increased 3 d after serum concentration reported
Gentamicin	Peak, 1.8 mg/L; trough, <0.5 mg/L	No change in dose
Gentamicin	Trough, 3.3 mg/L	Patient with renal failure; clinical pharmacy input not followed; additional dose given, with follow-up serum concentration 48 h after dose of 7.5 mg/L
Gentamicin	Trough, 1.8 mg/L	Patient with renal failure; next dose not given until 18 h after trough value obtained
Phenobarbital	Admission, 33.2 μmol/L (preoperative)	Maintenance dose increased but no loading dose given preoperatively; therapeutic serum concentration of 73.3 μmol/L measured 5 d after admission
Phenytoin	18.6 μmol/L	No loading dose given, no increase in maintenance dose
Phenytoin	27.7 μmol/L	Patient admitted for seizure activity; loading dose recommended but not given; no change in dose
Phenytoin	30.5 μmol/L	Level represented steady state (24th d of therapy); loading dose was given, but maintenance dose was not increased
Phenytoin	26.9 μmol/L	No change in dose; patient with seizure activity
Theophylline	9.4 μmol/L (repeated value)	No loading dose given; no change in infusion rate
Theophylline	Trough, 34.4 μmol/L	Sustained-release product; no change in dose (asthmatic)

samples with and without pharmacy input were compared. Without pharmacy input, errors occurred most often in sample collection (16%) and indication (15%). There was a 9% error rate for utilization of serum drug concentrations without pharmacy input.

Forty-five percent of the errors in indication were due to a serum drug concentration having been obtained even though a recent steady-state concentration was available and the patient's condition was clinically stable. Twenty-seven percent of the errors occurred when a serum concentration was drawn even though a recent dose was missed or the patient was not receiving the drug. Eighty-nine percent of sample collection errors (17/19) were due to inappropriate sample time in relation to the dose, duration of therapy, or both. Additional errors included incorrect rates of intravenous infusion and incomplete administration of intravenous doses. Twelve (86%) of 14 errors in utilization were due to the lack of a dosage adjustment after a nontherapeutic serum concentration (subtherapeutic or potentially toxic concentration) was obtained. The majority of these errors occurred in patients with serum concentrations below the normal therapeutic range who may have clinically benefited from an increase in their dosage (Table 3). Additional utilization errors included misinterpretation of the serum concentration based on a previous error and the improper use of a dosage form.

The overall evaluations of the 222 serum concentrations were as follows: appropriate, 110 (49.5%); inappropriate, 107 (48.2%); and unassessable, five (2.3%). In a subset of 100 serum concentrations that had no pharmacy input at any assessment level, 58% were inappropriate based on the overall evaluation. Table 4 lists the percentage of inappropriate serum drug concentrations for each drug studied. Of the most commonly used medications, digoxin, phenobarbital, and the aminoglycosides had the highest error rates. Aminoglycoside antibiotics composed the largest percentage of the total number of errors (32 of 107). Digoxin and aminoglycoside antibiotics were identified as having the largest error rates in the subset of serum concentrations without any pharmacy input.

Table 5 lists the cost analysis for inappropriate serum concentrations. The total cost of inappropriate serum drug concentrations for the 3 months studied was $3081.30, which was annualized to $12 325.20 for the services studied. Fifteen percent of this figure was due to serum drug concentrations with the sole error being lack of documentation of sample time.

COMMENT

Numerous studies in adult patients have evaluated TDM; however, little information is available specifically for the pediatric population.[12-14] Additionally, none of these previously reported pediatric studies assessed each of the four steps of the TDM process, and only one[14] evaluated more than three drugs. Our study design used a multilevel approach to review each of the four steps involved in the TDM process for medications commonly prescribed for pediatric patients. This method provided specific information regarding the successful completion of each step of the TDM process and allowed an evaluation of the overall appropriateness according to individual drug.

Although errors occurred at each assessment level, this study identified documentation as a major problem in the TDM process. Documentation is critical to evaluate the appropriateness of sample time and to utilize the laboratory value correctly. Although sample time was verbally established in approximately one half of all documentation errors, verbal establishment of a sample time is not acceptable from a quality assurance, accountability, or liability standpoint. In addition, without adequate documentation, retrospective drug audits may report a higher percentage of sampling time errors compared with concurrent audits. Makela et al[1] found a significant difference in the percentage of appropriate digoxin serum sampling times when they compared results of a retrospective (71.4%) vs a concurrent (87.9%) audit. In our study, the seemingly high rate of inappropriate documentation (37%) was actually lower than what has been previously

Table 4.—Percentage and Distribution of Inappropriate Serum Drug Concentrations

Drug	Frequency per Drug, No. (%)*	Frequency per Total Errors, No. (%)†
Theophylline	18/66 (27.3)	18/107 (16.8)
Aminoglycosides	32/59 (54.0)	32/107 (29.9)
Phenytoin	18/36 (50.0)	18/107 (16.8)
Phenobarbital	18/26 (69.0)	18/107 (16.8)
Digoxin	18/25 (72.0)	18/107 (16.8)
Valproic acid	1/3 (33.0)	1/107 (0.9)
Vancomycin	1/6 (17.0)	1/107 (0.9)
Carbamazepine	1/1 (100.0)	1/107 (0.9)

*Percentage inappropriate for each drug.
†Percentage inappropriate of total number of errors (n = 107).

Table 5.—Three-Month Cost Analysis of Inappropriate Serum Drug Concentrations

Drug	No.	Cost, $*
Aminoglycosides	32	638.40
Carbamazepine	1	33.60
Digoxin	18	529.20
Phenobarbital	18	623.70
Phenytoin	18	604.80
Theophylline	18	585.90
Valproic acid	1	35.70
Vancomycin	1	30.00
Total	**107**	**3081.30**

*Calculated by multiplying the laboratory charges for each specific drug by the number of inappropriate samples identified for the services studied.

reported. Only 18% of gentamicin serum concentration results were documented in the physicians' progress notes at a Veterans Affairs hospital.[2] Bollinger et al[12] reported that 44% of aminoglycoside and vancomycin serum sample times in pediatric patients were not documented. These samples were also considered inappropriate for the purposes of their audit.

Our rates of inappropriateness for indication, sample collection, and utilization are also consistent with error rates reported in the literature. Inappropriate or irrational indications for serum drug concentration determinations in adults have been reported to range from 10.8% to 49%.[1,3,4,8-10] (Only one of these studies included both pediatric and adult patients[3]; however, findings were not separated by age group.) Our finding of 15% inappropriate indications is well within the range of previously reported rates from adult studies. Likewise, our rate of inappropriate sample collection of 16% is within the observed 4% to 52% inappropriate sampling times from adult studies.[1-4,8,9]

In this present study, the lowest percentage of inappropriateness occurred at the utilization level. Appropriate utilization of serum drug concentrations have been reported to range from 22% to 98%.[1-4,8,13] Our higher rate of appropriate utilization (91%) may be due to the majority (67%) of serum concentrations being therapeutic and not requiring a dosage change. Slaughter et al[8] reported that 98% of digoxin and digitoxin serum concentrations were correctly utilized when a dosage change was not indicated. In contrast, 64% were correctly utilized when a dosage change was indicated (ie, in 36% the indicated dosage adjustment was not made). The errors that did occur in utilizing serum drug concentrations, in our study, could be associated with a less than optimal response to drug therapy, as suggested by Table 3. Our findings are also somewhat in contrast to those of other studies, which have reported a much lower appropriate use of serum drug concentrations. Only 22% of serum gentamicin concentration results were used appropriately in a study by Flynn et al.[2] Anderson et al[4] reported that results of 40% of gentamicin assays were ignored, and only 42% of nonignored correctly drawn samples were utilized appropriately.

On the basis of an overall evaluation, our model identified almost 50% of serum drug concentrations as inappropriate. This figure is also comparable with what is found in the adult literature. At a university medical center, results of a 2-month utilization review indicated that only 30% of serum theophylline samples complied with the overall set criteria.[3] Anderson et al[4] reported that approximately 20% of gentamicin serum assays in adults were appropriately drawn and correctly utilized.

It is important that, although approximately one half of serum concentrations were inappropriate (based on the overall evaluation), failure to obtain a serum concentration when one was indicated was not a problem at our institution. An indicated serum concentration was not drawn in only two of 43 cases where serum concentrations were not obtained.

In addition to identifying and targeting problems occurring at each level of TDM, the described method allows for targeting educational programs based on error rate per drug, per total errors, or by cost. Overall, this model identified three problem medications (digoxin, phenobarbital, and aminoglycosides) and also indicated that each of the five most frequently used drugs accounted for greater than 15% of the total amount of inappropriate serum drug concentrations. Future educational programs and specific drug utilization evaluation criteria can now be developed on the basis of these findings.

Studies in adults suggest several ways to improve the appropriateness of TDM. Levin et al[9] described an educational program for physicians, with concurrent reinforcement, that resulted in a significant increase in the appropriateness of indication, collection, utilization, and overall use of serum concentrations of four commonly prescribed medications. The lasting effects of an educational program, however, are unknown, and reinforcement or reeducation may be required. Additionally, physicians who may know how to perform TDM correctly may not be able to do so successfully due to constraints of time, workload, or other factors. Flynn et al[2] reported that although 93% of physicians surveyed knew the correct time to draw gentamicin serum concentrations, only 60% of gentamicin levels were properly labeled and drawn.

In addition to education, TDM may also be improved by delegating selected aspects of the TDM process to clinical pharmacists. Several studies[5-7] have shown an increase in appropriateness of sampling time by implementing pharmacy-controlled sampling time programs. Ambrose et al[5] demonstrated a significant reduction in inappropriateness (60% vs 1.9%) when sample times were scheduled by satellite pharmacists. The decrease in inappropriate serum concentrations resulted in a cost savings of approximately $500 000 for the 998-bed medical center. Additionally, Elenbaas et al[7] observed a 40% reduction in drug assays obtained per month with an estimated gross annual savings of $14 403, after institution of a program requiring a clinical pharmacists' authorization before serum drug assay determinations. Involvement of a clinical pharmacist at only one of the four steps of TDM does not necessarily prevent inappropriate serum drug concentration determinations. As identified by our multilevel method, errors made at other assessment levels may cause the drug concentration to be inappropriate.

Input by clinical pharmacists has also been reported to improve the rational use of serum drug concentrations. Pasko et al[18] reported appropriate utilization of tobramycin serum assays in 64% of cases without pharmacy input vs 90% of cases on services with active pharmacy participation. In a group of 75 pediatric patients, Illsley[13] found that no decrease in dose was made in 31% of patients with potentially toxic antibiotic serum concentrations. Some dosage reduction was indicated in one half of these cases. With pharmacy input, 64% of such cases received a dosage adjustment. In our study, the incidence of appropriateness at each of the three levels (indication, collection, and utilization) was significantly greater when pharmacists had input.

Multidisciplinary TDM services have also decreased the inappropriateness of serum drug concentrations. Koren et al[14] reported that the number of toxic serum concentrations of 13 different medications decreased at a pediatric hospital after implementation of a multidiscipline (physician and pharmacist) TDM service. A multidiscipline approach to TDM may be the most rational approach, as it permits a sharing of expertise among the health care professionals with a common goal of improving the quality of patient care.

Whether through the use of a multidisciplinary service, clinical pharmacokinetic service, or individual comprehensive clinical pharmacy coverage, a growing body of literature supports the cost benefit of the clinical pharmacist's involvement in the TDM process. Using a meta-analysis of 11 different studies, Reid et al[19] found that a clinical pharmacokinetic service appears to have a beneficial effect on the appropriateness of sample collection and utilization of serum drug concentrations.

The estimate of cost savings for our patients is a conservative one and only includes the cost of inappropriate serum concentrations. It does not include the cost saved due to appropriate TDM and enhanced drug therapy (shorter hospital stay, avoidance of repeated levels, avoidance of toxic reactions, etc). In a randomized, controlled, prospective study by Destache et al,[11] adult patients receiving aminoglycosides for gram-negative infections followed by a clinical pharmacokinetic service had a shorter hospital stay, a significantly shorter febrile period, a less expensive (lower) direct hospital cost per patient, and a higher number of adequate peak levels thanpatients not followed by the pharmacokinetic service. Projected annual net savings were estimated to be $2 220 540 for the institution based on 500 aminoglycoside recipients per year.

This study can also serve as a model method that could be used by a multidisciplinary team to develop specific drug utilization evaluation criteria to evaluate TDM further in pediatric patients.

CONCLUSIONS

Therapeutic drug monitoring is especially important in the pediatric population because of the number of drugs commonly prescribed in pediatrics that require monitoring of serum drug concentrations. The multilevel method described herein may be useful to evaluate TDM at other institutions and to target specific problem areas. The findings of this study also support the involvement of clinical pharmacists in the TDM process to decrease inappropriateness, improve the quality of patient care, and decrease drug monitoring costs.

References

1. Makela EH, Davis SK, Piveral K, et al. Effect of data collection method on results of serum digoxin concentration audit. *Am J Hosp Pharm.* 1988;45:126-130.
2. Flynn TW, Pevonka MP, Yost RL, Weber CE, Stewart RB. Use of serum gentamicin levels in hospitalized patients. *Am J Hosp Pharm.* 1978;35:806-808.
3. Guernsey BG, Ingrim NB, Hokanson JA, et al. A utilization review of theophylline assays: sampling patterns and use. *Drug Intell Clin Pharm.* 1984;18:906-912.
4. Anderson AC, Hodges GR, Barnes WG. Determination of serum gentamicin sulfate levels: ordering patterns and use as a guide to therapy. *Arch Intern Med.* 1976;136:785-787.
5. Ambrose PJ, Nitake M, Kildoo CW. Impact of pharmacist scheduling of blood-sampling times for therapeutic drug monitoring. *Am J Hosp Pharm.* 1988;45:380-382.
6. Greenlaw CW, Blough SS, Haugen RK. Aminoglycoside serum assays restricted through a pharmacy program. *Am J Hosp Pharm.* 1979;36:1080-1083.
7. Elenbaas RM, Payne VW, Bauman JL. Influence of clinical pharmacist consultations on the use of drug blood level tests. *Am J Hosp Pharm.* 1980;37:61-64.
8. Slaughter RL, Schneider PJ, Visconti JA. Appropriateness of the use of serum digoxin and digitoxin assays. *Am J Hosp Pharm.* 1978;35:1376-1379.
9. Levin B, Cohen SS, Birmingham PH. Effect of pharmacist intervention on the use of serum drug assays. *Am J Hosp Pharm.* 1981;38:845-851.
10. Floyd RA, Taketomo R. Serum drug level usage review: a clinical pharmacy service. *Drug Intell Clin Pharm.* 1979;13:44-45.
11. Destache CJ, Meyer SK, Bittner MJ, Hermann KG. Impact of a clinical pharmacokinetic service on patients treated with aminoglycosides. *Ther Drug Monit.* 1990;12:419-426.
12. Bollinger AM, So MH, Winter ME. Aminoglycoside and vancomycin pharmacokinetic monitoring in pediatric patients. *Am J Hosp Pharm.* 1989;46:1770-1771.
13. Illsley SS. Ongoing drug-use review through surveillance of serum antimicrobial-drug concentrations. *Am J Hosp Pharm.* 1988;45:2380-2381.
14. Koren G, Soldin SJ, MacLeod SM. Organization and efficacy of a therapeutic drug monitoring consultation service in a pediatric hospital. *Ther Drug Monit.* 1985;7:295-298.
15. Fox J, Hicks P, Feldman BR, Davis WJ, Feldman CH. Theophylline blood levels as a guide to intravenous therapy in children. *AJDC.* 1982;136:928-930.
16. Hatoum HT, Hutchinson RA, Witte KW, Newby P. Evaluation of the contribution of clinical pharmacists: inpatient care and cost reduction. *Drug Intell Clin Pharm.* 1988;22:252-259.
17. Finn AL, Taylor WJ, Kane WJ. General principles. In: Taylor WJ, Finn AL, eds. *Individualizing Drug Therapy: Practical Applications of Drug Monitoring.* New York, NY: Gross, Townsend, Frank Inc; 1981:1-30.
18. Pasko MT, Mylotto JM, Boh LE. Evaluation of the use of laboratory tests in monitoring tobramycin therapy. *Am J Hosp Pharm.* 1981;38:1956-1957.
19. Reid LD, McKenna DA, Horn JR. Meta-analysis of research of the effect of clinical pharmacokinetics services on therapeutic drug monitoring. *Am J Hosp Pharm.* 1989;46:945-951.

The Association of Pauciarticular Juvenile Arthritis and Myasthenia Gravis

John B. Glass, MD; Phyllis K. Sher, MD; Vanda A. Lennon, MD, PhD; Warren E. Regelmann, MD

• We encountered two children with fluorescent antinuclear antibody–positive pauciarticular juvenile arthritis who later developed myasthenia gravis. Acetylcholine receptor binding, blocking, and modulating antibodies, retrospectively tested on frozen serum, yielded negative results before the onset of myasthenic symptoms but all yielded strongly positive results coincident with the onset of weakness. In both children, myasthenia gravis responded to thymectomy, and one child had a beneficial response to plasmapheresis. Although, to our knowledge, only two patients with juvenile arthritis and myasthenia gravis have been described in the past, the presence of two additional children with both diseases in a single clinic population suggests that the association may be more prevalent than previously suspected.

(*AJDC.* 1991;145:1176-1180)

The coexistence in a patient of more than one autoimmune disease is not rare. The frequent association of myasthenia gravis (MG) and seropositive adult rheumatoid arthritis was one of the observations that led Simpson[1] to postulate about the autoimmune pathogenesis of MG in 1960. In contrast to MG and adult rheumatoid arthritis, juvenile arthritis (JA) has rarely been reported to coexist with other autoimmune diseases. Herein, we describe two children with pauciarticular JA who subsequently developed MG. Because of the occurrence of these disorders in a single clinic population within an 7-year period, we predict that the association may be more common than previously suspected.

PATIENTS AND METHODS

Patients were examined at the Pediatric Arthritis and Inflammatory Disease Clinic, the Pediatric Neurology Clinic, and the Pediatric Ophthalmology Clinic at the University of Minnesota Hospitals and Clinics, Minneapolis. Fluorescent antinuclear antibody (FANA) studies were performed with the use of mouse liver substrate and standard methods. Tests for acetylcholine receptor (AChR) binding, blocking, and modulating antibodies[2] and striational antibodies[3] were performed at Mayo Medical Laboratories, Rochester, Minn.

CLINICAL AND LABORATORY OBSERVATIONS

PATIENT 1.—This 6½-year-old white boy first presented to the University of Minnesota Hospitals and Clinics in July 1982 for a second opinion regarding arthritis. At age 18 months, he had onset of painful swelling in the right third-finger distal interphalangeal joint, the right knee, and the left ankle. Initial treatment with aspirin and tolmetin sodium was unsuccessful. A 1-year course of gold sodium thiomalate therapy beginning at age 3 years yielded excellent results for several months after discontinuation of this therapy. The medical history was otherwise normal, except for vernal rhinitis.

The patient's subsequent presentation to this institution was occasioned by the recurrence of arthritis in one finger joint, one knee, and one ankle. The hemogram was normal, the erythrocyte sedimentation rate was 42 mm/h (normal, 1 to 10 mm/h), serum third component of complement level was 2.61 g/L (normal, 0.97 to 2.24 g/L), total hemolytic complement was 52 U/mL (normal, 25 to 51 U/mL), and the FANA assay yielded positive results; he had no rheumatoid factor. The HLA-B locus could not be typed. He was diagnosed as having antinuclear antibody (ANA)–positive, pauciarticular JA. Ophthalmologic evaluation revealed photophobia and anterior uveitis of the left eye, and the patient was treated with topical steroid and anticholinergic medications. Joint symptoms were well controlled by modification of nonsteroidal anti-inflammatory drug therapy. The patient developed increased intraocular pressure that was unresponsive to medical therapy. A goniotomy of the left eye was necessary 29 months after his first visit for increased intraocular pressure that was unresponsive to medical therapy.

At age 9 years, the patient experienced gradual onset of generalized weakness, slurred speech, and difficulty swallowing, which were worse at the end of the day and which had progressed during a period of 8 weeks. The arthritis was quiescent at this time. Examination revealed bilateral ptosis and dysarthria. Proximal muscle strength was decreased and was graded as 4/5 by Medical Research Council criteria.[4] Serum creatinine phosphokinase and aldolase levels were normal. Anti–striated muscle, anti–smooth muscle, anti-thyroglobulin, and anti–microsomal antibodies were not detectable. Serum levels of IgG, IgA, and IgE were normal, and cryoglobulins were absent. Tests for AChR antibodies yielded positive results (Table 1). Electromyography showed decremental responses to repetitive nerve stimulation at low frequencies. This was corrected with edrophonium chloride, confirming the diagnosis of MG. He was initially treated with prednisone (up to 2 mg/kg per day) but expe-

Accepted for publication April 22, 1991.

From the Department of Pediatrics (Dr Glass), the Division of Pediatric Neurology, Department of Neurology (Dr Sher), and the Divisions of Pediatric Infectious Disease and Pulmonology, Department of Pediatrics (Dr Regelmann), University of Minnesota, Minneapolis; and the Departments of Immunology, Neurology, and Laboratory Medicine and Pathology Mayo Clinic, Rochester, Minn (Dr Lennon).

Reprint requests to the Division of Pediatric Neurology, Department of Neurology, University of Minnesota Medical School, Box 486, Mayo Building, Minneapolis, MN 55455 (Dr Sher).

Table 1.—Immunologic Studies in Patient 1*

Variable	Jul '82	Aug '82	Oct '82	Aug '83	Oct '84	Nov '84	Jan '85	Mar 26 '85	Apr '85	Aug '85	Nov '85	Jul '86	Dec '86	May '89
FANA (speckled pattern)	1:64	1:64	1:64	Negative	Onset of Weakness	Negative	. . .	Thymectomy	Negative	. . .	. . .	1:64	. . .	1:64
AChR Ab†														
Binding, nmol/L	0	. . .	0	. . .		35.8	19.9		32.8	17.0	4.21	13.5	21.9	29.0
Blocking, %	2	. . .	3	. . .		QNS	. . .		. . .	. . .	. . .	0	. . .	15
Modulating, %	0	. . .	0	. . .		96	. . .		. . .	. . .	. . .	35	. . .	5 g
Prednisone, mg/d	None	. . .	Ocular steroids only	. . .	None	None	60	. . .	20	5, plus ocular steroids	None	None	None	None

*FANA indicates fluorescent antinuclear antibody; QNS, sample quantity not sufficient.
†Acetylcholine receptor antibody (AChR Ab) binding reference range, 0.03 nmol/L or less; blocking reference range, 25% or less acetylcholine receptor blockade; and blockade modulating reference range, 20% or less acetylcholine receptor loss.

Table 2.—Immunologic Studies in Patient 2*

Variable	Jan '86	Jan '87	Feb '87	Aug '87	Jun '88	Sep 9 '88	Sep 15 '88	Sep 24 '88	Sep 25 '88	Sep 28 '88	Jan '89
FANA (speckled pattern)	1:64	1:64	1:64	Negative	Onset of Weakness	Negative	Plasmapheresis	. . .	Thymectomy	. . .	. . .
AChR Ab†											
Binding, nmol/L	. . .	0.00	. . .	0.03		86.1		6.82		10.6	64.2
Blocking, %	. . .	6	. . .	8		55		42		59	48
Modulating, %	. . .	6	. . .	0		62		90		83	88
Prednisone, mg/d	None	None	None	None	. . .	120	. . .	. . .	. . .	. . .	12.5

*FANA indicates fluorescent antinuclear antibody.
†Acetylcholine receptor antibody (AChR Ab) binding reference range, 0.03 nmol/L or less; blocking reference range, 25% or less acetylcholine receptor blockade; and modulating reference range, 20% or less acetylcholine receptor loss.

rienced persistent weakness. There were proportional reductions in the forced expiratory flow rate at 1 second from 95% to 61% of predicted value and in forced vital capacity from 92% to 77% of predicted. He underwent thymectomy 5 months after the diagnosis of MG and had an uncomplicated postoperative course. Histologic examination of the thymus revealed scattered germinal centers with no evidence of tumor. After thymectomy, he regained full strength, the forced expiratory flow rate at 1 second increased to 76%, and the forced vital capacity increased to 82% of predicted. He resumed normal activities with no further need for anticholinesterase medication.

Sixteen months after thymectomy, a recurrence of arthritis prompted reinstitution of anti-inflammatory medications.

Patient 2.—This 13½-year-old white girl presented in January 1986 with a 3-year history of intermittent pain and swelling in both wrists and ankles and occasional morning stiffness in the digits. The medical history also included autumnal rhinitis, reactive airway disease, and intermittent headaches.

She had arthralgias but not arthritic joints at presentation. Initial serologic studies revealed an erythrocyte sedimentation rate of 8 mm/h, normal third component of complement and total hemolytic complement levels, positive FANA assay results, and negative rheumatoid factor. Negative results included antibodies to mitochondria, smooth muscle, and immune complexes. The hematocrit value was normal, and there was mild neutropenia. Testing for HLA-B27 antigen yielded negative results. She was diagnosed as having ANA-positive pauciarticular JA. Arthritis recurred in both ankles and in one knee during the next 2 years and was controlled with nonsteroidal anti-inflammatory drugs. Periodic examinations with an ophthalmologic slit lamp yielded normal findings.

At age 16 years, the patient developed muscle weakness that was worse late in the day. She underwent evaluation at another institution, where a muscle biopsy demonstrated small to moderate lymphocytic infiltrates around arterioles and venules in the perimysial space, but serum creatinine phosphokinase and aldolase levels were normal. A diagnosis of polymyositis was made, and prednisone treatment was begun. Strength did not improve, and the prednisone dosage was increased to 120 mg/d. Three months later, the patient returned to the University of Minnesota Hospitals and Clinics, where examination revealed ptosis and substantial proximal muscle weakness. She was unable to fully extend her arms against gravity and could not walk well without support. Exertion exacerbated her symptoms. Immunoglobulin levels were normal, except for a mild elevation of the IgE level, and cryoglobulins and immune complexes were not detected. Electromyography showed decremental responses to repetitive stimulation, which resolved with edrophonium therapy. In addition, AChR antibodies were present in high concentrations (Table 2). The forced expiratory flow rate at 1 second was 68% of predicted, and the forced vital capacity was proportionately decreased to 66% of predicted.

Table 3.—Association of Juvenile Arthritis (JA) and Myasthenia Gravis (MG)*

Source	Age at Onset of JA, y	No. of Arthritic Joints in 1st 6 mo	Anterior Uveitis	FANA	Age at Onset of MG, y	Generalized/ Bulbar Weakness	AChR Ab Prior to Onset of MG	AChR Ab After Onset of MG
Present study, patient 1	1.5	3	+	Variable	9	+/+	−	+
Present study, patient 2	10	1-3	−	Variable	16	+/−	−	+
Aarli et al,[14] 1975	14	3	+	−	18	+/+	. . .	. . .
Denizot et al,[15] 1979	10	4	−	−	13	+/+	. . .	+

*FANA indicates fluorescent antinuclear antibody; AChR Ab, acetylcholine receptor antibody; plus sign, present; and minus sign, absent.

Weakness worsened rapidly, and the patient became nonambulatory. Three courses of plasmapheresis improved strength remarkably. Thymectomy was performed 3 weeks after diagnosis. The thymus was grossly and microscopically normal. Postoperatively, the patient developed *Staphylococcus aureus* sepsis with pleural and pericardial effusions that were treated successfully with antibiotics and with pleural and pericardial drainage. She recovered from these complications 3 weeks after the thymectomy. After three additional courses of plasmapheresis, her strength had improved considerably, and she was able to walk well. Eight weeks after thymectomy, the forced expiratory flow rate at 1 second had improved to 86% predicted, and the forced vital capacity had improved to 82% predicted. She required small doses of anticholinesterase medication to maintain normal strength but resumed normal activities and was able to play tennis. Six months later, weakness again increased, and anticholinesterase medication was poorly tolerated. She responded fairly well to repeated plasmapheresis, but high levels of AChR antibodies persisted. She has had no arthritis since the thymectomy was performed, and intermittent arthralgias are controlled with nonsteroidal anti-inflammatory drugs.

COMMENT

From 1982 to 1988, the Arthritis and Inflammatory Diseases Clinic actively followed 56 patients with all forms of JA. Of these, 26 (46%) had pauciarticular JA, a typical distribution of pauciarticular JA in the total juvenile rheumatoid arthritis population.[5] The two patients described herein with JA and MG account for 8% of the patients with pauciarticular JA. If only the 13 patients with pauciarticular JA at University of Minnesota Hospitals and Clinics who had positive ANA assay results are considered, the prevalence of MG in this population is 15%.

The coexistence of MG and other autoimmune diseases has been reported frequently.[6-11] In addition, MG has been documented in association with thyroidopathies, Raynaud's syndrome, systemic lupus erythematosus, adult seropositive rheumatoid arthritis, and other autoimmune diseases. The major association of JA and another putative autoimmune diseases is the observation of increased frequency of JA and insulin-dependent diabetes mellitus.[12,13] Seven of eight of those patients had the rheumatoid factor–positive polyarticular form of JA. The reported coexistence of the pauciarticular form of JA and another probable autoimmune disease is limited to only one child with JA and insulin-dependent mellitus[12] and two children with MG and JA.[14,15]

The coexistence of JA and MG in two children in a single clinic population is particularly surprising in light of the paucity of previous reports. This occurrence cannot be explained because of bias due to the referral of patients with complicated disease who already suffered from two diseases, because both children were patients at this institution for years before they developed their second autoimmune disease. It is also unlikely that the development of MG occurred secondary to medication. Patient 1 was treated with gold years before he developed MG; there is a single report of MG developing during chrysotherapy in an adult[16] in which the MG resolved after gold therapy was discontinued. The patient in that report had previously had an episode of MG associated with D-penicillamine therapy. Both patients described herein were treated with nonsteroidal anti-inflammatory drugs for arthritis. Patient 2 was also treated with inhaled β-agonists and systemic steroids for reactive airway disease and briefly with ergot derivatives for headaches. None of these medications has been implicated to induce MG. Neither of our patients had a history of treatment with D-penicillamine, the antiarthritic drug most commonly implicated to induce MG.[17]

Myasthenia gravis followed the onset of JA in two patients previously described. Aarli et al[14] described a Norwegian girl who at age 14 years presented with neck pain, arthritis in the left ankle and right great toe, and anterior uveitis who was diagnosed as having JA. At age 18 years, she became weak, and the diagnosis of MG was made by electromyography. The other patient, described by Denizot et al[15] in Switzerland, presented with arthritis in her knees and ankles at age 10 years but did not develop uveitis. Three years later, she developed MG, confirmed by electromyography and seropositivity for anti-AChR antibodies. Three years later, her MG responded well to thymectomy.

The clinical similarities between our patients and the two described previously are summarized in Table 3. All had clinical courses consistent with the pauciarticular subtype of JA.[18,19] It is possible that the patient described by Denizot et al may represent a case of adult seropositive arthritis presenting during childhood, because of the weakly positive rheumatoid factor. However, the lack of symmetrical multiple small-joint involvement favors the diagnosis of pauciarticular JA. Arthritis in these children was diagnosed 3 to 7 years before the onset of MG. The symptoms of MG were generalized in all children, and three of the four also had bulbar symptoms.[20] Each patient developed MG at a time when joint symptoms were quiescent.

The serologic data on our patients may shed light on some aspects of these diseases (Tables 1 and 2). Retrospective analysis of stored frozen serum from both of our patients revealed no evidence of AChR antibodies 2 to 3 years before the onset of weakness. The appearance of AChR binding and modulating antibodies in both patients and AChR blocking antibodies in patient 2 roughly coincided with the onset of myasthenic symptoms. This chronology is consistent with the known pathogenicity of AChR antibodies in MG. Although AChR antibodies are demonstrable in 90% or more of patients with MG during the course of their disease (provided that more than one type of serologic test is performed),[2] there still remains a subset of patients with acquired MG in whom AChR antibodies are not detectable with current laboratory measurements.[21]

Antinuclear antibodies were detected in both of our patients initially but became undetectable during the course of their disease. This conflicts with some reports in which patients with pauciarticular JA remain consistently ANA-positive throughout their disease course.[22] Antinuclear antibody is also not an uncommon finding in MG.[23] The disappearance of ANA occurred near the time of onset of weakness in both of our patients. The patients described by Aarli et al[14] and Denizot et al[15] were seronegative for ANA, but the number and timing of their ANA tests were not specified.

Currently recognized HLA associations do not explain the occurrence of these diseases in the same patient. The prevalence of HLA-B8 is increased in young white patients with MG,[24] but no form of JA has been associated with this HLA type. Some studies have indicated an association between pauciarticular JA and HLA-DR8 and HLA-DR6[25] and between ANA-positive pauciarticular JA with uveitis and HLA-DR5.[26-29] In our patients, HLA typing was not fully performed; they are not known to be related.

The family histories of our patients revealed the presence of other putative autoimmune diseases. The family history of patient 1 showed non–insulin dependent diabetes mellitus in both paternal and maternal lines (paternal grandmother, paternal great-grandparent, and maternal great-grandparent). Patient 1 also has a family history of arthritis, with onset in adulthood of both parental lines (mother, maternal grandmother, and paternal grandmother; severe arthritis in paternal great-aunt). Unfortunately, the form of arthritis in these relatives is unknown. Patient 2 has a family history of non–insulin dependent diabetes mellitus in the paternal line (father and gestational diabetes in paternal grandmother). The increased incidence of these diseases may suggest a familial link, particularly with non–insulin dependent diabetes mellitus.

The coexistence of MG and JA in two of our patients and in two previously described patients suggests a common defect at some level of the immune system. Myasthenia gravis is well described at the effector level and involves the binding of autoantibodies to AChRs at the myoneural end plate. This binding results in complement-mediated lysis of the end plate, increased degradation of AChR due to cross-linking of receptors, blocking of receptors, and cell-mediated immune attack.[30] Weakness results from insufficient functional postsynaptic AChR for depolarization to regularly exceed the threshold for triggering a muscle action potential.[31] The effector mechanism of JA is less well understood. Although several "marker" autoantibodies are associated with JA, no autoantibody has been demonstrated to be an effector of joint inflammation, nor has one been proved responsible for the uveitis that afflicts approximately 50% of patients with ANA-positive pauciarticular JA.[32,33] It seems unlikely that common epitopes would be shared by synovium and muscle, particularly since active synovitis disappeared with the onset of MG and the emergence of anti-AChR antibodies. The coexistence of JA with MG may suggest a role for as yet undefined specific autoantibodies in JA. A defect causing both diseases could ultimately reside at the immune regulatory level. In neither JA nor MG is an underlying immune regulatory defect clearly defined.[34,35]

Nothing in these patients' clinical course or laboratory findings might have predicted later development of MG. The importance in the reduction in FANA titer with the onset of MG has unclear significance as it was documented only in the two patients seen at our clinic. The lack of detectable AChR antibodies before the onset of weakness suggests that currently available serologic tests for MG would not predict the potential for development of MG in patients with JA. However, the sequential appearance of JA and MG, now documented in at least four patients, indicates that electromyography and serologic testing for AChR antibodies should be considered in any child with JA who complains of weakness.

The authors wish to thank Dr Youngki Kim for his assistance in performing fluorescent antinuclear antibody tests.

References

1. Simpson JA. Myasthenia gravis: a new hypothesis. *Scott Med J.* 1960;5:419-436.

2. Howard FM Jr, Lennon VA, Finley J, Matsumoto J, Elveback LR. Clinical correlations of antibodies that bind, block, or modulate human acetylcholine receptors in myasthenia gravis. *Ann N Y Acad Sci.* 1987;505:526-538.

3. Cikes N, Momoi MY, Williams CL, et al. Sriational autoantibodies: quantitative detection by immunoassay in myasthenia gravis, thymoma and recipients of D-penicillamine and allogeneic bone marrow. *Mayo Clin Proc.* 1988;63:474-481.

4. Riddoch BG, Bristow WR, Cairns HWB. Aids to the examination of the peripheral nervous system. In: *Medical Research Council Bulletin No. 45.* London, England: Her Majesty's Stationery Office; 1976:1.

5. Lindsley CB. Pauciarticular juvenile rheumatoid arthritis. In: Miller JJ III, ed. *Juvenile Rheumatoid Arthritis.* Littleton, Mass: PSG Publishing; 1979:135-147.

6. Oosterhuis HJGH, de Hass WHD. Rheumatic diseases in patients with myasthenia gravis: an epidemiological and clinical investigation. *Acta Neurol Scand.* 1968;44:219-227.

7. Simpson JA. Myasthenia gravis as an autoimmune disease: clinical aspects. *Ann N Y Acad Sci.* 1966;35:506-516.

8. Singer W, Sahay BM. Myasthenia gravis, Hashimoto's thyroiditis, and pernicious anemia. *BMJ.* 1966;1;904.

9. Branch CE Jr, Switft TR. Systemic lupus erythematosus, myasthenia gravis, and Ehlers-Danlos syndrome. *Ann Neurol.* 1978;4:374-375.

10. Goulon M. Estournet B, Tulliez M. Myasthenia gravis and associated diseases. *Int J Neurol.* 1980;14:61-72.

11. Somer H, Muller K, Kinnunen E. Myasthenia gravis associated with multiple sclerosis: an epidemiological survey and findings. *J Neurol Sci.* 1989;89:37-48.

12. Rudolf MCJ, Genel M, Tamborlane WV Jr, Dwyer JM. Juvenile rheumatoid arthritis in children with diabetes mellitus. *J Pediatr.* 1981;99:519-524.

13. Daugbjerg PS, Pedersen FK. Arthritis in a 15 year old boy with juvenile diabetes mellitus. *Dan Med Bull.* 1984;31:346-347.

14. Aarli JA, Milde E-J, Thungold S. Arthritis in myasthenia gravis. *J Neurol Neurosurg Psychiatry.* 1975;38:1048-1055.

15. Denizot M, Fulpius BW, Cox JN, Ferrier PE. Evolution clinique et biologique d'une myasthénie gràve après thymectomy chez une jeune fille de 13 ans. *Helv Paediatr Acta.* 1979;34:375-380.

16. Moore AP, Williams AC. Penicillamine-induced myasthenia reactivated by gold. *BMJ.* 1984;288:192.

17. Cooperative Systematic Studies of Rheumatic Diseases Group. Toxicity of longterm low-dose penicillamine therapy in rheumatoid arthritis. *J Rheumatol.* 1987;14:67-73.

18. Brewer EJ Jr, Bass JC, Cassidy JT, et al. Criteria for the classification of juvenile rheumatoid arthritis. *Bull Rheum Dis.* 1972-73;23:712-719.

19. Brewer EJ Jr, Bass JC, Baum J, et al. Current proposed revision of JRA criteria. *Arthritis Rheum.* 1977 suppl 20(2).

20. Fenichel GM. Clinical syndromes in myasthenia in infancy and adulthood: a review. *Arch Neurol.* 1978;35:97-103.

21. Lisak RP, Barchi RL. Myasthenia gravis. In: Walton JN, ed. *Major Problems in Neurology.* Philadelphia, Pa: WB Saunders Co; 1982;11:27-39, 110-156.

22. Rosenberg AM. The clinical association of antinuclear antibodies in juvenile rheumatoid arthritis. *Clin Immunol Immunopathol.* 1988;49:19-27.

23. White RG, Marshal AHE. The autoimmune response in myasthenia gravis. *Lancet.* 1962;2:120-123.

24. Schaller JG, Omenn GS. The histocompatibility system and human disease. *J Pediatr.* 1976;88:913-925.

25. Schaller JG, Hansen J. Early childhood pauciarticular juvenile rheumatoid arthritis: clinical and immunogenetic studies. *Arthritis Rheum.* 1982;25:S63.

26. Glass D, Litvin D, Wallace K, Chylack L, Garovoy M, Carpenter CB. Early-onset pauciarticular juvenile rheumatoid arthritis associated with human leukocyte antigen DRw-5, iritis and antinuclear antibody. *J Clin Invest.* 1980;66:426-429.

27. Suciu-Foca N, Jacobs J, Godfrey M, . HLA-DR5 in juvenile rheumatoid arthritis confined to a few points. *Lancet.* 1980;2:40.

28. Miller ML, Fraser PA, Jackson JM, et al. Inherited predisposition to iridocyclitis with juvenile rheumatoid arthritis: selectivity among HLA-DR5 haplotypes. *Proc Natl Acad Sci U S A.* 1984;81:3539-3542.

29. Hall PJ, Burman SJ, Laurent MR, et al. Genetic susceptibility to early pauciarticular juvenile chronic arthritis: a study of HLA and complement markers in 158 British patients. *Ann Rheum Dis.* 1986;45:464-474.

30. Ashizawa T, Appel SH. Immunopathological events at the endplate in myasthenia gravis. *Springer Semin Immunopathol.* 1985;8:209-233.

31. Lennon VA, Howard FM Jr. Serological diagnosis of myasthenia gravis. In: Nakamura RM, O'Sullivan MB, eds. *Clinical Laboratory Molecular Analysis.* New York, NY: Grune & Stratton; 1985:29-44.

32. Petty RE. Current knowledge of the etiology and pathogenesis of chronic uveitis accompanying juvenile rheumatoid arthritis. *Rheum Dis Clin North Am.* 1987;13:19-36.

33. Schaller JG, Szer I. Rheumatic disorders. In: Stiehm ER, ed. *Immunologic Disorders in Infants and Children.* Philadelphia, Pa: WB Saunders Co; 1989:551-559.

34. Lang BA, Shore A. A review of current concepts on the pathogenesis of juvenile rheumatoid arthritis. *J Rheumatol.* 1990;17(suppl 21):1-15.

35. Levinson AI, Lisak RP, Zweiman B, Kornstein M. Phenotypic and functional analysis of lymphocytes in myasthenia gravis. *Springer Semin Immunopathol.* 1985;8:177-196.

Epidemic Nephropathy in Children

Pentti Lautala, MD, Matti Uhari, MD

• Epidemic nephropathy, a form of hemorrhagic fever with renal syndrome, caused by the Puumala serotype of hantaviruses and occurring endemically in northern Scandinavia, was studied in 13 children. The clinical symptoms and signs were somewhat different from those reported in adults; none of our patients had hemorrhagic manifestations despite low thrombocyte counts. The most common presenting symptoms were fever, abdominal pain, and renal tenderness with oliguria followed by polyuria. The predominant laboratory findings were proteinuria and/or hematuria and elevated serum creatinine levels. Thrombocytopenia was a constant finding in the children in whom thrombocyte count was obtained. Most children had a decreased serum sodium concentration during the oliguric phase of the disease. All the children recovered, with no long-term renal disease. Epidemic nephropathy is an important alternative for differential diagnosis in children with findings suggesting nephritis, especially in endemic areas. An awareness and knowledge of this syndrome and an ability to diagnose it by means of a specific antibody measurement will probably improve our understanding of its epidemiologic features in children.

(*AJDC*. 1991;145:1181-1183)

Epidemic nephropathy (EN) is one of the worldwide group of hemorrhagic fevers with a renal syndrome[1-3] and is endemic to northern Scandinavia. The Puumala virus causing it is transmitted through the excrement of small rodents; the bank vole is the natural reservoir for the disease.[4] The annual incidence of EN varies markedly, with peaks occurring every third or fourth year, apparently depending on the cycle in vole populations.[5,6] The symptoms of EN are relatively uniform, with nonspecific clinical characteristics. It can be diagnosed by measuring antibodies to the Puumala virus by a fairly specific immunofluorescence technique from serum samples taken 2 weeks apart.[4]

Epidemic nephropathy has been reported to occur mainly in rural surroundings, among adult farm and forest workers, and has been thought to be rare among children. Thus, a recent series of 74 cases described by Settergren et al[7] included no patients under the age of 14 years. Since we have repeatedly diagnosed EN in children admitted to the Department of Pediatrics, University of Oulu (Finland), and since the disease is sometimes difficult to recognize, we decided to analyze the clinical and laboratory findings in our 13 patients under the age of 16 years with this diagnosis.

Accepted for publication May 13, 1991.

From the Department of Pediatrics, University of Oulu (Finland).
Reprint requests to Department of Pediatrics, University of Oulu, SF-90220 Oulu, Finland (Dr Lautala).

PATIENTS AND METHODS

Clinical and laboratory data were collected retrospectively on 13 children with the diagnosis of EN treated between 1977 and 1989. Eleven were treated in the Department of Pediatrics, University of Oulu, and two in other central hospitals in northern Finland.

All eight diagnoses made from 1982 to the present were based on the presence of specific serum antibodies to the Puumala virus. Patients with a fourfold or greater increase in this antibody titer or a titer of 1:160 or greater were accepted as serologically verified cases. The antibody measurements were done in the Department of Virology, University of Helsinki (Finland) for our routine clinical practice. Five children were treated before the antibody measurement technique was available, and their diagnosis was based on nonspecific clinical and laboratory findings indicating EN in the absence of evidence of any other renal disease.

Demographic data, presenting symptoms, clinical course data, and laboratory findings were extracted from the patient records.

RESULTS

The most common initial symptom in our patients was abdominal pain, occurring in all 13 patients. All of them had also had a period of oliguria, less than 4 days, followed by 2 to 3 days of polyuria in all patients. All except one patient had documented tenderness in the renal area. The mean duration of fever was 8.8 days (range, 4 to 20 days; median, 6 days). The maximum daily body temperature varied from 38.3°C to 40.5°C. Findings of conjunctivitis (five patients) and pharyngitis were also common. Symptoms suggesting nervous system involvement, including headache and behavioral changes noticed by the parents, were observed in eight patients. Neurologic symptoms occurred in five patients. Visual disturbances with impaired vision were common. The leading finding suggesting EN was proteinuria, which was found in all patients (Table). Ten of the patients had high blood pressure (>150/90 mm Hg). Thrombocytopenia was invariably present in the cases in which a thrombocyte count was obtained (Table). However, none of the patients had any hemorrhagic manifestations.

Microscopic hematuria (degree of hematuria measured from + to +++) was common, and the serum creatinine

Patient/Sex/Age, y	Year	Proteinuria	Creatinine, μmol/L	Sodium, mmol/L	Thrombocytes, X10⁹/L	AST, U/L†	ALT, U/L‡	CRP, mg/L
1/M/12.6	1977	+++	331	139	...	41	50	...
2/M/12.7	1977	+++	130	130	...	...	93	...
3/F/14.3	1977	+++	104	132	...	...	86	...
4/M/6.2	1981	+++	62	137	72	150	92	62
5/M/9.2	1981	+++	811	122	56	152	570	...
6/M/14.4	1984	+++	190	140	91	84	127	48
7/F/15.1	1984	++	211	142	84	35	145	84
8/F/9.3	1988	+++	314	129	87	...	...	69
9/M/12.7	1988	+++	179	125	47	94	78	40
10/F/12.9	1988	+++	400	131	39	121	81	21
11/M/15.3	1988	+++	178	134	59	93	112	62
12/M/8.7	1989	+++	80	136	80	18	19	14
13/M/15.9	1989	+++	601	133	83	54	36	51

Sex, Age, and Major Laboratory Findings of Children With Epidemic Nephropathy*

*Diagnosis in patients 1 through 5 was based solely on the clinical picture. AST indicates aspartate aminotransferase; ALT, alanine aminotransferase; CRP, C-reactive protein; and plus signs, degree of proteinuria.
†Normal, less than 35 U/L.
‡Normal, less than 40 U/L.

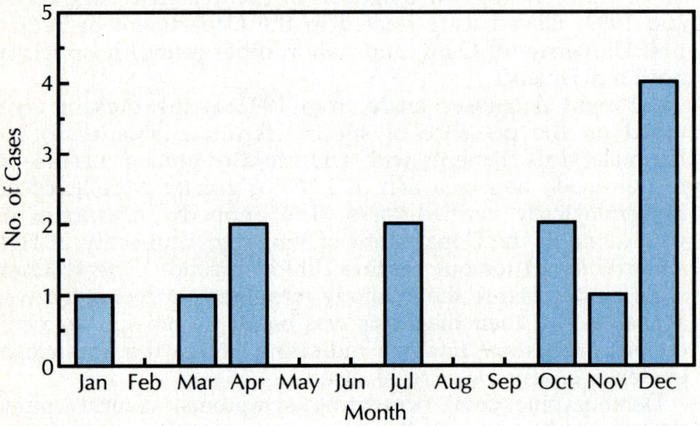

Monthly distribution of 13 cases of epidemic nephropathy.

level was elevated in all except one patient. Serum C-reactive protein level was only slightly elevated. Ten of the patients had elevated serum transaminase levels, and seven had low serum sodium concentrations.

Most cases of EN in children occurred in early winter (Figure), but there was a clear year-to-year variation in the incidence (Table). Winter 1988 to 1989 was exceptionally mild, which probably explains the high incidence of EN during the 2 successive years.

All patients recovered well and had normal serum creatinine and urine findings within 6 months of the onset of symptoms.

COMMENT

Anuria, oliguria, and other symptoms suggesting interstitial nephritis are rare in children[8] and inevitably lead to extensive examinations and diagnostic procedures. At least in endemic areas, EN should be considered as one possible differential diagnosis unless another cause is obvious. Initial symptoms may also resemble those of acute glomerulonephritis or hemolytic-uremic syndrome. However, EN is essentially an interstitial nephritis starting with a phase of oliguria followed by polyuria[9]. The duration of hematuria is usually short. None of our patients had any signs of hemolysis. The diagnosis of EN is now based on specific antibodies in the serum of patients with clinical symptoms suggestive of this disease.[7,10,11] The serologic diagnosis has been available since the detection of hantavirus-related antigen in bank voles (*Clethrionomys glariolus*).[4]

Epidemic nephropathy is a subtype of the hantavirus diseases.[12] There are several serologic variants of these viruses, of which the Hantaan virus is the prototype.[2,12] The variant occurring in Scandinavia, eastern Europe, and probably the Balkan countries is mild in its clinical course, and the infective agent is the Puumala virus.[4,13,14] Other variants with a similarly mild clinical disease occur in Europe, Japan, Southeast Asia, Africa, and the Pacific area, but the viruses have not been isolated. The clinical hantavirus disease has not been reported in North America, but there is evidence of the presence of these viruses. The most serious disease of this type is the Korean hemorrhagic fever.[2]

The annual variation in the incidence of EN has been shown to coincide with the population cycles of rodents carrying the virus.[6] It seems possible that there is some threshold in the number of infected rodents before the transmission of the virus to humans occurs. Similar epidemiologic characteristics, with years in which no cases occur in humans, have been observed with other zoonotic diseases.[15] The monthly distribution of our cases agrees with the suggested mode of transmission of the virus from the excrement of rodents via inhalation.[4] During early winter, the rodents invade cattle sheds and hay barns, thus providing infective material within the hay dust. Transmission in two of our patients occurred in spring, during the cleaning of recreational buildings.

Epidemic nephropathy is rare in children as a clinical disease leading to hospitalization,[13] but antibodies to the Puumala virus have been found in a high frequency in the population of endemic areas, suggesting that subclinical disease may be common.[6] During the last epidemic included in this survey (1988 to 1989), the incidence of EN in the adult population was markedly higher than that in children (at least 36 hospitalized cases during the 2 years). Yet there is no reason why children should not develop EN; they have many opportunities for exposure to the virus. The most probable explanation is that pediatricians do not recognize EN, so that it remains undiagnosed. We found a predominance of boys and of children living in rural areas among our patients, which probably reflects the more frequent contact with rodents.

Histologically, the renal involvement in EN is interstitial nephritis with variable evidence of medullary hemorrhage and tubular rupture.[9] If the diagnosis can be established serologically, there is no need for a renal biopsy. Epidemic nephropathy has a good prognosis with adequate supportive fluid therapy, and there is rarely any need for more active treatment, eg, dialysis.

In children, EN seems to be clinically somewhat different from that reported in adults.[7,9,13] About one third of the adult patients have had hemorrhagic manifestations, mainly epistaxis, whereas none of our patients had any kind of hemorrhage.[13] Conversely, the most common symptom in children was abdominal pain, which is not as frequently reported in adults.[13] About half of all adult patients have thrombocytopenia, which was a constant finding in the children in this study. Whether these discrepancies are due to differences in the interpretation of the symptoms and different selection of patients in childhood or to real differences in the manifestations of the disease cannot be answered on the basis of the present data.

The prognosis of EN in the present series was invariably good, with no permanent impairment of renal function. However, even when the prognosis is good, the clinical disease is a serious one and requires supportive fluid therapy, especially during the early hypotensive and oliguric phases. Fatal outcomes have been reported recently in two serologically confirmed cases in adults with no other underlying disease.[16] This report further underlines the need for careful clinical monitoring. These diseases can probably occur in a larger geographic area than is acknowledged at present, and they should be included in the differential diagnosis even in children.

References

1. Myhrman G. Nephropathia epidemica: a new infectious disease in northern Scandinavia. *Acta Med Scand.* 1951;140:52-56.

2. Hantavirus disease. *Lancet.* 1990;336:407-408. Editorial.

3. Lee HW, Lee PW, Lähdevirta J, Brummer-Korvenkontio M. Aetiological relation between Korean haemorrhagic fever and nephropathia epidemica. *Lancet.* 1979;1:186-187.

4. Brummer-Korvenkontio M, Vaheri A, Hovi T, et al. Nephropathia epidemica: detection of antigen in bank voles and serologic diagnosis of human disease. *J Infect Dis.* 1980;141:131-134.

5. Brummer-Korvenkontio M, Henttonen H, Vaheri A. Hemorrhagic fever with renal syndrome in Finland: ecology and virology of nephropathia epidemica. *Scand J Infect Dis Suppl.* 1982;36:88-91.

6. Nyström K. Incidence and prevalence of endemic benign (epidemic) nephropathy in AC country, Sweden, in relation to population density and prevalence of small rodents. *Acta Med Scand Suppl.* 1977;609:1-92.

7. Settergren B, Juto P, Trollfors B, et al. Clinical characteristics of nephropathia epidemica in Sweden: prospective study of 74 cases. *Rev Infect Dis.* 1989;11:921-927.

8. Burghard R, Brandis M, Hoyer PF, et al. Acute interstitial nephritis in childhood. *Eur J Pediatr.* 1984;142:103-110.

9. Lähdevirta J. Nephropathia epidemica in Finland: a clinical histological and epidemiological study. *Ann Clin Res Suppl.* 1971;8:1-154.

10. Settergren B, Juto P, Wadell G. Detection of specific serum immunoglobulin M in nephropathia epidemica (Scandinavian epidemic nephropathy) by a biotin-avidin-amplified immunofluorescence method. *J Clin Microbiol.* 1987;25:1134-1136.

11. Lähdevirta J, Savola J, Brummer-Korvenkontio M, et al. Clinical and serological diagnosis of nephropathia epidemica, the mild type of haemorrhagic fever with renal syndrome. *J Infect.* 1984;9:230-238.

12. Gajdusek DC. Muroid virus nephropathies and muroid viruses of the Hantaan virus group. *Scand J Infect Dis Suppl.* 1982;36:96-108.

13. Settergren B, Juto P, Trollfors B, et al. Haemorrhagic complications and other clinical findings in nephropathia epidemica in Sweden: a study of 355 serologically verified cases. *J Infect Dis.* 1988;157:380-382.

14. Niklasson B, Le Duc J. Isolation of nephropathia epidemica agent in Sweden. *Lancet.* 1984;1:1012-1013.

15. Uhari M, Syrjälä H, Salminen A. Tularemia in children caused by *Francisella tularensis* biovar *palaearctica. Pediatr Infect Dis J.* 1990;9:80-83.

16. Kauppila M, Kotilainen P, Lähdevirta J, et al. The first fatalities in serologically confirmed cases of nephropathia epidemica [in Finnish]. *Duodecim.* 1990;106:1103-1106.

Minor Malformations, Hyperactivity, and Learning Disabilities

Pasquale J. Accardo, MD; Terry Tomazic, PhD; Jill Morrow, MD; Carol Haake, EdD; Barbara Y. Whitman, PhD

• Standardized minor malformation scores have been reported to predict and identify children with attentional problems and hyperactivity. The reason why this marker works for only a subset of children with attention deficit hyperactivity disorder remains unclear. The dysmorphology scores on all children presenting for a multidisciplinary team evaluation of developmental disorders were examined for diagnostic correlations after children with chromosomal disorders and recognized dysmorphic syndromes were excluded. For 1233 subjects, the mean minor malformation score was 2.94 (SD=2.05). A significant association between minor malformation scores and IQ (mean=80.95, SD=23.67) was accounted for by the group with IQs greater than 100 exhibiting the higher dysmorphology scores. An analysis of variance revealed no significant association between minor malformation scores and hyperactivity or attention deficit disorder. Indeed, the presence of an attention deficit disorder yielded lower mean dysmorphology scores. When the minor malformation scores were compared for those subgroups of children with and without specific learning disabilities, the learning-disabled subjects had significantly higher dysmorphology scores. Minor dysmorphic features do not relate to the presence or absence of attentional problems or hyperactivity in referred children. Rather they appear to characterize that subpopulation of children with attention deficit disorder and learning disabilities as well as a group of learning-disabled children without attentional disorders.

(*AJDC*. 1991;145:1184-1187)

Minor dysmorphic features represent a frequent component of and provide helpful visual clues for the diagnosis of specific syndromes as well as the presence of major organ malformations.[1,2] However, even in the absence of identifiable syndromes, increased numbers of such minor dysmorphic features have been reported in mental retardation,[3-7] schizophrenia,[8-10] autism,[11-14] and cerebral palsy.[15] These minor malformations have been associated with prematurity,[16-19] and with prenatal and perinatal complications.[20-24] They can also be familial traits[20,25] and normal variations of no clinical significance. Most recent research has focused on their prominence in infant irritability,[23,26-29] attention,[30] hyperactivity,[22,31-41] and motor clumsiness,[40,42,43] with the implication that the monitoring of such minor dysmorphic features may provide an effective screening for at least a subgroup of children with attention deficit hyperactivity disorder (ADHD). In only two reports[24,44] has there been any suggestion that dysmorphic features might relate to learning disabilities (LDs) independently of intelligence or ADHD.

Thus, when a general pediatric population is surveyed, minor malformations are found to be associated positively with the presence of a variety of neurodevelopmental disabilities. However, most children with neurodevelopmental disorders do not exhibit elevated dysmorphology scores. The aim of this study is to look at the presence of minor dysmorphic features in a referral population and address the association between dysmorphology scores and specific neurodevelopmental diagnoses in such a population rather than reexamine the poor sensitivities and specificities of minor malformations as markers for the entire spectrum of developmental disabilities.[45,46]

SUBJECTS AND METHODS

During a 6-year period from 1981 to 1987, 1275 children presented to the Knights of Columbus Developmental Center at Cardinal Glennon Children's Hospital, St Louis, Mo, for multidisciplinary team evaluations of their developmental status. Chromosomal studies were performed when clinically indicated by history, physical findings, family genogram, and severity of developmental diagnosis. After recognized genetic syndromes and chromosomal disorders had been excluded, the remaining 1233 children had a mean age of 6.9 years (SD=3.9 years). Their ages ranged from 6 months through 24 years; only eight children were older than 18 years. There were 829 male subjects (67.2%) and 861 subjects (69.8%) were white. The mean full-scale IQ was 81.0 (SD=23.7). The Wechsler scales accounted for 48.1% of these scores, the Stanford-Binet scales accounted for 22.9%, and a variety of other tests accounted for the remainder. There were 338 children (27.4%) with IQs below 70, although only 23.8% were diagnosed as having mental retardation. Learning disability was diagnosed in 607 children (49.2%) by using a discrepancy model. An attention deficit disorder (ADD) without hyperactivity was present in 134 children (10.9%); an ADD with hyperactivity was present in 279 children (22.6%).[47] Both of these latter diagnoses were made in accordance with *Diagnostic and Statistical Manual of Mental Disorders, Third Edition* (*DSM-III*) criteria. Data were incomplete in 18 cases (1.5%); exclusion of these subjects from the analysis reduced the subject population to 1215 children.

A scoring of minor dysmorphic features was included as a routine part of each multidisciplinary assessment (Table). This was modified slightly from the original bat-

Accepted for publication April 8, 1991.

From the Department of Pediatrics, St Louis (Mo) University School of Medicine, Knights of Columbus Developmental Center, Cardinal Glennon Children's Hospital St. Louis.

Reprints not available.

Minor Dysmorphic Features

Electric hair
Hairwhorl abnormality
- Absent
- Multiple
- Poorly defined
- Clockwise
- Frontal

Head circumference greater than 1.5 SD above or below the mean for age
Epicanthal folds
Hypertelorism (increased inner canthal distance)
Low-set ears
Absent ear lobules (adherent lobes)
Other pinnae abnormalities
- Malformed
- Protuberant
- Flattened
- Rotated

Palate, high arched or steepled
Geographic tongue
Clinodactyly of fifth finger
Palmar crease abnormality
- Simian (single four-finger transverse crease)
- Sydney (proximal four-finger transverse crease)
- Other

Sandal gap deformity of the toes
Syndactyly of the toes, partial
Long middle toe

tery of Waldrop[48] by, for example, the addition of an extended distal transverse palmar crease, A_1, a_4, according to the schema of Dar et al.[49] (Because we are dealing with subgroup differences within a referral population, these minor alterations should not have any significant influence on subgroup comparisons.) Using a scoring system in which each individual malformation was given a score of 1 for present and 0 for absent, possible dysmorphology scores ranged from 0 to 20. (The maximum score was 20 because several items in the Table cannot coexist.) Analyses of variance were then performed to assess the relationship between actual dysmorphology scores and hyperactivity, ADD, LD, and IQ.

RESULTS

Dysmorphology scores in the 1233 children ranged from 0 to 11 with a mean of 2.94 (SD = 2.05). The effect of IQ on the presence of dysmorphic features was looked at for the 1192 children for whom dysmorphology scores and IQ were available. The IQ and mean (SE) dysmorphology scores for the IQ groups are as follows: IQ of 3 to 70 (n = 352), 2.93 (0.11); IQ of 71 to 100 (n = 589), 2.82 (0.08); and IQ of 101 to 142 (n = 251), 3.24 (0.13). The means for the first two IQ groups do not differ at the Scheffe .05 level. The group with low IQ scores (3 to 70) had a mean dysmorphology score not different from the mean score for the entire population. However, the mean dysmorphology score for those 251 children with IQs above 100 was 3.24 (SD = 2.08) and an analysis of variance showed this score to be significantly higher than the scores for those subgroups with IQs below 101 ($F[1,838] = 7.485$, $P = .006$).

The 407 children with ADD had a mean dysmorphology score of 2.89 (SD = 2.01); the 808 children without ADD

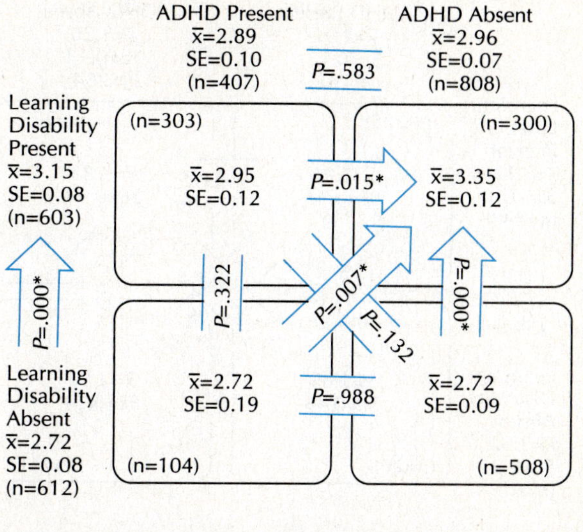

Fig 1.—*Minor dysmorphic features and learning disability/attention deficit hyperactivity disorder (ADHD) diagnoses in a referral population Asterisk indicates (P<.05).*

had a mean dysmorphology score of 2.96 (SD = 2.07). The difference between these means was not significant ($P = .58$).

With the 407 children with ADD, the 133 without hyperactivity had a mean dysmorphology score of 2.77 (SD = 1.95), and the 274 with hyperactivity had a mean dysmorphology score of 2.95 (SD = 2.03). An analysis of variance did not support this difference as significant ($P = .39$). When we restricted this analysis to the 353 children with ADD with IQs of 70 or above, the difference remained insignificant ($P = .11$). Because the dysmorphology scores in our population were highest in the subgroup with the highest IQ scores, we looked at the 263 children with ADD with IQs of 85 and greater. The 95 children with ADD without hyperactivity had a mean dysmorphology score of 2.78 (SD = 1.97), and the 165 children with ADD and hyperactivity had a mean dysmorphology score of 3.11 (SD = 2.02). This difference was not significant ($P = .20$).

The association between dysmorphology scores and the presence of LD was explored. The 612 children without LD (LD absent) had a mean dysmorphology score of 2.72 (SD = 2.03), and the 603 children with LD had a mean dysmorphology score of 3.15 (SD = 2.06). An analysis of variance found this difference to be significant ($F = 13.195$, $P = .0003$). Higher dysmorphology scores were associated not only with the presence of LD but also with the absence of ADHD (ADHD absent)—the absence of ADD with or without hyperactivity (Fig 1). Restricting the analysis to those 509 children aged 7 years and older and with IQs of 70 and above decreased the association with the presence of LD but maintained the association between higher dysmorphology scores and the absence of ADHD (Fig 2).

COMMENT

Suggested biologic markers for neurobehavioral disorders include physiologic correlates (eg, skin conductance, blood pressure, and heart rate responsiveness), electrophysiologic correlates (eg, evoked potentials, brain electrical activity mapping), biochemical correlates (eg, neurotransmitters), and dysmorphic features. The earliest attempt to systematize associations between human ap-

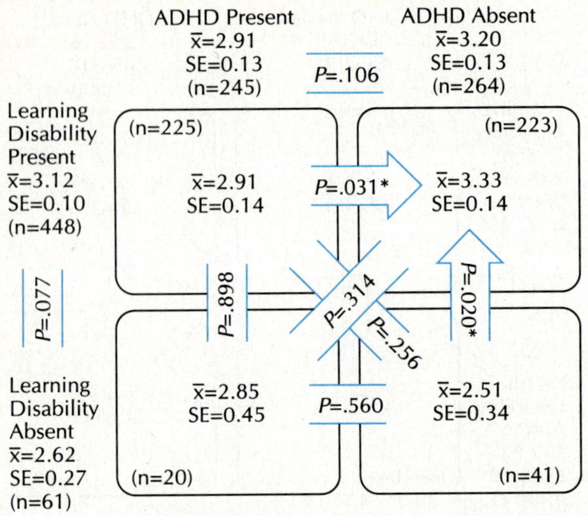

Fig 2.—*Minor dysmorphic features in referred children with ages of 7 years and older and IQs above 69). ADHD indicates attention deficit hyperactivity disorder; asterisk* $P<.05$.

pearance and character was Aristotle's *Physiognomia*.[50] Lavater (1741 to 1801) vastly expanded the catalogue of human traits under observation, and from his physiognomic studies the pseudosciences of palmistry and phrenology revitalized the search for external indicators of occult neurobehavioral abnormalities.[51-53] Syndrome identification in the last half of the 20th century has succeeded in salvaging selected components of this older physiognomic system but in a manner that focuses on diagnosis from patterns of dysmorphic features rather than the presence of single features.

While a single malformation such as increasingly severe degrees of microcephaly can be associated with a single developmental disability such as mental retardation,[54-57] microcephaly may also reflect the presence of LD[58] or language disorder[59] and can be present in nondisabled children. Abnormal scalp hair patterning has been associated with microcephaly,[60] ocular hypertelorism,[61] and underlying brain malformations.[62] Abnormal palmar crease patterns have been associated with Down's syndrome, congenital rubella,[63] hyperactivity,[64] and a variety of congenital disorders.[65,66] Other selected minor anomalies or "informative morphogenetic variants"[67] have been associated with major organ anomalies.[2]

In the area of developmental disabilities the current grouping of minor malformations[40,48] derives from the *petits signes mongoliens* or "microstigmata of Down syndrome."[68,69] With minor variations in the application of this standardized checklist, dysmorphology scores of less than 3 to 5 are usually considered to fall within the broad range of normal. Higher malformation scores have been interpreted as suggesting a morphogenetic disturbance occurring during the first trimester of fetal development and involving the ectodermal germ layer and its derivatives.

Perhaps the most commonly accepted clinical use of minor dysmorphic features is as a screening marker for ADHD. In our referral population the lack of any association with this group of disorders was striking. While a subtle bias in patient selection cannot be ruled out, the present results suggest that the earlier reports of an association between hyperactivity and minor dysmorphic features may have been secondary to an overreliance on preschool children in whom signs of ADHD reflected an underlying central processing deficit (LD or language disorder). This correlation with LD rather than with ADHD will need further investigation, especially with regard to LD subtypes. Another fruitful research direction should be provided by the study of asymmetric minor dysmorphic features.[70] While pursuing these lines of investigation, it should be remembered that these dysmorphic features are variations of normal as well as variations from normal.

Minor dysmorphic features do not relate to the presence of hyperactivity or attentional deficits in a referral population. They do appear to represent a nonspecific and nondiagnostic marker for LD in this group. Their low sensitivity and marked overlap with the dysmorphology scores of nondisabled children do not recommend their use for the screening or diagnosis of developmental disorders in a general pediatric population. However, in the presence of a developmental problem, high dysmorphology scores suggest an organic component to the cause and recommend a closer evaluation for the presence of a specific LD.

This work was supported in part by grants from Columbian Charities of Missouri, Kansas City.

References

1. Jones KL. *Smith's Recognizable Patterns of Human Malformation.* 4th ed. Philadelphia, Pa: WB Saunders Co; 1988.

2. Hoyme HE. Minor malformations: significant or insignificant? *AJDC.* 1987;141:947.

3. Burke NHM. Stigmata of degeneration in relation to mental deficiency. *Proc R Soc Med.* 1931;24:413-428.

4. Ireland WW. *On Idiocy and Imbecility.* London, England: J & A Churchill; 1877.

5. Penrose LS. *The Biology of Mental Defect.* London, England: Sidgwick & Jackson Ltd; 1949.

6. Smith DW, Bostian KE. Congenital anomalies associated with idiopathic mental retardation. *J Pediatr.* 1964;65:189-196.

7. Tredgold AF. *A Text-Book of Mental Deficiency (Amentia).* Baltimore, Md: William Wood & Co; 1908.

8. Green MF, Satz P, Soper HV, Kharaki F. Relationship between physical anomalies and age of onset of schizophrenia. *Am J Psychiatry.* 1987;144:666-667.

9. Gualtieri CT, Adams A, Shen CD, Loiselle D. Minor physical anomalies in alcoholic and schizophrenic adults and hyperactive and autistic children. *Am J Psychiatry.* 1982;139: 640-643.

10. Guy JD, Majorski LV, Wallace CJ, Guy MP. The incidence of minor physical anomalies in adult male schizophrenics. *Schizophr Bull.* 1983;9:571-582.

11. Campbell M, Geller B, Small AM, Petti TA, Ferris SH. Minor physical anomalies in young psychotic children. *Am J Psychiatry.* 1978;135:573-575.

12. Links PS. Minor physical anomalies in childhood autism, II: their relationship to maternal age. *J Autism Dev Disord.* 1980;10:287-292.

13. Links PS, Stockwell M, Abichandani F, Simeon J. Minor physical anomalies in childhood autism, I: their relationship to pre- and perinatal complications. *J Autism Dev Disord.* 1980;10: 273-285.

14. Walker HA. Incidence of minor physical anomalies in autism. *J Autism Child Schizophr.* 1977;7:165-176.

15. Miller G. Minor congenital anomalies and ataxic cerebral palsy. *Arch Dis Child.* 1989;64:557-562.

16. Drillien CM. Aetiology and outcome in low-birthweight infants. *Dev Med Child Neurol.* 1972;14:563-574.

17. Drillien C, Drummond M. *Developmental Screening and the Child With Special Needs.* Philadelphia, Pa: JB Lippincott; 1983.

18. Largo RH, Molinari L, Comenale Pinto L, Weber M, Duc G.

Language development of term and preterm children during the first five years of life. *Dev Med Child Neurol.* 1986;28: 333-350.
19. Simonds JF, Aston L. Behavioral assessment of premature, low-birthweight children a decade later. *Dev Med Child Neurol.* 1980;22:122-123.
20. Firestone P, Prabhu AN. Minor physical anomalies and obstetrical complications *J Abnorm Child Psychol.* 1983;11:207-216.
21. Largo RH, Pfister D, Molinari L, Kundi S, Lipp A, Duc G. Significance of prenatal, perinatal and postnatal factors in the development of AGA preterm infants at five to seven years. *Dev Med Child Neurol.* 1989;31:440-456.
22. Quinn PO, Rapoport JL. Minor physical anomalies and neurologic status in hyperactive boys. *Pediatrics.* 1974;53:742-747.
23. Rapoport JL, Pandoni C, Renfield M, Lake CR, Ziegler MG. Newborn dopamine β-hydroxylase, minor physical anomalies, and infant temperament. *Am J Psychiatry.* 1977;134:676-679.
24. Steg JP, Rapoport JL. Minor physical anomalies in normal, neurotic, learning disabled, and severely disturbed children. *J Autism Child Schizophr.* 1975;5:299-307.
25. Firestone P, Peters S, Rivier M, Knights RM. Minor physical anomalies in hyperactive, retarded and normal children and their families. *J Child Psychol Psychiatry.* 1978;19:155-160.
26. Burg C, Hart D, Quinn P, Rapoport JL. Newborn minor physical anomalies and prediction of infant behavior. *J Autism Child Schizophr.* 1978;8:427-439.
27. Burg C, Quinn P, Rapoport J. Clinical evaluation of one year old infants. *J Pediatr Psychol.* 1978;3:164-167.
28. Burg C, Rapoport J, Bartley L, Quinn PO, Timmins P. Newborn minor physical anomalies and problem behavior at age 3. *Am J Psychiatry.* 1980;137:791-796.
29. Quinn PO, Renfield M, Burg C, Rapoport JL. Minor physical anomalies. *J Am Acad Child Psychiatry.* 1977;16:662-669.
30. Schexnider VYR, Bell RQ, Shebilske WL, Quinn P. Habituation of visual attention in infants with minor physical anomalies. *Child Dev.* 1981;52:812-818.
31. Firestone P, Lewy F, Douglas VI. Hyperactivity and physical anomalies. *Can Psychiatr Assoc J.* 1976;21:23-26.
32. Fogel CA, Mednick SA, Michelsen N. Hyperactive behavior and minor physical anomalies. *Acta Psychiatr Scand.* 1985;72:551-556.
33. Gillberg C. Perceptual, motor and attentional deficits in Swedish primary school children: some child psychiatric aspects. *J Child Psychol Psychiatry.* 1983;24:377-403.
34. Gillberg C, Carlstrom G, Rasmussen P. Hyperkinetic disorder in seven-year-old children with perceptual, motor and attentional disorder deficits. *J Child Psychol Psychiatry.* 1983; 24:233-246.
35. Halverson CF Jr, Victor JB. Minor physical anomalies and problem behavior in elementary school children. *Child Dev.* 1976;47:281-285.
36. Jacklin C, Maccoby EE, Halverson CF. Minor physical anomalies and preschool behavior. *J Pediatr Psychol.* 1980;5: 199-205.
37. Rapoport JL, Quinn PO, Lamprecht F. Minor physical anomalies and plasma dopamine-beta-hydroxylase in hyperactive boys. *Am J Psychiatry.* 1974;131:386-390.
38. Waldrop MF, Bell RQ, Goering JD. Minor physical anomalies and inhibited behavior in elementary school girls. *J Child Psychol Psychiatry.* 1976;17:113-122.
39. Waldrop MF, Goering JD. Hyperactivity and minor physical anomalies in elementary school children. *Am J Orthopsychiatry.* 1971;41:602-607.
40. Waldrop MF, Halverson CF Jr. Minor physical anomalies and hyperactive behavior in young children. In: Hellmuth J, ed. *Exceptional Infant.* New York, NY: Brunner/Mazel Inc; 1971:2: 343-380.
41. Waldrop M, Pedersen F, Bell R. Minor physical anomalies and behavior in preschool children. *Child Dev.* 1968;39:391-400.
42. O'Donnell JP, O'Neill S, Staley A. Congenital correlates of distractibility. *J Abnorm Child Psychol.* 1979;7:465-470.
43. Paulsen KA, O'Donnell JP. Relationship between minor physical anomalies and 'soft signs' of brain damage. *Percept Mot Skills.* 1980;51:402.
44. Rosenberg JB, Weller GM. Minor physical anomalies and academic performance in young school children. *Dev Med Child Neurol.* 1973;15:131-135.
45. Krouse JP, Kauffman JM. Minor physical anomalies in exceptional children. *J Abnorm Child Psychol.* 1982;10:247-264.
46. Pomeroy JC, Sprafkin J, Gadow KD. Minor physical anomalies as a biologic marker for behavior disorders. *J Am Acad Child Adolesc Psychiatry.* 1988;27:466-473.
47. Accardo PJ, Blondis TA, Whitman BY. Disorders of attention and activity level in a referral population. *Pediatrics.* 1990; 85:426-431.
48. Waldrop MF. *Manual for Assessing Minor Physical Anomalies.* Bethesda, Md: National Institute of Mental Health; Laboratory of Developmental Psychology.
49. Dar H, Schmidt R, Nitowsky HM. Palmar crease variants and their clinical significance. *Pediatr Res.* 1977;11:103-108.
50. Loveday L, Forster ES, trans. Physiognomonics. In: Barnes J, ed. *The Complete Works of Aristotle: The Revised Oxford Translation.* Princeton, NJ: Princeton University Press; 1984;1:1237-1250.
51. Gilman SL. *Seeing the Insane.* New York, NY: John Wiley & Sons Inc; 1982.
52. Tytler G. *Physiognomy in the European Novel.* Princeton, NJ: Princeton University Press; 1982.
53. Wechsler J. *A Human Comedy: Physiognomy and Caricature in 19th Century Paris.* Chicago, Ill: University of Chicago Press; 1982.
54. Avery GB, Meneses L, Lodge A. The clinical significance of 'measurement microcephaly.' *AJDC.* 1972;123:214-217.
55. Martin HP. Microcephaly and mental retardation. *AJDC.* 1970;119:128-131.
56. O'Connell EJ, Feldt RH, Stickler GB. Head circumference, mental retardation, and growth failure. *Pediatrics.* 1965; 36:62-66.
57. Pryor HB, Thelander H. Abnormally small head size and intellect in children. *J Pediatr.* 1968;73:593-598.
58. Smith RD. Abnormal head circumference in learning-disabled children. *Dev Med Child Neurol.* 1981;23:626-632.
59. Accardo PJ, Whitman BY. Severe microcephaly with normal nonverbal intelligence. *Pediatr Rev Comm.* 1988;3:61-65.
60. Smith DW, Gong BT. Scalp-hair patterning . *Teratology.* 1974;9:17-34.
61. Smith DW, Cohen MM. Widow's peak scalp-hair anomaly and its relation to ocular hypertelorism. *Lancet.* 1973;2: 1127-1128.
62. Smith DW, Greely MJ. Unruly scalp hair in infancy . *Pediatrics.* 1978;61:783-785.
63. Purvis-Smith SG. The Sydney line: a significant sign in Down's syndrome. *Aus Paediatr J.* 1972;8:198-200.
64. Lerer RJ. Do hyperactive children tend to have abnormal palmar creases? report of a suggestive association. *Clin Pediatr.* 1977;16:645-647.
65. Johnson CF, Opitz E. The single palmar crease and its clinical significance in a child development clinic: observations and correlations. *Clin Pediatr.* 1971;10:392-403.
66. Johnson CF, Opitz E. Unusual palmar creases and unusual children . *Clin Pediatr.* 1973;12:101-112.
67. Pinsky L. Informative morphogenetic variants: minor congenital anomalies revisited. In: Kalter H, ed. *Issues and Reviews in Teratology.* New York, NY: Plenum Press; 1985;3:135-588.
68. Daryn E. Problems of children with 'diffuse brain damage.' *Arch Gen Psychiatry.* 1961;4:299-309.
69. Keizer DPR. Mongolism and other congenital abnormalities. *Lancet.* 1957;2:344-345.
70. Dlugosz LJ, Byers T, Msall M, Marshall J, Lesswing A, Cooke RA. Relationships between laterality of congenital upper limb reduction defects and school performance. *Clin Pediatr.* 1988;27:319-324.

Resident, Faculty, and Residency Program Development

An Integrated Approach Through Annual Retreats

Robert J. Winter, MD; Sharon M. Unti, MD; Jeffrey S. Rubenstein, MD; Fredric D. Burg, MD; James A. Stockman III, MD

• Retreats during residency training have evolved as an escape from the daily routine. Recognizing that the retreat format could also be used as a foundation for program design and personal development, we have designed annual retreats for each of the 3 years of pediatric residency training. The sessions vary in length and agenda, but serve as the basis for an ongoing effort fostering growth and maturation of the department and its component participants. The effectiveness of the program (and the morale of the residents) is greatly influenced by this program.

(*AJDC.* 1991;145:1191-1194)

Fostering program development and the development of program members is an ongoing challenge recognized by most faculty of academic pediatric departments and residency programs.[1-2] The complexity and size of many programs, the administrative burden in managing the day-to-day aspects of such programs, and the absence of personnel with the guidance and nurturing skills required for optimal development are typical dilemmas in large departments. All too often, this results in many "discretionary" issues remaining unresolved, wherein personal and program growth is neither structured nor planned, but occurs sporadically during intermittent crises. Before 1985, the program of the Department of Pediatrics of Northwestern University Medical School, Chicago, Ill, were no different.

To address this dilemma, we initiated a series of annual retreats for the pediatric house staff in 1986. Sponsorship was assumed by the Residency Committee (RC), a group of 20 residents and faculty charged with overall residency program development. Residents are selected for this committee by their peers; faculty are chosen by the program director based on evidence of their commitment to resident education. At the outset, we viewed the concept of retreats in a rather simplistic manner, assuming that benefit to the residents was assured merely because they were removed from the hospital routine for a time. As our experience with retreats increased, the RC recognized the substantial challenge attendant to organizing effective retreats and witnessed the power of them to influence and integrate all facets of the teaching programs of the department. The following description summarizes the sequence of retreats in place in our program and the effect they have on the issues of resident, faculty, and program development.

Accepted for publication April 4, 1991.

From the Department of Pediatrics, Northwestern University Medical School, and The Children's Memorial Hospital, Chicago, Ill (Drs Winter, Unti, Rubenstein, and Stockman), and the Department of Pediatrics, University of Pennsylvania School of Medicine, Philadelphia (Dr Burg).

Reprint requests to The Children's Memorial Hospital, Office of Medical Education, 2300 Children's Plaza, #18, Chicago, IL 60614 (Dr Winter).

DESIGN OF THE PROGRAM

Year 1

In February of the first year of training, a 28-hour retreat is held 90 miles from Chicago, Ill, at a rustic winter recreation area. Although the original intent of this session was to initiate discussion of issues setting the stage for the retreat of the second-year (PL-2) residents 7 months later, the present schedule of activities is designed to encourage interns to "bond" to one another in a manner not otherwise encouraged by the structure of the program except during the orientation period in late June. Considerable "bonding" of program leaders and house staff occurs as well. Residents' spouses and significant others meet at the local residence of one of the group members for a social function on the evening of the retreat. The retreat includes 22 residents, five faculty, and residency program leaders. The total cost is approximately $1000. The duties of the first-year (PL-1) residents are fulfilled by second- and third-year residents.

Impact of Retreats on Residency Committee Activity*								
	Before Retreat Program			After Retreat Program				
	1983	1984	1985	1986	1987	1988	1989	1990
Return of curriculum evaluation forms by residents at conclusion of rotation, % of all forms distributed	NA	NA	21	23	19	24	43	58
Submission of residency committee agenda items by residents, % of all items submitted	<1	<1	<1	3	5	28	42	63
Total No. of items on annual residency committee agenda	19	18	21	33	35	44	51	65

*NA indicates data not available.

Year 2

In September of the second year of residency, the "major" retreat of the program is held over 36 hours at a local resort. The agenda is intended to provide a balance between resident development, program development, and socialization. Spouses and significant others are invited for the reception and banquet Friday evening and stay overnight for the Saturday morning session, which is geared specifically to their interests and concerns. All 10 faculty who are also RC members attend, as do several faculty invited by the house staff in recognition of their teaching effectiveness. An outside facilitator (F.D.B.) also attends, supplementing approximately 22 residents, 15 faculty, and 25 spouses. Total cost is approximately $12 000. Funding for this (and all other retreats) comes from a bequest for medical education from a private donor. Third-year residents fulfill the duties of their junior colleagues.

Year 3

Just before beginning their senior, supervisory year (year 3) residencies, residents attend a 6-hour retreat held at a nearby university conference center. At this time, attention is focused on an agenda of issues related to teaching, leadership, and supervision. Twenty-five residents and faculty attend at a total cost of approximately $500. The intended impact of this retreat is reinforced by periodic meetings of the third-year (PL-3) residents during the third year of residency.

The impact of these retreats on the faculty and the residency program is closely related to the role the RC plays in these retreats. Charged with leadership in residency program development, the RC oversees all aspects of the program and is responsible for its success. As the success of the department reflects in large measure the success of the training program, the RC has a pivotal role that impacts the department and its programs. The RC organizes and conducts the retreats and uses information from them to improve all aspects of department teaching and leaders.

RESULTS OF THE PROGRAM

Year 1

This retreat has evolved into a social event only. The rejuvenating effect of being away as a group for 28 hours while PL-2 and PL-3 residents fulfill intern responsibilities is considerable. Morale and enthusiasm increase immeasurably, such that the absence of a program-oriented agenda is not a liability. It also is effective in producing a collegial relationship between program leaders and interns and sets the tone for their next retreat 7 months later.

Year 2

The format for this 2-day retreat, held Friday morning to Saturday afternoon, is designed to provide specific opportunities for resident development, program development, and faculty-resident-spouse interaction. The following are the major benefits of the retreat.

Resident Development.—In each of the retreats held so far, the opening session has been devoted to the process of giving and receiving feedback and evaluation, largely because we believe this is one area in need of continuous instruction, guidance, and reinforcement. We have consistently used a faculty-directed nominal group technique both as an icebreaker and to elicit examples of good and poor feedback. This not only sets the stage for the session, but also gives a clear message that comments during the retreat may be candid and forthright. The turf of the retreat, the residents quickly understand, is neutral. No holds are barred.

Following the nominal group technique, three consecutive feedback simulations are conducted in groups of six to eight residents each. In these groups, a resident provides feedback to simulators in scenarios illustrating interactions with nurses, students, fellow residents, and faculty. For example, one scenario requires a resident to play the role of an attending physician providing feedback to a psychologically impaired resident (played by the faculty simulator). Ample opportunity exists for commentary among group members and for summative discussion when the full group reconvenes before lunch. The willingness of house staff to give and request feedback, and their skill in doing so, has steadily increased over the last 4 years, as observed from narrative comments of students and faculty. The number of forms returned by faculty evaluating resident performance and documenting that face to face discussion of that evaluation occurred has increased threefold since beginning this process.

The other component of the agenda specifically designed to enhance resident development occurs Saturday morning as a combined session for residents, spouses, and faculty or as concurrent sessions for residents and faculty that are separate from sessions for spouses. The most successful combined sessions addressed personal commitment and time management and was led by an outside consultant invited for that purpose. The most successful concurrent sessions addressed the development of better teaching and role-modeling skills (residents and faculty) and the creation of a spouse support network (spouses and significant others).

Program Development.—The Friday afternoon session is reserved for resident critique of the training program. Led by the outside facilitator, the residents list all issues in the program they believe need to be addressed. Having completed the first year of training, these residents are in a very suitable position to provide such a critique. In this position, they are somewhat more detached and objective than during their internships. The group is asked to prioritize items on the list and select the four to six issues that most need attention. Three subgroups of residents then develop strategies for resolving two to three of these top-priority issues and reconvene before program leaders to present their recommendations.

This not only generates a critique of the program, but also encourages resident co-ownership of the program. Rather than developing a "gripe" list and giving it to the program director, this strategy empowers the residents to find solutions to the problems they have identified. By so doing, they understand the complexity of the issues and are enlisted to help find or be part of the solution. Since this modification has been adopted, there has been a noticeable shift from a "boss-employee" to a "co-ownership" relationship between the residents and program leaders. As a result, all participants have a much better understanding of exactly what it means to be colleagues of one another. Differences in age, experience, or coat color become less significant, and meaningful first-name relationships evolve more spontaneously.

The critique and the strategies developed to address issues raised by the critique become the substantive portion of the agenda for the RC for that academic year. As can be seen in the Table, before beginning this retreat program, the RC functioned virtually independently of the residents in creating an agenda for each academic year.

The RC agenda is reviewed 1 year later at the PL-2 retreat for the next cohort of residents, when the program director gives his annual "State of the Residency" report summarizing the progress of the program as reflected by how well each item on the previous year's agenda has been addressed. The development of an effective mechanism to provide feedback from residents to faculty is one example of an issue raised at the 1989 retreat and whose solution was implemented before the 1990 gathering. This reporting mechanism not only reminds residents that progress does occur, but it also forces program leaders to diligently ensure that the program progresses. The result is an ever improving residency program and consistent credibility of program leaders.

Faculty development also results from this portion of the retreat. Faculty attending the retreat convene by themselves Friday afternoon for a program critique session and participate in open discussion with house staff of faculty issues viewed as impediments to their learning and career development. As an outgrowth of this, the program has revised its method of providing feedback to faculty. Residents are now debriefed at the end of each rotation about their interactions with faculty by a program leader, and a written summary of resident comments is given to the attending physician. A copy of this summary is placed in the attending physician's permanent file. This program was begun in the 1989-1990 academic year; preliminary impressions of its effectiveness are very encouraging, although conclusive data concerning faculty behaviors will require several more years of observation.

Socialization.—Social activities occur at mealtimes, during breaks, at a 3-hour "free time" period, and during the Friday evening reception, banquet, and open bar. In addition, the recreation and entertainment facilities of the resort are open for resident use. This schedule, and inclusion of spouses/significant others, demonstrate to the residents the appreciation of the faculty for the residents and their contributions to the program and the institution.

Year 3

The retreat at the beginning of the third and final year of training is designed with the perspective that the residency program is only as good as the third-year residents. They set the tone for learning, patient care, and interpersonal interaction. If that tone is discordant, the ward entrusted to that resident will not run smoothly, and the deleterious impact on impressionable interns and medical students could be considerable.

With this in mind, an agenda has been developed by program leaders in which incoming third-year residents engage in small-group discussion and role-playing of issues of feedback, teaching, delegation of responsibility, use of consultants, communicating with referring physicians, and managing telephone requests for transport of critically ill children. Simulations are prepared and conducted by selected third-year residents. A copy of *The One Minute Manager*[3] is given to each resident as a reminder of the role they are about to assume. Although no dedicated time is reserved to review information from the PL-2 retreat in September, they are reminded that they are co-owners of the program and its structure. The clear intent of this retreat is that third-year residents enter their final year of training well prepared for the leadership roles entrusted to them.

Residency Program Development

A partial profile of the impact of these retreats on program function for the academic years 1983 through 1990 is shown in the Table. The data confirm that the residents have progressively become "co-owners" of the program and use the RC to address issues important to them and the residency program.

COMMENT

This report does not suggest that resident retreats are a novel idea. However, previously reported retreats[4-7] do not appear to have been as comprehensively integrated into the program as ours. Previous retreats have been described as predominantly educational and/or recreational[4,5] or as means of eliciting program critique.[6,7] By sponsoring an annual retreat for each group of residents, we have created a program that give continuity to the 3 years of residency training.

This retreat program provides a foundation for integrating both development of the residency program and development of residents and faculty. These efforts require some time and money, and do not assure success. They do, however, create an attitude, atmosphere, or commitment with which the day-to-day issues of personal and program development are more effectively resolved.

Precisely measuring the success of this retreat program by its outcomes is difficult, just as determining the ingredients for program or personal success are difficult. This residency program continues to strengthen, but it was strong before the retreats began. It is impossible to separate the influence on the program of individuals (the chairman, program director, and chief residents) from that of the retreats. Yet, as the result of this retreat program, most "discretionary" issues are given prompt and appropriate attention. A structure is firmly in place to foster an ongoing partnership between residents and program leaders. The "status quo" is certainly not maintained. Complacency has no more place in a residency program than in an individual physician.

One specific result of the retreats was the formation of the Medical Education Group, which meets weekly to discuss personal and program development. The Medical Education Group is the result of the department's commitment to medical education. It consists of the full-time program director and two other faculty with proven commitments to education who together spend about three quarters of their work time in medical education. The two chief residents are the remaining members of the group. Beginning in 1990, a 2-day retreat for group members was convened for program development. The incoming PL-2 and PL-3 chief residents participate in the retreat, in which they are oriented to the group and their active participation in the group is enlisted.

Resident and residency program development remain dynamic processes that should never become static. The success of the retreat program described in this report has highlighted the need to approach faculty development in a similar manner. Planning for an annual faculty retreat to address issues of teaching effectiveness, curricular development, and role modeling is under way.

References

1. Accreditation Council for Graduate Medical Education. *General Requirements of the Essentials of Accredited Residencies in Graduate Medical Education.* 76th ed. Chicago, Ill: American Medical Association; 1990.
2. Accreditation Council for Graduate Medical Education. *Program Information Form—Residency Review Committee for Pediatrics.* 76th ed. Chicago, Ill: American Medical Association; 1990.
3. Blanchard K, Johnson S. *The One Minute Manager.* New York, NY: Berkley Books; 1982.
4. Bergman AB, Rothenberg MB, Telzrow RW. A 'retreat' for pediatric interns. *Pediatrics.* 1979;64:529-532.
5. Schum TR, Rice TR, Chusid MJ, Blodgett FM. A retreat for first year house staff members. *J Med Educ.* 1982;57:568-569.
6. Moore SL. House officer retreats: a way to improve residency training programs. *Res Staff Physic.* 1979;25:105-108.
7. Alden ER, Holt C, Todd WA, Barko W. Pediatric retreat mode for planning. *Milit Med.* 1983;148:509-511.

In Other AMA Journals

ARCHIVES OF OTOLARYNGOLOGY—HEAD & NECK SURGERY

Microbiology of Chronic Sinusitis in Children

Peter W. Orobello, Jr, MD; Robert I. Park, MD; Laura J. Belcher, RN; Peyton Eggleston, MD; Howard M. Lederman, MD, PhD; James R. Banks, MD; John F. Modlin, MD; Robert M. Naclerio, MD
(*Arch Otolaryngol Head Neck Surg.* 1991;117:980-983)

Systemic Steroids for Otitis Media With Effusion in Children

Richard M. Rosenfeld, MD, MPH; Ellen M. Mandel, MD; Charles D. Bluestone, MD
(*Arch Otolaryngol Head Neck Surg.* 1991;117:984-989)

Language Screening as a Factor in the Management of the Pediatric Otolaryngic Patient: Effectiveness and Efficiency

Robert J. Ruben, MD
(*Arch Otolaryngol Head Neck Surg.* 1991;117:1021-1025)

Nodular Fasciitis of the Head and Neck in Children: A Deceptive Lesion

Laurence J. DiNardo, MD; Ralph F. Wetmore, MD; William P. Potsic, MD
(*Arch Otolaryngol Head Neck Surg.* 1991;117:1001-1002)

Hand Washing in Pediatric Ambulatory Settings

An Inconsistent Practice

Jacob A. Lohr, MD; David L. Ingram, MD; Sharon M. Dudley, MT; Elizabeth L. Lawton, RN, PNP; Leigh G. Donowitz, MD

• The first phase of this study was performed to determine the rate of breaks in hand washing technique by physicians in two pediatric ambulatory settings and to determine whether this technique was influenced by the physician's level of training. The second phase was performed to determine if reminding physicians to wash their hands would decrease the rate of breaks. A hand washing break in technique was defined as not washing hands before patient contact. The observations were made by medical students accompanying the providers. In the 496 encounters during the first phase, 254 breaks (51.2%) occurred. In the 293 encounters during the second phase, 150 (51.2%) breaks occurred. During both phases, the rates of hand washing breaks among the four groups of providers (residents in postgraduate years 1 through 3 and faculty) were similar. Breaks in hand washing technique occur at an unacceptably high rate in outpatient settings.

(*AJDC*. 1991;145:1198-1199)

Hand washing by physicians in a pediatric ambulatory setting should be standard practice. The first phase of this study was performed to determine the rate of breaks in hand washing technique by physicians in pediatric ambulatory settings and whether this rate was influenced by level of training or experience. The second phase of the study was performed to determine if reminding physicians of the importance of hand washing would decrease the rate of breaks.

SUBJECTS AND METHODS

Population

The University of Virginia (UVA), Charlottesville, general pediatric clinic annually sees approximately 12 500 patients who are younger than 16 years. The Wake Medical Center, Raleigh, NC, general pediatric clinic annually sees approximately 5500 patients who are younger than 18 years.

Accepted for publication February 4, 1991.

From the Department of Pediatrics, University of Virginia Children's Medical Center, Charlottesville (Drs Lohr and Donowitz and Mss Dudley and Lawton); and Department of Pediatrics, University of North Carolina, Chapel Hill (Dr Ingram). Dr Lohr is now with the University of North Carolina, Chapel Hill.

Reprints not available.

Facilities and Staffing

The UVA clinic has 16 examination rooms; each is equipped with a sink and bactericidal solution for hand washing. The Wake Medical Center clinic has 10 examination rooms; eight are equipped with sinks and bactericidal solution for hand washing, and two have sinks and hand washing solution outside the room.

The UVA and Wake Medical Center clinics are staffed by pediatric faculty and pediatric and family medicine residents.

Methods

A hand washing break in technique was defined as not washing hands before patient contact. The observations were made by medical students accompanying the providers during routine clinic hours and were made without the knowledge of the providers. The student documented resident year or faculty status and hand washing practice. Although the primary focus of the study was on hand washing before patient contact, hand washing practice after patient contact was also recorded.

The observations of the first phase of the study occurred during a 5-month period at UVA and Wake Medical Center. The observations of the second phase of the study occurred during a 7-month period only at UVA.

Before the second phase was initiated, two commercially printed signs stating "Good patient care includes good hand washing" were posted in highly visible places in the physicians' work room, the site of most patient care discussions and physician charting. In addition, the clinic faculty were informed that previous observations (they were not told what kind of observations) indicated that hand washing was not being practiced at an acceptable rate in the clinic and were encouraged to increase their personal rate of hand washing. Finally, at the beginning of each clinic rotation, the residents were reminded by the clinic head nurse of the importance of practicing good hand washing technique before any patient contact.

Statistical Methods

The rates of hand washing breaks among the four different physician provider groups (faculty and residents in postgraduate years 1 through 3) were compared using χ^2 analysis. The rates of hand washing breaks during the two phases of the study were likewise compared with a χ^2 analysis. A 95% confidence interval around the observed difference in hand washing breaks for the two study phases was calculated by standard methods.[1] The likelihood of having failed to detect a true 10% reduction in hand washing breaks during the second study phase was calculated by standard methods.[2]

Hand Washing Breaks in Technique by Physician Provider Groups*				
	Phase 1		Phase 2	
Provider Group	No. (%) of Breaks	No. of Encounters	No. (%) of Breaks	No. of Encounters
Faculty	125 (55.1)	227	42 (48.8)	86
PGY-3	29 (38.7)	75	33 (55.9)	59
PGY-2	43 (52.4)	82	23 (45.1)	51
PGY-1	57 (50.9)	112	52 (53.6)	97
Total	**254** (51.2)	**496**	**150** (51.2)	**293**

*Phase 1 was before physician providers were reminded of the importance of hand washing; Phase 2, after they were reminded of it. PGY indicates postgraduate year.

RESULTS

During the study's first phase, 496 patient encounters were monitored (Table). Collectively, all groups of physicians did not wash their hands before patient contact in 254 (51.2%) of the encounters. In 47 (9.5%) of the encounters (not shown in the Table), physicians who did not wash their hands before patient contact did wash after patient contact.

During the study's second phase, a total of 293 patient encounters were monitored (Table). Collectively, all groups of physicians did not wash their hands before patient contact in 150 (51.2%) of the encounters. In 33 (11.3%) of the encounters (not shown in the Table), physicians who did not wash their hands before patient contact did wash after patient contact.

The rates of hand washing breaks (not washing before patient contact) among the four different levels of provider (faculty and postgraduate years 1 through 3) were similar (Table; $\chi^2=2.1$, $df=3$, $P>.5$).

The rates of hand washing breaks during the two study phases were almost identical, with a minimal decrease of 0.02% during the second phase (95% confidence interval, −7.2% to 7.2%). Based on the study size and the observed rates of hand washing breaks, the likelihood of having failed to detect a true 10% reduction in hand washing breaks during the second phase was low ($P\ \beta<.005$).

COMMENT

Hand washing is the most effective available means of decreasing the transmission of potential bacterial and viral pathogens between patients and between staffs and patients.[3-6] The effectiveness of hand washing is enhanced by the use of one of several bacteriostatic or bactericidal agents that have been shown to decrease the permanent and transient bacterial flora on the hands of hospital personnel.[7-11] Although the risk of transmission of infectious agents is less well defined for clinic populations, the potential for spread of infection clearly exists, and means of interrupting transmission should be encouraged.

The first phase of this study in two pediatric general clinic settings shows that despite all of the historical knowledge of hand transmission of infectious pathogens and the availability of a bactericidal hand washing product, pediatric clinic faculty and residents fail to wash their hands more than 50% of the time before patient contact. This failure rate is less than that reported for pediatric inpatient units, where breaks in hand washing rates as high as 85% occur[12,13]; however, the rates in this study too are unacceptable.

The rates of breaks for faculty and for residents at different levels of training were not different in this study and imply that the use of hand washing does not increase with increased experience.

Disappointingly, the rates of breaks did not decrease significantly in the second phase of the study, demonstrating the ineffectiveness of the methods we chose to increase the use of hand washing.

Some might argue that hand washing after patient contact would be as acceptable as washing before patient contact. In only 9.5% of the encounters in the first phase of the study and 11.3% of the encounters in the second phase of the study did physicians who had not washed their hands before patient contact wash after patient contact.

Hand washing remains the most important method available for reducing the transmission of infectious pathogens. More effective methods for increasing its use must be identified and used in pediatric clinic settings.

We thank Gregory F. Hayden, MD, for his assistance with the statistical analysis of the data.

References

1. Fleiss JL. *Statistical Methods for Rates and Proportions.* New York, NY: John Wiley & Sons Inc; 1973:73-74.
2. Feinstein AR. *Clinical Biostatistics.* St Louis, Mo: CV Mosby Co; 1977:326-328.
3. Mortimer EA, Lipsitz PJ, Wolinsky E, et al. Transmission of staphylococci between newborns: importance of the hands of personnel. *AJDC.* 1962;104:289-295.
4. Steere AC, Mallison GF. Handwashing practices for the prevention of nosocomial infections. *Ann Intern Med.* 1975;83:683-690.
5. Knittle MA, Eitzman DV, Baer H. Role of hand contamination of personnel in the epidemiology of gram-negative nosocomial infections. *J Pediatr.* 1975;86:433-437.
6. Interview with Philip A. Pizzo. Isolation techniques in hospitals. *Pediatr Infect Dis.* 1983;2:94-98.
7. Lowbury EJL, Lilly HA, Bull JP. Disinfection of hands, removal of transient organisms. *Br Med J.* 1964;2:230-233.
8. Sprunt K, Redman W, Leidy G. Antibacterial effectiveness of routine hand washing. *Pediatrics.* 1973;52:264-271.
9. Larson E. Handwashing and skin physiologic and bacteriologic aspects. *Infect Control.* 1985;6:14-23.
10. Larson E, Leyden JJ, McGinley KJ, et al. Physiologic and microbiologic changes in skin related to frequent handwashing. *Infect Control.* 1986;7:59-63.
11. Morrison AJ, Gratz J, Cabezudo I, et al. The efficacy of several new hand washing agents for removing non-transient bacterial flora from hands. *Infect Control.* 1986;7:268-272.
12. Donowitz LG. Handwashing technique in a pediatric intensive care unit. *AJDC.* 1987;141:683-685.
13. Carvalho DM, Lopes JMA, Pellitteri M. Frequency and duration of hand washing in a neonatal intensive care unit. *Pediatr Infect Dis J.* 1989;8:179-180.

Immersion Events in Residential Swimming Pools

Evidence for an Experience Effect

Garen J. Wintemute, MD, MPH; Christiana Drake, PhD; Mona Wright

• ***Background.***—**Drowning and near-drowning in residential swimming pools are leading causes of morbidity and mortality for young children. We tested the hypothesis that the period immediately after a pool is acquired is a time of high risk for these events. This study was also designed to provide population-based data on swimming pool immersion events, regardless of severity.**

Methods.—**We conducted a mail survey of a probability sample of Sacramento County, California, households with in-ground swimming pools in January 1988; 80% of eligible subjects responded. Onset of exposure to a pool was defined as the month in which (1) the responding household had a pool installed, or (2) the responding household first occupied a residence with a pool. Exposures began in 1959 through 1987.**

Results.—**The home swimming pool immersion event rate was 11 per 1000 pool-years. The rate per 1000 pool-years was higher for the first 6 months of exposure than thereafter (0 to 6 months, 44; 7 to 24 months, 14; >24 months, seven), but 77% of events occurred outside the high-risk period. For households whose exposures began in 1984 through 1987, the immersion event rate was 51 per 1000 pool-years overall and 123 per 1000 pool-years for the first 6 months of pool exposure; these increases probably represent underreporting of earlier events. In this group, 48% of events occurred outside the high-risk period. The family swimming pool accounted for 91% of immersion events at the respondents' homes.**

Conclusions.—**The residential swimming pool is an important hazard for pool-owning households. The first 6 months of exposure constitute a high-risk period, but many immersion events occur later. Pool drowning prevention programs may focus on newly acquired swimming pools and their owners but should be as broad as possible to maximize their effectiveness.**

(*AJDC*. 1991;145:1200-1203)

Drowning and near-drowning in early childhood have become a leading focus of injury prevention efforts in the United States. This stems in part from the frequency and severity of these immersion injuries. In 1987, 652 children 1 to 4 years of age drowned in the United States.[1] For each child who drowns, three to four others are hospitalized after a near-drowning; as many as 20% of survivors suffer severe permanent disability.[2] The total annual economic losses due just to swimming pool drowning and near-drowning of young children are estimated to be $450 to $650 million.[3]

The need for, and potential success of, childhood drowning prevention efforts are enhanced by the fact that a proved intervention exists that will be effective in the majority of cases. From 52% to 85% of drownings and near-drownings among young children occur in residential swimming pools.[4-9] Four-sided fencing for residential swimming pools has been shown to reduce the incidence of these immersion injuries in case-control[10] and quasi-experimental[11-14] studies and is expected to prevent 50% to 90% of swimming pool immersion injuries if widely used.[10,13,15]

Pediatricians[16] and public health officials[17] have advocated mandatory fencing for residential swimming pools. A fencing requirement that extends to all residential pools could be justified by the epidemiology of childhood immersion injury: while children drown most frequently in their own home pools, a substantial minority drown at the homes of friends, neighbors, or relatives.[8,10] The model code drafted by the Consumer Product Safety Commission contains such a fencing requirement.[18]

However, a universal fencing requirement has limited public support in the United States. Although a number of jurisdictions have recently passed residential swimming pool fencing laws, these laws all contain significant exemptions. Some apply only to newly constructed pools; others exempt households without young children. A recent survey, conducted in a community with a high rate of swimming pool drownings, found only 18% of pool owners to be in support of a universal barrier requirement.[19]

The major purpose of this study was to help determine whether a universal fencing requirement is necessary. It may not be if an easily identifiable subset of households with swimming pools is at particularly high risk for childhood drowning and near-drowning. Specifically, we tested the hypothesis that there is an experience effect for immersion events in residential swimming pools. If such an effect exists, then the immersion event rate should be

Accepted for publication May 22, 1991.

From the Departments of Family Practice (Dr Wintemute and Ms Wright) and Statistics (Dr Drake), University of California, Davis, Sacramento.

Reprints not available.

Rate of Reported Swimming Pool Immersion Events per 1000 PY by Time Since Onset of Pool Exposure, Sacramento County, California*

Months Since Onset of Exposure	Events/1000 PY	95% CI
All Respondents		
0-6	44	25, 74
7-24	14	8, 25
>24	7	5, 10
Respondents With Exposure Beginning 1984-1987		
0-6	123	69, 220
7-24	25	11, 59
>24	36	12, 106

*PY indicates pool-years; CI, confidence interval.

high when exposure to a pool begins (when a pool is installed or when a household first occupies a residence with a pool) and should decline thereafter.

Our results are drawn from a probability sample of households with pools in a defined population. Therefore, the study also sought to determine the true risk of swimming pool and other immersion events, to rank swimming pools among the water hazards to which pool-owning households are exposed, and to expand our understanding of the epidemiology and course of these events.

DEFINITIONS

Immersion event is defined in this study as it was in the survey questionnaire, as "an event in which a person gets into trouble in the water and actually drowns, or might have drowned if they had not been rescued or managed to save themselves." *Immersion injury* is taken to mean any compromise of physical function or mental status resulting from an immersion event, however minor or transient. *Drownings* are fatal immersion injuries. *Near-drownings* are nonfatal immersion events; they do not necessarily involve immersion injury.

SUBJECTS AND METHODS

The data for this study were gathered by a survey of a probability sample of Sacramento County, California, households with in-ground pools, conducted January through April 1988. The survey methods have been described previously[19] and will be summarized herein. Households were selected by systematic sampling from a random starting point on a list of all Sacramento County building permits awarded for in-ground pool construction since 1959. Permits for multiple-dwelling and public pools were eliminated. Current owners were identified in County Assessor records; nonresident owners were excluded. The survey was conducted by mail, following the method developed by Dillman.[20,21] Eighty percent of eligible households responded. Only one question had more than 4% of responses missing.

Confidence intervals (CIs) for proportions and odds ratios (ORs) were calculated by the exact method. Immersion event rates were calculated on a pool-year (PY) basis, as our use of a mailed questionnaire did not permit us to gather detailed data on household composition over time for person-based rates. Rates were calculated for three periods of pool exposure: the first 6 months, 7 to 24 months, and beyond 24 months. Approximate CIs for these rates were derived by treating the number of events in each specified time interval (the numerator in the rate calculation) as a Poisson variable.[22]

Hazard rates for initial pool immersion events were also calculated. The hazard rate at time t (in this case, time since the onset of exposure to a pool) is the likelihood of the occurrence of the outcome of interest (here, a first immersion event) in the period immediately following t. Hazard rates permit more detailed analysis but may underestimate the true rate of outcomes, such as immersion events, which can occur more than once. The hazard rate is calculated using the life-table method and is a continuous function of time.

In calculating PY, we assumed that each pool contributed a half PY of exposure in the year exposure began. This assumption was justified by the survey results: 53% of exposures began in January through June, and 47% in July through December (74 households did not report this information).

Initial analysis revealed a substantial increase in the incidence of immersion events in the last 4 years of the study period, raising the possibility of artifact due to recall error. Rates were therefore recalculated for the 179 households whose exposures began in those years.

Results were rounded to whole numbers.

RESULTS

The 637 responding households contributed 5735 PY of exposure over the study period. During this time, 45 households (7%) (95% CI, 5%, 9%) reported a total of 61 swimming pool immersion events at home, for an overall rate of 11 events per 1000 PY (95% CI, 9, 14). Of these events, 74% (95% CI, 62%, 85%) involved children under 5 years of age; 73% (95% CI, 60%, 83%) involved boys; and 79% (95% CI, 66%, 88%) occurred during the summer (July through September).

The immersion event rate was substantially higher during the first 6 months of pool exposure than at any time thereafter (Table). This high initial risk was independent of previous pool exposure; households with a pool at their prior residence were as likely as others to report an early immersion event (OR=0.90; 95% CI, 0.25, 3.3). However, most reported pool immersion events (77%; 95% CI, 65%, 87%) occurred outside this high-risk period, and 57% (95% CI, 44%, 70%) occurred more than 2 years after the onset of exposure.

The existence of this initial high-risk period depended on the time of year in which exposure began. The hazard rate for the 412 pool exposures beginning in April through September (Figure) was high initially and fell to zero at 6 months (winter in the study area). The seasonal peaks seen thereafter in summer did not approach the rate of the first few months and did not recur after 3 years. When exposure began in October through March (Figure), the initial high-risk period was not observed, and the seasonal pattern was less well established.

The annual incidence of reported home pool immersion events increased substantially in the last years of the study period, with 66% of all such events and 79% of those occurring within 6 months of the onset of exposure occurring in 1984 through 1987. For households whose exposures began during those years, the overall immersion event rate was 51/1000 PY (95% CI, 33, 80). The rates for discrete exposure intervals are presented in the Table. Among these households, 42% of immersion events occurred outside the 6-month high-risk period.

The home swimming pool was by a wide margin the leading water hazard for responding households. Ninety-one percent (95% CI, 82%, 97%) of all immersion events at these households occurred in the swimming pool. For members of these households, immersion events in the family pool constituted 59% (95% CI, 45%, 72%) of all such events, whether occurring at home or elsewhere. For household members under the age of 5 years, 80% (95%

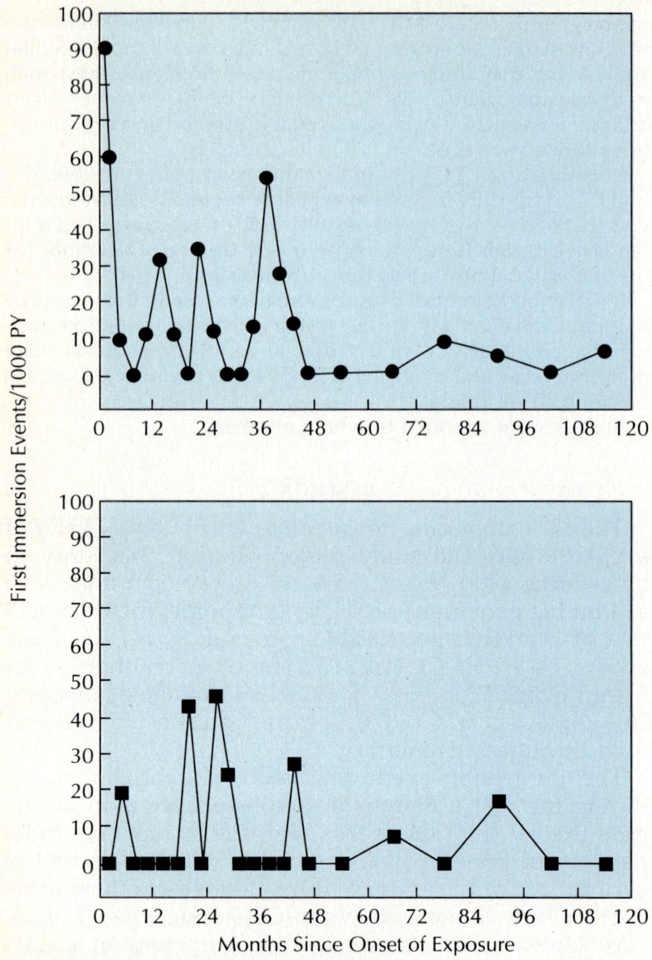

Hazard functions for first home swimming pool immersion events, Sacramento County, California. Top, Exposures beginning in April through September; bottom, exposures beginning in October through March. PY indicates pool-years.

CI, 63%, 92%) of all reported immersion events, whether at home or elsewhere, occurred in the family pool. Household members were not the only persons at risk, however. Nearly half (47%; 95% CI, 34%, 60%) of the persons suffering an immersion event in a responding household's pool were visitors.

Few events resulted in a reported immersion injury. Emergency resuscitation was needed in three cases. One child did not respond and was pronounced dead in the emergency department; one was hospitalized and "did fine"; one was discharged from the emergency department and subsequently suffered pneumonia. Two other children suffer persistent fear of water.

COMMENT

The first few months of exposure to a residential pool constitute a high-risk period, with immersion event rates three to five times higher than those for later periods. This is true even among households who lived with a pool at a prior residence.

The high-risk period is relatively brief. Over three fourths of immersion events for all respondents taken together, and over 40% of those for households with exposures beginning in the last 4 years of the study period, occurred after 6 months of pool exposure. Not surprisingly, the initial immersion event rate was high only when pool exposure began during a season when the pool was likely to be used.

The increased incidence of reported events in the final years of the study period, and the gradually increasing risk of first immersions during summers (Figure), are most likely the result of the underreporting of earlier events. To minimize such recall error, we initially planned to limit the study population to households whose pool exposures began within 5 years of the survey. Our eventual decision to use the entire building permit list as our sampling frame was supported by three findings. First, studies of the recall of life events[23-26] suggested that the salience of potentially lethal events, particularly those involving children, would minimize failure to recall. Second, accuracy of recall varies directly with the education and socioeconomic status of persons surveyed,[23] and an earlier survey[27] found that pool owners in the Sacramento area ranked high in both respects. Finally, when the questionnaire was tested, several subjects had detailed recollections of immersion events that had occurred many years previously.

Alternative explanations for this finding exist but seem much less likely. For example, children under 5 years of age may have become more numerous in the responding households in recent years. California's crude birth rate has increased linearly since 1972, however,[28] and the increase in immersion event rates began much later, in 1984. The intensity of pool use by young children (either household members or visitors) may have increased, or the quality of adult supervision may have declined. The absence of data make these untestable hypotheses; neither, in our view, is particularly plausible. Swimming pools may have become inherently more dangerous, thus allowing pool use of constant intensity to result in a higher rate of immersion events. However, data from both Sacramento County[8] and Australia[29] indicate that the drowning rate per in-ground pool has not increased over time.

Whatever its origin, the increase in reported immersion events in the years just before the survey suggests that results based on the experience of the entire population substantially underestimate the current rate of immersion events among households with pools. The overall immersion event rate for households with exposures beginning in 1984 or later, 51/1000 PY, was nearly five times greater than that for the entire study population.

A concurrent cohort study of households with pools would resolve this question. An inception cohort could be identified at the time pool exposure begins and contacted repeatedly, perhaps annually, to minimize loss of recall. Such a study could also gather data on the initial and evolving composition of exposed households, permitting immersion event rates to be calculated on a person-year basis.

IMPLICATIONS

For this population of residential pool owners, the home swimming pool is an important health hazard. The family pool accounts for nine of every 10 immersion events at the respondents' homes. For young children in these households, 80% of all immersion events, at home or elsewhere, occur in the home swimming pool.

Our findings suggest that residential pool fencing requirements and other drowning prevention programs should, at a minimum, include all households where pool exposures are just beginning. For example, a pool fencing requirement should at least apply both to newly constructed pools and to existing pools when they change ownership.

At the same time, it would be inappropriate to limit fencing requirements and other drowning-prevention efforts to these newly exposed households. Many, if not most, reported immersion events occurred outside the initial high-risk period. Nor would it be appropriate to limit fencing requirements to households with small children, as nearly half of those who suffer an immersion event in a home swimming pool are visitors.

The purpose of this study was to help assess the need for a universal pool fencing requirement, by determining whether a high-risk subset of households with pools could be selectively targeted for intervention. We conclude that newly exposed households do constitute such a population, but that fencing requirements will prevent the greatest number of drownings and near-drownings if they are extended to all residential swimming pools.

We thank Glen Koven of the Sacramento County Building Department for his cooperation, and Barbara Claire for assistance in executing the survey, assembling the data, and preparing the manuscript.

References

1. *Vital Statistics of the United States, 1987, II: Mortality P + A.* Hyattsville, Md: National Center for Health Statistics; 1990. US Dept of Health and Human Services publication PHS 90-1101.

2. Wintemute GJ. Childhood drowning and near-drowning in the United States. *AJDC.* 1990;144:663-669.

3. Zamula WW. *Social Cost of Drownings and Near-Drownings From Submersion Accidents Occurring to Children Under Five in Residential Swimming Pools.* Washington, DC: Directorate for Economic Analysis, US Consumer Product Safety Commission; 1987.

4. Pearn JH, Wong RYK, Brown J, Ching Y-C, Bart R, Hammar S. Drowning and near-drowning involving children: a five-year total population study from the city and county of Honolulu. *Am J Public Health.* 1979;69:450-454.

5. O'Carroll PW, Alkin E, Weiss B. Drowning mortality in Los Angeles County, 1976 to 1984. *JAMA.* 1988;260:380-383.

6. Quan L, Gore EJ, Wentz K, Allen J, Novack AH. Ten-year study of pediatric drownings and near-drownings in King County, Washington: lessons in injury prevention. *Pediatrics.* 1989;83:1035-1040.

7. Dietz PE, Baker SP. Drowning: epidemiology and prevention. *Am J Public Health.* 1974;64:303-312.

8. Wintemute GJ, Kraus JF, Teret SP, Wright M. Drowning in childhood and adolescence: a population-based study. *Am J Public Health.* 1987;77:830-832.

9. Flood TJ, Aickin M, Englender SJ, Tucker D. Child drownings and near drownings associated with swimming pools: Maricopa County, Arizona, 1988 and 1989. *MMWR.* 1990;39:441-442.

10. Present P. *Child Drowning Study: A Report on the Epidemiology of Drownings in Residential Pools to Children Under Age Five.* Washington, DC: Directorate for Epidemiology, US Consumer Product Safety Commission; 1987.

11. Hassall IB. Thirty-six consecutive under 5-year-old domestic swimming pool drownings. *Aust Paediatr J.* 1989;25:143-146.

12. Pearn JH, Nixon J, Wilke I. Freshwater drowning and near-drowning accidents involving children: a five-year total population study. *Med J Aust.* 1976;2:942-946.

13. Pearn JH, Thompson J. Drowning in the Australian Capitol Territory: a five-year total population study of immersion accidents. *Med J Aust.* 1977;1:130-133.

14. Milliner N, Pearn J, Guard R. Will fenced pools save lives? *Med J Aust.* 1980;2:510-511.

15. Pearn JH, Nixon J. Prevention of childhood drowning accidents. *Med J Aust.* 1977;1:616-618.

16. Orlowski JP. It's time for pediatricians to 'rally 'round the pool fence.' *Pediatrics.* 1989;83:1065-1066.

17. Division of Injury Control, Centers for Disease Control. Childhood injuries in the United States. *AJDC.* 1990;144:627-646.

18. *Residential Swimming Pool Barrier Code.* Washington, DC: US Consumer Product Safety Commission; 1989.

19. Wintemute GJ, Wright MA. Swimming pool owners' opinions of strategies for the prevention of drowning. *Pediatrics.* 1990;85:63-69.

20. Dillman DA. *Mail and Telephone Surveys.* New York, NY: John Wiley & Sons Inc; 1978.

21. Dillman DA. Mail and other self-administered questionnaires. In: Rossi DH, Wright JD, Anderson AB, eds. *Handbook of Survey Research.* Orlando, Fla: Academic Press Inc; 1983:359-377.

22. Kahn HA, Sempos CT. *Statistical Methods in Epidemiology.* New York, NY: Oxford University Press Inc; 1989:218.

23. *A Summary of Studies of Interviewing Methodology.* Rockville, Md: National Center for Health Statistics; 1977. US Dept of Health, Education, and Welfare publication HRA 77-1343.

24. Funch DP, Marshall JR. Measuring life stress: factors affecting fall-off in the reporting of life events. *J Health Soc Behav.* 1984;25:453-464.

25. Jenkins CD, Hurst MW, Rose RM. Life changes: do people really remember? *Arch Gen Psychiatry.* 1979;36:379-384.

26. Casey RL, Masuda M, Holmes TH. Quantitative study of recall of life events. *J Psychosom Res.* 1967;11:239-247.

27. *A Study to Evaluate SMUD's Swimming Pool Pump Load Management Program.* San Rafael, Calif: ADF Research; 1980.

28. *Vital Statistics of California, 1986.* Sacramento, Calif: Department of Health Services; 1988.

29. Pearn JH, Nixon J. Are swimming pools becoming more dangerous? *Med J Aust.* 1977;2:702-704.

Natural History of Hematuria Associated With Hypercalciuria in Children

Clotilde D. Garcia, MD; Leslie A. Miller, MLT; F. Bruder Stapleton, MD

• Hypercalciuria (HCU) is frequently found during the evaluation of children with hematuria; the long-term implications of untreated HCU in children are uncertain. Since 1981, we have identified HCU (urinary calcium, >0.1 mmol $\cdot kg^{-1} \cdot d^{-1}$) in 58 patients (41 male) with hematuria; 64% had gross hematuria and 74% had a relative with urolithiasis. Renal HCU was diagnosed in 19 patients and absorptive HCU in 24 patients. In 15 children, the calcium loading test was nondiagnostic. In nine patients (16%), urolithiasis developed, and in one patient, a renal calcification developed. These 10 patients (seven male) were older (10.1 vs 7.5 years) than the other 48 patients and initially presented with gross hematuria (nine of 10). All 10 patients had a family history of urolithiasis. The initial urinary calcium value was similar between the 10 patients with stones (0.15 mmol$\cdot kg^{-1} \cdot d^{-1}$) and the patients without stones (0.14 mmol$\cdot kg^{-1} \cdot d^{-1}$); five had absorptive HCU and four had renal HCU. At least one follow-up urinary calcium measurement was available for 23 patients who were not receiving thiazide therapy during 1 to 6 years after diagnosis (mean, 3.1 years). At 1-year follow-up, 12 of 17 patients had HCU and five had hematuria. Twenty-one patients were studied 2 to 3 years from diagnosis; 11 had HCU and eight had hematuria. After 4 years, six of seven patients had HCU and three had hematuria. We conclude that children with HCU and hematuria are at significant risk for urolithiasis, especially if they have gross hematuria and a family history of urolithiasis. Hypercalciuria may be episodic in children with hematuria, and factors other than urinary calcium concentration may be responsible for urinary bleeding.

(*AJDC.* 1991;145:1204-1207)

Hypercalciuria (HCU) is frequently found during the evaluation of children with hematuria. Moore et al,[1] Kalia et al,[2] and Roy et al[3] independently reported the association of unexplained hematuria with idiopathic HCU. In 1984, we reported that 23 (28%) of 83 consecutive children with isolated hematuria had HCU.[4] More recently, a multicenter trial showed that HCU was present in 76 (35%) of 215 children referred for evaluation of hematuria.[5]

The long-term implications of untreated HCU in children with hematuria are uncertain. In our original study, two children with HCU suffered calculi during a short observation period.[4] An increased risk for urolithiasis was found in children with HCU and hematuria in a report of the Southwest Pediatric Nephrology Study Group,[5] where stones developed in eight of 60 untreated children with HCU associated with hematuria. Although hydrochlorothiazide is known to reduce calciuria and to ameliorate hematuria in such patients,[2,4] the long-term risk-benefit ratio of diuretic therapy is unknown. In fact, confusion regarding appropriate treatment of children with hematuria associated with HCU exists owing to the absence of information concerning subsequent clinical manifestations.

To determine the natural history of untreated HCU and hematuria, we reviewed the records of a cohort of children with this association who have been followed up for at least 1 year. The objectives of this report are to examine the risk for urolithiasis and to determine whether HCU, hematuria, or both are episodic or constant in this population of children.

SUBJECTS AND METHODS

All children with hematuria, gross or microscopic (>5 red blood cells per high-power field on two consecutive urine examinations), who were also found to have HCU at LeBonheur Children's Medical Center, Memphis, Tenn, from July 1981 through 1986, were included in the study. Patients from previous reports[4,5] are included in this analysis. Hypercalciuria was defined as a urinary calcium excretion value of more than 0.1 mmol $\cdot kg^{-1} \cdot d^{-1}$ during an unrestricted diet on at least two occasions.[6,7] In each case, a thorough investigation failed to reveal alternative causes of hematuria.[4,5] A renal ultrasound examination was performed in the initial evaluation in all patients, and a computed tomographic examination was performed in 10 patients.

A family history of urolithiasis was sought from each patient and was considered positive if a sibling, parent, grandparent, or parental sibling had a history of urinary stone disease. No patient had a history of excessive intake of vitamin D or milk. In each patient, an effort to characterize the pathogenetic basis of HCU was attempted by performing an oral calcium loading test as previously described.[8,9] Renal HCU was defined as a fasting

Accepted for publication June 3, 1991.

From the Departments of Nephrology and Pediatrics (Dr Garcia), The Children's Hospital of Buffalo, State University of New York at Buffalo; and Department of Pediatrics, LeBonheur Children's Medical Center, Clinical Research Center, University of Tennessee, Memphis (Dr Stapleton and Ms Miller). Dr Stapleton is now with Children's Hospital of Buffalo, Buffalo, NY.

Reprint requests to Children's Hospital of Buffalo, 219 Bryant St, Buffalo, NY 14222 (Dr Stapleton).

Table 1.—Patients Identified With Hypercalciuria in Evaluation of Hematuria

Variable	Value
Total patients	58
Sex, M/F	41/17
Mean (±SE) age at diagnosis, y	8.0±0.4
Race, No. (%)	
W	56 (97)
B	1 (1.5)
Mixed	1 (1.5)
Family history of urolithiasis, No. (%)	43 (75)
Macroscopic hematuria, No. (%)	37 (64)
Mean (±SE) 24-h urinary calcium excretion, $mmol \cdot kg^{-1} \cdot d^{-1}$	0.145±0.01

Table 2.—Characteristics of 10 Patients With Urolithiasis or Calcification

	Stone	No Stone	*P*
Mean (±SE) age at diagnosis, y	10.1±1.0	7.6±3.2	.03
Sex, M/F	7/3	34/14	.61
Mean (±SE) urine calcium at diagnosis, $mmol \cdot kg^{-1} \cdot d^{-1}$	0.15±0.02	0.14±0.05	.3
Macroscopic hematuria	9	28	.06
Microscopic hematuria	1	20	. . .
Family history of urolithiasis	10	33	.04
Type of hypercalciuria			
Renal	4	15	.45
Absorptive	5	19	. . .
Indeterminate	1	14	. . .
Mean (±SE) parathyroid hormone, pmol/L	77.16±25.2	64.66±18.8	.09

urinary calcium–creatinine ratio (milligram per milligram) greater than 0.21. Absorptive HCU was defined as a normal fasting urinary calcium–creatinine ratio and a ratio greater than 0.27 after the oral calcium load.[9] When test data failed to meet the criteria for either renal or absorptive HCU, the patient was classified as indeterminate. During the observation period, none of the patients received thiazide therapy. All patients were advised to drink a volume of water equal to at least 1.5 to 2 times the recommended maintenance fluid intake as well as to eat no more than 3 g of sodium daily. Children with absorptive and indeterminate HCU were advised to limit dietary calcium to no more than 600 mg/d. Compliance with dietary manipulations was not assessed.

Blood samples obtained during the oral calcium loading test were assayed for serum levels of immunoreactive parathyroid hormone (INCSTAR Corp, Stillwater, Minn). Urinary calcium was analyzed by atomic absorption spectroscopy (Varian Associates, Palo Alto, Calif), and creatinine was determined with an analyzer (Beckman Creatinine Analyzer II, Beckman Instruments, Fullerton, Calif).

Patients were examined annually in the outpatient Clinical Research Center. In addition to a complete physical examination, a urinalysis was performed, and serum electrolyte, creatinine, calcium, parathyroid hormone, and phosphorous concentrations were determined. A 24-hour urine sample for calcium excretion and creatinine clearance was also obtained. A renal ultrasound examination was performed at annual visits. Acute symptoms were addressed by the urology or nephrology service.

Statistical analyses were performed with Student's *t* test for unpaired data, χ^2 analysis, or multivariate analysis. Data are presented as mean±SEM unless otherwise indicated.

RESULTS

Fifty-eight children with hematuria and HCU fulfilled the criteria for inclusion in the study. Clinical characteristics are given in Table 1. Most of the children were white boys. Forty-three (75%) of the children had a family history of urolithiasis (one was adopted). Thirty-seven (64%) of the patients presented with gross hematuria; the remainder had only microhematuria.

An oral calcium loading test demonstrated renal HCU in 19 patients (33%); 24 children (41%) were classified as having absorptive HCU. Fifteen children (26%) could not be classified based on their oral calcium loading test and were called indeterminate. The indeterminate group had a significant reduction in calcium excretion during a calcium-restricted diet similar to the group with absorptive HCU.

The 58 children have been followed up for a mean (±SEM) of 3.1±0.5 years, with a range of 1 to 6 years. During this follow-up period, nine children (16%) suffered urolithiasis that was not present in the initial studies. One child was found to have a urinary calcification on a computed tomographic study 1 month after the first evaluation; in this patient, the original and subsequent renal ultrasonographic evaluations were normal. The interval between the diagnosis of hematuria and HCU and the discovery of urolithiasis or calcification was 13.1±6 months, the range being 1 to 41 months.

The clinical and laboratory characteristics of the 10 patients in whom urolithiasis or calcification developed were compared with the characteristics of the 48 patients in whom stones did not develop (Table 2). The group with stones were older when initially evaluated for hematuria and presented with macroscopic hematuria. All had a family history of urolithiasis ($P<.04$ when compared with the group without stones). These patients were excluded from further follow-up analyses. All of these patients had persistent microscopic hematuria until the presentation of urolithiasis; only six had further episodes of gross hematuria before passing a urinary stone. Interval annual renal ultrasonographic examinations in the four children with urolithiasis after 1 year of follow-up were normal until clinical manifestations developed.

Follow-up data in 23 children without stones in whom 24-hour urine collections were available are shown in the Figure. Most patients were examined on multiple occasions. Marked variability in the presence and association of hematuria and HCU was observed in the patients. Hematuria did not recur in 11 patients following the initial episode, despite the continued presence of HCU in seven of these children. Among the 11 children without recurrence of hematuria, the initial diagnosis of absorptive HCU was assigned to seven of the children and of renal HCU to one patient, and three were in the indeterminate group. Hematuria was present at each annual evaluation in six (26%) of these 23 patients. Two of the patients with persistent hematuria had absorptive HCU, two had renal HCU, and two were in the indeterminate group. The follow-up data in the remaining six demonstrated hematuria (three with gross hematuria) at least once at the an-

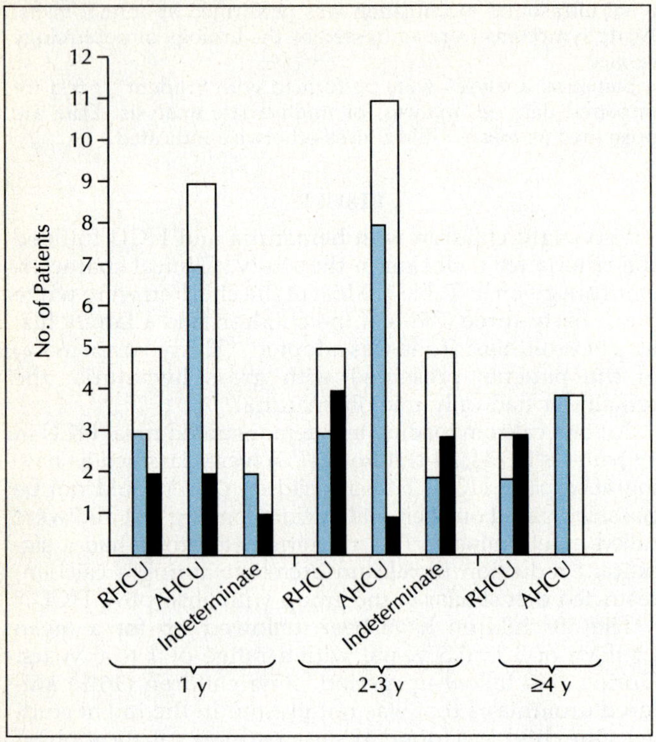

Clinical follow-up of patients with hematuria (solid bars) and hypercalciuria (tinted bars). Open bars indicate total patients; RHCU, renal hypercalciuria; and AHCU, absorptive hypercalciuria.

nual visit as well as a normal urinalysis result at another annual examination. Two of these patients had absorptive HCU, three had renal HCU, and one patient was in the indeterminate group. An alternative diagnosis of hematuria was found in one patient with absorptive HCU in whom a diagnosis of hereditary nephritis was assigned based on red blood cell casts and a family history of glomerular disease. This patient did not have a calculus and was excluded from the follow-up data analysis.

COMMENT

Whenever a new disease association is documented, a period of uncertainty exists for clinicians, who must evaluate and treat patients without knowledge of the long-term implications of the problem. The finding of HCU in children with unexplained hematuria presents such a dilemma. In this article, we offer some insights that may assist pediatricians who uncover this association during the evaluation of their patients. Clearly, an increased risk of urolithiasis exists in these children. Our study also shows that hematuria and HCU may be transient or episodic in many patients and may not always coincide.

Hypercalciuria is the most frequently identified metabolic abnormality associated with nephrolithiasis in adults and may account for up to 53% of all urinary stones in children.[10-15] In previous studies, we found that 51 (42%) of 122 children with urolithiasis and 17 (81%) of 21 children with otherwise unexplained calcium urolithiasis had idiopathic HCU.[9,11] In this study, we have demonstrated that 17% of the children with HCU and hematuria suffered urolithiasis or a calcification during a rather short follow-up period. Children who are at greatest risk for the development of urolithiasis tend to be older patients who have macroscopic hematuria at presentation and who also have a family history of urolithiasis. However, predictive indices were not forthcoming through the utilization of multivariate analyses. Age alone would have correctly identified seven of the 10 children with urolithiasis; on the other hand, 17 of the 48 children without stones (during the follow-up) would have been incorrectly assigned to the high-risk group. If gross hematuria is also included, eight of 10 patients with stones would have been predicted to have stones, yet nine children would have been incorrectly predicted to have stones. Perhaps with a longer observation period, these indices may prove more sensitive.

Because children with hematuria associated with HCU are at risk for future calculus formation, we suggest the general preventive measures of a large fluid intake and a reduction in dietary sodium intake. Moderate dietary calcium restriction is suggested for children with absorptive HCU, and supplemental vitamin D is discouraged. Thiazides are often recommended for patients with urolithiasis, especially secondary to HCU.[2,16,17] Our data failed to define sensitive and specific means for the clinical identification of children at greatest risk for development of urolithiasis. Furthermore, the inconsistent nature of hematuria and HCU during the follow-up period (without thiazide therapy) renders assessment of the efficiency of diuretic therapy speculative. Previously, we have documented that bone mineral density and growth are not impaired in untreated children with hematuria and HCU.[18] The pharmacological therapy most often recommended for HCU is thiazide therapy.[15,17] Clearly, long-term thiazide therapy has the well-known risk of electrolyte and other biochemical abnormalities.[19] Churchill and Taylor[20] have challenged the validity of studies reporting therapeutic efficacy for thiazide in urolithiasis. Because we believe the risk-benefit ratio of thiazide therapy in children with hematuria and HCU is inadequately characterized, we are hesitant to prescribe diuretic therapy. However, if diuretic therapy is considered, the first year following diagnosis seems to be a high-risk period, because half of the calculi developed within 12 months. Therefore, at least 1 year of therapy would be warranted.

Our data also suggest that oral calcium loading tests are not helpful in predicting subsequent urolithiasis and are often not diagnostic at the time of diagnosis. We do not recommend this test for the routine diagnostic evaluation of children with HCU unless the serum parathyroid hormone concentration is elevated.[21] Unless acute symptoms arise, annual follow-up evaluations are appropriate for children with HCU and hematuria. Follow-up renal ultrasonographic examinations were not helpful in detecting calculi in the absence of renal colic.

The etiology of hematuria in our patients with idiopathic HCU before the time that a renal calculus is clinically apparent remains unknown. Possible mechanisms might include interstitial inflammation, microscopic areas of nephrocalcinosis, or focal tubular damage from crystalluria.[3] We cannot exclude alternative etiologies of hematuria. Potential explanations for lack of correlation between urinary calcium excretion and hematuria during the follow-up period might include variations in fluid intake as well as other dietary variables. Although this study provides some insights into the natural history of HCU associated with hematuria, it is essential to gain a better understanding of the etiology of hematuria in children with HCU to develop acceptable methods of predicting stones and prescribing therapy.

References

1. Moore ES, Coe FL, McMann BY, Favus MY. Idiopathic hypercalciuria in children: prevalence and metabolic characteristics. *J Pediatr.* 1978;92:906-910.
2. Kalia A, Travis LB, Brouhard BH. The association of idiopathic hypercalciuria and asymptomatic gross hematuria in children. *J Pediatr.* 1981;99:716-719.
3. Roy S, Stapleton FB, Noe HN, Jerkins G. Hematuria preceding renal calculus formation in children with hypercalciuria. *J Pediatr.* 1981;99:712-715.
4. Stapleton FB, Roy S, Noe HN, Jerkins G. Hypercalciuria in children with hematuria. *N Engl J Med.* 1984;310:1345-1348.
5. Stapleton FB. Idiopathic hypercalciuria: association with isolated hematuria and risk for urolithiasis in children: the Southwest Pediatric Nephrology Study Group. *Kidney Int.* 1990;37:807-811.
6. Moore ES. Hypercalciuria in children. In: Berlyne GM, ed. *Contributions to Nephrology.* New York, NY: S Karger AG; 1981:20-32.
7. Ghazali S, Barratt TM. Urinary excretion of calcium and magnesium in children. *Arch Dis Child.* 1974;49:97-101.
8. Stapleton FB, Noe HN, Jerkins G, Roy S. Urinary excretion of calcium following an oral calcium loading test in healthy children. *Pediatrics.* 1982;69:594-597.
9. Stapleton FB, Noe HN, Jerkins G. Hypercalciuria in children with urolithiasis. *AJDC.* 1982;136:675-678.
10. Pak CYK, Britton F, Peterson R, et al. Ambulatory evaluation of nephrolithiasis: classification, clinical presentation and diagnostic criteria. *Am J Med.* 1980;69:19-28.
11. Stapleton FB, McKay CP, Noe HN. Urolithiasis in children: the role of hypercalciuria. *Pediatr Ann.* 1987; 16:980-992.
12. Walther PC, Lamm D, Kaplan GN. Pediatric urolithiasis: a 10-year review. *Pediatrics.* 1980;65:1068-1072.
13. Ghazali S, Barrett TM, Williams DI. Childhood urolithiasis in Britain. *AJDC.* 1973;48:291-295.
14. Choi H, Snyder HM, Duckett J. Urolithiasis in childhood: current management. *J Pediatr Surg.* 1987;22:158-164.
15. Pak CYK, Peters P, Hurt G, et al. Is selective therapy of recurrent nephrolithiasis possible? *Am J Med.* 1981;71:615-618.
16. Polinsky MS, Kaiser BA, Baluarte JH. Urolithiasis in children: the role of hypercalciuria. *Pediatr Ann.* 1987; 16:980-992.
17. Pak CYK. Medical management of nephrolithiasis in Dallas: update 1987. *J Urol.* 1988;140:461-467.
18. Stapleton FB, Jones DP, Miller LA. Evaluation of bone metabolism in children with hypercalciuria. *Semin Nephrol.* 1989;9:75-79.
19. McMahon FG. Thiazides. In: McMahon GM, ed. *Management of Essential Hypertension.* New York, NY: Fuhre Publishing Co; 1978:21-54.
20. Churchill DN, Taylor DW. Thiazides for patients with recurrent calcium stones: still an open question. *J Urol.* 1985;133:749-751.
21. Stapleton FB. Nephrolithiasis in children. *Pediatr Rev.* 1989;11:21-30.

In Other AMA Journals

ARCHIVES OF NEUROLOGY

The Epidemiology of Parkinson's Disease: A Case-Control Study of Young-Onset and Old-Onset Patients

Matthew Stern, MD; Eugene Dulaney; Stephen B. Gruber, PhD; Larry Golbe, MD; Mary Bergen, RN; Howard Hurtig, MD; Steve Gollomp, MD; Paul Stolley, MD, MPH
(*Arch Neurol.* 1991;48:903-907)

Lower Extremity Motor Evoked Potentials in Multiple Sclerosis

Seth M. Jones, MD; Leopold J. Streletz, MD; Vicki E. Raab, MD; Robert L. Knobler, MD, PhD; Kenneth M. Heilman, MD (*Arch Neurol.* 1991;48:944-948)

Classified Advertising

All classified advertising orders, correspondence and payments should be directed to: American Journal of Diseases of Children, P.O. Box 1510, Clearwater, Florida 34617. Our telephone numbers are: 800-237-9851; 813-443-7666. Please do not send classified ads, payments or related correspondence to the AMA headquarters in Chicago. This causes needless delay.

Inquiries about "BOX NUMBER" advertisements: All replies must be in writing and must cite the box number in the ad. Example: Box ____, c/o AJDC, P.O. Box 1510, Clearwater, Florida 34617. We are not permitted to divulge the identity of advertisers who wish their mail sent in care of American Journal of Diseases of Children .

CLASSIFIED INFORMATION

Regular Classified	1 Time	3 times or more*
Cost per word	$1.85	$1.70
Minimum ad: 20 words		per issue

In order to earn the three-time rate, your ad must be placed and prepaid at the same time for three or more issues.

Counting Words: Two initials are considered one word, each abbreviation is considered one word, and figures consisting of a dollar sign and five numerals or less are considered one word. Cities and states consisting of two words or more are counted as one word: i.e., "New York" and "Salt Lake City". Zip code is considered one word and must appear in all ads. Telephone number with area code is considered one word. When box numbers are used for replies, the words "Box____, c/o AJDC" are to be counted as three words.

Classified Display	1 Time	3 times or more*
Full page	$1,155	$1,005
Two-thirds page	985	856
One-half page	809	704
One-third page	638	554
One-sixth page	295	257
Column inch	80	65

Minimum display ad: one column inch
12-time and 24-time rates available on request.

Display Production Charge: The publication will pub-set advertisements upon request. The typesetting fee is 10% of the one-time ad cost shown above. Special requests will be billed to the advertiser and/or agency at the then prevailing rates.

Box Service

Available for all ads. The cost is $15.00 for the first issue only. Responses to your ad will be consolidated in our office and promptly mailed directly to you.

Closing Date

The 25th of the second month prior to the issue date. Example: The November issue closes September 25th. No ads can be cancelled after the closing date.

Send all copy, correspondence, production materials and payments to:

AMERICAN JOURNAL OF DISEASES OF CHILDREN

AJDC

Classified Department
P.O. Box 1510, Clearwater, Florida 34617

For assistance with your ad schedule call toll free:
800-237-9851 ◆ 813-443-7666

Professional Opportunities

IMMEDIATE OPENING for BC/BE pediatrician to associate with well-established, rapidly growing, 32-MD multi-specialty group. Located in the San Francisco Bay area in a growing community serving 170,000. Patients include both fee-for-service and prepaid health plan. Attractive compensation and benefits. Malpractice provided. California license required. Send CV to: Bart Bona, Administrator, Fairfield Medical Group, Caller Box 4020, Fairfield, CA 94533-0410. (707) 426-3911.

ROCHESTER, NEW YORK – Opportunity for a general pediatrician to develop their practice as part of the Rochester Medical Group pediatric department. Rochester Medical Group is a multi-specialty group practice which cares for fee-for-service as well as prepaid patients. In addition to full-time position, willing to consider part-time or job-share opportunities. Subspecialty interests possible. University affiliation encouraged. Competitive salary and benefits. Located in attractive metropolitan area with many cultural and recreational advantages. Send resume or call: Rochester Medical Group, P.C. Attention: James Tobin, MD, 800 Carter Street, Rochester, NY 14621. (716) 338-1400. EOE, M/F.

LARGE MULTI-SPECIALTY GROUP in northern Virginia area needs bilingual (Spanish) pediatrician to replace retiring physician of forty years. Send CV to: Medical Director, Falls Church Medical Center, 6060 Arlington Boulevard, Falls Church, VA 22044.

Professional Opportunities

PEDIATRICIAN – SEATTLE: Outstanding pediatric practice seeking an associate. Busy practice, affiliated with excellent 300-bed general hospital. Must be board-certified or board-eligible. Contact: Richard G. Wedig, Highline Hospital, 12844 Military Road South, Seattle, WA 98168. (206) 248-4561.

PHILADELPHIA – Two pediatricians seeking BE/BC third for growing practice in southwest Philadelphia. Full partnership opportunity after two years. Send CV to: Fredric Nelson, MD, 2801 Island Avenue, Philadelphia, PA 19153.

BC/BE PEDIATRICIAN NEEDED. Busy office practice. Guaranteed salary, benefits. Mountain local. CV to: Mike McCraley, Ogden Clinic, 4650 Harrison Boulevard, Ogden, UT 84403. (801) 479-4621.

PARTNER NEEDED IN 1992 for three physician practice. Join two BC pediatricians: a 1980 MD of University of Pittsburgh and residency at Children's Hospital, Pittsburgh and a 1984 MD of Pennsylvania State School of Medicine, Hershey and residency at the University of Chicago. Opportunity is close to New York and Ohio in the greater Lakeland area of Meadville, Pennsylvania. This college community is family oriented with excellent schools. First year guarantee and benefits. For further information call: (800) 283-8321, Extension 5705. Or send curriculum vitae to: Brenda Lewis, Meadville Medical Center, 1034 Grove Street, Meadville, PA 16335.

Pediatric Subspecialists

Developmental
Intensivist
Pulmonology
Hematology/Oncology
Neurology
Surgery
Neonatology

The University of South Dakota School of Medicine currently has openings for BE/BC pediatric subspecialties.

These are full-time academic positions ideally suited for the clinician scholar who wishes to develop and guide a program which will have a significant impact on the health care of children. Although our program is heavily slanted toward medical student education and patient care, the department encourages and provides ample resources for clinical and laboratory research.

Become part of a dynamic community where the economy (rated #1 nationally by Money Magazine), quality of life (#12), health care (#30), along with a growing population and a progressive educational systems make Sioux Falls an ideal place for your career and family life. South Dakota's four season climate welcomes endless recreational activities year-round.

Send CV or call:
Carl Hinson • (800) 468-3333

USD School of Medicine
1100 South Euclid, P.O. Box 5039
Sioux Falls, SD 57117

Competitive financial packages offered.
EOE/AAE.

Call for Abstracts

The American Pediatric Society and The Society for Pediatric Research announce that the abstract deadline for the 1992 Annual Meeting (May 4-7, 1992, Convention Center, Baltimore, Md) has been set as *January 3, 1992*. For further information, contact the APA Headquarters, 6728 Old McLean Village Dr, McLean, VA 22101 ([703]556-9222; FAX [703]556-8729), or the APS/SPR Association . . . . ([708]427-0205; FAX [708] 427-1305).

Sudden Cardiac Death

Sir.—The otherwise excellent review of sudden cardiac death in young athletes by McCaffrey and colleagues[1] is marred by misstatement of the inheritance of the long QT syndromes. The Jervell and Lange-Nielson syndrome[2] is autosomal recessive and accompanied by congenital deafness. The Romano-Ward syndrome[3,4] has an autosomal dominant inheritance and is accompanied by normal hearing. Many family studies have confirmed these patterns of inheritance.[5]

WILLIAM PEARL, MD
William Beaumont Army Medical Center
Division of Pediatric Cardiology
Box 70614
El Paso, TX 79920

1. McCaffrey FM, Braden DS, Strong WB. Sudden cardiac death in young athletes: a review. *AJDC.* 1991;145:177-183.
2. Jervell A, Lange-Nielson F. Congenital deaf-mutism: functional heart disease with prolongation of the QT interval and sudden death. *Am Heart J.* 1957;54: 59-68.
3. Romano C, Gemme G, Pangiglione R. Aritmie cardiache rare delleta pediatricia. *Clin Pediatr (Bologna).* 1963;45: 656-683.
4. Ward OC. New familial cardiac syndrome in children. *J Irish Med Assoc.* 1964;54:103-106.
5. Schwartz PJ. Idiopathic long QT syndrome: progress and questions. *Am Heart J.* 1985;109:399-411.

Staphylococcus aureus in Impetigo

Sir.—Demidovich et al[1] recently published the results of a study comparing penicillin, erythromycin, and cephalexin therapies for impetigo. This study has to be praised, since a lot of confusion still exists with regard to childhood impetigo. Two of their conclusions were that *Staphylococcus aureus* was the most common cause of impetigo in children in their population and that penicillin is an inadequate treatment for this infection.

Sixteen months earlier, I and a coauthor published our results of a study comparing amoxicillin with augmentin for the treatment of nonbullous impetigo.[2] In our population in southern Israel, *S aureus* was isolated from 100% of the patients, while additional streptococci were isolated from 29%. All 51 isolates of *S aureus* were resistant to penicillin; treatment failure was observed in five (20%) of 25 patients who received amoxicillin compared with none of those who received augmentin. Our conclusions, as follows, were similar to those expressed by Demidovich et al. "We conclude that in areas where *Staphylococcus aureus* is usually penicillin resistant, the empiric therapy of impetigo should include a drug that is active against both staphylococci and streptococci."[2]

It is surprising that our article, published in the same journal, was not cited in the report by Demidovich et al. Such a citation from a different geographical region could strengthen their conclusions.

RON DAGAN, MD
Pediatric Infectious Disease Unit
Soroka University Medical Center
PO Box 151
Beer-Sheva, Israel

1. Demidovich CW, Wittler RR, Ruff ME, Bass JW, Browning WC. Impetigo: current etiology and comparison of penicillin, erythromycin, and cephalexin therapies. *AJDC.* 1990;144:1313-1315.
2. Dagan R, Bar-David Y. Comparison of amoxicillin and clavulanic acid (Augmentin) for the treatment of nonbullous impetigo. *AJDC.* 1989;143:916-918.

In Reply.—I am sorry that we missed the report by Dagan and Bar-David. It was published a few months before our study was submitted for publication, so we did not find it in our review. We did cite two other recent studies from the southeastern and southwestern United States that showed, along with our study, that penicillin-resistant *Staphylococcus aureus* is emerging as the major pathogen implicated as the cause of impetigo in diverse areas of the United States. The report by Dagan and Bar-David, along with an extensive review of the cause of impetigo from numerous other reports summarized by Esterly et al[1] in a more recent issue of *AJDC*, confirms that this is a worldwide phenomenon. From these observations, it may be concluded that penicillin is no longer adequate for primary treatment of impetigo in most areas of the world.

JAMES W. BASS, MD
Department of Pediatrics
Tripler Army Medical Center
Honolulu, HI 96859-5000

1. Esterly NB, Nelson DB, Dunne WM. Impetigo. *AJDC.* 1991;145:125-126.

Treatment Withdrawal in Neonates

Sir.—The recent article by Young and Stevenson[1] describes the Stanford "individualized prognostic strategy" approach to aggressive support in the neonatal intensive care unit as the exception to the American norm. If this statement is indeed valid, it is a sad reflection on neonatal intensive care in the United States. The authors ask why there is such difficulty in stopping aggressive therapy, and suggest fear of litigation as a likely cause. Although such decision making is in an area of uncertainty, this should not prevent a decision from being reached. Physicians in training, particularly in acute care areas, must be taught that good clinical decisions cannot always be made with certainty. Clinical judgments are made in the best interest of the patient without any guarantee of certainty. The physician's responsibility must be to inform the family of the risks and benefits of treatment and to help formulate a plan to treat or to withdraw. If we continue to erode this responsibility or confuse it with medical paternalism, then we will become a profession of technicians rather than caring physicians. It is taking the easy way out to make a nondecision to treat every baby aggressively until multiple system failure develops on the respirator. As Campbell[2] has stated, "... taking these decisions are supreme tests of medical leadership." The acceptance of such decisions depends on mutual trusting that the doctors and the parents are putting the infant's interests above their own. If that trust does not exist within the neonatal intensive care unit, then the best interests of the infants will not be served. Surely "individualized prognostic strategy" simply means treating each patient and family with the care and dignity that they deserve and involves the practice of "close-up" ethics vs "distant" ethics as described by Duff.[3]

PAUL BYRNE, MB, CHB, FRCPC
R. WELCH, MB, CHB, MRCP
University of Alberta Hospitals
2C300 Walter V. Mackenzie Health Sciences Center
Edmonton, Alberta, Canada T6G 2R7

1. Young EWD, Stevenson DK. Limiting treatment for extremely premature low-birth-weight infants (500 to 750 g). *AJDC*. 1990;144:549-552.

2. Campbell AGM. Which infants should not receive intensive care? *AJDC*. 1982;136:569-571.

3. Duff RS. 'Close-up' versus 'distant' ethics: deciding the care of infants with poor prognosis. *Semin Perinatol*. 1987;11:244-253.

Exacerbation of Tinea Corporis During Treatment With 1% Clotrimazole/0.05% Betamethasone Diproprionate (Lotrisone)

Sir.—An 8-year-old girl with tinea corporis of the knee was treated with a combination product of 1% clotrimazole and 0.05% betamethasone diproprionate cream (Lotrisone). She had a prolonged course, with persistent pustules and inflammation that permanently scarred her knee. The histologic appearance was that of a Majocchi's granuloma, a fungal dermal abscess similar to a kerion. We postulate that the cause was local immunosuppression by the fluorinated steroid in this cream.

Patient Report.—Eleven weeks before presentation, an 8-year-old girl had played in a barn in which many cats made their home. Nine weeks before presentation, she developed an erythematous, ring-shaped, scaly lesion on her right knee, diagnosed by her family physician as "ringworm." A combination cream containing 1% clotrimazole and 0.05% betamethasone diproprionate was prescribed to be applied twice daily until the lesion resolved.

The cream was faithfully applied without occlusion for 9 weeks, but instead of resolving, the plaque enlarged, became bright red, boggy, pustular, tender, and covered with a serous exudate (Figure). The patient developed knee pain and had difficulty walking. She was brought to one of us (R.D.R.), and cellulitis was considered. The Lotrisone treatment was discontinued. A short course of oral cefadroxil monohydrate failed to heal the lesion.

The patient was seen in the Pediatric Dermatology Clinic at the Childrens Hospital Medical Center, Cincinnati, Ohio. Physical examination revealed a 10-cm tender, boggy, erythematous, pustular, exophytic plaque on the right knee. A diagnosis of tinea corporis with Majocchi's granuloma formation was made. A potassium hydroxide (KOH) preparation showed long branching septate hyphae and spores, and a culture of tissue obtained at skin biopsy yielded *Trichophyton mentagrophytes*. Histologic examination confirmed the presence of a dermal abscess with occasional yeast forms identified in the base of hair follicles.

The patient was treated with a course of oral microsize griseofulvin (15 mg/kg per

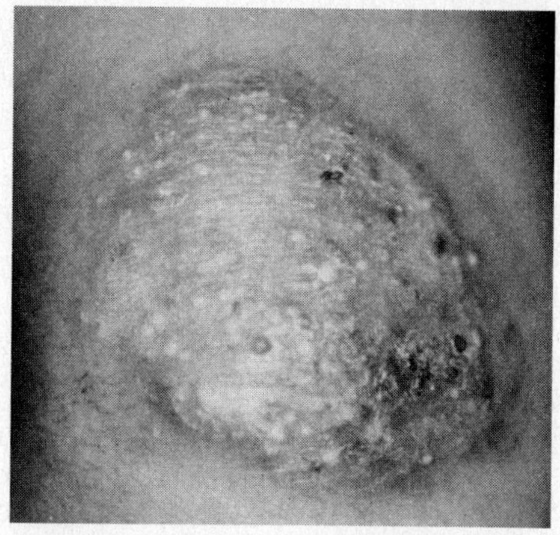

Majocchi's granuloma (fungal dermal abscess) on the right knee of an 8-year-old girl. The lesion developed during a 9-week treatment of tinea corporis with a combination product of 1% clotrimazole and 0.05% betamethasone diproprionate cream (Lotrisone).

day). Six weeks later, she walked without a limp but a culture was still positive for *T mentagrophytes*. At 8 weeks, the lesion had become flat, nearly flesh colored, and studded with 1- to 3-mm depressed scars at the sites of previous pustules. Fungal culture of the surface was sterile. Two and a half years later, the child has a permanently scarred knee.

Comment.—It is well documented that potent topical steroids applied alone may enhance fungal growth on the skin.[1,2] In one case report of an adverse effect of 1% clotrimazole/0.05% betamethasone diproprionate cream, an adult patient was not only unable to resolve a tinea corporis, but also developed significant striae from the combination's potent steroid. Simply switching to 1% clotrimazole cream (Lotrimin) afforded her brisk resolution of the tinea.[3] We describe this patient to alert physicians that combination creams containing both an antifungal and a potent fluorinated corticosteroid may enhance fungal growth to the point of Majocchi's granuloma formation.

The clinical and histologic appearance of our patient's knee lesion, ie, follicular pustules with intradermal abscess formation, was that of a Majocchi's granuloma. It is quite similar to a kerion, which is usually seen only on the scalp. We postulate that the potent anti-inflammatory action of the 0.05% betamethasone diproprionate in Lotrisone caused local immunosuppression such that both the antifungal activity of clotrimazole and local cell-mediated immunity were overwhelmed.

The steroid in Lotrisone is a class III fluorinated compound, betamethasone diproprionate (Diprosone).[4] Food and Drug Administration labeling for Lotrisone warns against its use for more than 2 weeks to treat tinea corporis and against use under occlusion. It is not approved for use in children under age 12 years. We suspect that few physicians and pharmacists are aware of, or inform patients of, these caveats.

Application of such a potent topical steroid to areas such as the perineum, especially with occlusion (eg, treating monilial diaper dermatitis) could potentially lead to cutaneous atrophy and stria formation. Systemic absorption of steroids from the perineum can be very high, leading to the possibility of adrenal suppression.[5]

Fluorinated topical steroid/antifungal combinations should not be used for conditions in which a simple topical antifungal, with or without the concomitant short-term use of a mild nonfluorinated topical steroid, would suffice.

Reprint requests to New Richmond Family Practice, 1050 Old US 52, New Richmond, OH 45157 (Dr Reynolds).

RONALD D. REYNOLDS, MD
New Richmond Family Practice
1050 Old US 52
New Richmond, OH 45157

SUSAN BOIKO, MD
Department of Dermatology
University of Cincinnati College of Medicine
Cincinnati, OH 45267

ANNE W. LUCKY, MD
Dermatology Clinic
Childrens Hospital Medical Center
Cincinnati, OH 45267

1. Jacobs PH. Majocchi's granuloma (due to therapy with steroid and occlusion). *Cutis*. 1986;38:23.
2. Ive FA, Marks R. Tinea incognito. *Br Med J*. 1968;3:149-152.
3. Barkey WF. Striae and persistent tinea corporis related to prolonged use of betamethasone diproprionate 0.05% cream/clotrimazole 1% cream (Lotrisone cream). *J Am Acad Dermatol*. 1987;17:518-519.
4. Cornell RC, Stoughton RB. The use of topical steroids in psoriasis. *Dermatol Clin N Am*. 1984;2:397-409.
5. Feldmann RJ, Maibach HI. Regional variation in percutaneous penetration of 14C cortisol in man. *J Invest Dermatol*. 1967;48:181-183.

Mediterranean Visceral Leishmaniasis: A Frequently Unrecognized Imported Disease

Sir.—Visceral leishmaniasis is endemic in countries surrounding the Mediterranean Sea. With mass tourism, nonresidents returning from this area are now also increasingly affected.[1,2] However, it appears from the literature that this diagnosis is often not considered in these patients, that numerous unnecessary investigations are performed, and that appropriate treatment of this potentially fatal infection is delayed or withheld.[3] This is clearly illustrated by the following report.

Patient Report.—A 10-month-old boy was referred to our department because of a persistent spiking fever of 3 weeks' duration that had not responded to oral treatment with amoxicillin and cefadroxil. Clinical investigation on admission revealed a fever of 40°C, marked hepatosplenomegaly, paleness, and slightly enlarged inguinal lymph nodes. Abnormal results of laboratory investigation were severe hypochromic anemia, leukopenia with neutropenia, thrombocytopenia, increased C-reactive protein levels, and positive results of a direct Coombs' test (Table). Roentgenograms of the chest and results of a tuberculin skin test as well as several blood and urine cultures, remained negative. Results of bone marrow aspiration showed generalized hypercellularity, normal megakaryocytes, a normal leukocyte series, and hypochromic erythroid hyperplasia. A computed tomographic scan showed bilateral accumulation of fluid in the middle ear and mastoid cavity. The diagnosis of mastoiditis was made, and intravenous treatment with sodium cefotaxime and amikacin sulfate was started. A blood transfusion was also performed.

During the following weeks, the clinical symptoms persisted, and the patient's general condition deteriorated. Laboratory investigation confirmed pancytopenia, a low serum albumin value, hypergammaglobulinemia, and increased C-reactive protein values, but now also revealed oligoclonal gammopathy, antinuclear antibodies, and increased circulating IgG immune complexes. Serum C3

Laboratory Values Associated With Leishmaniasis*

Sample Components	Component Values During Antimony Treatment at Week					Normal Values
	Week 1	3	5	7	Week 11	
Erythrocytes, $\times 10^{12}$/L	2.67	2.50	3.22	3.40	3.84	3.7-5.3
Hemoglobin, g/L	55	56	85	97	103	90-140
Leukocytes, $\times 10^{9}$/L	3.5	2.3	8.5	6.9	8.5	6.0-17.5
Neutrophils, $\times 10^{9}$/L	0.66	0.16	1.14	1.33	1.98	1.5-3.0
Platelets, $\times 10^{9}$/L	93	50	361	292	242	150-400
Albumin, g/L	40	27	38	42	47	40-50
Total protein, g/L	68	64	88	82	82	50-70
IgG, g/L	14.39	18.26	33.79	27.70	21.27	2.79-15.33
IgM, g/L	1.31	1.01	6.97	3.26	1.29	.22-1.47
CRP, g/L	.068	.1202	.0063	.0028	.0028	.0028
ANA	1/80	1/320	1/320	1/640	1/80	Negative

*CPR indicates C-reactive protein, and ANA, antinuclear antibodies. Albumin, total protein, IgG, IgM, CRP, and ANA values are from serum samples. ANA values are given as liters.

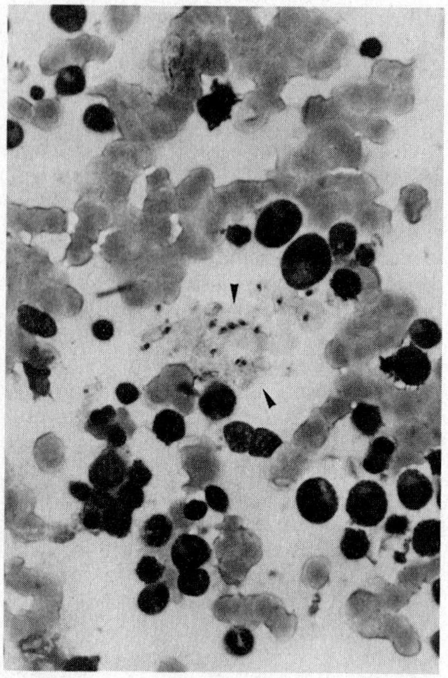

Photomicrograph of bone marrow aspirate showing amastigote forms of leishmania and disrupted macrophage (arrows) (May-Giemsa-Grünwald, original magnification ×1000).

and C4 and total hemolytic complement values were within normal limits, and results of extractable nuclear antigen, rheumatoid factor, and Rose-Waaler tests were negative. Still's disease was tentatively diagnosed, and treatment with oral aspirin (100 mg/kg of body weight per day) was started. This treatment lowered the patient's temperature and decreased the frequency of temperature spikes, but his general condition did not improve, and hepatosplenomegaly and pancytopenia persisted. Finally, attention was drawn to the fact that the family had spent 3 weeks in Barcelona, Spain, 8 months before the patient's admission to our facility and had regularly visited the beach. The previously performed bone marrow aspirate was carefully reinvestigated using a higher magnification (original magnification ×1200). Amastigote forms of *Leishmania* were seen extracellularly and within some macrophages (Figure). Intravenous sodium stibogluconate (Pentostam) was administered at a dose of 20 mg/kg of body weight per day for 30 days. Hepatosplenomegaly slowly regressed, but a residual splenomegaly of 5 cm persisted at the end of treatment. The patient's general condition markedly improved. C-reactive protein and peripheral blood cell values gradually normalized, but levels of antinuclear antibodies and serum IgG and IgM increased during treatment. Except for some flattening of T waves on electrocardiogram, no adverse reactions of therapy were seen.

Comment.—Mediterranean visceral leishmaniasis is caused by the protozoan *Leishmania donovani infantum* and is transmitted from animals, especially dogs, by the sand fly (*Phlebotomus* species). The disease affects mainly children; 80% of those affected are younger than age 5 years. The typical clinical presentation consists of persistent irregular fever, hepatosplenomegaly, hemolytic anemia (which is often severe), neutropenia, agranulocytosis with relative monocytosis, and thrombocytopenia that seldom causes a tendency to bleed[4] (pseudoleukemic pattern). Immunologic abnormalities such as positive results of direct Coombs' and Rose-Waaler tests and of tests to detect rheumatoid factor and antinuclear antibodies, increased levels of circulating immune complexes, and hypergammaglobulinemia have been observed.[5,6] The pathogenesis of these abnormalities has now been elucidated.[7,8]

Mediterranean visceral leishmaniasis has often been confused with other diseases with more or less similar clinical presentations, mainly, chronic bacterial or viral infections[9] and autoimmune diseases.[10] In many cases, malignant neoplasms were initially suspected. In others, pancytopenia was ascribed to the previous use of medications such as chloramphenicol.[11] Some patients underwent splenectomy for presumed idiopathic hypersplenism.[12,13] Leishmaniasis should be suspected in patients, mainly children, who visited Mediterranean countries and who present with one or more of the forementioned clinical symptoms, especially the pseudoleukemic pattern of hepatosplenomegaly and pancytopenia. It is important to note that incubation may vary from 3 months to more than 2 years, an aspect that was not considered in our patient. The diagnosis is based on the investigation of a bone marrow aspirate with the usual May-Giemsa-Grünwald or Giemsa stains using a magnification of at least ×1000. The ovoid protozoa appear in the cytoplasm of macrophages or extracellularly as clusters of 2- to 3-μm particles with large, eccentric, reddish nuclei, small kinetoplasts, and bluish cytoplasms. When a lower magnification is used, as in this case, or when experience with laboratory diagnosis of tropical conditions is lacking,[14] the protozoa may easily be mistaken for dust or inclusion bodies in the macrophages. The diagnosis can be confirmed with an indirect hemagglutination test, a complement fixation test, a highly sensitive indirect immunofluorescence antibody test, and highly specific immunoelectrophoretic techniques.[15]

The treatment of choice of Mediterranean visceral leishmaniasis is intramuscular or intravenous administration of pentavalent antimony compounds (either sodium stibogluconate [Pentostam] or meglumine antimoniate [Glucantine]) at a dose of 20 mg/kg of body weight per day for at least 14 days after negative results of bone marrow aspiration are obtained. Pentamidine, amphotericin B, and allopurinol may be used when antimony therapy is unsuccessful or contraindicated.[16] Treatment, such as blood transfusions and administration of antipyretic agents, should be given to alleviate symptoms. Splenectomy has been performed in drug-resistant cases.[17] In most instances, treatment with antimony results in resolution of fever, pancytopenia, and hepatosplenomegaly in that order. The latter, however, may persist for months. The immunologic abnormalities also disappear progressively, but hypergammaglobulinemia and autoimmune antibodies may persist for months. Postinfectious immunity is the rule, but relapses occur, mostly within 2 years.

Ludo M. Mahieu, MD
Karel J. Van Acker, MD, PhD
Department of Pediatrics
University Hospital of Antwerp
Wilrijkstraat 10
B-2650 Antwerpen, Belgium

1. Russo A, Russo Mancuso G, Battaglini CM, Schiliro G. Leishmaniasis, a worldwide disease. *Lancet.* 1986;1:451-452.

2. Filser TH, Heim ME, Kollmeier W, Heene DL. Visceral leishmaniasis in Europe. *Practitioner.* 1982;226:1559-1564.

3. Gottstein U, Steiner K, Hauk H, Klimaschewski G, Sedlmeyer I. Kala-Azar (viszerale Leishmaniose)—eine wichtige Krankheit nicht nur der Tropen. *Dtsch Med Wochenschr.* 1975;100:2022-2027.

4. Li Volti S, Fischer A, Musumeci S.

Hematological and serological aspects of Mediterranean kala-azar in infancy and childhood. *Acta Trop.* 1980;37:351-365.

5. Boel M, Gunawan J, Gillis F, et al. An unusual case of hepatosplenomegaly. *Acta Paediatr Belg.* 1981;34:97-102.

6. Hill FGH, Letsky EA. Infantile kala-azar in Britain. *BMJ.* 1975;2:354-355.

7. Galvao-Castro B, Ferreira JA, Marzochi KF, Marzochi MC, Coutinho SG, Lambert PH. Polyclonal B cell activation, circulating immune complexes and autoimmunity in human American visceral leishmaniasis. *Clin Exp Immunol.* 1984;56:58-66.

8. Böhme MW, Evans DA, Miles MA, Holborow EJ. Occurrence of autoantibodies to intermediate filament proteins in human visceral leishmaniasis and their induction by experimental polyclonal B-cell activation. *Immunology.* 1986;59:583-588.

9. Van de List-Nuver CJ, Sjamsoedin-Visser EJ, Hendrickx GF, Zegers BJ. Een patiënt met een vergrote lever en milt en piekende temperatuur. *Ned Tijdschr Geneeskd.* 1979;123:817-821.

10. Heilmann K, Döhnert G, Wohlenberg H. Tödlich verlaufende Leishmaniasis visceralis (Kala Azar) bei Mittelmeerurlaubern. *Dtsch Med Wochenschr.* 1971;96:36-38.

11. Van der Linde DL, Meuwissen OJ, Van Gorp LHM. Kala-Azar in Nederland. *Ned Tijdschr Geneeskd.* 1969;113:1413-1418.

12. Ornvold K, Carstensen H, Magnussen P, Nielsen MH, Pedersen FK. Kala-azar in a four-year-old child 18 months after brief exposure in Malta. *Acta Paediatr Scand.* 1989;78:650-652.

13. Baldus M, Schleiffer T, Brass H. Viszerale Leishmaniose (Kala-Azar): Eine seltene Differentialdiagnose bei Splenomegalie und Panzytopenie. *Dtsch Med Wochenschr.* 1989;114:1876-1881.

14. Boon DA, De Nef JJE, Kager PA. Grote milt, grote problemen. *Tijdschr Kindergeneeskd.* 1985;53:224-227.

15. Ridley DS. The laboratory diagnosis of tropical diseases with special reference to Britain: a review. *J Clin Pathol.* 1974;27:435-444.

16. Berman JD. Chemotherapy for leishmaniasis: biochemical mechanisms, clinical efficacy and future strategies. *Rev Infect Dis.* 1988;10:560-586.

17. Rees PH, Kager PA, Kyambi JM, Ayim EN, Bhatt KM. Splenectomy in kala azar. *Trop Geogr Med.* 1984;36:285-292.

Send Linus to Me

Sir.—I read about Friman's[1] research in the *Toronto Daily Star* and would like to explain how I get thumb-sucking children to stop. I teach parenting in a Toronto high school and direct a small on-site nursery laboratory center for 3-year-old children.

Thumb-sucking is discussed as something one does at home, in one's bed, usually when sleepy. I explain that since we have no bed at school, I will arrange a little corner as a bed, and if I see children sucking their thumbs, I let them rest there.

I ask the child, "Are you still sleepy, do you need to rest some more?" The response is usually "no," and the thumb comes out. The second time this happens I say, "I see you are still tired," and I lead the child to the "little bed" and say "When you are finished sucking your thumb, come back and join us." Thumb-sucking usually stops in 1 day. I do this in January, after the children have been in school 4 months.

I explain beforehand to the parents what I will do and try this method only with their consent. Parents are thrilled with this method because they usually have found the child unresponsive during thumb-sucking and are happy to have a real person around instead of a "zombie" kid.

I have been teaching this type of class for 16 years. During this time I have also led parent study groups using *Children: The Challenge,* by Dreikurs.[2]

I have confidence in this method and encourage physicians and parents to try it.

HARRIET SZONYI
336 St Clair Ave E
Toronto, Ontario,
Canada M4T 1P4

1. Friman PC. Concurrent habits: what would Linus do with his blanket if his thumb-sucking were treated? *AJDC.* 1990;144:1316-1318.

2. Dreikurs R. *Children: The Challenge.* Markham, Ontario: Fitzhenry & Whiteside; 1964.

In Reply.—I appreciate Szonyi's comments on her method of treating thumb-sucking, which certainly seems successful. Missing, of course, are supportive data, but she is not offering her comments as a scientific report. Should she need empirically derived support for her method, she need go no further than the nearest behavioral journal focused on analysis, modification, or therapy. Her method sounds similar to "time-out," a procedure involving contingent removal from reinforcing conditions. Time-out has been used effectively for a variety of child behavior problems and its use is often discussed in behavioral journals.

The primary advantage of the method I described is its privacy. Use of Szonyi's method makes a child's thumb-sucking and its treatment public. Given the potential risk that chronic thumb-sucking poses to self-esteem, a health care provider should weigh carefully the potential costs and benefits of such public intervention.

Finally, Szonyi's letter is something of a non sequitur because it addresses an issue that was not primary in my article, ie, treatment for thumb-sucking. The primary issue in my article was covariation between thumb-sucking and attachment to objects. The central question was what happens to attachment when thumb-sucking is treated? Still, I am interested in Szonyi's method. I would be even more interested in knowing what effect her treatment for thumb-sucking has on concurrent attachment in children who exhibit both behaviors.

PATRICK C. FRIMAN, PHD
Children's Hospital of
Philadelphia
Children's Seashore House
34th St & Civic Center Blvd
Philadelphia, PA 19104

A Markedly Immature Lecithin-Sphingomyelin Ratio at Term and Congenital Hypothyroidism

Sir.—A delay in pulmonary maturity and immature fetal lung profiles in infants born at term have been described in diabetic pregnancies.[1] This case report and review of neonatal screening results show that a markedly immature lecithin-sphingomyelin (L-S) ratio at term may be a prenatal marker for congenital hypothyroidism.

Patient Reports.—PATIENT 1.—A 25-

year-old gravida 2 woman with normal glucose screen results was admitted at 32 weeks' gestation with a diagnosis of a bleeding placenta previa. The bleeding resolved, and beginning at 35 weeks, weekly amniocentesis was performed for fetal lung profiles to ascertain pulmonary maturity as outlined by Kulovich et al.[2] The amniotic fluid L-S ratio never exceeded one and phosphatidyl glycerol was never detected. In spite of this, the infant was electively delivered at 40.5 weeks. The infant developed respiratory distress syndrome (RDS), which required intubation and mild ventilatory support. The thyrotropin level was 718 mU/L and the thyroxine (T_4) level was 15.2 nmol/L. The infant was diagnosed as having congenital hypothyroidism.

PATIENT 2.—A 25-year-old gravida 4 woman with normal prenatal glucose screen results underwent an amniocentesis for a fetal lung profile at 37 weeks' gestation because of a history of classic cesarean sections. The L-S ratio was markedly immature and measured on a weekly basis until 41 weeks. The ratio never exceeded 1.3, and phosphatidyl glycerol was not detected. The infant was delivered at 41.5 weeks and did not show any signs of respiratory distress. The thyrotropin level was 496 mU/L and the T_4 level was 60.5 nmol/L. The infant was diagnosed as having agenesis of the thyroid.

Comment.—There were 9188 live births at our institution between January 1, 1987, and December 1, 1989. Of those births, 7258 occurred after 37 weeks' gestation as defined by American College of Obstetricians and Gynecologists criteria.[3] Amniocentesis was performed on 204 of the 7258 term patients for assorted indications. Two of the 204 patients had markedly immature L-S ratios at term. The predictive value of the fetal lung profile for RDS at our institution was similar to that described by Kulovich et al.[1,2] Analysis of the neonatal blood screening performed by the Metabolic Unit of the Missouri Department of Health revealed two cases of abnormal T_4 and thyrotropin levels. Both of these patients were the infants with markedly immature fetal lung profiles. This suggests a correlation between a markedly low L-S ratio at term and congenital hypothyroidism.

Delayed fetal lung maturity has been well described in diabetic pregnancies. This delay can manifest itself as either a delay in the phospholipid maturity indexes or the development of RDS in the presence of a mature L-S ratio. Neonatal respiratory distress has also been described in an infant with a mature L-S ratio and present phosphatidyl glycerol.[4] This infant ultimately proved to have congenital hypothyroidism. Our data show that congenital hypothyroidism may also be associated with immature fetal lung maturation indexes at term. The role of thyroxine in the development of surfactant has been shown in a number of animal models.[5,6] This mechanism has been used to implement the acceleration of maturation of the fetal lung in utero. Intra-amniotic thyroxine and maternally administered protirelin (thyrotropin-releasing hormone) have been shown to accelerate the maturation of the fetal lung profile.[7,8]

Congenital hypothyroidism can have a devastating effect on the neurologic development of the fetus and neonate. Unfortunately, few infants affected with congenital hypothyroidism show overt signs at birth.[9] Newborn screening can take weeks between the initial testing and confirmation. This delay in diagnosis and treatment can significantly alter the potential intellectual development of the infant. Amniocentesis or percutaneous umbilical blood sampling as screening methods are not justified on the basis of their cost and risk for a disorder, with an incidence of one in 5000 births.

In summary, an immature L-S ratio accompanied by absent phosphatidyl glycerol can be indicative of potential congenital hypothyroidism. We do not recommend performing amniocentesis as a primary screening method in a low-risk patient. According to our data, if a markedly immature fetal lung profile is present at term, further workup is necessary to rule out congenital hypothyroidism.

GARY R. COHEN, MD
JAMES THORP, MD
JOHN D. YEAST, MD
BRUCE A. MEYER, MD
St Luke's Perinatal Center
University of Missouri—Kansas City
RICHARD O'KELL, MD
CANDACE MACY
Department of Laboratory Medicine
St Luke's Hospital
St Luke's Perinatal Center, OPC-2
44th and Wornall Rd
Kansas City, MO 64111

1. Kulovich M, Gluck L. The lung profile, II: complicated pregnancy. *Am J Obstet Gynecol.* 1979;135:64-70.

2. Kulovich M, Hallman M, Gluck L. The lung profile, I: normal pregnancy. *Am J Obstet Gynecol.* 1979;135:57-63.

3. American College of Obstetricians and Gynecologists. *Assessment of Fetal Maturity Prior to Repeat Cesarean Delivery or Elective Induction of Labor.* Washington, DC: American College of Obstetricians and Gynecologists Committee Opinions; 1989:72.

4. Anderson CS, Conrad L, Corder OL. Neonatal respiratory distress in the presence of amniotic fluid phosphatidylglycerol. *Am J Obstet Gynecol.* 1982;143:233.

5. Rooney SA, Gross I, Motoyama EK, et al. Effects of cortisol and thyroxine on fatty acid and phospholipid biosynthesis in fetal rabbit lung. *Physiologist.* 1974;17:323-325.

6. Smith BT, Torday JS. Factors affecting lecithin synthesis by fetal lung cells in culture. *Pediatr Res.* 1974;8:848-849.

7. Morales W, O'Brien W, Angel J, et al. Fetal lung maturation: the combined use of corticosteroids and thyrotropin releasing hormone. *Obstet Gynecol.* 1989;73:111-115.

8. Gonzales LK, Bullard PL. Glucocorticoid and thyroid hormone stimulation or phosphatidylcholine synthesis in cultured human fetal lung. *Pediatr Res.* 1984;18:310A.

9. Smith DW, Blizzard RM, Wilkins L. The mental prognosis in hypothyroidism in infancy and childhood: a review of 128 cases. *Pediatrics.* 1957;19:1011-1012.

Is Prophylaxis of Neonates With Intravenous Immunoglobulin Beneficial?

The human neonate, and especially the premature neonate, is uniquely susceptible to overwhelming bacterial infection. There are a variety of host defense abnormalities in neonates that aid in explaining this phenomenon, including deficiencies in specific antibodies, decreased levels of complement components, abnormalities in the function and number of neutrophils, and deficient T lymphocyte activity.[1] Until very recently, the only "gun" in the immunologist's or neonatologist's armamentarium for correcting these host defense abnormalities was immunoglobulin. This, coupled with the rather striking hypogammaglobulinemia observed in premature infants, led many investigators to examine the prophylactic role of immunoglobulin administration in preventing infections in neonates. Early anecdotal information or reports from small, uncontrolled trials suggested that the administration of intravenous immunoglobulin could prevent infection in premature infants weighing less than 1500 g.[1]

See also p 1233.

These early trials, which were conducted outside the United States, consisted of small numbers of patients (78 to 150), were not blinded or placebo-controlled, and often examined infections due to bacteria that are uncommon in US neonatal intensive care units. Thus, the results could not be extrapolated to use in this country. This prompted several large, controlled trials of the prophylactic use of intravenous immunoglobulin in neonates in the United States. To date, the preliminary reports of the results of these trials do not convincingly answer the question of the efficacy of intravenous immunoglobulin in the prophylaxis of bacterial infection. For instance, an initial report by Bussel and coworkers[2] of a double-blind, placebo-controlled trial of intravenous immunoglobulin in infants weighing less than 1300 g, as well as a verbal follow-up report at a recent National Institutes of Health Consensus Conference on intravenous immunoglobulin, failed to show a significant prophylactic effect against infection.

In contrast, Baker and associates,[3] in a large, multicenter, controlled trial (577 assessable patients), reported that the prophylactic administration of intravenous immunoglobulin to infants weighing 1500 g or less (500 mg/kg of body weight administered 3 to 7 days after birth, 1 week later, and then every 14 days) resulted in an overall reduction in infections of approximately 30%. Mortality was not significantly reduced in those given the immunoglobulin (3.5%) compared with those given the placebo (4.4%). There was, however, a reduction in hospital stay of 7 days (69 days in the group that received immunoglobulin vs 76 days in the group that received the placebo) and a significant reduction in severe necrotizing enterocolitis in immunoglobulin recipients. The most common microbial isolate in this study was *Staphylococcus epidermidis* (37%), followed by *Staphylococcus aureus* (20%). *Klebsiella* (14%) was the third most frequent isolate, while enterococci were fourth (11%).

More recently, Weisman and associates[4] described another large, multicenter, double-blind, placebo-controlled trial of the prophylactic use of intravenous immunoglobulin that involved 753 infants. They found that the administration of one dose of immunoglobulin (500 mg/kg of body weight) to preterm neonates delivered at 35 weeks' gestation or before resulted in no difference in the incidence of sepsis, total number of infections, incidence of necrotizing enterocolitis, or death due to sepsis. However, one could argue that the results may be due to the fact that only one dose of immunoglobulin was administered to the participants in this study.

The National Institutes of Health Neonatal Network is now conducting another randomized, controlled trial. Apparently, however, the placebo arm of this trial was eliminated because of some adverse effects observed in participants. Thus, there may be difficulties in the final interpretation of these data as well.

In this issue, the critically designed, expertly carried out, moderate-sized study (n=170) by Kinney and colleagues is presented.[5] These authors seem to have touched all of the bases in randomly selecting infants of different weights to blindly receive intravenous immunoglobulin (750 mg/kg of body weight) or a placebo. In contrast to the study by Weisman et al,[4] the infants in this trial received repeated doses of immunoglobulin (750 mg/kg of body weight) at 2-week intervals until discharge from the hospital. Even so, the authors found that the intravenous immunoglobulin did not affect the rate of systemic or localized infection. In addition, it did not affect the development of necrotizing enterocolitis, length of hospitalization, or use of antibiotics, assisted ventilation, or supplemental oxygen. Once again, the causes of both systemic and localized infections in patients who received intravenous immunoglobulin or a placebo in this study were not organisms usually associated with invasive neonatal disease, such as group B streptococci, *Escherichia coli* K1, or *Listeria monocytogenes*, but were coagulase-negative staphylococci, *S aureus*, and *Serratia marcescens*. The development of infection with these organisms is usually associated not with specific antibody deficiency but with indwelling catheters, respirators, and other invasive maneuvers so common in neonatal intensive care units. It is unlikely, therefore, that any study of intravenous immunoglobulin that focuses on the prevention of infection caused by these organisms will ever show a truly beneficial prophylactic effect. Furthermore, it may be impossible to design and conduct a study of the prophylactic effects of intravenous immunoglobulin large enough to show a beneficial effect on antibody-dependent, invasive, group B streptococcal, *E coli* K1, or *Listeria* infections given the low attack rate of these infections. An alternate and perhaps more successful strategy may be to employ standard intravenous immunoglobulin[1,6] or human monoclonal or hyperimmune intravenous immunoglobulin preparations[7] to treat, rather than prevent, invasive neonatal infections.

HARRY R. HILL, MD
Departments of Pediatrics and Pathology
University of Utah
50 N Medical Dr
Salt Lake City, UT 84132

References

1. Gonzales LA, Hill HR. The current status of intravenous gammaglobulin use in neonates. *Pediatr Infect Dis J.* 1989;8:315-322.

2. Bussel JB, LaGamma EF, Guiliano M. Intravenous gammaglobulin (IVIG) prophylaxis of late sepsis in VLBW infants: a randomized, placebo controlled trial. *Pediatr Res.* 1988;23:471A.

3. Baker CJ, Neonatal IVIG Collaborative Study Group. Multicenter trial of intravenous immunoglobulin (IVIG) to prevent late-onset infection in preterm infants: preliminary results. *Pediatr Res.* 1989;25:275A.

4. Weisman LE, Stoll B, Kueser T, et al. Intravenous immunoglobulin (IVIG) prophylaxis of late-onset septicemia in neonates. *Pediatr Res.* 1990;27:277A.

5. Kinney J, Mundorf L, Gleason C, et al. Efficacy and pharmacokinetics of intravenous IgG administration to high-risk neonates. *AJDC.* 1991;145:1233-1238.

6. Christensen RD, Brown MS, Hall DC, Lassiter HA, Hill HR. Effect of IVIG administration to neonates with clinical signs of early-onset sepsis on neutrophil kinetics and serum opsonic capacity. *J Pediatr.* 1991;118:606-614.

7. Hill HR, Gonzales LA, Knappe WA, Fischer GW, Kelsey DK, Raff HV. Comparative protective activity of human monoclonal and hyperimmune polyclonal antibody against group B streptococci. *J Infect Dis.* 1991;163:792-798.

In Other AMA Journals

ARCHIVES OF SURGERY

Is Early Prediction of Outcome in Severe Head Injury Possible?

Kenneth Waxman, MD; Michael J. Sundine, MD;
Ronald F. Young, MD (*Arch Surg.* 1991;126:1237-1242)

The Mangled Extremity: When to Amputate?

Markus S. Roessler, MD; David H. Wisner, MD;
James W. Holcroft, MD (*Arch Surg.* 1991;126:1243-1244)

Hepatic Vein and Retrohepatic Vena Caval Injuries in Children: Sternotomy First?

Steven L. Moulton, MD; Frank P. Lynch, MD;
Timothy G. Canty, MD; David L. Collions, MD; David B. Hoyt, MD
(*Arch Surg.* 1991;126:1262-1266)

The Impact of Liver Reductions in Pediatric Liver Transplantation

Carlos O. Esquivel, MD, PhD; Paul Nakazato, MD;
Kenneth Cox, MD; Waldo Concepcion, MD;
William Berquist, MD; Thomas R. Russell, MD
(*Arch Surg.* 1991;126:1278-1286)

Decortication for Childhood Empyema: The Primary Provider's Peccadillo

Andrew S. Kennedy, MD; Melisa Agness, MD;
Leonard Bailey, MD; John J. White, MD, CM
(*Arch Surg.* 1991;126:1287-1291)

Efficacy and Pharmacokinetics of Intravenous Immune Globulin Administration to High-Risk Neonates

Janet Kinney, MD; Lucinda Mundorf, RN; Christine Gleason, MD; Carlton Lee, PharmD;
Timothy Townsend, MD; Roshelle Thibault, RPh; Anna Nussbaum, MD; Helen Abby, PhD; Robert Yolken, MD

• *Objective.*—To determine whether intravenous immune globulin (IVIG) administration modifies the incidence of infections in high-risk neonates.

***Design.*—Randomized, double-blind study.**

***Setting.*—Neonatal intensive care unit at a tertiary care center.**

***Participants.*—A total of 170 infants were enrolled, 82 of whom received IVIG and 88 of whom received the placebo preparation. Infants were stratified by birth weight into one of three groups (category 1, those weighing less than 1000 g; category 2, those weighing between 1000 and 1500 g; and category 3, those weighing more than 1500 g).**

***Interventions.*—Intravenous immune globulin (750 mg/kg of body weight), or albumin placebo was administered within 72 hours of admission to the tertiary care center and every 14 days thereafter until discharge from the neonatal intensive care unit or age 3 months. Serum IgG levels were measured and data collected relating to the incidence of systemic and localized infections and to the course of hospitalization.**

***Measurements and Main Results.*—The administration of IVIG had no major side effects and resulted in higher serum IgG levels in infants in all birth weight categories compared with infants receiving the placebo. Systemic infections developed in five IVIG-treated infants and five placebo-treated infants. Administration of immunoglobulin had no significant effect on the rate of localized infections or necrotizing enterocolitis. It also did not affect hospital course of the infants as measured by length of hospitalization or the number of days on assisted ventilation, supplemental oxygen, or antibiotics was required.**

***Conclusions.*—The general administration of IVIG using this dosage regimen has limited effects on the clinical course of infants in a neonatal intensive care unit.**

(*AJDC.* 1991;145:1233-1238)

Infants admitted to a neonatal intensive care unit (NICU) are at high risk of infection. Premature infants are susceptible to infection because of many factors, including the relatively low level of immunoglobulins transferred across the placenta before the last month of gestation and the immature function of phagocytic cells.[1-4] Full-term infants in an NICU for an extended period may also be at risk of infections because of a rapid decline in maternally acquired antibodies and other factors related to their hospitalization.[1,5] Recently, preparations have become available that allow the intravenous administration of human immune globulins obtained from large pools of donors. These immune globulin preparations contain antibodies to a wide range of microorganisms that are potentially pathogenic in neonates.[6] However, studies measuring the actual effect of intravenous immune globulin (IVIG) administration on the course of hospitalization of infants in an intensive care setting during an extended period have generated conflicting data.[7-14]

We performed a randomized, double-blind trial to determine whether IVIG could be administered safely to infants and whether IVIG administration modifies the incidence of infections in infants in an NICU setting.

PATIENTS AND METHODS

Newborns admitted to the NICU at The Johns Hopkins Hospital, Baltimore, Md, were eligible for the study if they met the following criteria: (1) age less than 72 hours, (2) no severe metabolic disorders or congenital anomalies, (3) no receipt of immune globulin or blood products before enrollment, and (4) no receipt of blood products or immune globulin preparation by the mother within 2 weeks before delivery. The presence of early-onset sepsis or suspected sepsis did not eliminate an infant from the study. After informed consent was obtained, the study infants were enrolled and stratified by birth weight into three categories: those weighing less than 1000 g (category 1), 1000 to 1500 g (category 2), and more than 1500 g (category 3). Using a block randomization technique, infants in each birth weight

Accepted for publication July 15, 1991.

From the Eudowood Division of Infectious Diseases, Department of Pediatrics (Drs Kinney, Townsend, and Yolken and Ms Mundorf), Division of Neonatology, Department of Pediatrics (Dr Gleason), and the Department of Radiology (Dr Nussbaum), The Johns Hopkins School of Medicine; Department of Pharmacy Services, The Johns Hopkins Hospital (Dr Lee and Ms Thibault); and the Department of Biostatistics, The Johns Hopkins School of Hygiene and Public Health, Baltimore, Md (Dr Abby). Dr Townsend is now with the Divisions of Neonatology and Infectious Diseases, The Children's Mercy Hospital, University of Missouri, Kansas City School of Medicine.

Reprints not available.

stratum were assigned to receive either IVIG or placebo. Only the pharmacists knew of the infants' assignments to the IVIG or placebo group. This study was approved by the Joint Committee on Clinical Investigation of The Johns Hopkins Medical Institutions. It was overseen by an independent monitoring committee that confirmed the case definitions and determined the study end points.

An intravenous immune globulin, Gamimune-N (5% human immunoglobulin in 10% maltose [pH 4.5]) or placebo (0.1% albumin in 10% maltose) was administered intravenously to the infants within 72 hours of admission and every 14 days thereafter until discharge from the NICU or age 3 months. The IVIG was administered at a dose of 750 mg/kg of body weight, and placebo was prepared to be administered in a solution that had the same volume and appearance as the IVIG. Doses of IVIG and placebo were administered slowly using a syringe pump at an initial rate of 1 mL/kg of body weight per hour.

Detailed pharmacokinetic studies were performed involving selected infants enrolled in each weight category who received IVIG or placebo. Serum samples were obtained immediately before each infusion and 2, 3, and 7 days after infusion for up to three transfusions. In addition, cord blood samples were analyzed when available. The samples were analyzed using nephelometric methods to ascertain IgG concentration. The elimination (β) half-life was calculated using regression analysis (natural logarithm vs time). The volume of distribution was calculated using the noncompartmental model.[15]

Total IgG levels were also measured in each study infant before each infusion so that the preinfusion level of IgG could be ascertained. Preinfusion values were obtained for up to six infusions, and detailed time points were obtained for up to three infusions per infant. Levels were measured only while the infants were in the NICU.

Vital signs were monitored during infusions, and any adverse reaction or notable alteration in clinical status that occurred during or within 48 hours of the infusion was recorded. Levels of serum glucose were measured immediately before and 48 hours after the infusion using glucose oxidase strips (Chemstrips, Miles Laboratories, Elkhart, Ind). Oxygen saturation was monitored during the infusions using pulse oximetry. Gestational maturity was determined with clinical parameters using standard methods.[16]

Each episode of bacterial infection was recorded and categorized as systemic or localized. Systemic bacterial infections were defined when blood or cerebrospinal fluid cultures were positive for defined bacterial agents. The clinical significance of a blood culture positive for *Staphylococcus epidermidis* and other strains of staphylococci that do not produce coagulase is difficult to interpret with certainty in this patient population.[17,18] For this reason, a neonatologist and an infectious diseases attending physician not participating in the study and unaware of the treatment assignments reviewed each case in which a blood culture positive for coagulase-negative staphylococci was obtained. They considered an infant to have undergone systemic infection with coagulase-negative staphylococci if (1) the infant displayed signs and symptoms of sepsis and had two blood cultures positive for coagulase-negative staphylococci from at least two different blood sampling sites (including a central line) or from different days, or (2) the infant displayed signs and symptoms of sepsis, and one blood culture yielded pure coagulase-negative staphylococci within 24 hours of inoculation. Infants who had cultures positive for coagulase-negative staphylococci but who did not meet these criteria were not considered to have undergone systemic infection with coagulase-negative staphylococci. In addition, cultures positive for nonbacterial organisms such as *Candida albicans* were not included in the analysis of systemic bacterial infections.

Localized bacterial infections analyzed included tracheitis, urinary tract infections, wound infections, and conjunctivitis. Tracheitis was defined as the presence of purulent tracheal secretions coincident with the cultivation of a potential pathogen from endotracheal secretions associated with respiratory deterioration. A urinary tract infection was defined as the presence of more than 10 000 organisms on culture of a urine specimen obtained using a catheter or suprapubic puncture. A wound infection was characterized as the presence of a purulent discharge from a break in the skin and yielding of a microorganism from culture of the discharge. Conjunctivitis was defined as the presence of purulent discharge from the eye associated with the cultivation of a bacterial pathogen. In each case, an episode of localized infection was considered a separate event if it occurred at least 1 week before or after another episode involving the same mucosal surface. We did not attempt to systematically identify viral or fungal organisms in this study.

The infants were also evaluated to detect gastrointestinal disease, which was divided into three categories: necrotizing enterocolitis (NEC), suspected NEC, and gastroenteritis. Necrotizing enterocolitis and suspected NEC were defined according to the criteria of Bell et al.[19] Gastroenteritis was defined as an illness characterized by the passage of more than two loose, watery stools during two consecutive 8-hour periods or the passage of more than four loose, watery stools during 24 hours.[5]

In addition to the above determinations, we measured the number of days during which an antibiotic was administered to the infant after enrollment in the study, regardless of the culture results. We also determined the number of days during which an infant required assisted ventilation with a mechanical ventilator or continuous positive airway pressure device and the number of days during which an infant was administered supplemental oxygen using a face mask, nasal cannula, or hood in the absence of assisted ventilation. For these analyses, a day was recorded if the indicated therapy was administered at any time during 24 hours. The presence of intracranial hemorrhage was determined using ultrasound evaluations obtained during the first, second, and sixth weeks of life for infants born at less than 32 weeks' gestation and when clinically indicated for other infants.

The study was overseen by a study monitoring committee that included a neonatalogist, infectious disease specialist, and a statistician not participating in the study. The committee periodically reviewed the efficacy data and made decisions concerning the inclusion of cases of infection and the length of the study. The committee decided to terminate the study when they determined that a statistically significant difference in rates of infection could not be achieved in a reasonable period of time.

Statistical analyses were performed with the CSS Statistical Package (Statsoft Inc, San Francisco, Calif).

RESULTS

Study Population

Between May 1987 and April 1989, 187 infants were enrolled in the study. A total of 17 of the 187 infants originally enrolled were eliminated from the analysis for any of the following reasons: (1) infant was in the NICU less than 48 hours (n = 14); (2) infant received an exchange transfusion (n = 1); and (3) infant received the wrong study drug owing to pharmacy error (n = 2). Therefore, 170 infants completed the study. Of the 88 infants who received IVIG, 25 were in birth weight category 1; 29, category II; and 34, category 3. The birth weight distribution of the 82 infants receiving placebo was 24, 30, and 28 for categories 1, 2, and 3, respectively.

The demographic characteristics of participants in both groups were similar (Table 1). There were no statistically significant differences between the IVIG and placebo groups as a whole or within the birth weight groups for sex, race, type of delivery, gestational maturity, or mul-

Table 1.—Demographic Characteristics of Study Population*	No. (%) of Patients Receiving Immune Globulin	No. (%) of Patients Receiving a Placebo
Infant Characteristics		
Male	44 (50)	43 (51)
White	32 (36)	38 (45)
SVD	43 (51)	38 (45)
AGA	71 (81)	70 (83)
Multiple gestation	16 (18)	15 (18)
Maternal history before delivery		
Hypertension	14 (16)	9 (11)
Preeclampsia	14 (16)	9 (11)
Intrapartum fever	27 (31)	22 (26)
Premature ROM	43 (49)	51 (61)
Prolonged ROM	35 (40)	39 (35)

*$P>.1$ by χ^2 analysis for all demographic characteristics and administration of intravenous immune globulin or a placebo. SVD indicates spontaneous vaginal delivery; AGA, appropriate for gestational age; and ROM, rupture of membranes.

tiple gestation. There were also no differences between treatment groups for mean birth weight and Apgar scores. The distribution of maternal risk factors such as hypertension, preeclampsia, intrapartum fever, prematurity, and prolonged rupture of membranes was similar in the two treatment groups.

A total of 474 infusions were administered to 170 study infants as follows: 235 infusions to 88 infants in the IVIG group and 239 infusions to 82 infants in the placebo group. The mean number of infusions was 2.67 per infant in the IVIG group and 2.91 per infant in the placebo group. In category 1, an average of 4.44 infusions were administered per child in the placebo group and 4.45 infusions per child in the group receiving IVIG. No life-threatening reactions were noted to have been associated with the infusion of the IVIG or placebo preparations. Alteration in clinical status occurred several times during infusion and within 48 hours after infusion. These alterations included minor changes in respiratory, cardiac, and gastrointestinal function (Table 2). However, the frequency of these events in the infants receiving IVIG did not differ from that of the infants receiving placebo ($P>.2$ by Fisher's Exact Test for all comparisons). One infant who received IVIG developed a fever (38.5°C) after the fifth infusion and was not administered additional doses of the study drug. On retrospective review of the patient's chart, the fever was not believed to be attributable to IVIG. None of the other alterations in clinical status were judged to be of sufficient severity to warrant the withholding of subsequent infusions.

Pharmacokinetics

Serial IgG levels were measured 2, 3, 7, and 14 days after infusion in 35 of the infants who received IVIG. A total of 19 of these infants were in birth weight category 1, 10 infants were in birth weight category 2, and six were in birth weight category 3. Only infants from whom a complete set of blood specimens was obtained were included in the analysis. Data were obtained from up to three infusions per infant. The smaller number of infants studied in the higher birth weight categories is a reflection of their shorter length of stay in the NICU and of the fact that several of the infants enrolled were discharged before 14 days after infusion.

The mean preinfusion (trough) IgG levels for each weight category are depicted in Fig 1. Mean levels of IgG measured at birth or immediately before the first infusion were not different between IVIG and placebo groups. After administration of the study drug, mean IgG levels obtained before each subsequent dose were significantly higher in IVIG-treated neonates than in the infants receiving the placebo preparations for all birth weight groups ($P<.05$ by the Mann-Whitney *U* Test for all comparisons). The serum half-life of IVIG in the study infants was 18.1 days (95% confidence interval, 15.5 to 20.6 days). The volume of distribution of the IVIG was 0.082 L/kg of body weight (95% confidence interval, 0.074 to 0.090 L/kg). There were no statistically significant differences in serum half-life or volume of distribution among the birth weight categories. The mean levels of IgG during the 14 days after infusion are depicted in Fig 2.

Infections

Ten systemic bacterial infections were documented in 10 different infants evaluated during the study. Five of the episodes of systemic bacterial infection occurred in infants receiving IVIG, while five occurred in infants who received the placebo preparation. The difference in observed infection rates between the treatment groups was 0.4% (95% confidence interval, −6.7% to +7.5%). The five systemic infections in the infants receiving IVIG were detected using samples obtained on days 2, 5, 6, 9, and 13 after infusion. The five infections in the infants in the placebo group were detected on days 3, 5, 6, 9, and 14 after infusion.

Systemic infections in the infants receiving IVIG were caused by *Staphylococcus aureus* (n = 2), coagulase-negative staphylococci, *Escherichia coli*, and *Serratia marcescens*. Systemic bacterial infections in the neonates receiving placebo included coagulase-negative staphylococci (n = 2), *S aureus*, *S marcescens*, and *Enterobacter gergoviae*. Six of the 10 systemic bacterial infections occurred in infants with birth weights of less than 1000 g. These infections were also equally divided between the IVIG and placebo groups.

A total of 19 episodes of localized bacterial infection, as defined above, occurred in 17 infants during the study. Eleven of the localized infections occurred in 10 infants who had received IVIG, while eight localized infections were observed in seven infants who had received placebo. The sites of infection are enumerated in Table 3. The infections were caused by a wide range of microorganisms, including *S aureus*, coagulase-negative staphylococci, *Streptococcus faecalis*, *E coli*, *Moraxella catarrhalis*, *Pseudomonas aeruginosa*, *Klebsiella pneumoniae*, *S marcescens*, and *Acinetobacter baumannii* (formerly *A calcoaceticus*, biovar *anitratus*).

There were three cases of definite NEC and seven cases of suspected NEC. Four infants had gastroenteritis, as defined above, without signs of symptoms of NEC (Table 3). Thus, six infants with gastrointestinal symptoms had received IVIG and eight had not.

We also examined the effect of IVIG on the course of hospitalization of the infants (Table 4). Infants receiving IVIG were hospitalized for a mean of 43.1 days, while

Table 2.—Reactions Temporally Associated With Infusions of Intravenous Immune Globulin or a Placebo

	Birth Weight <1000 g		All Birth Weights	
	Intravenous Immune Globulin	Placebo	Intravenous Immune Globulin	Placebo
No. of infusions	111	107	225	239
No. of reactions				
Acidosis (pH<7.3)	7	2	9	3
Apnea	2	4	2	9
Tachypnea (>40 breaths/min)	5	1	5	1
Oxygen desaturation (<90%)	10	5	15	11
Fever (>38.5°C)	1	0	1	0
Lethargy	1	2	2	3
Tachycardia (>120 beats/min)	7	2	7	6
Bradycardia (<60 beats/min)	4	7	7	13
Emesis	2	2	2	5
Abdominal distention (>1 cm)	1	0	1	0
Hyperglycemia (>6.6 mmol/L [>120 mg/dL])	6	10	8	13
Hypoglycemia (<2.2 mmol/L [<40 mg/dL])	12	10	21	18

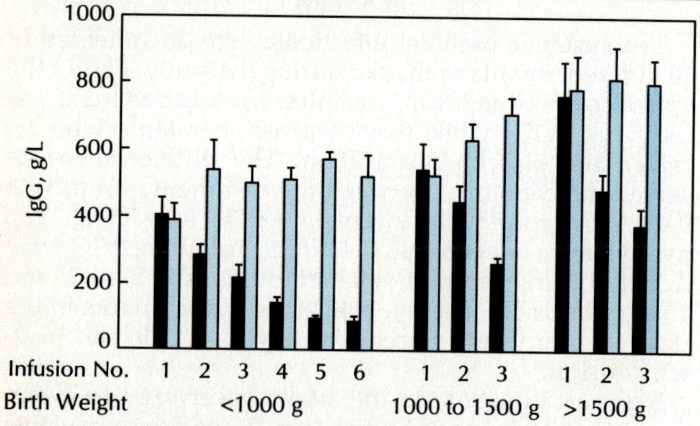

Fig 1.—*Trough serum immune globulin levels. The serum IgG levels were measured in all study infants before each infusion. The infusions were administered every 14 days while the infants were participating in the study. Values indicate the mean±95% confidence interval of the IgG levels measured in infants in the indicated birth weight strata. Solid bars indicate infants who received intravenous immune globulin (IVIG), and shaded bars, infants who received placebo. Numbers on the x axis indicate the infusion number before which the corresponding level was measured. Note that values for infusions 2 through 6 were obtained before the administration of IVIG or placebo.*

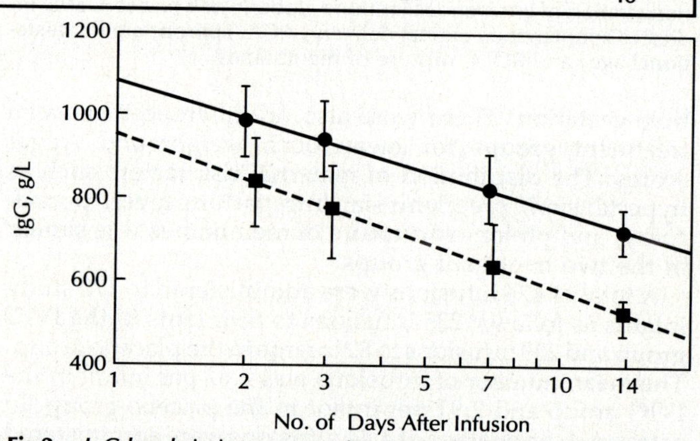

Fig 2.—*IgG levels in intravenous immune globulin–treated infants. Values are geometric means±95% confidence intervals of the IgG levels at the indicated times after infusion. Lines indicate the log-linear regression of the levels for infants weighing less than 1000 g at birth (squares; n=19) and infants weighing 1000 g or more at birth (circles; n=16). Values for up to three infusions were used for these analyses.*

those receiving placebo were hospitalized for a mean of 46.5 days (*P*>.2 by the Mann-Whitney *U* Test). Infants in the IVIG group received antibiotics for a mean of 9.4 days, while those in the placebo group received antibiotics for a mean of 9.2 days (*P*>.5 by the Mann-Whitney *U* Test). There were also no differences in the total number of days during which infants required supplemental oxygen therapy or assisted ventilation. Five infants in the IVIG group had evidence of intracranial hemorrhage as documented with cranial ultrasound examinations. Four of these cases were judged to be grade 3 or grade 4 hemorrhages. Seven patients receiving placebo had intracranial hemorrhage, and five of these were grade 3 or grade 4 hemorrhages.

Eight infants died during the study. Of these, four had received IVIG and four, placebo. Three of the deaths were directly associated with infection. Two of the infection-related mortalities occurred in the placebo group—one in an infant with staphylococcal-scalded skin syndrome and bacteremia due to *S aureus* and another in an infant with severe NEC and bacteremia with *E gergoviae*. The third infection-related death occurred in an infant who had received IVIG and who had bacteremia with *S marcescens*.

COMMENT

Our study indicates that IVIG can be administered safely to infants in an NICU and that IVIG administration results in higher levels of serum IgG. The pharmacokinetics in our IVIG-treated infants were similar to those reported by others.[20]

The administration of IVIG in a controlled, double-blinded fashion did not result in a decrease in the rate of systemic or localized microbial infection. We noted an incidence of systemic bacterial infection of 5.9% (ten of 170) among all study infants and of 12.2% (six of 49) among category 1 infants. Five infants in both the IVIG-treated group and the control group had culture-proven, systemic, bacterial infection. Eleven of the

Table 3.—Number of Episodes of Infection and Other Conditions Occurring in Neonates Receiving Intravenous Immune Globulin or a Placebo

	Patient Receiving Intravenous Immune Globulin (n=88)	Patients Receiving a Placebo (n=82)
Infections		
Systemic	5	5
Local	11	8
Tracheitis	4	4
Wound	3	0
Urinary	4	3
Eye	0	1
Total	**16**	**13**
Gastrointestinal conditions		
Definite necrotizing enterocolitis	1	2
Suspected necrotizing enterocolitis	3	4
Gastroenteritis	2	2
Total	**6**	**8**
Total	**22**	**21**

Table 4.—Effect of Intravenous Immune Globulin on Course of Hospitalization of High-Risk Neonates*

	Patients Receiving Intravenous Immune Globulin	Patients Receiving a Placebo
Hospital stay		
No.	88 (100)	82 (100)
Mean	43.1 (36.3-49.9)	46.5 (39.0-54.0)
Antibiotics		
No.	76 (86.4)	75 (91.5)
Mean	9.4 (7.7-11.1)	9.2 (7.2-11.1)
Assisted ventilation†		
No.	66 (75.0)	60 (73.2)
Mean	12.7 (8.7-16.7)	15.5 (10.0-21.0)
Supplemental oxygen‡		
No.	53 (60.2)	50 (61.0)
Mean	16.5 (10.7-22.4)	14.2 (9.4-19.0)

*Data are number (percent) of patients in the indicated category and the mean (95% confidence interval) of the infants in the category.

†Includes infants treated with mechanical ventilators or continuous positive airway pressure.

‡Includes infants not receiving assisted ventilation but receiving supplemental oxygen via nasal cannula, face mask, or hood.

IVIG-treated infants and eight infants in the placebo group developed local infections. There was no statistical difference between groups in the development of gastrointestinal illness, including NEC. In essence, we found that the administration of IVIG had no significant effect on the rate of systemic infection, localized infection, or NEC.

It is of note that the infants in our study population did not develop infections with organisms widely recognized as pathogens in neonates, such as group B streptococcus, enteric gram-negative rods or *Listeria monocytogenes*. Rather, the infecting microflora represented organisms commonly encountered in nosocomial infections in other inpatient intensive care populations, including a high rate of staphylococcal infections. The increased survival of high-risk infants results in long-term stays in intensive care settings and, subsequently, increased exposure to microflora and other environmental conditions that can lead to nosocomial infections.

The detection of infectious processes is a problem when studying any neonatal infection. While the identification of a pathogenic organism from a normally sterile body site, such as blood or cerebrospinal fluid, is a specific sign of infection, it is likely that microbiologic cultivation techniques do not detect all episodes of neonatal infection. This limitation is particularly a problem among low-birth-weight infants because repeated samples of large volumes of blood generally cannot be obtained. The frequent use of antibiotics in this population may also affect the rate of recovery of pathogenic microorganisms. Also, such methods will not detect anaerobic organisms and infections with nonbacterial agents, such as viruses or genital mycoplasmas.[21] It is possible that IVIG was affecting infectious processes in a way not evident from the analysis of blood cultures.

For this reason, we also examined the effect of IVIG on other parameters that might be related to infectious processes occurring in the study infants. We could find no effect of IVIG administration on the rate of localized bacterial infections, nor could we document an effect of IVIG on the incidence of NEC or other forms of gastrointestinal illness. Similarly, the administration of IVIG did not alter the number of days during which the infant was administered antibiotics by the attending physician. In addition, the administration of IVIG did not affect the length of hospitalization or the number of days in which assisted ventilation was required or supplemental oxygen was administered. Thus, we found no evidence that the administration of IVIG affected parameters that might be related to the occurrence of systemic or localized infectious processes.

Previous studies have presented contradictory findings concerning the effect of IVIG on the rate of infection in the NICU population. Some studies document a decrease in systemic infections,[8,9,12,14] while other studies show no significant affect on infection rate.[13] These differences might relate to the dosing regimens, constitution of the IVIG preparations, sample size, definition of infectious processes, or the incidence of the infections in the study populations. It is possible that the administration of IVIG at a higher dose or more frequent dosing interval or maintenance of a targeted level of IgG[22] would have more greatly affected the incidence of systemic infections. Likewise, a reduction in the incidence of infection might be observed in a population with a much higher incidence of infection or NEC.[8,9,12]

In essence, results of our study indicate that it is unlikely that the general administration of IVIG to neonates in an NICU setting with relatively low rates of infection will result in a substantial alteration in hospital course. In light of the cost of IVIG preparations, the routine administration of IVIG to all neonates in intensive care units cannot be recommended at this time. Additional efforts should be directed at the development of more specific therapies for the prevention of infectious complications in high-risk infants.

This work was supported by grant R01 DK 33089 from the National Institutes of Health, Bethesda, Md.

The authors thank Carol Baker, MD, and Robert T. Hall, MD, for their critical appraisal of the article and Miriam Budinger, MD, for her helpful suggestions.

References

1. Wilson CB. Immunologic basis for increased susceptibility of the neonate to infection. *J Pediatr.* 1986;108:1-12.

2. Speer CP, Gahr M, Wieland M, Eber S. Phagocytosis associated functions in neonatal monocyte derived macrophages. *Pediatr Res.* 19;24:213-216.

3. Gonzalez LA, Hill HR. The current status of intravenous gammaglobulin use in neonates. *Pediatr Infect Dis J.* 1989;8:315-322.

4. Cairo MS. Neonatal neutrophil host defence: prospects for immunologic enhancement during neonatal sepsis. *AJDC.* 1989;143:40-46.

5. Kinney JS, McCray E, Kaplan JE, et al. Risk factors associated with echovirus 11 infection in a hospital nursery. *J Pediatr Infect Dis.* 1986;5:192-197.

6. Baley JE. Neonatal sepsis: the potential for immunotherapy. *Clin Perinatol.* 1988;15:755-771.

7. Stabile A, Sopo SM, Romanelli V, Pastore M, Pesaresi MA. Intravenous immunoglobulin for prophylaxis of neonatal sepsis in premature infants. *Arch Dis Child.* 1988;63:441-443.

8. Haque KN, Zaidi MH, Haque SK, Bahakin DH, El-Hazmi M, El-Swailam M. Intravenous immunoglobulin for prevention of sepsis in preterm and low birth weight infants. *Pediatr Infect Dis.* 1986;5:622-625.

9. Chirico G, Rondini G, Plebani A, Chiara A, Massa M, Vaazio AG. Intravenous gamma globulin therapy for prophylaxis of infection in high-risk neonates. *J Pediatr.* 1987;110:437-442.

10. Christensen RD, Hardman T, Thornton J, Hill HR. A randomized, double-blind, placebo-controlled investigation of the safety of intravenous immune globulin administration to preterm neonates. *J Perinatol.* 1989;9:126-130.

11. Conray SP, Gillies DRN, Docherty A. Neonatal infection in premature infants and use of human immunoglobulin. *Arch Dis Child.* 1987;62:1252-1256.

12. Baker CJ, The Neonatal IVIG Collaborative Study Group. Multicenter trial of intravenous immunoglobulin (IVIG) to prevent late-onset infection in preterm infants: preliminary results. Presented before the Society for Pediatric Research; May 4, 1989; Washington, DC. Abstract.

13. Weisman LE, Stoll B, Kueser T, et al. Intravenous immunoglobulin (IVIG) prophylaxis of late-onset septicemia in neonates. Presented before the Society for Pediatric Research; May 8, 1990; Anaheim, Calif. Abstract.

14. Clapp DW, Kliegman RM, Baley JE, et al. Use of intravenously administered immune globulin to prevent nosocomial sepsis in low birth weight infants: report of a pilot study. *J Pediatr.* 1989;115:973-978.

15. Yamaska K, Nakagawa T, Uno T. Statistical moments in pharmacokinetics. *J Pharmacokinet.* 1978;6:547-558.

16. Battaglia F, Lubchenco LO. A practical classification of newborn infants by weight and gestational age. *J Pediatr.* 1967;71:159-163.

17. Fleer A, Senders RC, Visser MR, et al. Septicemia due to coagulase-negative staphylococci in a neonatal intensive care unit: clinical and bacteriological features and contaminated parenteral fluids as a source of sepsis. *Pediatr Infect Dis J.* 1983;2:426-431.

18. Noel GJ, Edelson PJ. Staphylococcus epidermidis bacteremia in neonates: further observations and the occurrence of focal infection. *Pediatrics.* 1984;74:832-837.

19. Bell MJ, Ternberg JL, Feigin RD, et al. Neonatal necrotizing enterocolitis: therapeutic decisions based upon clinical staging. *Ann Surg.* 1978;187:1-7.

20. Noya FJD, Rench MA, Courtney JT, Feldman S, Baker CJ. Pharmacokinetics of intravenous immunoglobulin in very low birthweight infants. *Pediatr Infect Dis J.* 1989;8:759-763.

21. Waites KB, Crouse DT, Philips JB, Canupp KC, Cassell GH. Ureaplasmal pneumonia and sepsis associated with persistent pulmonary hypertension of the newborn. *Pediatrics.* 1989;83:79-85.

22. Kyllonen KS, Clapp DW, Kliegman RM, et al. Dosage of intravenously administered immune globulin and dosing interval required to maintain target levels of immunoglobulin G in low birth weight infants. *J Pediatr.* 1989;11:1013-1021.

Vertical Transmission of Human Immunodeficiency Virus From Seronegative or Indeterminate Mothers

John P. Johnson, MD; Peter E. Vink, MD; Susan E. Hines, MS, C PNP; Barbara Robinson, RNC; John C. Davis, Jr, MD; Prasanna Nair, MD

• *Objective.*—To describe the identification of human immunodeficiency virus (HIV)–infected infants born to women who were seronegative or indeterminate during pregnancy.

***Research Design.*—Longitudinal cohort study.**

***Setting.*—Inner-city medical center.**

***Participants.*—A series of children born to women with histories of risk factors for HIV infection were followed up for studies of the natural history of HIV-infected infants. These children were identified through risk factor assessment of pregnant women presenting for obstetric care.**

***Interventions.*—Counseling and testing to detect HIV.**

***Results.*—Three women were retrospectively identified who were infected with HIV during pregnancy but whose test results showed them to be either seronegative or indeterminate. Two of these women transmitted HIV infection to their children. Subsequently, all three women were confirmed to be infected.**

***Conclusions.*—Standard serologic testing to detect HIV infection will not identify all infected pregnant women. Perinatal transmission of HIV can occur in women with negative results of enzyme-linked immunosorbent assay or indeterminate results of Western blot analysis during pregnancy.**

(*AJDC.* 1991;145:1239-1241)

In 1983, the first cases of acquired immunodeficiency syndrome in infants were presented.[1,2] Since then, the total number of cases of acquired immunodeficiency syndrome in the pediatric population has grown rapidly to more than 1300.[3] For each case of acquired immunodeficiency syndrome among children, many more children are infected with human immunodeficiency virus (HIV) but have mild or no apparent disease.[4-6] Because most cases of HIV infection in children have resulted from vertical transmission,[7] the Centers for Disease Control and the American College of Obstetrics have recommended the establishment of screening programs for women of childbearing age with risk factors for HIV infection.[8] These programs permit the counseling of women regarding HIV infection and pregnancy and the prospective identification of infants with perinatal exposure to HIV.[9]

Recent evidence suggests that not all infected women will be identified with HIV testing because the sensitivity of enzyme-linked immunosorbent assay (ELISA) testing in some at-risk individuals may be low. These individuals do not demonstrate seroconversion within the usual time, which has been ascribed to a long latency period after infection.[10] The transmission of HIV from seronegative or indeterminate persons by methods other than blood transfusion has not been previously demonstrated.[11] We discuss vertical transmission of HIV to infants born to women with risk factors for HIV infection who had negative or indeterminate responses to serologic tests to detect HIV.

PATIENT REPORTS

PATIENT 1.—A 36-year-old woman presented to the University of Maryland Obstetrical Clinic for prenatal care at 6 months' gestation. At that time, she was enrolled in a methadone maintenance program and admitted to a 10-year history of intravenous heroine and cocaine use. She complained of persistent nonproductive cough, night sweats, odynophagia, myalgias, and arthralgias. Results of physical examination revealed a thin woman with an enlarged, tender liver, a fundal height of 24 cm, white oral plaques, and esophageal erythema consistent with oral and possibly esophageal candidiasis. After written, informed consent was acquired, serum was obtained for HIV testing. Anti-HIV antibody determination by ELISA (DuPont, Wilmington, Del) revealed an OD_{405} value of 0.206, with the positive cutoff value being greater than 0.400.

She presented 6 weeks later in active labor with spontaneous rupture of membranes a few hours earlier. Her gestation was assessed to be 36⁴⁄₇ weeks by dates and 26⁶⁄₇ weeks by fundal height. Labor was uncomplicated and a female infant was vaginally delivered 3 hours later. Results of antibody ELISA were again negative, with a quantitative value of 0.107 and a positive cutoff value of 0.451.

Results of assessments during the infant's first year revealed episodes of oral and cutaneous candidiasis, atopic dermatitis, otitis media, delayed development, viral pneumonitis, *Staphylococcus epidermidis* septicemia, and hand-foot-and-mouth disease. At age 6 months, a coculture of the child's peripheral blood lymphocytes with donor lymphocytes revealed HIV antigen within 1 week. Attempts to locate the biologic mother of this child after delivery for confirmation of her virologic status were unsuccessful.

Accepted for publication June 9, 1991.

From the Department of Pediatrics, University of Maryland School of Medicine, Baltimore.

Reprint requests to the Division of Pediatric Immunology, School of Medicine, University of Maryland at Baltimore, 655 W Baltimore St, BRB, 10-027, Baltimore, MD 21201 (Dr Johnson).

Patient 2.—This patient presented to the University of Maryland Obstetric Clinic at 27 weeks' gestation. She admitted to sexual intercourse with a drug user and a history of multiple sexually transmitted diseases (gonorrhea and syphilis). Results of her physical examination were unremarkable except for a fundal height of 27 cm consistent with normal intrauterine pregnancy. Results of HIV ELISA were positive, while results of Western blot analysis were indeterminate. A second specimen was sent for analysis 2 weeks later and produced the same results. A third specimen, sent to the Red Cross 1 week after the second specimen, showed the patient to be positive by ELISA, while results of Western blot analysis showed her to be negative for HIV.

She presented 3 months later at term, with spontaneous onset of labor, and delivered a healthy male infant weighing 2940 g. Because of the difficulty in determining her serologic status (as recalled by the obstetric staff at that time), HIV testing was repeated. Results of both ELISA and Western blot analysis at this time showed her to be HIV positive; p24 antigen could not be detected in this specimen (HIV-1 p24 Core Profile ELISA DuPont, Boston, Mass). At age 15 months, the child was in good health and had no evidence of HIV infection.

Patient 3.—A 26-year-old woman presented to the obstetric clinic with intrauterine pregnancy of approximately 12 weeks' gestation. The patient admitted to intravenous drug use and sexual intercourse with intravenous drug users. Results of physical examination were unremarkable except for fundal height of 11 cm consistent with a 12-week intrauterine pregnancy. Results of HIV ELISA were positive, while results of Western blot analysis were indeterminate. An indeterminate result of the Western blot analysis was confirmed by the Maryland State Health Department. Four months later, ELISA was again performed and the results were positive. Results of another Western blot analysis showed the patient to be negative for HIV.

A vaginal delivery at 40 weeks' gestation produced a 2580-g, well-appearing female. At age 4 months, the child was noted to have hepatomegaly, splenomegaly, and an eczematoid skin rash. At ages 4 and 6 months, she was documented to have p24 serum antigenemia, with levels of 214 and 250 pg/mL, respectively.

In view of the findings in the child at age 6 months, the mother was reevaluated and confirmed at that time to be HIV seropositive by results of both ELISA and Western blot analysis. A serum specimen that had been collected and frozen at delivery was assayed and found to have 5.14 pg of p24 serum antigenemia per milliliter.

COMMENT

This report documents the retrospective identification of HIV infection in three pregnant women. Results of tests to detect HIV were indeterminate in two of the women, while the other woman was seronegative. Of even greater concern is that two of these women transmitted HIV to their children. Several explanations might account for the lack of confirmed seropositivity in these infected pregnant women: (1) the "window" period that follows infection with HIV and precedes seroconversion; (2) seroreversion, ie, the loss of HIV antibodies (this is usually seen in late symptomatic HIV infection, but has been described in asymptomatic individuals)[12]; (3) false-negative results of an antibody test; and (4) human error.

The window period of HIV infection is the time between exposure resulting in infection and the presence of detectable anti-HIV antibody. In approximately 95% of infected individuals, anti-HIV antibody is detectable within 6 months.[13] Patients 2 and 3 experienced complete seroconversion within 3 and 7 months of initial identification, respectively. Prolonged window periods lasting longer than 6 months were first reported in 1987.[10] Imagawa and colleagues[14] have prospectively described 31 (23%) of 133 men involved in high-risk activity who remained seronegative for up to 36 months after positive results of a culture to detect HIV. Wolinsky and colleagues[15] have prospectively shown a median of 18 months from positive results of polymerase chain reaction assay to Western blot analysis confirming the presence of HIV in 24 individuals and up to 42 months in two individuals. Latency has been suggested to explain why some individuals have such low titer antibody responses as to be undetectable. This phenomenon has been documented only in homosexual men, but it is reasonable to assume a similar phenomenon may occur in heterosexuals with risk factors for HIV related to intravenous drug use. Whether latency is more likely in pregnancy remains to be evaluated.

Patient 1 had physical findings suggestive of advanced disease, ie, oral and possibly esophageal candidiasis. The poor outcome of her pregnancy further suggests her ill health. Advanced disease has been associated with the loss of specific anti-HIV seroreactivity, ie, seroreversion. The loss of maternal anti-HIV antibody may permit the transmission of the virus, as has been demonstrated in other intrauterine infections with such viruses as varicella-zoster and rubella. The importance of anti-HIV antibody response has recently been demonstrated by the correlation of vertical transmission with an absence of maternal antibody against gp120.[16,17] Thus, seroreversion may increase the risk of vertical transmission.

Finally, human error and the test validity of Western blot analyses (which are often difficult to interpret) may be other mediating factors in the identification of HIV infection. Results of a survey of laboratories participating with the College of American Pathologists in performing Western blot analysis revealed only an 89.2% rate of correct identification of positive specimens. In another study by the Department of Defense comparing the performance of Western blot analysis in 19 laboratories, 10 laboratories failed the required proficiency panel at least once. Thus, there is still a lack of standardization in performing Western blot analyses and evaluating their results.[18,19]

The frequency of vertical HIV transmission from at-risk women shown to be HIV seronegative or indeterminate to their infants is uncertain. Long-term follow-up of both maternal and pediatric populations will be necessary to determine this. The identification of three such cases during 2 years from one program raises concern about ascertainment of HIV infection in pregnant, at-risk women. These cases suggest that, in women with histories or physical findings suggestive of HIV infection, a negative or indeterminate test result should be followed by a repeated test and/or other assays to detect infection (eg, peripheral blood coculture, polymerase chain reaction assay, or p24 antigen capture assay). It is remarkable that approximately half of the latently infected seronegative persons in the study by Ranki et al[10] were positive for p24 antigen.

It is certain that vertical transmission of HIV from at-risk women with seronegative or indeterminate results of anti-HIV antibody tests will occur, that obstetricians and pediatricians must be aware of maternal risk factors in addition to maternal serologic status, that women with risk factors should be tested several times during pregnancy (and with several assays), and that children born to seronegative, at-risk women should also be regarded as at risk for HIV infection.

This study was funded in part by grant DA04312 from the National Institute of Drug Abuse, Rockville, MD; grant NS26665 from the National Institute of Neurologic Disease and Communicative Disorders, Bethesda, MD; grant 90CA1318 from the US Department of Health and Human Services, Bethesda, MD; and the Bressler Research Committee and Medical Biotechnology Center of the University of Maryland at Baltimore.

References

1. Oleske J, Minnefor A, Cooper R Jr, et al. Immune deficiency syndrome in children. *JAMA.* 1983;249:2345-2349.

2. Rubinstein A, Sicklick M, Gupta A, et al. Acquired immunodeficiency with reversed T4/T8 ratios in infants born to promiscuous and drug addicted mothers. *JAMA.* 1983;249:2350-2359.

3. Centers for Disease Control. Update: acquired immunodeficiency syndrome. *MMWR.* 1989;38:229-252.

4. Scott GB, Fischel MA, Klimas N, et al. Immunodeficiency syndrome in children: evidence for both symptomatic and asymptomatic carriers. *JAMA.* 1985;253:363-366.

5. Pawha S, Kaplan M, Fikrig S, et al. Spectrum of human T cell lymphotropic virus type III infection in children. *JAMA.* 1986;225:2299-2305.

6. Rogers MF. AIDS in children: a review of the clinical, epidemiologic and public health aspects. *Pediatr Infect Dis J.* 1985;4:220-236.

7. Quinn TC. *The Global Epidemiology of AIDS: Report of the Surgeon General's Workshop in Children With HIV Infection and Their Families.* Washington, DC: Department of Health and Human Services; 1987:7-10.

8. Centers for Disease Control. Recommendations for assisting in the preventing of perinatal transmission of human T-lymphotropic virus type III/lymphadenopathy-associated virus and acquired immunodeficiency syndrome. *MMWR.* 1985:34:721-732.

9. Landesman SH, Minkoff H, Holman S, et al. Serosurvey of human immunodeficiency virus infection in participants: implications for HIV testing in programs of pregnant women. *JAMA.* 1987;258:2701-2703.

10. Ranki A, Valle S-L, Krohn M, et al. Long latency precedes overt seroconversion in sexually transmitted human immunodeficiency virus infection. *Lancet.* 1987;2:589-593.

11. Kleinman S, Seard K. Risks of human immunodeficiency virus (HIV) transmission by anti-HIV negative blood. *Transfusion.* 1988;28:499-501.

12. Farzadegan H, Polis MA, Wolinsky SM, et al. Loss of human immunodeficiency virus type 1 (HIV-1) antibodies with evidence of viral infection in asymptomatic homosexual men: a report from the multicenter AIDS cohort study. *Ann Intern Med.* 1988;108:785-790.

13. Horsburgh CR, Ou CY, Jason J, et al. Duration of human immunodeficiency virus infection before detection of antibody. *Lancet.* 1989;2:637-640.

14. Imagawa DT, Lee MH, Wolinsky SM, et al. Human immunodeficiency virus type 1 infection in homosexual men who remain seronegative for prolonged periods. *N Engl J Med.* 1989;320:1458-1462.

15. Wolinsky SM, Rinaldo CR, Kwok S, et al. Human immunodeficiency virus type 1 (HIV-1) infection a median of 18 months before a diagnostic Western blot. *Ann Intern Med.* 1989;111:961-972.

16. Devash Y, Calvelli T, Wood D, Reagan K, Rubenstein A. Vertical transmission of human immunodeficiency virus is correlated with the absence of high affinity/avidity maternal antibodies to gp120 principle neutralizing domain. *Proc Natl Acad Sci U S A.* 1990;87:3445-3449.

17. Rossi P, Moschese V, Broliden PA, et al. Presence of maternal antibodies to human immunodeficiency virus 1 envelope glycoprotein gp120 epitopes correlates with the infected status of children born to seropositive mothers. *Proc Natl Acad Sci U S A.* 1989;86:8055-8058.

18. Centers for Disease Control. Update: serologic testing for antibody to human immunodeficiency virus. *MMWR.* 1987;36:501-515.

19. Mortimer PP. The fallibility of HIV Western blot. *Lancet.* 1991;337:286-287.

CORRECTION

Incorrect Notations and Incomplete Footnote.— In the article titled "Evaluation of Intraosseous vs Intravenous Antibiotic Levels in a Porcine Model," published in the August issue of *AJDC* (1991;145:946-949), errors were made in the table and its footnote. On page 947, throughout the table, under the "Drug" column, the following notations should have been published C_{max} and T_{max}. The footnote for the Table was incomplete. It should have read as follows: "*Values are mean±SD. AUC indicates area under the plasma concentration time curve; C_{max}, maximum concentration; T_{max}, the time to peak plasma concentration; and NS, not significant."

Child Survival and Perinatal Infections With Human Immunodeficiency Virus

John V. Bennett, MD, Martha F. Rogers, MD

• A mathematical model was developed to assess the effect of various assumed prevalence rates of maternal human immunodeficiency virus (HIV) infection on perinatally acquired HIV infections and child survival. The model indicates that for children younger than 5 years, countries with low baseline mortality rates will experience greater relative increases in child mortality rates and larger proportions of HIV-caused deaths in children than countries with high mortality rates. It also suggests that perinatal HIV infection could become the most common cause of deaths in children in the developed world if maternal infection rates reach 2% to 3%. Rates of 25% to 30% would be needed to produce a similar effect in the developing world. Child survival gains in the last three decades in the developed world could be quickly erased at low levels of maternal HIV infection, but gains would not be completely offset in the developing world until more than 40% of mothers became infected with HIV. When basic demographic information and the maternal HIV infection rate are known, the model permits a direct assessment of infant and child mortality caused by HIV. It can also be used to estimate the prevalence of maternal HIV infection when values for all other variables are known.

(*AJDC*. 1991;145:1242-1247)

Over the past decade, human immunodeficiency virus (HIV) infection has spread throughout the world; over 150 countries have now reported cases to the World Health Organization. In the United States, Europe, and other developed countries, most women have become infected either through the abuse of intravenous drugs or by sexual contact with men who became infected through intravenous drug abuse. Women and children in these countries represent approximately 10% and 2%, respectively, of acquired immunodeficiency syndrome (AIDS) cases (World Health Organization Collaborating Centers). The overall seroprevalence of HIV among women in most developed countries is less than 1%,[1-3] but has exceeded 50% in subpopulations of intravenous drug-abusing women.[4] By contrast, in the developing countries of sub-Saharan Africa and the Caribbean, HIV has spread to women primarily through heterosexual contact, and the male-female ratio among infected persons is approximately 1:1.[5] The seroprevalence among pregnant women in some urban areas of these countries has exceeded 20%.[6]

Children acquire HIV infection primarily through perinatal exposure to their infected mothers. Between 20% and 40% of infants born to infected mothers appear to acquire HIV infection from their mothers[7-9]; one recent study reported a rate of 13%.[10] Many infected infants die in the first year of life as a consequence of this infection, and most are considered likely to succumb before their fifth birthday.[7-11] Early HIV-caused deaths are likely to occur more commonly among infected children in developing countries, where malnutrition and pulmonary and other infections are more likely, preventive measures such as immunoglobulin prophylaxis and zidovudine treatment are not available, and clinical treatment of illnesses is not optimal.

We selected infant and child mortality rates (MRs), as tallied by the United Nations Children's Fund in 1987,[12] for the baseline rates of 131 major countries of the world. We then sought to quantitate the effect of various assumed levels of maternal HIV infection on child survival. To do this, we used a mathematical model based on births, mother-to-infant transmission rates, and MRs for infants (defined as children between birth and age 1 year), 1- to 5-year-olds, and children younger than 5 years. Mortality rates were estimated for infants with and without HIV infection. This approach enabled us to compare the impact on childhood MRs in developing and developed countries with high and low baseline mortality rates, and to examine the potential for offsetting gains in child survival since 1960.

MATERIALS AND METHODS

Methods

Data and assumptions used in the mathematical model are detailed below and summarized in Table 1. To describe a country's MR for its children younger than 5 years, we used the following terms as defined by the United Nations Children's Fund: *very high, high, medium,* or *low.*

Accepted for publication August 14, 1991.

From The Task Force for Child Survival and Development, The Carter Center, Atlanta, Ga (Dr Bennett); Emory University School of Public Health, Atlanta (Dr Bennett); and the Division of Human Immunodeficiency Virus/Acquired Immunodeficiency Syndrome, Center for Infectious Diseases, Centers for Disease Control, Atlanta (Dr Rogers).

Reprint requests to The Task Force for Child Survival and Development, The Carter Center, One Copenhill, Atlanta, GA 30307 (Dr Bennett).

UNICEF Classification of MR for Children Under 5 Years Old (Deaths per 1000 Live Births)	No. of Countries	Median MR		Mother-to-Child Transmission Rate, %	% of HIV-Infected Infants Dying of All Causes by Age	
		Children<5 y Old	Infants		1 y	5 y
Very high (over 170)	33	209	129	40	50	85
High (95-170)	30	123	84	40	40	75
Medium (31-94)	29	60	45	30	25	60
Low (under 30)	39	13	10	30	15	50

Table 1.—Variables Used in Perinatal HIV Infection Model*

*UNICEF indicates United Nations Children's Fund; MR, mortality rate; and HIV, human immunodeficiency virus. All rates apply to 1000 live births. The *Very High* group includes Afghanistan, Mali, Mozambique, Angola, Sierra Leone, Malawi, Ethiopia, Guinea, Burkina Faso, Niger, Chad, Guinea-Bissau, Central African Republic, Somalia, Mauritania, Senegal, Rwanda, Kampuchea, People's Democratic Republic of Yemen, Bhutan, Nepal, Yemen, Burundi, Bangladesh, Benin, Madagascar, Sudan, United Republic of Tanzania, Nigeria, Bolivia, Haiti, Gabon, and Uganda; the *High* group, Pakistan, Zaire, Laos, Togo, Cameroon, India, Liberia, Ghana, Oman, Côte d'Ivoire, Lesotho, Zambia, Egypt, Peru, Libyan Arab Jamahiriya, Morocco, Indonesia, Congo, Kenya, Zimbabwe, Algeria, Honduras, Guatemala, Saudi Arabia, Nicaragua, Burma, South Africa, Turkey, Iraq, and Botswana; the *Medium* group, Islamic Republic of Iran, Vietnam, Ecuador, Brazil, El Salvador, Tunisia, Papua New Guinea, Dominican Republic, Philippines, Mexico, Colombia, Syrian Arab Republic, Paraguay, Mongolia, Jordan, Lebanon, Thailand, Albania, China, Sri Lanka, Venezuela, Guyana, Argentina, Panama, Democratic Republic of Korea, Republic of Korea, Malaysia, United Arab Emirates, and Uruguay; and the *Low* group, USSR, Mauritius, Romania, Yugoslavia, Chile, Trinidad and Tobago, Kuwait, Jamaica, Costa Rica, Bulgaria, Poland, Cuba, Hungary, Portugal, Greece, Czechoslovakia, Belgium, United States, New Zealand, Israel, Austria, Singapore, Italy, United Kingdom, Ireland, Germany, Denmark, Spain, Australia, France, Hong Kong, Canada, the Netherlands, Norway, Switzerland, Japan, Finland, and Sweden.

Information on perinatal HIV infections from the developing world is limited. A prospective study from 1987 to 1989 on mothers and newborns in Haiti, a country with a very high MR for children younger than 5 years in 1987,[12] showed HIV seropositivity in 443 (9.7%) of 4588 pregnant women.[13] At age 1 year, 23.4% of infants born to seropositive mothers had died, as had 10.8% of infants born to seronegative mothers. The vertical transmission rate of HIV was estimated at approximately 25%. These data indicate that about 61.2% of HIV-infected infants died in infancy since the observed overall mortality rate of 234 per 1000 live births in the cohort of children born to infected mothers = [the proportion of children infected with HIV (25%) × their MR (unknown)] + [the proportion of children not infected with HIV (75%) × their MR (108 per 1000 live births)].

In Zaire, a country with a high MR for the group younger than 5 years,[12] 468 infants born to seropositive mothers in 1986-1987 were followed up for 1 year[9]; 100 (21.4%) of the infants died. The study revealed a mother-to-child transmission rate of 39% and suggested that mothers in more advanced stages of HIV disease might be more likely to transmit the infection to their infants. If the infant MR (100)[14] for Zaire in 1986 is assumed to apply to the proportion of newborns not infected with HIV, then approximately 40% of the HIV-infected children can be inferred to have died in infancy.

No comparable studies have been reported from countries classified by the United Nations Children's Fund as having medium MR for children under 5 years old in 1987.

Several studies have been reported from highly developed European countries with a low MR for this age group (Table 2).[7,8,15] In addition to the mother-to-child transmission rates shown in Table 2, two other studies in the United States have also shown rates of about 30%.[16,17]

Based on the foregoing, a mother-to-child transmission frequency of 40% was assumed to apply to countries with very high or high MRs for children younger than 5 years. This vertical transmission rate is higher than that reported for Haiti,[13] and approximately equal to that reported for Zaire.[9] However, a bias reported in the Haitian study may have resulted in an artificially low estimate of vertical transmission.[13] We estimated that 50% of HIV-infected infants might die in infancy in countries with very high MRs for those younger than 5 years, and 40% might die in countries with high rates. Infant death rates are generally higher in countries with very high MRs for those younger than 5 years than in countries with high rates (Table 1), and deaths from HIV

Table 2.—Mother-to-Child Infection Studies in Highly Developed Countries*

Source, y	No. of HIV-Infected Children	No. (%) Dead in Infancy	Estimated Mother-to-Child HIV Transmission Rate, %
Blanche et al,[7] 1989	32	5 (15.6)	30
European Collaborative Study,[15] 1991	64	11 (17)	13
Italian Multicentre Study,[8] 1988	486	≥14 (≥8.5)	33

*HIV indicates human immunodeficiency virus.

infection in infancy might be expected to parallel baseline infant MRs.

Based on information for children younger than 5 years in countries with low MRs, a 30% mother-to-infant transmission rate was assumed for countries with medium and low MRs. For the 29 countries in the medium group, 25% of HIV-infected infants were assumed to die in infancy; for the 39 countries in the low group, 15% of HIV-infected infants were assumed to die in the first year of life.

Mortality in HIV-infected children who survive infancy has not been determined. However, because of the high frequency of symptomatic infections, mortality is likely to be substantial. The MR among HIV-infected children younger than 5 years is expected to increase as the overall MR for all children younger than 5 years in a country increases. We thus assumed that a total of 85%, 75%, 60%, and 50% of HIV-infected newborns would die before reaching age 5 years in the very high, high, medium, and low MR groups of children younger than 5 years, respectively. Among HIV-infected children who survive 1 year, these assumptions correspond with MRs of approximately 70%, 60%, 50%, and 40% in the very high, high, medium, and low MR categories, respectively, for children younger than 5 years.

The Mathematical Model

Maternal infection rates from 0% to 50% were applied to total births in 1987 for individual countries or groups of countries to obtain the number of births to mothers with and without HIV infection. We calculated the number of HIV-infected infants born

Table 3.—Application of the Mathematical Model for Countries With Very High Mortality (MR) Rates for Children Under 5 Years old (VHU5MR) at One Assumed Prevalence of Maternal Human Immunodeficieny Virus (HIV) Infection (1%)

Variable No.	Variable	No.	Calculation*
1	Births in 1987	24 695 000	. . .
2	Proportion of mothers infected with HIV	0.01	. . .
3	Births among HIV-infected mothers	246 950	No. 1 x No. 2
4	Newborns infected	98 780	No. 3 x 0.4 (the assumed vertical transmission rate in VHU5MR countries)
5	Births among uninfected women	24 448 050	No. 1 x (1.0 − No. 2)
6	Uninfected newborns	24 596 220	No. 5 + (No. 3 − No. 4)
	Deaths Among Uninfected Newborns		
7	Infant MR (129) in 1987	3 172 912	No. 6 x 129/1000 (the median infant mortality rate for VHU5MR in 1987)
8	1-5 year MR (80) in 1987	1 967 698	No. 6 x 80/1000 (the median 1- to 5-y MR for VHU5MR countries in 1987)
9	Total deaths before age 5 years for uninfected newborns	5 140 610	No. 7 + No. 8
10	Baseline death incidence from 1 to 5 y	0.092	No. 8 (baseline 1- to 5-y deaths in uninfected infants) ÷ [(No. 5 (uninfected infants) − No. 7 (baseline infant deaths in uninfected infants)]
	Deaths Among HIV-Infected Newborns		
11	Total 1st y among HIV infected	49 390	No. 4 (infected newborns) x 0.5 (the assumed total mortality for VHU5MR countries in first year of life)
12	1st y other causes	12 743	No. 4 (infected newborns) x 129/1000 live births (the 1987 median infant mortality for VHU5MR countries)
13	1st y HIV-caused	36 647	No. 11 (total infant deaths) − No. 12 (deaths from other causes in infants)
14	Total 1-5 y among HIV infected	34 573	No. 4 (infected newborns) x 0.35 (the assumed total mortality for VHU5MR countries from 1 to 5 y)
15	1-5 y causes other than HIV	4 536	[No. 4 (infected newborns) − No. 11 (infant deaths)] x No. 10 (baseline median 1 to 5 y mortality rate for VHU5MR countries)
16	1-5 y HIV-caused	30 037	No. 14 (total 1-5 year deaths) – No. 15 (deaths among 1- to 5-year-olds from other causes)
17	Total HIV-caused deaths before age 5 y in infected newborns	66 684	No. 13 (1st year HIV-caused) + No. 16 (1 to 5 y HIV-caused)
18	Total deaths from causes other than HIV before age 5 y in infected newborns	17 279	No. 12 (1st year other causes) + No. 15 (1 to 5 y other causes)
19	Total deaths before age 5 y in infected newborns	83 963	No. 17 + No. 18
20	Overall MR for children under 5 y	211.6	[(No. 9 + No. 19) ÷ No. 1] x 1000
	% of Children Dying Within 5 y		
21	HIV caused	0.3	(No. 17/No. 1) x 100
22	Non–HIV caused	20.9	[(No. 18 + No. 9) ÷ No. 1] x 100
23	% of deaths before age <5 y HIV caused	1.3	[No. 17 ÷ (No. 19 + No. 9)] x 100
24	Overall 1-5 y MR	81.1	[(No. 14 + No. 8) ÷ No. 1] x 1000

*Countries with very high MRs for children under 5 years were defined as those with 170 deaths per 1000 live births and higher. (Data for 1987 from UNICEF's *The State of the World's Children 1989.*[12]) The numbers refer to numbered lines on the left of the chart, which identify the value of the variable used in the equation.

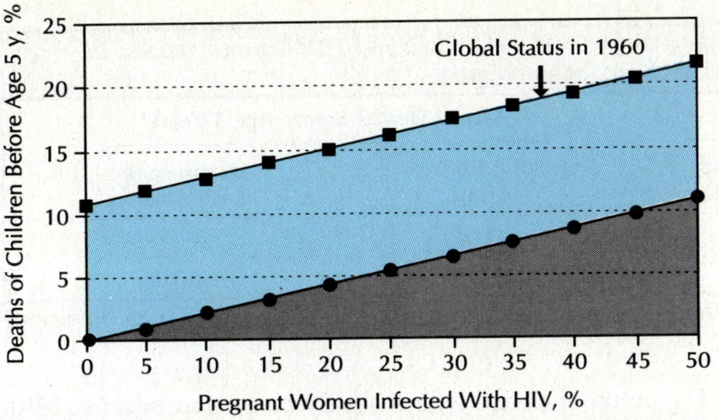

Fig 1.—*Global effect of various levels of maternal human immunodeficiency virus (HIV) infection on percentage of newborns dying within 5 years. Line with squares represents the total from all causes; line with plus signs, HIV-related causes.*

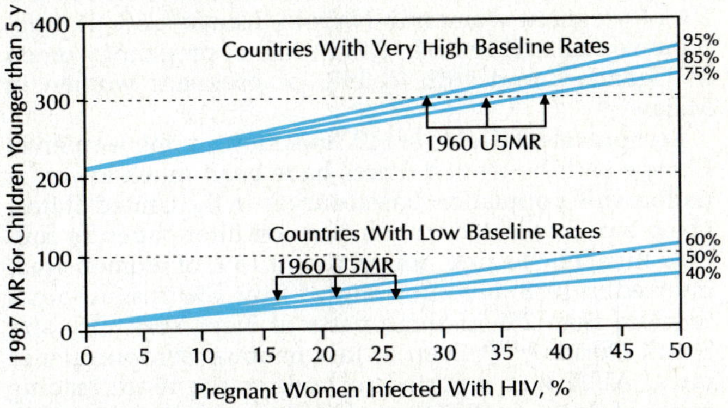

Fig 2.—*Mortality rates (MRs) for children younger than 5 years (U5MR) for 1987. Comparative impact of various levels of maternal human immunodeficiency virus (HIV) infection in countries with low vs very high baseline childhood MRs. (Overall mortality by age 5 years for HIV-infected children is also shown for +10% of the values assumed in Table 1.)*

to infected mothers in accordance with mother-to-child transmission rates for the MR group to which the country belonged in 1987 (Table 1). An example of the data and formulas used in a single application with an assumed maternal HIV infection prevalence of 1% is given in Table 3.

This example illustrates how the assumptions in Table 1, combined with baseline births, frequency of maternal HIV infection, infant MR, and MR for 1- to 5-year-olds in countries with very high rates of death among children younger than 5 years, can be used to establish changes in the overall MR for children younger than 5 years, the percentage of children dying within 5 years, the percentage of HIV-caused deaths in children younger than 5 years, and MRs for 1- to 5-year-olds.

RESULTS

On a global basis, HIV infection would account for about one third of all childhood deaths at a maternal HIV infection prevalence of 25% and would become the cause of most childhood deaths at a maternal prevalence of 45% (Fig 1). A global prevalence of 35% to 40% would be needed to offset the enormous global reductions in childhood mortality achieved from 1960 to 1987.

The impact of mortality from perinatal HIV infections will be far more evident among countries with low MRs for children younger than 5 years (Fig 2). For such countries, the MR for children younger than 5 years will double at a maternal HIV infection prevalence of about 9%, and will revert to average 1960 levels at maternal HIV in-

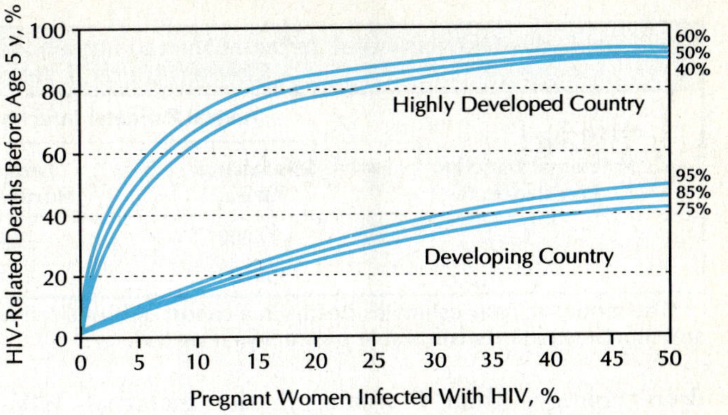

Fig 3.—*Percentage of human immunodeficiency virus (HIV)–caused deaths in children younger than 5 years. Impact of various levels of maternal HIV infection in two countries with widely differing baseline childhood mortalities. (Overall mortality by 5 years for HIV-infected children is also shown for ±10% of the values assumed for countries in their mortality rate grouping in Table 1.)*

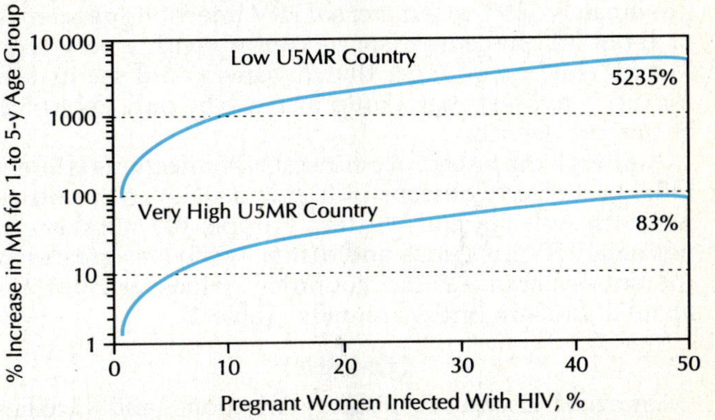

Fig 4.—*Comparison of percentage increase in mortality rates (MRs) for the 1- to 5-year age group between two countries with widely differing baseline childhood MRs. U5MR indicates MR for children under age 5 years; HIV, human immunodeficiency virus.*

fection levels of about 23%. In comparison, the MR for children younger than 5 years in countries with very high MRs for children younger than 5 years will not double until maternal infection prevalence exceeds 50%; about 35% of all pregnant women in these countries need to be infected with HIV to offset the enormous gains in child survival that have occurred since 1960. Countries in the high and medium MR groups for children younger than 5 years lie between these extremes.

Thus, if one compares the proportion of HIV-caused deaths of children in a highly developed European country (Sweden) with a developing sub-Saharan African country (Uganda), the impact of HIV will be relatively much greater in Sweden (Fig 3). The HIV infection would account for about one third of all deaths of children at a maternal HIV infection level of 2.4% in Sweden, and for more than half of all deaths of children at a prevalence of 4.8%. In contrast, HIV infection would account for one third of childhood deaths in Uganda at a maternal HIV infection level of 30%, and would not account for most childhood deaths until more than half of all pregnant women became infected with the virus.

Mortality rates for infants have exceeded those for 1- to 5-year-olds in all countries of the world since at least 1960. A reversal in this relationship, with the MR for the 1- to 5-year age group exceeding the MR for infants, is predicted for countries with low MRs for chil-

Table 4.—Distribution of Perinatal Human Immunodeficiency Virus (HIV) Infections and HIV-Caused Deaths in Children Under 5 Years Old by Geographic Region

	Annual Perinatal Infections		Annual Deaths Before Age 5 Years*	
Maternal Infection Prevalence, %	Sub-Saharan Africa	Europe and North America	Sub-Saharan Africa	Europe and North America
1	77 000	24 000	51 000	12 000
5	384 000	120 000	254 000	58 000

*The model actually estimates deaths in a cohort of births followed until age 5 years. Annual deaths will be identical if birth, infection, and mortality data remain stable over a 5-year period.

dren younger than 5 years, if the maternal HIV-infection prevalence reaches 10% to 15%.

The greatest predicted increase in death rates will be for the 1- to 5-year-olds in highly developed countries (Fig 4). In a country with a baseline MR for the 1- to 5-year age group of 3 per 1000 (a low MR for children younger than 5 years), the MR for 1- to 5-year-olds will increase by approximately 100% at a maternal HIV infection prevalence of about 3%. In comparison, a country with a very high MR for children younger than 5 years would see its MR for the 1- to 5-year age group increase by only about 5% at this prevalence.

Although the impact of perinatal HIV infections is likely to be particularly obvious in highly developed countries in North America and Western Europe, the numbers of perinatal HIV infections and deaths will be far greater in the sub-Saharan African countries, which account for about 20 million births annually (Table 4).

COMMENT

Diarrheal disease, respiratory infections, and vaccine-preventable deaths were the main causes of childhood mortality in 1987, with each responsible for about 30% of all childhood deaths worldwide.[12] While HIV infection is unlikely to surpass these diseases as the most common cause of death in children worldwide (ie, responsible for more than 30% of all childhood deaths), it is becoming an increasingly important cause of death in women and children in both developing and developed countries. Indeed, HIV infection has doubtlessly already emerged as the principal cause of death in some populations.

Chin et al[11] evaluated the effect of AIDS on MRs of children younger than 5 years at three different assumed levels of HIV infection of pregnant women in a single assumed population with a baseline MR of children younger than 5 years of 100 deaths per 1000 live births, a mother-to-infant HIV transmission rate of 25%, and an overall mortality rate of 80% in the first 5 years for HIV-infected newborns. The effect on outcome of altering the baseline MR for children younger than 5 years was not evaluated. At maternal HIV infection prevalence levels of 5%, 10%, and 20%, the death rates for children under 5 years old were predicted to increase by 9%, 18%, and 36%, respectively. We predicted comparable increases in the MRs for children younger than 5 years on a global basis (11%, 20% and 40%, respectively) for these maternal HIV infection prevalences.

Our model indicates that, in many areas, HIV infection has had a substantial effect on childhood rates of death. A population-based serosurvey in Rwanda found that 21% of urban women were infected with the HIV.[6] At this level, given Rwanda's overall baseline birth and mortality data for 1987, the child MR will have increased by 26%. The actual increase will probably be greater because MRs for children younger than 5 years tend to be lower in urban areas, and many additional deaths may result when these mothers' deaths produce large numbers of orphans.[18] Relatively high rates of maternal HIV infection have been reported from other African countries as well: 2% of pregnant women in Nairobi, Kenya[19]; 6% of pregnant women in Kinshasa, Zaire[9]; 14% of pregnant women in Uganda[20]; and 16% to 19% of pregnant women in Malawi.[21]

Seroprevalence rates of HIV infection among women in Europe and the United States have been much lower. A nationwide population-based survey in the United States, using blood collected from infants on filter paper for routine metabolic testing, found that 0.15% of women were infected in 1988, but rates ranged from 0% in some areas to more than 2% in some parts of New York City and South Florida.[1,22,23] Even at low national seroprevalence rates, AIDS was reported to rank as the ninth leading cause of death in 1987 for 1- to 5-year-old American children and to account for approximately 1.5% of all deaths in this age group.[24] Our model predicts that about 5% of all deaths in the United States in this age group will be caused by HIV infection at a maternal prevalence of 0.15%. The observed proportion of deaths due to the HIV infection may be lower than our predicted value because many HIV-attributable deaths may go unrecognized or be attributed to other causes.

Although we have applied the model only to countries, it can also be applied to subpopulations within countries when the childhood mortality and other variables of the population needed in the model can be estimated. In the United States, for instance, HIV infection disproportionately affects blacks and Hispanics,[25] groups already at higher risk of infant mortality.[26]

The greatest morbidity and mortality burden from perinatal HIV is expected in sub-Saharan Africa. Cases and number of deaths are larger, even at comparable rates of maternal HIV infection, because the number of births is greater and the mother-to-infant transmission frequency and MRs among children under 5 years old are higher. In addition, seroprevalence among pregnant women is also substantially higher in sub-Saharan Africa than in Europe and North America. Indeed, Preble[18] has estimated that HIV infection will cause as many as one half million deaths annually by the year 2000 in 10 Central and East African countries, should maternal HIV infection prevalence reach 30%. With the use of 1987 demographic data for these same countries and values in Table 1 appropriate for the MR for children younger than 5 years in each country, our model predicts about 650 000 HIV-caused deaths of children when the maternal HIV infection prevalence reaches this level. Even more deaths than this would be expected if increased numbers of births in the year 2000 were used in the model. Our estimated MRs for children younger than 5 years is higher than the maximum estimate of Preble[18] (235 and 189 per 1000 live births, respectively) for a maternal infection prevalence of 30% in these countries. These differences appear to derive largely from Preble's assuming a continuing decline in the MR for children younger than 5 years as projected before the advent of the AIDS epidemic. However, rates of non–HIV-related deaths of children may themselves increase consequent to the HIV epidemic, since the majority of children orphaned by HIV-caused deaths of their mothers will be uninfected but likely to experience sharply increased risks of death of uncertain magnitude. Also, access to and quality of care may decline for children not infected with the HIV in areas of high incidence of HIV infection as these areas become overburdened by HIV-caused illnesses. These factors may serve to offset any overall trend of improved child survival in children both with and without HIV infection.

With the use of 1987 data for Haiti and values appropriate for a country with a very high MR for children younger than 5 years, our model predicts an increase in the country's infant MR from 111 to 126, an 11.9% increase, at the observed maternal HIV infection prevalence of 9.7%. This is very close to the actual reported increase of 11.7% in the overall infant MR in this country.[13]

We believe our model can usefully evaluate the likely effect of HIV infection on infant and child survival in any population for which demographic information and a maternal HIV infection prevalence representative of that population are available. The model may also be helpful in estimating the value of single variables, including seroprevalence, when the values of all other variables can be specified.

We thank Terrel Hill, PhD, and Gareth Jones, United Nations Children's Fund, New York, NY, for making demographic information for countries of the world available to us. We also thank William H. Foege, MD, and Laurie Gavin, MPH, for their constructive comments on early drafts of the manuscript.

References

1. Gwinn M, Pappaioanou M, George JR, et al. Prevalence of HIV infection in childbearing women in the United States. *JAMA.* 1991;265:1704-1708.

2. Davison CF, Ades AE, Hudson CN, Peckham CS. Antenatal testing for human immunodeficiency virus. *Lancet.* 1989;2:1442-1444.

3. Herlitz C, Brorsson B. HIV testing in 25% of Swedish population aged 16-44. *Lancet.* 1989;2:386-387.

4. Hahn RA, Onorato IM, Jones TS, Dougherty J. Prevalence of HIV infection among intravenous drug users in the United States. *JAMA.* 1989;261:2677-2684.

5. Mann JM, Francis H, Quinn T, et al. Surveillance for AIDS in a central African city. *JAMA.* 1986;255:3255-3259.

6. Rwandan HIV Seroprevalence Study Group. Nationwide community-based serological survey of HIV-1 and other human retrovirus infections in a central African country. *Lancet.* 1989;1:941-943.

7. Blanche S, Rouzioux C, Moscato ML, et al. A prospective study of infants born to women seropositive for human immuno-deficiency virus type 1. *N Engl J Med.* 1989;320:1643-1648.

8. Italian Multicentre Study. Epidemiology, clinical features, and prognostic factors of paediatric HIV infection. *Lancet.* 1988;2:1043-1046.

9. Ryder RW, Nsa W, Hassig SE, et al. Perinatal transmission of the human immunodeficiency virus type 1 to infants of seropositive women in Zaire. *N Engl J Med.* 1989;320:1637-1642.

10. The European Collaborative Study. Mother to child transmission of HIV infection. *Lancet.* 1988;2:1039-1042.

11. Chin J, Sankaran G, Mann JM. Mother-to-infant transmission of HIV: an increasing global problem. In: Kessel E, Awan AK, eds. *Maternal and Child Care in Developing Countries.* Thun, Switzerland: OTT Publishers; 1989:299-305.

12. *The State of the World's Children 1989.* Oxford, England: Oxford University Press; 1990;94-95.

13. Halsey N, Boulos R, Holt E, et al. Transmission of HIV-1 infections from mothers to infants in Haiti. *JAMA.* 1990;264:2089-2092.

14. *The State of the World's Children 1988.* Oxford, England: Oxford University Press; 1989:64-65.

15. The European Collaborative Study. Children born to women with HIV-1 infection: maternal history and risk of transmission. *Lancet.* 1991;1:253-260.

16. Thomas PA, The New York City Perinatal HIV Transmission Collaborative Study Group. Early predictors and rate of perinatal HIV disease. Presented at the Fifth International Conference on AIDS; June 8, 1989; Montreal, Quebec.

17. Willoughby A, Mendez H, Goedert J, Berthaud M, Moroso G, Sunderland A. Presented at the Fifth International Conference on Aids; June 5, 1989; Montreal, Quebec.

18. Preble EA. Impact of HIV/AIDS on African Children. *Soc Sci Med.* 1990;31:671-680.

19. Piot P, Plummer FA, Rey MA, et al. Retrospective seroepidemiology of AIDS virus infection in Nairobi populations. *J Infect Dis.* 1987;155:1108-1112.

20. AIDS: a public health crisis. In: *Population Reports.* Baltimore, Md: The Johns Hopkins University; 1986:193-229.

21. Miotti PG, Dallabetta G, Ndovi E, Limoba G, Saah AJ, Chiphangwi J. HIV-1 and pregnant women: associated factors, prevalence, estimate of incidence and role in fetal wastage in central Africa. *AIDS.* 1990;4:733-736.

22. Hoff R, Berardi VP, Weiblen BJ, Mahoney-Trout L, Mitchell ML, Grady GF. Seroprevalence of human immunodeficiency virus among childbearing women. *N Engl J Med.* 1988;318:525-529.

23. Novick LF, Berns D, Stricof R, Pass K, Wethers J. HIV seroprevalence in newborns in New York state. *JAMA.* 1989;261:1745-1750.

24. Kilbourne BW, Buehler JW, Rogers MF. AIDS as a cause of death in children, adolescents, and young adults. *Am J Public Health.* 1990;80:499-500.

25. Rogers MF, Thomas PA, Starcher ET, Noa MC, Bush TJ, Jaffe HW. Acquired immunodeficiency syndrome in children: report of the Centers for Disease Control national surveillance, 1982 to 1985. *Pediatrics.* 1987;79:1008-1014.

26. National Center for Health Statistics. Advance report of final mortality statistics, 1987. Hyattsville, Md: National Center for Health Statistics, 1989. US Dept of Health and Human Services publication (PHS)89-1120.

Clinical and Endocrinologic Manifestations in Perinatally Human Immunodeficiency Virus Type 1–Infected Children Aged 5 Years or Older

Philippe Lepage, MD; Philippe Van de Perre, MD; Guy Van Vliet, MD, PhD; François Nsengumuremyi, MD; Christiaan Van Goethem, MD; Philippe Kestelyn, MD; Philippe Msellati, MD; Deo-Gratias Hitimana, MD

• Sixteen human immunodeficiency virus type 1 (HIV-1)–seropositive children aged 5 to 12 years (nine girls and seven boys), born to HIV-1–infected mothers, were diagnosed between 1984 and 1987 in Kigali, Rwanda. They were compared with a group of age- and sex-matched HIV-1–seronegative children consecutively selected from the outpatient department. Two subjects were asymptomatic. Chronic cough was the most frequent symptom (seven of 16 patients). The most common signs were short stature (12 of 16 patients), low weight for age (seven of 16 patients), chronic parotitis (eight of 16 patients), persistent generalized lymphadenopathy (seven of 16 patients), and pulmonary tuberculosis (four of 16 patients). Lymphoid interstitial pneumonitis was diagnosed on radiologic grounds in five of 16 patients. Evidence of perivasculitis in the fundus was noted in three of 16 patients. Two children died during the study period (mean duration of follow-up, 40 months; range, 27 to 62 months); none of the other children had life-threatening infection or loss of developmental milestones. Immunologic assessment in the 16 children revealed high levels of IgG, decreased $CD4^+/CD8^+$ ratio, and skin test anergy. Endocrinologic investigations revealed normal thyroid function and normal basal human growth hormone levels but low basal insulinlike growth factor I levels (0.21 ± 0.07 vs 0.44 ± 0.20 U/mL for controls). In Kigali, perinatally HIV-1–infected children surviving beyond 5 years of age often present with moderate signs and symptoms, principally pulmonary involvement, chronic parotitis, and persistent generalized lymphadenopathy. Short stature is the major clinical manifestation in these patients and may be due, in part, to low growth hormone secretion rather than to malnutrition.

(*AJDC*. 1991;145:1248-1251)

Most previous clinical and epidemiologic studies involving human immunodeficiency virus type 1 (HIV-1) in children have focused on infants and young children.[1-6] These patients were characterized by the severity of pediatric HIV-1 infection, including opportunistic infections, severe bacterial infections,[7,8] and neurologic involvement.[9,10] The broad spectrum of HIV-1 infection recognized in adult patients has also recently been described among pediatric patients, including patients with minor complaints or even "healthy carriers."[11-13] Based on mathematical modeling, Auger et al[14] have determined that the median incubation period for perinatally acquired acquired immunodeficiency syndrome (AIDS) was 4.8 years. Twenty percent of the infected newborns developed AIDS in the first year of life, with the remainder developing AIDS at a rate of 8% per year.[14] Thus, not all children infected perinatally with HIV-1 progress rapidly to AIDS. However, data regarding HIV-1 infected children are limited beyond infancy,[15-19] and follow-up information with relatively large series of children older than 5 years is lacking.

Herein, we describe our clinical experience with children perinatally infected with HIV-1 who survived longer than 5 years in Kigali, Rwanda.

PATIENTS AND METHODS

Selection of Patients

From 1984 to 1987, only 16 (3%) of 537 symptomatic HIV-1–infected children born to HIV-1–seropositive mothers who were diagnosed at the Pediatric Department of the Centre Hospitalier de Kigali were aged 5 years or older. These 16 children (patients) were enrolled prospectively after verbal consent was obtained from their mother or guardian. At the time of enrollment, their ages varied from 5 to 12 years (mean, 6.5 years); there were nine boys and seven girls. The mean follow-up at the time of this writing was 40 months (range, 27 to 62 months), during which time the children were clinically and biologically evaluated at least every 6 months. The patients were matched for age, sex, and ethnic origin with 16 HIV-1–seronegative subjects (controls). These

Accepted for publication April 22, 1991.

From the Departments of Pediatrics (Drs Lepage, Nsengumuremyi, Van Goethem, and Hitimana) and Ophthalmology (Dr Kestelyn), Centre Hospitalier de Kigali (Rwanda); the National Reference Laboratory, AIDS Control Program, Kigali (Dr Van de Perre); the Department of Pediatrics, Université Libre de Bruxelles (Belgium) (Dr Van Vliet); and INSERM, Unité 330, Bordeaux, France (Dr Msellati). Dr Van Vliet is now with the Research Center and Endocrine Service, Department of Pediatrics, Hôpital St Justine, Université de Montréal, Québec.

Reprint requests to 12, Eve Taille Cuvelier, 7000 Nous, Belgium (Dr Lepage).

control subjects were consecutively selected at the outpatient department, where they were seen for minor complaints.

Clinical Assessment

Clinical evaluation included regular chest roentgenography and eye fundus examinations. Short stature was defined as a height less than the fifth percentile for age and sex on the National Centre for Health Statistics' curves. Height SD scores and ratio of weight to the 50th percentile for chronologic age were calculated with use of the tables of Tanner et al[20] for British children.

Serologic Methods

All serum samples from the children, as well as the samples obtained from the mothers of the patients, were screened by a commercial immuonenzymatic assay (Vironostika, Organon Teknika, Boxtel, the Netherlands). Serum samples that were positive by immunoenzymatic assay were further confirmed by a commercial Western blot technique (Du Pont de Nemours, Wilmington, Del), in which a positive test was defined by the presence of at least one reactive band to a HIV-1 core protein (p17, p24, p55) plus at least one reactive band to an HIV-1 envelope protein (gp41, gp120, gp160).[21]

Immunologic Methods

Delayed-hypersensitivity skin testing was performed by means of seven recall antigens (Multitest, Bio Merieux, Narcy-L'Etoile, France), and the diameter of the induration was measured 3 days after exposure. Mononuclear cell subpopulations were quantified with an indirect immunofluorescent technique and monoclonal antibodies: OKT4 for helper-inducer T cells and OKT8 for suppressor-cytotoxic T cells (Ortho Diagnostic System, Raritan, NJ). Serum IgG, IgA, and IgM levels were measured by radial immunodiffusion (Nor Partigen, Behring, Narburg, Federal Republic of Germany).

Endocrinologic Methods

Levels of serum thyroid hormones and thyrotropin were measured with commercially available kits (Amersham, London, England), as was human growth hormone (GH) (Pharmacia, Uppsala, Sweden). The insulinlike growth factor I (IGF-I) level was measured by radioimmunoassay after acid-ethanol extraction (to decrease the interference of the binding proteins) with iodine 125–labeled IGF-I (Nichols, San Juan Capistrano, Calif) and a polyclonal antibody against synthetic IGF-I.[22]

Statistical Methods

Comparisons between the groups of children were performed with the Wilcoxon Rank-Sum test.

RESULTS

All of the patients were born to HIV-1–infected mothers. Six of the 16 mothers had died, five of them had died of AIDS as diagnosed by the World Health Organization's provisional clinical case definition of AIDS in adults. None of the 16 patients had a history of blood transfusion before the onset of signs or symptoms related to HIV-1 infection. Parenteral treatments had been performed at the Centre Hospitalier de Kigali and in the health centers surrounding the hospital, where sterilization of medical materials is routinely performed.

Clinical and Anthropometric Features

Two patients were asymptomatic. Chronic cough was the most frequently observed symptom (Table 1). The most common signs were short stature, chronic parotitis, persistent generalized lymphadenopathy, hepatosplenomegaly, and pulmonary tuberculosis (Table 1). Chronic otitis media, clubbing of the digits, herpes zoster infection, and chronic urticaria were also noted. Lymphoid interstitial pneumonitis was diagnosed on radiologic grounds (chronic diffuse bilateral micromodular infiltrate) in 31% of the patients. Evidence of perivasculitis on the fundus was noted in 19% of the patients. No patient had persistent oral thrush.

Table 1.—Clinical Manifestations in African Children Perinatally Infected by Human Immunodeficiency Virus Type 1 and Aged 5 Years or Older

Clinical Manifestation	No. (%) of Patients
Short stature*	12 (75)
Chronic cough	7 (44)
Chronic parotitis	8 (50)
Persistent generalized lymphadenopathy	7 (44)
Lymphoid interstitial pneumonitis	5 (31)
Hepatomegaly or hepatosplenomegaly	5 (31)
Pulmonary tuberculosis	4 (25)
Perivasculitis (in the fundus)	3 (19)
Chronic otitis media	2 (13)
Herpes zoster infection	2 (13)

*Height less than fifth percentile for age and sex (National Centre for Health Statistics curves).

The 16 patients had markedly shorter stature than controls (SD score, -2.5 ± 1.4 vs -0.4 ± 0.8; $P<.0001$), but the weight, expressed in percent of median weight for height age, was similar in both groups (96%±8% vs 94%±8%; $P>.5$). Height velocity, calculated in the 12 months preceding the more recent clinical evaluation, was 4.1±1.8 cm/y (SD of height velocity for age=–1.88±2.18 [SD] for age).

Two children died during the study period: one of AIDS and one of liver cirrhosis. None of the other children had life-threatening infection or loss of developmental milestones.

Immunologic Evaluation

Compared with controls, the 16 patients had an increased concentration of serum protein (10.2±0.9 vs 7.4±0.7 g/L; $P<.001$) and a decreased concentration of serum prealbumin (0.13±0.04 vs 0.18±0.03 g/L; $P<.01$). The serum concentration of IgG in the patients was statistically increased compared with controls (40.8±15.4 vs 16.9±11.9 g/L; $P<.01$).

Profound cell-mediated immune impairment was observed in the patients, with a dramatic decrease in the percentage of $CD4^+$ cells (13%±7% vs 39%±5% in controls; $P<.01$) and in the $CD4^+/CD8^+$ ratio (0.33±0.26 vs 1.82±0.35 in controls; $P<.01$). These patients also had a severe defect of delayed hypersensitivity, as measured by skin testing, with much smaller indurations (mean total induration, 4.5±3.1 mm vs 15.4±6.9 mm in controls; $P<.01$).

Endocrinologic Evaluation

Endocrinologic investigations were performed in 11 patients and in 11 matched controls. Mean levels of serum thyroid hormones and thyrotropin were similar among patients and seronegative controls (Table 2). Mean IGF-I concentrations were lower in patients compared with controls, while mean basal GH levels were similar (Table 2).

Table 2.—Endocrinologic Findings in African Children Perinatally Infected by Human Immunodeficiency Virus Type 1 and Aged 5 Years or Older*

	Patients (n=11)	Controls (n=11)	P
Thyrotropin, μU/mL	2.6 (1.3)	2.3 (0.9)	NS
T_3, mmol/L	2.99 (0.85)	2.36 (0.82)	NS
T_4, mmol/L	108 (32)	109 (27)	NS
IGF-I, U/L	219 (70)	440 (200)	.004
GH, μg/L	1.9 (1.5)	3.2 (3.6)	NS

*Values are means (SDs). T_3 indicates triiodothyronine; T_4, thyroxine; IGF-I, insulinlike growth factor-I; GH, basal plasma growth hormone; and NS, not significant.

COMMENT

These 16 patients with a prolonged, paucisymptomatic course of HIV-1 infection represented only 3% of the symptomatic HIV-1–infected children seen in our hospital from 1984 to 1987. None of the 14 survivors had life-threatening infection, neoplasia, or neurologic impairment during the study period (mean follow-up, 40 months). None had any other known risk factor for HIV-1 acquisition than having an HIV-1–seropositive mother (some of whom died of AIDS), strongly suggesting a maternally acquired infection.

Most of these children presented with signs such as chronic parotitis, generalized lymphadenopathy, and lymphoid interstitial pneumonitis. Previous studies[12,16,19] have shown that generalized lymphadenopathy and lymphoid interstitial pneumonitis are associated with a favorable outcome in HIV-1–infected children. These clinical features resemble the "diffuse infiltrative lymphocytosis syndrome" recently described in HIV-infected adults from New York by Itescu et al.[23] In these patients with the diffuse infiltrative lymphocytosis syndrome, the prevalence of HLA-DR5 subtype JVM—a phenotype more frequently encountered in black subjects than in white subjects—and the number of circulating $CD8^+$ cells was unusually high.[23] However, in our series, the number of circulating $CD8^+$ cells was not higher in the patients compared with pediatric patients with AIDS diagnosed at the Centre Hospitalier de Kigali (Rwanda) (data not shown).

Despite their clinical stability, these children had major immunologic dysfunctions of both their humoral and cell-mediated immune systems. The high level of circulating immunoglobulins, particularly of the IgG class, suggests an intense polyclonal B-cell activation in our patients. Usually, this B-cell abnormality is associated with a poor antibody response to new antigens.[24,25] We have recently shown[26] that 14 of the 16 patients had specific anti–HIV-1 IgM, which persisted during the entire study period, and that 11 of them had IgM antibodies directed to HIV-1 envelope proteins. It is not yet clear whether these specific IgM antibodies have protective characteristics. Severe cell-mediated impairment was manifested by low numbers of $CD4^+$ cells, decreased $CD4^+$/$CD8^+$ ratios, and skin test anergy.

The most striking clinical characteristic of these patients was short stature. Growth failure has recently been described in children with perinatal and postnatal HIV-1 infection,[27] but its mechanisms remain unknown. While malnutrition, chronic illness, and stress probably play a role, it is conceivable that endocrine factors contribute to the decreased growth. Indeed, Jospe and Powell[28] have recently described GH deficiency in an 8-year-old girl with perinatal HIV-1 infection. On the other hand, Laue et al[27] found low GH responses to two provocative stimuli in only one of nine children with AIDS and low IGF-I levels but normal GH levels in another child, suggesting that the endocrine features of this syndrome are heterogeneous. Five of nine patients in their study were receiving nutritional support (by either the enteral or parenteral route), and it is known that nutritional rehabilitation restores the low IGF-I levels of malnourished patients to normal.[29] Furthermore, the assay for IGF-I used by Laue et al does not involve prior extraction of plasma to remove IGF binding proteins, and this may lead to spuriously high IGF-I levels.[30] The HIV-1–infected patients described herein had a mean plasma IGF-I level after acid-ethanol extraction of less than 50% of that observed in a group of matched controls living in the same environment. This could be due to either nutritional factors or to a lower GH secretion in the HIV-1–infected children. Except for one child with liver cirrhosis, none of the 15 remaining patients had evidence of liver function abnormalities that could explain low levels of IGF-I. The fact that basal plasma GH levels were not elevated in the HIV-1–infected children together with the similar weight-for-height in both groups suggest that overt malnutrition is not the explanation for the lower IGF-I levels. Unfortunately, due to limited technical facilities in Rwanda, we were not able to perform pituitary stimulation tests, such as measurement of thyrotropin over time after stimulation with thyrotropin-releasing hormone or GH secretion after glucagon secretion. A definitive conclusion about the GH secretory status of these HIV-1–infected children would require formal testing of the pituitary GH reserve.

This work was supported in part by grant 3.4518.85 from the Fonds de la Recherche Scientifique Médicale, Brussels, Belgium (Dr Van Vliet).

We thank Pierre Bourdoux, MD, for determinations of levels of thyroid hormones and thyrotropin, Françoise Vertongen, MD, for albumin and prealbumin determinations, and Geneviève Art, MD, for technical assistance.

References

1. Oleske J, Minnefor A, Cooper R Jr, et al. Immune deficiency syndrome in children. *JAMA.* 1983;249:2345-2349.

2. Rubinstein A, Sicklick M, Gupta A, et al. Acquired immunodeficiency syndrome with reversed T4/T8 ratios in infants born to promiscuous and drug-addicted mothers. *JAMA.* 1983;249:2350-2356.

3. Joncas JH, Delage G, Chad Z, Lapointe N. Acquired (or congenital) immunodeficiency syndrome in infants born of Haïtian mothers. *N Engl J Med.* 1983;308:842.

4. Thomas P, Jaffe HW, Spira TJ, et al. Unexplained immunodeficiency in children. A surveillance report. *JAMA.* 1984;252:639-644.

5. Scott GB, Buck BE, Leterman JG, Bloom FL, Parks WP. Acquired immunodeficiency syndrome in infants. *N Engl J Med.* 1984;310:76-81.

6. Rogers MF, Thomas PA, Strarcher ET, Noa MC, Bush TJ, Jaffe HW. Acquired immunodeficiency syndrome in children: report of the Centers for Disease Control National Surveillance, 1982 to 1985. *Pediatrics.* 1987;79:1008-1017.

7. Bernstein LJ, Krieger BZ, Novick B, Sicklick MJ, Rubinstein A. Bacterial infection in the acquired immunodeficiency syndrome of children. *Pediatr Infect Dis.* 1985;4:472-475.

8. Krasinski K, Borkowski W, Bonk S, Lawrence R, Chandwani S. Bacterial infections in human immunodeficiency virus–infected children. *Pediatr Infect Dis J.* 1988;7:323-328.

9. Epstein LG, Sharer LR, Oleske JM, et al. Neurologic manifestations of human immunodeficiency virus infection in children. *Pediatrics.* 1986;78:678-687.
10. Belman AL, Diamond G, Dickson D, et al. Pediatric acquired immunodeficiency syndrome: neurologic syndromes. *AJDC.* 1988;142:29-35.
11. Jonckheer T, Levy J, Van de Perre P, et al. LAV/HTLV-III infection in children of African origin: experience in Belgium. *Eur J Pediatr.* 1986;145:511-516.
12. Parks W, Scott GB. An overview of pediatric AIDS: approaches to diagnosis and outcome assessment. In: Broder S, ed. *AIDS: Modern Concepts and Therapeutic Challenges.* New York, NY: Marcel Dekker Inc;1987:245-262.
13. Rubinstein A. Pediatric acquired immunodeficiency. In: Moss SJ, ed. *Pediatrics Update.* New York, NY: Elsevier Science Publishing Co Inc;1987:1-5.
14. Auger I, Thomas P, De Gruttola V, et al. Incubation period for pediatric AIDS. *Nature.* 1988;336:575-577.
15. Kelly DA, Hallett RJ, Saeed A, Morgan G, Levinsky RJ, Strobel. Prolonged survival and late presentation of vertically transmitted HIV infection in childhood. *Lancet.* 1987;1:806-807.
16. Kamani N, Lightman H, Leiderman I, Krilov LR. Pediatric acquired immunodeficiency syndrome–related complex: clinical and immunological features. *Pediatr Infect Dis J.* 1988;7:383-388.
17. Krasinski K, Borkowsky W, Holzman RS. Prognosis of human immunodeficiency virus infection in children and adolescents. *Pediatr Infect Dis J.* 1989;8:216-220.
18. Scott GB, Hutto C, Makuch RW, et al. Survival in children with perinatally acquired human immunodeficiency virus type 1 infection. *N Engl J Med.* 1989;321:1791-1796.
19. Blanche S, Tardieu M, Duliège AM, et al. Longitudinal study of 94 symptomatic infants with maternofetal HIV infection: evidence for a bimodal expression of clinical and biological symptoms. *AJDC.* 1990;144:1210-1215.
20. Tanner JW, Whitehouse RH, Takaishi M. Standards from birth to maturity for height, weight height velocity and weight velocity: British children, 1965: part 2. *Arch Dis Child.* 1966;41:613-635.
21. Centers for Disease Control. Interpretation and use of the Western blot assay for serodiagnosis of human immunodeficiency virus type 1 infection. *MMWR.* 1989;38:51-57.
22. Van Vliet G, Bosson D, Rummens E, Robyn C, Wolter R. Evidence against growth hormone releasing factor deficiency in children with idiopathic obesity. *Acta Endocrinol.* 1986; 279(suppl):410-414.
23. Itescu S, Brancato LJ, Winchester R. A sicca syndrome in HIV infection: association with HLA-DR5 and CD8 lymphocytosis. *Lancet.* 1989;2:466-468.
24. Bernstein LJ, Ochs HD, Wedgwood RJ, Rubinstein A. Defective humoral immunity in pediatric acquired immunodeficiency syndrome. *J Pediatr.* 1985;107:352-357.
25. Borkowsky W, Steele CJ, Grubman S, Moore T, La Russa P, Krasinski K. Antibody responses to bacterial toxoids in children infected with human immunodeficiency virus. *J Pediatr.* 1987;110:563-566.
26. Van de Pierre P, Lepage P, Simonon A, et al. Biological markers associated with prolonged survival in African children maternally infected by the human immunodeficiency virus type 1. *AIDS Res Hum Retroviruses.* In press.
27. Laue L, Pizzo PA, Butler K, Cutler GB. Growth and neuroendocrine dysfunction in children with acquired immunodeficiency syndrome. *J Pediatr.* 1990;117:541-545.
28. Jospe N, Powell KR. Growth hormone deficiency in an 8-year-old girl with human immunodeficiency virus infection. *Pediatrics.* 1990;86:309-312.
29. Clemons DR, Underwood LE, Dickerson RN, et al. Use of plasma somatomedin C/insulin-like growth factor-I measurement to monitor the response to nutritional repletion in malnourished patients. *Am J Clin Nutr.* 1985;41:191-198.
30. Relman AS. An error corrected, a conclusion withdrawn, and a lesson learned. *N Engl J Med.* 1990;323:1482-1483.

In Other AMA Journals

ARCHIVES OF SURGERY

Trauma During Pregnancy: A Review of 79 Cases

Thomas J. Esposito, MD, MPH; David R. Gens, MD; Lynn Gerber Smith, RN, MS; Ronald Scorpio, MD; Timothy Buchman, MD
(*Arch Surg.* 1991;126:1073-1078)

Trauma in Pregnancy: Predicting Pregnancy Outcome

David P. Kissinger, MD; Grace S. Rozycki, MD; John A Morris, Jr, MD; M. Margaret Knudson, MD; Wayne S. Copes, PhD; Sue M. Bass, ScM; H. Kendle Yates; Howard R. Champion, FRCS(Edin)
(*Arch Surg.* 1991;126:1079-1086)

Landmark study concludes: Enuretic children may lack diurnal rhythm of ADH common in non-enuretic children[1]

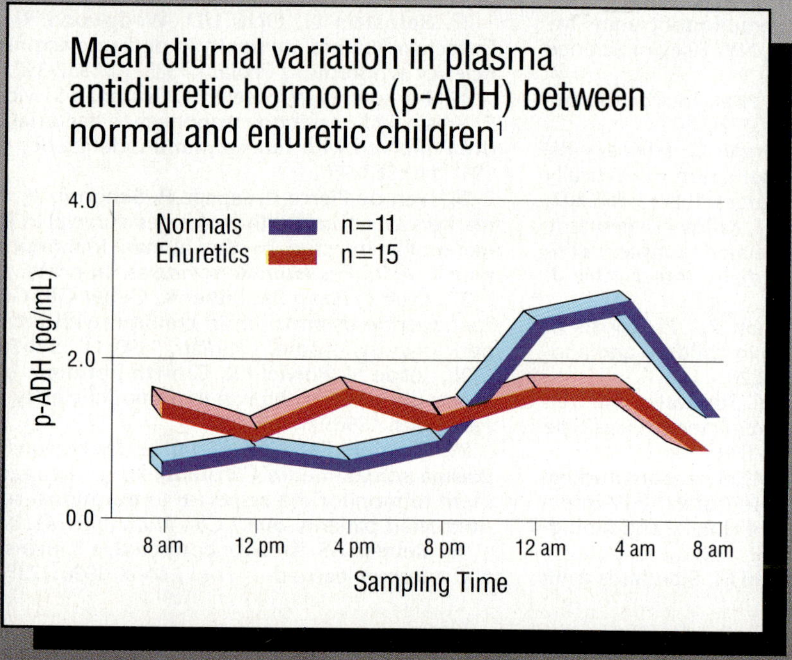

The ADH Deficit

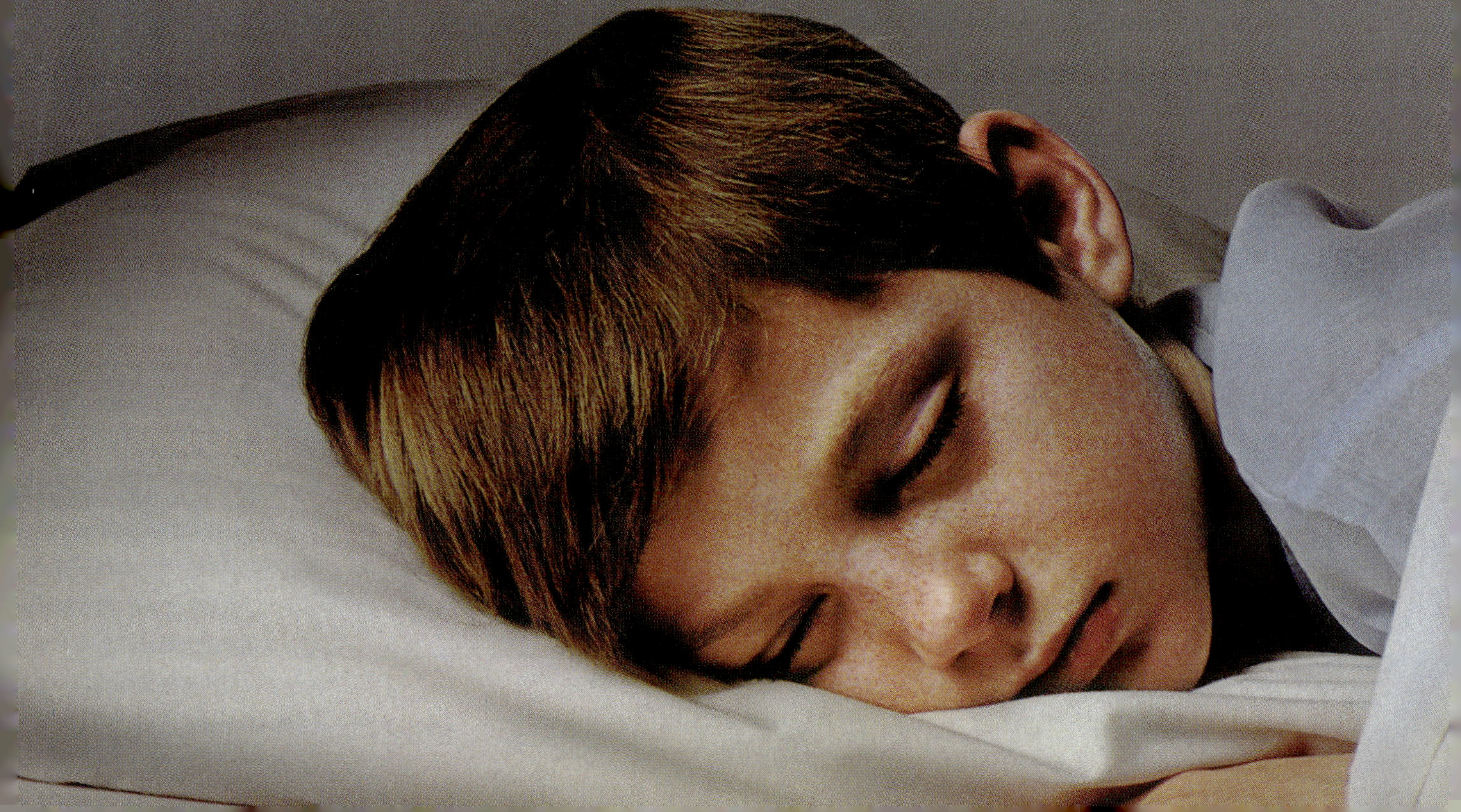

Comparison of a Computer Tutorial With Other Methods for Teaching Well-Newborn Care

Larry W. Desch, MD; Maria T. Esquivel, MD; Sharon K. Anderson, MA

• Research using a computer-assisted instructional program developed for teaching well-newborn care is described. Third-year medical students were randomly assigned during their week-long nursery rotation into three groups to study the acceptability and effectiveness of using the computer-assisted instructional lessons. Group A, the control group, was not required to complete any additional educational task. Group B was assigned specific reading material. Group C completed the microcomputer-based tutorial. (The term *tutorial* is often used interchangeably to describe the computer-assisted instructional program.) Both groups B and C improved dramatically on a posttest in comparison with group A. There was no statistically significant difference between groups B and C on the improvement from pretest to posttest scores. However, significantly less time was spent by group C completing the tutorial compared with the total time spent reading by group B. The results of this study provide further illustration of the feasibility and effectiveness of using a computer-assisted instructional program for medical student education.

(*AJDC.* 1991;145:1255-1258)

During the past 15 years, there has been nearly an exponential growth rate in the development of computer-assisted instruction (CAI) for medical education. Computer-assisted instruction has moved from mainframe computers to personal microcomputers, which often make use of additional devices such as laser videodisk players to enhance the quality of the instruction.[1,2] The field of CAI for medical education has improved so dramatically that many of the early CAI programs, although they are less than 10 years old, appear now to be very simplistic and, perhaps, naive compared with current medical CAI.[3]

The ease with which CAI can be produced has also improved markedly over the past several years. The cost of development has also decreased. For example, it is now possible to develop locally the laser videodisks for use with CAI programs. In addition, many types of "authoring systems" are available that can expedite the production of CAI programs. These authoring systems are computer programs that function as a "shell" program to speed up the process of developing CAI.[4,5]

This article summarizes the development and initial evaluation of a CAI program developed for teaching various basic aspects of well-newborn care. The CAI program was developed primarily for medical student education, but has also been intermittently used by pediatric residents. However, the data presented are concerned only with the use by medical students.

SUBJECTS AND METHODS

A commercially available authoring system was used to develop the neonatal tutorial. This system, called UNISON, was selected partially because of its relatively low cost and ease of use, but primarily because it, unlike most other authoring systems, does not require the payment of royalties for the distribution of programs developed with UNISON.[6] A microcomputer with two floppy disk drives was used to both develop and present the CAI program.

The CAI program that was produced consisted of several short lessons presenting basic material, such as steps in the physical examination of the newborn, as well as some presentations on therapeutic measures, such as treatment of hyperbilirubinemia. Questions about material previously presented by the program were also posed intermittently. The tutorial is primarily linear, but some branching can be done that includes optional review of previously presented material. Accompanying the tutorial is a small booklet containing pictures and graphic illustrations, which are used to demonstrate visually a number of findings such as mongolian spots.

Three groups of third-year medical students at the Univer-

Accepted for publication March 25, 1991.

From the Department of Child Health (Pediatrics) (Drs Desch and Esquivel); and the Division of Biostatistics, Department of Information Sciences, University of Missouri–Columbia School of Medicine (Ms Anderson).

Reprint requests to Department of Pediatrics, University of Wisconsin Medical School, 600 Highland Ave, Madison, WI 53792 (Dr Desch).

sity of Missouri–Columbia Medical School were selected during 1989 and 1990 to study the acceptability, effectiveness, and validity of using this neonatal CAI program. There were 26 students in each of these three groups. The well-nursery rotation for each group of the students lasted 1 week. All three groups were later subdivided into two subsets depending on whether they had taken their pediatrics rotation during the first half or the second half of their third year. This was done to determine whether there were any effects on the results obtained because the students had been exposed to clinical medical education for a longer period.

Participation by all of the subjects was purely voluntary and effort was made to ensure that the students did not believe that there would be positive or negative effects if they did or did not participate, respectively. Approval from the University of Missouri–Columbia School of Medicine's Institutional Review Board was obtained prior to the commencement of the project.

The third-year medical students who participated were selected into one of the three groups in a sequential random order. Attending physicians for these groups differed during the study periods; therefore, what was taught to them informally varied as well. Group A served as the true control group. These students were not given any additional educational intervention.

The second group, group B, was given specific instructions about the assigned reading that was required. A small paperback[7] was used for this reading material. Selected pages and, occasionally, particular paragraphs were listed as required reading. This textbook was not available to the students in the other groups. The students in group B were asked to keep track of their time spent reading. This group of students served as the attention-placebo group.

The students in group C served as the main experimental group. This group of students was given basic written instructions on how to use the microcomputer and was given the program on floppy disks and the accompanying book with pictures and diagrams. This group was also asked to keep track of their time spent working on the program. They were additionally requested to fill out an 11-item Likert scale questionnaire that asked questions about their interactions with the microcomputer and the CAI neonatal program. This scale will be described as an "acceptability index" in following discussions. The actual scale that was used has been published previously.[4]

Answers to questions on this scale helped to determine if the students believed, for example, that they "improved (their) knowledge about well-newborn care" and if the content of the tutorial was appropriate and understandable. Answers to other questions on the scale determined whether there were any problems with the use of the program and if the students appreciated the design features of the program, such as the brief quizzes presented and the ability to review.

In all three groups, a pretest and posttest were given to each student to complete. Both tests consisted of 20 multiple-choice questions (four choices each). Questions on the posttest were exactly the same as on the pretest, but were arranged in different order. The pretests for all groups were given shortly before the start of their nursery rotation or on the morning of the first day of the nursery rotation. The posttest was completed by the students on the last day of the rotation or the following day.

The questions that were used on the two tests were written, for the most part, so that the students could reflect on their experience rather than just recall facts. No questions were chosen that asked about material that was not specifically presented. Questions about topics that were of the most importance and were also likely topics to have been presented to the control group of students, for example, the etiology of hyperbilirubinemia, appeared on the survey. A convenience sample of five beginning third-year students was used to pilot test these questions. The mean score for this sample was 9.8.

The SAS statistical analysis computer program was used to organize and analyze the data using Kruskal-Wallis and Wilcoxon's rank sum nonparametric methods.[8]

Table 1.—Summary of Results in the Three Groups of Students*

	Group A (Control)	Group B (Book)	Group C (Computer)	P†
Pretest				
Mean (SD)	14.5 (2.00)	15.2 (2.61)	15.6 (2.16)	NS
Range	10-17	10-19	12-19	
Posttest				
Mean (SD)	16.7 (2.18)	18.8 (1.04)	19.4 (0.70)	.0001‡,§
Range	12-20	16-20	18-20	
Difference				
Mean (SD)	2.3 (1.31)	3.6 (2.22)	3.8 (2.09)	.0123‡,§
Range	0-5	(−1)-7	0-8	
Total time				
Mean (SD)	. . .	70.4 (8.2)	54.4 (7.9)	.0001
Range	. . .	60-85	45-70	
No.	. . .	14	17	

*The number of each was 26, except as indicated.

†Results from Kruskal-Wallis analysis. NS indicates not significant.

‡Post hoc analysis (using Wilcoxon's rank sum test): group B was significantly different from group A.

§Post hoc analysis: group C was significantly different from group A.

RESULTS

The results for the three groups are summarized in Table 1. Several students in groups B and C did not indicate the total time spent. However, the number missing is similar between the groups.

As was anticipated, groups B and C improved dramatically on their posttest in comparison with group A, in which no additional educational interventions were used. The results from Kruskal-Wallis nonparametric analysis demonstrated statistically significant ($P=.012$) differences in the change from pretest to posttest. Post hoc analysis revealed significant differences between group B and group A, as well as between group C and group A. Somewhat surprisingly, however, there was no statistically significant difference in the improvement from pretest to posttest scores between the group that was given assigned readings (group B) and the group using the computerized neonatal tutorial (group C). Group C demonstrated slightly better posttest scores as well as better improvement from pretest scores (19 vs 18 and 3.8 vs 3.6, respectively).

However, these two groups showed statistically significant differences in the time spent completing either the readings or the computerized tutorial ($P=.0001$). Group B spent a mean of 70 minutes, while group C spent about 20 minutes less time.

The data additionally demonstrate that there was a ceiling effect present that was not anticipated. Many students, especially those who took the pretest in the second half of their third year (first clinical year), achieved a relatively high score and, therefore, did not improve much on the posttest. Despite the ceiling effect, the different scores between the groups remain significant ($P=.0123$). The high pretest ceiling was not expected since the mean score from pilot testing of the test questions was 9.8.

Considering the subsets based on whether a student

Table 2.—Acceptability Index Results*

Question	First Half-Year Group (n=12), Mean (Range)	Second Half-Year Group (n=14), Mean (Range)
1	2.42 (2-3)	2.64 (2-3)
2	2.33 (2-3)	2.50 (2-3)
3	2.50 (2-3)	2.57 (2-3)
4	2.58 (2-3)	2.42 (2-3)
5	2.67 (2-3)	2.50 (2-3)
6	2.75 (2-4)	2.71 (2-3)
7	2.50 (2-3)	2.64 (2-3)
8	2.34 (1-3)	2.71 (2-4)
9	2.17 (2-3)	2.64 (2-3)
10	1.92 (1-3)	2.29 (2-3)
11	1.50 (1-2)	1.64 (1-2)

*Questions using 6-point Likert scale with 1 indicating "strongly agree" and 6 indicating "strongly disagree." Differences between groups were not statistically significant.

took the rotation in the first part of the year or the second part of the year, an analysis of all three groups yielded the following results. As expected, those students participating in the second half of their third year performed significantly better on the pretest (*P* values ranging from .0002 to .014). As previously mentioned, data analysis of the pretest and posttest difference vs the pretest demonstrated a strong ceiling effect, especially in the students in the second half-year groups. Comparison of the amount of time spent completing either the assigned reading or the computerized tutorial did not demonstrate any significant differences between the first half-year and the second half-year students (group B, $P=.265$; group C, $P=.433$).

The students who participated in the microcomputer tutorial also appeared to have enjoyed the experience and found it useful (Table 2). On the acceptability index, most of the means of the 11 items ranged between "agree" and "slightly agree," with one item listed between "strongly agree" and "agree." This highest score was in response to the item, "This program improved my knowledge about well-newborn care." The lowest mean score was in response to the item, "The text was easy to understand" (mean, 2.73). There were no statistically significant differences between the two half-year subsets on the results of the acceptability index.

COMMENT

As has been demonstrated by a number of authors, CAI for medical education is an important tool and one that will probably have increasing importance in the future.[3,9] In this study, which is one of the few to evaluate a computerized medical tutorial, the results illustrate the effectiveness of presenting specifically selected basic information to teach students. This is extremely important in situations in which the time spent during the clinical experience (in this case, a well-newborn nursery) is very limited. Other medical educators such as Schreiner et al[10] have had medical students use audiovisual materials to try to more efficiently teach in the well-newborn nursery.[10]

It was a common practice in the past, and may still be so in some instances, to tell medical students at the beginning of a clinical rotation to read a particular textbook. However, they often do not receive any guidance about what specific information may be important for them to learn. In this study, both the students who completed specific selected readings and those who spent time with a microcomputer learning selected information did comparably well. Those students who had no guidance for their learning experience did not show much, if any, improvement. However, it remains a possibility that the control group (group A) learned information that was not reflected in the posttest results.

The most important result of this study is that demonstrated by the time spent by students completing either the assigned reading or the microcomputer tutorial. The computer group spent nearly 20 minutes *less* time than the reading group. Obviously, had the reading group only been given the textbook to read without any guidance regarding specific paragraphs and pages, the time spent by the reading group would have been much greater. These students were requested to only read the indicated parts and to keep track of the time spent reading these specific pages and paragraphs. It is likely, as some students later admitted, that many students later read more of the book than was required.

Although the amount of this serendipitous learning was not evaluated, it may well be that the reading group picked up more useful information in this way. Some of the students who performed the computer tutorial or the readings also later requested to be able to read the textbook or to do the tutorial. It is uncertain whether the learning of these students was somehow enhanced when they followed up either the computer tutorial with reading or the reading with the tutorial. The investigators were pleased, however, that some students had been motivated into wanting to learn more.

It is possible that there may be some unreliability in the time reports given by the students in groups B and C. Alternative study designs were considered in planning the study, such as having a program coupled to the CAI program that would keep track of the time or possibly the use of hand-held stopwatches supplied to all the students. These ideas were rejected primarily because they were believed to be more intrusive or expensive and still subject to most of the same errors that may occur with self-report methods (eg, the student could leave the computer on, but not be using the CAI program). Both groups were allowed to have stops and starts. Using the CAI program, as well as the textbook, allowed students to end at any of several places, leave for any period of time, and start again later where they left off.

The time differential between groups might have been less if additional effort had gone into organizing the reading material. Passages of text could have been highlighted or underlined or other guides developed. It would have also been possible to prepare a programmed text with interspersed questions to stimulate learning. However, the effort required to perform such tasks would have been nearly that required to prepare the CAI program. In addition, the students who would use such a guide may not do as well comparatively since using computers, perhaps because it is still a novelty, frequently appears to be an additional enticement to learning new material.[9]

The use of an authoring system to develop the CAI program expedited its creation and made it possible for persons other than computer programmers to prepare the lesson. It may well be the current, most appropriate, and cost-effective way of preparing medical instructional programs, as well as some types of patient treatment simulations. The use of authoring systems allows a person with only a basic understanding of computers to develop an effective instructional program. It also allows, as was done with our CAI program, an easy way to add site-specific information to the program, as well as allowing alterations of the tutorial to be made as knowledge about diseases or treatments changes.

The issue of cost-effectiveness is often raised when there is an assessment of CAI. This was a specific concern with the development of the CAI program for this study, as it was entirely self-supported. Our assessment of this was very favorable, in terms of both time and money spent. The computer tutorial is equivalent to about 2 hours of didactic lecturing, and thus saves about 44 hours of faculty time per year, not including any preparation time for the faculty person. In regard to monetary concerns, the tutorial was primarily developed by a medical student working about 30 hours per week for 10 weeks. This student was hired at a total cost of $1500 as part of a summer research fellowship. He was not versed in the use of the authoring program prior to beginning work, and some of the time initially spent was in learning the system. However, additional time will be required to improve the CAI program in response to the feedback from the students.

The authoring system costs about $600, although some optional modules were purchased that were not actually used for this particular CAI program. The microcomputers used by the students were within a large microcomputer area in the medical library and are used for multiple purposes. This type of facility is becoming more commonplace, which improves on the overall cost-effectiveness of producing or acquiring CAI in that the cost of purchasing microcomputer equipment does not have to be figured into the total cost for one specific project.

CAI medical tutorials should work well as preliminary lessons that might be followed up by patient treatment simulations. The improvement of software and hardware for microcomputers in general and, specifically, the refinement of authoring systems recently and in the future, will allow more medical educators to be able to prepare these computerized lessons locally. The main advantage of this will be that these tutorials and simulations are more likely to suit individual teaching needs.

Although this study had a somewhat small number of subjects, CAI programs appear to promise to be increasingly important in medical education. It is also evident that the use of medical CAI programs are currently not being fully exploited. Current events, and likely future situations, appear to indicate that there will be further erosion of the time that clinical medical educators can spend in teaching. This is primarily because of increasing demands put on them for direct patient care. It is important, therefore, that time-saving and cost-effective measures be developed to ensure that the teaching of medical students does not suffer. The further development of CAI programs for medical education may be one way that students can be assured of having an efficient and individualized learning experience.

The authors wish to thank Brad Robison, MD, for his assistance in the development of the CAI tutorial.

References

1. Kumar K, Hodgins M. Use of interactive videodisc for teaching of pathology laboratory cases. *J Pathol.* 1990;160:145-149.
2. Blackman JA, Huntley JS. The pediatrician's guide to computer videodiscs. *Pediatrics.* 1984;74:543-547.
3. Piemme TE. Computer-assisted learning and evaluation in medicine. *JAMA.* 1988;260:367-372.
4. Desch LW. Use of commercial 'authoring systems' for medical education. *Med Educ.* 1986;20:417-423.
5. Kesnik B, Kidd MR. MATRIX: an authoring program for computer-assisted learning in medical education. In: Barber B, Cao D, Qin D, Wagner G, eds. *MEDINFO '89: Proceedings of the Sixth Conference on Medical Informatics.* Amsterdam, the Netherlands: North-Holland Publishing Co; 1989:1215.
6. Courseware Applications Inc. *UNISON Author Language Reference Manual.* Champaign, Ill: Courseware Applications Inc; 1988.
7. Coen RW, Koffler H. *Primary Care of the Newborn.* Boston, Mass: Little Brown & Co Inc; 1987.
8. SAS Institute Inc. *SAS User's Guide: Statistics.* 5th ed. Cary, NC: SAS Institute Inc; 1985.
9. Levy AH. Factors affecting computer-mediated instruction in medical education. *Methods Inf Med.* 1989;28:215-222.
10. Schreiner RL, Merk PL, Greene D, Greene S, Lein BE, Keener PA. A written and audiovisual educational program for students assigned to the normal newborn nursery. *J Med Educ.* 1980;55:628-630.

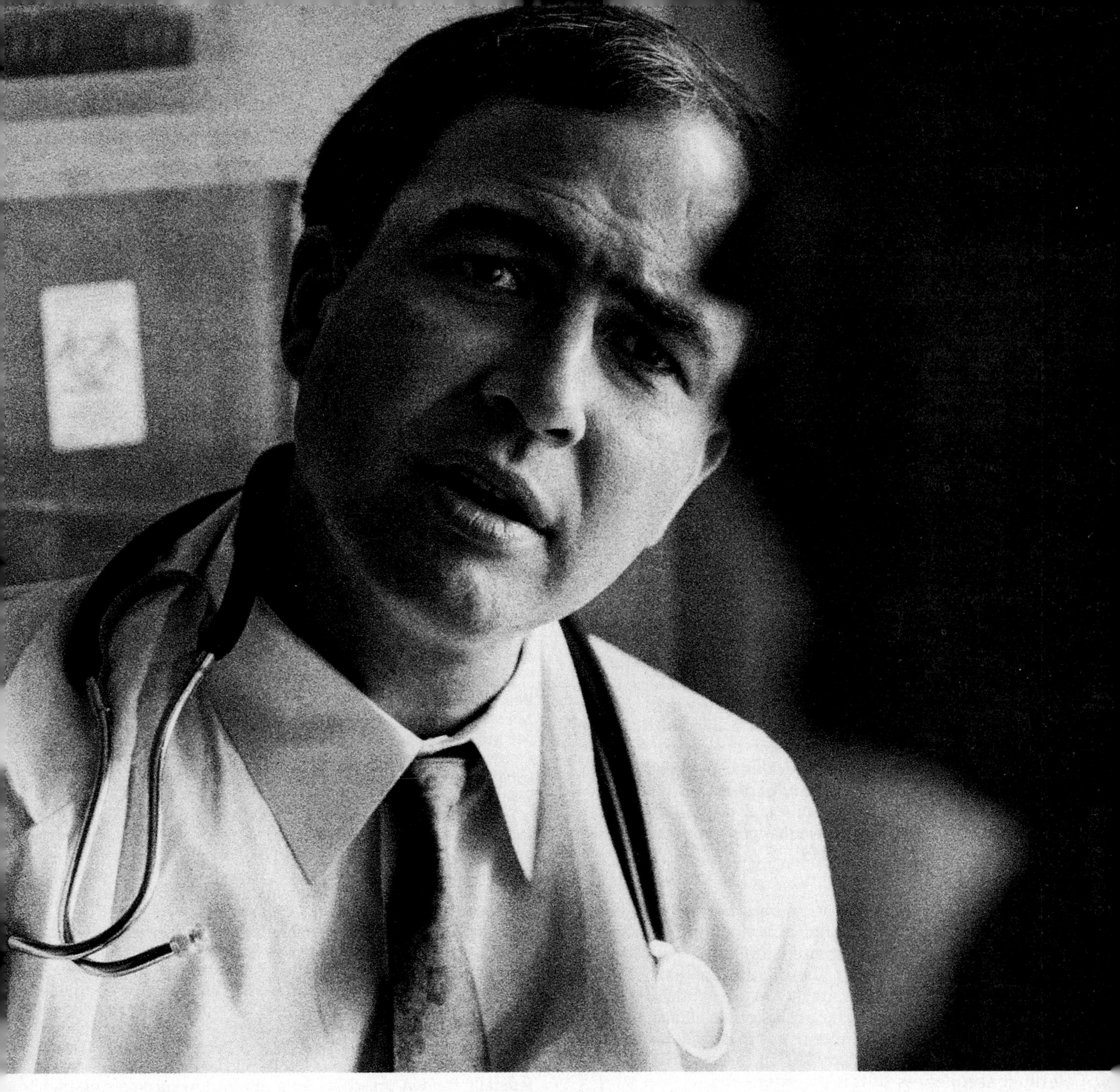

Obesity Among Mescalero Preschool Children

Association With Maternal Obesity and Birth Weight

Margaret M. Gallaher, MD; Fern R. Hauck, MD, MS; Miranda Yang-Oshida, RD, MPH; Mary K. Serdula, MD, MPH

• The prevalence of obesity among native American children ranks with the highest in the United States. However, little is known about associated risk factors for obesity among these children. We conducted a medical record review of 261 preschool children enrolled in the Mescalero Apache tribe to determine the prevalence of obesity and associated risk factors. The prevalence of obesity (weight for height >95th percentile) in this population was 19.5%. The prevalence of obesity (body mass index >95th percentile) in their mothers was 23%. Children with obese mothers were more than twice as likely to be obese than children of nonobese mothers. Children with a high birth weight were three times as likely to be obese as children of low or normal birth weight. The high prevalence of obesity may be due to both life-style and dietary patterns on the reservation. Family-based interventions are needed to prevent obesity and its long-term consequences in this population.

(*AJDC.* 1991;145:1262-1265)

Obesity among children is increasingly recognized as a significant nutritional disorder that is linked to orthopedic problems, hypertension, and psychosocial difficulties.[1-6] In addition, obese children may be more likely to become obese adults[7,8] who are at additional risk of morbidity. Obese adults are often resistant to interventions[9]; therefore, preventive measures targeted at children may be more successful in forestalling the long-term consequences of this disorder.

Data from the Pediatric Nutrition Surveillance System demonstrate that native American children have a higher prevalence of obesity than either black or white children.[10] Although some studies of predominantly white and black preschool children have identified risk factors for obesity, such as familial obesity,[11,12] socioeconomic status,[11-14] and small family size,[15] little is known about such factors among native American preschool children. Because the nutritionist (M. Y.-O.) for the Mescalero Apache tribe was concerned that a high proportion of children attending the well-child clinic was obese, we conducted a medical record review to determine the true extent of the problem, and as a first step in developing interventions to prevent obesity.

SUBJECTS AND METHODS

This study was conducted on the Mescalero Apache Reservation, which is situated on 460 000 acres in south central New Mexico. The chief sources of income on the reservation are timber sales, cattle farming, and recreational facilities. The per capita income was $1500 in 1988. As of 1988, 2893 were enrolled as tribal members and 295 (13.1%) children were under age 5 years.[16]

All primary health care for tribal members is provided at the Indian Health Service Hospital (Mescalero, NM), the only medical facility on the reservation. The hospital's medical records contain inpatient and outpatient records, including well-child visits and school physical examinations. It is estimated that at least 90% of the preschool children attend the well-child clinic.[16]

For inclusion in the study, children had to meet the following criteria: (1) born on or after January 1, 1983; (2) enrolled as a tribal member; (3) seen for a well-child visit in 1987 or 1988; (4) were age 1 to 5 years at the time of the well-child visit; and (5) mother's chart was available for review. From the child's medical record, we collected information on age, sex, number of siblings, birth order, birth weight, weight and height at the most recent well-child visit, and whether the child attended Head Start (a federally funded preschool program for low-income children). We also reviewed the mother's medical record for information on her age at the time of the child's birth, her most recent nonpregnant weight and height, her marital status, and whether she had ever been diagnosed as having diabetes. We obtained the mother's employment status from the tribal office.

Because siblings tend to have similar physical characteristics, only one child per family was included in the analysis to eliminate potential bias. Children were included in the study by alternately selecting the older and the younger child in families with two children, and alternately selecting the oldest, middle, and youngest child in families with three children. No families had more than three children who met the study criteria.

Using the ANTHRO software program,[17] anthropometric indices (weight for height [W/H] and height for age [H/A]) were calculated based on the National Center for Health Statistics (NCHS) reference population.[18,19] We defined obesity among the children as W/H above the 95th percentile, underweight as W/H below the 5th percentile, and short stature as H/A below the 5th percentile. Obesity among the mothers was defined as body

Accepted for publication August 14, 1991.

From the Division of Nutrition, Center for Chronic Disease Prevention and Health Promotion, Centers for Disease Control, Atlanta, Ga (Drs Gallaher, Hauck, and Serdula), and Mescalero Indian Health Service Hospital, Mescalero, NM (Ms Yang-Oshida).

Adapted from a presentation at the Epidemic Intelligence Service Conference, Atlanta, Ga, April 3, 1989.

Reprint requests to Division of Nutrition, Mail Stop K26, Centers for Disease Control, Atlanta, GA 30333 (Dr Serdula).

Age Distribution of Mescalero Apache Children and the Prevalence of Obesity in Children by Risk Factor

Risk Factor	No. (%) of Subjects	% Obese	Prevalence Ratio	95% Confidence Interval
Age of child, y				
5	20 (8)	20.0	0.9	(0.3, 2.3)
4	69 (26)	18.8	0.8	(0.4, 1.6)
3	49 (19)	18.4	0.8	(0.4, 1.7)
2	58 (22)	17.2	0.8	(0.4, 1.5)
1	65 (25)	23.1	1.0	Referent
Maternal obesity				
Yes	61	36.1	2.5	(1.6, 4.0)
No	200	14.5	1.0	Referent
Birth weight, g				
≥4000	36	36.1	3.0	(1.3, 6.8)
3000-3999	167	18.6	1.5	(0.7, 3.3)
2000-2999	58	12.1	1.0	Referent

mass index (weight divided by square of height) above the 95th percentile of women aged 20 to 29 years in the NHANESII reference population.[20]

The Epi Info computer program was used to calculate prevalence ratios (calculated in the same way as a relative risk) and 95% confidence intervals (CIs) for the prevalence ratios.[21] Variables significantly associated with obesity among the children by univariate analysis were further analyzed with logistic regression to determine the magnitude of their independent association with obesity.[22] Childhood obesity (present or absent) was the outcome variable in the logistic regression analysis. The magnitude and direction of the link between a child's obesity and the predictor variables were estimated by the odds ratio. Predictor variables included age (age 1 to 5 years), sex, birth weight (<3000 g, 3000 to 3999 g, or ≥4000 g), and maternal obesity (present or absent).

RESULTS

Of the 431 Mescalero children identified as meeting the age criteria, charts were located for 409 (95%). Of these, 377 preschool children had had a well-child visit in 1987 or 1988. Mothers' records were available and reviewed for 364 (97%) of the children. Excluding all but one child from each family left 261 children included in the analysis.

Fifty percent of the children were boys, eight (3%) had a birth weight below 2500 g, and 36 (14%) had a birth weight above 4000 g. Children aged 5 years made up the smallest proportion of the total study population (Table) because children receiving their last immunization at age 4 years would be discharged from the well-child clinic and would not return at age 5 years.

The overall prevalence of obesity among the children was 19.5% (n = 51), which is significantly greater than the expected prevalence of 5% based on the reference population ($P<.000001$, binomial distribution). In contrast, 1% of the children were underweight and 6% had short stature. Of the mothers, 61 (23%) were obese.

Obese children were 2.5 times more likely to have an obese mother than nonobese children (Table). Prevalence of obesity increased with increasing birth weight. No association existed between obesity and the age or sex of the child, number of siblings, or birth order, nor were maternal employment, maternal diabetes, marital status, or age closely connected with this condition.

In the logistic regression model, childhood obesity was significantly associated with maternal obesity and birth weight after adjustments were made for age and sex of the child. The adjusted odds ratio of obesity for children whose mothers were obese was 4.8 times (95% CI, 1.8 to 12.8) higher than that of children whose mothers were not obese. The adjusted odds ratio of obesity for children with a birth weight above 4000 g was 4.4 (95% CI, 1.3 to 15.4).

Among infants born to obese mothers, 24% were of high birth weight (>4000 g) compared with only 11% of infants born to nonobese mothers (prevalence ratio, 1.93; 95% CI, 1.16 to 3.23). Because birth weight and mother's obesity are shown here and in other studies to be closely related, we examined for the presence of multicollinearity between maternal obesity and birth weight in the logistic regression model. First, no change appeared in the magnitude of the odds ratios or the CIs around the odds ratios when the logistic regression model contained either one or both of the variables. Second, we calculated the correlation between maternal body mass index and infant birth weight as continuous variables; a correlation (r) of .05 (95% CI, −0.07 to 0.17) indicates a correlation not sufficient to cause problems with multicollinearity in the logistic regression model.

COMMENT

Compared with data from the NCHS reference populations (which were predominantly composed of white and black children), the prevalence of obesity among Mescalero children and their mothers was greater than expected. The prevalence of short stature was as expected, whereas that of low weight was lower than expected. These findings are consistent with those of the Pediatric Nutrition Surveillance System, which used the same criteria to define obesity, although the prevalence of obesity from the Pediatric Nutrition Surveillance System was somewhat lower (8% to 13%) among native Americans than in our study.[10]

The NCHS reference population is probably not the ideal population with which to compare native American children, as the standard is composed of predominantly white and black children. Little is known of the body composition of native American children and how this may influence comparisons with other ethnic groups. In a study of Peruvian children, high W/H (compared with the NCHS reference population) was associated with lower body fat and greater lean tissue hydration.[23] Until an appropriate reference is developed for native American children, as well as children of other ethnicities, the NCHS standard will continue to be used because it is both well-known and accessible to clinical practitioners.

Previous studies have identified risk factors for obesity among other populations of children, including familial obesity,[11,12] high birth weight,[24,25] low or high socioeconomic status,[11-14] and small family size.[15] Of the risk factors examined in our study, maternal obesity and high birth weight were most strongly associated with childhood obesity. The relationship between the weight class of parents and that of their child is well documented, and some studies have shown a stronger association between the weight class of the mother and obesity in the child compared with the father's weight class.[24,25] A study of Mexican-American preschool children found that mothers of obese children preferred a fatter baby, were "pushier" feeders, and were more likely to be obese themselves.[26] Based on our record review, we cannot assess maternal attitudes and perceptions of the child's weight or determine the magnitude of the contribution of common environmental factors and genetic factors to the link between maternal and child obesity. It is probable that dietary factors and low physical activity contribute to the overall high prevalence of obesity.

Obesity among the children was closely related to high birth weight. Studies have shown that obese women tend to have children of higher birth weight,[27-29] and that children with high birth weight are more likely to remain taller and heavier than children of lower birth weight,[30] which could explain this finding.

We did not find an association between child obesity and maternal employment, the only measure of socioeconomic status available by chart review. The Ten State Nutrition Survey showed a direct association between socioeconomic status and the prevalence of obesity among preschool children.[11] Other studies, which examined white preschool children only, found the opposite—that obesity was inversely related to socioeconomic status.[12,13] This population of native Americans may be too small and too homogeneous to detect differences in obesity due to socioeconomic status. Further studies are needed to clarify this issue among this and other native American populations.

In this study, W/H was chosen as the measure of obesity because it is the most practical and widely used and can be abstracted from existing medical records. Obesity, defined as an abnormally high proportion of body fat, can only be approximated by anthropometric measurements. The correlation between high W/H and obesity may be low among young children.[31] Weight for height cannot indicate whether increased weight is due to adiposity, increased muscularity, or edema. It is not known if the higher W/H in this population of native American children is due to an increase in body fat or a difference in body proportions. By defining obesity as W/H above the 95th percentile, we chose a definition that was extreme and, therefore, less likely to misclassify children as obese.

The strength of using record review in this population is that there is a single source of medical care, and attendance at the well-child clinic is high. However, there are several limitations to using a medical record review to determine risk factors for obesity. First, important contributing factors such as physical activity, diet composition, and the perception of the child's weight are not available from the medical record. Second, we did not have any information on the fathers of these native American preschoolers. Third, some degree of uncertainty was introduced by using charted measurements whose accuracy cannot be confirmed. However, we have no reason to believe that systematic measurement bias was operating during this study. Despite these limitations, the record review is a valuable first step in determining a baseline prevalence of and risk factors for obesity.

Further studies are needed to identify other potential risk factors for obesity to develop effective prevention strategies. The high prevalence of obesity among native American adults, with its associated high rates of diabetes and hypertension, is well documented.[32] Interventions are needed that focus on preventing obesity during childhood to avoid the long-term consequences of obesity in this population. Preschool children may be a desirable target population because they have regular contact with the medical system during well-baby visits. Given the high prevalence of obesity among the mothers and the strong association between child and maternal obesity, interventions targeted at the family rather than just the child may be most effective.

The opinions expressed in this article are those of the authors and do not necessarily reflect the views of the Indian Health Service.

The authors thank the Tribal Council, the record room staff at the Mescalero (NM) Indian Health Service Hospital, Robert Baldor, MD, and the Albuquerque (NM) Area Indian Health Service Office for their assistance in conducting this study.

References

1. Kelsey JL, Acheson RM, Keggi KJ. The body build of patients with slipped capital femoral epiphysis. *AJDC.* 1972;124:276-281.

2. Dietz WJ Jr, Gross WC, Kirkpatrick JA Jr. Blount disease (tibia vara): another skeletal disorder associated with childhood obesity. *J Pediatr.* 1982;101:735-737.

3. Lauer RM, Anderson AK, Beaglehole R, Burns TL. Factors related to tracking of blood pressure in children. *Hypertension.* 1984;6:307-314.

4. Rames LK, Clarke WR, Connor WE, Reiter MA, Lauer RM. Normal blood pressures and the evaluation of sustained blood pressure elevation in childhood: the Muscatine study. *Pediatrics.* 1978;61:245-251.

5. Gutin B, Basch C, Shea S, et al. Blood pressure, fitness and fatness in 5- and 6-year-old children. *JAMA.* 1990;264:1123-1127.

6. Monello LF, Mayer J. Obese adolescent girls: an interdisciplinary study of adolescent obesity. *J Pediatr.* 1972;13:35-39.

7. Charney E, Goodman HC, McBride M, et al. Childhood antecedents of adult obesity: do chubby infants become obese adults? *N Engl J Med.* 1976;295:6-9.

8. Stark D, Atkins E, Wolff DH, Douglas JWB. Longitudinal study of obesity in the National Survey of Health and Development. *BMJ.* 1981;283:12-17.

9. Stunkard AJ, Penick SB. Behavior modification in the treatment of obesity: the problem of maintaining weight loss. *Arch Gen Psychiatry.* 1979;36:801-806.

10. Centers for Disease Control. Nutrition surveillance. *CDC Surveillance Summaries.* 1983;32(No. 4SS):23-26.

11. Garn SM, Clark DC. Trends in fatness and the origins of obesity. *Pediatrics.* 1976;57:443-456.

12. Patterson RE, Typpo JT, Typpo MH, Krause GF. Factors related to obesity in preschool children. *J Am Diet Assoc.* 1986;86:1376-1381.

13. Stunkard A, d'Aquili E, Fox S, Filion RDL. Influence of social class on obesity and thinness in children. *JAMA.* 1972;221:579-583.

14. Ginsberg-Fellner F, Jagendorf LA, Carmel H, Harris T. Overweight and obesity in preschool children in New York City. *Am J Clin Nutr.* 1981;34:2236-2241.

15. Jacoby A, Altman DG, Cook J, Holland WW. Influence of some social and environmental factors on the nutrient intake and nutritional status of schoolchildren. *Br J Prev Soc Med.* 1975;29:116-120.

16. Mescalero Service Unit Profile, 1988. Available from: Albuquerque Area Office, Indian Health Service, Albuquerque, NM.

17. *ANTHRO: Anthropometry Software Program for the PC.* Atlanta, Ga: Division of Nutrition, Centers for Disease Control; 1988.

18. Dibley MJ, Goldsby JB, Staehling NW, Trowbridge FL. Development of normalized curves for the international growth reference: historical and technical considerations. *Am J Clin Nutr.* 1987;46:736-748.

19. Hamill PVV, Drizd TA, Johnson CL, Reed RB, Roche AF.

NCHS Growth Curves for Children Birth-18 Years, United States, November 1977. Rockville, Md: National Center for Health Statistics; 1977. Vital and Health Statistics 165 (series II), US Dept of Health, Education, and Welfare publication (PHS) 78-1650.

20. National Center for Health Statistics. *Plan and Operation of the Second National Health and Nutrition Examination Survey, 1976-1980.* Washington, DC: US Government Printing Office; 1981. Vital and Health Statistics 14 (series I), US Dept of Health and Human Services publication (PHS) 81-1213.

21. Dean AG, Dean JA, Burton AH, Dicker RC. Epi Info Version 5: a word processing, database, and statistics program for epidemiology on microcomputers. Stone Mountain, Ga: USD Inc; 1990.

22. McGee DL. Logress Version 2.0: a program for logistic regression on the IBM PC. *Am J Epidemiol.* 1986;124:702-705.

23. Trowbridge FL, Marks JS, Lopez de Romana G, Madrid S, Boutton TW, Klein PD. Body composition of Peruvian children with short stature and high weight-for-height, II: implications for the interpretation for weight-for-height as an indicator of nutritional status. *Am J Clin Nutr.* 1987;46:411-418.

24. Stunkard AJ, Sorensen TI, Hanis C, et al. An adoption study of human obesity. *N Engl J Med.* 1986;814:193-198.

25. Siervogel RM. Genetic and familial factors in human obesity. In: Krasnegor NA, Grave GD, Knetchener N, eds. *Childhood Obesity: A Biobehavioral Perspective*. Caldwell, NJ: Telford Press; 1988; 31-47.

26. Alexander MA, Blank JJ. Factors related to obesity in Mexican-American preschool children. *Image: J Nurs Scholarship.* 1988;20:79-82.

27. Garbaciak JA, Richter M, Miller S, Barton JJ. Maternal weight and pregnancy complications. *Am J Obstet Gynecol.* 1985;152:238-245.

28. Edwards LE, Dickes WF, Alton IR, Hakanson EY. Pregnancy in the massively obese: course, outcome, and obesity prognosis of the infant. *Am J Obstet Gynecol.* 1978;131:479-483.

29. Gross TL. Operative considerations in the obese pregnant patient. *Clin Perinatol.* 1983;10:411-421.

30. Binkin NJ, Yip R, Fleshood L, Trowbridge FL. Birthweight and childhood growth. *Pediatrics.* 1988;82:828-834.

31. Michielutte R, Diseker RA, Corbett WT, Schey HM, Ureda JR. The relationship between weight-height indices and the triceps skinfold measure among children age 5 to 12. *Am J Public Health.* 1984;74:604-606.

32. Jackson MY. Nutrition in American Indian health: past, present, and future. *J Am Diet Assoc.* 1986;86:1561-1565.

In Other AMA Journals

ARCHIVES OF NEUROLOGY

Monozygotic Twins With Seizures: Shared Characteristics

Rosalind A. Segal, Md, PhD; Catherine Chapman, MD; John Barlow, MD (*Arch Neurol.* 1991;48:1041-1045)

Isolated Congenital Hemianopia Caused by Prenatal Injury to the Optic Radiation

Nicola K. Ragge, MRCP, FCOphth; A. James Barkovich, MD; William F. Hoyt, MD; Scott R. Lambert, MD (*Arch Neurol.* 1991;48:1088-1091)

Serum Lipid Concentrations in Subjects With Phenylketonuria and Their Families

Terry J. DeClue, MD; Jim Davis, MD; Dawn M. Schocken, MPH; Ruth Kangas, RD; Steve A. Benford

• To determine if subjects with phenylketonuria receiving diets significantly lower in cholesterol and saturated fat had serum lipid concentrations different from those of their family members, we measured serum concentrations of total cholesterol, high-density lipoprotein cholesterol, and total triglycerides in the probands with phenylketonuria, their parents, and their siblings. Eleven adults (seven women and four men) and 16 children (eight girls and eight boys) were studied. Ten subjects (four girls and six boys) had phenylketonuria. Subjects with phenylketonuria consumed less cholesterol (0.02 vs 0.41 mmol/d) and fat (median, 21% vs 39.5% of total calories), and their diets had a higher ratio of polyunsaturated to saturated fatty acids (median, 2.0 vs 0.2) than did their siblings without phenylketonuria. The diet of the parents was similar to that of their offspring without phenylketonuria. No differences were noted between the subjects with phenylketonuria (consuming a diet lower in saturated fat and cholesterol) and their siblings without phenylketonuria in serum concentrations of total cholesterol (median, 3.34 vs 3.07 mmol/L); high-density lipoprotein cholesterol (median, 1.44 vs 1.37 mmol/L); low-density lipoprotein cholesterol (median, 1.44 vs 1.09 mmol/L); or triglycerides (median, 0.89 vs 0.54 mmol/L). We conclude that previously reported lipoprotein abnormalities noted between unrelated subjects with and without phenylketonuria may not be due to differences in dietary intake, but rather due to a (genetic) predisposition of the population with phenylketonuria toward lower serum lipid concentrations.

(*AJDC*. 1991;145:1266-1268)

Phenylketonuria (PKU) is an inborn error of metabolism secondary to a deficiency of phenylalanine hydroxylase. It is inherited as an autosomal recessive trait, and dietary intervention is the only treatment currently available. The basis of the PKU diet is to restrict phenylalanine intake early in life. To supply the recommended daily allowances of protein, carbohydrates, and fats, special casein hydrolysate formulas are used. As the patient ages, various low-protein solid food exchanges are added to the diet. Because of the reduction of animal protein in the patients' diet, they generally consume a lower percentage of calories from fat and cholesterol than does the general population.[1,2] It has been suggested that the PKU diet is responsible for the lower values of total cholesterol, low-density lipoprotein cholesterol (LDL-C), and high-density lipoprotein cholesterol (HDL-C) noted in the subject with PKU.[1-3] We evaluated lipoproteins in children with PKU and their families to determine if other (familial) factors might be responsible for these changes in serum total cholesterol.

Accepted for publication June 17, 1991.

From the Department of Pediatrics, University of South Florida Health Sciences Center.

Presented in part at the Southern Society for Pediatric Research Meeting, January 19, 1990; New Orleans, La.

Reprint requests to University of South Florida, MDC Box 45, 12901 Bruce B. Downs Blvd, Tampa, FL 33612-4799 (Dr DeClue).

SUBJECTS AND METHODS

Seven families with at least one child attending the PKU clinic at the University of South Florida were enrolled. Ten children (four girls and six boys) with PKU (median age, 7.3 years; range, 0.75 to 30 years) and six siblings without PKU (two girls and four boys; median age, 7.1 years; range, 5 to 17 years) were evaluated. Two subjects with PKU were older than 25 years (27 and 30 years) and had not been prescribed a phenylalanine-restricted diet at birth. At the time of the study, all subjects with PKU were receiving an appropriate phenylalanine-restricted diet. Eleven parents (seven women and four men) with a median age of 33 years (range, 24 to 48 years) were also studied. All subjects were euthyroid and none was obese. The study was reviewed and approved by the Institutional Review Board of the University of South Florida; informed consent was obtained from each family member before enrollment. Each subject studied completed a 3-day food diary before blood collection. The food diary was analyzed by a registered dietitian using Nutritionist III (N-Squared Computing, Silverton, Ore) for content of protein; carbohydrate; fat; cholesterol; and monounsaturated, polyunsaturated, and saturated fatty acids. The dietary information for each individual was averaged and reported as median and range for a 24-hour period.

On the day of blood collection, following an overnight fast, the subjects' heights and weights were measured and they were allowed to sit for 10 to 15 minutes before blood samples were collectied through an antecubital vein. Following collection, the serum was separated immediately. Serum concentrations of total cholesterol, HDL-C, triglycerides, and thyrotropin were measured in all subjects, and phenylalanine levels were determined in the probands with PKU. The serum sample for HDL-C was refrigerated at 4°C until assayed 48 to 72 hours after collection. Serum samples for analysis of total cholesterol, triglycerides, and thyrotropin were frozen at −70°C until assay. Total cholesterol, HDL-C, and triglyceride levels were measured at the University of Miami using nationally standardized methods previously de-

Subjects	No. of Subjects	Median (Range)				
		Protein	Carbohydrate	Fat	Cholesterol, mmol/d	P/S Ratio
Parents	8	20 (15-29)†	41.5 (28-63)†	38.5 (15-54)‡	0.63 (0.16-3.63)	0.59 (0.1-1.3)†
Children with PKU	7	11 (8-16)	68 (50-79)	21 (9-41)	0.02 (0.002-0.12)	2.0 (0.94-3.7)
Non-PKU children	4	15 (13-21)‡	46 (38-49)†	39.5 (38-42)†	0.41 (0.37-0.56)	0.2 (0.15-0.57)†

Table 1.—Dietary Analysis of Children With Phenylketonuria (PKU) and Their Family Members*

*Protein, carbohydrate, and fat values are percentages of total calories consumed per day. P/S indicates ratio of polyunsaturated to saturated fatty acids.
†$P<.005$ for children with PKU vs parents or non-PKU children.
‡$P<.05$ for children with PKU vs parents or non-PKU children.

Table 2.—Serum Lipid Concentrations*

Subjects	No. of Subjects	Median (Range)			
		Total Cholesterol mmol/L	HDL-C, mmol/L	LDL-C, mmol/L	Triglycerides, mmol/L
Parents	11	5.15 (2.96-6.63)	1.53 (0.78-3.12)	3.15 (0.42-4.73)	0.89 (0.15-2.40)
Children with PKU	10	3.34 (2.76-4.42)	1.44 (0.91-2.34)	1.44 (0.18-2.78)	0.89 (0.32-1.61)
Non-PKU children	6	3.07 (1.79-4.03)	1.37 (1.09-2.26)	1.09 (0.16-2.18)	0.54 (0.25-1.33)

*HDL-C and LDL-C indicate high-density and low-density lipoprotein cholesterol, respectively.

scribed.[4] Thyrotropin level was measured with a standard radioimmunoassay. Serum phenylalanine was measured using ion exchange chromatography with postcolumn triketohydrindene hydrate (Ninhydrin) detection. Statistical analyses were made using Student's *t* test.

RESULTS

The patients with PKU consumed significantly fewer calories from total fat and protein, but more calories from carbohydrates, than did their family members (Table 1). The subjects with PKU also consumed significantly less cholesterol in their diet, and the ratio of their polyunsaturated to saturated fatty acid intake was much higher. The diet of the parents was similar to that of the siblings without PKU; although the parents consumed more cholesterol, the difference was not statistically significant.

No differences were noted in serum concentrations of total cholesterol, HDL-C, LDL-C, and triglycerides between the subjects with PKU (consuming a diet significantly lower in cholesterol and higher in polyunsaturated fat) and their family members (Table 2). The serum concentrations of total cholesterol, LDL-C, and triglycerides in the parents were higher, but not statistically different, from the offspring with or without PKU. The HDL-C values were similar among all three groups. Thyrotropin levels were normal in all subjects. The mean (±SD) serum phenylalanine concentration in the patients with PKU was 365±242 μmol/L.

COMMENT

Previous investigators have reported that serum or plasma total cholesterol values were significantly lower in subjects with PKU than in unrelated control subjects without PKU.[1-3] Acosta et al[3] evaluated 93 children with PKU (23 children were not receiving a phenylalanine-restricted diet) and 30 normal control subjects and found that the total and free serum cholesterol values were lower in the children with PKU than in the normal subjects. Galluzzo et al[2] measured plasma levels of total cholesterol and HDL-C in 40 healthy, treated patients with PKU (triglycerides were measured in 30) and 150 sex- and age-matched control subjects. In this study, patients with PKU had significantly lower total cholesterol values than control subjects. There was no difference in HDL-C or triglyceride values, and LDL-C levels were not determined. Similarly, Schulpi and Scarpalezou[1] evaluated serum lipid concentrations in 20 Greek children with PKU and compared them with those in 200 matched healthy children. Significant differences were noted in triglyceride, total cholesterol, HDL-C, and very low density lipoprotein cholesterol concentrations, with the subjects with PKU having the more favorable profile. There was no difference in LDL-C levels between the two groups.

Recently, it has been noted that there is genetic heterogeneity in the response of serum lipid concentrations to alterations in the intake of cholesterol and saturated fat.[5] Sensitivity to dietary cholesterol varies among subjects, with the majority effectively compensating for increases in dietary cholesterol by feedback suppression of endogenous cholesterol synthesis, coupled with a reduction in dietary cholesterol fractional absorption. Hypothesizing that familial factors in addition to diet may affect serum lipid concentrations in individuals with PKU, we evaluated subjects with PKU and compared them with their parents and siblings without PKU.

Our study confirms that individuals with PKU receiving an appropriately low-phenylalanine diet consume significantly less cholesterol and a lower percentage of calories from fat in their diet. The majority of the fat consumed by our children with PKU consisted of polyunsaturated fatty acids. Diets high in polyunsaturated fatty acids lower HDL-C in subjects without PKU; however, no differences were noted in our study in HDL-C levels between groups. The small number of patients in this study does not reveal subtle changes that might occur in HDL-C between the various groups.

The greatest differences among the two sibling groups

was between serum concentrations of total cholesterol and HDL-C and total triglycerides. It is interesting that those children (without PKU) who consumed the largest amount of cholesterol and saturated fatty acids in their diet had lower serum total cholesterol and LDL-C concentrations. This is contrary to what one might expect since subjects consuming the highest amounts of dietary cholesterol are expected to have the higher serum total cholesterol concentrations. It is unlikely that age-related differences could account for the differences in serum cholesterol measurements between the siblings with and without PKU, since the subjects with PKU were of similar age. If the two oldest subjects with PKU are excluded in the analysis, the results are essentially the same (serum total cholesterol [n=8]: median, 3.46 mmol/L; range, 2.8 to 4.5 mmol/L). In view of this finding it is possible that the serum total cholesterol changes noted during variations in dietary intake are related to a threshold effect. For example, within genetically similar groups, unless a quantity of cholesterol above a certain threshold is consumed, the serum total cholesterol is unchanged. This would be in agreement with the findings of McNamara et al.[5]

Higher serum triglyceride values in children with PKU have been reported previously and have been suggested to be secondary to the significantly higher percentage of calories from carbohydrates consumed by the subject with PKU.[1] We noted similar findings in our study and agree that increasing the total percentage of calories from fat in the form of monounsaturated fatty acids in the diet (and lowering the polyunsaturated fatty acids and carbohydrates) may have a more favorable effect on serum HDL-C and LDL-C concentrations, as well as on serum triglyceride measurements.[6]

As a group, the families with PKU have favorable lipid profiles (Table 2). Of the seven families studied, one had familial combined hyperlipidemia. The proband with PKU was the only child in this family. Compared with the other siblings (with or without PKU), this child had the highest serum total cholesterol (4.4 mmol/L) and LDL-C (2.8 mmol/L) values. If this family is excluded from the analysis, there is no significant change in the overall results.

Subjects with PKU consume a diet that is less atherogenic than that of the general population. Previous studies have compared lipid profiles in children with PKU (demonstrating lower total cholesterol concentrations) to unrelated normal children without PKU.[1-3] It is likely that those studies were flawed in their comparisons because they did not control for possible genetic influence in cholesterol metabolism between the two groups. We did not demonstrate any differences in serum total cholesterol levels between children with or without PKU, although the subjects without PKU consumed 10 times more cholesterol and twice the fat in their diet. The highest total cholesterol and LDL-C measurement among the siblings studied was in a child with PKU from a family with familial combined hyperlipidemia. If the serum total cholesterol data from these children with PKU had been compared with data from children from the general population, the wrong conclusion would have been made (ie, that the lower cholesterol and fat in the diet is responsible for the lower serum total cholesterol values in the subjects with PKU). Our study suggests that genetic influences in cholesterol metabolism should be considered an important variable in interpreting total cholesterol data from children. Our data suggest that families with a child with PKU have lower serum total cholesterol values than the general population and that other factors (eg, familial combined hyperlipidemia) have a greater influence on cholesterol metabolism than diet.

We wish to thank Ronald Goldberg, MD, for measuring the lipoproteins, and Herbert H. Pomerance, MD, Allen W. Root, MD, and John I. Malone, MD, for their critical review of the article.

References

1. Schulpi KH, Scarpalezou A. Triglycerides, cholesterol, HDL, LDL, and VLDL cholesterol in serum of phenylketonuric children under dietary control. *Clin Pediatr.* 1989;28:466-469.
2. Galluzzo CR, Ortisi MY, Castelli L, Agostoni C, Longhi R. Plasma lipid concentration in 42 treated phenylketonuric children. *J Inherited Metab Dis.* 1985;8(suppl):129.
3. Acosta PB, Alfin-Slater RB, Koch R. Serum lipids in children with phenylketonuria (PKU). *J Am Diet Assoc.* 1973;63:631-635.
4. Allain CC, Poon LS, Chan CSG, Richmond W, Fu PC. Enzymatic determination of total serum cholesterol. *Clin Chem.* 1974;20:470-475.
5. McNamara DJ, Kolb R, Parker TS, Batwin H, et al. Heterogeneity of cholesterol homeostasis in man: response to changes in dietary fat quality and cholesterol quantity. *J Clin Invest.* 1987;79:1729-1739.
6. Mensink RP, Katan MB. Effect of monounsaturated fatty acids versus complex carbohydrates on high-density lipoproteins in healthy men and women. *Lancet.* 1987;1:122-125.

Adolescent Pelvic Examination

An Effective Practical Approach

Hyman C. Tolmas, MD

• The American Academy of Pediatrics has recommended that pediatric health care be extended through the adolescent years. Thus, there is a need to refamiliarize the physician with the pelvic examination. Formerly, workshops used simulated plastic models ("Ginny") to accomplish this goal. Such workshops have been conducted at the annual meeting of the American Academy of Pediatrics for several years. At the 1987 meeting in New Orleans, La, two workshops involving live models (gynecologic teaching assistants) were planned and implemented with great success. Following a didactic segment, each participant was given an opportunity to perform the pelvic examination with immediate feedback from the gynecologic teaching assistant as to the completeness and appropriateness of the pelvic examination. The immediate response of the attendees was overwhelmingly positive. A questionnaire was sent to the enrollees 8 months after the meeting to determine whether this experience had affected their attitude toward and approach to the pelvic examination. Eighty-three percent of questionnaires were returned with an affirmative response. This positive response suggested that such workshops be continued in an effort to reach as many pediatricians as possible.

(*AJDC*. 1991;145:1269-1271)

For several years, the Adolescent Health Section of the American Academy of Pediatrics has conducted workshops at the annual meeting that used the plastic "Ginny" models to teach the correct methods to perform a pelvic examination. Videotapes demonstrating the technique were used, and one or more moderators assisted participants with their examinations and answered questions.

The academy has placed special emphasis on adolescent health care.[1] Thus, pediatricians must learn or relearn how to perform pelvic examinations on adolescent patients. The gynecologic examination of an adolescent should not be a difficult experience for the patient, the parent, or the physician. The skills necessary to ensure a successful examination are attainable by any sensitive pediatrician willing to take the time to acquire them.[2] Historically, instruction in performance of the abdominal/pelvic examination in medical school and residency programs has been neglected. The objective of this workshop was to familiarize the pediatrician with the special needs of the adolescent gynecologic patient and to make him or her feel at ease while performing a screening examination of the female genitalia.

The use of live human models to teach the pelvic examination was originally introduced at a few medical centers beginning in 1971. Kretzschmar[3] reported his experience at the University of Iowa, Iowa City, employing trained volunteers called gynecology teaching associates (GTAs) to teach pelvic and breast examinations to medical students. This program proved to be an extremely effective method. Johnson[4] evaluated the impact of a similar system for a small group of students. The American Academy of Pediatrics first used the live teaching model at its annual meeting in 1986. Holzman et al[5] showed that students trained by professional simulated patients rated substantially better in psychomotor and interpersonal relations than did those taught by the mannequin or the physician preceptors techniques.

I presented the results of a carefully planned, hands-on workshop at the annual meeting of the American Academy of Pediatrics in 1987. I also presented the long-term effect as determined by questionnaire survey of the participants.

METHODS

Setting and Equipment

An appropriate setting is essential for adequate, "real-life" simulation of the examination milieu. Accordingly, the gynecologic clinic at Tulane Medical Center, New Orleans, La, was selected with provision of clinical examining rooms approximating the office setting of participants. In addition, classroom space was made available for the didactic sessions.

An adequate amount of supplies were provided for each examining room, eg, disposable gloves, specula, a mirror for patient education, a washbasin, laboratory equipment for the demonstration of Papanicolaou smears, and vaginal and cervical culture material for the preparation of microscopic slides. Visual aids were employed to explain pertinent concepts and to review anatomic relationships. A GTA acted as the overall moderator and supervisor for all the enrollees; she circulated among all examination sites.

Accepted for publication July 19, 1991.
From the Department of Pediatrics, Tulane University School of Medicine, New Orleans, La.
Reprint requests to 466 Crystal St, New Orleans, LA 70124 (Dr Tolmas).

Table 1.—Results of Evaluation by Participants*

Category	Score, Session 1/Session 2
Overall evaluation	4.63/4.64
Relevance to practice	4.57/4.64
Appropriateness of topic	4.63/4.76
Discussion	4.34/4.60
Handouts	4.41/4.52
Audiovisual	4.36/4.36

*Each session is evaluated on a scale of 1 to 5, with 5 being the highest score. The categories of evaluations and the scores received for each session are listed.

Faculty

Three physicians presented the didactic material. Two of these physicians were gynecologists, and the third was a physician trained in adolescent medicine.

Program

The 40 physicians were divided into two groups. One group attended lectures by faculty. Each of the three speakers presented a 15-minute discussion on one aspect of adolescent gynecology, eg, preliminary examination, sexually transmitted diseases, and sexuality. A question-and-answer period followed the discussion.

The second group was divided into smaller groups of four for instruction by the GTA in an examination room. Details of the pelvic examination were demonstrated, and each attendee performed an examination of a GTA. Several diagnostic studies (eg, wet mount) were also performed. The groups then switched; those who had been in the lectures performed examinations and vice versa.

A kit consisting of informative material was provided to each participant and included a group of published articles relating to adolescent gynecology.[6] Also distributed was a brief summary of the Gynecological Teaching Associates Program, a flow chart about contraceptive measures, and a detailed chart about oral contraceptives.

EVALUATION

The American Academy of Pediatrics distributed an evaluation form usually used as a yardstick to determine the effectiveness of any given workshop or seminar. We developed a specific questionnaire to evaluate certain aspects of the workshop.

The American Academy of Pediatrics received 38 responses to 40 questionnaires sent for the morning session and 25 responses to 26 questionnaires sent for the afternoon session. The ratings of the participants are listed in Table 1.

Among the comments by both session participants in response to a question about the most helpful aspects of the workshop were the following: "the hands-on experience," "graduate teaching assistants to teach the performance of the pelvic examination and actually performing the examination," "practicality and suitability for practice," "organization," "how to approach the adolescent patient and what to tell her," and "the discussion about the sexually abused child."

Among those comments listed in response to a question about the least helpful aspects of the workshop were as follows: "too many lectures in a short time," "lack of time," "too hurried," "should have more time for lectures," and "lectures should precede the practical examination."

Table 2.—Ratings of 55 Respondents (of 66 Attendees) Listed by Category*

Category	Score
Usefulness of workshop	9.3±0.99
Clarity and effectiveness of instructors	9.1±1.12
Material covered	8.9±1.13
Value of take-home kit	8.9±0.97
Effect on your practice	8.7±1.27
Value of gynecologic teaching assistant	9.8±0.54
Usefulness of doing actual vaginal examination	9.6±0.86

*Scores are mean±SD, with 10 being the highest score and 1 being the lowest.

Table 3.—Results of Follow-up Questionnaire

Question	Response, No. (%) Yes	No
Were you performing pelvic examinations on your adolescent patients where indicated before attending the workshop?	33 (70.2)	14 (29.8)
Do you feel more at ease doing a pelvic examination on your adolescent patients now?	44 (93.7)	1 (2.13)*
Do you discuss sexuality with your female adolescents?	38 (80.85)	5 (10.64)†
Do you perform cultures and/or Papanicolaou smears?	43 (91.49)	3 (6.38)‡
Do you believe that this type of workshop should continue to be a part of the annual meeting?	47 (100)	0 (0)

*Two respondents (4.26%) did not answer.
†Four respondents (8.51%) answered "sometimes."
‡One respondent (2.13%) did not answer.

The respondents suggested that the course be extended to a 3-hour format. The results of the evaluation are listed in Table 2.

The comments were generally positive (eg, "excellent workshop," "hands-on experience invaluable," "feel comfortable with live models," and "should be required in medical school"). However, the most frequent criticism was inadequate time. A few participants suggested that the didactic lectures lacked sufficient specifics regarding birth control, sexually transmitted diseases, relating to parents of teenagers, and the psychological aspects of sexuality. The GTAs received the most positive comments (eg, "excellent," "extraordinary teaching skills," and "the most useful lesson I have learned").

FOLLOW-UP RATINGS

In June 1988, a follow-up letter and questionnaire were sent to the participants in the adolescent pelvic examination workshop requesting that they be completed and returned. Of the 70 questionnaires sent, 47 (67%) were returned with the results shown in Table 3.

RESULTS

Of the 47 respondents, 37 were pediatricians in private practice (26 were in group practice, and 11 were in solo practice). The other 10 respondents were distributed as follows: pediatric child abuse (n=3), pediatric emergency room (n=1), family practice (n=1), resident in pediatrics (n=1), college health (n=2), and school health (n=2).

In response to the question, "Identify the type of setting for patient care" (eg, school health, private practice, and community clinic), the following answers were recorded: private practice (n=26), community clinic (n=6), multispecialty group (n=5), community/school health (n=2), sexual abuse clinic (n=2), large prepaid health plan (n=2), and hospital (n=4). Thirty-one answered affirmatively to the question "Do you perform pelvic examinations now?"

COMMENT

Gynecologic and contraceptive needs of teenagers were topics pediatricians had little need to consider in the past. Today, the pediatrician cares for a broader age group than in the past, necessitating knowledge and skills appropriate to this age group.[7,8] Learning the skills to perform the pelvic examination by the use of various plastic models of the breast, abdomen, and pelvis is inadequate. Plastic materials lack realistic pliability and resilience and the capacity for feedback about the accuracy of the examination. They also provide no sense of the potential discomfort that a patient may experience during the examination.[9]

An important component to adolescent gynecologic evaluation is the history obtained before the pelvic examination is performed. This should include family history; peer, school, and community involvement (social activities); and history of sexual activity and menstruation.

The first gynecologic examination is often of considerable importance for the female adolescent. She may feel pride, with a certain regret that she is leaving childhood behind. With sensitivity and careful planning, the physician will set the stage for a good physician-patient relationship that continues into adulthood.[10]

The program described herein, which utilizes live examinees, has been successful in refamiliarizing physicians with the need for pelvic examinations and ease with which they can be performed in the adolescent patient as judged by the positive responses of participants. There is a genuine need for evaluation procedures to measure the persistence of the learned skills and the adequacy of examinations in the actual practice of pediatric adolescent medicine.

References

1. Cohen MI. Importance, implementations, and impact of the adolescent medicine components of the report of the task force in pediatric education. *J Adolesc Health Care.* 1980;1:1-8.

2. Talbot CW. The gynecologic examination in the pediatric patient. *Pediatr Ann.* July 1986;15:501-508.

3. Kretzschmar LM. Evolution of the gynecologiy teaching associate: an education specialist. *Am J Obstet Gynecol.* 1978; 131:367-373.

4. Johnson GH. Teaching pelvic examinations to second year medical students using programmed patients. *Am J Obstet Gynecol.* 1975;121:714-717.

5. Holzman GB, Singleton D, Holmes TF, Maatch JL. Initial pelvic examination instruction: the effectiveness of three contemporary approaches. *Am J Obstet Gynecol.* 1977; 129:124-129.

6. Sanfilippo JS. Adolescent gynecologic practice. *Pediatr Ann.* July 1986;5:499-501.

7. Tyrer LD, Rothbart B, Anderson K. What every teen should know about contraceptives. *Contemporary Pediatr.* 1989;6:68-94.

8. McAnarney ER, Hendee WR. The prevention of adolescent pregnancy. *JAMA.* 1989;262:78-82.

9. Plauche WC, Baugniet-Nevrija W. Student's and physician's evaluations of gynecologic teaching associates programs. *J Med Educ.* 1985;60:870-875.

10. Leppert PC. Adolescent's first pelvic examination. *Contemp Obstet Gynecol.* 1986;28:76-92. Special Issue.

Current Trends in Pediatric Residency Training

Carol Carraccio, MD, Alice Ackerman, MD

• A spreading gap has developed between available pediatric level 1 positions and those filled through the National Resident Matching Program. To define which variables enhance a program's ability to match, we surveyed program directors of all categorical pediatric training programs. An 82% response rate showed that ability to match was positively associated with larger program size and offering of shared residency positions. A negative association was found between many benefits and ability to match. The call schedule and number of call-free elective months had no measurable effect. Factors that we were unable to investigate, such as geographic location and academic reputation, may also play a role. Our results emphasize the irrelevance of enhancing benefits as a way of making programs competitive. Our energies need to be directed at attracting junior medical students to a career in pediatrics rather than competing for fourth-year students applying to pediatric programs.

(*AJDC.* 1991;145:1272-1275)

During the last decade, the total number of pediatric residency positions offered through the National Resident Matching Program (NRMP) has increased steadily from 1808 in 1980, to 2068 in 1989, with a slight drop to 2052 in 1990 (Fig 1).[1,2] Although the percent of US graduates applying for these positions has remained constant, ranging from 9.2% to 10%, the absolute number of US graduates in the matching program showed a steady increase only through 1985, with a gradual decline from 1986 through 1990.[1,2] During the early 1970s, approximately 8500 active US students were participating in the match, with a continued increase to a peak of 14 849 in 1985. A gradual decline then ensued, with only 13 908 US seniors actively participating in the 1990 NRMP.[1,2] The spreading gap created by the increasing availability of positions and the declining number of US graduates filling these positions has led to more programs not filling through the NRMP. In 1986, 135 (65%) of the 209 categorical pediatric training programs participating in the NRMP completely filled all their available positions.[3] In 1987, this figure dropped to 61%.[4] In 1988, 1989, and 1990, 52%, 41%, and 53% of programs, respectively, completely filled through the NRMP.[5-7]

Accepted for publication April 22, 1991.

From the Department of Pediatrics, University of Maryland Medical Center, Baltimore.

Reprint requests to Department of Pediatrics, Room N5W56, University of Maryland, 22 S Greene St, Baltimore, MD 21201 (Dr Carraccio).

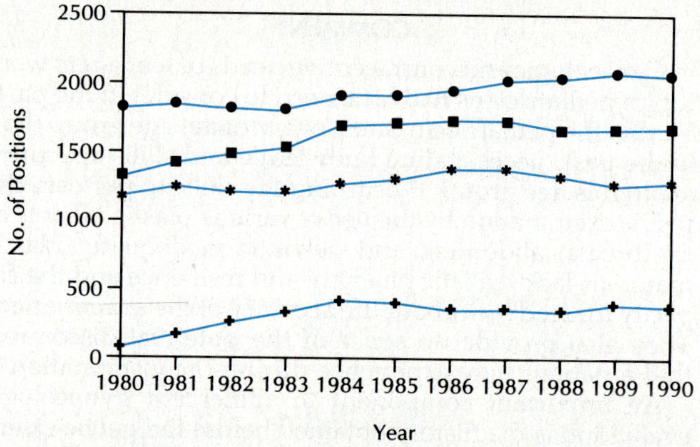

Fig 1.—*Positions available and filled by US (asterisks) and foreign medical graduates (pluses) through the National Resident Matching Program between 1980 and 1990. Plain line indicates positions available; line with squares, total filled.*

Between 1986 and 1990, the percent of the total positions filled by US graduates fell from 86.1% in 1986, to 80.0% in 1989, rising slightly in 1990, to 81.3%.[1,2] During each of the last 5 years, foreign medical graduates filled 15% to 20% of the total number of pediatric positions filled through the NRMP. The current situation has created a competitive climate among programs to attract applicants to fill pediatric residency training positions. We undertook this study to determine which factors, if any, contribute to the ability of programs to fill their available positions.

Purpose.—*This department is intended to share information concerning educational efforts in the broad field of pediatrics. We welcome studies on the following topics: undergraduate and graduate education in medicine and allied health occupations; continuing education of health professionals; education of patients and families; and health education for the general public, the community, and organizations that contribute to the promotion and improvement of the health of children.*

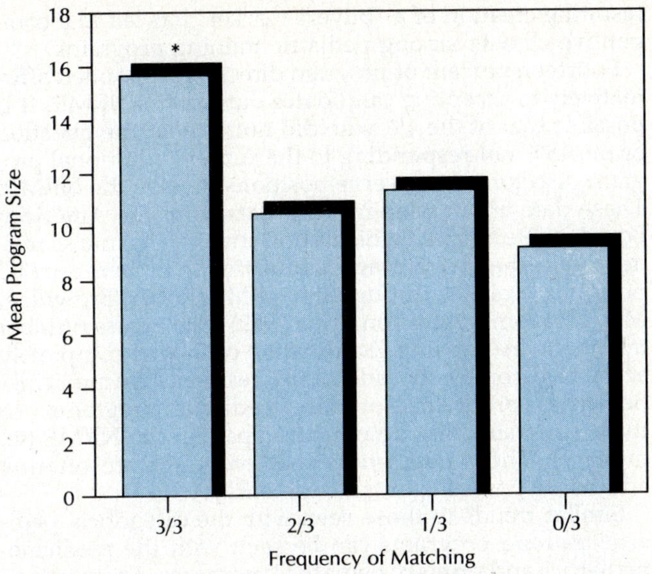

Fig 2.—*Mean number of pediatric level 1 positions in programs matching 3, 2, 1, or 0 of 3 years, 1987 through 1989. Asterisk indicates P<.05.*

MATERIALS AND METHODS

The 239 categorical pediatric residency training programs listed in the *1989-1990 Directory of Graduate Medical Education Programs*[8] were surveyed. We did not survey the 81 medicine-pediatrics, nine primary pediatrics, or two pediatrics-psychiatry–child psychiatry programs.[2] An anonymous questionnaire was sent to each program director requesting the following information: (1) total number of pediatric level 1 (PL1) positions; (2) whether the program matched for 1987, 1988, and 1989; (3) how many positions are reserved to be filled outside the NRMP; (4) the benefit package offered; (5) the frequency of night call in 1987, 1988, and 1989; (6) the number of shared residency positions; (7) the number of call-free elective months; and (8) the percent of male and female residents for each of the 3 study years. A second survey was sent to all programs 2 months after the first survey requesting program directors to respond if they had not previously done so.

The results were analyzed using Statistical Analysis Systems software. The data were separated into the following four groups for analysis: (1) those programs not filling their available positions in 1987, 1988, and 1989; (2) those programs filling 1 of the 3 years; (3) those programs filling 2 of the 3 years; and (4) those programs filling all available positions all 3 years. Analysis of variance and Tukey's test were used to determine whether significant differences in interval level variables existed among the groups. To analyze differences in categorical variables, the group matching 0 of 3 years was used as the reference, and all other groups were compared with it using a logistic regression model. We considered $P<.05$ to be significant.

RESULTS

One hundred fifty (63%) program directors responded on the first mailing. An additional 47 responded on the second mailing, for a total response rate of 82%.

Forty-five programs (23%) did not fill their available positions in the 1987, 1988, or 1989 NRMP. Forty programs (20%) filled all their positions 1 of 3 years, 37 (19%) filled 2 of 3 years, and 53 (27%) filled their positions 3 of 3 years. The remaining 11% either did not complete this information or indicated that they did not participate in the NRMP.

Fourteen percent of program directors, despite participation in the NRMP, reserved positions to be filled outside of the matching process. Further breakdown of the data showed 11% of those programs matching 0 of 3 years, 20% matching 1 of 3 years, 14% matching 2 of 3 years, and 8% matching 3 of 3 years in the reserved positions. Four percent of respondents did not answer this question.

A positive relationship existed between the size of the program and the number of years matched. Breakdown of the data showed a significant difference ($P<.0002$) in mean number of available PL1 positions in the programs matching 3 of 3 years (mean, 15.6) when compared with the groups matching 0, 1, and 2 of the 3 years (means of 9.1, 11.2, and 10.4), respectively (Fig 2). Ability to match favored the larger training programs. The number of benefits offered by programs matching 0, 1, 2, or 3 of the 3 study years is given in the Table. Further illustration of the significant relationships between frequency of matching and benefits can be seen in Fig 3. As noted in the "Materials and Methods" section, programs matching 0 of 3 years were used as the reference group. Reanalysis of the data using those programs matching 3 of 3 years as the reference group was exactly the same, with two minor exceptions. The first is that no significant difference was noted in life insurance for the programs that matched 2 of 3 years; the second is that the conference funds were no longer significant for the group that matched 1 of 3 years.

In looking at the number of programs adding benefits during the 3-year period, a significant difference was found in those programs matching 0 of 3 or 1 of 3 years vs 3 of 3 years ($P<.05$). Sixty-four percent and 79% of programs matching 0 of 3 years and 1 of 3 years, respectively, added new benefits, as compared with 17% of programs matching 3 of 3 years. In addition to those benefits listed in the Table, book allowances, retreats, maternity and paternity leave, and free access to MEDLINE were the most frequently cited additional benefits. Interestingly, $4 haircuts and $2 movies were also listed as benefits.

Number (Percent) of Pediatric Programs Offering Various Benefits

	Years Matching			
Benefit	0/3	1/3	2/3	3/3
Medical malpractice	45 (100)	40 (100)	37 (100)	53 (100)
Medical insurance	41 (91)	40 (100)	36 (97)	53 (100)
Dental insurance	34 (76)	30 (75)	25 (68)	40 (75)
Life insurance	38 (84)	31 (77)	23 (62)*	37 (70)
Disability	30 (67)	29 (72)	25 (68)	44 (83)
Vacation	45 (100)	40 (100)	37 (100)	53 (100)
Conference funds	42 (93)	30 (75)*	29 (78)	33 (62)†
Parking	41 (91)	28 (70)*	26 (70)*	25 (47)‡
Meals	33 (73)	34 (85)	32 (86)	42 (79)
Copying	43 (96)	38 (95)	34 (92)	52 (98)
Interview money	21 (47)	10 (25)*	9 (24)*	3 (5.7)‡

*$P<.05$ vs programs matching in none of the study years.
†$P<.01$ vs programs matching in none of the study years.
‡$P<.001$ vs programs matching in none of the study years.

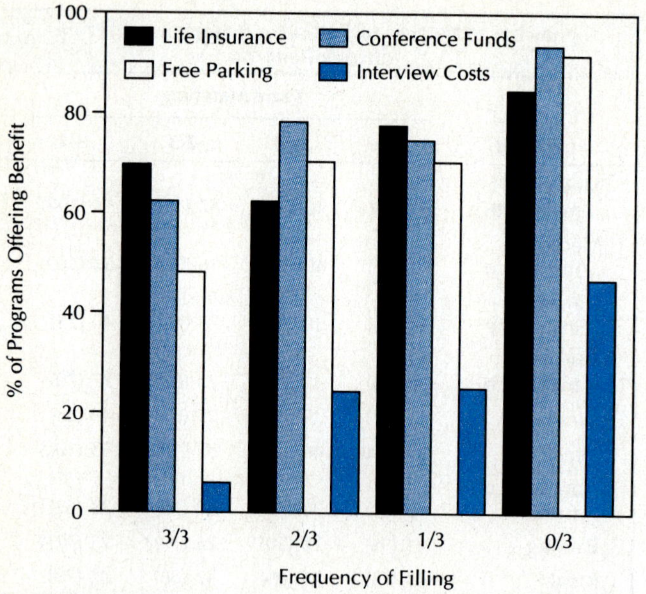

Fig 3.—*Percentage of programs offering various benefits vs matching 0, 1, 2, or 3 of 3 years, 1987 through 1989. See text for description of significant values.*

No significant differences were found in frequency of PL1 night call and the number of years matched. The mean frequency of call between the various groups ranged from every 3.37 to 3.55 nights for 1987, from 3.51 to 3.62 nights for 1988, and from 3.64 to 3.75 nights for 1989. The number of programs decreasing the frequency of the PL1 call between 1987 and 1989 ranged from 19% to 25%. No meaningful relationship between number of call-free elective months and ability to fill through the NRMP was detected. Forty-seven programs offered no call-free months, while 23, 26, and 22 programs offered 1, 2, and 3 call-free months, respectively. Ten programs had 6 call-free months, with the highest number cited being 11 call-free months in a 36-month period.

A positive relationship, however, was demonstrated between ability to match and whether a program offered shared residency positions. Only 23% of programs matching 0 of 3 years offered shared positions, in comparison with 43% of those matching 3 of 3 years ($P<.04$).

The percent male vs female residents was also analyzed in relation to whether a program matched 0, 1, 2, or 3 of the 3 study years. A significant difference in the percent male vs percent female residents was found between programs matching 0 of 3 years and those matching 1, 2, or 3 of the 3 years. The former group was composed of 53% males in comparison with the latter groups, in which the male representation accounted for 45%, 45%, and 44%, respectively.

COMMENT

In a recent commentary appearing in *Pediatrics*, James E. Strain, MD, executive director of the American Academy of Pediatrics, focuses on the career choices of medical students.[9] He brings to our attention the concerning figures generated by the NRMP regarding the increased number of available PL1 positions in the face of a decreasing number of US medical graduate residency applicants. This is reflected in the field of pediatrics by a widening of the gap created by the discrepancy between available PL1 positions and matched PL1 positions. The resulting creation of a "buyers market" has led to a competitive climate among pediatric training programs.

Fourteen percent of program directors responded affirmatively to accepting candidates outside the NRMP. It is possible that of the 4% who did not answer the question or the 18% not responding to the survey, additional program directors also reserve positions outside the NRMP. These data are in keeping with data from the American Board of Pediatrics, which show that many more residents take the In-Training Examination than there are PL1 positions available through the NRMP (Robert Brownlee, MD, oral communication, June 1989). The excess number taking the In-Training Examination cannot be completely accounted for by the additional residents in medicine-pediatrics programs, primary pediatric programs, or those programs that do not participate in the NRMP (ie, military). These data imply that programs are offering additional positions outside the NRMP.

Similar trends to those seen with the categorical pediatric training programs can be seen with the medicine-pediatrics and primary pediatrics programs. The percentage of available NRMP positions that actually filled was greatest for the years 1986 and 1987. In 1987, 81.1% of available medicine-pediatric positions filled as compared with 59.7% in 1990. Likewise, 95% of available primary pediatric positions filled in 1986 as compared with 80.5% in 1990.[2,10] Thus, increasing interest in other than categorical pediatric programs is not a factor in the declining interest in the categorical programs. In fact, there seems to be a widespread decline in interest for primary care specialties in general. During the first half of the last decade, there was an increasing number of positions available through the NRMP for both family practice and internal medicine. As with pediatrics, the percentage of positions being filled likewise increased until 1985-1986. The year 1987 heralded the beginning of a decline in the percent of matched positions, culminating in a 10% drop for both family practice and internal medicine during the last 5 years.[2] This compares with a 5% decline for pediatrics.[2] A decrease in the total number of senior medical students seeking training positions may account for a small portion of this decline. We also speculate that economics and life-style play important roles in the choice of a subspecialty career over a primary care career.

Our search for factors associated with an ability to match led us to the following profile. The larger the program is, the more likely it is to match. Although we did not collect data regarding type of program (ie, children's hospital vs university hospital vs community hospital), children's hospitals and university hospitals tend to have the larger programs. Programs matching all 3 years were more likely to offer shared residency positions. There seems to be a negative relationship between some of the benefits and ability to match. We interpret this to mean that programs that have a good track record for matching feel less compelled to offer such benefits as free parking, conference funds, interview money, and life insurance. Also, during the past 3 years the ability to match was associated with the addition of fewer benefits, again leading us to believe that the programs that have little or no difficulty matching do not feel pressured to improve their benefit package in contrast to those programs having greater difficulty filling their positions.

The PL1 call schedule had no influence on ability to match through the NRMP. This may be explained by the similarity among the four groups for mean frequency of PL1 nights on call. A meaningful relationship between the number of call-free elective months and ability to match could not be substantiated by our data. Most programs offer 0, 1, 2, or 3 call-free months despite a range of up to 11 call-free months.

The positive relationship between ability to match and the offering of shared residency positions may in some way be interrelated with program size and percentage of female residents, the latter two variables also being positively associated with ability to match. One may speculate that larger training programs have the flexibility to offer part-time or shared residency training positions and that this may be particularly appealing to women who have other family obligations.

The major problem with this descriptive study is that we may not have identified other variables that may have an influence on a program's ability to match. Geographic location may be a critical factor, but we did not evaluate this aspect. We thought that some program directors would be inhibited by our potential ability to trace the questionnaire to a specific program based on geographic location and size of the residency training program. The reputation of a program in the academic community may also bear a strong influence on ability to match, but there is no way to quantify this variable objectively.

In light of our findings, we contend that the focus of our efforts as pediatricians should not be to make our training programs more competitive in attracting fourth-year students interested in pediatrics but rather to influence the career choices of students early in medical school, thereby increasing the pool of medical students who enter pediatrics.

References

1. National Resident Matching Program. *National Resident Matching Program Data.* Evanston, Ill: National Resident Matching Program; April 1988.
2. National Resident Matching Program. *National Resident Matching Program Data.* Evanston, Ill: National Resident Matching Program; April 1990.
3. National Resident Matching Program. *National Resident Matching Program 1986 Results: Number of Applicants Sought and Number Matched for Each Hospital and Unfilled Programs by Specialty.* Evanston, Ill: National Resident Matching Program; March 1986.
4. National Resident Matching Program. *National Resident Matching Program 1987 Results: Number of Applicants Sought and Number Matched for Each Hospital and Unfilled Programs by Specialty.* Evanston, Ill: National Resident Matching Program; March 1987.
5. National Resident Matching Program. *National Resident Matching Program 1988 Results: Number of Applicants Sought and Number Matched for Each Hospital and Unfilled Programs by Specialty.* Evanston, Ill: National Resident Matching Program; March 1988.
6. National Resident Matching Program. *National Resident Matching Program 1989 Results: Number of Applicants Sought and Number Matched for Each Hospital and Unfilled Programs by Specialty.* Evanston, Ill: National Resident Matching Program; March 1989.
7. National Resident Matching Program. *National Resident Matching Program 1990 Results: Number of Applicants Sought and Number Matched for Each Hospital and Unfilled Programs by Specialty.* Evanston, Ill: National Resident Matching Program; March 1990.
8. *American Medical Association: 1989-1990 Directory of Graduate Medical Education Programs.* Chicago, Ill: American Medical Association; 1989.
9. Strain JE. The pediatrician as a role model in the career choice of medical students. *Pediatrics.* 1990;85:364-365.
10. National Resident Matching Program. *National Resident Matching Program Data.* Evanston, Ill: National Resident Matching Program; April 1989.

U.S. Postal Service

STATEMENT OF OWNERSHIP, MANAGEMENT AND CIRCULATION

Required by 39 U.S.C. 3685)

1A. Title of Publication	1B. PUBLICATION NO.	2. Date of Filing
AJDC - American Journal of Diseases of Children	0 1 9 6 8 0	09/30/91

3. Frequency of Issue	3A. No. of Issues Published Annually	3B. Annual Subscription Price
Monthly	12	$58.00

4. Complete Mailing Address of Known Office of Publication *(Street, City, County, State and ZIP+4 Code) (Not printers)*

515 N. State Street, Chicago, Cook, Illinois 60610

5. Complete Mailing Address of the Headquarters of General Business Offices of the Publisher *(Not printer)*

515 N. State Street, Chicago, Cook, Illinois 60610

6. Full Names and Complete Mailing Address of Publisher, Editor, and Managing Editor ***(This item MUST NOT be blank)***

Publisher *(Name and Complete Mailing Address)*

American Medical Association, 515 N. State Street, Chicago, Illinois 60610

Editor *(Name and Complete Mailing Address)*

Vincent A. Fulginiti, M.D., 515 N. State Street, Chicago, Illinois 60610

Managing Editor *(Name and Complete Mailing Address)*

Michael D. Springer, 515 N. State Street, Chicago, Illinois 60610

7. Owner *(If owned by a corporation, its name and address must be stated and also immediately thereunder the names and addresses of stockholders owning or holding 1 percent or more of total amount of stock. If not owned by a corporation, the names and addresses of the individual owners must be given. If owned by a partnership or other unincorporated firm, its name and address, as well as that of each individual must be given. If the publication is published by a nonprofit organization, its name and address must be stated.) (Item must be completed.)*

Full Name	Complete Mailing Address
American Medical Association	515 N. State Street, Chicago, IL 60610

8. Known Bondholders, Mortgagees, and Other Security Holders Owning or Holding 1 Percent or More of Total Amount of Bonds, Mortgages or Other Securities *(If there are none, so state)*

Full Name	Complete Mailing Address
None	

9. For Completion by Nonprofit Organizations Authorized To Mail at Special Rates *(DMM Section 423.12 only)*
The purpose, function, and nonprofit status of this organization and the exempt status for Federal income tax purposes *(Check one)*

(1) [X] Has Not Changed During Preceding 12 Months

(2) [ ] Has Changed During Preceding 12 Months

(If changed, publisher must submit explanation of change with this statement.)

10. Extent and Nature of Circulation *(See instructions on reverse side)*	Average No. Copies Each Issue During Preceding 12 Months	Actual No. Copies of Single Issue Published Nearest to Filing Date
A. Total No. Copies *(Net Press Run)*	10/90-09/91 41,042	09/91 40,501
B. Paid and/or Requested Circulation		
1. Sales through dealers and carriers, street vendors and counter sales	919	919
2. Mail Subscription *(Paid and/or requested)*	38,139	37,855
C. Total Paid and/or Requested Circulation *(Sum of 10B1 and 10B2)*	39,058	38,774
D. Free Distribution by Mail, Carrier or Other Means Samples, Complimentary, and Other Free Copies	-0-	-0-
E. Total Distribution *(Sum of C and D)*	39,058	38,774
F. Copies Not Distributed		
1. Office use, left over, unaccounted, spoiled after printing	1,984	1,727
2. Return from News Agents	-0-	-0-
G. TOTAL *(Sum of E, F1 and 2—should equal net press run shown in A)*	41,042	40,501

11. **I certify that the statements made by me above are correct and complete**

Signature and Title of Editor, Publisher, Business Manager, or Owner

[signature] Publisher

PS Form 3526, Feb. 1989 *(See instructions on reverse)*

Commotio Cordis

The Single, Most Common Cause of Traumatic Death in Youth Baseball

Thomas J. Abrunzo, MD

• Two cases of blunt chest trauma caused by a baseball are reported, including one death. At least one of these was in consequence of cardiac concussion or commotio cordis, an entity not described in the pediatric literature. Concussion of the heart is a functional injury, in contrast to cardiac contusion or cardiac rupture, which pertains to structural injury. However, a cardiac concussion appears more likely to have immediate, dire consequences than the structural injury of cardiac contusion. Both of the cases presented occurred in the Little League baseball setting. Blunt chest trauma is reported to cause two to three deaths in youth baseball each year. There appears to be an increased pediatric susceptibility to this type of injury. Unfortunately, these cases are quite resistant to resuscitative therapy. Devices and techniques for primary and secondary prevention exist, but have yet to be systematically verified and implemented.
(*AJDC.* 1991;145:1279-1282)

Clinically significant chest trauma in children is usually described in the setting of a major force, such as an automobile accident or fall from an extreme height.[1,2] There has been little recognition that youth sports present yet another route for fatal blunt cardiac injury, and even less recognition that these fatalities can occur in the absence of structural injury to the heart. The spectrum of blunt cardiac injury extends from a concussion ("a violent jar or shock")[3] to gross, structural disruption.[4,5] Unfortunately, a concussion can cause mortal injury as quickly as a ruptured ventricle. Published data regarding commotio cordis (CC) reveal current resuscitation attempts as uniformly unsuccessful. Successful resuscitation may involve the use of the precordial thump, a technique not generally recommended for children. Difficulties in resuscitating patients with this problem dramatize the importance of primary and secondary prevention, that is, avoiding exposure and early treatment, respectively. Two illustrative cases are presented.

PATIENT REPORTS

PATIENT 1.—The patient, a healthy 10-year-old boy, was a right-handed batter in the Little League for 9- to 12-year-old children. The pitcher was 9 years old and not remarkable for his pitching velocity, according to bystanders. There was informal, unsubstantiated consensus that he was throwing "about 30 mph." A pitch struck the batter in the left side of the chest and he was momentarily stunned. He fell to the ground and witnesses reported gasping respirations. A bystander found the carotid pulse to be present. However, the victim was almost immediately pale and cyanotic. Within about 30 seconds, the pulse was not felt and two-person cardiopulmonary resuscitation was begun by a nurse and paramedic bystander. Emergency medical services paramedics arrived at the scene within 8 minutes of the event. The victim was apneic, cyanotic, and the electrocardiogram was interpreted as fine ventricular fibrillation. His pupils were fixed and dilated. Serial defibrillations of 100 J, 100 J, and 200 J produced no change in rhythm. The boy's trachea was intubated and 0.5 mg of epinephrine was administered endotracheally. The rhythm continued in either fine ventricular fibrillation or asystole. The boy was transported by helicopter to our pediatric emergency department, receiving assisted ventilations and external cardiac compressions. On arrival in the emergency department, endotracheal tube placement was confirmed by auscultation and chest roentgenography. Cardiac rhythm was noted to be asystole. On physical examination, an approximately 3- to 4-cm crescentic ecchymosis just inferior and lateral to the left nipple was detected. As the patient was being evaluated, weight-estimated doses of

Accepted for publication March 28, 1991.

From Pediatric Emergency Services, St Joseph's Hospital, Tampa, Fla.

Reprint requests to 2706 Fountain Blvd, Tampa, FL 33609 (Dr Abrunzo).

Purpose.—*This section provides current information related to the medical needs of young athletes, as pertinent to counseling young athletes and their parents regarding sports participation and practices contributing to the health maintenance of the athlete, as well as current concepts in the prevention, diagnosis, and treatment of sports-related illnesses and injuries.*

Editorial Comment.—*Commotio cordis, a rarely described entity in the pediatric literature, is a distinct entity of which the pediatrician should be aware. The trauma may be lethal, but fortunately is rare. Because of its rarity, there should be no community outcry for increasing protective garb, eg, chest protectors, for youth baseball players. Life is a risk! We, unfortunately, do not live in a risk-free society. To attempt to make youth sports absolutely risk-free would be so expensive that no children or few children would benefit from the wonders of sports participation.*—W.B.S.

bicarbonate, epinephrine, atropine, and calcium were given; the dosages were repeated 5 minutes later. A continuous epinephrine infusion was ordered. A slow, wide-complex rhythm was generated. Pulse and blood pressure were absent. The pupils remained fixed and dilated. The patient was pronounced dead when no further cardiovascular or neurologic response to therapy was elicited. Autopsy revealed the heart to be free of gross or microscopic evidence of injury or congenital abnormality.

PATIENT 2.—An 11-year-old male baseball player was struck in the mid and upper sternum by a Little League regulation baseball thrown by another player during practice. The ball was "pegged hard" according to the victim's later recollection. Two adult witnesses reported the victim's immediate collapse. The boy fell forward, landing prone on the grass. Within 15 seconds, witnesses turned the patient supine, noting that his eyes were rolled back and his mouth was clenched, and that he did not respond to verbal and tactile stimuli. Urinary incontinence was evident. Cyanosis was not noted. His pulse rate was not evaluated. Witnesses attempted unsuccessfully to open the boy's clenched mouth. About 30 to 60 seconds into the event, attempts at cardiopulmonary resuscitation by chest compression were begun. After an estimated 10 compressions, the boy roused and became verbally responsive. He was found alert and responsive by emergency medical services personnel who arrived at the scene within 10 minutes of onset of the event. The boy arrived at our facility with normal, stable vital signs and normal mental status. Physical examination showed no external signs of chest trauma. The patient pointed to the mid and upper sternum as the site of chest impact, but denied pain or tenderness. No swelling, erythema, or ecchymosis was noted. Results of a cardiac examination, including inspection of the precordium, auscultatory evaluation of the first and second heart sounds, precordial and distal pulse palpation, jugular venous pulse, liver palpation, and examination for peripheral edema, were all negative. Electrocardiographic monitoring, venous access, and blood sampling for a complete blood cell count, electrolytes, and fractionated creatine kinase were ordered. The initial electrocardiogram showed minimal ST segment elevation, which was not present on an electrocardiogram done 24 hours later. The initial creatine kinase level was elevated to 396 U/L (normal range for age, 30 to 230 U/L). The initial creatine kinase–MB fraction level was 3.6 ng/mL, and at 24 hours after injury, 3.5 ng/mL (normal range, 0 to 7 ng/mL). An echocardiogram was reported as normal. The patient's medical history was significant for hospitalization at 5 years of age for episodes of "falling asleep in school." This evaluation, including electroencephalogram and Holter monitoring, revealed no abnormalities and the episodes did not recur. There was no family history of congenital heart disease, seizures, or premature death. The patient played youth football, basketball, and baseball without ever experiencing exertional syncope or near-syncope. He was discharged after an uneventful 3 days of observation. He was to be reevaluated in 2 weeks.

COMMENT

The US Consumer Product Safety Commission has generated data implicating ball impact to the chest as the single, most common cause of traumatic death in youth baseball.[6,7] However, these data appear not to have affected the community's main child health advocates—pediatricians.

Blunt cardiac injury in children has received little attention in the pediatric literature. Cardiac concussion is not even mentioned in standard texts in pediatrics,[8,9] pediatric cardiology,[10,11] pediatric surgery,[12] pediatric trauma,[13,14] pediatric intensive care,[15] or pediatric emergency medicine.[16]

The spectrum of blunt cardiac injury includes gross disruption of the anatomy, such as rupture of the ventricles, ventricular septum, chordae tendineae, or the cardiac valves; less severe damage causing contusion of myocardium, often involving elevation of serum cardiac enzymes and various electrocardiogram changes; and concussion or functional, nonstructural injury causing dysrhythmia.[4,5] This latter injury, known as CC, probably exists in a transient, benign form. Such cases are probably not generally recognized or subjected to medical analysis. Patient 2 appears to represent an incremental level of involvement, with objective, but self-limited signs and symptoms. Patient 1 represents an extreme manifestation of CC, a malignant, irreversible form resulting in death. The incidence of CC in the population is not known.

The pediatric patient is generally thought to be more susceptible to thoracic parenchymal injury after nonpenetrating trauma than the adult. Thoracic organs can be damaged in the absence of obvious injury to the skin or ribs. This is generally attributed to a thinner layer of soft tissue in the chest wall, and increased compliance of the immature rib cage.[17] These latter factors enhance direct transmission of force to the underlying parenchyma. In addition, neuromuscular immaturity with respect to injury avoidance makes the child more liable to injury in general.[18]

Seven recent case reports of fatal CC from sports projectiles such as a baseball, softball, hockey puck, and lacrosse ball were found in the medical literature.[19-24] All the reports describe collapse within seconds, unsuccessful resuscitation, and postmortem findings negative for structural cardiac damage. They involve both children and young adults. The baseball and softball cases do not appear to involve great force.

The resistance of dysrhythmias in CC to resuscitative efforts is puzzling. In many of the cases reported, resuscitation was unsuccessful even when begun immediately after the injury was sustained. Liedtke et al[25] suggested temporary alterations in coronary blood flow as a possible explanation for the cardiopathy of CC.

Experimental cardiac trauma studies suggest that relatively low levels of blunt injury induced only dysrhythmias; intermediate energy levels produced varying degrees of contusion associated with impairment of ventricular function; and the highest levels of energy were nearly always fatal, causing gross, structural cardiac disruption.[26] It seems that dysrhythmia is a specific manifestation of CC, not the response of an abnormal host to trivial chest injury. Lindsey et al,[27] drawing on the work of German and Russian investigators, compared the differential features of cardiac concussion and contusion (Table).

Of particular interest in the Table is the characteristic immediate onset, loss of consciousness, hypotension, and immediate disturbance of rhythm and conduction that marks CC as distinct from, and more dangerous than, cardiac contusion.

Therapy for the child who collapses after blunt chest trauma seems to be the same as for any other emergency: airway maintenance, assisted ventilations, chest compressions, and defibrillation, as indicated by electrocardiographic monitoring.[28] The lack of efficacy in the cases reviewed is disturbing. One might speculate on the possible use of the precordial thump. This maneuver is used for the adult victim of witnessed ventricular fibrillation.[29] Indeed, if ventricular fibrillation is the mechanism of death in CC, it seems reasonable to employ the precordial thump; if unsuccessful, immediate cardiopulmonary resuscitation should be instituted. In the past, the American Heart Association cautioned against the use of the pre-

Differential Features of Cardiac Concussion and Contusion		
Feature	**Concussion**	**Contusion**
Site of trauma	Precordial only	Chest, anywhere
Direction of force	Sternum to vertebra	Insignificant
Force	Sharp, not necessarily violent	Generally violent
Thoracic cage intact	Essential	Not essential
Onset	Immediate	Gradual
Course	Transitory	Lasting
Loss of consciousness	As a rule	Not characteristic
Blood pressure	Frequently drops	Normal; rarely up
Disturbances of rhythm and conduction	Characteristic, immediate	Absent or delayed
Changes in ST segment and T waves	Generally absent	Always present

cordial thump in children.[30] This is because of the infrequency of ventricular fibrillation as a presenting arrhythmia, the possibility of iatrogenic trauma to the heart, and the propensity for converting a benign rhythm to a malignant one. A different approach to children is not addressed in the most recent publication of advanced cardiac life support standards.[29] The precordial thump should be scientifically evaluated for its potential as emergency therapy for pediatric CC.

Trauma has long been recognized as the "Number 1 killer of children."[31] Sports-related death from injury is much less commonly observed.[32,33] While the pediatric medical literature generally acknowledges the nontraumatic cardiac causes of youth sports deaths,[34-38] traumatic cardiac death has not generated much interest. This is notwithstanding information from the US Consumer Product Safety Commission stating that in the 10-year period from 1973 to 1983, 51 children from age 5 to 14 years died of baseball-related injury, 23 of whom died of ball impact to the chest.[6] This would make ball impact to the chest the single, most common cause of traumatic death in youth baseball. Deaths are reported within and outside the formal Little League setting, suggesting that adult supervision is not always protective. If helmets and genital cups are a standard part of Little League equipment, the incidence and lethality of blunt chest trauma should also mandate consideration of protective equipment. Manufacturers have already marketed a "reduced injury factor" ball of lower mass and momentum than the standard ball (*Tampa Tribune*. March 29, 1990:1-C). Protective vests are also currently marketed (*Tampa Tribune*. April 26, 1990:3-B). The data available demand that more information be gathered and that protective devices be evaluated with the purpose of their implementation in youth baseball.[39,40]

SUMMARY

Commotio cordis or concussion of the heart is a distinct entity from cardiac contusion. It has received little attention as a source of pediatric mortality. It appears to be the single, most common cause of traumatic death in youth baseball. Although infrequent, its apparent resistance to therapy, high lethality, and prevalence in youth baseball indicate the aggressive implementation of prevention efforts.

The author acknowledges the assistance of Jerome Schulman, MD; Jean Mooney; the emergency department staff, and library staff of St Joseph's Hospital, Tampa, Fla, in the preparation of this manuscript.

References

1. Tellez DW, Hardin WD, Takahashi M, Miller J, Galvis AG, Mahour GH. Blunt cardiac injury in children. *J Pediatr Surg.* 1987;12:1123-1128.

2. Langer JC, Winthrop AL, Wesson DE, et al. Diagnosis and incidence of cardiac injury in children with blunt thoracic trauma. *J Pediatr Surg.* 1989;24:1091-1094.

3. Anderson DM, Patwell JM, Plaut K, McCullough K, eds. *Dorland's Illustrated Medical Dictionary.* 27th ed. Philadelphia, Pa: WB Saunders Co; 1985:370.

4. Tenzer ML. The spectrum of myocardial contusion: a review. *J Trauma.* 1985;5:620-627.

5. Cohn P, Braunwald E. Traumatic heart disease. In: Braunwald E, ed. *Heart Disease.* Philadelphia, Pa: WB Saunders Co; 1988:1535-1538.

6. Rutherford GW Jr, Kennedy J, McGhee L. *Hazard Analysis: Baseball and Softball Related Injuries to Children 5-14 Years of Age.* US Consumer Product Safety Commission; 1984.

7. King AI, Viano DC. *Baseball Related Chest Impact: Final Report to the Consumer Product Safety Commission.* US Consumer Product Safety Commission; 1986.

8. Behrman RE, Vaughan VC, Nelson WE. *Nelson Textbook of Pediatrics.* Philadelphia, Pa: WB Saunders Co; 1987.

9. Rudolph AM, ed. *Pediatrics.* East Norwalk, Conn: Appleton & Lange; 1987.

10. Moss AJ, Adams FH, Emmanouilides GC, Riemenschneider TA, eds. *Heart Disease in Infants, Children and Adolescents.* Baltimore, Md: Williams & Wilkins; 1989.

11. Anderson RH. *Pediatric Cardiology.* New York, NY: Churchill Livingstone Inc; 1987.

12. Welch KJ, Randolph JG, Ravitch MM, O'Neill JA, Rowe MI, eds. *Pediatric Surgery.* Chicago, Ill: Mosby–Year Book; 1986.

13. Mayer TA. *Emergency Management of Pediatric Trauma.* Philadelphia, Pa: WB Saunders Co; 1985.

14. Eichelberger MR, Pratsch GL, eds. *Pediatric Trauma Care.* Rockville, Md: Aspen Systems Corp; 1988.

15. Rogers MC, ed. *Textbook of Pediatric Intensive Care.* Baltimore, Md: Williams & Wilkins; 1987.

16. Fleisher GR, Ludwig S, eds. *Textbook of Pediatric Emergency Medicine.* Baltimore, Md: Williams & Wilkins; 1988.

17. Shoemaker WC, Thompson WL, Holbrook PR. *Textbook of Critical Care.* Philadelphia, Pa: WB Saunders Co; 1984.

18. Zuckerman BS, Duby JC. Developmental approach to injury prevention. *Pediatr Clin North Am.* 1985;32:17-29.

19. Dickman GL, Hassan A, Luckstead EF. Ventricular fibrillation following a baseball injury. *Phys Sportsmed.* 1978;6:85-86.

20. Green ED, Simson LR, Kellerman HH, Horowitz RN, Sturner WQ. Cardiac concussion following softball blow to the chest. *Ann Emerg Med.* 1980;9:155-157.

21. Froede RC, Lindsey D, Steinbronn K. Sudden unexpected death from cardiac concussion (commotio cordis) with unusual legal complications. *J Forensic Sci.* 1979;24:752-756.

22. Frazier M, Mirchandani H. Commotio cordis, revisited. *Am J Forensic Med Pathol.* 1984;5:249-251.

23. Karofsky PS. Death of a high school hockey player. *Phys Sportsmed.* 1990;18:99-103.

24. Edlich RF, Mayer NE, Fariss BL, et al. Commotio cordis in a lacrosse goalie. *J Emerg Med.* 1987;5:181-184.

25. Liedtke AJ, Allen RP, Nellis SH. Effects of blunt cardiac trauma on coronary vasomotion, perfusion, myocardial mechanics, and metabolism. *J Trauma.* 1980;20:777-785.

26. Lau VK, Viano DC, Doty DB. Experimental cardiac trauma: ballistics of a captive bolt pistol. *J Trauma.* 1982;21:39.

27. Lindsey D, Navin T, Finley PR. Transient elevation of serum creatine phosphokinase MB isoenzyme activity in drivers involved in auto accidents. *Chest.* 1978;74:15-18.
28. Chameides L, ed. *Textbook of Pediatric Advanced Life Support.* Dallas, Tex: American Heart Association; 1988.
29. Albarran-Sotelo R, Atkins JM, Bloom RS, et al. *Textbook of Advanced Cardiac Life Support.* Dallas, Tex: American Heart Association; 1987.
30. McIntyre KM, Lewis AJ, eds. *Textbook of Advanced Cardiac Life Support.* Dallas, Tex: American Heart Association; 1981.
31. Haller JA. Pediatric trauma: the number 1 killer of children. *JAMA.* 1983;245:47.
32. Goldberg B. Injury patterns in youth sports. *Phys Sportsmed.* 1989;17:175-186.
33. Mueller F, Blyth C. Epidemiology of sports injury in children. *Clin Sports Med.* 1982;1:343-352.
34. Maron BJ, Epstein SE, Roberts WC. Causes of sudden death in competitive athletes. *J Am Coll Cardiol.* 1986;7:204-214.
35. Maron BJ, Roberts WC, McAllister HA, Rosing DR, Epstein SE. Sudden death in young athletes. *Circulation.* 1980;62:218-229.
36. Topaz O, Edwards JE. Pathologic features of sudden death in children, adolescents and young adults. *Chest.* 1985;87:476-482.
37. Neuspiel DR, Kuller LH. Sudden and unexpected natural death in childhood and adolescents. *JAMA.* 1985;254:1321-1325.
38. Denfield SW, Garson A Jr. Sudden death in children and young adults. *Pediatr Clin North Am.* 1990;37:215-231.
39. Hale CJ. Protective equipment for baseball. *Phys Sportsmed.* 1979;7:59-63.
40. Ferstle J. Baseball deaths: unrecorded, preventable. *Phys Sportsmed.* 1978;6:21-22.

In Other AMA Journals

ARCHIVES OF SURGERY

Trauma During Pregnancy: A Review of 79 Cases

Thomas J. Esposito, MD, MPH; David R. Gens, MD; Lynn Gerber Smith, RN, MS; Ronald Scorpio, MD; Timothy Buchman, MD (*Arch Surg.* 1991;126:1073-1078)

Trauma in Pregnancy: Predicting Pregnancy Outcome

David P. Kissinger, MD; Grace S. Rozycki, MD; John A Morris, Jr, MD; M. Margaret Knudson, MD; Wayne S. Copes, PhD; Sue M. Bass, ScM; H. Kendle Yates; Howard R. Champion, FRCS(Edin) (*Arch Surg.* 1991;126:1079-1086)

Acellular Pertussis Vaccines

Efficacy and Evaluation of Clinical Case Definitions

William C. Blackwelder, PhD; Jann Storsaeter, MD; Patrick Olin, MD, PhD; Hans O. Hallander, MD, PhD

• The efficacy of two acellular pertussis vaccines was estimated for various clinical case definitions, with and without the requirement of culture confirmation, from a randomized trial in Sweden. Efficacy increased with duration of coughing spasms and when the case definition included whoops or whoops plus at least nine coughing spasms a day. After deletion of clinical cases not believed to be caused by pertussis, efficacies were closer to the higher values for culture-confirmed disease. Nonspecificity of the clinical criterion "21 days of coughing spasms with whoops" resulted in estimates of predictive value for pertussis of 85% for placebo recipients and 56% for vaccinees. We conclude that laboratory confirmation of suspected cases is needed in pertussis vaccine trials. A suggested case definition is 21 days or more of coughing spasms with confirmation by culture, serologic study, or household exposure to culture-confirmed pertussis.

(*AJDC.* 1991;145:1285-1289)

Reduced pertussis disease incidence in the Japanese population after the introduction of acellular pertussis vaccines in 1981 has been reported.[1] A randomized, double-blind, placebo-controlled trial of two acellular pertussis vaccines was conducted in Sweden during 1986 to 1987.[2] Estimated efficacy against any culture-confirmed pertussis disease was 54% (95% confidence interval, 26% to 72%) for a single-component vaccine and 69% (95% confidence interval, 47% to 82%) for a two-component vaccine; efficacy against culture-confirmed disease with a cough lasting more than 30 days was 80% and 79%, respectively. Unblinded posttrial passive surveillance yielded somewhat higher efficacy estimates. These higher estimates may be due to observer bias; on the other hand, the active surveillance during the double-blind trial may have detected milder cases that would have gone unrecognized under routine circumstances.[3]

No acellular pertussis vaccine has yet been licensed outside Japan, and further randomized trials of acellular vaccines are being planned. Some of these trials will compare acellular and whole-cell vaccines directly. The trials will be costly, requiring thousands of infants and several years to complete. Crucial to their success will be the case definition(s) used to determine the risk of pertussis disease.

We performed the present analysis (1) to assess the efficacy of the vaccines in the Swedish trial against clinical disease, using a variety of clinical case definitions; (2) to compare the estimates with those obtained when culture confirmation is also required; and (3) to explore the suitability for a future trial of a case definition based solely on clinical criteria.

SUBJECTS AND METHODS

The trial was approved by ethics committees at the Karolinska Institute, Stockholm, Sweden, and at Umeå, Uppsala, and Linköping universities, also in Sweden. Human subjects' clearances were obtained from the World Health Organization, Geneva, Switzerland, and the National Institute of Allergy and Infectious Diseases, Bethesda, Md. Oral informed consent was obtained from parents.

Clinical Methods

The methods of the trial have been described elsewhere.[2,4] The two acellular pertussis vaccines tested were developed at the National Institute of Health (JNIH) (Tokyo, Japan). Because there has been no routine immunization of infants against pertussis in Sweden since 1979, inclusion of a placebo group was considered ethical. Hence, infants aged 6 months to 1 year were randomized to receive two deep subcutaneous injections of a single-component (JNIH-7) or a two-component (JNIH-6) vaccine or placebo. The dose of each injection was 0.5 mL. The JNIH-7 vaccine contained 12 μg of protein nitrogen per milliliter of pertussis toxin (PT), and the JNIH-6 vaccine contained 7.5 μg per milliliter of PT and an equal amount of filamentous hemagglutinin (FHA). The first injection was given between February and April 1986, and the second injection was scheduled for 8 to 12 weeks later. After the second injection, study children were followed up in an active surveillance system either until the end of the study (August 1987) or until they had culture-confirmed pertussis disease. During follow-up, parents were told to call a study nurse if the study child coughed for more than 7 days, if whooping cough was diagnosed or suspected in any household member, or if any of certain specific symptoms (eg, whoops, coughing spasms, or cough with vomiting) occurred in any household member. Coughing spasms (paroxysmal cough) were

Accepted for publication June 24, 1991.

From the National Institute of Allergy and Infectious Diseases, Bethesda, Md (Dr Blackwelder), and the Department of Pediatrics, Karolinska Institute, Sachs' Children's Hospital (Drs Storsaeter and Olin), and the National Bacteriological Laboratory (Dr Hallander), Stockholm, Sweden.

Reprint requests to BHV, Drakenbergsgatan 39, S-117 41 Stockholm, Sweden (Dr Storsaeter).

defined as "sudden periodic attacks of coughing." A whoop was defined as a "sonorous and convulsive inspiratory sound following paroxysmal cough."

Study nurses were instructed to interview parents each month by telephone about possible pertussis in the household. When pertussis was suspected in a study child, clinical information and nasopharyngeal swabs were collected by a study nurse; swabs were collected again 1 week later if the child was still coughing and the first culture had been negative. In addition, in most cases, blood samples were obtained within 14 days after the onset of cough ("acute" specimen) and at least 6 weeks after the onset of cough ("convalescent" specimen). The household was monitored until the last day of coughing.

Randomization

Study participants were randomized into groups of eight within each of 13 study sites in a ratio of placebo to JNIH-6 vaccine to JNIH-7 vaccine of 2:3:3. It has been demonstrated that the randomization resulted in very similar distributions for various characteristics of study children and their families.[2]

Estimation of Risk and Efficacy

Risk of pertussis during 15 months of follow-up, beginning 30 days after the second injection of vaccine or placebo, was estimated for various case definitions with the use of the actuarial method.[5] This method involves division of the period of follow-up into smaller intervals (in our case, 30-day intervals) and calculation of overall risk from estimates for each interval, which account for unavailability for follow-up. Some children had more than one recorded episode. All recorded episodes were used in this analysis, but a child was counted as a case only once for any particular case definition. Vaccine efficacy was estimated by the usual formula: $1-p_v/p_u$, where p_v and p_u are estimated risks in vaccinated and unvaccinated children, respectively. Two-sided 95% confidence intervals for vaccine efficacy were obtained with use of a normal approximation for the natural logarithm of an observed proportion[6] and SEs were obtained from the actuarial analysis.

We calculated vaccine efficacy for clinical case definitions based on some combination of the following criteria: duration of coughing spasms (at least 1, 14, 21, 28, or 35 days), whoops, and nine or more coughing spasms on at least 1 day. The criterion for number of coughing spasms a day has been used previously as an indicator of moderate or severe disease.[7] Efficacy was also calculated when culture confirmation was required as part of the definition. In addition, we calculated efficacy against 21 days or more of coughing spasms with whoops after adjustment for nonpertussis disease, ie, cases that satisfied the clinical definition but could not be verified as being caused by pertussis infection by culture, serologic studies, or information concerning exposure.

An illness was considered a "nonpertussis case" if the culture was negative, if serologic data were available but no criterion for pertussis was met, and if there was no documented exposure to pertussis infection. Any of the following serologic criteria were considered verification of pertussis disease: a titer rise from acute to convalescent serum of at least two dilution steps by Chinese hamster ovary cell assay, which is specific for PT[8]; a 50% or greater increase in IgG antibody to PT or FHA as determined by enzyme-linked immunosorbent assay; or a 100% or greater increase in IgA antibody to PT or FHA as determined by enzyme-linked immunosorbent assay. The combination of these criteria was previously found to be nearly 100% sensitive in the detection of culture-positive pertussis disease.[4]

The proportion of nonpertussis cases was estimated by dividing the number of unverified cases by the number for which culture and serologic information was available. Estimation was performed separately for each study group (placebo, JNIH-7 vaccine, and JNIH-6 vaccine groups) and also for all vaccinees combined. The predictive value of the clinical case definition, or probability of pertussis given clinical disease, is a function of both the true attack rate and the probability of a false-positive result (ie, $1-$specificity).[9] If specificity is uniform in the study population but the attack rate is lower in vaccinees than in placebo recipients, then the predictive value will also be lower for vaccinees. Predictive value was estimated by subtracting the proportion of nonpertussis cases from 1. The estimate of predictive value was then multiplied by the actuarial estimate of risk, with the use of predictive value for all vaccinees combined in the adjustment for JNIH-7 and JNIH-6 vaccine recipients. The adjusted risks were used to obtain an adjusted estimate of efficacy.

Statistical Tests

Risk estimates and proportions of unverified cases were compared with the χ^2 test with continuity correction.[10] All *P* values reported correspond to two-tailed tests; $P<.05$ was considered statistically significant. No correction was made for multiple comparisons; hence, we would expect approximately 5% of the tests to be significant by chance alone.

RESULTS

Of 3801 infants who received the first trial injection, 3711 received two injections and were available for follow-up for pertussis beginning 30 days after the second injection: 923 received placebo, 1403 received the JNIH-7 vaccine, and 1385 received the JNIH-6 vaccine. Exactly one episode with coughing spasms was reported for 764 children, two episodes for 141 children, three episodes for 13 children, and four episodes for three children (n=921). Episodes with 21 days or more of spasms were reported for 319 children; the numbers of children with one, two, three, and four episodes were 299, 16, 3, and 1, respectively.

Table 1 gives risk estimates according to various clinical case definitions, with and without the requirement of culture confirmation, as well as point and interval estimates for vaccine efficacy. For both vaccines, but particularly the JNIH-7 vaccine, efficacy against coughing spasms of any duration was very low. Efficacy increased sharply for longer durations of coughing spasms. When whoops were added to the case definition, point estimates of efficacy increased, especially for the JNIH-7 vaccine. The addition of nine or more spasms on at least 1 day to the definition resulted in even higher efficacy estimates (data not shown).

Efficacy against clinical disease with 28 days or more of spasms and whoops was higher for the JNIH-7 than for the JNIH-6 vaccine (Table 1); the difference was statistically significant, both for all clinical disease and for culture-confirmed disease. However, no significant differences in efficacy were noted when whoops were not required in a case definition.

For illness with 21 days or more of coughing spasms, point estimates of efficacy were 27% for the JNIH-7 and 41% for the JNIH-6 vaccine (Table 1); the corresponding estimates for culture-confirmed disease were 75% and 81%, respectively. Similarly, for all other clinical case definitions as well, efficacy against culture-confirmed disease was higher than efficacy against any clinical disease, especially for illnesses with shorter durations of coughing spasms.

Among cases with 21 days or more of coughing spasms and whoops, the percentage that were not verified as pertussis by culture, serologic study, or exposure information was higher for JNIH-7 than JNIH-6 vaccine recipients, but the difference was not statistically significant

Table 1.—Estimates of Risk and Vaccine Efficacy											
	Placebo (n=923)		JNIH-7 Vaccine (n=1403)				JNIH-6 Vaccine (n=1385)				
Case Definition	No. of Cases	Risk, %†	No. of Cases	Risk, %†	VE, %‡	95% CI§	No. of Cases	Risk, %†	VE, %‡	95% CI§
				All Cases Meeting Clinical Criteria						
1	249	27.5	359	26.2	5	(−10, 17)	313	23.0	16	(3, 27)
14	151	16.7	213	15.5	7	(−13, 23)	176	13.0	22	(5, 36)
21	107	11.8	118	8.7	27	(6, 43)	94	7.0	41	(23, 55)
28	73	8.1	60	4.4	46	(24, 61)	65	4.8	41	(18, 57)
1W	70	7.8	52	3.8	51	(30, 65)	64	4.7	39	(16, 56)
14W	57	6.4	33	2.5	62	(41, 75)	40	3.0	53	(31, 69)
21W	46	5.1	26	1.9	62	(39, 76)	27	2.0	60	(37, 75)
28W	35	3.9	8	0.6	85	(68, 93)	22	1.6	58	(29, 75)
				Culture-Confirmed Cases Only						
1	39	4.3	23	1.7	60	(33, 76)	14	1.1	75	(54, 86)
14	37	4.1	15	1.2	72	(48, 84)	11	0.9	79	(59, 89)
21	35	3.9	12	1.0	75	(53, 87)	10	0.8	81	(61, 90)
28	31	3.5	6	0.5	86	(66, 94)	10	0.8	78	(56, 89)
1W	33	3.7	5	0.4	89	(72, 96)	7	0.5	85	(67, 94)
14W	32	3.6	4	0.3	91	(74, 97)	7	0.5	85	(66, 93)
21W	30	3.4	4	0.3	90	(73, 97)	7	0.5	84	(63, 93)
28W	26	2.9	0	0.0	100	. . .	7	0.5	82	(57, 92)

*1, 14, 21, and 28 indicate days of coughing spasms; W indicates whoops on at least 1 day.
†Risk of pertussis with the indicated case definition, estimated by the actuarial method.
‡VE indicates vaccine efficacy (point estimate).
§95% CI indicates 95% confidence interval for vaccine efficacy.

(P>.20). However, the percentage not verified was significantly higher among all vaccinees combined than among placebo recipients (P<.01). Predictive value was estimated as 85% for placebo recipients and 56% for vaccinees. The adjusted pertussis risk estimates for placebo, JNIH-7 vaccine, and JNIH-6 vaccine recipients were 4.4%, 1.1%, and 1.1%, respectively. The estimated risk of nonpertussis disease with 21 days or more of coughing spasms and whoops (ie, probability of a false-positive result) was similar for vaccinees (0.8%) and placebo recipients (0.7%). After adjustment for clinical cases not considered to be caused by pertussis, point estimates for vaccine efficacy were much closer to those for culture-confirmed disease. The adjusted estimates for 21 and 28 days of coughing spasms with whoops were 75% and 91%, respectively, for the JNIH-7 vaccine and 74% and 75%, respectively, for the JNIH-6 vaccine.

In the classification of disease as verified or not verified according to our criteria, four cases were questionable. One JNIH-6 vaccine recipient and one JNIH-7 vaccine recipient were considered to have possible pertussis and were therefore *not* classified as not verified, because the anti-FHA IgA level was greater than 15 ELISA (enzyme-linked immunosorbent assay) units in both acute or convalescent serum samples.[11] Two JNIH-7 vaccine recipients were considered to be unverified because of a positive culture for *Bordetella parapertussis* and no evidence of pertussis infection other than from FHA serologic study.

COMMENT

There is no single estimate of efficacy for these vaccines. Depending on the severity of clinical symptoms required in the case definition, and whether laboratory confirmation is required, we obtain a wide range of efficacy estimates. This dependence of estimated vaccine efficacy on case definition is one of numerous possible explanations for differing efficacy estimates from different studies.[12]

Efficacy against clinical disease with 28 or more days of coughing spasms and whoops was significantly higher for the JNIH-7 vaccine than for the JNIH-6 vaccine (Table 1). This result may be a chance occurrence or it may be an effect of the larger amount of PT per dose in the JNIH-7 vaccine, if whooping is a PT-associated symptom. There were no significant differences in vaccine efficacy when whoops were not required in a case definition. In an ongoing long-term follow-up of study children, a statistically significant difference has appeared in the opposite direction; efficacy against culture-confirmed pertussis with more than 30 days of cough was higher for the JNIH-6 vaccine than for the JNIH-7 vaccine.[3] Hence, we are unable to conclude that the single-component vaccine had any superiority over the two-component vaccine in protection against long-lasting illness.

For all clinical case definitions used in this analysis, higher vaccine efficacy estimates were obtained when culture confirmation was required. A lower probability of detecting a case (sensitivity) by culture in vaccinated than in unvaccinated children[13] may explain some of this dif-

Table 2.—Clinical Illnesses Not Verified as Pertussis

Case Definition*	Placebo Total	Placebo Complete Data†	Placebo No. (%) Not Verified‡	JNIH-7 Vaccine Total	JNIH-7 Vaccine Complete Data†	JNIH-7 Vaccine No. (%) Not Verified‡	JNIH-6 Vaccine Total	JNIH-6 Vaccine Complete Data†	JNIH-6 Vaccine No. (%) Not Verified‡
21W	46	41	6 (15)	26	21	11 (52)	27	18	6 (33)
28W	35	31	1 (3)	8	5	3 (60)	22	14	5 (36)

*21W and 28W indicate at least 21 or 28 days of coughing spasms with whoops.
†Values represent number with culture and serologic data (including one JNIH-7 vaccine recipient with no serology of, but a positive culture for *Bordetella parapertussis*).
‡"Not verified" values represent number with no evidence of pertussis disease from culture, serologic study, or exposure information, or with a positive culture for *B parapertussis*. Percentage refers to those with complete data.

ference, even though in the Swedish trial such a phenomenon appeared to occur mainly in disease with 21 days or less of coughing spasms.[4] The adjustment of estimated vaccine efficacy for nonpertussis cases suggests that the discrepancy was partially due to nonspecificity of the clinical criteria, as applied in this study. Other adjustment methods—eg, those based on a common estimate of specificity for the vaccine and placebo groups—yield the same qualitative result—that vaccine efficacy is underestimated by clinical case definitions.

One purpose of our analysis was to assess the validity for a future pertussis vaccine trial of a case definition based only on clinical criteria. Use of such a definition could entail less cost and effort than one requiring culture or other laboratory confirmation. A clinical case definition may be appropriate during an investigation of a pertussis outbreak or illness after household exposure, when the intensity of exposure would be relatively high for most individuals.[14] However, we found no clinical case definition that was sufficiently specific for pertussis in the Swedish trial; all of the clinical definitions used led to substantial underestimation of vaccine efficacy. The nonspecificity of clinical case definitions could be partly due to the reliance on parents and study nurses to ascertain disease. However, it was impractical to have a physician investigate each suspected case, and we would expect a similar situation in most large trials.

Similarly, when two vaccines are compared, a case definition with insufficient specificity can lead to considerable bias in the estimation of relative risk of pertussis.[9] If the vaccines have different efficacies, then inclusion of nonpertussis cases will bias relative risk estimates toward 1, tending to make vaccines appear more similar than they actually are. Our analysis suggests that a large proportion of episodes of coughing spasms among vaccinated children were not due to pertussis; this was true even for illnesses with 21 days or more of coughing spasms and whoops. Thus, we would not expect the predictive value for a clinical definition to be much greater than 50% in vaccinees without an unacceptable loss of sensitivity (Table 2). Such a low predictive value and the bias that could result during the estimation of relative risk[9] make a clinical case definition undesirable for a comparison of two pertussis vaccines.

Clearly, a vaccine trial confirmation of suspected pertussis cases is needed. However, the requirement of confirmation solely by culture may be insufficient. Culture may have a different sensitivity in vaccinated and unvaccinated children[4,13] and possibly, although less likely, with different vaccines as well. Moreover, culture lacks sensitivity.[15] Therefore, clinical criteria and culture confirmation should be used together with other laboratory criteria. The most practicable such criteria at present are based on serologic studies. Serologic criteria for diagnosis would have to be carefully determined; the specific criteria used in the Swedish trial, based on intra-assay variability for that laboratory,[4] may not be appropriate in a different setting. Whatever methods are used, it is important that they be chosen carefully, as serologic criteria as well as culture could have different sensitivities and thus introduce bias in the estimation of vaccine efficacy or relative risk.[9]

In future efficacy trials, vaccine efficacy should be estimated both for mild pertussis of short duration and for typical pertussis. For the assessment of efficacy against typical pertussis, a clinical criterion of 21 days or more of coughing spasms seems reasonable for many settings. This criterion is satisfied in 70% to 80% of cases in England and Wales notified to Public Health Laboratory Service, Communicable Disease Surveillance Centre, London, England (Mary Ramsay, MACP, written communication, January 16, 1991), and also appears to correspond to what is considered typical pertussis disease in young children in Sweden and elsewhere.[16,17] Thus, for trials of acellular pertussis vaccines, we suggest the following definition of typical pertussis: 21 days of coughing spasms with confirmation by culture, appropriate serologic techniques, or household exposure to culture-confirmed pertussis (World Health Organization meeting on pertussis case definitions, Geneva, Switzerland, January 10 through 11, 1991). Confirmation by laboratory methods or household exposure makes it unnecessary to require some additional clinical symptom, such as whoops or posttussive vomiting, to make the clinical criteria more specific for pertussis. However, because the sensitivity of either culture or serologic criteria could potentially differ in different vaccine or placebo groups, to determine the most appropriate estimate of vaccine efficacy or relative risk, useful information may be obtained from the estimate calculated with the clinical criteria only and estimates of specificity and predictive value of the clinical criteria (Elizabeth Miller, MB, BS, and Conor P. Farrington, PhD, World Health Organization meeting on pertussis case definitions, Geneva, Switzerland, January 10 through 11, 1991).

This investigation was supported by grant K89-16P-08450-02 from the Swedish Medical Research Council, Stockholm (Dr Storsaeter).

The authors thank Maria Deloria for computer programming assistance.

References

1. Kimura M, Kuno-Sakai H. Developments in pertussis immunisation in Japan. *Lancet.* 1990;2:30-32.

2. Ad Hoc Group for the Study of Pertussis Vaccines. Placebo-controlled trial of two acellular pertussis vaccines in Sweden: protective efficacy and adverse events. *Lancet.* 1988; 1:955-960.

3. Storsaeter J, Olin P. Relative efficacy of two acellular pertussis vaccines during three years of passive surveillance. *Vaccine.* In press.

4. Storsaeter J, Hallander H, Farrington CP, Olin P, Mollby R, Miller E. Secondary analyses of the efficacy of two acellular pertussis vaccines evaluated in a Swedish phase III trial. *Vaccine.* 1990;8:457-461.

5. Miller RG. *Survival Analysis.* New York, NY: John Wiley & Sons Inc; 1981.

6. Katz D, Baptista J, Azen SP, Pike MC. Obtaining confidence intervals for the risk ratio in cohort studies. *Biometrics.* 1978;34:469-474.

7. Grob PR, Crowder MJ, Robbins JF. Effect of vaccination on severity and dissemination of whooping cough. *Br Med J.* 1981;282:1925-1928.

8. Halperin SA, Bortolussi R, Kasina A, Wort AJ. Use of a Chinese hamster ovary cell cytotoxicity assay for the rapid diagnosis of pertussis. *J Clin Microbiol.* 1990;28:32-38.

9. Farrington CP. Quantifying misclassification bias in cohort studies of vaccine efficacy. *Stat Med.* 1990;9:1327-1337.

10. Armitage P. *Statistical Methods in Medical Research.* New York, NY: John Wiley & Sons Inc; 1971.

11. Hallander HO, Storsaeter J, Möllby R. Evaluation of serology and nasopharyngeal cultures for diagnosis of pertussis infection in a vaccine efficacy trial. *J Infect Dis.* 1991; 163:1046-1054.

12. Fine PEM, Clarkson JA. Reflections on the efficacy of pertussis vaccines. *Rev Infect Dis.* 1987;9:866-883.

13. Combined Scottish Study. Diagnosis of whooping cough: comparison of serological tests with isolation of *Bordetella pertussis. Br Med J.* 1970;4:637-639.

14. Patriarca PA, Biellik RJ, Sanden G, et al. Sensitivity and specificity of clinical case definitions for pertussis. *Am J Public Health.* 1988;78:833-836.

15. Onorato IM, Wassilak SGF. Laboratory diagnosis of pertussis: the state of the art. *Pediatr Infect Dis J.* 1987;6: 145-151.

16. Lautrop H. Whooping cough in Denmark during the period 1959-1974: experience with two prophylactic vaccination programmes. *Ugeskr Laeger.* 1976;138:1382-1389.

17. Bell JA. Pertussis prophylaxis with two doses of alum-precipitated vaccine. *Public Health Rep.* 1941;56:1535-1546.

In Other AMA Journals

ARCHIVES OF GENERAL PSYCHIATRY

Anxiety Disorders in Children and Their Families

Cynthia G. Last, PhD; Michel Lersen, PhD;
Alan Kazdin, PhD; Helen Orvaschel, PhD;
Sean Perrin, MS (*Arch Gen Psychiatry.* 1991;48:928-934)

Cognitive-Behavioral and Pharmacological Treatments of Social Phobia: A Controlled Study

Cheryl Shea Gelernter, PhD; Thomas W. Uhde, MD;
Peter Cimbolic, PhD; Diane B. Arnkoff, PhD;
Bernard J. Vittone, MD; Manuel E. Tancer, MD;
John J. Bartko, PhD (*Arch Gen Psychiatry.* 1991;48:938-944)

Cardiopulmonary Exercise Testing in Children Following Surgery for Tetralogy of Fallot

Teresa L. Tomassoni, PhD; Frank M. Galioto, Jr, MD; Paul Vaccaro, EdD

• The purpose of this study was to compare the cardiopulmonary responses at rest and during exercise of children following surgical correction of tetralogy of Fallot. The physiologic measurements assessed at rest and during maximal treadmill exercise included diffusing capacity of the lung for carbon monoxide, heart rate, oxygen consumption, minute ventilation, and cardiac output. Twenty children with repaired tetralogy of Fallot served as the study group, and 20 normal boys and girls served as controls. Subjects with tetralogy of Fallot had significantly lower values than those of control subjects for maximal cardiac output and somewhat lower values for diffusing capacity of the lung for carbon monoxide and heart rate. We conclude that the exercise cardiac function of children with surgically corrected tetralogy of Fallot is somewhat diminished compared with that of control children. This information is necessary to establish safe, yet effective exercise guidelines for this select population.

(*AJDC.* 1991;145:1290-1293)

Patients with surgically corrected tetralogy of Fallot (TF) have decreased resting mean values for vital capacity, total lung capacity, residual volume, and functional residual capacity.[1] Investigators who have examined the exercise response of children with surgically corrected TF reported abnormal hemodynamics during maximal exercise tests. They also reported a decreased duration in exercise time,[2] a diminished maximal oxygen consumption ($\dot{V}O_2max$),[1,3,4] a depressed cardiac output ($\dot{Q}$),[5] a low work capacity,[6] a low ventilatory threshold,[7] and a low reduced maximal heart rate (HR).[5,6,8] The reason for the decreased exercise capabilities is not fully understood. Early research suggested that the reduced exercise tolerance occurred even though pulmonary blood flow was assumed to be normal. It was attributed to a diminished functional capacity of the myocardium.[9,10] One group suggested that severe pulmonary regurgitation might cause reduced exercise capability.[11] Another group suggested that pulmonary vascular disease caused exercise intolerance in patients undergoing surgical correction of TF,[12] but this has not been supported by catheterization data collected after surgery. No study yet has measured the diffusing capacity of the lung for carbon monoxide (DLCO) during exercise in this population of boys and girls. This study is the first to integrate this parameter with catheterization data.

Based on the exercise responses noted during comprehensive exercise testing, information concerning long-term effects of surgery on exercise tolerance is needed to evaluate the benefits and to prescribe a safe level of recreational activity for patients who have undergone correction of TF. The purpose of this study was to compare the cardiorespiratory responses to exercise testing of control subjects and of patients who had undergone surgical repair of TF.

SUBJECTS AND METHODS

Forty boys and girls between ages 6 and 16 years participated in this study. The study group was composed of 20 patients (nine girls and 11 boys) who were undergoing routine postoperative evaluation for surgically repaired TF. Twenty children (nine girls and 11 boys) approximately matched by age, sex, and body surface area, who were free from any medical disorders and who were not participating in any physical training, volunteered to serve as control subjects. The purpose and procedures of this investigation were explained to the participants and their parents. Written informed consent was obtained for all the children, and the study was approved by the Institutional Human Subjects Review Board, of the Georgetown University Children's Medical Center in Washington, DC.

Laboratory Procedures

All exercise testing was performed in a medically equipped Exercise Physiology Laboratory of the Children's Medical Center. Graded exercise testing was performed on a motor-driven treadmill (Q-55, Quinton Instrument Co, Seattle, Wash). Blood pressure was measured with a mercury sphygmomanometer and a 12-lead electrocardiogram was obtained with a Quinton Q3000 controller. Each subject was allowed ample time to become familiar with breathing through a mouthpiece with a noseclip in place. The exercise protocol was a continuous multistage procedure with three minute stages. Children aged 8 years and older performed a standard Bruce protocol; younger children performed a modified version of this protocol, which consisted of two additional initial stages composed of 2.72 km at 0% grade and 2.72 km at 5% grade.

A medical gas analyzer (Marquette Gas Analysis Corp, St

Accepted for publication May 13, 1991.

From the Division of Pediatric Cardiology, Georgetown University Children's Medical Center, Washington, DC, (Drs Tomassoni and Galioto) and the Department of Physical Education, University of Maryland (College Park) (Dr Vaccaro).

Reprint requests to the Division of Pediatric Cardiology, Georgetown University Children's Medical Center, 3800 Reservoir Rd NW, Washington, DC 20007-2197 (Dr Tomassoni).

Table 1.—Physical Characteristics of Subjects*		
Variable	Tetralogy of Fallot	Controls
Age, y	9.93±2.88	10.22±2.48
Height, cm	136.07±19.55	139.98±13.52
Weight, kg	32.81±12.35	35.75±11.47
Body surface area, m^2	1.12±0.28	1.17±0.23

*Values are given as mean±SEM.

Table 2.—Catheterization Data for Subjects With Tetralogy of Fallot*

Subject No.	Intracardiac Pressures RA	RV	PA	LV	Angiography
1	3	60/4	20/8	. . .	Dilated, well-contracting RV
2	2	30/2	30/2	118/3	Dilated, fair RV contractility
3	3	30/6	26/10	120/80	Poor RV contractility
4	. . .	40/8	22/5	115/8	Normal RV contractility
5	5	46/8	32/8	115/. . .	Normal contractility
6	1	50/13	32/2	120/5	Good LV contractility
7	3	45/3	20/6	96/6	Left and right branch PS
8	2	42/5	24/4	100/. . .	Good RV and LV contractility
9	3	60/5	17/5	. . .	Good RV and LV contractility
10	3	30/5	30/10	100/. . .	Good RV contractility
11	2	30/4	20/5	110/6	Normal RV and LV contractility
12	. . .	70/. . .	20/8	. . .	. . .
13	2	60/3	15/5	120/0	Normal LV contractility
14	5	30/5	30/5	. . .	Good RV and LV contractility
15†	3	110/8	70/10	. . .	Good RV contractility
16	4	40/5	20/8	100/15	Good RV and LV contractility
17	2	35/0	25/0	95/. . .	Good RV and LV contractility
18	3	30/3	20/5	95/6	Diminished RV and LV contractility
19	3	60/4	. . .	. . .	Good RV contractility
20	2	40/5	24/8	100/10	Good RV and LV contractility

*LV indicates left ventricular; PA, pulmonary artery; PS, pulmonary stenosis; RA; right atrial, and RV, right ventricular.
†Surgical repair with conduit; all other patients had transannular outflow patches.

Louis, Mo 1100 Mass Spectrometer) and a pneumotachograph differential pressure transducer interfaced with a specially programmed minicomputer were used to measure gas concentrations for determination of respiratory variables. Baseline values for $\dot{Q}$ and DLCO were measured with the acetylene rebreathing method.[13-15]

During the exercise test, the blood pressure, HR, and electrocardiogram were monitored continuously. The subjects were encouraged to continue to exercise as long as possible to achieve maximal treadmill performance. At maximal exercise, measurements of each of the previously mentioned parameters were repeated. When testing was complete, these parameters were monitored for 5 minutes to provide for an adequate recovery period.

Statistical analysis consisted of Student's t tests to probe for significant differences between the control subjects and patients with TF in physiologic parameters measured at rest and at peak exercise. A P value of less than .05 was considered significant, and P value of less than .10 was suggestive of a trend. Physiologic measurements are presented as means±SEMs.

RESULTS

There were no significant differences in age, height, weight, or body surface area between the TF group and the control group (Table 1).

The 20 patients with TF had undergone surgery 2.0 to 12 years earlier (mean, 6.9 years) at a mean age of 34.7 months. Nineteen patients had right ventricular outflow tract reconstruction, which required a patch that extends across the pulmonary valve annulus. One patient had a conduit to establish continuity between the right ventricle and pulmonary artery. An electrocardiogram and echocardiogram revealed that all 20 patients had right bundle branch block and mild to moderate pulmonary insufficiency, respectively. Catheterization data are presented in Table 2. None of the subjects was symptomatic and all participated in regular physical education class in school.

There were no significant differences between the TF group and the control group in resting $\dot{V}O_2$, minute ventilation, $\dot{Q}$, DLCO, and HR (Table 3).

There were no significant differences between the two groups in peak exercise measures of $\dot{V}O_2$ and minute ventilation ($P>.05$) (Table 4). The mean peak exercise $\dot{Q}$ in the TF group was significantly lower than in the control group ($P<.05$). The DLCO and HR were suggestive of significance ($P<.10$).

Further statistical analyses were performed on the two groups after omitting six subjects, all of whom had high right ventricular pressures indicating residual pulmonary stenosis after repair of TF. By omitting these patients, the peak DLCO levels were significantly lower in the subjects with TF than in the control group ($P=.05$), while the difference in peak $\dot{Q}$ failed to reach significance ($P=.06$). These results indicate that residual problems with lung diffusion and $\dot{Q}$ exist even in those patients who are believed to have good operative results.

COMMENT

Postoperative catheterization data have demonstrated normal $\dot{Q}$ at rest in subjects with TF, provided that the repair has been technically successful.[5,16] Few studies have examined the $\dot{Q}$ response to exercise in subjects following surgical repair of TF. Those studies that are available support our finding of a lower $\dot{Q}$ in patients with surgically corrected TF than in healthy children.[1,3,5,8] Most catheterization-based studies did not evaluate patients during maximal activity. Some studies have revealed abnormal right heart hemodynamic responses at moderate exercise levels.[16,17] In this study, our data revealed poor $\dot{Q}$ dynamics in children after repair of TF during maximal treadmill exercise, while there were no detectable abnormalities at rest.

The mechanisms responsible for the diminished $\dot{Q}$ in patients with TF appear to be multidimensional and complex. Many patients who have undergone surgical repair of TF often develop significant pulmonary insufficiency

Table 3.—Group Means for Resting Physiologic Measurements*

Variable	Tetralogy of Fallot	Controls	P
$\dot{V}O_2$, L/min	0.23±0.02	0.27±0.02	.12
$\dot{V}O_2$, mL/kg per minute	7.91±0.81	8.59±1.14	.63
VE, L/min	10.82±0.52	9.55±0.70	.15
$\dot{Q}$, L/min	3.02±0.17	3.04±0.16	.94
DLCO, mL/mm Hg per minute	10.22±0.71	9.65±0.54	.53
RHR, beats per minute	94.1±2.16	92.9±2.44	.73

*Values are given as mean±SEM. $\dot{V}O_2$ indicates oxygen consumption; VE, minute ventilation; $\dot{Q}$, cardiac output; DLCO, diffusing capacity of the lung for carbon monoxide; and RHR, resting heart rate. N=20 except for control subjects' values of $\dot{V}O_2$ and VE.

Table 4.—Group Means for Peak Exercise Physiologic Measurements*

Variable	Tetralogy of Fallot	Controls	P
$\dot{V}O_2$, L/min	1.11±0.11	1.29±0.05	.17
$\dot{V}O_2$, mL/kg per minute	34.10±2.98	37.53±2.45	.38
VE, L/min	35.64±2.64	39.46±2.06	.26
$\dot{Q}$, L/min	6.11±0.42	7.51±0.44	.03
DLCO, mL/mm Hg per minute	14.01±0.88	16.14±0.81	.08
PHR, beats per minute	173.8±4.6	184.5±2.9	.056

*Values are given as mean±SEM. $\dot{V}O_2$ indicates oxygen consumption; VE, minute ventilation; $\dot{Q}$, cardiac output; DLCO, diffusing capacity of the lung for carbon monoxide; and PHR, peak heart rate. N=20 except for measures of $\dot{Q}$ and DLCO in the subjects with tetralogy of Fallot and $\dot{V}O_2$ and DLCO in control subjects.

across the reconstructed right ventricular outflow tract, thereby causing increases in right ventricular volume at rest and during exercise.[5,18] This elevated volume will magnify the right heart's filling pressure abnormalities as systemic venous return increases during exercise.[16] With resting elevation in end-diastolic volume in the right ventricle already using the Starling principle of cardiac reserve, further rises do not produce increases in stroke volume during exercise. Stroke volume also depends partially on the afterload resistance against which the ventricle must pump. Any residual pulmonary stenosis, which is often present in patients with TF, will increase this afterload. Inability to increase stroke volume during physical exertion inhibits the ability to increase $\dot{Q}$.[17] It has been demonstrated that in response to exercise of moderate intensity requiring a similar $\dot{V}O_2$, children with TF have higher arteriovenous oxygen differences than healthy children, thus compensating for the lower $\dot{Q}$.[8]

The mean maximal $\dot{V}O_2$ value in the control group was slightly lower than values in healthy children reported by other investigators, as summarized by Krahenbuhl et al.[19] The $\dot{V}O_2$max in the summary ranged from 1.25 L/min for 8-year-old children to 3.14 L/min for 15-year-old adolescents (33.4 to 63.2 mL/kg per minute). Other longitudinal studies have reported data for $\dot{V}O_2$max ranging from 42 to 56 mL/kg per minute for 7- to 15-year-old subjects.[20-24]

The mean maximal exercise $\dot{V}O_2$ value of patients with TF was not significantly different from that of the controls. This finding does not agree with some early reports that found lower exercise $\dot{V}O_2$ values in patients operated on for TF,[3,5,11,25] but it does agree with a recent study that did not find reduced $\dot{V}O_2$ values in children operated on for TF.[8] That recent study attributed the better $\dot{V}O_2$ response to the earlier age of primary repair and fewer residual defects.[8] All of the children in our study were operated on at or before the age of 6 years and had few residual defects, except for pulmonary insufficiency excluding one patient with residual obstructive problems who required another operation.

It is very difficult to compare our values for maximal exercise DLCO with those of others who have assessed DLCO in healthy children because different methods have been used to measure this variable. One previous study used the acetylene-helium rebreathing method to measure DLCO during exercise in children. A mean peak DLCO of 16.08 mL/mm Hg per minute (ranging from 12.87 to 20.47 mL/mm Hg per minute) was reported for healthy children aged 6 to 17 years.[26] No studies have been found that have measured maximal exercise values for DLCO in children following surgical repair of TF.

We believe that the slightly lower maximal exercise DLCO values achieved for patients operated on for TF compared with the controls in our study is due to a primary interstitial interface defect. Several investigators[27-29] have supported this theory of a diminished DLCO in subjects with TF. They suggest that pulmonary vascular changes occur as a result of either a decreased pulmonary blood flow or increased blood viscosity, which leads to thrombosis of small arteries that may form, occluding interstitial fibrotic bands. In our patients, cardiac catheterization following surgery revealed no evidence of pulmonary vascular obstructive disease, but catheterization data do not measure interstitial thickening.

These results emphasize the need to measure more than just $\dot{V}O_2$ in these patients because they have significant problems with DLCO and $\dot{Q}$ while having normal $\dot{V}O_2$.

The mean value for peak HR obtained in our study of the control subjects was slightly higher than that observed in the subjects with TF. It is difficult to compare these data with data in the literature as we report peak HR and only maximal values have been reported in the literature. When the generally accepted criteria for the attainment of the maximal effort are not met, the term *peak* is usually used.[30] In clinically tested children, a plateau of $\dot{V}O_2$ is usually not observed. Therefore, we report peak HR values. The maximal HR of healthy children and adolescents has been reported to range between 195 and 215 beats per minute.[31,32] The finding of a slightly lower peak HR in our subjects with TF compared with the reference group is in general agreement with other studies that have documented reduced maximal HR levels in patients following surgical repair of TF.[4-6,8,33] It has been suggested that this chronotropic limitation may be due to sinus node dysfunction as a result of the preoperative cyanosis.[8] Other explanations implicate pulmonary regurgitation or stenosis.[11] None of the patients who had surgery for TF in this study had severe pulmonary regurgitation, but six had significant residual stenosis.

CONCLUSION

We conclude that the cardiovascular system of children who have had surgery for TF is able to maintain proper functioning with the use of physiologic compensatory mechanisms during resting conditions. When the cardiorespiratory system is stressed by peak exercise, subjects with TF respond adversely because they have already used compensatory mechanisms to maintain normal resting values. The mean maximal $\dot{Q}$ is significantly lower than those of control subjects. Impaired gas exchange, when measured as DLCO during exercise in subjects with TF may be an inherent part of the pathophysiology of the defect or a complication of the palliative and surgical repairs.

This impairment in maximal $\dot{Q}$, DLCO, and HR should be considered when recommending exercise for patients who have been operated on to correct TF. We recommend that patients with impaired $\dot{Q}$ and/or lung-diffusing capacity avoid maximal effort during sports and advise participation in activities of only moderate intensity. Resting values of $\dot{Q}$, DLCO, and HR are deceiving, and the patient should undergo maximal exercise testing before participation in sports, especially on a competitive level.[34] Measurement of $\dot{Q}$, DLCO, and HR at peak exercise may uncover patients with exercise capacity not discerned at rest or on exercise testing that does not include measurements of these parameters.

References

1. Bjarke B. Spirometric data, pulmonary ventilation and gas exchange at rest and during exercise in adult patients with tetralogy of Fallot. *Scand J Respir Dis.* 1974;55:47-61.

2. Cumming GR. Maximal supine exercise hemodynamics after open heart surgery for Fallot's tetralogy. *Br Heart J.* 1979;41:683-691.

3. Mocellin R, Bastanier C, Buhlmeyer K. Exercise performance in children and adolescents after surgical repair of tetralogy of Fallot. *Eur J Cardiol.* 1976;4:367-374.

4. Wessel H, Cunningham W, Paul M, Bastanier C, Muster A, Idriss F. Exercise performance in tetralogy of Fallot after intracardiac repair. *J Thorac Cardiovasc Surg.* 1980;80:582-593.

5. Epstein S, Beiser D, Goldstein R, Rosing D, Redwood D, Morrow A. Hemodynamic abnormalities in response to mild and intense upright exercise following operative correction of an atrial septal defect of tetralogy of Fallot. *Circulation.* 1973;47:1065-1075.

6. James F, Kaplan S, Schwartz D, Chou T, Sandker M, Naylor V. Response to exercise in patients after total surgical correction of tetralogy of Fallot. *Circulation.* 1976;54:671-679.

7. Van der Hauwaert L, Reybrouck T. Exercise testing after repair of tetralogy of Fallot. *Congenital Heart Dis.* 1987;4:111-118.

8. Perrault H, Drblik S, Montigny M, et al. Comparison of cardiovascular adjustments to exercise in adolescents 8 to 15 years of age after correction of tetralogy of Fallot, ventricular septal defect or atrial septal defect. *Am J Cardiol.* 1989;64:213-217.

9. Crawford D, Simpson E, McIlroy M. Cardiopulmonary function in Fallot's tetralogy after palliative shunting operations. *Am Heart J.* 1967;74:463-472.

10. Davies H, Gazetopoulos N. Dyspnea in cyanotic congenital heart disease. *Br Heart J.* 1965;27:28-41.

11. Strieder D, Aziz K, Zaver A, Fellow K. Exercise tolerance after repair of tetralogy of Fallot. *Ann Thorac Surg.* 1975;19:397-405.

12. Marx G, Hicks R, Allen H, Goldberg S. Noninvasive assessment of hemodynamic responses to exercise in pulmonary regurgitation after operations to correct pulmonary outflow obstruction. *Am J Cardiol.* 1988;61:595-601.

13. Sackner MA, Greeneltch D, Heiman MS, Epstein S, Atkins N. Diffusing capacity, membrane diffusing capacity, capillary blood volume, pulmonary tissue volume, and cardiac output measured by a rebreathing technique. *Am Rev Respir Dis.* 1975;3:157-165.

14. Galioto FM, Clinton MA. Pediatric graded exercise testing. *Cardiovasc Physiol.* 1983;11:35-39.

15. Galioto FM. Exercise testing. In: Garson A, Bricker T, McNamara D, eds. *The Science and Practice of Pediatric Cardiology.* Philadelphia, Pa: Lea & Febiger; 1990:828-835.

16. Bristow JD, Kloster FE, Lees MH, Menashe VD, Griswold HE, Starr A. Serial cardiac catheterizations and exercise hemodynamics after correction of tetralogy of Fallot. *Circulation.* 1970;41:1057-1066.

17. Hirschfeld S, Tuboku-Metzger A, Borkat G, Ankeney J, Clayman J, Liebman J. Comparison of exercise and catheterization results following total surgical correction of tetralogy of Fallot. *J Thorac Cardiovasc Surg.* 1978;75:446-451.

18. Cumming JR. Recirculation times in exercising children. *J Appl Physiol: Respir Environ Exerc Physiol.* 1978;45:1005-1008.

19. Krahenbuhl GS, Skinner JS, Kohrt WM. Development aspects of maximal aerobic power in children. In: Terjung RL, ed. *Exercise and Sport Sciences Reviews.* New York, NY: Macmillan Publishing Co Inc; 1985:503-538.

20. Andersen KL, Selinger V, Rutenfranz J, Skrobak-Kaczynski J. Physical performance capacity of children in Norway: the rate of growth in maximal aerobic power and the influence of improved physical education of children in a rural community: population parameters in a rural community. *Eur J Appl Physiol.* 1976;35:49-58.

21. Hermansen L, Oseid S. Direct and indirect estimation of oxygen uptake in pre-pubertal boys. *Acta Paediatr Scand Suppl.* 1971;217:18-23.

22. Knuttgen HS. Aerobic capacity of adolescents. *J Appl Physiol.* 1967;22:655-658.

23. Kobayashi K, Kitamura K, Miura M, et al. Aerobic power as related to body growth and training in Japanese boys: a longitudinal study. *J Appl Physiol.* 1978;44:666-672.

24. Washington RL, Van Gundy JC, Cohen C, Sondheimer HM, Wolfe RR. Normal aerobic and anaerobic exercise data for North American school-age children. *J Pediatr.* 1988;12:223-233.

25. Rocchini AP. Hemodynamic abnormalities in response to supine exercise in patients after operative correction of tetralogy of Fallot after early childhood. *Am J Cardiol.* 1981;48:325-330.

26. Tomassoni TL, Galioto FM. Normal values for diffusing capacity of the lung for carbon monoxide (DL_{co}) at rest and during peak exercise in children of different ages. *Pediatr Exerc Sci.* 1988;1:82. Abstract.

27. McGaff CJ, Ross RS, Braunwald E. The development of elevated pulmonary vascular resistance in man following increased pulmonary blood flow from systemic-to-pulmonary anastomosis. *Am J Med.* 1962;33:201-212.

28. Paul MH, Miller RA, Potts WJ. Long-term results of aortic-pulmonary anastomosis for tetralogy of Fallot. *Circulation.* 1961;23:525-533.

29. Ross RS, Taussig H, Evans MH. Late hemodynamic complications of anastomotic surgery for the treatment of tetralogy of Fallot. *Circulation.* 1958;18:553-561.

30. McArdle W, Katch F, Katch V. *Exercise Physiology: Energy, Nutrition, and Human Performance.* 2nd ed. Philadelphia, Pa: Lea & Febiger; 1986:174.

31. Cumming GR, Everatt G, Hastman L. Bruce treadmill test in children: normal values in a clinic population. *Am J Cardiol.* 1978;41:69-75.

32. Bar-Or O. *Pediatric Sports Medicine for the Practitioner.* New York, NY: Springer-Verlag NY Inc; 1983:22-23.

33. Hurwitz R, Goldberg S. Maximal cardiac rate before and following repair of cardiac lesions. *J Sports Med Phys Fitness.* 1970;1:165-168.

34. Mitchell JH, Marion BJ, Epstein SE. 16th Bethesda Conference: Cardiovascular Abnormalities in the Athlete: Recommendation Regarding Eligibility for Competition. *J Am Coll Cardiol.* 1985;6:1186-1232.

Pediatric Germ Cell and Human Chorionic Gonadotropin–Producing Tumors

Clinical and Laboratory Features

Anna T. Englund, MD; Mitchell E. Geffner, MD; Ronald A. Nagel, MD; Barbara M. Lippe, MD; Glenn D. Braunstein, MD

• Germ cell tumors may cause various aberrations in pubertal development. In prepubertal boys, these tumors may secrete human chorionic gonadotropin, resulting in precocious puberty. Human chorionic gonadotropin and α-fetoprotein are both useful as germ cell tumor markers in the diagnosis and detection of recurrence. Pregnancy-specific β_1-glycoprotein, another oncoplacental antigen, has been used as a tumor marker for trophoblastic neoplasms, but not previously for human chorionic gonadotropin–producing tumors associated with precocious puberty. Patients with germ cell tumors may also have abnormal karyotypes. Herein, we describe six male pediatric patients with germ cell tumors and pubertal derangements seen during an 8-year period. We confirm the high incidence of associated sexual precocity, the usefulness of α-fetoprotein, human chorionic gonadotropin, and pregnancy-specific β_1-glycoprotein as tumor markers in the diagnosis and follow-up of these patients, and the occurrence of sex chromosomal abnormalities.

(*AJDC.* 1991;145:1294-1297)

Germ cell tumors occur rarely in children, but when present, they may cause abnormalities in puberty based on their anatomic location or due to the secretion of human chorionic gonadotropin (hCG). The most common hCG-secreting tumor causing precocious puberty is hepatoblastoma; however, germ cell tumors in various locations have also been reported to cause sexual precocity.[1-6] Human chorionic gonadotropin and α-fetoprotein (AFP) are two tumor markers that have been used in the diagnosis and treatment of these patients. Pregnancy-specific β_1-glycoprotein (SP-1), like hCG, is an oncoplacental protein that has been used as a marker for trophoblastic disease and various other neoplasms.[7,8] However, there are no reports concerning use of SP-1 as a tumor marker in patients with precocious puberty secondary to hCG-producing tumors. We describe six pediatric patients with germ cell tumors seen in our clinic during an 8-year period, in whom the usefulness of these tumor markers was investigated. Because of an association between germ cell tumors and Klinefelter's syndrome,[4,9-11] chromosomal analyses were also undertaken.

Accepted for publication June 3, 1991.

From the Department of Pediatrics, UCLA Medical Center (Drs Englund, Geffner, Nagel, and Lippe) and the Department of Medicine, Cedars-Sinai Medical Center, Los Angeles, Calif (Dr Braunstein).

Reprint requests to Department of Pediatrics, UCLA Medical Center, MDCC 22-315, 10833 Le Conte, Los Angeles, CA 90024 (Dr Englund).

PATIENTS AND METHODS

Patients

Between 1983 and 1990, five patients (all male) were referred to both the pediatric endocrinology and hematology services at UCLA Medical Center for evaluation of germ cell tumors with abnormalities in pubertal development. A sixth male patient is included who presented with precocious puberty associated with a hepatoblastoma. The clinical data of these patients are summarized in Table 1 and their laboratory data in Table 2.

Methods

Serum luteinizing hormone (LH) and follicle-stimulating hormone (FSH) concentrations were measured with radioimmunoassay (Amersham Corp, Arlington Heights, Ill). Testosterone was measured with standard radioimmunoassay. α-Fetoprotein was measured using an enzymatic immunoassay (Abbott Laboratories, Abbott Park, Ill); hCG, with an immunoradiometric assay (Hybritech Inc, San Diego, Calif); and SP-1, with radioimmunoassay as previously described.[12] Chromosomal karyotype was determined from peripheral lymphocytes, skin fibroblasts, and bone marrow using trypsin-Giemsa staining. A karyotype test was also performed on tumor tissue from patient 3. Bone age was determined from the standards of Greulich and Pyle.[13]

RESULTS

Patients 2, 3, and 6 clearly had precocious puberty and patient 5 had delayed puberty. While receiving therapy for growth hormone deficiency, patient 1 unexpectedly developed early pubertal changes, prompting an investigation that led to the discovery of his tumor.[3] The testicular volumes were small with respect to the degree of pubertal development in all patients except patient 2. Patients 2, 3, and 4 had germ cell tumors in the anterior mediastinum; patient 5, in the testicle; patient 1, in the

Table 1.—Clinical Data*

Patient No.	Age, y	Diagnosis	Ht Age,y	Ba, y	Test Vol, mL	Puberty
1	11.4	Suprasellar teratoma	8.8	10	4-5	Precocious; Tanner II
2	10.3	Anterior mediastinal teratoma/choriocarcinoma	11	16	15	Precocious; Tanner V
3	11.3	Anterior mediastinal yolk sac tumor	13	16-17	8-10	Precocious; Tanner V
4	15.9	Anterior mediastinal yolk sac tumor	18+	ND	5-6	Appropriate; Tanner V
5	18.5	L testicular seminoma	15	16	R 4; L 8-10	Delayed; Tanner III
6	1.5	Hepatoblastoma	1.7	1.5	4	Precocious; Tanner II

*Ht Age indicates the age at which the patient's height was at the 50th percentile; BA, bone age; Test Vol, testicular volume; R, right; L, left; ND, not done; and, Tanner, Tanner stage of genital/pubic hair development (II, early puberty; III, midpuberty; and V, adult).

Table 2.—Laboratory Data*

	Patient No.					
	1	2	3	4	5	6
hCG, IU/L						
Preoperative	33	1935	171	<5	100	110
Postoperative	<5	5	<5	ND	<5	6
AFP, μg/L						
Preoperative	<10	454	3000	7400	<4.8	1.1×10^6
Postoperative	ND	2.5	5.2	1.6	<4.8	9.6
SP-1, μg/L						
Preoperative	<5.7	9.95	<5.7	ND	ND	10.9
Postoperative	ND	<5.7	<5.7	ND	ND	<5.7
LH, IU/L†						
Preoperative	25	810	115	26	78	ND
Postoperative	<2	2	16	ND	13	ND
FSH, IU/L						
Preoperative	4	2	<2	39	<2	ND
Postoperative	<2	9	4	ND	48	ND
Testosterone, nmol/L						
Preoperative	18.2	33.6	19.3	3.0	35.0	44.4
Postoperative	<0.3	9.5	7.5	ND	14.5	<0.3
Karyotype	ND	46,XY‡§	46,XY‡§; 49,XXY,+8,+marker‖	46,XY/47,XXY‡	46,XY‡	ND

*hCG indicates human chorionic gonadotropin (normal, 0 to 5 IU/L); AFP, α-fetoprotein (normal, 0 to 6.6 μg/L); SP-1, pregnancy-specific β_1-glycoprotein (normal, <5.7 μg/L); LH, luteinizing hormone (normal adult male, 5.0 to 30 IU/L; prepubertal children, <5 IU/L); FSH, follicle-stimulating hormone (normal adult male, 2.5 to 16 IU/L; prepubertal children, <10 IU/L); and ND, not done. Normal testosterone levels are as follows: adult male, 12.1 to 35.7 nmol/L; prepubertal children, less than 0.3 nmol/L).

†False-positive increases in LH due to hCG.

‡Peripheral lymphocyte karyotype.

§Skin fibroblast karyotype.

‖Bone marrow and tumor tissue karyotype showed 49,XXY with an extra chromosome 8 and unidentified marker chromosomes (see text for explanation).

suprasellar region; and patient 6 had a hepatoblastoma. The bone age was advanced in two patients (patients 2 and 3) and appropriate for age in three others (patients 1, 5, and 6). The serum LH and testosterone levels were elevated before surgery in all patients, and decreased with therapy. The serum FSH level was low initially in all patients, except patient 4, who had Klinefelter's syndrome.

Tumor markers were useful in all patients. The hCG level was elevated in five of the six patients before surgery, and decreased with therapy. Patients 2, 3, 4, and 6 had elevated AFP levels; of the four patients in whom it was measured, SP-1 levels were elevated initially in patients 2 and 6, but decreased after surgery. However, hCG and AFP levels were also elevated in both patients in whom SP-1 was detected. Of the four patients tested, patients 3 and 4 had chromosomal mosaicism consistent with Klinefelter's syndrome. While mosaicism was detected with the routine peripheral lymphocyte chromosomal study of patient 4, the karyotype of patient 3 was normal in both peripheral blood and skin fibroblasts. However, analysis of bone marrow and tumor tissue from patient 3 revealed a mosaic Klinefelter karyotype as well as an additional chromosome 8 and an extra unidentified chromosomal marker. Fifty-six percent of the cells had 49 chromosomes (46,XXY, +8, +marker). Twenty-five cells had 48 chromosomes, all 46,XXY, but half with the +8 chromosome, and the other half with the +marker chromosome. The remaining cells had fewer than 48 chromosomes with similar changes, but random chromosome loss attributed to technical artifact.

COMMENT

Germ cell tumors may occur in the testis or ovary, or in a variety of extragonadal sites.[14] It is believed that the widespread location of germ cell tumors is due to aberrant migration in the fetus. While hepatoblastomas are not traditionally classified as germ cell tumors, reports on the structure of certain hepatoblastomas have shown multinucleated giant cells that stain positively for hCG and are morphologically similar to syncytiotrophoblastic cells.[6,15]

In pediatric patients, germ cell tumors often present with abnormalities in pubertal development. Paraneoplastic precocious puberty is caused by ectopic hormone production by a tumor, ie, hCG. Approximately 4% of boys with precocious puberty have hCG-producing tumors.[5] In a review of 35 cases of paraneoplastic precocious puberty, Navarro et al[4] noted that the most frequent cause was hepatoblastoma, followed by mediastinal teratoma, intracranial germ cell tumors, and, last, presacral and retroperitoneal carcinomas. All our patients had abnormalities in pubertal development. Three had tumors in the anterior mediastinum, while the other lesions occurred in the cranium, the testis, and the liver.

In patients with germ cell tumors, the early development of secondary sexual characteristics is due to stimulation of the testis by hCG causing secretion of testosterone without maturation of the hypothalamic-pituitary-testicular axis. This syndrome occurs almost exclusively in boys, although there have been reports of one affected girl.[16,17] Since hCG has LH-like biological activity (and cross-reactivity with the radioimmunoassay for LH), it is able to induce Leydig cell hyperplasia and testosterone secretion. However, Leydig cells do not constitute more than 25% of total testicular volume in the adult male.[1] Serum FSH levels are generally low in these patients, and therefore fail to stimulate Sertoli cell hyperplasia or spermatogenesis. For these reasons, boys with precocious puberty secondary to hCG production by tumors typically have only mildly enlarged testes, discordant with their degree of pubertal development.[18] Girls with hCG-producing tumors almost never develop precocious puberty, perhaps because the pulsatile secretion of both LH and FSH is required for follicular maturation.[2,4]

In patients with paraneoplastic precocious puberty, tumor markers such as AFP and hCG have been very helpful in diagnosis, monitoring of therapy, and detection of recurrence. α-Fetoprotein is a protein normally synthesized in fetal liver, gastrointestinal tract, and yolk sac; however, the postnatal detection of this protein may be indicative of abnormal secretion by a neoplasm. Human chorionic gonadotropin is normally synthesized by trophoblastic tissue of the placenta during pregnancy.[12,19] In our patients, either hCG or AFP levels were elevated at diagnosis and declined with therapy. Half of our patients had elevations of both tumor markers. We also report our results measuring SP-1, a protein that is normally secreted by the placental syncytiotrophoblast.[7,20] Although the function of SP-1 is not known, the concentration of this protein increases progressively throughout pregnancy until 36 weeks of gestation. Pregnancy-specific β_1-glycoprotein has been very useful as a tumor marker in the diagnosis and treatment of gestational trophoblastic diseases.[7,8,21-25] There have been many conflicting reports regarding the usefulness of SP-1 as a marker in other neoplasms such as testicular and ovarian germ cell tumors. Although many authors have described levels of serum SP-1 that parallel those of hCG, they do not offer any additional information.[17,26-29] However, there have been reports of cases of discordance between levels of serum SP-1 and hCG, suggesting that SP-1 alone can be a specific tumor marker.[30-33]

In our patients with germ cell tumors, the serum SP-1 concentration was elevated before surgery in two of the four patients in whom it was measured, and declined with therapy in both. It is noteworthy that the highest SP-1 level occurred in the patient with hepatoblastoma (patient 6). This supports the suggestion that hepatoblastomas may have syncytiotrophoblastic components. In our four patients in whom it was measured, SP-1 did not appear to have any advantage over hCG or AFP as a tumor marker.

There is a known association between Klinefelter's syndrome and anterior mediastinal tumors that secrete hCG.[4,9-11] Therefore, all our patients with tumors in this location underwent karyotyping. Patient 4, with an anterior mediastinal germ cell tumor, had mosaicism for Klinefelter's syndrome in peripheral blood lymphocytes. Patients 2 and 3, with tumors in this location, had normal chromosomes in peripheral blood and skin fibroblasts. However, patient 3 was shown to have Klinefelter's syndrome with a mosaic karyotype in the bone marrow and the tumor itself. Chromosome studies were not conducted on patients 1 and 6 since their tumor types (suprasellar teratoma and hepatoblastoma) are not known to be associated with karyotypic abnormalities. Thus, it is important to examine the chromosomal karyotype in a variety of tissues in male patients with anterior mediastinal germ cell tumors, regardless of their age or pubertal status.

This study was supported in part by the Hertzog Foundation, Los Angeles, Calif.

The karyotype test on tumor tissue from patient 3 was performed by Nancy Wang, PhD, University of Rochester (NY) Medical School.

References

1. Danon M, Weintraub BD, Kim SH, Scully RE, Crawford JD. Sexual precocity in a male due to thoracic polyembroma. *J Pediatr.* 1978;92:51-54.

2. Sklar CA, Conte FA, Kaplan SL, Grumbach MM. Human chorionic gonadotropin-secreting pineal tumor: relation to pathogenesis and sex limitation of sexual precocity. *J Clin Endocrinol Metab.* 1981;53:656-660.

3. Lippe BM, Edwards MS, Braunstein GD, Halks-Miller M. A nonmalignant teratoma secreting hCG: expanding the spectrum of ectopic hormone production. *J Pediatr.* 1984;105:765-768.

4. Navarro C, Corretger JM, Sancho A, Rovira J, Morales L. Paraneoplastic precocious puberty. *Cancer.* 1985;56:1725-1729.

5. Cheung PT, Low LCK. Case report: intracranial embryonal carcinoma and precocious puberty. *Aust Paediatr J.* 1987;23:201-203.

6. Heimann A, White PF, Riely CA, Ritchey AK, Flye MW, Barwick KW. Hepatoblastoma presenting as isosexual precocity. *J Clin Gastroenterol.* 1987;9:105-110.

7. Horne CHW, Towler CM. Pregnancy-specific β_1-glycoprotein: a review. *Obstet Gynecol Surv.* 1978;33:761-767.

8. Takayama M, Soma H, Isaka K, Okudera K, Ogawa T, Kikuchi K. Diagnostic reliability of simultaneous measurements of beta human chorionic gonadotropin and pregnancy-specific beta-1-glycoprotein in serum of patients with trophoblastic disease. *Gynecol Obstet Invest.* 1987;23:151-156.

9. Chaussain J, Lemerle J, Roger M, Canlorbe P, Job JC. Klinefelter syndrome, tumor, and sexual precocity. *J Pediatr.* 1980;97:607-609.
10. McNeil MM, Leong AS, Sage RE. Primary mediastinal embryonal carcinoma in association with Klinefelter's syndrome. *Cancer.* 1981;47:343-345.
11. Nichols CR, Heerema NA, Palmer C, Loehrer PJ, Williams SD, Einhorn LH. Klinefelter's syndrome associated with mediastinal germ cell neoplasms. *J Clin Oncol.* 1987;5:1290-1294.
12. Braunstein GD, Thompson R, Princler GL, McIntire KR. Trophoblastic proteins as tumor markers in nonseminomatous germ cell tumors. *Cancer.* 1986;57:1842-1845.
13. Greulich WW, Pyle SI. *Radiographic Atlas of Skeletal Development of the Hand and Wrist.* 2nd ed. Stanford, Calif: Stanford University Press; 1959.
14. Marsden HB, Birch JM, Swindell R. Germ cell tumors of childhood: a review of 137 cases. *J Clin Pathol.* 1981;34:879-883.
15. Watanabe I, Yamaguchi M, Kasai M. Histologic characteristics of gonadotropin-producing hepatoblastoma: a survey of seven cases from Japan. *J Pediatr Surg.* 1987;22:406-411.
16. Kubo O, Yamasaki N, Kamijo Y, Amano K, Kitamura K, Demura R. Human chorionic gonadotropin produced by ectopic pinealoma in a girl with precocious puberty. *J Neurosurg.* 1977;47:101-105.
17. Demura R, Demura H, Shizume K, Kubo O, Kitamura K. A female case of the hCG-producing ectopic pinealoma associated with precocious puberty. *Endocrinol Jpn.* 1976;23:215-219.
18. Pomarede R, Czernichow P, Finidori J, et al. Endocrine aspects and tumoral markers in intracranial germinoma: an attempt to delineate the diagnostic procedure in 14 patients. *J Pediatr.* 1982;101:374-378.
19. Skrabanek P, Kirrane J, Powell D. A unifying concept of chorionic gonadotropin production in malignancy. *Invest Cell Pathol.* 1979;2:75-85.
20. Sorensen S. Pregnancy-specific β_1-glycoprotein (SP_1): purification, characterization, quantification and clinical application in malignancies. *Tumor Biol.* 1984;5:275-302.
21. Lee JN, Salem HT, Al-Ani AT, et al. Circulating concentrations of specific placental proteins (human chorionic gonadotropin, pregnancy-specific beta-1 glycoprotein, and placental protein 5) in untreated gestational trophoblastic tumors. *Am J Obstet Gynecol.* 1981;139:702-704.
22. Than GN, Csaba IF, Bohn H, Szabo DG, Szalmasy M, Menczer G. Monitoring therapy in trophoblastic diseases by radioimmunoassay of pregnancy-specific β_1-glycoprotein and the β subunit of human chorionic gonadotropin. *Oncodevel Biol Med.* 1982;3:315-323.
23. Lee JN, Salem HT, Chard T, Huang SC, Ouyang PC. Circulating placental proteins (hCG, SP_1, and PP5) in trophoblastic disease. *Br J Obstet Gynecol.* 1982;89:69-72.
24. Szymendera JJ, Ploch E, Zalucka K, Sikorowa L, Kaminska JA, Gadek A. Gestational trophoblastic diseases: the ratio of choriogonadotropin to specific pregnancy protein, hCG/SP1, provides useful diagnostic and prognostic evidence. *Gynecol Oncol.* 1986;23:149-159.
25. Bocco JL, Panzetta G, Flury A, Patrito LC. Expression of pregnancy specific β_1-glycoprotein gene in human placenta and hydatiform mole. *Biochem Int.* 1989;18:999-1008.
26. Javadpour N, Utz M, Soares T. Immunocytochemical discordance in localization of pregnancy specific beta-1 glycoprotein, alpha-fetoprotein and human chorionic gonadotropin in testicular cancers. *J Urol.* 1980;124:615-616.
27. De Bruijn HWA, Sleijfer DT, Koops HS, Suurmeijer DTH, Marrink J, Ockhuizen T. Significance of human chorionic gonadotropin, alpha-fetoprotein, and pregnancy-specific beta-1-glycoprotein in the detection of tumor relapse and partial remission in 126 patients with nonseminomatous testicular germ cell tumors. *Cancer.* 1986;55:829-835.
28. Steffens J, Freidmann W, Nagel R. Immunohistochemical and radioimmunological determination of β-hCG and pregnancy-specific β_1-protein in seminomas. *Urol Int.* 1985;40:72-75.
29. Pulay T, Csomor S, Meszaros K, Szarka G, Csabay L, Szinnyai A. Significance of CEA, AFP, SP1 and hCG as tumor markers in ovarian carcinoma. *Neoplasma.* 1987;34:595-600.
30. Bagshawe KD, Lequin RM, Sizaret PH, Tatarinov YS. Pregnancy β_1 glycoprotein and chorionic gonadotrophin in serum of patients with trophoblastic and non-trophoblastic tumors. *Eur J Cancer.* 1978;14:1331-1335.
31. Lange PH, Bremner RD, Horne CHW, Vessella RL, Fraley EE. Is SP-1 a marker for testicular cancer? *Urology.* 1980;3:251-255.
32. Szymendera JJ, Zborzil J, Sikorowa L, Kaminska JA, Gadek A. Value of five tumor markers (AFP, CEA, hCG, hPL, and SP_1) in diagnosis and staging of testicular germ cell tumors. *Oncology.* 1981;38:222-229.
33. Suurmeijer AJH, de Bruijn HWA, Oosterhuis JW, Sleyfer DT, Koops HS, Fleuren GJ. Nonseminomatous germ cell tumors of the testis: immunohistochemical localization and serum levels of human chorionic gonadotropin (hCG) and pregnancy-specific beta-1 glycoprotein (SP-1); value of SP-1 as a tumor marker. *Oncodevel Biol Med.* 1982;3:409-422.

SPECIAL FEATURE

Radiological Case of the Month

William G. Bennett, MD (Contributor), *Beverly P. Wood, MD* (Section Editor)

A white boy born at 35 weeks' gestation was referred to Childrens Hospital of Los Angeles at age 4 days for evaluation of a mass palpated on the left side of the abdomen. The patient's mother was a gravida 1, para 1, 26-year-old whose prenatal course was complicated by gestational diabetes that was controlled with diet alone until 5 weeks before delivery, when it became necessary for her to self-administer subcutaneous insulin daily. Two days before admission, fetal movement ceased. On the second day of absent fetal movement, a nonstress test demonstrated mild decelerations in fetal heart rate thought to be secondary to fetal hypoxia. A transuterine ultrasound examination of the fetus was performed and demonstrated a mass in a left suprarenal location. On cesarean section, a 3600-g jaundiced boy was delivered.

Accepted for publication October 16, 1990.

Contributed from the Department of Radiology, Arkansas Children's Hospital, 800 Marshall St, Little Rock, AK 72202.

Reprint requests to the Department of Radiology, Box 81, Childrens Hospital of Los Angeles, 4650 Sunset Blvd, Los Angeles, CA 90054-0700 (Dr Wood).

The 1-minute and 5-minute Apgar scores were 7 and 9, respectively. Results of physical examination of the infant demonstrated a palpable left-upper-quadrant mass and jaundice. The total bilirubin level had risen from 200 µmol/L at birth to 320 µmol/L the day after birth and to 280 µmol/L the same day, but after phototherapy. The patient's urine was brown and contained numerous red blood cells. An abdominal ultrasound examination demonstrated a mass with a left suprarenal location displacing the left kidney inferiorly (Fig 1). The cortex of the kidney had hyperechoic streaks, and the pyramids were prominent (Fig 2). The right kidney and adrenal gland were normal.

The patient returned for a follow-up abdominal computed tomographic scan (Fig 3) and renal scan (Fig 4) 3 months after discharge. The left adrenal gland contained a few calcifications. However, the left kidney was markedly atrophic, nonenhancing, and only 2 cm long. The right kidney was normal in size and appearance, and the right adrenal gland was normal. The child was hypertensive but exhibited normal development.

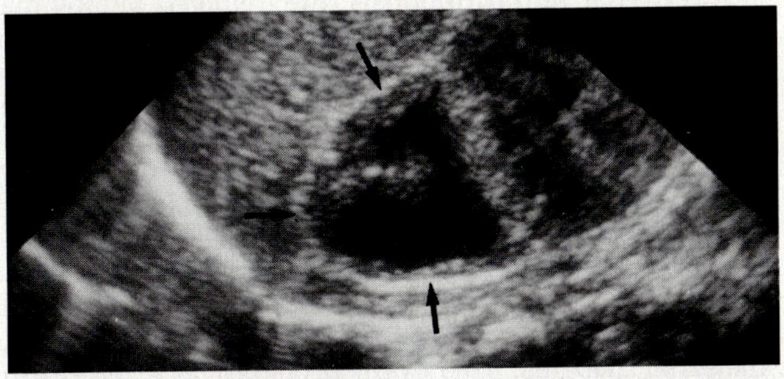

Figure 1.

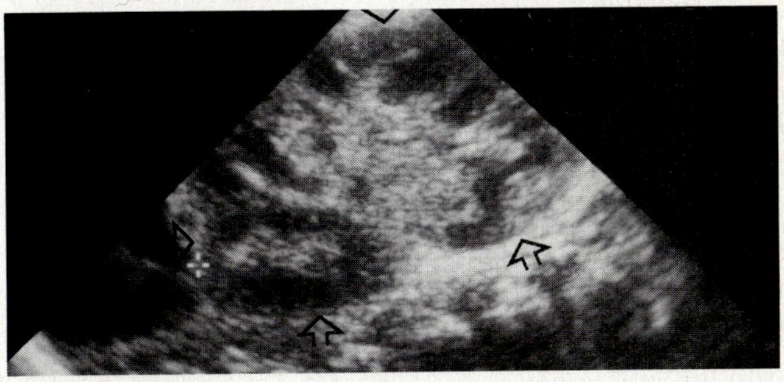

Figure 2.

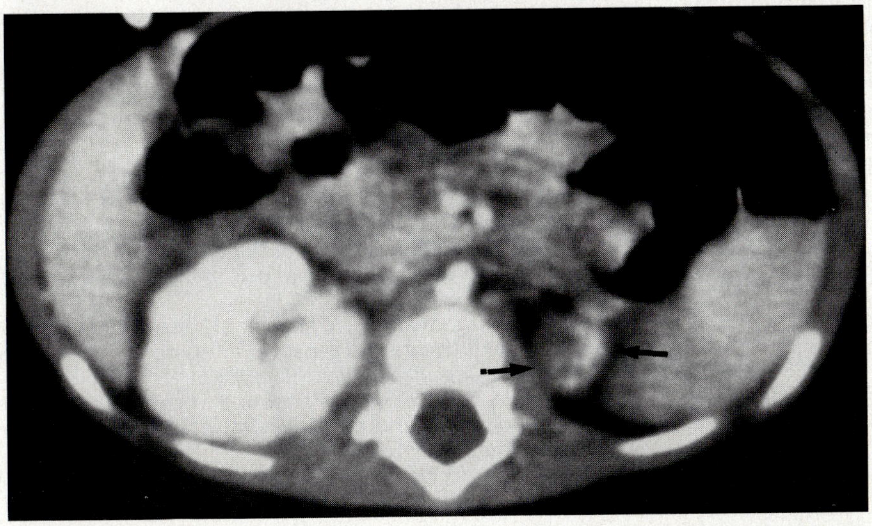

Figure 3.

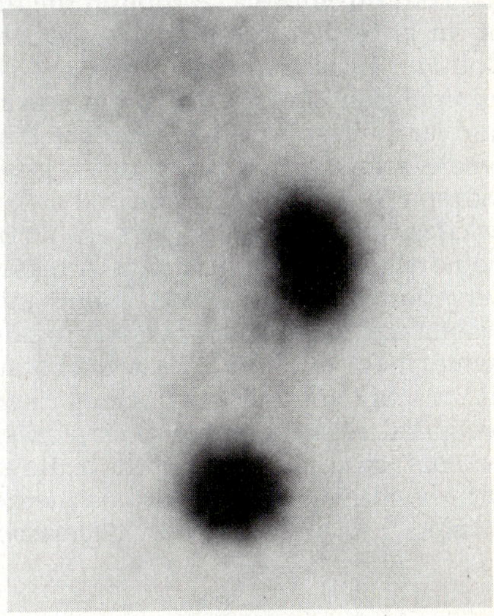

Figure 4.

Denouement and Discussion

Left Renal Vein Thrombosis and Left Adrenal Hemorrhage

Fig 1.—*Ultrasonogram of left suprarenal region shows mass with solid rim (arrows) and liquefied center.*

Fig 2.—*Ultrasonogram of left kidney (arrows) shows hyperechoic streaks in parenchyma.*

Fig 3.—*Computed tomogram at age 3 months shows tiny, atrophic left kidney (arrows).*

Fig 4.—*Renal scan at age 3 months shows no renal function in the left kidney.*

Adrenal hemorrhage is one of the less common causes of flank mass in neonates, the most common being renal masses such as hydronephrosis or multicystic dysplastic kidney.[1] There is an association between adrenal hemorrhage on the left side and ipsilateral renal vein thrombosis because of the anatomy of the left adrenal vein as a tributary of the left renal vein. Thrombus originating in the left adrenal vein may propagate into the left renal vein and even into the inferior vena cava.[2-4] On the right side, the renal and adrenal veins enter the inferior vena cava separately.

Adrenal hemorrhage in the neonate is associated with an infant who is large for gestational age, a breech delivery, sepsis, trauma, hypotension, hypovolemia, and hypoxemia. The clinical signs of adrenal hemorrhage are jaundice and a flank mass. The corresponding laboratory sign is elevated serum bilirubin values. Hematuria is not a feature of isolated adrenal hemorrhage but indicates renal vein thrombosis. Although the differential diagnosis of an adrenal mass includes neuroblastoma, serial abdominal ultrasound examinations demonstrate a solid adrenal gland followed by progressive central liquefaction and early resorption of adrenal hemorrhage within 2 weeks after birth, with complete resolution in 6 weeks. Adrenal function is unimpaired and residual dystrophic calcification frequently persists after resolution of the hemorrhage. Neuroblastoma increases in size during observation with serial ultrasound evaluation. Magnetic resonance imaging can help distinguish between adrenal hemorrhage and neuroblastoma because hemorrhage exhibits markedly increased signal intensity on T_1- and T_2-weighted sequences due to extracellular methemoglobin present within 72 hours of the acute event and persisting for several weeks afterward as methemoglobin is transformed into hematin, with decreased signal on T_1- and T_2-weighted images. Neuroblastoma exhibits heterogeneous intermediate signal intensity on T_1- and T_2-weighted images without significant change during the same time.

Renal vein thrombosis in the neonate is usually unilateral, and in most instances there is a history of hypoxia, sepsis, hypotension, or severe dehydration. There is an increased association with maternal diabetes, and thrombosis of the left renal vein is also associated with left adrenal hemorrhage. When both kidneys are affected, the infant presents with renal failure. When only one kidney is affected, the infant develops hematuria, proteinuria, and occasionally hypertension. The ultrasound findings vary from a normal appearance to enlargement of the kidney in the early stages, with a streaky increase of parenchymal echogenicity and loss of corticomedullary distinction. Later, results of radionuclide studies reveal poor or absent global renal perfusion, with poor excretion of tracer material. Serial radionuclide studies are helpful in monitoring return of function.

After renal vein thrombosis, the involved kidney may recover function if adequate collateral venous drainage is present or prompt recanalization of the renal vein occurs. If circulatory compromise persists, the involved kidney can respond by increasing renin production with resultant systemic hypertension, or the kidney may involute into an atrophic nonfunctioning kidney, usually without hypertension.

This neonate's adrenal hemorrhage was demonstrated in utero and was likely the result of hypoxia resulting from accelerated placental atherosclerosis in the presence of maternal diabetes. This event probably occurred during the 2 days before the nonstress test. Maternal diabetes and large infant size are predisposing factors in thrombosis of the left renal vein. This baby was large for gestational dates, which is consistent with poor control of maternal blood glucose levels.

References

1. Wofson BJ, Gainey MA, Faerber EN, Capitanio MA. Renal masses in children: an integrated imaging approach to diagnosi. *Urol Clin North Am.* 1985;4:755-769.

2. Lebowitz JM, Belman AB. Simultaneous idiopathic adrenal hemorrhage and renal vein thrombosis in the newborn. *J Urol.* 1983;3:574-576.

3. Brill PW, Jagannath A, Winchester P, Markisz JA, Zirinsky K. Adrenal hemorrhage and renal vein thrombosis in the newborn: MR imaging. *Radiology.* 1989;170(pt 1):95-98.

4. Bowen A, Smazal SF Jr. Ultrasound of coexisting right renal vein thrombosis and adrenal hemorrhage in a newborn. *J Clin Ultrasound.* 1981;9:511-513.

SPECIAL FEATURE

Picture of the Month

Philip R. Cohen, MD, Adelaide A. Hebert, MD (Contributors); *Murray Feingold, MD* (Editor for This Case); *Walter W. Tunnessen, Jr, MD* (Section Editor)

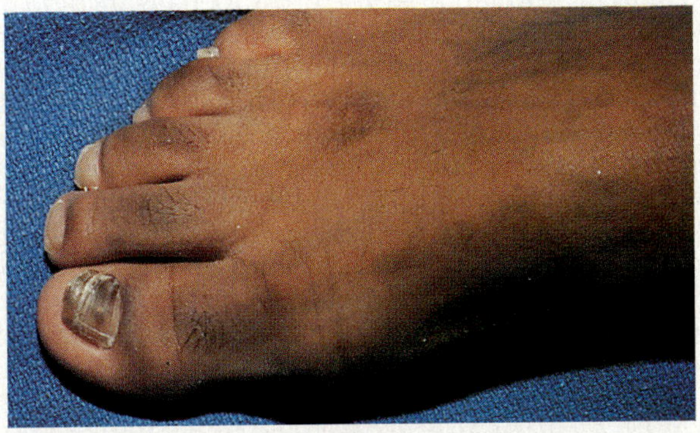

Figure 1.

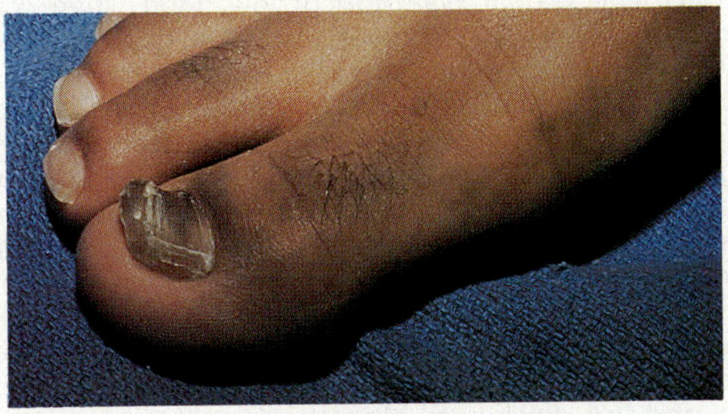

Figure 2.

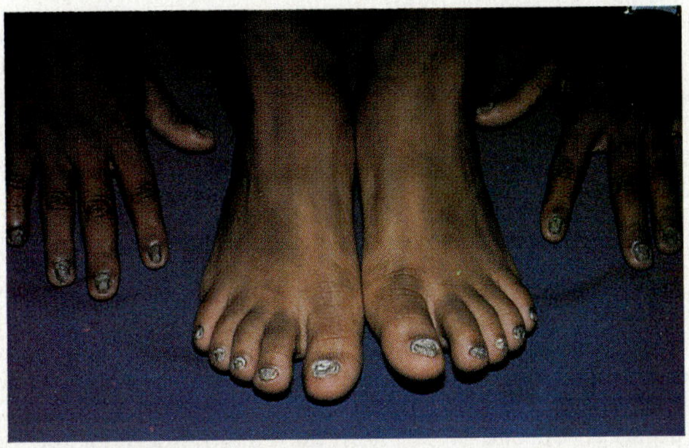

Figure 3.

The statements listed below are best associated with which of the figures: (*a*) This is a condition of autosomal-dominant inheritance affecting all nails. (*b*) This is a condition of autosomal-dominant inheritance affecting only one or two nails. (*c*) This is not a hereditary condition and affects all nails.

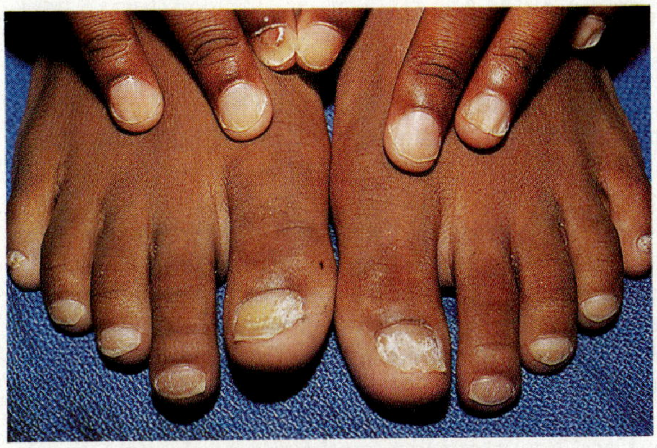

Figure 4.

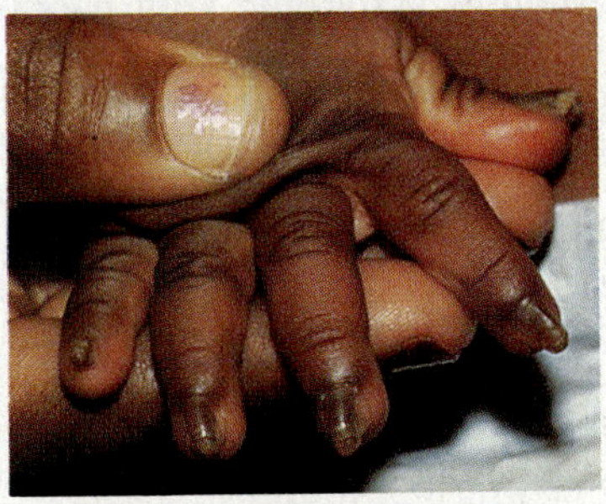

Figure 5.

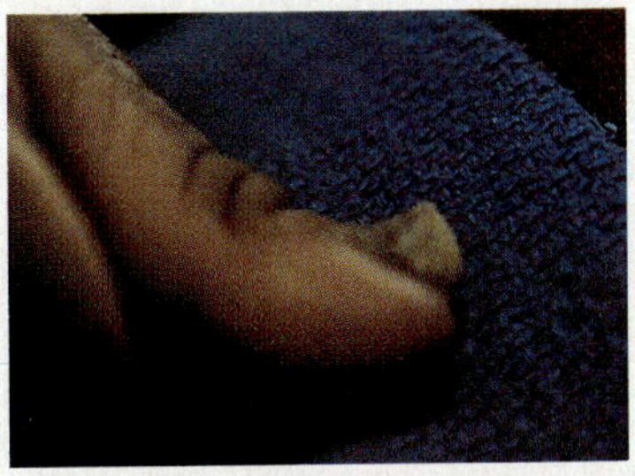

Figure 6.

Accepted for publication January 18, 1991.
Contributed from the Departments of Dermatology (Dr Cohen) and Pediatrics (Dr Hebert), University of Texas Medical School at Houston.
Reprint requests to National Birth Defects Center, Franciscan Children's Hospital, 30 Warren St, Brighton, MA 02135 (Dr Feingold).

Denouement and Discussion

Pachyonychia Congenita

Figs 1 and 2.—*A patient with congenital malalignment of the great toenail in which the right hallux nail is deviated in a lateral direction and has multiple transverse ridges on its surface.*

Figs 3 and 4.—*Thin, friable nails with loss of nail luster, multiple pits, excess longitudinal ridging, and distal notching that splits the nail into layers in a child with 20-nail dystrophy of childhood.*

Figs 5 and 6.—*Distal hypertrophy of the nails with marked subungual hyperkeratosis in a boy with pachyonychia congenita.*

(*a*) Pachyonychia congenita is a rare genodermatosis of autosomal-dominant inheritance with a high degree of penetrance and variable phenotypic expression. This disorder, first described by Jadassohn and Lewandowsky in 1906, has also been referred to as Jadassohn-Lewandowsky syndrome. The onychodystrophy typically appears within the first 6 months of life, and may be present at birth. It is characterized by hypertrophy and distal subungal hyperkeratosis of all nails. Secondary complications include nail shedding, chronic paronychial infections, and increased susceptibility to local traumatic injuries. The only effective treatment of the nail dystrophy has been surgical removal of the entire nail. Radical excision of the nail, nail bed, and nail matrix, followed by vigorous curretage and electrodessication of the bed and matrix with subsequent skin implantation at the site of the removed nail has provided good functional and esthetic results. In addition to onychodystrophy, mucosal and cutaneous manifestations associated with pachyonychia congenita include palmoplantar hyperkeratosis, leukokeratosis of the tongue and oral mucosa, follicular keratosis (especially on the elbows and knees), bullae and erosions on the palms and soles, natal or neonatal teeth, and angular cheilosis. Hair anomalies, corneal dyskeratosis, hoarseness, cataracts, mental retardation, and alopecia are less frequently noted features of pachyonychia congenita.

(*b*) Congenital malformation of the great toenails is an autosomal-dominant inherited onychodystrophy with variable expression that affects the nail of one or both halluces. The disorder is typically present at birth and characterized by lateral deviation of the nail with respect to the long axis of the phalanx. Transverse ridging is often present across the entire surface of the nail, and, less commonly, the nail may be discolored, thickened, shortened and/or onycholytic (characterized by loosening or separation of the nail from the nail bed). Complications of congenital malformation of the great toenails include ingrown toenails and hemionychogryphosis (a hooked or incurved nail). Although spontaneous improvement has been observed in a few children, the disorder usually persists into adulthood if not corrected earlier. Surgical realignment of the entire nail may be necessary for individuals with either marked nail deviation or condition-related disabling sequelae. The clinical differential diagnosis of congenital malformation of the great toenails may be made based on the presence of bacterial and candidal paronychia, ingrown toenails, congenital hypertrophy of the lateral nail folds of the hallux, dermatophyte infection, and onychogryphosis.

(*c*) In 1977, Hazelrigg et al described six healthy children with an onychodystrophy that uniformly affected the nails of all 20 digits: 20-nail dystrophy of childhood. There was no evidence of psoriasis vulgaris, lichen planus, alopecia areata, dermatitis, or ectodermal defects. Therefore, this condition was assumed to be idiopathic. In 20-nail dystrophy of childhood, the onychodystrophy is asymptomatic and appears insidiously. The nails are characterized by excessive longitudinal striations and loss of nail luster. The nails are thin, fragile, and have distal notching that splits the nails into layers. Regular manicuring and application of nail lacquer are the most effective palliative treatments. Similar features of this nail dystrophy have been noted in patients with lichen planus, alopecia areata, psoriasis vulgaris, and IgA deficiency. Hence, it is perhaps most appropriate to reserve the diagnosis of 20-nail dystrophy of childhood for children with idiopathic onychodystrophy that affects all of the nails.

The descriptive term for rough nails, trachyonychia, should be used when the nail changes traditionally found in 20-nail dystrophy of childhood are present in individuals with dermatologic or systemic illness that has also been associated with similar nail findings or in children or adults in whom less than all 20 nails are involved.

The Editors welcome contributions to Picture of the Month *and* Radiological Case of the Month. *Those who wish to contribute should send their manuscripts to Dr Tunnessen* (Picture of the Month), *The Children's Hospital of Philadelphia, 34th Street and Civic Center Blvd, Philadelphia, PA 19104, or Dr Wood* (Radiological Case of the Month), *Department of Radiology, Childrens Hospital of Los Angeles, 4650 Sunset Blvd, Los Angeles, CA 90027. Articles and photographs accepted for publication will bear the contributor's name. There is no charge for reproduction and printing of color illustrations.*

References

1. Feinstein A, Friedman J, Schewach-Millet M. Pachyonychia congenita. *J Am Acad Dermatol.* 1988;19:705-711.
2. Su WPD, Chun SI, Hammond DE, Gordon H. Pachyonychia congenita: a clinical study of 12 cases and review of the literature. *Pediatr Dermatol.* 1990;7:33-38.
3. Baran R, Bureau H. Congenital malalignment of the big toe-nail as a cause of ingrowing toe-nail in infancy: pathology and treatment (a study of thirty cases). *Clin Exp Dermatol.* 1983;8:619-623.
4. Harper KJ, Beer WE. Congenital malalignment of the great toe-nails—an inherited condition. *Clin Exp Dermatol.* 1986;11:514-516.
5. Hazelrigg DE, Duncan WC, Jarratt M. Twenty-nail dystrophy of childhood. *Arch Dermatol.* 1977;113:73-75.
6. Commens CA. Twenty nail dystrophy in identical twins. *Pediatr Dermatol.* 1988;5:117-119.

Direct Bilirubin Measurements in Jaundiced Term Newborns

A Reevaluation

Thomas B. Newman, MD, MPH; Sylvia Hope, PhD; David K. Stevenson, MD

• To investigate the usefulness of measuring direct bilirubin in jaundiced term newborns, we reviewed the outcome of 5255 such measurements on 2877 term (37 weeks' gestation) newborns in two hospitals. Direct bilirubin tests were ordered 15 times as often per infant at the University of California, San Francisco, as at Stanford (Calif) University, and the reported results were more than twice as high. In most of the 149 infants with high (>95th percentile) direct bilirubin levels, the high levels remained unexplained (52% of cases) or were due to apparent laboratory errors (21% of cases). Forty infants (27%) had conditions sometimes associated with high direct bilirubin levels. Elevation of direct bilirubin levels contributed to the diagnosis in only four of these infants. All had minor laboratory abnormalities that resolved spontaneously. Because of their low yield and poor specificity, direct bilirubin tests are seldom helpful in evaluating jaundice in term newborns.

(*AJDC*. 1991;145:1305-1309)

The evaluation of jaundice in newborns is one of the most common tasks in pediatrics. Many authorities recommend measuring the serum direct bilirubin in significantly jaundiced infants to distinguish between conjugated and unconjugated hyperbilirubinemia; algorithms for differential diagnosis of jaundice commonly begin with this step.[1-6] However, the "direct bilirubin" reported by many automated chemical analyzers may be a poor measure of the infant's actual conjugated bilirubin.[7-14]

Although the two terms are often used synonymously, *direct bilirubin* is not the same as *conjugated bilirubin*. Direct bilirubin refers to the bilirubin that reacts directly with diazotized sulfanilic acid (ie, without addition of an accelerating agent) in commonly used chemical assays. Conjugated bilirubin refers to bilirubin that has been made water soluble by binding with glucuronic acid in the liver. The amount of bilirubin that is called direct reacting depends on the concentration of conjugated bilirubin, but also on other factors, including the amount of time it is allowed to react, the concentration of various reagents, and the concentration of unconjugated bilirubin.[8] Unfortunately, in contrast to total bilirubin, for which interlaboratory standardization is available through the College of American Pathologists, there is no standardization of direct bilirubin measurements from laboratory to laboratory.

About 10% to 20% of term newborns develop significant jaundice,[15] but only about 0.04% develop pathologic conjugated hyperbilirubinemia.[16] Because direct bilirubin measurements tend to be least accurate in the presence of high unconjugated bilirubin levels, like those commonly found in newborns, measuring direct bilirubin in jaundiced infants could lead to many false-positive results.[17,18] The purposes of this study were to determine how commonly high direct bilirubin levels occur in infants who are and remain apparently well, to determine how commonly elevations of direct bilirubin are associated with previously unsuspected disease, and to develop guidelines for ordering and interpreting direct bilirubin measurements in jaundiced term newborns.

PATIENTS AND METHODS

Database

We used the Combined Patient Experience (COPE) database as the primary data source for this retrospective study. As has been described in previous reports,[19,20] the COPE database was created by merging computerized data from the clinical laboratory information systems, hospital census records, and hospital discharge abstracts at two hospitals: the University of California, San Francisco, Medical Center (UCSF), and the Stanford (Calif) University Medical Center. We supplemented the COPE database with data from the UCSF obstetrics department database and the Stanford Hospital Medical Information System (for length of stay, race, birth weight, and gestational age estimates). For infants born at UCSF in 1986 and 1987, the COPE database includes laboratory tests performed (at UCSF) after hospital discharge; for all other infants, outpatient data were available only by review of medical records.

Infants were included in the study if they were born and dis-

Accepted for publication May 13, 1991.

From the Division of General Pediatrics, Department of Pediatrics (Drs Newman and Hope), the Division of Clinical Epidemiology, Department of Epidemiology and Biostatistics (Dr Newman), and the Robert Wood Johnson Clinical Scholars Program (Dr Newman), School of Medicine, University of California, San Francisco, and the Division of Neonatology, Department of Pediatrics, School of Medicine, Stanford (Calif) University (Dr Stevenson).

Presented at the 31st Annual Meeting of the Ambulatory Pediatric Association, New Orleans, La, April 29, 1991.

Reprint requests to the Division of General Pediatrics, Box 0374, University of California, San Francisco, CA 94143 (Dr Newman).

Table 1.—Demographic Characteristics of Infants Born During the Study Period at Both Hospitals

	University of California, San Francisco 10/80-9/82	University of California, San Francisco 1/86-12/87	Stanford (Calif) University 1/86-6/87	Total
Total No. of births	2777	3001	5185	**10 963**
Term group				
No. of births at ≥ 37 weeks' gestation (% of all births)	2417 (87)	2614 (87)	4595 (89)	**9626** (88)
Mean ± SD birth weight, g	3427 ± 496	3435 ± 488	3486 ± 507	3457 ± 499
Length of stay, d				
Median	3	2	2	2
95th percentile	8	7	5	7
Race, No. (%) of infants				
White	1088 (45)	889 (34)	2343 (51)	4332 (45)
Asian	338 (14)	601 (23)	322 (7)	1251 (13)
Hispanic	242 (10)	183 (7)	597 (13)	1059 (11)
Black	193 (8)	157 (6)	368 (8)	674 (7)
Unknown/other	556 (23)	784 (30)	965 (21)	2310 (24)

charged during the periods covered by the COPE database: October 1, 1980, to September 30, 1982, and January 1, 1986, to December 31, 1987, at UCSF and January 1, 1986, to June 30, 1987, at Stanford. Premature infants (obstetrician's estimate at the time of maternal admission of less than 37 weeks' gestation) were excluded. Term infants who were small for gestational age and sick infants were not excluded. Based on reviews of medical records and nursery log books, we estimated that the UCSF database was close to 100% complete and the Stanford database was about 97% complete. The project was approved by the human subjects committees of both UCSF and Stanford.

Laboratory Methods

At UCSF, direct bilirubin was measured on either a DuPont Automated Chemical Analyzer (Dupont Instruments, Wilmington, Del) or a Coulter DACOS analyzer (Coulter Electronics, Hialeah, Fla). Both machines use a modification of the Jendrassik-Grof (diazotized sulfanilic acid) reaction; they were calibrated against each other daily. At Stanford, the Kodak Ektachem 700 (Eastman Kodak Co, Rochester, NY) was used. The Ektachem method measures conjugated (rather than direct) bilirubin using a multilayer slide technique. The conjugated bilirubin is assayed spectrophotometrically after it passes through a selective screening layer and complexes with a cationic polymer.[21]

Data Analysis

Our first task was to define what constitutes an abnormal direct bilirubin level. Textbook definitions generally range from 17 to 34 μmol/L.[5(p23),21-25] (To convert from micromoles per liter to milligrams per deciliter, divide the value by 17.10.) However, because the normal range depends on the analytic method used, we selected the maximum direct bilirubin level recorded for each infant, and arbitrarily defined as abnormal those values in the top 5% (of maximum recorded direct bilirubin levels) for their hospital of birth (≥39 μmol/L at UCSF; ≥17 μmol/L at Stanford). For all such infants, we reviewed the computerized laboratory data and medical records to determine the apparent reason (if any) for the elevation, using the following classifications:

Laboratory Error.—To classify an infant's high direct bilirubin level as due to laboratory error, we required that there be no diagnosis of hepatobiliary disease and that any aminotransferase levels measured be normal. Most of the apparent laboratory errors were isolated high values. To be so classified, there could be only a single abnormal value, and normal values at least 8.5 μmol/L less than the abnormal value had to have been obtained within 25 hours before and after the abnormal value. Other apparent laboratory errors were for miscellaneous reasons, including direct bilirubin levels exceeding the total bilirubin level (n = 2), specimens noted by the laboratory to be hemolyzed (n = 2), misplaced decimal points (n = 2), and mislabeled specimen (n = 1).

Associated Conditions.—This group included any infant not meeting the criteria for laboratory error, with either elevation of aminotransferase levels or a discharge diagnosis (confirmed by laboratory data or medical records review) of any significant hepatobiliary, gastrointestinal, renal, hematologic (except polycythemia), cardiovascular, metabolic (except infants of diabetic mothers), or infectious disease. The direct bilirubin was assumed to have potentially contributed to the diagnosis if its abnormality preceded the signs or diagnostic evaluation that led to the diagnosis, unless progress notes unambiguously indicated another reason for the evaluation.

Unexplained.—This group included all other infants. The high direct bilirubin level was considered to have resolved spontaneously if a return to well within the normal range (<90th percentile) was documented or if the infant was followed up in the outpatient clinic for at least 2 months without evidence of associated disease.

RESULTS

Demographic data on the 10 963 infants born at the two hospitals during the study periods are provided in Table 1. Both hospitals serve ethnically diverse populations, have high rates of preterm or low-birth-weight infants, and have short stays for term infants.

Ordering patterns and results for total and direct bilirubin levels are shown in Table 2 and Fig 1. Data for the two UCSF periods were similar and are combined in Table 2. There was a remarkable difference in the laboratory testing patterns of the two hospitals: infants born at UCSF were more than three times as likely to have total bilirubin measured at least once and more than 10 times as likely to have direct bilirubin measured at least once. The total number of direct bilirubin measurements per infant was 15 times higher at UCSF than at Stanford.

The mean, SD, and, in fact, the entire distributions of total bilirubin levels obtained at the two hospitals were practically identical. This surprising result suggests that the more selective total bilirubin testing at Stanford was based on factors other than the degree of jaundice.

In contrast, the median, 90th, and 95th percentiles for direct bilirubin at UCSF were more than twice as high as those at Stanford (for conjugated bilirubin), reflecting the

Table 2.—Measurements of Total and Direct Bilirubin in Term Infants at Two Hospitals*

	University of California, San Francisco (n=5031)	Stanford (Calif) University (n=4595)	Total (n=9626)
No. (%) of term infants with total bilirubin measured at least once	2786 (55)	753 (16)	3539
No. (%) of term infants with direct bilirubin measured at least once	2642 (53)	235 (5)	2877 (30)
Total No. of direct bilirubin tests	4948	307	5255
Mean (SD) maximum total bilirubin, μmol/L†	174 (63)	172 (62)	...
Maximum direct bilirubin percentiles, μmol/L†			
50	19	7	...
75	24	10	...
90	32	14	...
95	39	17	...
99	63	77	...

*At Stanford (but not at the University of California, San Francisco) direct bilirubin actually refers to conjugated bilirubin.
†To convert from micromoles per liter to milligrams per deciliter, divide the value by 17.10.

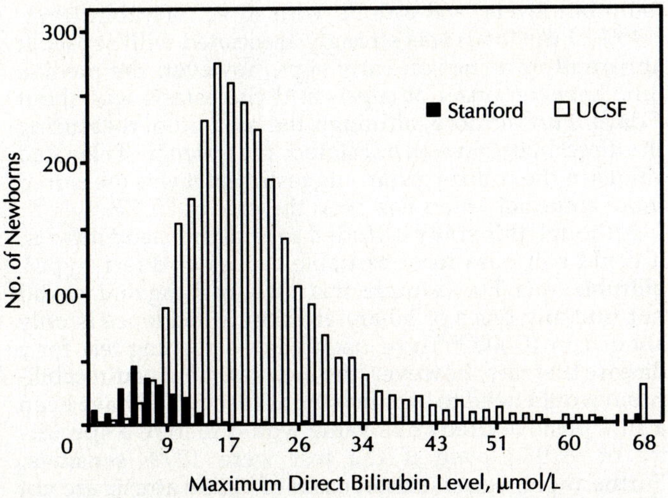

Fig 1.—*Maximum direct bilirubin levels for term infants born at Stanford (Calif) University (1986 to 1987) and at the University of California, San Francisco (UCSF) (1980 to 1982 and 1986 to 1987). To convert from micromoles per liter to milligrams per deciliter, divide values by 17.10.*

different measurement methods. The percentage of total bilirubin that was direct reacting at UCSF was similarly much higher than the percentage of conjugated bilirubin at Stanford.

Medical records were reviewed to determine possible reasons for direct bilirubin levels above the 95th percentile at each institution (Table 3). In most infants, the high direct bilirubin levels remained unexplained (52% of cases) or were due to an apparent laboratory error (21% of cases). Forty (27%) of the 149 infants with high direct

Table 3.—Reasons for Direct Bilirubin Levels Above the 95th Percentile Among Term Infants at University of California, San Francisco (n=140) and Stanford (n=9)*

Reason	No. (%) of Infants
Unexplained	
Resolved spontaneously, infant well	72 (48)
Well at discharge but no follow-up	6 (4)
Associated disease	
Direct bilirubin did not contribute to diagnosis†	
Isoimmunization	19 (13)
Sepsis or pneumonia	5 (3)
Congestive heart failure	5 (3)
Multiple anomalies	2 (1)
Pyloric stenosis	2 (1)
Extreme SGA, possible rubella‡	1 (1)
Hypothyroid (routine screening)	1 (1)
Choledochal cyst (prenatal sonography)	1 (1)
Direct bilirubin contributed to diagnosis	
Slightly high aminotransferase levels (<100 U/L)	3 (2)
Sludge in gallbladder	1 (1)
Laboratory error	
Isolated high value	24 (16)
Other	7 (5)

*At Stanford (but not at the University of California, San Francisco) direct bilirubin actually refers to conjugated bilirubin.
†Diagnosed from signs or symptoms, except as noted.
‡SGA indicates small for gestational age.

bilirubin levels had conditions that are at least occasionally associated with elevated conjugated bilirubin levels. However, the elevated direct bilirubin level did not lead to the diagnosis in any of these infants: most diagnoses were made before the direct bilirubin level was elevated, and most of the elevations were transient and of no apparent clinical significance. Four infants (3%) had findings identified apparently as a result of their direct hyperbilirubinemia. All had minor laboratory abnormalities that resolved spontaneously, including transient, slightly high (50 to 100 U/L) aminotransferase levels in three infants and "sludge" in the gallbladder in one infant.

Laboratory errors and unexplained elevations were frequent even at high levels of direct bilirubin (Fig 2). (The graph shows infants only at UCSF because seven of the nine infants at Stanford with maximum direct bilirubin values in the top 5% (for Stanford) had values less than 34 μmol/L) Use of a more restrictive cutoff resulted in little improvement in predictive value: of 30 infants with direct bilirubin values at or above the 99th percentile, only 11 (37%) had possibly associated conditions. Similarly, of 40 infants with direct or conjugated bilirubin levels exceeding the 95th percentile and comprising more than 30% of the total bilirubin, only 17 (42%) had possibly associated conditions. Thus, a more restrictive definition of direct hyperbilirubinemia was still associated with many apparently false-positive results.

We also investigated how often additional laboratory tests were ordered to evaluate direct hyperbilirubinemia. Only 23 (15%) of the 149 infants with high direct bilirubin levels had aminotransferase levels measured; levels were high in three well and 11 sick infants. Five infants received multiple serologic tests for congenital infection (no such infections were found), and three underwent serum protein electrophoresis, the results of which were normal. At least one infant underwent

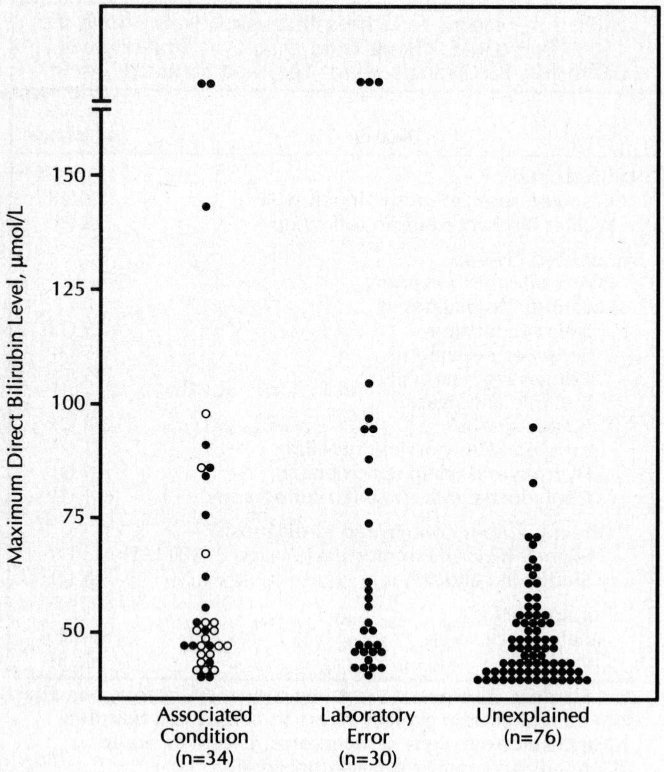

Fig 2.—*Distribution of the maximum direct bilirubin levels for infants born at the University of California, San Francisco (UCSF), with values in the top 5%, by apparent reason for the elevation. Open circles indicate infants in whom the elevation was attributed to isoimmunization; and solid circles, all other infants. To convert from micromoles per liter to milligrams per deciliter, divide values by 17.10.*

abdominal ultrasonography. Thus, additional tests were seldom performed; the usual response to high direct bilirubin levels was either to ignore them or to repeat them until they went down.

COMMENT

The COPE database allowed us to review results of more than 5000 determinations of direct bilirubin on 2877 infants at two hospitals. The striking findings were the marked variation in ordering patterns for this test at the two hospitals, the variation in the median and normal range for the different analytic methods, the high frequency of falsely positive results, and the absence of useful diagnostic information provided.

This study has some important limitations. Tests of direct bilirubin levels were ordered much more commonly at UCSF than at Stanford: the vast majority of infants (140 [94%] of 149) with documented high direct bilirubin levels were from UCSF. Since the analytic method at UCSF is particularly prone to errors, our results may not be generalizable to institutions using better methods. However, in a recent study, the DuPont ACA (used at UCSF) was the most popular machine, in use at 31% of the hospitals surveyed.[10] Clearly, clinicians interpreting results of direct bilirubin determinations need to be aware of the instrument used at their institution, as well as that instrument's accuracy and "normal range."

Our classification system for the high direct bilirubin values was necessarily arbitrary; we cannot say for sure that an isolated high direct bilirubin level was due to laboratory error, or that high values in infants with associated diseases were due to those diseases. However, in developing the classification scheme, we were very restrictive in the laboratory error and unexplained groups, and inclusive in the associated disease group.

This is illustrated by several diagnoses listed in Table 3. Pyloric stenosis, hypothyroidism, and even choledochal cysts are rarely associated with direct hyperbilirubinemia in the newborn period.[26-28] Thus, the elevations of direct bilirubin levels in infants in the associated condition category may have been largely coincidental. Among infants who had direct bilirubin measured, high values were only slightly more common in infants with a discharge diagnosis that would have qualified them for the associated condition category (97 [7.0%] of 1380 infants) than in infants with no such diagnosis (52 [3.5%] of 1497 infants). By including even questionable diagnoses in the associated disease category, we were giving the direct bilirubin measurement the benefit of the doubt in each case.

Similarly, in determining whether high direct bilirubin levels contributed to diagnoses, we required only that they could have contributed, not that they actually did. We were looking for instances in which direct bilirubin measurements led to diagnoses of unsuspected disease. Out of more than 5000 measurements of direct bilirubin, we found no such instances.

This study was limited to term infants, and most of those studied were well. It is likely that in a sicker population, a much greater proportion of the elevations of direct bilirubin would represent significant disease. For example, Wolf and Pohlandt,[29] in a recent case-control study of infants receiving parenteral nutrition, found that cholestasis (bilirubin levels >68 μmol/L with direct bilirubin levels >40% of the total) was strongly associated with sepsis. It apparently was not an early sign, however: the median time between onset of sepsis and cholestasis was about 7 days. Furthermore, although the method of measuring the direct bilirubin was not stated, the absence of elevated values in the control group suggests that it was measured more accurately than has been the case at UCSF.

Although this study included several thousand infants, it could still miss rare, treatable causes of direct hyperbilirubinemia. For example, it is not surprising that we did not find any cases of biliary atresia; its incidence is only about 1 in 10 000.[16] To be useful as a screening test for a disease that rare, however, the measurement of direct bilirubin would need to be much more specific. To have even a 10% positive predictive value would require a specificity of 99.9%, even if the test were 100% sensitive. Furthermore, because most cases of biliary atresia are not associated with cholestasis in the first few days of life,[16] direct bilirubin measurements would be insensitive as well as nonspecific. Finally, the prognosis for biliary atresia does not appear to worsen unless the diagnosis and surgery are delayed more than 2 months.[30,31] Thus, measurement of direct bilirubin in infants remaining jaundiced beyond the first week or two of life would be a more efficient strategy for detecting biliary atresia.

We do not know why tests of direct bilirubin were ordered so much less frequently at Stanford than at UCSF. While the charges for the test differed ($38 at Stanford vs $6 at UCSF), we doubt that the difference in frequency was due to the difference in charges. Rather, it is probably due to shorter stays at Stanford (leading to jaundice being noted in fewer infants), to differences in who decides to order the test (almost exclusively nurses and house staff at UCSF, compared with private pediatricians in about half the cases at Stanford), and differences in nursery traditions at the two institutions. At UCSF (before this study), tests of total and direct bilirubin were almost always ordered together, because treatment decisions were often based on the level of serum indirect bilirubin (ie, the total bilirubin level minus the direct bilirubin level), a practice recommended in many textbooks.[5,25,32]

Is this practice justified? We think usually not. Although automated analyzers provide a value that can be subtracted from the total bilirubin, it is a number that may have little relation to the infant's actual level of conjugated bilirubin. (Interestingly, the Kodak Ektachem, used with admirable restraint at Stanford, is one of the few machines that actually provides a good estimate of conjugated bilirubin.[8,13]) Thus, unless the test used provides an accurate reflection of conjugated bilirubin, treatment decisions should be based on total bilirubin and other evidence of cholestasis (eg, light stools or bilirubin in the urine).

In sick, jaundiced infants, or in any infants in whom cholestasis is suspected, measurement of serum direct bilirubin may be useful. Even then, however, visual examination of the stool and use of a dipstick in the infant's urine[33] may be as good. The infant's kidney can fractionate bilirubin better than most automated chemical analyzers.

Measurement of direct bilirubin is a poor screening test. Clinically inapparent, treatable causes of direct hyperbilirubinemia are rare, and many current methods of measuring direct bilirubin are inaccurate, leading to a high frequency of false-positive results. The practice of ordering a direct bilirubin test to make treatment decisions based on the indirect bilirubin level also generally cannot be justified unless the measurement of direct bilirubin is known to reflect conjugated bilirubin accurately. Our results suggest that measurements of direct bilirubin to evaluate jaundice in term newborns could be drastically reduced with no adverse effect on health.

This research was supported in part by grant MCJ-060573 from the Bureau of Maternal and Child Health, Health Resources and Services Administration, Department of Health and Human Services.

M. Jeffrey Maisels, MD, and Warren Browner, MD, MPH, provided helpful suggestions. The authors are indebted to the staff of the COPE project in the Department of Laboratory Medicine, University of California, San Francisco; the UCSF Department of Obstetrics and Gynecology; and the staff of the Stanford Hospital Medical Information System for providing us with data for this project.

References

1. Thaler MM. Jaundice in the newborn: algorithmic diagnosis of conjugated and unconjugated hyperbilirubinemia. *JAMA.* 1977;237:58-62.
2. Cloherty JP, Stark AR. *Manual of Neonatal Care.* 2nd ed. Boston, Mass: Little Brown & Co Inc; 1985:236.
3. White RD. Hyperbilirubinemia. In: Roberts KB, ed. *Manual of Clinical Problems in Pediatrics.* Boston, Mass: Little Brown & Co Inc; 1985:186-187.
4. Rosenthal P, Sinatra F. Jaundice in infancy. *Pediatr Rev.* 1989;11:79-85.
5. Cashore WJ. Neonatal hyperbilirubinemia. In: Oski FA, DeAngeles CD, Feigin RD, Warshaw JB, eds. *Principles and Practice of Pediatrics.* Philadelphia, Pa: JB Lippincott Co; 1990:401-405.
6. Rudolph AM, Hoffman JIE. *Pediatrics.* 18th ed. East Norwalk, Conn: Appleton & Lange; 1987:970-973.
7. Rosenthal P. The laboratory method as a variable in the diagnosis of hyperbilirubinemia. *AJDC.* 1987;141:1066.
8. Chan KM, Scott MG, Wu TW, Clouse RE, et al. Inaccurate values for direct bilirubin with some commonly used direct bilirubin procedures. *Clin Chem.* 1985;31:1560-1563.
9. Watkinson LR, St John A, Penberthy LA. Investigation into paediatric bilirubin analyses in Australia and New Zealand. *J Clin Pathol.* 1982;35:52-58.
10. Schreiner RL, Glick MR. Interlaboratory bilirubin variability. *Pediatrics.* 1982;69:277-281.
11. Mair B, Klempner LB. Abnormally high values for direct bilirubin in the serum of newborns as measured with the DuPont ACA. *Am J Clin Pathol.* 1987;87:642-644.
12. Pleasure JR. Bilirubin measurement problems. *Pediatrics.* 1988;82:808-809.
13. Ou C-N, Buffone GJ, Herr-Calomeni PJ, Finegold MJ, Shirey TL. Unconjugated hyperbilirubinemia is overestimated in neonates with cholestasis. *Am J Clin Pathol.* 1985;84:752-756.
14. Ou C-N, Buffone GJ, Herr-Calomeni PJ, Finegold MJ, Shirey TL. Conjugated bilirubin versus direct bilirubin in neonates. *Am J Clin Pathol.* 1986;85:613-616.
15. Newman TB, Easterling MJ, Goldman ES, Stevenson DK. Laboratory evaluation of jaundiced newborns: frequency, cost, and yield. *AJDC.* 1990;144:364-368.
16. Haber BA, Lake AM. Cholestatic jaundice in the newborn. *Clin Perinatol.* 1990;17:483-506.
17. Sackett DL, Haynes RB, Tugwell P. *Clinical Epidemiology: A Basic Science for Clinical Medicine.* Boston, Mass: Little Brown & Co Inc; 1985:139-158.
18. Fletcher RH, Fletcher SW, Wagner EH. *Clinical Epidemiology: The Essentials.* Baltimore, Md: Williams & Wilkins; 1982:67-73.
19. Kaplan EB, Sheiner LB, Boeckmann AJ, et al. The usefulness of preoperative laboratory screening. *JAMA.* 1985;253: 3576-3581.
20. Goldman ES, Easterling MJ, Sheiner L. Improving the homogeneity of diagnosis related groups by using clinical, laboratory, demographic, and discharge data. *Am J Public Health.* 1989;79:441-444.
21. Sykes E, Epstein E. Laboratory measurement of bilirubin. *Clin Perinatol.* 1990;17:397-416.
22. Behrman RE, Vaughan VC, eds. *Nelson Textbook of Pediatrics.* 13th ed. Philadelphia, Pa: WB Saunders Co; 1990:406.
23. Summit RL. *Comprehensive Pediatrics.* St Louis, Mo: Mosby–Year Book; 1990:346, 395.
24. Labrune P, Nyara A, Huguet P, Trivin F, Odievre M. Jaundice with hypertrophic pyloric stenosis: a possible manifestation of early Gilbert syndrome. *J Pediatr.* 1989;115:93-95.
25. Andres JM. Jaundice. In: Hoekelman RA, Blatman S, Nelson NM, Friedman SB, Seidel HM. *Primary Pediatric Care.* St Louis, Mo: Mosby–Year Book; 1987:1027.
26. Lippert MM. Pyloric stenosis presenting as severe prolonged jaundice: a case report. *S Afr Med J.* 1989;69:446-447.
27. Felber S, Sinatra F. Systemic disorders associated with neonatal cholestasis. *Semin Liver Dis.* 1987;7:108-118.
28. Hurst RW, MacGregor RS, Brookeman VA, Teates CD. Choledochal cyst: diagnosis in neonates. *South Med J.* 1988;81:1566-1568.
29. Wolf A, Pohlandt F. Bacterial infection: the main cause of acute cholestasis in newborn infants receiving short-term parenteral nutrition. *J Pediatr Gastroenterol Nutr.* 1989;8:297-303.
30. Hitch DC, Shikes RH, Lilly JR. Determinants of survival after Kasai's operation for biliary atresia using actuarial analysis. *J Pediatr Surg.* 1979;14:310-313.
31. Mieli-Vergani G, Howard ER, Portman B, Mowat AP. Late referral for biliary atresia—missed opportunities for surgical intervention. *Lancet.* 1986;1:421-423.
32. Gomella TL. Neonatology. *Basic Management, On Call Problems, Diseases, Drugs '88-'89.* East Norwalk, Conn: Appleton & Lange; 1988:422.
33. Maisels MJ. Bilirubin measurement problems. *Pediatrics.* 1988;82:809.

Bone Mineral Content of Healthy, Full-term Neonates

Effect of Race, Gender, and Maternal Cigarette Smoking

Pankaja S. Venkataraman, MBBS, James C. Duke, PhD

• In 238 healthy, full-term infants, we evaluated the effects of race, gender, and maternal cigarette smoking on the newborn radial bone mineral content. Sixty-one percent of the infants were male and 39% were female; 161 of 238 mothers were nonsmokers and 77 mothers were cigarette smokers. Bone mineral content was significantly correlated with birth weight, length, and head circumference. There were no significant race- and gender-related differences in neonatal bone mineral content. There was no significant difference in the bone mineral content, bone width, and bone density of the newborn at the left distal-third radius site among the infants of smokers compared with those of nonsmokers, and there was no correlation between neonatal bone mineral content and the number of cigarettes reportedly smoked per day by the mother.

(*AJDC*. 1991;145:1310-1312)

In a report from the United Kingdom in which the bone mineral content of the left forearm was measured, no significant differences were detected between Asian and white singleton newborns of greater than 35 weeks' gestational age and those of less than 2 weeks' postnatal age.[1] In reports from the United States, the bone mineral content of children has been shown to differ with race and gender,[2,3] with lower bone mineral content being observed in female children and in white children. However, we know of no studies that address the issue of whether such differences occur at birth.

The effect of cigarette smoking on the skeleton is varied. Smoking has been reported as a risk factor for development of osteoporosis in some studies,[4-13] but not in others.[14-17] In one study, bone mineral content of the radius was not significantly different between smokers and nonsmokers.[18] However, there was a significantly decreased response to menopausal hormonal therapy in smokers compared with nonsmokers.[19] The possible effects of maternal cigarette smoking on the bone mineral content of the neonate are not known. Hence, in healthy, full-term infants, we evaluated the hypothesis that bone mineral content at birth would be (1) higher in black infants than white infants, (2) higher in male infants than female infants, and 3) lower in infants born to cigarette smokers than in those born to nonsmokers.

Accepted for publication July 15, 1991.

From the Department of Pediatrics, University of Oklahoma Health Sciences Center, Oklahoma City.

Presented as a poster exhibit at the American Society for Bone and Mineral Research, Montreal, Quebec, September 12, 1989.

Reprint requests to Department of Pediatrics, University of Oklahoma Health Sciences Center, PO Box 26901 (2B307/CHO), Oklahoma City, OK 73190 (Dr Venkataraman).

SUBJECTS AND METHODS

Two hundred thirty-eight healthy, full-term infants delivered at Oklahoma Memorial Hospital, Oklahoma City, were studied. Informed consent was obtained from a parent in accordance with the University of Oklahoma Institutional Review Board regulations. All infants had weights appropriate for their gestational ages[20] and were free of major congenital malformations. History of maternal smoking was based on the mother's report of having smoked at least 10 cigarettes per day during pregnancy. All infants were studied during the first week of life, and bone mineral content was determined at the distal third of the left radius.

Sixty-one percent of the infants were male, and 39% were female. Race was assigned on the basis of parental identification; when there was ambiguity, data for these infants were excluded from analysis of race effects.

Bone mineral content was determined by photon absorption densitometry with the use of the single photon absorption densitometer (Lunar Radiation, Madison, Wis). The distal third of the left radius was scanned.[21-23] The coefficient of variation of the method is less than 7%.

Bone mineral content and bone width were measured, and bone density was computed as bone mineral content-bone width ratio.

Birth weights, lengths, and head circumferences were measured in all infants. The relationship of body weights and lengths to bone mineral content was also evaluated.

The data obtained were analyzed by means of *t* tests, Pearson's correlations, and regression analyses.[24] The SAS software was used. All data are given as mean±SD. Power was assessed for differences in bone mineral content between white male and female infants, black male and female infants, and infants born to cigarette smokers and nonsmokers.

RESULTS

Birth weights in male and female infants were 3,235±374 and 3208±353 g; length, 50.72±2.69 and 50.47±2.22 cm; and head circumference, 34.06±1.49 and 34.41±1.37 cm, respectively.

In all infants, bone mineral content at birth was positively correlated with birth weight, length, and head circumference with $r = .36$, $P < .0001$ for body weight;

Table 1.—Bone Mineralization in the Term Newborn Infant: Effect of Race and Gender*				
	Infant Group			
	White Male	White Female	Black Male	Black Female
N	65	51	50	23
Bone mineral content, g/cm	0.099±0.027	0.094±0.024	0.095±0.022	0.091±0.028
Bone width, cm	0.505±0.123	0.479±0.147	0.496±0.108	0.513±0.130

*Bone mineral content was not significantly different among black and white infants, nor by gender. Infants whose race could not clearly be defined are excluded here (hence the numbers given do not total 238).

Table 2.—Bone Mineral Content in Infants Categorized by Maternal Cigarette Smoking *		
	Smokers (n=77)	Nonsmokers (n=161)
Bone mineral content, g/cm	0.098±0.026	0.095±0.025
Bone width, cm	0.502±0.132	0.501±0.127
Bone density, g/cm²	0.194±0.031	0.194±0.038

*Bone mineral content, bone width, and bone density were not significantly different between the groups.

$r=.24$, $P<.0003$ for length at birth; and $r=.26$, $P<.0009$ for head circumference.

At the left distal-third radius site, the bone mineral content in male and female infants was 97.6±0.2 and 93±0.3 mg/cm, respectively (not significant). No significant differences were noted when infants were subgrouped by race. Bone mineral content and bone width were not significantly different between male and female infants at birth, or between white and black infants (Table 1).

There was no significant difference in bone mineral content, bone width, and bone density among infants delivered to smokers vs those of nonsmokers (group t test) (Table 2). Also, neonatal bone mineral content was not significantly correlated by regression analysis with the number of cigarettes smoked prenatally by the mothers.

The power assessment was computed based on a P value of .05 with β assumption of .1. For the data obtained in the present study, the power assessment for differences in mineral content between white male and female infants was 93%, that between black male and female infants, 90%; and that between infants born to smokers vs nonsmokers, 91%. The average power for all comparisons was 89%.

COMMENT

Previous studies in adults have documented the gender and racial[25,26] differences in bone mineral content and rate of bone loss with age. In a study of women aged 30 to 80 years, black women were found to have higher total body calcium content and higher radial bone mineral content than white women. The higher total body calcium content was observed even when corrections were made for body size.[27]

The skeletal development of black children has been reported to be advanced compared with that of white children, and body size is greater in black children than white children until adolescence.[26,28-30] In a study of skeletons, the bone density of skeletons from black Americans was found to be higher than that of age-matched white subjects,[31] and osteoporosis is less common in black than white subjects.[32-36]

Although in older children bone mineral content is higher in blacks than whites, and in male vs female children between the ages of 1 and 6 years,[2,3] it was previously unclear whether such differences exist at birth in healthy, full-term infants. In the present study, we found that the bone mineral content at birth did not differ significantly between white and black infants delivered at term gestation. Also, bone mineral content was not significantly different at birth among male and female infants. These findings suggest that although race- and gender-based differences in bone mineral content become apparent in the older child and in the adult, the in utero mineralization of the fetus is not significantly influenced by its race or gender. Our findings are consistent with those of previous reports from the United Kingdom in which there were no significant differences in radial bone mineral content as determined by photon absorption densitometry between white and Asian newborn infants,[1] suggesting that in those groups, ethnic differences are not present at birth.

Smoking has been suggested to decrease intestinal calcium absorption[18] and predispose to the development of skeletal demineralization.[4-13] Hence, smoking may influence the maternal skeleton and, indirectly, that of the offspring. In this study we determined that, in full-term infants, bone mineralization as determined at the distal-third radius site is not significantly altered by maternal cigarette smoking.

We are indebted to Sonja Ross and Suneela Bhoplay, MBBS, for technical assistance and to Linda Walling for secretarial assistance.

References

1. Congdon P, Horsman A, Kirby PA, Dibble J, Bashir T. Mineral content of the forearms of babies born to Asian and white mothers. *BMJ.* 1983;286:233-235.
2. Li J-Y, Specker BL, Ho M, Tsang RC. Bone mineral content in black and white children 1 to 6 years of age. *AJDC.* 1989;143:1346-1349.
3. Specker BL, Brazerol W, Tsang RC, Levin R, Searcy J, Steichen J. Bone mineral content in children 1 to 6 years of age: detectable differences after 4 years of age. *AJDC.* 1987;141: 343-344.
4. Daniell HW. Osteoporosis and smoking. *JAMA.* 1972;221: 509.
5. Daniell HW. Osteoporosis of the slender smoker. *Arch Intern Med.* 1976;136:298-304.
6. Daniell HW. Postmenopausal tooth loss: contributions to edentulism by osteoporosis and cigarette smoking. *Arch Intern Med.* 1983;143:1678-1682.
7. Williams AR, Weiss NS, Ure CL, et al. Effect of weight, smoking and estrogen use on the risk of hip and forearm fractures in postmenopausal women. *Obstet Gynecol.* 1982;60: 695-699.
8. Seeman E, Melton LJ, O'Fallon WM, et al. Risk factors for spinal osteoporosis in men. *Am J Med.* 1983;75:977-983.

9. Aloia JF, Cohn SH, Vaswani A, et al. Risk factors for postmenopausal osteoporosis. *Am J Med.* 1985;78:95-100.
10. Lindsay R. The influence of cigarette smoking on bone mass and bone loss. In: Deluca HF, ed. *Osteoporosis: Recent Advances in Pathogenesis and Treatment.* Baltimore, Md: University Park Press; 1981:481.
11. Mellstrom D, Rundgren A, Jagenburg R, et al. Tobacco smoking ageing and health among the elderly: a longitudinal population study of 70 year old men and an age cohort comparison. *Age Aging.* 1982;11:45-48.
12. McNair P, Christensen MS, Madsbad S, et al. Bone loss in patients with diabetes mellitus: effects of smoking. *Miner Electrolyte Metab.* 1980;3:94-97.
13. Hollo I, Gergely I, Boross M. Influence of heavy smoking upon the bone mineral content of the radius of the aged and effect of tobacco smoke on the sensitivity to calcitonin of rats. *Aktuel Gerontol.* 1979;9:365-368.
14. Paganini-Hill A, Ross RK, Gerkins VR, et al. Menopausal estrogen therapy and hip fractures. *Ann Intern Med.* 1981;95:28-31.
15. Kreiger N, Kelsey JL, Holford TR, et al. An epidemiologic study of hip fracture in postmenopausal women. *Am J Epidemiol.* 1982;116:141-148.
16. Aloia JF, Vaswani AN, Yeh JK, et al. Determinants of bone mass in postmenopausal women. *Arch Intern Med.* 1983;143:1700-1704.
17. Lindquist O, Bengtsson C, Hansson T, et al. Bone mineral content in relation to age and menopause in middle-aged women. *Scand J Clin Lab Invest.* 1981;41:215-223.
18. McDermott MT, Witte MC. Bone mineral content in smokers. *South Med J.* 1988;81:477-480.
19. Jensen J, Christiansen C. Effects of smoking on serum lipoproteins and bone mineral content during postmenopausal hormone replacement therapy. *Am J Obstet Gynecol.* 1988;159:820-825.
20. Brenner WE, Edelman DA, Hendricks CH. A standard of fetal growth for the United States of America. *Am J Obstet Gynecol.* 1976;126:555.
21. Cameron JR, Mazess RB, Sorenson JA. Precision and accuracy of bone mineral determination by direct photon absorptiometry. *Invest Radiol.* 1968;3:141-150.
22. Christiansen C, Rodbro P, Jenson H. Bone mineral content in the forearm measured by photon absorptiometry: principle and reliability. *Scand J Clin Lab Invest.* 1975;35:323-330.
23. Greer FR, Lane J, Weiner S, Mazess RB. An accurate and reproducible absorptiometric technique for determining bone mineral content in newborn infants. *Pediatr Res.* 1983;17:259-262.
24. Snedecor GW, Cochran GW, eds. *Statistical Methods.* 6th ed. Ames, Iowa: Iowa State University Press; 1967.
25. Garn SM. Bone loss and aging. In: Goldman R, ed. *Physiology and Pathology of Human Aging.* Orlando, Fla: Academic Press Inc; 1975:39-57.
26. Garn SM, Clark DC. Nutrition, growth, development and maturation: findings from the ten-state survey of 1968-70. *Pediatrics.* 1975;56:306-319.
27. Cohn SH, Abesamis C, Yasumura S, Aloia JF, Zanzi I, Ellis KJ. Comparative skeletal mass and radial bone mineral content in black and white women. *Metabolism.* 1977;26:171-178.
28. Owen GM, Lubin AH. Anthropometric differences between black and white preschool children. *AJDC.* 1973;126:168-169.
29. Garn SM, Sandusky ST, Nagy JM, McCann MB. Advanced skeletal development in low-income Negro children. *J Pediatr.* 1972;80:965-969.
30. Garn SM. Tendency toward greater stature in American black children. *AJDC.* 1973;126:164-166.
31. Trotter M, Broman GE, Peterson RR. Densities of bones of white and Negro skeletons. *J Bone Joint Surg Am.* 1960;42:50-58.
32. Bollet AJ, Engh G, Parson W. Epidemiology of osteoporosis. *Arch Intern Med.* 1965;116:191-194.
33. Engh G, Bollet AJ, Hardin G, Parson W. Epidemiology of osteoporosis. *J Bone Joint Surg Am.* 1968;50:557-562.
34. Gyepes M, Mellias HZ, Katz I. The low incidence of fracture of the hip in the Negro. *JAMA.* 1962;181:1073-1074.
35. Smith RW, Rizek J. Epidemiological studies of osteoporosis in women of Puerto Rico and southeastern Michigan with reference to age, race, national origin and other related or associated findings. *Clin Orthop.* 1966;45:31-48.
36. Smith RW, Eyler WR, Mellinger BC. On the incidence of senile osteoporosis. *Ann Intern Med.* 1960;52:773-781.

Correction

Incorrect Dose In the article entitled "Intraosseous Infusion of Dobutamine and Isoproterenol," published in the February issue of *AJDC* (1991;145:165-167), an error was made in the "Materials and Methods" section. On page 165, the first line of the fourth paragraph, in the right column, should have read as follows: "Dobutamine and isoproterenol were delivered at rates of 20 and 0.1 μg/kg per minute, respectively, intraosseously or intravenously."

Prevalence of Birth Defects Among Low-Birth-Weight Infants

A Population Study

Fatima Mili, MD, MPH; Larry D. Edmonds, MSPH; Muin J. Khoury, MD, PhD; Anne B. McClearn

• Major birth defects are diagnosed in about 3% to 4% of infants during their first year of life. Because many infants with birth defects have intrauterine growth retardation, are born prematurely, or both, the rate of birth defects undoubtedly varies according to the infant's birth weight. Nevertheless, the magnitude of such variation has not, to our knowledge, been adequately studied in well-defined populations. We analyzed data from the population-based Metropolitan Atlanta (Ga) Congenital Defects Program for 1978 through 1988. These data included information on 11 398 infants who were diagnosed with serious birth defects among 317 499 singleton live-born infants. Although the overall rate of birth defects was 3.6%, we observed a striking inverse relationship between the birth defects rate and the infants' birth weights. The birth defect rates were 16.2% for newborns weighing less than 1500 g at birth, 13.2% for newborns weighing from 1500 g to 1999 g, 6.2% for newborns weighing from 2000 g to 2499 g, 3.2% for newborns weighing from 2500 g to 3999 g, and 2.8% for newborns weighing 4000 g or more. Analyses by type of defect indicated that most birth defects were significantly associated with low birth weight. The higher risk of birth defects among low-birth-weight infants demonstrates that birth defects contribute to excess morbidity among low-birth-weight infants. Because of the overlap between birth defects and low birth weight, the prevention of low birth weight in the population depends greatly on a better recognition of the complex etiology of low birth weight and, in part, on the delineation of risk factors that influence the occurrence of birth defects.

(*AJDC.* 1991;145:1313-1318)

About 3% to 4% of infants are diagnosed with a major birth defect in their first year of life.[1] Because many infants with birth defects are born prematurely,[2] have intrauterine growth retardation,[3,4] or both, the rate of birth defects varies by birth weight. In a population-based study, Khoury et al[4] found a statistically significant higher risk of intrauterine growth retardation (birth weight below the race- and sex-specific 10th percentile limits for gestational age) among infants with serious birth defects (relative risk, 2.6). In population-based studies conducted in the United Kingdom,[5,6] 10% to 20% of stillborn and live-born infants weighing less than 2000 g at birth had birth defects. Investigators who obtained their information from hospital or vital records reported a high frequency of birth defects among infants with low or very low birth weight (<2500 g and <1500 g, respectively).[7-9] Case reports of infants with low and very low birth weight and specific birth defects have been frequently described in the literature: limb reduction,[10] esophageal atresia,[11-14] cleft lip and/or palate,[15,16] choanal atresia,[17] congenital heart disease,[18,19] neural tube defects[20-25] (particularly spina bifida[20,21] and anencephaly[22,23]), chromosomal disorders (including Down syndrome),[26-30] and various other syndromes.[31-39]

In this study, we present data on the rate of serious birth defects in the first year of life among low-birth-weight infants, using a population-based birth defects registry. The higher prevalence of birth defects among low-birth-weight infants has important implications for clinical care, etiologic research, and public health practice.

SUBJECTS AND METHODS

Study Population

The Metropolitan Atlanta Congenital Defects Program (MACDP) is an active surveillance system sponsored by the Centers for Disease Control, Emory University School of Medicine, and the Georgia Mental Health Institute (all located in Atlanta, Ga). Day-to-day program operations are the responsibility of the Centers for Disease Control. Created in October 1967, this program is designed to systematically collect data on all infants whose mothers reside in one of five counties in the metropolitan Atlanta area: Clayton, Cobb, DeKalb, Fulton, and Gwinnett. Subjects include live-born and stillborn infants (gestational age of at least 20 weeks or birth weight of 500 g or more) with major or serious structural defects diagnosed in the first year of life. Birth defects identified by prenatal diagnoses are excluded. Birth defects of interest include those that affect the child's survival, require substantial medical care, or cause marked physical or psychological handicap. Cases are ascertained from several sources: maternal and infant hospital medical records (20 hospi-

Accepted for publication July 15, 1991.

From the Birth Defects and Genetic Diseases Branch, Division of Birth Defects and Developmental Disabilities, Center for Environmental Health and Injury Control, Centers for Disease Control, Public Health Service, US Department of Health and Human Services, Atlanta, Ga.

Reprint requests to the Center for Environmental Health and Injury Control, Mail Stop F-29, Centers for Disease Control, 1600 Clifton Rd NE, Atlanta, GA 30333 (Mr Edmonds).

Table 1.—Rates of Major Birth Defects in Single Live Births by Birth Weight and Race From the Metropolitan Atlanta Congenital Defects Program, 1978-1988*

Birth Weight, g	Race	No. of Infants With Birth Defects	No. of Live Births	Rate of Major Birth Defects per 100 Live Births, %	Rate Ratio (95% Confidence Interval)
≤1499	White	277	1617	17.1	5.8 (5.2, 6.5)
	Other	429	2745	15.6	4.4 (4.0, 4.9)
	Total	**706**	**4362**	16.2	5.1 (4.8, 5.5)
1500-1999	White	280	1806	15.5	5.3 (4.7, 5.9)
	Other	297	2564	11.6	3.3 (2.9, 3.7)
	Total	**577**	**4370**	13.2	4.2 (3.8, 4.5)
2000-2499	White	438	6181	7.1	2.4 (2.2, 2.6)
	Other	446	8050	5.5	1.6 (1.4, 1.7)
	Total	**884**	**14 231**	6.2	2.0 (1.8, 2.1)
2500-3999	White	4723	160 236	2.9	1.0 (reference)
	Other	3622	102 630	3.5	1.0 (reference)
	Total	**8345**	**262 866**	3.2	1.0 (reference)
≥4000	White	674	24 780	2.7	0.9 (0.9, 1.0)
	Other	212	6890	3.1	0.9 (0.8, 1.0)
	Total	**886**	**31 670**	2.8	0.9 (0.8, 0.9)

*Birth defects considered secondary to prematurity are excluded among infants born weighing less than 2500 g (eg, patent ductus arterious, patent foramen ovale, pulmonary hypoplasia, hydrocephalus associated with intraventricular hemorrhage, and undescended testicles).

tals), local cytogenetic laboratories, specialty and genetic counseling clinics, and vital records. The surveillance system has been described in detail elsewhere.[40]

The MACDP is designed to collect data on major birth defects according to the six-digit Code for Reportable Congenital Anomalies, a modification of the British Pediatric Association Code, which itself is a modification of the ninth revision of the *International Classification of Diseases*. Since 1967, trained abstractors have collected data using standardized forms. These data include identification, demographic, clinical, and diagnostic information on the infant, as well as information on the mother's prior illnesses and pregnancy history. We excluded in our analyses the following defects for infants weighing less than 2500 g at birth because they were considered secondary to prematurity: patent ductus arteriosus, patent foramen ovale, pulmonary hypoplasia, hydrocephalus associated with intraventricular hemorrhage, and undescended testicles. The analysis was restricted to live-born singleton infants. We did not use data collected before 1978 because birth weight information was not complete among live-born infants. Between January 1, 1978, and December 31, 1988, MACDP monitored 317 499 neonates born live to mothers who reside in the metropolitan Atlanta area. Of these infants, 194 620 (61.3%) were white, and 122 879 (38.7%) were of other races. Among these infants, 11 398 (3.6%) singleton infants had serious birth defects.

Statistical Analysis

To determine the rate of birth defects in the first year of life among live-born singleton infants in five birth-weight categories (≤1499 g, 1500 g to 1999 g, 2000 g to 2499 g, 2500 g to 3999 g, and ≥4000 g), we analyzed data from the MACDP from 1978 through 1988 using Statistical Analysis Systems software.[41] The analyses were stratified according to race, maternal age (≤35 and >35 years), sex, and birth period (1978 to 1981, 1982 to 1985, and 1986 to 1988) as well as total number of defects and 37 specific types of defects. We determined birth defect rates by dividing the number of singleton live-born infants registered in the MACDP by the total number of singleton live births in five counties of the metropolitan Atlanta area during the same period. We calculated rate ratios by dividing the rate of birth defects for infants in each birth-weight category by that of infants weighing 2500 g to 3999 g, as well as the 95% confidence interval (CI) and corresponding two-tailed *P* value. To determine the significant interactions with demographic variables, we used the Breslow-Day test.[42,43] A significant test result suggests that the association between birth weight and birth defect varied across levels of the stratification variable. In the presence of interaction, we presented race-specific estimates for each category of the covariate. In the absence of interaction, we presented adjusted Mantel-Haenszel race-specific rate ratios.

RESULTS

Table 1 shows the rates of major birth defects among live-born singleton infants in different birth-weight categories according to race and the race-specific rate ratios adjusted for different demographic variables. The Figure summarizes the rates of birth defects by birth weight. Overall, 3.6% of the singleton infants born in Atlanta from 1978 through 1988 had major birth defects diagnosed in their first year of life. Low-birth-weight infants were at a 1.76-times higher risk of having birth defects than those weighing 2500 g to 3999 g (95% confidence interval, 1.7, 1.8). Infants weighing 4000 g or more were at a slightly lower risk of having birth defects than those weighing 2,500 g to 3,999 g. Stratified analyses by maternal age, birth period, and sex did not alter measures of rate ratio between birth weight and birth defects. Nevertheless, the magnitude of the rate ratio varied substantially across the different birth period categories among infants of other races weighing 1499 g or less or 2000 g to 2499 g, and between white male and white female infants weighing 4000 g or more.

As shown in Table 2, analyses by type of defect indicated that, with some exceptions, most specific birth defects were significantly associated with low birth weight. Incidences of the following birth defects were not statistically significantly increased among certain categories of low-birth-weight infants: choanal atresia, hypoplastic left heart, endocardial cushion defects, coarctation of aorta, esophageal atresia, bladder exstrophy, and Down syndrome in infants weighing 1499 g or less; transposition of great vessels in infants weighing 1499 g or less and 1500 g to 1999 g; common truncus in infants weighing 1500 g to 1999 g and 2000 g to 2499 g; pyloric stenosis and Hirschsprung's disease in infants weighing 1499 g or less, 1500 g to 1999 g, and 2000 g to 2499 g; and, finally, cataract in infants weighing 2000 g to 2499 g. In

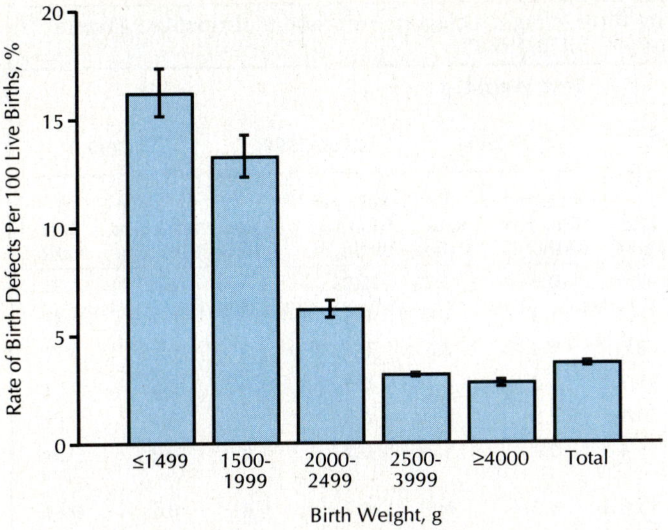

Rates of major birth defects in single live births by birth weight in Atlanta, Ga, from 1978 through 1988. Lines at tops of bars represent the 95% confidence interval around the rate.

addition, ventricular septal defect, endocardial cushion defects, reduction defects of limbs, Down syndrome, and congenital hip dislocation were the only defects significantly associated with the highest birth weight class. Their rate ratio was less than 1.0, except that congenital hip dislocation had a rate ratio of more than 1.0.

COMMENT

We have shown that although the overall rate of serious birth defects in these infants' first year of life is 3% to 4%, the rate of birth defects varies greatly across the different birth weight categories. From 16% to 17% of infants weighing less than 1500 g at birth had serious birth defects compared with about 3% of infants weighing 2500 g or more at birth.

A strength of our study is that Atlanta has operated a population-based birth defects registry since 1967. As an active surveillance system, MACDP maintains effective monitoring of all birth defects in infants regardless of their weight groups. In addition, the system includes multiple sources of ascertainment of serious birth defects in metropolitan Atlanta. Nevertheless, several potential limitations of this study should be considered. First, because data on gestational age have not been collected consistently among live-born infants in Atlanta, we could not directly evaluate rates of birth defects according to birth weight and gestational age. Second, our analyses are limited to live-born infants only, since stillborn infants are excluded from the denominator file (title containing the number of resident live births in the metropolitan Atlanta area). The rate of birth defects in stillborn infants may even be higher than that among live-born infants.[44] Third, some defects could more likely be detected in low-birth-weight infants (eg, cardiac defects) since sick infants tend to stay longer in the hospital. However, this type of detection bias is unlikely for severe and obvious birth defects such as neural tube defects, oral clefts, and diaphragmatic hernia. Finally, as shown in Table 1, infants of other races had lower rates of birth defects than white infants in the lower weight categories, which might reflect an underascertainment of birth defects among infants of other races.

These findings clearly suggest that low birth weight and birth defects are overlapping adverse perinatal outcomes that may share common pathogenic mechanisms. Two mechanisms may explain the association between low birth weight and birth defects: (1) birth defects can predispose infants to low birth weight if they lead to intrauterine growth retardation, preterm delivery, or both; and (2) low birth weight and birth defects may coexist because of common underlying factors.

The first mechanism suggests that the presence of birth defects is a risk factor for intrauterine growth retardation or preterm delivery. Serious birth defects are among a myriad of risk factors that contribute to intrauterine growth retardation or premature birth.[2,3,45] For example, infants with congenital heart malformations are at a higher risk of intrauterine growth retardation than those with or without other malformations.[18,19] Some researchers have suggested that hemodynamic factors, such as low oxygen saturation or perfusion, may contribute to the etiology of intrauterine growth retardation during fetal development and may be associated with some heart defects causing hypotrophy of organs such as the spleen, liver, kidneys, adrenals, and pancreas.[46] Analyses of the MACDP data[4] indicated that of 13 074 infants born with major birth defects in Atlanta between 1970 and 1984, 22.3% had intrauterine growth retardation (relative risk, 2.6; 95% CI, 2.5, 2.7); and of 48 defect categories evaluated in the analyses, 46 were associated with intrauterine growth retardation. The findings were particularly striking in infants with chromosomal anomalies (83.7% for infants with trisomy 18 syndrome; relative risk, 46) and anencephaly (73.3%; relative risk, 25). Furthermore, infants with multiple malformations were at a higher risk of having intrauterine growth retardation than those with isolated malformations. The risk increased substantially as the number of defects increased.

Likewise, birth defects could also be an important factor of premature birth. Fetal congenital malformations that seem to be associated with premature birth include anencephaly associated with polyhydramnios, renal agenesis associated with oligohydramnios, multiple congenital anomalies, and central nervous system anomalies.[2] Analyses of the MACDP showed that 21.3% of infants with birth defects are born prematurely (less than 37 weeks of gestation) compared with 5.6% of a random sample of all Atlanta infants (M.J.K. and A.B.M., Centers for Disease Control, unpublished data, 1990).

The second mechanism suggests that common factors may underlie the pathogenesis of low birth weight and birth defects. Some evidence indicates that embryologic and fetal growth are regulated by interactions between genes, environmental and nutritional components, fetal and placental hormones, and growth factors.[47,48] For example, birth weight correlates with fetal plasma levels of insulinlike growth factor I, although both insulinlike growth factors I and II increase gradually during fetal development up to birth.[47] Moreover, in teratogenesis, mechanisms that may be involved in the development of abnormal tissue include gene or chromosomal mutations, alteration of intercellular communication or membrane properties, and modulation of hormone receptors.[49] A well-established environmental risk factor for both birth defects and low birth weight is maternal consumption of alcohol during pregnancy.[50,51] Analyses of data from the MACDP, the Emory genetic clinics, and the Georgia Mental Health Institute showed that of 110 infants with

Table 2.—Rate of Specific Birth Defects in Single Live Births by Birth Weight Category From the Metropolitan Atlanta Congenital Defects Program, 1978-1988*

		Birth Weight, g									
		≤1499		1500-1999		2000-2499		2400-3999		≥4000	
Defect	No. of Cases	Rate per 1000 Live Births, %	Rate Ratio	Rate per 1000 Live Births, %	Rate Ratio	Rate per 1000 Live Births, %	Rate Ratio	Rate per 1000 Live Births, %	Rate Ratio	Rate per 1000 Live Births, %	Rate Ratio
Anencephaly	63	5.5	111.3	3.4	69.4	0.6	12.8	0.05	1.0	0.06	1.3†
Spina bifida	189	2.3	4.6	1.8	3.7	1.3	2.5	0.5	1.0	0.7	1.4†
Encephalocele	56	1.8	13.8	1.1	8.6	0.4	2.6	0.1	1.0	0.09	0.7†
Hydrocephalus	236	12.6	28.3	5.0	11.3	1.8	4.1	0.5	1.0	0.5	1.1†
Microcephalus	187	8.0	26.0	6.2	20.1	2.5	8.2	0.3	1.0	0.3	0.8†
Cataract	74	1.6	8.0	0.7	3.4	0.4	1.7†	0.2	1.0	0.2	0.9†
Anophthalnia and microphthalmia	116	3.7	16.1	3.4	15.0	1.5	6.5	0.2	1.0	0.1	0.6†
With or without cleft lip palate	310	3.9	4.7	5.0	6.1	1.7	2.0	0.8	1.0	0.9	1.1†
Cleft palate	155	3.0	7.5	3.2	8.1	1.2	3.0	0.4	1.0	0.2	0.6†
Choanal atresia	34	0.2	2.9†	0.5	5.7	0.5	6.2	0.08	1.0	0.09	1.2†
Ventricular septal defect	695	10.6	5.7	9.4	5.1	5.8	3.1	1.8	1.0	1.3	0.8
Tetralogy of Fallot	110	0.9	3.3	1.8	6.5	1.1	3.7	0.3	1.0	0.3	1.0†
Transposition of great vessels	148	0.7	1.6†	0.9	2.1†	0.8	1.9	0.4	1.0	0.4	1.0†
Hypoplastic left heart	102	0.7	2.5†	1.6	5.9	0.7	2.6	0.3	1.0	0.4	1.3†
Common truncus	24	0.5	6.7	0.2	3.3†	0.2	3.1†	0.07	1.0	0.0	0.0
Endocardial cushion defects	108	0.2	0.7†	1.1	3.7	1.2	3.8	0.3	1.0	0.09	0.3
Coarctation of aorta	122	0.5	1.3†	1.4	3.8	0.7	2.0	0.4	1.0	0.3	0.9†
Esophageal atresia	69	0.5	3.5†	4.1	31.8	1.0	7.6	0.1	1.0	0.03	0.2†
Small intestinal atresia	55	2.3	25.1	2.1	22.6	0.8	8.5	0.09	1.0	0.03	0.3†
Anorectal atresia	111	2.5	11.0	2.8	12.0	1.4	6.2	0.2	1.0	0.3	1.1†
Pyloric stenosis	445	0.7	0.5†	0.9	0.7	1.1	0.8†	1.4	1.0	1.6	1.2†
Hirschsprung's disease	51	0.0	0.0	0.0	0.0	0.1	0.8†	0.2	1.0	0.2	0.9†
Diaphragmatic hernia	64	0.7	3.9	0.7	3.9	0.4	2.4	0.2	1.0	0.2	1.0†
Omphalocele	73	0.7	4.3	2.3	14.3	0.8	4.8	0.2	1.0	0.2	1.4†
Gastroschisis	60	1.6	16.2	2.5	25.4	1.1	10.7	0.1	1.0	0.03	0.3†
Renal agenesis	87	3.4	33.5	5.0	49.0	1.3	13.0	0.1	1.0	0.1	1.2†
Cystic kidneys	96	1.2	5.6	3.0	14.5	1.4	6.8	0.2	1.0	0.1	0.6†
Bladder exstrophy	6	0.0	0.0	0.2	12.0	0.0	0.0	0.02	1.0	0.0	0.0
Hypospadias	919	8.5	3.3	8.5	3.3	5.6	2.2	2.6	1.0	2.6	1.0†
Anomalies of renal pelvis and ureter	187	3.7	8.2	2.8	6.2	1.8	3.9	0.5	1.0	0.5	1.2†
Clubfoot	858	9.4	3.8	8.9	3.6	4.6	1.8	2.5	1.0	2.0	0.8†
Reduction defects of limbs	136	2.5	8.0	3.7	11.7	1.7	5.4	0.3	1.0	0.09	0.3
Polydactyly	732	5.0	2.3	6.4	3.0	3.8	1.8	2.2	1.0	2.0	0.9†
Congenital hip dislocation	220	1.6	2.7	1.8	3.1	1.4	2.4	0.6	1.0	0.9	1.5
Down syndrome	300	1.4	1.6†	2.1	2.4	3.4	4.0	0.9	1.0	0.4	0.5
Trisomy 13	27	0.5	8.6	0.9	17.2	0.4	7.9	0.05	1.0	0.03	0.6†
Trisomy 18	46	2.8	120.5	3.4	150.4	0.9	40.0	0.02	1.0	0.0	0.0

*Birth defects considered secondary to prematurity are excluded among infants weighing less than 2500 g (eg, patent ductus arteriosus, patent foramen ovale, pulmonary hypoplasia, hydrocephalus associated with intraventricular hemorrhage, and undescended testicles).
†Not statistically significant.

fetal alcohol syndrome or fetal alcohol effect (diagnosed according to a scoring scheme developed by the Georgia Mental Health Institute), about 84% have low birth weight (M. L. Martin, and A.B.M., Centers for Disease Control, unpublished data, 1990). In addition, of 550 live-born cases reported in the literature worldwide,[52] 77% had low birth weight.

Finally, these findings have implications for clinical care, surveillance, and prevention. First, birth defects contribute to increased morbidity and mortality among low-birth-weight infants and are often associated with costly medical and surgical care that compounds medical problems related to low birth weight. These data are consistent with a recent analysis of National Center for Health Statistics data for the 1983 US birth cohort, indicating that the contribution of birth defects to infant mortality is relatively high among infants born weighing less than 2500 g.[53] The proportional mortality due to birth defects was 30% to 50% among those weighing 1500 g to 2499 g, compared with 20% to 30% among those weighing 2500 g or more.

Second, an increasing number of statewide programs are conducting or planning birth defect surveillance activities. Because low-birth-weight infants are at high risk for birth defects, targeting medical records of low-birth-weight infants should improve the overall ascertainment of birth defects in the population. Lastly, because a substantial proportion of low-birth-weight infants have associated birth defects, public health prevention strategies should include the complex etiology and pathogenesis of low birth weight and attempt to better delineate and prevent risk factors that influence the occurrence of birth defects.

References

1. Centers for Disease Control. *Congenital Malformations Surveillance Report. January 1982-December 1985.* Atlanta, Ga: US Dept of Health and Human Services; 1988.

2. Creasy RK. Preterm labor and delivery. In: Creasy RK, Resnik R, eds. *Maternal and Fetal Medicine: Principles and Practice.* Philadelphia, Pa: WB Saunders Co; 1984:415-443.

3. Creasy RK, Resnik R. Intrauterine growth retardation. In: Creasy RK, Resnik R, eds. *Maternal and Fetal Medicine: Principles and Practice.* Philadelphia, Pa: WB Saunders Co; 1984:491-510.

4. Khoury MJ, Erickson JD, Cordero JF, McCarthy BJ. Congenital malformations and intrauterine growth retardation: a population study. *Pediatrics.* 1988;82:83-90.

5. Powell TG, Pharoah POD, Cooke RWI. Congenital defects and the care of low birthweight infants. *Early Hum Dev.* 1988;16:173-183.

6. Alberman E, Benson J, Kani W. Disabilities in survivors of low birthweight. *Arch Dis Child.* 1985;60:913-919.

7. Fortune DW, Kitchen WH. Malformations in infants of very low birth weight. *Med J Aust.* 1977;1:239-242.

8. Drillien CM. Aetiology and outcome in low-birthweight infants. *Dev Med Child Neurol.* 1972;14:563-574.

9. Babson SG, Osterud HT, Thompson H. The congenitally malformed, IX: congenital malformation and the low birth weight infant. *Northwest Med.* 1966;65:729-732.

10. Calzolari E, Manservigi D, Garani GP, Cocchi G, Magnani C, Milan M. Limb reduction defects in Emilia Romagna, Italy: epidemiology and genetic study in 173 109 consecutive births. *J Med Genet.* 1990;27:353-357.

11. Ein SH, Shandling B, Wesson D, Filler RM. Esophageal atresia with distal tracheosophageal fistula: associated anomalies and prognosis in the 1980s. *J Pediatr Surg.* 1989;24:1055-1059.

12. Sapin E, Kurzenne JY, Bargy F, et al. Esophageal atresia in the new-born weighing less than 2000 grams: based upon 37 cases. *Chir Pediatr.* 1988;29:247-251.

13. Rickham PP. Infants with esophageal atresia weighing under 3 pounds. *J Pediatr Surg.* 1981;16(suppl 1):595-598.

14. Cozzi F, Wilkinson AW. Low birthweight babies with oesophageal atresia or tracheo-oesophageal fistula. *Arch Dis Child.* 1975;50:791-795.

15. Seth AK, McWilliams BJ. Weight gain in children with cleft palate from birth to two years. *Cleft Palate J.* 1988;25:146-150.

16. Rintala AE, Gylling U. Birth weight of infants with cleft lip and palate. *Scand J Plast Reconstr Surg.* 1967;1:109-112.

17. Takehara H, Hino M, Kameoka K, Okada A, Komi N, Ueda T. A case of congenital choanal atresia with extreme low birth weight baby. *Tokushima J Exp Med.* 1987;34:107-111.

18. Levin DL, Stanger P, Kitterman JA, Heymann MA. Congenital heart disease in low birth weight infants. *Circulation.* 1975;52:500-503.

19. Levy RJ, Rosenthal A, Fyler DC, Nadas AS. Birthweight of infants with congenital heart disease. *AJDC.* 1978;132:249-254.

20. Wald NJ, Cuckle HS, Boreham J, Althouse R. Birth weight of infants with spina bifida cystica. *Br J Obstet Gynaecol.* 1980;87:578-581.

21. Burns JK. Birth-weight distribution patterns in relation to estimated duration of pregnancy in normal infants, spina bifida and Down's syndrome. *J Physiol.* 1973;230:50P-51P.

22. Honnebier WJ, Swaab DF. The influence of anencephaly upon intrauterine growth of fetus and placenta and upon gestation length. *J Obstet Gynaecol Br Commonw.* 1973;80:577-588.

23. Milic AB, Adamsons K. The relationship between anencephaly and prolonged pregnancy. *J Obstet Gynaecol Br Commonw.* 1969;76:102-111.

24. Stoll C, Dott B, Roth MP, Alembik Y. Etiologic and epidemiologic aspects of neural tube defects. *Arch Fr Pediatr.* 1988;45:617-622.

25. Kulkarni ML, Mathew MA, Reddy V. The range of neural tube defects in southern India. *Arch Dis Child.* 1989;64:201-204.

26. Pueschel SM, Rothman KJ, Ogilby JD. Birth weight of children with Down's syndrome. *Am J Ment Defic.* 1976;80:442-445.

27. Anderson NG. A five year study of small for dates infants for chromosomal abnormalities. *Aust Paediatr J.* 1976;12:19-23.

28. Kucera J, Dolezalova V. Prenatal development of malformed fetuses at 28-42 weeks of gestational age (anencephalus, hydrocephalus, Down's syndrome, cleft lip and palate, and hypospadias). *Biol Neonate.* 1973;22:319-324.

29. Chen ATL, Chan YK, Falek A. The effects of chromosome abnormalities on birth weight in man, II: autosomal defects. *Hum Hered.* 1972;22:209-224.

30. Chen ATL, Sergovich FR, McKim JS, Barr ML, Gruber D. Chromosome studies in full-term, low-birth–weight, mentally retarded patients. *J Pediatr.* 1970;76:393-398.

31. Tokugawa K, Ueda K, Fukushige J. Congenital rubella syndrome in the Ryukyu islands: birth-weight and physical status before two years of age. *Acta Paediatr Jpn.* 1987;29:155-159.

32. Spiers PS, Wang L. Short pregnancy interval, low birthweight, and the sudden infant death syndrome. *Am J Epidemiol.* 1976;104:15-21.

33. Hunter AGW, Woerner SJ, Montalvo-Hicks LDC, et al. The Bowen-Conradi syndrome: a highly lethal autosomal recessive syndrome of microcephaly, micrognathia, low birth weight, and joint deformities. *Am J Med Genet.* 1979;3:269-279.

34. Adams JM, Gordon LP, Dutton RV, Rosenberg HS, Rudolph AJ. Leprechaunism (Donohue's syndrome) in a low birth weight infant. *South Med J.* 1977;70:998-1001.

35. Majewski F, Michaelis R, Moosmann K, Bierich JR. A rare type of low birthweight dwarfism: the Dubowitz syndrome. *Eur J Pediatr.* 1975;120:283-292.

36. Miller JD, McKusick VA, Malvaux P, Temtamy S, Salinas C. The 3-M syndrome: a heritable low birthweight dwarfism.

Birth Defects. 1975;11:39-47.
37. Christian JC, Johnson VP, Biegel AA, Gresham EL, Rosenberg GJ. Sisters with low birth weight, dwarfism, congenital anomalies, and dysgammaglobulinemia. *AJDC.* 1971;122:529-534.
38. Penchaszadeh VB. Low birthweight dwarfism. *Birth Defects.* 1971;7:303-304.
39. Ostergaard GZ, Tommerup N. The 8p-syndrome. *Ann Genet.* 1989;32:87-91.
40. Edmonds LD, Layde PM, James LM, Flynt JW, Erickson JD, Oakley GP Jr. Congenital malformations surveillance: two American systems. *Int J Epidemiol.* 1981;10:247-252.
41. *SAS User's Guide: Statistics.* Version 5 ed. Cary, NC: SAS Institute Inc; 1985.
42. Breslow NE, Day NE. Classical methods of analysis of grouped data. In: Breslow NE, Day NE, eds. *Statistical Methods in Cancer Research, II: The Analysis of Case-Control Studies.* Lyon, France: International, Agency for Research on Cancer scientific publication 32; 1980:121-159.
43. Stratified analysis. In: Kleinbaum DG, Kupper LL, Morgenstern H, eds. *Epidemiologic Research.* New York, NY: Van Nostrand Reinhold Co; 1982:373-374.
44. Incidence of congenital anomalies. In: Winter RM, Knowles SAS, Bieber FR, Baraitser M, eds. *The Malformed Fetus and Stillbirth.* New York, NY: John Wiley & Sons Inc; 1988:9-11.
45. Kliegman RM, Behrman RE. The high risk infant. In: *Nelson Textbook of Pediatrics.* 13th ed. Philadelphia, Pa: WB Saunders Co; 1987:373-385.
46. Naeye RL. Unsuspected organ abnormalities associated with congenital heart disease. *Am J Pathol.* 1965;47:905-915.
47. Milner RDG, Hill DJ. Fetal growth signals. *Arch Dis Child.* 1989;64:53-57.
48. Milner RDG, Hill DJ. Interaction between endocrine and paracrine peptides in prenatal growth control. *Eur J Pediatr.* 1987;146:113-122.
49. Vainio H. Carcinogenesis and teratogenesis may have common mechanisms. *Scand J Work Environ Health.* 1989;15:13-17.
50. Fetal alcohol effects. In: Jones KJ, ed. *Smith's Recognizable Patterns of Human Malformation.* Philadelphia, Pa: WB Saunders Co; 1988:491-494.
51. Day NL, Jasperse D, Richardson G, et al. Prenatal exposure to alcohol: effect on infant growth and morphologic characteristics. *Pediatrics.* 1989;84:536-541.
52. Abel EL. Diagnostic features of fetal alcohol syndrome. In: *Fetal Alcohol Syndrome.* Oradell, NJ: Medical Economics Books; 1990:55.
53. Centers for Disease Control. Contribution of birth defects to infant mortality among racial/ethnic minority groups, United States, 1983. *MMWR.* 1990;39(suppl 3):1-12.

In Other AMA Journals

ARCHIVES OF INTERNAL MEDICINE

Increasing Impact of Obesity on Serum Lipids and Lipoproteins in Young Adults: The Bogalusa Heart Study

Wendy A. Wattigney, MS; David W. Harsha, PhD; Santhanur R. Srinivasan, PhD; Larry S. Webber, PhD; Gerald S. Berenson, MD
(*Arch Intern Med.* 1991;151:2017-2022)

Substantial Improvement in Compliance With Universal Precautions in an Emergency Department Following Institution of Policy

Gabor D. Kelen, MD; Gary B. Green, MD; David A. Hexter, MD; Dewitt C. Fortenberry, MD; Eric Taylor, MD; Deborah H. Fleetwood, RN; Keith T. Sivertson, MD
(*Arch Intern Med.* 1991;151:2051-2056)

Sudden Deaths and Apparent Life-Threatening Events in Hospitalized Neonates Presumed to Be Healthy

David J. Burchfield, MD, D. Jim Rawlings, MD

• We describe 10 apparently healthy newborns who were patients in a level 1 nursery and were found by caregivers to be limp, apneic, and requiring resuscitation. All patients were between ages 15 hours and 3½ days, products of term gestations, and of appropriate weight for gestational age. Prenatal or perinatal complications were present in nine of the 10 patients; in no patient was the complication considered a risk for serious, late-onset neonatal problems. All patients had been examined by a physician and were deemed to be in good health before the apparent life-threatening event. Subsequent to the event, each patient required positive pressure ventilation and seven patients received chest compressions. Five patients died. Autopsies were performed on four of the five patients and in none was an adequate explanation for death established. Intrathoracic petechiae were found in one patient whose sibling had died of sudden infant death syndrome at age 11 weeks. Evaluation of the five survivors failed to determine a cause for the episodes. Of the five survivors, one had normal results of developmental examination at age 6 months, while the remaining four survivors had severe neurologic impairment at age 1 year. Apparent life-threatening events occur in hospitalized newborns presumed to be normal and may be a manifestation of early sudden infant death syndrome or early near-miss sudden infant death syndrome.

(*AJDC.* 1991;145:1319-1322)

Sudden infant death syndrome (SIDS) is recognized as the largest single cause of postneonatal infant mortality, with a peak incidence between ages 2 and 4 months, followed by a rapid decline in frequency by age 6 months.[1-3] When studied, 1% to 3% of cases of SIDS were found to occur during the first 2 weeks of life.[3-5] Many investigators excluded this age group from their epidemiologic studies[6-14] because of possible undetected perinatal events that may have led to the death. A diagnosis of SIDS during the first 2 postnatal weeks is often regarded with suspicion because of either the low incidence or the lack of inclusion in epidemiologic studies.

Accepted for publication June 17, 1991.

From the Department of Pediatrics, Division of Neonatology, University of Florida College of Medicine, Gainesville (Dr Burchfield) and Jacksonville (Dr Rawlings).

Reprint requests to Department of Pediatrics, Division of Neonatology, University of Florida College of Medicine, PO Box 100296, Gainesville, FL 32610-0296 (Dr Burchfield).

Between October 1985 and April 1990, 10 newborns were cared for in our neonatal intensive care units who were less than age 3½ days and had been found "limp and lifeless" or apneic by their caregivers in a level 1 newborn nursery. All the patients had been examined by a physician and were considered healthy. In our judgment, these events are best ascribed to SIDS or apparent life-threatening events (ALTEs) during the early neonatal period. We describe these 10 newborns to highlight that ALTEs occasionally occur in the early newborn period.

MATERIALS AND METHODS

The Regional Perinatal Intensive Care Unit at Shands Hospital in Gainesville, Fla, is a 20-bed, level 3 nursery with a mean of 760 patients admitted annually. Approximately 40% of the patients are transferred in; most transferees live within the 16-county area that is served by hospitals with level 1 nurseries. The Citywide Neonatology Program in Jacksonville, Fla, has 40 level 3 beds with a mean of 960 patients admitted annually. Of these patients, approximately 15% are transferred, primarily from level 1 and 2 nurseries within Jacksonville and five surrounding counties. Each patient in this report was either born at one of the level 3 hospitals and was initially cared for in the normal newborn nursery or was transferred to the level 3 hospital from a referring hospital following an acute event. All prenatal and perinatal data were obtained retrospectively from the patients' and their mothers' hospital records. In addition, all survivors were examined at age 6 months, and four of the five survivors were again examined at age 12 months in the State of Florida prospective longitudinal follow-up program of high-risk neonates.

PATIENT REPORT

A 4.03-kg white male neonate was born at 40 weeks' gestation to a healthy 19-year-old primigravida who had had frequent prenatal care. She smoked approximately 10 cigarettes each day and had mild pre-eclampsia treated with bedrest. She went into spontaneous labor 36 hours before delivery, with spontaneous rupture of the amniotic membranes 20 hours before delivery. She received meperidine hydrochloride (25 mg) and promethazine hydrochloride (10 mg) 5 hours before delivery. The mother received general anesthesia for a cesarean section due to cephalopelvic disproportion. The newborn received an Apgar score of 8/9 at 1 and 5 minutes. Resuscitation included nasopharyngeal suctioning for light meconium-stained fluid. Physical examination of the newborn revealed a weight in the 95th percentile. Results of the remainder of the examination were normal. The newborn had blood glucose values (Chemstrip bG, Boehringer Mannheim Corp, Indianapolis, Ind) of 2.2 mmol/L at ages 0.5, 2, and 4 hours. The newborn received formula by mouth begin-

Table 1.—Maternal and Perinatal Data*							
Patient No.	Maternal Age, y	Race	Gravity	Parity (F-P-A-L)	Syphilis Serology	Health, Pregnancy, L & D Complications	Type of Delivery
1	21	B	8	3-0-4-3	Nonreactive	Previous sudden infant death syndrome at 11 wk; fluid leak 4-6 wk; foul smell at delivery; nuchal cord	Spontaneous vaginal delivery
2	22	W	2	0-0-1-0	Nonreactive	Thick meconium in fluid; cords clear to inspection; 10% abruption	Spontaneous vaginal delivery, w/vacuum
3	27	W	2	0-0-1-0	Nonreactive	Elective abortion at 8 wk; glucosuria, normal glucose tolerance test result; light meconium	Spontaneous vaginal delivery w/vacuum
4	28	B	1	0-0-0-0	Reactive	Mild essential hypertension; pre-eclampsia	Cesarean section
5	32	W	1	0-0-0-0	Nonreactive	Thin meconium; failure to progress	Cesarean section
6	17	W	1	0-0-0-0	. . .	15% abruption	Spontaneous vaginal delivery
7	18	W	1	0-0-0-0	. . .	Smoked 1 pack of cigarettes per day; marijuana use	Spontaneous vaginal delivery, low
8	19	W	1	0-0-0-0	Nonreactive	Smoked ½ pack of cigarettes per day; mild pre-eclampsia	Cesarean section
9	21	W	2	1-0-0-1	Nonreactive	Normal	Spontaneous vaginal delivery
10	19	W	1	0-0-0-0	. . .	Decreased fetal movement near term; glucosuria, normal glucose tolerance test result	Spontaneous vaginal delivery, low forceps

*F-P-A-L indicates full term, premature, abortions, living; L & D, labor and delivery.

ning at age 6 hours and was fed 30 mL to 60 mL per feeding. The newborn was examined at age 14 hours by a pediatrician and was considered healthy. He nursed well from a bottle throughout the first 32 hours of life. At age 36 hours, routine nursing care was documented. About 10 minutes later, a nurse found the newborn in the bassinet limp, cyanotic, and without a detectable heart rate. She immediately administered assisted ventilation with bag and mask, and began chest compressions. The newborn's trachea was intubated and the heart rate returned to greater than 100 beats per minute within 2 minutes. However, spontaneous respiration did not return for 45 minutes. Plasma electrolyte levels were within normal limits and plasma glucose was 13.5 mmol/L following resuscitation. No abnormalities were found on a chest film. Blood was obtained for aerobic and anaerobic culture and the newborn was transferred to the Regional Perinatal Intensive Care Unit at Shands Hospital. The patient had a seizure during the transfer and was administered phenobarbital (40 mg/kg) intravenously. Further treatment included fluid restriction, hyperventilation, antibiotics, and nitroprusside for severe hypertension with lactic acidosis. Computed tomography of the brain performed within 12 hours of the event revealed no structural abnormalities or abnormal collections of blood. Blood cultures obtained after the event were sterile. Results of serum amino acid profile were within normal limits. Other than irregular respiratory efforts, the newborn had no evidence of brain-stem function for 7 days and artificial ventilation was withdrawn. Autopsy revealed hypoxic-ischemic damage to the brain, but no developmental defects were noted.

RESULTS

Table 1 summarizes maternal and perinatal data for each of the 10 patients who experienced ALTEs. Ellipses indicate that no information was available for that category. Nine of the 10 pregnancies had some complicating factor prenatally or ante partum but in no case was the complication considered a risk for serious, late-onset neonatal problems. Reactive serologic results occurred in one mother who received treatment for syphilis 1 year previously. No evidence of syphilis in the newborn was evident at autopsy.

Table 2 summarizes postnatal data for each case. Ellipses indicate that documentation was too vague to obtain specific times. All newborns were examined by a pediatrician or family practitioner before the ALTE and were considered healthy. The "Last Fed" and "Last Seen" columns in Table 2 record the times that the staff interacted with the patients. All patients had sucked formula or breast milk within 6 hours of the event except patient 8, who drank glucose water 3 times before the event. The patients' ages at the time of the ALTE ranged from 15.3 to 76.5 hours. Six of the ALTEs took place between 3 AM and 6 AM. The rest were interspersed throughout the day.

All newborns required assisted ventilation and seven of the 10 required chest compressions. Autopsies were performed on four of the five who died. Patient 1, whose sibling had died of SIDS, had thymic and pulmonary petechiae. The other autopsies revealed no abnormalities. Patient 6 died at age 21.7 hours and had a postmortem blood culture that yielded coagulase-negative *Staphylococcus*. He had a normal white blood cell count and differential count, normal cerebrospinal fluid study results, no growth on his urine culture, and no evidence of focal infection at autopsy. These facts suggest that this bacterium was not an overwhelming pathogen in the newborn. Coagulase-negative *Staphylococcus* has been a common contaminant in that particular nursery and has been identified as a pathogen only infrequently, usually in chronically stressed premature infants with in-dwelling central catheters.

Immediate postevent arterial blood gas measurements were available for nine of the 10 patients (Table 2). Metabolic acidosis of moderate to severe degree was uniformly present. The $PaCO_2$ and PaO_2 values varied, perhaps in part due to the amount of ventilation and oxygenation provided during initial resuscitation.

Table 2.—Postnatal Data

Patient No.	Sex	Apgar at 1 min/5 min	Gestational Age, wk	Weight, g	Time, min* Last Fed	Last Seen	Postnatal Age, h	Arterial Blood Gas pH	PCO_2	PO_2	BE†	Outcome
1	F	3/8	40	3465	−175	−175	17.5	6.82	40	90	−29	Died; autopsy revealed thymic and pulmonary petechiae; focal choroid plexus hemorrhage
2	F	8/9	39	3125	. . .	−15	76.5	6.95	23	317	−27	Died; organ donor; no autopsy; removed from ventilator
3	F	9/9	39	3490	−175	−15	15.3	6.74	38	309	−32	Lived; normal evaluation at age 6 mo.
4	M	9/10	40	3949	. . .	−75	69.0	6.95	126	46	−13	Died; autopsy revealed normal findings
5	M	9/10	39	3900	−60	−60	17.3	6.88	18	474	−22	Lived; severe neurologic impairment
6	M	8/9	41	3550	−347	−37	21.7	. . .	. . .	. . .	. . .	Died; autopsy revealed normal findings
7	F	8/10	40	3025	−126	−126	27.3	7.04	20	443	−24	Lived; severe neurologic impairment
8	M	8/9	40	4028	−285	−10	36.5	6.97	23	641	−27	Died; autopsy revealed normal findings
9	M	9/9	39	3550	−240	−10	36.5	7.27	22	372	−10.6	Lived; severe neurologic impairment
10	M	8/9	39	3200	−259	−19	36.7	6.85	65	80	−20.1	Lived; severe neurologic impairment

*Last Fed and Last Seen show time before apparent life-threatening event.
†BE indicates base excess and is expressed in milliequivalent per liter.

Survivors had extensive but unrevealing diagnostic evaluations that included sterile blood cultures, normal cranial computed tomograms, normal serum electrolyte levels, normal electrocardiograms, no reducing substance in the urine, and normal amino acid profile in either serum or urine or both. Of the five survivors, four were severely neurologically impaired at age 1 year. At age 6 months, patient 3 scored within normal ranges on all aspects of the Bayley Scales of Infant Development. This patient's family moved out of state, so the patient could not be evaluated at age 1 year.

COMMENT

We describe 10 newborns who suffered an ALTE during the early newborn period. We believe that these newborns demonstrated no signs or symptoms of ill health and that their admission to and care provided in a level 1 or "normal newborn" nursery was warranted. Postresuscitation and/or autopsy studies did not identify causes for the events.

Because the 10 neonates were born in five different cities and because we cannot be certain that no similar cases occurred in these cities, the incidence of early neonatal ALTEs cannot be defined. Polberger and Svenningsen[15] described 13 neonates who suffered either early SIDS or early near-miss SIDS. Ten of these newborns were born at the authors' institution, which allowed them to establish an incidence of early SIDS or early near-miss SIDS in their hospital of 0.50 per 1000 full-term infant births. Four of the 13 neonates were later proven to have bacterial sepsis and two had anemia. However, seven of the neonates had no identifiable cause for their life-threatening or life-taking episodes.

Six of the 10 patients described herein experienced their ALTE in the early morning. In the study by Polberger and Svenningsen, all 13 neonates experienced their ALTE between 11 PM and 6 AM. These findings are consistent with the epidemiology of SIDS occurring in the early morning.[4,16]

The characteristic SIDS event is quiet, sudden, unexpected, and life-threatening. Autopsy reveals no anatomic cause for the demise, and may show mild pulmonary congestion, inflammation, or intrathoracic petechiae.[3,16] Since nine of the 10 patients in this study were in nurseries and under professional care at the time they experienced an ALTE, the circumstances surrounding these events are well documented. The patients fit into the diagnostic category of SIDS or ALTE, despite their early postnatal age. Because the frequency of SIDS is known to be quite low during the first 2 weeks of extrauterine life, the closer to birth that such an event occurs, the greater is the tendency to view a diagnosis of SIDS with suspicion. When faced with a patient who presents with an ALTE during the first hours or days of life, the physician should diligently seek known causes of severe apnea and bradycardia, especially treatable ones. If death occurs, a complete postmortem examination should be performed. If no cause of death is found, it is important to classify the event as SIDS and not to rule out this diagnosis based on the age of the patient. Pediatric caregivers who might be involved with similar cases should know that neonates may have an unexplained ALTE in the early newborn period.

References

1. Hunt CE, Brouillette RT. Sudden infant death syndrome: 1987 perspective. *J Pediatr.* 1987;110:669-677.
2. Mellins RB, Haddad GG. Sudden infant death syndrome. In: Behrman RE, Vaughan VC, Nelson WE, eds. *Nelson Textbook of Pediatrics.* Philadelphia, Pa: WB Saunders Co; 1987:1480-1482.
3. Beckwith JB. *The Sudden Infant Death Syndrome.* Rockville, Md; Public Health Service Office of Maternal and Child Health;1976. US Dept of Health, Education, and Welfare publication HSA 76-5137.
4. Brooks JG. Apnea of infancy and sudden infant death syndrome. *AJDC.* 1982;136:1012-1023.
5. Fedrick J. Sudden unexpected death in infants in the Oxford Record Linkage area: an analysis with respect to time and place. *Br J Prev Soc Med.* 1973;27:217-224.
6. Irgens LM, Skajaerven R, Peterson DR. Prospective assessment of recurrence risk in sudden infant death syndrome siblings. *J Pediatr.* 1984;104:349-351.
7. Biering-Sorenson F, Jorgensen T, Hilden J. Sudden infant death syndrome in Copenhagen 1956-1971, II: social factors and morbidity. *Acta Paediatr Scand.* 1979;68:1-9.
8. Naeye RL, Ladis B, Drage JS. Sudden infant death syndrome: a prospective study. *AJDC.* 1976;130:1207-1210.
9. Froggatt P, Lynas MA, Marshall TK. Sudden death in babies: epidemiology. *Am J Cardiol.* 1968;22:457-468.
10. Kraus JF, Borhani NO. Post-neonatal sudden unexplained death in California: a cohort story. *Am J Epidemiol.* 1972;95:497-510.
11. Peterson DR. Sudden, unexplained death in infants: an epidemiologic study. *Am J Epidemiol.* 1966;84:478-482.
12. Nelson KE, Greenberg MA, Mufson MA, Moses VK. The sudden infant death syndrome and epidemic viral disease. *Am J Epidemiol.* 1975;101:423-430.
13. Froggatt P, Lynas MA, MacKenzie G. Epidemiology of sudden unexpected death in infants ('cot death') in Northern Ireland. *Br J Prev Soc Med.* 1971;25:119-134.
14. Standfast SJ, Jereb S, Janerich DT. The epidemiology of sudden infant death in upstate New York. *JAMA.* 1979;241:1121-1124.
15. Polberger S, Svenningsen NW. Early neonatal sudden infant death and near death of full term infants in maternity wards. *Acta Paediatr Scand.* 1985;74:861-866.
16. Valdés-Dapena MA. Sudden and unexpected death in infancy: a review of the world literature 1954-1966. *Pediatrics.* 1967;39:123-138.

In Other AMA Journals

ARCHIVES OF OPHTHALMOLOGY

Pigmented Paravenous Retinochoroidal Atrophy: Discordant Expression in Monozygotic Twins

Kent W. Small, MD, W. Banks Anderson, Jr, MD
(*Arch Ophthalmol.* 1991;109:1408-1410)

How Much of Neonatal Encephalopathy Is due to Birth Asphyxia?

Karin B. Nelson, MD, Alan Leviton, MD

• In the literature on neonatal encephalopathy, the pervasive assumption is that once infants with major malformations or infections have been excluded, most of the remaining cases are due to birth asphyxia. Assessing the proportion of neonatal encephalopathy that is due to asphyxia during birth is difficult because of problems in defining asphyxia and neonatal encephalopathy and in recognizing the cause of neonatal neurologic illness. Available evidence indicates that neonatal neurologic signs are not strongly related to obstetric complications, signs of fetal distress, or biochemical markers usually considered to indicate perinatal asphyxia. Most studies that have sought positive evidence of independent markers of intrapartum asphyxia have found them to be absent in a large majority of neurologically symptomatic neonates. We conclude that the proportion of neonatal encephalopathy that is asphyxial in origin is not known but warrants examination, especially in view of the probable need in the near future to identify, on the basis of *evidence available in the first hour or so of life*, suitable candidates for clinical trials of powerful but risky treatments of birth asphyxia.

(*AJDC.* 1991;145:1325-1331)

Intrapartum asphyxia severe enough to produce irreversible brain injury in the term infant is regularly followed by signs of neurologic illness in the neonatal period.[1-3] Neonatal encephalopathy (NE) is a clinically defined syndrome of disturbed neurologic function in the earliest days of life in the term infant, manifested by difficulty with initiating and maintaining respiration, depression of tone and reflexes, subnormal level of consciousness, and often by seizures.[4] Other names for this syndrome, such as hypoxic-ischemic encephalopathy (HIE) and postasphyxial encephalopathy, suggest that this syndrome almost always follows recent asphyxia (or hypoxia or ischemia or some combination of these), especially during birth.

Is it true that NE is usually due to asphyxia? This question gains a fresh urgency because new treatments intended to prevent death or long-term neurologic deficits from birth asphyxia are on the horizon.[5-10] These powerful and potentially risky therapies will require an ability to identify—and identify very rapidly—infants whose problems are truly secondary to asphyxia at birth and serious enough to warrant some risk in their treatment.

In this article, we review the knowledge base currently available for assessing the fraction of NE that is due to asphyxia at birth and ask how well predictors of neonatal asphyxia that are *available within the first hour or two of life* permit us to recognize seriously asphyxiated infants who might be candidates for immediate intervention for birth asphyxia.

DEFINITIONS OF BIRTH ASPHYXIA AND THEIR USE AS PREREQUISITES TO DEFINITIONS OF NE

Asphyxia

A major initial problem in assessing the relationship between NE and asphyxia is the lack of generally accepted and operationally defined measures of hypoxia, ischemia, or asphyxia. Asphyxia has been defined as "the depletion of oxygen and the accumulation of carbon dioxide leading to acidosis."[11] What level of oxygen depletion, carbon dioxide accumulation, or acidosis warrants the term asphyxia?

Defects in oxygenation may be accompanied by hypoperfusion and lead to tissue ischemia. Levels of oxygen or carbon dioxide in the brain are not measured directly. Most investigators of asphyxia in the newborn human have employed instead a variety of the following clinical markers to suggest the presence of asphyxia: meconium in the amniotic fluid, fetal bradycardia, abnormal patterns of fetal heart rate, abnormalities on blood flow studies or neuroimaging, or biochemical markers. Towell[12] has discussed the range and variability of these markers. The different approaches of investigators who have implicated asphyxia and fetal distress adds to the confusion (Table 1).

NE

In 1976, Sarnat and Sarnat[2] described 21 depressed newborns with an encephalopathy following fetal distress, but they did not provide neurologic criteria for inclusion in the sample. Each infant had an Apgar score less than 6 at 1 or 5 minutes or "a well-defined episode of fetal

Accepted for publication June 3, 1991.

From the Neuroepidemiology Branch, National Institute of Neurological Disorders and Stroke, Bethesda, Md (Dr Nelson), and Children's Hospital, and Harvard Medical School, Boston, Mass (Dr Leviton).

Reprint requests to 7550 Wisconsin Ave, Room 700, Bethesda, MD 20892 (Dr Nelson).

Table 1.—Intranatal or Immediate Postnatal Requirements for Diagnoses of Newborn Encephalopathy

Neonatal encephalopathy
Sarnat and Sarnat,[2] 1976
One of two criteria
Well-defined episode of fetal distress (not defined)
Apgar score, ≤4 at 1 or 5 min
Hypoxic encephalopathy
Volpe,[27] 1981
Not defined
Finer et al,[14] 1981
One of three criteria
Abnormal heart rate pattern (not defined)
Apgar score, ≤4 at 1 or 5 min
Need for immediate resuscitation or intubation
Amiel-Tison and Ellison, 1986*
One of four criteria
Fetal heart rate, <120 or >160 beats per min once (?) if by auscultation, prolonged (not defined) if by electronic monitoring
Repetitive heart rate decelerations (not defined)
Presence of meconium
Apgar score, <6 at 5 min
Postasphyxial encephalopathy
Levene et al,[17] 1986
Diagnosis of "birth asphyxia" plus "good evidence (not defined) that asphyxia was the cause of neurological disturbance"
Postasphyxia score
Lipper et al,[16] 1986
Apgar score, <6 plus one of the following
Bradycardia (not defined)
Variable or late heart rate decelerations (how many?)
Loss of beat-to-beat variability of fetal heart rate
Scalp or a cord pH, <7.2
Need for resuscitation
Meconium aspiration

*Dev Med Child Neurol. 1986;28:671-678.

distress" that was not further defined although case descriptions suggest that fetal distress was inferred on the basis of intubation at birth, fetal bradycardia or tachycardia during labor, in utero passage of meconium, or precipitous delivery.

Also in 1976, Ziegler and colleagues[13] described a group of term neonates with an encephalopathy ("cerebral distress syndrome") that was not related to malformation, infection, or erythroblastosis. They defined neonatal asphyxia in these infants by delay of the first cry (>2.5 minutes), low Apgar score, levels of pH or lactic acid, or need for resuscitation. The frequency of these characteristics among infants free of neonatal neurologic abnormalities is rarely reported.

Starting from variously preselected clinical samples, subsequent authors have discussed HIE without a definition[9] or with definitions that were vague[14-16] or circular.[17,18] Elements of the diagnosis for many workers have been electronic fetal-monitoring (EFM) characteristics and measures of acid-base balance; thus, they have built into the definition of NE a relationship to the characteristics that they take to be markers of asphyxia, thereby preventing an examination of the association between asphyxia and encephalopathy. Few workers specify unambiguous, objective, noncircular, and reproducible definitions or selection criteria by which to recognize infants with NE attributable to hypoxia, ischemia, or asphyxia.

Table 2.—Similarity of Characteristics Often Taken to Define 'Birth Asphyxia' and 'HIE'*

Characteristics	Birth Asphyxia	HIE
Depression of		
Tone†	+	+
Reflexes†		
Suck	+	+
Swallow	. . .	+
Moro's	+	+
Respiration†		
Difficulty with initiating repiration	+	. . .
Difficulty with maintaining respiration	. . .	+
Pulse rate†	+	. . .
Circulation/color†	+	. . .
Lethargy, stupor, coma	(+)	+
Seizure	. . .	+

*HIE indicates hypoxic-ischemic encephalopathy; plus sign, yes; and parenthetic plus sign, implicit but not explicit.
†Low Apgar score components.

Similarities Between the Putative *Cause* and the *Effect*

Another wrinkle in the logic of HIE is that the characteristics of the putative *cause,* ie, asphyxia, have a great deal in common with the characteristics of the putative *effect,* ie, NE (Table 2). The characteristics most often cited as markers of asphyxia are low Apgar scores and the component elements of low Apgar scores, including hypotonia, poor reflex responsivity, difficulty or delay with initiating and maintaining respiration, and bradycardia, and other abnormalities of the fetal heart rate, or the presence of meconium. The characteristics of NE are hypotonia, poor reflex responsivity (which can include autonomic reflex dysfunction), difficulty with maintaining respiration, and seizures. Consciousness, not examined as part of the Apgar score, might be assumed to be depressed in the apneic and very hypotonic infant. Thus, most of the characteristics cited are shared by putative cause and putative effect.

The Apgar score is a rapid standardized measure of neurologic depression during the first minutes of life. Low Apgar scores may be the result of drugs or toxins, immaturity, or infection,[19-21] or these scores may be associated with such antecedents, as low socioeconomic status, route of delivery, high parity,[22] maternal alcohol use,[23] and maternal illnesses, including coagulopathy, pulmonary tuberculosis, and hypothyroidism.[24] Low Apgar scores are unlikely to be causes of morbidity, but rather the results of prior causes. Indeed, they may be the earliest postnatal manifestations of an encephalopathy that is already present at birth.

If low Apgar scores and their correlates are part of the syndrome of NE and not acceptable as explanations for the NE, then to establish the cause of the encephalopathy requires identification of antecedents that are not part of the outcome.

ARE INDICATORS OF ASPHYXIA REGULARLY PRESENT IN NEONATES WITH ENCEPHALOPATHY?

Clinical Abnormalities of Labor and Delivery

If the majority of NE is truly secondary to birth asphyxia, then one might reasonably expect that "anoxigenic" obstetric complications would be powerful predictors of NE. Ziegler et al[13] and Amiel-Tison[25] described obstetric abnormalities in a substantial proportion of infants with NE, but they did not compare the frequency of the same factors in asymptomatic newborns. Neither group of investigators found symptomatic newborns to have a different outcome, depending on whether obstetric problems were identified. A Finnish report[26] observed diverse cerebral symptoms in the newborn to be associated with diverse characteristics of pregnancy, labor, and the newborn period; the proportion of infants who were premature and the overlap in risk factors were not stated. Volpe[27] noted that 30% of infants with encephalopathy, described as hypoxic-ischemic, had had no recognized abnormalities during labor.

At least one birth complication or sign of fetal distress (meconium in the amniotic fluid or fetal heart rate below 100 beats per minute) occurred in 74% of infants whose birth weight was greater than 2500 g and who had three or more signs compatible with NE, and in 61% of infants who had no signs of NE.[3] This is a difference, but not a great difference. Among infants in the same study whose births were uncomplicated and who showed no signs of fetal distress, 2.9% manifested sustained neonatal abnormalities consistent with NE, compared with a rate of 3.3% among infants with one or more birth complications or signs of fetal distress.

Obstetric Optimality Scores

Prechtl,[28] noting the weakness of the relationship between obstetric complications and neonatal neurologic morbidity and an "impression that complications do not operate as risk factors if they occur in isolation," invented an optimality measure. With the use of the Prechtl and Beintema neonatal neurologic examination and the Prechtl optimality concept, Touwen and coworkers[29] found that the obstetric characteristics that distinguished best between neurologically optimal and nonoptimal neonates were maternal proteinuria, prenatal care, gestational age, time to first cry, Apgar score, and transfer to a neonatal special care unit. None of these factors is best described as a complication of birth, and none of the complications examined proved to be important predictors of neonatal neurologic syndromes.

In the studies examined, some problem in pregnancy or birth was common but far from universal in the histories of children with neonatal neurologic symptoms, but birth problems were also fairly common in children free of neonatal symptoms. The limited evidence available does not document a powerful association of intrapartum complications with signs of NE.

Classic Signs of Fetal Distress

Meconium in the amniotic fluid and fetal bradycardia are the classic signs of fetal distress. Two reports that apparently overlapped in study population[30,31] indicated that half of term infants with neonatal seizures had meconium staining of the amniotic fluid, compared with 11% to 25% of controls. In other studies, the presence of meconium in the amniotic fluid was not related to neonatal neurologic abnormality[26,32] or pH.[32] Steer et al[33] found the major predictor of meconium in the amniotic fluid to be gestational age, and they observed so little coherence among the various measures that are usually taken to constitute "fetal distress" that they questioned the existence of such an entity.

The presence of meconium or of fetal bradycardia (heart rate <100 beats per minute) was associated with an increase in risk of cerebral palsy only in the small minority of infants whose Apgar score was low,[34] suggesting that neither meconium nor moderate bradycardia alone is a marker of serious fetal compromise.

Altshuler and Hyde[35] reported that meconium itself can induce constriction of umbilical and placental vessels sufficient to cause vascular necrosis of the placenta. The possibility that some component regularly or occasionally present in meconium may itself be injurious warrants further evaluation.

EFM

Electronic fetal (heart rate) monitoring in labor was introduced to help reduce the probability of intrapartum fetal death. Some obstetricians also offered the hope that EFM would permit medical attendants to recognize asphyxia early, enabling preventive interventions to "rescue" affected fetuses and thus prevent cerebral palsy and sharply decrease the frequency of mental retardation.[36] However, EFM does not appear to be superior to intermittent auscultation in decreasing neonatal morbidity.[37,38]

In the Dublin (Ireland) randomized clinical trial of fetal monitoring, infants who were assigned randomly to intermittent auscultation or to EFM with or without an option for fetal scalp pH did not differ in the rate of Apgar scores below 4 at 1 or 5 minutes.[39] In another study, EFM did not predict low 5-minute Apgar scores.[40]

Visser[41] reported that among growth-retarded fetuses, results of neonatal examination correlated better with heart rate patterns that were recorded before labor began than with intrapartum abnormalities. This and the repeated finding of an association between congenital anomalies and EFM abnormalities[42-44] are in keeping with the view that in some infants, EFM abnormalities reflect preexisting intracranial abnormalities.

A recent study has noted a relationship between late decelerations in the first stage of labor and neonatal neurologic status, but it did not report predictive values.[45] The sample for that study was selected by virtue of medical concern for the infants, and it is not clear that the analyses included birth weight or gestational age as potential confounders. A higher rate of neonatal seizures was seen in the intermittently auscultated group than in the EFM group in one study.[39] The seizure excess was limited to the relatively small subset of infants who were born after lengthy labors that were augmented with oxytocin, an observation that warrant examination in a fresh study.[46] Seven other studies have not shown that fetal heart rate monitoring lowers the risk of neonatal seizures.[37,38] In infants who were randomly assigned to EFM or intermittent auscultation, neonatal morbidity and developmental status were comparable at the age of 9 months.[47] The rate of later cerebral palsy was not lower in electronically monitored than in auscultated infants in two studies,[38,48] and it was, in fact, significantly higher among monitored preterm infants in one of these.[38] If this observation is confirmed, then an explanation should be sought. One possibility is that intra-amniotic infection, an important risk factor for cerebral palsy, may be more common in infants exposed to lengthy internal fetal monitoring.[49]

Acid-Base Measures

Some authors view umbilical artery acidosis or buffer base deficit as the best readily available marker of systemic hypoxia that occurs during the later stages of labor.[50] However, accumulated experience from a number of studies indicates that most infants with encephalopathy are not acidotic.[51-54] For example, in term infants with persistent hypotonia, 81% had pH_{ua} values over 7.15,[54] and cord blood gas measurements explained less than 1% of the variance in the score on a standardized neonatal neurologic examination.[30] In addition, most acidotic infants are not encephalopathic.[32,55,56]

Sykes and colleagues[57] in Oxfordshire, England, suggested that since pH and Apgar score were not strongly correlated, Apgar scoring should be abandoned. Follow-up of their cohort indicated no relationship between pH and measures of neurologic and psychologic function at the age of 4.5 years.[58]

It seems likely that with pH as with Apgar scores,[59,60] only extremely depressed scores are associated with an increase in risk of unfavorable neurologic outcome. Among 32 835 births with birth weights greater than 2500 g, the risk of death, neonatal seizures, or need for intensive care was increased only when the umbilical artery pH was below 7.05. Most of the risk was with pH below 7.00, and even at that level, the majority of infants had no neonatal complications.[61] Furthermore, preexisting vulnerabilities may interact with factors that produce acidosis in determining outcome: of 23 very acidotic infants (pH <7.00 with metabolic component; 1- and 5-minute Apgar scores ≤3), the only two who were symptomatic as neonates were infants with severe prenatal problems.[55]

In the light of these findings, we conclude as others have that the relationship of pH or base deficit to neonatal or to long-term neurologic disability does not appear to be strong.

Neonatal Seizures

Neonatal seizures are a part of the NE syndrome in its moderate or severe forms[4] and may indicate serious risk of adverse outcome.[62] But neonatal seizures are a heterogeneous group of disorders. Among neonatal seizures is a benign familial variety for which a gene locus may have been identified[63] and conditions of very unfavorable outlook, not related to asphyxia.[64] Many studies do not distinguish neonatal seizures that occur in isolation in infants who are otherwise well, or with only transient metabolic dysfunction, from seizures accompanied by other evidence of encephalopathy or by evidence of involvement of organs other than the central nervous system.

Some infants who are thought to have clinical seizures may not display electroencephalographic evidence of these, and electrical seizures are not necessarily accompanied by clinically recognizable manifestations.[18] It is not known whether clinical features or electroencephalographic characteristics are better predictors of handicap in surviving infants.

In series of infants with neonatal seizures, meconium staining of the amniotic fluid was absent in 28% to 53%,[30,31,65,66] and acidosis was absent in 60%.[67] In addition, intubation was not needed at birth by 65%, and 89% did not need subsequent ventilatory support.[68] Thus, even broad definitions of asphyxia or hypoxia were not met by most newborns with otherwise unexplained seizures.

The literature has stressed that most "asphyxial" seizures occur early.[30,67] The inference has been drawn[31] that most early seizures are therefore asphyxial. In one large study, of all the children with seizures in the nursery period, three quarters had them in the first 48 hours of life.[62] However, 61% of seizures in the first 2 days occurred in infants with Apgar scores of 7 or higher. "Thus, although depressed infants tended to have seizures early, about half of early neonatal seizures were in nondepressed infants."[62]

The more energetic the workup of newborn seizures, the more likely it is that nonasphyxial causes will be identified. For example, in a group of young children whose epilepsy began with neonatal seizures as early as 2 hours of age, positron emission tomography identified lesions that were later shown on neuropathologic examination to reflect defects in neuronal migration.[69] Even very early seizures, as well as continuing neurologic morbidity, can be the result of neuroanatomic defects that are present in the infant since the middle trimester of fetal life.

OTHER FEATURES THAT MAY BE HELPFUL IN RECOGNIZING WHEN NE IS ASPHYXIAL

Multisystem Involvement

In term newborns, the kidney and myocardium may be at least as vulnerable as the brain to impaired blood flow and oxygenation.[70-72] Impairment of systemic blood flow sufficient to damage the brain regularly also damages other organs in addition. Infants with NE but without multisystem involvement are unlikely to have their encephalopathy on the basis of intrapartum asphyxia. Perlman and Tack[73] reported that sustained oliguria and an elevated urinary β_2-microglobulin level (reflecting a renal origin of the oliguria) were predictors of neonatal seizures or cranial ultrasound abnormality, as well as of later abnormal neurologic status. However, encephalopathy with seizures accompanied by hematuria or oliguria and involvement of other organs, including gastrointestinal, genitourinary, and other systems, as well as the brain, can occur with embolization or coagulopathy,[74,75] thrombosis, or infectious (see below) or other conditions, so this constellation is not specific to asphyxial injury.

Other Markers

A variety of indicators have been described, including biochemical,[76-80] electroencephalographic,[2,81-83] and evoked potentials,[84] neuroimaging, including ultrasound[85,86] and magnetic resonance imaging,[87-89] magnetic resonance spectroscopy and near-infrared spectroscopy,[90-92] and impaired regulation of cerebral blood flow.[92-94] Many of these techniques are not widely available, and few can identify abnormalities as soon after delivery as will be required for therapies directed at prevention of consequences of birth asphyxia.

WHAT ELSE CAN CAUSE SIGNS OF NE?

Many features of the NE that are so commonly attributed to asphyxia, such as neonatal hypotonia,[95] difficulty with feeding,[96] and neonatal respiratory delay,[97] may have other explanations. In congenital myotonic dystrophy[98] and in the Prader-Willi syndrome,[99] for example, abnormalities of pregnancy and birth and low Apgar scores, hypotonia, poor suck, and need for respiratory assistance are relatively frequent. Focal cerebral infarction,[100] metabolic disorders of a wide variety,[101] and trauma[102] can produce many of the same signs. Diagnoses of birth asphyxia are often made clinically in infants with these other conditions.

Chorioamnionitis is associated with low Apgar scores[23,24] and prolonged labor[103] and perhaps with progressive metabolic acidosis, although evidence on this last point is not consistent. Chorioamnionitis is a risk factor for cystic lesions on ultrasound that are in turn important predictors of cerebral palsy.[104] Organisms that cause chorioamnionitis may be fastidious and evade routine bacteriologic identification and be recognized only by means of histology.[105,106] Chorioamnionitis is also a precursor of neonatal sepsis, which can produce systemic and neurologic illness, including neonatal seizures. Since infection can mimic so many of the features of HIE, the distinction between infectious and asphyxial encephalopathic illnesses in the neonate, and a judgment as to the contribution of each if both are present, may be difficult.

For these and other disorders, differential diagnosis rests on recognition of specific features that are not always prominent in the newborn, even if carefully sought. Although many of these conditions are uncommon individually, no one knows what proportion of all HIE that they represent.

NE AND THE FOURTH DIMENSION[107]: HOW QUICKLY AFTER BIRTH CAN A CONFIDENT CONCLUSION BE REACHED THAT A SEVERE INSULT HAS OCCURRED AND THAT ASPHYXIA IS ITS BASIS?

A number of investigators[2,13,65,108] have written that infants who have truly suffered cerebral injury due to asphyxia at birth display a characteristic evolution of signs over time. These observations are reasonably consistent and of great importance to understanding NE. However, this evolution has not yet been captured and quantified in a formulation that permits its predictive use.[4] Furthermore, and a critical problem for planning for future studies of early therapeutic interventions, most of the characteristics that permit a confident recognition of the severity of NE, and perhaps of an asphyxial origin, are features of the clinical course that cannot be recognized until many hours or days after birth. Yet, most currently proposed interventions must take place very soon after delivery.

COMMENT

The signs of NE are nonspecific. Birth asphyxia sufficient to produce NE is not easy to distinguish from other causes as events unfold in the early minutes and hours after delivery. The markers that are often used as indicators of asphyxia, such as low Apgar scores and their correlates, including hypotonia and delayed respiration, are not specific to asphyxia and may themselves be early evidence of encephalopathy predating birth, or of other kinds of neonatal illness. The usual measures of perinatal asphyxia do not correlate well with one another and are not good predictors of neurologic condition even within the neonatal period.

Most severely asphyxiated children who survive are later clinically normal.[59,60,109] Agents proposed for treating birth asphyxia are powerful and possess risks that are known from animal testing, with effects in the human that are not fully predictable. Proposers of clinical trials of new therapies for birth asphyxia will be under a strong obligation to judge that the treatment is not worse than the disease.

For future clinical trials of agents for birth asphyxia, then, it will be necessary to select as candidates infants who are at high risk of encephalopathy, neonatal and subsequent, because of asphyxia. It will probably be necessary to make decisions about magnitude and cause of risk on the basis of information in hand within the first hour or two of life. To what extent is that feasible today? In preparation for the anticipated clinical trials for birth asphyxia, we recommend consideration of tests of the predictive validity of clinical and technologic markers specific to asphyxia that are available soon after birth.

References

1. Christensen E, Melchior JC. *Cerebral Palsy: A Clinical and Neuropathological Study: Clinics in Developmental Medicine No. 25.* London, England: Heinemann Medical Books Ltd; 1967:117.
2. Sarnat HB, Sarnat MS. Neonatal encephalopathy following fetal distress: a clinical and electroencephalographic study. *Arch Neurol.* 1976;33:696-705.
3. Nelson KB, Ellenberg JH. The asymptomatic newborn and risk of cerebral palsy. *AJDC.* 1987;141:1333-1335.
4. Leviton A, Nelson KB. Neonatal encephalopathy: problems with definitions and classifications. *Pediatric Neurol.* In press.
5. Hattori H, Morin AM, Schwartz PH, Fujikawa DG, Wasterlan CG. Posthypoxic treatment with MK-801 reduces hypoxic-ischemic damage in the neonatal rat. *Neurology.* 1989;39:713-718.
6. Sheardown MJ, Nielsen EO, Hansen AJ, Jacobsen P, Honore T. 2,3-Dihydroxy-6-nitro-7-sulfamoyl-benzo(F) quinoxaline: a neuroprotectant for cerebral ischemia. *Science.* 1990;247:571-577.
7. Palmer C, Vannucci RC, Towfighi J. Reduction of perinatal hypoxic-ischemic brain damage with allopurinol. *Pediatr Res.* 1990;27:332-336.
8. Espinoza MI, Parer JT. Mechanisms of asphyxial brain damage, and possible pharmacologic interventions, in the fetus. *Am J Obstet Gynecol.* 1991;164:1582-1591.
9. Vannucci RC. Current and potentially new management strategies for perinatal hypoxic-ischemic encephalopathy. *Pediatrics.* 1990;85:961-968.
10. McDonald JW, Johnston MV. Physiological and pathophysiological roles of excitatory amino acids during central nervous system development. *Brain Res Rev.* 1990;15:41-70.
11. Boehm JJ. Resuscitation of the newborn and prevention of asphyxia. In: Sciarra JJ, ed. *Maternal and Fetal Medicine: Gynecology and Obstetrics.* New York, NY: Harper & Row Publishers Inc; 1981;2:1-11.
12. Towell ME. The rationale for biochemical monitoring of the fetus. *J Perinat Med.* 1988;16(suppl 1):55-70.
13. Ziegler AL, Calame A, Marchand C, Passera M, Reymond-Goni I, Prod'hom LS. Cerebral distress in full-term newborns and its prognostic value: a follow-up study of 90 infants. *Helv Paediatr Acta.* 1976;31:299-317.
14. Finer NN, Robertson CM, Richards RT, Pinnell LE, Peters KL. Hypoxic-ischemic encephalopathy in term neonates: perinatal factors and outcome. *J Pediatr.* 1981;98:112-117.
15. Roland EH, Jan JE, Hill A, Wong PK. Cortical visual impairment following birth asphyxia. *Pediatr Neurol.* 1986;2: 133-137.
16. Lipper EG, Voorhies TM, Ross G, Vannucci RC, Auld PAM. Early predictors of one-year outcome for infants asphyxiated at birth. *Dev Med Child Neurol.* 1986;28:303-309.
17. Levene MI, Kornberg J, Williams THC. The incidence and severity of post-asphyxial encephalopathy in full-term infants. *Early Hum Dev.* 1985;11:21-26.
18. Mizrahi EM, Kellaway P. Characterization and classification of neonatal seizures. *Neurology.* 1987;37:1837-1844.
19. Committee on Fetus and Newborn, American Academy of Pediatrics. Use and abuse of the Apgar score. *Pediatrics.*

1986;78:1148-1149.
20. Hankins GDV, Snyder RR, Yeomans ER. Umbilical arterial and venous acid-base and blood gas values and the effect of chorioamnionitis on those values in a cohort of preterm infants. *Am J Obstet Gynecol.* 1991;164:1261-1264.
21. Maberry MC, Ramin SM, Gilstrap LC, Leveno KJ, Dax JS. Intrapartum asphyxia in pregnancies complicated by intra-amniotic infection. *Obstet Gynecol.* 1990;76:351-354.
22. Burt RD, Vaughan TL, Daling JR. Evaluating the risks of cesarean section: low Apgar score in repeat C-section and vaginal deliveries. *Am J Public Health.* 1988;78:1312-1314.
23. Streissguth AP, Barr HM, Martin DC. Offspring effects and pregnancy complications related to self-reported maternal alcohol use. *Dev Pharmacol Ther.* 1982;5:21-32.
24. Friedman EA, Neff RD. *Labor and Delivery: Impact on Offspring.* Littleton, Mass: PSG Publishing Co Inc; 1987:202-239.
25. Amiel-Tison C. Neurological morbidity in term infants as an indicator of safe obstetrical practice. In: Kubli F, Patel N, Schmidt W, Linderkam O, eds. *Perinatal Events and Mental Handicap.* New York, NY: Springer-Verlag NY Inc; 1988:175-191.
26. Piekkala P, Kero P, Erkkola R, Sillanpaa M. Perinatal events and neonatal morbidity: an analysis of 5380 cases. *Early Hum Dev.* 1986;13:249-268.
27. Volpe JJ. *Neurology of the Newborn.* Philadelphia, Pa: WB Saunders Co; 1981.
28. Prechtl HFR. The optimality concept. *Early Hum Dev.* 1980;4:201-205.
29. Touwen BCL, Huisjes HJ, Jurgens-van der Zee AD, Bierman-van Eendenburg MEC, Smrkovsky M, Olinga AA. Obstetrical condition and neonatal neurological morbidity: an analysis with the help of the optimality concept. *Early Hum Dev.* 1980;4:207-228.
30. Derham RJ, Matthews TG, Clarke TA. Early seizures indicate quality of perinatal care. *Arch Dis Child.* 1985;60:809-813.
31. Curtis PD, Matthews TG, Clarke TA, et al. Neonatal seizures: the Dublin Collaborative Study. *Arch Dis Child.* 1988;63:1065-1068.
32. Dijxhoorn MJ, Visser GHA, Fidler VJ, Touwen BCL, Huisjes HJ. Apgar score, meconium and acidaemia at birth in relation to neonatal neurological abnormality in term infants. *Br J Obstet Gynaecol.* 1986;93:217-222.
33. Steer PH, Eigbe F, Lissauer TJ, Beard RW. Interrelationships among abnormal cardiotocograms in labor, meconium staining of the amniotic fluid, arterial cord blood pH, and Apgar scores. *Obstet Gynecol.* 1989;74:715-721.
34. Nelson KB, Ellenberg JH. Obstetric complications as risk factors for cerebral palsy or seizure disorders. *JAMA.* 1984;251:1843-1848.
35. Altshuler G, Hyde S. Meconium-induced vasocontraction: a potential cause of cerebral and other fetal hypoperfusion and of poor pregnancy outcome. *J Child Neurol.* 1989;4:137-142.
36. Quilligan EJ, Paul RH. Fetal monitoring: is it worth it? *Obstet Gynecol.* 1975;45:96-100.
37. Institute of Medicine. *Medical Professional Liability and the Delivery of Obstetrical Care.* Washington, DC: National Academic Press; 1989.
38. Shy KK, Luthy DA, Bennett FC, et al. Effects of electronic fetal heart rate monitoring, as compared with periodic auscultation, on the neurologic development of premature infants. *N Engl J Med.* 1990;322:588-593.
39. MacDonald D, Grant A, Sheridan-Pereira M, Boylan P, Chalmers I. The Dublin randomized controlled trial of intrapartum fetal heart rate monitoring. *Am J Obstet Gynecol.* 1985;152:524-539.
40. McCusker J, Harris DR, Hosmer DW Jr. Association of electronic fetal monitoring during labor with cesarean section rate and with neonatal morbidity and mortality. *Am J Public Health.* 1988;78:1170-1174.
41. Visser GHA. Abnormal antepartum fetal heart rate patterns and subsequent handicap. *Ballieres Clin Obstet Gynaecol.* 1988;2:117-124.
42. Garite TJ, Linzey EM, Freeman RK, Dorchester W. Fetal heart rate patterns and fetal distress in fetuses with congenital anomalies. *Obstet Gynecol.* 1979;53:716-720.
43. Didolkar SM, Mutch M. Major/multiple congenital anomalies and intrapartum fetal heart rate patterns. *South Dakota Med.* 1979;32:5-9.
44. Biale U, Brawer-Ostrovsky Y, Insler V. Fetal heart rate tracings in fetuses with congenital malformations. *J Reprod Med.* 1985;30:43-47.
45. Ellison PH, Foster M, Sheridan-Pereira M, MacDonald D. Electronic fetal heart monitoring, auscultation, and neonatal outcome. *Am J Obstet Gynecol.* 1991;164:1281-1289.
46. Haverkamp AD. Oxytocin, neonatal seizures, and other insights derived from the Dublin trial. *Birth.* 1986;13:188-189.
47. Langendoerfer S, Haverkamp AD, Murphy J, et al. Pediatric followup-up of a randomized controlled trial of intrapartum fetal monitoring techniques. *J Pediatr.* 1980;97:103-107.
48. Grant A, O'Brien N, Joy M-T, Hennessy E, MacDonald D. Cerebral palsy among children born during the Dublin randomised trial of intrapartum monitoring. *Lancet.* 1989;2:1233-1236.
49. Newton ER, Prihoda TJ, Gibbs RS. Logistic regression analysis of risk factors for intra-amniotic infection. *Obstet Gynecol.* 1989;73:571-575.
50. Low JA. The role of blood gas and acid-base assessment in the diagnosis of intrapartum fetal asphyxia. *Am J Obstet Gynecol.* 1988;159:1235-1240.
51. Visser GHA, Dijxhoorn MJ. Intrapartum cardiotocogram, Apgar score and acidaemia at birth: relationship to neonatal neurological morbidity. In: Kubli F, Patel N, Schmidt W, Linderkamp O, eds. *Perinatal Events and Brain Damage in Surviving Children.* New York, NY: Springer-Verlag NY Inc; 1988:168-174.
52. Jurgens-van der Zee AD, Bierman-van Eendenburg MEC, Fidler VJ, et al. Preterm birth, growth retardation and acidaemia in relation to neurologic abnormality of the newborn. *Early Hum Dev.* 1979;3:141-154.
53. Huisjes HJ, Touwen BCL, Hoekstra J, v Woerden-Blanksma JT, et al. Obstetrical-neonatal neurological relationship: a replication study. *Eur J Obstet Gynecol Reprod Biol.* 1980;10:247-256.
54. Gilstrap LC III, Leveno KJ, Burris J, Williams ML, Little BB. Diagnosis of birth asphyxia on the basis of fetal pH, Apgar score, and newborn cerebral dysfunction. *Am J Obstet Gynecol.* 1989;161:825-830.
55. Winkler CL, Hauth JC, Tucker JM, Owsen J, Brumfield CG. Neonatal complications at term as related to the degree of umbilical artery acidemia. *Am J Obstet Gynecol.* 1991;164:637-641.
56. Fee SC, Malee K, Deddish R, Minogue JP, Socol ML. Severe acidosis and subsequent neurologic status. *Am J Obstet Gynecol.* 1990;162:802-806.
57. Sykes GS, Molloy PM, Johnson P, et al. Do Apgar scores indicate asphyxia? *Lancet.* 1982;1:494-496.
58. Dennis J, Johnson A, Mutch L, Yudkin P, Johnson P. Acid-base status at birth and neurodevelopmental outcome at four and one-half years. *Am J Obstet Gynecol.* 1989;161:213-220.
59. Nelson KB, Ellenberg JH. Apgar scores as predictors of chronic neurologic disability. *Pediatrics.* 1981;68:36-44.
60. Seidman DS, Paz I, Laor A, Gale R, Stevenson DK, Danon YL. Apgar scores and cognitive performance at 17 years of age. *Obstet Gynecol.* 1991;77:875-878.
61. Goldaber K, Gilstrap L, Leveno K, Dax J. Pathologic fetal acidemia. *Soc Perinatal Obstet Am J Obstet Gynecol.* 1991;164(pt 2):251. Abstract.
62. Ellenberg JH, Nelson KB. Cluster of perinatal events identifying infants at high risk for death or disability. *J Pediatr.* 1988;113:546-552.
63. Leppert M, Anderson VE, Quattlebaum T, et al. Benign familial neonatal convulsions linked to genetic markers on chromosome 20. *Nature.* 1989;337:647-648.
64. Clarke M, Gill J, Noronha M, McKinlay I. Early infantile epileptic encephalopathy with suppression burst: Ohtahara

syndrome. *Dev Med Child Neurol.* 1987;29:520-528.
65. Patterson CA, Graves WL, Bugg G, Sasso SC, Brann AW. Antenatal and intrapartum factors associated with the occurrence of seizures in the term infant. *Obstet Gynecol.* 1989;74:361-365.
66. Keegan KA, Waffarn F, Quilligan EJ. Obstetric characteristics and fetal heart rate patterns of infants who convulse during the newborn period. *Am J Obstet Gynecol.* 1985;153:732-737.
67. Minchom P, Niswander K, Chalmers I, et al. Antecedents and outcome of very early neonatal seizures in infants born at or after term. *Br J Obstet Gynaecol.* 1987;94:431-439.
68. Dennis J, Chalmers I. Very early neonatal seizure rate—a possible epidemiological indicator of the quality of perinatal care. *Br J Obstet Gynaecol.* 1982;89:418-426.
69. Chugani HT, Shewmon DA, Peacock WJ, Shields WD, Mazziotta JC, Phelps ME. Surgical treatment of intractable neonatal-onset seizures: the role of positron emission tomography. *Neurology.* 1988;38:1178-1188.
70. Kojima T, Kobayashi T, Matsuzaki S, Iwase S, Kobayashi Y. Effects of perinatal asphyxia and myoglobinuria on development of acute neonatal renal failure. *Arch Dis Child.* 1985;60:908-912.
71. Kabra SK, Saxena S, Sharma U. Myocardial dysfunction in birth asphyxia. *Indian J Pediatr.* 1988;55:416-419.
72. Laing I, Brown JK, Harkness RA. Clinical and biochemical assessments of damage due to perinatal asphyxia: a double blind trial of a quantitative method. *J Clin Pathol.* 1988;41:247-252.
73. Perlman JM, Tack ED. Acute systemic organ injury in term infants after asphyxia. *AJDC.* 1989;143:617-620.
74. Szymonowicz W, Preston H, Yu VY. The surviving monozygotic twin. *Arch Dis Child.* 1986;61:454-458.
75. Patten RM, Mack LA, Nyberg DA, Filly RA. Twin embolization syndrome: prenatal sonographic detection and significance. *Radiology.* 1989;173:685-689.
76. Ruth V, Autti-Ramo I, Granstrom M-L, Korkman M, Raivio KO. Prediction of perinatal brain damage by cord plasma vasopressin, erythropoietin, and hypoxanthine values. *J Pediatr.* 1988;113:880-885.
77. Saugstad OD. Hypoxanthine as an indicator of hypoxia: its role in health and disease through free radical production. *Pediatr Res.* 1988;23:143-150.
78. Fernandez F, Quero J, Verdu A, Ferreiros MC, Daimiel E, Roche MC. LDH isoenzymes in CSF in the diagnosis of neonatal brain damage. *Acta Neurol Scand.* 1986;74:30-33.
79. Dalens B, Bezou M-J, Coulet M, Raynaud E-J. Fibrin-fibrinogen degradation products in cerebrospinal fluid as an indicator of neonatal brain damage. *Acta Neurol Scand.* 1981; 64:81-87.
80. Smith A, Prakash P, Nesbitt J, McIntosh N. The vasopressin response to severe birth asphyxia. *Early Hum Dev.* 1990;22:119-129.
81. Takeuchi T, Watanabe K. The EEG evolution and neurological prognosis of perinatal hypoxia [in] neonates. *Brain Dev.* 1989;11:115-120.
82. Holmes G, Rowe J, Hafford J, et al. Prognostic value of the electroencephalogram in neonatal asphyxia. *EEG Clin Neurophysiol.* 1982;53:60-72.
83. Bell AH, McClure BG, Hicks EM. Power spectral analysis of the EEG of term infants following birth asphyxia. *Dev Med Child Neurol.* 1990;32:990-998.
84. Hakamada S, Watanabe K, Hara K, et al. The evolution of visual and auditory evoked potentials in infants with perinatal disorder. *Brain Dev.* 1981;3:339-344.
85. Babcock DS, Ball W. Postasphyxial encephalopathy in full-term infants: ultrasound diagnosis. *Radiology.* 1983;148: 417-423.
86. Kreusser KL, Schmidt RE, Shackelford GD, Volpe JJ. Value of ultrasound for identification of acute hemorrhagic necrosis of thalamus and basal ganglia in an asphyxiated term infant. *Ann Neurol.* 1984;16:361-363.
87. McArdle CB, Richardson CJ, Hayden CK, Nicholas DA, Amparo EG. Abnormalities of the neonatal brain: MR imaging, II: hypoxic-ischemic brain injury. *Radiology.* 1987;163:395-403.
88. Barkovich AJ, Truwit CL. Brain damage from perinatal asphyxia: correlation of MR findings with gestational age. *AJNR.* 1990;11:1087-1096.
89. Keeney SE, Adcock EW, McArdle CB. Prospective observations of 100 high-risk neonates by high-field (1.5 tesla) magnetic resonance imaging of the central nervous system, II: lesions associated with hypoxic-ischemic encephalopathy. *Pediatrics.* 1991;87:431-438.
90. Wyatt JS, Edwards AD, Azzopardi D, Reynolds EOR. Magnetic resonance and near infrared spectroscopy for investigation of perinatal hypoxic-ischaemic brain injury. *Arch Dis Child.* 1989;64:953-963.
91. Laptook AR, Corbett RJT, Uauy R, Mize C, Mendelsohn D, Nunnally RL. Use of ^{31}P magnetic resonance spectroscopy to characterize evolving brain damage after perinatal asphyxia. *Neurology.* 1989;39:709-712.
92. Levene MI, Fenton AC, Evans DH, Archer LNJ, Shortland DB, Gibson NA. Severe birth asphyxia and abnormal cerebral blood-flow velocity. *Dev Med Child Neurol.* 1989;31:427-434.
93. Pryds O, Greisen G, Lou H, Friis-Hansen B. Vasoparalysis associated with brain damage in asphyxiated term infants. *J Pediatr.* 1990;117:119-125.
94. Mujsce DJ, Christensen MA, Vannucci RCA. Cerebral blood flow and edema in perinatal hypoxic-ischemic brain damage. *Pediatr Res.* 1990;27:450-453.
95. Fenichel GM. The newborn with poor muscle tone. *Semin Perinatol.* 1982;6:68-88.
96. Fenichel GM. *Clinical Pediatric Neurology: A Signs and Symptoms Approach.* Philadelphia, Pa: WB Saunders Co; 1988.
97. Brazy JE, Kinney HC, Oakes WJ. Central nervous system structural lesions causing apnea at birth. *J Pediatr.* 1987; 111:163-175.
98. Rutherford MA, Heckmatt JZ, Dubowitz V. Congenital myotonic dystrophy: respiratory function at birth determines survival. *Arch Dis Child.* 1989;64:191-195.
99. Wharton RH, Bresnan MJ. Neonatal respiratory depression and delay in diagnosis in Prader-Willi syndrome. *Dev Med Child Neurol.* 1989;31:231-236.
100. Levy SR, Abaroms IF, Marshall PC, Rosquete EE. Seizures and cerebral infarction in the full-term newborn. *Ann Neurol.* 1985;17:366-370.
101. Kyllerman M, Blomstrand S, Mansson J-E, Conradi NG, Hindmarsh T. Central nervous system malformations and white matter changes in pseudo-neonatal adrenoleukodystrophy. *Neuropediatrics.* 1990;21:199-201.
102. Lanska MJ, Roessmann V, Wiznitzer M. Magnetic resonance imaging in cervical cord injury. *Pediatrics.* 1990;85:760-764.
103. Mueller-Heubach E, Rubinstein DN, Schwarz SS. Histologic chorioamnionitis and preterm delivery in different patient populations. *Obstet Gynecol.* 1990;75:622-626.
104. Bejar R, Coen RW, Merritt TA, et al. Focal necrosis of the white matter (periventricular leukomalacia): sonographic, pathologic and electroencephalographic features. *Am J Neuroradiol.* 1986;7:1073-1080.
105. Benirschke K, Robb JA. Infectious causes of fetal death. *Clin Obstet Gynecol.* 1987;30:284-294.
106. Zlatnik FJ, Gellhaus TM, Benda JA, Koontz FP, Burmeister LF. Histologic chorioamnionitis, microbial infection, and prematurity. *Obstet Gyencol.* 1990;76:355-359.
107. Prensky AL. Time—a fourth dimension for encephalopathies. *N Engl J Med.* 1984;310:1527-1528.
108. Hill A, Volpe JJ. Perinatal asphyxia: clinical aspects. *Clin Perinatol.* 1989;16:435-457.
109. Jain L, Ferre C, Vidyasagar D, Nath S, Sheftel D. Cardiopulmonary resuscitation of apparently stillborn infants: survival and long-term outcome. *J Pediatr.* 1991;118:778-782.

Call for Abstracts

The American Pediatric Society and The Society for Pediatric Research announce that the abstract deadline for the 1992 Annual Meeting (May 4-7, 1992, Convention Center, Baltimore, Md) has been set as *January 3, 1992*. For further information, contact the APA Headquarters, 6728 Old McLean Village Dr, McLean, VA 22101 ([703]556-9222; FAX [703]556-8729), or the APS/SPR Association ([708]427-0205; FAX [708] 427-1305).

1992 Pediatric Cardiology Examination

The American Board of Pediatrics will administer the Certifying Examination in Pediatric Cardiology on Tuesday, August 11, 1992, in three US cities.

Applications are available now. Registration will continue through January 31, 1992. The application fee for the examination is $1150, but applications postmarked after December 31, 1991, must include an additional $200 late fee. New applications postmarked after January 31 *cannot be accepted* for the 1992 examination.

Each application will be considered individually and must be acceptable to the Sub-board of Pediatric Cardiology. Please contact the American Board of Pediatrics for eligibility requirements.

Reregistration materials will be mailed to eligible candidates on January 2. The reregistration fee is $1050. Please direct inquiries to the American Board of Pediatrics, 111 Silver Cedar Ct, Chapel Hill, NC 27514-1651 ([919] 929-0461).

1992 Pediatric Hematology-Oncology Examination

The American Board of Pediatrics will administer the Certifying Examination in Pediatric Hematology-Oncology Tuesday, August 11, 1992, in three US cities.

Applications are available now. Registration will continue through January 31. The application fee for the examination is $1150, but applications postmarked after December 31, 1991, must include an additional $200 late fee. New applications postmarked after January 31 *cannot be accepted* for the 1992 examination.

Each application will be considered individually and must be acceptable to the Sub-board of Pediatric Hematology-Oncology. Please contact the American Board of Pediatrics for eligibility requirements.

Reregistration materials will be mailed to eligible candidates on January 2. The reregistration fee is $1050. Please direct inquiries to the American Board of Pediatrics, 111 Silver Cedar Ct, Chapel Hill, NC 27514-1651 ([919] 929-0461).

The 1992 General Pediatrics Certifying Examination of the American Board of Pediatrics

The 1992 General Pediatrics Certifying Examination will be administered Tuesday and Wednesday, October 27 and 28, 1992, in various cities throughout the United States and Canada.

For new applicants, regular registration begins December 2, 1991, and continues through March 2, 1992. The registration fee is $1050. The registration fee must accompany the completed application material and be *postmarked* by March 2. On December 2, 1991, application material will be sent to qualified residents at their training program addresses. However, any resident who does not receive the material by mid-December should request the material directly from the American Board of Pediatrics. A three-part partial payment plan will be available for *new* applicants only. The deadline for participation in that plan is January 13; details will be included in the application material. Late registration for new applicants begins March 3. The late registration fee is $1250, which includes a $200 nonrefundable late fee. The final deadline for receipt of applications from new applicants is May 1.

In mid-February, reregistration material will be mailed to active candidates who meet the examination requirements. Those who do not meet the examination requirement of having a copy of their permanent, unrestricted license on file will not be sent the reregistration material. Regular reregistration begins February 17 and continues through April 17. Qualified individuals who do not receive the material by March 2 should request the material directly from the American Board of Pediatrics. The reregistration fee is $950. The reregistration fee must accompany the completed reregistration form and be *postmarked* by April 17. Late reregistration begins April 18. The late reregistration fee is $1150, which includes a $200 nonrefundable late fee. The final deadline for receipt of reregistration material is May 1, 1992.

Site assignment is based on the date of receipt of the application or the reregistration material. Seating may be limited at some sites, so early registration is suggested. Correspondence to the American Board of Pediatrics should be sent to 111 Silver Cedar Ct, Chapel Hill, NC 27514-1651 ([919] 929-0461).

Medical Management of Postobstructive Polyuria

Sir.—Obstructive uropathy can be complicated by a defect in urinary concentrating ability that results in marked losses of water and electrolytes after relief of the obstruction. We describe a neonate with posterior

Laboratory Values During Hospitalization*

Day of Hospitalization	Sodium, mmol/L	Potassium, mmol/L	Chloride, mmol/L	Bicarbonate, mmol/L	Urea Nitrogen, mmol/L	Creatinine, µmol/L	Osmolality, mOsm/kg
1	116	5.9	88	9	15	513	110
2	142	4.2	106	15	10	248	110
3	146	5.6	109	20	1.1	44	62
4	138	4.6	99	22	0.4	53	84

*Values for osmalality are from urine; all other values are from serum.

urethral valves who had a marked postobstructive diuresis. Hydrochlorothiazide and indomethacin were used to prevent dehydration. The defect in urine concentration and polyuria recurred on discontinuation of indomethacin and hydrochlorothiazide therapy, but improved after therapy with both drugs was restarted.

Patient Report.—A 6-day-old neonate was admitted for evaluation of abdominal distention, decreased urine output, swelling of the penis and scrotum, and poor feeding, which began 1 day before admission to the hospital. He was born at 37 weeks' gestation by normal spontaneous vaginal delivery after normal pregnancy and labor. He was discharged from the hospital at age 2 days. Results of physical examination showed marked distention and tenderness of the abdomen, with swelling of the penis and scrotum. No abdominal masses were found on palpation. He had poor capillary refill, a blood pressure of 80/50 mm Hg, and a pulse of 140 beats per minute. On admission, serum electrolyte values were as follows: sodium, 116 mmol/L; potassium, 5.9 mmol/L; chloride, 88 mmol/L; (with serum) bicarbonate, 9 mmol/L; urea nitrogen, 15 mmol/L; and creatinine, 513 µmol/L.

Placing a urinary catheter resulted in increased urine output and prompt improvement of abdominal distention and scrotal swelling. Perfusion and serum electrolyte values improved with intravenous administration of 20 mL of normal saline per kilogram of body weight, followed by intravenous administration of a 0.2% sodium chloride and 0.2% sodium bicarbonate solution. Serum electrolyte concentrations 24 hours after admission were as follows: sodium, 142 mmol/L; potassium, 4.2 mmol/L; chloride, 106 mmol/L; bicarbonate, 15 mmol/L; urea nitrogen (with serum), 18 mmol/L; and serum creatinine, 248 µmol/L. Urine osmolality was 110 mOsm/kg, and serum osmolality was 301 mOsm/kg. Abdominal ultrasonography study and avoiding cystourethrogram revealed bilateral hydroureteronephrosis; a dilated, thick-walled bladder; a dilated posterior urethra; and bilateral severe reflux. A urine culture yielded a coagulase-positive

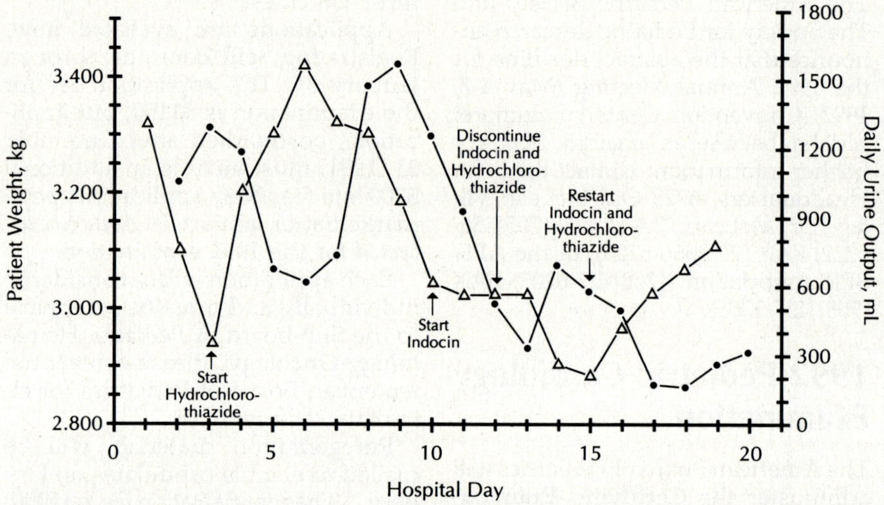

Daily weight (triangles) and daily urine output (dot) measured in relation to the use of indomethacin and hydrochlorothiazide.

Staphylococcus, which was treated with intravenous antibiotics.

After 48 hours of urinary drainage and intravenous administration of fluids to replace urinary and insensible fluid losses, the serum creatinine concentration decreased to 44 µmol/L, and the serum electrolyte concentrations were normal. The Table shows the serum electrolyte, urea nitrogen, creatinine, and urine osmolality values during the patient's initial 4 days in the hospital. Although these values remained essentially unchanged throughout the remainder of the hospitalization, urine output continued to increase, reaching a maximum of 1600 mL/d (21 mL/kg per hour) 9 days after relief of obstruction. This was associated with progressive weight loss and dehydration. Administration of hydrochlorothiazide (1 mg/kg twice daily) to increase proximal tubular reabsorption of sodium and water resulted in only transient improvement in the polyuria until indomethacin (1 mg/kg twice daily) was added (Figure). This led to stabilization of weight and marked reduction in urine output to normal levels (4.8 mL/kg per hour). Discontinuing these medications 2 days later resulted in recurrence of the polyuria in association with weight loss and mild dehydration. Subsequent treatment with indomethacin and hydrochlorothiazide again resulted in a prompt response, with a decrease in urine output to normal amounts and stabilization of weight. As mentioned, no changes in serum creatinine or electrolyte values were noted during this time. After 1 week, hydrochlorothiazide therapy was discontinued, and urine output did not increase. After 2 months of normal growth and development (the patient was in the 25th percentile for height and 20th percentile for weight for his age), indomethacin was discontinued, and the polyuria did not recur.

Comment.—A period of postobstructive diuresis often occurs after relief of urinary tract obstruction and this can be associated with a decrease in the ability to maximally concentrate urine.[1-5] This impairment of the ability to concentrate urine after the initial period of postobstructive diuresis is usually transient, and most patients regain the ability to concentrate urine appropriately days to months after relief of obstruction.[2,3] A number of factors appear to contribute to postobstructive diuresis. Intravascular volume is often expanded before relief of the obstruction, and a physiologic diuresis would be expected to occur after relief of obstruction.[6] Accumulation of natriuretic factors in response to the volume expansion may also play a role in postobstructive diuresis.[7] In addition, obstruction results in the accumulation of urea, which may also induce a postobstructive solute diuresis, with large losses of sodium and water.[8] Finally, there may[4] or may not[3] be a relationship between obstruction complicated by urinary tract infection and impaired ability to concentrate urine. Although data on the relative involvement of each of these factors in humans are lacking, the pathogenesis of postobstructive diuresis is probably multifactorial.

Although there may be multiple defects in distal tubular function, the return of normal function to individual areas of the distal tubule can vary. The ability to maximally concentrate urine, which is a function of the most distal segment of the nephron, should, therefore, also be the most vulnerable to increased intrapelvic pressure.[9] A group of infants who, after relief of urinary tract obstruction, had an initial defect in aldosterone responsiveness in association with polyuria were studied by Heijden et al.[10] The excessive urinary sodium losses improved in most of the patients, but in some patients polyuria persisted for as long as 10 years after surgical relief of the obstruction. This was thought to be caused by collecting tubule unresponsiveness to antidiuretic hormone.

The clinical findings of polyuria, hypotonic urine, dehydration, and unresponsiveness to administration of exogenous antidiuretic hormone are the hallmarks of nephrogenic diabetes insipidus. This phenomenon may persist for years in some patients with postobstructive nephropathy. Conventional therapy has included sodium restriction and use of thiazide diuretics. This treatment causes a decrease in extracellular fluid volume, which leads to a mild reduction in glomerular filtration rate. As a result, proximal tubular reabsorption of sodium and water is increased, and because less water is delivered to the distal nephron, urine output is reduced.[1] More recently, however, prostaglandin synthetase inhibitors have also been found to be effective in the treatment of hereditary nephrogenic diabetes insipidus[11-14] and in one case of postobstructive acquired nephrogenic diabetes insipidus.[2]

Prostaglandin synthetase inhibitors may improve renal concentrating ability in patients with postobstructive nephropathy by inhibition of the prostaglandin-mediated suppression of adenylate cyclase and by an antidiuretic hormone–independent mechanism, such as an increase in medullary tonicity.[11] By inhibiting medullary prostaglandin synthesis, the inhibitors increase cyclic adenosine monophosphate production by the kidney[2] and enhance antidiuretic hormone responsiveness.[15] Prostaglandin synthetase inhibitors also increase solute reabsorption in the medullary segment of the thick ascending limb of Henle's loop.[16] This increased sodium reabsorption results in less distal sodium and water delivery, so that fractional free water clearance is reduced, and the urine-plasma osmolar ratio is increased. The net result is a decrease in urine output.[12] Prostaglandin synthetase inhibitors may also decrease glomerular filtration rate and thereby decrease solute delivery to the tubule. It is also possible that increased urea retention plays a role in the antidiuresis associated with the use of indomethacin.[11]

Several investigators have studied the use of thiazide diuretics and prostaglandin synthetase inhibitors, individually and simultaneously, in the treatment of nephrogenic diabetes insipidus.[2,11-14,17] Most of these studies involved patients with congenital nephrogenic diabetes insipidus. However, Davidai et al[2] described the case of a 5-year-old child with posterior urethral valves who had persistent marked postobstructive polyuria (6200 mL of urine excreted per day) with an inability to produce a urine concentration of higher than 59 mOsm/Kg. Treatment with indomethacin corrected the increased urinary excretion of prostaglandin E_2, increased renal adenosine monophosphate production, and resulted in partial improvement in the urinary concentrating defect. Subsequent addition of a thiazide to the treatment regimen restored the child's urinary concentrating ability. The additive effect of thiazides and indomethacin in the treatment of children with congenital nephrogenic diabetes insipidus has also been reported.[14] Although the use of prostaglandin synthetase inhibitors in children with nephrogenic diabetes insipidus has been previously reported,[18-21] we could not find reports of their use in neonates with obstructive uropathy.

The response of our patient to hydrochlorothiazide and indomethacin (Figure) demonstrates the effectiveness of this combination in the treatment of postobstructive nephrogenic diabetes insipidus. Initial treatment with hydrochlorothiazide resulted in a transient weight gain and decrease in urine output. However, the addition of indomethacin resulted in stabilization of weight and a marked reduction in urine output. This was not likely due to a decrease in glomerular filtration rate, as the serum creatinine concentration remained stable when indomethacin was added to therapy. Efficacy of therapy was further documented by the recurrence of polyuria and weight loss after discontinuation of the medications and subsequent improvement after reinstitution of therapy.

Few data exist concerning the use of indomethacin and hydrochlorothiazide in neonates with acquired nephrogenic diabetes insipidus. Although no controlled trials regarding the use of indomethacin and hydrochlorothiazide in this setting have been reported, this case demonstrates their effectiveness in the treatment of postobstructive polyuria in neonates. It is unclear whether increased prostaglandin production is the primary cause of this disorder or merely a secondary response to another primary renal insult. However, the use of indomethacin, in combination with hydrochlorothiazide, may be a safe and effective treatment for infants and children with persistent postobstructive polyuria.

William E. Smoyer, MD
Division of Nephrology
Children's Hospital of Philadelphia
34th Street and Civic Center Boulevard
Philadelphia, PA 19104

The author would like to thank Bernard S. Kaplan, MBBCh, for his critical review of this article.

1. Glassberg KI. Current issues regarding posterior valves. *Urol Clin North Am.* 1985;12:175-185.

2. Davidai G, Alon U, Jaffe M, Hochberg Z. Post obstructive urinary concentrating defect: a case study in the role of prostaglandins. *Acta Paediatr Scand.* 1987;76:999-1002.

3. Kekomaki M, Reunanen M, Vilkki P. Desaminocysteine-d-arginine vasopressin test in the evaluation and postoperative followup of obstructed kidneys in infancy and childhood. *J Urol.* 1982;128:981-983.

4. Nilsson S, Aurell M, Bratt CG. Maximum urinary concentration ability in patients with idiopathic hydronephrosis. *Br J Urol.* 1979;51:432-436.

5. Beck N, Webster SK. Impaired urinary concentrating ability and vasopressin-dependent cyclic AMP in postobstructive kidneys. *Kidney Int.* 1975; 8:455A.

6. Klahr S. Pathophysiology of obstructive nephropathy. *Kidney Int.* 1983;23:414-426.

7. Harris RH, Yarger WE. The pathogenesis of post-obstructive diuresis: the role of circulating natriuretic and diuretic factors, including urea. *J Clin Invest.* 1975;56:880-887.

8. Maher JF, Schreiner GE, Waters JT. Osmotic diuresis due to retained urea after release of obstructive uropathy. *N Engl J Med.* 1963;268:1099-1104.

9. Wilson DR. Pathophysiology of obstructive nephropathy. *Kidney Int.* 1980;18:281-292.

10. Heijden AJVD, Versteegh FGA, Wolff ED, Sukhai RN, Scholtmeijer RJ. Acute tubular dysfunction in infants with obstructive uropathy. *Acta Paediatr Scand.* 1985;74:589-594.

11. Libber S, Harrison H, Spector D. Treatment of nephrogenic diabetes insipidus with prostaglandin synthesis inhibitors. *J Pediatr.* 1986;108:305-311.

12. Usberti M, Pecoraro C, Federico S, et al. Mechanism of action of indomethacin in tubular defects. *Pediatrics.* 1985;75:501-507.

13. Monn E. Prostaglandin synthetase inhibitors in the treatment of nephrogenic diabetes insipidus. *Acta Paediatr Scand.* 1981;70:39-42.

14. Monnens L, Jonkman A, Thomas C. Response to indomethacin and hydrochlorothiazide in nephrogenic diabetes insipidus. *Clin Sci.* 1984;66:709-715.

15. Anderson RJ, Berl T, McDonald KM, Schrier RW. Evidence for an in vivo antagonism between vasopressin and prostaglandin in the mammalian kidney. *J Clin Invest.* 1975;56:420-426.

16. Kaojarern S, Chennavasin P, Anderson S, Brater DC. Nephron site of effect of nonsteroidal anti-inflammatory drugs on solute excretion in humans. *Am J Physiol.* 1983;244:F134-F139.

17. Alon U, Chan JCM. Hydrochlorothiazide-amiloride in the treatment of congenital nephrogenic diabetes insipidus. *Am J Nephrol.* 1985;5:9-13.

18. Usberti M, Dechaux M, Guillot M, et al. Renal prostaglandin E_2 in nephrogenic diabetes insipidus: effects of inhibition of prostaglandin synthesis by indomethacin. *J Pediatr.* 1980;97:476-478.

19. Fichman MP, Speckart P, Zia P, Lee A. Antidiuretic response to prostaglandin inhibition in nephrogenic diabetes insipidus. *Clin Res.* 1976;24:161A.

20. Anderson O, Jacobsen BB. The renin-aldosterone system in nephrogenic diabetes insipidus and the influence of hydrochlorothiazide and indomethacin. *Acta Paediatr Scand.* 1983; 72:717-720.

21. Rosen GH, Klein-Schwartz W, Medani CR. Indomethacin for nephrogenic diabetes insipidus in a four-week-old infant. *Clin Pharm.* 1986;5:254-256.

A Third Pattern of Disease Progression in Children Infected With Human Immunodeficiency Virus

Sir.—We read with interest the article by Blanche et al[1] on infants with perinatally acquired human immunodeficiency virus (HIV) infection. We too have noted a bimodal pattern of HIV-related disease in our pediatric patients with acquired immunodeficiency syndrome (AIDS).[2] In the last few years we have become aware of a third pattern of HIV infection in children, namely, severe manifestations of disease early in life that lessen over the next 5 to 10 years without antiretroviral therapy. This pattern is illustrated in the following patient reports of three HIV-infected children born to drug-abusing mothers.

Patient Reports.—PATIENT 1.—A 10-year-old black twin boy was born between 34 and 36 weeks' gestation. He weighed 1520 g at birth. His Apgar scores were 8/9 at 1 and 5 minutes. The boy had an uncomplicated neonatal course and was discharged after 2 weeks weighing 1950 g. Within his first 10 months of life he had six admissions, two of them prolonged, for diarrhea, dehydration, bronchiolitis, failure to thrive, and developmental delay. He had no opportunistic infections at this time. By age 2 years, the failure to thrive and developmental delay began to improve. By age 4 years, he developed lymphocytic interstitial pneumonia (Centers for Disease Control [CDC] Class P2C) by clinical criteria.[3,4] At this writing, he had growth retardation, mild right heart failure secondary to chronic pneumonitis, and infection with *Mycobacterium avium-intracellulare* (his first opportunistic infection), putting him in CDC Class P2D1 as well.[4] Until recently, the boy attended school with his uninfected twin and did very well. One year he had perfect school attendance.

PATIENT 2.—A 5-year-old black girl had been admitted at age 4 months for pneumonia. No lung biopsy was performed and no pathogen was ever isolated. She responded clinically to empirically administered sulfamethoxazole and trimethoprim. The infant was hospitalized again at age 5 months for vomiting and diarrhea; during this hospitalization she was treated for an *Escherichia coli* urinary tract infection. At age 8 months, she had developmental delay, thrush, hepatosplenomegaly, and lymphadenopathy. At age 9 months, she was hospitalized again for vomiting and diarrhea. She has developed lymphocytic interstitial pneumonitis (CDC Class P2C),[3,4] but at this writing had no other acute illnesses (aside from otitis media) in the previous four years, and was developmentally normal.

PATIENT 3.—A 3½-year-old black boy was born with a ventricular septal defect. He had congestive heart failure at age 1 month necessitating hospitalization and therapy with digitalis. At ages 6 and 8 months, he was admitted for aseptic meningitis. At age 11 months, he was admitted for pneumonia, at which time he was noted to have diffuse lymphadenopathy. At age 13 months, the boy was admitted for *Salmonella* osteomyelitis of the left shoulder. Lymphadenopathy and thrush were noted during a physical examination. Hemoglobin electrophoresis showed type AA. After being successfully treated for his osteomyelitis, he had no further hospitalizations or serious infections, and at this writing was classified as CDC Class P2A.

Comment.—These cases highlight the difficulty of predicting early in life who among our HIV-infected infants will have the "rapid" form of the disease[1,2] and who will not. Failure to identify opportunistic infections in these HIV-infected children with multiple hospitalizations under age 1 year appears to be a critical prognostic sign.

BEN Z. KATZ, MD
JAMES G. MCNAMARA, MD
Yale University School of Medicine
Department of Pediatrics
333 Cedar St
New Haven, CT 06510-8064

1. Blanche S, Tardieu M, Duliege A-M, et al. Longitudinal study of 94

symptomatic infants with perinatally acquired human immunodeficiency virus infection: evidence for a bimodal expression of clinical and biological symptoms. *AJDC.* 1990;144:1210-1215.

2. Katz BZ. Natural history and clinical management of the infant born to a mother infected with human immunodeficiency virus. *Semin Perinatol.* 1989;13:27-34.

3. Centers for Disease Control. Revision of the case definition of acquired immunodeficiency syndrome for national reporting—United States. *MMWR.* 1985;34:373-375.

4. Centers for Disease Control. Classification system for HIV infection in children under 13 years of age. *MMWR.* 1987;36:225-236.

In Reply.—We fully agree with the comments by Drs Katz and McNamara regarding the various types of disease progressions in children infected with (HIV). Indeed, some patients with a "borderline" or an unusual progression might not perfectly fit into our description of a "bimodal population" of children according to the progression of the disease.[1] We followed up a child, perinatally infected with HIV, who, at age 4 months, developed *Pneumocystis carinii* pneumonia. Three years later she was well, with no neurologic impairment or secondary infection. Her most recent CD4 cell count was over 1.5 × 109/L, and the results of her in vitro lymphocyte proliferation tests became progressively normal, showing an association between the clinical and immunologic improvements. In most cases of HIV-infected children, there is a correlation between the severity of the symptoms and the impairment of the immune system or the intensity of the viral load. However, it is more important and useful to show the prognostic value of these tests when performed early in life, before the occurrence of symptoms. Rodgers et al[2] suggested that the outcome of the disease was worse for children with a positive polymerase chain reaction test for HIV-DNA rapidly after birth, than for those whose polymerase chain reaction test result became positive later in life. However, our experience is slightly different. Finally, more recent techniques such as quantitative DNA polymerase chain reaction, plasma viral culture, and RNA polymerase chain reaction are under evaluation in infants, and together with the assessment of the immune function, might bring valuable prognostic information. This will become more helpful with the development of treatment protocols in newborns.

STEPHANE BLANCHE, MD
ANNE-MARIE DULIEGE, MD
CHRISTINE ROUZIOUX, MD
FRANÇOISE LE DEIST, MD
KEN FUKUNAGA, MD
MAURIZIO CANIGLIA, MD
CHRISTINE JACOMET, MD
CLAUDE GRISCELLI, MD
Pediatric Immunology Division,
INSERM U 132,
and Virology Unit
Hopital Necker
149 rue de Sèvres
75015 Paris, France
MARC TARDIEU, MD
Pediatric Neurology Division,
INSERM U 56
ANTOINE MESSIAH, PHD
Epidemiology Division,
INSERM U 292
Bicêtre Hospital
Paris, France

1. Blanche S, Tardieu M, Duliege A-M, et al. Longitudinal study of 94 symptomatic infants with perinatally acquired immunodeficiency virus infection: evidence for a bimodal expression of clinical and biological symptoms. *AJDC.* 1990;144:1210-1215.

2. Rodgers M, Ou CY, Rayfield M, et al. Use of the PCR for early detection of the proviral sequences of HIV in infants born to seropositive mothers. *N Engl J Med.* 1989;320:1649-1654.

Hydrocele in Kawasaki Disease: Importance in Early Recognition of Atypical Disease

Sir.—Kawasaki disease (KD) is an acute febrile mucocutaneous vasculitis of unknown cause occurring in infants and children.[1] Diagnostic criteria for KD have been defined by the Centers for Disease Control[2] and are shown in Table 1. In the last decade, cases of atypical KD (AKD) have been reported that do not meet these criteria, but that have a very high coronary artery complication rate and mortality.[3-13] These coronary complications can safely be prevented with intravenous immunoglobulin if administered within 10 days of the beginning of illness.[14-16] In AKD, diagnosis is often delayed, preventing this effective early therapy.[3-13] We report five cases of KD (the first three of which are atypical cases) with development of a hydrocele by 10 days after illness began. To our knowledge, this is the first report of hydrocele with KD, and these findings may aid in early diagnosis and treatment of AKD. The diagnosis of hydrocele was made by the same infectious diseases consultant between 1980 and 1990. During this time, 44 cases of KD were reported at our hospital; 28 occurred in males, six of whom had AKD.

Table 1.—Diagnostic Criteria for Kawasaki Disease

Fever for ≥5 days
Presence of four of the following five conditions:
Bilateral conjunctival injection
Change(s) in the mucous membranes of the upper respiratory tract, such as reddened pharynx, reddened lips, dry fissured lips, and strawberry tongue
Changes of the peripheral extremities, such as peripheral edema, peripheral erythema, and desquamation
Rash, primarily truncal (polymorphous, but nonvesicular)
Cervical lymph glands ≥1.5 cm
Illness unexplained by other known disease processes

Patient Reports.—PATIENT 1.—A previously well 10-month-old Chinese boy presented with a 4-day history of fever unresponsive to amoxicillin, irritability, and diarrhea, and a 2-day history of truncal rash with perineal accentuation. Initial examination revealed an irritable infant with a temperature of 38.3°C, generalized rash, and shotty cervical lymphadenopathy. Results of the remainder of the examination were normal. Two days after admission to the hospital, an asymptomatic, transilluminating, moderate-sized, noncommunicating hydrocele of the left testicle developed. There was no inflammation or tenderness. Six days after admission, results of an echocardiogram revealed an aneurysm of the left coronary artery. After therapy with intravenous immunoglobulin (400 mg/kg of body weight per day) and aspirin (100

Table 2.—Patient Summary*

Patient No.	Age, mo	No. of CDC Criteria Fulfilled	Day of Illness on Which Desquamation Occurred	Aneurysm Occurred (Location)	Hydrocele Occurred (Location)	Treatment Was Given	ESR mm/h
1	10	2	12	10 (LCA)	6 (left testicle)	10	76
2	11	4	12	8 (LCA)	10 (right testicle)	8	108
3	23	4	13	None	6 (right testicle)	10	23
4	36	5	None	None	7 (left testicle)	7	114
5	44	5	9	None	10 (left testicle)	9	75

*CDC indicates Centers for Disease Control; ESR, erythrocyte sedimentation rate; and LCA, left coronary artery.

mg/kg of body weight per day) was started, fever and mood improved within 24 hours. On day 8 of his hospital stay, periungual desquamation occurred. Follow-up 1 week later showed complete resolution of the hydrocele.

PATIENT 2.—A previously well 11-month-old white boy presented with a 5-day history of a rectal temperature of up to 40.8°C and generalized rash with perineal accentuation. He was irritable and anorexic. He had a mild cough and clear rhinorrheal discharge for 3 days. Results of initial examination revealed an irritable infant with a temperature of 39.2°C, nonexudative pharyngitis, truncal rash, palmar erythema, and foot edema. Results of the rest of the examination were normal. Results of an echocardiogram on day 3 of hospitalization revealed proximal left coronary artery dilatation of 4.0 mm. Administration of intravenous immunoglobulin (400 mg/kg of body weight per day) and aspirin (100 mg/kg of body weight per day) was followed by resolution of fever and improved mood by the next day. Five days after admission to the hospital, a transilluminating, small, noncommunicating hydrocele of the right testicle developed that was not present on admission; this hydrocele was asymptomatic and nontender, with no inflammation. On day 7 of the hospital stay, periungual desquamation occurred. Follow-up 1 week later showed complete resolution of the hydrocele.

PATIENT 3.—A 23-month-old white boy presented with a 6-day history of a temperature of up to 39°C, unresponsiveness to amoxicillin, and generalized rash, and a 2-day history of red, cracked lips and red eyes. Results of initial examination revealed a febrile child with a temperature of 39.4°C, clear rhinorrheal discharge, bilateral nonexudative conjunctivitis, erythematous cracked lips, strawberry tongue, generalized rash with perineal accentuation and desquamation, and a transilluminating small hydrocele of the right testicle. The hydrocele was noncommunicating and asymptomatic, with no inflammation. Results of an echocardiogram were normal. The patient's temperature returned to normal after intravenous immunoglobulin (400mg/kg of body weight per day) and aspirin (100 mg/kg of body weight per day) were administered on day 4 of hospitalization. Periungual desquamation occurred on day 7 of the hospital stay. Records from hospital admissions at ages 5, 6, and 12 months and a parental report of the child's health history did not reveal hydrocele. On 2-week follow-up, the hydrocele had resolved.

PATIENT 4.—A previously well 3-year-old American Indian boy presented with a 7-day history of fever, cervical lymphadenopathy with tenderness, red eyes, red tongue, and arthralgias. He was unresponsive to amoxicillin, which was substituted with erythromycin ethylsuccinate andsulfisoxazole after development of a generalized rash. Results of initial examination revealed a temperature of 38.6°C; bilateral nonexudative conjunctivitis; dry, erythematous cracked lips; a red tongue; bilateral cervical lymphadenopathy with tenderness; indurated edema of the hands and feet; a desquamating perineal rash, and a transilluminating small hydrocele of the left testicle (which had not occurred previously by parental report). The noncommunicating hydrocele was nontender, with no inflammation. Results of an echocardiogram were normal. Treatment with intravenous immunoglobulin (400 mg/kg of body weight per day) and aspirin (100 mg/kg of body weight per day) on admission resulted in resolution of fever the next day. Results of a follow-up examination revealed complete resolution of the hydrocele.

PATIENT 5.—A previously well white boy aged 3 years 8 months presented with a 7-day history of fever that was unresponsive to amoxicillin and a generalized rash. For 4 days before admission to the hospital, he had red eyes and a red tongue. Results of initial examination revealed a rectal temperature of 39.5°C, irritability, bilateral nonexudative conjunctivitis, strawberry tongue, rash, and hepatomegaly. Results of the rest of the examination were normal. Periungual desquamation occurred on day 2 of hospitalization, and a transilluminating moderate-sized hydrocele of the left testicle developed on day 4. The hydrocele was communicating, and asymptomatic with no inflammation. Results of an echocardiogram were normal. He was treated with aspirin (100 mg/kg of body weight per day) on day 2 of hospitalization, with resolution of the fever by day 5. The hydrocele was surgically excised 2 years later.

Other diagnoses were excluded for these patients based on negative results of the following tests (if indicated): complete blood cell count; urinalysis; lumbar puncture; bacterial cultures of blood, urine, throat, and cerebrospinal fluid; viral cultures of stool, throat, nasopharynx, and cerebrospinal fluid; viral serologic tests, including the monospot test; antistreptolysin-O titer; tests to identify antinuclear antibody and rheumatoid factor; chest roentgenogram; abdominal ultrasound; and measurement of immunoglobulins.

Comment.—Although initially thought to be a benign febrile illness in children,[1] KD has been found to have significant complications, a mortality rate of up to 2%,[1] and a coronary artery aneurysm or ectasia rate of 15% to 25%.[15] Most of these coronary dilatations have resolved on follow-up angiography and echocardiography, but vessel wall abnormalities often persist[17,18]; the ultimate fate of patients with these coronary abnormalities, including risk for future ischemic heart disease, is unknown.[1] In fact, there are several reports of myocardial infarction or sudden death months to years after an illness suggestive of KD.[19-25] Administration of intravenous immunoglobulin combined with high-dose salicylate therapy is known to significantly decrease the coronary complication rate.[14,15] The ultimate long-term benefits of this therapy are yet to be defined.[16] No published studies have been conducted that suggest a benefit of therapy if begun after the 10th day of illness.[14-16]

In the last decade, there have been many reports of KD that does not satisfy the diagnostic criteria of the condition, but that are complicated by a high rate of coronary abnormalities (90%) or mortality (35%).[3-13] In most of these atypical cases, diagnosis was made late in the disease process, when results of echocardiography or autopsy revealed coronary dilatation or aneurysm. For effective early intravenous immunoglobulin therapy in these cases, diagnostic clues before the 10th day of illness are needed. Reported herein are five patients (Table 2) with KD in whom hydrocele developed by day 10 of illness. The first three patients had AKD. In all but one patient, there was complete resolution of hydrocele within 2 weeks of the acute illness. To our knowledge, the finding of hydrocele in KD has not been previously reported. A possible mechanism for development of hydrocele is suggested by reports of a high incidence of spermatic cord and testicular arteritis discovered at autopsy of subjects with KD.[26-28]

In 1976, Tanaka et al[26] reported testicular arteritis in five (23%) of 22 autopsies of subjects with KD and in four (36%) of 11 autopsies of infants with KD. Infantile periarteritis nodosa and KD are now considered the same disease,[26,28-30] and studies of infantile periarteritis nodosa have reported a high incidence of testicular or spermatic cord arteritis at autopsy: three (25%) of 12 in a 1963 review[27] and nine (60%) of 15 in a 1977 review.[28] The 1977 review by Landing and Larson reported hydrocele in eight (75%) of 12 infants with infantile periarteritis nodosa.[28] In fact, in Henoch-Schönlein purpura[31] and classic adult polyarteritis nodosa,[32] testicular arteritis is not uncommon, and hydrocele has been reported with these conditions. This may be a sympathetic effusion resulting from the underlying arteritis inflammation.

Although the finding of hydrocele in KD needs to be confirmed in prospective studies, we suggest that development of a hydrocele during an acute febrile illness is suggestive of KD, and that identifying hydrocele may aid in the early diagnosis and effective treatment of KD. Hydrocele is a particularly useful sign of possible disease in infants with atypical presentations of Kawasaki disease.

Amin Kabani, MD, FRCPC
Ari Joffe, MD
Taj Jadavji, MD, FRCPC, FAAP
Departments of Pediatrics, Microbiology, and Infectious Disease
Alberta Children's Hospital
1820 Richmond Rd SW
University of Calgary
Calgary, Alberta,
Canada T2T 5C7

1. Rowley A, Gonzalez-Crussi F, Shulman S. Kawasaki syndrome. *Rev Infect Dis.* 1988;10:1-15.

2. Centers for Disease Control. Kawasaki disease—New York. *MMWR.* 1980;29:61-63.

3. Levy M, Koren G. Atypical Kawasaki disease: analysis of clinical presentation and diagnostic clues. *Pediatr Infect Dis J.* 1990;9:122-126.

4. Reller M, Decristofaro J, Schwartz D. Coronary aneurysms in a patient with atypical Kawasaki syndrome and a streptococcal infection. *Pediatr Cardiol.* 1984;5:205-208.

5. Canter C, Bower R, Strauss A. Atypical Kawasaki disease with aortic aneurysm. *Pediatrics.* 1981;68:885-888.

6. Friedman A. An atypical presentation of Kawasaki syndrome in an infant. *Pediatr Dermatol.* 1988;5:120-122.

7. Rowley A, Gonzalez-Crussi F, Gidding S, Duffy E, Shulman S. Incomplete Kawasaki disease with coronary artery involvement. *J Pediatr.* 1987;110:409-413.

8. Burns J, Wiggins J, Toews W, et al. Clinical spectrum of Kawasaki disease in infants younger than 6 months of age. *J Pediatr.* 1986;109:759-763.

9. Schuh S, Laxer R, Smallhorn J, Hilliard R, Rowe R. Kawasaki disease with atypical presentation. *Pediatr Infect Dis.* 1988;3:201-203.

10. Kleiman MB, Passo MH. Incomplete Kawasaki disease with facial nerve paralysis and coronary artery involvement. *Pediatr Infect Dis J.* 1988;7:301-302.

11. Avner J, Shaw K, Chin A. Atypical presentation of Kawasaki disease with early development of giant coronary artery aneurysms. *J Pediatr.* 1989;114:605-606.

12. Krapf R, Zimmerman A, Stocker F. Lethal vasculitis of coronary arteries in a neonate and two infants: possible neonatal variant of MLNS/IPN complex? *Helv Pediatr Acta.* 1981;36:589-598.

13. Sonobe T, Kawasaki T. Atypical Kawasaki disease. *Prog Clin Biol Res.* 1987;250:367-378.

14. Furusho K, Nakano H, Shinomiya K, et al. High-dose intravenous gamma globulin for Kawasaki disease. *Lancet.* 1984;2:1055-1058.

15. Newburger J, Takahashi M, Burns J, et al. The treatment of Kawasaki syndrome with intravenous gammaglobulin. *N Engl J Med.* 1986;315:341-347.

16. Rauch A. Kawasaki syndrome: issues in etiology and treatment. *Adv Pediatr Infect Dis.* 1989;4:163-182.

17. Kato H, Ichinose E, Yoshioka F, et al. Fate of coronary aneurysms in Kawasaki disease: serial coronary angiography and long term follow-up study. *Am J Cardiol.* 1982;49:1758-1766.

18. Kato H, Inoue O, Akagi T. Kawasaki disease: cardiac problems and management. *Pediatr Review.* 1988;9: 209-217.

19. Gorgels A, Braat S, Becker A, et al. Multiple aneurysms of the coronary arteries as a cause of sudden death in childhood. *Am J Cardiol.* 1986;57:1193-1194.

20. Tang P, Segal A. Polyarteritis nodosa of infancy: fatal late complication. *JAMA.* 1971;217:1666-1670.

21. Liddicoat JF, Bekassy SM, O'Donnell MJ, Debakey ML. Coronary artery aneurysm in a 9 year old child. *Surgery.* 1974;76:845-847.

22. Flugelman M, Hasin Y, Bassan M, Leor R, Gotsman M. Acute myocardial infarction 14 years after an acute episode of Kawasaki disease. *Am J Cardiol.* 1983;52:427-428.

23. Kohr R. Progressive asymptomatic coronary artery disease as a late fatal sequelae of Kawasaki disease. *J Pediatr.* 1986;2:256-259.

24. Pounder D. Coronary artery aneurysms presenting as sudden death 14 years after Kawasaki disease in infancy. *Arch Pathol Lab Med.* 1985;109:874-876.

25. McMartin D, Stone A, Franch R. Multiple coronary artery aneurysms in a child with angina pectoris. *N Engl J Med.* 1974;290:669-670.

26. Tanaka N, Sekimoto K, Naoe S. Kawasaki disease: relationship with infantile periarteritis nodosa. *Arch Pathol Lab Med.* 1976;100:81-86.

27. Roberts FB, Fetterman GH. Polyarteritis nodosa in infancy. *J Pediatr.* 1963;63:519-529.

28. Landing BH, Larson EJ. Are infantile periarteritis nodosa with coronary artery involvement and fatal mucocutaneous lymph node syndrome the same?: comparison of 20 patients from North America with patients from Hawaii and Japan. *Pediatrics.* 1977;59:651-662.

29. Melish ME, Hicks R, Larson EJ. Mucocutaneous lymph node syndrome in the United States. *AJDC.* 1976; 130:599-607.

30. Fetterman G. Mucocutaneous lymph node syndrome (MLNS): a disease widespread in Japan which demands our attention. *Pediatrics.* 1974;54:268-270.

31. Khan AU, Williams TH, Malek RS. Acute scrotal swelling in Henoch-Schönlein syndrome. *Urology.* 1977; 10:139-141.

32. Roy JB, Hamblin DW, Brown CH. Periarteritis nodosa of epididymis. *Urology.* 1977;10:62-63.

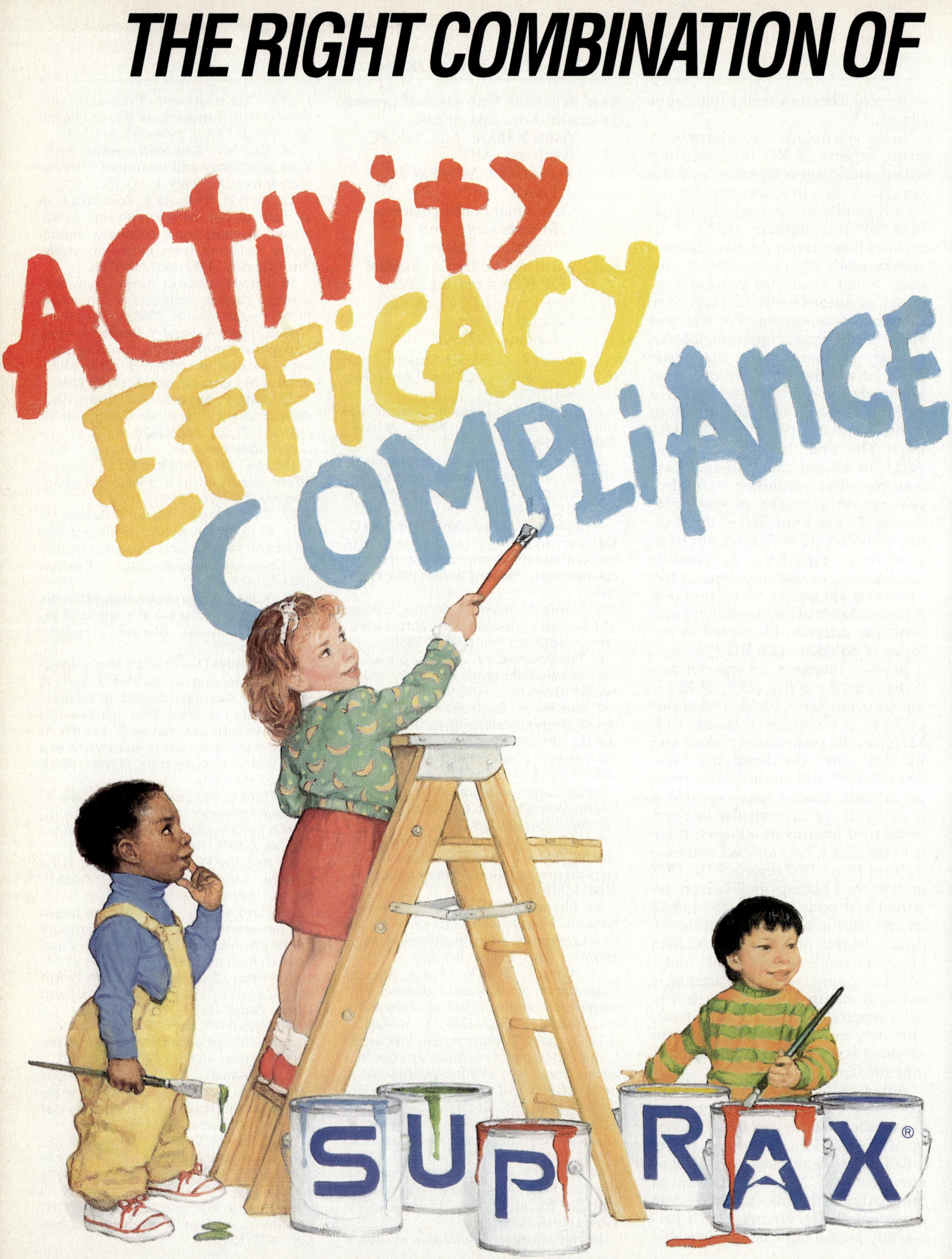
THE RIGHT COMBINATION OF
Activity
Efficacy
Compliance
SUPRAX®

ONCE-A-DAY

SUPRAX®

cefixime/Lederle

Oral Suspension 100 mg/5 mL

8 mg/kg/day

NOW AVAILABLE IN COST-EFFECTIVE 75 mL BOTTLE

References: 1. Nash DR, Flanagan C, Steele LC, et al. Comparison of the activity of cefixime and activities of other oral antibiotics against adult clinical isolates of *Moraxella (Branhamella) catarrhalis* containing BRO-1 and BRO-2 and *Haemophilus influenzae. Antimicrob Agents Chemother.* 1991;35:192-194. **2.** Schentag JJ. Pharmacokinetic profiles as predictors of therapeutic success. In: *Respiratory Infections: Therapeutic Considerations in a Dynamic Environment.* Lederle Laboratories; 1990. Data on file. Lederle Laboratories, Pearl River, NY. **3.** Jones RN, Barry AL. Antimicrobial activity, spectrum, and recommendations for disk diffusion susceptibility testing of ceftibuten (7432-S; SCH 39720), a new orally administered cephalosporin. *Antimicrob Agents Chemother.* 1988; 32(10):1576-1582. **4.** Pichichero ME. Cefixime multicenter national otitis media study. In: *The Contemporary Treatment of Otitis Media.* Lederle Laboratories; 1990. Data on file. Lederle Laboratories, Pearl River, NY. **5.** Cockburn J, Gibberd RW, Reid AL, et al. Determinants of non-compliance with short term antibiotic regimens. *Br Med J,* 1987;295:814-818. **6.** Ruff ME, Schotik DA, Bass JW, et al. Antimicrobial drug suspensions: a blind comparison of taste of fourteen common pediatric drugs. *Pediatr Infect Dis J.* 1991;10:30-33.

Brief Summary

SUPRAX® Cefixime

Please see package insert for full Prescribing Information.

INDICATIONS AND USAGE

Otitis Media caused by *Haemophilus influenzae* (beta-lactamase positive and negative strains), *Moraxella (Branhamella) catarrhalis* (most of which are beta-lactamase positive), and *Streptococcus pyogenes.**

Note: For information on otitis media caused by *Streptococcus pneumoniae,* see **CLINICAL STUDIES** section.

Acute Bronchitis and Acute Exacerbations of Chronic Bronchitis caused by *S pneumoniae* and *H influenzae* (beta-lactamase positive and negative strains).

Perform culture and susceptibility studies to determine causative organism and its susceptibility to SUPRAX. Therapy may begin while waiting for study results and may be adjusted when results are known.

Pharyngitis and Tonsillitis caused by *S pyogenes.*

Note: Penicillin is the usual drug of choice in the treatment of *S pyogenes* infections, including the prophylaxis of rheumatic fever. SUPRAX is generally effective in the eradication of *S pyogenes* from the nasopharynx; however, data establishing the efficacy of SUPRAX in the subsequent prevention of rheumatic fever are not available.

Uncomplicated Urinary Tract Infections caused by *Escherichia coli* and *Proteus mirabilis.*

*Efficacy for this organism was studied in fewer than ten patients with otitis media.

CLINICAL STUDIES

In clinical trials of otitis media in nearly 400 children between the ages of 6 months and 10 years, *S pneumoniae* was isolated from 47% of the patients, *H influenzae* from 34%, *B catarrhalis* from 15%, and *S pyogenes* from 4%.

The overall response rate of *S pneumoniae* to cefixime was approximately 10% lower and that of *H influenzae* or *B catarrhalis* approximately 7% higher (12% when beta-lactamase positive strains of *H influenzae* are included) than the response rates of these organisms to the active control drugs.

In these studies, patients were randomized and treated with either cefixime at dose regimens of 4 mg/kg bid or 8 mg/kg qd, or with a standard antibiotic regimen. Sixty-nine to 70% of the patients in each group had resolution of signs and symptoms of otitis media when evaluated 2 to 4 weeks posttreatment, but persistent effusion was found in 15% of the patients. When evaluated at the completion of therapy, 17% of patients receiving cefixime and 14% of patients receiving effective comparative drugs (18% including those patients who had *H influenzae* resistant to the control drug and who received the control antibiotic) were considered to be treatment failures. By the 2- to 4-week follow-up, a total of 30% to 31% of patients had evidence of either treatment failure or recurrent disease.

Bacteriological Outcome of Otitis Media at 2- to 4-Weeks Posttherapy
Based on Repeat Middle Ear Fluid Culture or Extrapolation from Clinical Outcome

Organism	Cefixime(a) 4 mg/kg bid	Cefixime(a) 8 mg/kg qd	Control(a) drugs
Streptococcus pneumoniae	48/70 (69%)	18/22 (82%)	82/100 (82%)
Haemophilus influenzae beta-lactamase negative	24/34 (71%)	13/17 (76%)	23/34 (68%)
Haemophilus influenzae beta-lactamase positive	17/22 (77%)	9/12 (75%)	1/1(b)
Moraxella (Branhamella) catarrhalis	26/31 (84%)	5/5	18/24 (75%)
Streptococcus pyogenes	5/5	3/3	6/7
All Isolates	120/162 (74%)	48/59 (81%)	130/166 (78%)

(a) Number eradicated/number isolated.

(b) An additional 20 beta-lactamase positive strains of *H influenzae* were isolated, but were excluded from this analysis because they were resistant to the control antibiotic. In 19 of these the clinical course could be assessed, and a favorable outcome occurred in 10. When these cases are included in the overall bacteriological evaluation of therapy with the control drugs, 140/185 (76%) of pathogens were considered to be eradicated.

Tablets should not be substituted for suspension when treating otitis media.

CONTRAINDICATIONS

Known allergy to cephalosporins.

WARNINGS

BEFORE THERAPY WITH SUPRAX IS INSTITUTED, CAREFUL INQUIRY SHOULD BE MADE TO DETERMINE WHETHER THE PATIENT HAS HAD PREVIOUS HYPERSENSITIVITY REACTIONS TO CEPHALOSPORINS, PENICILLINS, OR OTHER DRUGS. IF THIS PRODUCT IS TO BE GIVEN TO PENICILLIN-SENSITIVE PATIENTS, CAUTION SHOULD BE EXERCISED BECAUSE CROSS-HYPERSENSITIVITY AMONG BETA-LACTAM ANTIBIOTICS HAS BEEN CLEARLY DOCUMENTED AND MAY OCCUR IN UP TO 10% OF PATIENTS WITH A HISTORY OF PENICILLIN ALLERGY. IF AN ALLERGIC REACTION TO SUPRAX OCCURS, DISCONTINUE THE DRUG. SERIOUS, ACUTE HYPERSENSITIVITY REACTIONS MAY REQUIRE TREATMENT WITH EPINEPHRINE AND OTHER EMERGENCY MEASURES, INCLUDING OXYGEN, INTRAVENOUS FLUIDS, INTRAVENOUS ANTIHISTAMINES, CORTICOSTEROIDS, PRESSOR AMINES, AND AIRWAY MANAGEMENT, AS CLINICALLY INDICATED.

Administer cautiously to allergic patients.

Treatment with broad-spectrum antibiotics alters the normal flora of the colon and may permit overgrowth of clostridia. Studies indicate that a toxin produced by *Clostridium difficile* is a primary cause of severe antibiotic-associated diarrhea including pseudomembranous colitis. Pseudomembranous colitis has been reported with the use of SUPRAX and other broad-spectrum antibiotics (including macrolides, semisynthetic penicillins, and cephalosporins). It is important to consider this diagnosis in patients who develop diarrhea in association with antibiotic use. Symptoms of pseudomembranous colitis may occur during or after antibiotic treatment and may range in severity from mild to life threatening. Mild cases usually respond to drug discontinuation alone. Moderate-to-severe cases should be managed with fluid, electrolyte, and protein supplementation. When the colitis is not relieved by drug discontinuance, or when it is severe, oral vancomycin is the drug of choice for antibiotic-associated pseudomembranous colitis produced by *C difficile.* Other causes of colitis should be excluded.

PRECAUTIONS

General: Prolonged use may result in overgrowth of nonsusceptible organisms. If superinfection occurs, take appropriate measures.

Carefully monitor patients on dialysis. Adjust dosage of SUPRAX in patients with renal impairment and those undergoing continuous ambulatory peritoneal dialysis and hemodialysis. (See **DOSAGE AND ADMINISTRATION.**)

Prescribe cautiously in patients with a history of gastrointestinal disease, particularly colitis.

Drug Interactions: No significant drug interactions have been reported to date.

Drug/Laboratory Test Interactions: A false-positive reaction for ketones in the urine may occur with tests using nitroprusside but not with those using nitroferricyanide.

SUPRAX administration may result in a false-positive reaction for glucose in the urine using Clinitest®,** Benedict's solution, or Fehling's solution. Use glucose tests based on enzymatic glucose oxidase reactions (such as Clinistix®** or Tes-Tape®**).

A false-positive direct Coombs test has been reported during treatment with other cephalosporin antibiotics; therefore, it should be recognized that a positive Coombs test may be due to the drug.

Carcinogenesis, Mutagenesis, Impairment of Fertility: Although no lifetime animal studies have been conducted to evaluate carcinogenic potential, no mutagenic potential of SUPRAX was found in standard laboratory tests. Reproductive studies revealed no fertility impairment in rats at doses up to 125 times the adult therapeutic dose.

Usage in Pregnancy: *Pregnancy Category B:* Reproduction studies have been performed in mice and rats at doses up to 400 times the human dose and have revealed no evidence of harm to the fetus due to SUPRAX.

There are no adequate and well-controlled studies in pregnant women. Because animal reproduction studies are not always predictive of human response, this drug should be used during pregnancy only if clearly needed.

Labor and Delivery: SUPRAX has not been studied for use during labor and delivery. Treatment should only be given if clearly needed.

Nursing Mothers: It is not known whether SUPRAX is excreted in human milk. Consider discontinuing nursing temporarily during treatment with this drug.

Pediatric Use: Safety and effectiveness of SUPRAX in children aged less than 6 months have not been established.

The incidence of gastrointestinal adverse reactions, including diarrhea and loose stools, in pediatric patients receiving the suspension, was comparable to adult patients receiving tablets.

ADVERSE REACTIONS

Most adverse reactions observed in clinical trials were of a mild and transient nature. Less than four percent (3.8%) of patients in the US trials discontinued therapy because of drug-related adverse reactions. Commonly seen adverse reactions in US trials of the tablet formulation were gastrointestinal events, which were reported in 30% of adult patients on either the bid or the qd regimen. Clinically mild gastrointestinal side effects occurred in 20% of all patients, moderate events occurred in 9% of all patients, and severe adverse reactions occurred in 2% of all patients. Individual event rates included diarrhea 16%, loose or frequent stools 6%, abdominal pain 3%, nausea 7%, dyspepsia 3%, and flatulence 3%. The incidence of gastrointestinal adverse reactions, including diarrhea and loose stools, in pediatric patients receiving the suspension was comparable to adult patients receiving tablets.

Symptoms usually responded to symptomatic therapy or ceased when SUPRAX was discontinued.

Several patients developed severe diarrhea and/or documented pseudomembranous colitis, and a few required hospitalization.

The following adverse reactions have been reported following the use of SUPRAX. Incidence rates were less than 1 in 50 (less than 2%), except as noted above for gastrointestinal events.

Gastrointestinal: Diarrhea, loose stools, abdominal pain, dyspepsia, nausea, and vomiting. Several cases of documented pseudomembranous colitis were identified during the studies. The onset of pseudomembranous colitis symptoms may occur during or after therapy.

Hypersensitivity Reactions: Skin rashes, urticaria, drug fever, and pruritus. Erythema multiforme, Stevens-Johnson syndrome, and serum sickness have been reported rarely.

Hepatic: Transient elevations in SGPT, SGOT, and alkaline phosphatase.

Renal: Transient elevations in BUN or creatinine.

Central Nervous System: Headaches 3%; dizziness.

Hemic and Lymphatic Systems: Transient thrombocytopenia, leukopenia, and eosinophilia. Prolongation in prothrombin time was seen rarely.

Other: Genital pruritus, vaginitis, candidiasis.

The following adverse reactions and altered laboratory tests have been reported for cephalosporin-class antibiotics:

Adverse Reactions: Allergic reactions including anaphylaxis, toxic epidermal necrolysis, superinfection, renal dysfunction, toxic nephropathy, hepatic dysfunction, including cholestasis, aplastic anemia, hemolytic anemia, hemorrhage.

Several cephalosporins have been implicated in triggering seizures, particularly in patients with renal impairment when the dosage was not reduced (see **DOSAGE AND ADMINISTRATION** and **OVERDOSAGE**). If seizures associated with drug therapy occur, discontinue drug. Administer anticonvulsant therapy if clinically indicated.

Abnormal Laboratory Tests: Positive direct Coombs test, elevated bilirubin, elevated LDH, pancytopenia, neutropenia, agranulocytosis.

OVERDOSAGE

Gastric lavage may be indicated; otherwise, no specific antidote exists. Cefixime is not removed in significant quantities from the circulation by hemodialysis or peritoneal dialysis. Adverse reactions in small numbers of healthy adult volunteers receiving single doses up to 2 g of SUPRAX did not differ from the profile seen in patients treated at the recommended doses.

**Clinitest and Clinistix are registered trademarks of Ames Division, Miles Laboratories, Inc. Tes-Tape is a registered trademark of Eli Lilly and Company.

Rev. 5/91
10753-91

LEDERLE LABORATORIES DIVISION
American Cyanamid Company, Pearl River, NY 10965
Under License of **Fujisawa Pharmaceutical Co., Ltd.,** Osaka, Japan

Lederle

Lederle Laboratories
A Division of American Cyanamid Company
Wayne, New Jersey 07470

Under License of
Fujisawa Pharmaceutical Co., Ltd.
Osaka, Japan

ROSS LABORATORIES
COLUMBUS, OHIO 43216
Division of Abbott Laboratories, USA

THE EDITORIAL BOARD SPEAKS. . . .

"Grampa, Can I Get Something That I'd Like?"

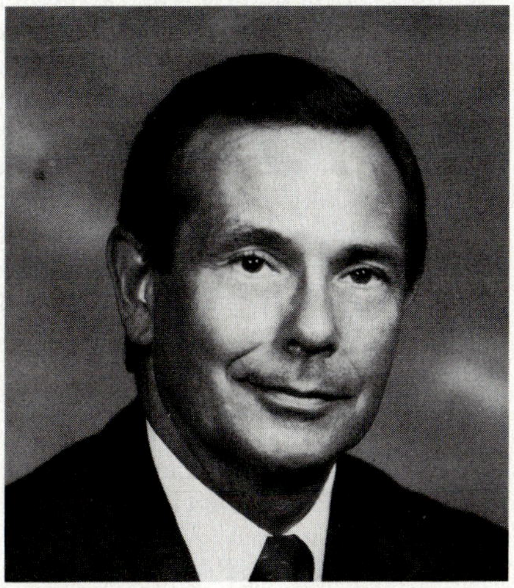

William B. Strong, MD

"Grampa, can I get something that I'd like" hit me like a Mike Tyson uppercut to the solar plexus. The sports metaphor is intentional. I enjoy sports participation more than as a spectator.

Max is my grandson; he's only age 4½ years. He knocked me out in Toys "R" Us with the above question. I rarely see my daughter Beth and her three children since they live in New Hampshire. This past April, I was really looking forward to seeing them. I dreamt and fantasized about how much fun we were going to have playing together. Until now, its been mainly with blocks and Legos. Legos are my favorite. Well, it was spring and I thought it would be fun to play catch and bat a ball with Max and Caroline, his sister. Will is still a bit young for baseball; he's only age 18 months. So, after I arrived for my 2-day visit and settled in, I inventoried all the kids' toys. No baseball paraphernalia! It was time to go to Toys "R" Us for some baseball gloves and a tee-ball set. Boy! Were we going to have fun! Grampa was in hog heaven. "Max, how'd you like this glove?" "What about you, Caroline?" "What color ball should we get?" "*We need* a light bat so nobody gets hurt." It happened after we (I) made some super selections and were headed toward the sales counter. That's when Max chopped me down. Trailing on my left side, he threw a sneak punch. POW! It took a moment for me to catch my breath, to get my defenses up. But what defense is there for a little boy who innocently looks up at you and asks "Now grampa, can I get something that I'd like?" What a fantastic lesson; one that I espouse every day as a pediatrician, but was blinded by my own selfish desires. Sure, I wanted these for the children. STOP! Examine that last sentence. It began "*I wanted,*" not what Max and Caroline wanted. All Max wanted was a little truck. Max got his truck and I got an incredible lesson, and one that I hope I never forget. Thanks, Max.

I do not believe this little vignette is a unique experience. How often do we do for others what we would want them to do for us rather than doing for them what they want to be done for them?

THE PEDIATRIC FORUM

Tiny Tim Remembered

Sir.—Of all the haunting images that moved the hardened heart of Ebenezer Scrooge on that infamous Christmas Eve, the picture of Tiny Tim seemed to touch him most deeply. Tiny Tim, perhaps the most pathetic yet endearing character in Dickens' story, *A Christmas Carol,* suffered from a crippling condition. "Alas for Tiny Tim, he bore a little crutch and had his limbs supported by an iron frame." Sitting by the fire after Christmas dinner, Bob Cratchit held Tim's ". . . withered little hand in his, as if he loved the child, and wished to keep him by his side, and dreaded that he might be taken from him."

Dickens has little more to say about the boy's illness. Tim might have had any one of a number of congenital abnormalities of his limbs. In an age before corrective surgery and prosthesis, he was likely destined to remain a cripple for life. Tiny Tim's condition, however, was more serious. The Ghost of Christmas Present observed to Scrooge: "I see a vacant seat in the poor chimney corner, and a crutch without an owner carefully preserved. If these shadows remain unaltered by the Future, the child will die." Even the most casual Dickens reader must occasionally wonder about the nature of this crippling, eventually fatal disease.

In 1843, when Dickens wrote *A Christmas Carol,* approximately one half of the English population was affected with tuberculosis. It was the single greatest cause of death and disease in the western world.[1] It was particularly common among families of the lower classes. Tuberculosis tended to pass from one generation to the next in families during the winter months when the house was closed against the cold and parents huddled with their children for warmth.[1] It is possible that Bob or Mrs Cratchit had tuberculosis, and passed it on to Tiny Tim, who developed a pulmonary infection initially. He may have experienced hematogenous spread because of malnutrition and altered immunity. (It was not easy to feed a family of eight on 15 "bob" a week.) Bone and joint complications accompany primary pulmonary tuberculosis in as many as 5% of children, according to a relatively recent review.[2] It is easy to imagine that these complications occurred more commonly 150 years ago.

Tuberculous spondylitis was first described by Percivall Pott in 1779.[3] The thoracic vertebrae are the most commonly affected, and the majority of cases in children occur between the ages of 3 and 10 years.[4] Patients experience pain and stiffness, followed by wasting, fatigue, and fever. Degeneration of the spine leads to shortened trunk height as the ribs descend into the pelvis, perhaps the reason Tim was "Tiny."[4] Paraplegia accompanies tuberculosis of the spine, with involvement of the midthoracic vertebrae in as many as 25% of patients.[4] Death occurs if the tuberculosis abscess ruptures through the dura and drains into the spinal canal.[4]

Tiny Tim did not die, because Scrooge changed his ways and became "a second father" to him. Ebenezer could have paid for Tiny Tim to be moved to a sanatorium like the "Royal Sea Bathing Infirmary for Scrofula" in Margate, England, which was started in 1791.[1] There, Tiny Tim would have enjoyed good hygienic conditions, rest, and adequate nutrition and recumbency in the fresh salt air. He would have been fitted with a custom fixative apparatus such as the Davis spinal assistant.[5] Thus, he would have recovered some of his leg function and experienced remission of his disease.

There are many possible causes for Tiny Tim's affliction. Other forms of hematogenous osteomyelitis or septic arthritis can cause a crippling fatal condition. Diseases such as these, however, cause a child to be acutely ill, and hardly energetic enough to accompany his father to church as Tim did that Christmas. A myelomeningocele could cause a crippling condition like the one that affected Tiny Tim. Death in a child with this defect could result from urosepsis—a complication of a neurogenic bladder—or from erosion of the skin above the defect, and meningitis. Leukemia with bone involvement could lead to a crippling, fatal condition. One expects the victim to appear more sick than Tim. In the case of this malignancy, one also has to assume that Tim experienced a spontaneous remission after Scrooge's reformation.[6]

Nutritional deficiences represent another group of possible causes for Tiny Tim's malady. Scurvy, a deficiency of vitamin C, might account for his symptoms. This deficiency, first described by Sir Thomas Barlow in the late 19th century, causes painful, swollen legs, pseudoparalysis, fractures of the epiphyseal plates, weakness, lethargy, and arthralgias. Children with scurvy may also have visceral and oropharyngeal bleeding. Death may occur after cerebral hemorrhage.[7] The patients described by Barlow were younger than Tim, between 6 and 15 months of age in most instances.[7] More importantly, scurvy did not occur in the very poor, since potatoes were a major source of dietary starch.[7] Potatoes were a part of the Cratchits' diet. They feasted on goose, apple sauce, and potatoes that Christmas Eve. Without a doubt, this meal was better than their average daily fare. However, only one medium-sized potato a day is required to prevent the clinical manifestations of scurvy.[8]

Tiny Tim could also have suffered from vitamin D–deficient rickets. The burning of fossil fuels during the 19th century blackened the skies over European and American cities. Air pollution filtered out the sunlight and caused epidemic rickets.[6] In the most advanced stages, rickets can cause deformity of the thoracic cage, such as pigeon breast and kyphoscoliosis, as well as bowed legs, knock-knees, and coxa vara. Even when severely affected, children with rickets are usually not crippled; and rickets alone would rarely be fatal.[9]

Tuberculosis was common in Dickens' England. Many of his contemporaries suffered from the disease. In literature, it was pictured as a tragic yet romantic, gradually wasting process that affected rich and poor alike. The prevalence of tuberculosis and its popularity as a literary theme may have influenced Dickens' portrayal of Tiny Tim's affliction.[1]

One hopes that a physician of this decade would never allow Tim's condition to progress to such an advanced state. Tuberculosis would be suspected if this sickly, anergic boy with pneumonia were referred to a medical center. The diagnosis would be made quickly by gastric lavage and Ziehl-Neelsen stain, or bronchoalveolar lavage with tuberculostearic acid assay, before the onset of secondary hematogenous spread. The incidence of tuberculosis is on the rise, especially in areas of poverty. The practitioner of today would do well to heed the words of a somber Bob Cratchit: "I am sure we shall none of us forget poor Tiny Tim, shall we?"

MAJ Charles W. Callahan, Jr, DO, MC, USAR
Section of Pulmonary Medicine
St Christopher's Hospital for Children
Philadelphia, PA 19134

The opinions expressed by the author are not to be construed as being official or as reflecting the views of the Department of the Army or the Department of Defense.

I thank Howard Panitch, MD, and Daniel Schidlow, MD, for their assistance with the manuscript.

1. Dubos J, Dubos R. *The White Plague.* Boston, Mass: Little Brown & Co Inc; 1952.
2. Lincoln EM, Sewell EM. *Tuberculosis in Children.* New York, NY: McGraw-Hill International Book Co; 1963.
3. Aegerter E, Kirkpatrick JA, eds. *Orthopedic Disease.* 4th ed. Philadelphia, Pa: WB Saunders Co; 1975.
4. Ferguson AB, ed. *Orthopedic Surgery in Infancy and Childhood.* 2nd ed. Baltimore, Md: Williams & Wilkins; 1963.
5. Roberts AS. Pott's disease. In: Keating JM, ed. *Cyclopedia of the Diseases of Children.* Philadelphia, Pa: JB Lippincott; 1890.
6. Rudolph AM, Hoffman JI, eds. *Pediatrics.* East Norwalk, Conn: Appleton & Lange; 1987.
7. Evens PR. Infantile scurvy: the centenary of Barlow's disease. *BMJ.* 1983; 287:1862-1863.
8. Shil ME, Young VR, eds. *Modern Nutrition in Health and Disease.* 7th ed. Philadelphia, Pa: Lea & Febiger; 1984.
9. Suskind RM, ed. *Textbook of Pediatric Nutrition.* New York, NY: Raven Press; 1981.

Cautionary Note on the Use of Empiric Ceftriaxone for Suspected Bacteremia

Empiric use of parenteral ceftriaxone sodium is becoming increasingly prevalent in the treatment of suspected occult bacteremia in young, highly febrile children who lack an apparent focal infection other than presumed viral upper respiratory tract infection. This strategy has begun to pervade clinical practice in the absence of any published data to prove its efficacy. The authors of two recent exercises in decision analysis conclude that empiric antimicrobial therapy is the most cost-effective and clinically beneficial treatment strategy and recommend its use.[1,2] We write to express concern and urge caution in adopting this approach lest it further complicate the difficult task of treating occult bacteremia by requiring a more extensive evaluation and generating a potentially ambiguous database.

Occult bacteremia is a relatively common problem in pediatric patients, occurring most often in children between ages 3 and 36 months with temperatures of at least 38.9°C. Numerous reports have identified an incidence of bacteremia in approximately 3% to 6% of patients from both the private and public sectors.[3-5] By far, the most common bacterial species associated with occult bacteremia is *Streptococcus pneumoniae*. Much less frequently, *Haemophilus influenzae* type b and *Neisseria meningitidis* are implicated. Young age and high fever are risk factors for bacteremia. The presence of various clinical or laboratory features, such as seizures or elevated sedimentation rate or white blood cell count, may further increase the likelihood of bacteremia. However, no single feature or combination of clinical or laboratory parameters identifies all patients with bacteremia at the time of initial presentation. Accordingly, some authorities have made the controversial recommendation to routinely obtain blood cultures from all children at risk for occult bacteremia in the hope of achieving an early diagnosis.[6]

The outcome of patients with occult bacteremia is influenced by a number of factors, including the host, the pathogen, and perhaps the empiric initiation of antimicrobial therapy. In many patients, bacteremia clears spontaneously; in others, a focal infection, such as otitis media or pneumonia, develops within the next 24 to 48 hours, thereby directing the initiation of specific therapy in an acceptably timely fashion. Some patients remain persistently bacteremic while others develop serious focal infections, including meningitis, the latter approximately 4% of the time.[7] The prime rationale for empirically treating all patients with suspected occult bacteremia is prevention, if possible, of this most serious complication—meningitis.

This leads us to ask two questions: (1) Are blood cultures essential in treating patients with suspected occult bacteremia? (2) Will empiric therapy successfully prevent the development of serious complications of bacteremia? Review of medical records of patients with occult bacteremia seen at the Yale–New Haven (Conn) Hospital showed that nine of 21 patients with serious focal complications or persistent bacteremia returned to the emergency department because of continued symptoms and signs before notification about positive blood cultures.[8] Furthermore, a study regarding the usefulness of blood cultures employing decision analysis technique implied that a "no blood culture" strategy had the highest utility.[9] Accordingly, argument can be made for the treatment of patients at risk for occult bacteremia without obtaining blood cultures at the first encounter; when feasible, careful follow-up and comprehensive reevaluation of patients who fail to improve under observation are a viable and perhaps preferable alternative.

Data addressing the success of empiric therapy in preventing serious complications of bacteremia are scant. The results of a recently published study, which prospectively evaluated oral antimicrobial therapy in the treatment of suspected bacteremia, were disappointing.[10] Only modest benefits in terms of fever reduction and clinical improvement were associated with presumptive therapy. Major infectious morbidity was not averted in the children who received antibiotic therapy.

Will ceftriaxone sodium be effective in preventing meningitis if it is used empirically in patients with presumptive bacteremia? On the basis of limited clinical data,[11,12] we presume that one or two doses of ceftriaxone will produce a serum level sufficient to sterilize the bloodstream of *S pneumoniae*, *H influenzae* type b, and *N meningitidis*, and to prevent seeding of the meninges in most patients. It is likely that empiric therapy would also sterilize a recently inoculated cerebrospinal fluid, although such a regimen may not suffice to adequately treat established meningitis. The significant potential benefit achieved by parenteral ceftriaxone in patients with occult bacteremia would be the elimination of four cases of meningitis among every 100 patients with occult bacteremia.

Realizing such a benefit would require the treatment of 2500 patients with suspected occult bacteremia. Nevertheless, a decision regarding the routine use of parenteral ceftriaxone in patients at risk for occult bacteremia requires a balanced consideration of potential problems as well as benefits.

Aside from the obvious potential liabilities associated with treating large numbers of nonbacteremic patients with an antibiotic (eg, allergic, idiosyncratic, or other adverse reactions), other important adverse consequences are associated with the strategy of presumptive therapy. If physicians elect the routine empiric treatment of young children with suspected bacteremia (ie, all infants and children between ages 3 and 36 months with a temperature of at least 38.9°C), they would be appropriately expected to obtain blood and urine cultures (the latter by suprapubic aspiration or catheterization) from all such patients before initiating treatment. A lumbar puncture would also be required for any patient whose clinical status mandated excluding a diagnosis of unsuspected early meningitis before antibiotics were given. If a blood culture is reported to be positive, it will be necessary to obtain another blood culture and, frequently, to repeat lumbar puncture to assess whether bacteremia had resolved and whether an occult, partially treated meningitis had developed. Although the routine use of blood cultures is a controversial issue, using ceftriaxone sodium as empiric therapy mandates the necessity of obtaining blood cultures (generating laboratory costs and patient discomfort) and subjects many bacteremic infants and children treated in this way to at least one, or in some cases two, lumbar punctures.

Some patients with suspected occult bacteremia will be initially reported as having blood cultures containing "gram-positive cocci." Approximately 40% to 50% of these isolates will prove to be contaminants.[3,13] Many of these gram-positive cocci will ultimately be identified as coagulase-negative staphylococci and, as such, will be eventually dismissed as contaminants. However, patients will frequently be recalled to the hospital, have blood cultures repeated, and be hospitalized for parenteral therapy of presumed serious infection until the identity and significance of the blood culture isolates are clarified. Occasionally, *Staphylococcus aureus* will be isolated. Unfortunately, in such instances, it may not be possible to clarify the significance of such an isolate simply by repeating the blood culture. If the second blood culture is sterile, it may be unclear whether the original isolate represents a contaminant or a partially treated pathogen. In some such circumstances, bone scans or echocardiograms will be performed to locate presumed staphylococcal infection. Furthermore, when blood cultures prove to be positive and patients are subsequently recalled to the hospital, it puts us in the somewhat paradoxical situation of admitting the "well" child to the hospital after having sent the "sick" child home 24 hours earlier. If presumptive therapy had not been used in such children, decisions concerning treatment would have been based on clinical appearance, without concerns about the confounding impact of partial therapy.

Another dilemma will unfold when a patient whose blood culture is negative returns 24 hours after having received parenteral ceftriaxone looking sicker or unimproved. According to a recent study, there may be a 50% risk of failing to detect bacteremia when only a single blood culture is obtained.[14] Unfortunately, the value of a repeated blood culture done at this time will have been obviated by the prior partial treatment. Equally problematic is the situation in which the initial urine culture is reported to contain two or three bacterial species or a colony count of ambiguous significance. Although contamination of urine specimens obtained by suprapubic aspiration or catheterization is infrequent, "clean-catch" or "bagged" specimens are more likely to have been obtained for culture when clinical suspicion of urinary tract infection is relatively low. Again, a repeated urine culture will be of little value in clarifying the situation because the ceftriaxone will surely have eradicated a true pathogen or obscured a contaminant. The significance of the bacteriuria cannot be established and the need for radiographic evaluation of the urinary tract will be difficult to determine. Again, had presumptive therapy been withheld, the database could easily have been clarified.

Philosophically, the most troublesome aspect of the routine use of empiric ceftriaxone for suspected occult bacteremia is that it may lead to a less thoughtful approach to treatment of the patient. Until now, we have individually considered the disposition of patients at risk for occult bacteremia. When particularly worried (when sepsis seemed a more likely possibility), we have hospitalized such patients for observation or presumptive treatment until laboratory results became available. In those few patients, the "complete" sepsis evaluation was properly undertaken (including suprapubic bladder aspiration or urethral catheterization) and easily justified. In the remaining febrile children, we used carefully scheduled follow-up, often without blood culture, to ensure further clinical and laboratory evaluation as individually warranted. The current availability of a powerful, broad-spectrum, long-acting antimicrobial agent should not tempt us to adopt strategies based on the routine use of an unproved therapy, which may further complicate the treatment of febrile children, who, for the most part, are not bacteremic.

Ellen R. Wald, MD
Barry Dashefsky, MD
Children's Hospital of Pittsburgh
Department of Pediatrics
One Children's Place
3705 Fifth Ave
at DeSoto Street
Pittsburgh, PA 15213-2583

References

1. Downs SM, McNutt RA, Margolis PA. Management of infants at risk for occult bacteremia: a decision analysis. *J Pediatr.* 1991;118:11-21.
2. Lieu TA, Schwartz JS, Jaffe DM, Fleisher GR. Strategies for diagnosis and treatment of children at risk for occult bacteremia: clinical effectiveness and cost-effectiveness. *J Pediatr.* 1991;118:21-29.
3. Teele DW, Pelton SI, Grant MJA, et

al. Bacteremia in febrile children under 2 years of age: results of cultures of blood of 600 consecutive febrile children seen in a 'walk-in' clinic. *J Pediatr.* 1975;87:227-230.

4. McGowan JE, Bratton L, Klein JO, Finland M. Bactermia in febrile children seen in a 'walk-in' clinic. *N Engl J Med.* 1973;288:1309-1312.

5. Baron MA, Fink HD. Bacteremia in private pediatric practice. *Pediatrics.* 1980;66:171-175.

6. Teele DW, Marshall R, Klein JO. Unsuspected bacteremia in young children. *Pediatr Clin North Am.* 1979; 26:773-784.

7. Bratton L, Teele DW, Klein JO. Outcome of unsuspected pneumococcemia in children not initially admitted to the hospital. *J Pediatr.* 1977;90:703-706.

8. Alario AJ, Nelson EW, Shapiro ED. Blood cultures in the management of febrile outpatients later found to have bacteremia. *J Pediatr.* 1989;115:195-199.

9. Kramer MS, Lane DA, Mills EL. Should blood cultures be obtained in the evaluation of young febrile children without evident focus of bacterial infection? A decision analysis of diagnostic management strategies. *Pediatrics.* 1989;84:18-27.

10. Jaffe DM, Tanz RR, Davis AT, et al. Antibiotic administration to treat possible occult bacteremia in febrile children. *N Engl J Med.* 1987;317:1175-1180.

11. McCarthy CA, Powell KR, Jaskiewicz JA, et al. Outpatient management of selected infants younger than two months of age evaluated for possible sepsis. *Pediatr Infect Dis J.* 1990;9:385-389.

12. Baskin MN, Fleisher GR, O'Rourke EJ. Outpatient management of febrile infants 28 to 90 days of age with intramuscular ceftriaxone. *AJDC.* 1988;142:391.

13. Isaacman DJ, Karasic RB. Lack of effect of changing needles on contamination of blood cultures. *Pediatr Infect Dis J.* 1990;9:274-278.

14. Isaacman DJ, Karasic RB. Utility of collecting blood cultures through newly inserted intravenous catheters. *Pediatr Infect Dis J.* 1990;9:815-818.

Adolescents With Chronic Illness

The article by Newacheck et al in this issue of *AJDC* improves our understanding of the epidemiology and prevalence of chronic illness in adolescence and defines some of the physical limitations and behavioral consequences of chronic illness. A striking finding is the apparently high rate of chronic illness in this age group, approaching one in three adolescents aged 10 to 17 years. Data available in this study do not allow determination of the physiological severity of these chronic conditions; however, other studies[1,2] suggest that about 10% to 20% of children with chronic illness have severe conditions of the type likely to have a daily impact on the child's life.

Thus, the data presented in the article by Newacheck et al suggest that 3% to 6% of adolescents have severe long-term illnesses, consistent with other work indicating similar rates of health disability among adolescents.[3] Of great import is the finding that these rates are similar to those for younger children (using the same data set) and that most of these chronic health conditions are compatible with long life. Thus, the very large majority of adolescents with chronic illnesses will survive to adulthood, and one can predict similar or even higher rates of chronic illness among young adults. The secondary physical and behavioral problems faced by adolescents with chronic illness, as described by Newacheck et al, may have as great an impact on their ability to function as adults as does their primary health condition.

As the authors point out, adolescence is a time of great stress made more difficult by the presence of a chronic health condition. Although adolescents face many complex tasks, two merit special attention for adolescents with chronic illnesses: the development of autonomy and formation of personal identity. Chronic illnesses often create special dependency needs, such as physical therapy for the person with arthritis or cystic fibrosis and help with pulmonary toilet for a person dependent on a respirator or with a tracheostomy. Developing satisfactory autonomy in the context of maintaining significant physical dependency can be very difficult for many adolescents. Further, the tendency of parents and clinicians alike to label children by their disease (eg, "diabetics," "cystics," or "leukemics") often allows the disease, its consequences, and treatments to obscure the underlying child or adolescent. For some, the disease becomes their identity.

Exclusive attention to the disease limits attention to other areas important to adolescence (eg, growth and physical development, sexuality, athletics, and interpersonal relationships). Limiting expectations to disease-related issues limits opportunities for adolescents to develop more appropriate and well-rounded identities as young people with a future, despite having a severe chronic illness. In general, adolescents with chronic illnesses face the *same* developmental tasks as adolescents without illness, and it is important not to label these adolescents as special or different in these tasks. Particular barriers (such as physical barriers for adolescents with mobility impairments or disincentives for employers to shoulder potentially higher health insurance premiums) may hinder the employment progress of young adults with chronic illnesses, but the basic task of increasing independence remains the same.

The prevalence data presented by Newacheck et al must be interpreted carefully. The authors knowingly chose a very broad definition of a chronic health condition: one that was present in the previous 12 months and first noted at least 3 months prior to the interview, except for certain conditions that are considered chronic, regardless of their duration prior to the time of interview (such as asthma, heart disease, or leukemia). Thus, an adolescent with a swimmer's ear in the year before the interview and a middle ear infection at some time during early childhood might be considered to have a chronic illness.

Furthermore, parental reports may be inaccurate, especially in regard to such conditions as respiratory allergies, asthma, or heart diseases. For this last category, the estimates seem high, and one wonders whether parental interpretations of heart murmurs affected the response rates. Other condition-specific rates are surprising. Most studies of recurrent middle ear disease, for example, indicate a significantly higher prevalence among boys than girls, and the rates for anemia are higher than recent estimates from the Centers for Disease Control.

As the authors clearly explain, the rates reported here likely represent the upper limits of prevalence. It would have been interesting had the authors compared rates using broader and narrower definitions of chronic illness, yet the use of this data set requires certain difficult decisions, and Newacheck and colleagues chose wisely. Even if the high rates reported here are twice those of reality, their estimates still document a sizeable burden of chronic illness in this age group and the need for efforts to diminish the long-term consequences of chronic illness.

This study suggests two important further lines of research. First, what are the implications of physical limitations and behavioral consequences for the transition of adolescents with chronic illnesses to adulthood?[4] How does this population compare with its counterparts without illness with respect to educational attainment, entering the job market, development of permanent relationships and families, and dependence on public institutions? Do adolescents with physical limitations or behavior problems face greater burdens or barriers than those without such limitations? Does identification and treatment of these behavioral problems improve these outcomes?

The second important line of research is to explore the mechanisms by which chronic illness appears to place adolescents at higher risk of behavior problems. The current study does not report differences by condition groups with respect to the increased risk of behavior problems, but other studies[5] suggest that the increased behavioral risks relate not to the specific health condition but rather to the fact of having a chronic illness, regardless of the specific diagnosis. Severity of illness also does not predict well the risk of behavior problems.[6] In the current study, an increasing number of conditions was associated with a greater risk of behavior problems, suggesting that adolescents with more severe conditions may face higher risks. Yet, severity is very difficult to measure, especially across illnesses.[7]

Further, although the increased risk of behavior problems is clearly significant, both statistically and clinically, data presented by Newacheck and colleagues support the notion that most adolescents with chronic illnesses are psychologically healthy. What factors aid those adolescents to do well despite the burdens and tasks created by their chronic illness? How do self-esteem, parental factors, family structure, education, and social and health programs help to encourage this resilience? A clearer understanding of the roles of these many factors in influencing resilience and risk will help direct pediatric clinical attention to the most promising areas of prevention and intervention in the future.

Given the data presented by Newacheck et al, the need to assess physical and behavioral functioning in the context of developmentally appropriate pediatric care for adolescents with chronic illnesses seems increasingly clear. Helping to insure that chronic illness interferes as little as possible with the normal tasks and transitions of adolescence is a particularly important pediatric responsibility.

JAMES M. PERRIN, MD
Harvard Medical School
Children's Service
Massachusetts General Hospital
Fruit St
Boston, MA 02114

References

1. Hobbs N, Perrin JM, Ireys HT. *Chronically Ill Children and Their Families.* San Francisco, Calif: Jossey-Bass; 1985:38-43.
2. Gortmaker S, Sappenfield W. Chronic childhood disorders: prevalence and impact. *Pediatr Clin North Am.* 1984;31:3-18.
3. Newacheck PW. Adolescents with special health needs: prevalence, severity, and access to health services. *Pediatrics.* 1989;84:872-881.
4. Pless IB, Wadsworth MEJ. Long-term effects of chronic illness on young adults. In: Stein REK, ed. *Caring for Children with Chronic Illness.* New York, NY: Springer Publishing Co Inc; 1989:147-158.
5. Stein REK, Jessop DJ. What diagnosis does not tell: the case for a noncategorical approach to chronic illness in children. *Soc Sci Med.* 1989;29:769-778.
6. Perrin JM, Maclean WE, Perrin EC. Parents' perception of health status and psychological adjustment of children with asthma. *Pediatrics.* 1989;83:26-30.
7. Stein REK, Perrin EC, Pless IB, et al. Severity of illness: concepts and measurements. *Lancet.* 1987;2:1506-1509.

The Evolution of Surgical Treatment for Congenital Cardiac Disease

The goals of reparative surgical therapy for any disease are to restore function and life expectancy to normal. The development of cardiopulmonary bypass and the implementation of techniques of reparative surgery for patients with congenital cardiovascular malformations in the 1950s and 1960s introduced the reality of reparative surgery in patients with otherwise fatal cardiovascular disease. Attention was initially focused on ensuring survival through the surgical procedure and in the early postoperative period. As the number of patients with "repaired" congenital cardiovascular disease increased, long-term follow-up of these patients became possible. The report by Morris and Menashe[1] in the *Journal of the*

American Medical Association analyzes long-term survival and the cause of late death after repair of eight common congenital cardiovascular malformations. This cohort of patients included all children from the state of Oregon who underwent reparative surgery for one of these congenital cardiac defects before age 18 years. The authors conclude that surgical repair of many congenital cardiovascular malformations is associated with lingering cardiac mortality and morbidity, particularly in patients with aortic stenosis, coarctation of the aorta, and transposition of the great arteries.

This report is notable for chronicling the evolution of the surgical treatment for congenital cardiac disease since the late 1950s. To that end, the authors note that the age at surgery and hospital mortality generally has diminished substantially during the last 30 years of cardiac surgery in Oregon. The causes of late mortality were described by these authors as primarily due to disturbances of cardiac rhythm, progressive ventricular dysfunction, and fixed pulmonary vascular obstructive disease resulting in pulmonary hypertension. As a report of long-term survival after reparative surgery for several common congenital cardiovascular malformations, this article is excellent and deserves further study.

This report leaves several unanswered questions that are central to the understanding of optimal treatment of patients with congenital heart disease. First, it could be expected that a group of patients with unusual or particularly severe malformations was excluded from surgical therapy or underwent only palliative surgery. To fully define the altered natural history of a congenital cardiovascular malformation, all patients with this diagnosis should be included in any evaluation, irrespective of surgical intervention. Second, one of the major strengths of this article is that the significant majority of patients were operated on at one institution, primarily under the leadership of one surgeon. This also proves to be a drawback in the interpretation of the information presented, since any single surgical group may have a greater or lesser degree of expertise in the surgical repair of certain malformations. Finally, the statistical analysis of the various groups of patients undergoing surgical therapy, as well as their late follow-up, may be made more robust with more sophisticated statistical analytic techniques (eg, hazard functions for death).

Many factors have contributed to improved survival after surgical repair of congenital cardiac disease. Perhaps foremost among them is our increased understanding of fetal and neonatal physiologic characteristics. This has led to an increased understanding of the natural history of many cardiovascular malformations, and has stimulated the development of medications specifically designed to alter natural postnatal physiologic changes (ie, prostaglandins to maintain patency of the ductus arteriosus). Our more profound understanding of neonatal physiologic features has permitted the development of techniques of intraoperative (ie, anesthetic) and postoperative treatment specifically designed for patients with congenital cardiac disease. Our complete understanding of anatomy has led to innovative surgical techniques and instrumentation that permit reparative surgery even in the very young. In many centers, reparative surgery is currently being offered early in life in patients with even the most complex congenital cardiovascular malformations.

There are numerous examples of the changes in surgical practice these advances have permitted. In spite of a calculated 20-year survival of 80% for an atrial inversion operation in certain hands, anatomical repair of transposition of the great arteries (arterial switch procedure) has become increasingly popular due to the well-documented incidence of atrial arrhythmias as well as progressive right ventricular dysfunction with atrial inversion procedures.[2] Furthermore, fewer palliative procedures are being performed on patients with tetralogy of Fallot, and earlier reparative surgery is being offered in most centers. This may have a favorable impact on long-term survival because of preservation of ventricular function.[3] In patients with coarctation of the aorta, the single most important determinant of survival and freedom from persistent hypertension after repair is the age at operation. With increasing experience in relatively newer surgical techniques (eg, extended end-to-end anastomosis), it is quite possible that the incidence of restenosis and persistent hypertension after repair may be minimized in the long term. Of particular note in this subgroup of patients is the fact that the most common cause of death in patients undergoing repair of coarctation is progressive coronary artery disease.

An important issue raised by the authors of the current report[1] is the somewhat disquieting incidence of pulmonary hypertension, congestive heart failure, and ventricular arrhythmias leading to late death. A significant fraction of these patients may have had residual anatomic lesions, best treated with reoperation, or may have undergone surgical repair after irreversible physiologic changes occurred. Therefore, the findings of this historical review regarding postoperative morbidity and mortality may not be applicable and appropriate for patients undergoing corrective surgery today. Fundamental to the improved treatment of patients with congenital cardiovascular disease are the precepts of early detection, early reparative surgery, thoughtful and appropriate postoperative treatment, and meticulous long-term follow-up. It is only with a combination of all of these factors that long-term patient function and survival can be maximized.

JOHN D. PIGOTT, MD
Department of Surgery
Tulane University School of Medicine
New Orleans, LA 70112

References

1. Morris CD, Menashe VD. 25-year mortality after surgical repair of congenital heart defect in childhood: a population-based cohort study. *JAMA*. In press..

2. Williams WG, Trusler GA, Kirklin JW, et al. Early and late results of a protocol for simple transposition leading to an atrial switch (Mustard) repair. *J Thorac Cardiovasc Surg*. 1988;95:717-726.

3. Borow KM, Keane JF, Castaneda AR, Freed MD. Systemic ventricular function in patients with tetralogy of Fallot, ventricular septal defect and transposition of the great arteries repaired during infancy. *Circulation*. 1981;64:878-885.

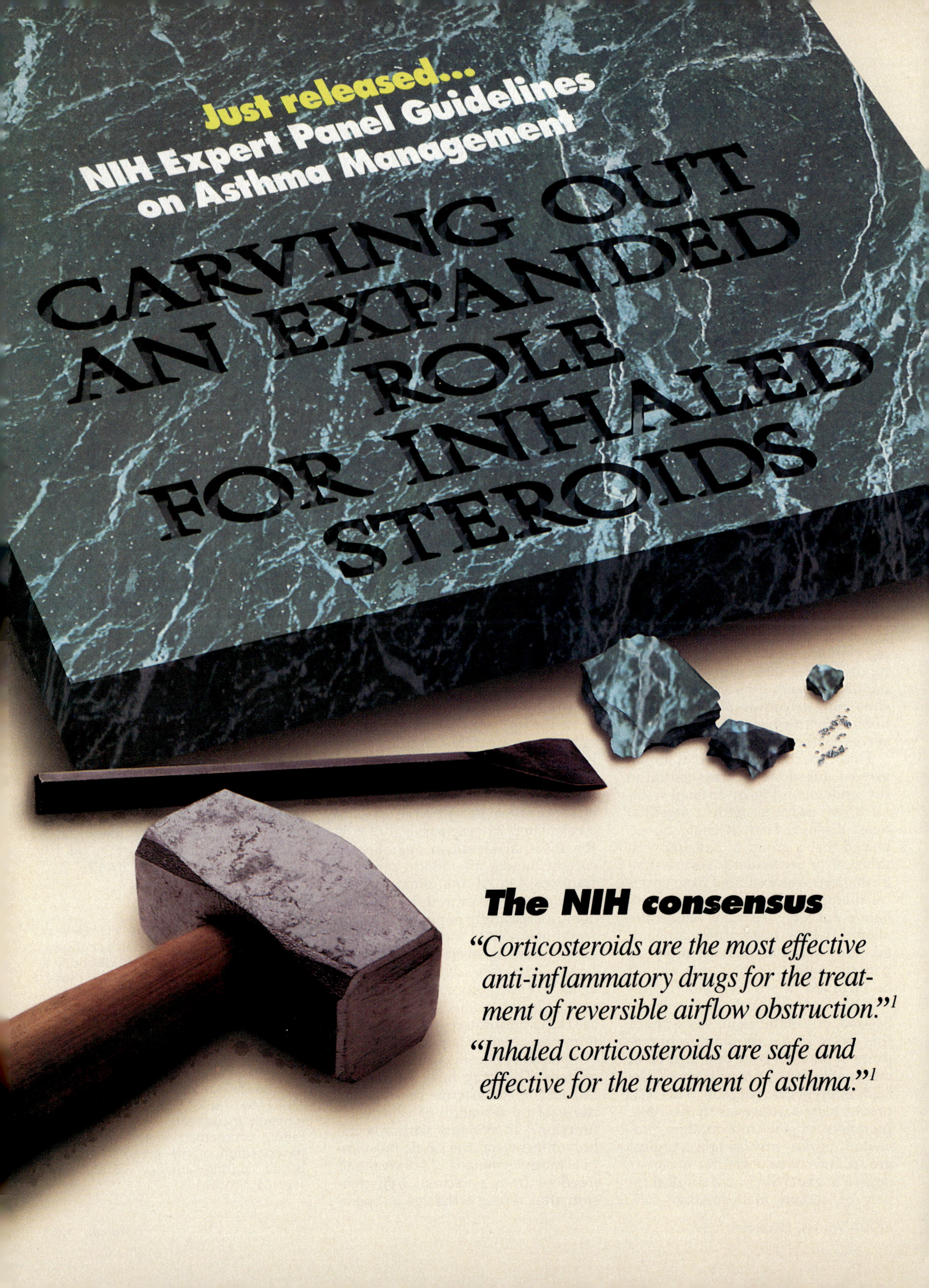
Just released...
NIH Expert Panel Guidelines
on Asthma Management
CARVING OUT
AN EXPANDED
ROLE
FOR INHALED
STEROIDS
The NIH consensus
"Corticosteroids are the most effective anti-inflammatory drugs for the treatment of reversible airflow obstruction."[1]
"Inhaled corticosteroids are safe and effective for the treatment of asthma."[1]

Prevalence and Impact of Chronic Illness Among Adolescents

Paul W. Newacheck, DrPH; Margaret A. McManus, MHS; Harriette B. Fox, MSS

A sample of 7465 persons aged 10 to 17 years from the 1988 National Health Interview Survey on Child Health was used to assess the prevalence and impact of chronic conditions in adolescents. We defined a condition as chronic if it was first noted more than 3 months before the interview or a condition that ordinarily would be of lengthy duration, such as arthritis or heart disease. An estimated 31.5% of US adolescents were reported to have one or more chronic conditions. The most commonly reported chronic conditions included respiratory allergies, asthma, and frequent or severe headaches. Chronic conditions had widely varying impact on adolescent activity levels. On average, adolescents with chronic conditions experienced 3.4 bed days and 4.4 school absence days related to their chronic conditions in the year before the interview. Adolescents with chronic conditions were also reported to experience 35% more behavioral problems than their counterparts without chronic conditions. Adolescents with multiple chronic conditions had substantially more bed days, school absence days, and behavioral problems than adolescents with a single chronic condition. Implications of these findings are discussed.

(*AJDC.* 1991;145:1367-1373)

Adolescence is a period of major transition in physical, psychologic, and social development. Normal adolescent development can be extremely variable in terms of height, weight, sexual maturation, identity formation (eg, increasing independence from family), intellectual ability, and psychologic development. Health status also varies among adolescents, but most appear quite healthy when traditional health status measures are used. For example, most adolescents are reported to be in excellent or very good health; they suffer from fewer acute illnesses than their younger counterparts, and their mortality rates are low compared with those of adults. However, a significant portion of this population suffers from developmental and transitional stresses, adverse consequences of risk-taking behaviors, and other morbidities, including chronic illness.[1-5]

Chronic physical and mental illnesses are an important contributor to adolescent morbidity. National survey data indicate that approximately 6% of US adolescents suffer from chronic illnesses that result in some limitation of activity or disability.[6] There is also evidence to suggest that the burden of chronic illness has been growing for adolescents. Specifically, advances in diagnosis and treatment have dramatically changed mortality rates for both children and adolescents with chronic conditions, with the result being that many adolescents with life-threatening chronic conditions now survive into adulthood.

For example, in 1940, the median length of survival for children with cystic fibrosis was 2 years; in 1970, it rose to 15 years, and in 1990 the mean life expectancy was 28 years (S.C. Fitzsimmons, PhD, unpublished data, 1991, Cystic Fibrosis Patient Registry, Cystic Fibrosis Foundation, Bethesda, Md). While not as dramatic, sizable improvements in longevity have also been demonstrated for certain forms of leukemia and heart conditions.[7] There is also evidence, although it is somewhat controversial, of an increase in the prevalence of severe, but generally not life-threatening conditions, such as asthma, orthopedic impairments, and visual and hearing problems among children and adolescents.[8]

For those with no significant health problems, the biologic, psychologic and social transitions that accompany adolescence are stressful, but for the less fortunate adolescent with a chronic illness this period of transition can impose added burdens, ranging from excessive dependence on families to low self-esteem. Previous studies have demonstrated a clear association between presence of chronic physical conditions and behavioral problems among adolescents.[9] Indeed, the increasing burden of chronic physical illnesses referenced above may be both a cause and a consequence of psychologic and behavioral problems among adolescents.

Despite renewed concern over the plight of chronically ill adolescents, relatively little is known about the prevalence of chronic conditions or their impact. Previous studies have combined children and adolescents, focused on subgroups of the adolescent population (eg, younger adolescents or disabled adolescents), or relied on clinic populations or localized samples that may not be gener-

Accepted for publication May 20, 1991.

From the Institute for Health Policy Studies, School of Medicine, University of California at San Francisco (Dr Newacheck); McManus Health Policy Inc, Washington, DC (Ms McManus); and Fox Health Policy Consultants, Washington, DC (Ms Fox).

Reprint requests to the Institute for Health Policy Studies, School of Medicine, University of California at San Francisco, San Francisco, CA 94143-0936 (Dr Newacheck).

alizable. No recent studies provide a profile of adolescent chronic conditions.

Release of the 1988 National Health Interview Survey (NHIS) on Child Health permits a new and current assessment of the prevalence and impact of chronic conditions among adolescents. We used this nationally representative data set to provide estimates of the prevalence of a variety of chronic conditions among adolescents aged 10 to 17 years; describe the impact of chronic conditions, especially multiple chronic conditions, on adolescent activity levels; and investigate the relationship between chronic conditions and behavioral problems among adolescents.

SUBJECTS AND METHODS

The NHIS is a continuing nationwide household survey conducted by the US Bureau of the Census for the National Center for Health Statistics.[10] The sample is designed to be representative of the civilian noninstitutional population. Each year interviews are conducted in approximately 45 000 households, including about 135 000 persons. This makes the NHIS the largest general- purpose health survey conducted in the United States.

In 1988, a special supplemental questionnaire on child and adolescent health was included in the survey. This supplemental questionnaire is similar to one that was fielded for the first time in 1981. The 1988 questionnaire, like its predecessor, covered a range of topics relevant to child health, including child care, pregnancy and birth, sleep habits, behavioral problems, developmental problems, other health problems, and use of health services. This questionnaire was administered for one randomly selected child or adolescent in each household. Interviews were completed for 91% of all eligible children and adolescents, resulting in a sample of 17 110 persons ranging in age from newborn to 17 years.[11] We used the entire sample of 7465 adolescents aged 10 to 17 years for this analysis.

Of particular importance for our purposes was the inclusion of a detailed checklist of childhood health problems in the supplement. Respondents were read this extensive list of conditions and asked whether the sample adolescent had any of these conditions during the previous 12 months. In this manner, prevalence estimates could be derived for more than 50 distinct adolescent health conditions, including such diverse conditions as urinary tract infections, asthma, and cerebral palsy, but excluding minor acute illnesses, such as colds, influenza, and minor injuries. The conditions included in the checklist were primarily those of a physical nature. Mental health conditions were largely excluded from the checklist due to past underreporting of such conditions in household interviews.

The large sample combined with this lengthy checklist provided an opportunity to examine adolescent health problems in a more comprehensive fashion than was possible from past national surveys. In particular, data on the impact of checklist conditions were collected for the first time. These data permit analyses of the impact of chronic conditions on adolescent activity levels and analyses of hospital and ambulatory care use for different types of childhood chronic conditions.

We asked a panel of eight pediatricians to review the checklist conditions to determine whether any should be excluded from our analysis of chronic conditions. Where a majority of the pediatricians considered a checklist condition not to be chronic, it was eliminated. Eight conditions were eliminated in this fashion, including pneumonia, repeated tonsillitis, mononucleosis, meningitis, urinary tract infection, seizures with fever, enuresis, and conditions requiring surgery but not otherwise specified. We then classified the remaining conditions according to chronicity using conventions similar to those developed by the Division of Health Interview Statistics of the National Center for Health Statistics.[10]

Specifically, a condition was considered chronic if the respondent indicated it was first noticed more than 3 months before the interview or it was a type of condition that ordinarily has a duration of more than 3 months. Examples of conditions that are considered chronic regardless of their time of onset include diabetes, heart conditions, and arthritis. Because no severity criteria were used, this approach to defining chronic illness leads to inclusion of a large number of conditions. Still, we think the definition is useful, particularly for providing an upper-bound estimate of the size of the chronically ill child population.

To enable a manageable analysis and presentation, conditions were grouped into 19 broader categories, including five impairment groupings and 14 disease groupings. The categorization scheme is based on grouping conditions that are clinically related while taking into account sample size limitations. The disease categorization includes conditions with active disease. Impairments are chronic or permanent defects, usually static in nature, that result from disease, injury, or congenital malformation. The overall categorization scheme and condition groupings are illustrated in Table 1.

In addition to the checklist of child health conditions, NHIS respondents were also asked an extensive series of structured questions concerning adolescent behavioral problems. The 26 questions dealt with specific problem behaviors present during the year before the interview and were derived from the Achenbach Behavior Problems checklist and other child behavior scales.[12-14] Using the checklist results, we scored adolescents according to a behavioral problems index with five subscales originally developed by Zill.[15]

The subscales include from four to six items and represent some of the more common syndromes of problem behaviors among adolescents. The five subscales include the following: (1) antisocial behavior; (2) anxiety and depressed mood; (3) hyperactive behavior; (4) headstrong behavior; and (5) peer conflict and social withdrawal. Using data from the predecessor 1981 survey, the internal consistency reliability of the overall index was found to be α equals .91 for adolescents. The α coefficients for the subscales ranged from .70 to .76.[15]

Since the behavioral problem subscales contain a variable number of items, the results presented here have been converted into index or ratio scores. In addition, because different sets of questions were used for sample persons younger than 12 years and those aged 12 years and older, we restricted our analysis to the population aged 12 years and older.

In reviewing the NHIS results presented here, one should keep in mind that the results are based on household interviews, not clinical tests or medical examinations. In the case of adolescents, an adult member of the household knowledgeable about the adolescent's health, usually the mother, served as the respondent. Thus, the NHIS results represent the mother's or other adult's *perception* of the adolescent's health. Although great effort was made to ensure accurate reporting, the information obtained might be inaccurate because the respondent might have been unaware of relevant information, have forgotten it, or have been unwilling to report certain types of information. For example, parents might be unwilling to report certain potentially "embarrassing" or stigmatic conditions, such as behavioral problems.

The results of our analysis are presented in simple tabular form. The observations were weighted according to the inverse of their sampling probabilities so that the estimates presented reflect national population totals. Standard errors were calculated using software that accounts for the complex sample design of the NHIS.[16,17] Relative SEs were obtained by dividing the SE of the estimate by the estimate itself. Readers should interpret estimates with large SEs with caution. This especially applies to estimates for conditions of comparatively low prevalence, such as cerebral palsy, juvenile diabetes, and sickle cell disease.

RESULTS

Prevalence

Of an estimated 27.2 million adolescents aged 10 to 17 years in the United States, 31.5%, or 8.6 million, had one or more chronic conditions in 1988, according to the NHIS (Table 2). The majority of adolescents with chronic condi-

Table 1.—Chronic Conditions

Condition Category	Checklist Conditions
Impairments	
Musculoskeletal	Missing limbs, fingers, or toes*; permanent impairment*; stiffness or deformity of back or side, limbs, fingers, or toes*
Deafness and hearing loss	Deafness or trouble hearing in one ear*; deafness or trouble hearing in both ears*
Blindness and visual impairment	Blindness in one eye*; blindness in both eyes*; crossed eyes*; any other trouble seeing*
Speech defects	Stammering or stuttering; any other speech defect
Cerebral palsy	Cerebral palsy*
Disease	
Diabetes	Diabetes*
Sickle cell disease	Sickle cell anemia*
Anemia	Anemia
Asthma	Asthma*
Eczema and skin allergies	Eczema or any other skin allergy*
Epilepsy and seizures	Epilepsy or convulsions without fever*
Arthritis	Arthritis or other joint problem*
Heart disease	Congenital heart disease*; any other heart disease or condition*
Frequent ear infections	Frequent or repeated ear infections
Frequent diarrhea/bowel trouble	Frequent or repeated diarrhea or colitis; any other persistent bowel trouble
Digestive allergies	Any food or digestive allergy
Frequent or severe headaches	Frequent or severe headaches, including migraines
Other	Mononucleosis; hepatitis; meningitis; rheumatic fever*; seizures associated with fever; other bone, cartilage, muscle, or tendon problem; conditions requiring surgery; conditions lasting more than 3 months

*Condition deemed chronic regardless of date of onset; other conditions deemed chronic if first noted more than 3 months before the interview.

Table 2.—Prevalence of Chronic Conditions Among US Adolescents

No. of Chronic Conditions	n	No. per 100 Adolescents	SE	Population Estimate
0	5098	68.5	0.7	18 621 000
1	1585	21.3	0.5	5 776 000
2	539	7.0	0.4	1 910 000
≥3	243	3.2	0.3	875 000

Table 3.—Prevalence of Chronic Conditions Among US Adolescents According to Sociodemographic Characteristics

Characteristic	Prevalence of Chronic Conditions per 100 Adolescents	SE	Population Estimate
Age, y			
All ages	31.5	0.7	8 561 000
10 to 13	31.0	0.9	4 138 000
14 to 17	31.9	0.9	4 423 000
Sex			
M	32.1	1.0	4 453 000
F	30.9	0.9	4 108 000
Race and ethnicity			
White	34.8	0.8	6 576 000
Black	23.7	1.5	981 000
Hispanic	24.0	2.4	723 000
Other	25.5	2.9	282 000
Poverty status			
At or below poverty level	30.1	1.9	1 184 000
Above poverty level	32.4	0.8	7 026 000
Region			
Northeast	31.5	1.2	1 548 000
Midwest	33.0	1.2	2 353 000
South	28.0	1.4	2 673 000
West	35.5	1.5	1 988 000
Residence			
Central city	28.8	1.2	2 247 000
Suburbs	32.4	1.0	4 171 000
Nonmetropolitan	32.8	1.3	2 143 000

tions had only one such condition, but a significant minority were afflicted with multiple chronic conditions. Specifically, 7% of all adolescents were reported to have two chronic conditions and 3% had three or more conditions. Put another way, nearly one third of adolescents with chronic conditions had multiple conditions.

Prevalence of chronic conditions was surprisingly similar among adolescents with widely different sociodemographic characteristics (Table 3). The overall prevalence of chronic conditions was almost identical between younger adolescents, aged 10 to 13 years, and older adolescents, aged 14 to 17 years, as well as between boys and girls. Table 3 reveals that there was also little difference in the overall prevalence of chronic conditions by poverty status. Some modest differences are apparent by region and residence. Specifically, chronic conditions were more prevalent in the West than in the South ($P<.01$) and among adolescents living in suburban and rural areas

Table 4.—Age and Sex Differences in Prevalence of Chronic Conditions

Condition	All Adolescents	Cases per 1000 US Adolescents: Age, y: 10 to 13	14 to 17	Sex: M	F
All children with conditions	315.0	310.4	319.3	320.5	309.1
Impairment					
Musculoskeletal impairments	20.9	13.6	28.0	20.2	21.7
Deafness and hearing loss	17.0	18.9	15.2	20.6	13.3
Blindness and visual impairment	16.0	17.2	14.8	12.5	19.6
Speech defects	18.9	23.6	14.5	26.6	10.9
Cerebral palsy	1.2*	0.5*	1.8*	0.9*	1.4*
Disease					
Diabetes	1.5*	0.8*	2.2*	2.4*	0.6*
Sickle cell disease	0.9*	0.6*	1.2*	0.9*	1.0*
Anemia	5.8	4.6	6.9	3.0	8.6
Asthma	46.8	48.7	44.9	51.2	42.1
Respiratory allergies	130.3	127.6	132.8	139.9	120.2
Eczema and skin allergies	35.2	32.9	37.5	31.6	39.1
Epilepsy and seizures	3.3	2.7*	3.8*	2.1*	4.5*
Arthritis	8.7	5.3	11.9	8.1	9.3
Heart disease	17.4	14.8	19.8	19.0	15.7
Frequent or repeated ear infections	33.6	41.8	25.8	32.6	34.7
Frequent diarrhea/bowel trouble	9.6	8.6	10.6	10.1	9.0
Digestive allergies	21.1	26.7	15.8	22.2	20.0
Frequent or severe headaches	45.8	40.3	51.2	41.1	50.8
Other	30.0	21.2	38.5	27.3	32.8

*Relative SE exceeds 30% of estimate value.

compared with central city areas ($P<.05$). Larger differences are apparent by race and ethnicity. Specifically, chronic conditions were reported much more frequently for whites than for blacks ($P<.01$), Hispanics ($P<.01$), and other minority adolescents ($P<.01$).

Prevalence estimates for 19 categories of chronic conditions are shown in Table 4. Respiratory allergies (eg, hay fever) ranked as the leading chronic condition, affecting 13% of all adolescents. Asthma ranked second, affecting 5% of all adolescents. The third and fourth ranking conditions, headaches and skin conditions, were substantially less prevalent, each affecting fewer than 5% of US adolescents in 1988. The fifth leading condition affecting adolescents was recurrent ear infections.

Although little difference was apparent in the overall prevalence of chronic conditions among younger and older adolescents, substantial differences in the prevalence of individual conditions by age can be seen in Table 4. For example, speech defects and digestive allergies were almost twice as prevalent among younger adolescents ($P<.05$), while musculoskeletal impairments and arthritis were at least twice as prevalent among older adolescents ($P<.01$). Clearly, the illness burden is substantially different for younger and older adolescents even if the overall prevalence of chronic conditions is similar for the two age groups.

Like the pattern for age, the absence of an overall prevalence difference by gender masks a number of substantial condition-specific prevalence differentials (Table 4). For example, boys were reported to be more than twice as likely as girls to have speech defects ($P<.01$). Girls were more than twice as likely as boys to be reported to have anemia ($P<.05$).

Impact on Activities

The impact of chronic conditions on adolescent activity levels is shown in Table 5. On average, adolescents with one or more chronic conditions spent 3.4 days ill in bed and missed 4.4 days from school in the year before the interview due to their chronic conditions. These restricted activity days are entirely attributable to chronic conditions and are in addition to those caused by acute illnesses. Hence, they reflect the added illness burden faced by children with chronic conditions. Nationally, a total of 29 million bed days and 38 million school absence days were attributable to adolescent chronic conditions in 1988. The largest number of bed days and school loss days were reported for adolescents afflicted with arthritis, asthma, and heart disease. However, it should be noted that the precision of bed day and school loss day estimates is limited for many of the conditions shown in Table 5.

The last column of Table 5 shows the percentage of adolescents reported to have experienced limitation of activity due to chronic conditions. Adolescents who are limited in their activities include those who are unable to attend school, those limited in the amount or kind of school activities they can engage in, and adolescents who are limited in extracurricular activities, such as sports or

Table 5.—Impact of Chronic Conditions on US Adolescents

Condition	Mean No. of Bed Days	Mean No. of School Absence Days	% of Adolescents With Limitation of Activity
All children with chronic conditions	3.4	4.4	15.7
Impairment			
Musculoskeletal impairments	1.3*	2.7*	35.5
Deafness and hearing loss†	...	...	29.5
Blindness and visual impairment†	...	...	21.5
Speech defects†	...	...	41.2
Cerebral palsy	3.7*	3.7*	100.0
Disease			
Diabetes	0.7*	0.4*	18.8*
Sickle cell disease	0.5*	0.4*	20.6*
Anemia	1.4*	1.4*	18.4*
Asthma	3.2	4.6	28.8
Respiratory allergies	0.7	1.3	12.1
Eczema and skin allergies†	...	...	12.9
Epilepsy and seizures	3.8*	3.7*	74.4
Arthritis	4.0*	3.5*	24.6
Heart disease	2.4*	1.6*	23.0
Frequent or repeated ear infections	1.5	2.3	15.7
Frequent diarrhea/bowel trouble	0.7*	1.4	32.2
Digestive allergies	0.4	1.0	21.9
Frequent or severe headaches	3.2	3.6	17.0
Other	3.5	4.0	22.8

*Relative SE exceeds 30% of estimate value.
†Information on bed days and school absences was not obtained for these conditions.

after-school work. Overall, 16% of adolescents with chronic conditions were reported to be limited in their activities. The percentage of adolescents with limitation of activity ranged from a low of 12% for adolescents with respiratory and skin allergies to a high of 100% for adolescents with cerebral palsy.

One might expect adolescents with more than one chronic condition to experience greater restriction of their activities compared with adolescents with only a single chronic condition. This is indeed the case, as is shown in Table 6. Adolescents with two chronic conditions had almost twice as many bed days and school absence days as adolescents with only one condition ($P<.05$). They were also more than twice as likely to be reported as being limited in their activities ($P<.01$). Adolescents with three or more chronic conditions had about twice as many days ill in bed ($P<.01$) and lost from school ($P<.05$) as adolescents with two chronic health problems. Similarly, they were much more likely than their counterparts with two conditions to be limited in their activities ($P<.05$). Hence, the detrimental impact of chronic conditions on adolescent activity levels increases substantially with the number of conditions reported.

Impact on Behavior

Adolescents with chronic conditions are more likely than their counterparts without chronic conditions to experience behavioral problems (Table 7). Based on the Behavioral Problems Index, adolescents aged 12 to 17 years with one or more chronic conditions had 35% more behavioral problems than adolescents with no chronic conditions ($P<.01$). Chronically ill adolescents scored higher than adolescents without chronic conditions on each of the five subscales shown in Table 7 ($P<.01$), especially the subscale reflecting peer conflict and social withdrawal. This later subscale included these four items: (1) trouble getting along with other children; (2) not being liked by other children; (3) being withdrawn; and (4) feeling that others are out to get him or her.

There is also a clear progressive relationship between the number of chronic conditions and the number of behavioral problems reported. Adolescents with one chronic condition were reported to have 23% more behavioral problems on average than adolescents with no chronic conditions ($P<.01$). Adolescents with two chronic conditions experienced 45% more behavioral problems than adolescents with no chronic conditions ($P<.01$), and those with three or more chronic conditions had 82% more behavioral problems than adolescents without chronic conditions ($P<.01$). Similar relationships were found for each of the subscales. Again, the most powerful association between chronic conditions and behavioral problems is apparent for the peer conflict and social withdrawal subscale. Adolescents with three or more chronic conditions scored more than twice as high on this subscale as adolescents with no chronic conditions ($P<.01$).

COMMENT

A substantial number of adolescents aged 10 to 17 years are affected by chronic conditions. According to the NHIS on Child Health, as many as 8.6 million or 31.5% of adolescents had one or more chronic conditions in 1988. This

Table 6.—Impact of Multiple Chronic Conditions on US Adolescents

No. of Chronic Conditions	Mean No. of Bed Days	Mean No. of School Absence Days	% of Adolescents With Limitation of Activity
1	2.5	3.0	9.9
2	3.9	5.8	24.4
≥3	8.0	8.9	35.1

Table 7.—Association Between Chronic Conditions and Behavioral Problems Among US Adolescents

	Behavioral Problem Index Ratios					
No. of Chronic Conditions	Total	Anxiety and Depressed Mood	Headstrong	Antisocial	Hyperactive	Peer Conflict and Social Withdrawal
0	1.00	1.00	1.00	1.00	1.00	1.00
≥1	1.35	1.40	1.29	1.21	1.31	1.64
1	1.23	1.29	1.21	1.13	1.21	1.39
2	1.45	1.51	1.36	1.20	1.46	1.86
≥3	1.82	1.79	1.59	1.73	1.67	2.57

estimate is quite similar to the 30.8% prevalence estimate derived for children younger than age 10 years using the same survey data set and definition of chronic illness.[18]

Surprisingly few differences were found in the overall prevalence of chronic conditions among adolescents by age, gender, and poverty status. In contrast, the survey results revealed significant variation in prevalence of chronic conditions by race and ethnicity. Further assessment is needed to determine if these results are attributable to reporting or interviewer biases, since they differ from previous studies of adolescents with severe chronic conditions. For example, one previous study of adolescents with activity-limiting chronic conditions showed no difference in prevalence for whites and minorities.[6]

The National Center for Health Statistics has conducted no studies of how reliably childhood chronic conditions are reported in NHIS interviews. However, previous comparisons of NHIS interview results with medical records among adults indicate that chronic conditions with some impact on a person's activities and conditions associated with recent medical encounters are generally accurately reported in household interviews, but conditions with little functional impact are frequently underreported when compared with physician records. The most recent study of NHIS interviewing methods found that between 35% and 45% of conditions were underreported, while between 8% and 12% of conditions were overreported compared with medical records. Those conditions most likely to be underreported include conditions related to the urinary and reproductive systems, mental illness, and cancer.[19,20]

The prevalence estimates presented in this article do not take severity into account. Consequently, not all of the conditions categorized as chronic are likely to be of clinical or personal significance. Indeed, most of these conditions had apparently quite mild impact on adolescent activity levels. For example, 84% of adolescents with chronic conditions had no long-term limitations in their activities as a result of their chronic conditions.

While modest overall, the impact of chronic illness, as measured by days spent in bed, school absence days, and limitation of activity, varied by specific impairment or disease. Respiratory allergies, the most common chronic conditions among adolescents, tended to have relatively minor impact on children's activities, while cerebral palsy, one of the least common conditions, tended to have quite severe impact on adolescents. Adolescents with respiratory allergies had below-average rates of bed days, school absences, and limitation of activity. They were reported to have less than 1 bed day per year and fewer than one in eight adolescents were reported to be limited in their activities. Adolescents with cerebral palsy were reported to have above-average rates of bed days, and the entire sample was reported to experience some limitation of activity.

Although not shown in the Tables, we also found tremendous variation in bed days and school absence days among adolescents with the same condition. Similar results have been found in other studies of childhood chronic conditions, leading some researchers to conclude that there may be as much variation in severity within disease categories as between disease categories.[21] These results indicate that there is a need to identify new ways of accurately measuring the impact of chronic illness besides simply identifying the presence or absence of a chronic condition or the type of chronic condition.

In addition to their impact on physical activities, chronic conditions were associated with a variety of behavioral problems, including anxiety, depression, hyperactivity, peer conflict, and social withdrawal, as well as behaviors reflecting antisocial tendencies. Although all of those types of problem behaviors were more common among adolescents with chronic conditions than adolescents without chronic conditions, the analysis revealed that behavioral problems related to peer conflict and social withdrawal were especially pronounced among adolescents with chronic illness. These findings are similar to those reported in an earlier study of the relationship between chronic physical conditions and behavioral problems using the 1981 NHIS on Child Health and underscore the importance of increased attention on the part of pediatricians and other child health professionals to the behavioral problems of chronically ill adolescents.[9]

Up until now little has been known about the impact of multiple chronic conditions on adolescents. Results from this study indicate that about 10% of US adolescents suffer from multiple chronic conditions. The impact of multiple conditions on adolescents, measured in terms of restricted activity days, limitation of activity, and behavioral problems, is substantially greater than the impact experienced by adolescents with a single chronic condition. For instance, adolescents with three or more conditions spent more than twice as many days in bed and out of school and were more than three times as likely to suffer from limitation of activity as those adolescents with only one chronic condition. In addition, adolescents with multiple chronic conditions were significantly more apt to experience behavioral problems, especially those related to peer conflict and social withdrawal.

Pediatric health care providers serving adolescents need to be especially sensitive to the greater needs of adolescents with multiple chronic conditions. The results of this analysis clearly underscore the need to focus additional attention on adolescents with multiple conditions. Further efforts by child health professionals are needed to address early intervention, to promote coordinated service provision systems that integrate health and mental health services, and to develop improved private and public benefit plans that take into account the greater intensity of health services required by adolescents with multiple conditions.

It is important, too, for other professionals serving adolescents to be familiar with the special situation of those with chronic conditions, particularly those with multiple chronic conditions. Teachers, guidance counselors, mental health professionals, and others need to understand that the normal social and developmental challenges of adolescence are especially difficult for this population. Achieving separation from parents, establishing satisfying peer group relationships, and planning for college or work are among the tasks that may require sustained and coordinated input from various professionals.

Ideally, adolescents with multiple or severe chronic conditions would be served by multidisciplinary teams able to support them through transitional periods. Achieving this goal, however, requires that greater attention be devoted to adolescents with special needs in basic and continuing education programs for professionals who serve them. It also requires that the salary and reimbursement structures for compensating these professionals be altered to provide financial incentives for collaborative and consultative activities.

This study was supported in part by grants MCH-067031-01 and MCH-067026-01 from the Maternal and Child Health Bureau. Additional support was provided by the National Institute for Disability and Rehabilitation Research through the Center For Children With Chronic Illness and Disability. Data were provided by the National Center for Health Statistics. The authors appreciate the helpful suggestions of the Research Consortium on Chronic Illness in Childhood and thank Helen Gonzales for preparing the manuscript.

References

1. Blum R. Contemporary threats to adolescent health in the United States. *JAMA*. 1987;257:3390-3395.

2. Tonkin RS. Adolescent risk-taking behavior. *J Adolesc Health Care*. 1987;8:213-220.

3. Klerman LV, Kovar MG, Brown SS. Adolescents: health status and needed services. In: *Better Health for Our Children: A National Strategy*. Washington, DC; 1981. US Dept of Health and Human Services PHS publication 79-55071.

4. Garell DC. Beyond survival of the fittest . Presented at the National Invitational Conference on Health Futures of Adolescents; April 1986; Daytona Beach, Fla.

5. US Dept of Education and Dept of Health and Human Services. Conference on youth with disability: the transition years, June 20-22, 1984; Wayzata, Minn. *J Adolesc Health Care*. 1985;6:77-184.

6. Newacheck PW. Adolescents with special health needs . *Pediatrics*. 1989;84:872-881.

7. Gortmaker SL. Demography of chronic childhood diseases. In: Hobbs N, Perrin J, eds. *Issues in the Care of Children with Chronic Illness*. San Francisco, Calif: Jossey-Bass; 1985:135-154.

8. Newacheck PW, Budetti PP, Halfon N. Trends in activity-limiting chronic conditions among children. *Am J Public Health*. 1986;76:178-184.

9. Gortmaker SL, Walker DK, Weitzman M, Sobol AM. Chronic conditions, socioeconomic risks, and behavioral problems in children and adolescents. *Pediatrics*. 1990;85:267-276.

10. Adams PF, Hardy AM. Current estimates from the National Health Interview Survey: United States, 1988. *Vital Health Stat 10*. 1989. Document No. 173.

11. Bloom B. *Health Insurance and Medical Care: Health of our Nation's Children, United States, 1988*. Advance data from *Vital and Health Statistics*; Hyattsville, Md: National Center for Health Statistics; 1990. No. 188.

12. Achenbach TS, Edelbrock CS. Behavioral problems and competencies reported by parents of normal and disturbed children aged four through sixteen. *Monogr Soc Res Child Dev. 1981: 46.*

13. Graham PJ, Rutter ML. The reliability and validity of the psychiatric assessment of the child, II: interview with the parent. *Br J Psychiatry*. 1968;114:581-592.

14. Rutter M, Tizard J, Whitmore K. *Education, Health and Behaviour*. New York, NY: Longman Inc; 1970.

15. Zill N. *Behavior Problem Scales Developed From the 1981 Child Health Supplement to the National Health Interview Survey*. Washington, DC: Child Trends Inc; November 25, 1985.

16. Shah BV. *SESUDAAN: Standard Errors Program for Computing of Standardized Rates from Sample Survey Data*. Research Triangle Park, NC: Research Triangle Institute; April 1981.

17. Shah BV. *RTIFREQS: Program to Compute Weighted Frequencies, Percentages, and Their Standard Errors*. Research Triangle Park, North Carolina: Research Triangle Institute; October 1982.

18. Newacheck PW, Taylor W. *Childhood Chronic Illness: Prevalence, Severity and Impact*. Altanta, Ga: Report for the Office of Program Planning and Evaluation, Centers for Disease Control; December 1990.

19. National Center for Health Statistics. *Interview Data on Chronic Conditions Compared With Information Derived From Medical Records*. Washington, DC: US Government Printing Office; 1967. Series 2, No. 23. PHS publication 1000.

20. Javine TB. *Reporting Chronic Conditions in the National Health Interview Survey: A Review of Findings From Evaluation Studies and Methodological Tests*. Washington, DC: US Government Printing Office; 1985. A report prepared under Department of Health and Human Services, Government Printing Office 85A046165001D.

21. Stein REK, Jessop DJ. A noncategorical approach to chronic childhood illness. *Public Health Rep*. 1982;97:355-362.

The Role of Corticosteroid Therapy in Children With Pneumococcal Meningitis

William A. Kennedy, MD; Martha Jean Hoyt, RN; George H. McCracken, Jr, MD

• The records of 97 infants and children with pneumococcal meningitis treated in Dallas, Tex, from 1984 to 1990 were reviewed to determine whether corticosteroid therapy improved disease outcome as has been demonstrated in patients with *Haemophilus* meningitis. Forty-one patients received corticosteroid therapy, 39 of whom were given dexamethasone in the conventional 4-day regimen. There were no significant differences in the demographic and clinical characteristics of steroid- and non–steroid-treated patients. In addition, there were no significant differences between treatment groups with regard to presence of seizures, subdural effusions, hydrocephalus, and positive cerebrospinal fluid cultures 24 hours after the start of treatment. When steroid therapy was given before or concurrently with antibiotic therapy, none of 30 steroid-treated vs 16 of 52 non–steroid-treated patients developed evidence of neurologic or cardiovascular instability after the first parenteral antibiotic dose was given. Among 86 survivors examined, significantly fewer steroid-treated patients had an adverse neurologic long-term outcome, including hearing impairment, compared with non–steroid-treated patients (four of 35 vs 14 of 43). This was also true for those patients with overwhelming meningeal infection. We believe that corticosteroid therapy is also beneficial in infants and children with pneumococcal meningitis.

(*AJDC.* 1991;145:1374-1378)

The incidence of pneumococcal meningitis in the United States is approximately 1.1 cases per 100 000 population. It is more common in children, with a peak incidence of 30 cases per 100 000 in infants 3 to 5 months of age.[1] In our institution, *Streptococcus pneumoniae* accounted for 10% of the 2766 cases of bacterial meningitis in infants and children treated from 1969 through 1990. *Haemophilus influenzae* was the most common meningeal pathogen. The 10% case-fatality and 20% to 30% morbidity rates in children with pneumococcal meningitis have changed very little in the past 30 years despite the availability of more potent antibiotics that have high cerebrospinal fluid (CSF) bactericidal activity.[1,2]

In experimental pneumococcal meningitis, bacterial lysis resulting from antibiotic therapy causes release into CSF of cell wall fragments that are responsible for local induction of proinflammatory cytokines, including interleukin 1 and tumor necrosis factor.[3,4] These and other inflammatory proteins promote a destructive leukocyte–cerebral capillary endothelial cell interaction, platelet-mediated thrombosis, and cytotoxic, interstitial, and vasogenic cerebral edema.[5,6] These events cause increased blood-brain barrier permeability to leukocytes and to low-molecular-weight serum proteins and can alter cerebral blood flow. In the rabbit pneumococcal meningitis model, anticytokine antibodies reduced CSF leukocytosis and brain edema,[6] whereas monoclonal antibodies to CD11/CD18 leukocyte receptors involved in endothelial adhesion markedly reduced recruitment of leukocytes into the CSF, brain edema, and mortality in treated animals compared with untreated animals.[7] As in the experimental *H influenzae* meningitis model,[8,9] dexamethasone therapy markedly reduced the meningeal leukocyte mass,[10] brain edema, CSF pressure, and lactate concentrations[11] in experimental pneumococcal meningitis.

Because of the similarities in the molecular pathophysiologic activity and modulatory effects of dexamethasone therapy in these two experimental meningitis models, it seemed reasonable to assume that dexamethasone therapy might be effective in infants and children with pneumococcal meningitis, as it has been demonstrated in Dallas and Costa Rican children with meningitis caused predominantly by *H influenzae*.[12,13] We reviewed our experience with 97 infants and children with pneumococcal meningitis, 41 of whom received corticosteroid therapy.

PATIENTS AND METHODS

The records of all patients admitted to either Parkland Memorial Hospital or Children's Medical Center, Dallas, Tex, with pneumococcal meningitis from January 1984 through September 1990 were reviewed. Of the 98 patients admitted, 27 were enrolled in one of three double-blind, placebo-controlled trials of dexamethasone therapy; 23 were enrolled in prospective evaluations of antimicrobial agents; and the remaining 47 patients either declined entry, had received antibiotic therapy for more than 1 day before admission, or were enrolled at a time when no studies were being conducted, and one patient was not included because the dexamethasone was given orally. A final total of 97

Accepted for publication August 28, 1991.

From the Department of Pediatrics, University of Texas Southwestern Medical Center, Dallas, Tex.

Reprint requests to the Department of Pediatrics, University of Texas Southwestern Medical Center, 5323 Harry Hines Blvd, F3-202A, Dallas, TX 75235-9063 (Dr McCracken).

Table 1.—Patient Characteristics on Admission to the Hospital*

Characteristic	Treatment Groups: Steroid (n=41)	No Steroid (n=56)
Mean±SD age, y (range)	16.0±17.3 (2-72)	20.8±32.8 (2-180)
Age <6 mo	14 (34)	22 (39)
Sex		
M	21	28
F	20	28
Race or ethnic group		
White	21	22
Black	10	20
Hispanic	8	13
Other	2	1
Estimated duration of meningeal symptoms before admission, h	39.7±22.9	39.5±38.8
Pretreatment with oral antibiotics	13 (32)	12 (22)
Seizures before admission	13 (32)	11 (20)
Coma on admission	6/39 (15)	7/53 (13)
Shock on admission	3/40 (8)	5/55 (9)
Sepsis syndrome on admission	12/40 (30)	22/55 (40)
Relatively penicillin-resistant organisms	2/41 (5)	0/56 (0)

*Values are mean±SD or number of patients/total number (percent). There were no statistically significant differences in characteristics between treatment groups.

Table 2.—Hospital Course and Response to Therapy for Patients in the Two Treatment Groups*

Characteristic	Treatment Groups: Steroid (n=41)	No Steroid (n=56)	*P*
Fever duration, d	2.6±2.7	3.6±3.3	.035
Incidence of 2° fever	14/27 (38)	10/50 (20)	.11
Thrombocytopenia†	9/39 (23)	9/55 (16)	.58
Anemia‡	27 (66)	32 (57)	.51
Hypocalcemia§	4 (10)	5 (9)	1.0
Hyponatremia‖	8/39 (21)	15/55 (27)	.61
Relative neutropenia¶	6 (15)	5/55 (9)	.52
Seizures	19 (46)	22/55 (40)	.68
Subdural effusions	7 (17)	9 (16)	.88
Hydrocephalus	1 (2)	2 (4)	1.00
Positive blood culture	33/35 (94)	42/46 (91)	.69
Positive cerebrospinal fluid culture at 24-48 h	2/30 (7)	0/35 (0)	.21
Deaths during treatment	4 (10)	5 (9)	1.00

*Values are mean±SD or number of patients/total number (percent).

†Thrombocytopenia was defined as platelet count less than 150×10^9/L.

‡Anemia was defined as a hemoglobin or hematocrit value less than 2 SDs from the mean for age.

§Hypocalcemia was defined as a serum total calcium level less than 2.24 mmol/L.

‖Hyponatremia was difined as a serum sodium value less than 130 mmol/L.

¶Relative neutropenia was defined as a white blood cell count less than 2 SDs from the mean for age or equivalent neutrophil count.

patients were included in the study, all of whom received therapy for a minimum of 10 days with cefotaxime, ceftriaxone, cefuroxime, ampicillin, or penicillin or more than one of these drugs. Thirty-nine patients received parenterally administered dexamethasone (0.15 mg/kg per dose every 6 hours for 4 days), one received methylprednisolone for 7 days, and one patient was given dexamethasone for 2 days.

Patients were diagnosed as having pneumococcal meningitis based on their clinical condition and results of CSF examination and a CSF culture that yielded *S pneumoniae* in 92 cases. If the patient was pretreated with parenterally administered antibiotics, either a positive blood culture or a positive CSF latex agglutination test result was required. Cerebrospinal fluid samples obtained at diagnosis and approximately 24 hours later from most patients were sent to the laboratory for routine tests and culture.

Management of patients was consistent throughout the 6-year study period. Patients underwent neurologic examinations daily while in the hospital, 6 weeks after discharge, and again at the 4- to 12-month follow-up visit or later. A brain-stem evoked response (BSER) audiologic examination was performed when therapy was discontinued and again 2 to 6 months later if results were abnormal. The BSER audiograms were interpreted by experienced pediatric audiologists. An absence of wave V response at 30 to 40 dB was considered mild, at 50 to 60 dB was considered moderate, at 70 dB was considered moderate-severe, at 80 to 100 dB was considered severe, and at greater than 100 dB was considered severe-profound hearing loss.[12,13] Only bilateral moderate or greater sensory neural hearing loss was considered evidence of substantial hearing loss.

Because BSER audiograms were not obtained in 12 patients, the physicians' findings of speech and language acquisition and grossly normal hearing in the patients at 4 years or longer after diagnosis were considered evidence that substantial permanent hearing loss had not occurred.

Statistical analyses were performed to detect differences between independent group proportions with a χ^2 or Fisher's Exact Test and between means with a Student t test or Mann-Whitney *U* test, when appropriate.[14] Only two-tailed *P* values less than or equal to .05 were considered significant.

RESULTS

Patient Characteristics

Among the 97 patients, 44% were white, 32% were black, 22% were Hispanic, and 2% were other races, reflecting the general patient population served by the two hospitals in Dallas. The male-to-female ratio was 1:1. Sixty-four percent of the patients were younger than 1 year, and only 18% were older than 2 years. Forty-six patients had concomitant otitis media, seven had pneumonia, one had buccal cellulitis, one had periorbital cellulitis, two had maxillary sinusitis, and one had suppurative arthritis. No differences were noted in case-fatality rates or in neurologic outcome in those who presented with a focus of infection in addition to the central nervous system compared with those who did not.

On admission, 34 patients had evidence of sepsis syndrome as defined by Jacobs et al[15] and modified for age

(Table 1). On admission or shortly thereafter, approximately 8% of the patients had septic shock, defined as the presence of sepsis syndrome and a blood pressure less than 2 SDs from the mean for age.

Forty-one patients received parenteral corticosteroid therapy in addition to antibiotic therapy, 13 of whom had been enrolled in one of the randomized, placebo-controlled trials.[12,13] Fifty-six patients did not receive steroid therapy, 14 of whom had been enrolled in one of the placebo-controlled trials. From 1984 through 1987, 10 of the 41 steroid-treated and 44 of the 56 non–steroid-treated patients were examined ($P<.001$). The only treatment difference identified in those admitted earlier in the study was that a larger number were initially treated with ampicillin or penicillin plus chloramphenicol or with cefuroxime compared with cefotaxime or ceftriaxone, which were used later. All of the 35 non–steroid-treated and 28 of the 30 steroid-treated patients who underwent second lumbar punctures had sterile CSF cultures after 24 hours of therapy (Table 2). There were no statistically significant differences between steroid- and non–steroid-treated patients with regard to clinical and laboratory characteristics on admission to the hospital (Table 1). Two patients had relatively penicillin-resistant organisms (minimum inhibitory concentration, 0.1 to 1.0 μg/mL) and had received several courses of orally administered β-lactam antibiotics for recurrent otitis media before admission. Both were treated with parenterally administered cephalosporin from the outset, and follow-up CSF cultures at approximately 24 hours after diagnosis were sterile.

Hospital Course and Response to Therapy

Dexamethasone administration was associated with a marked reduction in total duration of fever, defined as a maximal rectal temperature greater than 38.2°C after the day of admission (Table 2). There were no significant differences between steroid- and non–steroid-treated patients with regard to routine laboratory studies, presence of seizures, subdural effusions, hydrocephalus requiring a shunt, positive second CSF cultures 24 to 48 hours after the onset of treatment, or case-fatality rates in the hospital (Table 1).

Results of the CSF examinations at the time of admission were similar for the two groups; at 24 to 48 hours, however, those who received dexamethasone therapy had a significantly higher mean (±SD) glucose concentration compared with that in non–steroid-treated patients (3.8±1.4 vs 2.2±1.1 mmol/L, $P<.001$). The mean protein concentrations in the second CSF samples of steroid-treated patients were lower than those of non–steroid-treated patients, but the difference was not statistically significant (0.87±0.58 vs 1.0±1.9 g/L, $P=.12$). The mean number of white blood cells in the second samples was similar for both groups.

Complications

Four patients each in the steroid- and non–steroid-treated groups had clinically evident gastrointestinal bleeding, and three patients in each group required a blood transfusion. However, two patients in each group had evidence of blood loss before diagnosis and treatment. Two patients with gastrointestinal bleeding died; both were from the non–steroid-treated group. One death was related to disseminated intravascular coagulation, and in the other death, neurologic deterioration occurred after the first parenteral antibiotic dose. All patients with clinically apparent gastrointestinal bleeding had an altered sensorium, either semicoma or coma, on admission, and all but one had evidence of sepsis syndrome or septic shock, as defined previously.[15]

Cerebrovascular Instability.—Five (14%) of 35 assessable patients in the steroid-treated group and 16 (31%) of 52 assessable patients in the non–steroid-treated group ($P=.132$) developed evidence of cerebrovascular instability after initiation of parenteral antibiotic therapy. Cerebrovascular instability was defined as a change in neurologic and/or cardiovascular condition within 6 hours of initiation of parenteral antibiotic therapy and included a change in cardiovascular vital signs from normal for age to meeting the definition of sepsis syndrome/shock,[15] a change in neurologic condition from being alert to semiconscious, or the development of a first seizure. All five of the steroid-treated patients developed cerebrovascular instability after the start of antibiotic therapy and before the first dose of steroid was administered. By contrast, none of 30 patients who received steroid therapy before or concurrently with antibiotic therapy developed cerebrovascular instability (0 of 30 vs 16 of 52 treated with antibiotics alone, $P=.0003$).

Nine (9%) of 97 patients died during hospitalization, four in the steroid-treated group and five in the non–steroid-group (Table 2). Two other patients died, one at 2 months and the other at 6 months after completion of treatment; neither had received steroid treatment. Death occurred significantly more often in patients who developed cerebrovascular instability (24% [5/21] vs 1.5% [1/68]; $P=.0025$).

Overwhelming Meningeal Infection.—Twenty-seven patients had evidence of overwhelming meningeal infection, defined by a white blood cell count less than 0.075×10^9/L of CSF and more than an average of 10 organisms per high-power field on gram-stained smears of CSF observed at the time of diagnosis.[16,17] These patients were sicker than those without evidence of overwhelming meningeal infection, as indicated by laboratory studies, altered states of consciousness, and the presence of septic shock, cerebrovascular instability, and gross gastrointestinal bleeding (Table 3). They accounted for two thirds of the deaths and had a significantly increased incidence of seizures and permanent bilateral moderate or greater hearing loss. Of the survivors of overwhelming meningeal infection, one of eight steroid-treated patients compared with seven of 13 non–steroid-treated patients had moderate or greater bilateral hearing loss ($P=.085$). The one steroid-treated patient had severe neurologic damage and BSER evidence of bilateral hearing loss before dexamethasone therapy was administered 31 hours after the first parenteral dose of antibiotic.

Neurologic Outcome

There was a consistent trend of fewer neurologic abnormalities in the steroid-treated group on examinations at 6 weeks and 6 months after illness (Table 4). In addition, bilateral moderate or greater hearing loss occurred less often in steroid-treated patients compared with non–steroid-treated patients ($P=.13$).

There were significantly fewer patients with an overall adverse neurologic outcome, including hearing impairment, in those who received steroid therapy compared with those who did not (four [11%] of 35 vs 14 [33%] of 43; $P=.033$) (Table 4). The presence of seizures controlled

Table 3.—Characteristics of Patients With Overwhelming Meningeal Infection in Pneumococcal Meningitis*

	Overwhelming Meningeal Infection		
Characteristic	Present (n=27)	Absent (n=65)	*P*
Steroid therapy	11 (41)	28 (43)	.98
Admission cerebrospinal fluid white blood cell count, ×10⁹/L	0.216±0.210	3.087±3.770	<.001
Coma	8 (30)	5/60 (8)	.024
Altered state of consciousness†	22 (81)	25/60 (42)	.001
Shock	6 (22)	2/63 (3)	.008
Cerebrovascular instability	10/25 (40)	10/61 (16)	.038
Gastrointestinal bleeding	5 (19)	3 (5)	.045
Relative neutropenia	7/26 (27)	3 (5)	.005
Thrombocytopenia	10/26 (38)	7 (11)	.006
Seizures	19 (70)	20/64 (31)	.001
Died in hospital	6 (22)	3 (5)	.017
Long-term neurologic sequelae	4/20 (20)	5/54 (9)	.241
Bilateral moderate or greater hearing loss	8 (30)	4/56 (7)	.016
Total adverse outcome‡	9 (33)	8/56 (14)	.085

*Values are number of patients/total number (percent) or mean±SD. The definitions of some characteristics are given in Table 1 or the text. "Overwhelming meningeal infection" is defined in Scheld et al,[16] Weiss,[17] or the text.

†Altered state of consciousness includes lethargy with decreased responsiveness, semiconsciousness, and coma.

‡Total adverse outcome includes patients with one or more neurologic abnormalities, including bilateral moderate or greater hearing loss.

by medication and isolated hydrocephalus in patients who had normal motor and intellectual development were not included in these figures.

COMMENT

The use of systemic corticosteroids as adjunctive therapy for bacterial meningitis in infants and children was shown in double-blind, placebo-controlled trials in Dallas and Costa Rica to modulate meningeal inflammation and lumbar CSF pressure and to substantially improve long-term outcome in those with disease caused principally by *H influenzae*.[12,13] Because of the inevitable reduction in the incidence of *H influenzae* meningitis resulting from vaccination with the conjugated *Haemophilus* vaccines in early infancy, it is likely that a predominance of pneumococcal meningitis will be seen in the future. The paucity of data concerning dexamethasone therapy in these latter patients prompted our review of the Dallas experience with steroid treatment for pneumococcal meningitis.

Table 4.—Neurologic and Audiologic Outcome in Infants and Children With Pneumococcal Meningitis*

	Treatment Groups		
Characteristic	Steroid (n=37)†	No Steroid (n=49)†	*P*
Neurologic‡			
6-wk follow-up	3/34 (9)	6/38 (16)	.49
4-6 mo or longer follow-up	2/35 (6)	7/43 (16)	.18
Audiologic§			
Bilateral moderate or greater hearing loss	3/35 (9)	10/47 (21)	.14
Total adverse outcome‖	4/35 (11)¶	14/43 (33)¶	.033

*Values are number with sequela/number examined (percent).

†Numbers represent survivors who were available for follow-up.

‡Excludes hearing impairment, transient ataxia, and seizures controlled by medication.

§Patients with abnormal brain-stem evoked response examination results at discharge or at 6 weeks' follow-up were reexamined at 4 to 6 months or later to confirm impairment (see text).

‖Includes patients with one or more neurologic abnormalities, including bilateral moderate or greater hearing loss.

¶Three patients received dexamethasone sodium phosphate therapy more than 24 hours after initiation of antibiotic treatment. If they are excluded from analysis (see text), the rates of total neurologic sequelae were three (9%) of 32 vs 14 (33%) of 43 ($P=.025$) for steroid- and non–steroid-treated patients, respectively.

Because the basic pathophysiologic mechanisms of meningeal inflammation in experimental pneumococcal and *Haemophilus* meningitis are similar,[3,5,6,8,17,18] it was not surprising that dexamethasone had similar antiinflammatory effects in both models, as determined by CSF pressure, brain edema, cytokine concentrations, and the conventional CSF indexes of inflammation.[5,19] This was also the case in our analysis of the effects of corticosteroid treatment on CSF inflammatory indexes and CSF interleukin 1 β and tumor necrosis factor α concentrations in patients with pneumococcal and *Haemophilus* meningitis enrolled in the placebo-controlled, double-blind trials.[12,13]

The results of our retrospective study suggest strongly that corticosteroid therapy, especially when administered within 24 hours of starting parenteral antibiotic therapy, benefits neurologic and audiologic outcome in infants and children with pneumococcal meningitis. The percentage of survivors with any adverse outcome was markedly smaller in patients given steroid therapy within 24 hours of initiating parenteral antibiotic therapy compared with those who never received steroid therapy (three [9%] of 32 vs 14 [33%] 43; $P=.025$). It also appeared that steroid-treated patients with overwhelming pneumococcal meningeal infection[16,17] fared better on follow-up neurologic and audiologic examinations and that fewer steroid-treated patients developed evidence of cerebrovascular instability after initiation of parenteral antibiotic therapy compared with non–steroid-treated patients (0 of 30 vs 16 [31%] of 52; $P=.0003$). Five steroid-treated patients developed cerebrovascular instability before steroids were administered, underscoring the importance of providing steroid therapy before or concurrently with antibiotic therapy.[9,13] Our results are consistent with those of Girgis et al,[20] who demonstrated markedly lower rates of death and hearing impairment in 52 dexamethasone-treated compared with 54 non–steroid-treated children, adolescents, and adults with pneumococcal meningitis.

However, the data substantiating a beneficial effect on outcome from meningitis caused principally by *H influenzae* were derived from prospective, double-blind, placebo-controlled trials,[12,13] whereas the data from our study were retrospectively gathered, although more than half of the patients had been prospectively enrolled in therapeutic trials.[12,21] Although a placebo-controlled, double-blind study of dexamethasone therapy in pneumococcal meningitis would be ideal, we believe that the risk-benefit ratio is favorable and that dexamethasone therapy should be considered for use in infants and children with pneumococcal meningitis until results of such a study, if undertaken, are available.

References

1. Wenger JD, Hightower AW, Facklam RR, Gaventa S, Broome CV. Bacterial meningitis in the United States, 1986: report of a multistate surveillance study. *J Infect Dis.* 1990;162:1316-1323.
2. Pedersen FK, Henricksen J. Pneumococcal meningitis and bacteremia in Danish children, 1969-1978. *Acta Pathol Microbiol Immunol Scand.* 1983;91:129-134. Section B.
3. Tuomanen E, Tomasz A, Henstetler B, Zak O. The relative role of bacterial cell wall and capsule in the induction of inflammation in pneumococcal meningitis. *J Infect Dis.* 1985;151:535-540.
4. Tuomanen E, Hengstler B, Rich R, et al. Nonsteroidal antiinflammatory agents in the therapy for experimental pneumococcal meningitis. *J Infect Dis.* 1987;155:985-990.
5. Täuber MG, Khayam-Bashi H, Sande MA. Effects of ampicillin and corticosteroids on brain water content, cerebrospinal fluid pressure and cerebrospinal fluid lactate levels in experimental pneumococcal meningitis. *J Infect Dis.* 1985;151:528-534.
6. Saukkonen K, Sande S, Coieffe C, et al. The role of cytokines in the generation of inflammation and tissue damage in experimental gram-positive meningitis. *J Exp Med.* 1990;171:439-448.
7. Tuomanen EI, Saukkonen K, Sande S, Coiffe C, Wright SD. Reduction of inflammation, tissue damage, and mortality in bacterial meningitis in rabbits treated with monoclonal antibodies against adhesion-promoting receptors of leukocytes. *J Exp Med.* 1989;170:959-968.
8. Syrogiannopoulos GA, Hansen EJ, Erwin AL, et al. *Haemophilus influenzae* type b lipooligosaccharide induces meningeal inflammation. *J Infect Dis.* 1988;157:237-244.
9. Mustafa MM, Ramilo O, Mertsola J, et al. Modulation of inflammation and cachectin activity in relation to treatment of experimental *Haemophilus influenzae* type b meningitis. *J Infect Dis.* 1989;160:818-825.
10. Nolan CM, McAllister CK, Walters E, Beatty HN. Experimental pneumococcal meningitis, IV: the effect of methyl prednisolone on meningeal inflammation. *J Lab Clin Med.* 1978;91:979-988.
11. Täuber MG, Sande MA. Pathogenesis of bacterial meningitis: contributions of lactate and protein in experimental meningitis. *J Infect Dis.* 1988;157:456-459.
12. Lebel MH, Freij BJ, Syrogiannopoulos GA, et al. Dexamethasone therapy for bacterial meningitis: results of two double-blind, placebo-controlled trials. *N Engl J Med.* 1988;3:964-971.
13. Odio CM, Faingezicht I, Paris M, et al. The beneficial effects of early dexamethasone administration in infants and children with bacterial meningitis. *N Engl J Med.* 1991;324:1525-1531.
14. Zar JH. *Biostatistical Analysis.* 2nd ed. Englewood Cliffs, NJ: Prentice-Hall International Inc; 1984:62-71, 390-375.
15. Jacobs RF, Sowell MK, Moss MM, Fiser DH. Septic shock in children: bacterial etiologies and temporal relationships. *Pediatr Infect Dis J.* 1990;9:196-200.
16. Scheld WM, Giampaolo C, Beat J, Savory J, Willis MR, Sande MA. Cerebrospinal fluid prognostic indices in experimental pneumococcal meningitis. *J Lab Clin Med.* 1982;100:218-229.
17. Weiss W, Figueroa W, Shapiro WH, Flippen HF. Prognostic factors in pneumococcal meningitis. *Arch Intern Med.* 1967;120:517-524.
18. Sáez-Llorens X, Ramilo O, Mustafa M, Mertsola J, McCracken GH. Molecular pathophysiology of bacterial meningitis: current concepts and therapeutic implications. *J Pediatr.* 1990;116:671-684.
19. Syrogiannopoulos GA, Olsen KD, Reisch JS, McCracken GH. Dexamethasone in the treatment of experimental *Haemophilus influenzae* type b meningitis. *J Infect Dis.* 1987;155:213-219.
20. Girgis NI, Zoheir F, Mikhail IA, et al. Dexamethasone treatment for bacterial meningitis in children and adults. *Pediatr Infect Dis J.* 1989;8:848-851.
21. Lebel M, Hoyt MJ, Waagner DC, Rollins NK, Finitzo T, McCracken GH. Magnetic resonance imaging and dexamethasone therapy for bacterial meningitis. *AJDC.* 1989;143:301-306.

Haemophilus b Disease After Vaccination With *Haemophilus* b Polysaccharide or Conjugate Vaccine

Carl E. Frasch, PhD; Elizabeth E. Hiner, RPh; Thomas P. Gross, MD, MPh

• The reported frequency of invasive *Haemophilus influenzae* type b disease occurring within 1 year after immunization was compared in American children who received either Praxis Biologics' *Haemophilus* b polysaccharide vaccine or Connaught Laboratories' *Haemophilus* b conjugate vaccine during the first year of distribution. All domestic cases reported to the Food and Drug Administration or the Centers for Disease Control were included in the study. An estimated 4.5 million and 2.0 million doses of polysaccharide and conjugate vaccines were administered, respectively. Approximately three cases of early-onset disease (disease developing less than 15 days after vaccination) per million doses were reported for the polysaccharide compared with four cases per million doses for the conjugate vaccine. There were 30.7 reported vaccine failures per million doses of the polysaccharide vaccine compared with 9.0 per million doses of the conjugate vaccine, a 3.4-fold difference. The reporting rate ratios (cases of vaccine failure to cases of early-onset disease) for the polysaccharide and conjugate were 11.5 and 2.3, respectively, a fivefold difference. Thus, compared with recipients of the polysaccharide vaccine, vaccine failures reported among recipients of the conjugate vaccine were 80% fewer than expected.

(*AJDC.* 1991;145:1379-1382)

Haemophilus influenzae is the causative agent of a spectrum of human diseases, the most serious of which is meningitis. Other invasive infections caused by this organism include pneumonia, epiglottitis, cellulitis, and septic arthritis. Nearly all invasive disease caused by *H influenzae* in children is due to capsular type b, one of six capsular types.[1] The estimated annual incidence of *Haemophilus* b disease in children younger than age 2 years in the United States is about 100 per 100 000.[2]

The low incidence of *Haemophilus* b disease in older children and adults correlates with the presence of serum bactericidal antibodies.[3] Antibodies to the type b capsular polysaccharide, which is composed of ribose ribitol phosphate, are bactericidal and opsonic.[4,5] A 1974 efficacy trial with a *Haemophilus* b polysaccharide vaccine showed significant protection for children aged 18 months and older.[6] Based on this finding, a *Haemophilus* b polysaccharide vaccine was licensed in April 1985 for use in children aged 24 months and older. However, protective effectiveness of the polysaccharide vaccine in the United States was less than expected.[7,8] An improved polysaccharide-protein conjugate vaccine for protection against *H influenzae* type b was licensed in December 1987 for use in children aged 18 months and older.

Reporting of unexpected adverse events after administration of *Haemophilus* b vaccines has been strongly encouraged.[9] Failure of vaccines to protect against *Haemophilus* b disease is a reportable adverse event. Adverse events are generally reported to the Food and Drug Administration (FDA), but may be reported to the Centers for Disease Control (CDC). Reports submitted to the FDA are primarily from manufacturers or health care providers[10] and are entered into the Spontaneous Reporting System, a computerized database. Adverse events reported to the FDA and CDC were used in an earlier study[11] to describe the spectrum of disease due to *H influenzae* type b occurring in polysaccharide-vaccinated children.

In this study, we compare the frequency of reported invasive disease occurring within 1 year after immunization in American children who received either the *Haemophilus* b polysaccharide (PRP, Praxis Biologics Inc, Rochester, NY) or the *Haemophilus* b conjugate (PRP-D, Connaught Laboratories Inc, Swiftwater, Pa) vaccine any time during the first year of the products' distribution. The first year was chosen for both products because during this time only one manufacturer's product was on the market.

PATIENTS AND METHODS

The first year of distribution of PRP was defined as May 1, 1985, through April 30, 1986, and the first year for PRP-D was defined as January 1, 1988, through December 31, 1988. Children vaccinated in the United States during these times who developed *Haemophilus* b disease within 1 year of immunization were eligible for our study and were included if their disease was reported to the FDA or CDC. Thus, each vaccinated child was allotted equal time (365 days) to develop disease. In a similar study by Nelson and Granoff,[12] this was

Accepted for publication August 30, 1991.

From the Division of Bacterial Products, Center for Biologics Evaluation and Research (Dr Frasch and Ms Hiner), and the Division of Epidemiology and Surveillance, Center for Drug Evaluation and Research (Dr Gross), Food and Drug Administration, Bethesda, Md.

This article contains the professional views of the authors and does not constitute the official position of the Food and Drug Administration.

Reprint requests to the Division of Bacterial Products, Center for Biologics Evaluation and Research, HFB-640, 8800 Rockville Pike, Bethesda, MD 20892 (Dr Frasch).

Table 1.—*Haemophilus* b Disease Occurring Within 1 Year of Immunization With Connaught Laboratories' *Haemophilus* b Conjugate Vaccine*

Patient No.	Sex	No. of Days Between Vaccination and Disease Onset	Disease	State	Age at Immunization, mo	Surveillance
1	M	1	Septicemia	Minn	32	A
2	M	2	Meningitis	Wash	18	P
3	F	2	Meningitis	Calif	29	A
4	M	3	Cellulitis	Mich	17	P
5	F	4	Septicemia	Ga	26	P
6	F	4	Meningitis	Ore	23	P
7	M	6	Meningitis	Ohio	20	P
8	M	14	Meningitis	Mass	18	P
9	M	25	Meningitis	Calif	19	P
10	M	35	Meningitis	Pa	19	P
11	F	50	Meningitis	Conn	19	A
12	F	59	Meningitis	Mont	17	P
13	F	65	Meningitis	Calif	27	A
14	NS	91	Pneumonia	Wis	18	P
15	M	116	Meningitis	Fla	15	P
16	M	119	Septicemia	Calif	46	A
17	NS	128	Meningitis	Tenn	37	A
18	NS	140	Meningitis	Ill	18	P
19	NS	143	Cellulitis	Okla	23	A
20	F	174	Meningitis	Calif	18	A
21	NS	176	Cellulitis	Calif	18	A
22	M	220	Septicemia	Tex	29	A
23	F	261	Cellulitis	Minn	23	A
24	F	290	Meningitis	Calif	18	A
25	F	321	Meningitis	Tenn	19	A
26	M	353	Epiglottitis	Okla	23	A

*NS indicates not specified; A, active; and P, passive. Included under active surveillance are six reports from the Centers for Disease Control and eight reports from parts of the United States considered to be under more active surveillance than usual.

not the case, as only those vaccinated children who developed disease within the first 13 months of distribution of the applied vaccine could have been included if their disease had been reported. Thus, children vaccinated 10 months into a vaccine's first 13 months of distribution would have to have developed disease in 3 months to be included in their study.

Other study methods and case definitions are as described by Hiner and Frasch.[11] Cases of disease developing in children less than 15 days after immunization were counted as early-onset cases of the disease, not as vaccine failures. The child's age at immunization was determined when possible from the date of birth and was recorded as the last full month of age. When the birth date was not available, the age at vaccination indicated on the report was used. The number of days between vaccination and disease onset was calculated based on the reported dates of immunization and hospital admission. The two manufacturers provided estimates of amounts of vaccine distributed and administered.

RESULTS

There were 150 cases of *Haemophilus* b disease reported in children who received PRP, and these 150 cases are a subset of cases presented in our earlier paper.[11] Twenty-six cases of *Haemophilus* b disease were reported after immunization with PRP-D (Table 1). Another case of early-onset disease was reported after PRP-D vaccination in a 19-month-old infant, but was not included because the child resided in British Columbia. Twenty cases (77%) were reported by physicians and/or the manufacturer, but, of these, eight were considered to be from areas of active surveillance.[8,13-15] Six reports (23%) obtained from the CDC were from an active surveillance study of meningitis.[16] In comparison, 16 (11%) of 150 reports of cases of disease after PRP vaccination originally reported by Granoff et al[17] were from active surveillance studies. Two (25%) of the eight PRP-D–associated cases of early-onset disease and 12 (67%) of 18 PRP-D vaccine failures were considered to have been reported from areas of active surveillance. There were no cases of early-onset disease associated with PRP among the active surveillance reports.

Approximately 60% of cases of both early-onset disease and vaccine failure after receipt of PRP-D involved meningitis compared with 54% of cases of PRP vaccine failures (Table 2). Approximately 75% fewer cases of epiglottitis developed in patients with PRP-D vaccine failure (6%) compared with patients with PRP vaccine failure (25%). There was no important difference between the mean or median age at immunization of children who experienced early-onset disease or vaccine failures in the PRP or PRP-D groups, but there was a median age difference of 6 months between administration of the two vaccines (Table 3).

Table 4 compares the rates of reported *Haemophilus* b disease within 1 year after immunization with PRP and PRP-D. Praxis Biologics reported that during the first year of distribution approximately 4.5 million doses of PRP had been administered (about 70% of distributed vaccine). Connaught Laboratories reported that 2.0 million doses of PRP-D had been administered during its first year (about 60% of distributed vaccine). There were 2.7 reported cases of early-onset disease per million doses of PRP compared with 4.0 cases per million doses of PRP-D. The rate of reported PRP-D vaccine failures was about 30% that of PRP. The reporting rate ratios (cases of vaccine failure to cases of early-onset disease) for PRP and PRP-D were 11.4 (30.7:2.7) and 2.3 (9.0:4.0), respectively, demonstrating a fivefold difference. Excluding reports from active surveillance areas for both vaccines resulted in a 10.2-fold difference in the rate ratios.

Table 2.—Distribution of Disease in Patients With Early-Onset Disease and Vaccine Failures After *Haemophilus* b Vaccination*

	Polysaccharide		Conjugate	
Disease	Early-Onset Disease	Vaccine Failure	Early-Onset Disease	Vaccine Failure
Meningitis	4 (33)	75 (54)	5 (62)	11 (61)
Epiglottitis	3 (25)	34 (25)	0	1 (6)
Cellulitis	1 (8)	10 (7)	1 (13)	3 (17)
Pneumonia	0	8 (6)	0	1 (6)
Bacteremia	2 (17)	6 (4)	2 (25)	2 (11)
Other	2 (17)	5 (4)	0	0
Total	**12 (100)**	**138 (100)**	**8 (100)**	**18 (101)**

*Values are number (percentage) of cases developing less than 15 days after vaccination. Percentages may not total 100 owing to rounding.

Table 3.—Age at Immunization of Vaccinated Children Who Later Developed *Haemophilus* b Disease

	Age at Immunization, mo					
	Early-Onset Disease			Vaccine Failure		
Vaccine	Median	Mean	Range	Median	Mean	Range
Polysaccharide	24	27.4	22-41	25	29.1	16-60
Conjugate	22	22.2	17-32	19	22.8	15-47

COMMENT

We compared the frequency of reported *Haemophilus* b disease occurring within 1 year after immunization in children vaccinated with either PRP or PRP-D anytime during the first year of the vaccines' distribution when PRP was the only *Haemophilus* b vaccine available and when PRP-D was the only *Haemophilus* b conjugate available. Cases were reported from both active and passive surveillance systems. Because the dynamics of reporting in these two systems are different, examining their separate effects was important. By excluding reports from active surveillance, the reporting rate ratio difference increased from fivefold to tenfold. We also noted that cases occurring more than 3 months after immunization with PRP-D were much more likely to be reported by active surveillance.

The median age at immunization for the PRP and PRP-D vaccine recipients who experienced vaccine failure was 25 months and 19 months, respectively, but it is unclear whether this difference can fully account for the lower incidence of epiglottitis after vaccination with PRP-D. The peak age for occurrence of epiglottitis is approximately 30 months.[18]

In an approach similar to that of Nelson and Granoff,[12] but using reporting rates rather than reported numbers, we determined that the reported rate of vaccine failures in PRP-D recipients would have to be 46.0 per million doses administered for the vaccine failure–early-onset disease rate ratios in PRP-D and PRP recipients to be the same (PRP-D, 46.0:4.0 [11.5]; PRP, 30.7:2.7 [11.4]). Given the number of PRP-D doses administered (2.0 million), the rate of 46.0 per million would correspond to 92 vaccine failures among those who received PRP-D. However, only 18 cases were reported, or 80% fewer than expected. These data and the 3.4-fold fewer vaccine failures per million doses suggest that PRP-D is more effective than PRP. These calculations are based on the assumption that no cases of early-onset disease result from the transient decrease in antibody that occurs in the first few days after immunization.[19]

Because underreporting of cases of both early-onset disease and vaccine failure is certain and the number of vaccine doses administered is an approximation, the derived reporting rates of disease after immunization are only crude estimates of the true incidence. The reporting rate ratios, however, remain unchanged even if vaccine exposure changed because both the numerator and the denominator of the rate ratio are equally affected. Underreporting becomes a more important issue in considering potential biases in this study.

Potential biases include a relative overreporting of early-onset disease after PRP-D vaccination or a relative

Table 4.—Comparison of Reported Rates of *Haemophilus* b Disease in Children Who Received Polysaccharide or Conjugate Vaccine During the First Year of the Vaccine's Distribution

			Haemophilus b Disease, No. of Cases Per Million Doses (No. of Cases)			
Vaccine	No. of Doses Distributed, Millions	No. of Doses Administered, Millions (% of Doses Distributed)	Early-Onset Disease	Vaccine Failure	Total	Rate Ratio*
Polysaccharide	6.4	4.5 (70)	2.7 (12)	30.7 (138)	**33.4 (150)**	11.4
Conjugate	3.3	2.0 (61)	4.0 (8)	9.0 (18)	**13.0 (26)**	2.3

*Ratio of rate of vaccine failure to rate of development of early-onset disease.

underreporting of PRP-D vaccine failures. Given the nature of invasive *Haemophilus* b disease, it is unlikely that PRP-D-associated cases of early-onset disease would be preferentially reported compared with PRP-associated cases. Regarding the latter bias, given the extent of publicity and discussion in the last half of 1987 and into 1988 after studies of the efficacy of the PRP vaccines,[7,8] heightened interest in the efficacy of the conjugate vaccines would likely have stimulated reporting of vaccine failures. Thus, comparative underreporting of PRP-D vaccine failures seems unlikely. However, such a bias might have existed if children vaccinated with PRP-D had been allotted less time to develop disease than children vaccinated with PRP. This could have occurred if (1) to be included in the study, vaccinated children who developed disease would have had to have experienced disease onset within the first year of distribution of the applied vaccine, and (2) PRP-D had been used more extensively during the last half of its first year of distribution than PRP was during its first distribution year. Importantly, the variation in overall use of PRP-D vs PRP during their first year of distribution did not have to be accounted for with our study design because all vaccinated children were allotted 365 days to develop disease.

The first conjugate vaccine, PRP-D, was introduced in 1987. It was licensed based on its superior immunogenicity compared with PRP. The reported effectiveness of PRP in American children has been estimated in a series of postmarketing case-control studies.[7,8,20] The effectiveness estimates ranged from 50% to 88% for most of these studies. Recent case-control studies of PRP-D have shown its effectiveness to be 100% (95% confidence interval [CI], 72% to 100%) in Minnesota[21] and 88% (95% CI, 49% to 97%) in Los Angeles County, California.[15]

Based on the data presented and considering potential reporting biases, the PRP-D conjugate vaccine appears to be more effective than the polysaccharide in children aged 18 months or older. This is consistent with the results of the above cited case-control studies. *Haemophilus* b conjugate vaccines produced by Praxis Biologics and Merck Sharp & Dohme, West Point, Pa, have been recently licensed for use in children beginning at age 2 months.[22]

We thank Jay Wenger, MD, Special Pathogens Branch, Centers for Disease Control, Atlanta, Ga, for providing reports of *Haemophilus* b disease in vaccinated children.

References

1. Pittman M. Variation and type specificity in the bacterial species *Haemophilus influenzae*. *J Exp Med*. 1931;53:471-492.

2. Sherry B, Emanuel I, Kronmal RA, et al. Interannual variation of the incidence of *Haemophilus influenzae* type b meningitis. *JAMA*. 1989;261:1924-1929.

3. Fothergill LD, Wright J. Influenzal meningitis: relation of age incidence to the bactericidal power of blood against the causal organism. *J Immunol*. 1933;24:273-284.

4. Schneerson R, Rodrigues LP, Parke JC, Robbins JB. Immunity to disease caused by *Haemophilus influenzae* type b, 2: specificity and some biologic characteristics of 'natural,' infection-acquired, and immunization-induced antibodies to the capsular polysaccharide of *Haemophilus influenzae* type b. *J Immunol*. 1971;107:1081-1089.

5. Anderson P, Johnston RB Jr, Smith DH. Human serum activities against *Haemophilus influenzae* type b. *J Clin Invest*. 1972;51:31-38.

6. Peltola H, Hayhty H, Sivonen A, Makela PH. *Haemophilus influenzae* type b capsular polysaccharide vaccine in children: a double blind study of 100 000 vaccinees 3 months to 5 years of age in Finland. *Pediatrics*. 1977;60:730-737.

7. Harrison LH, Broome CV, Hightower AW, *Haemophilus* Vaccine Efficacy Study Group. *Haemophilus influenzae* type b polysaccharide vaccine: an efficacy study. *Pediatrics*. 1989;84:255-261.

8. Shapiro ED, Murphy TV, Wald ER, Brady CA. The protective efficacy of *Haemophilus* b polysaccharide vaccine. *JAMA*. 1988;260:1419-1422.

9. FDA workshop on *Haemophilus* b polysaccharide vaccine: a preliminary report. *MMWR*. 1987;36:529-531.

10. Turner WT, Milstein JB, Fiach GA, et al. The processing of adverse reaction reports at FDA. *Drug Info J*. 1986;20:147-150.

11. Hiner EE, Frasch CE. Spectrum of disease due to *Haemophilus influenzae* type b occurring in vaccinated children. *J Infect Dis*. 1988;158:343-348.

12. Nelson WL, Granoff DM. Protective efficacy of *Haemophilus influenzae* type b polysaccharide-diphtheria toxoid-conjugate vaccine. *AJDC*. 1990;144:292-295.

13. Black BB, Schinfield HR, Haitt RA, Fireman BH, The Kaiser Permanente Pediatric Vaccine Study Group. Efficacy of *Haemophilus influenzae* type b capsular polysaccharide vaccine. *Pediatr Infect Dis J*. 1988;7:149-156.

14. Murphy TV, Osterholm MT, Pierson LM, et al. Prospective surveillance of *Haemophilus influenzae* type b disease in Dallas County, Texas, and in Minnesota. *Pediatrics*. 1987;79:173-179.

15. Greenberg DP, Vadheim CM, Christenson P, et al. Protective efficacy of *Haemophilus influenzae* type b polysaccharide and conjugate vaccines in children 18 months of age and older. *JAMA*. 1991;265:987-992.

16. Wenger JD, Hightower AW, Facklam RR, Gaventa S, Broome CV, the Bacterial Meningitis Study Group. Bacterial meningitis in the United States, 1986: report of a multistate surveillance study. *J Infect Dis*. 1990;162:1316-1323.

17. Granoff DM, Shackelford PG, Suarez BK, et al. *Haemophilus influenzae* type b disease in children vaccinated with type b polysaccharide vaccine. *N Engl J Med*. 1986;315:1584-1590.

18. Todd JK, Bruhn FW. Severe *Haemophilus influenzae* infections: spectrum of disease. *AJDC*. 1975;129:607-611.

19. Marchant CD, Band E, Froeshle JE, McVerry PH. Depression of anticapsular antibody after immunization with *Haemophilus influenzae* type b polysaccharide-diphtheria conjugate vaccine. *Pediatr Infect Dis J*. 1989;8:508-511.

20. Osterholm MT, Rambeck JH, White KE, et al. Lack of efficacy of *Haemophilus* b polysaccharide vaccine in Minnesota. *JAMA*. 1988;260:1423-1428.

21. Osterholm MT. Efficacy of *Haemophilus* b plain polysaccharide (PRP) vaccine and conjugate vaccine in Minnesota. In: *Abstracts of the 29th Interscience Conference on Antimicrobial Agents and Chemotherapy*. Houston, Tex: American Society for Microbiology; 1989. Abstract 449A.

22. Centers for Disease Control. *Haemophilus* b conjugate vaccines for the prevention of *Haemophilus influenzae* type b disease among infants and children two months of age and older: recommendations of the immunization practices advisory committee (ACIP). *MMWR*. 1991;40:RR-1.

Comparison of Maternal and Newborn Serologic Tests for Syphilis

Sarah A. Rawstron, MB, BS, Kenneth Bromberg, MD

• *Objective.*—**To compare the cord blood, newborn serum, and maternal serum for the diagnosis of congenital syphilis.**

Design.—**Retrospective chart review.**

Setting.—**Kings County Hospital Center, Brooklyn, NY.**

Patients.—**Three hundred forty-eight mother-newborn pairs with positive syphilis serology.**

Measurements and Results.—**One hundred fifteen newborns (33%) had rapid plasma reagin tests of cord blood that were nonreactive. Their mothers had positive serologic findings. There were 10% false-positive cord blood samples (cord blood rapid plasma reagin tests reactive, newborn serum rapid plasma reagin tests nonreactive) and 5% false-negative cord blood samples (cord rapid plasma reagin tests nonreactive, newborn serum rapid plasma reagin tests reactive). Thirty-three newborns had congenital syphilis. Seven newborns had cord titers fourfold higher than their mothers'; only four of these newborns had congenital syphilis. Maternal serology is superior to cord blood analysis for identifying newborns at risk of congenital syphilis.**

(*AJDC.* 1991;145:1383-1388)

Congenital syphilis has reached epidemic proportions in New York State. In response to this outbreak, the state requires that all newborns have their cord blood tested for syphilis.[1] According to state law, maternal blood tested at delivery is an acceptable alternative to cord blood. Do the two samples provide similar information? Only limited comparisons of mother's and newborn's serology results at delivery[2,3] are available. These studies suggest that cord blood serology is inferior to maternal blood serology for the detection of congenital syphilis.

Although there is said to be a large experience with serology results in the diagnosis of congenital syphilis, recommendations and statements about syphilis serology results in the newborn period are based on anecdotal information and unpublished data. For instance, the Centers for Disease Control, Atlanta, Ga, suggests syphilis serologic testing on a newborn's serum rather than on the cord blood because of fewer false-positive results on serum samples,[4] but data are not available to support or refute these findings. A recently adopted diagnostic criterion for congenital syphilis[5] is a newborn's titer that is four times as great as that of the maternal titer at delivery. Evidence for the usefulness of this ratio has not been published.

Because only limited studies or anecdotal information on the association between cord blood and maternal blood syphilis serologies were available, cord blood, maternal serum, and newborn serum syphilis serology results were reviewed at this institution to determine if (1) a rapid plasma reagin test (RPR; Becton Dickinson Microbiology Systems, Cockeysville, Md) performed on cord blood identified newborns with congenital syphilis, (2) the ratio of newborn cord blood RPR to maternal blood RPR was helpful in the diagnosis of congenital syphilis, and (3) an RPR performed on newborn serum was superior to an RPR performed on cord blood.

Accepted for publication July 22, 1991.

From the Division of Pediatric Infectious Diseases, Department of Pediatrics, Children's Medical Center of Brooklyn (Kings County Hospital Center, and SUNY Health Science Center at Brooklyn).

Reprint requests to the Department of Pediatrics, SUNY Health Science Center at Brooklyn, Box 49, 450 Clarkson Ave, Brooklyn, NY 11203 (Dr Rawstron).

PATIENTS, MATERIALS, AND METHODS

In Kings County Hospital Center, Brooklyn, NY, an RPR test is performed on the cord blood of almost all newborns and on blood obtained from almost all mothers at delivery. A positive RPR is confirmed with the use of a fluorescent treponemal antibody absorption test (FTA-ABS; Clinical Sciences, Whippany, NJ). Quality control of the RPR test is performed twice a day. The RPR test was reproducible within one tube dilution when 2 months' of tests were reviewed.

All RPR tests performed on women who gave birth at Kings County Hospital from January 1988 to November 1989 were reviewed. Mother-newborn pairs were identified by finding a positive RPR in any serum specimen from either member of the pair. Specimens that were sent for RPR testing were maternal serum, newborn's cord blood, or serum of a newborn during the first days of life. Additional newborn testing was only done on a second newborn serum specimen and not further testing of the serum from the clotted cord blood. The diagnosis of congenital syphilis was based on the following modified guidelines established by the Centers for Disease Control:[5,6]

The definition for congenital syphilis includes confirmed or presumptive categories. The Centers for Disease Control defines *confirmed cases* of congenital syphilis as infants in whom *Treponema pallidum* is identified by dark-field microscopy, fluorescent antibody, or other specific stains in specimens from lesions, placenta, umbilical cord, or autopsy material. The Centers for Disease Control defines *presumptive cases* of congenital syphilis as either of the following:

A. An infant whose mother had untreated or inadequately treated syphilis at delivery, regardless of findings in the infant; or

B. Any infant or child who has a reactive treponemal test for syphilis and any one of the following:

1. any evidence of congenital syphilis on physical examination (signs in an infant less than age 2 years may include hepatosplenomegaly, characteristic skin rash, condyloma lata, snuffles, jaundice (syphilitic hepatitis), pseudoparalysis, or edema (nephrotic syndrome); or

2. any evidence of congenital syphilis on long-bone radiograph; or

3. reactive cerebrospinal fluid (CSF) VDRL; or

4. elevated CSF cell count or protein level (without other cause); or

5. quantitative nontreponemal serologic titers that are fourfold higher than the mother's (both drawn at birth); or

6. reactive test for FTA-ABS-19S-IgM antibody.

The definition of congenital syphilis used in this study included only confirmed and presumptive B:1,2,3 categories. Newborns were included in group B1 with any of the following signs or symptoms: hepatosplenomegaly, hepatitis, characteristic rash, or lymphadenopathy. *Hepatitis* was defined as hyperbilirubinemia with an indirect bilirubin level greater than 17 μmol/L, or an aspartate aminotransferase level greater than 75 U/L. Newborns were not excluded from the diagnosis of congenital syphilis if they had nonreactive (NR) cord blood titers. A diagnosis of congenital syphilis was not made on the inadequacy of maternal therapy alone (presumptive group A) since only some of these newborns have congenital syphilis. Categories B:4, 5, and 6 were also excluded. Category B4 was excluded since the values given for abnormal CSF white blood cell count ($>0.005 \times 10^9$/L) and protein level (>0.40 g/L)[5] are well within normal for newborns.[7] Category B5 was excluded since this definition was being evaluated. Category B6 was excluded since no newborns had this test performed.

The diagnosis of confirmed congenital syphilis was made based on a positive immunofluorescence test for *T pallidum* using rabbit antiserum in an indirect immunofluorescent antigen test. After November 1988, all newborns born to mothers with positive RPRs received parenteral penicillin (either intravenous penicillin G or intramuscular penicillin G procaine) for 10 days.

RESULTS

Of the 9421 newborns born during the 22-month study period, there were 429 (5%) mother-newborn pairs with positive RPR results in either one of the pair. Four hundred eight had medical records available for review. Twenty-eight were excluded from analysis because the FTA-ABS was either negative (11) or not done (17), leaving 380 (89%) mother-newborn pairs with positive FTA-ABS results. Of the 380 pairs, 14 (3.7%) had discordant FTA-ABS results between members of the pair but were still included in the analysis.

Only 348 (91.6%) of the 380 mother-newborn pairs could be evaluated for comparison of maternal and newborn serologic findings since five newborns had no cord blood samples sent for analysis, and 27 mothers had no maternal serum samples sent for analysis. These 348 pairs were the basis for the analysis.

RANGE OF TITERS

The range of RPR titers seen in all specimens was similar: cord serum NR to 1:2048, newborn serum NR to 1:1024, and maternal serum NR to 1:1024. Significant discordance between titers was assumed, based on usual practice, if titers differed by more than or equal to two tube dilutions (fourfold). Analysis of the 348 mother-newborn pairs included 171 pairs where there were both newborn cord, serum, and maternal samples for comparison. The results for mother-newborn pairs with RPR-positive results were analyzed separately from those with any RPR NR results (Figure).

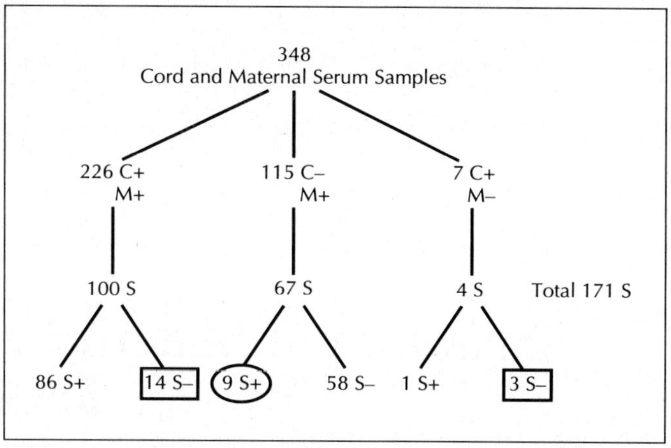

Analysis of 348 cord and maternal serum samples. C indicates cord serum; M, maternal serum; S, newborn serum; plus sign, RPR (rapid plasma reagin) positive; minus sign, RPR nonreactive; boxed items, cord blood RPR false positives; and circled item, cord blood RPR false negatives.

Analysis of RPR-Positive Serum Samples

Comparison of RPR-Positive Cord and Maternal Serum Samples.—There were 226 (65%) pairs with RPR-positive cord and maternal serum samples (Table 1). The majority of cord blood samples (136 of 226 or 60%) were within two dilutions of maternal titer.

Comparison of RPR-Positive Newborn and Maternal Serum Samples.—One hundred seventy-one pairs of newborn serum and maternal titers were available for comparison, but only 95 (55.6%) of these newborn serum samples were RPR positive when maternal RPR was also RPR positive. The majority of the specimens (54 of 95 or 57%) were fourfold lower (two or more dilutions lower) than the maternal titer (Table 1).

Comparison of RPR-Positive Cord and Newborn Serum Samples.—Only 87 (51%) of 171 samples of both newborn cord and newborn serum were RPR positive. There were few differences between titers when both cord and newborn serum samples were RPR positive. Most (79 of 87 or 91%) cord and newborn serum samples were within two tube dilutions of each other. Three newborns had cord blood that was four times higher than the newborn serum titer, and five newborns had newborn serum that was four times higher than the cord titer.

Analysis of Serum Samples With RPR Nonreactive Samples

Comparison of Cord and Maternal Serum Samples Where One Sample Is Nonreactive.—There were 115 newborns (33%) whose cord blood samples were RPR NR when maternal serum samples were positive. There were seven newborns (2%) with RPR-positive cord blood samples whose mothers had RPR NR serum samples.

Comparison of Newborn Serum With Maternal Serum.—*Group With RPR NR Cord Blood Samples.*—Sixty-seven (58%) of the 115 newborns who had RPR NR cord blood samples and RPR-positive maternal serum had additional newborn serum samples sent for clarification of titers. Nine of these serum samples were RPR positive (Table 1). These nine included eight with newborn serum

Table 1.—Comparison of Fourfold Difference in RPR-Reactive Mother-Newborn Serum Sample Pairs*

	Fourfold Lower	Same†	Fourfold Higher	Total
Cord vs maternal	83 (12)	136 (13)	7 (4)	**226 (29)**
Serum vs maternal	54 (4)	39 (5)	2 (1)	**95 (10)**

*RPR indicates rapid plasma reagin. Numbers in parentheses denote newborns with congenital syphilis. Ten had serum samples taken that were RPR positive and a total of 29 had newborn cord and maternal serum samples that were RPR positive.

†Newborn titer within two tube dilutions of maternal titer.

samples two dilutions or more higher than the cord blood sample (1:2 to 1:32), and one with newborn and cord titers within two dilutions (newborn titer 1:1).

Group With RPR NR Maternal Serum.—There were seven newborns with positive cord RPR and NR maternal RPR. Additional newborn serum samples were sent for analysis on four newborns and only one remained positive (cord and newborn serum titer 1:16), with three becoming NR (cord titers 1:1 to 1:2). The mother's serum samples on these newborns were unavailable for further testing so it is unknown if any maternal specimens were NR due to the prozone phenomenon.

Group With RPR NR Newborn Serum.—The group with positive RPR in both maternal and cord serum samples had additional newborn serum samples sent for analysis on 100 (44%) of 226. Fourteen of these newborns, who initially had RPR-positive cord serum samples (titers 1:1 to 1:8), had additional newborn serum samples that were NR.

False-Positive and False-Negative Cord Serum Samples

If newborn serum specimens are taken to be the true-positive samples, then the number of false-positive cord RPR tests was 17 (10%) of 171. The number of false-negative cord RPR tests was nine (5%) of 171.

Newborns With Congenital Syphilis

Thirty-three newborns with congenital syphilis in the group of 348 pairs had cord and maternal titers available for comparison; of these, 13 had cord, newborn serum, and maternal titers available for comparison. Cord titers ranged from NR to 1:2048. However, after November 1988, all newborns at risk were treated for congenital syphilis; therefore, more newborns may have had congenital syphilis since asymptomatic newborns may not be detected with routine testing. Twenty-nine newborns had RPR-positive cord blood samples, and four newborns had RPR NR cord blood samples at delivery.

The diagnosis of congenital syphilis was made using the criteria already mentioned. Table 2 contains information on the newborns with congenital syphilis. Eleven newborns had only abnormal roentgenographic findings, five had only a positive CSF VDRL, and six had both findings. Some of these newborns also had other manifestations of congenital syphilis such as hepatosplenomegaly, rash, and hepatitis. Three newborns only had hepatosplenomegaly as their manifestation of congenital syphilis, and seven newborns had hepatitis as their sole manifestation of congenital syphilis. Four newborns had confirmed congenital syphilis, and 29 had presumptive congenital syphilis.

The four newborns with confirmed congenital syphilis had *T pallidum* identified with immunofluorescence techniques in either nasopharyngeal or umbilical smears. Two of these had positive CSF VDRL alone. One had a positive CSF VDRL and abnormal roentgenographic findings, and one had abnormal roentgenographic findings alone.

The four newborns with NR cord blood samples had findings compatible with presumptive congenital syphilis. Three of them had evidence of congenital syphilis at birth (patients 2, 19, and 32) and one did not (patient 16). The newborn who did not have evidence of congenital syphilis at birth (patient 16) had no additional newborn serum samples sent for analysis and was not evaluated for congenital syphilis at birth. The newborn received no therapy and returned at age 4 months with florid congenital syphilis and a titer of 1:512. This patient is the subject of a previous report.[8] Comparison of RPR-positive infant and maternal titers is included in Table 1.

Analysis of Newborn Cord Serum Titer Four Times Higher Than Maternal Titer in RPR-Positive Specimens

Among newborns and mothers with positive syphilis tests, there were seven newborns whose cord serum titer was four times higher than their mothers' at delivery (Table 3). Only four of these had evidence of congenital syphilis. The other three did not have evidence of congenital syphilis; however, they did not undergo a full evaluation since none had roentgenograms performed, and only one had a lumbar puncture performed. Therefore, the number with congenital syphilis could have been higher. Another five newborns had cord serum titers four times higher than their mothers' (1:2 to 1:16), but their mothers had NR RPR serologic findings. None of these newborns had any evidence of congenital syphilis, and they were not included in the analysis of newborn cord serum titer four times higher than maternal titer since only one member of the pair had RPR-positive serologic findings.

All those with congenital syphilis whose titers were fourfold higher than their mothers' had titers of 1:1024 or greater. However, all newborns in the analysis with titers of 1:1024 or greater had congenital syphilis. Sensitivity and specificity of cord titer fourfold maternal titer are four (12%) of 33 and 312 (99%) of 315, respectively. The positive predictive value is four (57%) of seven and the negative predictive value is 312 (91%) of 341.

Analysis of Newborn Serum Titer Fourfold Maternal

Only three newborns had newborn serum titers fourfold higher than maternal titers. One newborn (Table 2, patient 10) had evidence of congenital syphilis. One newborn with newborn cord and serum titer of 1:16 and maternal titer RPR NR had no evidence of congenital syphilis. The third newborn had a cord titer of 1:16, serum titer of 1:128, maternal titer of 1:16, and no evidence of congenital syphilis; however, no roentgenograms were obtained.

COMMENT

These data confirm that RPR testing of newborn's cord serum fails to identify many mother-newborn pairs who are at risk for syphilis. One third of newborns whose mothers have positive syphilis serologic findings will have RPR NR cord blood samples. Our data are similar to those of Miller et al,[2] who, in 1960, found that 66% of 221 infants born to mothers with positive syphilis serologic

Table 2.—33 Newborns With Congenital Syphilis*

Patient No.	Rapid Plasma Reagin: Cord	Serum	Maternal	Symptoms	Roentgenogram	CSF VDRL	IFA
1	1:64	1:64	1:128	−	+	+	+
2	NR	NR	1:32	P	ND	−	ND
3	1:8	ND	1:32	P	−	−	ND
4	1:256	1:128	1:1024	−	−	+	+
5	1:512	1:512	1:512	R,H,S	ND	ND	ND
6	1:256	ND	1:256	−	+	ND	ND
7	1:64	1:64	1:256	H,P	ND	−	ND
8	1:64	1:64	1:128	−	+	+	ND
9	1:2048	ND	1:256	R,H,S,P	+	+	ND
10	1:1024	1:1024	1:256	−	+	+	−
11	1:64	ND	1:128	R,H,S,P,L	+	+	ND
12	1:32	ND	1:512	−	+	−	−
13	1:256	ND	1:256	H,S,P	+	+	ND
14	1:1	NR	1:2	−	+	−	+
15	1:64	ND	1:64	−	+	−	ND
16	NR	ND	1:16	−	ND	ND	ND
17	1:32	ND	1:256	H,P	+	ND	ND
18	1:8	1:2	1:32	H,P	−	ND	ND
19	NR	ND	1:2	P	ND	−	ND
20	1:32	ND	1:64	R,H,S	+	−	ND
21	1:16	1:16	1:128	−	ND	+	+
22	1:128	ND	1:1024	−	−	+	ND
23	1:64	ND	1:128	H,S,P	+	−	ND
24	1:4	ND	1:32	P	ND	−	ND
25	1:16	ND	1:128	R,H,S	+	−	ND
26	1:32	1:64	1:128	R,H,S	−	ND	ND
27	1:1024	ND	1:128	H,S	ND	ND	ND
28	1:2048	ND	1:64	R,H,S	−	+	ND
29	1:4	ND	1:32	P	−	−	ND
30	1:512	ND	1:512	H,S,P	+	−	ND
31	1:16	ND	1:32	−	ND	+	ND
32	NR	NR	1:8	−	+	ND	ND
33	1:8	1:8	1:8	−	+	ND	ND

*CSF VDRL indicates cerebrospinal fluid Venereal Disease Research Laboratory Test; IFA, immunofluorescent *Treponena pallidum* antigen detection test; NR, nonreactive; ND, not done; P, hepatitis; R, rash; H, hepatomegaly; S, splenomegaly; L, lymphadenopathy; plus sign, positive or abnormal; and minus sign, negative or abnormal.

findings had positive serologic tests for syphilis and/or *T pallidum* immobilizing antibody at birth.

While the aim of cord blood testing is to identify newborns with congenital syphilis, the real goal of the screening program should be to identify mothers with syphilis and therefore also their newborns. If the mother has syphilis then the newborn is at risk of congenital syphilis.

Many of these women do not have prenatal care,[9] and their first screening for syphilis is at delivery. The hospitalization at delivery may be the only chance for treatment of the mother and prevention of further syphilitic pregnancies. Even if a woman has had prenatal care, one should not rely on a previous negative syphilis serologic finding during the pregnancy to determine maternal infection at delivery.[10]

Screening the mother's serum alone would miss few newborns. In our series, seven newborns whose maternal titers were RPR NR had RPR-positive cord serum samples. However, additional newborn serum testing only confirmed RPR positivity in one of the four newborns who were retested. It is possible that some of these mothers had false-negative results due to the prozone phenomenon, although we were unable to test this hypothesis since further testing on maternal serum could not be performed. The prozone phenomenon is a false-negative nontreponemal serologic test that can occur when undiluted serum containing high antibody titers is tested. Diluting the specimen solves this problem. The prozone phenomenon has been responsible for misdiagnosis of syphilis in pregnant women,[11] and clinicians should be

Patient No.	Titer: Cord	Titer: Newborn	Titer: Maternal	Symptoms of Syphilis	Roentgenograms	CSF VDRL
1	1:4	1:2	1:1	−	ND	ND
2	1:8	ND	1:2	−	ND	ND
3	1:512	ND	1:32	−	ND	−
4†,‡	1:1024	ND	1:128	+	ND	ND
5†	1:1024	1:1024	1:256	−	+	+
6†	1:2048	ND	1:256	+	+	+
7†	1:2048	ND	1:64	+	+	+

Table 3.—Newborns With Cord Serum Titer Four Times Their Mothers'*

*CSF indicates cerebrospinal fluid; ND, not done; minus sign, negative or normal; and plus sign, positive or abnormal.
†Newborns with congenital syphilis.
‡Patient died.

aware that many laboratories do not routinely dilute serum specimens for screening purposes.

Although maternal serology is superior to cord or newborn serum serology, it still may be of benefit to send both maternal and newborn specimens for analysis at delivery. This would provide a fail-safe mechanism in case the maternal specimen is not tested or the mother's specimen was negative due to the prozone phenomenon. This approach has been effective at Kings County Hospital.

Comparison of cord serologic results with newborn serum serologic results yielded more false-positive cord serologic results (10%) than false-negative cord serologic (5%) results. However, the correlation between cord and newborn serum samples results was very good when both specimens were RPR positive, with 91% of the cord and newborn serum samples being within two tube dilutions of one another. The problems with false-positive and false-negative cord results emphasize that the diagnosis of congenital syphilis should not rely on testing of the newborn, but on testing of the mother. Regardless of whether a newborn has positive or NR serologic results, if the mother has syphilis and needs treatment, the newborn needs treatment as well.[12] Since these data suggest that newborn serum testing is not clearly better than cord serum testing, it seems prudent to perform RPR testing on cord rather than newborn serum since it is easier to collect cord blood samples. Additional newborn specimens can be sent in individual cases for clarification of titers as necessary. A newborn should not be discharged from the nursery before the results of the maternal serologic test are available.[5]

Published reports are consistent with the finding that newborns with congenital syphilis can have NR nontreponemal antibodies at birth. In 1933, Roberts[13] found that 37% of a group of 273 newborns with congenital syphilis had an NR Wassermann reaction on cord blood. Mascola et al,[14] investigating 50 newborns with congenital syphilis, found five of 50 newborns had NR serologic findings at birth. More recently, Cohen[12] described seven of 154 newborns with congenital syphilis whose mothers were RPR positive and in whom cord blood was NR. Most newborns with congenital syphilis and NR cord RPRs will have mothers with positive serologic results and so will be identified if maternal screening is performed.

There will always be some newborns and mothers who are so recently infected that they both have NR tests at delivery. In a series of 22 mothers who were delivered of newborns with congenital syphilis, Taber and Huber[3] had six mother-newborn pairs with NR nontreponemal serologic results on both members of the pair. Similarly, Dorfman and Glaser[15] had four mother-newborn pairs in their series who had both NR maternal and cord serology at delivery. The newborns later became symptomatic with congenital syphilis. No serum screening test will identify these mother-newborn pairs.

Our data confirm the belief that a newborn's titer that is fourfold higher than the maternal titer at delivery may be useful in making the diagnosis of congenital syphilis. However, this ratio is not absolutely diagnostic of congenital syphilis. Although this ratio is included in reviews[16] and has been used as a diagnostic criterion for congenital syphilis,[5] there are few data to support its use in the diagnosis of congenital syphilis. Taber and Huber[3] found two of 45 newborns in their series with titers that were fourfold higher than their mothers'. Only one of these newborns had congenital syphilis. Mascola et al[14] had three of 50 newborns with congenital syphilis who had cord titers fourfold higher than their mothers'. Similarly, Srinivasan et al[17] found that only one of eight newborns with congenital syphilis had a titer fourfold higher than the mother's at birth.[17] Our data indicate that it is not a sensitive or predictive test. Only four of the seven newborns with titers fourfold higher than their mothers' had obvious congenital syphilis. However, the three newborns without congenital syphilis did not have all possible tests performed, so the number with congenital syphilis could have been higher. The height of the titer may be more useful than the ratio of cord and maternal titers. All newborns with titers higher than 1:1024 had congenital syphilis, and all of them also had titers fourfold higher than maternal. The newborns with titers lower than 1:1024 and titers fourfold maternal did not have congenital syphilis.

Definitions of congenital syphilis have varied widely in the past few years.[4,5,18] Congenital syphilis was strictly defined in this study to avoid overdiagnosis, and the number of newborns with congenital syphilis was probably higher than the 33 described herein. Use of *T pallidum*-specific IgM Western blot[19] and *T pallidum* immunofluorescent antigen detection tests may provide better identification of infected newborns in the future.

A newborn serum specimen that is fourfold higher than maternal at delivery suggests congenital syphilis but should not be the only criterion used to make the diagnosis. Most newborns with this titer ratio had obvious symptoms, and all had abnormal findings that enabled the diagnosis of congenital syphilis to be made without the use of this ratio.

Syphilis screening used at delivery should identify the largest number of infected mothers and their newborns. Cord screening is inadequate in that one third of infants and mothers will be missed. Using both maternal and newborn screening at delivery is the best way to identify infected mothers and newborns. Newborn cord and additional newborn serum specimens both have problems with false-positive and false-negative results, but cord blood is easier to obtain and is therefore preferable.

This work was aided by clinical research grant 6-FY90-570 from The March of Dimes Birth Defects Foundation, White Plains, NY.

The authors thank Laurence Finberg, MD, and William McCormack, MD, for their helpful comments in the production of this manuscript.

References

1. Umbilical Cord Blood Testing. In: *Official Compilation of Codes*. Albany, NY: Lenz & Riecker Inc; 1989. Rules and regulations of the State of New York, title 10, subpart 69-2.
2. Miller JL, Meyer PG, Parrott NA, Hill JH. A study of the biologic falsely positive reactions for syphilis in children. *J Pediatr.* 1960;57:548-552.
3. Taber LH, Huber TW. Congenital syphilis. *Prog Clin Biol Res.* 1975;3:183-190.
4. Centers for Disease Control. Guidelines for the prevention and control of congenital syphilis. *MMWR.* 1988;37(suppl S-1):1-13.
5. Centers for Disease Control. 1989 sexually transmitted disease treatment guidelines. *MMWR.* 1989;38(suppl S-8):5-15.
6. Zenker P. New case definition for congenital syphilis reporting. *Sex Transm Dis.* 1991;18:44-45.
7. Sarff LD, Platt LH, McCracken G. Cerebrospinal fluid evaluation in neonates: comparison of high-risk infants with and without meningitis. *J Pediatr.* 1976;88:473-477.
8. Rawstron SA, Bromberg K. Failure of recommended maternal therapy to prevent congenital syphilis. *Sex Transm Dis.* 1991;18:102-106.
9. Centers for Disease Control. Congenital syphilis: New York City, 1986-1988. *MMWR.* 1989;38:825-829.
10. Mascola L, Pelosi R, Blount JH, Binkin NJ, Alexander CE, Cates W Jr. Congenital syphilis: why is it still occurring? *JAMA.* 1984;252:1719-1722.
11. Berkowitz KM, Stampf K, Baxi L, Fox HE. False negative screening tests for syphilis in pregnant women. *N Engl J Med.* 1990;322:270-271.
12. Cohen DA. Congenital syphilis. *N Engl J Med.* 1991;324:1063-1064.
13. Roberts MH. Congenital syphilis. *AJDC.* 1933;45:463-474.
14. Mascola L, Pelosi R, Blount JH, Alexander CE, Cates W Jr. Congenital syphilis revisited. *AJDC.* 1985;139:575-580.
15. Dorfman DH, Glaser JH. Congenital syphilis in infants after the newborn period. *N Engl J Med.* 1990;323:1299-1302.
16. Ikeda MK, Jenson HB. Evaluation and treatment of congenital syphilis. *J Pediatr.* 1990;117:843-852.
17. Srinivasan G, Ramanurthy RS, Bharathi A, Voora S, Pildes R. Congenital syphilis: a diagnostic and therapeutic dilemma. *Pediatr Infect Dis J.* 1983;2:436-441.
18. Rathbun KC. Congenital syphilis: a proposal for improved surveillance, diagnosis, and treatment. *Sex Transm Dis.* 1983;10:102-107.
19. Sanchez PJ, McCracken GH, Wendel GD, Olsen K, Threlkeld N, Norgard MV. Molecular analysis of the fetal IgM response to *Treponema pallidum* antigens: implications for improved serodiagnosis of congenital syphilis. *J Infect Dis.* 1989;159:508-517.

How Are Pediatric Training Programs Preparing Residents for Practice?

Larrie W. Greenberg, MD; Pamela Getson, PhD; Cynthia Brasseux; Evan G. Pattishall III, MD; Sudesh Kataria, MD; Glen S. Bartlett, MD, PhD; Susan B. Tully, MD; Daniel Shea, MD

• The majority of pediatric residents continue to choose a career in practice on completion of their training. Despite knowing residents' career preferences, many training programs have focused on inpatient tertiary care at the expense of primary care. Perhaps this reflects service needs and the significant technology and extensive information resulting in the growth of pediatric subspecialties. To determine the spectrum of didactic and clinical experiences pediatric training programs offer residents to prepare them for managing a practice, we conducted a survey of pediatric training program directors in 1988. Although the majority of residency programs have a practice management curriculum, the number of hours devoted to this area is minimal. In addition, a significant number of residents are not experiencing a community office rotation. This survey indicates the need to develop a practice management curriculum if trainees are to be prepared for choosing the right career and for being competitive in practice.

(*AJDC.* 1991;145:1389-1392)

Preparing pediatric residents for careers in primary care practice has not been a major emphasis in most medical training programs.[1,2] During the 1960s and 1970s, residency training focused on inpatient tertiary and subspecialty care, with primary care almost exclusively addressed within the confines of medical centers that serve an urban, poor population. Residents received little exposure to community pediatric resources and personnel outside the hospital.

The changing face of pediatric practice from the 1980s through the 1990s has been shaped by increased competition for patients, government regulations, rising costs of inpatient care, and other forces such as managed care. These changes have resulted in new career opportunities in primary care for residents. Since the majority of residents who complete their training continue to choose a career in practice, many programs have recently recognized the need to incorporate education about community practice into the curricula to prepare residents for this career path.

The purpose of this survey was to determine what pediatric training programs are doing to prepare residents to manage a practice more effectively. The need for a survey addressing this issue was based on three criteria: (1) practitioners believe that their training did not adequately prepare them for practice[3]; (2) the majority of pediatric residents are involved in general pediatrics after completing residency; and (3) residents need to be exposed to practice by means of didactic and practical experiences to make informed career choices.[4]

To determine what didactic and clinical experiences pediatric training programs offer residents to prepare them for managing a practice, a survey was conducted of all pediatric training program directors in 1988. Members of the Education Committee of the Ambulatory Pediatric Association and representatives from the American Academy of Pediatrics assisted in the development of the survey questionnaire, which was mailed in March and June 1988 to all approved pediatric training programs. The questionnaire requested detailed information on whether each program included a curriculum devoted to practice management, and solicited information on didactic and clinical experiences, the settings for training, and faculty who were included in the program. Statistical analyses were performed using either descriptive statistics or analysis of variance (ANOVA) F tests, Students t tests, and χ^2 tests, as appropriate, for either discontinuous or continuous and normally distributed variables. All tests for significance were two-tailed, and the criterion for significance was $\alpha = .05$.

Accepted for publication July 5, 1991.

From the Education Committee of the Ambulatory Pediatric Association (Drs Greenberg, Pattishall, Kataria, Bartlett, and Tully), McLean, VA, and Children's National Medical Center (Drs Greenberg and Getson and Ms Brasseux), and the Department of Pediatrics, George Washington University School of Medicine (Drs Greenberg and Getson), Washington, DC. Dr Shea is president of the American Academy of Pediatrics, Elk Grove Village, Ill.

Reprint requests to Children's National Medical Center, the Office of Medical Education, 111 Michigan Ave NW, Washington, DC 20010 (Dr Greenberg).

Purpose.—*This department is intended to share information concerning educational efforts in the broad field of pediatrics. We welcome studies on the following topics: undergraduate and graduate education in medicine and allied health occupations; continuing education of health professionals; education of patients and families; and health education for the general public, the community, and organizations that contribute to the promotion and improvement of the health of children.*

Table 1.—Curriculum Hours in Practice Management*

Teaching Format	Resident Year	No. of Hours Mean±SD	Median	Range
Didactic	PL-1 (n=78)	4.6±5.4	3.0	0-20
	PL-2 (n=79)	5.0±4.9	3.0	0-20
	PL-3 (n=92)	7.8±8.5	4.5	0-50
Clinical experience	PL-1 (n=49)	31.9±4.0	0.0	0-360
	PL-2 (n=63)	55.0±81.8	10.0	0-360
	PL-3 (n=72)	79.5±79.2	4.0	0-400

*n indicates number of programs; PL, pediatric level.

RESULTS

Of the 233 resident training program directors surveyed, 137 (59%) responded after two mailings; their responses are included in the data presented.

Program Information

Survey respondents represented pediatric residency programs that included pediatric departments of university hospitals (38%), children's hospitals (21%), university-affiliated community hospitals (29%), non–university-affiliated community hospitals (3%), the military (7%), and unspecified programs (2%). Residency program directors stated that 59% of graduates in the previous 5 years had entered pediatric practice, 25% selected academic medicine, 12% entered the military or the public health service, 2% opted for research, and 2% chose other miscellaneous fields. Of those graduates completing their residency program in June 1987, 45% chose direct entry into pediatric practice, 29% opted for a fellowship with intent to enter academic medicine, 10% opted for a fellowship with intent to enter practice, while the smallest attributed selections were in the fields of military or public health (12%). Four percent of respondents chose other fields.

Curriculum and Education Issues

Two thirds of the resident program directors stated that their curriculum specifically included experiences designed to prepare residents for entry into the practice setting. Content areas reportedly offered included career decisions; establishing, joining, or managing a practice; community involvement; continuing medical education; participation in professional organizations; professional interests; and personal life-style. For most of the content areas listed, there was a progressively increased involvement of residents during the 3-year training period.

Program directors were asked to delineate the number of curriculum hours devoted to practice management at each residency level and in which format these presentations were offered (Table 1). The opportunities for clinical experiences increased progressively with the residency level and represented the major emphasis of time in the curricula. The number of didactic hours was limited, but increased slightly as residents progressed through their pediatric training. At pediatric level 1 (PL-1), six programs assigned more than 100 hours of clinical experience as did 13 programs at pediatric level 2 (PL-2) and 25 programs at pediatric level 3 (PL-3), causing the distribution and mean values to be positively skewed.

The survey also determined who provided instruction and the mode of presentation (Table 2). Examination of the survey responses revealed that full-time and voluntary faculty provided most of the teaching, and business consultants and hospital administrators also provided didactic presentations.

When program directors were asked how they chose the teaching faculty for practice management programs, 14 (12.3%) of 114 stated that they accepted all full-time and community volunteers; 55 (48.2%) said that they evaluated each prospective volunteer; and 78 (68.4%) declared that they recruited specific faculty. Some program directors used more than one approach.

A majority of the management programs offered experiences in community practice settings; in fact, 116 programs included elective (55%) or mandatory (38%) practice experiences in their curricula. Eight programs (7%) offered both elective and mandatory office experiences. In those in which the opportunity was elective, a mean of 2.8%, 17.5%, and 26.2% of PL-1s, PL-2s, and PL-3s, respectively, chose this option as part of their residency program.

The average length of time a resident spent in a community practice varied with the level of training (Table 3). Opportunities for this experience increased with training level and were most available to PL-2s and PL-3s ($P=.0001$). The most frequently reported amount of time available to these residents was a range of 1 to 4 weeks in an office setting.

Programs offered community office rotations to residents in a variety of practice settings: group practices, health maintenance organizations, health departments, school health programs, solo practices, and the military. Group and solo practices were predictably most frequently used, but health departments played a surprisingly large role, as did health maintenance organizations.

Seventy-four percent of the faculty members were generally informed of the curricular objectives, that is, what to teach. The day-to-day expectations and responsibilities of the resident in the practice setting included accompanying the practitioner on hospital rounds (67.8%), observing only (8.5%), observing and providing patient care (86.4%), and only providing patient care (6%).

Ninety-one percent of the programs required preceptors to complete written evaluations of each resident's performance, but only 69% required written evaluations of the experience and of the preceptor by the resident. Of those having measured responses, the program directors believed that the majority of both residents and preceptors considered the experience very good to excellent. Training program directors noted the major strengths of the office rotation were faculty commitment and resources, clinical setting, practical experience, curriculum, and resident-faculty relationship. Faculty commitment and resources, in addition to the physical setting of the experience, were rated the top two strengths.

Separate ANOVA F tests with post hoc comparisons were used to compare either hours of didactic or clinical experience assigned to pediatric level residents across different program types. A statistically significantly different number of hours was noted for PL-1s across practice settings ($P=.0178$). Post hoc comparisons indicated that the number of didactic hours offered to PL-1 residents was similar among university-affiliated community hospitals, children's hospitals, and pediatric departments in university hospitals; however, the number of didactic hours was

Table 2.—Faculty, Format, and Time Spent in Practice Management Curriculum

Faculty	Total Time Spent, % Mean ± SD	Median	Range	Teaching Format, (%)
Practice management consultants	11.4±23.9	0	0-100	Didactic (100)
Business consultants	8.0±20.0	0	0-100	Didactic (100)
Full-time faculty	37.8±33.2	30	0-100	Didactic (65; practice (25); both (10)
Voluntary	38.0±32.3	40	0-100	Didactic (48); practice (25); both (27)
Hospital administration	4.7±9.8	0	0-50	Didactic (100)

Table 3.—Time Spent in an Office*

Resident Year†	Amount of Time, % of Residents: None	1 d	1-5 d	1-4 wk	>4 wk
PL-1 (n=84)	65	6	4	13	12
PL-2 (n=104)	38	4	10	29	19
PL-3 (n=121)	12	2	7	57	22

*$P=.0001$; $\chi^2=78.167$.
†PL indicates pediatric level.

Table 4.—Percentage of Office Experience Hours in the Pediatric Level 1 (n=48)

Institutional Setting	Amount of Time, % of Residents: None	1-3 h	4-8 h	>8 h
Children's hospitals (n=8)	100	0	0	0
Pediatric departments (n=21)	62	0	19	19
Military (n=6)	33	0	0	67
Community hospital, university-affiliated (n=13)	61	8	0	31
Community hospital, non–university-affiliated (n=0)	0	0	0	0

Table 5.—Time Spent in Elective and Mandatory Office Experiences by Pediatric Level (PL)

Resident Year	Amount of Time, No. of Residents: <1 month	>1 month	P	χ^2
PL-1 (n=67)				
Elective	38	1	<.01	9.480
Mandatory	20	8		
PL-2 (n=84)				
Elective	43	5	<.01	6.693
Mandatory	24	12		
PL-3 (n=98)				
Elective	57	5	<.001	17.903
Mandatory	20	16		

significantly higher for military residency programs. No statistical differences were found among the types of residency programs and number of didactic hours for PL-2 and PL-3 residents. Similarly, no statistical differences were noted for the number of clinical hours offered among the types of residency programs for PL-1 and PL-2 residents. Although based on the report of only 48 hospitals, pediatric departments, military, and university-affiliated community hospital programs were more likely to involve PL-1s in a limited office experience than residency programs at children's hospitals. Table 4 shows categorical summaries of the reported hours. For PL-3 residents, there was a significant difference in the number of hours offered between military training programs and university-affiliated or children's hospital programs, with the number of clinical hours offered for PL-3s in military programs being significantly higher ($P=.0459$).

Results of the *t* tests showed that differences in the number of full-time or general/ambulatory pediatric faculty were not statistically significantly different between those programs that did and those programs that did not prepare residents for practice. Similarly, time spent in an office setting did not differ significantly between these groups. The number of residents in a training program also did not differ between programs with and without a practice management or office experience curriculum. Results of a χ^2 analysis indicated no statistically significant relationship between whether a program offered a curriculum and included time in an office setting. A significant ($P=.0103$) relationship exists between program curriculum type and office experience (elective or mandatory), with those programs without specific practice curricula more likely offering outside experience as an elective rather than a mandatory part of the program. In programs in which residents spent less time (<1 month) in offices, there was more likely to be an elective experience with each of the pediatric resident levels (PL-1, $P=.0021$; PL-2, $P=.0097$; and PL-3, $P=.0001$). For all pediatric residents, rotations of more than a month were more likely to be mandatory (Table 5). The requirement for preceptor evaluations was no more likely to occur in elective office rotations than in mandatory office rotations; however, residents' evaluations were more likely to be required for mandatory programs ($\chi^2=4.4$; $P=.0360$). No statistical relationship existed between the residents' and preceptors' evaluations of the rotation and the amount of time spent in an office setting as reported by resident training directors. The reported evaluations of the preceptors and residents were highly statistically correlated ($r=.78$, $P<.001$).

COMMENT

The practice of pediatrics has undergone major transformation. As an example, infants with failure to thrive may have been routinely hospitalized in the past, but now are often assessed and treated as outpatients. Diagnosis-related groups have mandated shorter hospital stays, changed reimbursement procedures, and shifted care to the home, clinics, health departments, and private pediatric offices. Other influencing variables include uncompensated care, the focus on tertiary care, high operational costs in medical centers, and competition among trainees for patients in university-based programs. These forces, among others, have stimulated the academic community to reexamine how care and training have traditionally been offered and to open new partnerships with resources in the community.

Program directors confirmed that in the previous 5 years, a majority of their graduates continued to enter practice. Finding that two thirds of the resident program directors have curricula that specifically address preparing a resident for practice was more than was anticipated. We postulated that those programs with a practice management curriculum would have a larger number of residents in the program, but this assumption was not supported statistically. While the number of residents in a program is not a critical factor, scheduling, enlisting faculty, and agreeing on core curriculum are key variables that must be considered in the development of this curriculum.

The major responsibility for teaching the curriculum is assumed by full-time and voluntary faculty, but programs do involve nonmedical personnel in teaching didactic issues as they pertain to practice. Although it was hypothesized that those departments with large numbers of general/ambulatory faculty would more likely have curricula addressing practice management, this was not the case for either didactic or practice experiences. The incorporation of this program into the curriculum may be more dependent on an individual or core group of faculty who assume leadership and advisory roles in this area.

Our data confirm that a greater emphasis is given to practice management in the military than in other training programs. This focus perhaps reflects requirements of military residents on their completion of training, ie, that they administer and provide care in a military health care facility. The military health system is structured and consistent across different service branches and resembles a pre-paid health maintenance organization. In this setting, there is no need for residents to spend time in private offices because their needs are met from within the program.

Not unexpectedly, the survey documents that a number of residency programs still do not offer any experience to residents in an office setting outside the medical center. This is in spite of the fact that in the American Medical Association's *Directory of Graduate Medical Education Programs*, the section on pediatrics states that certain aspects of ambulatory care deserve special attention, such as office electives or preceptorships, and the implementation of such experiences would be an important consideration in the accreditation review.[5] Thirty-nine percent of programs do not include an office rotation for PL-2s and it is precisely at this level that residents are trying to make informed career decisions. More programs are involved in the office concept as the PL-3 year is approached, but this timing can create confusion for residents when there are pressures to make an earlier career decision, such as committing to a fellowship in their second year of training.

Those programs with formal curricula tend to offer more didactic information during the PL-1 year than other levels of training and an increasing amount of practical experience, with progression through the PL-2 and PL-3 years. However, on average, the actual number of curricular hours offered at each resident level of training is minimal, at best, with median values even lower. Two major factors were related to whether an office experience was mandatory or elective: the presence of a curriculum, and the resident spending 1 month or more in an office. Both of these factors demonstrate a commitment on the part of the training program to this concept.

The variety of practice settings used by residency programs is impressive, from traditional solo or group practices to health departments and health maintenance organizations. As the practice of medicine becomes more complex and the delivery of health care changes, residents will need to observe these differences first-hand to make their career plans and consider their career options. Examining their priorities and seeing how these best fit with what is available in practice options are more likely to result in career satisfaction.

Although there may be some sampling bias in that we did not follow up with nonresponders, this survey documents that the majority of residency training programs have at least some curricula to prepare residents to enter pediatric practice. The problem is that the number of hours devoted to practice management is generally minimal, considering the number of trainees who choose practice for their career. In addition, a significant number of residents are not experiencing a community office rotation, which when offered in the curriculum, is rated highly. Participation in the office setting can assist residents in determining if practice is the most desirable career path. Finally, this study indicates the need to develop a meaningful curriculum in practice management if graduates of residency programs in the 1990s are going to be prepared for and competitive in pediatric practice. For those programs planning to implement a practice management curriculum, a number of models have been described.[6-11] Reaching a consensus on a core curriculum in this area from organizations such as the Ambulatory Pediatric Association, American Academy of Pediatrics, and the Association of Medical School Pediatric Department Chairmen would be an important contribution.

References

1. Kotak D, Palermo AM. Pediatric primary care in hospitals. In: O'Shea JS, ed. *Effectiveness of Pediatric Primary Care*. Lexington, Mass: Collamore Press; 1988:75-92.

2. Roemer MI. *Ambulatory Health Services in America*. Rockville, Md: Aspen Systems Corp; 1981:7.

3. Task Force on Pediatric Education. *The Future of Pediatric Education*. Evanston, Ill: American Academy of Pediatrics; 1978.

4. Greenberg LW, Jewett LS, Einhorn AH, Leibowitz ZB, Cohen LF. Career counseling practices in pediatric residency training programs. *AJDC*. 1990;144:497-501.

5. *1990-1991 Directory of Graduate Medical Education Programs*. Chicago, Ill: American Medical Association; 1990:95.

6. Greenberg LW. Teaching primary care pediatrics to pediatric residents through an office rotation. *J Med Educ*. 1979; 54:340-342.

7. Altemeier WA III, St Petery L, Scheibler GL. The demonstration of private practice to pediatric residents through an office rotation. *J Med Educ*. 1976;51:138-140.

8. McKay RJ Jr. The academic pediatrician and the practicing pediatrician. *AJDC*. 1985;139:39-40.

9. Reeb KG. Education of residents in the pediatric office. *Pediatr Clin North Am*. 1981;28:601-615.

10. Sargent JR, Osborn LM. Resident training in community pediatricians' offices. *AJDC*. 1990;144:1356-1359.

11. Mankad VN, Shell RT. Development of a model practice for pediatric residents: economic and administrative considerations. *Clin Pediatr*. 1982;21:519-524

Breathing Patterns and Heart Rates at Ages 6 Weeks and 2 Years

Christian F. Poets, MD; Valerie A. Stebbens; John R. Alexander, MSc, FSS MIS; David P. Southall, MD, FRCP

• Forty-two randomly selected, full-term, healthy infants underwent 24-hour electrocardiographic recordings and breathing movements at about ages 6 weeks (median age, 43 days; range, 34 to 61 days) and 2 years (median age, 26 months; range, 21 to 35 months). The number and duration of apneic pauses of 3.6 seconds or longer were analyzed. Periodic apnea was defined as a sequence of three or more apneic pauses, each separated by fewer than 20 breaths. All other apneic pauses were defined as isolated. Median heart rates and respiratory rates, which were measured during regular breathing, decreased from 137/min and 35/min to 98/min and 21/min, respectively. The total duration of periodic apnea remained unchanged (median, 0.06 min/h vs 0.05 min/h). Although the median frequency of all isolated apneic pauses decreased from 3.6/h to 2.5/h, the number of those that were longer than 6 seconds increased from 0.37/h to 0.80/h, leading to an increase in the proportion of these pauses, among all isolated apneic pauses, from 10% at age 6 weeks to 32% at age 2 years. Only one apneic pause in one infant at age 6 weeks, but eight pauses in six children at age 2 years, were longer than 15 seconds. A knowledge of such normal variability in the duration of apneic pauses in older infants and young children is essential for the interpretation of pneumograms and alarms while monitoring breathing movements.

(*AJDC.* 1991;145:1393-1396)

Many studies have analyzed heart rates and breathing patterns in infancy[1-5] and found that the frequency of apneic pauses during the first 6 months of life decreases with age. It has been suggested that this decrease indicates a maturational process in the respiratory center of the brain stem. Data to follow this process into childhood have not been available.

Long-term recordings of respiration and heart rate (pneumograms) are used to identify an abnormal regulation of breathing in infants who are considered at risk of sudden death. Based on normative data obtained in full-term infants in their first 6 months of life, the finding of prolonged apneic pauses in these recordings is widely considered to indicate a potentially dangerous abnormality in the regulation of respiration.[6-8] The definition of prolonged apneic pauses varies. While many authors follow that of the American Academy of Pediatrics, which defined a prolonged apneic pause as a cessation in breathing movements of 20 seconds or longer,[8] others regard any apneic pause longer than 15 seconds as prolonged.[6,9,10] As a result, an alarm threshold of 10 to 20 seconds is used in most home monitors, which detect an absence of breathing movements.[11-13]

Prospective population-based studies, however, have failed to show that prolonged apneic pauses are more frequent in infants who subsequently die of sudden infant death syndrome.[14] Moreover, there is little knowledge about normal breathing patterns beyond the first 6 months of life. In this study, 24-hour electrocardiographic recordings and abdominal wall movements were performed sequentially in 42 healthy, full-term infants at about ages 6 weeks and 2 years.

SUBJECTS AND METHODS

Forty-two full-term subjects were selected at random from a population-based sample who had undergone an initial recording at about age 6 weeks as part of a prospective study of sudden infant death syndrome.[14] For the purpose of this study, parental consent was given to an additional recording in this subgroup at age 2 years. Parents were reassured that the aim of the study was the acquisition of normal data, and that the recording would not interfere with the normal care of their child. Of the 42 children studied, 22 were male. Their birth weights ranged from 2500 g to 4560 g (median, 3350 g), and gestational age at birth from 38 weeks to 42 weeks (median, 40 weeks).

Recordings were performed in the children's homes between 34 days and 61 days (median, 43 days) and between ages 21 months and 35 months (median, 26 months). Recordings were performed only if the child was in good health, that is, free of major symptoms or disease. At the time of the 6-week recording, three infants were reported to have colic, and four were reported to have a cold (cough and/or sniffles). At the time of the second recording, 10 children were reported to have a cold.

All subjects underwent 24-hour recordings of their heart rates (from a modified lead I configuration) and breathing movements (Graseby pressure capsule). These signals were recorded on a portable cassette recorder (Medilog 1, Oxford Medical Systems, Oxford, England). The recordings were set up by a research worker and terminated by the parents about

Accepted for publication June 10, 1991.

From the Department of Pediatrics, National Heart & Lung Institute, London (Drs Poets and Southall, and Mrs Stebbens), and the Department of Statistics, Hazleton UK Ltd, Harrogate, England (Dr Alexander).

Reprint requests to the Department of Pediatrics, National Heart & Lung Institute, Dovehouse Street, London SW3 6HP, England (Dr Southall).

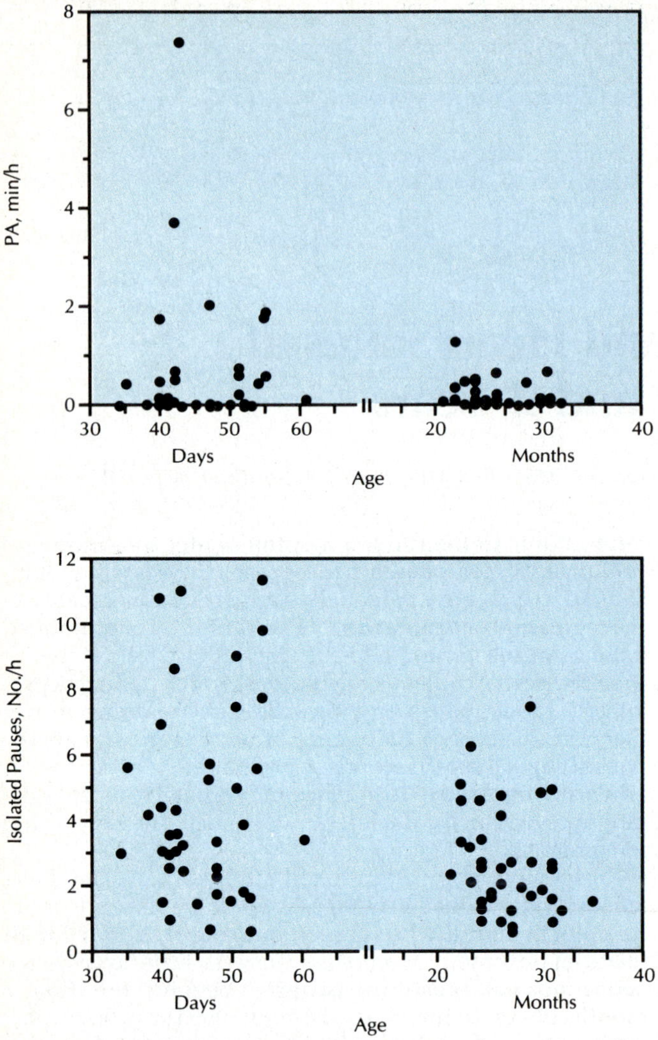

Duration of periodic apnea (PA) in minutes per hour of recording (top), and number of isolated apneic pauses of 3.6 seconds or longer per hour of recording (bottom), related to age at the time of the recording. Note the different units on the x axis.

24 hours later. The ability of the pressure capsule transducer to provide accurate information on breathing patterns has been verified by comparison with simultaneous recordings using impedance pneumography, respiratory inductance, and jacket plethysmography.[15]

The recordings were replayed with an ink jet chart recorder (Mingograf 34T, Siemens-Elema, Stockholm, Sweden) at a speed of 1.2 s/mm. Printouts were analyzed by three workers who were blind to the source of the data. Periods of regular and nonregular breathing patterns were defined as described previously.[5] In summary, regular breathing is a reproducible pattern in which breathing movements are steady in rate and amplitude. Periods not conforming to this definition were classified as nonregular. Heart and respiratory rates were analyzed at the middle of each period of regular breathing for 6 seconds and 1 minute, respectively, at least 10 seconds away from apneic pauses or sighs, and averaged for the whole recording. Pauses in breathing movements of 3.6 seconds or longer were counted and their durations measured. These apneic pauses were grouped according to their duration, that is, 3.6 seconds to 6 seconds, 6.1 seconds to 12 seconds, or greater than 12 seconds. Periodic apnea was defined as a sequence of three or more apneic pauses, with each pause separated by fewer than 20 breaths.[5] All apneic pauses appearing out of such sequences were regarded as isolated. The term periodic apnea was chosen rather than periodic breathing, as the latter includes recurrent episodes of hypoventilation,[5] which were not included in this analysis.

Comparison of Variables Measured at Ages 6 Weeks and 2 Years*

Variable	Median (Range) 6 wk	Median (Range) 2 y	*P*
Respiratory rate, breaths/min	35 (23-51)	21 (15-31)	<.001
Heart rate, beats/min	137 (96-159)	98 (73-120)	<.001
Duration of PA, min/h	0.06 (0.0-7.4)	0.05 (0.0-1.3)	NS
No. of pauses in PA/h	0.2 (0.0-23.9)	0.2 (0.0-3.8)	NS
% of pauses in PA 3.6 - 6.0 s	85 (40-100)	77 (50-100)	NS
% of pauses in PA 6.1 - 12.0 s	13 (0-60)	19 (0-50)	NS
% of pauses in PA >12.0 s	0 (0-3)	0 (0-25)	NS
No. of isolated pauses per hour	3.6 (0.7-11.5)	2.5 (0.6-7.5)	<.01
% of isolated pauses 3.6 - 6.0 s	89 (64-100)	65 (37-90)	<.001
% of isolated pauses 6.1 - 12.0 s	10 (0-36)	32 (10-57)	<.001
% of isolated pauses >12 s	0 (0-3)	0 (0-13)	<.001
Duration of longest pause overall, s	9.0 (6.0-18.0)	12.6 (7.2-19.2)	<.001

**P* values were obtained using the Wilcoxon Signed Rank Test; PA indicates periodic apnea, and NS, not significant.

Results are presented as means and SDs or medians and ranges for each variable, with frequencies per hour of recording. Comparisons between values obtained at ages 6 weeks and 2 years were performed using Wilcoxon's Signed Rank Test. Correlations were assessed using Spearman's rank correlation coefficient.

RESULTS

The mean duration of the initial recording was 22.4 hours (SD, 1.1 hour), and of the second recording, 21.0 hours (SD, 2.3 hours). The mean duration of regular breathing was 3.7 hours (SD, 0.9 hour) at about age 6 weeks, and 3.3 hours (SD, 1.8 hours) at age 2 years. The initial and follow-up recordings did not show a significant difference in any of the variables studied between subjects with and without a cold ($P>.05$, Mann-Whitney *U* test). There was also no evidence that, within the range of ages at each recording, age affected the results (Figure). Therefore, results for both the initial and follow-up recordings are presented without regard to age or the presence of a cold, and are summarized in the Table.

Heart and respiratory rates were significantly lower at age 2 years. Every recording contained apneic pauses. In their initial recordings, 29 infants (69%) showed periodic apnea; this proportion remained almost constant, with 67% of the recordings (28) obtained at age 2 years containing such episodes. Neither the number of pauses during periodic apnea nor the proportion of time spent in this pattern changed significantly. However, at age 6 weeks, there was a small number of infants with extremely long-summed durations of periodic apnea. By age 2 years, most of these extreme values were not seen (Figure). The proportion of periodic apneic pauses longer than 6 seconds was higher at age 2 years than at age 6 weeks; however, these differences were not significant.

The frequency of isolated apneic pauses was significantly lower at about age 2 years ($P<.01$). Again, this distribution was more skewed at age 6 weeks than at age 2 years (Figure). In contrast, the mean duration of these pauses was longer, as expressed by the increase in the proportion of isolated apneic pauses with durations of more than 6 seconds. Thus, the overall trend in the frequency of isolated apneic pauses to decrease was reversed for the group of pauses of 6.1 seconds to 12 seconds, whose median frequency more than doubled from 0.37/h at age 6 weeks to 0.80/h at age 2 years ($P<.02$). Moreover, the median duration of the longest apneic pause (isolated or periodic) observed in each recording was significantly longer at age 2 years than at age 6 weeks ($P<.001$). In the initial recording, one infant exhibited an apneic pause longer than 15 seconds. In the second recording, six children had a total of eight pauses of greater than 15 seconds in duration.

The frequency of isolated apneic pauses was directly proportional to that of periodic apneic pauses in both the initial and follow-up recordings ($r=.91$ and .80, respectively; $P<.0001$). Thus, at both ages, the subjects with high numbers of isolated apneic pauses also showed more periodic apnea. There was also a significant correlation between individual values at the initial and follow-up recordings for the number of pauses in periodic apnea ($r=.37$, $P<.02$), but not for heart or respiratory rates ($r=.20$ and .12, respectively; $P>.05$), or isolated apneic pauses ($r=.26$, $P=.09$).

COMMENT

This study highlights some of the changes that occur in respiratory patterns between early infancy and early childhood. However, our data address only respiratory rates and pauses in abdominal wall movements. The recording technique used cannot detect such phenomena as obstructive, mixed, or expiratory apnea. Our findings at about age 6 weeks are comparable with those in other studies[1-5] that show a nonnormal distribution of apneic pause frequency and duration of periodic apnea with a wide scattering of values (Figure). However, comparability of absolute figures for apneic pause frequency with those of other studies is limited due to different definitions of apneic pauses. Data concerning respiratory patterns at age 2 years are not available to compare with our findings. Our data remain statistically significant even when adjustment is made for the increased probability of a false-positive result due to multiple tests of significance. Even after making the most conservative adjustments to the *P* values (Bonferroni adjustment), all of the results remain highly significant ($P<.01$).

The proportion of children exhibiting periodic apnea and the median duration of this pattern remained almost constant between the two ages. However, there was a much narrower range in the duration of periodic apnea at age 2 years (Figure). During the first 6 months of life, Carse et al[1] included pauses of 2 seconds or longer in their analysis and found a significant decrease in periodic apnea. In contrast, the study by Richards et al[5] showed that the duration of periodic apnea decreased significantly only between the first and sixth week of life, and remained constant thereafter, whereas Hoppenbrouwers et al[3] analyzed pauses of 3 seconds to 6 seconds and found stable values for periodic apnea during the entire first 6 months of life. From the data in this study, it may be speculated that in the majority of the children, the proportion of time spent in periodic apnea did not change substantially between the second month and the second year of life.

The decreasing number of isolated apneic pauses with age corresponds with results of developmental studies of apneic pause frequency during infancy.[1-3] However, both the proportion of apneic pauses of more than 6 seconds and their absolute number, as well as the duration of the longest apneic pause, were higher at age 2 years than at age 6 weeks. Moreover, apneic pauses longer than 15 seconds, a duration widely considered as abnormal in infancy[6,9,10] and rare in our own group when studied initially, appeared more frequently in the older age group. A tendency for apneic pauses of more than 6 seconds to increase in frequency during the second half of the first 6 months of life, associated with a decreasing frequency of shorter pauses, has been described by Richards et al.[5] These authors also found a positive correlation between age and increasing duration of the longest pause beyond the first month of life.

The present data cannot be used to explain why the duration of apneic pauses increases with age. This increase may be related to the decrease in the respiratory rate, which, together with the activity of lung reflexes, such as the Hering-Breuer lung inflation reflex,[16] may result in longer pauses since the average number of "missed breaths" during an apneic pause remains constant. However, these speculations require further investigation.

Clinically, the finding of pauses of up to 19 seconds in healthy infants is important in relation to the interpretation of pneumograms performed in this age group. Parental reports of alarms occurring on breathing movement detectors used for home monitoring in young children should also be interpreted with caution. As mentioned above, most monitors alarm after breathing movements have not been sensed for 10 seconds to 20 seconds (this interval being derived from studies on young infants). A proportion of infants at risk of sudden death are monitored beyond their first year of life, and the retention of an alarm setting for a 20-second apneic pause will result in alarms from normal respiratory phenomena. Further support for the latter has been given by data from a recent study by Weese-Mayer et al,[17] who performed event recordings of heart rate and breathing movements in infants and children at risk of sudden infant death syndrome. They found an increase in the number of apneic pauses longer than 15 seconds with increasing age, with apneic pauses of 25 seconds or longer becoming a frequent event in children older than age 5 years.

These results suggest that the common definition of an "abnormal" apneic pause duration is too simplistic since it does not account for age. From a physiologic viewpoint, the effect of an apneic pause on blood gas homeostasis must be more important than the duration of the pause. Therefore, future studies on respiratory pathophysiology in infants and young children should include continuous measurements of oxygenation. This approach may provide more direct information about potentially dangerous respiratory pathophysiology.

Dr Poets' research was funded by Deutsche Forschungsgemeinschaft, Bonn, Germany; Mrs Valerie Stebbens by the Nuffield Foundation, London, England; and Dr Southall's by the Royal Brompton National Heart & Lung Hospitals, London, England; and Nellcor Inc, Hayward, Calif.

The authors gratefully acknowledge the support of the British Heart Foundation, London, England; the Foundation for the Study of Infant Deaths, London, England; and the people of Doncaster and Brighton, England, for their support of data collection; Vivian G. Taylor for data management; and Jackie Kelly, Pauline Mills, and Wendy Yates for data analysis.

References

1. Carse EA, Wilkinson AR, Whyte PL, Henderson-Smart DJ, Johnson P. Oxygen and carbon dioxide tensions, breathing and heart rate in normal infants during the first six months of life. *J Dev Physiol.* 1981;3:85-100.

2. Flores-Guevara R, Sternberg B, Guidasci S, Durupt N, Monod N. Respiratory pauses and periodic breathing assessed by cardiopneumography in normal infants and in SIDS-siblings. *Neuropediatrics.* 1986;17:59-62.

3. Hoppenbrouwers T, Hodgman JE, Harper RM, Hofmann E, Sterman MB, McGinty DJ. Polygraphic studies of normal infants during the first six months of life, III: incidence of apnea and periodic breathing. *Pediatrics.* 1977;60:418-425.

4. Hunt CE, Brouillette RT, Hanson D, David RJ, Stein IM, Weissbluth M. Home pneumograms in normal infants. *J Pediatr.* 1985;106:551-555.

5. Richards JM, Alexander JR, Shinebourne EA, de Swiet M, Wilson AJ, Southall DP. Sequential 22-hour profiles of breathing patterns and heart rate in 110 full-term infants during their first 6 months of life. *Pediatrics.* 1984;74:763-777.

6. Steinschneider A. Prolonged apnea and the sudden infant death syndrome: clinical and laboratory observations. *Pediatrics.* 1972;50:646-654.

7. Rigatto H. Apnea. *Pediatr Clin North Am.* 1982;29:1105-1116.

8. Little GA, Ariagno RB, Beckwith B, et al. Task Force on Prolonged Infantile Apnea; prolonged infantile apnea: 1985. *Pediatrics.* 1985;76:129-131.

9. Muttitt SC, Finer NN, Tierney AJ, Rossmann J. Neonatal apnea: diagnosis by nurse versus computer. *Pediatrics.* 1988; 82:713-720.

10. Oren J, Kelly D, Shannon DC. Identification of a high-risk group for sudden infant death syndrome among infants who were resuscitated for sleep apnea. *Pediatrics.* 1986;77:495-499.

11. Rahilly PM, Symonds PF. Simplified pneumographic monitoring of infants at risk from sudden infant death syndrome. *Arch Dis Child.* 1984;59:351-355.

12. Benetele KHP, Albani M, Schulte FJ. Apnoe-Heimüberwachung von Kindern mit erhöhtem Risiko für den plötzlichen Kindstod (SIDS). *Monatsschr Kinderheilkd.* 1986; 134:5-9.

13. Foundation of the Study of Infant Death and the British Paediatric Respiratory Group. Apnoea monitors and sudden infant death. *Arch Dis Child.* 1985;60:76-80.

14. Southall DP, Richards JM, de Swiet M, et al. Identification of infants destined to die unexpectedly during infancy: evaluation of predictive importance of prolonged apnoea and disorders of cardiac rhythm or conduction. *BMJ.* 1983;286:1092-1096.

15. Richards JM. A comparison of recordings obtained using the pressure capsule transducer with those obtained using jacket plethysmography, ribcage and abdominal inductance plethysmography and transthoracic impedance pneumography. In: *Long-term Recordings of Heart Rates and Breathing Patterns of Full-Term Infants During Their First Six Months of Life: Their Possible Relevance to the Sudden Infant Death Syndrome.* London, England: University of London; 1987. Thesis.

16. Rabette PS, Stocks J, Costeloe K. Persistence of the Hering-Breuer reflex beyond the neonatal period. *Eur Respir J.* 1990;3:309. Abstract.

17. Weese-Mayer DE, Morrow AS, Conway LP, Brouillette RT, Silvestri JM. Assessing clinical significance of apnea exceeding fifteen seconds with event recording. *J Pediatr.* 1990; 117:568-574.

Pictures From the Heart

A 7-year-old hemophiliac boy with acquired immunodeficiency syndrome asked his mother why a young friend had recently died. She replied, "You never have to lose somebody you really love. You can keep them with you always in your heart." She continued, "Did you know your heart can take pictures, and they are the best kind because you can take them at the most special moments, and nobody has those same pictures but you."

Oyler C. *Go Toward the Light.* New York, NY: New American Library; 1990:58-59.

Cardiac Care for Infants

Determinants of Hospital Charges for Acute Care

Gail D. Pearson, MD, ScD; Langford Kidd, MD, FRCP; Timothy M. Beittel; Catherine A. Neill, MD, FRCP

• We analyzed hospital use and inpatient charges retrospectively for infants hospitalized at a tertiary referral center in the first year of life for cardiac disease. For 93 infants hospitalized between August 1987 and June 1989, there were 1.8 admissions per patient, with a median stay of 14 days; 24.7% required more than 28 days of acute inpatient care. Total hospital charges (excluding professional fees) in the first year of life were $3 417 612, which represents $36 749 per infant and $35 386 per survivor. Reimbursement totaled 93.2% of charges. Multivariate analysis revealed that complex disease, surgery, and length of stay in the intensive care unit were significantly associated with increased charges, while extracardiac anomalies, birth weight, outcome, and type of insurance were not. The economic benefits of averting infant death outweigh the associated costs by as much as 5.4 to 1. We conclude that current treatment of most infants with cardiac disease is both effective and economically beneficial.

(*AJDC.* 1991;145:1397-1400)

Changes in the management of cardiac disease in infancy during the past 20 years have resulted in a majority of definitive surgical procedures being performed before a child's first birthday[1,2] and thus a concomitant reduction in subsequent operations and hospitalizations. This change has implications for the pattern of expenditures for pediatric cardiac disease in infants. In recent years, attention has been drawn repeatedly to the issues of cost and access to medical care and, more recently, to the question of access to care for children with cardiac disease.[3] It is valuable, therefore, to determine the magnitude of hospital expenditures for infants younger than 1 year with cardiac disease, which in turn allows estimation of the relationship between costs and benefits associated with infant cardiac disease. To do this, we analyzed hospital use and inpatient charges at a tertiary referral center for infants hospitalized for cardiac disease in the first year of life, and we report our findings herein.

Accepted for publication June 24, 1991.

From the Division of Pediatric Cardiology, The Johns Hopkins Hospital, Baltimore, Md.

Presented in part at the Mid-Atlantic Pediatric Cardiology Society Meeting, Bethesda, Md, May 17, 1991.

Reprint requests to the Division of Pediatric Cardiology, The Johns Hopkins Hospital, Brady 516, 600 N Wolfe St, Baltimore, MD 21205 (Dr Neill).

PATIENTS AND METHODS

The present study is part of a larger investigation of determinants of outcome in hospitalized infants with heart disease.[4] Infants admitted to The Johns Hopkins Hospital Children's Center, Baltimore, Md, in 1988 with cardiac disease were identified retrospectively. Information concerning other admissions between birth and 1 year of age was obtained for these infants, thus generating a complete record of inpatient care during the first year of life, which spanned the period from August 1987 through June 1989 for this cohort. Preterm infants with isolated persistent ductus arteriosus were excluded. Only those infants who received all care in the first year of life at The Johns Hopkins Hospital were included, so that data on charges would be comparable for the cohort.

The following patient data were obtained: race, sex, birth weight, source of medical insurance, charges for inpatient care, type of surgery if applicable, number of admissions, total number of days in the hospital and intensive care unit during the first year of life, cardiac diagnoses, extracardiac defect(s), and outcome at 1 year of age. Cardiac disease was classified as complex or noncomplex[4] based on a spectrum of severity. Complex defects comprised those in which there were not two adequately functioning ventricles, including hypoplastic left- and right-heart syndromes, septal malalignment, outflow atresia, and cardiomyopathy. Extracardiac anomalies included chromosomal abnormalities, mendelian and other syndromes, and other major anomalies. Charges for inpatient care for each patient (excluding professional fees), as well as source and amount of reimbursement, were obtained from The Johns Hopkins Hospital Billing Department.

Statistical analysis was performed with the Mann-Whitney *U* test, coefficient of determination, and multivariate techniques. A multiple linear regression model was constructed to examine the effect of each independent variable on total charges, while holding the remaining covariates constant. The following independent variables were entered into the regression equation: complexity of the lesion, presence of extracardiac anomalies, surgery, birth weight, type of insurance, length of stay in the intensive care unit, and 1-year outcome. Length of hospital stay was not included in the model because of the high degree of correlation between this variable and length of stay in the intensive care unit. All tests of significance were two-tailed and were based on rejecting the null hypothesis at the $P = .05$ level.

Approval for the project was granted by the Joint Committee on Clinical Investigation of The Johns Hopkins University School of Medicine and The Johns Hopkins Hospital, Baltimore.

Characteristic	No. (%) of Patients
Complex disease	31 (33.3)
Extracardiac anomaly	29 (31.2)
Both complex disease and extracardiac anomaly	10 (10.8)
1-y mortality	24 (25.8)
Surgery	
Patients	66 (71.0)
Procedures	88 (94.6)

Table 1.—Characteristics of Study Patients (N=93)

RESULTS

Complete data were available for a total of 93 patients who met the study criteria. Characteristics of these infants are presented in Table 1. As shown, 31 patients (33.3%) had complex cardiac disease, 29 (31.2%) had one or more extracardiac anomalies, and 10 (10.8%) had both complex disease and extracardiac anomalies. The infant mortality rate in the total cohort was 25.8% (24/93). A total of 66 patients (71.0%) had undergone 88 surgical procedures, or 0.9 procedure per study patient and 1.3 procedures per patient who underwent surgery.

Hospital admissions totaled 167, or 1.8 per patient, with a median length of stay of 14 days (range, 1 to 241 days). Twenty-three infants (24.7%) required more than 28 days of acute inpatient care during the first year of life. Of the 2679 total hospital days, 1642 (61.3%) were spent in intensive care units.

Data concerning hospital charges are shown in the Figure. Total hospital charges (excluding professional fees) in the first year of life were $3 417 612, which represents $36 749 per infant (range, $1003 to $306 043). Hospital charges are separated by The Johns Hopkins Hospital into eight categories. Routine care charges (for basic room, board, and nursing) accounted for 52.1% of the total ($1 776 188). The second largest component of total charges was laboratory charges (10.2%; $350 086); this component includes charges for respiratory care, such as ventilators and blood gas analyses. Other charges were for medical and surgical supplies (8.6%; $294 867), physical therapy (7.5%; $255 849), operating room time and supplies (6.8%; $234 345), radiologic procedures (5.8%; $198 921), pharmacy supplies (4.7%; $160 542), and blood and related products (4.3%; $146 814).

Table 2 presents information about the source and amount of reimbursement for these charges. The total amount of reimbursement, $3 185 322, represents 93.2% of total charges, leaving 6.8% as unreimbursed care. Medical Assistance was the largest single third-party payer, with 36.7% of total reimbursement, followed by "other sources," which included commercial insurers and self-payment (35.5%) and Blue Cross (27.4%). CHAMPUS accounted for less than 1% of total reimbursement.

Mean charges for infants with complex cardiac disease were 53.2% higher than for infants with noncomplex disease ($47 820 vs $31 213), but this difference did not reach statistical significance (Mann-Whitney *U*, 810; *P*=.22). Similarly, mean charges for infants with extracardiac anomalies were 69.1% higher than for infants without such anomalies ($51 123 vs $30 235); this difference was statistically significant (Mann Whitney *U*, 679; *P*=.04). If

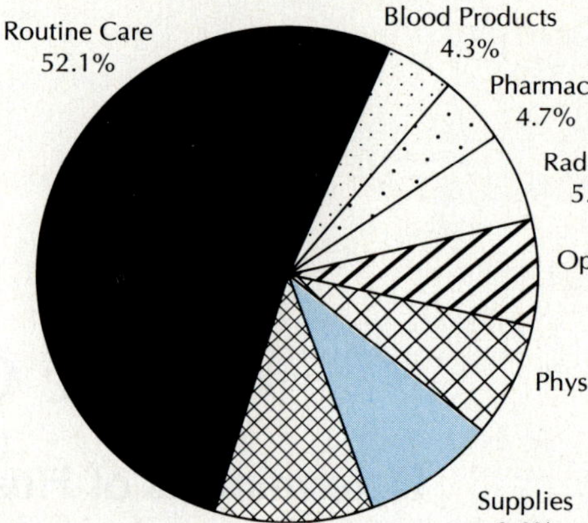

Breakdown of hospital charges. Total hospital charges were $3 417 612.

Table 2.—Source and Amount of Reimbursement

Source of Reimbursement	Amount, $	% of Charges
Medical Assistance	1 168 059	34.2
Blue Cross	871 716	25.5
CHAMPUS	13 367	0.4
Other (commercial, self-pay)	1 132 180	33.1
Total Reimbursement	**3 185 322**	**93.2**

the mean charges for infants with neither complex cardiac disease nor extracardiac anomalies are compared with those for other study infants, even more striking differences emerge. Infants with neither complex disease nor anomalies had mean charges 61.1% lower than those for other infants ($20 345 vs $53 013; Mann-Whitney *U*, 682; *P*=.003).

For infants who died before age 1 year, mean charges were $40 664, compared with survivors for whom mean charges were $35 386, a 14.9% difference (Mann-Whitney *U*, 800; *P*=.8). Another, more conservative way to assess costs of care is to attribute all hospital charges incurred by the 93 study infants to be of the 69 survivors. When this is done, the mean charge per survivor is calculated to be $49 531.

Undergoing one or more surgical procedures significantly affected mean charges ($46 708 vs $12 402; Mann-Whitney *U*, 299; *P*<.0001). Length of hospital stay was highly correlated with charges (r^2=.9470; *P*<.0001), as was length of stay in the intensive care unit (r^2=.9299; P<.0001).

Results of the multiple linear regression analysis are shown in Table 3, which includes variable estimates for each independent variable, the *t* value for each variable estimate, and the F value and r^2 for the model. The F value indicates that the model as a whole is statistically significant (ie, significantly different in explanatory ability from having no model), and the r^2 value indicates that the independent variables together explain approximately 90% of the variance in the dependent variable, charges. As

Table 3.—Results of Multiple Linear Regression Analysis (Dependent Variable Is Hospital Charges) ($F=117.54$ and $r^2=.9006$)

Independent Variable	Variable Estimate	t for Null Hypothesis (Variable = 0*)
Complex disease (1 = yes)	+7531.36	2.062†
Surgery (1 = yes)	+20,464.21	5.104‡
Days spent in intensive care unit	+1472.93	23.395‡
Extracardiac anomalies (1 = yes)	−1751.47	−0.448
Outcome (1 = yes)	−1260.53	−0.292
Birth weight, g	+2.46	0.950
Insurance (1 = private)	−6371.15	−1.644

*t Test value when testing the null hypothesis that the variable does not differ significantly from zero.
†$P<.05$.
‡$P<.0001$.

shown, complex disease was significantly associated with increased charges in this model, but extracardiac anomalies were not, in contrast to the univariate results. Surgery and length of stay in the intensive care unit also were significantly associated with increased charges, while the remaining variables showed no significant association.

COMMENT

In a population of infants with cardiac disease requiring hospitalization in the first year of life, we found that nearly 75% survived and that the mean first-year hospital expenditure (excluding professional fees) was $36 749 for all infants and $35 386 per survivor. Data regarding professional fees were difficult to obtain retrospectively and hence were not included in the formal analysis. Some information was available, however, for 60 of the 93 study infants, for whom hospital charges were $2 408 939, estimated cardiology fees were $150 612, and estimated surgery fees were $148 050 (40 of the 60 underwent surgery). Thus, for infants undergoing surgery, the average professional fee was $6200, representing an additional approximately 15% addition to the mean hospital charge. Data available for 58 of the 60 patients indicated that the average reimbursement rate for professional fees was approximately 47%, in sharp contrast to the rate for hospital charges. Future prospective studies should include more detailed analysis of professional fees charged and of reimbursement rates. It is evident that although physician fees are an important component of overall costs to the family and society, their omission from the present analysis would not bias the overall conclusions.

The benefit of saving a life often is quantified in terms of the economic benefit that individual can be expected to contribute to society during a productive lifetime. For children younger than 1 year, the present value of lifetime earnings has been conservatively estimated at $191 184 (based on means for men and women).[5] Employing this figure, we estimate the economic benefits of averting death in infancy for the 69 survivors to be $13 191 696 compared with total hospital expenditures of $2 441 634, yielding a benefit-to-cost ratio of 5.4 to 1. A number of caveats must be mentioned in interpreting this figure. First, the hospital expenditures are charges, not costs, although charges are likely to exceed costs, making our estimate conservative. Second, the expenditures include only those for acute care for survivors in the first year of life. Other costs for subsequent acute or chronic medical care are excluded, leading to possible underestimation of chronic medical care costs for infants with extracardiac anomalies, including Down's syndrome. Third, the value of the benefits assumes that all first-year survivors enjoy the productive life expectancy of the average worker. This view may be optimistic, but most recent survivors of cardiac operations performed during early infancy have normal or optimal cardiac health.[6] Even if the medical care expenses are doubled and the estimated societal contribution is halved, however, the benefit-to-cost ratio remains greater than 1 (1.4 to 1). Furthermore, these calculations ignore the inestimable psychological benefit to the family of averting an infant death.

The magnitude of hospital charges reported herein is consistent with results from studies that have examined the costs and benefits of cardiac care[6,7] as well as other technologically intensive medical interventions, such as neonatal intensive care[8,9] and extracorporeal membrane oxygenation.[10] In a study from the New England Regional Infant Cardiac Program concerning the cost of hospital care for infants with cardiac disease, Fyler[11] reported that the cost per patient younger than 1 year was estimated to be $9000, and the cost per survivor was approximately $18 000 (in 1979 dollars). If Fyler's estimated costs are inflated to 1988 dollars,[12] the costs per patient and per survivor would be $18 480 and $36 954, respectively. Fyler's cost analysis, like ours, was based on hospital bills rendered. In our study, mean charges per patient were $36 749, considerably higher than Fyler's adjusted costs. This discrepancy can be explained in large part by differences in surgical management of infants between the late 1970s and the present. In Fyler's population, there was 0.55 surgical procedure per patient younger than 1 year. In contrast, in our study, there was 0.9 surgical procedure per patient younger than 1 year, which reflects the trend toward earlier repair. In our multivariate model, undergoing surgery represented an increase in charges of $20 464, so that the difference in surgery alone could explain a substantial portion of the difference between Fyler's figures and those reported herein.

In contrast to the mean expenditure per patient, the mean expenditure per first-year survivor in our study ($35 386) is lower than the estimated cost (in 1988 dollars) per survivor in Fyler's cohort ($36 749). This almost certainly reflects the emerging paradigm for many newborns with serious heart disease, which is early, definitive surgical repair, followed by a relatively uncomplicated recovery. Moreover, the survivors in our cohort are likely to be infants with more complex lesions, so the lower contemporary expenditures are even more remarkable.

Results of our multivariate analysis emphasized the influence of complex disease, surgery, and length of stay in the intensive care unit on hospital charges. These factors are interrelated in that infants with complex disease are more likely to undergo multiple surgical procedures, and thus spend more days in the intensive care unit, but the regression analysis showed them each to be independently associated with charges as well. From a health policy perspective, this analysis suggests that efforts to prevent the birth of infants with complex cardiac disease may result in reduced expenditures.

Our data concerning expenditures reflect only those infants who required hospitalization in the first year of life. Current practice patterns that emphasize outpatient management whenever possible, including outpatient cardiac catheterization, mean that many infants no longer require hospitalization for diagnosis and management. Thus, for example, infants born with small or moderate-sized ventricular septal defects, the most frequent cardiac lesion, are not represented in our study. If all infants with structural cardiac lesions were in the denominator in our study, the cost per cardiac infant would be reduced substantially.

The expenditure data presented herein represent charges incurred only in the first year of life. Given the pattern of early repair for correctable lesions, the majority of charges should occur in the first year of life, ideally with only routine follow-up subsequently. Of the 93 patients, only 11 (with complex disease) had not yet undergone a definitive surgical procedure by age 1 year. Nevertheless, estimates of the total hospital expenditures associated with cardiac disease in childhood require long-term follow-up of the cohort. Future analyses of professional fees and hospital charges for both acute and chronic care in the long term are warranted.

Congenital anomalies are the fifth-ranking cause of premature death in the United States, and cardiac malformations account for 44% of this burden.[13] The cost to society of premature death is quantified by the concept of years of potential life lost, which represents lost economic productivity. In this context, although the cost per survivor may seem high, it is considerably lower than the estimated $191 184 in lost productivity to society for each infant death. We conclude that the current approach of early definitive repair of cardiac defects in a major tertiary care center is beneficial in both therapeutic and economic terms. Further studies concerning long-term expenditures are needed, particularly in infants with complex defects not amenable to one-stage repair, and concerning the long-term quality of life and productivity of surviving infants.

References

1. Benson DW. Changing profile of congenital heart disease. *Pediatrics.* 1989;83:790-791.
2. Kirklin JW. The movement of cardiac surgery to the very young. In: Crupi G, Parenzan L, Anderson RH, eds. *Perspectives in Pediatric Cardiology.* Mount Kisco, NY: Futura Publishing Co Inc; 1989;2:3-20.
3. Allen HD, Taubert KA, Deckelbaum RJ, et al. Poverty and cardiac disease in children. *AJDC.* 1991;145:550-553.
4. Pearson GD, Neill CA, Beittel TM, Kidd L. Determinants of outcome in hospitalized infants with congenital heart disease. *Am J Cardiol.* 1991;68:1055-1059.
5. Max W, Rice DP, MacKenzie EJ. The lifetime cost of injury. *Inquiry.* 1990;27:332-343.
6. Watson DC, Bradley LM, Midgley FM, Scott LP. Costs and results of cardiac operations in infants less than 4 months old. *J Thorac Cardiovasc Surg.* 1986;91:667-673.
7. Hoffman JIE. Incidence, mortality and natural history. In: Anderson RH, Macartney FJ, Shinebourne EA, Tynan M, eds. *Paediatric Cardiology.* New York, NY: Churchill Livingstone Inc; 1987:3-14.
8. Walker D-JB, Vohr BR, Oh W. Economic analysis of regionalized neonatal care for very low-birth-weight infants in the state of Rhode Island. *Pediatrics.* 1985;76:69-74.
9. Pomerance JJ, Ukrainski CT, Ukra T, Henderson DH, Nash AH, Meredith JL. Cost of living for infants weighing 1,000 grams or less at birth. *Pediatrics.* 1978;61:908-910.
10. Pearson GD, Short BL. An economic analysis of extracorporeal membrane oxygenation. *J Intensive Care Med.* 1987; 2:116-120.
11. Fyler DC. Congenital heart disease. In: Hobbs N, Perrin JM, eds. *Issues in the Care of Children With Chronic Illness.* San Francisco, Calif: Jossey-Bass; 1985:261-281.
12. US Department of Labor, Bureau of Labor Statistics. *CPI Detailed Report.* January 1989.
13. Clark EB, Takao A. Overview: a focus for research in cardiovascular development. In: Clark EB, Takao A, ed. *Developmental Cardiology: Morphogenesis and Function.* Mount Kisco, NY: Futura Publishing Co Inc; 1990:3-12.

Taurine Decreases Fecal Fatty Acid and Sterol Excretion in Cystic Fibrosis

A Randomized Double-blind Trial

Lesley J. Smith, MD; Florence Lacaille, MD; Guy Lepage, MSc; Nancy Ronco, RT; André Lamarre, MD; Claude C. Roy, MD

• Patients with cystic fibrosis may still have a significant degree of steatorrhea despite adequate pancreatic enzyme supplementation. Taurine is a conditionally essential amino acid that possibly improves the micellar phase of fat digestion. Thirteen children with cystic fibrosis and a significant degree of steatorrhea (>13 g/d) were enrolled in a randomized double-blind crossover study of taurine (30 mg/kg per day) in contrast to placebo for two successive 4-month periods. No difference was noted in height and weight velocity, lung function, vitamin A level, and essential fatty acid status. Twelve of the 13 patients showed a decrease in fecal fatty acid excretion (26.5±2.6 g/24 h vs 15.4±2.5 g/24 h), affecting mainly saturates and monounsaturates, and a decrease in total sterol excretion (1492.6±303 mg/24 h vs 1211.7±213.8 mg/24 h) while ingesting taurine. Taurine may be a useful adjunct in patients with cystic fibrosis and severe steatorrhea.

(*AJDC.* 1991;145:1401-1404)

As a result of studies showing an interdependence between pulmonary disease, pancreatic insufficiency, and nutrition in relation to survival in cystic fibrosis, greater emphasis is now being placed on nutritional supplements and optimal correction of the maldigestion and malabsorption of nutrients.[1]

We recently observed that nearly 25% of our patients still have a significant degree (>15 g/d) of steatorrhea despite optimal amounts of Pancrease (pancrelipase).[2] It therefore is evident that there are still shortcomings of current modalities of treatment. Having previously reported that the lipolytic phase defect secondary to pancreatic lipase and bicarbonate deficiency is compounded by impairment of the micellar phase of digestion,[3,4] we reasoned that the increased ratio of glycine to taurine-conjugated bile acids secondary to large fecal losses of bile acids[5,6] could contribute to fat malabsorption.

Accepted for publication April 8, 1991.

From the Department of Pediatrics, Hôpital Ste-Justine and the Université de Montréal, Quebec.

Reprint requests to Gastroenterology and Nutrition Unit, Hôpital Ste-Justine, 3175 Ste-Catherine Rd, Montréal, Québec, Canada H3T 1C5 (Dr Roy).

Taurine-conjugated bile acids have theoretical advantages over glycine conjugates. Their lower pKa (1.8 vs 3.8 to 4.3) keeps them soluble in the acidic duodenum of patients with pancreatic insufficiency.[7] In contrast to glycine conjugates, which are, in part, passively absorbed in the proximal jejunum, taurine conjugates are mostly absorbed in the ileum.[8] Taurine is said to be a "conditionally essential" nutrient since needs cannot be met[9] when taurine intake is inadequate[10] or when bile acid, and therefore, taurine losses are increased as in cystic fibrosis.[11]

So far, four studies have been conducted to test the hypothesis that taurine supplementation could improve fat absorption. Three articles stated that taurine was effective particularly in patients with more severe steatorrhea,[12-14] while the only double-blind study failed to show an effect.[15] We herein confirm our earlier reports[12,13] in a double-blind randomized trial targeted to patients with a significant degree of fat malabsorption.

PATIENTS AND METHODS

Of 33 patients initially screened, 13 (six boys and seven girls) with a mean age of 11.5 years (6.2 to 20.3 years) were included in the study with documentation of a fecal fatty acid excretion in excess of 13 g/d while receiving pancreatic enzyme supplements (pancrelipase). Relevant anthropometric, pulmonary function, and biochemical data are shown in Table 1. None of these patients had evidence of liver disease according to results of tests to check bilirubin, aspartate aminotransferase, γ-glutamyltransferase, and cholylglycine levels, and according to echography. Anthropometric data showed that there was little evidence of growth impairment or malnutrition. However, there was evidence of deficiency of vitamin A as well as essential fatty acid as assessed with ratios previously reported as the most reliable indexes of essential fatty acid deficiency.[16] Dietary records of fat intake were kept by parents and checked by the clinic dietitian. Fat intake averaged 103±13 g/d. The average fat excretion was 27 g with a range of 15 g/d to 51 g/d. The study protocol was approved by the Ethics Committee of Hôpital Ste-Justine (Montreal, Quebec), and consent was obtained from the parents.

The 13 patients were randomly assigned to receive either recrystallized taurine (McNeil Pharmaceutical, Springhouse, Pa) or placebo during an initial 4-month period after which each patient received the alternate supplement during the second 4-month period. Taurine capsules (285 mg each) and placebo (lactose) were prepared by McNeil Pharmaceutical, Spring

Table 1.—Clinical and Biological Characteristics of the Patients at Entry in the Study*

Patient No./ Sex/Age, y	Anthropometric Data: Height, % Expected	Weight for Height, % Expected	Shwachman Score	FEF	γ-GT, U/L	Vitamin A, mg/L	α-Tocopherol Total Lipids, mg/g	Fatty Acid Ratios†: 20:3 n9 / 20:4 n6	n7 Family / 18:2 n6
1/M/8.2	103	98	98	. . .	8	0.18	2.02	0.057	0.298
2/F/8.7	98	95	90	49	19	0.27	. . .	0.051	0.226
3/F/11.6	98	98	88	112	20	0.32	1.01	0.163	0.771
4/F/11.9	100	94	87	112	10	0.47	1.69	0.054	0.294
5/F/14.9	98	97	87	75	23	0.34	0.60	0.042	0.308
6/F/20.3	96	134	94	89	9	0.69	1.53	0.05	0.375
7/M/6.3	101	104	92	84	9	0.27	1.90	0.111	0.496
8/M/12	94	100	91	101	8	0.34	0.35	0.067	0.380
9/M/15.7	101	87	96	115	13	0.36	2.02	0.035	0.235
10/F/10.9	88	91	75	. . .	8	0.25	1.25	0.064	0.407
11/F/10.1	100	95	96	95	21	0.35	2.02	0.033	0.201
12/M/10.8	95	92	82	91	11	0.34	1.56	0.066	0.366
13/M/7.9	88	87	82	82	10	0.37	2.60	0.033	0.291
Mean ± SE	97 ± 1.3	97.8 ± 3.3	89.1 ± 1.8	91.4 ± 5.8	13 ± 5.6	0.35 ± 0.034	1.55 ± 0.19	0.064 ± 0.01	0.358 ± 0.041
Normal values, (Mean ± SEM)	100 ± 5	100 ± 5	100	100 ± 5	13 ± 10	0.55 ± 0.25	1.44 ± 0.06	0.016 ± 0.006	0.11 ± 0.025

*FEF indicates forced expiratory flow between 25% and 75% of expired vital capacity as percentage of expected value for age; and γ-GT, γ-glutamyl transpeptidase. The mean ± SE age of the patients in the study is 11.5 ± 1 years.
†Eicosanoic/arachidic acid (17); and family of n7 fatty acids/linoleic acid (17).

House, Pa, and coded before they were sent to the hospital pharmacy responsible for issuing them to the patients at the time of their regular clinic visits along with pancrelipase capsules, tocopherol acetate (Aquasol E, 200 IU/d), and the daily multivitamin supplement of vitamin A (4000 IU), vitamin D (400 IU), and vitamin C (75 mg). During the two experimental periods, no change was made in the type (pancrelipase) and number of capsules or in the vitamin supplementation program. Six of the 13 patients were administered cloxacillin during the duration of the study. Taurine (30 mg/kg per day) or placebo was administered in fractionated dosages at the same time as pancreatic supplements.

At the end of each treatment period, a questionnaire was given to each parent to be completed before the child's next clinic visit. Total energy and fat intake, frequency and consistency of bowel movements, and whether there was any abdominal pain were recorded. Seventy-two–hour stool and 24-hour urine collections were obtained at the end of each 4-month period. Stools were frozen on evacuation. At the time of clinic appointments, anthropometric data were recorded, a blood sample was obtained, and pulmonary function tests were repeated.

Stool homogenates were used for the gas-liquid chromatography determination of fatty acids as well as neutral and acidic sterols.[12] Stool nitrogen was measured with a modification of the Kjeldahl procedure.[17] Blood collected after an overnight fast in test tubes containing ethylenediaminetetraacetic acid were used for gas-liquid chromatography measurements of fatty acids.[16] Vitamin A levels were determined with spectrophotometry and α-tocopherol levels with high-pressure liquid chromatography.[18] Values for α-tocopherol were expressed in milligrams per gram of total lipids.[19] Urinary taurine was determined with ion exchange chromatography on sulfonated polystyrene beads linked to divinyl benzene using an LKB Alpha Plus 4151 analyzer (LKB Instruments Inc, Gaithersburg, Md) and a Hewlett-Packard 3392 A integrator (Hewlett-Packard Co, Palo Alto, Calif).[20]

All results, unless otherwise specified, were expressed as mean±SE. The response to taurine supplementation was evaluated using paired and unpaired Student's *t* tests as described in the analysis of crossover designs.[21]

RESULTS

The questionnaires that were completed by the parents failed to show a change in the appetite and fat intake of the 13 patients. With regard to digestive symptoms, there was an improvement in the number and consistency of stools as well as a disappearance of abdominal pain in four patients who received taurine supplements, while placebo reportedly produced an improvement in two patients. No difference in height and weight velocities could be documented as a result of taurine supplementation, and no change could be detected in lung function. There was good compliance with the protocol as all patients increased their urinary excretion of taurine. The mean excretion (micromole per millimole of creatinine) was 56.0±6.9 with placebo and 414.3±31.2 with taurine supplementation.

The percentage of fat absorption was improved by taurine supplementation (75%±3% vs 86%±2%, $P<.01$). Twelve of the 13 patients showed a decrease in fecal fatty acid excretion (Figure). The overall improvement of more than 40% in fatty acid excretion was highly significant ($P<.005$), but it affected mainly saturated fatty acids (C16:0, C18:0) and the monounsaturate, oleic acid (C18:1, n9); the difference in the mean excretion of linoleic acid was only marginally significant ($P<.1$) (Table 2). Despite the decrease in the loss of lipid nutrients caused by taurine supplements, it failed to improve vitamin A levels and the ratios of fatty acids used as indicators of essential fatty acid deficiency.

As expected, there was a close correlation between fecal fatty acids and nitrogen excretion. However, a paired *t* test ($P<.1$) did not show a statistical difference in nitrogen excretion between the taurine (2.44±0.33 g/24 h) and the placebo (3.04±0.44 g/24 h) treatment periods. The effect of taurine on sterol excretion is shown in Table 3. Al-

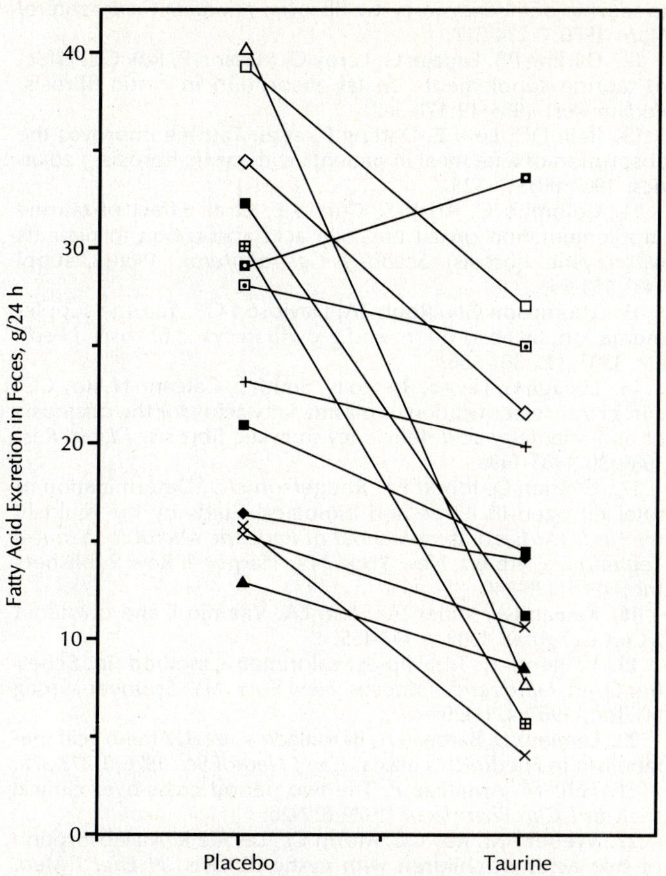

Individual response of fecal fat excretion obtained from 3-day stool collections carried out following 4 months of treatment with placebo and taurine. Twelve of the 13 patients responded to taurine supplementation (P<.005 by paired t test).

Table 2.—Effect of Taurine on the Total and Pattern of Excreted Fatty Acids (n=13)*

Treatment	16:0	18:0	18:1 (n=9)	18:2 (n=6)	Total Fatty Acid Excretion
Placebo	7.5±0.8	7.7±1.6	5.4±1.0	2.4±0.8	26.5±2.6
Taurine	4.8±0.7	4.3±1.2	2.8±0.6	0.9±0.2	15.4±2.5
Paired *t* test	*P*<.05	*P*<.05	*P*<.05	*P*<.1	*P*<.005

*The individual fatty acids account for nearly 90% of the total fatty acids excreted in the stools. Values are given as mean±SE and are expressed in grams per 24 h.

Table 3.—Effect of Taurine on Sterol Excretion (n=13)*

Treatment	Neutral Sterols	Acidic Sterols	Total
Placebo	645.9±155.8	846.7±156.1	1492.6±303.0
Taurine	509.5±97.3	702.2±126.8	1211.7±213.8
Paired *t* test	NS	NS	*P*<.05

*Values are given as mean±SE and expressed in milligrams per 24 h. NS indicates not statistically significant.

though no difference was observed in neutral and acidic sterols (bile acids) taken separately, total sterol excretion decreased significantly ($P<.05$) during the taurine treatment period. In addition, there was a close relationship between bile acid loss and fatty acid malabsorption ($y=41.5x-200.8$, $r=.73$, $P<.01$).

COMMENT

This study has shown that a taurine supplement of 30 mg/kg per day administered during a 4-month period in a double-blind crossover trial had an insignificant effect on gastrointestinal manifestations, but led to a significant decrease in both fatty acid and sterol excretion.

Our initial report[12] had shown a more modest effect of taurine, but we had noted (as have others since)[14] that patients with cystic fibrosis and more severe steatorrhea are more likely to ameliorate their condition with the use of taurine supplements. Because of these earlier findings obtained in open trials and in view of a double-blind study conducted in Australia reporting no effect of taurine,[15] we decided to adopt a double-blind randomized design to test the effect of taurine in patients who had significant gastrointestinal manifestations and a significant degree of steatorrhea while receiving a high-energy diet and a liberal intake of lipids.

The reduction in fecal fatty acid excretion coupled with an improvement of fat absorption was impressive. It confirms our earlier findings,[12] as well as those of a study performed in Italy,[14] but is at odds with a double-blind protocol carried out in Australia. The reason for this may well be that patients for that study had a wide range (48% to 96%) of fat absorption. Only seven of their 20 patients had a moderately severe degree (75.6%±15.6%) of fat malabsorption.[15]

Because taurine supplementation also decreased total sterol excretion, it can therefore be expected to exert a favorable influence on the interruption of the enterohepatic circulation of bile acids.[22] However, in these 13 patients with no evidence of growth impairment or clinical malnutrition, taurine had no effect on growth velocity or weight gain. We recently reported that there was a good correlation between essential fatty acid deficiency and fecal fatty acid loss.[23] However, the present study failed to show an amelioration of the plasma essential fatty acid patterns despite a 40% decrease in steatorrhea. On the other hand, the present findings confirm our initial study[12] that showed that taurine does not appear to improve the absorption of polyunsaturated fatty acid. Its effect is mainly directed to the nonpolar saturates and monounsaturates, which require a higher concentration of bile acids for their incorporation into micelles and are taken up more slowly by the absorptive apparatus than polyunsaturates.[22]

Besides the well characterized role of taurine for the conjugation of bile acids in the liver,[24] taurine is present in muscle in quantities exceeding those of all other amino acids.[25] Taurine has been shown to play a key role in the myocardium,[26] to stabilize muscle intracellular membranes,[27] and to protect against proteolysis of muscle structural proteins.[28] However, a recent study testing the hypothesis that taurine deficiency could contribute to the increased breakdown of proteins in cystic fibrosis failed to show that taurine had any effect on whole-body protein flux, synthesis, and catabolism.[29]

In the treatment of pancreatic steatorrhea, the challenge is to deliver enough active enzymes to a digestive-absorptive apparatus with a pH close to neutrality. Several factors may be responsible for the persistence of a significant degree of steatorrhea in any patient treated with pancreatic enzymes: the potency and dosage of the pancreatic enzyme preparation, the acid-secreting status of the patient, and the patient's capacity to compensate for the bile acid loss associated with maldigestion of nutrients.[30] The present findings suggest that a hepatic pool of taurine sufficient to maintain a normal glycine-taurine ratio of conjugated bile acids may be an additional factor.

Further studies will be required to define the effect of taurine supplementation on the absorption of lipids and on the metabolism of bile salts before recommending its general use. However, we can conclude from this study, from others published so far,[12-14] and from our experience over the past few years that taurine is a safe and effective adjuvant in patients with severe steatorrhea who fail to respond to pancreatic enzyme supplements. Only longer periods of treatment will allow conclusions on its effects on nutritional status, growth, and pulmonary function.

This study was supported by the Canadian Cystic Fibrosis Foundation (CCFF) and by McNeil Pharmaceutical, Springhouse, Pa. Dr Smith was the recipient of a CCFF Research Fellowship, and Dr Lacaille received a grant from the Association Française pour la Lutte Contre la Mucoviscidose.

We thank Ronald Sokol, MD, and Iris Osberg of the Pediatric Clinical Center, University of Colorado Health Sciences Center, Denver, for determination of α-tocopherol and total lipid levels. We also thank Robert Giguère, MD, of the Pediatric Department at the University of Sherbrooke, Quebec, for urinary taurine measurements, and Danielle St-Cyr Huot for typing the manuscript.

References

1. Roy CC, Weber AM. Nutrition of the child with cystic fibrosis. In: Walker WA, Watkins JB, eds. *Nutrition in Pediatrics.* Boston, Mass: Little Brown & Co Inc; 1985:463-484.

2. Roy CC, Weber AM, Lepage G, Smith L, Levy E. Digestive and absorptive phase anomalies associated with the exocrine pancreatic insufficiency of cystic fibrosis. *J Pediatr Gastroenterol Nutr.* 1988;7(suppl 1):S1-S7.

3. Zentler-Munro PL, Fitzpatrick WJF, Batten JC, Northfield TC. Effect of intrajejunal acidity on aqueous phase bile acid and lipid concentrations in pancreatic steatorrhea due to cystic fibrosis. *Gut.* 1984;25:500-507.

4. Weber AM, Roy CC. Bile acid metabolism in cystic fibrosis. *Acta Paediatr Scand.* 1985;317(suppl):9-15.

5. Roy CC, Weber AM, Morin CL, et al. Abnormal biliary lipid composition in cystic fibrosis. *N Engl J Med.* 1977;297:1301-1305.

6. Harries JT, Muller DPR, McCollumn JPK, Lipson A, Rowe E, Norman AP. Intestinal bile salts in cystic fibrosis. *Arch Dis Child.* 1979;54:19-24.

7. Regan PT, Malagelada JR, Dimagno EP, Go VLW. Reduced intraluminal bile acid concentrations and fat maldigestion in pancreatic insufficiency: correction by treatment. *Gastroenterology.* 1979;77:285-289.

8. Krag E, Phillips SF. Active and passive bile acids absorption in man. *J Clin Invest.* 1974;53:1686-1694.

9. Gaull GE. Taurine in human milk: growth modulator or conditionally essential amino acid? *J Pediatr Gastroenterol Nutr.* 1983;2(suppl):S266-S271.

10. Ament ME, Geggel HS, Heckenlively JR, Martin DA, Kopple J. Taurine supplementation in infants receiving long-term total parenteral nutrition. *J Am Coll Nutr.* 1986;5:127-135.

11. Thompson GN. Excessive fecal taurine loss predisposes to taurine deficiency in cystic fibrosis. *J Pediatr Gastroenterol Nutr.* 1988;7:214-217.

12. Darling PB, Lepage G, Leroy C, Masson P, Roy CC. Effect of taurine supplements on fat absorption in cystic fibrosis. *Pediatr Res.* 1985;19:578-582.

13. Belli DC, Levy E, Darling P, et al. Taurine improves the absorption of a fat meal in patients with cystic fibrosis. *Pediatrics.* 1987;80:517-523.

14. Colombo C, Arlati S, Curcio L, et al. Effect of taurine supplementation on fat and bile acid absorption in patients with cystic fibrosis. *Scand J Gastroenterol.* 1988;23(suppl 143):151-156.

15. Thompson GN, Robb TA, Davidson GP. Taurine supplementation, fat absorption, and growth in cystic fibrosis. *J Pediatr.* 1987;111:501-506.

16. Lepage G, Levy E, Ronco N, Smith L, Galéano N, Roy CC. Direct transesterification of plasma fatty acids for the diagnosis of essential fatty acid deficiency in cystic fibrosis. *J Lipid Res.* 1989;30:1483-1490.

17. O'Brien D, Ibbott FA, Rodgerson DO. Determination of total nitrogen in tissue and biological fluids by the Kjeldahl method. In: *Laboratory Manual of Pediatric Microbiochemical Techniques.* 4th ed. New York, NY: Harper & Row Publishers Inc; 1968:238-240.

18. Kaplan LA, Miller JA, Stein EA. Vitamin E and carotene. *J Clin Lab Anal.* 1987;1:147-155.

19. Wagener H. Total lipids: calorimetric method. In: Schettler G, ed. *Lipids and Lipidoses.* New York, NY: Springer-Verlag NY Inc; 1967:421-429.

20. Lemieux B, Barbeau A, Beroniade V, et al. Amino acid metabolism in Friedreich's ataxia. *Can J Neurol Sci.* 1976;3:373-378.

21. Hills M, Armitage P. The two period cross-over clinical trial. *Br J Clin Pharmacol.* 1979;8:7-20.

22. Weber AM, Roy CC, Morin CL, Lasalle R. Malabsorption of bile acids in children with cystic fibrosis. *N Engl J Med.* 1973;289:1001-1005.

23. Lacaille F, Smith LJ, Lepage G, et al. The severity of essential fatty acid deficiency in cystic fibrosis is related to steatorrhea rather than to nutritional status. Presented at the joint meeting of ESPGAN/NASPGN; May 25, 1990; Amsterdam, the Netherlands. Abstract.

24. Hayes KC, Sturman JA. Taurine in metabolism. *Annu Rev Nutr.* 1981;1:401-425.

25. Nyhan WL, Yujnovsky M, Wheeler RF. Amino acids and cell growth. In: Check D, ed. *Human Growth.* Philadelphia, Pa: Lea & Febiger; 1968:396-416.

26. Pion PD, Kittleson MD, Rogers QR, Morriss JG. Myocardial failure in cats associated with low plasma taurine: a reversible cardiomyopathy. *Science.* 1987;237:764-768.

27. Huxtable R, Bressler R. Effect of taurine on a muscle intracellular membrane. *Biochim Biophys Acta.* 1973;323:573-583.

28. Iwata H, Baba A. Specific increase of taurine in denervated skeletal muscle. In: Oja SS, Ahtee L, Koutro P, Paasonen MK, eds. *Taurine: Biological Actions and Clinical Perspective.* New York, NY: Alan R Liss Inc; 1985:397-405.

29. Thompson GN, Thomas FM. Protein metabolism in cystic fibrosis: responses to malnutrition and taurine supplementation. *Am J Clin Nutr.* 1987;46:606-613.

30. Leroy C, Lepage G, Morin CL, Bertrand JM, Dufour-Larue O, Roy CC. Effect of dietary fat and residues on fecal loss of sterols and on their microbial degradation in cystic fibrosis. *Dig Dis Sci.* 1986;31:911-918.

Respirosonography in Infants With Acute Bronchiolitis

Asher Tal, MD; Ignacio Sanchez, MD; Hans Pasterkamp, MD

• Respirosonography was used to analyze lung sounds and breathing patterns in 16 infants with acute bronchiolitis who were treated with nebulized salbutamol (albuterol). Wheezing was measured as a proportion of respiratory time (time spent wheezing [T_w]/total time [T_{tot}]). A decrease of 10% or greater in T_w/T_{tot} or a reduction in T_w/T_{tot} to less than 2% was considered a positive response to salbutamol. Seven infants responded to the salbutamol, and nine did not. In responders, T_w/T_{tot} decreased from 47%±26% to 20%±25% (mean±SD), and the respiratory rate decreased from 65±8 to 57±7 breaths per minute. In nonresponders, mean T_w/T_{tot} either did not change or increased, and there was no significant change in respiratory rate (53±10 breaths per minute before salbutamol inhalation and 56±9 breaths per minute after salbutamol inhalation). Complex repetitive waveforms, different from the sinusoidal waveforms of typical wheezing, were observed in 14 of 16 infants. Our findings add supportive evidence to the clinical impression that some infants with bronchiolitis respond to salbutamol. Respirosonography provides a noninvasive method for objective clinical assessment of young, wheezy children.

(*AJDC*. 1991;145:1405-1410)

Wheezing is a common clinical sign of obstructive airway disease. Wheezes are musical adventitious lung sounds that originate from oscillating airway walls and depend on a critical airflow rate, a critical flutter frequency, and some degree of airway geometry distortion.[1] Several respiratory illnesses during infancy that are associated with airflow obstruction (ie, bronchiolitis, infantile asthma, bronchopulmonary dysplasia, and cystic fibrosis), are accompanied by wheezing. The role of bronchial hyperresponsiveness in the pathogenesis of these conditions is not yet clear. It has been shown that infants with histories of recurrent wheezing episodes may develop airflow obstruction after bronchial provocation with inhaled histamine[2] or nebulized distilled water.[3] However, clinical airway obstruction may not be relieved with nebulized bronchodilators, which indicates a more complex pathogenesis of airway obstruction in infantile asthma.[4] While some studies have reported a lack of efficacy of bronchodilators in the treatment of acute wheezing,[5,6] others have found a beneficial effect.[7-9] Generally, pediatricians evaluate the potential role of a bronchodilator by clinically assessing a wheezy infant before and after administration of a trial dose to establish therapeutic benefit before further use.[10]

Objective assessment of the response to bronchodilators in patients in this age group is difficult. Most bedside lung function measurements are impractical in infants with acute wheezing. These techniques require sedation, which causes problems in acutely sick infants.[11] Therefore, the evaluation of a trial dose of a bronchodilator is usually subjective, being based on changes in respiratory rate, use of accessory muscles, inspiratory-expiratory ratio, presence of cyanosis, and estimation of the severity of wheezing.[12] However, subjective wheeze assessment is flawed by interobserver and intraobserver variability.[13]

Computer-aided analysis of recorded lung sounds is useful as an objective and noninvasive approach to the clinical assessment of wheezy infants. Wheezes present as sharp peaks in the power spectrum that can be detected and measured with automated analysis.[14] In a previous investigation of older asthmatic children before and after exercise,[15] we documented a correlation between the proportion of time spent wheezing and the degree of airway obstruction measured by forced expiratory volume in 1 second (FEV_1), maximum midexpiratory airflow, and specific airway conductance. In the present study, we used digital respirosonography[16] in infants with acute airway obstruction to assess changes in wheeze characteristics before and after bronchodilator treatment. This pilot project was undertaken to define acoustic characteristics of wheezing in infants and to evaluate a potential role for lung sound analysis as a noninvasive method of assessing airway responsiveness in young children.

SUBJECTS AND METHODS

Subjects

Infants younger than age 2 years who were admitted to the Children's Hospital in Winnipeg, Manitoba, between November 1, 1989, and March 15, 1990, with a clinical diagnosis of acute bronchiolitis were studied. Patients for whom salbutamol (albuterol) inhalations were part of the prescribed treatment were included after informed parental consent was obtained. Infants with cystic fibrosis, congenital heart disease, or congenital anomalies of the respiratory system were excluded. Routine vi-

Accepted for publication August 18, 1991.

From the Department of Pediatrics, Ben Gurion University, Beersheba, Israel (Dr Tal), and the Department of Pediatrics and Child Health, University of Manitoba, Winnipeg (Drs Sanchez and Pasterkamp).

Presented at the 56th Annual Scientific Assembly, American College of Chest Physicians, Toronto, Ontario, October 25, 1990.

Reprint requests to AE103-671 William Ave, Winnipeg, Manitoba, Canada R3E 0Z2 (Dr Pasterkamp).

Table 1.—Characteristics of Infants With Acute Bronchiolitis*

Patient No.	Sex/Age, mo	Virus	Associated Problems	No. of Previous Wheezing Episodes
1	M/11	None	FHxA	1
2†	F/1.5	None	BPD	0
3†	M/5	RSV	BPD	>3
4†	F/12	RSV	BPD	>3
5	M/8	Adeno 3	BPD, FHxA	0
6	M/3	RSV	None	0
7	F/21	None	None	0
8	M/10	None	None	0
9	M/15	RSV	None	0
10†	F/6	RSV	FHxA	0
11†	M/1	RSV	None	0
12	M/6	None	FHxA	0
13†	M/23	None	FHxA	1
14	M/5	None	None	1
15†	M/13	None	None	2
16	M/10	Influenza A	FHxA	0

*FHxA indicates family history of asthma; BPD, bronchopulmonary dysplasia; RSV, respiratory syncytial virus; and adeno 3, adenovirus type 3.

†Patients who responded to bronchodilator administration.

ral studies were performed. The personal and family history of asthma, allergies, wheezing episodes, and respiratory tract infections were noted. This study was approved by the Faculty Committee on the Use of Human Subjects in Research.

Study Protocol

Lung sounds were recorded immediately before and 10 to 15 minutes after one salbutamol inhalation. A dose of 0.03 mL of nebulizer solution per kilogram of body weight is routinely used in our institution. The 0.5% nebulizer solution contains 0.9% saline that is added to a total volume of 2 mL. The solution is administered via a face mask with 5 L of oxygen per minute. All patients were awake during lung sound recording. Most of them were resting comfortably on a parent's lap or in bed. Studies performed after salbutamol administration were always conducted with the patient in the same position as before inhalation.

Recording and Analysis of Respiratory Sounds

Lung sounds were recorded as previously described[16]: a contact transducer (EMT25C, Elema/Siemens, Iselin, NJ) was attached with double-sided adhesive rings to the anterior or posterior upper chest on the right or to the posterior upper chest on the left. The recording site depended on the patient's most comfortable position during the study. The position of the sound transducer remained unchanged before and after treatment. Respiration signals from the rib cage and abdomen were obtained with uncalibrated respiratory inductive plethysmography (Respitrace TM, Ambulatory Monitoring Inc, Ardsley, NY). Sound and respiration signals were simultaneously recorded on a four-channel frequency modulation instrumentation recorder (3960B, Hewlett Packard, Waltham, Mass).

On playback, the sounds were first low-pass filtered with a sixth-order Butterworth filter at 1200 Hz to avoid aliasing during sampling. The signals were played through an analog-to-digital converter (Data Translation 2801a, Marlborough, Mass) into a personal computer compatible with a PC/AT (IBM, Chicago, Ill). The sampling rate was 5120 Hz per channel. A customized computer program[16] was used for data acquisition, analysis, and display. Fast-Fourier transformation was applied to 1024 data points at 100-ms intervals. This resulted in a 50% overlap into adjacent 100-ms segments, allowing the application of a Hanning window to the data with no loss of information.

Digital respirosonograms were produced from the resulting power spectra. Any particular 100-ms segment could be highlighted and viewed in detail in both the time and the frequency domains, and any part of the data could be selected for digital-to-analog conversion and playback through a loudspeaker or headphones.

For each infant, 10 to 15 seconds of continuous lung sounds before and after salbutamol administration were chosen for analysis. The selection of sound from the recording was based on absence of artifacts such as movement, crying, and environmental noise. Consecutive segments of 100 ms were marked as wheezing or normal based on (1) the distinct peaks in the frequency domain, (2) periodic waveform appearance in the time domain, and (3) auditory verification on playback. Wheezing was measured as a proportion of total respiratory time (time spent wheezing [T_w]/total time [T_{tot}]). The average peak frequency of the wheezing (avgF_w) was computed for each recording. Respiratory rate and ventilatory timing components (inspiration-expiration ratio) were measured from the plethysmographic signals. We arbitrarily defined a decrease of 10% or greater in T_w/T_{tot} or a reduction in T_w/T_{tot} to less than 2% as positive responses to salbutamol.

We used unpaired, two-tailed Student's *t* tests to compare the T_w/T_{tot}, avgF_w, respiratory rate, and inspiration-expiration ratios of responders with those of nonresponders. We also compared results before and after salbutamol administration using paired *t* tests. Statistical significance was accepted as $P<.05$. The data are presented as means±SDs.

RESULTS

Sixteen infants (12 boys) with a mean age of 9.4 months (range, 1 to 23 months) were enrolled in this study. Results of viral studies revealed the presence of a virus in half the infants. Six infants had respiratory syncytial virus; one, adenovirus type 3; and one, influenza A. Four of the infants also had histories of bronchopulmonary dysplasia. Asthma was present in first-degree relatives of six patients, and six patients had histories of wheezing episodes (Table 1).

Based on our definition of a 10% or greater reduction in T_w/T_{tot} or a reduction in T_w/T_{tot} to less than 2% after salbutamol administration, seven infants were classified as responders and nine as nonresponders (Fig 1). Patient characteristics, such as age, gender, family history of asthma, and presence of viruses were not markedly different between the two groups (Table 2). Responders had a significant decrease in respiratory rate (from 65±8 to 57±7 breaths per minute; $P<.05$) after salbutamol administration, whereas respiratory rate in nonresponders remained essentially unchanged (from 53±10 to 56±9 breaths per minute; Fig 2). The inspiration-expiration ratio was similar in both groups (0.7±0.2 and 0.7±0.1, in responders and nonresponders, respectively), and did not change after salbutamol administration in either group. In responders, T_w/T_{tot} decreased from 47%±26% to 20%±25%, with no significant change in avgF_w (230±5 Hz and 255±101 Hz, before and after salbutamol inhalation, respectively). By definition, nonresponders had an unchanged or even greater T_w/T_{tot} after treatment compared with pretreatment values (31%±13% vs 38%±12%), but their avgF_w decreased significantly from 271±64 Hz to 206±21 Hz after treatment ($P<.03$; Fig 3). In four children, T_w/T_{tot} increased 10% or greater after salbutamol administration (Fig 1). There was no significant difference in res-

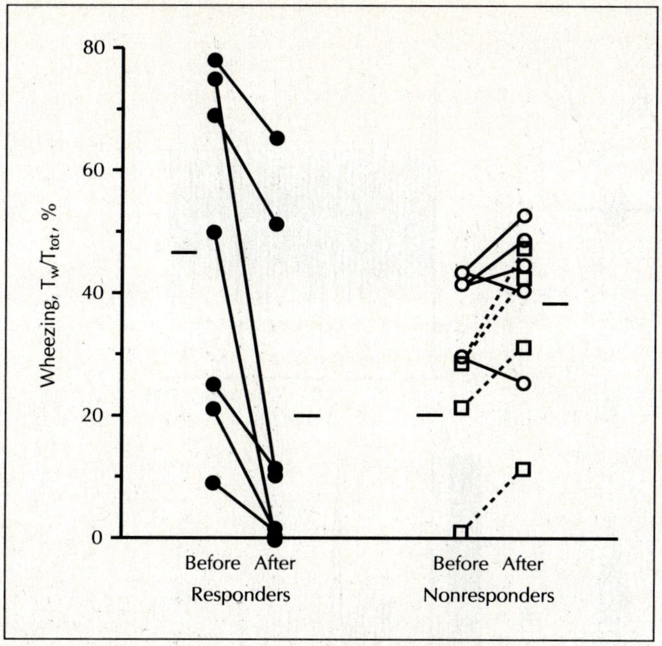

Fig 1.—*Changes in time spent wheezing (T_w)/total time (T_{tot}) before and after salbutamol inhalation. Group means are indicated by horizontal lines. Among nonresponders, patients with less than a 10% increase in T_w/T_{tot} are indicated by open circles and solid lines, while those with increases in T_w/T_{tot} of 10% or more are shown by open squares and dashed lines.*

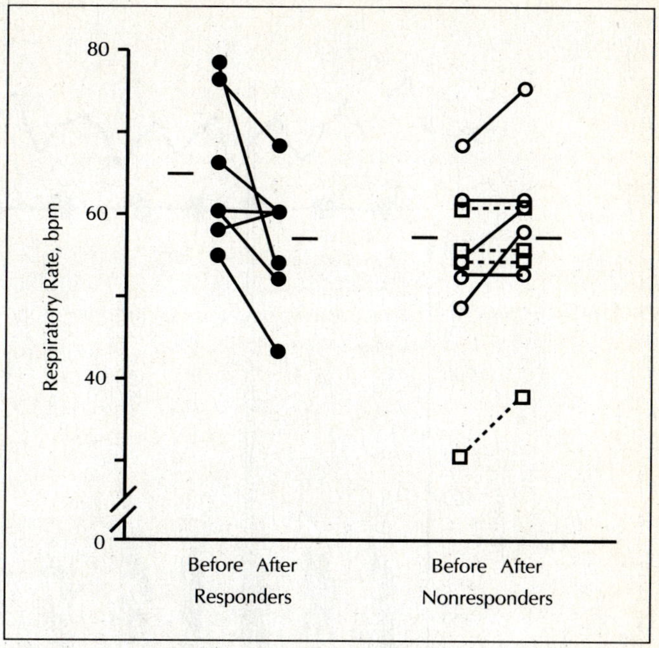

Fig 2.—*Changes in respiratory rate before and after salbutamol inhalation (bpm indicates breaths per minute). Among nonresponders, patients with a paradoxical increase in wheezing of 10% or greater are indicated by open squares and dashed lines.*

Table 2.—Characteristics of Responders and Non-Responders Before and After Bronchodilator Administration*

	Responders (n=7)		Nonresponders (n=9)	
Characteristic	**Before**	**After**	**Before**	**After**
Respiratory rate, breaths per minute	64.7±8.4	56.7±7.3†	53.3±9.9	56.4±9.2
Inspiration-expiration ratio	0.7±0.1	0.7±0.1	0.7±0.1	0.7±0.1
T_w/T_{tot}, %	47±26	20±25	31±13	38±12
avgF_w, Hz	230±35	255±101	271±64†‡	206±21

*The mean age (range) was 8.8 months (1 to 23 months) in responders and 9.9 months (3 to 21 months) in nonresponders. Values are means±SEMs. T_w/T_{tot} indicates time spent wheezing divided by total time, and avgF_w, average peak frequency of wheezing.

†*P*<.05.

‡Data from one patient were excluded.

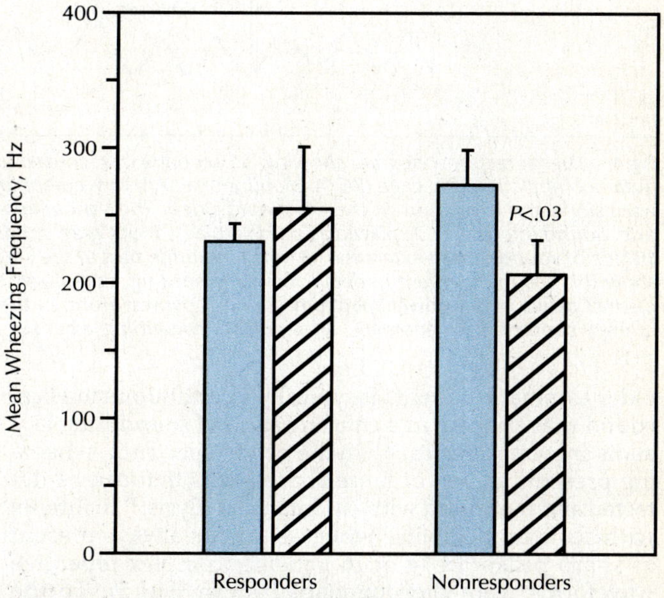

Fig 3.—*Changes (mean±SEM) in wheezing frequency before (shaded bars) and after (hatched bars) salbutamol inhalation. One patient (number 9, Table 1) was excluded from the nonresponders.*

piratory rate after inhalation in these four patients (Fig 2). In one patient (number 9, Table 1) who underwent evaluation on admission, salbutamol caused an increase in T_w/T_{tot} from 1% before treatment to 11% after treatment. Because wheezing was almost absent before therapy, this patient's data were excluded from the comparison of avgF_w between responders and nonresponders (Fig 3). Sinusoidal waveforms of typical wheezing were easily identified (Fig 4), but complex repetitive waveforms were present in 14 of the 16 infants (Fig 5).

COMMENT

Wheezing in infancy is not well defined. Although the term *wheezy infant* is commonly used to characterize young patients with a variety of obstructive lung diseases, we are not aware of published data that describe the acoustic characteristics of adventitious lung sounds in this age group. Recent advances in computer technology have made it possible for acoustic measurements of respiration to be conveniently performed using a personal computer.[16]

We used a customized computer program (Respiration Acoustics Laboratory Environment, Medi-Wave Inc, Winnipeg, Manitoba) for digital respirosonography and found that wheezes in infants have different acoustic characteristics than those in older patients. Wheezing in

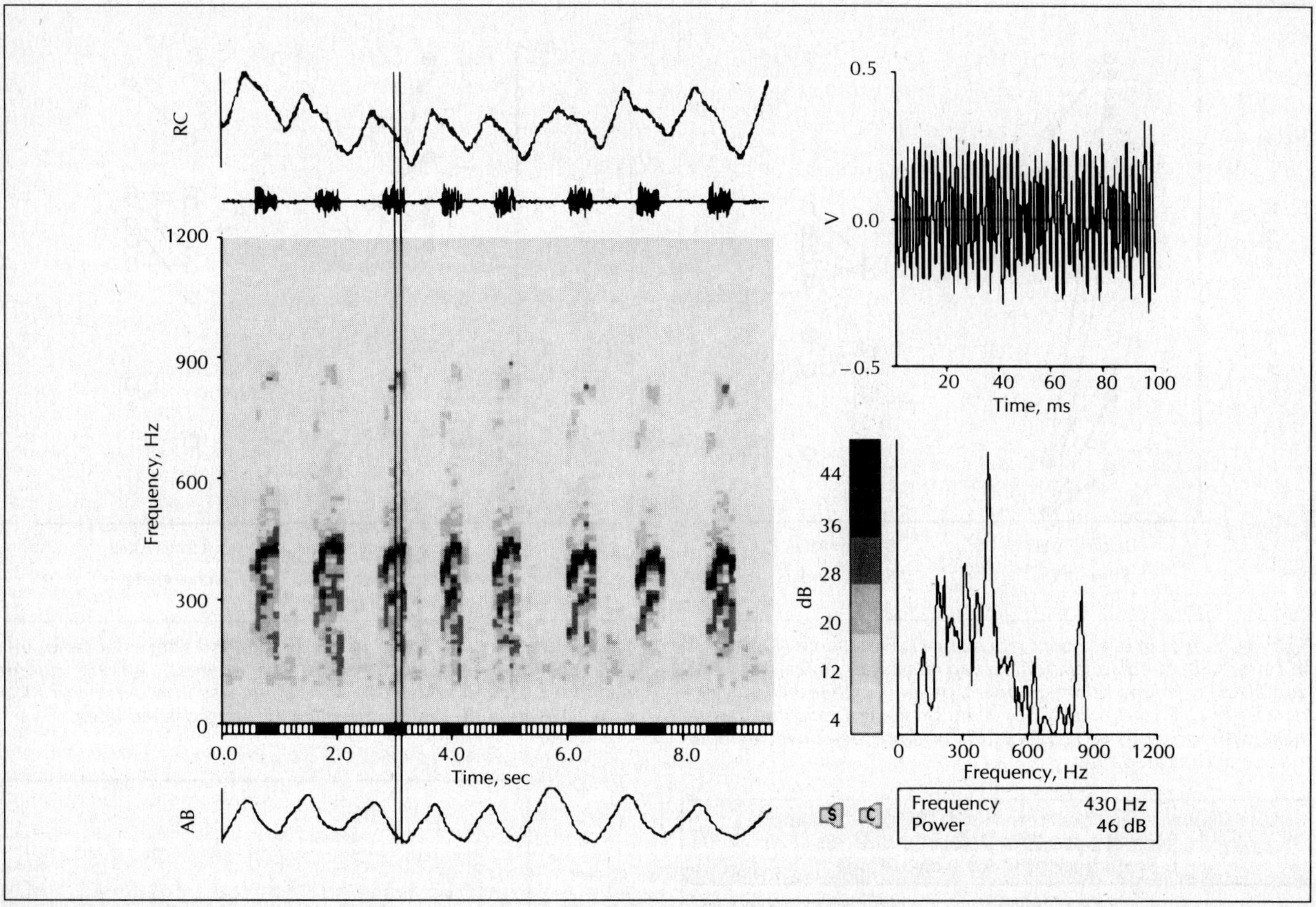

Fig 4.—*Digital respirosonogram showing 9.5 seconds of recorded lung sounds and breathing patterns from patient 8 (Table 1) before salbutamol inhalation. Rib cage (RC) and abdominal (AB) movement are plotted at the top and bottom, respectively. Inspiration is on the upward slope and expiration on the downward slope. The sonogram shows time on the horizontal axis and sound frequency on the vertical axis. Sound intensity is displayed as shades (black, loud; gray, medium; and white, low). The vertical double bar at 3.1 seconds highlights 100 ms of sound during expiration. A time amplitude plot of the sound wave (top right) and the respective Fourier spectrum (bottom right) show this 100-ms segment in detail. Typical wheezing, commonly seen in older patients with asthma, is present in this infant. There are distinct peaks in the power spectrum, a sinusoidal waveform in the time domain, and a concentration of sound intensity in a narrow frequency band on the sonogram. All segments containing wheezes are shaded in gray on the horizontal axis.*

older asthmatic patients is typically a continuous musical sound that appears as a concentration of sound intensity at distinct frequencies.[14,17] In the power spectrum, wheezing presents as one or more sharp peaks that can be detected and measured with automated analysis.[18] In infants with acute bronchiolitis, wheezes did not always present as sharp peaks. In 14 of 16 patients, complex repetitive waveforms were the dominant pattern (Fig 5). To the subjective listener, these sounds appear less musical and more raspy and are frequently concurrent with coarse crackles. Therefore, automated wheeze characterization with fast-Fourier transformation, based only on the detection of spectral peaks, is unreliable in infants. In addition to power spectral analysis, we studied lung sounds in the time domain with expanded waveform analysis.[19] We found that a combination of waveform assessment in the time domain, peak detection in the frequency domain, and auditory verification on playback, were necessary to characterize and measure wheezing in young infants.

Baughman and Loudon[14] analyzed lung sounds of adult patients with acute asthma. They used T_w/T_{tot} as an acoustic parameter that indicated the severity of airway obstruction and found a significant correlation between FEV_1 and T_w/T_{tot}. In asthmatic children with postexertional asthma, we also observed a significant correlation between T_w/T_{tot} and severity of airway obstruction as measured considering FEV_1, maximum midexpiratory airflow, and specific airway conductance.[15] In the present study, we documented a decrease in T_w/T_{tot} of 10% or greater or a reduction in T_w/T_{tot} to less than 2% after salbutamol inhalation in seven of the 16 infants. We chose this definition of a positive response to salbutamol because a change in T_w/T_{tot} of 10% or greater would likely be noticed on subjective auscultation[13] and because false-positive wheeze detection using spectral characterization has occurred in fewer than 3% of patients tested in our laboratory.[18] In our study, the significantly lower respiratory rate of patients who wheezed less after salbutamol inhalation also indicates less airflow obstruction. There is no evidence that wheeze duration depends on respiratory rate. If there were a relationship between breathing pattern and duration of wheeze, one would expect rapid, shallow breathing to produce less wheezing than slower and deeper breathing because wheeze generation requires critical transpulmonary pressures and airway deformation.[1]

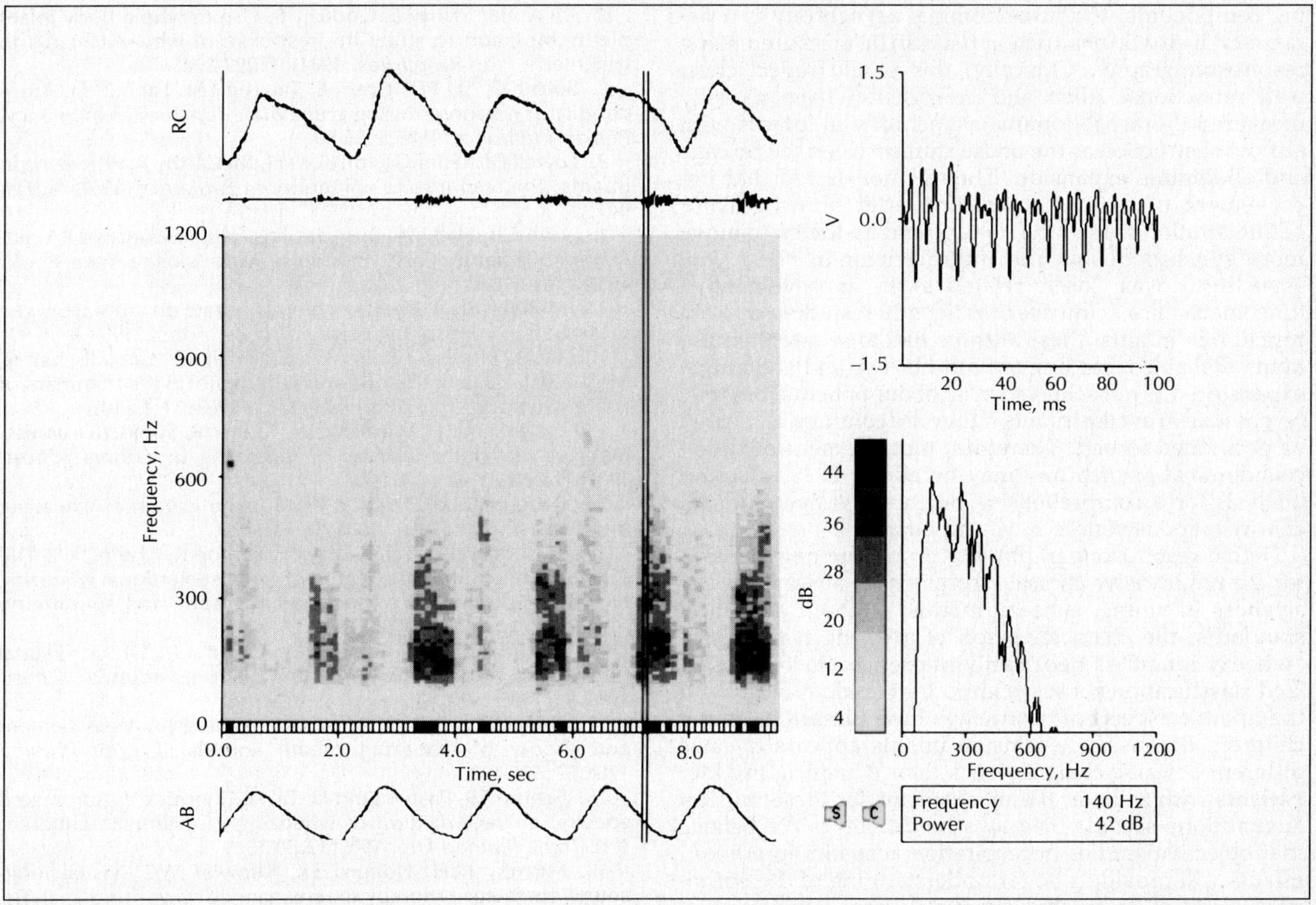

Fig 5.—*Digital respirosonogram as described in Fig 4 showing 9.5 seconds of recorded lung sounds and breathing patterns from patient 13 (Table 1) before salbutamol inhalation. The vertical double bar at 7.3 seconds points to a 100-ms segment of wheezing during expiration. The time amplitude display (top right) shows a complex repetitive wave form. The Fourier spectrum (bottom right) has fewer distinct peaks than that in Fig 4. One hundred-millisecond time intervals during which wheezing occurred are marked in gray on the horizontal axis.*

The efficacy of inhaled bronchodilators in infants with acute bronchiolitis is still controversial.[4,6] Although the relationship between airway hyperresponsiveness in infancy and symptomatic airway disease is not well determined, recent studies[7-9,20] indicate that many infants with wheezing will improve if treated with bronchodilators regardless of whether they are classified as having asthma, bronchiolitis, or wheezing-associated respiratory illness.[21]

Some infants may experience a paradoxical deterioration in lung function after salbutamol inhalation.[22,23] We found significantly increased wheezing after salbutamol inhalation in four of 16 infants. The respiratory rate remained unchanged after salbutamol inhalation in three of these four infants. In very severe airflow obstruction, normal lung sounds may be of very low intensity, and wheezing may be absent. Under these circumstances, improvement after bronchodilator administration may be accompanied by wheezing. However, these infants had normal vesicular lung sound intensity before inhalation. By both clinical and respirosonographic analysis, these patients did not improve after salbutamol inhalation, but whether increased wheezing reflected a paradoxical response remains unclear.

Baughman and Loudon[14] found that adult subjects with asthma and increased FEV_1 after bronchodilator administration experienced a reduction in the sound frequency of the highest pitched wheeze.[14] It is not clear from their data whether a reduction of T_w/T_{tot} in their patients correlated with the reduction in wheeze frequency. In a previous study,[15] we could not demonstrate a relationship between T_w/T_{tot} and wheeze frequency. In our present study of wheezy infants, we found that, after salbutamol inhalation, four of the responders had a reduction in $avgF_w$, two showed an increase in $avgF_w$, and one had no wheezing. It is interesting that wheeze frequency decreased after salbutamol inhalation even among nonresponders (seven of nine patients). At present, it is unclear whether a reduction in wheeze frequency indicates an improvement in the airflow obstruction or is caused by another mechanism.

The graphic display of lung sounds and respiration curves from the rib cage and abdomen shown in Figs 4 and 5 contains most parameters commonly used in the clinical scoring of wheezy infants. In fact, only the patient's oxygenation, which is generally addressed in clinical scores through an assessment of cyanosis, cannot be derived from the parameters recorded in our study. While oximetry is useful for the initial assessment of severity in bronchiolitis,[24,25] it may not reflect improvement after treatment.[20] In older children with asthma, we found that oxygen saturation may actually decrease immediately after salbutamol inhalation.[26]

In addition to the respiratory rate and ventilatory timing components, thoracoabdominal asynchrony is a parameter of airway obstruction that can be measured using respirosonography. Clinically, this would reflect chest wall retractions. Allen and coworkers[27] have recently measured thoracoabdominal asynchrony in infants with airflow obstruction as the phase shift between the rib cage and abdominal expansion. They demonstrated that improvement of airflow obstruction after bronchodilator administration caused the rib cage and abdomen to move more synchronously. The improvement in chest wall asynchrony was closely related to an improvement in lung mechanics. However, as in other studies of lung function in infants, these authors had to sedate their patients. Reliable recording of both rib cage and abdominal expansion was not achieved in all of our patients, but may be possible in awake infants if they are comfortably seated or positioned in bed. Therefore, measurement of thoracoabdominal asynchrony may be added to lung sound analysis for a comprehensive but noninvasive study of airway responsiveness in young infants.

Digital respirosonography is a promising new method for the noninvasive clinical assessment of airway responsiveness in young, wheezy infants. Without acoustical standards, the characterization of a young patient as a "wheezy infant" is necessarily imprecise. Such generalized classifications obscure important epidemiologic and therapeutic aspects of obstructive lung disease in young children. Because wheezing in infants appears to have different acoustic characteristics than wheezing in older patients with asthma, the mechanisms for these musical adventitious sounds may also be different. We believe that objective studies of respiration acoustics in wheezy infants will provide a better understanding of the pathophysiology of obstructive airway diseases developing at this young age.

This study was supported by the Children's Hospital of Winnipeg Research Foundation and the Manitoba Health Research Council, Winnipeg.

We thank Victor Chernick, MD, for his helpful suggestions and review of our article and Doris Jensen for secretarial support.

References

1. Gavrieli N, Kelly KB, Grotberg JB, Loring SH. Critical pressures required for generation of forced expiratory wheezes. *J Appl Physiol.* 1989;66:1136-1142.
2. Prendiville A, Green S, Silverman M. Bronchial responsiveness to histamine in wheezy infants. *Thorax.* 1987;42:92-99.
3. O'Callaghan C, Milner AD, Swarbrick A. Nebulized salbutamol does have a protective effect on airways in children under 1 year old. *Arch Dis Child.* 1988;63:479-483.
4. Silverman M. Airway responsiveness in infancy. *Clin Exp Allergy.* 1989;19:345-348.
5. Phelan PD, Williams HE. Sympathomimetic drugs in acute viral bronchiolitis. *Pediatrics.* 1969;44:493-497.
6. Lenny W, Milner AD. At what age do bronchodilator drugs work? *Arch Dis Child.* 1978;53:532-535.
7. Tal A, Bar Yishay E, Godfrey S. Use of whole body infant plethysmograph to study the response of wheezy infants to treatment. *Prog Respir Res.* 1981;17:299-300.
8. Soto ME, Sly PD, Urem E, Taussig LM, Landau LI. Bronchodilator response during acute viral bronchiolitis in infancy. *Pediatr Pulmonol.* 1985;2:85-90.
9. Lowell DI, Lister G, Von Koss H, McCarthy P. Wheezing in infants: the response to epinephrine. *Pediatrics.* 1987;79:939-945.
10. Hall CB, Hall WJ. Bronchiolitis. In: Hoekelman RA, ed. *Primary Pediatric Care.* St Louis, Mo: Mosby–Year Book; 1987:1161-1164.
11. Mallol J, Sly P. Effect of chloral hydrate on arterial oxygen saturation in wheezy infants. *Pediatr Pulmonol.* 1988;5:96-99.
12. Tal A, Bavilski, Yohai D, Bearman JE, Gorodischer R, Moses SW. Dexamethasone and salbutamol in the treatment of acute wheezing in infants. *Pediatrics.* 1983;71:13-18.
13. Pasterkamp H, Wiebicke W, Fenton R. Subjective assessment vs computer analysis of wheezing in asthma. *Chest.* 1987;91:376-381.
14. Baughman RP, Loudon RG. Quantification of wheezing in acute asthma. *Chest.* 1984;86:718-722.
15. Pasterkamp H, Tal A, Leahy F, Fenton R, Chernick V. The effect of anticholinergic treatment on postexertional wheezing in asthma studied by phonopneumography and spirometry. *Am Rev Respir Dis.* 1985;132:16-21.
16. Pasterkamp H, Carson C, Daien D, Oh Y. Digital respirosonography: new images of lung sounds. *Chest.* 1989;96:1405-1412.
17. Gavrieli N, Palti Y, Alroy G, Grotberg JB. Measurement and theory of wheezing breath sounds. *J Appl Physiol.* 1984;57:481-492.
18. Fenton TR, Pasterkamp H, Tal A, Chernick V. Automated spectral characterization of wheezing in asthmatic children. *IEEE Trans Biomed Eng.* 1985;32:50-55.
19. Murphy RLH, Holford SK, Knowler WC. Visual lung-sound characterization by time-expanded wave-form analysis. *N Engl J Med.* 1977;296:968-971.
20. Klassen TP, Rowe PC, Sutcliffe T, Ropp LJ, McDowell IW, Li MM. Randomized trial of salbutamol in acute bronchiolitis. *J Pediatr.* 1991;118:807-811.
21. Milburn WH. Bronchodilator treatment of wheezing infants. *Pediatr Rev.* 1990;11:287.
22. Prendiville A, Green S, Silverman M. Paradoxical response to nebulized salbutamol in wheezy infants: assessment by partial expiratory flow-volume curves. *Thorax.* 1987;42:86-91.
23. Hughes DM, LeSouef PN, Landau LI. Effect of salbutamol on respiratory mechanics in bronchiolitis. *Pediatr Res.* 1987;22:83-86.
24. Mulholland EK, Olinsky A, Shann FA. Clinical findings and severity of acute bronchiolitis. *Lancet.* 1990;335:1259-1261.
25. Shaw KN, Bell LM, Sherman NH. Outpatient assessment of infants with bronchiolitis. *AJDC.* 1991;145:151-155.
26. Tal A, Pasterkamp H, Leahy F. Arterial oxygen desaturation following salbutamol inhalation in acute asthma. *Chest.* 1984;86:868-869.
27. Allen JL, Wolfson MR, McDowell K, Shaffer TH. Thoracoabdominal asynchrony in infants with airflow obstruction. *Am Rev Respir Dis.* 1990;141:337-342.

Neuroblastoma Screening Data

An Epidemiologic Analysis

Steven N. Goodman, MD, MHS, PhD

• Neuroblastoma is one of the most common malignant neoplasms in children under age 5 years. Little progress has been made in the prognosis of advanced stage disease in the past three decades. Since the development in the 1960s of a simple urine test to detect neuroblastoma metabolites, there has been hope that mortality from this disease could be reduced by early detection via mass screening of young infants. Encouraging reports from Japan on mass screening programs instituted in the 1970s have been appearing in the medical literature since 1982, resulting in widespread interest in screening. This article applies standard epidemiologic criteria for screening evaluations to the Japanese reports. We find that the data needed to definitively assess the value of screening were not a part of those reports and that the benefits claimed from the reported data could be due to overdiagnosis. In addition, the most recent Japanese data, combined with recent advances in biologic understanding of neuroblastoma, show that screening at age 6 months may not detect tumors with poor prognoses. Even if it could, it is uncertain whether those outcomes could be substantially altered by earlier diagnosis. Although a final verdict on the value of neuroblastoma screening is not yet possible, these neuroblastoma studies are an excellent example of how screening results must be viewed with extreme caution in the absence of age-specific, population-based incidence and mortality rates.

(*AJDC.* 1991;145:1415-1422)

Neuroblastoma, one of the most common cancers of early childhood, ranks in incidence just below leukemias and approximately equal to brain tumors among children younger than 5 years.[1] In spite of intensive research and new chemotherapeutic regimens, long-term survival from advanced-stage disease has stayed relatively constant at about 10% to 20% in the past three decades.[2-4] Since the development in the 1960s of a simple urine spot test for the excreted metabolites of neuroblastoma, there has been hope that the mortality from this childhood cancer could be reduced through screening.[5] The basic rationale for such screening was simple: the tumor was thought to be present at birth, and both early stage and young age were associated with excellent prognosis. If the tumor could be detected biochemically at an age when there was known to be excellent survival, we should, in theory, be able to prevent the mortality usually accompanying clinical presentation at a later age. This offered the first possibility that a potentially fatal pediatric disease could be detected and cured via mass screening after the neonatal period.

This reasoning led Japanese investigators to institute experimental screening programs in Japan in the early 1970s. These programs were expanded to eight Japanese regions by the end of that decade, in a consortium known as the Japanese Mass Screening Study Group (MSSG). The first English language report on the Kyoto (Japan) experience was published by Sawada et al[6] in 1982. This, along with later encouraging reports on the apparent successes of the Japanese screening, led to great enthusiasm for the test both inside and outside that country. By 1985, the results were deemed so convincing within Japan that neuroblastoma screening in 6-month-old infants became recommended as part of their well-child care program, with each prefecture administering its own program.

With increasing awareness of the Japanese experience, scientists in North America and Europe began to call for an examination of neuroblastoma screening in settings outside Japan.[2] Although one such trial is currently under way in Canada[7] and another proposed for Britain,[8] there have been calls in both the medical literature and lay press for the institution of mass screening (*Palm Beach Post*. June 7, 1990:D1).[9] There also have been anecdotal reports of pediatricians and informed laypeople pressuring regional health departments or taking on themselves the task of organizing local screening programs.

This ground swell was based mainly on the perception that the Japanese screening programs were an unqualified success. This existed partially because of an absence of close examinations of the screening data using well-established epidemiologic criteria. Starting in the late 1980s, investigators began publishing cautions that the data were far from conclusive.[10-12] This article will show the basis for those cautions in detail by applying standard epidemiologic criteria to those data, and demonstrate the importance of such analyses in preventing premature implementation of mass screening technologies.

Accepted for publication March 7, 1991.
From the Division of Biostatistics, Department of Oncology, The Johns Hopkins University School of Medicine, Baltimore, Md.
Reprint requests to The Johns Hopkins University, 550 N Broadway, Suite 1103, Baltimore, MD 21205 (Dr Goodman).

BACKGROUND

Neuroblastoma is thought to be an embryonal tumor, present at birth and arising from cells in the sympathetic nervous system. Most tumors arise from the adrenal medulla and become clinically detectable as abdominal masses. Annual incidence in the United States based on Surveillance, Epidemiology, End Results (SEER) data for 1973 to 1982 was 8.5 per million children under age 15 years (95% confidence interval, 7.6 to 9.4 per million), with 85% of this incidence occurring before age 4 years, and 96% by age 9 years.[13] Incidence rates from 6.6 to 10.6 per million children have been reported in other countries, with the age pattern being similar in all regions.

It has long been recognized that age and stage have strong, independent effects on prognosis, with survival exceeding 90% in young, early-stage infants and dropping below 20% in older, late-stage cases.[14,15] This supports the notion that neuroblastoma is a congenital malignancy that grows from birth, and the longer before it is "caught," the worse the prognosis due to older age and/or more advanced stage. Neuroblastoma has at least one form that is known to spontaneously regress.[16,17] One autopsy study found neuroblastomalike cells in 30% of newborns who died of other causes.[18]

Several discoveries during the past 7 years about the molecular biology of neuroblastoma showed that this simple conceptual model relating age, growth, spread, and prognosis was flawed. Brodeur et al[19] reported in 1984 that amplification of the proto-oncogene N-*myc* had a very strong correlation with survival independent of stage and age. That same year, Look et al[20] reported that DNA ploidy had a strong relationship with prognosis, and this was confirmed in subsequent research.[21-27] Bourhis et al[28] found that once DNA ploidy and N-*myc* status were determined in a multivariate analysis of neuroblastoma prognosis, age no longer had an independent effect on prognosis. Most importantly, in addition to improving statistical prediction, such biologic markers have a potentially close link to basic mechanisms of oncogenesis.[29,30]

These reports, along with succeeding confirmatory research, have led to the suggestion that neuroblastoma may include two types of disease. The first is a true congenital tumor that is growing at birth, probably slowly, and is of the good prognostic type, usually presenting at a young age as a mass, without extension or metastases. The second type may lie dormant until an activation step occurs at later ages, then growing quickly and aggressively, often having metastasized by the time the primary mass is detected.[10,11]

The Japanese neuroblastoma screening program conducted urine tests on infants at age 6 months. Initially, only vanillylmandelic acid (VMA) levels were tested using a qualitative "spot test," based on a color change of treated paper.[5] Later, some districts increased test sensitivity by adding a thin-layer chromatography test for homovanillic acid (HVA) levels.[31] Most recently, some regions have used high-performance liquid chromatography (HPLC), the most sensitive of the three methods for testing levels of both VMA and HVA.[32,33]

THE SCREENING DATA

The data from the original Japanese reports are summarized herein in the order in which they were published, to give some sense of how perceptions of neuroblastoma screening were formed. The emphases in these summaries are not always those of the authors. The main focus in most of the articles from Japan was on the excellent outcomes of screened cases, and on the rates of false-negative and -positive test results, which were thought to represent the main "costs" incurred by the test. Here, the focus is on the observed incidence rates and prevalence of positive results among those screened. These are then compared with expected rates in the epidemiologic analysis that follows.

There have been many reports since 1984 on the Japanese screening experience, some of them overlapping; six of the most important are summarized in the Table. The first study was that by Sawada et al[6] on screening experience in Kyoto from 1974 to 1979, using the spot test. They reported that the test identified four patients out of 78 331 infants screened at age 6 months (a prevalence of 1 in 19 500).

Two years later, Sawada et al[34] analyzed all patients treated at Kyoto University from 1962 to 1982. Stage, age, and survival were reported for 35 patients identified before screening started in 1974, and the 22 patients identified after that time. The proportion of patients identified at a young age or early stage was greater in the screened cohort than in the earlier unscreened one, and survival rates were much higher. However, 16 of the 22 patients from the screening period were detected clinically and not through the test, so the shift to diagnosis at earlier ages and stages was partially attributed to an indirect effect of screening: greater awareness among Kyoto pediatricians of the need for good abdominal examinations, with consequent increased clinical recognition. The number of cases annually was virtually constant throughout the entire period: 2.9 per year between 1962 and 1973 and 2.8 per year between 1974 and 1982. In a separate study, Sawada et al[35] reported that the Kyoto incidence rate, including the screened cases, was 13.3 cases per million person-years for children under age 15 years, and 93 cases per million person-years for infants under age 1 year.

The next major screening report was in 1984, the first from the MSSG.[36] The previously described Kyoto cohort made up 42% of the infants screened in this report. This study reported approximately the same prevalence of true positive results as had the Kyoto studies—16 in 281 939 cases, or about 1 per 18 000 infants. However, two regions that used modified testing procedures had very high prevalences (1 in 6400 and 1 in 4000), providing all but one of the cases found outside Kyoto.[37] As in the previous reports, screened cases had excellent prognoses. In 1986, an update by the MSSG added nine new cases, and showed a continued prevalence of 1 in 19 000 infants, with excellent outcomes.[38] In April 1985 the Japanese government recommended that all local governments develop mass screening programs.

The most influential study appeared in 1987, in which Nishi et al[39] reported on the Sapporo (Japan) screening program. The city of Sapporo commenced screening in 1981, but the surrounding prefecture of Hokkaido did not have a program. In both regions, pediatric cancer cases were reported to the same children's cancer registry that had been in place since 1969. Nishi et al compared neuroblastoma cases in the two regions before (1969-1980) and during (1981-1984) testing in Sapporo.

Figure 1, derived from the data of Nishi et al,[39] summarizes their most important result. Briefly, the age and

Summary of Characteristics and Results of Main Published Japanese Reports on Neuroblastoma Screening, 1982-1990*

Source, y	Source of Screened Population	Method of Detecting Unscreened or Missed Screened Cases	Source of Comparison Population	Type of Test	Size of Screened Population	No. of Cases/ No. Screened/ No. Missed at Clinical Presentation	Prevalance of True-Positives in Screened Population	Primary Outcomes
Sawada et al,[6] (1982)	11 Health centers in Kyoto, 1973-1979	Not stated	None	VMA Spot test	78 331	4/1/?	1/15 700	Good survival of screening-detected patients
Sawada et al,[34] (1984)	8 Districts in Japan (MSSG), including Kyoto	Not stated	None	Several methods, mainly qualitative[38]	281 939	16/6/?	1/17 600	Favorable age/stage of screened cases, and good short-term survival
Sawada et al,[36] (1984)	Kyoto, 1974-1982	Patients treated at Kyoto University	Kyoto, 1962-1974	VMA Spot test	117 103	6/1/16	1/16 700	Improvement of survival, age, and stage of 22 patients found in screening era (6 via screening) compared with prescreening era
Nishi et al,[39] (1987)	Sapporo, 1981-1984	Pediatric tumor registry	Sapporo, 1969-1980; Hokkaido, 1969-1980, 1981-1984	Spot for VMA, TLC for HVA	73 226	11/4/1	1/4900	Dramatic favorable shift in age and stage distribution, with improved survival (20%-90%) comparing Sapporo before-after screening and concurrently with Hokkaido
Sawada et al,[41] (1988)	MSSG, 9 regions, 1981-1986	Unstated, different in each region	Case from JPSR, 1971-1976, and USCCSG	Several methods, mainly qualitative	Not stated	89/?/?	1/15 500-1/18 800	Good age/stage distribution and survival compared with USCCSG reports and JPSR; median tumor weight, 50g, 70% of abdominal neuroblastomas palpable after screening
Naito et al,[43] (1990)	Sapporo and Hokkaido, 1981-1989 (Hokkaido started screen in 1987)	Patients undergoing surgery at two hospitals (? 60% of total)	Sapporo and Hokkaido, 1972-1980	1981-1984, Same as Nishi et al,[39] 1984-1989, HPLC	Unknown	27/?/23	Unknown	Improvement in stage and resectability of screened tumors and improved 5-year survival of screening era cases, compared with cases in prescreening era (67% vs 23%)

*VMA indicates vanillylmandelic acid; MSSG, Mass Screening Study Group; TLC, thin-layer chromatography; HVA, homovanillic acid; JPSR, Japanese Pediatric Surgery Registry; USCCSG, US Children's Cancer Study Group; and HPLC, high-performance liquid chromatography.

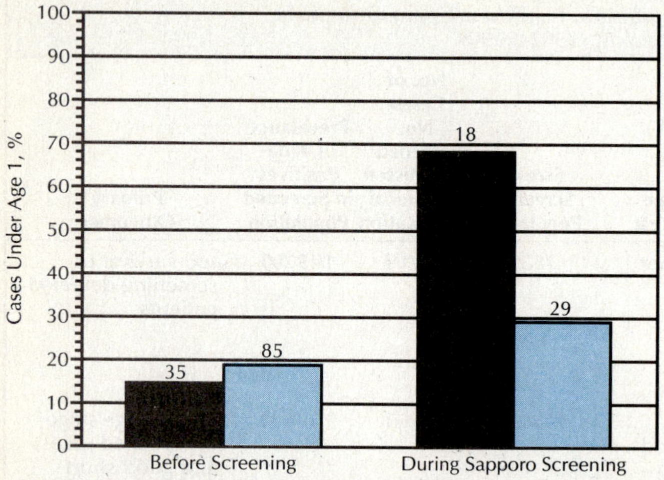

Fig 1.—*Percentage of neuroblastoma cases in patients under age 1 year in Sapporo, Japan (solid bars), and Hokkaido, Japan (shaded bars), before screening was started (1969 to 1980) and during screening in Sapporo (1981 to 1984). Numbers above bars indicate the total number of cases. Based on data from Nishi et al.*[39]

stage distribution of cases was similar between Sapporo and Hokkaido in the years before screening, but after screening commenced in Sapporo, cases in that city showed a dramatic shift to younger ages and earlier stages. The long-term survival rate increased from 25% to 90% in Sapporo but was unchanged in Hokkaido. Eleven of the 18 cases in Sapporo in this latter period were identified through screening. Of 73 226 infants screened, 15 (1 per 4900) tested positive and had the disease. Four additional infants initially tested negative, but were diagnosed with neuroblastoma after age 6 months, for a total neuroblastoma risk of 1 per 3900 in this cohort.

Later in 1987, Sawada et al[40] reported that after the January 1985 shift to the more sensitive HPLC screening in Kyoto, the prevalence of positive results increased from 1 in 17 800 to 1 in 5000; however, the reason for the apparent increase was uncertain.

In 1988, a report by the MSSG on 89 screening-detected cases (which included the 25 previously reported cases) showed continued good outcomes. Prevalence among screened infants was 1 in 15 000 to 18 000. Of 80 patients with abdominal neuroblastoma, 70% had palpable masses, although 50% of the total had tumors that weighed less than 50 g.[41]

With the adoption of testing throughout Japan, the possibility of another natural experiment like that conducted by Nishi et al diminished. However, in 1989, they compared results from districts still using low-sensitivity detection methods with those from Sapporo, which had used the high-sensitivity HPLC since 1984.[42] The screening prevalence was 1 in 5500 in Sapporo and 1 in 24 630 in the low-sensitivity districts. The median size of the tumors found in Sapporo was less than half of those in the other districts (24 vs 60 g); the median metabolite levels in Sapporo were half of those in the other regions; and the percentage of cases in stage I was double (40% vs 20%). They concluded, " . . . more patients with a small tumor must have been missed in the districts of qualitative methods."

In 1990, Naito et al[43] extended the 1987 data of Nishi et al[39] based on screening in Sapporo, and reported a dramatic improvement in surgical mortality and prognosis among screened cases in Sapporo and Hokkaido (where screening started in 1987) detected through March 1989. The 5-year survival rate improved from 23% in the prescreening era to 67% during screening, based on approximately 50 cases in each group. They concluded that while screening still had problems related to cost, false-negative results, and HVA/VMA cutoff values, " . . . this program is steadily improving the prognosis for neuroblastoma. Because of these results we suggest that the efforts to perfect and implement such programs elsewhere will similarly have a positive impact on outcome from neuroblastoma." Commenting on this article, a noted US pediatrician commented, "I cannot understand why screening for neuroblastoma in infants has not become routine in the US. . . . I would suspect that there are other pilot studies which will eventually be reported. I would argue that there is no reason to wait."[9]

More recently, data from Sawada et al show a continuation of previous patterns. Of 337 cases detected by screening through 1988 by the MSSG, 58% had tumors of less than 50 g, and 52% of the 293 abdominal neuroblastomas were palpable. In Kyoto, the prevalence stayed as high through 1988 as it had been in the 1987 report, eight cases in 36 000 screened (1 in 4600). This corresponded with a shift to younger patients and increase of 5-year survival rate from 17% in the prescreening period to 55% and 85% during low-sensitivity and high-sensitivity screening, respectively (Tadashi Sawada, MD, personal communication, March 1990).

EPIDEMIOLOGIC ASSESSMENT

Did these reports provide strong evidence that screening could improve the prognosis for neuroblastoma? We will attempt to answer this by applying standard epidemiologic criteria to these data. The four basic epidemiologic biases that all studies of early disease detection or screening can be subject to are as follows: referral bias, detection bias, lead-time bias, and length-time bias.[44,45] Each one will be discussed in relation to the neuroblastoma screening data.

Referral (Selection) Bias

This bias is produced when the screened population is self-selected or chosen by the investigator so that their prognosis, once the disease is recognized, is better than that of the unscreened population. It is evaluated by examining the process and outcome of screening selection. There should be no known prognostic factors that are unbalanced between the screened and unscreened populations. No strong demographic or environmental risk factors for neuroblastoma have yet been identified,[13] nor are any such factors (aside from age) known to be associated with prognosis. Thus it is unlikely that the screened populations could self-select to have either different neuroblastoma risk than the unscreened group or a better prognosis once disease was identified.

Detection (Overdiagnosis) Bias

This bias occurs when screening detects disease that would never have presented clinically, ie, it would have spontaneously regressed and never been noticed if not for the test.

The only way to definitively assess overdiagnosis is by comparing age-specific and overall disease incidence rates between screened and unscreened populations or before and after screening in the same population. An incidence rate is the ratio of new cases to the number at risk during a specific time interval. Unfortunately, the number at risk is often difficult to define, and in none of the screening reports except that by Sawada et al[35] were incidence rates determined on a combined screened and unscreened population.

However, two indexes from these reports can be used as crude surrogates for incidence rates. The first is the annual number of cases in a defined geographic region. To draw any conclusions from such numbers, it has to be assumed that the population at risk is constant, and the reporting mechanisms are reliable and unbiased. If these conditions apply, the annual number of cases should be proportional to the annual incidence rate.

The second index is the prevalence of screening-detected disease among all those tested. Its relationship to incidence rates is not simple. Presumably, a screening-detected case is one that would have presented at a later age if the patient had not been screened. Therefore, with perfect screening, the proportion of infants in whom the disease is detected at the time of screening (prevalence of disease in the screened cohort) should be equal to the proportion of the cohort that would eventually have presented clinically at later ages (cumulative risk of disease beyond the screening age). If more cases are detected through screening than we would expect to detect clinically at and beyond the screening age, overdiagnosis is a likely explanation.

The subsequent analysis will show that both of those surrogate measures suggest that more infants were diagnosed with high-sensitivity screening than would have developed the disease later, making it possible that a certain proportion of them would have naturally regressed.

Screening Prevalence.—Sawada et al[35] reported in 1984 that the incidence rate in Japan for children under age 15 years was 8.2 per million per year. This is equivalent to a total neuroblastoma risk for the first 15 years of life of about $15 \times 8.2 \times 10^{-6}$, or 1 in 8130. Since about 25% of all cases occur before the screening age of 6 months, the prevalence of cases at the time of screening should be about $0.75 \times (1/8130)$, or 1 in 10 840. If the test had a sensitivity of 75%, we should have expected the Japanese researchers to find neuroblastoma in approximately 1 per 14 000 infants tested.

The earliest reports were consistent with these numbers, showing a prevalence of 1 in 15 000 to 18 000 among screened infants, using the qualitative VMA spot test, with a sensitivity of about 75%.[39,46] However, the addition of more sensitive testing methods increased the prevalence of positive results to 1 in 5000 in both Sapporo and Kyoto, suggesting that the number of cases diagnosed with those techniques might have been twofold to threefold higher than would have presented clinically without screening. The prevalence based on the total Japanese screening experience has so far not appeared excessive, because cumulative reports have included the early qualitatively tested populations, and many prefectures still use low-sensitivity tests.[41]

Number of Cases per Year.—Several years of screening should result in an increase in the number of cases diagnosed before age 1 year by exactly the same amount as the decrease in the number diagnosed after that age. If the test overdiagnoses tumors, the increased number of cases in the first year of life will be greater than the reduction at older ages.

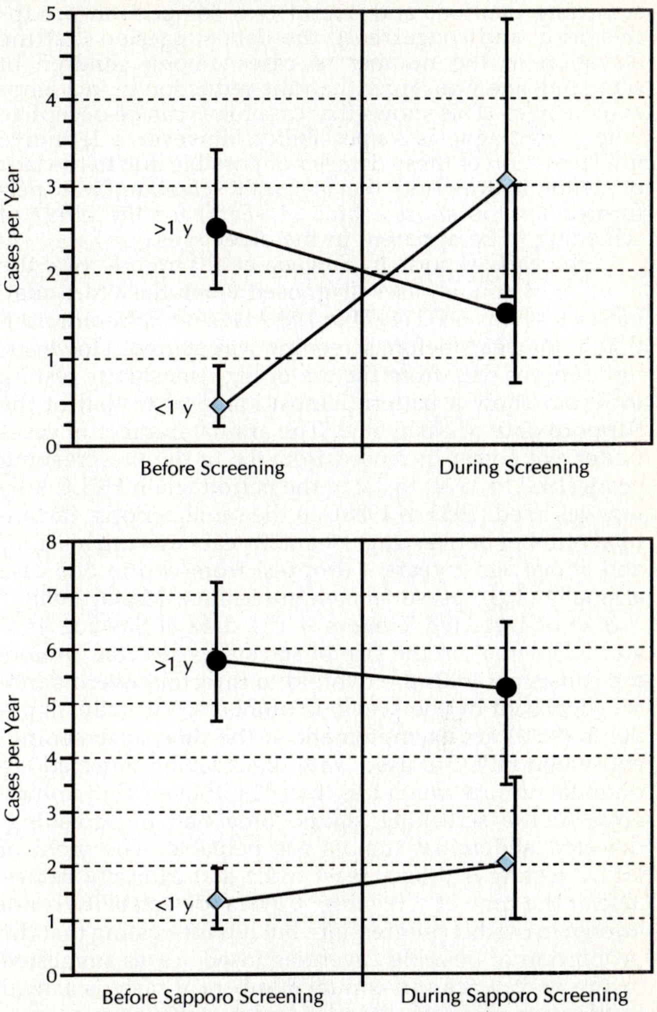

Fig 2.—*Annual number of neuroblastoma cases, by age, in Sapporo (top) and Hokkaido (bottom) during the years before screening (1969 to 1980) and during screening in Sapporo (1981 to 1984). Error bars represent 95% confidence intervals. Based on data from Nishi et al.*[39]

This shift to younger ages is what Nishi et al[39] claimed to have demonstrated in 1987 (Fig 1). Figure 2 redisplays the numbers from Fig 1, presented now as annual number of cases, with 95% confidence intervals. This figure shows that an interpretation different from that in the original article was also supported by these data. Looking first at data from Hokkaido, where there was no screening, we see a minimal, nonsignificant change in the annual number of cases in both age categories before and during the Sapporo screening periods. In Sapporo, where the prevalence of positive results was high, the pattern was quite different. Among children over age 1 year, there was a statistically nonsignificant decrease of about 1 case per year after the onset of screening. Among those under age 1 year, there was a statistically significant increase of 2.5 cases per year, a sevenfold change. There was only minimal statistical evidence that the rate in older children had changed, and even if change were real, it was less than the statistically significant increase among the younger children.

Thus, we find that in a study with probably good case ascertainment (through a single tumor registry), sensitive screening method, and use of two comparison groups (historical and concurrent), the data suggested that the elevation in the number of cases among children of screening age was larger than the reduction in incidence at older ages. This shows that case totals can be deceptive when overdiagnosis is a possibility. However, a definitive interpretation of these data is not possible due to the lack of denominators and the fact that screening was performed for too short a time (4 years) for the effect of screening to be apparent in the older ages.

In the early reports by Sawada et al[34] from Kyoto, the number of annual cases diagnosed when the VMA qualitative test was used (1974 to 1982) was not different from that in the years before screening was started. However, more recent data from the era of high-sensitivity testing in Kyoto show a pattern almost identical to that of the Sapporo data of Nishi et al. The annual number of cases under age 1 year increased from 0.6 in the prescreening years (1962 to 1974) to 3.2 in the period when HPLC testing was used (1983 to 1988). In the same periods, the annual number between ages 1 and 2 years was unchanged, and above age 2 years it dropped from two to one case annually (T.S., personal communication, March 1990).

Size of Detected Tumors.—The data of Sawada et al and Nishi et al on the size of screening-detected tumors are consistent with the twofold to threefold overdiagnosis suggested by the previous numbers. Virtually all patients (96%) are asymptomatic at the time of screening, and when HPLC is used, 75% of screening detected abdominal tumors weigh less than 50 g.[42] Even with knowledge of the screening status, only half of screening-detected abdominal tumors are palpable. The yield of HPLC testing is thus at least twice that clinically detectable at the time of screening. Clinical detectability is not known to predict progression, but it is interesting that the proportion of possible "overdiagnosed" cases suggested by the prevalence and annual numbers of cases is similar to the proportion of clinically undetectable ones.

A finding of overdiagnosis does not eliminate the possibility that a screening program might be of benefit if it can be determined that the prognosis of nonoverdiagnosed cases is improved by earlier detection. However, overdiagnosis injects another serious cost (ie, unnecessary treatment of overdiagnosed cases) into the cost-benefit equation.

Lead-Time Bias

This bias exists when the survival of the screened patients from the time of diagnosis appears longer only because their conditions were diagnosed earlier; they still die at the same age they would have without the early diagnosis.

The purpose of screening is to either reduce overall mortality rates or shift the age-specific mortality to older ages. If there is lead-time bias, age-specific mortality rates will remain constant even though survival time after diagnosis appears longer. Lead-time bias "slides" survival curves over, ie, they show the same long-term survival, but with a longer period of low mortality at the beginning.

In both the before-after comparisons of Sawada et al and the parallel comparisons of Nishi et al, long-term survival was substantially better in screened cases than in those detected clinically (approximately 90% vs 20% to 30%), a difference that cannot be produced by lead-time bias. The 55% 5-year survival rate of the Kyoto cases during the qualitative screening period (1974 to 1982) was better than the 20% survival rate before screening, but it was comparable with the survival rates from the United States and Denmark at that time,[3,11,47] suggesting a contribution of improved medical care. However, medical care could not explain the concurrent Sapporo-Hokkaido comparison, in which all cases were treated in the same hospital at the same time. However, the survival curve approach cannot be used in the presence of overdiagnosis, since this will "pad" the screened cases with patients with good prognoses who would not have been included in these curves without the screen, making it appear as though something more than a time-shift has occurred. In such a situation, only age-specific mortality rates can be used, which were not reported.

Length-Time Bias

This effect occurs if the timing of screening in some way selects for cases with better prognoses. It derives its name from the situation in which a test preferentially picks up patients with slower-growing tumors with the longest preclinical detection phase, because faster-growing disease will be more likely to have been clinically recognized before screening.

This is a difficult bias to assess because the good outcome of the screening-detected tumors is usually ascribed to early detection and not to the selection of less aggressive cases. Its presence is strongly suggested when, even after controlling for other biases, screening-detected cases appear to do well without a concomitant change in age-specific mortality rates. If screening is repeated periodically, such as with Papanicolaou smears and mammograms, this effect diminishes and the outcome of initial and later screens can be compared. Alternatively, if there is any intrinsic biologic marker of disease aggressiveness, this can be used to evaluate whether screening-detected cases are qualitatively different from those later detected with symptoms.

With the finding of N-*myc* amplification and diploidy as strong negative prognostic factors, neuroblastoma is one of the unusual diseases in which this bias can be directly assessed. It is known that there is a strong association between young age and good prognostic markers among those that present clinically.[28-30,48] If screening detected tumors that would have presented at older ages, we would expect the proportion of screening-detected cases with bad prognostic markers to be higher than among those that clinically present at the same age. If a length-bias or similar effect were operating, another pattern would appear: screened cases would have the same fraction of favorable prognostic markers (or higher, if there is overdiagnosis) than those that present clinically at the same age.

This latter pattern is what has been shown clearly among the screened cases studied so far. There have been several studies comparing genetic markers among screening-detected cases, clinically detected cases under age 1 year, and those that presented clinically at older ages.[21,49-51] All of the studies show that both screening-detected cases and young clinical cases have a high percentage of good prognostic markers, and no screening case has yet been reported with N-*myc* amplification. These patients have had excellent survival. In contrast, those who presented clinically at older ages have had very poor prognostic markers and their long-term survival has been correspondingly poor. The

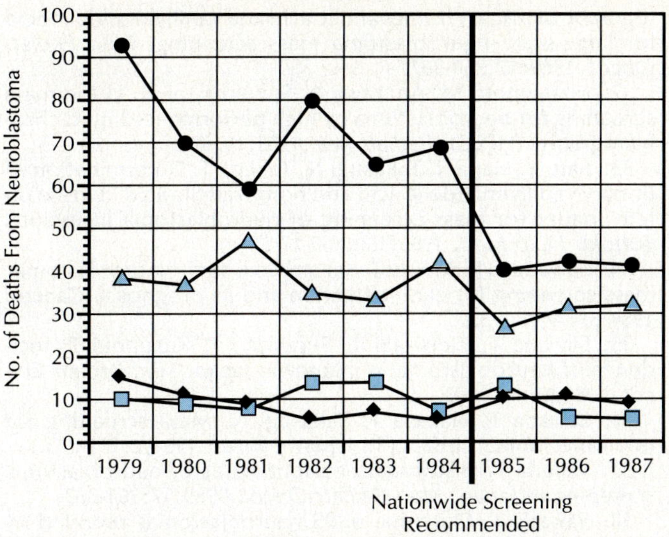

Fig 3.—*Annual number of deaths from neuroblastoma according to death certificates issued by the Japanese Ministry of Law between 1979 and 1987. Screening started in individual districts before 1985, and is being phased in nationally since then (see text). Squares represent newborns; circles, children between ages 1 and 4 years; triangles, children between ages 5 and 9 years; and diamonds, children less than age 10 years.*

authors of the largest study of this type concluded that screening at age 6 months missed most of the poor prognosis neuroblastomas.[51]

This evidence suggests that many of the screening detected cases are not ones that in the absence of screening would later become poor prognostic cases. If true, this would weaken the primary rationale for screening. However, if an untreated tumor of good prognostic genotype could evolve into one of poor prognostic genotype, the observed patterns would not be evidence that screening was missing poor prognosis tumors. Brodeur et al[52] addressed the question by following up 60 patients being treated for neuroblastoma, and found none whose N-*myc* amplification changed with relapse or progression, even under the selective pressure of chemotherapy. This is further support for the contention that the known age/stage pattern of prognosis and disease may be the manifestation of the two distinctly different biologic processes.

Whatever biases may be operating, the final, definitive measure of the benefit of screening is the difference in age-specific mortality rates between screened and unscreened populations, preferably compared concurrently. As yet, no such data have been reported from Japan or elsewhere, although the Canadian project will provide such numbers.[7] The data of Dr Tadashi Sawada (personal communication, March 1990) on the number of deaths from neuroblastoma reported in Japan through 1987 are the only related numbers available at this time (Fig 3). The sudden decrease in the number of cases in the 1- to 4-year age group in 1985 is both intriguing and puzzling. It is difficult to attribute this entirely to mass screening, since it was recommended but not immediately instituted nationwide in 1985. Screening was performed in a number of districts before that time; however, it takes at least 3½ years for the effect of screening at 6 months to be fully apparent in a 1- to 4-year age group. Since neither a denominator nor completeness of the reporting mechanism is known, it is not possible to know at this time what this pattern represents, or if it will continue.

CONCLUSION

The Japanese neuroblastoma screening studies were an ambitious and exciting attempt to examine the potential of a new technology to reduce mortality from an often fatal pediatric disease. However, the application of rigorous epidemiologic criteria to the Japanese neuroblastoma screening data might have tempered early enthusiasm. As has occurred in the United States for other childhood diseases,[53] this enthusiasm resulted in pressure to institute neuroblastoma screening programs. A formal epidemiologic analysis would have drawn attention away from false-negative and false-positive rates and the survival of detected cases, and instead highlighted the importance of missing data (incidence and mortality rates) that are critical to the evaluation of biases that can produce an illusion of screening benefit. It would have raised the possibility of twofold to threefold overdiagnosis, and could have suggested the presence of a length-time effect. In the absence of mortality rates, recent studies based on genetic prognostic markers have provided strong evidence that high-sensitivity screening preferentially detects cases that would have had excellent prognoses even if they had later presented clinically. At this time, there are few data on the effect of advancing the time of diagnosis within biologic prognostic categories, so the effect of using different, or multiple, screening ages is not known. The status of neuroblastoma screening is very uncertain at this time, and further data from Japan, as well as Canada, are needed to determine whether screening is harmful or beneficial, and at what individual and societal cost.

This work was supported in part by grants from the Maryland Children's Cancer Foundation, Baltimore, and the CSX Corporation, Baltimore.

We thank Tadashi Sawada, MD, for graciously supplying Japanese screening data through 1988 and granting permission for its use.

References

1. Young J, Reis L, Silverberg E, Horm J, Miller R. Cancer incidence, survival, and mortality for children younger than age 15 years. *Cancer.* 1986;58:598-602.

2. Woods W, Tuchman M. Neuroblastoma: the case for screening infants in North America. *Pediatrics.* 1987;79:869-873.

3. Carlsen N, Schroeder H, Bro P, et al. Neuroblastoma treated at the four major child oncologic clinics in Denmark 1943-80: an evaluation of 180 cases. *Med Pediatr Oncol.* 1985;13:180-186.

4. Kinnier Wilson L, Draper G. Neuroblastoma, its natural history and prognosis: a study of 487 cases. *BMJ.* 1974;3:301-307.

5. LaBrosse EH. Biochemical diagnosis of neuroblastoma: use of a urine spot test. *Proc Am Assoc Cancer Res.* 1968;9:39.

6. Sawada T, Todo S, Fujita K, Iino S, Imashuku S, Kusunoki T. Mass screening of neuroblastoma in infancy. *AJDC.* 1982;136:710-712.

7. Tuchman M, Lemieux B, Auray-Blais C, et al. Screening for neuroblastoma in North America: preliminary results from the Quebec project. *Pediatrics.* 1990;86:765-773.

8. Craft A, Dale G, McGill A, Seviour J, Spence E. Biochemical screening for neuroblastoma in infants: a feasibility study. *Med Pediatr Oncol.* 1989;17:373-378.

9. Gellis S. Isn't it time for mass screening of infants for neuroblastoma? *Pediatr Notes.* 1990;14:39.

10. Mauer A. Screening for neuroblastoma. *J Pediatr.* 1988;112:576-577.

11. Tuchman M, Lemieux B, Woods WB. Screening for neuroblastoma in infants: investigate or implement? *Pediatrics.* 1990;86:791-793.

12. Murphy S, Cohn S, Craft A, et al. Do children benefit from mass screening for neuroblastoma? consensus statement for the American Cancer Society Workshop on Neuroblastoma Screening. *Lancet.* 1991;337:344-346.

13. Davis S, Rogers M, Prendergrass T. The incidence and epidemiologic characteristics of neuroblastoma in the United States. *Am J Epidemiol.* 1987;126:1063-1074.

14. Breslow N, McCann B. Statistical estimation of prognosis for children with neuroblastoma. *Cancer Res.* 1971;31:2098-2103.

15. Coldman A, Fryer C, Elwood J, Sonley M. Influence of age at diagnosis, stage, tumor site, and sex on prognosis. *Cancer.* 1980;46:1896-1901.

16. Evans A, Chatten J, D'Angio G, Gerson J, Robinson J, Schnauffer L. A review of 17 IV-S neuroblastoma patients at the children's hospital of Philadelphia. *Cancer.* 1989;45:833-839.

17. Haas D, Ablin A, Miller C, et al. Complete pathologic maturation and regression of stage IV-S neuroblastoma without treatment. *Cancer.* 1988;62:818-825.

18. Beckwith J, Perrin E. In situ neuroblastomas: a contribution to the natural history of neural crest tumors. *Am J Pathol.* 1963;43:1089-1104.

19. Brodeur G, Seeger R, Schwab M, Varmus HE, Bishop JM. Amplification of n-*myc* in untreated human neuroblastomas correlates with advanced disease stage. *Science.* 1984;224:1121-1124.

20. Look A, Hayes F, Noitschke R, McWilliams N, Green A. Cellular DNA content as a predictor of response to chemotherapy in infants with unresectable neuroblastoma. *N Engl J Med.* 1984;311:231-235.

21. Hayashi Y, Inaba T, Hanada R, Yamamoto K. Chromosome findings and prognosis in 15 patients with neuroblastoma found by VMA mass screening. *J Pediatr.* 1988;112:567-571.

22. Kaneko Y, Kanda N, Maseki N, et al. Different karyotypic patterns in early and advanced stage neuroblastomas. *Cancer Res.* 1987;47:311-318.

23. Oppedal B, Storm-Mathisen I, Lie S, Brandtzaeb P. Prognostic factors in neuroblastoma: clinical, histopathologic, and immunohistochemical features and DNA ploidy in relation to prognosis. *Cancer.* 1988;62:772-780.

24. Nakagawara A. Genomic aspects of neuroblastomas in children under one year of age. In: D'Angio G, Evans A, Knudson A, Seeger R, eds. *The Fifth Symposium on Neuroblastoma Research.* Philadelphia, Pa: The Children's Hospital of Pennsylvania; 1990:47.

25. Nakagawara A, Ikeda K, Tsuda T, Higashi K. Biological characteristics of n-*myc* amplified neuroblastoma in patients over one year of age. *Adv Neuroblastoma Res.* 1988;2:31-39.

26. Nakagawara A, Ikeda K, Tsuda T, Higashi K. N-*myc* oncogene amplification and prognostic factors of neuroblastoma in children. *J Pediatr Surg.* 1987;22:895-898.

27. Tsuda T, Obara M, Hirano H, et al. Analysis of n-*myc* amplification in relation to disease stage and histologic types in human neuroblastomas. *Cancer.* 1987;60:820-826.

28. Bourhis J, Benard J, Wilson G, et al. Prognostic value of ploidic index and N-*myc* DNA amplification in 59 neuroblastomas. In: D'Angio G, Evans A, Knudson A, Seeger R, eds. *The Fifth Symposium on Neuroblastoma Research.* Philadelphia, Pa: The Children's Hospital of Pennsylvania; 1990:10.

29. Brodeur G. Clinical significance of genetic rearrangements in human neuroblastomas. *Clin Chem.* 1989;35/7B:B38-B42.

30. Brodeur G. The involvement of oncogenes and suppressor genes in human neoplasia. *Adv Pediatr.* 1987;34:1-44.

31. Auray-Blais C, Giguere R, Lemieux B. Thin-layer chromatography of urinary homovanillic acid and vanillylmandelic acid for large-scale neuroblastoma mass screening. *Med Pediatr Oncol.* 1989;17:364-367.

32. Matsumoto M, Anazawa A, Suzuki K, et al. Urine mass screening for neuroblastoma by high performance liquid chromatography (HPLC). *Pediatr Res.* 1985;19:625.

33. Sato Y, Hanai J, Takasugi N, Takeda T. Determination of urinary vanillylmandelic acid and homovanillic acid in urine on filter paper for mass screening of neuroblastoma in infants. *Tohoku J Exp Med.* 1986;150:169-174.

34. Sawada T, Kidowaki T, Sakamoto I, et al. Neuroblastoma: mass screening for early detection and its prognosis. *Cancer.* 1984;53:2731-2735.

35. Sawada T, Kidowaki T, Sugimoto T, Kusunoki T. Incidence of neuroblastoma in infancy in Japan. *Med Pediatr Oncol.* 1984;12:101-103.

36. Sawada T, Nakaza T, Takasugi N. Mass screening for neuroblastoma in infants in Japan. *Lancet.* 1984;2:271-273.

37. Takeda T. History and current status of neuroblastoma screening in Japan. *Med Pediatr Oncol.* 1989;17:361-363.

38. Sawada T. Outcome of 25 neuroblastomas revealed by mass screening in Japan. *Lancet.* 1986;1:377.

39. Nishi M, Miyake H, Takeda T, et al. Effects of the mass screening of neuroblastoma in Sapporo City. *Cancer.* 1987;60:433-436.

40. Sawada T, Kawakatu H, Sugimoto T. Screening for neuroblastoma. *Lancet.* 1987;2:1204.

41. Sawada T, Sugimoto T, Matsumura T, Tunoda A, Takeda T, et al. Mass screening for neuroblastoma in infancy. In: *Advances in Neuroblastoma Research 2.* New York, NY: Alan R Liss Inc; 1988:525-534.

42. Nishi M, Hirotsugo M, Takeda T, et al. Cases of neuroblastoma missed by the mass screening programs. *Pediatr Res.* 1989;26:603-607.

43. Naito H, Sasaki M, Yamashiro K, et al. Improvement in prognosis of neuroblastoma through mass population screening. *J Pediatr Surg.* 1990;25:245-248.

44. Cole P, Morrison AS. Basic issues in population screening for Cancer. *J Natl Cancer Inst.* 1980;64:1263-1272.

45. Miller A. Screening for cancer: issues and future directions. *J Chronic Dis.* 1986;39:1067-1077.

46. Sawada T, Kawakatus H, Sugimoto T, et al. Neuroblastoma mass screening in infancy in Kyoto, Japan. *Indian J Pediatr.* 1987;54:874-882.

47. Kramer S, Meadows A, Jarnett P, Evans A. Incidence of childhood cancer: experience of a decade in a population-based registry. *J Natl Cancer Inst.* 1983;70:49-55.

48. Evans A, D'Angio G, Propert K, Anderson J, Hahn H-W. Prognostic factors in neuroblastoma. *Cancer.* 1987;59:1853-1859.

49. Kaneko Y, Maseki N, Sakurai M, et al. Chromosomes and screening for neuroblastoma. *Lancet.* 1988;1:174-175.

50. Ishimoto K, Kiyokawa N, Ohya T, Miyano T, Shinohara T, Sera Y. Biological analysis of neuroblastoma in mass screened negative cases. In: D'Angio G, Evans A, Knudson A, Seeger R, eds. *The Fifth Symposium on Neuroblastoma Research.* Philadelphia, Pa: The Children's Hospital of Pennsylvania; 1990:117.

51. Kaneko K, Kanda N, Maseki N, et al. Current urinary mass screening for catecholamine metabolites at 6 months of age may be detecting only a small portion of high-risk neuroblastomas: a chromosome and N-*myc* amplification study. *J Clin Oncol.* 1990;8:2005-2013.

52. Brodeur G, Hayes A, Green A, et al. Consistent n-*myc* copy number in simultaneous or consecutive neuroblastoma samples from sixty individual patients. *Cancer Res.* 1987;47:4248-4253.

53. Holtzman NA. What drives neonatal screening programs? *N Engl J Med.* 1991;325:802-804.

Value of Subject Height in Predicting Lower Esophageal Sphincter Location

Annamaria Staiano, MD, Ray E. Clouse, MD

• Subject height and lower esophageal sphincter location were determined in 213 children and adults to determine whether the anthropometric variable could be used to accurately predict sphincter location across all age ranges. The upper margin of the lower esophageal sphincter was determined with a nasally placed manometry catheter. Height was highly predictive of lower esophageal sphincter location across all subject groups ($r^2 = .96$) and in the youngest subset of subjects (≤2 years of age, $r^2 = .88$). The predictive ability of height remained significant but progressively decreased in the four older subject groups (>2 and ≤10 years of age, $r^2 = .74$; >10 and ≤20 years of age, $r^2 = .66$; >20 and ≤40 years, $r^2 = .58$; and >40 years, $r^2 = .49$). The regression equation that described subjects 2 years of age or younger ($L = 0.22[H] + 4.92$, where L is the location in centimeters from the nares and H is the height in centimeters) correctly predicted lower esophageal sphincter location within 1.0 cm in 90% of these subjects. In the older subject groups, predicted lower esophageal sphincter location was in error by greater than 2 cm in 25% to 35% of the subjects, even when age group–specific regression equations were used. Decreased predictive ability related to both increasing age and increasing height. We conclude that lower esophageal sphincter location can be predicted from height in subjects up to 2 years of age. The prediction is sufficiently accurate in this age group to allow placement of pH probes without manometric measurements.

(*AJDC.* 1991;145:1424-1427)

Prolonged intraesophageal pH monitoring is being increasingly used in children and adults to diagnose and treat gastroesophageal reflux disease.[1,2] Proper placement of the pH probe in relation to the lower esophageal sphincter (LES) is essential for correct interpretation of the study results. Manometry has become the established standard for determination of the proximal margin of the LES, but this procedure can add considerable expense and patient discomfort if manometric studies are not otherwise required. In 1979, Strobel and colleagues[3] demonstrated that esophageal length correlates well with subject height in children. To our knowledge, this observation has not been reproduced, the accuracy of such a correlation in relation to age groups is unknown, and the use of a calculation based on height is rarely employed despite its potential advantages. Herein, we examine the relationship of subject height to LES location (manometric determination) in groups of patients ranging from younger than 2 to older than 40 years to determine the potential value of this measurement for the placement of intraluminal pH probes.

Accepted for publication May 13, 1991.

From the Department of Pediatrics, University of Naples (Italy) (Dr Staiano), and the Division of Gastroenterology, Washington University School of Medicine, St Louis, Mo (Dr Clouse).

Reprint requests to the Digestive Disease Clinical Center, One Barnes Hospital Plaza, St Louis, MO 63110 (Dr Clouse).

SUBJECTS AND METHODS

Manometric tracings and clinical records from the University of Naples (Italy) and Washington University School of Medicine, St Louis, Mo, were reviewed to identify subjects for this study. Consecutive subjects who had been referred for evaluation of esophageal symptoms or symptoms potentially indicative of gastroesophageal reflux from 1987 through 1990 were included until at least 20 subjects collectively in each of five age groups were found (age ≤2 years, age >2 years and ≤10 years, age >10 years and ≤20 years, age >20 years and ≤40 years, and age >40 years). Patients who had undergone manometry but in whom the LES had not been traversed were excluded, as were neurologically impaired children and other subjects in whom accurate height measurements could not be obtained.

Esophageal manometry was performed similarly at the two institutions according to previously reported methods.[4,5] A transnasal triple-lumen manometry catheter with a 2.4-mm outside diameter was used for children younger than 10 years, and a catheter assembly with a 3.8-mm outside diameter was used for older subjects. Recording ports were spaced at 2- and 5-cm intervals along the smaller- and larger-diameter catheters, respectively. The manometry catheters were perfused with a low-compliance pneumohydraulic perfusion device. In subjects of all ages, the proximal margin of the LES was determined as the highest position recording from a high-pressure zone as the catheter was withdrawn in a stepwise fashion (0.5-cm steps in children younger than 15 years; 1.0-cm steps in all other subjects). Location was averaged from all three lumina, and this position was recorded in centimeters from the nares. The length in infants (subjects younger than 2 years) was measured by two observers with the child in the supine position on a board with a vertical support for the head and an adjustable vertical support for the feet. For the purpose of consistency, infant length will be referred to herein as height. Heights in older subjects were measured with a movable anthropometer while standing without shoes. Height measurements were compared with published population standards for children and adults.[6,7]

Table 1.—Clinical Characteristics of the Subjects				
Age Group, y	No.	Gender M/F	Median Age, y (Range)	Median Height, cm (Range)
≤2	72	46/26	0.5 (0.1-1.7)	63 (52-94)
>2-≤10	31	22/9	5.2 (2.2-9.2)	107 (76-135)
>10-≤20	20	12/8	13.0 (10.5-20.0)	155.5 (118-182)
>20-≤40	32	13/19	34.0 (21.0-40.0)	169.5 (152-188)
>40	58	22/36	57.5 (41.1-89.0)	168 (152-191)

Herein, grouped data are presented as the median and range. Linear regression equations were determined for predicting LES location from subject height, and the coefficient of determination (r^2), reflecting the overall variation of one variable (height) in relation to another (LES location), was calculated to compare the relationships for each age group. Significance levels less than .05 were required.

RESULTS

A total of 213 subjects were included in the study. Characteristics of the subjects in each of the five age groups are shown in Table 1. The third group (>10 and ≤20 years) contained the fewest subjects, because indications for manometry or pH monitoring are infrequent in this age subset. On average, each group fell within 15 percentiles of the general population means of height for age (median percentile for each group: ≤2 years, 36th percentile; >2 to ≤10 years, 36th percentile; >10 to ≤20 years, 39th percentile; >20 to ≤40 years, 51st percentile; and >40 years, 40th percentile).

The scatter diagram and regression line showing the relationship of LES location to height for all subjects is shown in Fig 1. It is apparent from this figure that the relationship is better for younger subjects of lesser height than for the older subjects of greater height. Separate regression equations predicting LES location from height were calculated for each age group (Table 2). All r^2 values derived from these equations were highly significant ($P<.001$ for each), but the prediction deteriorated with increasing age. Actual LES locations were compared with predicted locations for the subjects in each group to determine the accuracy of the estimate in this reference population (Table 3). For the youngest group, predicted LES location was within 1 cm of the actual LES location in more than 90% of cases and was within 1.5 cm in all subjects. In contrast, predicted LES location fell within 2 cm of the actual LES location in only 64.5% to 74.1% of subjects in the four older age groups. Ninety percent or more of subjects were included in the groups between 2 and 40 years of age, only if a variation of 3 cm or less was permitted. Because the clinical utility of the equations to predict LES location from height appeared to be restricted to the youngest age group, a separate scatterplot with the regression line and 95% confidence intervals is shown for this group in Fig 2.

Regression equations were also calculated separately for male and female subjects within each age group. The relationship between height and LES location remained significant for both male and female subjects when all subjects and the two subgroups aged 10 years or younger were considered (all subjects: $r^2=.96$ for each gender; age ≤2 years: $r^2=.86$ for female subjects, $r^2=.88$ for male subjects; age >2 and ≤10 years: $r^2=.74$ for each gender; $P<.001$ for each). In the three older age groups, the relationship appeared to be stronger for female subjects than for male subjects (age >10 and ≤20 years: $r^2=.81$ for female subjects and $r^2=.62$ for male subjects; age >20 and ≤40 years: $r^2=.62$ for female subjects and $r^2=.52$ for male subjects; age >40 years: $r^2=.61$ for female subjects and $r^2=.23$ for male subjects), although r^2 values were significantly different from zero within each subgroup ($P<.05$ for each).

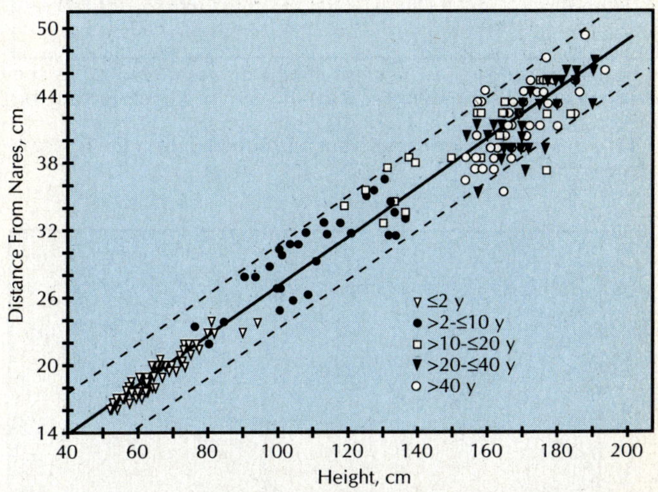

Fig 1.—*Relationship between subject height and distance to the lower esophageal sphincter from the nares, as determined with manometry. The dashed lines outline the 95% confidence band for predicting lower esophageal sphincter location at any specific height* (r=.98).

Table 2.—Regression Equations for Predicting Lower Esophageal Sphincter Location* From Subject Height			
Age Group, y	Regression Equation†	r^2‡	SE of the Estimate
≤2	L=0.22(H) + 4.92	.88	0.71
>2-≤10	L=0.20(H) + 8.53	.74	2.26
>10-≤20	L=0.16(H) + 15.61	.66	2.49
>20-≤40	L=0.23(H) + 3.93	.58	2.05
>40	L=0.24(H) + 2.98	.49	2.22
All subjects	L=0.23(H) + 4.71	.96	1.91

*Location of lower esophageal sphincter was measured as the distance to the lower esophageal sphincter in centimeters from the nares.

†L indicates lower esophageal sphincter location in centimeters from the nares; H, subject height in centimeters.

‡$P<.001$ for each.

COMMENT

These data demonstrate the striking accuracy with which height is predictive of LES location (determined as

Table 3.—Precision of the Regression Equations in Predicting Lower Esophageal Sphincter Location* When Applied to the Study Subjects

	Difference in Predicted and Measured Locations, No. (%)			
Age Group, y	≤1 cm	≤1.5 cm†	≤2 cm	≤3 cm
≤2	65 (90)	72 (100)	72 (100)	72 (100)
>2-≤10	9 (31)	15 (48)	20 (65)	28 (90)
>10-≤20	6 (30)	...	13 (65)	19 (95)
>20-≤40	9 (28)	...	21 (66)	29 (91)
>40	23 (40)	...	43 (74)	51 (88)

*Location of lower esophageal sphincter was measured as the distance to the lower esophageal sphincter in centimeters from the nares.

†The 0.5-cm measurements were performed only in the first two age groups.

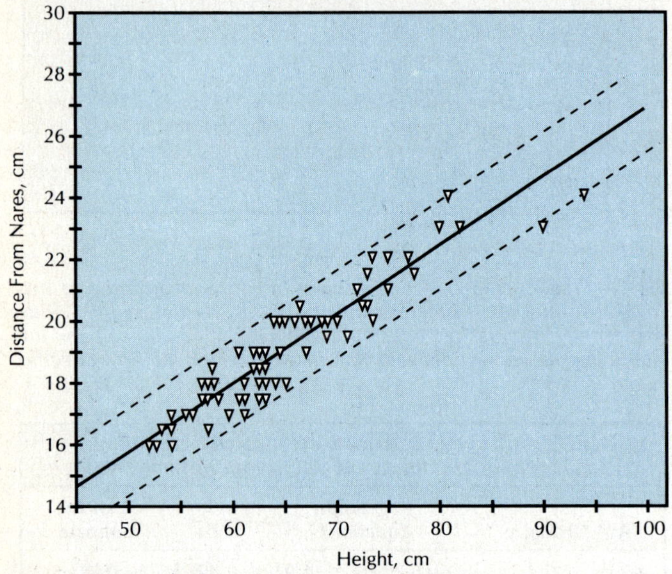

Fig 2.—*Scatterplot and regression equation predicting lower esophageal sphincter location (L) (distance from nares) from subject height (H) (or length) in the youngest subject group (age ≤2 years). The equation L = 0.22(H) + 4.92 was used to form the solid line. The dashed lines outline the 95% confidence band for predicting lower esophageal sphincter location at any specific height.*

the distance to the LES from the nares) across all age groups. However, the precision decreases as subject height increases, even during childhood, and significantly deteriorates in adults. This observation is particularly true for male subjects. A single regression equation ($L = 0.22[H] + 4.92$) describing the relationship of height (H) and LES location (L) in subjects aged 2 years or younger will accurately identify the location of the LES within 1.0 cm in more than 90% of subjects. A similar accuracy is not found in older subjects, even when regression equations defined solely by the age category are used.

Strobel and coworkers[3] first examined this important relationship in children undergoing evaluation for suspected gastroesophageal reflux (all subjects <20 years). Earlier reports described an association of esophageal length with age,[8,9] but the association was found to be more directly related to subject height than age, an interrelated variable. The regression equation $L = 0.252(H) + 5$ was derived by Strobel et al to determine the location of the LES with a transnasal catheter. Strobel et al suggested that a calculation of LES location could obviate the need for manometry before pH probe placement for the Tuttle test, a then-popular test for the diagnosis of gastroesophageal reflux in children.

Prolonged intraluminal pH monitoring is becoming an important tool for diagnosis and management of gastroesophageal reflux and its complications in all age groups. Fluoroscopy, manometry, and pH step-up on probe withdrawal into the esophagus have been utilized to appropriately identify the location of the LES. Although the last of these techniques could be most easily utilized with no additional equipment or morbidity, the technique is not sufficiently accurate to be used with confidence.[10] Manometry (in children and adults) and fluoroscopy (in children) are now routinely employed.[1,11-13] Since publication of the report by Strobel et al,[3] many studies of intraluminal pH recording in children have been published, but the method of LES localization based on subject height has rarely been utilized in research reports, and only then has been utilized in conjunction with fluoroscopy.[14,15] We suspect that this is related to several factors, including (1) the lack of data reproducing the original findings, (2) the fact that transoral catheters were used for the youngest children and that these measurements were used in calculating the regression equations, and (3) underrecognition of the method. A recent review suggests that the calculation of LES location for pH probe placement is beginning to gain some acceptance in clinical practice.[16]

Herein, we have expanded on the original observations in children and have explored the relationship between height and LES location in adults. Only transnasal manometry catheters were employed, and the most proximal region rather than the midpoint of the LES was determined; these methods are more applicable to pH probe positioning for prolonged monitoring. Thus, our regression equations could be considered more applicable by other investigators and clinicians, although they have not yet been applied prospectively to confirm validity. We derived a very similar equation for young subjects to that of Strobel and colleagues,[3] a finding that would support the reproducibility of this method. Placement of a manometry probe simply to locate the LES before pH monitoring is particularly undesirable in the youngest subject group, as the manometry studies provide little additional information in this subset of subjects. The error in LES location with use of the regression equation is sufficiently small in children aged 2 years or younger to strongly advocate the use of calculated esophageal lengths as a standard method to determine probe placement. Gastroesophageal reflux and the need for 24-hour pH monitoring are also particularly important in these young children.[1,14,17,18]

We were unable to show that height remained a good predictor of LES location with advancing age. Although data are not specifically provided, the relationship between height and LES location was poorer even in the younger and older subsets of the 2- to 10-year age group, as suggested by Fig 1. Deterioration of the relationship in adults could be explained by the occurrence of hiatal hernia or a shortened esophagus from esophagitis that would be expected to increase with age. However, such disorders would bias the relationship toward decreasing esophageal length with age, and no such bias was observed (Fig 1). As worsening predictive precision appeared even in the older children and adolescents, it seems more likely that the relationship between visceral and skeletal growth only remains strong in infancy and early childhood. Considering that pH probes are placed 3 to 5 cm above the LES in children and adults (87% of the length from the nares to the LES in children and 5 cm above the LES in adults), placement error should be less than 2 cm, even in older subjects. Prospective evaluation of 24-hour pH monitoring results with the use of calculated vs measured LES location would actually be necessary to determine the adequacy of the simpler technique. The error in estimated LES location in the subjects older than 2 years, however, was unfortunately sufficient that this technique cannot be recommended at present for pH probe placement in any but the youngest patients, unless no other method is available.

The authors thank Maria Rosaria Andreotti, MD, and Mary Fahy, LPN, for performing the motility studies and Debbie Smith, PhD, Division of Biostatistics, Washington University School of Medicine, St Louis, Mo, for her assistance with the statistical analyses.

References

1. Cucchiara S, Staiano A, Gobio Casali L, Boccieri A, Paone F. Value of the 24 hour intraesophageal pH monitoring in children. *Gut.* 1990;31:129-133.

2. Ogorek CP, Risher RS. Detection and treatment of gastroesophageal reflux disease. *Gastroenterol Clin North Am.* 1989;18:293-313.

3. Strobel CT, Byrne WJ, Ament ME, Euler AR. Correlation of esophageal lengths in children with height: application to the Tuttle test without prior esophageal manometry. *J Pediatr.* 1979;94:81-84.

4. Cucchiara S, Staiano A, Di Lorenzo C, et al. Esophageal motor abnormalities in children with gastroesophageal reflux and peptic esophagitis. *J Pediatr.* 1986;108:907-910.

5. Clouse RE, Staiano A. Contraction abnormalities of the esophageal body in patients referred for manometry: a new approach to manometric classification. *Dig Dis Sci.* 1983;28:784-791.

6. Hamill PVV, Drizd TA, Johnson CL, Reed RB, Roche AF, Moore WM. Physical growth: National Center for Health Statistics percentiles. *Am J Clin Nutr.* 1979;32:607-629.

7. Abraham S, Johnson C, Najjar MF. *Weight by Height and Age for Adults 18-74 Years: United States, 1971-1974.* Washington, DC: Government Printing Office; 1979:1-11. US Dept of Health, Education, and Welfare. Vital and Health Statistics, Series 11, publication 211.

8. Holinger PH. The esophagus. In: Vaughan VC, McKay RJ, eds. *Nelson Textbook of Pediatrics.* Philadelphia, Pa: WB Saunders Co; 1975:803.

9. Jackson C, Jackson CL. Notes on the anatomy and physiology of the esophagus. *Bronchoesophagology.* Philadelphia, Pa: WB Saunders Co; 1950:229.

10. Marples MI, Mughal M, Baucewicz J. Can an oesophageal pH electrode be accurately positioned without manometry. In: Siewert JR, Holscher AH, eds. *Diseases of the Esophagus.* New York, NY: Springer-Verlag NY Inc; 1987:789-791.

11. Vandeplas Y, Sacré L. Continuous 24 hour esophageal pH monitoring in 285 asymptomatic infants (from 0 to 15 months old). *J Pediatr Gastroenterol Nutr.* 1987;6:220-224.

12. Emde C, Garner A, Blum AL. Technical aspects of intraluminal pH-metry in man: current status and recommendations. *Gut.* 1987;22:1177-1188.

13. Vandeplas Y, Helven R, Goyvaerts H, Sacré L. Reproducibility of continuous 24 hour esophageal pH monitoring in infants and children. *Gut.* 1990;31:374-377.

14. Colson DJ, Campbell CA, Wright VA, Watson BW. Predictive value of oesophageal pH variables in children with gastro-oesophageal reflux. *Gut.* 1990;31:370-373.

15. Orenstein SR. Effect of nonnutritive sucking in infant gastroesophageal reflux. *Pediatr Res.* 1988;24:38-40.

16. Sutphen JL. Pediatric gastroesophageal reflux disease. *Gastroenterol Clin North Am.* 1990;19:617-629.

17. Black DD, Haggitt RC, Orenstein SR, Whitington PF. Esophagitis in infants: morphometric histological diagnosis and correlation with measures of gastroesophageal reflux. *Gastroenterology.* 1990;98:1408-1414.

18. Orenstein SR. Prone positioning in infant gastroesophageal reflux: is elevation of the head worth the trouble? *J Pediatr.* 1990;117:184-187.

Trimethoprim-Sulfamethoxazole Oral Desensitization in Hemophiliacs Infected With Human Immunodeficiency Virus With a History of Hypersensitivity Reactions

Morris Kletzel, MD; Suzanne Beck, MD; Joe Elser, MD; Nikki Shock, MSS; Wesley Burks, MD

• Hemophiliacs infected with human immunodeficiency virus with a history of hypersensitivity reaction to a combination product of trimethoprim and sulfamethoxazole were desensitized orally. Six of the seven patients included in the study successfully completed the desensitization protocol and received trimethoprim-sulfamethoxazole for 5 to 7 months after desensitization (mean length of treatment, 5.7 months) for prophylaxis of *Pneumocystis carinii* pneumonia. The small number of patients and the short follow-up allow us to suggest that oral desensitization may be an effective and inexpensive means to treat hemophiliacs infected with human immunodeficiency virus with trimethoprim-sulfamethoxazole as prophylaxis against *Pneumocystis carinii* pneumonia.

(*AJDC.* 1991;145:1428-1429)

All patients infected with human immunodeficiency virus (HIV) with CD4 cell counts of less than 0.20×10^9/L are at risk of developing *Pneumocystis carinii* pneumonia (PCP).[1] Major efforts have been made to prevent this infection. Several methods have been tried, including the use of a combination product of trimethoprim and sulfamethoxazole, aerosolized pentamidine, dapsone-trimethoprim, intravenous pentamidine,[2] and others. Patients with HIV infection have an increased frequency of hypersensitivity reactions to several drugs, including trimethoprim-sulfamethoxazole.[3,4] The possibility of oral desensitization with trimethoprim-sulfamethoxazole prompted the study in HIV-infected patients with clotting disorders.

PATIENTS AND METHODS

Patients with clotting disorders followed up at the Arkansas Hemophilia Center, Little Rock, who had a history of hypersensitivity to trimethoprim-sulfamethoxazole were included in the study. All developed hypersensitivity reactions to trimethoprim-sulfamethoxazole ranging from erythema multiforme to minor respiratory difficulty and edema. Informed consent was obtained from seven patients, six of whom were male. The age range was 7 to 33 years, with a mean age of 19.3 years. The six males all had severe factor VIII deficiency, and the female had type III von Willebrand's disease. All patients were HIV positive and their CD4 cell counts were less than 0.2×10^9/L when they were included in this study. The Table shows the clinical characteristics of these patients. Patients who had a history of exfoliative dermatitis or Stevens-Johnson syndrome were not included in this trial.

All patients were hospitalized at the time this procedure was attempted. We used a regimen modified from that suggested by Yango and colleagues.[5] Pediatric suspension of trimethoprim-sulfamethoxazole (Bactrim) was administered orally every 8 hours beginning with 1/10 000 of the desired total daily dose and progressing through serial dilutions of 1/5000, 1/1000, 1/500, 1/100, 1/50, and 1/10. Subsequently, the desired dosage was administered orally twice per day. If mild skin rashes developed, the patients were treated with antihistamines. The procedure was terminated with the development of systemic symptoms or exanthems involving the mucous membranes. Epinephrine and resuscitative equipment were kept readily available.

RESULTS

Five patients tolerated the procedure well without complications. Of the two remaining patients, one (patient 6) developed an erythematous rash that responded well to antihistamine therapy. Patient 1 developed an urticarial rash that responded partially to antihistamine therapy; the protocol was stopped inadvertently, but was subsequently restarted and completed successfully. All patients except patient 3 continued to receive trimethoprim-sulfamethoxazole for 5 to 7 months after desensitization; the mean length of treatment was 5.7 months. The patient who discontinued trimethoprim-sulfamethoxazole treatment had poorly complied with the dosage regimen and thus missed several doses. He then developed an urticarial rash, forcing the discontinuation of the drug, and was treated with aerosolized pentamidine. A second attempt to desensitize this patient failed due to the development of urticaria.

COMMENT

Trimethoprim-sulfamethoxazole is an effective and inexpensive means of preventing PCP. In a randomized study, patients with Kaposi's sarcoma and no history of opportunistic infections were assigned to receive trimethoprim-sulfamethoxazole vs placebo. None of the patients in the trimethoprim-sulfamethoxazole group developed PCP, while 16 (53%) of 30 patients in the control group developed PCP. Fifteen (50%) of the 30 patients in the trimethoprim-sulfamethoxazole group developed adverse reactions, including nausea, vomiting, pruritus, erythroderma, fever, and leukopenia.[3]

Recent studies have documented that the frequency of allergic reactions to drugs is increased in patients with HIV infection despite the compromise of their immune status.[5,6] Because trimethoprim-sulfamethoxazole is one of the drugs of choice for prophylaxis and treatment of PCP, development of a safe and effective protocol for desensitization is of prime clinical importance.

Sullivan et al[7] has shown that oral desensitization to penicillin is effective and relatively safe. Further evidence of successful oral desensitization to trimethoprim-sulfamethoxa-

Accepted for publication July 8, 1991.

From the Department of Pediatrics, University of Arkansas for Medical Sciences and Arkansas Children's Hospital, Little Rock. Dr Kletzel is now with the Department of Pediatrics, Children's Memorial Hospital, Chicago, Ill.

Reprint requests to Northwestern University, Children's Memorial Hospital, 2300 Children's Plaza, Chicago, IL 60614 (Dr Kletzel).

Clinical Characteristics of Patients Infected With HIV With Clotting Disorders Who Develop Hypersensitivity Reactions to Trimethoprim-Sulfamethoxazole*

Patient No./ Age, y/Sex	Factor Deficient	Absolute CD4 Count, $\times 10^9$/L	CD4/CD8 Ratio	Type of Reaction	Other Medications at the Time of Reaction
1/7/M	VIII severe	0.021	0.05	Rash	Zidovudine
2/24/M	VIII severe	0.019	0.2	Rash	Zidovudine
3/15/M	VIII severe	0.049	0.2	Rash	Zidovudine
4/33/M	VIII severe	0.023	0.05	Rash	Zidovudine
5/15/M	VIII severe	0.017	0.05	Rash, dyspnea	Zidovudine
6/15/M	VIII severe	0.079	0.08	Rash, swelling	Zidovudine, tetracycline
7/21/F	VWD/III	0.199	0.5	Rash	Zidovudine

*HIV indicates human immunodeficiency virus; and VWD, von Willebrand's disease.

zole with subsequent intravenous administration of the drug was described by Finegold.[8] Several investigators have successfully reported oral desensitization to sulfasalazine.[9,10] Based on previous work, this approach is appealing since oral administration of trimethoprim-sulfamethoxazole is less likely to provoke a systemic reaction than parenteral administration.[11]

The mechanism of desensitization to trimethoprim-sulfamethoxazole and penicillin may be similar, although these immunologic changes have not been clearly described. Antigen-specific mast-cell desensitization has been proposed by some authors. Sullivan[12] and Stark et al[13] reported the conversion of positive penicillin skin test results to negative results following oral desensitization with penicillin; however, the skin test results to irrelevant antigens remained unaffected. Further work by this group demonstrated that the mast cells retain their ability to react to some antigens, while the response to other antigens was deleted. This suggested an independent regulation and sensitivity of each antigen IgE antibody system.[12] Following desensitization, the persistence of other IgE-mediated signals indicates that tachyphylaxis to mediators such as histamine or mediator depletion does not play a significant role in the clinical response. It is not known whether adverse reactions to trimethoprim-sulfamethoxazole are IgE mediated. The successful desensitization suggests that mediator depletion does occur in these patients. Whether IgE plays a role in this process remains to be fully elucidated.

The role of antigen-specific IgG as a blocking antibody in protection against further IgE-mediated drug reactions has not been fully described. Immunoglobulin G may bind the allergenic epitopes of the drug and thus prevent binding to the mast cell.

The prevention of PCP in HIV-infected individuals has become a standard of care. The method used for prevention depends on the individual's tolerance to different treatment regimens. All the approaches produce a certain degree of adverse reactions. Aerosolized pentamidine produces coughing in 36% of patients and wheezing in 11% of patients,[14] while with trimethoprim-sulfamethoxazole the main adverse reactions include hypersensitivity, gastrointestinal intolerance, and marrow suppression.[3] The use of trimethoprim-sulfamethoxazole in our view offers several advantages, including low cost, ease of administration in all ages, and its broad spectrum to prevent other bacterial infections. The use of trimethoprim-sulfamethoxazole as the first-line prophylactic therapy for PCP in HIV-infected patients with CD4 cell counts of less than 0.2×10^9/L is a reasonable one.

The small numbers and short follow-up allow us to suggest that oral desensitization with trimethoprim-sulfamethoxazole may be an effective and inexpensive means to again treat patients infected with HIVwith trimethoprim-sulfamethoxazole as prophylaxis against PCP. Further studies on larger groups of patients are needed to evaluate safety, efficacy, and the mechanism of response.

This study was supported in part by grant MCJ-052002-01-0 from the Office of Maternal and Child Health.

The authors gratefully acknowledge Patty Whaley and Lisa Jones for their help in the preparation of this manuscript.

References

1. DeVita VT Jr, Broder S, Fauci AS, Kovaci JA, Chabner BA. Developmental therapeutics and the acquired immunodeficiency syndrome. *Ann Intern Med.* 1987;106:568-581.

2. Glatt AE, Chirgwin K, Landesman SH. Current concepts: treatment of infections associated with human immunodeficiency virus. *N Engl J Med.* 1988;318:1439-1448.

3. Fischl MA, Dickinson GM, LaVoie L. Safety and efficacy of sulfamethoxasole and trimethoprim chemoprophylaxis for pneumocystis carinii pneumonia in AIDS. *JAMA.* 1988; 259:1185-1189.

4. Jaffe HS, Abrams DI, Ammann AJ, Lewis BJ, Golden JA. Complications of clotrimoxazole use in the treatment of AIDS associated *Pneumocystis carinii* pneumonia in homosexual men. *Lancet.* 1983;2:1109-1111.

5. Yango C, Kim K, Evans R. Oral desensitization to trimethoprim sulfamethoxazole in pediatric patients. Presented at the American Academy of Pediatrics; October 1990; Atlanta, Ga.

6. Gordin FM, Simon GL, Wofsy CB, Mills J. Adverse reactions to trimetroprim-sulfamethoxasole in patients with acquired immune deficiency syndrome. *Ann Intern Med.* 1984;100:495-499.

7. Sullivan TJ, Yecies LD, Shatz GS, Parker CW, Wedner HJ. Desensitization of patients allergic to penicillin using orally administered B-lactam antibiotics. *J Allergy Clin Immunol.* 1982;69:275-282.

8. Finegold I. Oral desensitization to trimetoprim-sulfamethoxasole in a patient with acquired immune deficiency syndrome. *J Allergy Clin Immunol.* 1986;78:905-908.

9. Taffet SL, Daz KM. Desensitization of patients with inflammatory bowel disease to sulfasalasine. *Am J Med.* 1982;73:520-524.

10. Purdy BH, Phillips DM, Summers RW. Desensitization for sulfasalasine skin rash. *Ann Intern Med.* 1984;100:512-514.

11. Herman R, Jick H. Cutaneous reaction rates to penicillins oral versus parenteral. *Cutis.* 1979;24:232-234.

12. Sullivan TJ. Antigen-specific desensitization of patients allergic to penicillin. *J Allergy Clin Immunol.* 1982;69:500-508.

13. Stark BJ, Earl HS, Gross GN, Lumbry WR, Goodman EL, Sullivan TJ. Acute and chronic desensitization of penicillin in allergic patients using oral penicillin. *J Allergy Clin Immunol.* 1987;73:523-532.

14. Leoung GS, Feigal DW Jr, Montgomery AB, et al. Aerosolized pentamidine for prophylaxis against pneumocystis carinii pneumonia. *N Engl J Med.* 1990;323:769-775.

Occult Cocaine Exposure in Children

Norman M. Rosenberg, DO; Kathleen L. Meert, MD; Stephen R. Knazik, DO;
Hugh Yee, PhD; Ralph E. Kauffman, MD

• We determined the prevalence of cocaine and cannabinoid exposure among young children presenting to an urban pediatric emergency department without signs or symptoms suggestive of the exposure. The study included 460 children between 1 and 60 months of age in whom urinalysis was required for investigation of routine pediatric complaints. Anonymously and without informed consent, an aliquot of urine was screened for cocaine metabolite (benzoylecgonine) and 11- or Δ-9-tetrahydrocannabinol-9 carboxylic acid with the enzyme multiplied immunoassay technique. Positive specimens were rescreened with a radioimmunoassay and confirmed with gas chromatography/mass spectrometry, if a sufficient quantity of urine was available. Benzoylecgonine was identified in 25 patients (5.4%) by both screening techniques. Enough urine was available for confirmatory testing in eight patients, and all eight urine specimens contained benzoylecgonine. Neither 11- nor Δ-9-tetrahydrocannabinol-9 carboxylic acid was detected in any patient. We documented the magnitude of the problem of occult passive cocaine exposure in young children living in an urban environment. Such exposure has serious implications for the assessment of outcomes in postnatal follow-up studies of prenatally exposed children as well as potential risks to children living in household environments where occult cocaine exposure occurs.

(*AJDC.* 1991;145:1430-1432)

Cocaine use in the United States has increased dramatically during the past decade. The National Institutes on Drug Abuse reported that in 1986 cocaine became the most frequent cause of drug-related emergency department visits.[1] Changing trends in drugs of abuse among a pediatric population were studied by Soldin et al,[2] who described a decline in the use of cannabis but a rise in the use of cocaine from 1986 to 1988. Cocaine exposure among certain pediatric subpopulations has been emphasized in the literature. These include adolescents,[3] breast-fed infants,[4] and neonates born to addicted mothers.[5,6] Recent reports have identified cocaine toxicity among non–breast-fed infants and toddlers.[7,8] Accidental ingestion and passive inhalation of free-base cocaine vapors are putative mechanisms of intoxication in this age group. Little is known regarding the prevalence of asymptomatic or unsuspected cocaine exposure in young children. Our purpose was to determine the prevalence of cocaine and cannabinoid exposure among young children presenting to an urban pediatric emergency department without signs or symptoms suggestive of the exposure.

Accepted for publication June 17, 1991.

From the Department of Pediatrics (Drs Rosenberg, Meert, Knazik, and Kauffman), Children's Hospital of Michigan, Wayne State University School of Medicine, and Damon Clinical Laboratory (Dr Lee), Detroit (Mich) Medical Center.

Presented at the Society for Pediatric Research meeting, New Orleans, La, April 28, 1991, and at the American Academy of Pediatrics meeting, New Orleans, October 27, 1991.

Reprint requests to Director of Emergency Services, Children's Hospital of Michigan, 3901 Beaubien Blvd, Detroit, MI 48201 (Dr Rosenberg).

PATIENTS AND METHODS

Our study was conducted in the emergency department of the Children's Hospital of Michigan, Detroit, an urban pediatric teaching hospital, during the period from October 1989 to December 1990. Children included were those between 1 and 60 months of age in whom urinalysis was required for investigation of one of the following chief complaints: fever, abdominal pain, genitourinary symptoms, blunt trauma, crying/fussiness, vomiting, diarrhea, or failure to thrive. Patients were excluded if exposure to drugs of abuse was suspected by history or physical examination. Anonymously and without informed consent, an aliquot of urine was tested for benzoylecgonine (BE), the major metabolite of cocaine, and 11- or Δ-9-tetrahydrocannabinol-9 carboxylic acid (THC). Anonymity was maintained by assigning a code number to each specimen that was cross-referenced to a data sheet that contained no patient identification information. This study was approved by the Children's Hospital of Michigan Institutional Review Board.

Urine samples were first screened with the enzyme multiplied immunoassay technique (EMIT) (Syva Corp, Palo Alto, Calif) with a minimal detection sensitivity of 50 μg/L. Samples that were positive by EMIT were rescreened with a radioimmunoassay (RIA) (Abuscreen, Roche Diagnostic System, Mont Clair, NJ) that had the same sensitivity. Urine was considered positive for BE or THC only when the drug was detected by both EMIT and RIA. Confirmation of positive specimens was performed with gas chromatography/mass spectrometry (GC/MS) when a sufficient quantity of urine was available.[9]

Patient data recorded included the chief complaint, age, presence or absence of breast-feeding, day of the week at presentation, current medications, and residential zip code.

A sample size of 400 patients was calculated based on an estimated cocaine exposure rate of 1%, with an accuracy of 1% and 95% confidence. Demographics were assessed with χ^2 analysis for nominal variables and an independent t test for continuous variables.

RESULTS

During the period of this study, 76 362 patients were cared for in the Children's Hospital of Michigan emergency department. Departmental statistics revealed that 90% of these patients were black, 8% were white, and 2% belonged to other races. Eighty percent were Medicaid or uninsured patients, while 20% had private medical insurance. Ninety-seven percent resided in Wayne County, Michigan, which encompasses the city of Detroit, while 3% resided in outlying counties. Therefore, the population from which our study sample was drawn consists of children between 1 and 60 months of age, who are predominantly black, who are covered by Medicaid or are uninsured, and who reside in an urban environment. Of this total population of patients, 460 (0.6%) were included in our study.

The cocaine metabolite BE was identified in 25 (5.4%) of 460 patients by both EMIT and RIA. Sufficient urine was available for GC/MS confirmation in eight patients, and all eight samples contained BE. The urine of one patient also contained intact cocaine, as determined by GC/MS confirmation. Neither 11- nor Δ-9-tetrahydrocannabinol-9 carboxylic acid was detected in any patient.

There was no difference in age between those patients who were positive or negative for BE (20±18 vs 21±17 months, $P=.7$). No cocaine-exposed patients were breast-fed. By history, six of the BE-positive patients were taking medications consisting of semisynthetic penicillins and/or acetaminophen; neither of these drugs interfere with BE or THC assays. No significant relationship was found between the day of the week and the percentage of patients exposed to cocaine ($\chi^{2=6.3,}$ $P=.4$).

Patients were enrolled in the study from a catchment area of 78 zip codes. Of these, BE-positive urines were identified in 13 zip code areas. Cocaine exposure tended to be concentrated within three zip codes, in each of which more than 20% of samples obtained were positive. Demographic characteristics of these three zip code areas combined include a racial distribution of 93% black, 6% white, and 1% other; a sex distribution of 46% male and 54% female; a median age of 28.9 years, with 11% of the population younger than 6 years; a median annual household income of $18 713; and a median number of years of school completed of 11.9.[10]

COMMENT

Our study demonstrated the magnitude of the problem of unsuspected cocaine exposure in young urban children. Hicks et al[11] previously reported 2.8% urine positivity for BE and 0% positivity for THC among 0- to 5-year-old children not suspected to have been exposed to drugs. Kharasch et al[12] found 2.5% of urine samples also obtained from children in whom drug exposure was not suspected in the same age group to be positive for BE. Our higher prevalence rate of 5.4% compared with the other studies may be due, in part, to lowering the threshold concentration for a positive screening test from 80 µg/L to 50 µg/L or greater. Although lowering the threshold concentration will reduce the probability of false-negative results, it also may increase the risk of false-positive results. However, this is unlikely, as specimens were only designated as positive when BE could be identified by both the EMIT and the RIA. Also, for all positive urine samples in which sufficient quantity was available, the presence of BE was confirmed by GC/MS.

Possible routes of exposure among the infants and toddlers studied include accidental ingestion, intentional administration, and passive inhalation of cocaine vapors. Passage of cocaine from mother to infant via breast milk has been described; however, none of our BE-positive patients were breast-fed. Cocaine may be detected in the urine of newborns up to 3 to 5 days following delivery if exposure occurs in utero.[13] All children in this study were older than 1 month of age, eliminating in utero exposure as a possible mechanism contributing to the high prevalence rate. No history of accidental ingestion or intentional administration of the drug was obtained from any of the patients included in our study. Also, no patient had signs or symptoms of drug intoxication as have been described with cocaine ingestion.[14,15] We speculate that passive inhalation of vapors when free-base cocaine is smoked by adult caretakers is the likely mechanism of exposure in these young children.

More than 300 000 infants are born annually to women who use cocaine during pregnancy.[16] Longitudinal studies of these infants have demonstrated abnormal respiratory patterns,[17] sudden infant death syndrome,[18] visual impairment,[19] abnormal motor development,[20] poor reading and mathematical skills,[21] and impaired social and emotional development.[22] Although the possible contribution of continued environmental exposure to the observed problems in these infants is unknown, many of these infants live in an environment where adults regularly use cocaine. A "kindling" phenomenon has been described in which the central nervous system becomes sensitized following repeated exposure to cocaine.[23] Eventually, central nervous system stimulation occurs in response to relatively low levels of the drug. It is possible that continued environmental exposure to cocaine may influence the results of long-term follow-up studies of infants exposed to cocaine in utero. This should be considered in future follow-up studies of such infants.

The prevalence of unsuspected cocaine exposure in infants and toddlers revealed by our study is indeed alarming. Physicians must be aware of this high-risk pediatric subpopulation, particularly those who practice in areas where cocaine use is epidemic. Parental education concerning the possibility of inhalational cocaine exposure may be important. However, the potential deleterious effects of such exposure remain to be determined.

This work was funded in part by the European Endorsement Fund of the Children's Hospital of Michigan (Dr Meert).

References

1. National Institute on Drug Abuse. *Data From the Drug Abuse Warning Network (DAWN).* Washington, DC: 1987; US Dept of Health and Human Services publication 87-1530. Series 1, No. 6.

2. Soldin S, Gutierrez A, Boeckx R, Hicks JM. Changing trends in drugs of abuse in a pediatric population over the period 1986 to 1988. *Pediatr Pathol.* 1990;10:467-468.

3. Shannon M, Lacouture PG, Roa J, Woolf A. Cocaine exposure among children seen at a pediatric hospital. *Pediatrics.* 1989;83:337-342.

4. Chasnoff IJ, Lewis DE, Squires L. Cocaine intoxication in a breast-fed infant. *Pediatrics.* 1987;80:836-838.

5. Chasnoff IJ. Cocaine: effects on pregnancy and the neo-

nate. In: Chasnoff IJ, ed. *Drugs, Alcohol, Pregnancy and Parenting*. Lancaster, United Kingdom: Kluwer Academic Publishers; 1988:97-103.

6. Chasnoff IJ, Burns WJ, Schnoll SH, Burns KA. Cocaine use in pregnancy. *N Engl J Med.* 1985;313:666-669.

7. Dinnies JD, Darr CD, Saulys AJ. Cocaine toxicity in toddlers. *AJDC.* 1990;14:743-744.

8. Bateman DA, Heagarty MC. Passive freebase cocaine ('crack') inhalation by infants and toddlers. *AJDC.* 1989;143:25-27.

9. Taylor RW, Jain NC. Simultaneous identification of cocaine and benzoyl ecgonine using solid phase extraction and gas chromatography/mass spectrometry. *J Anal Toxicol.* 1987;11:65-66.

10. *Epidemiological Characteristics.* Detroit, Mich: Inforum, Wayne State University; 1990.

11. Hicks JM, Morales A, Soldin SJ. Drugs of abuse in a pediatric outpatient population. *Clin Chem.* 1990;36:1256-1257.

12. Kharasch S, Vinci R, Glotzer D, Sargent J, Weitzman M. Unsuspected cocaine exposure in young children. *AJDC.* 1991;145:204-206.

13. Halstead AC, Godolphin W, Lockitch G, Segal S. Timing of specimen collection is crucial in urine screening of drug-dependent mothers and new borns. *Clin Biochem.* 1988;21:59-61.

14. Riggs D, Weibley RE. Acute toxicity from oral ingestion of crack cocaine: a report of four cases. *Pediatr Emerg Care.* 1990;6:24-26.

15. Rivkin M, Gilmore HE. Generalized seizures in an infant due to environmentally acquired cocaine. *Pediatrics.* 1989;84:1100-1101.

16. Chasnoff IJ. Drug use in women: establishing a standard of care. *Ann N Y Acad Sci.* 1989;562:208-210.

17. Chasnoff IJ, Hunt CE, Kletter R, Kaplan D. Prenatal cocaine exposure is associated with respiratory pattern abnormalities. *AJDC.* 1989;143:583-587.

18. Durand DJ, Espinoza AM, Nickerson BG. Association between prenatal cocaine exposure and sudden infant death syndrome. *J Pediatr.* 1990;117:909-911.

19. Dixon S, Coen R, Crutchfield S. Visual dysfunction in cocaine exposed infants. *Pediatr Res.* 1987;21:1112A. Abstract.

20. Scheider J, Chasnoff IJ. Motor assessment of cocaine exposed infants. *Pediatr Res.* 1987;21:68A. Abstract.

21. Hill RM, Tennyso LM. Maternal drug therapy: effect on fetal and neonatal growth and neurobehavior. *Neurotoxicology.* 1986;7:121-139.

22. Rodning C, Beckwith L, Howard J. Prenatal exposure to drugs: behavioral distortions reflecting CNS impairment. *Neurotoxicology.* 1989;10:629-634.

23. Weiss RD, Mirin SM. *Cocaine.* Washington DC: American Psychiatric Press; 1987:48-49.

The Incidence of Prenatal Brain Injury

A series of 165 brains of infants who were stillborn or who died shortly after birth were examined to identify the incidence and nature of prenatal brain damage. Forty-four percent of the stillborn infants showed evidence of brain damage thought to be related to circulatory disorders, primarily ischemic damage to cerebral white matter. Of 90 liveborn infants, 36% had prenatal ischemic damage.

Once again, a modern neuropathologic study has shown that prenatal factors are probably far more important in causation of cerebral palsy than previously assumed.

Squier M, Keeling JW. The incidence of prenatal brain injury. *Neuropathol Appl Neurobiol.* 1991;17:29-38.

Frequency of Infections Associated With Implanted Systems vs Cuffed, Tunneled Silastic Venous Catheters in Patients With Acute Leukemia

Carlos Severien, MD, John D. Nelson, MD

• A total of 75 central venous catheters were used for prolonged chemotherapy in 39 children with acute lymphocytic leukemia and 21 patients with acute myelocytic leukemia. Infection rates were 2.2 per 1000 catheter days with the use of cuffed, tunneled, single-lumen Silastic catheters, 2.0 per 1000 catheter days with cuffed, tunneled, double-lumen Silastic catheters, and 0.5 per 1000 catheter days with the use of implanted venous access systems. Eighty-one percent of catheter sepsis episodes were successfully treated without removal of the catheter. All tunnel infections required withdrawal of the catheter for cure. The microorganisms were gram-positive bacteria in 15%, gram-negative bacteria in 7%, and fungi in 4%. Coagulase-negative staphylococci and *Pseudomonas aeruginosa* were the most commonly isolated organisms. Three of six fatal sepsis episodes were caused by disseminated fungal infections. We conclude that the use of intracorporeal venous catheter systems in patients with acute lymphocytic leukemia is associated with a lower infection rate than that with cuffed, tunneled Silastic single- or double-lumen catheters and that most septicemias can be cured with antimicrobial therapy without removal of the catheter.

(*AJDC.* 1991;145:1433-1438)

Since the introduction of cuffed, tunneled Silastic catheters by Broviac et al[1] in 1973 and Hickman et al[2] in 1979, the treatment of pediatric oncology patients requiring prolonged central venous access for total parenteral nutrition and intensive chemotherapy has markedly improved. However, catheter-related infections are a major problem in pediatric patients with cancer. In addition, thrombotic occlusions, dislocations, and other mechanical complications are common. Meticulous care in regular sterile gauze dressing changes and daily heparin-saline flushes of the external catheter seems to be critical for reducing the incidence of catheter complications during hospital or outpatient management.

In recent years, totally implanted central venous catheter systems have been employed in children with malignant disease for prolonged chemotherapy. Reported infection rates suggest that intracorporeal venous access systems may be associated with a lower risk of infection than external venous catheters. However, studies with implanted catheter systems in pediatric oncology patients are scarce, and the various neoplastic diseases usually included may be associated with different infection rates. Children with leukemia are at a particular high risk for infection. Neutropenia, whether related to the primary disease or a consequence of chemotherapy, seems to be the most important predisposing factor.[3-5] In addition, qualitative abnormalities of neutrophil function, including defects of chemotaxis, phagocytosis, or bactericidal activity, have been described even with a normal number of circulating leukocytes.[6-8]

We reviewed the experience during a 7½-year period with intracorporeal venous access systems and cuffed, tunneled single- or double-lumen Silastic catheters in our pediatric patients with acute lymphocytic and myelocytic leukemia.

Accepted for publication June 10, 1991.

From the Department of Pediatrics, University of Texas Southwestern Medical Center, Dallas.

Reprints not available.

MATERIALS AND METHODS

Hospital and outpatient records of the Oncology Division of Children's Medical Center at Dallas, University of Texas, were reviewed to identify all patients with acute leukemia selected for insertion of a central venous catheter for chemotherapy between January 1983 and July 1990. Catheters were inserted, with the patient under general anesthesia in the operating room, by external jugular, cephalic, or facial vein cutdown or subclavian puncture. Cuffed, tunneled venous catheters were inserted according to described methods[9] and included 20-F Cook double-lumen catheters. In addition, five noncuffed catheters, consisting of two percutaneous plastic, two Silastic, and one unspecified central venous catheters, were placed. Sterile film and iodophor solution dressings were applied to the exit site wound. The catheter care protocol consisted of cleaning and disinfection of the exit site twice a week by the nursing personnel and by the parents at home after being instructed in catheter care by the nursing staff. Capped catheters were filled with heparin-saline solution (100 U/mL) daily and after infusion.

Twenty-five Port-a-Cath and one Mediport systems were implanted for central venous access. Fluoroscopy was used to confirm the position of the tip of each catheter after placement. Thereafter, the reservoir and catheter were flushed with heparinized saline once every month and after each use for chemotherapy. Medical records of all patients were studied for sex, race, age at diagnosis of leukemia, and classification of leukemia

Table 1.—Study of 75 Central Venous Catheters in 60 Pediatric Patients With Acute Leukemia

Type of Catheter	No.	Duration, d: Range	Duration, d: Total	No. of Catheter-Related Infections: Septic	Local	Both	No. of Infections/ 1000 Catheter Days	Other Complications, No.: Malposition	Occlusion	Leak
Tunneled, cuffed, single-lumen Silastic	19	6-1207	5477	9	3	0	2.2	4	3	1
Tunneled, cuffed, double-lumen Silastic	26	4-962	6570	10	1	2	2.0	1	4	0
Implanted venous access system	25	7-1062	9611	4	1	0	0.5	1	0	1
Other*	6	32-629	1382	0	1	0	0.7	0	1	0
Total	**75**	**4-1207**	**23 040**	**23**	**6**	**2**	1.3	**6**	**8**	**2**

*Two percutaneous plastic catheters, one percutaneous noncuffed, nontunneled Silastic catheter, one tunneled, noncuffed Silastic catheter, and one unspecified catheter.

as lymphocytic and myelocytic. Catheter duration was defined as the time interval from the day of insertion to the day of withdrawal of the catheter, death of the patient, or last hospital visit during the study period with the catheter infection. The end of the infection-free interval also included the day of catheter removal for reasons other than infection, death of the patient with an uninfected catheter, or the last hospital visit with the catheter still in use.

Nonquantitative blood cultures from a peripheral vein and from the catheter were performed in conventional blood culture broth when sepsis was suspected. Sepsis was classified as catheter related when fever (temperature, >38°C) and at least one positive culture of blood, whether from peripheral veins, through the catheter, or both, was present and no other focus could be identified as a source of septicemia. Sepsis was considered to be cured when clinical signs resolved and at least one blood culture during or after treatment was negative. Neutropenia at the presentation of the infection was defined as an absolute granulocyte count of less than 500/mm^3.

Empiric parenteral antibiotic therapy was started immediately in the neutropenic febrile patient after the cultures were taken. Nonneutropenic patients were hospitalized and treated either when sepsis was suspected or when a positive blood culture was obtained. Catheter-related local infections at the exit site, in the tunnel, or in the subcutaneous pocket required for definition that progressive cutaneous or subcutaneous inflammatory signs with or without exudate were present.

Chemotherapy according to the Dallas–Fort Worth Pediatric Oncology Group protocols for lymphocytic and myelocytic leukemia was given to the majority of patients. The induction and consolidation phases represented periods of approximately 1 and 3 months, respectively, when the patients received more immunosuppressive treatment than during the following maintenance phase of chemotherapy.

Statistical analysis was performed by Wilcoxon signed rank test for two independent samples. $P<.05$ was considered significant.

RESULTS

Seventy-five central venous catheters were inserted for chemotherapy in 60 children with acute leukemia. There were 46 catheters in 39 patients with acute lymphocytic leukemia and 29 catheters in 21 children with acute myelocytic leukemia. At diagnosis, the mean age of the 33 boys and 27 girls was 6½ years, with a range of 8 months to 16 years. There were 47 white, five black, and eight Hispanic children. A single catheter was inserted in 49 patients (82%), two catheters were placed in nine patients (15%), one patient required three catheters, and one patient required five catheters.

Thirty-two catheters were removed, 14 catheters remained in place until death, and 29 catheters were still in use at the last hospital visit. Of the 75 central venous catheters implanted for chemotherapy, 19 were cuffed, tunneled, single-lumen catheters; 26 were cuffed, tunneled, double-lumen catheters; 25 were implanted venous access systems; and five were noncuffed catheters.

Nineteen cuffed, tunneled, single-lumen catheters were placed in patients at a mean age of 77 months, with a mean duration of 288 days. Nine were removed, five remained in place until death, and five were still in use at the last hospital visit. Of 26 cuffed, tunneled, double-lumen catheters implanted at a mean age of 82 months, with a mean duration of 253 days, 15 catheters were removed, five remained in place until death, and six were still functioning. Of 25 intracorporeal venous access devices placed at a mean age of 81 months, with a mean duration of 384 days, 17 were still in use, five had been removed, and three were in place when the patients died.

Of the 32 central venous catheters that required removal (43%), seven had thrombotic occlusions, nine had catheter-related infections, and 16 were removed for other reasons (dislocation, leakage, or end of chemotherapy). Of the seven episodes of thrombotic occlusions, only one episode was reversible after flushing with urokinase. The interval between placement and obstruction of the catheter ranged from 4 to 164 days, with a mean of 66 days. No thrombotic obstruction was reported in intracorporeal venous access systems. The incidence of catheter-related mechanical complications other than infections was 1.46 per 1000 catheter days in cuffed, tunneled, single-lumen catheters; 0.76 per 1000 catheter days in cuffed, tunneled, double-lumen catheters; and 0.21 per 1000 catheter days in implanted catheter systems (Table 1).

Overall, 30 septic episodes occurred in 26 patients during central venous catheter use. Fifteen patients (68%) had one, six patients two, and one patient three sepsis episodes. According to the source of infection, the distribution of the 60 patients with central venous catheters was as follows. Thirty patients (50%) had no catheter-related infection or non–catheter-related sepsis; 25 patients (42%) had catheter-related infections (septic and/or local) only; one patient had a local catheter-related episode and a non–catheter-related septic episode; and three patients (5%) had only non–catheter-related septic episodes.

Of the 27 patients with catheter-related infections, 20 (74%) had sepsis, five (19%) had local catheter infections, and two (7%) had combined sepsis and local infections. Five children with five septic episodes had identified

Table 2.—Organisms Isolated From Blood and Catheter Exit Site in 30 Patients				
	No.			
	Catheter-Related Infections			
Organism	Sepsis	Local	Non–Catheter-Related Sepsis	Total
Gram-positive bacteria				
Coagulase-negative staphylococci	5 (1*)	1*	0	**6**
Staphylococcus aureus	4	3 (1,* 2†)	0	**7**
Streptococcus, viridans group	2	0	0	**2**
Other streptococci	1	0	0	**1**
Bacillus species	2	0	0	**2**
Clostridium butyricum	1	0	0	**1**
Total	**15**	**4**	**0**	**19**
Gram-negative bacteria				
Pseudomonas aeruginosa	5	1*	0	**6**
Klebsiella pneumoniae	2 (1*)	0	1	**3**
Enterobacter aerogenes	0	1*	0	**1**
Shigella species	0	0	1*	**1**
Citrobacter freundii	0	0	1*	**1**
Escherichia coli	0	0	1	**1**
Haemophilus influenzae, type b	0	0	1	**1**
Total	**7**	**2**	**5**	**14**
Fungi				
Candida tropicalis	2	0	1	**3**
Candida albicans	1	0	0	**1**
Candida parapsilosis	1	0	0	**1**
Total	**4**	**0**	**1**	**5**

*Mixed culture.
†Combined septic and exit wound infection.

sources other than the catheter: perianal abscess (*Escherichia coli*), perirectal abscess (mixed culture of *Shigella* species and *Citrobacter freundii*), pneumonia in two patients (*Haemophilus influenzae* type b and *Klebsiella pneumoniae*), and erosive esophagitis (*Candida tropicalis*).

Local catheter infections consisted of two exit wound infections, two tunnel infections, one exit wound and tunnel infection, and one pocket infection. Neutropenia and fever were present in half of the episodes. In only two of the six cases could organisms be isolated: *Pseudomonas aeruginosa* and a mixed culture of *Staphylococcus aureus*, coagulase-negative staphylococci, and *Enterobacter aerogenes*. The infection-free interval ranged from 2 to 564 days. Five of six local catheter infections occurred during the induction or consolidation phase of chemotherapy. Oral antibiotic therapy was given to one patient, and five patients received intravenous antibiotic treatment for 7 to 28 days. Removal of the catheter was required for cure of three tunnel infections and one exit wound infection. In two episodes of combined sepsis and local infection, *Staphylococcus aureus* was isolated and intravenous antibiotic treatment was given for 7 and 28 days; removal of the catheter was required for successful treatment in one case. The infection-free interval was 70 and 41 days, and both infections occurred during the consolidation phase of chemotherapy.

Twenty-two patients had 25 septic episodes without an identified source other than the catheter. Peripheral-vein and catheter blood cultures were positive in 14 episodes, catheter blood culture only in seven cases, and peripheral blood culture only in four episodes. Gram-positive bacteria were isolated in 58%, gram-negative bacteria in 27%, and fungi in 15% of cases (Table 2). Coagulase-negative staphylococci and *P aeruginosa* were the most frequently isolated single organisms. Neutropenia was present in 19 (76%) of 25 septic episodes. Seventeen (68%) of the 25 episodes occurred during the induction or consolidation phase of chemotherapy.

Although the infection rate for cuffed, tunneled Silastic catheters was higher in acute myelocytic than in lymphocytic leukemia, with 2.6 vs 1.7 infections per 1000 catheter days, the difference was not statistically significant ($P = .25$). Twenty-six catheters used in 21 patients with myelocytic leukemia at a mean age of 94 months had a total duration of 5450 days, whereas 19 catheters inserted in 16 patients with lymphocytic leukemia at a mean age of 61 months had a total duration of 6597 days. Twenty-four intracorporeal venous access systems implanted in 23 children with acute lymphocytic leukemia at a mean age of 80 months had a total duration of 9604 days and 0.3 infection per 1000 catheter days. This was a significantly lower infection rate ($P = .025$) than that for cuffed, tunneled Silastic catheters used in patients with acute lymphocytic leukemia. Only one Port-a-Cath was placed in a child with acute myelocytic leukemia.

Overall, seven (50%) of 14 catheter-related infections in

Table 3.—Studies of Totally Implanted Central Venous Access Devices in Pediatric Oncology Patients

Source, y	Location	No. of Patients	No. of Catheters	No. of Infections/ 1000 Catheter Days
Pegelow et al,[11] 1986	Miami, Fla	15	16	0.97
McGovern et al,[13] 1985	San Antonio, Tex	39	NI*	0.4
McDowell et al,[10] 1986	Liverpool, England	12	12	2.3
Shulman et al,[12] 1987	Houston, Tex	31	33	0.66
Present report	Dallas, Tex	24	25	0.52

*No information.

Table 4.—Studies of Cuffed, Tunneled Silastic Catheters in Pediatric Oncology Patients

Source, y	Location	No. of Patients	No. of Catheters	No. of Infections/ 1000 Catheter Days
Merrit et al,[14] 1981	Los Angeles, Calif	18	21	2.21
Shapiro et al,[15] 1982	Pittsburgh, Pa	27	31	2.68*
Darbyshire et al,[16] 1985	Bristol, England	36	49	6.99
King et al,[17] 1985	Columbus, Ohio	88	NI†	1.37*
Gilman et al,[18] 1986	Morgantown, WVa	16	21	1.33
Cairo et al,[19] 1986	Irvine, Calif	46	53	3.40
Johnson et al,[20] 1986	Nashville, Tenn	64	70	2.84
Hartman and Shochat,[21] 1987	Stanford, Calif	50	63	2.56
Viscoli et al,[22] 1988	Genoa, Italy/London, England	145	157	0.68
Present report	Dallas, Tex	37	46	2.07

*Catheter-related local infections not determined.
†No information.

patients with acute lymphocytic leukemia and 15 (87%) of 17 infectious episodes in patients with acute myelocytic leukemia occurred during the induction and consolidation phases of chemotherapy.

Intravenous antibiotic therapy was given for a mean duration of 10 days. The infection-free interval in the 50 uninfected catheters was 15 733 days, with a mean of 314 days; in the 25 infected catheters, it was 3473 days, with a mean of 139 days. After four patients who died of sepsis were excluded, 17 (81%) of the remaining 21 catheter-related septic episodes were cured without removal of the catheter. In four septic episodes with isolation of *S aureus*, *Bacillus* species, *P aeuruginosa*, and *C tropicalis*, the central venous catheter required removal to cure the infection.

Fourteen patients died during the study period, six in association with sepsis and one with pneumonia. *Candida tropicalis* was isolated from the lung culture of the patient with pneumonia. In two of six fatal septic episodes, a perirectal abscess (*Shigella* species) and an erosive esophagitis (*C tropicalis*) were found at autopsy. Disseminated fungal infections were responsible for three and gram-negative organisms for the other three of the fatal infections. The sepsis-free interval was variable and ranged from 25 to 315 days. Neutropenia was present in all fatal episodes, and two of three occurred during the induction or consolidation phase of chemotherapy.

COMMENT

Sepsis and pocket infection rates of implanted venous access systems in this study were in the lower range of comparable studies,[10-12] which showed 0.49, 0.53, and 1.89 septic episodes and 0.0, 0.47, and 0.49 pocket infections per 1000 catheter days, respectively. In three of four studies, the overall catheter infection rate in pediatric oncology patients receiving chemotherapy through totally implanted venous access systems was lower than one per 1000 catheter days[10-13] (Table 3). However, in one study an infection rate of 2.3 per 1000 catheter days was found,[10] suggesting that different factors, such as catheter care, intensity of catheter use, and hospital vs home therapy, might contribute to a higher infection rate. No mortality related to sepsis was reported.

Studies with cuffed, tunneled Silastic catheters in pediatric oncology patients[14-22] (Table 4) showed infection rates between 0.68 and 3.4 per 1000 catheter days[14,16,19,21,22] with the exception of one report of 6.99 infections per 1000 catheter days.[16]

Successful antimicrobial therapy with the vascular catheter kept in place occurred in 81% of septic episodes and in 63% of all infections related to central venous catheters. In nine studies with pediatric cancer patients and cuffed, tunneled Silastic catheters, between 57% and 100% of catheter infections were treated and cured without removal of the catheter.[16-19,21,23] However, some investigators considered catheter sepsis cured only if the same organism did not recur after completion of antibiotic therapy. Difficulty in clearing tunnel infections without removing the catheter has been reported by several investigators and may reflect poor antibiotic penetration or lack of drainage.[24,25] *Candida* and *Bacillus* species, isolated in two of our septic episodes that required catheter removal for cure, are traditionally considered difficult to eradicate with the catheter kept in place.[17,25-28] *Candida* species have the ability to adhere to host cells and plastic surfaces, and, on electron microscopy, naturally infected catheters show adherent *Candida* enmeshed with fibrin strands.[29] Persistent adherence and colonization of catheters may be facilitated by reduced phagocyte activity in this microenvironment.[29,30]

Although the infection of the catheter lumen or tunnel might occur during implantation or by hematogenous seeding from bacteremia,[31] the mechanism of contamination of these devices is not always clear. Coagulase-negative staphylococci, a frequent cause of catheter-related septic and local infections, are able to produce an extracellular slime substance that limits penetration of antibiotics and drastically reduces the inflammatory host response, facilitating bacteriologic growth at the inner and outer slime surface.[20,32-34] Although coagulase-negative staphylococci are common contaminants in blood cultures, even a single isolation of this organism in a patient with a central venous catheter must be taken seriously,[35-37] especially in neutropenic patients.[5,28,38-40]

Some investigators have noted a change in the spectrum of microorganisms isolated from blood of oncology patients using central venous catheters rather than peripheral venous catheters in the last 10 to 15 years.[41-43] This study showed no consistent predominance or shift to gram-positive organisms in septicemia during a 7½-year period. However, the limited number of blood isolates allows no definite conclusions.

The clinical diagnosis of central venous catheter sepsis in pediatric oncology patients is difficult. There is a wide variation in categorizing a septic infection as catheter related. Some studies have counted all febrile episodes, all bacteremia, or all culture-proved septic infections. Most have required that there be no evidence of an alternative focus of infection.[17,19,21,44] Although the distinction between catheter-related and non–catheter-related septicemia may not be critical for the choice of antimicrobial therapy, some investigators have recommended quantitative blood cultures drawn through the catheter and from a peripheral vein to permit a more precise diagnosis and facilitate the decision of the clinician about whether catheter sepsis might be successfully treated without removal of the catheter.[27,41] The use of comparative quantitative blood cultures currently represents the most accurate method for identifying catheter-related sepsis; however, appropriate processing of such cultures depends on careful collaboration with the clinical microbiology laboratory.

In terms of mechanical complications of cuffed, tunneled Silastic catheters, comparable studies in pediatric oncology patients showed rates between 0.23 and 2.21 thrombotic occlusions per 1000 catheter days.[16,19,21,22] Thrombosis occlusion rates in three studies[11-13] with implanted venous access devices in pediatric oncology patients ranged from 0.3 to 0.53 per 1000 catheter days, and one report showed no occlusion during 2117 catheter days.

We conclude that implanted venous catheter systems in pediatric patients with leukemia not only offer advantages in terms of catheter care and psychological acceptability but also have substantially lower infection rates and longer duration than cuffed, tunneled Silastic catheters in patients with acute lymphocytic leukemia. Whether this is also true for patients with acute myelocytic leukemia remains to be analyzed in future studies. We believe that intracorporeal venous access devices should be preferred in all children with acute lymphocytic leukemia considered for chemotherapy through a central venous catheter.

References

1. Broviac JW, Cole JJ, Scribner BH. A silicone rubber atrial catheter for prolonged parenteral alimentation. *Surg Gynecol.* 1973;136:602-606.
2. Hickman RO, Buckner CD, Clift RA, et al. A modified right atrial catheter for access to the venous system in marrow transplant recipients. *Surg Gynecol Obstet.* 1979;148:871-875.
3. Bodey GP, Buckley MS, Sathe YS, et al. Quantitative relationship between circulating leukocytes and infection in patients with acute leukemia. *Ann Intern Med.* 1966;64:328-340.
4. De Clerck Y, De Clerck D, Rivard GE, et al. Septicemia in children with leukemia. *Can Med Assoc J.* 1978;118:1523-1526.
5. Wade JC, Schimpff SC, Newman KA, et al. *Staphylococcus epidermidis:* an increasing cause of infection in patients with granulocytopenia. *Ann Intern Med.* 1982;97:503-508.
6. Holland JF, Senn H, Banerjee T. Quantitative studies of localized leukocyte mobilization in acute leukemia. *Blood.* 1971;37:449-511.
7. Rosner F, Valmont I, Kozinn PJ. Leukocyte function in patient with leukemia. *Cancer.* 1970;25:835-842.
8. Strauss RR, Paul BB, Jacobs AA. The metabolic and phagocytic activities of leukocytes from children with acute leukemia. *Cancer Res.* 1970;30:80-88.
9. Reed WP, Newman KA, de Jongh C. Prolonged venous access for chemotherapy by means of the Hickman catheter. *Cancer.* 1983;52:185-192.
10. Mc Dowell HP, Hart CA, Martin J. Implantable subcutaneous venous catheters. *Arch Dis Child.* 1986;61:1037-1038.
11. Pegelow CH, Narvaez M, Toledano SR, et al. Experience with a totally implantable venous device in children. *AJDC.* 1986;140:69-71.
12. Shulman RJ, Rahman S, Mahoney D, et al. A totally implanted venous access system used in pediatric patients with cancer. *J Clin Oncol.* 1987;5:137-140.
13. McGovern B, Solenberger R, Reed K. A totally implanted venous access system for long-term chemotherapy in children. *J Pediatr Surg.* 1985;20:725-727.
14. Merrit RJ, Ennis CE, Andrassy RJ, et al. Use of Hickman right atrial catheter in pediatric oncology patients. *JPEN J Parenter Enteral Nutr.* 1981;5:83-85.
15. Shapiro ED, Wald ER, Nelson KA, et al. Broviac catheter related bacteremia in oncology patients. *AJDC.* 1982;136:679-681.
16. Darbyshire PJ, Weightman NC, Speller DCE. Problems associated with indwelling central venous catheters. *Arch Dis Child.* 1985;60:129-134.
17. King DR, Komer M, Hoffman J, et al. Broviac catheter sepsis: the natural history of an iatrogenic infection. *J Pediatr Surg.* 1985;20:728-733.
18. Gilman PA, Palmer TF, Hraborsky EE. The use of right atrial catheters in pediatric cancer patients. *W V Med J.* 1986;82:37-41.
19. Cairo MS, Spooner S, Sowden L, et al. Long-term indwelling multipurpose Silastic catheter in pediatric cancer patients treated with aggressive chemotherapy. *J Clin Oncol.* 1986;4:784-788.
20. Johnson GM, Lee DA, Regelman WE, et al. Interference with granulocyte function by *Staphylococcus epidermidis* slime. *Infect Immun.* 1986;54:13-20.
21. Hartman GE, Shochat SJ. Management of septic complications associated with Silastic catheters in childhood malignancy. *Pediatr Infect Dis J.* 1987;6:1042-1047.
22. Viscoli C, Van der Auwere P, Meunier F. Gram-positive infections in granulocytopenic patients: an important issue? *J Antimicrob Chemother.* 1988;21(suppl C):149-155.
23. Viscoli C, Garaventa A, Boni L, et al. Role of Broviac catheters in infections in children with cancer. *Pediatr Infect Dis.* 1988;7:556-560.
24. Hiemenz J, Skelton J, Pizzo PA. Perspective on the man-

agement of catheter related infections in cancer patients. *Pediatr Infect Dis J.* 1986;5:6-11.
25. Newman K, Tenney J, Reed W, et al. Infectious and noninfectious complications of Hickman catheters. In: Program and abstracts of the 27th Interscience Conference on Antimicrobial Agents and Chemotherapy; October 4-7, 1987; Washington, DC. Abstract 345.
26. Eppes SC, Trautman JL, Gutman LT. Outcome of treatment of candidemia in children whose central catheters were removed or retained. *Pediatr Infect Dis J.* 1989;8:99-104.
27. Flynn PM, Shennep JL, Stokes DC, et al. In situ management of confirmed central venous catheter-related bacteremia. *Pediatr Infect Dis J.* 1987;6:729-734.
28. Weber TR, West KW, Grosfeld JL. Broviac central venous catheterization in infants and children. *Am J Surg.* 1983;145:202-204.
29. Rotrosen D, Calderone RA, Edwards JE Jr. Adherence of *Candida* species to host tissue and plastic surface. *Rev Infect Dis.* 1986;8:73-75.
30. Locci R, Peters G, Pulverer G. Microbial colonization of prosthetic devices, IV: scanning electron microscopy of intravenous catheters invaded by yeast. *Zentralbl Bakteriol Hyg B.* 1981;173:419-424.
31. Pfaller MA, Herwaldt LA. Laboratory, clinical and epidemiological aspects of coagulase-negative staphylococci. *Clin Microbiol Rev.* 1988;1:281-299.
32. Fishman M. Microbial adherence and infection-clinical relevance. *Infect Control.* 1986;7:181-184.
33. Gray ED, Peters G, Verstegen M, Regelman WE. Effect of extracellular slime substance from *Staphylococcus epidermidis* immune response. *Lancet.* 1984;1:365-367.
34. Peters G, Locci R, Pulverer G. Adherence and growth of coagulase-negative staphylococci on surface of intravenous catheters. *J Infect Dis.* 1982;141:479-482.
35. Dominguez de Villota E, Algora-Weber A, Millan I, et al. Early evaluation of coagulase-negative staphylococcus in blood samples of intensive care patients. *Intensive Care Med.* 1987;13:390-394.
36. Martin MA, Pfaller MA, Wenzel RP. Coagulase-negative staphylococcal bacteremia: mortality and hospital stay. *Ann Intern Med.* 1989;110:9-16.
37. Ponce de Leon S, Wenzel RP. Hospital-acquired bloodstream infections with *Staphylococcus epidermidis. Am J Med.* 1984;77:639-644.
38. Baltimore RS. Is it real or is it a contaminant? A guide to the interpretation of blood cultures. *AJDC.* 1987;141:241-242.
39. Del Favero A, Menichetti F, Bucanave G, et al. Septicaemia due to gram-positive cocci in cancer patients. *J Antimicrob Chemother.* 1988;21(suppl C):157-165.
40. Sanz MA, Suck M, Rafecas FJ, et al. *Staphylococcus epidermidis* infections in acute myeloblastic leukemia patients fitted with Hickman catheters. *Lancet.* 1983;2:1191-1192.
41. Kiehn TE, Armstrong D. Changes in the spectrum of organisms causing bacteremia and fungemia in immunocompromised patients due to venous access devices. *Eur J Microbiol Infect Dis.* 1990;9:869-872.
42. Lowder JN, Hillard ML, Herzig RH. Bacteremia and fungemia in oncology patients with central venous catheters. *Arch Intern Med.* 1982;142:1456-1459.
43. Pizzo PA, Ladish S, Simon RM, et al. Increasing incidence of gram-positive sepsis in cancer patients. *Med Pediatr Oncol.* 1978;5:241-244.
44. Johnson PR, Decker MD, Edwards KM, et al. Frequency of Broviac catheter infections in pediatric oncology patients. *J Infect Dis.* 1986;154:570-578.

Mismatch Between Pediatric Training and Pediatric Practice: An Australian View

A questionnaire was sent in 1985 to 232 Australian pediatricians asking whether they had seen an increase or decrease in "the new morbidity" in the previous 5 years. Striking increases were reported in numbers of patients presenting with behavior problems, developmental delay, learning and school problems, and adolescent health and behavior problems. While the pediatricians considered their training in the traditional subspecialty areas of infectious disease, respiratory medicine, and gastroenterology to have been appropriate, they believed their training in the new morbidity areas had been inadequate, especially in behavioral pediatrics, adolescent medicine, parental counseling, and the care of children with chronic handicaps.

Oberklaid F. Mismatch between pediatric training and pediatric practice. *Lancet.* 1991;337:920.

SPECIAL FEATURE

Radiological Case of the Month

Michael P. Mah, MD; Jonathan S. Fain, MD; Sue L. Hall, MD (Contributors);
Beverly P. Wood, MD (Section Editor)

A male newborn, born at 41 weeks' gestation and weighing 3230 g, presented on the first day of life with complex cyanotic heart disease, including the following signs: double-outlet right ventricle, mitral atresia with hypoplastic left ventricle, and hypoplastic aortic arch with coarctation. He was transferred to a level-3 nursery at age 12 days. He underwent pulmonary artery banding, repair of the coarctation of the aorta, and ligation of a patent ductus arteriosus. Congestive heart failure continued after surgery, and the patient was maintained on total parenteral nutrition administered through a double-lumen femoral venous catheter that had been placed during surgery. Eleven days after surgery, he was pale, poorly perfused, and tachypneic.

A septic workup was performed and cultures of blood, urine, and cerebrospinal fluid were obtained. Attempted lumbar puncture using a 22-gauge spinal needle, introduced at the L3-4 interspace, yielded 4 mL of milky white fluid. Cefotaxime and vancomycin therapy was started immediately. The following laboratory values were obtained from the lumbar puncture specimen: glucose, 1268 mmol/L; protein, 4.8 g/L; red blood cell count, 132×10^6/L; and white blood cell count, 99×10^6/L. Gram staining was negative for organisms and bacterial antigens representing *Neisseria meningitidis* (groups A, B, C, Y, and W135), *Streptococcus pneumoniae, Haemophilus influenzae* (type b), and group B *Streptococcus*. Total parenteral nutrition consisting of 22.5% dextrose and 20% lipid emulsion, which was infused into one of the two lumens of his femoral venous catheter, was discontinued. A low-osmolality contrast medium was injected into the same lumen of the femoral line and a frontal roentgenogram obtained (Fig 1). Forty-five minutes later, a contrast medium was again injected, with the results shown in Fig 2. The femoral venous line was removed. A lumbar puncture 3 days later yielded normal cerebrospinal fluid. The patient was eventually discharged without apparent neurologic or infectious sequelae.

From the Departments of Pediatrics (Drs Mah and Hall) and Pathology (Dr Fain), University of California-Los Angeles Medical Center, Los Angeles, CA.
Reprint requests to the Department of Radiology, Box 81, Childrens Hospital of Los Angeles, 4650 Sunset Blvd, Los Angeles, CA 90054-0700 (Dr Wood).

Figure 1.

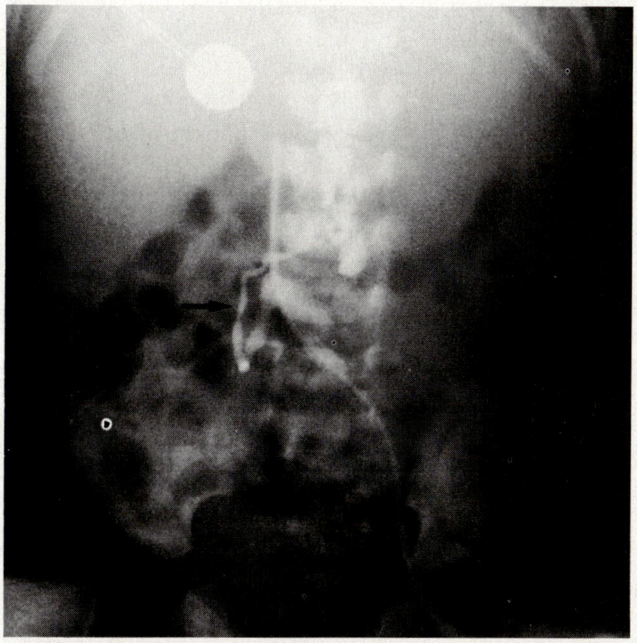

Figure 2.

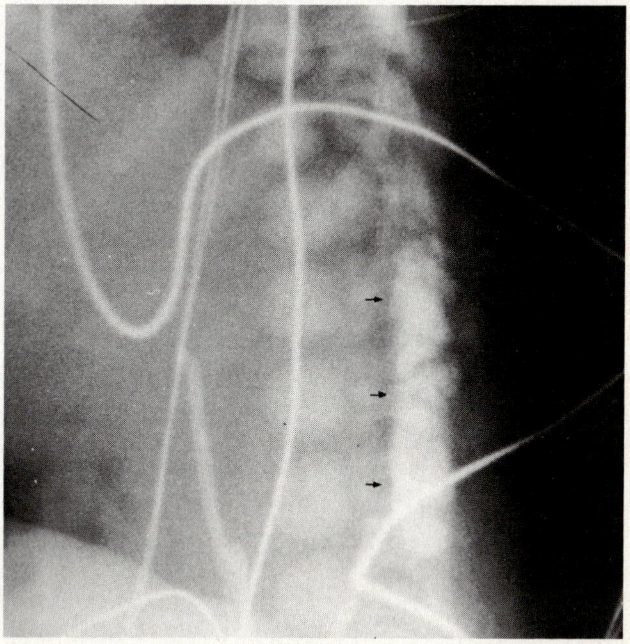

Denouement and Discussion

Intravenous Hyperalimentation Fluid Obtained With Lumbar Puncture: An Unusual Complication of a Central Venous Catheter

Fig 1.—*Frontal roentgenogram of abdomen shows retrograde flow of contrast medium from the inferior vena cava through a lumbar vein (arrow) into the epidural venous plexus.*

Fig 2.—*Lateral abdominal roentgenogram demonstrates contrast medium located in the epidural venous plexus (arrows) anterior to the subarachnoid space.*

Central venous catheters are important for adequate medical management of severely ill neonates and children. Although usually safe, complications of central venous catheters do occur. Reported complications include pneumothorax, hydrothorax, pulmonary embolus, sepsis, caval thrombosis, and intracardiac catheter-tip thrombus formation.[1] This case represents an unusual complication. There was preferential flow of total parenteral nutrition from the side port of the central venous catheter into a lumbar vein, with consequent progression into and distension of the epidural venous plexus. This complication was attributed to catheter thrombosis. The recovery of "milky cerebrospinal fluid" from the lumbar puncture constituted recovery of total parenteral nutrition from the venous plexus superficial to and surrounding the spinal canal. The cerebrospinal fluid contained no contrast material, as distinguished with roentgenography.

To our knowledge, there is one previous report[2] of a lumbar puncture yielding milky fluid with an extremely high glucose and protein content in an infant receiving hyperalimentation. That case differs from ours in that a postmortem barium study showed the catheter had entered an ascending lumbar vein. Free barium extravasated into the epidural space and retroperitoneum. As in our case, roentgenography did not demonstrate entry of the contrast medium into the cerebrospinal fluid.

A markedly elevated level of protein and glucose from a lumbar puncture specimen in an infant receiving central venous hyperalimentation should alert the physician to the possibility that a misplaced or thrombosed catheter has allowed retrograde venous flow of parenteral fluid into the epidural venous plexus surrounding the spinal canal. Both this case and the previous report illustrate the importance of confirming catheter position by injection of the catheter as part of a roentgenographic contrast study.

References

1. Ross P Jr, Ehrenkranz R, Kleinman CS, Seashore JH. Thrombus associated with central venous catheters in infants and children. *J Pediatr Surg.* 1989;24:253-256.

2. Kelly MA, Finer NN, Dunbar LG. Fatal neurologic complication of parenteral feeding through a central vein catheter. *AJDC.* 1984;138:352-353.

SPECIAL FEATURE

Picture of the Month

Walter W. Tunnessen, Jr, MD (Contributor and Section Editor)

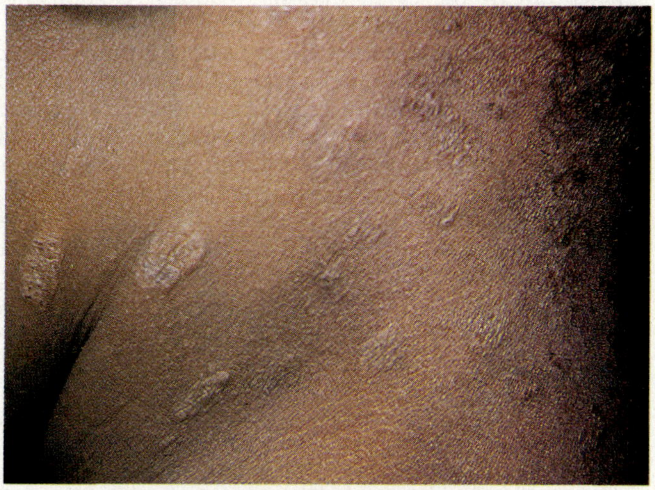

Figure 1.

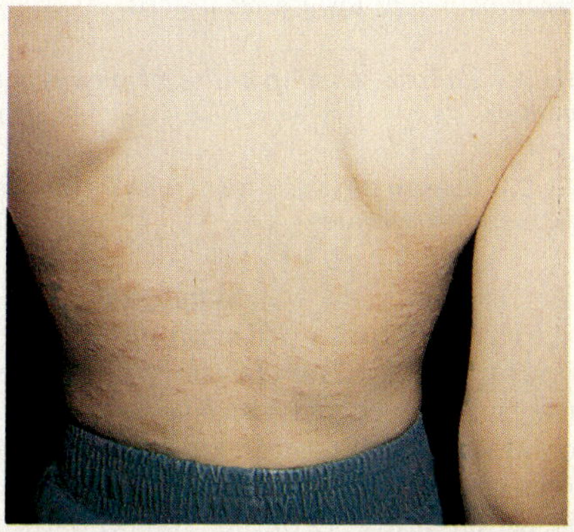

Figure 2.

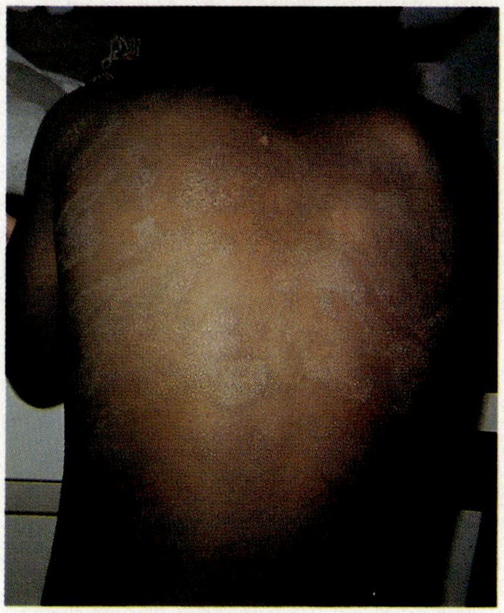

Figure 3.

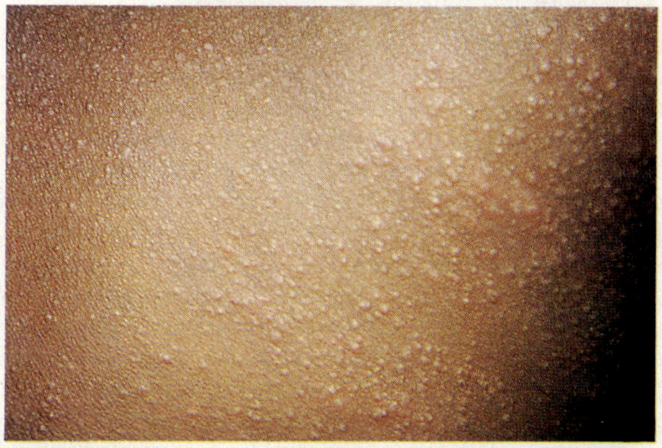

Figure 4.

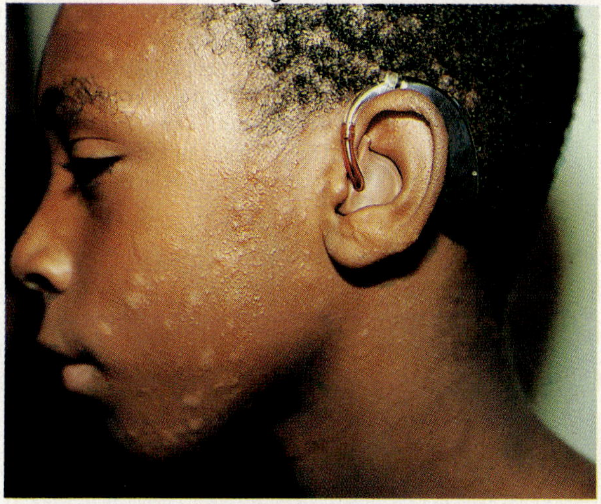

Figure 5.

Accepted for publication March 15, 1991.
Contributed from the Department of Pediatrics, School of Medicine, University of Pennsylvania, Philadelphia.
Reprint requests to the Children's Hospital of Philadelphia, 34th St and Civic Center Blvd, Philadelphia, PA 19104 (Dr Tunnessen).

Denouement and Discussion

Pityriasis Rosea

Fig 1.—*Typical, ovoid plaques of pityriasis rosea with fine scales.*

Fig 2.—*Multiple pink plaques of pityriasis rosea are arranged in lines of skin cleavage, producing a fir-tree type of configuration.*

Fig 3.—*Giant, confluent plaques of pityriasis rosea bear little resemblance to the classic lesions.*

Fig 4.—*Diffuse, small papules of pityriasis rosea obscure a larger plaque.*

Fig 5.—*Inverse pityriasis rosea with lesions primarily located on the face and extremities.*

Manifestations

Pityriasis rosea (PR) commonly occurs in children and young adults. The classic appearance, ovoid plaques arranged with their long axes following skin cleavage lines, creating a pine-bough or fir-tree configuration, is easily recognized by most physicians. The rash of this disorder is much more variable than most suspect, resulting in missed diagnoses, unnecessary laboratory tests, and referral to dermatologists. The figures illustrate the typical lesions and some of the variability seen with this common eruption.

The label applied to dermatologic disorders often describes the clinical picture. Pityriasis means a fine scale and rosea means pink. The rash, then, is characterized by pink lesions with fine scales. The lesions of pityriasis rosea occur most commonly on the trunk. A single lesion, the herald patch, may precede the appearance of the secondary rash by 7 to 14 days. The patch occurs most frequently on the trunk and may be as large as 10 cm in diameter. Its prevalence is varied, but it probably precedes the diffuse rash in less than 50% of cases.

The typical, later appearing lesions are elliptical and average 1 cm in diameter. They are macular or slightly raised plaquelike lesions with pink or brownish bases. The fine scales covering the lesion may be made more apparent with light scratching. Papules of 1 to 2 mm may be so prominent that the plaques are "concealed." The typical fir-tree configuration of the rash is best appreciated by observing the back from a distance of 1.2 to 1.8 m.

The Editors welcome contributions to Picture of the Month *and* Radiological Case of the Month. *Those who wish to contribute should send their manuscripts to Dr Tunnessen* (Picture of the Month), *The Children's Hospital of Philadelphia, 34th Street and Civic Center Blvd, Philadelphia, PA 19104, or Dr Wood* (Radiological Case of the Month), *Department of Radiology, Childrens Hospital of Los Angeles, 4650 Sunset Blvd, Los Angeles, CA 90027. Articles and photographs accepted for publication will bear the contributor's name. There is no charge for reproduction and printing of color illustrations.*

Coalescent gigantic plaques may also conceal the fir-tree pattern. Lesions sometimes can have an urticarial nature. Vesicular or bullous forms are rarely recognized as PR. The appearance of the palms and soles may be similar to that of subjects with dyshidrosis, or there may be a varicellalike appearance if the vesicles are widespread.[1] A rare hemorrhagic character and an erythema multiforme–like appearance have been described.[2,3] Oral lesions of various types, including erythematous plaques, hemorrhagic puncta, and ulcers, have also been reported.[4]

Two unusual patterns of PR are noteworthy. The typical secondary lesions appear over areas generally spared, such as the face and extremities, and remarkable sparing of the trunk occurs in the inverse type of PR. There is also a less commonly recognized localized form producing lesions that may occur only on the lower abdomen, the inguinal area, one axilla, the neck, or one part of the face.

The prolonged course of PR needs to be explained to affected patients. The secondary rash generally develops over 2 weeks, persists for another 2 weeks, and fades over another 2 weeks for an average duration of 6 weeks. However, lesions have persisted for as long as 3 to 4 months.

The lesions of PR are most frequently confused with tinea corporis, nummular eczema, and drug eruptions. Guttate psoriasis and tinea versicolor occasionally may have similar presentations. The rash of secondary syphilis may almost be indistinguishable from PR, in which case serologic testing may be necessary for proper diagnosis.

Pityriasis rosea is more common in the fall, winter, and spring. About 75% of cases occur in subjects aged 10 to 35 years, but a 3-month-old has been reported to have this rash. The cause of PR is unknown, but it is believed to be the result of an infectious, probably viral, process. Small epidemics and family outbreaks have been reported. There are usually no prodromal symptoms to call attention to the disorder. Recurrences are uncommon, probably occurring in less than 3% of affected individuals. There is no reason to exclude children with PR from school.

Treatment

The most common symptom associated with PR is pruritus, which occurs in up to 75% of those affected. Because the disorder is self-limited, pruritus is generally the only symptom that requires attention, and then only if the individual is uncomfortable. Some recommend a mild topical steroid or an emollient with 0.25% menthol to control this symptom. An oral antipruritic agent is rarely required.

References

1. Parsons JM. Pityriasis rosea update: 1986. *J Am Acad Dermatol.* 1986;15:159-167.
2. Paller AS, Esterly NB, Lucky AW, Millstone EB, Higgins TP. Hemorrhagic pityriasis rosea: an unusual variant. *Pediatrics.* 1982;70:357-359.
3. Friendman SJ. Pityriasis rosea with erythema multiform-like lesions. *J Am Acad Dermatol.* 1988;17:135-136.
4. Kay MH, Rapini RP, Fritz KA. Oral lesions in pityriasis rosea. *Arch Dermatol.* 1985;121:1449-1451.

AMERICAN JOURNAL OF
DISEASES OF CHILDREN

AJDC

Index to

Volume 145

January through December 1991

Editor
Vincent A. Fulginiti, MD
American Journal of Diseases of Children
Dean's Office, Room 1529
Tulane University, School of Medicine
1430 Tulane Ave, New Orleans, LA 70112

Associate Editors
Thomas G. Storch, MD
New Orleans, La
William W. Waring, MD
New Orleans, La

Book Review Editor
Peggy C. Ferry, MD
Tucson, Ariz

Administrative Assistant
Joann M. Quane
New Orleans, La

Secretary
Laura Martin
Tucson, Ariz

Editorial Board

AUTHOR INDEX TO VOLUME 145

In this Index in alphabetical order are listed names of authors of all articles and letters. Full citation is given under first author only; reference is made from joint authors. Names which begin with a prefix are entered under the prefix. The month is given as a two letter notation in parentheses.

A

Abby H see Kinney J
Abrunzo TJ: Commotio cordis: the single, most common cause of traumatic death in youth baseball, 1279 (No)
Acampora D see Forsyth BW
Accardo PJ, Tomazic T, Morrow J, Haake C, Whitman BY: Minor malformations, hyperactivity, and learning disabilities, 1184 (Oc)
Ackerman A see Carraccio C
Adger H Jr see Duggan AK
Adler R see Bergman AS; Wong VK
Aguirre Vila-Coro A see Dominguez R
Ajuriaguerra M de, Radvanyi-Bouvet M-F, Huon C, Moriette G: Gastroesophageal reflux and apnea in prematurely born infants during wakefulness and sleep, 1132 (Oc)
Al-Salem AH, Grant C: Hypoplastic left upper lobe, 821 (Jy)
Aladjem M see Eshel G
Alagille D see Gottrand F
Alexander JR see Poets CF
Allan WC see Marro PJ
Allen HD: Mitral valve prolapse: back to the basics, 1095 (Oc)
Allen HD, Burg F, Levine H, Starfield B, Greenberg LW, eds: Educational interventions, 79 (Ja), 161 (Fe), 299 (Mr), 449 (Ap), 639 (Je), 757 (Jy), 881 (Au), 1002 (Se), 1125, 1191 (Oc), 1255, 1272 (No), 1389 (De)
Allen HD, Taubert KA, Deckelbaum RJ, Driscoll D, Dunnigan A, Gidding SS, Herndon P, Kavey R-EW, Mullins C, Snider AR, Strong WB, Washington R: Poverty and cardiac disease in children, 550 (My)
Allison JW, Stephenson CA, Angtuaco TL, Glasier CM: Tuberous sclerosis with myocardial and central nervous system involvement at birth, 471 (Ap)
AMA Board of Trustees: Use of infant walkers, 933 (Au)
Amoruso LP see Maynard EC
Anderson SK see Desch LW
Andreotti M-R see Staiano A
Angelus P see Scott SM
Angtuaco TL see Allison JW
Antonson DL see Hart MH
Antonucci DL see Charney EB
Apple RD see Greer FR
Arden MR, Budow L, Bunnell DW, Nussbaum MP, Shenker IR, Jacobson MS: Alkaline urine is associated with eating disorders (letter) 28 (Ja)
Arden MR, Nussbaum MP, Jacobson MS: Association of alkaline urine with eating disorders (letter) 1091 (Oc)
Arensman FW see Treiber FA
Arola M see Heikkinen T
Avner JR, Henretig FM, McAneney CM: Acquired methemoglobinemia: the relationship of cause to course of illness, 144:1229(No); correction, 145:158 (Fe)
Azen CG, Koch R, Friedman EG, Berlow S, Coldwell J, Krause W, Matalon R, McCabe E, O'Flynn M, Peterson R, Rouse B, Valle D, Scott CR, Sigman B, Warner R: Intellectual development in 12-year-old children treated for phenylketonuria, 35 (Ja)

B

Backstrom C see Scott SM
Bader M: Your child's best friend: TV or not TV? (letter) 963 (Se)
Bahakim HM see Haque KN
Baker CJ see Landers S
Baker RB: Anal fissure produced by examination for sexual abuse (letter) 848 (Au)
Baldwin V see Rotschild A
Balfour IC, Drimmer AM, Nouri S, Pennington DG, Hemkens CL, Harvey LL: Pediatric cardiac rehabilitation, 627 (Je)
Ball A see Davidson M
Baranowski T see Bee DE
Barash V see Eshel G
Barka N see Ruderman JW
Barnes N see Parker RM
Barness LA: Health care for uninsured and underinsured children (letter)1086 (Oc)
Barnett SE see Niebuhr VN
Baroncelli GI see Saggese G
Barr J see Eshel G
Bartlett GS see Greenberg LW
Bartley DL see Piatt JP
Barton LL see Hoddy DM; Rathore MH
Bass JW: *Staphylococcus aureus* in impetigo (letter) 1223 (No)
Bass M: Fallacy of the hemorrhagic shock and encephalopathy syndrome (letter) 718 (Jy)
Bastian JF see Wilson NW
Bauer CR see Schwersenski J
Bautista D see Ward SLD
Bays J, Jenny C: Anal fissure produced by examination for sexual abuse (letter) 849 (Au)
Beachler MP: Improving health care for underserved infants, children, and adolescents: the Robert Wood Johnson Foundation's experience, 565 (My)
Bean XD see Ward SLD
Beck S see Kletzel M
Bedrick AD: Eighty-hour workweek and residency programs: closing arguments (letter) 846 (Au)
Pediatric perspectives: vistas and vantage points, 256 (Mr)
Bedrick AD, ed: Pediatric perspectives, 314 (Mr)
Bee DE, Baranowski T, Rassin DK, Richardson CJ, Mikrut W: Breast-feeding initiation in a triethnic population, 306 (Mr)
Behrman RE, Larson CS: Health care for pregnant women and young children, 572 (My)
Beittel TM see Pearson GD
Belamarich PF see Starc TJ
Bell LM see Shaw KN
Benford SA see DeClue TJ
Bennett FC see Luchi JM
Bennett JV, Rogers MF: Child survival and perinatal infections with human immunodeficiency virus, 1242 (No)
Bennett WG: Left renal vein thrombosis and left adrenal hemorrhage, 1299 (No)
Berger LR: Exhibitor 'giveaways': a curmudgeon's view (letter) 427 (Ap)
Bergman AS, Adler R: Support services for pediatric trainees: a survey of training program directors, 1002 (Se)
Berkowitz CD: Serving the underserved: impact on resident education, 544 (My)
Berlow S see Azen CG
Berman ER see Thilo EH
Bernard O see Gottrand F
Bernasconi S see Volta C
Bernstein HH see Rothstein EP
Bertelloni S see Saggese G
Berwick M see Bolognia JL
Bhowmick SK, Johnson KR, Rettig KR: Rickets caused by vitamin D deficiency in breast-fed infants in the southern United States, 127 (Fe)
Bilello JF, O'Hair KC, Kirby WC, Moore JW: Intraosseous infusion of dobutamine and isoproterenol, 165 (Fe); correction, 1312 (No)
Binet A see Kooh SW
Black SB, Cherry JD, Shinefield HR, Fireman B, Christenson P, Lampert D: Apparent decreased risk of invasive bacterial disease after heterologous childhood immunization, 746 (Jy)
Blackwelder WC, Storsaeter J, Olin P, Hallander HO: Acellular pertussis vaccines: efficacy and evaluation of clinical case definitions, 1285 (No)
Blanche S, Duliege A-M, Rouzioux C, Le Deist F, Fukunaga K, Caniglia M, Jacomet C, Griscelli C, Tardieu M: Third pattern of disease progression in children infected with human immunodeficiency virus (letter) 1348 (De)
Blanchette VS, Hume HA, Levy GJ, Luban NLC, Strauss RG: Guidelines for auditing pediatric blood transfusion practices, 787 (Jy)
Blank S see Blum BB
Blum BB, Blank S: Children's services in an era of budget deficits, 575 (My)
Blum RW see Story M
Bohan TP see Dominguez R
Boiko S see Reynolds RD
Bolognia JL, Berwick M, Fine JA, Simpson P, Jasmin M: Sun protection in newborns: a comparison of educational methods, 1125 (Oc)
Bonadio WA, Smith DS, Madagame E, Machi J, Kini N: *Escherichia coli* bacteremia in children: a review of 91 cases in 10 years, 671 (Je)
Bowen J, Fenton T, Rappaport L: Stimulant medication and attention deficit-hyperactivity disorder: the child's perspective, 291 (Mr)
Boyce WT, Chesterman EA, Winkleby MA: Psychosocial predictors of maternal and infant health among adolescent mothers, 267 (Mr)
Boyd AS:
Condylomata acuminata: still usually a sexually transmitted disease in children (letter) 601 (Je)
Diagnosis of child sexual abuse in children with genital warts (letter) 126 (Fe)
Boyd MT see Roberts RL
Braden DS see McCaffrey FM
Brasseux C see Greenberg LW
Braunstein GD see Englund AT
Braunstein H, Thomas S, Ito R, Jarman C: Response of seronegative adults to measles immunization (letter) 969 (Se)
Brent RL: Comments on life after residency (letter) 597 (Je)
Bromberg K see Rawstron SA
Brookfield E see Tayel S
Bross-Soriano D see Mota-Hernández F
Brown GW: Buddy, can you paradigm?, 727 (Jy)
More on the *P value* (letter) 249 (Mr)
Browner WS see Newman TB
Bryson SM see Lui K
Buchanan GR see Jonsson OG
Buckley S see Ward SLD
Budow L see Arden MR
Buffkin DC see Reller MD
Bulkow L see Davidson M
Bunnell DW see Arden MR
Burchfield DJ, Rawlings DJ: Sudden deaths and apparent life-threatening events in hospitalized neonates presumed to be healthy, 1319 (No)
Burg F see Allen HD
Burg FD see Winter RJ
Burks W see Kletzel M
Butler MG, Hassell S: Antley-Bixler syndrome, 701 (Je)
Byrne P, Welch R: Treatment withdrawal in neonates (letter) 1223 (No)
Byrt T: *P* values (letter) 250 (Mr)

C

Cabral H see Zuckerman B
Calderazzi A see Saggese G
Callahan CW Jr: Tiny Tim remembered, 1355 (De)
Calligaro ILS see Kraus DM
Caniglia M see Blanche S
Carey JC see Kershisnik MM
Carithers HA, Margileth AM: Cat-scratch disease: acute encephalopathy and other neurologic manifestations, 98 (Ja)
Carraccio C, Ackerman A: Current trends in pediatric residency training, 1272 (No)
Carson BS see Thilo EH
Carter G, Park JW, Tarvin C: Clavicular fractures in neonates (letter)251 (Mr)
Carzoli RP, Murphy SP, Hammer-Knisely J, Houy J: Evaluation of auditory brain-stem response in full-term infants of cocaine-abusing mothers, 1013 (Se)
Chacko MR see Sugerman ST
Chan GM: Dietary calcium and bone mineral status of children and adolescents, 631 (Je)
Chan JCM see Hanna JD
Chang C-H see Moore EC
Chapin J see Davidson EC Jr
Charney EB, Melchionni JB, Antonucci DL: Ventriculitis in newborns with myelomeningocele, 287 (Mr)
Cheng TL: House staff work hours and moonlighting: what do residents want?: a survey of pediatric residents in California, 1104 (Oc)
Cherry JD see Black SB; Davidson M; Kimura M
Cherry JD: Vaccine myth and physician handouts (letter) 426 (Ap)
Chesterman EA see Boyce WT
Chitayat D see Rotschild A
Christenson P see Black SB; Davidson M
Christoffel K see Retsky J
Claude S see Secord E
Cleveland WW: Redoing the health care quilt: patches or whole cloth?, 499 (My)
Clouse RE see Staiano A
Cohen F see Moore EC
Cohen GR, Thorp J, Yeast JD, Meyer BA, O'Kell R, Macy C: Markedly immature lecithin-sphingomyelin ratio at term and congenital hypothyroidism (letter)1227 (No)
Cohen PR, Hebert AA: Pachyonychia congenita, 1301 (No)
Colasurdo MA see Reller MD
Coldwell J see Azen CG
Comerci GD: Fasting Girls: The History of Anorexia Nervosa (Book Review)146 (Fe)
Conway EE Jr, Singer LP: Hemorrhagic shock and encephalopathy: an entity similar to heatstroke (letter) 720 (Jy)
Corazziari E see Staiano A
Corrigan JJ Jr see Glasser L; Tarantino MD
Costello S see Lui K
Coulter DM: More on the *P value* (letter) 249 (Mr)
Craven CM see Kershisnik MM
Crosby WM: Studies in fetal malnutrition, 871 (Au)
Cuevas D see Cuevas L
Cuevas L, Yeh TF, John EG, Cuevas D, Plides RS: Effect of low-dose dopamine infusion on cardiopulmonary and renal status in premature newborns with respiratory distress syndrome, 799 (Jy)
Cutting GR see McColley SA

D

Dagan R: *Staphylococcus aureus* in impetigo (letter) 1223 (No)
Daigler GE, Welliver RC, Stapleton FB: New York State health code 405 update (letter) 428 (Ap)
Danon YL see Seidman DS
Dashefsky B see Wald ER
Davidson BL see Ing DJ
Davidson EC Jr, Gibbs CE, Chapin J: Challenge of care for the poor and underserved in the United States: an American College of Obstetricians and Gynecologists perspective on access to care for underserved women, 546 (My)
Davidson M, Letson GW, Ward JI, Ball A, Bulkow L, Christenson P, Cherry JD: DTP immunization and susceptibility to infectious diseases: is there a relationship?, 750 (Jy)
Davis H see Treiber FA
Davis J see DeClue TJ
Davis JC Jr see Johnson JP
Davis JH: Health care for uninsured and underinsured children (letter)1085 (Oc)
Davis MW see Roberts RL
Dean JM: Pediatric Intensive Care, ed 2 (Book Review) 175 (Fe)
DeAngelis C: Women in medicine: fantasies, dreams, myths, and realities, 49 (Ja)
DeBeukelaer MM see Tayel S
Deckelbaum RJ see Allen HD; Starc TJ
DeClue TJ, Davis J, Schocken DM, Kangas R, Benford SA: Serum lipid concentrations in subjects with phenylketonuria and their families, 1266 (No)
Deforest A see Ridgway D
Deguchi M see Kimura M
Delepoulle F see Leclerc F
Dell RB see Starc TJ
Desch LW, Esquivel MT, Anderson SK: Comparison of a computer tutorial with other methods for teaching well-newborn care, 1255 (No)
Deshpande JK see Stoddard JJ
Dietz WH see Segal KR
DiGaudio KM, Msall ME: Guidelines for safe transportation of children in wheelchairs, 653 (Je)
DiMauro S see Eshel G
Ditchek S see Schaeffer AV
DiTraglia J: Family physicians and neonatology (letter) 963 (Se)
Dobrin-Seckler BE see Starc TJ
Dodd DA see Johns KJ
Dodge PR see Keating JP
Dominguez R, Aguirre Vila-Coro A, Slopis JM, Bohan TP: Brain and ocular abnormalities in infants with in utero exposure to cocaine and other street drugs, 688 (Je)
Donner J see DuRant RH
Donowitz LG see Lohr JA
Dornbusch SM see Hammer LD
Doughty RA see Weiss JC
Doughty RA, Williams PD, Seashore CN: Chief resident training: developing leadership skills for future medical leaders, 639 (Je)
Downing GJ, Horner SR, Kilbride HW: Characteristics of perinatal cocaine-exposed infants with necrotizing enterocolitis (letter) 26 (Ja)
Drake C see Wintemute GJ
Dransfield DA see Marro PJ
Drimmer AM see Balfour IC
Driscoll D see Allen HD
Dudley SM see Lohr JA
Duggan AK, Adger H Jr, McDonald EM, Stokes EJ, Moore R: Detection of alcoholism in hospitalized children and their families, 613 (Je)
Duke JC see Venkataraman PS
Duliege A-M see Blanche S
Duncan BR see Glasser L
Dunkle LM see Rathore MH
Dunn K see Horner AA
Dunne WM Jr see Esterly NB
Dunnigan A see Allen HD
Dupee CR: Hyperpyrexia, hemorrhagic shock and encephalopathy, and creatinine phosphokinase (letter) 719 (Jy)
DuRant RH, Pendergrast RA, Donner J, Seymore C, Gaillard G: Adolescents'attrition from school-sponsored sports, 1119 (Oc)

E

Edelman DS: Laparoscopic cholecystectomy under continuous epidural anesthesia in patients with cystic fibrosis (letter) 723 (Jy)
Edmonds LD see Mili F
Ehrlich R see Tayel S
Einarson TR see Sharav T
Eisenberg CSL see Melzer-Lange M
Elser J see Kletzel M
Elster AB: New initiatives in adolescent health promotion, 495 (My)
Englund AT, Geffner ME, Nagel RA, Lippe BM, Braunstein GD: Pediatric germ cell and human chorionic gonadotropin-producing tumors: clinical and laboratory features, 1294 (No)
Erdman S see Hart MH
Ervin MG see Padilla G
Eshel G, Lahat E, Fried K, Barr J, Barash V, Gutman A, DiMauro S, Aladjem M: Autosomal recessive lethal infantile cytochrome C oxidase deficiency, 661 (Je)
Eskola J see Käyhty H; Nohynek H
Esquivel MT see Desch LW
Esterly NB, Nelson DB, Dunne WM Jr: Impetigo, 125 (Fe)

F

Faden H, Grossi M: Acute osteomyelitis in children: reassessment of etiologic agents and their clinical characteristics, 65 (Ja)
Faigel HC: Gilding the lily (letter) 849 (Au)
Fain JS see Mah MP
Farooki Z see Moore EC
Farrow JA: Youth alienation as an emerging pediatric health care issue, 491 (My)
Farrow JA, Schwartz RH, Vanderleeuw J: Tattooing behavior in adolescence: a comparison study, 184 (Fe)
Faye-Petersen OM, Knisely AS: Neural arch stenosis and spinal cord injury in thanatophoric dysplasia, 87 (Ja)
Feingold M: Syringomas in Down syndrome (letter) 966 (Se)
Feingold M, ed: Picture of the month, 113 (Ja), 211 (Fe), 341 (Mr), 473 (Ap), 701 (Je), 1047 (Se), 1301 (No)
Feman SS see Johns KJ
Fenton T see Bowen J
Ferry PC: Current Concepts in Childhood Spinal Muscular Atrophy (Book Review) 462 (Ap)
HL Mencken Baby Book (Book Review) 817 (Jy)
Part-time Peg: who, me?, 852 (Au)
Pediatric legal medicine: a new venture, 255 (Mr)
Seizures and Epilepsy in Childhood: A Guide for Parents (Book Review) 539 (My)
Ferry PC, ed: Pediatric legal medicine, 275 (Mr), 1153 (Oc)
Fields AI, Rosenblatt A, Pollack MM, Kaufman J: Home care cost-effectiveness for respiratory technology-dependent children, 729 (Jy)
Fikar CR, Koslap-Petraco M: What about gay teenagers? (letter) 252 (Mr)
Finberg L see Saavedra JM
Finberg L: How much iron is enough? (letter) 598 (Je)
Water intoxication: a prevalent problem in the inner city, 981 (Se)
Fine JA see Bolognia JL
Fingerhut LA see Kleinman JC
Fink HW: Formula companies and the medical profession (letter) 1088 (Oc)
Finkelstein JA see Parker RM
Fireman B see Black SB
Fischer H see Schneider JR
Fisher P see Friedman DE
Forrest T see Treiber FA
Forsyth BW, Shapiro ED, Horwitz RI, Viscoli CM, Acampora D: Misdiagnosis of Reye's-like illness (letter) 964 (Se)
Forsythe AB see Schatz M
Fox HB see Newacheck PW
Fraley JK see Landers S
Francom S see Jaimovich DG
Frasch CE, Hiner EE, Gross TP: *Haemophilus* b disease after vaccination with *Haemophilus* b polysaccharide or conjugate vaccine, 1379 (De)
Freed GL, Landers S, Schanler RJ: Practical guide to successful breast-feeding management, 917 (Au)
Fried K see Eshel G
Fried LE see Needlman R
Friedman AD see Rathore MH
Friedman DE, Pines RJ, Shelley M, Fisher P, Silberbach GM: Acropustulosis of infancy, 341 (Mr)
Friedman EG see Azen CG
Friman PC: Send Linus to me (letter) 1227 (No)
Thumb-sucking (letter) 846 (Au)
Fukunaga K see Blanche S
Fulginiti VA: *AJDC* is 80 years old: from pedology to pediatrics, 11 (Ja)
Diphtheria and tetanus toxoids and pertussis vaccine litigation (letter) 425 (Ap)
Far from the ideal: the plight of poor children in the United States, 489 (My)
More on a myth (letter) 717 (Jy)
Vaccine myth and physician handouts (letter) 427 (Ap)
Furfaro S, Gauthier M, Lacroix J, Nadeau D, Lafleur L, Mathews S: Arterial catheter-related infections in children: a 1-year cohort analysis, 1037 (Se)

G

Gaillard G see DuRant RH
Gale R see Seidman DS
Galil A see Goldstein E
Galioto FM Jr see Tomassoni TL
Gallaher MM, Hauck FR, Yang-Oshida M, Serdula MK: Obesity among Mescalero preschool children: association with maternal obesity and birth weight, 1262 (No)
Garcia CD, Miller LA, Stapleton FB: Natural history of hematuria associated with hypercalciuria in children, 1204 (Oc)
Garcia RE, Moodie DS: Lipoprotein profiles in hypercholesterolemic children, 147 (Fe); correction, 515 (My)
Garty B-Z, Kauli R, Livni E, Laron Z, Nitzan M: Myopathy associated with ketoconazole treatment (letter) 970 (Se)
Gauthier F see Gottrand F
Gauthier M see Furfaro S
Geddes KM see Pittard WB III
Geffner ME see Englund AT
Gersony WM see Starc TJ
Gertner JM see Wilson DM
Getson P see Greenberg LW
Ghizzoni L see Volta C
Giacola GP: Congenital syphilis, 1045 (Se)
Giardino A, Giardino E: Resident and nurse practitioners: responding to education and patient care needs (letter) 843 (Au)
Giardino E see Giardino A
Gibbs CE see Davidson EC Jr
Gidding SS see Allen HD
Gilstrap LC III see Little B
Girone JAC see Rothstein EP
Glasier CM see Allison JW
Glaspy JA see Roberts RL
Glass JB, Sher PK, Lennon VA, Regelmann WE: Association of pauciarticular juvenile arthritis and myasthenia gravis, 1176 (Oc)
Glass RI see Ing DJ
Glasser L see Tarantino MD
Glasser L, Duncan BR, Corrigan JJ Jr: Measurement of serum granulocyte colony-stimulating factor in a patient with congenital agranulocytosis (Kostmann's syndrome), 925 (Au)
Glasson M see Kozlowski K
Gleason C see Kinney J
Glotzer D see Kharasch SJ
Goetzman BW: Priorities in academic pediatrics (letter) 845 (Au)
Goldenring JM: Condylomata acuminata: still usually a sexually transmitted disease in children (letter) 600 (Je)
Goldstein E, Porter B, Galil A: Neurodevelopmental outcome of offspring of the diabetic mother: need for further research (letter) 602 (Je)
Gonzalez-Heydrich J, Kerner JA Jr, Steiner H: Testing the psychogenic vomiting diagnosis: four pediatric patients, 913 (Au)
Gooding A see Wilson NW
Goodman SN: Neuroblastoma screening data: an epidemiologic analysis, 1415 (De)
Gorlick GM: Word choice (letter) 724 (Jy)
Gottrand F, Bernard O, Hadchouel M, Pariente D, Gauthier F, Alagille D: Late cholangitis after successful surgical repair of biliary atresia, 213 (Fe)
Grant C see Al-Salem AH
Gratton TL see Specker BL
Greenberg LW see Allen HD
Greenberg LW, Getson P, Brasseux C, Pattishall EG III, Kataria S, Bartlett GS, Tully SB, Shea D: How are pediatric training programs preparing residents for practice?, 1389 (De)
Greer FR, Apple RD:
Formula companies and the medical profession (letter) 1090 (Oc)
Physicians, formula companies, and advertising: a historical perspective, 282 (Mr)
Griscelli C see Blanche S
Groothuis JR: Introduction to Clinical Resarch, 945 (Au)
Gross TP see Frasch CE
Grossi M see Faden H
Grosso J see Myer CM III
Grunebaum M see Laron Z
Gunn WJ, Pinsky PF, Sacks JJ, Schonberger LB: Injuries and poisonings in out-of-home child care and home care, 779 (Jy)
Gutgesell ME: Safety of a preadolescent basketball program, 1023 (Se)
Gutman A see Eshel G
Gutman LT, Herman-Giddens M, Prose NS: Diagnosis of child sexual abuse in children with genital warts (letter) 126 (Fe)
Gutman LT, St Claire K, Herman-Giddens M, McKinney RE Jr: Child sexual abuse and human immunodeficiency virus transmission (letter) 847 (Au)
Gutman LT, St Claire KK, Weedy C, Herman-Giddens ME, Lane BA, Niemeyer JG, McKinney RE Jr: Human immunodeficiency virus transmission by child sexual abuse, 137 (Fe)

H

Haake C see Accardo PJ
Hadchouel M see Gottrand F
Haggerty RJ: Care of the poor and underserved in America: older adolescents: a group at special risk, 569 (My)
Hall SL see Mah MP
Hallander HO see Blackwelder WC
Halonen P see Heikkinen T; Nohynek H
Hammer LD, Kraemer HC, Wilson DM, Ritter PL, Dornbusch SM: Standardized percentile curves of body-mass index for children and adolescents, 259 (Mr)
Hammer LD, Wilson DM, Kraemer HC, Ritter PL, Dornbusch SM: Obesity and body-mass index (letter) 972 (Se)

Hammer-Knisely J see Carzoli RP
Handelsman E, Voulalas D: Albuterol inhalations in acute chest syndrome (letter) 603 (Je)
Hanna JD, Niimi K, Chan JCM: X-linked hypophosphatemia: genetic and clinical correlates, 865 (Au)
Hansen EJ see Mertsola J
Haque KN, Bahakim HM: Percentile curves for various hematologic measurements at birth in Arab preterm babies of different gestational ages, 645 (Je)
Harden KM see Schatz M
Harris GD see Saavedra JM
Harris LJ see Story M
Hart MH, Kaufman SS, Vanderhoof JA, Erdman S, Linder J, Markin RS, Kruger R, Antonson DL: Neonatal hepatitis and extrahepatic biliary atresia associated with cytomegalovirus infection in twins, 302 (Mr)
Harvey LL see Balfour IC
Hassell S see Butler MG
Hatoum HT see Kraus DM
Hauck FR see Gallaher MM
Heagarty MC: Pediatric acquired immunodeficiency syndrome, poverty, and national priorities, 527 (My)
Hebert AA see Cohen PR
Hecker JA: Health care for uninsured and underinsured children (letter)1086 (Oc)
Hegenbarth MA see Melzer-Lange M
Heikkinen T, Ruuskanen O, Waris M, Ziegler T, Arola M, Halonen P: Influenza vaccination in the prevention of acute otitis media in children, 445 (Ap)
Hemkens CL see Balfour IC
Hennes HM, Lee MB, Rimm AA, Shapiro DL: Surfactant replacement therapy in respiratory distress syndrome: meta-analysis of clinical trials of single-dose surfactant extracts, 102 (Ja)
Hennessy JR see Tayel S
Henretig FM see Avner JR
Hergenroeder AC see Sugerman ST
Hergenroeder AC: Obesity and body-mass index (letter) 972 (Se)
Herman-Giddens M see Gutman LT
Herman-Giddens ME see Gutman LT
Herndon P see Allen HD
Hess KW: Fetal alcohol syndrome: misplaced emphasis (letter) 721 (Jy)
Hicks JM see Rifai N
Hickson GB see White BD
Hill HR: Is prophylaxis of neonates with intravenous immunoglobulin beneficial?, 1229 (No)
Himes JH see Story M
Hiner EE see Frasch CE
Hines SE see Johnson JP
Hinman AR: What will it take to fully protect all American children with vaccines?, 559 (My)
Hipp TJ see Rothstein EP
Hitimana D-G see Lepage P
Ho ML see Specker BL
Hochberg Z see Rudolf MCJ
Hockenberry-Eaton MJ see van Hoff J
Hoddy DM, Barton LL: Puncture wound-induced *Achromobacter xylosoxidans* osteomyelitis of the foot (letter) 599 (Je)
Hoffman CP see Schatz M
Hollis BW see Pittard WB III
Holloway MK, Wason S, Willging JP, Meyer CM III: Pediatric case of Eagle's syndrome, 339 (Mr)
Holmes JH see Parker RM
Hong R: Word choice (letter) 724 (Jy)
Hope S see Newman TB
Horiuchi K see Kimura M
Horner AA, Dunn K, Stiehm ER: Penile vasculitis with impending necrosis treated with prostaglandin E_1 infusion (letter) 604 (Je)
Horner SR see Downing GJ
Horwitz RI see Forsyth BW
Houy J see Carzoli RP
Hoyt MJ see Kennedy WA
Hu H: 50-year follow-up of childhood plumbism: hypertension, renal function, and hemoglobin levels among survivors, 681 (Je)
Hue V see Leclerc F
Hulsey TC see Pittard WB III
Hume HA see Blanchette VS
Huon C see Ajuriaguerra M de
Hurt H see Vera LA
Hutchison HT see Opala G
Hutter JJ see van Hoff J

I

Ing DJ, Glass RI, Woods PA, Simonetti M, Pallansch MA, Wilcox WD, Davidson BL, Sievert AJ: Immunogenicity of tetravalent rhesus rotavirus vaccine administered with buffer and oral polio vaccine, 892 (Au)
Ingram DL see Lohr JA
Iosefsohn M see Rifai N
Irwin DB see Lui K
Isomura S see Kimura M
Ito R see Braunstein H

J

Jackson JC see Luchi JM
Jacobs NM: Pneumococcal osteomyelitis and arthritis in children: a hospital series and literature review, 70 (Ja)
Jacobs SE: Priorities in academic pediatrics (letter) 845 (Au)
Jacobson AD see Piatt JP
Jacobson MS see Arden MR
Jacomet C see Blanche S
Jadavji T see Kabani A
Jaffe D see Retsky J
Jaimovich DG, Kumar A, Francom S: Evaluation of intraosseus vs intravenous antibiotic levels in a porcine model, 946 (Au); correction, 1241 (No)
Jardine DS: Reexpansion pulmonary edema (letter) 1092 (Oc)
Jarman C see Braunstein H
Jasmin M see Bolognia JL
Jenny C see Bays J
Jeter MA see Tarantino MD
Joffe A see Kabani A
John EG see Cuevas L
Johns JA see Johns KJ
Johns KJ, Johns JA, Feman SS, Dodd DA: Retinopathy of prematurity in infants with cyanotic congenital heart disease, 200 (Fe)
Johnson CL see Rothstein EP
Johnson J see Waller KS
Johnson JD: Tell the whole story, 135 (Fe)
Johnson JP, Vink PE, Hines SE, Robinson B, Davis JC Jr, Nair P: Vertical transmission of human immunodeficiency virus from seronegative or indeterminate mothers, 1239 (No)
Johnson KR see Bhowmick SK
Johnston RB Jr: Poverty and the health of American children: implications for academic pediatrics, 507 (My)
Jonsson OG, Buchanan GR: Chronic neutropenia during childhood: a 13-year experience in a single institution, 232 (Fe)
Joorabchi B: Objective structured clinical examination in a pediatric residency program, 757 (Jy)
Joseph PR, Rosenfeld W:
Clavicular fractures in neonates (letter) 252 (Mr)
Clavicular fractures in neonates: frequency vs significance (letter) 251 (Mr)
Jung AL see Kershisnik MM

K

Kabani A, Joffe A, Jadavji T: Hydrocele in Kawasaki disease: importance in early recognition of atypical disease (letter) 1348 (De)
Kallen RJ: Paleonephrology and reflux nephropathy: from the 'big bang' to end-stage renal disease, 860 (Au)
Kamei R: Difficult Diagnosis in Pediatrics (Book Review) 541 (My)
Kamiya H see Kimura M
Kangas R see DeClue TJ
Karanko V see Käyhty H
Kataria S see Greenberg LW
Kato T see Kimura M
Katz BZ, McNamara JG: Third pattern of disease progression in children infected with human immunodeficiency virus (letter) 1347 (De)
Kauffman RE see Rosenberg NM
Kaufman J see Fields AI
Kaufman SS see Hart MH
Kauli R see Garty B-Z
Kavey R-EW see Allen HD
Käyhty H, Eskola J, Peltola H, Rönnberg P-R, Kela E, Karanko V, Saarinen L: Antibody responses to 4 *Haemophilus influenzae* type b conjugate vaccines, 223 (Fe)
Keating JP, Schears GJ, Dodge PR: Oral water intoxication in infants: an American epidemic, 985 (Se)
Kela E see Käyhty H
Kennedy WA see Mertsola J
Kennedy WA, Hoyt MJ, McCracken GH Jr: Role of corticosteroid therapy in children with pneumococcal meningitis, 1374 (De)
Kerner JA Jr see Gonzalez-Heydrich J
Kershisnik MM, Craven CM, Jung AL, Carey JC, Knisely AS: Osteochondrodysplasia in Fryns syndrome, 656 (Je)
Kessen W see Nelson EW
Kestelyn P see Lepage P
Kharasch SJ, Glotzer D, Vinci R, Weitzman M, Sargent J: Unsuspected cocaine exposure in young children, 204 (Fe)
Khoury MJ see Mili F
Kidd L see Pearson GD
Kilbride HW see Downing GJ
Kim KS see Wong VK
Kimura M, Kuno-Sakai H, Sato Y, Kamiya H, Nii R, Isomura S, Horiuchi K, Kato T, Deguchi M, Saikusa H, Mortimer EA Jr, Cherry JD: Comparative trial of the reactogenicity and immunogenicity of Takeda acellular pertussis vaccine combined with tetanus and diphtheria toxoids: outcome in 3- to 8-month old infants, 9- to 23-month-old infants and children, and 24- to 30-month-old children, 734 (Jy)
Kini N see Bonadio WA
Kinney J, Mundorf L, Gleason C, Lee C, Townsend T, Thibault R, Nussbaum A, Abby H, Yolken R: Efficacy and pharmacokinetics of intravenous immune globulin administration to high-risk neonates, 1233 (No)
Kirby WC see Bilello JF
Kirschner BS: Health care for uninsured and underinsured children (letter) 1085 (Oc)
Kleemola M see Nohynek H
Kleinman JC, Fingerhut LA, Prager K: Differences in infant mortality by race, nativity status, and other maternal characteristics, 194 (Fe)
Kletzel M, Beck S, Elser J, Shock N, Burks W: Trimethoprim-sulfamethoxazole oral desensitization in hemophiliacs infected with human immunodeficiency virus with a history of hypersensitivity reactions, 1428 (De)
Klinger B see Laron Z
Knazik SR see Rosenberg NM
Knisely AS see Faye-Petersen OM; Kershisnik MM
Koch R see Azen CG
Kohl S: Challenge of care for the poor child: the research agenda, 542 (My)
Kohn G see Shamir R
Kooh SW, Binet A: Partial hypoparathyroidism: a variant of transient congenital hypoparathyroidism, 877 (Au)
Korsch BM see Serwint JR
Koslap-Petraco M see Fikar CR
Kozinetz CA: Sexual maturation and blood pressure levels of a biracial sample of girls, 142 (Fe)
Kozlowski K, Glasson M: Thorn-induced pseudotumor of the tibia, 1159 (Oc)
Kraemer HC see Hammer LD
Kraus DM, Calligaro ILS, Hatoum HT: Multilevel model to assess appropriateness of pediatric serum drug concentrations, 1171 (Oc)
Krause W see Azen CG
Kruger R see Hart MH
Krugman RD: Child abuse and neglect: critical first steps in response to a national emergency: the report of the US Advisory Board on Child Abuse and Neglect, 513 (My)
Kumar A see Jaimovich DG
Kuno-Sakai H see Kimura M
Kurczynski TW see Tayel S

L

Lacaille F see Smith LJ
Lacroix J see Furfaro S
Lafleur L see Furfaro S
Lahat E see Eshel G
Laine E see Nohynek H
Lamarre A see Smith LJ
Lampe R see Weiss JC
Lampert D see Black SB
Landau H see Sharav T
Landers S see Freed GL
Landers S, Moise AA, Fraley JK, Smith EOB, Baker CJ: Factors associated with umbilical catheter-related sepsis in neonates, 675 (Je)
Landi TM see Specker BL
Lane BA see Gutman LT
Laor A see Seidman DS
Laron Z see Garty B-Z
Laron Z, Klinger B, Grunebaum M: Laron-type dwarfism, 473 (Ap)
Larson CS see Behrman RE
Lascari AD: Improvement of leukemic hyperleukocytosis with only fluid and allopurinol therapy (letter) 969 (Se)
Lautala P, Uhari M: Epidemic nephropathy in children, 1181 (Oc)
Lawton EL see Lohr JA
Le Deist F see Blanche S
Leake RD see Padilla G
Lebenthal E see Reif S
Leclerc F, Hue V, Martinot A, Delepoulle F: Scoring systems for accurate prognosis of patients with meningococcal infections (letter) 1090 (Oc)
Lee C see Kinney J
Lee MB see Hennes HM
Lee PDK see Wilson DM
Leinonen M see Nohynek H
Lennon VA see Glass JB
Lepage G see Smith LJ
Lepage P, Van de Perre P, Van Vliet G, Nsengumuremyi F, Van Goethem C, Kestelyn P, Msellati P, Hitimana D-G: Clinical and endocrinologic manifestations in perinatally human immunodeficiency virus type 1-infected children aged 5 years or older, 1248 (No)
Letson GW see Davidson M
Leung AKC see Robson WLM
Levine H see Allen HD
Levine M see Tayel S
Leviton A see Nelson KB
Levy GJ see Blanchette VS
Lewy JE: Jack Metcoff festschrift, 851 (Au)
Li S see Saavedra JM
Linder J see Hart MH
Ling E see Rotschild A
Linn LS see Opala G
Linn S see Rudolf MCJ
Lippe BM see Englund AT

Little B, Gilstrap LC III, Snell LM, Rosenfeld CR: Fetal alcohol syndrome: misplaced emphasis (letter) 721 (Jy)
Livni E see Garty B-Z
Loening-Baucke V: Lichen sclerosus et atrophicus in children, 1058 (Se)
Lohr JA, Ingram DL, Dudley SM, Lawton EL, Donowitz LG: Hand washing in pediatric ambulatory settings: an inconsistent practice, 1198 (Oc)
Lokietz H: Diphtheria and tetanus toxoids and pertussis vaccine litigation (letter) 425 (Ap)
Loughead JL, Mimouni F, Schilling S: Lowe's syndrome, 113 (Ja)
Luban NLC see Blanchette VS
Lubicky JP: Thumb-sucking (letter) 845 (Au)
Luchi JM, Bennett FC, Jackson JC: Predictors of neurodevelopmental outcome following bronchopulmonary dysplasia, 813 (Jy)
Lucky AW see Reynolds RD
Lui K, Bryson SM, Irwin DB, Costello S: Evaluation of Bayesian forecasting for individualized gentamicin dosage in infants weighing 1000 g or less, 463 (Ap)
Lynch TP: Vaccine myth and physician handouts (letter) 426 (Ap)

M

Mabry CC: Status report on phenylketonuria treatment: 1990, 33 (Ja)
MacDonald DI: Parental alcoholism: a neglected pediatric responsibility, 609 (Je)
Machi J see Bonadio WA
Macy C see Cohen GR
Madagame E see Bonadio WA
Madore DV see Rothstein EP
Mah MP, Fain JS, Hall SL: Intravenous hyperalimentation fluid obtained with lumbar puncture: an unusual complication of a central venous catheter, 1439 (De)
Mahieu LM, Van Acker KJ: Mediterranean visceral leishmaniasis: a frequently unrecognized imported disease (letter) 1225 (No)
Marcus R see Wilson DM
Margileth AM see Carithers HA
Markin RS see Hart MH
Marro PJ, Dransfield DA, Mott SH, Allan WC: Posthemorrhagic hydrocephalus: use of an intravenous-type catheter for cerebrospinal fluid drainage, 1141 (Oc)
Marshall GS see Ponder D
Martinot A see Leclerc F
Mason MH see Udow M
Matalon R see Azen CG
Mathews S see Furfaro S
Maurer HM: Growing neglect of American children, 540 (My)
Mayer JE Jr: Development, growth, and cardiac surgery, 33 (Ja)
Maynard EC see Zuckerman B
Maynard EC, Amoruso LP, Oh W: Meconium for drug testing, 650 (Je)
McAnarney E: Complex problem: complex solutions, 429 (Ap)
McAneney CM see Avner JR
McCabe E see Azen CG
McCaffrey FM, Braden DS, Strong WB: Sudden cardiac death in young athletes: a review, 177 (Fe)
McCarthy PL see Nelson EW
McClearn AB see Mili F
McColley SA, Rosenstein BJ, Cutting GR: Differences in expression of cystic fibrosis in blacks and whites, 94 (Ja)
McCormick DP see Niebuhr VN
McCracken GH Jr see Kennedy WA; Mertsola J
McDonald EM see Duggan AK
McDonald RW see Reller MD
McIntyre FL: Family physicians and neonatology (letter) 963 (Se)
McIntyre L see Schwersenski J
McKinney RE Jr see Gutman LT
McManus MA see Newacheck PW
McNamara JG see Katz BZ
Meert KL see Rosenberg NM
Melchionni JB see Charney EB
Mellins ED see Sherry DD
Melzer-Lange M, Wyatt D, Walsh-Kelly C, Smith D, Hegenbarth MA, Eisenberg CSL: Improved speed and accuracy of calculations with a programmable calculator in pediatric emergency scenarios, 264 (Mr)
Mendoza JC, Wilkerson SA, Reese AH: Follow-up of patients who underwent arterial switch repair for transposition of the great arteries, 40 (Ja)
Mengarda G see Radetti G
Mertsola J, Kennedy WA, Waagner D, Sáez-Llorens X, Olsen K, Hansen EJ, McCracken GH Jr: Endotoxin concentrations in cerebrospinal fluid correlate with clinical severity and neurologic outcome of *Haemophilus influenzae* type b meningitis, 1099 (Oc)
Metzker A see Shamir R
Meyer BA see Cohen GR
Meyer CM III see Holloway MK
Mikrut W see Bee DE
Mili F, Edmonds LD, Khoury MJ, McClearn AB: Prevalence of birth defects among low-birth-weight infants: a population study, 1313 (No)
Miller LA see Garcia CD
Miller ML, White PH: Challenge of caring for indigent children with rheumatologic diseases, 554 (My)
Miller RM see Serwint JR
Mimouni F see Loughead JL
Moise AA see Landers S
Monteleone JA: Child sexual abuse and human immunodeficiency virus transmission (letter) 847 (Au)
Moodie DS see Garcia RE
Moore EC, Cohen F, Farooki Z, Chang C-H: Focal scleroderma and severe cardiomyopathy: patient report and brief review, 229 (Fe)
Moore JW see Bilello JF
Moore R see Duggan AK
Morelli JG, Tan OT, Weston WL: Treatment of ulcerated hemangiomas with pulsed tunable dye laser, 1062 (Se)
Moriette G see Ajuriaguerra M de
Morley DS see Needlman R
Morris AH see Wilson DM
Morrow J see Accardo PJ
Mortimer EA Jr see Kimura M
Mota-Hernández F, Bross-Soriano D, Pérez-Ricardez ML, Velásquez-Jones L: Rice solution and World Health Organization solution by gastric infusion for high stool output diarrhea, 937 (Au)
Mott SH see Marro PJ
Msall ME see DiGaudio KM
Msellati P see Lepage P
Mullins C see Allen HD
Mundorf L see Kinney J
Murphy SP see Carzoli RP
Musante L see Treiber FA
Muto G see Volta C
Myer CM III, Grosso J: Gilding the lily (letter) 849 (Au)

N

Nadeau D see Furfaro S
Nagel RA see Englund AT
Nair P see Johnson JP
Needlman R, Fried LE, Morley DS, Taylor S, Zuckerman B: Clinic-based intervention to promote literacy: a pilot study, 881 (Au)
Neill CA see Pearson GD
Nelson DB see Esterly NB
Nelson EW, Van Cleve S, Swartz MK, Kessen W, McCarthy PL: Improving the use of early follow-up care after emergency department visits: a randomized trial, 440 (Ap)
Nelson JD see Severien C
Nelson KB, Leviton A: How much of neonatal encephalopathy is due to birth asphyxia?, 1325 (No)
Nelson WE: Regional pediatric approach to the epidemic of social ills within our cities, 505 (My)
Newacheck PW, McManus MA, Fox HB: Prevalence and impact of chronic illness among adolescents, 1367 (De)
Newman J: Formula companies and the medical profession (letter) 1089 (Oc)
Newman TB, Browner WS: Multiple comparisons and *P* values (letter) 250 (Mr)
Newman TB, Hope S, Stevenson DK: Direct bilirubin measurements in jaundiced term newborns: a reevaluation, 1305 (No)
Newton C see Secord E
Niebuhr VN, McCormick DP, Barnett SE: School health training during pediatric residency, 79 (Ja)
Niemeyer JG see Gutman LT
Nii R see Kimura M
Niimi K see Hanna JD
Nitzan M see Garty B-Z
Nohynek H, Eskola J, Laine E, Halonen P, Ruutu P, Saikku P, Kleemola M, Leinonen M: Causes of hospital-treated acute lower respiratory tract infection in children, 618 (Je)
Norgard MV see Sánchez PJ
Nouri S see Balfour IC
Nsengumuremyi F see Lepage P
Nussbaum A see Kinney J
Nussbaum MP see Arden MR

O

O'Connor DW see Sulkes SB
O'Flynn M see Azen CG
O'Hair KC see Bilello JF
O'Halloran MJ: Clavicular fractures in neonates: frequency vs significance (letter) 251 (Mr)
O'Kell R see Cohen GR
Oh W see Maynard EC
Olin P see Blackwelder WC
Olsen K see Mertsola J
Opala G, Winter S, Vance C, Vance H, Hutchison HT, Linn LS: Effect of valproic acid on plasma carnitine levels, 999 (Se)

P

Padilla G, Ervin MG, Ross MG, Leake RD: Vasopressin levels in infants during the course of aseptic and bacterial meningitis, 991 (Se)
Pallansch MA see Ing DJ
Parcel GS see Sugerman ST
Pariente D see Gottrand F
Park JW see Carter G
Park-Moore B see Thilo EH
Parker RM, Rescorla LA, Finkelstein JA, Barnes N, Holmes JH, Stolley PD: Survey of the health of homeless children in Philadelphia shelters, 520 (My)
Pasterkamp H see Tal A
Patterson K see van Hoff J
Pattishall EG III see Greenberg LW
Payne CM see Tarantino MD
Pearl W: Sudden cardiac death (letter) 1223 (No)
Pearson GD, Kidd L, Beittel TM, Neill CA: Cardiac care for infants: determinants of hospital charges for acute care, 1397 (De)
Pearson SJ: Health care for uninsured and underinsured children (letter)1085 (Oc)
Peltola H see Käyhty H
Pendergrast RA see DuRant RH
Pennington DG see Balfour IC
Pérez-Ricardez ML see Mota-Hernández F
Perri G see Saggese G
Perrin JM: Adolescents with chronic illness, 1361 (De)
Peter JB see Ruderman JW
Peterson B see Wilson NW
Peterson R see Azen CG
Phang MS see Rotschild A
Piatt JP, Bartley DL, Jacobson AD, Rimsza ME: Practice management training for pediatric residents, 299 (Mr)
Pidcock FS: Child welfare: the phantom of the health care system (letter)843 (Au)
Pigott JD: Evolution of surgical treatment for congenital cardiac disease, 1362 (De)
Pines RJ see Friedman DE
Pinsky PF see Gunn WJ
Pittard WB III, Geddes KM, Hulsey TC, Hollis BW: How much vitamin D for neonates?, 1147 (Oc)
Pittschieler K see Radetti G
Plides RS see Cuevas L
Poets CF, Stebbens VA, Alexander JR, Southall DP: Breathing patterns and heart rates at ages 6 weeks and 2 years, 1393 (De)
Pollack MM see Fields AI
Ponder D, Marshall GS, Rabalais GP: Visceral larva migrans, 699 (Je)
Porter B see Goldstein E
Prager K see Kleinman JC
Prose NS see Gutman LT
Pruitt AW: Losing time, 607 (Je)
Puterman ML see Rotschild A

Q

Quagliata R see Wong VK
Quarmby VE see Wilson DM

R

Rabalais GP see Ponder D
Radetti G, Rizza F, Mengarda G, Pittschieler K: Adipsic hypernatremia in 2 sisters, 321 (Mr)
Radvanyi-Bouvet M-F see Ajuriaguerra M de
Ranco N see Smith LJ
Rappaport L see Bowen J
Rassin DK see Bee DE
Rathore MH, Friedman AD, Barton LL, Dunkle LM: Herpes zoster oticus (letter) 722 (Jy)
Rawlings DJ see Burchfield DJ
Rawstron SA, Bromberg K: Comparison of maternal and infant serologic tests for syphilis, 1383 (De)
Reese AH see Mendoza JC
Regelmann WE see Glass JB
Reif S, Sloven DG, Lebenthal E: Gallstones in children: characterization by age, etiology, and outcome, 105 (Ja)
Reiter EO see Wilson DM
Reller MD, Buffkin DC, Colasurdo MA, Rice MJ, McDonald RW: Ductal patency in neonates with respiratory distress syndrome: a randomized surfactant trial, 1017 (Se)
Rescorla LA see Parker RM
Resnick M see Story M
Retsky J, Jaffe D, Christoffel K: Skateboarding injuries in children: a second wave, 188 (Fe)
Rettig KR see Bhowmick SK
Reynolds RD, Boiko S, Lucky AW: Exacerbation of tinea corporis during treatment with 1% clotrimazole/0.05% betamethasone diproprionate (Lotrisone)(letter) 1224 (No)
Ricci LR: Photographing the physically abused child, principles and practice, 275 (Mr)
Rice MJ see Reller MD
Richardson CJ see Bee DE
Ridgway D, Wolff LJ, Deforest A: Immunization response varies with intensity of acute lymphoblastic leukemia therapy, 887 (Au)
Rifai N, Iosefsohn M, Hicks JM: Cholesterol testing in the physician's office: accuracy assessment (letter) 1087 (Oc)
Rimm AA see Hennes HM
Rimsza ME see Piatt JP
Ritter PL see Hammer LD

Rizza F see Radetti G
Roberts RL, Szelc CM, Scates SM, Boyd MT, Soderstrom KM, Davis MW, Glaspy JA: Neutropenia in an extremely premature infant treated with recombinant human granulocyte colony-stimulating factor, 808 (Jy)
Robinson B see Johnson JP
Robson WLM, Leung AKC: Association of alkaline urine with eating disorders (letter) 1091 (Oc)
Rogers C see Scott SM
Rogers MF see Bennett JV
Rogers WB: How much iron is enough? (letter) 598 (Je)
Rollins CJ: Parenteral nutrition in infants and children: basic principles and practical guidelines, 1025 (Se)
Roman J Jr: More on a myth (letter) 717 (Jy)
Rönnberg P-R see Käyhty H
Roscelli JD: 'H' in hemorrhagic shock and encephalopathy syndrome (letter) 720 (Jy)
Rosenberg NM, Meert KL, Knazik SR, Yee H, Kauffman RE: Occult cocaine exposure in children, 1430 (De)
Rosenblatt A see Fields AI
Rosenfeld CR see Little B
Rosenfeld RG see Wilson DM
Rosenfeld W see Joseph PR
Rosenstein BJ see McColley SA
Rosenwinkel K see Story M
Ross MG see Padilla G
Rothstein EP, Schiller RP, Girone JAC, Hipp TJ, Souder RL, Bernstein HH, Madore DV, Johnson CL, Smith DH: Response of 7- to 15-month-old infants to sequential immunization with *Haemophilus influenzae* type b-CRM_{197}conjugate and polysaccharide vaccines, 898 (Au)
Rotschild A, Chitayat D, Puterman ML, Phang MS, Ling E, Baldwin V: Optimal positioning of endotracheal tubes for ventilation of preterm infants, 1007 (Se)
Rouse B see Azen CG
Rouzioux C see Blanche S
Rowland TW: Effects of obesity on aerobic fitness in adolescent females, 764 (Jy)
Roy CC see Smith LJ
Rubenstein JS see Winter RJ
Rubinstein A see Schwartz LJ
Ruderman JW, Barka N, Peter JB, Stiehm ER: Antibody response to MMR vaccination in children who received IVIG as neonates (letter) 425 (Ap)
Rudolf MCJ, Zadik Z, Linn S, Hochberg Z: Seasonal variation in growth during growth hormone therapy, 769 (Jy)
Ruff ME, Southgate WM: Neonatal appendicitis with perforation, 111 (Ja)
Rutstein RM: Predicting risk of *Pneumocystis carinii* pneumonia in human immunodeficiency virus-infected children, 922 (Au)
Ruuskanen O see Heikkinen T
Ruutu P see Nohynek H
Ryals BD: Major congenital neurologic malformations (letter) 30 (Ja)

S

Saarinen L see Käyhty H
Saavedra JM, Harris GD, Li S, Finberg L: Capillary refilling (skin turgor) in the assessment of dehydration, 296 (Mr)
Sacks JJ see Gunn WJ
Saenger P see Schwartz LJ
Sáez-Llorens X see Mertsola J
Saggese G, Bertelloni S, Baroncelli GI, Perri G, Calderazzi A: Mineral metabolism and calcitriol therapy in idiopathic juvenile osteoporosis, 457 (Ap)
Saikku P see Nohynek H
Saikusa H see Kimura M
Sanchez I see Tal A
Sánchez PJ, Wendel GD, Norgard MV: Congenital syphilis associated with negative results of maternal serologic tests at delivery (letter) 967 (Se)
Sandstead HH: Zinc deficiency: a public health problem?, 853 (Au)
Sargent J see Kharasch SJ
Sato Y see Kimura M
Saunders BS see Schatz M
Scates SM see Roberts RL
Schaeffer AV, Ditchek S: Current social practices leading to water intoxication in infants (letter) 27 (Ja)
Schanler RJ see Freed GL
Schatz M, Zeiger RS, Hoffman CP, Saunders BS, Harden KM, Forsythe AB: Increased transient tachypnea of the newborn in infants with asthmatic mothers, 156 (Fe)
Schears GJ see Keating JP
Schiller RP see Rothstein EP
Schilling S see Loughead JL
Schink JC: Nintendo enuresis (letter) 1094 (Oc)
Schmitt B: Clinic attending: teaching strategies for patient encounters, 977 (Se)
Schneider JR, Fischer H: Acrodermatitis enteropathica, 211 (Fe)
Schocken DM see DeClue TJ
Schonberger LB see Gunn WJ
Schoumacher RA: Saving money with home care, 725 (Jy)
Schuetz S see Ward SLD
Schwartz LJ, St Louis Y, Wu R, Wiznia A, Rubinstein A, Saenger P: Endocrine function in children with human immunodeficiency virus infection, 330 (Ja)
Schwartz RH see Farrow JA
Schwartz RH: Legalization of drugs of abuse and the pediatrician, 1153 (Oc)
Schwersenski J, McIntyre L, Bauer CR: Lumbar puncture frequency and cerebrospinal fluid analysis in the neonate, 54 (Ja)
Scott CR see Azen CG
Scott SM, Rogers C, Angelus P, Backstrom C: Effect of necrotizing enterocolitis on urinary epidermal growth factor levels, 804 (Jy); correction, 982 (Se)
Seashore CN see Doughty RA
Secord E, Claude S, Newton C: War souvenir poisoning (letter) 724 (Jy)
Segal KR, Dietz WH: Physiologic responses to playing a video game, 1034 (Se)
Sehgal S see Ward SLD
Seidman DS, Laor A, Gale R, Stevenson DK, Danon YL: Longitudinal study of birth weight and being overweight in late adolescence, 782 (Jy)
Selbst SM see Tesoro LJ
Serdula MK see Gallaher MM
Serwint JR, Miller RM, Korsch BM: Influenza type A and B infections in hospitalized pediatric patients: who should be immunized?, 623 (Je)
Severien C, Nelson JD: Frequency of infections associated with implanted systems vs cuffed, tunneled silastic venous catheters in patients with acute leukemia, 1433 (De)
Seymore C see DuRant RH
Shamir R, Kohn G, Metzker A: Nevus flammeus: discordance in monozygotic twins, 85 (Ja)
Shapiro DL see Hennes HM
Shapiro ED see Forsyth BW
Sharav T, Landau H, Zadik Z, Einarson TR: Age-related patterns of thyroid-stimulating hormone response to thyrotropin-releasing hormone stimulation in Down syndrome, 172 (Fe)
Shaw KN, Bell LM, Sherman NH: Outpatient assessment of infants with bronchiolitis, 151 (Fe)
Shea D see Greenberg LW
Shea S see Starc TJ
Shelley M see Friedman DE
Shenker IR see Arden MR
Sher PK see Glass JB
Sherman NH see Shaw KN
Sherry DD, Mellins ED, Wedgwood RJ: Decreasing severity of chronic uveitis in children with pauciarticular arthritis, 1026 (Se)
Shinefield HR see Black SB
Shock N see Kletzel M
Sievert AJ see Ing DJ
Sigman B see Azen CG
Silberbach GM see Friedman DE
Simonetti M see Ing DJ
Simpson P see Bolognia JL
Singer LP see Conway EE Jr
Slopis JM see Dominguez R
Sloven DG see Reif S
Smith D see Melzer-Lange M
Smith DH see Rothstein EP
Smith DS see Bonadio WA
Smith EOB see Landers S
Smith LJ, Lacaille F, Lepage G, Ranco N, Lamarre A, Roy CC: Taurine decreases fecal fatty acid and sterol excretion in cystic fibrosis: a randomized double-blind trial, 1401 (De)
Smith RE see Strong WB
Smith VK see Udow M
Smoyer WE: Medical management of postobstructive polyuria (letter) 1345 (De)
Snell LM see Little B
Snider AR see Allen HD
Soderstrom KM see Roberts RL
Souder RL see Rothstein EP
Southall DP see Poets CF
Southgate WM see Ruff ME
Spaggiari R see Volta C
Specker BL, Tsang RC, Ho ML, Landi TM, Gratton TL: Low serum calcium and high parathyroid hormone levels in neonates fed 'humanized' cow's milk-based formula, 941 (Au)
St Claire K see Gutman LT
St Claire KK see Gutman LT
St Louis Y see Schwartz LJ
Stahlman MT: Improving health care provision to neonates in the United States, 510 (My)
Staiano A, Clouse RE: Value of subject height in predicting lower esophageal sphincter location, 1424 (De)
Staiano A, Corazziari E, Andreotti M-R, Clouse RE: Esophageal motility in children with Hirschsprung's disease, 310 (Mr)
Stanitski CL see Strong WB
Stapleton FB see Daigler GE; Garcia CD
Starc TJ, Belamarich PF, Shea S, Dobrin-Seckler BE, Dell RB, Gersony WM, Deckelbaum RJ: Family history fails to identify many children with severe hypercholesterolemia, 61 (Ja)
Starfield B see Allen HD
Stebbens VA see Poets CF
Steiner H see Gonzalez-Heydrich J
Stephenson CA see Allison JW
Stevenson DK see Newman TB; Seidman DS
Stiehm ER see Horner AA; Ruderman JW
Stiehm ER: Your child's best friend: TV or not TV, 257 (Mr)
Your child's best friend: TV or not TV? (letter) 963 (Se)
Stockman JA III see Winter RJ
Stoddard JJ, Deshpande JK: Acute glossitis and bacteremia caused by *Streptococcus pneumoniae*: case report and review (letter) 598 (Je)
Stokes EJ see Duggan AK
Stolley PD see Parker RM
Storsaeter J see Blackwelder WC
Story M, Rosenwinkel K, Himes JH, Resnick M, Harris LJ, Blum RW: Demographic and risk factors associated with chronic dieting in adolescents, 994 (Se)
Strain JE: American Academy of Pediatrics response to the growing health needs of children, 536 (My)
Strauss RG see Blanchette VS
Strauss RG: Transfusion therapy in neonates, 904 (Au)
Strong WB see Allen HD; McCaffrey FM; Treiber FA
Strong WB: Grampa, can I get something that I'd like?, 1355 (De)
Strong WB, Stanitski CL, Smith RE, Wilmore JH, eds: Sports medicine, 177 (Fe), 665 (Je), 764 (Jy), 1023 (Se), 1119 (Oc), 1223, 1279 (No)
Sugerman ST, Hergenroeder AC, Chacko MR, Parcel GS: Acquired immunodeficiency syndrome and adolescents: knowledge, attitudes, and behaviors of runaway and homeless youths, 431 (Ap)
Sulkes SB, O'Connor DW: Lead poisoning in children with developmental disabilities (letter) 602 (Je)
Swartz MK see Nelson EW
Szelc CM see Roberts RL
Szonyi H: Send Linus to me (letter) 1227 (No)

T

Tal A, Sanchez I, Pasterkamp H: Respirosonography in infants with acute bronchiolitis, 1405 (De)
Tan OT see Morelli JG
Tanji JL: Tracking of elevated blood pressure values in adolescent athletes at 1-year follow-up, 665 (Je)
Tarantino MD, Corrigan JJ Jr, Glasser L, Payne CM, Jeter MA: Variant form of thrombasthenia, 1053 (Se)
Tardieu M see Blanche S
Tarvin C see Carter G
Taubert KA see Allen HD
Tayel S, Kurczynski TW, Levine M, Brookfield E, Ehrlich R, Hennessy JR, DeBeukelaer MM: Marfanoid children: etiologic heterogeneity and cardiac findings, 90 (Ja)
Taylor S see Needlman R
Tenenbein M, Yatscoff RW: Total iron-binding capacity in iron poisoning: is it useful?, 437 (Ap)
Terndrup TE, Wong A: Influence of otitis media on the correlation between rectal and auditory canal temperatures, 75 (Ja)
Tesoro LJ, Selbst SM: Factors affecting outcome in meningococcal infections, 218 (Fe)
Theriot R see White BD
Thibault R see Kinney J
Thilo EH, Park-Moore B, Berman ER, Carson BS: Oxygen saturation by pulse oximetry in healthy infants at an altitude of 1610 m (5280 ft): what is normal?, 1137 (Oc)
Thomas S see Braunstein H
Thorp J see Cohen GR
Todd DJ: Gallstones in children (letter) 971 (Se)
Tolmas HC: Adolescent pelvic examination: an effective practical approach, 1269 (No)
Tomassoni TL, Galioto FM Jr, Vaccaro P: Cardiopulmonary exercise testing in children following surgery for tetralogy of Fallot, 1290 (No)
Tomazic T see Accardo PJ
Townsend T see Kinney J
Treiber FA, Strong WB, Arensman FW, Forrest T, Davis H, Musante L: Family history of myocardial infarction and hemodynamic responses to exercise in young black boys, 1029 (Se)
Tsang RC see Specker BL
Tully SB see Greenberg LW
Tunnessen WW Jr: Henoch-Schönlein Purpura, 823 (Jy)
Juvenile dermatomyositis, 1161 (Oc)
Pityriasis rosea, 1441 (De)
Tunnessen WW Jr, ed: Picture of the month, 473 (Ap), 701 (Je), 823 (Jy), 1047 (Se), 1161 (Oc), 1301 (No), 1441 (De)

U

Udow M, Smith VK, Mason MH: Caring program for children: the Michigan experience, 579 (My)
Uhari M see Lautala P
Unti SM see Winter RJ

V

Vaccaro P see Tomassoni TL
Valdez RB see Wood D
Valle D see Azen CG
Van Acker KJ see Mahieu LM
Van Cleve S see Nelson EW

Van de Perre P see Lepage P
Van Dyke RB: Pediatric human immunodeficiency virus infection and the acquired immunodeficiency syndrome: a health care crisis of children and families, 529 (My)
Van Goethem C see Lepage P
van Hoff J, Hockenberry-Eaton MJ, Patterson K, Hutter JJ: Survey of antiemetic use in children with cancer, 773 (Jy)
Van Vliet G see Lepage P
Vance C see Opala G
Vance H see Opala G
Vanderhoof JA see Hart MH
Vanderleeuw J see Farrow JA
Velásquez-Jones L see Mota-Hernández F
Venkataraman PS, Duke JC: Bone mineral content of healthy, full-term neonates: effect of race, gender, and maternal cigarette smoking, 1310 (No)
Vera LA, Zaeri N, Hurt H: Subcutaneous fat necrosis of the newborn, 1047 (Se)
Villani MA see Wells JJ
Vinci R see Kharasch SJ
Vink PE see Johnson JP
Virdis R see Volta C
Viscoli CM see Forsyth BW
Volta C, Ghizzoni L, Muto G, Spaggiari R, Virdis R, Bernasconi S: Effectiveness of growth-promoting therapies: comparison among growth hormone, clonidine, and levodopa, 168 (Fe)
Voulalas D see Handelsman E

W

Waagner D see Mertsola J
Wachsman L see Ward SLD
Wald ER, Dashefsky B: Cautionary note on the use of empiric ceftriaxone for suspected bacteremia, 1359 (De)
Waller KS, Johnson J: Cavitary pneumonia due to *Arcanobacterium hemolyticum*, 209 (Fe)
Walsh-Kelly C see Melzer-Lange M
Warburton D see Ward SLD
Ward JI see Davidson M
Ward SLD, Schuetz S, Wachsman L, Bean XD, Bautista D, Buckley S, Sehgal S, Warburton D: Elevated plasma norepinephrine levels in infants of substance-abusing mothers, 44 (Ja)
Waris M see Heikkinen T
Warner R see Azen CG
Washington R see Allen HD
Wason S see Holloway MK
Wedgwood RJ see Sherry DD
Weedy C see Gutman LT
Weiss JC, Doughty RA, Lampe R: Pediatric program director: an analysis of the role and its problems, 449 (Ap)
Weitzman M see Kharasch SJ
Welch R see Byrne P
Welliver RC see Daigler GE
Wells JJ, Villani MA: Parental drinking habits (letter) 1087 (Oc)
Wendel GD see Sánchez PJ
Weston WL see Morelli JG
White BD, Hickson GB, Theriot R, Zaner RM: Medical ethics issues survey of residents in 5 pediatric training programs, 161 (Fe)
White PH see Miller ML
Whitman BY see Accardo PJ
Wilcox WD see Ing DJ
Wilkerson SA see Mendoza JC
Willging JP see Holloway MK
Williams PD see Doughty RA
Wilmore JH see Strong WB
Wilson DM see Hammer LD
Wilson DM, Lee PDK, Morris AH, Reiter EO, Gertner JM, Marcus R, Quarmby VE, Rosenfeld RG: Growth hormone therapy in hypophosphatemic rickets, 1165 (Oc)
Wilson NW, Gooding A, Peterson B, Bastian JF: Anergy in pediatric head trauma patients, 326 (Mr)
Winkleby MA see Boyce WT
Wintemute GJ, Drake C, Wright M: Immersion events in residential swimming pools: evidence for an experience effect, 1200 (Oc)
Winter RJ, Unti SM, Rubenstein JS, Burg FD, Stockman JA III: Resident, faculty, and residency program development: an integrated approach through annual retreats, 1191 (Oc)
Winter S see Opala G
Wiswell TE: Major congenital neurologic malformations (letter) 30 (Ja)
Wiznia A see Schwartz LJ
Wolff LJ see Ridgway D
Wong A see Terndrup TE
Wong VK, Quagliata R, Adler R, Kim KS: Dose-related immunogenicity of *Haemophilus influenzae* type b capsular polysaccharide—*Neisseria meningitidis* outer membrane protein conjugate vaccine, 742 (Jy)
Wood BP, ed: Radiological case of the month, 111 (Ja), 209 (Fe), 339 (Mr), 471 (Ap), 699 (Je), 821 (Jy), 1045 (Se), 1159 (Oc), 1299 (No), 1439 (De)
Wood D, Valdez RB: Barriers to medical care for homeless families compared with housed poor families, 1109 (Oc)
Woods PA see Ing DJ
Wright JD: Children in and of the streets: health, social policy, and the homeless young, 516 (My)
Wright M see Wintemute GJ
Wu R see Schwartz LJ
Wyatt D see Melzer-Lange M
Wyllie E: Cortical resection for children with epilepsy: perspectives in pediatrics, 314 (Mr)

Y

Yang-Oshida M see Gallaher MM
Yatscoff RW see Tenenbein M
Yeast JD see Cohen GR
Yee H see Rosenberg NM
Yeh TF see Cuevas L
Yolken R see Kinney J

Z

Zadik Z see Rudolf MCJ; Sharav T
Zaeri N see Vera LA
Zaner RM see White BD
Zeiger RS see Schatz M
Ziegler T see Heikkinen T
Zuckerman B see Needlman R
Zuckerman B, Maynard EC, Cabral H: Preliminary report of prenatal cocaine exposure and respiratory distress syndrome in premature infants, 696 (Je)

SUBJECT INDEX TO VOLUME 145

The following index is an alphabetical list of significant subjects presented in this volume. Books reviewed are listed alphabetically by first author under the heading "BOOK REVIEWS." The month is given as a two letter notation in parentheses.

A

Abdomen, Acute
Neonatal appendicitis with perforation [Ruff] 111 (Ja)
Abdominal Pain
Gallstones in children: characterization by age, etiology, and outcome [Reif] 105 (Ja)
Abnormalities
Chronic neutropenia during childhood: a 13-year experience in a single institution [Jonsson] 232 (Fe)
Elevated plasma norepinephrine levels in infants of substance-abusing mothers [Ward] 44 (Ja)
Hypoplastic left upper lobe [Al-Salem] 821 (Jy)
Major congenital neurologic malformations (letter) [Ryals] 30 (Ja)
Markedly immature lecithin-sphingomyelin ratio at term and congenital hypothyroidism (letter) [Cohen] 1227 (No)
Measurement of serum granulocyte colony-stimulating factor in a patient with congenital agranulocytosis (Kostmann's syndrome) [Glasser] 925 (Au)
Minor malformations, hyperactivity, and learning disabilities [Accardo] 1184 (Oc)
Neuroblastoma screening data: an epidemiologic analysis [Goodman] 1415 (De)
Pachyonychia congenita [Cohen] 1301 (No)
Partial hypoparathyroidism: a variant of transient congenital hypoparathyroidism [Kooh] 877 (Au)
Prevalence of birth defects among low-birth-weight infants: a population study [Mili] 1313 (No)
Sudden cardiac death in young athletes: a review [McCaffrey] 177 (Fe)
Tuberous sclerosis with myocardial and central nervous system involvement at birth [Allison] 471 (Ap)
Abnormalities, Drug-Induced
Characteristics of perinatal cocaine-exposed infants with necrotizing enterocolitis (letter) [Downing] 26 (Ja)
Abnormalities, Multiple
Antley-Bixler syndrome [Butler] 701 (Je)
Autosomal recessive lethal infantile cytochrome C oxidase deficiency [Eshel] 661 (Je)
Brain and ocular abnormalities in infants with in utero exposure to cocaine and other street drugs [Dominguez] 688 (Je)
Neural arch stenosis and spinal cord injury in thanatophoric dysplasia [Faye-Petersen] 87 (Ja)
Osteochondrodysplasia in Fryns syndrome [Kershisnik] 656 (Je)
Abortion
Challenge of care for the poor and underserved in the United States: an American College of Obstetricians and Gynecologists perspective on access to care for underserved women [Davidson] 546 (My)
Improving health care provision to neonates in the United States [Stahlman] 510 (My)
Abscess
Exacerbation of tinea corporis during treatment with 1% clotrimazole/0.05% betamethasone diproprionate (Lotrisone) (letter) [Reynolds] 1224 (No)
Gilding the lily (letter) [Faigel] (reply) [Myer] 849 (Au)
Absenteeism
Prevalence and impact of chronic illness among adolescents [Newacheck] 1367 (De)
Accident Prevention
Immersion events in residential swimming pools: evidence for an experience effect [Wintemute] 1200 (Oc)
Skateboarding injuries in children: a second wave [Retsky] 188 (Fe)
Use of infant walkers [AMA Board of Trustees] 933 (Au)
Accidental Falls
Use of infant walkers [AMA Board of Trustees] 933 (Au)
Accidents
Immersion events in residential swimming pools: evidence for an experience effect [Wintemute] 1200 (Oc)
War souvenir poisoning (letter) [Secord] 724 (Jy)
Accidents, Home
Injuries and poisonings in out-of-home child care and home care [Gunn] 779 (Jy)
Acetylcholine Receptors see Receptors, Cholinergic
Achalasia, Esophageal see Esophageal Achalasia
Achievement
Intellectual development in 12-year-old children treated for phenylketonuria [Azen] 35 (Ja)
Women in medicine: fantasies, dreams, myths, and realities [DeAngelis] 49 (Ja)
Achromobacter see Alcaligenes
Acidosis
Acquired methemoglobinemia: the relationship of cause to course of illness [Avner] 144:1229 (No); correction, **145:**158 (Fe)
Acidosis, Diabetic
Improved speed and accuracy of calculations with a programmable calculator in pediatric emergency scenarios [Melzer-Lange] 264 (Mr)
Acquired Immunodeficiency Syndrome
Acquired immunodeficiency syndrome and adolescents: knowledge, attitudes, and behaviors of runaway and homeless youths [Sugerman] 431 (Ap)
Child survival and perinatal infections with human immunodeficiency virus [Bennett] 1242 (No)
Pediatric acquired immunodeficiency syndrome, poverty, and national priorities [Heagarty] 527 (My)
Pediatric human immunodeficiency virus infection and the acquired immunodeficiency syndrome: a health care crisis of children and families [Van Dyke] 529 (My)
Acrodermatitis
Acrodermatitis enteropathica [Schneider] 211 (Fe)
Activities of Daily Living
Adolescents with chronic illness [Perrin] 1361 (De)
Prevalence and impact of chronic illness among adolescents [Newacheck] 1367 (De)
Adenosine Triphosphate
Variant form of thrombasthenia [Tarantino] 1053 (Se)
Adenovirus Infections
Causes of hospital-treated acute lower respiratory tract infection in children [Nohynek] 618 (Je)

Adipose Tissue
Effects of obesity on aerobic fitness in adolescent females [Rowland] 764 (Jy)
Administration, Oral
Trimethoprim-sulfamethoxazole oral desensitization in hemophiliacs infected with human immunodeficiency virus with a history of hypersensitivity reactions [Kletzel] 1428 (De)
Administration, Topical
Exacerbation of tinea corporis during treatment with 1% clotrimazole/0.05% betamethasone diproprionate (Lotrisone) (letter) [Reynolds] 1224 (No)
Impetigo [Esterly] 125 (Fe)
Administrative Personnel
Chief resident training: developing leadership skills for future medical leaders [Doughty] 639 (Je)
Pediatric program director: an analysis of the role and its problems [Weiss] 449 (Ap)
Women in medicine: fantasies, dreams, myths, and realities [DeAngelis] 49 (Ja)
Administrators see Administrative Personnel
Adolescence
Adolescent pelvic examination: an effective practical approach [Tolmas] 1269 (No)
Adolescents with chronic illness [Perrin] 1361 (De)
Alkaline urine is associated with eating disorders (letter) [Arden] 28 (Ja)
Children in and of the streets: health, social policy, and the homeless young [Wright] 516 (My)
Dietary calcium and bone mineral status of children and adolescents [Chan] 631 (Je)
Effects of obesity on aerobic fitness in adolescent females [Rowland] 764 (Jy)
Far from the ideal: the plight of poor children in the United States [Fulginiti] 489 (My)
Health care for uninsured and underinsured children (letter) [Kirschner] 1085 (Oc)
Longitudinal study of birth weight and being overweight in late adolescence [Seidman] 782 (Jy)
New initiatives in adolescent health promotion [Elster] 495 (My)
Prevalence and impact of chronic illness among adolescents [Newacheck] 1367 (De)
Sexual maturation and blood pressure levels of a biracial sample of girls [Kozinetz] 142 (Fe)
Standardized percentile curves of body-mass index for children and adolescents [Hammer] 259 (Mr)
Sudden cardiac death in young athletes: a review [McCaffrey] 177 (Fe)
Tracking of elevated blood pressure values in adolescent athletes at 1-year follow-up [Tanji] 665 (Je)
Zinc deficiency: a public health problem? [Sandstead] 853 (Au)
Adolescent Behavior
Acquired immunodeficiency syndrome and adolescents: knowledge, attitudes, and behaviors of runaway and homeless youths [Sugerman] 431 (Ap)
Adolescents with chronic illness [Perrin] 1361 (De)
Adolescents' attrition from school-sponsored sports [DuRant] 1119 (Oc)
Complex problem: complex solutions [McAnarney] 429 (Ap)
Demographic and risk factors associated with chronic dieting in adolescents [Story] 994 (Se)
Detection of alcoholism in hospitalized children and their families [Duggan] 613 (Je)
Improving health care provision to neonates in the United States [Stahlman] 510 (My)
Legalization of drugs of abuse and the pediatrician [Schwartz] 1153 (Oc)
Losing time [Pruitt] 607 (Je)
Pediatric human immunodeficiency virus infection and the acquired immunodeficiency syndrome: a health care crisis of children and families [Van Dyke] 529 (My)
Prevalence and impact of chronic illness among adolescents [Newacheck] 1367 (De)
Tattooing behavior in adolescence: a comparison study [Farrow] 184 (Fe)
What about gay teenagers? (letter) [Fikar] 252 (Mr)
Your child's best friend: TV or not TV? (letter) [Bader] (reply) [Stiehm] 963 (Se)
Adolescent, Institutionalized
Losing time [Pruitt] 607 (Je)
Adolescent Medicine
Care of the poor and underserved in America: older adolescents: a group at special risk [Haggerty] 569 (My)
Challenge of care for the poor and underserved in the United States: an American College of Obstetricians and Gynecologists perspective on access to care for underserved women [Davidson] 546 (My)
Improving health care for underserved infants, children, and adolescents: the Robert Wood Johnson Foundation's experience [Beachler] 565 (My)
New initiatives in adolescent health promotion [Elster] 495 (My)
Adolescent Psychology
Acquired immunodeficiency syndrome and adolescents: knowledge, attitudes, and behaviors of runaway and homeless youths [Sugerman] 431 (Ap)
Adolescents with chronic illness [Perrin] 1361 (De)
Adolescents' attrition from school-sponsored sports [DuRant] 1119 (Oc)
Complex problem: complex solutions [McAnarney] 429 (Ap)
Demographic and risk factors associated with chronic dieting in adolescents [Story] 994 (Se)
Losing time [Pruitt] 607 (Je)
Prevalence and impact of chronic illness among adolescents [Newacheck] 1367 (De)
Psychosocial predictors of maternal and infant health among adolescent mothers [Boyce] 267 (Mr)
Tattooing behavior in adolescence: a comparison study [Farrow] 184 (Fe)
What about gay teenagers? (letter) [Fikar] 252 (Mr)
Youth alienation as an emerging pediatric health care issue [Farrow] 491 (My)
Adrenal Cortex Hormones
Exacerbation of tinea corporis during treatment with 1% clotrimazole/0.05% betamethasone diproprionate (Lotrisone) (letter) [Reynolds] 1224 (No)
Role of corticosteroid therapy in children with pneumococcal meningitis [Kennedy] 1374 (De)
Survey of antiemetic use in children with cancer [van Hoff] 773 (Jy)
Adrenoceptors see Receptors, Adrenergic
Advertising
Exhibitor "giveaways": a curmudgeon's view (letter) [Berger] 427 (Ap)
Formula companies and the medical profession (letters) [Fink, Newman] 1088, 1089, (reply) [Greer] 1090 (Oc)
Physicians, formula companies, and advertising: a historical perspective [Greer] 282 (Mr)
Aerobic Exercise see Exercise
Age Factors
Acute osteomyelitis in children: reassessment of etiologic agents and their clinical characteristics [Faden] 65 (Ja)
Age-related patterns of thyroid-stimulating hormone response to thyrotropin-releasing hormone stimulation in Down syndrome [Sharav] 172 (Fe)
Breathing patterns and heart rates at ages 6 weeks and 2 years [Poets] 1393 (De)
Comparative trial of the reactogenicity and immunogenicity of Takeda acellular pertussis vaccine combined with tetanus and diphtheria toxoids: outcome in 3- to 8-month old infants, 9- to 23-month-old infants and children, and 24- to 30-month-old children [Kimura] 734 (Jy)
Demographic and risk factors associated with chronic dieting in adolescents [Story] 994 (Se)
Differences in infant mortality by race, nativity status, and other maternal characteristics [Kleinman] 194 (Fe)
Dose-related immunogenicity of *Haemophilus influenzae* type b capsular polysaccharide—*Neisseria meningitidis* outer membrane protein conjugate vaccine [Wong] 742 (Jy)
Lumbar puncture frequency and cerebrospinal fluid analysis in the neonate [Schwersenski] 54 (Ja)
Outpatient assessment of infants with bronchiolitis [Shaw] 151 (Fe)
Skateboarding injuries in children: a second wave [Retsky] 188 (Fe)
Standardized percentile curves of body-mass index for children and adolescents [Hammer] 259 (Mr)
Sudden cardiac death in young athletes: a review [McCaffrey] 177 (Fe)
Agglutinins
Comparative trial of the reactogenicity and immunogenicity of Takeda acellular pertussis vaccine combined with tetanus and diphtheria toxoids: outcome in 3- to 8-month old infants, 9- to 23-month-old infants and children, and 24- to 30-month-old children [Kimura] 734 (Jy)
Agranulocytosis
Measurement of serum granulocyte colony-stimulating factor in a patient with congenital agranulocytosis (Kostmann's syndrome) [Glasser] 925 (Au)
Agriculture
Paleonephrology and reflux nephropathy: from the 'big bang' to end-stage renal disease [Kallen] 860 (Au)
Agriculture Department (U.S.)
Oral water intoxication in infants: an American epidemic [Keating] 985 (Se)
AIDS-Related Complex
Clinical and endocrinologic manifestations in perinatally human immunodeficiency virus type 1-infected children aged 5 years or older [Lepage] 1248 (No)
Alaska
DTP immunization and susceptibility to infectious diseases: is there a relationship? [Davidson] 750 (Jy)
Legalization of drugs of abuse and the pediatrician [Schwartz] 1153 (Oc)
Albuterol
Albuterol inhalations in acute chest syndrome (letter) [Handelsman] 603 (Je)
Respirosonography in infants with acute bronchiolitis [Tal] 1405 (De)
Alcaligenes
Puncture wound-induced *Achromobacter xylosoxidans* osteomyelitis of the foot (letter) [Hoddy] 599 (Je)
Alcohol Drinking
Fetal alcohol syndrome: misplaced emphasis (letter) [Hess] (reply) [Little] 721 (Jy)
Parental drinking habits (letter) [Wells] 1087 (Oc)
Alcoholism
Detection of alcoholism in hospitalized children and their families [Duggan] 613 (Je)
Parental alcoholism: a neglected pediatric responsibility [MacDonald] 609 (Je)
Alienation, Social see Social Alienation
Alkaline Phosphatase
Growth hormone therapy in hypophosphatemic rickets [Wilson] 1165 (Oc)
Alkalosis
Alkaline urine is associated with eating disorders (letter) [Arden] 28 (Ja)
Association of alkaline urine with eating disorders (letter) [Robson] (reply) [Arden] 1091 (Oc)
Allergy see Hypersensitivity
Allopurinol
Improvement of leukemic hyperleukocytosis with only fluid and allopurinol therapy (letter) [Lascari] 969 (Se)
Alopecia
Acrodermatitis enteropathica [Schneider] 211 (Fe)
Alpha Fetoproteins
Major congenital neurologic malformations (letter) [Ryals] 30 (Ja)
Pediatric germ cell and human chorionic gonadotropin-producing tumors: clinical and laboratory features [Englund] 1294 (No)
Alprostadil
Penile vasculitis with impending necrosis treated with prostaglandin E_1 infusion (letter) [Horner] 604 (Je)
Altitude
Oxygen saturation by pulse oximetry in healthy infants at an altitude of 1610 m (5280 ft): what is normal? [Thilo] 1137 (Oc)
Ambulatory Care
Barriers to medical care for homeless families compared with housed poor families [Wood] 1109 (Oc)
Cholesterol testing in the physician's office: accuracy assessment (letter) [Rifai] 1087 (Oc)
Hand washing in pediatric ambulatory settings: an inconsistent practice [Lohr] 1198 (Oc)
Outpatient assessment of infants with bronchiolitis [Shaw] 151 (Fe)
Ambulatory Pediatric Association
1991 Annual Meeting, 26 (Ja), 125 (Fe), 249 (Mr), 425 (Ap)
31st annual meeting April 29-May 3, 1991, New Orleans, La, program 365-382; abstracts 383-423, 365 (Ap)
Serving the underserved: impact on resident education [Berkowitz] 544 (My)
American Academy of Pediatrics
American Academy of Pediatrics response to the growing health needs of children [Strain] 536 (My)
Exhibitor "giveaways": a curmudgeon's view (letter) [Berger] 427 (Ap)
Physicians, formula companies, and advertising: a historical perspective [Greer] 282 (Mr)
Practice management training for pediatric residents [Piatt] 299 (Mr)
American Association of Blood Banks
Guidelines for auditing pediatric blood transfusion practices [Blanchette] 787 (Jy)
American College of Obstetricians and Gynecologists
Challenge of care for the poor and underserved in the United States: an American College of Obstetricians and Gynecologists perspective on access to care for underserved women [Davidson] 546 (My)
AMERICAN JOURNAL OF DISEASES OF CHILDREN
AJDC is 80 years old: from pedology to pediatrics [Fulginiti] 11 (Ja)
Pediatric legal medicine: a new venture [Ferry] 255 (Mr)
Pediatric perspectives: vistas and vantage points [Bedrick] 256 (Mr)
American Medical Association
New initiatives in adolescent health promotion [Elster] 495 (My)
Physicians, formula companies, and advertising: a historical perspective [Greer] 282 (Mr)
American Pediatric Society
1991 Annual Meeting, 26 (Ja), 125 (Fe), 249 (Mr), 425 (Ap)
Call for abstracts, 1085 (Oc), 1223 (No), 1345 (De)
Aminoglycosides
Multilevel model to assess appropriateness of pediatric serum drug concentrations [Kraus] 1171 (Oc)
Amoxicillin
Staphylococcus aureus in impetigo (letter) [Dagan] (reply) [Bass] 1223 (No)
Ampicillin
Ventriculitis in newborns with myelomeningocele [Charney] 287 (Mr)
Anabolic Steroids
Tracking of elevated blood pressure values in adolescent athletes at 1-year follow-up [Tanji] 665 (Je)
Analeptics
Stimulant medication and attention deficit-hyperactivity disorder: the child's perspective [Bowen] 291 (Mr)
Anemia, Hemolytic
Gallstones in children: characterization by age, etiology, and outcome [Reif] 105 (Ja)
Anemia, Hypochromic
How much iron is enough? (letter) [Rogers] (reply) [Finberg] 598 (Je)
Anemia, Sickle Cell
Albuterol inhalations in acute chest syndrome (letter) [Han-

delsman] 603 (Je)
Anesthesia, Epidural
Laparoscopic cholecystectomy under continuous epidural anesthesia in patients with cystic fibrosis (letter) [Edelman] 723 (Jy)
Anoxemia
Outpatient assessment of infants with bronchiolitis [Shaw] 151 (Fe)
Retinopathy of prematurity in infants with cyanotic congenital heart disease [Johns] 200 (Fe)
Anoxia
How much of neonatal encephalopathy is due to birth asphyxia? [Nelson] 1325 (No)
Anthropometry
Optimal positioning of endotracheal tubes for ventilation of preterm infants [Rotschild] 1007 (Se)
Antibiotic Resistance see Drug Resistance, Microbial
Antibiotics
Evaluation of intraosseus vs intravenous antibiotic levels in a porcine model [Jaimovich] 946 (Au); correction, 1241 (No)
Factors associated with umbilical catheter-related sepsis in neonates [Landers] 675 (Je)
Role of corticosteroid therapy in children with pneumococcal meningitis [Kennedy] 1374 (De)
Ventriculitis in newborns with myelomeningocele [Charney] 287 (Mr)
Antibodies, Antinuclear
Association of pauciarticular juvenile arthritis and myasthenia gravis [Glass] 1176 (Oc)
Antibody Formation
Antibody response to MMR vaccination in children who received IVIG as neonates (letter) [Ruderman] 425 (Ap)
Antibody responses to 4 *Haemophilus influenzae* type b conjugate vaccines [Käyhty] 223 (Fe)
Comparative trial of the reactogenicity and immunogenicity of Takeda acellular pertussis vaccine combined with tetanus and diphtheria toxoids: outcome in 3- to 8-month old infants, 9- to 23-month-old infants and children, and 24- to 30-month-old children [Kimura] 734 (Jy)
Dose-related immunogenicity of *Haemophilus influenzae* type b capsular polysaccharide—*Neisseria meningitidis* outer membrane protein conjugate vaccine [Wong] 742 (Jy)
Antibody-Toxin Conjugates see Immunotoxins
Anticonvulsants
Effect of valproic acid on plasma carnitine levels [Opala] 999 (Se)
Antiemetics
Survey of antiemetic use in children with cancer [van Hoff] 773 (Jy)
Antiepileptic Agents see Anticonvulsants
Antigens, CD4
Predicting risk of *Pneumocystis carinii* pneumonia in human immunodeficiency virus-infected children [Rutstein] 922 (Au)
Antihistaminics, Classical see Histamine H1 Receptor Blockaders
Antimony
Mediterranean visceral leishmaniasis: a frequently unrecognized imported disease (letter) [Mahieu] 1225 (No)
Antley-Bixler Syndrome
Antley-Bixler syndrome [Butler] 701 (Je)
Anus
Acquired immunodeficiency syndrome and adolescents: knowledge, attitudes, and behaviors of runaway and homeless youths [Sugerman] 431 (Ap)
Anal fissure produced by examination for sexual abuse (letter) [Baker] 848, (reply) [Bays] 849 (Au)
Lichen sclerosus et atrophicus in children [Loening-Baucke] 1058 (Se)
Aortic Valve Insufficiency
Marfanoid children: etiologic heterogeneity and cardiac findings [Tayel] 90 (Ja)
Apgar Score
How much of neonatal encephalopathy is due to birth asphyxia? [Nelson] 1325 (No)
Apnea
Breathing patterns and heart rates at ages 6 weeks and 2 years [Poets] 1393 (De)
Gastroesophageal reflux and apnea in prematurely born infants during wakefulness and sleep [Ajuriaguerra] 1132 (Oc)
Sudden deaths and apparent life-threatening events in hospitalized neonates presumed to be healthy [Burchfield] 1319 (No)
Apnea, Obstructive see Sleep Apnea Syndromes
Appendicitis
Neonatal appendicitis with perforation [Ruff] 111 (Ja)
Arcanobacterium hemolyticum
Cavitary pneumonia due to *Arcanobacterium hemolyticum* [Waller] 209 (Fe)
Arm Injuries
Skateboarding injuries in children: a second wave [Retsky] 188 (Fe)
Arrhythmia
Sudden cardiac death (letter) [Pearl] 1223 (No)
Sudden cardiac death in young athletes: a review [McCaffrey] 177 (Fe)
Arteries
Arterial catheter-related infections in children: a 1-year cohort analysis [Furfaro] 1037 (Se)
Arteriovenous Malformations
Evolution of surgical treatment for congenital cardiac disease [Pigott] 1362 (De)
Arthritis, Infectious
Pneumococcal osteomyelitis and arthritis in children: a hospital series and literature review [Jacobs] 70 (Ja)
Arthritis, Juvenile Rheumatoid
Association of pauciarticular juvenile arthritis and myasthenia gravis [Glass] 1176 (Oc)
Challenge of caring for indigent children with rheumatologic diseases [Miller] 554 (My)
Decreasing severity of chronic uveitis in children with pauciarticular arthritis [Sherry] 1026 (Se)
Asphyxia Neonatorum
How much of neonatal encephalopathy is due to birth asphyxia? [Nelson] 1325 (No)
Asthma
Improved speed and accuracy of calculations with a programmable calculator in pediatric emergency scenarios [Melzer-Lange] 264 (Mr)
Increased transient tachypnea of the newborn in infants with asthmatic mothers [Schatz] 156 (Fe)
Prevalence and impact of chronic illness among adolescents [Newacheck] 1367 (De)
Asystole see Heart Arrest
Atelectasis
Outpatient assessment of infants with bronchiolitis [Shaw] 151 (Fe)
Atherosclerosis, Coronary see Coronary Arteriosclerosis
Athletic Injuries
Adolescents' attrition from school-sponsored sports [DuRant] 1119 (Oc)
Commotio cordis: the single, most common cause of traumatic death in youth baseball [Abrunzo] 1279 (No)
Safety of a preadolescent basketball program [Gutgesell] 1023 (Se)
Skateboarding injuries in children: a second wave [Retsky] 188 (Fe)
Athletics see Sports
Atropine
War souvenir poisoning (letter) [Secord] 724 (Jy)
Attention Deficit Disorder with Hyperactivity
Minor malformations, hyperactivity, and learning disabilities [Accardo] 1184 (Oc)
Stimulant medication and attention deficit-hyperactivity disorder: the child's perspective [Bowen] 291 (Mr)
Attitude of Health Personnel
House staff work hours and moonlighting: what do residents want?: a survey of pediatric residents in California [Cheng] 1104 (Oc)
Attitude to Health
Health care for uninsured and underinsured children (letter) [Barness] 1086 (Oc)
Auditory Canal, External see Ear Canal
Authorship
Tell the whole story [Johnson] 135 (Fe)
Autoimmune Diseases
Association of pauciarticular juvenile arthritis and myasthenia gravis [Glass] 1176 (Oc)
Chronic neutropenia during childhood: a 13-year experience in a single institution [Jonsson] 232 (Fe)

B

Bacteremia see Septicemia
Bacterial Infections
Apparent decreased risk of invasive bacterial disease after heterologous childhood immunization [Black] 746 (Jy)
Causes of hospital-treated acute lower respiratory tract infection in children [Nohynek] 618 (Je)
Cautionary note on the use of empiric ceftriaxone for suspected bacteremia [Wald] 1359 (De)
Cavitary pneumonia due to *Arcanobacterium hemolyticum* [Waller] 209 (Fe)
DTP immunization and susceptibility to infectious diseases: is there a relationship? [Davidson] 750 (Jy)
Efficacy and pharmacokinetics of intravenous immune globulin administration to high-risk neonates [Kinney] 1233 (No)
Frequency of infections associated with implanted systems vs cuffed, tunneled silastic venous catheters in patients with acute leukemia [Severien] 1433 (De)
Is prophylaxis of neonates with intravenous immunoglobulin beneficial? [Hill] 1229 (No)
Late cholangitis after successful surgical repair of biliary atresia [Gottrand] 213 (Fe)
Lumbar puncture frequency and cerebrospinal fluid analysis in the neonate [Schwersenski] 54 (Ja)
Neutropenia in an extremely premature infant treated with recombinant human granulocyte colony-stimulating factor [Roberts] 808 (Jy)
Pneumococcal osteomyelitis and arthritis in children: a hospital series and literature review [Jacobs] 70 (Ja)
Vasopressin levels in infants during the course of aseptic and bacterial meningitis [Padilla] 991 (Se)
Ventriculitis in newborns with myelomeningocele [Charney] 287 (Mr)
Bacterial Vaccines
Response of 7- to 15-month-old infants to sequential immunization with *Haemophilus influenzae* type b-CRM$_{197}$ conjugate and polysaccharide vaccines [Rothstein] 898 (Au)
Bacteriuria
Cautionary note on the use of empiric ceftriaxone for suspected bacteremia [Wald] 1359 (De)
Balkan Nephropathy
Epidemic nephropathy in children [Lautala] 1181 (Oc)
Baseball
Commotio cordis: the single, most common cause of traumatic death in youth baseball [Abrunzo] 1279 (No)
Basilar Bone see Occipital Bone
Basketball
Safety of a preadolescent basketball program [Gutgesell] 1023 (Se)
Basophils
Percentile curves for various hematologic measurements at birth in Arab preterm babies of different gestational ages [Haque] 645 (Je)
Bayes Theorem
Evaluation of Bayesian forecasting for individualized gentamicin dosage in infants weighing 1000 g or less [Lui] 463 (Ap)
Behavior
Buddy, can you paradigm? [Brown] 727 (Jy)
Betamethasone
Exacerbation of tinea corporis during treatment with 1% clotrimazole/0.05% betamethasone diproprionate (Lotrisone) (letter) [Reynolds] 1224 (No)
Bias (Epidemiology)
Neuroblastoma screening data: an epidemiologic analysis [Goodman] 1415 (De)
Biliary Atresia
Late cholangitis after successful surgical repair of biliary atresia [Gottrand] 213 (Fe)
Neonatal hepatitis and extrahepatic biliary atresia associated with cytomegalovirus infection in twins [Hart] 302 (Mr)
Bilirubin
Direct bilirubin measurements in jaundiced term newborns: a reevaluation [Newman] 1305 (No)
Biological Markers
Effect of necrotizing enterocolitis on urinary epidermal growth factor levels [Scott] 804 (Jy); correction, 982 (Se)
Minor malformations, hyperactivity, and learning disabilities [Accardo] 1184 (Oc)
Biopsy
Misdiagnosis of Reye's-like illness (letter) [Forsyth] 964 (Se)
Birth Control see Family Planning
Birth Injuries
Clavicular fractures in neonates (letter) [Carter] 251, (reply) [Joseph] 252 (Mr)
Clavicular fractures in neonates: frequency vs significance (letter) [O'Halloran] (reply) [Joseph] 251 (Mr)
How much of neonatal encephalopathy is due to birth asphyxia? [Nelson] 1325 (No)
Birth Weight
Factors associated with umbilical catheter-related sepsis in neonates [Landers] 675 (Je)
Longitudinal study of birth weight and being overweight in late adolescence [Seidman] 782 (Jy)
Obesity among Mescalero preschool children: association with maternal obesity and birth weight [Gallaher] 1262 (No)
Prevalence of birth defects among low-birth-weight infants: a population study [Mili] 1313 (No)
Studies in fetal malnutrition [Crosby] 871 (Au)
Blacks
Adolescents' attrition from school-sponsored sports [DuRant] 1119 (Oc)
Breast-feeding initiation in a triethnic population [Bee] 306 (Mr)
Demographic and risk factors associated with chronic dieting in adolescents [Story] 994 (Se)
Differences in expression of cystic fibrosis in blacks and whites [McColley] 94 (Ja)
Differences in infant mortality by race, nativity status, and other maternal characteristics [Kleinman] 194 (Fe)
Family history of myocardial infarction and hemodynamic responses to exercise in young black boys [Treiber] 1029 (Se)
Rickets caused by vitamin D deficiency in breast-fed infants in the southern United States [Bhowmick] 127 (Fe)
Sexual maturation and blood pressure levels of a biracial sample of girls [Kozinetz] 142 (Fe)
Blood Cell Count
Percentile curves for various hematologic measurements at birth in Arab preterm babies of different gestational ages [Haque] 645 (Je)
Blood Chemical Analysis
Elevated plasma norepinephrine levels in infants of substance-abusing mothers [Ward] 44 (Ja)
Multiple comparisons and *P* values (letter) [Newman] 250 (Mr)
Blood Donors
Transfusion therapy in neonates [Strauss] 904 (Au)
Blood Plasma see Plasma
Blood Platelets
Elevated plasma norepinephrine levels in infants of sub-

stance-abusing mothers [Ward] 44 (Ja)
Guidelines for auditing pediatric blood transfusion practices [Blanchette] 787 (Jy)
Transfusion therapy in neonates [Strauss] 904 (Au)
Variant form of thrombasthenia [Tarantino] 1053 (Se)
Blood Pressure
Family history of myocardial infarction and hemodynamic responses to exercise in young black boys [Treiber] 1029 (Se)
Pediatric cardiac rehabilitation [Balfour] 627 (Je)
Physiologic responses to playing a video game [Segal] 1034 (Se)
Sexual maturation and blood pressure levels of a biracial sample of girls [Kozinetz] 142 (Fe)
Tracking of elevated blood pressure values in adolescent athletes at 1-year follow-up [Tanji] 665 (Je)
Blood Sedimentation
Factors affecting outcome in meningococcal infections [Tesoro] 218 (Fe)
Blood Transfusion
Guidelines for auditing pediatric blood transfusion practices [Blanchette] 787 (Jy)
Transfusion therapy in neonates [Strauss] 904 (Au)
Blue Cross
Caring program for children: the Michigan experience [Udow] 579 (My)
Blue Shield
Caring program for children: the Michigan experience [Udow] 579 (My)
Body Fluids
Association of alkaline urine with eating disorders (letter) [Robson] (reply) [Arden] 1091 (Oc)
Body Height
Clinical and endocrinologic manifestations in perinatally human immunodeficiency virus type 1-infected children aged 5 years or older [Lepage] 1248 (No)
Effectiveness of growth-promoting therapies: comparison among growth hormone, clonidine, and levodopa [Volta] 168 (Fe)
Follow-up of patients who underwent arterial switch repair for transposition of the great arteries [Mendoza] 40 (Ja)
Optimal positioning of endotracheal tubes for ventilation of preterm infants [Rotschild] 1007 (Se)
Sexual maturation and blood pressure levels of a biracial sample of girls [Kozinetz] 142 (Fe)
Standardized percentile curves of body-mass index for children and adolescents [Hammer] 259 (Mr)
Value of subject height in predicting lower esophageal sphincter location [Staiano] 1424 (De)
Body Image
Demographic and risk factors associated with chronic dieting in adolescents [Story] 994 (Se)
Body Mass Index
Obesity and body-mass index (letter) [Hergenroeder] (reply) [Hammer] 972 (Se)
Standardized percentile curves of body-mass index for children and adolescents [Hammer] 259 (Mr)
Body Temperature
Influence of otitis media on the correlation between rectal and auditory canal temperatures [Terndrup] 75 (Ja)
Body Weight
Follow-up of patients who underwent arterial switch repair for transposition of the great arteries [Mendoza] 40 (Ja)
Longitudinal study of birth weight and being overweight in late adolescence [Seidman] 782 (Jy)
Obesity and body-mass index (letter) [Hergenroeder] (reply) [Hammer] 972 (Se)
Optimal positioning of endotracheal tubes for ventilation of preterm infants [Rotschild] 1007 (Se)
Sexual maturation and blood pressure levels of a biracial sample of girls [Kozinetz] 142 (Fe)
Standardized percentile curves of body-mass index for children and adolescents [Hammer] 259 (Mr)
Tracking of elevated blood pressure values in adolescent athletes at 1-year follow-up [Tanji] 665 (Je)
Bonding (Psychology) see Object Attachment
Bone and Bones
Dietary calcium and bone mineral status of children and adolescents [Chan] 631 (Je)
Osteochondrodysplasia in Fryns syndrome [Kershisnik] 656 (Je)
Bone Density
Bone mineral content of healthy, full-term neonates: effect of race, gender, and maternal cigarette smoking [Venkataraman] 1310 (No)
Dietary calcium and bone mineral status of children and adolescents [Chan] 631 (Je)
Bone Marrow
Evaluation of intraosseus vs intravenous antibiotic levels in a porcine model [Jaimovich] 946 (Au); correction, 1241 (No)
Intraosseous infusion of dobutamine and isoproterenol [Bilello] 165 (Fe); correction, 1312 (No)
Bone Mineral Content see Bone Density
Bone Mineralization see Calcification, Physiologic
BOOK REVIEWS
Brumberg JJ: Fasting Girls: The History of Anorexia Nervosa, 146 (Fe)
DeAngelis C: Introduction to Clinical Resarch, 945 (Au)
Freeman JM, Vining EPG, Pillas DJ: Seizures and Epilepsy in Childhood: A Guide for Parents, 539 (My)
Markel H, Oski FA: HL Mencken Baby Book, 817 (Jy)
Merlini L, Granata C, Dubowitz V, eds: Current Concepts in Childhood Spinal Muscular Atrophy, 462 (Ap)
Nussbaum E, ed: Pediatric Intensive Care, ed 2, 175 (Fe)
Ramanujam TM, ed: Parenteral nutrition in infants and children: basic principles and practical guidelines, 1025 (Se)
Stockman JA III, ed: Difficult Diagnosis in Pediatrics, 541 (My)
Books
Clinic-based intervention to promote literacy: a pilot study [Needlman] 881 (Au)
Bradycardia
Gastroesophageal reflux and apnea in prematurely born infants during wakefulness and sleep [Ajuriaguerra] 1132 (Oc)
Sudden deaths and apparent life-threatening events in hospitalized neonates presumed to be healthy [Burchfield] 1319 (No)
Brain
Brain and ocular abnormalities in infants with in utero exposure to cocaine and other street drugs [Dominguez] 688 (Je)
Brain Diseases
Fallacy of the hemorrhagic shock and encephalopathy syndrome (letter) [Bass] 718 (Jy)
'H' in hemorrhagic shock and encephalopathy syndrome (letter) [Roscelli] 720 (Jy)
Hemorrhagic shock and encephalopathy: an entity similar to heatstroke (letter) [Conway] 720 (Jy)
Hyperpyrexia, hemorrhagic shock and encephalopathy, and creatinine phosphokinase (letter) [Dupee] 719 (Jy)
Brain Injuries
How much of neonatal encephalopathy is due to birth asphyxia? [Nelson] 1325 (No)
Breast Feeding
Breast-feeding initiation in a triethnic population [Bee] 306 (Mr)
Formula companies and the medical profession (letters) [Fink, Newman] 1088, 1089, (reply) [Greer] 1090 (Oc)
Physicians, formula companies, and advertising: a historical perspective [Greer] 282 (Mr)
Practical guide to successful breast-feeding management [Freed] 917 (Au)
Rickets caused by vitamin D deficiency in breast-fed infants in the southern United States [Bhowmick] 127 (Fe)
Bristol Myers
Physicians, formula companies, and advertising: a historical perspective [Greer] 282 (Mr)
Bronchiolitis
Causes of hospital-treated acute lower respiratory tract infection in children [Nohynek] 618 (Je)
Outpatient assessment of infants with bronchiolitis [Shaw] 151 (Fe)
Respirosonography in infants with acute bronchiolitis [Tal] 1405 (De)
Bronchopulmonary Dysplasia
Predictors of neurodevelopmental outcome following bronchopulmonary dysplasia [Luchi] 813 (Jy)
Buffers
Immunogenicity of tetravalent rhesus rotavirus vaccine administered with buffer and oral polio vaccine [Ing] 892 (Au)
Burnout, Professional
Pediatric program director: an analysis of the role and its problems [Weiss] 449 (Ap)

C

C-Reactive Protein
Scoring systems for accurate prognosis of patients with meningococcal infections (letter) [Leclerc] 1090 (Oc)
Calcidiol see 25-Hydroxycholecalciferol 1-Hydroxylase
Calcifediol
How much vitamin D for neonates? [Pittard] 1147 (Oc)
Calcification, Pathologic see Calcinosis
Calcification, Physiologic
Mineral metabolism and calcitriol therapy in idiopathic juvenile osteoporosis [Saggese] 457 (Ap)
Calcinosis
Pediatric case of Eagle's syndrome [Holloway] 339 (Mr)
Calcitriol
Growth hormone therapy in hypophosphatemic rickets [Wilson] 1165 (Oc)
Mineral metabolism and calcitriol therapy in idiopathic juvenile osteoporosis [Saggese] 457 (Ap)
X-linked hypophosphatemia: genetic and clinical correlates [Hanna] 865 (Au)
Calcium
Dietary calcium and bone mineral status of children and adolescents [Chan] 631 (Je)
Low serum calcium and high parathyroid hormone levels in neonates fed 'humanized' cow's milk-based formula [Specker] 941 (Au)
Natural history of hematuria associated with hypercalciuria in children [Garcia] 1204 (Oc)
Partial hypoparathyroidism: a variant of transient congenital hypoparathyroidism [Kooh] 877 (Au)
Calculators, Programmable see Computers
Canada
Redoing the health care quilt: patches or whole cloth? [Cleveland] 499 (My)
Candidiasis, Chronic Mucocutaneous
Myopathy associated with ketoconazole treatment (letter) [Garty] 970 (Se)
Cannabinoids
Occult cocaine exposure in children [Rosenberg] 1430 (De)
Capillaries
Capillary refilling (skin turgor) in the assessment of dehydration [Saavedra] 296 (Mr)
Carbamazepine
Effect of valproic acid on plasma carnitine levels [Opala] 999 (Se)
Carbon Monoxide
Cardiopulmonary exercise testing in children following surgery for tetralogy of Fallot [Tomassoni] 1290 (No)
Cardiac Output
Cardiopulmonary exercise testing in children following surgery for tetralogy of Fallot [Tomassoni] 1290 (No)
Family history of myocardial infarction and hemodynamic responses to exercise in young black boys [Treiber] 1029 (Se)
Cardiology
Poverty and cardiac disease in children [Allen] 550 (My)
Cardiomyopathies see Myocardial Diseases
Cardiomyopathy, Hypertrophic
Sudden cardiac death in young athletes: a review [McCaffrey] 177 (Fe)
Cardiopulmonary Arrest see Heart Arrest
Cardiopulmonary Bypass
Development, growth, and cardiac surgery [Mayer] 33 (Ja)
Cardiopulmonary Resuscitation see Resuscitation
Cardiovascular Diseases
Evolution of surgical treatment for congenital cardiac disease [Pigott] 1362 (De)
Pediatric cardiac rehabilitation [Balfour] 627 (Je)
Cardiovascular System
Cardiopulmonary exercise testing in children following surgery for tetralogy of Fallot [Tomassoni] 1290 (No)
Effect of low-dose dopamine infusion on cardiopulmonary and renal status in premature newborns with respiratory distress syndrome [Cuevas] 799 (Jy)
Effects of obesity on aerobic fitness in adolescent females [Rowland] 764 (Jy)
Family history of myocardial infarction and hemodynamic responses to exercise in young black boys [Treiber] 1029 (Se)
Role of corticosteroid therapy in children with pneumococcal meningitis [Kennedy] 1374 (De)
Career Choice
Current trends in pediatric residency training [Carraccio] 1272 (No)
Part-time Peg: who, me? [Ferry] 852 (Au)
Priorities in academic pediatrics (letter) [Jacobs] (reply) [Goetzman] 845 (Au)
Carnitine
Effect of valproic acid on plasma carnitine levels [Opala] 999 (Se)
Case Report
Thumb-sucking (letter) [Lubicky] 845, (reply) [Friman] 846 (Au)
Cat-Scratch Disease
Cat-scratch disease: acute encephalopathy and other neurologic manifestations [Carithers] 98 (Ja)
Catecholamines
Elevated plasma norepinephrine levels in infants of substance-abusing mothers [Ward] 44 (Ja)
Cathartics
Association of alkaline urine with eating disorders (letter) [Robson] (reply) [Arden] 1091 (Oc)
Demographic and risk factors associated with chronic dieting in adolescents [Story] 994 (Se)
Catheterization
Factors associated with umbilical catheter-related sepsis in neonates [Landers] 675 (Je)
Posthemorrhagic hydrocephalus: use of an intravenous-type catheter for cerebrospinal fluid drainage [Marro] 1141 (Oc)
Catheterization, Central Venous
Escherichia coli bacteremia in children: a review of 91 cases in 10 years [Bonadio] 671 (Je)
Frequency of infections associated with implanted systems vs cuffed, tunneled silastic venous catheters in patients with acute leukemia [Severien] 1433 (De)
Intravenous hyperalimentation fluid obtained with lumbar puncture: an unusual complication of a central venous catheter [Mah] 1439 (De)
Catheterization, Peripheral
Arterial catheter-related infections in children: a 1-year cohort analysis [Furfaro] 1037 (Se)
Catheters, Indwelling
Frequency of infections associated with implanted systems vs cuffed, tunneled silastic venous catheters in patients with acute leukemia [Severien] 1433 (De)
CD4 Antigens see Antigens, CD4
Cefotaxime
Evaluation of intraosseus vs intravenous antibiotic levels in

a porcine model [Jaimovich] 946 (Au); correction, 1241 (No)
Ceftriaxone
Cautionary note on the use of empiric ceftriaxone for suspected bacteremia [Wald] 1359 (De)
Celiac Disease
Taurine decreases fecal fatty acid and sterol excretion in cystic fibrosis: a randomized double-blind trial [Smith] 1401 (De)
Centers for Disease Control (U.S.)
Vaccine myth and physician handouts (letter) [Lynch] 426, (replies) [Cherry, Fulginiti] 426, 427 (Ap)
Central Nervous System
Tuberous sclerosis with myocardial and central nervous system involvement at birth [Allison] 471 (Ap)
Central Nervous System Stimulants see Analeptics
Central Venous Catheterization see Catheterization, Central Venous
Cephalometry
Follow-up of patients who underwent arterial switch repair for transposition of the great arteries [Mendoza] 40 (Ja)
Cerebral Cortex
Cortical resection for children with epilepsy: perspectives in pediatrics [Wyllie] 314 (Mr)
Cerebral Hemorrhage
Posthemorrhagic hydrocephalus: use of an intravenous-type catheter for cerebrospinal fluid drainage [Marro] 1141 (Oc)
Predictors of neurodevelopmental outcome following bronchopulmonary dysplasia [Luchi] 813 (Jy)
Cerebral Ventricles
Posthemorrhagic hydrocephalus: use of an intravenous-type catheter for cerebrospinal fluid drainage [Marro] 1141 (Oc)
Predictors of neurodevelopmental outcome following bronchopulmonary dysplasia [Luchi] 813 (Jy)
Ventriculitis in newborns with myelomeningocele [Charney] 287 (Mr)
Cerebrospinal Fluid
Endotoxin concentrations in cerebrospinal fluid correlate with clinical severity and neurologic outcome of *Haemophilus influenzae* type b meningitis [Mertsola] 1099 (Oc)
Lumbar puncture frequency and cerebrospinal fluid analysis in the neonate [Schwersenski] 54 (Ja)
Posthemorrhagic hydrocephalus: use of an intravenous-type catheter for cerebrospinal fluid drainage [Marro] 1141 (Oc)
Cerebrospinal Fluid Shunts
Posthemorrhagic hydrocephalus: use of an intravenous-type catheter for cerebrospinal fluid drainage [Marro] 1141 (Oc)
Cerebrovascular Disorders
Endocrine function in children with human immunodeficiency virus infection [Schwartz] 330 (Mr)
Cervical Vertebrae
Neural arch stenosis and spinal cord injury in thanatophoric dysplasia [Faye-Petersen] 87 (Ja)
Osteochondrodysplasia in Fryns syndrome [Kershisnik] 656 (Je)
Chemical Warfare
War souvenir poisoning (letter) [Secord] 724 (Jy)
Chest see Thorax
Child
Antibody responses to 4 *Haemophilus influenzae* type b conjugate vaccines [Käyhty] 223 (Fe)
Children in and of the streets: health, social policy, and the homeless young [Wright] 516 (My)
Far from the ideal: the plight of poor children in the United States [Fulginiti] 489 (My)
Guidelines for safe transportation of children in wheelchairs [DiGaudio] 653 (Je)
Mineral metabolism and calcitriol therapy in idiopathic juvenile osteoporosis [Saggese] 457 (Ap)
Occult cocaine exposure in children [Rosenberg] 1430 (De)
Predicting risk of *Pneumocystis carinii* pneumonia in human immunodeficiency virus-infected children [Rutstein] 922 (Au)
Safety of a preadolescent basketball program [Gutgesell] 1023 (Se)
Survey of the health of homeless children in Philadelphia shelters [Parker] 520 (My)
Child Abuse
Child abuse and neglect: critical first steps in response to a national emergency: the report of the US Advisory Board on Child Abuse and Neglect [Krugman] 513 (My)
Medical ethics issues survey of residents in 5 pediatric training programs [White] 161 (Fe)
Photographing the physically abused child, principles and practice [Ricci] 275 (Mr)
Child Abuse, Sexual
Anal fissure produced by examination for sexual abuse (letter) [Baker] 848, (reply) [Bays] 849 (Au)
Child abuse and neglect: critical first steps in response to a national emergency: the report of the US Advisory Board on Child Abuse and Neglect [Krugman] 513 (My)
Child sexual abuse and human immunodeficiency virus transmission (letter) [Monteleone] (reply) [Gutman] 847 (Au)
Condylomata acuminata: still usually a sexually transmitted disease in children (letter) [Goldenring] 600, (reply) [Boyd] 601 (Je)
Diagnosis of child sexual abuse in children with genital warts (letter) [Gutman] (reply) [Boyd] 126 (Fe)
Human immunodeficiency virus transmission by child sexual abuse [Gutman] 137 (Fe)
Child Behavior
Buddy, can you paradigm? [Brown] 727 (Jy)
Detection of alcoholism in hospitalized children and their families [Duggan] 613 (Je)
Nintendo enuresis (letter) [Schink] 1094 (Oc)
Your child's best friend: TV or not TV? (letter) [Bader] (reply) [Stiehm] 963 (Se)
Child Care
Injuries and poisonings in out-of-home child care and home care [Gunn] 779 (Jy)
Women in medicine: fantasies, dreams, myths, and realities [DeAngelis] 49 (Ja)
Child Day Care Centers
Injuries and poisonings in out-of-home child care and home care [Gunn] 779 (Jy)
Child Development
Buddy, can you paradigm? [Brown] 727 (Jy)
Development, growth, and cardiac surgery [Mayer] 33 (Ja)
Dietary calcium and bone mineral status of children and adolescents [Chan] 631 (Je)
Follow-up of patients who underwent arterial switch repair for transposition of the great arteries [Mendoza] 40 (Ja)
Intellectual development in 12-year-old children treated for phenylketonuria [Azen] 35 (Ja)
Minor malformations, hyperactivity, and learning disabilities [Accardo] 1184 (Oc)
Neurodevelopmental outcome of offspring of the diabetic mother: need for further research (letter) [Goldstein] 602 (Je)
Predictors of neurodevelopmental outcome following bronchopulmonary dysplasia [Luchi] 813 (Jy)
Standardized percentile curves of body-mass index for children and adolescents [Hammer] 259 (Mr)
Survey of the health of homeless children in Philadelphia shelters [Parker] 520 (My)
Child Development Disorders
Lead poisoning in children with developmental disabilities (letter) [Sulkes] 602 (Je)
Zinc deficiency: a public health problem? [Sandstead] 853 (Au)
Child Development Disorders, Specific see Child Development Disorders
Child Health Services
American Academy of Pediatrics response to the growing health needs of children [Strain] 536 (My)
Barriers to medical care for homeless families compared with housed poor families [Wood] 1109 (Oc)
Cardiac care for infants: determinants of hospital charges for acute care [Pearson] 1397 (De)
Caring program for children: the Michigan experience [Udow] 579 (My)
Challenge of care for the poor child: the research agenda [Kohl] 542 (My)
Challenge of caring for indigent children with rheumatologic diseases [Miller] 554 (My)
Children's services in an era of budget deficits [Blum] 575 (My)
Family physicians and neonatology (letter) [McIntyre] (reply) [DiTraglia] 963 (Se)
Far from the ideal: the plight of poor children in the United States [Fulginiti] 489 (My)
Growing neglect of American children [Maurer] 540 (My)
Health care for pregnant women and young children [Behrman] 572 (My)
Health care for uninsured and underinsured children (letters)
[Davis, Kirschner, Pearson, Hecker, Barness] 1085, 1086 (Oc)
Home care cost-effectiveness for respiratory technology-dependent children [Fields] 729 (Jy)
Improving health care for underserved infants, children, and adolescents: the Robert Wood Johnson Foundation's experience [Beachler] 565 (My)
Improving the use of early follow-up care after emergency department visits: a randomized trial [Nelson] 440 (Ap)
Pediatric acquired immunodeficiency syndrome, poverty, and national priorities [Heagarty] 527 (My)
Pediatric human immunodeficiency virus infection and the acquired immunodeficiency syndrome: a health care crisis of children and families [Van Dyke] 529 (My)
Pediatric legal medicine: a new venture [Ferry] 255 (Mr)
Poverty and cardiac disease in children [Allen] 550 (My)
Poverty and the health of American children: implications for academic pediatrics [Johnston] 507 (My)
Priorities in academic pediatrics (letter) [Jacobs] (reply) [Goetzman] 845 (Au)
Redoing the health care quilt: patches or whole cloth? [Cleveland] 499 (My)
Regional pediatric approach to the epidemic of social ills within our cities [Nelson] 505 (My)
Resident and nurse practitioners: responding to education and patient care needs (letter) [Giardino] 843 (Au)
Saving money with home care [Schoumacher] 725 (Jy)
Serving the underserved: impact on resident education [Berkowitz] 544 (My)
Tiny Tim remembered [Callahan] 1355 (De)
What will it take to fully protect all American children with vaccines? [Hinman] 559 (My)
Child, Hospitalized
Child welfare: the phantom of the health care system (letter) [Pidcock] 843 (Au)
Detection of alcoholism in hospitalized children and their families [Duggan] 613 (Je)
Child Neglect see Child Abuse
Child Nutrition
Children in and of the streets: health, social policy, and the homeless young [Wright] 516 (My)
Child Nutrition Disorders
Zinc deficiency: a public health problem? [Sandstead] 853 (Au)
Child, Preschool
Child survival and perinatal infections with human immunodeficiency virus [Bennett] 1242 (No)
Clinic-based intervention to promote literacy: a pilot study [Needlman] 881 (Au)
Health care for pregnant women and young children [Behrman] 572 (My)
Injuries and poisonings in out-of-home child care and home care [Gunn] 779 (Jy)
Obesity among Mescalero preschool children: association with maternal obesity and birth weight [Gallaher] 1262 (No)
Survey of the health of homeless children in Philadelphia shelters [Parker] 520 (My)
Unsuspected cocaine exposure in young children [Kharasch] 204 (Fe)
Child Psychiatry
Buddy, can you paradigm? [Brown] 727 (Jy)
Child Psychology
Buddy, can you paradigm? [Brown] 727 (Jy)
Grampa, can I get something that I'd like? [Strong] 1355 (De)
Send Linus to me (letter) [Szonyi] (reply) [Friman] 1227 (No)
Stimulant medication and attention deficit-hyperactivity disorder: the child's perspective [Bowen] 291 (Mr)
Survey of the health of homeless children in Philadelphia shelters [Parker] 520 (My)
Testing the psychogenic vomiting diagnosis: four pediatric patients [Gonzalez-Heydrich] 913 (Au)
Thumb-sucking (letter) [Lubicky] 845, (reply) [Friman] 846 (Au)
Child Rearing
Comments on life after residency (letter) [Brent] 597 (Je)
Complex problem: complex solutions [McAnarney] 429 (Ap)
Your child's best friend: TV or not TV [Stiehm] 257 (Mr)
Child Welfare
Child welfare: the phantom of the health care system (letter) [Pidcock] 843 (Au)
Chloramphenicol
Evaluation of intraosseus vs intravenous antibiotic levels in a porcine model [Jaimovich] 946 (Au); correction, 1241 (No)
Chlorides
Association of alkaline urine with eating disorders (letter) [Robson] (reply) [Arden] 1091 (Oc)
Cholangitis
Late cholangitis after successful surgical repair of biliary atresia [Gottrand] 213 (Fe)
Cholecystectomy
Gallstones in children: characterization by age, etiology, and outcome [Reif] 105 (Ja)
Laparoscopic cholecystectomy under continuous epidural anesthesia in patients with cystic fibrosis (letter) [Edelman] 723 (Jy)
Cholelithiasis
Gallstones in children: characterization by age, etiology, and outcome [Reif] 105 (Ja)
Gallstones in children (letter) [Todd] 971 (Se)
Laparoscopic cholecystectomy under continuous epidural anesthesia in patients with cystic fibrosis (letter) [Edelman] 723 (Jy)
Cholesterol
Cholesterol testing in the physician's office: accuracy assessment (letter) [Rifai] 1087 (Oc)
Serum lipid concentrations in subjects with phenylketonuria and their families [DeClue] 1266 (No)
Chronic Disease
Adolescents with chronic illness [Perrin] 1361 (De)
Chronic neutropenia during childhood: a 13-year experience in a single institution [Jonsson] 232 (Fe)
Prevalence and impact of chronic illness among adolescents [Newacheck] 1367 (De)
Classification
Buddy, can you paradigm? [Brown] 727 (Jy)
Clavicle
Clavicular fractures in neonates (letter) [Carter] 251, (reply) [Joseph] 252 (Mr)
Clavicular fractures in neonates: frequency vs significance (letter) [O'Halloran] (reply) [Joseph] 251 (Mr)
Clinical Competence
Objective structured clinical examination in a pediatric residency program [Joorabchi] 757 (Jy)

Clinical Pharmacy Service see Pharmacy Service, Hospital
Clinical Trial Overviews see Meta-Analysis
Clinical Trials
Antibody responses to 4 *Haemophilus influenzae* type b conjugate vaccines [Käyhty] 223 (Fe)
Comparative trial of the reactogenicity and immunogenicity of Takeda acellular pertussis vaccine combined with tetanus and diphtheria toxoids: outcome in 3- to 8-month old infants, 9- to 23-month-old infants and children, and 24- to 30-month-old children [Kimura] 734 (Jy)
Effectiveness of growth-promoting therapies: comparison among growth hormone, clonidine, and levodopa [Volta] 168 (Fe)
Pediatric human immunodeficiency virus infection and the acquired immunodeficiency syndrome: a health care crisis of children and families [Van Dyke] 529 (My)
Clonidine
Effectiveness of growth-promoting therapies: comparison among growth hormone, clonidine, and levodopa [Volta] 168 (Fe)
Seasonal variation in growth during growth hormone therapy [Rudolf] 769 (Jy)
Clotrimazole
Exacerbation of tinea corporis during treatment with 1% clotrimazole/0.05% betamethasone diproprionate (Lotrisone) (letter) [Reynolds] 1224 (No)
Cocaine
Brain and ocular abnormalities in infants with in utero exposure to cocaine and other street drugs [Dominguez] 688 (Je)
Characteristics of perinatal cocaine-exposed infants with necrotizing enterocolitis (letter) [Downing] 26 (Ja)
Child welfare: the phantom of the health care system (letter) [Pidcock] 843 (Au)
Elevated plasma norepinephrine levels in infants of substance-abusing mothers [Ward] 44 (Ja)
Evaluation of auditory brain-stem response in full-term infants of cocaine-abusing mothers [Carzoli] 1013 (Se)
Meconium for drug testing [Maynard] 650 (Je)
Occult cocaine exposure in children [Rosenberg] 1430 (De)
Preliminary report of prenatal cocaine exposure and respiratory distress syndrome in premature infants [Zuckerman] 696 (Je)
Unsuspected cocaine exposure in young children [Kharasch] 204 (Fe)
Codeine
Meconium for drug testing [Maynard] 650 (Je)
Coitus
Acquired immunodeficiency syndrome and adolescents: knowledge, attitudes, and behaviors of runaway and homeless youths [Sugerman] 431 (Ap)
Colon
Esophageal motility in children with Hirschsprung's disease [Staiano] 310 (Mr)
Colorado
Oxygen saturation by pulse oximetry in healthy infants at an altitude of 1610 m (5280 ft): what is normal? [Thilo] 1137 (Oc)
Commerce
Physicians, formula companies, and advertising: a historical perspective [Greer] 282 (Mr)
Commotio Cordis
Commotio cordis: the single, most common cause of traumatic death in youth baseball [Abrunzo] 1279 (No)
Community Health Services
American Academy of Pediatrics response to the growing health needs of children [Strain] 536 (My)
Comprehensive Health Care
Redoing the health care quilt: patches or whole cloth? [Cleveland] 499 (My)
Computer-Assisted Instruction
Comparison of a computer tutorial with other methods for teaching well-newborn care [Desch] 1255 (No)
Computers
Improved speed and accuracy of calculations with a programmable calculator in pediatric emergency scenarios [Melzer-Lange] 264 (Mr)
Condylomata acuminata
Condylomata acuminata: still usually a sexually transmitted disease in children (letter) [Goldenring] 600, (reply) [Boyd] 601 (Je)
Diagnosis of child sexual abuse in children with genital warts (letter) [Gutman] (reply) [Boyd] 126 (Fe)
Congenital Defects see Abnormalities
Continuity of Patient Care
Eighty-hour workweek and residency programs: closing arguments (letter) [Bedrick] 846 (Au)
Contraception
Complex problem: complex solutions [McAnarney] 429 (Ap)
Contraceptive Devices
Acquired immunodeficiency syndrome and adolescents: knowledge, attitudes, and behaviors of runaway and homeless youths [Sugerman] 431 (Ap)
Contusions
Safety of a preadolescent basketball program [Gutgesell] 1023 (Se)
Convulsions
Cat-scratch disease: acute encephalopathy and other neurologic manifestations [Carithers] 98 (Ja)
Water intoxication: a prevalent problem in the inner city [Finberg] 981 (Se)
Coronary Arteriosclerosis
Lipoprotein profiles in hypercholesterolemic children [Garcia] 147 (Fe); correction, 515 (My)
Sudden cardiac death in young athletes: a review [McCaffrey] 177 (Fe)
Coronary Artery Disease see Coronary Disease
Coronary Disease
Evolution of surgical treatment for congenital cardiac disease [Pigott] 1362 (De)
Family history fails to identify many children with severe hypercholesterolemia [Starc] 61 (Ja)
Family history of myocardial infarction and hemodynamic responses to exercise in young black boys [Treiber] 1029 (Se)
Sudden cardiac death in young athletes: a review [McCaffrey] 177 (Fe)
Coronary Vessels
Sudden cardiac death in young athletes: a review [McCaffrey] 177 (Fe)
CORRECTIONS
Acquired methemoglobinemia: the relationship of cause to course of illness [Avner] **144**:1229 (No); correction, **145**:158 (Fe)
Effect of necrotizing enterocolitis on urinary epidermal growth factor levels [Scott] 804 (Jy); correction, 982 (Se)
Evaluation of intraosseus vs intravenous antibiotic levels in a porcine model [Jaimovich] 946 (Au); correction, 1241 (No)
Intraosseous infusion of dobutamine and isoproterenol [Bilello] 165 (Fe); correction, 1312 (No)
Lipoprotein profiles in hypercholesterolemic children [Garcia] 147 (Fe); correction, 515 (My)
Corticosteroids see Adrenal Cortex Hormones
Cortisol see Hydrocortisone
Cost Benefit Analysis
Cardiac care for infants: determinants of hospital charges for acute care [Pearson] 1397 (De)
Home care cost-effectiveness for respiratory technology-dependent children [Fields] 729 (Jy)
Cost Control
Children's services in an era of budget deficits [Blum] 575 (My)
Saving money with home care [Schoumacher] 725 (Jy)
Cost Effectiveness see Cost Benefit Analysis
Costs and Cost Analysis
Multilevel model to assess appropriateness of pediatric serum drug concentrations [Kraus] 1171 (Oc)
Cranial Nerve Diseases
Cat-scratch disease: acute encephalopathy and other neurologic manifestations [Carithers] 98 (Ja)
Creatine Kinase
Hyperpyrexia, hemorrhagic shock and encephalopathy, and creatinine phosphokinase (letter) [Dupee] 719 (Jy)
Creatine Phosphokinase see Creatine Kinase
Creatinine
Effect of necrotizing enterocolitis on urinary epidermal growth factor levels [Scott] 804 (Jy); correction, 982 (Se)
50-year follow-up of childhood plumbism: hypertension, renal function, and hemoglobin levels among survivors [Hu] 681 (Je)
Hyperpyrexia, hemorrhagic shock and encephalopathy, and creatinine phosphokinase (letter) [Dupee] 719 (Jy)
Crime
Legalization of drugs of abuse and the pediatrician [Schwartz] 1153 (Oc)
Tattooing behavior in adolescence: a comparison study [Farrow] 184 (Fe)
Criminal Law
Legalization of drugs of abuse and the pediatrician [Schwartz] 1153 (Oc)
Crippled see Handicapped
Cross Infection
Anergy in pediatric head trauma patients [Wilson] 326 (Mr)
Arterial catheter-related infections in children: a 1-year cohort analysis [Furfaro] 1037 (Se)
Influenza type A and B infections in hospitalized pediatric patients: who should be immunized? [Serwint] 623 (Je)
Cultural Evolution
Paleonephrology and reflux nephropathy: from the 'big bang' to end-stage renal disease [Kallen] 860 (Au)
Cyanosis
Acquired methemoglobinemia: the relationship of cause to course of illness [Avner] **144**:1229(No); correction, **145**:158 (Fe)
Retinopathy of prematurity in infants with cyanotic congenital heart disease [Johns] 200 (Fe)
Cystic Fibrosis
Differences in expression of cystic fibrosis in blacks and whites [McColley] 94 (Ja)
Laparoscopic cholecystectomy under continuous epidural anesthesia in patients with cystic fibrosis (letter) [Edelman] 723 (Jy)
Taurine decreases fecal fatty acid and sterol excretion in cystic fibrosis: a randomized double-blind trial [Smith] 1401 (De)
Cysts
Adipsic hypernatremia in 2 sisters [Radetti] 321 (Mr)
Cytochrome C Oxidase see Cytochrome Oxidase
Cytochrome Oxidase
Autosomal recessive lethal infantile cytochrome C oxidase deficiency [Eshel] 661 (Je)
Cytomegaloviruses
Guidelines for auditing pediatric blood transfusion practices [Blanchette] 787 (Jy)
Neonatal hepatitis and extrahepatic biliary atresia associated with cytomegalovirus infection in twins [Hart] 302 (Mr)
Transfusion therapy in neonates [Strauss] 904 (Au)

D

Data Analysis, Statistical see Data Interpretation, Statistical
Data Interpretation, Statistical
Child sexual abuse and human immunodeficiency virus transmission (letter) [Monteleone] (reply) [Gutman] 847 (Au)
Child survival and perinatal infections with human immunodeficiency virus [Bennett] 1242 (No)
Diagnosis of child sexual abuse in children with genital warts (letter) [Gutman] (reply) [Boyd] 126 (Fe)
More on the *P value* (letter) [Coulter] (reply) [Brown] 249 (Mr)
Multiple comparisons and *P* values (letter) [Newman] 250 (Mr)
Neuroblastoma screening data: an epidemiologic analysis [Goodman] 1415 (De)
P values (letter) [Byrt] 250 (Mr)
Death, Sudden
Sudden cardiac death (letter) [Pearl] 1223 (No)
Sudden cardiac death in young athletes: a review [McCaffrey] 177 (Fe)
Decision Making
Treatment withdrawal in neonates (letter) [Byrne] 1223 (No)
Deferoxamine
Total iron-binding capacity in iron poisoning: is it useful? [Tenenbein] 437 (Ap)
Deficiency Diseases
Alkaline urine is associated with eating disorders (letter) [Arden] 28 (Ja)
Zinc deficiency: a public health problem? [Sandstead] 853 (Au)
Deglutition
Esophageal motility in children with Hirschsprung's disease [Staiano] 310 (Mr)
Dehydration
Acquired methemoglobinemia: the relationship of cause to course of illness [Avner] **144**:1229(No); correction, **145**:158 (Fe)
Capillary refilling (skin turgor) in the assessment of dehydration [Saavedra] 296 (Mr)
Differences in expression of cystic fibrosis in blacks and whites [McColley] 94 (Ja)
Water intoxication: a prevalent problem in the inner city [Finberg] 981 (Se)
Delivery
Congenital syphilis associated with negative results of maternal serologic tests at delivery (letter) [Sánchez] 967 (Se)
Vertical transmission of human immunodeficiency virus from seronegative or indeterminate mothers [Johnson] 1239 (No)
Delivery of Health Care
Challenge of care for the poor and underserved in the United States: an American College of Obstetricians and Gynecologists perspective on access to care for underserved women [Davidson] 546 (My)
Challenge of caring for indigent children with rheumatologic diseases [Miller] 554 (My)
Children's services in an era of budget deficits [Blum] 575 (My)
Far from the ideal: the plight of poor children in the United States [Fulginiti] 489 (My)
Improving health care provision to neonates in the United States [Stahlman] 510 (My)
New initiatives in adolescent health promotion [Elster] 495 (My)
Pediatric acquired immunodeficiency syndrome, poverty, and national priorities [Heagarty] 527 (My)
Redoing the health care quilt: patches or whole cloth? [Cleveland] 499 (My)
Regional pediatric approach to the epidemic of social ills within our cities [Nelson] 505 (My)
Youth alienation as an emerging pediatric health care issue [Farrow] 491 (My)
Dependency (Psychology)
Adolescents with chronic illness [Perrin] 1361 (De)
Dermatitis
Acrodermatitis enteropathica [Schneider] 211 (Fe)
Dermatomyositis
Challenge of caring for indigent children with rheumatologic diseases [Miller] 554 (My)
Juvenile dermatomyositis [Tunnessen] 1161 (Oc)
Desensitization, Immunologic
Trimethoprim-sulfamethoxazole oral desensitization in hemophiliacs infected with human immunodeficiency virus with a history of hypersensitivity reactions [Kletzel] 1428 (De)
Desmopressin

Adipsic hypernatremia in 2 sisters [Radetti] 321 (Mr)
Developing Countries
Child survival and perinatal infections with human immunodeficiency virus [Bennett] 1242 (No)
Formula companies and the medical profession (letter) [Newman] 1089, (reply) [Greer] 1090 (Oc)
Dexamethasone
Endotoxin concentrations in cerebrospinal fluid correlate with clinical severity and neurologic outcome of *Haemophilus influenzae* type b meningitis [Mertsola] 1099 (Oc)
Role of corticosteroid therapy in children with pneumococcal meningitis [Kennedy] 1374 (De)
Survey of antiemetic use in children with cancer [van Hoff] 773 (Jy)
Dextroamphetamine
Stimulant medication and attention deficit-hyperactivity disorder: the child's perspective [Bowen] 291 (Mr)
Diabetes Mellitus
Neurodevelopmental outcome of offspring of the diabetic mother: need for further research (letter) [Goldstein] 602 (Je)
Diagnosis
Anal fissure produced by examination for sexual abuse (letter) [Baker] 848, (reply) [Bays] 849 (Au)
Buddy, can you paradigm? [Brown] 727 (Jy)
Causes of hospital-treated acute lower respiratory tract infection in children [Nohynek] 618 (Je)
Clavicular fractures in neonates (letter) [Carter] 251, (reply) [Joseph] 252 (Mr)
Clavicular fractures in neonates: frequency vs significance (letter) [O'Halloran] (reply) [Joseph] 251 (Mr)
Clinic attending: teaching strategies for patient encounters [Schmitt] 977 (Se)
Congenital syphilis [Giacola] 1045 (Se)
Detection of alcoholism in hospitalized children and their families [Duggan] 613 (Je)
Diagnosis of child sexual abuse in children with genital warts (letter) [Gutman] (reply) [Boyd] 126 (Fe)
Direct bilirubin measurements in jaundiced term newborns: a reevaluation [Newman] 1305 (No)
Fetal alcohol syndrome: misplaced emphasis (letter) [Hess] (reply) [Little] 721 (Jy)
Gilding the lily (letter) [Faigel] (reply) [Myer] 849 (Au)
Henoch-Schönlein Purpura [Tunnessen] 823 (Jy)
Hydrocele in Kawasaki disease: importance in early recognition of atypical disease (letter) [Kabani] 1348 (De)
Juvenile dermatomyositis [Tunnessen] 1161 (Oc)
Marfanoid children: etiologic heterogeneity and cardiac findings [Tayel] 90 (Ja)
Mediterranean visceral leishmaniasis: a frequently unrecognized imported disease (letter) [Mahieu] 1225 (No)
Mitral valve prolapse: back to the basics [Allen] 1095 (Oc)
Outpatient assessment of infants with bronchiolitis [Shaw] 151 (Fe)
Parental alcoholism: a neglected pediatric responsibility [MacDonald] 609 (Je)
Sudden cardiac death in young athletes: a review [McCaffrey] 177 (Fe)
Vertical transmission of human immunodeficiency virus from seronegative or indeterminate mothers [Johnson] 1239 (No)
Diagnosis, Differential
Epidemic nephropathy in children [Lautala] 1181 (Oc)
Fallacy of the hemorrhagic shock and encephalopathy syndrome (letter) [Bass] 718 (Jy)
Gallstones in children (letter) [Todd] 971 (Se)
'H' in hemorrhagic shock and encephalopathy syndrome (letter) [Roscelli] 720 (Jy)
Hemorrhagic shock and encephalopathy: an entity similar to heatstroke (letter) [Conway] 720 (Jy)
Hyperpyrexia, hemorrhagic shock and encephalopathy, and creatinine phosphokinase (letter) [Dupee] 719 (Jy)
Testing the psychogenic vomiting diagnosis: four pediatric patients [Gonzalez-Heydrich] 913 (Au)
Diagnostic Errors
Misdiagnosis of Reye's-like illness (letter) [Forsyth] 964 (Se)
Mitral valve prolapse: back to the basics [Allen] 1095 (Oc)
Diagnostic Tests, Routine
Cholesterol testing in the physician's office: accuracy assessment (letter) [Rifai] 1087 (Oc)
Diarrhea
Acrodermatitis enteropathica [Schneider] 211 (Fe)
Diarrhea, Infantile
Capillary refilling (skin turgor) in the assessment of dehydration [Saavedra] 296 (Mr)
Rice solution and World Health Organization solution by gastric infusion for high stool output diarrhea [Mota-Hernández] 937 (Au)
Dickens, Charles
Tiny Tim remembered [Callahan] 1355 (De)
Diet
Dietary calcium and bone mineral status of children and adolescents [Chan] 631 (Je)
Zinc deficiency: a public health problem? [Sandstead] 853 (Au)
Diet, Reducing
Demographic and risk factors associated with chronic dieting in adolescents [Story] 994 (Se)
Diet Therapy
Intellectual development in 12-year-old children treated for phenylketonuria [Azen] 35 (Ja)
Paleonephrology and reflux nephropathy: from the 'big bang' to end-stage renal disease [Kallen] 860 (Au)
Serum lipid concentrations in subjects with phenylketonuria and their families [DeClue] 1266 (No)
Status report on phenylketonuria treatment: 1990 [Mabry] 33 (Ja)
Digoxin
Multilevel model to assess appropriateness of pediatric serum drug concentrations [Kraus] 1171 (Oc)
Dihydroxycholecalciferols
Mineral metabolism and calcitriol therapy in idiopathic juvenile osteoporosis [Saggese] 457 (Ap)
Dihydroxyvitamins D see Dihydroxycholecalciferols
Diphenhydramine
Survey of antiemetic use in children with cancer [van Hoff] 773 (Jy)
Diphtheria-Tetanus-Pertussis Vaccine
Apparent decreased risk of invasive bacterial disease after heterologous childhood immunization [Black] 746 (Jy)
Diphtheria and tetanus toxoids and pertussis vaccine litigation (letter) [Lokietz] (reply) [Fulginiti] 425 (Ap)
DTP immunization and susceptibility to infectious diseases: is there a relationship? [Davidson] 750 (Jy)
Vaccine myth and physician handouts (letter) [Lynch] 426, (replies) [Cherry, Fulginiti] 426, 427 (Ap)
Diphtheria Toxoid
Comparative trial of the reactogenicity and immunogenicity of Takeda acellular pertussis vaccine combined with tetanus and diphtheria toxoids: outcome in 3- to 8-month old infants, 9- to 23-month-old infants and children, and 24- to 30-month-old children [Kimura] 734 (Jy)
Immunization response varies with intensity of acute lymphoblastic leukemia therapy [Ridgway] 887 (Au)
Vaccine myth and physician handouts (letter) [Lynch] 426, (replies) [Cherry, Fulginiti] 426, 427 (Ap)
Diuresis
Medical management of postobstructive polyuria (letter) [Smoyer] 1345 (De)
Diuretics
Association of alkaline urine with eating disorders (letter) [Robson] (reply) [Arden] 1091 (Oc)
Demographic and risk factors associated with chronic dieting in adolescents [Story] 994 (Se)
Diuretics, Thiazide
Medical management of postobstructive polyuria (letter) [Smoyer] 1345 (De)
DNA, Recombinant
Neutropenia in an extremely premature infant treated with recombinant human granulocyte colony-stimulating factor [Roberts] 808 (Jy)
Word choice (letter) [Gorlick] (reply) [Hong] 724 (Jy)
Dobutamine
Intraosseous infusion of dobutamine and isoproterenol [Bilello] 165 (Fe); correction, 1312 (No)
Documentation
Multilevel model to assess appropriateness of pediatric serum drug concentrations [Kraus] 1171 (Oc)
Domperidone
Survey of antiemetic use in children with cancer [van Hoff] 773 (Jy)
Dopamine
Effect of low-dose dopamine infusion on cardiopulmonary and renal status in premature newborns with respiratory distress syndrome [Cuevas] 799 (Jy)
Elevated plasma norepinephrine levels in infants of substance-abusing mothers [Ward] 44 (Ja)
Dose-Response Relationship, Immunologic
Antibody response to MMR vaccination in children who received IVIG as neonates (letter) [Ruderman] 425 (Ap)
Double-Blind Method
Taurine decreases fecal fatty acid and sterol excretion in cystic fibrosis: a randomized double-blind trial [Smith] 1401 (De)
Down's Syndrome
Age-related patterns of thyroid-stimulating hormone response to thyrotropin-releasing hormone stimulation in Down syndrome [Sharav] 172 (Fe)
Syringomas in Down syndrome (letter) [Feingold] 966 (Se)
Drainage
Posthemorrhagic hydrocephalus: use of an intravenous-type catheter for cerebrospinal fluid drainage [Marro] 1141 (Oc)
Drowning
Immersion events in residential swimming pools: evidence for an experience effect [Wintemute] 1200 (Oc)
Drug Abuse see Substance Abuse
Drug Administration Routes
Evaluation of intraosseus vs intravenous antibiotic levels in a porcine model [Jaimovich] 946 (Au); correction, 1241 (No)
Intraosseous infusion of dobutamine and isoproterenol [Bilello] 165 (Fe); correction, 1312 (No)
Drug Industry
Exhibitor "giveaways": a curmudgeon's view (letter) [Berger] 427 (Ap)
Drug Resistance, Microbial
Impetigo [Esterly] 125 (Fe)
Drug Therapy
Improved speed and accuracy of calculations with a programmable calculator in pediatric emergency scenarios [Melzer-Lange] 264 (Mr)
Survey of antiemetic use in children with cancer [van Hoff] 773 (Jy)
Drug Therapy, Combination
Effect of valproic acid on plasma carnitine levels [Opala] 999 (Se)
Drug Utilization
Multilevel model to assess appropriateness of pediatric serum drug concentrations [Kraus] 1171 (Oc)
DSM-III
Buddy, can you paradigm? [Brown] 727 (Jy)
Ductus Arteriosus, Patent
Ductal patency in neonates with respiratory distress syndrome: a randomized surfactant trial [Reller] 1017 (Se)
Dwarfism
Laron-type dwarfism [Laron] 473 (Ap)
Dyes
Treatment of ulcerated hemangiomas with pulsed tunable dye laser [Morelli] 1062 (Se)

E

Eagle's Syndrome
Pediatric case of Eagle's syndrome [Holloway] 339 (Mr)
Ear Canal
Influence of otitis media on the correlation between rectal and auditory canal temperatures [Terndrup] 75 (Ja)
Ear Diseases
Herpes zoster oticus (letter) [Rathore] 722 (Jy)
Eating Disorders
Alkaline urine is associated with eating disorders (letter) [Arden] 28 (Ja)
Association of alkaline urine with eating disorders (letter) [Robson] (reply) [Arden] 1091 (Oc)
Demographic and risk factors associated with chronic dieting in adolescents [Story] 994 (Se)
Echocardiography
Marfanoid children: etiologic heterogeneity and cardiac findings [Tayel] 90 (Ja)
Economics, Hospital
Cardiac care for infants: determinants of hospital charges for acute care [Pearson] 1397 (De)
Economics, Medical
Children's services in an era of budget deficits [Blum] 575 (My)
Far from the ideal: the plight of poor children in the United States [Fulginiti] 489 (My)
Formula companies and the medical profession (letter) [Newman] 1089, (reply) [Greer] 1090 (Oc)
Health care for uninsured and underinsured children (letter) [Barness] 1086 (Oc)
Improving health care provision to neonates in the United States [Stahlman] 510 (My)
Redoing the health care quilt: patches or whole cloth? [Cleveland] 499 (My)
Edema
Subcutaneous fat necrosis of the newborn [Vera] 1047 (Se)
EDITORIAL BOARD SPEAKS
Buddy, can you paradigm? [Brown] 727 (Jy)
Clinic attending: teaching strategies for patient encounters [Schmitt] 977 (Se)
Complex problem: complex solutions [McAnarney] 429 (Ap)
Grampa, can I get something that I'd like? [Strong] 1355 (De)
Losing time [Pruitt] 607 (Je)
Mitral valve prolapse: back to the basics [Allen] 1095 (Oc)
Part-time Peg: who, me? [Ferry] 852 (Au)
Tell the whole story [Johnson] 135 (Fe)
Your child's best friend: TV or not TV [Stiehm] 257 (Mr)
Education
Clinic-based intervention to promote literacy: a pilot study [Needlman] 881 (Au)
Your child's best friend: TV or not TV? (letter) [Bader] (reply) [Stiehm] 963 (Se)
Education, Medical
Comparison of a computer tutorial with other methods for teaching well-newborn care [Desch] 1255 (No)
Improved speed and accuracy of calculations with a programmable calculator in pediatric emergency scenarios [Melzer-Lange] 264 (Mr)
Poverty and the health of American children: implications for academic pediatrics [Johnston] 507 (My)
Education, Medical, Continuing
Adolescent pelvic examination: an effective practical approach [Tolmas] 1269 (No)
Hand washing in pediatric ambulatory settings: an inconsistent practice [Lohr] 1198 (Oc)
Education, Medical, Graduate
Chief resident training: developing leadership skills for future medical leaders [Doughty] 639 (Je)
Clinic attending: teaching strategies for patient encounters [Schmitt] 977 (Se)
Current trends in pediatric residency training [Carraccio] 1272 (No)
Eighty-hour workweek and residency programs: closing arguments (letter) [Bedrick] 846 (Au)
Hand washing in pediatric ambulatory settings: an inconsistent practice [Lohr] 1198 (Oc)

How are pediatric training programs preparing residents for practice? [Greenberg] 1389 (De)
Medical ethics issues survey of residents in 5 pediatric training programs [White] 161 (Fe)
Objective structured clinical examination in a pediatric residency program [Joorabchi] 757 (Jy)
Pediatric program director: an analysis of the role and its problems [Weiss] 449 (Ap)
Practice management training for pediatric residents [Piatt] 299 (Mr)
Resident and nurse practitioners: responding to education and patient care needs (letter) [Giardino] 843 (Au)
Resident, faculty, and residency program development: an integrated approach through annual retreats [Winter] 1191 (Oc)
School health training during pediatric residency [Niebuhr] 79 (Ja)
Serving the underserved: impact on resident education [Berkowitz] 544 (My)
Support services for pediatric trainees: a survey of training program directors [Bergman] 1002 (Se)
Educational Achievement see Educational Status
EDUCATIONAL INTERVENTIONS
Chief resident training: developing leadership skills for future medical leaders [Doughty] 639 (Je)
Clinic-based intervention to promote literacy: a pilot study [Needlman] 881 (Au)
Comparison of a computer tutorial with other methods for teaching well-newborn care [Desch] 1255 (No)
Current trends in pediatric residency training [Carraccio] 1272 (No)
How are pediatric training programs preparing residents for practice? [Greenberg] 1389 (De)
Medical ethics issues survey of residents in 5 pediatric training programs [White] 161 (Fe)
Objective structured clinical examination in a pediatric residency program [Joorabchi] 757 (Jy)
Pediatric program director: an analysis of the role and its problems [Weiss] 449 (Ap)
Practice management training for pediatric residents [Piatt] 299 (Mr)
Resident, faculty, and residency program development: an integrated approach through annual retreats [Winter] 1191 (Oc)
School health training during pediatric residency [Niebuhr] 79 (Ja)
Sun protection in newborns: a comparison of educational methods [Bolognia] 1125 (Oc)
Support services for pediatric trainees: a survey of training program directors [Bergman] 1002 (Se)
Educational Measurement
Objective structured clinical examination in a pediatric residency program [Joorabchi] 757 (Jy)
Educational Status
Adolescents' attrition from school-sponsored sports [DuRant] 1119 (Oc)
Breast-feeding initiation in a triethnic population [Bee] 306 (Mr)
Differences in infant mortality by race, nativity status, and other maternal characteristics [Kleinman] 194 (Fe)
Tattooing behavior in adolescence: a comparison study [Farrow] 184 (Fe)
Efficiency
Children's services in an era of budget deficits [Blum] 575 (My)
Tell the whole story [Johnson] 135 (Fe)
Elasticity
Capillary refilling (skin turgor) in the assessment of dehydration [Saavedra] 296 (Mr)
Emergency Medical Services
Improved speed and accuracy of calculations with a programmable calculator in pediatric emergency scenarios [Melzer-Lange] 264 (Mr)
Intraosseous infusion of dobutamine and isoproterenol [Bilello] 165 (Fe); correction, 1312 (No)
Emergency Service, Hospital
Barriers to medical care for homeless families compared with housed poor families [Wood] 1109 (Oc)
Improving the use of early follow-up care after emergency department visits: a randomized trial [Nelson] 440 (Ap)
Emigration and Immigration
Differences in infant mortality by race, nativity status, and other maternal characteristics [Kleinman] 194 (Fe)
Employment
Care of the poor and underserved in America: older adolescents: a group at special risk [Haggerty] 569 (My)
Health care for uninsured and underinsured children (letter) [Kirschner] 1085 (Oc)
House staff work hours and moonlighting: what do residents want?: a survey of pediatric residents in California [Cheng] 1104 (Oc)
Losing time [Pruitt] 607 (Je)
Encephalitis
Cat-scratch disease: acute encephalopathy and other neurologic manifestations [Carithers] 98 (Ja)
Diphtheria and tetanus toxoids and pertussis vaccine litigation (letter) [Lokietz] (reply) [Fulginiti] 425 (Ap)
More on a myth (letter) [Roman] (reply) [Fulginiti] 717 (Jy)
Vaccine myth and physician handouts (letter) [Lynch] 426, (replies) [Cherry, Fulginiti] 426, 427 (Ap)
Endemic Nephropathy, Balkan see Balkan Nephropathy
Endocrine Glands
Endocrine function in children with human immunodeficiency virus infection [Schwartz] 330 (Mr)
Endotoxins
Endotoxin concentrations in cerebrospinal fluid correlate with clinical severity and neurologic outcome of *Haemophilus influenzae* type b meningitis [Mertsola] 1099 (Oc)
Hemorrhagic shock and encephalopathy: an entity similar to heatstroke (letter) [Conway] 720 (Jy)
Energy Expenditure see Energy Metabolism
Energy Metabolism
Physiologic responses to playing a video game [Segal] 1034 (Se)
Enterocolitis, Necrotizing see Enterocolitis, Pseudomembranous
Enterocolitis, Pseudomembranous
Characteristics of perinatal cocaine-exposed infants with necrotizing enterocolitis (letter) [Downing] 26 (Ja)
Effect of necrotizing enterocolitis on urinary epidermal growth factor levels [Scott] 804 (Jy); correction, 982 (Se)
Enuresis
Nintendo enuresis (letter) [Schink] 1094 (Oc)
Enzyme Tests
Juvenile dermatomyositis [Tunnessen] 1161 (Oc)
Eosinophils
Percentile curves for various hematologic measurements at birth in Arab preterm babies of different gestational ages [Haque] 645 (Je)
Epidemiologic Methods
Neuroblastoma screening data: an epidemiologic analysis [Goodman] 1415 (De)
Epidermal Growth Factor see Epidermal Growth Factor-Urogastrone
Epidermal Growth Factor-Urogastrone
Effect of necrotizing enterocolitis on urinary epidermal growth factor levels [Scott] 804 (Jy); correction, 982 (Se)
Epilepsy
Cortical resection for children with epilepsy: perspectives in pediatrics [Wyllie] 314 (Mr)
Epilepsy, Focal
Cortical resection for children with epilepsy: perspectives in pediatrics [Wyllie] 314 (Mr)
Epinephrine
Elevated plasma norepinephrine levels in infants of substance-abusing mothers [Ward] 44 (Ja)
Epistaxis
Safety of a preadolescent basketball program [Gutgesell] 1023 (Se)
Equipment and Supplies
Photographing the physically abused child, principles and practice [Ricci] 275 (Mr)
Equipment Safety
Use of infant walkers [AMA Board of Trustees] 933 (Au)
Erythrocyte Count
Percentile curves for various hematologic measurements at birth in Arab preterm babies of different gestational ages [Haque] 645 (Je)
Erythrocyte Sedimentation see Blood Sedimentation
Erythrocytes
Guidelines for auditing pediatric blood transfusion practices [Blanchette] 787 (Jy)
Transfusion therapy in neonates [Strauss] 904 (Au)
Erythromycin
Impetigo [Esterly] 125 (Fe)
Escherichia coli Infections
Escherichia coli bacteremia in children: a review of 91 cases in 10 years [Bonadio] 671 (Je)
Esophageal Achalasia
Testing the psychogenic vomiting diagnosis: four pediatric patients [Gonzalez-Heydrich] 913 (Au)
Esophageal Motility Disorders
Esophageal motility in children with Hirschsprung's disease [Staiano] 310 (Mr)
Esophageal Sphincter see Esophagogastric Junction
Esophagogastric Junction
Esophageal motility in children with Hirschsprung's disease [Staiano] 310 (Mr)
Value of subject height in predicting lower esophageal sphincter location [Staiano] 1424 (De)
Ethics, Medical
Medical ethics issues survey of residents in 5 pediatric training programs [White] 161 (Fe)
Treatment withdrawal in neonates (letter) [Byrne] 1223 (No)
Ethnic Groups
Breast-feeding initiation in a triethnic population [Bee] 306 (Mr)
Prevalence and impact of chronic illness among adolescents [Newacheck] 1367 (De)
Ethosuximide
Effect of valproic acid on plasma carnitine levels [Opala] 999 (Se)
Evaluation Studies
Support services for pediatric trainees: a survey of training program directors [Bergman] 1002 (Se)
Evoked Potentials, Auditory, Brain Stem
Evaluation of auditory brain-stem response in full-term infants of cocaine-abusing mothers [Carzoli] 1013 (Se)
Evoked Responses, Auditory, Brain Stem see Evoked Potentials, Auditory, Brain Stem
Exercise
Effects of obesity on aerobic fitness in adolescent females [Rowland] 764 (Jy)
Family history of myocardial infarction and hemodynamic responses to exercise in young black boys [Treiber] 1029 (Se)
Pediatric cardiac rehabilitation [Balfour] 627 (Je)
Exercise Test
Cardiopulmonary exercise testing in children following surgery for tetralogy of Fallot [Tomassoni] 1290 (No)
Effects of obesity on aerobic fitness in adolescent females [Rowland] 764 (Jy)
Family history of myocardial infarction and hemodynamic responses to exercise in young black boys [Treiber] 1029 (Se)
Pediatric cardiac rehabilitation [Balfour] 627 (Je)
Exhibits
Exhibitor 'giveaways': a curmudgeon's view (letter) [Berger] 427 (Ap)
Extracorporeal Membrane Oxygenation
Poverty and the health of American children: implications for academic pediatrics [Johnston] 507 (My)
Eye Abnormalities
Brain and ocular abnormalities in infants with in utero exposure to cocaine and other street drugs [Dominguez] 688 (Je)

F

Face
Antley-Bixler syndrome [Butler] 701 (Je)
Facial Neoplasms
Syringomas in Down syndrome (letter) [Feingold] 966 (Se)
Facial Nerve
Herpes zoster oticus (letter) [Rathore] 722 (Jy)
Facial Paralysis
Herpes zoster oticus (letter) [Rathore] 722 (Jy)
Factor VIII
Guidelines for auditing pediatric blood transfusion practices [Blanchette] 787 (Jy)
Factor IX
Guidelines for auditing pediatric blood transfusion practices [Blanchette] 787 (Jy)
Faculty, Medical
Clinic attending: teaching strategies for patient encounters [Schmitt] 977 (Se)
Hand washing in pediatric ambulatory settings: an inconsistent practice [Lohr] 1198 (Oc)
Medical ethics issues survey of residents in 5 pediatric training programs [White] 161 (Fe)
Part-time Peg: who, me? [Ferry] 852 (Au)
Pediatric program director: an analysis of the role and its problems [Weiss] 449 (Ap)
Priorities in academic pediatrics (letter) [Jacobs] (reply) [Goetzman] 845 (Au)
Regional pediatric approach to the epidemic of social ills within our cities [Nelson] 505 (My)
Resident, faculty, and residency program development: an integrated approach through annual retreats [Winter] 1191 (Oc)
Tell the whole story [Johnson] 135 (Fe)
Fallot's Tetralogy see Tetralogy of Fallot
Falls, Accidental see Accidental Falls
Family
Barriers to medical care for homeless families compared with housed poor families [Wood] 1109 (Oc)
Challenge of caring for indigent children with rheumatologic diseases [Miller] 554 (My)
Child abuse and neglect: critical first steps in response to a national emergency: the report of the US Advisory Board on Child Abuse and Neglect [Krugman] 513 (My)
Comments on life after residency (letter) [Brent] 597 (Je)
Detection of alcoholism in hospitalized children and their families [Duggan] 613 (Je)
Family history fails to identify many children with severe hypercholesterolemia [Starc] 61 (Ja)
Family history of myocardial infarction and hemodynamic responses to exercise in young black boys [Treiber] 1029 (Se)
Grampa, can I get something that I'd like? [Strong] 1355 (De)
Guidelines for safe transportation of children in wheelchairs [DiGaudio] 653 (Je)
Health care for pregnant women and young children [Behrman] 572 (My)
Human immunodeficiency virus transmission by child sexual abuse [Gutman] 137 (Fe)
Medical ethics issues survey of residents in 5 pediatric training programs [White] 161 (Fe)
Occult cocaine exposure in children [Rosenberg] 1430 (De)
Pediatric acquired immunodeficiency syndrome, poverty, and national priorities [Heagarty] 527 (My)
Pediatric human immunodeficiency virus infection and the acquired immunodeficiency syndrome: a health care crisis of children and families [Van Dyke] 529 (My)
Survey of the health of homeless children in Philadelphia shelters [Parker] 520 (My)
Tattooing behavior in adolescence: a comparison study [Farrow] 184 (Fe)

Testing the psychogenic vomiting diagnosis: four pediatric patients [Gonzalez-Heydrich] 913 (Au)
Tracking of elevated blood pressure values in adolescent athletes at 1-year follow-up [Tanji] 665 (Je)
Your child's best friend: TV or not TV? (letter) [Bader] (reply) [Stiehm] 963 (Se)
Youth alienation as an emerging pediatric health care issue [Farrow] 491 (My)
Family Planning
Challenge of care for the poor and underserved in the United States: an American College of Obstetricians and Gynecologists perspective on access to care for underserved women [Davidson] 546 (My)
Family Practice
Family physicians and neonatology (letter) [McIntyre] (reply) [DiTraglia] 963 (Se)
Fat Necrosis
Subcutaneous fat necrosis of the newborn [Vera] 1047 (Se)
Fatty Acids
Taurine decreases fecal fatty acid and sterol excretion in cystic fibrosis: a randomized double-blind trial [Smith] 1401 (De)
Fatty Acids, Unsaturated
Serum lipid concentrations in subjects with phenylketonuria and their families [DeClue] 1266 (No)
Feces
Rice solution and World Health Organization solution by gastric infusion for high stool output diarrhea [Mota-Hernández] 937 (Au)
Taurine decreases fecal fatty acid and sterol excretion in cystic fibrosis: a randomized double-blind trial [Smith] 1401 (De)
Fees and Charges
Cardiac care for infants: determinants of hospital charges for acute care [Pearson] 1397 (De)
Fetal Alcohol Syndrome
Fetal alcohol syndrome: misplaced emphasis (letter) [Hess] (reply) [Little] 721 (Jy)
Fetal Development
Studies in fetal malnutrition [Crosby] 871 (Au)
Fetal Distress
How much of neonatal encephalopathy is due to birth asphyxia? [Nelson] 1325 (No)
Fetal Growth Retardation
Prevalence of birth defects among low-birth-weight infants: a population study [Mili] 1313 (No)
Fetal Monitoring
How much of neonatal encephalopathy is due to birth asphyxia? [Nelson] 1325 (No)
Fetus
Nevus flammeus: discordance in monozygotic twins [Shamir] 85 (Ja)
Fever
'H' in hemorrhagic shock and encephalopathy syndrome (letter) [Roscelli] 720 (Jy)
Hemorrhagic shock and encephalopathy: an entity similar to heatstroke (letter) [Conway] 720 (Jy)
Hydrocele in Kawasaki disease: importance in early recognition of atypical disease (letter) [Kabani] 1348 (De)
Hyperpyrexia, hemorrhagic shock and encephalopathy, and creatinine phosphokinase (letter) [Dupee] 719 (Jy)
Fibroma
Thorn-induced pseudotumor of the tibia [Kozlowski] 1159 (Oc)
Fingersucking
Send Linus to me (letter) [Szonyi] (reply) [Friman] 1227 (No)
Thumb-sucking (letter) [Lubicky] 845, (reply) [Friman] 846 (Au)
Finland
Causes of hospital-treated acute lower respiratory tract infection in children [Nohynek] 618 (Je)
Epidemic nephropathy in children [Lautala] 1181 (Oc)
Fluid Therapy
Improved speed and accuracy of calculations with a programmable calculator in pediatric emergency scenarios [Melzer-Lange] 264 (Mr)
Improvement of leukemic hyperleukocytosis with only fluid and allopurinol therapy (letter) [Lascari] 969 (Se)
Rice solution and World Health Organization solution by gastric infusion for high stool output diarrhea [Mota-Hernández] 937 (Au)
Fluorescent Antinuclear Antibodies see Antibodies, Antinuclear
Food, Fortified
How much iron is enough? (letter) [Rogers] (reply) [Finberg] 598 (Je)
Rickets caused by vitamin D deficiency in breast-fed infants in the southern United States [Bhowmick] 127 (Fe)
Food, Supplemented see Food Fortified
Foot
Puncture wound-induced *Achromobacter xylosoxidans* osteomyelitis of the foot (letter) [Hoddy] 599 (Je)
Foot Dermatoses
Acropustulosis of infancy [Friedman] 341 (Mr)
Football
Adolescents' attrition from school-sponsored sports [Durant] 1119 (Oc)
Foramen Magnum
Neural arch stenosis and spinal cord injury in thanatophoric dysplasia [Faye-Petersen] 87 (Ja)
Forecasting
Evaluation of Bayesian forecasting for individualized gentamicin dosage in infants weighing 1000 g or less [Lui] 463 (Ap)
Optimal positioning of endotracheal tubes for ventilation of preterm infants [Rotschild] 1007 (Se)
Predictors of neurodevelopmental outcome following bronchopulmonary dysplasia [Luchi] 813 (Jy)
Foreign Bodies
Pediatric case of Eagle's syndrome [Holloway] 339 (Mr)
Thorn-induced pseudotumor of the tibia [Kozlowski] 1159 (Oc)
Forensic Medicine
Pediatric legal medicine: a new venture [Ferry] 255 (Mr)
Photographing the physically abused child, principles and practice [Ricci] 275 (Mr)
Foundations
Improving health care for underserved infants, children, and adolescents: the Robert Wood Johnson Foundation's experience [Beachler] 565 (My)
Fractures
Clavicular fractures in neonates (letter) [Carter] 251, (reply) [Joseph] 252 (Mr)
Clavicular fractures in neonates: frequency vs significance (letter) [O'Halloran] (reply) [Joseph] 251 (Mr)
Mineral metabolism and calcitriol therapy in idiopathic juvenile osteoporosis [Saggese] 457 (Ap)
Use of infant walkers [AMA Board of Trustees] 933 (Au)
Fresh Frozen Plasma see Plasma
Fringe Benefits see Salaries and Fringe Benefits
Frontal Lobe
Cortical resection for children with epilepsy: perspectives in pediatrics [Wyllie] 314 (Mr)
Fryns Syndrome
Osteochondrodysplasia in Fryns syndrome [Kershisnik] 656 (Je)
Fungus Diseases see Mycoses

G

Gallstones see Cholelithiasis
Gastroenteritis
Acquired methemoglobinemia: the relationship of cause to course of illness [Avner] **144**:1229(No); correction, **145**:158 (Fe)
Gastroesophageal Reflux
Gastroesophageal reflux and apnea in prematurely born infants during wakefulness and sleep [Ajuriaguerra] 1132 (Oc)
Value of subject height in predicting lower esophageal sphincter location [Staiano] 1424 (De)
Gastrointestinal Motility
Esophageal motility in children with Hirschsprung's disease [Staiano] 310 (Mr)
Gastrointestinal System
Escherichia coli bacteremia in children: a review of 91 cases in 10 years [Bonadio] 671 (Je)
Hemorrhagic shock and encephalopathy: an entity similar to heatstroke (letter) [Conway] 720 (Jy)
Genetics
Nevus flammeus: discordance in monozygotic twins [Shamir] 85 (Ja)
Genetics, Medical
Differences in expression of cystic fibrosis in blacks and whites [McColley] 94 (Ja)
Pediatric perspectives: vistas and vantage points [Bedrick] 256 (Mr)
X-linked hypophosphatemia: genetic and clinical correlates [Hanna] 865 (Au)
Genital Warts see Condylomata acuminata
Genitalia
Anal fissure produced by examination for sexual abuse (letter) [Baker] 848, (reply) [Bays] 849 (Au)
Gentamicins
Evaluation of Bayesian forecasting for individualized gentamicin dosage in infants weighing 1000 g or less [Lui] 463 (Ap)
Ventriculitis in newborns with myelomeningocele [Charney] 287 (Mr)
Gerber Food Company
Physicians, formula companies, and advertising: a historical perspective [Greer] 282 (Mr)
Germ Cells
Pediatric germ cell and human chorionic gonadotropin-producing tumors: clinical and laboratory features [Englund] 1294 (No)
Gestational Age
Outpatient assessment of infants with bronchiolitis [Shaw] 151 (Fe)
Percentile curves for various hematologic measurements at birth in Arab preterm babies of different gestational ages [Haque] 645 (Je)
Giardiasis
Testing the psychogenic vomiting diagnosis: four pediatric patients [Gonzalez-Heydrich] 913 (Au)
Glomerular Filtration Rate
Effect of low-dose dopamine infusion on cardiopulmonary and renal status in premature newborns with respiratory distress syndrome [Cuevas] 799 (Jy)
Paleonephrology and reflux nephropathy: from the 'big bang' to end-stage renal disease [Kallen] 860 (Au)
Glomerulonephritis, Focal Sclerosing see Glomerulosclerosis, Focal
Glomerulosclerosis, Focal
Paleonephrology and reflux nephropathy: from the 'big bang' to end-stage renal disease [Kallen] 860 (Au)
Glossitis
Acute glossitis and bacteremia caused by *Streptococcus pneumoniae:* case report and review (letter) [Stoddard] 598 (Je)
Glucagon
Endocrine function in children with human immunodeficiency virus infection [Schwartz] 330 (Mr)
Gonadotropins, Chorionic
Pediatric germ cell and human chorionic gonadotropin-producing tumors: clinical and laboratory features [Englund] 1294 (No)
Government Agencies
Redoing the health care quilt: patches or whole cloth? [Cleveland] 499 (My)
Graft vs Host Disease
Guidelines for auditing pediatric blood transfusion practices [Blanchette] 787 (Jy)
Gram-Negative Bacteria
Frequency of infections associated with implanted systems vs cuffed, tunneled silastic venous catheters in patients with acute leukemia [Severien] 1433 (De)
Gram-Positive Bacteria
Frequency of infections associated with implanted systems vs cuffed, tunneled silastic venous catheters in patients with acute leukemia [Severien] 1433 (De)
Granulocyte Colony-Stimulating Factor
Measurement of serum granulocyte colony-stimulating factor in a patient with congenital agranulocytosis (Kostmann's syndrome) [Glasser] 925 (Au)
Neutropenia in an extremely premature infant treated with recombinant human granulocyte colony-stimulating factor [Roberts] 808 (Jy)
Granulocytes
Guidelines for auditing pediatric blood transfusion practices [Blanchette] 787 (Jy)
Transfusion therapy in neonates [Strauss] 904 (Au)
Granuloma
Exacerbation of tinea corporis during treatment with 1% clotrimazole/0.05% betamethasone dipropionate (Lotrisone) (letter) [Reynolds] 1224 (No)
Great Britain
Legalization of drugs of abuse and the pediatrician [Schwartz] 1153 (Oc)
Growth
Development, growth, and cardiac surgery [Mayer] 33 (Ja)
Dietary calcium and bone mineral status of children and adolescents [Chan] 631 (Je)
Effectiveness of growth-promoting therapies: comparison among growth hormone, clonidine, and levodopa [Volta] 168 (Fe)
Endocrine function in children with human immunodeficiency virus infection [Schwartz] 330 (Mr)
Follow-up of patients who underwent arterial switch repair for transposition of the great arteries [Mendoza] 40 (Ja)
Growth hormone therapy in hypophosphatemic rickets [Wilson] 1165 (Oc)
Seasonal variation in growth during growth hormone therapy [Rudolf] 769 (Jy)
Growth Hormone, Pituitary see Somatotropin
Gynecology
Adolescent pelvic examination: an effective practical approach [Tolmas] 1269 (No)
Challenge of care for the poor and underserved in the United States: an American College of Obstetricians and Gynecologists perspective on access to care for underserved women [Davidson] 546 (My)

H

Habits
Send Linus to me (letter) [Szonyi] (reply) [Friman] 1227 (No)
Thumb-sucking (letter) [Lubicky] 845, (reply) [Friman] 846 (Au)
Haemophilus influenzae
Acute osteomyelitis in children: reassessment of etiologic agents and their clinical characteristics [Faden] 65 (Ja)
Antibody responses to 4 *Haemophilus influenzae* type b conjugate vaccines [Käyhty] 223 (Fe)
Causes of hospital-treated acute lower respiratory tract infection in children [Nohynek] 618 (Je)
Dose-related immunogenicity of *Haemophilus influenzae* type b capsular polysaccharide—*Neisseria meningitidis* outer membrane protein conjugate vaccine [Wong] 742 (Jy)
DTP immunization and susceptibility to infectious diseases: is there a relationship? [Davidson] 750 (Jy)
Endotoxin concentrations in cerebrospinal fluid correlate with clinical severity and neurologic outcome of *Haemophilus influenzae* type b meningitis [Mertsola] 1099 (Oc)
Haemophilus b disease after vaccination with *Haemophilus* b polysaccharide or conjugate vaccine [Frasch] 1379 (De)
Immunization response varies with intensity of acute lym-

phoblastic leukemia therapy [Ridgway] 887 (Au)
Pneumococcal osteomyelitis and arthritis in children: a hospital series and literature review [Jacobs] 70 (Ja)
Response of 7- to 15-month-old infants to sequential immunization with *Haemophilus influenzae* type b-CRM$_{197}$ conjugate and polysaccharide vaccines [Rothstein] 898 (Au)
Hand Dermatoses
Acropustulosis of infancy [Friedman] 341 (Mr)
Handicapped
Guidelines for safe transportation of children in wheelchairs [DiGaudio] 653 (Je)
Tiny Tim remembered [Callahan] 1355 (De)
Handwashing
Hand washing in pediatric ambulatory settings: an inconsistent practice [Lohr] 1198 (Oc)
Hantaan Virus see Hemorrhagic Fever Virus, Epidemic
Head Injuries
Anergy in pediatric head trauma patients [Wilson] 326 (Mr)
Skateboarding injuries in children: a second wave [Retsky] 188 (Fe)
Use of infant walkers [AMA Board of Trustees] 933 (Au)
Headache
Prevalence and impact of chronic illness among adolescents [Newacheck] 1367 (De)
Health Care Coalitions
Caring program for children: the Michigan experience [Udow] 579 (My)
Health Care Rationing
Redoing the health care quilt: patches or whole cloth? [Cleveland] 499 (My)
Treatment withdrawal in neonates (letter) [Byrne] 1223 (No)
Health Education
Acquired immunodeficiency syndrome and adolescents: knowledge, attitudes, and behaviors of runaway and homeless youths [Sugerman] 431 (Ap)
Sun protection in newborns: a comparison of educational methods [Bolognia] 1125 (Oc)
Health Manpower
Health care for uninsured and underinsured children (letter) [Pearson] 1085 (Oc)
Resident and nurse practitioners: responding to education and patient care needs (letter) [Giardino] 843 (Au)
Health Policy
American Academy of Pediatrics response to the growing health needs of children [Strain] 536 (My)
Challenge of care for the poor and underserved in the United States: an American College of Obstetricians and Gynecologists perspective on access to care for underserved women [Davidson] 546 (My)
Children in and of the streets: health, social policy, and the homeless young [Wright] 516 (My)
Children's services in an era of budget deficits [Blum] 575 (My)
Growing neglect of American children [Maurer] 540 (My)
Health Promotion
New initiatives in adolescent health promotion [Elster] 495 (My)
Health Services Accessibility
American Academy of Pediatrics response to the growing health needs of children [Strain] 536 (My)
Barriers to medical care for homeless families compared with housed poor families [Wood] 1109 (Oc)
Challenge of care for the poor and underserved in the United States: an American College of Obstetricians and Gynecologists perspective on access to care for underserved women [Davidson] 546 (My)
Challenge of caring for indigent children with rheumatologic diseases [Miller] 554 (My)
Far from the ideal: the plight of poor children in the United States [Fulginiti] 489 (My)
Growing neglect of American children [Maurer] 540 (My)
Poverty and cardiac disease in children [Allen] 550 (My)
Redoing the health care quilt: patches or whole cloth? [Cleveland] 499 (My)
What will it take to fully protect all American children with vaccines? [Hinman] 559 (My)
Health Services Research
Challenge of care for the poor child: the research agenda [Kohl] 542 (My)
Improving health care for underserved infants, children, and adolescents: the Robert Wood Johnson Foundation's experience [Beachler] 565 (My)
Poverty and the health of American children: implications for academic pediatrics [Johnston] 507 (My)
Health Status
Survey of the health of homeless children in Philadelphia shelters [Parker] 520 (My)
Hearing Disorders
Evaluation of auditory brain-stem response in full-term infants of cocaine-abusing mothers [Carzoli] 1013 (Se)
Hearing Loss, Partial
Role of corticosteroid therapy in children with pneumococcal meningitis [Kennedy] 1374 (De)
Hearing Loss, Sensorineural
Evaluation of auditory brain-stem response in full-term infants of cocaine-abusing mothers [Carzoli] 1013 (Se)
Heart Arrest
Improved speed and accuracy of calculations with a programmable calculator in pediatric emergency scenarios [Melzer-Lange] 264 (Mr)
Intraosseous infusion of dobutamine and isoproterenol [Bilello] 165 (Fe); correction, 1312 (No)
Sudden cardiac death (letter) [Pearl] 1223 (No)
Sudden cardiac death in young athletes: a review [McCaffrey] 177 (Fe)
Heart Defects, Congenital
Development, growth, and cardiac surgery [Mayer] 33 (Ja)
Evolution of surgical treatment for congenital cardiac disease [Pigott] 1362 (De)
Retinopathy of prematurity in infants with cyanotic congenital heart disease [Johns] 200 (Fe)
Tuberous sclerosis with myocardial and central nervous system involvement at birth [Allison] 471 (Ap)
Heart Diseases
Cardiac care for infants: determinants of hospital charges for acute care [Pearson] 1397 (De)
Evolution of surgical treatment for congenital cardiac disease [Pigott] 1362 (De)
Lipoprotein profiles in hypercholesterolemic children [Garcia] 147 (Fe); correction, 515 (My)
Poverty and cardiac disease in children [Allen] 550 (My)
Heart Injuries
Commotio cordis: the single, most common cause of traumatic death in youth baseball [Abrunzo] 1279 (No)
Heart Murmurs
Ductal patency in neonates with respiratory distress syndrome: a randomized surfactant trial [Reller] 1017 (Se)
Heart Rate
Breathing patterns and heart rates at ages 6 weeks and 2 years [Poets] 1393 (De)
Cardiopulmonary exercise testing in children following surgery for tetralogy of Fallot [Tomassoni] 1290 (No)
Physiologic responses to playing a video game [Segal] 1034 (Se)
Heat Exhaustion
Fallacy of the hemorrhagic shock and encephalopathy syndrome (letter) [Bass] 718 (Jy)
Hemorrhagic shock and encephalopathy: an entity similar to heatstroke (letter) [Conway] 720 (Jy)
Hyperpyrexia, hemorrhagic shock and encephalopathy, and creatinine phosphokinase (letter) [Dupee] 719 (Jy)
Hemagglutinins
Comparative trial of the reactogenicity and immunogenicity of Takeda acellular pertussis vaccine combined with tetanus and diphtheria toxoids: outcome in 3- to 8-month old infants, 9- to 23-month-old infants and children, and 24- to 30-month-old children [Kimura] 734 (Jy)
Hemangioma
Treatment of ulcerated hemangiomas with pulsed tunable dye laser [Morelli] 1062 (Se)
Hematocrit
Percentile curves for various hematologic measurements at birth in Arab preterm babies of different gestational ages [Haque] 645 (Je)
Transfusion therapy in neonates [Strauss] 904 (Au)
Hematologic Tests
Cautionary note on the use of empiric ceftriaxone for suspected bacteremia [Wald] 1359 (De)
Effect of valproic acid on plasma carnitine levels [Opala] 999 (Se)
50-year follow-up of childhood plumbism: hypertension, renal function, and hemoglobin levels among survivors [Hu] 681 (Je)
Multilevel model to assess appropriateness of pediatric serum drug concentrations [Kraus] 1171 (Oc)
Percentile curves for various hematologic measurements at birth in Arab preterm babies of different gestational ages [Haque] 645 (Je)
Third pattern of disease progression in children infected with human immunodeficiency virus (letter) [Katz] 1347, (reply) [Blanche] 1348 (De)
Total iron-binding capacity in iron poisoning: is it useful? [Tenenbein] 437 (Ap)
Vertical transmission of human immunodeficiency virus from seronegative or indeterminate mothers [Johnson] 1239 (No)
Hematuria
Natural history of hematuria associated with hypercalciuria in children [Garcia] 1204 (Oc)
Hemodynamics
Family history of myocardial infarction and hemodynamic responses to exercise in young black boys [Treiber] 1029 (Se)
Pediatric cardiac rehabilitation [Balfour] 627 (Je)
Hemoglobins
50-year follow-up of childhood plumbism: hypertension, renal function, and hemoglobin levels among survivors [Hu] 681 (Je)
Percentile curves for various hematologic measurements at birth in Arab preterm babies of different gestational ages [Haque] 645 (Je)
Hemophilia
Trimethoprim-sulfamethoxazole oral desensitization in hemophiliacs infected with human immunodeficiency virus with a history of hypersensitivity reactions [Kletzel] 1428 (De)
Hemorrhage
Left renal vein thrombosis and left adrenal hemorrhage [Bennett] 1299 (No)
Hemorrhage, Cerebral see Cerebral Hemorrhage
Hemorrhagic Fever Virus, Epidemic
Epidemic nephropathy in children [Lautala] 1181 (Oc)
Henoch Purpura see Purpura, Schoenlein-Henoch
Hepatitis
Neonatal hepatitis and extrahepatic biliary atresia associated with cytomegalovirus infection in twins [Hart] 302 (Mr)
Hepatitis, Viral, Non-A, Non-B
Transfusion therapy in neonates [Strauss] 904 (Au)
Hereditary Diseases
Acrodermatitis enteropathica [Schneider] 211 (Fe)
Autosomal recessive lethal infantile cytochrome C oxidase deficiency [Eshel] 661 (Je)
Evolution of surgical treatment for congenital cardiac disease [Pigott] 1362 (De)
Laron-type dwarfism [Laron] 473 (Ap)
Lowe's syndrome [Loughead] 113 (Ja)
Osteochondrodysplasia in Fryns syndrome [Kershisnik] 656 (Je)
Pachyonychia congenita [Cohen] 1301 (No)
Sudden cardiac death (letter) [Pearl] 1223 (No)
Herpes Zoster
Herpes zoster oticus (letter) [Rathore] 722 (Jy)
Hidradenoma
Syringomas in Down syndrome (letter) [Feingold] 966 (Se)
Hirschsprung Disease
Esophageal motility in children with Hirschsprung's disease [Staiano] 310 (Mr)
Hispanic Americans
Breast-feeding initiation in a triethnic population [Bee] 306 (Mr)
Histamine H1 Receptor Blockaders
Survey of antiemetic use in children with cancer [van Hoff] 773 (Jy)
History
Physicians, formula companies, and advertising: a historical perspective [Greer] 282 (Mr)
History of Medicine
AJDC is 80 years old: from pedology to pediatrics [Fulginiti] 11 (Ja)
Studies in fetal malnutrition [Crosby] 871 (Au)
HIV
Acquired immunodeficiency syndrome and adolescents: knowledge, attitudes, and behaviors of runaway and homeless youths [Sugerman] 431 (Ap)
Pediatric acquired immunodeficiency syndrome, poverty, and national priorities [Heagarty] 527 (My)
Pediatric human immunodeficiency virus infection and the acquired immunodeficiency syndrome: a health care crisis of children and families [Van Dyke] 529 (My)
Transfusion therapy in neonates [Strauss] 904 (Au)
HIV-1
Clinical and endocrinologic manifestations in perinatally human immunodeficiency virus type 1-infected children aged 5 years or older [Lepage] 1248 (No)
HIV Infections
Child survival and perinatal infections with human immunodeficiency virus [Bennett] 1242 (No)
Clinical and endocrinologic manifestations in perinatally human immunodeficiency virus type 1-infected children aged 5 years or older [Lepage] 1248 (No)
Predicting risk of *Pneumocystis carinii* pneumonia in human immunodeficiency virus-infected children [Rutstein] 922 (Au)
Trimethoprim-sulfamethoxazole oral desensitization in hemophiliacs infected with human immunodeficiency virus with a history of hypersensitivity reactions [Kletzel] 1428 (De)
Vertical transmission of human immunodeficiency virus from seronegative or indeterminate mothers [Johnson] 1239 (No)
HIV Seropositivity
Child sexual abuse and human immunodeficiency virus transmission (letter) [Monteleone] (reply) [Gutman] 847 (Au)
Clinical and endocrinologic manifestations in perinatally human immunodeficiency virus type 1-infected children aged 5 years or older [Lepage] 1248 (No)
Human immunodeficiency virus transmission by child sexual abuse [Gutman] 137 (Fe)
Vertical transmission of human immunodeficiency virus from seronegative or indeterminate mothers [Johnson] 1239 (No)
HIV Seroprevalence
Child survival and perinatal infections with human immunodeficiency virus [Bennett] 1242 (No)
HLA Antigens
Association of pauciarticular juvenile arthritis and myasthenia gravis [Glass] 1176 (Oc)
Holidays
Parental drinking habits (letter) [Wells] 1087 (Oc)
Home Care Services
Home care cost-effectiveness for respiratory technology-dependent children [Fields] 729 (Jy)
Saving money with home care [Schoumacher] 725 (Jy)
Home Nursing
Home care cost-effectiveness for respiratory technology-dependent children [Fields] 729 (Jy)

Saving money with home care [Schoumacher] 725 (Jy)
Homeless Persons
Acquired immunodeficiency syndrome and adolescents: knowledge, attitudes, and behaviors of runaway and homeless youths [Sugerman] 431 (Ap)
Barriers to medical care for homeless families compared with housed poor families [Wood] 1109 (Oc)
Children in and of the streets: health, social policy, and the homeless young [Wright] 516 (My)
Survey of the health of homeless children in Philadelphia shelters [Parker] 520 (My)
Youth alienation as an emerging pediatric health care issue [Farrow] 491 (My)
Homosexuality
What about gay teenagers? (letter) [Fikar] 252 (Mr)
Hormones, Synthetic
Effectiveness of growth-promoting therapies: comparison among growth hormone, clonidine, and levodopa [Volta] 168 (Fe)
Hospital Administrators
Support services for pediatric trainees: a survey of training program directors [Bergman] 1002 (Se)
Hospital Departments
Fetal alcohol syndrome: misplaced emphasis (letter) [Hess] (reply) [Little] 721 (Jy)
Hospitalization
Child welfare: the phantom of the health care system (letter) [Pidcock] 843 (Au)
Hospitals
Pediatric human immunodeficiency virus infection and the acquired immunodeficiency syndrome: a health care crisis of children and families [Van Dyke] 529 (My)
Hospitals, Military
Major congenital neurologic malformations (letter) [Ryals] 30 (Ja)
Hospitals, Teaching
Eighty-hour workweek and residency programs: closing arguments (letter) [Bedrick] 846 (Au)
House staff work hours and moonlighting: what do residents want?: a survey of pediatric residents in California [Cheng] 1104 (Oc)
Resident and nurse practitioners: responding to education and patient care needs (letter) [Giardino] 843 (Au)
Support services for pediatric trainees: a survey of training program directors [Bergman] 1002 (Se)
Hydrocele
Hydrocele in Kawasaki disease: importance in early recognition of atypical disease (letter) [Kabani] 1348 (De)
Hydrocephalus
Posthemorrhagic hydrocephalus: use of an intravenous-type catheter for cerebrospinal fluid drainage [Marro] 1141 (Oc)
Hydrochlorothiazide
Medical management of postobstructive polyuria (letter) [Smoyer] 1345 (De)
Hydrocortisone
Endocrine function in children with human immunodeficiency virus infection [Schwartz] 330 (Mr)
Hydrogen-Ion Concentration
Alkaline urine is associated with eating disorders (letter) [Arden] 28 (Ja)
Association of alkaline urine with eating disorders (letter) [Robson] (reply) [Arden] 1091 (Oc)
Gastroesophageal reflux and apnea in prematurely born infants during wakefulness and sleep [Ajuriaguerra] 1132 (Oc)
How much of neonatal encephalopathy is due to birth asphyxia? [Nelson] 1325 (No)
Value of subject height in predicting lower esophageal sphincter location [Staiano] 1424 (De)
25-Hydroxycholecalciferol 1-Hydroxylase
How much vitamin D for neonates? [Pittard] 1147 (Oc)
25-Hydroxyvitamin D 3 see Calcifediol
Hydroxyzine
Survey of antiemetic use in children with cancer [van Hoff] 773 (Jy)
Hyperalimentation, Parenteral see Parenteral Hyperalimentation
Hypercholesterolemia
Family history fails to identify many children with severe hypercholesterolemia [Starc] 61 (Ja)
Lipoprotein profiles in hypercholesterolemic children [Garcia] 147 (Fe); correction, 515 (My)
Hyperlipidemia
Family history fails to identify many children with severe hypercholesterolemia [Starc] 61 (Ja)
Hypernatremia
Adipsic hypernatremia in 2 sisters [Radetti] 321 (Mr)
Water intoxication: a prevalent problem in the inner city [Finberg] 981 (Se)
Hypersensitivity
Predicting risk of *Pneumocystis carinii* pneumonia in human immunodeficiency virus-infected children [Rutstein] 922 (Au)
Prevalence and impact of chronic illness among adolescents [Newacheck] 1367 (De)
Trimethoprim-sulfamethoxazole oral desensitization in hemophiliacs infected with human immunodeficiency virus with a history of hypersensitivity reactions [Kletzel] 1428 (De)
Hypersensitivity, Delayed
Anergy in pediatric head trauma patients [Wilson] 326 (Mr)
Hypertension
50-year follow-up of childhood plumbism: hypertension, renal function, and hemoglobin levels among survivors [Hu] 681 (Je)
Sexual maturation and blood pressure levels of a biracial sample of girls [Kozinetz] 142 (Fe)
Tracking of elevated blood pressure values in adolescent athletes at 1-year follow-up [Tanji] 665 (Je)
Hypertonic Saline Solution see Saline Solution, Hypertonic
Hypocalcemia
Low serum calcium and high parathyroid hormone levels in neonates fed 'humanized' cow's milk-based formula [Specker] 941 (Au)
Partial hypoparathyroidism: a variant of transient congenital hypoparathyroidism [Kooh] 877 (Au)
Hyponatremia
Differences in expression of cystic fibrosis in blacks and whites [McColley] 94 (Ja)
Oral water intoxication in infants: an American epidemic [Keating] 985 (Se)
Hypoparathyroidism
Partial hypoparathyroidism: a variant of transient congenital hypoparathyroidism [Kooh] 877 (Au)
Hypophosphatemia, Familial
Growth hormone therapy in hypophosphatemic rickets [Wilson] 1165 (Oc)
X-linked hypophosphatemia: genetic and clinical correlates [Hanna] 865 (Au)
Hypotension
Escherichia coli bacteremia in children: a review of 91 cases in 10 years [Bonadio] 671 (Je)
Hypothalamic Neoplasms
Adipsic hypernatremia in 2 sisters [Radetti] 321 (Mr)
Hypothermia, Induced
Development, growth, and cardiac surgery [Mayer] 33 (Ja)
Hypothyroidism
Endocrine function in children with human immunodeficiency virus infection [Schwartz] 330 (Mr)
Markedly immature lecithin-sphingomyelin ratio at term and congenital hypothyroidism (letter) [Cohen] 1227 (No)
Hypoxemia see Anoxemia
Hypoxia see Anoxia

I

IgG
Efficacy and pharmacokinetics of intravenous immune globulin administration to high-risk neonates [Kinney] 1233 (No)
Predicting risk of *Pneumocystis carinii* pneumonia in human immunodeficiency virus-infected children [Rutstein] 922 (Au)
Immersion
Immersion events in residential swimming pools: evidence for an experience effect [Wintemute] 1200 (Oc)
Immunity, Cellular
Anergy in pediatric head trauma patients [Wilson] 326 (Mr)
Immunity, Humoral see Antibody Formation
Immunization
Apparent decreased risk of invasive bacterial disease after heterologous childhood immunization [Black] 746 (Jy)
DTP immunization and susceptibility to infectious diseases: is there a relationship? [Davidson] 750 (Jy)
Growing neglect of American children [Maurer] 540 (My)
Immunization response varies with intensity of acute lymphoblastic leukemia therapy [Ridgway] 887 (Au)
Response of seronegative adults to measles immunization (letter) [Braunstein] 969 (Se)
Vaccine myth and physician handouts (letter) [Lynch] 426, (replies) [Cherry, Fulginiti] 426, 427 (Ap)
What will it take to fully protect all American children with vaccines? [Hinman] 559 (My)
Immunization, Passive
Antibody response to MMR vaccination in children who received IVIG as neonates (letter) [Ruderman] 425 (Ap)
Immunization Schedule
Immunogenicity of tetravalent rhesus rotavirus vaccine administered with buffer and oral polio vaccine [Ing] 892 (Au)
Response of 7- to 15-month-old infants to sequential immunization with *Haemophilus influenzae* type b-CRM_{197} conjugate and polysaccharide vaccines [Rothstein] 898 (Au)
Immunoenzyme Techniques
Causes of hospital-treated acute lower respiratory tract infection in children [Nohynek] 618 (Je)
Immunoglobulin Therapy see Immunization, Passive
Immunoglobulins
Antibody response to MMR vaccination in children who received IVIG as neonates (letter) [Ruderman] 425 (Ap)
Efficacy and pharmacokinetics of intravenous immune globulin administration to high-risk neonates [Kinney] 1233 (No)
Is prophylaxis of neonates with intravenous immunoglobulin beneficial? [Hill] 1229 (No)
Immunologic Deficiency Syndromes
Escherichia coli bacteremia in children: a review of 91 cases in 10 years [Bonadio] 671 (Je)
Word choice (letter) [Gorlick] (reply) [Hong] 724 (Jy)
Immunosuppression
Anergy in pediatric head trauma patients [Wilson] 326 (Mr)
Immunotoxins
Antibody responses to 4 *Haemophilus influenzae* type b conjugate vaccines [Käyhty] 223 (Fe)
Dose-related immunogenicity of *Haemophilus influenzae* type b capsular polysaccharide—*Neisseria meningitidis* outer membrane protein conjugate vaccine [Wong] 742 (Jy)
Haemophilus b disease after vaccination with *Haemophilus* b polysaccharide or conjugate vaccine [Frasch] 1379 (De)
Response of 7- to 15-month-old infants to sequential immunization with *Haemophilus influenzae* type b-CRM_{197} conjugate and polysaccharide vaccines [Rothstein] 898 (Au)
Impetigo
Impetigo [Esterly] 125 (Fe)
Staphylococcus aureus in impetigo (letter) [Dagan] (reply) [Bass] 1223 (No)
Inappropriate ADH Syndrome
Vasopressin levels in infants during the course of aseptic and bacterial meningitis [Padilla] 991 (Se)
Incentives see Motivation
Income
Women in medicine: fantasies, dreams, myths, and realities [DeAngelis] 49 (Ja)
Indians, North American
DTP immunization and susceptibility to infectious diseases: is there a relationship? [Davidson] 750 (Jy)
Obesity among Mescalero preschool children: association with maternal obesity and birth weight [Gallaher] 1262 (No)
Indigency, Medical see Medical Indigency
Indomethacin
Ductal patency in neonates with respiratory distress syndrome: a randomized surfactant trial [Reller] 1017 (Se)
Medical management of postobstructive polyuria (letter) [Smoyer] 1345 (De)
Infant
Acellular pertussis vaccines: efficacy and evaluation of clinical case definitions [Blackwelder] 1285 (No)
Acropustulosis of infancy [Friedman] 341 (Mr)
Age-related patterns of thyroid-stimulating hormone response to thyrotropin-releasing hormone stimulation in Down syndrome [Sharav] 172 (Fe)
Antibody responses to 4 *Haemophilus influenzae* type b conjugate vaccines [Käyhty] 223 (Fe)
Autosomal recessive lethal infantile cytochrome C oxidase deficiency [Eshel] 661 (Je)
Brain and ocular abnormalities in infants with in utero exposure to cocaine and other street drugs [Dominguez] 688 (Je)
Capillary refilling (skin turgor) in the assessment of dehydration [Saavedra] 296 (Mr)
Cardiac care for infants: determinants of hospital charges for acute care [Pearson] 1397 (De)
Cautionary note on the use of empiric ceftriaxone for suspected bacteremia [Wald] 1359 (De)
Challenge of care for the poor and underserved in the United States: an American College of Obstetricians and Gynecologists perspective on access to care for underserved women [Davidson] 546 (My)
Comparative trial of the reactogenicity and immunogenicity of Takeda acellular pertussis vaccine combined with tetanus and diphtheria toxoids: outcome in 3- to 8-month old infants, 9- to 23-month-old infants and children, and 24- to 30-month-old children [Kimura] 734 (Jy)
Comparison of maternal and infant serologic tests for syphilis [Rawstron] 1383 (De)
Effect of necrotizing enterocolitis on urinary epidermal growth factor levels [Scott] 804 (Jy); correction, 982 (Se)
Elevated plasma norepinephrine levels in infants of substance-abusing mothers [Ward] 44 (Ja)
Fallacy of the hemorrhagic shock and encephalopathy syndrome (letter) [Bass] 718 (Jy)
Focal scleroderma and severe cardiomyopathy: patient report and brief review [Moore] 229 (Fe)
'H' in hemorrhagic shock and encephalopathy syndrome (letter) [Roscelli] 720 (Jy)
Hemorrhagic shock and encephalopathy: an entity similar to heatstroke (letter) [Conway] 720 (Jy)
Hydrocele in Kawasaki disease: importance in early recognition of atypical disease (letter) [Kabani] 1348 (De)
Hyperpyrexia, hemorrhagic shock and encephalopathy, and creatinine phosphokinase (letter) [Dupee] 719 (Jy)
Immunogenicity of tetravalent rhesus rotavirus vaccine administered with buffer and oral polio vaccine [Ing] 892 (Au)
Improving health care for underserved infants, children, and adolescents: the Robert Wood Johnson Foundation's experience [Beachler] 565 (My)
Influenza type A and B infections in hospitalized pediatric patients: who should be immunized? [Serwint] 623 (Je)
Injuries and poisonings in out-of-home child care and home care [Gunn] 779 (Jy)
Intraosseous infusion of dobutamine and isoproterenol [Bilello] 165 (Fe); correction, 1312 (No)
Left renal vein thrombosis and left adrenal hemorrhage [Bennett] 1299 (No)
Measurement of serum granulocyte colony-stimulating fac-

tor in a patient with congenital agranulocytosis (Kostmann's syndrome) [Glasser] 925 (Au)
Mediterranean visceral leishmaniasis: a frequently unrecognized imported disease (letter) [Mahieu] 1225 (No)
Neuroblastoma screening data: an epidemiologic analysis [Goodman] 1415 (De)
Outpatient assessment of infants with bronchiolitis [Shaw] 151 (Fe)
Pediatric human immunodeficiency virus infection and the acquired immunodeficiency syndrome: a health care crisis of children and families [Van Dyke] 529 (My)
Pneumococcal osteomyelitis and arthritis in children: a hospital series and literature review [Jacobs] 70 (Ja)
Respirosonography in infants with acute bronchiolitis [Tal] 1405 (De)
Response of 7- to 15-month-old infants to sequential immunization with *Haemophilus influenzae* type b-CRM_{197} conjugate and polysaccharide vaccines [Rothstein] 898 (Au)
Role of corticosteroid therapy in children with pneumococcal meningitis [Kennedy] 1374 (De)
Third pattern of disease progression in children infected with human immunodeficiency virus (letter) [Katz] 1347, (reply) [Blanche] 1348 (De)
Treatment of ulcerated hemangiomas with pulsed tunable dye laser [Morelli] 1062 (Se)
Unsuspected cocaine exposure in young children [Kharasch] 204 (Fe)
Vasopressin levels in infants during the course of aseptic and bacterial meningitis [Padilla] 991 (Se)
Vertical transmission of human immunodeficiency virus from seronegative or indeterminate mothers [Johnson] 1239 (No)

Infant Care
Comparison of a computer tutorial with other methods for teaching well-newborn care [Desch] 1255 (No)

Infant Equipment
Use of infant walkers [AMA Board of Trustees] 933 (Au)

Infant Food
Current social practices leading to water intoxication in infants (letter) [Schaeffer] 27 (Ja)
Formula companies and the medical profession (letters) [Fink, Newman] 1088, 1089, (reply) [Greer] 1090 (Oc)
How much iron is enough? (letter) [Rogers] (reply) [Finberg] 598 (Je)
Low serum calcium and high parathyroid hormone levels in neonates fed 'humanized' cow's milk-based formula [Specker] 941 (Au)
Oral water intoxication in infants: an American epidemic [Keating] 985 (Se)
Physicians, formula companies, and advertising: a historical perspective [Greer] 282 (Mr)
Water intoxication: a prevalent problem in the inner city [Finberg] 981 (Se)

Infant Health Services see Child Health Services

Infant, Low Birth Weight
Evaluation of Bayesian forecasting for individualized gentamicin dosage in infants weighing 1000 g or less [Lui] 463 (Ap)
Factors associated with umbilical catheter-related sepsis in neonates [Landers] 675 (Je)
Growing neglect of American children [Maurer] 540 (My)
How much vitamin D for neonates? [Pittard] 1147 (Oc)
Predictors of neurodevelopmental outcome following bronchopulmonary dysplasia [Luchi] 813 (Jy)
Prevalence of birth defects among low-birth-weight infants: a population study [Mili] 1313 (No)

Infant Mortality
Child survival and perinatal infections with human immunodeficiency virus [Bennett] 1242 (No)
Differences in infant mortality by race, nativity status, and other maternal characteristics [Kleinman] 194 (Fe)
Far from the ideal: the plight of poor children in the United States [Fulginiti] 489 (My)
Growing neglect of American children [Maurer] 540 (My)
Sudden deaths and apparent life-threatening events in hospitalized neonates presumed to be healthy [Burchfield] 1319 (No)
Surfactant replacement therapy in respiratory distress syndrome: meta-analysis of clinical trials of single-dose surfactant extracts [Hennes] 102 (Ja)

Infant, Newborn
Antibody response to MMR vaccination in children who received IVIG as neonates (letter) [Ruderman] 425 (Ap)
Bone mineral content of healthy, full-term neonates: effect of race, gender, and maternal cigarette smoking [Venkataraman] 1310 (No)
Breathing patterns and heart rates at ages 6 weeks and 2 years [Poets] 1393 (De)
Child welfare: the phantom of the health care system (letter) [Pidcock] 843 (Au)
Clavicular fractures in neonates (letter) [Carter] 251, (reply) [Joseph] 252 (Mr)
Clavicular fractures in neonates: frequency vs significance (letter) [O'Halloran] (reply) [Joseph] 251 (Mr)
Development, growth, and cardiac surgery [Mayer] 33 (Ja)
Direct bilirubin measurements in jaundiced term newborns: a reevaluation [Newman] 1305 (No)
Efficacy and pharmacokinetics of intravenous immune globulin administration to high-risk neonates [Kinney] 1233 (No)
Evaluation of auditory brain-stem response in full-term infants of cocaine-abusing mothers [Carzoli] 1013 (Se)
Factors associated with umbilical catheter-related sepsis in neonates [Landers] 675 (Je)
Follow-up of patients who underwent arterial switch repair for transposition of the great arteries [Mendoza] 40 (Ja)
Guidelines for auditing pediatric blood transfusion practices [Blanchette] 787 (Jy)
How much vitamin D for neonates? [Pittard] 1147 (Oc)
Improving health care provision to neonates in the United States [Stahlman] 510 (My)
Increased transient tachypnea of the newborn in infants with asthmatic mothers [Schatz] 156 (Fe)
Is prophylaxis of neonates with intravenous immunoglobulin beneficial? [Hill] 1229 (No)
Low serum calcium and high parathyroid hormone levels in neonates fed 'humanized' cow's milk-based formula [Specker] 941 (Au)
Lumbar puncture frequency and cerebrospinal fluid analysis in the neonate [Schwersenski] 54 (Ja)
Markedly immature lecithin-sphingomyelin ratio at term and congenital hypothyroidism (letter) [Cohen] 1227 (No)
Meconium for drug testing [Maynard] 650 (Je)
Medical ethics issues survey of residents in 5 pediatric training programs [White] 161 (Fe)
Medical management of postobstructive polyuria (letter) [Smoyer] 1345 (De)
Neonatal appendicitis with perforation [Ruff] 111 (Ja)
Neonatal hepatitis and extrahepatic biliary atresia associated with cytomegalovirus infection in twins [Hart] 302 (Mr)
Neutropenia in an extremely premature infant treated with recombinant human granulocyte colony-stimulating factor [Roberts] 808 (Jy)
Oxygen saturation by pulse oximetry in healthy infants at an altitude of 1610 m (5280 ft): what is normal? [Thilo] 1137 (Oc)
Partial hypoparathyroidism: a variant of transient congenital hypoparathyroidism [Kooh] 877 (Au)
Predictors of neurodevelopmental outcome following bronchopulmonary dysplasia [Luchi] 813 (Jy)
Subcutaneous fat necrosis of the newborn [Vera] 1047 (Se)
Sudden deaths and apparent life-threatening events in hospitalized neonates presumed to be healthy [Burchfield] 1319 (No)
Sun protection in newborns: a comparison of educational methods [Bolognia] 1125 (Oc)
Transfusion therapy in neonates [Strauss] 904 (Au)
Tuberous sclerosis with myocardial and central nervous system involvement at birth [Allison] 471 (Ap)
Ventriculitis in newborns with myelomeningocele [Charney] 287 (Mr)

Infant, Newborn, Diseases
Fetal alcohol syndrome: misplaced emphasis (letter) [Hess] (reply) [Little] 721 (Jy)

Infant Nutrition
How much vitamin D for neonates? [Pittard] 1147 (Oc)
Practical guide to successful breast-feeding management [Freed] 917 (Au)
Rickets caused by vitamin D deficiency in breast-fed infants in the southern United States [Bhowmick] 127 (Fe)

Infant, Premature
Ductal patency in neonates with respiratory distress syndrome: a randomized surfactant trial [Reller] 1017 (Se)
Effect of low-dose dopamine infusion on cardiopulmonary and renal status in premature newborns with respiratory distress syndrome [Cuevas] 799 (Jy)
Gastroesophageal reflux and apnea in prematurely born infants during wakefulness and sleep [Ajuriaguerra] 1132 (Oc)
Neutropenia in an extremely premature infant treated with recombinant human granulocyte colony-stimulating factor [Roberts] 808 (Jy)
Optimal positioning of endotracheal tubes for ventilation of preterm infants [Rotschild] 1007 (Se)
Osteochondrodysplasia in Fryns syndrome [Kershisnik] 656 (Je)
Percentile curves for various hematologic measurements at birth in Arab preterm babies of different gestational ages [Haque] 645 (Je)
Posthemorrhagic hydrocephalus: use of an intravenous-type catheter for cerebrospinal fluid drainage [Marro] 1141 (Oc)
Predictors of neurodevelopmental outcome following bronchopulmonary dysplasia [Luchi] 813 (Jy)
Preliminary report of prenatal cocaine exposure and respiratory distress syndrome in premature infants [Zuckerman] 696 (Je)
Prevalence of birth defects among low-birth-weight infants: a population study [Mili] 1313 (No)
Retinopathy of prematurity in infants with cyanotic congenital heart disease [Johns] 200 (Fe)
Transfusion therapy in neonates [Strauss] 904 (Au)

Infant Walkers see Infant Equipment

Infant Welfare
Psychosocial predictors of maternal and infant health among adolescent mothers [Boyce] 267 (Mr)

Influenza Vaccine
Haemophilus b disease after vaccination with *Haemophilus* b polysaccharide or conjugate vaccine [Frasch] 1379 (De)
Influenza type A and B infections in hospitalized pediatric patients: who should be immunized? [Serwint] 623 (Je)
Influenza vaccination in the prevention of acute otitis media in children [Heikkinen] 445 (Ap)

Influenza Viruses Type A see Orthomyxoviruses Type A

Informed Consent
Vaccine myth and physician handouts (letter) [Lynch] 426, (replies) [Cherry, Fulginiti] 426, 427 (Ap)

Infusions, Intravenous
Efficacy and pharmacokinetics of intravenous immune globulin administration to high-risk neonates [Kinney] 1233 (No)
Intraosseous infusion of dobutamine and isoproterenol [Bilello] 165 (Fe); correction, 1312 (No)
Is prophylaxis of neonates with intravenous immunoglobulin beneficial? [Hill] 1229 (No)

Injections, Intravenous
Evaluation of intraosseus vs intravenous antibiotic levels in a porcine model [Jaimovich] 946 (Au); correction, 1241 (No)

Inositol Hexaphosphate see Phytic Acid

Institutional Management Teams
Chief resident training: developing leadership skills for future medical leaders [Doughty] 639 (Je)

Insulin-Like Growth Factor I
Endocrine function in children with human immunodeficiency virus infection [Schwartz] 330 (Mr)
Laron-type dwarfism [Laron] 473 (Ap)
Seasonal variation in growth during growth hormone therapy [Rudolf] 769 (Jy)

Insurance Benefits
Current trends in pediatric residency training [Carraccio] 1272 (No)

Insurance, Health
American Academy of Pediatrics response to the growing health needs of children [Strain] 536 (My)
Barriers to medical care for homeless families compared with housed poor families [Wood] 1109 (Oc)
Caring program for children: the Michigan experience [Udow] 579 (My)
Challenge of care for the poor and underserved in the United States: an American College of Obstetricians and Gynecologists perspective on access to care for underserved women [Davidson] 546 (My)
Health care for pregnant women and young children [Behrman] 572 (My)
Redoing the health care quilt: patches or whole cloth? [Cleveland] 499 (My)

Intelligence
Intellectual development in 12-year-old children treated for phenylketonuria [Azen] 35 (Ja)
Neurodevelopmental outcome of offspring of the diabetic mother: need for further research (letter) [Goldstein] 602 (Je)

Intensive Care, Neonatal
Efficacy and pharmacokinetics of intravenous immune globulin administration to high-risk neonates [Kinney] 1233 (No)
Improving health care provision to neonates in the United States [Stahlman] 510 (My)
Medical ethics issues survey of residents in 5 pediatric training programs [White] 161 (Fe)
Pediatric perspectives: vistas and vantage points [Bedrick] 256 (Mr)
Treatment withdrawal in neonates (letter) [Byrne] 1223 (No)

Internship and Residency
Chief resident training: developing leadership skills for future medical leaders [Doughty] 639 (Je)
Clinic attending: teaching strategies for patient encounters [Schmitt] 977 (Se)
Comments on life after residency (letter) [Brent] 597 (Je)
Current trends in pediatric residency training [Carraccio] 1272 (No)
Eighty-hour workweek and residency programs: closing arguments (letter) [Bedrick] 846 (Au)
Hand washing in pediatric ambulatory settings: an inconsistent practice [Lohr] 1198 (Oc)
House staff work hours and moonlighting: what do residents want?: a survey of pediatric residents in California [Cheng] 1104 (Oc)
How are pediatric training programs preparing residents for practice? [Greenberg] 1389 (De)
Medical ethics issues survey of residents in 5 pediatric training programs [White] 161 (Fe)
New York State health code 405 update (letter) [Daigler] 428 (Ap)
Objective structured clinical examination in a pediatric residency program [Joorabchi] 757 (Jy)
Pediatric program director: an analysis of the role and its problems [Weiss] 449 (Ap)
Poverty and the health of American children: implications for academic pediatrics [Johnston] 507 (My)
Practice management training for pediatric residents [Piatt] 299 (Mr)
Priorities in academic pediatrics (letter) [Jacobs] (reply) [Goetzman] 845 (Au)

Resident and nurse practitioners: responding to education and patient care needs (letter) [Giardino] 843 (Au)
Resident, faculty, and residency program development: an integrated approach through annual retreats [Winter] 1191 (Oc)
School health training during pediatric residency [Niebuhr] 79 (Ja)
Serving the underserved: impact on resident education [Berkowitz] 544 (My)
Support services for pediatric trainees: a survey of training program directors [Bergman] 1002 (Se)
Interpersonal Relations
Chief resident training: developing leadership skills for future medical leaders [Doughty] 639 (Je)
Comments on life after residency (letter) [Brent] 597 (Je)
Intestinal Perforation
Neonatal appendicitis with perforation [Ruff] 111 (Ja)
Intracranial Pressure
Posthemorrhagic hydrocephalus: use of an intravenous-type catheter for cerebrospinal fluid drainage [Marro] 1141 (Oc)
Intraoperative Complications
Development, growth, and cardiac surgery [Mayer] 33 (Ja)
Intrauterine Growth Retardation see Fetal Growth Retardation
Intravenous Infusions see Infusions, Intravenous
Intubation, Gastrointestinal
Rice solution and World Health Organization solution by gastric infusion for high stool output diarrhea [Mota-Hernández] 937 (Au)
Intubation, Intratracheal
Optimal positioning of endotracheal tubes for ventilation of preterm infants [Rotschild] 1007 (Se)
Ipecac
Demographic and risk factors associated with chronic dieting in adolescents [Story] 994 (Se)
Iron
How much iron is enough? (letter) [Rogers] (reply) [Finberg] 598 (Je)
Total iron-binding capacity in iron poisoning: is it useful? [Tenenbein] 437 (Ap)
Iron Deficiency Anemia see Anemia, Hypochromic
Isoproterenol
Intraosseous infusion of dobutamine and isoproterenol [Bilello] 165 (Fe); correction, 1312 (No)
Israel
Longitudinal study of birth weight and being overweight in late adolescence [Seidman] 782 (Jy)
Seasonal variation in growth during growth hormone therapy [Rudolf] 769 (Jy)
Italy
Legalization of drugs of abuse and the pediatrician [Schwartz] 1153 (Oc)

J

Jacobi, Abraham
AJDC is 80 years old: from pedology to pediatrics [Fulginiti] 11 (Ja)
Japan
Comparative trial of the reactogenicity and immunogenicity of Takeda acellular pertussis vaccine combined with tetanus and diphtheria toxoids: outcome in 3- to 8-month old infants, 9- to 23-month-old infants and children, and 24- to 30-month-old children [Kimura] 734 (Jy)
Neuroblastoma screening data: an epidemiologic analysis [Goodman] 1415 (De)
Jaundice
Gallstones in children: characterization by age, etiology, and outcome [Reif] 105 (Ja)
Jaundice, Neonatal
Direct bilirubin measurements in jaundiced term newborns: a reevaluation [Newman] 1305 (No)
Practical guide to successful breast-feeding management [Freed] 917 (Au)
Jervell-Lange Nielsen Syndrome see Long QT Syndrome
Jurisprudence
Diphtheria and tetanus toxoids and pertussis vaccine litigation (letter) [Lokietz] (reply) [Fulginiti] 425 (Ap)

K

Kawasaki Disease see Mucocutaneous Lymph Node Syndrome
Ketoconazole
Myopathy associated with ketoconazole treatment (letter) [Garty] 970 (Se)
Kidney
Effect of low-dose dopamine infusion on cardiopulmonary and renal status in premature newborns with respiratory distress syndrome [Cuevas] 799 (Jy)
50-year follow-up of childhood plumbism: hypertension, renal function, and hemoglobin levels among survivors [Hu] 681 (Je)
Kidney Concentrating Ability
Medical management of postobstructive polyuria (letter) [Smoyer] 1345 (De)
Kidney Diseases
Paleonephrology and reflux nephropathy: from the 'big bang' to end-stage renal disease [Kallen] 860 (Au)
Kidney Failure, Acute
50-year follow-up of childhood plumbism: hypertension, renal function, and hemoglobin levels among survivors [Hu] 681 (Je)
Kidney Failure, Chronic
Paleonephrology and reflux nephropathy: from the 'big bang' to end-stage renal disease [Kallen] 860 (Au)
Knee
Exacerbation of tinea corporis during treatment with 1% clotrimazole/0.05% betamethasone diproprionate (Lotrisone) (letter) [Reynolds] 1224 (No)
Knee Injuries
Adolescents' attrition from school-sponsored sports [DuRant] 1119 (Oc)
Kostmann's Syndrome see Agranulocytosis

L

Labor Stage, Second
Clavicular fractures in neonates (letter) [Carter] 251, (reply) [Joseph] 252 (Mr)
Clavicular fractures in neonates: frequency vs significance (letter) [O'Halloran] (reply) [Joseph] 251 (Mr)
Laboratories
Cholesterol testing in the physician's office: accuracy assessment (letter) [Rifai] 1087 (Oc)
Lactation
Practical guide to successful breast-feeding management [Freed] 917 (Au)
Language
Word choice (letter) [Gorlick] (reply) [Hong] 724 (Jy)
Laparoscopy see Peritoneoscopy
Laparotomy
Neonatal appendicitis with perforation [Ruff] 111 (Ja)
Laron-Type Dwarfism see Dwarfism
Larva Migrans, Visceral
Visceral larva migrans [Ponder] 699 (Je)
Lasers
Treatment of ulcerated hemangiomas with pulsed tunable dye laser [Morelli] 1062 (Se)
Laxatives see Cathartics
Lead
50-year follow-up of childhood plumbism: hypertension, renal function, and hemoglobin levels among survivors [Hu] 681 (Je)
Lead Poisoning
50-year follow-up of childhood plumbism: hypertension, renal function, and hemoglobin levels among survivors [Hu] 681 (Je)
Lead poisoning in children with developmental disabilities (letter) [Sulkes] 602 (Je)
Leadership
Chief resident training: developing leadership skills for future medical leaders [Doughty] 639 (Je)
Learning
Comparison of a computer tutorial with other methods for teaching well-newborn care [Desch] 1255 (No)
Women in medicine: fantasies, dreams, myths, and realities [DeAngelis] 49 (Ja)
Learning Disorders
Minor malformations, hyperactivity, and learning disabilities [Accardo] 1184 (Oc)
Lecithins see Phosphatidylcholines
Leg Injuries
Skateboarding injuries in children: a second wave [Retsky] 188 (Fe)
LEGAL MEDICINE
Legalization of drugs of abuse and the pediatrician [Schwartz] 1153 (Oc)
Photographing the physically abused child, principles and practice [Ricci] 275 (Mr)
Legislation
Guidelines for safe transportation of children in wheelchairs [DiGaudio] 653 (Je)
House staff work hours and moonlighting: what do residents want?: a survey of pediatric residents in California [Cheng] 1104 (Oc)
Legalization of drugs of abuse and the pediatrician [Schwartz] 1153 (Oc)
Skateboarding injuries in children: a second wave [Retsky] 188 (Fe)
Leishmania donovani
Mediterranean visceral leishmaniasis: a frequently unrecognized imported disease (letter) [Mahieu] 1225 (No)
Leishmaniasis, Visceral
Mediterranean visceral leishmaniasis: a frequently unrecognized imported disease (letter) [Mahieu] 1225 (No)
Leukemia, Lymphoblastic, Acute see Leukemia, Lymphocytic, Acute
Leukemia, Lymphocytic, Acute
Frequency of infections associated with implanted systems vs cuffed, tunneled silastic venous catheters in patients with acute leukemia [Severien] 1433 (De)
Immunization response varies with intensity of acute lymphoblastic leukemia therapy [Ridgway] 887 (Au)
Improvement of leukemic hyperleukocytosis with only fluid and allopurinol therapy (letter) [Lascari] 969 (Se)
Leukemia, Myelocytic, Acute
Frequency of infections associated with implanted systems vs cuffed, tunneled silastic venous catheters in patients with acute leukemia [Severien] 1433 (De)
Improvement of leukemic hyperleukocytosis with only fluid and allopurinol therapy (letter) [Lascari] 969 (Se)
Leukocyte Count
Factors affecting outcome in meningococcal infections [Tesoro] 218 (Fe)
Improvement of leukemic hyperleukocytosis with only fluid and allopurinol therapy (letter) [Lascari] 969 (Se)
Percentile curves for various hematologic measurements at birth in Arab preterm babies of different gestational ages [Haque] 645 (Je)
Leukocytosis
Improvement of leukemic hyperleukocytosis with only fluid and allopurinol therapy (letter) [Lascari] 969 (Se)
Levodopa
Effectiveness of growth-promoting therapies: comparison among growth hormone, clonidine, and levodopa [Volta] 168 (Fe)
Liability, Legal
Diphtheria and tetanus toxoids and pertussis vaccine litigation (letter) [Lokietz] (reply) [Fulginiti] 425 (Ap)
More on a myth (letter) [Roman] (reply) [Fulginiti] 717 (Jy)
Redoing the health care quilt: patches or whole cloth? [Cleveland] 499 (My)
Vaccine myth and physician handouts (letter) [Lynch] 426, (replies) [Cherry, Fulginiti] 426, 427 (Ap)
Lichen Sclerosus et Atrophicus
Lichen sclerosus et atrophicus in children [Loening-Baucke] 1058 (Se)
Life Support Care
Medical ethics issues survey of residents in 5 pediatric training programs [White] 161 (Fe)
Ligaments
Pediatric case of Eagle's syndrome [Holloway] 339 (Mr)
Linkage (Genetics)
Lowe's syndrome [Loughead] 113 (Ja)
Lip
Optimal positioning of endotracheal tubes for ventilation of preterm infants [Rotschild] 1007 (Se)
Lipopolysaccharides
Endotoxin concentrations in cerebrospinal fluid correlate with clinical severity and neurologic outcome of *Haemophilus influenzae* type b meningitis [Mertsola] 1099 (Oc)
Hemorrhagic shock and encephalopathy: an entity similar to heatstroke (letter) [Conway] 720 (Jy)
Lipoproteins, HDL Cholesterol
Lipoprotein profiles in hypercholesterolemic children [Garcia] 147 (Fe); correction, 515 (My)
Serum lipid concentrations in subjects with phenylketonuria and their families [DeClue] 1266 (No)
Lipoproteins, LDL Cholesterol
Lipoprotein profiles in hypercholesterolemic children [Garcia] 147 (Fe); correction, 515 (My)
Serum lipid concentrations in subjects with phenylketonuria and their families [DeClue] 1266 (No)
Literacy Programs see Education
Literature
Tiny Tim remembered [Callahan] 1355 (De)
Liver
Misdiagnosis of Reye's-like illness (letter) [Forsyth] 964 (Se)
Long QT Syndrome
Sudden cardiac death (letter) [Pearl] 1223 (No)
Sudden cardiac death in young athletes: a review [McCaffrey] 177 (Fe)
Lorazepam
Survey of antiemetic use in children with cancer [van Hoff] 773 (Jy)
Lowe Syndrome see Oculocerebrorenal Syndrome
Lumbar Puncture see Spinal Puncture
Lung
Hypoplastic left upper lobe [Al-Salem] 821 (Jy)
Lung Capacity, Total see Total Lung Capacity
Lung Diseases
Influenza type A and B infections in hospitalized pediatric patients: who should be immunized? [Serwint] 623 (Je)
Lupus Erythematosus, Systemic
Challenge of caring for indigent children with rheumatologic diseases [Miller] 554 (My)
Lymphadenopathy Syndrome see AIDS-Related Complex
T-Lymphocyte Subsets
Anergy in pediatric head trauma patients [Wilson] 326 (Mr)
Lymphocytes
Elevated plasma norepinephrine levels in infants of substance-abusing mothers [Ward] 44 (Ja)
Percentile curves for various hematologic measurements at birth in Arab preterm babies of different gestational ages [Haque] 645 (Je)
B-Lymphocytes
Anergy in pediatric head trauma patients [Wilson] 326 (Mr)
T-Lymphocytes
Anergy in pediatric head trauma patients [Wilson] 326 (Mr)

M

Magic
Word choice (letter) [Gorlick] (reply) [Hong] 724 (Jy)
Magnetic Resonance Spectroscopy see Nuclear Magnetic Resonance
Malnutrition see Nutrition Disorders
Management Teams, Institutional see Institutional Management Teams
Manometry
Esophageal motility in children with Hirschsprung's disease [Staiano] 310 (Mr)
Marfan Syndrome
Marfanoid children: etiologic heterogeneity and cardiac findings [Tayel] 90 (Ja)
Sudden cardiac death in young athletes: a review [McCaffrey] 177 (Fe)
Marijuana Abuse
Meconium for drug testing [Maynard] 650 (Je)
Markers, Biological see Biological Markers
Marriage
Comments on life after residency (letter) [Brent] 597 (Je)
Differences in infant mortality by race, nativity status, and other maternal characteristics [Kleinman] 194 (Fe)
Maryland
Home care cost-effectiveness for respiratory technology-dependent children [Fields] 729 (Jy)
Mass Screening
Lipoprotein profiles in hypercholesterolemic children [Garcia] 147 (Fe); correction, 515 (My)
Neuroblastoma screening data: an epidemiologic analysis [Goodman] 1415 (De)
Mast Cells
Trimethoprim-sulfamethoxazole oral desensitization in hemophiliacs infected with human immunodeficiency virus with a history of hypersensitivity reactions [Kletzel] 1428 (De)
Mastitis
Practical guide to successful breast-feeding management [Freed] 917 (Au)
Maternal Behavior
Breast-feeding initiation in a triethnic population [Bee] 306 (Mr)
Maternal-Fetal Exchange
Brain and ocular abnormalities in infants with in utero exposure to cocaine and other street drugs [Dominguez] 688 (Je)
Elevated plasma norepinephrine levels in infants of substance-abusing mothers [Ward] 44 (Ja)
Meconium for drug testing [Maynard] 650 (Je)
Preliminary report of prenatal cocaine exposure and respiratory distress syndrome in premature infants [Zuckerman] 696 (Je)
Maternal Health Services
American Academy of Pediatrics response to the growing health needs of children [Strain] 536 (My)
Challenge of care for the poor and underserved in the United States: an American College of Obstetricians and Gynecologists perspective on access to care for underserved women [Davidson] 546 (My)
Differences in infant mortality by race, nativity status, and other maternal characteristics [Kleinman] 194 (Fe)
Far from the ideal: the plight of poor children in the United States [Fulginiti] 489 (My)
Fetal alcohol syndrome: misplaced emphasis (letter) [Hess] (reply) [Little] 721 (Jy)
Growing neglect of American children [Maurer] 540 (My)
Health care for pregnant women and young children [Behrman] 572 (My)
Improving health care provision to neonates in the United States [Stahlman] 510 (My)
Redoing the health care quilt: patches or whole cloth? [Cleveland] 499 (My)
Maternal Welfare
Psychosocial predictors of maternal and infant health among adolescent mothers [Boyce] 267 (Mr)
Mead Johnson Company
Physicians, formula companies, and advertising: a historical perspective [Greer] 282 (Mr)
Measles Vaccine
Antibody response to MMR vaccination in children who received IVIG as neonates (letter) [Ruderman] 425 (Ap)
Apparent decreased risk of invasive bacterial disease after heterologous childhood immunization [Black] 746 (Jy)
Response of seronegative adults to measles immunization (letter) [Braunstein] 969 (Se)
Meconium
Meconium for drug testing [Maynard] 650 (Je)
Medicaid
American Academy of Pediatrics response to the growing health needs of children [Strain] 536 (My)
Barriers to medical care for homeless families compared with housed poor families [Wood] 1109 (Oc)
Home care cost-effectiveness for respiratory technology-dependent children [Fields] 729 (Jy)
Poverty and cardiac disease in children [Allen] 550 (My)
Redoing the health care quilt: patches or whole cloth? [Cleveland] 499 (My)
Medical Audit
Guidelines for auditing pediatric blood transfusion practices [Blanchette] 787 (Jy)
Medical History Taking
Family history fails to identify many children with severe hypercholesterolemia [Starc] 61 (Ja)
Medical Indigency
Barriers to medical care for homeless families compared with housed poor families [Wood] 1109 (Oc)
Caring program for children: the Michigan experience [Udow] 579 (My)
Challenge of caring for indigent children with rheumatologic diseases [Miller] 554 (My)
Health care for uninsured and underinsured children (letter) [Davis] 1085 (Oc)
Redoing the health care quilt: patches or whole cloth? [Cleveland] 499 (My)
Medical Staff, Hospital
Fetal alcohol syndrome: misplaced emphasis (letter) [Hess] (reply) [Little] 721 (Jy)
Medically Underserved Area
Challenge of care for the poor and underserved in the United States: an American College of Obstetricians and Gynecologists perspective on access to care for underserved women [Davidson] 546 (My)
Health care for uninsured and underinsured children (letter) [Pearson] 1085 (Oc)
Serving the underserved: impact on resident education [Berkowitz] 544 (My)
Medication Errors
Multilevel model to assess appropriateness of pediatric serum drug concentrations [Kraus] 1171 (Oc)
Mediterranean Sea
Mediterranean visceral leishmaniasis: a frequently unrecognized imported disease (letter) [Mahieu] 1225 (No)
Megacolon
Esophageal motility in children with Hirschsprung's disease [Staiano] 310 (Mr)
Meningitis
Cautionary note on the use of empiric ceftriaxone for suspected bacteremia [Wald] 1359 (De)
Lumbar puncture frequency and cerebrospinal fluid analysis in the neonate [Schwersenski] 54 (Ja)
Meningitis, Aseptic
Vasopressin levels in infants during the course of aseptic and bacterial meningitis [Padilla] 991 (Se)
Meningitis, Haemophilus
Endotoxin concentrations in cerebrospinal fluid correlate with clinical severity and neurologic outcome of *Haemophilus influenzae* type b meningitis [Mertsola] 1099 (Oc)
Role of corticosteroid therapy in children with pneumococcal meningitis [Kennedy] 1374 (De)
Vasopressin levels in infants during the course of aseptic and bacterial meningitis [Padilla] 991 (Se)
Meningitis, Meningococcal
Factors affecting outcome in meningococcal infections [Tesoro] 218 (Fe)
Vasopressin levels in infants during the course of aseptic and bacterial meningitis [Padilla] 991 (Se)
Meningitis, Pneumococcal
Role of corticosteroid therapy in children with pneumococcal meningitis [Kennedy] 1374 (De)
Meningococcal Infections
Factors affecting outcome in meningococcal infections [Tesoro] 218 (Fe)
Scoring systems for accurate prognosis of patients with meningococcal infections (letter) [Leclerc] 1090 (Oc)
Meningomyelocele
Ventriculitis in newborns with myelomeningocele [Charney] 287 (Mr)
Mental Disorders
Factors affecting outcome in meningococcal infections [Tesoro] 218 (Fe)
Mental Retardation
Lead poisoning in children with developmental disabilities (letter) [Sulkes] 602 (Je)
Mentors
Women in medicine: fantasies, dreams, myths, and realities [DeAngelis] 49 (Ja)
Meta-Analysis
Surfactant replacement therapy in respiratory distress syndrome: meta-analysis of clinical trials of single-dose surfactant extracts [Hennes] 102 (Ja)
Metabolic Diseases
Autosomal recessive lethal infantile cytochrome C oxidase deficiency [Eshel] 661 (Je)
Metabolism
Mineral metabolism and calcitriol therapy in idiopathic juvenile osteoporosis [Saggese] 457 (Ap)
Metcoff, Jack
Jack Metcoff festschrift [Lewy] 851 (Au) Studies in fetal malnutrition [Crosby] 871 (Au)
Methemoglobinemia
Acquired methemoglobinemia: the relationship of cause to course of illness [Avner] **144**:1229(No); correction, **145**:158 (Fe)
Methylphenidate
Stimulant medication and attention deficit-hyperactivity disorder: the child's perspective [Bowen] 291 (Mr)
Metoclopramide
Survey of antiemetic use in children with cancer [van Hoff] 773 (Jy)
Mexican Americans see Hispanic Americans
Michigan
Caring program for children: the Michigan experience [Udow] 579 (My)
Microscopy, Electron
Misdiagnosis of Reye's-like illness (letter) [Forsyth] 964 (Se)
Milk
Current social practices leading to water intoxication in infants (letter) [Schaeffer] 27 (Ja)
How much iron is enough? (letter) [Rogers] (reply) [Finberg] 598 (Je)
Low serum calcium and high parathyroid hormone levels in neonates fed 'humanized' cow's milk-based formula [Specker] 941 (Au)
Milk, Human
Low serum calcium and high parathyroid hormone levels in neonates fed 'humanized' cow's milk-based formula [Specker] 941 (Au)
Minerals
Mineral metabolism and calcitriol therapy in idiopathic juvenile osteoporosis [Saggese] 457 (Ap)
Minority Groups
Barriers to medical care for homeless families compared with housed poor families [Wood] 1109 (Oc)
Breast-feeding initiation in a triethnic population [Bee] 306 (Mr)
Pediatric human immunodeficiency virus infection and the acquired immunodeficiency syndrome: a health care crisis of children and families [Van Dyke] 529 (My)
What will it take to fully protect all American children with vaccines? [Hinman] 559 (My)
Youth alienation as an emerging pediatric health care issue [Farrow] 491 (My)
Mitochondria
Autosomal recessive lethal infantile cytochrome C oxidase deficiency [Eshel] 661 (Je)
Mitral Valve Prolapse
Marfanoid children: etiologic heterogeneity and cardiac findings [Tayel] 90 (Ja)
Mitral valve prolapse: back to the basics [Allen] 1095 (Oc)
Sudden cardiac death in young athletes: a review [McCaffrey] 177 (Fe)
Models, Statistical
Child survival and perinatal infections with human immunodeficiency virus [Bennett] 1242 (No)
Monitoring, Physiologic
Effects of obesity on aerobic fitness in adolescent females [Rowland] 764 (Jy)
Monocytes
Percentile curves for various hematologic measurements at birth in Arab preterm babies of different gestational ages [Haque] 645 (Je)
Moonlighting see Employment
Morphine
Meconium for drug testing [Maynard] 650 (Je)
Mortality
Child survival and perinatal infections with human immunodeficiency virus [Bennett] 1242 (No)
Commotio cordis: the single, most common cause of traumatic death in youth baseball [Abrunzo] 1279 (No)
Escherichia coli bacteremia in children: a review of 91 cases in 10 years [Bonadio] 671 (Je)
Evolution of surgical treatment for congenital cardiac disease [Pigott] 1362 (De)
Factors affecting outcome in meningococcal infections [Tesoro] 218 (Fe)
Follow-up of patients who underwent arterial switch repair for transposition of the great arteries [Mendoza] 40 (Ja)
Mothers
Bone mineral content of healthy, full-term neonates: effect of race, gender, and maternal cigarette smoking [Venkataraman] 1310 (No)
Child survival and perinatal infections with human immunodeficiency virus [Bennett] 1242 (No)
Clinical and endocrinologic manifestations in perinatally human immunodeficiency virus type 1-infected children aged 5 years or older [Lepage] 1248 (No)
Comparison of maternal and infant serologic tests for syphilis [Rawstron] 1383 (De)
Complex problem: complex solutions [McAnarney] 429 (Ap)
Differences in infant mortality by race, nativity status, and other maternal characteristics [Kleinman] 194 (Fe)
Elevated plasma norepinephrine levels in infants of substance-abusing mothers [Ward] 44 (Ja)
Increased transient tachypnea of the newborn in infants with asthmatic mothers [Schatz] 156 (Fe)
Obesity among Mescalero preschool children: association with maternal obesity and birth weight [Gallaher] 1262 (No)
Pediatric human immunodeficiency virus infection and the acquired immunodeficiency syndrome: a health care crisis of children and families [Van Dyke] 529 (My)
Sun protection in newborns: a comparison of educational methods [Bolognia] 1125 (Oc)
Survey of the health of homeless children in Philadelphia

shelters [Parker] 520 (My)
Vertical transmission of human immunodeficiency virus from seronegative or indeterminate mothers [Johnson] 1239 (No)
Motivation
Health care for uninsured and underinsured children (letter) [Barness] 1086 (Oc)
Mucocutaneous Lymph Node Syndrome
Hydrocele in Kawasaki disease: importance in early recognition of atypical disease (letter) [Kabani] 1348 (De)
Sudden cardiac death in young athletes: a review [McCaffrey] 177 (Fe)
Mumps Vaccine
Antibody response to MMR vaccination in children who received IVIG as neonates (letter) [Ruderman] 425 (Ap)
Apparent decreased risk of invasive bacterial disease after heterologous childhood immunization [Black] 746 (Jy)
Mupirocin
Impetigo [Esterly] 125 (Fe)
Mutation
Differences in expression of cystic fibrosis in blacks and whites [McColley] 94 (Ja)
Myasthenia Gravis
Association of pauciarticular juvenile arthritis and myasthenia gravis [Glass] 1176 (Oc)
Mycoplasma pneumoniae
Causes of hospital-treated acute lower respiratory tract infection in children [Nohynek] 618 (Je)
Mycoses
Frequency of infections associated with implanted systems vs cuffed, tunneled silastic venous catheters in patients with acute leukemia [Severien] 1433 (De)
Myelomeningocele see Meningomyelocele
Myocardial Diseases
Focal scleroderma and severe cardiomyopathy: patient report and brief review [Moore] 229 (Fe)
Myocardial Infarction
Family history of myocardial infarction and hemodynamic responses to exercise in young black boys [Treiber] 1029 (Se)
Myocarditis
Sudden cardiac death in young athletes: a review [McCaffrey] 177 (Fe)
Myositis
Myopathy associated with ketoconazole treatment (letter) [Garty] 970 (Se)

N

Nails
Capillary refilling (skin turgor) in the assessment of dehydration [Saavedra] 296 (Mr)
Nails, Malformed
Pachyonychia congenita [Cohen] 1301 (No)
Narcotics
Elevated plasma norepinephrine levels in infants of substance-abusing mothers [Ward] 44 (Ja)
National Health Insurance, United States
Redoing the health care quilt: patches or whole cloth? [Cleveland] 499 (My)
Regional pediatric approach to the epidemic of social ills within our cities [Nelson] 505 (My)
National Health Programs
Redoing the health care quilt: patches or whole cloth? [Cleveland] 499 (My)
Natriuresis
Effect of low-dose dopamine infusion on cardiopulmonary and renal status in premature newborns with respiratory distress syndrome [Cuevas] 799 (Jy)
Nausea
Survey of antiemetic use in children with cancer [van Hoff] 773 (Jy)
Near Drowning
Immersion events in residential swimming pools: evidence for an experience effect [Wintemute] 1200 (Oc)
Neck
Skateboarding injuries in children: a second wave [Retsky] 188 (Fe)
Necrosis
Penile vasculitis with impending necrosis treated with prostaglandin E_1 infusion (letter) [Horner] 604 (Je)
Neisseria meningitidis
Dose-related immunogenicity of *Haemophilus influenzae* type b capsular polysaccharide—*Neisseria meningitidis* outer membrane protein conjugate vaccine [Wong] 742 (Jy)
Neonatal Intensive Care see Intensive Care, Neonatal
Neonatology
Treatment withdrawal in neonates (letter) [Byrne] 1223 (No)
Neoplasms
Survey of antiemetic use in children with cancer [van Hoff] 773 (Jy)
Nephrons
Paleonephrology and reflux nephropathy: from the 'big bang' to end-stage renal disease [Kallen] 860 (Au)
Nephropathy, Balkan see Balkan Nephropathy
Nervous System Diseases
Major congenital neurologic malformations (letter) [Ryals] 30 (Ja)
Nestlé-Carnation
Physicians, formula companies, and advertising: a historical perspective [Greer] 282 (Mr)
Netherlands
Legalization of drugs of abuse and the pediatrician [Schwartz] 1153 (Oc)
Neural Tube Defects
Major congenital neurologic malformations (letter) [Ryals] 30 (Ja)
Neuritis
Cat-scratch disease: acute encephalopathy and other neurologic manifestations [Carithers] 98 (Ja)
Neuroblastoma
Neuroblastoma screening data: an epidemiologic analysis [Goodman] 1415 (De)
Neurologic Manifestations
Cat-scratch disease: acute encephalopathy and other neurologic manifestations [Carithers] 98 (Ja)
Development, growth, and cardiac surgery [Mayer] 33 (Ja)
Endotoxin concentrations in cerebrospinal fluid correlate with clinical severity and neurologic outcome of *Haemophilus influenzae* type b meningitis [Mertsola] 1099 (Oc)
Fallacy of the hemorrhagic shock and encephalopathy syndrome (letter) [Bass] 718 (Jy)
Follow-up of patients who underwent arterial switch repair for transposition of the great arteries [Mendoza] 40 (Ja)
'H' in hemorrhagic shock and encephalopathy syndrome (letter) [Roscelli] 720 (Jy)
Role of corticosteroid therapy in children with pneumococcal meningitis [Kennedy] 1374 (De)
Neuromuscular Diseases
Autosomal recessive lethal infantile cytochrome C oxidase deficiency [Eshel] 661 (Je)
Neuropsychological Tests
Development, growth, and cardiac surgery [Mayer] 33 (Ja)
Neurodevelopmental outcome of offspring of the diabetic mother: need for further research (letter) [Goldstein] 602 (Je)
Predictors of neurodevelopmental outcome following bronchopulmonary dysplasia [Luchi] 813 (Jy)
Neuroses see Neurotic Disorders
Neurotic Disorders
Testing the psychogenic vomiting diagnosis: four pediatric patients [Gonzalez-Heydrich] 913 (Au)
Neutropenia
Chronic neutropenia during childhood: a 13-year experience in a single institution [Jonsson] 232 (Fe)
Escherichia coli bacteremia in children: a review of 91 cases in 10 years [Bonadio] 671 (Je)
Frequency of infections associated with implanted systems vs cuffed, tunneled silastic venous catheters in patients with acute leukemia [Severien] 1433 (De)
Measurement of serum granulocyte colony-stimulating factor in a patient with congenital agranulocytosis (Kostmann's syndrome) [Glasser] 925 (Au)
Neutropenia in an extremely premature infant treated with recombinant human granulocyte colony-stimulating factor [Roberts] 808 (Jy)
Neutrophils
Measurement of serum granulocyte colony-stimulating factor in a patient with congenital agranulocytosis (Kostmann's syndrome) [Glasser] 925 (Au)
Percentile curves for various hematologic measurements at birth in Arab preterm babies of different gestational ages [Haque] 645 (Je)
Transfusion therapy in neonates [Strauss] 904 (Au)
Nevus
Nevus flammeus: discordance in monozygotic twins [Shamir] 85 (Ja)
New York
New York State health code 405 update (letter) [Daigler] 428 (Ap)
Nipples
Practical guide to successful breast-feeding management [Freed] 917 (Au)
Nomenclature
Acellular pertussis vaccines: efficacy and evaluation of clinical case definitions [Blackwelder] 1285 (No)
Fallacy of the hemorrhagic shock and encephalopathy syndrome (letter) [Bass] 718 (Jy)
'H' in hemorrhagic shock and encephalopathy syndrome (letter) [Roscelli] 720 (Jy)
Norepinephrine
Elevated plasma norepinephrine levels in infants of substance-abusing mothers [Ward] 44 (Ja)
Nose
Optimal positioning of endotracheal tubes for ventilation of preterm infants [Rotschild] 1007 (Se)
Nosocomial Infections see Cross Infection
Nuclear Magnetic Resonance
X-linked hypophosphatemia: genetic and clinical correlates [Hanna] 865 (Au)
Nurse-Patient Relations
Improving the use of early follow-up care after emergency department visits: a randomized trial [Nelson] 440 (Ap)
Nurse Practitioners
Improving the use of early follow-up care after emergency department visits: a randomized trial [Nelson] 440 (Ap)
Resident and nurse practitioners: responding to education and patient care needs (letter) [Giardino] 843 (Au)
Nursing
Home care cost-effectiveness for respiratory technology-dependent children [Fields] 729 (Jy)
Saving money with home care [Schoumacher] 725 (Jy)
Nutrition
Obesity and body-mass index (letter) [Hergenroeder] (reply) [Hammer] 972 (Se)
Nutrition Disorders
Studies in fetal malnutrition [Crosby] 871 (Au)

O

Obesity
Effects of obesity on aerobic fitness in adolescent females [Rowland] 764 (Jy)
Longitudinal study of birth weight and being overweight in late adolescence [Seidman] 782 (Jy)
Obesity among Mescalero preschool children: association with maternal obesity and birth weight [Gallaher] 1262 (No)
Obesity and body-mass index (letter) [Hergenroeder] (reply) [Hammer] 972 (Se)
Standardized percentile curves of body-mass index for children and adolescents [Hammer] 259 (Mr)
Object Attachment
Resident, faculty, and residency program development: an integrated approach through annual retreats [Winter] 1191 (Oc)
Send Linus to me (letter) [Szonyi] (reply) [Friman] 1227 (No)
Thumb-sucking (letter) [Lubicky] 845, (reply) [Friman] 846 (Au)
Obstetrics
Challenge of care for the poor and underserved in the United States: an American College of Obstetricians and Gynecologists perspective on access to care for underserved women [Davidson] 546 (My)
Fetal alcohol syndrome: misplaced emphasis (letter) [Hess] (reply) [Little] 721 (Jy)
Occipital Bone
Osteochondrodysplasia in Fryns syndrome [Kershisnik] 656 (Je)
Oculocerebrorenal Syndrome
Lowe's syndrome [Loughead] 113 (Ja)
Office Management
Practice management training for pediatric residents [Piatt] 299 (Mr)
Office Visits
Cholesterol testing in the physician's office: accuracy assessment (letter) [Rifai] 1087 (Oc)
Oligosaccharides
Response of 7- to 15-month-old infants to sequential immunization with *Haemophilus influenzae* type b-CRM_{197} conjugate and polysaccharide vaccines [Rothstein] 898 (Au)
Opiates see Narcotics
Opportunistic Infections
Third pattern of disease progression in children infected with human immunodeficiency virus (letter) [Katz] 1347, (reply) [Blanche] 1348 (De)
Oregon
Legalization of drugs of abuse and the pediatrician [Schwartz] 1153 (Oc)
Orthomyxoviruses Type A
Influenza type A and B infections in hospitalized pediatric patients: who should be immunized? [Serwint] 623 (Je)
Influenza vaccination in the prevention of acute otitis media in children [Heikkinen] 445 (Ap)
Orthomyxoviruses Type B
Influenza type A and B infections in hospitalized pediatric patients: who should be immunized? [Serwint] 623 (Je)
Osmolar Concentration
Water intoxication: a prevalent problem in the inner city [Finberg] 981 (Se)
Osmoregulation see Water-Electrolyte Balance
Osteocalcin
Growth hormone therapy in hypophosphatemic rickets [Wilson] 1165 (Oc)
Osteochondrodysplasias
Neural arch stenosis and spinal cord injury in thanatophoric dysplasia [Faye-Petersen] 87 (Ja)
Osteochondrodysplasia in Fryns syndrome [Kershisnik] 656 (Je)
Osteomyelitis
Acute osteomyelitis in children: reassessment of etiologic agents and their clinical characteristics [Faden] 65 (Ja)
Pneumococcal osteomyelitis and arthritis in children: a hospital series and literature review [Jacobs] 70 (Ja)
Puncture wound-induced *Achromobacter xylosoxidans* osteomyelitis of the foot (letter) [Hoddy] 599 (Je)
Osteoporosis
Mineral metabolism and calcitriol therapy in idiopathic juvenile osteoporosis [Saggese] 457 (Ap)
Otitis Media
Influence of otitis media on the correlation between rectal and auditory canal temperatures [Terndrup] 75 (Ja)
Influenza vaccination in the prevention of acute otitis media in children [Heikkinen] 445 (Ap)
Outpatients

Improving the use of early follow-up care after emergency department visits: a randomized trial [Nelson] 440 (Ap)
Oximetry
Outpatient assessment of infants with bronchiolitis [Shaw] 151 (Fe)
Oxygen saturation by pulse oximetry in healthy infants at an altitude of 1610 m (5280 ft): what is normal? [Thilo] 1137 (Oc)
Oxygen
Oxygen saturation by pulse oximetry in healthy infants at an altitude of 1610 m (5280 ft): what is normal? [Thilo] 1137 (Oc)
Oxygen Consumption
Pediatric cardiac rehabilitation [Balfour] 627 (Je) Physiologic responses to playing a video game [Segal] 1034 (Se)
Oxygen Inhalation Therapy
Home care cost-effectiveness for respiratory technology-dependent children [Fields] 729 (Jy)
Predictors of neurodevelopmental outcome following bronchopulmonary dysplasia [Luchi] 813 (Jy)

P

Pain
Gallstones in children: characterization by age, etiology, and outcome [Reif] 105 (Ja)
Paleontology
Paleonephrology and reflux nephropathy: from the 'big bang' to end-stage renal disease [Kallen] 860 (Au)
Pancreatitis
Gallstones in children: characterization by age, etiology, and outcome [Reif] 105 (Ja)
Papillomaviruses
Condylomata acuminata: still usually a sexually transmitted disease in children (letter) [Goldenring] 600, (reply) [Boyd] 601 (Je)
Paralysis
Tiny Tim remembered [Callahan] 1355 (De)
Parathyroid Hormones
Low serum calcium and high parathyroid hormone levels in neonates fed 'humanized' cow's milk-based formula [Specker] 941 (Au)
Partial hypoparathyroidism: a variant of transient congenital hypoparathyroidism [Kooh] 877 (Au)
Parent-Child Relations
Comments on life after residency (letter) [Brent] 597 (Je)
Detection of alcoholism in hospitalized children and their families [Duggan] 613 (Je)
Parental alcoholism: a neglected pediatric responsibility [MacDonald] 609 (Je)
Parenteral Feeding
Gallstones in children: characterization by age, etiology, and outcome [Reif] 105 (Ja)
Parenteral Hyperalimentation
Factors associated with umbilical catheter-related sepsis in neonates [Landers] 675 (Je)
Intravenous hyperalimentation fluid obtained with lumbar puncture: an unusual complication of a central venous catheter [Mah] 1439 (De)
Parents
Clinic attending: teaching strategies for patient encounters [Schmitt] 977 (Se)
Clinic-based intervention to promote literacy: a pilot study [Needlman] 881 (Au)
Detection of alcoholism in hospitalized children and their families [Duggan] 613 (Je)
Improving the use of early follow-up care after emergency department visits: a randomized trial [Nelson] 440 (Ap)
Parental alcoholism: a neglected pediatric responsibility [MacDonald] 609 (Je)
Parental drinking habits (letter) [Wells] 1087 (Oc)
Stimulant medication and attention deficit-hyperactivity disorder: the child's perspective [Bowen] 291 (Mr)
Parity
Differences in infant mortality by race, nativity status, and other maternal characteristics [Kleinman] 194 (Fe)
Parotitis
Clinical and endocrinologic manifestations in perinatally human immunodeficiency virus type 1-infected children aged 5 years or older [Lepage] 1248 (No)
Patient Compliance
Improving the use of early follow-up care after emergency department visits: a randomized trial [Nelson] 440 (Ap)
Patients
Adolescents with chronic illness [Perrin] 1361 (De)
PEDIATRIC LEGAL MEDICINE
Legalization of drugs of abuse and the pediatrician [Schwartz] 1153 (Oc)
Photographing the physically abused child, principles and practice [Ricci] 275 (Mr)
Pediatric Nursing
Resident and nurse practitioners: responding to education and patient care needs (letter) [Giardino] 843 (Au)
PEDIATRIC PERSPECTIVES
Cortical resection for children with epilepsy: perspectives in pediatrics [Wyllie] 314 (Mr)
Pediatric perspectives: vistas and vantage points [Bedrick] 256 (Mr)
Pediatrics
Adolescent pelvic examination: an effective practical approach [Tolmas] 1269 (No)
AJDC is 80 years old: from pedology to pediatrics [Fulginiti] 11 (Ja)
American Academy of Pediatrics response to the growing health needs of children [Strain] 536 (My)
Buddy, can you paradigm? [Brown] 727 (Jy)
Care of the poor and underserved in America: older adolescents: a group at special risk [Haggerty] 569 (My)
Chief resident training: developing leadership skills for future medical leaders [Doughty] 639 (Je)
Child abuse and neglect: critical first steps in response to a national emergency: the report of the US Advisory Board on Child Abuse and Neglect [Krugman] 513 (My)
Clinic attending: teaching strategies for patient encounters [Schmitt] 977 (Se)
Comparison of a computer tutorial with other methods for teaching well-newborn care [Desch] 1255 (No)
Current trends in pediatric residency training [Carraccio] 1272 (No)
Detection of alcoholism in hospitalized children and their families [Duggan] 613 (Je)
Eighty-hour workweek and residency programs: closing arguments (letter) [Bedrick] 846 (Au)
Family physicians and neonatology (letter) [McIntyre] (reply) [DiTraglia] 963 (Se)
Fetal alcohol syndrome: misplaced emphasis (letter) [Hess] (reply) [Little] 721 (Jy)
Formula companies and the medical profession (letters) [Fink, Newman] 1088, 1089, (reply) [Greer] 1090 (Oc)
Health care for uninsured and underinsured children (letters) [Kirschner, Pearson] 1085 (Oc)
House staff work hours and moonlighting: what do residents want?: a survey of pediatric residents in California [Cheng] 1104 (Oc)
How are pediatric training programs preparing residents for practice? [Greenberg] 1389 (De)
Jack Metcoff festschrift [Lewy] 851 (Au)
Medical ethics issues survey of residents in 5 pediatric training programs [White] 161 (Fe)
More on a myth (letter) [Roman] (reply) [Fulginiti] 717 (Jy)
New York State health code 405 update (letter) [Daigler] 428 (Ap)
Objective structured clinical examination in a pediatric residency program [Joorabchi] 757 (Jy)
Parental alcoholism: a neglected pediatric responsibility [MacDonald] 609 (Je)
Part-time Peg: who, me? [Ferry] 852 (Au)
Pediatric human immunodeficiency virus infection and the acquired immunodeficiency syndrome: a health care crisis of children and families [Van Dyke] 529 (My)
Pediatric legal medicine: a new venture [Ferry] 255 (Mr)
Pediatric perspectives: vistas and vantage points [Bedrick] 256 (Mr)
Pediatric program director: an analysis of the role and its problems [Weiss] 449 (Ap)
Poverty and cardiac disease in children [Allen] 550 (My)
Poverty and the health of American children: implications for academic pediatrics [Johnston] 507 (My)
Practical guide to successful breast-feeding management [Freed] 917 (Au)
Practice management training for pediatric residents [Piatt] 299 (Mr)
Priorities in academic pediatrics (letter) [Jacobs] (reply) [Goetzman] 845 (Au)
Regional pediatric approach to the epidemic of social ills within our cities [Nelson] 505 (My)
Resident, faculty, and residency program development: an integrated approach through annual retreats [Winter] 1191 (Oc)
School health training during pediatric residency [Niebuhr] 79 (Ja)
Serving the underserved: impact on resident education [Berkowitz] 544 (My)
Support services for pediatric trainees: a survey of training program directors [Bergman] 1002 (Se)
Youth alienation as an emerging pediatric health care issue [Farrow] 491 (My)
Peer Group
Tattooing behavior in adolescence: a comparison study [Farrow] 184 (Fe)
Pelvis
Adolescent pelvic examination: an effective practical approach [Tolmas] 1269 (No)
Penicillin Resistance
Staphylococcus aureus in impetigo (letter) [Dagan] (reply) [Bass] 1223 (No)
Penile Diseases
Penile vasculitis with impending necrosis treated with prostaglandin E_1 infusion (letter) [Horner] 604 (Je)
Pennsylvania
Regional pediatric approach to the epidemic of social ills within our cities [Nelson] 505 (My)
Peptic Ulcer
Differences in expression of cystic fibrosis in blacks and whites [McColley] 94 (Ja)
Periodicals
AJDC is 80 years old: from pedology to pediatrics [Fulginiti] 11 (Ja)
Peripheral Nerve Diseases
Cat-scratch disease: acute encephalopathy and other neurologic manifestations [Carithers] 98 (Ja)
Peripheral Resistance see Vascular Resistance
Peritoneoscopy
Laparoscopic cholecystectomy under continuous epidural anesthesia in patients with cystic fibrosis (letter) [Edelman] 723 (Jy)
Personality Development
Adolescents with chronic illness [Perrin] 1361 (De)
Personnel Selection
Priorities in academic pediatrics (letter) [Jacobs] (reply) [Goetzman] 845 (Au)
Pertussis Toxins
Comparative trial of the reactogenicity and immunogenicity of Takeda acellular pertussis vaccine combined with tetanus and diphtheria toxoids: outcome in 3- to 8-month old infants, 9- to 23-month-old infants and children, and 24- to 30-month-old children [Kimura] 734 (Jy)
Pertussis Vaccine
Acellular pertussis vaccines: efficacy and evaluation of clinical case definitions [Blackwelder] 1285 (No)
Comparative trial of the reactogenicity and immunogenicity of Takeda acellular pertussis vaccine combined with tetanus and diphtheria toxoids: outcome in 3- to 8-month old infants, 9- to 23-month-old infants and children, and 24- to 30-month-old children [Kimura] 734 (Jy)
More on a myth (letter) [Roman] (reply) [Fulginiti] 717 (Jy)
Vaccine myth and physician handouts (letter) [Lynch] 426, (replies) [Cherry, Fulginiti] 426, 427 (Ap)
Petechiae see Purpura
pH see Hydrogen-Ion Concentration
Pharmacology, Clinical
Multilevel model to assess appropriateness of pediatric serum drug concentrations [Kraus] 1171 (Oc)
Pharynx
Gilding the lily (letter) [Faigel] (reply) [Myer] 849 (Au)
Phenobarbital
Effect of valproic acid on plasma carnitine levels [Opala] 999 (Se)
Multilevel model to assess appropriateness of pediatric serum drug concentrations [Kraus] 1171 (Oc)
Phenothiazines
Survey of antiemetic use in children with cancer [van Hoff] 773 (Jy)
Phenotype
Differences in expression of cystic fibrosis in blacks and whites [McColley] 94 (Ja)
Phenylalanine
Intellectual development in 12-year-old children treated for phenylketonuria [Azen] 35 (Ja)
Status report on phenylketonuria treatment: 1990 [Mabry] 33 (Ja)
Phenylalanine Hydroxylase
Status report on phenylketonuria treatment: 1990 [Mabry] 33 (Ja)
Phenylketonuria
Intellectual development in 12-year-old children treated for phenylketonuria [Azen] 35 (Ja)
Serum lipid concentrations in subjects with phenylketonuria and their families [DeClue] 1266 (No)
Status report on phenylketonuria treatment: 1990 [Mabry] 33 (Ja)
Phenytoin
Effect of valproic acid on plasma carnitine levels [Opala] 999 (Se)
Philadelphia
Child welfare: the phantom of the health care system (letter) [Pidcock] 843 (Au)
Survey of the health of homeless children in Philadelphia shelters [Parker] 520 (My)
Philadelphia Pediatric Society
Regional pediatric approach to the epidemic of social ills within our cities [Nelson] 505 (My)
Phosphates
Growth hormone therapy in hypophosphatemic rickets [Wilson] 1165 (Oc)
X-linked hypophosphatemia: genetic and clinical correlates [Hanna] 865 (Au)
Phosphatidylcholines
Markedly immature lecithin-sphingomyelin ratio at term and congenital hypothyroidism (letter) [Cohen] 1227 (No)
Phosphatidylglycerols
Markedly immature lecithin-sphingomyelin ratio at term and congenital hypothyroidism (letter) [Cohen] 1227 (No)
Phosphorus
Low serum calcium and high parathyroid hormone levels in neonates fed 'humanized' cow's milk-based formula [Specker] 941 (Au)
Photography
Photographing the physically abused child, principles and practice [Ricci] 275 (Mr)
Photosensitivity Disorders
Gallstones in children (letter) [Todd] 971 (Se)
Physical Examination
Adolescent pelvic examination: an effective practical approach [Tolmas] 1269 (No)
Anal fissure produced by examination for sexual abuse (letter) [Baker] 848, (reply) [Bays] 849 (Au)
Clinic attending: teaching strategies for patient encounters [Schmitt] 977 (Se)
Outpatient assessment of infants with bronchiolitis [Shaw] 151 (Fe)

Physical Fitness
Effects of obesity on aerobic fitness in adolescent females [Rowland] 764 (Jy)
Physiologic responses to playing a video game [Segal] 1034 (Se)
Physician-Patient Relations
Treatment withdrawal in neonates (letter) [Byrne] 1223 (No)
Physician Shortage Area see Medically Underserved Area
Physicians
Chief resident training: developing leadership skills for future medical leaders [Doughty] 639 (Je)
Comments on life after residency (letter) [Brent] 597 (Je)
Detection of alcoholism in hospitalized children and their families [Duggan] 613 (Je)
Eighty-hour workweek and residency programs: closing arguments (letter) [Bedrick] 846 (Au)
Formula companies and the medical profession (letter) [Newman] 1089, (reply) [Greer] 1090 (Oc)
Hand washing in pediatric ambulatory settings: an inconsistent practice [Lohr] 1198 (Oc)
House staff work hours and moonlighting: what do residents want?: a survey of pediatric residents in California [Cheng] 1104 (Oc)
Jack Metcoff festschrift [Lewy] 851 (Au)
Medical ethics issues survey of residents in 5 pediatric training programs [White] 161 (Fe)
Parental alcoholism: a neglected pediatric responsibility [MacDonald] 609 (Je)
Priorities in academic pediatrics (letter) [Jacobs] (reply) [Goetzman] 845 (Au)
Regional pediatric approach to the epidemic of social ills within our cities [Nelson] 505 (My)
Physicians' Assistants
Resident and nurse practitioners: responding to education and patient care needs (letter) [Giardino] 843 (Au)
Physicians' Offices
Practice management training for pediatric residents [Piatt] 299 (Mr)
Physicians, Women
Part-time Peg: who, me? [Ferry] 852 (Au)
Support services for pediatric trainees: a survey of training program directors [Bergman] 1002 (Se)
Women in medicine: fantasies, dreams, myths, and realities [DeAngelis] 49 (Ja)
Phytic Acid
Zinc deficiency: a public health problem? [Sandstead] 853 (Au)
Pica
Lead poisoning in children with developmental disabilities (letter) [Sulkes] 602 (Je)
PICTURE OF THE MONTH
Acrodermatitis enteropathica [Schneider] 211 (Fe)
Acropustulosis of infancy [Friedman] 341 (Mr)
Antley-Bixler syndrome [Butler] 701 (Je)
Henoch-Schönlein Purpura [Tunnessen] 823 (Jy)
Juvenile dermatomyositis [Tunnessen] 1161 (Oc)
Laron-type dwarfism [Laron] 473 (Ap)
Lowe's syndrome [Loughead] 113 (Ja)
Pachyonychia congenita [Cohen] 1301 (No)
Pityriasis rosea [Tunnessen] 1441 (De)
Subcutaneous fat necrosis of the newborn [Vera] 1047 (Se)
Pituitary Gland
Endocrine function in children with human immunodeficiency virus infection [Schwartz] 330 (Mr)
Pityriasis
Pityriasis rosea [Tunnessen] 1441 (De)
Plants
Thorn-induced pseudotumor of the tibia [Kozlowski] 1159 (Oc)
Plasma
Guidelines for auditing pediatric blood transfusion practices [Blanchette] 787 (Jy)
Plasmapheresis
Association of pauciarticular juvenile arthritis and myasthenia gravis [Glass] 1176 (Oc)
Platelet Aggregation
Variant form of thrombasthenia [Tarantino] 1053 (Se)
Platelet Count
Percentile curves for various hematologic measurements at birth in Arab preterm babies of different gestational ages [Haque] 645 (Je)
Platelet Membrane Glycoproteins
Variant form of thrombasthenia [Tarantino] 1053 (Se)
Platelets see Blood Platelets
Play and Playthings
Grampa, can I get something that I'd like? [Strong] 1355 (De)
Nintendo enuresis (letter) [Schink] 1094 (Oc)
Physiologic responses to playing a video game [Segal] 1034 (Se)
Pleural Effusion
Reexpansion pulmonary edema (letter) [Jardine] 1092 (Oc)
Pneumococcal Infections
Pneumococcal osteomyelitis and arthritis in children: a hospital series and literature review [Jacobs] 70 (Ja)
Pneumocystis carinii Pneumonia see Pneumonia, Pneumocystis carinii
Pneumonia
Causes of hospital-treated acute lower respiratory tract infection in children [Nohynek] 618 (Je)
Cavitary pneumonia due to *Arcanobacterium hemolyticum* [Waller] 209 (Fe)
Pneumonia, Pneumocystis carinii
Predicting risk of *Pneumocystis carinii*
pneumonia in human immunodeficiency virus-infected children [Rutstein] 922 (Au)
Trimethoprim-sulfamethoxazole oral desensitization in hemophiliacs infected with human immunodeficiency virus with a history of hypersensitivity reactions [Kletzel] 1428 (De)
Pneumonitis, Interstitial see Pulmonary Fibrosis
Pneumothorax
Reexpansion pulmonary edema (letter) [Jardine] 1092 (Oc)
Surfactant replacement therapy in respiratory distress syndrome: meta-analysis of clinical trials of single-dose surfactant extracts [Hennes] 102 (Ja)
Poisoning
Fallacy of the hemorrhagic shock and encephalopathy syndrome (letter) [Bass] 718 (Jy)
Injuries and poisonings in out-of-home child care and home care [Gunn] 779 (Jy)
Total iron-binding capacity in iron poisoning: is it useful? [Tenenbein] 437 (Ap)
War souvenir poisoning (letter) [Secord] 724 (Jy)
Poliovirus Vaccine, Oral
Apparent decreased risk of invasive bacterial disease after heterologous childhood immunization [Black] 746 (Jy)
Immunogenicity of tetravalent rhesus rotavirus vaccine administered with buffer and oral polio vaccine [Ing] 892 (Au)
Polymerase Chain Reaction
Third pattern of disease progression in children infected with human immunodeficiency virus (letter) [Katz] 1347, (reply) [Blanche] 1348 (De)
Polysaccharides
Antibody responses to 4 *Haemophilus influenzae* type b conjugate vaccines [Käyhty] 223 (Fe)
Dose-related immunogenicity of *Haemophilus influenzae* type b capsular polysaccharide—*Neisseria meningitidis* outer membrane protein conjugate vaccine [Wong] 742 (Jy)
Haemophilus b disease after vaccination with *Haemophilus* b polysaccharide or conjugate vaccine [Frasch] 1379 (De)
Response of 7- to 15-month-old infants to sequential immunization with *Haemophilus influenzae* type b-CRM_{197} conjugate and polysaccharide vaccines [Rothstein] 898 (Au)
Polyuria
Medical management of postobstructive polyuria (letter) [Smoyer] 1345 (De)
Porphyria
Gallstones in children (letter) [Todd] 971 (Se)
Postoperative Care
Cardiopulmonary exercise testing in children following surgery for tetralogy of Fallot [Tomassoni] 1290 (No)
Follow-up of patients who underwent arterial switch repair for transposition of the great arteries [Mendoza] 40 (Ja)
Postoperative Complications
Gallstones in children: characterization by age, etiology, and outcome [Reif] 105 (Ja)
Late cholangitis after successful surgical repair of biliary atresia [Gottrand] 213 (Fe)
Postpartum Period see Puerperium
Potassium
Paleonephrology and reflux nephropathy: from the 'big bang' to end-stage renal disease [Kallen] 860 (Au)
Poverty
American Academy of Pediatrics response to the growing health needs of children [Strain] 536 (My)
Barriers to medical care for homeless families compared with housed poor families [Wood] 1109 (Oc)
Care of the poor and underserved in America: older adolescents: a group at special risk [Haggerty] 569 (My)
Challenge of care for the poor and underserved in the United States: an American College of Obstetricians and Gynecologists perspective on access to care for underserved women [Davidson] 546 (My)
Challenge of care for the poor child: the research agenda [Kohl] 542 (My)
Challenge of caring for indigent children with rheumatologic diseases [Miller] 554 (My)
Children in and of the streets: health, social policy, and the homeless young [Wright] 516 (My)
Children's services in an era of budget deficits [Blum] 575 (My)
Far from the ideal: the plight of poor children in the United States [Fulginiti] 489 (My)
Growing neglect of American children [Maurer] 540 (My)
Health care for uninsured and underinsured children (letter) [Pearson] 1085 (Oc)
Oral water intoxication in infants: an American epidemic [Keating] 985 (Se)
Pediatric acquired immunodeficiency syndrome, poverty, and national priorities [Heagarty] 527 (My)
Poverty and cardiac disease in children [Allen] 550 (My)
Poverty and the health of American children: implications for academic pediatrics [Johnston] 507 (My)
Water intoxication: a prevalent problem in the inner city [Finberg] 981 (Se)
Practice Management, Medical
How are pediatric training programs preparing residents for practice? [Greenberg] 1389 (De)
Practice management training for pediatric residents [Piatt] 299 (Mr)
Predictive Value of Tests
Predicting risk of *Pneumocystis carinii*
pneumonia in human immunodeficiency virus-infected children [Rutstein] 922 (Au)
Prednisone
Focal scleroderma and severe cardiomyopathy: patient report and brief review [Moore] 229 (Fe)
Pregnancy
Child survival and perinatal infections with human immunodeficiency virus [Bennett] 1242 (No)
Elevated plasma norepinephrine levels in infants of substance-abusing mothers [Ward] 44 (Ja)
Increased transient tachypnea of the newborn in infants with asthmatic mothers [Schatz] 156 (Fe)
Support services for pediatric trainees: a survey of training program directors [Bergman] 1002 (Se)
Vertical transmission of human immunodeficiency virus from seronegative or indeterminate mothers [Johnson] 1239 (No)
Women in medicine: fantasies, dreams, myths, and realities [DeAngelis] 49 (Ja)
Pregnancy Complications
Zinc deficiency: a public health problem? [Sandstead] 853 (Au)
Pregnancy in Adolescence
Challenge of care for the poor and underserved in the United States: an American College of Obstetricians and Gynecologists perspective on access to care for underserved women [Davidson] 546 (My)
Complex problem: complex solutions [McAnarney] 429 (Ap)
Differences in infant mortality by race, nativity status, and other maternal characteristics [Kleinman] 194 (Fe)
Gallstones in children: characterization by age, etiology, and outcome [Reif] 105 (Ja)
Growing neglect of American children [Maurer] 540 (My)
Improving health care provision to neonates in the United States [Stahlman] 510 (My)
Psychosocial predictors of maternal and infant health among adolescent mothers [Boyce] 267 (Mr)
Pregnancy in Diabetes
Neurodevelopmental outcome of offspring of the diabetic mother: need for further research (letter) [Goldstein] 602 (Je)
Pregnancy-Specific beta 1-Glycoprotein
Pediatric germ cell and human chorionic gonadotropin-producing tumors: clinical and laboratory features [Englund] 1294 (No)
Prejudice
Women in medicine: fantasies, dreams, myths, and realities [DeAngelis] 49 (Ja)
Prenatal Care
Complex problem: complex solutions [McAnarney] 429 (Ap)
Practical guide to successful breast-feeding management [Freed] 917 (Au)
Studies in fetal malnutrition [Crosby] 871 (Au)
Prenatal Diagnosis
Congenital syphilis associated with negative results of maternal serologic tests at delivery (letter) [Sánchez] 967 (Se)
Major congenital neurologic malformations (letter) [Ryals] 30 (Ja)
Prenatal Exposure Delayed Effects
Brain and ocular abnormalities in infants with in utero exposure to cocaine and other street drugs [Dominguez] 688 (Je)
Evaluation of auditory brain-stem response in full-term infants of cocaine-abusing mothers [Carzoli] 1013 (Se)
Preoperative Care
Ventriculitis in newborns with myelomeningocele [Charney] 287 (Mr)
Prevalence
Adolescents with chronic illness [Perrin] 1361 (De)
Prevalence and impact of chronic illness among adolescents [Newacheck] 1367 (De)
Preventive Health Services
Acquired immunodeficiency syndrome and adolescents: knowledge, attitudes, and behaviors of runaway and homeless youths [Sugerman] 431 (Ap)
American Academy of Pediatrics response to the growing health needs of children [Strain] 536 (My)
Apparent decreased risk of invasive bacterial disease after heterologous childhood immunization [Black] 746 (Jy)
Differences in infant mortality by race, nativity status, and other maternal characteristics [Kleinman] 194 (Fe)
Efficacy and pharmacokinetics of intravenous immune globulin administration to high-risk neonates [Kinney] 1233 (No)
Improving health care provision to neonates in the United States [Stahlman] 510 (My)
Influenza vaccination in the prevention of acute otitis media in children [Heikkinen] 445 (Ap)
New initiatives in adolescent health promotion [Elster] 495 (My)
What about gay teenagers? (letter) [Fikar] 252 (Mr)
Primary Health Care

American Academy of Pediatrics response to the growing health needs of children [Strain] 536 (My)
Prisoners
Losing time [Pruitt] 607 (Je)
Prisons
Losing time [Pruitt] 607 (Je)
Private Practice
Regional pediatric approach to the epidemic of social ills within our cities [Nelson] 505 (My)
Probability
More on the *P value* (letter) [Coulter] (reply) [Brown] 249 (Mr)
Multiple comparisons and *P* values (letter) [Newman] 250 (Mr)
P values (letter) [Byrt] 250 (Mr)
Productivity see Efficiency
Professional Practice
Comments on life after residency (letter) [Brent] 597 (Je)
Prognosis
Factors affecting outcome in meningococcal infections [Tesoro] 218 (Fe)
Scoring systems for accurate prognosis of patients with meningococcal infections (letter) [Leclerc] 1090 (Oc)
Third pattern of disease progression in children infected with human immunodeficiency virus (letter) [Katz] 1347, (reply) [Blanche] 1348 (De)
Treatment withdrawal in neonates (letter) [Byrne] 1223 (No)
Program Evaluation
Comparison of a computer tutorial with other methods for teaching well-newborn care [Desch] 1255 (No)
Current trends in pediatric residency training [Carraccio] 1272 (No)
How are pediatric training programs preparing residents for practice? [Greenberg] 1389 (De)
Resident, faculty, and residency program development: an integrated approach through annual retreats [Winter] 1191 (Oc)
School health training during pediatric residency [Niebuhr] 79 (Ja)
Prostaglandin E1 see Alprostadil
Prostaglandin Synthase
Medical management of postobstructive polyuria (letter) [Smoyer] 1345 (De)
Prostaglandin Synthetase see Prostaglandin Synthase
Prostitution
Acquired immunodeficiency syndrome and adolescents: knowledge, attitudes, and behaviors of runaway and homeless youths [Sugerman] 431 (Ap)
Protoporphyrins
Gallstones in children (letter) [Todd] 971 (Se)
Pruritus
Pityriasis rosea [Tunnessen] 1441 (De)
Pseudomonas aeruginosa
Acute osteomyelitis in children: reassessment of etiologic agents and their clinical characteristics [Faden] 65 (Ja)
Differences in expression of cystic fibrosis in blacks and whites [McColley] 94 (Ja)
Pseudotumor, Inflammatory see Fibroma
Psychology
Women in medicine: fantasies, dreams, myths, and realities [DeAngelis] 49 (Ja)
Psychophysiologic Disorders
Testing the psychogenic vomiting diagnosis: four pediatric patients [Gonzalez-Heydrich] 913 (Au)
Psychosocial Support Systems see Social Support
Psychosomatic Disorders see Psychophysiologic Disorders
Puberty, Precocious
Pediatric germ cell and human chorionic gonadotropin-producing tumors: clinical and laboratory features [Englund] 1294 (No)
Public Health
Child abuse and neglect: critical first steps in response to a national emergency: the report of the US Advisory Board on Child Abuse and Neglect [Krugman] 513 (My)
Children in and of the streets: health, social policy, and the homeless young [Wright] 516 (My)
Legalization of drugs of abuse and the pediatrician [Schwartz] 1153 (Oc)
New initiatives in adolescent health promotion [Elster] 495 (My)
Poverty and the health of American children: implications for academic pediatrics [Johnston] 507 (My)
What will it take to fully protect all American children with vaccines? [Hinman] 559 (My)
Youth alienation as an emerging pediatric health care issue [Farrow] 491 (My)
Zinc deficiency: a public health problem? [Sandstead] 853 (Au)
Public Policy
Children in and of the streets: health, social policy, and the homeless young [Wright] 516 (My)
Children's services in an era of budget deficits [Blum] 575 (My)
Public Relations
American Academy of Pediatrics response to the growing health needs of children [Strain] 536 (My)
Puerperium
Practical guide to successful breast-feeding management [Freed] 917 (Au)
Pulmonary Diffusing Capacity
Cardiopulmonary exercise testing in children following surgery for tetralogy of Fallot [Tomassoni] 1290 (No)
Pulmonary Diseases see Lung Diseases
Pulmonary Edema
Effect of low-dose dopamine infusion on cardiopulmonary and renal status in premature newborns with respiratory distress syndrome [Cuevas] 799 (Jy)
Reexpansion pulmonary edema (letter) [Jardine] 1092 (Oc)
Pulmonary Fibrosis
Clinical and endocrinologic manifestations in perinatally human immunodeficiency virus type 1-infected children aged 5 years or older [Lepage] 1248 (No)
Pulse Oximetry see Oximetry
Purpura
Factors affecting outcome in meningococcal infections [Tesoro] 218 (Fe)
Scoring systems for accurate prognosis of patients with meningococcal infections (letter) [Leclerc] 1090 (Oc)
Purpura, Schoenlein-Henoch
Henoch-Schönlein Purpura [Tunnessen] 823 (Jy)

Q

Quality of Health Care
Resident and nurse practitioners: responding to education and patient care needs (letter) [Giardino] 843 (Au)

R

Racial Stocks
Barriers to medical care for homeless families compared with housed poor families [Wood] 1109 (Oc)
Bone mineral content of healthy, full-term neonates: effect of race, gender, and maternal cigarette smoking [Venkataraman] 1310 (No)
Prevalence and impact of chronic illness among adolescents [Newacheck] 1367 (De)
Radiography
Differences in expression of cystic fibrosis in blacks and whites [McColley] 94 (Ja)
RADIOLOGICAL CASE OF THE MONTH
Cavitary pneumonia due to *Arcanobacterium hemolyticum* [Waller] 209 (Fe)
Congenital syphilis [Giacola] 1045 (Se)
Gilding the lily (letter) [Faigel] (reply) [Myer] 849 (Au)
Hypoplastic left upper lobe [Al-Salem] 821 (Jy)
Intravenous hyperalimentation fluid obtained with lumbar puncture: an unusual complication of a central venous catheter [Mah] 1439 (De)
Left renal vein thrombosis and left adrenal hemorrhage [Bennett] 1299 (No)
Neonatal appendicitis with perforation [Ruff] 111 (Ja)
Pediatric case of Eagle's syndrome [Holloway] 339 (Mr)
Thorn-induced pseudotumor of the tibia [Kozlowski] 1159 (Oc)
Tuberous sclerosis with myocardial and central nervous system involvement at birth [Allison] 471 (Ap)
Visceral larva migrans [Ponder] 699 (Je)
Radius
Bone mineral content of healthy, full-term neonates: effect of race, gender, and maternal cigarette smoking [Venkataraman] 1310 (No)
Randomized Controlled Trials
Acellular pertussis vaccines: efficacy and evaluation of clinical case definitions [Blackwelder] 1285 (No)
Ductal patency in neonates with respiratory distress syndrome: a randomized surfactant trial [Reller] 1017 (Se)
Efficacy and pharmacokinetics of intravenous immune globulin administration to high-risk neonates [Kinney] 1233 (No)
Immunogenicity of tetravalent rhesus rotavirus vaccine administered with buffer and oral polio vaccine [Ing] 892 (Au)
Impetigo [Esterly] 125 (Fe)
Improving the use of early follow-up care after emergency department visits: a randomized trial [Nelson] 440 (Ap)
Taurine decreases fecal fatty acid and sterol excretion in cystic fibrosis: a randomized double-blind trial [Smith] 1401 (De)
Reading
Clinic-based intervention to promote literacy: a pilot study [Needlman] 881 (Au)
Comparison of a computer tutorial with other methods for teaching well-newborn care [Desch] 1255 (No)
Receptors, Adrenergic, Alpha
Elevated plasma norepinephrine levels in infants of substance-abusing mothers [Ward] 44 (Ja)
Receptors, Adrenergic, Beta
Elevated plasma norepinephrine levels in infants of substance-abusing mothers [Ward] 44 (Ja)
Receptors, Cholinergic
Association of pauciarticular juvenile arthritis and myasthenia gravis [Glass] 1176 (Oc)
Rectum
Influence of otitis media on the correlation between rectal and auditory canal temperatures [Terndrup] 75 (Ja)
Refusal to Treat
Medical ethics issues survey of residents in 5 pediatric training programs [White] 161 (Fe)
Treatment withdrawal in neonates (letter) [Byrne] 1223 (No)
Regional Health Planning
Regional pediatric approach to the epidemic of social ills within our cities [Nelson] 505 (My)
Regurgitation, Aortic Valve see Aortic Valve Insufficiency
Rehabilitation
Pediatric cardiac rehabilitation [Balfour] 627 (Je)
Rehydration Solutions
Rice solution and World Health Organization solution by gastric infusion for high stool output diarrhea [Mota-Hernández] 937 (Au)
Rehydration, Oral see Fluid Therapy
Religion
Medical ethics issues survey of residents in 5 pediatric training programs [White] 161 (Fe)
Tattooing behavior in adolescence: a comparison study [Farrow] 184 (Fe)
Renal Veins
Left renal vein thrombosis and left adrenal hemorrhage [Bennett] 1299 (No)
Research
More on the *P value* (letter) [Coulter] (reply) [Brown] 249 (Mr)
Multiple comparisons and *P* values (letter) [Newman] 250 (Mr)
Neurodevelopmental outcome of offspring of the diabetic mother: need for further research (letter) [Goldstein] 602 (Je)
P values (letter) [Byrt] 250 (Mr)
Priorities in academic pediatrics (letter) [Jacobs] (reply) [Goetzman] 845 (Au)
Tell the whole story [Johnson] 135 (Fe)
Research Design
Status report on phenylketonuria treatment: 1990 [Mabry] 33 (Ja)
Thumb-sucking (letter) [Lubicky] 845, (reply) [Friman] 846 (Au)
Research Support
Challenge of care for the poor child: the research agenda [Kohl] 542 (My)
Improving health care for underserved infants, children, and adolescents: the Robert Wood Johnson Foundation's experience [Beachler] 565 (My)
Residency, Medical see Internship and Residency
Respiration
Breathing patterns and heart rates at ages 6 weeks and 2 years [Poets] 1393 (De)
Outpatient assessment of infants with bronchiolitis [Shaw] 151 (Fe)
Respiration, Artificial
Optimal positioning of endotracheal tubes for ventilation of preterm infants [Rotschild] 1007 (Se)
Predictors of neurodevelopmental outcome following bronchopulmonary dysplasia [Luchi] 813 (Jy)
Respiration Disorders
Albuterol inhalations in acute chest syndrome (letter) [Handelsman] 603 (Je)
Respirators see Ventilators, Mechanical
Respiratory Distress Syndrome
Ductal patency in neonates with respiratory distress syndrome: a randomized surfactant trial [Reller] 1017 (Se)
Effect of low-dose dopamine infusion on cardiopulmonary and renal status in premature newborns with respiratory distress syndrome [Cuevas] 799 (Jy)
Pediatric perspectives: vistas and vantage points [Bedrick] 256 (Mr)
Preliminary report of prenatal cocaine exposure and respiratory distress syndrome in premature infants [Zuckerman] 696 (Je)
Surfactant replacement therapy in respiratory distress syndrome: meta-analysis of clinical trials of single-dose surfactant extracts [Hennes] 102 (Ja)
Respiratory Function Tests
Cardiopulmonary exercise testing in children following surgery for tetralogy of Fallot [Tomassoni] 1290 (No)
Respiratory Insufficiency
Albuterol inhalations in acute chest syndrome (letter) [Handelsman] 603 (Je)
Increased transient tachypnea of the newborn in infants with asthmatic mothers [Schatz] 156 (Fe)
Neural arch stenosis and spinal cord injury in thanatophoric dysplasia [Faye-Petersen] 87 (Ja)
Respiratory Sounds
Increased transient tachypnea of the newborn in infants with asthmatic mothers [Schatz] 156 (Fe)
Respirosonography in infants with acute bronchiolitis [Tal] 1405 (De)
Respiratory Syncytial Viruses
Causes of hospital-treated acute lower respiratory tract infection in children [Nohynek] 618 (Je)
Outpatient assessment of infants with bronchiolitis [Shaw] 151 (Fe)
Respiratory System
Differences in expression of cystic fibrosis in blacks and whites [McColley] 94 (Ja)
Respiratory Tract Diseases
Prevalence and impact of chronic illness among adolescents [Newacheck] 1367 (De)
Respiratory Tract Infections

Causes of hospital-treated acute lower respiratory tract infection in children [Nohynek] 618 (Je)
Cautionary note on the use of empiric ceftriaxone for suspected bacteremia [Wald] 1359 (De)
Influenza vaccination in the prevention of acute otitis media in children [Heikkinen] 445 (Ap)
Resuscitation
Intraosseous infusion of dobutamine and isoproterenol [Bilello] 165 (Fe); correction, 1312 (No)
Retinitis
Cat-scratch disease: acute encephalopathy and other neurologic manifestations [Carithers] 98 (Ja)
Retinopathy of Prematurity
Retinopathy of prematurity in infants with cyanotic congenital heart disease [Johns] 200 (Fe)
REVIEWERS
1990 reviewers for *AJDC,* 115 (Ja)
Reye's Syndrome
Misdiagnosis of Reye's-like illness (letter) [Forsyth] 964 (Se)
Rheumatology
Challenge of caring for indigent children with rheumatologic diseases [Miller] 554 (My)
Rice
Rice solution and World Health Organization solution by gastric infusion for high stool output diarrhea [Mota-Hernández] 937 (Au)
Rickets
Growth hormone therapy in hypophosphatemic rickets [Wilson] 1165 (Oc)
Rickets caused by vitamin D deficiency in breast-fed infants in the southern United States [Bhowmick] 127 (Fe)
Ringworm see Tinea
Risk Factors
Acquired immunodeficiency syndrome and adolescents: knowledge, attitudes, and behaviors of runaway and homeless youths [Sugerman] 431 (Ap)
Apparent decreased risk of invasive bacterial disease after heterologous childhood immunization [Black] 746 (Jy)
Child sexual abuse and human immunodeficiency virus transmission (letter) [Monteleone] (reply) [Gutman] 847 (Au)
Demographic and risk factors associated with chronic dieting in adolescents [Story] 994 (Se)
Differences in infant mortality by race, nativity status, and other maternal characteristics [Kleinman] 194 (Fe)
DTP immunization and susceptibility to infectious diseases: is there a relationship? [Davidson] 750 (Jy)
Escherichia coli bacteremia in children: a review of 91 cases in 10 years [Bonadio] 671 (Je)
Factors associated with umbilical catheter-related sepsis in neonates [Landers] 675 (Je)
Human immunodeficiency virus transmission by child sexual abuse [Gutman] 137 (Fe)
Increased transient tachypnea of the newborn in infants with asthmatic mothers [Schatz] 156 (Fe)
Influenza type A and B infections in hospitalized pediatric patients: who should be immunized? [Serwint] 623 (Je)
Longitudinal study of birth weight and being overweight in late adolescence [Seidman] 782 (Jy)
Obesity among Mescalero preschool children: association with maternal obesity and birth weight [Gallaher] 1262 (No)
Outpatient assessment of infants with bronchiolitis [Shaw] 151 (Fe)
Predicting risk of *Pneumocystis carinii* pneumonia in human immunodeficiency virus-infected children [Rutstein] 922 (Au)
Rickets caused by vitamin D deficiency in breast-fed infants in the southern United States [Bhowmick] 127 (Fe)
Studies in fetal malnutrition [Crosby] 871 (Au)
Vaccine myth and physician handouts (letter) [Lynch] 426, (replies) [Cherry, Fulginiti] 426, 427 (Ap)
Vertical transmission of human immunodeficiency virus from seronegative or indeterminate mothers [Johnson] 1239 (No)
What about gay teenagers? (letter) [Fikar] 252 (Mr)
Ristocetin
Variant form of thrombasthenia [Tarantino] 1053 (Se)
Robert Wood Johnson Foundation
Improving health care for underserved infants, children, and adolescents: the Robert Wood Johnson Foundation's experience [Beachler] 565 (My)
Rodentia
Epidemic nephropathy in children [Lautala] 1181 (Oc)
Roentgenography see Radiography
Romano-Ward Syndrome see Long QT Syndrome
Rotaviruses
Immunogenicity of tetravalent rhesus rotavirus vaccine administered with buffer and oral polio vaccine [Ing] 892 (Au)
Rubella Vaccine
Antibody response to MMR vaccination in children who received IVIG as neonates (letter) [Ruderman] 425 (Ap)
Apparent decreased risk of invasive bacterial disease after heterologous childhood immunization [Black] 746 (Jy)
Rural Health
Health care for uninsured and underinsured children (letter) [Pearson] 1085 (Oc)
Rwanda
Clinical and endocrinologic manifestations in perinatally human immunodeficiency virus type 1-infected children aged 5 years or older [Lepage] 1248 (No)

S

Safety
Guidelines for safe transportation of children in wheelchairs [DiGaudio] 653 (Je)
Safety of a preadolescent basketball program [Gutgesell] 1023 (Se)
Use of infant walkers [AMA Board of Trustees] 933 (Au)
Salaries and Fringe Benefits
Current trends in pediatric residency training [Carraccio] 1272 (No)
Health care for uninsured and underinsured children (letter) [Pearson] 1085 (Oc)
Salbutamol see Albuterol
Saline Solution, Hypertonic
Oral water intoxication in infants: an American epidemic [Keating] 985 (Se)
Water intoxication: a prevalent problem in the inner city [Finberg] 981 (Se)
Saudi Arabia
Percentile curves for various hematologic measurements at birth in Arab preterm babies of different gestational ages [Haque] 645 (Je)
School Health Services
School health training during pediatric residency [Niebuhr] 79 (Ja)
Schools
Guidelines for safe transportation of children in wheelchairs [DiGaudio] 653 (Je)
Scleroderma, Circumscribed
Focal scleroderma and severe cardiomyopathy: patient report and brief review [Moore] 229 (Fe)
Seasons
Seasonal variation in growth during growth hormone therapy [Rudolf] 769 (Jy)
Seizures
How much of neonatal encephalopathy is due to birth asphyxia? [Nelson] 1325 (No)
Pediatric perspectives: vistas and vantage points [Bedrick] 256 (Mr)
Self Concept
Send Linus to me (letter) [Szonyi] (reply) [Friman] 1227 (No)
Self Esteem see Self Concept
Septicemia
Acute glossitis and bacteremia caused by *Streptococcus pneumoniae*: case report and review (letter) [Stoddard] 598 (Je)
Cautionary note on the use of empiric ceftriaxone for suspected bacteremia [Wald] 1359 (De)
Escherichia coli bacteremia in children: a review of 91 cases in 10 years [Bonadio] 671 (Je)
Factors associated with umbilical catheter-related sepsis in neonates [Landers] 675 (Je)
Frequency of infections associated with implanted systems vs cuffed, tunneled silastic venous catheters in patients with acute leukemia [Severien] 1433 (De)
Neutropenia in an extremely premature infant treated with recombinant human granulocyte colony-stimulating factor [Roberts] 808 (Jy)
Serum Albumin
Guidelines for auditing pediatric blood transfusion practices [Blanchette] 787 (Jy)
Sex Behavior
Acquired immunodeficiency syndrome and adolescents: knowledge, attitudes, and behaviors of runaway and homeless youths [Sugerman] 431 (Ap)
Improving health care provision to neonates in the United States [Stahlman] 510 (My)
Sex Chromosome Abnormalities
Pediatric germ cell and human chorionic gonadotropin-producing tumors: clinical and laboratory features [Englund] 1294 (No)
Sex Education
Acquired immunodeficiency syndrome and adolescents: knowledge, attitudes, and behaviors of runaway and homeless youths [Sugerman] 431 (Ap)
Complex problem: complex solutions [McAnarney] 429 (Ap)
Sex Factors
Bone mineral content of healthy, full-term neonates: effect of race, gender, and maternal cigarette smoking [Venkataraman] 1310 (No)
Cat-scratch disease: acute encephalopathy and other neurologic manifestations [Carithers] 98 (Ja)
Demographic and risk factors associated with chronic dieting in adolescents [Story] 994 (Se)
Gallstones in children: characterization by age, etiology, and outcome [Reif] 105 (Ja)
Lichen sclerosus et atrophicus in children [Loening-Baucke] 1058 (Se)
Safety of a preadolescent basketball program [Gutgesell] 1023 (Se)
Standardized percentile curves of body-mass index for children and adolescents [Hammer] 259 (Mr)
Women in medicine: fantasies, dreams, myths, and realities [DeAngelis] 49 (Ja)
Sex Maturation
Sexual maturation and blood pressure levels of a biracial sample of girls [Kozinetz] 142 (Fe)
Sexual Intercourse see Coitus
Sexual Partners
Acquired immunodeficiency syndrome and adolescents: knowledge, attitudes, and behaviors of runaway and homeless youths [Sugerman] 431 (Ap)
Sexually Transmitted Diseases, Viral
Condylomata acuminata: still usually a sexually transmitted disease in children (letter) [Goldenring] 600, (reply) [Boyd] 601 (Je)
Human immunodeficiency virus transmission by child sexual abuse [Gutman] 137 (Fe)
Shock
Factors affecting outcome in meningococcal infections [Tesoro] 218 (Fe)
Scoring systems for accurate prognosis of patients with meningococcal infections (letter) [Leclerc] 1090 (Oc)
Shock, Hemorrhagic
Fallacy of the hemorrhagic shock and encephalopathy syndrome (letter) [Bass] 718 (Jy)
'H' in hemorrhagic shock and encephalopathy syndrome (letter) [Roscelli] 720 (Jy)
Hemorrhagic shock and encephalopathy: an entity similar to heatstroke (letter) [Conway] 720 (Jy)
Hyperpyrexia, hemorrhagic shock and encephalopathy, and creatinine phosphokinase (letter) [Dupee] 719 (Jy)
SIADH see Inappropriate ADH Syndrome
Silastics see Silicone Elastomers
Silicone Elastomers
Frequency of infections associated with implanted systems vs cuffed, tunneled silastic venous catheters in patients with acute leukemia [Severien] 1433 (De)
Skating
Skateboarding injuries in children: a second wave [Retsky] 188 (Fe)
Skeleton
Antley-Bixler syndrome [Butler] 701 (Je)
Skin
Capillary refilling (skin turgor) in the assessment of dehydration [Saavedra] 296 (Mr)
Skin Diseases
Pityriasis rosea [Tunnessen] 1441 (De)
Skin Neoplasms
Sun protection in newborns: a comparison of educational methods [Bolognia] 1125 (Oc)
Skin Ulcer
Treatment of ulcerated hemangiomas with pulsed tunable dye laser [Morelli] 1062 (Se)
Skinfold Thickness
Obesity and body-mass index (letter) [Hergenroeder] (reply) [Hammer] 972 (Se)
Skull
Antley-Bixler syndrome [Butler] 701 (Je)
Sleep
Gastroesophageal reflux and apnea in prematurely born infants during wakefulness and sleep [Ajuriaguerra] 1132 (Oc)
Sleep Apnea Syndromes
Gastroesophageal reflux and apnea in prematurely born infants during wakefulness and sleep [Ajuriaguerra] 1132 (Oc)
Smoking
Bone mineral content of healthy, full-term neonates: effect of race, gender, and maternal cigarette smoking [Venkataraman] 1310 (No)
Social Alienation
Youth alienation as an emerging pediatric health care issue [Farrow] 491 (My)
Social Behavior
Buddy, can you paradigm? [Brown] 727 (Jy)
Social Discrimination see Prejudice
Social Environment
Clinic-based intervention to promote literacy: a pilot study [Needlman] 881 (Au)
Social Policy see Public Policy
Social Support
Psychosocial predictors of maternal and infant health among adolescent mothers [Boyce] 267 (Mr)
Social Work
Barriers to medical care for homeless families compared with housed poor families [Wood] 1109 (Oc)
Societies, Medical
Regional pediatric approach to the epidemic of social ills within our cities [Nelson] 505 (My)
Society for Pediatric Research
1991 Annual Meeting, 26 (Ja), 125 (Fe), 249 (Mr), 425 (Ap)
Call for abstracts, 1085 (Oc), 1223 (No), 1345 (De)
Challenge of care for the poor child: the research agenda [Kohl] 542 (My)
Socioeconomic Factors
Barriers to medical care for homeless families compared with housed poor families [Wood] 1109 (Oc)
Breast-feeding initiation in a triethnic population [Bee] 306 (Mr)
Care of the poor and underserved in America: older adolescents: a group at special risk [Haggerty] 569 (My)
Child welfare: the phantom of the health care system (letter) [Pidcock] 843 (Au)
Complex problem: complex solutions [McAnarney] 429 (Ap)

Far from the ideal: the plight of poor children in the United States [Fulginiti] 489 (My)
Health care for uninsured and underinsured children (letter) [Hecker] 1086 (Oc)
Human immunodeficiency virus transmission by child sexual abuse [Gutman] 137 (Fe)
Improving health care provision to neonates in the United States [Stahlman] 510 (My)
Occult cocaine exposure in children [Rosenberg] 1430 (De)
Psychosocial predictors of maternal and infant health among adolescent mothers [Boyce] 267 (Mr)
Regional pediatric approach to the epidemic of social ills within our cities [Nelson] 505 (My)
Sexual maturation and blood pressure levels of a biracial sample of girls [Kozinetz] 142 (Fe)
Survey of the health of homeless children in Philadelphia shelters [Parker] 520 (My)
Tattooing behavior in adolescence: a comparison study [Farrow] 184 (Fe)
Your child's best friend: TV or not TV? (letter) [Bader] (reply) [Stiehm] 963 (Se)
Youth alienation as an emerging pediatric health care issue [Farrow] 491 (My)
Sodium
Association of alkaline urine with eating disorders (letter) [Robson] (reply) [Arden] 1091 (Oc)
Paleonephrology and reflux nephropathy: from the 'big bang' to end-stage renal disease [Kallen] 860 (Au)
Sodium Chloride
Water intoxication: a prevalent problem in the inner city [Finberg] 981 (Se)
Somatomedin C see Insulin-Like Growth Factor I
Somatotropin
Effectiveness of growth-promoting therapies: comparison among growth hormone, clonidine, and levodopa [Volta] 168 (Fe)
Endocrine function in children with human immunodeficiency virus infection [Schwartz] 330 (Mr)
Growth hormone therapy in hypophosphatemic rickets [Wilson] 1165 (Oc)
Seasonal variation in growth during growth hormone therapy [Rudolf] 769 (Jy)
Spasm
Acellular pertussis vaccines: efficacy and evaluation of clinical case definitions [Blackwelder] 1285 (No)
Special Supplemental Food Program for Women, Infants, and Children
Oral water intoxication in infants: an American epidemic [Keating] 985 (Se)
Specialties, Medical
Family physicians and neonatology (letter) [McIntyre] (reply) [DiTraglia] 963 (Se)
Women in medicine: fantasies, dreams, myths, and realities [DeAngelis] 49 (Ja)
Sphingomyelins
Markedly immature lecithin-sphingomyelin ratio at term and congenital hypothyroidism (letter) [Cohen] 1227 (No)
Spinal Canal
Neural arch stenosis and spinal cord injury in thanatophoric dysplasia [Faye-Petersen] 87 (Ja)
Spinal Cord Injuries
Neural arch stenosis and spinal cord injury in thanatophoric dysplasia [Faye-Petersen] 87 (Ja)
Spinal Puncture
Cautionary note on the use of empiric ceftriaxone for suspected bacteremia [Wald] 1359 (De)
Intravenous hyperalimentation fluid obtained with lumbar puncture: an unusual complication of a central venous catheter [Mah] 1439 (De)
Lumbar puncture frequency and cerebrospinal fluid analysis in the neonate [Schwersenski] 54 (Ja)
Posthemorrhagic hydrocephalus: use of an intravenous-type catheter for cerebrospinal fluid drainage [Marro] 1141 (Oc)
Spinal Stenosis
Neural arch stenosis and spinal cord injury in thanatophoric dysplasia [Faye-Petersen] 87 (Ja)
Spondylitis
Tiny Tim remembered [Callahan] 1355 (De)
Sports
Adolescents' attrition from school-sponsored sports [DuRant] 1119 (Oc)
Sports Medicine
Adolescents' attrition from school-sponsored sports [DuRant] 1119 (Oc)
Commotio cordis: the single, most common cause of traumatic death in youth baseball [Abrunzo] 1279 (No)
Effects of obesity on aerobic fitness in adolescent females [Rowland] 764 (Jy)
Safety of a preadolescent basketball program [Gutgesell] 1023 (Se)
Sudden cardiac death (letter) [Pearl] 1223 (No)
Sudden cardiac death in young athletes: a review [McCaffrey] 177 (Fe)
Tracking of elevated blood pressure values in adolescent athletes at 1-year follow-up [Tanji] 665 (Je)
Sprains and Strains
Safety of a preadolescent basketball program [Gutgesell] 1023 (Se)
Staphylococcal Infections
Factors associated with umbilical catheter-related sepsis in neonates [Landers] 675 (Je)
Staphylococcus
Frequency of infections associated with implanted systems vs cuffed, tunneled silastic venous catheters in patients with acute leukemia [Severien] 1433 (De)
Staphylococcus aureus
Acute osteomyelitis in children: reassessment of etiologic agents and their clinical characteristics [Faden] 65 (Ja)
Impetigo [Esterly] 125 (Fe)
Staphylococcus aureus in impetigo (letter) [Dagan] (reply) [Bass] 1223 (No)
State Government
Children's services in an era of budget deficits [Blum] 575 (My)
Statistical Models see Models, Statistical
Statistics
More on the *P value* (letter) [Coulter] (reply) [Brown] 249 (Mr)
Multiple comparisons and *P* values (letter) [Newman] 250 (Mr)
P values (letter) [Byrt] 250 (Mr)
Steatorrhea see Celiac Disease
Sterols
Taurine decreases fecal fatty acid and sterol excretion in cystic fibrosis: a randomized double-blind trial [Smith] 1401 (De)
Streptococcal Infections
Neutropenia in an extremely premature infant treated with recombinant human granulocyte colony-stimulating factor [Roberts] 808 (Jy)
Streptococcus agalactiae
Neutropenia in an extremely premature infant treated with recombinant human granulocyte colony-stimulating factor [Roberts] 808 (Jy)
Streptococcus Group A see Streptococcus pyogenes
Streptococcus pneumoniae
Acute glossitis and bacteremia caused by *Streptococcus pneumoniae*: case report and review (letter) [Stoddard] 598 (Je)
Causes of hospital-treated acute lower respiratory tract infection in children [Nohynek] 618 (Je)
DTP immunization and susceptibility to infectious diseases: is there a relationship? [Davidson] 750 (Jy)
Hypoplastic left upper lobe [Al-Salem] 821 (Jy)
Influenza vaccination in the prevention of acute otitis media in children [Heikkinen] 445 (Ap)
Streptococcus pyogenes
Impetigo [Esterly] 125 (Fe)
Stress, Psychological
Pediatric program director: an analysis of the role and its problems [Weiss] 449 (Ap)
Psychosocial predictors of maternal and infant health among adolescent mothers [Boyce] 267 (Mr)
Support services for pediatric trainees: a survey of training program directors [Bergman] 1002 (Se)
Students
Adolescents' attrition from school-sponsored sports [DuRant] 1119 (Oc)
Students, Medical
Comparison of a computer tutorial with other methods for teaching well-newborn care [Desch] 1255 (No)
Current trends in pediatric residency training [Carraccio] 1272 (No)
Poverty and the health of American children: implications for academic pediatrics [Johnston] 507 (My)
Substance Abuse
Acquired immunodeficiency syndrome and adolescents: knowledge, attitudes, and behaviors of runaway and homeless youths [Sugerman] 431 (Ap)
Brain and ocular abnormalities in infants with in utero exposure to cocaine and other street drugs [Dominguez] 688 (Je)
Child welfare: the phantom of the health care system (letter) [Pidcock] 843 (Au)
Elevated plasma norepinephrine levels in infants of substance-abusing mothers [Ward] 44 (Ja)
Evaluation of auditory brain-stem response in full-term infants of cocaine-abusing mothers [Carzoli] 1013 (Se)
Legalization of drugs of abuse and the pediatrician [Schwartz] 1153 (Oc)
Meconium for drug testing [Maynard] 650 (Je)
Occult cocaine exposure in children [Rosenberg] 1430 (De)
Preliminary report of prenatal cocaine exposure and respiratory distress syndrome in premature infants [Zuckerman] 696 (Je)
Survey of the health of homeless children in Philadelphia shelters [Parker] 520 (My)
Tattooing behavior in adolescence: a comparison study [Farrow] 184 (Fe)
Third pattern of disease progression in children infected with human immunodeficiency virus (letter) [Katz] 1347, (reply) [Blanche] 1348 (De)
Unsuspected cocaine exposure in young children [Kharasch] 204 (Fe)
Substance Abuse Detection
Meconium for drug testing [Maynard] 650 (Je)
Sudden Infant Death
Elevated plasma norepinephrine levels in infants of substance-abusing mothers [Ward] 44 (Ja)
Sudden deaths and apparent life-threatening events in hospitalized neonates presumed to be healthy [Burchfield] 1319 (No)
Suicide
What about gay teenagers? (letter) [Fikar] 252 (Mr)
Sulfamethoxazole
Puncture wound-induced *Achromobacter xylosoxidans* osteomyelitis of the foot (letter) [Hoddy] 599 (Je)
Sunlight
Rickets caused by vitamin D deficiency in breast-fed infants in the southern United States [Bhowmick] 127 (Fe)
Sun protection in newborns: a comparison of educational methods [Bolognia] 1125 (Oc)
Sunscreening Agents
Sun protection in newborns: a comparison of educational methods [Bolognia] 1125 (Oc)
Surface-Active Agents
Ductal patency in neonates with respiratory distress syndrome: a randomized surfactant trial [Reller] 1017 (Se)
Pediatric perspectives: vistas and vantage points [Bedrick] 256 (Mr)
Surfactant replacement therapy in respiratory distress syndrome: meta-analysis of clinical trials of single-dose surfactant extracts [Hennes] 102 (Ja)
Surfactants see Surface-Active Agents
Surgery, Operative
Cortical resection for children with epilepsy: perspectives in pediatrics [Wyllie] 314 (Mr)
Evolution of surgical treatment for congenital cardiac disease [Pigott] 1362 (De)
Survival
Child survival and perinatal infections with human immunodeficiency virus [Bennett] 1242 (No)
Evolution of surgical treatment for congenital cardiac disease [Pigott] 1362 (De)
Swallowing see Deglutition
Sweat Gland Neoplasms
Syringomas in Down syndrome (letter) [Feingold] 966 (Se)
Sweden
Acellular pertussis vaccines: efficacy and evaluation of clinical case definitions [Blackwelder] 1285 (No)
Swimming Pools
Immersion events in residential swimming pools: evidence for an experience effect [Wintemute] 1200 (Oc)
Swine
Evaluation of intraosseus vs intravenous antibiotic levels in a porcine model [Jaimovich] 946 (Au); correction, 1241 (No)
Intraosseous infusion of dobutamine and isoproterenol [Bilello] 165 (Fe); correction, 1312 (No)
Sympathetic Nervous System
Elevated plasma norepinephrine levels in infants of substance-abusing mothers [Ward] 44 (Ja)
Syncope
Sudden cardiac death in young athletes: a review [McCaffrey] 177 (Fe)
Syphilis, Congenital
Congenital syphilis [Giacola] 1045 (Se)
Congenital syphilis associated with negative results of maternal serologic tests at delivery (letter) [Sánchez] 967 (Se)
Syphilis Serodiagnosis
Comparison of maternal and infant serologic tests for syphilis [Rawstron] 1383 (De)
Syringes
War souvenir poisoning (letter) [Secord] 724 (Jy)
Syringoma, Chondroid see Hidradenoma
Systole
Family history of myocardial infarction and hemodynamic responses to exercise in young black boys [Treiber] 1029 (Se)
Systolic Click-Murmur Syndrome see Mitral Valve Prolapse

T

Tachypnea see Respiratory Insufficiency
Tattooing
Tattooing behavior in adolescence: a comparison study [Farrow] 184 (Fe)
Taurine
Taurine decreases fecal fatty acid and sterol excretion in cystic fibrosis: a randomized double-blind trial [Smith] 1401 (De)
Teaching
Clinic attending: teaching strategies for patient encounters [Schmitt] 977 (Se)
Technology
Gilding the lily (letter) [Faigel] (reply) [Myer] 849 (Au)
Word choice (letter) [Gorlick] (reply) [Hong] 724 (Jy)
Television
Your child's best friend: TV or not TV? (letter) [Bader] (reply) [Stiehm] 963 (Se)
Your child's best friend: TV or not TV [Stiehm] 257 (Mr)
Temporal Bone
Pediatric case of Eagle's syndrome [Holloway] 339 (Mr)
Temporal Lobe
Cortical resection for children with epilepsy: perspectives in pediatrics [Wyllie] 314 (Mr)
Tetanus Toxoid
Comparative trial of the reactogenicity and immunogenic-

ity of Takeda acellular pertussis vaccine combined with tetanus and diphtheria toxoids: outcome in 3- to 8-month old infants, 9- to 23-month-old infants and children, and 24- to 30-month-old children [Kimura] 734 (Jy)
Immunization response varies with intensity of acute lymphoblastic leukemia therapy [Ridgway] 887 (Au)
Vaccine myth and physician handouts (letter) [Lynch] 426, (replies) [Cherry, Fulginiti] 426, 427 (Ap)
Tetany
Low serum calcium and high parathyroid hormone levels in neonates fed 'humanized' cow's milk-based formula [Specker] 941 (Au)
Tetralogy of Fallot
Cardiopulmonary exercise testing in children following surgery for tetralogy of Fallot [Tomassoni] 1290 (No)
Texas
Acquired immunodeficiency syndrome and adolescents: knowledge, attitudes, and behaviors of runaway and homeless youths [Sugerman] 431 (Ap)
Thiazide Diuretics see Diuretics, Thiazide
Thinking
Women in medicine: fantasies, dreams, myths, and realities [DeAngelis] 49 (Ja)
Thirst
Adipsic hypernatremia in 2 sisters [Radetti] 321 (Mr)
Thorax
Albuterol inhalations in acute chest syndrome (letter) [Handelsman] 603 (Je)
Commotio cordis: the single, most common cause of traumatic death in youth baseball [Abrunzo] 1279 (No)
Thrombasthenia
Variant form of thrombasthenia [Tarantino] 1053 (Se)
Thrombocytes see Blood Platelets
Thrombocytopenia
Epidemic nephropathy in children [Lautala] 1181 (Oc)
Thrombophlebitis
Left renal vein thrombosis and left adrenal hemorrhage [Bennett] 1299 (No)
Thrombosis, Venous see Thrombophlebitis
Thumbsucking see Fingersucking
Thymectomy
Association of pauciarticular juvenile arthritis and myasthenia gravis [Glass] 1176 (Oc)
Thyroid Stimulating Hormone see Thyrotropin
Thyrotropin
Age-related patterns of thyroid-stimulating hormone response to thyrotropin-releasing hormone stimulation in Down syndrome [Sharav] 172 (Fe)
Endocrine function in children with human immunodeficiency virus infection [Schwartz] 330 (Mr)
Thyrotropin-Releasing Hormone
Age-related patterns of thyroid-stimulating hormone response to thyrotropin-releasing hormone stimulation in Down syndrome [Sharav] 172 (Fe)
Thyroxine
Endocrine function in children with human immunodeficiency virus infection [Schwartz] 330 (Mr)
Tibia
Thorn-induced pseudotumor of the tibia [Kozlowski] 1159 (Oc)
Time
Arterial catheter-related infections in children: a 1-year cohort analysis [Furfaro] 1037 (Se)
Tinea
Exacerbation of tinea corporis during treatment with 1% clotrimazole/0.05% betamethasone diproprionate (Lotrisone) (letter) [Reynolds] 1224 (No)
Tobramycin
Evaluation of intraosseus vs intravenous antibiotic levels in a porcine model [Jaimovich] 946 (Au); correction, 1241 (No)
Tomography, X-Ray Computed
Gilding the lily (letter) [Faigel] (reply) [Myer] 849 (Au)
Total Lung Capacity
Cardiopulmonary exercise testing in children following surgery for tetralogy of Fallot [Tomassoni] 1290 (No)
Total Parenteral Nutrition see Parenteral Hyperalimentation
Toxin Conjugates see Immunotoxins
Toxocara
Visceral larva migrans [Ponder] 699 (Je)
Trachea
Optimal positioning of endotracheal tubes for ventilation of preterm infants [Rotschild] 1007 (Se)
Tracheostomy
Home care cost-effectiveness for respiratory technology-dependent children [Fields] 729 (Jy)
Transport of Wounded and Sick see Transportation of Patients
Transportation of Patients
Guidelines for safe transportation of children in wheelchairs [DiGaudio] 653 (Je)
Transposition of Great Vessels
Development, growth, and cardiac surgery [Mayer] 33 (Ja)
Follow-up of patients who underwent arterial switch repair for transposition of the great arteries [Mendoza] 40 (Ja)
Travel
Mediterranean visceral leishmaniasis: a frequently unrecognized imported disease (letter) [Mahieu] 1225 (No)
Treatment Refusal
Medical ethics issues survey of residents in 5 pediatric training programs [White] 161 (Fe)
Triglycerides
Lipoprotein profiles in hypercholesterolemic children [Garcia] 147 (Fe); correction, 515 (My)
Serum lipid concentrations in subjects with phenylketonuria and their families [DeClue] 1266 (No)
Triiodothyronine
Endocrine function in children with human immunodeficiency virus infection [Schwartz] 330 (Mr)
Trimethoprim
Puncture wound-induced *Achromobacter xylosoxidans* osteomyelitis of the foot (letter) [Hoddy] 599 (Je)
Trimethoprim-Sulfamethoxazole Combination
Predicting risk of *Pneumocystis carinii* pneumonia in human immunodeficiency virus-infected children [Rutstein] 922 (Au)
Trimethoprim-sulfamethoxazole oral desensitization in hemophiliacs infected with human immunodeficiency virus with a history of hypersensitivity reactions [Kletzel] 1428 (De)
Tuberculosis, Pulmonary
Clinical and endocrinologic manifestations in perinatally human immunodeficiency virus type 1-infected children aged 5 years or older [Lepage] 1248 (No)
Tiny Tim remembered [Callahan] 1355 (De)
Tuberous Sclerosis
Tuberous sclerosis with myocardial and central nervous system involvement at birth [Allison] 471 (Ap)
Tumor Markers, Biological
Pediatric germ cell and human chorionic gonadotropin-producing tumors: clinical and laboratory features [Englund] 1294 (No)
Twins
Neonatal hepatitis and extrahepatic biliary atresia associated with cytomegalovirus infection in twins [Hart] 302 (Mr)
Nevus flammeus: discordance in monozygotic twins [Shamir] 85 (Ja)

U

Ultrasonic Diagnosis see Ultrasonography
Ultrasonography
Mitral valve prolapse: back to the basics [Allen] 1095 (Oc)
Umbilical Arteries
Factors associated with umbilical catheter-related sepsis in neonates [Landers] 675 (Je)
Umbilical Veins
Factors associated with umbilical catheter-related sepsis in neonates [Landers] 675 (Je)
United States
Challenge of care for the poor and underserved in the United States: an American College of Obstetricians and Gynecologists perspective on access to care for underserved women [Davidson] 546 (My)
Child abuse and neglect: critical first steps in response to a national emergency: the report of the US Advisory Board on Child Abuse and Neglect [Krugman] 513 (My)
Children in and of the streets: health, social policy, and the homeless young [Wright] 516 (My)
Far from the ideal: the plight of poor children in the United States [Fulginiti] 489 (My)
Growing neglect of American children [Maurer] 540 (My)
Improving health care provision to neonates in the United States [Stahlman] 510 (My)
Urban Health
Occult cocaine exposure in children [Rosenberg] 1430 (De)
Pediatric acquired immunodeficiency syndrome, poverty, and national priorities [Heagarty] 527 (My)
Pediatric human immunodeficiency virus infection and the acquired immunodeficiency syndrome: a health care crisis of children and families [Van Dyke] 529 (My)
Regional pediatric approach to the epidemic of social ills within our cities [Nelson] 505 (My)
What will it take to fully protect all American children with vaccines? [Hinman] 559 (My)
Urethral Obstruction
Medical management of postobstructive polyuria (letter) [Smoyer] 1345 (De)
Urinary Calculi
Natural history of hematuria associated with hypercalciuria in children [Garcia] 1204 (Oc)
Urinary Tract
Medical management of postobstructive polyuria (letter) [Smoyer] 1345 (De)
Urinary Tract Infections
Escherichia coli bacteremia in children: a review of 91 cases in 10 years [Bonadio] 671 (Je)
Paleonephrology and reflux nephropathy: from the 'big bang' to end-stage renal disease [Kallen] 860 (Au)
Urine
Alkaline urine is associated with eating disorders (letter) [Arden] 28 (Ja)
Association of alkaline urine with eating disorders (letter) [Robson] (reply) [Arden] 1091 (Oc)
Effect of low-dose dopamine infusion on cardiopulmonary and renal status in premature newborns with respiratory distress syndrome [Cuevas] 799 (Jy)
Meconium for drug testing [Maynard] 650 (Je)
Natural history of hematuria associated with hypercalciuria in children [Garcia] 1204 (Oc)
Vasopressin levels in infants during the course of aseptic and bacterial meningitis [Padilla] 991 (Se)
Urine Concentrating Ability see Kidney Concentrating Ability
Urolithiasis see Urinary Calculi
Uveitis
Decreasing severity of chronic uveitis in children with pauciarticular arthritis [Sherry] 1026 (Se)

V

Vaccines
Antibody responses to 4 *Haemophilus influenzae* type b conjugate vaccines [Käyhty] 223 (Fe)
Dose-related immunogenicity of *Haemophilus influenzae* type b capsular polysaccharide—*Neisseria meningitidis* outer membrane protein conjugate vaccine [Wong] 742 (Jy)
Vaccines, Synthetic
Acellular pertussis vaccines: efficacy and evaluation of clinical case definitions [Blackwelder] 1285 (No)
Comparative trial of the reactogenicity and immunogenicity of Takeda acellular pertussis vaccine combined with tetanus and diphtheria toxoids: outcome in 3- to 8-month old infants, 9- to 23-month-old infants and children, and 24- to 30-month-old children [Kimura] 734 (Jy)
Valproic Acid
Effect of valproic acid on plasma carnitine levels [Opala] 999 (Se)
Vancomycin
Evaluation of intraosseus vs intravenous antibiotic levels in a porcine model [Jaimovich] 946 (Au); correction, 1241 (No)
Varicella-Zoster Virus
Herpes zoster oticus (letter) [Rathore] 722 (Jy)
Vascular Resistance
Family history of myocardial infarction and hemodynamic responses to exercise in young black boys [Treiber] 1029 (Se)
Vasculitis
Penile vasculitis with impending necrosis treated with prostaglandin E_1 infusion (letter) [Horner] 604 (Je)
Vasoconstriction
Brain and ocular abnormalities in infants with in utero exposure to cocaine and other street drugs [Dominguez] 688 (Je)
Vasopressin, Deamino-Arginine see Desmopressin
Vasopressins
Adipsic hypernatremia in 2 sisters [Radetti] 321 (Mr)
Vasopressin levels in infants during the course of aseptic and bacterial meningitis [Padilla] 991 (Se)
Ventilation, Mechanical see Respiration, Artificial
Ventilators, Mechanical
Home care cost-effectiveness for respiratory technology-dependent children [Fields] 729 (Jy)
Saving money with home care [Schoumacher] 725 (Jy)
Vesico-Ureteral Reflux
Paleonephrology and reflux nephropathy: from the 'big bang' to end-stage renal disease [Kallen] 860 (Au)
Video Games see Play and Playthings
Vital Capacity
Differences in expression of cystic fibrosis in blacks and whites [McColley] 94 (Ja)
Vitamin D
How much vitamin D for neonates? [Pittard] 1147 (Oc)
Rickets caused by vitamin D deficiency in breast-fed infants in the southern United States [Bhowmick] 127 (Fe)
X-linked hypophosphatemia: genetic and clinical correlates [Hanna] 865 (Au)
Vocal Cords
Optimal positioning of endotracheal tubes for ventilation of preterm infants [Rotschild] 1007 (Se)
Voluntary Health Agencies
Challenge of caring for indigent children with rheumatologic diseases [Miller] 554 (My)
Vomiting
Alkaline urine is associated with eating disorders (letter) [Arden] 28 (Ja)
Association of alkaline urine with eating disorders (letter) [Robson] (reply) [Arden] 1091 (Oc)
Demographic and risk factors associated with chronic dieting in adolescents [Story] 994 (Se)
Gallstones in children: characterization by age, etiology, and outcome [Reif] 105 (Ja)
Survey of antiemetic use in children with cancer [van Hoff] 773 (Jy)
Testing the psychogenic vomiting diagnosis: four pediatric patients [Gonzalez-Heydrich] 913 (Au)

W

Wakefulness
Gastroesophageal reflux and apnea in prematurely born infants during wakefulness and sleep [Ajuriaguerra] 1132 (Oc)
Walking
Effects of obesity on aerobic fitness in adolescent females [Rowland] 764 (Jy)

War
War souvenir poisoning (letter) [Secord] 724 (Jy)
Warts, Genital see Condylomata acuminata
Washington
Decreasing severity of chronic uveitis in children with pauciarticular arthritis [Sherry] 1026 (Se)
Water-Electrolyte Balance
Adipsic hypernatremia in 2 sisters [Radetti] 321 (Mr)
Water Intoxication
Current social practices leading to water intoxication in infants (letter) [Schaeffer] 27 (Ja)
Oral water intoxication in infants: an American epidemic [Keating] 985 (Se)
Water intoxication: a prevalent problem in the inner city [Finberg] 981 (Se)
Weight Lifting
Tracking of elevated blood pressure values in adolescent athletes at 1-year follow-up [Tanji] 665 (Je)
Weight Loss
Demographic and risk factors associated with chronic dieting in adolescents [Story] 994 (Se)
West Indies
Current social practices leading to water intoxication in infants (letter) [Schaeffer] 27 (Ja)
Wheelchairs
Guidelines for safe transportation of children in wheelchairs [DiGaudio] 653 (Je)
Wheezing see Respiratory Sounds
Whites
Breast-feeding initiation in a triethnic population [Bee] 306 (Mr)
Differences in expression of cystic fibrosis in blacks and whites [McColley] 94 (Ja)
Differences in infant mortality by race, nativity status, and other maternal characteristics [Kleinman] 194 (Fe)
Sexual maturation and blood pressure levels of a biracial sample of girls [Kozinetz] 142 (Fe)
Standardized percentile curves of body-mass index for children and adolescents [Hammer] 259 (Mr)
Whooping Cough
Acellular pertussis vaccines: efficacy and evaluation of clinical case definitions [Blackwelder] 1285 (No)
Women
Effects of obesity on aerobic fitness in adolescent females [Rowland] 764 (Jy)
Pediatric human immunodeficiency virus infection and the acquired immunodeficiency syndrome: a health care crisis of children and families [Van Dyke] 529 (My)
Women in medicine: fantasies, dreams, myths, and realities [DeAngelis] 49 (Ja)
Women, Working
Women in medicine: fantasies, dreams, myths, and realities [DeAngelis] 49 (Ja)
Women's Health Services
Challenge of care for the poor and underserved in the United States: an American College of Obstetricians and Gynecologists perspective on access to care for underserved women [Davidson] 546 (My)
Work
Part-time Peg: who, me? [Ferry] 852 (Au)
Resident and nurse practitioners: responding to education and patient care needs (letter) [Giardino] 843 (Au)
Work Schedule Tolerance
Eighty-hour workweek and residency programs: closing arguments (letter) [Bedrick] 846 (Au)
House staff work hours and moonlighting: what do residents want?: a survey of pediatric residents in California [Cheng] 1104 (Oc)
New York State health code 405 update (letter) [Daigler] 428 (Ap)
Support services for pediatric trainees: a survey of training program directors [Bergman] 1002 (Se)
World Health Organization
Formula companies and the medical profession (letter) [Newman] 1089, (reply) [Greer] 1090 (Oc)
Rice solution and World Health Organization solution by gastric infusion for high stool output diarrhea [Mota-Hernández] 937 (Au)
Wounds and Injuries
Commotio cordis: the single, most common cause of traumatic death in youth baseball [Abrunzo] 1279 (No)
Injuries and poisonings in out-of-home child care and home care [Gunn] 779 (Jy)
Use of infant walkers [AMA Board of Trustees] 933 (Au)
Wounds, Penetrating
Puncture wound-induced *Achromobacter xylosoxidans* osteomyelitis of the foot (letter) [Hoddy] 599 (Je)

X

X Chromosome
Lowe's syndrome [Loughead] 113 (Ja)
X-linked hypophosphatemia: genetic and clinical correlates [Hanna] 865 (Au)

Z

Zinc
Acrodermatitis enteropathica [Schneider] 211 (Fe)
Zinc deficiency: a public health problem? [Sandstead] 853 (Au)